17th Edition

HARRISON'S

Principles of INTERNAL MEDICINE

EDITORS OF PREVIOUS EDITIONS

T. R. Harrison
Editor-in-Chief, Editions 1, 2, 3, 4, 5

W. R. Resnick
Editor, Editions 1, 2, 3, 4, 5

M. M. Wintrobe
Editor, Editions 1, 2, 3, 4, 5
Editor-in-Chief, Editions 6, 7

G. W. Thorn
Editor, Editions 1, 2, 3, 4, 5, 6, 7
Editor-in-Chief, Edition 8

R. D. Adams
Editor, Editions 2, 3, 4, 5, 6, 7, 8, 9, 10

P. B. Beeson
Editor, Editions 1, 2

I. L. Bennett, Jr.
Editor, Editions 3, 4, 5, 6

E. Braunwald
Editor, Editions 6, 7, 8, 9, 10, 12, 13, 14, 16
Editor-in-Chief, Editions 11, 15

K. J. Isselbacher
Editor, Editions 6, 7, 8, 10, 11, 12, 14
Editor-in-Chief, Editions 9, 13

R. G. Petersdorf
Editor, Editions 6, 7, 8, 9, 11, 12, 13
Editor-in-Chief, Edition 10

J. D. Wilson
Editor, Editions 9, 10, 11, 13, 14
Editor-in-Chief, Edition 12

J. B. Martin
Editor, Editions 10, 11, 12, 13, 14

A. S. Fauci
Editor, Editions 11, 12, 13, 15, 16
Editor-in-Chief, Edition 14

R. Root
Editor, Edition 12

D. L. Kasper
Editor, Editions 13, 14, 15
Editor-in-Chief, Edition 16

S. L. Hauser
Editor, Editions 14, 15, 16

D. L. Longo
Editor, Editions 14, 15, 16

J. L. Jameson
Editor, Editions 15, 16

GASTROENTEROLOGY AND HEPATOLOGY

HEMATOLOGY AND ONCOLOGY

INFECTIOUS DISEASES AND HIV/AIDS

NEPHROLOGY

NEUROLOGY AND PSYCHIATRY

PULMONARY

SYSTEMIC PRESENTATIONS

17th Edition

HARRISON'S Principles of INTERNAL MEDICINE

EDITORS

Anthony S. Fauci, MD
Chief, Laboratory of Immunoregulation; Director,
National Institute of Allergy and Infectious Diseases,
National Institutes of Health, Bethesda

Eugene Braunwald, MD
Distinguished Hersey Professor of Medicine,
Harvard Medical School; Chairman, TIMI Study Group,
Brigham and Women's Hospital, Boston

Dennis L. Kasper, MD
William Ellery Channing Professor of Medicine,
Professor of Microbiology and Molecular Genetics,
Harvard Medical School; Director, Channing Laboratory,
Department of Medicine, Brigham and Women's Hospital, Boston

Stephen L. Hauser, MD
Robert A. Fishman Distinguished Professor and Chairman,
Department of Neurology, University of California,
San Francisco, San Francisco

Dan L. Longo, MD
Scientific Director, National Institute on Aging,
National Institutes of Health, Bethesda and Baltimore

J. Larry Jameson, MD, PhD
Professor of Medicine;
Vice-President for Medical Affairs and Lewis Landsberg Dean,
Northwestern University Feinberg School of Medicine, Chicago

Joseph Loscalzo, MD, PhD
Hersey Professor of the Theory and Practice of Medicine,
Harvard Medical School; Chairman, Department of Medicine;
Physician-in-Chief, Brigham and Women's Hospital, Boston

VOLUME I

McGraw Hill Medical

New York Chicago San Francisco Lisbon London Madrid Mexico City
New Delhi San Juan Seoul Singapore Sydney Toronto

The McGraw·Hill Companies

Note: Dr. Fauci's and Dr. Longo's works as editors and authors were performed outside the scope of their employment as U.S. government employees. These works represent their personal and professional views and not necessarily those of the U.S. government.

Harrison's
PRINCIPLES OF INTERNAL MEDICINE
Seventeenth Edition

2 3 4 5 6 7 8 9 0 DOWDOW 12 11 10 9

Single Edition Set ISBN 978-0-07-146633-2; MHID 0-07-146633-9
Single Edition Book ISBN 978-0-07-159991-7; MHID 0-07-159991-6

Two Volume Set ISBN 978-0-07-147691-1; MHID 0-07-147691-1
Volume 1 ISBN 978-0-07-147692-8; MHID 0-07-147692-X
Volume 2 ISBN 978-0-07-147693-5; MHID 0-07-147693-8

DVD ISBN 978-0-07-159990-0; MHID 0-07-159990-8

FOREIGN LANGUAGE EDITIONS

Arabic (13e): McGraw-Hill Libri Italia srl (1996)
Chinese Long Form (15e): McGraw-Hill International Enterprises, Inc., Taiwan
Chinese Short Form (15e): McGraw-Hill Education (Asia), Singapore
Croatian (16e): Placebo, Split, Croatia
French (16e): Medecine-Sciences Flammarion, Paris, France
German (16e): ABW Wissenschaftsverlagsgesellschaft mbH, Berlin, Germany
Greek (16e): Parissianos, S.A., Athens, Greece
Italian (16e): The McGraw-Hill Companies, Srl, Milan, Italy
Japanese (16e): MEDSI-Medical Sciences International Ltd, Tokyo, Japan
Korean (16e): McGraw-Hill Korea, Inc., Seoul, Korea
Polish (14e): Czelej Publishing Company, Lubin, Poland (2000)
Portuguese (16e): McGraw-Hill Interamericana do Brazil, Rio de Janeiro, Brazil
Romanian (14e): Teora Publishers, Bucharest, Romania (2000)
Serbian (15e): Publishing House Romanov, Bosnia & Herzegovina, Republic of Serbska
Spanish (16e): McGraw-Hill Interamericana de Espana S.A., Madrid, Spain
Turkish (15e): Nobel Tip Kitabevleri, Ltd., Istanbul, Turkey
Vietnamese (15e): McGraw-Hill Education (Asia), Singapore

This book was set in Minion, Myriad, and Dax by Silverchair Science + Communications, Inc. The editors were James Shanahan and Mariapaz Ramos Englis; editorial assistant was Jenna Esposito. The production director was Phil Galea and production manager was Catherine Saggese. The index was prepared by Barbara Littlewood. The text designer was Alan Barnett of alan barnett design; cover design was by David Dell'Accio. The medical illustrator was Daniel Knopsnyder.

RR Donnelley was printer and binder.

Library of Congress Cataloging-in-Publication Data

Harrison's principles of internal medicine. -- 17th ed. / editors, Anthony S. Fauci ... [et al.].
p. ; cm.
Includes bibliographical references and index.
ISBN-13: 978-0-07-146633-2 (hardcover : v. 2 : alk. paper)
ISBN-10: 0-07-146633-9 (hardcover : v. 2 : alk. paper)
ISBN-13: 978-0-07-147691-1 (hardcover : set : v. 2 : alk. paper)
ISBN-10: 0-07-147691-1 (hardcover : set : v. 2 : alk. paper) 1. Internal medicine. I. Fauci, Anthony S.,
II. Title: Principles of internal medicine.
[DNLM: 1. Internal Medicine. WB 115 H322 2008]
RC46.H333 2008
616--dc22

2007012181

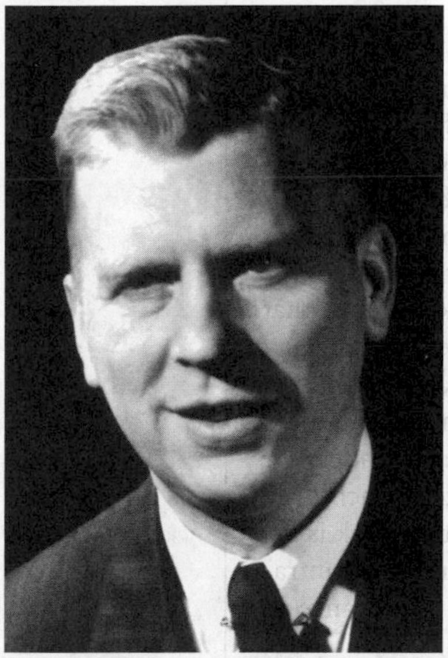

George W. Thorn
1906–2004

George W. Thorn was an editor of the first seven editions and Editor-in-Chief of the eighth edition. As a founding editor, he had an enormous impact on *Harrison's* and thereby on the education of countless thousands of physicians and medical students. His incisiveness, inventiveness, and originality, coupled with his broad knowledge of clinical medicine and medical science and his unswerving dedication to the application of techniques of contemporary science to the advancement of clinical medicine, played a vital role in the original organization of this textbook.

George Thorn began his remarkable career in endocrinologic research as a medical student at the University of Buffalo School of Medicine. Following a stint in general practice, which subsequently served him well as an educator, clinical investigator, and consultant, he obtained research training and held faculty positions at several institutions. In 1942, at the age of 36, he became Hersey Professor of the Theory and Practice of Physic (Medicine) at Harvard Medical School and Physician-in-Chief at Brigham and Women's. During the three decades in which he filled these positions with distinction, he created one of the first modern academic medical units where the education of physician-scientists, the highest standards of clinical care, and the conduct of exciting clinical research were inextricably intertwined and mutually reinforcing. Thorn's personal investigative interests focused on the adrenal cortex and the kidney. He developed techniques for the diagnosis of adrenal disease that are still in wide use. He characterized salt-losing nephritis and catalyzed the development of renal dialysis and the work that led to the development of renal transplantation.

George Thorn played many leadership roles in medicine and medical science. As a member of the governing board of the Massachusetts Institute of Technology (MIT) he was instrumental in the development of the Harvard-MIT program in Health Science and Technology. He was the founder, Director, and then President of the Howard Hughes Medical Institute, which became a major world force in the conduct of fundamental biomedical research under his leadership.

Thorn has influenced most profoundly a number of institutions: Harvard, the Brigham, MIT, and the Hughes Institute. To these and to *Harrison's*, he brought a unique blend of ebullience, imagination, curiosity, personal leadership, good humor, warmth, and compassion, which inspired generations of Harvard medical students, Brigham residents and research fellows, Hughes investigators, and editorial colleagues. The present Editors are pleased to express their admiration for this medical giant and beloved friend by dedicating this seventeenth edition of *Harrison's* to George W. Thorn, one of the founders of this book.

THE EDITORS

NOTICE

COVER ILLUSTRATIONS

(1) **Figure 222-10.** Three-dimensional reconstruction of a CT angiogram demonstrating a normal main left coronary artery arising from the aorta and its two branches, the left anterior descending artery (left) and the left circumflex artery (right).

(2) Computer rendition of chains of *Streptococcus pneumoniae* bacteria. This gram-positive oval-shaped bacterium is one of the causes of pneumonia. Although found living harmlessly in the body, *S. pneumoniae* can cause dangerous opportunistic infections of the lung. *(Credit: Hybrid Medical Animation/Photo Researchers, Inc.)*

(3) Three-dimensional representation of blood cells.

(4) Illustration of a myelinated axon with sodium channels clustered at the nodes of Ranvier where axonal depolarization occurs; this event results in saltatory conduction, with nerve impulse jumping from one node to the next.

(5) **Figure 364-15A.** A CT perfusion mean transit–time map showing delayed perfusion of the left middle cerebral artery distribution.

CONTENTS

PART 6 Oncology and Hematology

SECTION 1 NEOPLASTIC DISORDERS

SECTION 2 HEMATOPOIETIC DISORDERS

SECTION 3 DISORDERS OF HEMOSTASIS

PART 7 Infectious Diseases

SECTION 1 BASIC CONSIDERATIONS IN INFECTIOUS DISEASES

SECTION 2 CLINICAL SYNDROMES: COMMUNITY-ACQUIRED INFECTIONS

CONTENTS

CONTENTS

PART 10 Disorders of the Respiratory System

SECTION 1 DIAGNOSIS OF RESPIRATORY DISORDERS

SECTION 2 DISEASES OF THE RESPIRATORY SYSTEM

PART 11 Critical Care Medicine

SECTION 1 RESPIRATORY CRITICAL CARE

SECTION 2 SHOCK AND CARDIAC ARREST

SECTION 3 NEUROLOGIC CRITICAL CARE

SECTION 4 ONCOLOGIC EMERGENCIES

PART 12 Disorders of the Kidney and Urinary Tract

PART 13 Disorders of the Gastrointestinal System

SECTION 1 DISORDERS OF THE ALIMENTARY TRACT

SECTION 2 LIVER AND BILIARY TRACT DISEASE

SECTION 3 DISORDERS OF THE PANCREAS

PART 14 Disorders of the Immune System, Connective Tissue, and Joints

SECTION 1 THE IMMUNE SYSTEM IN HEALTH AND DISEASE

SECTION 2 DISORDERS OF IMMUNE-MEDIATED INJURY

SECTION 3 DISORDERS OF THE JOINTS AND ADJACENT TISSUES

PART 15 Endocrinology and Metabolism

SECTION 1 ENDOCRINOLOGY

SECTION 2 DISORDERS OF BONE AND MINERAL METABOLISM

SECTION 3 DISORDERS OF INTERMEDIARY METABOLISM

PART 16 Neurologic Disorders

SECTION 1 DIAGNOSIS OF NEUROLOGIC DISORDERS

SECTION 2 DISEASES OF THE CENTRAL NERVOUS SYSTEM

SECTION 3 NERVE AND MUSCLE DISORDERS

SECTION 4 CHRONIC FATIGUE SYNDROME

SECTION 5 PSYCHIATRIC DISORDERS

SECTION 6 ALCOHOLISM AND DRUG DEPENDENCY

PART 17 Poisoning, Drug Overdose, and Envenomation

PART 18 e-Chapters from International Advisory Editors

For complete text for these chapters, see Harrison's, 17e, DVD

Chapter e1 The Safety and Quality of Health Care

A number of interventions that have been demonstrated to improve the safety and quality of care are available today and should be used more widely in clinical practice. Other interventions are undergoing evaluation, and still others are being developed in parallel with new technologies such as electronic health records systems. Many interventions will require changing the structure of care—for example, moving to a more team-oriented approach and ensuring that patients are more involved in their own care. Payers and the general public are now demanding better information about safety and quality as well as better performance in these areas. The clear implication is that these domains will need to be addressed directly by providers. Thus, physicians must learn about these two domains, how they can be improved, and the relative strengths and limitations of our current ability to measure them.

Chapter e2 Economic Considerations in the Practice of Medicine

Physicians need to develop and maintain an understanding of this topic and to reflect that understanding in their professional behavior. Covered in this chapter are the many causes of rising health care costs, with new technology being the main one; the ways in which insurance coverage (including Medicare and Medicaid) can drive demand for health care services; the influence of health professionals, hospitals, and the pharmaceutical and device industries on the supply of health care; and the different strategies available for cost control. With health care spending in the United States at >16% of the gross domestic product (as of 2005), this chapter should be of interest to all physicians.

Chapter e3 Racial and Ethnic Disparities in Health Care

This chapter illustrates how such disparities persist in spite of the great improvements in overall health and life expectancy. Many graphs and bar charts document the nature, extent, and root causes of differences in health care for minorities. These causes include social determinants, lack of access, complexity of the health care system, stereotyping, and patient-level factors such as mistrust. Key recommendations to bring about improvement are given, as is advice to the individual health care provider (e.g., being aware of disparities, practicing culturally competent care, avoiding stereotyping, and working to build trust).

Chapter e4 Ethical Issues in Clinical Medicine

This chapter discusses fundamental ethical guidelines, patients who lack decision-making capacity, decisions about life-sustaining interventions, conflicts of interest, and just allocation of resources. The chapter helps the physician to follow two fundamental but frequently conflicting ethical principles: respecting patient autonomy and acting in the patient's best interest. Also discussed are assessment of a patient's capacity to make medical decisions, choice of a surrogate, and standards for surrogate decision-making; care of dying patients, do-not-resuscitate orders, and decisions about when to withdraw or withhold life-sustaining interventions; and the risks of financial incentives, gifts from pharmaceutical companies, fear of treating HIV-infected patients, and reporting medical errors. The less-experienced physician will gain confidence in dealing with these perplexing and, at times, emotionally draining issues.

Chapter e5 Atlas of Rashes Associated with Fever

This chapter presents high-quality images of a variety of rashes that have an infectious etiology and are commonly associated with fever. Even the most astute and experienced clinician is often diagnostically challenged by a patient with fever and rash, given the broad differential diagnosis. This atlas will help the physician to rapidly narrow the differential, promptly recognize key features, and administer appropriate and sometimes life-saving therapy.

Chapter e6 Memory Loss

This chapter discusses the formation of both long- and short-term memories. Long-term memory is divided into declarative and nondeclarative memory; the former is further subdivided into semantic and episodic memories. Nondeclarative memory is subdivided into skills and habits (procedural memory), priming, conditioning, and nonassociative learning. Also covered are the associated anatomic substrates for each. Lesions in any of these associated areas cause deficits in storing, retaining, and retrieving information. Short-term, or working, memory relies on different regions of the brain, and lesions that disrupt their structure or function can be devastating. Testing of working memory can be effectively performed at the bedside. More detailed testing of memory should probably be done by a neuropsychologist, neuropsychiatrist, or behavioral neurologist.

Chapter e7 Atlas of Oral Manifestations of Disease

This atlas presents numerous outstanding photographs illustrating many oral conditions that indicate clinical disease either in the mouth or elsewhere. There is significant clinical value in examining the oral cavity for signs of disease, as the health status of the oral cavity is connected to cardiovascular disease and diabetes mellitus.

Chapter e8 Approach to the Patient with a Heart Murmur

This chapter provides comprehensive coverage of heart murmurs (systolic, diastolic, and continuous), their major attributes, and their response to bedside maneuvers, detected by auscultation. Together with the history, clinical context, and associated findings, this information allows the clinician to construct a differential diagnosis to guide the need for and urgency of further testing, such as echocardiography, transesophageal echocardiography, or cardiac CT or MRI.

Chapter e9 Atlas of Urinary Sediments and Renal Biopsies

This chapter illustrates key diagnostic features of selected kidney diseases, using light microscopy, immunofluorescence, and electron microscopy. Common urinalysis findings are also documented. The chapter amplifies the physician's knowledge of disorders of the kidney and urinary tract.

Chapter e10 Atlas of Skin Manifestations of Internal Disease

The atlas provides pictures of a selected group of inflammatory skin eruptions and neoplastic conditions, illustrating (1) common skin diseases and lesions, (2) nonmelanoma skin cancer, (3) melanoma and pigmented lesions, (4) infectious diseases and the skin, (5) immunologically mediated skin disease, and (6) skin manifestations of internal disease. Physicians frequently have to decide whether a cutaneous process is confined to the skin—a pure dermatologic event—or whether it is a manifestation of internal disease relating to the patient's overall medical condition, given the marked rise in both melanoma and nonmelanoma skin cancer.

Chapter e11 Atlas of Hematology and Analysis of Peripheral Blood Smears

This atlas gives many examples of both normal and abnormal blood smears and a guide to blood smear interpretation. A normal peripheral blood smear is shown, as are normal granulocytes, monocytes, eosinophils, basophils, plasma cells, and bone marrow. Abnormal smears illustrate the defects found in conditions such as iron-deficiency anemia, sickle cell anemia, aplastic anemia, metastatic cancer, erythroid hyperplasia, acute myeloid and lymphoblastic leukemias, chronic myeloid and lymphoid leukemias, adult T cell leukemia, follicular lymphoma, and Burkitt's lymphoma, among others.

Chapter e12 Thymoma

The chapter begins with a brief overview of the composition and function of the thymus and lists the various abnormalities that can occur. A thymoma develops when epithelial cells in the thymus become neoplastic. A link to myasthenia gravis (MG) is noted; about 30% of patients with a thymoma have MG, and MG patients have a high incidence of thymic abnormalities. Thymomas may be associated with other conditions (e.g., pure red cell aplasia) but to a lesser degree. Staging and histologic classification are presented. Early-stage disease is treated by surgical resection, with or without postoperative radiation. A multimodality approach is taken in late-stage disease: neoadjuvant chemotherapy followed by surgery, radiation therapy, and additional consolidation chemotherapy.

Chapter e13 Late Consequences of Cancer and Its Treatment

This chapter discusses the long-term consequences of successful cancer treatment. Some problems may be related to the cancer itself or to the normal aging process, but many are caused by therapy, whether surgery, radiation, or chemotherapy. There may also be associated psychosocial problems. The consequences are covered in two ways—by organ system and by cancer type. It is now apparent that monitoring of cancer survivors is a critical component of their overall health care and that some aspects of primary treatment should be modified, where possible, to reduce later consequences.

Chapter e14 Laboratory Diagnosis of Infectious Diseases

The chapter documents the evolution of methods used in the clinical microbiology laboratory to detect and identify viral, bacterial, fungal, and parasitic agents and to determine the antibiotic susceptibility of bacterial and fungal pathogens. Detection methods range from microscopic visualization, aided by a variety of stains, to systems that detect and amplify biologic signals. Identification methods include both classic biochemical phenotyping and more sophisticated methods such as gas chromatography and nucleic acid tests. Perhaps most useful to the nonspecialist is the large table giving clear and precise instructions for collection and transport of specimens to the laboratory for culture.

Chapter e15 Infectious Complications of Burns and Bites

This chapter details the consequences of breaches in the skin from animal bites and scratches, which allow the inoculation of microorganisms into deeper, susceptible host tissues, and from burns, which may cause massive destruction of the integument and derangements in humoral and cellular immunity. The patient's own flora and organisms from the hospital environment can cause infections in burn injuries, and the frequency of infection parallels the extent and severity of the injury. Immunosuppression resulting from severe burns also puts patients at risk of infections, as do the necessary manipulations for clinical care. The risks of infection, both local and systemic, that can result from the variety of microorganisms involved in an animal or human bite are detailed. The treatment section covers wound management, antibiotic therapy for established infection and for prophylactic purposes, and rabies and tetanus prophylaxis.

Chapter e16 Laboratory Diagnosis of Parasitic Infections

This chapter emphasizes the importance of the history and epidemiology of a patient's illness. Tables provide clear information on the geographic distribution, transmission, anatomic locations, and methods employed for the diagnosis of flatworm, roundworm, and protozoal infections. These tables should help the physician select the appropriate body fluid or biopsy site for microscopic examination. Other tables give information about the identification of parasites in samples from specific anatomic locations. Also listed are parasites frequently associated with eosinophilia and the serologic and molecular tests currently available for parasitic infections.

Chapter e17 Pharmacology of Agents Used to Treat Parasitic Infections

This chapter deals exclusively with the pharmacologic properties of the agents used to treat infections due to parasites. Information on these agents' major toxicities, spectrum of activity, and safety for use during pregnancy and lactation is presented in Chap. 201.

Chapter e18 Atlas of Blood Smears of Malaria and Babesiosis

This chapter provides both thin and thick blood films for *Plasmodium falciparum*, *P. vivax*, *P. ovale*, and *P. malariae*. The thick film allows detection of densities as low as 50 parasites per microliter, with great sensitivity; the thin film is better for speciation and provides useful prognostic information in severe falciparum malaria. One thin blood film showing trophozoites of *Babesia* is included.

Chapter e19 Atlas of Electrocardiography

This chapter shows electrocardiograms to supplement those used in Chap. 221. The interpretations emphasize findings of specific teaching value.

Chapter e20 Atlas of Noninvasive Cardiac Imaging

This chapter provides "real-time" image clips, as they are viewed in clinical practice, as well as additional static images. Noninvasive cardiac imaging is essential to the diagnosis and management of patients with known or suspected cardiovascular disease. This atlas supplements Chap. 222, which describes the principles and clinical applications of these important techniques.

Chapter e21 Atlas of Cardiac Arrhythmias

This chapter shows electrocardiograms to supplement those used in Chaps. 225 and 226. The interpretations emphasize findings of specific teaching value.

Chapter e22 Atlas of Atherosclerosis

The atlas consists of six videos that highlight some of the current understanding of atherosclerosis. Topics include pulse pressure, plaque instability, rudiments of the clinically important lipoproteins, formation and complications of atherosclerotic plaques, mechanisms of atherogenesis, and metabolic derangements that underlie the metabolic syndrome. Videos e22-2, e22-3, e22-5, and e22-6 were written and developed by Peter Libby, MD, and CCG Metamedia, Inc (Boris Polinsky, lead animator; Ralph Bonheim, science writer) for Changes and Challenges in Cardiovascular Protection, a Special CME Activity for Physicians. Created under an unrestricted educational grant from Merck & Co., Inc. Copyright © 2002, Cardinal Health; used with permission.

Chapter e23 Atlas of Percutaneous Revascularization

The atlas presents seven case studies ranging from cardiogenic shock with left main coronary artery obstruction to percutaneous aortic valve replacement. The cases are illustrated by a selection of electrocardiograms, videos of angiograms, graphs, and CT scans, providing a good teaching tool.

Chapter e24 Atlas of Chest Imaging

The atlas is a collection of chest x-rays and CT scans illustrative of specific major findings, which are categorized by those of volume loss, loss of parenchyma, interstitial processes, alveolar processes, bronchiectasis, pleural abnormalities, nodules and masses, and pulmonary vascular abnormalities.

Chapter e25 Video Atlas of Gastrointestinal Endoscopy

This atlas demonstrates endoscopic findings in a variety of infectious, inflammatory, vascular, and neoplastic conditions. The premalignant conditions of Barrett's esophagus and colonic polyps are also illustrated. At the end of the chapter are several video clips demonstrating endoscopic treatment modalities for gastrointestinal bleeding, polyps, and biliary stones.

Chapter e26 Atlas of Liver Biopsies

The atlas gives examples of common morphologic features of acute and chronic liver disorders—some involving the lobular areas and others the portal tracts. Liver biopsy is thought to represent the "gold standard" for assessing the degree of liver injury and fibrosis. Other important histologic features include those found in hepatic steatosis, injury of bile ducts in the portal tract, plasma cell infiltration, and portal inflammation affecting portal veins.

Chapter e27 Primary Immunodeficiencies Associated with or Secondary to Other Diseases

The tables in this chapter add to the information given in Chap. 310 by listing (1) the primary immunodeficiencies associated with or secondary to other conditions, and (2) the genes or genetic loci associated with primary immunodeficiencies.

Chapter e28 Atlas of Clinical Imaging in the Vasculitic Diseases

The atlas enhances the information given in Chap. 319 by images illustrating features associated with vasculitic syndromes such as Wegener's granulomatosis, Churg-Strauss syndrome, polyarteritis nodosa, and giant cell and Takayasu's arteritis. The images have been made using mainly CT scans and arteriograms.

Chapter e29 Atlas of Clinical Manifestations of Metabolic Diseases

The atlas provides a visual survey of selected metabolic disorders, which can be used to facilitate learning and thereby enhance the recognition and care of patients with these disorders. The study of metabolic diseases has been invaluable for advancing understanding of human genetics, leading to novel approaches to therapy such as screening programs, blood and organ transplantation, gene therapy, and enzyme replacement.

Chapter e30 Atlas of Neuroimaging

This atlas comprises 29 cases to assist the clinician caring for patients with neurologic symptoms. The majority of the images are MRIs; other techniques used are MR and conventional angiography and CT scans. Many neurologic diseases are illustrated, such as tuberculosis of the central nervous system (CNS), neurosyphilis, CNS aspergillosis, neurosarcoid, middle cerebral artery stenosis, CNS vasculitis, Huntington's disease, and acute transverse myelitis.

Chapter e31 Electrodiagnostic Studies of Nervous System Disorders: EEG, Evoked Potentials, EMG

This chapter covers the two main techniques for electrodiagnosis of neurologic symptoms: the electroencephalogram (EEG) and the electromyogram (EMG). Evoked potentials (sensory, cognitive, and motor) are also covered. The EEG is most useful in evaluating patients with suspected epilepsy but is also helpful in assessing coma and as a noninvasive screening tool for focal structural abnormalities of the brain. EMG enables disorders of the motor units to be detected and characterized as neurogenic or myopathic, and the findings may provide a guide to the severity of an acute nerve disorder or, in chronic or degenerative disorders, whether the process is active or progressive—important for prognosis. Nerve conduction studies, which complement the EMG, are also covered.

Chapter e32 Technique of Lumbar Puncture

This chapter covers the procedure of lumbar puncture (LP) in detail (with illustrations), from indications for imaging and laboratory studies prior to LP, analgesia, positioning, and the procedure itself (including dealing with complications that may arise during LP). Also included is a section on the main complication of LP—the post-LP headache—and its causes and therapy and strategies to avoid it.

Chapter e33 Special Issues in Inpatient Neurologic Consultation

This chapter provides coverage of neurologic diseases and syndromes that are common reasons for inpatient consultation but that are not covered elsewhere in the text. Detailed here are central nervous system dysfunction (hyperperfusion states, post–cardiac bypass brain injury, and post–solid organ transplant injury); common neurologic complications of electrolyte disturbances (hyper- and hyponatremia, hyperosmolality, hypo- and hyperkalemia, and disturbances of calcium and magnesium); and peripheral nervous system dysfunction (including entrapment and obstetric neuropathies).

Chapter e34 Heavy Metal Poisoning

This chapter provides specific information about the four main heavy metals that pose a significant threat to health via occupational and environmental exposures: lead, mercury, arsenic, and cadmium. A table clearly details the main sources, metabolism, toxic effects produced, diagnosis, and appropriate therapy for poisoning from these metals. Other metals covered, though not in the table, are copper, selenium, aluminum, chromium, manganese, and thallium.

Chapter e35 Poisoning and Drug Overdosage

This chapter provides comprehensive coverage of the dose-related adverse effects following exposure to chemicals, drugs, or other xenobiotics. The section on diagnosis gives thorough coverage of the physical examination, laboratory assessment, electrocardiographic and radiologic studies, and toxicologic analysis. The treatment section gives detailed coverage of the general principles of care, supportive care, prevention of poison absorption, enhancement of poison elimination, administration of antidotes, and prevention of reexposure. Pathophysiologic features and treatment of specific toxic syndromes and poisonings are presented in tabular form.

Chapter e36 Pulmonary Biomarkers in COPD

There has been increasing interest in using pulmonary biomarkers to understand and monitor the inflammation in the respiratory tracts of patients with COPD. A biomarker refers to any molecule or material (e.g., cells and tissue) that reflects the disease process. This chapter covers topics on bronchial biopsies, bronchoalveolar lavage, and sputum, among others.

Chapter e37 Chagas' Disease: Advances in Diagnosis and Management

Chagasic cardiomyopathy is the major complication resulting from infection by *Trypanosoma cruzi*. This infection is related to the close proximity between humans and triatomines carrying *T. cruzi*. This chapter discusses laboratory diagnosis and both etiologic and complementary treatments for the disease.

Chapter e38 The Polypill

Several risk factors contribute to causing atherosclerotic coronary artery disease, and some of these can be reduced by a variety of drugs. This chapter discusses the advantages and disadvantages of combining these drugs into one pill, the so-called polypill. The advantages include convenience of delivery, inclusion of all drugs thought to be essential for prevention, low cost, and possible enhanced compliance; disadvantages include possible overtreatment of low-risk patients, undertreatment of high-risk patients, and side effects from one or more components.

The authors emphasize that the role of a polypill in secondary and high-risk prevention is still speculative, and more trials need to be carried out. The polypill's greatest risk appears to be that both patients and physicians may give up on eliminating smoking and modifying sedentary lifestyles and unhealthy diets—tried and true risk-modification techniques.

Chapter e39 Mitochondrial DNA and Heritable Traits and Diseases

The structure and function of mitochondrial DNA (mtDNA) are discussed in depth in this chapter, which includes the proposition that the total cumulative burden of somatic mtDNA mutations acquired with age may contribute to aging and common age-related disturbances. Also included are an overview of the clinical and pathologic features of human mtDNA diseases and their presentations (enhanced by useful tables) and a discussion of the role of mtDNA mutations in the metabolic syndrome, type 2 diabetes mellitus, and neurodegenerative diseases in particular. Genetic counseling and treatment for mtDNA diseases round out the discussion.

INTERNATIONAL ADVISORY EDITORS

Oded Abramsky, MD, PhD
Professor and Head, Department of Neurology, Hebrew University Hadassah Medical School, Jerusalem, Israel

Peter J. Barnes, MA, DM, DSc
Professor and Head of Thoracic Medicine, National Heart & Lung Institute; Head of Respiratory Medicine, Imperial College London; Honorary Consultant Physician, Royal Brompton Hospital, London

Professor Dame Carol Black
Royal College of Physicians, Regents Park, London, United Kingdom

John Funder, MD
Professor, Prince Henry's Institute of Medical Research, Clayton, Victoria, Australia

Professor Donald Metcalf
Professor Emeritus, The Royal Melbourne Hospital, Victoria, Australia

Jose Antonio F. Ramires, MD, PhD
Heard Professor of Cardiology; General Director of the Heart Institute-INCOR, University of São Paulo Medical School, Brazil

Professor Philippe J. Sansonetti
Unité de Pathogénie Microbienne Moléculaire, INSERM U786 Institut Pasteur, Paris, France

Karl Skorecki, MD
Annie Chutick Professor and Chair in Medicine (Nephrology); Director, Rappaport Research Institute, Technion-Israel Institute of Technology; Director of Medicine and Research Development, Ramban Medical Center, Haifa, Israel

Professor K. Srinath Reddy
Professor and Head, Department of Cardiology, All India Institute of Medical Sciences, Ansari Nagar, New Delhi, India

George Stingl, MD
Department of Dermatology, Medical University of Vienna, Wahringer Gurtel 18-20, Vienna, Austria

Professor Nicholas J. White
Professor of Tropical Medicine, Oxford University, United Kingdom; Mahidol University, Bangkok, Thailand

Numbers in brackets refer to the chapters written or co-written by the contributor.

James L. Abbruzzese, MD
Chair and Professor, GI Medical Oncology; Associate Medical Director, GI and Endoscope Center, Ofc/EVP; University of Texas, MD Anderson Cancer Center, Houston [95]

Elias Abrutyn, MD†
Professor of Medicine and Public Health, Drexel University College of Medicine, Philadelphia [133, 134]

John C. Achermann, MD
Lecturer in Endocrinology, UCL Institute of Child Health, University College, London, United Kingdom [343]

John W. Adamson, MD
Clinical Professor of Medicine, UCSD Cancer Center, Hematology/Oncology, University of California at San Diego, La Jolla [58, 98]

Anthony A. Amato, MD
Associate Professor of Neurology, Harvard Medical School; Chief, Divison of Neuromuscular Diseases, Department of Neurology, Brigham and Women's Hospital, Boston [382]

Michael J. Aminoff, MD, DSc
Professor of Neurology, School of Medicine, University of California, San Francisco, San Francisco [23, 25, e31]

Neil M. Ampel, MD
Professor of Medicine, University of Arizona; Staff Physician, SAVAHCS, Tucson [193]

Jennifer Anderson, MD
Clinical Fellow, Department of Newborn Medicine, Children's Hospital of Boston, Boston [69]

Kenneth C. Anderson, MD
Kraft Family Professor of Medicine, Harvard Medical School; Chief, Division of Hematologic Neoplasia, Dana-Farber Cancer Institute, Boston [106, 107]

Elliott M. Antman, MD
Professor of Medicine, Harvard Medical School; Director, Samuel L. Levine Cardiac Unit, and Senior Investigator, TIMI Study Group, Brigham and Women's Hospital, Boston [237, 239]

Frederick R. Appelbaum, MD
Member and Director, Clinical Research Division, Fred Hutchinson Cancer Research Center; Professor and Head, Division of Medical Oncology, University of Washington School of Medicine, Seattle [108]

†Deceased.

Gordon L. Archer, MD
Professor of Medicine and Microbiology/Immunology; Associate Dean for Research, School of Medicine, Virginia Commonwealth University, Richmond [127]

Valder Arruda, MD, PhD
Associate Professor of Pediatrics, University of Pennsylvania School of Medicine, Division of Hematology, The Children's Hospital of Philadelphia, Philadelphia [110]

Arthur K. Asbury, MD
Van Meter Professor of Neurology Emeritus, Philadelphia [25, 380]

John R. Asplin, MD
Clinical Associate, Department of Medicine, University of Chicago; Medical Director, Litholink Corporation, Chicago [281]

Kenneth H. Astrin, MD
Associate Professor, Department of Human Genetics, Mount Sinai School of Medicine of New York University, New York [352]

John C. Atherton, MD
Professor of Gastroenterology; Director, Wolfson Digestive Diseases Centre, University of Nottingham, United Kingdom [144]

Jane C. Atkinson, DDS
Program Director, Clinical Trials Program, Center for Clinical Research, National Institute of Dental and Craniofacial Research, National Institutes of Health, Bethesda [e7]

Paul S. Auerbach, MD, MS
Clinical Professor, Department of Surgery, Division of Emergency Medicine, Stanford University School of Medicine, Stanford [391]

K. Frank Austen, MD
AstraZeneca Professor of Respiratory and Inflammatory Diseases, Harvard Medical School; Director, Inflammation & Allergic Diseases Research Section, Division of Rheumatology, Immunology & Allergy, Brigham and Women's Hospital, Boston [311]

Eric H. Awtry, MD
Assistant Professor of Medicine, Boston University School of Medicine, Boston [233, 234]

Bruce R. Bacon, MD
James F. King Endowed Chair in Gastroenterology; Professor of Internal Medicine, Division of Gastroenterology & Hepatology, St. Louis [302, 303]

Lindsey R. Baden, MD
Assistant Professor of Medicine, Harvard Medical School, Boston [171]

Kamal F. Badr, MD
Professor and Dean, School of Medicine, Lebanese American University, Byblos, Lebanon [280]

Donald S. Baim, MD
Professor of Medicine, Harvard Medical School; Executive Vice President, Chief Medical and Scientific Officer, Boston Scientific Corporation, Natick [223, 240, e23]

John R. Balmes, MD
Professor of Medicine, University of California, San Francisco; Chief, Division of Occupational and Environmental Medicine, San Francisco General Hospital; Professor of Environmental Health Sciences, School of Public Health, University of California, Berkeley [250]

Robert L. Barbieri, MD
Kate Macy Ladd Professor of Obstetrics, Gynecology and Reproductive Biology, Harvard Medical School, Boston [7]

Joanne M. Bargman, MD
Professor of Medicine, University of Toronto; Director, Peritoneal Dialysis Program, and Co-Director, Combined Renal-Rheumatology Lupus Clinic, University Health Network, Toronto [274]

Tamar F. Barlam, MD
Associate Professor of Medicine, Boston University School of Medicine, Boston [115, 140]

Peter J. Barnes, MA, DM, DSc
Professor and Head of Thoracic Medicine, National Heart & Lung Institute; Head of Respiratory Medicine, Imperial College London; Honorary Consultant Physician, Royal Brompton Hospital, London [248, e37]

Miriam J. Baron, MD
Instructor in Medicine, Harvard Medical School, Boston [121]

Kenneth J. Bart, MD, MPH, MSHPM
Professor Emeritus, Epidemiology and Biostatistics, San Diego State University, San Diego; Consultant, National Vaccine Program Office, Office of the Secretary, Department of Health and Human Services, Washington [116]

Shari S. Bassuk, ScD
Epidemiologist, Division of Preventive Medicine, Brigham and Women's Hospital, Boston [342]

David W. Bates, MD, MSc
Professor of Medicine, Harvard Medical School; Chief, General Medical Division, Brigham and Women's Hospital; Medical Director, Clinical and Qualitative Analysis Program, Partners Healthcare System, Boston [e1]

Robert P. Baughman, MD
Professor of Medicine, Cincinnati [322]

M. Flint Beal, MD
Anne Parrish Titzel Professor and Chair, Department of Neurology and Neuroscience, Weill Medical College of Cornell University; Neurologist-in-Chief, New York Presbyterian Hospital, New York [360, 371]

Nicholas J. Beeching, FFTM (RCPS Glas) DCH, DTM&H
Senior Lecturer in Infectious Diseases, Liverpool School of Tropical Medicine, University of Liverpool; Consultant and Clinical Lead, Tropical and Infectious Disease Unit, Royal Liverpool University Hospital, Liverpool, United Kingdom [150]

Robert S. Benjamin, MD
Professor of Medicine; Chairman, Department of Sarcoma Medical Oncology, The University of Texas MD Anderson Cancer Center, Houston [94]

Edward J. Benz, Jr., MD
Richard and Susan Smith Professor of Medicine; Professor of Pediatrics; Professor of Pathology, Harvard Medical School; President and CEO, Dana-Farber Cancer Institute; Director, Dana-Farber/Harvard Cancer Center, Boston [99]

Jean Bergounioux, MD
Medical Doctor of Pediatrics, Unité de Pathogénie Microbienne Moléculaire, Paris [147]

Joseph R. Betancourt, MD, MPH
Director, The Disparities Solutions Center, Massachusetts General Hospital; Assistant Professor of Medicine, Harvard Medical School [e3]

Shalender Bhasin, MD
Chief and Professor, Department of Endocrinology, Diabetes, & Nutrition, Boston University, Boston [340]

Atul K. Bhan, MBBS, MD
Professor of Pathology, Harvard Medical School; Director of the Immunopathology Unit, Department of Pathology, Massachusetts General Hospital, Boston [e26]

David R. Bickers, MD
Carl Truman Nelson Professor and Chair, Department of Dermatology, College of Physicians and Surgeons, Columbia University Medical Center, New York [57]

Henry J. Binder, MD
Professor of Medicine; Professor of Cellular & Molecular Physiology, Yale University, New Haven [288]

Thomas D. Bird, MD
Professor, Neurology and Medicine, University of Washington; Research Neurologist, Geriatric Research Education and Clinical Center, VA Puget Sound Health Care System, Seattle [365]

William R. Bishai, MD, PhD
Professor of Medicine, The Johns Hopkins School of Medicine, Baltimore [131]

Bruce R. Bistrian, MD, PhD
Chief, Clinical Nutrition, Beth Israel Deaconess Medical Center; Professor of Medicine, Harvard Medical School, Boston [73]

Martin J. Blaser, MD
Frederick H. King Professor of Internal Medicine; Chair, Department of Medicine; Professor of Microbiology, New York University School of Medicine, New York [144, 148]

Clara D. Bloomfield, MD
Distinguished University Professor; William G. Pace III Professor of Cancer Research, Cancer Scholar and Senior Advisor, The Ohio State University Comprehensive Cancer Center and Arthur G. James Cancer Hospital and Richard J. Solove Research Institute, Columbus [104]

Richard S. Blumberg, MD
Professor of Medicine, Harvard Medical School; Chief, Division of Gastroenterology, Hepatology and Endoscopy, Brigham and Women's Hospital, Boston [289]

David Blumenthal, MD, MPP
Samuel O. Their Professor of Medicine; Professor of Health Care Policy, Harvard Medical School; Director, Institute for Health Policy, Massachusetts General Hospital/Partners HealthCare System, Boston [e3]

Jean L. Bolognia, MD
Professor of Dermatology, Yale Medical School [54]

George J. Bosl, MD
Chairman, Department of Medicine, Memorial Sloan-Kettering Cancer Center; Professor of Medicine, Joan and Sanford I Weill Medical College of Cornell University, New York [92]

Richard C. Boucher, Jr., MD
William Rand Kenan Professor of Medicine, University of North Carolina at Chapel Hill; Director, University of Carolina Cystic Fibrosis Center, Chapel Hill [253]

Eugene Braunwald, MD, MA (Hon), ScD (Hon)
Distinguished Hersey Professor of Medicine, Harvard Medical School; Chairman, TIMI Study Group, Brigham and Women's Hospital, Boston [1, 35, 36, 217, 219, 220, 230–232, 237–239, e8]

Irwin M. Braverman, MD
Professor of Dermatology, Yale University School of Medicine, New Haven [54]

Otis Webb Brawley, MD
Professor, Hematology, Oncology, Medicine & Epidemiology, Emory University; Chief Medical Officer, American Cancer Society, Atlanta [78]

Joel G. Breman, MD, DTPH
Senior Scientific Advisor, Fogarty International Center, National Institutes of Health, Bethesda [203, e18]

Barry M. Brenner, MD, AM, DSc (Hon), DMSc (Hon), Dipl (Hon)
Samuel A. Levine Professor of Medicine, Harvard Medical School; Director Emeritus, Renal Division, Brigham and Women's Hospital, Boston [45, 46, 279, 280, 283]

George J. Brewer, MD
Morton S. and Henrietta K. Sellner Active Emeritus Professor of Human Genetics; Active Emeritus Professor of Internal Medicine, University of Michigan Medical School, Ann Arbor [354]

F. Richard Bringhurst, MD
Senior Vice President for Medicine and Research Management , Massachusetts General Hospital; Associate Professor of Medicine, Harvard Medical School, Boston [346]

Kevin E. Brown, MD
Consultant Medical Virologist, Health Protection Agency, London [177]

Robert H. Brown, Jr., MD, DPhil
Neurologist, Massachusetts General Hospital; Professor of Neurology, Harvard Medical School, Boston [369, 382]

H. R. Büller, MD
Professor of Medicine; Chairman, Department of Vascular Medicine, Academic Medical Center, Amsterdam [111]

David M. Burns, MD
Professor Emeritus, Department of Family and Preventive Medicine, University of California, San Diego School of Medicine, San Diego [390]

Michael J. Burns, MD
Assistant Professor of Medicine, Harvard Medical School, Boston [e35]

Joan R. Butterton, MD
Assistant Clinical Professor of Medicine, Harvard Medical School; Clinical Associate in Medicine, Massachusetts General Hospital, Boston [122]

John C. Byrd, MD
D. Warren Brown Professor of Leukemia Research Professor; Co-Director of Hematologic Malignancies, Division of Hematology and Oncology, Arthur G. James Cancer Hospital, Columbus [104]

Stephen B. Calderwood, MD
Morton N. Swartz, MD Academy Professor of Medicine (Microbiology and Molecular Genetics), Harvard Medical School; Chief, Division of Infectious Diseases, Massachusetts General Hospital, Boston [122]

Michael V. Callahan, MD, DTM&H (UK), MSPH
Clinical Associate Physician, Division of Infectious Diseases, Massachusetts General Hospital; Program Manager, Biodefense, Defense Advanced Research Project Agency (DARPA), United States Department of Defense, Washington [19]

Michael Camilleri, MD
Atherton and Winifred W. Bean Professor; Professor of Medicine and Physiology, Mayo Clinic College of Medicine, Rochester [40]

Grant L. Campbell, MD, PhD
Division of Vector-Borne Infectious Diseases, National Center for Infectious Diseases, Centers for Disease Control and Prevention, U.S. Public Health Service, Laporte [152]

Christopher P. Cannon, MD
Associate Professor of Medicine, Harvard Medical School; Associate Physician, Cardiovascular Division, Senior Investigator, TIMI Study Group, Brigham and Women's Hospital, Boston [238]

Jonathan R. Carapetis, MBBS, PhD
Director, Menzies School of Health Research; Professor, Charles Darwin University, Australia [315]

Mark Carlson, MD, MA
Chief Medical Officer and Senior Vice President, Clinical Affairs, St. Jude Medical, Sylmar; Adjunct Professor of Medicine, Case Western Reserve University, Cleveland[21]

Charles B. Carpenter, MD
Professor of Medicine, Harvard Medical School; Senior Physician, Brigham and Women's Hospital, Boston [276]

Brian I. Carr, MD, PhD
Professor of Medicine, Thomas Jefferson University; Director of the Liver Tumor Program, Kimmel Cancer Center, Philadelphia [88]

Lisa B. Caruso, MD, MPH
Assistant Professor of Medicine, Boston Medical Center, Boston [9]

Arturo Casadevall, MD, PhD
Professor of Microbiology and Immunology and of Medicine; Chair, Department of Microbiology and Immunology, Albert Einstein College of Medicine, New York [195]

Agustin Castellanos, MD
Professor of Medicine; Director, Clinical Electrophysiology, University of Miami Miller School of Medicine, Miami [267]

Stanley W. Chapman, MD
Professor of Medicine and Microbiology; Director, Division of Infectious Diseases; Vice-Chair for Academic Affairs, Department of Medicine, University of Mississippi School of Medicine, Jackson [194, 199]

Vinay Chaudhry, MD
Professor and Vice Chair, The Johns Hopkins University School of Medicine; Co-Director, EMG Laboratory, Johns Hopkins Hospital, Baltimore [379]

Lan X. Chen, MD
Clinical Assistant Professor of Medicine, University of Pennsylvania, Penn Presbyterian Medical Center & Philadelphia Veteran Affairs Medical Center, Philadelphia [327]

Yuan-Tsong Chen, MD
Distinguished Research Fellow and Director, Institute of Biomedical Sciences, Academia Sinica, Taiwan [356]

Glenn M. Chertow, MD
Professor of Medicine, Epidemiology and Biostatistics, University of California, San Francisco School of Medicine; Director, Clinical Services, Division of Nephrology, University of California, San Francisco Medical Center, San Francisco [273, 275]

John S. Child, MD
Director, Ahmanson-UCLA Adult Congenital Heart Disease Center; Streisand Professor of Medicine and Cardiology, David Geffen School of Medicine at UCLA, Los Angeles [229]

Yu Jo Chua, MBBS
Research Fellow (Medical Oncology), Royal Marsden Hospital, London [89]

Raymond T. Chung, MD
Associate Professor of Medicine, Harvard Medical School; Director of Hepatology, Massachusetts General Hospital; Medical Director, Liver Transplant Program, Massachusetts General Hospital, Boston [304]

Fredric L. Coe, MD
Professor of Medicine, University of Chicago, Chicago [281]

Jeffrey I. Cohen, MD
Chief, Medical Virology Section, Laboratory of Clinical Infectious Diseases, National Institute of Allergy and Infectious Diseases, National Institutes of Health, Bethesda [174, 184]

Ronit Cohen-Poradosu, MD
Channing Laboratory, Brigham and Women's Hospital, Boston [157]

Francis Collins, MD, PhD
Director, National Human Genome Research Institute, National Institutes of Health, Bethesda [79]

Wilson S. Colucci, MD
Thomas J. Ryan Professor of Medicine, Boston University School of Medicine; Chief, Cardiovascular Medicine, Boston University Medical Center, Boston [233, 234]

Max D. Cooper, MD
Professor of Medicine, Pediatrics, Microbiology, and Pathology, The University of Alabama at Birmingham, Birmingham [310, e27]

Michael J. Corbel, PhD, DSc(Med), FIBiol
Head, Division of Bacteriology, National Institute for Biological Standards and Control, Potters Bar, United Kingdom [150]

Lawrence Corey, MD
Professor of Medicine and Laboratory Medicine; Chair of Medical Virology, University of Washington; Head, Program in Infectious Diseases, Fred Hutchinson Cancer Research Center, Seattle [172]

Felicia Cosman, MD
Associate Professor of Clinical Medicine, Columbia University College of Physicians and Surgeons; Medical Director, Clinical Research Center, Helen Hayes Hospital, West Haverstraw, New York [348]

Mark A. Creager, MD
Professor of Medicine, Harvard Medical School; Simon C. Fireman Scholar in Cardiovascular Medicine; Director, Vascular Center, Brigham and Women's Hospital, Boston [242, 243]

Philip E. Cryer, MD
Irene E. and Michael M. Karl Professor of Endocrinology and Metabolism in Medicine, Washington University, St. Louis [339]

David Cunningham, MD
Professor of Cancer Medicine, Institute of Cancer Research; Consultant Medical Oncologist, Head of Gastrointestinal Unit, Royal Marsden Hospital, London [89]

John J. Cush, MD
Director of Clinical Rheumatology, Baylor Research Institute; Professor of Medicine and Rheumatology, Baylor University Medical Center, Dallas [325]

Malwina Czarny-Ratajczak, PhD
Research Assistant Professor, Center for Gene Therapy, Tulane University Health Sciences Center, Tulane University, New Orleans [357]

Charles A. Czeisler, MD, PhD
Baldino Professor of Sleep Medicine, and Director, Division of Sleep Medicine, Harvard Medical School; Chief, Division of Sleep Medicine, Department of Medicine, Brigham and Women's Hospital, Boston [28]

Marinos C. Dalakas, MD
Professor of Neurology; Chief, Neuromuscular Diseases Section, NINDS, National Institute of Health, Bethesda [383]

Josep Dalmau, MD, PhD
Professor of Neurology, Division Neuro-Oncology, Department of Neurology, Philadelphia [97]

Daniel F. Danzl, MD
Professor and Chair, Department of Emergency Medicine, University of Louisville School of Medicine, Louisville [20]

Emily Darby, MD
Senior Fellow, Division of Infectious Diseases, University of Washington, Seattle [153]

Robert B. Daroff, MD
Gilbert W. Humphrey Professor of Neurology and Interim Chair, Department of Neurology, Case Western Reserve University School of Medicine and University Hospitals Case Medical Center, Cleveland [22]

Charles E. Davis, MD
Professor of Pathology and Medicine Emeritus, University of California San Diego School of Medicine; Director Emeritus, Microbiology Laboratory, University of California San Diego Medical Center, San Diego [e16]

Mahlon R. DeLong, MD
Timmie Professor of Neurology, Emory University School of Medicine, Atlanta [366]

John Del Valle, MD
Professor and Senior Associate Chair of Graduate Medical Education, Department of Internal Medicine, Division of Gastroenterology, University of Michigan Health System, Ann Arbor [287]

Marie B. Demay, MD
Associate Professor of Medicine, Harvard Medical School; Associate Physician, Massachusetts General Hospital, Boston [346]

Bradley M. Denker, MD
Associate Professor of Medicine, Harvard Medical School; Physician, Brigham and Women's Hospital; Chief of Nephrology, Harvard Vanguard Medical Associates, Boston [45]

David W. Denning, MBBS
Professor of Medicine and Medical Mycology, University of Manchester; Director, Regional Mycology Laboratory, Manchester Education and Research Centre, Wythenshawe Hospital, Manchester, United Kingdom [197]

David T. Dennis, MD, MPH
Faculty Affiliate, Department of Microbiology, Immunology and Pathology, Colorado State University; Medical Epidemiologist, Division of Influenza, Centers for Disease Control and Prevention, Atlanta [152, 165]

Robert J. Desnick, MD, PhD
Professor and Chair, Department of Genetics and Genomic Sciences, Mount Sinai School of Medicine of New York University, New York [352]

Betty Diamond, MD
Chief, Autoimmune Disease Center, The Feinstein Institute for Medical Research, New York [312]

Jules L. Dienstag, MD
Carl W. Walter Professor of Medicine and Dean for Medical Education, Harvard Medical School; Physician, Gastrointestinal Unit, Massachusetts General Hospital, Boston [298–300, 304, e26]

William P. Dillon, MD
Professor of Radiology, Neurology, and Neurosurgery; Vice-Chair, Department of Radiology; Chief, Neuroradiology, University of California, San Francisco [362, e30]

Charles A. Dinarello, MD
Professor of Medicine, University of Colorado Health Science Center, Denver [17]

Robert G. Dluhy, MD
Program Director, Fellowship in Endocrinology; Professor of Medicine, Brigham and Women's Hospital, Harvard Medical School; Associate Editor, New England Journal of Medicine, Boston [336]

Raphael Dolin, MD
Maxwell Finland Professor of Medicine (Microbiology and Molecular Genetics); Dean for Academic and Clinical Programs, Harvard Medical School, Boston [171, 179, 180]

Neil J. Douglas, MD
Professor of Respiratory and Sleep Medicine, University of Edinburgh; Honorary Consultant Physician, Royal Infirmary of Edinburgh, United Kingdom [259]

Daniel B. Drachman, MD
Professor of Neurology & Neuroscience; WW Smith Charitable Trust Professor of Neuroimmunology, The Johns Hopkins University School of Medicine, Baltimore [381]

David F. Driscoll, PhD
Assistant Professor of Medicine, Harvard Medical School, Boston [73]

Thomas D. DuBose, Jr., MD
Tinsley R. Harrison Professor and Chair of Internal Medicine; Professor of Physiology and Pharmacology, Wake Forest University School of Medicine, Winston-Salem [48]

J. Stephen Dumler, MD
Professor, Division of Medical Microbiology, Department of Pathology, The Johns Hopkins University School of Medicine and Immunology, The Johns Hopkins University Bloomberg School of Public Health, Baltimore [167]

Andrea E. Dunaif, MD
Charles F. Kettering Professor of Medicine and Chief, Division of Endocrinology, Metabolism, and Molecular Medicine, Northwestern University Feinberg School Medicine, Chicago [6]

Samuel C. Durso, MD, MBA
Associate Professor of Medicine, Clinical Director, Division of Geriatric Medicine and Gerontology, The Johns Hopkins University School of Medicine, Baltimore [32, e7]

Janice P. Dutcher, MD
Professor, New York Medical College; Associate Director, Our Lady of Mercy Cancer Center, Bronx [270]

Johanna Dwyer, DSc, RD
Professor of Medicine and Community Health, Tufts University School of Medicine and Friedman School of Nutrition Science and Policy; Senior Scientist Jean Mayer Human Nutrition Research Center on Aging at Tufts; Director of the Frances Stern Nutrition Center, Tufts-New England Medical Center Hospital, Boston [70]

Jeffery S. Dzieczkowski, MD
Physician, St. Alphonsus Regional Medical Center; Medical Director, Coagulation Clinic, Saint Alphonsus Medical Group/Internal Medicine, Boise [107]

Kim A. Eagle, MD
Albion Walter Hewlett Professor of Internal Medicine, Chief of Clinical Cardiology and Director, University of Michigan Cardiovascular Center, University of Michigan, Ann Arbor [8]

Robert H. Eckel, MD
Professor of Medicine, Division of Endocrinology, Metabolism and Diabetes, Division of Cardiology; Professor of Physiology and Biophysics; Charles A. Boettcher II Chair in Atherosclerosis; Program Director, Adult General Clinical Research Center, University of Colorado at Denver and Health Sciences Center; Director Lipid Clinic, University Hospital, Aurora [236]

John E. Edwards, Jr., MD
Chief, Division of Infectious Diseases, Harbor/University of California, Los Angeles Medical Center; Professor of Medicine, David Geffen School of Medicine at the University of California, Los Angeles, Torrance [191, 196]

David A. Ehrmann, MD
Professor of Medicine; Associate Director, University of Chicago General Clinical Research Center, Chicago [50]

Ezekiel J. Emanuel, MD, PhD
Chair, Department of Bioethics, The Warren G. Magnuson Clinical Center, National Institutes of Health, Bethesda [11]

Linda L. Emanuel, MD, PhD
Buehler Professor of Medicine; Director, Buehler Center on Aging, Health & Society, Northwestern University Feinberg School of Medicine, Chicago [11]

Joey English, MD, PhD
Assistant Professor of Neurology, University of California, San Francisco, San Francisco [364]

John W. Engstrom, MD
Professor of Neurology; Clinical Chief of Service; Neurology Residency Program Director, University of California, San Francisco, San Francisco [16, 370]

Paul Farmer, MD, PhD
Maude and Lillian Presley Professor of Medical Anthropology, Department of Social Medicine, Harvard Medical School; Associate Chief, Division of Social Medicine and Health Inequalities, Brigham and Women's Hospital; Co-Founder, Partners In Health, Boston [2]

Anthony S. Fauci, MD, DSc (Hon), DM&S (Hon), DHL (Hon), DPS (Hon), DLM (Hon), DMS (Hon)
Chief, Laboratory of Immunoregulation; Director, National Institute of Allergy and Infectious Diseases, National Institutes of Health, Bethesda [1, 181, 182, 214, 308, 319, e28]

Murray J. Favus, MD
Professor of Medicine, Interim Head, Endocrine Section; Director, Bone Section, University of Chicago Pritzker School of Medicine, Chicago [281, 349]

David T. Felson, MD, MPH
Professor of Medicine and Epidemiology; Chief, Clinical Epidemiology Unit, Boston University, Boston [326]

Robert G. Fenton, MD, PhD
Staff Clinician, National Institute on Aging, National Institutes of Health, Baltimore [80]

Howard L. Fields, MD, PhD
Professor of Neurology; Director, Wheeler Center for Neurobiology of Addiction, University of California, San Francisco, San Francisco [12]

Gregory A. Filice, MD
Professor of Medicine, University of Minnesota; Chief, Infectious Disease Section, Minneapolis Veterans Affairs Medical Center, Minneapolis [155]

Robert Finberg, MD
Professor and Chair, Department of Medicine, University of Massachusetts Medical School, Worcester [82, 126]

Joyce Fingeroth, MD
Associate Professor of Medicine, Harvard Medical School, Boston [126]

Daniel J. Fink, MD, MPH
Associate Professor of Clinical Pathology, College of Physicians and Surgeons, Columbia University, New York [Appendix]

Jeffrey S. Flier, MD
Caroline Shields Walker Professor of Medicine, Harvard Medical School; Dean of the Faculty of Medicine, Harvard School of Medicine, Boston [74]

Agnes B. Fogo, MD
Professor of Pathology, Medicine and Pediatrics; Director, Renal/EM Division, Department of Pathology, Vanderbilt University Medical Center, Nashville [e9]

Sonia Friedman, MD
Assistant Professor of Medicine, Harvard Medical School; Associate Physician, Brigham and Women's Hospital, Boston [289]

Andre D. Furtado, MD
Associate Specialist at the Department of Radiology, Neuroradiology Section, University of California, San Francisco, San Francisco [e30]

Robert F. Gagel, MD
Professor of Medicine and Head, Division of Internal Medicine, University of Texas MD Anderson Cancer Center, Houston [345]

John I. Gallin, MD
Director, The Warren G. Magnuson Clinical Center, National Institutes of Health, Bethesda [61]

J. Michael Gaziano, MD, MPH
Chief, Division of Aging, Brigham and Women's Hospital; Director, Massachusetts Veterans Epidemiology, Research and Information Center (MAVERIC) and Geriatric Research, Education and Clinical Center (GRECC), Boston VA Healthcare System; Associate Professor of Medicine, Harvard Medical School, Boston [218]

Thomas A. Gaziano, MD, MSc
Instructor in Medicine, Harvard Medical School; Associate Physician of Cardiovascular Medicine, Brigham and Women's Hospital, Boston [218]

Susan L. Gearhart, MD
Assistant Professor of Colorectal Surgery and Oncology, The Johns Hopkins University School of Medicine, Baltimore [291, 292, 293, 294]

Robert H. Gelber, MD
Scientific Director, Leonard Wood Memorial Leprosy Research Center, Cebu, Philippines; Clinical Professor of Medicine and Dermatology, University of California, San Francisco, San Francisco [159]

Jeffrey A. Gelfand, MD
Professor of Medicine, Harvard Medical School; Physician, Department of Medicine, Massachusetts General Hospital, Boston [19, 204]

Alfred L. George, MD
Grant W. Liddle Professor of Medicine and Pharmacology; Chief, Division of Genetic Medicine, Department of Medicine, Vanderbilt University, Nashville [271]

Dale N. Gerding, MD
Assistant Chief of Staff for Research, Hines VA Hospital, Hines; Professor, Stritch School of Medicine, Loyola University, Maywood [123]

Anne Gershon, MD
Professor of Pediatrics, Columbia University College of Physicians and Surgeons, New York [185–187]

Marc Ghany, MD
Staff Physician, Liver Diseases Branch, National Institute of Diabetes and Digestive and Kidney Diseases, National Institutes of Health, Bethesda [295]

Raymond J. Gibbons, MD
Arthur M. and Gladys D. Gray Professor of Medicine, Mayo Clinic College of Medicine; Consultant, Cardiovascular Diseases, Mayo Clinic, Rochester [222, e20]

Bruce C. Gilliland,† MD
Professor of Medicine and Laboratory Medicine, University of Washington School of Medicine, Seattle [321, 329–331]

Roger I. Glass, MD, PhD
Director, Fogarty International Center; Associate Director for International Research, National Institutes of Health, Bethesda [183]

Eli Glatstein, MD
Morton M. Kligerman Professor and Vice Chairman, Clinical Director, Department of Radiation Oncology, University of Pennsylvania Medical Center, Philadelphia [216]

Robert M. Glickman, MD
Professor of Medicine, New York University School of Medicine, New York [44]

James F. Glockner, MD
Assistant Professor of Radiology, Mayo Clinic College of Medicine, Rochester [222]

Peter J. Goadsby, MD, PhD, DSc
Professor of Clinical Neurology, Institute of Neurology, Queen Square London; Professor of Neurology, Department of Neurology, University of California, San Francisco, San Francisco [15]

Ary L. Goldberger, MD
Professor of Medicine, Harvard Medical School; Associate Director, Division of Interdisciplinary Medicine and Biotechnology, Beth Israel Deaconess Medical Center, Boston [221, e19, e21]

Samuel Z. Goldhaber, MD
Professor of Medicine, Harvard Medical School; Director, Venous Thromboembolism Research Group, Director, Anticoagulation Service, and Senior Staff Cardiologist, Department of Medicine, Brigham and Women's Hospital, Boston [256]

†Deceased.

Ralph Gonzales, MD, MSPH
Professor of Medicine, Epidemiology and Biostatistics, University of California, San Francisco, San Francisco [31]

Douglas S. Goodin, MD
Professor of Neurology, University of California, San Francisco, San Francisco [375]

Raj K. Goyal, MD
Mallinckrodt Professor of Medicine, Harvard Medical School, Boston; Physician, VA Boston Healthcare and Beth Israel Deaconess Medical Center, West Roxbury [38, 286]

Gregory A. Grabowski, MD
The A. Graeme Mitchell Chair of Human Genetics; Professor, University of Cincinnati College of Medicine, Department of Pediatrics; Director, Division of Human Genetics, Cincinnati Children's Hospital Medical Center, Cincinnati [355]

Norton J. Greenberger, MD
Clinical Professor of Medicine, Harvard Medical School; Senior Physician, Brigham and Women's Hospital, Boston [305–307]

David E. Griffith, MD
Professor of Medicine; William A. and Elizabeth B. Moncrief Distinguished Professor, University of Texas Health Center, Tyler [161]

Rasim Gucalp, MD
Professor of Clinical Medicine, Albert Einstein College of Medicine, Montefiore Medical Center, Bronx [270]

Chadi A. Hage, MD
Assistant Professor of Medicine, Indiana University School of Medicine, Roudebush VA Medical Center, Pulmonary-Critical Care and Infectious Diseases, Indianapolis [192]

Bevra Hannahs Hahn, MD
Professor of Medicine; Chief of Rheumatology; Vice Chair, Department of Medicine, David Geffen School of Medicine, University of California, Los Angeles, Los Angeles [313]

Janet E. Hall, MD
Associate Professor of Medicine, Harvard Medical School; Associate Physician, Massachusetts General Hospital, Boston [51, 341]

Jesse B. Hall, MD
Professor of Medicine, Anesthesia & Critical Care; Section Chief, Pulmonary and Critical Care Medicine, University of Chicago, Chicago [261]

Scott A. Halperin, MD
Professor of Pediatrics and of Microbiology and Immunology, Dalhousie University, Halifax, Nova Scotia [142]

Raymond C. Harris, Jr., MD
Ann and Roscoe R. Robinson Professor of Medicine; Chief, Division of Nephrology & Hypertension, Department of Medicine, Vanderbilt University, Nashville [272]

Gavin Hart, MD, MPH
Director, STD Services, Royal Adelaide Hospital; Clinical Associate Professor, School of Medicine, Flinders University, Adelaide, South Australia, Australia [154]

Rudy Hartskeerl, PhD
Head, FAO/OIE, World Health Organization and National Leptospirosis Reference Centre, KIT Biomedical Research, Royal Tropical Institute, Amsterdam, The Netherlands [164]

William L. Hasler, MD
Professor of Medicine, Division of Gastroenterology, University of Michigan Health System, Ann Arbor [39, 284]

Terry J. Hassold, PhD
Eastlick Distinguished Professor, Washington State University, Pullman [63]

Joshua Hauser, MD
Assistant Professor of Medicine and Palliative Care; Assistant Director of the Beuler Center on Aging, Northwestern University, Chicago [11]

Stephen L. Hauser, MD
Robert A. Fishman Distinguished Professor and Chairman, Department of Neurology, University of California, San Francisco, San Francisco [1, 360, 361, 371, 372, 375, 380, e32]

Barton F. Haynes, MD
Frederic M. Hanes Professor of Medicine and Immunology, Departments of Medicine and Immunology; Director, Duke Human Vaccine Institute, Duke University School of Medicine, Durham [308]

Douglas C. Heimburger, MD, MS
Professor of Nutrition Sciences; Professor of Medicine; Director, Clinical Nutrition Fellowship Program, University of Alabama at Birmingham, Birmingham [72]

J. Claude Hemphill III, MD, MAS
Associate Professor of Clinical Neurology and Neurological Surgery, University of California, San Francisco; Director, Neurocritical Care Program, San Francisco General Hospital, San Francisco [269]

Patrick H. Henry, MD
Adjunct Clinical Professor of Medicine, University of Iowa, Iowa City [60]

Barbara L. Herwaldt, MD, MPH
Medical Epidemiologist, Division of Parasitic Diseases, Centers for Disease Control and Prevention, Atlanta [205]

Katherine A. High, MD
William H. Bennett Professor of Pediatrics, University of Pennsylvania School of Medicine; Investigator, Howard Hughes Medical Institute, The Children's Hospital of Philadelphia, Philadelphia [65, 110]

Martin S. Hirsch, MD
Professor of Medicine, Harvard Medical School; Professor of Immunology and Infectious Diseases, Harvard School of Public Health; Physician, Massachusetts General Hospital, Boston [175]

Helen H. Hobbs, MD
Investigator, Howard Hughes Medical Institute; Professor of Internal Medicine and Molecular Genetics, University of Texas Southwestern Medical Center, Dallas [350]

Judith S. Hochman, MD
Harold Synder Family Professor of Cardiology; Clinical Chief, the Leon H. Charney Division of Cardiology; New York University School of Medicine; Director, Cardiovascular Clinical Research, New York [226]

Elizabeth L. Hohmann, MD
Associate Professor of Medicine and Infectious Diseases, Harvard Medical School, Massachusetts General Hospital, Boston [132]

A. Victor Hoffbrand, DM
Emeritus Professor of Haematology, Royal Free and University College, London [100]

Steven M. Holland, MD
Senior Investigator and Head, Immunopathogenesis Unit, Clinical Pathophysiology Section, Laboratory of Host Defenses, National Institute of Allergy and Infectious Diseases, National Institutes of Health, Bethesda [61]

King K. Holmes, MD, PhD
William H. Foege Chair, Department of Global Health; Director, Center for AIDS and STD; Professor of Medicine and Global Health, University of Washington; Head, Infectious Diseases, Harborview Medical Center, Seattle [124]

Jay H. Hoofnagle, MD
Director, Liver Diseases Research Branch, Division of Digestive Diseases and Nutrition, National Institute of Diabetes and Digestive and Kidney Diseases, National Institutes of Health, Bethesda [295]

Robert J. Hopkin, MD
Assistant Professor of Clinical Pediatrics, The University of Cincinnati College of Medicine; Division and Program in Human Genetics, Cincinnati Children's Hospital Research Foundation, Cincinnati [355]

Jonathan C. Horton, MD, PhD
William F. Hoyt Professor of Neuro-Ophthalmology; Professor of Ophthalmology, Neurology, and Physiology, University of California, San Francisco, San Francisco [29]

Howard Hu, MD, MPH, ScD
NSF International Chair, Department of Environmental Health Sciences; Professor of Environmental Health, Epidemiology and Medicine, University of Michigan Schools of Public Health and Medicine, Ann Arbor [e34]

Gary W. Hunninghake, MD
Sterba Professor of Medicine; Director, Division of Pulmonary, Critical Care and Occupational Medicine; Director, Institute for Clinical and Translational Science; Director, Graduate Program in Translational Biomedicine; Senior Associate Dean for Clinical and Translational Science, Iowa City [249]

Sharon A. Hunt, MD
Professor, Cardiovascular Medicine, Stanford University, Palo Alto [228]

Charles G. Hurst, MD
Chief, Chemical Casualty Care Division, United States Medical Research Institute of Chemical Defense, Maryland [215]

Steven E. Hyman, MD
Provost, Harvard University; Professor of Neurobiology, Harvard Medical School, Boston [385]

David H. Ingbar, MD
Professor of Medicine, Physiology & Pediatrics; Director, Pulmonary, Allergy, Critical Care & Sleep Division; Executive Director, Center for Lung Science & Health, University of Minnesota School of Medicine; Co-Director, Medical ICU & Respiratory Care, University of Minnesota Medical Center, Fairview [266]

Edward P. Ingenito, MD, PhD
Assistant Professor, Harvard Medical School, Boston [263]

Mark A. Israel, MD
Professor of Pediatrics and Genetics, Dartmouth Medical School; Director, Norris Cotton Cancer Center, Dartmouth-Hitchcock Medical Center, Lebanon [374]

Alan C. Jackson, MD, FRCPC
Professor of Medicine (Neurology) and of Medical Microbiology, University of Manitoba; Section Head of Neurology, Winnipeg Regional Health Authority, Winnipeg, Manitoba, Canada [188]

Richard F. Jacobs, MD, FAAP
President, Arkansas Children's Hospital Research Institute; Horace C. Cabe Professor of Pediatrics, University of Arkansas for Medical Sciences, College of Medicine, Little Rock [151]

J. Larry Jameson, MD, PhD
Professor of Medicine; Vice President for Medical Affairs and Lewis Landsberg Dean, Northwestern University Feinberg School of Medicine, Chicago [1, 62, 64, 96, 332, 333, 335, 340, 343, e29]

Robert T. Jensen, MD
Chief, Digestive Diseases Branch, National Institute of Diabetes, Digestive and Kidney Diseases, National Institutes of Health, Bethesda [344]

Camilo Jimenez, MD
Assistant Professor, Department of Endocrine Neoplasia & Hormonal Disorders, The University of Texas, MD Cancer Center, Houston [345]

Eric C. Johannsen, MD
Assistant Professor, Department of Medicine, Harvard Medical School; Associate Physician, Division of Infectious Diseases, Brigham and Women's Hospital, Boston [188]

Bruce E. Johnson, MD
Director, Lowe Center for Thoracic Oncology, Department of Medical Oncology; Dana-Farber Cancer Institute, Department of Medicine, Brigham and Women's Hospital; Professor of Medicine, Harvard Medical School, Boston [96]

James R. Johnson, MD
Professor of Medicine, University of Minnesota, Minneapolis [143]

Stuart Johnson, MD
Associate Professor, Stritch School of Medicine, Loyola University, Maywood; Staff Physician, Hines VA Hospital, Hines [123]

S. Claiborne Johnston, MD, PhD
Professor, Neurology; Professor, Epidemiology and Biostatistics; Director, University of California, San Francisco Stroke Service, San Francisco [364]

S. Andrew Josephson, MD
Assistant Clinical Professor of Neurology, University of California, San Francisco, San Francisco [26, e33]

Jorge L. Juncos, MD
Associate Professor of Neurology, Emory University School of Medicine; Director of Neurology, Wesley Woods Hospital, Atlanta [366]

Eric Kandel, MD
University Professor; Fred Kavli Professor and Director, Kavli Institute for Brain Sciences; Senior Investigator, Howard Hughes Medical Institute, Columbia University, New York [385]

Marshall M. Kaplan, MD
Professor of Medicine, Tufts University School of Medicine; Chief Emeritus, Division of Gastroenterology, Tufts-New England Medical Center, Boston [43, 296]

Adolf W. Karchmer, MD
Professor of Medicine, Harvard Medical School, Boston [118]

Dennis L. Kasper, MD, MA (Hon)
William Ellery Channing Professor of Medicine, Professor of Microbiology and Molecular Genetics, Harvard Medical School; Director, Channing Laboratory, Department of Medicine, Brigham and Women's Hospital, Boston [1, 113, 115, 121, 135, 140, 157]

Lloyd H. Kasper, MD
Professor of Medicine and Microbiology/Immunology; Co-Director, Program in Immunotherapeutics, Dartmouth Medical Schoool, Lebanon [207]

Daniel Kastner, MD, PhD
Chief, Genetics and Genomic Section, National Institute of Arthritis and Musculoskeletal and Skin Diseases, National Institutes of Health, Bethesda [323]

Elaine T. Kaye, MD
Clinical Assistant Professor of Dermatology, Harvard Medical School; Assistant in Medicine, Department of Medicine, Children's Hospital Medical Center, Boston [18, e5]

Kenneth M. Kaye, MD
Associate Professor of Medicine, Harvard Medical School; Associate Physician, Division of Infectious Diseases, Brigham and Women's Hospital, Boston [18, e5]

Jack A. Kessler, MD
Davis Professor of Stem Cell Biology; Chairman, Davis Department of Neurology, Northwestern University Feinberg School of Medicine, Chicago [67]

Gerald T. Keusch, MD
Associate Provost and Associate Dean for Global Health, Boston University School of Medicine, Boston [116, 149]

Jay S. Keystone, MD, FRCPC
Professor of Medicine, University of Toronto; Staff Physician, Centre for Travel and Tropical Medicine, Toronto General Hospital, Toronto [117]

Sundeep Khosla, MD
Professor of Medicine and Physiology, Mayo Clinic College of Medicine, Rochester [47]

Elliott Kieff, MD, PhD
Harriet Ryan Albee Professor of Medicine and Microbiology and Molecular Genetics, Harvard Medical School; Senior Physician, Brigham and Women's Hospital, Boston [170]

Jim Yong Kim, MD, PhD
Chief, Division of Social Medicine and Health Inequalities, Brigham and Women's Hospital; Director and Professor, François Xavier-Bagnoud Center for Health and Human Rights, Harvard School of Public Health; Professor of Social Medicine and Chair, Department of Social Medicine, Harvard Medical School, Boston [2]

Talmadge E. King, Jr., MD
Constance B. Wofsy Distinguished Professor and Interim Chair, Department of Medicine, University of California, San Francisco, San Francisco [255]

Louis V. Kirchhoff, MD, MPH
Professor, Departments of Internal Mediciene and Epidemiology, University of Iowa; Staff Physician, Department of Veterans Affairs Medical Center, Iowa City [206]

Joel N. Kline, MD, MSc
Professor, Internal Medicine and Occupational & Environmental Health; Director, University of Iowa Asthma Center, Iowa City [249]

Minoru S. H. Ko, MD, PhD
Senior Investigator & Chief, Developmental Genomics & Aging Section, Laboratory of Genetics, National Institute on Aging, NIH, Baltimore [66]

Barbara A. Konkle, MD
Professor of Medicine and Hematology/Oncology, University of Pennsylvania; Director, Penn Comprehensive Hemophilia and Thrombosis Program, Philadelphia [59, 109]

Peter Kopp, MD
Associate Professor, Division of Endocrinology, Metabolism and Molecular Science, Northwestern University Feinberg School of Medicine, Chicago [62]

Walter J. Koroshetz, MD
Deputy Director, National Institute of Neurological Disorders and Stroke, National Institutes of Health, Bethesda [377]

Theodore A. Kotchen, MD
Associate Dean for Clinical Research; Director, General Clinical Research Center, Medical College of Wisconsin, Wisconsin [241]

Phyllis E. Kozarsky, MD
Professor of Medicine, Infectious Diseases; Co-Director, Travel and Tropical Medicine, Emory University School of Medicine, Atlanta [117]

Barnett S. Kramer, MD, MPH
Associate Director for Disease Prevention, Office of the Director, National Institutes of Health, Bethesda [78]

Stephen M. Krane, MD
Persis, Cyrus and Marlow B. Harrison Distinguished Professor of Medicine, Harvard Medical School, Massachusetts General Hospital, Boston [346]

Alexander Kratz, MD, PhD, MPH
Assistant Professor of Clinical Pathology, Columbia University College of Physicians and Surgeons; Associate Director, Core Laboratory, Columbia University Medical Center, New York-Presbyterian Hospital; Director, Allen Pavilion Laboratory, New York [Appendix]

John P. Kress, MD
Associate Professor of Medicine, Section of Pulmanary and Critical Care, University of Chicago, Chicago [261]

Patricia A. Kritek, MD, EdM
Instructor in Medicine, Harvard Medical School; Co-Director, Harvard Pulmonary and Critical Care Medicine Fellowship, Brigham and Women's Hospital, Boston [e24]

Henry M. Kronenberg, MD
Chief, Endocrine Unit, Massachusetts General Hospital; Professor of Medicine, Harvard Medical School, Boston [346]

Robert F. Kushner, MD
Professor of Medicine, Northwestern University Feinberg School of Medicine, Chicago [75]

Loren Laine, MD
Professor of Medicine, Keck School of Medicine, University of Southern California, Los Angeles [42]

Anil K. Lalwani, MD
Mendik Foundation Professor and Chairman, Department of Otolaryngology; Professor, Department of Pediatrics; Professor, Department of Physiology and Neuroscience, New York University School of Medicine, New York [30]

H. Clifford Lane, MD
Clinical Director; Director, Division of Clinical Research; Deputy Director, Clinical Research and Special Projects; Chief, Clinical and Molecular Retrovirology Section, Laboratory of Immunoregulation, National Institute of Allergy and Infectious Diseases, National Institutes of Health, Bethesda [182, 214]

Carol A. Langford, MD, MHS
Associate Professor of Medicine; Director, Center for Vasculitis Care and Research, Department of Rheumatic and Immunologic Diseases, Cleveland Clinic, Cleveland [319, 321, 329–331, e28]

Wei C. Lau, MD
Associate Professor; Medical Director, Cardiovascular Center Operating Rooms; Director, Adult Cardiovascular Anesthesiology, Ann Arbor [8]

Thomas J. Lawley, MD
William P. Timmie Professor of Dermatology; Dean, Emory University School of Medicine, Atlanta [52, 23, 55, e10]

Thomas H. Lee, MD
Professor of Medicine, Harvard Medical School; Chief Executive Officer, Partners Community Health Care, Inc; Network President, Partners Health Care, Boston [13]

Bruce D. Levy, MD
Associate Professor of Medicine, Harvard Medical School; Pulmonary and Critical Care Medicine, Brigham and Women's Hospital, Boston [262]

Julia B. Lewis, MD
Professor of Medicine, Division of Nephrology and Hypertension, Department of Medicine, Vanderbilt University School of Medicine, Nashville [277]

Peter Libby, MD
Mallinckrodt Professor of Medicine, Harvard Medical School; Chief, Cardiovascular Medicine, Brigham and Women's Hospital, Boston [217, 235, e22]

Richard W. Light, MD
Professor of Medicine, Vanderbilt University, Nashville [257]

Christopher H. Linden, MD
Professor, Department of Emergency Medicine, Division of Medical Toxicology, University of Massachusetts Medical School, Worcester [e35]

Robert Lindsay, MD, PhD
Professor of Clinical Medicine, Columbia University College of Physicians and Surgeons; Chief, Internal Medicine, Helen Hayes Hospital, West Havershaw, New York [348]

Marc E. Lippman, MD
Professor and Chair, Department of Medicine, University of Miami Leonard M. Miller School of Medicine, Miami [86]

Peter E. Lipsky, MD
Chief, Autoimmunity Branch, National Institute of Arthritis, Musculoskeletal, and Skin Diseases, National Institutes of Health, Department of Health and Human Services, Bethesda [312, 314, 325]

David A. Lipson, MD
Assistant Professor of Medicine, Pulmonary, Allergy & Critical Care Division, University of Pennsylvania Medical Center, King of Prussia [34, 345]

Kathleen D. Liu, MD, PhD, MCR
Assistant Professor, Division of Nephrology, San Francisco [273, 275]

Bernard Lo, MD
Professor of Medicine; Director, Program in Medical Ethics, University of California, San Francisco, San Francisco [e4]

Dan L. Longo, MD
Scientific Director, National Institute on Aging, National Institutes of Health, Bethesda and Baltimore [1, 58, 60, 68, 77, 80, 81, 105, 106, 181, e11–e13]

Nicola Longo, MD, PhD
Professor of Pediatrics; Chief, Division of Medical Genetics, Department of Pediatrics, University of Utah, Salt Lake City [358, 359]

Joseph Loscalzo, MD, PhD, MA (Hon)
Hersey Professor of the Theory and Practice of Medicine, Harvard Medical School; Chairman, Department of Medicine, Physician-in-Chief, Brigham and Women's Hospital, Boston [1, 36, 37, 217, 237, 242, 243]

Phillip A. Low, MD
Robert D and Patricia E Kern Professor of Neurology, Mayo Clinic College of Medicine, Rochester [370]

Daniel H. Lowenstein, MD
Professor of Neurology; Director, University of California, San Francisco Epilepsy Center; Associate Dean for Clinical/Translational Research, San Francisco [361, 363]

Elyse E. Lower, MD
Professor of Medicine, University of Cincinnati, Cincinnati [322]

Franklin D. Lowy, MD, PhD
Professor of Medicine and Pathology, Columbia University, College of Physicians & Surgeons, New York [129]

Sheila A. Lukehart, PhD
Professor of Medicine, University of Washington, Seattle [162, 163]

Lucio Luzzatto, MD, PhD
Professor of Hematology, University of Florence; Scientific Director, Instituto Toscano Tumori (ITT), Firenze, Italy [101]

Lawrence C. Madoff, MD
Associate Professor of Medicine, Harvard Medical School, Boston [113, 135, 328, e15]

James H. Maguire, MD, MPH
Professor and Director, International Health Division, Department of Epidemiology and Preventive Medicine, University of Maryland School of Medicine, Baltimore [392]

Adel A. F. Mahmoud, MD, PhD
Professor, Molecular Biology, Princeton University, Princeton [212]

Ronald V. Maier, MD
Jane and Donald D. Trunkey Professor and Vice Chair, Surgery, University of Washington; Surgeon-in-Chief, Harborview Medical Center, Seattle [264]

Mark E. Malliard, MD
Associate Professor and Chief, Division of Gastroenterology and Hepatology, Omaha [301]

Scott Manaker, MD, PhD
Associate Professor of Medicine and Pharmacology, Pulmonary and Critical Care Division, Department of Medicine, University of Pennsylvania, Philadelphia [247]

Hanna Mandel, MD
Director, Metabolic Disease Unit, Rambam Medical Health Care Campus, Haifa, Israel [e39]

Lionel A. Mandell, MD
Professor of Medicine, McMaster University, Hamilton, Ontario [251]

Douglas L. Mann, MD
Professor of Medicine, Molecular Physiology and Biophysics; Chief, Section of Cardiology, Baylor College of Medicine, St. Luke's Episcopal Hospital and Texas Heart Institute, Houston [227]

JoAnn E. Manson, MD, DrPH
Professor of Medicine and the Elizabeth Fay Brigham Professor of Women's Health, Harvard Medical School; Chief, Division of Preventive Medicine, Brigham and Women's Hospital, Boston [342]

Eleftheria Maratos-Flier, MD
Associate Professor of Medicine, Harvard Medical School; Chief, Obesity Section, Joslin Diabetes Center, Boston [74]

Francis Marchlinski, MD
Professor of Medicine; Director of Cardiac Electrophysiology, University of Pennsylvania Health System, University of Pennsylvania School of Medicine, Philadelphia [226]

Daniel B. Mark, MD, MPH
Professor of Medicine, Duke University Medical Center; Director, Outcomes Research, Duke Clinical Research Institute, Durham [3]

Thomas Marrie, MD
Professor, Department of Medicine; Dean, Faculty of Medicine and Dentistry, University of Alberta, Edmonton, Alberta [167]

Gary J. Martin, MD
Raymond J. Langenbach MD Professor of Medicine; Vice Chairman for Faculty Affairs and Education, Department of Medicine, Northwestern University Feinberg School of Medicine, Chicago [4]

Joseph B. Martin, MD, PhD, MA (Hon)
Dean Emeritus of the Faculty of Medicine, Edward R. and Anne G. Lefler Professor of Neurobiology, Harvard Medical School, Boston [12, 361]

Robert J. Mayer, MD
Stephen B. Kay Family Professor of Medicine, Harvard Medical School, Dana-Farber Cancer Institute, Boston [87]

Alexander J. McAdam, MD, PhD
Medical Director, Infectious Diseases Diagnostic Division, Children's Hospital, Boston; Assistant Professor, Department of Pathology, Harvard Medical School, Boston [e14]

Calvin O. McCall, MD
Associate Professor of Dermatology, Virginia Commonwealth University Medical Center, Richmond [53]

William M. McCormack, MD
Distinguished Teaching Professor of Medicine; Chief, Infectious Disease Division, SUNY Downstate Medical Center, Brooklyn [168]

Kevin T. McVary, MD
Associate Professor of Urology, Northwestern University Feinberg School of Medicine, Chicago [49]

Nancy K. Mello, PhD
Professor of Psychology (Neuroscience), Harvard Medical School, Boston [389]

Shlomo Melmed, MD
Senior Vice President, Academic Affairs; Associate Dean, Cedars Sinai Medical Center, David Geffen School of Medicine at UCLA, Los Angeles [333]

David Meltzer, MD, PhD
Associate Professor, Departments of Medicine and Economics, Harris School of Public Policy; Director of the Center for Health and the Social Sciences, The University of Chicago, Chicago [e2]

Jerry R. Mendell, MD
Professor of Pediatrics, Neurology and Pathology, The Ohio State University; Director, Center for Gene Therapy, The Research Institute at Nationwide Children's Hospital, Columbus [382]

Jack H. Mendelson,† MD
Professor of Psychiatry (Neuroscience), Harvard Medical School, Belmont [389]

M.-Marsel Mesulam, MD
Director, Cognitive Neurology and Alzheimer's Disease Center; Dunbar Professor of Neurology and Psychiatry, Northwestern University Feinberg School of Medicine, Chicago [27]

Susan Miesfeldt, MD
Medical Oncology Medical Director, Cancer Risk and Prevention Clinic, Maine Medical Cancer and Maine Center for Cancer Medicine & Blood Disorders, Portland [64]

Edgar L. Milford, MD
Associate Professor of Medicine, Harvard Medical School; Director, Tissue Typing Laboratory, Brigham and Women's Hospital, Boston [276]

Bruce L. Miller, MD
AW and Mary Margaret Clausen Distinguished Professor of Neurology, University of California, San Francisco School of Medicine, San Francisco [26, 365, 378, e6]

Mark Miller, MD
Associate Director for Research, National Institutes of Health, Bethesda [116]

Samuel I. Miller, MD
Professor of Genome Sciences, Medicine, and Microbiology, University of Washington, Seattle [146]

John D. Minna, MD
Professor, Internal Medicine and Pharmacology; Director, Hamon Center for Therapeutic Oncology Research, University of Texas Southwestern Medical Center, Dallas [85]

Thomas A. Moore, MD
Clinical Professor and Associate Program Director, Department of Medicine, University of Kansas School of Medicine, Wichita [201, e17]

Pat J. Morin, PhD
Senior Investigator, Laboratory of Cellular and Molecular Biology, National Institute on Aging, National Institutes of Health, Bethesda [79]

Robert J. Motzer, MD
Attending Physician, Department of Medicine, Memorial Sloan-Kettering Cancer Center; Professor of Medicine, Weill Medical College of Cornell University, New York [90, 92]

Haralampos M. Moutsopoulos, MD
Professor and Chair, Department of Pathophysiology, School of Medicine, National University of Athens, Greece [317, 320]

Robert S. Munford, MD
Jan and Henri Bromberg Chair in Internal Medicine, University of Texas Southwestern Medical Center, Dallas [265]

Nikhil C. Munshi, MD
Associate Director, Jerome Lipper Multiple Myeloma Center, Dana-Farber Cancer Institute, Boston VA Health Care System; Associate Professor, Harvard Medical School, Boston [106]

John R. Murphy, PhD
Professor of Medicine and Microbiology; Chief, Section of Molecular Medicine, Boston University School of Medicine, Boston [131]

Timothy F. Murphy, MD
UB Distinguished Professor, Department of Medicine and Microbiology; Chief, Infectious Diseases, State Univerity of New York, Buffalo [139]

Joseph A. Murray, MD
Professor of Medicine, Division of Gastroenterology and Hepatology, The Mayo Clinic, Rochester [40]

Daniel M. Musher, MD
Chief, Infectious Disease Section, Michael E. DeBakey Veterans Affairs Medical Center; Professor of Medicine and Professor of Molecular Virology and Microbiology, Baylor College of Medicine, Houston [128, 138]

Mark B. Mycyk, MD
Assistant Professor of Emergency Medicine; Director of Clinical Toxicology and Toxicological Research, Northwestern University Feinberg School of Medicine, Chicago [e35]

Robert J. Myerberg, MD
Professor of Medicine and Physiology; AHA Chair in Cardiovascular Research, University of Miami Miller School of Medicine, Miami [267]

Nitish Naik, MD, DS
Department of Cardiology, All India Institute of Medical Sciences, Ansari Nagar, New Delhi, India [e38]

Eric G. Neilson, MD
Hugh J. Morgan Professor of Medicine and Cell Biology, Physician-in-Chief, Vanderbilt University Hospital; Chairman, Department of Medicine, Vanderbilt University School of Medicine, Nashville [271, 272, 277, e9]

Gerald T. Nepom, MD, PhD
Director, Benaroya Research Institute at Virginia Mason; Professor, University of Washington School of Medicine, Seattle [309]

Hartmut P. H. Neumann, MD
Head, Section Preventative Medicine, Department of Nephrology and General Medicine, Albert-Ludwigs-University of Freiburg, Germany [337]

Jonathan Newmark, MD, Colonel, Medical Corps, US Army
Deputy Joint Program Executive Officer, Medical Systems, Joint Program Executive Office for Chemical/Biological Defense, US Department of Defense Chemical Casualty Care; Consultant to the US Army Surgeon General; Adjunct Professor, Neurology, F. Edward Hébert School of Medicine, Uniformed Services University of the Health Sciences, Falls Church [215]

Rick A. Nishimura, MD
Judd and Mary Morris Leighton Professor of Cardiovascular Diseases; Professor of Medicine, Mayo Clinic College of Medicine, Rochester [222, e20]

Robert L. Norris, MD
Associate Professor, Department of Surgery, Division of Emergency Medicine, Stanford University School of Medicine, Stanford [391]

Thomas B. Nutman, MD
Head, Helminth Immunology Section; Head, Clinical Parasitology Unit; Laboratory of Parasitic Diseases, National Institute of Allergy and Infectious Diseases, National Insitutes of Health, Bethesda [210, 211]

Richard J. O'Brien, MD
Head of Scientific Evaluation, Foundation for Innovative New Diagnostics, Geneva, Switzerland [158]

Patrick O'Gara, MD
Associate Professor of Medicine, Harvard Medical School; Director, Clinical Cardiology, Brigham and Women's Hospital, Boston [230, e8]

Robert A. O'Rourke, MD
Distinguished Professor of Medicine Emeritus, University of Texas Health Science Center, San Antonio [220]

C. Warren Olanow, MD
Henry P. and Georgette Goldschmidt Professor and Chairman of the Department of Neurology, Professor of Neuroscience, The Mount Sinai School of Medicine, New York [367]

Andrew B. Onderdonk, PhD
Professor of Pathology, Harvard Medical School and Brigham and Women's Hospital, Boston [e14]

Chung Owyang, MD
Professor of Internal Medicine, H. Marvin Pollard Collegiate Professor; Chief, Division of Gastroenterology, University of Michigan Health System, Ann Arbor [284, 290]

Umesh D. Parashar, MBBS, MPH
Lead, Enteric and Respiratory Viruses Team, Epidemiology Branch, Division of Viral Diseases, National Center for Immunization and Respiratory Diseases, Centers for Disease Control and Prevention, Atlanta [183]

Jeffrey Parsonnet, MD
Associate Professor of Medicine and Microbiology, Dartmouth Medical School, Lebanon [120]

Parul S. Patel, MD
Transplant Neurologist, California Pacific Medical Center, San Francisco [278]

Shreyaskumar R. Patel, MD
Professor of Medicine, Deputy Chairman, Department of Sarcoma Medical Oncology, University of Texas, Houston [94]

Gustav Paumgartner, MD
Professor of Medicine, University of Munich, Munich, Germany [305]

David A. Pegues, MD
Professor of Medicine, Division of Infectious Diseases, David Geffen School of Medicine at UCLA, Los Angeles [146]

Florencia Pereyra, MD
Instructor in Medicine, Harvard Medical School; Division of Infectious Disease, Brigham and Women's Hospital, Boston [e15]

Michael C. Perry, MD, MS
Professor and Director, Division of Hematology/Medical Oncology, Department of Internal Medicine, Nellie B. Smith Chair of Oncology, University of Missouri-Columbia School of Medicine, Columbia [e13]

Michael A. Pesce, PhD
Clinical Professor of Pathology, Columbia University College of Physicians and Surgeons; Director of Specialty Laboratory, New York Presbyterian Hospital, Columbia University Medical Center, New York [Appendix]

Clarence J. Peters, MD
John Sealy Distinguished University Chair in Tropical and Emerging Virology, Director for Biodefense, Center for Biodefense and Emerging Infectious Diseases, University of Texas Medical Branch in Galveston, Galveston [189, 190]

Eliot A. Phillipson, MD
Professor, Department of Medicine, University of Toronto, Toronto [258]

Gerald B. Pier, PhD
Professor of Medicine (Microbiology and Molecular Genetics), Harvard Medical School; Microbiologist, Brigham and Women's Hospital, Boston [114]

Ronald E. Polk, PharmD
Chair, Department of Pharmacy, Professor of Pharmacy and Medicine, School of Pharmacy, Virginia Commonwealth University, Richmond [127]

Richard J. Pollack, MD
Research Associate in Immunology and Infectious Diseases, Harvard School of Public Health, Boston [392]

Reuven Porat, MD
Professor of Medicine; Director, Internal Medicine, Tel Aviv Sourasky Medical Center, Sackler Faculty of Medicine, Tel Aviv University, Tel Aviv [17]

Daniel A. Portnoy, PhD
Professor of Biochemistry and Molecular Biology, Department of Molecular and Cell Biology, University of California, Berkeley [132]

John T. Potts, Jr., MD
Jackson Distinguished Professor of Clinical Medicine, Harvard Medical School; Director of Research and Physician-in-Chief Emeritus, Massachusetts General Hospital, Charlestown [347]

Lawrie W. Powell, MD, PhD
Professor of Medicine, The University of Queensland and The Royal Brisbane and Women's Hospital, Brisbane, Queensland, Australia [351]

Alvin C. Powers, MD
Joe C. Davis Chair in Biomedical Science; Professor of Medicine, Molecular Physiology and Biophysics; Director, Vanderbilt Diabetes Research and Training Center; Director, Vanderbilt Diabetes Center, Nashville [338]

Daniel S. Pratt, MD
Assistant Professor of Medicine, Harvard Medical School; Director, Liver-Billary-Pancreas Center, Massachusetts General Hospital, Boston [43, 296]

Darwin J. Prockop, MD, PhD
Director of Center for Gene Therapy and Professor of Biochemistry, Tulane Health Sciences Center, New Orleans [357]

Stanley B. Prusiner, MD
Director, Institute for Neurodegenerative Diseases; Professor, Department of Neurology; Professor, Department of Biochemistry and Biophysics, University of California, San Francisco, San Francisco [378]

Daniel J. Rader, MD
Cooper-McClure Professor of Medicine, University of Pennsylvania School of Medicine, Philadelphia [350]

Roshini Rajapaksa, MD, BA
Assistant Professor, Department of Medicine, Gastroenterology, New York University Medical Center School of Medicine and Hospitals Center, New York [44]

Sanjay Ram, MD
Assistant Professor of Medicine, Division of Infectious Diseases and Immunology, University of Massachusetts Medical School, Worcester [137]

Jose A. F. Ramires
Head Professor of Cardiology; University of São Paulo Medical School and Heart Institute-INCOR, São Paulo, Brazil [e37]

Reuben Ramphal, MD
Professor, Division of Infectious Diseases, Department of Medicine, University of Florida College of Medicine, Gainesville [145]

Neil H. Raskin, MD
Professor of Neurology, University of California, San Francisco, San Francisco [15]

Mario C. Raviglione, MD
Director, StopTB Department, World Health Organization, Geneva [158]

K. Srinath Reddy, MD, DM, MSC
Department of Cardiology, All India Institute of Medical Sciences, Ansari Nagar, New Delhi, India [e38]

Sharon L. Reed, MD
Professor of Pathology and Medicine; Director, Microbiology and Virology Laboratories, University of California, San Diego Medical Center, San Diego [202, e16]

Richard C. Reichman, MD
Professor of Medicine and of Microbiology and Immunology; Director, Infectious Diseases Division, University of Rochester School of Medicine, Rochester [178]

Carol M. Reife, MD
Clinical Associate Professor of Medicine, Jefferson Medical College, Philadelphia [41]

John J. Reilly, Jr., MD
Associate Professor of Medicine, Harvard Medical School; Vice Chairman, Integrative Services, Department of Medicine, Brigham and Women's Hospital, Boston [254, e24]

John T. Repke, MD
University Professor and Chairman, Department of Obstetrics and Gynecology, Penn State University College of Medicine; Obstetrician-Gynecologist-In-Chief, The Milton S. Hershey Medical Center, Hershey [7]

Victor I. Reus, MD
Professor, Department of Psychiatry, University of California, San Francisco School of Medicine; Attending Physician, Langley Porter Hospital and Clinics, San Francisco [386]

Peter A. Rice, MD
Professor of Medicine, Division of Infectious Diseases and Immunology, University of Massachusetts Medical School, Worcester [137]

Stuart Rich, MD
Professor of Medicine, Section of Cardiology, University of Chicago, Chicago [244]

Gary S. Richardson, MD
Assistant Professor of Psychiatry, Case Western Reserve University, Cleveland; Senior Research Scientist, Sleep Disorders and Research Center, Henry Ford Hospital, Detroit [28]

Elizabeth Robbins, MD
Associate Clinical Professor, University of California, San Francisco, San Francisco [e32]

Gary L. Robertson, MD
Emeritus Professor of Medicine, Northwestern University Feinberg School of Medicine, Chicago [334]

Daniel M. Roden, MD
Professor of Medicine and Pharmacology, Assistant Vice-Chancellor for Personalized Medicine, Vanderbilt University, Nashville [5]

James A. Romano, Jr., PhD, DABT
Senior Principal Life Specialist, Science Applications International Corporation, Frederick [215]

Karen L. Roos, MD
John and Nancy Nelson Professor of Neurology, Indiana University School of Medicine, Indianapolis [376]

Allan H. Ropper, MD
Executive Vice-Chair, Department of Neurology, Brigham and Women's Hospital, Harvard Medical School, Boston [268, 372, 373]

Ilene M. Rosen, MD, MSc
Associate Director, Internal Medical Residency Program; Assistant Professor of Clinical Medicine, University of Pennsylvania School of Medicine, Philadelphia [246]

Roger N. Rosenberg, MD
Zale Distinguished Chair and Professor of Neurology, Department of Neurology, University of Texas Southwestern Medical Center, Dallas [368]

F. R. Rosendaal, MD
Professor of Clinical Epidemiology; Chairman, Department of Clinical Epidemiology, and Department of Thrombosis and Hemostasis, Leiden University Medical Center, The Netherlands [111]

Myrna R. Rosenfeld, MD, PhD
Associate Professor of Neurology, Division Neuro-Oncology, Department of Neurology, University of Pennsylvania, Philadelphia [97]

Jean-Claude Roujeau, MD
Professor of Dermatology, Hôpital Henri Mondor, Université Paris XII, Créteil, France [56]

Ambuj Roy, MD, DM
Department of Cardiology, All India Institute of Medical Sciences, Ansari Nagar, New Delhi, India [e38]

Michael A. Rubin, MD, PhD
Assistant Professor of Medicine, Division of Epidemiology and Infectious Diseases, Department of Internal Medicine, University of Utah School of Medicine, Salt Lake City [31]

Robert M. Russell, MD
Director, Jean Mayer USDA Human Nutrition Research Center on Aging at Tufts University; Professor of Medicine and Nutrition, Tufts University, Boston [71]

Thomas A. Russo, MD, CM
Professor of Medicine and Microbiology, State University of New York, Buffalo [143, 156]

Miguel Sabria, MD, PhD
Professor of Medicine, Autonomous University of Barcelona; Chief, Infectious Diseases Section, Germans Trias i Pujol Hospital, Barcelona, Spain [141]

Stephen M. Sagar, MD
Professor of Neurology, Case Western Reserve School of Medicine; Director of Neuro-Oncology, Ireland Cancer Center, University Hospitals of Cleveland, Cleveland [374]

David J. Salant, MD
Professor of Medicine, Pathology, and Laboratory Medicine, Boston University School of Medicine; Chief, Section of Nephrology, Boston Medical Center, Boston [278]

Martin A. Samuels, MD, DSc (Hon)
Chairman, Department of Neurology, Brigham and Women's Hospital; Professor of Neurology, Harvard Medical Center, Boston [e33]

Merle A. Sande,† MD
Professor of Medicine, University of Washington School of Medicine; President, Academic Alliance Foundation, Seattle [31]

Philippe Sansonetti
Professeur à l'Institut Pasteur, Paris, France [147]

Edward A. Sausville, MD, PhD
Professor of Medicine; Associate Director for Clinical Research, Marlene & Stewart Greenebaum Cancer Center, University of Maryland, Baltimore [81]

†Deceased.

Mohamed H. Sayegh, MD
Director, Warren E. Grupe and John P. Morill Chair in Transplantation Medicine; Professor of Medicine and Pediatrics, Harvard Medical School, Boston [276]

David T. Scadden, MD
Gerald and Darlene Jordan Professor of Medicine, Harvard University; Co-Chair, Department of Stem Cell and Regenerative Biology, Harvard University, Boston [68]

Howard I. Scher, MD
Professor of Medicine, Weill Medical College of Cornell University; D. Wayne Calloway Chair in Urologic Oncology; Chief, Genitourinary Oncology Service, Memorial Sloan-Kettering Cancer Center, New York [90, 91]

Joan H. Schiller, MD
Professor of Medicine and Hematology/Oncology, University of Texas Southwestern Medical School; Simmons Comprehensive Cancer Center, Dallas [85]

Harry W. Schroeder, Jr., MD, PhD
Professor of Medicine, Microbiology, and Genetics, The University of Alabama, Birmingham [310, e27]

Marc A. Schuckit, MD
Distinguished Professor of Psychiatry, School of Medicine, University of California, San Diego; Director, Alcohol Research Center, VA San Diego Healthcare System, San Diego [387, 388]

H. Ralph Schumacher, MD
Professor of Medicine, University of Pennsylvania School of Medicine, Philadelphia [327]

Gordon E. Schutze, MD
Professor of Pediatrics and Pathology, University of Arkansas for Medical Sciences, College of Medicine; Chief, Pediatric Infectious Diseases, Arkansas Children's Hospital, Little Rock [151]

Stuart Schwartz, PhD
Professor of Human Genetics, Medicine and Pathology, University of Chicago, Chicago [63]

Richard M. Schwartzstein, MD
Professor of Medicine, Harvard Medical School; Associate Chair, Pulmonary and Critical Care Medicine; Vice-President for Education, Beth Israel Deaconess Medical Center, Boston [33]

Julian L. Seifter, MD
Physician, Brigham and Women's Hospital; Associate Professor of Medicine, Harvard Medical School, Boston [283]

David C. Seldin, MD, PhD
Professor of Medicine and Microbiology; Director, Amyloid Treatment and Research Program Section of Hematology-Oncology, Department of Medicine, Boston University School of Medicine and Boston Medical Center, Boston [324]

Andrew P. Selwyn, MA, MD
Professor of Medicine, Harvard Medical School, Boston [237]

Steven D. Shapiro, MD
Jack D. Myers Professor and Chair, University of Pittsburgh, Pittsburgh [254, 262]

William Silen, MD
Johnson and Johnson Distinguished Professor of Surgery, Emeritus, Harvard Medical School, Boston [14, 293, 294]

Rebecca A. Silliman, MD, PhD
Professor of Medicine and Epidemiology, Boston University Schools of Medicine and Public Health; Chief, Section of Geriatrics, Boston University Medical Center, Boston [9]

Edwin K. Silverman, MD, PhD
Associate Professor of Medicine, Harvard Medical School, Brigham and Women's Hospital, Boston [254]

Gary G. Singer, MD
Assistant Professor of Clinical Medicine, Washington University School of Medicine, St. Louis [46]

Martha Skinner, MD
Professor of Medicine, Boston University School of Medicine; Director, Special Projects, Amyloid Treatment and Research Program, Boston [324]

Karl Skorecki, MD
Annie Chutick Professor in Medicine (Nephrology); Director, Rappaport Research Institute, Director of Medical and Research Development, Rambam Medical Health Care Campus, Haifa, Israel [274, e39]

Wade S. Smith, MD, PhD
Professor of Neurology, Daryl R. Gress Endowed Chair of Neurocritical Care and Stroke; Director, University of California, San Francisco Neurovascular Service, San Francisco [269, 364]

A. George Smulian, MB, BCh
Associate Professor, University of Cincinnati College of Medicine; Chief, Infectious Disease Section, Cincinnati VA Medical Center, Cincinnati [200]

Arthur J. Sober, MD
Professor, Department of Dermatology, Harvard Medical School; Associate Chief, Department of Dermatology, Massachusetts General Hospital, Boston [83]

Kelly A. Soderberg, PhD, MPH
Director, Program Management, Duke Human Vaccine Institute, Duke University School of Medicine, Durham [308]

Michael F. Sorrell, MD
Robert L. Grissom Professor of Medicine, University of Nebraska Medical Center, Omaha [301]

David H. Spach, MD
Professor of Medicine, Division of Infectious Diseases, University of Washington, Seattle [153]

Peter Speelman, MD, PhD
Professor of Medicine and Infectious Diseases; Head, Division of Infectious Diseases, Tropical Medicine and AIDS; Department of Internal Medicine, Academic Medical Center, University of Amsterdam, The Netherlands [164]

Frank E. Speizer, MD
Edward H. Kass Professor of Medicine, Harvard Medical School, Channing Laboratory, Department of Medicine, Brigham and Women's Hospital, Boston [250]

Jerry L. Spivak, MD
Professor of Medicine, The Johns Hopkins University School of Medicine; Attending Physician, Johns Hopkins Hospital, Baltimore [103]

Andrei C. Sposito
Professor of Medicine, University of Basilia Medical School, Basilia, Brazil [e37]

Walter E. Stamm, MD
Professor of Medicine; Head, Division of Allergy and Infectious Diseases, University of Washington School of Medicine, Seattle [169, 282]

Allen C. Steere, MD
Professor of Medicine, Harvard Medical School, Boston [166]

Robert S. Stern, MD
Dermatologist-in-Chief; Carl J. Herzog Professor of Medicine, Harvard Medical School, Boston [56]

Dennis L. Stevens, MD, PhD
Chief, Infectious Diseases Section, Veteran Affairs Medical Center, Boise; Professor of Medicine, University of Washington School of Medicine, Seattle [119]

Stephen E. Straus,† MD
Senior Investigator, Laboratory of Clinical Investigation, National Institute of Allergy and Infectious Diseases; Director, National Center for Complementary and Alternative Medicine, National Institutes of Health, Bethesda [10, 384]

Lewis Sudarsky, MD
Associate Professor of Neurology, Harvard Medical School; Director of Movement Disorders, Brigham and Women's Hospital, Boston [24]

Alan M. Sugar, MD
Professor of Medicine, Boston University School of Medicine; Medical Director, Infectious Diseases Clinical Services, HIV/AIDS Program, and Infection Control, Cape Cod Healthcare, Hyannis [198]

Donna C. Sullivan, PhD
Associate Professor of Medicine and Microbiology, Division of Infectious Diseases, Department of Medicine, University of Mississippi School of Medicine, Jackson [194, 199]

†Deceased.

Paolo M. Suter, MD, MS
Professor of Medicine, Medical Policlinic, Zurich, Switzerland [71]

Morton N. Swartz, MD
Professor of Medicine, Harvard Medical School; Chief, Jackson Firm Medical Service and Infectious Disease Unit, Massachusetts General Hospital, Boston [377]

A. Jamil Tajik, MD
Thomas J. Watson, Jr., Professor; Professor of Medicine and Pediatrics; Chairman (Emeritus), Zayed Cardiovascular Center, Mayo Clinic, Rochester, Minnesota; Consultant, Cardiovascular Division, Mayo Clinic, Scottsdale [222, e20]

Joel D. Taurog, MD
Professor of Internal Medicine, William M. and Gatha Burnett Professor for Arthritis Research, University of Texas Southwestern Medical Center, Dallas [318]

Stephen F. Templeton, MD
Clinical Assistant Professor of Dermatology, Emory University School of Medicine, Atlanta [e10]

Gregory Tino, MD
Associate Professor of Medicine, University of Pennsylvania School of Medicine; Chief, Pulmonary Clinical Service Hospital of the University of Pennsylvania, Philadelphia [252]

Zelig A. Tochner, MD
Associate Professor of Radiation Oncology; Clinical Director, Proton Therapy Project, University of Pennsylvania, Philadelphia [216]

Gordon F. Tomaselli, MD
David J. Carver Professor of Medicine, Vice Chairman, Department of Medicine for Research, The Johns Hopkins University, Baltimore [224, 225]

Mark Topazian, MD
Associate Professor of Medicine, Mayo College of Medicine, Rochester [285, e25]

Phillip P. Toskes, MD
Professor of Medicine, Division of Gastroenterology, Hepatology and Nutrition, University of Florida College of Medicine, Gainesville [306, 307]

Jeffrey M. Trent, PhD
President and Scientific Director, Translational Genomics Research Institute, Phoenix [79]

Elbert P. Trulock, MD
Professor of Medicine, Rosemary and I. Jerome Flance Professor of Pulmonary Medicine, Washington University School of Medicine, St. Louis [260]

Hensin Tsao, MD
Assistant Professor of Dermatology, Harvard Medical School; Clinical Director, Melanoma Genetics Program, Massachusetts General Hospital, Boston [83]

Kenneth L. Tyler, MD
Reuler-Lewin Family Professor of Neurology and Professor of Medicine and Microbiology, University of Colorado Health Sciences Center; Chief, Neurology Service, Denver Veterans Affairs Medical Center, Denver [376]

Joseph P. Vacanti, MD
John Homan Professor of Surgery, Harvard Medical School; Surgeon-in-Chief, Massachusetts General Hospital for Children, Boston [69]

Edouard Vannier, PhD
Assistant Professor, Department of Medicine, Division of Infectious Diseases, Tufts–New England Medical Center and Tufts University School of Medicine, Boston [204]

Gauri R. Varadhachary, MD
Associate Professor, Department of Gastrointestinal Medical Oncology, University of Texas MD Anderson Cancer Center, Houston [95]

John Varga, MD
Hughes Professor of Medicine, Northwestern University Feinberg School of Medicine, Chicago [316]

Indre V. Viskontas, PhD
Department of Neurology, Memory and Aging Center, University of California, San Francisco, San Francisco [e6]

Bert Vogelstein, MD
Director, Ludwig Center for Cancer Genetics & Therapeutics; Investigator, Howard Hughes Medical Institute; Clayton Professor for Oncology & Pathology, The Johns Hopkins University School of Medicine, Baltimore [79]

Everett E. Vokes, MD
Director, Section of Hematology/Oncology; Vice Chairman for Clinical Research, Department of Medicine; Deputy Director, Cancer Research Center; John E. Ultmann Professor of Medicine and Radiation and Cellular Oncology, University of Chicago School of Medicine, Chicago [84]

Tamara J. Vokes, MD
Associate Professor, Section of Endocrinology, University of Chicago, Chicago [349]

C. Fordham von Reyn, MD
Professor of Medicine (Infectious Disease) and International Health; Director, DARDAR International Programs, Dartmouth Medical School, Lebanon [160]

Matthew K. Waldor, MD, PhD
Professor of Medicine (Microbiology and Molecular Genetics), Channing Laboratory, Brigham and Women's Hospital, Harvard Medical School, Boston [149]

David H. Walker, MD
The Carnage and Martha Walls Distinguished University Chair in Tropical Diseases; Professor and Chairman, Department of Pathology; Executive Director, Center for Biodefense and Emerging Infectious Disease, University of Texas Medical Branch, Galveston [167]

Richard J. Wallace, Jr., MD
Chairman, Department of Microbiology, University of Texas Health Center at Tyler, Tyler [161]

B. Timothy Walsh, MD
Professor of Psychiatry, College of Physicians & Surgeons, Columbia University; Director, Eating Disorders Research Unit, New York Psychiatric Institute, New York [76]

Peter D. Walzer, MD, MSc
Associate Chief of Staff for Research, Cincinnati VA Medical Center; Professor of Medicine, University of Cincinnati College of Medicine, Cincinnati [200]

Fred Wang, MD
Professor of Medicine, Harvard Medical School, Boston [170, 176]

Carl V. Washington, Jr., MD
Associate Professor of Dermatology, Emory University School of Medicine; Co-Director, Dermatologic Surgery Unit, The Emory Clinic, Atlanta [83]

Anthony P. Weetman, MD, DSc
Professor of Medicine and Dean of the School of Medicine and Biomedical Sciences, University of Sheffield, Sheffield, United Kingdom [335]

Steven E. Weinberger, MD
Senior Vice President for Medical Education Division, American College of Physicians; Senior Lecturer on Medicine, Harvard Medical School; Adjunct Professor of Medicine, University of Pennsylvania School of Medicine, Philadelphia [34, 245–247, 252]

Robert A. Weinstein, MD
Professor of Medicine, Rush University Medical Center; Chairman, Infectious Diseases, Cook County Hospital; Chief Operating Officer, CORE Center, Chicago [125]

Jeffrey I. Weitz, MD
Professor of Medicine and Biochemistry, McMaster University; Director, Henderson Research Centre, Heart and Stroke Foundation/J. Fraser Mustard Chair in Cardiovascular Research; Canada Research Chair (Tier1) in Thrombosis; Career Investigator, Heart and Stroke Foundation of Canada [112]

Peter F. Weller, MD
Professor of Medicine, Harvard Medical School; Co-Chief, Infectious Diseases Division; Chief, Allergy and Inflammation Division; Vice-Chair for Research, Department of Medicine, Beth Israel Deaconess Medical Center, Boston [208–211, 213]

Michael R. Wessels, MD
Professor of Pediatrics and Medicine (Microbiology and Molecular Genetics), Harvard Medical School; Chief, Division of Infectious Diseases, Children's Hospital, Boston [130]

Lee M. Wetzler, MD
Professor of Medicine, Associate Professor of Microbiology, Boston University School of Medicine, Boston [136]

Meir Wetzler, MD
Professor of Medicine, Roswell Park Cancer Institute, Buffalo [104]

L. Joseph Wheat, MD
President and Director, MiraVista Diagnostics and MiraBella Technology, Indianapolis [192]

A. Clinton White, Jr., MD
The Paul R. Stalnaker, MD, Distinguished Professor of Internal Medicine; Director, Infectious Disease Division, Department of Internal Medicine, University of Texas Medical Branch, Galveston [213]

Nicholas J. White, DSc
Professor of Tropical Medicine, Oxford University, United Kingdom; Mahidol University, Bangkok, Thailand [203, e18]

Richard J. Whitley, MD
Loeb Scholar in Pediatrics, Professor of Pediatrics, Microbiology, Medicine, and Neurosurgery, University of Alabama, Birmingham [173]

Gordon H. Williams, MD
Professor of Medicine, Harvard Medical School; Chief, Cardiovascular Endocrinology Section, Brigham and Women's Hospital, Boston [336]

John W. Winkleman, MD, PhD
Assistant Professor of Psychiatry, Harvard Medical School; Medical Director, Sleep Health Center, Brigham and Women's Hospital, Boston [28]

Bruce U. Wintroub, MD
Professor and Chair of Dermatology, Department of Dermatology; Vice Dean, School of Medicine Dean's Office, University of California, San Francisco, San Francisco [56]

Allan W. Wolkoff, MD
Professor of Medicine and Anatomy and Structural Biology; Director, Belfer Institute for Advanced Biomedical Studies; Associate Chair of Medicine for Research; Chief, Division of Hepatology, Albert Einstein College of Medicine, Bronx [297]

Louis Michel Wong-Kee-Song, MD
Assistant Professor of Medicine, Division of Gastroenterology and Hepatology, Mayo College of Medicine, Rochester [285, e25]

Robert L. Wortmann, MD
Dartmouth-Hitchcock Medical Center, Lebanon [353]

Richard Wunderink, MD
Professor, Division of Pulmonary and Critical Care, Department of Medicine, Northwestern University Feinberg School of Medicine; Director, Medical Intensive Care Unit, Northwestern Memorial Hospital, Chicago [251]

Joshua Wynne, MD, MBA, MPH
Executive Associate Dean, Professor of Medicine, University of North Dakota School of Medicine and Health Sciences, Grand Forks [231]

Kim B. Yancey, MD
Professor and Chair, Department of Dermatology, University of Texas, Southwestern, Dallas [52, 55]

Janet A. Yellowitz, DMD, MPH
Associate Professor; Director, Geriatric Dentistry, The Johns Hopkins University School of Medicine, Baltimore [e7]

Neal S. Young, MD
Chief, Hematology Branch, National Heart, Lung, and Blood Institute, National Institutes of Health, Bethesda [102]

Robert C. Young, MD
Chancellor, Fox Chase Cancer Center, Philadelphia [93]

Alan S. L. Yu, MB, BChir
Associate Professor of Medicine, Physiology and Biophysics, University of Southern California Keck School of Medicine, Los Angeles [279]

Victor L. Yu, MD
Professor of Medicine, University of Pittsburgh, Pittsburgh [141]

PREFACE

The first edition of *Harrison's Principles of Internal Medicine* was published almost 60 years ago. Over the decades, the field of internal medicine has evolved greatly and has incorporated the spectacular advances that have occurred in the science of medicine into its armamentarium of diagnosis, prevention, and treatment. This textbook has evolved simultaneously to keep step with these advances while at the same time maintaining an appreciation of the art of medicine and the principles underlying the optimal care of the patient. In shaping and revising this latest edition, the Editors have committed themselves to making the textbook an invaluable resource for students and practitioners coping with the demands of modern medicine.

From the standpoint of physical appearance, one of the most striking elements of the textbook is the number of new and updated figures. The seventeenth edition features 300 additional illustrations (20% more than the previous edition); with the new illustrations included on the enclosed DVD, this edition has approximately 800 more images, a 60% increase in the course of just one edition. Many images have been redrawn by graphic artists working closely with the authors and editors to illustrate complex concepts, pathways, and algorithms in a clear and compelling manner. The seventeenth edition also features many additional plain film, CT, MRI, and ultrasound images, in recognition of the increased use of radiologic diagnosis in general medical practice. The notably increased use of pathologic and clinical photographs completes our concerted approach to a more robustly illustrated edition of *Harrison's*.

The seventeenth edition of *Harrison's* has a full-color format that draws from and extends the excellent appearance of the sixteenth edition to make the content more accessible and pleasant to read. The placement of color illustrations within the chapters rather than in the separate atlas was very favorably received by our sixteenth edition readers and has been continued in the current edition. Many changes to the design of this edition have been made in order to speed the reader's navigation through the textual and visual materials. For example, tables have been shaded for ease of reading, citations in tables and illustrations are now more instantly notable and in color, and our Treatment sections in each chapter have been redesigned to allow even faster access. The new global icons call greater attention to key epidemiologic and clinical differences in the practice of medicine throughout the world.

Evolving information technology enables us to broaden and deepen the nature, format, and medium of content included under the *Harrison's* name. Purchase of this textbook now includes a DVD, which has allowed the editors to expand the content in *Harrison's* by the use of "e-chapters," 39 in number. In addition to new chapters in traditional narrative format, the DVD includes a number of diagnostic and procedural atlases, which readers should find enormously helpful. The DVD also includes dozens of motion video clips of endoscopic and cardiac imaging. These diagnostic approaches have become central to the practice of medicine, and the video clips show crystal-clear depictions of abnormal anatomy, function, and results.

Globalization of economies and trade has had an enormous impact on nations throughout the world, both developing and developed. This phenomenon has underscored the reality of the globalization of medicine. In this regard, as this textbook is widely used by students and practitioners throughout the world and as we in the United States are more frequently confronted with issues related to global health, a special emphasis has been placed in this edition on global health in individual chapters together with an over-arching view presented by Dr. Kim and Dr. Farmer in a new chapter entitled "Global Issues in Medicine." We have highlighted, where appropriate, regional differences in the prevalence, approach, and treatment of diseases that need to be considered for delivery of the highest-quality medical care possible in various geographic settings. These are only highlights of the changes that the Editors hope will make the new *Harrison's* a helpful tool, not only for the student who needs an expert source of basic knowledge in internal medicine, but also for the pressured practitioner who needs a clear, concise, and balanced distillation of the best information on which to base daily clinical decisions.

The seventeenth edition has been enriched by the addition of a new editor, Joseph Loscalzo, MD, PhD, who joined with our most senior editor Eugene Braunwald, MD, in contributing to and/or editing of chapters in the Parts on Disorders of the Cardiovascular System, Disorders of the Respiratory System, and Disorders of the Kidney and Urinary Tract. The addition of Dr. Loscalzo provides a smooth editorial transition in preparation for the upcoming retirement from *Harrison's* of Dr. Braunwald who has served as an esteemed editor for 12 editions.

Part 1, "Introduction to Clinical Medicine," contains a new chapter that lays the framework for appreciating the global issues in medicine and the variations in disease incidence and patterns throughout the world. It sets the stage for the discussion in individual chapters of global issues related to specific diseases, a novel feature in this edition. In addition, there are e-chapters on quality and safety issues in patient care, economics of health care delivery, ethics in clinical medicine, and health care disparities. The last chapter addresses the evidence for racial and ethnic disparities in health care in the United States and globally and offers a variety of approaches for minimizing them.

Part 2, "Cardinal Manifestations and Presentation of Diseases," serves as a comprehensive introduction to clinical medicine as well as a practical guide to the care of patients with these manifestations. Each section focuses on a particular group of disorders, examining the concepts of pathophysiology and differential diagnosis that must be considered in caring for patients with these common clinical presentations. Major symptoms are reviewed and correlated with specific disease states, and clinical approaches to patients presenting with these symptoms are summarized. There are eleven new chapters in this Part. Every chapter that appeared in the sixteenth edition has been updated, and two chapters have new authors. Among the e-chapters are atlases of rashes associated with fever; oral manifestations of disease; renal biopsies and urinary sediments; skin manifestations of internal disease; and peripheral blood and bone marrow. A new chapter on Hypercalcemia and Hypocalcemia provides a succinct overview of the causes, clinical presentations, and management of these conditions as a complement to the more extensive discussion of these topics in Part 15, "Endocrinology and Metabolism." New chapters discuss common clinical presentations such as menstrual disorders and pelvic pain, the pathogenesis and treatment of headache, the clinical approach to imbalance, and the causes of confusion and delirium.

Part 3, "Genetics and Disease," has been extensively updated, reflecting the remarkable impact of the human genome project and its implications for clinical medicine. The material included in this edition is strongly geared toward clinical practice, in which genetic information increasingly comes into play. A new chapter on gene transfer in clinical medicine addresses the principles and strategies for this novel, but still experimental, therapeutic area.

Part 4, "Regenerative Medicine," is a new part initiated for this edition. It contains chapters on Stem Cell Biology, Applications of Stem Cell Biology in Clinical Medicine, Hematopoietic Stem Cells, and Tissue Engineering. These chapters summarize the state of the science in these emerging fields and outline the future directions for clinical applications of stem cell biology in regenerative medicine.

Part 5, "Nutrition," covers topics critical to clinical medicine, whether dealing with undernutrition in the context of chronic starvation or acute illness or the implications of overfeeding in industrialized nations. New authors with global expertise in nutrition have prepared the chapters on protein-energy malnutrition and enteral and parenteral nutrition therapy. A new chapter on the Management of Obesity and a complementary chapter on the Biology of Obesity address the explosion of new knowledge about pathways that regulate body weight and composition and the urgent need to provide effective means to prevent and treat the global epidemic of obesity and its complications.

The core of *Harrison's* continues to encompass the disorders of the organ systems and is contained in Parts 6 through 17. These sections include succinct accounts of the pathophysiology of diseases involving the major organ systems as well as infectious diseases, with an emphasis on clinical manifestations, diagnostic procedures, differential diagnosis, and treatment strategies and guidelines.

Part 6, "Oncology and Hematology," includes 11 chapters by new authors, including a completely revised section on Disorders of Hemostasis. A new e-chapter on Thymoma has also been added. As novel therapies are being added at a record pace to the armamentarium for oncologic and hematologic disorders, the mechanisms of action, pharmacology, clinical uses, and toxicities of these new agents have been included. Recent progress in the treatment of renal cell cancer, colorectal cancer, and breast cancer is highlighted. Revised chapters include the impact of genetic factors on cancer development and the use of gene expression data to define prognostic disease subsets.

Part 7, "Infectious Diseases," presents an overview of the latest information on disease epidemiology, pathogenesis, and genetics while focusing on the needs of clinicians who must accurately diagnose and treat infections under time pressure and cost constraints. Abundant illustrations offer key information in an easily accessible format to assist clinicians with these challenges. The expert authors of each chapter make specific recommendations regarding therapeutic regimens, including the drug(s) of choice, doses, durations, and alternatives. Current trends in antimicrobial resistance are discussed fully in light of their impact on therapeutic choices. In line with the international emphasis of this edition, the infectious diseases section includes expanded information on disease prevalences, distributions, features, and management in different regions of the world.

A total of 17 chapters have been completely rewritten by new authors, covering the latest advances in the management of important diseases such as pneumonia, shigellosis, and rabies and of infections due to *Pseudomonas*, *Bartonella*, *Listeria*, corynebacteria, and parvovirus. The section on fungal infections is entirely new and encompasses the expertise of current authorities on specific mycoses. Health care–associated infections, an area of enormous significance in terms of patient care in general and antimicrobial resistance in particular, are addressed by Robert Weinstein in a thorough, highly practical chapter. Another topic of ever-increasing importance—infections with gram-negative enteric bacilli, including *Escherichia coli*—is dealt with by Thomas Russo and James Johnson in a substantially reworked and updated chapter. The superb chapter on human papillomaviruses by Richard Reichman includes the latest information and recommendations regarding the recently licensed and widely publicized HPV vaccine. Finally, the chapter on HIV infection and AIDS by Anthony S. Fauci and H. Clifford Lane has once again been completely revised, with an emphasis on therapeutic strategies. This chapter is widely considered to be a classic in the field; its clinically pragmatic focus in combination with its comprehensive and analytical approach to the pathogenesis of HIV disease has led to its use as the sole complete reference on HIV/AIDS in medical schools.

New in this edition is a chapter on babesiosis, an important emerging infection that can cause severe disease in immunodeficient and elderly patients. Three additional new chapters of substantial clinical relevance appear in the electronic version of the textbook: an atlas of rashes associated with fever, an atlas of blood smears showing the various stages of the parasites causing malaria and babesiosis, and a chapter detailing the pharmacology of antiparasitic agents.

Terrorist attacks in various forms have become a frightening reality throughout the world. Important among these is the threat of bioterror attacks involving microbes or their toxins, chemicals, and radiation. This has become of particular concern in light of the anthrax attacks in the United States shortly after the September 11, 2001, airplane attacks on the World Trade Center in New York City and the Pentagon in Washington, DC. In the sixteenth edition, the editors developed a new Part on Bioterrorism and Clinical Medicine. Part 8 in the current edition has been updated with descriptions of the most recent countermeasures that have been developed as part of the United States preparedness plan against bioterror attacks. Edited by *Harrison's* Anthony S. Fauci, these chapters are written succinctly and include easily readable charts, tables, and algorithms; their goal is to confer an understanding of the pathogenesis, diagnosis, treatment, and prognosis of the diseases in question.

Part 9, "Disorders of the Cardiovascular System," is now co-edited by two of the most preeminent experts in the field, Eugene Braunwald and Joseph Loscalzo, the newest addition to the team of *Harrison* editors. There are new chapters on the epidemiology of cardiovascular disease with an overview of the global nature of the growing pandemic, the basic biology of the cardiovascular system (written by Braunwald, Libby, and Loscalzo), and principles of electrophysiology. A new chapter on the metabolic syndrome summarizes the clinical features and complications of this disorder, which reflects the rapidly rising prevalence of obesity and insulin resistance. In addition, there are new e-chapters that provide atlases of basic electrocardiography, arrhythmias, noninvasive imaging, and percutaneous revascularization. Finally, every chapter has been revised to reflect the latest information on approaches to the diagnosis and treatment of specific cardiovascular diseases, and eight of these chapters have been written by new authors.

Part 10, "Disorders of the Respiratory System," includes a new e-chapter on chest imaging that provides an atlas of chest radiographs and computed tomographic studies of a wide range of chest diseases. In addition, three chapters have been written by new authors, including a superb chapter on asthma by Peter Barnes and an excellent chapter on pneumonia by Lionel Mandell.

With advances in health care delivery and pressures aimed at cost containment, critical care units account for a growing percentage of hospital beds. Part 11, "Critical Care Medicine," was first introduced as a separate Part for the sixteenth edition of *Harrison's*. It is devoted to the provision of optimal care in this medical setting of growing importance and deals with four main areas: respiratory critical care, shock and cardiac arrest, neurologic critical care, and a new section on oncologic emergencies.

Part 12, "Disorders of the Kidney and Urinary Tract," has undergone extensive revision and reorganization under the guidance of new editor Joseph Loscalzo. There is an outstanding new chapter on the cellular and molecular biology of the kidney by Eric Neilson, as well as a new e-chapter atlas of urinary sediments and renal pathology. In addition to a thorough updating of each revised chapter, five have new authors who bring a unique, contemporary perspective to their subject.

Part 13, "Disorders of the Gastrointestinal System," includes two new atlases of endoscopic findings, both static photographs and movies. New chapters have been added on mesenteric vascular insufficiency and common disorders of the colon and ano-rectum, and new authors have written two other chapters. The chapter on Cirrhosis and Its Complications has been completely rewritten by a new author, Bruce Bacon, who is also the new author for the chapter on Infiltrative, Genetic, and Metabolic Diseases Affecting the Liver. An Atlas of Liver Biopsies has been added as a new e-chapter.

Part 14, "Disorders of the Immune System, Connective Tissue, and Joints," has been extensively revised. The chapter on Introduction to the Immune System has been thoroughly updated. It has become a classic in its field and is often used as the textbook of immunology in postgraduate and medical school courses. This chapter combines an in-depth description and analysis of the principles of basic immunology with an easy flow into the application of these principles to clinical disease states. Its description of the relationship of innate to adaptive immunity is a model for understanding the intricacies of the human immune system. A new e-chapter written by Max Cooper on Primary Immunodeficiencies Associated with or Secondary to Other Diseases has been added to complement his printed book chapter on Primary Immunodeficiencies. The chapter on Systemic Sclerosis (Scleroderma) and Related Disorders has been rewritten by a new author. An Atlas of Clinical Imaging in the Vasculitis Syndromes has been added as a new e-chapter. The chapters on Sarcoidosis, Amyloidosis, Osteoarthritis, and Gout and Other Crystal Arthropathies have been rewritten by new authors. A highly skilled, academic, and clinical rheumatologist (Carol Langford) has joined the team as an author and has co-authored the chapters on the Vasculitis Syndromes, Relapsing Polychondritis, Fibromyalgia, and Arthritis Associated with Systemic Disease and Other Arthritides.

Part 15, "Endocrinology and Metabolism," includes several new authors, including those for the chapter on pheochromocytoma, which highlights recent advances in the genetic causes of these catecholamine-secreting tumors, as well as updated strategies for diagnosis and management. The chapter on the Ovary has a new author who integrates traditional hypothalamic-pituitary regulation of the menstrual cycle with the identification of multiple ovarian growth factors that regulate follicle development. Identification of these pathways has provided insight into the causes of premature ovarian failure and infertility. There have been rapid changes in the clinical management of many endocrine diseases, especially diabetes, lipoprotein disorders, and the menopause. These and other chapters have been updated extensively. A new Atlas of Metabolic Disorders has been added as an e-chapter.

Part 16, "Neurologic Disorders," has been extensively rewritten to highlight the many advances that have taken place in the understanding, diagnosis, treatment, and prevention of neurologic and psychiatric diseases. Notable are new chapters on essential tremor and movement disorders, peripheral neuropathy, and neurologic problems in hospitalized patients. Many illustrative neuroimaging figures appear throughout the section, and a new atlas of neuroimaging findings has been added. Knowledge of the dementias, Parkinson's disease, and related neurodegenerative disorders has been transformed by new findings from genetics, modular imaging, cell biology, and clinical research. The very latest information has been included, providing a practical guide to diagnosis and appropriate use of the latest treatments. New therapies are also revolutionizing the care of patients with stroke and multiple sclerosis, and these are also discussed in an evidence-based fashion that will be useful to all practitioners and not only to specialists. Another new chapter, authored by Stephen Hyman and Eric Kandel, reviews progress in deciphering the pathogenesis of common psychiatric disorders and discusses the remaining challenges to development of more effective treatments.

Part 17, "Poisoning, Drug Overdose, and Envenomation," focuses on topics most relevant to internal medicine.

Part 18 is a new feature to *Harrison's* and represents four brand new e-chapters from our International Advisory Editors. Dr. Peter Barnes addresses the emerging use of pulmonary biomarkers in COPD. This state of the art summary will be useful to clinicians and researchers alike. Chagas' disease continues to cause significant morbidity in Central and South America, and the long period between infection and cardiovascular complications can make the etiologic aspects of its diagnosis difficult. The cardiovascular pathologies and sequelae, as well as current approaches to diagnosis and treatment, are clearly described by Dr. Sposito and Dr. Ramires. Chapter e38 by Dr. Reddy, Dr. Naik, and Dr. Roy addresses the potential benefits and challenges of a polypill for multiple cardiovascular risk factors, an issue of global interest in light of increases in cardiovascular disease worldwide. Interest in the mitochondrial role in human health and disease has advanced considerably in recent years, and Chapter e39 by Dr. Skorecki and Dr. Mandel sets forth the current understanding of the role of the mitochondria in a large number of diseases and approaches to diagnosis and treatment.

Within the last 10 years, the *Harrison's* collection of publications has expanded as information delivery technology has evolved. *Harrison's Online (HOL)* is now one of the standard informational resources used in medical centers throughout the United States. In addition to the full content of the parent text, HOL offers frequent updates from and links to the emerging scientific and clinical literature; an expanded collection of reference citations; audio recordings and Podcasts of lectures by authorities in the various specialties of medicine; and other helpful supplementary materials such as a complete database of pharmacologic therapeutics, self-assessment questions for examination and board review; and an expanded collection of clinical photographs. The brand new "e-chapters" on the enclosed DVD, including the video clips of cardiac and endoscopic imaging, are also available on *HOL*. Future iterations of *HOL* will include expanded use of such supplementary multimedia materials to illustrate further key concepts and clinical approaches discussed in the parent text.

In 2006, in recognition of the increasing time pressures placed on clinicians and the increasing use of electronic medical records systems, *Harrison's Practice of Medicine (HP)* made its debut. *HP* is a comprehensive database of specific clinical topics built from the ground up to provide authoritative guidance quickly at the point of care. *HP* is highly structured so that physicians and other health professionals can access the most salient features of any one of more than 700 diseases and clinical presentations within minutes. This innovative new application is updated regularly and includes fully integrated, detailed information on brand name and generic drugs. In addition, hyperlinks throughout *HP* enable quick access to the primary literature via PubMed. *HP* is available via the Internet and on PDA; samples of approximately 20 core topics from *HP* are included on the DVD packaged within this book.

The print publications within the *Harrison's* family are being revised for publication in new editions. The *Harrison's Manual of Medicine* is widely used by students and clinicians worldwide and, like the parent text, is available in print and digital formats. The PDA version of the *Harrison's Manual* provides full text coverage, the full complement of illustrations and tables from the print edition, and extensive cross-referencing between terms. In view of the requirements for continuing education for licensure and relicensure as well as emphasis on certification and recertification, a revision of the *Harrison's Self-Assessment and Board Review* will be published with this edition. This volume is again in the capable hands of Dr. Charles Wiener from Johns Hopkins. It consists of several hundred questions based on the seventeenth edition of *Harrison's*, along with answers and explanations for the answers.

Taken as a portfolio, *Harrison's* is now available in a wide variety of formats suitable for all levels of medical education and practice, and for all varieties of health care settings. It is gratifying that, whether in print or digital formats, the content within *Harrison's* remains so widely used and referenced by students and clinicians throughout medicine and health care across the globe.

We wish to express our appreciation to our many associates and colleagues, who, as experts in their fields, have offered us constructive criticisms and helpful suggestions. We acknowledge especially the contributions of the following individuals: Arv Vanagunas, Laura Kulik, Pat Lynch, Sundeep Khosla, Michael Bray, Mark D. Carlson, Daniel H. Lowenstein, Lawrence C. Madoff, Chung Owyang, Alice Pau, Mary Wright, and Gregory K. Folkers.

We thank in particular Kenneth and Elaine Kaye and Lindsey Baden, who gathered many high-quality illustrations of infectious disease manifestations. We also express our gratitude to Eileen J. Scott, who has applied her editorial expertise to the past six editions of *Harrison's*, and Alan Barnett, the text designer for this edition. This book could not have been edited without the dedicated help of our co-workers in the editorial offices of the individual editors. We are especially indebted to Patricia L. Duffey, Gregory K. Folkers, Sarah Matero, Julie B. McCoy, Elizabeth Robbins, Kathryn Saxon, Marie Scurti, Stephanie Tribuna, Karl Cremieux, and Kristina Shontz.

Finally, we continue to be highly indebted to the outstanding members of the McGraw-Hill organization: Mariapaz Ramos Englis, Senior Managing Editor, who will be retiring after serving the book and its Editors so well for four editions; Phil Galea and Catherine Saggese, Production Director and Manager, respectively; Jenna Esposito, the Editorial Assistant for this edition; James Halston, Digital Editing Manager; James F. Shanahan, Executive Editor; and Martin J. Wonsiewicz, Publisher, who recently left McGraw-Hill after serving as an extremely effective partner to the Editors for 10 years. They are an effective team who have given the Editors constant encouragement and sage advice. They have been instrumental in guiding the many changes instituted with this edition of *Harrison's* and in bringing this volume to fruition in a timely manner.

THE EDITORS

1 The Practice of Medicine

The Editors

THE MODERN-DAY PHYSICIAN

No greater opportunity, responsibility, or obligation can fall to the lot of a human being than to become a physician. In the care of the suffering, [the physician] needs technical skill, scientific knowledge, and human understanding.… Tact, sympathy, and understanding are expected of the physician, for the patient is no mere collection of symptoms, signs, disordered functions, damaged organs, and disturbed emotions. [The patient] is human, fearful, and hopeful, seeking relief, help, and reassurance.

–*Harrison's Principles of Internal Medicine*, 1950

The practice of medicine has changed in significant ways since the first edition of this book appeared in 1950. The advent of molecular biology with its enormous implications for the biological sciences (the sequencing of the human genome), sophisticated new imaging techniques, and advances in bioinformatics and information technology have contributed to an explosion of scientific information that has fundamentally changed the way we define, diagnose, treat, and prevent disease. This explosion of scientific knowledge is not at all static as it continues to intensify with time.

The widespread use of electronic medical records and the Internet have altered the way we practice medicine and exchange information. As today's physician struggles to integrate the copious amounts of scientific knowledge into everyday practice, it is important to remember that the ultimate goal of medicine is to treat the patient. Despite more than 50 years of scientific advances since the first edition of this text, it is critical to underscore that cultivating the intimate relationship that exists between physician and patient still lies at the heart of successful patient care.

The Science and Art of Medicine Science-based technology and deductive reasoning form the foundation for the solution to many clinical problems. Spectacular advances in biochemistry, cell biology, and genomics, coupled with newly developed imaging techniques, allow access to the innermost parts of the cell and provide a window to the most remote recesses of the body. Revelations about the nature of genes and single cells have opened the portal for formulating a new molecular basis for the physiology of systems. Increasingly, we are understanding how subtle changes in many different genes can affect the function of cells and organisms. We are beginning to decipher the complex mechanisms by which genes are regulated. We have developed a new appreciation of the role of stem cells in normal tissue function and in the development of cancer, degenerative disease, and other disorders. The knowledge gleaned from the science of medicine has already improved and undoubtedly will further improve our understanding of complex disease processes and provide new approaches to disease treatment and prevention. Yet skill in the most sophisticated application of laboratory technology and in the use of the latest therapeutic modality alone does not make a good physician.

When a patient poses challenging clinical problems, an effective physician must be able to identify the crucial elements in a complex history and physical examination, to order the appropriate laboratory tests, and to extract the key results from the crowded computer printouts of data to determine whether to "treat" or to "watch." Deciding whether a clinical clue is worth pursuing or should be dismissed as a "red herring" and weighing whether a proposed treatment entails a greater risk than the disease itself are essential judgments that the skilled clinician must make many times each day. This combination of medical knowledge, intuition, experience, and judgment defines the ***art of medicine***, which is as necessary to the practice of medicine as is a sound scientific base.

CLINICAL SKILLS

History-Taking The written history of an illness should include all the facts of medical significance in the life of the patient. Recent events should be given the most attention. The patient should, at some early point, have the opportunity to tell his or her own story of the illness without frequent interruption and, when appropriate, receive expressions of interest, encouragement, and empathy from the physician. Any event related by the patient, however trivial or seemingly irrelevant, may provide the key to solving the medical problem. In general, only patients who feel comfortable will offer complete information, and thus putting the patient at ease to the greatest extent possible contributes substantially to obtaining an adequate history.

An informative history is more than an orderly listing of symptoms; by listening to patients and noting the way in which they describe their symptoms, physicians can gain valuable insight into the problem. Inflections of voice, facial expression, gestures, and attitude, i.e., "body language," may reveal important clues to the meaning of the symptoms to the patient. Because patients vary in their medical sophistication and ability to recall facts, the reported medical history should be corroborated whenever possible. The social history can also provide important insights into the types of diseases that should be considered. The family history not only identifies rare Mendelian disorders within a family but often reveals risk factors for common disorders such as coronary heart disease, hypertension, or asthma. A thorough family history may require input from multiple relatives to ensure completeness and accuracy. However, once recorded, it can be readily updated. The process of history-taking provides an opportunity to observe the patient's behavior and to watch for features to be pursued more thoroughly during the physical examination.

The very act of eliciting the history provides the physician with the opportunity to establish or enhance the unique bond that forms the basis for the ideal patient-physician relationship. This process helps the physician develop an appreciation of the patient's perception of the illness, the patient's expectations of the physician and the health care system, and the financial and social implications of the illness to the patient. Although current health care settings may impose time constraints on patient visits, it is important not to rush the history-taking since the patient may get the impression that what he or she is relating is not of importance to the physician and therefore may hold back relevant information. The confidentiality of the patient-physician relationship cannot be overemphasized.

Physical Examination The purpose of the physical examination is to identify the physical signs of disease. The significance of these objective indications of disease is enhanced when they confirm a functional or structural change already suggested by the patient's history. At times, however, the physical signs may be the only evidence of disease.

The physical examination should be performed methodically and thoroughly, with consideration for the patient's comfort and modesty. Although attention is often directed by the history to the diseased organ or part of the body, the examination of a new patient must extend from head to toe in an objective search for abnormalities. Unless the physical examination is systematic and performed in a consistent manner from patient to patient, important segments may be inadvertently omitted. The results of the examination, like the details of the history, should be recorded at the time they are elicited, not hours later when they are subject to the distortions of memory. Skill in physical diagnosis is acquired with experience, but it is not merely technique that determines success in eliciting signs of disease. The detection of a few scattered petechiae, a faint diastolic murmur, or a small mass in the abdomen is not a question of keener eyes and ears or more sensitive fingers, but of a mind alert to these findings. Because physical findings can change with time, the physical examination should be repeated as frequently as the clinical situation warrants. Because a large number of highly sensitive diagnostic tests are available, particularly imaging techniques, it may be tempting to put less emphasis on the physical examination. Indeed, many patients are seen for the first time after a series of diagnostic tests have already been performed and the results known. This should not deter the physician from performing a thorough physical examination since clinical findings are often present that have "escaped" the barrage of preexamination diagnostic tests.

Diagnostic Studies We have become increasingly reliant on a wide array of laboratory tests to solve clinical problems. However, accumulated laboratory data do not relieve the physician from the responsibility of carefully observing, examining, and studying the patient. It is also essential to appreciate the limitations of diagnostic tests. By virtue of their impersonal quality, complexity, and apparent precision, they often gain an aura of authority regardless of the fallibility of the tests themselves, the instruments used in the tests, and the individuals performing or interpreting them. Physicians must weigh the expense involved in the laboratory procedures relative to the value of the information they are likely to provide.

Single laboratory tests are rarely ordered. Rather, physicians generally request "batteries" of multiple tests, which often prove useful. For example, abnormalities of hepatic function may provide the clue to such nonspecific symptoms as generalized weakness and increased fatigability, suggesting the diagnosis of chronic liver disease. Sometimes a single abnormality, such as an elevated serum calcium level, points to a particular disease, such as hyperparathyroidism or underlying malignancy.

The thoughtful use of screening tests, such as low-density lipoprotein cholesterol, may be quite useful. A group of laboratory determinations can be carried out conveniently on a single specimen at relatively low cost. Screening tests are most informative when directed toward common diseases or disorders and when their results indicate the need for other useful tests or interventions that may be costly to perform. On the one hand, biochemical measurements, together with simple laboratory examinations such as blood count, urinalysis, and sedimentation rate, often provide a major clue to the presence of a pathologic process. On the other hand, the physician must learn to evaluate occasional abnormalities among the screening tests that may not necessarily connote significant disease. An in-depth workup following a report of an isolated laboratory abnormality in a person who is otherwise well is almost invariably wasteful and unproductive. Among the more than 40 tests that are routinely performed as screening, it would not be unusual for one or two of them to be slightly abnormal. If there is no suspicion of an underlying illness, these tests are ordinarily repeated to ensure that the abnormality does not represent a laboratory error. If an abnormality is confirmed, it is important to consider its potential significance in the context of the patient's condition and other test results.

The development of technically improved imaging studies with greater sensitivity and specificity is one of the most rapidly advancing areas of medicine. These tests provide remarkably detailed anatomic information that can be a pivotal factor in medical decision-making. Ultrasonography, a variety of isotopic scans, CT, MRI, and positron emission tomography have benefited patients by supplanting older, more invasive approaches and opening new diagnostic vistas. Cognizant of their capabilities and the rapidity with which they can lead to a diagnosis, it is tempting to order a battery of imaging studies. All physicians have had experiences in which imaging studies turned up findings leading to an unexpected diagnosis. Nonetheless, patients must endure each of these tests, and the added cost of unnecessary testing is substantial. A skilled physician must learn to use these powerful diagnostic tools judiciously, always considering whether the results will alter management and benefit the patient.

PRINCIPLES OF PATIENT CARE

Evidence-Based Medicine Evidence-based medicine refers to the concept that clinical decisions are formally supported by data, preferably data that are derived from prospectively designed, randomized, controlled clinical trials. This is in sharp contrast to anecdotal experience, which may often be biased. Unless they are attuned to the importance of using larger, more objective studies for making decisions, even the most experienced physicians can be influenced by recent encounters with selected patients. Evidence-based medicine has become an increasingly important part of the routine practice of medicine and has led to the publication of a number of practice guidelines.

Practice Guidelines Professional organizations and government agencies are developing formal clinical-practice guidelines to aid physicians and other caregivers in making diagnostic and therapeutic decisions that are evidence-based, cost-effective, and most appropriate to a particular patient and clinical situation. As the evidence base of medicine increases, guidelines can provide a useful framework for managing patients with particular diagnoses or symptoms. They can protect patients—particularly those with inadequate health care benefits—from receiving substandard care. Guidelines can also protect conscientious caregivers from inappropriate charges of malpractice and society from the excessive costs associated with the overuse of medical resources. There are, however, caveats associated with clinical practice guidelines since they tend to oversimplify the complexities of medicine. Furthermore, groups with differing perspectives may develop divergent recommendations regarding issues as basic as the need for periodic sigmoidoscopy in middle-aged persons. Finally, guidelines do not—and cannot be expected to—account for the uniqueness of each individual and his or her illness. The physician's challenge is to integrate into clinical practice the useful recommendations offered by experts without accepting them blindly or being inappropriately constrained by them.

Medical Decision-Making Medical decision-making is an important responsibility of the physician and occurs at each stage of the diagnostic and treatment process. It involves the ordering of additional tests, requests for consults, and decisions regarding treatment and prognosis. This process requires an in-depth understanding of the pathophysiology and natural history of disease. As described above, medical decision-making should be evidence-based so that patients derive the full benefit of the scientific knowledge available to physicians. Formulating a differential diagnosis requires not only a broad knowledge base but also the ability to assess the relative probabilities of various diseases. Application of the scientific method, including hypothesis formation and data collection, is essential to the process of accepting or rejecting a particular diagnosis. Analysis of the differential diagnosis is an iterative process. As new information or test results are acquired, the group of disease processes being considered can be contracted or expanded appropriately.

Despite the importance of evidence-based medicine, much of medical decision-making relies on good clinical judgment—a process that is difficult to quantify or even to assess qualitatively. Physicians must use their knowledge and experience as a basis for weighing known factors along with the inevitable uncertainties and the need to use sound judgment; this is particularly important when a relevant evidence base is not available. Several quantitative tools may be invaluable in synthesizing the available information, including diagnostic tests, Bayes' theorem, and multivariate statistical models. *Diagnostic tests* serve to reduce uncertainty about a diagnosis or prognosis in a particular individual and to help the physician decide how best to manage that individual's condition. The battery of diagnostic tests complements the history and the physical examination. The accuracy of a given test is ascertained by determining its sensitivity (true positive rate) and specificity (true negative rate) as well as the predictive value of a positive and negative result. *Bayes' theorem* uses information on a test's sensitivity and specificity, in conjunction with the pretest probability of a diagnosis, to determine mathematically the posttest probability of the diagnosis. More complex clinical problems can be approached with *multivariate statistical models*, which generate highly accurate information even when multiple factors are acting individually or together to affect disease risk, progression, or response to treatment. Studies comparing the performance of statistical models with that of expert clinicians have documented equivalent accuracy, although the models tend to be more consistent. Thus, multivariate statistical models may be particularly helpful to less experienced clinicians. See Chap. 3 for a more thorough discussion of decision-making in clinical medicine.

Electronic Medical Records Our growing reliance on computers and the strength of information technology are playing an increasingly important role in medicine. Laboratory data are accessed almost universally through computers. Many medical centers now have electronic medical records, computerized order entry, and bar-coded tracking of medications. Some of these systems are interactive and provide reminders or warn of potential medical errors. In many ways, the health care system has lagged behind other industries in the adoption of information technology. Electronic medical records have extraordinary potential for providing rapid access to clinical information, imaging studies, laboratory results, and medications. This type of information is invaluable for ongoing efforts to enhance quality and improve patient safety. Ideally, patient records should be easily transferred across the health care system, providing reliable access to relevant data and historic information. However, technology limitations and concerns about privacy and cost continue to limit a broad-based utilization of electronic health records in most clinical settings. It should also be emphasized that information technology is merely a tool and can never replace the clinical decisions that are best made by the physician. In this regard, clinical knowledge and an understanding of the patient's needs, supplemented by quantitative tools, still seem to represent the best approach to decision-making in the practice of medicine.

Evaluation of Outcomes Clinicians generally use *objective* and readily measurable parameters to judge the outcome of a therapeutic intervention. For example, findings on physical or laboratory examination—such as the blood pressure level, the patency of a coronary artery on an angiogram, or the size of a mass on a radiologic examination—can provide critically important information. However, patients usually seek medical attention for *subjective* reasons; they wish to obtain relief from pain, to preserve or regain function, and to enjoy life. The components of a patient's health status or quality of life can include bodily comfort, capacity for physical activity, personal and professional function, sexual function, cognitive function, and overall perception of health. Each of these important areas can be assessed by means of structured interviews or specially designed questionnaires. Such assessments also provide useful parameters by which the physician can judge the patient's subjective view of his or her disability and the response to treatment, particularly in chronic illness. The practice of medicine requires consideration and integration of both objective and subjective outcomes.

Women's Health and Disease Although past epidemiologic studies and clinical trials have often focused predominantly on men, more recent studies have included more women, and some, like the Women's Health Initiative, have exclusively addressed women's health issues. Significant gender differences exist in diseases that afflict both men and women. Much is still to be learned in this arena, and ongoing studies should enhance our understanding of the mechanisms of gender differences in the course and outcome of certain diseases. For a more complete discussion of women's health, see Chap. 6.

Care of the Elderly The relative proportion of elderly individuals in the populations of developed nations has been growing considerably over the past few decades and will continue to grow. In this regard, the practice of medicine will continue to be greatly influenced by the health care needs of this growing elderly population. The physician must understand and appreciate the decline in physiologic reserve associated with aging; the diminished responses of the elderly to vaccinations such as those against influenza; the different responses of the elderly to common diseases; and disorders that occur commonly with aging, such as depression, dementia, frailty, urinary incontinence, and fractures. For a more complete discussion of medical care for the elderly, see Chap. 9.

Errors in the Delivery of Health Care A report from the Institute of Medicine called for an ambitious agenda to reduce medical-error rates and improve patient safety by designing and implementing fundamental changes in health care systems. Adverse drug reactions occur in at least 5% of hospitalized patients, and the incidence increases with use of a large number of drugs. No matter what the clinical situation, it is the responsibility of the physician to use powerful therapeutic measures wisely, with due regard for their beneficial action, potential dangers, and cost. It is also the responsibility of hospitals and health care organizations to develop systems to reduce risk and ensure patient safety. Medication errors can be reduced through the use of ordering systems that eliminate misreading of handwriting. Implementation of infection-control systems, enforcement of hand-washing protocols, and careful oversight of antibiotic use can minimize complications of nosocomial infections.

The Role of the Physician in the Informed Consent of the Patient The fundamental principles of medical ethics require physicians to act in the patient's best interest and to respect the patient's autonomy. This is particularly relevant to the issue of informed consent. Most patients possess only limited medical knowledge and must rely on their physicians for advice. Physicians must respect their patients' autonomy, fully discussing the alternatives for care and the risks, benefits, and likely consequences of each alternative.

Patients are required to sign a consent form for essentially any diagnostic or therapeutic procedure. In such cases, it is particularly important for the patient to understand clearly the risks and benefits of these procedures; this is the definition of *informed consent.* It is incumbent on the physician to explain the procedures in a clear and understandable manner and to ascertain that the patient comprehends both the nature of the procedure and the attendant risks and benefits. The dread of the unknown, inherent in hospitalization, can be mitigated by such explanations.

The Approach to Grave Prognoses and Death No problem is more distressing than the diagnosis of an incurable disease, particularly when premature death is inevitable. What should the patient and family be told? What measures should be taken to maintain life? What can be done to maintain the quality of life?

Although some would argue otherwise, there is no ironclad rule that the patient must immediately be told "everything," even if the patient is an adult with substantial family responsibilities. How much is told at a given point in time should depend on the individual's ability to deal with the possibility of imminent death; often this capacity grows with time, and, whenever possible, gradual rather than abrupt disclosure is the best strategy. A wise and insightful physician is often guided by an understanding of what a patient wants to know and when he or she wants to know it. The patient's religious beliefs may also be taken into consideration. The patient must be given an opportunity to talk with the physician and ask questions. Patients may find it easier to share their feelings about death with their physician, who is likely to be more objective and less emotional, than with family members. As William Osler wrote, "One thing is certain; it is not for you to don the black cap and, assuming the judicial function, take hope away from any patient." Even when the patient directly inquires, "Am I dying?" the physician must attempt to determine whether this is a request for information or for reassurance. Only open communication between the patient and the physician can resolve this question and guide the physician in what to say and how to say it.

The physician should provide or arrange for emotional, physical, and spiritual support and must be compassionate, unhurried, and open. There is much to be gained by the laying on of hands. Pain should be adequately controlled, human dignity maintained, and isolation from family and close friends avoided. These aspects of care tend to be overlooked in hospitals, where the intrusion of life-sustaining apparati can so easily detract from attention to the whole person and encourage concentration instead on the life-threatening disease, against which the battle will ultimately be lost in any case. In the face of terminal illness, the goal of medicine must shift from *cure* to *care*, in the broadest sense of the term. In offering care to the dying patient, the physician must be prepared to provide information to family members and to deal with their grief and sometimes their feelings of guilt. It is important for the doctor to assure the family that everything possible has been done. For a more complete discussion of end-of-life care, see Chap. 11.

THE PATIENT-PHYSICIAN RELATIONSHIP

> *The significance of the intimate personal relationship between physician and patient cannot be too strongly emphasized, for in an extraordinarily large number of cases both the diagnosis and treatment are directly dependent on it. One of the essential qualities of the clinician is interest in humanity, **for the secret of the care of the patient is in caring for the patient**.*
>
> –Francis W. Peabody, 1881–1927

Physicians must never forget that patients are individual human beings with problems that all too often transcend their physical complaints. They are not "cases" or "admissions" or "diseases." This point is particularly important in this era of high technology in clinical medicine. Most patients are anxious and fearful. Physicians should instill confidence and should be reassuring but should never be arrogant. A professional attitude, coupled with warmth and openness, can do much to alleviate anxiety and to encourage patients to share all aspects of their medical history. Whatever the patient's attitude, the physician needs to consider the setting in which an illness occurs—in terms not only of the patients themselves but also of their familial, social, and cultural backgrounds. The ideal patient-physician relationship is based on thorough knowledge of the patient, on mutual trust, and on the ability to communicate.

The Dichotomy of Inpatient and Outpatient Internal Medicine The hospital environment has transformed dramatically over the past few decades. In more recent times, emergency departments and critical care units have evolved to identify and manage critically ill patients, allowing them to survive formerly fatal diseases. There is increasing pressure to reduce the length of stay in the hospital and to manage complex disorders in the outpatient setting. This transition has been driven not only by efforts to reduce costs but also by the availability of new outpatient technologies, such as imaging and percutaneous infusion catheters for long-term antibiotics or nutrition, and by evidence that outcomes are often improved by minimizing inpatient hospitalization. Hospitals now consist of multiple distinct levels of care, such as the emergency department, procedure rooms, overnight observation units, critical care units, and palliative care units, in addition to traditional medical beds. A consequence of this differentiation has been the emergence of new specialties such as emergency medicine, intensivists, hospitalists, and end-of-life care. Moreover, these systems frequently involve "hand-offs" from the outpatient to the inpatient environment, from the critical care unit to a general medicine floor, and from the hospital to the outpatient environment. Clearly, one of the important challenges in internal medicine is to maintain continuity of care and information flow during these transitions, which threaten the traditional one-to-one relationship between patient and physician. In the current environment, teams of physicians, specialists, and other health care professionals have often replaced the personal interaction between doctor and patient. The patient can benefit greatly from effective collaboration among a number of health care professionals; however, *it is the duty of the patient's principal or primary physician to provide cohesive guidance through an illness.* In order to meet this challenge, the primary physician must be familiar with the techniques, skills, and objectives of specialist physicians and allied health professionals. The primary physician must ensure that the patient will benefit from scientific advances and from the expertise of specialists when they are needed, while still retaining responsibility for the major decisions concerning diagnosis and treatment.

Appreciation of the Patient's Hospital Experience The hospital is an intimidating environment for most individuals. Hospitalized patients find themselves surrounded by air jets, buttons, and glaring lights; invaded by tubes and wires; and beset by the numerous members of the health care team—nurses, nurses' aides, physicians' assistants, social workers, technologists, physical therapists, medical students, house officers, attending and consulting physicians, and many others. They may be transported to special laboratories and imaging facilities replete with blinking lights, strange sounds, and unfamiliar personnel; they may be left unattended for periods of time; they may be obliged to share a room with other patients who have their own health problems. It is little wonder that patients may lose their sense of reality. Physicians who can appreciate the hospital experience from the patient's perspective and make an effort to develop a strong personal relationship with the patient whereby they may guide the patient through this experience can make a stressful situation more tolerable.

Trends in the Delivery of Health Care: A Challenge to the Humane Physician Many trends in the delivery of health care tend to make medical care impersonal. These trends, some of which have been mentioned already, include (1) vigorous efforts to reduce the escalating costs of health care; (2) the growing number of managed-care programs, which are intended to reduce costs but in which the patient may have little choice in selecting a physician or in seeing that physician consistently; (3) increasing reliance on technological advances and computerization for many aspects of diagnosis and treatment; (4) the need for numerous physicians to be involved in the care of most patients who are seriously ill; and (5) an increased number of malpractice suits, some of which are justifiable because of medical errors, but others of which reflect an unrealistic expectation on the part of many patients that their disease will be cured or that complications will not occur during the course of complex illnesses or procedures.

Given these changes in the medical care system, it is a major challenge for physicians to maintain the *humane* aspects of medical care. The American Board of Internal Medicine, working together with the American College of Physicians–American Society of Internal Medicine and the European Federation of Internal Medicine, has published a *Charter on Medical Professionalism* that underscores three main principles in physicians' contract with society: (1) the primacy of patient welfare, (2) patient autonomy, and (3) social justice. Medical schools have also increased their emphasis on physician professionalism in recent years (Fig. 1-1). The humanistic qualities of a physician must encompass integrity, respect, and compassion. Availability, the expression of sincere concern, the willingness to take the time to explain all aspects of the illness, and a nonjudgmental attitude when dealing with patients whose cultures, lifestyles, attitudes, and values differ from those of the physician are just a few of the characteristics of the humane physician. Every physician will, at times, be challenged by patients who evoke strongly negative or positive emotional responses. Physicians should be alert to their own reactions to such patients and situations and should consciously monitor and control their behavior so that the patient's best interest remains the principal motivation for their actions at all times.

An important aspect of patient care involves an appreciation of the patient's "quality of life," a subjective assessment of what each patient values most. Such an assessment requires detailed, sometimes intimate knowledge of the patient, which can usually be obtained only through deliberate, unhurried, and often repeated conversations. Time pressures will always threaten these interactions, but they should not diminish the importance of understanding and seeking to fulfill the priorities of the patient.

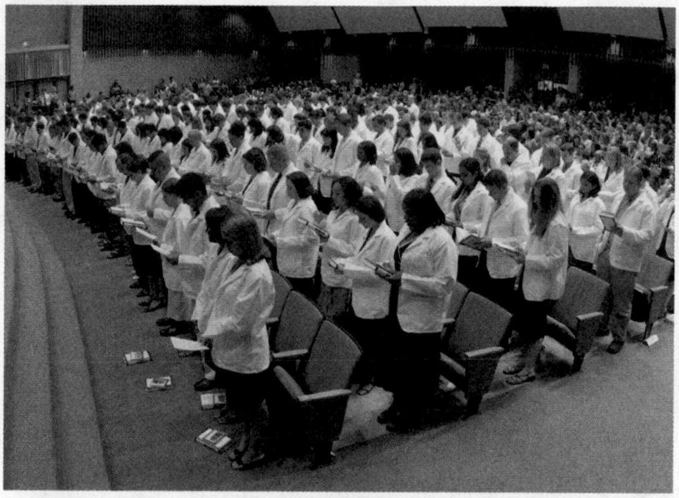

FIGURE 1-1 A typical "white coat" ceremony in medical school where students are introduced to the responsibilities of patient care. *(Courtesy of The University of Texas Health Science Center at San Antonio; with permission.)*

THE TWENTY-FIRST CENTURY PHYSICIAN: EXPANDING FRONTIERS

The Era of Genomics In the spring of 2003, the complete sequencing of the human genome was announced, officially ushering in the genomic era. However, even before this landmark accomplishment, the practice of medicine had been evolving as a result of the insights gained from an understanding of the human genome as well as the genomes of a wide variety of microbes, whose genetic sequences were becoming widely available as a result of the breathtaking advances in sequencing techniques and informatics. Examples of the latter include the identification of a novel coronavirus as the etiologic agent of the severe acute respiratory syndrome (SARS) and the tracking of the evolution of a potentially pandemic influenza virus found in birds. Today, gene expression profiles are being used to guide therapy and inform prognosis for a number of diseases; the use of genotyping is providing a new means to assess the risk of certain diseases as well as variation in response to a number of drugs; we are understanding better the role of certain genes in the causality of certain common conditions such as obesity and allergies. Despite these advances, we are still in the infancy of understanding and utilizing the complexities of genomics in the diagnosis, prevention, and treatment of disease. Our task is complicated by the fact that phenotypes are generally determined not by genes alone but by the interplay of genetic and environmental factors. Indeed, we have just begun to scratch the surface of possibilities that the era of genomics will provide to the practice of medicine.

The rapidity of these advances may seem overwhelming to the practicing physician. However, he or she has an important role to play in ensuring that these powerful technologies and sources of new information are applied with sensitivity and intelligence to the patient. Since genomics is such a rapidly evolving field, physicians and other health care professionals must continue to educate themselves so that they can apply this new knowledge to the benefit of their patients' health and well-being. Genetic testing requires wise counsel based on an understanding of the value and limitations of the tests as well as the implications of their results for specific individuals. For a more complete discussion of genetic testing, see Chap. 64.

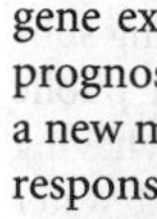

The Globalization of Medicine Physicians should be cognizant of diseases and health care services beyond local boundaries. Global travel has implications for disease spread, and it is not uncommon for diseases endemic to certain regions to be seen in other regions after a patient has traveled and returned from these regions. Patients have broader access to unique expertise or clinical trials at distant medical centers, and the cost of travel may be offset by the quality of care at these distant locations. As much as any other factor influencing global aspects of medicine, the Internet has transformed the transfer of medical information throughout the world. This change has been accompanied by the transfer of technological skills through telemedicine and international consultation for radiologic images and pathologic specimens. For a complete discussion of global issues, see Chap. 2.

Medicine on the Internet On the whole, the Internet has had a very positive effect on the practice of medicine; a wide range of information is available to physicians and patients through personal computers almost instantaneously at any time and from anywhere in the world. This medium holds enormous potential for delivering up-to-date information, practice guidelines, state-of-the-art conferences, journal contents, textbooks (including this text), and direct communications with other physicians and specialists, thereby expanding the depth and breadth of information available to the physician about the diagnosis and care of patients. Most medical journals are now accessible online, providing rapid and comprehensive sources of information. This medium also serves to lessen the information gap felt by physicians and health care providers in remote areas of the world by bringing them into direct and instant contact with the latest developments in medical care.

Patients, too, are turning to the Internet in increasing numbers to acquire information about their illnesses and therapies and to join Internet-based support groups. Physicians are increasingly faced with the prospect of dealing with patients who arrive with sophisticated information about their illness. In this regard, physicians are challenged in a positive way to keep themselves abreast of the latest relevant information while serving as an "editor" for the patients as they navigate through this seemingly endless source of information.

A critically important caveat is that virtually anything can be published on the Internet, with easy circumvention of the peer-review process that is an essential feature of quality publications. Physicians or patients who search the Internet for medical information must be aware of this danger. Notwithstanding this limitation, appropriate use of the Internet is revolutionizing information access for physicians and patients and in this regard is a great benefit that was not available to our predecessors.

Public Expectations and Accountability The level of knowledge and sophistication regarding health issues on the part of the general public has grown rapidly over the past few decades. As a result, expectations of the health care system in general and of physicians in particular have risen. Physicians are expected to master rapidly advancing fields (the *science* of medicine) while considering their patients' unique needs (the *art* of medicine). Thus, physicians are held accountable not only for the technical aspects of the care that they provide but also for their patients' satisfaction with the delivery and costs of care.

In many parts of the world, physicians are increasingly expected to account for the way in which they practice medicine by meeting certain standards prescribed by federal and local governments. The hospitalization of patients whose health care costs are reimbursed by the government and other third parties is subjected to utilization review. Thus, the physician must defend the cause for and duration of a patient's hospitalization if it falls outside certain "average" standards. Authorization for reimbursement is increasingly based on documentation of the nature and complexity of an illness, as reflected by recorded elements of the history and physical examination. There is a growing "pay for performance" movement, which seeks to link reimbursement to quality of care. The goal of this movement is to improve standards of health care and to contain spiraling health care costs. Physicians are also expected to give evidence of their continuing competence through mandatory continuing education, patient-record audits, maintenance of certification, or relicensing.

Medical Ethics and New Technologies The rapid pace of technological advances has profound implications for medical applications far beyond their traditional roles to prevent, treat, and cure disease. Cloning, genetic engineering, gene therapy, human-computer interfaces, nanotechnology, and designer drugs have the potential to modify inherited predispositions to disease, select desired characteristics in embryos, augment "normal" human performance, replace failing tissues, and substantially prolong life span. Because of their unique training, physicians have a responsibility to help shape the debate concerning the appropriate uses of, and limits that should be placed on, these new techniques.

The Physician as Perpetual Student It becomes all too apparent from the time we graduate from medical school that as physicians our lot is that of the "perpetual student" and the mosaic of our knowledge and experiences is eternally unfinished. This concept can be at the same time exhilarating and anxiety-provoking. It is exhilarating because we will continue to expand our knowledge that can be applied to our patients; it is anxiety-provoking because we realize that we will never know as much as we want or need to know. At best, we will translate this latter feeling into energy to continue to improve ourselves and realize our potential as physicians. In this regard, it is the responsibility of a physician to pursue new knowledge continually by reading, attending conferences and courses, and consulting colleagues and the Internet. This is often a difficult task for a busy practitioner; however, such a commitment to continued learning is an integral part of being a physician and must be given the highest priority.

Research, Teaching, and the Practice of Medicine The title *doctor* is derived from the Latin *docere*, "to teach," and physicians should share information and medical knowledge with colleagues, with students of medicine and related professions, and with their patients. The practice of medicine is dependent on the sum total of medical knowledge, which in turn is based on an unending chain of scientific discovery, clinical observation, analysis, and interpretation. Advances in medicine depend on the acquisition of new information through research, and improved medical care requires the transmission of this information. As part of broader societal responsibilities, the physician should encourage patients to participate in ethical and properly approved clinical investigations if they do not impose undue hazard, discomfort, or inconvenience. On the other hand, physicians engaged in clinical research must be alert to potential conflicts of interest between their research goals and their obligations to individual patients; the best interests of the patient must always take priority.

> *To wrest from nature the secrets which have perplexed philosophers in all ages, to track to their sources the causes of disease, to correlate the vast stores of knowledge, that they may be quickly available for the prevention and cure of disease—these are our ambitions.*
>
> –William Osler, 1849–1919

FURTHER READINGS

BLANK L et al: Medical professionalism in the new millennium: A physician charter 15 months later. Ann Intern Med 138:839, 2003

COUNCIL ON GRADUATE MEDICAL EDUCATION: *Thirteenth Report: Physician Education for a Changing Health Care Environment.* US Department of Health and Human Services, March 1999

GUTTMACHER AE, COLLINS FS: Welcome to the genomic era. N Engl J Med 349:996, 2003

LUDMERER KM, JOHNS MME: Reforming graduate medical eduction. JAMA 294:1083, 2005

STRAUS SE et al: Teaching evidence-based medicine skills can change practice in a community hospital. J Gen Intern Med 20:340, 2005

2 Global Issues in Medicine

Jim Yong Kim, Paul Farmer

WHY GLOBAL HEALTH?

Global health, it has been noted, is not a discipline; it is, rather, a collection of problems. No single review can do much more than lay out the leading problems faced in applying evidence-based medicine in settings of great poverty or across national boundaries. In this chapter, we first introduce the major international bodies engaged in addressing these problems; identify the more significant barriers to improving the health of people who to date have not, by and large, had access to modern medicines; and summarize population-based data regarding the most common health problems faced by people living in poverty. Examining specific problems—notably AIDS (Chap. 182), but also tuberculosis (TB, Chap. 158), malaria (Chap. 203), severe acute respiratory syndrome (SARS; Chap. 179), and key noncommunicable diseases—helps to sharpen the discussion of barriers to prevention, diagnosis, and care as well as means of overcoming them. We next discuss global health equity, drawing on notions of social justice that once were central to international public health but have fallen out of favor over the past several decades. We close by acknowledging the importance of cost-effectiveness analysis linked to national economic data, while at the same time underlining the need to address disparities of disease risk and access to care.

HISTORY OF GLOBAL HEALTH INSTITUTIONS

Concern about health across national boundaries dates back many centuries, predating the Black Plague and other pandemics. Before the advent of germ theory, when epidemic disease began to be understood to be the result of microbes rather than of "miasmas" or the wrath of a divine being, the chief social responses to such epidemics often included accusations that this or that human group was responsible for propagating the affliction in question. Similarly inaccurate and ineffective beliefs abounded when the arrival of European colonists led to catastrophic outbreaks of communicable diseases among indigenous populations in the Americas, and these viewpoints continued to hold sway during subsequent pandemics of cholera. Many historians trace modern public health and epidemiology to the day in 1851 when Dr. John Snow, having discerned the link between cholera outbreaks in London and water sources used by the afflicted populace, removed the handle of the Broad Street water pump. Thus one cholera epidemic was stopped, but it would still be years before the etiology of cholera was discovered.

A proper understanding of etiology was necessary to the birth not only of epidemiology but also of efforts to apply public health measures across administrative boundaries; indeed, without agreement upon etiology and case definitions, there could be no sound metrics upon which to base either assessments of disease burden or effective interventions. The close of the nineteenth century marked the birth and rapid growth of microbiology and the development of some of the first effective vaccines, which, along with measures to promote sanitation, were for decades the mainstay of modern public health. Before the development of effective antibiotics in the mid-twentieth century, international health endeavors consisted largely of the transnational application of a small number of lessons learned from local or regional campaigns. Perhaps the first organization founded explicitly to tackle cross-border health issues was the Pan American Sanitary Bureau, which was formed by 11 countries in the Americas in 1902. The primary goal of what was later to become the Pan American Health Organization was the control of infectious diseases across the Americas. Of special concern was yellow fever, which had been running a deadly course through much of South and Central America and posed a threat to the construction of the Panama Canal. The identification of a mosquito vector in 1901 led public and private health authorities to focus on mosquito control; a vaccine was developed in the 1930s.

Even in the early heyday of vaccine development, no global institutions tackled the health problems of the world's poor. Colonial powers did address (with varying degrees of effectiveness and sources of motivation) the ranking infectious killers in regions now known as the developing world, but universal standards or even aspirations for international public health and medicine were still far in the future. Although the League of Nations concerned itself with health issues such as malaria in the early twentieth century, and although various organs of the nascent United Nations—including the United Nations Development Program and the United Nations Children's Fund (UNICEF)—also addressed health issues, the World Health Organization (WHO) was the first truly global health institution. Since its founding in 1948, the WHO has witnessed dramatic shifts in population health and in its own stature as the premier global health institution. In line with a long-standing focus on communicable diseases that readily cross administrative and political borders, leaders in global health, under the aegis of the WHO, initiated the effort that led to what some see as the greatest success in international health: the eradication of smallpox. Historians of the smallpox campaign note the preconditions that made eradication possible: international consensus regarding the potential for success, an effective vaccine, and the apparent lack of a nonhuman reservoir for the often-lethal and highly infectious etiologic agent. The primary obstacle was the lack of effective delivery mechanisms for the vaccine in settings of poverty, where health personnel were scarce and health systems weak. Close collaborations across administrative and political borders were clearly necessary. Naysayers were surprised when the smallpox eradication campaign, which engaged public health officials throughout the world, proved successful at the height of the Cold War.

The optimism born of the world's first successful disease-eradication campaign invigorated the international health community, if only briefly. Global consensus regarding the right to primary health care for all was reached at the International Conference on Primary Health Care in Alma-Ata (in what is now Kazakhstan) in 1978. However, the declaration of this collective vision was not followed by substantial funding, nor did the apparent consensus reflect universal commitment to the right to health care. Moreover, as is too often the case, success paradoxically weakened commitment. Basic-science research that might lead to effective vaccines and therapies for TB and malaria faltered in the latter decades of the twentieth century after these diseases were brought under control in the affluent countries where most such research is conducted. U.S. Surgeon General William H. Stewart declared in the late 1960s that it was time to "close the book on infectious diseases," and attention was turned to the main health problems of countries that had already undergone an "epidemiological transition"; that is, the focus shifted from premature deaths due to infectious diseases toward deaths from complications of chronic noncommunicable diseases, including malignancies and complications of heart disease.

In 1982, the visionary leader of UNICEF, James P. Grant, frustrated by the lack of action around the Health for All initiative announced in Alma-Ata, launched a "child survival revolution" focused on four inexpensive interventions collectively known by the acronym GOBI: growth monitoring; oral rehydration; breast-feeding; and immunizations for TB, diphtheria, whooping cough, tetanus, polio, and measles. GOBI, which was later expanded to GOBI-FFF (to include *f*emale education, *f*ood, and *f*amily planning), was controversial from the start, but Grant's advocacy led to enormous improvements in the health of poor children worldwide. The Expanded Programme on Immunization was especially successful and is thought to have raised the proportion of children worldwide who were receiving critical vaccines by more than threefold—i.e., from <20% to almost 80% (the target level).

For many reasons (including, perhaps, the success of the UNICEF-led campaign for child survival), the influence of the WHO waned during the 1980s. In the early 1990s, many observers argued that, with its vastly superior financial resources and close if unequal relationships with the governments of poor countries, the World Bank had eclipsed the WHO as the most important multilateral institution working in the area of health. One of the stated goals of the World Bank was to help poor countries identify "cost-effective" interventions worthy of international public support. At the same time, the World Bank encouraged many of these nations to reduce public expenditures in health and education as part of (later discredited) structural adjustment programs (SAPs), which were imposed as a condition for access to credit and assistance through international financial institutions such as the Bank and the International Monetary Fund (IMF). One trend related, at least in part, to these expenditure-reduction policies was the resurgence in Africa of many diseases that colonial regimes had brought under control, including malaria, trypanosomiasis, and schistosomiasis. Tuberculosis, an eminently curable disease, remained the world's leading infectious killer of adults. Half a million women per year died in childbirth during the last decade of the twentieth century, and few of the world's largest philanthropic or funding institutions focused on global health.

AIDS, first described in 1981, precipitated a change. In the United States, the advent of this newly described infectious killer marked the culmination of a series of events that discredited the grand talk of "closing the book" on infectious diseases. In Africa, which would emerge as the global epicenter of the pandemic, HIV disease further weakened TB control programs, while malaria continued to take as many lives as ever. At the dawn of the twenty-first century, these three diseases alone killed an estimated 6 million people each year. New research, new policies, and new funding mechanisms were called for. Some of the requisite innovations have emerged in the past few years. The leadership of the WHO has been challenged by the rise of institutions such as the Global Fund to Fight AIDS, Tuberculosis, and Malaria; the Joint United Nations Program on HIV/AIDS (UNAIDS); and the Bill & Melinda Gates Foundation and by bilateral efforts such as the U.S. President's Emergency Plan for AIDS Relief (PEPFAR). Yet with its 193 member states and 147 country offices, the WHO remains preeminent in matters relating to the cross-border spread of infectious and other health threats. In the aftermath of the SARS epidemic of 2003, the International Health Regulations—which provide a legal foundation for the WHO's direct investigation of a wide range of global health problems, including pandemic influenza, in any member state—were strengthened and brought into force in May 2007.

Even as attention to and resources for health problems in resource-poor settings grow, the lack of coherence in and among global health institutions may seriously undermine efforts to forge a more comprehensive and effective response. While UNICEF had great success in launching and sustaining the child survival revolution, the end of James Grant's term at UNICEF upon his death in 1995 was followed by a lamentable shift of focus away from immunizations; predictably, coverage dropped. The WHO has gone through two recent leadership transitions and is still woefully underfunded despite the ever-growing need to engage a wider and more complex range of health issues. In another instance of the paradoxical impact of success, the rapid growth of the Gates Foundation, while clearly one of the most important developments in the history of global health, has led other foundations to question the wisdom of continuing to invest their more modest resources in this field. We may indeed be living in what some have called "the golden age of global health," but leaders of major organizations such as the WHO, the Global Fund, UNICEF, UNAIDS, and the Gates Foundation must work together to design an effective architecture that will make the most of the extraordinary opportunities that now exist. To this end, new and old players in global health must invest heavily in *discovery* (relevant basic science); in the *development* of new tools (preventive, diagnostic, and therapeutic); and in a new science of implementation, or *delivery*.

THE ECONOMICS OF GLOBAL HEALTH

Political and economic concerns have often guided global health interventions. As mentioned previously, early efforts to control yellow fever were tied to the completion of the Panama Canal. However, the precise nature of the link between economics and health remains a matter for debate. Some economists and demographers argue that economic development is the key to improving the health status of populations, while others maintain that ill health is the chief barrier to development in poor countries. In either case, investment in health care, and especially in the control of communicable diseases, should lead to increased productivity. The question is where to find the necessary resources to start the predicted "virtuous cycle."

International financial institutions, including the World Bank and the IMF, have counseled limited investments and the capping of social expenditures in health and education. The socioeconomic argument was that a balanced budget and a "friendly investment climate"—that is, privatization, deregulation, decreased trade barriers, devalued currencies, and debt repayment—would favor development and thus improve health outcomes. The limitations on social-sector spending recommended for many poor countries by the World Bank and the IMF from the 1970s through the 1990s tended to confirm the opposite view. In the poorest countries, already-tiny health-sector budgets were further constricted. Moreover, health-sector spending in many poor countries channeled a majority of resources toward city hospitals that served mostly élites who were able to pay; consequently, in the past quarter-century, little spending went toward addressing the problems that most affected poor people in poor countries.

Since 1999, spurred by the leadership of the Gates Foundation and the growing interest in addressing novel and persistent challenges such as AIDS, spending on health in poor countries has increased, with $40 billion in new funds earmarked for the discovery and development of drugs and diagnostics targeting diseases of the poor; for comprehensive responses to the AIDS, TB, and malaria epidemics; for vaccine development and delivery; and even for improved methods of data collection in resource-poor settings. Nevertheless, in order to reach the United Nations' Millennium Development Goals, which include targets for poverty reduction, universal primary education, and gender equality, spending in the health sector will have to be further increased and sustained. To determine by how much and for how long, it is imperative that we improve our ability to assess the global burden of disease (GBD) and to plan interventions that more precisely match the need, which is glaring but often poorly understood. Refining metrics is an important task for global health: only recently have we had solid assessments of the GBD. Such assessments may serve as preliminaries or as correctives to effective interventions among the poor.

LIFE EXPECTANCY AND GLOBAL BURDEN OF DISEASE

Since the late 1980s, serious efforts have been made to calculate the GBD. The first GBD study, conducted in 1990, laid the foundation for the first report on *Disease Control Priorities in Developing Countries* (DCP1) and for the World Bank's 1993 World Development Report entitled *Investing in Health*. These efforts represented a major advance in our understanding of health status in developing countries. *Investing in Health* has been especially influential: it familiarized a broad audience with cost-effectiveness analysis for specific health interventions and with the notion of disability-adjusted life years (DALYs). The DALY, which has become a standard measure of the impact of a specific health condition on a population, combines in a single measure both absolute years of life lost and years lost due to disability for incident cases of a condition.

The second GBD analysis was carried out on health data from 2001. The latter report reflects growth in the available data on health in the poorest countries and in our capacity to measure the impact of specific conditions on a population. Yet, even in 2001, only 107 of 192 nations surveyed had reliable information on the causes of deaths within their own borders. It is essential to expand efforts to collect the most basic health data; this task falls to the WHO, national governments, and certain academic institutions. The lack of complete data has led to considerable uncertainty in estimates of overall mortality. The level of uncertainty ranges from as low as 1% for estimates of all-cause mortality in developed countries to well over 50% for disability resulting from diseases for which surveillance mechanisms are incomplete. As analytic methods and data quality have improved, however, important trends can be identified in a comparison of GBD estimates from 1990 and 2001.

Of the 56 million deaths worldwide in 2001, one-third were due to communicable diseases, maternal and perinatal conditions, and nutritional deficiencies. While the proportion of all deaths attributable to these causes was unchanged from 1990, the share of all deaths due to the communicable disease HIV/AIDS grew from just 2% to an astonishing 14%. If these deaths were excluded, the fraction of all deaths related to communicable diseases, maternal and perinatal conditions, and nutritional deficiencies dropped from one-third to one-fifth. Of the deaths making up that one-fifth of the total figure, 97% occurred in middle- and low-income countries. The leading cause of death among adults in 2001 was ischemic heart disease, accounting for 17.3% of all deaths in high-income countries and for 11.8% in middle- and low-income countries. In second place was cerebrovascular disease, which accounted for 9.9% of deaths in high-income countries and for 9.5% of deaths in middle- and low-income countries. While the third leading cause of death in high-income countries was tracheal, bronchial, and lung cancers (which accounted for 5.8% of all deaths), these conditions do not even register in the top 10 places in middle- and low-income countries. Of the 10 leading causes of death in poorer countries, 5 were communicable diseases; in high-income countries, however, only 1 communicable disease—lower respiratory infection—was ranked among the top 10 causes of death.

Nearly 20% (10.6 million) of the 56 million dead in 2001 were children <5 years of age who died of acute respiratory infections, measles, diarrhea, malaria, and HIV/AIDS (Fig. 2-1). Of these deaths, 99% occurred in middle- and low-income countries, and fully 40% occurred in sub-Saharan Africa. If stillbirths are counted, the number of childhood deaths rises to 13.5 million worldwide (~25% of all deaths worldwide), of which more than half (i.e., one-eighth of all deaths) occurred before the first birthday. Between 1990 and 2001, under-five childhood mortality dropped by ≥30% in high-income countries, Latin America, the Caribbean, the Middle East, North Africa, and the middle- and low-income countries of Europe and Central Asia. Notably, the total number of deaths from diarrheal diseases dropped from 2.4 million in 1990 to 1.6 million in 2001, probably as a result of the increased use of oral rehydration therapy in poor countries. Malaria and HIV infection were the only two conditions for which childhood death rates increased between 1990 and 2001.

Among persons 15–59 years of age (Fig. 2-2), noncommunicable diseases accounted for more than half of all deaths in all regions except South Asia and sub-Saharan Africa, where communicable diseases, maternal and perinatal conditions, and nutritional deficiencies together accounted for one-third and two-thirds of all deaths, respectively. The 15- to 59-year-olds with noncommunicable conditions in low- and middle-income countries faced a 30% greater risk of death from their conditions than did their peers in high-income countries. In this age group, injuries accounted for 25% of all deaths; Europe and Central Asia registered even higher rates, with injuries accounting for one-third of all deaths. Overall, death rates in this age group declined between 1990 and 2001 in all regions except Europe and Central Asia, where cardiovascular diseases and injuries have caused increased mortality, and sub-Saharan Africa, where the impact of HIV/AIDS in this age cohort has been particularly devastating.

Noncommunicable diseases accounted for almost 60% of all deaths in 2001 but, because of the later onset of these diseases, accounted for only 40% of years of life lost. In contrast, because they occur more often in younger people, injuries accounted for 12% of years of life lost but for only 9% of deaths. Overall, males had an 11% higher death rate than females as well as a 15% higher rate of years of life lost; these figures reflect the earlier age of death of males worldwide. Notably, almost half of the disease burden in middle- and low-income countries in 2001 derived from noncommunicable disease—an increase of 10% since 1990.

Compared with years of life lost, there is greater uncertainty in calculating years of life lived with disability for specific conditions. Best estimates from 2001 reveal that, while the prevalence of diseases common in older populations (e.g., dementia and musculoskeletal disease) was higher in high-income countries, the disability experienced as a result of cardiovascular diseases, chronic respiratory diseases, and the long-term impact of communicable diseases was greater in low- and middle-income countries. Thus, predictably, in most low- and middle-income

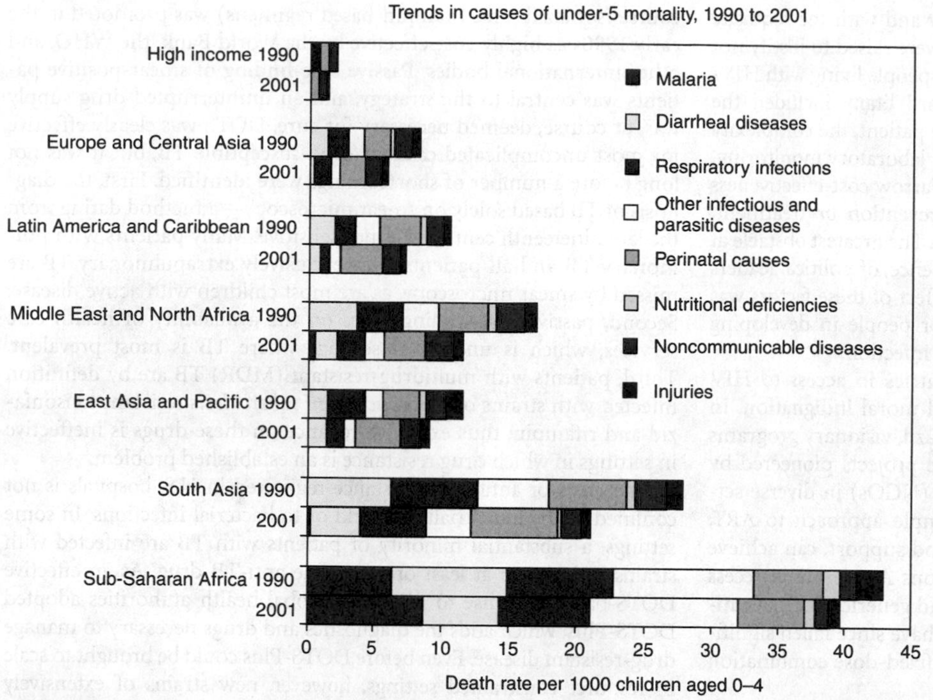

FIGURE 2-1 Death rates among children from birth through 4 years of age, by disease group and region, in 1990 and 2001. Cause-specific death rates for 1990, estimated from Murray and Lopez (1996), may not be completely comparable to those for 2001 because of changes in data availability and methods as well as some approximations in mapping 1990 estimates to the 2001 regions of East Asia and Pacific, South Asia, and Europe and Central Asia. For all geographic regions, high-income countries are excluded and are shown as a single group at the top of the graph. The geographic regions therefore refer to low- and middle-income countries only. *(Reprinted from Lopez et al, with permission from Elsevier.)*

countries, people both lived shorter lives and experienced disability and poor health for a greater proportion of their lives. Indeed, 45% of the overall burden of disease occurred in South Asia and sub-Saharan Africa, which together comprise only one-third of the global population.

In its analysis of risk factors for ill health, the GBD project found that undernutrition was the leading cause of loss of DALYs in both 1990 and 2001. In an era that has seen obesity become a major health concern in so many developed countries, the persistence of undernutrition is surely cause for great consternation. Our inability to feed the hungry indicts many years of failed development projects and must be addressed as a problem of the highest priority. Indeed, no health care initiative, however generously funded and scientifically justified, will be effective without adequate nutrition.

The GBD analysis was used as the basis for the second edition of *Disease Control Priorities in Developing Countries* (DCP2). Published in 2006, DCP2 is a document of stunning breadth and ambition, providing cost-effectiveness analyses for >100 interventions and including 21 chapters focused on strategies for strengthening health systems. Cost-effectiveness analyses that compare two relatively equal interventions and facilitate the best choices under constraint are important; however, as both resources and ambitions for global health grow, cost-effectiveness analyses (particularly those based on past conditions) must not hobble the increased worldwide commitment to provide resources and accessible services to all who need them. To illustrate this point, we turn in greater detail to AIDS, which has become, in the course of the last three decades, the world's leading infectious cause of death during adulthood.

AIDS

Chapter 182 provides an overview of the AIDS epidemic in the world today. Here we will limit ourselves to a discussion of AIDS in the developing world. Lessons learned in tackling AIDS in resource-constrained settings are highly relevant to discussions of other chronic diseases, including noncommunicable diseases, for which effective therapies have been developed. We highlight several of these lessons below.

In the United States, the availability of highly active antiretroviral therapy (ART) for AIDS has transformed this disease from an inescapably fatal destruction of cell-mediated immunity into a manageable chronic illness. In developing countries, treatment has been offered more broadly only since 2003, and only in the summer of 2006 did the number of patients receiving treatment exceed 25% of the number who currently need it. (It remains to be seen how many of

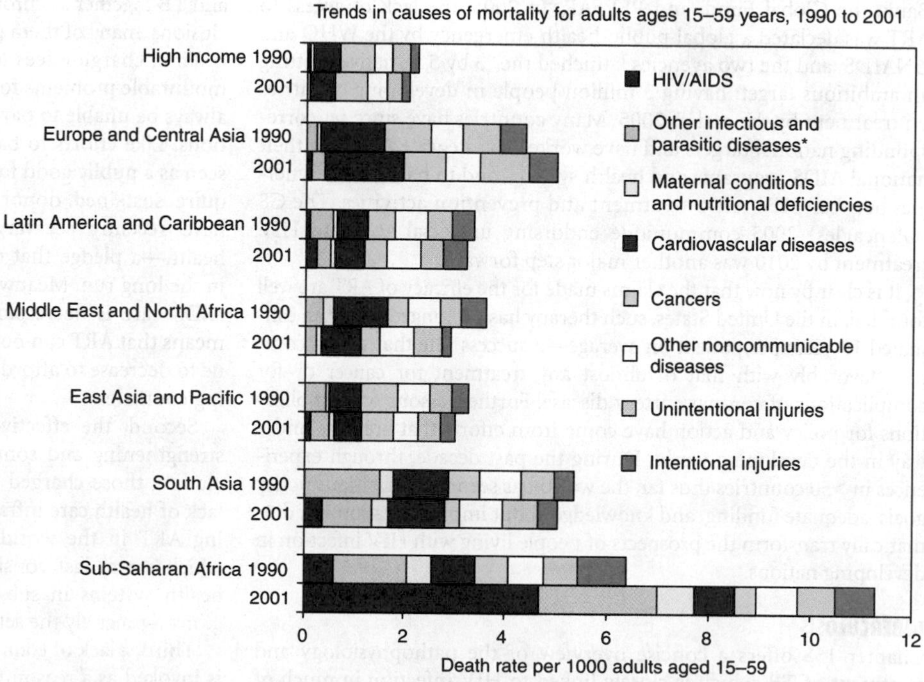

FIGURE 2-2 Death rates among persons 15–59 years old, by disease group and region, in 1990 and 2001. *Includes respiratory infections. Cause-specific death rates for 1990, estimated from Murray and Lopez (1996), may not be completely comparable to those for 2001 because of changes in data availability and methods as well as some approximations in mapping 1990 estimates to the 2001 regions of East Asia and Pacific, South Asia, and Europe and Central Asia. For all geographic regions, high-income countries are excluded and are shown as a single group at the top of the graph. The geographic regions therefore refer to low- and middle-income countries only. *(Reprinted from Lopez et al, with permission from Elsevier.)*

these fortunate few are receiving ART regularly and with the requisite social support.) Before 2003, many arguments were raised to justify not moving forward rapidly with ART programs for people living with HIV/AIDS in resource-limited settings. The standard litany included the price of therapy compared to the poverty of the patient, the complexity of the intervention, the lack of infrastructure for laboratory monitoring, and the lack of trained health care providers. Narrow cost-effectiveness arguments that created false dichotomies—prevention *or* treatment, rather than both—too often went unchallenged. The greatest obstacle at the time was the ambivalence, if not outright silence, of political leaders and experts in public health. The cumulative effect of these factors was to condemn to death tens of millions of poor people in developing countries who had become ill as a result of HIV infection.

The inequity between rich and poor countries in access to HIV treatment has rightly given rise to widespread moral indignation. In several middle-income countries, including Brazil, visionary programs have bridged the access gap. Other innovative projects pioneered by international nongovernmental organizations (NGOs) in diverse settings have clearly established that a very simple approach to ART, based on intensive community engagement and support, can achieve remarkable results. In 2000, the United Nations Accelerating Access Initiative finally brought the research-based and generic pharmaceutical industries into play, and AIDS drug prices have since fallen significantly. At the same time, easier-to-administer fixed-dose combination drugs have become more widely available.

Building on these lessons, the WHO advocated a public health approach to the treatment of people with AIDS in resource-limited settings. This approach, which was derived from models of care pioneered by the NGO Partners In Health and other groups, proposed standard first-line treatment regimens based on a simple five-drug formulary, with a more complex (and, up to now, more expensive) set of second-line options in reserve. Common clinical protocols were standardized, and intensive training packages for health and community workers were developed and implemented in many countries. These efforts were supported by unprecedented funding through the World Bank, the Global Fund, and PEPFAR. In 2003, the lack of access to ART was declared a global public-health emergency by the WHO and UNAIDS, and the two agencies launched the "3 by 5 initiative," setting an ambitious target: having 3 million people in developing countries on treatment by the end of 2005. Many countries have since set corresponding national targets and have worked to integrate ART into their national AIDS programs and health systems and to harness the synergies between HIV/AIDS treatment and prevention activities. The G8 (Gleneagles) 2005 communiqué endorsing universal access to HIV treatment by 2010 was another major step forward.

It is clear by now that the claims made for the efficacy of ART are well founded: in the United States, such therapy has prolonged life by an estimated 13 years per patient on average—a success rate that would compare favorably with that of almost any treatment for cancer or for complications of coronary artery disease. Further lessons with implications for policy and action have come from efforts that are now under way in the developing world. During the past decade, through experiences in >50 countries thus far, the world has seen that ambitious policy goals, adequate funding, and knowledge about implementation can dramatically transform the prospects of people living with HIV infection in developing nations.

TUBERCULOSIS

Chapter 158 offers a concise overview of the pathophysiology and treatment of TB, which is closely linked to HIV infection in much of the world. Indeed, a substantial proportion of the resurgence of TB registered in southern Africa may be attributed to HIV co-infection. Even before the advent of HIV, however, it was estimated that fewer than half of all cases of TB in developing countries were ever diagnosed, much less treated.

Primarily because of the common failure to diagnose and treat TB, international authorities devised a single strategy to reduce the burden of disease. The DOTS strategy (*d*irectly *o*bserved *t*herapy using *s*hort-course isoniazid- and rifampin-based regimens) was promoted in the early 1990s as highly cost-effective by the World Bank, the WHO, and other international bodies. Passive case-finding of smear-positive patients was central to the strategy, and an uninterrupted drug supply was, of course, deemed necessary for cure. DOTS was clearly effective for most uncomplicated cases of drug-susceptible TB, but it was not long before a number of shortcomings were identified. First, the diagnosis of TB based solely on smear microscopy—a method dating from the late nineteenth century—is not sensitive. Many patients with pulmonary TB and all patients with exclusively extrapulmonary TB are missed by smear microscopy, as are most children with active disease. Second, passive case-finding relies on the availability of health care services, which is uneven in settings where TB is most prevalent. Third, patients with multidrug-resistant (MDR) TB are by definition infected with strains of *Mycobacterium tuberculosis* resistant to isoniazid and rifampin; thus exclusive reliance on these drugs is ineffective in settings in which drug resistance is an established problem.

The crisis of antibiotic resistance registered in U.S. hospitals is not confined to the industrialized world or to bacterial infections. In some settings, a substantial minority of patients with TB are infected with strains resistant to at least one first-line anti-TB drug. As an effective DOTS-based response to MDR TB, global health authorities adopted DOTS-Plus, which adds the diagnostics and drugs necessary to manage drug-resistant disease. Even before DOTS-Plus could be brought to scale in resource-constrained settings, however, new strains of extensively drug-resistant (XDR) *M. tuberculosis* began to threaten the success of TB control programs in already-beleaguered South Africa, for example, where high rates of HIV infection have led to a doubling of TB incidence over the past decade.

TUBERCULOSIS AND AIDS AS CHRONIC DISEASES: LESSONS LEARNED

Strategies effective against MDR TB have implications for the management of drug-resistant HIV infection and even drug-resistant malaria, which, through repeated infections and a lack of effective therapy, has become a chronic disease in parts of Africa. Indeed, examining AIDS and TB together as chronic diseases allows us to draw a number of conclusions, many of them pertinent to global health in general (Fig. 2-3).

First, charging fees for AIDS prevention and care will pose insurmountable problems for people living in poverty, many of whom will always be unable to pay even modest amounts for services or medications. Like efforts to battle airborne TB, such services might best be seen as a public good for public health. Initially, this approach will require sustained donor contributions, but many African countries have recently set targets for increased national investments in health—a pledge that could render ambitious programs sustainable in the long run. Meanwhile, as local investments increase, the price of AIDS care is decreasing. The development of generic medications means that ART can now cost <\$0.50 (U.S.) per day, and costs continue to decrease to affordable levels for public health bodies in developing countries.

Second, the effective scale-up of pilot projects will require the strengthening and sometimes rebuilding of health care systems, including those charged with delivering primary care. In the past, the lack of health care infrastructure has been cited as a barrier to providing ART in the world's poorest regions; however, AIDS resources, which are at last considerable, may be marshaled to rebuild public health systems in sub-Saharan Africa and other HIV-burdened regions—precisely the settings in which TB is resurgent.

Third, a lack of trained health care personnel, most notably doctors, is invoked as a reason for the failure to treat AIDS in poor countries. The lack is real, and the "brain drain," which is discussed below, continues. However, one reason doctors leave Africa is that they lack the tools to practice their trade there. AIDS funding provides an opportunity not only to recruit physicians and nurses to underserved regions but also to train community health workers to supervise care for AIDS and many other diseases within their home villages and neighborhoods. Such training should be undertaken even in places where physicians are abundant, since community-based, closely supervised care

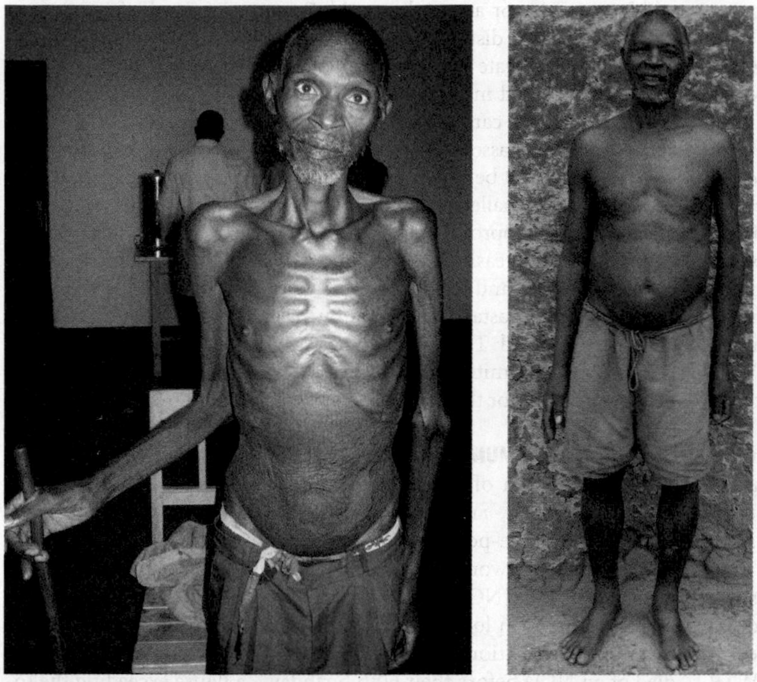

FIGURE 2-3 An HIV/TB co-infected patient in Rwanda, before (***left***) and after (***right***) 6 months of treatment.

represents the highest standard of care for chronic disease, whether in the First World or the Third.

Fourth, extreme poverty makes it difficult for many patients to comply with therapy for chronic diseases, whether communicable or not. Indeed, poverty in its many dimensions is far and away the greatest barrier to the scale-up of treatment and prevention programs. It is possible to remove many of the social and economic barriers to adherence, but only with what are sometimes termed "wrap-around services": food supplements for the hungry, help with transportation to clinics, child care, and housing. In many rural regions of Africa, hunger is the major coexisting condition in patients with AIDS or TB, and these consumptive diseases cannot be treated effectively without adequate caloric intake.

Finally, there is a need for a renewed basic-science commitment to the discovery and development of vaccines; of more reliable, less expensive diagnostic tools; and of new classes of therapeutic agents. This need applies not only to the three leading infectious killers—against none of which an effective vaccine exists—but also to many other neglected diseases of poverty.

MALARIA

We turn now to the world's third largest infectious killer, which has taken its greatest toll among children, especially African children, living in poverty.

The Cost of Malaria Malaria's human toll is enormous. An estimated 250 million people suffer from malarial disease each year, and the disease annually kills between 1 million and 2.5 million people, mostly pregnant women and children under the age of 5. The poor disproportionately suffer the consequences of malaria: 58% of malaria deaths occur in the poorest 20% of the world's population, and 90% are registered in sub-Saharan Africa. The differential magnitude of this mortality burden is greater than that associated with any other disease. Likewise, the morbidity differential is greater for malaria than for diseases caused by other pathogens, as documented in a study from Zambia that revealed a 40% greater prevalence of parasitemia among children under 5 in the poorest quintile than in the richest.

Despite suffering the greatest consequences of malaria, the poor are precisely those least able to access effective prevention and treatment tools. Economists describe the complex interactions between malaria and poverty from an opposite but complementary perspective: they delineate ways in which malaria arrests economic development both for individuals and for whole nations. Microeconomic analyses focusing on direct and indirect costs estimate that malaria may consume up to 10% of a household's annual income. A Ghanaian study that categorized the population by income group highlighted the regressive nature of this cost: the burden of malaria represents only 1% of a wealthy family's income but 34% of a poor household's income.

At the national level, macroeconomic analyses estimate that malaria may reduce the per capita gross national product of a disease-endemic country by 50% relative to that of a nonmalarial country. The causes of this drag include high fertility rates, impaired cognitive development of children, decreased schooling, decreased saving, decreased foreign investment, and restriction of worker mobility. Given this enormous cost, it is little wonder that an important review by the economists Sachs and Malaney concludes that "where malaria prospers most, human societies have prospered least."

Rolling Back Malaria In part because of differences in vector distribution and climate, resource-rich countries offer few blueprints for malaria control and treatment that are applicable in tropical (and resource-poor) settings. In 2001, African heads of state endorsed the WHO Roll Back Malaria (RBM) campaign, which prescribes strategies appropriate for sub-Saharan African countries. RBM recommends a three-pronged strategy to reduce malaria-related morbidity and mortality: the use of insecticide-treated bed nets (ITNs), combination antimalarial therapy, and indoor residual spraying.

ITNs are an efficacious and cost-effective public health intervention. A meta-analysis of controlled trials indicates that malaria incidence is reduced by 50% among persons who sleep under ITNs compared with that among those who do not use nets at all. Even untreated nets reduce malaria incidence by one-quarter. On an individual level, the utility of ITNs extends beyond protection from malaria. Several studies suggest that all-cause mortality is reduced among children under 5 to a greater degree than can be attributed to the reduction in malarial disease alone. Morbidity (specifically that due to anemia) predisposing children to diarrheal and respiratory illnesses and pregnant women to the delivery of low-birth-weight infants is also reduced in populations using ITNs. In some areas, ITNs offer a supplemental benefit by preventing transmission of lymphatic filariasis, cutaneous leishmaniasis, Chagas' disease, and tick-borne relapsing fever. At the community level, investigators suggest that the use of an ITN in just one household may reduce the number of mosquito bites in households up to several hundred meters away. The cost of ITNs per DALY saved is estimated at \$10–\$38 (U.S.), which qualifies ITNs as a "very efficient use of resources and [a] good candidate for public subsidy."[1]

Some RBM programs have had limited success, but overall the burden of malarial disease has continued to grow. In fact, annual malaria-attributable mortality increased between 1999 and 2003. While the RBM campaign's own report from that year is quick to note that morbidity and mortality data-collection methods in sub-Saharan Africa are inadequate and indicators may thus lag behind actual outcomes of ongoing campaigns, they nevertheless acknowledge that "RBM is acting against a background of increasing malaria burden."

Limited success in scaling-up ITN coverage reflects the inadequately acknowledged economic barriers that prevent the destitute sick from accessing critical preventive technologies. Despite proven efficacy and what are considered "reasonable costs," the 2003 RBM report reveals disappointing levels of ITN coverage. In 28 African countries surveyed, only 1.3% (range, 0.2–4.9%) of households owned at least one ITN, and <2% of children slept under an ITN. Why has the RBM campaign failed to achieve its goals? Do Africans not want to use bed nets? Do they not

---

[1]Nuwaha F: The challenge of chloroquine-resistant malaria in sub-Saharan Africa. Health Policy Plan 16:1, 2001.

recognize malaria as a health risk? Or have project managers and donors miscalculated most Africans' ability to obtain bed nets?

These are not rhetorical questions. The RBM strategy initially emphasized the importance of commercial markets as sources of ITNs for African populations. A precedent supporting this emphasis is the prior existence in countries such as Madagascar and Mali of local markets for untreated bed nets. Presumably, therefore, a demand for bed nets existed prior to the RBM campaign, as did a distribution system with points of sale. However, even with the application of subsidized social marketing strategies, this market approach has not resulted in large increases in coverage during the first years of the RBM campaign. Several studies have attempted to define willingness to pay (WTP) and actual payment for ITNs in African countries and thereby to determine why market-based strategies have been unsuccessful. Policy-makers often use WTP figures to determine appropriate pricing for social marketing projects and to project revenue and demand. A cross-sectional study in a rural Nigerian community administered two questionnaires, 1 month apart, to examine community members' WTP for ITNs, actual purchase of ITNs (with the second questionnaire accompanied by the opportunity to buy a subsidized ITN), and factors (such as socioeconomic status and recent history of malarial illness) contributing to hypothetical and actual ITN purchase. Among the 453 persons answering both surveys, the poorest quintile perceived a greater risk of malaria than the other quintiles (27.3% vs. 12.9–21.6%, $p < .05$). However, the poorest quintile was least likely to own a net, purchase a net, or express a hypothetical WTP. Even the most well-off quintile was willing to pay only 51% of the government-set price for an ITN. This finding suggests that even the relatively well-off may not be willing or able to pay for bed nets at set prices. The authors of this study concluded that reliance on the sale of nets alone may prove inadequate and that further studies are needed to define the degrees to which costs can be lowered and/or demand increased.

A 2002 study in highland Kenya compared the attitudes of people living in homesteads provided with heavily subsidized ITNs ($n = 190$) with those of residents of households that had no ITNs and had not been targeted by other health care initiatives ($n = 200$). Of all households, 97% expressed willingness to pay for ITNs. However, only 4% of those willing to pay offered spontaneously to meet the suggested price of 350 Kenyan shillings. After being prompted that "nets are expensive," 26% of respondents expressed willingness to pay the full price. This study did not offer nets for sale; therefore, the number of nets that would actually have been purchased is unknown. However, the study did contextualize the hypothetical WTP for ITNs by comparing their cost with other household costs: the price of one ITN is equal to the cost of sending three children to primary school for a year. By placing the nets' relative cost in context, the authors of this study call into question the likelihood that families in this district, over half of whom fall below the Kenyan poverty line, would actually be able to purchase ITNs.

Given the documented barriers to purchasing ITNs, especially among the poorest of the poor, many researchers and development professionals involved in malaria programs have called for the free distribution of ITNs, comparing their importance as a public health measure with that of childhood vaccination. The adoption of free ITN distribution strategies has been limited, however, by concerns about their feasibility and potential ITN misuse (for example, as nets for fishing). Evidence from a targeted free-distribution program discounts both concerns. In 2001, a Kenyan program sponsored by UNICEF sought to distribute 70,000 ITNs to pregnant women through antenatal clinics. Within 12 weeks, >50% of the ITNs had reached their intended recipients. A 1-year follow-up evaluation of 294 women who had received bed nets while pregnant—152 women from a high-transmission area and 142 from a low-transmission area—revealed that 84% of women in the high-transmission area used the ITNs throughout pregnancy. One year later, 77% continued to use the bed nets. In the low-transmission area, 57% of women used the ITNs during pregnancy, and 46% continued to use them a year later. These results contradict suppositions that free nets may not be used because recipients do not value them.

Given the scope and magnitude of the challenge posed by malaria, it is unlikely that any one strategy will work for every region or population within a country or across the world. Encouraging results from an employer-based ITN distribution system in Kenya highlight the potential role of public-private partnerships. Potential synergies between antimalaria programs and measles vaccine campaigns or possibly lymphatic filariasis eradication campaigns have been reported or suggested. Concerns about discomfort associated with sleeping under ITNs or about insecticide toxicities must be addressed through educational campaigns.

Meeting the challenge of malaria control will continue to require careful study of appropriate preventive and therapeutic strategies in the context of our increasingly sophisticated molecular understanding of the pathogen, vector, and host. However, an appreciation for the economic and structural devastation wrought by malaria—like that inflicted by diarrhea, AIDS, and TB—on the most vulnerable populations should heighten our commitment to the critical analysis of ways to implement proven strategies for the prevention and treatment of these diseases.

CHRONIC NONCOMMUNICABLE DISEASES

While the burden of communicable diseases—especially HIV infection, tuberculosis, and malaria—still accounts for the majority of deaths in resource-poor regions such as sub-Saharan Africa, close to 60% of all deaths worldwide in 2005 were due to chronic noncommunicable diseases (NCDs). Moreover, 80% of deaths attributable to NCDs occurred in low- and middle-income countries, where 85% of the global population lives. In 2005, 8.5 million people in the world died of an NCD before their 60th birthday—a figure exceeding the total number of deaths due to AIDS, TB, and malaria combined. By 2020, NCDs will account for 80% of the GBD and for 7 of every 10 deaths in developing countries. The recent rise in resources for and attention to communicable diseases is both welcome and long overdue, but developing countries are already carrying a "double burden" of communicable and noncommunicable diseases.

Cardiovascular Disease Unlike TB, HIV infection, and malaria—diseases caused by single pathogens that damage multiple organs—cardiovascular diseases reflect injury to a single organ system downstream of a variety of insults. The burden of chronic cardiovascular disease in low-income countries represents one consequence of decades of health system neglect; furthermore, cardiovascular research and investment have long focused on the ischemic conditions that are increasingly common in high- and middle-income countries. Meanwhile, despite awareness of its health impact during the early twentieth century, cardiovascular damage in response to infection and malnutrition has fallen out of view until recently.

The perception of cardiovascular diseases as a problem of elderly populations in middle- and high-income countries has contributed to their neglect by global health institutions. Even in Eastern Europe and Central Asia, where the collapse of the Soviet Union was followed by a catastrophic surge in cardiovascular disease deaths (mortality rates from ischemic heart disease nearly doubled between 1991 and 1994 in Russia, for example), the modest flows of overseas development assistance to the health sector focused on the communicable causes that accounted for <1 in 20 excess deaths during this period.

Predictions of an imminent rise in the share of deaths and disabilities due to NCDs in developing countries have led to calls for preventive policies to restrict tobacco use, improve diet, and increase exercise alongside the prescription of multidrug regimens for persons with high levels of vascular risk. Although this agenda could do much to prevent pandemic NCD, it will do little to help those with established heart disease stemming from non-atherogenic pathologies.

The epidemiology of heart failure reflects inequalities in risk factor prevalence and treatment. Heart failure as a consequence of pericardial, myocardial, endocardial, or valvular injury accounts for as many as 1 in 10 admissions to hospitals around the world. Countries have reported a remarkably similar burden of this condition at the health system level since the 1950s, but the causes of heart failure and the age of the people affected vary with resources and ecology. In populations with a high human-development index, coronary artery disease and hypertension among the elderly account for most cases of heart failure. Among the world's poorest billion people, however, heart failure reflects poverty-driven exposure of children and young adults to rheumatogenic strains of streptococci and cardiotropic microorganisms (e.g., HIV, *Trypanosoma cruzi*, enteroviruses, *M. tuberculosis*), untreated high blood pressure, and nutrient deficiencies. The mechanisms of other causes of heart failure common in these populations—such as idiopathic dilated cardiomyopathy, peripartum cardiomyopathy, and endomyocardial fibrosis—remain unclear.

Of the 2.3 million annual cases of pediatric rheumatic heart disease, nearly half occur in sub-Saharan Africa. This disease leads to more than 33,000 cases of endocarditis, 252,000 strokes, and 680,000 deaths per year—almost all in developing countries. Researchers in Ethiopia have reported annual death rates as high as 12.5% in rural areas. In part because the prevention of rheumatic heart disease has not advanced since the disappearance of this disease in wealthy countries, no part of sub-Saharan Africa has yet eradicated rheumatic heart disease despite examples of success in Costa Rica, Cuba, and some Caribbean nations.

Strategies to eliminate rheumatic heart disease may depend on active case-finding confirmed by echocardiography among high-risk groups as well as efforts to extend access to surgical interventions among children with advanced valvular damage. Partnerships between established surgical programs and areas with limited or nonexistent facilities may help develop capacity and provide care to patients who would otherwise suffer an early and painful death. A long-term goal is the establishment of regional centers of excellence equipped to provide consistent, accessible, high-quality services.

In stark contrast to the extraordinary lengths to which patients in wealthy countries will go to treat ischemic cardiomyopathy, young patients with nonischemic cardiomyopathies in resource-poor settings have received little attention. These conditions account for as many as 25–30% of admissions for heart failure in sub-Saharan Africa and include poorly understood entities such as peripartum cardiomyopathy (which has an incidence in rural Haiti of 1 per 300 live births) and HIV cardiomyopathy. Multidrug regimens that include heart failure beta-blockers, ACE inhibitors, and other neurohormonal antagonists can dramatically reduce mortality risk and improve quality of life for these patients. Lessons learned in the scale-up of chronic care for HIV infection and TB may be illustrative as progress is made in establishing means to deliver cardiac therapies over a background of careful fluid management with diuretic drugs.

Because systemic investigation of the causes of stroke and heart failure in sub-Saharan Africa has begun only recently, little is known about the impact of elevated blood pressure in this portion of the continent. Modestly elevated blood pressure in the absence of tobacco use in populations with low rates of obesity may confer little risk of adverse events in the short run. In contrast, persistently elevated blood pressure above 180/110 goes largely undetected, untreated, and uncontrolled in this setting. In the Framingham cohort of men 45–74 years old, the prevalence of blood pressures above 210/120 declined from 1.8% in the 1950s to 0.1% in the 1990s with the introduction of effective antihypertensive agents. While debate continues about appropriate screening strategies and treatment thresholds, rural health centers staffed by nonphysicians must quickly gain access to essential antihypertensive medications.

In 1960, Paul Dudley White and colleagues reported on the prevalence of cardiovascular disease in the region near the Albert Schweitzer Hospital in Lambaréné, Gabon. Although the group found little evidence of myocardial infarction, they concluded that "*the high prevalence of mitral stenosis* [sic] is astonishing. . . . We believe strongly that it is a duty to help bring to these sufferers the benefits of better penicillin prophylaxis and of cardiac surgery when indicated. The same responsibility exists for those with correctable congenital cardiovascular defects."[2] Leaders from tertiary centers in sub-Saharan Africa and elsewhere have continued to call for prevention and treatment of the cardiovascular conditions of the poor. The reconstruction of health services in response to pandemic infectious disease offers an opportunity to identify and treat patients with organ damage and to undertake the prevention of cardiovascular and other chronic conditions of poverty.

[2]Miller DC et al: Survey of cardiovascular disease among Africans in the vicinity of the Albert Schweitzer Hospital in 1960. Am J Cardiol 19:432, 1962.

Cancer Low- and middle-income countries accounted for 53% and 56%, respectively, of the 10 million cases and 7 million deaths due to cancer in 2000. By 2020, the total number of new cancer cases will rise by 29% in developed countries and by 73% in developing countries. Also by 2020, overall mortality from cancer will increase by 104%, and the increase will be fivefold higher in developing than in developed countries. "Western" lifestyle changes will be responsible for the increased incidence of cancers of the breast, colon, and prostate, but historic realities, sociocultural and behavioral factors, genetics, and poverty itself will also have a profound impact on cancer-related mortality and morbidity. While infectious causes are responsible for <10% of cancers in developed countries, they account for 25% of all malignancies in low- and middle-income countries. Infectious causes of cancer such as human papillomavirus (cervical cancer), hepatitis B virus (liver cancer), and *Helicobacter pylori* (stomach cancer) will continue to have a much larger impact in developing countries. Environmental and dietary factors, such as indoor air pollution and high-salt diets, also help account for increased rates of certain cancers (e.g., lung and stomach cancers). Tobacco use (both smoking and chewing) is the most important source of increased mortality from lung and oral cancers. In contrast to decreasing tobacco use in many developed countries, the number of smokers is growing in developing countries, especially among women and young people.

For many reasons, outcomes of malignancies are far worse in developing countries than in developed nations. Overstretched health systems in poor countries simply are not capable of early detection; 80% of patients already have incurable malignancies at diagnosis. Treatment of cancers is available for only a very small number of mostly wealthy citizens in the majority of poor countries, and, even when treatment is available, the range and quality of services are often substandard.

Diabetes The International Diabetes Federation reports that the number of diabetics in the world is expected to increase from 194 million in 2003 to 330 million by 2030, when 3 of every 4 sufferers will live in developing countries. Because diabetics are far more frequently under the age of 65 in developing nations, the complications of micro- and macrovascular disease take a far greater toll. In 2005, an estimated 1.1 million people died of diabetes-related illnesses, and >80% of these deaths occurred in low- and middle-income countries.

Obesity and Tobacco Use In 2004, the WHO released its Global Strategy on Diet, Physical Activity and Health, which focused on the population-wide promotion of healthy diet and regular physical activity in an effort to reduce the growing global problem of overweight and obesity. Passing this strategy at the World Health Assembly proved difficult because of strong opposition from the food industry and from a number of WHO member states, including the United States. While globalization has had many positive effects, one negative aspect has been the growth in both developed and developing countries of well-financed lobbies that have aggressively promoted unhealthy dietary changes and increased consumption of alcohol and tobacco. Foreign direct investment in tobacco, beverage, and food products in developing countries reached $327 million in 2002—a figure nearly five times greater than the amount spent during that year to address NCDs by bilateral funding agencies, the WHO, and the World Bank combined.

The Three Pillars of Prevention The WHO estimates that 80% of all cases of cardiovascular disease and type 2 diabetes as well as 40% of all cancers can be prevented through the three pillars of healthy diet, physical activity, and avoidance of tobacco. While there is some evidence that population-based measures can have some impact on these behaviors, it is sobering to note that increasing obesity levels have not been successfully reversed in any population, including those of high-income countries with robust diet industries. Nonetheless, in Mauritius, for example, a single policy measure that changed the type of cooking oil available to the population led to a fall in mean serum cholesterol levels. Tobacco avoidance may be the most important and most difficult behavioral modification of all. In the twentieth century, 100 million people died worldwide of tobacco-related diseases; it is projected that >1 billion people will die of these diseases in the twenty-first century, with the vast majority of these deaths in developing countries. Today, 80% of the world's 1.2 billion smokers live in low- and middle-income countries, and, while tobacco consumption is falling in most developed countries, it continues to rise at a rate of ~3.4% per year in developing countries. The WHO's Framework Convention on Tobacco Control was a major advance, committing all of its signatories to a set of policy measures that have been shown to reduce tobacco consumption. However, most developing countries have continued to take a passive approach to the control of smoking.

ENVIRONMENTAL HEALTH

In a recent publication that examined how specific diseases and injuries are affected by environmental risk, the WHO determined that ~24% of the total GBD, one-third of the GBD among children, and 23% of all deaths are due to modifiable environmental factors. Many of these factors lead to deaths from infectious diseases; others lead to deaths from malignancies. Increasingly, etiology and nosology are difficult to parse. As much as 94% of diarrheal disease, which is linked to unsafe drinking water and poor sanitation, can be attributed to environmental factors. Risk factors such as indoor air pollution due to use of solid fuels, exposure to second-hand tobacco smoke, and outdoor air pollution account for 20% of lower respiratory infections in developed countries and for as many as 42% of such infections in developing countries. Various forms of unintentional injury and malaria top the list of health problems to which environmental factors contribute. Some 4 million children die every year from causes related to unhealthy environments, and the number of infant deaths due to environmental factors in developing countries is 12 times that in developed countries.

MENTAL HEALTH

The WHO reports that some 450 million people worldwide are affected by mental, neurologic, or behavioral problems at any given time and that ~873,000 people die by suicide every year. Major depression is the leading cause of lost DALYs in the world today. One in four patients visiting a health service has at least one mental, neurologic, or behavioral disorder, but most of these disorders are neither diagnosed nor treated. Most low- and middle-income countries devote <1% of their already-paltry health expenditures to mental health.

Increasingly effective therapies exist for many of the major causes of mental disorder. Effective treatments for many neurologic diseases, including seizure disorders, have long been available. One of the greatest barriers to delivery of such therapies is the paucity of skilled personnel. Most sub-Saharan African countries have only a handful of psychiatrists, for example; most of them practice in cities and are unavailable within the public sector or to patients living in poverty. Of the few patients who are fortunate enough to see a psychiatrist or neurologist, fewer still are able to adhere to treatment regimens: several surveys of already-diagnosed patients ostensibly receiving daily therapy have revealed that, among the poor, few can take their medications as prescribed. The same barriers that prevent the poor from having reliable access to insulin or ART also prevent them from benefiting from antidepressant, antipsychotic, and antiepileptic agents. To alleviate this problem, some authorities are proposing the training of health workers to provide community-based adherence support, counseling services, and referrals for patients in need of mental health services.

World Mental Health: Problems and Priorities in Low-Income Countries offers a comprehensive analysis of the burden of mental, behavioral, and social problems in low-income countries and relates the mental health consequences of social forces such as violence, dislocation, poverty, and the disenfranchisement of women to current economic, political, and environmental concerns.

HEALTH SYSTEMS AND THE "BRAIN DRAIN"

A significant and oft-invoked barrier to effective health care in resource-poor settings is the lack of medical personnel. In what is termed the *brain drain*, many physicians and nurses emigrate from their home countries to pursue opportunities abroad, leaving behind health systems that are understaffed and ill-equipped to deal with the epidemic diseases that ravage local populations. The WHO recommends a minimum of 20 physicians and 100 nurses per 100,000 persons, but recent reports from that organization and others confirm that many countries, especially in sub-Saharan Africa, fall far short of those target numbers. More than half of these countries register fewer than 10 physicians per 100,000 population. In contrast, the United States and Cuba register 279 and 596 doctors per 100,000 population, respectively. Similarly, the majority of sub-Saharan African countries do not have even half of the WHO-recommended minimum number of nurses. In addition to these appalling national aggregates, further inequalities in health care staffing exist *within* countries. Rural-urban disparities in health care personnel mirror disparities of both wealth and health. In 1992, the poorest districts in southern Africa reported 5.5 doctors, 188.1 nurses, and 0.5 pharmacists per 100,000 population. The same survey found, in the richest districts, 35.6 doctors, 375.3 nurses, and 5.4 pharmacists per 100,000 population. Nearly 90% of Malawi's population is rural, but >95% of clinical officers were at urban facilities, and 47% of nurses were at tertiary care facilities. Even community health workers, trained to provide first-line services to rural populations, often transfer to urban districts. In 1989 in Kenya, for example, there were only 138 health workers per 100,000 persons in the rural North Eastern Province, whereas there were 688 per 100,000 in Nairobi.

In addition to inter- and intranational transfer of personnel, the AIDS epidemic contributes to personnel shortages across Africa. Although data on the prevalence of HIV infection among health professionals are scarce, the available numbers suggest substantial and adverse impacts on an already-overburdened health sector. In 1999, it was estimated that 17–32% of health care workers in Botswana had HIV disease, and this number is expected to increase in the coming years. A recent study that examined the fates of a small cohort of Ugandan physicians found that at least 22 of the 77 doctors who graduated from Makerere University Medical School in 1984 had died by 2004—most, presumably, of AIDS. Similar numbers have been registered in South Africa, where a small study by the Human Sciences Research Council found an HIV seroprevalence among health professionals similar to that among the general population—in this case, 15.7% of all health care workers surveyed. The shortage of medical personnel in the areas hardest hit by HIV has profound implications for prevention and treatment efforts in these regions. The cycle of health-sector impoverishment, brain drain, and lack of personnel to fill positions when they are available conspires against ambitious programs to bring ART to persons living with both AIDS and poverty. The president of Botswana recently declared that one of his country's main obstacles to rapid expansion of HIV/AIDS treatment is "a dearth of doctors, nurses, pharmacists, and other health workers."[3] In South Africa, the departure of nearly 600 pharmacists in 2001, coupled with standing vacancies for 32,000 nurses, has put continued strain on that relatively affluent country's ability to respond to calls for expanded treatment programs. In Malawi, only 28% of established nursing posts are filled. Furthermore, the education of medical trainees is jeopardized as the ranks of the health and academic communities continue to shrink as a result of migration or disease. The long-term implications are sobering.

A proper biosocial analysis of the brain drain reminds us that the flight of health personnel—almost always, as most reviews suggest, from poor to less-poor regions—is not simply a question of desire for more equitable remuneration. Epidemiologic trends and access to the tools of the trade are also relevant, as are working conditions in general. In many settings now losing skilled health personnel, the advent of HIV has led to a sharp rise in TB incidence; in the eyes of health care providers, other

[3]Dugger C: Botswana's brain drain cripples war on AIDS. New York Times A10 (13 November 2003).

opportunistic infections have also become insuperable challenges. Together, these forces have conspired to render the provision of proper care impossible, as the comments of a Kenyan medical resident suggest: "Regarding HIV/AIDS, it is impossible to go home and forget about it. Even the simplest opportunistic infections we have no drugs for. Even if we do, there is only enough for a short course. It is impossible to forget about it. . . . Just because of the numbers, I am afraid of going to the floors. It is a nightmare thinking of going to see the patients. You are afraid of the risk of infection, diarrhea, urine, vomit, blood. . . . It is frightening to think about returning."[4] Another resident noted, "Before training we thought of doctors as supermen. . . . [Now] we are only mortuary attendants."[5] Nurses and other providers are, of course, similarly affected.

Given the difficult conditions under which these health care personnel work, is it any surprise when the U.S. government's appointed Global AIDS Coordinator notes that there are more Ethiopian physicians practicing in Chicago than in all of Ethiopia? In Zambia, only 50 of the 600 doctors trained since the country's independence in 1964 remain in their home country. Nor is it surprising that a 1999 survey of medical students in Ghana in their final year of training revealed that 40 of 43 students planned to leave the country upon graduation. When providing care for the sick becomes a nightmare for those at the beginning of clinical training, physician burn-out soon follows among those who carry on in settings of impoverishment. In the public-sector institutions put in place to care for the poorest people, the confluence of epidemic disease, lack of resources with which to respond, and unrealistically high user fees has led to widespread burn-out among health workers. Patients and their families are those who pay most dearly for provider burn-out, just as they bear the burden of disease and—with the introduction of user fees—much of the cost of responding, however inadequately, to new epidemics and persistent plagues.

CONCLUSION: TOWARD A SCIENCE OF IMPLEMENTATION

Public-health strategies draw largely on quantitative methods—from epidemiology and biostatistics, but also from economics. Clinical practice, including internal medicine, draws on a rapidly expanding knowledge base but remains focused on individual patient care; clinical interventions are rarely population-based. In fact, neither public-health nor clinical approaches alone will prove adequate in addressing the problems of global health. There is a long way to go before evidence-based internal medicine is applied effectively among the world's poor. Complex infectious diseases such as AIDS and TB have proven difficult but not impossible to manage; drug resistance and a lack of effective health systems have further complicated such work. Beyond communicable disease, in the arena of chronic diseases (e.g., cardiovascular disease), global health is a nascent endeavor. Efforts to address any one of these problems in settings of great scarcity need to be integrated into broader efforts to strengthen failing health systems and to alleviate the growing personnel crisis within these systems.

For these reasons, scholarly work and practice in the field once known as international health and now often designated *global health equity* are changing rapidly. Such work is still informed by the tension between clinical practice and population-based interventions, between analysis and action. Once metrics are refined, how might they inform efforts to lessen the premature morbidity and mortality registered among the world's poor? As in the nineteenth century, human rights perspectives have proven helpful in turning attention to the problems of the destitute sick; such perspectives may also inform strategies of delivering care equitably. A number of university hospitals are developing training programs for physicians with interests in global health. In medical schools across the United States and in other wealthy countries, interest in global health has been exploding. An informal survey at Harvard Medical School in 2006 revealed that nearly one-quarter of the 160 entering students either had significant global health experience or were planning a career in global health. A similar sea-change among trainees has been reported at other medical schools. Half a century or even a decade ago, such high levels of interest would have been unimaginable.

Persistent epidemics, improved metrics, and growing interest have only recently been matched by an unprecedented investment in addressing the health problems of poor people in the developing world. Ours is a moment of opportunity. To ensure that the opportunity is not wasted, the basic facts need to be laid out for specialists and laypeople alike. More than 12 million people die each year simply because they live in poverty. An absolute majority of these premature deaths occur in Africa, with the poorer regions of Asia not far behind. Most of these deaths occur because the world's poorest do not have access to the fruits of science. They include deaths from vaccine-preventable illness; deaths during childbirth; deaths from infectious diseases that might be cured with access to antibiotics and other essential medicines; deaths from malaria that would have been prevented by bed nets and access to therapy; and deaths from water-borne illnesses. Other excess mortality is attributable to the inadequacy of efforts to develop new tools. Those funding the discovery and development of new tools typically neglect the concurrent need for strategies to make them available to the poor. Indeed, some would argue that the biggest challenge facing those who seek to address this outcome gap is the lack of practical means of distribution in the regions most heavily affected.

The development of tools must be followed in short order by their equitable distribution. When new preventive and therapeutic tools are developed without concurrent attention to delivery or implementation, we face what are sometimes termed *perverse effects:* even as new tools are developed, inequalities of outcome—less morbidity and mortality among those who can afford access, with sustained high morbidity and mortality among those who cannot—will grow in the absence of an equity plan to deliver the tools to those most at risk. Preventing such a future is the most important goal of global health.

FURTHER READINGS

COHEN J: The new world of global health. Science 311:162, 2006

DESJARLAIS R et al (eds): *World Mental Health: Problems and Priorities in Low-Income Countries*. New York, Oxford University Press, 1995

FARMER PE: *Infections and Inequalities: The Modern Plagues*, 2d ed. Berkeley, University of California Press, 2001

———: From "marvelous momentum" to healthcare for all. Response to Garrett L: The challenge of global health. Foreign Affairs 86:155, 2007

FAUCI AS et al: Emerging infectious diseases: A 10-year perspective from the National Institute of Allergy and Infectious Diseases. Emerg Infect Dis 11:519, 2005

GARRETT L: The challenge of global health. Foreign Affairs 86:14, 2007

HOTEZ PJ et al: Neglected tropical diseases and HIV/AIDS. Lancet 368:1865, 2006

JAMISON DT et al (eds): *Disease Control Priorities in Developing Countries*, 2d ed. Washington, DC, Oxford University Press and The World Bank, 2006

KIM JY et al (eds): *Dying for Growth: Global Inequality and the Health of the Poor*. Monroe, ME, Common Courage Press, 2000

LOPEZ AD et al: Global and regional burden of disease and risk factors, 2001: Systematic analysis of population health data. Lancet 367:1747, 2006

MURRAY CJL, LOPEZ AD (eds): The global burden of disease: A comprehensive assessment of mortality and disability from diseases, injuries, and risk factors in 1990 and projected to 2020. Cambridge, MA, Harvard University Press, 1996

SACHS J, MALANEY O: The economic and social burden of malaria. Nature 415:680, 2002

WORLD BANK: *World Development Report 1993: Investing in Health*. New York, Oxford University Press, 1993

WORLD HEALTH ORGANIZATION: *Macroeconomics and Health: Investing in Health for Economic Development*. Geneva, Commission on Macroeconomics and Health, 2001

———: *World Health Report 2006: Working Together for Health*. Geneva, World Health Organization, 2006

[4]Raviola G et al: HIV, disease plague, demoralization, and "burnout": Resident experience of the medical profession in Nairobi, Kenya. Cult Med Psychiatry 26:55, 2002.
[5]Ibid.

3 Decision-Making in Clinical Medicine

Daniel B. Mark

To the medical student who requires 2 h to collect a patient's history and perform a physical examination, and several additional hours to organize them into a coherent presentation, the experienced clinician's ability to reach a diagnosis and decide on a management plan in a fraction of the time seems extraordinary. While medical knowledge and experience play a significant role in the senior clinician's ability to arrive at a differential diagnosis and plan quickly, much of the process involves skill in clinical decision-making. The first goal of this chapter is to provide an introduction to the study of clinical reasoning.

Equally bewildering to the student are the proper use of diagnostic tests and the integration of the results into the clinical assessment. The novice medical practitioner typically uses a "shotgun" approach to testing, hoping to hit a target without knowing exactly what that target is. The expert, on the other hand, usually has a specific target in mind and efficiently adjusts the testing strategy to it. The second goal of this chapter is to review briefly some of the crucial basic statistical concepts that govern the proper interpretation and use of diagnostic tests. Quantitative tools available to assist in clinical decision-making will also be discussed.

Evidence-based medicine is the term used to describe the integration of the best available research evidence with clinical judgment and experience in the care of patients. The third goal of this chapter is to provide a brief overview of some of the tools of evidence-based medicine.

CLINICAL DECISION-MAKING

CLINICAL REASONING

The most important clinical actions are not procedures or prescriptions but the judgments from which all other aspects of clinical medicine flow. In the modern era of large randomized trials and evidence-based medicine, it is easy to overlook the importance of this elusive mental activity and focus instead on the algorithmic practice guidelines constructed to improve care. One reason for this apparent neglect is that much more research has been done on how doctors *should* make decisions (e.g., using a Bayesian model, discussed below) than on how they actually *do*. Thus, much of what we know about clinical reasoning comes from empirical studies of nonmedical problem-solving behavior.

Despite the great technological advances of medicine over the last century, uncertainty still plays a pivotal role in all aspects of medical decision-making. We may know that a patient does not have long to live, but we cannot be certain how long. We may prescribe a potent new receptor blocker to reverse the course of a patient's illness, but we cannot be certain that the therapy will achieve the desired result and that result alone. Uncertainty in medical outcomes creates the need for probabilities and other mathematical/statistical tools to help guide decision-making. (These tools are reviewed later in the chapter.)

Uncertainty is compounded by the information overload that characterizes modern medicine. Today's experienced clinician needs close to 2 million pieces of information to practice medicine. Doctors subscribe to an average of seven journals, representing over 2500 new articles each year. Computers offer the obvious solution both for management of information and for better quantitation and management of the daily uncertainties of medical care. While the technology to computerize medical practice is available, many practical problems remain to be solved before patient information can be standardized and integrated with medical evidence on a single electronic platform.

The following three examples introduce the subject of clinical reasoning:

- A 46-year-old man presents to his internist with a chief complaint of hemoptysis. The physician knows that the differential diagnosis of hemoptysis includes over 100 different conditions, including cancer and tuberculosis. The examination begins with some general background questions, and the patient is asked to describe his symptoms and their chronology. By the time the examination is completed, and even before any tests are run, the physician has formulated a working diagnostic hypothesis and planned a series of steps to test it. In an otherwise healthy and nonsmoking patient recovering from a viral bronchitis, the doctor's hypothesis would be that the acute bronchitis is responsible for the small amount of blood-streaked sputum the patient observed. In this case, a chest x-ray may provide sufficient reassurance that a more serious disorder is not present.
- A second 46-year-old patient with the same chief complaint who has a 100-pack-year smoking history, a productive morning cough, and episodes of blood-streaked sputum may generate the principal diagnostic hypothesis of carcinoma of the lung. Consequently, along with the chest x-ray, the physician obtains a sputum cytology examination and refers this patient for fiberoptic bronchoscopy.
- A third 46-year-old patient with hemoptysis who is from a developing country is evaluated with an echocardiogram as well, because the physician thinks she hears a soft diastolic rumbling murmur at the apex on cardiac auscultation, suggesting rheumatic mitral stenosis.

These three simple vignettes illustrate two aspects of expert clinical reasoning: (1) the use of cognitive shortcuts as a way to organize the complex unstructured material that is collected in the clinical evaluation, and (2) the use of diagnostic hypotheses to consolidate the information and indicate appropriate management steps.

THE USE OF COGNITIVE SHORTCUTS

Cognitive shortcuts or rules of thumb, sometimes referred to as *heuristics*, can help solve complex problems, of the sort encountered daily in clinical medicine, with great efficiency. Clinicians rely on three basic types of heuristics. When assessing a particular patient, clinicians often weigh the probability that this patient's clinical features match those of the class of patients with the leading diagnostic hypotheses being considered. In other words, the clinician is searching for the diagnosis for which the patient appears to be a representative example; this cognitive shortcut is called the *representativeness heuristic*.

It may take only a few characteristics from the history for an expert clinician using the representativeness heuristic to arrive at a sound diagnostic hypothesis. For example, an elderly patient with new-onset fever, cough productive of copious sputum, unilateral pleuritic chest pain, and dyspnea is readily identified as fitting the pattern for acute pneumonia, probably of bacterial origin. Evidence of focal pulmonary consolidation on the physical examination will increase the clinician's confidence in the diagnosis because it fits the expected pattern of acute bacterial pneumonia. Knowing this allows the experienced clinician to conduct an efficient, directed, and therapeutically productive patient evaluation since there may be little else in the history or physical examination of direct relevance. The inexperienced medical student or resident, who has not yet learned the patterns most prevalent in clinical medicine, must work much harder to achieve the same result and is often at risk of missing the important clinical problem in a sea of compulsively collected but unhelpful data.

However, physicians using the representativeness heuristic can reach erroneous conclusions if they fail to consider the underlying prevalence of two competing diagnoses (i.e., the prior, or pretest, probabilities). Consider a patient with pleuritic chest pain, dyspnea, and a low-grade fever. A clinician might consider acute pneumonia and acute pulmonary embolism to be the two leading diagnostic alternatives. Using the representativeness heuristic, the clinician might judge both diagnostic candidates to be equally likely, although to do so would be wrong if pneumonia was much more prevalent in the underlying population. Mistakes may also result from a failure to consider that a pattern based on a small number of prior observations will likely be less reliable than one based on larger samples.

A second commonly used cognitive shortcut, the *availability heuristic*, involves judgments made on the basis of how easily prior similar cases or outcomes can be brought to mind. For example, the experienced clinician may recall 20 elderly patients seen over the past few years who presented with painless dyspnea of acute onset and were found to have acute myocardial infarction. The novice clinician may spend valuable time seeking a pulmonary cause for the symptoms before considering and then confirming the cardiac diagnosis. In this situation, the patient's clinical pattern does not fit the expected pattern of acute myocardial infarction, but experience with this atypical presentation, and the ability to recall it, can help direct the physician to the diagnosis.

Errors with the availability heuristic can come from several sources of recall bias. For example, rare catastrophes are likely to be remembered with a clarity and force out of proportion to their value, and recent experience is, of course, easier to recall and therefore more influential on clinical judgments.

The third commonly used cognitive shortcut, the *anchoring heuristic*, involves estimating a probability by starting from a familiar point (the anchor) and adjusting to the new case from there. Anchoring can be a powerful tool for diagnosis but is often used incorrectly. For example, a clinician may judge the probability of coronary artery disease (CAD) to be very high after a positive exercise thallium test, because the prediction has been anchored to the test result ("positive test = high probability of CAD"). Yet, as discussed below, this prediction would be inaccurate if the clinical (pretest) picture of the patient being tested indicates a low probability of disease (e.g., a 30-year-old woman with no risk factors). As illustrated in this example, anchors are not necessarily the same as the pretest probability (see "Measures of Disease Probability and Bayes' Theorem," below).

DIAGNOSTIC HYPOTHESIS GENERATION

Cognitive scientists studying the thought processes of expert clinicians have observed that clinicians group data into packets, or "chunks," which are stored in their memories and manipulated to generate diagnostic hypotheses. Because short-term memory can typically hold only 7–10 items at a time, the number of packets that can be actively integrated into hypothesis-generating activities is similarly limited. The cognitive shortcuts discussed above play a key role in the generation of diagnostic hypotheses, many of which are discarded as rapidly as they are formed.

A diagnostic hypothesis sets a context for diagnostic steps to follow and provides testable predictions. For example, if the enlarged and quite tender liver felt on physical examination is due to acute hepatitis (the hypothesis), certain specific liver function tests should be markedly elevated (the prediction). If the tests come back normal, the hypothesis may need to be discarded or substantially modified.

One of the factors that make teaching diagnostic reasoning difficult is that expert clinicians do not follow a fixed pattern in patient examinations. From the outset, they are generating, refining, and discarding diagnostic hypotheses. The questions they ask in the history are driven by the hypotheses they are working with at the moment. Even the physical examination is driven by specific questions rather than a preordained checklist. While the student is palpating the abdomen of the alcoholic patient, waiting for a finding to strike him, the expert clinician is on a focused search mission. Is the spleen enlarged? How big is the liver? Is it tender? Are there any palpable masses or nodules? Each question focuses the attention of the examiner to the exclusion of all other inputs until answered, allowing the examiner to move on to the next specific question.

Negative findings are often as important as positive ones in establishing and refining diagnostic hypotheses. Chest discomfort that is not provoked or worsened by exertion in an active patient reduces the likelihood that chronic ischemic heart disease is the underlying cause. The absence of a resting tachycardia and thyroid gland enlargement reduces the likelihood of hyperthyroidism in a patient with paroxysmal atrial fibrillation.

The acuity of a patient's illness can play an important role in overriding considerations of prevalence and other issues described above. For example, clinicians are taught to consider aortic dissection routinely as a possible cause of acute severe chest discomfort along with myocardial infarction, even though the typical history of dissection is different from myocardial infarction and dissection is far less prevalent (Chap. 242). This recommendation is based on the recognition that a relatively rare but catastrophic diagnosis like aortic dissection is very difficult to make unless it is explicitly considered. If the clinician fails to elicit any of the characteristic features of dissection by history and finds equivalent blood pressures in both arms and no pulse deficits, he or she may feel comfortable in discarding the aortic dissection hypothesis. If, however, the chest x-ray shows a widened mediastinum, the hypothesis may be reinstated and a diagnostic test ordered [e.g., thoracic computed tomography (CT) scan, transesophageal echocardiogram] to evaluate it more fully. In nonacute situations, the prevalence of potential alternative diagnoses should play a much more prominent role in diagnostic hypothesis generation.

Generation of Diagnostic Hypotheses Because the generation and evaluation of appropriate diagnostic hypotheses is a skill that not all clinicians possess to an equal degree, errors in this process can occur; in the patient with serious acute illness, these may lead to tragic consequences. Consider the following hypothetical example. A 45-year-old male patient with a 3-week history of a "flulike" upper respiratory infection (URI) presented to his physician with symptoms of dyspnea and a productive cough. Based on the presenting complaint, the clinician pulled out a "URI Assessment Form" to improve quality and efficiency of care. The physician quickly completed the examination components outlined on this structured form, noting in particular the absence of fever and a clear chest examination. He then prescribed an antibiotic for presumed bronchitis, showed the patient how to breathe into a paper bag to relieve his "hyperventilation," and sent him home with the reassurance that his illness was not serious. After a sleepless night with significant dyspnea unrelieved by breathing into a bag, the patient developed nausea and vomiting and collapsed. He was brought into the Emergency Department in cardiac arrest and could not be resuscitated. Autopsy showed a posterior wall myocardial infarction and a fresh thrombus in an atherosclerotic right coronary artery. What went wrong? The clinician decided, even before starting the history, that the patient's complaints were not serious. He therefore felt confident that he could perform an abbreviated and focused examination using the URI assessment protocol rather than considering the full range of possibilities and performing appropriate tests to confirm or refute his initial hypotheses. In particular, by concentrating on the "URI," the clinician failed to elicit the full dyspnea history, which would have suggested a far more serious disorder, and neglected to search for other symptoms that could have directed him to the correct diagnosis.

This example illustrates how patients can diverge from textbook symptoms and the potential consequences of being unable to adapt the diagnostic process to real-world challenges. The expert, while recognizing that common things occur commonly, approaches each evaluation on high alert for clues that the initial diagnosis may be wrong. Patients often provide information that "does not fit" with any of the leading diagnostic hypotheses being considered. Distinguishing real clues from false trails can only be achieved by practice and experience. A less-experienced clinician who tries to be too efficient (as in the above example) can make serious errors. Use of a rapid systematic clinical survey of symptoms and organ systems can help prevent the clinician from overlooking important but inapparent clues.

MAJOR INFLUENCES ON CLINICAL DECISION-MAKING

More than a decade of research on variations in clinician practice patterns has shed much light on forces that shape clinical decisions. The use of heuristic "shortcuts," as detailed above, provides a partial explanation, but several other key factors play an important role in shaping diagnostic hypotheses and management decisions. These factors can be grouped conceptually into three overlapping categories: (1) factors related to physicians' personal characteristics and practice style, (2) factors related to the practice setting, and (3) factors related to economic incentives.

Factors Related to Practice Style One of the key roles of the physician in medical care is to serve as the patient's agent to ensure that necessary care is provided at a high level of quality. Factors that influence this role include the physician's knowledge, training, and experience. It is obvious that physicians cannot practice evidence-based medicine (EBM; described later in the chapter) if they are unfamiliar with the evidence. As would be expected, specialists generally know the evidence in their field better than do generalists. Surgeons may be more enthusiastic about recommending surgery than medical doctors because their belief in the beneficial effects of surgery is stronger. For the same reason, invasive cardiologists are much more likely to refer chest pain patients for diagnostic catheterization than are noninvasive cardiologists or generalists. The physician beliefs that drive these different practice styles are based on personal experience, recollection, and interpretation of the available medical evidence. For example, heart failure specialists are much more likely than generalists to achieve target angiotensin-converting enzyme (ACE) inhibitor therapy in their heart failure patients because they are more familiar with what the targets are (as defined by large clinical trials), have more familiarity with the specific drugs (including dosages and side effects), and are less likely to overreact to foreseeable problems in therapy such as a rise in creatinine levels or symptomatic hypotension. Other intriguing research has shown a wide distribution of acceptance times of antibiotic therapy for peptic ulcer disease following widespread dissemination of the "evidence" in the medical literature. Some gastroenterologists accepted this new therapy before the evidence was clear (reflecting, perhaps, an aggressive practice style), and some gastroenterologists lagged behind (a conservative practice style, associated in this case with older physicians). As a group, internists lagged several years behind gastroenterologists.

The opinion of influential leaders can also have an important effect on practice patterns. Such influence can occur at both the national level (e.g., expert physicians teaching at national meetings) and the local level (e.g., local educational programs, "curbside consultations"). Opinion leaders do not have to be physicians. When conducting rounds with clinical pharmacists, physicians are less likely to make medication errors and more likely to use target levels of evidence-based therapies.

The patient's welfare is not the only concern that drives clinical decisions. The physician's perception about the risk of a malpractice suit resulting from either an erroneous decision or a bad outcome creates a style of practice referred to as *defensive medicine*. This practice involves using tests and therapies with very small marginal returns to preclude future criticism in the event of an adverse outcome. For example, a 40-year-old woman who presents with a long-standing history of intermittent headache and a new severe headache along with a normal neurologic examination has a very low likelihood of structural intracranial pathology. Performance of a head CT or magnetic resonance imaging (MRI) scan in this situation would constitute defensive medicine. On the other hand, the results of the test could provide reassurance to an anxious patient.

Practice Setting Factors Factors in this category relate to the physical resources available to the physician's practice and the practice environment. *Physician-induced demand* is a term that refers to the repeated observation that physicians have a remarkable ability to accommodate to and employ the medical facilities available to them. One of the foundational studies in outcomes research showed that physicians in Boston had an almost 50% higher hospital admission rate than did physicians in New Haven, despite there being no obvious differences in the health of the cities' inhabitants. The physicians in New Haven were not aware of using fewer hospital beds for their patients, nor were the Boston physicians aware of using less stringent criteria to admit patients. In both cities, physicians unconsciously adopted their practice styles to the available level of hospital beds.

Other environmental factors that can influence decision-making include the local availability of specialists for consultations and procedures, "high tech" facilities such as angiography suites, a heart surgery program, and MRI machines.

Economic Incentives Economic incentives are closely related to the other two categories of practice-modifying factors. Financial issues can exert both stimulatory and inhibitory influences on clinical practice. In general, physicians are paid on a fee-for-service, capitation, or salary basis. In fee-for-service, the more the physician does, the more the physician gets paid. The economic incentive in this case is to do more. When fees are reduced (discounted fee-for-service), doctors tend to increase the number of services billed for. Capitation, in contrast, provides a fixed payment per patient per year, encouraging physicians to take on more patients but to provide each patient with fewer services. Expensive services are more likely to be affected by this type of incentive than inexpensive preventive services. Salary compensation plans pay physicians the same regardless of the amount of clinical work performed. The incentive here is to see fewer patients.

In summary, expert clinical decision-making can be appreciated as a complex interplay between cognitive devices used to simplify large amounts of complex information interacting with physician biases reflecting education, training, and experience, all of which are shaped by powerful, sometimes perverse, external forces. In the next section, a set of statistical tools and concepts that can assist in making clinical decisions in the presence of uncertainty are reviewed.

QUANTITATIVE METHODS TO AID CLINICAL DECISION-MAKING

The process of medical decision-making can be divided into two parts: (1) defining the available courses of action and estimating the likely outcomes with each, and (2) assessing the desirability of the outcomes. The former task involves integrating key information about the patient along with relevant evidence from the medical literature to create the structure of a decision. The remainder of this chapter will review some quantitative tools available to assist the clinician in these activities.

QUANTITATIVE MEDICAL PREDICTIONS

Diagnostic Testing: Measures of Test Accuracy The purpose of performing a test on a patient is to reduce uncertainty about the patient's diagnosis or prognosis and to aid the clinician in making management decisions. Although diagnostic tests are commonly thought of as laboratory tests (e.g., measurement of serum amylase level) or procedures (e.g., colonoscopy or bronchoscopy), any technology that changes our understanding of the patient's problem qualifies as a diagnostic test. Thus, even the history and physical examination can be considered a form of diagnostic test. In clinical medicine, it is common to reduce the results of a test to a dichotomous outcome, such as positive or negative, normal or abnormal. In many cases, this simplification results in the waste of useful information. However, such simplification makes it easier to demonstrate some of the quantitative ways in which test data can be used.

The accuracy of diagnostic tests is defined in relation to an accepted "gold standard," which is presumed to reflect the true state of the patient (Table 3-1). To define the diagnostic performance of a new test, an appropriate population must be identified (ideally patients in whom the new test would be used) and both the new and the gold standard tests are applied to all subjects. The results of the two tests are then compared. The *sensitivity* or *true-positive rate* of the new test is the proportion of patients with disease (defined by the gold standard) who have a positive (new) test. This measure reflects how well the test identifies patients with disease. The proportion of patients with disease who have a negative test is the *false-negative rate* and is calculated as 1 – sensitivity. The proportion of patients without disease who have a negative test is the *specificity* or *true-negative rate*. This measure reflects how well the test correctly identifies patients without disease. The proportion of patients without disease who have a positive test is the *false-positive rate*, calculated as 1 – specificity. A perfect test would have a sensitivity of 100% and a specificity of 100% and would completely separate patients with disease from those without it.

Calculating sensitivity and specificity requires selection of a decision value for the test to define the threshold value at or above which the test is considered "positive." For any given test, as this cut point is moved to

TABLE 3-1 MEASURES OF DIAGNOSTIC TEST ACCURACY

	Disease Status	
Test Result	**Present**	**Absent**
Positive	True-positive (*TP*)	False-positive (*FP*)
Negative	False-negative (*FN*)	True-negative (*TN*)
Identification of Patients with Disease		
True-positive rate (sensitivity) = *TP*/(*TP*+*FN*)		
False-negative rate = *FN*/(*TP*+*FN*)		
True-positive rate = 1 – false-negative rate		
Identification of Patients without Disease		
True-negative rate (specificity) = *TN*/(*TN*+*FP*)		
False-positive rate = *FP*/(*TN*+*FP*)		
True-negative rate = 1 – false-positive rate		

TABLE 3-2 MEASURES OF DISEASE PROBABILITY

Pretest probability of disease = probability of disease before test is done. May use population prevalence of disease or more patient-specific data to generate this probability estimate.

Posttest probability of disease = probability of disease accounting for both pretest probability and test results. Also called predictive value of the test.

Bayes' theorem: Computational version:

$$\text{Posttest probability} = \frac{\text{Pretest probability} \times \text{test sensitivity}}{\text{Pretest probability} \times \text{test sensitivity} + (1 - \text{pretest probability}) \times \text{test false-positive rate}}$$

Example [with a pretest probability of 0.50 and a "positive" diagnostic test result (test sensitivity = 0.90, test specificity = 0.90)]:

$$\text{Posttest probability} = \frac{(0.50)(0.90)}{(0.50)(0.90) + (0.50)(0.10)} = 0.90$$

improve sensitivity, specificity typically falls and vice versa. This dynamic tradeoff between more accurate identification of subjects with disease versus those without disease is often displayed graphically as a receiver operating characteristic (ROC) curve (Fig. 3-1). An ROC curve plots sensitivity (*y*-axis) versus 1 – specificity (*x*-axis). Each point on the curve represents a potential cut point with an associated sensitivity and specificity value. The area under the ROC curve is often used as a quantitative measure of the information content of a test. Values range from 0.5 (no diagnostic information at all, test is equivalent to flipping a coin) to 1.0 (perfect test).

In the testing literature, ROC areas are often used to compare alternative tests that can be used for a particular diagnostic problem (Fig. 3-1). The test with the highest area (i.e., closest to 1.0) is presumed to be the most accurate. However, ROC curves are not a panacea for evaluation of diagnostic test utility. Like Bayes' theorem (discussed below), they are typically focused on only one possible test parameter (e.g., ST-segment response in a treadmill exercise test) to the exclusion of other potentially relevant data. In addition, ROC area comparisons do not simulate the way test information is actually used in clinical practice. Finally, biases in the underlying population used to generate the ROC curves (e.g., related to an unrepresentative test sample) can bias the ROC area and the validity of a comparison among tests.

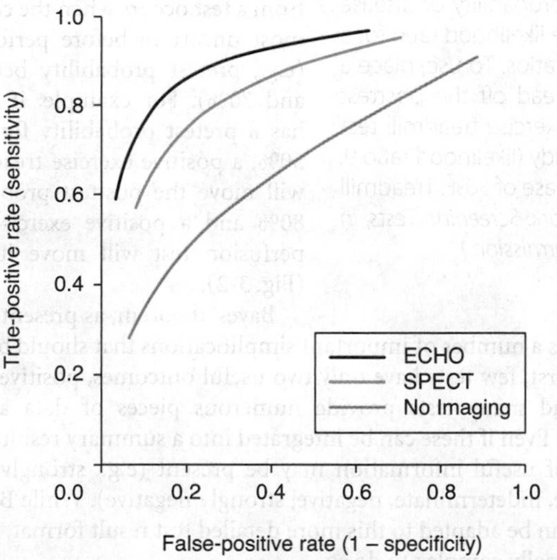

FIGURE 3-1 The receiver operating characteristic (ROC) curves for three diagnostic exercise tests for detection of CAD: exercise ECG, exercise SPECT, and exercise echo. Each ROC curve illustrates the trade-off that occurs between improved test sensitivity (accurate detection of patients with disease) and improved test specificity (accurate detection of patients without disease), as the test value defining when the test turns from "negative" to "positive" is varied. A 45° line would indicate a test with no information (sensitivity = specificity at every test value). The area under each ROC curve is a measure of the information content of the test. Moving to a test with a larger ROC area (e.g., from exercise ECG to exercise echo) improves diagnostic accuracy. However, these curves are not measured in the same populations and the effect of referral biases on the results cannot easily be discerned. *(From KE Fleischmann et al: JAMA 280:913, 1998, with permission.)*

Measures of Disease Probability and Bayes' Theorem Unfortunately, there are no perfect tests; after every test is completed, the true disease state of the patient remains uncertain. Quantitating this residual uncertainty can be done with Bayes' theorem. This theorem provides a simple mathematical way to calculate the posttest probability of disease from three parameters: the pretest probability of disease, the test sensitivity, and the test specificity (Table 3-2). The pretest probability is a quantitative expression of the confidence in a diagnosis before the test is performed. In the absence of more relevant information, it is usually estimated from the prevalence of the disease in the underlying population. For some common conditions, such as coronary artery disease (CAD), nomograms and statistical models have been created to generate better estimates of pretest probability from elements of the history and physical examination. The posttest probability, then, is a revised statement of the confidence in the diagnosis, taking into account what was known both before and after the test.

The term *predictive value* is often used as a synonym for the posttest probability. Unfortunately, clinicians commonly misinterpret reported predictive values as intrinsic measures of test accuracy. Studies of diagnostic tests compound the confusion by calculating predictive values on the same sample used to measure sensitivity and specificity. Since all posttest probabilities are a function of the prevalence of disease in the tested population, such calculations are clinically irrelevant unless the test is subsequently applied to populations with the same disease prevalence. For these reasons, the term *predictive value* is best avoided in favor of the more informative *posttest probability*.

To understand conceptually how Bayes' theorem estimates the posttest probability of disease, it is useful to examine a nomogram version of Bayes' theorem (Fig. 3-2). In this nomogram, the accuracy of the diagnostic test in question is summarized by the *likelihood ratio*, which is defined as the ratio of the probability of a given test result (e.g., "positive" or "negative") in a patient with disease to the probability of that result in a patient without disease.

For a positive test, the likelihood ratio is calculated as the ratio of the true-positive rate to the false-positive rate [or sensitivity/(1 – specificity)]. For example, a test with a sensitivity of 0.90 and a specificity of 0.90 has a likelihood ratio of 0.90/(1 – 0.90), or 9. Thus, for this hypothetical test, a "positive" result is 9 times more likely in a patient with the disease than in a patient without it. Most tests in medicine have likelihood ratios for a positive result between 1.5 and 20. Higher values are associated with tests that are more accurate at identifying patients with disease, with values of 10 or greater of particular note. If sensitivity is excellent but specificity is less so, the likelihood ratio will be substantially reduced (e.g., with a 90% sensitivity but a 60% specificity, the likelihood ratio is 2.25).

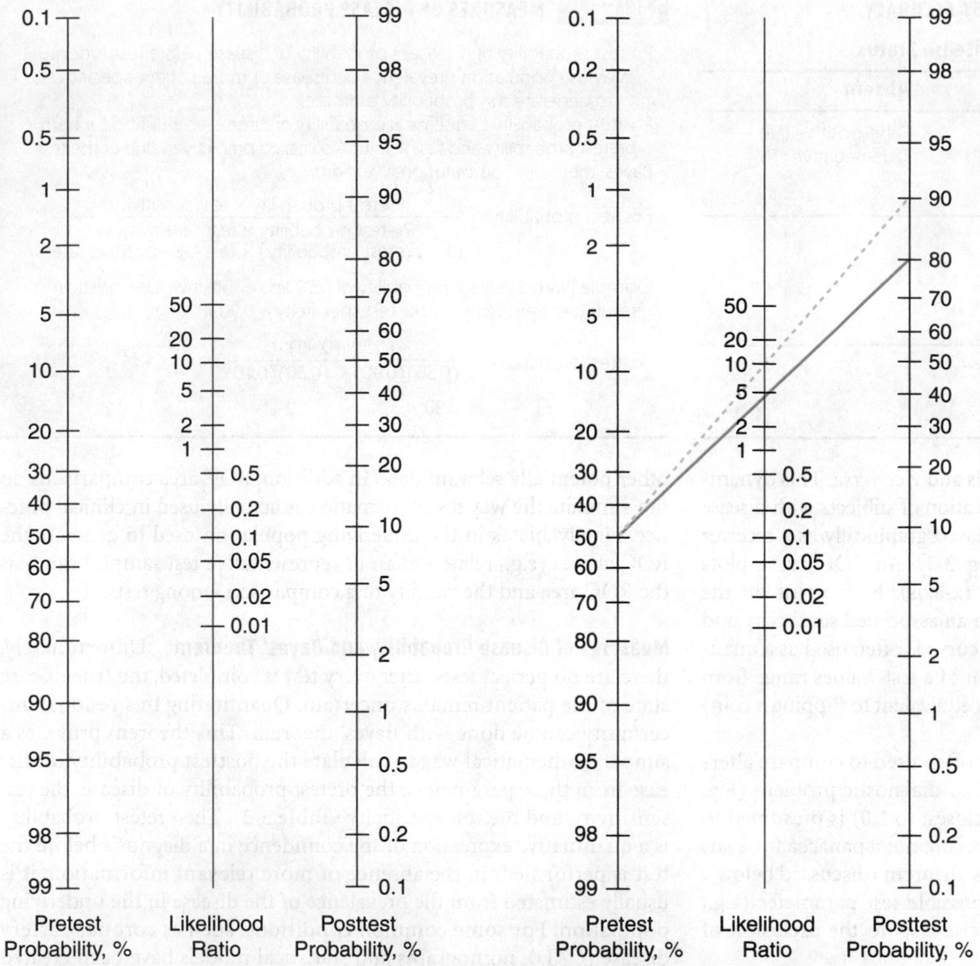

FIGURE 3-2 Nomogram version of Bayes' Theorem used to predict the posttest probability of disease (right-hand scale) using the pretest probability of disease (left-hand scale) and the likelihood ratio for a positive test (middle scale). See text for information on calculation of likelihood ratios. To use, place a straightedge connecting the pretest probability and the likelihood ratio and read off the posttest probability. The right-hand part of the figure illustrates the value of a positive exercise treadmill test (likelihood ratio 4, green line) and a positive exercise thallium SPECT perfusion study (likelihood ratio 9, broken yellow line) in the patient with a pretest probability of coronary artery disease of 50%. Treadmill results shown in solid line; thallium perfusion results in dashed line. *(From DB Mark: Screening Tests, in Atlas of Cardiovascular Risk Factors. Philadelphia, Current Medicine, LLC, 2006, with permission.)*

For a negative test, the corresponding likelihood ratio is the ratio of the false negative rate to the true negative rate [or (1 – sensitivity)/specificity]. The smaller the likelihood ratio (i.e., closer to 0) the better the test performs at ruling out disease. The hypothetical test we considered above with a sensitivity of 0.9 and a specificity of 0.9 would have a likelihood ratio for a negative test result of (1 – 0.9)/0.9 of 0.11, meaning that a negative result is almost 10 times more likely if the patient is disease-free than if he has disease.

Applications to Diagnostic Testing in CAD Consider two tests commonly used in the diagnosis of CAD, an exercise treadmill and an exercise single photon emission CT (SPECT) myocardial perfusion imaging test (Chap. 222). Meta-analysis has shown a positive treadmill ST-segment response to have an average sensitivity of 66% and an average specificity of 84%, yielding a likelihood ratio of 4.1 [0.66/(1 – 0.84)]. If we use this test on a patient with a pretest probability of CAD of 10%, the posttest probability of disease following a positive result rises to only about 30%. If a patient with a pretest probability of CAD of 80% has a positive test result, the posttest probability of disease is about 95%.

The exercise SPECT myocardial perfusion test is a more accurate test for the diagnosis of CAD. For our purposes, assume that the finding of a reversible exercise-induced perfusion defect has both a sensitivity and specificity of 90%, yielding a likelihood ratio for a positive test of 9.0 [0.90/(1 – 0.90)]. If we again test our low pretest probability patient and he has a positive test, using Fig. 3-2 we can demonstrate that the posttest probability of CAD rises from 10 to 50%. However, from a decision-making point of view, the more accurate test has not been able to improve diagnostic confidence enough to change management. In fact, the test has moved us from being fairly certain that the patient did not have CAD to being completely undecided (a 50:50 chance of disease). In a patient with a pretest probability of 80%, using the more accurate exercise SPECT test raises the posttest probability to 97% (compared with 95% for the exercise treadmill). Again, the more accurate test does not provide enough improvement in posttest confidence to alter management, and neither test has improved much upon what was known from clinical data alone.

If the pretest probability is low (e.g., 20%), even a positive result on a very accurate test will not move the posttest probability to a range high enough to rule in disease (e.g., 80%). Conversely, with a high pretest probability, a negative test will not adequately rule out disease. Thus, the largest gain in diagnostic confidence from a test occurs when the clinician is most uncertain before performing it (e.g., pretest probability between 30 and 70%). For example, if a patient has a pretest probability for CAD of 50%, a positive exercise treadmill test will move the posttest probability to 80% and a positive exercise SPECT perfusion test will move it to 90% (Fig. 3-2).

Bayes' theorem, as presented above, employs a number of important simplifications that should be considered. First, few tests have only two useful outcomes, positive or negative, and many tests provide numerous pieces of data about the patient. Even if these can be integrated into a summary result, multiple levels of useful information may be present (e.g., strongly positive, positive, indeterminate, negative, strongly negative). While Bayes' theorem can be adapted to this more detailed test result format, it is computationally complex to do so.

Finally, it has long been asserted that sensitivity and specificity are prevalence-independent parameters of test accuracy, and many texts still make this statement. This statistically useful assumption, however, is clinically simplistic. A treadmill exercise test, for example, has a sensitivity in a population of patients with one-vessel CAD of around 30%, whereas its sensitivity in severe three-vessel CAD approaches 80%. Thus, the best estimate of sensitivity to use in a particular decision will often vary, depending on the distribution of disease stages present in the tested population. A hospitalized population typically has a higher prevalence of disease and in particular a higher prevalence of more advanced disease than an outpatient population. As a consequence, test sensitivity will tend to be higher in hospitalized patients, whereas test specificity will be higher in outpatients.

Statistical Prediction Models Bayes' theorem, as presented above, deals with a clinical prediction problem that is unrealistically simple relative to most problems a clinician faces. Prediction models, based on multivariable statistical models, can handle much more complex problems and substantially enhance predictive accuracy for specific situations. Their particular advantage is the ability to take into account many overlapping pieces of information and assign a relative weight to each based on its unique contribution to the prediction in question. For example, a logistic regression model to predict the probability of CAD takes into account all of the relevant independent factors from the clinical examination and diagnostic testing instead of the small handful of data that clinicians can manage in their heads or with Bayes' theorem. However, despite this strength, the models are too complex computationally to use without a calculator or computer (although this limit may be overcome once medicine is practiced from a fully computerized platform).

To date, only a handful of prediction models have been properly validated. The importance of independent validation in a population separate from the one used to develop the model cannot be overstated. An unvalidated prediction model should be viewed with the same skepticism appropriate for a new drug or medical device that has not been through rigorous clinical trial testing.

When statistical models have been compared directly with expert clinicians, they have been found to be more consistent, as would be expected, but not significantly more accurate. Their biggest promise, then, would seem to be to make less-experienced clinicians more accurate predictors of outcome.

DECISION SUPPORT TOOLS

DECISION SUPPORT SYSTEMS

Over the past 35 years, many attempts have been made to develop computer systems to help clinicians make decisions and manage patients. Conceptually, computers offer a very attractive way to handle the vast information load that today's physicians face. The computer can help by making accurate predictions of outcome, simulating the whole decision process, or providing algorithmic guidance. Computer-based predictions using Bayesian or statistical regression models inform a clinical decision but do not actually reach a "conclusion" or "recommendation." Artificial intelligence systems attempt to simulate or replace human reasoning with a computer-based analogue. To date, such approaches have achieved only limited success. Reminder or protocol-directed systems do not make predictions but use existing algorithms, such as practice guidelines, to guide clinical practice. In general, however, decision support systems have shown little impact on practice. Reminder systems, although not yet in widespread use, have shown the most promise, particularly in correcting drug dosing and in promoting adherence to guidelines. The full impact of these approaches will only be evaluable when computers are fully integrated into medical practice.

DECISION ANALYSIS

Compared with the methods discussed above, decision analysis represents a completely different approach to decision support. Its principal application is in decision problems that are complex and involve a substantial risk, a high degree of uncertainty in some key area, or an idiosyncratic feature that does not "fit" the available evidence. Five general steps are involved. First, the decision problem must be clearly defined. Second, the elements of the decision must be made explicit. This involves specifying the alternatives being considered, their relevant outcomes, the probabilities attached to each outcome, and the relative desirability (called "utility") of each outcome. Cost can also be assigned to each branch of the decision tree, allowing calculation of cost effectiveness. Typically, the data to populate a decision model are derived from the literature, from unpublished sources, from expert opinion and from other secondary sources. Third, the decision model must be "evaluated" to determine the net long-term health benefits and costs of each strategy being considered. Fourth, the incremental health benefits and costs of the more effective strategies must be calculated. Finally, extensive sensitivity analyses must be used to examine the effects on the results of varying the starting assumptions through plausible alternative values.

An example decision tree created to evaluate strategies for screening for human immunodeficiency virus (HIV) infection is shown in Fig. 3-3. Up to 20,000 new cases of HIV infection are believed to be caused each year in the United States by infected individuals who are unaware of their illness. In addition, about 40% of HIV-positive patients progress to AIDS within a year of their diagnosis. Early identification offers the opportunity both to prevent progression to AIDS through use of serial CD4 counts and measurements of viral load linked to selective use of combination antiretroviral therapy and to encourage reduction of risky sexual behavior.

The Centers for Disease Control and Prevention (CDC) proposed in 2003 that routine HIV testing should be a part of standard medical care. In a decision-model exploration of this proposed strategy compared with usual care, assuming a 1% prevalence of unidentified HIV infection in the population, routine screening of a cohort of 43-year-old men and women increased life expectancy by 5.5 days and cost $194 per subject screened. The cost-effectiveness ratio for screening relative to usual care was $15,078 per quality-adjusted life year. Results were sensitive to assumptions about the effectiveness of behavior modification on subsequent sexual behavior, the benefits of early therapy of HIV infection and the prevalence and incidence of HIV infection in the population targeted. This model, which required over 75 separate data points, provides novel insights into a clinical management problem that has not been subjected to a randomized clinical trial.

The process of building and evaluating decision models is generally too complex for use in real-time clinical management. The potential for this tool therefore lies in the development of a set of published models addressing a particular decision or policy area that can serve to highlight key pressure points in the problem. Although many published models tend to focus excessively on providing an "answer," their better role is to enhance understanding of the most important questions that deserve particular attention in clinical decision-making.

EVIDENCE-BASED MEDICINE

The "art of medicine" is traditionally defined as a practice combining medical knowledge (including scientific evidence), intuition, and judgment in the care of patients (Chap. 1). Evidence-based medicine (EBM) updates this construct by placing a much-greater emphasis on the processes by which the clinician gains knowledge of the most up-to-date and relevant clinical research. The key processes of EBM can be summarized in four steps:

1. Formulating the management question to be answered
2. Searching the literature and on-line databases for applicable research data

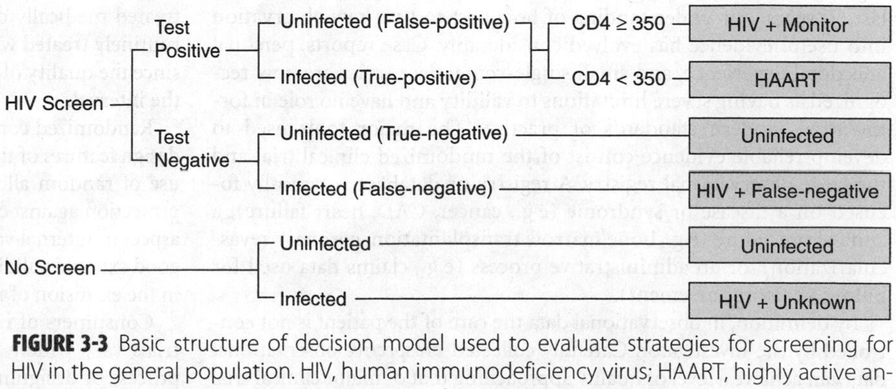

FIGURE 3-3 Basic structure of decision model used to evaluate strategies for screening for HIV in the general population. HIV, human immunodeficiency virus; HAART, highly active antiretroviral therapy. *(Figure provided courtesy of G. Sanders; with permission.)*

TABLE 3-3 SELECTED TOOLS FOR FINDING THE EVIDENCE IN EVIDENCE-BASED MEDICINE

Name	Description	Web Address	Availability
Evidence-Based Medicine Reviews	Comprehensive electronic database that combines and integrates: 1. The Cochrane Database of Systematic Reviews 2. ACP Journal Club 3. The Database of Abstracts of Reviews of Effectiveness	http://www.ovid.com	Subscription required; available through medical center libraries and other institutions
Cochrane Library	Collection of EBM databases including The Cochrane Database of Systematic Reviews—full text articles reviewing specific health care topics	http://www.cochrane.org	Subscription required; abstracts of systematic reviews available free online; some countries have funding to provide free access to all residents
ACP Journal Club	Collection of summaries of original studies and systematic reviews; published bimonthly; all data since 1991 available on Web site, updated yearly	http://www.acpjc.org	Subscription required
Clinical Evidence	Monthly updated directory of concise overviews of common clinical interventions	http://www.clinicalevidence.com	Subscription required; free access for UK and for developing countries
MEDLINE	National Library of Medicine database with citations back to 1966	http://www.nlm.nih.gov	Free via Internet

Note: ACP, American College of Physicians; EBM, evidence-based medicine.

3. Appraising the evidence gathered with regard to its validity and relevance
4. Integrating this appraisal with knowledge about the unique aspects of the patient (including preferences)

Steps 2 and 3 are the heart of EBM as it is currently used in practice. The process of searching the world's research literature and appraising the quality and relevance of studies thus identified can be quite time-consuming and requires skills and training that most clinicians do not possess. Thus, the best starting point for most EBM searches is the identification of recent systematic overviews of the problem in question (Table 3-3).

Generally, the EBM tools listed in Table 3-3 provide access to research information in one of two forms. The first, primary research reports, is the original peer-reviewed research work that is published in medical journals. Initial access to this information in an EBM search may be gained through MEDLINE, which provides access to a huge amount of data in abstract form. However, it is often difficult, using MEDLINE, to locate reports that are on point in a sea of irrelevant or unhelpful information and being reasonably certain that important reports have not been overlooked. The second form, systematic reviews, comprehensively summarizes the available evidence on a particular topic up to a certain date and provides the interpretation of the reviewer. Explicit criteria are used to find all the relevant scientific research and grade its quality. The prototype for this kind of resource is the Cochrane Database of Systematic Reviews. One of the key components of a systematic review is a meta-analysis. In the next two sections, we will review some of the major types of clinical research reports available in the literature and the process of aggregating those data into meta-analyses.

Sources of Evidence: Clinical Trials and Registries The notion of learning from observation of patients is as old as medicine itself. Over the last 50 years, our understanding of how best to turn raw observation into useful evidence has evolved considerably. Case reports, personal anecdotal experience, and small single-center case series are now recognized as having severe limitations to validity and have no role in formulating modern standards of practice. The major tools used to develop reliable evidence consist of the randomized clinical trial and the large observational registry. A registry or database is typically focused on a disease or syndrome (e.g., cancer, CAD, heart failure), a clinical procedure (e.g., bone marrow transplantation, coronary revascularization), or an administrative process (e.g., claims data used for billing and reimbursement).

By definition, in observational data the care of the patient is not controlled by the investigator. Carefully collected *prospective* observational data can achieve a level of quality approaching that of major clinical trial data. At the other end of the spectrum, data collected retrospectively (e.g., chart review) are limited in form and content to what previous observers thought was important to record, which may not serve the research question under study particularly well. Data not specifically collected for research (e.g., claims data) will often have important limitations that cannot be overcome in the analysis phase of the research. Advantages to observational data include the ability to capture a broader population than is typically represented in clinical trials. In addition, observational data are the primary source of evidence for questions where a randomized trial cannot or will not be performed. For example, it may be difficult to randomize patients to test diagnostic or therapeutic strategies that are unproven but widely accepted in practice. In addition, we cannot randomize patients to a gender, racial/ethnic group, socioeconomic status, or country of residence. We are also not willing to randomize patients to a potentially harmful intervention, such as smoking or overeating to develop obesity.

The major difference between a well-done clinical trial and a well-done prospective observational study of a particular management strategy is the lack of protection from treatment selection bias in the latter. The underlying concept in the use of observational data to compare diagnostic or therapeutic strategies is that there is enough uncertainty in practice that similar patients will be managed differently by different physicians. In short, the assumption is that there is an element of randomness (in the sense of disorder rather than in the formal statistical sense) to clinical management. In such cases, statistical models can be used to adjust for important imbalances and "level the playing field" so that a fair comparison among treatment options can be made. When management is clearly not random (e.g., all eligible left main coronary artery disease patients are referred for coronary bypass surgery), the problem may be too confounded for statistical correction, and observational data may not provide reliable evidence.

In general, use of concurrent controls is vastly preferable to historical controls. For example, comparison of current surgical management of left main coronary artery disease with left main patients treated medically during the 1970s (the last time these patients were routinely treated with medicine alone) would be extremely misleading since the quality of "medical therapy" has made huge improvements in the interval.

Randomized controlled clinical trials include the careful prospective design features of the best observational data studies but also include the use of random allocation of treatment. This design provides the best protection against confounding due to treatment selection bias (a major aspect of internal validity). However, the randomized trial may not have good external validity if the process of recruitment into the trial resulted in the exclusion of many potentially eligible subjects.

Consumers of medical evidence need to be aware that randomized trials vary widely in their quality and applicability to practice. The process of designing such a trial often involves a great many compromises. For example, trials designed to gain FDA approval for an investigational drug or device will need to address certain regulatory requirements that may result in a different trial design from what practicing clinicians would find useful.

Meta-Analysis The Greek prefix *meta* signifies something at a later or higher stage of development. Meta-analysis is research done on research data for the purpose of combining and summarizing the available evidence quantitatively. Although it can be used to combine nonrandomized studies, meta-analysis is most valuable when used to summarize all of the randomized trials on a particular therapeutic problem. Ideally, unpublished trials should be identified and included to avoid publication bias (i.e., "positive" trials are more likely to be published). Furthermore, some of the best meta-analyses obtain and analyze the raw patient-level data from the individual trials rather than working only with what is available in the published reports of each trial. Not all published meta-analyses are reliable sources of evidence on a particular problem. Their methodology must be carefully scrutinized to ensure proper study design and analysis. The results of a well-done meta-analysis are likely to be most persuasive if it includes at least several large-scale, properly performed randomized trials. In cases where the available trials are small or poorly done, meta-analysis should not be viewed as a remedy for the deficiency in primary trial data.

Meta-analyses typically focus on summary measures of relative treatment benefit, such as odds ratios or relative risks. Clinicians should also examine what absolute risk reduction (ARR) can be expected from the therapy. A useful summary metric of absolute treatment benefit is the number needed to treat (NNT) to prevent one adverse outcome event (e.g., death, stroke). NNT is simply 1/ARR. For example, if a hypothetical therapy reduced mortality over a 5-year follow-up by 33% (the relative treatment benefit) from 12% (control arm) to 8% (treatment arm), the absolute risk reduction would be 12% – 8% = 4% and the NNT = $^1/_4$ or 25. Thus, we would need to treat 25 patients for 5 years to prevent 1 death. If we applied our hypothetical treatment to a lower-risk population, say with a 6% 5-year mortality, the 33% relative treatment benefit would reduce absolute mortality by 2% (from 6 to 4%) and the NNT for the same therapy in this different group of patients would be 50. Although not always made explicit, comparisons of NNT estimates from different studies need to take account of the duration of follow-up used to create each estimate.

Clinical Practice Guidelines According to the 1990 Institute of Medicine definition, clinical practice guidelines are "systematically developed statements to assist practitioner and patient decisions about appropriate health care for specific clinical circumstances." This definition provides emphasis to several crucial features of modern guideline development. First, guidelines are created using the tools of EBM. In particular, the core of the development process is a systematic literature search followed by a review of the relevant peer-reviewed literature. Second, guidelines are usually focused around a clinical disorder (e.g., adult diabetes, stable angina pectoris) or a health care intervention (e.g., cancer screening). Third, guidelines are intended to "assist" decision-making, not to define explicitly what decisions should be made in a particular situation. The primary objective is to improve the quality of medical care by identifying areas where care should be standardized, based on compelling evidence.

Guidelines are narrative documents constructed by an expert panel whose composition is often chosen by interested professional organizations. These panels vary in the degree to which they represent all relevant stakeholders. The guideline documents consist of a series of specific management recommendations, a summary indication of the quantity and quality of evidence supporting each recommendation, and a narrative discussion of the recommendations. Many recommendations have little or no supporting evidence and, thus, reflect the expert consensus of the guideline panel. In part to protect against errors by individual panels, the final step in guideline construction is peer review, followed by a final revision in response to the critiques provided.

Guidelines are closely tied to the process of quality improvement in medicine through their identification of evidence-based best practices. Such practices can be used as quality indicators. Examples include the proportion of acute MI patients who receive aspirin upon admission to a hospital and the proportion of heart-failure patients with depressed ejection fraction who are on an ACE inhibitor. Routine measurement and reporting of such quality indicators can produce selective improvements in quality, since many physicians prefer not to be outliers.

CONCLUSIONS

In this era of EBM, it is tempting to think that all the difficult decisions practitioners face have been or soon will be solved and digested into practice guidelines and computerized reminders. However, EBM provides practitioners with an ideal rather than a finished set of tools with which to manage patients. The significant contribution of EBM has been to promote the development of more powerful and user-friendly EBM tools that can be accessed by the busy practitioners. This is an enormously important contribution that is slowly changing the way medicine is practiced. One of the repeated admonitions of EBM pioneers has been to replace reliance on the local "gray-haired expert" (who may be often wrong but is rarely in doubt) with a systematic search for and evaluation of the evidence. But EBM has not eliminated the need for subjective judgments. Each systematic review or clinical practice guideline presents the interpretation of "experts" whose biases remain largely invisible to the review's consumers. In addition, meta-analyses cannot generate evidence where there are no adequate randomized trials, and most of what clinicians confront in practice will never be thoroughly tested in a randomized trial. For the foreseeable future, excellent clinical reasoning skills and experience supplemented by well-designed quantitative tools and a keen appreciation for individual patient preferences will continue to be of paramount importance in the professional life of medical practitioners.

FURTHER READINGS

BALK EM et al: Correlation of quality measures with estimates of treatment effect in meta-analyses of randomized controlled trials. JAMA 287:2973, 2002

DEL MAR C et al: *Clinical Thinking: Evidence, Communication and Decision Making.* Malden, Mass., Blackwell, 2006

GRIMES DA et al: Refining clinical diagnosis with likelihood ratios. Lancet 365:1500, 2005

HAYNES RB et al: *Clinical Epidemiology: How to Do Clinical Practice Research.* Philadelphia, Lippincott Williams & Wilkins, 2006

PETERSON ED et al: Association between hospital process performance and outcomes among patients with acute coronary syndromes JAMA 295:1912, 2006

REILLY BM et al: Translating clinical research into clinical practice: Impact of using prediction rules to make decisions. Ann Intern Med 144:201, 2006

SANDERS GD et al: Cost-effectiveness of screening for HIV in the era of highly active antiretroviral therapy. N Engl J Med 352:570, 2005

4 Screening and Prevention of Disease

Gary J. Martin

A primary goal of health care is to prevent disease or to detect it early enough that intervention will be more effective. Strategies for disease screening and prevention are driven by evidence that testing and intervention are practical and effective. Currently most screening tests are readily available and inexpensive. Examples include tests that are biochemical (e.g., cholesterol, glucose), physiologic (e.g., blood pressure, growth curves), radiologic (e.g., mammogram, bone densitometry), or tissue specimens (e.g., Pap smear, fine-needle aspirations). In the future, it is anticipated that genetic testing will play an increasingly important role for predicting disease risk (Chap. 64). However, such tests are not widely used except for individuals at risk for high-penetrance genes based on family or ethnic history (e.g., *BRCA1*, *BRCA2*). The identification of low-penetrance but high-frequency genes that cause common disorders such as diabetes, hypertension, or macular degeneration offers the possibility of new genetic tests. However, any new screening test, whether based on genetic or other methods, must be subjected to rigorous evaluation of its sensitivity, specificity, impact on disease, and cost-effectiveness. Physicians and patients are continuously introduced to new screening tests, often in advance of complete evaluation. For example, the use of whole-body CT imaging has been advocated as a means to screen for a variety of disorders. Though appealing in concept, there is currently no evidence to justify this approach, which is associated with high cost and a substantial risk of false-positive results.

This chapter will review the basic principles of screening and prevention in the primary care setting. Recommendations for specific disorders, such as cardiovascular disease, diabetes, or cancer, are provided in the chapters dedicated to these topics.

BASIC PRINCIPLES OF SCREENING

In general, screening is most effective when applied to relatively common disorders that carry a large disease burden (Table 4-1). The five leading causes of mortality in the United States are heart diseases, malignant neoplasms, accidents, cerebrovascular diseases, and chronic obstructive pulmonary disease. Thus, many prevention strategies are targeted at these conditions. From a global health perspective, these same conditions are priorities, but malaria, malnutrition, AIDS, tuberculosis, and violence carry a heavy disease burden (Chap. 2).

A primary goal of screening is the early detection of a risk factor or disease at a stage when it can be corrected or cured. For example, most cancers have a better prognosis when identified as premalignant lesions or when they are still resectable. Similarly, early identification of hypertension or hyperlipidemia allows therapeutic interventions that reduce the long-term risk of cardiovascular or cerebrovascular events. However, early detection does not necessarily influence survival. For example, in some studies of lung cancer screening, tumors are identified at an earlier stage, but overall mortality does not differ between screened and unscreened populations. The apparent improvement in 5-year survival rates can be attributed to the detection of smaller tumors rather than a real change in clinical course after diagnosis. Similarly, the detection of prostate cancer may not lead to a mortality difference because the disease is often indolent and competing morbidities, such as coronary artery disease, may ultimately cause mortality (Chap. 78).

Disorders with a long latency period increase the potential gains associated with detection. For example, cancer of the cervix has a long latency between dysplasia and invasive carcinoma, providing an opportunity for detection by routine screening. It is hoped that the introduction of new papilloma virus vaccines will provide additional disease prevention, ultimately reducing the reliance on screening for cervical cancer. For colon cancer, an adenomatous polyp progresses to invasive cancer over 4–12 years, providing an opportunity to detect early lesions by fecal occult blood testing (FOBT) or endoscopy. On the other hand, breast cancer screening in premenopausal women is more challenging because of the relatively short interval between development of a localized breast cancer and metastasis to regional nodes (estimated to be ~12 months).

METHODS OF MEASURING HEALTH BENEFITS

It is not practical to perform all possible screening procedures. For example, screening for laryngeal cancer in smokers is not currently recommended. It is necessary to examine the strength of evidence in favor of screening measures relative to the cost and risk of false-positive tests. For example, should ultrasound be used to screen for ovarian cancer in average-risk women? It is currently estimated that the unnecessary laparotomies triggered by finding benign ovarian masses would actually cause more harm than the benefit derived from detecting the occasional curable ovarian cancer.

A variety of endpoints are used to assess the potential gain from screening and prevention interventions:

1. *The number of subjects screened to alter the outcome in one individual.* It is estimated, for example, that 731 women ages 65–69 would need to be screened by dual-energy x-ray absorptiometry (DEXA) and then treated appropriately to prevent one hip fracture from osteoporosis.
2. *The absolute and relative impact of screening on disease outcome.* A meta-analysis of Swedish mammography trials (ages 40–70) found that ~1.2 fewer women per thousand would die from breast cancer if they were screened over a 12-year period. By comparison, ~3 lives per 1000 might be saved from colon cancer in a population (ages 50–75) screened with annual FOBT over a 13-year period. Based on this analysis, colon cancer screening may actually save more women's lives than mammography. The impact of FOBT (8.8/1000 versus 5.9/1000) might be stated either as 3 lives per 1000 or as a 30% reduction in colon cancer death; thus, it is important to consider both the relative and absolute impact on numbers of lives saved.
3. *The cost per year of life saved* is used to assess the effectiveness of many screening and prevention strategies. Typically, strategies that cost <$30,000–50,000 per year of life saved are considered "cost-effective" (Chap. 3). For example, using alendronate to treat 65-year-old women with osteoporosis approaches this threshold of approximately $30,000 per year of life saved.
4. *Increase in average life expectancy for a population.* Predicted increases in life expectancy for various screening procedures are listed in Table 4-2. It should be noted, however, that the life-expectancy increase is an average that applies to a population and not to an individual. In reality, the vast majority of the screened population does not derive any benefit and possibly incurs a slight risk from false-positive results. A small subset of patients, however, will benefit greatly from being screened. For example, Pap smears do not benefit the 98% of women who never develop cancer of the cervix. However, for the 2% who would develop localized cervical cancer, Pap smears may add as much as 25 years to their lives. Some studies suggest that a 1-month gain of life expectancy is a reasonable goal for a population-based preventive strategy.

The U.S. Preventive Services Task Force (USPSTF) provides recommendations for evidence-based screening (Table 4-3). In addition to these population-based guidelines, it is reasonable to consider family and social history to identify individuals with special risk (*www.ahrq.gov/clinic/uspstfix.htm*). For example, when there is a significant family history of breast, colon, or prostate cancer, it is prudent to initiate screening about 10 years before the age when the youngest

TABLE 4-1 LIFETIME CUMULATIVE RISK

Breast cancer for women	10%
Colon cancer	6%
Cancer of the cervix for women[a]	2%
Domestic violence for women	Up to 15%
Hip fracture for Caucasian women	16%

[a]Assuming an unscreened population.

TABLE 4-2 ESTIMATED AVERAGE INCREASE IN LIFE EXPECTANCY FOR A POPULATION

Screening Procedure	Average Increase
Mammography:	
Women, 40–50 years	0–5 days
Women, 50–70 years	1 month
Pap smears, age 18–65	2–3 months
Screening treadmill for a 50-year-old (asymptomatic) man	8 days
PSA and digital rectal exam for a man >50 years	Up to 2 weeks
Getting a 35-year-old smoker to quit	3–5 years
Beginning regular exercise for a 40-year-old man (30 min 3 times a week)	9 months to 2 years

Note: PSA, prostate-specific antigen.

family member developed cancer. Screening should also be considered for many other common disorders pending the development of further evidence. Three examples are screening for diabetes (using fasting blood glucose), domestic violence, and coronary artery disease in intermediate-risk asymptomatic individuals.

Cost-Effectiveness Screening techniques must be cost-effective if they are to be applied to large populations. Costs include not only the expense of testing but also time away from work and potential risks. When the risk-to-benefit ratio is less favorable, it is useful to provide information to patients and factor their perspectives into the decision-making process. For example, many expert groups, including the USPSTF, recommend an individualized discussion about prostate cancer screening, as the decision-making process is complex and relies heavily on personal issues. Although the early detection of prostate cancer may intuitively seem desirable, risks include false-positive results that can lead to anxiety and unnecessary surgery. Potential complications from surgery and radiation treatment include erectile dysfunction, urinary incontinence, and bowel dysfunction. Some men may decline screening, while others may be more willing to accept the risks of an early-detection strategy.

TABLE 4-4 COUNSELING TO PREVENT DISEASE

Topic	Chapter Reference
Tobacco cessation	390
Drug and alcohol use	387, 388
Nutrition to maintain caloric balance and vitamin intake	70
Calcium intake in women >18 years	348
Folic acid: Women of childbearing age	71
Oral health	32
Aspirin use to prevent cardiovascular disease in selected men >40 years and women >50 years	235
Chemoprevention of breast cancer in women at high risk	86
STDs and HIV prevention	124, 182
Physical activity	
Sun exposure	57
Injury prevention (loaded handgun, seat belts, bicycle helmet)	
Issues in the elderly	9
Polypharmacy	
Fall prevention	
Hot water heater <120°	
Vision, hearing, dental evaluations	
Immunizations (pneumococcal, influenza)	

Note: STDs, sexually transmitted diseases.

Another example of shared decision-making is the choice of colon cancer screening techniques (Chap. 78). In controlled studies, the use of annual FOBT reduces colon cancer deaths by 15–30%. Flexible sigmoidoscopy reduces colon cancer deaths by ~60%. Colonoscopy offers the same, or greater, benefit than flexible sigmoidoscopy, but its use incurs additional costs and risks. These screening procedures have not been directly compared in the same population, but the estimated cost to society is similar: $10,000–25,000 per year of life saved. Thus, while one patient may prefer the ease of preparation, less time disruption, and the lower risk of flexible sigmoidoscopy, others may prefer the sedation and thoroughness of colonoscopy.

When considering the impact of screening tests, it is important to recognize that tobacco and alcohol use, diet, and exercise comprise the vast majority of factors that influence preventable deaths in developed countries. Perhaps the single greatest preventive health care measure is to help patients quit smoking (Chap. 390).

TABLE 4-3 CLINICAL PREVENTIVE SERVICES FOR NORMAL-RISK ADULTS RECOMMENDED BY THE U.S. PREVENTIVE SERVICES TASK FORCE

Test or Disorder	Population,[a] Years	Frequency	Chapter Reference
Blood pressure, height and weight	>18	Periodically	74
Cholesterol	Men > 35	Every 5 years	235
	Women > 45	Every 5 years	
Diabetes	>45 or earlier, if there are additional risk factors	Every 3 years	338
Pap smear[b]	Within 3 years of onset of sexual activity or 21–65	Every 1–3 years	78
Chlamydia	Women 18–25	Every 1–2 years	169
Mammography[a]	Women > 40	Every 1–2 years	78, 86
Colorectal cancer[a]	>50		78, 87
fecal occult blood and/or		Every year	
sigmoidoscopy or		Every 5 years	
colonoscopy		Every 10 years	
Osteoporosis	Women > 65; >60 at risk	Periodically	348
Abdominal aortic aneurysm (ultrasound)	Men 65–75 who have ever smoked	Once	
Alcohol use	>18	Periodically	387
Vision, hearing	>65	Periodically	29, 30
Adult immunization			116, 117
Tetanus-diptheria (Td)	>18	Every 10 years	
Varicella (VZV)	Susceptibles only, >18	Two doses	
Measles, mumps, rubella (MMR)	Women, childbearing age	One dose	
Pneumococcal	>65	One dose	
Influenza	>50	Yearly	
Human papillomavirus (HPV)	Up to age 26	If not done prior	

[a]Screening is performed earlier and more frequently when there is a strong family history. Randomized, controlled trials have documented that fecal occult blood testing (FOBT) confers a 15 to 30% reduction in colon cancer mortality. Although randomized trials have not been performed for sigmoidoscopy or colonoscopy, well-designed case-control studies suggest similar or greater efficacy relative to FOBT.

[b]In the future, Pap smear frequency may be influenced by HPV testing and the HPV vaccine.

Note: Prostate-specific antigen (PSA) testing is capable of enhancing the detection of early-stage prostate cancer, but evidence is inconclusive that it improves health outcomes. PSA testing is recommended by several professional organizations and is widely used in clinical practice, but it is not currently recommended by the U.S. Preventive Services Task Force (Chap. 81).

Source: Adapted from the U.S. Preventive Services Task Force, 2005. *Guide to Clinical Prevention Services*, 3d ed. *http://www.ahrq.gov/clinic/uspstfix.htm*

COMMONLY ENCOUNTERED ISSUES

Despite compelling evidence that prevention strategies can have major health care benefits, implementation of these services is challenging because of competing demands on physician and patient time and because of gaps in health care reimbursement. Moreover, efforts to reduce disease risk frequently involve behavior changes (e.g., weight loss, exercise, seatbelts) or managing addictive conditions (e.g., tobacco and alcohol use) that are often recalcitrant to intervention. Public education and economic incentives are often useful, in addition to counseling by health care providers (Table 4-4).

A number of techniques can assist the physician with the growing number of recommended screening tests. An appropriately configured electronic health record can provide reminder systems that make it easier for physicians to track and meet guidelines. Some systems provide patients with secure access to their medical records, providing an additional means to enhance adherence to routine screening. Systems that provide nurses and other staff with standing orders are effective for smoking prevention and immunizations. The Agency for Healthcare Research and Quality and the Centers for Disease Control and Prevention have developed flow sheets as part of their "Put Prevention into Practice" program (*http://www.ahcpr.gov/clinic/ppipix.htm*). Age-specific recommendations for screening and counseling are summarized in Table 4-5.

A routine health care examination should be performed every 1–3 years before age 50 and every year thereafter. History should include medication use (prescription and nonprescription), allergies, dietary history, use of alcohol and tobacco, sexual practices, and a thorough family history, if not obtained previously. Routine measurements should include assessments of height, weight (body mass index), and blood pressure, in addition to the relevant physical examination. The increasing incidence of skin cancer underscores the importance of screening for suspicious skin lesions. Hearing and vision should be tested after age 65, or earlier if the patient describes difficulties. Other gender- and age-specific examinations are listed in Table 4-3. Counseling and instruction about self-examination (e.g., skin, breast) can be provided during the routine examination.

Many patients see a physician for ongoing care of chronic illnesses, and this visit provides an opportunity to include a "measure of prevention" for other health problems. For example, the patient seen for management of hypertension or diabetes can have breast cancer screening incorporated into one visit and a discussion about colon cancer screening at the next visit. Other patients may respond more favorably to a clearly defined visit that addresses all relevant screening and prevention interventions. Because of age or comorbidities, it may be appropriate in some patients to abandon certain screening and prevention activities, although there are fewer data about when to "sunset" these services. The risk of certain cancers, like cancer of the cervix, ultimately declines, and it is reasonable to cease Pap smears after about age 65 if previous recent Pap smears have been negative. For breast, colon, and prostate cancer, it is reasonable to reevaluate the need for screening after about age 75. For some older patients with advanced diseases such as severe chronic obstructive pulmonary disease or congestive heart failure or who are immobile, the benefit of some screening procedures is low, and other priorities emerge when life expectancy is <10 years. This shift in focus needs to be done tactfully and allows greater focus on the conditions likely to impact quality and length of life.

TABLE 4-5 AGE-SPECIFIC CAUSES OF MORTALITY AND CORRESPONDING PREVENTATIVE OPTIONS

Age Group	Leading Causes of Age-Specific Mortality	Screening Prevention Interventions to Consider for Each Specific Population
15–24	1. Accident 2. Homicide 3. Suicide 4. Malignancy 5. Heart disease	• Counseling on routine seat belt use, bicycle/motorcycle/ATV helmets (1) • Counseling on diet and exercise (5) • Discuss dangers of alcohol use while driving, swimming, boating (1) • Ask about vaccination status (tetanus, diphtheria, hepatitis B, MMR, rubella, varicella, meningitis, HPV) • Ask about gun use and/or gun possession (2,3) • Assess for substance abuse history including alcohol (2,3) • Screen for domestic violence (2,3) • Screen for depression and/or suicidal/homicidal ideation (2,3) • Pap smear for cervical cancer screening, discuss STD prevention (4) • Recommend skin, breast, and testicular self-exams (4) • Recommend UV light avoidance and regular sun screen use (4) • Measurement of blood pressure, height, weight and body mass index (5) • Discuss health risks of tobacco use, consider emphasis of cosmetic and economic issues to improve quit rates for younger smokers (4,5) • *Chlamydia* screening and contraceptive counseling for sexually active females • HIV, hepatitis B, and syphilis testing if there is high-risk sexual behavior(s) or any prior history of sexually transmitted disease
25–44	1. Accident 2. Malignancy 3. Heart disease 4. Suicide 5. Homicide 6. HIV	*As above plus consider the following:* • Readdress smoking status, encourage cessation at every visit (2,3) • Obtain detailed family history of malignancies and begin early screening/prevention program if patient is at significant increased risk (2) • Assess all cardiac risk factors (including screening for diabetes and hyperlipidemia) and consider primary prevention with aspirin for patients at >3% 5-year risk of a vascular event (3) • Assess for chronic alcohol abuse, risk factors for viral hepatitis, or other risks for development of chronic liver disease • Begin breast cancer screening with mammography at age 40 (2)
45–64	1. Malignancy 2. Heart disease 3. Accident 4. Diabetes mellitus 5. Cerebrovascular disease 6. Chronic lower respiratory disease 7. Chronic liver disease and cirrhosis 8. Suicide	• Consider prostate cancer screen with annual PSA and digital rectal exam at age 50 (or possibly earlier in African Americans or patients with family history) (1) • Begin colorectal cancer screening at age 50 with either fecal occult blood testing, flexible sigmoidoscopy, or colonoscopy (1) • Reassess vaccination status at age 50 and give special consideration to vaccines against *Streptococcus pneumoniae*, influenza, tetanus, and viral hepatitis • Consider screening for coronary disease in higher risk patients (2,5)
≥65	1. Heart disease 2. Malignancy 3. Cerebrovascular disease 4. Chronic lower respiratory disease 5. Alzheimer's disease 6. Influenza and pneumonia 7. Diabetes mellitus 8. Kidney disease 9. Accidents 10. Septicemia	*As above plus consider the following:* • Readdress smoking status, encourage cessation at every visit (1,2,3) • One-time ultrasound for AAA in men 65–75 who have ever smoked • Consider pulmonary function testing for all long-term smokers to assess for development of chronic obstructive pulmonary disease (3,7) • Vaccinate all smokers against influenza and *S. pneumoniae* at age 50 (6) • Screen all postmenopausal women (and all men with risk factors) for osteoporosis • Reassess vaccination status at age 65, emphasis on influenza and *S. pneumoniae* (3,7) • Screen for dementia and depression (5) • Screen for visual and hearing problems, home safety issues, and elder abuse (9)

Note: The numbers in parentheses refer to areas of risk in the mortality column affected by the specified intervention.
Abbreviations: MMR, measles-mumps-rubella; HPV, human papilloma virus; STD, sexually transmitted disease; UV, ultraviolet; PSA, prostate-specific antigen; AAA, abdominal aortic aneurysm.

ACKNOWLEDGMENTS

The author is grateful to Dan Evans, MD, for contributions to this topic in Harrison's Manual of Medicine.

FURTHER READINGS

BARRETT-CONNOR E et al: The rise and fall of menopausal hormone therapy. Annu Rev Public Health 26:115, 2005

FENTON JJ et al: Delivery of cancer screening: How important is the preventive health examination? Arch Intern Med 167(6):580, 2007

GREENLAND P et al: Coronary artery calcium score combined with Framingham score for risk prediction in asymptomatic individuals. JAMA 291:210, 2004

RANSOHOFF DF, SANDLER RS: Clinical practice: Screening for colorectal cancer. N Engl J Med 346:40, 2002

U.S. PREVENTIVE SERVICES TASK FORCE: Clinical preventive services for normal-risk adults. Put prevention into practice. Agency for Healthcare Research and Quality, Rockville, MD, January 2003. Available at *www.ahrq.gov/ppip/adulttm.htm*

WRIGHT JC, WEINSTEIN MC: Gains in life expectancy from medical interventions—standardizing data on outcomes. N Engl J Med 339:380, 1998

5 Principles of Clinical Pharmacology

Dan M. Roden

Drugs are the cornerstone of modern therapeutics. Nevertheless, it is well recognized among physicians and among the lay community that the outcome of drug therapy varies widely among individuals. While this variability has been perceived as an unpredictable, and therefore inevitable, accompaniment of drug therapy, this is not the case. The goal of this chapter is to describe the principles of clinical pharmacology that can be used for the safe and optimal use of available and new drugs.

Drugs interact with specific target molecules to produce their beneficial and adverse effects. The chain of events between administration of a drug and production of these effects in the body can be divided into two components, both of which contribute to variability in drug actions. The first component comprises the processes that determine drug delivery to, and removal from, molecular targets. The resultant description of the relationship between drug concentration and time is termed *pharmacokinetics*. The second component of variability in drug action comprises the processes that determine variability in drug actions despite equivalent drug delivery to effector drug sites. This description of the relationship between drug concentration and effect is termed *pharmacodynamics*. As discussed further below, pharmacodynamic variability can arise as a result of variability in function of the target molecule itself or of variability in the broad biologic context in which the drug-target interaction occurs to achieve drug effects.

Two important goals of the discipline of clinical pharmacology are (1) to provide a description of conditions under which drug actions vary among human subjects; and (2) to determine mechanisms underlying this variability, with the goal of improving therapy with available drugs as well as pointing to new drug mechanisms that may be effective in the treatment of human disease. The first steps in the discipline were empirical descriptions of the influence of disease X on drug action Y or of individuals or families with unusual sensitivities to adverse drug effects. These important descriptive findings are now being replaced by an understanding of the molecular mechanisms underlying variability in drug actions. Thus, the effects of disease, drug coadministration, or familial factors in modulating drug action can now be reinterpreted as variability in expression or function of specific genes whose products determine pharmacokinetics and pharmacodynamics. Nevertheless, it is the personal interaction of the patient with the physician or other health care provider that first identifies unusual variability in drug actions; maintained alertness to unusual drug responses continues to be a key component of improving drug safety.

Unusual drug responses, segregating in families, have been recognized for decades and initially defined the field of *pharmacogenetics*. Now, with an increasing appreciation of common polymorphisms across the human genome, comes the opportunity to reinterpret descriptive mechanisms of variability in drug action as a consequence of specific DNA polymorphisms, or sets of DNA polymorphisms, among individuals. This approach defines the nascent field of *pharmacogenomics*, which may hold the opportunity of allowing practitioners to integrate a molecular understanding of the basis of disease with an individual's genomic makeup to prescribe personalized, highly effective, and safe therapies.

INDICATIONS FOR DRUG THERAPY

It is self-evident that the benefits of drug therapy should outweigh the risks. Benefits fall into two broad categories: those designed to alleviate a symptom and those designed to prolong useful life. An increasing emphasis on the principles of evidence-based medicine and techniques such as large clinical trials and meta-analyses have defined benefits of drug therapy in specific patient subgroups. Establishing the balance between risk and benefit is not always simple: for example, therapies that provide symptomatic benefits but shorten life may be entertained in patients with serious and highly symptomatic diseases such as heart failure or cancer. These decisions illustrate the continuing highly personal nature of the relationship between the prescriber and the patient.

Some adverse effects are so common and so readily associated with drug therapy that they are identified very early during clinical use of a drug. On the other hand, serious adverse effects may be sufficiently uncommon that they escape detection for many years after a drug begins to be widely used. The issue of how to identify rare but serious adverse effects (that can profoundly affect the benefit-risk perception in an individual patient) has not been satisfactorily resolved. Potential approaches range from an increased understanding of the molecular and genetic basis of variability in drug actions to expanded postmarketing surveillance mechanisms. None of these have been completely effective, so practitioners must be continuously vigilant to the possibility that unusual symptoms may be related to specific drugs, or combinations of drugs, that their patients receive.

Beneficial and adverse reactions to drug therapy can be described by a series of dose-response relations (Fig. 5-1). Well-tolerated drugs

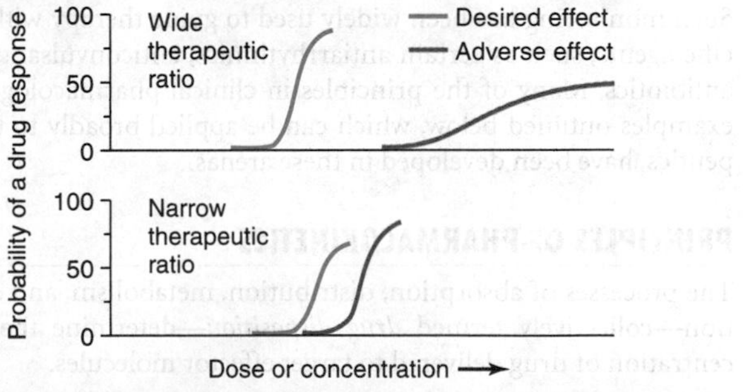

FIGURE 5-1 The concept of a therapeutic ratio. Each panel illustrates the relationship between increasing dose and cumulative probability of a desired or adverse drug effect. ***Top.*** A drug with a wide therapeutic ratio, i.e., a wide separation of the two curves. ***Bottom.*** A drug with a narrow therapeutic ratio; here, the likelihood of adverse effects at therapeutic doses is increased because the curves are not well separated. Further, a steep dose-response curve for adverse effects is especially undesirable, as it implies that even small dosage increments may sharply increase the likelihood of toxicity. When there is a definable relationship between drug concentration (usually measured in plasma) and desirable and adverse effect curves, concentration may be substituted on the abscissa. Note that not all patients necessarily demonstrate a therapeutic response (or adverse effect) at any dose, and that some effects (notably some adverse effects) may occur in a dose-independent fashion.

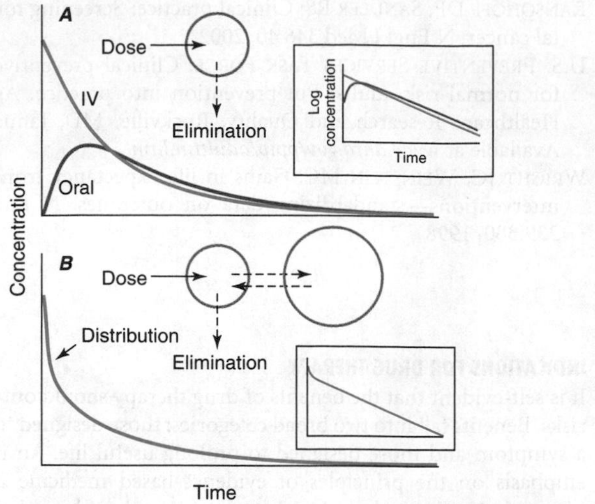

FIGURE 5-2 Idealized time-plasma concentration curves after a single dose of drug. ***A.*** The time course of drug concentration after an instantaneous IV bolus or an oral dose in the one-compartment model shown. The area under the time-concentration curve is clearly less with the oral drug than the IV, indicating incomplete bioavailability. Note that despite this incomplete bioavailability, concentration after the oral dose can be higher than after the IV dose at some time points. The inset shows that the decline of concentrations over time is linear on a log-linear plot, characteristic of first-order elimination, and that oral and IV drug have the same elimination (parallel) time course. ***B.*** The decline of central compartment concentration when drug is distributed both to and from a peripheral compartment and eliminated from the central compartment. The rapid initial decline of concentration reflects not drug elimination but distribution.

demonstrate a wide margin, termed the *therapeutic ratio, therapeutic index*, or *therapeutic window*, between the doses required to produce a therapeutic effect and those producing toxicity. In cases where there is a similar relationship between plasma drug concentration and effects, monitoring plasma concentrations can be a highly effective aid in managing drug therapy by enabling concentrations to be maintained above the minimum required to produce an effect and below the concentration range likely to produce toxicity. Such monitoring has been widely used to guide therapy with specific agents, such as certain antiarrhythmics, anticonvulsants, and antibiotics. Many of the principles in clinical pharmacology and examples outlined below, which can be applied broadly to therapeutics, have been developed in these arenas.

PRINCIPLES OF PHARMACOKINETICS

The processes of absorption, distribution, metabolism, and excretion—collectively termed *drug disposition*—determine the concentration of drug delivered to target effector molecules.

ABSORPTION

Bioavailability When a drug is administered orally, subcutaneously, intramuscularly, rectally, sublingually, or directly into desired sites of action, the amount of drug actually entering the systemic circulation may be less than with the intravenous route (Fig. 5-2*A*). The fraction of drug available to the systemic circulation by other routes is termed *bioavailability*. Bioavailability may be <100% for two reasons: (1) absorption is reduced, or (2) the drug undergoes metabolism or elimination prior to entering the systemic circulation.

When a drug is administered by a nonintravenous route, the peak concentration occurs later and is lower than after the same dose given by rapid intravenous injection, reflecting absorption from the site of administration (Fig. 5-2). The extent of absorption may be reduced because a drug is incompletely released from its dosage form, undergoes destruction at its site of administration, or has physicochemical properties such as insolubility that prevent complete absorption from its site of administration. Slow absorption is deliberately designed into "slow-release" or "sustained-release" drug formulations in order to minimize variation in plasma concentrations during the interval between doses.

"First-Pass" Effect When a drug is administered orally, it must transverse the intestinal epithelium, the portal venous system, and the liver prior to entering the systemic circulation (Fig. 5-3). Once a drug enters the enterocyte, it may undergo metabolism, be transported into the portal vein, or undergo excretion back into the intestinal lumen. Both excretion into the intestinal lumen and metabolism decrease systemic bioavailability. Once a drug passes this enterocyte barrier, it may also be taken up into the hepatocyte, where bioavailability can be further limited by metabolism or excretion into the bile. This elimination in intestine and liver, which reduces the amount of drug delivered to the systemic circulation, is termed *presystemic elimination*, or *first-pass elimination*.

Drug movement across the membrane of any cell, including enterocytes and hepatocytes, is a combination of passive diffusion and active transport, mediated by specific drug uptake and efflux molecules. The drug transport molecule that has been most widely studied is P-glycoprotein, the product of the normal expression of the *MDR1* gene. P-glycoprotein is expressed on the apical aspect of the enterocyte and on the canalicular aspect of the hepatocyte (Fig. 5-3); in both locations, it serves as an efflux pump, thus limiting availability of drug to the systemic circulation. P-glycoprotein is also an important component of the blood-brain barrier, discussed further below.

Drug metabolism generates compounds that are usually more polar and hence more readily excreted than parent drug. Metabolism takes place predominantly in the liver but can occur at other sites such as kidney, intestinal epithelium, lung, and plasma. "Phase I" metabolism involves chemical modification, most often oxidation accomplished by members of the cytochrome P450 (CYP) monooxygenase superfamily. CYPs that are especially important for drug metabolism (Table 5-1)

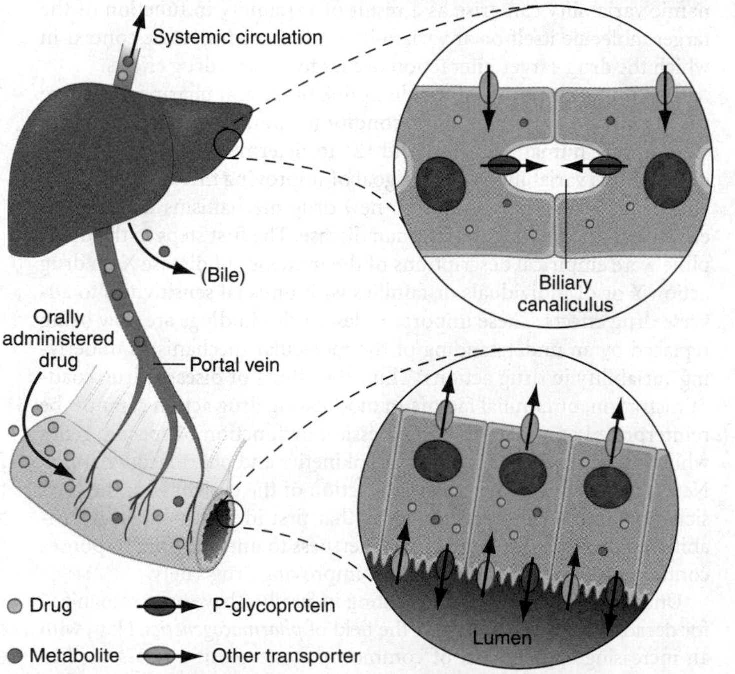

FIGURE 5-3 Mechanism of presystemic clearance. After drug enters the enterocyte, it can undergo metabolism, excretion into the intestinal lumen, or transport into the portal vein. Similarly, the hepatocyte may accomplish metabolism and biliary excretion prior to the entry of drug and metabolites to the systemic circulation. *[Adapted by permission from DM Roden, in DP Zipes, J Jalife (eds): Cardiac Electrophysiology: From Cell to Bedside, 4th ed. Philadelphia, Saunders, 2003. Copyright 2003 with permission from Elsevier.]*

TABLE 5-1 MOLECULAR PATHWAYS MEDIATING DRUG DISPOSITION

Molecule	Substrates[a]	Inhibitors[a]
CYP3A	Calcium channel blockers	Amiodarone
	Antiarrhythmics (lidocaine, quinidine, mexiletine)	Ketoconazole, itraconazole
	HMG-CoA reductase inhibitors ("statins"; see text)	Erythromycin, clarithromycin
	Cyclosporine, tacrolimus	Ritonavir
	Indinavir, saquinavir, ritonavir	
CYP2D6[b]	Timolol, metoprolol, carvedilol	Quinidine (even at ultra-low doses)
	Phenformin	Tricyclic antidepressants
	Codeine	Fluoxetine, paroxetine
	Propafenone, flecainide	
	Tricyclic antidepressants	
	Fluoxetine, paroxetine	
CYP2C9[b]	Warfarin	Amiodarone
	Phenytoin	Fluconazole
	Glipizide	Phenytoin
	Losartan	
CYP2C19[b]	Omeprazole	
	Mephenytoin	
Thiopurine S-methyltransferase[b]	6-Mercaptopurine, azathioprine	
N-acetyltransferase[b]	Isoniazid	
	Procainamide	
	Hydralazine	
	Some sulfonamides	
UGT1A1[b]	Irinotecan	
Pseudocholinesterase[b]	Succinylcholine	
P-glycoprotein	Digoxin	Quinidine
	HIV protease inhibitors	Amiodarone
	Many CYP3A substrates	Verapamil
		Cyclosporine
		Itraconazole
		Erythromycin

[a]Inhibitors affect the molecular pathway, and thus may affect substrate.
[b]Clinically important genetics variants described.
A listing of CYP substrates, inhibitors, and inducers is maintained at *http://medicine.iupui.edu/flockhart/table.htm.*

include CYP3A4, CYP3A5, CYP2D6, CYP2C9, CYP2C19, CYP1A2, and CYP2E1, and each drug may be a substrate for one or more of these enzymes. "Phase II" metabolism involves conjugation of specific endogenous compounds to drugs or their metabolites. The enzymes that accomplish phase II reactions include glucuronyl-, acetyl-, sulfo- and methyltransferases. Drug metabolites may exert important pharmacologic activity, as discussed further below.

Clinical Implications of Altered Bioavailability Some drugs undergo near-complete presystemic metabolism and thus cannot be administered orally. Nitroglycerin cannot be used orally because it is completely extracted prior to reaching the systemic circulation. The drug is therefore used by the sublingual or transdermal routes, which bypass presystemic metabolism.

Some drugs with very extensive presystemic metabolism can still be administered by the oral route, using much higher doses than those required intravenously. Thus, a typical intravenous dose of verapamil is 1–5 mg, compared to the usual single oral dose of 40–120 mg. Administration of low-dose aspirin can result in exposure of cyclooxygenase in platelets in the portal vein to the drug, but systemic sparing because of first-pass aspirin deacylation in the liver. This is an example of presystemic metabolism being exploited to therapeutic advantage.

DISTRIBUTION AND ELIMINATION

Most pharmacokinetic processes are first-order; i.e., the rate of the process depends on the amount of drug present. Clinically important exceptions are discussed below (see "Principles of Dose Selection"). In the simplest pharmacokinetic model (Fig. 5-2*A*), a drug bolus is administered instantaneously to a central compartment, from which drug elimination occurs as a first-order process. The first-order nature of drug elimination leads directly to the relationship describing drug concentration (*C*) at any time (*t*) following the bolus:

$$C = (\text{dose}/V_c) \cdot e^{(-0.69t/t_{1/2})}$$

where V_c is the volume of the compartment into which drug is delivered and $t_{1/2}$ is elimination half-life. As a consequence of this relationship, a plot of the logarithm of concentration vs time is a straight line (Fig. 5-2*A*, inset). *Half-life* is the time required for 50% of a first-order process to be complete. Thus, 50% of drug elimination is accomplished after one drug-elimination half-life, 75% after two, 87.5% after three, etc. In practice, first-order processes such as elimination are near-complete after four–five half-lives.

In some cases, drug is removed from the central compartment not only by elimination but also by distribution into peripheral compartments. In this case, the plot of plasma concentration vs time after a bolus may demonstrate two (or more) exponential components (Fig. 5-2*B*). In general, the initial rapid drop in drug concentration represents not elimination but drug distribution into and out of peripheral tissues (also first-order processes), while the slower component represents drug elimination; the initial precipitous decline is usually evident with administration by intravenous but not other routes. Drug concentrations at peripheral sites are determined by a balance between drug distribution to and redistribution from peripheral sites, as well as by elimination. Once the distribution process is near-complete (four to five distribution half-lives), plasma and tissue concentrations decline in parallel.

Clinical Implications of Half-Life Measurements The elimination half-life not only determines the time required for drug concentrations to fall to near-immeasurable levels after a single bolus; it is also the key determinant of the time required for steady-state plasma concentrations to be achieved after any change in drug dosing (Fig. 5-4). This applies to the initiation of chronic drug therapy (whether by multiple oral doses or by continuous intravenous infusion), a change in chronic drug dose or dosing interval, or discontinuation of drug.

Steady state describes the situation during chronic drug administration when the amount of drug administered per unit time equals drug eliminated per unit time. With a continuous intravenous infusion, plasma concentrations at steady state are stable, while with chronic oral drug administration, plasma concentrations vary during the dosing interval but the time-concentration profile between dosing intervals is stable (Fig. 5-4).

DRUG DISTRIBUTION

In a typical 70-kg human, plasma volume is ~3 L, blood volume is ~5.5 L, and extracellular water outside the vasculature is ~9 L. The volume of distribution of drugs extensively bound to plasma proteins but not to tissue components approaches plasma volume; warfarin is an example. By contrast, for drugs highly bound to tissues, the volume of distribution can be far greater than any physiologic space. For example, the volume of distribution of digoxin and tricyclic antidepressants is hundreds of liters, obviously exceeding total-body volume. Such drugs are not readily removed by dialysis, an important consideration in overdose.

Clinical Implications of Drug Distribution Digoxin accesses its cardiac site of action slowly, over a distribution phase of several hours. Thus,

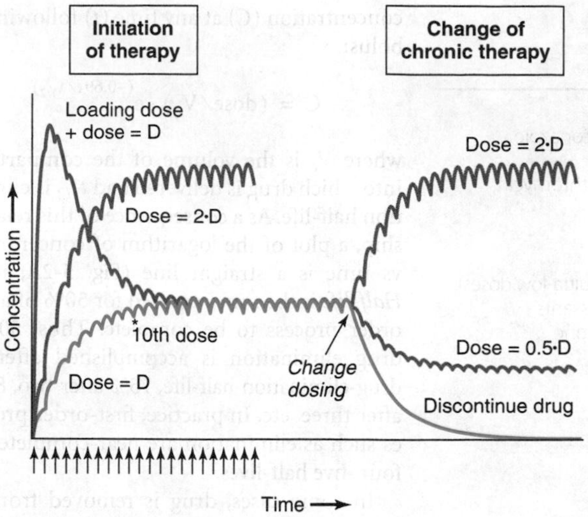

FIGURE 5-4 Drug accumulation to steady state. In this simulation, drug was administered (arrows) at intervals = 50% of the elimination half-life. Steady state is achieved during initiation of therapy after ~5 elimination half-lives, or 10 doses. A loading dose did not alter the eventual steady state achieved. A doubling of the dose resulted in a doubling of the steady state but the same time course of accumulation. Once steady state is achieved, a change in dose (increase, decrease, or drug discontinuation) results in a new steady state in ~5 elimination half-lives. *[Adapted by permission from DM Roden, in DP Zipes, J Jalife (eds): Cardiac Electrophysiology: From Cell to Bedside, 4th ed. Philadelphia, Saunders, 2003. Copyright 2003 with permission from Elsevier.]*

after an intravenous dose, plasma levels fall, but those at the site of action increase over hours. Only when distribution is near-complete does the concentration of digoxin in plasma reflect pharmacologic effect. For this reason, there should be a 6–8 h wait after administration before plasma levels of digoxin are measured as a guide to therapy.

Animal models have suggested, and clinical studies are confirming, that limited drug penetration into the brain, the "blood-brain barrier," often represents a robust P-glycoprotein–mediated efflux process from capillary endothelial cells in the cerebral circulation. Thus, drug distribution into the brain may be modulated by changes in P-glycoprotein function.

LOADING DOSES For some drugs, the indication may be so urgent that the time required to achieve steady-state concentrations may be too long. Under these conditions, administration of "loading" dosages may result in more rapid elevations of drug concentration to achieve therapeutic effects earlier than with chronic maintenance therapy (Fig. 5-4). Nevertheless, the time required for true steady state to be achieved is still determined only by elimination half-life. This strategy is only appropriate for drugs exhibiting a defined relationship between drug dose and effect.

Disease can alter loading requirements: in congestive heart failure, the central volume of distribution of lidocaine is reduced. Therefore, lower-than-normal loading regimens are required to achieve equivalent plasma drug concentrations and to avoid toxicity.

RATE OF INTRAVENOUS ADMINISTRATION Although the simulations in Fig. 5-2 use a single intravenous bolus, this is very rarely appropriate in practice because side effects related to transiently very high concentrations can result. Rather, drugs are more usually administered orally or as a slower intravenous infusion. Some drugs are so predictably lethal when infused too rapidly that special precautions should be taken to prevent accidental boluses. For example, solutions of potassium for intravenous administration >20 meq/L should be avoided in all but the most exceptional and carefully monitored circumstances. This minimizes the possibility of cardiac arrest due to accidental increases in infusion rates of more concentrated solutions.

While excessively rapid intravenous drug administration can lead to catastrophic consequences, transiently high drug concentrations after intravenous administration can occasionally be used to advantage. The use of midazolam for intravenous sedation, for example, depends upon its rapid uptake by the brain during the distribution phase to produce sedation quickly, with subsequent egress from the brain during the redistribution of the drug as equilibrium is achieved.

Similarly, adenosine must be administered as a rapid bolus in the treatment of reentrant supraventricular tachycardias (Chap. 226) to prevent elimination by very rapid ($t_{1/2}$ of seconds) uptake into erythrocytes and endothelial cells before the drug can reach its clinical site of action, the atrioventricular node.

PLASMA PROTEIN BINDING

Many drugs circulate in the plasma partly bound to plasma proteins. Since only unbound (free) drug can distribute to sites of pharmacologic action, drug response is related to the free rather than the total circulating plasma drug concentration.

Clinical Implications of Altered Protein Binding For drugs that are normally highly bound to plasma proteins (>90%), small changes in the extent of binding (e.g., due to disease) produce a large change in the amount of unbound drug, and hence drug effect. The acute-phase reactant α_1-acid glycoprotein binds to basic drugs, such as lidocaine or quinidine, and is increased in a range of common conditions, including myocardial infarction, surgery, neoplastic disease, rheumatoid arthritis, and burns. This increased binding can lead to reduced pharmacologic effects at therapeutic concentrations of total drug. Conversely, conditions such as hypoalbuminemia, liver disease, and renal disease can decrease the extent of drug binding, particularly of acidic and neutral drugs, such as phenytoin. Here, plasma concentration of free drug is increased, so drug efficacy and toxicity are enhanced if total (free + bound) drug concentration is used to monitor therapy.

CLEARANCE

When drug is eliminated from the body, the amount of drug in the body declines over time. An important approach to quantifying this reduction is to consider that drug concentration at the beginning and end of a time period are unchanged, and that a specific volume of the body has been "cleared" of the drug during that time period. This defines clearance as volume/time. Clearance includes both drug metabolism and excretion.

Clinical Implications of Altered Clearance • ***ADJUSTING DRUG DOSAGES*** While elimination half-life determines the time required to achieve steady-state plasma concentrations (C_{ss}), the *magnitude* of that steady state is determined by clearance (Cl) and dose alone. For a drug administered as an intravenous infusion, this relationship is

$$Css = \text{dosing rate}/Cl \quad \text{or} \quad \text{dosing rate} = Cl \times Css$$

When drug is administered orally, the average plasma concentration within a dosing interval ($C_{avg,ss}$) replaces C_{ss}, and bioavailability (F) must be included:

$$F \times \text{dosing rate} = Cl \times C_{avg,ss}$$

Genetic variants, drug interactions, or diseases that reduce the activity of drug-metabolizing enzymes or excretory mechanisms may lead to decreased clearance and hence a requirement for downward dose adjustment to avoid toxicity. Conversely, some drug interactions and genetic variants increase CYP expression, and hence increased drug dosage may be necessary to maintain a therapeutic effect.

THE CONCEPT OF HIGH-RISK PHARMACOKINETICS When drugs utilize a single pathway exclusively for elimination, any condition that inhibits that pathway (be it disease-related, genetic, or due to a drug interaction) can lead to dramatic changes in drug concentrations and thus increase the risk of concentration-related drug toxicity. For example, administration of drugs that inhibit P-glycoprotein reduces digoxin clearance, since P-glycoprotein is the major mediator of digoxin elimination; the risk of digoxin toxicity is high with this drug interaction unless digoxin dosages are reduced. Conversely, when drugs undergo elimination by multiple drug metabolizing or excretory pathways, absence of one pathway (due to a genetic variant or drug interaction) is much less likely to have a large impact on drug concentrations or drug actions.

ACTIVE DRUG METABOLITES

From an evolutionary point of view, drug metabolism probably developed as a defense against noxious xenobiotics (foreign substances, e.g., from plants) to which our ancestors inadvertently exposed themselves. The organization of the drug uptake and efflux pumps and the location of drug metabolism in the intestine and liver prior to drug entry to the systemic circulation (Fig. 5-3) support this idea of a primitive protective function.

However, drug metabolites are not necessarily pharmacologically inactive. Metabolites may produce effects similar to, overlapping with, or distinct from those of the parent drug. For example, *N*-acetylprocainamide (NAPA) is a major metabolite of the antiarrhythmic procainamide. While it exerts antiarrhythmic effects, its electrophysiologic properties differ from those of the parent drug. Indeed, NAPA accumulation is the usual explanation for marked QT prolongation and torsades des pointes ventricular tachycardia (Chap. 226) during therapy with procainamide. Thus, the common laboratory practice of adding procainamide to NAPA concentrations to estimate a total therapeutic effect is inappropriate.

Prodrugs are inactive compounds that require metabolism to generate active metabolites that mediate the drug effects. Examples include many angiotensin-converting enzyme (ACE) inhibitors, the angiotensin receptor blocker losartan, the antineoplastic irinotecan, and the analgesic codeine (whose active metabolite morphine probably underlies the opioid effect during codeine administration). Drug metabolism has also been implicated in bioactivation of procarcinogens and in generation of reactive metabolites that mediate certain adverse drug effects (e.g., acetaminophen hepatotoxicity, discussed below).

PRINCIPLES OF PHARMACODYNAMICS

Once a drug accesses a molecular site of action, it alters the function of that molecular target, with the ultimate result of a drug effect that the patient or physician can perceive. For drugs used in the urgent treatment of acute symptoms, little or no delay is anticipated (or desired) between the drug-target interaction and the development of a clinical effect. Examples of such acute situations include vascular thrombosis, shock, malignant hypertension, or status epilepticus.

For many conditions, however, the indication for therapy is less urgent, and a delay between the interaction of a drug with its pharmacologic target(s) and a clinical effect is common. Pharmacokinetic mechanisms that can contribute to such a delay include uptake into peripheral compartments or accumulation of active metabolites. Commonly, the clinical effect develops as a downstream consequence of the initial molecular effect the drug produces. Thus, administration of a proton-pump inhibitor or an H_2-receptor blocker produces an immediate increase in gastric pH but ulcer healing that is delayed. Cancer chemotherapy inevitably produces delayed therapeutic effects, often long after drug is undetectable in plasma and tissue. Translation of a molecular drug action to a clinical effect can thus be highly complex and dependent on the details of the pathologic state being treated. These complexities have made pharmacodynamics and its variability less amenable than pharmacokinetics to rigorous mathematical analysis. Nevertheless, some clinically important principles can be elucidated.

A drug effect often depends on the presence of underlying pathophysiology. Thus, a drug may produce no action or a different spectrum of actions in unaffected individuals compared to patients. Further, concomitant disease can complicate interpretation of response to drug therapy, especially adverse effects. For example, high doses of anticonvulsants such as phenytoin may cause neurologic symptoms, which may be confused with the underlying neurologic disease. Similarly, increasing dyspnea in a patient with chronic lung disease receiving amiodarone therapy could be due to drug, underlying disease, or an intercurrent cardiopulmonary problem. Thus the presence of chronic lung disease may alter the risk-benefit ratio in a specific patient to argue against the use of amiodarone.

The concept that a drug interacts with a specific molecular receptor does not imply that the drug effect will be constant over time, even if stable drug and metabolite concentrations are maintained. The drug-receptor interaction occurs in a complex biologic milieu that it can vary to modulate the drug effect. For example, ion channel blockade by drugs, an important anticonvulsant and antiarrhythmic effect, is often modulated by membrane potential, itself a function of factors such as extracellular potassium or local ischemia. Thus, the effects of these drugs may vary depending on the external milieu. Receptors may be up- or down-regulated by disease or by the drug itself. For example, β-adrenergic blockers upregulate β-receptor density during chronic therapy. While this effect does not usually result in resistance to the therapeutic effect of the drugs, it may produce severe agonist–mediated effects (such as hypertension or tachycardia) if the blocking drug is abruptly withdrawn.

PRINCIPLES OF DOSE SELECTION

The desired goal of therapy with any drug is to maximize the likelihood of a beneficial effect while minimizing the risk of adverse effects. Previous experience with the drug, in controlled clinical trials or in postmarketing use, defines the relationships between dose (or plasma concentration) and these dual effects and provides a starting point for initiation of drug therapy.

Figure 5-1 illustrates the relationships among dose, plasma concentrations, efficacy, and adverse effects and carries with it several important implications:

1. *The target drug effect should be defined when drug treatment is started.* With some drugs, the desired effect may be difficult to measure objectively, or the onset of efficacy can be delayed for weeks or months; drugs used in the treatment of cancer and psychiatric disease are examples. Sometimes a drug is used to treat a symptom, such as pain or palpitations, and here it is the patient who will report whether the selected dose is effective. In yet other settings, such as anticoagulation or hypertension, the desired response is more readily measurable.
2. *The nature of anticipated toxicity often dictates the starting dose.* If side effects are minor, it may be acceptable to start at a dose highly likely to achieve efficacy and downtitrate if side effects occur. However, this approach is rarely if ever justified if the anticipated toxicity is serious or life-threatening; in this circumstance, it is more appropriate to initiate therapy with the lowest dose that may produce a desired effect.
3. *The above considerations do not apply if these relationships between dose and effects cannot be defined.* This is especially relevant to some adverse drug effects (discussed in further detail below) whose development is not readily related to drug dose.
4. *If a drug dose does not achieve its desired effect, a dosage increase is justified only if toxicity is absent and the likelihood of serious toxicity is small.* For example, a small percentage of patients with strong seizure foci require plasma levels of phenytoin >20 μg/mL to control seizures. Dosages to achieve this effect may be appropriate, if tolerated. Conversely, clinical experience with flecainide suggests that levels >1000 ng/mL, or dosages >400 mg/d, may be associated with an increased risk of sudden death; thus dosage increases beyond these limits are ordinarily not appropriate, even if the higher dosage appears tolerated.

Other mechanisms that can lead to failure of drug effect should also be considered; drug interactions and noncompliance are common examples. This is one situation in which measurement of plasma drug concentrations, if available, can be especially useful. Noncompliance is an especially frequent problem in the long-term treatment of diseases such as hypertension and epilepsy, occurring in ≥25% of patients in therapeutic environments in which no special effort is made to involve patients in the responsibility for their own health. Multidrug regimens with multiple doses per day are especially prone to noncompliance.

Monitoring response to therapy, by physiologic measures or by plasma concentration measurements, requires an understanding of the relationships between plasma concentration and anticipated effects. For example, measurement of QT interval is used during treatment with sotalol or dofetilide to avoid marked QT prolongation that can herald serious arrhythmias. In this setting, evaluating the electrocardiogram at the time of anticipated peak plasma concentration and effect (e.g., 1–2 h postdose at steady state) is most appropriate. Maintained high aminoglycoside levels carry a risk of nephrotoxicity, so dosages should be adjusted on the basis of plasma concentrations measured at trough (predose). On the other hand, ensuring aminoglycoside efficacy is accomplished by adjusting dosage so that peak drug concentrations are above a minimal antibacterial concentration. For dose adjustment of other drugs (e.g., anticonvulsants), concentration should be measured at its lowest during the dosing interval, just prior to a dose at steady state (Fig. 5-4), to ensure a maintained therapeutic effect.

CONCENTRATION OF DRUGS IN PLASMA AS A GUIDE TO THERAPY

Factors such as interactions with other drugs, disease-induced alterations in elimination and distribution, and genetic variation in drug disposition combine to yield a wide range of plasma levels in patients given the same dose. Hence, if a predictable relationship can be established between plasma drug concentration and beneficial or adverse drug effect, measurement of plasma levels can provide a valuable tool to guide selection of an optimal dose. This is particularly true when there is a narrow range between the plasma levels yielding therapeutic and adverse effects, as with digoxin, theophylline, some antiarrhythmics, aminoglycosides, cyclosporine, and anticonvulsants. On the other hand, if drug access to important sites of action outside plasma is highly variable, monitoring plasma concentration may not provide an accurate guide to therapy (Fig. 5-5A).

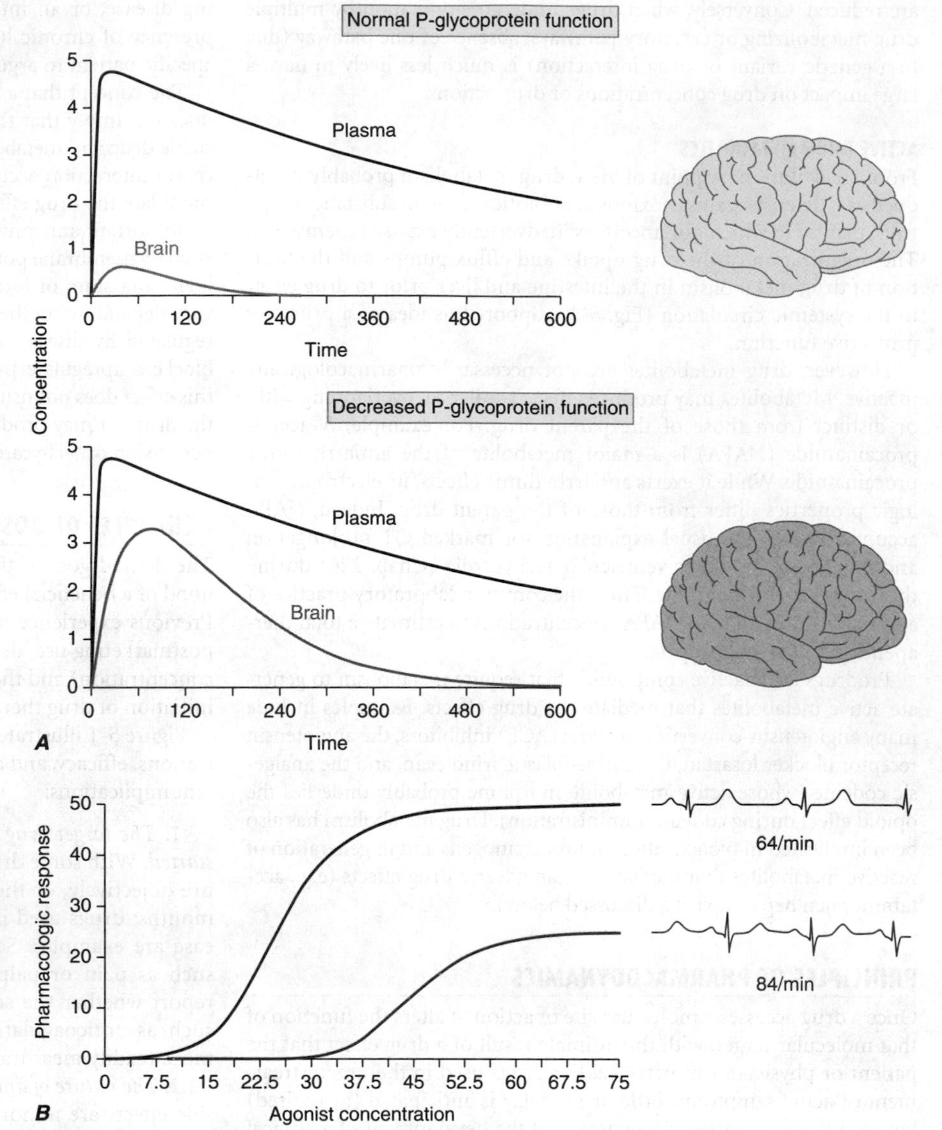

FIGURE 5-5 ***A.*** The efflux pump P-glycoprotein excludes drugs from the endothelium of capillaries in the brain, and so constitutes a key element of the blood-brain barrier. Thus, reduced P-glycoprotein function (e.g., due to drug interactions or genetically determined variability in gene transcription) increases penetration of substrate drugs into the brain, even when plasma concentrations are unchanged. ***B.*** The graph shows an effect of a β_1-receptor polymorphism on receptor function in vitro. Patients with the hypofunctional variant may display greater heart-rate slowing or blood pressure lowering on exposure to receptor blocking agents.

The common situation of first-order elimination implies that average, maximum, and minimum steady-state concentrations are related linearly to the dosing rate. Accordingly, the maintenance dose may be adjusted on the basis of the ratio between the desired and measured concentrations *at steady state*; for example, if a doubling of the steady-state plasma concentration is desired, the dose should be doubled. In some cases, elimination becomes saturated at high doses, and the process then occurs at a fixed amount per unit time (zero order). For drugs with this property (e.g., phenytoin and theophylline), plasma concentrations change disproportionately more than the alteration in the dosing rate. In this situation, changes in dose should be small to minimize the degree of unpredictability, and plasma concentration monitoring should be used to ensure that dose modification achieves the desired level.

DETERMINATION OF MAINTENANCE DOSE

An increase in dosage is usually best achieved by changing the drug dose but not the dosing interval, e.g., by giving 200 mg every 8 h instead of 100 mg every 8 h. However, this approach is acceptable only if the resulting maximum concentration is not toxic and the trough value does not fall below the minimum effective concentration for an undesirable period of time. Alternatively, the steady state may be changed by altering the frequency of intermittent dosing but not the size of each dose. In this case, the magnitude of the fluctuations around the average steady-state level will change—the shorter the dosing interval, the smaller the difference between peak and trough levels.

Fluctuation within a dosing interval is determined by the relationship between the dosing interval and the drug's half-life. If the dosing interval is equal to the drug's half-life, fluctuation is about twofold, which is usually acceptable. With drugs that have a low therapeutic ratio, dosage changes should be conservative (<50% dose change) and not more frequent than every three–four half-lives. Other drugs, such as many antihypertensives, have little dose-related toxicity, so the therapeutic ratio is large. Even if drug is eliminated rapidly, it can be given infrequently. Thus, 75 mg of captopril will result in reduced blood pressure for up to 12 h, even though captopril elimination half-life is about 2 h; this is because the dose raises the concentration of drug in plasma many times higher than the threshold for its pharmacologic effect.

EFFECTS OF DISEASE ON DRUG CONCENTRATION AND RESPONSE

RENAL DISEASE

Renal excretion of parent drug and metabolites is generally accomplished by glomerular filtration and by specific drug transporters, only now being identified. If a drug or its metabolites are primarily excreted through the kidneys and increased drug levels are associated with adverse effects, drug dosages must be reduced in patients with renal dysfunction to avoid toxicity. The antiarrhythmics dofetilide and sotalol undergo predominant renal excretion and carry a risk of QT prolongation and arrhythmias if doses are not reduced in renal disease. Thus, in end-stage renal disease, sotalol can be given as 40 mg after dialysis (every second day), compared to the usual daily dose, 80–120 mg every 12 h. The narcotic analgesic meperidine undergoes extensive hepatic metabolism, so that renal failure has little effect on its plasma concentration. However, its metabolite, normeperidine, does undergo renal excretion, accumulates in renal failure, and probably accounts for the signs of central nervous system excitation, such as irritability, twitching, and seizures, that appear when multiple doses of meperidine are administered to patients with renal disease. Protein binding of some drugs (e.g., phenytoin) may be altered in uremia, so measuring free drug concentration may be desirable.

In non-end-stage renal disease, changes in renal drug clearance are generally proportional to those in creatinine clearance, which may be measured directly or estimated from the serum creatinine (Chap. 272). This estimate, coupled with the knowledge of how much drug is normally excreted renally vs nonrenally, allows an estimate of the dose adjustment required. In practice, most decisions involving dosing adjustment in patients with renal failure use published recommended adjustments in dosage or dosing interval based on the severity of renal dysfunction indicated by creatinine clearance. Any such modification of dose is a first approximation and should be followed by plasma concentration data (if available) and clinical observation to further optimize therapy for the individual patient.

LIVER DISEASE

In contrast to the predictable decline in renal clearance of drugs in renal insufficiency, the effects of diseases like hepatitis or cirrhosis on drug disposition range from impaired to increased drug clearance, in an unpredictable fashion. Standard tests of liver function are not useful in adjusting doses. First-pass metabolism may decrease—and thus oral bioavailability increases—as a consequence of disrupted hepatocyte function, altered liver architecture, and portacaval shunts. The oral availability for high-first-pass drugs such as morphine, meperidine, midazolam, and nifedipine is almost doubled in patients with cirrhosis, compared to those with normal liver function. Therefore the size of the oral dose of such drugs should be reduced in this setting.

HEART FAILURE AND SHOCK

Under conditions of decreased tissue perfusion, the cardiac output is redistributed to preserve blood flow to the heart and brain at the expense of other tissues (Chap. 227). As a result, drugs may be distributed into a smaller volume of distribution, higher drug concentrations will be present in the plasma, and the tissues that are best perfused (the brain and heart) will be exposed to these higher concentrations. If either the brain or heart is sensitive to the drug, an alteration in response will occur. As well, decreased perfusion of the kidney and liver may impair drug clearance. Thus, in severe congestive heart failure, in hemorrhagic shock, and in cardiogenic shock, response to usual drug doses may be excessive, and dosage reduction may be necessary. For example, the clearance of lidocaine is reduced by about 50% in heart failure, and therapeutic plasma levels are achieved at infusion rates of 50% or less than those usually required. The volume of distribution of lidocaine is also reduced, so loading regimens should be reduced.

DRUG USE IN THE ELDERLY

In the elderly, multiple pathologies and medications used to treat them result in more drug interactions and adverse effects. Aging also results in changes in organ function, especially of the organs involved in drug disposition. Initial doses should be less than the usual adult dosage and should be increased slowly. The number of medications, and doses per day, should be kept as low as possible.

Even in the absence of kidney disease, renal clearance may be reduced by 35–50% in elderly patients. Dosage adjustments are therefore necessary for drugs that are eliminated mainly by the kidneys. Because muscle mass and therefore creatinine production are reduced in older individuals, a normal serum creatinine concentration can be present even though creatinine clearance is impaired; dosages should be adjusted on the basis of creatinine clearance, as discussed above. Aging also results in a decrease in the size of, and blood flow to, the liver and possibly in the activity of hepatic drug-metabolizing enzymes; accordingly, the hepatic clearance of some drugs is impaired in the elderly. As with liver disease, these changes are not readily predicted.

Elderly patients may display altered drug sensitivity. Examples include increased analgesic effects of opioids, increased sedation from benzodiazepines and other CNS depressants, and increased risk of bleeding while receiving anticoagulant therapy, even when clotting parameters are well controlled. Exaggerated responses to cardiovascular drugs are also common because of the impaired responsiveness of normal homeostatic mechanisms. Conversely, the elderly display decreased sensitivity to β-adrenergic receptor blockers.

Adverse drug reactions are especially common in the elderly because of altered pharmacokinetics and pharmacodynamics, the frequent use of multidrug regimens, and concomitant disease. For example, use of long half-life benzodiazepines is linked to the occurrence of hip fractures in elderly patients, perhaps reflecting both a risk of falls from these drugs (due to increased sedation) and the increased incidence of osteoporosis in elderly patients. In population surveys of the noninstitutionalized elderly, as many as 10% had at least one adverse drug reaction in the previous year.

GENETIC DETERMINANTS OF THE RESPONSE TO DRUGS

PRINCIPLES OF GENETIC VARIATION AND HUMAN TRAITS

(See also Chaps. 62 and 64) Variants in the human genome resulting in variation in level of expression or function of molecules important for pharmacokinetics and pharmacodynamics are increasingly recognized. These may be mutations (very rare variants, often associated with disease) or polymorphisms, variants that are much more common in a population. Variants may occur at a single nucleotide [known as single nucleotide polymorphism (SNP)] or involve insertion or deletion of one or more nucleotides. They may be in the exons (coding regions) or introns (noncoding intervening sequences). Exonic polymorphisms may or may not alter the encoded protein, and variant proteins may or may not display altered function. Similarly, polymorphisms in intronic regions may or may not alter gene expression and protein level.

As variation in the human genome is increasingly well documented, associations are being described between polymorphisms and various traits (including response to drug therapy). Some of these rely on well-developed chains of evidence, including in vitro studies demonstrating variant protein function, familial aggregation of the variant allele with the trait, and association studies in large populations. In other cases, the associations are less compelling. Identifying "real" associations is one challenge that must be overcome before the concept of genotyping to identify optimal drugs (or dosages) in individual patients prior to prescribing can be considered for widespread clinical practice. Nevertheless, the appeal of using genomic information to guide therapy is considerable.

Rates of drug efficacy and adverse effects often vary among ethnic groups. Many explanations for such differences are plausible; genomic approaches have now established that functionally important variants determining differences in drug response often display differing distributions among ethnic groups. This finding may have importance for drug use among ethnic groups, as well as in drug development.

GENETICALLY DETERMINED DRUG DISPOSITION AND VARIABLE EFFECTS

The concept that genetically determined variations in drug metabolism might be associated with variable drug levels, and hence effect, was advanced at the end of the nineteenth century, and the first exam-

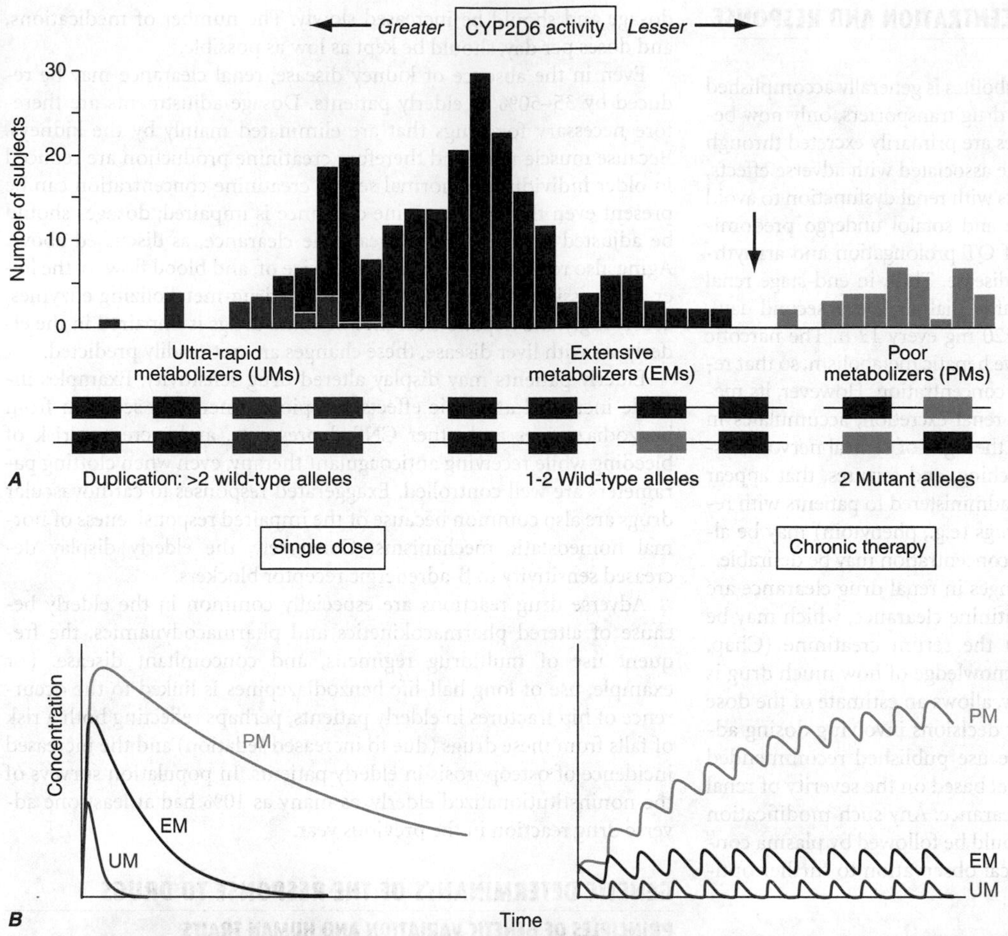

FIGURE 5-6 ***A.*** CYP2D6 metabolic activity was assessed in 290 subjects by administration of a test dose of a probe substrate and measurement of urinary formation of the CYP2D6-generated metabolite. The heavy arrow indicates a clear antimode, separating poor metabolizer subjects (PMs, green), with two loss-of-function CYP2D6 alleles, indicated by the intron-exon structures below the bar chart. Individuals with one or two functional alleles are grouped together as extensive metabolizers (EMs, blue). Also shown are ultrarapid metabolizers (UMs), with 2–12 functional copies of the gene (red), displaying the greatest enzyme activity. *(Adapted by permission from M-L Dahl et al: J Pharmacol Exp Ther 274:516, 1995.)* ***B.*** These simulations show the predicted effects of CYP2D6 genotype on disposition of a substrate drug. With a single dose (*left*), there is an inverse "gene-dose" relationship between the number of active alleles and the areas under the time-concentration curves (smallest in UM subjects; highest in PM subjects); this indicates that clearance is greatest in UM subjects. In addition, elimination half-life is longest in PM subjects. The right panel shows that these single dose differences are exaggerated during chronic therapy: steady-state concentration is much higher in PM subjects (decreased clearance), as is the time required to achieve steady state (longer elimination half-life).

ples of familial clustering of unusual drug responses due to this mechanism were noted in the mid-twentieth century. Clinically important genetic variants have been described in multiple molecular pathways of drug disposition (Table 5-1). A distinct multimodal distribution of drug disposition (as shown in Fig. 5-6) argues for a predominant effect of variants in a single gene in the metabolism of that substrate. Individuals with two alleles (variants) encoding for nonfunctional protein make up one group, often termed *poor metabolizers* (PM phenotype); many variants can produce such a loss of function, complicating the use of genotyping in clinical practice. Individuals with one functional allele make up a second (*intermediate metabolizers*) and may or may not be distinguishable from those with two functional alleles (*extensive metabolizers*, EMs). *Ultra-rapid metabolizers* with especially high enzymatic activity (occasionally due to gene duplication; Fig. 5-6) have also been described for some traits. Many drugs in widespread use can inhibit specific drug disposition pathways (Table 5-1), and so EM individuals receiving such agents can respond like PM patients (*phenocopying*). Polymorphisms in genes encoding drug uptake or drug efflux transporters may be another contributor to variability in drug delivery to target sites and, hence, drug effects. However, loss-of-function alleles in these genes have not yet been described.

CYP Variants CYP3A4 is the most abundant hepatic and intestinal CYP and is also the enzyme responsible for metabolism of the greatest number of drugs in therapeutic use. CYP3A4 activity is highly variable (up to an order of magnitude) among individuals, but the underlying mechanisms are not yet well understood. A closely related gene, encoding CYP3A5 (which shares substrates with CYP3A4), does display loss-of-function variants, especially in African-derived populations. CYP3A refers to both enzymes.

CYP2D6 is second to CYP3A4 in the number of commonly used drugs that it metabolizes. CYP2D6 is polymorphically distributed, with about 7% of European- and African-derived populations (but very few Asians) displaying the PM phenotype (Fig. 5-6). Dozens of loss-of-function variants in the CYP2D6 gene have been described; the PM phenotype arises in individuals with two such alleles. In addition, ultrapid metabolizers with multiple functional copies of the CYP2D6 gene have been identified, particularly among northern Africans.

CYP2D6 represents the main metabolic pathway for a number of drugs (Table 5-1). Codeine is biotransformed by CYP2D6 to the potent active metabolite morphine, so its effects are blunted in PMs and exaggerated in ultrarapid metabolizers. In the case of drugs with beta-blocking properties metabolized by CYP2D6, including ophthalmic timolol and the sodium channel–blocking antiarrhythmic propafenone, PM subjects display greater signs of beta blockade (including bradycardia and bronchospasm) than EMs. Further, in EM subjects, propafenone elimination becomes zero-order at higher doses; so, for example, a tripling of the dose may lead to a tenfold increase in drug concentration. The oral hypoglycemic agent phenformin was withdrawn because it occasionally caused profound lactic acidosis; this likely arose as a result of high concentrations in CYP2D6 PMs. Ultrapid metabolizers may require very high dosages of tricyclic antidepressants to achieve a therapeutic effect and, with codeine, may display transient euphoria and nausea due to very rapid generation of morphine. Tamoxifen undergoes CYP2D6-mediated biotransformation to an active metabolite, so its efficacy may be in part related to this polymorphism. In addition, the widespread use of selective serotonin reuptake inhibitors (SSRIs) to treat tamoxifen-related hot flashes may also alter the drug's effects since many SSRIs (fluoxetine, paroxetine) are also CYP2D6 inhibitors.

The PM phenotype for CYP2C19 is common (20%) among Asians and rarer (3–5%) in European-derived populations. The impact of polymorphic CYP2C19-mediated metabolism has been demonstrated with the proton pump inhibitor omeprazole, where ulcer cure rates with "standard" dosages were markedly lower in EM patients (29%) than in PMs (100%). Thus, understanding the importance of this polymorphism would have been important in developing the drug, and knowing a patient's CYP2C19 genotype should improve therapy.

There are common allelic variants of *CYP2C9* that encode proteins with loss of catalytic function. These variant alleles are associated increased rates of neurologic complications with phenytoin and of hypoglycemia with glipizide. The angiotensin-receptor blocker losartan is a prodrug that is bioactivated by CYP2C9; as a result, PMs and those receiving inhibitor drugs may display little response to therapy.

Transferase Variants One of the most extensively studied phase II polymorphisms is the PM trait for thiopurine S-methyltransferase (TPMT). TPMT bioinactivates the antileukemic drug 6-mercaptopurine. Further, 6-mercaptopurine is itself an active metabolite of the immunosuppressive azathioprine. Homozygotes for alleles encoding the inactive TPMT (1 in 300 individuals) predictably exhibit severe and potentially fatal pancytopenia on standard doses of azathioprine or 6-mercaptopurine. On the other hand, homozygotes for fully functional alleles may display less anti-inflammatory or antileukemic effect with the drugs.

N-acetylation is catalyzed by hepatic *N*-acetyl transferase (NAT), which represents the activity of two genes, *NAT-1* and *NAT-2*. Both enzymes transfer an acetyl group from acetyl coenzyme A to the drug; NAT-1 activity is generally constant, while polymorphisms in *NAT-2* result in individual differences in the rate at which drugs are acetylated and thus define "rapid acetylators" and "slow acetylators." Slow acetylators make up ~50% of European- and African-derived populations but are less common among Asians.

Slow acetylators have an increased incidence of the drug-induced lupus syndrome during procainamide and hydralazine therapy and of hepatitis with isoniazid. Induction of CYPs (e.g., by rifampin) also increases the risk of isoniazid-related hepatitis, likely reflecting generation of reactive metabolites of acetylhydrazine, itself an isoniazid metabolite.

Individuals homozygous for a common promoter polymorphism that reduces transcription of uridine diphosphate glucuronosyltransferase (*UGT1A1*) have benign hyperbilirubinemia (Gilbert's syndrome; Chap. 297). This variant has also been associated with diarrhea and increased bone marrow depression with the antineoplastic prodrug irinotecan, whose active metabolite is normally detoxified by this UGT1A1-mediated glucuronidation.

VARIABILITY IN THE MOLECULAR TARGETS WITH WHICH DRUGS INTERACT

As molecular approaches identify specific gene products as targets of drug action, polymorphisms that alter the expression or function of these drug targets—and thus modulate their actions in patients—are also being recognized. Multiple polymorphisms identified in the β_2-adrenergic receptor appear to be linked to specific phenotypes in asthma and congestive heart failure, diseases in which β_2-receptor function might be expected to determine prognosis. Polymorphisms in the β_2-receptor gene have also been associated with response to inhaled β_2-receptor agonists, while those in the β_1-adrenergic receptor gene have been associated with variability in heart rate slowing and blood pressure lowering (Fig. 5-5*B*). In addition, in heart failure, a common polymorphism in the β_1-adrenergic receptor gene has been implicated in variable clinical outcome during therapy with the beta blocker bucindolol. Response to the 5-lipoxygenase inhibitor zileuton in asthma has been linked to polymorphisms that determine the expression level of the 5-lipoxygenase gene. Herceptin, which potentiates anthracycline-related cardiotoxicity, is ineffective in breast cancers that do not express the herceptin receptor; thus, "genotyping" the tumor is a mechanism to avoid potentially toxic therapy in patients who would derive no benefit.

Drugs may also interact with genetic pathways of disease, to elicit or exacerbate symptoms of the underlying conditions. In the porphyrias, CYP inducers are thought to increase the activity of enzymes proximal to the deficient enzyme, exacerbating or triggering attacks (Chap. 352). Deficiency of glucose-6-phosphate dehydrogenase (G6PD), most often in individuals of African or Mediterranean descent, increases risk of hemolytic anemia in response to primaquine and a number of other drugs that do not cause hemolysis in patients with normal amounts of the enzyme (Chap. 101). Patients with mutations in the ryanodine receptor, which controls intracellular calcium in skeletal muscle and other tissues, may be asymptomatic until exposed to certain general anesthetics, which trigger the syndrome of malignant hyperthermia. Certain antiarrhythmics and other drugs can produce marked QT prolongation and torsades des pointes (Chap. 226), and in some patients this adverse effect represents unmasking of previously subclinical congenital long QT syndrome.

POLYMORPHISMS THAT MODULATE THE BIOLOGIC CONTEXT WITHIN WHICH THE DRUG-TARGET INTERACTIONS OCCUR

The interaction of a drug with its molecular target is translated into a clinical action in a complex biologic milieu that is itself often perturbed by disease. Thus, polymorphisms that determine variability in this biology may profoundly influence drug response, although the genes involved are not themselves directly targets of drug action. Polymorphisms in genes important for lipid homeostasis (such as the ABCA1 transporter and the cholesterol ester transport protein) modulate response to 3-hydroxymethylglutaryl-CoA (HMG-CoA) reductase inhibitors, "statins." In one large study, the combination of diuretic use combined with a variant in the adducin gene (encoding a cytoskeletal protein important for renal tubular sodium absorption) decreased stroke or myocardial infarction risk, while neither factor alone had an effect. Common polymorphisms in ion channel genes that are not themselves the target of QT-prolonging drugs may nevertheless influence the extent to which those drugs affect the electrocardiogram and produce arrhythmias. These findings not only point to new mechanisms for understanding drug action, but also can be used for drug development. For example, a set of polymorphisms in the gene encoding 5-lipoxygenase activating protein (FLAP) has been identified as a risk factor for myocardial infarction in an Icelandic population, and an initial clinical trial of a FLAP inhibitor was conducted only in subjects with the high risk allele.

MULTIPLE VARIANTS MODULATING DRUG EFFECTS

As this discussion makes clear, for each drug with a defined mechanism of action and disposition pathways, a set of "candidate genes," in which polymorphisms may mediate variable clinical responses, can be identified. Indeed, polymorphisms in multiple genes have been associated with variability in the effect of a single drug. CYP2C9 loss-of-function variants are associated with a requirement for lower maintenance doses of the vitamin K antagonist anticoagulant warfarin. In rarer (<2%) individuals homozygous for these variant alleles, maintenance warfarin dosages may be difficult to establish, and the risk of bleeding complications appears increased. In addition to *CYP2C9*, variants in the promoter region of *VKORC1*, encoding a vitamin K epoxide reductase, predict warfarin dosages; these promoter variants are in tight *linkage disequilibrium*, i.e. genotyping at one polymorphic site within this *haplotype block* provides reliable information on the identity of genotypes at other linked sites (Chap. 62). Thus, variability in response to warfarin can be linked to both coding region polymorphisms in CYP2C9 and promoter haplotypes in the warfarin target *VKORC1*.

As genotyping technologies improve and data sets of patients with well-documented drug responses are accumulated, it is becoming possible to interrogate hundreds of polymorphisms in dozens of candidate genes. This approach has been applied to implicate linked noncoding polymorphisms in the HMG-CoA reductase gene as predicting efficacy of HMG-CoA reductase inhibitors, and in variants in the gene-encoding corticotrophin-releasing hormone receptor 1 as predicting efficacy of inhaled steroids in asthma.

Technologies are now evolving to interrogate hundreds of thousands of SNPs across the genome, or to rapidly resequence each patient's genome. These approaches, which have been applied to identify new genes modulating disease susceptibility (Chap. 62), may be applicable to the problem of identifying genomic predictors of variable drug effects.

PROSPECTS FOR INCORPORATING GENETIC INFORMATION INTO CLINICAL PRACTICE

The examples of associations between specific genotypes and drug responses raise the tantalizing prospect that patients will undergo routine genotyping for loci known to modulate drug levels or response prior to receiving a prescription. Indeed, clinical tests for some of the polymorphisms described above, including those in *TPMT*, *UGT1A1*, *CYP2D6*, and *CYP2C19*, have been approved by the U.S. Food and Drug Administration (FDA). The twin goals are to identify patients likely to exhibit adverse effects and those most likely to respond well. Obstacles that must be overcome before this vision becomes a reality include replication of even the most compelling associations, demonstrations of cost-effectiveness, development of readily useable genotyping technologies, and ethical issues involved in genotyping. While these barriers seem daunting, the field is very young and evolving rapidly. Indeed, one major result of understanding of the role of genetics in drug action has been improved screening of drugs during the development process to reduce the likelihood of highly variable metabolism or unanticipated toxicity (such as torsades des pointes).

TABLE 5-2 DRUGS WITH A HIGH RISK OF GENERATING PHARMACOKINETIC INTERACTIONS

Drug	Mechanism	Examples
Antacids Bile acid sequestrants	Reduced absorption	Antacids/tetracyclines Cholestryamine/digoxin
Proton pump inhibitors H_2-receptor blockers	Altered gastric pH	Ketoconazole absorption decreased
Rifampin Carbamazepine Barbiturates Phenytoin St. John's wort Glutethimide	Induction of hepatic metabolism	Decreased concentration and effects of warfarin quinidine cyclosporine losartan oral contraceptives methadone
Tricyclic antidepressants Fluoxetine Quinidine	Inhibitors of CYP2D6	Increased β-blockade Decreased codeine effect
Cimetidine	Inhibitor of multiple CYPs	Increased concentration and effects of warfarin theophylline phenytoin
Ketoconazole, itraconazole Erythromycin, clarithromycin Calcium channel blockers Ritonavir	Inhibitor of CYP3A	Increased concentration and toxicity of some HMG-CoA reductase inhibitors cyclosporine cisapride, terfenadine (now withdrawn) Increased concentration and effects of indinavir (with ritonavir) Decreased clearance and dose requirement for cyclosporine (with calcium channel blockers)
Allopurinol	Xanthine oxidase inhibitor	Azathioprine and 6-mercaptopurine toxicity
Amiodarone	Inhibitor of many CYPs and of P-glycoprotein	Decreased clearance (risk of toxicity) for warfarin digoxin quinidine
Gemfibrazol (and other fibrates)	CYP3A inhibition	Rhabdomyolysis when co-prescribed with some HMG-CoA reductase inhibitors
Quinidine Amiodarone Verapamil Cyclosporine Itraconazole Erythromycin	P-glycoprotein inhibition	Risk of digoxin toxicity
Phenylbutazone Probenecid Salicylates	Inhibition of renal tubular transport	Salicylates → increased risk of methotrexate toxicity

INTERACTIONS BETWEEN DRUGS

Drug interactions can complicate therapy by increasing or decreasing the action of a drug; interactions may be based on changes in drug disposition or in drug response in the absence of changes in drug levels. *Interactions must be considered in the differential diagnosis of any unusual response occurring during drug therapy.* Prescribers should recognize that patients often come to them with a legacy of drugs acquired during previous medical experiences, often with multiple physicians who may not be aware of all the patient's medications. A meticulous drug history should include examination of the patient's medications and, if necessary, calls to the pharmacist to identify prescriptions. It should also address the use of agents not often volunteered during questioning, such as over-the-counter (OTC) drugs, health food supplements, and topical agents such as eye drops. Lists of interactions are available from a number of electronic sources. While it is unrealistic to expect the practicing physician to memorize these, certain drugs consistently run the risk of generating interactions, often by inhibiting or inducing specific drug elimination pathways. Examples are presented below and in Table 5-2. Accordingly, when these drugs are started or stopped, prescribers must be especially alert to the possibility of interactions.

PHARMACOKINETIC INTERACTIONS CAUSING DECREASED DRUG EFFECTS

Gastrointestinal absorption can be reduced if a drug interaction results in drug binding in the gut, as with aluminum-containing antacids, kaolin-pectin suspensions, or bile acid sequestrants. Drugs such as histamine H_2 receptor antagonists or proton pump inhibitors that alter gastric pH may decrease the solubility and hence absorption of weak bases such as ketoconazole.

Expression of some genes responsible for drug elimination, notably *CYP3A* and *MDR1*, can be markedly increased by "inducing" drugs, such as rifampin, carbamazepine, phenytoin, St. John's wort, and glutethimide and by smoking, exposure to chlorinated insecticides such as DDT (CYP1A2), and chronic alcohol ingestion. Administration of inducing agents lowers plasma levels over 2–3 weeks as gene expression is increased. If a drug dose is stabilized in the presence of an inducer that is subsequently stopped, major toxicity can occur as clearance returns to preinduction levels and drug concentrations rise. Individuals vary in the extent to which drug metabolism can be induced, likely through genetic mechanisms.

Interactions that inhibit the bioactivation of prodrugs will similarly decrease drug effects. The analgesic effect of codeine depends on its metabolism to morphine via CYP2D6. Thus, the CYP2D6 inhibitor quinidine reduces the analgesic efficacy of codeine in EMs.

Interactions that decrease drug delivery to intracellular sites of action can decrease drug effects: tricyclic antidepressants can blunt the antihypertensive effect of clonidine by decreasing its uptake into adrenergic neurons. Reduced CNS penetration of multiple HIV protease inhibitors (with the attendant risk of facilitating viral replication in a sanctuary site) appears attributable to P-glycoprotein-mediated exclusion of the drug from the CNS; indeed, inhibition of P-glycoprotein has been proposed as a therapeutic approach to enhance drug entry to the CNS (Fig. 5-5A).

PHARMACOKINETIC INTERACTIONS CAUSING INCREASED DRUG EFFECTS

The most common mechanism here is inhibition of drug elimination. In contrast to induction, new protein synthesis is not involved, and the effect develops as drug and any inhibitor metabolites accumulate (a function of their elimination half-lives). Since shared substrates of a single enzyme can compete for access to the active site of the protein, many CYP substrates can also be considered inhibitors. However, some drugs are especially potent as inhibitors (and occasionally may not even be substrates) of specific drug-elimination pathways, and so it is in the use of these agents that clinicians must be most alert to the potential for interactions (Table 5-2). Commonly implicated interacting drugs of this type include cimetidine, erythromycin and some other macrolide antibiotics (clarithromycin but not azithromycin), ketoconazole and other azole antifungals, the antiretroviral agent ritonavir, and high concentrations of grapefruit juice (Table 5-2). The consequences of such interactions will depend on the drug whose elimination is being inhibited; high-risk drugs are those for which alternate pathways of elimination are not available and for which drug accumulation increases the risk of serious toxicity (see "The Concept of High-Risk Pharmacokinetics," above). Examples include CYP3A inhibitors increasing the risk of cyclosporine toxicity or of rhabdomyolysis with some HMG-CoA reductase inhibitors (lovastatin, simvastatin, atorvastatin), and P-glycoprotein inhibitors increasing risk of digoxin toxicity.

Phenytoin, an inducer of many systems, including CYP3A, inhibits CYP2C9. CYP2C9 metabolism of losartan to its active metabolite is inhibited by phenytoin, with potential loss of antihypertensive effect.

The antiviral ritonavir is a very potent CYP3A4 inhibitor that has been added to anti-HIV regimens, not because of its antiviral effects but because it decreases clearance, and hence increases efficacy, of other anti-HIV agents. Grapefruit (but not orange) juice inhibits CYP3A, especially at high doses; patients receiving drugs where even modest CYP3A inhibition may increase the risk of adverse effects (e.g., cyclosporine, some HMG-CoA reductase inhibitors) should therefore avoid grapefruit juice.

CYP2D6 is markedly inhibited by quinidine, a number of neuroleptic drugs (chlorpromazine and haloperidol), and the SSRIs fluoxetine and paroxetine. Clinical consequences of fluoxetine's interaction with CYP2D6 substrates may not be apparent for weeks after the drug is started, because of its very long half-life and slow generation of a CYP2D6-inhibiting metabolite.

6-Mercaptopurine, the active metabolite of azathioprine, is metabolized not only by TPMT but also by xanthine oxidase. When allopurinol, a potent inhibitor of xanthine oxidase, is administered with standard doses of azathioprine or 6-mercaptopurine, life-threatening toxicity (bone marrow suppression) can result.

A number of drugs are secreted by the renal tubular transport systems for organic anions. Inhibition of these systems can cause excessive drug accumulation. Salicylate, for example, reduces the renal clearance of methotrexate, an interaction that may lead to methotrexate toxicity. Renal tubular secretion contributes substantially to the elimination of penicillin, which can be inhibited (to increase its therapeutic effect) by probenecid. Similarly, inhibition of the tubular cation transport system by cimetidine decreases the renal clearance of dofetilide and of procainamide and its active metabolite NAPA.

DRUG INTERACTIONS NOT MEDIATED BY CHANGES IN DRUG DISPOSITION

Drugs may act on separate components of a common process to generate effects greater than either has alone. Antithrombotic therapy with combinations of antiplatelet agents (glycoprotein IIb/IIIa inhibitors, aspirin, clopidogrel) and anticoagulants (warfarin, heparins) are often used in the treatment of vascular disease, although such combinations carry an increased risk of bleeding.

Nonsteroidal anti-inflammatory drugs (NSAIDs) cause gastric ulcers, and in patients treated with warfarin, the risk of bleeding from a peptic ulcer is increased almost threefold by concomitant use of an NSAID.

Indomethacin, piroxicam, and probably other NSAIDs antagonize the antihypertensive effects of β-adrenergic receptor blockers, diuretics, ACE inhibitors, and other drugs. The resulting elevation in blood pressure ranges from trivial to severe. This effect is not seen with aspirin and sulindac but has been found with the cyclooxygenase 2 (COX-2) inhibitor celecoxib.

Torsades des pointes during administration of QT-prolonging antiarrhythmics (quinidine, sotalol, dofetilide) occur much more frequently in patients receiving diuretics, probably reflecting hypokalemia. In vitro, hypokalemia not only prolongs the QT interval in the absence of drug but also potentiates drug block of ion channels that results in QT prolongation. Also, some diuretics have direct electrophysiologic actions that prolong QT.

The administration of supplemental potassium leads to more frequent and more severe hyperkalemia when potassium elimination is reduced by concurrent treatment with ACE inhibitors, spironolactone, amiloride, or triamterene.

The pharmacologic effects of sildenafil result from inhibition of the phosphodiesterase type 5 isoform that inactivates cyclic GMP in the vasculature. Nitroglycerin and related nitrates used to treat angina produce vasodilation by elevating cyclic GMP. Thus, coadministration of these nitrates with sildenafil can cause profound hypotension, which can be catastrophic in patients with coronary disease.

Sometimes, combining drugs can increase overall efficacy and/or reduce drug-specific toxicity. Such therapeutically useful interactions are described in chapters dealing with specific disease entities, elsewhere in this text.

ADVERSE REACTIONS TO DRUGS

The beneficial effects of drugs are coupled with the inescapable risk of untoward effects. The morbidity and mortality from these untoward effects often present diagnostic problems because they can involve every organ and system of the body; these may be mistaken for signs of underlying disease.

Adverse reactions can be classified in two broad groups. One type results from exaggeration of an intended pharmacologic action of the drug, such as increased bleeding with anticoagulants or bone marrow suppression with antineoplastics. The other type of adverse reactions ensues from toxic effects unrelated to the intended pharmacologic actions. The latter effects are often unanticipated (especially with new drugs) and frequently severe and result from recognized as well as undiscovered mechanisms.

Drugs may increase the frequency of an event that is common in a general population, and this may be especially difficult to recognize; the increase in myocardial infarctions with the COX-2 inhibitor rofecoxib is an excellent example. Drugs can also cause rare and serious adverse effects, such as hematologic abnormalities, arrhythmias, or hepatic or renal dysfunction. Prior to regulatory approval and marketing, new drugs are tested in relatively few patients who tend to be less sick and to have fewer concomitant diseases than those patients who subsequently receive the drug therapeutically. Because of the relatively small number of patients studied in clinical trials and the selected nature of these patients, rare adverse effects are generally not detected prior to a drug's approval, and physicians therefore need to be cautious in the prescription of new drugs and alert for the appearance of previously unrecognized adverse events.

Elucidating mechanisms underlying adverse drug effects can assist development of safer compounds or allow a patient subset at especially high risk to be excluded from drug exposure. National adverse reaction reporting systems, such as those operated by the FDA (suspected adverse reactions can be reported online at *http://www.fda.gov/medwatch/report/hcp.htm*) and the Committee on Safety of Medicines in Great Britain, can prove useful. The publication or reporting of a newly recognized adverse reaction can in a short time stimulate many similar such reports of reactions that previously had gone unrecognized.

Occasionally, "adverse" effects may be exploited to develop an entirely new indication for a drug. Unwanted hair growth during minoxidil treatment of severely hypertensive patients led to development of the drug for hair growth. Sildenafil was initially developed as an antianginal, but its effects to alleviate erectile dysfunction not only led to a new drug indication but also to increased understanding of the role of type 5 phosphodiesterase in erectile tissue. These examples further reinforce the concept that prescribers must remain vigilant to the possibility that unusual symptoms may reflect unappreciated drug effects.

Some 25–50% of patients make errors in self-administration of prescribed medicines, and these errors can be responsible for adverse drug effects. Similarly, patients commit errors in taking OTC drugs by not reading or following the directions on the containers. Physicians must recognize that providing directions with prescriptions does not always guarantee compliance.

In hospital, drugs are administered in a controlled setting, and patient compliance is, in general, ensured. Errors may occur nevertheless—the wrong drug or dose may be given or the drug may be given to the wrong patient—and improved drug distribution and administration systems are addressing this problem.

EPIDEMIOLOGY

Patients receive, on average, 10 different drugs during each hospitalization. The sicker the patient, the more drugs are given, and there is a corresponding increase in the likelihood of adverse drug reactions. When <6 different drugs are given to hospitalized patients, the probability of an adverse reaction is ~5%, but if >15 drugs are given, the probability is >40%. Retrospective analyses of ambulatory patients have revealed adverse drug effects in 20%. Serious adverse reactions are also well recognized with "herbal" remedies and OTC compounds: examples include kava-associated hepatotoxicity, L-tryptophan-associated eosinophilia-myalgia, and phenylpropanolamine-associated stroke, each of which has caused fatalities.

A small group of widely used drugs accounts for a disproportionate number of reactions. Aspirin and other NSAIDs, analgesics, digoxin, anticoagulants, diuretics, antimicrobials, glucocorticoids, antineoplastics, and hypoglycemic agents account for 90% of reactions, although the drugs involved differ between ambulatory and hospitalized patients.

TOXICITY UNRELATED TO A DRUG'S PRIMARY PHARMACOLOGIC ACTIVITY

Cytotoxic Reactions Drugs or more commonly reactive metabolites generated by CYPs can covalently bind to tissue macromolecules (such as proteins or DNA) to cause tissue toxicity. Because of the reactive nature of these metabolites, covalent binding often occurs close to the site of production, typically the liver.

The most common cause of drug-induced hepatotoxicity is acetaminophen overdosage. Normally, reactive metabolites are detoxified by combining with hepatic glutathione. When glutathione becomes exhausted, the metabolites bind instead to hepatic protein, with resultant hepatocyte damage. The hepatic necrosis produced by the ingestion of acetaminophen can be prevented or attenuated by the administration of substances such as *N*-acetylcysteine that reduce the binding of electrophilic metabolites to hepatic proteins. The risk of acetaminophen-related hepatic necrosis is increased in patients receiving drugs such as phenobarbital or phenytoin that increase the rate of drug metabolism or ethanol that exhaust glutathione stores. Such toxicity has even occurred with therapeutic dosages, so patients at risk through these mechanisms should be warned.

Immunologic Mechanisms Most pharmacologic agents are small molecules with low molecular weights (<2000) and thus are poor immunogens. Generation of an immune response to a drug therefore usually requires in vivo activation and covalent linkage to protein, carbohydrate, or nucleic acid.

Drug stimulation of antibody production may mediate tissue injury by several mechanisms. The antibody may attack the drug when the drug is covalently attached to a cell and thereby destroy the cell. This occurs in penicillin-induced hemolytic anemia. Antibody-drug-antigen complexes may be passively adsorbed by a bystander cell, which is then destroyed by activation of complement; this occurs in quinine- and quinidine-induced thrombocytopenia. Heparin-induced thrombocytopenia arises when antibodies against complexes of platelet factor 4 peptide and heparin generate immune complexes that activate platelets; thus, the thrombocytopenia is accompanied by "paradoxical" thrombosis and is treated with thrombin inhibitors. Drugs or their reactive metabolites may alter a host tissue, rendering it antigenic and eliciting autoantibodies. For example, hydralazine and procainamide (or their reactive metabolites) can chemically alter nuclear material, stimulating the formation of antinuclear antibodies and occasionally causing lupus erythematosus. Drug-induced pure red cell aplasia (Chap. 102) is due to an immune-based drug reaction. Red cell formation in bone marrow cultures can be inhibited by phenytoin and purified IgG obtained from a patient with pure red cell aplasia associated with phenytoin.

Serum sickness (Chap. 311) results from the deposition of circulating drug-antibody complexes on endothelial surfaces. Complement activation occurs, chemotactic factors are generated locally, and an inflammatory response develops at the site of complex entrapment. Arthralgias, urticaria, lymphadenopathy, glomerulonephritis, or cerebritis may result. Foreign proteins (vaccines, streptokinase, therapeutic antibodies) and antibiotics are common causes. Many drugs, particularly antimicrobial agents, ACE inhibitors, and aspirin, can elicit anaphylaxis with production of IgE, which binds to mast cell membranes. Contact with a drug antigen initiates a series of biochemical events in the mast cell and results in the release of mediators that can produce the characteristic urticaria, wheezing, flushing, rhinorrhea, and (occasionally) hypotension.

Drugs may also elicit cell-mediated immune responses. Topically administered substances may interact with sulfhydryl or amino groups in the skin and react with sensitized lymphocytes to produce the rash characteristic of contact dermatitis. Other types of rashes may also result from the interaction of serum factors, drugs, and sensitized lymphocytes.

DIAGNOSIS AND TREATMENT OF ADVERSE DRUG REACTIONS

The manifestations of drug-induced diseases frequently resemble those of other diseases, and a given set of manifestations may be produced by different and dissimilar drugs. Recognition of the role of a drug or drugs in an illness depends on appreciation of the possible adverse reactions to drugs in any disease, on identification of the temporal relationship between drug administration and development of the illness, and on familiarity with the common manifestations of the drugs. Many associations between particular drugs and specific reactions have been described, but there is always a "first time" for a novel association, and any drug should be suspected of causing an adverse effect if the clinical setting is appropriate.

Illness related to a drug's intended pharmacologic action is often more easily recognized than illness attributable to immune or other mechanisms. For example, side effects such as cardiac arrhythmias in patients receiving digitalis, hypoglycemia in patients given insulin, and bleeding in patients receiving anticoagulants are more readily related to a specific drug than are symptoms such as fever or rash, which may be caused by many drugs or by other factors.

Electronic sources of adverse drug reactions can be useful. However, exhaustive compilations often provide little sense of perspective in terms of frequency and seriousness, which can vary considerably among patients.

Eliciting a drug history from patients is important for diagnosis. Attention must be directed to OTC drugs and herbal preparations as well as to prescription drugs. Each type can be responsible for adverse drug effects, and adverse interactions may occur between OTC drugs and prescribed drugs. Loss of efficacy of oral contraceptives or cyclosporine by concurrent use of St. John's wort are examples. In addition, it is common for patients to be cared for by several physicians, and duplicative, additive, counteractive, or synergistic drug combinations may therefore be administered if the physicians are not aware of the patients' drug histories. Every physician should determine what drugs a patient has been taking, for the previous month or two ideally, before prescribing any medications. Medications stopped for inefficacy or adverse effects should be documented to avoid pointless and potentially dangerous reexposure. A frequently overlooked source of additional drug exposure is topical therapy; for example, a patient complaining of bronchospasm may not mention that an ophthalmic beta blocker is being used unless specifically asked. A history of previous adverse drug effects in patients is common. Since these patients have shown a predisposition to drug-induced illnesses, such a history should dictate added caution in prescribing drugs.

Laboratory studies may include demonstration of serum antibody in some persons with drug allergies involving cellular blood elements, as in agranulocytosis, hemolytic anemia, and thrombocytopenia. For example, both quinine and quinidine can produce platelet agglutination in vitro in the presence of complement and the serum from a patient who has developed thrombocytopenia following use of this drug. Biochemical abnormalities such as G6PD deficiency, serum pseudocholinesterase level, or genotyping may also be useful in diagnosis, often after an adverse effect has occurred in the patient or a family member.

Once an adverse reaction is suspected, discontinuation of the suspected drug followed by disappearance of the reaction is presumptive evidence of a drug-induced illness. Confirming evidence may be sought by cautiously reintroducing the drug and seeing if the reaction reappears. However, that should be done only if confirmation would be useful in the future management of the patient and if the attempt would not entail undue risk. With concentration-dependent adverse reactions, lowering the dosage may cause the reaction to disappear, and raising it may cause the reaction to reappear. When the reaction is thought to be allergic, however, readministration of the drug may be hazardous, since anaphylaxis may develop. Readministration is unwise under these conditions unless no alternative drugs are available and treatment is necessary.

If the patient is receiving many drugs when an adverse reaction is suspected, the drugs likeliest to be responsible can usually be identified; this should include both potential culprit agents as well as drugs that alter their elimination. All drugs may be discontinued at once or, if this is not practical, discontinued one at a time, starting with the ones most suspect, and the patient observed for signs of improvement. The time needed for a concentration-dependent adverse effect to disappear depends on the time required for the concentration to fall below the range associated with the adverse effect; that, in turn, depends on the initial blood level and on the rate of elimination or metabolism of the drug. Adverse effects of drugs with long half-lives or those not directly related to serum concentration may take a considerable time to disappear.

SUMMARY

Modern clinical pharmacology aims to replace empiricism in the use of drugs with therapy based on in-depth understanding of factors that determine an individual's response to drug treatment. Molecular pharmacology, pharmacokinetics, genetics, clinical trials, and the educated prescriber all contribute to this process. No drug response should ever be termed *idiosyncratic*; all responses have a mechanism whose understanding will help guide further therapy with that drug or successors. This rapidly expanding understanding of variability in drug actions makes the process of prescribing drugs increasingly daunting for the practitioner. However, fundamental principles should guide this process:

- The benefits of drug therapy, however defined, should always outweigh the risk.
- The smallest dosage necessary to produce the desired effect should be used.
- The number of medications and doses per day should be minimized.
- Although the literature is rapidly expanding, accessing it is becoming easier; tools such as computers and hand-held devices to search databases of literature and unbiased opinion will become increasingly commonplace.
- Genetics play a role in determining variability in drug response and may become a part of clinical practice.
- Prescribers should be particularly wary when adding or stopping specific drugs that are especially liable to provoke interactions and adverse reactions.
- Prescribers should use only a limited number of drugs, with which they are thoroughly familiar.

FURTHER READINGS

BAILEY DG, DRESSER GK: Interactions between grapefruit juice and cardiovascular drugs. Am J Cardiovasc Drugs 4:281, 2004

CHASMAN DI et al: Pharmacogenetic study of statin therapy and cholesterol reduction. JAMA 291:2821, 2004

EICHELBAUM M et al: Pharmacogenomics and individualized drug therapy. Annu Rev Med 57:119, 2006

GURWITZ JH: Serious adverse drug effects—Seeing the trees through the forest. N Engl J Med 354:1413, 2006

HAKONARSON H et al: Effects of a 5-lipoxygenase-activating protein inhibitor on biomarkers associated with risk of myocardial infarction: a randomized trial. JAMA 293:2245, 2005

JOHNSON JA, TURNER ST: Hypertension pharmacogenomics: Current status and future directions. Curr Opin Mol Ther 7:218, 2005

KIM RB: Transporters and drug discovery: Why, when, and how. Mol Pharm 3:26, 2006

LIGGETT SB et al: A polymorphism within a conserved β_1-adrenergic receptor motif alters cardiac function and β-blocker response in human heart failure. Proc Natl Acad Sci USA 103:11288–11293, 2006

NAVARRO VJ, SENIOR JR: Drug-related hepatotoxicity. N Engl J Med 354:731, 2006

PIRMOHAMED M et al: Adverse drug reactions as cause of admission to hospital: Prospective analysis of 18,820 patients. Br Med J 329:15, 2004

RIEDER MJ et al: Effect of VKORC1 haplotypes on transcriptional regulation and warfarin dose. N Engl J Med 352:2285, 2005

RODEN DM: Drug-induced prolongation of the QT Interval. N Engl J Med 350:1013, 2004

——— et al: Pharmacogenomics: challenges and opportunities. Ann Intern Med, 145:745, 2006

SHU Y et al: Evolutionary conservation predicts function of variants of the human organic cation transporter, OCT1. Proc Natl Acad Sci USA 100:5902, 2003

WEISS ST et al: Asthma steroid pharmacogenetics: A study strategy to identify replicated treatment responses. Proc Am Thorac Soc 1:364, 2004

6 Women's Health

Andrea Dunaif

The study of biologic differences between sexes has emerged as a distinct scientific discipline. A report from the Institute of Medicine (IOM) found that sex has a broad impact on biologic and disease processes and succinctly concluded: sex matters. The National Institutes of Health established the Office of Research on Women's Health in 1990 to develop an agenda for future research in the field. In parallel, women's health has become a distinct clinical discipline with a focus on disorders that are disproportionately represented in women. The integration of women's health into internal medicine and other specialties has been accompanied by novel approaches to health care delivery, including greater attention to patient education and involvement in disease prevention and medical decision-making.

The IOM report recommended the term *sex difference* to describe biologic processes that differ between males and females and *gender difference* for features related to social influences. Disorders highlighted here are reviewed in detail in other chapters.

DISEASE RISK: REALITY AND PERCEPTION

The leading causes of death are the same in women and men: (1) heart disease, (2) cancer, and (3) cerebrovascular disease (Table 6-1; Fig.

TABLE 6-1 DEATHS AND PERCENT OF TOTAL DEATHS FOR THE 15 LEADING CAUSES OF DEATH BY SEX IN THE UNITED STATES, 2003

	Women			Men		
Cause of Death	Rank	Deaths	Total Deaths, %	Rank	Deaths	Total Deaths, %
Diseases of heart	1	348,994	28.0	1	336,095	28.0
Malignant neoplasms	2	268,912	21.6	2	287,990	24.0
Cerebrovascular diseases	3	96,263	7.7	4	61,426	5.1
Chronic lower respiratory diseases	4	65,668	5.3	5	60,714	5.1
Alzheimer's disease	5	45,122	3.6	10	18,335	1.5
Diabetes mellitus	6	38,781	3.1	6	35,438	2.9
Accidents	7	38,745	3.1	3	70,532	5.9
Influenza, pneumonia	8	36,385	2.9	7	28,778	2.4
Nephritis, nephrotic syndrome, nephrosis	9	21,972	1.8	9	20,481	1.7
Septicemia	10	19,082	1.5	12	14,987	1.2
Essential (primary) hypertension, hypertensive renal disease	11	13,727	1.1	15	8,213	0.7
Chronic liver disease, cirrhosis	12	9,591	0.8	11	17,912	1.5
Parkinson's disease	13	7,817	0.6	14	10,180	0.8
Intentional self-harm (suicide)	14	6,281	0.5	8	25,203	2.1
Assault (homicide)	15	3,850	0.3	13	13,882	1.2

Source: Data from Centers for Disease Control and Prevention: National Vital Statistics Reports, Vol. 54, No. 13, April 19, 2006, Table 12, *http://www.cdc.gov/nchs/data/nvsr/nvsr54/nvsr54_13.pdf.*

6-1). The leading cause of cancer death, lung cancer, is the same in both sexes, with higher mortality rates than breast, colon, and prostate cancer combined. Breast cancer is the second leading cause of cancer death in women, but it causes about 60% fewer deaths than lung cancer. Men are substantially more likely to die from suicide, homicide, and accidents than women.

Women's risk for many diseases increases at menopause, which occurs at a median age of 51.4 years. In the industrialized world, women spend one-third of their lives in the postmenopausal period. Estrogen levels fall abruptly at menopause, inducing a variety of physiologic and metabolic responses. Rates of cardiovascular disease increase and bone density begins to decrease rapidly after menopause. In the United States, women live on average about 5 years longer than men, with a life expectancy at birth in 2004 of 80.4 years, compared to 75.2 years in men. Elderly women outnumber elderly men, so that age-related conditions, such as hypertension, have a female preponderance. However, the difference in life expectancy between men and women has decreased an average of 0.1 year every year since 1980, and, if this convergence in mortality figures continues, it is projected that mortality rates will be similar by 2054.

Women's perception of disease risk is often inaccurate. Public awareness campaigns have resulted in almost 50% of U.S. women knowing that cardiovascular disease is the leading cause of death in women. Nevertheless, the condition they fear most is breast cancer, despite the fact that death rates from breast cancer have been falling since the 1990s. In any given decade of life, a woman's risk for breast cancer never exceeds 1 in 34. Although a woman's lifetime risk of developing breast cancer if she lives past 85 years is about 1 in 9, it is much more likely that she will die from cardiovascular disease than from breast cancer. In other words, many elderly women have breast cancer but die from other causes. Similarly, a minority of women are aware that lung cancer is the leading cause of cancer death in women. These misconceptions are unfortunate as they perpetuate inadequate attention to modifiable risk factors, such as dyslipidemia, hypertension, and cigarette smoking.

Physicians are also less likely to recognize women's risk for cardiovascular disease. A survey of physicians in 2004 found that women with intermediate risk for cardiovascular disease, according to Framingham risk score, were significantly more likely to be assigned to a lower risk category than men with similar risk profiles. Moreover, when presented with actors portraying patients with chest pain, physicians' estimates for probability of coronary heart disease (CHD) were significantly lower for women than for men and lower for black women than for white women. These perceptions on the part of both the patient and her physician lead to important differences in cardiac care.

SEX DIFFERENCES IN HEALTH AND DISEASE

ALZHEIMER'S DISEASE

(See also Chap. 365) Alzheimer's disease (AD) affects approximately twice as many women as men. Because the risk for AD increases with age, part of this sex difference is accounted for by the fact that women live longer than men. However, additional factors likely contribute to the increased risk for AD in women, including sex differences in brain size, structure, and functional organization. There is emerging evidence for sex-specific differences in gene expression, not only for genes on the X and Y chromosomes but also for some autosomal genes. Estrogens have pleiotropic genomic and nongenomic effects on the central nervous system, including neurotrophic actions in key areas involved in cognition and memory. Women with AD have lower endogenous estrogen levels compared to women without AD. These observations have led to the hypothesis that estrogen is neuroprotective.

Some studies have suggested that estrogen administration improves cognitive function in nondemented postmenopausal women as well as in women with AD, and several observational studies have suggested that postmenopausal hormone therapy (PHT) may decrease the risk of AD. However, recent placebo-controlled trials have found no improvement in disease progression or cognitive function after up to 15 months of PHT in women with AD. Further, the Women's Health Initiative Memory Study (WHIMS), an ancillary study in the Women's Health Initiative (WHI), found no benefit compared to placebo of estrogen alone [combined continuous equine estrogen (CEE), 0.625 mg qd] or estrogen with progestin [CEE, 0.625 mg qd, and medroxyprogesterone acetate (MPA), 2.5 mg qd] on cognitive function or the development of dementia in women 65 years and older. Indeed, there was a significantly increased risk for both dementia and mild cognitive impairment in women receiving hormone therapy. The possible explanations for the discrepant results between the observational studies and the randomized clinical trials remain unclear (Chap. 342).

CORONARY HEART DISEASE

(See also Chap. 237) There are major sex differences in CHD, the leading cause of death in men and women in developed countries. CHD death rates have been falling in men over the past 30 years, but they have been increasing in women. Since 1984, more women than men have died of cardiovascular disease. Gonadal steroids have major effects on the cardiovascular system and lipid metabolism. Estrogen increases high-density lipoprotein (HDL) and lowers low-density lipoprotein (LDL), whereas androgens have the opposite effect. Estrogen has direct vasodilatory effects on the vascular endothelium, enhances insulin sensitivity, and has antioxidant properties. There is a striking increase in CHD after both natural and surgical menopause suggesting that endogenous estrogens are cardioprotective. Women also have longer QT intervals on electrocardiograms, which increases their susceptibility to certain arrhythmias. Animal studies suggest that the sex difference in QT interval duration is caused by sex steroid effects on cardiac repolarization, in part related to their effects on cardiac voltage-gated potassium channels; there is a lower density of the

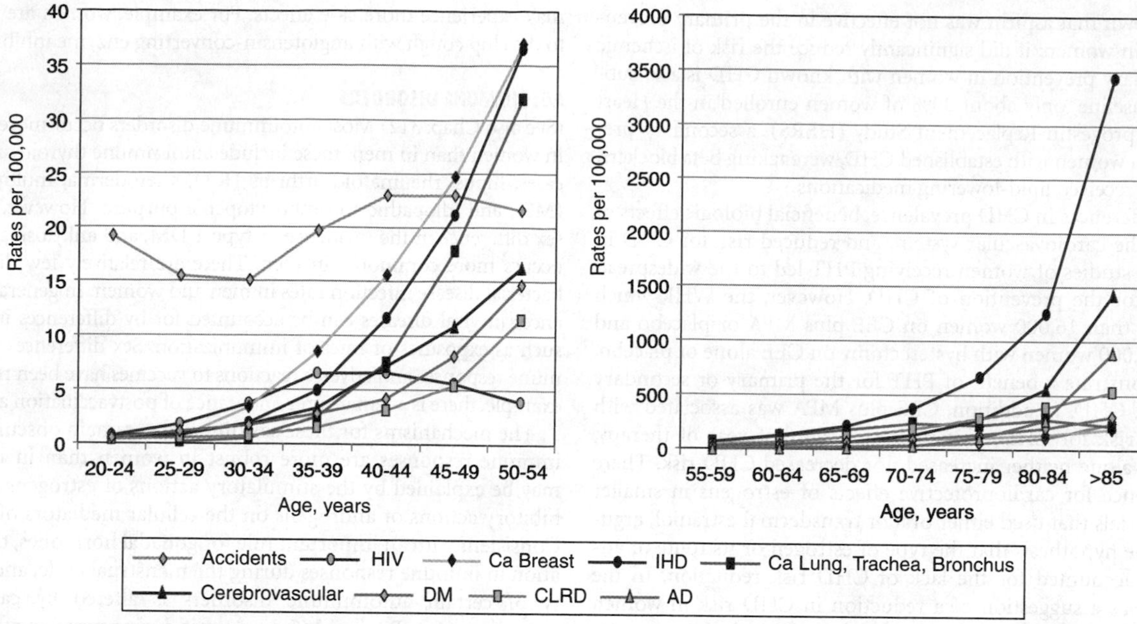

FIGURE 6-1 Death rates per 100,000 population for 2003 by 5-year age groups in U.S. women. Note that the scale of the *y*-axis is increased in the graph on the right compared to that on the left. Accidents and HIV/AIDS are the leading causes of death in young women 20–34 years of age. Accidents, breast cancer, and ischemic heart disease (IHD) are the leading causes of death in women 35–44 years of age. Breast cancer is the leading cause of death in women 45–49 years of age, and IHD becomes the leading cause of death in women beginning at 50 years of age. In older women, IHD remains the leading cause of death, cerebrovascular disease becomes the second leading cause of death, and lung cancer is the leading cause of cancer-related deaths. AD, Alzheimer's disease; Ca, cancer; CLRD, chronic lower respiratory disease; DM, diabetes mellitus. *(Data adapted from Centers for Disease Control and Prevention, www.cdc.gov/nchs/data/statab/Mortfinal2003_worktable210r.pdf.)*

rapid component (I_{Kr}) of the delayed rectifier potassium current (I_K) in females.

CHD presents differently in women, who are usually 10–15 years older than their male counterparts and are more likely to have comorbidities such as hypertension, congestive heart failure, and diabetes mellitus (DM). In the Framingham study, angina was the most frequent initial symptom of CHD in women, whereas myocardial infarction was the most frequent initial presentation in men. Women more often have atypical symptoms, such as nausea, vomiting, indigestion, and upper back pain.

Women with myocardial infarction are more likely to present with cardiac arrest or cardiogenic shock, whereas men are more likely to present with ventricular tachycardia. Further, younger women with myocardial infarction are more likely to die than men of similar age, with women under 50 experiencing twice the mortality rate of men, even after adjustment for differences in disease severity and management. Indeed, the younger the woman, the greater the risk of death from myocardial infarction compared to men (Fig. 6-2).

Physicians are less likely to suspect heart disease in women with chest pain and less likely to perform diagnostic and therapeutic cardiac procedures in women. In addition, there are sex differences in the accuracy of certain diagnostic procedures. The exercise electrocardiogram has substantial false-positive as well as false-negative rates in women compared to men. Women are less likely to receive therapies such as angioplasty, thrombolytic therapy, coronary artery bypass grafts (CABGs), beta blockers, or aspirin. There are also sex differences in outcomes when women with CHD do receive therapeutic interventions. Women undergoing CABG surgery have more advanced disease, a higher perioperative mortality rate, less relief of angina, and less graft patency; however, 5- and 10-year survival rates are similar. Women undergoing percutaneous transluminal coronary angioplasty have lower rates of initial angiographic and clinical success than men, but they also have a lower rate of restenosis and a better long-term outcome. Women may benefit less and have more frequent serious bleeding complications from thrombolytic therapy than do men. Factors such as older age, more comorbid conditions, and more severe CHD in women at the time of events or procedures appear to account in part for the observed sex differences.

Elevated cholesterol levels, hypertension, smoking, obesity, low HDL cholesterol levels, DM, and lack of physical activity are important risk factors for CHD in both men and women. Total triglyceride levels are an independent risk factor for CHD in women but not in men. Low HDL cholesterol and DM are more important risk factors for CHD in women than in men. Smoking is an important risk factor for CHD in women—it accelerates atherosclerosis, exerts direct negative effects on cardiac function, and is associated with an earlier age of menopause. Cholesterol-lowering drugs are equally effective in men and women for primary and secondary prevention of CHD. However, because of perceptions that women are at lower risk for CHD, they receive fewer interventions for modifiable risk factors than do men. In contrast to men, randomized

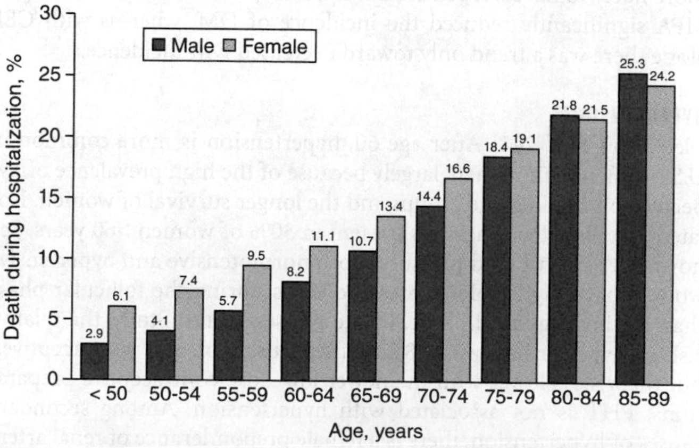

FIGURE 6-2 Rates of death during hospitalization for myocardial infarction among women and men according to age. The overall mortality rate during hospitalization was 16.7% among women and 11.5% among men but was twice the rate in women <50 years compared to men in the same age range. The interaction between sex and age was significant ($p < .001$). *(From V Vaccarino et al: N Engl J Med 341:217, 1999; with permission.)*

trials have shown that aspirin was not effective in the primary prevention of CHD in women; it did significantly reduce the risk of ischemic stroke. Secondary prevention in women with known CHD is also suboptimal. At baseline, only about 30% of women enrolled in the Heart and Estrogen/progestin Replacement Study (HERS), a secondary prevention trial in women with established CHD, were taking beta blockers, and only 45% received lipid-lowering medications.

The sex differences in CHD prevalence, beneficial biologic effects of estradiol on the cardiovascular system, and reduced risk for CHD in observational studies of women receiving PHT led to the widespread use of PHT for the prevention of CHD. However, the WHI, which studied more than 16,000 women on CEE plus MPA or placebo and more than 10,000 women with hysterectomy on CEE alone or placebo, did not demonstrate a benefit of PHT for the primary or secondary prevention of CHD. In addition, CEE plus MPA was associated with an increased risk for CHD, particularly in the first year of therapy, whereas CEE alone neither increased nor decreased CHD risk. There was no evidence for cardioprotective effects of estrogens in smaller randomized trials that used either oral or transdermal estradiol, arguing against the hypothesis that the type of estrogen or its route of administration accounted for the lack of CHD risk reduction. In the WHI, there was a suggestion of a reduction in CHD risk in women ages 50–59 at baseline who received CEE alone. This finding suggests that the time at which PHT is initiated is critical for cardioprotection and is consistent with the "timing hypothesis." According to this hypothesis, PHT has differential effects depending on the stage of atherosclerosis; adverse effects are seen with advanced, unstable lesions. This hypothesis is currently under investigation in randomized clinical trials. PHT is discussed further in Chap. 342.

DIABETES MELLITUS

(See also Chap. 338) Women are more sensitive to insulin than men. Despite this, the prevalence of type 2 DM is similar in men and women. There is a sex difference in the relationship between endogenous androgen levels and DM risk: higher bioavailable testosterone levels are associated with increased risk in women, whereas lower bioavailable testosterone levels are associated with increased risk in men. Polycystic ovary syndrome and gestational DM—common conditions in premenopausal women—are associated with a significantly increased risk for type 2 DM. Premenopausal women with DM lose the cardioprotective effect of female sex and have identical rates of CHD to those in males. These women have impaired endothelial function and reduced coronary vasodilatory responses, which may predispose to cardiovascular complications. In individuals with DM, women have a greater risk for myocardial infarction than men. Women with DM are more likely to have left ventricular hypertrophy. In the WHI, CEE plus MPA significantly reduced the incidence of DM, whereas with CEE alone there was a trend only toward decreased DM incidence.

HYPERTENSION

(See also Chap. 241) After age 60, hypertension is more common in U.S. women than in men, largely because of the high prevalence of hypertension in older age groups and the longer survival of women. Isolated systolic hypertension is present in 30% of women >60 years. Sex hormones affect blood pressure. Both normotensive and hypertensive women have higher blood pressure levels during the follicular phase than during the luteal phase. In the Nurses Health Study, the relative risk of hypertension was 1.8 in current users of oral contraceptives, but this risk is lower with the newer low-dose contraceptive preparations. PHT is not associated with hypertension. Among secondary causes of hypertension, there is a female preponderance of renal artery fibromuscular dysplasia.

The benefits of treatment for hypertension have been dramatic in both women and men. In a meta-analysis of the effects of hypertension treatment, the Individual Data Analysis of Antihypertensive Intervention Trial found a reduction of risk for stroke and for major cardiovascular events in women. The effectiveness of various antihypertensive drugs appears to be comparable in women and men; however, women may experience more side effects. For example, women are more likely to develop cough with angiotensin-converting enzyme inhibitors.

AUTOIMMUNE DISORDERS

(See also Chap. 312) Most autoimmune disorders occur more commonly in women than in men; these include autoimmune thyroid and liver diseases, lupus, rheumatoid arthritis (RA), scleroderma, multiple sclerosis (MS), and idiopathic thrombocytopenic purpura. However, there is no sex difference in the incidence of type 1 DM, and ankylosing spondylitis occurs more commonly in men. There are relatively few differences in bacterial disease infection rates in men and women. In general, sex differences in viral diseases can be accounted for by differences in behaviors, such as exposures or rates of immunization. Sex differences in both immune responses and adverse reactions to vaccines have been reported. For example, there is a female preponderance of postvaccination arthritis.

The mechanisms for these sex differences remain obscure. Adaptive immune responses are more robust in women than in men, which may be explained by the stimulatory actions of estrogens and the inhibitory actions of androgens on the cellular mediators of immunity. Consistent with an important role for gonadal hormones, there is variation in immune responses during the menstrual cycle, and the activity of certain autoimmune disorders is altered by castration or pregnancy (e.g., RA and MS may remit during pregnancy). Nevertheless, the majority of studies show that exogenous estrogens and progestins in the form of PHT or oral contraceptives do not alter autoimmune disease incidence or activity. Exposure to fetal antigens, including circulating fetal cells that persist in certain tissues, has been speculated to increase the risk of autoimmune responses. There is clearly an important genetic component to autoimmunity, as indicated by the familial clustering and HLA association of many such disorders. However, HLA types are not sexually dimorphic.

HIV INFECTION

(See also Chap. 182) Women account for almost 50% of the 40 million persons infected with HIV-1 worldwide. AIDS is an important cause of death in younger women (Fig. 6-1). Heterosexual contact with an at-risk partner is the fastest-growing transmission category, and women are more susceptible to HIV infection than men. This increased susceptibility is in part accounted for by an increased prevalence of sexually transmitted diseases in women. Some studies have suggested that hormonal contraceptives may increase the risk of HIV transmission. Progesterone has been shown to increase susceptibility to infection in nonhuman primate models of HIV. Women are also more likely to be infected by multiple variants of the virus than men. Women with HIV have more rapid decreases in their CD4 cell counts than men. Compared with men, HIV-infected women more frequently develop candidiasis, but Kaposi's sarcoma is less common than in men.

Other sexually transmitted diseases, such as chlamydial infection and gonorrhea, are important causes of infertility in women, and papilloma virus infection predisposes to cervical cancer.

OBESITY

(See also Chap. 75) The prevalence of obesity is higher in women than in men. However, according to a recent study by the Agency for Healthcare Research and Quality, >80% of patients undergoing bariatric surgery are women. Pregnancy and menopause are risk factors for obesity. There are major sex differences in body fat distribution. Women characteristically have gluteal and femoral or gynoid pattern of fat distribution, whereas men typically have a central or android pattern. Gonadal steroids appear to be the major regulators of fat distribution through a number of direct effects on adipose tissue. Studies in humans also suggest that gonadal steroids play a role in modulating food intake and energy expenditure.

In men and women, upper-body obesity characterized by increased visceral fat is associated with an increased risk for cardiovascular disease and DM. In women, endogenous androgen levels are positively associated with upper-body obesity, and androgen administration increases visceral fat. In contrast, there is an inverse relationship between endogenous androgen levels and central obesity in men. Further, androgen administration decreases visceral fat in centrally obese men. The reasons for these sex differences in the relationship between visceral fat and androgens are unknown. Obesity increases a woman's risk for certain cancers, in particular postmenopausal breast and endometrial cancer, in part because adipose tissue provides an extragonadal source of estrogen through aromatization of circulating adrenal and ovarian androgens, especially the conversion of androstenedione to estrone. Obesity increases the risk of infertility, miscarriage, and complications of pregnancy.

OSTEOPOROSIS

(See also Chap. 348) Osteoporosis is about five times more common in postmenopausal women than in age-matched men, and osteoporotic hip fractures are a major cause of morbidity in elderly women. Men accumulate more bone mass and lose bone more slowly than women. Sex differences in bone mass are found as early as infancy. Calcium intake, vitamin D, and estrogen all play important roles in bone formation and bone loss. Particularly during adolescence, calcium intake is an important determinant of peak bone mass. Vitamin D deficiency is surprisingly common in elderly women, occurring in >40% of women living in northern latitudes. Receptors for estrogens and androgens have been identified in bone. Estrogen deficiency is associated with increased osteoclast activity and a decreased number of bone-forming units, leading to net bone loss. The aromatase enzyme, which converts androgens to estrogens, is also present in bone. Recent studies show that estrogen is an important determinant of bone mass in men (derived from the aromatization of androgens) as well as in women.

PHARMACOLOGY

On average, women have lower body weights, smaller organs, higher percent body fat, and lower total-body water than men. There are also important sex differences in drug action and metabolism that are not accounted for by these differences in body size and composition. Gonadal steroids alter the binding and metabolism of a number of drugs. Further, menstrual cycle phase and pregnancy can alter drug action. Two-thirds of cases of drug-induced torsades des pointes, a rare, life-threatening ventricular arrhythmia, occur in women because they have a longer, more vulnerable QT interval. These drugs, which include certain antihistamines, antibiotics, antiarrhythmics, and antipsychotics, can prolong cardiac repolarization by blocking cardiac voltage-gated potassium channels, particularly I_{Kr}. Women require lower doses of neuroleptics to control schizophrenia. Women awaken from anesthesia faster than men given the same doses of anesthetics. Women also take more medications than men, including over-the-counter formulations and supplements. The greater use of medications combined with these biologic differences may account for the reported higher frequency of adverse drug reactions in women than in men.

PSYCHOLOGICAL DISORDERS

(See also Chap. 386) Depression, anxiety, and affective and eating disorders (bulimia and anorexia nervosa) are more common in women than in men. Epidemiologic studies from both developed and developing nations consistently find major depression to be twice as common in women as in men, with the sex difference becoming evident in early adolescence. Depression occurs in 10% of women during pregnancy and in 10–15% of women during the postpartum period. There is a high likelihood of recurrence of postpartum depression with subsequent pregnancies. The incidence of major depression diminishes after age 45 years and does not increase with the onset of menopause. Depression in women appears to have a worse prognosis than in men; episodes last longer, and there is a lower rate of spontaneous remission. Schizophrenia and bipolar disorders occur at equal rates in men and women, although there may be sex differences in symptoms.

Both biologic and social factors account for the greater prevalence of depressive disorders in women. Men have higher levels of the neurotransmitter serotonin. Gonadal steroids also affect mood, and fluctuations during the menstrual cycle have been linked to symptoms of premenstrual syndrome. Sex hormones differentially affect the hypothalamic-pituitary-adrenal responses to stress. Testosterone appears to blunt cortisol responses to corticotropin-releasing hormone. Both low and high levels of estrogen can activate the hypothalamic-pituitary-adrenal axis.

SLEEP DISORDERS

(See also Chap. 28) There are striking sex differences in sleep and its disorders. During sleep, women have an increased amount of slow-wave activity, differences in timing of delta activity, and an increase in the number of sleep spindles. Testosterone modulates neural control of breathing and upper airway mechanics. Men have a higher prevalence of sleep apnea. Testosterone administration to hypogonadal men as well as to women increases apneic episodes during sleep. Women with the hyperandrogenic disorder polycystic ovary syndrome have an increased prevalence of obstructive sleep apnea, and apneic episodes are positively correlated with their circulating testosterone levels. In contrast, progesterone accelerates breathing, and, in the past, progestins were used for treatment of sleep apnea.

SUBSTANCE ABUSE AND TOBACCO

(See also Chaps. 387 and 390) Substance abuse is more common in men than in women. However, one-third of Americans who suffer from alcoholism are women. Women alcoholics are less likely to be diagnosed than men. A greater proportion of men than women seek help for alcohol and drug abuse. Men are more likely to go to an alcohol or drug treatment facility, while women tend to approach a primary care physician or mental health professional for help under the guise of a psychosocial problem. Late-life alcoholism is more common in women than men. On average, alcoholic women drink less than alcoholic men but exhibit the same degree of impairment. Blood alcohol levels are higher in women than in men after drinking equivalent amounts of alcohol, adjusted for body weight. This greater bioavailability of alcohol in women is due to both the smaller volume of distribution and the slower gastric metabolism of alcohol secondary to lower activity of gastric alcohol dehydrogenase than is the case in men. In addition, alcoholic women are more likely to abuse tranquilizers, sedatives, and amphetamines. Women alcoholics have a higher mortality rate than do nonalcoholic women and alcoholic men. Women also appear to develop alcoholic liver disease and other alcohol-related diseases with shorter drinking histories and lower levels of alcohol consumption. Alcohol abuse also poses special risks to a woman, adversely affecting fertility and the health of the baby (fetal alcohol syndrome). Even moderate alcohol use increases the risk of breast cancer, hypertension, and stroke in women.

More men than women smoke tobacco, but the prevalence of smoking is declining faster in men than in women. Smoking markedly increases the risk of cardiovascular disease in premenopausal women and is also associated with a decrease in the age of menopause. Women who smoke are more likely to develop chronic obstructive pulmonary disease and lung cancer than men and at lower levels of tobacco exposure.

VIOLENCE AGAINST WOMEN

Domestic violence is the most common cause of physical injury in women, exceeding the combined incidence of all other types of injury (such as from rape, mugging, and auto accidents). Sexual assault is one of the most common crimes against women. One in five adult women in the United States reports having experienced sexual assault during her lifetime. Adult women are much more likely to be raped by a spouse, ex-spouse, or acquaintance than by a stranger. Domestic violence may be an unrecognized feature of certain clinical presentations such as chronic abdominal pain, headaches, substance abuse, and eating disorders, in addition to more obvious manifestations such as trauma.

SUMMARY

Women's health is now a mature discipline, and the importance of sex differences in biologic processes is well-recognized. It is clear that understanding the mechanisms of these differences will have an impact on both women's and men's health. For example, estrogen is now recognized as an important regulator of bone density in men as well as in women. Elucidating the biology of sex hormone action has resulted in the design of drugs with tissue-specific hormone agonist and antagonist effects. These discoveries will make it feasible to selectively modulate the actions of sex hormones in both women and men to prevent and treat disease.

FURTHER READINGS

HSIA J et al: Conjugated equine estrogens and coronary heart disease: The Women's Health Initiative. Arch Intern Med 166:357, 2006

MENDELSOHN ME, KARAS RH: Molecular and cellular basis of cardiovascular gender differences. Science 308:1583, 2005

MOSCA L et al: National Study of Physician Awareness and Adherence to Cardiovascular Disease Prevention Guidelines. Circulation 111:499, 2005

RIDKER PM et al: A randomized trial of low-dose aspirin in the primary prevention of cardiovascular disease in women. N Engl J Med 352:1293, 2005

Special Section Women's Health. Science 308:1569, 2005

TURGEON JL et al: Hormone therapy: Physiological complexity belies therapeutic simplicity. Science 304:1269, 2004

WIZEMANN TM, PARDUE M-L (eds): *Exploring the Biological Contributions to Human Health: Does Sex Matter?* Washington, DC, National Academy of Sciences, 2001

7 Medical Disorders during Pregnancy

Robert L. Barbieri, John T. Repke

Approximately 4 million births occur in the United States each year. A significant proportion of these are complicated by one or more medical disorders. Three decades ago, many medical disorders were contraindications to pregnancy. Advances in obstetrics, neonatology, obstetric anesthesiology, and medicine have increased the expectation that pregnancy will result in an excellent outcome for both mother and fetus despite most of these conditions. Successful pregnancy requires important physiologic adaptations, such as a marked increase in cardiac output. Medical problems that interfere with the physiologic adaptations of pregnancy increase the risk for poor pregnancy outcome; conversely, in some instances pregnancy may adversely impact an underlying medical disorder.

HYPERTENSION (See also Chap. 241)

In pregnancy, cardiac output increases by 40%, most of which is due to an increase in stroke volume. Heart rate increases by ~10 beats/min during the third trimester. In the second trimester of pregnancy, systemic vascular resistance decreases and this is associated with a fall in blood pressure. During pregnancy, a blood pressure of 140/90 mmHg is considered to be abnormally elevated and is associated with an increase in perinatal morbidity and mortality. In all pregnant women, the measurement of blood pressure should be performed in the sitting position, because for many the lateral recumbent position is associated with a blood pressure lower than that recorded in the sitting position. The diagnosis of hypertension requires the measurement of two elevated blood pressures, at least 6 h apart. Hypertension during pregnancy is usually caused by preeclampsia, chronic hypertension, gestational hypertension, or renal disease.

PREECLAMPSIA

Approximately 5–7% of all pregnant women develop *preeclampsia*, the new onset of hypertension (blood pressure >140/90 mmHg) and proteinuria (>300 mg/24 h) after 20 weeks of gestation. Although the precise placental factors that cause preeclampsia are unknown, the end result is vasospasm and endothelial injury in multiple organs. Excessive placental secretion of a soluble fms-like tyrosine kinase 1, a naturally occurring vascular endothelial growth factor antagonist, and decreased secretion of placental growth factor may contribute to the endothelial dysfunction, hypertension, and proteinuria observed in preeclampsia. Glomerular endothelial cells demonstrate swelling and encroach on the vascular lumen. Preeclampsia is associated with abnormalities of cerebral circulatory autoregulation, which increase the risk of stroke at near-normal blood pressures. Risk factors for the development of preeclampsia include nulliparity, diabetes mellitus, a history of renal disease or chronic hypertension, a prior history of preeclampsia, extremes of maternal age (>35 years or <15 years), obesity, factor V Leiden mutation, angiotensinogen gene T235, G20210A prothrombin gene mutation, antiphospholipid antibody syndrome, and multiple gestation.

Severe preeclampsia is the presence of new-onset hypertension and proteinuria accompanied by central nervous system (CNS) dysfunction (headaches, blurred vision, seizures, coma), marked elevations of blood pressure (>160/110 mmHg), severe proteinuria (>5 g/24 h), oliguria or renal failure, pulmonary edema, hepatocellular injury (ALT > 2 × the upper limits of normal), thrombocytopenia (platelet count < 100,000/L), or disseminated intravascular coagulation. Women with *mild preeclampsia* are those with the diagnosis of new-onset hypertension, proteinuria, and edema without evidence of severe preeclampsia. The HELLP (*h*emolysis, *e*levated *l*iver enzymes, *l*ow *p*latelets) syndrome is a special subgroup of severe preeclampsia and is a major cause of morbidity and mortality in this disease. The presence of platelet dysfunction and coagulation disorders further increases the risk of stroke.

℞ PREECLAMPSIA

Preeclampsia resolves within a few weeks after delivery. For pregnant women with preeclampsia prior to 37 weeks' gestation, delivery reduces the mother's morbidity but exposes the fetus to the risk of premature delivery. The management of preeclampsia is challenging because it requires the clinician to balance the health of both mother and fetus simultaneously and to make management decisions that afford both the best opportunities for infant survival. In general, prior to term, women with *mild* preeclampsia can be managed conservatively with bed rest, close monitoring of blood pressure and renal function, and careful fetal surveillance. For women with *severe* preeclampsia, delivery is recommended unless the patient is eligible for expectant management in a tertiary hospital setting. Expectant management of severe preeclampsia remote from term affords some benefits for the fetus with significant risks for the mother.

The definitive treatment of preeclampsia is delivery of the fetus and placenta. For women with severe preeclampsia, aggressive management of blood pressures > 160/110 mmHg reduces the risk of cerebrovascular accidents. Intravenous labetalol or hydralazine are the drugs most commonly used to manage preeclampsia. Intravenous hydralazine may be associated with more episodes of maternal hypotension than labetalol. Alternative agents such as calcium channel blockers may be used. Elevated arterial pressure should be reduced slowly to avoid hypotension and a decrease in blood flow to the fetus. *Angiotensin-converting enzyme (ACE) inhibitors as well as angiotensin-receptor blockers should be avoided in the second and third trimesters of pregnancy because of their adverse effects on fetal development.* Pregnant women treated with ACE inhibitors often develop oligohydramnios, which may be caused by decreased fetal renal function.

Magnesium sulfate is the treatment of choice for the prevention and treatment of eclamptic seizures. Two large randomized clinical trials have demonstrated the superiority of magnesium sulfate over phenytoin and diazepam, and a recent large randomized clinical trial has demonstrated the efficacy of magnesium sulfate in reducing the risk of seizure and possibly reducing the risk of maternal death. Magnesium may prevent seizures by interacting with *N*-methyl-D-aspartate (NMDA) receptors in the CNS. Given the difficulty of predicting eclamptic seizures on the basis of disease severity, it is recommended that once the decision to proceed with delivery is made, all patients carrying a diagnosis of preeclampsia be treated with magnesium sulfate (see **Regimens**, below).

REGIMENS FOR THE ADMINISTRATION OF MAGNESIUM SULFATE FOR SEIZURE PROPHYLAXIS IN WOMEN IN LABOR WITH PREECLAMPSIA

Intramuscular	Intravenous
10 g (5 g IM deep in each buttock)[a]	6-g bolus over 15 min 1–3 g/h by continuous infusion pump
5 g IM deep q4h, alternating sides	May be mixed in 100 mL crystalloid; if given by intravenous push, make up as 20% solution; push at maximum rate of 1 g/min 40-g $MgSO_4{\cdot}7H_2O$ in 1000 mL Ringers lactate; run at 25–75 mL/h (1–3 g/h)[a]

[a]Made up as 50% solution

CHRONIC ESSENTIAL HYPERTENSION

Pregnancy complicated by chronic essential hypertension is associated with intrauterine growth restriction and increased perinatal mortality. Pregnant women with chronic hypertension are at increased risk for superimposed preeclampsia and abruptio placenta. Women with chronic hypertension should have a thorough prepregnancy evaluation, both to identify remediable causes of hypertension and to ensure that the prescribed antihypertensive agents are not associated with an adverse outcome of pregnancy (e.g., ACE inhibitors, angiotensin-receptor blockers). α-Methyldopa, labetalol, and nifedipine are the most commonly used medications for the treatment of chronic hypertension in pregnancy. Baseline evaluation of renal function is necessary to help differentiate the effects of chronic hypertension versus superimposed preeclampsia should the hypertension worsen during pregnancy. There are no convincing data that demonstrate that treatment of mild chronic hypertension improves perinatal outcome.

GESTATIONAL HYPERTENSION

This is the development of elevated blood pressure during pregnancy or in the first 24 h post partum in the absence of preexisting chronic hypertension and other signs of preeclampsia. Uncomplicated gestational hypertension that does not progress to preeclampsia has not been associated with adverse pregnancy outcome or adverse long-term prognosis.

RENAL DISEASE (See also Chaps. 272 and 280)

Normal pregnancy is characterized by an increase in glomerular filtration rate and creatinine clearance. This occurs secondary to a rise in renal plasma flow and increased glomerular filtration pressures. Patients with underlying renal disease and hypertension may expect a worsening of hypertension during pregnancy. If superimposed preeclampsia develops, the additional endothelial injury results in a capillary leak syndrome that may make the management of these patients challenging. In general, patients with underlying renal disease and hypertension benefit from aggressive management of blood pressure. Preconception counseling is also essential for these patients so that accurate risk assessment can occur prior to the establishment of pregnancy and important medication changes and adjustments can be made. In general, a prepregnancy serum creatinine level <133 μmol/L (<1.5 mg/dL) is associated with a favorable prognosis. When renal disease worsens during pregnancy, close collaboration between the nephrologist and the maternal-fetal medicine specialist is essential so that decisions regarding delivery can be weighed in the context of sequelae of prematurity for the neonate versus long-term sequelae for the mother with respect to future renal function.

CARDIAC DISEASE

VALVULAR HEART DISEASE

(See also Chap. 230) This is the most common cardiac problem complicating pregnancy.

Mitral Stenosis This is the valvular disease most likely to cause death during pregnancy. The pregnancy-induced increase in blood volume, cardiac output, and tachycardia can increase the transmitral pressure gradient and cause pulmonary edema in women with mitral stenosis. Pregnancy associated with long-standing mitral stenosis may result in pulmonary hypertension. Sudden death has been reported when hypovolemia has been allowed to occur in this condition. Careful control of heart rate, especially during labor and delivery, minimizes the impact of tachycardia and reduced ventricular filling times on cardiac function. Pregnant women with mitral stenosis are at increased risk for the development of atrial fibrillation and other tachyarrhythmias. Medical management of severe mitral stenosis and atrial fibrillation with digoxin and beta blockers is recommended. Balloon valvulotomy can be carried out during pregnancy.

Mitral Regurgitation and Aortic Regurgitation and Stenosis These are generally well tolerated during pregnancy. The pregnancy-induced decrease in systemic vascular resistance reduces the risk of cardiac failure with these conditions. As a rule, mitral valve prolapse does not present problems for the pregnant patient, and aortic stenosis, unless very severe, is well tolerated. In the most severe cases of aortic stenosis, limitation of activity or balloon valvuloplasty may be indicated.

CONGENITAL HEART DISEASE

(See also Chap. 229) The presence of a congenital cardiac lesion in the mother increases the risk of congenital cardiac disease in the newborn. Prenatal screening of the fetus for congenital cardiac disease with ultrasound is recommended. Atrial or ventricular septal defect is usually well tolerated during pregnancy in the absence of pulmonary hypertension, provided that the woman's prepregnancy cardiac status is favorable. Use of air filters on IV sets during labor and delivery in patients with intracardiac shunts is generally recommended.

OTHER CARDIAC DISORDERS

Supraventricular tachycardia (Chap. 226) is a common cardiac complication of pregnancy. Treatment is the same as in the nonpregnant patient, and fetal tolerance of medications such as adenosine and calcium channel blockers is acceptable. When necessary, electrocardioversion may be performed and is generally well tolerated by mother and fetus.

Peripartum cardiomyopathy (Chap. 231) is an uncommon disorder of pregnancy associated with myocarditis, and its etiology remains unknown. Treatment is directed toward symptomatic relief and improvement of cardiac function. Many patients recover completely; others are left with a progressive dilated cardiomyopathy. Recurrence in a subsequent pregnancy has been reported, and women should be counseled to avoid pregnancy after a diagnosis of peripartum cardiomyopathy.

SPECIFIC HIGH-RISK CARDIAC LESIONS

Marfan Syndrome (See also Chap. 357) This is an autosomal dominant disease, associated with a high risk of maternal morbidity. Approximately 15% of pregnant women with Marfan syndrome develop a major cardiovascular manifestation during pregnancy, with almost all women surviving. An aortic root diameter <40 mm is considered to be associated with a favorable outcome of pregnancy. Prophylactic therapy with beta blockers has been advocated, although large-scale clinical trials in pregnancy have not been performed.

Pulmonary Hypertension (See also Chap. 244) Maternal mortality in the setting of severe pulmonary hypertension is high, and primary pulmonary hypertension is a contraindication to pregnancy. Termination of pregnancy may be advisable in these circumstances to preserve the life of the mother. In the Eisenmenger syndrome, i.e., the combination of pulmonary hypertension with right-to-left shunting due to congenital abnormalities (Chap. 229), maternal and fetal death occur frequently. Systemic hypotension may occur after blood loss, prolonged Valsalva maneuver, or regional anesthesia; sudden death secondary to hypotension is a dreaded complication. Management of these patients is challenging, and invasive hemodynamic monitoring during labor and delivery is generally recommended.

In patients with pulmonary hypertension, vaginal delivery is less stressful hemodynamically than cesarean section, which should be reserved for accepted obstetric indications.

DEEP VENOUS THROMBOSIS AND PULMONARY EMBOLISM (See also Chap. 256)

A hypercoagulable state is characteristic of pregnancy, and deep venous thrombosis (DVT) occurs in about 1 in 2000 pregnancies. Pulmonary embolism is one of the most common causes of maternal death in the United States. In pregnant women, DVT occurs much more commonly in the left leg than in the right leg, due to the compression of the left iliac vein by the iliac artery and the uterus. Activated protein C resistance caused by the factor V Leiden mutation increases the risk for DVT and pulmonary embolism during pregnancy. Approximately 25% of women with DVT during pregnancy carry the factor V Leiden allele. The presence of the factor V Leiden mutation also increases the risk for severe preeclampsia. Additional genetic mutations associated with DVT during pregnancy include the prothrombin G20210A mutation (heterozygotes and homozygotes) and the methylenetetrahydrofolate reductase C677T mutation (homozygotes).

Rx DEEP VENOUS THROMBOSIS

Aggressive diagnosis and management of DVT and suspected pulmonary embolism optimize the outcome for mother and fetus. In general, all diagnostic and therapeutic modalities afforded the nonpregnant patient should be utilized in pregnancy. Anticoagulant therapy with low-molecular-weight heparin (LMWH) or unfractionated heparin is indicated in pregnant women with DVT. LMWH may be associated with an increased risk of epidural hematoma in women receiving an epidural anesthetic in labor. One approach to this problem is to switch from LMWH to unfractionated heparin before the anticipated delivery date. Warfarin therapy is contraindicated in the first trimester due to its association with fetal chondrodysplasia punctata. In the second and third trimesters, warfarin may cause fetal optic atrophy and mental retardation. When DVT occurs in the postpartum period, LMWH therapy for 7–10 days may be followed by warfarin therapy for 3–6 months. Warfarin is not contraindicated in breast-feeding women.

ENDOCRINE DISORDERS

DIABETES MELLITUS

(See also Chap. 338) In pregnancy, the fetoplacental unit induces major metabolic changes, the purpose of which is to shunt glucose and amino acids to the fetus while the mother uses ketones and triglycerides to fuel her metabolic needs. These metabolic changes are accompanied by maternal insulin resistance, caused in part by placental production of steroids, a growth hormone variant, and placental lactogen. Although pregnancy has been referred to as a state of "accelerated starvation," it is better characterized as "accelerated ketosis." In pregnancy, after an overnight fast, plasma glucose is lower by 0.8–1.1 mmol/L (15–20 mg/dL) than in the nonpregnant state. This is due to the use of glucose by the fetus. In early pregnancy, fasting may result in circulating glucose concentrations in the range of 2.2 mmol/L (40 mg/dL) and may be associated with symptoms of hypoglycemia. In contrast to the decrease in maternal glucose concentration, plasma hydroxybutyrate and acetoacetate levels rise to two to four times normal after a fast.

Rx DIABETES MELLITUS IN PREGNANCY

Pregnancy complicated by diabetes mellitus is associated with higher maternal and perinatal morbidity and mortality rates. Preconception counseling and treatment are important for the diabetic patient contemplating pregnancy and can reduce the risk of congenital malformations and improve pregnancy outcome. Folate supplementation reduces the incidence of fetal neural tube defects, which occur with greater frequency in fetuses of diabetic mothers. In addition, optimizing glucose control during key periods of organogenesis reduces other congenital anomalies including sacral agenesis, caudal dysplasia, renal agenesis, and ventricular septal defect.

Once pregnancy is established, glucose control should be managed more aggressively than in the nonpregnant state. In addition to dietary changes, this requires more frequent blood glucose monitoring and often involves additional injections of insulin or conversion to an insulin pump. Fasting blood glucose levels should be maintained at <5.8 mmol/L (<105 mg/dL) with no values >7.8 mmol/L (140 mg/dL). Commencing in the third trimester, regular surveillance of maternal glucose control as well as assessment of fetal growth (obstetric sonography) and fetoplacental oxygenation (fetal heart rate monitoring or biophysical profile) optimizes pregnancy outcome. Pregnant diabetic patients without vascular disease are at greater risk for delivering a macrosomic fetus, and attention to fetal growth via clinical and ultrasound examinations is important. Fetal macrosomia is associated with an increased risk of maternal and fetal birth trauma. Pregnant women with diabetes have an increased risk of developing preeclampsia, and those with vascular disease are at greater risk for developing intrauterine growth restriction, which is associated with an increased risk of fetal and neonatal death. Excellent pregnancy outcomes in patients with diabetic nephropathy and proliferative retinopathy have been reported with aggressive glucose control and intensive maternal and fetal surveillance.

Glycemic control may become more difficult to achieve as pregnancy progresses due to an increase in insulin resistance. Because of delayed pulmonary maturation of the fetuses of diabetic mothers, early delivery should be avoided unless there is biochemical evidence of fetal lung maturity. In general, efforts to control glucose and maintain the pregnancy until the estimated date of delivery result in the best overall outcome for both mother and newborn.

GESTATIONAL DIABETES

All pregnant women should be screened for gestational diabetes unless they are in a low-risk group. Women at low risk for gestational diabetes are those <25 years of age; those with a body mass index < 25 kg/m^2, no maternal history of macrosomia or gestational diabetes, and no diabetes in a first-degree relative; and those not members of a high-risk ethnic group (African American, Hispanic, Native American). A typical two-step strategy for establishing the diagnosis of gestational diabetes involves administration of a 50-g oral glucose challenge with a single serum glucose measurement at 60 min. If the plasma glucose is <7.8 mmol/L (<140 mg/dL), the test is considered normal. Serum glucose > 7.8 mmol/L (>140 mg/dL) warrants administration of a 100-g oral glucose challenge with serum glucose measurements obtained in the fasting state, and at 1, 2, and 3 h. Normal values are plasma glucose concentrations <5.8 mmol/L (<105 mg/dL), 10.5 mmol/L (190 mg/dL), 9.1 mmol/L (165 mg/dL), and 8.0 mmol/L (145 mg/dL), respectively. Some centers have adopted more conservative criteria, using <7.5 mmol/L (<135 mg/dL) as the screening threshold, and values of <5.3 mmol/L (<95 mg/dL), <10 mmol/L (<180 mg/dL), <8.6 mmol/L (<155 mg/dL), and <7.8 mmol/L (<140 mg/dL) as the upper norms for a 3-h glucose tolerance test.

Pregnant women with gestational diabetes are at increased risk of preeclampsia, delivering infants who are large for their gestational age, and birth lacerations. Their fetuses are at risk of hypoglycemia and birth trauma (brachial plexus) injury.

Rx GESTATIONAL DIABETES

Treatment of gestational diabetes with a two-step strategy of dietary intervention followed by insulin injections if diet alone does not adequately control blood sugar [fasting glucose < 5.6 mmol/L (<100 mg/dL) and 2-h post-prandial <7.0 mmol/L (<126 mg/dL)] is associated with a decreased risk of birth trauma for the fetus. More recently the use of the oral hypoglycemic agent glyburide has become popular for managing gestational diabetes refractory to nutritional management. More data on the safety and efficacy of glyburide for the management of gestational diabetes are needed before it supplants insulin as the treatment agent of choice. For women with gestational diabetes, within the 10 years after the index pregnancy there is a 40% risk of being diagnosed with diabetes. All women with a history of gestational diabetes should be counseled about prevention strategies and evaluated regularly for diabetes.

THYROID DISEASE

(See also Chap. 335) In pregnancy, the estrogen-induced increase in thyroxine-binding globulin causes an increase in circulating levels of total T_3 and total T_4. The normal range of circulating levels of free T_4, free T_3, and thyroid-stimulating hormone (TSH) remain unaltered by pregnancy.

The thyroid gland normally enlarges during pregnancy. Maternal hyperthyroidism occurs at a rate of ~2 per 1000 pregnancies and is generally well tolerated by pregnant women. Clinical signs and symptoms should alert the physician to the occurrence of this disease. Many of the physiologic adaptations to pregnancy may mimic subtle signs of hyperthyroidism. Although pregnant women are able to tolerate mild hyperthyroidism without adverse sequelae, more severe hyperthyroidism can cause spontaneous abortion or premature labor, and thyroid storm is associated with a significant risk of maternal mortality.

Rx HYPERTHYROIDISM IN PREGNANCY

Hyperthyroidism in pregnancy should be aggressively evaluated and treated. The treatment of choice is propylthiouracil. Because it crosses the placenta, the minimum effective dose should be used to maintain free T_4 in the upper normal range. Methimazole crosses the placenta to a greater degree than propylthiouracil and has been associated with fetal aplasia cutis. Radioiodine should not be used during pregnancy, either for scanning or treatment, because of effects on the fetal thyroid. In emergent circumstances, additional treatment with beta blockers and a saturated solution of potassium iodide may be necessary. Hyperthyroidism is most difficult to control in the first trimester of pregnancy and easiest to control in the third trimester.

The goal of therapy for *hypothyroidism* is to maintain the serum TSH in the normal range, and thyroxine is the drug of choice. Children born to women with an elevated serum TSH (and a normal total thyroxine) during pregnancy have impaired performance on neuropsychologic tests. During pregnancy, the dose of thyroxine required to keep the TSH in the normal range rises. In one study, the mean replacement dose of thyroxine required to maintain the TSH in the normal range was 0.1 mg daily before pregnancy, and it increased to 0.15 mg daily during pregnancy. Since the increased thyroxine requirement occurs as early as the fifth week of pregnancy, one approach is to increase the thyroxine dose by 30% as soon as pregnancy is diagnosed and then adjust the dose by serial measurement of TSH.

HEMATOLOGIC DISORDERS

Pregnancy has been described as a state of physiologic anemia. Part of the reduction in hemoglobin concentration is dilutional, but iron and folate deficiencies are the major causes of correctable anemia during pregnancy.

In populations at high risk for hemoglobinopathies (Chap. 99), hemoglobin electrophoresis should be performed as part of the prenatal screen. Hemoglobinopathies can be associated with increased maternal and fetal morbidity and mortality. Management is tailored to the specific hemoglobinopathy and is generally the same for both pregnant and nonpregnant women. Prenatal diagnosis of hemoglobinopathies in the fetus is readily available and should be discussed with prospective parents either prior to or early in pregnancy.

Thrombocytopenia occurs commonly during pregnancy. The majority of cases are benign gestational thrombocytopenias, but the differential diagnosis should include immune thrombocytopenia (Chap. 109) and preeclampsia. Maternal thrombocytopenia may also be caused by catastrophic obstetric events such as retention of a dead fetus, sepsis, abruptio placenta, and amniotic fluid embolism.

NEUROLOGIC DISORDERS

Headache appearing during pregnancy is usually due to migraine (Chap. 15), a condition that may worsen, improve, or be unaffected by pregnancy. A new or worsening headache, particularly if associated with visual blurring, may signal eclampsia (above) or pseudotumor cerebri (benign intracranial hypertension; Chap. 29); diplopia due to a sixth nerve palsy suggests pseudotumor cerebri. The risk of seizures in patients with epilepsy increases in the postpartum period but not consistently during pregnancy; management is discussed in Chap. 363. The risk of stroke is generally thought to increase during pregnancy because of a hypercoagulable state; however, studies suggest that the period of risk occurs primarily in the postpartum period and that both ischemic and hemorrhagic strokes may occur at this time. Guidelines for use of heparin therapy are summarized above (see "Deep Venous Thrombosis and Pulmonary Embolism"); warfarin is teratogenic and should be avoided.

The onset of a new movement disorder during pregnancy suggests chorea gravidarum, a variant of Sydenham's chorea associated with rheumatic fever and streptococcal infection (Chap. 315); the chorea may recur with subsequent pregnancies. Patients with preexisting multiple sclerosis (Chap. 375) experience a gradual decrease in the risk of relapses as pregnancy progresses and, conversely, an increase in attack risk during the postpartum period. Beta interferons should *not* be administered to pregnant MS patients, but moderate or severe relapses can be safely treated with pulse glucocorticoid therapy. Finally, certain tumors, particularly pituitary adenoma and meningioma (Chap. 374), may manifest during pregnancy because of accelerated growth, possibly driven by hormonal factors.

Peripheral nerve disorders associated with pregnancy include Bell's palsy (idiopathic facial paralysis, Chap. 379), which is approximately threefold more likely to occur during the third trimester and immediate postpartum period than in the general population. Therapy with glucocorticoids should follow the guidelines established for nonpregnant patients. Entrapment neuropathies are common in the later stages of pregnancy, presumably as a result of fluid retention. Carpal tunnel syndrome (median nerve) presents as pain and paresthesia in the hand, often worse at night, and later with weakness in the thenar muscles. Treatment is generally conservative; wrist splints may be helpful, and glucocorticoid injections or surgical section of the carpal tunnel can usually be postponed. Meralgia paresthetica (lateral femoral cutaneous nerve) consists of pain and numbness in the lateral aspect of the thigh without weakness. Patients are usually reassured to learn that these symptoms are benign and can be expected to remit spontaneously after the pregnancy has been completed.

Judicious use of neuroimaging procedures is reasonable during pregnancy. Some centers require that formal consent be obtained from pregnant patients before MRI scans are administered. Experimental data indicate that high-field-strength MRI may be teratogenic to rodents; however, studies in pregnant MRI technicians have failed to show any risk to the fetus, even with chronic exposure. The paramagnetic MRI contrast agent gadolinium is usually not administered, particularly during the first trimester, because it crosses the blood-brain barrier. CT scanning of the brain is also considered safe, particularly as the procedure is fast, little radioactive scatter is produced, and pelvic contents are easily shielded; iodinated contrast media should be avoided whenever possible.

GASTROINTESTINAL AND LIVER DISEASE

Up to 90% of pregnant women experience nausea and vomiting during the first trimester of pregnancy. Occasionally, hyperemesis gravidarum requires hospitalization to prevent dehydration, and sometimes parenteral nutrition is required.

Crohn's disease may be associated with exacerbations in the second and third trimesters. Ulcerative colitis is associated with disease exacerbations in the first trimester and during the early postpartum period. Medical management of these diseases during pregnancy is identical to the management in the nonpregnant state (Chap. 289).

Exacerbation of gall bladder disease is commonly observed during pregnancy. In part this may be due to pregnancy-induced alteration in the metabolism of bile and fatty acids. Intrahepatic cholestasis of pregnancy is generally a third-trimester event. Profound pruritus may accompany this condition, and it may be associated with increased fetal mortality. It has been suggested that placental bile salt deposition may contribute to progressive uteroplacental insufficiency. Therefore, regular fetal surveillance should be undertaken once the diagnosis of intrahepatic cholestasis is made. Favorable results with ursodiol have been reported.

Acute fatty liver is a rare complication of pregnancy. Frequently confused with the HELLP syndrome (see "Preeclampsia," above) and severe preeclampsia, the diagnosis of acute fatty liver of pregnancy may be facilitated by imaging studies and laboratory evaluation. Acute fatty liver of pregnancy is generally characterized by markedly increased levels of bilirubin and ammonia and by hypoglycemia. Management of acute fatty liver of pregnancy is supportive; recurrence in subsequent pregnancies has been reported.

All pregnant women should be screened for hepatitis B. This information is important for pediatricians after delivery of the infant. All infants receive hepatitis B vaccine. Infants born to mothers who are carriers of hepatitis B surface antigen should also receive hepatitis B immune globulin as soon after birth as possible and preferably within the first 72 h. Screening for hepatitis C is recommended for individuals at high risk for exposure.

INFECTIONS

BACTERIAL INFECTIONS

Other than bacterial vaginosis, the most common bacterial infections during pregnancy involve the urinary tract (Chap. 282). Many pregnant women have asymptomatic bacteriuria, most likely due to stasis caused by progestational effects on ureteral and bladder smooth muscle and later in pregnancy due to compression effects of the enlarging uterus. In itself, this condition is not associated with an adverse outcome of pregnancy. However, if asymptomatic bacteriuria is left untreated, symptomatic pyelonephritis may occur. Indeed, ~75% of cases of pregnancy-associated pyelonephritis are the result of untreated asymptomatic bacteriuria. All pregnant women should be screened with a urine culture for asymptomatic bacteriuria at the first prenatal visit. Subsequent screening with nitrite/leukocyte esterase strips is indicated for high-risk women, such as those with sickle cell trait or a history of urinary tract infections. All women with positive screens should be treated.

Abdominal pain and fever during pregnancy create a clinical dilemma. The diagnosis of greatest concern is intrauterine amniotic infection. While amniotic infection most commonly follows rupture of the membranes, this is not always the case. In general, antibiotic therapy is not recommended as a temporizing measure in these circumstances. If intrauterine infection is suspected, induced delivery with concomitant antibiotic therapy is generally indicated. Intrauterine amniotic infection is most often caused by pathogens such as *Escherichia coli* and group B streptococcus. In high-risk patients at term or in preterm patients, routine intrapartum prophylaxis of group B streptococcal (GBS) disease is recommended. Penicillin G and ampicillin are the drugs of choice. In penicillin-allergic patients, clindamycin is recommended. For the reduction of neonatal morbidity due to GBS, universal screening of pregnant women for GBS between 35 and 37 weeks gestation with intrapartum antibiotic treatment of infected women is recommended.

Postpartum infection is a significant cause of maternal morbidity and mortality. While rare after vaginal delivery, postpartum endomyometritis develops in 5% of patients having elective repeat cesarean section and in 25% of patients after emergency cesarean section following prolonged labor. Prophylactic antibiotics should be given to all patients undergoing cesarean section. As most cases of postpartum endomyometritis are polymicrobial, broad-spectrum antibiotic coverage with a penicillin, aminoglycoside, and metronidazole is recommended (Chap. 157). Most cases resolve within 72 h. Women who do not respond to antibiotic treatment for postpartum endomyometritis should be evaluated for septic pelvic thrombophlebitis. Imaging studies may be helpful in establishing the diagnosis, which is primarily a clinical diagnosis of exclusion. Patients with septic pelvic thrombophlebitis generally have tachycardia out of proportion to their fever and respond rapidly to intravenous administration of heparin.

All patients are screened prenatally for gonorrhea and chlamydial infections, and the detection of either should result in prompt treatment. Ceftriaxone and azithromycin are the agents of choice (Chaps. 137 and 169).

VIRAL INFECTIONS

Cytomegalovirus Infection Viral infection in pregnancy presents a significant challenge. The most common cause of congenital viral infection in the United States is cytomegalovirus (CMV) (Chap. 175). As many as 50–90% of women of childbearing age have antibodies to CMV, but only rarely does CMV reactivation result in neonatal infection. More commonly, primary CMV infection during pregnancy creates a risk of congenital CMV. No currently accepted treatment of CMV during pregnancy has been demonstrated to protect the fetus effectively. Moreover, it is impossible to predict which fetus will sustain life-threatening CMV infection. Severe CMV disease in the newborn is characterized most often by petechiae, hepatosplenomegaly, and jaundice. Chorioretinitis, microcephaly, intracranial calcifications, hepatitis, hemolytic anemia, and purpura may also develop. CNS involvement, resulting in the development of psychomotor, ocular, auditory, and dental abnormalities over time, has been described.

Rubella (See also Chap. 186) Rubella virus is a known teratogen; first-trimester rubella carries a high risk of fetal anomalies, though the risk decreases significantly later in pregnancy. Congenital rubella may be diagnosed by percutaneous umbilical blood sampling with the detection of IgM antibodies in fetal blood. All pregnant women should be screened for their immune status to rubella. Indeed, all women of childbearing age, regardless of pregnancy status, should have their immune status for rubella verified and be immunized if necessary. The incidence of congenital rubella in the United States is extremely low.

Herpesvirus (See also Chap. 172) The acquisition of genital herpes during pregnancy is associated with spontaneous abortion, prematurity, and congenital and neonatal herpes. A recent cohort study of pregnant women without evidence of previous herpes infection demonstrated that ~2% of the women acquired a new herpes infection during the pregnancy. Approximately 60% of the newly infected women had no clinical symptoms. Infection occurred equally in all three trimesters. If herpes seroconversion occurred early in pregnancy, the risk of transmission to the newborn was very low. In women who acquired genital herpes shortly before delivery, the risk of transmission was high. The risk of active genital herpes lesions at term can be reduced by prescribing acyclovir for the last 4 weeks of pregnancy to women who have had their first episode of genital herpes during the pregnancy.

Herpesvirus infection in the newborn can be devastating. Disseminated neonatal herpes carries with it high mortality and morbidity rates from CNS involvement. It is recommended that pregnant women with active genital herpes lesions at the time of presentation in labor be delivered by cesarean section.

Parvovirus (See also Chap. 177) Parvovirus infection (human parvovirus B19) may occur during pregnancy. It rarely causes sequelae, but susceptible women infected during pregnancy may be at risk for fetal hydrops secondary to erythroid aplasia and profound anemia.

HIV Infection (See also Chap. 182) The predominant cause of HIV infection in children is transmission of the virus from the mother to the newborn during the perinatal period. Exposures, which increase the risk of mother-to-child transmission, include vaginal delivery, preterm delivery, trauma to the fetal skin, and maternal bleeding. Additionally, recent infection with high maternal viral load, low maternal CD4+ T cell count, prolonged labor, prolonged length of membrane rupture, and the presence of other genital tract infections, such as syphilis or herpes, increase the risk of transmission. Breast-feeding may also transmit HIV to the newborn and is therefore contraindicated in most developed countries for HIV-infected mothers. There is no clear evidence to suggest that the course of HIV disease is altered by pregnancy. There is also no clear evidence to suggest that uncomplicated HIV disease adversely impacts pregnancy other than by its inherent infection risk.

Rx HIV INFECTION IN PREGNANCY

The majority of cases of mother-to-child (vertical) transmission of HIV-1 occur during the intrapartum period. Mechanisms of vertical transmission include infection after rupture of the membranes and direct contact of the fetus with infected secretions or blood from the maternal genital tract. Zidovudine (ZDV) administered during pregnancy and labor and to the newborn reduces the risk of vertical transmission by 70%. Cesarean section is associated with additional risk reduction compared to vaginal delivery, especially in women with a viral load >1000 copies/mL. Regardless of the mode of delivery, intrapartum ZDV should be provided.

SUMMARY

Maternal mortality has decreased steadily during the past 70 years. The maternal death rate has decreased from nearly 600/100,000 live births in 1935 to 8/100,00 live births in 2002. The most common causes of maternal death in the United States today are, in decreasing order of frequency, pulmonary embolism, obstetric hemorrhage, hypertension, sepsis, cardiovascular conditions including peripartum cardiomyopathy, and ectopic pregnancy. With improved diagnostic and therapeutic modalities as well as with advances in the treatment of infertility, more patients with medical complications will be seeking, and be in need of, complex obstetric care. Improving outcome of pregnancy in these women will be best obtained by assembling a team of internists, specialists in maternal-fetal medicine (high-risk obstetrics), and anesthesiologists to counsel these patients about the risks of pregnancy and to plan their treatment prior to conception. The importance of preconception counseling cannot be overstated. It is the responsibility of all physicians caring for women in the reproductive age group to assess their patient's reproductive plans as part of their overall health evaluation.

FURTHER READINGS

ALEXANDER EK et al: Timing and magnitude of increases in levothyroxine requirements during pregnancy in women with hypothyroidism. N Engl J Med 351:292, 2005

BATES SM et al: Use of antithrombotic agents during pregnancy: The Seventh ACCP Conference on antithrombotic and thrombolytic therapy. Chest 126:627S, 2004

BUCHANAN TA, XIANG AH: Gestational diabetes mellitus. J Clin Invest 115:485, 2005

CROWTHER CA et al: Effect of treatment of gestational diabetes mellitus on pregnancy outcomes. N Engl J Med 352:2477, 2005

DENEUX-THARAUX C et al: Underreporting of pregnancy-related mortality in the United States and Europe. Obstet Gynecol 106:684, 2005

KAAJA RJ, GREER IA: Manifestations of chronic disease during pregnancy. JAMA 294:2751, 2005

LEVINE RJ: Circulating angiogenic factors and the risk of preeclampsia. N Engl J Med 350:672, 2004

MAGEE LA et al: Hydralazine for treatment of severe hypertension in pregnancy: Meta-analysis. BMJ 327:955, 2003

SIBAI BM: Chronic hypertension in pregnancy. Obstet Gynecol 100:369, 2002

THE MAGPIE TRIAL COLLABORATIVE GROUP: Do women with pre-eclampsia, and their babies, benefit from magnesium sulfate? The Magpie Trial: A randomised placebo-controlled trial. Lancet 359:1877, 2002

8 Medical Evaluation of the Surgical Patient

Wei C. Lau, Kim A. Eagle

Over 40 million persons undergo noncardiac surgical procedures in the United States annually. Cardiovascular and pulmonary complications continue to account for major morbidity and mortality in such patients. Emerging evidence-based practices dictate that the internist should perform an individualized evaluation of the surgical patient to provide an accurate preoperative risk assessment and stratification in order to guide optimum perioperative risk-reduction strategies. This chapter reviews cardiovascular and pulmonary preoperative risk assessment, targeting intermediate- and high-risk patients to strategically guide perioperative therapies in order to improve outcome. It also reviews perioperative management and prophylaxis of diabetes mellitus, endocarditis, and venous thromboembolism.

ANESTHETICS

Mortality is extremely low with safe delivery of modern anesthesia, especially in low-risk patients undergoing low-risk surgery (Table 8-1). Inhaled anesthetics have predictable circulatory and respiratory effects; all decrease arterial pressure in a dose-dependent manner by reducing sympathetic tone, causing systemic vasodilation, myocardial depression, and decreased cardiac output. Inhaled anesthetics also cause respiratory depression with diminished responses to both hypercapnia and hypoxemia in a dose-dependent manner, and they have a variable effect on heart rate. In combination with neuromuscular blockade, inhaled anesthetic agents also cause reduction in functional residual lung capacity due to loss of diaphragmatic and intercostal muscle function. This decreases lung volume, which may lead to atelectasis in the dependent lung regions and, in turn, may result in arterial hypoxemia from ventilation-perfusion mismatch as well as an increased risk of postoperative pulmonary complications.

Several meta-analyses have examined the safety of general (inhaled) and neuroaxial (epidural or spinal) anesthesia and found that overall mortality was lower in patients receiving neuroaxial anesthesia. Lower rates of venous thrombosis, pulmonary embolism, pneumonia, and respiratory depression were also observed in patients who were provided neuroaxial anesthesia. However, there were no significant differences in cardiac events between the two approaches. A combination of neuroaxial blockade and general anesthesia is useful when it is desired to reduce general anesthesia requirements. Evidence from a meta-analysis of randomized controlled trials also supports postoperative epidural analgesia for the purpose of pain relief for more than 24 h.

EVALUATION OF INTERMEDIATE- TO HIGH-RISK PATIENTS

Simple, standardized preoperative screening questionnaires, such as the one shown in Table 8-2, have been developed for the purpose of identifying patients at intermediate or high risk who would benefit from a more detailed clinical evaluation. Evaluation of such patients for operation should always begin with a thorough history and physical examination and with a 12-lead resting ECG, in accordance with the American College of Cardiology/American Heart Association (ACC/AHA) guideline recommendations. The history should focus on symptoms of occult cardiac or pulmonary disease. The urgency of the surgery should be determined, as true emergent procedures are associ-

TABLE 8-1 SURGERY: GRADATION OF RISK OF COMMON NONCARDIAC SURGICAL PROCEDURES

Higher	• Emergent major operations, especially elderly • Aortic and other noncarotid major vascular surgery (endovascular and nonendovascular) • Prolonged surgery associated with large fluid shift and/or blood loss
Intermediate	• Major thoracic surgery • Major abdominal surgery • Carotid endarterectomy surgery • Head/neck surgery • Orthopedic surgery • Prostate surgery
Lower	• Eye, skin, and superficial surgery • Endoscopic procedures

Source: From KA Eagle et al.

ated with an unavoidably higher morbidity and mortality. Preoperative laboratory testing should be carried out only for specific clinical conditions based on the clinical examination. Thus, healthy patients of any age undergoing elective surgical procedures without coexisting medical conditions should not require any testing unless the degree of surgical stress may result in unusual changes from the baseline state.

PREOPERATIVE CARDIAC RISK ASSESSMENT

Assessment of exercise tolerance in the prediction of in-hospital perioperative risk is most helpful in patients who self-report worsening exercise-induced cardiopulmonary symptoms, those who may benefit from noninvasive or invasive cardiac testing regardless of scheduled surgical procedure, and those with known coronary artery disease (CAD) or with multiple risk factors who are able to exercise. For predicting perioperative events, poor exercise tolerance has been defined as the inability to walk four blocks or climb two flights of stairs at a normal pace or to meet a metabolic equivalent (MET) level of four (e.g., carrying objects of 15–20 lb, playing golf or doubles tennis) because of the development of dyspnea, angina, or excessive fatigue (Table 8-3).

TABLE 8-2 STANDARDIZED PREOPERATIVE QUESTIONNAIRES[a]

1. Age, weight, height
2. Are you:
   Female and 55 years of age or older or male and 45 years of age of older?
   If yes, are you also 70 years of age or older?
3. Do you take anticoagulant ("blood thinners") medications?
4. Do you have or have you had any of the following heart related conditions?
   Heart disease
   Heart attack within the last 6 months
   Angina (chest pain)
   Irregular heartbeat
   Heart failure
5. Do you have or have you ever had any of the following?
   Rheumatoid arthritis
   Kidney disease
   Liver disease
   Diabetes
6. Do you get short of breath when you lie flat?
7. Are you currently on oxygen treatment?
8. Do you have a chronic cough that produces any discharge or fluid?
9. Do you have lung problems or diseases?
10. Have you or any member of your family ever had a problem with any anesthesia other than nausea?
    If yes, describe:
11. If female, is it possible that you could be pregnant?
    Pregnancy test:
    Please list date of last menstrual period:

[a]University of Michigan Health System patient information report. Patients who answer yes to any of questions 2–9 should receive a more detailed clinical evaluation.

Source: Adapted from KK Tremper, P Benedict: Anesthesiology 92:1212, 2000; with permission.

TABLE 8-3 FUNCTIONAL STATUS

	Higher	• Difficulty with adult activities of daily living
	↑	• Cannot walk four blocks or up two flights of stairs or unable to meet a MET level of 4
Risk		• Inactive but no limitation
	↓	• Active: easily does vigorous tasks
	Lower	• Performs regular vigorous exercises

Source: From KA Eagle et al.

Previous studies have prospectively compared several cardiac risk indices. Given its accuracy and simplicity, the revised cardiac risk index (RCRI) (Table 8-4) is favored. The RCRI relies on the presence or absence of six identifiable predictive factors, which include high-risk surgery, ischemic heart disease, congestive heart failure, cerebrovascular disease, diabetes mellitus, and renal dysfunction. Each of these predictors is assigned one point. The risk of major cardiac events—defined as myocardial infarction, pulmonary edema, ventricular fibrillation or primary cardiac arrest, and complete heart block—can then be predicted. Based on the presence of none, one, two, three, or more of these clinical predictors, the rate of development of one of these major cardiac events is estimated to be 0.5, 1, 5, and 10%, respectively (Fig. 8-1). RCRI 0 has 0.4–0.5% risk of cardiac events; RCRI 1 has 0.9–1.3%; RCRI 2 has 4–6.6%; and RCRI ≥3 has 9–11% risk of cardiac events. The clinical utility of the RCRI is to identify patients with three or more predictors who are at higher risk (≥10%) for cardiac complications, and who may benefit from further risk stratification with noninvasive cardiac testing or initiation of preoperative preventive medical management.

PREOPERATIVE NONINVASIVE CARDIAC TESTING FOR RISK STRATIFICATION

There is little evidence to support widespread application of preoperative noninvasive cardiac testing for all patients undergoing major surgery. Rather, a selective approach based on clinical risk categorization appears to be both useful clinically and cost-effective. There is potential benefit in identifying asymptomatic but high-risk patients, such as those with left main or left main–equivalent CAD, or those with three-vessel CAD with poor left ventricular function who may benefit from coronary revascularization (Chap. 237). However, evidence does not support aggressive attempts to identify patients at intermediate risk with asymp-

TABLE 8-4 REVISED CARDIAC RISK INDEX CLINICAL MARKERS

High-risk surgical procedures
- Vascular surgery
- Major intraperitoneal or intrathoracic procedures

Ischemic heart disease
- History of myocardial infarction
- Current angina considered to be ischemic
- Requiring sublingual nitroglycerin
- Positive exercise test
- Pathological Q-waves on ECG
- History of PTCA and/or CABG with current angina considered to be ischemic

Congestive heart failure
- Left ventricular failure by physical examination
- History of paroxysmal nocturnal dyspnea
- History of pulmonary edema
- S3 gallop on cardiac auscultation
- Bilateral rales on pulmonary auscultation
- Pulmonary edema on chest x-ray

Cerebrovascular disease
- History of transient ischemic attack
- History of cerebrovascular accident

Diabetes mellitus
- Treatment with insulin

Chronic renal insufficiency
- Serum creatinine >2 mg/dL

Note: ECG, electrocardiogram; PTCA, percutaneous transluminal coronary angioplasty; CABG, coronary artery bypass grafting.

Source: Adapted from TH Lee et al, with permission.

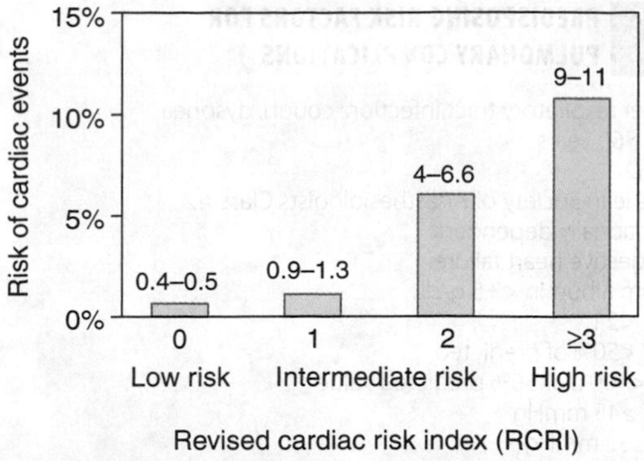

FIGURE 8-1 Risk stratification based on the Revised Cardiac Risk Index. Derivation and prospective validation of a simple index for prediction of cardiac risk of major noncardiac surgery. Cardiac events include myocardial infarction, pulmonary edema, ventricular fibrillation, cardiac asystole, and complete heart block. *(Adapted from TH Lee et al, with permission.)*

tomatic but advanced coronary artery disease, since coronary revascularization appears to offer little advantage over medical therapy.

An RCRI score ≥3 in patients with severe myocardial ischemia on stress testing should lead to consideration of coronary revascularization prior to noncardiac surgery. Noninvasive cardiac testing is most appropriate if it is anticipated that in the event of a strongly positive test a patient will meet guidelines for coronary angiography and coronary revascularization. Pharmacologic stress tests are more useful than exercise testing in patients with functional limitations. Dobutamine echocardiography and persantine, adenosine or dobutamine nuclear perfusion testing (Chap. 222) have excellent negative predictive values (near 100%) but poor positive predictive values (< 20%) for identification of patients at risk for perioperative myocardial infarction or death. Thus, a negative study is reassuring, but a positive study is a relatively weak predictor of a "hard" perioperative cardiac event. A stepwise approach is illustrated in Fig. 8-2.

RISK MODIFICATION USING PREVENTIVE STRATEGIES TO REDUCE CARDIAC RISK

Perioperative Coronary Revascularization Currently, potential options for reducing perioperative cardiovascular risk include coronary artery revascularization and/or perioperative medical preventive therapies

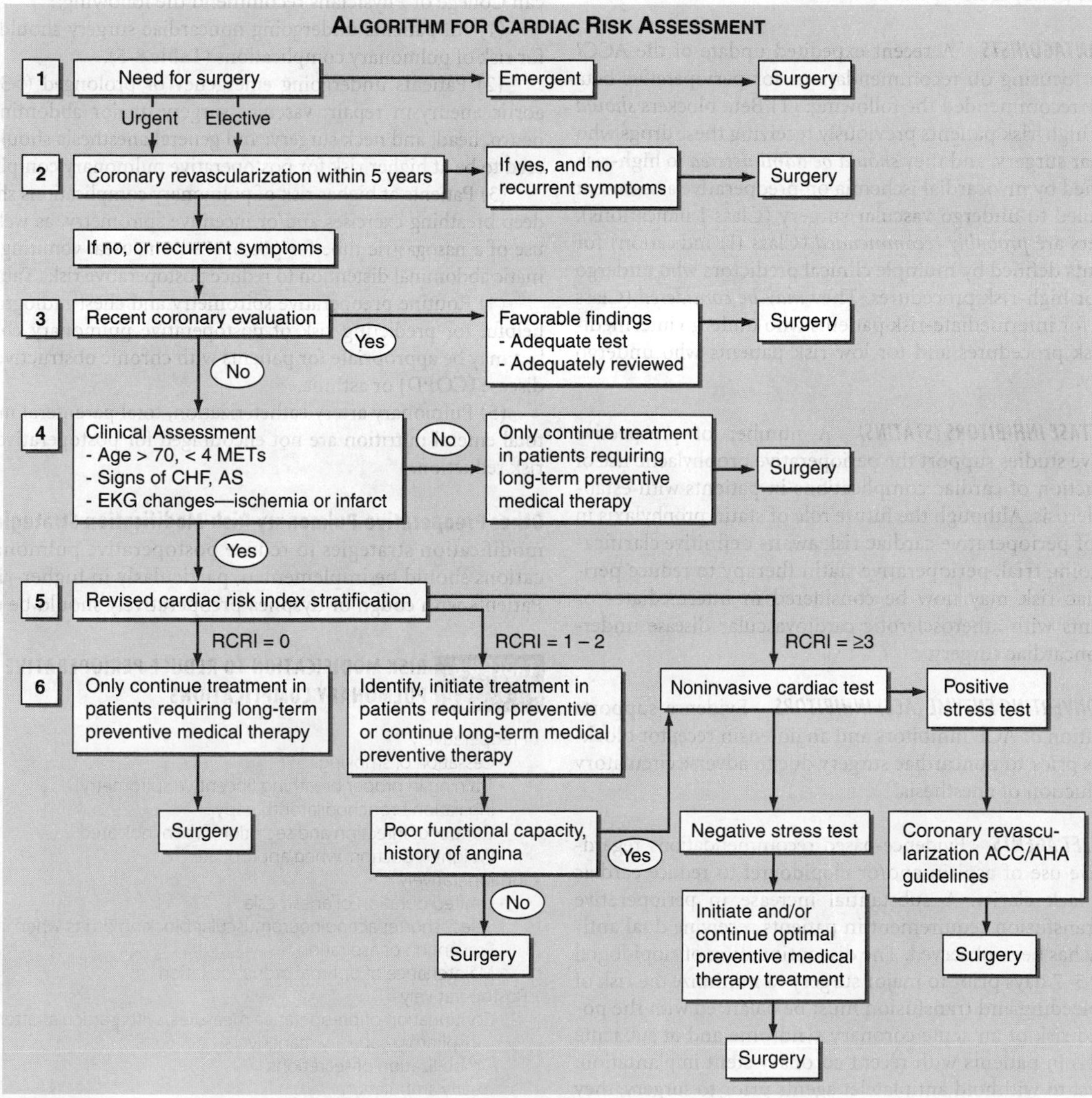

FIGURE 8-2 Composite algorithm for cardiac risk assessment and stratification in patients undergoing noncardiac surgery. Stepwise clinical evaluation: [1] Emergency surgery; [2] Prior coronary revascularization; [3] Prior coronary evaluation; [4] Clinical assessment; [5] Revised cardiac risk index; [6] Risk modification strategies. Preventative medical therapy = beta blocker and statin therapy. RCRI, revised cardiac risk index. *(Adapted from KA Eagle et al and TH Lee et al.)*

(Chap. 237). *Prophylactic* coronary revascularization with either coronary artery bypass grafting (CABG) or percutaneous coronary intervention (PCI) provides no short- or midterm survival benefit for patients *without* left main CAD or three-vessel CAD in the presence of poor left ventricular systolic function. Although PCI is associated with lower procedural risk than is CABG in the perioperative setting, the placement of a coronary artery stent in a short period of time prior to noncardiac surgery may increase the risk of bleeding during surgery if dual antiplatelet therapy (aspirin and clopidogrel) is administered, or it increases the perioperative risk of myocardial infarction and cardiac death due to stent thrombosis if such therapy is withdrawn prematurely (Chap. 240). It is recommended that, if possible, noncardiac surgery be delayed 4–6 weeks after placement of a bare metal coronary stent and 3–6 months after a drug-eluting stent. For patients who *must* undergo noncardiac surgery early (first few days to 4 weeks) after PCI, simple balloon angioplasty without stent placement appears to be a reasonable alternative, since dual antiplatelet therapy is not necessary in such patients.

PERIOPERATIVE MEDICAL PREVENTIVE THERAPIES Perioperative preventive medical therapy with β-adrenergic antagonists, HMG-CoA reductase inhibitors (statins), and aspirin has the goal of reducing perioperative adrenergic stimulation, ischemia, and inflammation, which are triggered during the perioperative period.

β-ADRENERGIC ANTAGONISTS A recent expedited update of the ACC/AHA guideline focusing on recommendations for perioperative beta blocker therapy recommended the following: (1) Beta blockers *should be continued* in high-risk patients previously receiving these drugs who undergo vascular surgery, and they *should be administered* to high-risk patients identified by myocardial ischemia on preoperative assessment who are scheduled to undergo vascular surgery (Class I indications). (2) Beta blockers are *probably recommended* (Class IIa indication) for high-risk patients defined by multiple clinical predictors who undergo intermediate- or high-risk procedures. They *may be considered* (Class IIb indication) for intermediate-risk patients who undergo intermediate- or high-risk procedures and for low-risk patients who undergo vascular surgery.

HMG-COA REDUCTASE INHIBITORS (STATINS) A number of prospective and retrospective studies support the perioperative prophylactic use of statins for reduction of cardiac complications in patients with established atherosclerosis. Although the future role of statin prophylaxis in the reduction of perioperative cardiac risk awaits definitive clarification by an ongoing trial, perioperative statin therapy to reduce perioperative cardiac risk may now be considered in intermediate- or high-risk patients with atherosclerotic cardiovascular disease undergoing major noncardiac surgery.

ANGIOTENSIN-CONVERTING ENZYME (ACE) INHIBITORS Evidence supports the discontinuation of ACE inhibitors and angiotensin receptor blockers for 24 hours prior to noncardiac surgery due to adverse circulatory effects after induction of anesthesia.

ORAL ANTIPLATELET AGENTS Evidence-based recommendations regarding perioperative use of aspirin and/or clopidogrel to reduce cardiac risk currently lack clarity. A substantial increase in perioperative bleeding and transfusion requirement in patients receiving dual antiplatelet therapy has been observed. The discontinuation of clopidogrel and aspirin for 5–7 days prior to major surgery to minimize the risk of perioperative bleeding and transfusion must be balanced with the potential increased risk of an acute coronary syndrome and of subacute stent thrombosis in patients with recent coronary stent implantation. If clinicians elect to withhold antiplatelet agents prior to surgery, they should be restarted as soon as possible postoperatively.

CALCIUM CHANNEL BLOCKERS Evidence is lacking to support the use of calcium channel blockers as a prophylactic strategy to decrease perioperative risk in major noncardiac surgery.

TABLE 8-5 PREDISPOSING RISK FACTORS FOR PULMONARY COMPLICATIONS

1. Upper respiratory tract infection: cough, dyspnea
2. Age >60 years
3. COPD
4. American Society of Anesthesiologists Class ≥2
5. Functionally dependent
6. Congestive heart failure
7. Serum albumin <3.5 g/dL
8. FEV_1 <2 L
9. MVV <50% of predicted
10. PEF <100 L or 50% predicted value
11. P_{CO_2} ≥45 mmHg
12. P_{O_2} ≤50 mmHg

Note: COPD, chronic obstructive pulmonary disease; FEV_1, forced expiratory volume in one second; MVV, maximum voluntary ventilation; PEF, peak expiratory flow rate; P_{CO_2}, partial pressure of carbon dioxide; P_{O_2}, partial pressure of oxygen.
Source: Modified from GW Smetana et al and from DN Mohr et al: Postgrad Med 100:247, 1996, with permission.

PREOPERATIVE PULMONARY ASSESSMENT

Perioperative pulmonary complications occur frequently and lead to significant morbidity and mortality. The guidelines from the American College of Physicians recommend the following:

(1) All patients undergoing noncardiac surgery should be assessed for risk of pulmonary complications (Table 8-5).

(2) Patients undergoing emergency or prolonged (>3 h) surgery; aortic aneurysm repair; vascular surgery; major abdominal, thoracic, neuro, head, and neck surgery; and general anesthesia should be considered to be at higher risk for postoperative pulmonary complications.

(3) Patients at higher risk of pulmonary complications should receive deep breathing exercises and/or incentive spirometry, as well as selective use of a nasogastric tube for postoperative nausea, vomiting, or symptomatic abdominal distention to reduce postoperative risk (Table 8-6).

(4) Routine preoperative spirometry and chest radiography are less helpful for predicting risk of postoperative pulmonary complications, but may be appropriate for patients with chronic obstructive pulmonary disease (COPD) or asthma.

(5) Pulmonary artery catheterization, total parenteral nutrition, and total enteral nutrition are not encouraged for postoperative pulmonary risk reduction.

Other Preoperative Pulmonary Risk-Modification Strategies Risk-modification strategies to reduce postoperative pulmonary complications should be implemented, particularly in higher-risk patients. Patients with cough or dyspnea preoperatively should be evaluated to

TABLE 8-6 RISK MODIFICATION TO REDUCE PERIOPERATIVE PULMONARY COMPLICATIONS

Preoperatively
- Cessation of smoking
- Training in proper breathing (incentive spirometry)
- Inhalation bronchodilator therapy
- Control of infection and secretion, when indicated
- Weight reduction, when appropriate

Intraoperatively
- Limited duration of anesthesia
- Select shorter acting neuromuscular blocking drugs when indicated
- Prevention of aspiration
- Maintenance of optimal bronchodilation

Postoperatively
- Continuation of preoperative measures, with particular attention to
  - inspiratory capacity maneuvers
  - mobilization of secretions
  - early ambulation
  - encouragement of coughing
  - selective use of a nasogastric tube
  - adequate pain control without excessive narcotics

Source: From VA Lawrence et al and from WF Dunn, PD Scanlon, Mayo Clin Proc 68:371, 1993, with permission.

determine the underlying cause of these symptoms. Patients who smoke should be counseled to quit for at least 8 weeks prior to elective surgery. Patients with asthma or COPD can be given steroids and bronchodilators pre- and postoperatively to optimize pulmonary function. Bacterial pulmonary infection should be treated preoperatively.

DIABETES MELLITUS

(See also Chap. 338) Many patients with diabetes mellitus have significant symptomatic or asymptomatic CAD and may have silent myocardial ischemia due to autonomic dysfunction. Evidence supports intensive perioperative glycemic control to achieve near-normal glucose levels (90–110 mg/dL) versus moderate glycemic control (120–200 mg/dL), using insulin infusion. This practice must be balanced against the risk of hypoglycemic complications. Oral hypoglycemic agonists should be held on the morning of operation. Perioperative hyperglycemia should be treated with intravenous infusion of short-acting insulin or subcutaneous sliding-scale insulin. Patients who are diet-controlled may proceed to surgery with close postoperative monitoring.

PROPHYLAXIS FOR INFECTIVE ENDOCARDITIS

(See also Chap. 118) Perioperative prophylactic antibiotics should be administered to patients with congenital or valvular heart disease, prosthetic valves, mitral valve prolapse, or other cardiac abnormalities in accordance with ACC/AHA practice guidelines.

PROPHYLAXIS OF VENOUS THROMBOEMBOLISM

(See also Chap. 256) Perioperative prophylaxis of venous thromboembolism should follow established guidelines of the American College of Chest Physicians. Aspirin is not supported as a single agent for thromboprophylaxis. Low-dose unfractionated heparin (≤5000 units subcutaneous bid), low-molecular-weight heparin (e.g., enoxaparin 30 mg bid or 40 mg od) or a pentasaccharide (fondaparinux 2.5 mg od) for patients at moderate risk, and unfractionated heparin (5000 units subcutaneous tid) for patients at high risk. Graduated compression stockings and pneumatic compression devices are useful supplements to anticoagulant therapy.

FURTHER READINGS

EAGLE KA et al: ACC/AHA guideline update for perioperative cardiovascular evaluation for noncardiac surgery—executive summary: A report of the American College of Cardiology/American Heart Association Task Force on Practice Guidelines (Committee to Update the 1996 Guidelines on Perioperative Cardiovascular Evaluation for Noncardiac Surgery). J Am Coll Cardiol 39:542, 2002

FLEISHER LA et al: ACC/AHA 2006 guideline update for perioperative cardiovascular evaluation for noncardiac surgery: Focused update on perioperative beta-blocker therapy. A report of the American College of Cardiology/American Heart Association Task Force on Practice Guidelines (writing committee to update the 2002 guidelines on perioperative cardiovascular evaluation for noncardiac surgery). J Am Coll Cardiol 47:2343, 2006

GEERTS WH et al: Prevention of venous thromboembolism: The Seventh ACCP Conference on Antithrombotic and Thrombolytic Therapy. Chest 126(Suppl 3):338S, 2004

LAWRENCE VA et al: Strategies to reduce postoperative pulmonary complications after noncardiothoracic surgery: Systematic review for the American College of Physicians. Ann Intern Med 144:596, 2006

LEE TH et al: Derivation and prospective validation of a simple index for prediction of cardiac risk of major noncardiac surgery. Circulation 100:1043, 1999

LINDENAUER PK et al: Perioperative beta-blocker therapy and mortality after major noncardiac surgery. N Engl J Med 353:349, 2005

MCFALLS EO et al: Coronary-artery revascularization before elective major vascular surgery. N Engl J Med 351:2795, 2004

QASEEM A et al: Risk assessment for and strategies to reduce perioperative pulmonary complications for patients undergoing noncardiothoracic surgery: A guideline from the American College of Physicians. Ann Intern Med 144:575, 2006

SMETANA GW et al: Preoperative pulmonary risk stratification for noncardiothoracic surgery: Systematic review for the American College of Physicians. Ann Intern Med 144:581, 2006

9 Geriatric Medicine

Lisa B. Caruso, Rebecca A. Silliman

AGING

Aging is the progressive, universal decline first in functional reserve and then in function that occurs in organisms over time. Aging is heterogeneous. It varies widely in different individuals and in different organs within a particular individual. Aging is not a disease; however, the risk of developing disease is increased, often dramatically, as a function of age. The biochemical composition of tissues changes with age; physiologic capacity decreases, the ability to maintain homeostasis in adapting to stressors declines, and vulnerability to disease processes increases with age. After maturation, mortality rate increases exponentially with age.

DEMOGRAPHY OF AGING

Populations worldwide are aging. Improvements in environmental (e.g., clean water and improved sanitation) and behavioral (nutrition, reduced risk exposures) factors and the treatment and prevention of infectious diseases are largely responsible for the 30-year increase in life expectancy since 1900. In the United States, by 2030, 1 person in 5 will be >65 years. Old people are not evenly distributed geographically. Half of older people in the United States live in nine states, led by California, Florida, New York, and Texas.

GLOBAL AGING

Between 2000 and 2030, the number of older adults worldwide is expected to increase from 420 to 974 million. At present 59% of older adults live in the developing countries of Africa, Asia, Latin America, the Caribbean, and Oceania. The developing world has the largest absolute number of older adults and is experiencing the largest percentage increase.

Only 13% of those ≥80 years live in the United States; over 40% of those ≥80 years live in Asia. Embedded within these figures are additional critically important factors. Women outlive men; only 15% of centenarians are men. Men also remarry more frequently than do women; consequently, older women are frequently single and live alone. Women are more likely to have inadequate financial resources. Women also spend a greater portion of their surviving years being disabled than do men. In the United States, rates of disability decreased during the 1980s and 1990s, but the epidemics of obesity and physical inactivity may reverse these trends. A further concern for countries that already have high proportions of older adults (e.g., Japan, Sweden, Greece, and Italy, whose citizens >65 are 17–18% of their population) is the ratio of the >65 age group to the 15- to 64-year age group—the so-called dependency ratio. This ratio currently ranges from 22% in Europe to 6% in Africa but is expected to rise to >50% in Europe by 2050, with all other areas of the world exceeding 25% by 2050, except Africa.

LIFE EXPECTANCY

Often life-extending therapies are not offered to older patients because of an underestimate of life expectancy. Figure 9-1 shows average life expectancy as a function of age together with values for the lowest and highest quartiles of the population. White women currently have the highest life expectancy. Black women and white men have nearly identical life expectancies, and black men have the poorest life expectancy. At age 85 years, racial differences in life expectancy largely disappear. The average 75-year-

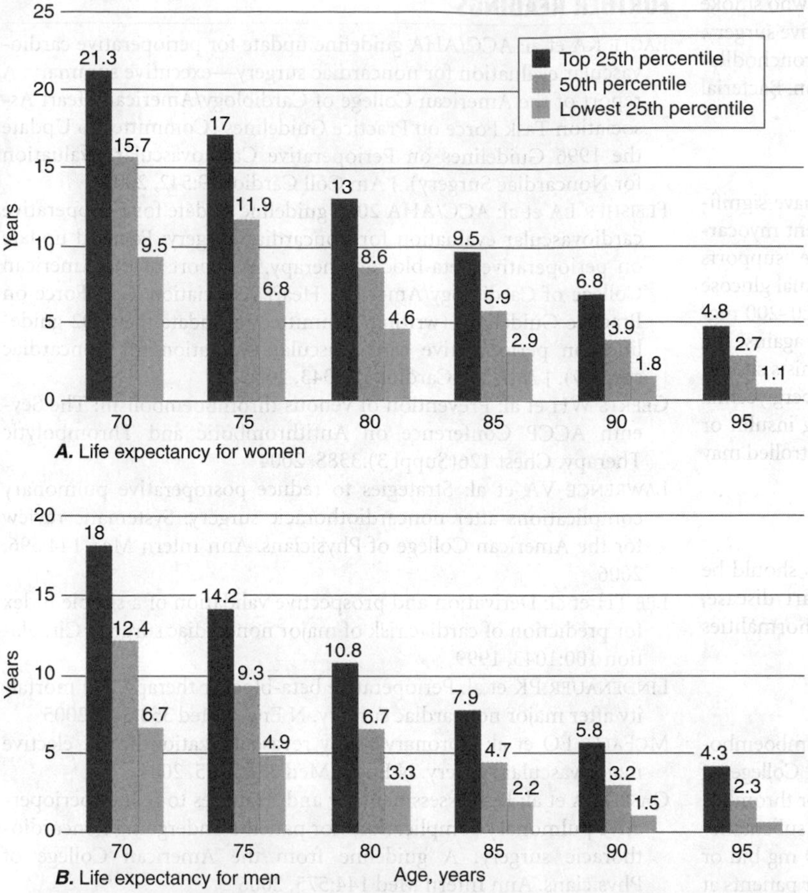

FIGURE 9-1 Upper, middle, and lower quartiles of life expectancy for women and men at selected ages. *(From LC Walter, KE Covinsky, JAMA 285:2751, 2001.)*

old is expected to live to age 86 and the average 85-year-old to age 91. Furthermore, where the issue has been examined, age is not a factor in determining the efficacy of a particular intervention. Thus, age alone generally should not be used to withhold life-extending interventions.

BIOLOGY OF AGING

As we age, we become increasingly unlike one another. For any variable one can measure, the variation in the distribution of values in a population increases with age. While the mean value may trend up or down, the age-related increase in the range of values is striking testimony to the diverse manifestations of the aging process. In addition, homeostatic mechanisms are slower to respond to stressors and take longer to restore normal function as we age. The ability to maintain stable function in the face of a change in the environment is called *allostasis* and it declines with age.

One problem as we age is nosologic; when is a particular change considered a normal age-related alteration and when does it become a disease? Ideas about the range of normal for a particular age continue to evolve. At one time, a 75-year-old with a blood pressure of 170/90 mmHg might have been considered to have an age-related increase in systolic blood pressure that did not require intervention. However, we now know that such a reading is a reflection of increased vascular stiffness, one of the most important risk factors for cardiovascular morbidity and mortality. Similarly, follow-up of individuals with fasting serum glucose levels of 6.1–6.7 mmol/L (110–120 mg/dL) have shown them to be at increased risk of diabetes complications. Accordingly impaired glucose metabolism is now defined as a fasting glucose level > 6.1 mmol/L (>110 mg/dL). Thus, the indications for interventions to alter natural history have changed and will continue to change as we learn more about aging.

Whether age-related changes that produce an aging phenotype have a common origin in a global process that alters cell or organ function or have heterogeneous contributions in different systems or different individuals is unclear. Studies of aging (*gerontology*) are aimed at understanding the cellular and molecular basis of age-related changes and have two ultimate therapeutic goals: preserving function as long as possible and extending life span. These two goals may not be linked.

The lack of model systems for studying aging has hampered progress. For many years, researchers have studied replicative senescence of normal cells in culture. Why do normal cells have a finite replicative potential in vitro and why do cells from older individuals undergo fewer divisions than cells from younger individuals? Many have hoped that insights from such studies would reveal information about the aging process. However, the link between the failure of cells to divide in a synthetic culture medium and the aging phenotype of a whole organism is tenuous, at best. The body tissues with the greatest replicative potential should identify the organs most susceptible to age-related defective replication. In humans, these organs are the lining of the small intestine and the hematopoietic system. In the absence of disease, no age-related problem is caused by the inability of cells to replicate. Old people do not run out of absorptive surface in the small intestine or fail to make blood cells. Better in vitro models of aging are needed.

Experimental aging studies rely heavily on manipulation of life span in intact organisms such as worms, flies, and rodents. Such studies have revealed important insights. Alteration of genes involved in DNA repair often leads to premature aging. Alteration of genes involved in insulin signaling often leads to life extension. In the worm, life extension can be accomplished by alteration of gene expression in a single tissue, neurons. Calorie restriction (at least 30% lower than an ad lib diet) increases both average and maximal life span in a wide range of species. In several species, interventions associated with increased life span activate the expression of one or more of a family of genes, called *sirtuins*, that function by silencing the expression of certain other genes. However, these and other important observations have not yet led to a complete picture of the molecular basis of aging. Some ideas are summarized in Table 9-1.

Additional insights about aging may be derived by understanding the clinical syndromes that produce a premature aging phenotype, the so-called segmental progerias. These syndromes are rare inherited disorders that mimic normal aging imperfectly. They include Werner

TABLE 9-1 SOME THEORIES OF AGING

Hypothesis	How It May Work
Genetic	Aging is a genetic program activated in post-reproductive life when an individual's evolutionary mission is accomplished
Oxidative stress	Accumulation of oxidative damage to DNA, proteins, and lipids interferes with normal function and produces a decrease in stress responses
Mitochondrial dysfunction	A common deletion in mitochondrial DNA with age compromises function and alters cell metabolic processes and adaptability to environmental change
Hormonal changes	The decline and loss of circadian rhythm in secretion of some hormones produces a functional hormone deficiency state
Telomere shortening	Aging is related to a decline in the ability of cells to replicate
Defective host defenses	The failure of the immune system to respond to infectious agents and the overactivity of natural immunity create vulnerability to environmental stresses
Accumulation of senescent cells	Renewing tissues become dysfunctional through loss of ability to renew

syndrome, Bloom syndrome, Cockayne syndrome, Hutchinson-Gilford progeria, and Rothmund-Thomson syndrome. Hutchinson-Gilford progeria involves a mutation in lamin A, a component of the nuclear envelope. The symptoms have an onset in early childhood, and median survival is only about 13 years. All the other well-studied progeria syndromes involve mutations in DNA helicases, which are involved in DNA repair and recombination. The syndromes have features of accelerated aging and are associated with an increased risk of cancers. Werner syndrome has accelerated atherosclerosis as a prominent feature. Whether these conditions can reveal secrets of normal aging is not yet clear. However, they suggest that the maintenance of the integrity of the genome is a vulnerable function that can lead to premature aging if it is performed suboptimally.

Genetics and Exceptional Longevity Just as genetics is revealing information about premature aging, family studies may also identify features of delayed or successful aging. Twin studies suggest that ~30% of the variation in longevity can be attributed to genetic factors, with the remainder being attributable to environmental and behavioral factors. Long life span runs in families, and studies of centenarians and their offspring may define particularly adaptive phenotypes. For example, centenarians are less likely to be carriers of the apolipoprotein E ε4 allele, which is associated both with risk for heart disease and Alzheimer's disease. Ashkenazi Jewish centenarians and their offspring have been found to have larger high-density lipoprotein (HDL) and low-density lipoprotein (LDL) particle sizes; a lower prevalence of hypertension, cardiovascular disease, and the metabolic syndrome; and a greater likelihood of carrying an atheroprotective variant of the cholesteryl ester transfer protein gene. As studies of genetically more homogeneous populations such as those in Iceland and Sardinia progress, additional genetic contributions to healthy aging may be identified.

Frailty, Disabilty, and Comorbid Illness Frailty is defined as a clinical syndrome in which three or more of the following are present: unintentional weight loss of ≥4.5 kg (≥10 lb) in the past year (reflecting poor nutrition, catabolic metabolism, and sarcopenia), feeling exhausted (poor endurance), poor grip strength (weakness), slow walking speed, and low physical activity. Frailty overlaps with disability and comorbid illness but is not synonymous with them. Frailty is associated with a high risk of falls, disability, and death. It is unknown whether frailty is a single clinical syndrome or multiple syndromes and whether it has a central cause or multiple causes. Frail patients often share many physical and biochemical characteristics, and studies are underway to assess whether the syndrome or parts of it are responsive to interventions.

CHRONIC DISEASES AND THEIR IMPLICATIONS

The incidence, prevalence, and burden of chronic diseases increase with age, and this increased burden of disease is also associated with an increased risk of disability and decreased ability to recover from disability once it occurs.

The Global Perspective In 2005, chronic diseases accounted for 20 million deaths worldwide among those ≥70 years. The major disease contributors were cardiovascular disease (30%), cancer (13%), chronic respiratory disease (7%), and diabetes mellitus (2%). These diseases, driven to a large extent by tobacco use and obesity, are not concentrated in the developed world; rather, they are a large and growing problem in developing/low-income countries that lack the resources to prevent and manage chronic diseases and their consequences.

General Considerations Hypertension and diabetes mellitus are two common chronic conditions whose prevalence increases with age. In the United States, the National Health and Nutrition Examination Survey estimates that the prevalence of hypertension is between 60 and 84% and the prevalence of diabetes mellitus is between 18 and 21% in adults >65 years. The prevalence of both hypertension and diabetes is projected to increase substantially based on the demographics of aging and obesity. Moreover, rates of uncontrolled blood pressure in older adults are increasing, not decreasing. Both hypertension and diabetes accelerate functional decline in older adults, with hypertension accelerating cognitive decline and diabetes accelerating physical decline. Diabetes is also associated with a greater risk and severity of urinary incontinence (UI) and of falls in older women. Moreover, diabetes and stroke are the conditions most consistently associated with a diminished capacity for functional recovery in the aged.

The incidence of most cancers and cancer-specific mortality both increase with age. The age-adjusted incidence of cancer is ten times higher in the 65+ population than in those <65, and the age-adjusted cancer mortality is 15-fold higher. As a result, the incidence of cancer is expected to increase disproportionately in relation to overall population growth, and this trend is observed in countries throughout the world. Moreover, the majority of cancer survivors (>60%) are 65+ years of age.

In 2000, the leading causes of death among older Americans were heart disease (33%), cancer (22%), and cerebrovascular disease (8%). The death rate from heart disease has continued to decline; in 2006, cancer was the leading cause of death in persons <85 years. The management of chronic disease in older adults is particularly challenging. As examples, both hypertension and diabetes are established risk factors for micro- and macrovascular disease. Randomized clinical trials have demonstrated treatment efficacy, and guidelines for therapy are well established. Yet substantial evidence indicates that both conditions are inadequately treated, particularly in older adults with comorbidity. A portion of the problem is related to the fact that most clinical trials omit patients with comorbidities, making their results difficult to extrapolate to older patients with comorbid illness who are taking several other medications. The risks of drug-drug or drug-food interactions increase as a function of the number of medications used and patient age. In addition, the physician must take into account the impact of the disease and its treatment on the quality of life. Here, current functional status and rate of previous decline are helpful factors in estimating the level of functioning to which the patient may return. In concert with patient preferences and life goals, this information can help physicians and patients make decisions that are optimal at the individual patient level.

One attempt to develop an evidence-based quality of care framework for older adults cared for in ambulatory settings has been the Assessing Care of Vulnerable Elders (ACOVE) project. Designed to inform the care of persons >65 years who are at high risk for death or functional decline over a 2-year period, based on age, self-rated health, self-report of physical capability, and functional limitations, the ACOVE indicators cover 22 topics, including diseases, syndromes, impairments, and clinical situations that are prevalent, have strong influence on health/quality of life, and are amenable to available interventions. The tool has drawbacks. The indicators are generally focused on the care of one disease or condition at a time, and the total number of indicators is overwhelmingly large (236). However, it appears that better quality of care is associated with improved survival. Better strategies to target clusters of interventions to those who will benefit most are needed.

APPROACH TO: The Geriatric Patient

FUNCTIONAL ASSESSMENT While the geriatric patient may have multiple chronic illnesses, functional status is the best indicator of prognosis and longevity. Functional status is defined as how well a person is able to provide for his or her own daily needs. Changes in function may signal a medical illness, advancing cognitive impairment, changes in social support, depression, substance abuse, or a combination of these. These changes should not be accepted as "just part of getting old." Documentation of a patient's baseline functional status is essential so that changes can be identified and addressed.

TABLE 9-2 SUGGESTED BRIEF GERIATRIC ASSESSMENT INSTRUMENTS

Domain	Instrument	Sensitivity	Specificity	Time (min)	Cutpoint	Comments
Cognition						
Dementia	MMSE	79–100%[a]	46–100%	9	<24[b]	Widely studied and accepted
	Timed time and change test	94–100%	37–46%	<2	<3 s for time and <10 s for change	Sensitive and quick
Delirium	CAM	94–100%	90–95%	<5		Sensitive and easy to apply
Affective disorders	GDS 5-question form	97%	85%	1	2	Rapid screen
Visual impairment	Snellen chart	"Gold standard"	"Gold standard"	2	Inability to read at 20/40 line	Universally used
Hearing impairment	Whispered voice	80–90%	70–89%	0.5	50% correct	No special equipment needed
	Pure tone audiometry	94–100%	70–94%	<5	Inability to hear >2 of 4 40-db tones (0.5, 1, 2, and 3 kHz)	Can be performed by trained office staff
Dental health	DENTAL[c]	82%	90%	<2 (estimated)	Score >2	
Nutritional status	Weight loss of >4.5 kg (>10 lb) in 6 months or weight <45 kg (<100 lb)	65–70%	87–88%		Yes to either	
Gait and balance	"Timed Get Up and Go" test	88%	94%	<1	>20s	Requires no special equipment

[a]Some studies have found lower sensitivities, but most studies of dementia subjects fall in this range.
[b]Cutoff is dependent on a number of variables including age, education, and racial or ethnic background.
[c]KA Atchinson, TA Dolan. Development of the geriatric oral health assessment index. J Dent Educ 11:680, 1990; with permission.

Note: MMSE, Mini-Mental Status Examination; CAM, confusion assessment method; GDS, geriatric depression scale.
Source: From CK Cassel et al. *Geriatric Medicine: An Evidence-Based Approach*, 4th ed. New York, Springer-Verlag, 2003; with permission.

Table 9-2 lists some suggested brief screening strategies for assessing functional status.

The first opportunity to assess the functional status of an older adult is when the patient is greeted and taken for a short walk into an examination room. In what way is the greeting received? Does the patient need assistance in getting out of a chair? Does he or she use an assistive device, such as a cane or walker? What is the patient's gait speed? How stable is the patient's gait? Is the patient fatigued after a short walk? These observations provide important initial information about how chronic illnesses affect the life of an older adult.

The basic activities of daily living (ADLs), which comprise activities essential for physical independence, and the instrumental activities of daily living (IADLs), which are necessary for independence in the community, are the most commonly used tools to assess functional status. The ADLs are dressing, bathing, feeding, toileting, transferring, and ambulating. The IADLs are money management, medication administration, using transportation, using the telephone, shopping, housekeeping, and meal preparation. These activities should be reviewed with the patient at the initial encounter and at periodic intervals. Cognitive deficits and psychosocial factors, however, may invalidate a patient's self-report, requiring the assistance of a third party for an accurate assessment. When functional deficits are identified, services provided by community (formal) or familial (informal) supports can be implemented to help the older adult continue to live in the least restrictive setting possible.

Other dimensions of the geriatric functional assessment include assessments of gait and balance, cognition, vision and hearing, dental and nutritional health, and driving ability. The Timed Get Up and Go Test is a valid clinical measure of balance in older adults. The patient is observed and timed as he or she rises from a chair, walks 3 m, turns around, and returns to sit down in the chair. A healthy older adult should be able to complete the test in <10 s. Difficulty performing this test is associated with increased fall risk and warrants further evaluation of mobility.

The screening tools to assess cognition in the older adult assist in identifying dementia and delirium, two common geriatric syndromes, both of which have a major effect on the functional status of the older adult. In addition, history-taking can be inaccurate and misleading if cognitive impairment is not recognized before a medical evaluation. The Mini-Mental State Examination (MMSE) is the most commonly used test to assess cognitive function (Chap. 26). The Mini-Cog assessment instrument is an alternative to the MMSE and may be superior in assessing culturally diverse populations. The Mini-Cog consists of repeating three unrelated words, followed by a clock-drawing test (CDT) showing a specific time. The times 11:10 or 8:20 are often used. The patient is then asked to recall the three words. The patient receives one point for each recalled word after the CDT and two points for a normal clock. A score of 0–2 is a positive screen for dementia.

Delirium can cause loss of independence, prolonged hospitalizations, and increased health care costs and can be life threatening. It is often undiagnosed by health care providers and not recognized as a symptom of other medical illnesses. The Confusion Assessment Method (CAM) is highly sensitive and specific for identifying delirium. Delirium is diagnosed when the confusional state is both (1) acute in onset with a fluctuating course and (2) associated with inattention, and either (3) manifested by disorganized thinking or (4) an altered level of consciousness. Simple tests of attention include having the patient repeat a series of numbers or stating the months of the year backwards.

While specialists perform full vision and hearing assessments, any provider caring for an older adult should be able to screen for deficits in these areas because they commonly present in older patients, they can lead to loss of patient independence, and they often result from treatable conditions. Basic tests for visual acuity such as the handheld Jaeger card for testing near vision and the wall-mounted Snellen chart for testing far vision are the tests most commonly used in office-based practices. Visual impairment is defined as being unable to read the 20/40 line or worse. Visual acuity itself has not been associated with increased fall risk in most studies; however, binocular vision, depth perception, and contrast sensitivity contribute to postural stability and object recognition. Hearing impairment can lead to decreased physical function, depression, and social isolation. The whisper test and testing with a handheld audioscope are used frequently as screening tests. To perform the whisper test, the examiner covers the opposite ear of the patient being tested, exhales completely, and then whispers an easily answered question from a distance of 60 cm (2 ft) from the ear being tested. Treatment of hearing loss with amplification by a hearing aid has been shown to improve quality of life. Patients demonstrating vision or hearing impairment should be referred for full ophthalmologic and audiologic evaluation. Hearing and vision impairment together are associated with lower functional status than either impairment alone.

Malnutrition is not uncommon in older adults and is associated with increased mortality, morbidity, and admission to nursing homes. In community-dwelling adults, the following definitions of malnutrition may be used: (1) involuntary weight loss [e.g., ≥4.5 kg (≥10 lb) over 6 months, ≥4% over 1 year], (2) abnormal body mass index [BMI: weight/height^2 (in kg/m^2) (e.g., BMI < 22 or BMI > 27], (3) hypoalbuminemia [e.g., ≤38 g/L (≤3.8 g/dL)], (4) hypocholesterolemia [e.g., <4.1 mmol/L (<160 mg/dL)], or (5) specific vitamin or micronutrient deficiency (e.g., vitamin B_{12}). When any one of these is present, a multidimensional assessment should be undertaken. The clinician should review the patient's access to food. Are there economic or other barriers to receiving high-quality food? Are there dental problems that might interfere with eating such as loose dentures, missing teeth, or other oral pathology? Many medical illnesses interfere with digestion or absorption of food, increase nutritional requirements, or require dietary restrictions. Is the patient unable to shop, prepare meals, or feed him- or herself? Does the patient have cultural habits or food preferences that could affect his or her nutritional status? Poor appetite may be related to medications, medical illnesses, or depression.

For many older adults, being independent depends on driving an automobile. However, the traffic violation rate per driver is increased in both teenagers and older drivers. One study has identified poor design copying on the MMSE, fewer blocks walked, and more foot abnormalities as the best predictors of adverse driving events. While a patient can undergo a formal driving assessment, often done by rehabilitation experts, the clinician can also indirectly assess a patient's driving skills by performing vision, cognition, and motor assessments in the office. Making the decision that an older adult is no longer able to drive is often done by the patient, but when the patient has limited insight into his or her physical and/or cognitive impairments, family, friends, health care providers, and sometimes government employees are responsible for keeping the older patient, as well as other drivers, safe.

GERIATRIC SYNDROMES

Geriatric syndrome refers to a symptom presentation that is common in older adults; most are multifactorial in origin. Several of these topics are covered in more detail elsewhere in the text.

Dementia and Delirium Dementia is a syndrome of progressive decline in which multiple intellectual abilities deteriorate, causing both cognitive and functional impairment. While dementia is a state of chronic confusion, delirium is an acute state of confusion. It is important to differentiate delirium from dementia. Early identification and treatment of the underlying causes of delirium can improve outcomes. Delirium may be the only manifestation of a life-threatening illness in the older adult. Both dementia and delirium are characterized by disorientation, memory impairment, paranoia, hallucinations, emotional lability, and sleep-wake cycle reversal. Key features of delirium are acute onset, impaired attention, and an altered level of consciousness. Dementia and delirium are described more fully in Chaps. 365 and 26, respectively.

The main goals of care of a patient with dementia are to maintain an optimal quality of life and to maximize cognitive and physical functioning. Therefore, when an older patient presents with cognitive impairment, a key goal is to identify and treat reversible causes of cognitive impairment, such as infections, electrolyte abnormalities, vitamin deficiencies, thyroid disease, substance abuse, medication, and psychiatric illnesses. The clinician must then ask key questions: (1) Is the patient safe in the community? (2) Is the patient able to perform his or her own ADLs and IADLs? (3) What assistance is needed to maximize the patient's functioning in his or her living situation? The patient may not be able to answer these questions accurately, so an objective, cognitively intact informant will be helpful.

If the patient has dangerous behaviors, such as leaving the stove on or getting lost, a plan of care involving increased patient supervision should be put in place. As dementia progresses, more caregiving services, both formal and informal, will need to be added to support the patient in the community. *Formal caregivers* are paid care providers. Examples are visiting nurses, home health aides who assist with personal hygiene, homemakers who assist with housework and meal preparation, Meals-on-Wheels, adult day programs, state aging services, and hospice services. *Informal caregivers* are persons who provide an older adult with unpaid care. Examples are family members, friends, neighbors, or church members.

The primary caregiver of a patient with dementia may need more physician support than the patient. Caring for a disabled spouse or parent is associated with an increased risk of depression or anxiety. Caregivers experiencing mental or emotional strain have an increased risk of dying compared to non-caregivers. Predictors of nursing home admission for patients with Alzheimer's disease include aggression, assault, paranoia, nighttime wandering, and loss of capacity to recognize the caregiver. Adult day care and respite programs may help to alleviate some caregiver burden. Support groups, through organizations such as the Alzheimer's Association, can also help to educate caregivers and decrease stress.

When patients with dementia exhibit agitated behaviors, medical illnesses, such as infections, pain syndromes, and drug side effects, must be ruled out as causes. These behaviors are, however, often part of a dementing illness. If the agitated behavior is harmful to the patient or others and does not respond to non-pharmacologic therapies, such as redirecting the patient, providing a calm environment, or familiar surroundings, then low doses of psychotropic medication may be helpful. Antipsychotics, anxiolytics, or antidepressants can be used, depending on the type of symptoms. Low-dose risperidone (0.25–1.5 mg/d) or olanzapine (2.5–10 mg/d) can be used if a patient has upsetting delusions or hallucinations. Antidepressants such as citalopram (10–30 mg/d) can be used for depressive symptoms. Patients on antipsychotics should be monitored closely for the development of extrapyramidal side effects, such as tremor, rigidity, and bradykinesia. The lowest dose possible should be used; dosage reductions should be attempted, if possible, at 6-month intervals. Sometimes, as cognitive functioning worsens, patients will no longer have the psychoses or the depression causing the agitated behaviors.

Falls This discussion of falls excludes falls occurring from seizure, stroke, syncope, or an insurmountable environmental hazard (Chap. 24). Fall rates and risk of injury from falls increase with age. Annually, ~30% of community dwelling adults >65 years fall, while 50% of individuals >80 years fall. Injuries in 20–30% of fallers reduce subsequent mobility and independence, with 3–5% of falls resulting in fracture. Falling is an independent risk factor for nursing home placement. Often the occurrence of a fall does not come to the attention of the health care provider. Given fall frequency and resulting morbidity and mortality from falling in older adults, all older patients should have a fall risk assessment and be asked about falls in the past year.

While most falls are multifactorial, falling is sometimes a symptom of another disease, such as an infection or neurologic disorder, or a medication side effect. In addition, age-related physiologic changes contribute to fall risk. These include decreased proprioception, increased postural sway, and declines in baroreflex sensitivity resulting in orthostatic hypotension. The evaluation of a fall should begin with a history, including the circumstances at the time of the fall, any associated symptoms, and a thorough medication review of both prescription and over-the-counter medications. The physical examination should include postural vital signs, vision evaluation, gait and balance testing, and a musculoskeletal evaluation of joint stability and range of motion. An environmental assessment of the patient's home by a visiting nurse or other health care provider can reveal additional hazards that can increase fall risk, such as clutter, loose carpets, and poor lighting.

Interventions designed to reduce fall rates must also preserve mobility and independence. Physical restraint use has been found to be strongly associated with increased fall risk and increased risk for serious injury from a fall in nursing home residents. The major risk factors for falls are shown in Table 9-3. Several factors associated with increased risk for falling include low creatinine clearance [<1.1 mL/s (< 65 mL/min)], low serum 25-hydroxyvitamin D levels (< 39 nmol/L) and high serum parathyroid hormone levels, insomnia, and fear of falling. Table 9-3 also outlines suggested interventions targeted at common fall risk factors. General exercise and balance training; t'ai chi; psychotropic medication elimination; and multidisciplinary, multifactorial, risk factor screening and intervention have been shown to reduce fall risk.

TABLE 9-3 RECOMMENDED COMPONENTS OF CLINICAL ASSESSMENT AND MANAGEMENT FOR OLDER PERSONS LIVING IN THE COMMUNITY WHO ARE AT RISK FOR FALLING

Assessment and Risk Factor	Management
Circumstances of previous falls[a]	Changes in environment and activity to reduce the likelihood of recurrent falls
Medication use High-risk medications (e.g., benzodiazepines, other sleeping medications, neuroleptics, antidepressants, anticonvulsants, or class IA antiarrhythmics)[a,b,c] Four or more medications[c]	Review and reduction of medications
Vision[a] Acuity <20/60 Decreased depth perception Decreased contrast sensitivity Cataracts	Ample lighting without glare; avoidance of multifocal glasses while walking; referral to an ophthalmologist
Postural blood pressure (after ≥5 min in a supine position, immediately after standing, and 2 min after standing)[c] ≥20 mmHg (or ≥20%) drop in systolic pressure, with or without symptoms, either immediately or after 2 min of standing	Diagnosis and treatment of underlying cause, if possible; review and reduction of medications; modification of salt restriction; adequate hydration; compensatory strategies (e.g., elevation of head of bed, rising slowly, or dorsiflexion exercises); pressure stockings; pharmacologic therapy if the above strategies fail
Balance and gait[b,c] Patient's report or observation of unsteadiness Impairment on brief assessment (e.g., the Get-Up and Go test or performance-oriented assessment of mobility)	Diagnosis and treatment of underlying cause, if possible; reduction of medications that impair balance; environmental interventions; referral to physical therapist for assistive devices and for gait and progressive balance training
Targeted neurologic examination Impaired proprioception[a] Impaired cognition[a] Decreased muscle strength[b,c]	Diagnosis and treatment of underlying cause, if possible; increase in proprioceptive input (with an assistive device or appropriate footwear that encases the foot and has a low heel and thin sole); reduction of medications that impede cognition; awareness on the part of caregivers of cognitive deficits; reduction of environmental risk factors; referral to physical therapist for gait, balance, and strength training
Targeted musculoskeletal examination: examination of legs (joints and range of motion) and examination of feet[a]	Diagnosis and treatment of the underlying cause, if possible; referral to physical therapist for strength, range-of-motion, and gait and balance training and for assistive devices; use of appropriate footwear; referral to podiatrist
Targeted cardiovascular examination[b] Syncope Arrhythmia (if there is known cardiac disease, an abnormal electrocardiogram, and syncope)	Referral to cardiologist; carotid-sinus massage (in the case of syncope)
Home-hazard evaluation after hospital discharge[b,c]	Removal of loose rugs and use of nightlights; nonslip bath-mats, and stair rails; other interventions as necessary

[a]Recommendation of this assessment is based on observational data that the finding is associated with an increased risk of falling.
[b]Recommendation of this assessment is based on one or more randomized controlled trials of a single intervention.
[c]Recommendation of this assessment is based on one or more randomized controlled trials of a multifactorial intervention strategy that included this component.
Source: ME Tinetti: N Engl J Med 348:45, 2003; with permission.

Urinary Incontinence UI is a major problem for older adults, afflicting up to 30% of community-dwelling elders and 50% of nursing home residents. Up to age 80 years, UI affects women twice as commonly as men; after age 80, the sexes are equally affected. In addition to the great impact of UI on a patient's well-being, including embarrassment, social isolation, and depression, UI is also a risk factor for nursing home placement. While certainly not a normal part of aging, advanced age, functional impairment, dementia, obesity, smoking, affective disorder, constipation, certain medical illnesses (such as chronic obstructive pulmonary disease and heart failure), and a history of pelvic surgery are associated with UI. UI is often due to a combination of these risk factors.

Older patients must be asked directly whether they have symptoms of UI, since only half of community-dwelling women with incontinence will discuss their incontinence with a health care provider. UI can then be determined to be either *transient* or *established*, although "transient" UI may be misdiagnosed as "established" if left untreated. The "DRIIIPP" mnemonic (Table 9-4) is very useful when evaluating a patient for reversible conditions that may cause or contribute to UI. If these conditions are identified and treated, the older adult benefits from relief of UI and symptoms of other comorbidities.

Leaking of urine occurs in four ways. The bladder can be limited in its ability to empty *or* in its ability to store urine; or one or both of the urethral sphincters may be unable to allow storage of urine *or* to allow passage of urine. Impairments can exist in one or in several of the urine storage mechanisms of the lower urinary tract. Four classifications of established UI have been proposed based on this understanding of the lower urinary tract: stress incontinence, urge incontinence, mixed stress and urge incontinence, and overflow incontinence.

Stress incontinence, which is rare in men, results when the urethral sphincter mechanisms are inadequate to hold urine during bladder filling. Patients describe symptoms of leaking small amounts of urine during activities that increase intraabdominal pressure, such as coughing, laughing, sneezing, lifting, or standing up. Patient history is very sensitive (0.906) but not very specific (0.511) in diagnosing stress incontinence. A stress test in the office can be performed by having the patient stand with a full bladder and cough. The test is positive if urine leakage coincides with the cough. An involuntary bladder contraction induced by the cough may cause leakage several seconds after the cough. The most common causes of stress incontinence in women are insufficient pelvic support due to childbearing, gynecologic surgery, and the decreased effects of estrogen on tissues of the lower urinary tract. Surgical interventions are the most effective treatments; pelvic muscle exercises can be helpful, although treatment failure is higher in patients who have two or more leakages per day.

Urge incontinence, also known as detrusor overactivity (DO), is characterized by uninhibited bladder contractions and is the most common form of UI in older adults. Patients often describe symptoms of an uncontrollable need to void. Urinary frequency and nocturnal incontinence are common, particularly accompanied by loss of larger urine

TABLE 9-4 REVERSIBLE CONDITIONS ASSOCIATED WITH URINARY INCONTINENCE

*D*elirium
*R*estricted mobility—illness, injury, gait disorder, restraint
*I*nfection—acute, symptomatic urinary tract infection
*I*nflammation—atrophic vaginitis
*I*mpaction—of feces
*P*olyuria—diabetes, caffeine intake, volume overload
*P*harmaceuticals—diuretics, α-adrenergic agonists or antagonists, anticholinergic agents (psychotropics, antidepressants, anti-Parkinsonians)

Source: After DB Reuben et al.

volumes (>100 mL). Urge incontinence may be idiopathic, associated with lesions of the central nervous system, such as a stroke, or be due to bladder irritation from infection, stones, or tumors. The term *detrusor hyperactivity with impaired contractility* (DHIC) is a type of urge incontinence characterized by involuntary bladder contractions with a weak detrusor muscle leading to incomplete emptying of the bladder. The diagnosis is primarily based on a patient's symptoms in the absence of urinary retention and the leakage of urine with stress maneuvers.

Measurement of postvoid residual (PVR) should be part of an incontinence evaluation in all patients. Under sterile conditions, the patient's bladder is catheterized 5–10 min after the patient has voided. Generally, a PVR > 200 mL suggests detrusor underactivity or obstruction. The patient should be referred for further urologic evaluation.

Initial treatment of urge incontinence should be bladder retraining by encouraging the patient to void every 2 h or based on the patient's symptom frequency. The patient can also try urgency control by sitting or standing quietly while focusing on allowing the urgency to pass before slowly walking to the bathroom to void. If the patient has no incontinence for 2 days, the voiding interval can be increased by 30–60 minutes until the patient is only voiding every 3–4 h. The anticholinergic drugs, oxybutinin and tolterodine, which cause bladder relaxation, can be added to this therapy. Their use in older adults may be limited by anticholinergic symptoms such as urinary retention, confusion, constipation, and dry mouth. Patients using tolterodine have a reduced risk of dry mouth and fewer withdrawals due to side effects, but the efficacy of oxybutinin and tolterodine is similar.

Mixed incontinence refers to UI where symptoms of both stress and urge incontinence are present. A simple, quick questionnaire consisting of three incontinence questions (3IQ) may help to classify urge and stress incontinence in women in the primary care setting. Question one asks if the patient has leaked urine in the past 3 months. Question two familiarizes patients with types of incontinence: stress, urge, or other. Question three asks the patient for the category of incontinence based on her symptoms during the past 3 months: stress, urge, mixed, or other. The 3IQ improved the likelihood of a positive diagnosis of urge incontinence (+likelihood ratio of 3.29) and of stress incontinence (+likelihood ratio of 2.13).

Overflow incontinence is due to either bladder outlet obstruction or an atonic bladder. Male patients, but rarely females, may complain of dribbling after voiding, an incessant urge to urinate, or straining to urinate. On physical examination, patients may have a palpable distended bladder. Prostatic hypertrophy, prostate cancer, and urethral strictures are the most common causes of overflow incontinence in men, while a cystocele can cause this problem in women. Detrusor atonicity or underactivity can be caused by spinal cord disease, autonomic neuropathy of diabetes, alcoholism, vitamin B_{12} deficiency, Parkinson's disease, tabes dorsalis, or chronic outlet obstruction. Urodynamic testing is helpful in distinguishing urethral obstruction from detrusor underactivity. The most effective treatment for bladder outlet obstruction is surgical removal of the obstruction. Intermittent or indwelling catheterization may be required for nonoperative candidates with obstruction or for patients with detrusor underactivity. For men who have benign prostatic hypertrophy (BPH) and are not in retention, α-adrenergic blockers such as terazosin, doxazosin, or tamulosin can decrease symptoms of urinary frequency and nocturia. Finasteride, a 5α-reductase inhibitor, may be useful in combination with doxazosin for decreasing lower urinary tract symptoms due to BPH in men with a total prostate volume of ≥25 mL.

The diagnosis of *functional incontinence* describes individuals who have UI and have either cognitive or functional impairments which limit their ability to toilet themselves. However, other treatable causes of UI may be missed if one assumes dementia or immobility is the cause of UI in these patients.

Pressure Ulcers Pressure ulcers, also known as pressure sores, bedsores, or decubitus ulcers, occur in older patients with reduced mobility. A pressure ulcer occurs when increased pressure between skin and a bony prominence produces tissue necrosis. While pressure ulcers can occur anywhere, 80% of pressure ulcers occur over the heels, lateral malleoli, sacrum, ischia, and greater trochanters. Shear forces, causing stretching and angulation of blood vessels, and frictional forces, causing separation of the epidermal or dermal layers, can also lead to tissue necrosis and open ulceration. Moisture can increase friction leading to maceration and superficial skin erosions.

Reported incidence data for the United States vary widely by site of care: general acute care, 0.4–38%; long-term care, 2.2–23.9%; and home care, 0–17%. Prevalence rates range from 10–18% in general acute care, 2.3–28% in long-term care, and 0–29% in home care. In older adults and nursing home residents, the development of a pressure ulcer increases mortality by fourfold. Osteomyelitis and sepsis are important, morbid complications of pressure ulcers.

The notion that all pressure ulcers are preventable is controversial. While repositioning patients at risk for developing pressure ulcers every 2 h and providing bedbound patients mattresses with pressure-relieving capabilities are standard interventions to prevent pressure ulcers, other immutable risk factors may ultimately contribute to skin breakdown in certain patients. Major risk factors associated with the development of pressure ulcers are listed in Table 9-5.

When an ulcer is identified, one must try to identify its etiology. Pressure ulcers lie at sites of pressure. Diabetic ulcers can also be caused by pressure in extremities compromised by neuropathy and vascular disease, including both large and small blood vessels. Venous stasis ulcers develop on the lower extremities with or without edema due to incompetent valves of the veins. Arterial ischemic ulcers develop at sites of decreased blood flow. Since adequate blood supply is necessary for tissue to heal, assessment of pulses and ankle-brachial indices (ABI) for ulcers of the lower extremities can provide prognostic information. An ABI of <0.4 is associated with a low likelihood of wound healing. If the patient is not a surgical candidate for revascularization, the goal of care must be to keep the wound free of infection and to alleviate any related patient discomfort.

When an ulcer is identified as a pressure ulcer, the ulcer should be staged so that the appropriate therapy may be instituted. The staging in

TABLE 9-5 MAJOR RISK FACTORS ASSOCIATED WITH THE DEVELOPMENT OF PRESSURE ULCERS IN THE OLDER ADULT

Alterations in sensation or response to discomfort
Degenerative neurologic disease
Cerebrovascular disease
Central nervous system (CNS) injury
Depression
Drugs that adversely affect alertness
Alterations in mobility
Neurologic disease/injury
Fractures
Pain
Restraints
Significant changes in weight (≥5% in 30 days or ≥10% in the previous 180 days)
Protein-calorie undernutrition
Edema
Incontinence
Bowel and bladder

Source: From American Medical Directors Association (AMDA): *Pressure Ulcers*. Columbia, MD, American Medical Directors Association, 1996.

TABLE 9-6 STAGING SYSTEM FOR PRESSURE ULCERS

Stage 1	Nonblanchable erythema of intact skin, or dislocation, edema, induration, and warmth over a bony prominence among patients with darker skin; the heralding lesion of skin ulceration.
Stage 2	Partial thickness skin loss involving epidermis, dermis, or both. The ulcer is superficial and presents clinically as an abrasion, blister, or shallow crater.
Stage 3	Full thickness skin loss involving damage to, or necrosis of, subcutaneous tissue that may extend down to, but not through, fascia. The ulcer presents clinically as a deep crater with or without undermining adjacent tissue.
Stage 4	Full thickness skin loss with extensive destruction, tissue necrosis or damage to muscle, bone, or supporting structures (e.g., tendon, joint capsule). Undermining and sinus tracts also may be associated with Stage 4 pressure ulcers.

Source: From American Medical Directors Association (AMDA): *Pressure Ulcers.* Columbia, MD, American Medical Directors Association, 1996.

Table 9-6 is based on a system developed in 1989 by the National Pressure Ulcer Advisory Panel. Nonblanching erythema constitutes vascular damage and hemorrhage. Stage 1 ulcers can progress to stage 4 ulcers in as little as a day or two, depending on how deeply the necrosis extends. Once a hard, dark eschar develops, the ulcer cannot be staged until the necrotic tissue is removed. Three major steps in pressure ulcer management lead to wound healing: debridement, cleansing, and dressing. *Debridement*, either surgical or chemical, is necessary to remove necrotic tissue to allow new granulation tissue to grow. Necrotic tissue can also contain bacteria that impede wound healing. *Cleansing* the wound helps to lower bacteria counts. Normal saline is best, as its use protects new granulation tissue. In foul-smelling, infected wounds, bacteriocidal agents such as 1% povidine-iodine, 0.25% acetic acid, or 0.5% sodium hypochlorite (Dakin's solution) can be used as disinfectants, but not for more than a week at a time as they are cytotoxic to fibroblasts and delay wound healing. A discussion of which *dressing* to use is beyond the scope of this chapter, but the choice of a dressing should be based on the ulcer stage, whether or not local infection is present, whether or not excessive exudate is present, and whether continued debridement is necessary. Management of pressure ulcers should be interdisciplinary involving physicians, nurses, wound care specialists, occupational or physical therapists, and nutritionists. Usually, stage 1 and 2 pressure ulcers heal in days to weeks, whereas healing of stage 3 and 4 ulcers may be seen at 2–4 weeks, but they often take many months to heal.

PREVENTION AND HEALTHY AGING

Central to the care of older adults is the prevention of functional decline, accidents, and the development of new diseases or worsening of prevalent ones. When asked, most older adults identify maintenance of independence as their top priority. Thus, although the U.S. Preventive Services Task Force (USPSTF) has 30 recommendations for primary and secondary disease prevention in older adults, those most likely to help elders achieve their goal of maintaining independence are emphasized here. Specific discussions of vision and hearing, safe driving, and falls risk are discussed elsewhere in this chapter.

Nutrition Adequate nutrition is fundamental to healthy aging. In general, energy requirements decrease with age due to a decline in lean body mass and decreased physical activity. Despite this decrease, older adults may be at risk of undernutrition due to medication side effects; functional, visual, or cognitive impairment; oral disease, swallowing disorders, or loss of smell/taste; depression and social isolation; and chronic illnesses.

Although the proportional requirements of protein, fat, and carbohydrates do not change with age, calories from carbohydrate sources gradually substitute for those from fat. To maintain adequate caloric intake and also promote cardiovascular health, substitution of monounsaturated (olive oil, canola oil, peanuts, avocados, nuts, seeds), omega-3 (sardines, mackerel, salmon, tuna, flounder, haddock), and omega-6 (liquid vegetable oils) fatty acids (the so-called "Mediterranean Diet") for *trans* fatty acids may be beneficial. As older adults tend to have lower intakes of both dietary fiber and fluids, increased intake of both should be encouraged, particularly as antidotes for age-related constipation. Although vitamin requirements do not change with age, older adults are particularly prone to inadequate intake of vitamins D and B_{12} and calcium, and supplementation should be considered.

Functional Decline There are 14 million noninstitutionalized older adults with functional disabilities, with a greater proportion of women being disabled (43%) than men (40%). Exercise improves body composition, psychological well-being, and disease outcomes, and reduces risk of injurious falls. Physical and cognitive exercise may also reduce the risk of dementia. Even the most sedentary of individuals appear to benefit from increasing physical activity. All patients should be asked about their level of physical activity, e.g., the number of days during an average week that they spend at least 15 min walking, bicycling, swimming, weight training, etc. An exercise prescription may be beneficial. It should consider flexibility, endurance, strength, and balance but should be preceded by attention to musculoskeletal problems, footwear, and risk factors for cardiovascular disease. Guidelines for such a prescription are shown in Table 9-7.

An exercise program should be initiated gradually. Increasingly, community organizations provide supervised group programs. The National Institute on Aging also has a range of on-line and video resources for older adults.

Accident Prevention In addition to exercise, attention to accident prevention is critical. Falls risk assessment is addressed above. In addition, exercise, particularly directed at balance, resistance, and aerobic training, decreases risk. Seatbelt use should be encouraged. Per mile driven, older adults are at highest risk of serious injury or death as a result of motor vehicle accidents. Assessment of the ability to drive safely is critical to motor vehicle safety (see above). With many older adults riding bicycles, motorcycles, and mopeds, patients should be encouraged to use helmets. Head injuries are common among riders and are particularly devastating to older adults; helmets mitigate this risk.

Although moderate alcohol consumption has been associated with many salutary effects, it is not without consequences for older adults who, because of age-related changes in alcohol distribution, increased brain sensitivity to its effects, and the potential for medication-alcohol interactions, are at risk for alcohol side effects at lower levels of consumption than their younger counterparts. When the definition of at least 12 drinks per year is used, 29% of older adults are classified as regular consumers: 40% of men and 21% of women. The National Institute on Alcohol Abuse and Alcoholism recommends that both men and women aged ≥65 consume no more than three drinks in a day and no more than seven drinks in a week, while the American Geriatrics Society recommends no more than two drinks on any single drinking occasion. Lower drinking limits or abstinence is recommended for those who take medications that interact with alcohol or who have a health condition exacerbated by alcohol. An approach to screening for heavy drinking is first to ask about heavy drinking days in the past year. If a man reports that he consumed five or more drinks in a day, or a woman reports that she consumed four or more drinks in a day, further questioning is warranted. The 10-item AUDIT (Alcohol Use Disorders Identification Test) is a validated strategy for identifying unhealthy drinking.

DISEASE PREVENTION AND EARLY DETECTION

Immunizations Although vaccine efficacy declines with age, the risks of no vaccination far outweigh the consequences of less than complete protection. Influenza vaccination is thus recommended annually, and all adults ≥65 should receive the pneumococcal vaccine at least once. In addition, a one-time revaccination should be given if the original vaccination was ≥5 years earlier and persons were ≤65 years at the time of primary vaccination. Tetanus vaccinations should be administered every 10 years.

TABLE 9-7 RECOMMENDATIONS FOR OPTIMAL AGING AND PREVENTION AND TREATMENT OF DISEASE IN OLDER ADULTS

Modality	Resistance Training	Cardiovascular Endurance Training	Flexibility Training	Balance Training
Dose				
Frequency	2–3 days/week	3–7 days/week	1–7 days/week	3–7 days/week
Volume	1–3 sets of 8–12 repetitions, 8–10 major muscle groups	20–60 min per session	Major muscle groups 1 sustained stretch (20 s) of each	1–2 sets of 4–10 different exercises emphasizing dynamic postures[a]
Intensity	15–18 on Perceived Exertion Scale (70–80% 1 RM), 6 s/repetition, 1–2 min rest between sets	12–14 on Perceived Exertion Scale (50–60% heart rate reserve or maximal exercise capacity)	Progressive neuromuscular facilitation technique[b]	Progressive difficulty as tolerated, at the level that is not yet mastered[c]
Requirements for safety and maximal efficacy	Slow speed, no ballistic movements, day of rest between sessions Good form, no substitution of muscles No breath holding, Valsalva maneuver Increase weight progressively to maintain relative intensity at high load If possible, power training (high-velocity, high-loading) provides benefits of increased strength, power, endurance, balance, and bone density	Low-impact activity if arthritis present; high impact more potent for bone remodeling Weight-bearing, best include hills/stairs if possible Increase workload progressively to maintain relative intensity Perceived exertion better than monitoring pulse to gauge intensity May accumulate short bouts (10 min) of exercise to reach volume goal One hour/week high-intensity endurance exercise equivalent to 3–4 hours/week moderate-intensity endurance exercise for cardiovascular/metabolic benefits	Static rather than ballistic stretching Stretch warmed muscles after other exercises are complete, as part of cool-down	Safe environment or monitoring Dynamic as well as static modes of training Gradual increase in difficulty as competence is demonstrated

[a]Examples of balance enhancing activities include t'ai chi movements, standing yoga or ballet movements, tandem walking, standing on one leg, stepping over objects, climbing up and down steps slowly, turning, standing on heels and toes, walking on compliant surface such as foam mattresses, maintaining balance on moving vehicle such as bus or train, and dual tasking (addition of a cognitive distractor such as naming animals while balancing), etc.
[b]Proprioceptive neuromuscular facilitation involves stretching as far as possible, then relaxing the involved muscles, then attempting to stretch further, and finally holding the maximal stretch position for at least 20 s.
[c]Intensity is increased by decreasing the base of support (e.g., progressing from standing on two feet while holding onto the back of a chair to standing on one foot with no hand support); by decreasing other sensory input (e.g., closing eyes or standing on a foam pillow); or by perturbing the center of mass (e.g., holding a heavy object out to one side while maintaining balance, standing on one leg while lifting other leg out behind body, or leaning forward as far as possible without falling or moving feet).
Note: 1 RM, one repetition maximum that is a measure of maximal dynamic strength: the maximal weight one can lift with a particular muscle group one time in good form; the Perceived Exertion Scale of is a self rating of how hard one's body is working.
Source: From MAF Singh: J Gerontol: Med Sci 57A:M274, 2002; with permission.

Bone Health Some 70% of women ≥80 years have osteoporosis. Given this substantial risk, the significant morbidity and mortality associated with osteoporotic fractures, and the proven efficacy of bisphosphonates in increasing bone mineral density and preventing fractures, all women >65 years should receive dual-energy x-ray absorptiometry (DEXA) screening at least once. The most appropriate interval between screening tests has not been determined, although a minimum of 2 years is recommended to reliably measure a change in bone density. Although routine measurement of vitamin D levels is not recommended, women who are at high risk for deficiency by virtue of dietary insufficiency and/or lack of sun exposure should be considered for screening.

Cancer Screening The effect of cancer screening is not evident for at least 3–5 years; thus, screening is not likely to be of benefit in persons with a limited life expectancy. Individual values and preferences are clearly also important considerations.

BREAST CANCER The incidence of breast cancer increases with age and peaks in the eighth decade. The sensitivity and specificity of mammography reaches its maximum in the ninth decade. Over 25% of breast cancer deaths occur in women ≥80 years. These facts suggest that mammographic screening would be of benefit in older women; however, only two clinical trials have examined the efficacy of mammographic screening in women ≥70 years, and both were inconclusive. The best supporting observational evidence comes from two Surveillance, Epidemiology, and End Results Medicare studies that found an association between screening mammography and decreased breast cancer mortality. Mammography screening in the 2 years preceding a diagnosis of breast cancer eliminated the age-related disparities in size and stage of the breast tumor at diagnosis.

Annual clinical breast examination (CBE) is a potentially attractive screening alternative to mammography, since the postmenopausal atrophy of breast tissue improves CBE sensitivity in older women compared to younger women. It is also less uncomfortable and cheaper than a mammogram. However, it should be used to complement mammographic screening and reserved as a stand alone strategy only for women who refuse or cannot undergo mammography.

PROSTATE CANCER Prostate cancer screening in older men is a particularly challenging topic as many more older men die with prostate cancer than from it. Nonetheless, 92% of prostate cancer deaths occur in men who are >65 years. Although prostate cancer can be detected earlier via prostate-specific antigen testing, mortality from prostate cancer has not been reduced as a result of screening. The U.S. Preventive Services Task Force has concluded that evidence to recommend for or against screening is lacking. Other organizations such as the American Cancer Society and American Urological Society recommend screening among those with at least a 10-year life expectancy. The matter is complicated by the fact that techniques to treat prostate cancer often greatly affect quality of life. Furthermore, we are not able to reliably predict whether a particular prostate cancer is life-threatening. Given the uncertainties, PSA screening should be reserved for the most robust of older men and only after a thorough discussion of the arguments for and against screening.

COLORECTAL CANCER Annual or biennial fecal occult blood testing (FOBT) reduces mortality in those up to age 80. Other screening options include sigmoidoscopy (every 5 years), FOBT and sigmoidoscopy (every 5 years), double-contrast barium enema (every 5–10 years), and colonoscopy (every 10 years). No one method has been shown to be superior, and all methods are cost effective. Digital rectal examination (DRE) alone or with a FOBT is not recommended (though DRE is used to screen for prostate cancer). The choice of a colorectal cancer screening strategy is based on many considerations, including procedure risk. Colonoscopy might seem the most attractive option; the colon can be completely visualized and biopsies taken if the examination is positive. If the examination is negative, it does not need to be repeated for 10 years. However, adequate preparation requires lower extremity strength and mobility, and the ability to tolerate substantial fluid losses. Furthermore, the procedure has a small risk of bowel perforation or bleeding. Yet about half of colon cancers occur beyond the reach of a sigmoidoscope.

LUNG CANCER Although lung cancer is also a leading killer, no screening interventions have been shown to be effective.

Disease Risk Modification Longitudinal studies are providing evidence that risk factor modification, especially smoking cessation and blood pressure reduction, particularly in mid-life but also up to age 75, results in greater gains in life-years than do medical and surgical therapies, especially in men. In addition, lower levels of risk factors in mid-life are associated with survival free of major morbidity to age 85. Although lifestyle modifications in mid-life are important, modifications even late in life may make a difference. A person is never too old to benefit from smoking cessation.

Older adults are also at risk for obesity, which is becoming more common among successive birth cohorts. Among men, 33.4% of those 65–74 years are obese compared to 20.4% among those >75 years. For women, the comparable figures are 38.8% and 25.1%. Weight loss in obese older adults has the potential advantage of improving mobility and decreasing the severity of comorbidities. Nonetheless, it should be pursued cautiously and be coupled with aerobic and resistance training, since many obese persons are relatively sarcopenic. No data confirm the efficacy and safety of pharmacotherapies for obesity in older persons. Although bariatric surgery has higher perioperative morbidity/mortality in older adults, if successful it can also result in improvements in the severity of comorbidities.

FURTHER READINGS

BROWN JS et al: The sensitivity and specificity of a simple test to distinguish between urge and stress urinary incontinence. Ann Intern Med 144:715, 2006

CASSEL CK et al (eds): *Geriatric Medicine: An Evidence-Based Approach*, 4th ed. New York, Springer-Verlag, 2003

KIRKLAND JL et al: Adipogenesis and aging: Does aging make fat go MAD? Exp Gerontol 37:757, 2002

PERLS T, TERRY D: Understanding the determinants of exceptional longevity. Ann Intern Med 139:445, 2003

REUBEN DB et al: *Geriatrics At Your Fingertips: 2006–2007*, 8th ed. New York: The American Geriatrics Society, 2006

TINETTI ME et al: Potential pitfalls of disease-specific guidelines for patients with multiple conditions. N Engl J Med 351:2870, 2004

WALTER LC et al: Screening for colorectal, breast, and cervical cancer in the elderly: A review of the evidence. Am J Med 118:1078, 2005

10 Complementary and Alternative Medicine

Stephen E. Straus†

BACKGROUND

Medicine, not long ago the domain of solitary generalists and their nurse assistants, now engages scores of specialists and allied professionals—radiation physicists, cytologists, nurse practitioners, psychiatric social workers, dental hygienists, and many more—who wield tools of unprecedented ability to extend life and sustain its quality. This evolution of the health care system has been achieved, in part, by a formidable enterprise of critical observation and formal investigation that disproves some once-accepted practices and stimulates emergence of new approaches that compete for acceptance. One need only peruse the serial editions of this textbook to comprehend the scope of these changes.

Other factors have also affected evolutionary changes in medicine. Immigration and related demographic changes yield increasingly diverse populations who value their own health traditions. The public's expectations of health and the nature of the health care system itself have been altered by unprecedented access to sources of information, goods, and services; the disposable income to afford them; and a patchwork quilt of regulations and laws that constrain medical practice on the one hand and facilitate increased choice in health care on the other. The emergence of complementary and alternative medicine is one manifestation of these changes in health care.

DEFINITIONS

In every generation, medical practices exist that are not accepted by the mainstream: they are viewed with suspicion and dismissed as implausible or irrational. For a time, approaches that evoked some appeal, but which had not been thoroughly tested, were deemed *unconventional*. Over the past decade or so, they have been called *complementary and alternative medicine* (CAM), to reflect their use as adjuncts to or as substitutes for more generally accepted practices, respectively. CAM does not encompass practices that have yet to be translated fully from the laboratory into the clinic or practices that were well studied and disproved, but which manage to sustain some public appeal. Rather, CAM entails approaches with surprising pervasiveness, many of which can claim at least some evidentiary support. Until recently, CAM could also be defined as practices that are neither widely taught in medical schools nor reimbursed. However, medical students increasingly seek and receive some instruction about CAM, while third-party payers have identified in CAM a marketing tool to attract new, well-heeled clients. In the past few years, another term has been coined—*integrative medicine*—to suggest encouragingly that some CAM approaches, and the practitioners who deliver them, will be shown worthy of being added to the health care repertoire.

SCOPE

The myriad practices and products that encompass CAM (Table 10-1) can be organized into five somewhat overlapping domains. Special diets, high doses of vitamins and minerals, and extracts of animal or botanical products are grouped together as *biologically based* CAM approaches. Massage, osteopathic and chiropractic manipulation, and cranial-sacral therapies are grouped as *manipulative and body-based* CAM approaches. Diverse forms of meditation, spirituality, and various uses of hypnosis are CAM approaches that attempt to harness brain pathways to affect health and behavior. All three of these CAM domains have well-accepted analogues in conventional medicine—low-fat, low-cholesterol diets; physical therapy; and psychotherapy, to name but a few.

A fourth CAM domain is known as *energy medicine*, to reflect its exploitation of veritable or putative energy fields. Today, magnets are increasingly popular health products. Over 2000 years ago, however, while Greek physicians believed that health requires a balance of vital humors, Asian practitioners postulated the flow and balance of vital energies and described tools to restore them. Acupuncture aims to correct energies that flow through special meridians, or channels. Reiki, a Japanese approach, and healing touch, a modern variant, purport to diagnose and correct one's energy by passing the hands of an adept therapist over the patient.

†Deceased. Dr. Straus was a contributor to *Harrison's* since the 13th edition. He died on May 14, 2007.

TABLE 10-1 SOME COMPLEMENTARY AND ALTERNATIVE MEDICAL PRACTICES

Type	Description
Acupuncture	A Chinese medical practice that involves the insertion of hair-thin needles into nonanatomic energy channels, called meridians
Alexander technique	A movement therapy that emphasizes efficient use of muscles to relieve pain, decrease skeletal strain, and improve posture
Anthroposophic medicine	A spiritually based system of medicine that incorporates herbs, homeopathy, diet, and a movement therapy called eurythmy
Aromatherapy	The use of essential plant oils (distilled concentrates) in massage, baths, or inhalation
Ayurvedic medicine	The major East Indian traditional medicine system, utilizing pulse and tongue diagnosis; treatment includes diet, exercise, herbs, oil massages, and elimination regimens (utilizing emetics, diarrheals, etc.)
Bach flower remedies	Dilute flower infusions used to treat emotional conditions
Biofeedback	The use of machinery that translates physiologic processes into audio or visual signals
Chiropractic	Adjustments of spinal vertebrae in an effort to affect neuromuscular function
Cranial-sacral therapy	Gentle manipulation of the cranium and spine
Curanderismo	A spiritual healing tradition common in Mexican-American communities that utilizes ritual cleansing, herbs and incantations
Dance therapy	Therapeutic method that uses movement to facilitate emotional expression and release
Feldenkrais bodywork	Highly structured movement sequences that emphasize proper head positioning
Guided imagery	The use of imagination to invoke specific images that are hoped to affect physiologic function
Hydropathy	Treatment utilizing water at various temperatures, sometimes aerated or under pressure, sometimes with added salts or other substances
Hypnosis	The induction of an altered state of mind within which a subject becomes receptive to specific suggestions
Massage	The use of specific gliding and kneading strokes and friction to achieve muscle relaxation
Meditation	A process by which one tries to achieve awareness without thought
Music therapy	Singing, playing instruments, or listening to music
Naturopathy	A mixture of modalities that may include herbs, homeopathy, acupuncture, hydropathy, diet, and exercise
Native American medicine	Diverse systems, many of which incorporate prayer, chant, music, healing ceremonies, counseling, herbs, laying on of hands, and smudging (ritual cleansing with smoke from sacred plants)
Osteopathy	A medical field incorporating manipulative techniques for correcting abnormalities of the musculoskeletal system
Reflexology/zone therapy	Manual stimulation of points on the hands or feet, believed to affect distant organs
Rolfing/structural integration	A manual therapy that attempts to realign the body by deep tissue manipulation of fasciae
Shiatsu/acupressure	Finger pressure at points along nonanatomic meridians
Siddha medicine	An East Indian medical system (prevalent among Tamil-speaking people) utilizing breathing techniques, incantations, herbs, and muppu (a tri-salt preparation)
T'ai chi ch'aun	Chinese dancelike exercises described as a "moving meditation"
Therapeutic touch	Secular version of the laying on hands, described as a "healing meditation"
Tibetan medicine	A medical system that utilizes diagnosis by pulse and urine examination; therapies include herbs, diet, and massage
Traditional Chinese medicine	A medical system that utilizes examination of the tongue and pulses for diagnosis and acupuncture, herbal mixtures, massage, exercise, and diet
Trager bodywork	Light massage combined with gentle passive movements to help patients maximize freedom of movement
Unani medicine	An East Indian medical system, derived from Persian medicine, practiced primarily in the Muslim community; also called "hikmat"
Yoga	An Indian practice that includes postures (asanas), breathing exercises (pranayama), and cleansing practices (kriyas)

The fifth domain, termed *alternative systems of medicine*, combines elements of the four other domains and aims to provide primary approaches to all health needs, rather than just adjunctive solutions to them. Western variants include practices developed by Native Americans, homeopathy, and naturopathic medicine. Eastern variants such as Ayurvedic medicine of India, traditional Chinese medicine, and Tibetan medicine are rich in their use of meditative exercises and herbal products.

PATTERNS OF USE

Despite its enormous success in prolonging life and sustaining its quality, contemporary western biomedicine has features that discourage some patients: many diseases, especially chronic ones, are neither curable nor well palliated; existing treatments can impose serious adverse reactions; and provision of care is fragmented and impersonal. CAM, despite lack of proof of efficacy, appeals to many because its practitioners are optimistic, and they invest the time to speak with and touch their patients. CAM empowers patients to make their own health choices, its natural products are believed to be inherently healthier and safer than synthetic ones, and care is provided in a "holistic" fashion, meaning that the broader medical, social, and emotional contexts of illness are considered in designing the treatment plan.

The first large survey by Eisenberg in 1993 surprised the medical community by showing that >30% of Americans use CAM approaches. Many studies since then have extended these conclusions by surveying specific demographic groups and patient populations. The Centers for Disease Control and Prevention (CDC) study of nearly 31,000 American adults revealed that in 2002 36% had used one or more modalities, with spiritual approaches, herbal medicine, chiropractic, and massage being the most prevalent. Over 1% underwent acupuncture treatment that year. Surveys among patients with cancer showed that 30 to 86% used CAM, with highest rates in those with more advanced disease and undergoing aggressive treatments. Similarly, among AIDS patients, 36 to 91% are reported to use CAM. In devastating chronic illnesses like these, CAM is called upon to provide hope of cures when conventional medicine cannot, to extend life, to ameliorate treatment side effects, and to provide emotional and physical comfort. While somewhat subject to vagaries of definition as to what counts as a CAM treatment, surveys have shown that Americans are willing to pay for these services out of pocket, with an estimated $7 billion each year on vitamins and mineral supplements, $4 billion on herbals and other natural products, and nearly $4 billion more on sports supplements. Eisenberg reported that total CAM expenditures in 1997 approached $30 billion, with more visits to practitioners for CAM services than to physicians in general.

FIELDS OF PRACTICE

Osteopathic Medicine Founded in 1892 in the American heartland by the physician Andrew Taylor Still, osteopathic medicine was based originally on the belief that manipulation of soft tissue and bone can correct a wide range of diseases of the musculoskeletal and other organ systems. Over the ensuing century, osteopathy evolved progressively towards conventional (allopathic) medicine. Today, the training, practice, credentialing, licensure, and reimbursement of osteopathic physicians is virtually indistinguishable from those of allopathic physicians, with 4 years of osteopathic medical school followed by specialty and subspecialty training and certification by organizations such as the American Board of Internal Medicine. Some osteopathic physicians continue to practice spinal manipulation, primarily as a tool to address specific musculoskeletal complaints.

Chiropractic Medicine In 1895, Daniel David Palmer founded in Missouri the first school of chiropractic medicine to teach manipulation of the spine. Palmer believed that subluxations, or partial dislocations of vertebrae, cause disease by impinging on key nerve roots. Today, chiropractors undertake 5 years of training in basic and relevant clinical sciences. Increasingly, they complete additional postgraduate training in radiology and outpatient therapeutics, primarily of musculoskeletal conditions, although within the discipline there are factions that continue to perform manipulation for many other pathologic entities. Chiropractors also advise on nutrition, exercise, and other health maintenance approaches. Over 70,000 doctors of chiropractic medicine are licensed to practice in the United States.

Acupuncture A venerable component of traditional Chinese medicine, acupuncture emerged in recent decades as a free-standing clinical discipline. Over 3000 American physicians have acquired targeted postgraduate training that permits them to practice acupuncture in over 40 states and the District of Columbia. Over 4000 non-MDs have taken far more extended training, leading to licensure to practice independently or under the supervision of a physician.

Massage Therapy Drawing upon millennia of empirical knowledge, some 80 American schools instruct students in an array of the soft tissue manipulative approaches that constitute massage. Thirty-one states and the District of Columbia license trainees to perform therapeutic massage.

Naturopathic Medicine Twelve states license practitioners of naturopathy, a discipline that emerged in central Europe in the late eighteenth century. That conventional treatments of the day were usually ineffective, if not overtly harmful, stimulated the search for safer and more "natural" approaches—naturopathy is one of them. The concept underlying this discipline is that the body possesses powerful mechanisms for self-healing that a properly instructed practitioner could harness. About 1400 naturopathic physicians have completed 4 years of education in basic and clinical sciences and are licensed to manage a predominantly outpatient population. Conventional and unconventional diagnostic tests and medications are prescribed with an emphasis on relatively low doses of drugs, herbal medicines, special diets, and exercises.

Homeopathic Medicine The late eighteenth century also witnessed the emergence of homeopathy, another discipline that arose at least in part as a reaction to the toxicity inherent to many of the allopathic approaches of the day. Homeopathy was developed by Samuel Hahnemann, a German physician, who postulated that substances that cause particular side effects in a well person may be used to treat or prevent such symptoms in an ill person if administered in miniscule amounts—what is known as "the doctrine of similars." For example, contact with poison ivy (*Rhus toxicodendron*) causes susceptible persons to experience an itchy, blistering rash. Homeopathy espouses administration of highly diluted extracts of poison ivy to treat other blistering, pruritic eruptions such as varicella. During the early nineteenth century, the then-nascent field of homeopathy used blinded tests on volunteers, presaging wider use of placebo-controlled trials, to "prove" which materials were the most able to induce or relieve symptoms. By the mid-nineteenth century homeopathy had gained considerable presence in the American medical establishment and may, in fact, have facilitated the development of immunization and allergen desensitization, both of which utilize very small quantities of materials to elicit measurable biologic outcomes. Today, however, homeopathy is accepted less fully in the United States than in some other countries: it is the largest of all CAM practices in the United Kingdom, Germany, and France and is widely used in India. In America, only three states currently license the practice of homeopathy. The relative decline of homeopathy relates, at least in part, to the field's inability to articulate a rational mechanism as to why products that are diluted more than 10^{60}-fold, greater than Avogadro's number, could incite biologic effects. Nonetheless, homeopathic remedies are readily available and commonly recommended by naturopathic physicians and other licensed and unlicensed practitioners.

Other Disciplines There are numerous other CAM practices, among which some involve formal training, such as that leading to a Doctorate of Oriental Medicine, or extended apprenticeships, as in learning herbal medicine. Unfortunately, most of the other fields have not agreed upon practice standards, credentialing processes, requirements for continuing education, or external accountability.

REGULATION

As indicated above, some CAM disciplines are carefully regulated. CAM products, however, are not strongly regulated. Herbal medicines, and dietary supplements more generally, occupy a unique regulatory status that affords the public remarkable freedom of choice but also many undesired challenges, summarized below.

Elements of virtually all traditional healing approaches, herbal medicines were presumed safe long before the implementation of stringent drug regulations by the U.S. Food and Drug Administration (FDA). In 1994, the United States Congress passed the Dietary Supplements Health and Education Act (DSHEA) that permits sale of dietary supplements "over-the-counter," as it were, but without the requirement imposed on manufacturers of prescription or conventional over-the-counter drugs to prove their products to be safe and effective before marketing. Supplements can be removed by the FDA from the market only if they are proven to be hazardous. Purveyors of dietary supplements cannot claim them to prevent or treat any disease. They can, however, claim that they maintain "normal structure and function" of body systems. For example, a product cannot claim to treat arthritis, but it can claim to maintain "normal joint health."

Homeopathic products predate FDA drug regulations and are sold with no requirement that they be proven effective. It would be reasonable to assume, however, given the extent to which homeopathic products are diluted, that most of them are safe.

SAFETY

Despite their lack of apparent toxicities, homeopathic products, like all other CAM products and practices, do convey one type of risk, namely, that individuals will pursue them in lieu of more conventional modalities that are proven to be beneficial. Members of the public have considerable freedom to determine what is in their own best interest, even if those decisions deny them effective treatment, although the courts have found the rights of parents to withhold treatment of their children to be limited in instances of life-threatening illnesses. Investigators have a broad ethical obligation to not withhold proven treatments for serious illnesses for the sake of testing unproven ones.

Additional risks are imposed by the use of other CAM approaches: injuries inflicted by a practice, inherent toxicities of the modality, and interference by the modality with more conventional treatments.

Injury Physical and manipulative interventions can harm patients. In past decades, reused acupuncture needles transmitted hepatitis B virus infection; today, the standard of care requires disposable needles. Aggressive massage can cause soft tissue injuries. Spinal manipulation of patients with unrecognized vertebral lesions has been associated with cord injuries, and cervical manipulation has been associated with stroke. These appear to be rare events.

Inherent Toxicity While the public may believe that "natural" equates with "safe," it is abundantly clear that natural products can be toxic.

Misidentification of medicinal mushrooms has led to liver failure. Contamination of tryptophan supplements caused the eosinophilia-myalgia syndrome. Herbal products containing particular species of *Aristolochia* were associated with genitourinary malignancies. In 2001, extracts of kava, long used by Pacific Islanders for its mild anxiolytic and sedative properties, were associated with fulminant liver failure. A number of products, including the popular *Ginkgo biloba*, are known to prolong bleeding times and have been associated with postoperative hemorrhage. Among the most controversial of dietary supplements is *Ephedra sinica*, or ma huang, a product used in traditional Chinese medicine for short-term treatment of asthma and bronchial congestion. The scientific basis for these indications was revealed when ephedra was shown to contain the ephedrine alkaloids, especially ephedrine and pseudoephedrine. With the promulgation of the DSHEA regulations, supplements containing ephedra and herbs rich in caffeine sold widely in the U.S. marketplace, because of their claims to promote weight loss and to enhance athletic performance. Reports of severe and fatal adverse events associated with use of ephedra-containing products led to an evidence-based review of the data surrounding them, and finally, in 2004, the FDA banned their sale in the United States.

Herbal-Drug Interactions The constituents of a few natural products are toxic; others are known to interfere with the metabolism of lifesaving drugs. This effect was illustrated most compellingly with the demonstration in 2000 that consumption of St.-John's-wort interferes with the bioavilability of the HIV protease inhibitor indinavir. Later studies showed its similar interference with metabolism of topoisomerase inhibitors such as irinotecan, with cyclosporine, and with many other drugs. The breadth of interference stems from the ability of hyperforin in St.-John's-wort to upregulate expression of the pregnane X receptor, a promiscuous nuclear regulatory factor that promotes the expression of many hepatic oxidative, conjugative, and efflux enzymes engaged in drug and food metabolism.

ACQUIRING EVIDENCE

CAM evolved through an entirely different epistemologic framework than contemporary biomedicine. Empirical observations of individual patients constitute the primary evidentiary base on which CAM practices are guided and taught. Nonetheless, over the past few decades, thousands of studies have been performed of various CAM approaches, including hundreds of trials involving herbals, acupuncture, or homeopathy. To date, very few CAM approaches have been proved effective. Several factors contribute to this lack of convincing evidence. The vast majority of CAM studies have been seriously flawed by lack of appropriate controls, bias on the part of the investigators, small sample sizes, reliance on highly subjective and nonvalidated measures of benefit, and by inappropriate statistical tests.

In addition, a series of methodologic issues challenge even the better-designed CAM studies. No uniform practice guidelines exist, and the herbal products marketed in the United States are highly variable in quality and composition. Some CAM practices are not amenable to blinding. For example, both the patient and the practitioner would know if spinal manipulation had been performed. These problems are not unique to CAM, as they also complicate attempts to study conventional practices such as psychotherapy or surgery. Efforts are now being made to randomize patients to other equally demanding control interventions, and acupuncture at traditional needling points is being compared to needling at what are arguably irrelevant points.

Even with ongoing improvements in study design and conduct, issues of belief stand in the way of comprehending and accepting the results of some CAM studies. Many physicians are reluctant to believe positive outcomes of clinical approaches that have not emerged through the classic experimental paradigm by which drugs and biologic agents are developed, namely, the orderly progression from preclinical testing through serial phases of clinical trials. More importantly, it is difficult to accept results that are counterintuitive or whose underlying mechanism still defies rational explanation. As suggested above, an example of this dilemma involves studies of homeopathy. Some clinical trials of homeopathy for asthma, infantile diarrhea, and other common conditions reported positive results. Two systematic reviews of homeopathy trials gleaned an overall favorable impression of the clinical trials data, concluding that the treatments were more beneficial than placebo. Even the best trials and these reviews have been criticized on methodologic grounds. It remains unclear what evidence could compel a change in belief about the benefits of homeopathy when there remain no cogent explanations for how substances diluted beyond the point at which only solute remains could exert physiologic effects.

By contrast, while methodologic problems continue to plague acupuncture trials, belief has been growing even in academic centers that acupuncture may be effective. The emerging acceptance of acupuncture results, in part, from its widespread availability and use in the United States today, even within the walls of major medical centers where it is used as an ancillary approach to pain management. Yet, its acceptance appears to stem from more than just its communal appeal. Since the mid-1970s, biochemical and imaging studies began to yield evidence that needling can trigger release of endogenous opioids that bind to specific receptors in the very brain regions that mediate the beneficial effects of narcotic analgesics.

EXISTING EVIDENCE

While it is difficult to conclude decisively that a particular CAM approach lacks any merit, it is quite feasible to discern that its effect size, or degree of benefit, is too small or inconsistent to be worth pursuing further. Over the past century, many once unconventional medical approaches failed—one need only think back to the exotic electrical devices, procedures, and tonics that fell out of fashion. Two questions are often asked: (1) Whether any of the more contemporary CAM modalities deserve to be rejected? (2) Whether data showing them to be ineffective would change anyone's mind about using them?

The case of laetrile is instructive. This extract of apricot seeds was touted in the 1970s as a cure for solid tumors. Thousands crossed the Mexican border to secure laetrile for their own use. The lack of any positive preclinical data discouraged oncologists from agreeing at first to study laetrile, until public pressure required that an answer be obtained. Two studies in the 1980s showed no benefit of laetrile treatment. Today, some continue to seek the product, but the numbers are vastly smaller than before meaningful data were obtained. A similar fate befell a cocktail of drugs used for cancer patients through the 1970s and 1980s by Dr. Luigi DiBella in Italy, once large studies revealed it to have no detectable impact on the course of a variety of advanced cancers.

In contrast, modalities that have been well tested and found ineffective are still in fairly common practice. For example, the renowned biochemist Linus Pauling proclaimed vitamin C able to effectively treat and even prevent the common cold. Several high-quality studies failed to demonstrate clinically important effects of vitamin C in preventing or treating viral colds. The early studies were criticized for using too little of the vitamin, yet doses that well exceeded its bioavailability also proved negative. Nonetheless, ingestion of extra vitamin C remains a common habit of individuals who perceive the onset of cold symptoms. For most people, this practice is wasteful but not harmful; however, people with iron overload (either hemochromatosis or chronic transfusion requirement) can be damaged by vitamin C, which generates free radicals in the setting of iron excess.

Despite the failure of some CAM approaches, early studies have yielded positive or at least encouraging data for a number of them. Good sources of information include the Natural Medicines Comprehensive Database (*www.NaturalDatabase.com*) and National Institutes of Health (NIH) websites such as *http://ods.od.nih.gov*; *http://nccam.nih.gov/health/* and *http://www3.cancer.gov/occam/information.html.*

Vitamins/Minerals

- *Vitamin A:* Large studies in a number of developing nations proved that vitamin A deficiency is prevalent and associated with increased risks of mortality in young children. Prospective trials showed that ingestion of 100,000 to 200,000 IU of vitamin A twice a year reduces the overall death rate in early childhood and possibly also the progression of HIV/AIDS significantly.

- *Folic acid:* Rates of neural tube defects in newborns are significantly diminished by folate food supplementation.
- *Folic acid, vitamin B_6, and vitamin B_{12}:* Some high-quality randomized, double-blind, controlled trials suggested that this vitamin combination lowers serum homocysteine levels, but this has not lowered the risk of cardiovascular end points.
- *Vitamins C and E, β-carotene, and zinc:* A large randomized controlled trial showed that these supplements combined reduce the progression of age-related macular degeneration.

Even vitamins and minerals, which are presumed safe in moderate doses, can have unexpected adverse effects. Two large controlled trials of β-carotene for prevention of cancer or retinal diseases found increased rates of lung cancer in those randomized to the supplement. Ongoing large prospective trials are seeking benefits from ingestion of supplements on rates of prostate cancer (vitamin E and selenium) and Alzheimer's disease (vitamin E).

Herbals and Other Natural Products

- *Glucosamine and/or chondroitin sulfate:* Systematic surveys of smaller controlled trials led to a large multicenter trial that concluded that these products are superior to placebo in improving performance and slowing the narrowing of the joint space in patients with moderate to severely painful and disabling osteoarthritis of the knee. It remains uncertain whether their use also slows degradation of joint cartilage.
- *Ginkgo biloba:* Americans spent nearly $250 million on this herbal product in 2000. The literature shows no evidence that it improves cognition, but over 3000 older Americans currently participate in a randomized blinded trial to ascertain whether its use can reduce the rate of onset and progression of dementia.
- *Saw palmetto (Serenoa repens) and African plum (Pygeum africanum):* Each of these botanicals has been advocated for aging men to obtain symptomatic relief treatment of benign prostatic hyperplasia. Sales of saw palmetto are growing, with an estimated $131 million spent on the product consumed by Americans in 2000. However, clinical trials have shown that saw palmetto is ineffective in this setting.
- *St.-John's-wort (Hypericum perforatum):* Among the most popular herbal products worldwide, numerous small studies and systematic reviews suggested it to benefit patients with a wide range of depressive syndromes. High-quality, randomized, placebo-controlled trials found St.-John's-wort to not be superior to placebo for treatment of major depression of moderate severity, a spectrum of illness that clearly warrants professional evaluation and treatment.
- *Echinacea species: Echinacea* roots are widely used to treat or prevent respiratory infections, with over $200 million in sales in 2000. Although in vitro studies have shown that *Echinacea* constituents stimulate humoral and cellular immune responses, systematic reviews of the clinical trials have not concluded that they are beneficial.

Other Modalities

- *Acupuncture:* A frequently cited NIH-led consensus development conference in 1997 concluded that acupuncture relieves nausea from chemotherapy and pain following extraction of molars. Some subsequent studies confirmed these earlier impressions regarding acute nausea and vomiting, but the data regarding pain management have been mixed, with little evidence that it benefits neuropathic pain. A well-conducted study reported in 2004, however, concluded that acupuncture provides significant adjunctive relief for patients with osteoarthritis of the knee.
- *Mind-body medicine:* Clinical trials support the use of biofeedback for incontinence, headache, and stroke rehabilitation. Hypnosis may be beneficial in relieving pain due to minor surgical interventions, chemotherapy-associated nausea, and irritable bowel syndrome.
- *Spinal manipulation:* Systematic reviews of some well-designed trials concluded that chiropractic or osteopathic manipulation provides significant improvement for patients with uncomplicated acute back pain. No proof exists that they are superior to, or more cost-effective than, other conventional approaches, nor do they alter the long-term outcome.

SUMMARY

An array of unproven modalities will always be used by the patients under our care. Physicians must approach each encounter as an opportunity to better understand their patient's beliefs and expectations and use those insights to help guide their personal health care practices in a constructive way. Many of these choices are entirely innocuous and can be accommodated in the context of the established diagnostic and therapeutic interventions. Some of these choices should be actively discouraged. Along the way, scientific evidence will drive many CAM approaches out of favor. Some modalities will garner sufficient support to become part of mainstream care: the next generation of physicians will never know they were once controversial.

FURTHER READINGS

ADAMS M, JEWELL AP: The use of complementary and alternative medicine by cancer patients. Int Semin Surg Oncol 4:10, 2007

BARNES PM et al: Complementary and alternative medicine use among adults: United States, 2002. Adv Data 27:1, 2004

BENT S et al: Saw palmetto for benign prostatic hyperplasia. N Engl J Med 354: 557, 2006

BERMAN B et al: Effectiveness of acupuncture as adjunctive therapy in osteoarthritis of the knee: A randomized, controlled trial. Ann Intern Med 141: 120, 2004

DE SMET PA: Herbal remedies. N Engl J Med 347:2046, 2002

EISENBERG DM et al: Trends in alternative medicine use in the United States, 1990–1997: Results of a follow-up national survey. JAMA 280:1569, 1998

KAPTCHUK TJ: Acupuncture: Theory, efficacy and practice. Ann Intern Med 136:374, 2002

KINSEL JF, STRAUS SE: Complementary and alternative therapeutics: Rigorous research is needed to support claims. Annu Rev Pharmacol Toxicol 43:463, 2003

11 Palliative and End-of-Life Care

Ezekiel J. Emanuel, Joshua Hauser, Linda L. Emanuel

EPIDEMIOLOGY

In 2003, 2,448,288 individuals died in the United States (Table 11-1). Over 70% of all deaths occur in those >65 years of age. The epidemiology of mortality is similar in most developed countries; cardiovascular diseases and cancer are the predominant causes of death, a marked change since 1900, when heart disease caused ~8% of all deaths and cancer accounted for <4% of all deaths. In 2003, AIDS accounted for <1% of all deaths, although among those age 35–44, it remains a leading cause of death.

It is estimated that in developed countries ~70% of all deaths are preceded by a disease or condition such that it is reasonable to plan for dying in the foreseeable future. Cancer has served as the paradigm for terminal care, but it is not the only type of illness with a recognizable and predictable terminal phase. Since heart failure, chronic obstructive pulmonary disease (COPD), chronic liver failure, dementia, and many

TABLE 11-1 TEN LEADING CAUSES OF DEATH IN THE UNITED STATES AND BRITAIN

	United States			Britain	
Cause of Death	**Number of Deaths**	**Percent of Total**	**Number of Deaths Among People ≥65 Years of Age**	**Number of Deaths**	**Percent of Total**
All deaths	2,448,288	100	1,804,373	538,254	100
Heart disease	685,089	28	563,390	129,009	24
Cancer	556,902	22.7	388,390	135,955	25.3
Stroke	157,689	6.4	138,134	57,808	10.7
Chronic obstructive pulmonary disease	126,382	5.2	109,139	27,905	5.2
Accidents	109,277	4.5	34,335	10,979	2
Diabetes	74,219	3	54,919	6316	1.2
Pneumonia/influenza	65,163	2.7	57,670	34,477	6.4
Alzheimer's disease	63,457	2.6	62,814	5055	0.9
Nephritis, nephritic syndrome, nephrosis	42,453	1.7	35,254	3287	0.6
Septicemia	34,069	1.3	26,445	2206	0.4

Source: National Center for Health Statistics (2003) *http://www.cdc.gov/nchs*; National Statistics (Great Britain, 2003) *http://www.statistics.gov.uk*.

other conditions have recognizable terminal phases, a systematic approach to end-of-life care should be part of all medical specialties. Many patients with illness-related suffering can also benefit from palliative care, regardless of prognosis. Ideally, palliative care should be considered as a part of comprehensive care for all patients.

Over the past few decades in the United States, a significant change in the site of death has occurred that coincides with patient and family preferences. Nearly 60% of Americans died as inpatients in hospitals in 1980. By 2000, the trend was reversing, with ~40% of Americans dying as hospital inpatients (Fig. 11-1). This shift has been most dramatic for those dying from cancer and COPD and for younger and very old individuals. In the past decade, it is associated with the increased use of hospice care; in 2005, ~33% of all decedents in the United States received such care. Cancer patients currently constitute ~50% of hospice users, with ~60% of all terminal cancer patients receiving hospice care. About 70% of patients receiving hospice care die out of the hospital. In addition, with shortening of hospital stays, many serious conditions are being treated at home or on an outpatient basis. Consequently, providing optimal palliative and end-of-life care requires ensuring that appropriate services are available in a variety of settings, including noninstitutional settings.

HOSPICE AND THE PALLIATIVE CARE FRAMEWORK

Central to this type of care is an interdisciplinary team approach that typically encompasses pain and symptom management, spiritual and psychological care for the patient, and support for family caregivers during the patient's illness and the bereavement period.

Terminally ill patients have a wide variety of advanced diseases, often with multiple symptoms demanding relief, and require noninvasive therapeutic regimens to be delivered in flexible care settings. Fundamental to ensuring quality palliative and end-of-life care is a focus on four broad domains: (1) physical symptoms; (2) psychological symptoms; (3) social needs that include interpersonal relationships, caregiving, and economic concerns; and (4) existential or spiritual needs.

A comprehensive assessment screens for and evaluates needs in each of these four domains. Goals for care are established in discussion with the patient and/or family based on the assessment in each of these domains. Interventions are then aimed at improving or managing symptoms and needs. While physicians are responsible for certain especially technical interventions, and for coordinating the interventions, they cannot be responsible for providing all of them. Since failing to address any one of the domains is likely to preclude a good death, a well coordinated, effectively communicating interdisciplinary team takes on special importance in end-of-life care. Depending on the setting, critical members of the interdisciplinary team will include physicians, nurses, social workers, chaplains, nurse's aides, physical therapists, bereavement counselors, and volunteers.

ASSESSMENT AND CARE PLANNING

Comprehensive Assessment Standardized methods for conducting a comprehensive assessment focus on evaluating the patient's condition in all four domains affected by illness: physical, psychological, social, and spiritual. The assessment of physical and mental symptoms should follow a modified version of the traditional medical history and physical examination that emphasizes symptoms. Questions should aim at elucidating symptoms and discerning sources of suffering and gauging how much these symptoms interfere with the patient's quality of life. Standardized assessment is critical. Currently, there are 21 symptom assessment instruments for cancer alone. Instruments with good psychometric properties that assess a wide range of symptoms include the Memorial Symptom Assessment Scale (MSAS), the Rotterdam Symptom Checklist, the Worthing Chemotherapy Questionnaire, and the Computerized Symptom Assessment Instrument. These are long and may be useful for initial clinical or for research assessments. Shorter instruments are useful for patients whose performance status does not permit comprehensive assessments. Suitable shorter instruments include the Condensed Memorial Symptom Assessment Scale, the Edmonton Symptom Assessment System, the M.D. Anderson Symptom Assessment Inventory, and the Symptom Distress Scale. Using such instruments ensures that the assessment is comprehensive and does not just focus on pain and a few other physical symptoms. Invasive tests are best avoided in end-of-life care, and even minimally invasive tests should be carefully evaluated for their benefit-to-burden ratio for the patient. Aspects of the physical examination that are uncomfortable and unlikely to yield useful information can also be omitted.

Regarding social needs, health care providers should assess the status of important relationships, financial burdens, care-giving needs, and access to medical care. Relevant questions will include: *How often is there someone to feel close to? How has this illness been for your family? How has it affected your relationships? How much help do you need with things like getting meals or getting around? How much trouble do you have getting the medical care you need?* In the area of existential needs,

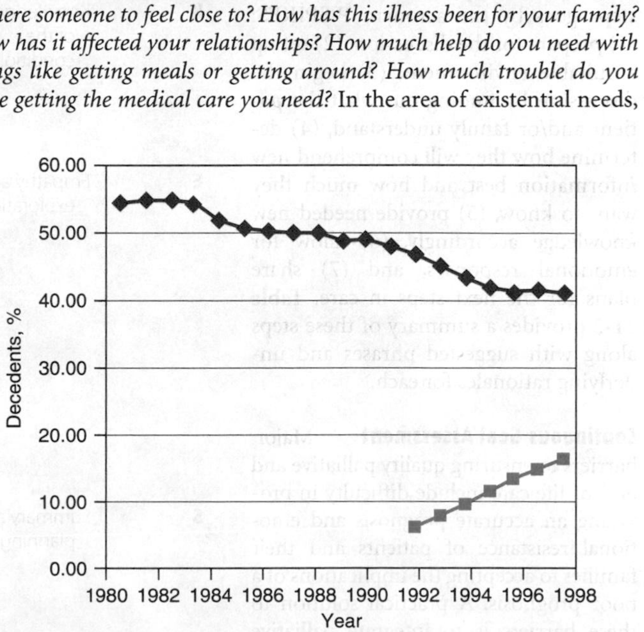

FIGURE 11-1 Graph showing trends in the site of death in the past two decades. ◆, percentage of hospital inpatient deaths; ■, percentage of decendents enrolled in a hospice.

providers should assess distress and the patient's sense of being emotionally and existentially settled and of finding purpose or meaning. Helpful assessment questions can include: *How much are you able to find meaning since your illness began? What things are most important to you at this stage?* In addition, it can be helpful to ask about how well the patient perceives his or her care to be: *How much do you feel your doctors and nurses respect you? How clear is the information from us about what to expect regarding your illness? How much do you feel that the medical care you are getting fits with your goals?* If concern is detected in any of these areas, deeper evaluative questions are warranted.

Communication Especially when an illness is life-threatening, there are many emotionally charged and potentially conflict-creating moments, collectively called "bad news" situations, in which empathic and effective communication skills are essential. These moments include communicating to the patient and/or family about a terminal diagnosis, the patient's prognosis, any treatment failures, deemphasizing efforts to cure and prolong life while focusing more on symptom management and palliation, advance care planning, and the patient's death.

Just as surgeons plan and prepare for major operations or investigators rehearse a presentation of research results, physicians and health care providers caring for patients with significant or advanced illness can develop a practiced approach to sharing important information and planning interventions. In addition, families identify as important both how well the physician was prepared to deliver bad news and the setting in which it was delivered. For instance, 27% of families making critical decisions for patients in an intensive care unit (ICU) desired better and more private physical space to communicate with physicians, and 48% found having clergy present reassuring.

An organized and effective procedure for communicating bad news with seven steps goes by the acronym P-SPIKES: (1) ***p***repare for the discussion, (2) ***s***et up a suitable environment, (3) begin the discussion by finding out what the ***pa***tient and/or family understand, (4) determine how they will comprehend new ***i***nformation best and how much they want to know, (5) provide needed new ***k***nowledge accordingly, (6) allow for ***e***motional responses, and (7) ***s***hare plans for the next steps in care. Table 11-2 provides a summary of these steps along with suggested phrases and underlying rationales for each.

Continuous Goal Assessment Major barriers to ensuring quality palliative and end-of-life care include difficulty in providing an accurate prognosis and emotional resistance of patients and their families to accepting the implications of a poor prognosis. A practical solution to these barriers is to integrate palliative care with curative care regardless of prognosis. With this approach, palliative care no longer conveys the message of failure, having no more treatments, or "giving up hope." Fundamental to integrating palliative care with curative therapy is to include continuous goal assessment as part of the routine patient reassessment that occurs at most patient-physician encounters.

Goals for care are numerous, ranging from cure of a specific disease, to prolonging life, to relief of a symptom, to delaying the course of an incurable disease, to adapting to progressive disability without disrupting the family, to finding peace of mind or personal meaning, to dying in a manner that leaves loved ones with positive memories. Discernment of goals for care can be approached through a seven-step protocol: (1) ensure that medical and other information is as complete as reasonably possible and understood by all relevant parties (see above); (2) explore what the patient and/or family are hoping for while identifying relevant and realistic goals; (3) share all the options with the patient and family; (4) respond with empathy as they adjust to changing expectations; (5) make a plan, emphasizing what can be done toward the realistic

TABLE 11-2 ELEMENTS OF COMMUNICATING BAD NEWS—THE P-SPIKES APPROACH

Acronym	Steps	Aim of the Interaction	Preparations, Questions, or Phrases
P	Preparation	Mentally prepare for the interaction with the patient and/or family.	Review what information needs to be communicated. Plan how you will provide emotional support. Rehearse key steps and phrases in the interaction.
S	Setting of the interaction	Ensure the appropriate setting for a serious and potentially emotionally charged discussion.	Ensure patient, family, and appropriate social supports are present. Devote sufficient time. Ensure privacy and prevent interruptions by people or beeper. Bring a box of tissues.
P	Patient's perception and preparation	Begin the discussion by establishing the baseline and whether the patient and family can grasp the information. Ease tension by having the patient and family contribute.	Start with open-ended questions to encourage participation. Possible phrases to use: *What do you understand about your illness?* *When you first had symptom X, what did you think it might be?* *What did Dr. X tell you when he sent you here?* *What do you think is going to happen?*
I	Invitation and information needs	Discover what information needs the patient and/or family have and what limits they want regarding the bad information.	Possible phrases to use: *If this condition turns out to be something serious, do you want to know?* *Would you like me to tell you all the details of your condition? If not, then who would you like me to talk to?*
K	Knowledge of the condition	Provide the bad news or other information to the patient and/or family sensitively.	Do not just dump the information on the patient and family. Check for patient and family understanding. Possible phrases to use: *I feel badly to have to tell you this, but...* *Unfortunately, the tests showed...* *I'm afraid the news is not good...*
E	Empathy and exploration	Identify the cause of the emotions—e.g., poor prognosis. Empathize with the patient and/or family's feeling. Explore by asking open-ended questions.	Strong feelings in reaction to bad news are normal. Acknowledge what the patient and family are feeling. Remind them such feelings are normal, even if frightening. Give them time to respond. Remind patient and family you won't abandon them. Possible phrases to use: *I imagine this is very hard for you to hear.* *You look very upset. Tell me how you are feeling.* *I wish the news were different.* *We'll do whatever we can to help you.*
S	Summary and planning	Delineate for the patient and the family the next steps, including additional tests or interventions.	It is the unknown and uncertain that can increase anxiety. Recommend a schedule with goals and landmarks. Provide your rationale for the patient and/or family to accept (or reject). If the patient and/or family are not ready to discuss the next steps, schedule a follow-up visit.

Source: Adapted from Buckman.

goals; (6) follow through with the plan; and (7) review and revise this plan periodically, considering at every encounter whether the goals of care should be reviewed with the patient and/or family. Each of these steps need not be followed in rote order, but together they provide a helpful framework for interactions with patients and their families about goals for care. It can be especially challenging if a patient or family member has difficulty letting go of an unrealistic goal. One strategy is to help them refocus on more realistic goals, and also suggest that, while hoping for the best, it is still prudent to plan for other outcomes as well.

TABLE 11-3 STEPS IN ADVANCE CARE PLANNING

Step	Goals to be Achieved and Measures to Cover	Useful Phrases or Points to Make
Introducing advance care planning	Ask the patient what he or she knows about advance care planning and if he or she has already completed an advanced care directive. Indicate that you as a physician have completed advance care planning. Indicate that you try to perform advance care planning with all patients regardless of prognosis. Explain the goals of the process as empowering the patient and ensuring you and the proxy understand the patient's preferences. Provide the patient relevant literature including the advance care directive that you prefer to use. Recommend the patient identify a proxy decision-maker who should attend the next meeting.	*I'd like to talk with you about something I try to discuss with all my patients. It's called advance care planning. In fact, I feel that this is such an important topic that I have done this myself. Are you familiar with advance care planning or living wills?* *Have you thought about the type of care you would want if you ever became too sick to speak for yourself? That is the purpose of advance care planning.* *There is no change in health that we have not discussed. I am bringing this up now because it is sensible for everyone, no matter how well or ill, old or young.* Have many copies of advance care directives available, including in the waiting room, for patients and families. Know resources for state-specific forms (available at *www.nhpco.org*).
Structured discussion of scenarios and patient	Affirm that the goal of the process is to follow the patient's wishes if the patient loses decision-making capacity. Elicit the patient's overall goals related to health care. Elicit the patient's preferences for specific interventions in a few salient and common scenarios. Help the patient define the threshold for withdrawing and withholding interventions. Define the patient's preference for the role of the proxy.	Use a structured worksheet with typical scenarios. Begin the discussion with persistent vegetative state and consider other scenarios, such as recovery from an acute event with serious disability, asking the patient about his or her preferences regarding specific interventions, such as ventilators, artificial nutrition, and CPR, and then proceeding to less-invasive interventions, such as blood transfusions and antibiotics.
Review the patient's preferences	After the patient has made choices of interventions, review them to ensure they are consistent and the proxy is aware of them.	
Document the patient's preferences	Formally complete the advance care directive and have witness sign it. Provide a copy for the patient and the proxy. Insert a copy into the patient's medical record and summarize in a progress note.	
Update the directive	Periodically, and with major changes in health status, review the directive with the patient and make any modifications.	
Apply the directive	The directive goes into effect only when the patient becomes unable to make medical decisions for him- or herself. Re-read the directive to be sure about its content. Discuss your proposed actions based on the directive with the proxy.	

Note: CPR, cardiopulmonary resuscitation.

Advance Care Planning • ***PRACTICES*** Advance care planning is a process of planning for future medical care in case the patient becomes incapable of making medical decisions. Ideally, such planning would occur before a health care crisis or the terminal phase of an illness. Unfortunately, diverse barriers prevent this. While 80% of Americans endorse advance care planning and completing living wills, only 29% have actually done so. Most patients expect physicians to initiate advance care planning and will wait for physicians to broach the subject. Patients also wish to discuss advance care planning with their families. Yet patients with unrealistic expectations are significantly more likely to prefer aggressive treatments. Fewer than one-third of health care providers have completed advance care planning for themselves. Hence, a good first step is for health care providers to complete advance care planning for themselves. This makes providers aware of the critical choices in the process and the issues that are especially charged and allows them to tell their patients truthfully that they have done advance planning themselves.

Steps in effective advance care planning center on (1) introducing the topic, (2) structuring a discussion, (3) reviewing plans that have been discussed by the patient and family, (4) documenting the plans, (5) updating them periodically, and (6) implementing the advance care directives (Table 11-3). Two of the main barriers to advance care planning are problems in raising the topic and structuring a succinct discussion. Raising the topic can be done efficiently as a routine matter, noting that it is recommended for all patients, analogous to purchasing insurance or estate planning. Almost all of the most difficult cases have involved unexpected, acute episodes of brain damage in young individuals.

Structuring a focused discussion is a central communication skill. Identify the health care proxy and recommend his or her involvement in the advance care planning process. Select a worksheet, preferably one that has been evaluated and demonstrated to produce reliable and valid expressions of patient preferences, and orient the patient and proxy to it. Such worksheets exist for both general and disease-specific situations. Discuss with the patient and proxy one scenario as an example to demonstrate how to think about the issues. It is often helpful to begin with a scenario in which the patient is likely to have settled preferences for care, such as being in a persistent vegetative state. Once the patient's preferences for interventions in this scenario are determined, suggest that the patient and proxy discuss and complete the worksheet for the others. If appropriate, suggest they involve other family members in the discussion. On a return visit, go over the patient's preferences, checking and resolving any inconsistencies. After having the patient and proxy sign the document, place it in the medical chart and be sure that copies are provided to relevant family members and care sites. Since patients' preferences can change, these documents need to be reviewed periodically.

TYPES OF DOCUMENTS Advance care planning documents are of two broad types. The first includes living wills or instructional directives; these are advisory documents that describe the types of decisions that should direct care. Some are more specific, delineating different scenarios and interventions for the patient to choose from. Among these, some are for general use and others are designed for use by patients with a specific type of disease, such as cancer or HIV. Less specific directives can be general statements of not wanting life-sustaining interventions or forms that describe the values that should guide specific terminal care decisions. The second type of advance directive allows the designation of a health care proxy (sometimes also referred to as a durable attorney for health care) who is an individual selected by the patient to make decisions. The choice is not either/or; a combined directive that includes a living will and designates a proxy is often used, and the directive should clearly indicate whether the specified patient preferences or the proxy's choice takes precedence if they conflict.

A potentially misleading distinction relates to statutory as opposed to advisory documents. Statutory documents are drafted to fulfill relevant state laws. Advisory documents are drafted to reflect the patient's wishes. Both are legal, the first under state law, and the latter under common or constitutional law.

LEGAL ASPECTS As of 2006, 48 states and the District of Columbia had enacted living will legislation. Many states have their own statutory forms. Massachusetts and Michigan do not have living will laws, although both have health care proxy laws. In 25 states, the laws state that the living will is not valid if a woman is pregnant. However, like all other states except Alaska, these states have enacted durable power of attorney for health care laws that permit patients to designate a proxy decision-maker with authority to terminate life-sustaining treatments. Only in Alaska does the law prohibit proxies from terminating life-sustaining treatments.

The U.S. Supreme Court has ruled that patients have a constitutional right to decide about refusing and terminating medical interventions, including life-sustaining interventions, and that mentally incompetent patients can exercise this right by providing "clear and convincing evidence" of their preferences. Since advance care directives permit patients to provide such evidence, commentators agree that they are constitutionally protected. Most commentators believe that a state is required to honor any clear advance care directive, whether or not it is written on an "official" form. Many states have enacted laws to explicitly honor out-of-state directives. If a patient is not using a statutory form, then it might be advisable to attach a statutory form to the advance care directive being used. State-specific forms are readily available free of charge for health care providers and patients and families through the website of the National Hospice and Palliative Care Organization (*http://www.nhpco.org*).

INTERVENTIONS

PHYSICAL SYMPTOMS AND THEIR MANAGEMENT

Great emphasis has been placed on addressing dying patients' pain. Some institutions have made pain assessment a fifth vital sign to emphasize its importance. This has also been advocated by large health care systems, such as the Veterans' Administration and accrediting bodies such as the Joint Commission on the Accreditation of Health Care Organizations (JCAHO). Although this embrace of pain as the fifth vital sign has been symbolically important, no data document that it has changed pain management practices. While good palliative care requires good pain management, it also requires more. The frequency of symptoms varies by disease and other factors. The most common physical and psychological symptoms among all terminally ill patients include pain, fatigue, insomnia, anorexia, dyspnea, depression, anxiety, and nausea and vomiting. In the last days of life, terminal delirium is also common. Assessments of patients with advanced cancer have shown that patients experienced an average of 11.5 different physical and psychological symptoms (Table 11-4).

Evaluations to determine the etiology of these symptoms can usually be limited to the history and physical examination. In some cases, radiologic or other diagnostic examinations will provide sufficient benefit in directing optimal palliative care to warrant the risks, potential discomfort, and inconvenience especially to the seriously ill patient. Only a few of the common symptoms presenting difficult management issues will be addressed in this chapter. Additional information on the management of other symptoms, such as nausea and vomiting, insomnia, and diarrhea can be found in Chaps. 39 and 77, Chap. 28, and Chap. 40, respectively.

TABLE 11-4 COMMON PHYSICAL AND PSYCHOLOGICAL SYMPTOMS OF TERMINALLY ILL PATIENTS

Physical Symptoms	Psychological Symptoms
Pain	Anxiety
Fatigue and weakness	Depression
Dyspnea	Hopelessness
Insomnia	Meaninglessness
Dry mouth	Irritability
Anorexia	Impaired concentration
Nausea and vomiting	Confusion
Constipation	Delirium
Cough	Loss of libido
Swelling of arms or legs	
Itching	
Diarrhea	
Dysphagia	
Dizziness	
Fecal and urinary incontinence	
Numbness/tingling in hands/feet	

Pain • ***FREQUENCY*** The frequency of pain among terminally ill patients varies widely. Substantial pain occurs in 36–90% of patients with advanced cancer. In the SUPPORT study of hospitalized patients with diverse conditions and an estimated survival of ≤6 months, 22% reported moderate to severe pain, and caregivers of these patients noted that 50% had similar levels of pain during the last few days of life.

ETIOLOGY *Nociceptive pain* is the result of direct mechanical or chemical stimulation of nociceptors and normal neural signaling to the brain. It tends to be localized, aching, throbbing, and cramping. The classic example is bone metastases. *Visceral pain* is caused by nociceptors in gastrointestinal, respiratory, and other organ systems. It is a deep or colicky type of pain classically associated with pancreatitis, myocardial infarction, or tumor invasion of viscera. *Neuropathic pain* arises from disordered nerve signals. It is described by patients as burning, electrical, or shocklike pain. Classic examples are post-stroke pain, tumor invasion of the brachial plexus, and herpetic neuralgia.

ASSESSMENT Pain is a subjective experience. Depending upon the patient's circumstances, perspective, and physiologic condition, the same physical lesion or disease state can produce different levels of reported pain and need for pain relief. Systematic assessment includes eliciting the following: (1) type: throbbing, cramping, burning, etc. (2) periodicity: continuous, with or without exacerbations, or incident; (3) location; (4) intensity; (5) modifying factors; (6) effects of treatments; (7) functional impact; and (8) impact on patient. Several validated pain assessment measures may be used, such as the Visual Analogue Scale, the Brief Pain Inventory, and the pain component of one of the more comprehensive symptom assessment instruments. Frequent reassessments are essential to assess the effects of interventions.

INTERVENTIONS Interventions for pain must be tailored to each individual with the goal of preempting chronic pain and relieving breakthrough pain. At the end of life, there is rarely reason to doubt the patient's report of pain. Pain medications are the cornerstone of management. If these are failing and nonpharmacologic interventions—including radiotherapy, anesthetic or neurosurgical procedures, such as peripheral nerve blocks or epidural medications—are required, a pain consultation is appropriate.

Pharmacologic interventions follow the World Health Organization three-step approach involving nonopioid analgesics, mild opioids, and strong opioids, with or without adjuvants (Chap. 12). Nonopioid analgesics, especially nonsteroidal anti-inflammatory drugs (NSAIDs), are the initial treatments for mild pain. They work primarily by inhibiting peripheral prostaglandins, reducing inflammation, but may also have central nervous system (CNS) effects. They have a ceiling effect. Ibuprofen, up to 1600 mg/d qid, has a minimal risk of bleeding and renal impairment and is a good initial choice. In patients with a history of severe gastrointestinal (GI) or other bleeding, it should be avoided. In patients with a history of mild gastritis or gastroesophageal reflux disease (GERD), acid-lowering therapy, such as a proton-pump inhibitor, should be used. Acetaminophen is an alternative in patients with a history of GI bleeding and can be used safely at up to 4 g/d, qid. In patients with liver dysfunction due to metastases or other causes or in patients with heavy alcohol use, doses should be reduced.

If nonopioid analgesics are insufficient, then opioids should be introduced. They work by interacting with mu opioid receptors in the CNS to activate pain-inhibitory neurons; most are receptor antagonists. The mixed agonist/antagonist opioids useful for post-acute pain should not be used for the chronic pain in end-of-life care. Weak opioids, such as codeine, can be used initially. However, if these are escalated and fail to relieve pain, then strong opioids, such as morphine 5–10 mg every 4 h, should be used. Nonopioid analgesics should be combined with opioids because they potentiate the effect of opioids.

For continuous pain, opioids should be administered on a regular, around-the-clock basis consistent with their duration of analgesia. They should not be provided only when the patient experiences pain; the goal is to prevent patients from experiencing pain. Patients should also be provided rescue medication, such as liquid morphine, for breakthrough pain that should generally be 20% of the baseline dose. Patients should be informed that using the rescue medication does not obviate their taking the next standard dose of pain medication. If after 24 h the patient's pain remains uncontrolled and recurs before the next dose, requiring the patient to utilize the rescue medication, the daily opioid dose can be increased by the total dose of rescue medications used by the patient, or by 50% for moderate pain and 100% for severe pain of the standing opioid daily dose.

It is inappropriate to start with extended-release preparations. Instead, an initial focus on using short-acting preparations in order to determine how much is required in the first 24–48 h will allow clinicians to determine opioid needs. Once pain relief is obtained with short-acting preparations, then switch to extended-release preparations. Even with a stable extended-release preparation regimen, the patient may have incident pain, such as during movement or dressing changes. Short-acting preparations should be taken before such predictable episodes. Although less common, patients may have "end-of-dose failure" with long-acting opioids, meaning that they develop pain after 8 h in the case of an every 12-h medication. In these cases, a trial of giving an every 12-h medication every 8 h is appropriate.

Because of differences in opioid receptors, cross-tolerance among opioids is incomplete and patients may experience different side effects with different opioids. Therefore, if a patient is not experiencing pain relief or is experiencing too many side effects, change to another opioid preparation is appropriate. When switching, begin with 50–75% of the published equianalgesic dose of the new opioid.

Unlike NSAIDs, opioids have no ceiling effect; therefore, there is no maximum dose no matter how many milligrams the patient is receiving. The appropriate dose is the dose needed to achieve pain relief. This is an important point for clinicians to explain to patients and families. Addiction or excessive respiratory depression is extremely unlikely in the terminally ill; fear of these side effects should neither prevent escalating opioid medications when the patient is experiencing insufficient pain relief nor justify using opioid antagonists.

Opioid side effects should be anticipated and treated preemptively. Nearly all patients experience constipation that can be debilitating (see below). Failure to prevent constipation often results in noncompliance with opioid therapy. Methylnaltrexone is a drug that targets opioid- induced constipation by blocking peripheral opioid receptors but not central receptors for analgesia. In placebo-controlled trials, it has been shown to cause laxation within 24 h of administration. As with the use of opioids, about a third of patients using methylnaltrexone experience nausea and vomiting, but unlike constipation, tolerance develops, usually within a week. Therefore, when beginning opioids, an antiemetic, such as metoclopramide or a serotonin antagonist, is often prescribed prophylactically and stopped after 1 week. Olanzapine has also been shown to have anti-nausea properties and can also be effective in countering delirium or anxiety, with the advantage of some weight gain.

Drowsiness, a common side effect of opioids, also usually abates within a week. During this period, drowsiness can be treated with psychostimulants, such as dextroamphetamine, methylphenidate, or modafinil. Modafinil has the advantage of every day dosing. Pilot reports suggest that donepezil may also be helpful for opiate-induced drowsiness, as well as relieving fatigue and anxiety. Metabolites of morphine and most opioids are cleared renally; doses may need to be adjusted for patients with renal failure.

Seriously ill patients with chronic pain relief rarely if ever become addicted. Suspicion of addiction should not be a reason to withhold pain medications from terminally ill patients. Patients and families may withhold prescribed opioids for fear of addiction or dependence. Physicians and health care providers should reassure patients and families that the patient will not become addicted to opioids if used as prescribed for pain relief; this fear should not prevent the patient from taking the medications around the clock. However, diversion of drugs for use by other family members or illicit sale may occur. It may be necessary to advise the patient and caregiver about secure storage of opioids. Contract writing with the patient and family can help. If that fails, transfer to a safe facility may be necessary.

Tolerance is the need for increasing medication dosage for the same pain relief without a change in disease. In the case of patients with advanced disease, the need for increasing opioid dosage for pain relief is usually caused by disease progression rather than tolerance. Physical dependence is indicated by symptoms from the abrupt withdrawal of opioids and should not be confused with addiction.

Adjuvant analgesic medications are nonopioids that potentiate the analgesic effects of opioids. They are especially important in the management of neuropathic pain. Gabapentin, an anticonvulsant initially studied in the setting of herpetic neuralgia, is now the first-line treatment for neuropathic pain from a variety of causes. It is begun at 100–300 mg bid or tid, with 50–100% dose increments every 3 days. Usually 900–3600 mg/d in two or three doses is effective. One potential side effect to be aware of is confusion and drowsiness, especially in the elderly. Other effective adjuvant medications include pregabalin, which has the same mechanism of action as gabapentin but is more efficiently absorbed from the GI tract. Lamotrigine is a novel agent whose mechanism of action is unknown, but it has shown effectiveness. It is recommended to begin at 25–50 mg/d increasing to 100 mg/d. Carbamazepine, a first-generation agent, has been proven effective in randomized trials for neuropathic pain. Other potentially effective anticonvulsant adjuvants include topiramate (25–50 mg qd or bid rising to 100–300 mg/d) and oxcarbazepine (75–300 mg bid, rising to 1200 mg bid). Glucocorticoids, preferably dexamethasone given once a day, can be useful in reducing inflammation that causes pain while elevating mood, energy, and appetite. Its main side effects include confusion, sleep difficulties, and fluid retention. Glucocorticoids are especially effective for bone pain and abdominal pain from distention of the GI tract or liver. Other drugs, including clonidine and baclofen, can be effective in pain relief. These drugs are adjuvants and should generally be used in conjunction with—not instead of—opioids. Methadone, carefully dosed because of unpredictable half-life in many patients, has activity at the *N*-methyl D-aspartamate (NMDA) receptor and is useful for complex pain syndromes and neuropathic pain. It is generally reserved for cases when first-line opioids (morphine, oxycodone, hydromorphone) are either ineffective or unavailable.

Radiation therapy can treat bone pain from single metastatic lesions. Bone pain from multiple metastases can be amenable to radiopharmaceuticals, such as strontium 89 and samarium 153. Bisphosphonates [such as pamidronate (90 mg every 4 weeks)] and calcitonin (200 IU intranasally once or twice a day) also provide relief from bone pain but have onset of action of days.

Constipation • ***FREQUENCY*** Constipation is reported in up to 90% of terminally ill patients.

ETIOLOGY While hypercalcemia and other factors can cause constipation, it is most frequently a predictable consequence of the use of opioids for the relief of pain and dyspnea and of tricyclic antidepressants, from their anticholinergic effects, as well as of the inactivity and poor diet that are common among seriously ill patients. If untreated, constipation can cause substantial pain and vomiting and is also associated with confusion and delirium. Whenever opioids and other medications known to cause constipation are used, preemptive treatment for constipation should be instituted.

TABLE 11-5 MEDICATIONS FOR THE MANAGEMENT OF CONSTIPATION

Intervention	Dose	Comment
Stimulant laxatives		These agents directly stimulate peristalsis and may reduce colonic absorption of water.
Prune juice	120–240 mL/d	
Senna (Senokot)	2–8 tablets PO bid	
Bisacodyl	5–15 mg/d PO, PR	Work in 6–12 h.
Osmotic laxatives		These agents are not absorbed. They attract and retain water in the gastrointestinal tract.
Lactulose	15–30 mL PO q4–8h	Lactulose may cause flatulence and bloating.
Magnesium hydroxide (Milk of Magnesia)	15–30 mL/d PO	
Magnesium citrate	125–250 mL/d PO	Lactulose works in 1 day; magnesium products in 6 h.
Stool softeners		These agents work by increasing water secretion and as detergents increasing water penetration into the stool.
Sodium docusate (Colace)	300–600 mg/d PO	
Calcium docusate	300–600 mg/d PO	Work in 1–3 days.
Suppositories and enemas		
Bisacodyl	10–15 PR qd	
Sodium phosphate enema	PR qd	Fixed dose, 4.5 oz, Fleet's.

ASSESSMENT Establish the patient's previous bowel habits, including the frequency, consistency, and volume. Abdominal and rectal examinations should be performed to exclude impaction or acute abdomen. Radiographic assessments beyond a simple flat plate of the abdomen in cases where obstruction is suspected are rarely necessary.

INTERVENTION While physical activity, adequate hydration, and dietary treatments with fiber can be helpful, each is limited in its effectiveness for most seriously ill patients, and fiber may exacerbate problems in the setting of dehydration and if impaired motility is the etiology. Fiber is contraindicated in the presence of opioid use. Stimulant and osmotic laxatives, stool softeners, fluids, and enemas are the mainstays of therapy (Table 11-5). When preventing constipation from opioids and other medications, a combination of a laxative and stool softener (such as senna and docusate) should be used. If after several days of treatment a bowel movement has not occurred, a rectal examination to remove impacted stool and to place a suppository is necessary. For patients with impending bowel obstruction or gastric stasis, octreotide to reduce secretions can be helpful. For patients in whom the suspected mechanism is dysmotility, metoclopramide can be helpful.

Nausea • ***FREQUENCY*** Up to 70% of patients with advanced cancer have nausea, defined as the subjective sensation of wanting to vomit.

ETIOLOGY Nausea and vomiting are both caused by stimulation at one of four sites: the GI tract, the vestibular system, the chemoreceptor trigger zone (CTZ), and the cerebral cortex. Medical treatments of nausea are aimed at receptors at each of these sites: The GI tract contains mechanoreceptors, chemoreceptors, and 5-hydroxytryptamine type 3 (5-HT3) receptors; the vestibular system likely contains histamine and acetylcholine receptors; and the CTZ contains chemoreceptors, dopamine type 2 receptors, and 5-HT3 receptors. An example of nausea that is most likely mediated by the cortex is anticipatory nausea before a dose of chemotherapy or other noxious stimuli.

Specific causes of nausea include metabolic changes (liver failure, uremia from renal failure, hypercalcemia), bowel obstruction, constipation, infection, GERD, vestibular disease, brain metastases, medications (including antibiotics, NSAIDs, proton-pump inhibitors, opioids, chemotherapy), and radiation therapy. Anxiety can also contribute to nausea.

INTERVENTION Medical treatment of nausea is directed at the anatomic and receptor-mediated cause that a careful history and physical examination reveals. When a single specific cause is not found, many advocate beginning treatment with dopamine antagonists such as haloperidol or prochlorperazine. Prochlorperazine is usually more sedating than haloperidol. When decreased motility is suspected, metoclopramide can be an effective treatment. When inflammation of the GI tract is suspected, glucocorticoids such as dexamethasone are an appropriate treatment. For post-chemotherapy and -radiation therapy nausea, one of the 5-HT3 receptor antagonists (ondansetron, granisetron, dolasetron) is recommended. When a vestibular cause (such as "motion sickness" or labyrinthitis) is suspected, antihistamines such as meclizine (whose primary side effect is drowsiness) or anticholinergics such as scopolamine can be effective. In anticipatory nausea, a benzodiazepine such as lorazepam is indicated. As with antihistamines, drowsiness and confusion are the main side effects.

Dyspnea • ***FREQUENCY*** Dyspnea is a subjective experience of being short of breath. Nearly 75% of dying patients experience dyspnea at some point in their illness. Dyspnea is among the most distressing of physical symptoms and can be even more distressing than pain.

ASSESSMENT As with pain, dyspnea is a subjective experience that may not correlate with objective measures of P_{O_2}, P_{CO_2}, or respiratory rate. Consequently, measurements of oxygen saturation through pulse oximetry or blood gases are rarely helpful in guiding therapy. Potentially reversible or treatable causes of dyspnea include infection, pleural effusions, pulmonary emboli, pulmonary edema, asthma, or tumor encroachment on the airway. However, the risk-benefit ratio of the diagnostic and therapeutic interventions for patients with little time left to live must be carefully considered before undertaking diagnostic steps. Frequently, the specific etiology cannot be identified, and dyspnea is the consequence of progression of the underlying disease that cannot be treated. The anxiety caused by dyspnea and the choking sensation can significantly exacerbate the underlying dyspnea in a negatively reinforcing cycle.

INTERVENTIONS When reversible or treatable etiologies are diagnosed, they should be treated as long as the side effects of treatment, such as repeated drainage of effusions or anticoagulants, are less burdensome than the dyspnea itself. More aggressive treatments, such as stenting a bronchial lesion may be warranted if it is clear that the dyspnea is due to tumor invasion at that site and if the patient and family understand the risks of such a procedure. Usually, treatment will be symptomatic (Table 11-6). Low-dose opioids reduce the sensitivity of the central respiratory center and the sensation of dyspnea. If patients are not receiving opioids, weak opioids can be initiated; if patients are already receiving opioids, then morphine or other strong opioids should be used. Controlled trials do not support the use of nebulized opioids for dyspnea at the end of life. Phenothiazines and chlorpromazine may be helpful when combined with opioids. Benzodiazepines can be helpful if anxiety is present but should be neither first-line therapy nor used alone in the treatment of dyspnea. If the patient has a history of COPD or asthma, inhaled bronchodilators and glucocorticoids may also be helpful. If the patient has pulmonary edema due to heart failure, di-

TABLE 11-6 MEDICATIONS FOR THE MANAGEMENT OF DYSPNEA

Intervention	Dose	Comments
Weak opioids		For patients with mild dyspnea
Codeine (or codeine with 325 mg acetaminophen)	30 mg PO q4h	For opioid-naïve patient
Hydrocodone	5 mg PO q4h	
Strong opioids		For opioid-naïve patients with moderate to severe dyspnea
Morphine	5–10 mg PO q4h	
	30–50% of baseline opioid dose q4h	For patients already taking opioids for pain or other symptoms
Oxycodone	5–10 mg PO q4h	
Hydromorphone	1–2 mg PO q4h	
Anxiolytics		Give a dose every hour until the patient is relaxed, then provide a dose for maintenance
Lorazepam	0.5–2.0 mg PO/SL/IV qh then q4–6h	
Clonazepam	0.25–2.0 mg PO q12h	
Midazolam	0.5 mg IV q15min	

uresis with a medication such as furosemide is indicated. Excess secretions can be dried with scopolamine, transdermally or intravenously. Oxygen can be used, although it may only be an expensive placebo. For some families and patients, oxygen is distressing; for some it is reassuring. More general interventions that medical staff can do include: sitting the patient upright, removing smoke or other irritants such as perfume, ensuring a supply of fresh air with sufficient humidity, and minimizing other factors that can increase anxiety.

Fatigue • ***FREQUENCY*** More than 90% of terminally ill patients experience fatigue and/or weakness. Fatigue is frequently cited as among the most distressing of symptoms.

ETIOLOGY The multiple causes of fatigue in the terminally ill can be categorized as resulting from the underlying disease; from disease-induced factors, such as tumor necrosis factor and other cytokines; and from secondary factors such as dehydration, anemia, infection, hypothyroidism, and drug side effects. Apart from low caloric intake, loss of muscle mass and changes in muscle enzymes may play an important role in fatigue of terminal illness. The importance of changes in the CNS, especially the reticular activating system, have been hypothesized based on reports of fatigue in patients receiving cranial radiation, experiencing depression, or with chronic pain in the absence of cachexia or other physiologic changes. Finally, depression and other causes of psychological distress can contribute to fatigue.

ASSESSMENT Fatigue is subjective; objective changes, even in body mass, may be absent. Consequently, assessment must rely on patient self-reporting. Scales used to measure fatigue, such as the Edmonton Functional Assessment Tool, the Fatigue Self-Report scales, or the Rhoten Fatigue scale, are usually appropriate for research rather than clinical purposes. In clinical practice, a simple performance assessment such as the Karnofsky Performance Status or the Eastern Cooperative Oncology Group's question "How much of the day does the patient spend in bed?" may be the best measure. In this 0–4 performance status assessment, a 0 = normal activity; 1 = symptomatic without being bedridden; 2 = requiring some, but <50%, bed time; 3 = bedbound more than half the day; and 4 = bedbound all the time. Such a scale allows for assessment over time and correlates with overall disease severity and prognosis.

INTERVENTIONS At the end of life, fatigue will not be "cured." The goal is to ameliorate it and help patients and families to adjust expectations. Behavioral interventions should be utilized to avoid blaming the patient for inactivity and to educate both the family and patient that the underlying disease causes physiologic changes producing low energy levels. Understanding that the problem is physiologic not psychological can help to alter expectations regarding the patient's level of physical activity. Practically, this may mean reducing routine activities, such as housework and cooking, or social events outside the house, and making it acceptable to receive guests lying on a couch. At the same time, institution of exercise regimens and physical therapy can raise endorphins, reduce muscle wasting, and reduce the risk of depression. In addition, ensuring good hydration without worsening edema may help reduce fatigue. Discontinuing medications that worsen fatigue may help, including cardiac medications, benzodiazepines, certain antidepressants or opioids, if pain is well-controlled.

Only a few pharmacologic interventions target fatigue and weakness. Glucocorticoids can increase energy and enhance mood. Dexamethasone is preferred for its once-a-day dosing and minimal mineralocorticoid activity. Benefit, if any, will usually be seen within the first month. Psychostimulants, such as dextroamphetamine (5–10 mg PO) and methylphenidate (2.5–5 mg PO), may also enhance energy levels, although a randomized trial did not show methylphenidate beneficial compared to placebo in cancer fatigue. Dosages should be given in the morning and at noon to minimize the risk of counterproductive insomnia. Modafinil, developed for narcolepsy, has shown some promise in the treatment of fatigue and has the advantage of once-daily dosing. Its precise role in the fatigue at the end of life is yet to be determined. Anecdotal evidence suggests that L-carnitine might improve fatigue, depression, and sleep disruption.

PSYCHOLOGICAL SYMPTOMS AND THEIR MANAGEMENT

Depression • ***FREQUENCY*** Depression at the end of life presents an apparently paradoxical situation. Many people believe that depression is normal among seriously ill patients because they are dying. People frequently say "wouldn't you be depressed?" However, depression is not a necessary part of terminal illness and can contribute to needless suffering. While sadness, anxiety, anger, and irritability are normal responses to a serious condition, they are typically of modest intensity and transient. Persistent sadness and anxiety and the physically disabling symptoms that these can lead to are abnormal and suggestive of major depression. While as many as 75% of terminally ill patients experience depressive symptoms, <25% of terminally ill patients have major depression.

ETIOLOGY Previous history of depression, family history of depression or bipolar disorder, and prior suicide attempts are associated with increased risk for depression among terminally ill patients. Other symptoms, such as pain and fatigue, are associated with higher rates of depression; uncontrolled pain can exacerbate depression, and depression can cause patients to be more distressed by pain. Many medications used in the terminal stages, including glucocorticoids, and some anticancer agents, such as tamoxifen, interleukin 2, interferon α, and vincristine, are also associated with depression. Some terminal conditions, such as pancreatic cancer, certain strokes, and heart failure have been reported to be associated with higher rates of depression, although this is controversial. Finally, depression may be attributable to grief over the loss of a role or function, social isolation, or loneliness.

ASSESSMENT Diagnosing depression among seriously ill patients is complicated because many of the vegetative symptoms in the DSM-IV criteria for clinical depression—insomnia, anorexia and weight loss, fatigue, decreased libido, and difficulty concentrating—are associated with the dying process itself. The assessment of depression in seriously ill patients should therefore focus on the dysphoric mood, helplessness, hopelessness, and lack of interest and enjoyment and concentration in normal activities. The single questions "how often do you feel downhearted and blue?" (more than a good bit of the time or similar responses) or "do you feel depressed most of the time?" are appropriate for screening.

Certain conditions may be confused with depression. Endocrinopathies, such as hypothyroidism or Cushing's syndrome, electrolyte abnormalities such as hypercalcemia, and akathisia, especially from dopamine-blocking antiemetics such as metoclopramide and prochlorperazine, can mimic depression and should be excluded.

INTERVENTIONS Physicians must treat any physical symptom, such as pain, that may be causing or exacerbating depression. Fostering adaptation to the many losses that the patient is experiencing can also be helpful. Nonpharmacologic interventions, including group or individual psychological counseling, and behavioral therapies, such as relaxation or imagery, can be helpful, especially in combination with drug therapy.

Pharmacologic interventions remain the core of therapy. The same medications are used to treat depression in terminally ill as in non-terminally ill patients. Psychostimulants may be preferred for patients with a poor prognosis or for those with fatigue or opioid-induced somnolence. Psychostimulants are comparatively fast acting, working within a few days, instead of the weeks required for selective serotonin reuptake inhibitors (SSRIs). Dextroamphetamine or methylphenidate should be started at 2.5–5.0 mg in the morning and at noon, the same starting dosages used for treating fatigue. The dose can be escalated up to 15 mg bid. Modafinil is started at 100 mg qd and can be increased to 200 mg if there is no effect at the lower dose. Pemoline is a nonamphetamine psychostimulant with minimal abuse potential. It is also effective as an antidepressant beginning at 18.75 mg in the morning and at noon. Because it can be absorbed through the buccal mucosa, it is preferred for patients with intestinal obstruction or dysphagia. If used for prolonged periods, liver function must be monitored. The psychostimulants can also be combined with more traditional antidepressants, while waiting for the latter to become effective, and then tapered after a few weeks if necessary. Psychostimulants have side effects, particularly initial anxiety, insomnia, and rarely paranoia, which may necessitate lowering the dose or discontinuing treatment.

Mirtazapine, an antagonist at the postsynaptic serotonin receptors, is a promising psychostimulant. It should be started at 7.5 mg before bed. It has sedating, antiemetic and anxiolytic properties with few drug interactions. Its side effect of weight gain may also be beneficial for seriously ill patients; it is available in orally disintegrating tablets.

For patients with a prognosis of several months or longer, SSRIs, including fluoxetine, sertraline, paroxetine and citalopram, and serotonin-noradrenaline reuptake inhibitors, such as venlafaxine, are the preferred treatment because of their efficacy and comparatively few side effects. Because low doses of these medications may be effective for seriously ill patients, use half the usual starting dose for healthy adults. The starting dose for fluoxetine is 10 mg once a day. In most cases, once-a-day dosing is possible. The choice of which SSRI to use should be driven by (1) the patient's past success or failure with the specific medication, and (2) the most favorable side effect profile for that specific agent. For instance, for a patient in whom fatigue is a major symptom, a more activating SSRI (fluoxetine) would be appropriate. For a patient in whom anxiety and sleeplessness are major symptoms, a more sedating SSRI (paroxetine) would be appropriate.

Atypical antidepressants are recommended only in selected circumstances, usually with the assistance of a specialty consultation. Trazodone can be an effective antidepressant but is sedating and can cause orthostatic hypotension and, rarely, priapism. Therefore, it should be used only when a sedating effect is desired and is often used for patients with insomnia, at a dose starting at 25 mg. In addition to its antidepressant effects, bupropion is energizing, making it useful for depressed patients suffering from fatigue. However, it can cause seizures, preventing its use for patients with a risk of CNS neoplasms or terminal delirium. Finally, alprazolam, a benzodiazepine, starting at 0.25–1.0 mg tid, can be effective in seriously ill patients suffering from a combination of anxiety and depression. While it is potent and works quickly, it has many drug interactions and may cause delirium, especially among very ill patients, because of its strong binding to the benzodiazepine–GABA receptor complex.

Unless used as adjuvants for the treatment of pain, tricyclic antidepressants are not recommended. Similarly, the monoamine oxidase (MAO) inhibitors are not recommended because of their side effects and dangerous drug interactions.

Delirium • ***FREQUENCY*** In the weeks or months before death, delirium is uncommon, although it may be significantly underdiagnosed. However, delirium becomes relatively common in the hours and days immediately before death. Up to 85% of patients dying from cancer may experience terminal delirium.

ETIOLOGY Delirium is a global cerebral dysfunction characterized by alterations in cognition and consciousness. It is frequently preceded by anxiety, changes in sleep patterns (especially reversal of day and night), and decreased attention. In contrast to dementia, delirium has an acute onset, fluctuating consciousness and inattention, and is reversible, although reversibility may be more theoretical than real for patients near death. Delirium may occur in a patient with dementia; indeed, patients with dementia are more vulnerable to delirium.

Causes of delirium include metabolic encephalopathy arising from liver or renal failure, hypoxemia, or infection; electrolyte imbalances such as hypercalcemia; paraneoplastic syndromes; dehydration; and primary brain tumors, brain metastases, or leptomeningeal spread of tumor. Commonly, among dying patients, delirium can be caused by side effects of treatments, including radiation for brain metastases, and medications, including opioids, glucocorticoids, anticholinergic drugs, antihistamines, antiemetics, benzodiazepines, and chemotherapeutic agents. The etiology may be multifactorial; e.g., dehydration may exacerbate opioid-induced delirium.

ASSESSMENT Delirium should be recognized in any terminally ill patient with new onset of disorientation, impaired cognition, somnolence, fluctuating levels of consciousness, or delusions with or without agitation. Delirium must be distinguished from acute anxiety and depression, as well as dementia. The central distinguishing feature is altered consciousness, which is not usually noted in anxiety, depression, and dementia. Although "hyperactive" delirium characterized by overt confusion and agitation is likely more common, patients should also be assessed for "hypoactive" delirium characterized by sleep-wake reversal and decreased alertness.

In some cases, use of formal assessment tools such as the Mini-Mental Status Examination (which does not distinguish delirium from dementia) or the Delirium Rating Scale (which does distinguish delirium from dementia) may be helpful in distinguishing delirium from other processes. The patient's list of medications must be carefully evaluated. Nonetheless, a reversible etiologic factor for delirium is found in fewer than half of terminally ill patients. Because most terminally ill patients experiencing delirium will be very close to death and may be at home, extensive diagnostic evaluations, such as lumbar punctures or neuroradiologic examinations, are usually inappropriate.

INTERVENTIONS One of the most important objectives of terminal care is to provide terminally ill patients the lucidity to say goodbye to the people they love. Delirium, especially with agitation during the final days, is distressing to family and caregivers. A strong determinant of bereavement difficulties is witnessing a difficult death. Thus, terminal delirium should be treated aggressively.

At the first sign of delirium, such as day-night reversal with slight changes in mentation, let the family know that it is time to be sure that everything they want to have said has been said. The family should be informed that delirium is common just before death.

If medications are suspected of being a cause of the delirium, then unnecessary agents should be discontinued. Other potentially reversible causes such as constipation, urinary retention, and metabolic abnormalities should be treated. Supportive measures aimed at providing a familiar environment should be instituted, including restricting visits only to individuals with whom the patient is familiar and eliminating new experiences; orienting the patient, if possible, by providing a clock and calendar; and gently correcting the patient's hallucinations or cognitive mistakes.

Pharmacologic management focuses on the use of neuroleptics and, in the extreme, anesthetics (Table 11-7). Haloperidol remains first-line therapy. Usually, patients can be controlled with a low dose (1–3 mg/d),

TABLE 11-7 MEDICATIONS FOR THE MANAGEMENT OF DELIRIUM

Interventions	Dose
Neuroleptics	
Haloperidol	0.5–5 mg q2–12h, PO/IV/SC/IM
Thioridazine	10–75 mg q4–8h, PO
Chlorpromazine	12.5–50 mg q4–12h, PO/IV/IM
Atypical neuroleptics	
Olanzapine	2.5–5 mg qd or bid, PO
Risperidone	1–3 mg q12h, PO
Anxiolytics	
Lorazepam	0.5–2 mg q1–4h, PO/IV/IM
Midazolam	1–5 mg/h continuous infusion, IV/SC
Anesthetics	
Propofol	0.3–2.0 mg/h continuous infusion, IV

usually given every 6 h, although some may require as much as 20 mg/d. It can be administered PO, SC, or IV. IM injections should not be used, except when it is the only way to get a patient under control. Olanzapine, an atypical neuroleptic, has shown significant effectiveness in completely resolving delirium in cancer patients. It has other beneficial effects for terminally ill patients, including antinausea, antianxiety, and weight gain. It is useful for patients with longer anticipated life expectancy because it is less likely to cause dysphoria and has a lower risk of dystonic reactions. Also, because it is metabolized through multiple pathways, it can be used in patients with hepatic and renal dysfunction. Olanzapine has the disadvantage that it is only available orally and that it takes a week to reach steady state. The usual dose is 2.5–5 mg PO bid. Chlorpromazine (10–25 mg every 4–6 h) can be useful if sedation is desired and can be administered IV or PR in addition to PO. Dystonic reactions resulting from dopamine blockade are a side effect of neuroleptics, although they are reported to be rare when used to treat terminal delirium. If patients develop dystonic reactions, benztropine should be administered. Neuroleptics may be combined with lorazepam to reduce agitation when the delirium is the result of alcohol or sedative withdrawal.

If no response to first-line therapy is seen, a specialty consultation should be obtained with a change to a different medication. If patients fail to improve after a second neuroleptic, then sedation with an anesthetic such as propofol or continuous-infusion midazolam may be necessary. By some estimates, at the very end of life as many as 25% of patients experiencing delirium, especially restless delirium with myoclonus or convulsions, may require sedation.

Physical restraints should be used with great reluctance only when the patient's violence is threatening to self or others. If used, their appropriateness should be reevaluated frequently.

Insomnia • ***FREQUENCY*** Sleep disorders, defined as either difficulty initiating sleep or maintaining sleep, sleep difficulty at least 3 nights a week or sleep difficulty that causes impairment of daytime functioning, occurs in between 19 and 63% of patients with advanced cancer.

ETIOLOGY Patients with cancer may have changes in sleep efficiency such as an increase in stage I sleep. Other etiologies of insomnia are coexisting physical illness, such as thyroid disease, or coexisting psychological illnesses, such as depression and anxiety. Medications, including antidepressants, psychostimulants, steroids, and β agonists, are significant contributors to sleep disorders, as are caffeine and alcohol. Multiple over-the-counter medications contain caffeine and antihistamines, which can contribute to sleep disorders.

ASSESSMENT Assessment should include specific questions concerning sleep onset, sleep maintenance, and early morning wakening as these will provide clues to the causative agents and to management. Patients should be asked about previous sleep problems, screened for depression and anxiety, and asked about symptoms of thyroid disease. Caffeine and alcohol are prominent causes of sleep problems, and a careful history of these substances should be obtained. Both excessive use and withdrawal from alcohol can be causes of sleep problems.

INTERVENTIONS The mainstays of intervention include improvement of sleep hygiene (encouraging regular time for sleep, decreased nighttime distractions, elimination of caffeine and other stimulants and alcohol), intervention to treat anxiety and depression, and finally treatment for the insomnia itself. For patients with depression who have insomnia and anxiety, a sedating antidepressant such as mirtazapine can be helpful. In the elderly, trazodone, beginning at 25 mg at nighttime, is an effective sleep aid at doses lower than its antidepressant effect. Zolpidem may have a decreased incidence of delirium in patients compared with traditional benzodiazepines, but this has not been clearly established. When benzodiazepines are prescribed, short-acting ones (such as lorazepam) are favored over longer-acting (such as diazepam). Patients who receive these medications should be observed for signs of increased confusion and delirium.

SOCIAL NEEDS AND THEIR MANAGEMENT

Financial Burdens • ***FREQUENCY*** Dying can impose substantial economic strains on patients and families, causing distress. In the United States, with one of the least comprehensive health insurance systems among the developed countries, ~20% of terminally ill patients and their families spend >10% of family income on health care costs over and above health insurance premiums. Between 10 and 30% of families sell assets, use savings, or take out a mortgage to pay for the patient's health care costs. Nearly 40% of terminally ill patients in the United States report that the cost of their illness is a moderate or great economic hardship for their family.

The patient is likely to reduce and stop working. In 20% of cases, a family member of the terminally ill patient also stops working to provide care. The major underlying causes of economic burden are related to poor physical functioning and care needs, such as the need for housekeeping, nursing, and personal care. More debilitated patients and poor patients experience greater economic burdens.

INTERVENTION This economic burden should not be ignored as a private matter. It has been associated with a number of adverse health outcomes, including preferring comfort care over life-prolonging care as well as consideration of euthanasia or physician-assisted suicide. Economic burdens increase the psychological distress of families and caregivers of terminally ill patients, and poverty is associated with many adverse health outcomes. Assistance from a social worker, early on if possible, to ensure access to all available benefits may be helpful. Many patients, families, and health care providers are unaware of options for long-term care insurance, respite care, the Family Medical Leave Act (FMLA), and other sources of assistance. Some of these options (such as respite care) may be part of a formal hospice program but others (such as the FMLA) do not require enrollment in a hospice program.

Relationships • ***FREQUENCY*** Settling personal issues and closing the narrative of lived relationships are universal needs. When asked if sudden death or death after an illness is preferable, respondents often initially select the former but soon change to the latter as they reflect on the importance of saying goodbye. Bereaved family members who have not had the chance to say goodbye often have a more difficult grief process.

INTERVENTIONS Care of seriously ill patients requires efforts to facilitate the types of encounters and time spent with family and friends that are necessary to meet these needs. Family and close friends may need to be accommodated with unrestricted visiting hours, which may include sleeping near the patient even in otherwise regimented institutional settings. Physicians and other health care providers may be able to facilitate and resolve strained interactions between the patient and other family members. Assistance for patients and family members who are unsure about how to create or help preserve memories, whether by providing materials such as a scrap book or memory box or by offering them suggestions and informational resources, can be deeply appreciated. Taking photographs and creating videos can be especially helpful to terminally ill patients who have younger children or grandchildren.

Family Caregivers • *FREQUENCY* Caring for seriously ill patients places a heavy burden on families. Families are frequently required to provide transportation and homemaking as well as other services. Typically, paid professionals such as home health nurses and hospice workers supplement family care; only about a quarter of all care giving is exclusively paid professional assistance. The trend toward more out-of-hospital deaths will increase reliance on families for end-of-life care. Increasingly, family members are being called upon to provide physical care (such as moving and bathing patients) and medical care (such as assessing symptoms and giving medications) in addition to emotional care and support.

Three-quarters of family caregivers of terminally ill patients are women—wives, daughters, and even sisters. Since many are widowed, women themselves tend to be able to rely less on family for caregiving assistance and may need more paid assistance. About 20% of terminally ill patients report substantial unmet needs for nursing and personal care. The impact of caregiving on family caregivers is substantial: both bereaved and current caregivers have a higher mortality compared to non-caregiving controls.

INTERVENTIONS It is imperative to inquire about unmet needs and to try to ensure those needs are met either through the family or paid professional services when possible. Community assistance through houses of worship or other community groups can often be mobilized by one or two phone calls from the medical team to someone the patient or family identifies. Sources of support specifically for family caregivers should be identified through local sources or nationally through groups such as the National Family Caregivers Association (*www.nfcacares.org*), the American Cancer Society (*www.cancer.org*), and the Alzheimer's Association (*www.alz.org*).

EXISTENTIAL NEEDS AND THEIR MANAGEMENT

FREQUENCY Religion and spirituality are often important to dying patients. Nearly 70% of patients report becoming more religious or spiritual when they became terminally ill, and many find comfort in various religious or spiritual practices such as prayer. However, ~20% of terminally ill patients become less religious, frequently feeling cheated or betrayed by becoming terminally ill. For other patients, the need is for existential meaning and purpose that is distinct from and may even be antithetical to religion or spirituality. When asked, patients and family caregivers frequently report wanting their professional caregivers to be more attentive to religion and spirituality.

ASSESSMENT Health care providers are often hesitant about involving themselves in the religious, spiritual, and existential experiences of their patients, because it may seem private or not relevant to the current illness. But physicians and other members of the care team should be able to at least detect spiritual and existential needs. Screening questions have been developed for a physician's spiritual history taking. Spiritual distress can amplify other types of suffering and even masquerade as intractable physical pain, anxiety, or depression. The screening questions in the comprehensive assessment are usually sufficient. Deeper evaluation and intervention are rarely appropriate for the physician unless no other member of a care team is available or suitable. Pastoral care providers may be helpful, whether from the medical institution or the patient's own community.

INTERVENTIONS Precisely how religious practices, spirituality, and existential explorations can be facilitated and improve end-of-life care is not well established. What is clear is that for physicians, one main intervention is to inquire about the role and importance of spirituality and religion in a patient's life. This will help a patient feel heard and help physicians to identify specific needs. In one study, only 36% of respondents indicated that a clergy member would be comforting. Nevertheless, the increase in religious and spiritual interest among a substantial fraction of dying patients suggests inquiring of individual patients how this need can be addressed.

MANAGING THE LAST STAGES

WITHDRAWING AND WITHHOLDING LIFE-SUSTAINING TREATMENT

LEGAL ASPECTS For centuries, it has been deemed ethical to withhold or withdraw life-sustaining interventions. The current legal consensus is that patients have a constitutional and common law right to refuse medical interventions. Courts have also held that incompetent patients have a right to refuse medical interventions. For patients who are incompetent and terminally ill and who have not completed an advance care directive, next of kin can exercise this right, although this may be restricted in some states depending how clear and convincing the evidence is of the patient's preferences. Courts have limited families' ability to terminate life-sustaining treatments from patients who are conscious, incompetent, but not terminally ill. In theory, patients' right to refuse medical therapy can be limited by four countervailing interests: (1) preservation of life, (2) prevention of suicide, (3) protection of third parties such as children, and (4) preserving the integrity of the medical profession. In practice, these interests almost never override the right of competent patients and incompetent patients who have left explicit and advance care directives.

Regarding incompetent patients who either appointed a proxy without specific indications of their wishes or who never completed an advance care directive, three criteria have been suggested to guide the decision to terminate medical interventions. First, some commentators suggest that ordinary care should be administered but extraordinary care could be terminated. Because the ordinary/extraordinary distinction is too vague, courts and commentators widely agree that it should not be used to justify decisions about stopping treatment. Second, many courts have advocated use of the substituted-judgment criterion, which holds that the proxy decision-makers should try to imagine what the incompetent patient would do if he or she were competent. However, multiple studies indicate that many proxies, even close family members, cannot accurately predict what the patient would have wanted. Therefore, substituted judgment becomes more of a guessing game than a way of fulfilling the patient's wishes. Finally, the best-interests criterion holds that proxies should evaluate treatments by balancing their benefits and risks and select those treatments in which the benefits maximally outweigh the burdens of treatment. Clinicians have a clear and crucial role in this by carefully and dispassionately explaining the known benefits and burdens of specific treatments. Yet, even when information is as clear as possible, different individuals can have very different views of what is in the patient's best interests, and families may have disagreements or even overt conflicts. This criterion has been criticized because no single way exists of determining the balance between benefits and burdens; it depends on a patient's personal values. As a matter of practice, physicians rely on family members to make decisions that they feel are best and object only if these decisions seem to demand treatments that the physicians consider not beneficial.

PRACTICES Withholding and withdrawing acutely life-sustaining medical interventions from terminally ill patients are now standard practice. More than 90% of American patients die without cardiopulmonary resuscitation (CPR), and just as many forgo other potentially life-sustaining interventions. For instance, during 1987–1988 in ICUs, CPR was performed 49% of the time, but only 10% of the time in 1992–1993. On average, 3.8 interventions, such as vasopressors and transfusions, were stopped for each dying ICU patient. However, practices vary widely among hospitals and ICUs, suggesting an important element of physician preferences rather than objective data.

Mechanical ventilation may be the most challenging intervention to withdraw. The two approaches are *terminal extubation*, which is the removal of the endotracheal tube, and *terminal weaning*, which is the gradual reduction of the FI_{O_2} or ventilator rate. One-third of ICU physicians prefer to use the terminal wean technique, while 13% extubate; the majority of physicians utilize both techniques. Some recommend terminal weaning because patients do not develop upper airway obstruction and the distress caused by secretions or stridor; however, terminal weaning can also prolong the dying process and not allow a patient's family to be with him or her unencumbered by an endotracheal tube. To ensure comfort for conscious or semiconscious patients before withdrawal of the ventilator, neuromuscular blocking agents should be terminated and sedatives and analgesics administered. Removing the neuromuscular blocking agents permits patients to show discomfort, facilitating the titration of sedatives and analgesics; it also permits interactions between patients and their families. A common practice is to inject a bolus of midazolam (2–4 mg) or lorazepam (2–4 mg) before withdrawal, followed by 5–10 mg of morphine and continuous infusion of morphine (50% of the bolus dose per hour) during weaning. In patients who have significant upper airway secretions, IV scopolamine at a rate of 100 μg/h can be administered. Additional boluses of morphine or increases in the infusion rate should be administered for respiratory distress or signs of pain. Higher doses will be needed for patients already receiving sedatives and opioids. Families need to be reassured about treatments for common symptoms after withdrawal of ventilatory support such as dyspnea or agitation and warned about the uncertainty of length of survival after withdrawal of ventilatory support: up to 10% of patients unexpectedly survive for 1 day or more after mechanical ventilation is stopped.

FUTILE CARE

Beginning in the late 1980s, some commentators argued that physicians could terminate futile treatments demanded by families of terminally ill patients. Although no objective definition or standard of futility exists, several categories have been proposed. Physiologic futility means that an intervention will have no physiologic effect. Some have defined qualitative futility as those that "fail to end a patient's total dependence on intensive medical care." Quantitative futility occurs "when physicians conclude (either through personal experience, experiences shared with colleagues, or consideration of reported empiric data) that in the last 100 cases, a medical treatment has been useless." The term conceals subjective value judgments about when a treatment is "not beneficial." Deciding whether a treatment that obtains an additional 6 weeks of life or a 1% survival advantage confers benefit depends upon patients' preferences and goals. Furthermore, physicians' predictions of when treatments were futile deviated markedly from the quantitative definition. When residents thought CPR was quantitatively futile, more than one in five patients had a >10% chance of survival to hospital discharge. Quantitative futility rarely applies in ICU settings. Many commentators reject using futility as a criterion of withdrawing care, preferring instead to consider futility situations as ones that represent conflict that can benefit from careful negotiation between families and health care providers.

Some hospitals have enacted "unilateral DNR" policies to allow clinicians to provide a do-not-resuscitate order in cases where consensus cannot be reached with families and medical opinion is that resuscitation would be futile if attempted. This type of a policy is not a replacement for careful and patient communication and negotiation, but recognizes that agreement cannot always be reached. Texas, Virginia, Maryland, and California and have enacted so-called medical futility laws that provide physicians a "safe harbor" from liability if they terminate life-sustaining treatments over the wishes of the patient's family. For instance, in Texas when a disagreement about terminating interventions between the medical team and family has not been resolved by an ethics consultation, then the hospital is supposed to try to facilitate transfer of the patient to another institution willing to provide treatment. If this fails after 10 days, then the hospital and physician may unilaterally withdraw treatments determined to be futile. The family may appeal to a state court. Early data suggest the law increases futility consultations for the ethics committee and that while most families concur with withdrawal, about 10–15% of families refuse to withdraw treatment. Approximately 12 cases have gone to court in Texas in 7 years after adoption of the law.

EUTHANASIA AND PHYSICIAN-ASSISTED SUICIDE

Euthanasia and physician-assisted suicide are defined in Table 11-8. Terminating life-sustaining care and providing opioid medications to manage symptoms have long been considered ethical by the medical profession and legal by courts and should not be confused with euthanasia or physician-assisted suicide.

LEGAL ASPECTS Euthanasia is legal in the Netherlands and Belgium. Euthanasia was legalized in the Northern Territory of Australia but then repealed. Euthanasia is not legal in any state in the United States. Physician-assisted suicide is legal in Oregon but only if multiple criteria are met and then only after a process that includes a 15-day waiting period. In Switzerland, a layperson can legally assist suicide. In all other countries and all other states in the United States, physician-assisted suicide and euthanasia are illegal explicitly or by common law.

PRACTICES Fewer than 10–20% of terminally ill patients actually consider euthanasia and/or physician-assisted suicide for themselves. In the Netherlands and Oregon, >70% of patients utilizing these interventions are dying of cancer; <5% of deaths by euthanasia or physician-assisted suicide involve patients with AIDS or amyotrophic lateral sclerosis. In the Netherlands, if all legal and illegal acts are grouped, euthanasia and physician-assisted suicide account for 3.5% of all deaths. In Oregon, ~0.1% of patients die by physician-assisted suicide, although this may be an underestimate.

Pain is not a primary motivator for patients' requests for or interest in euthanasia and/or physician-assisted suicide. Among the first patients to receive physician-assisted suicide in Oregon, only 1 patient of 15 had inadequate pain control compared to 15 of 43 patients in a control group experiencing inadequate pain relief. Depression, hopelessness, and, more profoundly, concerns about loss of dignity or autonomy or being a burden on family members, appear to be primary factors motivating a desire for euthanasia or physician-assisted suicide. A study from the Netherlands showed that depressed terminally ill cancer patients were four times more likely to request euthanasia, and confirmed that uncontrolled pain was not associated with greater interest in euthanasia.

Euthanasia and physician-assisted suicide are no guarantee of a painless, quick death. Data from the Netherlands indicate that in as many as 20% of cases technical and other problems arose, including patients waking from coma, not becoming comatose, regurgitating medications, and a prolonged time to death. Problems were significantly more common in physician-assisted suicide, sometimes requiring the physician to intervene and provide euthanasia.

Whether practicing in a setting where euthanasia is legal or not, over a career, between 12 and 54% of physicians will receive a request for euthanasia or physician-assisted suicide from a patient. Competency in dealing with such a request is crucial. While challenging, such a request can also be a chance to address intense suffering. After receiving a request for euthanasia and/or physician-assisted suicide, health care providers should carefully clarify the request with empathic, open-ended questions to help elucidate the underlying cause for the request such as: "What makes you

TABLE 11-8 DEFINITIONS OF ASSISTED SUICIDE AND EUTHANASIA

Term	Definition	Legal Status
Voluntary active euthanasia	Intentionally administering medications or other interventions to cause the patient's death with the patient's informed consent	Netherlands Belgium
Involuntary active euthanasia	Intentionally administering medications or other interventions to cause the patient's death when the patient was competent to consent but did not—e.g., the patient may not have been asked	Nowhere
Passive euthanasia	Withholding or withdrawing life-sustaining medical treatments from a patient to let him or her die (terminating life-sustaining treatments)	Everywhere
Physician-assisted suicide	A physician provides medications or other interventions to a patient with the understanding that the patient can use them to commit suicide	Oregon Netherlands Belgium Switzerland

want to consider this option?" Endorsing either moral opposition or moral support for the act tends to be counterproductive, either lending an impression of being judgmental or of endorsing the idea that the patient's life is worthless. Health care providers must reassure the patient of continued care and commitment. The patient should be educated about alternative, less controversial options, such as symptom management and withdrawing any unwanted treatments; the reality of euthanasia and/or physician-assisted suicide, since the patient may have misconceptions about their effectiveness; and also the legal implications of the choice. Depression, hopelessness, and other symptoms of psychological distress as well as physical suffering and economic burdens are likely factors motivating the request, and such factors should be assessed and treated aggressively. After these interventions and clarification of options, most patients proceed with another approach, declining life-sustaining interventions, possibly including refusal of nutrition and hydration.

CARE DURING THE LAST HOURS

Most laypersons have limited experiences with the actual dying process and death. They frequently do not know what to expect of the final hours, and afterwards. The family and other caregivers must be prepared, especially if the plan is for the patient to die at home.

Patients in the last days of life typically experience extreme weakness and fatigue and become bedbound; this can lead to pressure sores. The issue of turning patients who are near the end of life, however, must be balanced against the potential discomfort that movement may cause. Patients stop eating and drinking with drying of mucosal membranes and dysphagia. Careful attention to oral swabbing, lubricants for lips, and use of artificial tears can provide a form of care to substitute for attempts at feeding the patient. With loss of the gag reflex and dysphagia, patients may also experience accumulation of oral secretions, producing noises during respiration sometimes called "the death rattle." Scopolamine can reduce the secretions. Patients also experience changes in respiration with periods of apnea or Cheyne-Stokes breathing. Decreased intravascular volume and cardiac output cause tachycardia, hypotension, peripheral coolness, and livedo reticularis (skin mottling). Patients can have urinary and, less frequently, fecal incontinence. Changes in consciousness and neurologic function generally lead to two different paths to death (Fig. 11-2).

Each of these terminal changes can cause patients and families distress, requiring reassurance and targeted interventions (Table 11-9). Informing families that these changes might occur, and even providing them an information sheet, can help to preempt problems and minimize distress. Understanding that patients stop eating because they are dying, not dying because they have stopped eating, can reduce family and caregiver anxiety. Similarly, informing the family and caregivers that the "death rattle" may occur and that it is not indicative of suffocation or choking can reduce their worry from the breathing sounds.

Families and caregivers may also feel guilty about stopping treatments, fearing that they are "killing" the patient. This may lead to demands for interventions that may be ineffective. In such cases, the physician should remind the family and caregivers about the inevitability of events and the palliative goals. Interventions may prolong the dying process and cause discomfort. Physicians should also emphasize that withholding treatments is both legal and ethical, and that the family members are not the cause of the patient's death. This reassurance may need to be provided multiple times.

Hearing and touch are said to be the last senses to stop functioning. Whether this is the case or not, families and caregivers can be encouraged to communicate with the dying patient. Encouraging them to talk directly to the patient, even if he or she is unconscious, and hold the patient's hand or demonstrate affection in other ways can be an effective way to channel their urge "to do something" for the patient.

When the plan is for the patient to die at home, the physician must inform the family and caregivers how to determine that the patient has died. The cardinal signs are cessation of cardiac function and respiration; the pupils become fixed; the body becomes cool; muscles relax; and incontinence may occur. Remind the family and caregivers that the eyes may remain open even when the patient has died because the retroorbital fat pad may be depleted, permitting the orbit to fall posteriorly, which makes it difficult for the eyelids to cover the eyeball.

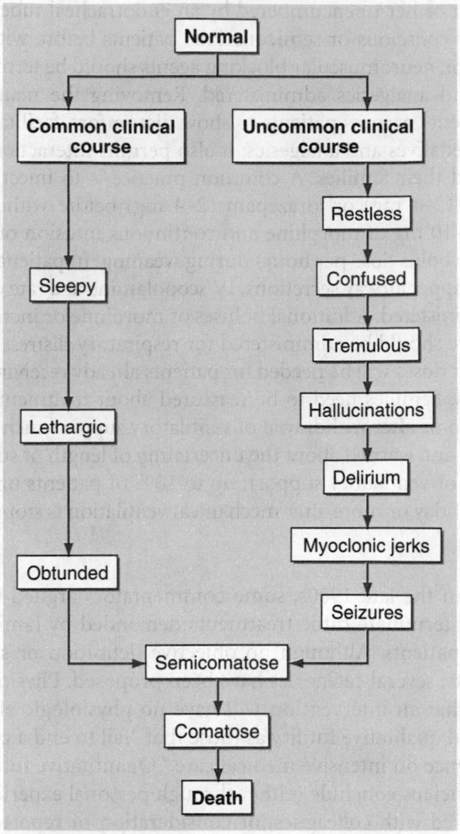

FIGURE 11-2 Common and uncommon clinical courses in the last days of terminally ill patients. *(Adapted from FD Ferris et al: Module 4: Palliative care, in Comprehensive Guide for the Care of Persons with HIV Disease. Toronto: Mt. Sinai Hospital and Casey Hospice, 1995, at www.cpsonline.info/content/resources/hivmodule4.html.)*

The physician should establish a plan for who the family or caregivers will contact when the patient is dying or has died. Without a plan, they may panic and call 911, unleashing a cascade of unwanted events from arrival of emergency personnel and resuscitation to hospital admission. The family and caregivers should be instructed to contact the hospice (if one is involved), the covering physician, or the on-call member of the palliative care team. They should also be told that the medical examiner need not be called, unless the state requires it for all deaths. Unless foul play is suspected, the health care team need not contact the medical examiner either.

Just after the patient dies, even the best-prepared family may experience shock and loss and be emotionally distraught. They need time to assimilate the event and be comforted. Health care providers may find it meaningful to write a bereavement card or letter to the family. The purpose is to communicate about the patient, perhaps emphasizing the patient's virtues, the honor it was to care for the patient, and express concern for the family's hardship. Some physicians attend the funerals of their patients. While this is beyond any medical obligation, the presence of the physician can be a source of support to the grieving family and provides an opportunity for closure for the physician.

Death of a spouse is a strong predictor of poor health, and even mortality, for the surviving spouse. It may be important to alert the spouse's physician about the death to be aware of symptoms that might require professional attention.

PALLIATIVE CARE SERVICES: HOW AND WHERE

Determining the best approach to providing palliative care to patients will depend upon patient preferences, the availability of caregivers and specialized services in close proximity, institutional resources, and re-

TABLE 11-9 MANAGING CHANGES IN THE PATIENT'S CONDITION DURING THE FINAL DAYS AND HOURS

Changes in the Patient's Condition	Potential Complication	Family's Possible Reaction and Concern	Advice and Intervention
Profound fatigue	Bedbound with development of pressure ulcers that are prone to infection, malodor, and pain, and joint pain	Patient is lazy and giving up.	Reassure family and caregivers that terminal fatigue will not respond to interventions and should not be resisted. Use an air mattress if necessary.
Anorexia	None	Patient is giving up; patient will suffer from hunger and will starve to death.	Reassure family and caregivers that the patient is not eating because he or she is dying; not eating at the end of life does not cause suffering or death. Forced feeding, whether oral, parenteral, or enteral, does not reduce symptoms or prolong life.
Dehydration	Dry mucosal membranes (see below)	Patient will suffer from thirst and die of dehydration.	Reassure family and caregivers that dehydration at the end of life does not cause suffering because patients lose consciousness before any symptom distress. Intravenous hydration can worsen symptoms of dyspnea by pulmonary edema and peripheral edema as well as prolong dying process.
Dysphagia	Inability to swallow oral medications needed for palliative care		Do not force oral intake. Discontinue unnecessary medications that may have been continued including antibiotics, diuretics, anti-depressants, and laxatives. If swallowing pills is difficult, convert essential medications (analgesics, antiemetics, anxiolytics, and psychotropics) to oral solutions, buccal, sublingual, or rectal administration.
"Death rattle"—noisy breathing		Patient is choking and suffocating.	Reassure the family and caregivers that this is caused by secretions in the oropharynx and the patient is not choking. Reduce secretions with scopolamine (0.2–0.4 mg SC q4h or 1–3 patches q3d) Reposition patient to permit drainage of secretions. Do not suction. Suction can cause patient and family discomfort, and is usually ineffective.
Apnea, Cheyne-Stokes respirations, dyspnea		Patient is suffocating.	Reassure family and caregivers that unconscious patients do not experience suffocation or air hunger. Apneic episodes are frequently a premorbid change. Opioids or anxiolytics may be used for dyspnea. Oxygen is unlikely to relieve dyspneic symptoms and may prolong the dying process.
Urinary or fecal incontinence	Skin breakdown if days until death Potential transmission of infectious agents to caregivers	Patient is dirty, malodorous, and physically repellent.	Remind family and caregivers to use universal precautions. Frequent changes of bedclothes and bedding. Use diapers, urinary catheter, or rectal tube if diarrhea or high urine output.
Agitation or delirium	Day/night reversal Hurt self or caregivers	Patient is in horrible pain and going to have a horrible death.	Reassure family and caregivers that agitation and delirium do not necessarily connote physical pain. Depending upon the prognosis and goals of treatment, consider evaluating for causes of delirium and modify medications. Manage symptoms with haloperidol, chlorpromazine, diazepam, or midazolam.
Dry mucosal membranes	Cracked lips, mouth sores, and candidiasis can also cause pain. Odor	Patient may be malodorous, physically repellent.	Use baking soda mouthwash or saliva preparation q15–30min. Use topical nystatin for candidiasis. Coat lips and nasal mucosa with petroleum jelly q60–90min. Use ophthalmic lubricants q4h or artificial tears q30min.

imbursement. Hospice is a leading, but not the only, model of palliative care services. In the United States, the vast majority of hospice care is provided in residential homes. By 2002, just over 20% of hospice was provided in nursing homes. In the United States, Medicare pays for hospice services under Part A, the hospital insurance part of reimbursement. Two physicians must certify that the patient has a prognosis of ≤6 months, if the disease runs its usual course. Prognoses are probabilistic by their nature; patients are not required to die within 6 months but rather to have a condition from which half the individuals with it would not be alive within 6 months. Patients sign a hospice enrollment form that states their intent to forgo curative services related to their terminal illness, but they can still receive medical services for other comorbid conditions. Patients can also withdraw enrollment and re-enroll later; the hospice Medicare benefit can be revoked later to secure traditional Medicare benefits. Payments to the hospice are per diem (or capitated), not fee-for-service. Payments are intended to cover physician services for the medical direction of the care team; regular home care visits by registered nurses and licensed practical nurses; home health aid and homemaker services; chaplain services; social work services; bereavement counseling; and medical equipment, supplies, and medications. No specific therapy is excluded and the goal is for each therapy to be considered for its symptomatic (as opposed to disease-modifying) effect. Additional clinical care, including services of the primary physician, is covered by Medicare Part B, even while the hospice Medicare benefit is in place.

By 2005, the mean length of enrollment in a hospice was 59 days, with the median being 26 days. Such short stays create barriers to establishing high-quality palliative services in patients' homes and also place financial strains on hospice providers since the initial assessments are resource intensive. Physicians should initiate early referrals to the hospice to allow more time for patients to receive palliative care.

Hospice care has been the main way of securing palliative services for terminally ill patients. However, efforts are now being made to ensure continuity of palliative care across settings and through time. Palliative care services are becoming available as consultative services and more rarely as palliative care units in hospitals, in day care and other outpatient settings, and in nursing homes. Palliative care consultations for non-hospice patients can be billed as for other consultations under Medicare

Part B, the physician reimbursement part. Many believe palliative care should be offered to patients regardless of their prognosis. A patient, his or her family, and physicians should not have to make a "curative vs. palliative care" decision because it is rarely possible to make such a decisive switch to embracing mortality.

FUTURE DIRECTIONS

OUTCOME MEASURES

Care near the end of life cannot be measured by most of the available validated outcome measures since palliative care does not consider death a bad outcome. Similarly, the family and patients receiving end-of-life care may not desire the elements elicited in current quality-of-life measurements. Symptom control, enhanced family relationships, and quality of bereavement are difficult to measure and are rarely the primary focus of carefully developed or widely used outcome measures. Nevertheless, outcomes are as important in end-of-life care as in any other field of medical care. Specific end-of-life care instruments are being developed both for assessment, such as The Brief Hospice Inventory and NEST (*n*eeds near the *e*nd of life *s*creening *t*ool), and for outcome measures, such as the Palliative Care Outcomes Scale, and for prognosis, such as the Palliative Prognostic Index. The field of end-of-life care is entering an era of evidence-based practice and continuous improvement through clinical trials.

FURTHER READINGS

Web Sites

Education in Palliative and End of Life Care (EPEC): *http://www.epec.net*

End of Life—Palliative Education Resource Center: *http://www.eperc.mcw.edu*

National Hospice and Palliative Care Organization (including state-specific advance directives): *http://www.nhpco.org*

NCCN: The National Comprehensive Cancer Network palliative care guidelines: *http://www.nccn.org*

Center to Advance Palliative Care: *http://www.capc.org*

Family Caregiver Alliance: *http://www.caregiver.org*

National Family Caregivers Association: *http://www.nfcacares.org/*

The Medical Directive: *http://www.medicaldirective.org*

American Academy of Hospice and Palliative Medicine: *www.aahpm.org*

Books

American Society of Clinical Oncology: *Optimizing Cancer Care—The Importance of Symptom Management.* vols 1 and 2. Alexandria, VA, ASCO, 2001

Buckman R: *How to Break Bad News: A Guide for Health Care Professionals.* Baltimore, Johns Hopkins University Press, 1992

Articles

Christakis NA, Allison PD: Mortality after the hospitalization of a spouse. N Engl J Med 354:719, 2006.

Emanuel L et al, for the Palliative Care Guidelines Group of the American Hospice Foundation: Integrating palliative care into disease management guidelines. Journal of Palliative Medicine 7:774, 2004

Kapo J et al: Palliative care for the older adult. J Palliat Med 10:185, 2007

Lynn J: Serving patients who may die soon and their families: The role of hospice and other services. JAMA 285:925, 2001

Meisel A et al, for the American College of Physicians–American Society of Internal Medicine End-of-Life Care Consensus Panel: Seven legal barriers to end-of-life care: Myths, realities, and grains of truth. JAMA 284:2495, 2000

Murray SA et al: Illness trajectories and palliative care. BMJ 330:1007, 2005

PART 2: Cardinal Manifestations and Presentation of Diseases

SECTION 1 PAIN

12 Pain: Pathophysiology and Management

Howard L. Fields, Joseph B. Martin

The task of medicine is to preserve and restore health and to relieve suffering. Understanding pain is essential to both these goals. Because pain is universally understood as a signal of disease, it is the most common symptom that brings a patient to a physician's attention. The function of the pain sensory system is to protect the body and maintain homeostasis. It does this by detecting, localizing, and identifying tissue-damaging processes. Since different diseases produce characteristic patterns of tissue damage, the quality, time course, and location of a patient's pain complaint and the location of tenderness provide important diagnostic clues and are used to evaluate the response to treatment. Once this information is obtained, it is the obligation of the physician to provide rapid and effective pain relief.

THE PAIN SENSORY SYSTEM

Pain is an unpleasant sensation localized to a part of the body. It is often described in terms of a penetrating or tissue-destructive process (e.g., stabbing, burning, twisting, tearing, squeezing) and/or of a bodily or emotional reaction (e.g., terrifying, nauseating, sickening). Furthermore, any pain of moderate or higher intensity is accompanied by anxiety and the urge to escape or terminate the feeling. These properties illustrate the duality of pain: it is both sensation and emotion. When acute, pain is characteristically associated with behavioral arousal and a stress response consisting of increased blood pressure, heart rate, pupil diameter, and plasma cortisol levels. In addition, local muscle contraction (e.g., limb flexion, abdominal wall rigidity) is often present.

PERIPHERAL MECHANISMS

The Primary Afferent Nociceptor A peripheral nerve consists of the axons of three different types of neurons: primary sensory afferents, motor neurons, and sympathetic postganglionic neurons (Fig. 12-1). The cell bodies of primary sensory afferents are located in the dorsal root ganglia in the vertebral foramina. The primary afferent axon bifurcates to send one process into the spinal cord and the other to innervate tissues. Primary afferents are classified by their diameter, degree of myelination, and conduction velocity. The largest-diameter fibers, A-beta (Aβ), respond maximally to light touch and/or moving stimuli; they are present primarily in nerves that innervate the skin. In normal individuals, the activity of these fibers does not produce pain. There are two other classes of primary afferents: the small-diameter myelinated A-delta (Aδ) and the unmyelinated (C fiber) axons (Fig. 12-1). These fibers are present in nerves to the skin and to deep somatic and visceral structures. Some tissues, such as the cornea, are innervated only by Aδ and C afferents. Most Aδ and C afferents respond maximally only to intense (painful) stimuli and produce the subjective experience of pain when they are electrically stimulated; this defines them as *primary afferent nociceptors* (*pain receptors*). The ability to detect painful stimuli is completely abolished when Aδ and C axons are blocked.

Individual primary afferent nociceptors can respond to several different types of noxious stimuli. For example, most nociceptors respond to heating, intense cold, intense mechanical stimuli such as a pinch, and application of irritating chemicals including ATP, serotonin, bradykinin and histamine.

Sensitization When intense, repeated, or prolonged stimuli are applied to damaged or inflamed tissues, the threshold for activating primary afferent nociceptors is lowered and the frequency of firing is higher for all stimulus intensities. Inflammatory mediators such as bradykinin, nerve growth factor, some prostaglandins, and leukotrienes contribute to this process, which is called *sensitization*. In sensitized tissues, normally innocuous stimuli can produce pain. Sensitization is a clinically important process that contributes to tenderness, soreness, and hyperalgesia. A striking example of sensitization is sunburned skin, in which severe pain can be produced by a gentle slap on the back or a warm shower.

Sensitization is of particular importance for pain and tenderness in deep tissues. Viscera are normally relatively insensitive to noxious mechanical and thermal stimuli, although hollow viscera do generate significant discomfort when distended. In contrast, when affected by a disease process with an inflammatory component, deep structures such as joints or hollow viscera characteristically become exquisitely sensitive to mechanical stimulation.

A large proportion of Aδ and C afferents innervating viscera are completely insensitive in normal noninjured, noninflamed tissue. That is, they cannot be activated by known mechanical or thermal stimuli and are not spontaneously active. However, in the presence of inflammatory mediators, these afferents become sensitive to mechanical stimuli. Such afferents have been termed *silent nociceptors*, and

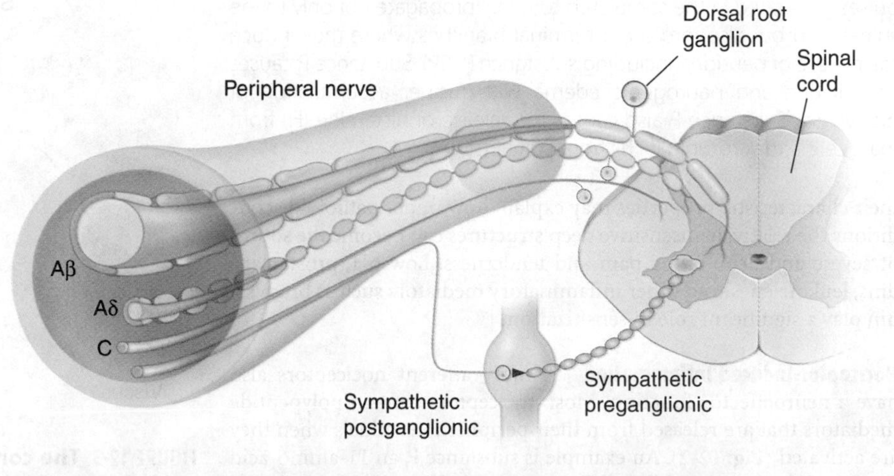

FIGURE 12-1 Components of a typical cutaneous nerve. There are two distinct functional categories of axons: primary afferents with cell bodies in the dorsal root ganglion, and sympathetic postganglionic fibers with cell bodies in the sympathetic ganglion. Primary afferents include those with large-diameter myelinated (Aβ), small-diameter myelinated (Aδ), and unmyelinated (C) axons. All sympathetic postganglionic fibers are unmyelinated.

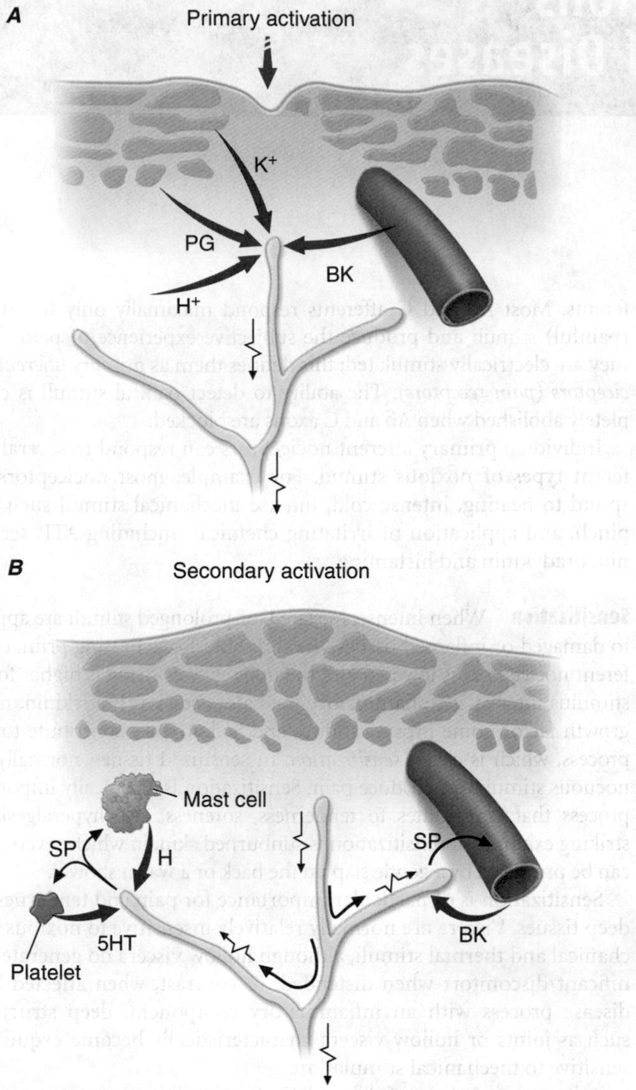

FIGURE 12-2 Events leading to activation, sensitization, and spread of sensitization of primary afferent nociceptor terminals. ***A.*** Direct activation by intense pressure and consequent cell damage. Cell damage induces lower pH (H^+) and leads to release of potassium (K^+) and to synthesis of prostaglandins (PG) and bradykinin (BK). Prostaglandins increase the sensitivity of the terminal to bradykinin and other pain-producing substances. ***B.*** Secondary activation. Impulses generated in the stimulated terminal propagate not only to the spinal cord but also into other terminal branches where they induce the release of peptides, including substance P (SP). Substance P causes vasodilation and neurogenic edema with further accumulation of bradykinin. Substance P also causes the release of histamine (H) from mast cells and serotonin (5HT) from platelets.

their characteristic properties may explain how under pathologic conditions the relatively insensitive deep structures can become the source of severe and debilitating pain and tenderness. Low pH, prostaglandins, leukotrienes, and other inflammatory mediators such as bradykinin play a significant role in sensitization.

Nociceptor-Induced Inflammation Primary afferent nociceptors also have a neuroeffector function. Most nociceptors contain polypeptide mediators that are released from their peripheral terminals when they are activated (Fig. 12-2). An example is substance P, an 11-amino-acid peptide. Substance P is released from primary afferent nociceptors and has multiple biologic activities. It is a potent vasodilator, degranulates mast cells, is a chemoattractant for leukocytes, and increases the production and release of inflammatory mediators. Interestingly, depletion of substance P from joints reduces the severity of experimental arthritis. Primary afferent nociceptors are not simply passive messengers of threats to tissue injury but also play an active role in tissue protection through these neuroeffector functions.

CENTRAL MECHANISMS

The Spinal Cord and Referred Pain The axons of primary afferent nociceptors enter the spinal cord via the dorsal root. They terminate in the dorsal horn of the spinal gray matter (Fig. 12-3). The terminals of primary afferent axons contact spinal neurons that transmit the pain signal to brain sites involved in pain perception. When primary afferents are activated by noxious stimuli, they release neurotransmitters from their terminals that excite the spinal cord neurons. The major neurotransmitter they release is glutamate, which rapidly excites dorsal horn neurons. Primary afferent nociceptor terminals also release peptides, including substance P and calcitonin gene-related peptide, which produce a slower and longer-lasting excitation of the dorsal horn neurons. The axon of each primary afferent contacts many spinal neurons, and each spinal neuron receives convergent inputs from many primary afferents.

The convergence of sensory inputs to a single spinal pain-transmission neuron is of great importance because it underlies the phenomenon of referred pain. All spinal neurons that receive input from the viscera and deep musculoskeletal structures also receive input from the skin. The convergence patterns are determined by the spinal segment of the dorsal root ganglion that supplies the afferent innervation of a structure. For example, the afferents that supply the central diaphragm are derived from the third and fourth cervical dorsal root ganglia. Primary afferents with cell bodies in these same ganglia supply the skin of the shoulder and lower neck. Thus, sensory inputs from both the shoulder skin and the central diaphragm converge on pain-transmission neurons in the third and fourth cervical spinal segments. *Because of this convergence and the fact that the spinal neurons are most often activated by inputs from the skin, activity evoked in spinal neurons by input from deep structures is mislocalized by the patient to a place that is roughly coextensive with the region of skin innervated by the same spinal segment.* Thus, inflammation near the central diaphragm is usually reported as discomfort near the shoulder. This spatial displacement of pain sensation from the site of the injury that produces it is known as *referred pain.*

Ascending Pathways for Pain A majority of spinal neurons contacted by primary afferent nociceptors send their axons to the contralateral thalamus. These axons form the contralateral spinothalamic tract, which lies in the anterolateral white matter of the spinal cord, the lateral edge of the medulla, and the lateral pons and midbrain. The spinothalamic pathway is crucial for pain sensation in humans. Interruption of this pathway produces permanent deficits in pain and temperature discrimination.

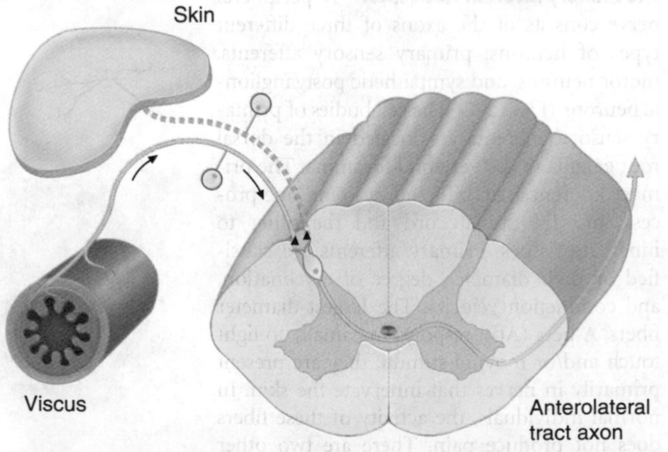

FIGURE 12-3 The convergence-projection hypothesis of referred pain. According to this hypothesis, visceral afferent nociceptors converge on the same pain-projection neurons as the afferents from the somatic structures in which the pain is perceived. The brain has no way of knowing the actual source of input and mistakenly "projects" the sensation to the somatic structure.

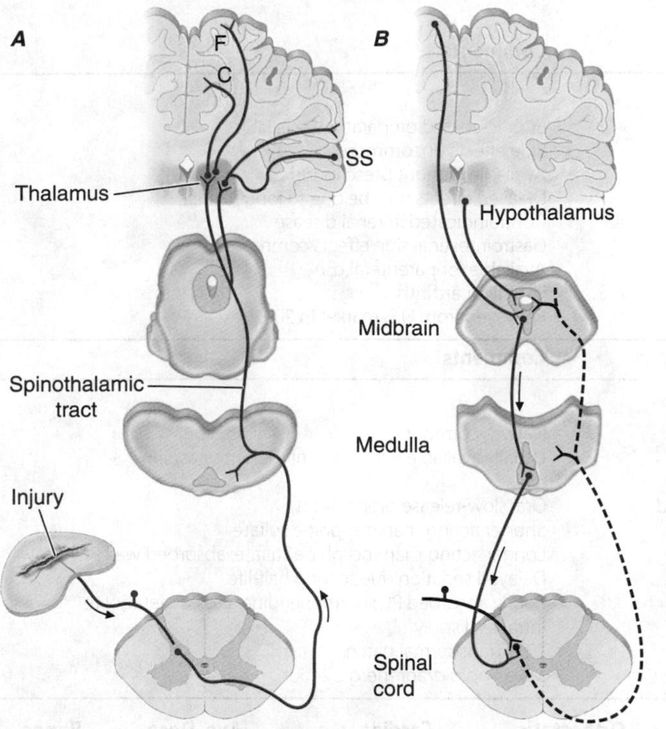

FIGURE 12-4 Pain transmission and modulatory pathways. *A.* Transmission system for nociceptive messages. Noxious stimuli activate the sensitive peripheral ending of the primary afferent nociceptor by the process of transduction. The message is then transmitted over the peripheral nerve to the spinal cord, where it synapses with cells of origin of the major ascending pain pathway, the spinothalamic tract. The message is relayed in the thalamus to the anterior cingulate (C), frontal insular (F), and somatosensory cortex (SS). ***B.*** Pain-modulation network. Inputs from frontal cortex and hypothalamus activate cells in the midbrain that control spinal pain-transmission cells via cells in the medulla.

Spinothalamic tract axons ascend to several regions of the thalamus. There is tremendous divergence of the pain signal from these thalamic sites to broad areas of the cerebral cortex that subserve different aspects of the pain experience (Fig. 12-4). One of the thalamic projections is to the somatosensory cortex. This projection mediates the purely sensory aspects of pain, i.e., its location, intensity, and quality. Other thalamic neurons project to cortical regions that are linked to emotional responses, such as the cingulate gyrus and other areas of the frontal lobes, including the insular cortex. These pathways to the frontal cortex subserve the affective or unpleasant emotional dimension of pain. This affective dimension of pain produces suffering and exerts potent control of behavior. Because of this dimension, fear is a constant companion of pain.

PAIN MODULATION

The pain produced by injuries of similar magnitude is remarkably variable in different situations and in different individuals. For example, athletes have been known to sustain serious fractures with only minor pain, and Beecher's classic World War II survey revealed that many soldiers in battle were unbothered by injuries that would have produced agonizing pain in civilian patients. Furthermore, even the suggestion of relief can have a significant analgesic effect (placebo). On the other hand, many patients find even minor injuries (such as venipuncture) frightening and unbearable, and the expectation of pain has been demonstrated to induce pain without a noxious stimulus.

The powerful effect of expectation and other psychological variables on the perceived intensity of pain implies the existence of brain circuits that can modulate the activity of the pain-transmission pathways. One of these circuits has links in the hypothalamus, midbrain, and medulla, and it selectively controls spinal pain-transmission neurons through a descending pathway (Fig. 12-4).

Human brain imaging studies have implicated this pain-modulating circuit in the pain-relieving effect of attention, suggestion, and opioid analgesic medications. Furthermore, each of the component structures of the pathway contains opioid receptors and is sensitive to the direct application of opioid drugs. In animals, lesions of the system reduce the analgesic effect of systemically administered opioids such as morphine. Along with the opioid receptor, the component nuclei of this pain-modulating circuit contain endogenous opioid peptides such as the enkephalins and β-endorphin.

The most reliable way to activate this endogenous opioid-mediated modulating system is by prolonged pain and/or fear. There is evidence that pain-relieving endogenous opioids are released following surgical procedures and in patients given a placebo for pain relief.

Pain-modulating circuits can enhance as well as suppress pain. Both pain-inhibiting and pain-facilitating neurons in the medulla project to and control spinal pain-transmission neurons. Since pain-transmission neurons can be activated by modulatory neurons, it is theoretically possible to generate a pain signal with no peripheral noxious stimulus. In fact, human functional imaging studies have demonstrated increased activity in this circuit during migraine headache. A central circuit that facilitates pain could account for the finding that pain can be induced by suggestion or enhanced by expectation, and it could provide a framework for understanding how psychological factors can contribute to chronic pain.

NEUROPATHIC PAIN

Lesions of the peripheral or central nervous pathways for pain typically result in a loss or impairment of pain sensation. Paradoxically, damage to or dysfunction of these pathways can produce pain. For example, damage to peripheral nerves, as occurs in diabetic neuropathy, or to primary afferents, as in herpes zoster, can result in pain that is referred to the body region innervated by the damaged nerves. Though rare, pain may also be produced by damage to the central nervous system, particularly the spinothalamic pathway or thalamus. Such neuropathic pains are often severe and are notoriously intractable to standard treatments for pain.

Neuropathic pains typically have an unusual burning, tingling, or electric shock–like quality and may be triggered by very light touch. These features are rare in other types of pain. On examination, a sensory deficit is characteristically present in the area of the patient's pain. Hyperpathia is also characteristic of neuropathic pain; patients often complain that the very lightest moving stimuli evoke exquisite pain (allodynia). In this regard it is of clinical interest that a topical preparation of 5% lidocaine in patch form is effective for patients with postherpetic neuralgia who have prominent allodynia.

A variety of mechanisms contribute to neuropathic pain. As with sensitized primary afferent nociceptors, damaged primary afferents, including nociceptors, become highly sensitive to mechanical stimulation and begin to generate impulses in the absence of stimulation. There is evidence that this increased sensitivity and spontaneous activity is due to an increased concentration of sodium channels. Damaged primary afferents may also develop sensitivity to norepinephrine. Interestingly, spinal cord pain-transmission neurons cut off from their normal input may also become spontaneously active. Thus, both central and peripheral nervous system hyperactivity contribute to neuropathic pain.

Sympathetically Maintained Pain Patients with peripheral nerve injury can develop a severe burning pain (causalgia) in the region innervated by the nerve. The pain typically begins after a delay of hours to days or even weeks. The pain is accompanied by swelling of the extremity, periarticular osteoporosis, and arthritic changes in the distal joints. The pain is dramatically and immediately relieved by blocking the sympathetic innervation of the affected extremity. Damaged primary afferent nociceptors acquire adrenergic sensitivity and can be activated by stimulation of the sympathetic outflow. A similar syndrome called *reflex sympathetic dystrophy* can be produced without obvious nerve damage by a variety of injuries, including fractures of bone, soft tissue trauma, myocardial infarction, and stroke (Chap. 370). Although the pathophysiology of this condition is poorly understood, the pain and the signs of inflammation are rapidly relieved by blocking the sympathetic nervous

TABLE 12-1 DRUGS FOR RELIEF OF PAIN

Generic Name	Dose, mg	Interval	Comments
Nonnarcotic Analgesics: Usual Doses and Intervals			
Acetylsalicylic acid	650 PO	q 4 h	Enteric-coated preparations available
Acetaminophen	650 PO	q 4 h	Side effects uncommon
Ibuprofen	400 PO	q 4–6 h	Available without prescription
Naproxen	250–500 PO	q 12 h	Delayed effects may be due to long half-life
Fenoprofen	200 PO	q 4–6 h	Contraindicated in renal disease
Indomethacin	25–50 PO	q 8 h	Gastrointestinal side effects common
Ketorolac	15–60 IM/IV	q 4–6 h	Available for parenteral use
Celecoxib	100–200 PO	q 12–24 h	Useful for arthritis
Valdecoxib	10–20 PO	q12–24 h	Removed from U.S. market in 2005

Generic Name	Parenteral Dose, mg	PO Dose, mg	Comments
Narcotic Analgesics: Usual Doses and Intervals			
Codeine	30–60 q 4 h	30–60 q 4 h	Nausea common
Oxycodone	—	5–10 q 4–6 h	Usually available with acetaminophen or aspirin
Morphine	10 q 4 h	60 q 4 h	
Morphine sustained release	—	30–200 bid to tid	Oral slow-release preparation
Hydromorphone	1–2 q 4 h	2–4 q 4 h	Shorter acting than morphine sulfate
Levorphanol	2 q 6–8 h	4 q 6–8 h	Longer acting than morphine sulfate; absorbed well PO
Methadone	10 q 6–8 h	20 q 6–8 h	Delayed sedation due to long half-life
Meperidine	75–100 q 3–4 h	300 q 4 h	Poorly absorbed PO; normeperidine a toxic metabolite
Butorphanol	—	1–2 q 4 h	Intranasal spray
Fentanyl	25–100 μg/h	—	72 h Transdermal patch
Tramadol	—	50–100 q 4–6 h	Mixed opioid/adrenergic action

Generic Name	Uptake Blockade 5-HT	Uptake Blockade NE	Sedative Potency	Anticholinergic Potency	Orthostatic Hypotension	Cardiac Arrhythmia	Ave. Dose, mg/d	Range, mg/d
Antidepressants[a]								
Doxepin	++	+	High	Moderate	Moderate	Less	200	75–400
Amitriptyline	++++	++	High	Highest	Moderate	Yes	150	25–300
Imipramine	++++	++	Moderate	Moderate	High	Yes	200	75–400
Nortriptyline	+++	++	Moderate	Moderate	Low	Yes	100	40–150
Desipramine	+++	++++	Low	Low	Low	Yes	150	50–300
Venlafaxine	+++	++	Low	None	None	No	150	75–400
Duloxetine	+++	+++	Low	None	None	No	40	30–60

Generic Name	PO Dose, mg	Interval	Generic Name	PO Dose, mg	Interval
Anticonvulsants and Antiarrhythmics[a]					
Phenytoin	300	daily/qhs	Clonazepam	1	q 6 h
Carbamazepine	200–300	q 6 h	Gabapentin[b]	600–1200	q 8 h
Oxcarbazine	300	bid	Pregabalin	150–600	bid

[a]Antidepressants, anticonvulsants, and antiarrhythmics have not been approved by the U.S. Food and Drug Administration (FDA) for the treatment of pain.

[b]Gabapentin in doses up to 1800 mg/d is FDA approved for postherpetic neuralgia.

Note: 5-HT, serotonin; NE, norepinephrine.

system. This implies that sympathetic activity can activate undamaged nociceptors when inflammation is present. Signs of sympathetic hyperactivity should be sought in patients with posttraumatic pain and inflammation and no other obvious explanation.

℞ ACUTE PAIN

The ideal treatment for any pain is to remove the cause; thus, diagnosis should always precede treatment planning. Sometimes treating the underlying condition does not immediately relieve pain. Furthermore, some conditions are so painful that rapid and effective analgesia is essential (e.g., the postoperative state, burns, trauma, cancer, sickle cell crisis). Analgesic medications are a first line of treatment in these cases, and all practitioners should be familiar with their use.

ASPIRIN, ACETAMINOPHEN, AND NONSTEROIDAL ANTI-INFLAMMATORY AGENTS (NSAIDS) These drugs are considered together because they are used for similar problems and may have a similar mechanism of action (**Table 12-1**). All these compounds inhibit cyclooxygenase (COX), and, except for acetaminophen, all have anti-inflammatory actions, especially at higher dosages. They are particularly effective for mild to moderate headache and for pain of musculoskeletal origin.

Since they are effective for these common types of pain and are available without prescription, COX inhibitors are by far the most commonly used analgesics. They are absorbed well from the gastrointestinal tract and, with occasional use, have only minimal side effects. With chronic use, gastric irritation is a common side effect of aspirin and NSAIDs and is the problem that most frequently limits the dose that can be given. Gastric irritation is most severe with aspirin, which may cause erosion and ulceration of the gastric mucosa leading to bleeding or perforation. Because aspirin irreversibly acetylates platelets and thereby interferes with coagulation of the blood, gastrointestinal bleeding is a particular risk. Increased age and history of gastrointestinal disease increase the risks of aspirin and NSAIDs. In addition to NSAIDs' well-known gastrointestinal toxicity, nephrotoxicity is a significant problem for patients using them on a chronic basis, and patients at risk for renal insufficiency should be monitored closely. NSAIDs also cause an increase in blood pressure in a significant number of individuals. Long-term treatment with NSAIDs requires regular blood pressure monitoring and treatment if necessary. Although toxic to the liver when taken in a high dose, acetaminophen rarely produces gastric irritation and does not interfere with platelet function.

The introduction of a parenteral form of NSAID, ketorolac, extends the usefulness of this class of compounds in the management of acute severe pain. Ketorolac is sufficiently potent and rapid in onset to supplant opioids for many patients with acute severe headache and musculoskeletal pain.

There are two major classes of COX: COX-1 is constitutively expressed, and COX-2 is induced in the inflammatory state. COX-2–selective drugs have moderate analgesic potency and produce less gastric irritation than the nonselective COX inhibitors. It is not yet clear whether the use of COX-2–selective drugs is associated with a lower risk of nephrotoxicity compared to nonselective NSAIDs. On the other hand, COX-2–selective drugs offer a significant benefit in the management of acute postoperative pain because they do not affect blood coagulation. This is a situation in which the nonselective COX inhibitors would be contraindicated because they impair platelet-mediated blood clotting and are thus associated with increased bleeding at the operative site. COX-2 inhibitors, including celecoxib (Celebrex), and valdecoxib (Bextra), are associated with increased cardiovascular risk. It is possible that this is a class effect of NSAIDs, excluding aspirin. These drugs are contraindicated in patients in the immediate period after coronary artery bypass surgery and should be used with caution in patients having a history of or significant risk factors for cardiovascular disease.

OPIOID ANALGESICS Opioids are the most potent pain-relieving drugs currently available. Furthermore, of all analgesics, they have the broadest range of efficacy, providing the most reliable and effective method for rapid pain relief. Although side effects are common, they are usually not serious except for respiratory depression and can be reversed rapidly with the narcotic antagonist naloxone. The physician should not hesitate to use opioid analgesics in patients with acute severe pain. **Table 12-1** lists the most commonly used opioid analgesics.

Opioids produce analgesia by actions in the central nervous system. They activate pain-inhibitory neurons and directly inhibit pain-transmission neurons. Most of the commercially available opioid analgesics act at the same opioid receptor (μ-receptor), differing mainly in potency, speed of onset, duration of action, and optimal route of administration. Although the dose-related side effects (sedation, respiratory depression, pruritus, constipation) are similar among the different opioids, some side effects are due to accumulation of nonopioid metabolites that are unique to individual drugs. One striking example of this is normeperidine, a metabolite of meperidine. Normeperidine produces hyperexcitability and seizures that are not reversible with naloxone. Normeperidine accumulation is increased in patients with renal failure.

The most rapid relief with opioids is obtained by intravenous administration; relief with oral administration is significantly slower. Common side effects include nausea, vomiting, constipation, and sedation. The most serious side effect is respiratory depression. Patients with any form of respiratory compromise must be kept under close observation following opioid administration; an oxygen saturation monitor may be useful. The opioid antagonist naloxone should be readily available. Opioid effects are dose-related, and there is great variability among patients in the doses that relieve pain and produce side effects. Because of this, initiation of therapy requires titration to optimal dose and interval. The most important principle is to provide adequate pain relief. This requires determining whether the drug has adequately relieved the pain and the duration of the relief. *The most common error made by physicians in managing severe pain with opioids is to prescribe an inadequate dose. Since many patients are reluctant to complain, this practice leads to needless suffering*. In the absence of sedation at the expected time of peak effect, a physician should not hesitate to repeat the initial dose to achieve satisfactory pain relief.

An innovative approach to the problem of achieving adequate pain relief is the use of patient-controlled analgesia (PCA). PCA requires a device that can deliver a baseline continuous dose of an opioid drug, as well as preprogrammed additional doses whenever the patient pushes a button. The patient can then titrate the dose to the optimal level. This approach is used most extensively for the management of postoperative pain, but there is no reason why it should not be used for any hospitalized patient with persistent severe pain. PCA is also used for short-term home care of patients with intractable pain, such as that caused by metastatic cancer.

Because of patient variability in analgesia requirement, intravenous PCA is generally begun after the patient's pain has been controlled. The bolus dose of the drug (typically 1 mg morphine or 40 μg fentanyl) can then be delivered repeatedly as needed. To prevent overdosing, PCA devices are programmed with a lockout period after each demand dose is delivered (5–10 min) and a limit on the total dose delivered per hour. While some have advocated the use of a simultaneous background infusion of the PCA drug, this increases the risk of respiratory depression and has not been shown to increase the overall efficacy of the technique.

Many physicians, nurses, and patients have a certain trepidation about using opioids that is based on an exaggerated fear of addiction. In fact, there is a vanishingly small chance of patients becoming addicted to narcotics as a result of their appropriate medical use.

The availability of new routes of administration has extended the usefulness of opioid analgesics. Most important is the availability of spinal administration. Opioids can be infused through a spinal catheter placed either intrathecally or epidurally. By applying opioids directly to the spinal cord, regional analgesia can be obtained using a relatively low total dose. In this way, such side effects as sedation, nausea, and respiratory depression can be minimized. This approach has been used extensively in obstetric procedures and for lower-body postoperative pain. Opioids can also be given intranasally (butorphanol), rectally, and transdermally (fentanyl), thus avoiding the discomfort of frequent injections in patients who cannot be given oral medication. The fentanyl transdermal patch has the advantage of providing fairly steady plasma levels, which maximizes patient comfort.

Opioid and COX Inhibitor Combinations When used in combination, opioids and COX inhibitors have additive effects. Because a lower dose of each can be used to achieve the same degree of pain relief, and their side effects are nonadditive, such combinations can be used to lower the severity of dose-related side effects. Fixed-ratio combinations of an opioid with acetaminophen carry a special risk. Dose escalation as a result of increased severity of pain or decreased opioid effect as a result of tolerance may lead to levels of acetaminophen that are toxic to the liver.

CHRONIC PAIN

Managing patients with chronic pain is intellectually and emotionally challenging. The patient's problem is often difficult to diagnose; such patients are demanding of the physician's time and often appear emotionally distraught. The traditional medical approach of seeking an obscure organic pathology is usually unhelpful. On the other hand, psychological evaluation and behaviorally based treatment paradigms are frequently helpful, particularly in the setting of a multidisciplinary pain-management center.

There are several factors that can cause, perpetuate, or exacerbate chronic pain. First, of course, the patient may simply have a disease that is characteristically painful for which there is presently no cure. Arthritis, cancer, migraine headaches, fibromyalgia, and diabetic neuropathy are examples of this. Second, there may be secondary perpetuating factors that are initiated by disease and persist after that disease has resolved. Examples include damaged sensory nerves, sympathetic efferent activity, and painful reflex muscle contraction. Finally, a variety of psychological conditions can exacerbate or even cause pain.

There are certain areas to which special attention should be paid in the medical history. Because depression is the most common emotional disturbance in patients with chronic pain, patients should be questioned about their mood, appetite, sleep patterns, and daily activity. A simple standardized questionnaire, such as the Beck Depression Inventory, can be a useful screening device. It is important to remember that major depression is a common, treatable, and potentially fatal illness.

Other clues that a significant emotional disturbance is contributing to a patient's chronic pain complaint include: pain that occurs in multiple unrelated sites; a pattern of recurrent, but separate, pain problems beginning in childhood or adolescence; pain beginning at a time of emotional trauma, such as the loss of a parent or spouse; a history of physical or sexual abuse; and past or present substance abuse.

On examination, special attention should be paid to whether the patient guards the painful area and whether certain movements or postures are avoided because of pain. Discovering a mechanical component to the pain can be useful both diagnostically and therapeutically. Painful areas should be examined for deep tenderness, noting whether this is localized to muscle, ligamentous structures, or joints. Chronic myofascial pain is very common, and in these patients deep palpation may reveal highly localized trigger points that are firm bands or knots in muscle. Relief of the pain following injection of local anesthetic into these trigger points supports the diagnosis. A neuropathic component to the pain is indicated by evidence of nerve damage, such as sensory impairment, exquisitely sensitive skin, weakness and muscle atrophy, or loss of deep tendon reflexes. Evidence suggesting sympathetic nervous system involvement includes the presence of diffuse swelling, changes in skin color and temperature, and hypersensitive skin and joint tenderness compared with the normal side. Relief of the pain with a sympathetic block is diagnostic.

A guiding principle in evaluating patients with chronic pain is to assess both emotional and organic factors before initiating therapy. Addressing these issues together, rather than waiting to address emotional issues after organic causes of pain have been ruled out, improves compliance in part because it assures patients that a psychological evaluation does not mean that the physician is questioning the validity of their complaint. Even when an organic cause for a patient's pain can be found, it is still wise to look for other factors. For example, a cancer patient with painful bony metastases may have additional pain due to nerve damage and may also be depressed. Optimal therapy requires that each of these factors be looked for and treated.

℞ CHRONIC PAIN

Once the evaluation process has been completed and the likely causative and exacerbating factors identified, an explicit treatment plan should be developed. An important part of this process is to identify specific and realistic functional goals for therapy, such as getting a good night's sleep, being able to go shopping, or returning to work. A multidisciplinary approach that utilizes medications, counseling, physical therapy, nerve blocks, and even surgery may be required to improve the patient's quality of life. There are also some newer, relatively invasive procedures that can be helpful for some patients with intractable pain. These procedures include implanting intraspinal cannulae to deliver morphine or intraspinal electrodes for spinal stimulation. There are no set criteria for predicting which patients will respond to these procedures. They are generally reserved for patients who have not responded to conventional pharmacologic approaches. Referral to a multidisciplinary pain clinic for a full evaluation should precede any invasive procedures. Such referrals are clearly not necessary for all chronic pain patients. For some, pharmacologic management alone can provide adequate relief.

ANTIDEPRESSANT MEDICATIONS The tricyclic antidepressants [amitriptyline, imipramine, nortriptyline, desipramine (TCAs; Table 12-1)] are extremely useful for the management of patients with chronic pain. Although developed for the treatment of depression, the tricyclics have a spectrum of dose-related biologic activities that include the production of analgesia in a variety of clinical conditions. Although the mechanism is unknown, the analgesic effect of TCAs has a more rapid onset and occurs at a lower dose than is typically required for the treatment of depression. Furthermore, patients with chronic pain who are not depressed obtain pain relief with antidepressants. There is evidence that tricyclic drugs potentiate opioid analgesia, so they may be useful adjuncts for the treatment of severe persistent pain such as occurs with malignant tumors. **Table 12-2** lists some of the painful conditions that respond to tricyclics. TCAs are of particular value in the management of neuropathic pain such as occurs in diabetic neuropathy and postherpetic neuralgia, for which there are few other therapeutic options.

The TCAs that have been shown to relieve pain have significant side effects (Table 12-1; Chap. 386). Some of these side effects, such as orthostatic hypotension, drowsiness, cardiac conduction delay, memory impairment, constipation, and urinary retention, are particularly problematic in elderly patients, and several are additive to the side effects of opioid analgesics. The serotonin-selective reuptake inhibitors such as fluoxetine (Prozac) have fewer and less serious side effects than TCAs, but they are much less effective for relieving pain. It is of interest that venlafaxine (Effexor) and duloxetine (Cymbalta), which are nontricyclic antidepressants that block both serotonin and norepinephrine reuptake, appear to retain most of the pain-relieving effect of TCAs with a side-effect profile more like that of the serotonin-selective reuptake inhibitors. These drugs may be particularly useful in patients who cannot tolerate the side effects of tricyclics.

TABLE 12-2 PAINFUL CONDITIONS THAT RESPOND TO TRICYCLIC ANTIDEPRESSANTS

Postherpetic neuralgia[a]
Diabetic neuropathy[a]
Tension headache[a]
Migraine headache[a]
Rheumatoid arthritis[a,b]
Chronic low back pain[b]
Cancer
Central post-stroke pain

[a]Controlled trials demonstrate analgesia.
[b]Controlled studies indicate benefit but not analgesia.

ANTICONVULSANTS AND ANTIARRHYTHMICS These drugs are useful primarily for patients with neuropathic pain. Phenytoin (Dilantin) and carbamazepine (Tegretol) were first shown to relieve the pain of trigeminal neuralgia. This pain has a characteristic brief, shooting, electric shock–like quality. In fact, anticonvulsants seem to be helpful largely for pains that have such a lancinating quality. Newer anticonvulsants, gabapentin (Neurontin) and pregabalin (Lyrica), are effective for a broad range of neuropathic pains.

Antiarrhythmic drugs such as low-dose lidocaine and mexiletine (Mexitil) can also be effective for neuropathic pain. These drugs block the spontaneous activity of damaged primary afferent nociceptors.

CHRONIC OPIOID MEDICATION The long-term use of opioids is accepted for patients with pain due to malignant disease. Although opioid use for chronic pain of nonmalignant origin is controversial, it is clear that for many such patients opioid analgesics are the best available option. This is understandable since opioids are the most potent and have the broadest range of efficacy of any analgesic medications. Although addiction is rare in patients who first use opioids for pain relief, some degree of tolerance and physical dependence are likely with long-term use. Therefore, before embarking on opioid therapy, other options should be explored, and the limitations and risks of opioids should be explained to the patient. It is also important to point out that some opioid analgesic medications have mixed agonist-antagonist properties (e.g., pentazocine and butorphanol). From a practical standpoint, this means that they may worsen pain by inducing an abstinence syndrome in patients who are physically dependent on other opioid analgesics.

With long-term outpatient use of orally administered opioids, it is desirable to use long-acting compounds such as levorphanol, methadone, or sustained-release morphine (Table 12-1). Transdermal fentanyl is another excellent option. The pharmacokinetic profile of these drug preparations enables prolonged pain relief, minimizes side effects such as sedation that are associated with high peak plasma levels, and reduces the likelihood of rebound pain associated with a rapid fall in plasma opioid concentration. Constipation is a virtually universal side effect of opioid use and should be treated expectantly.

TREATMENT OF NEUROPATHIC PAIN It is important to individualize treatment for patients with neuropathic pain. Several general principles should guide therapy: the first is to move quickly to provide relief; a second is to minimize drug side effects. For example, in patients with postherpetic neuralgia and significant cutaneous hypersensitivity, topical lidocaine (Lidoderm patches) can provide immediate relief without side effects. Anticonvulsants (gabapentin or pregabalin, see above) or antidepressants can be used as first-line drugs for patients with neuropathic pain. Antiarrhythmic drugs such as lidocaine and mexiletene can be effective (see above). There is no consensus on which class of drug should be used as a first-line treatment for any chronically painful condition. However, because relatively high doses of anticonvulsants are required for pain relief, sedation is very common. Sedation is also a problem with the tricyclic antidepressants but is much less of a problem with serotonin/norepinephrine reuptake inhibitors (SNRIs, e.g., venlafaxine and duloxetine). Thus, in the elderly or in those patients whose daily activities require high-level mental activity, these drugs should be considered as the first line. In contrast, opioid medications should be used as a second- or third-line drug class. While highly effective for many painful conditions, opioids are sedating, and their effect tends to lessen over time, leading to dose escalation and, occasionally, a worsening of pain due to physical dependence. Drugs of different classes can be used in combination to optimize pain control.

It is worth emphasizing that many patients, especially those with chronic pain, seek medical attention primarily because they are suffering and because only physicians can provide the medications required for pain relief. A primary responsibility of all physicians is to minimize the physical and emotional discomfort of their patients. Familiarity with pain mechanisms and analgesic medications is an important step toward accomplishing this aim.

FURTHER READINGS

CRAIG AD: How do you feel? Interoception: The sense of the physiological condition of the body. Nat Rev Neurosci 8:655, 2002

FIELDS HL: Should we be reluctant to prescribe opioids for chronic nonmalignant pain? Pain 129:233, 2007

KELTNER JR et al: Isolating the modulatory effect of expectation on pain transmission: A functional magnetic resonance imaging study. J Neurosci 26:4437, 2006

MACINTYRE PE: Safety and efficacy of patient-controlled analgesia. Br J Anaesth 87:36, 2001

WAGER TD et al: Placebo-induced changes in FMRI in the anticipation and experience of pain. Science 303:1162, 2004

13 Chest Discomfort

Thomas H. Lee

Chest discomfort is one of the most common challenges for clinicians in the office or emergency department. The differential diagnosis includes conditions affecting organs throughout the thorax and abdomen, with prognostic implications that vary from benign to life-threatening (Table 13-1). Failure to recognize potentially serious conditions such as acute ischemic heart disease, aortic dissection, tension pneumothorax, or pulmonary embolism can lead to serious complications, including death. Conversely, overly conservative management of low-risk patients leads to unnecessary hospital admissions, tests, procedures, and anxiety.

CAUSES OF CHEST DISCOMFORT

Myocardial Ischemia and Injury Myocardial ischemia occurs when the oxygen supply to the heart is not sufficient to meet metabolic needs. This mismatch can result from a decrease in oxygen supply, a rise in demand, or both. The most common underlying cause of myocardial ischemia is obstruction of coronary arteries by atherosclerosis; in the presence of such obstruction, transient ischemic episodes are usually precipitated by an increase in oxygen demand as a result of physical exertion. However, ischemia can also result from psychological stress, fever, or large meals or from compromised oxygen delivery due to anemia, hypoxia, or hypotension. Ventricular hypertrophy due to valvular heart disease, hypertrophic cardiomyopathy, or hypertension can predispose the myocardium to ischemia because of impaired penetration of blood flow from epicardial coronary arteries to the endocardium.

ANGINA PECTORIS (See also Chap. 237) The chest discomfort of myocardial ischemia is a visceral discomfort that is usually described as a heaviness, pressure, or squeezing (Table 13-2). Other common adjectives for anginal pain are burning and aching. Some patients deny any "pain" but may admit to dyspnea or a vague sense of anxiety. The word "sharp" is sometimes used by patients to describe intensity rather than quality.

The location of angina pectoris is usually retrosternal; most patients do not localize the pain to any small area. The discomfort may radiate to the neck, jaw, teeth, arms, or shoulders, reflecting the common origin in the posterior horn of the spinal cord of sensory neurons supplying the heart and these areas. Some patients present with aching in sites of radiated pain as their only symptoms of ischemia. Occasional patients report epigastric distress with ischemic episodes. Less common is radiation to below the umbilicus or to the back.

TABLE 13-1 DIFFERENTIAL DIAGNOSES OF PATIENTS ADMITTED TO HOSPITAL WITH ACUTE CHEST DISCOMFORT RULED NOT MYOCARDIAL INFARCTION

Diagnosis	Percent
Gastroesophageal disease[a]	42
Gastroesophageal reflux	
Esophageal motility disorders	
Peptic ulcer	
Gallstones	
Ischemic heart disease	31
Chest wall syndromes	28
Pericarditis	4
Pleuritis/pneumonia	2
Pulmonary embolism	2
Lung cancer	1.5
Aortic aneurysm	1
Aortic stenosis	1
Herpes zoster	1

[a]In order of frequency.

Source: P Fruergaard et al: Eur Heart J 17:1028, 1996.

Stable angina pectoris usually develops gradually with exertion, emotional excitement, or after heavy meals. Rest or treatment with sublingual nitroglycerin typically leads to relief within several minutes. In contrast, pain that is fleeting (lasting only a few seconds) is rarely ischemic in origin. Similarly, pain that lasts for several hours is unlikely to represent angina, particularly if the patient's electrocardiogram (ECG) does not show evidence of ischemia.

Anginal episodes can be precipitated by any physiologic or psychological stress that induces tachycardia. Most myocardial perfusion occurs during diastole, when there is minimal pressure opposing coronary artery flow from within the left ventricle. Since tachycardia decreases the percentage of the time in which the heart is in diastole, it decreases myocardial perfusion.

UNSTABLE ANGINA AND MYOCARDIAL INFARCTION (See also Chaps. 238 and 239) Patients with these acute ischemic syndromes usually complain of symptoms similar in quality to angina pectoris, but more prolonged and severe. The onset of these syndromes may occur with the patient at rest, or awakened from sleep, and sublingual nitroglycerin may lead to transient or no relief. Accompanying symptoms may include diaphoresis, dyspnea, nausea, and light-headedness.

The physical examination may be completely normal in patients with chest discomfort due to ischemic heart disease. Careful auscultation during ischemic episodes may reveal a third or fourth heart sound, reflecting myocardial systolic or diastolic dysfunction. A transient murmur of mitral regurgitation suggests ischemic papillary muscle dysfunction. Severe episodes of ischemia can lead to pulmonary congestion and even pulmonary edema.

OTHER CARDIAC CAUSES Myocardial ischemia caused by hypertrophic cardiomyopathy or aortic stenosis leads to angina pectoris similar to that caused by coronary atherosclerosis. In such cases, a loud systolic murmur or other findings usually suggest that abnormalities other than coronary atherosclerosis may be contributing to the patient's symptoms. Some patients with chest pain and normal coronary angiograms have functional abnormalities of the coronary circulation, ranging from coronary spasm visible on coronary angiography to abnormal vasodilator responses and heightened vasoconstrictor responses. The term "cardiac syndrome X" is used to describe patients with angina-like chest pain and ischemic-appearing ST-segment depression during stress despite normal coronary arteriograms. Some data indicate that many such patients have limited changes in coronary flow in response to pacing stress or coronary vasodilators. Despite the possibility that chest pain may be due to myocardial ischemia in such patients, their prognosis is excellent.

Pericarditis (See also Chap. 232) The pain in pericarditis is believed to be due to inflammation of the adjacent parietal pleura, since most of the pericardium is believed to be insensitive to pain. Thus, infectious pericarditis, which usually involves adjoining pleural surfaces, tends to be associated with pain, while conditions that cause only local inflammation (e.g., myocardial infarction or uremia) and cardiac tamponade tend to result in mild or no chest pain.

TABLE 13-2 TYPICAL CLINICAL FEATURES OF MAJOR CAUSES OF ACUTE CHEST DISCOMFORT

Condition	Duration	Quality	Location	Associated Features
Angina	More than 2 and less than 10 min	Pressure, tightness, squeezing, heaviness, burning	Retrosternal, often with radiation to or isolated discomfort in neck, jaw, shoulders, or arms—frequently on left	Precipitated by exertion, exposure to cold, psychologic stress S_4 gallop or mitral regurgitation murmur during pain
Unstable angina	10–20 min	Similar to angina but often more severe	Similar to angina	Similar to angina, but occurs with low levels of exertion or even at rest
Acute myocardial infarction	Variable; often more than 30 min	Similar to angina but often more severe	Similar to angina	Unrelieved by nitroglycerin May be associated with evidence of heart failure or arrhythmia
Aortic stenosis	Recurrent episodes as described for angina	As described for angina	As described for angina	Late-peaking systolic murmur radiating to carotid arteries
Pericarditis	Hours to days; may be episodic	Sharp	Retrosternal or toward cardiac apex; may radiate to left shoulder	May be relieved by sitting up and leaning forward Pericardial friction rub
Aortic dissection	Abrupt onset of unrelenting pain	Tearing or ripping sensation; knifelike	Anterior chest, often radiating to back, between shoulder blades	Associated with hypertension and/or underlying connective tissue disorder, e.g., Marfan syndrome Murmur of aortic insufficiency, pericardial rub, pericardial tamponade, or loss of peripheral pulses
Pulmonary embolism	Abrupt onset; several minutes to a few hours	Pleuritic	Often lateral, on the side of the embolism	Dyspnea, tachypnea, tachycardia, and hypotension
Pulmonary hypertension	Variable	Pressure	Substernal	Dyspnea, signs of increased venous pressure including edema and jugular venous distention
Pneumonia or pleuritis	Variable	Pleuritic	Unilateral, often localized	Dyspnea, cough, fever, rales, occasional rub
Spontaneous pneumothorax	Sudden onset; several hours	Pleuritic	Lateral to side of pneumothorax	Dyspnea, decreased breath sounds on side of pneumothorax
Esophageal reflux	10–60 min	Burning	Substernal, epigastric	Worsened by postprandial recumbency Relieved by antacids
Esophageal spasm	2–30 min	Pressure, tightness, burning	Retrosternal	Can closely mimic angina
Peptic ulcer	Prolonged	Burning	Epigastric, substernal	Relieved with food or antacids
Gallbladder disease	Prolonged	Burning, pressure	Epigastric, right upper quadrant, substernal	May follow meal
Musculoskeletal disease	Variable	Aching	Variable	Aggravated by movement May be reproduced by localized pressure on examination
Herpes zoster	Variable	Sharp or burning	Dermatomal distribution	Vesicular rash in area of discomfort
Emotional and psychiatric conditions	Variable; may be fleeting	Variable	Variable; may be retrosternal	Situational factors may precipitate symptoms Anxiety or depression often detectable with careful history

The adjacent parietal pleura receives its sensory supply from several sources, so the pain of pericarditis can be experienced in areas ranging from the shoulder and neck to the abdomen and back. Most typically, the pain is retrosternal and is aggravated by coughing, deep breaths, or changes in position—all of which lead to movements of pleural surfaces. The pain is often worse in the supine position and relieved by sitting upright and leaning forward. Less common is a steady aching discomfort that mimics acute myocardial infarction.

Diseases of the Aorta (See also Chap. 242) *Aortic dissection* is a potentially catastrophic condition that is due to spread of a subintimal hematoma within the wall of the aorta. The hematoma may begin with a tear in the intima of the aorta or with rupture of the vasa vasorum within the aortic media. This syndrome can occur with trauma to the aorta, including motor vehicle accidents or medical procedures in which catheters or intraaortic balloon pumps damage the intima of the aorta. Nontraumatic aortic dissections are rare in the absence of hypertension and/or conditions associated with deterioration of the elastic or muscular components of the media within the aorta's wall. Cystic medial degeneration is a feature of several inherited connective tissue diseases, including Marfan and Ehlers-Danlos syndromes. About half of all aortic dissections in women under 40 years of age occur during pregnancy.

Almost all patients with acute dissections present with severe chest pain, although some patients with chronic dissections are identified without associated symptoms. Unlike the pain of ischemic heart disease, symptoms of aortic dissection tend to reach peak severity immediately, often causing the patient to collapse from its intensity. The classic teaching is that the adjectives used to describe the pain reflect the process occurring within the wall of the aorta—"ripping" and "tearing"—but more recent data suggest that the most common presenting complaint is sudden onset of severe, sharp pain. The location often correlates with the site and extent of the dissection. Thus, dissections that begin in the ascending aorta and extend to the descending aorta tend to cause pain in the front of the chest that extends into the back, between the shoulder blades.

Physical findings may also reflect extension of the aortic dissection that compromises flow into arteries branching off the aorta. Thus, loss of a pulse in one or both arms, cerebrovascular accident, or paraplegia can all be catastrophic consequences of aortic dissection. Hematomas that extend proximally and undermine the coronary arteries or aortic valve apparatus may lead to acute myocardial infarction or acute aortic insufficiency. Rupture of the hematoma into the pericardial space leads to pericardial tamponade.

Another abnormality of the aorta that can cause chest pain is a *thoracic aortic aneurysm*. Aortic aneurysms are frequently asymptomatic but can cause chest pain and other symptoms by compressing adjacent structures. This pain tends to be steady, deep, and sometimes severe.

Pulmonary Embolism (See also Chap. 256) Chest pain due to pulmonary embolism is believed to be due to distention of the pulmonary artery or infarction of a segment of the lung adjacent to the pleura. Massive pulmonary emboli may lead to substernal pain that is suggestive of acute myocardial infarction. More commonly, smaller emboli lead to focal pulmonary infarctions that cause pain that is lateral and pleuritic. Associated symptoms include dyspnea and, occasionally, hemoptysis. Tachycardia is usually present. Although not always present, certain characteristic ECG changes can support the diagnosis.

Pneumothorax (See also Chap. 257) Sudden onset of pleuritic chest pain and respiratory distress should lead to consideration of spontaneous pneumothorax, as well as pulmonary embolism. Such events may occur without a precipitating event in persons without lung disease, or as a consequence of underlying lung disorders.

Pneumonia or Pleuritis (See also Chaps. 251 and 257) Lung diseases that damage and cause inflammation of the pleura of the lung usually cause a sharp, knifelike pain that is aggravated by inspiration or coughing.

Gastrointestinal Conditions (See also Chap. 286) Esophageal pain from acid reflux from the stomach, spasm, obstruction, or injury can be difficult to discern from myocardial syndromes. Acid reflux typically causes a deep burning discomfort that may be exacerbated by alcohol, aspirin, or some foods; this discomfort is often relieved by antacid or other acid-reducing therapies. Acid reflux tends to be exacerbated by lying down and may be worse in early morning when the stomach is empty of food that might otherwise absorb gastric acid.

Esophageal spasm may occur in the presence or absence of acid reflux and leads to a squeezing pain indistinguishable from angina. Prompt relief of esophageal spasm is often provided by antianginal therapies such as sublingual nifedipine, further promoting confusion between these syndromes. Chest pain can also result from injury to the esophagus, such as a Mallory-Weiss tear caused by severe vomiting.

Chest pain can result from diseases of the gastrointestinal tract below the diaphragm, including *peptic ulcer disease, biliary disease*, and *pancreatitis*. These conditions usually cause abdominal pain as well as chest discomfort; symptoms are not likely to be associated with exertion. The pain of ulcer disease typically occurs 60 to 90 min after meals, when postprandial acid production is no longer neutralized by food in the stomach. Cholecystitis usually causes a pain that is described as aching, occurring an hour or more after meals.

Neuromusculoskeletal Conditions *Cervical disk disease* can cause chest pain by compression of nerve roots. Pain in a dermatomal distribution can also be caused by *intercostal muscle cramps* or by *herpes zoster*. Chest pain symptoms due to herpes zoster may occur before skin lesions are apparent.

Costochondral and *chondrosternal syndromes* are the most common causes of anterior chest musculoskeletal pain. Only occasionally are physical signs of costochondritis such as swelling, redness, and warmth (Tietze's syndrome) present. The pain of such syndromes is usually fleeting and sharp, but some patients experience a dull ache that lasts for hours. Direct pressure on the chondrosternal and costochondral junctions may reproduce the pain from these and other musculoskeletal syndromes. Arthritis of the shoulder and spine and bursitis may also cause chest pain. Some patients who have these conditions and myocardial ischemia blur and confuse symptoms of these syndromes.

Emotional and Psychiatric Conditions As many as 10% of patients who present to emergency departments with acute chest discomfort have panic disorder or other emotional conditions. The symptoms in these populations are highly variable, but frequently the discomfort is described as visceral tightness or aching that lasts more than 30 min. Some patients offer other atypical descriptions, such as pain that is fleeting, sharp, and/or localized to a small region. The ECG in patients with emotional conditions may be difficult to interpret if hyperventilation causes ST-T-wave abnormalities. A careful history may elicit clues of depression, prior panic attacks, somatization, agoraphobia, or other phobias.

APPROACH TO THE PATIENT: Chest Discomfort

The evaluation of the patient with chest discomfort must accommodate two goals—determining the diagnosis and assessing the safety of the immediate management plan. The latter issue is often dominant when the patient has acute chest discomfort, such as patients seen in the emergency department. In such settings, the clinician must focus first on identifying patients who require aggressive interventions to diagnose or manage potentially life-threatening conditions, including acute ischemic heart disease, acute aortic dissection, pulmonary embolism, and tension pneumothorax. If such conditions are unlikely, the clinician must address questions such as the safety of discharge to home, admission to a non-coronary care unit facility, or immediate exercise testing. Table 13-3 displays a sequence of questions that can be used in the evaluation of the patient with chest discomfort, with the diagnostic entities that are most important for consideration at each stage of the evaluation.

TABLE 13-3 CONSIDERATIONS IN THE ASSESSMENT OF THE PATIENT WITH CHEST DISCOMFORT

1. Could the chest discomfort be due to an acute, potentially life-threatening condition that warrants immediate hospitalization and aggressive evaluation?	
Acute ischemic heart disease	Pulmonary embolism
Aortic dissection	Spontaneous pneumothorax
2. If not, could the discomfort be due to a chronic condition likely to lead to serious complications?	
Stable angina	
Aortic stenosis	
Pulmonary hypertension	
3. If not, could the discomfort be due to an acute condition that warrants specific treatment?	
Pericarditis	
Pneumonia/pleuritis	
Herpes zoster	
4. If not, could the discomfort be due to another treatable chronic condition?	
Esophageal reflux	Cervical disk disease
Esophageal spasm	Arthritis of the shoulder or spine
Peptic ulcer disease	Costochondritis
Gallbladder disease	Other musculoskeletal disorders
Other gastrointestinal conditions	Anxiety state

ACUTE CHEST DISCOMFORT In patients with acute chest discomfort, the clinician must first assess the patient's respiratory and hemodynamic status. If either is compromised, initial management should focus on stabilizing the patient before the diagnostic evaluation is pursued. If, however, the patient does not require emergent interventions, then a focused history, physical examination, and laboratory evaluation should be performed to assess the patient's risk of life-threatening conditions.

Clinicians who are seeing patients in the office setting should not assume that they do not have acute ischemic heart disease, even if the prevalence may be lower. Malpractice litigation related to myocardial infarctions that were missed during office evaluations is becoming increasingly common, and ECGs were not performed in many such cases. The prevalence of high-risk patients seen in office settings may be increasing due to congestion in emergency departments.

In either setting, the *history* should include questions about the quality and location of the chest discomfort (Table 13-2). The patient should also be asked about the nature of onset of the pain and its duration. Myocardial ischemia is usually associated with a gradual intensification of symptoms over a period of minutes. Pain that is fleeting or that lasts hours without being associated with electrocardiographic changes is not likely to be ischemic in origin. Although the presence of risk factors for coronary artery disease may heighten concern for this diagnosis, the absence of such risk factors does not lower the risk for myocardial ischemia enough to be used to justify a decision to discharge a patient.

Wide radiation of chest pain increases probability that pain is due to myocardial infarction. Radiation of chest pain to the left arm is common with acute ischemic heart disease, but radiation to the right arm is also highly consistent with this diagnosis. Figure 13-1 shows estimates derived from several studies of the impact of various clinical features from the history on the probability that a patient has an acute myocardial infarction.

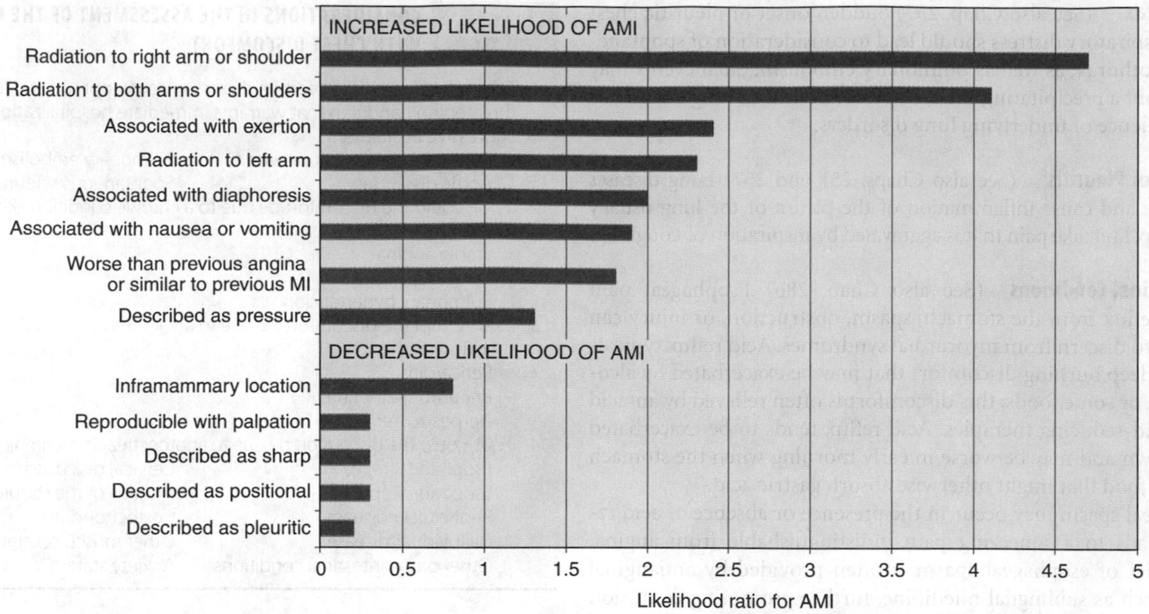

FIGURE 13-1 Impact of chest pain characteristics on odds of acute myocardial infarction (AMI). *(Figure prepared from data in Swap and Nagurney.)*

Right shoulder pain is also common with acute cholecystitis, but this syndrome is usually accompanied by pain that is located in the abdomen rather than chest. Chest pain that radiates between the scapulae raises the question of aortic dissection.

The *physical examination* should include evaluation of blood pressure in both arms and of pulses in both legs. Poor perfusion of a limb may be due to an aortic dissection that has compromised flow to an artery branching from the aorta. Chest auscultation may reveal diminished breath sounds; a pleural rub; or evidence of pneumothorax, pulmonary embolism, pneumonia, or pleurisy. Tension pneumothorax may lead to a shift in the trachea from the midline, away from the side of the pneumothorax. The cardiac examination should seek pericardial rubs, systolic and diastolic murmurs, and third or fourth heart sounds. Pressure on the chest wall may reproduce symptoms in patients with musculoskeletal causes of chest pain; it is important that the clinician ask the patient if the chest pain syndrome is being completely reproduced before drawing too much reassurance that more serious underlying conditions are not present.

An *ECG* is an essential test for adults with chest discomfort that is not due to an obvious traumatic cause. In such patients, the presence of electrocardiographic changes consistent with ischemia or infarction (Chap. 221) is associated with high risks of acute myocardial infarction or unstable angina (Table 13-4); such patients should be admitted to a unit with electrocardiographic monitoring and the capacity to respond to a cardiac arrest. The absence of such changes does not exclude acute ischemic heart disease, but the risk of life-threatening complications is low for patients with normal electrocardiograms or only nonspecific ST-T-wave changes. If these patients are not considered appropriate for immediate discharge, they are often candidates for early or immediate exercise testing.

Markers of myocardial injury are often obtained in the emergency department evaluation of acute chest discomfort. The most commonly used markers are creatine kinase (CK), CK-MB, and the cardiac troponins (I and T). Rapid bedside assays of the cardiac troponins have been developed and shown to be sufficiently accurate to predict prognosis and guide management. Some data support the use of other markers, such as serum myoglobin, C-reactive protein (CRP), placental growth factor, myeloperoxidase, and B-type natriuretic peptide (BNP); their roles are the subject of ongoing research. Single values of any of these markers do not have high sensitivity for acute myocardial infarction or for prediction of complications. Hence, decisions to discharge patients home should not be made on the basis of single negative values of these tests.

Provocative tests for coronary artery disease are not appropriate for patients with ongoing chest pain. In such patients, rest myocardial perfusion scans can be considered; a normal scan reduces the likelihood of coronary artery disease and can help avoid admission of low-risk patients to the hospital. Promising early results suggest that 64-slice CT and cardiac MRI may be of sufficient accuracy for diagnosis of coronary disease that these technologies may become widely used for patients with acute chest pain in whom the diagnosis is not clear.

Clinicians frequently employ therapeutic trials with sublingual nitroglycerin or antacids or, in the stable patient seen in the office setting, a proton pump inhibitor. A common error is to assume that a response to any of these interventions clarifies the diagnosis. While such information is often helpful, the patient's response may be due to the placebo effect. Hence, myocardial ischemia should never be considered excluded solely because of a response to antacid therapy. Similarly, failure of nitroglycerin to relieve pain does not exclude the diagnosis of coronary disease.

TABLE 13-4 PREVALENCE OF MYOCARDIAL INFARCTION AND UNSTABLE ANGINA AMONG SUBSETS OF PATIENTS WITH ACUTE CHEST DISCOMFORT IN THE EMERGENCY DEPARTMENT

	Prevalence	
Finding	**Myocardial Infarction, %**	**Unstable Angina, %**
ST elevation (≥1 mm) or Q waves on ECG not known to be old	79	12
Ischemia or strain on ECG not known to be old (ST depression ≥1 mm or ischemic T waves)	20	41
None of the preceding ECG changes but a prior history of angina or myocardial infarction (history of heart attack or nitroglycerin use)	4	51
None of the preceding ECG changes and no prior history of angina or myocardial infarction (history of heart attack or nitroglycerin use)	2	14

Note: ECG, electrocardiogram.
Unpublished data from Brigham and Women's Hospital Chest Pain Study, 1997–1999.

If the patient's history or examination is consistent with aortic dissection, imaging studies to evaluate the aorta must be pursued promptly because of the high risk of catastrophic complications with this condition. Appropriate tests include a chest CT scan with contrast, MRI, or transesophageal echocardiography.

Acute pulmonary embolism should be considered in patients with respiratory symptoms, pleuritic chest pain, hemoptysis, or a history of venous thromboembolism or coagulation abnormalities. Initial tests usually include CT angiography or a lung scan, which are sometimes combined with lower extremity venous ultrasound or D-dimer testing.

If patients with acute chest discomfort show no evidence of life-threatening conditions, the clinician should then focus on serious chronic conditions with the potential to cause major complications, the most common of which is stable angina. Early use of exercise electrocardiography, stress echocardiography, or stress perfusion imaging for such patients, whether in the office or the emergency department, is now an accepted management strategy for low-risk patients. Exercise testing is not appropriate, however, for patients who (1) report pain that is believed to be ischemic occurring at rest or (2) have electrocardiographic changes not known to be old that are consistent with ischemia.

Patients with sustained chest discomfort who do not have evidence for life-threatening conditions should be evaluated for evidence of conditions likely to benefit from acute treatment (Table 13-3). Pericarditis may be suggested by the history, physical examination, and ECG (Table 13-2). Clinicians should carefully assess blood pressure patterns and consider echocardiography in such patients to detect evidence of impending pericardial tamponade. Chest x-rays can be used to evaluate the possibility of pulmonary disease.

GUIDELINES AND CRITICAL PATHWAYS FOR ACUTE CHEST DISCOMFORT

Guidelines for the initial evaluation for patients with acute chest pain have been developed by the American College of Cardiology, American Heart Association, and other organizations. These guidelines recommend performance of an ECG for virtually all patients with chest pain who do not have an obvious noncardiac cause of their pain, and performance of a chest x-ray for patients with signs or symptoms consistent with congestive heart failure, valvular heart disease, pericardial disease, or aortic dissection or aneurysm.

The American College of Cardiology/American Heart Association guidelines on exercise testing support its use in low-risk patients presenting to the emergency department, as well as in selected intermediate-risk patients. However, these guidelines emphasize that exercise tests should be performed only after patients have been screened for high-risk features or other indicators for hospital admission.

Many medical centers have adopted critical pathways and other forms of guidelines to increase efficiency and to expedite the treatment of patients with high-risk acute ischemic heart disease syndromes. These guidelines emphasize the following strategies:

- Rapid identification and treatment of patients for whom emergent reperfusion therapy, either via percutaneous coronary interventions or thrombolytic agents, is likely to lead to improved outcomes.
- Triage to non-coronary care unit monitored facilities such as intermediate-care units or chest pain units of patients with a low risk for complications, such as patients without new ischemic changes on their ECGs and without ongoing chest pain. Such patients can usually be safely observed in non-coronary care unit settings, undergo early exercise testing, or be discharged home. Risk stratification can be assisted through use of prospectively validated multivariate algorithms that have been published for acute ischemic heart disease and its complications.
- Shortening lengths of stay in the coronary care unit and hospital. Recommendations regarding the minimum length of stay in a monitored bed for a patient who has no further symptoms have decreased in recent years to 12 h or less if exercise testing or other risk stratification technologies are available.

NONACUTE CHEST DISCOMFORT

The management of patients who do not require admission to the hospital or who no longer require inpatient observation should seek to identify the cause of the symptoms and the likelihood of major complications. Noninvasive tests for coronary disease serve both to diagnose this condition and to identify patients with high-risk forms of coronary disease who may benefit from revascularization. Gastrointestinal causes of chest pain can be evaluated via endoscopy or radiology studies, or with trials of medical therapy. Emotional and psychiatric conditions warrant appropriate evaluation and treatment; randomized trial data indicate that cognitive therapy and group interventions lead to decreases in symptoms for such patients.

FURTHER READINGS

BRENNAN M-L et al: Prognostic value of myeloperoxidase in patients with chest pain. N Engl J Med 349:1595, 2003

GIBBONS RJ et al: ACC/AHA 2002 guideline update for exercise testing. A report of the American College of Cardiology/American Heart Association Task Force on Practice Guidelines (Committee on Exercise Testing). Available at *www.acc.org/qualityandscience/clinical/guidelines/exercise/dirindex.htm*. Accessed on January 22, 2006

GIBSON PB et al: Low event rate for stress-only perfusion imaging in patients evaluated for chest pain. J Am Coll Cardiol 39:999, 2002

HEESCHEM C et al: Prognostic value of placental growth factor in patients with chest pain. JAMA 291:435, 2004

KWONG RY et al: Detecting acute coronary syndrome in the emergency department with cardiac magnetic resonance imaging. Circulation 197:531, 2003

LEBER AW et al: Quantification of obstructive and nonobstructive coronary lesions of 64-slice computed tomography. J Am Coll Cardiol 46:147, 2005

SWAP CJ, NAGURNEY JT: Value and limitations of chest pain history in the evaluation of patients with suspected acute coronary syndromes. JAMA 294:2623, 2005

TONG KL et al: Myocardial contrast echocardiography versus Thrombolysis in Myocardial Infarction score in patients presenting to the emergency department with chest pain and a nondiagnostic electrocardiogram. J Am Coll Cardiol 46:928, 2005

TSAI TT et al: Acute aortic syndromes. Circulation 205:3802, 2005

14 Abdominal Pain

William Silen

The correct interpretation of acute abdominal pain is challenging. Since proper therapy may require urgent action, the unhurried approach suitable for the study of other conditions is sometimes denied. Few other clinical situations demand greater judgment, because the most catastrophic of events may be forecast by the subtlest of symptoms and signs. A meticulously executed, detailed history and physical examination are of great importance. The etiologic classification in Table 14-1, although not complete, forms a useful basis for the evaluation of patients with abdominal pain.

The diagnosis of "acute or surgical abdomen" is not an acceptable one because of its often misleading and erroneous connotation. The most obvious of "acute abdomens" may not require operative intervention, and the mildest of abdominal pains may herald an urgently correctable lesion. Any patient with abdominal pain of recent onset requires early and thorough evaluation and accurate diagnosis.

Inflammation of the Parietal Peritoneum The pain of parietal peritoneal inflammation is steady and aching in character and is located directly over the inflamed area, its exact reference being possible because it is transmitted by somatic nerves supplying the parietal peritoneum. The intensity of the pain is dependent on the type and amount of material to which the peritoneal surfaces are exposed in a given time period. For example, the sudden release into the peritoneal cavity of a small quantity of *sterile* acid gastric juice causes much more pain than the same amount of grossly contaminated neutral feces. Enzymatically active pancreatic juice incites more pain and inflammation than does the same amount of sterile bile containing no potent enzymes. Blood and urine are often so bland as to go undetected if their contact with the peritoneum has not been sudden and massive. In the case of bacterial contamination, such as in pelvic inflammatory disease, the pain is frequently of low intensity early in the illness until bacterial multiplication has caused the elaboration of irritating substances.

The rate at which the irritating material is applied to the peritoneum is important. Perforated peptic ulcer may be associated with entirely different clinical pictures dependent only on the rapidity with which the gastric juice enters the peritoneal cavity.

The pain of peritoneal inflammation is invariably accentuated by pressure or changes in tension of the peritoneum, whether produced by palpation or by movement, as in coughing or sneezing. The patient with peritonitis lies quietly in bed, preferring to avoid motion, in contrast to the patient with colic, who may writhe incessantly.

Another characteristic feature of peritoneal irritation is tonic reflex spasm of the abdominal musculature, localized to the involved body segment. The intensity of the tonic muscle spasm accompanying peritoneal inflammation is dependent on the location of the inflammatory process, the rate at which it develops, and the integrity of the nervous system. Spasm over a perforated retrocecal appendix or perforated ulcer into the lesser peritoneal sac may be minimal or absent because of the protective effect of overlying viscera. A slowly developing process often greatly attenuates the degree of muscle spasm. Catastrophic abdominal emergencies such as a perforated ulcer may be associated with minimal or no detectable pain or muscle spasm in obtunded, seriously ill, debilitated elderly patients or in psychotic patients.

Obstruction of Hollow Viscera The pain of obstruction of hollow abdominal viscera is classically described as intermittent, or colicky. Yet the lack of a truly cramping character should not be misleading, because distention of a hollow viscus may produce steady pain with only very occasional exacerbations. It is not nearly as well localized as the pain of parietal peritoneal inflammation.

The colicky pain of obstruction of the small intestine is usually periumbilical or supraumbilical and is poorly localized. As the intestine becomes progressively dilated with loss of muscular tone, the colicky nature of the pain may diminish. With superimposed strangulating obstruction, pain may spread to the lower lumbar region if there is traction on the root of the mesentery. The colicky pain of colonic obstruction is of lesser intensity than that of the small intestine and is often located in the infraumbilical area. Lumbar radiation of pain is common in colonic obstruction.

Sudden distention of the biliary tree produces a steady rather than colicky type of pain; hence the term *biliary colic* is misleading. Acute distention of the gallbladder usually causes pain in the right upper quadrant with radiation to the right posterior region of the thorax or to the tip of the right scapula, and distention of the common bile duct is often associated with pain in the epigastrium radiating to the upper part of the lumbar region. Considerable variation is common, however, so that differentiation between these may be impossible. The typical subscapular pain or lumbar radiation is frequently absent. Gradual dilatation of the biliary tree, as in carcinoma of the head of the pancreas, may cause no pain or only a mild aching sensation in the epigastrium or right upper quadrant. The pain of distention of the pancreatic ducts is similar to that described for distention of the common bile duct but, in addition, is very frequently accentuated by recumbency and relieved by the upright position.

TABLE 14-1 SOME IMPORTANT CAUSES OF ABDOMINAL PAIN

Pain Originating in the Abdomen
Parietal peritoneal inflammation
Bacterial contamination
Perforated appendix or other perforated viscus
Pelvic inflammatory disease
Chemical irritation
Perforated ulcer
Pancreatitis
Mittelschmerz
Mechanical obstruction of hollow viscera
Obstruction of the small or large intestine
Obstruction of the biliary tree
Obstruction of the ureter
Vascular disturbances
Embolism or thrombosis
Vascular rupture
Pressure or torsional occlusion
Sickle cell anemia
Abdominal wall
Distortion or traction of mesentery
Trauma or infection of muscles
Distension of visceral surfaces, e.g. by hemorrhage
Hepatic or renal capsules
Inflammation of a viscus
Appendicitis
Typhoid fever
Typhlitis
Pain Referred from Extraabdominal Source
Cardiothoracic
Acute myocardial infarction
Myocarditis, endocarditis, pericarditis
Congestive heart failure
Pneumonia
Pulmonary embolus
Pleurodynia
Pneumothorax
Empyema
Esophageal disease, spasm, rupture, inflammation
Genitalia
Torsion of the testis
Metabolic Causes
Diabetes
Uremia
Hyperlipidemia
Hyperparathyroidism
Acute adrenal insufficiency
Familial Mediterranean fever
Porphyria
C'1 esterase inhibitor deficiency (angioneurotic edema)
Neurologic/Psychiatric Causes
Herpes zoster
Tabes dorsalis
Causalgia
Radiculitis from infection or arthritis
Spinal cord or nerve root compression
Functional disorders
Psychiatric disorders
Toxic Causes
Lead poisoning
Insect or animal envenomations
Black widow spiders
Snake bites
Uncertain Mechanisms
Narcotic withdrawal
Heat stroke

Obstruction of the urinary bladder results in dull suprapubic pain, usually low in intensity. Restlessness without specific complaint of pain may be the only sign of a distended bladder in an obtunded patient. In contrast, acute obstruction of the intravesicular portion of the ureter is characterized by severe suprapubic and flank pain that radiates to the penis, scrotum, or inner aspect of the upper thigh. Obstruction of the ureteropelvic junction is felt as pain in the costovertebral angle, whereas obstruction of the remainder of the ureter is associated with flank pain that often extends into the same side of the abdomen.

Vascular Disturbances A frequent misconception, despite abundant experience to the contrary, is that pain associated with intraabdominal vascular disturbances is sudden and catastrophic in nature. The pain of embolism or thrombosis of the superior mesenteric artery or that of impending rupture of an abdominal aortic aneurysm certainly may be severe and diffuse. Yet, just as frequently, the patient with occlusion of the superior mesenteric artery has only mild continuous diffuse pain for 2 or 3 days before vascular collapse or findings of peritoneal inflammation appear. The early, seemingly insignificant discomfort is caused by hyperperistalsis rather than peritoneal inflammation. Indeed, absence of tenderness and rigidity in the presence of continuous, diffuse pain in a patient likely to have vascular disease is quite characteristic of occlusion of the superior mesenteric artery. Abdominal pain with radiation to the sacral region, flank, or genitalia should always signal the possible presence of a rupturing abdominal aortic aneurysm. This pain may persist over a period of several days before rupture and collapse occur.

Abdominal Wall Pain arising from the abdominal wall is usually constant and aching. Movement, prolonged standing, and pressure accentuate the discomfort and muscle spasm. In the case of hematoma of the rectus sheath, now most frequently encountered in association with anticoagulant therapy, a mass may be present in the lower quadrants of the abdomen. Simultaneous involvement of muscles in other parts of the body usually serves to differentiate myositis of the abdominal wall from an intraabdominal process that might cause pain in the same region.

REFERRED PAIN IN ABDOMINAL DISEASES

Pain referred to the abdomen from the thorax, spine, or genitalia may prove a vexing diagnostic problem, because diseases of the upper part of the abdominal cavity such as acute cholecystitis or perforated ulcer are frequently associated with intrathoracic complications. A most important, yet often forgotten, dictum is that the possibility of intrathoracic disease must be considered in every patient with abdominal pain, especially if the pain is in the upper part of the abdomen. Systematic questioning and examination directed toward detecting myocardial or pulmonary infarction, pneumonia, pericarditis, or esophageal disease (the intrathoracic diseases that most often masquerade as abdominal emergencies) will often provide sufficient clues to establish the proper diagnosis. Diaphragmatic pleuritis resulting from pneumonia or pulmonary infarction may cause pain in the right upper quadrant and pain in the supraclavicular area, the latter radiation to be distinguished from the referred subscapular pain caused by acute distention of the extrahepatic biliary tree. The ultimate decision as to the origin of abdominal pain may require deliberate and planned observation over a period of several hours, during which repeated questioning and examination will provide the diagnosis or suggest the appropriate studies.

Referred pain of thoracic origin is often accompanied by splinting of the involved hemithorax with respiratory lag and decrease in excursion more marked than that seen in the presence of intraabdominal disease. In addition, apparent abdominal muscle spasm caused by referred pain will diminish during the inspiratory phase of respiration, whereas it is persistent throughout both respiratory phases if it is of abdominal origin. Palpation over the area of referred pain in the abdomen also does not usually accentuate the pain and in many instances actually seems to relieve it. Thoracic disease and abdominal disease frequently coexist and may be difficult or impossible to differentiate. For example, the patient with known biliary tract disease often has epigastric pain during myocardial infarction, or biliary colic may be referred to the precordium or left shoulder in a patient who has suffered previously from angina pectoris. For an explanation of the radiation of pain to a previously diseased area, see Chap. 12.

Referred pain from the spine, which usually involves compression or irritation of nerve roots, is characteristically intensified by certain motions such as cough, sneeze, or strain and is associated with hyperesthesia over the involved dermatomes. Pain referred to the abdomen from the testes or seminal vesicles is generally accentuated by the slightest pressure on either of these organs. The abdominal discomfort is of dull aching character and is poorly localized.

METABOLIC ABDOMINAL CRISES

Pain of metabolic origin may simulate almost any other type of intraabdominal disease. Several mechanisms may be at work. In certain instances, such as hyperlipidemia, the metabolic disease itself may be accompanied by an intraabdominal process such as pancreatitis, which can lead to unnecessary laparotomy unless recognized. C1 esterase deficiency associated with angioneurotic edema is often associated with episodes of severe abdominal pain. Whenever the cause of abdominal pain is obscure, a metabolic origin always must be considered. Abdominal pain is also the hallmark of familial Mediterranean fever (Chap. 323).

The problem of differential diagnosis is often not readily resolved. The pain of porphyria and of lead colic is usually difficult to distinguish from that of intestinal obstruction, because severe hyperperistalsis is a prominent feature of both. The pain of uremia or diabetes is nonspecific, and the pain and tenderness frequently shift in location and intensity. Diabetic acidosis may be precipitated by acute appendicitis or intestinal obstruction, so if prompt resolution of the abdominal pain does not result from correction of the metabolic abnormalities, an underlying organic problem should be suspected. Black widow spider bites produce intense pain and rigidity of the abdominal muscles and back, an area infrequently involved in intraabdominal disease.

NEUROGENIC CAUSES

Causalgic pain may occur in diseases that injure sensory nerves. It has a burning character and is usually limited to the distribution of a given peripheral nerve. Normal stimuli such as touch or change in temperature may be transformed into this type of pain, which is frequently present in a patient at rest. The demonstration of irregularly spaced cutaneous pain spots may be the only indication of an old nerve lesion underlying causalgic pain. Even though the pain may be precipitated by gentle palpation, rigidity of the abdominal muscles is absent, and the respirations are not disturbed. Distention of the abdomen is uncommon, and the pain has no relationship to the intake of food.

Pain arising from spinal nerves or roots comes and goes suddenly and is of a lancinating type (Chap. 16). It may be caused by herpes zoster, impingement by arthritis, tumors, herniated nucleus pulposus, diabetes, or syphilis. It is not associated with food intake, abdominal distention, or changes in respiration. Severe muscle spasm, as in the gastric crises of tabes dorsalis, is common but is either relieved or is not accentuated by abdominal palpation. The pain is made worse by movement of the spine and is usually confined to a few dermatomes. Hyperesthesia is very common.

Pain due to functional causes conforms to none of the aforementioned patterns. Mechanism is hard to define. Irritable bowel syndrome (IBS) is a functional gastrointestinal disorder characterized by abdominal pain and altered bowel habits. The diagnosis is made on the basis of clinical criteria (Chap. 290) and after exclusion of demonstrable structural abnormalities. The episodes of abdominal pain are often brought on by stress, and the pain varies considerably in type and location. Nausea and vomiting are rare. Localized tenderness and muscle spasm are inconsistent or absent. The causes of IBS or related functional disorders are not known.

APPROACH TO THE PATIENT: Abdominal Pain

Few abdominal conditions require such urgent operative intervention that an orderly approach need be abandoned, no matter how ill the patient. Only those patients with exsanguinating intraabdominal hemorrhage (e.g., ruptured aneurysm) must be rushed to the operating room immediately, but in such instances only a few minutes are required to assess the critical nature of the problem. Under these circumstances, all obstacles must be swept aside, adequate venous access for fluid replacement obtained, and the operation begun. Many patients of this type have died in the radiology department or the emergency room while awaiting such unnecessary examinations as electrocardiograms or abdominal films. *There are no contraindications to operation when massive intraabdominal hemorrhage is present.* Fortunately, this situation is relatively rare. These comments do not pertain to gastrointestinal hemorrhage, which can often be managed by other means (Chap. 42).

Nothing will supplant an orderly, painstakingly *detailed history*, which is far more valuable than any laboratory or radiographic examination. This kind of history is laborious and time-consuming, making it not especially popular, even though a reasonably accurate diagnosis can be made on the basis of the history alone in the majority of cases. Computer-aided diagnosis of abdominal pain provides no advantage over clinical assessment alone. In cases of *acute* abdominal pain, a diagnosis is readily established in most instances, whereas success is not so frequent in patients with *chronic* pain. IBS is one of the most common causes of abdominal pain and must always be kept in mind (Chap. 290). The location of the pain can assist in narrowing the differential diagnosis (see Table 14-2); however, the *chronological sequence of events* in the patient's history is often more important than emphasis on the location of pain. If the examiner is sufficiently open-minded and unhurried, asks the proper questions, and listens, the patient will usually provide the diagnosis. Careful attention should be paid to the extraabdominal regions that may be responsible for abdominal pain. An accurate menstrual history in a female patient is essential. Narcotics or analgesics should *not* be withheld until a definitive diagnosis or a definitive plan has been formulated; obfuscation of the diagnosis by adequate analgesia is unlikely.

In the examination, simple critical inspection of the patient, e.g., of facies, position in bed, and respiratory activity, may provide valuable clues. The amount of information to be gleaned is directly proportional to the *gentleness* and thoroughness of the examiner. Once a patient with peritoneal inflammation has been examined brusquely, accurate assessment by the next examiner becomes almost impossible. Eliciting rebound tenderness by sudden release of a deeply palpating hand in a patient with suspected peritonitis is cruel and unnecessary. The same information can be obtained by gentle percussion of the abdomen (rebound tenderness on a miniature scale), a maneuver that can be far more precise and localizing. Asking the patient to cough will elicit true rebound tenderness without the need for placing a hand on the abdomen. Furthermore, the forceful demonstration of rebound tenderness will startle and induce protective spasm in a nervous or worried patient in whom true rebound tenderness is not present. A palpable gallbladder will be missed if palpation is so brusque that voluntary muscle spasm becomes superimposed on involuntary muscular rigidity.

As in history taking, sufficient time should be spent in the examination. Abdominal signs may be minimal but nevertheless, if accompanied by consistent symptoms, may be exceptionally meaningful. Abdominal signs may be virtually or totally absent in cases of pelvic peritonitis, so careful *pelvic and rectal examinations are mandatory in every patient with abdominal pain.* Tenderness on pelvic or rectal examination in the absence of other abdominal signs can be caused by operative indications such as perforated appendicitis, diverticulitis, twisted ovarian cyst, and many others.

Much attention has been paid to the presence or absence of peristaltic sounds, their quality, and their frequency. Auscultation of the abdomen is one of the least revealing aspects of the physical examination of a patient with abdominal pain. Catastrophes such as strangulating small intestinal obstruction or perforated appendicitis may occur in the presence of normal peristaltic sounds. Conversely, when the proximal part of the intestine above an obstruction becomes markedly distended and edematous, peristaltic sounds may lose the characteristics of borborygmi and become weak or absent, even when peritonitis is not present. It is usually the severe chemical peritonitis of sudden onset that is associated with the truly silent abdomen. Assessment of the patient's state of hydration is important.

Laboratory examinations may be of great value in assessment of the patient with abdominal pain, yet with few exceptions they rarely establish a diagnosis. Leukocytosis should never be the single deciding factor as to whether or not operation is indicated. A white blood cell count >20,000/μL may be observed with perforation of a viscus, but pancreatitis, acute cholecystitis, pelvic inflammatory disease, and intestinal infarction may be associated with marked leukocytosis. A normal white blood cell count is not rare in cases of perforation of abdominal viscera. The diagnosis of anemia may be more helpful than the white blood cell count, especially when combined with the history.

The urinalysis may reveal the state of hydration or rule out severe renal disease, diabetes, or urinary infection. Blood urea nitrogen, glucose, and serum bilirubin levels may be helpful. Serum amylase levels may be increased by many diseases other than pancreatitis, e.g., perforated ulcer, strangulating intestinal obstruction, and acute cholecystitis; thus, elevations of serum amylase do not rule out the need for an operation. The determination of the serum lipase may have greater accuracy than that of the serum amylase.

Plain and upright or lateral decubitus radiographs of the abdomen may be of value in cases of intestinal obstruction, perforated ulcer, and a variety of other conditions. They are usually unnecessary in patients with acute appendicitis or strangulated external hernias. In rare instances, barium or water-soluble contrast study of the upper part of the gastrointestinal tract may demonstrate partial intestinal obstruction that may elude diagnosis by other means. If there is any question of obstruction of the colon, oral administration of barium sulfate should be avoided. On the other hand, in cases of suspected colonic obstruction (without perforation), contrast enema may be diagnostic.

In the absence of trauma, peritoneal lavage has been replaced as a diagnostic tool by ultrasound, CT, and laparoscopy. Ultrasonog-

TABLE 14-2 DIFFERENTIAL DIAGNOSES OF ABDOMINAL PAIN BY LOCATION

Right Upper Quadrant	Epigastric	Left Upper Quadrant
Cholecystitis	Peptic ulcer disease	Splenic infarct
Cholangitis	Gastritis	Splenic rupture
Pancreatitis	GERD	Splenic abscess
Pneumonia/empyema	Pancreatitis	Gastritis
Pleurisy/pleurodynia	Myocardial infarction	Gastric ulcer
Subdiaphragmatic abscess	Pericarditis	Pancreatitis
Hepatitis	Ruptured aortic aneurysm	Subdiaphragmatic abscess
Budd-Chiari syndrome	Esophagitis	
Right Lower Quadrant	**Periumbilical**	**Left Lower Quadrant**
Appendicitis	Early appendicitis	Diverticulitis
Salpingitis	Gastroenteritis	Salpingitis
Inguinal hernia	Bowel obstruction	Inguinal hernia
Ectopic pregnancy	Ruptured aortic aneurysm	Ectopic pregnancy
Nephrolithiasis		Nephrolithiasis
Inflammatory bowel disease		Irritable bowel syndrome
Mesenteric lymphadenitis		Inflammatory bowel disease
Typhlitis		
Diffuse Nonlocalized Pain		
Gastroenteritis	Diabetes	
Mesenteric ischemia	Malaria	
Bowel obstruction	Familial Mediterranean fever	
Irritable bowel syndrome	Metabolic diseases	
Peritonitis	Psychiatric disease	

raphy has proved to be useful in detecting an enlarged gallbladder or pancreas, the presence of gallstones, an enlarged ovary, or a tubal pregnancy. Laparoscopy is especially helpful in diagnosing pelvic conditions, such as ovarian cysts, tubal pregnancies, salpingitis, and acute appendicitis. Radioisotopic scans (HIDA) may help differentiate acute cholecystitis from acute pancreatitis. A CT scan may demonstrate an enlarged pancreas, ruptured spleen, or thickened colonic or appendiceal wall and streaking of the mesocolon or mesoappendix characteristic of diverticulitis or appendicitis.

Sometimes, even under the best circumstances with all available aids and with the greatest of clinical skill, a definitive diagnosis cannot be established at the time of the initial examination. Nevertheless, despite lack of a clear anatomic diagnosis, it may be abundantly clear to an experienced and thoughtful physician and surgeon that on clinical grounds alone operation is indicated. Should that decision be questionable, watchful waiting with repeated questioning and examination will often elucidate the true nature of the illness and indicate the proper course of action.

FURTHER READINGS

CERVERO F, LAIRD JM: Visceral pain. Lancet 353:2145, 1999

JONES PF: Suspected acute appendicitis: Trends in management over 30 years. Br J Surg 88:1570, 2001

LYON C, CLARK DC: Diagnosis of acute abdominal pain in older patients. Am Fam Physician 74:1537, 2006

SILEN W: Cope's Early Diagnosis of the Acute Abdomen, 21st ed, New York and Oxford: Oxford University Press, 2005

TAIT IS et al: Do patients with abdominal pain wait unduly long for analgesia? J R Coll Surg Edinb 44:181, 1999

15 Headache

Peter J. Goadsby, Neil H. Raskin

Headache is among the most common reasons that patients seek medical attention. Diagnosis and management is based on a careful clinical approach that is augmented by an understanding of the anatomy, physiology, and pharmacology of the nervous system pathways that mediate the various headache syndromes.

GENERAL PRINCIPLES

A classification system developed by the International Headache Society characterizes headache as primary or secondary (Table 15-1). *Primary headaches* are those in which headache and its associated features are the disorder in itself, whereas *secondary headaches* are those caused by exogenous disorders. Primary headache often results in considerable disability and a decrease in the patient's quality of life. Mild secondary headache, such as that seen in association with upper respiratory tract infections, is common but rarely worrisome. Life-threatening headache is relatively uncommon, but vigilance is required in order to recognize and appropriately treat patients with this category of head pain.

ANATOMY AND PHYSIOLOGY OF HEADACHE

Pain usually occurs when peripheral nociceptors are stimulated in response to tissue injury, visceral distension, or other factors (Chap. 12). In such situations, pain perception is a normal physiologic response mediated by a healthy nervous system. Pain can also result when pain-producing pathways of the peripheral or central nervous system (CNS) are damaged or activated inappropriately. Headache may originate from either or both mechanisms. Relatively few cranial structures are pain-producing; these include the scalp, middle meningeal artery, dural sinuses, falx cerebri, and proximal segments of the large pial arteries. The ventricular ependyma, choroid plexus, pial veins, and much of the brain parenchyma are not pain-producing.

TABLE 15-1 COMMON CAUSES OF HEADACHE

Primary Headache		Secondary Headache	
Type	**%**	**Type**	**%**
Migraine	16	Systemic infection	63
Tension-type	69	Head injury	4
Cluster	0.1	Vascular disorders	1
Idiopathic stabbing	2	Subarachnoid hemorrhage	<1
Exertional	1	Brain tumor	0.1

Source: After J Olesen et al: *The Headaches*. Philadelphia, Lippincott, Williams & Wilkins, 2005.

The key structures involved in primary headache appear to be

- the large intracranial vessels and dura mater
- the peripheral terminals of the trigeminal nerve that innervate these structures
- the caudal portion of the trigeminal nucleus, which extends into the dorsal horns of the upper cervical spinal cord and receives input from the first and second cervical nerve roots (the trigeminocervical complex)
- the pain modulatory systems in the brain that receive input from trigeminal nociceptors

The innervation of the large intracranial vessels and dura mater by the trigeminal nerve is known as the *trigeminovascular system*. Autonomic symptoms, such as *lacrimation* and *nasal congestion*, are prominent in the trigeminal autonomic cephalalgias, including cluster headache and paroxysmal hemicrania, and may also be seen in migraine. These autonomic symptoms reflect activation of cranial parasympathetic pathways, and functional imaging studies indicate that vascular changes in migraine and cluster headache, when present, are similarly driven by these cranial autonomic systems. Migraine and other primary headache types are not "vascular headaches"; these disorders do not reliably manifest vascular changes, and treatment outcomes cannot be predicted by vascular effects.

CLINICAL EVALUATION OF ACUTE, NEW-ONSET HEADACHE

The patient who presents with a new, severe headache has a differential diagnosis that is quite different from the patient with recurrent headaches over many years. In new-onset and severe headache, the probability of finding a potentially serious cause is considerably greater than in recurrent headache. Patients with recent onset of pain require prompt evaluation and often treatment. Serious causes to be considered include meningitis, subarachnoid hemorrhage, epidural or subdural hematoma, glaucoma, and purulent sinusitis. When worrisome symptoms and signs are present (Table 15-2), rapid diagnosis and management is critical.

TABLE 15-2 HEADACHE SYMPTOMS THAT SUGGEST A SERIOUS UNDERLYING DISORDER

"Worst" headache ever
First severe headache
Subacute worsening over days or weeks
Abnormal neurologic examination
Fever or unexplained systemic signs
Vomiting that precedes headache
Pain induced by bending, lifting, cough
Pain that disturbs sleep or presents immediately upon awakening
Known systemic illness
Onset after age 55
Pain associated with local tenderness, e.g., region of temporal artery

A complete neurologic examination is an essential first step in the evaluation. In most cases, patients with an abnormal examination or a history of recent-onset headache should be evaluated by a CT or MRI study. As an initial screening procedure for intracranial pathology in this setting, CT and MRI methods appear to be equally sensitive. In some circumstances a lumbar puncture (LP) is also required, unless a benign etiology can be otherwise established. A general evaluation of acute headache might include the investigation of cardiovascular and renal status by blood pressure monitoring and urine examination; eyes by fundoscopy, intraocular pressure measurement, and refraction; cranial arteries by palpation; and cervical spine by the effect of passive movement of the head and by imaging.

The psychological state of the patient should also be evaluated since a relationship exists between head pain and depression. Many patients in chronic daily pain cycles become depressed, although depression itself is rarely a cause of headache. Drugs with antidepressant actions are also effective in the prophylactic treatment of both tension-type headache and migraine.

Underlying recurrent headache disorders may be activated by pain that follows otologic or endodontic surgical procedures. Thus, pain about the head as the result of diseased tissue or trauma may reawaken an otherwise quiescent migrainous syndrome. Treatment of the headache is largely ineffective until the cause of the primary problem is addressed.

Serious underlying conditions that are associated with headache are described below. Brain tumor is a rare cause of headache and even less commonly a cause of severe pain. The vast majority of patients presenting with severe headache have a benign cause.

SECONDARY HEADACHE

The management of secondary headache focuses on diagnosis and treatment of the underlying condition.

MENINGITIS

Acute, severe headache with stiff neck and fever suggests meningitis. LP is mandatory. Often there is striking accentuation of pain with eye movement. Meningitis can be easily mistaken for migraine in that the cardinal symptoms of pounding headache, photophobia, nausea, and vomiting are present. **Meningitis is discussed in Chaps. 376 and 377.**

INTRACRANIAL HEMORRHAGE

Acute, severe headache with stiff neck but without fever suggests subarachnoid hemorrhage. A ruptured aneurysm, arteriovenous malformation, or intraparenchymal hemorrhage may also present with headache alone. Rarely, if the hemorrhage is small or below the foramen magnum, the head CT scan can be normal. Therefore, LP may be required to definitively diagnose subarachnoid hemorrhage. **Intracranial hemorrhage is discussed in Chap. 269.**

BRAIN TUMOR

Approximately 30% of patients with brain tumors consider headache to be their chief complaint. The head pain is usually nondescript—an intermittent deep, dull aching of moderate intensity, which may worsen with exertion or change in position and may be associated with nausea and vomiting. This pattern of symptoms results from migraine far more often than from brain tumor. The headache of brain tumor disturbs sleep in about 10% of patients. Vomiting that precedes the appearance of headache by weeks is highly characteristic of posterior fossa brain tumors. A history of amenorrhea or galactorrhea should lead one to question whether a prolactin-secreting pituitary adenoma (or the polycystic ovary syndrome) is the source of headache. Headache arising de novo in a patient with known malignancy suggests either cerebral metastases or carcinomatous meningitis, or both. Head pain appearing abruptly after bending, lifting, or coughing can be due to a posterior fossa mass (or a Chiari malformation). **Brain tumors are discussed in Chap. 374.**

TEMPORAL ARTERITIS

(See also Chaps. 29 and 319) Temporal (giant cell) arteritis is an inflammatory disorder of arteries that frequently involves the extracranial carotid circulation. It is a common disorder of the elderly; its annual incidence is 77 per 100,000 individuals ages 50 and older. The average age of onset is 70 years, and women account for 65% of cases. About half of patients with untreated temporal arteritis develop blindness due to involvement of the ophthalmic artery and its branches; indeed, the ischemic optic neuropathy induced by giant cell arteritis is the major cause of rapidly developing bilateral blindness in patients >60 years. Because treatment with glucocorticoids is effective in preventing this complication, prompt recognition of the disorder is important.

Typical presenting symptoms include headache, polymyalgia rheumatica (Chap. 319), jaw claudication, fever, and weight loss. Headache is the dominant symptom and often appears in association with malaise and muscle aches. Head pain may be unilateral or bilateral and is located temporally in 50% of patients but may involve any and all aspects of the cranium. Pain usually appears gradually over a few hours before peak intensity is reached; occasionally, it is explosive in onset. The quality of pain is only seldom throbbing; it is almost invariably described as dull and boring, with superimposed episodic stabbing pains similar to the sharp pains that appear in migraine. Most patients can recognize that the origin of their head pain is superficial, external to the skull, rather than originating deep within the cranium (the pain site for migraineurs). Scalp tenderness is present, often to a marked degree; brushing the hair or resting the head on a pillow may be impossible because of pain. Headache is usually worse at night and often aggravated by exposure to cold. Additional findings may include reddened, tender nodules or red streaking of the skin overlying the temporal arteries, and tenderness of the temporal or, less commonly, the occipital arteries.

The erythrocyte sedimentation rate (ESR) is often, though not always, elevated; a normal ESR does not exclude giant cell arteritis. A temporal artery biopsy followed by treatment with prednisone 80 mg daily for the first 4–6 weeks should be initiated when clinical suspicion is high. The prevalence of migraine among the elderly is substantial, considerably higher than that of giant cell arteritis. Migraineurs often report amelioration of their headaches with prednisone; thus, caution must be used when interpreting the therapeutic response.

GLAUCOMA

Glaucoma may present with a prostrating headache associated with nausea and vomiting. The headache often starts with severe eye pain. On physical examination, the eye is often red with a fixed, moderately dilated pupil. **Glaucoma is discussed in Chap. 29.**

PRIMARY HEADACHE SYNDROMES

Primary headaches are disorders in which headache and associated features occur in the absence of any exogenous cause (Table 15-1). The most common are migraine, tension-type headache, and cluster headache.

MIGRAINE HEADACHE

Migraine, the second most common cause of headache, afflicts approximately 15% of women and 6% of men. It is usually an episodic headache that is associated with certain features such as sensitivity to light, sound, or movement; nausea and vomiting often accompany the headache. A useful description of migraine is a benign and recurring syndrome of headache associated with other symptoms of neurologic dysfunction in varying admixtures (Table 15-3). Migraine can often be recognized by its activators, referred to as *triggers*.

The brain of the migraineur is particularly sensitive to environmental and sensory stimuli; migraine-prone patients do not habituate easily to sensory stimuli. This sensitivity is amplified in females during the menstrual cycle. Headache can be initiated or amplified by various triggers, including glare, bright lights, sounds, or other afferent stimulation; hunger; excess stress; physical exertion; stormy weather or barometric pressure changes; hormonal fluctuations during menses; lack of or excess sleep; and alcohol or other chemical stimulation. Knowledge of a patient's susceptibility to specific triggers can be useful in management strategies involving lifestyle adjustments.

TABLE 15-3 SYMPTOMS ACCOMPANYING SEVERE MIGRAINE ATTACKS IN 500 PATIENTS

Symptom	Patients Affected, %
Nausea	87
Photophobia	82
Lightheadedness	72
Scalp tenderness	65
Vomiting	56
Visual disturbances	36
Photopsia	26
Fortification spectra	10
Paresthesias	33
Vertigo	33
Alteration of consciousness	18
Syncope	10
Seizure	4
Confusional state	4
Diarrhea	16

Source: From NH Raskin, *Headache*, 2d ed. New York, Churchill Livingston, 1988; with permission.

Pathogenesis The sensory sensitivity that is characteristic of migraine is probably due to dysfunction of monoaminergic sensory control systems located in the brainstem and thalamus (Fig. 15-1).

Activation of cells in the trigeminal nucleus results in the release of vasoactive neuropeptides, particularly calcitonin gene-related peptide (CGRP), at vascular terminations of the trigeminal nerve. Recently, antagonists of CGRP have shown some early promise in the therapy of migraine. Centrally, the second-order trigeminal neurons cross the midline and project to ventrobasal and posterior nuclei of the thalamus for further processing. Additionally, there are projections to the periaqueductal gray and hypothalamus, from which reciprocal descending systems have established anti-nociceptive effects. Other brainstem regions likely to be involved in descending modulation of trigeminal pain include the nucleus locus coeruleus in the pons and the rostroventromedial medulla.

Pharmacologic and other data point to the involvement of the neurotransmitter 5-hydroxytryptamine (5-HT; also known as serotonin) in migraine. Approximately 50 years ago, methysergide was found to antagonize certain peripheral actions of 5-HT and was introduced as the first drug capable of preventing migraine attacks. The triptans are designed to selectively stimulate subpopulations of 5-HT receptors; at least 14 different 5-HT receptors exist in humans. The triptans are potent agonists of 5-HT_{1B}, 5-HT_{1D}, and 5-HT_{1F} receptors and are less potent at the 5-HT_{1A} receptor. A growing body of data indicates that the antimigraine efficacy of the triptans relates to their ability to stimulate $5\text{-HT}_{1B/1D}$ receptors, which are located on both blood vessels and nerve terminals.

Data also support a role for dopamine in the pathophysiology of certain subtypes of migraine. Most migraine symptoms can be induced by dopaminergic stimulation. Moreover, there is dopamine receptor hypersensitivity in migraineurs, as demonstrated by the induction of yawning, nausea, vomiting, hypotension, and other symptoms of a migraine attack by dopaminergic agonists at doses that do not affect nonmigraineurs. Dopamine receptor antagonists are effective therapeutic agents in migraine, especially when given parenterally or concurrently with other antimigraine agents.

Migraine genes identified by studying families with familial hemiplegic migraine (FHM) reveal involvement of ion channels, suggesting that alterations in membrane excitability can predispose to migraine. Mutations involving the $Ca_v2.1$ (P/Q) type voltage-gated calcium channel *CACNA1A* gene are now known to cause FHM 1; this mutation is responsible for about 50% of FHM. Mutations in the Na^+-K^+ATPase *ATP1A2* gene, designated FHM 2, are responsible for about 20% of FHM. Mutations in the neuronal voltage-gated sodium channel *SCN1A* cause FHM 3. Functional neuroimaging has suggested that brainstem regions in migraine (Fig. 15-2) and the posterior hypothalamic gray matter region close to the human circadian pacemaker cells of the suprachiasmatic nucleus in cluster headache (Fig. 15-3) are good candidates for specific involvement in primary headache.

Diagnosis and Clinical Features Diagnostic criteria for migraine headache are listed in Table 15-4. A high index of suspicion is required to diagnose migraine: the migraine aura, consisting of visual disturbances with flashing lights or zigzag lines moving across the visual field or of other neurologic symptoms, is reported in only 20–25% of patients. A headache diary can often be helpful in making the diagnosis; this is also helpful in assessing disability and the frequency of treatment for acute attacks. Patients with episodes of migraine that occur daily or near-daily are considered to have chronic migraine (see "Chronic Daily Headache," below). Migraine must be differentiated from tension-type headache (discussed below), the most common primary headache syndrome seen in clinical practice. *Migraine at its most basic level is headache with associated features, and tension-type headache is headache that is featureless. Most patients with disabling headache probably have migraine.*

Patients with acephalgic migraine experience recurrent neurologic symptoms, often with nausea or vomiting, but with little or no headache. Vertigo can be prominent; it has been estimated that one-third of patients referred for vertigo or dizziness have a primary diagnosis of migraine.

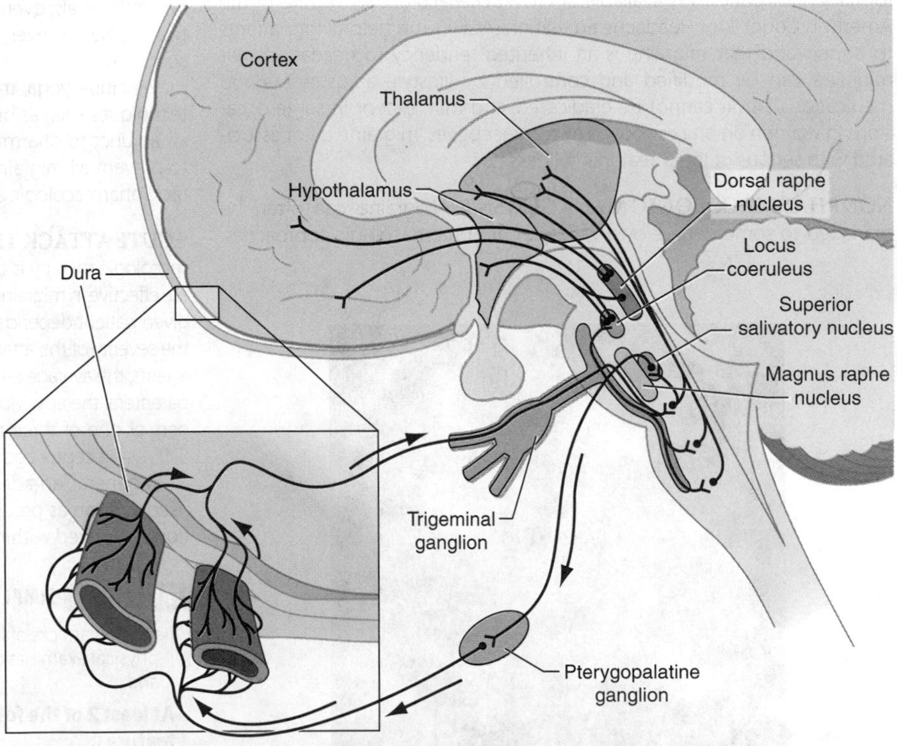

FIGURE 15-1 Brainstem pathways that modulate sensory input. The key pathway for pain in migraine is the trigeminovascular input from the meningeal vessels, which passes through the trigeminal ganglion and synapses on second-order neurons in the trigeminocervical complex. These neurons in turn project in the quintothalamic tract and, after decussating in the brainstem, synapse on neurons in the thalamus. Important modulation of the trigeminovascular nociceptive input comes from the dorsal raphe nucleus, locus coeruleus, and nucleus raphe magnus.

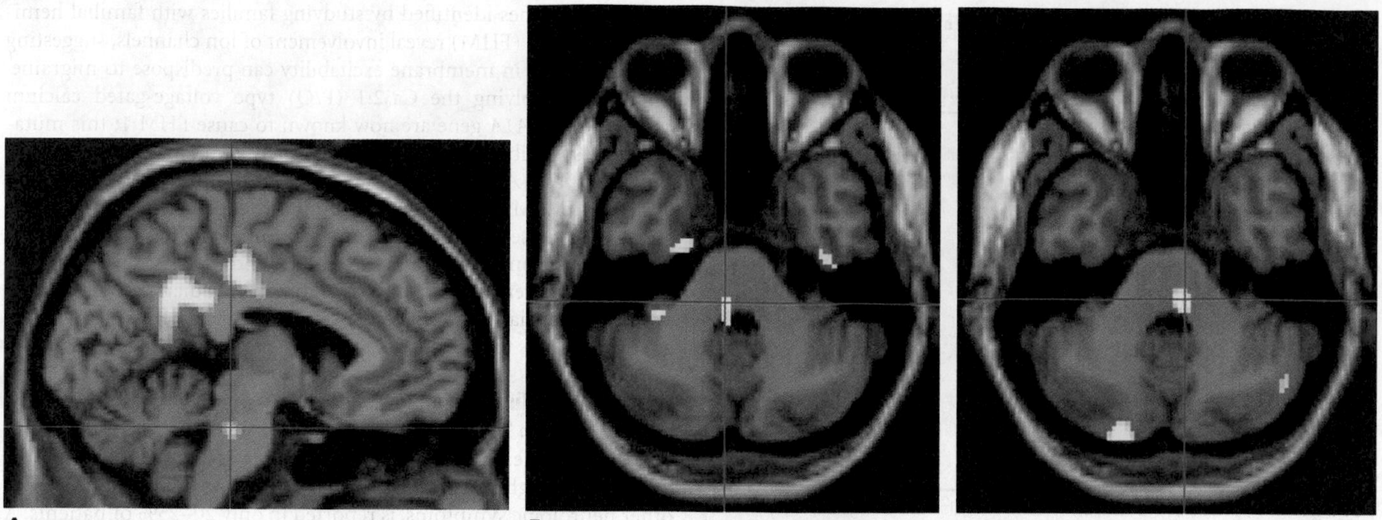

FIGURE 15-2 Positron emission tomography (PET) activation in migraine. In spontaneous attacks of episodic migraine (***A***) there is activation of the region of the dorsolateral pons (intersection of dark blue lines); an identical pattern is found in chronic migraine (not shown). This area, which includes the noradrenergic locus coeruleus, is fundamental to the expression of migraine. Moreover, lateralization of changes in this region of the brainstem correlates with lateralization of the head pain in hemicranial migraine; the scans shown in panels ***B*** and ***C*** are of patients with acute migraine headache on the right and left side, respectively. *(From S Afridi et al: Arch Neurol 62:1270, 2005; Brain 128:932, 2005.)*

℞ MIGRAINE HEADACHES

Once a diagnosis of migraine has been established, it is important to assess the extent of a patient's disease and disability. The Migraine Disability Assessment Score (MIDAS) is a well-validated, easy-to-use tool (Fig. 15-4).

Patient education is an important aspect of migraine management. Information for patients is available at *www.achenet.org*, the website of the American Council for Headache Education (ACHE). It is helpful for patients to understand that migraine is an inherited tendency to headache; that migraine can be modified and controlled by lifestyle adjustments and medications, but it cannot be eradicated; and that, except in some occasions in women on oral estrogens or contraceptives, migraine is not associated with serious or life-threatening illnesses.

NONPHARMACOLOGIC MANAGEMENT Migraine can often be managed to some degree by a variety of nonpharmacologic approaches. Most patients benefit by the identification and avoidance of specific headache triggers. A regulated lifestyle is helpful, including a healthful diet, regular exercise, regular sleep patterns, avoidance of excess caffeine and alcohol, and avoidance of acute changes in stress levels.

The measures that benefit a given individual should be used routinely since they provide a simple, cost-effective approach to migraine management. Patients with migraine do not encounter more stress than headache-free individuals; overresponsiveness to stress appears to be the issue. Since the stresses of everyday living cannot be eliminated, lessening one's response to stress by various techniques is helpful for many patients. These may include yoga, transcendental meditation, hypnosis, and conditioning techniques such as biofeedback. For most patients, this approach is, at best, an adjunct to pharmacotherapy. Nonpharmacologic measures are unlikely to prevent all migraine attacks. When these measures fail to prevent an attack, pharmacologic approaches are then needed to abort an attack.

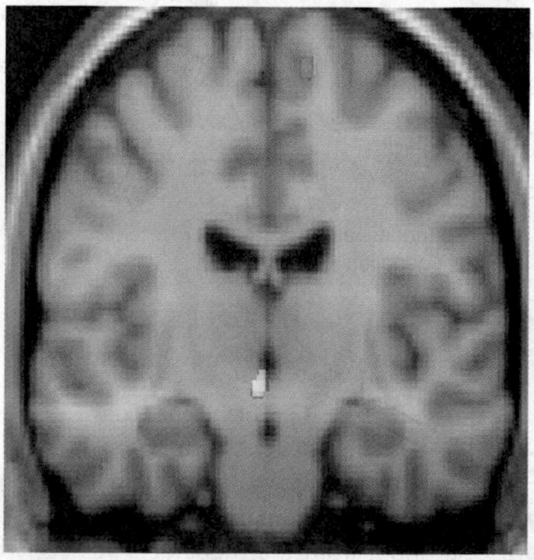

FIGURE 15-3 Posterior hypothalamic gray matter activation on positron emission tomography (PET) in a patient with acute cluster headache. Posterior hypothalamic gray matter activation on positron emission tomography (PET) in a patient with acute cluster headache. *(From A May et al: Lancet 352:275, 1998.)*

ACUTE ATTACK THERAPIES FOR MIGRAINE The mainstay of pharmacologic therapy is the judicious use of one or more of the many drugs that are effective in migraine (Table 15-5). The selection of the optimal regimen for a given patient depends on a number of factors, the most important of which is the severity of the attack. Mild migraine attacks can usually be managed by oral agents; the average efficacy rate is 50–70%. Severe migraine attacks may require parenteral therapy. Most drugs effective in the treatment of migraine are members of one of three major pharmacologic classes: anti-inflammatory agents, $5HT_{1B/1D}$ receptor agonists, and dopamine receptor antagonists.

In general, an adequate dose of whichever agent is chosen should be used as soon as possible after the onset of an attack. If additional medication is required within 60 min because symptoms return or have not abat-

TABLE 15-4 SIMPLIFIED DIAGNOSTIC CRITERIA FOR MIGRAINE

Repeated attacks of headache lasting 4–72 h in patients with a normal physical examination, no other reasonable cause for the headache, and:

At least 2 of the following features:	Plus at least 1 of the following features:
Unilateral pain	Nausea/vomiting
Throbbing pain	Photophobia and phonophobia
Aggravation by movement	
Moderate or severe intensity	

Source: Adapted from the International Headache Society Classification (Headache Classification Committee of the International Headache Society, 2004).

***MIDAS Questionnaire**

INSTRUCTIONS: Please answer the following questions about ALL headaches you have had over the last 3 months. Write zero if you did not do the activity in the last 3 months.

1. On how many days in the last 3 months did you miss work or school because of your headaches? .... ____ days
2. How many days in the last 3 months was your productivity at work or school reduced by half or more because of your headaches *(do not include days you counted in question 1 where you missed work or school)*? .... ____ days
3. On how many days in the last 3 months did you **not** do household work because of your headaches? .... ____ days
4. How many days in the last 3 months was your productivity in household work reduced by half or more because of your headaches *(do not include days you counted in question 3 where you did not do household work)*? .... ____ days
5. On how many days in the last 3 months did you miss family, social, or leisure activities because of your headaches? .... ____ days

A. On how many days in the last 3 months did you have a headache? *(If a headache lasted more than one day, count each day.)* .... ____ days

B. On a scale of 0–10, on average how painful were these headaches? *(Where 0 = no pain at all, and 10 = pain as bad as it can be.)* .... ____

*Migraine Disability Assessment Score
(Questions 1–5 are used to calculate the MIDAS score.)
Grade I—Minimal or Infrequent Disability: 0–5
Grade II—Mild or Infrequent Disability: 6–10
Grade III—Moderate Disability: 11–20
Grade IV—Severe Disability: > 20

FIGURE 15-4 MIDAS Questionnaire.

ed, the initial dose should be increased for subsequent attacks. Migraine therapy must be individualized; a standard approach for all patients is not possible. A therapeutic regimen may need to be constantly refined until one is identified that provides the patient with rapid, complete, and consistent relief with minimal side effects (Table 15-6).

Nonsteroidal Anti-Inflammatory Drugs (NSAIDs) Both the severity and duration of a migraine attack can be reduced significantly by anti-inflammatory agents (Table 15-5). Indeed, many undiagnosed migraineurs are self-treated with nonprescription NSAIDs. A general consensus is that NSAIDs are most effective when taken early in the migraine attack. However, the effectiveness of anti-inflammatory agents in migraine is usually less than optimal in moderate or severe migraine attacks. The combination of acetaminophen, aspirin, and caffeine has been approved for use by the U.S. Food and Drug Administration (FDA) for the treatment of mild to moderate migraine. The combination of aspirin and metoclopramide has been shown to be equivalent to a single dose of sumatriptan. Important side effects of NSAIDs include dyspepsia and gastrointestinal irritation.

5-HT$_1$ AGONISTS Oral Stimulation of 5-HT$_{1B/1D}$ receptors can stop an acute migraine attack. Ergotamine and dihydroergotamine are nonselective receptor agonists, while the triptans are selective 5-HT$_{1B/1D}$ receptor agonists. A variety of triptans (e.g., naratriptan, rizatriptan, eletriptan, sumatriptan, zolmitriptan, almotriptan, frovatriptan) are now available for the treatment of migraine.

Each drug in the triptan class has similar pharmacologic properties but varies slightly in terms of clinical efficacy. Rizatriptan and eletriptan are the most efficacious of the triptans currently available in the United States. Sumatriptan and zolmitriptan have similar rates of efficacy as well as time to onset, whereas naratriptan and frovatriptan are the slowest-acting and least efficacious. Clinical efficacy appears to be related more to the t_{max} (time to peak plasma level) than to the potency, half-life, or bioavailability. This observation is consistent with a large body of data indicating that faster-acting analgesics are more effective than slower-acting agents.

Unfortunately, monotherapy with a selective oral 5-HT$_{1B/1D}$ agonist does not result in rapid, consistent, and complete relief of migraine in all patients. Triptans are not effective in migraine with aura unless given after the aura is completed and the headache initiated. Side effects are common though often mild and transient. Moreover, 5-HT$_{1B/1D}$ agonists are contraindicated in individuals with a history of cardiovascular and cerebrovascular disease. Recurrence of headache is another important limitation of triptan use and occurs at least occasionally in most patients.

Ergotamine preparations offer a nonselective means of stimulating 5-HT$_1$ receptors. A nonnauseating dose of ergotamine should be sought since a dose that provokes nausea is too high and may intensify head pain. Except for a sublingual formulation of ergotamine, oral formulations of ergotamine also contain 100 mg caffeine (theoretically to enhance ergotamine absorption and possibly to add additional analgesic activity). The average oral ergotamine dose for a migraine attack is 2 mg. Since the clinical studies demonstrating the efficacy of ergotamine in migraine predated the clinical trial methodologies used with the triptans, it is difficult to assess the clinical efficacy of ergotamine versus the triptans. In general, ergotamine appears to have a much higher incidence of nausea than triptans, but less headache recurrence.

Nasal The fastest-acting nonparenteral antimigraine therapies that can be self-administered include nasal formulations of dihydroergotamine (Migranal), zolmitriptan (Zomig nasal), or sumatriptan. The nasal sprays result in substantial blood levels within 30–60 min. Although in theory nasal sprays might provide faster and more effective relief of a migraine attack than oral formulations, their reported efficacy is only approximately 50–60%.

Parenteral Parenteral administration of drugs such as dihydroergotamine and sumatriptan is approved by the FDA for the rapid relief of a migraine attack. Peak plasma levels of dihydroergotamine are achieved 3 min after intravenous dosing, 30 min after intramuscular dosing, and 45 min after subcutaneous dosing. If an attack has not already peaked, subcutaneous or intramuscular administration of 1 mg dihydroergotamine suffices for about 80–90% of patients. Sumatriptan, 6 mg subcutaneously, is effective in ~70–80% of patients.

DOPAMINE ANTAGONISTS Oral Oral dopamine antagonists should be considered as adjunctive therapy in migraine. Drug absorption is impaired during migraine because of reduced gastrointestinal motility. Delayed absorption occurs even in the absence of nausea and is related to the severity of the attack and not its duration. Therefore, when oral NSAIDs and/or triptan agents fail, the addition of a dopamine antagonist such as metoclopramide, 10 mg, should be considered to enhance gastric absorption. In addition, dopamine antagonists decrease nausea/vomiting and restore normal gastric motility.

Parenteral Parenteral dopamine antagonists (e.g., chlorpromazine, prochlorperazine, metoclopramide) can also provide significant acute relief of migraine; they can be used in combination with parenteral 5-HT$_{1B/1D}$ agonists. A common intravenous protocol used for the treatment of severe migraine is the administration over 2 min of a mixture of 5 mg of prochlorperazine and 0.5 mg of dihydroergotamine.

OTHER MEDICATIONS FOR ACUTE MIGRAINE Oral The combination of acetaminophen, dichloralphenazone, and isometheptene, one to two capsules, has been classified by the FDA as "possibly" effective in the treatment of migraine. Since the clinical studies demonstrating the efficacy of this combination analgesic in migraine predated the clinical trial methodologies used with the triptans, it is difficult to compare the efficacy of this sympathomimetic compound to other agents.

Nasal A nasal preparation of butorphanol is available for the treatment of acute pain. As with all narcotics, the use of nasal butorphanol should be limited to a select group of migraineurs, as described below.

Parenteral Narcotics are effective in the acute treatment of migraine. For example, intravenous meperidine (50–100 mg) is given frequently in the emergency room. This regimen "works" in the sense that the pain of migraine is eliminated. However, this regimen is clearly suboptimal for patients with recurrent headache. Narcotics do not treat the underlying headache mechanism; rather, they act to alter the pain sensation. Moreover, in patients taking oral narcotics such as oxycodone or hydrocodone, narcotic addiction can greatly con-

TABLE 15-5 TREATMENT OF ACUTE MIGRAINE

Drug	Trade Name	Dosage
Simple Analgesics		
Acetaminophen, aspirin, caffeine	Excedrin Migraine	Two tablets or caplets q6h (max 8 per day)
NSAIDs		
Naproxen	Aleve, Anaprox, generic	220–550 mg PO bid
Ibuprofen	Advil, Motrin, Nuprin, generic	400 mg PO q3–4h
Tolfenamic acid	Clotam Rapid	200 mg PO. May repeat x 1 after 1–2 h
5-HT$_1$ Agonists		
Oral		
Ergotamine	Ergomar	One 2 mg sublingual tablet at onset and q$1/2$h (max 3 per day, 5 per week)
Ergotamine 1 mg, caffeine 100 mg	Ercaf, Wigraine	One or two tablets at onset, then one tablet q$1/2$h (max 6 per day, 10 per week)
Naratriptan	Amerge	2.5 mg tablet at onset; may repeat once after 4 h
Rizatriptan	Maxalt Maxalt-MLT	5–10 mg tablet at onset; may repeat after 2 h (max 30 mg/d)
Sumatriptan	Imitrex	50–100 mg tablet at onset; may repeat after 2 h (max 200 mg/d)
Frovatriptan	Frova	2.5 mg tablet at onset, may repeat after 2 h (max 5 mg/d)
Almotriptan	Axert	12.5 mg tablet at onset, may repeat after 2 h (max 25 mg/d)
Eletriptan	Relpax	40 or 80 mg
Zolmitriptan	Zomig Zomig Rapimelt	2.5 mg tablet at onset; may repeat after 2 h (max 10 mg/d)
Nasal		
Dihydroergotamine	Migranal Nasal Spray	Prior to nasal spray, the pump must be primed 4 times; 1 spray (0.5 mg) is administered, followed in 15 min by a second spray
Sumatriptan	Imitrex Nasal Spray	5–20 mg intranasal spray as 4 sprays of 5 mg or a single 20 mg spray (may repeat once after 2 h, not to exceed a dose of 40 mg/d)
Zolmitriptan	Zomig	5 mg intranasal spray as one spray (may repeat once after 2 h, not to exceed a dose of 10 mg/d)
Parenteral		
Dihydroergotamine	DHE-45	1 mg IV, IM, or SC at onset and q1h (max 3 mg/d, 6 mg per week)
Sumatriptan	Imitrex Injection	6 mg SC at onset (may repeat once after 1 h for max of 2 doses in 24 h)
Dopamine Antagonists		
Oral		
Metoclopramide	Reglan,[a] generic[a]	5–10 mg/d
Prochlorperazine	Compazine,[a] generic[a]	1–25 mg/d
Parenteral		
Chlorpromazine	Generic[a]	0.1 mg/kg IV at 2 mg/min; max 35 mg/d
Metoclopramide	Reglan,[a] generic	10 mg IV
Prochlorperazine	Compazine,[a] generic[a]	10 mg IV
Other		
Oral		
Acetaminophen, 325 mg, *plus* dichloralphenazone, 100 mg, *plus* isometheptene, 65 mg	Midrin, Duradrin, generic	Two capsules at onset followed by 1 capsule q1h (max 5 capsules)
Nasal		
Butorphanol	Stadol[a]	1 mg (1 spray in 1 nostril), may repeat if necessary in 1–2 h
Parenteral		
Narcotics	Generic[a]	Multiple preparations and dosages; see Table 12-1

[a]Not all drugs are specifically indicated by the FDA for migraine. Local regulations and guidelines should be consulted.
Note: Antiemetics (e.g., domperidone 10 mg or ondansetron) or prokinetics (e.g., metoclopramide 10 mg) are sometimes useful adjuncts.
Abbreviations: NSAIDs, nonsteroidal anti-inflammatory drugs; 5-HT, 5-hydroxytryptamine.

fuse the treatment of migraine. Narcotic craving and/or withdrawal can aggravate and accentuate migraine. Therefore, it is recommended that narcotic use in migraine be limited to patients with severe, but infrequent, headaches that are unresponsive to other pharmacologic approaches.

MEDICATION-OVERUSE HEADACHE

Acute attack medications, particularly codeine or barbiturate-containing compound analgesics, have a propensity to aggravate headache frequency and induce a state of refractory daily or near-daily headache called *medication-overuse headache*. This condition is likely not a separate headache entity but a reaction of the migraine patient to a particular medicine. Migraine patients who have two or more headache days a week should be cautioned about frequent analgesic use (see "Chronic Daily Headache," below).

PREVENTIVE TREATMENTS FOR MIGRAINE

Patients with an increasing frequency of migraine attacks, or with attacks that are either unresponsive or poorly responsive to abortive treatments, are good candidates for preventive agents. In general, a preventive medication should be considered in the subset of patients with five or more attacks a month. Significant side effects are associated with the use of many of these agents; furthermore, determination of dose can be difficult since the recommended doses have been derived for conditions other than migraine. The mechanism of action of these drugs is unclear; it seems likely that the brain sensitivity that underlies migraine is modified. Patients are usually started on a low dose of a chosen treatment; the dose is then gradually increased, up to a reasonable maximum to achieve clinical benefit.

Drugs that have the capacity to stabilize migraine are listed in **Table 15-7**. Drugs must be taken daily, and there is usually a lag of at least 2–12 weeks before an effect is seen. The drugs that have been approved by the FDA for the prophylactic treatment of migraine include propranolol, timolol, sodium valproate, topiramate, and methysergide (not available in the United States). In addition, a number of other drugs appear to display prophylactic efficacy. This group includes amitriptyline, nortriptyline, flunarizine, phenelzine, gabapentin, topiramate, and cyproheptadine. Phenelzine and methysergide are usually reserved for recalcitrant cases because of their serious potential side effects. Phenelzine is a monoamine oxidase inhibitor (MAOI); therefore, tyramine-containing foods, decongestants, and meperidine are contraindicated. Methysergide may cause retroperitoneal or cardiac valvular fibrosis when it is used for >6 months, and thus monitoring is required for patients using this drug; the risk of fibrosis is about 1:1500 and is likely to reverse after the drug is stopped.

The probability of success with any one of the antimigraine drugs is 50–75%. Many patients are managed adequately with low-dose amitriptyline, propranolol, topiramate, gabapentin, or valproate. If these agents fail or lead to unacceptable side effects, second-line agents such as methysergide or phenelzine can be used. Once effective stabilization is achieved, the drug is continued for 5–6 months and then slowly tapered to assess the continued need. Many patients are able to discontinue medication and experience fewer and milder attacks for long periods, suggesting that these drugs may alter the natural history of migraine.

TENSION-TYPE HEADACHE

Clinical Features

The term *tension-type headache* (TTH) is commonly used to describe a chronic head-pain syndrome characterized by bilateral tight, bandlike discomfort. The pain typically builds slowly,

TABLE 15-6 CLINICAL STRATIFICATION OF ACUTE SPECIFIC MIGRAINE TREATMENTS

Clinical Situation	Treatment Options
Failed NSAIDS/analgesics	**First tier** Sumatriptan 50 mg or 100 mg PO Almotriptan 12.5 mg PO Rizatriptan 10 mg PO Eletriptan 40 mg PO Zolmitriptan 2.5 mg PO **Slower effect/better tolerability** Naratriptan 2.5 mg PO Frovatriptan 2.5 mg PO **Infrequent headache** Ergotamine 1–2 mg PO Dihydroergotamine nasal spray 2 mg
Early nausea or difficulties taking tablets	Zolmitriptan 5 mg nasal spray Sumatriptan 20 mg nasal spray Rizatriptan 10 mg MLT wafer
Headache recurrence	Ergotamine 2 mg (most effective PR/usually with caffeine) Naratriptan 2.5 mg PO Almotriptan 12.5 mg PO Eletriptan 40 mg
Tolerating acute treatments poorly	Naratriptan 2.5 mg Almotriptan 12.5 mg
Early vomiting	Zolmitriptan 5 mg nasal spray Sumatriptan 25 mg PR Sumatriptan 6 mg SC
Menses-related headache	**Prevention** Ergotamine PO at night Estrogen patches **Treatment** Triptans Dihydroergotamine nasal spray
Very rapidly developing symptoms	Zolmitriptan 5 mg nasal spray Sumatriptan 6 mg SC Dihydroergotamine 1 mg IM

fluctuates in severity, and may persist more or less continuously for many days. The headache may be episodic or chronic (present >15 days per month).

A useful clinical approach is to diagnose TTH in patients whose headaches are completely without accompanying features such as nausea, vomiting, photophobia, phonophobia, osmophobia, throbbing, and aggravation with movement. Such an approach neatly separates migraine, which has one or more of these features and is the main differential diagnosis, from TTH. However, the International Headache Society's definition of TTH allows an admixture of nausea, photophobia, or phonophobia in various combinations, illustrating the difficulties in distinguishing these two clinical entities. Patients whose headaches fit the TTH phenotype and who have migraine at other times, along with a family history of migraine, migrainous illnesses of childhood, or typical migraine triggers to their migraine attacks, may be biologically different from those who have TTH headache with none of the features.

Pathophysiology The pathophysiology of TTH is incompletely understood. It seems likely that TTH is due to a primary disorder of CNS pain modulation alone, unlike migraine, which involves a more generalized disturbance of sensory modulation. Data suggest a genetic contribution to TTH, but this may not be a valid finding: given the current diagnostic criteria, the studies undoubtedly included many migraine patients. The name *tension-type headache* implies that pain is a product of *nervous tension*, but there is no clear evidence for tension as an etiology. Muscle contraction has been considered to be a feature that distinguishes TTH from migraine, but there appear to be no differences in contraction between the two headache types.

℞ TENSION-TYPE HEADACHE

The pain of TTH can generally be managed with simple analgesics such as acetaminophen, aspirin, or NSAIDs. Behavioral approaches including relaxation can also be effective. Clinical studies have demonstrated that triptans in pure TTH are not helpful, although triptans are effective in TTH when the patient also has migraine. For chronic TTH, amitriptyline is the only proven treatment (Table 15-7); other tricyclics, selective serotonin reuptake inhibitors, and the benzodiazepines have not been shown to be effective. There is no evidence for the efficacy of acupuncture. Placebo controlled trials of botulinum toxin type A in chronic TTH have not shown benefit.

TRIGEMINAL AUTONOMIC CEPHALALGIAS, INCLUDING CLUSTER HEADACHE

The trigeminal autonomic cephalalgias (TACs) are a group of primary headaches that includes cluster headache, paroxysmal hemicrania, and SUNCT (*s*hort-lasting *u*nilateral *n*euralgiform headache attacks with *c*onjunctival injection and *t*earing). TACs are characterized by relatively short-lasting attacks of head pain associated with cranial autonomic symptoms, such as lacrimation, conjunctival injection, or nasal congestion (Table 15-8). Pain is usually severe and may occur more than once a day. Because of the associated nasal congestion or rhinorrhea, patients are often misdiagnosed with "sinus headache" and treated with decongestants, which are ineffective.

TACs must be differentiated from short-lasting headaches that do not have prominent cranial autonomic syndromes, notably trigeminal neuralgia, primary stabbing headache, and hypnic headache. The cycling pattern and length, frequency, and timing of attacks are useful in classifying patients. Patients with TACs should undergo pituitary imaging and pituitary function tests as there is an excess of TAC presentations in patients with pituitary tumor–related headache.

Cluster Headache Cluster headache is a rare form of primary headache with a population frequency of 0.1%. The pain is deep, usually retroorbital, often excruciating in intensity, nonfluctuating, and explosive in quality. A core feature of cluster headache is periodicity. At least one of the daily attacks of pain recurs at about the same hour each day for the duration of a cluster bout. The typical cluster headache patient has daily bouts of one to two attacks of relatively short-duration unilateral pain for 8–10 weeks a year; this is usually followed by a pain-free interval that averages 1 year. Cluster headache is characterized as chronic when there is no period of sustained remission. Patients are generally perfectly well between episodes. Onset is nocturnal in about 50% of patients, and men are affected three times more often than women. Patients with cluster headache tend to move about during attacks, pacing, rocking, or rubbing their head for relief; some may even become aggressive during attacks. This is in sharp contrast to patients with migraine, who prefer to remain motionless during attacks.

Cluster headache is associated with ipsilateral symptoms of cranial parasympathetic autonomic activation: conjunctival injection or lacrimation, rhinorrhea or nasal congestion, or cranial sympathetic dysfunction such as ptosis. The sympathetic deficit is peripheral and likely to be due to parasympathetic activation with injury to ascending sympathetic fibers surrounding a dilated carotid artery as it passes into the cranial cavity. When present, photophobia and phonophobia are far more likely to be unilateral and on the same side of the pain, rather than bilateral, as is seen in migraine. This phenomenon of unilateral photophobia/phonophobia is characteristic of TACs. Cluster headache is likely to be a disorder involving central pacemaker neurons in the region of the posterior hypothalamus (Fig. 15-2).

℞ CLUSTER HEADACHE

The most satisfactory treatment is the administration of drugs to prevent cluster attacks until the bout is over. However, treatment of acute attacks is required for all cluster headache patients at some time.

ACUTE ATTACK TREATMENT Cluster headache attacks peak rapidly, and thus a treatment with quick onset is required. Many patients with acute cluster headache respond very well to oxygen inhalation. This should be given as 100% oxygen at 10–12 L/min for 15–20 min. It appears that high flow and high oxygen content are important. Sumatriptan 6 mg subcutaneously is rapid in onset and will usually shorten an attack to 10–15 min; there is no evidence of tachyphylaxis. Sumatriptan (20 mg) and zolmitriptan (5 mg) nasal sprays are both effective in acute cluster head-

TABLE 15-7 PREVENTIVE TREATMENTS IN MIGRAINE[a]

Drug	Dose	Selected Side Effects
Pizotifen[b]	0.5–2 mg qd	Weight gain Drowsiness
Beta blocker		
Propranolol	40–120 mg bid	Reduced energy Tiredness Postural symptoms *Contraindicated in asthma*
Tricyclics		
Amitriptyline	10–75 mg at night	Drowsiness
Dothiepin	25–75 mg at night	
Nortriptyline	25–75 mg at night	***Note:*** Some patients may only need a total dose of 10 mg, although generally 1–1.5 mg/kg body weight is required
Anticonvulsants		
Topiramate	25–200 mg/d	Paresthesias Cognitive symptoms Weight loss Glaucoma Caution with nephrolithiasis
Valproate	400–600 mg bid	Drowsiness Weight gain Tremor Hair loss Fetal abnormalities Hematologic or liver abnormalities
Gabapentin	900–3600 mg qd	Dizziness Sedation
Serotonergic drugs		
Methysergide	1–4 mg qd	Drowsiness Leg cramps Hair loss Retroperitoneal fibrosis (1-month drug holiday is required every 6 months)
Flunarizine[b]	5–15 mg qd	Drowsiness Weight gain Depression Parkinsonism
No convincing evidence from controlled trials		
Verapamil		
Controlled trials demonstrate *no effect*		
Nimodipine		
Clonidine		
SSRIs: fluoxetine		

[a]Commonly used preventives are listed with reasonable doses and common side effects. Not all listed medicines are approved by the FDA; local regulations and guidelines should be consulted.
[b]Not available in the United States.

ache, offering a useful option for patients who may not wish to self-inject daily. Oral sumatriptan is not effective for prevention or for acute treatment of cluster headache.

PREVENTIVE TREATMENTS (Table 15-9) The choice of a preventive treatment in cluster headache depends in part on the length of the bout. Patients with long bouts or those with chronic cluster headache require medicines that are safe when taken for long periods. For patients with relatively short bouts, limited courses of oral glucocorticoids or methysergide (not available in the United States) can be very useful. A 10-day course of prednisone, beginning at 60 mg daily for 7 days and followed by a rapid taper, may interrupt the pain bout for many patients. When ergotamine (1–2 mg) is used, it is most effective when given 1–2 h before an expected attack. Patients who use ergotamine daily must be educated regarding the early symptoms of ergotism, which may include vomiting, numbness, tingling, pain, and cyanosis of the limbs; a weekly limit of 14 mg should be adhered to. Lithium (600–900 mg qd) appears to be particularly useful for the chronic form of the disorder.

Many experts favor verapamil as the first-line preventive treatment for patients with chronic cluster headache or prolonged bouts. While verapamil compares favorably with lithium in practice, some patients require verapamil doses far in excess of those administered for cardiac disorders. The initial dose range is 40–80 mg twice daily; effective doses may be as high as 960 mg/d. Side effects such as constipation and leg swelling can be problematic. Of paramount concern, however, is the cardiovascular safety of verapamil, particularly at high doses. Verapamil can cause heart block by slowing conduction in the atrioventricular node, a condition that can be monitored by following the PR interval on a standard EKG. Approximately 20% of patients treated with verapamil develop EKG abnormalities, which can be observed with doses as low as 240 mg/d; these abnormalities can worsen over time in patients on stable doses. A baseline EKG is recommended for all patients. The EKG is repeated 10 days after a dose change in those patients whose dose is being increased above 240 mg daily. Dose increases are usually made in 80-mg increments. For patients on long-term verapamil, EKG monitoring every 6 months is advised.

NEUROSTIMULATION THERAPY When medical therapies fail in chronic cluster headache, neurostimulation therapy strategies can be employed. Deep-brain stimulation of the region of the posterior hypothalamic gray matter has proven successful in a substantial proportion of patients. Favorable results have also been reported with the less-invasive approach of occipital nerve stimulation.

Paroxysmal Hemicrania Paroxysmal hemicrania (PH) is characterized by frequent unilateral, severe, short-lasting episodes of headache. Like cluster headache, the pain tends to be retroorbital but may be experienced all over the head and is associated with autonomic phe-

TABLE 15-8 CLINICAL FEATURES OF THE TRIGEMINAL AUTONOMIC CEPHALALGIAS

	Cluster Headache	Paroxysmal Hemicrania	SUNCT
Gender	M>F	F=M	F~M
Pain			
Type	Stabbing, boring	Throbbing, boring, stabbing	Burning, stabbing, sharp
Severity	Excruciating	Excruciating	Severe to excruciating
Site	Orbit, temple	Orbit, temple	Periorbital
Attack frequency	1/alternate day–8/d	1–40/d (>5/d for more than half the time)	3–200/d
Duration of attack	15–180 min	2–30 min	5–240 s
Autonomic features	Yes	Yes	Yes (prominent conjunctival injection and lacrimation)[a]
Migrainous features[b]	Yes	Yes	Yes
Alcohol trigger	Yes	No	No
Cutaneous triggers	No	No	Yes
Indomethacin effect	—	Yes[c]	No
Abortive treatment	Sumatriptan injection or nasal spray Oxygen	No effective treatment	Lidocaine (IV)
Prophylactic treatment	Verapamil Methysergide Lithium	Indomethacin	Lamotrigine Topiramate Gabapentin

[a]If conjunctival injection and tearing not present, consider SUNA.
[b]Nausea, photophobia, or phonophobia; photophobia and phonophobia are typically unilateral on the side of the pain.
[c]Indicates complete response to indomethacin.
Note: SUNCT, short-lasting *u*nilateral *n*euralgiform headache attacks with *c*onjunctival injection and *t*earing.

TABLE 15-9 PREVENTIVE MANAGEMENT OF CLUSTER HEADACHE

Short-Term Prevention	Long-Term Prevention
Episodic Cluster Headache	Episodic Cluster Headache & Prolonged Chronic Cluster Headache
Prednisone 1 mg/kg up to 60 mg qd, tapering over 21 days	Verapamil 160–960 mg/d
Methysergide 3–12 mg/d	Lithium 400–800 mg/d
Verapamil 160–960 mg/d	Methysergide 3–12 mg/d
Greater occipital nerve injection	Topiramate[a] 100–400 mg/d
	Gabapentin[a] 1200–3600 mg/d
	Melatonin[a] 9–12 mg/d

[a]Unproven but of potential benefit.

nomena such as lacrimation and nasal congestion. Patients with remissions are said to have episodic PH, while those with the nonremitting form are said to have chronic PH. The essential features of PH are: unilateral, very severe pain; short-lasting attacks (2–45 min); very frequent attacks (usually more than five a day); marked autonomic features ipsilateral to the pain; rapid course (<72 h); and excellent response to indomethacin. In contrast to cluster headache, which predominantly affects males, the male:female ratio in PH is close to 1:1.

Indomethacin (25–75 mg tid), which can completely suppress attacks of PH, is the treatment of choice. Although therapy may be complicated by indomethacin-induced gastrointestinal side effects, currently there are no consistently effective alternatives. Topiramate is helpful in some cases. Piroxicam has been used, although it is not as effective as indomethacin. Verapamil, an effective treatment for cluster headache, does not appear to be useful for PH. In occasional patients, PH can coexist with trigeminal neuralgia (PH-tic syndrome); similar to cluster-tic syndrome, each component may require separate treatment.

Secondary PH has been reported with lesions in the region of the sella turcica, including arteriovenous malformation, cavernous sinus meningioma, and epidermoid tumors. Secondary PH is more likely if the patient requires high doses (>200 mg/d) of indomethacin. In patients with apparent bilateral PH, raised CSF pressure should be suspected. It is important to note that indomethacin reduces CSF pressure. When a diagnosis of PH is considered, MRI is indicated to exclude a pituitary lesion.

SUNCT/SUNA SUNCT is a rare primary headache syndrome characterized by severe, unilateral orbital or temporal pain that is stabbing or throbbing in quality. Diagnosis requires at least 20 attacks, lasting for 5–240 s; ipsilateral conjunctival injection and lacrimation should be present. In some patients conjunctival injection or lacrimation are missing, and the diagnosis of SUNA (*s*hort-lasting *u*nilateral *n*euralgiform headache attacks with cranial *a*utonomic symptoms) has been suggested.

DIAGNOSIS The pain of SUNCT/SUNA is unilateral and may be located anywhere in the head. Three basic patterns can be seen: single stabs, which are usually short-lived; groups of stabs; or a longer attack comprising many stabs between which the pain does not completely resolve, thus giving a "saw-tooth" phenomenon with attacks lasting many minutes. Each pattern may be seen in the context of an underlying continuous head pain. Characteristics that lead to a suspected diagnosis of SUNCT are the cutaneous (or other) triggerability of attacks, a lack of refractory period to triggering between attacks, and the lack of a response to indomethacin. Apart from trigeminal sensory disturbance, the neurologic examination is normal in primary SUNCT.

The diagnosis of SUNCT is often confused with trigeminal neuralgia (TN) particularly in first-division TN (Chap. 371). Minimal or no cranial autonomic symptoms and a clear refractory period to triggering indicate a diagnosis of TN.

SECONDARY (SYMPTOMATIC) SUNCT SUNCT can be seen with posterior fossa or pituitary lesions. All patients with SUNCT/SUNA should be evaluated with pituitary function tests and a brain MRI with pituitary views.

TABLE 15-10 CLASSIFICATION OF CHRONIC DAILY HEADACHE

Primary		
>4 h Daily	**<4 h Daily**	**Secondary**
Chronic migraine[a]	Chronic cluster headache[b]	Posttraumatic Head injury Iatrogenic Postinfectious
Chronic tension-type headache[a]	Chronic paroxysmal hemicrania	Inflammatory, such as Giant cell arteritis Sarcoidosis Behçet's syndrome
Hemicrania continua[a]	SUNCT/SUNA	Chronic CNS infection
New daily persistent headache[a]	Hypnic headache	Medication-overuse headache[a]

[a]May be complicated by analgesic overuse.
[b]Some patients may have headache > 4 h per day.
Note: SUNCT, *s*hort-lasting *u*nilateral *n*euralgiform headache attacks with *c*onjunctival injection and *t*earing; SUNA, *s*hort-lasting *u*nilateral *n*euralgiform headache *a*ttacks with cranial autonomic symptoms.

Rx SUNCT/SUNA

ABORTIVE THERAPY Therapy of acute attacks is not a useful concept in SUNCT/SUNA since the attacks are of such short duration. However, intravenous lidocaine, which arrests the symptoms, can be used in hospitalized patients.

PREVENTIVE THERAPY Long-term prevention to minimize disability and hospitalization is the goal of treatment. The most effective treatment for prevention is lamotrigine, 200–400 mg/d. Topiramate and gabapentin may also be effective. Carbamazepine, 400–500 mg/d, has been reported by patients to offer modest benefit.

Surgical approaches such as microvascular decompression or destructive trigeminal procedures are seldom useful and often produce long-term complications. Greater occipital nerve injection has produced limited benefit in some patients. Mixed success with occipital nerve stimulation has been observed. Complete control with deep-brain stimulation of the posterior hypothalamic region was reported in a single patient. For intractable cases, short-term prevention with intravenous lidocaine can be effective.

CHRONIC DAILY HEADACHE

The broad diagnosis of chronic daily headache (CDH) can be applied when a patient experiences headache on 15 days or more per month. CDH is not a single entity; it encompasses a number of different headache syndromes, including chronic TTH as well as headache secondary to trauma, inflammation, infection, medication overuse, and other causes (Table 15-10). Population-based estimates suggest that about 4% of adults have daily or near-daily headache. Daily headache may be primary or secondary, an important consideration in guiding management of this complaint.

APPROACH TO THE PATIENT: Chronic Daily Headache

The first step in the management of patients with CDH is to diagnose any underlying condition (Table 15-10). For patients with primary headaches, diagnosis of the headache type will guide therapy. Preventive treatments such as tricyclics, either amitriptyline or doxepin at doses up to 1 mg/kg, are very useful in patients with CDH. Tricyclics are started in low doses (10–25 mg) daily and may be given 12 h before the expected time of awakening in order to avoid excess morning sleepiness. Anticonvulsants, such as topiramate, valproate, and gabapentin, are also useful in migraineurs. Flunarizine can also be very effective for some patients, as can methysergide or phenelzine.

MANAGEMENT OF MEDICALLY INTRACTABLE DISABLING CHRONIC DAILY HEADACHE The management of medically intractable headache is difficult. At this time, the only promising approach is occipital nerve stimulation, which appears to modulate thalamic processing in migraine and has shown promise in both chronic cluster headache and hemicrania continua (see below). Clinical trials using botulinum toxin in chronic migraine have failed to show any objective benefit.

MEDICATION-OVERUSE HEADACHE Overuse of analgesic medication for headache can aggravate headache frequency and induce a state of refractory daily or near-daily headache called *medication-overuse headache*. A proportion of patients who stop taking analgesics will experience substantial improvement in the severity and frequency of their headache. However, even after cessation of analgesic use, many patients continue to have headache, although they may feel clinically improved in some way, especially if they have been using codeine or barbiturates regularly. The residual symptoms probably represent the underlying headache disorder.

Management of Medication Overuse: Outpatients For patients who overuse medications, it is essential that analgesic use be reduced and eliminated. One approach is to reduce the medication dose by 10% every 1–2 weeks. Immediate cessation of analgesic use is possible for some patients, provided there is no contraindication. Both approaches are facilitated by the use of a medication diary maintained during the month or two before cessation; this helps to identify the scope of the problem. A small dose of an NSAID such as naproxen, 500 mg bid if tolerated, will help relieve residual pain as analgesic use is reduced. NSAID overuse is not usually a problem for patients with daily headache when the dose is taken once or twice daily; however, overuse problems may develop with more frequent dosing schedules. Once the patient has substantially reduced analgesic use, a preventive medication should be introduced. It must be emphasized that *preventives generally do not work in the presence of analgesic overuse.* The most common cause of unresponsiveness to treatment is the use of a preventive when analgesics continue to be used regularly. For some patients, discontinuing analgesics is very difficult; often the best approach is to directly inform the patient that some degree of pain is inevitable during this initial period.

Management of Medication Overuse: Inpatients Some patients will require hospitalization for detoxification. Such patients have typically failed efforts at outpatient withdrawal or have a significant medical condition, such as diabetes mellitus, which would complicate withdrawal as an outpatient. Following admission to the hospital, acute medications are withdrawn completely on the first day, in the absence of a contraindication. Antiemetics and fluids are administered as required; clonidine is used for opiate withdrawal symptoms. For acute intolerable pain during the waking hours aspirin, 1 g (not approved in United States) intravenously, is useful. Intramuscular chlorpromazine can be helpful at night; patients must be adequately hydrated. If the patient does not improve within 3–5 days, a course of intravenous dihydroergotamine (DHE) can be employed. DHE, administered every 8 h for 3 consecutive days, can induce a significant remission that allows a preventive treatment to be established. 5-HT_3 antagonists, such as ondansetron or granisetron, are often required with DHE to prevent significant nausea.

NEW DAILY PERSISTENT HEADACHE New daily persistent headache (NDPH) is a clinically distinct syndrome; its causes are listed in Table 15-11.

TABLE 15-11 DIFFERENTIAL DIAGNOSIS OF NEW DAILY PERSISTENT HEADACHE

Primary	Secondary
Migrainous-type	Subarachnoid hemorrhage
Featureless (tension-type)	Low CSF volume headache
	Raised CSF pressure headache
	Posttraumatic headache[a]
	Chronic meningitis

[a]Includes postinfectious forms.

Clinical Presentation The patient with NDPH presents with headache on most if not all days; the onset is recent and clearly recalled by the patient. The headache usually begins abruptly, but onset may be more gradual; evolution over 3 days has been proposed as the upper limit for this syndrome. Patients typically recall the exact day and circumstances of the onset of headache; the new, persistent head pain does not remit. The first priority is to distinguish between a primary and a secondary cause of this syndrome. Subarachnoid hemorrhage is the most serious of the secondary causes and must be excluded either by history or appropriate investigation (Chap. 269).

Secondary NDPH ***Low CSF Volume Headache*** In these syndromes, head pain is positional: it begins when the patient sits or stands upright and resolves upon reclining. The pain, which is occipitofrontal, is usually a dull ache but may be throbbing. Patients with chronic low CSF volume headache typically present with a history of headache from one day to the next that is generally not present on waking but worsens during the day. Recumbency usually improves the headache within minutes, but it takes only minutes to an hour for the pain to return when the patient resumes an upright position.

The most common cause of headache due to persistent low CSF volume is CSF leak following lumbar puncture (LP). Post-LP headache usually begins within 48 h but may be delayed for up to 12 days. Its incidence is between 10 and 30%. Beverages with caffeine may provide temporary relief. Besides LP, index events may include epidural injection or a vigorous Valsalva maneuver, such as from lifting, straining, coughing, clearing the eustachian tubes in an airplane, or multiple orgasms. Spontaneous CSF leaks are well recognized, and the diagnosis should be considered whenever the headache history is typical, even when there is no obvious index event. As time passes from the index event, the postural nature may become less apparent; cases in which the index event occurred several years before the eventual diagnosis have been recognized. Symptoms appear to result from low volume rather than low pressure: although low CSF pressures, typically 0–50 mmH_2O, are usually identified, a pressure as high as 140 mmH_2O has been noted with a documented leak. Postural orthostatic tachycardia syndrome [POTS (Chap. 370)] can present with orthostatic headache similar to low CSF volume headache and is a diagnosis that needs consideration here.

When imaging is indicated to identify the source of a presumed leak, an MRI with gadolinium is the initial study of choice (Fig. 15-5). A striking pattern of diffuse meningeal enhancement is so typical that in the appropriate clinical context the diagnosis is established. Chiari malformations may sometimes be noted on MRI; in such cases surgery to decompress the posterior fossa usually worsens the headache. The source of CSF leakage may be identified by spinal MRI, by CT myelogram, or with ^{111}In-DTPA CSF studies; in the absence of a directly identified site of leakage, early emptying of ^{111}In-DTPA tracer into the bladder or slow progress of tracer across the brain suggests a CSF leak.

Initial treatment for low CSF volume headache is bed rest. For patients with persistent pain, intravenous caffeine (500 mg in 500 mL saline administered over 2 h) is often very effective. An EKG to screen for arrhythmia should be performed before administration. It is reasonable to administer at least two infusions of caffeine before embarking on additional tests to identify the source of the CSF leak. Since intravenous caffeine is safe and can be curative, it spares many patients the need for further investigations. If unsuccessful, an abdominal binder may be helpful. If a leak can be identified, an autologous blood patch is usually curative. A blood patch is also effective for post-LP headache; in this setting the location is empirically determined to be the site of the LP. In patients with intractable pain, oral theophylline is a useful alternative; however, its effect is less rapid than caffeine.

Raised CSF Pressure Headache Raised CSF pressure is well recognized as a cause of headache. Brain imaging can often reveal the

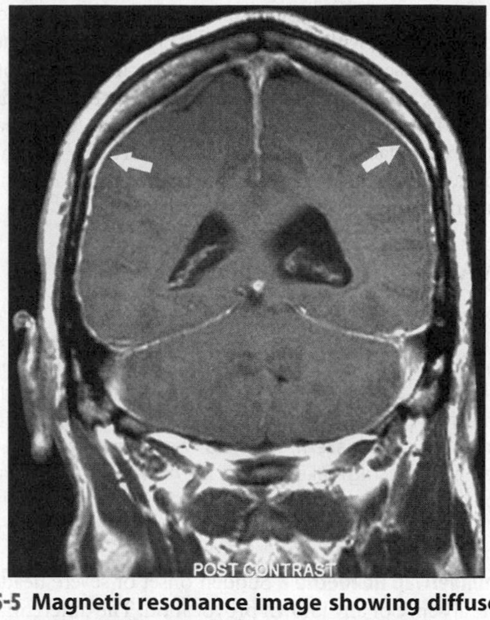

FIGURE 15-5 Magnetic resonance image showing diffuse meningeal enhancement after gadolinium administration in a patient with low CSF volume headache.

cause, such as a space-occupying lesion. NDPH due to raised CSF pressure can be the presenting symptom for patients with idiopathic intracranial hypertension (pseudotumor cerebri) without visual problems, particularly when the fundi are normal. Persistently raised intracranial pressure can trigger chronic migraine. These patients typically present with a history of generalized headache that is present on waking and improves as the day goes on. It is generally worse with recumbency. Visual obscurations are frequent. The diagnosis is relatively straightforward when papilledema is present, but the possibility must be considered even in patients without fundoscopic changes. Formal visual-field testing should be performed even in the absence of overt ophthalmic involvement. Headache on rising in the morning or nocturnal headache is also characteristic of obstructive sleep apnea or poorly controlled hypertension.

Evaluation of patients suspected to have raised CSF pressure requires brain imaging. It is most efficient to obtain an MRI, including an MR venogram as the initial study. If there are no contraindications, the CSF pressure should be measured by LP; this should be done when the patient is symptomatic so that both the pressure and the response to removal of 20–30 mL of CSF can be determined. An elevated opening pressure and improvement in headache following removal of CSF is diagnostic.

Initial treatment is with acetazolamide (250–500 mg bid); the headache may improve within weeks. If ineffective, topiramate is the next treatment of choice; it has many actions that may be useful in this setting, including carbonic anhydrase inhibition, weight loss, and neuronal membrane stabilization, likely mediated via effects on phosphorylation pathways. Severely disabled patients who do not respond to medical treatment require intracranial pressure monitoring and may require shunting.

Post-Traumatic Headache A traumatic event can trigger a headache process that lasts for many months or years after the event. The term *trauma* is used in a very broad sense: headache can develop following an injury to the head, but it can also develop after an infectious episode, typically viral meningitis, a flulike illness, or a parasitic infection. Complaints of dizziness, vertigo, and impaired memory can accompany the headache. Symptoms may remit after several weeks or persist for months and even years after the injury. Typically the neurologic examination is normal and CT or MRI studies are unrevealing. Chronic subdural hematoma may on occasion mimic this disorder. In one series, one-third of patients with NDPH reported headache beginning after a transient flulike illness characterized by fever, neck stiffness, photophobia, and marked malaise. Evaluation reveals no apparent cause for the headache. There is no convincing evidence that persistent Epstein-Barr infection plays a role in this syndrome. A complicating factor is that many patients undergo LP during the acute illness; iatrogenic low CSF volume headache must be considered in these cases. Post-traumatic headache may also be seen after carotid dissection and subarachnoid hemorrhage, and following intracranial surgery. The underlying theme appears to be that a traumatic event involving the pain-producing meninges can trigger a headache process that lasts for many years.

Treatment is largely empirical. Tricyclic antidepressants, notably amitriptyline, and anticonvulsants such as topiramate, valproate, and gabapentin, have been used with reported benefit. The MAOI phenelzine may also be useful in carefully selected patients. The headache usually resolves within 3–5 years, but it can be quite disabling.

Primary NDPH Primary NDPH occurs in both males and females. It can be of the migrainous type, with features of migraine, or it can be featureless, appearing as new-onset TTH (Table 15-11). Migrainous features are common and include unilateral headache and throbbing pain; each feature is present in about one-third of patients. Nausea, photophobia, and/or phonophobia occur in about half of patients. Some patients have a previous history of migraine; however, the proportion of NDPH sufferers with preexisting migraine is no greater than the frequency of migraine in the general population. At 24 months, ~86% of patients are headache-free. Treatment of migrainous-type primary NDPH consists of using the preventive therapies effective in migraine (Table 15-7). Featureless NDPH is one of the primary headache forms most refractory to treatment. Standard preventive therapies can be offered but are often ineffective.

OTHER PRIMARY HEADACHES

Hemicrania Continua The essential features of hemicrania continua are moderate and continuous unilateral pain associated with fluctuations of severe pain; complete resolution of pain with indomethacin; and exacerbations that may be associated with autonomic features, including conjunctival injection, lacrimation, and photophobia on the affected side. The age of onset ranges from 11 to 58 years; women are affected twice as often as men. The cause is unknown.

℞ HEMICRANIA CONTINUA

Treatment consists of indomethacin; other NSAIDs appear to be of little or no benefit. The intramuscular injection of 100 mg indomethacin has been proposed as a diagnostic tool; administration with a placebo injection has been recommended. Alternatively, a trial of oral indomethacin, starting with 25 mg tid, then 50 mg tid, and then 75 mg tid, can be given. Up to 2 weeks may be necessary to assess whether a dose has a useful effect. Topiramate can be helpful in some patients. Occipital nerve stimulation may have a role in patients with hemicrania continua who are unable to tolerate indomethacin.

Primary Stabbing Headache The essential features of primary stabbing headache are stabbing pain confined to the head or, rarely, the face, lasting from 1 to many seconds or minutes and occurring as a single stab or a series of stabs; absence of associated cranial autonomic features; absence of cutaneous triggering of attacks; and a pattern of recurrence at irregular intervals (hours to days). The pains have been variously described as "ice-pick pains" or "jabs and jolts." They are more common in patients with other primary headaches, such as migraine, the TACs, and hemicrania continua.

℞ PRIMARY STABBING HEADACHE

The response of primary stabbing headache to indomethacin (25–50 mg two to three times daily) is usually excellent. As a general rule the symptoms wax and wane, and after a period of control on indomethacin, it is appropriate to withdraw treatment and observe the outcome.

Primary Cough Headache Primary cough headache is a generalized headache that begins suddenly, lasts for several minutes, and is precipitated by coughing; it is preventable by avoiding coughing or other precipitating events, which can include sneezing, straining, laughing, or stooping. In all patients with this syndrome serious etiologies must be excluded before a diagnosis of "benign" primary cough headache can be established. A Chiari malformation or any lesion causing obstruction of CSF pathways or displacing cerebral structures can be the cause of the head pain. Other conditions that can present with cough or exertional headache as the initial symptom include cerebral aneurysm, carotid stenosis, and vertebrobasilar disease. Benign cough headache can resemble benign exertional headache (below), but patients with the former condition are typically older.

Rx PRIMARY COUGH HEADACHE

Indomethacin 25–50 mg two to three times daily is the treatment of choice. Some patients with cough headache obtain pain relief with LP; this is a simple option when compared to prolonged use of indomethacin, and it is effective in about one-third of patients. The mechanism of this response is unclear.

Primary Exertional Headache Primary exertional headache has features resembling both cough headache and migraine. It may be precipitated by any form of exercise; it often has the pulsatile quality of migraine. The pain, which can last from 5 min to 24 h, is bilateral and throbbing at onset; migrainous features may develop in patients susceptible to migraine. Primary exertional headache can be prevented by avoiding excessive exertion, particularly in hot weather or at high altitude.

The mechanism of primary exertional headache is unclear. Acute venous distension likely explains one syndrome, the acute onset of headache with straining and breath holding, as in weightlifter's headache. As exertion can result in headache in a number of serious underlying conditions, these must be considered in patients with exertional headache. Pain from angina may be referred to the head, probably by central connections of vagal afferents, and may present as exertional headache (cardiac cephalgia). The link to exercise is the main clinical clue that headache is of cardiac origin. Pheochromocytoma may occasionally cause exertional headache. Intracranial lesions and stenosis of the carotid arteries are other possible etiologies.

Rx PRIMARY EXERTIONAL HEADACHE

Exercise regimens should begin modestly and progress gradually to higher levels of intensity. Indomethacin at daily doses from 25 to 150 mg is generally effective in benign exertional headache. Indomethacin (50 mg), ergotamine (1 mg orally), dihydroergotamine (2 mg by nasal spray), or methysergide (1–2 mg orally given 30–45 min before exercise) are useful prophylactic measures.

Primary Sex Headache Sex headache is precipitated by sexual excitement. The pain usually begins as a dull bilateral headache which suddenly becomes intense at orgasm. The headache can be prevented or eased by ceasing sexual activity before orgasm. Three types of sex headache are reported: a dull ache in the head and neck that intensifies as sexual excitement increases; a sudden, severe, explosive headache occurring at orgasm; and a postural headache developing after coitus that resembles the headache of low CSF pressure. The latter arises from vigorous sexual activity and is a form of low CSF pressure headache. Headaches developing at the time of orgasm are not always benign; 5–12% of cases of subarachnoid hemorrhage are precipitated by sexual intercourse. Sex headache is reported by men more often than women and may occur at any time during the years of sexual activity. It may develop on several occasions in succession and then not trouble the patient again, even without an obvious change in sexual activity. In patients who stop sexual activity when headache is first noticed, the pain may subside within a period of 5 min to 2 h. In about half of patients, sex headache will subside within 6 months. About half of patients with sex headache have a history of exertional headaches, but there is no excess of cough headache. Migraine is probably more common in patients with sex headache.

Rx PRIMARY SEX HEADACHE

Benign sex headaches recur irregularly and infrequently. Management can often be limited to reassurance and advice about ceasing sexual activity if a mild, warning headache develops. Propranolol can be used to prevent headache that recurs regularly or frequently, but the dosage required varies from 40 to 200 mg/d. An alternative is the calcium channel-blocking agent diltiazem, 60 mg tid. Ergotamine (1 mg) or indomethacin (25–50 mg) taken about 30–45 min prior to sexual activity can also be helpful.

Primary Thunderclap Headache Sudden onset of severe headache may occur in the absence of any known provocation. The differential diagnosis includes the sentinel bleed of an intracranial aneurysm, cervicocephalic arterial dissection, and cerebral venous thrombosis. Headaches of explosive onset may also be caused by the ingestion of sympathomimetic drugs or of tyramine-containing foods in a patient who is taking MAOIs, or they may be a symptom of pheochromocytoma. Whether thunderclap headache can be the presentation of an unruptured cerebral aneurysm is uncertain. When neuroimaging studies and LP exclude subarachnoid hemorrhage, patients with thunderclap headache usually do very well over the long term. In one study of patients whose CT scans and CSF findings were negative, ~15% had recurrent episodes of thunderclap headache, and nearly half subsequently developed migraine or tension-type headache.

The first presentation of any sudden-onset severe headache should be vigorously investigated with neuroimaging (CT or, when possible, MRI with MR angiography) and CSF examination. Formal cerebral angiography should be reserved for those cases in which no primary diagnosis is forthcoming and for clinical situations that are particularly suggestive of intracranial aneurysm. Reversible segmental cerebral vasoconstriction may be seen in primary thunderclap headache without an intracranial aneurysm. In the presence of posterior leukoencephalopathy, the differential diagnosis includes cerebral angiitis, drug toxicity (cyclosporine, intrathecal methotrexate/cytarabine, pseudoephedrine, or cocaine), posttransfusion effects, and postpartum angiopathy. Treatment with nimodipine may be helpful, although by definition the vasoconstriction of primary thunderclap headache resolves spontaneously.

Hypnic Headache This headache syndrome typically begins a few hours after sleep onset. The headaches last from 15 to 30 min and are typically moderately severe and generalized, although they may be unilateral and can be throbbing. Patients may report falling back to sleep only to be awakened by a further attack a few hours later; up to three repetitions of this pattern occur through the night. Daytime naps can also precipitate head pain. Most patients are female, and the onset is usually after age 60. Headaches are bilateral in most, but may be unilateral. Photophobia or phonophobia and nausea are usually absent. The major secondary consideration in this headache type is poorly controlled hypertension; 24-h blood pressure monitoring is recommended to detect this treatable condition.

Rx HYPNIC HEADACHE

Patients with hypnic headache generally respond to a bedtime dose of lithium carbonate (200–600 mg). For those intolerant of lithium, verapamil (160 mg) or methysergide (1–4 mg at bedtime) may be alternative strategies. One to two cups of coffee or caffeine, 60 mg orally, at bedtime may be effective in approximately one-third of patients. Case reports suggest that flunarizine, 5 mg nightly, can be effective.

FURTHER READINGS

COHEN AS et al: Trigeminal autonomic cephalalgias: Current and future treatments. Headache 47:969, 2007

GOADSBY PJ: Is medication-overuse headache a distinct biological entity? Nat Clin Pract Neurol 2:401, 2006

HEADACHE CLASSIFICATION COMMITTEE OF THE INTERNATIONAL HEADACHE SOCIETY: The international classification of headache disorders (second edition). Cephalalgia 24:1, 2004

LANCE JW, GOADSBY PJ: *Mechanism and Management of Headache.* New York, Elsevier, 2005

LEVY M et al: The clinical characteristics of headache in patients with pituitary tumours. Brain 128:1921, 2005

OLESEN J et al: *The Headaches.* Philadelphia, Lippincott, Williams & Wilkins, 2005

16 Back and Neck Pain

John W. Engstrom

The importance of back and neck pain in our society is underscored by the following: (1) the cost of back pain in the United States is ~$100 billion annually, including direct health care expenses plus costs due to loss of productivity; (2) back symptoms are the most common cause of disability in those <45 years; (3) low back pain is the second most common reason for visiting a physician in the United States; and (4) ~1% of the U.S. population is chronically disabled because of back pain.

ANATOMY OF THE SPINE

The anterior portion of the spine consists of cylindrical vertebral bodies separated by intervertebral disks and held together by the anterior and posterior longitudinal ligaments. The intervertebral disks are composed of a central gelatinous nucleus pulposus surrounded by a tough cartilaginous ring, the annulus fibrosis; disks are responsible for 25% of spinal column length (Figs. 16-1 and 16-2). The disks are largest in the cervical and lumbar regions where movements of the spine are greatest. The disks are elastic in youth and allow the bony vertebrae to move easily upon each other. Elasticity is lost with age. The function of the anterior spine is to absorb the shock of body movements such as walking and running.

The posterior portion of the spine consists of the vertebral arches and seven processes. Each arch consists of paired cylindrical pedicles anteriorly and paired laminae posteriorly. The vertebral arch gives rise to two transverse processes laterally, one spinous process posteriorly, plus two superior and two inferior articular facets. The apposition of a superior and inferior facet constitutes a *facet joint.* The functions of the posterior spine are to protect the spinal cord and nerves within the spinal canal and to stabilize the spine by providing sites for the attachment of muscles and ligaments. The contraction of muscles attached to the spinous and transverse processes produces a system of pulleys and levers that results in flexion, extension, and lateral bending movements of the spine.

Nerve root injury (*radiculopathy*) is a common cause of neck, arm, low back, and leg pain (Figs. 25-2 and 25-3). The nerve roots exit at a level above their respective vertebral bodies in the cervical region (the C7 nerve root exits at the C6-C7 level) and below their respective vertebral bodies in the thoracic and lumbar regions (the T1 nerve root exits at the T1-T2 level). The cervical nerve roots follow a short intraspinal course before exiting. By contrast, because the spinal cord ends at the vertebral L1 or L2 level, the lumbar nerve roots follow a long intraspinal course and can be injured anywhere from the upper lumbar spine to their exit at the intervertebral foramen. For example, disk herniation at the L4-L5 level commonly produces compression of the traversing S1 nerve root (Fig. 16-3).

Pain-sensitive structures in the spine include the periosteum of the vertebrae, dura, facet joints, annulus fibrosus of the intervertebral disk, epidural veins, and the posterior longitudinal ligament. Disease of these diverse structures may explain many cases of back pain without nerve root compression. The nucleus pulposus of the intervertebral disk is not pain-sensitive under normal circumstances. Pain sensation is conveyed partially by the sinuvertebral nerve that arises from the spinal nerve at each spine segment and reenters the spinal canal through the intervertebral foramen at the same level. The lumbar and cervical spine possess the greatest potential for movement and injury.

APPROACH TO THE PATIENT: Back Pain

TYPES OF BACK PAIN Understanding the type of pain experienced by the patient is the essential first step. Attention is also focused on identification of risk factors for serious underlying diseases; the majority of these are due to radiculopathy, fracture, tumor, infection, or referred pain from visceral structures (Table 16-1).

Local pain is caused by stretching of pain-sensitive structures that compress or irritate sensory nerve endings. The site of the pain is near the affected part of the back.

Pain referred to the back may arise from abdominal or pelvic viscera. The pain is usually described as primarily abdominal or pelvic but is accompanied by back pain and usually unaffected by posture. The patient may occasionally complain of back pain only.

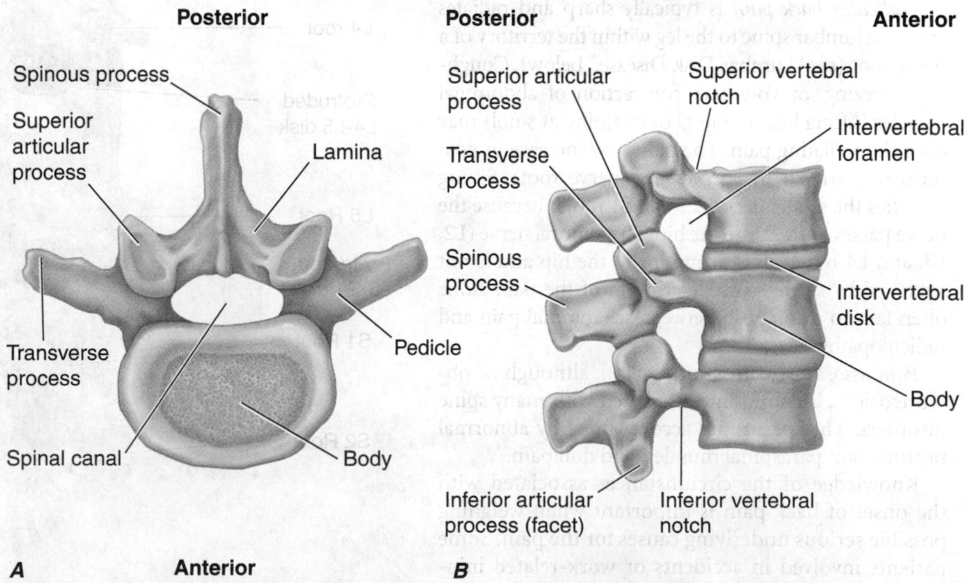

FIGURE 16-1 Vertebral anatomy. *(From A Gauthier Cornuelle, DH Gronefeld: Radiographic Anatomy Positioning. New York, McGraw-Hill, 1998; with permission.)*

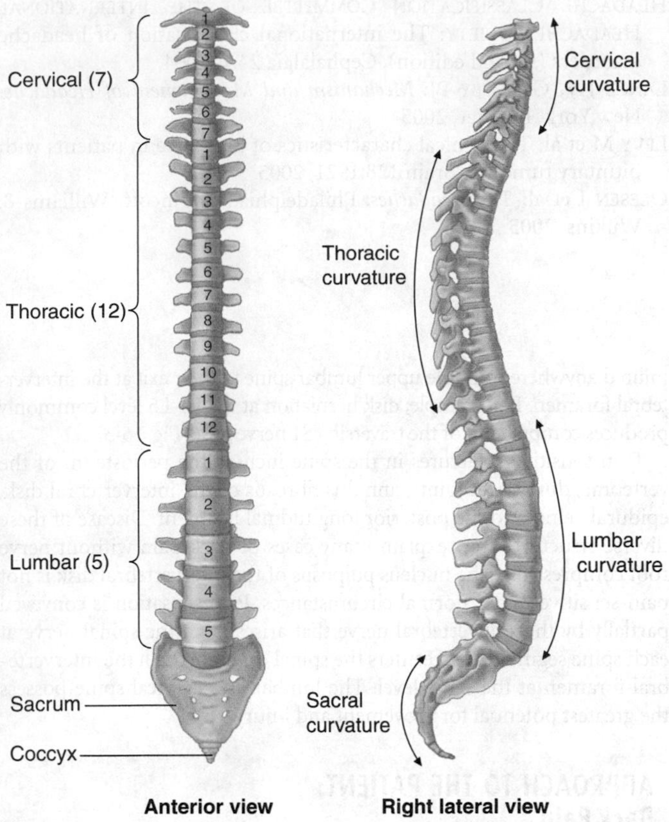

FIGURE 16-2 Spinal column. *(From: A Gauthier Cornuelle, DH Gronefeld: Radiographic Anatomy Positioning. New York, McGraw-Hill, 1998; with permission.)*

Pain of spine origin may be located in the back or referred to the buttocks or legs. Diseases affecting the upper lumbar spine tend to refer pain to the lumbar region, groin, or anterior thighs. Diseases affecting the lower lumbar spine tend to produce pain referred to the buttocks, posterior thighs, or rarely the calves or feet. Provocative injections into pain-sensitive structures of the lumbar spine may produce leg pain that does not follow a dermatomal distribution. This "sclerotomal" pain may explain some cases of back and leg pain without evidence of nerve root compression.

Radicular back pain is typically sharp and radiates from the lumbar spine to the leg within the territory of a nerve root (see "Lumbar Disk Disease," below). Coughing, sneezing, or voluntary contraction of abdominal muscles (lifting heavy objects or straining at stool) may elicit the radiating pain. The pain may increase in postures that stretch the nerves and nerve roots. Sitting stretches the sciatic nerve (L5 and S1 roots) because the nerve passes posterior to the hip. The femoral nerve (L2, L3, and L4 roots) passes anterior to the hip and is not stretched by sitting. The description of the pain alone often fails to distinguish between sclerotomal pain and radiculopathy.

Pain associated with muscle spasm, although of obscure origin, is commonly associated with many spine disorders. The spasms are accompanied by abnormal posture, taut paraspinal muscles, and dull pain.

Knowledge of the circumstances associated with the onset of back pain is important when weighing possible serious underlying causes for the pain. Some patients involved in accidents or work-related injuries may exaggerate their pain for the purpose of compensation or for psychological reasons.

EXAMINATION OF THE BACK A physical examination that includes the abdomen and rectum is advisable. Back pain referred from visceral organs may be reproduced during palpation of the abdomen [pancreatitis, abdominal aortic aneurysm (AAA)] or percussion over the costovertebral angles (pyelonephritis).

The normal spine has cervical and lumbar lordosis, and a thoracic kyphosis. Exaggeration of these normal alignments may result in hyperkyphosis of the thoracic spine or hyperlordosis of the lumbar spine. Inspection may reveal a lateral curvature of the spine (scoliosis) or an asymmetry in the paraspinal muscles, suggesting muscle spasm. Back pain of bony spine origin is often reproduced by palpation or percussion over the spinous process of the affected vertebrae.

Forward bending is often limited by paraspinal muscle spasm; the latter may flatten the usual lumbar lordosis. Flexion of the hips is normal in patients with lumbar spine disease, but flexion of the lumbar spine is limited and sometimes painful. Lateral bending to the side opposite the injured spinal element may stretch the damaged tissues, worsen pain, and limit motion. Hyperextension of the spine (with the patient prone or standing) is limited when nerve root compression, facet joint pathology, or other bony spine disease is present.

Pain from hip disease may mimic pain of lumbar spine disease. Hip pain can be reproduced by internal and external rotation at the hip with the knee and hip in flexion (Patrick sign) and by tapping the heel with the examiner's palm while the leg is extended.

With the patient lying flat, passive flexion of the extended leg at the hip stretches the L5 and S1 nerve roots and the sciatic nerve. Passive dorsiflexion of the foot during the maneuver adds to the stretch. While flexion to at least 80° is normally possible without causing pain, tight hamstring muscles are a source of pain in some patients. The *straight leg–raising (SLR)* test is positive if the maneuver reproduces the patient's usual back or limb pain. Eliciting the SLR sign in the sitting position may help determine if the finding is reproducible. The patient may describe pain in the low back, buttocks, posterior thigh, or lower leg, but the key feature is reproduction of the patient's usual pain. The *crossed*

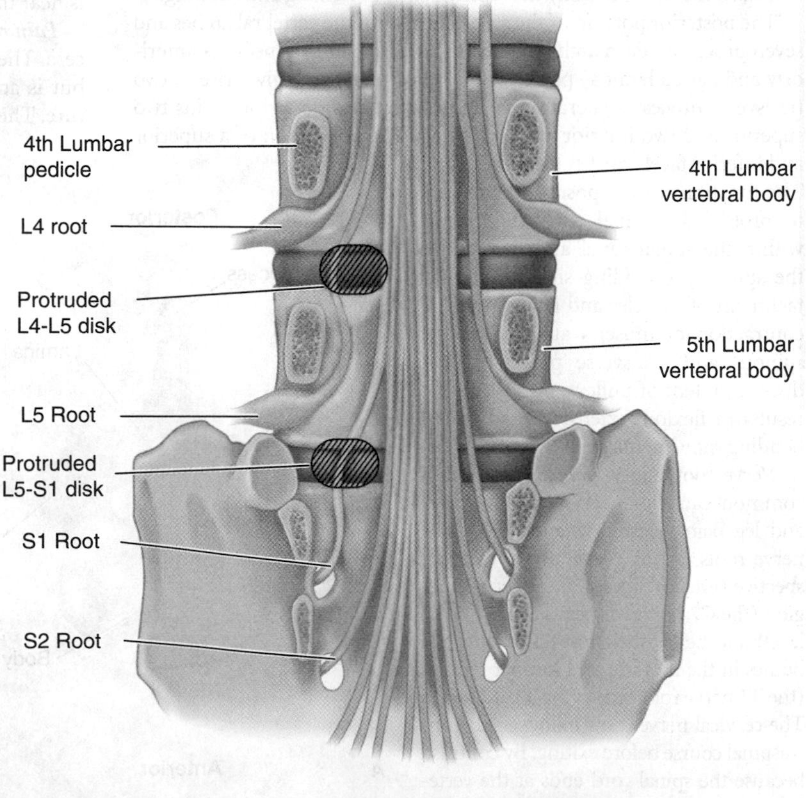

FIGURE 16-3 Compression of L5 and S1 roots by herniated disks. *(From: RD Adams et al: Principles of Neurology, 8th ed. New York, McGraw-Hill, 2005; with permission.)*

TABLE 16-1 ACUTE LOW BACK PAIN: RISK FACTORS FOR AN IMPORTANT STRUCTURAL CAUSE

History
- Pain worse at rest or at night
- Prior history of cancer
- History of chronic infection (esp. lung, urinary tract, skin)
- History of trauma
- Incontinence
- Age > 50 years
- Intravenous drug use
- Glucocorticoid use
- History of a rapidly progressive neurologic deficit

Examination
- Unexplained fever
- Unexplained weight loss
- Percussion tenderness over the spine
- Abdominal, rectal, or pelvic mass
- Patrick's sign or heel percussion sign
- Straight leg or reverse straight-leg raising signs
- Progressive focal neurologic deficit

SLR sign is positive when flexion of one leg reproduces the pain in the opposite leg or buttocks. The crossed SLR sign is less sensitive but more specific for disk herniation than the SLR sign. The nerve or nerve root lesion is always on the side of the pain. The *reverse SLR sign* is elicited by standing the patient next to the examination table and passively extending each leg with the knee fully extended. This maneuver, which stretches the L2-L4 nerve roots and the femoral nerve, is considered positive if the patient's usual back or limb pain is reproduced.

The neurologic examination includes a search for focal weakness or muscle atrophy, focal reflex changes, diminished sensation in the legs, and signs of spinal cord injury. The examiner should be alert to the possibility of breakaway weakness, defined as fluctuating strength during muscle testing. Breakaway weakness may be due to pain or a combination of pain and underlying true weakness. Breakaway weakness without pain is due to lack of effort. In uncertain cases, electromyography (EMG) can determine whether or not true weakness is present. Findings with specific nerve root lesions are shown in Table 16-2 and are discussed below.

LABORATORY, IMAGING, AND EMG STUDIES Routine laboratory studies are rarely needed for the initial evaluation of nonspecific acute (<3 months duration) low back pain (ALBP). If risk factors for a serious underlying cause are present, then laboratory studies [complete blood count (CBC), erythrocyte sedimentation rate (ESR), urinalysis] are indicated.

CT scanning is superior to routine x-rays for the detection of fractures involving posterior spine structures, craniocervical and craniothoracic junctions, C1 and C2 vertebrae, bone fragments within the spinal canal, or malalignment; CT scans are increasingly used as a primary screening modality for moderate to severe trauma. In the absence of risk factors, these imaging studies are rarely helpful in nonspecific ALBP. MRI and CT-myelography are the radiologic tests of choice for evaluation of most serious diseases involving the spine. MRI is superior for the definition of soft tissue structures, whereas CT-myelography provides optimal imaging of the lateral recess of the spinal canal and bony lesions and is tolerated by claustrophobic patients. While the added diagnostic value of modern neuroimaging is significant, there is concern that these studies may be overutilized in patients with ALBP.

Electrodiagnostic studies can be used to assess the functional integrity of the peripheral nervous system (**Chap. e30**). Sensory nerve conduction studies are normal when focal sensory loss is due to nerve root damage because the nerve roots are proximal to the nerve cell bodies in the dorsal root ganglia. The diagnostic yield of needle EMG is higher than that of nerve conduction studies for radiculopathy. Denervation changes in a myotomal (segmental) distribution are detected by sampling multiple muscles supplied by different nerve roots and nerves; the pattern of muscle involvement indicates the nerve root(s) responsible for the injury. Needle EMG provides objective information about motor nerve fiber injury when the clinical evaluation of weakness is limited by pain or poor effort. EMG and nerve conduction studies will be normal when only limb pain or sensory nerve root injury or irritation is present.

TABLE 16-2 LUMBOSACRAL RADICULOPATHY—NEUROLOGIC FEATURES

Lumbosacral Nerve Roots	Examination Findings: Reflex	Sensory	Motor	Pain Distribution
L2[a]	—	Upper anterior thigh	Psoas (hip flexion)	Anterior thigh
L3[a]	—	Lower anterior thigh Anterior knee	Psoas (hip flexion) Quadriceps (knee extension) Thigh adduction	Anterior thigh, knee
L4[a]	Quadriceps (knee)	Medial calf	Quadriceps (knee extension)[b] Thigh adduction Tibialis anterior (foot dorsiflexion)	Knee, medial calf Anterolateral thigh
L5[c]	—	Dorsal surface—foot Lateral calf	Peroneii (foot eversion)[b] Tibialis anterior (foot dorsiflexion) Gluteus medius (hip abduction) Toe dorsiflexors	Lateral calf, dorsal foot, posterolateral thigh, buttocks
S1[c]	Gastrocnemius/soleus (ankle)	Plantar surface—foot Lateral aspect—foot	Gastrocnemius/soleus (foot plantar flexion)[b] Abductor hallucis (toe flexors)[b] Gluteus maximus (hip extension)	Bottom foot, posterior calf, posterior thigh, buttocks

[a]Reverse straight leg–raising sign present—see "Examination of the Back."
[b]These muscles receive the majority of innervation from this root.
[c]Straight leg–raising sign present—see "Examination of the Back."

CAUSES OF BACK PAIN (Table 16-3)

CONGENITAL ANOMALIES OF THE LUMBAR SPINE

Spondylolysis is a bony defect in the pars interarticularis (a segment near the junction of the pedicle with the lamina) of the vertebra; the etiology may be a stress fracture in a congenitally abnormal segment. The defect (usually bilateral) is best visualized on oblique projections in plain x-rays, CT scan, or single photon emission CT (SPECT) bone scan and occurs in the setting of a single injury, repeated minor injuries, or growth. Although frequently asymptomatic, it is the most common cause of persistent low back pain in adolescents and is often activity-related.

Spondylolisthesis is the anterior slippage of the vertebral body, pedicles, and superior articular facets, leaving the posterior elements behind. Spondylolisthesis can be associated with spondylolysis, congenital anomalies of the lumbosacral junction, infection, osteoporosis, tumor, trauma, prior surgery, or degenerative spine disease. It occurs more frequently in women. The slippage may be asymptomatic or may cause low back pain and hamstring tightness, nerve root injury (the L5 root most frequently), or symptomatic spinal stenosis. Tenderness may be elicited near the segment that has "slipped" forward (most often L4 on L5 or occasionally L5 on S1). A "step" may be present on deep palpation of the posterior elements of the segment above the spondylolisthetic joint. The trunk may be shortened and the abdomen protu-

TABLE 16-3 CAUSES OF BACK AND NECK PAIN

Congenital/developmental	Spondylolysis and spondylolisthesis[a]
	Kyphoscoliosis[a]
	Spina bifida occulta[a]
	Tethered spinal cord[a]
Minor trauma	Strain or sprain
	Whiplash injury[b]
Fractures	Traumatic—falls, motor vehicle accidents
	Atraumatic—osteoporosis, neoplastic infiltration, exogenous steroids
Intervertebral disk herniation	
Degenerative	Disk-osteophyte complex
	Internal disk disruption
	Spinal stenosis with neurogenic claudication[a]
	Uncovertebral joint disease[b]
	Atlantoaxial joint disease (e.g., rheumatoid arthritis)[a]
Arthritis	Spondylosis
	Facet or sacroiliac arthropathy
	Autoimmune (e.g., anklyosing spondylitis, Reiter's syndrome)
Neoplasms—metastatic, hematologic, primary bone tumors	
Infection/inflammation	Vertebral osteomyelitis
	Spinal epidural abscess
	Septic disk
	Meningitis
	Lumbar arachnoiditis[a]
Metabolic	Osteoporosis—hyperparathyroidism, immobility
	Osteosclerosis (e.g., Paget's disease)
Vascular	Abdominal aortic aneurysm
	Vertebral artery dissection[b]
Other	Referred pain from visceral disease
	Postural
	Psychiatric, malingering, chronic pain syndromes

[a]Low back pain only.
[b]Neck pain only.

berant as a result of extreme forward displacement of L4 on L5; in severe cases cauda equina syndrome (CES) may occur (see below). Surgery is considered for symptoms persisting for >1 year that do not respond to conservative measures (e.g., rest, physical therapy). Surgery is usually indicated for cases with progressive neurologic deficit, abnormal gait or postural deformity, slippage > 50%, or scoliosis.

Spina bifida occulta is a failure of closure of one or several vertebral arches posteriorly; the meninges and spinal cord are normal. A dimple or small lipoma may overlie the defect. Most cases are asymptomatic and discovered incidentally during evaluation for back pain.

Tethered cord syndrome usually presents as a progressive cauda equina disorder (see below), although myelopathy may also be the initial manifestation. The patient is often a young adult who complains of perineal or perianal pain, sometimes following minor trauma. Neuroimaging studies reveal a low-lying conus (below L1-L2) and a short and thickened filum terminale.

TRAUMA

A patient complaining of back pain and inability to move the legs may have a spinal fracture or dislocation, and, with fractures above L1, spinal cord compression. Care must be taken to avoid further damage to the spinal cord or nerve roots by immobilizing the back pending results of x-rays.

Sprains and Strains The terms *low back sprain, strain,* or *mechanically induced muscle spasm* refer to minor, self-limited injuries associated with lifting a heavy object, a fall, or a sudden deceleration such as in an automobile accident. These terms are used loosely and do not clearly describe a specific anatomic lesion. The pain is usually confined to the lower back, and there is no radiation to the buttocks or legs. Patients with paraspinal muscle spasm often assume unusual postures.

Traumatic Vertebral Fractures Most traumatic fractures of the lumbar vertebral bodies result from injuries producing anterior wedging or compression. With severe trauma, the patient may sustain a fracture-dislocation or a "burst" fracture involving the vertebral body and posterior elements. Traumatic vertebral fractures are caused by falls from a height (a pars interarticularis fracture of the L5 vertebra is common), sudden deceleration in an automobile accident, or direct injury. Neurologic impairment is common, and early surgical treatment is indicated. In victims of blunt trauma, CT scans of the chest, abdomen, or pelvis can be reformatted to detect associated vertebral fractures.

LUMBAR DISK DISEASE

This is a common cause of chronic or recurrent low back and leg pain (Figs. 16-3 and 16-4). Disk disease is most likely to occur at the L4-L5 and L5-S1 levels, but upper lumbar levels are involved occasionally. The cause is often unknown; the risk is increased in overweight individuals. Disk herniation is unusual prior to age 20 and is rare in the fibrotic disks of the elderly. Degeneration of the nucleus pulposus and the annulus fibrosus increases with age and may be asymptomatic or painful. Genetic factors may play a role in predisposing some patients to disk degeneration. The pain may be located in the low back only or referred to the leg, buttock, or hip. A sneeze, cough, or trivial movement may cause the nucleus pulposus to prolapse, pushing the frayed and weakened annulus posteriorly. With severe disk disease, the nucleus may protrude through the annulus (herniation) or become extruded to lie as a free fragment in the spinal canal.

The mechanism by which intervertebral disk injury causes back pain is controversial. The inner annulus fibrosus and nucleus pulposus are normally devoid of innervation. Inflammation and production of proinflammatory cytokines within the protruding or ruptured disk may trigger or perpetuate back pain. Ingrowth of nociceptive (pain) nerve fibers into inner portions of a diseased disk may be responsible for chronic "diskogenic" pain. Nerve root injury (radiculopathy) from disk herniation may be due to compression, inflammation, or both; pathologically, demyelination and axonal loss are usually present.

Symptoms of a ruptured disk include back pain, abnormal posture, limitation of spine motion (particularly flexion), or radicular pain. A dermatomal pattern of sensory loss or a reduced or absent deep ten-

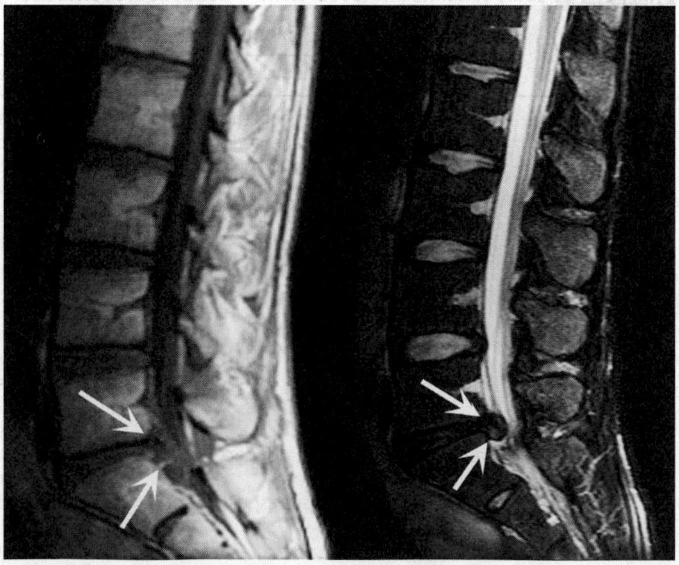

FIGURE 16-4 MRI of lumbar herniated disk; left S1 radiculopathy. Sagittal T1-weighted image on the left with arrows outlining disk margins. Sagittal T2 image on the right reveals a protruding disk at the L5-S1 level (*arrows*), which displaces the central thecal sac.

don reflex is more suggestive of a specific root lesion than is the pattern of pain. Motor findings (focal weakness, muscle atrophy, or fasciculations) occur less frequently than focal sensory or reflex changes. Symptoms and signs are usually unilateral, but bilateral involvement does occur with large central disk herniations that compress multiple descending nerve roots within the spinal canal. Clinical manifestations of specific nerve root lesions are summarized in Table 16-2. There is suggestive evidence that lumbar disk herniation with a nonprogressive nerve root deficit can be managed nonsurgically. The size of the disk protrusion may naturally decrease over time.

The differential diagnosis covers a variety of serious and treatable conditions, including epidural abscess, hematoma, or tumor. Fever, constant pain uninfluenced by position, sphincter abnormalities, or signs of spinal cord disease suggest an etiology other than lumbar disk disease. Bilateral absence of ankle reflexes can be a normal finding in old age or a sign of bilateral S1 radiculopathy. An absent deep tendon reflex or focal sensory loss may indicate injury to a nerve root, but other sites of injury along the nerve must also be considered. For example, an absent knee reflex may be due to a femoral neuropathy or an L4 nerve root injury. A loss of sensation over the foot and lateral lower calf may result from a peroneal or lateral sciatic neuropathy or an L5 nerve root injury. Focal muscle atrophy may reflect a nerve root or peripheral nerve injury, an anterior horn cell disease, or disuse.

An MRI scan or CT-myelogram is necessary to establish the location and type of pathology. Spinal MRI yields exquisite views of intraspinal and adjacent soft tissue anatomy. Bony lesions of the lateral recess or intervertebral foramen are optimally visualized by CT-myelography. The correlation of neuroradiologic findings to symptoms, particularly pain, is not simple. Contrast-enhancing tears in the annulus fibrosus or disk protrusions are widely accepted as common sources of back pain; however, many studies have found that most asymptomatic adults have similar findings. Asymptomatic disk protrusions are also common and may enhance with contrast. Furthermore, in patients with known disk herniation treated either medically or surgically, persistence of the herniation 10 years later had no relationship to the clinical outcome. In summary, MRI findings of disk protrusion, tears in the annulus fibrosus, or contrast enhancement are common incidental findings that, by themselves, should not dictate management decisions for patients with back pain.

There are four indications for intervertebral disk surgery: (1) progressive motor weakness from nerve root injury demonstrated on clinical examination or EMG, (2) bowel or bladder disturbance or other signs of spinal cord compression, (3) incapacitating nerve root pain despite conservative treatment for 4 weeks at a minimum, and (4) recurrent incapacitating pain despite conservative treatment. The latter two criteria are more subjective and less well established than the others. Surgical treatment should also be considered if steady pain and/or neurologic findings do not substantially improve over 4–12 weeks.

The usual surgical procedure is a partial hemilaminectomy with excision of the prolapsed disk. Fusion of the involved lumbar segments should be considered only if significant spinal instability is present (i.e., degenerative spondylolisthesis or isthmic spondylolysis). Over a recent 5-year period, the number of lumbar fusion procedures performed in the United States more than doubled, for uncertain reasons. There are no large prospective, randomized trials comparing fusion to other types of surgical intervention. In one study, patients with persistent low back pain despite an initial diskectomy fared no better with spine fusion than with a conservative regimen of cognitive intervention and exercise.

Cauda equina syndrome (CES) signifies an injury of multiple lumbosacral nerve roots within the spinal canal. Low back pain, weakness and areflexia in the legs, saddle anesthesia, and loss of bladder function may occur. The problem must be distinguished from disorders of the lower spinal cord (conus medullaris syndrome), acute transverse myelitis (Chap. 372), and Guillain-Barré syndrome (Chap. 380). Combined involvement of the conus medullaris and cauda equina can occur. CES is commonly due to a ruptured lumbosacral intervertebral disk, lumbosacral spine fracture, hematoma within the spinal canal (e.g., following lumbar puncture in patients with coagulopathy), compressive tumor, or other mass lesion. Treatment options include surgical decompression, sometimes urgently in an attempt to restore or preserve motor or sphincter function, or radiotherapy for metastatic tumors (Chap. 374).

DEGENERATIVE CONDITIONS

Lumbar spinal stenosis describes a narrowed lumbar spinal canal. *Neurogenic claudication* is the usual symptom, consisting of back and buttock or leg pain induced by walking or standing and relieved by sitting. Symptoms in the legs are usually bilateral. Lumbar stenosis, by itself, is frequently asymptomatic, and the correlation between the severity of symptoms and degree of stenosis of the spinal canal is poor. Unlike vascular claudication, symptoms are often provoked by standing without walking. Unlike lumbar disk disease, symptoms are usually relieved by sitting. Focal weakness, sensory loss, or reflex changes may occur when spinal stenosis is associated with radiculopathy. Severe neurologic deficits, including paralysis and urinary incontinence, occur rarely. Spinal stenosis can be acquired (75%), congenital, or due to a combination of these factors. Congenital forms (achondroplasia, idiopathic) are characterized by short, thick pedicles that produce both spinal canal and lateral recess stenosis. Acquired factors that contribute to spinal stenosis include degenerative diseases (spondylosis, spondylolisthesis, scoliosis), trauma, spine surgery, metabolic or endocrine disorders (epidural lipomatosis, osteoporosis, acromegaly, renal osteodystrophy, hypoparathyroidism), and Paget's disease. MRI provides the best definition of the abnormal anatomy (Fig. 16-5).

Conservative treatment of symptomatic spinal stenosis includes nonsteroidal anti-inflammatory drugs (NSAIDs), exercise programs, and symptomatic treatment of acute pain episodes. Surgical therapy is considered when medical therapy does not relieve symptoms sufficiently to allow for activities of daily living or when significant focal neurologic signs are present. Most patients with neurogenic claudication treated surgically experience at least 75% relief of back and leg pain. Up to 25% develop recurrent stenosis at the same spinal level or an adjacent level 5 years after the initial surgery; recurrent symptoms usually respond to a second surgical decompression.

Facet joint hypertrophy can produce unilateral radicular symptoms or signs due to bony compression; symptoms are often indistinguishable from disk-related radiculopathy. Stretch signs, focal motor weakness, hyporeflexia, or dermatomal sensory loss may be present. Hypertrophic superior or inferior facets can be visualized by x-rays, CT, or MRI. Surgical foraminotomy results in long-term relief of leg and back pain in 80–90% of these patients. The usefulness of therapeutic facet joint blocks for pain has not been rigorously studied.

ARTHRITIS

Spondylosis, or osteoarthritic spine disease, typically occurs in later life and primarily involves the cervical and lumbosacral spine. Patients of-

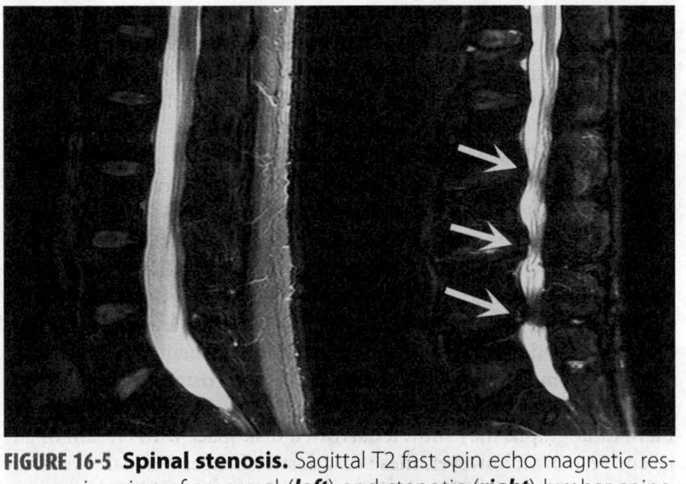

FIGURE 16-5 Spinal stenosis. Sagittal T2 fast spin echo magnetic resonance imaging of a normal (***left***) and stenotic (***right***) lumbar spine, revealing multifocal narrowing (*arrows*) of the cerebrospinal fluid spaces surrounding the nerve roots within the thecal sac.

ten complain of back pain that is increased with movement and associated with stiffness. The relationship between clinical symptoms and radiologic findings is usually not straightforward. Pain may be prominent when x-ray, CT, or MRI findings are minimal, and large osteophytes can be seen in asymptomatic patients. Radiculopathy occurs when hypertrophied facets and osteophytes compress nerve roots in the lateral recess or intervertebral foramen. Osteophytes arising from the vertebral body may cause or contribute to central spinal canal stenosis. Disc degeneration may also play a role in reducing the cross-sectional area of the intervertebral foramen; the descending pedicle may compress the exiting nerve root. Rarely, osteoarthritic changes in the lumbar spine are sufficient to compress the cauda equina.

Ankylosing Spondylitis (See also Chap. 318) This distinctive arthritic spine disease typically presents with the insidious onset of low back and buttock pain. Patients are often males below age 40. Associated features include morning back stiffness, nocturnal pain, pain unrelieved by rest, an elevated ESR, and the histocompatibility antigen HLA-B27. Onset at a young age and back pain improving with exercise are characteristic. Loss of the normal lumbar lordosis and exaggeration of thoracic kyphosis develop as the disease progresses. Inflammation and erosion of the outer fibers of the annulus fibrosus at the point of contact with the vertebral body are followed by ossification and bony growth that bridges adjacent vertebral bodies and reduces spine mobility in all planes. Radiologic hallmarks are periarticular destructive changes, sclerosis of the sacroiliac joints, and bridging of vertebral bodies to produce the fused "bamboo spine."

Stress fractures through the spontaneously ankylosed posterior bony elements of the rigid, osteoporotic spine may produce focal pain, spinal instability, spinal cord compression, or CES. Atlantoaxial subluxation with spinal cord compression occasionally occurs. Ankylosis of the ribs to the spine and a decrease in the height of the thoracic spine may compromise respiratory function. For many patients, therapy with anti-tumor necrosis factor agents is effective in reducing disease activity. Similar to ankylosing spondylitis, restricted movements may accompany Reiter's syndrome, psoriatic arthritis, and chronic inflammatory bowel disease.

NEOPLASMS

(See also Chap. 374) Back pain is the most common neurologic symptom in patients with systemic cancer and may be the presenting symptom. The cause is usually vertebral metastases. Metastatic carcinoma (breast, lung, prostate, thyroid, kidney, gastrointestinal tract), multiple myeloma, and non-Hodgkin's and Hodgkin's lymphomas frequently involve the spine. Cancer-related back pain tends to be constant, dull, unrelieved by rest, and worse at night. By contrast, mechanical low back pain usually improves with rest. Plain x-rays may or may not show destructive lesions in one or several vertebral bodies without disk space involvement. MRI, CT, and CT-myelography are the studies of choice when spinal metastasis is suspected. MRI is preferred, but the most rapidly available procedure is best because the patient's condition may worsen quickly. Fewer than 5% of patients who are nonambulatory at the time of diagnosis ever regain the ability to walk, thus early diagnosis is crucial.

INFECTIONS/INFLAMMATION

Vertebral osteomyelitis is usually caused by staphylococci, but other bacteria or tuberculosis (Pott's disease) may be responsible. The primary source of infection is usually the urinary tract, skin, or lungs. Intravenous drug use is a well-recognized risk factor. Whenever pyogenic osteomyelitis is found, the possibility of bacterial endocarditis should be considered. Back pain exacerbated by motion and unrelieved by rest, spine tenderness over the involved spine segment, and an elevated ESR are the most common findings in vertebral osteomyelitis. Fever or an elevated white blood cell count is found in a minority of patients. Plain radiographs may show a narrowed disk space with erosion of adjacent vertebrae; however, these diagnostic changes may take weeks or months to appear. MRI and CT are sensitive and specific for osteomyelitis; CT may be more readily available in emergency settings and better tolerated by some patients with severe back pain.

Spinal epidural abscess (Chap. 372) presents with back pain (aggravated by movement or palpation) and fever. Signs of nerve root injury or spinal cord compression may be present. The abscess may track over multiple spinal levels and is best delineated by spine MRI.

Lumbar adhesive arachnoiditis with radiculopathy is due to fibrosis following inflammation within the subarachnoid space. The fibrosis results in nerve root adhesions, and presents as back and leg pain associated with motor, sensory, or reflex changes. Causes of arachnoiditis include multiple lumbar operations, chronic spinal infections, spinal cord injury, intrathecal hemorrhage, myelography (rare), intrathecal injection of glucocorticoids or anesthetics, and foreign bodies. The MRI shows clumped nerve roots located centrally or adherent to the dura peripherally, or loculations of cerebrospinal fluid within the thecal sac. Clumped nerve roots may also occur with demyelinating polyneuropathy or neoplastic infiltration. Treatment is usually unsatisfactory. Microsurgical lysis of adhesions, dorsal rhizotomy, and dorsal root ganglionectomy have been tried, but outcomes have been poor. Dorsal column stimulation for pain relief has produced varying results. Epidural injections of glucocorticoids have been of limited value.

METABOLIC CAUSES

Osteoporosis and Osteosclerosis Immobilization or underlying conditions such as osteomalacia, hyperparathyroidism, hyperthyroidism, multiple myeloma, metastatic carcinoma, or glucocorticoid use may accelerate osteoporosis and weaken the vertebral body, leading to compression fractures and pain. The most common causes of nontraumatic vertebral body fractures are postmenopausal (type 1) or senile (type 2) osteoporosis (Chap. 348). Compression fractures occur in up to half of patients with severe osteoporosis, and those who sustain a fracture have a 4.5-fold increased risk for recurrence. The sole manifestation of a compression fracture may be localized back pain or radicular pain exacerbated by movement and often reproduced by palpation over the spinous process of the affected vertebra. The clinical context, neurologic signs, and x-ray appearance of the spine establish the diagnosis. Antiresorptive drugs including bisphosphonates (e.g., alendronate), transdermal estrogen, and tamoxifen have been shown to reduce the risk of osteoporotic fractures. Fewer than one-third of patients with prior compression fractures are adequately treated for osteoporosis despite the increased risk for future fractures; rates of primary prevention among individuals at risk, but without a history of fracture, are even less. Compression fractures above the midthoracic region suggest malignancy; if tumor is suspected, a bone biopsy or diagnostic search for a primary tumor is indicated. **For a complete discussion of diagnosis and management of osteoporosis, see Chap. 348.**

Interventions [percutaneous vertebroplasty (PVP), kyphoplasty] exist for osteoporotic compression fractures associated with debilitating pain. Candidates for PVP have midline back pain, palpation tenderness over the spinous process of the affected vertebral body, <80% loss of vertebral body height, and onset of symptoms within the prior 4 months. The PVP technique consists of injection of polymethylmethacrylate, under fluoroscopic guidance, into the affected vertebral body. Kyphoplasty adds the inflation of a balloon in the vertebral body prior to the injection of cement. Rare complications can include extravasation of cement into the epidural space (resulting in myelopathy) or fatal pulmonary embolism from migration of cement into paraspinal veins. Approximately three-quarters of patients who meet selection criteria have reported enhanced quality of life. Relief of pain following PVP has also been reported in patients with vertebral metastases, myeloma, or hemangiomas.

Osteosclerosis, an abnormally increased bone density often due to Paget's disease, is readily identifiable on routine x-ray studies and may or may not produce back pain. Spinal cord or nerve root compression may result from bony encroachment. **For further discussion of these bone disorders, see Chaps. 347–349.**

REFERRED PAIN FROM VISCERAL DISEASE

Diseases of the thorax, abdomen, or pelvis may refer pain to the posterior portion of the spinal segment that innervates the diseased organ. Occasionally, back pain may be the first and only manifestation. Upper abdominal diseases generally refer pain to the lower thoracic or upper lumbar region (eighth thoracic to the first and second lumbar vertebrae), lower abdominal diseases to the mid-lumbar region (second to fourth lumbar vertebrae), and pelvic diseases to the sacral region. Local signs (pain with spine palpation, paraspinal muscle spasm) are absent, and little or no pain accompanies routine movements of the spine.

Low Thoracic or Lumbar Pain with Abdominal Disease Peptic ulcers or tumors of the posterior wall of the stomach or duodenum typically produce epigastric pain (Chaps. 87 and 287), but midline back or paraspinal pain may occur if retroperitoneal extension is present. Fatty foods are more likely to induce back pain associated with biliary disease. Diseases of the pancreas produce back pain to the right of the spine (head of the pancreas involved) or to the left (body or tail involved). Pathology in retroperitoneal structures (hemorrhage, tumors, pyelonephritis) produces paraspinal pain that radiates to the lower abdomen, groin, or anterior thighs. A mass in the iliopsoas region often produces unilateral lumbar pain with radiation toward the groin, labia, or testicles. The sudden appearance of lumbar pain in a patient receiving anticoagulants suggests retroperitoneal hemorrhage.

Isolated low back pain occurs in 15–20% of patients with a contained rupture of an abdominal aortic aneurysm (AAA). The classic clinical triad of abdominal pain, shock, and back pain occurs in <20% of patients. Two of these three features are present in two-thirds of patients, and hypotension is present in half. The typical patient is an elderly male smoker with back pain. Frequently, the diagnosis is initially missed because the symptoms and signs can be nonspecific. Common misdiagnoses include nonspecific back pain, diverticulitis, renal colic, sepsis, and myocardial infarction. A careful abdominal examination revealing a pulsatile mass (present in 50–75% of patients) is an important physical finding. Patients with suspected AAA should be evaluated with abdominal ultrasound, CT, or MRI (Chap. 242).

Inflammatory bowel disorders (colitis, diverticulitis) or cancers of the colon may produce lower abdominal pain, midlumbar back pain, or both. The pain may have a beltline distribution around the body. A lesion in the transverse or proximal descending colon may refer pain to the mid or left back at the L2-L3 level. Lesions of the sigmoid colon may refer pain to the upper sacral or midline suprapubic regions or left lower quadrant of the abdomen.

Sacral Pain with Gynecologic and Urologic Disease Pelvic organs rarely cause low back pain, except for gynecologic disorders involving the uterosacral ligaments. The pain is referred to the sacral region. Endometriosis or uterine cancers may invade the uterosacral ligaments. Pain associated with endometriosis is typically premenstrual and often continues until it merges with menstrual pain. Uterine malposition may cause uterosacral ligament traction (retroversion, descensus, and prolapse)or produce sacral pain after prolonged standing.

Menstrual pain may be felt in the sacral region. The poorly localized, cramping pain can radiate down the legs. Pain due to neoplastic infiltration of nerves is typically continuous, progressive in severity, and unrelieved by rest at night. Less commonly, radiation therapy of pelvic tumors may produce sacral pain from late radiation necrosis of tissue or nerves. Low back pain that radiates into one or both thighs is common in the last weeks of pregnancy.

Urologic sources of lumbosacral back pain include chronic prostatitis, prostate cancer with spinal metastasis (Chap. 91), and diseases of the kidney and ureter. Lesions of the bladder and testes do not usually produce back pain. Infectious, inflammatory, or neoplastic renal diseases may produce ipsilateral lumbosacral pain, as can renal artery or vein thrombosis. Paraspinal lumbar pain may be a symptom of ureteral obstruction due to nephrolithiasis.

OTHER CAUSES OF BACK PAIN

Postural Back Pain There is a group of patients with nonspecific chronic low back pain (CLBP) in whom no anatomic lesion can be found despite exhaustive investigation. These individuals complain of vague, diffuse back pain with prolonged sitting or standing that is relieved by rest. The physical examination is unrevealing except for "poor posture." Imaging studies and laboratory evaluations do not identify a specific cause. Exercises to strengthen the paraspinal and abdominal muscles are sometimes helpful.

Psychiatric Disease CLBP may be encountered in patients who seek financial compensation; in malingerers; or in those with concurrent substance abuse, chronic anxiety states, or depression. Many patients with CLBP have a history of psychiatric illness (depression, anxiety, substance abuse) or childhood trauma (physical or sexual abuse) that antedates the onset of back pain. Preoperative psychological assessment has been used to exclude patients with marked psychological impairments that predict a poor surgical outcome.

Unidentified The cause of low back pain occasionally remains unclear. Some patients have had multiple operations for disk disease but have persistent pain and disability. The original indications for surgery may have been questionable, with back pain only, no definite neurologic signs, or a minor disk bulge noted on CT or MRI. Scoring systems based upon neurologic signs, psychological factors, physiologic studies, and imaging studies have been devised to minimize the likelihood of unsuccessful surgery.

Rx BACK PAIN

ACUTE LOW BACK PAIN (ALBP) ALBP is defined as pain of <3 months' duration. Full recovery can be expected in 85% of adults with ALBP without leg pain. Most have purely "mechanical" symptoms (i.e., pain that is aggravated by motion and relieved by rest).

Observational studies have been used to justify a minimalist approach to this problem. These studies share a number of limitations: (1) a true placebo control group is often lacking; (2) patients who consult different provider groups (generalists, orthopedists, neurologists) are assumed to have similar etiologies for their back pain; (3) no information is provided about the details of treatment; and (4) no attempt to tabulate structural causes of ALBP is made.

The algorithms for the treatment of back pain **(Fig. 16-6)** draw from published clinical practice guidelines (CPGs). However, since CPGs are based on incomplete evidence, guidelines should not substitute for clinical judgment.

The initial assessment excludes serious causes of spine pathology that require urgent intervention, including infection, cancer, and trauma. Risk factors for a serious cause of ALBP are shown in Table 16-1. Laboratory studies are unnecessary if risk factors are absent. Plain spine films or CT are rarely indicated in the first month of symptoms unless a spine fracture is suspected.

Clinical trials have shown no benefit of >2 days of bed rest for uncomplicated ALBP. There is evidence that bed rest is also ineffective for patients with sciatica or for acute back pain with signs of nerve root injury. Similarly, traction is not effective for ALBP. Possible advantages of early ambulation for ALBP include maintenance of cardiovascular conditioning, improved disk and cartilage nutrition, improved bone and muscle strength, and increased endorphin levels. One trial of early vigorous exercise was negative, but the value of less vigorous exercise or other exercise programs are unknown. Early resumption of normal physical activity (without heavy manual labor) is likely to be beneficial.

Proof is lacking to support the treatment of acute back and neck pain with acupuncture, transcutaneous electrical nerve stimulation, massage, ultrasound, diathermy, magnets, or electrical stimulation. Cervical collars can be modestly helpful by limiting spontaneous and reflex neck movements that exacerbate pain. Evidence regarding the efficacy of ice is lacking; heat may provide a short-term reduction in pain and disability. These interventions are optional given the lack of negative evidence, low cost, and low risk. Biofeedback has not been studied rigorously. Facet joint, trigger point, and ligament injections are not recommended for acute treatment.

A role for modification of posture has not been validated by rigorous clinical studies. As a practical matter, temporary suspension of activity known to increase mechanical stress on the spine (heavy lifting, prolonged sitting, bending or twisting, straining at stool) may be helpful.

Education is an important part of treatment. Satisfaction and the likelihood of follow-up increase when patients are educated about prognosis,

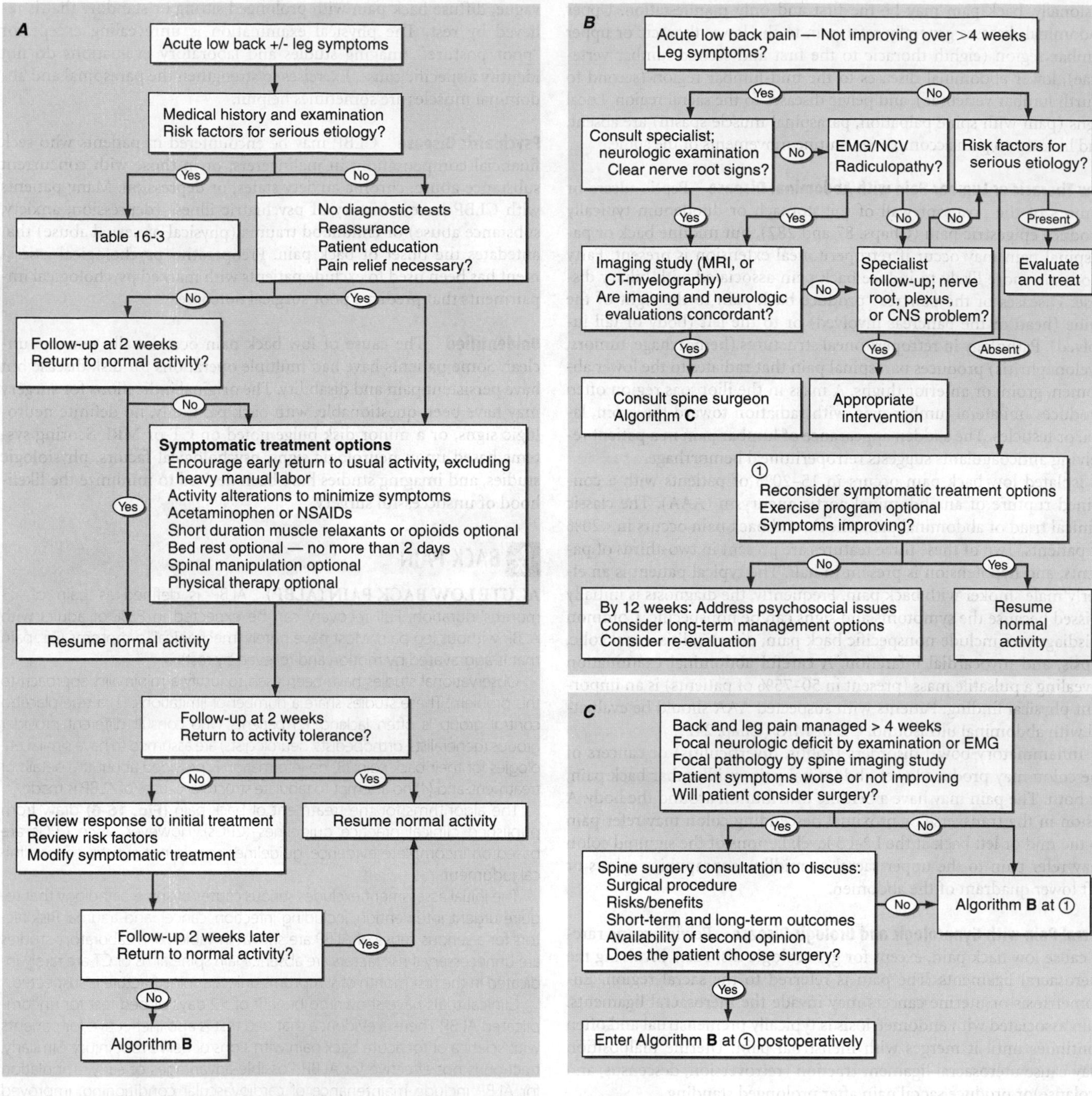

FIGURE 16-6 Algorithms for management of acute low back pain, age ≥ 18 years. ***A.*** Symptoms <3 months, first 4 weeks. ***B.*** Management weeks 4–12. ①, entry point from Algorithm *C* postoperatively or if patient declines surgery. ***C.*** Surgical options. (NSAIDs, nonsteroidal anti-inflammatory drugs; CBC, complete blood count; ESR, erythrocyte sedimentation rate; UA, urinalysis; EMG, electromyography; NCV, nerve conduction velocity studies; MRI, magnetic resonance imaging; CT, computed tomography; CNS, central nervous system.)

treatment methods, activity modifications, and strategies to prevent future exacerbations. In one study, patients who felt they did not receive an adequate explanation for their symptoms wanted further diagnostic tests. Evidence for the efficacy of structured education programs ("back school") is inconclusive; there is modest evidence for a short-term benefit, but evidence for a long-term benefit is lacking. Randomized studies of back school for primary prevention of low back injury and pain have failed to demonstrate any benefit.

NSAIDs and acetaminophen (see Table 12-1) are effective over-the-counter agents for ALBP. Muscle relaxants (cyclobenzaprine, 10 mg PO qhs as initial dose, up to 10 mg PO tid) provide short-term (4–7 days) benefit, particularly at night if sleep is affected, but drowsiness limits daytime use. Opioid analgesics are no more effective than NSAIDs or acetaminophen for initial treatment of ALBP, nor do they increase the likelihood of return to work. Short-term use of opioids may be necessary in patients unresponsive to or intolerant of acetaminophen or NSAIDs. There is no evidence to support the use of oral glucocorticoids or tricyclic antidepressants for ALBP.

Epidural glucocorticoids may occasionally produce short-term pain relief in ALBP with radiculopathy, but proof is lacking for pain relief beyond 1 month. Epidural glucocorticoids, anesthetics, or opioids are not indicated in the initial treatment of ALBP without radiculopathy. Diagnostic nerve root blocks have been advocated to determine if pain originates from a specific nerve root. However, improvement may result even when the nerve root is not responsible for the pain; this may occur as a placebo effect, from a pain-generating lesion located distally along the peripheral nerve, or from anesthesia of the sinuvertebral nerve. Therapeutic nerve root blocks with injection of glucocorticoids and a local anesthetic should be considered only after conservative measures fail, particularly when temporary relief of pain is necessary.

A short course of lumbar spinal manipulation or physical therapy (PT) for symptomatic relief of uncomplicated ALBP is a reasonable option. Prospective,

TABLE 16-4 CERVICAL RADICULOPATHY—NEUROLOGIC FEATURES

Cervical Nerve Roots	Examination Findings			
	Reflex	Sensory	Motor	Pain Distribution
C5	Biceps	Over lateral deltoid	Supraspinatus[a] (initial arm abduction) Infraspinatus[a] (arm external rotation) Deltoid[a] (arm abduction) Biceps (arm flexion)	Lateral arm, medial scapula
C6	Biceps	Thumb, index fingers Radial hand/forearm	Biceps (arm flexion) Pronator teres (internal forearm rotation)	Lateral forearm, thumb, index finger
C7	Triceps	Middle fingers Dorsum forearm	Triceps[a] (arm extension) Wrist extensors[a] Extensor digitorum[a] (finger extension)	Posterior arm, dorsal forearm, lateral hand
C8	Finger flexors	Little finger Medial hand and forearm	Abductor pollicis brevis (abduction D1) First dorsal interosseous (abduction D2) Abductor digiti minimi (abduction D5)	4th and 5th fingers, medial forearm
T1	Finger flexors	Axilla and medial arm	Abductor pollicis brevis (abduction D1) First dorsal interosseous (abduction D2) Abductor digiti minimi (abduction D5)	Medial arm, axilla

[a]These muscles receive the majority of innervation from this root.

randomized studies are difficult to perform in part because there is no consensus about what constitutes an adequate placebo control. Specific PT or chiropractic protocols that may provide benefit have not been fully defined.

CHRONIC LOW BACK PAIN CLBP, defined as pain lasting >12 weeks, accounts for 50% of total back pain costs. Risk factors include obesity, female gender, older age, prior history of back pain, restricted spinal mobility, pain radiating into a leg, high levels of psychological distress, poor self-rated health, minimal physical activity, smoking, job dissatisfaction, and widespread pain. Combinations of these premorbid factors have been used to predict which individuals with ALBP are likely to develop CLBP. The initial approach to these patients is similar to that for ALBP. Treatment of this heterogeneous group of patients is directed toward the underlying cause when known; the ultimate goal is to restore function to the maximum extent possible.

Many conditions that produce CLBP can be identified by a combination of neuroimaging and electrophysiologic studies. Spine MRI and CT-myelography are almost always the imaging techniques of choice. Imaging studies should be performed only in circumstances when the results are likely to influence management.

Injection studies can be used diagnostically to help determine the anatomic source of back pain. Reproduction of the patient's typical pain with diskography has been used as evidence that a specific disk is the pain generator. Pain relief following a foraminal nerve root block or glucocorticoid injection into a facet has been similarly used as evidence that the facet joint or nerve root is the source. However, the possibility that the injection response was a placebo effect or due to systemic absorption of the glucocorticoids is usually not considered. The value of these procedures in the treatment of CLBP or in the selection of candidates for surgery is largely unknown despite their widespread use. The value of thermography in the assessment of radiculopathy also has not been rigorously studied.

The diagnosis of nerve root injury is most secure when the history, examination, results of imaging studies, and the EMG are concordant. The correlation between CT and EMG for localization of nerve root injury is between 65 and 73%. Up to one-third of asymptomatic adults have a disk protrusion detected by CT or MRI scans. Thus, surgical intervention based solely upon radiologic findings increases the likelihood of an unsuccessful outcome.

An unblinded study in patients with chronic sciatica found that surgery could hasten relief of symptoms by ~2 months; however, at 1 year there was no advantage of surgery over conservative medical therapy, and nearly all patients (95%) in both groups made a full recovery regardless of the treatment approach.

CLBP can be treated with a variety of conservative measures. Acute and subacute exacerbations are managed with NSAIDs and comfort measures. There is no good evidence to suggest that one NSAID is more effective than another. Bed rest should not exceed 2 days. Activity tolerance is the primary goal, while pain relief is secondary. Exercise programs can reverse atrophy in paraspinal muscles and strengthen extensors of the trunk. Intensive physical exercise or "work hardening" regimens (under the guidance of a physical therapist) have been effective in returning some patients to work, improving walking distances, and diminishing pain. The benefit can be sustained with home exercise regimens. It is difficult to endorse one specific exercise or PT regimen given the heterogeneous nature of this patient group. The role of manipulation, back school, or epidural steroid injections in the treatment of CLBP is unproven. There is no strong evidence to support the use of acupuncture or traction. A reduction in sick leave days, long-term health care utilization, and pension expenditures may offset the initial expense of multidisciplinary treatment programs. Studies of hydrotherapy for CLBP have yielded mixed results; however, given its low risk and cost, hydrotherapy can be considered as a treatment option. Transcutaneous electrical nerve stimulation (TENS) has not been adequately studied in CLBP.

PAIN IN THE NECK AND SHOULDER (Table 16-4)

Neck pain, which usually arises from diseases of the cervical spine and soft tissues of the neck, is common (4.6% of adults in one study). Neck pain arising from the cervical spine is typically precipitated by movement and may be accompanied by focal tenderness and limitation of motion. Pain arising from the brachial plexus, shoulder, or peripheral nerves can be confused with cervical spine disease, but the history and examination usually identify a more distal origin for the pain. Cervical spine trauma, disk disease, or spondylosis may be asymptomatic or painful and can produce a myelopathy, radiculopathy, or both. The nerve roots most commonly affected are C7 and C6.

TRAUMA TO THE CERVICAL SPINE

Trauma to the cervical spine (fractures, subluxation) places the spinal cord at risk for compression. Motor vehicle accidents, violent crimes, or falls account for 87% of spinal cord injuries (Chap. 372). Immediate immobilization of the neck is essential to minimize further spinal cord injury from movement of unstable cervical spine segments. A CT scan is the diagnostic procedure of choice for detection of acute fractures. Following major trauma to the cervical spine, injury to the vertebral arteries is common; most lesions are asymptomatic and can be visualized by MRI and angiography.

Whiplash injury is due to trauma (usually automobile accidents) causing cervical musculoligamental sprain or strain due to hyperflexion or hyperextension. This diagnosis should not be applied to patients with fractures, disk herniation, head injury, focal neurologic findings, or altered consciousness. Imaging of the cervical spine is not cost-effective acutely but is useful to detect disk herniations when symptoms persist for >6 weeks following the injury. Severe initial symptoms have been associated with a poor long-term outcome.

CERVICAL DISK DISEASE

Herniation of a lower cervical disk is a common cause of neck, shoulder, arm, or hand pain or tingling. Neck pain, stiffness, and a range of motion limited by pain are the usual manifestations. A herniated cervical disk is responsible for ~25% of cervical radiculopathies. Extension and lateral rotation of the neck narrows the ipsilateral intervertebral foramen and may reproduce radicular symptoms (Spurling's sign). In young persons, acute nerve root compression from a ruptured cervical disk is often due to trauma. Cervical disk herniations are usually posterolateral near the lateral recess and intervertebral foramen. Typical patterns of reflex, sensory, and motor changes that accompany specific cervical nerve root lesions are summarized in Table 16-4; however, (1) overlap in function between adjacent nerve roots is common, (2) symptoms and signs may be evident in only part of the injured nerve root territory, and (3) the location of pain is the most variable of the clinical features.

CERVICAL SPONDYLOSIS

Osteoarthritis of the cervical spine may produce neck pain that radiates into the back of the head, shoulders, or arms, or may be the source of headaches in the posterior occipital region (supplied by the C2-C4 nerve roots). Osteophytes, disk protrusions, and hypertrophic facet or uncovertebral joints may compress one or several nerve roots at the intervertebral foramina (Fig. 16-7); this compression accounts for 75% of cervical radiculopathies. The roots most commonly affected are C7 and C6. Narrowing of the spinal canal by osteophytes, ossification of the posterior longitudinal ligament (OPLL), or a large central disk may compress the cervical spinal cord. Combinations of radiculopathy and myelopathy may also be present. Spinal cord involvement is suggested by Lhermitt's symptom, an electrical sensation elicited by neck flexion and radiating down the spine from the neck. When little or no neck pain accompanies cord compression, the diagnosis may be confused with amyotrophic lateral sclerosis (Chap. 369), multiple sclerosis (Chap. 375), spinal cord tumors, or syringomyelia (Chap. 372). The possibility of cervical spondylosis should be considered even when the patient presents with symptoms or signs in the legs only. MRI is the study of choice to define the anatomic abnormalities, but plain CT is adequate to assess bony spurs, foraminal narrowing, or OPLL. EMG and nerve conduction studies can localize and assess the severity of the nerve root injury.

OTHER CAUSES OF NECK PAIN

Rheumatoid arthritis (RA) (Chap. 314) of the cervical apophyseal joints produces neck pain, stiffness, and limitation of motion. In advanced RA, synovitis of the atlantoaxial joint (C1-C2; Fig. 16-2) may damage the transverse ligament of the atlas, producing forward displacement of the atlas on the axis (atlantoaxial subluxation). Radiologic evidence of atlantoaxial subluxation occurs in 30% of patients with RA. Not surprisingly, the degree of subluxation correlates with the severity of erosive disease. When subluxation is present, careful assessment is important to identify early signs of myelopathy. Occasional patients develop high spinal cord compression leading to quadriparesis, respiratory insufficiency, and death. Surgery should be considered when myelopathy or spinal instability is present.

Ankylosing spondylitis can cause neck pain and less commonly atlantoaxial subluxation; surgery may be required to prevent spinal cord compression. Acute *herpes zoster* presents as acute posterior occipital or neck pain prior to the outbreak of vesicles. *Neoplasms* metastatic to the cervical spine, *infections* (osteomyelitis and epidural abscess), and *metabolic bone diseases* may be the cause of neck pain. Neck pain may also be referred from the heart with coronary artery ischemia (cervical angina syndrome).

THORACIC OUTLET

The thoracic outlet contains the first rib, the subclavian artery and vein, the brachial plexus, the clavicle, and the lung apex. Injury to these structures may result in postural or movement-induced pain around the shoulder and supraclavicular region. *True neurogenic thoracic outlet syndrome* (TOS) results from compression of the lower trunk of the brachial plexus or ventral rami of the C8 or T1 nerve roots by an anomalous band of tissue connecting an elongate transverse process at C7 with the first rib. Signs include weakness of intrinsic muscles of the hand and diminished sensation on the palmar aspect of the fourth and fifth digits. EMG and nerve conduction studies confirm the diagnosis. Treatment consists of surgical resection of the anomalous band. The weakness and wasting of intrinsic hand muscles typically does not improve, but surgery halts the insidious progression of weakness. *Arterial TOS* results from compression of the subclavian artery by a cervical rib; the compression results in poststenotic dilatation of the artery and thrombus formation. Blood pressure is reduced in the affected limb, and signs of emboli may be present in the hand. Neurologic signs are absent. Ultrasound can confirm the diagnosis noninvasively. Treatment is with thrombolysis or anticoagulation (with or without embolectomy) and surgical excision of the cervical rib compressing the subclavian artery or vein. *Disputed TOS* includes a large number of patients with chronic arm and shoulder pain of unclear cause. The lack of sensitive and specific findings on physical examination or laboratory markers for this condition frequently results in diagnostic uncertainty. The role of surgery in disputed TOS is controversial. Multidisciplinary pain management is a conservative approach, although treatment is often unsuccessful.

BRACHIAL PLEXUS AND NERVES

Pain from injury to the brachial plexus or peripheral nerves of the arm can occasionally mimic pain of cervical spine origin. Neoplastic infiltration of the lower trunk of the brachial plexus may produce shoulder pain radiating down the arm, numbness of the fourth and fifth fingers, and weakness of intrinsic hand muscles innervated by the ulnar and median nerves. Postradiation fibrosis (most commonly from treatment of breast cancer) may produce similar findings, although pain is less often present. A Pancoast tumor of the lung (Chap. 85) is another cause and should be considered, especially when a Horner's syndrome is present. *Suprascapular neuropathy* may produce severe shoulder pain, weakness, and wasting of the supraspinatous and infraspinatous muscles. *Acute brachial neuritis* is often confused with radiculopathy; the acute onset of severe shoulder or scapular pain is followed over days to weeks by weakness of the proximal arm and shoulder girdle muscles innervated by the upper brachial plexus. The onset is often preceded by an infection. The suprascapular and long thoracic nerves are most often affected; the latter results in a winged scapula. Brachial neuritis may also present as an isolated paralysis of the diaphragm. Complete recovery occurs in 75% of patients after 2 years and in 89% after 3 years.

Occasional cases of carpal tunnel syndrome produce pain and paresthesias extending into the forearm, arm, and shoulder resembling a

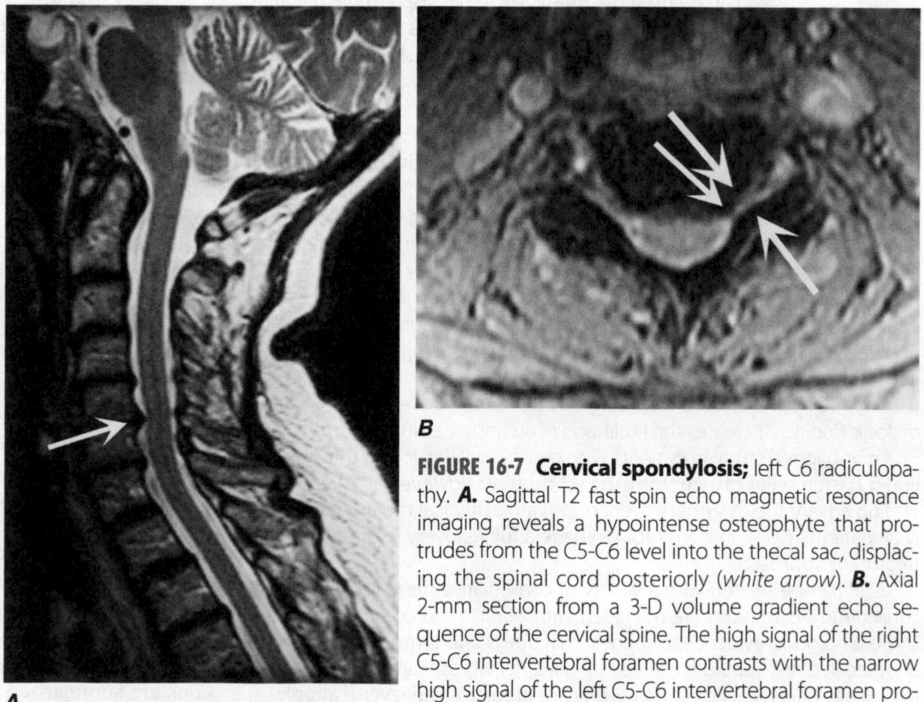

A

B

FIGURE 16-7 Cervical spondylosis; left C6 radiculopathy. ***A.*** Sagittal T2 fast spin echo magnetic resonance imaging reveals a hypointense osteophyte that protrudes from the C5-C6 level into the thecal sac, displacing the spinal cord posteriorly (*white arrow*). ***B.*** Axial 2-mm section from a 3-D volume gradient echo sequence of the cervical spine. The high signal of the right C5-C6 intervertebral foramen contrasts with the narrow high signal of the left C5-C6 intervertebral foramen produced by osteophytic spurring (*arrows*).

C5 or C6 root lesion. Lesions of the radial or ulnar nerve can mimic a radiculopathy at C7 or C8, respectively. EMG and nerve conduction studies can accurately localize lesions to the nerve roots, brachial plexus, or peripheral nerves. **For further discussion of peripheral nerve disorders, see Chap. 379.**

SHOULDER

Pain arising from the shoulder can on occasion mimic pain from the spine. If symptoms and signs of radiculopathy are absent, then the differential diagnosis includes mechanical shoulder pain (tendonitis, bursitis, rotator cuff tear, dislocation, adhesive capsulitis, and cuff impingement under the acromion) and referred pain (subdiaphragmatic irritation, angina, Pancoast tumor). Mechanical pain is often worse at night, associated with local shoulder tenderness and aggravated by abduction, internal rotation, or extension of the arm. Pain from shoulder disease may radiate into the arm or hand, but sensory, motor, and reflex changes are absent.

℞ NECK PAIN

There are few well-designed clinical trials that address optimal treatment of neck pain or cervical radiculopathy. Relief of pain, prevention of recurrence, and improved neurologic function are reasonable goals. Symptomatic treatment includes the use of analgesic medications and/or a soft cervical collar. Most treatment recommendations reflect anecdotal experience, case series, or conclusions derived from studies of the lumbar spine. Controlled studies of oral prednisone or transforaminal glucocorticoid injections have not been performed. Reasonable indications for cervical disk surgery include a progressive radicular motor deficit, pain that fails to respond to conservative management and limits activities of daily living, or cervical spinal cord compression. Surgical management of herniated cervical disks usually consists of an anterior approach with diskectomy followed by anterior interbody fusion. A simple posterior partial laminectomy with diskectomy is an acceptable alternative approach. Another surgical approach involves implantation of an artificial disk; in one prospective trial, outcomes after 2 years favored the implant over a traditional anterior cervical discectomy with fusion. The artificial disk is not yet approved for general use in the United States. The risk of subsequent radiculopathy or myelopathy at cervical segments adjacent to the fusion is ~3% per year and 26% per decade. Although this risk is sometimes portrayed as a late complication of surgery, it may also reflect the natural history of degenerative cervical disk disease.

Nonprogressive cervical radiculopathy due to a herniated cervical disk may be treated conservatively, even if a focal neurologic deficit is present, with a high rate of success. However, if the cervical radiculopathy is due to bony compression from cervical spondylosis, then surgical decompression is generally indicated to forestall the progression of neurologic signs.

Cervical spondylotic myelopathy is typically managed with either anterior decompression and fusion or laminectomy in order to forestall progression of the myelopathy known to occur in 20–30% of untreated patients. However, one prospective study comparing surgery vs. conservative treatment for mild cervical spondylotic myelopathy showed no difference in outcome after 2 years of follow-up.

FURTHER READINGS

ATLAS SJ, NARDIN RA: Evaluation and treatment of low back pain: An evidence-based approach to clinical care. Muscle Nerve 27:265, 2003

BAGLEY LJ: Imaging of spinal trauma. Radiol Clin North Am 44:1, 2006

CASSIDY JD et al: Effect of eliminating compensation for pain and suffering on the outcome of insurance claims for whiplash injury. N Engl J Med 342:1179, 2000

CAVALIER R et al: Spondylolysis and spondylolisthesis in children and adolescents: Diagnosis, natural history, and non-surgical management. J Am Acad Orthop Surg 14:417, 2006

COWAN JA JR et al: Changes in the utilization of spinal fusion in the United States. Neurosurgery 59:1, 2006

GORBACH C et al: Therapeutic efficacy of facet joint blocks. AJR Am J Roentgenol 186:5, 2006

MUMMANENI PV et al: Clinical and radiographic analysis of cervical disk arthroplasty compared with allograft fusion: A randomized controlled clinical trial. J Neurosurg Spine 6:198, 2007

PEUL WC et al: Surgery versus prolonged conservative treatment for sciatica. N Engl J Med 356:2245, 2007

VAN ALFEN N, VAN ENGELEN BG: The clinical spectrum of neuralgic amyotrophy in 246 cases. Brain 129:438, 2006

WEINSTEIN JN et al: Surgical versus nonsurgical treatment for lumbar degenerative spondylolisthesis. N Engl J Med 356:2257, 2007

——— et al: Surgical vs nonoperative treatment for lumbar disc herniation. The spine patient outcomes research trial (SPORT): A randomized trial. JAMA 296:2441, 2006

SECTION 2 ALTERATIONS IN BODY TEMPERATURE

17 Fever and Hyperthermia

Charles A. Dinarello, Reuven Porat

Body temperature is controlled by the hypothalamus. Neurons in both the preoptic anterior hypothalamus and the posterior hypothalamus receive two kinds of signals: one from peripheral nerves that transmit information from warmth/cold receptors in the skin and the other from the temperature of the blood bathing the region. These two types of signals are integrated by the thermoregulatory center of the hypothalamus to maintain normal temperature. In a neutral temperature environment, the metabolic rate of humans produces more heat than is necessary to maintain the core body temperature at 37°C.

A normal body temperature is ordinarily maintained, despite environmental variations, because the hypothalamic thermoregulatory center balances the excess heat production derived from metabolic activity in muscle and the liver with heat dissipation from the skin and lungs. According to studies of healthy individuals 18–40 years of age, the mean oral temperature is 36.8° ± 0.4°C (98.2° ± 0.7°F), with low levels at 6 A.M. and higher levels at 4–6 P.M. The maximum normal oral temperature is 37.2°C (98.9°F) at 6 A.M. and 37.7°C (99.9°F) at 4 P.M.; these values define the 99th percentile for healthy individuals. In light of these studies, *an A.M. temperature of >37.2°C (>98.9°F) or a P.M. temperature of >37.7°C (>99.9°F) would define a fever.* The normal daily temperature variation is typically 0.5°C (0.9°F). However, in some individuals recovering from a febrile illness, this daily variation can be as great as 1.0°C. During a febrile illness, the diurnal variation is usually maintained but at higher, febrile levels. The daily temperature variation appears to be fixed in early childhood; in contrast, elderly individuals can exhibit a reduced ability to develop fever, with only a modest fever even in severe infections.

Rectal temperatures are generally 0.4°C (0.7°F) higher than oral readings. The lower oral readings are probably attributable to mouth breathing, which is a factor in patients with respiratory infections and rapid breathing. Lower-esophageal temperatures closely reflect core temperature. Tympanic membrane (TM) thermometers measure radiant heat from the tympanic membrane and nearby ear canal and display that absolute value (unadjusted mode) or a value automatically calculated from the absolute reading on the basis of nomograms relating the radiant temperature measured to actual core temperatures obtained in clinical studies (adjusted mode). These measurements, although convenient, may be more variable than directly determined oral or rectal values. Studies in adults show that readings are lower with unadjusted-mode than with adjusted-mode TM thermometers and that unadjusted-mode TM values are 0.8°C (1.6°F) lower than rectal temperatures.

In women who menstruate, the A.M. temperature is generally lower in the 2 weeks before ovulation; it then rises by ~0.6°C (1°F) with ovulation and remains at that level until menses occur. Body temperature can be elevated in the postprandial state. Pregnancy and endocrinologic dysfunction also affect body temperature.

FEVER VERSUS HYPERTHERMIA

FEVER

Fever is an elevation of body temperature that exceeds the normal daily variation and occurs *in conjunction with an increase in the hypothalamic set point* (e.g., from 37°C to 39°C). This shift of the set point from "normothermic" to febrile levels very much resembles the resetting of the home thermostat to a higher level in order to raise the ambient temperature in a room. Once the hypothalamic set point is raised, neurons in the vasomotor center are activated and vasoconstriction commences. The individual first notices vasoconstriction in the hands and feet. Shunting of blood away from the periphery to the internal organs essentially decreases heat loss from the skin, and the person feels cold. For most fevers, body temperature increases by 1°–2°C. Shivering, which increases heat production from the muscles, may begin at this time; however, shivering is not required if heat conservation mechanisms raise blood temperature sufficiently. Nonshivering heat production from the liver also contributes to increasing core temperature. In humans, behavioral adjustments (e.g., putting on more clothing or bedding) help raise body temperature by decreasing heat loss.

The processes of heat conservation (vasoconstriction) and heat production (shivering and increased nonshivering thermogenesis) continue until the temperature of the blood bathing the hypothalamic neurons matches the new thermostat setting. Once that point is reached, the hypothalamus maintains the temperature at the febrile level by the same mechanisms of heat balance that function in the afebrile state. When the hypothalamic set point is again reset downward (in response to either a reduction in the concentration of pyrogens or the use of antipyretics), the processes of heat loss through vasodilation and sweating are initiated. Loss of heat by sweating and vasodilation continues until the blood temperature at the hypothalamic level matches the lower setting. Behavioral changes (e.g., removal of clothing) facilitate heat loss.

A fever of >41.5°C (>106.7°F) is called *hyperpyrexia*. This extraordinarily high fever can develop in patients with severe infections but most commonly occurs in patients with central nervous system (CNS) hemorrhages. In the preantibiotic era, fever due to a variety of infectious diseases rarely exceeded 106°F, and there has been speculation that this natural "thermal ceiling" is mediated by neuropeptides functioning as central antipyretics.

In rare cases, the hypothalamic set point is elevated as a result of local trauma, hemorrhage, tumor, or intrinsic hypothalamic malfunction. The term *hypothalamic fever* is sometimes used to describe elevated temperature caused by abnormal hypothalamic function. However, most patients with hypothalamic damage have *sub*normal, not *supra*normal, body temperatures.

HYPERTHERMIA

Although most patients with elevated body temperature have fever, there are circumstances in which elevated temperature represents not fever but hyperthermia (Table 17-1). Hyperthermia is characterized by an uncontrolled increase in body temperature that exceeds the body's ability to lose heat. The setting of the hypothalamic thermoregulatory center is unchanged. In contrast to fever in infections, hyperthermia does not involve pyrogenic molecules (see "Pyrogens," below). Exogenous heat exposure and endogenous heat production are two mechanisms by which hyperthermia can result in dangerously high internal temperatures. Excessive heat production can easily cause hyperthermia despite physiologic and behavioral control of body temperature.

TABLE 17-1 CAUSES OF HYPERTHERMIA SYNDROMES

Heat Stroke
Exertional: Exercise in higher-than-normal heat and/or humidity Nonexertional: Anticholinergics, including antihistamines; antiparkinsonian drugs; diuretics; phenothiazines
Drug-Induced Hyperthermia
Amphetamines, cocaine, phencyclidine (PCP), methylenedioxymethamphetamine (MDMA; "ecstasy"), lysergic acid diethylamide (LSD), salicylates, lithium, anticholinergics, sympathomimetics
Neuroleptic Malignant Syndrome
Phenothiazines; butyrophenones, including haloperidol and bromperidol; fluoxetine; loxapine; tricyclic dibenzodiazepines; metoclopramide; domperidone; thiothixene; molindone; withdrawal of dopaminergic agents
Serotonin Syndrome
Selective serotonin reuptake inhibitors (SSRIs), monoamine oxidase inhibitors (MAOIs), tricyclic antidepressants
Malignant Hyperthermia
Inhalational anesthetics, succinylcholine
Endocrinopathy
Thyrotoxicosis, pheochromocytoma
Central Nervous System Damage
Cerebral hemorrhage, status epilepticus, hypothalamic injury

Source: After FJ Curley, RS Irwin, JM Rippe et al (eds): *Intensive Care Medicine*, 3d ed. Boston, Little, Brown, 1996.

For example, work or exercise in hot environments can produce heat faster than peripheral mechanisms can lose it.

Heat stroke in association with a warm environment may be categorized as exertional or nonexertional. *Exertional heat stroke* typically occurs in individuals exercising at elevated ambient temperatures and/or humidities. In a dry environment and at maximal efficiency, sweating can dissipate ~600 kcal/h, requiring the production of >1 L of sweat. Even in healthy individuals, dehydration or the use of common medications (e.g., over-the-counter antihistamines with anticholinergic side effects) may precipitate exertional heat stroke. *Nonexertional heat stroke* typically occurs in either very young or elderly individuals, particularly during heat waves. According to the Centers for Disease Control and Prevention, there were 7000 deaths attributed to heat injury in the United States from 1979 to 1997. The elderly, the bedridden, persons taking anticholinergic or antiparkinsonian drugs or diuretics, and individuals confined to poorly ventilated and non-air-conditioned environments are most susceptible.

Drug-induced hyperthermia has become increasingly common as a result of the increased use of prescription psychotropic drugs and illicit drugs. Drug-induced hyperthermia may be caused by monoamine oxidase inhibitors (MAOIs), tricyclic antidepressants, and amphetamines and by the illicit use of phencyclidine (PCP), lysergic acid diethylamide (LSD), methylenedioxymethamphetamine (MDMA, "ecstasy"), or cocaine.

Malignant hyperthermia occurs in individuals with an inherited abnormality of skeletal-muscle sarcoplasmic reticulum that causes a rapid increase in intracellular calcium levels in response to halothane and other inhalational anesthetics or to succinylcholine. Elevated temperature, increased muscle metabolism, muscle rigidity, rhabdomyolysis, acidosis, and cardiovascular instability develop within minutes. This rare condition is often fatal. The *neuroleptic malignant syndrome* occurs in the setting of neuroleptic agent use (antipsychotic phenothiazines, haloperidol, prochlorperazine, metoclopramide) or the withdrawal of dopaminergic drugs and is characterized by "lead-pipe" muscle rigidity, extrapyramidal side effects, autonomic dysregulation, and hyperthermia. This disorder appears to be caused by the inhibition of central dopamine receptors in the hypothalamus, which results in increased heat generation and decreased heat dissipation. The *serotonin syndrome*, seen with selective serotonin uptake inhibitors (SSRIs), MAOIs, and other serotonergic medications, has many overlapping features, including hyperthermia, but may be distinguished by the presence of diarrhea, tremor, and myoclonus rather than the lead-pipe rigidity of the neuroleptic malignant syndrome. Thyrotoxicosis and pheochromocytoma can also cause increased thermogenesis.

It is important to distinguish between fever and hyperthermia since hyperthermia can be rapidly fatal and characteristically does not respond to antipyretics. In an emergency situation, however, making this distinction can be difficult. For example, in systemic sepsis, fever (hyperpyrexia) can be rapid in onset, and temperatures can exceed 40.5°C. Hyperthermia is often diagnosed on the basis of the events immediately preceding the elevation of core temperature—e.g., heat exposure or treatment with drugs that interfere with thermoregulation. In patients with heat stroke syndromes and in those taking drugs that block sweating, the skin is hot but dry, whereas in fever the skin can be cold as a consequence of vasoconstriction. Antipyretics do not reduce the elevated temperature in hyperthermia, whereas in fever—and even in hyperpyrexia—adequate doses of either aspirin or acetaminophen usually result in some decrease in body temperature.

PATHOGENESIS OF FEVER

PYROGENS

The term *pyrogen* is used to describe any substance that causes fever. *Exogenous* pyrogens are derived from outside the patient; most are microbial products, microbial toxins, or whole microorganisms. The classic example of an exogenous pyrogen is the lipopolysaccharide (endotoxin) produced by all gram-negative bacteria. Pyrogenic products of gram-positive organisms include the enterotoxins of *Staphylococcus aureus* and the group A and B streptococcal toxins, also called *superantigens*. One staphylococcal toxin of clinical importance is that associated with isolates of *S. aureus* from patients with toxic shock syndrome. These products of staphylococci and streptococci cause fever in experimental animals when injected intravenously at concentrations of 1–10 μg/kg. Endotoxin is a highly pyrogenic molecule in humans: when injected intravenously into volunteers, a dose of 2–3 ng/kg produces fever, leukocytosis, acute-phase proteins, and generalized symptoms of malaise.

PYROGENIC CYTOKINES

Cytokines are small proteins (molecular mass, 10,000–20,000 Da) that regulate immune, inflammatory, and hematopoietic processes. For example, the elevated leukocytosis seen in several infections with an absolute neutrophilia is the result of the cytokines interleukin (IL) 1 and IL-6. Some cytokines also cause fever; formerly referred to as *endogenous pyrogens*, they are now called *pyrogenic cytokines*. The pyrogenic cytokines include IL-1, IL-6, tumor necrosis factor (TNF), ciliary neurotropic factor (CNTF), and interferon (IFN) α. (IL-18, a member of the IL-1 family, does not appear to be a pyrogenic cytokine.) Other pyrogenic cytokines probably exist. Each cytokine is encoded by a separate gene, and each pyrogenic cytokine has been shown to cause fever in laboratory animals and in humans. When injected into humans, IL-1 and TNF produce fever at low doses (10–100 ng/kg); in contrast, for IL-6, a dose of 1–10 μg/kg is required for fever production.

A wide spectrum of bacterial and fungal products induce the synthesis and release of pyrogenic cytokines, as do viruses. However, fever can be a manifestation of disease in the absence of microbial infection. For example, inflammatory processes, trauma, tissue necrosis, or antigen-antibody complexes can induce the production of IL-1, TNF, and/or IL-6, which—individually or in combination—trigger the hypothalamus to raise the set point to febrile levels.

ELEVATION OF THE HYPOTHALAMIC SET POINT BY CYTOKINES

During fever, levels of prostaglandin E_2 (PGE_2) are elevated in hypothalamic tissue and the third cerebral ventricle. The concentrations of PGE_2 are highest near the circumventricular vascular organs (organum vasculosum of lamina terminalis)—networks of enlarged capillaries surrounding the hypothalamic regulatory centers. Destruction of these organs reduces the ability of pyrogens to produce fever. Most studies in animals have failed to show, however, that pyrogenic cytokines pass from the circulation into the brain itself. Thus, it appears that both exogenous and endogenous pyrogens interact with the endothelium of these capillaries and that this interaction is the first step in initiating fever—i.e., in raising the set point to febrile levels.

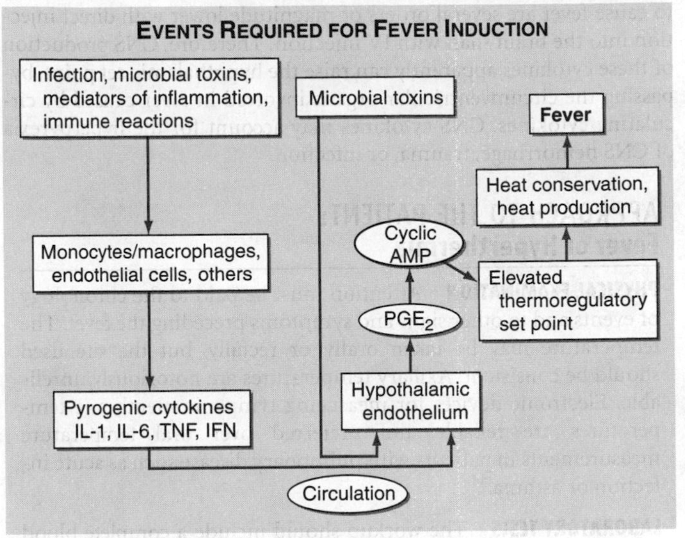

FIGURE 17-1 Chronology of events required for the induction of fever. AMP, adenosine 5′-monophosphate; IFN, interferon; IL, interleukin; PGE_2, prostaglandin E_2; TNF, tumor necrosis factor.

The key events in the production of fever are illustrated in Fig. 17-1. As has been mentioned, several cell types can produce pyrogenic cytokines. Pyrogenic cytokines such as IL-1, IL-6, and TNF are released from the cells and enter the systemic circulation. Although the systemic effects of these circulating cytokines lead to fever by inducing the synthesis of PGE_2, they also induce PGE_2 in peripheral tissues. The increase in PGE_2 in the periphery accounts for the nonspecific myalgias and arthralgias that often accompany fever. It is thought that some systemic PGE_2 escapes destruction by the lung and gains access to the hypothalamus via the internal carotid. However, it is the elevation of PGE_2 in the brain that starts the process of raising the hypothalamic set point for core temperature.

There are four receptors for PGE_2, and each signals the cell in different ways. Of the four receptors, the third (EP-3) is essential for fever: when the gene for this receptor is deleted in mice, no fever follows the injection of IL-1 or endotoxin. Deletion of the other PGE_2 receptor genes leaves the fever mechanism intact. Although PGE_2 is essential for fever, it is not a neurotransmitter. Rather, the release of PGE_2 from the brain side of the hypothalamic endothelium triggers the PGE_2 receptor on glial cells, and this stimulation results in the rapid release of cyclic adenosine 5′-monophosphate (cyclic AMP), which is a neurotransmitter. As shown in Fig. 17-1, the release of cyclic AMP from the glial cells activates neuronal endings from the thermoregulatory center that extend into the area. The elevation of cyclic AMP is thought to account for changes in the hypothalamic set point either directly or indirectly (by inducing the release of neurotransmitters). Distinct receptors for microbial products are located on the hypothalamic endothelium. These receptors are called *Toll-like receptors* and are similar in many ways to IL-1 receptors. The direct activation of Toll-like receptors also results in PGE_2 production and fever.

PRODUCTION OF CYTOKINES IN THE CNS

Several viral diseases produce active infection in the brain. Glial and possibly neuronal cells synthesize IL-1, TNF, and IL-6. CNTF is also synthesized by neural as well as neuronal cells. What role in the production of fever is played by these cytokines produced in the brain itself? In experimental animals, the concentrations of cytokine required to cause fever are several orders of magnitude lower with direct injection into the brain than with IV injection. Therefore, CNS production of these cytokines apparently can raise the hypothalamic set point, bypassing the circumventricular organs involved in fever caused by circulating cytokines. CNS cytokines may account for the hyperpyrexia of CNS hemorrhage, trauma, or infection.

APPROACH TO THE PATIENT: Fever or Hyperthermia

PHYSICAL EXAMINATION Attention must be paid to the chronology of events and to other signs and symptoms preceding the fever. The temperature may be taken orally or rectally, but the site used should be consistent. Axillary temperatures are notoriously unreliable. Electronic devices for measuring tympanic membrane temperatures are reliable and preferred over oral temperature measurements in patients with pulmonary disease such as acute infection or asthma.

LABORATORY TESTS The workup should include a complete blood count; a differential count should be performed manually or with an instrument sensitive to the identification of eosinophils, juvenile or band forms, toxic granulations, and Döhle bodies, the last three of which are suggestive of bacterial infection. Neutropenia may be present with some viral infections.

Measurement of circulating cytokines in patients with fever is of little use since levels of pyrogenic cytokines in the circulation often are below the detection limit of the assay or do not coincide with the fever. Although some studies have shown correlations between circulating IL-6 levels and peak febrile elevations, the most valuable measurements in patients with fever are C-reactive protein level and erythrocyte sedimentation rate. These markers of pathologic processes are particularly helpful in identifying disease in patients with small elevations in body temperature.

FEVER IN RECIPIENTS OF ANTICYTOKINE THERAPY As of this writing, more than 750,000 patients in the United States are receiving chronic anticytokine therapy for Crohn's disease, rheumatoid arthritis, or psoriasis. Does such therapy mask infection by preventing fever? With the increasing use of anticytokines to reduce the activity of IL-1, IL-6, IL-12, and TNF, the effect of these agents on the febrile response must be considered.

The blocking of cytokine activity has the distinct clinical drawback of lowering the level of host defenses against both routine bacterial and opportunistic infections. The opportunistic infections reported in patients given neutralizing antibodies to TNF-α (infliximab or adalimumab) are similar to those reported in the HIV-1-infected population (e.g., new infection with or reactivation of *Mycobacterium tuberculosis*, with dissemination). A soluble receptor for TNF, etanercept, is also associated with opportunistic infections but less so than the neutralizing antibodies.

In nearly all reported cases of infection associated with anticytokine therapy, fever is among the presenting signs. However, the extent to which the febrile response is reduced in these patients remains unknown. Fever in a patient who develops an infection during anticytokine treatment is likely to be due to the direct action of microbial products on the hypothalamic thermoregulatory center, with induction of PGE_2. For example, blocking the activity of IL-1 or TNF during experimental endotoxin-induced fever in volunteers does not affect the febrile response.

Rx FEVER AND HYPERTHERMIA

THE DECISION TO TREAT FEVER Most fevers are associated with self-limited infections, such as common viral diseases. The use of antipyretics is not contraindicated in these infections: there is no significant clinical evidence that antipyretics delay the resolution of viral or bacterial infections, nor is there evidence that fever facilitates recovery from infection or acts as an adjuvant to the immune system. In fact, peripheral PGE_2 production is a potent immunosuppressant. In short, treatment of fever and its symptoms does no harm and does not slow the resolution of common viral and bacterial infections.

However, in bacterial infections, withholding antipyretic therapy can be helpful in evaluating the effectiveness of a particular antibiotic therapy, particularly in the absence of cultural identification of the infecting organism. The routine use of antipyretics can mask an inadequately treated bacterial infection. Withholding antipyretics in some cases may facilitate the diagnosis of an unusual febrile disease. For example, the usual times of peak and trough temperatures may be reversed in typhoid fever and disseminated tuberculosis. Temperature-pulse dissociation (relative bradycardia) occurs in typhoid fever, brucellosis, leptospirosis, some drug-induced fevers, and factitious fever. In newborns, the elderly, patients with chronic renal failure, and patients taking glucocorticoids, fever may not be present despite infection, or core temperature may be hypothermic. Hypothermia is often observed in patients with septic shock.

Some infections have characteristic patterns in which febrile episodes are separated by intervals of normal temperature. For example, *Plasmodium vivax* causes fever every third day, whereas fever occurs every fourth day with *P. malariae*. Other relapsing fevers are related to *Borrelia* infections, with days of fever followed by a several-day afebrile period and then a relapse of days of fever. In the Pel-Ebstein pattern, fever lasting 3–10 days is followed by afebrile periods of 3–10 days; this pattern can be classic for Hodgkin's disease and other lymphomas. In cyclic neutropenia, fevers occur every 21 days and accompany the neutropenia. There is no periodicity of fever in patients with familial Mediterranean fever.

Recurrent fever is documented at some point in most autoimmune diseases and all autoinflammatory diseases. The autoinflammatory diseases include adult and juvenile Still's disease, familial Mediterranean fever, hyper-IgD syndrome, familial cold-induced autoinflammatory syndrome, neonatal-onset multisystem autoinflammatory disease, Blau syndrome, Schnitzler syndrome, Muckle-Wells syndrome, and TNF receptor–associated periodic syndrome. Besides recurrent fevers, neutrophilia and serosal inflammation characterize these diseases. The fevers associated with these illnesses are dramatically reduced by blocking of IL-1β activity. Anticytokines therefore reduce fever in autoimmune and autoinflammatory diseases. Although fevers in autoinflammatory diseases are mediated by IL-1β, patients also respond to antipyretics.

MECHANISMS OF ANTIPYRETIC AGENTS The reduction of fever by lowering of the elevated hypothalamic set point is a direct function of reducing the level of PGE_2 in the thermoregulatory center. The synthesis of PGE_2 depends on the constitutively expressed enzyme cyclooxygenase. The substrate for cyclooxygenase is arachidonic acid released from the cell membrane, and this release is the rate-limiting step in the synthesis of PGE_2. Therefore, inhibitors of cyclooxygenase are potent antipyretics. The antipyretic potency of various drugs is directly correlated with the inhibition of brain cyclooxygenase. Acetaminophen is a poor cyclooxygenase inhibitor in peripheral tissue and lacks noteworthy anti-inflammatory activity; in the brain, however, acetaminophen is oxidized by the p450 cytochrome system, and the oxidized form inhibits cyclooxygenase activity. Moreover, in the brain, the inhibition of another enzyme, COX-3, by acetaminophen may account for the antipyretic effect of this agent. However, COX-3 is not found outside the CNS.

Oral aspirin and acetaminophen are equally effective in reducing fever in humans. Nonsteroidal anti-inflammatory drugs (NSAIDs) such as ibuprofen and specific inhibitors of COX-2 are also excellent antipyretics. Chronic, high-dose therapy with antipyretics such as aspirin or any NSAID does not reduce normal core body temperature. Thus, PGE_2 appears to play no role in normal thermoregulation.

As effective antipyretics, glucocorticoids act at two levels. First, similar to the cyclooxygenase inhibitors, glucocorticoids reduce PGE_2 synthesis by inhibiting the activity of phospholipase A_2, which is needed to release arachidonic acid from the cell membrane. Second, glucocorticoids block the transcription of the mRNA for the pyrogenic cytokines. Limited experimental evidence indicates that ibuprofen and COX-2 inhibitors reduce IL-1-induced IL-6 production and may contribute to the antipyretic activity of NSAIDs.

REGIMENS FOR THE TREATMENT OF FEVER The objectives in treating fever are first to reduce the elevated hypothalamic set point and second to facilitate heat loss. Reducing fever with antipyretics also reduces systemic symptoms of headache, myalgias, and arthralgias.

Oral aspirin and NSAIDs effectively reduce fever but can adversely affect platelets and the gastrointestinal tract. Therefore, acetaminophen is preferred to all of these agents as an antipyretic. In children, acetaminophen must be used because aspirin increases the risk of Reye's syndrome. If the patient cannot take oral antipyretics, parenteral preparations of NSAIDs and rectal suppository preparations of various antipyretics can be used.

Treatment of fever in some patients is highly recommended. Fever increases the demand for oxygen (i.e., for every increase of 1°C over 37°C, there is a 13% increase in oxygen consumption) and can aggravate preexisting cardiac, cerebrovascular, or pulmonary insufficiency. Elevated temperature can induce mental changes in patients with organic brain disease. Children with a history of febrile or nonfebrile seizure should be aggressively treated to reduce fever, although it is unclear what triggers the febrile seizure and there is no correlation between absolute temperature elevation and onset of a febrile seizure in susceptible children.

In hyperpyrexia, the use of cooling blankets facilitates the reduction of temperature; however, cooling blankets should not be used without oral antipyretics. In hyperpyretic patients with CNS disease or trauma, reducing core temperature mitigates the ill effects of high temperature on the brain.

TREATING HYPERTHERMIA A high core temperature in a patient with an appropriate history (e.g., environmental heat exposure or treatment with anticholinergic or neuroleptic drugs, tricyclic antidepressants, succinylcholine, or halothane) along with appropriate clinical findings (dry skin, hallucinations, delirium, pupil dilation, muscle rigidity, and/or elevated levels of creatine phosphokinase) suggests hyperthermia. Attempts to lower the already normal hypothalamic set point are of little use. Physical cooling with sponging, fans, cooling blankets, and even ice baths should be initiated immediately in conjunction with the administration of IV fluids and appropriate pharmacologic agents (see below). If insufficient cooling is achieved by external means, internal cooling can be achieved by gastric or peritoneal lavage with iced saline. In extreme circumstances, hemodialysis or even cardiopulmonary bypass with cooling of blood may be performed.

Malignant hyperthermia should be treated immediately with cessation of anesthesia and IV administration of dantrolene sodium. The recommended dose of dantrolene is 1–2.5 mg/kg given intravenously every 6 h for at least 24–48 h—until oral dantrolene can be administered, if needed. Procainamide should also be administered to patients with malignant hyperthermia because of the likelihood of ventricular fibrillation in this syndrome. Dantrolene at similar doses is indicated in the neuroleptic malignant syndrome and in drug-induced hyperthermia and may even be useful in the hyperthermia of the serotonin syndrome and thyrotoxicosis. The neuroleptic malignant syndrome may also be treated with bromocriptine, levodopa, amantadine, or nifedipine or by induction of muscle paralysis with curare and pancuronium. Tricyclic antidepressant overdose may be treated with physostigmine.

ACKNOWLEDGMENT

The substantial contributions of Jeffrey A. Gelfand to this chapter in previous editions are gratefully acknowledged.

FURTHER READINGS

De Koning HD et al: Beneficial response to anakinra and thalidomide in Schnitzler's syndrome. Ann Rheum Dis 65:542, 2006

Dinarello CA: Infection, fever, and exogenous and endogenous pyrogens: Some concepts have changed. J Endotoxin Res 10:202, 2004

Hawkins PN et al: Spectrum of clinical features in Muckle-Wells syndrome and response to anakinra. Arthritis Rheum 50:607, 2004

Hoffman HM et al: Prevention of cold-associated acute inflammation in familial cold autoinflammatory syndrome by interleukin-1 receptor antagonist. Lancet 364:1779, 2004

Keane J et al: Tuberculosis associated with infliximab, a tumor necrosis factor-α-neutralizing agent. N Engl J Med 345:1098, 2001

Pascual V et al: Role of interleukin-1 (IL-1) in the pathogenesis of systemic onset juvenile idiopathic arthritis and clinical response to IL-1 blockade. J Exp Med 201:1479, 2005

Simon A, van der Meer JW: Pathogenesis of familial periodic fever syndromes or hereditary autoinflammatory syndromes. Am J Physiol Regul Integr Comp Physiol 292:R86, 2007

——— et al: Beneficial response to interleukin-1 receptor antagonist in TRAPS. Am J Med 117:208, 2004

Wallis RS et al: Differential effects of TNF blockers on TB immunity. Ann Rheum Dis 64(Suppl3):132, 2005

——— et al: Granulomatous infectious diseases associated with tumor necrosis factor antagonists. Clin Infect Dis 38:1261, 2004

18 Fever and Rash

Elaine T. Kaye, Kenneth M. Kaye

The acutely ill patient with fever and rash often presents a diagnostic challenge for physicians. The distinctive appearance of an eruption in concert with a clinical syndrome may facilitate a prompt diagnosis and the institution of life-saving therapy or critical infection-control interventions. **Representative images of many of the rashes discussed in this chapter are included in Chap. e5.**

APPROACH TO THE PATIENT: Fever and Rash

A thorough history of patients with fever and rash includes the following relevant information: immune status, medications taken within the previous month, specific travel history, immunization status, exposure to domestic pets and other animals, history of animal (including arthropod) bites, existence of cardiac abnormalities, presence of prosthetic material, recent exposure to ill individuals, and exposure to sexually transmitted diseases. The history should also include the site of onset of the rash and its direction and rate of spread.

A thorough physical examination entails close attention to the rash, with an assessment and precise definition of its salient features. First, it is critical to determine the *type* of lesions that make up the eruption. *Macules* are flat lesions defined by an area of changed color (i.e., a blanchable erythema). *Papules* are raised, solid lesions <5 mm in diameter; *plaques* are lesions >5 mm in diameter with a flat, plateau-like surface; and *nodules* are lesions >5 mm in diameter with a more rounded configuration. *Wheals* (urticaria, hives) are papules or plaques that are pale pink and may appear annular (ringlike) as they enlarge; classic (nonvasculitic) wheals are transient, lasting only 24–48 h in any defined area. *Vesicles* (<5 mm) and *bullae* (>5 mm) are circumscribed, elevated lesions containing fluid. *Pustules* are raised lesions containing purulent exudate; vesicular processes such as varicella or herpes simplex may evolve to pustules. *Nonpalpable purpura* is a flat lesion that is due to bleeding into the skin; if <3 mm in diameter, the purpuric lesions are termed *petechiae*; if >3 mm, they are termed *ecchymoses*. *Palpable purpura* is a raised lesion that is due to inflammation of the vessel wall (vasculitis) with subsequent hemorrhage. An *ulcer* is a defect in the skin extending at least into the upper layer of the dermis, and an *eschar* (tâche noire) is a necrotic lesion covered with a black crust.

Other pertinent features of rashes include their *configuration* (i.e., annular or target), the *arrangement* of their lesions, and their *distribution* (i.e., central or peripheral). **For further discussion, see Chaps. 52, 54, and 115.**

CLASSIFICATION OF RASH

This chapter reviews rashes that reflect systemic disease, but it does not include localized skin eruptions (i.e., cellulitis, impetigo) that may also be associated with fever (Chap. 119). Rashes are classified herein on the basis of the morphology and distribution of lesions. For practical purposes, this classification system is based on the most typical disease presentations. However, morphology may vary as rashes evolve, and the presentation of diseases with rashes is subject to many variations (Chap. 54). For instance, the classic petechial rash of Rocky Mountain spotted fever (RMSF; Chap. 167) may initially consist of blanchable erythematous macules distributed peripherally; at times, the rash associated with RMSF may not be predominantly acral, or a rash may not develop at all.

Diseases with fever and rash may be classified by type of eruption: centrally distributed maculopapular, peripheral, confluent desquamative erythematous, vesiculobullous, urticarial, nodular, purpuric, ulcerated, or eschar (**Table 18-1**). For a more detailed discussion of each disease associated with a rash, the reader is referred to the chapter dealing with that specific disease. (Reference chapters are cited in the text and listed in Table 18-1.)

TABLE 18-1 DISEASES ASSOCIATED WITH FEVER AND RASH

Disease	Etiology	Description	Group Affected/ Epidemiologic Factors	Clinical Syndrome	Chapter
Centrally Distributed Maculopapular Eruptions					
Acute meningococcemia[a]	—	—	—	—	136
Rubeola (measles, first disease)	Paramyxovirus	Discrete lesions that become confluent as rash spreads from hairline downward, sparing palms and soles; lasts ≥3 days; Koplik's spots	Nonimmune individuals	Cough, conjunctivitis, coryza, severe prostration	185
Rubella (German measles, third disease)	Togavirus	Spreads from hairline downward, clearing as it spreads; Forschheimer spots	Nonimmune individuals	Adenopathy, arthritis	186
Erythema infectiosum (fifth disease)	Human parvovirus B19	Bright-red "slapped-cheek" appearance followed by lacy reticular rash that waxes and wanes over 3 weeks; rarely, papular-purpuric "gloves-and-socks" syndrome on hands and feet	Most common in children aged 3–12 years; occurs in winter and spring	Mild fever; arthritis in adults; rash following resolution of fever	177
Exanthem subitum (roseola, sixth disease)	Human herpesvirus 6	Diffuse maculopapular eruption (sparing face); resolves within 2 days	Usually affects children <3 years old	Rash following resolution of fever; similar to Boston exanthem (echovirus 16)	175
Primary HIV infection	HIV	Nonspecific diffuse macules and papules; may be urticarial; oral or genital ulcers in some cases	Individuals recently infected with HIV	Pharyngitis, adenopathy, arthralgias	182
Infectious mononucleosis	Epstein-Barr virus	Diffuse maculopapular eruption (10–15% of cases; 90% if ampicillin is given); urticaria in some cases; periorbital edema (50%); palatal petechiae (25%)	Adolescents, young adults	Hepatosplenomegaly, pharyngitis, cervical lymphadenopathy, atypical lymphocytosis, heterophile antibody	174
Other viral exanthems	Echoviruses 2, 4, 9, 11, 16, 19, and 25; coxsackieviruses A9, B1, and B5; etc.	Skin findings mimicking rubella or measles	Affect children more commonly than adults	Nonspecific viral syndromes	184
Exanthematous drug-induced eruption	Drugs (antibiotics, anticonvulsants, diuretics, etc.)	Intensely pruritic, bright-red macules and papules, symmetric on trunk and extremities; may become confluent	Occurs 2–3 d after exposure in previously sensitized individuals; otherwise, after 2–3 weeks (but can occur anytime, even shortly after drug is discontinued)	Variable findings: fever and eosinophilia	56
Epidemic typhus	*Rickettsia prowazekii*	Maculopapular eruption appearing in axillae, spreading to trunk and later to extremities; usually spares face, palms, soles; evolves from blanchable macules to confluent eruption with petechiae; rash evanescent in recrudescent typhus (Brill-Zinsser disease)	Exposure to body lice; occurrence of recrudescent typhus as relapse after 30–50 years	Headache, myalgias; 10–40% mortality if untreated; milder clinical presentation in recrudescent form	167
Endemic (murine) typhus	*Rickettsia typhi*	Maculopapular eruption, usually sparing palms, soles	Exposure to rat or cat fleas	Headache, myalgias	167
Scrub typhus	*Orientia tsutsugamushi*	Diffuse macular rash starting on trunk; eschar at site of mite bite	Endemic in South Pacific, Australia, Asia; transmitted by mites	Headache, myalgias, regional adenopathy; mortality up to 30% if untreated	167
Rickettsial spotted fevers	*Rickettsia conorii* (boutonneuse fever), *Rickettsia australis* (North Queensland tick typhus), *Rickettsia sibirica* (Siberian tick typhus), and others	Eschar common at bite site; maculopapular (rarely, vesicular and petechial) eruption on proximal extremities, spreading to trunk and face	Exposure to ticks; *R. conorii* in Mediterranean region, India, Africa; *R. australis* in Australia; *R. sibirica* in Siberia, Mongolia	Headache, myalgias, regional adenopathy	167

(continued)

TABLE 18-1 DISEASES ASSOCIATED WITH FEVER AND RASH (CONTINUED)

Disease	Etiology	Description	Group Affected/ Epidemiologic Factors	Clinical Syndrome	Chapter
Human monocytotropic ehrlichiosis[b]	*Ehrlichia chaffeensis*	Maculopapular eruption (40% of cases), involves trunk and extremities; may be petechial	Tick-borne; most common in U.S. Southeast, southern Midwest, and mid-Atlantic regions	Headache, myalgias, leukopenia	167
Leptospirosis	*Leptospira interrogans*	Maculopapular eruption; conjunctivitis; scleral hemorrhage in some cases	Exposure to water contaminated with animal urine	Myalgias; aseptic meningitis; *fulminant form*: icterohemorrhagic fever (Weil's disease)	164
Lyme disease	*Borrelia burgdorferi*	Papule expanding to erythematous annular lesion with central clearing (erythema chronicum migrans or ECM; average diameter, 15 cm), sometimes with concentric rings, sometimes with indurated or vesicular center; multiple secondary ECM lesions in some cases	Bite of tick vector	Headache, myalgias, chills, photophobia occurring acutely; CNS disease, myocardial disease, arthritis weeks to months later in some cases	166
Typhoid fever	*Salmonella typhi*	Transient, blanchable erythematous macules and papules, 2–4 mm, usually on trunk (rose spots)	Ingestion of contaminated food or water (rare in U.S.)	Variable abdominal pain and diarrhea; headache, myalgias, hepatosplenomegaly	146
Dengue fever[c]	Dengue virus (4 serotypes; flaviviruses)	Rash in 50% of cases; initially diffuse flushing; midway through illness, onset of maculopapular rash, which begins on trunk and spreads centrifugally to extremities and face; pruritus, hyperesthesia in some cases; after defervescence, petechiae on extremities in some cases	Occurs in tropics and subtropics; transmitted by mosquito	Headache, musculoskeletal pain ("breakbone fever"); leukopenia; occasionally biphasic ("saddleback") fever	189
Rat-bite fever (sodoku)	*Spirillum minus*	Eschar at bite site; then blotchy violaceous or red-brown rash involving trunk and extremities	Rat bite; primarily found in Asia; rare in U.S.	Regional adenopathy, recurrent fevers if untreated	...
Relapsing fever	*Borrelia* species	Central rash at end of febrile episode; petechiae in some cases	Exposure to ticks or body lice	Recurrent fever, headache, myalgias, hepatosplenomegaly	165
Erythema marginatum (rheumatic fever)	Group A *Streptococcus*	Erythematous annular papules and plaques occurring as polycyclic lesions in waves over trunk, proximal extremities; evolving and resolving within hours	Patients with rheumatic fever	Pharyngitis preceding polyarthritis, carditis, subcutaneous nodules, chorea	315
Systemic lupus erythematosus	Autoimmune disease	Macular and papular erythema, often in sun-exposed areas; discoid lupus lesions (local atrophy, scale, pigmentary changes); periungual telangiectasis; malar rash; vasculitis sometimes causing urticaria, palpable purpura; oral erosions in some cases	Most common in young to middle-aged women; flares precipitated by sun exposure	Arthritis; cardiac, pulmonary, renal, hematologic, and vasculitic disease	313
Still's disease	Autoimmune disease	Transient 2- to 5-mm erythematous papules appearing at height of fever on trunk, proximal extremities; lesions evanescent	Children and young adults	High spiking fever, polyarthritis, splenomegaly; erythrocyte sedimentation rate, >100 mm/h	331
Arcanobacterial pharyngitis	*Arcanobacterium (Corynebacterium) haemolyticum*	Diffuse, erythematous, maculopapular eruption involving trunk and proximal extremities; may desquamate	Children and young adults	Exudative pharyngitis, lymphadenopathy	131
Peripheral Eruptions					
Chronic meningococcemia, disseminated gonococcal infection[a], human parvovirus B19 infection[g]	—	—	—	—	136, 137, 177
Rocky Mountain spotted fever	*Rickettsia rickettsii*	Rash beginning on wrists and ankles and spreading centripetally; appears on palms and soles later in disease; lesion evolution from blanchable macules to petechiae	Tick vector; widespread but more common in southeastern and southwest-central U.S.	Headache, myalgias, abdominal pain; mortality up to 40% if untreated	167

(continued)

TABLE 18-1 DISEASES ASSOCIATED WITH FEVER AND RASH (CONTINUED)

Disease	Etiology	Description	Group Affected/ Epidemiologic Factors	Clinical Syndrome	Chapter
Secondary syphilis	*Treponema pallidum*	Coincident primary chancre in 10% of cases; copper-colored, scaly papular eruption, diffuse but prominent on palms and soles; rash never vesicular in adults; condyloma latum, mucous patches, and alopecia in some cases	Sexually transmitted	Fever, constitutional symptoms	162
Atypical measles	Paramyxovirus	Maculopapular eruption beginning on distal extremities and spreading centripetally; may evolve into vesicles or petechiae; edema of extremities; Koplik's spots absent	Individuals contracting measles who received killed measles vaccine in 1963–1967 in U.S. without subsequent live vaccine	Headache, nodular pneumonia	185
Hand-foot-and-mouth disease	Coxsackievirus A16 most common cause	Tender vesicles, erosions in mouth; 0.25-cm papules on hands and feet with rim of erythema evolving into tender vesicles	Summer and fall; primarily children <10 years old; multiple family members	Transient fever	184
Erythema multiforme	Drugs, infection, idiopathic causes	Target lesions (central erythema surrounded by area of clearing and another rim of erythema) up to 2 cm; symmetric on knees, elbows, palms, soles; may become diffuse; may involve mucosal surfaces; life-threatening in maximal form (Stevens-Johnson syndrome)	Drug intake (i.e., sulfa, phenytoin, penicillin); herpes simplex virus or *Mycoplasma pneumoniae* infection	Varies with predisposing factor	—[d]
Rat-bite fever (Haverhill fever)	*Streptobacillus moniliformis*	Maculopapular eruption over palms, soles, and extremities; tends to be more severe at joints; eruption sometimes becoming generalized; may be purpuric; may desquamate	Rat bite, ingestion of contaminated food	Myalgias; arthritis (50%); fever recurrence in some cases	. . .
Bacterial endocarditis	*Streptococcus, Staphylococcus*, etc.	*Subacute course*: Osler's nodes (tender pink nodules on finger or toe pads); petechiae on skin and mucosa; splinter hemorrhages. *Acute course* (*Staphylococcus aureus*): Janeway lesions (painless erythematous or hemorrhagic macules, usually on palms and soles)	Abnormal heart valve, intravenous drug use	New heart murmur	118
Confluent Desquamative Erythemas					
Scarlet fever (second disease)	Group A *Streptococcus* (pyrogenic exotoxins A, B, C)	Diffuse blanchable erythema beginning on face and spreading to trunk and extremities; circumoral pallor; "sandpaper" texture to skin; accentuation of linear erythema in skin folds (Pastia's lines); enanthem of white evolving into red "strawberry" tongue; desquamation in second week	Most common in children aged 2–10 years; usually follows group A streptococcal pharyngitis	Fever, pharyngitis, headache	130
Kawasaki disease	Idiopathic causes	Rash similar to scarlet fever (scarlatiniform) or erythema multiforme; fissuring of lips, strawberry tongue; conjunctivitis; edema of hands, feet; desquamation later in disease	Children <8 years	Cervical adenopathy, pharyngitis, coronary artery vasculitis	54, 319
Streptococcal toxic shock syndrome	Group A *Streptococcus* (associated with pyrogenic exotoxin A and/or B or certain M types)	When present, rash often scarlatiniform	May occur in setting of severe group A streptococcal infections, such as necrotizing fasciitis, bacteremia, pneumonia	Multiorgan failure, hypotension; 30% mortality rate	130
Staphylococcal toxic shock syndrome	*S. aureus* (toxic shock syndrome toxin 1, enterotoxin B or C)	Diffuse erythema involving palms; pronounced erythema of mucosal surfaces; conjunctivitis; desquamation 7–10 days into illness	Colonization with toxin-producing *S. aureus*	Fever >39°C (102°F), hypotension, multi-organ dysfunction	129
Staphylococcal scalded-skin syndrome	*S. aureus*, phage group II	Diffuse tender erythema, often with bullae and desquamation; Nikolsky's sign	Colonization with toxin-producing *S. aureus*; occurs in children <10 years old (termed "Ritter's disease" in neonates) or adults with renal dysfunction	Irritability; nasal or conjunctival secretions	129

(continued)

TABLE 18-1 DISEASES ASSOCIATED WITH FEVER AND RASH (CONTINUED)

Disease	Etiology	Description	Group Affected/ Epidemiologic Factors	Clinical Syndrome	Chapter
Exfoliative erythroderma syndrome	Underlying psoriasis, eczema, drug eruption, mycosis fungoides	Diffuse erythema (often scaling) interspersed with lesions of underlying condition	Usually occurs in adults over age 50; more common in men	Fever, chills (i.e., difficulty with thermoregulation); lymphadenopathy	53, 56
Stevens-Johnson syndrome (SJS), toxic epidermal necrolysis (TEN)	Drugs, other causes (infection, neoplasm, graft-vs.-host disease)	Diffuse erythema or target-like lesions progressing to bullae, with sloughing and necrosis of entire epidermis; Nikolsky's sign. *TEN:* maximal form of SJS. *SJS:* maximal form of erythema multiforme	Uncommon in children; more common in patients with HIV infection or graft-vs.-host disease	Dehydration, sepsis sometimes resulting from lack of normal skin integrity; 25% mortality	56
Vesiculobullous Eruptions					
Hand-foot-and-mouth syndrome[e]; staphylococcal scalded-skin syndrome; toxic epidermal necrolysis[f]	—	—	—	—	—[d]
Varicella (chickenpox)	Varicella-zoster virus	Macules (2–3 mm) evolving into papules, then vesicles (sometimes umbilicated), on an erythematous base ("dewdrops on a rose petal"); pustules then forming and crusting; lesions appearing in crops; may involve scalp, mouth; intensely pruritic	Usually affects children; 10% of adults susceptible; most common in late winter and spring	Malaise; generally mild disease in healthy children; more severe disease with complications in adults and immunocompromised children	173
Pseudomonas "hot-tub" folliculitis	*Pseudomonas aeruginosa*	Pruritic, erythematous follicular, papular, vesicular, or pustular lesions that may involve axillae, buttocks, abdomen, and especially areas occluded by bathing suits; can manifest as tender isolated nodules on palmar or plantar surfaces (the latter designated "*Pseudomonas* hot-foot syndrome")	Bathers in hot tubs or swimming pools; occurs in outbreaks	Earache, sore eyes and/or throat; generally self-limited	145
Variola (smallpox)	Variola major virus	Red macules on tongue, palate evolving to papules and vesicles; skin macules evolving to papules, then vesicles, then pustules over 1 week, with subsequent lesion crusting; lesions initially appearing on face and spreading centrifugally from trunk to extremities; differs from varicella in that (1) skin lesions in any given area are at same stage of development and (2) there is a prominent distribution of lesions on face and extremities (including palms, soles) as opposed to prominent rash on trunk	Nonimmune individuals exposed to smallpox	Prodrome of fever, headache, backache, myalgias; vomiting in 50% of cases	214
Primary herpes simplex virus (HSV) infection	HSV	Erythema rapidly followed by hallmark *grouped vesicles* that may evolve into pustules; painful lesions that may ulcerate, especially on mucosal surfaces; lesions at site of inoculation: commonly gingivostomatitis for HSV-1 and genital lesions for HSV-2; recurrent disease milder (e.g., herpes labialis does not involve oral mucosa)	Primary infection most common in children and young adults for HSV-1 and in sexually active young adults for HSV-2; no fever in recurrent infection	Regional lymphadenopathy	172

(continued)

Disease	Etiology	Description	Group Affected/ Epidemiologic Factors	Clinical Syndrome	Chapter
Disseminated herpesvirus infection	Varicella-zoster virus or HSV	Generalized vesicles that can evolve to pustules and ulcerations; individual lesions similar for varicella-zoster and HSV. *Zoster cutaneous dissemination*: >25 lesions extending outside involved dermatome. *HSV*: extensive, progressive mucocutaneous lesions in some cases; HSV lesions sometimes disseminate in eczematous skin (eczema herpeticum); HSV visceral dissemination may occur with only limited skin lesions	Immunosuppressed individuals, eczema	Visceral organ involvement (especially liver) in some cases	172, 173, 376
Rickettsialpox	*Rickettsia akari*	Eschar found at site of mite bite; generalized rash involving face, trunk, extremities; may involve palms and soles; <100 papules and plaques (2–10 mm); tops of lesions develop vesicles that may evolve into pustules	Seen in urban settings; transmitted by mouse mites	Headache, myalgias, regional adenopathy; mild disease	167
Disseminated *Vibrio vulnificus* infection	*V. vulnificus*	Erythematous lesions evolving into hemorrhagic bullae and then into necrotic ulcers	Patients with cirrhosis, diabetes, renal failure; exposure by ingestion of contaminated saltwater seafood	Hypotension; 50% mortality	149
Ecthyma gangrenosum	*P. aeruginosa*, other gram-negative rods, fungi	Indurated plaque evolving into hemorrhagic bulla or pustule that sloughs, resulting in eschar formation; erythematous halo; most common in axillary, groin, perianal regions	Usually affects neutropenic patients; occurs in up to 28% of individuals with *Pseudomonas* bacteremia	Clinical signs of sepsis	145
Urticarial Eruptions					
Urticarial vasculitis	Serum sickness, often due to infection (including hepatitis B viral, enteroviral, parasitic), drugs (including penicillins, sulfonamides, salicylates, barbiturates); connective tissue disease; idiopathic causes	Erythematous, circumscribed areas of edema; occasionally indurated; pruritic or burning; lesions sometimes purpuric; individual lesions lasting up to 5 days	In serum sickness, occurs 8–14 days after antigen exposure in nonsensitized individuals; may occur within 36 h in sensitized individuals	Malaise, lymphadenopathy, myalgias, arthralgias	319[d]
Nodular Eruptions					
Disseminated infection	Fungi (e.g., candidiasis, histoplasmosis, cryptococcosis, sporotrichosis, coccidioidomycosis); mycobacteria	Subcutaneous nodules (up to 3 cm); fluctuance, draining common with mycobacteria; necrotic nodules (extremities, periorbital or nasal regions) common with *Aspergillus*, *Mucor*	Immunocompromised hosts (i.e., bone marrow transplant recipients, patients undergoing chemotherapy, HIV-infected patients, alcoholics)	Features vary with organism	—[d]
Erythema nodosum (septal panniculitis)	Infections (e.g., streptococcal, fungal, mycobacterial, yersinial); drugs (e.g., sulfas, penicillins, oral contraceptives); sarcoidosis; idiopathic causes	Large, violaceous, nonulcerative, subcutaneous nodules; exquisitely tender; usually on lower legs but also on upper extremities	More common in females 15–30 years old	Arthralgias (50%); features vary with associated condition	—[d]
Sweet's syndrome (acute febrile neutrophilic dermatosis)	Yersinial infection; lymphoproliferative disorders; idiopathic causes	Tender red or blue edematous nodules giving impression of vesiculation; usually on face, neck, upper extremities; when on lower extremities, may mimic erythema nodosum	More common in women and in persons 30–60 years old; 20% of cases associated with malignancy (men and women equally affected in this group)	Headache, arthralgias, leukocytosis	54
Bacillary angiomatosis	*Bartonella henselae* or *Bartonella quintana*	Many forms, including erythematous, smooth vascular nodules; friable, exophytic lesions; erythematous plaques (may be dry, scaly); subcutaneous nodules (may be erythematous)	Usually in HIV infection	Peliosis of liver and spleen in some cases; lesions may involve multiple organs; bacteremia	153

(continued)

TABLE 18-1 DISEASES ASSOCIATED WITH FEVER AND RASH (CONTINUED)

Disease	Etiology	Description	Group Affected/ Epidemiologic Factors	Clinical Syndrome	Chapter
Purpuric Eruptions					
Rocky Mountain spotted fever, rat-bite fever, endocarditis[e]; epidemic typhus[g]; dengue fever[c]; human parvovirus B19 infection[g]	—	—	—	—	—[d]
Acute meningococcemia	*Neisseria meningitidis*	Initially pink maculopapular lesions evolving into petechiae; petechiae rapidly becoming numerous, sometimes enlarging and becoming vesicular; trunk, extremities most commonly involved; may appear on face, hands, feet; may include purpura fulminans reflecting disseminated intravascular coagulation (see below)	Most common in children, individuals with asplenia or terminal complement component deficiency (C5-C8)	Hypotension, meningitis (sometimes preceded by upper respiratory infection)	136
Purpura fulminans	Severe disseminated intravascular coagulation	Large ecchymoses with sharply irregular shapes evolving into hemorrhagic bullae and then into black necrotic lesions	Individuals with sepsis (e.g., involving *N. meningitidis*), malignancy, or massive trauma; asplenic patients at high risk for sepsis	Hypotension	136, 265
Chronic meningococcemia	*N. meningitidis*	Variety of recurrent eruptions, including pink maculopapular; nodular (usually on lower extremities); petechial (sometimes developing vesicular centers); purpuric areas with pale blue-gray centers	Individuals with complement deficiencies	Fevers, sometimes intermittent; arthritis, myalgias, headache	136
Disseminated gonococcal infection	*Neisseria gonorrhoeae*	Papules (1–5 mm) evolving over 1–2 days into hemorrhagic pustules with gray necrotic centers; hemorrhagic bullae occurring rarely; lesions (usually fewer than 40) distributed peripherally near joints (more commonly on upper extremities)	Sexually active individuals (more often females), some with complement deficiency	Low-grade fever, tenosynovitis, arthritis	137
Enteroviral petechial rash	Usually echovirus 9 or coxsackievirus A9	Disseminated petechial lesions (may also be maculopapular, vesicular, or urticarial)	Often occurs in outbreaks	Pharyngitis, headache; aseptic meningitis with echovirus 9	184
Viral hemorrhagic fever	Arboviruses and arenaviruses	Petechial rash	Residence in or travel to endemic areas or other virus exposure	Triad of fever, shock, hemorrhage from mucosa or gastrointestinal tract	189, 190
Thrombotic thrombocytopenic purpura/hemolytic-uremic syndrome	Idiopathic, *Escherichia coli* O157:H7 (Shiga toxin), drugs	Petechiae	Individuals with *E. coli* O157:H7 gastroenteritis (especially children), cancer chemotherapy, HIV infection, autoimmune diseases; pregnant/postpartum women	Fever (not always present), hemolytic anemia, thrombocytopenia, renal dysfunction, neurologic dysfunction; coagulation studies normal	54, 101, 109, 143, 147
Cutaneous small-vessel vasculitis (leukocytoclastic vasculitis)	Infections (including group A *Streptococcus*, viral hepatitis), drugs, chemicals, food allergens, idiopathic causes	Palpable purpuric lesions appearing in crops on legs or other dependent areas; may become vesicular or ulcerative; usually resolve over 3–4 weeks	Occurs in a wide spectrum of diseases, including connective tissue disease, cryoglobulinemia, malignancy, Henoch-Schönlein purpura (HSP); more common in children	Fever, malaise, arthralgias, myalgias; systemic vasculitis in some cases; renal, joint, and gastrointestinal involvement commonly seen in HSP	54

(continued)

TABLE 18-1 DISEASES ASSOCIATED WITH FEVER AND RASH (CONTINUED)

Disease	Etiology	Description	Group Affected/ Epidemiologic Factors	Clinical Syndrome	Chapter
Eruptions with Ulcers and/or Eschars					
Scrub typhus, rickettsial spotted fevers, rat-bite fever[g]; rickettsialpox, ecthyma gangrenosum[h]	—	—	—	—	—[d]
Tularemia	*Francisella tularensis*	Ulceroglandular form: erythematous, tender papule evolves into necrotic, tender ulcer with raised borders; in 35% of cases, eruptions (maculopapular, vesiculopapular, acneiform, urticarial, erythema nodosum, or erythema multiforme) may occur	Exposure to ticks, biting flies, infected animals	Fever, headache, lymphadenopathy	151
Anthrax	*Bacillus anthracis*	Pruritic papule enlarging and evolving into a 1- by 3-cm painless ulcer surrounded by vesicles and then developing a central eschar with edema; residual scar	Exposure to infected animals or animal products or other exposure to anthrax spores	Lymphadenopathy, headache	214

[a]See "Purpuric eruptions."
[b]In human granulocytotropic ehrlichiosis, or anaplasmosis (caused by *Anaplasma phagocytophila*; most common in the upper midwestern and northeastern regions of the United States), rash is rare.
[c]See "Viral hemorrhagic fever" under "Purpuric eruptions" for dengue hemorrhagic fever/dengue shock syndrome.
[d]See etiology-specific chapters.
[e]See "Peripheral eruptions."
[f]See "Confluent desquamative erythemas."
[g]See "Centrally distributed maculopapular eruptions."
[h]See "Vesiculobullous eruptions."

CENTRALLY DISTRIBUTED MACULOPAPULAR ERUPTIONS

Centrally distributed rashes, in which lesions are primarily truncal, are the most common type of eruption. The rash of *rubeola* (measles) starts at the hairline 2–3 days into the illness and moves down the body, sparing the palms and soles (Chap. 185). It begins as discrete erythematous lesions, which become confluent as the rash spreads. Koplik's spots (1- to 2-mm white or bluish lesions with an erythematous halo on the buccal mucosa) are pathognomonic for measles and are generally seen during the first 2 days of symptoms. They should not be confused with Fordyce's spots (ectopic sebaceous glands), which have no erythematous halos and are found in the mouth of healthy individuals. Koplik's spots may briefly overlap with the measles exanthem.

Rubella (German measles) also spreads from the hairline downward; unlike that of measles, however, the rash of rubella tends to clear from originally affected areas as it migrates, and it may be pruritic (Chap. 186). Forchheimer spots (palatal petechiae) may develop but are nonspecific since they also develop in mononucleosis (Chap. 174) and scarlet fever (Chap. 130). Postauricular and suboccipital adenopathy and arthritis are common among adults with German measles. Exposure of pregnant women to ill individuals should be avoided, as rubella causes severe congenital abnormalities. Numerous strains of enteroviruses (Chap. 184), primarily echoviruses and coxsackieviruses, cause nonspecific syndromes of fever and eruptions that may mimic rubella or measles. Patients with infectious mononucleosis caused by Epstein-Barr virus (Chap. 174) or with primary infection caused by HIV (Chap. 182) may exhibit pharyngitis, lymphadenopathy, and a nonspecific maculopapular exanthem.

The rash of *erythema infectiosum* (fifth disease), which is caused by human parvovirus B19, primarily affects children 3–12 years old; it develops after fever has resolved as a bright blanchable erythema on the cheeks ("slapped cheeks") with perioral pallor (Chap. 177). A more diffuse rash (often pruritic) appears the next day on the trunk and extremities and then rapidly develops into a lacy reticular eruption that may wax and wane (especially with temperature change) over 3 weeks. Adults with fifth disease often have arthritis, and fetal hydrops can develop in association with this condition in pregnant women.

Exanthem subitum (roseola) is caused by human herpesvirus 6 and is most common among children <3 years of age (Chap. 175). As in erythema infectiosum, the rash usually appears after fever has subsided. It consists of 2- to 3-mm rose-pink macules and papules that rarely coalesce, occur initially on the trunk and sometimes on the extremities (sparing the face), and fade within 2 days.

Although drug reactions have many manifestations, including urticaria, exanthematous *drug-induced eruptions* (Chap. 56) are most common and are often difficult to distinguish from viral exanthems. Eruptions elicited by drugs are usually more intensely erythematous and pruritic than viral exanthems, but this distinction is not reliable. A history of new medications and an absence of prostration may help to distinguish a drug-related rash from an eruption of another etiology. Rashes may persist for up to 2 weeks after administration of the offending agent is discontinued. Certain populations are more prone than others to drug rashes. Of HIV-infected patients, 50–60% develop a rash in response to sulfa drugs; 90% of patients with mononucleosis due to Epstein-Barr virus develop a rash when given ampicillin.

Rickettsial illnesses (Chap. 167) should be considered in the evaluation of individuals with centrally distributed maculopapular eruptions. The usual setting for *epidemic typhus* is a site of war or natural disaster in which people are exposed to body lice. A diagnosis of recrudescent typhus should be considered in European immigrants to the United States. However, an indigenous form of typhus, presumably transmitted by flying squirrels, has been reported in the southeastern United States. *Endemic typhus* or *leptospirosis* (the latter caused by a spirochete; Chap. 164) may be seen in urban environments where rodents proliferate. Outside the United States, other rickettsial diseases cause a spotted-fever syndrome and should be considered in residents of or travelers to endemic areas. Similarly, *typhoid fever*, a nonrickettsial disease caused by *Salmonella typhi* (Chap. 146), is usually acquired during travel outside the United States. Dengue fever, caused by a mosquito-transmitted flavivirus, occurs in tropical and subtropical regions of the world (Chap. 189).

Some centrally distributed maculopapular eruptions have distinctive features. Erythema chronicum migrans (ECM), the rash of Lyme disease (Chap. 166), typically manifests as singular or multiple annular plaques. Untreated ECM lesions usually fade within a month but may persist for more than a year. *Erythema marginatum*, the rash of acute rheumatic fever (Chap. 315), has a distinctive pattern of enlarging and shifting transient annular lesions.

Collagen vascular diseases may cause fever and rash. Patients with *systemic lupus erythematosus* (Chap. 313) typically develop a sharply defined, erythematous eruption in a butterfly distribution on the cheeks (malar rash) as well as many other skin manifestations. *Still's disease* (Chap. 331) manifests as an evanescent salmon-colored rash on the trunk and proximal extremities that coincides with fever spikes.

PERIPHERAL ERUPTIONS

These rashes are alike in that they are most prominent peripherally or begin in peripheral (acral) areas before spreading centripetally. Early diagnosis and therapy are critical in RMSF (Chap. 167) because of its grave prognosis if untreated. Lesions evolve from macular to petechial, start on the wrists and ankles, spread centripetally, and appear on the palms and soles only later in the disease. The rash of *secondary syphilis* (Chap. 162), which may be generalized but is prominent on the palms and soles, should be considered in the differential diagnosis of pityriasis rosea, especially in sexually active patients. *Atypical measles* (Chap. 185) is seen in individuals contracting measles who received the killed measles vaccine between 1963 and 1967 in the United States and who were not subsequently protected with the live vaccine. *Hand-foot-and-mouth disease* (Chap. 184), most commonly caused by coxsackievirus A16, is distinguished by tender vesicles distributed peripherally and in the mouth; outbreaks commonly occur within families. The classic target lesions of *erythema multiforme* (EM) appear symmetrically on the elbows, knees, palms, soles, and face. In severe cases, these lesions spread diffusely and involve mucosal surfaces. Stevens-Johnson syndrome is considered a maximal form of erythema multiforme and is life-threatening. Lesions may develop on the hands and feet in *endocarditis* (Chap. 118).

CONFLUENT DESQUAMATIVE ERYTHEMAS

These eruptions consist of diffuse erythema frequently followed by desquamation. The eruptions caused by group A *Streptococcus* or *Staphylococcus aureus* are toxin mediated. *Scarlet fever* (Chap. 130) usually follows pharyngitis; patients have a facial flush, a "strawberry" tongue, and accentuated petechiae in body folds (Pastia's lines). *Kawasaki disease* (Chaps. 54 and 319) presents in the pediatric population as fissuring of the lips, a strawberry tongue, conjunctivitis, adenopathy, and sometimes cardiac abnormalities. *Streptococcal toxic shock syndrome* (Chap. 130) manifests with hypotension, multiorgan failure, and often a severe group A streptococcal infection (e.g., necrotizing fasciitis). *Staphylococcal toxic shock syndrome* (Chap. 129) also presents with hypotension and multiorgan failure, but usually only *S. aureus* colonization—not a severe *S. aureus* infection—is documented. *Staphylococcal scalded-skin syndrome* (Chap. 129) is seen primarily in children and in immunocompromised adults. Generalized erythema is often evident during the prodrome of fever and malaise; profound tenderness of the skin is distinctive. In the exfoliative stage, the skin can be induced to form bullae with light lateral pressure (Nikolsky's sign). In a mild form, a scarlatiniform eruption mimics scarlet fever, but the patient does not exhibit a strawberry tongue or circumoral pallor. In contrast to the staphylococcal scalded-skin syndrome, in which the cleavage plane is superficial in the epidermis, *toxic epidermal necrolysis* (Chap. 56), a maximal variant of Stevens-Johnson syndrome, involves sloughing of the entire epidermis, resulting in severe disease. *Exfoliative erythroderma syndrome* (Chaps. 53 and 56) is a serious reaction associated with systemic toxicity that is often due to eczema, psoriasis, mycosis fungoides, or a severe drug reaction.

VESICULOBULLOUS ERUPTIONS

Varicella (Chap. 173) is highly contagious, often occurring in winter or spring. At any point in time, within a given region of the body, varicella lesions are in different stages of development. In immunocompromised hosts, varicella vesicles may lack the characteristic erythematous base or may appear hemorrhagic. Lesions of *Pseudomonas* "hot-tub" folliculitis (Chap. 145) are also pruritic and may appear similar to those of varicella. However, hot-tub folliculitis generally occurs in outbreaks after bathing in hot tubs or swimming pools, and lesions occur in regions occluded by bathing suits. Lesions of *variola* (smallpox; Chap. 214) also appear similar to those of varicella but are all at the same stage of development in a given region of the body. Variola lesions are most prominent on the face and extremities, while varicella lesions are most prominent on the trunk. Herpes simplex virus infection (Chap. 172) is characterized by hallmark grouped vesicles on an erythematous base. Primary herpes infection is accompanied by fever and toxicity, while recurrent disease is milder. *Rickettsialpox* (Chap. 167) is often documented in urban settings and is characterized by vesicles. It can be distinguished from varicella by an eschar at the site of the mouse-mite bite and the papule/plaque base of each vesicle. Disseminated *Vibrio vulnificus* infection (Chap. 149) or *ecthyma gangrenosum* due to *Pseudomonas aeruginosa* (Chap. 145) should be considered in immunosuppressed individuals with sepsis and hemorrhagic bullae.

URTICARIAL ERUPTIONS

Individuals with classic urticaria ("hives") usually have a hypersensitivity reaction without associated fever. In the presence of fever, urticarial eruptions are usually due to *urticarial vasculitis* (Chap. 319). Unlike individual lesions of classic urticaria, which last up to 48 h, these lesions may last up to 5 days. Etiologies include serum sickness (often induced by drugs such as penicillins, sulfas, salicylates, or barbiturates), connective-tissue disease (e.g., systemic lupus erythematosus or Sjögren's syndrome), and infection (e.g., with hepatitis B virus, enteroviruses, or parasites). Malignancy may be associated with fever and chronic urticaria (Chap. 54).

NODULAR ERUPTIONS

In immunocompromised hosts, nodular lesions often represent disseminated infection. Patients with disseminated *candidiasis* (often due to *Candida tropicalis*) may have a triad of fever, myalgias, and eruptive nodules (Chap. 196). Disseminated *cryptococcosis* lesions (Chap. 195) may resemble molluscum contagiosum (Chap. 176). Necrosis of nodules should raise the suspicion of *aspergillosis* (Chap. 197) or *mucormycosis* (Chap. 198). *Erythema nodosum* presents with exquisitely tender nodules on the lower extremities. *Sweet's syndrome* (Chap. 54) should be considered in individuals with multiple nodules and plaques, often so edematous that they give the appearance of vesicles or bullae. Sweet's syndrome may affect either healthy individuals or persons with lymphoproliferative disease.

PURPURIC ERUPTIONS

Acute meningococcemia (Chap. 136) classically presents in children as a petechial eruption, but initial lesions may appear as blanchable macules or urticaria. RMSF should be considered in the differential diagnosis of acute meningococcemia. *Echovirus 9 infection* (Chap. 184) may mimic acute meningococcemia; patients should be treated as if they have bacterial sepsis since prompt differentiation of these conditions may be impossible. Large ecchymotic areas of *purpura fulminans* (Chaps. 136 and 265) reflect severe underlying disseminated intravascular coagulation, which may be due to infectious or noninfectious causes. The lesions of *chronic meningococcemia* (Chap. 136) may have a variety of morphologies, including petechial. Purpuric nodules may develop on the legs and resemble erythema nodosum but lack its exquisite tenderness. Lesions of *disseminated gonococcemia* (Chap. 137) are distinctive, sparse, countable hemorrhagic pustules, usually located near joints. The lesions of chronic meningococcemia and those of gonococcemia may be indistinguishable in terms of appearance and distribution. *Viral hemorrhagic fever* (Chaps. 189 and 190) should be considered in patients with an appropriate travel history and a petechial rash. *Thrombotic thrombocytopenic purpura* (Chaps. 54, 101, and 109) and *hemolytic-uremic syndrome* (Chaps. 109, 143, and 147) are closely related and are noninfectious causes of fever and petechiae. *Cutaneous small-vessel vasculitis* (*leukocytoclastic vasculitis*) typically manifests as palpable purpura and has a wide variety of causes (Chap. 54).

ERUPTIONS WITH ULCERS OR ESCHARS

The presence of an ulcer or eschar in the setting of a more widespread eruption can provide an important diagnostic clue. For example, the presence of an eschar may suggest the diagnosis of scrub typhus or rickettsialpox (Chap. 167) in the appropriate setting. In other illnesses (e.g., anthrax; Chap. 214), an ulcer or eschar may be the only skin manifestation.

FURTHER READINGS

CHERRY JD: Contemporary infectious exanthems. Clin Infect Dis 16:199, 1993

———: Cutaneous manifestations of systemic infections, in *Textbook of Pediatric Infectious Diseases*, vol. 1, 4th ed, RD Feigin, JD Cherry (eds). Philadelphia, Saunders, 1998, pp 713–737

EICHENFIELD LF et al (eds): *Textbook of Neonatal Dermatology*. Philadelphia, Saunders, 2001

FREEDBERG IM et al (eds): *Fitzpatrick's Dermatology in General Medicine*, 6th ed. New York, McGraw-Hill, 2003

LEVIN S, GOODMAN LJ: An approach to acute fever and rash (AFR) in the adult. Curr Clin Top Infect Dis 15:19, 1995

PALLER AS, MANCINI AJ (eds): *Hurwitz Clinical Pediatric Dermatology*, 3d ed. Philadelphia, Elsevier Saunders, 2006

SCHLOSSBERG D: Fever and rash. Infect Dis Clin North Am 10:101, 1996

WEBER DJ et al: The acutely ill patient with fever and rash, in *Principles and Practice of Infectious Diseases*, vol 1, 6th ed, GL Mandell et al (eds). Philadelphia, Elsevier Churchill Livingstone, 2005, pp 729–746

WENNER HA: Virus diseases associated with cutaneous eruptions. Prog Med Virol 16:269, 1973

WOLFF K, JOHNSON RAJ: *Fitzpatrick's Color Atlas and Synopsis of Clinical Dermatology*, 5th ed. New York, McGraw-Hill, 2005

19 Fever of Unknown Origin

Jeffrey A. Gelfand, Michael V. Callahan

DEFINITION AND CLASSIFICATION

Fever of unknown origin (FUO) was defined by Petersdorf and Beeson in 1961 as (1) temperatures of >38.3°C (>101°F) on several occasions; (2) a duration of fever of >3 weeks; and (3) failure to reach a diagnosis despite 1 week of inpatient investigation. While this classification has stood for more than 30 years, Durack and Street have proposed a new system for classification of FUO: (1) classic FUO; (2) nosocomial FUO; (3) neutropenic FUO; and (4) FUO associated with HIV infection.

Classic FUO corresponds closely to the earlier definition of FUO, differing only with regard to the prior requirement for 1 week's study in the hospital. The newer definition is broader, stipulating three outpatient visits or 3 days in the hospital without elucidation of a cause or 1 week of "intelligent and invasive" ambulatory investigation. In *nosocomial FUO*, a temperature of ≥38.3°C (≥101°F) develops on several occasions in a hospitalized patient who is receiving acute care and in whom infection was not manifest or incubating on admission. Three days of investigation, including at least 2 days' incubation of cultures, is the minimum requirement for this diagnosis. *Neutropenic FUO* is defined as a temperature of ≥38.3°C (≥101°F) on several occasions in a patient whose neutrophil count is <500/μL or is expected to fall to that level in 1–2 days. The diagnosis of neutropenic FUO is invoked if a specific cause is not identified after 3 days of investigation, including at least 2 days' incubation of cultures. *HIV-associated FUO* is defined by a temperature of ≥38.3°C (≥101°F) on several occasions over a period of >4 weeks for outpatients or >3 days for hospitalized patients with HIV infection. This diagnosis is invoked if appropriate investigation over 3 days, including 2 days' incubation of cultures, reveals no source.

Adoption of these categories of FUO in the literature has allowed a more rational compilation of data regarding these disparate groups. In the remainder of this chapter, the discussion will focus on classic FUO in the adult unless otherwise specified.

CAUSES OF CLASSIC FUO

Table 19-1 summarizes the findings of several large studies of FUO carried out since the advent of the antibiotic era, including a prospective study of 167 adult patients with FUO encompassing all eight university hospitals in the Netherlands and using a standardized protocol in which the first author reviewed every patient. Coincident with the widespread use of antibiotics, increasingly useful diagnostic technologies—both noninvasive and invasive—have been developed. Newer studies reflect not only changing patterns of disease but also the impact of diagnostic techniques that make it possible to eliminate many patients with specific illness from the FUO category. The ubiquitous use of potent broad-spectrum antibiotics may have decreased the number of infections causing FUO. The wide availability of ultrasonography, CT, MRI, radionuclide scanning, and positron emission tomography (PET) scanning has enhanced the detection of localized infections and of occult neoplasms and lymphomas in patients previously thought to have FUO. Likewise, the widespread availability of highly specific and sensitive immunologic testing has reduced the number of undetected cases of systemic lupus erythematosus and other autoimmune diseases.

Infections, especially extrapulmonary tuberculosis, remain the leading diagnosable cause of FUO. Prolonged mononucleosis syndromes caused by Epstein-Barr virus, cytomegalovirus (CMV), or HIV are conditions whose consideration as a cause of FUO is sometimes confounded by delayed antibody responses. Intraabdominal abscesses (sometimes poorly localized) and renal, retroperitoneal, and paraspinal abscesses continue to be difficult to diagnose. Renal malacoplakia, with submucosal plaques or nodules involving the urinary tract, may cause FUO and is often fatal if untreated. It is associated with intracellular bacterial infection, is seen most often in patients with defects of intracellular bacterial killing, and is treated with fluoroquinolones or trimethoprim-sulfamethoxazole. Occasionally, other organs may be involved. Osteomyelitis, especially where prosthetic devices have been implanted, and infective endocarditis must be considered. Although true culture-negative infective endocarditis is rare, one may be misled by slow-growing organisms of the HACEK group (*Haemophilus aphrophilus*, *Actinobacillus actinomycetemcomitans*, *Cardiobacterium hominis*, *Eikenella corrodens*, and *Kingella kingae*; Chap. 140), *Bartonella* spp. (previously *Rochalimaea*), *Legionella* spp., *Coxiella burnetii*, *Chlamydophila psittaci*, and fungi. Prostatitis, dental abscesses, sinusitis, and cholangitis continue to be sources of occult fever.

Fungal disease, most notably histoplasmosis involving the reticuloendothelial system, may cause FUO. FUO with headache should

TABLE 19-1 CLASSIC FUO IN ADULTS

Authors (Year of Publication)	Years of Study	No. of Cases	Infections (%)	Neoplasms (%)	Noninfectious Inflammatory Diseases (%)	Miscellaneous Causes (%)	Undiagnosed Causes (%)
Petersdorf and Beeson (1961)	1952–1957	100	36	19	19[a]	19[a]	7
Larson and Featherstone (1982)	1970–1980	105	30	31	16[a]	11[a]	12
Knockaert and Vanneste (1992)	1980–1989	199	22.5	7	23[a]	21.5[a]	25.5
de Kleijn et al. (1997, Part I)	1992–1994	167	26	12.5	24	8	30

[a]Authors' raw data retabulated to conform to altered diagnostic categories.
Source: Modified from de Kleijn et al., 1997 (Part I).

prompt examination of spinal fluid for *Cryptococcus neoformans*. Malaria (which may result from transfusion, the failure to take a prescribed prophylactic agent, or infection with a drug-resistant strain) continues to be a cause, particularly of asynchronous FUO. A related protozoan infection, babesiosis, may cause FUO and is increasing in geographic distribution and in incidence, especially among the elderly and immunosuppressed.

In most earlier series, neoplasms were the next most common cause of FUO after infections (Table 19-1). In more recent series, a decrease in the percentage of FUO cases due to malignancy was attributed to improvement in diagnostic technologies—in particular, high-resolution tomography, MRI, PET scanning, and tumor antigen assays. This observation does not diminish the importance of considering neoplasia in the initial diagnostic evaluation of a patient with fever. A number of patients in these series had temporal arteritis, adult Still's disease, drug-related fever, and factitious fever. In recent series, ~25–30% of cases of FUO have remained undiagnosed. The general term *noninfectious inflammatory diseases* applies to systemic rheumatologic or vasculitic diseases such as polymyalgia rheumatica, lupus, and adult Still's disease as well as to granulomatous diseases such as sarcoidosis and Crohn's and granulomatous hepatitis.

In the elderly, multisystem disease is the most frequent cause of FUO, giant-cell arteritis being the leading etiologic entity in this category. In patients >50 years of age, this disease accounts for 15–20% of FUO cases. Tuberculosis is the most common infection causing FUO in the elderly, and colon cancer is an important cause of FUO with malignancy in this age group.

Many diseases have been grouped in the various studies as "miscellaneous." On this list are drug fever, pulmonary embolism, factitious fever, the hereditary periodic fever syndromes (familial Mediterranean fever, hyper-IgD syndrome, tumor necrosis factor receptor–associated periodic syndrome, familial cold urticaria, and the Muckle-Wells syndrome), and Fabry disease.

A drug-related etiology must be considered in any case of prolonged fever. Any febrile pattern may be elicited by a drug. Virtually all classes of drugs cause fever, but antimicrobial agents (especially β-lactam antibiotics), cardiovascular drugs (e.g., quinidine), antineoplastic drugs, and drugs acting on the central nervous system (e.g., phenytoin) are particularly common causes.

It is axiomatic that, as the duration of fever increases, the likelihood of an infectious cause decreases, even for the more indolent infectious etiologies (e.g., brucellosis, paracoccidioidomycosis, malaria due to *Plasmodium malariae*). In a series of 347 patients referred to the National Institutes of Health from 1961 to 1977, only 6% had an infection (Table 19-2). A significant proportion (9%) had factitious fevers—i.e., fevers due either to false elevations of temperature or to self-induced disease. A substantial number of these factitious cases were in young women in the health professions. It is worth noting that 8% of the patients with prolonged fevers (some of whom had completely normal liver function studies) had granulomatous hepatitis, and 6% had adult Still's disease. After prolonged investigation, 19% of cases still had no specific diagnosis. A total of 27% of patients had no actual fever during inpatient observation or had an exaggerated circadian temperature rhythm without chills, elevated pulse, or other abnormalities.

More than 200 conditions may be considered in the differential diagnosis of classic FUO in adults; the most common of these are listed in Table 19-3. This list applies strictly to the United States. Geographic considerations are paramount. For example, in Japan, human T cell lymphotropic virus type I is a consideration; in China, infection plays a greater role and tuberculosis is prominent; and in Spain, visceral leishmaniasis may be a more common cause of FUO. The frequency of global travel underscores the need for a detailed travel history, and the continuing emergence of new infectious diseases makes this listing potentially incomplete. The possibility of international and domestic terrorist activity involving the intentional release of infectious agents, many of which cause illnesses presenting with prolonged fever, underscores the need for obtaining an insightful environmental, occupational, and professional history, with early notification of public health authorities in cases of suspicious etiology (Chap. 214).

TABLE 19-2 CAUSES OF FUO LASTING >6 MONTHS

Cause	Cases, %
None identified	19
Miscellaneous causes	13
Factitious causes	9
Granulomatous hepatitis	8
Neoplasm	7
Still's disease	6
Infection	6
Collagen vascular disease	4
Familial Mediterranean fever	3
No fever[a]	27

[a]No actual fever observed during 2–3 weeks of inpatient observation. Includes patients with exaggerated circadian rhythm.

Source: From a study of 347 patients referred to the National Institutes of Health from 1961 to 1977 with a presumptive diagnosis of FUO of >6 months' duration (R Aduan et al. Prolonged fever of unknown origin. Clin Res 26:558A, 1978).

SPECIALIZED DIAGNOSTIC STUDIES

Classic FUO A stepwise flow chart depicting the diagnostic workup and therapeutic management of FUO is provided in Fig. 19-1. In this flow chart, reference is made to "potentially diagnostic clues," as outlined by de Kleijn and colleagues; these clues may be key findings in the history (e.g., travel), localizing signs, or key symptoms. Certain specific diagnostic maneuvers become critical in dealing with prolonged fevers. If factitious fever is suspected, electronic thermometers should be used, temperature-taking should be supervised, and simultaneous urine and body temperatures should be measured. Thick blood smears should be examined for *Plasmodium*; thin blood smears, prepared with proper technique and quality stains and subjected to expert microscopy, should be used to speciate *Plasmodium* and to identify *Babesia*, *Trypanosoma*, *Leishmania*, *Rickettsia*, and *Borrelia*. Any tissue removed during prior relevant surgery should be reexamined; slides should be requested, and, if need be, paraffin blocks of fixed pathologic material should be reexamined and additional special studies performed. Relevant x-rays should be reexamined; reviewing of prior radiologic reports may be insufficient. Serum should be set aside in the laboratory as soon as possible and retained for future examination for rising antibody titers.

Febrile agglutinins is a vague term that in most laboratories refers to serologic studies for salmonellosis, brucellosis, and rickettsial diseases. These studies are seldom useful, having low sensitivity and variable specificity. Multiple blood samples (no fewer than three and rarely more than six, including samples for anaerobic culture) should be cultured in the laboratory for at least 2 weeks to ensure that any HACEK group organisms that may be present have ample time to grow (Chap. 140). Lysis-centrifugation blood culture techniques should be employed in cases where prior antimicrobial therapy or fungal or atypical mycobacterial infection is suspected. Blood culture media should be supplemented with L-cysteine or pyridoxal to assist in the isolation of nutritionally variant streptococci. It should be noted that sequential cultures positive for multiple organisms may reflect self-injection of contaminated substances. Urine cultures, including cultures for mycobacteria, fungi, and CMV, are indicated. In the setting of recurrent fevers with lymphocytic meningitis (Mollaret's meningitis), cerebrospinal fluid can be tested for herpesvirus, with use of the polymerase chain reaction (PCR) to amplify and detect viral nucleic acid (Chap. 172). A recent report described a highly multiplexed oligonucleotide microarray using PCR amplification and containing probes for all recognized vertebrate virus species and for 135 bacterial, 73 fungal, and 63 parasitic genera and species. The eventual clinical validation of such microarrays will further diminish rates of undiagnosed FUO of infectious etiology.

In any FUO workup, the erythrocyte sedimentation rate (ESR) should be determined. Striking elevation of the ESR and anemia of chronic disease are frequently seen in association with giant-cell arteritis

TABLE 19-3 CAUSES OF FUO IN ADULTS IN THE UNITED STATES

Infections

- Localized pyogenic infections
  - Appendicitis
  - Cat-scratch disease
  - Cholangitis
  - Cholecystitis
  - Dental abscess
  - Diverticulitis/abscess
  - Lesser sac abscess
  - Liver abscess
  - Mesenteric lymphadenitis
  - Osteomyelitis
  - Pancreatic abscess
  - Pelvic inflammatory disease
  - Perinephric/intrarenal abscess
  - Prostatic abscess
  - Renal malacoplakia
  - Sinusitis
  - Subphrenic abscess
  - Suppurative thrombophlebitis
  - Tuboovarian abscess
- Intravascular infections
  - Bacterial aortitis
  - Bacterial endocarditis
  - Vascular catheter infection
- Systemic bacterial infections
  - Bartonellosis
  - Brucellosis
  - *Campylobacter* infection
  - Cat-scratch disease/bacillary angiomatosis (*B. henselae*)
  - Gonococcemia
  - Legionnaires' disease
  - Leptospirosis
  - Listeriosis
  - Lyme disease
  - Melioidosis
  - Meningococcemia
  - Rat-bite fever
  - Relapsing fever
  - Salmonellosis
  - Syphilis
  - Tularemia
  - Typhoid fever
  - Vibriosis
  - *Yersinia* infection
- Mycobacterial infections
  - *M. avium/M. intracellulare* infections
  - Other atypical mycobacterial infections
  - Tuberculosis
- Other bacterial infections
  - Actinomycosis
  - Bacillary angiomatosis
  - Nocardiosis
  - Whipple's disease
- Rickettsial infections
  - Anaplasmosis
  - Ehrlichiosis
  - Murine typhus
  - Q fever
  - Rickettsialpox
  - Rocky Mountain spotted fever
- Mycoplasmal infections
- Chlamydial infections
  - Lymphogranuloma venereum
  - Psittacosis
  - TWAR (*C. pneumoniae*) infection
- Viral infections
  - Colorado tick fever
  - Coxsackievirus group B infection
  - Cytomegalovirus infection
  - Dengue
  - Epstein-Barr virus infection
  - Hepatitis A, B, C, D, and E
  - Human herpesvirus 6 infection
  - Human immunodeficiency virus infection
  - Lymphocytic choriomeningitis
  - Parvovirus B19 infection
- Fungal infections
  - Aspergillosis
  - Blastomycosis
  - Candidiasis
  - Coccidioidomycosis
  - Cryptococcosis
  - Histoplasmosis
  - Mucormycosis
  - Paracoccidioidomycosis
  - *Pneumocystis* infection
  - Sporotrichosis
- Parasitic infections
  - Amebiasis
  - Babesiosis
  - Chagas' disease
  - Leishmaniasis
  - Malaria
  - Strongyloidiasis
  - Toxocariasis
  - Toxoplasmosis
  - Trichinosis
- Presumed infections, agent undetermined
  - Kawasaki's disease (mucocutaneous lymph node syndrome)
  - Kikuchi's necrotizing lymphadenitis

Neoplasms

- Malignant
  - Colon cancer
  - Gall bladder carcinoma
  - Hepatoma
  - Hodgkin's lymphoma
  - Immunoblastic T-cell lymphoma
  - Leukemia
  - Lymphomatoid granulomatosis
  - Malignant histiocytosis
  - Non-Hodgkin's lymphoma
  - Pancreatic cancer
  - Renal cell carcinoma
  - Sarcoma
- Benign
  - Atrial myxoma
  - Castleman's disease
  - Renal angiomyolipoma

Habitual Hyperthermia

(Exaggerated circadian rhythm)

Collagen Vascular/Hypersensitivity Diseases

- Adult Still's disease
- Behçet's disease
- Erythema multiforme
- Erythema nodosum
- Giant-cell arteritis/polymyalgia rheumatica
- Hypersensitivity pneumonitis
- Hypersensitivity vasculitis
- Mixed connective-tissue disease
- Polyarteritis nodosa
- Relapsing polychondritis
- Rheumatic fever
- Rheumatoid arthritis
- Schnitzler's syndrome
- Systemic lupus erythematosus
- Takayasu's aortitis
- Weber-Christian disease
- Wegener's granulomatosis

Granulomatous Diseases

- Crohn's disease
- Granulomatous hepatitis
- Midline granuloma
- Sarcoidosis

Miscellaneous Conditions

- Aortic dissection
- Drug fever
- Gout
- Hematomas
- Hemoglobinopathies
- Laennec's cirrhosis
- PFPA syndrome: periodic fever, adenitis, pharyngitis, aphthae
- Postmyocardial infarction syndrome
- Recurrent pulmonary emboli
- Subacute thyroiditis (de Quervain's)
- Tissue infarction/necrosis

Inherited and Metabolic Diseases

- Adrenal insufficiency
- Cyclic neutropenia
- Deafness, urticaria, and amyloidosis
- Fabry disease
- Familial cold urticaria
- Familial Mediterranean fever
- Hyperimmunoglobulinemia D and periodic fever
- Muckle-Wells syndrome
- Tumor necrosis factor receptor–associated periodic syndrome
- Type V hypertriglyceridemia

Thermoregulatory Disorders

- Central
  - Brain tumor
  - Cerebrovascular accident
  - Encephalitis
  - Hypothalamic dysfunction
- Peripheral
  - Hyperthyroidism
  - Pheochromocytoma

Factitious Fevers

"Afebrile" FUO (<38.3°C)

Source: Modified from RK Root, RG Petersdorf, in JD Wilson et al (eds): *Harrison's Principles of Internal Medicine*, 12th ed. New York, McGraw-Hill, 1991.

or polymyalgia rheumatica—common causes of FUO in patients >50 years of age. Still's disease is suggested by elevations of ESR, leukocytosis, and anemia and is often accompanied by arthralgias, polyserositis (pleuritis, pericarditis), lymphadenopathy, splenomegaly, and rash. The C-reactive protein level may be a useful cross-reference for the ESR and is a more sensitive and specific indicator of an "acute-phase" inflammatory metabolic response. Antinuclear antibody, antineutrophil cytoplasmic antibody, rheumatoid factor, and serum cryoglobulins should be measured to rule out other collagen vascular diseases and vasculitis. Elevated levels of angiotensin-converting enzyme in serum may point to sarcoi-

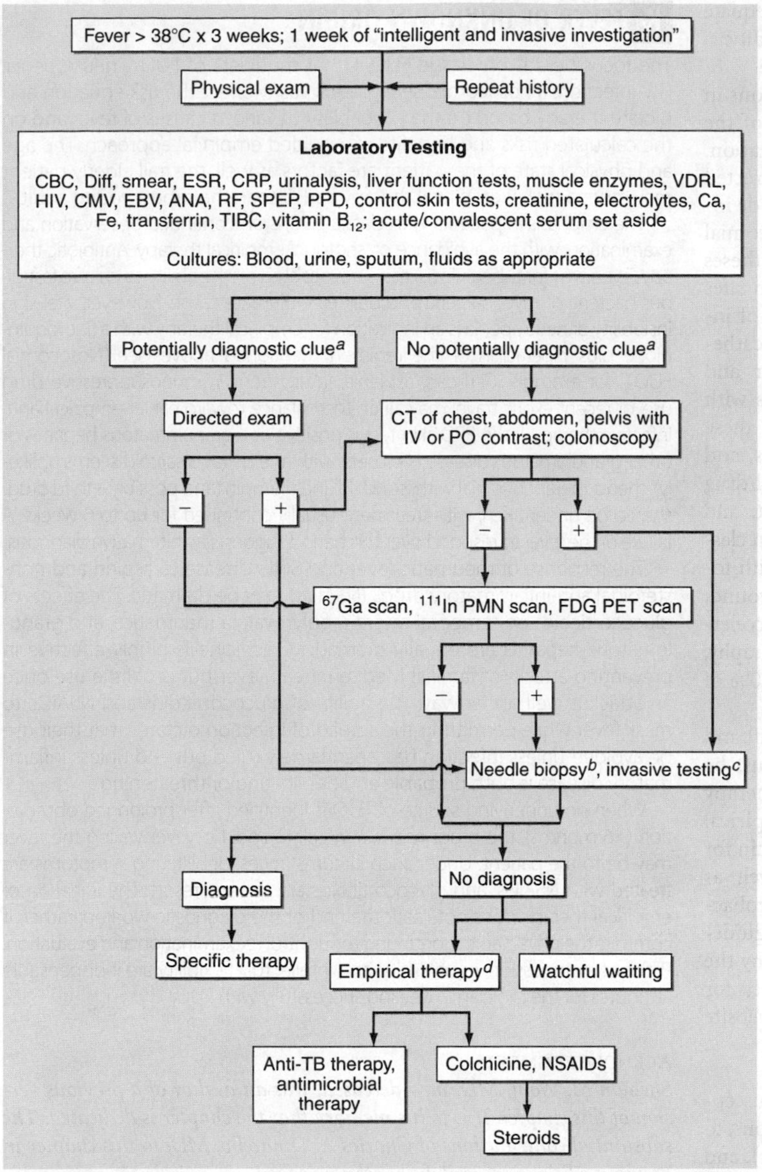

FIGURE 19-1 Approach to the patient with classic FUO. [a]"Potentially diagnostic clues," as outlined by de Kleijn and colleagues (1997, Part II), may be key findings in the history, localizing signs, or key symptoms. ANA, antinuclear antibody; CBC, complete blood count; CMV, cytomegalovirus; CRP, C-reactive protein; CT, computed tomography; Diff, differential; EBV, Epstein-Barr virus; ESR, erythrocyte sedimentation rate; FDG, fluorodeoxyglucose F18; NSAIDs, nonsteroidal anti-inflammatory drugs; PET, positron emission tomography; PMN, polymorphonuclear leukocyte; PPD, purified protein derivative; RF, rheumatoid factor; SPEP, serum protein electrophoresis; TB, tuberculosis; TIBC, total iron-binding capacity; VDRL, Venereal Disease Research Laboratory test. [b]Needle biopsy of liver as well as any other tissue indicated by "potentially diagnostic clues." [c]Invasive testing could involve laparoscopy. [d]Empirical therapy is a last resort, given the good prognosis of most patients with FUO persisting without a diagnosis.

dosis. With rare exceptions, the intermediate-strength purified protein derivative (PPD) skin test should be used to screen for tuberculosis in patients with classic FUO. Concurrent control tests, such as the mumps skin test antigen (Aventis-Pasteur, Swiftwater, PA), should be employed. It should be kept in mind that both the PPD skin test and control tests may yield negative results in miliary tuberculosis, sarcoidosis, Hodgkin's disease, malnutrition, or AIDS.

Noninvasive procedures should include an upper gastrointestinal contrast study with small-bowel follow-through and colonoscopy to examine the terminal ileum and cecum. Colonoscopy is especially strongly indicated in the elderly. Chest x-rays should be repeated if new symptoms arise. Sputum should be induced with an ultrasonic nebulizer for cultures and cytology. If there are pulmonary signs or symptoms, bronchoscopy with bronchoalveolar lavage for cultures and cytology should be considered. High-resolution spiral CT of the chest and abdomen should be performed with both IV and oral contrast. If a spinal or paraspinal lesion is suspected, however, MRI is preferred. MRI may be superior to CT in demonstrating intraabdominal abscesses and aortic dissection, but the relative utility of MRI and CT in the diagnosis of FUO is unknown. At present, abdominal CT with contrast should be used unless MRI is specifically indicated. Arteriography may be useful for patients in whom systemic necrotizing vasculitis is suspected. Saccular aneurysms may be seen, most commonly in renal or hepatic vessels, and may permit diagnosis of arteritis when biopsy is difficult. Ultrasonography of the abdomen is useful for investigation of the hepatobiliary tract, kidneys, spleen, and pelvis. Echocardiography may be helpful in an evaluation for bacterial endocarditis, pericarditis, nonbacterial thrombotic endocarditis, and atrial myxomas. Transesophageal echocardiography is especially sensitive for these lesions.

Radionuclide scanning procedures using technetium (Tc) 99m sulfur colloid, gallium (Ga) 67 citrate, or indium (In) 111–labeled leukocytes may be useful in identifying and/or localizing inflammatory processes. In one study, Ga scintigraphy yielded useful diagnostic information in almost one-third of cases, and it was suggested that this procedure might actually be used before other imaging techniques if no specific organ is suspected of being abnormal. It is likely that PET scanning, which provides quicker results (hours vs days), will prove even more sensitive and specific than ^{67}Ga scanning in FUO. ^{99m}Tc bone scan should be undertaken to look for osteomyelitis or bony metastases; ^{67}Ga scan may be used to identify sarcoidosis (Chap. 322) or *Pneumocystis* infection (Chap. 200) in the lungs or Crohn's disease (Chap. 289) in the abdomen. ^{111}In-labeled white blood cell (WBC) scan may be used to locate abscesses. With these scans, false-positive and false-negative findings are common. Fluorodeoxyglucose F18 (FDG) PET scanning appears to be superior to other forms of nuclear imaging. The FDG used in PET scans accumulates in tumors and at sites of inflammation and has even been shown to accumulate reliably at sites of vasculitis. Where available, FDG PET scanning should therefore be chosen over ^{67}Ga scanning in the diagnosis of FUO.

Biopsy of the liver and bone marrow should be considered in the workup of FUO if the studies mentioned above are unrevealing and if fever is prolonged. Granulomatous hepatitis has been diagnosed by liver biopsy, even when liver enzymes are normal and no other diagnostic clues point to liver disease. All biopsy specimens should be cultured for bacteria, mycobacteria, and fungi. Likewise, in the absence of clues pointing to the bone marrow, bone marrow biopsy (not simple aspiration) for histology and culture has yielded diagnoses late in the workup. When possible, a section of the tissue block should be retained for further sections or stains. PCR technology makes it possible in some cases to identify and speciate mycobacterial DNA in paraffin-embedded, fixed tissues at some research centers. Thus, in some cases, a retrospective diagnosis can be made on the basis of studies of long-fixed pathologic tissues. In a patient over age 50 (or occasionally in a younger patient) with the appropriate symptoms and laboratory findings, "blind biopsy" of one or both temporal arteries may yield a diagnosis of arteritis. Tenderness or decreased pulsation, if noted, should guide the selection of a site for biopsy. Lymph node biopsy may be helpful if nodes are enlarged, but inguinal nodes are often palpable and are seldom diagnostically useful.

Exploratory laparotomy has been performed when all other diagnostic procedures fail but has largely been replaced by imaging and guided-biopsy techniques. Laparoscopic biopsy may provide more adequate guided sampling of lymph nodes or liver, with less invasive morbidity.

Nosocomial FUO (See also Chap. 125) The primary considerations in diagnosing nosocomial FUO are the underlying susceptibility of the patient coupled with the potential complications of hospitalization. The original surgical or procedural field is the place to begin a directed physical and laboratory examination for abscesses, hematomas, or infected foreign bodies. More than 50% of patients with nosocomial FUO are infected. Intravascular lines, septic phlebitis, and prostheses are all suspect. In this setting, the best approach is to focus on sites where occult infections may be sequestered, such as the sinuses of intubated patients or a prostatic abscess in a man with a urinary catheter. *Clostridium difficile* colitis may be associated with fever and leukocytosis before the onset of diarrhea. In ~25% of patients with nosocomial FUO, the fever has a noninfectious cause. Among these causes are acalculous cholecystitis, deep-vein thrombophlebitis, and pulmonary embolism. Drug fever, transfusion reactions, alcohol/drug withdrawal, adrenal insufficiency, thyroiditis, pancreatitis, gout, and pseudogout are among the many possible causes to consider. As in classic FUO, repeated meticulous physical examinations, coupled with focused diagnostic techniques, are imperative. Multiple blood, wound, and fluid cultures are mandatory. The pace of diagnostic tests is accelerated, and the threshold for procedures—CT scans, ultrasonography, ^{111}In WBC scans, noninvasive venous studies—is low. Even so, 20% of cases of nosocomial FUO may go undiagnosed.

Like diagnostic measures, therapeutic maneuvers must be swift and decisive, as many patients are already critically ill. IV lines must be changed (and cultured), drugs stopped for 72 h, and empirical therapy started if bacteremia is a threat. In many hospital settings, empirical antibiotic coverage for nosocomial FUO now includes vancomycin for coverage of methicillin-resistant *Staphylococcus aureus* as well as broad-spectrum gram-negative coverage with piperacillin/tazobactam, ticarcillin/clavulanate, imipenem, or meropenem. Practice guidelines covering many of these issues have been published jointly by the Infectious Diseases Society of America (IDSA) and the Society for Critical Care Medicine and can be accessed on the IDSA website (*www.journals.uchicago.edu/IDSA/guidelines*).

Neutropenic FUO (See also Chap. 82) Neutropenic patients are susceptible to focal bacterial and fungal infections, to bacteremic infections, to infections involving catheters (including septic thrombophlebitis), and to perianal infections. *Candida* and *Aspergillus* infections are common. Infections due to herpes simplex virus or CMV are sometimes causes of FUO in this group. While the duration of illness may be short in these patients, the consequences of untreated infection may be catastrophic; 50–60% of febrile neutropenic patients are infected, and 20% are bacteremic. The IDSA has published extensive practice guidelines covering these critically ill neutropenic patients; these guidelines appear on the website cited in the previous section. In these patients, severe mucositis, quinolone prophylaxis, colonization with methicillin-resistant *S. aureus*, obvious catheter-related infection, or hypotension dictates the use of vancomycin plus ceftazidime, cefepime, or a carbapenem with or without an aminoglycoside to provide empirical coverage for bacterial sepsis.

HIV-Associated FUO HIV infection alone may be a cause of fever. Infection due to *Mycobacterium avium* or *Mycobacterium intracellulare*, tuberculosis, toxoplasmosis, CMV infection, *Pneumocystis* infection, salmonellosis, cryptococcosis, histoplasmosis, non-Hodgkin's lymphoma, and (of particular importance) drug fever are all possible causes of FUO. Mycobacterial infection can be diagnosed by blood cultures and by liver, bone marrow, and lymph node biopsies. Chest CT should be performed to identify enlarged mediastinal nodes. Serologic studies may reveal cryptococcal antigen, and ^{67}Ga scan may help identify *Pneumocystis* pulmonary infection. FUO has an infectious etiology in >80% of HIV-infected patients, but drug fever and lymphoma remain important considerations. Treatment of HIV-associated FUO depends on many factors and is discussed in Chap. 182.

℞ FEVER OF UNKNOWN ORIGIN

The focus here is on classic FUO. Other modifiers of FUO—neutropenia, HIV infection, a nosocomial setting—all vastly affect the risk equation and dictate therapy based on the probability of various causes of fever and on the calculated risks and benefits of a guided empirical approach. The age and physical state of the patient are factors as well: the frail elderly patient may merit a trial of empirical therapy earlier than the robust young adult.

The emphasis in patients with classic FUO is on continued observation and examination, with the avoidance of "shotgun" empirical therapy. Antibiotic therapy (even that for tuberculosis) may irrevocably alter the ability to culture fastidious bacteria or mycobacteria and delineate ultimate cause. However, vital-sign instability or neutropenia is an indication for empirical therapy with a fluoroquinolone plus piperacillin or the regimen mentioned above (see "Nosocomial FUO"), for example. Cirrhosis, asplenia, intercurrent immunosuppressive drug use, or recent exotic travel may all tip the balance toward earlier empirical anti-infective therapy. If the PPD skin test is positive or if granulomatous hepatitis or other granulomatous disease is present with anergy (and sarcoid seems unlikely), then a therapeutic trial with isoniazid and rifampin (and possibly a third drug) should be undertaken, with treatment usually continued for up to 6 weeks. A failure of the fever to respond over this period suggests an alternative diagnosis.

The response of rheumatic fever and Still's disease to aspirin and nonsteroidal anti-inflammatory drugs (NSAIDs) may be dramatic. The effects of glucocorticoids on temporal arteritis, polymyalgia rheumatica, and granulomatous hepatitis are equally dramatic. Colchicine is highly effective in preventing attacks of familial Mediterranean fever but is of little use once an attack is well under way. The ability of glucocorticoids and NSAIDs to mask fever while permitting the spread of infection dictates that their use be avoided unless infection has been largely ruled out and unless inflammatory disease is both probable and debilitating or threatening.

When no underlying source of FUO is identified after prolonged observation (>6 months), the prognosis is generally good, however vexing the fever may be to the patient. Under such circumstances, debilitating symptoms are treated with NSAIDs, and glucocorticoids are the last resort. The initiation of empirical therapy does not mark the end of the diagnostic workup; rather, it commits the physician to continued thoughtful reexamination and evaluation. Patience, compassion, equanimity, and intellectual flexibility are indispensable attributes for the clinician in dealing successfully with FUO.

ACKNOWLEDGMENTS

Sheldon M. Wolff, MD, now deceased, was an author of a previous version of this chapter. It is to his memory that the chapter is dedicated. The substantial contributions of Charles A. Dinarello, MD, to this chapter in previous editions are gratefully acknowledged.

FURTHER READINGS

BLEEKER-ROVERS CP et al: A prospective multicenter study on fever of unknown origin: The yield of a structured diagnostic protocol. Medicine 86:26, 2007

DE KLEIJN EM et al: Fever of unknown origin (FUO): I. A prospective multicenter study of 167 patients with FUO, using fixed epidemiologic entry criteria. Medicine 76:392, 1997

——— et al: Fever of unknown origin (FUO): II. Diagnostic procedures in a prospective multicenter study of 167 patients. Medicine 76:401, 1997

GOTO M et al: A retrospective review of 226 hospitalized patients with fever. Intern Med 46:17, 2007

HIRSCHMANN JV: Fever of unknown origin in adults. Clin Infect Dis 24:291, 1997

HUGHES WT et al: 2002 guidelines for the use of antimicrobial agents in neutropenic patients with cancer. Clin Infect Dis 34:730, 2002

KNOCKAERT DC et al: Fever of unknown origin in adults: 40 years on. J Intern Med 253:263, 2003

MOURAD O et al: A comprehensive evidence-based approach to fever of unknown origin. Arch Intern Med 163:545, 2003

O'GRADY NP et al: Practice guidelines for evaluating new fever in critically ill adult patients. Clin Infect Dis 26:1042, 1998

ZENONE T: Fever of unknown origin in adults: Evaluation of 144 cases in a non-university hospital. Scand J Infect Dis 38:632, 2006

20 Hypothermia and Frostbite

Daniel F. Danzl

HYPOTHERMIA

Accidental hypothermia occurs when there is an unintentional drop in the body's core temperature below 35°C (95°F). At this temperature, many of the compensatory physiologic mechanisms to conserve heat begin to fail. *Primary accidental hypothermia* is a result of the direct exposure of a previously healthy individual to the cold. The mortality rate is much higher for those patients who develop *secondary hypothermia* as a complication of a serious systemic disorder.

CAUSES

Primary accidental hypothermia is geographically and seasonally pervasive. Although most cases occur in the winter months and in colder climates, it is surprisingly common in warmer regions as well. Multiple variables make individuals at the extremes of age, the elderly and neonates, particularly vulnerable to hypothermia (Table 20-1). The elderly have diminished thermal perception and are more susceptible to immobility, malnutrition, and systemic illnesses that interfere with heat generation or conservation. Dementia, psychiatric illness, and socioeconomic factors often compound these problems by impeding adequate measures to prevent hypothermia. Neonates have high rates of heat loss because of their increased surface-to-mass ratio and their lack of effective shivering and adaptive behavioral responses. In addition, malnutrition can contribute to heat loss because of diminished subcutaneous fat and because of depleted energy stores used for thermogenesis.

Individuals whose occupations or hobbies entail extensive exposure to cold weather are at increased risk for hypothermia. Military history is replete with hypothermic tragedies. Hunters, sailors, skiers, and climbers also are at great risk of exposure, whether it involves injury, changes in weather, or lack of preparedness.

Ethanol causes vasodilatation (which increases heat loss), reduces thermogenesis and gluconeogenesis, and may impair judgment or lead to obtundation. Phenothiazines, barbiturates, benzodiazepines, cyclic antidepressants, and many other medications reduce centrally mediated vasoconstriction. Up to 25% of patients admitted to an intensive care unit because of drug overdose are hypothermic. Anesthetics can block the shivering responses; their effects are compounded when patients are not covered adequately in the operating or recovery rooms.

Several types of endocrine dysfunction can lead to hypothermia. Hypothyroidism—particularly when extreme, as in myxedema coma—reduces the metabolic rate and impairs thermogenesis and behavioral responses. Adrenal insufficiency and hypopituitarism also increase susceptibility to hypothermia. Hypoglycemia, most commonly caused by insulin or oral hypoglycemic drugs, is associated with hypothermia, in part the result of neuroglycopenic effects on hypothalamic function. Increased osmolality and metabolic derangements associated with uremia, diabetic ketoacidosis, and lactic acidosis can lead to altered hypothalamic thermoregulation.

TABLE 20-1 RISK FACTORS FOR HYPOTHERMIA

Age extremes	Endocrine-related
Elderly	Diabetes mellitus
Neonates	Hypoglycemia
Environmental exposure	Hypothyroidism
Occupational	Adrenal insufficiency
Sports-related	Hypopituitarism
Inadequate clothing	Neurologic-related
Immersion	Cerebrovascular accident
Toxicologic & pharmacologic	Hypothalamic disorders
Ethanol	Parkinson's disease
Phenothiazines	Spinal cord injury
Barbiturates	Multisystem
Carcinomatosis	Trauma
Anesthetics	Sepsis
Neuromuscular blockers	Shock
Antidepressants	Hepatic or renal failure
Insufficient fuel	Burns and exfoliative dermatologic disorders
Malnutrition	Immobility or debilitation
Marasmus	
Kwashiorkor	

Neurologic injury from trauma, cerebrovascular accident, subarachnoid hemorrhage, or hypothalamic lesions increases susceptibility to hypothermia. Agenesis of the corpus callosum, or Shapiro syndrome, is one cause of episodic hypothermia, characterized by profuse perspiration followed by a rapid fall in temperature. Acute spinal cord injury disrupts the autonomic pathways that lead to shivering and prevents cold-induced reflex vasoconstrictive responses.

Hypothermia associated with sepsis is a poor prognostic sign. Hepatic failure causes decreased glycogen stores and gluconeogenesis, as well as a diminished shivering response. In acute myocardial infarction associated with low cardiac output, hypothermia may be reversed after adequate resuscitation. With extensive burns, psoriasis, erythrodermas, and other skin diseases, increased peripheral blood flow leads to excessive heat loss.

THERMOREGULATION

Heat loss occurs through five mechanisms: radiation (55–65% of heat loss), conduction (10–15% of heat loss, but much greater in cold water), convection (increased in the wind), respiration, and evaporation (which are affected by the ambient temperature and the relative humidity).

The preoptic anterior hypothalamus normally orchestrates thermoregulation (Chap. 17). The immediate defense of thermoneutrality is via the autonomic nervous system, whereas delayed control is mediated by the endocrine system. Autonomic nervous system responses include the release of norepinephrine, increased muscle tone, and shivering, leading to thermogenesis and an increase in the basal metabolic rate. Cutaneous cold thermoreception causes direct reflex vasoconstriction to conserve heat. Prolonged exposure to cold also stimulates the thyroid axis, leading to an increased metabolic rate.

CLINICAL PRESENTATION

In most cases of hypothermia, the history of exposure to environmental factors, such as prolonged exposure to the outdoors without adequate clothing, makes the diagnosis straightforward. In urban settings, however, the presentation is often more subtle and other disease processes, toxin exposures, or psychiatric diagnoses should be considered.

After initial stimulation by hypothermia, there is progressive depression of all organ systems. The timing of the appearance of these clinical manifestations varies widely (Table 20-2). Without knowing the core temperature, it can be difficult to interpret other vital signs. For example, a tachycardia disproportionate to the core temperature suggests secondary hypothermia resulting from hypoglycemia, hypovolemia, or a toxin overdose. Because carbon dioxide production declines progressively, the respiratory rate should be low; persistent hyperventilation suggests a central nervous system (CNS) lesion or one of the organic acidoses. A markedly depressed level of consciousness in a patient with mild hypothermia should raise suspicion of an overdose or CNS dysfunction due to infection or trauma.

Physical examination findings can also be altered by hypothermia. For instance, the assumption that areflexia is solely attributable to hypothermia can obscure and delay the diagnosis of a spinal cord lesion. Patients with hypothermia may be confused or combative; these symptoms abate more rapidly with rewarming than with the use of restraints. A classic example of maladaptive behavior in patients with hypothermia is paradoxical undressing, which involves the inappropriate removal of clothing in response to a cold stress. The cold-induced ileus and abdominal rectus spasm can mimic, or mask, the presentation of an acute abdomen (Chap. 14).

When a patient in hypothermic cardiac arrest is first discovered, cardiopulmonary resuscitation is indicated, unless (1) a do-not-resuscitate status is verified, (2) obviously lethal injuries are identified, or

TABLE 20-2 PHYSIOLOGIC CHANGES ASSOCIATED WITH ACCIDENTAL HYPOTHERMIA

Severity	Body Temperature	Central Nervous System	Cardiovascular	Respiratory	Renal and Endocrine	Neuromuscular
Mild	35°C (95°F)–32.2°C (90°F)	Linear depression of cerebral metabolism; amnesia; apathy; dysarthria; impaired judgment; maladaptive behavior	Tachycardia, then progressive bradycardia; cardiac-cycle prolongation; vasoconstriction; increase in cardiac output and blood pressure	Tachypnea, then progressive decrease in respiratory minute volume; declining oxygen consumption; bronchorrhea; bronchospasm	Diuresis; increase in catecholamines, adrenal steroids, triiodothyronine and thyroxine; increase in metabolism with shivering	Increased preshivering muscle tone, then fatiguing
Moderate	<32.2°C (90°F)–28°C (82.4°F)	EEG abnormalities; progressive depression of level of consciousness; pupillary dilatation; paradoxical undressing; hallucinations	Progressive decrease in pulse and cardiac output; increased atrial and ventricular arrhythmias; suggestive (J-wave) ECG changes	Hypoventilation; 50% decrease in carbon dioxide production per 8°C drop in temperature; absence of protective airway reflexes	50% increase in renal blood flow; renal autoregulation intact; impaired insulin action	Hyporeflexia; diminishing shivering-induced thermogenesis; rigidity
Severe	<28°C (82.4°F)	Loss of cerebrovascular autoregulation; decline in cerebral blood flow; coma; loss of ocular reflexes; progressive decrease in EEG	Progressive decrease in blood pressure, heart rate, and cardiac output; re-entrant dysrhythmias; maximum risk of ventricular fibrillation; asystole	Pulmonic congestion and edema; 75% decrease in oxygen consumption; apnea	Decrease in renal blood flow parallels decrease in cardiac output; extreme oliguria; poikilothermia; 80% decrease in basal metabolism	No motion; decreased nerve-conduction velocity; peripheral areflexia; no corneal or oculocephalic reflexes

Source: Modified from RR Kempainen, DD Brunette: Resp. Care 49:192, 2004.

(3) the depression of a frozen chest wall is not possible. As the resuscitation proceeds, the prognosis is grave if there is evidence of widespread cell lysis, as reflected by potassium levels > 10 mmol/L (10 meq/L). Other findings that may preclude continuing resuscitation include a core temperature < 10–12°C, a pH < 6.5, or evidence of intravascular thrombosis with a fibrinogen value < 0.5 g/L (<50 mg/dL). The decision to terminate resuscitation before rewarming the patient past 33°C should be predicated on the type and severity of the precipitants of hypothermia. There are no validated prognostic indicators for recovery from hypothermia. A history of asphyxia with secondary cooling is the most important negative predictor of survival.

DIAGNOSIS AND STABILIZATION

Hypothermia is confirmed by measuring the core temperature, preferably at two sites. Rectal probes should be placed to a depth of 15 cm and not adjacent to cold feces. A simultaneous esophageal probe should be placed 24 cm below the larynx; it may read falsely high during heated inhalation therapy. Relying solely on infrared tympanic thermography is not advisable.

After a diagnosis of hypothermia is established, cardiac monitoring should be instituted, along with attempts to limit further heat loss. If the patient is in ventricular fibrillation, one defibrillation attempt (2 J/kg) should be administered. If the rhythm does not convert, rewarm the patient to 30–32°C before repeating defibrillation attempts. Supplemental oxygenation is always warranted, since tissue oxygenation is adversely affected by the leftward shift of the oxyhemoglobin dissociation curve. Pulse oximetry may be unreliable in patients with vasoconstriction. If protective airway reflexes are absent, gentle endotracheal intubation should be performed. Adequate pre-oxygenation will prevent ventricular arrhythmias. Although cardiac pacing for hypothermic bradydysrhythmias is rarely indicated, the transthoracic technique is preferable.

Insertion of a gastric tube prevents dilatation secondary to decreased bowel motility. Indwelling bladder catheters facilitate monitoring of cold-induced diuresis. Dehydration is commonly encountered with chronic hypothermia, and most patients benefit from a bolus of crystalloid. Normal saline is preferable to lactated Ringer's solution, as the liver in hypothermic patients inefficiently metabolizes lactate. The placement of a pulmonary artery catheter risks perforation of the less compliant pulmonary artery. Insertion of a central venous catheter into the cold right atrium should be avoided, since this can precipitate arrhythmias.

Arterial blood gases should not be corrected for temperature (Chap. 48). An uncorrected pH of 7.42 and a P_{CO_2} of 40 mmHg reflects appropriate alveolar ventilation and acid-base balance at any core temperature. Acid-base imbalances should be corrected gradually, since the bicarbonate buffering system is inefficient. A common error is overzealous hyperventilation in the setting of depressed CO_2 production. When the P_{CO_2} decreases 10 mmHg at 28°C, it doubles the pH increase of 0.08 that occurs at 37°C.

The severity of anemia may be underestimated because the hematocrit increases 2% for each 1°C drop in temperature. White blood cell sequestration and bone marrow suppression are common, potentially masking an infection. Although hypokalemia is more common in chronic hypothermia, hyperkalemia also occurs; the expected electrocardiographic changes can be obscured by hypothermia. Patients with renal insufficiency, metabolic acidoses, or rhabdomyolysis are at greatest risk for electrolyte disturbances.

Coagulopathies are common because cold inhibits the enzymatic reactions required for activation of the intrinsic cascade. In addition, thromboxane B_2 production by platelets is temperature-dependent, and platelet function is impaired. The administration of platelets and fresh frozen plasma is, therefore, not effective. The prothrombin or partial thromboplastin times or INR (international normalized ratio) reported by the laboratory appear deceptively normal and contrast with the observed in vivo coagulopathy. This contradiction occurs because all coagulation tests are routinely performed at 37°C, and the enzymes are thus rewarmed.

REWARMING STRATEGIES

The key initial decision is whether to rewarm the patient passively or actively. *Passive external rewarming* simply involves covering and insulating the patient in a warm environment. With the head also covered, the rate of rewarming is usually 0.5° to 2.0°C per hour. This technique is ideal for previously healthy patients who develop acute, mild primary accidental hypothermia. The patient must have sufficient glycogen to support endogenous thermogenesis.

The application of heat directly to the extremities of patients with chronic severe hypothermia should be avoided because it can induce peripheral vasodilatation and precipitate core temperature "afterdrop"—a response characterized by a continual decline in the core temperature after removal of the patient from the cold. Truncal heat application reduces the risk of afterdrop.

Active rewarming is necessary under the following circumstances: core temperature < 32°C (poikilothermia), cardiovascular instability, age extremes, CNS dysfunction, hormone insufficiency, or suspicion of secondary hypothermia. *Active external rewarming* is best accomplished with forced-air heating blankets. Other options include radiant heat sources and hot packs. Monitoring a patient with hypothermia in a heated tub is extremely difficult. Electric blankets should be avoided because vasoconstricted skin is easily burned.

There are numerous widely available *active core rewarming* options. Airway rewarming with heated humidified oxygen (40°–45°C) is a convenient option via mask or endotracheal tube. Although airway rewarming provides less heat than some other forms of active core rewarming, it eliminates respiratory heat loss and adds 1°–2°C to the overall rewarming rate. Crystalloids should be heated to 40°–42°C, but the quantity of heat provided is significant only during massive volume resuscitation. The most efficient method for heating and delivering fluid or blood is with a countercurrent in-line heat exchanger. Heated irrigation of the gastrointestinal tract or bladder transfers minimal heat because of the limited available surface area. These methods should be reserved for patients in cardiac arrest and then used in combination with all available active rewarming techniques. Closed thoracic lavage is far more efficient in severely hypothermic patients with cardiac arrest. The hemithoraces are irrigated through two large-bore thoracostomy tubes that are inserted into the hemithoraces. Thoracostomy tubes should not be placed in the left chest of a spontaneously perfusing patient for purposes of rewarming. Peritoneal lavage with the dialysate at 40°–45°C efficiently transfers heat when delivered through two catheters with outflow suction. Like peritoneal dialysis, standard hemodialysis is especially useful for patients with electrolyte abnormalities, rhabdomyolysis, or toxin ingestions.

Extracorporeal blood rewarming options (Table 20-3) should be considered in severely hypothermic patients, especially those with *primary accidental hypothermia*. Cardiopulmonary bypass should be considered in nonperfusing patients without documented contraindications to resuscitation. Circulatory support may be the only effective option in patients with completely frozen extremities, or those with significant tissue destruction coupled with rhabdomyolysis. There is no evidence that extremely rapid rewarming improves survival in perfusing patients. The best strategy is usually a combination of passive, truncal active, and active core rewarming techniques.

TABLE 20-3 OPTIONS FOR EXTRACORPOREAL BLOOD REWARMING

Extracorporeal Rewarming (ECR) Technique	Considerations
Venovenous (VV)	Circuit—CV catheter to CV or peripheral catheter No oxygenator/circulatory support Flow rates 150–400 mL/min ROR 2°–3°C/h
Hemodialysis (HD)	Circuit—single or dual vessel cannulation Stabilizes electrolyte or toxicologic abnormalities Exchange cycle volumes 200–500 mL/min ROR 2°–3°C/h
Continuous arteriovenous rewarming (CAVR)	Circuit—percutaneous 8.5 Fr femoral catheters Requires BP 60 mmHg systolic No perfusionist/pump/anticoagulation Flow rates 225–375 mL/min ROR 3°–4°C/h
Cardiopulmonary bypass (CPB)	Circuit—full circulatory support with pump and oxygenator Perfusate-temperature gradient (5°–10°C) Flow rates 2–7 L/min (ave. 3–4) ROR up to 9.5°C/h

Note: BP, blood pressure; CV, central venous; ROR, rate of rewarming.

Rx HYPOTHERMIA

When a patient is hypothermic, target organs and the cardiovascular system respond minimally to most medications. Moreover, cumulative doses can cause toxicity during rewarming because of increased binding of drugs to proteins, and impaired metabolism and excretion. As an example, the administration of repeated doses of digoxin or insulin would be ineffective while the patient is hypothermic, and the residual drugs are potentially toxic during rewarming.

Achieving a mean arterial pressure of at least 60 mmHg should be an early objective. If the hypotension does not respond to crystalloid/colloid infusion and rewarming, low-dose dopamine (2–5 μg/kg per min) support should be considered. Perfusion of the vasoconstricted cardiovascular system may also be improved with low-dose IV nitroglycerin.

Atrial arrhythmias should initially be monitored without intervention, as the ventricular response will be slow, and unless preexistent, most will convert spontaneously during rewarming. The role of prophylaxis and treatment of ventricular arrhythmias is problematic. Preexisting ventricular ectopy may be suppressed by hypothermia and reappear during rewarming. None of the class I agents has proved to be safe and efficacious. When available, bretylium tosylate was the class III ventricular antiarrhythmic of choice. There is no evidence that amiodarone is safe.

Initiating empirical therapy for adrenal insufficiency is usually not warranted unless there is a history suggesting steroid dependence, hypoadrenalism, or a failure to rewarm with standard therapy. The administration of parenteral levothyroxine to euthyroid patients with hypothermia, however, is potentially hazardous. Because laboratory results can be delayed and confounded by the presence of the sick euthyroid syndrome (Chap. 335), historic clues or physical findings suggestive of hypothyroidism should be sought. When myxedema is the cause of hypothermia, the relaxation phase of the Achilles reflex is prolonged more than the contraction phase.

Hypothermia obscures most of the symptoms and signs of infection, notably fever and leukocytosis. Shaking rigors from infection may be mistaken for shivering. Except in mild cases, extensive cultures and repeated physical examinations are essential. Unless an infectious source is identified, empirical antibiotic prophylaxis is most warranted in the elderly, neonates, and immunocompromised patients.

Preventive measures should be discussed with high-risk individuals, such as the elderly or people whose work frequently exposes them to extreme cold. The importance of layered clothing and headgear, adequate shelter, increased caloric intake, and the avoidance of ethanol should be emphasized, along with access to rescue services.

FROSTBITE

Peripheral cold injuries include both freezing and nonfreezing injuries to tissue. Tissue freezes quickly when in contact with thermal conductors such as metal or volatile solutions. Other predisposing factors include constrictive clothing or boots, immobility, or vasoconstrictive medications. Frostbite occurs when the tissue temperature drops below 0°C. Ice crystal formation subsequently distorts and destroys the cellular architecture. Once the vascular endothelium is damaged, stasis progresses rapidly to microvascular thrombosis. After the tissue thaws, there is progressive dermal ischemia. The microvasculature begins to collapse, arteriovenous shunting increases tissue pressures, and edema forms. Finally, thrombosis, ischemia, and superficial necrosis appear. The development of mummification and demarcation may take weeks to months.

CLINICAL PRESENTATION

The initial presentation of frostbite can be deceptively benign. The symptoms always include a sensory deficiency affecting light touch, pain, and temperature perception. The acral areas and distal extremities are the most common insensate areas. Some patients complain of a clumsy or "chunk of wood" sensation in the extremity.

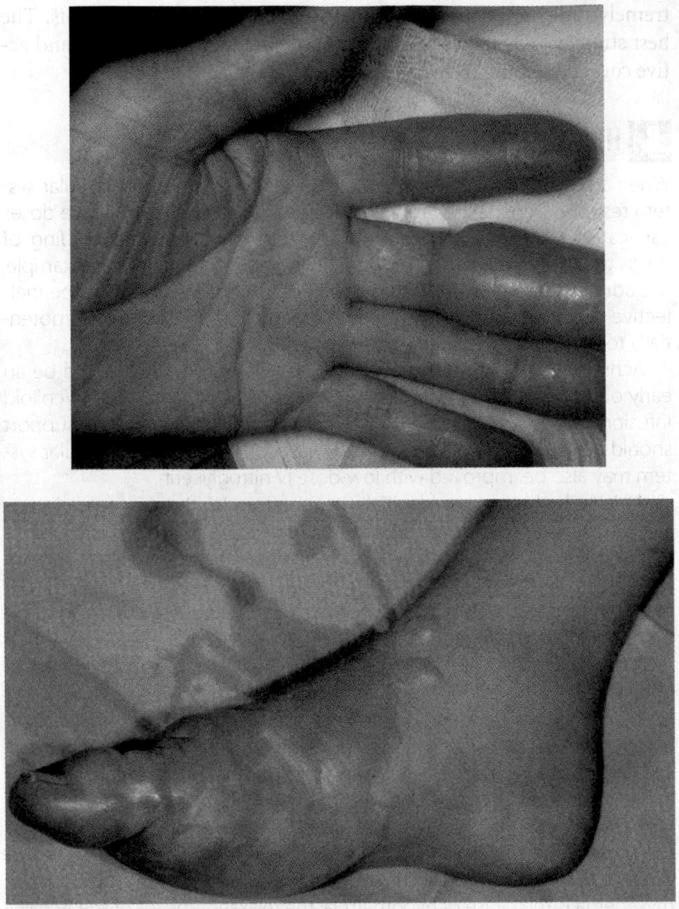

FIGURE 20-1 Frostbite with vesiculation, surrounded by edema and erythema.

Deep frostbitten tissue can appear waxy, mottled, yellow, or violaceous-white. Favorable presenting signs include some warmth or sensation with normal color. The injury is often superficial if the subcutaneous tissue is pliable or if the dermis can be rolled over boney prominences.

Clinically, it is most practical to classify frostbite as superficial or deep. Superficial does not entail tissue loss. Classically, frostbite is retrospectively graded like a burn. First-degree frostbite causes only anesthesia and erythema. The appearance of superficial vesiculation surrounded by edema and erythema is considered second degree (**Fig. 20-1**). Hemorrhagic vesicles reflect a serious injury to the microvasculature and indicate third-degree frostbite. Fourth-degree injuries damage subcuticular, muscular, and osseous tissues.

The two most common nonfreezing peripheral cold injuries are *chilblain (pernio)* and *immersion (trench) foot*. Chilblain results from neuronal and endothelial damage induced by repetitive exposure to dry cold. Young females, particularly those with a history of Raynaud's phenomenon, are at greatest risk. Persistent vasospasticity and vasculitis can cause erythema, mild edema, and pruritus. Eventually plaques, blue nodules, and ulcerations develop. These lesions typically involve the dorsa of the hands and feet. In contrast, immersion (trench) foot results from repetitive exposure to wet cold above the freezing point. The feet initially appear cyanotic, cold, and edematous. The subsequent development of bullae is often indistinguishable from frostbite. This vesiculation rapidly progresses to ulceration and liquefaction gangrene. Patients with milder cases complain of hyperhidrosis, cold sensitivity, and painful ambulation for many years.

℞ FROSTBITE

Frozen tissue should be rapidly and completely thawed by immersion in circulating water at 37°–40°C. Rapid rewarming often produces an initial hyperemia. The early formation of large clear distal blebs is more favorable than smaller proximal dark hemorrhagic blebs. A common error is the premature termination of thawing, since the reestablishment of perfusion is intensely painful. Parenteral narcotics will be necessary with deep frostbite. If cyanosis persists after rewarming, the tissue compartment pressures should be monitored carefully.

Numerous experimental antithrombotic and vasodilatory treatment regimens have been evaluated. There is no conclusive evidence that dextran, heparin, steroids, calcium channel blockers, hyperbaric oxygen, or prostaglandin inhibitors salvage tissue. A treatment protocol for frostbite is summarized in **Table 20-4**.

Unless infection develops, any decision regarding debridement or amputation should be deferred until there is clear evidence of demarcation, mummification, and sloughing. Magnetic resonance angiography may demonstrate the line of demarcation earlier than clinical demarcation. The most common symptomatic sequelae reflect neuronal injury and the persistently abnormal sympathetic tone, including paresthesias, thermal misperception, and hyperhidrosis. Delayed findings include nail deformities, cutaneous carcinomas, and epiphyseal damage in children.

Management of the chilblain syndrome is usually supportive. With refractory perniosis, alternatives include nifedipine, steroids, or limaprost, a prostaglandin E_1 analogue.

TABLE 20-4 TREATMENT FOR FROSTBITE

Before Thawing	During Thawing	After Thawing
Remove from environment	Consider parenteral analgesia and ketorolac	Gently dry and protect part; elevate; pledgets between toes, if macerated
Prevent partial thawing and refreezing	Administer ibuprofen, 400 mg PO	If clear vesicles are intact, aspirate sterilely; if broken, debride and dress with antibiotic or sterile aloe vera ointment
Stabilize core temperature and treat hypothermia	Immerse part in 37°–40°C (thermometer-monitored) circulating water containing an antiseptic soap until distal flush (10–45 min)	Leave hemorrhagic vesicles intact to prevent dessication and infection
Protect frozen part—no friction or massage	Encourage patient to gently move part	Continue ibuprofen 400 mg PO (12 mg/kg per day) q8–12h
Address medical or surgical conditions	If pain is refractory, reduce water temperature to 35°–37°C and administer parenteral narcotics	Consider tetanus and streptococcal prophylaxis; elevate part Hydrotherapy at 37°C Consider phenoxybenzamine in severe cases

FURTHER READINGS

Brieva J et al: Severe hypothermia: Challenging normal physiology. Anesth Intensive Care 33:662, 2005

Danzl DF: Accidental hypothermia, in *Rosen's Emergency Medicine: Concepts and Clinical Practice*, 6th ed, J Marx et al (eds). St. Louis, Mosby, 2006, p 2236

Ervasti O et al: The occurrence of frostbite and its risk factors in young men. Int J Circumpolar Health 63:71, 2004

Giesbrecht GG: Cold stress, near drowning and accidental hypothermia: A review. Aviat Space Environ Med 71:733, 2000

Jurkovich GJ: Environmental cold-induced injury. Surg Clin North Am 87(1):247, viii, 2007

Kempainen RR, Brunette DD: The evaluation and management of accidental hypothermia. Respir Care 49:192, 2004

Vassal T et al: Severe accidental hypothermia treated in an ICU: Prognosis and outcome. Chest 120:1998, 2001

SECTION 3 NERVOUS SYSTEM DYSFUNCTION

21 Syncope

Mark D. Carlson

Syncope, a transient loss of consciousness and postural tone due to reduced cerebral blood flow, is associated with spontaneous recovery. It may occur suddenly, without warning, or may be preceded by symptoms of faintness ("presyncope"). These symptoms include lightheadedness, dizziness, a feeling of warmth, diaphoresis, nausea, and visual blurring occasionally proceeding to transient blindness. Presyncopal symptoms vary in duration and may increase in severity until loss of consciousness occurs, or they may resolve prior to loss of consciousness if the cerebral ischemia is corrected. The differentiation of syncope from seizure is an important, sometimes difficult, diagnostic problem.

Syncope may be benign when it occurs as a result of normal cardiovascular reflex effects on heart rate and vascular tone, or serious when due to a life-threatening cardiac arrhythmia. Syncope may occur as a single event or may be recurrent. Recurrent, unexplained syncope, particularly in an individual with structural heart disease, is associated with a high risk of death (40% mortality within 2 years).

PATHOPHYSIOLOGY

Under normal circumstances systemic blood pressure is regulated by a complex process that includes the musculature, venous valves, autonomic nervous system, and renin-aldosterone-angiotensin system. Knowledge of these processes is important to understanding the pathophysiology of syncope. Approximately three-fourths of the systemic blood volume is contained in the venous bed, and any interference in venous return may lead to a reduction in cardiac output. Cerebral blood flow can be maintained if cardiac output and systemic arterial vasoconstriction compensate, but when these adjustments fail, hypotension with resultant cerebral underperfusion to less than half of normal results in syncope. Normally, the pooling of blood in the lower parts of the body is prevented by (1) pressor reflexes that induce constriction of peripheral arterioles and venules, (2) reflex acceleration of the heart by means of aortic and carotid reflexes, and (3) improvement of venous return to the heart by activity of the muscles of the limbs. Tilting a normal person upright on a tilt table causes some blood to accumulate in the lower limbs and diminishes cardiac output slightly; this may be followed by a slight transitory fall in systolic blood pressure. However, in a patient with defective vasomotor reflexes, upright tilt may produce an abrupt and sustained fall in blood pressure, precipitating a faint.

CAUSES OF SYNCOPE

Transiently decreased cerebral blood flow is usually due to one of three general mechanisms: disorders of vascular tone or blood volume, cardiovascular disorders including obstructive lesions and cardiac arrhythmias, or cerebrovascular disease (Table 21-1). Not infrequently, however, the cause of syncope is multifactorial.

DISORDERS OF VASCULAR TONE OR BLOOD VOLUME

Disorders of vascular tone or blood volume that can cause syncope include the reflex syncopes and a number of conditions resulting in orthostatic intolerance. The reflex syncopes—including neurocardiogenic syncope, situational syncope, and carotid sinus hypersensitivity—share common autonomic nervous system pathophysiologic mechanisms: a cardioinhibitory component (e.g., bradycardia due to increased vagal activity), a vasodepressor component (e.g., inappropriate vasodilatation due to sympathetic withdrawal), or both.

Neurocardiogenic (Vasovagal and Vasodepressor) Syncope The term *neurocardiogenic* is generally used to encompass both vasovagal and vasodepressor syncope. Strictly speaking, vasovagal syncope is associated with both sympathetic withdrawal (vasodilatation) and increased parasympathetic activity (bradycardia), whereas vasodepressor syncope is associated with sympathetic withdrawal alone.

These forms of syncope are the common faint that may be experienced by normal persons; they account for approximately half of all episodes of syncope. Neurocardiogenic syncope is frequently recurrent and commonly precipitated by a hot or crowded environment, alcohol, extreme fatigue, severe pain, hunger, prolonged standing, and emotional or stressful situations. Episodes are often preceded by a presyncopal prodrome lasting seconds to minutes, and rarely occur in the supine position. The individual is usually sitting or standing and experiences

TABLE 21-1 CAUSES OF SYNCOPE

I. Disorders of Vascular Tone or Blood Volume
- A. Reflex syncopes
  1. Neurocardiogenic
  2. Situational
     - Cough
     - Micturition
     - Defecation
     - Valsalva
     - Deglutition
  3. Carotid sinus hypersensitivity
- B. Orthostatic hypotension
  1. Drug-induced (antihypertensive or vasodilator drugs)
  2. Pure autonomic failure (idiopathic orthostatic hypotension)
  3. Multisystem atrophies
  4. Peripheral neuropathy (diabetic, alcoholic, nutritional, amyloid)
  5. Physical deconditioning
  6. Sympathectomy
  7. Decreased blood volume

II. Cardiovascular Disorders
- A. Structural and obstructive causes
  1. Pulmonary embolism
  2. Pulmonary hypertension
  3. Atrial myxoma
  4. Mitral valvular stenosis
  5. Myocardial disease (massive acute myocardial infarction)
  6. Left ventricular myocardial restriction or constriction
  7. Pericardial constriction or tamponade
  8. Aortic outflow tract obstruction
  9. Aortic valvular stenosis
  10. Hypertrophic obstructive cardiomyopathy
- B. Cardiac arrhythmias
  1. Bradyarrhythmias
     - a. Sinus bradycardia, sinoatrial block, sinus arrest, sick-sinus syndrome
     - b. Atrioventricular block
  2. Tachyarrhythmias
     - a. Supraventricular tachycardia with structural cardiovascular disease
     - b. Atrial fibrillation with the Wolff-Parkinson-White syndrome
     - c. Atrial flutter with 1:1 atrioventricular conduction
     - d. Ventricular tachycardia

III. Cerebrovascular Disease
- A. Vertebrobasilar insufficiency
- B. Basilar artery migraine

IV. Other Disorders that May Resemble Syncope
- A. Metabolic
  1. Hypoxia
  2. Anemia
  3. Diminished carbon dioxide due to hyperventilation
  4. Hypoglycemia
- B. Psychogenic
  1. Anxiety attacks
  2. Hysterical fainting
- C. Seizures

weakness, nausea, diaphoresis, lightheadedness, blurred vision, and often a forceful heartbeat with tachycardia followed by cardiac slowing and decreasing blood pressure prior to loss of consciousness. The individual appears pale or ashen; in dark-skinned individuals, the pallor may only be notable in the conjunctivae and lips. Patients with a gradual onset of presyncopal symptoms have time to protect themselves against injury; in others, syncope occurs suddenly, without warning.

The depth and duration of unconsciousness vary. Sometimes the patient remains partly aware of the surroundings, or there may be complete unresponsiveness. The unconscious patient usually lies motionless, with skeletal muscles relaxed, but a few clonic jerks of the limbs and face may occur. Sphincter control is usually maintained, in contrast to a seizure. The pulse may be feeble or apparently absent, the blood pressure low or undetectable, and breathing may be almost imperceptible. The duration of unconsciousness is rarely longer than a few minutes if the conditions that provoke the episode are reversed. Once the patient is placed in a horizontal position, the strength of the pulse improves, color begins to return to the face, breathing becomes quicker and deeper, and consciousness is restored. Some patients may experience a sense of residual weakness after regaining consciousness, and rising too soon may precipitate another faint. Unconsciousness may be prolonged if an individual remains upright; thus, it is essential that individuals with vasovagal syncope assume a recumbent position as soon as possible. Although usually benign, neurocardiogenic syncope can be associated with prolonged asystole and hypotension, resulting in hypoxic-ischemic injury.

Neurocardiogenic syncope often occurs in the setting of increased peripheral sympathetic activity and venous pooling. Under these conditions, vigorous myocardial contraction of a relatively empty left ventricle is thought to activate myocardial mechanoreceptors and vagal afferent nerve fibers that inhibit sympathetic activity and increase parasympathetic activity. The resultant vasodilatation and bradycardia induce hypotension and syncope. Although the reflex involving myocardial mechanoreceptors is the mechanism usually accepted as responsible for neurocardiogenic syncope, other reflexes may also be operative. Patients with transplanted (denervated) hearts have experienced cardiovascular responses identical to those present during neurocardiogenic syncope. This should not be possible if the response depends solely on the reflex mechanisms described above, unless the transplanted heart has become reinnervated. Moreover, neurocardiogenic syncope often occurs in response to stimuli (fear, emotional stress, or pain) that may not be associated with venous pooling in the lower extremities, which suggests a cerebral component to the reflex.

As distinct from the peripheral mechanisms, the central nervous system (CNS) mechanisms responsible for neurocardiogenic syncope are uncertain, but a sudden surge in central serotonin levels may contribute to the sympathetic withdrawal. Endogenous opiates (endorphins) and adenosine are also putative participants in the pathogenesis.

Situational Syncope A variety of activities, including cough, deglutition, micturition, and defecation, are associated with syncope in susceptible individuals. Like neurocardiogenic syncope, these syndromes may involve a cardioinhibitory response, a vasodepressor response, or both. Cough, micturition, and defecation are associated with maneuvers (such as Valsalva's, straining, and coughing) that may contribute to hypotension and syncope by decreasing venous return. Increased intracranial pressure secondary to the increased intrathoracic pressure may also contribute by decreasing cerebral blood flow.

Cough syncope typically occurs in men with chronic bronchitis or chronic obstructive lung disease during or after prolonged coughing fits. Micturition syncope occurs predominantly in middle-aged and older men, particularly those with prostatic hypertrophy and obstruction of the bladder neck; loss of consciousness usually occurs at night during or immediately after voiding. Deglutition syncope and defecation syncope occur in men and women. Deglutition syncope may be associated with esophageal disorders, particularly esophageal spasm. In some individuals, particular foods and carbonated or cold beverages initiate episodes by activating esophageal sensory receptors that trigger reflex sinus bradycardia or atrioventricular (AV) block. Defecation syncope is probably secondary to Valsalva's maneuver in older individuals with constipation.

Carotid Sinus Hypersensitivity Syncope due to carotid sinus hypersensitivity is precipitated by pressure on the carotid sinus baroreceptors, which are located just cephalad to the bifurcation of the common carotid artery. This typically occurs in the setting of shaving, a tight collar, or turning the head to one side. Carotid sinus hypersensitivity occurs predominantly in men ≥50 years old. Activation of carotid sinus baroreceptors gives rise to impulses carried via the nerve of Hering, a branch of the glossopharyngeal nerve, to the medulla in the brainstem. These afferent impulses activate efferent sympathetic nerve fibers to the heart and blood vessels, cardiac vagal efferent nerve fibers, or both. In patients with carotid sinus hypersensitivity, these responses may cause sinus arrest or AV block (a cardioinhibitory response), vasodilatation (a vasodepressor response), or both (a mixed response). The underlying mechanisms responsible for the carotid sinus hypersensitivity are not clear, and validated diagnostic criteria do not exist.

Postural (Orthostatic) Hypotension Orthostatic intolerance can result from hypovolemia or from disturbances in vascular control. The latter may occur due to agents that affect the vasculature or due to primary or secondary abnormalities of autonomic control. Sudden rising from a recumbent position or standing quietly are precipitating circumstances. *Orthostatic hypotension may be the cause of syncope in up to 30% of the elderly; polypharmacy with antihypertensive or antidepressant drugs is often a contributor in these patients.*

Postural syncope may occur in otherwise normal persons with defective postural reflexes. Pure autonomic failure (formerly called *idiopathic postural hypotension*) is characterized by orthostatic hypotension, syncope and near syncope, neurocardiogenic bladder, constipation, heat intolerance, inability to sweat, and erectile dysfunction (Chap. 370). The disorder is more common in men than women and typically begins between the ages of 50 and 75 years.

Orthostatic hypotension, often accompanied by disturbances in sweating, impotence, and sphincter difficulties, is also a primary feature of a variety or other autonomic nervous system disorders (Chap. 370). Among the most common causes of neurogenic orthostatic hypotension are chronic diseases of the peripheral nervous system that involve postganglionic unmyelinated fibers (e.g., diabetic, nutritional, and amyloid polyneuropathy). Much less common are the multiple system atrophies; these are CNS disorders in which orthostatic hypotension is associated with (1) parkinsonism (Shy-Drager syndrome), (2) progressive cerebellar degeneration, or (3) a more variable parkinsonian and cerebellar syndrome (Chap. 366). A rare, acute postganglionic dysautonomia may represent a variant of Guillain-Barré syndrome (Chap. 380); a related disorder, autoimmune autonomic neuropathy, is associated with autoantibodies to the ganglionic acetylcholine receptor.

There are several additional causes of postural syncope: (1) after physical deconditioning (such as after prolonged illness with recumbency, especially in elderly individuals with reduced muscle tone) or after prolonged weightlessness, as in space flight; (2) after sympathectomy that has abolished vasopressor reflexes; and (3) in patients receiving antihypertensive or vasodilator drugs and those who are hypovolemic because of diuretics, excessive sweating, diarrhea, vomiting, hemorrhage, or adrenal insufficiency.

Glossopharyngeal Neuralgia Syncope due to glossopharyngeal neuralgia (Chap. 371) is preceded by pain in the oropharynx, tonsillar fossa, or tongue. Loss of consciousness is usually associated with asystole rather than vasodilatation. The mechanism is thought to involve activation of afferent impulses in the glossopharyngeal nerve that terminate in the nucleus solitarius of the medulla and, via collaterals, activate the dorsal motor nucleus of the vagus nerve.

CARDIOVASCULAR DISORDERS

Cardiac syncope results from a sudden reduction in cardiac output, caused most commonly by a cardiac arrhythmia. In normal individuals, heart rates between 30 and 180 beats/min do not reduce cerebral blood flow, especially if the person is in the supine position. As the heart rate decreases, ventricular filling time and stroke volume increase to maintain normal cardiac output. At rates <30 beats/min, stroke volume can no longer increase to compensate adequately for the decreased heart rate. At rates greater than ~180 beats/min, ventricular filling time is inadequate to maintain adequate stroke volume. In either case, cerebral hypoperfusion and syncope may occur. Upright posture; cerebrovascular disease; anemia; loss of atrioventricular synchrony; and coronary, myocardial, or valvular disease all reduce the tolerance to alterations in rate.

Bradyarrhythmias (Chap. 225) may occur as a result of an abnormality of impulse generation (e.g., sinoatrial arrest) or impulse conduction (e.g., AV block). Either may cause syncope if the escape pacemaker rate is insufficient to maintain cardiac output. Syncope due to bradyarrhythmias may occur abruptly, without presyncopal symptoms, and recur several times daily. Patients with *sick sinus syndrome* may have sinus pauses (>3 s), and those with syncope due to high-degree AV block (*Stokes-Adams-Morgagni syndrome*) may have evidence of conduction system disease (e.g., prolonged PR interval, bundle branch block). However, the arrhythmia is often transitory, and the surface electrocardiogram or continuous electrocardiographic monitor (Holter monitor) taken later may not reveal the abnormality. The *bradycardia-tachycardia syndrome* is a common form of sinus node dysfunction in which syncope generally occurs as a result of marked sinus pauses, some following termination of paroxysms of atrial tachyarrhythmias. Drugs are a common cause for bradyarrhythmias, particularly in patients with underlying structural heart disease. Digoxin, β-adrenergic receptor antagonists, calcium channel blockers, and many antiarrhythmic drugs may suppress sinoatrial node impulse generation or slow AV nodal conduction.

Syncope due to a *tachyarrhythmia* (Chap. 226) is usually preceded by palpitation or lightheadedness but may occur abruptly with no warning symptoms. *Supraventricular tachyarrhythmias* are unlikely to cause syncope in individuals with structurally normal hearts but may do so if they occur in patients with (1) heart disease that also compromises cardiac output, (2) cerebrovascular disease, (3) a disorder of vascular tone or blood volume, or (4) a rapid ventricular rate. These tachycardias result most commonly from paroxysmal atrial flutter, atrial fibrillation, or reentry involving the AV node or accessory pathways that bypass part or all of the AV conduction system. Patients with *Wolff-Parkinson-White syndrome* may experience syncope when a very rapid ventricular rate occurs due to reentry across an accessory AV connection.

In patients with structural heart disease, ventricular tachycardia is a common cause of syncope, particularly in those with a prior myocardial infarction. Patients with aortic valvular stenosis and hypertrophic obstructive cardiomyopathy are also at risk for ventricular tachycardia. Individuals with abnormalities of ventricular repolarization (prolongation of the QT interval) are at risk to develop polymorphic ventricular tachycardia (torsades des pointes). Those with the inherited form of this syndrome often have a family history of sudden death in young individuals. Genetic markers can identify some patients with familial long-QT syndrome, but the clinical utility of these markers remains unproven. Drugs (i.e., certain antiarrhythmics and erythromycin) and electrolyte disorders (i.e., hypokalemia, hypocalcemia, hypomagnesemia) can prolong the QT interval and predispose to torsades des pointes. Antiarrhythmic medications may precipitate ventricular tachycardia, particularly in patients with structural heart disease.

In addition to arrhythmias, syncope may also occur with a variety of structural cardiovascular disorders. Episodes are usually precipitated when the cardiac output cannot increase to compensate adequately for peripheral vasodilatation. Peripheral vasodilatation may be appropriate, such as following exercise, or may occur due to inappropriate activation of left ventricular mechanoreceptor reflexes, as occurs in aortic outflow tract obstruction (aortic valvular stenosis or hypertrophic obstructive cardiomyopathy). Obstruction to forward flow is the most common reason that cardiac output cannot increase. Pericardial tamponade is a rare cause of syncope. Syncope occurs in up to 10% of patients with massive pulmonary embolism and may occur with exertion in patients with severe primary pulmonary hypertension. The cause is an inability of the right ventricle to provide appropriate cardiac output in the presence of obstruction or increased pulmonary vascular resistance. Loss of consciousness is usually accompanied by other symptoms such as chest pain and dyspnea. Atrial myxoma, a prosthetic valve thrombus, and, rarely, mitral stenosis may impair left ventricular filling, decrease cardiac output, and cause syncope.

CEREBROVASCULAR DISEASE

Cerebrovascular disease alone rarely causes syncope but may lower the threshold for syncope in patients with other causes. The vertebrobasilar arteries, which supply brainstem structures responsible for maintaining consciousness, are usually involved when cerebrovascular disease causes or contributes to syncope. An exception is the rare patient with tight bilateral carotid stenosis and recurrent syncope, often precipitated by standing or walking. Most patients who experience lightheadedness or syncope due to cerebrovascular disease also have symptoms of focal neurologic ischemia, such as arm or leg weakness, diplopia, ataxia, dysarthria, or sensory disturbances. Basilar artery migraine is a rare disorder that causes syncope in adolescents.

DIFFERENTIAL DIAGNOSIS

ANXIETY ATTACKS AND HYPERVENTILATION SYNDROME

Anxiety, such as occurs in panic attacks, is frequently interpreted as a feeling of faintness or dizziness resembling presyncope. However, the symptoms are not accompanied by facial pallor and are not relieved by recumbency. The diagnosis is made on the basis of the associated symptoms such as a feeling of impending doom, air hunger, palpitations, and tingling of the fingers and perioral region. Attacks can often be reproduced by hyperventilation, resulting in hypocapnia, alkalosis, increased cerebrovascular resistance, and decreased cerebral blood flow. The release of epinephrine also contributes to the symptoms.

SEIZURES

A seizure may be heralded by an aura, which is caused by a focal seizure discharge and hence has localizing significance (Chap. 363). The aura is usually followed by a rapid return to normal or by a loss of consciousness. Injury from falling is frequent in a seizure and rare in syncope, since only in generalized seizures are protective reflexes abolished instantaneously. Sustained tonic-clonic movements are characteristic of convulsive seizures, but brief clonic, or tonic-clonic, seizure-like activity can accompany fainting episodes. The period of unconsciousness in seizures tends to be longer than in syncope. Urinary incontinence is frequent in seizures and rare in syncope. The return of consciousness is prompt in syncope and slow after a seizure. Mental confusion, headache, and drowsiness are common sequelae of seizures, whereas physical weakness with a clear sensorium characterizes the postsyncopal state. Repeated spells of unconsciousness in a young person at a rate of several per day or month are more suggestive of epilepsy than syncope. See Table 363-7 for a comparison of seizures and syncope.

HYPOGLYCEMIA

Severe hypoglycemia is usually due to a serious disease such as a tumor of the islets of Langerhans or advanced adrenal, pituitary, or hepatic disease; or to excessive administration of insulin.

HYSTERICAL FAINTING

The attack is usually unattended by an outward display of anxiety. Lack of change in pulse and blood pressure or color of the skin and mucous membranes distinguish it from the vasodepressor faint.

APPROACH TO THE PATIENT: Syncope

The diagnosis of syncope is often challenging. The cause may only be apparent at the time of the event, leaving few, if any, clues when the patient is seen later by the physician. The physician should think first of those causes that constitute a therapeutic emergency, including massive internal hemorrhage or myocardial infarction, which may be painless, and cardiac arrhythmias. In elderly persons, a sudden faint, without obvious cause, should arouse the sus-

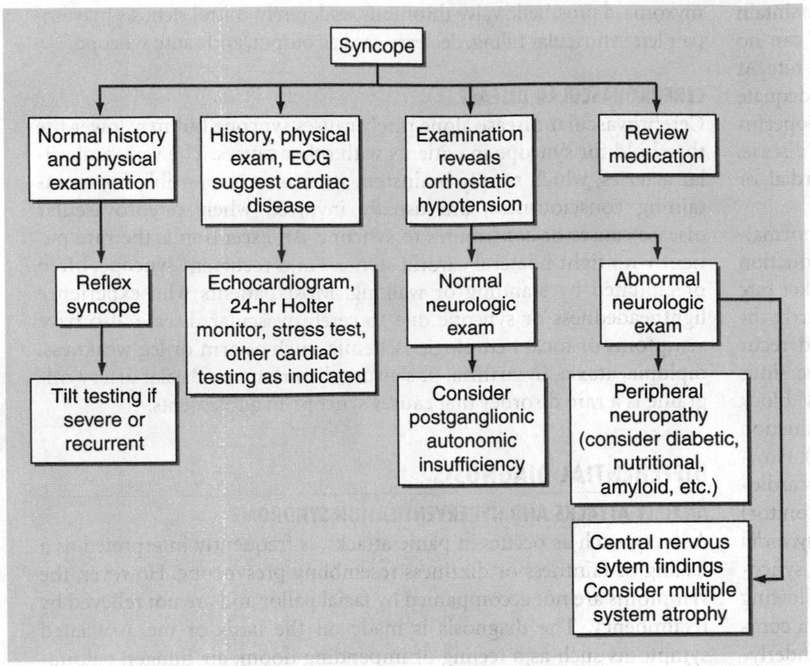

FIGURE 21-1 Approach to the patient with syncope.

picion of complete heart block or a tachyarrhythmia, even though all findings are negative when the patient is seen.

Figure 21-1 depicts an algorithmic approach to syncope. A careful history is the most important diagnostic tool, both to suggest the correct cause and to exclude important potential causes (Table 21-1). The nature of the events and their time course immediately prior to, during, and after an episode of syncope often provide valuable etiologic clues. Loss of consciousness in particular situations, such as during venipuncture or micturition or with volume depletion, suggests an abnormality of vascular tone. The position of the patient at the time of the syncopal episode is important; syncope in the supine position is unlikely to be vasovagal and suggests an arrhythmia or a seizure. Syncope due to carotid sinus syndrome may occur when the individual is wearing a shirt with a tight collar, turning the head (turning to look while driving in reverse), or manipulating the neck (as in shaving). The patient's medications must be noted, including nonprescription drugs or health store supplements, with particular attention to recent changes.

The physical examination should include evaluation of heart rate and blood pressure in the supine, sitting, and standing positions. In patients with unexplained recurrent syncope, an attempt to reproduce an attack may assist in diagnosis. Anxiety attacks induced by hyperventilation can be reproduced readily by having the patient breathe rapidly and deeply for 2–3 min. Cough syncope may be reproduced by inducing the Valsalva's maneuver. Carotid sinus massage should generally be avoided, unless carotid ultrasound is negative for atheroma, because its diagnostic specificity is unknown and it may provoke a transient ischemic attack (TIA) or stroke in individuals with carotid atheromas.

DIAGNOSTIC TESTS The choice of diagnostic tests should be guided by the history and the physical examination. Measurements of serum electrolytes, glucose, and the hematocrit are usually indicated. Cardiac enzymes should be evaluated if myocardial ischemia is suspected. Blood and urine toxicology screens may reveal the presence of alcohol or other drugs. In patients with possible adrenocortical insufficiency, plasma aldosterone and mineralocorticoid levels should be obtained.

Although the surface electrocardiogram is unlikely to provide a definitive diagnosis, it may provide clues to the cause of syncope *and should be performed in almost all patients*. The presence of conduction abnormalities (PR prolongation and bundle branch block) suggests a bradyarrhythmia, whereas pathologic Q waves or prolongation of the QT interval suggests a ventricular tachyarrhythmia. Inpatients should undergo continuous electrocardiographic monitoring; outpatients should wear a Holter monitor for 24–48 h. Whenever possible, symptoms should be correlated with the occurrence of arrhythmias. Continuous electrocardiographic monitoring may establish the cause of syncope in as many as 15% of patients. Cardiac event monitors may be useful in patients with infrequent symptoms, particularly in patients with presyncope. An implantable event monitor may be necessary for patients with extremely infrequent episodes. The presence of a late potential on a signal-averaged electrocardiogram is associated with increased risk for ventricular tachyarrhythmias in patients with a prior myocardial infarction. Low-voltage (visually inapparent) T wave alternans is also associated with development of sustained ventricular arrhythmias.

Invasive cardiac electrophysiologic testing provides diagnostic and prognostic information regarding sinus node function, AV conduction, and supraventricular and ventricular arrhythmias (Chaps. 225 and 226). Prolongation of the sinus node recovery time (>1500 ms) is a specific finding (85–100%) for diagnosis of sinus node dysfunction but has a low sensitivity; continuous electrocardiographic monitoring is usually more effective for diagnosing this abnormality. Prolongation of the HV interval and conduction block below the His bundle indicate that His-Purkinje disease may be responsible for syncope. Programmed stimulation for ventricular arrhythmias is most useful in patients who have experienced a myocardial infarction; the sensitivity and specificity of this technique is lower in patients with normal hearts or those with heart disease other than coronary artery disease.

Upright tilt table testing is indicated for recurrent syncope, a single syncopal episode that caused injury, or a single syncopal event in a "high-risk" setting (pilot, commercial vehicle driver, etc.), whether or not there is a history of preexisting heart disease or prior vasovagal episodes. In susceptible patients, upright tilt at an angle between 60° and 80° for 30–60 min induces a vasovagal episode. The protocol can be shortened if upright tilt is combined with administration of drugs that cause venous pooling or increase adrenergic stimulation (isoproterenol, nitroglycerin, edrophonium, or adenosine). The sensitivity and specificity of tilt-table testing is difficult to ascertain because of the lack of validated criteria. Moreover, the reflexes responsible for vasovagal syncope can be elicited in most, if not all, individuals given the appropriate stimulus. The specificity of tilt-table testing has been reported to be near 90%, but it is lower when pharmacologic provocation is employed. The reported sensitivity of the test ranges between 20 and 74%, the variability due to differences in populations studied, techniques used, and the absence of a true "gold standard" against which to compare test results. The reproducibility (in a time ranging from several hours to weeks) is 80–90% for an initially positive response, but may be less for an initially negative response (ranging from 30 to 90%).

A variety of other tests may be useful to determine the presence of structural heart disease that may cause syncope. The echocardiogram with Doppler examination detects valvular, myocardial, and pericardial abnormalities. The echocardiogram is the "gold standard" for the diagnosis of hypertrophic cardiomyopathy and atrial myxoma. Cardiac cine MRI provides an alternative noninvasive modality that may be useful for patients in whom diagnostic-quality echocardiographic images cannot be obtained. This test is also indicated for patients suspected of having arrhythmogenic right ventricular dysplasia or right ventricular outflow tract ventricular tachycardia. Both are associated with right ventricular structural abnormalities that are better visualized on MR imaging than by echocardiogram. Exercise testing may detect ischemia or exercise-induced arrhythmias. In some patients, cardiac catheterization may be necessary to diagnose the presence or severity of coronary artery disease or valvular abnormalities. Ultrafast CT scan, ventilation-perfusion scan, or pulmonary angiography is indicated in patients in whom syncope may be due to pulmonary embolus.

In cases of possible cerebrovascular syncope, neuroimaging tests may be indicated, including Doppler ultrasound studies of the carotid and vertebrobasilar systems, MRI, magnetic resonance angiography, and x-ray angiography of the cerebral vasculature (Chap. 364). Electroencephalography is indicated if seizures are suspected.

℞ SYNCOPE

The treatment of syncope is directed at the underlying cause. This discussion will focus on disorders of autonomic control. **Arrhythmias are discussed in Chaps. 225 and 226, valvular heart diseases in Chap. 230, and cerebrovascular disorders in Chap. 364.**

Certain precautions should be taken regardless of the cause of syncope. At the first sign of symptoms, patients should make every effort to avoid injury should they lose consciousness. Patients with frequent episodes, or those who have experienced syncope without warning symptoms, should avoid situations in which sudden loss of consciousness might result in injury (e.g., climbing ladders, swimming alone, operating heavy machinery, driving). Patients should lower their head to the extent possible and preferably should lie down. Lowering the head by bending at the waist should be avoided because it may further compromise venous return to the heart. When appropriate, family members or other close contacts should be educated as to the problem. This will ensure appropriate therapy and may prevent delivery of inappropriate therapy (chest compressions associated with cardiopulmonary resuscitation) that may inflict trauma.

Patients who have lost consciousness should be placed in a position that maximizes cerebral blood flow, offers protection from trauma, and secures the airway. Whenever possible, the patient should be placed supine with the head turned to the side to prevent aspiration and the tongue from blocking the airway. Assessment of the pulse and direct cardiac auscultation may assist in determining if the episode is associated with a bradyarrhythmia or a tachyarrhythmia. Clothing that fits tightly around the neck or waist should be loosened. Peripheral stimulation, such as sprinkling cold water on the face, may be helpful. Patients should not be given anything by mouth or be permitted to rise until the sense of physical weakness has passed.

Patients with vasovagal syncope should be instructed to avoid situations or stimuli that have caused them to lose consciousness and to assume a recumbent position when premonitory symptoms occur. These behavioral modifications alone may be sufficient for patients with infrequent and relatively benign episodes of vasovagal syncope, particularly when loss of consciousness occurs in response to a specific stimulus. Tilt training (standing and leaning against a wall for progressively longer periods each day) has been used with limited success, particularly for patients with orthostatic intolerance. Episodes associated with intravascular volume depletion may be prevented by salt and fluid loading prior to provocative events.

Drug therapy may be necessary when vasovagal syncope is resistant to the above measures, when episodes occur frequently, or when syncope is associated with a significant risk for injury. β-Adrenergic receptor antagonists (metoprolol, 25–50 mg bid; atenolol, 25–50 mg qd; or nadolol, 10–20 mg bid; all starting doses), the most widely used agents, mitigate the increase in myocardial contractility that stimulates left ventricular mechanoreceptors and also block central serotonin receptors. Serotonin reuptake inhibitors (paroxetine, 20–40 mg qd; or sertraline, 25–50 mg qd), appear to be effective for some patients. Bupropion SR (150 mg qd), another antidepressant, has also been used with success. β-Adrenergic receptor antagonists and serotonin reuptake inhibitors are well tolerated and are often used as first-line agents for younger patients. Hydrofludrocortisone (0.1–0.2 mg qd), a mineralocorticoid, promotes sodium retention, volume expansion, and peripheral vasoconstriction by increasing β-receptor sensitivity to endogenous catecholamines. Hydrofludrocortisone is useful for patients with intravascular volume depletion and for those who also have postural hypotension. Proamatine (2.5–10 mg bid or tid), an α-agonist, has been used as a first-line agent for some patients. In a randomized controlled trial, proamatine was more effective than placebo in preventing syncope during an upright tilt-test. However, in some patients, proamatine and hydrofludrocortisone may increase resting supine systemic blood pressure, which may be problematic for those with hypertension.

Disopyramide (150 mg bid), a vagolytic antiarrhythmic drug with negative inotropic properties, and transdermal scopolamine, another vagolytic, have been used to treat vasovagal syncope, as have theophylline and ephedrine. Side effects associated with these drugs have limited their use for this indication. Disopyramide is a type 1A antiarrhythmic drug and should be used with great caution, if at all, in patients who are at risk for ventricular arrhythmias.

Although several clinical trials have suggested that pharmacologic therapy for neurocardiogenic syncope is effective, the few long-term prospective randomized controlled trials have yielded mixed results. In the Prevention of Syncope Trial (POST), metoprolol was ineffective in patients <42 years of age but decreased the incidence of syncope in patients >42, raising the possibility that there may be significant age-related differences in response to pharmacologic therapy.

Studies of permanent pacing for neurocardiogenic syncope have also yielded mixed results. Dual-chamber cardiac pacing may be effective for patients with frequent episodes of vasovagal syncope, particularly for those with prolonged asystole associated with vasovagal episodes. Pacemakers that can be programmed to transiently pace at a high rate (90–100 beats/min) after a profound drop in the patient's intrinsic heart rate are most effective.

Patients with orthostatic hypotension should be instructed to rise slowly and systematically (supine to seated, seated to standing) from the bed or a chair. Movement of the legs prior to rising facilitates venous return from the lower extremities. Whenever possible, medications that aggravate the problem (vasodilators, diuretics, etc.) should be discontinued. Elevation of the head of the bed [20–30 cm (8–12 in.)] and use of compression stockings may help.

Additional therapeutic modalities include salt loading and a variety of pharmacologic agents including sympathomimetic amines, monamine oxidase inhibitors, beta blockers, and levodopa. The treatment of orthostatic hypotension secondary to central or peripheral disorders of the autonomic nervous system is discussed in Chap. 370.

Glossopharyngeal neuralgia is treated with carbamazepine, which is effective for syncope as well as for pain. Patients with carotid sinus hypersensitivity should be instructed to avoid clothing and situations that stimulate carotid sinus baroreceptors. They should turn their entire body, rather than just their head, when looking to the side. Those with intractable syncope due to the cardioinhibitory response to carotid sinus stimulation should undergo permanent pacemaker implantation.

Patients with syncope should be hospitalized when there is a possibility that the episode may have resulted from a life-threatening abnormality or if recurrence with significant injury seems likely. These individuals should be admitted to a bed with continuous electrocardiographic monitoring. Patients who are known to have a normal heart and for whom the history strongly suggests vasovagal or situational syncope may be treated as outpatients if the episodes are neither frequent nor severe.

FURTHER READINGS

GRUBB BP: Neurocardiogenic syncope and related disorders of orthostatic intolerance. Circulation 111:2997, 2005

———, OLSHANSKY B (eds): *Syncope: Mechanisms and Management*, 2d ed. Malden, Mass., Blackwell Futura, 2005

KAPOOR WN: Current evaluation in management of syncope. Circulation 106:1606, 2002

KAUFMAN H et al: Midodrine in neurally mediated syncope: A double-blind, randomized, crossover study. Ann Neurol 52:342, 2002

KAUFMANN H, BHATTACHARYA K: Diagnosis and treatment of neurally mediated syncope. Neurologist 8:175, 2002

KERR SRJ et al: Carotid sinus hypersensitivity in asymptomatic older persons: Implications for diagnosis of syncope and falls. Arch Intern Med 166:515, 2006

MAISEL W, STEBENSON W: Syncope—getting to the heart of the matter. N Engl J Med 347:931, 2002

SOTERIADES E et al: Incidence and prognosis of syncope. N Engl J Med 347:878, 2002

STRICKBERGER SA et al: AHA/ACCF scientific statement on the evaluation of syncope: From the American Heart Association Councils on Clinical Cardiology, Cardiovascular Nursing, Cardiovascular Disease in the Young, and Stroke, and the Quality of Care and Outcomes Research Interdisciplinary Working Group; and the American College of Cardiology Foundation: In collaboration with the Heart Rhythm Society: Endorsed by the American Autonomic Society. Circulation 113(2):316, 2006

VAN DIJK N et al: Quality of life within one year following presentation after transient loss of consciousness. Am J Cardio 100:672, 2007

22 Dizziness and Vertigo

Robert B. Daroff

Dizziness is a common and often vexing symptom. Patients use the term to encompass a variety of sensations, including those that seem semantically appropriate (e.g., lightheadedness, faintness, spinning, giddiness) and those that are misleadingly inappropriate, such as mental confusion, blurred vision, headache, or tingling. Moreover, some individuals with gait disorders caused by peripheral neuropathy, myelopathy, spasticity, parkinsonism, or cerebellar ataxia complain of "dizziness" despite the absence of vertigo or other abnormal cephalic sensations. In this context, the term *dizziness* is being used to describe disturbed ambulation. There may be mild associated lightheadedness, particularly with impaired sensation from the feet or poor vision; this is known as *multiple-sensory-defect dizziness* and occurs in elderly individuals who complain of dizziness only when walking. Decreased position sense (secondary to neuropathy or myelopathy) and poor vision (from cataracts or retinal degeneration) create an overreliance on the aging vestibular apparatus. A less precise but sometimes comforting designation to patients is *benign dysequilibrium of aging*. Thus, a careful history is necessary to determine exactly what a patient who states, "Doctor, I'm dizzy," is experiencing. After eliminating the misleading symptoms or gait disturbance, "dizziness" usually means either *faintness* (presyncope) or *vertigo* (an illusory or hallucinatory sense of movement of the body or environment, most often a feeling of spinning). Operationally, after obtaining the history, dizziness may be classified into three categories: (1) faintness, (2) vertigo, and (3) miscellaneous head sensations.

FAINTNESS

Prior to an actual faint (syncope), there are often prodromal presyncopal symptoms (faintness) reflecting ischemia to a degree insufficient to impair consciousness. These include lightheadedness, "dizziness" without true vertigo, a feeling of warmth, diaphoresis, nausea, and visual blurring occasionally proceeding to blindness. Presyncopal symptoms vary in duration and may increase in severity until loss of consciousness occurs or may resolve prior to loss of consciousness if the cerebral ischemia is corrected. Faintness and syncope are discussed in detail in Chap. 21.

VERTIGO

Vertigo is usually due to a disturbance in the vestibular system. The end organs of this system, situated in the bony labyrinths of the inner ears, consist of the three semicircular canals and the otolithic apparatus (utricle and saccule) on each side. The canals transduce angular acceleration, while the otoliths transduce linear acceleration and the static gravitational forces that provide a sense of head position in space. The neural output of the end organs is conveyed to the vestibular nuclei in the brainstem via the eighth cranial nerves. The principal projections from the vestibular nuclei are to the nuclei of cranial nerves III, IV, and VI; spinal cord; cerebral cortex; and cerebellum. The vestibuloocular reflex (VOR) serves to maintain visual stability during head movement and depends on direct projections from the vestibular nuclei to the sixth cranial nerve (abducens) nuclei in the pons and, via the medial longitudinal fasciculus, to the third (oculomotor) and fourth (trochlear) cranial nerve nuclei in the midbrain. These connections account for the nystagmus (to-and-fro oscillation of the eyes) that is an almost invariable accompaniment of vestibular dysfunction. The vestibular nerves and nuclei project to areas of the cerebellum (primarily the flocculus and nodulus) that modulate the VOR. The vestibulospinal pathways assist in the maintenance of postural stability. Projections to the cerebral cortex, via the thalamus, provide conscious awareness of head position and movement.

The vestibular system is one of three sensory systems subserving spatial orientation and posture; the other two are the visual system (retina to occipital cortex) and the somatosensory system that conveys peripheral information from skin, joint, and muscle receptors. The three stabilizing systems overlap sufficiently to compensate (partially or completely) for each other's deficiencies. Vertigo may represent either physiologic stimulation or pathologic dysfunction in any of the three sensory systems.

Physiologic Vertigo This occurs in normal individuals when (1) the brain is confronted with an intersensory mismatch among the three stabilizing sensory systems; (2) the vestibular system is subjected to unfamiliar head movements to which it is unadapted, such as in seasickness; (3) unusual head/neck positions, such as the extreme extension when painting a ceiling; or (4) following a spin. Intersensory mismatch explains carsickness, height vertigo, and the visual vertigo most commonly experienced during motion picture chase scenes; in the latter, the visual sensation of environmental movement is unaccompanied by concomitant vestibular and somatosensory movement cues. *Space sickness*, a frequent transient effect of active head movement in the weightless zero-gravity environment, is another example of physiologic vertigo.

Pathologic Vertigo This results from lesions of the visual, somatosensory, or vestibular systems. Visual vertigo is caused by new or incorrect eyeglasses or by the sudden onset of an extraocular muscle paresis with diplopia; in either instance, central nervous system (CNS) compensation rapidly counteracts the vertigo. Somatosensory vertigo, rare in isolation, is usually due to a peripheral neuropathy or myelopathy that reduces the sensory input necessary for central compensation when there is dysfunction of the vestibular or visual systems.

The most common cause of pathologic vertigo is vestibular dysfunction involving either its end organ (labyrinth), nerve, or central connections. The vertigo is associated with jerk nystagmus and is frequently accompanied by nausea, postural unsteadiness, and gait ataxia. Since vertigo increases with rapid head movements, patients tend to hold their heads still.

LABYRINTHINE DYSFUNCTION This causes severe rotational or linear vertigo. When rotational, the hallucination of movement, whether of environment or self, is directed away from the side of the lesion. The fast phases of nystagmus beat away from the lesion side, and the tendency to fall is toward the side of the lesion, particularly in darkness or with the eyes closed.

Under normal circumstances, when the head is straight and immobile, the vestibular end organs generate a tonic resting firing frequency that is equal from the two sides. With any rotational acceleration, the anatomic positions of the semicircular canals on each side necessitate an increased firing rate from one and a commensurate decrease from the other. This change in neural activity is ultimately projected to the cerebral cortex, where it is summed with inputs from the visual and somatosensory systems to produce the appropriate conscious sense of rotational movement. After cessation of prolonged rotation, the firing frequencies of the two end organs reverse; the side with the initially increased rate decreases, and the other side increases. A sense of rotation in the opposite direction is experienced; since there is no actual head movement, this hallucinatory sensation is *physiologic postrotational vertigo*.

Any disease state that changes the firing frequency of an end organ, producing unequal neural input to the brainstem and ultimately the cerebral cortex, causes vertigo. The symptom can be conceptualized as the cortex inappropriately interpreting the abnormal neural input as indicating actual head rotation. Transient abnormalities produce short-lived symptoms. With a fixed unilateral deficit, central compensatory mechanisms ultimately diminish the vertigo. Since compensation depends on the plasticity of connections between the vestibular nuclei and the cerebellum, patients with brainstem or cerebellar disease have diminished adaptive capacity, and symptoms may persist indefinitely. Compensation is always inadequate for severe fixed bilateral lesions despite normal cerebellar connections; these patients are permanently symptomatic when they move their heads.

Acute unilateral labyrinthine dysfunction is caused by infection, trauma, and ischemia. Often, no specific etiology is uncovered, and the nonspecific terms *acute labyrinthitis, acute peripheral vestibulopathy*, or *vestibular neuritis* are used to describe the event. The vertiginous attacks are brief and leave the patient with mild vertigo for several days. Infection with herpes simplex virus type 1 has been implicated. It is impossible to predict whether a patient recovering from the first bout of vertigo will have recurrent episodes.

Labyrinthine ischemia, presumably due to occlusion of the labyrinthine branch of the internal auditory artery, may be the sole manifestation of vertebrobasilar insufficiency (Chap. 364); patients with this syndrome present with the abrupt onset of severe vertigo, nausea, and vomiting, but without tinnitus or hearing loss.

Acute bilateral labyrinthine dysfunction is usually the result of toxins such as drugs or alcohol. The most common offending drugs are the aminoglycoside antibiotics that damage the hair cells of the vestibular end organs and may cause a permanent disorder of equilibrium.

Recurrent unilateral labyrinthine dysfunction, in association with signs and symptoms of cochlear disease (progressive hearing loss and tinnitus), is usually due to Ménière's disease (Chap. 30). When auditory manifestations are absent, the term *vestibular neuronitis* denotes recurrent monosymptomatic vertigo. Transient ischemic attacks of the posterior cerebral circulation (vertebrobasilar insufficiency) only infrequently cause recurrent vertigo without concomitant motor, sensory, visual, cranial nerve, or cerebellar signs (Chap. 364).

Positional vertigo is precipitated by a recumbent head position, either to the right or to the left. Benign paroxysmal positional (or positioning) vertigo (BPPV) of the posterior semicircular canal is particularly common. Although the condition may be due to head trauma, usually no precipitating factors are identified. It generally abates spontaneously after weeks or months. The vertigo and accompanying nystagmus have a distinct pattern of latency, fatigability, and habituation that differs from the less common central positional vertigo (Table 22-1) due to lesions in and around the fourth ventricle. Moreover, the pattern of nystagmus in posterior canal BPPV is distinctive. When supine, with the head turned to the side of the offending ear (bad ear down), the lower eye displays a large-amplitude torsional nystagmus, and the upper eye has a lesser degree of torsion combined with upbeating nystagmus. If the eyes are directed to the upper ear, the vertical nystagmus in the upper eye increases in amplitude. Mild dysequilibrium when upright may also be present.

A *perilymphatic fistula* should be suspected when episodic vertigo is precipitated by Valsalva or exertion, particularly upon a background of a stepwise progressive sensory-neural hearing loss. The condition is usually caused by head trauma or barotrauma or occurs after middle ear surgery.

TABLE 22-1 BENIGN PAROXYSMAL POSITIONAL VERTIGO AND CENTRAL POSITIONAL VERTIGO

Features	BPPV	Central
Latency[a]	3–40 s	None: immediate vertigo and nystagmus
Fatigability[b]	Yes	No
Habituation[c]	Yes	No
Intensity of vertigo	Severe	Mild
Reproducibility[d]	Variable	Good

[a]Time between attaining head position and onset of symptoms.
[b]Disappearance of symptoms with maintenance of offending position.
[c]Lessening of symptoms with repeated trials.
[d]Likelihood of symptom production during any examination session.

TABLE 22-2 FEATURES OF PERIPHERAL AND CENTRAL VERTIGO

Sign or Symptom	Peripheral (Labyrinth)	Central (Brainstem or Cerebellum)
Direction of associated nystagmus	Unidirectional; fast phase opposite lesion[a]	Bidirectional or unidirectional
Purely horizontal nystagmus without torsional component	Uncommon	Common
Vertical or purely torsional nystagmus	Never present	May be present
Visual fixation	Inhibits nystagmus and vertigo	No inhibition
Severity of vertigo	Marked	Often mild
Direction of spin	Toward fast phase	Variable
Direction of fall	Toward slow phase	Variable
Duration of symptoms	Finite (minutes, days, weeks) but recurrent	May be chronic
Tinnitus and/or deafness	Often present	Usually absent
Associated CNS abnormalities	None	Extremely common (e.g., diplopia, hiccups, cranial neuropathies, dysarthria)
Common causes	BPPV, infection (labyrinthitis), Ménière's, neuronitis, ischemia, trauma, toxin	Vascular, demyelinating, neoplasm

[a]In Ménière's disease, the direction of the fast phase is variable.

VERTIGO OF VESTIBULAR NERVE ORIGIN This occurs with diseases that involve the nerve in the petrous bone or the cerebellopontine angle. Although less severe and less frequently paroxysmal, it has many of the characteristics of labyrinthine vertigo. The adjacent auditory division of the eighth cranial nerve is usually affected, which explains the frequent association of vertigo with unilateral tinnitus and hearing loss. The most common cause of eighth cranial nerve dysfunction is a tumor, usually a schwannoma (*acoustic neuroma*) or a meningioma. These tumors grow slowly and produce such a gradual reduction of labyrinthine output that central compensatory mechanisms can prevent or minimize the vertigo; auditory symptoms are the most common manifestations.

CENTRAL VERTIGO Lesions of the brainstem or cerebellum can cause acute vertigo, but associated signs and symptoms usually permit distinction from a labyrinthine etiology (Table 22-2). Occasionally, an acute lesion of the vestibulocerebellum may present with monosymptomatic vertigo indistinguishable from a labyrinthopathy.

Vertigo may be a manifestation of a migraine aura (Chap. 15), but some patients with migraine have episodes of vertigo unassociated with their headaches. Antimigrainous treatment should be considered in such patients with otherwise enigmatic vertiginous episodes.

Vestibular epilepsy, vertigo secondary to temporal lobe epileptic activity, is rare and almost always intermixed with other epileptic manifestations.

PSYCHOGENIC VERTIGO This is sometimes called phobic postural vertigo and is usually a concomitant of panic attacks (Chap. 386) or agoraphobia (fear of large open spaces, crowds, or leaving the safety of home). It should be suspected in patients so "incapacitated" by their symptoms that they adopt a prolonged housebound status. Most patients with organic vertigo attempt to function despite their discomfort. Organic vertigo is accompanied by nystagmus; a psychogenic etiology is almost certain when nystagmus is absent during a vertiginous episode. The symptoms often develop after an episode of acute labyrinthine dysfunction.

MISCELLANEOUS HEAD SENSATIONS

This designation is used, primarily for purposes of initial classification, to describe dizziness that is neither faintness nor vertigo. Cephalic ischemia or vestibular dysfunction may be of such low intensity that the usual symptomatology is not clearly identified. For example, a small decrease in blood pressure or a slight vestibular imbalance may cause sensations different from distinct faintness or vertigo but that may be identified properly by provocative testing techniques (see below). Other causes of dizziness in this category are hyperventilation syndrome, hypoglycemia, and the somatic symptoms of a clinical depression; these patients should all have normal neurologic examinations and vestibular function tests. Depressed patients often insist that the depression is "secondary" to the dizziness.

APPROACH TO THE PATIENT: Dizziness and Vertigo

The most important diagnostic tool is a detailed history focused on the meaning of "dizziness" to the patient. Is it faintness (presyncope)? Is there a sensation of spinning? If either of these is affirmed and the neurologic examination is normal, appropriate investigations for the multiple causes of cephalic ischemia, presyncope (Chap. 21), or vestibular dysfunction are undertaken.

When the meaning of "dizziness" is uncertain, provocative tests may be helpful. These office procedures simulate either cephalic ischemia or vestibular dysfunction. Cephalic ischemia is obvious if the dizziness is duplicated during maneuvers that produce orthostatic hypotension. Further provocation involves the Valsalva maneuver, which decreases cerebral blood flow and should reproduce ischemic symptoms.

Hyperventilation is the cause of dizziness in many anxious individuals; tingling of the hands and face may be absent. Forced hyperventilation for 1 min is indicated for patients with enigmatic dizziness and normal neurologic examinations.

The simplest provocative test for vestibular dysfunction is rapid rotation and abrupt cessation of movement in a swivel chair. This always induces vertigo that the patients can compare with their symptomatic dizziness. The intense induced vertigo may be unlike the spontaneous symptoms, but shortly thereafter, when the vertigo has all but subsided, a lightheadedness supervenes that may be identified as "my dizziness." When this occurs, the dizzy patient, originally classified as suffering from "miscellaneous head sensations," is now properly diagnosed as having mild vertigo secondary to a vestibulopathy.

Patients with symptoms of positional vertigo should be appropriately tested (Table 22-1). A final provocative and diagnostic vestibular test, requiring the use of Frenzel eyeglasses (self-illuminated goggles with convex lenses that blur out the patient's vision, but allow the examiner to see the eyes greatly magnified), is vigorous head shaking in the horizontal plane for about 10 s. If nystagmus develops after the shaking stops, even in the absence of vertigo, vestibular dysfunction is demonstrated. The maneuver can then be repeated in the vertical plane. If the provocative tests establish the dizziness as a vestibular symptom, an evaluation of vestibular vertigo is undertaken.

EVALUATION OF PATIENTS WITH PATHOLOGIC VESTIBULAR VERTIGO

The evaluation depends on whether a central etiology is suspected (Table 22-2). If so, MRI of the head is mandatory. Such an examination is rarely helpful in cases of recurrent monosymptomatic vertigo with a normal neurologic examination. Typical BPPV requires no investigation after the diagnosis is made (Table 22-1).

Vestibular function tests serve to (1) demonstrate an abnormality when the distinction between organic and psychogenic is uncertain, (2) establish the side of the abnormality, and (3) distinguish between peripheral and central etiologies. The standard test is electronystagmography (calorics), where warm and cold water (or air) are applied, in a prescribed fashion, to the tympanic membranes, and the slow-phase velocities of the resultant nystagmus from the two are compared. A velocity decrease from one side indicates hypofunction ("canal paresis"). An inability to induce nystagmus with ice water denotes a "dead labyrinth." Some institutions have the capability of quantitatively determining various aspects of the VOR using computer-driven rotational chairs and precise oculographic recording of the eye movements.

TABLE 22-3 TREATMENT OF VERTIGO

Agent[a]	Dose[b]
Antihistamines	
Meclizine	25–50 mg 3 times/day
Dimenhydrinate	50 mg 1–2 times/day
Promethazine[c]	25–50-mg suppository or IM
Benzodiazepines	
Diazepam	2.5 mg 1–3 times/day
Clonazepam	0.25 mg 1–3 times/day
Phenothiazines	
Prochlorperazine[c]	5 mg IM or 25 mg suppository
Anticholinergic[d]	
Scopolamine transdermal	Patch
Sympathomimetics[d]	
Ephedrine	25 mg/d
Combination preparations[d]	
Ephedrine and promethazine	25 mg/d of each
Exercise therapy	
Repositioning maneuvers[e]	
Vestibular rehabilitation[f]	
Other	
Diuretics or low-salt (1 g/d) diet[g]	
Antimigrainous drugs[h]	
Inner ear surgery[i]	
Glucocorticoids[c]	100 mg/d for 3 days, tapered by 20 mg every 3 days

[a]All listed drugs are U.S. Food and Drug Administration approved, but most are not approved for the treatment of vertigo.
[b]Usual oral (unless otherwise stated) starting dose in adults; maintenance dose can be reached by a gradual increase.
[c]For acute vertigo only.
[d]For motion sickness only.
[e]For benign paroxysmal positional vertigo.
[f]For vertigo other than Ménière's and positional.
[g]For Ménière's disease.
[h]For migraine-associated vertigo (see Chap. 15 for a listing of prophylactic antimigrainous drugs).
[i]For perilymphatic fistula and refractory cases of Ménière's disease.

CNS disease can produce dizzy sensations of all types. Consequently, a neurologic examination is always required even if the history or provocative tests suggest a cardiac, peripheral vestibular, or psychogenic etiology. Any abnormality on the neurologic examination should prompt appropriate neurodiagnostic studies.

Rx VERTIGO

Treatment of acute vertigo consists of bed rest (1–2 days maximum) and vestibular suppressant drugs such as antihistaminics (meclizine, dimenhydrinate, promethazine), tranquilizers with GABA-ergic effects (diazepam, clonazepam), phenothiazines (prochlorperazine), or glucocorticoids (**Table 22-3**). If the vertigo persists beyond a few days, most authorities advise ambulation in an attempt to induce central compensatory mechanisms, despite the short-term discomfort to the patient. Chronic vertigo of labyrinthine origin may be treated with a systematized vestibular rehabilitation program to facilitate central compensation.

Posterior semicircular canal BPPV, the most common type, is often self-limited but, when persistent, may respond dramatically to specific repositioning exercise programs designed to empty particulate debris from the canal. One of these exercises, the Epley procedure, is graphically demonstrated, in four languages, on a website for use in both physicians' offices and self-treatment (*www.charite.de/ch/neuro/vertigo.html*).

Prophylactic measures to prevent recurrent vertigo are variably effective. Antihistamines are commonly utilized but are of limited value. Ménière's disease may respond to a diuretic or, more effectively, to a very low salt diet (1 g/d). Recurrent episodes of migraine-associated vertigo should be treated with antimigrainous therapy (Chap. 15). There are a variety of inner ear surgical procedures for refractory Ménière's disease, but these are only rarely necessary.

Psychogenic ("phobic postural") vertigo is best treated with cognitive-behavioral therapy.

Helpful websites for both physicians and vertigo patients are: *www.iVertigo.net* and *www.tchain.com*.

Global Considerations There are no epidemiologic studies indicating an increased frequency of specific types of vertigo in different geographical areas. However, whereas BPPV of the posterior semicircular canal is overwhelmingly the most common form of positional vertigo in most countries, there seems to be an unusually large number of reports of horizontal (lateral) BPPV from Italy and Korea.

FURTHER READINGS

DIETERICH M: Dizziness. The Neurologist 10:154, 2004

HALMAGI GM: Diagnosis and management of vertigo. Clin Med 5:159, 2005

LEIGH RJ, ZEE DS: *Neurology of Eye Movement*, 4th ed. New York, Oxford, 2006, pp 76–79; 559–597

STRUPP M et al: Methylprednisolone, valacyclovir, or the combination for vestibular neuritis. N Engl J Med 351:354, 2004

———, BRANDT T: Pharmacological advances in the treatment of neuro-otological and eye movement disorders. Curr Opin Neurol 19:33, 2006

WHITE J et al: Canalith repositioning for benign paroxysmal positional vertigo. Otol Neurotol 26:704, 2005

ZINGLER VC et al: Causative factors and epidemiology of bilateral vestibulopathy in 255 patients. Ann Neurol 61:524, 2007

23 Weakness and Paralysis

Michael J. Aminoff

Normal motor function involves integrated muscle activity that is modulated by the activity of the cerebral cortex, basal ganglia, cerebellum, and spinal cord. Motor system dysfunction leads to weakness or paralysis, which is discussed in this chapter, or to ataxia (Chap. 368) or abnormal movements (Chap. 367). The mode of onset, distribution, and accompaniments of weakness help to suggest its cause.

Weakness is a reduction in the power that can be exerted by one or more muscles. Increased fatigability or limitation in function due to pain or articular stiffness is often confused with weakness by patients. *Increased fatigability* is the inability to sustain the performance of an activity that should be normal for a person of the same age, gender, and size. Increased time is sometimes required for full power to be exerted, and this *bradykinesia* may be misinterpreted as weakness. Severe proprioceptive sensory loss may also lead to complaints of weakness because adequate feedback information about the direction and power of movements is lacking. Finally, *apraxia,* a disorder of planning and initiating a skilled or learned movement unrelated to a significant motor or sensory deficit (Chap. 27), is sometimes mistaken for weakness by inexperienced medical staff.

Paralysis indicates weakness that is so severe that the muscle cannot be contracted at all, whereas *paresis* refers to weakness that is mild or moderate. The prefix "hemi-" refers to one half of the body, "para-" to both legs, and "quadri-" to all four limbs. The suffix "-plegia" signifies severe weakness or paralysis.

Weakness or paralysis is typically accompanied by other neurologic abnormalities that help to indicate the site of the responsible lesion. These include changes in tone, muscle bulk, muscle stretch reflexes, and cutaneous reflexes (Table 23-1).

Tone is the resistance of a muscle to passive stretch. Central nervous system (CNS) abnormalities that cause weakness generally produce *spasticity*, an increase in tone associated with disease of upper motor neurons. Spasticity is velocity-dependent, has a sudden release after reaching a maximum (the "clasp-knife" phenomenon), and predominantly affects the antigravity muscles (i.e., upper-limb flexors and lower-limb extensors). Spasticity is distinct from rigidity and paratonia, two other types of hypertonia. *Rigidity* is increased tone that is present throughout the range of motion (a "lead pipe" or "plastic" stiffness) and affects flexors and extensors equally; it sometimes has a cogwheel quality that is enhanced by voluntary movement of the contralateral limb (reinforcement). Rigidity occurs with certain extrapyramidal disorders such as Parkinson's disease. *Paratonia* (or *gegenhalten*) is increased tone that varies irregularly in a manner that may seem related to the degree of relaxation, is present throughout the range of motion, and affects flexors and extensors equally; it usually results from disease of the frontal lobes. Weakness with *decreased tone* (*flaccidity*) or normal tone occurs with disorders of *motor units.* A motor unit consists of a single lower motor neuron and all of the muscle fibers that it innervates.

TABLE 23-1 SIGNS THAT DISTINGUISH ORIGIN OF WEAKNESS

Sign	Upper Motor Neuron	Lower Motor Neuron	Myopathic
Atrophy	None	Severe	Mild
Fasciculations	None	Common	None
Tone	Spastic	Decreased	Normal/decreased
Distribution of weakness	Pyramidal/regional	Distal/segmental	Proximal
Tendon reflexes	Hyperactive	Hypoactive/absent	Normal/hypoactive
Babinski's sign	Present	Absent	Absent

Muscle bulk is generally unaffected in patients with upper motor neuron lesions, although mild disuse atrophy may eventually occur. By contrast, atrophy is often conspicuous when a lower motor neuron lesion is responsible for weakness and may also occur with advanced muscle disease.

Muscle stretch (tendon) reflexes are usually increased with upper motor neuron lesions, although they may be decreased or absent for a variable period immediately after onset of an acute lesion. This is usually—but not invariably—accompanied by abnormalities of *cutaneous reflexes* (such as superficial abdominals; Chap. 361) and, in particular, by an extensor plantar (Babinski) response. The muscle stretch reflexes are depressed in patients with lower motor neuron lesions when there is direct involvement of specific reflex arcs. The stretch reflexes are generally preserved in patients with myopathic weakness except in advanced stages, when they are sometimes attenuated. In disorders of the neuromuscular junction, the intensity of the reflexes may be affected by preceding voluntary activity of affected muscles—such activity may lead to enhancement of initially depressed reflexes in Lambert-Eaton myasthenic syndrome and, conversely, to depression of initially normal reflexes in myasthenia gravis (Chap. 381).

The distinction of *neuropathic* (lower motor neuron) from *myopathic* weakness is sometimes difficult clinically, although distal weakness is likely to be neuropathic and symmetric proximal weakness myopathic. *Fasciculations* (visible or palpable twitch within a muscle due to the spontaneous discharge of a motor unit) and early atrophy indicate that weakness is neuropathic.

PATHOGENESIS

Upper Motor Neuron Weakness This pattern of weakness results from disorders that affect the upper motor neurons or their axons in the cerebral cortex, subcortical white matter, internal capsule, brainstem, or spinal cord (Fig. 23-1). Such lesions produce weakness through decreased activation of the lower motor neurons. In general, distal muscle groups are affected more severely than proximal ones, and axial movements are spared unless the lesion is severe and bilateral. With corticobulbar involvement, weakness is usually observed only in the lower face and tongue; extraocular, upper facial, pharyngeal, and jaw muscles are almost always spared. With bilateral corticobulbar lesions, *pseudobulbar palsy* often develops: dysarthria, dysphagia, dysphonia, and emotional

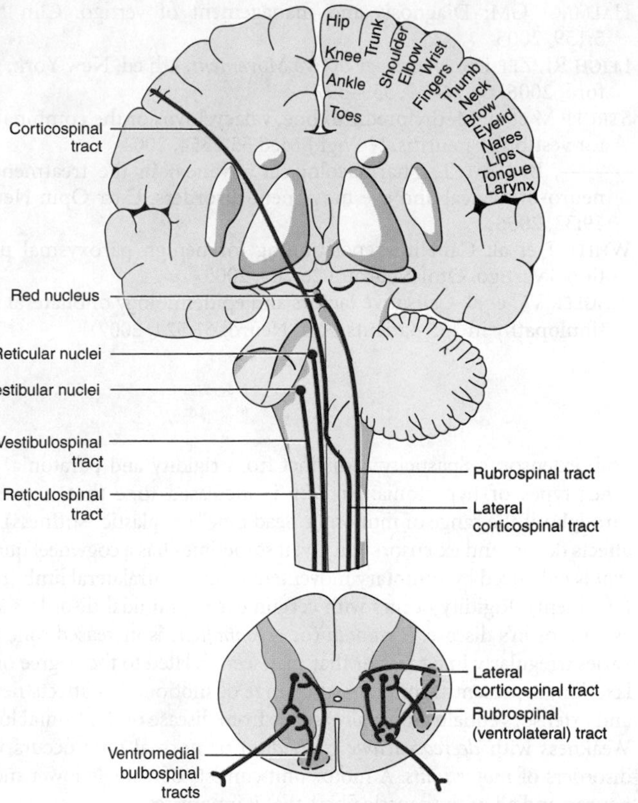

FIGURE 23-1 The corticospinal and bulbospinal upper motor neuron pathways. Upper motor neurons have their cell bodies in layer V of the primary motor cortex (the precentral gyrus, or Brodmann's area 4) and in the premotor and supplemental motor cortex (area 6). The upper motor neurons in the primary motor cortex are somatotopically organized as illustrated on the right side of the figure.

Axons of the upper motor neurons descend through the subcortical white matter and the posterior limb of the internal capsule. Axons of the *pyramidal* or *corticospinal system* descend through the brainstem in the cerebral peduncle of the midbrain, the basis pontis, and the medullary pyramids. At the cervicomedullary junction, most pyramidal axons decussate into the contralateral corticospinal tract of the lateral spinal cord, but 10–30% remain ipsilateral in the anterior spinal cord. Pyramidal neurons make direct monosynaptic connections with lower motor neurons. They innervate most densely the lower motor neurons of hand muscles and are involved in the execution of learned, fine movements. Corticobulbar neurons are similar to corticospinal neurons but innervate brainstem motor nuclei.

Bulbospinal upper motor neurons influence strength and tone but are not part of the pyramidal system. The descending *ventromedial bulbospinal pathways* originate in the tectum of the midbrain (tectospinal pathway), the vestibular nuclei (vestibulospinal pathway), and the reticular formation (reticulospinal pathway). These pathways influence axial and proximal muscles and are involved in the maintenance of posture and integrated movements of the limbs and trunk. The descending *ventrolateral bulbospinal pathways*, which originate predominantly in the red nucleus (rubrospinal pathway), facilitate distal limb muscles. The bulbospinal system is sometimes referred to as the *extrapyramidal upper motor neuron system*. In all figures, nerve cell bodies and axon terminals are shown, respectively, as closed circles and forks.

lability accompany bilateral facial weakness and a brisk jaw jerk. Spasticity accompanies upper motor neuron weakness but may not be present in the acute phase. Upper motor neuron lesions also affect the ability to perform rapid repetitive movements. Such movements are slow and coarse, but normal rhythmicity is maintained. Finger-nose-finger and heel-knee-shin maneuvers are performed slowly but adequately.

Lower Motor Neuron Weakness This pattern results from disorders of cell bodies of lower motor neurons in the brainstem motor nuclei and the anterior horn of the spinal cord, or from dysfunction of the axons of these neurons as they pass to skeletal muscle (Fig. 23-2). Weakness is due to a decrease in the number of muscle fibers that can be activated, through a loss of α motor neurons or disruption of their connections to muscle. Loss of γ motor neurons does not cause weakness but decreases tension on the muscle spindles, which decreases muscle tone and attenuates the stretch reflexes elicited on examination. An absent stretch reflex suggests involvement of spindle afferent fibers.

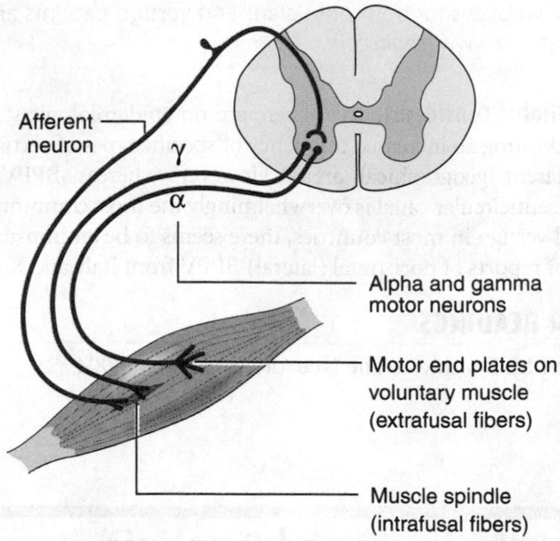

FIGURE 23-2 Lower motor neurons are divided into α and γ types. The larger α motor neurons are more numerous and innervate the extrafusal muscle fibers of the motor unit. Loss of α motor neurons or disruption of their axons produces lower motor neuron weakness. The smaller, less numerous γ motor neurons innervate the intrafusal muscle fibers of the muscle spindle and contribute to normal tone and stretch reflexes. The α motor neuron receives direct excitatory input from corticomotoneurons and primary muscle spindle afferents. The α and γ motor neurons also receive excitatory input from other descending upper motor neuron pathways, segmental sensory inputs, and interneurons. The α motor neurons receive direct inhibition from Renshaw cell interneurons, and other interneurons indirectly inhibit the α and γ motor neurons.

A tendon reflex requires the function of all illustrated structures. A tap on a tendon stretches muscle spindles (which are tonically activated by γ motor neurons) and activates the primary spindle afferent neurons. These stimulate the α motor neurons in the spinal cord, producing a brief muscle contraction, which is the familiar tendon reflex.

When a motor unit becomes diseased, especially in anterior horn cell diseases, it may spontaneously discharge, producing *fasciculations* that may be seen or felt clinically or recorded by electromyography (EMG). When α motor neurons or their axons degenerate, the denervated muscle fibers may also discharge spontaneously. These single muscle fiber discharges, or *fibrillation potentials,* cannot be seen or felt but can be recorded with EMG. If lower motor neuron weakness is present, recruitment of motor units is delayed or reduced, with fewer than normal activated at a given discharge frequency. This contrasts with weakness of upper motor neuron type, in which a normal number of motor units is activated at a given frequency but with a diminished maximal discharge frequency.

Myopathic Weakness Myopathic weakness is produced by disorders of the muscle fibers. Disorders of the neuromuscular junctions also produce weakness, but this is variable in degree and distribution and is influenced by preceding activity of the affected muscle. At a muscle fiber, if the nerve terminal releases a normal number of acetylcholine molecules presynaptically and a sufficient number of postsynaptic acetylcholine receptors are opened, the end plate reaches threshold and thereby generates an action potential that spreads across the muscle fiber membrane and into the transverse tubular system. This electrical excitation activates intracellular events that produce an energy-dependent contraction of the muscle fiber (excitation-contraction coupling).

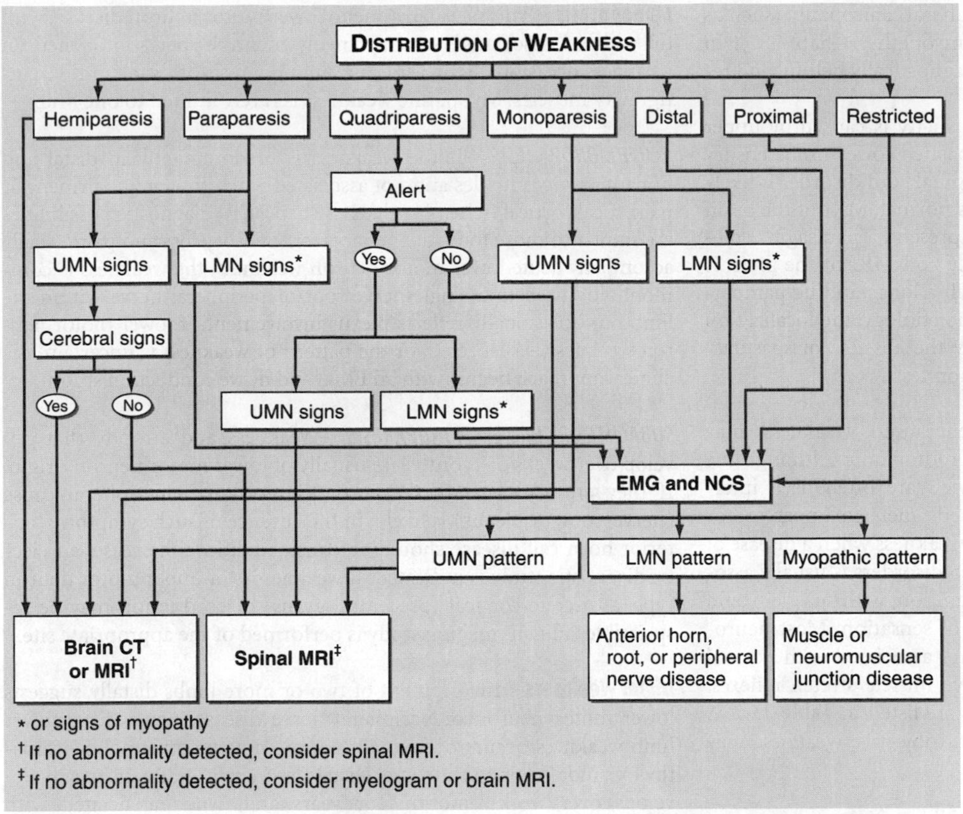

FIGURE 23-3 An algorithm for the initial workup of a patient with weakness. EMG, electromyography; LMN, lower motor neuron; NCS, nerve conduction studies; UMN, upper motor neuron.

Myopathic weakness is produced by a decrease in the number or contractile force of muscle fibers activated within motor units. With muscular dystrophies, inflammatory myopathies, or myopathies with muscle fiber necrosis, the number of muscle fibers is reduced within many motor units. On EMG, the size of each motor unit action potential is decreased, and motor units must be recruited more rapidly than normal to produce the desired power. Some myopathies produce weakness through loss of contractile force of muscle fibers or through relatively selective involvement of the type II (fast) fibers. These may not affect the size of individual motor unit action potentials and are detected by a discrepancy between the electrical activity and force of a muscle.

Diseases of the neuromuscular junction, such as myasthenia gravis, produce weakness in a similar manner, but the loss of muscle fibers is functional (due to inability to activate them) rather than related to muscle fiber loss. The number of muscle fibers that are activated varies over time, depending on the state of rest of the neuromuscular junctions. Thus, fatigable weakness is suggestive of myasthenia gravis or other disorders of the neuromuscular junction.

Hemiparesis Hemiparesis results from an upper motor neuron lesion above the midcervical spinal cord; most such lesions are above the foramen magnum. The presence of other neurologic deficits helps to localize the lesion. Thus, language disorders, cortical sensory disturbances, cognitive abnormalities, disorders of visual-spatial integration, apraxia, or seizures point to a cortical lesion. Homonymous visual field defects reflect either a cortical or a subcortical hemispheric lesion. A "pure motor" hemiparesis of the face, arm, or leg is often due to a small, discrete lesion in the posterior limb of the internal capsule, cerebral peduncle, or upper pons. Some brainstem lesions produce "crossed paralyses," consisting of ipsilateral cranial nerve signs and contralateral hemiparesis (Chap. 364). The absence of cranial nerve signs or facial weakness suggests that a hemiparesis is due to a lesion in the high cervical spinal cord, especially if associated with ipsilateral loss of proprioception and contralateral loss of pain and temperature sense (the Brown-Séquard syndrome).

Acute or episodic hemiparesis usually results from ischemic or hemorrhagic stroke, but may also relate to hemorrhage occurring into brain tumors or as a result of trauma; other causes include a focal structural lesion or inflammatory process as in multiple sclerosis, abscess, or sarcoidosis. Evaluation begins immediately with a CT scan of the brain (Fig. 23-3) and laboratory studies. If the CT is normal and an ischemic stroke is unlikely, MRI of the brain or cervical spine is performed.

Subacute hemiparesis that evolves over days or weeks has an extensive differential diagnosis. A common cause is subdural hematoma, especially in elderly or anticoagulated patients, even when there is no history of trauma. Infectious possibilities include cerebral abscess, fungal granuloma or meningitis, and parasitic infection. Weakness from primary and metastatic neoplasms may evolve over days to weeks. AIDS may present with subacute hemiparesis due to toxoplasmosis or primary CNS lymphoma. Noninfectious inflammatory processes, such as multiple sclerosis or, less commonly, sarcoidosis, merit consideration. If the brain MRI is normal and there are no cortical and hemispheric signs, MRI of the cervical spine should be undertaken.

Chronic hemiparesis that evolves over months is usually due to a neoplasm or vascular malformation, a chronic subdural hematoma, or a degenerative disease. If an MRI of the brain is normal, the possibility of a foramen magnum or high cervical spinal cord lesion should be considered.

Paraparesis An intraspinal lesion at or below the upper thoracic spinal cord level is most commonly responsible, but a paraparesis may also result from lesions at other locations that disturb upper motor neurons (especially parasagittal intracranial lesions) and lower motor neurons [anterior horn cell disorders, cauda equina syndromes due to involvement of nerve roots derived from the lower spinal cord (Chap. 372), and peripheral neuropathies].

Acute paraparesis may not be recognized as due to spinal cord disease at an early stage if the legs are flaccid and areflexic. Usually, however, there is sensory loss in the legs with an upper level on the trunk; a dissociated sensory loss suggestive of a central cord syndrome; or exaggerated stretch reflexes in the legs with normal reflexes in the arms. It is important to image the spinal cord (Fig. 23-3). Compressive lesions (particularly epidural tumor, abscess, or hematoma, but also a prolapsed intervertebral disk and vertebral involvement by malignancy or infection), spinal cord infarction (proprioception is usually spared), an arteriovenous fistula or other vascular anomaly, and transverse myelitis, are among the possible causes (Chap. 372).

Diseases of the cerebral hemispheres that produce acute paraparesis include anterior cerebral artery ischemia (shoulder shrug is also affected), superior sagittal sinus or cortical venous thrombosis, and acute hydrocephalus. If upper motor neuron signs are associated with drowsiness, confusion, seizures, or other hemispheric signs, MRI of the brain should be undertaken.

Paraparesis may result from a cauda equina syndrome, for example, following trauma to the low back, a midline disk herniation, or an intraspinal tumor; although sphincters are affected, hip flexion is often spared, as is sensation over the anterolateral thighs. Rarely, paraparesis is caused by a rapidly evolving anterior horn cell disease (such as poliovirus or West Nile virus infection), peripheral neuropathy (such as Guillain-Barré syndrome; Chap. 380) or myopathy (Chap. 382). In such cases, electrophysiologic studies are diagnostically helpful and refocus the subsequent evaluation.

Subacute or chronic paraparesis with spasticity is caused by upper motor neuron disease. When there is associated lower-limb sensory loss and sphincter involvement, a chronic spinal cord disorder is likely (Chap. 372). If an MRI of the spinal cord is normal, MRI of the brain may be indicated. If hemispheric signs are present, a parasagittal meningioma or chronic hydrocephalus is likely and MRI of the brain is the initial test. In the rare situation in which a longstanding paraparesis has a lower motor neuron or myopathic etiology, the localization is usually suspected on clinical grounds by the absence of spasticity and confirmed by EMG and nerve conduction tests.

Quadriparesis or Generalized Weakness Generalized weakness may be due to disorders of the CNS or of the motor unit. Although the terms *quadriparesis* and *generalized weakness* are often used interchangeably, quadriparesis is commonly used when an upper motor neuron cause is suspected, and generalized weakness when a disease of the motor unit is likely. Weakness from CNS disorders is usually associated with changes in consciousness or cognition, with spasticity and brisk stretch reflexes, and with alterations of sensation. Most neuromuscular causes of generalized weakness are associated with normal mental function, hypotonia, and hypoactive muscle stretch reflexes. The major causes of intermittent weakness are listed in Table 23-2. A patient with generalized fatigability without objective weakness may have the chronic fatigue syndrome (Chap. 384).

ACUTE QUADRIPARESIS Acute quadriparesis with onset over minutes may result from disorders of upper motor neurons (e.g., anoxia, hypotension, brainstem or cervical cord ischemia, trauma, and systemic metabolic abnormalities) or muscle (electrolyte disturbances, certain inborn errors of muscle energy metabolism, toxins, or periodic paralyses). Onset over hours to weeks may, in addition to the above, be due to lower motor neuron disorders. Guillain-Barré syndrome (Chap. 380) is the most common lower motor neuron weakness that progresses over days to 4 weeks; the finding of an elevated protein level in the cerebrospinal fluid is helpful but may be absent early in the course.

In obtunded patients, evaluation begins with a CT scan of the brain. If upper motor neuron signs are present but the patient is alert, the initial test is usually an MRI of the cervical cord. If weakness is lower motor neuron, myopathic, or uncertain in origin, the clinical approach begins with blood studies to determine the level of muscle enzymes and electrolytes and an EMG and nerve conduction study.

SUBACUTE OR CHRONIC QUADRIPARESIS When quadriparesis due to upper motor neuron disease develops over weeks, months, or years, the distinction between disorders of the cerebral hemispheres, brainstem, and cervical spinal cord is usually possible clinically. An MRI is obtained of the clinically suspected site of pathology. EMG and nerve conduction studies help to distinguish lower motor neuron disease (which usually presents with weakness that is most profound distally) from myopathic weakness, which is typically proximal.

TABLE 23-2 CAUSES OF EPISODIC GENERALIZED WEAKNESS

1. Electrolyte disturbances, e.g., hypokalemia, hyperkalemia, hypercalcemia, hypernatremia, hyponatremia, hypophosphatemia, hypermagnesemia
2. Muscle disorders
   a. Channelopathies (periodic paralyses)
   b. Metabolic defects of muscle (impaired carbohydrate or fatty acid utilization; abnormal mitochondrial function)
3. Neuromuscular junction disorders
   a. Myasthenia gravis
   b. Lambert-Eaton myasthenic syndrome
4. Central nervous system disorders
   a. Transient ischemic attacks of the brainstem
   b. Transient global cerebral ischemia
   c. Multiple sclerosis

Monoparesis This is usually due to lower motor neuron disease, with or without associated sensory involvement. Upper motor neuron weakness occasionally presents as a monoparesis of distal and nonantigravity muscles. Myopathic weakness is rarely limited to one limb.

ACUTE MONOPARESIS If the weakness is predominantly in distal and nonantigravity muscles and not associated with sensory impairment or pain, focal cortical ischemia is likely (Chap. 364); diagnostic possibilities are similar to those for acute hemiparesis. Sensory loss and pain usually accompany acute lower motor neuron weakness; the weakness is commonly localized to a single nerve root or peripheral nerve within the limb but occasionally reflects plexus involvement. If lower motor neuron weakness is suspected, or the pattern of weakness is uncertain, the clinical approach begins with an EMG and nerve conduction study.

SUBACUTE OR CHRONIC MONOPARESIS Weakness and atrophy that develop over weeks or months are usually of lower motor neuron origin. If they are associated with sensory symptoms, a peripheral cause (nerve, root, or plexus) is likely; in the absence of such symptoms, anterior horn cell disease should be considered. In either case, an electrodiagnostic study is indicated. If weakness is of upper motor neuron type, a discrete cortical (precentral gyrus) or cord lesion may be responsible, and an imaging study is performed of the appropriate site.

Distal Weakness Involvement of two or more limbs distally suggests lower motor neuron or peripheral nerve disease. Acute distal lower limb weakness occurs occasionally from an acute toxic polyneuropathy or cauda equina syndrome. Distal symmetric weakness usually develops over weeks, months, or years and, when associated with numbness, is due to metabolic, toxic, hereditary, degenerative, or inflammatory diseases of peripheral nerves (Chap. 379). Anterior horn cell disease may begin distally but is typically asymmetric and without accompanying numbness (Chap. 369). Rarely, myopathies present with distal weakness (Chap. 382). Electrodiagnostic studies help to localize the disorder (Fig. 23-3).

Proximal Weakness Myopathy often produces symmetric weakness of the pelvic or shoulder girdle muscles (Chap. 382). Diseases of the neuromuscular junction [such as myasthenia gravis (Chap. 381)], may present with symmetric proximal weakness often associated with ptosis, diplopia, or bulbar weakness and fluctuating in severity during the day. Extreme fatigability present in some cases of myasthenia gravis may even suggest episodic weakness, but strength rarely returns fully to normal. In anterior horn cell disease proximal weakness is usually asymmetric, but may be symmetric if familial. Numbness does not occur with any of these diseases. The evaluation usually begins with determination of the serum creatine kinase level and electrophysiologic studies.

Weakness in a Restricted Distribution Weakness may not fit any of the above patterns, being limited, for example, to the extraocular, hemifacial, bulbar, or respiratory muscles. If unilateral, restricted weakness is usually due to lower motor neuron or peripheral nerve disease, such as in a facial palsy (Chap. 379) or an isolated superior oblique muscle paresis (Chap. 382). Weakness of part of a limb is usually due to a peripheral nerve lesion such as carpal tunnel syndrome or another entrapment neuropathy. Relatively symmetric weakness of extraocular or bulbar muscles is usually due to a myopathy (Chap. 382) or neuromuscular junction disorder (Chap. 381). Bilateral facial palsy with areflexia suggests Guillain-Barré syndrome (Chap. 380). Worsening of relatively symmetric weakness with fatigue is characteristic of neuromuscular junction disorders. Asymmetric bulbar weakness is usually due to motor neuron disease. Weakness limited to respiratory muscles is uncommon and is usually due to motor neuron disease, myasthenia gravis, or polymyositis/dermatomyositis (Chap. 383).

ACKNOWLEDGMENT

Richard K. Olney, MD, was the author of this chapter in previous editions, and his contributions in the last three editions of Harrison's are appreciated.

24 Gait and Balance Disorders

Lewis Sudarsky

PREVALENCE, MORBIDITY, AND MORTALITY

Gait and balance problems are common in the elderly and contribute to the risk of falls and injury. Gait disorders have been described in 15% of individuals over the age of 65. By age 80, one person in four will use a mechanical aid to assist ambulation. Among those 85 and older, the prevalence of gait abnormality approaches 40%. In epidemiologic studies, gait disorders are consistently identified as a major risk factor for falls and injury.

A substantial number of older persons report insecure balance and experience falls and fear of falling. Prospective studies indicate that 20–30% of those over age 65 fall each year, and the proportion is even higher in hospitalized elderly and nursing home patients. Each year 8% of individuals >75 suffer a serious fall-related injury. Hip fractures often result in hospitalization and nursing home admission. For each person who is physically disabled, there are others whose functional independence is constrained by anxiety and fear of falling. Nearly one in five of elderly individuals voluntarily limit their activity because of fear of falling. With loss of ambulation, there is a diminished quality of life and increased morbidity and mortality.

ANATOMY AND PHYSIOLOGY

Upright bipedal gait depends on the successful integration of postural control and locomotion. These functions are widely distributed in the central nervous system. The biomechanics of bipedal walking are complex, and the performance is easily compromised by injury at any level. Command and control centers in the brainstem, cerebellum, and forebrain modify the action of spinal pattern generators to promote stepping. While a form of "fictive locomotion" can be elicited from quadrupedal animals after spinal transection, this capacity is limited in primates. Step generation in primates is dependent on locomotor centers in the pontine tegmentum, midbrain, and subthalamic region. Locomotor synergies are executed through the reticular formation and descending pathways in the ventromedial spinal cord. Cerebral control provides a goal and purpose for walking and is involved in avoidance of obstacles and adaptation of locomotor programs to context and terrain.

Postural control requires the maintenance of the center of mass over the base of support through the gait cycle. Unconscious postural adjustments maintain standing balance: long latency responses are measurable in the leg muscles, beginning 110 ms after a perturbation. Forward motion of the center of mass provides propulsive force for stepping, but failure to maintain the center of mass within stability limits results in falls. The anatomic substrate for dynamic balance has not been well defined, but the vestibular nucleus and midline cerebellum contribute to balance control in animals. Human patients with damage to these structures have impaired balance with standing and walking.

Standing balance depends on good quality sensory information about the position of the body center with respect to the environment, support surface, and gravitational forces. Sensory information for postural control is primarily generated by the visual system, the vestibular system, and by proprioceptive receptors in the muscle spindles and joints. A healthy redundancy of sensory afferent information is generally available, but loss of two of the three pathways is sufficient to compromise standing balance. Balance disorders in older individuals sometimes result from multiple insults in the peripheral sensory systems (e.g., visual loss, vestibular deficit, peripheral neuropathy), critically degrading the quality of afferent information needed for balance stability.

Older patients with mental status abnormalities and dementia from neurodegenerative diseases appear to be particularly prone to falls and injury. Frailty, muscle weakness, and deconditioning undoubtedly contribute to the risk. There is a growing literature on the use of attentional resources to manage locomotion. The ability to walk while attending to a cognitive task (dual tasking) may be particularly compromised in older adults with a history of falls. Walking is generally considered to be unconscious and automatic, but older patients with deficits in executive function may be unable to manage the attention needed for dynamic balance when distracted.

DISORDERS OF GAIT

The heterogeneity of gait disorders observed in clinical practice reflects the large network of neural systems involved in the task. There is the potential for abnormalities to develop, and walking is vulnerable to neurologic disease at every level. Gait disorders have been classified descriptively, based on the abnormal physiology and biomechanics. One problem with this approach is that many failing gaits look fundamentally similar. This overlap reflects common patterns of adaptation to threatened balance stability and declining performance. *The gait disorder observed clinically must be viewed as the product of a neurologic deficit and a functional adaptation.* Unique features of the failing gait are often overwhelmed by the adaptive response. Some of the common patterns of abnormal gait are summarized below. Gait disorders can also be classified by etiology, as listed in Table 24-1.

Cautious Gait The term *cautious gait* is used to describe the patient who walks with an abbreviated stride and lowered center of mass, as if walking on a slippery surface. This disorder is both common and nonspecific. It is, in essence, an adaptation to a perceived postural threat. A fear of falling may be associated. In one study, this disorder was observed in more than one-third of older patients with a higher level gait disturbance. Physical therapy often improves walking to the degree that follow-up observation may reveal a more specific underlying disorder.

Stiff-Legged Gait Spastic gait is characterized by stiffness in the legs, an imbalance of muscle tone, and a tendency to circumduct and scuff the feet. The disorder reflects compromise of corticospinal command and overactivity of spinal reflexes. The patient may walk on his or her toes. In extreme instances, the legs cross due to increased tone in the adductors. Upper motor neuron signs are present on physical examination. Shoes often reflect an uneven pattern of wear across the outside. The disorder may be cerebral or spinal in origin.

Myelopathy from cervical spondylosis is a common cause of spastic or spastic-ataxic gait. Demyelinating disease and trauma are the leading causes of myelopathy in younger patients. In a chronic progressive myelopathy of unknown cause, workup with laboratory and imaging tests may establish a diagnosis of multiple sclerosis. A family history should suggest hereditary spastic paraplegia (HSP). Genetic testing is now available for some of the common HSP mutations. Tropical spastic paraparesis related to the retrovirus HTLV-I is endemic in parts of the Caribbean and South America. A structural lesion, such as tumor or spinal vascular malformation, should be excluded with appropriate testing. Spinal cord disorders are discussed in detail in Chap. 372.

With cerebral spasticity asymmetry is common, involvement of the upper extremities is usually observed, and dysarthria is often an associated feature. Common causes include vascular disease (stroke), multiple sclerosis, and perinatal injury to the nervous system (cerebral palsy).

Other stiff-legged gaits include dystonia (Chap. 382) and stiff-person syndrome. Dystonia is a disorder characterized by sustained muscle con-

TABLE 24-1 ETIOLOGY OF GAIT DISORDER

	Cases	Percent
Sensory deficits	22	18.3
Myelopathy	20	16.7
Multiple infarcts	18	15.0
Parkinsonism	14	11.7
Cerebellar degeneration	8	6.7
Hydrocephalus	8	6.7
Toxic/metabolic	3	2.5
Psychogenic	4	3.3
Other	6	5.0
Unknown cause	17	14.2
Total	120	100%

Source: Reproduced with permission from Masdeu et al.

tractions, resulting in repetitive twisting movements and abnormal posture. It often has a genetic basis. Dystonic spasms produce plantar flexion and inversion of the feet, sometimes with torsion of the trunk. In autoimmune stiff-person syndrome, there is exaggerated lordosis of the lumbar spine and overactivation of antagonist muscles, which restricts trunk and lower limb movement and results in a wooden or fixed posture.

Parkinsonism and Freezing Gait Parkinson's disease (Chap. 366) is common, affecting 1% of the population >55. The stooped posture and shuffling gait are characteristic and distinctive features. Patients sometimes accelerate (festinate) with walking or display retropulsion. There may be difficulty with gait initiation (freezing) and a tendency to turn en bloc. Imbalance and falls may develop as the disease progresses over years. Other progressive neurodegenerative disorders may also involve a freezing gait; these include progressive supranuclear palsy, multiple system atrophy, corticobasal degeneration, and primary pallidal degeneration. Such patients with atypical parkinsonian syndromes frequently present with axial stiffness, postural instability, and a shuffling gait but tend to lack the characteristic pill-rolling tremor of Parkinson's disease. Falls within the first year suggest the possibility of progressive supranuclear palsy.

Hyperkinetic movement disorders also produce characteristic and recognizable disturbances in gait. In Huntington's disease (Chap. 367), the unpredictable occurrence of choreic movements gives the gait a dancing quality. Tardive dyskinesia is the cause of many odd, stereotypic gait disorders seen in chronic psychiatric patients.

Frontal Gait Disorder Frontal gait disorder, sometimes known as "gait apraxia," is common in the elderly and has a variety of causes. Typical features include a wide base of support, short stride, shuffling along the floor, and difficulty with starts and turns. Many patients exhibit difficulty with gait initiation, descriptively characterized as the "slipping clutch" syndrome or "gait ignition failure." The term *lower body parkinsonism* is also used to describe such patients. Strength is generally preserved, and patients are able to make stepping movements when not standing and maintaining balance at the same time. This disorder is a higher level motor control disorder, as opposed to an apraxia.

The most common cause of frontal gait disorder is vascular disease, particularly subcortical small-vessel disease. Lesions are frequently found in the deep frontal white matter and centrum ovale. Gait disorder may be the salient feature in hypertensive patients with ischemic lesions of the deep hemisphere white matter (Binswanger's disease). The clinical syndrome includes mental change (variable in degree), dysarthria, pseudobulbar affect (emotional disinhibition), increased tone, and hyperreflexia in the lower limbs.

Communicating hydrocephalus in the adult also presents with a gait disorder of this type. Other features of the diagnostic triad (mental change, incontinence) may be absent in the initial stages. MRI demonstrates ventricular enlargement, an enlarged flow void about the aqueduct, and a variable degree of periventricular white matter change. A lumbar puncture or dynamic test is necessary to confirm the presence of hydrocephalus.

Cerebellar Gait Ataxia Disorders of the cerebellum have a dramatic impact on gait and balance. Cerebellar gait ataxia is characterized by a wide base of support, lateral instability of the trunk, erratic foot placement, and decompensation of balance when attempting to walk tandem. Difficulty maintaining balance when turning is often an early feature. Patients are unable to walk tandem heel to toe, and display truncal sway in narrow-based or tandem stance. They show considerable variation in their tendency to fall in daily life.

Causes of cerebellar ataxia in older patients include stroke, trauma, tumor, and neurodegenerative disease, including multiple system atrophy (Chaps. 366 and 370) and various forms of hereditary cerebellar degeneration (Chap. 368). MRI demonstrates the extent and topography of cerebellar atrophy. A short expansion at the site of the fragile X mutation (fragile X pre-mutation) has been associated with gait ataxia in older men. Alcoholic cerebellar degeneration can be screened by history and often confirmed by MRI.

Sensory Ataxia As reviewed above, balance depends on high-quality afferent information from the visual and the vestibular systems and proprioception. When this information is lost or degraded, balance during locomotion is impaired and instability results. The sensory ataxia of tabetic neurosyphilis is a classic example. The contemporary equivalent is the patient with neuropathy affecting large fibers. Vitamin B_{12} deficiency is a treatable cause of large-fiber sensory loss in the spinal cord and peripheral nervous system. Joint position and vibration sense are diminished in the lower limbs. The stance in such patients is destabilized by eye closure; they often look down at their feet when walking and do poorly in the dark. Patients have been described with imbalance from bilateral vestibular loss, caused by disease or by exposure to ototoxic drugs. Table 24-2 compares sensory ataxia with cerebellar ataxia and frontal gait disorder. Some patients exhibit a syndrome of imbalance from the combined effect of multiple sensory deficits. Such patients, often elderly and diabetic, have disturbances in proprioception, vision, and vestibular sense that impair postural support.

Neuromuscular Disease Patients with neuromuscular disease often have an abnormal gait, occasionally as a presenting feature. With distal weakness (peripheral neuropathy) the step height is increased to compensate for foot drop, and the sole of the foot may slap on the floor during weight acceptance. Neuropathy may be associated with a degree of sensory imbalance, as described above. Patients with myopathy or muscular dystrophy more typically exhibit proximal weakness. Weakness of the hip girdle may result in a degree of excess pelvic sway during locomotion.

Toxic and Metabolic Disorders Alcohol intoxication is the most common cause of acute walking difficulty. Chronic toxicity from medications and metabolic disturbances can impair motor function and gait. Mental status changes may be present, and examination may reveal asterixis or myoclonus. Static equilibrium is disturbed, and such patients are easily thrown off balance. Disequilibrium is particularly evident in patients with chronic renal disease and those with hepatic failure, in whom asterixis may impair postural support. Sedative drugs, especially neuroleptics and long-acting benzodiazepines, affect postural control and increase the risk for falls. These disorders are important to recognize because they are often treatable.

Psychogenic Gait Disorder Psychogenic disorders are common in outpatient practice, and the presentation often involves gait. Some patients with extreme anxiety or phobia walk with exaggerated caution with abduction of the arms, as if walking on ice. This inappropriately overcautious gait differs in degree from the gait of the patient who is insecure and making adjustments for imbalance. Depressed patients exhibit primarily slowness, a manifestation of psychomotor retardation, and lack of purpose in their stride. Hysterical gait disorders are among the most spectacular encountered. Odd gyrations of posture with wastage of muscular energy (astasia-abasia), extreme slow mo-

TABLE 24-2 FEATURES OF CEREBELLAR ATAXIA, SENSORY ATAXIA, AND FRONTAL GAIT DISORDERS

	Cerebellar Ataxia	Sensory Ataxia	Frontal Gait
Base of support	Wide-based	Narrow base, looks down	Wide-based
Velocity	Variable	Slow	Very slow
Stride	Irregular, lurching	Regular with path deviation	Short, shuffling
Romberg	+/–	Unsteady, falls	+/–
Heel→ shin	Abnormal	+/–	Normal
Initiation	Normal	Normal	Hesitant
Turns	Unsteady	+/–	Hesitant, multistep
Postural instability	+	+++	++++ Poor postural synergies getting up from a chair
Falls	Late event	Frequent	Frequent

tion, and dramatic fluctuations over time may be observed in patients with somatoform disorders and conversion reaction.

APPROACH TO THE PATIENT: Slowly Progressive Disorder of Gait

When reviewing the history it is helpful to inquire about the onset and progression of disability. Initial awareness of an unsteady gait often follows a fall. Stepwise evolution or sudden progression suggest vascular disease. Gait disorder may be associated with urinary urgency and incontinence, particularly in patients with cervical spine disease or hydrocephalus. It is always important to review the use of alcohol and medications that affect gait and balance. Information on localization derived from the neurologic examination can be helpful to narrow the list of possible diagnoses.

Gait observation provides an immediate sense of the patient's degree of disability. Characteristic patterns of abnormality are sometimes observed, though failing gaits often look fundamentally similar. Cadence (steps/min), velocity, and stride length can be recorded by timing a patient over a fixed distance. Watching the patient get out of a chair provides a good functional assessment of balance.

Brain imaging studies may be informative in patients with an undiagnosed disorder of gait. MRI is sensitive for cerebral lesions of vascular or demyelinating disease and is a good screening test for occult hydrocephalus. Patients with recurrent falls are at risk for subdural hematoma. Many elderly patients with gait and balance difficulty have white matter abnormalities in the periventricular region and centrum semiovale. While these lesions may be an incidental finding, a substantial burden of white matter disease will ultimately impact cerebral control of locomotion.

DISORDERS OF BALANCE

Balance is the ability to maintain equilibrium: a state in which opposing physical forces cancel. In physiology, this is taken to mean the ability of the organism to control the center of mass with respect to gravity and the support surface. In reality, no one is aware of what or where the center of mass is, but everyone, including gymnasts, figure skaters, and platform divers, move so as to manage it. Imbalance implies a disturbance of equilibrium. Disorders of balance present with difficulty maintaining posture standing and walking and with a subjective sense of disequilibrium, a form of dizziness.

The cerebellum and vestibular system organize antigravity responses needed to maintain the upright posture. As reviewed above, these responses are physiologically complex, and the anatomic representation is not well understood. Failure, resulting in disequilibrium, can occur at several levels: cerebellar, vestibular, somatosensory, and higher level disequilibrium. Patients with hereditary ataxia or alcoholic cerebellar degeneration do not generally complain of dizziness, but balance is visibly impaired. Neurologic examination will reveal a variety of cerebellar signs. Postural compensation may prevent falls early on, but falls inevitably occur with disease progression. The progression of a neurodegenerative ataxia is often measured by the number of years to loss of stable ambulation. Vestibular disorders have symptoms and signs in three categories: vertigo, the subjective appreciation or illusion of movement; nystagmus, a vestibulo-oculomotor sign; and poor balance, an impairment of vestibulo-spinal function. Not every patient has all manifestations. Patients with vestibular deficits related to ototoxic drugs may lack vertigo or obvious nystagmus, but balance is impaired on standing and walking, and the patient cannot navigate in the dark. Laboratory testing is available to explore vestibulo-oculomotor and vestibulo-spinal deficits.

Somatosensory deficits also produce imbalance and falls. There is often a subjective sense of insecure balance and fear of falling. Postural control is compromised by eye closure (Romberg's sign); these patients also have difficulty navigating in the dark. A dramatic example is the patient with autoimmune subacute sensory neuropathy, sometimes a paraneoplastic disorder (Chap. 97). Compensatory strategies enable such patients to walk in the virtual absence of proprioception, but the task requires active visual monitoring. Patients with higher level disorders of equilibrium have difficulty maintaining balance in daily life and may present with falls. There may be reduced awareness of balance impairment. Classic examples include patients with progressive supranuclear palsy and normal pressure hydrocephalus. Patients on sedating medications are also in this category. In prospective studies, cognitive impairment and the use of sedative medications substantially increase the risk for falls.

TABLE 24-3 RISK FACTORS FOR FALLS, A META-ANALYSIS: SUMMARY OF SIXTEEN CONTROLLED STUDIES

Risk Factor	Mean RR (OR)	Range
Weakness	4.9	1.9–10.3
Balance deficit	3.2	1.6–5.4
Gait disorder	3.0	1.7–4.8
Visual deficit	2.8	1.1–7.4
Mobility limitation	2.5	1.0–5.3
Cognitive impairment	2.4	2.0–4.7
Impaired functional status	2.0	1.0–3.1
Postural hypotension	1.9	1.0–3.4

Note: RR, relative risks from prospective studies; OR, odds ratios from retrospective studies.
Source: Reprinted from Masdeu et al, with permission.

FALLS

Falls are a common event, particularly among the elderly. Modest changes in balance function have been described in fit older subjects as a result of normal aging. Subtle deficits in sensory systems, attention, and motor reaction time contribute to the risk, and environmental hazards abound. Epidemiologic studies have identified a number of risk factors for falls, summarized in Table 24-3. A fall is not a neurologic problem, nor reason for referral to a specialist, but there are circumstances in which neurologic evaluation is appropriate. In a classic study, 90% of fall events occurred among 10% of individuals, a group known as *recurrent fallers*. Some of these are frail older persons with chronic diseases. Recurrent falls sometimes indicate the presence of serious balance impairment. Syncope, seizure, or falls related to loss of consciousness require appropriate evaluation and treatment (Chaps. 21 and 363).

The descriptive classification of falls is as difficult as the classification of gait disorders, for many of the same reasons. Postural control systems are widely distributed, and a number of disease-related abnormalities occur. Unlike gait problems that are apparent on observation, falls are rarely observed in the office. The patient and family may have limited information about what triggered the fall. Injuries can complicate the physical examination. While there is no standard nosology of falls, common patterns can be identified.

Slipping, Tripping, and "Mechanical Falls" Slipping on icy pavement, tripping on obstacles, and falls related to obvious environmental factors are often termed *mechanical falls*. They occasionally occur in healthy individuals with good balance compensation. Frequent tripping falls raise suspicion about an underlying neurologic deficit. Patients with spasticity, leg weakness, or foot drop experience tripping falls.

Weakness and Frailty Patients who lack strength in antigravity muscles have difficulty rising from a chair, fatigue easily when walking, and have difficulty maintaining their balance after a perturbation. These patients are often unable to get up after a fall and may be on the floor for an hour or more before help arrives. Deconditioning of this sort is often treatable. Resistance strength training can increase muscle mass and leg strength in people in their 80s and 90s.

Drop Attacks and Collapsing Falls Drop attacks are sudden collapsing falls without loss of consciousness. Patients who collapse from lack of postural tone present a diagnostic challenge. The patient may report that his or her legs just gave out underneath; the family may describe the patient as "collapsing in a heap." Orthostatic hypotension may be a factor in some such falls. Asterixis or epilepsy may impair postural support. A colloid cyst of the third ventricle can present with intermittent obstruction of the foramen of Monroe, resulting in a drop attack. While collapsing falls are more common in older patients with vascular risk factors, they should not be confused with vertebrobasilar ischemic attacks.

Toppling Falls Some patients maintain tone in antigravity muscles but fall over like a tree trunk, as if postural defenses had disengaged. There may be a consistent direction to such falls. The patient with cerebellar pathology may lean and topple over toward the side of the lesion. Patients with lesions of the vestibular system or its central pathways may experience lateral pulsion and toppling falls. Patients with progressive supranuclear palsy often fall over backwards. Falls of this nature occur in patients with advanced Parkinson's disease once postural instability has developed.

Gait Freezing Another fall pattern in Parkinson's disease and related disorders is the fall due to freezing of gait. The feet stick to the floor and the center of mass keeps moving, resulting in a disequilibrium from which the patient cannot recover. This can result in a forward fall. Gait freezing can also occur as the patient attempts to turn and change direction. Similarly, the patient with Parkinson's disease and festinating gait may find his feet unable to keep up, resulting in a forward fall.

Falls Related to Sensory Deficit Patients with somatosensory, visual, or vestibular deficits are prone to falls. These patients have particular difficulty dealing with poor illumination or walking on uneven ground. These patients often express subjective imbalance, apprehension, and fear of falling. Deficits in joint position and vibration sense are apparent on physical examination.

Rx INTERVENTIONS TO REDUCE THE RISK OF FALLS AND INJURY

Efforts should be made to define the etiology of the gait disorder and mechanism of the falls. Standing blood pressure should be recorded. Specific treatment may be possible, once a diagnosis is established. Therapeutic intervention is often recommended for older patients at substantial risk for falls, even if no neurologic disease is identified. A home visit to look for environmental hazards can be helpful. A variety of modifications may be recommended to improve safety, including improved lighting and the installation of grab bars and nonslip surfaces.

Rehabilitation interventions attempt to improve muscle strength and balance stability and to make the patient more resistant to injury. High-intensity resistance strength training with weights and machines is useful to improve muscle mass, even in frail older patients. Improvements are realized in posture and gait, which should translate to reduced risk of falls and injury. The goal of sensory balance training is to improve balance stability. Measurable gains can be achieved in a few weeks of training, and benefits can be maintained over 6 months by a 10- to 20-min home exercise program. This strategy is particularly successful in patients with vestibular and somatosensory balance disorders. The Yale Health and Aging study used a strategy of targeted, multiple risk factor abatement to reduce falls in the elderly. Prescription medications were adjusted, and home-based exercise programs were tailored to the patient's need, based on an initial geriatric assessment. The program realized a 44% reduction in falls, compared with a control group of patients who had periodic social visits.

FURTHER READINGS

BRONSTEIN A et al: *Clinical Disorders of Balance, Posture and Gait.* London, Arnold Press, 2003

GANZ DA et al: Will my patient fall? JAMA 297:77, 2007

MASDEU J et al: *Gait Disorders of Aging: With Special Reference to Falls.* Boston, Little Brown, 1995

SNIJDERS AH et al: Neurological gait disorders in elderly people: Clinical approach and classification. Lancet Neurol 6:63, 2007

SPRINGER S et al: Dual-tasking effects on gait variability: The role of aging, falls, and executive function. Mov Disord 21:950, 2006

SUDARSKY L: Gait disorders in the elderly. N Engl J Med 322:1441, 1990

TINETTI ME: Preventing falls in elderly persons. N Engl J Med 348:42, 2003

25 Numbness, Tingling, and Sensory Loss

Michael J. Aminoff, Arthur K. Asbury

Normal somatic sensation reflects a continuous monitoring process, little of which reaches consciousness under ordinary conditions. By contrast, disordered sensation, particularly when experienced as painful, is alarming and dominates the sufferer's attention. Physicians should be able to recognize abnormal sensations by how they are described, know their type and likely site of origin, and understand their implications.

POSITIVE AND NEGATIVE SYMPTOMS

Abnormal sensory symptoms may be divided into two categories, positive and negative. The prototypical positive symptom is tingling (pins-and-needles); other positive sensory phenomena include altered sensations that are described as pricking, bandlike, lightning-like shooting feelings (lancinations), aching, knifelike, twisting, drawing, pulling, tightening, burning, searing, electrical, or raw feelings. Such symptoms are often painful.

Positive phenomena usually result from trains of impulses generated at sites of lowered threshold or heightened excitability along a peripheral or central sensory pathway. The nature and severity of the abnormal sensation depend on the number, rate, timing, and distribution of ectopic impulses and the type and function of nervous tissue in which they arise. Because positive phenomena represent excessive activity in sensory pathways, they are not necessarily associated with a sensory deficit (loss) on examination.

Negative phenomena represent loss of sensory function and are characterized by diminished or absent feeling, often experienced as numbness, and by abnormal findings on sensory examination. In disorders affecting peripheral sensation, it is estimated that at least half the afferent axons innervating a given site are lost or functionless before a sensory deficit can be demonstrated by clinical examination. This threshold varies according to how rapidly function is lost in sensory nerve fibers. If the rate of loss is slow, lack of cutaneous feeling may be unnoticed by the patient and difficult to demonstrate on examination, even though few sensory fibers are functioning; if rapid, both positive and negative phenomena are usually conspicuous. Subclinical degrees of sensory dysfunction may be revealed by sensory nerve conduction studies or somatosensory evoked potentials (**Chap. e31**).

Whereas sensory symptoms may be either positive or negative, sensory signs on examination are always a measure of negative phenomena.

TERMINOLOGY

Words used to characterize sensory disturbance are descriptive and based on convention. Paresthesias and dysesthesias are general terms used to denote positive sensory symptoms. The term *paresthesias* typically refers to tingling or pins-and-needles sensations but may include a wide variety of other abnormal sensations, except pain; it sometimes implies that the abnormal sensations are perceived spontaneously. The more general term *dysesthesias* denotes all types of abnormal sensations, including painful ones, regardless of whether a stimulus is evident.

Another set of terms refers to sensory abnormalities found on examination. *Hypesthesia* or *hypoesthesia* refers to a reduction of cutaneous sensation to a specific type of testing such as pressure, light touch, and warm or cold stimuli; *anesthesia,* to a complete absence of skin sensation to the same stimuli plus pinprick; and *hypalgesia* or *analgesia* to reduced or absent pain perception (nociception), such as perception of the pricking quality elicited by a pin. *Hyperesthesia* means pain or increased sensitivity in response to touch. Similarly, *allodynia* describes the situation in which a nonpainful stimulus, once perceived, is experienced as painful, even excruciating. An example is elicitation of a painful sensation by application of a vibrating tuning fork. *Hyperalgesia* denotes severe pain in response to a mildly noxious stimulus, and *hyperpathia*, a broad term, encompasses all the phenomena described by hyperesthesia, allodynia, and hyperalgesia. With hyperpathia, the threshold for a sensory stimulus is increased and perception is delayed, but once felt, is unduly painful.

Disorders of deep sensation, arising from muscle spindles, tendons, and joints, affect proprioception (position sense). Manifestations include imbalance (particularly with eyes closed or in the dark), clumsiness of precision movements, and unsteadiness of gait, which are referred to collectively as *sensory ataxia*. Other findings on examination usually, but not invariably, include reduced or absent joint position and vibratory sensibility and absent deep tendon reflexes in the affected limbs. Romberg's sign is positive, which means that the patient sways markedly or topples when asked to stand with feet close together and eyes closed. In severe states of deafferentation involving deep sensation, the patient cannot walk or stand unaided or even sit unsupported. Continuous involuntary movements (*pseudoathetosis*) of the outstretched hands and fingers occur, particularly with eyes closed.

ANATOMY OF SENSATION

Cutaneous afferent innervation is conveyed by a rich variety of receptors, both naked nerve endings (nociceptors and thermoreceptors) and encapsulated terminals (mechanoreceptors). Each type of receptor has its own set of sensitivities to specific stimuli, size and distinctness of receptive fields, and adaptational qualities. Much of the knowledge about these receptors has come from the development of techniques to study single intact nerve fibers intraneurally in awake, unanesthetized human subjects. It is possible not only to record from but also to stimulate single fibers in isolation. A single impulse, whether elicited by a natural stimulus or evoked by electrical microstimulation in a large myelinated afferent fiber may be both perceived and localized.

Afferent fibers of all sizes in peripheral nerve trunks traverse the dorsal roots and enter the dorsal horn of the spinal cord (Fig. 25-1). From there the smaller fibers take a different route to the parietal cortex than the larger fibers. The polysynaptic projections of the smaller fibers (unmyelinated and small myelinated), which subserve mainly nociception, temperature sensibility, and touch, cross and ascend in the opposite anterior and lateral columns of the spinal cord, through the brainstem, to the ventral posterolateral (VPL) nucleus of the thalamus, and ultimately project to the postcentral gyrus of the parietal cortex (Chap. 12). This is the *spinothalamic pathway* or *anterolateral system*. The larger fibers, which subserve tactile and position sense and kinesthesia, project rostrally in the posterior column on the same side of the spinal cord and make their first synapse in the gracile or cuneate nucleus of the lower medulla. Axons of the second-order neuron decussate and ascend in the medial lemniscus located medially in the medulla and in the tegmentum of the pons and midbrain and synapse in the VPL nucleus; the third-order neurons project to parietal cortex. This large-fiber system is referred to as the *posterior column–medial lemniscal pathway* (lemniscal, for short). Note that although the lemniscal and the anterolateral pathways both project up the spinal cord to the thalamus, it is the (crossed) anterolateral pathway that is referred to as the *spinothalamic tract*, by convention.

Although the fiber types and functions that make up the spinothalamic and lemniscal systems are relatively well known, many other fibers, particularly those associated with touch, pressure, and position sense, ascend in a diffusely distributed pattern both ipsilaterally and contralaterally in the anterolateral quadrants of the spinal cord. This explains why a complete lesion of the posterior columns of the spinal cord may be associated with little sensory deficit on examination.

EXAMINATION OF SENSATION

The main components of the sensory examination are tests of primary sensation (pain, touch, vibration, joint position, and thermal sensation; Table 25-1).

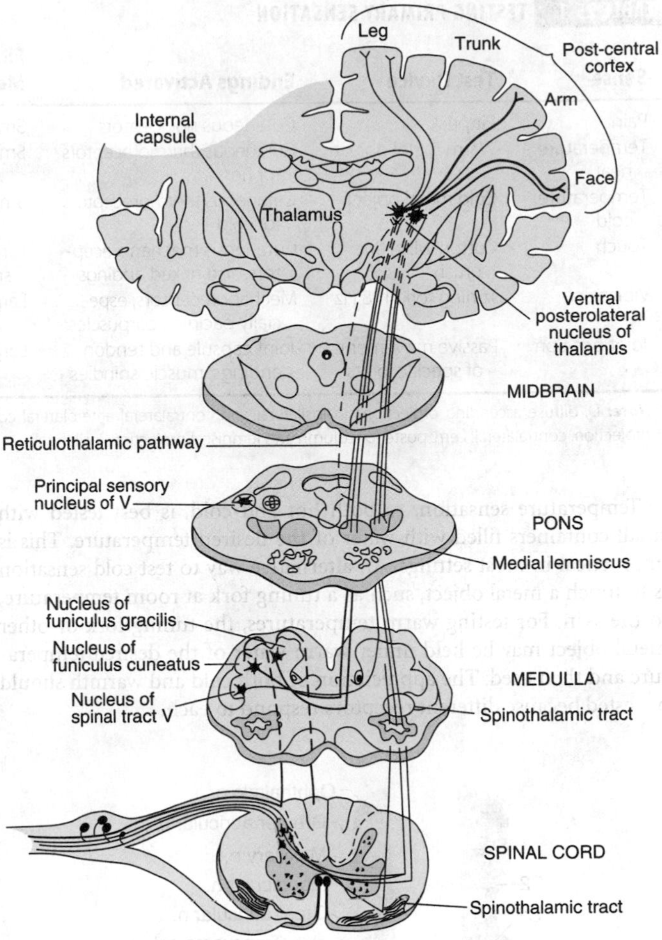

FIGURE 25-1 The main somatosensory pathways. The spinothalamic tract (pain, thermal sense) and the posterior column–lemniscal system (touch, pressure, joint position) are shown. Offshoots from the ascending anterolateral fasciculus (spinothalamic tract) to nuclei in the medulla, pons, and mesencephalon and nuclear terminations of the tract are indicated. *(From AH Ropper, RH Brown, in Adams and Victor's Principles of Neurology, 8th ed. New York, McGraw-Hill, 2007.)*

Some general principles pertain. The examiner must depend on patient responses, particularly when testing cutaneous sensation (pin, touch, warm, or cold), which complicates interpretation. Further, examination may be limited in some patients. In a stuporous patient, for example, sensory examination is reduced to observing the briskness of withdrawal in response to a pinch or other noxious stimulus. Comparison of response on one side of the body to the other is essential. In the alert but uncooperative patient, it may not be possible to examine cutaneous sensation, but some idea of proprioceptive function may be gained by noting the patient's best performance of movements requiring balance and precision. Frequently, patients present with sensory symptoms that do not fit an anatomic localization and that are accompanied by either no abnormalities or gross inconsistencies on examination. The examiner should then consider whether the sensory symptoms are a disguised request for help with psychological or situational problems. Discretion must be used in pursuing this possibility. Finally, sensory examination of a patient who has no neurologic complaints can be brief and consist of pinprick, touch, and vibration testing in the hands and feet plus evaluation of stance and gait, including the Romberg maneuver. Evaluation of stance and gait also tests the integrity of motor and cerebellar systems.

Primary Sensation (See Table 25-1) The sense of pain is usually tested with a clean pin, asking the patient to focus on the pricking or unpleasant quality of the stimulus and not just the pressure or touch sensation elicited. Areas of hypalgesia should be mapped by proceeding radially from the most hypalgesic site (Figs. 25-2 and 25-3).

TABLE 25-1 TESTING PRIMARY SENSATION

Sense	Test Device	Endings Activated	Fiber Size Mediating	Central Pathway
Pain	Pinprick	Cutaneous nociceptors	Small	SpTh, also D
Temperature, heat	Warm metal object	Cutaneous thermoreceptors for hot	Small	SpTh
Temperature, cold	Cold metal object	Cutaneous thermoreceptors for cold	Small	SpTh
Touch	Cotton wisp, fine brush	Cutaneous mechanoreceptors, also naked endings	Large and small	Lem, also D and SpTh
Vibration	Tuning fork, 128 Hz	Mechanoreceptors, especially pacinian corpuscles	Large	Lem, also D
Joint position	Passive movement of specific joints	Joint capsule and tendon endings, muscle spindles	Large	Lem, also D

Note: D, diffuse ascending projections in ipsilateral and contralateral anterolateral columns; SpTh, spinothalamic projection, contralateral; Lem, posterior column and lemniscal projection, ipsilateral.

Temperature sensation, to both hot and cold, is best tested with small containers filled with water of the desired temperature. This is impractical in most settings. An alternative way to test cold sensation is to touch a metal object, such as a tuning fork at room temperature, to the skin. For testing warm temperatures, the tuning fork or other metal object may be held under warm water of the desired temperature and then used. The appreciation of both cold and warmth should be tested because different receptors respond to each.

Touch is usually tested with a wisp of cotton or a fine camelhair brush. In general, it is better to avoid testing touch on hairy skin because of the profusion of sensory endings that surround each hair follicle.

Joint position testing is a measure of proprioception, one of the most important functions of the sensory system. With the patient's eyes closed, joint position is tested in the distal interphalangeal joint of the great toe and fingers. If errors are made in recognizing the direction of passive movements, more proximal joints are tested. A test of proximal joint position sense, primarily at the shoulder, is performed by asking the patient to bring the two index fingers together with arms extended and eyes closed. Normal individuals can do this accurately, with errors of 1 cm or less.

The sense of vibration is tested with a tuning fork that vibrates at 128 Hz. Vibration is usually tested over bony points, beginning distally; in the feet, it is tested over the dorsal surface of the distal phalanx of the big toes and at the malleoli of the ankles, and in the hands dorsally at the distal phalanx of the fingers. If abnormalities are found, more proximal sites can be examined. Vibratory thresholds at the same site in the patient and the examiner may be compared for control purposes.

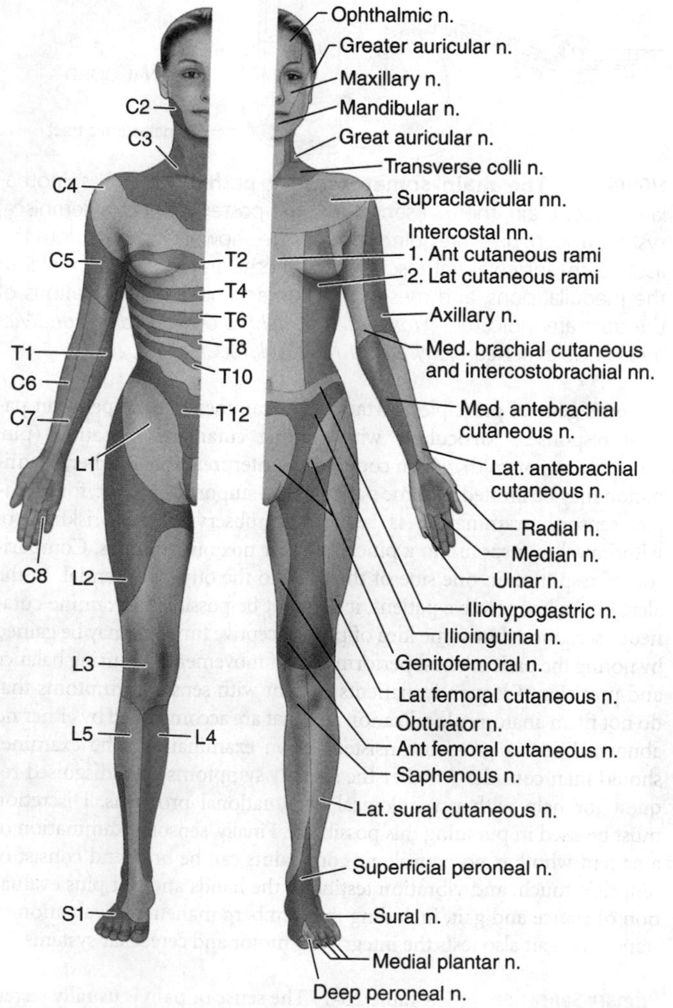

FIGURE 25-2 Anterior view of dermatomes (*left*) and cutaneous areas (*right*) supplied by individual peripheral nerves. *(Modified from MB Carpenter and J Sutin, in Human Neuroanatomy, 8th ed, Baltimore, Williams & Wilkins, 1983.)*

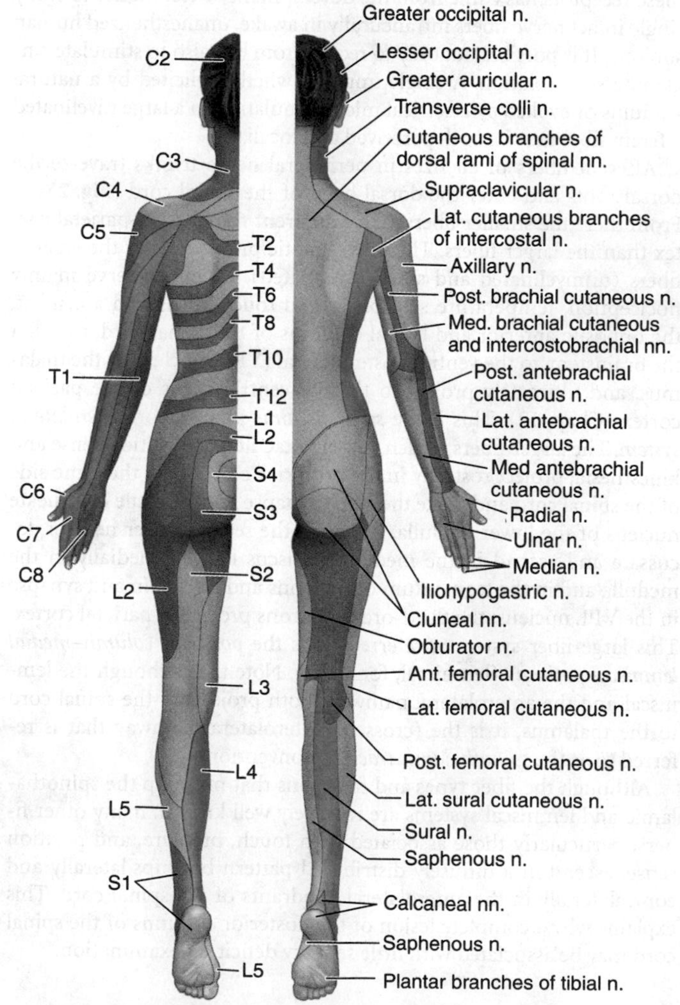

FIGURE 25-3 Posterior view of dermatomes (*left*) and cutaneous areas (*right*) supplied by individual peripheral nerves. *(Modified from MB Carpenter and J Sutin, in Human Neuroanatomy, 8th ed, Baltimore, Williams & Wilkins, 1983.)*

Quantitative Sensory Testing Effective sensory testing devices are now available commercially. Quantitative sensory testing is particularly useful for serial evaluation of cutaneous sensation in clinical trials. Threshold testing for touch and vibratory and thermal sensation is the most widely used application.

Cortical Sensation The most commonly used tests of cortical function are two-point discrimination, touch localization, and bilateral simultaneous stimulation and tests for graphesthesia and stereognosis. Abnormalities of these sensory tests, in the presence of normal primary sensation in an alert cooperative patient, signify a lesion of the parietal cortex or thalamocortical projections to the parietal lobe. If primary sensation is altered, these cortical discriminative functions will usually be abnormal also. Comparisons should always be made between analogous sites on the two sides of the body because the deficit with a specific parietal lesion is likely to be unilateral. Interside comparisons are important for all cortical sensory testing.

Two-point discrimination is tested by special calipers, the points of which may be set from 2 mm to several centimeters apart and then applied simultaneously to the site to be tested. The pulp of the fingertips is a common site to test; a normal individual can distinguish about 3-mm separation of points there.

Touch localization is performed by light pressure for an instant with the examiner's fingertip or a wisp of cottonwool; the patient, whose eyes are closed, is required to identify the site of touch with the fingertip. *Bilateral simultaneous stimulation* at analogous sites (e.g., the dorsum of both hands) can be carried out to determine whether the perception of touch is extinguished consistently on one side or the other. The phenomenon is referred to as *extinction*. *Graphesthesia* means the capacity to recognize with eyes closed letters or numbers drawn by the examiner's fingertip on the palm of the hand. Once again, interside comparison is of prime importance. Inability to recognize numbers or letters is termed *agraphesthesia*.

Stereognosis refers to the ability to identify common objects by palpation, recognizing their shape, texture, and size. Common standard objects, such as a key, paper clip, or coins, are best used. Patients with normal stereognosis should be able to distinguish a dime from a penny and a nickel from a quarter without looking. Patients should only be allowed to feel the object with one hand at a time. If they are unable to identify it in one hand, it should be placed in the other for comparison. Individuals unable to identify common objects and coins in one hand and who can do so in the other are said to have *astereognosis* of the abnormal hand.

LOCALIZATION OF SENSORY ABNORMALITIES

Sensory symptoms and signs can result from lesions at almost any level of the nervous system from parietal cortex to the peripheral sensory receptor. Noting the distribution and nature of sensory symptoms and signs is the most important way to localize their source. Their extent, configuration, symmetry, quality, and severity are the key observations.

Dysesthesias without sensory findings by examination may be difficult to interpret. To illustrate, tingling dysesthesias in an acral distribution (hands and feet) can be systemic in origin, e.g., secondary to hyperventilation, or induced by a medication such as acetazolamide. Distal dysesthesias can also be an early event in an evolving polyneuropathy or may herald a myelopathy, such as from vitamin B_{12} deficiency. Sometimes distal dysesthesias have no definable basis. In contrast, dysesthesias that correspond to a particular peripheral nerve territory denote a lesion of that nerve trunk. For instance, dysesthesias restricted to the fifth digit and the adjacent one-half of the fourth finger on one hand reliably point to disorder of the ulnar nerve, most commonly at the elbow.

Nerve and Root In focal nerve trunk lesions severe enough to cause a deficit, sensory abnormalities are readily mapped and generally have discrete boundaries (Figs. 25-2 and 25-3). Root ("radicular") lesions are frequently accompanied by deep, aching pain along the course of the related nerve trunk. With compression of a fifth lumbar (L5) or first sacral (S1) root, as from a ruptured intervertebral disc, sciatica (radicular pain relating to the sciatic nerve trunk) is a frequent manifestation (Chap. 16). With a lesion affecting a single root, sensory deficits may be minimal or absent because adjacent root territories overlap extensively.

With polyneuropathies, sensory deficits are generally graded, distal, and symmetric in distribution (Chap. 379). Dysesthesias, followed by numbness, begin in the toes and ascend symmetrically. When dysesthesias reach the knees, they have usually also appeared in the fingertips. The process appears to be nerve length–dependent, and the deficit is often described as "stocking-glove" in type. Involvement of both hands and feet also occurs with lesions of the upper cervical cord or the brainstem, but an upper level of the sensory disturbance may then be found on the trunk and other evidence of a central lesion may be present, such as sphincter involvement or signs of an upper motor neuron lesion (Chap. 23). Although most polyneuropathies are pansensory and affect all modalities of sensation, selective sensory dysfunction according to nerve fiber size may occur. Small-fiber polyneuropathies are characterized by burning, painful dysesthesias with reduced pinprick and thermal sensation but sparing of proprioception, motor function, and deep tendon reflexes. Touch is involved variably; when spared, the sensory pattern is referred to as exhibiting *sensory dissociation*. Sensory dissociation may occur with spinal cord lesions as well as small-fiber neuropathies. Large-fiber polyneuropathies are characterized by vibration and position sense deficits, imbalance, absent tendon reflexes, and variable motor dysfunction but preservation of most cutaneous sensation. Dysesthesias, if present at all, tend to be tingling or bandlike in quality.

Spinal Cord (See also Chap. 372) If the spinal cord is transected, all sensation is lost below the level of transection. Bladder and bowel function are also lost, as is motor function. Hemisection of the spinal cord produces the Brown-Séquard syndrome, with absent pain and temperature sensation contralaterally and loss of proprioceptive sensation and power ipsilaterally below the lesion (see Figs. 25-1 and 372-1).

Numbness or paresthesias in both feet may arise from a spinal cord lesion; this is especially likely when the upper level of the sensory loss extends to the trunk. When all extremities are affected, the lesion is probably in the cervical region or brainstem unless a peripheral neuropathy is responsible. The presence of upper motor neuron signs (Chap. 23) supports a central lesion; a hyperesthetic band on the trunk may suggest the level of involvement.

A dissociated sensory loss can reflect spinothalamic tract involvement in the spinal cord, especially if the deficit is unilateral and has an upper level on the torso. Bilateral spinothalamic tract involvement occurs with lesions affecting the center of the spinal cord, such as in syringomyelia. There is a dissociated sensory loss with impairment of pinprick and temperature appreciation but relative preservation of light touch, position sense, and vibration appreciation.

Dysfunction of the posterior columns in the spinal cord or of the posterior root entry zone may lead to a bandlike sensation around the trunk or a feeling of tight pressure in one or more limbs. Flexion of the neck sometimes leads to an electric shock–like sensation that radiates down the back and into the legs (Lhermitte's sign) in patients with a cervical lesion affecting the posterior columns, such as from multiple sclerosis, cervical spondylosis, or recent irradiation to the cervical region.

Brainstem Crossed patterns of sensory disturbance, in which one side of the face and the opposite side of the body are affected, localize to the lateral medulla. Here a small lesion may damage both the ipsilateral descending trigeminal tract and ascending spinothalamic fibers subserving the opposite arm, leg, and hemitorso (see "Lateral medullary syndrome" in Fig. 364-10). A lesion in the tegmentum of the pons and midbrain, where the lemniscal and spinothalamic tracts merge, causes pansensory loss contralaterally.

Thalamus Hemisensory disturbance with tingling numbness from head to foot is often thalamic in origin but can also arise from the anterior parietal region. If abrupt in onset, the lesion is likely to be due to a small stroke (lacunar infarction), particularly if localized to the thalamus. Occasionally, with lesions affecting the VPL nucleus or adjacent white matter, a syndrome of thalamic pain, also called *Déjerine-Roussy* *syndrome*, may ensue. The persistent, unrelenting unilateral pain is often described in dramatic terms.

Cortex With lesions of the parietal lobe involving either the cortex or subjacent white matter, the most prominent symptoms are contralateral hemineglect, hemi-inattention, and a tendency not to use the affected hand and arm. On cortical sensory testing (e.g., two-point discrimination, graphesthesia), abnormalities are often found but primary sensation is usually intact. Anterior parietal infarction may present as a pseudothalamic syndrome with contralateral loss of primary sensation from head to toe. Dysesthesias or a sense of numbness may also occur, and rarely, a painful state.

Focal Sensory Seizures These are generally due to lesions in the area of the postcentral or precentral gyrus. The principal symptom of focal sensory seizures is tingling, but additional, more complex sensations may occur, such as a rushing feeling, a sense of warmth, or a sense of movement without detectable motion. Symptoms typically are unilateral; commonly begin in the arm or hand, face, or foot; and often spread in a manner that reflects the cortical representation of different bodily parts, as in a Jacksonian march. Duration of seizures is variable; they may be transient, lasting only for seconds, or persist for an hour or more. Focal motor features may supervene, often becoming generalized with loss of consciousness and tonic-clonic jerking.

26 Confusion and Delirium

S. Andrew Josephson, Bruce L. Miller

Confusion, a mental and behavioral state of reduced comprehension, coherence, and capacity to reason, is one of the most common problems encountered in medicine, accounting for a large number of emergency department visits, hospital admissions, and inpatient consultations. *Delirium*, a term used to describe an acute confusional state, remains a major cause of morbidity and mortality, contributing billions of dollars yearly to health care costs in the United States alone. Delirium often goes unrecognized despite clear evidence that it is usually the cognitive manifestation of serious underlying medical or neurologic illness.

CLINICAL FEATURES OF DELIRIUM

A multitude of terms are used to describe delirium, including encephalopathy, acute brain failure, acute confusional state, and postoperative or intensive care unit (ICU) psychosis. Delirium has many clinical manifestations, but essentially it is defined as a relatively acute decline in cognition that fluctuates over hours or days. The hallmark of delirium is a deficit of attention, although all cognitive domains—including memory, executive function, visuospatial tasks, and language—are variably involved. Associated symptoms may include altered sleep-wake cycles, perceptual disturbances such as hallucinations or delusions, affect changes, and autonomic findings including heart rate and blood pressure instability.

Delirium is a clinical diagnosis that can only be made at the bedside. Two broad clinical categories of delirium have been described, hyperactive and hypoactive subtypes, based on differential psychomotor features. The cognitive syndrome associated with severe alcohol withdrawal remains the classic example of the hyperactive subtype, featuring prominent hallucinations, agitation, and hyperarousal, often accompanied by life-threatening autonomic instability. In striking contrast is the hypoactive subtype of delirium, exemplified by opiate intoxication, in which patients are withdrawn and quiet, with prominent apathy and psychomotor slowing.

This dichotomy between subtypes of delirium is a useful construct, but patients often fall somewhere along a spectrum between the hyperactive and hypoactive extremes, sometimes fluctuating from one to the other within minutes. Therefore, clinicians must recognize the broad range of presentations of delirium in order to identify all patients with this potentially reversible cognitive disturbance. Hyperactive patients, such as those with delirium tremens, are easily recognized by their characteristic severe agitation, tremor, hallucinations, and autonomic instability. Patients who are quietly disturbed are more often overlooked on the medical wards and in the ICU, yet multiple studies suggest that this under-recognized hypoactive subtype is associated with worse outcomes.

The reversibility of delirium is emphasized because many etiologies, such as systemic infection and medication effects, can be easily treated. However, the long-term cognitive effects of delirium remain largely unknown and understudied. Some episodes of delirium continue for weeks, months, or even years. The persistence of delirium in some patients and its high recurrence rate may be due to inadequate treatment of the underlying etiology for the syndrome. In some instances, delirium does not disappear because there is underlying permanent neuronal damage. Even after an episode of delirium resolves, there may still be lingering effects of the disorder. A patient's recall of events after delirium varies widely, ranging from complete amnesia to repeated reexperiencing of the frightening period of confusion in a disturbing manner, similar to what is seen in patients with posttraumatic stress disorder.

RISK FACTORS

An effective primary prevention strategy for delirium begins with identification of patients at highest risk, including those preparing for elective surgery or being admitted to the hospital. Although no single validated scoring system has been widely accepted as a screen for asymptomatic patients, there are multiple well-established risk factors for delirium.

The two most consistently identified risks are older age and baseline cognitive dysfunction. Individuals who are over age 65 or exhibit low scores on standardized tests of cognition develop delirium upon hospitalization at a rate approaching 50%. Whether age and baseline cognitive dysfunction are truly independent risk factors is uncertain. Other predisposing factors include sensory deprivation, such as preexisting hearing and visual impairment, as well as indices for poor overall health, including baseline immobility, malnutrition, and underlying medical or neurologic illness.

In-hospital risks for delirium include the use of bladder catheterization, physical restraints, sleep and sensory deprivation, and the addition of three or more new medications. Avoiding such risks remains a key component of delirium prevention as well as treatment. Surgical and anesthetic risk factors for the development of postoperative delirium include specific procedures such as those involving cardiopulmonary bypass and inadequate or excessive treatment of pain in the immediate postoperative period.

The relationship between delirium and dementia (Chap. 365) is complicated by significant overlap between these two conditions, and it is not always simple to distinguish between the two. Dementia and preexisting cognitive dysfunction serve as major risk factors for delirium, and at least two-thirds of cases of delirium occur in patients with coexisting underlying dementia. A form of dementia with parkinsonism, termed *dementia with Lewy bodies*, is characterized by a fluctuating course, prominent visual hallucinations, parkinsonism, and an attentional deficit that clinically resembles hyperactive delirium. Delirium in the elderly often reflects an insult to the brain that is vulnerable due to an underlying neurodegenerative condition. Therefore, the development of delirium sometimes heralds the onset of a previously unrecognized brain disorder.

EPIDEMIOLOGY

Delirium is a common disease, but its reported incidence has varied widely based on the criteria used to define the disorder. Estimates of delirium in hospitalized patients range from 14 to 56%, with higher rates reported for elderly patients and patients undergoing hip surgery. Older patients in the ICU have especially high rates of delirium ranging from 70 to 87%. The condition is not recognized in up to one-third of delirious inpatients, and the diagnosis is especially problematic in the ICU environment where cognitive dysfunction is often difficult to appreciate in the setting of serious systemic illness and sedation. Delirium in the ICU should be viewed as an important manifestation of organ dysfunction not unlike liver, kidney, or heart failure.

Outside of the acute hospital setting, delirium occurs in nearly two-thirds of patients in nursing homes and in over 80% of those at the end of life. These estimates emphasize the remarkably high frequency of this cognitive syndrome in older patients, a population expected to grow in the upcoming decade with the aging of the "baby boom" generation.

In previous decades an episode of delirium was viewed as a transient condition that carried a benign prognosis. Delirium has now been clearly associated with substantial morbidity and increased mortality, and is increasingly recognized as a sign of serious underlying illness. Recent estimates of in-hospital mortality among delirious patients have ranged from 25 to 33%, a rate that is similar to patients with sepsis. Patients with an in-hospital episode of delirium have a higher mortality in the months and years following their illness compared with age-matched nondelirious hospitalized patients. Delirious hospitalized patients have a longer length of stay, are more likely to be discharged to a nursing home, and are more likely to experience subsequent episodes of delirium; as a result, this condition has enormous economic implications.

PATHOGENESIS

The pathogenesis and anatomy of delirium are incompletely understood. The attentional deficit that serves as the neuropsychological hallmark of delirium appears to have a diffuse localization with the brainstem, thalamus, prefrontal cortex, thalamus, and parietal lobes. Rarely, focal lesions such as ischemic strokes have led to delirium in otherwise healthy persons; right parietal and medial dorsal thalamic lesions have been reported most commonly, stressing the relevance of these areas to delirium pathogenesis. In most cases, delirium results from widespread disturbances in cortical and subcortical regions, rather than a focal neuroanatomic cause. Electroencephalogram (EEG) data in persons with delirium usually show symmetric slowing, a nonspecific finding supporting diffuse cerebral dysfunction.

Deficiency of acetylcholine often plays a key role in delirium pathogenesis. Medications with anticholinergic properties can precipitate delirium in susceptible individuals, and therapies designed to boost cholinergic tone such as cholinesterase inhibitors have, in small trials, been shown to relieve symptoms of delirium. Dementia patients are susceptible to episodes of delirium, and those with Alzheimer's pathology are known to have a chronic cholinergic deficiency state due to degeneration of acetylcholine-producing neurons in the basal forebrain. Another common dementia associated with decreased acetylcholine levels, dementia with Lewy bodies, clinically mimics delirium in some patients. Other neurotransmitters are also likely involved in this diffuse cerebral disorder. For example, increases in dopamine can also lead to delirium. Patients with Parkinson's disease treated with dopaminergic medications can develop a delirious-like state that features visual hallucinations, fluctuations, and confusion. In contrast, reducing dopaminergic tone with dopamine antagonists such as typical and atypical antipsychotic medications has long been recognized as effective symptomatic treatment in patients with delirium.

Not all individuals exposed to the same insult will develop signs of delirium. A low dose of an anticholinergic medication may have no cognitive effects on a healthy young adult but may produce a florid delirium in an elderly person with known underlying dementia. However, an extremely high dose of the same anticholinergic medication may lead to delirium even in healthy young persons. This concept of delirium developing as the result of an insult in predisposed individuals is currently the most widely accepted pathogenic construct. Therefore, if a previously healthy individual with no known history of cognitive illness develops delirium in the setting of a relatively minor insult such as elective surgery or hospitalization, then an unrecognized underlying neurologic illness such as a neurodegenerative disease, multiple previous strokes, or another diffuse cerebral cause should be considered. In this context, delirium can be viewed as the symptom resulting from a "stress test for the brain" induced by the insult. Exposure to known inciting factors such as systemic infection or offending drugs can unmask a decreased cerebral reserve and herald a serious underlying and potentially treatable illness.

TABLE 26-1 THE CONFUSION ASSESSMENT METHOD (CAM) DIAGNOSTIC ALGORITHM

The diagnosis of delirium requires the presence of features 1 and 2 and of *either* 3 or 4.[a]

Feature 1: Acute onset and fluctuating course

This feature is satisfied by positive responses to these questions: Is there evidence of an acute change in mental status from the patient's baseline? Did the (abnormal) behavior fluctuate during the day—that is, tend to come and go—or did it increase and decrease in severity?

Feature 2: Inattention

This feature is satisfied by a positive response to this question: Did the patient have difficulty focusing attention—for example, was easily distractible—or have difficulty keeping track of what was being said?

Feature 3: Disorganized thinking

This feature is satisfied by a positive response to this question: Was the patient's thinking disorganized or incoherent, such as rambling or irrelevant conversation, unclear or illogical flow of ideas, or unpredictable switching from subject to subject?

Feature 4: Altered level of consciousness

This feature is satisfied by any answer other than "alert" to this question: Overall, how would you rate this patient's level of consciousness: alert (normal), vigilant (hyperalert), lethargic (drowsy, easily aroused), stupor (difficult to arouse), or coma (unarousable)?

[a]Information is usually obtained from a reliable reporter, such as a family member, caregiver, or nurse.

Source: Modified from Inouye SK et al: Ann Intern Med 113:941, 1990.

APPROACH TO THE PATIENT: Delirium

As the diagnosis of delirium is clinical and made at the bedside, a careful history and physical examination is necessary when evaluating patients with possible confusional states. Screening tools can aid physicians and nurses in identifying patients with delirium, including the Confusion Assessment Method (CAM) (Table 26-1); the Organic Brain Syndrome Scale; the Delirium Rating Scale; and, in the ICU, the Delirium Detection Score and the ICU version of the CAM. These scales are based on criteria from the American Psychiatric Association's *Diagnostic and Statistical Manual of Mental Disorders* (DSM) or the World Health Organization's International Classification of Diseases (ICD). Unfortunately, these scales themselves do not identify the full spectrum of patients with delirium. All patients who are acutely confused should be presumed delirious regardless of their presentation due to the wide variety of possible clinical features. A course that fluctuates over hours or days and may worsen at night (termed *sundowning*) is typical but not essential for the diagnosis. Observation of the patient will usually reveal an altered level of consciousness or a deficit of attention. Other hallmark features that may be present in the delirious patient include alteration of sleep-wake cycles, thought disturbances such as hallucinations or delusions, autonomic instability, and changes in affect.

HISTORY It may be difficult to elicit an accurate history in delirious patients who have altered levels of consciousness or impaired attention. Information from a collateral source such as a spouse or other family member is therefore invaluable. The three most important pieces of history include the patient's baseline cognitive function, the time course of the present illness, and current medications.

Premorbid cognitive function can be assessed through the collateral source or, if needed, via a review of outpatient records. Delirium by definition represents a change that is relatively acute, usually over hours to days, from a cognitive baseline. As a result, an acute confusional state is nearly impossible to diagnose without some knowledge of baseline cognitive function. Without this information, many patients with dementia or depression may be mistaken as delirious during a single initial evaluation. Patients with a more hypoactive, apathetic presentation with psychomotor slowing may only be identified as being different from baseline through conversations with family members. A number of validated instruments have been shown to accurately diagnose cognitive dysfunction using a collateral source including the modified Blessed Dementia Rating Scale and Clinical Dementia Rating (CDR). Baseline cognitive impairment is common in patients with delirium. Even when no such history of cognitive impairment is elicited, there should still be a high suspicion for previously unrecognized underlying neurologic disorder.

Establishing the time course of cognitive change is important not only to make a diagnosis of delirium but also to correlate the onset of the illness with potentially treatable etiologies such as recent medication changes or symptoms of systemic infection.

Medications remain a common cause of delirium, especially those compounds with anticholinergic or sedative properties. It is estimated that nearly one-third of all cases of delirium are secondary to medications, especially in the elderly. Medication histories should include all prescription as well as over-the-counter and herbal substances taken by the patient and any recent changes in dosing or formulation, including substitution of generics for brand-name medications.

Other important elements of the history include screening for symptoms of organ failure or systemic infection, which often contributes to delirium in the elderly. A history of illicit drug use, alcoholism, or toxin exposure is common in younger delirious patients. Finally, asking the patient and collateral source about other symptoms that may accompany delirium, such as depression or hallucinations, may help identify potential therapeutic targets.

PHYSICAL EXAMINATION The general physical examination in a delirious patient should include a careful screening for signs of infection such as fever, tachypnea, pulmonary consolidation, heart murmur, or stiff neck. The patient's fluid status should be assessed; both dehydration and fluid overload with resultant hypoxia have been associated with delirium, and each is usually easily rectified. The appearance of the skin can be helpful, showing jaundice in hepatic encephalopathy, cyanosis in hypoxia, or needle tracks in patients using intravenous drugs.

The neurologic examination requires a careful assessment of mental status. Patients with delirium often present with a fluctuating course; therefore the diagnosis can be missed when relying on a single time point of evaluation. Some but not all patients exhibit the characteristic pattern of sundowning, a worsening of their condition in the evening. In these cases, assessment only during morning rounds may be falsely reassuring.

An altered level of consciousness ranging from hyperarousal to lethargy to coma is present in most patients with delirium and can be easily assessed at the bedside. In the patient with a relatively normal level of consciousness, a screen for an attentional deficit is in order, as this deficit is the classic neuropsychological hallmark of delirium. Attention can be assessed while taking a history from the patient. Tangential speech, a fragmentary flow of ideas, or inability to follow complex commands often signifies an attentional problem. Formal neuropsychological tests to assess attention exist, but a simple bedside test of digit span forward is quick and fairly sensitive. In this task, patients are asked to repeat successively longer random strings of digits beginning with two digits in a row. Average adults can repeat a string of between five to seven digits before faltering; a digit span of four or less usually indicates an attentional deficit unless hearing or language barriers are present.

More formal neuropsychological testing can be extraordinarily helpful in assessing the delirious patient, but it is usually too cumbersome and time-consuming in the inpatient setting. A simple Mini Mental Status Examination (MMSE) (see Table 365-5) can provide some information regarding orientation, language, and visuospatial skills; however, performance of some tasks on the MMSE such as spelling "world" backwards or serial subtraction of digits will be impaired by delirious patients' attentional deficits alone and are therefore unreliable.

The remainder of the screening neurologic examination should focus on identifying new focal neurologic deficits. Focal strokes or mass lesions in isolation are rarely the cause of delirium, but patients with underlying extensive cerebrovascular disease or neurodegenerative conditions may not be able to cognitively tolerate even relatively small new insults. Patients should also be screened for additional signs of neurodegenerative conditions such as parkinsonism, which is seen not only in idiopathic Parkinson's disease but also in other dementing conditions such as Alzheimer's disease, dementia with Lewy bodies, and progressive supranuclear palsy. The presence of multifocal myoclonus or asterixis on the motor examination is nonspecific but usually indicates a metabolic or toxic etiology of the delirium.

ETIOLOGY Some etiologies can be easily discerned through a careful history and physical examination, while others require confirmation with laboratory studies, imaging, or other ancillary tests. A large, diverse group of insults can lead to delirium, and the cause in many patients is often multifactorial. Common etiologies are listed in Table 26-2.

Prescribed, over-the-counter, and herbal medications are common precipitants of delirium. Drugs with anticholinergic properties, narcotics, and benzodiazepines are especially frequent offenders, but nearly any compound can lead to cognitive dysfunction in a predisposed patient. While an elderly patient with baseline dementia may become delirious upon exposure to a relatively low dose of a medication, other less-susceptible individuals may only become delirious with very high doses of the same medication. This observation emphasizes the importance of correlating the timing of recent medication changes, including dose and formulation, with the onset of cognitive dysfunction.

TABLE 26-2 COMMON ETIOLOGIES OF DELIRIUM

- Toxins
  - Prescription medications: especially those with anticholinergic properties, narcotics and benzodiazepines
  - Drugs of abuse: alcohol intoxication and alcohol withdrawal, opiates, ecstasy, LSD, GHB, PCP, ketamine, cocaine
  - Poisons: inhalants, carbon monoxide, ethylene glycol, pesticides
- Metabolic conditions
  - Electrolyte disturbances: hypoglycemia, hyperglycemia, hyponatremia, hypernatremia, hypercalcemia, hypocalcemia, hypomagnesemia
  - Hypothermia and hyperthermia
  - Pulmonary failure: hypoxemia and hypercarbia
  - Liver failure/hepatic encephalopathy
  - Renal failure/uremia
  - Cardiac failure
  - Vitamin deficiencies: B_{12}, thiamine, folate, niacin
  - Dehydration and malnutrition
  - Anemia
- Infections
  - Systemic infections: urinary tract infections, pneumonia, skin and soft tissue infections, sepsis
  - CNS infections: meningitis, encephalitis, brain abscess
- Endocrinologic conditions
  - Hyperthyroidism, hypothyroidism
  - Hyperparathyroidism
  - Adrenal insufficiency
- Cerebrovascular disorders
  - Global hypoperfusion states
  - Hypertensive encephalopathy
  - Focal ischemic strokes and hemorrhages: especially nondominant parietal and thalamic lesions
- Autoimmune disorders
  - CNS vasculitis
  - Cerebral lupus
- Seizure-related disorders
  - Nonconvulsive status epilepticus
  - Intermittent seizures with prolonged post-ictal states
- Neoplastic disorders
  - Diffuse metastases to the brain
  - Gliomatosis cerebri
  - Carcinomatous meningitis
- Hospitalization
- Terminal end of life delirium

Abbreviations: LSD, lysergic acid diethylamide; GHB, γ-hydroxybutyrate; PCP, phencyclidine; CNS, central nervous system.

In younger patients especially, illicit drugs and toxins are common causes of delirium. In addition to more classic drugs of abuse, the recent rise in availability of so-called club drugs, such as methylenedioxymethamphetamine (MDMA, ecstasy), γ-hydroxybutyrate (GHB), and the PCP-like agent ketamine, has led to an increase in delirious young persons presenting to acute care settings. Many common prescription drugs such as oral narcotics and benzodiazepines are now often abused and readily available on the street. Alcohol intoxication with high serum levels can cause confusion, but more commonly it is withdrawal from alcohol that leads to a classic hyperactive delirium. Alcohol and benzodiazepine withdrawal should be considered in all cases of delirium as even patients who drink only a few servings of alcohol every day can experience relatively severe withdrawal symptoms upon hospitalization.

Metabolic abnormalities such as electrolyte disturbances of sodium, calcium, magnesium, or glucose can cause delirium, and mild derangements can lead to substantial cognitive disturbances in susceptible individuals. Other common metabolic etiologies include liver and renal failure, hypercarbia and hypoxia, vitamin deficiencies of thiamine and B_{12}, autoimmune disorders including CNS vasculitis, and endocrinopathies such as thyroid and adrenal disorders.

Systemic infections often cause delirium, especially in the elderly. A common scenario involves the development of an acute cognitive decline in the setting of a urinary tract infection in a patient with baseline dementia. Pneumonia, skin infections such as cellulitis, and frank sepsis can also lead to delirium. This so-called septic encephalopathy, often seen in the ICU, is likely due to the release of proinflammatory cytokines and their diffuse cerebral effects. CNS infections such as meningitis, encephalitis, and abscess are less-common etiologies of delirium; however, given the high mortality associated with these conditions when not treated quickly, clinicians must always maintain a high index of suspicion.

In some susceptible individuals, exposure to the unfamiliar environment of a hospital can lead to delirium. This etiology usually occurs as part of a multifactorial delirium and should be considered a diagnosis of exclusion after all other causes have been thoroughly investigated. Many primary prevention and treatment strategies for delirium involve relatively simple methods to address those aspects of the inpatient setting that are most confusing.

Cerebrovascular etiologies are usually due to global hypoperfusion in the setting of systemic hypotension from heart failure, septic shock, dehydration, or anemia. Focal strokes in the right parietal lobe and medial dorsal thalamus can rarely lead to a delirious state. A more common scenario involves a new focal stroke or hemorrhage causing confusion in a patient who has decreased cerebral reserve. In these individuals, it is sometimes difficult to distinguish between cognitive dysfunction resulting from the new neurovascular insult itself and delirium due to the infectious, metabolic, and pharmacologic complications that can accompany hospitalization after stroke.

Because a fluctuating course is often seen in delirium, intermittent seizures may be overlooked when considering potential etiologies. Both nonconvulsive status epilepticus as well as recurrent focal or generalized seizures followed by post-ictal confusion can cause delirium; EEG remains essential for this diagnosis. Seizure activity spreading from an electrical focus in a mass or infarct can explain global cognitive dysfunction caused by relatively small lesions.

It is very common for patients to experience delirium at the end of life in palliative care settings. This condition, sometimes described as *terminal restlessness*, must be identified and treated aggressively as it is an important cause of patient and family discomfort at the end of life. It should be remembered that these patients may also be suffering from more common etiologies of delirium such as systemic infection.

LABORATORY AND DIAGNOSTIC EVALUATION A cost-effective approach to the diagnostic evaluation of delirium allows the history and physical examination to guide tests. No established algorithm for workup will fit all delirious patients due to the staggering number of potential etiologies, but one step-wise approach is detailed in Table 26-3. If a clear precipitant is identified early, such as an offending medication, then little further workup is required. If, however, no likely etiology is uncovered with initial evaluation, an aggressive search for an underlying cause should be initiated.

TABLE 26-3 STEP-WISE EVALUATION OF A PATIENT WITH DELIRIUM

Initial evaluation
History with special attention to medications (including over-the-counter and herbals)
General physical examination and neurologic examination
Complete blood count
Electrolyte panel including calcium, magnesium, phosphorus
Liver function tests including albumin
Renal function tests
First-tier further evaluation guided by initial evaluation
Systemic infection screen
Urinalysis and culture
Chest radiograph
Blood cultures
Electrocardiogram
Arterial blood gas
Serum and/or urine toxicology screen (perform earlier in young persons)
Brain imaging with MRI with diffusion and gadolinium (preferred) or CT
Suspected CNS infection: lumbar puncture following brain imaging
Suspected seizure-related etiology: electroencephalogram (EEG) (if high suspicion should be performed immediately)
Second-tier further evaluation
Vitamin levels: B_{12}, folate, thiamine
Endocrinologic laboratories: thyroid-stimulating hormone (TSH) and free T4; cortisol
Serum ammonia
Sedimentation rate
Autoimmune serologies: antinuclear antibodies (ANA), complement levels; p-ANCA, c-ANCA
Infectious serologies: rapid plasmin reagin (RPR); fungal and viral serologies if high suspicion; HIV antibody
Lumbar puncture (if not already performed)
Brain MRI with and without gadolinium (if not already performed)

Note: p-ANCA, perinuclear antineutrophil cytoplasmic antibody; c-ANCA, cytoplasmic antineutrophil cytoplasmic antibody.

Basic screening labs, including a complete blood count, electrolyte panel, and tests of liver and renal function, should be obtained in all patients with delirium. In elderly patients, screening for systemic infection, including chest radiography, urinalysis and culture, and possibly blood cultures, is important. In younger individuals, serum and urine drug and toxicology screening may be appropriate early in the workup. Additional laboratory tests addressing other autoimmune, endocrinologic, metabolic, and infectious etiologies should be reserved for patients in whom the diagnosis remains unclear after initial testing.

Multiple studies have demonstrated that brain imaging in patients with delirium is often unhelpful. However, if the initial workup is unrevealing, most clinicians quickly move toward imaging of the brain in order to exclude structural causes. A noncontrast CT scan can identify large masses and hemorrhages but is otherwise relatively insensitive for discovering an etiology of delirium. The ability of MRI to identify most acute ischemic strokes as well as to provide neuroanatomic detail that gives clues to possible infectious, inflammatory, neurodegenerative, and neoplastic conditions makes it the test of choice. Since MRI techniques are limited by availability, speed of imaging, patient cooperation, and contraindications to magnetic exposure, many clinicians begin with CT scanning and proceed to MRI if the etiology of delirium remains elusive.

Lumbar puncture (LP) must be obtained immediately, after appropriate neuroimaging, in all patients in whom CNS infection is suspected. Spinal fluid examination can also be useful in identifying inflammatory and neoplastic conditions as well as in the diagnosis of hepatic encephalopathy through elevated CSF glutamine levels. As a result, LP should be considered in any delirious patient with a negative workup. EEG does not have a routine role in the workup of delirium, but it remains invaluable if seizure-related etiologies are considered.

Management of delirium begins with treatment of the underlying inciting factor (e.g., patients with systemic infections should be given appropriate antibiotics and underlying electrolyte disturbances judiciously corrected). These treatments often lead to prompt resolution of delirium. Blindly targeting the symptoms of delirium pharmacologically only serves to prolong the time patients remain in the confused state and may mask important diagnostic information.

Relatively simple methods of supportive care can be highly effective in treating patients with delirium. Reorientation by the nursing staff and family combined with visible clocks, calendars, and outside-facing windows can reduce confusion. Sensory isolation should be prevented by providing glasses and hearing aids to those patients who need them. Sundowning can be addressed to a large extent through vigilance to appropriate sleep-wake cycles. During the day, a well-lit room should be accompanied by activities or exercises to prevent napping. At night, a quiet, dark environment with limited interruptions by staff can assure proper rest. These sleep-wake cycle interventions are especially important in the ICU setting as the usual constant 24-h activity commonly provokes delirium. Attempting to mimic the home environment as much as possible has also been shown to help treat and even prevent delirium. Visits from friends and family throughout the day minimize the anxiety associated with the constant flow of new faces of staff and physicians. Allowing hospitalized patients to have access to home bedding, clothing, and nightstand objects makes the hospital environment less foreign and therefore less confusing. Simple standard nursing practices such as maintaining proper nutrition and volume status as well as managing incontinence and skin breakdown also help to alleviate discomfort and resulting confusion.

In some instances, patients pose a threat to their own safety or to the safety of staff members, and acute management is required. Bed alarms and personal sitters are more effective and much less disorienting than physical restraints. Chemical restraints should be avoided, but, when necessary, very-low-dose typical or atypical antipsychotic medications administered on an as-needed basis are effective. The recent association of atypical antipsychotic use in the elderly with increased mortality underscores the importance of using these medications judiciously and only as a last resort. Benzodiazepines are not as effective as antipsychotics and often worsen confusion via their sedative properties. Although many clinicians still use benzodiazepines to treat acute confusion, their use should be limited only to cases in which delirium is caused by alcohol or benzodiazepine withdrawal.

PREVENTION

Given the high morbidity associated with delirium and the tremendously increased health care costs that accompany it, development of an effective strategy to prevent delirium in hospitalized patients is extremely important. Successful identification of high-risk patients is the first step, followed by initiation of appropriate interventions. One trial randomized more than 850 elderly inpatients to simple standardized protocols used to manage risk factors for delirium, including cognitive impairment, immobility, visual impairment, hearing impairment, sleep deprivation, and dehydration. Significant reductions in the number and duration of episodes of delirium were observed in the treatment group, but unfortunately delirium recurrence rates were unchanged. All hospitals and health care systems should work toward developing standardized protocols to address common risk factors with the goal of decreasing the incidence of delirium.

ACKNOWLEDGMENT

In the previous edition, Allan H. Ropper contributed to a section on acute confusional states that was incorporated into this current chapter.

FURTHER READINGS

ELY EW et al: Delirium as a predictor of mortality in mechanically ventilated patients in the intensive care unit. JAMA 291:1753, 2004

INOUYE SK: Delirium in older persons. N Engl J Med 354:1157, 2006

——— et al: A multicomponent intervention to prevent delirium in hospitalized older patients. N Engl J Med 340:669, 1999

KALISVAART KJ et al: Risk factors and prediction of postoperative delirium in elderly hip-surgery patients: Implementation and validation of a medical risk factor model. J Am Geriatr Soc 54:817, 2006

YOUNG J, INOUYE SK: Delirium in older people. BMJ 334:842, 2007

27 Aphasia, Memory Loss, and Other Focal Cerebral Disorders

M.-Marsel Mesulam

The cerebral cortex of the human brain contains ~20 billion neurons spread over an area of 2.5 m^2. The *primary sensory* areas provide an obligatory portal for the entry of sensory information into cortical circuitry, whereas the *primary motor* areas provide final common pathways for coordinating complex motor acts. The primary sensory and motor areas constitute 10% of the cerebral cortex. The rest is subsumed by unimodal, heteromodal, paralimbic, and limbic areas, collectively known as the *association cortex* (Fig. 27-1). The association cortex mediates the integrative processes that subserve cognition, emotion, and behavior. A systematic testing of these mental functions is necessary for the effective clinical assessment of the association cortex and its diseases.

According to current thinking, there are no centers for "hearing words," "perceiving space," or "storing memories." Cognitive and behavioral functions (domains) are coordinated by intersecting *large-scale neural networks* that contain interconnected cortical and subcortical components. The network approach to higher cerebral function has at least four implications of clinical relevance: (1) a single domain such as language or memory can be disrupted by damage to any one of several areas, as long as these areas belong to the same network; (2) damage confined to a single area can give rise to multiple deficits, involving the functions of all networks that intersect in that region; (3) damage to a network component may give rise to minimal or transient deficits if other parts of the network undergo compensatory reorganization; and (4) individual anatomic sites within a network display a relative (but not absolute) specialization for different behavioral aspects of the relevant function. Five anatomically defined large-scale networks are most relevant to clinical practice: a perisylvian network for language; a parietofrontal network for spatial cognition; an occipitotemporal network for face and object recognition; a limbic network for retentive memory; and a prefrontal network for attention and behavior.

THE LEFT PERISYLVIAN NETWORK FOR LANGUAGE: APHASIAS AND RELATED CONDITIONS

Language allows the communication and elaboration of thoughts and experiences by linking them to arbitrary symbols known as words. The neural substrate of language is composed of a distributed network centered in the perisylvian region of the *left* hemisphere. The posterior pole of this network is located at the temporoparietal junction and includes a region known as *Wernicke's area*. An essential function of Wernicke's area is to transform sensory inputs into their lexical representations so that these can establish the distributed associations that give the word its meaning. The anterior pole of the language network is located in the inferior frontal gyrus and includes a region known as *Broca's area*. An essential function of this area is to transform lexical representations into their articulatory sequences so that the words can be uttered in the form of spoken language. The sequencing function of Broca's area also appears to involve the ordering of words into sentences that contain a meaning-appropriate *syntax* (grammar). Wernicke's and Broca's areas are interconnected with each other and with additional perisylvian, temporal, prefrontal, and posterior parietal regions, making up a neural network subserving the various aspects of lan-

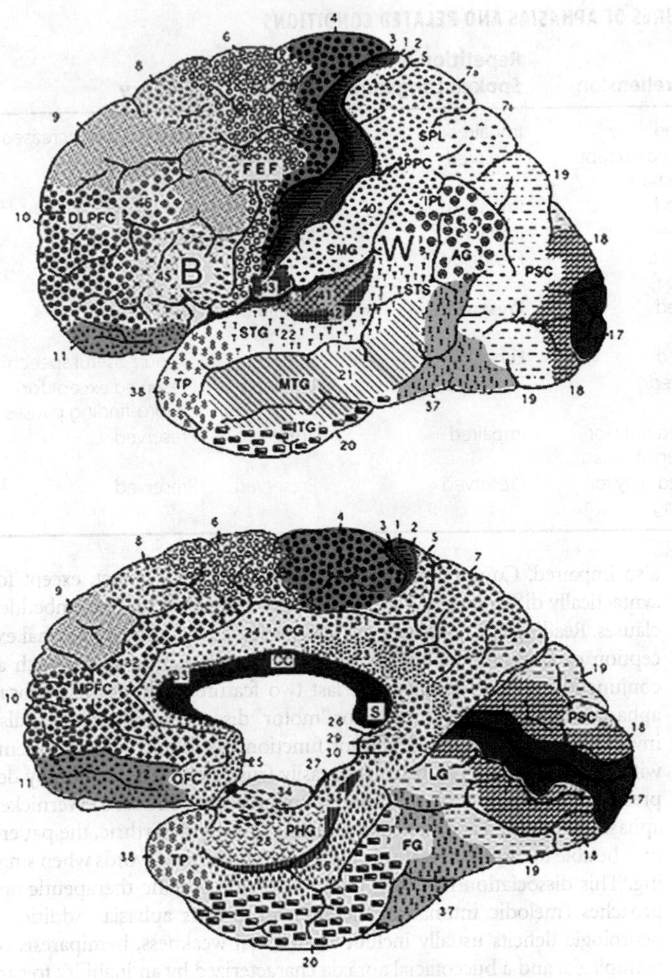

FIGURE 27-1 Lateral *(top)* and medial *(bottom)* views of the cerebral hemispheres. The numbers refer to the Brodmann cytoarchitectonic designations. Area 17 corresponds to the primary visual cortex, 41–42 to the primary auditory cortex, 1–3 to the primary somatosensory cortex, and 4 to the primary motor cortex. The rest of the cerebral cortex contains association areas. AG, angular gyrus; B, Broca's area; CC, corpus callosum; CG, cingulate gyrus; DLPFC, dorsolateral prefrontal cortex; FEF, frontal eye fields (premotor cortex); FG, fusiform gyrus; IPL, inferior parietal lobule; ITG, inferior temporal gyrus; LG, lingual gyrus; MPFC, medial prefrontal cortex; MTG, middle temporal gyrus; OFC, orbitofrontal cortex; PHG, parahippocampal gyrus; PPC, posterior parietal cortex; PSC, peristriate cortex; SC, striate cortex; SMG, supramarginal gyrus; SPL, superior parietal lobule; STG, superior temporal gyrus; STS, superior temporal sulcus; TP, temporopolar cortex; W, Wernicke's area.

guage function. Damage to any one of these components or to their interconnections can give rise to language disturbances (*aphasia*). Aphasia should be diagnosed only when there are deficits in the formal aspects of language such as naming, word choice, comprehension, spelling, and syntax. Dysarthria and mutism do not, by themselves, lead to a diagnosis of aphasia. The language network shows a left hemisphere dominance pattern in the vast majority of the population. In ~90% of right handers and 60% of left handers, aphasia occurs only after lesions of the left hemisphere. In some individuals no hemispheric dominance for language can be discerned, and in some others (including a small minority of right handers) there is a right hemisphere dominance for language. A language disturbance occurring after a right hemisphere lesion in a right hander is called *crossed aphasia.*

CLINICAL EXAMINATION

The clinical examination of language should include the assessment of naming, spontaneous speech, comprehension, repetition, reading, and writing. A deficit of naming (*anomia*) is the single most common finding in aphasic patients. When asked to name common objects (pencil or wristwatch), the patient may fail to come up with the appropriate word, may provide a circumlocutious description of the object ("the thing for writing"), or may come up with the wrong word (*paraphasia*). If the patient offers an incorrect but legitimate word ("pen" for "pencil"), the naming error is known as a *semantic paraphasia*; if the word approximates the correct answer but is phonetically inaccurate ("plentil" for "pencil"), it is known as a *phonemic paraphasia.* Asking the patient to name body parts, geometric shapes, and component parts of objects (lapel of coat, cap of pen) can elicit mild forms of anomia in patients who can otherwise name common objects. In most anomias, the patient cannot retrieve the appropriate name when shown an object but can point to the appropriate object when the name is provided by the examiner. This is known as a one-way (or retrieval-based) naming deficit. A two-way naming deficit exists if the patient can neither provide nor recognize the correct name, indicating the presence of a language comprehension impairment. *Spontaneous speech* is described as "fluent" if it maintains appropriate output volume, phrase length, and melody or as "nonfluent" if it is sparse, halting, and average utterance length is below four words. The examiner should also note if the speech is paraphasic or circumlocutious; if it shows a relative paucity of substantive nouns and action verbs versus function words (prepositions, conjunctions); and if word order, tenses, suffixes, prefixes, plurals, and possessives are appropriate. *Comprehension* can be tested by assessing the patient's ability to follow conversation, by asking yes-no questions ("Can a dog fly?", "Does it snow in summer?") or asking the patient to point to appropriate objects ("Where is the source of illumination in this room?"). Statements with embedded clauses or passive voice construction ("If a tiger is eaten by a lion, which animal stays alive?") help to assess the ability to comprehend complex syntactic structure. Commands to close or open the eyes, stand up, sit down, or roll over should not be used to assess overall comprehension since appropriate responses aimed at such axial movements can be preserved in patients who otherwise have profound comprehension deficits.

Repetition is assessed by asking the patient to repeat single words, short sentences, or strings of words such as "No ifs, ands, or buts." The testing of repetition with tongue-twisters such as "hippopotamus" or "Irish constabulary" provides a better assessment of dysarthria and palilalia than aphasia. Aphasic patients may have little difficulty with tongue-twisters but have a particularly hard time repeating a string of function words. It is important to make sure that the number of words does not exceed the patient's attention span. Otherwise, the failure of repetition becomes a reflection of the narrowed attention span rather than an indication of an aphasic deficit. *Reading* should be assessed for deficits in reading aloud as well as comprehension. *Writing* is assessed for spelling errors, word order, and grammar. *Alexia* describes an inability to either read aloud or comprehend single words and simple sentences; *agraphia* (or dysgraphia) is used to describe an acquired deficit in the spelling or grammar of written language.

The correspondence between individual deficits of language function and lesion location does not display a rigid one-to-one relationship and should be conceptualized within the context of the distributed network model. Nonetheless, the classification of aphasias of acute onset into specific clinical syndromes helps to determine the most likely anatomic distribution of the underlying neurologic disease and has implications for etiology and prognosis (Table 27-1). The syndromes listed in Table 27-1 are most applicable to aphasias caused by cerebrovascular accidents (CVA). They can be divided into "central" syndromes, which result from damage to the two epicenters of the language network (Broca's and Wernicke's areas), and "disconnection" syndromes, which arise from lesions that interrupt the functional connectivity of these centers with each other and with the other components of the language network. The syndromes outlined below are idealizations; pure syndromes occur rarely.

Wernicke's Aphasia Comprehension is impaired for spoken and written language. Language output is fluent but is highly paraphasic and circumlocutious. The tendency for paraphasic errors may be so pronounced that it leads to strings of neologisms, which form the basis of what is known as "jargon aphasia." Speech contains large numbers of function words (e.g., prepositions, conjunctions) but few substantive nouns or verbs that refer to specific actions. The output is therefore voluminous but uninformative. For example, a patient attempts to describe how his wife accidentally threw away something important, perhaps his dentures: "We don't need it anymore, she says. And with it when that was downstairs was my teeth-tick . . . a . . . den . . . dentith . . . my dentist. And they happened to be in that bag . . . see? How could this have happened? How could a thing like this happen...So she says we won't need it anymore...I didn't think we'd use it. And now if I have any problems anybody coming a month from now, 4 months from now, or 6 months from now, I have a new dentist. Where my two . . . two little pieces of dentist that I use . . . that I . . . all gone. If she throws the whole thing away . . . visit some friends of hers and she can't throw them away."

TABLE 27-1 CLINICAL FEATURES OF APHASIAS AND RELATED CONDITIONS

	Comprehension	Repetition of Spoken Language	Naming	Fluency
Wernicke's	Impaired	Impaired	Impaired	Preserved or increased
Broca's	Preserved (except grammar)	Impaired	Impaired	Decreased
Global	Impaired	Impaired	Impaired	Decreased
Conduction	Preserved	Impaired	Impaired	Preserved
Nonfluent (motor) transcortical	Preserved	Preserved	Impaired	Impaired
Fluent (sensory) transcortical	Impaired	Preserved	Impaired	Preserved
Isolation	Impaired	Echolalia	Impaired	No purposeful speech
Anomic	Preserved	Preserved	Impaired	Preserved except for word-finding pauses
Pure word deafness	Impaired only for spoken language	Impaired	Preserved	Preserved
Pure alexia	Impaired only for reading	Preserved	Preserved	Preserved

Gestures and pantomime do not improve communication. The patient does not seem to realize that his or her language is incomprehensible and may appear angry and impatient when the examiner fails to decipher the meaning of a severely paraphasic statement. In some patients this type of aphasia can be associated with severe agitation and paranoid behaviors. One area of comprehension that may be preserved is the ability to follow commands aimed at axial musculature. The dissociation between the failure to understand simple questions ("What is your name?") in a patient who rapidly closes his or her eyes, sits up, or rolls over when asked to do so is characteristic of Wernicke's aphasia and helps to differentiate it from deafness, psychiatric disease, or malingering. Patients with Wernicke's aphasia cannot express their thoughts in meaning-appropriate words and cannot decode the meaning of words in any modality of input. This aphasia therefore has expressive as well as receptive components. Repetition, naming, reading, and writing are also impaired.

The lesion site most commonly associated with Wernicke's aphasia is the posterior portion of the language network and tends to involve at least parts of Wernicke's area. An embolus to the inferior division of the middle cerebral artery, and to the posterior temporal or angular branches in particular, is the most common etiology (Chap. 364). Intracerebral hemorrhage, severe head trauma, or neoplasm are other causes. A coexisting right hemi- or superior quadrantanopia is common, and mild right nasolabial flattening may be found, but otherwise the examination is often unrevealing. The paraphasic, neologistic speech in an agitated patient with an otherwise unremarkable neurologic examination may lead to the suspicion of a primary psychiatric disorder such as schizophrenia or mania, but the other components characteristic of acquired aphasia and the absence of prior psychiatric disease usually settle the issue. Some patients with Wernicke's aphasia due to intracerebral hemorrhage or head trauma may improve as the hemorrhage or the injury heals. In most other patients, prognosis for recovery is guarded.

Broca's Aphasia Speech is nonfluent, labored, interrupted by many word-finding pauses, and usually dysarthric. It is impoverished in function words but enriched in meaning-appropriate nouns and verbs. Abnormal word order and the inappropriate deployment of *bound morphemes* (word endings used to denote tenses, possessives, or plurals) lead to a characteristic agrammatism. Speech is telegraphic and pithy but quite informative. In the following passage, a patient with Broca's aphasia describes his medical history: "I see . . . the dotor, dotor sent me . . . Bosson. Go to hospital. Dotor . . . kept me beside. Two, tee days, doctor send me home."

Output may be reduced to a grunt or single word ("yes" or "no"), which is emitted with different intonations in an attempt to express approval or disapproval. In addition to fluency, naming and repetition are also impaired. Comprehension of spoken language is intact, except for syntactically difficult sentences with passive voice structure or embedded clauses. Reading comprehension is also preserved, with the occasional exception of a specific inability to read small grammatical words such as conjunctions and pronouns. The last two features indicate that Broca's aphasia is not just an "expressive" or "motor" disorder and that it may also involve a comprehension deficit for function words and syntax. Patients with Broca's aphasia can be tearful, easily frustrated, and profoundly depressed. Insight into their condition is preserved, in contrast to Wernicke's aphasia. Even when spontaneous speech is severely dysarthric, the patient may be able to display a relatively normal articulation of words when singing. This dissociation has been used to develop specific therapeutic approaches (melodic intonation therapy) for Broca's aphasia. Additional neurologic deficits usually include right facial weakness, hemiparesis or hemiplegia, and a buccofacial apraxia characterized by an inability to carry out motor commands involving oropharyngeal and facial musculature (e.g., patients are unable to demonstrate how to blow out a match or suck through a straw). Visual fields are intact. The cause is most often infarction of Broca's area (the inferior frontal convolution; "B" in Fig. 27-1) and surrounding anterior perisylvian and insular cortex, due to occlusion of the superior division of the middle cerebral artery (Chap. 364). Mass lesions including tumor, intracerebral hemorrhage, or abscess may also be responsible. Small lesions confined to the posterior part of Broca's area may lead to a nonaphasic and often reversible deficit of speech articulation, usually accompanied by mild right facial weakness. When the cause of Broca's aphasia is stroke, recovery of language function generally peaks within 2–6 months, after which time further progress is limited.

Global Aphasia Speech output is nonfluent, and comprehension of spoken language is severely impaired. Naming, repetition, reading, and writing are also impaired. This syndrome represents the combined dysfunction of Broca's and Wernicke's areas and usually results from strokes that involve the entire middle cerebral artery distribution in the left hemisphere. Most patients are initially mute or say a few words, such as "hi" or "yes." Related signs include right hemiplegia, hemisensory loss, and homonymous hemianopia. Occasionally, a patient with a lesion in Wernicke's area will present with a global aphasia that soon resolves into Wernicke's aphasia.

Conduction Aphasia Speech output is fluent but paraphasic, comprehension of spoken language is intact, and repetition is severely impaired. Naming and writing are also impaired. Reading aloud is impaired, but reading comprehension is preserved. The lesion sites spare Broca's and Wernicke's areas but may induce a functional disconnection between the two so that lexical representations formed in Wernicke's area and adjacent regions cannot be conveyed to Broca's area for assembly into corresponding articulatory patterns. Occasionally, a Wernicke's area lesion gives rise to a transient Wernicke's aphasia that rapidly resolves into a conduction aphasia. The paraphasic output in conduction aphasia interferes with the ability to express meaning, but this deficit is not nearly as severe as the one displayed by patients with Wernicke's aphasia. Associated neurologic signs in conduction aphasia vary according to the primary lesion site.

Nonfluent Transcortical Aphasia (Transcortical Motor Aphasia) The features are similar to Broca's aphasia, but repetition is intact and agrammatism may be less pronounced. The neurologic examination may be otherwise intact, but a right hemiparesis can also exist. The lesion site disconnects the intact language network from prefrontal areas of the brain and usually involves the anterior watershed zone between anterior and middle cerebral artery territories or the supplementary motor cortex in the territory of the anterior cerebral artery.

Fluent Transcortical Aphasia (Transcortical Sensory Aphasia) Clinical features are similar to those of Wernicke's aphasia, but repetition is intact. The lesion site disconnects the intact core of the language network from other temporoparietal association areas. Associated neurologic findings may include hemianopia. Cerebrovascular lesions (e.g., infarctions in the posterior watershed zone) or neoplasms that involve the temporoparietal cortex posterior to Wernicke's area are the most common causes.

Isolation Aphasia This rare syndrome represents a combination of the two transcortical aphasias. Comprehension is severely impaired, and there is no purposeful speech output. The patient may parrot fragments of heard conversations (*echolalia*), indicating that the neural mechanisms for repetition are at least partially intact. This condition represents the pathologic function of the language network when it is isolated from other regions of the brain. Broca's and Wernicke's areas tend to be spared, but there is damage to the surrounding frontal, parietal, and temporal cortex. Lesions are patchy and can be associated with anoxia, carbon monoxide poisoning, or complete watershed zone infarctions.

Anomic Aphasia This form of aphasia may be considered the "minimal dysfunction" syndrome of the language network. Articulation, comprehension, and repetition are intact, but confrontation naming, word finding, and spelling are impaired. Speech is enriched in function words but impoverished in substantive nouns and verbs denoting specific actions. Language output is fluent but paraphasic, circumlocutious, and uninformative. The lesion sites can be anywhere within the left hemisphere language network, including the middle and inferior temporal gyri. *Anomic aphasia is the single most common language disturbance seen in head trauma, metabolic encephalopathy, and Alzheimer's disease.*

Pure Word Deafness The most common causes are either bilateral or left-sided middle cerebral artery strokes affecting the superior temporal gyrus. The net effect of the underlying lesion is to interrupt the flow of information from the unimodal auditory association cortex to Wernicke's area. Patients have no difficulty understanding written language and can express themselves well in spoken or written language. They have no difficulty interpreting and reacting to environmental sounds since primary auditory cortex and subcortical auditory relays are intact. Since auditory information cannot be conveyed to the language network, however, it cannot be decoded into lexical representations and the patient reacts to speech as if it were in an alien tongue that cannot be deciphered. Patients cannot repeat spoken language but have no difficulty naming objects. In time, patients with pure word deafness teach themselves lip reading and may appear to have improved. There may be no additional neurologic findings, but agitated paranoid reactions are frequent in the acute stages. Cerebrovascular lesions are the most frequent cause.

Pure Alexia without Agraphia This is the visual equivalent of pure word deafness. The lesions (usually a combination of damage to the left occipital cortex and to a posterior sector of the corpus callosum—the splenium) interrupt the flow of visual input into the language network. There is usually a right hemianopia, but the core language network remains unaffected. The patient can understand and produce spoken language, name objects in the left visual hemifield, repeat, and write. However, the patient acts as if illiterate when asked to read even the simplest sentence because the visual information from the written words (presented to the intact left visual hemifield) cannot reach the language network. Objects in the left hemifield may be named accurately because they activate nonvisual associations in the right hemisphere, which, in turn, can access the language network through transcallosal pathways anterior to the splenium. Patients with this syndrome may also lose the ability to name colors, although they can match colors. This is known as a *color anomia*. The most common etiology of pure alexia is a vascular lesion in the territory of the posterior cerebral artery or an infiltrating neoplasm in the left occipital cortex that involves the optic radiations as well as the crossing fibers of the splenium. Since the posterior cerebral artery also supplies medial temporal components of the limbic system, the patient with pure alexia may also experience an amnesia, but this is usually transient because the limbic lesion is unilateral.

Aphemia There is an acute onset of severely impaired fluency (often mutism), which cannot be accounted for by corticobulbar, cerebellar, or extrapyramidal dysfunction. Recovery is the rule and involves an intermediate stage of hoarse whispering. Writing, reading, and comprehension are intact, so this is not a true aphasic syndrome. Partial lesions of Broca's area or subcortical lesions that undercut its connections with other parts of the brain may be present. Occasionally, the lesion site is on the medial aspects of the frontal lobes and may involve the supplementary motor cortex of the left hemisphere.

Apraxia This generic term designates a complex motor deficit that cannot be attributed to pyramidal, extrapyramidal, cerebellar, or sensory dysfunction and that does not arise from the patient's failure to understand the nature of the task. The form that is most frequently encountered in clinical practice is known as *ideomotor apraxia*. Commands to perform a specific motor act ("cough," "blow out a match") or to pantomime the use of a common tool (a comb, hammer, straw, or toothbrush) in the absence of the real object cannot be followed. The patient's ability to comprehend the command is ascertained by demonstrating multiple movements and establishing that the correct one can be recognized. Some patients with this type of apraxia can imitate the appropriate movement (when it is demonstrated by the examiner) and show no impairment when handed the real object, indicating that the sensorimotor mechanisms necessary for the movement are intact. Some forms of ideomotor apraxia represent a disconnection of the language network from pyramidal motor systems: commands to execute complex movements are understood but cannot be conveyed to the appropriate motor areas, even though the relevant motor mechanisms are intact. *Buccofacial apraxia* involves apraxic deficits in movements of the face and mouth. *Limb apraxia* encompasses apraxic deficits in movements of the arms and legs. Ideomotor apraxia is almost always caused by lesions in the left hemisphere and is commonly associated with aphasic syndromes, especially Broca's aphasia and conduction aphasia. Its presence cannot be ascertained in patients with language comprehension deficits. The ability to follow commands aimed at axial musculature ("close the eyes," "stand up") is subserved by different pathways and may be intact in otherwise severely aphasic and apraxic patients. Patients with lesions of the anterior corpus callosum can display a special type of ideomotor apraxia confined to the left side of the body. Since the handling of real objects is not impaired, ideomotor apraxia, by itself, causes no major limitation of daily living activities.

Ideational apraxia refers to a deficit in the execution of a goal-directed sequence of movements in patients who have no difficulty executing the individual components of the sequence. For example, when asked to pick up a pen and write, the sequence of uncapping the pen, placing the cap at the opposite end, turning the point toward the writing surface, and writing may be disrupted, and the patient may be seen trying to write with the wrong end of the pen or even with the removed cap. These motor sequencing problems are usually seen in the context of confusional states and dementias rather than focal lesions associated with aphasic conditions. *Limb-kinetic apraxia* involves a clumsiness in the actual use of tools that cannot be attributed to sensory, pyramidal, extrapyramidal, or cerebellar dysfunction. This condition can emerge in the context of focal premotor cortex lesions or *corticobasal ganglionic degeneration.*

Gerstmann's Syndrome The combination of *acalculia* (impairment of simple arithmetic), *dysgraphia* (impaired writing), *finger anomia* (an inability to name individual fingers such as the index or thumb), and *right-left confusion* (an inability to tell whether a hand, foot, or arm of the patient or examiner is on the right or left side of the body) is known as Gerstmann's syndrome. In making this diagnosis it is important to establish that the finger and left-right naming deficits are not part of a more generalized anomia and that the patient is not otherwise aphasic. When Gerstmann's syndrome is seen in isolation, it is commonly associated with damage to the inferior parietal lobule (especially the angular gyrus) in the left hemisphere.

Aprosodia Variations of melodic stress and intonation influence the meaning and impact of spoken language. For example, the two statements "He *is* clever." and "He is *clever*?" contain an identical word choice and syntax but convey vastly different messages because of differences in the intonation and stress with which the statements are uttered. This aspect of language is known as *prosody.* Damage to perisylvian areas in the right hemisphere can interfere with speech prosody and can lead to syndromes of aprosodia. Damage to right hemisphere regions corresponding to Wernicke's area can selectively impair decoding of speech prosody, whereas damage to right hemisphere regions corresponding to Broca's area yields a greater impairment in the ability to introduce meaning-appropriate prosody into spoken language. The latter deficit is the most common type of aprosodia identified in clinical practice—the patient produces grammatically correct language with accurate word choice but the statements are uttered in a monotone that interferes with the ability to convey the intended stress and affect. Patients with this type of aprosodia give the mistaken impression of being depressed or indifferent.

Subcortical Aphasia Damage to subcortical components of the language network (e.g., the striatum and thalamus of the left hemisphere) can also lead to aphasia. The resulting syndromes contain combinations of deficits in the various aspects of language but rarely fit the specific patterns described in Table 27-1. In a patient with a CVA, an anomic aphasia accompanied by dysarthria or a fluent aphasia with hemiparesis should raise the suspicion of a subcortical lesion site.

Progressive Aphasias In clinical practice, acquired aphasias are most commonly encountered in one of two contexts: CVAs and degenerative diseases. Aphasias caused by CVAs start suddenly and display maximal deficits at the onset. The underlying lesion is relatively circumscribed and associated with a total loss of neural function at the lesion site. These are the "classic" aphasias described above where relatively reproducible relationships between lesion site and aphasia pattern can be discerned. Aphasias caused by neurodegenerative diseases have an insidious onset and relentless progression so that the symptomatology changes over time. Since the neuronal loss within the areas encompassed by the neurodegeneration is partial and since it tends to include multiple components of the language network, distinctive clinical patterns and clinico-anatomic correlations are less obvious.

Dementia is a generic term used to designate a neurodegenerative disease that impairs intellect and behavior to the point where customary daily living activities become compromised (Chap. 365). Alzheimer's disease is the single most common cause of dementia. The neuropathology of Alzheimer's disease causes the earliest and most profound neuronal loss in memory-related parts of the brain such as the entorhinal cortex and the hippocampus. This is why progressive forgetfulness for recent events and experiences is the cardinal feature of Alzheimer's disease. In time, the neuronal pathology in Alzheimer's disease spreads to the language network and a progressive aphasia, usually of the anomic type, becomes added to the progressive amnesia. There are other patterns of dementia, however, where neurodegeneration initially targets the language rather than memory network of the brain, leading to the emergence of a progressive aphasia that becomes the most prominent aspect of the clinical picture during the initial phases of the disease. Primary progressive aphasia (PPA) is the most widely recognized syndrome with this pattern of selective language impairment.

CLINICAL PRESENTATION AND DIAGNOSIS OF PPA The patient with PPA comes to medical attention because of word-finding difficulties, abnormal speech patterns, and spelling errors of recent onset. PPA is diagnosed when other mental faculties such as memory for daily events, visuospatial skills (assessed by tests of drawing and face recognition), and comportment (assessed by history obtained from a third party) remain relatively intact; when language is the major area of dysfunction for the first few years of the disease; and when structural brain imaging does not reveal a specific lesion, other than atrophy, to account for the language deficit. Impairments in other cognitive functions may also emerge, but the language dysfunction remains the most salient feature and deteriorates most rapidly throughout the illness.

LANGUAGE IN PPA The language impairment in PPA varies from patient to patient. Some patients cannot find the right words to express thoughts; others cannot understand the meaning of heard or seen words; still others cannot name objects in the environment. The language impairment can be fluent (that is, with normal articulation, flow, and number of words per utterance) or nonfluent. The single most common sign of primary progressive aphasia is anomia, manifested by an inability to come up with the right word during conversation and/or an inability to name objects shown by the examiner. Many patients remain in an anomic phase through most of the disease and experience a gradual intensification of word-finding deficits to the point of near-mutism. Others, however, proceed to develop distinct forms of agrammatism and/or word comprehension deficits. The agrammatism consists of inappropriate word order and misuse of small grammatical words. One patient, for example, sent the following e-mail to her daughter: "I will come my house in your car and drive my car into chicago. . . . You will back get your car and my car park in my driveway. Love, Mom." Comprehension deficits, if present, start with an occasional inability to understand single low-frequency words and gradually progress to encompass the comprehension of conversational speech.

The impairments of syntax, comprehension, naming, or writing in PPA are no different from those seen in aphasias of cerebrovascular causes. However, they form slightly different patterns. According to a classification proposed by Gorno-Tempini and colleagues, three variants of PPA can be recognized: an agrammatical variant characterized by poor fluency and impaired syntax, a semantic variant characterized by preserved fluency and syntax but poor single word comprehension, and a logopenic variant characterized by preserved syntax and comprehension but frequent word-finding pauses during spontaneous speech. The agrammatical variant is also known as *progressive nonfluent aphasia* and displays similarities to Broca's aphasia. However, dysarthria is usually absent. The semantic variant of PPA is also known as *semantic dementia* and displays similarities to Wernicke's aphasia, but the comprehension difficulty tends to be milder. The most obvious difference between aphasias caused by CVA and those caused by neurodegenerative disease is the post-stroke improvement in CVA-related aphasias, leading to a progressive crystallization of the subtypes listed in Table 27-1, versus the gradual deterioration that leads to a loss of syndromic specificity as the disease progresses.

PATHOPHYSIOLOGY Patients with PPA display progressive atrophy (indicative of neuronal loss), electroencephalographic slowing, decreased blood flow (measured by single photon emission CT) and decreased glucose utilization (measured by positron emission tomography) that are most pronounced within the language network of the brain. The abnormalities may remain confined to left hemisphere perisylvian and anterior temporal cortices for many years. The clinical focality of primary progressive aphasia is thus matched by the anatomic selectivity of the underlying pathologic process.

The three variants display overlapping distributions of neuronal loss but the agrammatical variant is most closely associated with atrophy in the anterior parts of the language network (where Broca's area is located), the semantic variant with atrophy in the temporal components of the language network, and the logopenic variant with atrophy in the temporoparietal component of the language network. The relationship between poor language comprehension and damage to Wernicke's area, which is a feature of CVA-related aphasias, is not present in PPA. Instead, poor comprehension is most closely associated with neuronal loss in the lateral and anterior temporal cortex.

NEUROPATHOLOGY Approximately 30% of patients have shown the microscopic pathology of Alzheimer's disease, presumably with an atypical distribution of lesions. In the majority of cases, the neuropathology falls within the family of frontotemporal lobar degenerations (FTLD) and displays various combinations of focal neuronal loss, gliosis, tau-positive inclusions, Pick bodies, and tau-negative ubiquitin inclusions (Chap. 365). Familial forms of PPA with tau-negative ubiquinated inclusions have recently been linked to mutations of the progranulin gene on chromosome 17. Apolipoprotein E and prion protein genotyping has shown differences between patients with typical clinical patterns of Alzheimer's disease and those with a diagnosis of PPA. The intriguing possibility has been raised that a personal or family history of dyslexia may be a risk factor for primary progressive aphasia, at least in some patients, suggesting that this disease may arise on a background of genetic or developmental vulnerability affecting language-related areas of the brain.

THE PARIETOFRONTAL NETWORK FOR SPATIAL ORIENTATION: NEGLECT AND RELATED CONDITIONS

HEMISPATIAL NEGLECT

Adaptive orientation to significant events within the extrapersonal space is subserved by a large-scale network containing three major cortical components. The *cingulate cortex* provides access to a limbic-motivational mapping of the extrapersonal space, the *posterior parietal cortex* to a sensorimotor representation of salient extrapersonal events, and the *frontal eye fields* to motor strategies for attentional behaviors (Fig. 27-2). Subcortical components of this network include the striatum and the thalamus. Contralesional hemispatial neglect represents one outcome of damage to any of the cortical or subcortical components of this network. *The traditional view that hemispatial neglect always denotes a parietal lobe lesion is inaccurate.* In keeping with this anatomic organization, the clinical manifestations of neglect display three behavioral components: sensory events (or their mental representations) within the neglected hemispace have a lesser impact on overall awareness; there is a paucity of exploratory and orienting acts directed toward the neglected hemispace; and the patient behaves as if the neglected hemispace was motivationally devalued.

According to one model of spatial cognition, the right hemisphere directs attention within the *entire* extrapersonal space, whereas the left hemisphere directs attention mostly within the contralateral right hemispace. Consequently, unilateral left hemisphere lesions do not give rise to much contralesional neglect since the global attentional mechanisms of the right hemisphere can compensate for the loss of the *contralaterally* directed attentional functions of the left hemisphere. Unilateral right hemisphere lesions, however, give rise to severe contralesional left hemispatial neglect because the unaffected left hemisphere does not contain ipsilateral attentional mechanisms. This model is consistent with clinical experience, which shows that contralesional neglect is more common, severe, and lasting after damage to the right hemisphere than after damage to the left hemisphere. Severe neglect for the right hemispace is rare, even in left handers with left hemisphere lesions.

Patients with severe neglect may fail to dress, shave, or groom the left side of the body; may fail to eat food placed on the left side of the tray; and may fail to read the left half of sentences. When the examiner draws a large circle [12–15 cm (5–6 in.) in diameter] and asks the patient to place the numbers 1–12 as if the circle represented the face of a clock, there is a tendency to crowd the numbers on the right side and leave the left side empty. When asked to copy a simple line drawing, the patient fails to copy detail on the left; and when asked to write, there is a tendency to leave an unusually wide margin on the left.

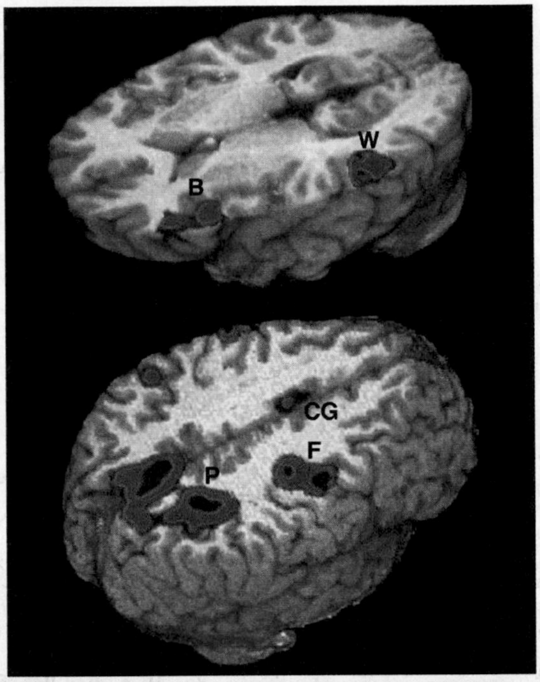

FIGURE 27-2 Functional magnetic resonance imaging of language and spatial attention in neurologically intact subjects. The dark areas show regions of task-related significant activation. (*Top*) The subjects were asked to determine if two words were synonymous. This language task led to the simultaneous activation of the two epicenters of the language network, Broca's area (B) and Wernicke's area (W). The activations are exclusively in the left hemisphere. (*Bottom*) The subjects were asked to shift spatial attention to a peripheral target. This task led to the simultaneous activation of the three epicenters of the attentional network, the posterior parietal cortex (P), the frontal eye fields (F), and the cingulate gyrus (CG). The activations are predominantly in the right hemisphere. (*Courtesy of Darren Gitelman, MD; with permission.*)

Two bedside tests that are useful in assessing neglect are *simultaneous bilateral stimulation* and *visual target cancellation*. In the former, the examiner provides either unilateral or simultaneous bilateral stimulation in the visual, auditory, and tactile modalities. Following right hemisphere injury, patients who have no difficulty detecting unilateral stimuli on either side experience the bilaterally presented stimulus as coming only from the right. This phenomenon is known as *extinction* and is a manifestation of the sensory-representational aspect of hemispatial neglect. In the target detection task, targets (e.g., As) are interspersed with foils (e.g., other letters of the alphabet) on a 21.5 × 28.0 cm (8.5 × 11 in.) sheet of paper and the patient is asked to circle all the targets. A failure to detect targets on the left is a manifestation of the exploratory deficit in hemispatial neglect (Fig. 27-3A). Hemianopia, by itself, does not interfere with performance in this task since the patient is free to turn the head and eyes to the left. The normal tendency in target detection tasks is to start from the left upper quadrant and move systematically in horizontal or vertical sweeps. Some patients show a tendency to start the process from the right and proceed in a haphazard fashion. This represents a subtle manifestation of left neglect, even if the patient eventually manages to detect all the appropriate targets. Some patients with neglect may also deny the existence of hemiparesis and may even deny ownership of the paralyzed limb, a condition known as *anosognosia*.

Cerebrovascular lesions and neoplasms in the right hemisphere are the most common causes of hemispatial neglect. Depending on the

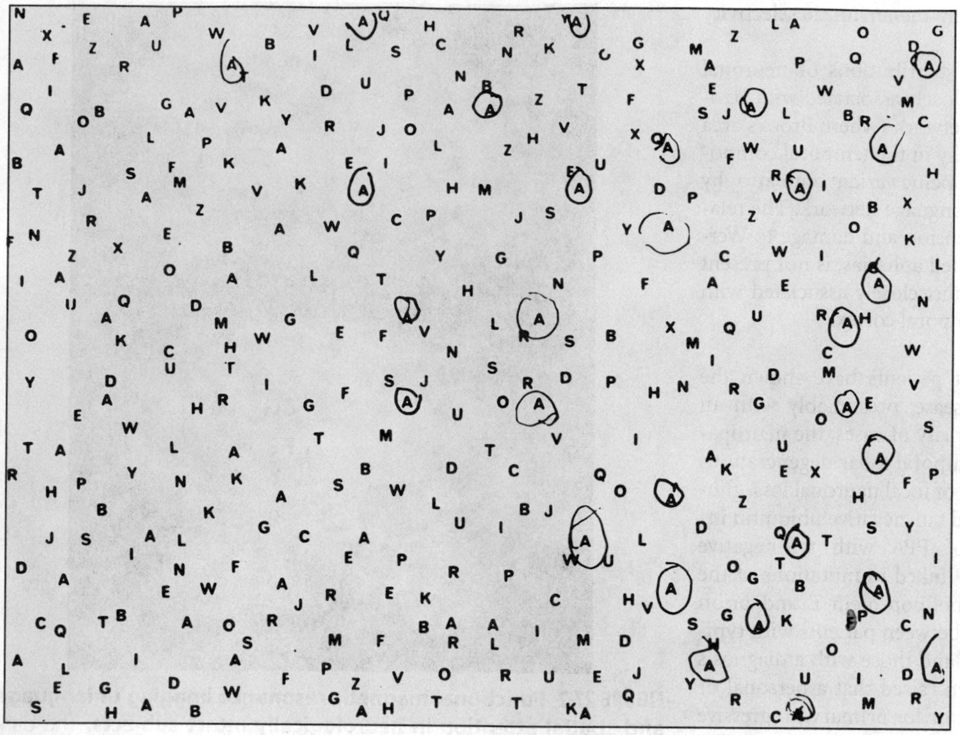

A

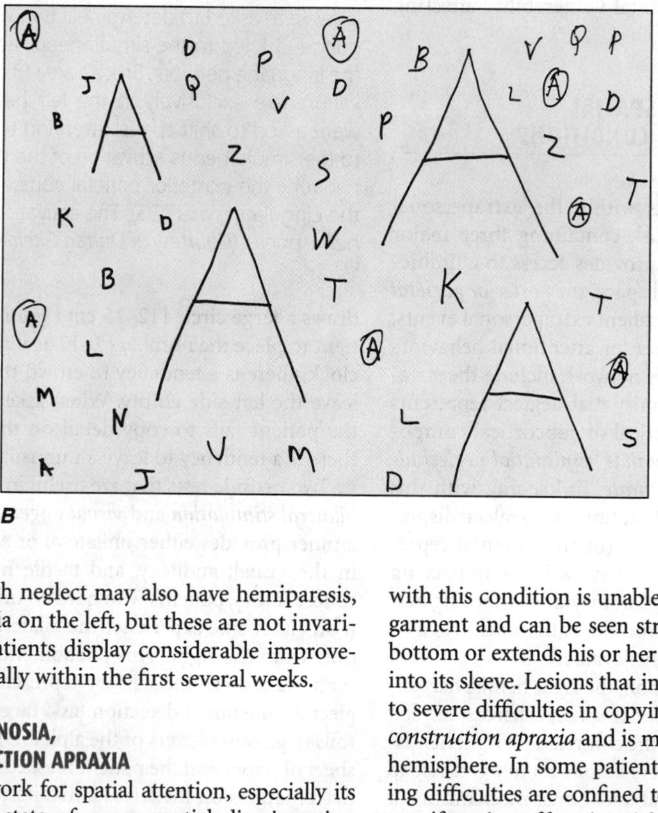

B

FIGURE 27-3 Evidence of left hemispatial neglect and simultanagnosia. ***A.*** A 47-year-old man with a large frontoparietal lesion in the right hemisphere was asked to circle all the As. Only targets on the right are circled. This is a manifestation of left hemispatial neglect. ***B.*** A 70-year-old woman with a 2-year history of degenerative dementia was able to circle most of the small targets but ignored the larger ones. This is a manifestation of simultanagnosia.

site of the lesion, the patient with neglect may also have hemiparesis, hemihypesthesia, and hemianopia on the left, but these are not invariant findings. The majority of patients display considerable improvement of hemispatial neglect, usually within the first several weeks.

BÁLINT'S SYNDROME, SIMULTANAGNOSIA, DRESSING APRAXIA, AND CONSTRUCTION APRAXIA

Bilateral involvement of the network for spatial attention, especially its parietal components, leads to a state of severe spatial disorientation known as *Bálint's syndrome.* Bálint's syndrome involves deficits in the orderly visuomotor scanning of the environment (*oculomotor apraxia*) and in accurate manual reaching toward visual targets (*optic ataxia*). The third and most dramatic component of Bálint's syndrome is known as *simultanagnosia* and reflects an inability to integrate visual information in the center of gaze with more peripheral information. The patient gets stuck on the detail that falls in the center of gaze without attempting to scan the visual environment for additional information. The patient with simultanagnosia "misses the forest for the trees." Complex visual scenes cannot be grasped in their entirety, leading to severe limitations in the visual identification of objects and scenes. For example, a patient who is shown a table lamp and asked to name the object may look at its circular base and call it an ash tray. Some patients with simultanagnosia report that objects they look at may suddenly vanish, probably indicating an inability to look back at the original point of gaze after brief saccadic displacements. Movement and distracting stimuli greatly exacerbate the difficulties of visual perception. Simultanagnosia can sometimes occur without the other two components of Bálint's syndrome.

A modification of the letter cancellation task described above can be used for the bedside diagnosis of simultanagnosia. In this modification, some of the targets (e.g., As) are made to be much larger than the others [7.5–10 cm vs 2.5 cm (3–4 in. vs 1 in.) in height], and all targets are embedded among foils. Patients with simultanagnosia display a counterintuitive but characteristic tendency to miss the larger targets (Fig. 27-3*B*). This occurs because the information needed for the identification of the larger targets cannot be confined to the immediate line of gaze and requires the integration of visual information across a more extensive field of view. The greater difficulty in the detection of the larger targets also indicates that poor acuity is not responsible for the impairment of visual function and that the problem is central rather than peripheral. Bálint's syndrome results from bilateral dorsal parietal lesions; common settings include watershed infarction between the middle and posterior cerebral artery territories, hypoglycemia, sagittal sinus thrombosis, or atypical forms of Alzheimer's disease. In patients with Bálint's syndrome due to stroke, bilateral visual field defects (usually inferior quadrantanopias) are common.

Another manifestation of bilateral (or right-sided) dorsal parietal lobe lesions is *dressing apraxia.* The patient with this condition is unable to align the body axis with the axis of the garment and can be seen struggling as he or she holds a coat from its bottom or extends his or her arm into a fold of the garment rather than into its sleeve. Lesions that involve the posterior parietal cortex also lead to severe difficulties in copying simple line drawings. This is known as a *construction apraxia* and is much more severe if the lesion is in the right hemisphere. In some patients with right hemisphere lesions, the drawing difficulties are confined to the left side of the figure and represent a manifestation of hemispatial neglect; in others, there is a more universal deficit in reproducing contours and three-dimensional perspective. Dressing apraxia and construction apraxia represent special instances of a more general disturbance in spatial orientation.

THE OCCIPITOTEMPORAL NETWORK FOR FACE AND OBJECT RECOGNITION: PROSOPAGNOSIA AND OBJECT AGNOSIA

Perceptual information about faces and objects is initially encoded in primary (striate) visual cortex and adjacent (upstream) peristriate visual association areas. This information is subsequently relayed first to the downstream visual association areas of occipitotemporal cortex and then to other heteromodal and paralimbic areas of the cerebral cortex. Bilateral lesions in the fusiform and lingual gyri of the occipitotemporal cortex disrupt this process and interfere with the ability of otherwise intact perceptual information to activate the distributed multimodal associations that lead to the recognition of faces and objects. The resultant face and object recognition deficits are known as *prosopagnosia* and *visual object agnosia*.

The patient with prosopagnosia cannot recognize familiar faces, including, sometimes, the reflection of his or her own face in the mirror. This is not a perceptual deficit since prosopagnosic patients can easily tell if two faces are identical or not. Furthermore, a prosopagnosic patient who cannot recognize a familiar face by visual inspection alone can use auditory cues to reach appropriate recognition if allowed to listen to the person's voice. The deficit in prosopagnosia is therefore modality-specific and reflects the existence of a lesion that prevents the activation of otherwise intact multimodal templates by relevant visual input. Damasio has pointed out that the deficit in prosopagnosia is not limited to the recognition of faces but that it can also extend to the recognition of individual members of larger generic object groups. For example, prosopagnosic patients characteristically have no difficulty with the generic identification of a face as a face or of a car as a car, but they cannot recognize the identity of an individual face or the make of an individual car. This reflects a visual recognition deficit for proprietary features that characterize individual members of an object class. When recognition problems become more generalized and extend to the generic identification of common objects, the condition is known as visual object agnosia. In contrast to prosopagnosic patients, those with object agnosia cannot recognize a face as a face or a car as a car.

It is important to distinguish visual object agnosia from anomia. The patient with anomia cannot name the object but can describe its use. In contrast, the patient with visual agnosia is unable either to name a visually presented object or to describe its use. The characteristic lesions in prosopagnosia and visual object agnosia consist of bilateral infarctions in the territory of the posterior cerebral arteries. Associated deficits can include visual field defects (especially superior quadrantanopias) or a centrally based color blindness known as *achromatopsia*. Rarely, the responsible lesion is unilateral. In such cases, prosopagnosia is associated with lesions in the right hemisphere and object agnosia with lesions in the left.

THE LIMBIC NETWORK FOR MEMORY: AMNESIAS

Limbic and paralimbic areas (such as the hippocampus, amygdala, and entorhinal cortex), the anterior and medial nuclei of the thalamus, the medial and basal parts of the striatum, and the hypothalamus collectively constitute a distributed network known as the *limbic system*. The behavioral affiliations of this network include the coordination of emotion, motivation, autonomic tone, and endocrine function. An additional area of specialization for the limbic network, and the one which is of most relevance to clinical practice, is that of declarative (conscious) memory for recent episodes and experiences. A disturbance in this function is known as an *amnestic state*. In the absence of deficits in motivation, attention, language, or visuospatial function, the clinical diagnosis of a persistent global amnestic state is always associated with bilateral damage to the limbic network, usually within the hippocampo-entorhinal complex or the thalamus.

Although the limbic network is the site of damage for amnestic states, it is almost certainly not the storage site for memories. Memories are stored in widely distributed form throughout the cerebral cortex. The role attributed to the limbic network is to bind these distributed fragments into coherent events and experiences that can sustain conscious recall. Damage to the limbic network does not necessarily destroy memories but interferes with their conscious (declarative) recall in coherent form. The individual fragments of information remain preserved despite the limbic lesions and can sustain what is known as *implicit memory*. For example, patients with amnestic states can acquire new motor or perceptual skills, even though they may have no conscious knowledge of the experiences that led to the acquisition of these skills.

The memory disturbance in the amnestic state is multimodal and includes retrograde and anterograde components. The *retrograde amnesia* involves an inability to recall experiences that occurred before the onset of the amnestic state. Relatively recent events are more vulnerable to retrograde amnesia than more remote and more extensively consolidated events. A patient who comes to the emergency room complaining that he cannot remember his identity but who can remember the events of the previous day is almost certainly not suffering from a neurologic cause of memory disturbance. The second and most important component of the amnestic state is the *anterograde amnesia*, which indicates an inability to store, retain, and recall new knowledge. Patients with amnestic states cannot remember what they ate a few minutes ago or the details of an important event they may have experienced a few hours ago. In the acute stages, there may also be a tendency to fill in memory gaps with inaccurate, fabricated, and often implausible information. This is known as *confabulation*. Patients with the amnestic syndrome forget that they forget and tend to deny the existence of a memory problem when questioned.

The patient with an amnestic state is almost always disoriented, especially to time. Accurate temporal orientation and accurate knowledge of current news rule out a major amnestic state. The anterograde component of an amnestic state can be tested with a list of four to five words read aloud by the examiner up to five times or until the patient can immediately repeat the entire list without intervening delay. In the next phase of testing, the patient is allowed to concentrate on the words and to rehearse them internally for 1 min before being asked to recall them. Accurate performance in this phase indicates that the patient is motivated and sufficiently attentive to hold the words online for at least 1 min. The final phase of the testing involves a retention period of 5–10 min, during which the patient is engaged in other tasks. Adequate recall at the end of this interval requires offline storage, retention, and retrieval. Amnestic patients fail this phase of the task and may even forget that they were given a list of words to remember. Accurate recognition of the words by multiple choice in a patient who cannot recall them indicates a less severe memory disturbance that affects mostly the retrieval stage of memory. The retrograde component of an amnesia can be assessed with questions related to autobiographical or historic events. The anterograde component of amnestic states is usually much more prominent than the retrograde component. In rare instances, usually associated with temporal lobe epilepsy or benzodiazepine intake, the retrograde component may dominate.

The assessment of memory can be quite challenging. Bedside evaluations may only detect the most severe impairments. Less severe memory impairments, as in the case of patients with temporal lobe epilepsy, mild head injury, or early dementia, require quantitative evaluations by neuropsychologists. Confusional states caused by toxic-metabolic encephalopathies and some types of frontal lobe damage interfere with attentional capacity and lead to secondary memory impairments, even in the absence of any limbic lesions. This sort of memory impairment can be differentiated from the amnestic state by the presence of additional impairments in the attention-related tasks described below in the section on the frontal lobes.

Many neurologic diseases can give rise to an amnestic state. These include tumors (of the sphenoid wing, posterior corpus callosum, thalamus, or medial temporal lobe), infarctions (in the territories of the anterior or posterior cerebral arteries), head trauma, herpes simplex encephalitis, Wernicke-Korsakoff encephalopathy, paraneoplastic limbic encephalitis, and degenerative dementias such as Alzheimer's or Pick's disease. The one common denominator of all these diseases is that they lead to the bilateral lesions within one or more components in the limbic network, most commonly the hippocampus, entorhinal cortex, the mammillary bodies of the hypothalamus, and the limbic thalamus. Occasionally, unilateral left-sided lesions can give rise to an amnestic state, but the memory disorder tends to be transient. Depending on the nature and distribution of the underlying neurologic disease, the patient may also have visual field deficits, eye movement limitations, or cerebellar findings.

Transient global amnesia is a distinctive syndrome usually seen in late middle age. Patients become acutely disoriented and repeatedly ask who they are, where they are, what they are doing. The spell is characterized by anterograde amnesia (inability to retain new information) and a retrograde amnesia for relatively recent events that occurred before the onset. The syndrome usually resolves within 24–48 h and is followed by the filling-in of the period affected by the retrograde amnesia, although there is persistent loss of memory for the events that occurred during the ictus. Recurrences are noted in ~20% of patients. Migraine, temporal lobe seizures, and transient ischemic events in the posterior cerebral territory have been postulated as causes of transient global amnesia. The absence of associated neurologic findings may occasionally lead to the incorrect diagnosis of a psychiatric disorder.

THE PREFRONTAL NETWORK FOR ATTENTION AND BEHAVIOR

Approximately one-third of all the cerebral cortex in the human brain is located in the frontal lobes. The frontal lobes can be subdivided into motor-premotor, dorsolateral prefrontal, medial prefrontal, and orbitofrontal components. The terms *frontal lobe syndrome* and *prefrontal cortex* refer only to the last three of these four components. These are the parts of the cerebral cortex that show the greatest phylogenetic expansion in primates and especially in humans. The dorsolateral prefrontal, medial prefrontal, and orbitofrontal areas, and the subcortical structures with which they are interconnected (i.e., the head of the caudate and the dorsomedial nucleus of the thalamus), collectively make up a large-scale network that coordinates exceedingly complex aspects of human cognition and behavior.

The prefrontal network plays an important role in behaviors that require an integration of thought with emotion and motivation. There is no simple formula for summarizing the diverse functional affiliations of the prefrontal network. Its integrity appears important for the simultaneous awareness of context, options, consequences, relevance, and emotional impact so as to allow the formulation of adaptive inferences, decisions, and actions. Damage to this part of the brain impairs mental flexibility, reasoning, hypothesis formation, abstract thinking, foresight, judgment, the online (attentive) holding of information, and the ability to inhibit inappropriate responses. Behaviors impaired by prefrontal cortex lesions, especially those related to the manipulation of mental content, are often referred to as "executive functions."

Even very large bilateral prefrontal lesions may leave all sensory, motor, and basic cognitive functions intact while leading to isolated but dramatic alterations of personality and behavior. The most common clinical manifestations of damage to the prefrontal network take the form of two relatively distinct syndromes. In the *frontal abulic syndrome*, the patient shows a loss of initiative, creativity, and curiosity and displays a pervasive emotional blandness and apathy. In the *frontal disinhibition syndrome*, the patient becomes socially disinhibited and shows severe impairments of judgment, insight, and foresight. The dissociation between intact cognitive function and a total lack of even rudimentary common sense is striking. Despite the preservation of all essential memory functions, the patient cannot learn from experience and continues to display inappropriate behaviors without appearing to feel emotional pain, guilt, or regret when such behaviors repeatedly lead to disastrous consequences. The impairments may emerge only in real-life situations when behavior is under minimal external control and may not be apparent within the structured environment of the medical office. Testing judgment by asking patients what they would do if they detected a fire in a theater or found a stamped and addressed envelope on the road is not very informative since patients who answer these questions wisely in the office may still act very foolishly in the more complex real-life setting. The physician must therefore be prepared to make a diagnosis of frontal lobe disease on the basis of historic information alone even when the office examination of mental state may be quite intact.

The abulic syndrome tends to be associated with damage to the dorsolateral prefrontal cortex, and the disinhibition syndrome with the medial prefrontal or orbitofrontal cortex. These syndromes tend to arise almost exclusively after bilateral lesions, most frequently in the setting of head trauma, stroke, ruptured aneurysms, hydrocephalus, tumors (including metastases, glioblastoma, and falx or olfactory groove meningiomas), or focal degenerative diseases. Unilateral lesions confined to the prefrontal cortex may remain silent until the pathology spreads to the other side. The emergence of developmentally primitive reflexes, also known as frontal release signs, such as grasping (elicited by stroking the palm) and sucking (elicited by stroking the lips) are seen primarily in patients with large structural lesions that extend into the premotor components of the frontal lobes or in the context of metabolic encephalopathies. The vast majority of patients with prefrontal lesions and frontal lobe behavioral syndromes do not display these reflexes.

Damage to the frontal lobe disrupts a variety of attention-related functions including working memory (the transient online holding of information), concentration span, the scanning and retrieval of stored information, the inhibition of immediate but inappropriate responses, and mental flexibility. The capacity for focusing on a trend of thought and the ability to voluntarily shift the focus of attention from one thought or stimulus to another can become impaired. Digit span (which should be seven forward and five reverse) is decreased; the recitation of the months of the year in reverse order (which should take less than 15 s) is slowed; and the fluency in producing words starting with a, f, or s that can be generated in 1 min (normally ≥12 per letter) is diminished even in nonaphasic patients. Characteristically, there is a progressive slowing of performance as the task proceeds; e.g., the patient asked to count backwards by 3s may say "100, 97, 94, . . . 91, . . . 88," etc., and may not complete the task. In "go–no-go" tasks (where the instruction is to raise the finger upon hearing one tap but to keep it still upon hearing two taps), the patient shows a characteristic inability to keep still in response to the "no-go" stimulus; mental flexibility (tested by the ability to shift from one criterion to another in sorting or matching tasks) is impoverished; distractibility by irrelevant stimuli is increased; and there is a pronounced tendency for impersistence and perseveration.

These attentional deficits disrupt the orderly registration and retrieval of new information and lead to *secondary* memory deficits. Such memory deficits can be differentiated from the *primary* memory impairments of the amnestic state by showing that they improve when the attentional load of the task is decreased. Working memory (also known as immediate memory) is an attentional function based on the temporary online holding of information. It is closely associated with the integrity of the prefrontal network and the ascending reticular activating system. Retentive memory, on the other hand, depends on the stable (offline) storage of information and is associated with the integrity of the limbic network. The distinction of the underlying neural mechanisms is illustrated by the observation that severely amnestic patients who cannot remember events that occurred a few minutes ago may have intact if not superior working memory capacity as shown in tests of digit span.

Lesions in the caudate nucleus or in the dorsomedial nucleus of the thalamus (subcortical components of the prefrontal network) can also produce a frontal lobe syndrome. This is one reason why the mental state changes associated with degenerative basal ganglia diseases, such as Parkinson's or Huntington's disease, may take the form of a frontal lobe syndrome. Because of its widespread connections with other regions of association cortex, one essential computational role of the prefrontal network is to function as an integrator, or "orchestrator," for other networks. Bilateral multifocal lesions of the cerebral hemispheres, none of which are individually large enough to cause specific cognitive deficits such as aphasia or neglect, can collectively interfere with the connectivity and integrating function of the prefrontal cortex. A frontal lobe syndrome is the single most common behavioral profile associated with a variety of bilateral multifocal brain diseases including metabolic encephalopathy, multiple sclerosis, vitamin B_{12} deficiency, and others. In fact, the vast majority of patients with the clinical diagnosis of a frontal lobe syndrome tend to have lesions that do not involve prefrontal cortex but involve either the subcortical components of the prefrontal network or its connections with other parts of the brain. In order to avoid making a diagnosis of "frontal lobe syndrome" in a patient with no evidence of frontal cortex disease, it is advisable to use the diagnostic term *frontal network syndrome*, with the understanding that the responsible lesions can lie anywhere within this distributed network.

The patient with frontal lobe disease raises potential dilemmas in differential diagnosis: the abulia and blandness may be misinterpreted as depression, and the disinhibition as idiopathic mania or acting-out. Appropriate intervention may be delayed while a treatable tumor keeps expanding. An informed approach to frontal lobe disease and its behavioral manifestations may help to avoid such errors.

CARING FOR THE PATIENT WITH DEFICITS OF HIGHER CEREBRAL FUNCTION

Some of the deficits described in this chapter are so complex that they may bewilder not only the patient and family but also the physician. It is imperative to carry out a systematic clinical evaluation in order to characterize the nature of the deficits and explain them in lay terms to the patient and family. Such an explanation can allay at least some of the anxieties, address the mistaken impression that the deficit (e.g., social disinhibition or inability to recognize family members) is psychologically motivated, and lead to practical suggestions for daily living activities. The consultation of a skilled neuropsychologist may aid in the formulation of diagnosis and management. Patients with simultanagnosia, for example, may benefit from the counterintuitive instruction to stand back when they cannot find an item so that a greater search area falls within the immediate field of gaze. Some patients with frontal lobe disease can be extremely irritable and abusive to spouses and yet display all the appropriate social graces during the visit to the medical office. In such cases, the history may be more important than the bedside examination in charting a course of treatment.

Reactive depression is common in patients with higher cerebral dysfunction and should be treated. These patients may be sensitive to the usual doses of antidepressants or anxiolytics and deserve a careful titration of dosage. Brain damage may cause a dissociation between feeling states and their expression, so that a patient who may superficially appear jocular could still be suffering from an underlying depression that deserves to be treated. In many cases, agitation may be controlled with reassurance. In other cases, treatment with sedating antidepressants may become necessary. The use of neuroleptics for the control of agitation should be reserved for refractory cases since extrapyramidal side effects are frequent in patients with coexisting brain damage.

Spontaneous improvement of cognitive deficits due to acute neurologic lesions is common. It is most rapid in the first few weeks but may continue for up to 2 years, especially in young individuals with single brain lesions. The mechanisms for this recovery are incompletely understood. Some of the initial deficits appear to arise from remote dysfunction (diaschisis) in parts of the brain that are interconnected with the site of initial injury. Improvement in these patients may reflect, at least in part, a normalization of the remote dysfunction. Other mechanisms may involve functional reorganization in surviving neurons adjacent to the injury or the compensatory use of homologous structures, e.g., the right superior temporal gyrus with recovery from Wernicke's aphasia. In some patients with large lesions involving Broca's and Wernicke's areas, only Wernicke's area may show contralateral compensatory reorganization (or bilateral functionality), giving rise to a situation where a lesion that should have caused a global aphasia becomes associated with a residual Broca's aphasia. Prognosis for recovery from aphasia is best when Wernicke's area is spared. Cognitive rehabilitation procedures have been used in the treatment of higher cortical deficits. There are few controlled studies, but some do show a benefit of rehabilitation in the recovery from hemispatial neglect and aphasia. Some types of deficits may be more prone to recovery than others. For example, patients with nonfluent aphasias are more likely to benefit from speech therapy than patients with fluent aphasias and comprehension deficits. In general, lesions that lead to a denial of illness (e.g., anosognosia) are associated with cognitive deficits that are more resistant to rehabilitation. The recovery from higher cortical dysfunction is rarely complete. Periodic neuropsychological assessment is necessary for quantifying the pace of the improvement and for generating specific recommendations for cognitive rehabilitation, modifications in the home environment, and the timetable for returning to school or work.

In general medical practice, most patients with deficits in higher cognitive functions will be suffering from dementia. There is a mistaken belief that dementias are anatomically diffuse and that they cause global cognitive impairments. This is only true at the terminal stages. During most of the clinical course, dementias are exquisitely selective with respect to anatomy and cognitive pattern. Alzheimer's disease, for example, causes the greatest destruction in medial temporal areas belonging to the memory network and is clinically characterized by a correspondingly severe amnesia. There are other dementias where memory is intact. Frontal lobe dementia results from a selective degeneration of the frontal lobe and leads to a gradual dissolution of behavior and complex attention. Primary progressive aphasia is characterized by a gradual atrophy of the left perisylvian language network and leads to a progressive dissolution of language that can remain isolated for up to 10 years. An enlightened approach to the differential diagnosis and treatment of these patients requires an understanding of the principles that link neural networks to higher cerebral functions.

FURTHER READINGS

CATANI M, FFYCHTE H: The rises and falls of disconnection syndromes. Brain 128:2224, 2005

CRUTS M et al: Null mutations in progranulin cause ubiquitin-positive frontotemporal dementia linked to chromosome 17q21. Nature 442:916, 2006

GITELMAN DR et al: A large-scale distributed network for covert spatial attention. Further anatomical delineation based on stringent behavioral and cognitive controls. Brain 122:1093, 1999

HEISS W-D et al: Differential capacity of left and right hemispheric areas for compensation of poststroke aphasia. Ann Neurol 45:430, 1999

HILLIS AE: Aphasia: Progress in the last quarter of a century. Neurology 69:200, 2007

KNIBB JA et al: Clinical and pathological characterization of progressive aphasia. Ann Neurol 59:156, 2006

LEIGUARDA RC, MARSDEN CD: Limb apraxias: Higher-order disorders of sensorimotor integration. Brain 123:860, 2000

LI X et al: Prion protein codon 129 genotype is altered in primary progressive aphasia. Ann Neurol 58:858, 2005

MESULAM M-M: Behavioral neuroanatomy: Large-scale networks, association cortex, frontal syndromes, the limbic system and hemispheric specializations, in *Principles of Behavioral and Cognitive Neurology*, 2d ed, M-M Mesulam (ed). New York, Oxford University Press, 2000, pp 1–120

———: Current concepts: Primary progressive aphasia—a language-based dementia. New Engl J Med 348:1535, 2003

———: The human frontal lobes: Transcending the default mode through contingent encoding, in *Principles of Frontal Lobe Function*, DT Stuss, RT Knight (eds). New York, Oxford University Press, 2002, pp 8–30

SUMMERFIELD JJ et al: Orienting attention based on long-term memory experience. Neuron 49:905, 2006

28 Sleep Disorders

Charles A. Czeisler, John W. Winkelman, Gary S. Richardson

Disturbed sleep is among the most frequent health complaints physicians encounter. More than one-half of adults in the United States experience at least intermittent sleep disturbances. For most, it is an occasional night of poor sleep or daytime sleepiness. However, the Institute of Medicine estimates that 50–70 million Americans suffer from a chronic disorder of sleep and wakefulness, which can lead to serious impairment of daytime functioning. In addition, such problems may contribute to or exacerbate medical or psychiatric conditions. Thirty years ago, many such complaints were treated with hypnotic medications without further diagnostic evaluation. Since then, a distinct class of sleep and arousal disorders has been identified.

PHYSIOLOGY OF SLEEP AND WAKEFULNESS

Most adults sleep 7–8 h per night, although the timing, duration, and internal structure of sleep vary among healthy individuals and as a

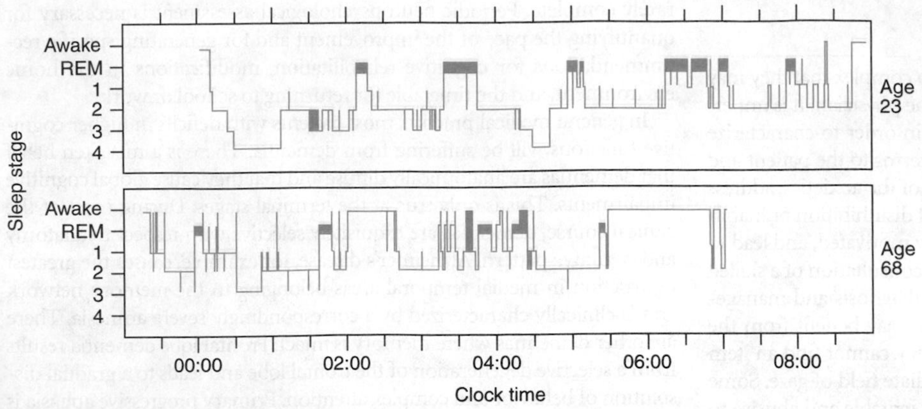

FIGURE 28-1 Stages of REM sleep (solid bars), the four stages of NREM sleep, and wakefulness over the course of the entire night for representative young and older adult men. Characteristic features of sleep in older people include reduction of slow-wave sleep, frequent spontaneous awakenings, early sleep onset, and early morning awakening. *(From the Division of Sleep Medicine, Brigham and Women's Hospital.)*

function of age. At the extremes, infants and the elderly have frequent interruptions of sleep. In the United States, adults of intermediate age tend to have one consolidated sleep episode per day, although in some cultures sleep may be divided into a mid-afternoon nap and a shortened night sleep. Two principal systems govern the sleep-wake cycle: one actively generates sleep and sleep-related processes and another times sleep within the 24-h day. Either intrinsic abnormalities in these systems or extrinsic disturbances (environmental, drug- or illness-related) can lead to sleep or circadian rhythm disorders.

STATES AND STAGES OF SLEEP

States and stages of human sleep are defined on the basis of characteristic patterns in the electroencephalogram (EEG), the electrooculogram (EOG—a measure of eye-movement activity), and the surface electromyogram (EMG) measured on the chin and neck. The continuous recording of this array of electrophysiologic parameters to define sleep and wakefulness is termed *polysomnography*.

Polysomnographic profiles define two states of sleep: (1) rapid-eye-movement (REM) sleep, and (2) non-rapid-eye-movement (NREM) sleep. NREM sleep is further subdivided into four stages, characterized by increasing arousal threshold and slowing of the cortical EEG. REM sleep is characterized by a low-amplitude, mixed-frequency EEG similar to that of NREM stage 1 sleep. The EOG shows bursts of REM similar to those seen during eyes-open wakefulness. Chin EMG activity is absent, reflecting the brainstem-mediated muscle atonia that is characteristic of that state.

ORGANIZATION OF HUMAN SLEEP

Normal nocturnal sleep in adults displays a consistent organization from night to night (Fig. 28-1). After sleep onset, sleep usually progresses through NREM stages 1–4 within 45–60 min. Slow-wave sleep (NREM stages 3 and 4) predominates in the first third of the night and comprises 15–25% of total nocturnal sleep time in young adults. The percentage of slow-wave sleep is influenced by several factors, most notably age (see below). Prior sleep deprivation increases the rapidity of sleep onset and both the intensity and amount of slow-wave sleep.

The first REM sleep episode usually occurs in the second hour of sleep. More rapid onset of REM sleep in a young adult (particularly if <30 min) may suggest pathology such as endogenous depression, narcolepsy, circadian rhythm disorders, or drug withdrawal. NREM and REM alternate through the night with an average period of 90–110 min (the "ultradian" sleep cycle). Overall, REM sleep constitutes 20–25% of total sleep, and NREM stages 1 and 2 are 50–60%.

Age has a profound impact on sleep state organization (Fig. 28-1). Slow-wave sleep is most intense and prominent during childhood, decreasing sharply at puberty and across the second and third decades of life. After age 30, there is a progressive decline in the amount of slow-wave sleep, and the amplitude of delta EEG activity comprising slow-wave sleep is profoundly reduced. The depth of slow-wave sleep, as measured by the arousal threshold to auditory stimulation, also decreases with age. In the otherwise healthy older person, slow-wave sleep may be completely absent, particularly in males.

A different age profile exists for REM sleep than for slow-wave sleep. In infancy, REM sleep may comprise 50% of total sleep time, and the percentage is inversely proportional to developmental age. The amount of REM sleep falls off sharply over the first postnatal year as a mature REM-NREM cycle develops; thereafter, REM sleep occupies a relatively constant percentage of total sleep time.

NEUROANATOMY OF SLEEP

Experimental studies in animals have variously implicated the medullary reticular formation, the thalamus, and the basal forebrain in the generation of sleep, while the brainstem reticular formation, the midbrain, the subthalamus, the thalamus, and the basal forebrain have all been suggested to play a role in the generation of wakefulness or EEG arousal.

Current models suggest that the capacity for sleep and wakefulness generation is distributed along an axial "core" of neurons extending from the brainstem rostrally to the basal forebrain. A cluster of γ-aminobutyric acid (GABA) and galaninergic neurons in the ventrolateral preoptic (VLPO) hypothalamus is selectively activated coincident with sleep onset. These neurons project to and inhibit multiple distinct wakefulness centers including the tuberomammilary (histaminergic) nucleus that are important to the ascending arousal system, indicating that the hypothalamic VLPO neurons play a key executive role in sleep regulation.

Specific regions in the pons are associated with the neurophysiologic correlates of REM sleep. Small lesions in the dorsal pons result in the loss of the descending muscle inhibition normally associated with REM sleep; microinjections of the cholinergic agonist carbachol into the pontine reticular formation appear to produce a state with all of the features of REM sleep. These experimental manipulations are mimicked by pathologic conditions in humans and animals. In narcolepsy, for example, abrupt, complete, or partial paralysis (cataplexy) occurs in response to a variety of stimuli. In dogs with this condition, physostigmine, a central cholinesterase inhibitor, increases the frequency of cataplectic attacks, while atropine decreases their frequency. Conversely, in REM sleep behavior disorder (see below), patients suffer from incomplete motor inhibition during REM sleep, resulting in involuntary, occasionally violent movement during REM sleep.

NEUROCHEMISTRY OF SLEEP

Early experimental studies that focused on the raphe nuclei of the brainstem appeared to implicate serotonin as the primary sleep-promoting neurotransmitter, while catecholamines were considered to be responsible for wakefulness. Simple neurochemical models have given way to more complex formulations involving multiple parallel waking systems. Pharmacologic studies suggest that histamine, acetylcholine, dopamine, serotonin, and noradrenaline are all involved in wake promotion. In addition, pontine cholinergic neurotransmission is known to play a role in REM sleep generation. The alerting influence of caffeine implicates adenosine, whereas the hypnotic effect of benzodiazepines and barbiturates suggests a role for endogenous ligands of the $GABA_A$ receptor complex. A newly characterized neuropeptide, hypocretin (orexin), has recently been implicated in the pathophysiology of narcolepsy (see below), but its role in normal sleep regulation remains to be defined.

A variety of sleep-promoting substances have been identified, although it is not known whether they are involved in the endogenous sleep-wake regulatory process. These include prostaglandin D_2, delta

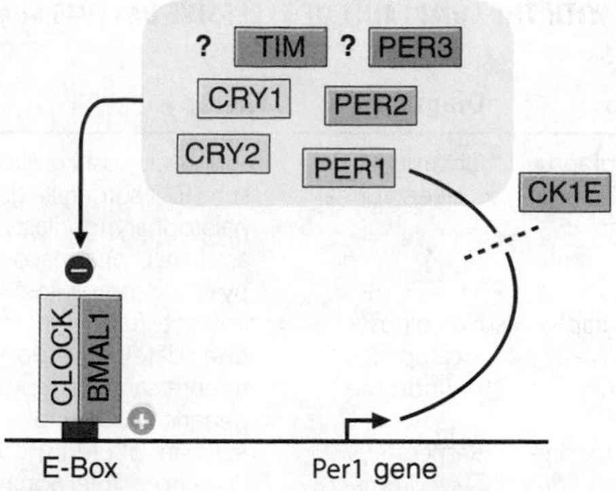

FIGURE 28-2 Model of the molecular feedback loop at the core of the mammalian circadian clock. The positive element of the feedback loop (+) is the transcriptional activation of the *Per1* gene (and probably other clock genes) by a heterodimer of the transcription factors CLOCK and BMAL1 (also called MOP3) bound to an E-box DNA regulatory element. The *Per1* transcript and its product, the clock component PER1 protein, accumulate in the cell cytoplasm. As it accumulates, the PER1 protein is recruited into a multiprotein complex thought to contain other circadian clock component proteins such as cryptochromes (CRYs), Period proteins (PERs), and others. This complex is then transported into the cell nucleus (across the dotted line), where it functions as the negative element in the feedback loop (–) by inhibiting the activity of the CLOCK-BMAL1 transcription factor heterodimer. As a consequence of this action, the concentration of PER1 and other clock proteins in the inhibitory complex falls, allowing CLOCK-BMAL1 to activate transcription of *Per1* and other genes and begin another cycle. The dynamics of the 24-h molecular cycle are controlled at several levels, including regulation of the rate of PER protein degradation by casein kinase-1 epsilon (CK1E). Additional limbs of this genetic regulatory network, omitted for the sake of clarity, are thought to contribute stability. Question marks denote putative clock proteins, such as Timeless (TIM), as yet lacking genetic proof of a role in the mammalian clock mechanism. *(Copyright Charles J. Weitz, Ph.D., Department of Neurobiology, Harvard Medical School.)*

sleep–inducing peptide, muramyl dipeptide, interleukin 1, fatty acid primary amides, and melatonin. The hypnotic effect of these substances is commonly limited to NREM or slow-wave sleep, although peptides that increase REM sleep have also been reported. Many putative "sleep factors," including interleukin 1 and prostaglandin D_2, are immunologically active as well, suggesting a link between immune function and sleep-wake states.

PHYSIOLOGY OF CIRCADIAN RHYTHMICITY

The sleep-wake cycle is the most evident of the many 24-h rhythms in humans. Prominent daily variations also occur in endocrine, thermoregulatory, cardiac, pulmonary, renal, gastrointestinal, and neurobehavioral functions. At the molecular level, endogenous circadian rhythmicity is driven by self-sustaining transcriptional/translational feedback loops (Fig. 28-2). In evaluating a daily variation in humans, it is important to distinguish between those rhythmic components passively evoked by periodic environmental or behavioral changes (e.g., the increase in blood pressure and heart rate upon assumption of the upright posture) and those actively driven by an endogenous oscillatory process (e.g., the circadian variation in plasma cortisol that persists under a variety of environmental and behavioral conditions).

While it is now recognized that many peripheral tissues in mammals have circadian clocks that regulate diverse physiologic processes, these independent tissue-specific oscillations are coordinated by a central neural pacemaker located in the suprachiasmatic nuclei (SCN) of the hypothalamus. Bilateral destruction of these nuclei results in a loss of the endogenous circadian rhythm of locomotor activity, which can be restored only by transplantation of the same structure from a donor animal. The genetically determined period of this endogenous neural oscillator, which averages ~24.2 h in humans, is normally synchronized to the 24-h period of the environmental light-dark cycle. Small differences in circadian period underlie variations in diurnal preference, with the circadian period shorter in individuals who typically rise early compared to those who typically go to bed late. Entrainment of mammalian circadian rhythms by the light-dark cycle is mediated via the retinohypothalamic tract, a monosynaptic pathway that links specialized, photoreceptive retinal ganglion cells directly to the SCN. Humans are exquisitely sensitive to the resetting effects of light, particularly at the blue end (~460–480 nm) of the visible spectrum.

The timing and internal architecture of sleep are directly coupled to the output of the endogenous circadian pacemaker. Paradoxically, the endogenous circadian rhythms of sleep tendency, sleepiness, and REM sleep propensity all peak near the habitual wake time, just after the nadir of the endogenous circadian temperature cycle, whereas the circadian wake propensity rhythm peaks 1–3 h before the habitual bedtime. These rhythms are thus timed to oppose the homeostatic decline of sleep tendency during the habitual sleep episode and the rise of sleep tendency throughout the usual waking day, respectively. Misalignment of the output of the endogenous circadian pacemaker with the desired sleep-wake cycle can, therefore, induce insomnia, decreased alertness, and impaired performance evident in night-shift workers and airline travelers.

BEHAVIORAL CORRELATES OF SLEEP STATES AND STAGES

Polysomnographic staging of sleep correlates with behavioral changes during specific states and stages. During the transitional state between wakefulness and sleep (stage 1 sleep), subjects may respond to faint auditory or visual signals without "awakening." Memory incorporation is inhibited at the onset of NREM stage 1 sleep, which may explain why individuals aroused from that transitional sleep stage frequently deny having been asleep. Such transitions may intrude upon behavioral wakefulness after sleep deprivation, notwithstanding attempts to remain continuously awake (see "Shift-Work Disorder," below).

Awakenings from REM sleep are associated with recall of vivid dream imagery >80% of the time. The reliability of dream recall increases with REM sleep episodes occurring later in the night. Imagery may also be reported after NREM sleep interruptions, though these typically lack the detail and vividness of REM sleep dreams. The incidence of NREM sleep dream recall can be increased by selective REM sleep deprivation, suggesting that REM sleep and dreaming per se are not inexorably linked.

PHYSIOLOGIC CORRELATES OF SLEEP STATES AND STAGES

All major physiologic systems are influenced by sleep. Changes in cardiovascular function include a decrease in blood pressure and heart rate during NREM and particularly during slow-wave sleep. During REM sleep, phasic activity (bursts of eye movements) is associated with variability in both blood pressure and heart rate mediated principally by the vagus. Cardiac dysrhythmias may occur selectively during REM sleep. Respiratory function also changes. In comparison to relaxed wakefulness, respiratory rate becomes more regular during NREM sleep (especially slow-wave sleep) and tonic REM sleep and becomes very irregular during phasic REM sleep. Minute ventilation decreases in NREM sleep out of proportion to the decrease in metabolic rate at sleep onset, resulting in a higher P_{CO_2}.

Endocrine function also varies with sleep. Slow-wave sleep is associated with secretion of growth hormone, while sleep in general is associated with augmented secretion of prolactin. Sleep has a complex effect on the secretion of luteinizing hormone (LH): during puberty, sleep is associated with increased LH secretion, whereas sleep in the postpubertal female inhibits LH secretion in the early follicular phase of the menstrual cycle. Sleep onset (and probably slow-wave sleep) is associated with inhibition of thyroid-stimulating hormone and of the adrenocorticotropic hormone–cortisol axis, an effect that is superimposed on the prominent circadian rhythms in the two systems.

The pineal hormone melatonin is secreted predominantly at night in both day- and night-active species, reflecting the direct modulation of pineal activity by the circadian pacemaker through a circuitous neural pathway from the SCN to the pineal gland. Melatonin secretion is not dependent upon the occurrence of sleep, persisting in individuals kept awake at night. In addition, exogenous melatonin increases sleepiness and increases sleep duration when administered to healthy adults attempting to sleep during daylight hours, at a time when endogenous melatonin levels are low. The efficacy of melatonin as a sleep-promoting therapy for patients with insomnia is currently not known.

Sleep is also accompanied by alterations of thermoregulatory function. NREM sleep is associated with an attenuation of thermoregulatory responses to either heat or cold stress, and animal studies of thermosensitive neurons in the hypothalamus document an NREM-sleep-dependent reduction of the thermoregulatory set-point. REM sleep is associated with complete absence of thermoregulatory responsiveness, effectively resulting in functional poikilothermy. However, the potential adverse impact of this failure of thermoregulation is blunted by inhibition of REM sleep by extreme ambient temperatures.

TABLE 28-1 EVALUATION OF THE PATIENT WITH THE COMPLAINT OF EXCESSIVE DAYTIME SOMNOLENCE

Findings on History and Physical Examination	Diagnostic Evaluation	Diagnosis	Therapy
Obesity, snoring, hypertension	Polysomnography with respiratory monitoring	Obstructive sleep apnea	Continuous positive airway pressure; ENT surgery (e.g., uvulopalatopharyngoplasty); dental appliance; pharmacologic therapy (e.g., protriptyline); weight loss
Cataplexy, hypnogogic hallucinations, sleep paralysis, family history	Polysomnography with multiple sleep latency testing	Narcolepsy-cataplexy syndrome	Stimulants (e.g., modafinil, methylphenidate); REM-suppressant antidepressants (e.g., protriptyline); genetic counseling
Restless legs, disturbed sleep, predisposing medical condition (e.g., iron deficiency or renal failure)	Assesment for predisposing medical conditions	Restless legs syndrome	Treatment of predisposing condition, if possible; dopamine agonists (e.g., pramipexole, ropinirole)
Disturbed sleep, predisposing medical conditions (e.g., asthma) and/or predisposing medical therapies (e.g., theophylline)	Sleep-wake diary recording	Insomnias (see text)	Treatment of predisposing condition and/or change in therapy, if possible; behavioral therapy; short-acting benzodiazepine receptor agonist (e.g., zolpidem)

Note: ENT, ears, nose, throat; REM, rapid eye movement; EMG, electromyogram.

DISORDERS OF SLEEP AND WAKEFULNESS

APPROACH TO THE PATIENT: Sleep Disorders

Patients may seek help from a physician because of one of several symptoms: (1) an acute or chronic inability to initiate or maintain sleep adequately at night (insomnia); (2) chronic fatigue, sleepiness, or tiredness during the day; or (3) a behavioral manifestation associated with sleep itself. Complaints of insomnia or excessive daytime sleepiness should be approached as symptoms (much like fever or pain) of underlying disorders. Knowledge of the differential diagnosis of these presenting complaints is essential to identify any underlying medical disorder. Only then can appropriate treatment, rather than nonspecific approaches (e.g., over-the-counter sleeping aids), be applied. Diagnoses of exclusion, such as primary insomnia, should be made only after other diagnoses have been ruled out. Table 28-1 outlines the diagnostic and therapeutic approach to the patient with a complaint of excessive daytime sleepiness.

A careful history is essential. In particular, the duration, severity, and consistency of the symptoms are important, along with the patient's estimate of the consequences of the sleep disorder on waking function. Information from a friend or family member can be invaluable; some patients may be unaware of, or will underreport, such potentially embarrassing symptoms as heavy snoring or falling asleep while driving. Patients with excessive sleepiness should be advised to avoid all driving until effective therapy has been achieved.

Completion by the patient of a day-by-day sleep-work-drug log for at least 2 weeks can help the physician better understand the nature of the complaint. Work times and sleep times (including daytime naps and nocturnal awakenings) as well as drug and alcohol use, including caffeine and hypnotics, should be noted each day.

Polysomnography is necessary for the diagnosis of specific disorders such as narcolepsy and sleep apnea and may be of utility in other settings as well. In addition to the three electrophysiologic variables used to define sleep states and stages, the standard clinical polysomnogram includes measures of respiration (respiratory effort, air flow, and oxygen saturation), anterior tibialis EMG, and electrocardiogram.

EVALUATION OF INSOMNIA

Insomnia is the complaint of inadequate sleep; it can be classified according to the nature of sleep disruption and the duration of the complaint. Insomnia is subdivided into difficulty falling asleep (*sleep onset insomnia*), frequent or sustained awakenings (*sleep maintenance insomnia*), early morning awakenings (*sleep offset insomnia*), or persistent sleepiness/fatigue despite sleep of adequate duration (*nonrestorative sleep*). Similarly, the duration of the symptom influences diagnostic and therapeutic considerations. An insomnia complaint lasting one to several nights (within a single episode) is termed *transient insomnia* and is typically the result of situational stress or a change in sleep schedule or environment (e.g., jet lag disorder). *Short-term insomnia* lasts from a few days to 3 weeks. Disruption of this duration is usually associated with more protracted stress, such as recovery from surgery or short-term illness. *Long-term insomnia*, or *chronic insomnia*, lasts for months or years and, in contrast with short-term insomnia, requires a thorough evaluation of underlying causes (see below). Chronic insomnia is often a waxing and waning disorder, with spontaneous or stressor-induced exacerbations.

An occasional night of poor sleep, typically in the setting of stress or excitement about external events, is both common and without lasting consequences. However, persistent insomnia can lead to impaired daytime function, injury due to accidents, and the development of major depression. In addition, there is emerging evidence that individuals with chronic insomnia have increased utilization of health care resources, even after controlling for co-morbid medical and psychiatric disorders.

All insomnias can be exacerbated and perpetuated by behaviors that are not conducive to initiating or maintaining sleep. *Inadequate sleep hygiene* is characterized by a behavior pattern prior to sleep or a bedroom environment that is not conducive to sleep. Noise or light in the bedroom can interfere with sleep, as can a bed partner with periodic limb movements during sleep or one who snores loudly. Clocks can heighten the anxiety about the time it has taken to fall asleep. Drugs that act on the central nervous system, large meals, vigorous exercise, or hot showers just before sleep may all interfere with sleep onset. Many individuals participate in stressful work-related activities in the evening, producing a state incompatible with sleep onset. In preference to hypnotic medications, patients should be counseled to avoid stressful activities before bed, develop a soporific bedtime ritual, and to prepare and reserve the bedroom environment for sleeping. Consistent, regular rising times should be maintained daily, including weekends.

PRIMARY INSOMNIA

Many patients with chronic insomnia have no clear, single identifiable underlying cause for their difficulties with sleep. Rather, such patients often have multiple etiologies for their insomnia, which may evolve over the years. In addition, the chief sleep complaint may change over time, with initial insomnia predominating at one point, and multiple awakenings or nonrestorative sleep occurring at other times. Subsyndromal psychiatric disorders (e.g., anxiety and mood complaints), negative conditioning to the sleep environment (psychophysiologic insomnia, see below), amplification of the time spent awake (paradoxical insomnia), physiologic hyperarousal, and poor sleep hygiene (see above) may all be present. As these processes may be both causes and consequences of chronic insomnia, many individuals will have a progressive course to their symptoms in which the severity is proportional to the chronicity, and much of the complaint may persist even after effective treatment of the initial inciting etiology. Treatment of insomnia is often directed to each of the putative contributing factors: behavior therapies for anxiety and negative conditioning (see below), pharmacotherapy and/or psychotherapy for mood/anxiety disorders, and an emphasis on maintenance of good sleep hygiene.

If insomnia persists after treatment of these contributing factors, empirical pharmacotherapy is often used on a nightly or intermittent basis. A variety of sedative compounds are used for this purpose. Alcohol and antihistamines are the most commonly used nonprescription sleep aids. The former may help with sleep onset but is associated with sleep disruption during the night and can escalate into abuse, dependence, and withdrawal in the predisposed individual. Antihistamines may be of benefit when used intermittently but often produce rapid tolerance and may have multiple side effects (especially anticholinergic), which limit their use, particularly in the elderly. Benzodiazepine-receptor agonists are the most effective and well-tolerated class of medications for insomnia. The broad range of half-lives allows flexibility in the duration of sedative action. The most commonly prescribed agents in this family are zaleplon (5–20 mg), with a half-life of 1–2 h; zolpidem (5–10 mg) and triazolam (0.125–0.25 mg), with half-lives of 2–3 h; eszopiclone (1–3 mg), with a half-life of 5.5–8 h; and temazepam (15–30 mg) and lorazepam (0.5–2 mg), with half-lives of 6–12 h. Generally, side effects are minimal when the dose is kept low and the serum concentration is minimized during the waking hours (by using the shortest-acting, effective agent). Recent data suggest that at least one benzodiazepine receptor agonist (eszopiclone) continues to be effective for 6 months of nightly use. However, longer durations of use have not been evaluated, and it is unclear whether this is true of other agents in this class. Moreover, with even brief continuous use of benzodiazepine-receptor agonists, rebound insomnia can occur upon discontinuation. The likelihood of rebound insomnia and tolerance can be minimized by short durations of treatment, intermittent use, or gradual tapering of the dose. For acute insomnia, nightly use of a benzodiazepine receptor agonist for a maximum of 2–4 weeks is advisable. For chronic insomnia, intermittent use is recommended, unless the consequences of untreated insomnia outweigh concerns regarding chronic use. Benzodiazepine receptor agonists should be avoided, or used very judiciously, in patients with a history of substance or alcohol abuse. The heterocyclic antidepressants (trazodone, amitriptyline, and doxepin) are the most commonly prescribed alternatives to benzodiazepine receptor agonists due to their lack of abuse potential and lower cost. Trazodone (25–100 mg) is used more commonly than the tricyclic antidepressants as it has a much shorter half-life (5–9 h), has much less anticholinergic activity (sparing patients, particularly the elderly, constipation, urinary retention, and tachycardia), is associated with less weight gain, and is much safer in overdose. The risk of priapism is small (~1 in 10,000).

Psychophysiologic Insomnia Persistent *psychophysiologic insomnia* is a behavioral disorder in which patients are preoccupied with a perceived inability to sleep adequately at night. This sleep disorder begins like any other acute insomnia; however, the poor sleep habits and sleep-related anxiety ("insomnia phobia") persist long after the initial incident. Such patients become hyperaroused by their own efforts to sleep or by the sleep environment, and the insomnia becomes a conditioned or learned response. Patients may be able to fall asleep more easily at unscheduled times (when not trying) or outside the home environment. Polysomnographic recording in patients with psychophysiologic insomnia reveals an objective sleep disturbance, often with an abnormally long sleep latency; frequent nocturnal awakenings; and an increased amount of stage 1 transitional sleep. Rigorous attention should be paid to improving sleep hygiene, correction of counterproductive, arousing behaviors before bedtime, and minimizing exaggerated beliefs regarding the negative consequences of insomnia. Behavioral therapies are the treatment modality of choice, with intermittent use of medications. When patients are awake for >20 min, they should read or perform other relaxing activities to distract themselves from insomnia-related anxiety. In addition, bedtime and wake time should be scheduled to restrict time in bed to be equal to their perceived total sleep time. This will generally produce sleep deprivation, greater sleep drive, and, eventually, better sleep. Time in bed can then be gradually expanded. In addition, methods directed towards producing relaxation in the sleep setting (e.g., meditation, muscle relaxation) are encouraged.

Adjustment Insomnia (Acute Insomnia) This typically develops after a change in the sleeping environment (e.g., in an unfamiliar hotel or hospital bed) or before or after a significant life event, such as a change of occupation, loss of a loved one, illness, or anxiety over a deadline or examination. Increased sleep latency, frequent awakenings from sleep, and early morning awakening can all occur. Recovery is generally rapid, usually within a few weeks. Treatment is symptomatic, with intermittent use of hypnotics and resolution of the underlying stress. *Altitude insomnia* describes a sleep disturbance that is a common consequence of exposure to high altitude. Periodic breathing of the Cheyne-Stokes type occurs during NREM sleep about half the time at high altitude, with restoration of a regular breathing pattern during REM sleep. Both hypoxia and hypocapnia are thought to be involved in the development of periodic breathing. Frequent awakenings and poor quality sleep characterize altitude insomnia, which is generally worse on the first few nights at high altitude but may persist. Treatment with acetazolamide can decrease time spent in periodic breathing and substantially reduce hypoxia during sleep.

COMORBID INSOMNIA

Insomnia Associated with Mental Disorders Approximately 80% of patients with psychiatric disorders describe sleep complaints. There is considerable heterogeneity, however, in the nature of the sleep disturbance both between conditions and among patients with the same condition. *Depression* can be associated with sleep onset insomnia, sleep maintenance insomnia, or early morning wakefulness. However, hypersomnia occurs in some depressed patients, especially adolescents and those with either bipolar or seasonal (fall/winter) depression (Chap. 386). Indeed, sleep disturbance is an important vegetative sign of depression and may commence before any mood changes are perceived by the patient. Consistent polysomnographic findings in depression include decreased REM sleep latency, lengthened first REM sleep episode, and shortened first NREM sleep episode; however, these findings are not specific for depression, and the extent of these changes varies with age and symptomatology. Depressed patients also show decreased slow-wave sleep and reduced sleep continuity.

In *mania* and *hypomania*, sleep latency is increased and total sleep time can be reduced. Patients with *anxiety disorders* tend not to show the changes in REM sleep and slow-wave sleep seen in endogenously depressed patients. *Chronic alcoholics* lack slow-wave sleep, have decreased amounts of REM sleep (as an acute response to alcohol), and have frequent arousals throughout the night. This is associated with impaired daytime alertness. The sleep of chronic alcoholics may remain disturbed for years after discontinuance of alcohol usage. Sleep architecture and physiology are disturbed in *schizophrenia* (with a decreased amount of stage 4 sleep and a lack of augmentation of REM sleep following REM sleep deprivation); chronic schizophrenics often show day-night reversal, sleep fragmentation, and insomnia.

Insomnia Associated with Neurologic Disorders A variety of neurologic diseases result in sleep disruption through both indirect, nonspecific mechanisms (e.g., pain in cervical spondylosis or low back pain) or by impairment of central neural structures involved in the generation and control of sleep itself. For example, *dementia* from any cause has long been associated with disturbances in the timing of the sleep-wake cycle, often characterized by nocturnal wandering and an exacerbation of symptomatology at night (so-called sundowning).

Epilepsy may rarely present as a sleep complaint (Chap. 363). Often the history is of abnormal behavior, at times with convulsive movements during sleep. The differential diagnosis includes REM sleep behavior disorder, sleep apnea syndrome, and periodic movements of sleep (see above). Diagnosis requires nocturnal polysomnography with a full EEG montage. Other neurologic diseases associated with abnormal movements, such as *Parkinson's disease, hemiballismus, Huntington's chorea*, and *Tourette syndrome* (Chap. 366), are also associated with disrupted sleep, presumably through secondary mechanisms. However, the abnormal movements themselves are greatly reduced during sleep. Headache syndromes (*migraine* or *cluster headache*) may show sleep-associated exacerbations (Chap. 15) by unknown mechanisms.

Fatal familial insomnia is a rare hereditary disorder caused by degeneration of anterior and dorsomedial nuclei of the thalamus. Insomnia is a prominent early symptom. Patients develop progressive autonomic dysfunction, followed by dysarthria, myoclonus, coma, and death. The pathogenesis is a mutation in the prion gene (Chap. 378).

Insomnia Associated with Other Medical Disorders A number of medical conditions are associated with disruptions of sleep. The association is frequently nonspecific, e.g., sleep disruption due to chronic pain from rheumatologic disorders. Attention to this association is important in that sleep-associated symptoms are often the presenting or most bothersome complaint. Treatment of the underlying medical problem is the most useful approach. Sleep disruption can also result from the use of medications such as glucocorticoids (see below).

One prominent association is between sleep disruption and *asthma*. In many asthmatics there is a prominent daily variation in airway resistance that results in marked increases in asthmatic symptoms at night, especially during sleep. In addition, treatment of asthma with theophylline-based compounds, adrenergic agonists, or glucocorticoids can independently disrupt sleep. When sleep disruption is a side effect of asthma treatment, inhaled glucocorticoids (e.g., beclomethasone) that do not disrupt sleep may provide a useful alternative.

Cardiac ischemia may also be associated with sleep disruption. The ischemia itself may result from increases in sympathetic tone as a result of sleep apnea. Patients may present with complaints of nightmares or vivid, disturbing dreams, with or without awareness of the more classic symptoms of angina or of the sleep disordered breathing. Treatment of the sleep apnea may substantially improve the angina and the nocturnal sleep quality. *Paroxysmal nocturnal dyspnea* can also occur as a consequence of sleep-associated cardiac ischemia that causes pulmonary congestion exacerbated by the recumbent posture.

Chronic obstructive pulmonary disease is also associated with sleep disruption, as is *cystic fibrosis, menopause, hyperthyroidism, gastroesophageal reflux, chronic renal failure*, and *liver failure*.

Medication-, Drug-, or Alcohol-Dependent Insomnia Disturbed sleep can result from ingestion of a wide variety of agents. Caffeine is perhaps the most common pharmacologic cause of insomnia. It produces increased latency to sleep onset, more frequent arousals during sleep, and a reduction in total sleep time for up to 8–14 h after ingestion. Even small amounts of coffee can significantly disturb sleep in some patients; therefore, a 1- to 2-month trial without caffeine should be attempted in patients with these symptoms. Similarly, alcohol and nicotine can interfere with sleep, despite the fact that many patients use them to relax and promote sleep. Although alcohol can increase drowsiness and shorten sleep latency, even moderate amounts of alcohol increase awakenings in the second half of the night. In addition, alcohol ingestion prior to sleep is contraindicated in patients with sleep apnea because of the inhibitory effects of alcohol on upper airway muscle tone. Acutely, amphetamines and cocaine suppress both REM sleep and total sleep time, which return to normal with chronic use. Withdrawal leads to a REM sleep rebound. A number of prescribed medications can produce insomnia. Antidepressants, sympathomimetics, and glucocorticoids are common causes. In addition, severe rebound insomnia can result from the acute withdrawal of hypnotics, especially following the use of high doses of benzodiazepines with a short half-life. For this reason, hypnotic doses should be low to moderate and prolonged drug tapering is encouraged.

RESTLESS LEGS SYNDROME (RLS)

Patients with this sensory-motor disorder report an irresistible urge to move the legs, or sometimes the upper extremities, that is often associated with a creepy-crawling or aching dysesthesias deep within the affected limbs. For most patients with RLS, the dysesthesias and restlessness are much worse in the evening or night compared to the daytime and frequently interfere with the ability to fall asleep. The symptoms appear with inactivity and are temporarily relieved by movement. In contrast, paresthesias secondary to peripheral neuropathy persist with activity. The severity of this chronic disorder may wax and wane over time and can be exacerbated by sleep deprivation, caffeine, alcohol, serotonergic antidepressants, and pregnancy. The prevalence is 1–5% of young to middle-age adults and 10–20% of those >60 years. There appear to be important differences in RLS prevalence among racial groups, with higher prevalence in those of Northern European ancestry. Roughly one-third of patients (particularly those with an early age of onset) will have multiple affected family members. At least three separate chromosomal loci have been identified in familial RLS, though no gene has been identified to date. Iron deficiency and renal failure may cause RLS, which is then considered secondary RLS. The symptoms of RLS are exquisitely sensitive to dopaminergic drugs (e.g., pramipexole 0.25–0.5 mg q8PM or ropinirole 0.5–4.0 mg q8PM), which are the treatments of choice. Opiods, benzodiazepines, and gabapentin may also be of therapeutic value. Most patients with restless legs also experience periodic limb movements of sleep, although the reverse is not the case.

PERIODIC LIMB MOVEMENT DISORDER (PLMD)

Periodic limb movements of sleep (PLMS), previously known as *nocturnal myoclonus*, consists of stereotyped, 0.5- to 5.0-s extensions of the great toe and dorsiflexion of the foot, which recur every 20–40 s during NREM sleep, in episodes lasting from minutes to hours, as documented by bilateral surface EMG recordings of the anterior tibialis on polysomnography. PLMS is the principal objective polysomnographic finding in 17% of patients with insomnia and 11% of those with excessive daytime somnolence (Fig. 28-3). It is often unclear whether it is an incidental finding or the cause of disturbed sleep. When deemed to be the latter, PLMS is called PLMD. PLMS occurs in a wide variety of sleep disorders (including narcolepsy, sleep apnea, REM sleep behavior disorder, and various forms of insomnia) and may be associated with frequent arousals and an increased number of sleep-stage transitions. The pathophysiology is not well understood, though individuals with high spinal transections can exhibit periodic leg movements during sleep, suggesting the existence of a spinal generator. Treatment options include dopaminergic medications or benzodiazepines.

EVALUATION OF DAYTIME SLEEPINESS

Daytime impairment due to sleep loss may be difficult to quantify for several reasons. First, sleepiness is not necessarily proportional to subjectively assessed sleep deprivation. In obstructive sleep apnea, for example, the repeated brief interruptions of sleep associated with resumption of respiration at the end of apneic episodes result in daytime sleepiness, despite the fact that the patient may be unaware of the sleep fragmentation. Second, subjective descriptions of waking impairment vary from patient to patient. Patients may describe themselves as "sleepy," "fatigued," or "tired" and may have a clear sense of the meaning of those terms, while others may use the same terms to describe a completely different condition. Third, sleepiness, particularly when profound, may affect judgment in a manner analogous to ethanol, such that subjective awareness of the condition and the consequent cognitive and motor impairment is reduced. Finally, patients may be reluctant to admit that sleepiness is a problem, both because they are generally unaware of what constitutes normal alertness and because sleepiness is generally viewed pejoratively, ascribed more often to a deficit in motivation than to an inadequately addressed physiologic sleep need.

Specific questioning about the occurrence of sleep episodes during normal waking hours, both intentional and unintentional, is necessary to determine the extent of the adverse effects of sleepiness on a patient's day-

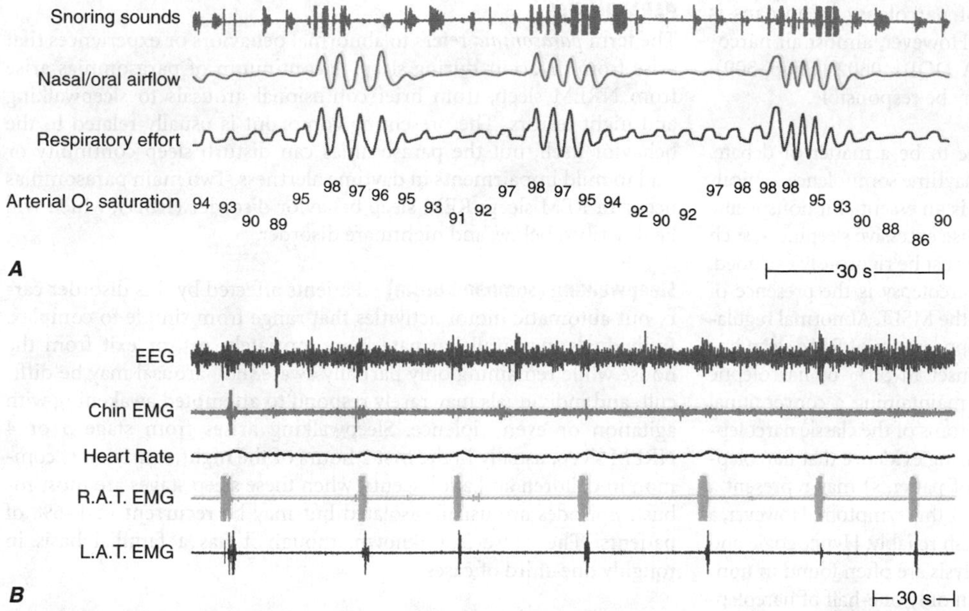

FIGURE 28-3 Polysomnographic recordings of *(A)* obstructive sleep apnea and *(B)* periodic limb movement of sleep. Note the snoring and reduction in air flow in the presence of continued respiratory effort, associated with the subsequent oxygen desaturation (upper panel). Periodic limb movements occur with a relatively constant intermovement interval and are associated with changes in the EEG and heart rate acceleration (lower panel). Abbreviations: R.A.T., right anterior tibialis; L.A.T., left anterior tibialis. *(From the Division of Sleep Medicine, Brigham and Women's Hospital.)*

time function. Specific areas to be addressed include the occurrence of inadvertent sleep episodes while driving or in other safety-related settings, sleepiness while at work or school (and the relationship of sleepiness to work and school performance), and the effect of sleepiness on social and family life. Driving is particularly hazardous for patients with increased sleepiness. Reaction time is equally impaired by 24 h of sleep loss as by a blood alcohol level of 0.10 g/dL. More than half of Americans admit to driving when drowsy. An estimated 250,000 motor vehicle crashes per year are due to drowsy drivers, thus causing 20% of all serious crash injuries. Drowsy driving legislation, aimed at improving education of all drivers about the hazards of driving drowsy and establishing sanctions comparable to those for drunk driving, is pending in several states. Screening for sleep disorders, provision of an adequate number of safe highway rest areas, maintenance of unobstructed shoulder rumble strips, and strict enforcement and compliance monitoring of hours-of-service policies are needed to reduce the risk of sleep-related transportation crashes. Evidence for significant daytime impairment [in association either with the diagnosis of a primary sleep disorder, such as narcolepsy or sleep apnea, or with imposed or self-selected sleep-wake schedules (see "Shift-Work Disorder," below)] raises the issue of the physician's responsibility to notify motor vehicle licensing authorities of the increased risk of sleepiness-related vehicle accidents. As with epilepsy, legal requirements vary from state to state, and existing legal precedents do not provide a consistent interpretation of the balance between the physician's responsibility and the patient's right to privacy. At a minimum, physicians should document discussions with the patient regarding the increased risk of operating a vehicle, as well as a recommendation that driving be suspended until successful treatment or a schedule modification can be instituted.

The distinction between fatigue and sleepiness can be useful in the differentiation of patients with complaints of fatigue or tiredness in the setting of disorders such as fibromyalgia (Chap. 329), chronic fatigue syndrome (Chap. 384), or endocrine deficiencies such as hypothyroidism (Chap. 335) or Addison's disease (Chap. 336). While patients with these disorders can typically distinguish their daytime symptoms from the sleepiness that occurs with sleep deprivation, substantial overlap can occur. This is particularly true when the primary disorder also results in chronic sleep disruption (e.g., sleep apnea in hypothyroidism) or in abnormal sleep (e.g., fibromyalgia).

While clinical evaluation of the complaint of excessive sleepiness is usually adequate, objective quantification is sometimes necessary. Assessment of daytime functioning as an index of the adequacy of sleep can be made with the multiple sleep latency test (MSLT), which involves repeated measurement of sleep latency (time to onset of sleep) under standardized conditions during a day following quantified nocturnal sleep. The average latency across four to six tests (administered every 2 h across the waking day) provides an objective measure of daytime sleep tendency. Disorders of sleep that result in pathologic daytime somnolence can be reliably distinguished with the MSLT. In addition, the multiple measurements of sleep onset may identify direct transitions from wakefulness to REM sleep that are suggestive of specific pathologic conditions (e.g., narcolepsy).

NARCOLEPSY

Narcolepsy is both a disorder of the ability to sustain wakefulness voluntarily and a disorder of REM sleep regulation (Table 28-2). The classic "narcolepsy tetrad" consists of excessive daytime somnolence plus three specific symptoms related to an intrusion of REM sleep characteristics (e.g., muscle atonia, vivid dream imagery) into the transition between wakefulness and sleep: (1) sudden weakness or loss of muscle tone without loss of consciousness, often elicited by emotion (cataplexy); (2) hallucinations at sleep onset (hypnogogic hallucinations) or upon awakening (hypnopompic hallucinations); and (3) muscle paralysis upon awakening (sleep paralysis). The severity of cataplexy varies, as patients may have two to three attacks per day or per decade. Some patients with objectively confirmed narcolepsy (see below) may show no evidence of cataplexy. In those with cataplexy, the extent and duration of an attack may also vary, from a transient sagging of the jaw lasting a few seconds to rare cases of flaccid paralysis of the entire voluntary musculature for up to 20–30 min. Symptoms of narcolepsy typically begin in the second decade, although the onset ranges from ages 5–50. Once established, the disease is chronic without remissions. Secondary forms of narcolepsy have been described (e.g., after head trauma).

Narcolepsy affects about 1 in 4000 people in the United States and appears to have a genetic basis. Recently, several convergent lines of evidence suggest that the hypothalamic neuropeptide hypocretin (orexin) is involved in the pathogenesis of narcolepsy: (1) a mutation in the hypocretin receptor 2 gene has been associated with canine narcolepsy; (2) hypocretin "knockout" mice that are genetically unable to produce this neuropeptide exhibit behavioral and electrophysiologic features resembling human narcolepsy; and (3) cerebrospinal fluid levels of hypocretin are reduced in most patients who have narcolepsy

TABLE 28-2 PREVALENCE OF SYMPTOMS IN NARCOLEPSY

Symptom	Prevalence, %
Excessive daytime somnolence	100
Disturbed sleep	87
Cataplexy	76
Hypnagogic hallucinations	68
Sleep paralysis	64
Memory problems	50

Source: Modified from TA Roth, L Merlotti in SA Burton et al (eds), *Narcolepsy 3rd International Symposium: Selected Symposium Proceedings*, Chicago, Matrix Communications, 1989.

 with cataplexy. The inheritance pattern of narcolepsy in humans is more complex than in the canine model. However, almost all narcoleptics with cataplexy are positive for HLA DQB1*0602 (Chap. 309), suggesting that an autoimmune process may be responsible.

Diagnosis The diagnostic criteria continue to be a matter of debate. Certainly, objective verification of excessive daytime somnolence, typically with MSLT mean sleep latencies <8 min, is an essential if nonspecific diagnostic feature. Other conditions that cause excessive sleepiness, such as sleep apnea or chronic sleep deprivation, must be rigorously excluded. The other objective diagnostic feature of narcolepsy is the presence of REM sleep in at least two of the naps during the MSLT. Abnormal regulation of REM sleep is also manifested by the appearance of REM sleep immediately or within minutes after sleep onset in 50% of narcoleptic patients, a rarity in unaffected individuals maintaining a conventional sleep-wake schedule. The REM-related symptoms of the classic narcolepsy tetrad are variably present. There is increasing evidence that narcoleptics with cataplexy (one-half to two-thirds of patients) may represent a more homogeneous group than those without this symptom. However, a history of cataplexy can be difficult to establish reliably. Hypnogogic and hypnopompic hallucinations and sleep paralysis are often found in nonnarcoleptic individuals and may be present in only one-half of narcoleptics. Nocturnal sleep disruption is commonly observed in narcolepsy but is also a nonspecific symptom. Similarly, a history of "automatic behavior" during wakefulness (a trancelike state during which simple motor behaviors persist) is not specific for narcolepsy and serves principally to corroborate the presence of daytime somnolence.

Rx NARCOLEPSY

The treatment of narcolepsy is symptomatic. Somnolence is treated with wake-promoting therapeutics. Modafinil is now the drug of choice, principally because it is associated with fewer side effects than older stimulants and has a long half-life; 200–400 mg is given as a single daily dose. Older drugs such as methylphenidate (10 mg bid to 20 mg qid) or dextroamphetamine (10 mg bid) are still used as alternatives, particularly in refractory patients. These latter medications are now available in slow-release formulations, extending their duration of action and allowing once daily dosing.

Treatment of the REM-related phenomena cataplexy, hypnogogic hallucinations, and sleep paralysis requires the potent REM sleep suppression produced by antidepressant medications. The tricyclic antidepressants [e.g., protriptyline (10–40 mg/d) and clomipramine (25–50 mg/d)] and the selective serotonin reuptake inhibitors (SSRIs) [e.g., fluoxetine (10–20 mg/d)] are commonly used for this purpose. Efficacy of the antidepressants is limited largely by anticholinergic side effects (tricyclics) and by sleep disturbance and sexual dysfunction (SSRIs). Alternatively, gamma hydroxybutyrate (GHB), given at bed time, and 4 h later, is effective in reducing daytime cataplectic episodes. Adequate nocturnal sleep time and planned daytime naps (when possible) are important preventative measures.

SLEEP APNEA SYNDROMES

Respiratory dysfunction during sleep is a common, serious cause of excessive daytime somnolence as well as of disturbed nocturnal sleep. An estimated 2–5 million individuals in the United States have a reduction or cessation of breathing for 10–150 s, from thirty to several hundred times every night during sleep. These episodes may be due to either an occlusion of the airway (*obstructive sleep apnea*), absence of respiratory effort (*central sleep apnea*), or a combination of these factors (*mixed sleep apnea*) (Fig. 28-3). Failure to recognize and treat these conditions appropriately may lead to impairment of daytime alertness, increased risk of sleep-related motor vehicle accidents, hypertension and other serious cardiovascular complications, and increased mortality. Sleep apnea is particularly prevalent in overweight men and in the elderly, yet it is estimated to remain undiagnosed in 80–90% of affected individuals. This is unfortunate since effective treatments are available. **Readers are referred to Chap. 259 for a comprehensive review of the diagnosis and treatment of patients with these conditions.**

PARASOMNIAS

The term *parasomnia* refers to abnormal behaviors or experiences that arise from or occur during sleep. A continuum of parasomnias arise from NREM sleep, from brief confusional arousals to sleepwalking and night terrors. The presenting complaint is usually related to the behavior itself, but the parasomnias can disturb sleep continuity or lead to mild impairments in daytime alertness. Two main parasomnias occur in REM sleep: REM sleep behavior disorder (RBD), which will be described below, and nightmare disorder.

Sleepwalking (Somnambulism) Patients affected by this disorder carry out automatic motor activities that range from simple to complex. Individuals may walk, urinate inappropriately, eat, or exit from the house while remaining only partially aware. Full arousal may be difficult, and individuals may rarely respond to attempted awakening with agitation or even violence. Sleepwalking arises from stage 3 or 4 NREM sleep, usually in the first 2 hours of the night, and is most common in children and adolescents, when these sleep stages are most robust. Episodes are usually isolated but may be recurrent in 1–6% of patients. The cause is unknown, though it has a familial basis in roughly one-third of cases.

Sleep Terrors This disorder, also called *pavor nocturnus*, occurs primarily in young children during the first several hours after sleep onset, in stages 3 and 4 of NREM sleep. The child suddenly screams, exhibiting autonomic arousal with sweating, tachycardia, and hyperventilation. The individual may be difficult to arouse and rarely recalls the episode on awakening in the morning. Parents are usually reassured to learn that the condition is self-limited and benign and that no specific therapy is indicated. Both sleep terrors and sleepwalking represent abnormalities of arousal. In contrast, *nightmares* occur during REM sleep and cause full arousal, with intact memory for the unpleasant episode.

Sleep Bruxism Bruxism is an involuntary, forceful grinding of teeth during sleep that affects 10–20% of the population. The patient is usually unaware of the problem. The typical age of onset is 17–20 years, and spontaneous remission usually occurs by age 40. Sex distribution appears to be equal. In many cases, the diagnosis is made during dental examination, damage is minor, and no treatment is indicated. In more severe cases, treatment with a rubber tooth guard is necessary to prevent disfiguring tooth injury. Stress management or, in some cases, biofeedback can be useful when bruxism is a manifestation of psychological stress. There are anecdotal reports of benefit using benzodiazepines.

Sleep Enuresis Bedwetting, like sleepwalking and night terrors, is another parasomnia that occurs during sleep in the young. Before age 5 or 6, nocturnal enuresis should probably be considered a normal feature of development. The condition usually improves spontaneously by puberty, has a prevalence in late adolescence of 1–3%, and is rare in adulthood. In older patients with enuresis a distinction must be made between primary and secondary enuresis, the latter being defined as bedwetting in patients who have previously been fully continent for 6–12 months. Treatment of primary enuresis is reserved for patients of appropriate age (>5 or 6 years) and consists of bladder training exercises and behavioral therapy. Urologic abnormalities are more common in primary enuresis and must be assessed by urologic examination. Important causes of secondary enuresis include emotional disturbances, urinary tract infections or malformations, cauda equina lesions, epilepsy, sleep apnea, and certain medications. Symptomatic pharmacotherapy is usually accomplished with desmopressin (0.2 mg qhs), oxybutynin chloride (5–10 mg qhs) or imipramine (10–50 mg qhs).

Miscellaneous Parasomnias Other clinical entities may be characterized as a parasomnia or a sleep-related movement disorder in that they occur selectively during sleep and are associated with some degree of sleep disruption. Examples include *jactatio capitis nocturna* (nocturnal headbanging, rhythmic movement disorder), confusional arousals, sleep-related eating disorder, and nocturnal leg cramps.

REM Sleep Behavior Disorder (RBD) RBD is a rare condition that is distinct from other parasomnias in that it occurs during REM sleep. It primarily afflicts men of middle age or older, many of whom have an existing, or developing, neurologic disease. Approximately one-half of patients with RBD will develop Parkinson's disease (Chap. 366) within 10–20 years. Presenting symptoms consist of agitated or violent behavior during sleep, as reported by a bed partner. In contrast to typical somnambulism, injury to the patient or bed partner is not uncommon, and, upon awakening, the patient reports vivid, often unpleasant, dream imagery. The principal differential diagnosis is nocturnal seizures, which can be excluded with polysomnography. In RBD, seizure activity is absent on the EEG, and disinhibition of the usual motor atonia is observed in the EMG during REM sleep, at times associated with complex motor behaviors. The pathogenesis is unclear, but damage to brainstem areas mediating descending motor inhibition during REM sleep may be responsible. In support of this hypothesis are the remarkable similarities between RBD and the sleep of animals with bilateral lesions of the pontine tegmentum in areas controlling REM sleep motor inhibition. Treatment with clonazepam (0.5–1.0 mg qhs) provides sustained improvement in almost all reported cases.

CIRCADIAN RHYTHM SLEEP DISORDERS

A subset of patients presenting with either insomnia or hypersomnia may have a disorder of sleep *timing* rather than sleep *generation*. Disorders of sleep timing can be either organic (i.e., due to an intrinsic defect in the circadian pacemaker or its input from entraining stimuli) or environmental (i.e., due to a disruption of exposure to entraining stimuli from the environment). Regardless of etiology, the symptoms reflect the influence of the underlying circadian pacemaker on sleep-wake function. Thus, effective therapeutic approaches should aim to entrain the oscillator at an appropriate phase.

Jet Lag Disorder More than 60 million persons experience transmeridian air travel annually, which is often associated with excessive daytime sleepiness, sleep onset insomnia, and frequent arousals from sleep, particularly in the latter half of the night. Gastrointestinal discomfort is common. The syndrome is transient, typically lasting 2–14 d depending on the number of time zones crossed, the direction of travel, and the traveler's age and phase-shifting capacity. Travelers who spend more time outdoors reportedly adapt more quickly than those who remain in hotel rooms, presumably due to bright (outdoor) light exposure. Avoidance of antecedent sleep loss and obtaining nap sleep on the afternoon prior to overnight travel greatly reduces the difficulty of extended wakefulness. Laboratory studies suggest that sub-milligram doses of the pineal hormone melatonin can enhance sleep efficiency, but only if taken when endogenous melatonin concentrations are low (i.e., during biologic daytime), and that melatonin may induce phase shifts in human rhythms. A large-scale clinical trial evaluating the safety and efficacy of melatonin as a treatment for jet lag disorder and other circadian sleep disorders is needed.

Shift-Work Disorder More than 7 million workers in the United States regularly work at night, either on a permanent or rotating schedule. In addition, each week millions more elect to remain awake at night to meet deadlines, drive long distances, or participate in recreational activities. This results in both sleep loss and misalignment of the circadian rhythm with respect to the sleep-wake cycle.

Studies of regular night-shift workers indicate that the circadian timing system usually fails to adapt successfully to such inverted schedules. This leads to a misalignment between the desired work-rest schedule and the output of the pacemaker and in disturbed daytime sleep in most individuals. Sleep deprivation, increased length of time awake prior to work, and misalignment of circadian phase produce decreased alertness and performance, increased reaction time, and increased risk of performance lapses, thereby resulting in greater safety hazards among night workers and other sleep-deprived individuals. Sleep disturbance nearly doubles the risk of a fatal work accident. Additional problems include higher rates of cancer and of cardiac, gastrointestinal, and reproductive disorders in chronic night-shift workers.

Sleep onset is associated with marked attenuation in perception of both auditory and visual stimuli and lapses of consciousness. The sleepy individual may thus attempt to perform routine and familiar motor tasks during the transition state between wakefulness and sleep (stage 1 sleep) in the absence of adequate processing of sensory input from the environment. Motor vehicle operators are especially vulnerable to sleep-related accidents since the sleep-deprived driver or operator often fails to heed the warning signs of fatigue. Such attempts to override the powerful biologic drive for sleep by the sheer force of will can yield a catastrophic outcome when sleep processes intrude involuntarily upon the waking brain. Such sleep-related attentional failures typically last only seconds but are known on occasion to persist for longer durations. These frequent brief intrusions of stage 1 sleep into behavioral wakefulness are a major component of the impaired psychomotor performance seen with sleepiness. There is a significant increase in the risk of sleep-related, fatal-to-the-driver highway crashes in the early morning and late afternoon hours, coincident with bimodal peaks in the daily rhythm of sleep tendency.

Medical housestaff constitute another group of workers at risk for accidents and other adverse consequences of lack of sleep and misalignment of the circadian rhythm. Recent research has demonstrated that the practice of scheduling interns and residents to work shifts of 30 consecutive hours both doubles the risk of attentional failures among intensive care unit interns working at night and significantly increases the risk of serious medical errors in intensive care units. Moreover, working for >24 h consecutively increases the risk of needlestick injuries and more than doubles the risk of motor vehicle crashes on the commute home. Some 20% of hospital interns report making a fatigue-related mistake that injured a patient, and 5% admit making a mistake that results in the death of a patient.

From 5–10% of individuals scheduled to work at night or in the early morning hours have much greater than average difficulties remaining awake during night work and sleeping during the day; these individuals are diagnosed with chronic and severe shift-work disorder (SWD). Patients with this disorder have a level of excessive sleepiness during night work and insomnia during day sleep that the physician judges to be clinically significant; the condition is associated with an increased risk of sleep-related accidents and with some of the illnesses associated with night-shift work. Patients with chronic and severe SWD are profoundly sleepy at night. In fact, their sleep latencies during night work average just 2 min, comparable to mean sleep latency durations of patients with narcolepsy or severe daytime sleep apnea.

Rx SHIFT-WORK DISORDER

Caffeine is frequently used to promote wakefulness. However, it cannot forestall sleep indefinitely, and it does not shield users from sleep-related performance lapses. Postural changes, exercise, and strategic placement of nap opportunities can sometimes temporarily reduce the risk of fatigue-related performance lapses. Properly timed exposure to bright light can facilitate rapid adaptation to night-shift work.

While many techniques (e.g., light treatment) used to facilitate adaptation to night shift work may help patients with this disorder, modafinil is the only therapeutic intervention that has ever been evaluated as a treatment for this specific patient population. Modafinil (200 mg, taken 30–60 min before the start of each night shift) is approved by the U.S. Food and Drug Administration as a treatment for the excessive sleepiness during night work in patients with SWD. Although treatment with modafinil significantly increases sleep latency and reduces the risk of lapses of attention during night work, SWD patients remain excessively sleepy at night, even while being treated with modafinil.

Safety programs should promote education about sleep and increase awareness of the hazards associated with night work. The goal should be to minimize both sleep deprivation and circadian disruption. Work schedules should be designed to minimize: (1) exposure to night work, (2) the frequency of shift rotation so that shifts do not rotate more than once every 2–3 weeks, (3) the number of consecutive night shifts, and (4) the duration of night shifts. Shift durations of >16 h should be universally recognized as increasing the risk of sleep-related errors and performance lapses to a level that is unacceptable in nonemergency circumstances.

Delayed Sleep Phase Disorder Delayed sleep phase disorder is characterized by: (1) reported sleep onset and wake times intractably later than desired, (2) actual sleep times at nearly the same clock hours daily, and (3) essentially normal all-night polysomnography except for delayed sleep onset. Patients exhibit an abnormally delayed endogenous circadian phase, with the temperature minimum during the constant routine occurring later than normal. This delayed phase could be due to: (1) an abnormally long, genetically determined intrinsic period of the endogenous circadian pacemaker; (2) an abnormally reduced phase-advancing capacity of the pacemaker; or (3) an irregular prior sleep-wake schedule, characterized by frequent nights when the patient chooses to remain awake well past midnight (for social, school, or work reasons). In most cases, it is difficult to distinguish among these factors, since patients with an abnormally long intrinsic period are more likely to "choose" such late-night activities because they are unable to sleep at that time. Patients tend to be young adults. This self-perpetuating condition can persist for years and does not usually respond to attempts to reestablish normal bedtime hours. Treatment methods involving bright-light phototherapy during the morning hours or melatonin administration in the evening hours show promise in these patients, although the relapse rate is high.

Advanced Sleep Phase Disorder Advanced sleep phase disorder (ASPD) is the converse of the delayed sleep phase syndrome. Most commonly, this syndrome occurs in older people, 15% of whom report that they cannot sleep past 5 A.M., with twice that number complaining that they wake up too early at least several times per week. Patients with ASPD experience excessive daytime sleepiness during the evening hours, when they have great difficulty remaining awake, even in social settings. Typically, patients awaken from 3–5 A.M. each day, often several hours before their desired wake times. In addition to age-related ASPD, an early-onset familial variant of this condition has also been reported. In one such family, autosomal dominant ASPD was due to a missense mutation in a circadian clock component (PER2, as shown in Fig. 28-2) that altered the circadian period. Patients with ASPD may benefit from bright-light phototherapy during the evening hours, designed to reset the circadian pacemaker to a later hour.

Non-24-Hour Sleep-Wake Disorder This condition can occur when the maximal phase-advancing capacity of the circadian pacemaker is not adequate to accommodate the difference between the 24-h geophysical day and the intrinsic period of the pacemaker in the patient. Alternatively, patients' self-selected exposure to artificial light may drive the circadian pacemaker to a >24-h schedule. Affected patients are not able to maintain a stable phase relationship between the output of the pacemaker and the 24-h day. Such patients typically present with an incremental pattern of successive delays in sleep onsets and wake times, progressing in and out of phase with local time. When the patient's endogenous rhythms are out of phase with the local environment, insomnia coexists with excessive daytime sleepiness. Conversely, when the endogenous rhythms are in phase with the local environment, symptoms remit. The intervals between symptomatic periods may last several weeks to several months. Blind individuals unable to perceive light are particularly susceptible to this disorder. Nightly low-dose (0.5 mg) melatonin administration has been reported to improve sleep and, in some cases, to induce synchronization of the circadian pacemaker.

MEDICAL IMPLICATIONS OF CIRCADIAN RHYTHMICITY

Prominent circadian variations have been reported in the incidence of acute myocardial infarction, sudden cardiac death, and stroke, the leading causes of death in the United States. Platelet aggregability is increased after arising in the early morning hours, coincident with the peak incidence of these cardiovascular events. A better understanding of the possible role of circadian rhythmicity in the acute destabilization of a chronic condition such as atherosclerotic disease could improve the understanding of the pathophysiology.

Diagnostic and therapeutic procedures may also be affected by the time of day at which data are collected. Examples include blood pressure, body temperature, the dexamethasone suppression test, and plasma cortisol levels. The timing of chemotherapy administration has been reported to have an effect on the outcome of treatment. Few physicians realize the extent to which routine measures are affected by the time (or sleep/wake state) when the measurement is made.

In addition, both the toxicity and effectiveness of drugs can vary during the day. For example, more than a fivefold difference has been observed in mortality rates following administration of toxic agents to experimental animals at different times of day. Anesthetic agents are particularly sensitive to time-of-day effects. Finally, the physician must be increasingly aware of the public health risks associated with the ever-increasing demands made by the duty-rest-recreation schedules in our round-the-clock society.

FURTHER READINGS

FLEMONS WW: Clinical practice. Obstructive sleep apnea. N Engl J Med 347:498, 2002

PACK AI et al: Risk factors for excessive sleepiness in older adults. Ann Neurol 59:893, 2006

SCAMMELL TE: The neurobiology, diagnosis, and treatment of narcolepsy. Ann Neurol 53:154, 2003

SILBER MH: Clinical practice. Chronic insomnia. N Engl J Med 353:803, 2005

SECTION 4 DISORDERS OF EYES, EARS, NOSE, AND THROAT

29 Disorders of the Eye

Jonathan C. Horton

THE HUMAN VISUAL SYSTEM

The visual system provides a supremely efficient means for the rapid assimilation of information from the environment to aid in the guidance of behavior. The act of seeing begins with the capture of images focused by the cornea and lens upon a light-sensitive membrane in the back of the eye, called the *retina*. The retina is actually part of the brain, banished to the periphery to serve as a transducer for the conversion of patterns of light energy into neuronal signals. Light is absorbed by photopigment in two types of receptors: rods and cones. In the human retina there are 100 million rods and 5 million cones. The rods operate in dim (scotopic) illumination. The cones function under daylight (photopic) conditions. The cone system is specialized for color perception and high spatial resolution. The majority of cones are located within the macula, the portion of the retina serving the central 10° of vision. In the middle of the macula a small pit termed the *fovea*, packed exclusively with cones, provides best visual acuity.

Photoreceptors hyperpolarize in response to light, activating bipolar, amacrine, and horizontal cells in the inner nuclear layer. After processing of photoreceptor responses by this complex retinal circuit, the flow of sensory information ultimately converges upon a final common pathway: the ganglion cells. These cells translate the visual image impinging upon the retina into a continuously varying barrage of action potentials that propagates along the primary optic pathway to visual centers within the brain. There are a million ganglion cells in each retina, and hence a million fibers in each optic nerve.

Ganglion cell axons sweep along the inner surface of the retina in the nerve fiber layer, exit the eye at the optic disc, and travel through the optic nerve, optic chiasm, and optic tract to reach targets in the brain. The majority of fibers synapse upon cells in the lateral geniculate body, a thalamic relay station. Cells in the lateral geniculate body project in turn to the primary visual cortex. This massive afferent retinogeniculocortical sensory pathway provides the neural substrate for visual perception. Although the lateral geniculate body is the main target of the retina, separate classes of ganglion cells project to other subcortical visual nuclei involved in different functions. Ganglion cells that mediate pupillary constriction and circadian rhythms are light sensitive, owing to a novel visual pigment, melanopsin. Pupil responses are mediated by input to the pretectal olivary nuclei in the midbrain. The pretectal nuclei send their output to the Edinger-Westphal nuclei, which in turn provide parasympathetic innervation to the iris sphincter via an interneuron in the ciliary ganglion. Circadian rhythms are timed by a retinal projection to the suprachiasmatic nucleus. Visual orientation and eye movements are served by retinal input to the superior colliculus. Gaze stabilization and optokinetic reflexes are governed by a group of small retinal targets known collectively as the *brainstem accessory optic system*.

The eyes must be rotated constantly within their orbits to place and maintain targets of visual interest upon the fovea. This activity, called *foveation*, or looking, is governed by an elaborate efferent motor system. Each eye is moved by six extraocular muscles, supplied by cranial nerves from the oculomotor (III), trochlear (IV), and abducens (VI) nuclei. Activity in these ocular motor nuclei is coordinated by pontine and midbrain mechanisms for smooth pursuit, saccades, and gaze stabilization during head and body movements. Large regions of the frontal and parietooccipital cortex control these brainstem eye movement centers by providing descending supranuclear input.

CLINICAL ASSESSMENT OF VISUAL FUNCTION

REFRACTIVE STATE

In approaching the patient with reduced vision, the first step is to decide whether refractive error is responsible. In *emmetropia*, parallel rays from infinity are focused perfectly upon the retina. Sadly, this condition is enjoyed by only a minority of the population. In *myopia*, the globe is too long, and light rays come to a focal point in front of the retina. Near objects can be seen clearly, but distant objects require a diverging lens in front of the eye. In *hyperopia*, the globe is too short, and hence a converging lens is used to supplement the refractive power of the eye. In *astigmatism*, the corneal surface is not perfectly spherical, necessitating a cylindrical corrective lens. In recent years it has become possible to correct refractive error with the excimer laser by performing LASIK (laser in situ keratomileusis) to alter the curvature of the cornea.

With the onset of middle age, *presbyopia* develops as the lens within the eye becomes unable to increase its refractive power to accommodate upon near objects. To compensate for presbyopia, the emmetropic patient must use reading glasses. The patient already wearing glasses for distance correction usually switches to bifocals. The only exception is the myopic patient, who may achieve clear vision at near simply by removing glasses containing the distance prescription.

Refractive errors usually develop slowly and remain stable after adolescence, except in unusual circumstances. For example, the acute onset of diabetes mellitus can produce sudden myopia because of lens edema induced by hyperglycemia. Testing vision through a pinhole aperture is a useful way to screen quickly for refractive error. If the visual acuity is better through a pinhole than with the unaided eye, the patient needs a refraction to obtain best corrected visual acuity.

VISUAL ACUITY

The Snellen chart is used to test acuity at a distance of 6 m (20 ft). For convenience, a scale version of the Snellen chart, called the Rosenbaum card, is held at 36 cm (14 in) from the patient (Fig. 29-1). All subjects should be able to read the 6/6 m (20/20 ft) line with each eye

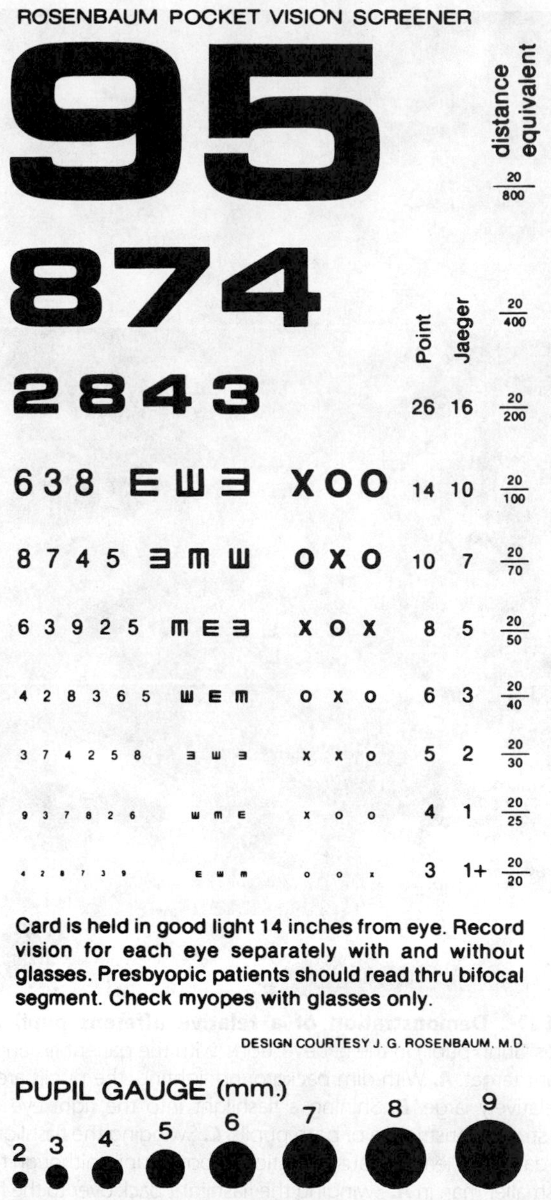

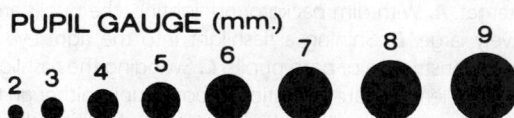

FIGURE 29-1 The Rosenbaum card is a miniature, scale version of the Snellen chart for testing visual acuity at near. When the visual acuity is recorded, the Snellen distance equivalent should bear a notation indicating that vision was tested at near, not at 6 m (20 ft), or else the Jaeger number system should be used to report the acuity.

using their refractive correction, if any. Patients who need reading glasses because of presbyopia must wear them for accurate testing with the Rosenbaum card. If 6/6 (20/20) acuity is not present in each eye, the deficiency in vision must be explained. If worse than 6/240 (20/800), acuity should be recorded in terms of counting fingers, hand motions, light perception, or no light perception. Legal blindness is defined by the Internal Revenue Service as a best corrected acuity of 6/60 (20/200) or less in the better eye, or a binocular visual field subtending 20° or less. For driving the laws vary by state, but most require a corrected acuity of 6/12 (20/40) in at least one eye for unrestricted privileges. Patients with a homonymous hemianopia should not drive.

PUPILS

The pupils should be tested individually in dim light with the patient fixating on a distant target. If they respond briskly to light, there is no need to check the near response, because isolated loss of constriction (miosis) to accommodation does not occur. For this reason, the ubiquitous abbreviation PERRLA (pupils equal, round, and reactive to light and accommodation) implies a wasted effort with the last step.

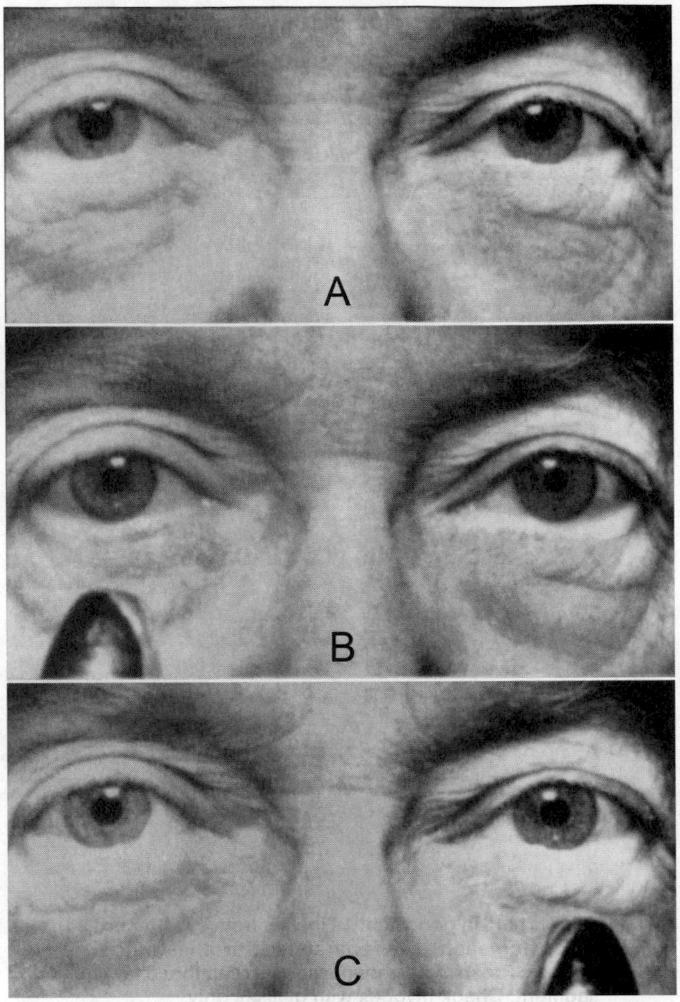

FIGURE 29-2 Demonstration of a relative afferent pupil defect (Marcus Gunn pupil) in the left eye, done with the patient fixating upon a distant target. ***A.*** With dim background lighting, the pupils are equal and relatively large. ***B.*** Shining a flashlight into the right eye evokes equal, strong constriction of both pupils. ***C.*** Swinging the flashlight over to the damaged left eye causes dilation of both pupils, although they remain smaller than in ***A.*** Swinging the flashlight back over to the healthy right eye would result in symmetric constriction back to the appearance shown in ***B.*** Note that the pupils always remain equal; the damage to the left retina/optic nerve is revealed by weaker bilateral pupil constriction to a flashlight in the left eye compared with the right eye. *(From P Levatin, Arch Ophthalmol 62:768, 1959.)*

However, it is important to test the near response if the light response is poor or absent. Light-near dissociation occurs with neurosyphilis (Argyll Robertson pupil), lesions of the dorsal midbrain (obstructive hydrocephalus, pineal region tumors), and after aberrant regeneration (oculomotor nerve palsy, Adie's tonic pupil).

An eye with no light perception has no pupillary response to direct light stimulation. If the retina or optic nerve is only partially injured, the direct pupillary response will be weaker than the consensual pupillary response evoked by shining a light into the other eye. This *relative afferent pupillary defect* (Marcus Gunn pupil) can be elicited with the swinging flashlight test (Fig. 29-2). It is an extremely useful sign in retrobulbar optic neuritis and other optic nerve diseases, where it may be the sole objective evidence for disease.

Subtle inequality in pupil size, up to 0.5 mm, is a fairly common finding in normal persons. The diagnosis of essential or physiologic anisocoria is secure as long as the relative pupil asymmetry remains constant as ambient lighting varies. Anisocoria that increases in dim light indicates a sympathetic paresis of the iris dilator muscle. The triad of miosis with ipsilateral ptosis and anhidrosis constitutes *Horner's syndrome*, although anhidrosis is an inconstant feature. Brainstem stroke, carotid dissection, or neoplasm impinging upon the sympathetic chain are occasionally identified as the cause of Horner's syndrome, but most cases are idiopathic.

Anisocoria that increases in bright light suggests a parasympathetic palsy. The first concern is an oculomotor nerve paresis. This possibility is excluded if the eye movements are full and the patient has no ptosis or diplopia. Acute pupillary dilation (mydriasis) can occur from damage to the ciliary ganglion in the orbit. Common mechanisms are infection (herpes zoster, influenza), trauma (blunt, penetrating, surgical), or ischemia (diabetes, temporal arteritis). After denervation of the iris sphincter the pupil does not respond well to light, but the response to near is often relatively intact. When the near stimulus is removed, the pupil redilates very slowly compared with the normal pupil, hence the term *tonic pupil.* In *Adie's syndrome*, a tonic pupil occurs in conjunction with weak or absent tendon reflexes in the lower extremities. This benign disorder, which occurs predominantly in healthy young women, is assumed to represent a mild dysautonomia. Tonic pupils are also associated with Shy-Drager syndrome, segmental hypohidrosis, diabetes, and amyloidosis. Occasionally, a tonic pupil is discovered incidentally in an otherwise completely normal, asymptomatic individual. The diagnosis is confirmed by placing a drop of dilute (0.125%) pilocarpine into each eye. Denervation hypersensitivity produces pupillary constriction in a tonic pupil, whereas the normal pupil shows no response. Pharmacologic dilation from accidental or deliberate instillation of anticholinergic agents (atropine, scopolamine drops) into the eye can also produce pupillary mydriasis. In this situation, normal strength (1%) pilocarpine causes no constriction.

Both pupils are affected equally by systemic medications. They are small with narcotic use (morphine, heroin) and large with anticholinergics (scopolamine). Parasympathetic agents (pilocarpine, demecarium bromide) used to treat glaucoma produce miosis. In any patient with an unexplained pupillary abnormality, a slit-lamp examination is helpful to exclude surgical trauma to the iris, an occult foreign body, perforating injury, intraocular inflammation, adhesions (synechia), angle-closure glaucoma, and iris sphincter rupture from blunt trauma.

EYE MOVEMENTS AND ALIGNMENT

Eye movements are tested by asking the patient with both eyes open to pursue a small target such as a penlight into the cardinal fields of gaze. Normal ocular versions are smooth, symmetric, full, and maintained in all directions without nystagmus. Saccades, or quick refixation eye movements, are assessed by having the patient look back and forth between two stationary targets. The eyes should move rapidly and accurately in a single jump to their target. Ocular alignment can be judged by holding a penlight directly in front of the patient at about 1 m. If the eyes are straight, the corneal light reflex will be centered in the middle of each pupil. To test eye alignment more precisely, the cover test is useful. The patient is instructed to gaze upon a small fixation target in the distance. One eye is covered suddenly while observing the second eye. If the second eye shifts to fixate upon the target, it was misaligned. If it does not move, the first eye is uncovered and the test is repeated on the second eye. If neither eye moves, the eyes are aligned orthotropically. If the eyes are orthotropic in primary gaze but the patient complains of diplopia, the cover test should be performed with the head tilted or turned in whatever direction elicits diplopia. With practice the examiner can detect an ocular deviation (heterotropia) as small as 1–2° with the cover test. Deviations can be measured by placing prisms in front of the misaligned eye to determine the power required to neutralize the fixation shift evoked by covering the other eye.

STEREOPSIS

Stereoacuity is determined by presenting targets with retinal disparity separately to each eye using polarized images. The most popular office tests measure a range of thresholds from 800–40 seconds of arc. Normal stereoacuity is 40 seconds of arc. If a patient achieves this level of stereoacuity, one is assured that the eyes are aligned orthotropically and that vision is intact in each eye. Random dot stereograms have no monocular depth cues and provide an excellent screening test for strabismus and amblyopia in children.

COLOR VISION

The retina contains three classes of cones, with visual pigments of differing peak spectral sensitivity: red (560 nm), green (530 nm), and blue (430 nm). The red and green cone pigments are encoded on the X chromosome; the blue cone pigment on chromosome 7. Mutations of the blue cone pigment are exceedingly rare. Mutations of the red and green pigments cause congenital X-linked color blindness in 8% of males. Affected individuals are not truly color blind; rather, they differ from normal subjects in how they perceive color and how they combine primary monochromatic lights to match a given color. Anomalous trichromats have three cone types, but a mutation in one cone pigment (usually red or green) causes a shift in peak spectral sensitivity, altering the proportion of primary colors required to achieve a color match. Dichromats have only two cone types and will therefore accept a color match based upon only two primary colors. Anomalous trichromats and dichromats have 6/6 (20/20) visual acuity, but their hue discrimination is impaired. Ishihara color plates can be used to detect red-green color blindness. The test plates contain a hidden number, visible only to subjects with color confusion from red-green color blindness. Because color blindness is almost exclusively X-linked, it is worth screening only male children.

The Ishihara plates are often used to detect acquired defects in color vision, although they are intended as a screening test for congenital color blindness. Acquired defects in color vision frequently result from disease of the macula or optic nerve. For example, patients with a history of optic neuritis often complain of color desaturation long after their visual acuity has returned to normal. Color blindness can also occur from bilateral strokes involving the ventral portion of the occipital lobe (cerebral achromatopsia). Such patients can perceive only shades of gray and may also have difficulty recognizing faces (prosopagnosia). Infarcts of the dominant occipital lobe sometimes give rise to color anomia. Affected patients can discriminate colors, but they cannot name them.

VISUAL FIELDS

Vision can be impaired by damage to the visual system anywhere from the eyes to the occipital lobes. One can localize the site of the lesion with considerable accuracy by mapping the visual field deficit by finger confrontation and then correlating it with the topographic anatomy of the visual pathway (Fig. 29-3). Quantitative visual field mapping is performed by computer-driven perimeters (Humphrey, Octopus) that present a target of variable intensity at fixed positions in the visual field (Fig. 29-3*A*). By generating an automated printout of light thresholds, these static perimeters provide a sensitive means of detecting scotomas in the visual field. They are exceedingly useful for serial assessment of visual function in chronic diseases such as glaucoma or pseudotumor cerebri.

The crux of visual field analysis is to decide whether a lesion is before, at, or behind the optic chiasm. If a scotoma is confined to one eye, it must be due to a lesion anterior to the chiasm, involving either the optic nerve or retina. Retinal lesions produce scotomas that correspond optically to their location in the fundus. For example, a superior-nasal retinal detachment results in an inferior-temporal field cut. Damage to the macula causes a central scotoma (Fig. 29-3*B*).

Optic nerve disease produces characteristic patterns of visual field loss. Glaucoma selectively destroys axons that enter the superotemporal or inferotemporal poles of the optic disc, resulting in arcuate scotomas shaped like a Turkish scimitar, which emanate from the blind spot and curve around fixation to end flat against the horizontal meridian (Fig. 29-3*C*). This type of field defect mirrors the arrangement of the nerve fiber layer in the temporal retina. Arcuate or nerve fiber layer scotomas also occur from optic neuritis, ischemic optic neuropathy, optic disc drusen, and branch retinal artery or vein occlusion.

Damage to the entire upper or lower pole of the optic disc causes an altitudinal field cut that follows the horizontal meridian (Fig. 29-3*D*). This pattern of visual field loss is typical of ischemic optic neuropathy but also occurs from retinal vascular occlusion, advanced glaucoma, and optic neuritis.

About half the fibers in the optic nerve originate from ganglion cells serving the macula. Damage to papillomacular fibers causes a cecocentral scotoma encompassing the blind spot and macula (Fig. 29-3*E*). If the damage is irreversible, pallor eventually appears in the temporal portion of the optic disc. Temporal pallor from a cecocentral scotoma may develop in optic neuritis, nutritional optic neuropathy, toxic optic neuropathy, Leber's hereditary optic neuropathy, and compressive optic neuropathy. It is worth mentioning that the temporal side of the optic disc is slightly more pale than the nasal side in most normal individuals. Therefore, it can sometimes be difficult to decide whether the temporal pallor visible on fundus examination represents a pathologic change. Pallor of the nasal rim of the optic disc is a less equivocal sign of optic atrophy.

At the optic chiasm, fibers from nasal ganglion cells decussate into the contralateral optic tract. Crossed fibers are damaged more by compression than uncrossed fibers. As a result, mass lesions of the sellar region cause a temporal hemianopia in each eye. Tumors anterior to the optic chiasm, such as meningiomas of the tuberculum sella, produce a junctional scotoma characterized by an optic neuropathy in one eye and a superior-temporal field cut in the other eye (Fig. 29-3*G*). More symmetric compression of the optic chiasm by a pituitary adenoma (Fig. 333-4), meningioma, craniopharyngioma, glioma, or aneurysm results in a bitemporal hemianopia (Fig. 29-3*H*). The insidious development of a bitemporal hemianopia often goes unnoticed by the patient and will escape detection by the physician unless each eye is tested separately.

It is difficult to localize a postchiasmal lesion accurately, because injury anywhere in the optic tract, lateral geniculate body, optic radiations, or visual cortex can produce a homonymous hemianopia, i.e., a temporal hemifield defect in the contralateral eye and a matching nasal hemifield defect in the ipsilateral eye (Fig. 29-3*I*). A unilateral postchiasmal lesion leaves the visual acuity in each eye unaffected, although the patient may read the letters on only the left or right half of the eye chart. Lesions of the optic radiations tend to cause poorly matched or incongruous field defects in each eye. Damage to the optic radiations in the temporal lobe (Meyer's loop) produces a superior quadrantic homonymous hemianopia (Fig. 29-3*J*), whereas injury to the optic radiations in the parietal lobe results in an inferior quadrantic homonymous hemianopia (Fig. 29-3*K*). Lesions of the primary visual cortex give rise to dense, congruous hemianopic field defects. Occlusion of the posterior cerebral artery supplying the occipital lobe is a frequent cause of total homonymous hemianopia. Some patients with hemianopia after occipital stroke have macular sparing, because the macular representation at the tip of the occipital lobe is supplied by collaterals from the middle cerebral artery (Fig. 29-3*L*). Destruction of both occipital lobes produces cortical blindness. This condition can be distinguished from bilateral prechiasmal visual loss by noting that the pupil responses and optic fundi remain normal.

DISORDERS

RED OR PAINFUL EYE

Corneal Abrasions These are seen best by placing a drop of fluorescein in the eye and looking with the slit lamp using a cobalt-blue light. A penlight with a blue filter will suffice if no slit lamp is available. Damage to the corneal epithelium is revealed by yellow fluorescence of the exposed basement membrane underlying the epithelium. It is important to check for foreign bodies. To search the conjunctival fornices, the lower lid should be pulled down and the upper lid everted. A foreign body can be removed with a moistened cotton-tipped applicator after placing a drop of topical anesthetic, such as proparacaine, in the eye. Alternatively, it may be possible to flush the foreign body from the eye by irrigating copiously with saline or artificial tears. If the corneal epithelium has been abraded, antibiotic ointment and a patch should be applied to the eye. A drop of an intermediate-acting cycloplegic, such as cyclopentolate hydrochloride 1%, helps to reduce pain by relaxing the ciliary body. The eye should be reexamined the next day. Minor abrasions may not require patching and cycloplegia.

Subconjunctival Hemorrhage This results from rupture of small vessels bridging the potential space between the episclera and conjunctiva. Blood dissecting into this space can produce a spectacular red eye, but vision is not affected and the hemorrhage resolves without treatment. Subconjunctival hemorrhage is usually spontaneous but can occur from blunt trauma, eye rubbing, or vigorous coughing. Occasionally it is a clue to an underlying bleeding disorder.

Pinguecula This is a small, raised conjunctival nodule at the temporal or nasal limbus. In adults such lesions are extremely common and have little significance, unless they become inflamed (pingueculitis). A *pterygium* resembles a pinguecula but has crossed the limbus to encroach upon the corneal surface. Removal is justified when symptoms of irritation or blurring develop, but recurrence is a common problem.

Blepharitis This refers to inflammation of the eyelids. The most common form occurs in association with acne rosacea or seborrheic dermatitis. The eyelid margins are usually colonized heavily by staphylococci. Upon close inspection, they appear greasy, ulcerated, and crusted with scaling debris that clings to the lashes. Treatment consists of warm compresses, strict eyelid hygiene, and topical antibiotics such as *erythromycin*. An external *hordeolum* (sty) is caused by staphylococcal infection of the superficial accessory glands of Zeis or Moll located in the eyelid margins. An internal hordeolum occurs after suppurative infection of the oil-secreting meibomian glands within the tarsal plate of the eyelid. Systemic antibiotics, usually tetracyclines, are sometimes necessary for treatment of meibomian gland inflammation (meibomitis) or chronic, severe blepharitis. A *chalazion* is a painless, granulomatous inflammation of a meibomian gland that produces a pealike nodule within the eyelid. It can be incised and drained, or injected with glucocorticoids. Basal cell, squamous cell, or meibomian gland carcinoma should be suspected for any nonhealing, ulcerative lesion of the eyelids.

Dacrocystitis An inflammation of the lacrimal drainage system, this can produce epiphora (tearing) and ocular injection. Gentle pressure over the lacrimal sac evokes pain and reflux of mucus or pus from the tear puncta. Dacrocystitis usually occurs after obstruction of the lacrimal system. It is treated with topical and systemic antibiotics, followed by probing or surgery to reestablish patency. *Entropion* (inversion of the eyelid) or *ectropion* (sagging or eversion of the eyelid) can also lead to epiphora and ocular irritation.

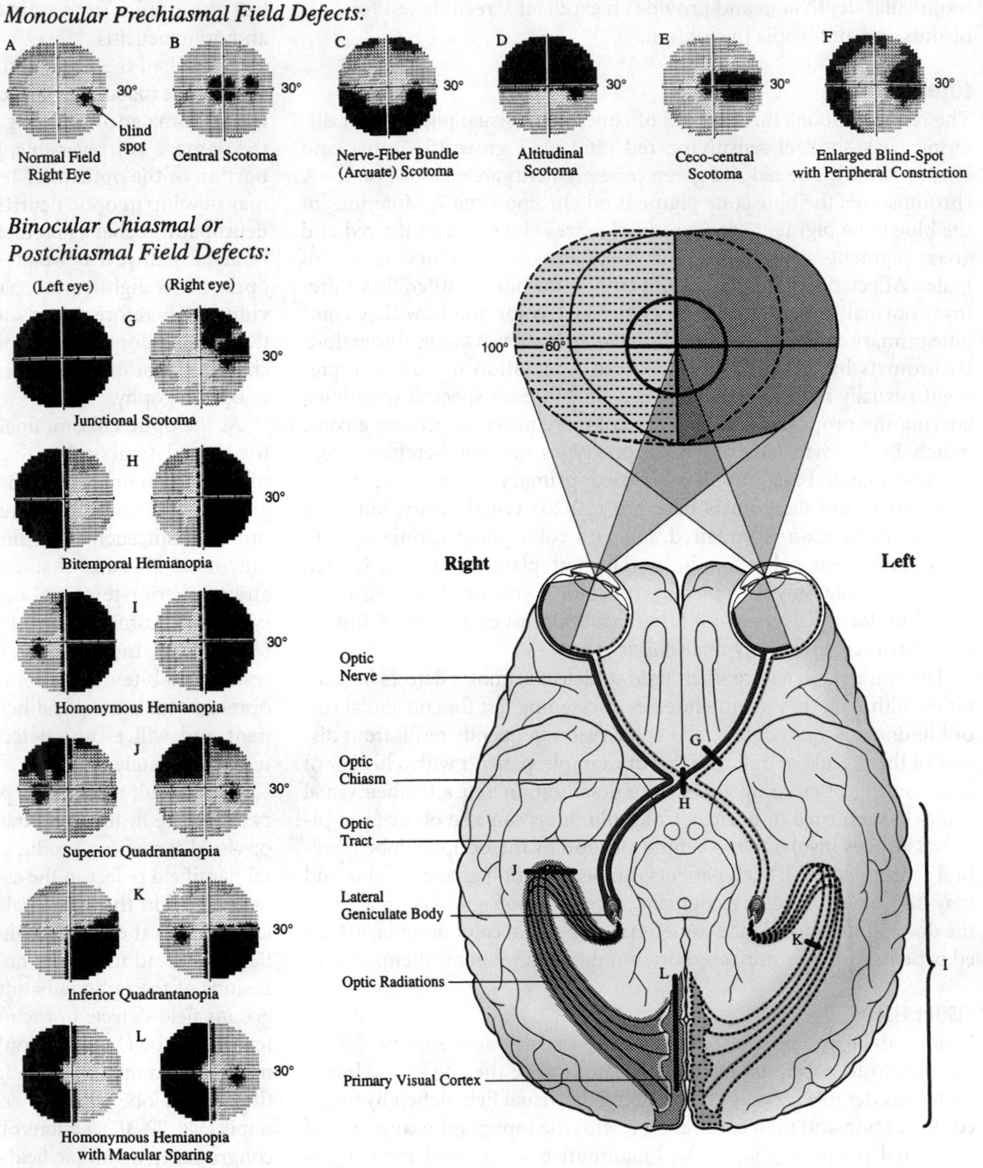

FIGURE 29-3 Ventral view of the brain, correlating patterns of visual field loss with the sites of lesions in the visual pathway. The visual fields overlap partially, creating 120° of central binocular field flanked by a 40° monocular crescent on either side. The visual field maps in this figure were done with a computer-driven perimeter (Humphrey Instruments, Carl Zeiss, Inc.). It plots the retinal sensitivity to light in the central 30° using a gray scale format. Areas of visual field loss are shown in black. The examples of common monocular, prechiasmal field defects are all shown for the right eye. By convention, the visual fields are always recorded with the left eye's field on the left, and the right eye's field on the right, just as the patient sees the world.

Conjunctivitis This is the most common cause of a red, irritated eye. Pain is minimal, and the visual acuity is reduced only slightly. The most common viral etiology is adenovirus infection. It causes a watery discharge, mild foreign-body sensation, and photophobia. Bacterial infection tends to produce a more mucopurulent exudate. Mild cases of infectious conjunctivitis are usually treated empirically with broad-spectrum topical ocular antibiotics, such as sulfacetamide 10%, polymixin-bacitracin-neomycin, or trimethoprim-polymixin combination. Smears and cultures are usually reserved for severe, resistant, or recurrent cases of conjunctivitis. To prevent contagion, patients should be admonished to wash their hands frequently, not to touch their eyes, and to avoid direct contact with others.

Allergic Conjunctivitis This condition is extremely common and often mistaken for infectious conjunctivitis. Itching, redness, and epiphora are typical. The palpebral conjunctiva may become hypertropic with giant excrescences called cobblestone papillae. Irritation from contact lenses or any chronic foreign body can also induce formation of cobblestone papillae. *Atopic conjunctivitis* occurs in subjects with atopic dermatitis or asthma. Symptoms caused by allergic conjunctivitis can be alleviated with cold compresses, topical vasoconstrictors, antihistamines, and mast cell stabilizers such as cromolyn sodium. Topical glucocorticoid solutions provide dramatic relief of immune-mediated forms of conjunctivitis, but their long-term use is ill-advised because of the complications of glaucoma, cataract, and secondary infection. Topical nonsteroidal anti-inflammatory agents (NSAIDs) such as ketorolac tromethamine are a better alternative.

Keratoconjunctivitis Sicca Also known as dry eye, it produces a burning, foreign-body sensation, injection, and photophobia. In mild cases the eye appears surprisingly normal, but tear production measured by wetting of a filter paper (Schirmer strip) is deficient. A variety of systemic drugs, including antihistaminic, anticholinergic, and psychotropic medications, result in dry eye by reducing lacrimal secretion. Disorders that involve the lacrimal gland directly, such as sarcoidosis or Sjögren's syndrome, also cause dry eye. Patients may develop dry eye after radiation therapy if the treatment field includes the orbits. Problems with ocular drying are also common after lesions affecting cranial nerves V or VII. Corneal anesthesia is particularly dangerous, because the absence of a normal blink reflex exposes the cornea to injury without pain to warn the patient. Dry eye is managed by frequent and liberal application of artificial tears and ocular lubricants. In severe cases the tear puncta can be plugged or cauterized to reduce lacrimal outflow.

Keratitis This is a threat to vision because of the risk of corneal clouding, scarring, and perforation. Worldwide, the two leading causes of blindness from keratitis are trachoma from chlamydial infection and vitamin A deficiency related to malnutrition. In the United States, contact lenses play a major role in corneal infection and ulceration. They should not be worn by anyone with an active eye infection. In evaluating the cornea, it is important to differentiate between a superficial infection (*keratoconjunctivitis*) and a deeper, more serious ulcerative process. The latter is accompanied by greater visual loss, pain, photophobia, redness, and discharge. Slit-lamp examination shows disruption of the corneal epithelium, a cloudy infiltrate or abscess in the stroma, and an inflammatory cellular reaction in the anterior chamber. In severe cases, pus settles at the bottom of the anterior chamber, giving rise to a hypopyon. Immediate empirical antibiotic therapy should be initiated after corneal scrapings are obtained for Gram's stain, Giemsa stain, and cultures. Fortified topical antibiotics are most effective, supplemented with subconjunctival antibiotics as required. A fungal etiology should always be considered in the patient with keratitis. Fungal infection is common in warm humid climates, especially after penetration of the cornea by plant or vegetable material.

Herpes Simplex The *herpes viruses* are a major cause of blindness from keratitis. Most adults in the United States have serum antibodies to herpes simplex, indicating prior viral infection (Chap. 172). Primary ocular infection is generally caused by herpes simplex type 1, rather than type 2. It manifests as a unilateral follicular blepharoconjunctivitis, easily confused with adenoviral conjunctivitis unless telltale vesicles appear on the periocular skin or conjunctiva. A dendritic pattern of corneal epithelial ulceration revealed by fluorescein staining is pathognomonic for herpes infection but is seen in only a minority of primary infections. Recurrent ocular infection arises from reactivation of the latent herpes virus. Viral eruption in the corneal epithelium may result in the characteristic herpes dendrite. Involvement of the corneal stroma produces edema, vascularization, and iridocyclitis. Herpes keratitis is treated with topical antiviral agents, cycloplegics, and oral acyclovir. Topical glucocorticoids are effective in mitigating corneal scarring but must be used with extreme caution because of the danger of corneal melting and perforation. Topical glucocorticoids also carry the risk of prolonging infection and inducing glaucoma.

Herpes Zoster Herpes zoster from reactivation of latent varicella (chickenpox) virus causes a dermatomal pattern of painful vesicular dermatitis. Ocular symptoms can occur after zoster eruption in any branch of the trigeminal nerve but are particularly common when vesicles form on the nose, reflecting nasociliary (V1) nerve involvement (Hutchinson's sign). Herpes zoster ophthalmicus produces corneal dendrites, which can be difficult to distinguish from those seen in herpes simplex. Stromal keratitis, anterior uveitis, raised intraocular pressure, ocular motor nerve palsies, acute retinal necrosis, and postherpetic scarring and neuralgia are other common sequelae. Herpes zoster ophthalmicus is treated with antiviral agents and cycloplegics. In severe cases, glucocorticoids may be added to prevent permanent visual loss from corneal scarring.

Episcleritis This is an inflammation of the episclera, a thin layer of connective tissue between the conjunctiva and sclera. Episcleritis resembles conjunctivitis but is a more localized process and discharge is absent. Most cases of episcleritis are idiopathic, but some occur in the setting of an autoimmune disease. *Scleritis* refers to a deeper, more severe inflammatory process, frequently associated with a connective tissue disease such as rheumatoid arthritis, lupus erythematosus, polyarteritis nodosa, Wegener's granulomatosis, or relapsing polychondritis. The inflammation and thickening of the sclera can be diffuse or nodular. In anterior forms of scleritis, the globe assumes a violet hue and the patient complains of severe ocular tenderness and pain. With posterior scleritis the pain and redness may be less marked, but there is often proptosis, choroidal effusion, reduced motility, and visual loss. Episcleritis and scleritis should be treated with NSAIDs. If these agents fail, topical or even systemic glucocorticoid therapy may be necessary, especially if an underlying autoimmune process is active.

Uveitis Involving the anterior structures of the eye, this is also called *iritis* or *iridocyclitis*. The diagnosis requires slit-lamp examination to identify inflammatory cells floating in the aqueous humor or deposited upon the corneal endothelium (keratic precipitates). Anterior uveitis develops in sarcoidosis, ankylosing spondylitis, juvenile rheumatoid arthritis, inflammatory bowel disease, psoriasis, Reiter's syndrome, and Behçet's disease. It is also associated with herpes infections, syphilis, Lyme disease, onchocerciasis, tuberculosis, and leprosy. Although anterior uveitis can occur in conjunction with many diseases, no cause is found to explain the majority of cases. For this reason, laboratory evaluation is usually reserved for patients with recurrent or severe anterior uveitis. Treatment is aimed at reducing inflammation and scarring by judicious use of topical glucocorticoids. Dilation of the pupil reduces pain and prevents the formation of synechiae.

Posterior Uveitis This is diagnosed by observing inflammation of the vitreous, retina, or choroid on fundus examination. It is more likely than anterior uveitis to be associated with an identifiable systemic disease. Some patients have panuveitis, or inflammation of both the anterior and posterior segments of the eye. Posterior uveitis is a manifestation of autoimmune diseases such as sarcoidosis, Behçet's disease, Vogt-Koyanagi-Harada syndrome, and inflammatory bowel disease (Fig. 29-4). It also accompanies diseases such as toxoplasmosis, onchocerciasis, cysticercosis, coccidioidomycosis, toxocariasis, and histoplasmosis; infections caused by organisms such as *Candida*, *Pneumocystis carinii*, *Cryptococcus*, *Aspergillus*, herpes, and cytomegalovirus (see Fig. 175-1); and other diseases such as syphilis, Lyme disease, tuberculosis, cat-scratch disease, Whipple's disease, and brucellosis. In multiple sclerosis, chronic inflammatory changes can develop in the extreme periphery of the retina (pars planitis or intermediate uveitis).

Acute Angle-Closure Glaucoma This is a rare and frequently misdiagnosed cause of a red, painful eye. Susceptible eyes have a shallow anterior chamber, either because the eye has a short axial length (hyperopia) or a lens enlarged by the gradual development of cataract. When the pupil becomes mid-dilated, the peripheral iris blocks aqueous outflow via the anterior chamber angle and the intraocular pressure rises

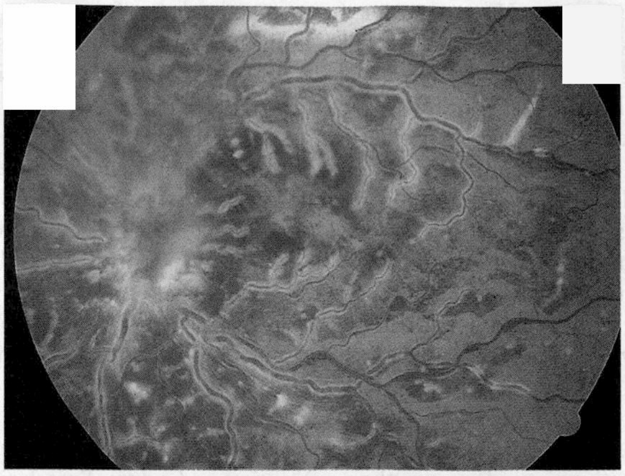

FIGURE 29-4 Retinal vasculitis, uveitis, and hemorrhage in a 32-year-old woman with Crohn's disease. Note that the veins are frosted with a white exudate. Visual acuity improved from 20/400 to 20/20 following treatment with intravenous methylprednisolone.

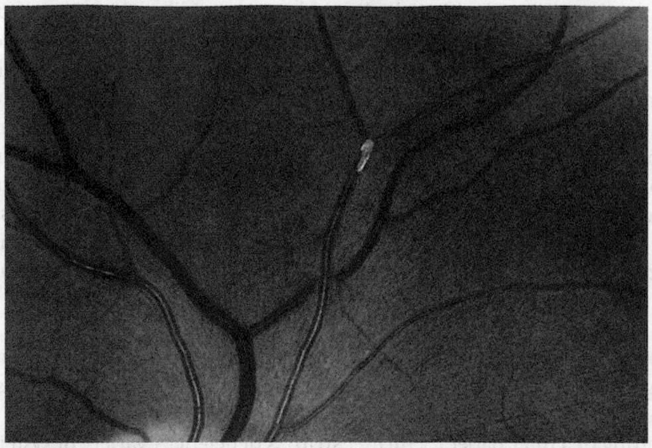

FIGURE 29-5 Hollenhorst plaque lodged at the bifurcation of a retinal arteriole proves that a patient is shedding emboli from either the carotid artery, great vessels, or heart.

abruptly, producing pain, injection, corneal edema, obscurations, and blurred vision. In some patients, ocular symptoms are overshadowed by nausea, vomiting, or headache, prompting a fruitless workup for abdominal or neurologic disease. The diagnosis is made by measuring the intraocular pressure during an acute attack or by observing a narrow chamber angle by means of a specially mirrored contact lens. Acute angle closure is treated with acetazolamide (PO or IV), topical beta blockers, prostaglandin analogues, α_2-adrenergic agonists, and pilocarpine to induce miosis. If these measures fail, a laser can be used to create a hole in the peripheral iris to relieve pupillary block. Many physicians are reluctant to dilate patients routinely for fundus examination because they fear precipitating an angle-closure glaucoma. The risk is actually remote and more than outweighed by the potential benefit to patients of discovering a hidden fundus lesion visible only through a fully dilated pupil. Moreover, a single attack of angle closure after pharmacologic dilation rarely causes any permanent damage to the eye and serves as an inadvertent provocative test to identify patients with narrow angles who would benefit from prophylactic laser iridectomy.

Endophthalmitis This occurs from bacterial, viral, fungal, or parasitic infection of the internal structures of the eye. It is usually acquired by hematogenous seeding from a remote site. Chronically ill, diabetic, or immunosuppressed patients, especially those with a history of indwelling IV catheters or positive blood cultures, are at greatest risk for endogenous endophthalmitis. Although most patients have ocular pain and injection, visual loss is sometimes the only symptom. Septic emboli, from a diseased heart valve or a dental abscess, that lodge in the retinal circulation can give rise to endophthalmitis. White-centered retinal hemorrhages (Roth's spots) are considered pathognomonic for subacute bacterial endocarditis, but they also appear in leukemia, diabetes, and many other conditions. Endophthalmitis also occurs as a complication of ocular surgery, occasionally months or even years after the operation. An occult penetrating foreign body or unrecognized trauma to the globe should be considered in any patient with unexplained intraocular infection or inflammation.

TRANSIENT OR SUDDEN VISUAL LOSS

Amaurosis Fugax This term refers to a transient ischemic attack of the retina (Chap. 364). Because neural tissue has a high rate of metabolism, interruption of blood flow to the retina for more than a few seconds results in *transient monocular blindness*, a term used interchangeably with amaurosis fugax. Patients describe a rapid fading of vision like a curtain descending, sometimes affecting only a portion of the visual field. Amaurosis fugax usually occurs from an embolus that becomes stuck within a retinal arteriole (Fig. 29-5). If the embolus breaks up or passes, flow is restored and vision returns quickly to normal without permanent damage. With prolonged interruption of blood flow, the inner retina suffers infarction. Ophthalmoscopy reveals zones of whitened, edematous retina following the distribution of branch retinal arterioles. Complete occlusion of the central retinal artery produces arrest of blood flow and a milky retina with a cherry-red fovea (Fig. 29-6). Emboli are composed of either cholesterol (Hollenhorst plaque), calcium, or platelet-fibrin debris. The most common source is an atherosclerotic plaque in the carotid artery or aorta, although emboli can also arise from the heart, especially in patients with diseased valves, atrial fibrillation, or wall motion abnormalities.

In rare instances, amaurosis fugax occurs from low central retinal artery perfusion pressure in a patient with a critical stenosis of the ipsilateral carotid artery and poor collateral flow via the circle of Willis. In this situation, amaurosis fugax develops when there is a dip in systemic blood pressure or a slight worsening of the carotid stenosis. Sometimes there is contralateral motor or sensory loss, indicating concomitant hemispheric cerebral ischemia.

Retinal arterial occlusion also occurs rarely in association with retinal migraine, lupus erythematosus, anticardiolipin antibodies (Fig. 29-6), anticoagulant deficiency states (protein S, protein C, and antithrombin III deficiency), pregnancy, IV drug abuse, blood dyscrasias, dysproteinemias, and temporal arteritis.

Marked *systemic hypertension* causes sclerosis of retinal arterioles, splinter hemorrhages, focal infarcts of the nerve fiber layer (cotton-wool spots), and leakage of lipid and fluid (hard exudate) into the macula (Fig. 29-7). In hypertensive crisis, sudden visual loss can result

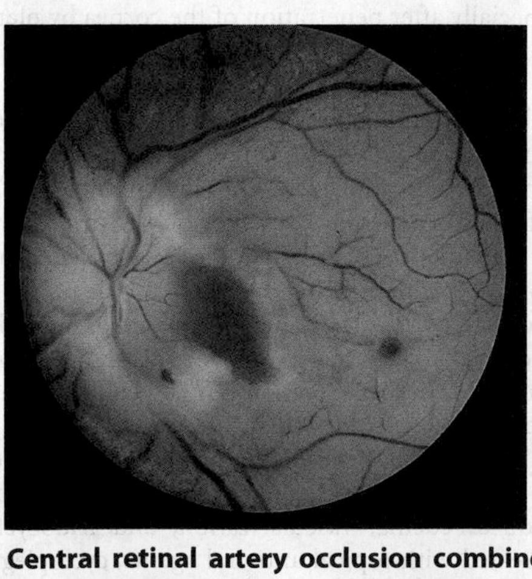

FIGURE 29-6 Central retinal artery occlusion combined with ischemic optic neuropathy in a 19-year-old woman with an elevated titer of anticardiolipin antibodies. Note the orange dot (rather than cherry red) corresponding to the fovea and the spared patch of retina just temporal to the optic disc.

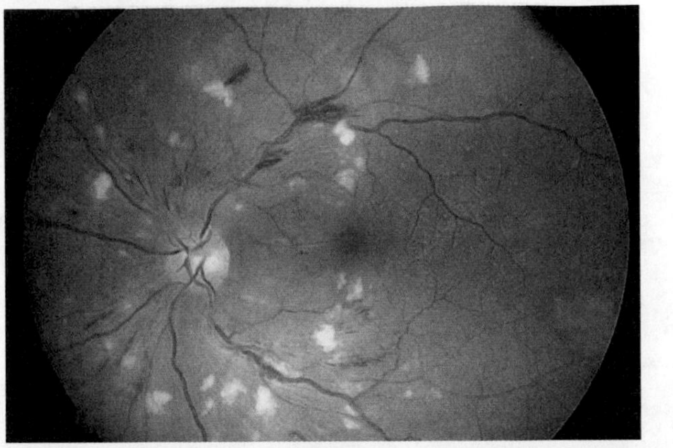

FIGURE 29-7 Hypertensive retinopathy with scattered flame (splinter) hemorrhages and cotton-wool spots (nerve fiber layer infarcts) in a patient with headache and a blood pressure of 234/120.

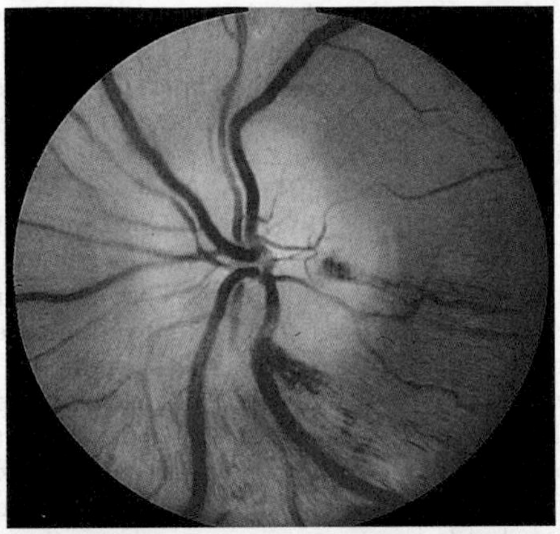

FIGURE 29-9 Anterior ischemic optic neuropathy from temporal arteritis in a 78-year-old woman with pallid disc swelling, hemorrhage, visual loss, myalgia, and an erythrocyte sedimentation rate of 86 mm/h.

from vasospasm of retinal arterioles and retinal ischemia. In addition, acute hypertension may produce visual loss from ischemic swelling of the optic disc. Patients with acute hypertensive retinopathy should be treated by lowering the blood pressure. However, the blood pressure should not be reduced precipitously, because there is a danger of optic disc infarction from sudden hypoperfusion.

Impending *branch* or *central retinal vein occlusion* can produce prolonged visual obscurations that resemble those described by patients with amaurosis fugax. The veins appear engorged and phlebitic, with numerous retinal hemorrhages (Fig. 29-8). In some patients, venous blood flow recovers spontaneously, while others evolve a frank obstruction with extensive retinal bleeding ("blood and thunder" appearance), infarction, and visual loss. Venous occlusion of the retina is often idiopathic, but hypertension, diabetes, and glaucoma are prominent risk factors. Polycythemia, thrombocythemia, or other factors leading to an underlying hypercoagulable state should be corrected; aspirin treatment may be beneficial.

Anterior Ischemic Optic Neuropathy (AION) This is caused by insufficient blood flow through the posterior ciliary arteries supplying the optic disc. It produces painless, monocular visual loss that is usually sudden, although some patients have progressive worsening. The optic disc appears swollen and surrounded by nerve fiber layer splinter hemorrhages (Fig. 29-9). AION is divided into two forms: arteritic and nonarteritic. The nonarteritic form of AION is most common. No specific cause can be identified, although diabetes and hypertension are frequent risk factors. No treatment is available. About 5% of patients, especially those over age 60, develop the arteritic form of AION in conjunction with giant cell (temporal) arteritis (Chap. 319). It is urgent to recognize arteritic AION so that high doses of glucocorticoids can be instituted immediately to prevent blindness in the second eye. Symptoms of polymyalgia rheumatica may be present; the sedimentation rate and C-reactive protein level are usually elevated. In a patient with visual loss from suspected arteritic AION, temporal artery biopsy is mandatory to confirm the diagnosis. Glucocorticoids should be started immediately, without waiting for the biopsy to be completed. The diagnosis of arteritic AION is difficult to sustain in the face of a negative temporal artery biopsy, but such cases do occur rarely.

Posterior Ischemic Optic Neuropathy This is an infrequent cause of acute visual loss, induced by the combination of severe anemia and hypotension. Cases have been reported after major blood loss during surgery, exsanguinating trauma, gastrointestinal bleeding, and renal dialysis. The fundus usually appears normal, although optic disc swelling develops if the process extends far enough anteriorly. Vision can be salvaged in some patients by prompt blood transfusion and reversal of hypotension.

Optic Neuritis This is a common inflammatory disease of the optic nerve. In the Optic Neuritis Treatment Trial (ONTT), the mean age of patients was 32 years, 77% were female, 92% had ocular pain (especially with eye movements), and 35% had optic disc swelling. In most patients, the demyelinating event was retrobulbar and the ocular fundus appeared normal on initial examination (Fig. 29-10), although optic disc pallor slowly developed over subsequent months.

Virtually all patients experience a gradual recovery of vision after a single episode of optic neuritis, even without treatment. This rule is so reliable that failure of vision to improve after a first attack of optic

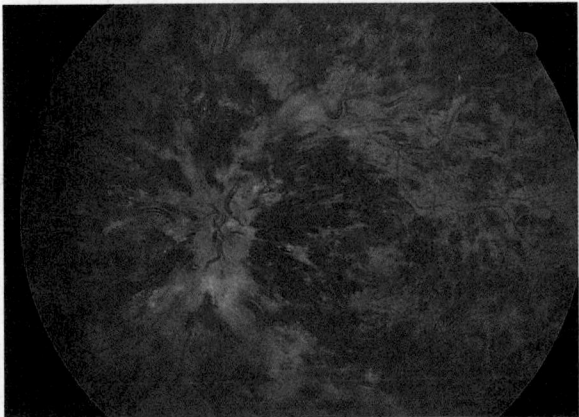

FIGURE 29-8 Central retinal vein occlusion can produce massive retinal hemorrhage ("blood and thunder"), ischemia, and vision loss.

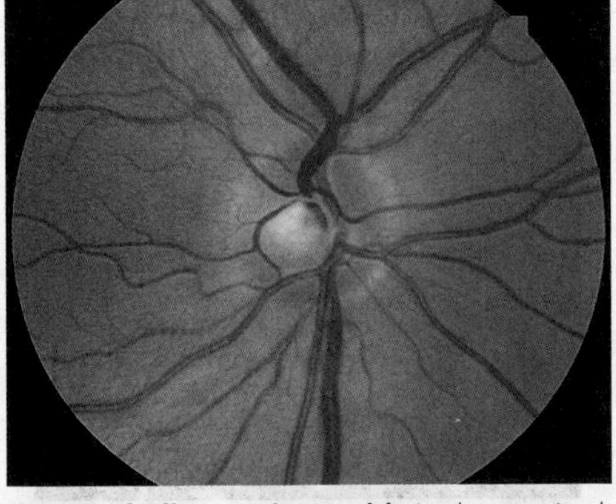

FIGURE 29-10 Retrobulbar optic neuritis is characterized by a normal fundus examination initially, hence the rubric, "the doctor sees nothing, and the patient sees nothing." Optic atrophy develops after severe or repeated attacks.

 neuritis casts doubt upon the original diagnosis. Treatment with high-dose IV methylprednisolone (250 mg every 6 h for 3 days) followed by oral prednisone (1 mg/kg per day for 11 days) makes no difference in final acuity (measured 6 months after the attack), but the recovery of visual function occurs more rapidly.

For some patients, optic neuritis remains an isolated event. However, the ONTT showed that the 10-year cumulative probability of developing clinically definite multiple sclerosis following optic neuritis is 38%. In patients with two or more demyelinating plaques on brain magnetic resonance (MR) imaging, treatment with interferon beta-1a can retard the development of more lesions. In summary, an MR scan is recommended in every patient with a first attack of optic neuritis. When visual loss is severe (worse than 20/100), treatment with intravenous followed by oral glucocorticoids hastens recovery. If multiple lesions are present on the MR scan, treatment with interferon β-1a should be considered.

Leber's Hereditary Optic Neuropathy This disease usually affects young men, causing gradual, painless, severe, central visual loss in one eye, followed weeks or months later by the same process in the other eye. Acutely, the optic disc appears mildly plethoric with surface capillary telangiectases, but no vascular leakage on fluorescein angiography. Eventually optic atrophy ensues. Leber's optic neuropathy is caused by a point mutation at codon 11778 in the mitochondrial gene encoding nicotinamide adenine dinucleotide dehydrogenase (NADH) subunit 4. Additional mutations responsible for the disease have been identified, most in mitochondrial genes encoding proteins involved in electron transport. Mitochondrial mutations causing Leber's neuropathy are inherited from the mother by all her children, but usually only sons develop symptoms. There is no treatment.

Toxic Optic Neuropathy This can result in acute visual loss with bilateral optic disc swelling and central or cecocentral scotomas. Such cases have been reported to result from exposure to ethambutol, methyl alcohol (moonshine), ethylene glycol (antifreeze), or carbon monoxide. In toxic optic neuropathy, visual loss can also develop gradually and produce optic atrophy (Fig. 29-11) without a phase of acute optic disc edema. Many agents have been implicated as a cause of toxic optic neuropathy, but the evidence supporting the association for many is weak. The following is a partial list of potential offending drugs or toxins: disulfiram, ethchlorvynol, chloramphenicol, amiodarone, monoclonal anti-CD3 antibody, ciprofloxacin, digitalis, streptomycin, lead, arsenic, thallium, D-penicillamine, isoniazid, emetine, and sulfonamides. Deficiency states, induced either by starvation, malabsorption, or alcoholism, can lead to insidious visual loss. Thiamine, vitamin B_{12}, and folate levels should be checked in any patient with unexplained, bilateral central scotomas and optic pallor.

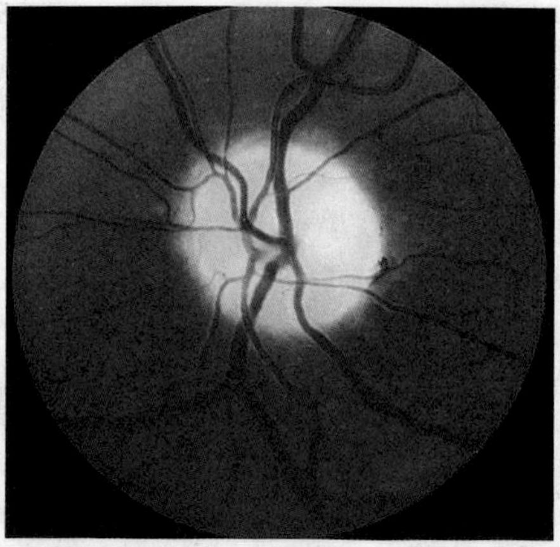

FIGURE 29-11 Optic atrophy is not a specific diagnosis, but refers to the combination of optic disc pallor, arteriolar narrowing, and nerve fiber layer destruction produced by a host of eye diseases, especially optic neuropathies.

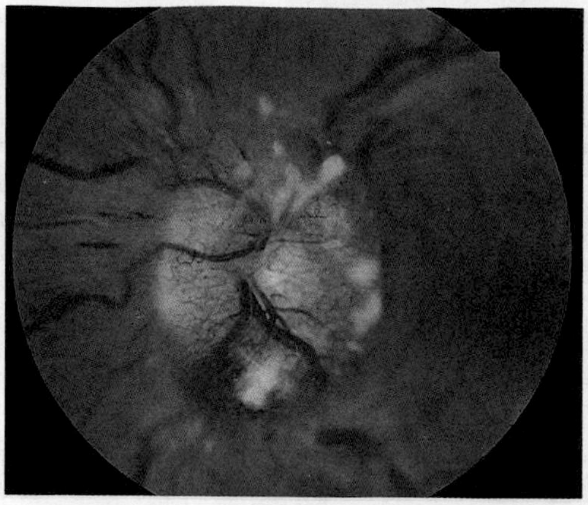

FIGURE 29-12 Papilledema means optic disc edema from raised intracranial pressure. This obese young woman with pseudotumor cerebri was misdiagnosed as a migraineur until fundus examination was performed, showing optic disc elevation, hemorrhages, and cotton-wool spots.

Papilledema This connotes bilateral optic disc swelling from raised intracranial pressure (Fig. 29-12). Headache is a frequent, but not invariable, accompaniment. All other forms of optic disc swelling, e.g., from optic neuritis or ischemic optic neuropathy, should be called "optic disc edema." This convention is arbitrary but serves to avoid confusion. Often it is difficult to differentiate papilledema from other forms of optic disc edema by fundus examination alone. Transient visual obscurations are a classic symptom of papilledema. They can occur in only one eye or simultaneously in both eyes. They usually last seconds but can persist longer. Obscurations follow abrupt shifts in posture or happen spontaneously. When obscurations are prolonged or spontaneous, the papilledema is more threatening. Visual acuity is not affected by papilledema unless the papilledema is severe, longstanding, or accompanied by macular edema and hemorrhage. Visual field testing shows enlarged blind spots and peripheral constriction (Fig. 29-3*F*). With unremitting papilledema, peripheral visual field loss progresses in an insidious fashion while the optic nerve develops atrophy. In this setting, reduction of optic disc swelling is an ominous sign of a dying nerve rather than an encouraging indication of resolving papilledema.

Evaluation of papilledema requires neuroimaging to exclude an intracranial lesion. MR angiography is appropriate in selected cases to search for a dural venous sinus occlusion or an arteriovenous shunt. If neuroradiologic studies are negative, the subarachnoid opening pressure should be measured by lumbar puncture. An elevated pressure, with normal cerebrospinal fluid, points by exclusion to the diagnosis of *pseudotumor cerebri* (idiopathic intracranial hypertension). The majority of patients are young, female, and obese. Treatment with a carbonic anhydrase inhibitor such as acetazolamide lowers intracranial pressure by reducing the production of cerebrospinal fluid. Weight reduction is vital but often unsuccessful. If acetazolamide and weight loss fail, and visual field loss is progressive, a shunt should be performed without delay to prevent blindness. Occasionally, emergency surgery is required for sudden blindness caused by fulminant papilledema.

Optic Disc Drusen These are refractile deposits within the substance of the optic nerve head (Fig. 29-13). They are unrelated to drusen of the retina, which occur in age-related macular degeneration. Optic disc drusen are most common in people of northern European descent. Their diagnosis is obvious when they are visible as glittering particles upon the surface of the optic disc. However, in many patients they are hidden beneath the surface, producing pseudo-papilledema. It is important to recognize optic disc drusen to avoid an unnecessary evaluation for papilledema. Ultrasound or CT scanning is sensitive for detection of buried optic disc drusen because they contain calcium. In most patients, optic disc drusen are an incidental, innocuous finding, but they can produce visual obscurations. On perimetry they give rise

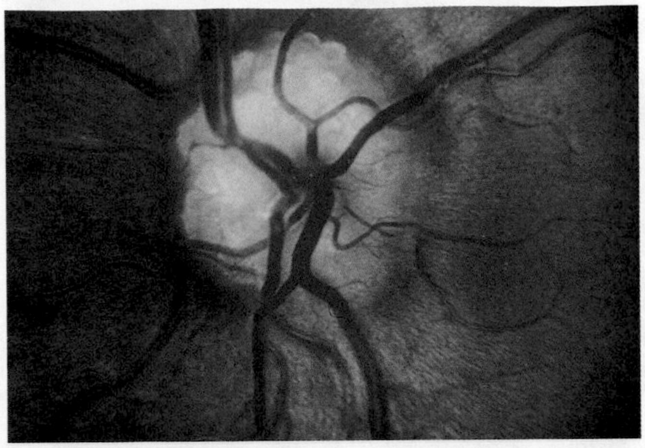

FIGURE 29-13 **Optic disc drusen** are calcified deposits of unknown etiology within the optic disc. They are sometimes confused with papilledema.

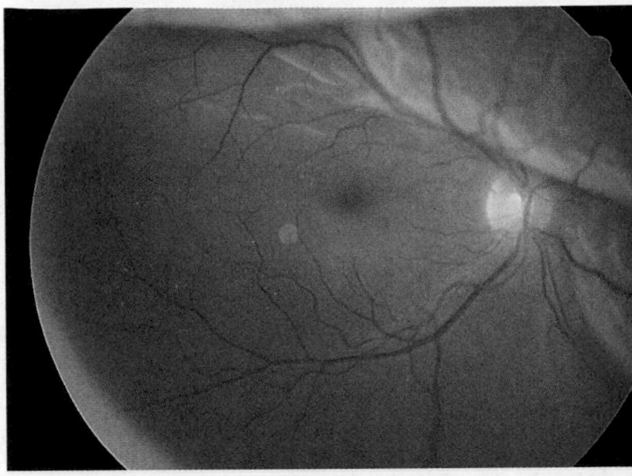

FIGURE 29-14 **Retinal detachment** appears as an elevated sheet of retinal tissue with folds. In this patient the fovea was spared, so acuity was normal, but a superior detachment produced an inferior scotoma.

to enlarged blind spots and arcuate scotomas from damage to the optic disc. With increasing age, drusen tend to become more exposed on the disc surface as optic atrophy develops. Hemorrhage, choroidal neovascular membrane, and AION are more likely to occur in patients with optic disc drusen. No treatment is available.

Vitreous Degeneration This occurs in all individuals with advancing age, leading to visual symptoms. Opacities develop in the vitreous, casting annoying shadows upon the retina. As the eye moves, these distracting "floaters" move synchronously, with a slight lag caused by inertia of the vitreous gel. Vitreous traction upon the retina causes mechanical stimulation, resulting in perception of flashing lights. This photopsia is brief and confined to one eye, in contrast to the bilateral, prolonged scintillations of cortical migraine. Contraction of the vitreous can result in sudden separation from the retina, heralded by an alarming shower of floaters and photopsia. This process, known as *vitreous detachment*, is a frequent involutional event in the elderly. It is not harmful unless it damages the retina. A careful examination of the dilated fundus is important in any patient complaining of floaters or photopsia to search for peripheral tears or holes. If such a lesion is found, laser application can forestall a retinal detachment. Occasionally a tear ruptures a retinal blood vessel, causing vitreous hemorrhage and sudden loss of vision. On attempted ophthalmoscopy the fundus is hidden by a dark red haze of blood. Ultrasound is required to examine the interior of the eye for a retinal tear or detachment. If the hemorrhage does not resolve spontaneously, the vitreous can be removed surgically. Vitreous hemorrhage also occurs from the fragile neovascular vessels that proliferate on the surface of the retina in diabetes, sickle cell anemia, and other ischemic ocular diseases.

Retinal Detachment This produces symptoms of floaters, flashing lights, and a scotoma in the peripheral visual field corresponding to the detachment (Fig. 29-14). If the detachment includes the fovea, there is an afferent pupil defect and the visual acuity is reduced. In most eyes, retinal detachment starts with a hole, flap, or tear in the peripheral retina (rhegmatogenous retinal detachment). Patients with peripheral retinal thinning (lattice degeneration) are particularly vulnerable to this process. Once a break has developed in the retina, liquified vitreous is free to enter the subretinal space, separating the retina from the pigment epithelium. The combination of vitreous traction upon the retinal surface and passage of fluid behind the retina leads inexorably to detachment. Patients with a history of myopia, trauma, or prior cataract extraction are at greatest risk for retinal detachment. The diagnosis is confirmed by ophthalmoscopic examination of the dilated eye.

Classic Migraine (See also Chap. 15) This usually occurs with a visual aura lasting about 20 min. In a typical attack, a small central disturbance in the field of vision marches toward the periphery, leaving a transient scotoma in its wake. The expanding border of migraine scotoma has a scintillating, dancing, or zig-zag edge, resembling the bastions of a fortified city, hence the term *fortification spectra*. Patients' descriptions of fortification spectra vary widely and can be confused with amaurosis fugax. Migraine patterns usually last longer and are perceived in both eyes, whereas amaurosis fugax is briefer and occurs in only one eye. Migraine phenomena also remain visible in the dark or with the eyes closed. Generally they are confined to either the right or left visual hemifield, but sometimes both fields are involved simultaneously. Patients often have a long history of stereotypic attacks. After the visual symptoms recede, headache develops in most patients.

Transient Ischemic Attacks Vertebrobasilar insufficiency may result in acute homonymous visual symptoms. Many patients mistakenly describe symptoms in their left or right eye, when in fact they are occurring in the left or right hemifield of both eyes. Interruption of blood supply to the visual cortex causes a sudden fogging or graying of vision, occasionally with flashing lights or other positive phenomena that mimic migraine. Cortical ischemic attacks are briefer in duration than migraine, occur in older patients, and are not followed by headache. There may be associated signs of brainstem ischemia, such as diplopia, vertigo, numbness, weakness, or dysarthria.

Stroke This occurs when interruption of blood supply from the posterior cerebral artery to the visual cortex is prolonged. The only finding on examination is a homonymous visual field defect that stops abruptly at the vertical meridian. Occipital lobe stroke is usually due to thrombotic occlusion of the vertebrobasilar system, embolus, or dissection. Lobar hemorrhage, tumor, abscess, and arteriovenous malformation are other common causes of hemianopic cortical visual loss.

Factitious (Functional, Nonorganic) Visual Loss This is claimed by hysterics or malingerers. The latter comprise the vast majority, seeking sympathy, special treatment, or financial gain by feigning loss of sight. The diagnosis is suspected when the history is atypical, physical findings are lacking or contradictory, inconsistencies emerge on testing, and a secondary motive can be identified. In our litigious society, the fraudulent pursuit of recompense has spawned an epidemic of factitious visual loss.

CHRONIC VISUAL LOSS

Cataract This is a clouding of the lens sufficient to reduce vision. Most cataracts develop slowly as a result of aging, leading to gradual impairment of vision. The formation of cataract occurs more rapidly in patients with a history of ocular trauma, uveitis, or diabetes mellitus. Cataracts are acquired in a variety of genetic diseases, such as myotonic dystrophy, neurofibromatosis type 2, and galactosemia. Radiation therapy and glucocorticoid treatment can induce cataract as a side effect. The cataracts associated with radiation or glucocorticoids have a typical posterior subcapsular location. Cataract can be detected by noting an impaired red reflex when viewing light reflected from the fundus with an ophthalmoscope or by examining the dilated eye using the slit lamp.

The only treatment for cataract is surgical extraction of the opacified lens. Over a million cataract operations are performed each year in the United States. The operation is generally done under local anesthesia on an outpatient basis. A plastic or silicone intraocular lens is placed within the empty lens capsule in the posterior chamber, substituting for the natural lens and leading to rapid recovery of sight. More than 95% of patients who undergo cataract extraction can expect an improvement in vision. In some patients, the lens capsule remaining in the eye after cataract extraction eventually turns cloudy, causing secondary loss of vision. A small opening is made in the lens capsule with a laser to restore clarity.

Glaucoma This is a slowly progressive, insidious optic neuropathy, usually associated with chronic elevation of intraocular pressure. In Americans of African descent it is the leading cause of blindness. The mechanism whereby raised intraocular pressure injures the optic nerve is not understood. Axons entering the inferotemporal and superotemporal aspects of the optic disc are damaged first, producing typical nerve fiber bundle or arcuate scotomas on perimetric testing. As fibers are destroyed, the neural rim of the optic disc shrinks and the physiologic cup within the optic disc enlarges (Fig. 29-15). This process is referred to as pathologic "cupping." The cup-to-disc diameter is expressed as a ratio, e.g., 0.2/1. The cup-to-disc ratio ranges widely in normal individuals, making it difficult to diagnose glaucoma reliably simply by observing an unusually large or deep optic cup. Careful documentation of serial examinations is helpful. In the patient with physiologic cupping, the large cup remains stable, whereas in the patient with glaucoma it expands relentlessly over the years. Detection of visual field loss by computerized perimetry also contributes to the diagnosis. Finally, most patients with glaucoma have raised intraocular pressure. However, many patients with typical glaucomatous cupping and visual field loss have intraocular pressures that apparently never exceed the normal limit of 20 mmHg (so-called low-tension glaucoma).

In acute angle-closure glaucoma, the eye is red and painful due to abrupt, severe elevation of intraocular pressure. Such cases account for only a minority of glaucoma cases: most patients have open, anterior chamber angles. The cause of raised intraocular pressure in open angle glaucoma is unknown, but it is associated with gene mutations in the heritable forms.

Glaucoma is usually painless (except in angle-closure glaucoma). Foveal acuity is spared until end-stage disease is reached. For these reasons, severe and irreversible damage can occur before either the patient or physician recognizes the diagnosis. Screening of patients for glaucoma by noting the cup-to-disc ratio on ophthalmoscopy and by measuring intraocular pressure is vital. Glaucoma is treated with topical adrenergic agonists, cholinergic agonists, beta blockers, and prostaglandin analogues. Occasionally, systemic absorption of beta blocker from eye drops can be sufficient to cause side effects of bradycardia, hypotension, heart block, bronchospasm, or depression. Topical or oral carbonic anhydrase inhibitors are used to lower intraocular pressure by reducing aqueous production. Laser treatment of the trabecular meshwork in the anterior chamber angle improves aqueous outflow from the eye. If medical or laser treatments fail to halt optic nerve damage from glaucoma, a filter must be constructed surgically (trabeculectomy) or a valve placed to release aqueous from the eye in a controlled fashion.

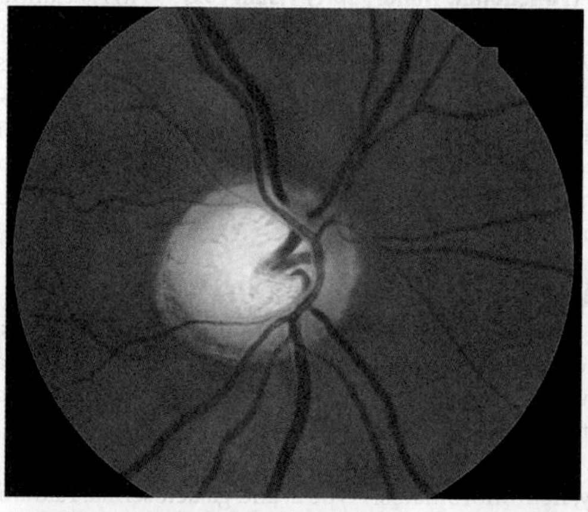

FIGURE 29-15 Glaucoma results in "cupping" as the neural rim is destroyed and the central cup becomes enlarged and excavated. The cup-to-disc ratio is about 0.7/1.0 in this patient.

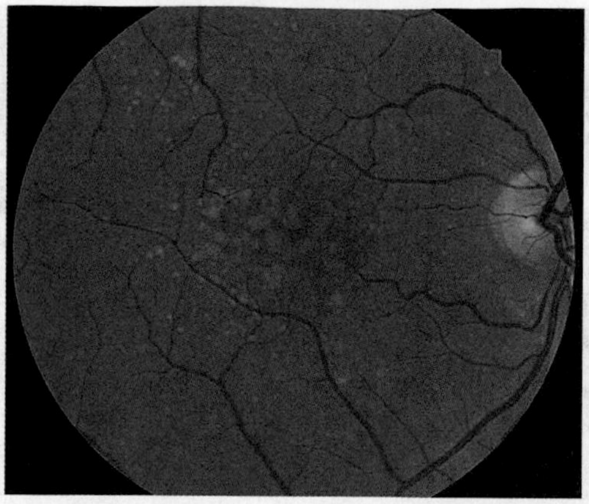

FIGURE 29-16 Age-related macular degeneration begins with the accumulation of drusen within the macula. They appear as scattered yellow subretinal deposits.

Macular Degeneration This is a major cause of gradual, painless, bilateral central visual loss in the elderly. The old term, "senile macular degeneration," misinterpreted by many patients as an unflattering reference, has been replaced with "age-related macular degeneration." It occurs in a nonexudative (dry) form and an exudative (wet) form. Inflammation may be important in both forms of macular degeneration; recent genetic data indicates that susceptibility is associated with variants in the gene for complement factor H, an inhibitor of the alternative complement pathway. The nonexudative process begins with the accumulation of extracellular deposits, called drusen, underneath the retinal pigment epithelium. On ophthalmoscopy, they are pleomorphic but generally appear as small discrete yellow lesions clustered in the macula (Fig. 29-16). With time they become larger, more numerous, and confluent. The retinal pigment epithelium becomes focally detached and atrophic, causing visual loss by interfering with photoreceptor function. Treatment with vitamins C and E, beta carotene, and zinc may retard dry macular degeneration.

Exudative macular degeneration, which develops in only a minority of patients, occurs when neovascular vessels from the choroid grow through defects in Bruch's membrane into the potential space beneath the retinal pigment epithelium. Leakage from these vessels produces elevation of the retina and pigment epithelium, with distortion (metamorphopsia) and blurring of vision. Although onset of these symptoms is usually gradual, bleeding from subretinal choroidal neovascular membranes sometimes causes acute visual loss. The neovascular membranes can be difficult to see on fundus examination because they are beneath the retina. Fluorescein or indocyanine green angiography is extremely useful for their detection. Neovascular membranes are treated with either photodynamic therapy or intraocular injection of vascular endothelial growth factor antagonists. Surgical attempts to remove subretinal membranes in age-related macular degeneration have not improved vision in most patients. However, outcomes have been more encouraging for patients with choroidal neovascular membranes from ocular histoplasmosis syndrome.

Major or repeated hemorrhage under the retina from neovascular membranes results in fibrosis, development of a round (disciform) macular scar, and permanent loss of central vision.

Central Serous Chorioretinopathy This primarily affects males between the ages of 20 and 50. Leakage of serous fluid from the choroid causes small, localized detachment of the retinal pigment epithelium and the neurosensory retina. These detachments produce acute or chronic symptoms of metamorphopsia and blurred vision when the macula is involved. They are difficult to visualize with a direct ophthalmoscope because the detached retina is transparent and only slightly elevated. Diagnosis of central serous chorioretinopathy is made easily by fluorescein angiography, which shows dye streaming into the subretinal space. The cause of central serous chorioretinopathy is unknown. Symptoms may resolve spontaneously if the retina reattaches, but recurrent detachment is common. Laser photocoagulation has benefited some patients with this condition.

Diabetic Retinopathy A rare disease until 1921, when the discovery of insulin resulted in a dramatic improvement in life expectancy for patients with diabetes mellitus, it is now a leading cause of blindness in the United States. The retinopathy of diabetes takes years to develop but eventually appears in nearly all cases. Regular surveillance of the dilated fundus is crucial for any patient with diabetes. In advanced diabetic retinopathy, the proliferation of neovascular vessels leads to blindness from vitreous hemorrhage, retinal detachment, and glaucoma (see Fig. 338-9). These complications can be avoided in most patients by administration of panretinal laser photocoagulation at the appropriate point in the evolution of the disease. For further discussion of the manifestations and management of diabetic retinopathy, see Chap. 338.

Retinitis Pigmentosa This is a general term for a disparate group of rod and cone dystrophies characterized by progressive night blindness, visual field constriction with a ring scotoma, loss of acuity, and an abnormal electroretinogram (ERG). It occurs sporadically or in an autosomal recessive, dominant, or X-linked pattern. Irregular black deposits of clumped pigment in the peripheral retina, called *bone spicules* because of their vague resemblance to the spicules of cancellous bone, give the disease its name (Fig. 29-17). The name is actually a misnomer because retinitis pigmentosa is not an inflammatory process. Most cases are due to a mutation in the gene for rhodopsin, the rod photopigment, or in the gene for peripherin, a glycoprotein located in photoreceptor outer segments. Vitamin A (15,000 IU/day) slightly retards the deterioration of the ERG in patients with retinitis pigmentosa but has no beneficial effect on visual acuity or fields. Some forms of retinitis pigmentosa occur in association with rare, hereditary systemic diseases (olivopontocerebellar degeneration, Bassen-Kornzweig disease, Kearns-Sayre syndrome, Refsum's disease). Chronic treatment with chloroquine, hydroxychloroquine, and phenothiazines (especially thioridazine) can produce visual loss from a toxic retinopathy that resembles retinitis pigmentosa.

Epiretinal Membrane This is a fibrocellular tissue that grows across the inner surface of the retina, causing metamorphopsia and reduced visual acuity from distortion of the macula. A crinkled, cellophane-like membrane is visible on the retinal examination. Epiretinal membrane is most common in patients over 50 years of age and is usually unilateral. Most cases are idiopathic, but some occur as a result of hypertensive retinopathy, diabetes, retinal detachment, or trauma. When visual acuity is reduced to the level of about 6/24 (20/80), vitrectomy and surgical peeling of the membrane to relieve macular puckering are recommended. Contraction of an epiretinal membrane sometimes gives rise to a *macular hole*. Most macular holes, however, are caused by local vitreous traction within the fovea. Vitrectomy can improve acuity in selected cases.

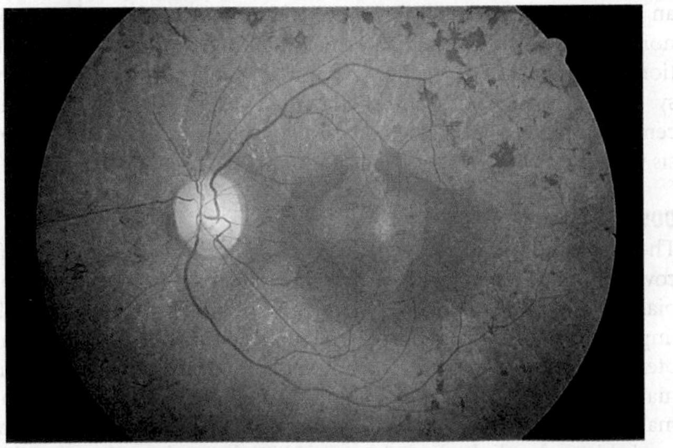

FIGURE 29-17 Retinitis pigmentosa with black clumps of pigment in the retinal periphery known as "bone spicules." There is also atrophy of the retinal pigment epithelium, making the vasculature of the choroid easily visible.

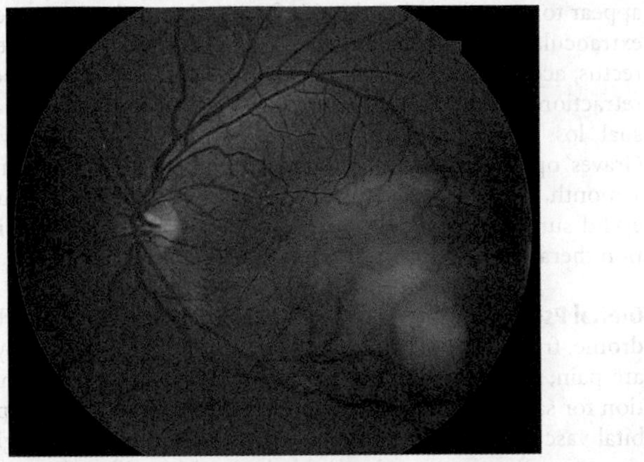

FIGURE 29-18 Melanoma of the choroid, appearing as an elevated dark mass in the inferior temporal fundus, just encroaching upon the fovea.

Melanoma and Other Tumors Melanoma is the most common primary tumor of the eye (Fig. 29-18). It causes photopsia, an enlarging scotoma, and loss of vision. A small melanoma is often difficult to differentiate from a benign choroidal nevus. Serial examinations are required to document a malignant pattern of growth. Treatment of melanoma is controversial. Options include enucleation, local resection, and irradiation. *Metastatic tumors* to the eye outnumber primary tumors. Breast and lung carcinoma have a special propensity to spread to the choroid or iris. Leukemia and lymphoma also commonly invade ocular tissues. Sometimes their only sign on eye examination is cellular debris in the vitreous, which can masquerade as a chronic posterior uveitis. *Retrobulbar tumor* of the optic nerve (meningioma, glioma) or *chiasmal tumor* (pituitary adenoma, meningioma) produces gradual visual loss with few objective findings, except for optic disc pallor. Rarely, sudden expansion of a pituitary adenoma from infarction and bleeding (*pituitary apoplexy*) causes acute retrobulbar visual loss, with headache, nausea, and ocular motor nerve palsies. In any patient with visual field loss or optic atrophy, CT or MR scanning should be considered if the cause remains unknown after careful review of the history and thorough examination of the eye.

PROPTOSIS

When the globes appear asymmetric, the clinician must first decide which eye is abnormal. Is one eye recessed within the orbit (*enophthalmos*) or is the other eye protuberant (*exophthalmos*, or *proptosis*)? A small globe or a Horner's syndrome can give the appearance of enophthalmos. True enophthalmos occurs commonly after trauma, from atrophy of retrobulbar fat, or fracture of the orbital floor. The position of the eyes within the orbits is measured using a Hertel exophthalmometer, a hand-held instrument that records the position of the anterior corneal surface relative to the lateral orbital rim. If this instrument is not available, relative eye position can be judged by bending the patient's head forward and looking down upon the orbits. A proptosis of only 2 mm in one eye is detectable from this perspective. The development of proptosis implies a space-occupying lesion in the orbit, and usually warrants CT or MR imaging.

Graves' Ophthalmopathy This is the leading cause of proptosis in adults (Chap. 335). The proptosis is often asymmetric and can even appear to be unilateral. Orbital inflammation and engorgement of the extraocular muscles, particularly the medial rectus and the inferior rectus, account for the protrusion of the globe. Corneal exposure, lid retraction, conjunctival injection, restriction of gaze, diplopia, and visual loss from optic nerve compression are cardinal symptoms. Graves' ophthalmopathy is treated with oral prednisone (60 mg/d) for 1 month, followed by a taper over several months, topical lubricants, eyelid surgery, eye muscle surgery, or orbital decompression. Radiation therapy is not effective.

Orbital Pseudotumor This is an idiopathic, inflammatory orbital syndrome, frequently confused with Graves' ophthalmopathy. Symptoms are pain, limited eye movements, proptosis, and congestion. Evaluation for sarcoidosis, Wegener's granulomatosis, and other types of orbital vasculitis or collagen-vascular disease is negative. Imaging often shows swollen eye muscles (orbital myositis) with enlarged tendons. By contrast, in Graves' ophthalmopathy the tendons of the eye muscles are usually spared. The Tolosa-Hunt syndrome may be regarded as an extension of orbital pseudotumor through the superior orbital fissure into the cavernous sinus. The diagnosis of orbital pseudotumor is difficult. Biopsy of the orbit frequently yields nonspecific evidence of fat infiltration by lymphocytes, plasma cells, and eosinophils. A dramatic response to a therapeutic trial of systemic glucocorticoids indirectly provides the best confirmation of the diagnosis.

Orbital Cellulitis This causes pain, lid erythema, proptosis, conjunctival chemosis, restricted motility, decreased acuity, afferent pupillary defect, fever, and leukocytosis. It often arises from the paranasal sinuses, especially by contiguous spread of infection from the ethmoid sinus through the lamina papyracea of the medial orbit. A history of recent upper respiratory tract infection, chronic sinusitis, thick mucous secretions, or dental disease is significant in any patient with suspected orbital cellulitis. Blood cultures should be obtained, but they are usually negative. Most patients respond to empirical therapy with broad-spectrum IV antibiotics. Occasionally, orbital cellulitis follows an overwhelming course, with massive proptosis, blindness, septic cavernous sinus thrombosis, and meningitis. To avert this disaster, orbital cellulitis should be managed aggressively in the early stages, with immediate imaging of the orbits and antibiotic therapy that includes coverage of methicillin-resistant *Staphylococcus aureus*. Prompt surgical drainage of an orbital abscess or paranasal sinusitis is indicated if optic nerve function deteriorates despite antibiotics.

Tumors Tumors of the orbit cause painless, progressive proptosis. The most common primary tumors are hemangioma, lymphangioma, neurofibroma, dermoid cyst, adenoid cystic carcinoma, optic nerve glioma, optic nerve meningioma, and benign mixed tumor of the lacrimal gland. Metastatic tumor to the orbit occurs frequently in breast carcinoma, lung carcinoma, and lymphoma. Diagnosis by fine-needle aspiration followed by urgent radiation therapy can sometimes preserve vision.

Carotid Cavernous Fistulas With anterior drainage through the orbit these produce proptosis, diplopia, glaucoma, and corkscrew, arterialized conjunctival vessels. Direct fistulas usually result from trauma. They are easily diagnosed because of the prominent signs produced by high-flow, high-pressure shunting. Indirect fistulas, or dural arteriovenous malformations, are more likely to occur spontaneously, especially in older women. The signs are more subtle and the diagnosis is frequently missed. The combination of slight proptosis, diplopia, enlarged muscles, and an injected eye is often mistaken for thyroid ophthalmopathy. A bruit heard upon auscultation of the head, or reported by the patient, is a valuable diagnostic clue. Imaging shows an enlarged superior ophthalmic vein in the orbits. Carotid cavernous shunts can be eliminated by intravascular embolization.

PTOSIS

Blepharoptosis This is an abnormal drooping of the eyelid. Unilateral or bilateral ptosis can be congenital, from dysgenesis of the levator palpebrae superioris, or from abnormal insertion of its aponeurosis into the eyelid. Acquired ptosis can develop so gradually that the patient is unaware of the problem. Inspection of old photographs is helpful in dating the onset. A history of prior trauma, eye surgery, contact lens use, diplopia, systemic symptoms (e.g., dysphagia or peripheral muscle weakness), or a family history of ptosis should be sought. Fluctuating ptosis that worsens late in the day is typical of myasthenia gravis. Examination should focus upon evidence for proptosis, eyelid masses or deformities, inflammation, pupil inequality, or limitation of motility. The width of the palpebral fissures is measured in primary gaze to quantitate the degree of ptosis. The ptosis will be underestimated if the patient compensates by lifting the brow with the frontalis muscle.

Mechanical Ptosis This occurs in many elderly patients from stretching and redundancy of eyelid skin and subcutaneous fat (dermatochalasis). The extra weight of these sagging tissues causes the lid to droop. Enlargement or deformation of the eyelid from infection, tumor, trauma, or inflammation also results in ptosis on a purely mechanical basis.

Aponeurotic Ptosis This is an acquired dehiscence or stretching of the aponeurotic tendon, which connects the levator muscle to the tarsal plate of the eyelid. It occurs commonly in older patients, presumably from loss of connective tissue elasticity. Aponeurotic ptosis is also a frequent sequela of eyelid swelling from infection or blunt trauma to the orbit, cataract surgery, or hard contact lens usage.

Myogenic Ptosis The causes of *myogenic ptosis* include myasthenia gravis (Chap. 381) and a number of rare myopathies that manifest with ptosis. The term *chronic progressive external ophthalmoplegia* refers to a spectrum of systemic diseases caused by mutations of mitochondrial DNA. As the name implies, the most prominent findings are symmetric, slowly progressive ptosis and limitation of eye movements. In general, diplopia is a late symptom because all eye movements are reduced equally. In the *Kearns-Sayre* variant, retinal pigmentary changes and abnormalities of cardiac conduction develop. Peripheral muscle biopsy shows characteristic "ragged-red fibers." *Oculopharyngeal dystrophy* is a distinct autosomal dominant disease with onset in middle age, characterized by ptosis, limited eye movements, and trouble swallowing. *Myotonic dystrophy*, another autosomal dominant disorder, causes ptosis, ophthalmoparesis, cataract, and pigmentary retinopathy. Patients have muscle wasting, myotonia, frontal balding, and cardiac abnormalities.

Neurogenic Ptosis This results from a lesion affecting the innervation to either of the two muscles that open the eyelid: Müller's muscle or the levator palpebrae superioris. Examination of the pupil helps to distinguish between these two possibilities. In Horner's syndrome, the eye with ptosis has a smaller pupil and the eye movements are full. In an oculomotor nerve palsy, the eye with the ptosis has a larger, or a normal, pupil. If the pupil is normal but there is limitation of adduction, elevation, and depression, a pupil-sparing oculomotor nerve palsy is likely (see next section). Rarely, a lesion affecting the small, central subnucleus of the oculomotor complex will cause bilateral ptosis with normal eye movements and pupils.

DOUBLE VISION (DIPLOPIA)

The first point to clarify is whether diplopia persists in either eye after covering the opposite eye. If it does, the diagnosis is monocular diplopia. The cause is usually intrinsic to the eye and therefore has no dire implications for the patient. Corneal aberrations (e.g., keratoconus, pterygium), uncorrected refractive error, cataract, or foveal traction may give rise to monocular diplopia. Occasionally it is a symptom of malingering or psychiatric disease. Diplopia alleviated by covering one eye is binocular diplopia and is caused by disruption of ocular alignment. Inquiry should be made into the nature of the double vision (purely side-by-side versus partial vertical displacement of images), mode of onset, duration, intermittency, diurnal variation, and associated neurologic or systemic symptoms. If the patient has diplopia while being examined, motility testing should reveal a deficiency corresponding to the patient's symptoms. However, subtle limitation of ocular excursions is often difficult to detect. For example, a patient with a slight left abducens nerve paresis may appear to have full eye movements, despite a complaint of horizontal diplopia upon looking to the left. In this situation, the cover test provides a more sensitive method for demonstrating the ocular misalignment. It should be conducted in primary gaze, and then with the head turned and tilted in each direction. In the above example, a cover test with the head turned to the right will maximize the fixation shift evoked by the cover test.

Occasionally, a cover test performed in an asymptomatic patient during a routine examination will reveal an ocular deviation. If the eye movements are full and the ocular misalignment is equal in all directions of gaze (concomitant deviation), the diagnosis is strabismus. In this condition, which affects about 1% of the population, fusion is disrupted in infancy or early childhood. To avoid diplopia, vision is suppressed from the nonfixating eye. In some children, this leads to impaired vision (amblyopia, or "lazy" eye) in the deviated eye.

Binocular diplopia occurs from a wide range of processes: infectious, neoplastic, metabolic, degenerative, inflammatory, and vascular. One must decide if the diplopia is neurogenic in origin or due to restriction of globe rotation by local disease in the orbit. Orbital pseudotumor, myositis, infection, tumor, thyroid disease, and muscle entrapment (e.g., from a blowout fracture) cause restrictive diplopia. The diagnosis of restriction is usually made by recognizing other associated signs and symptoms of local orbital disease in conjunction with imaging.

Myasthenia Gravis (See also Chap. 381) This is a major cause of diplopia. The diplopia is often intermittent, variable, and not confined to any single ocular motor nerve distribution. The pupils are always normal. Fluctuating ptosis may be present. Many patients have a purely ocular form of the disease, with no evidence of systemic muscular weakness. The diagnosis can be confirmed by an IV edrophonium injection or by an assay for antiacetylcholine receptor antibodies. Negative results from these tests do not exclude the diagnosis. *Botulism* from food or wound poisoning can mimic ocular myasthenia.

After restrictive orbital disease and myasthenia gravis are excluded, a lesion of a cranial nerve supplying innervation to the extraocular muscles is the most likely cause of binocular diplopia.

Oculomotor Nerve The third cranial nerve innervates the medial, inferior, and superior recti; inferior oblique; levator palpebrae superioris; and the iris sphincter. Total palsy of the oculomotor nerve causes ptosis, a dilated pupil, and leaves the eye "down and out" because of the unopposed action of the lateral rectus and superior oblique. This combination of findings is obvious. More challenging is the diagnosis of early or partial oculomotor nerve palsy. In this setting, any combination of ptosis, pupil dilation, and weakness of the eye muscles supplied by the oculomotor nerve may be encountered. Frequent serial examinations during the evolving phase of the palsy help ensure that the diagnosis is not missed. The advent of an oculomotor nerve palsy with a pupil involvement, especially when accompanied by pain, suggests a compressive lesion, such as a tumor or circle of Willis aneurysm. Neuroimaging should be obtained, along with a CT or MR angiogram. Occasionally, a catheter arteriogram must be done to exclude an aneurysm.

A lesion of the oculomotor nucleus in the rostral midbrain produces signs that differ from those caused by a lesion of the nerve itself. There is bilateral ptosis because the levator muscle is innervated by a single central subnucleus. There is also weakness of the contralateral superior rectus, because it is supplied by the oculomotor nucleus on the other side. Occasionally both superior recti are weak. Isolated nuclear oculomotor palsy is rare. Usually neurologic examination reveals additional signs to suggest brainstem damage from infarction, hemorrhage, tumor, or infection.

Injury to structures surrounding fascicles of the oculomotor nerve descending through the midbrain has given rise to a number of classic eponymic designations. In *Nothnagel's syndrome*, injury to the superior cerebellar peduncle causes ipsilateral oculomotor palsy and contralateral cerebellar ataxia. In *Benedikt's syndrome*, injury to the red nucleus results in ipsilateral oculomotor palsy and contralateral tremor, chorea, and athetosis. *Claude's syndrome* incorporates features of both the aforementioned syndromes, by injury to both the red nucleus and the superior cerebellar peduncle. Finally, in *Weber's syndrome*, injury to the cerebral peduncle causes ipsilateral oculomotor palsy with contralateral hemiparesis.

In the subarachnoid space the oculomotor nerve is vulnerable to aneurysm, meningitis, tumor, infarction, and compression. In cerebral herniation the nerve becomes trapped between the edge of the tentorium and the uncus of the temporal lobe. Oculomotor palsy can also occur from midbrain torsion and hemorrhages during herniation. In the cavernous sinus, oculomotor palsy arises from carotid aneurysm, carotid cavernous fistula, cavernous sinus thrombosis, tumor (pituitary adenoma, meningioma, metastasis), herpes zoster infection, and the Tolosa-Hunt syndrome.

The etiology of an isolated, pupil-sparing oculomotor palsy often remains an enigma, even after neuroimaging and extensive laboratory testing. Most cases are thought to result from microvascular infarction of the nerve, somewhere along its course from the brainstem to the orbit. Usually the patient complains of pain. Diabetes, hypertension, and vascular disease are major risk factors. Spontaneous recovery over a period of months is the rule. If this fails to occur, or if new findings develop, the diagnosis of microvascular oculomotor nerve palsy should be reconsidered. Aberrant regeneration is common when the oculomotor nerve is injured by trauma or compression (tumor, aneurysm). Miswiring of sprouting fibers to the levator muscle and the rectus muscles results in elevation of the eyelid upon downgaze or adduction. The pupil also constricts upon attempted adduction, elevation, or depression of the globe. Aberrant regeneration is not seen after oculomotor palsy from microvascular infarct and hence vitiates that diagnosis.

Trochlear Nerve The fourth cranial nerve originates in the midbrain, just caudal to the oculomotor nerve complex. Fibers exit the brainstem dorsally and cross to innervate the contralateral superior oblique. The principal actions of this muscle are to depress and to intort the globe. A palsy therefore results in hypertropia and excyclotorsion. The cyclotorsion is seldom noticed by patients. Instead, they complain of vertical diplopia, especially upon reading or looking down. The vertical diplopia is also exacerbated by tilting the head toward the side with the muscle palsy, and alleviated by tilting it away. This "head tilt test" is a cardinal diagnostic feature.

Isolated trochlear nerve palsy occurs from all the causes listed above for the oculomotor nerve, except aneurysm. The trochlear nerve is particularly apt to suffer injury after closed head trauma. The free edge of the tentorium is thought to impinge upon the nerve during a concussive blow. Most isolated trochlear nerve palsies are idiopathic and hence diagnosed by exclusion as "microvascular." Spontaneous improvement occurs over a period of months in most patients. A base-down prism (conveniently applied to the patient's glasses as a stick-on Fresnel lens) may serve as a temporary measure to alleviate diplopia. If the palsy does not resolve, the eyes can be realigned by weakening the inferior oblique muscle.

Abducens Nerve The sixth cranial nerve innervates the lateral rectus muscle. A palsy produces horizontal diplopia, worse on gaze to the side of the lesion. A nuclear lesion has different consequences, because the abducens nucleus contains interneurons that project via the medial longitudinal fasciculus to the medial rectus subnucleus of the contralateral oculomotor complex. Therefore, an abducens nuclear lesion produces a complete lateral gaze palsy, from weakness of both the ipsilateral lateral rectus and the contralateral medial rectus. *Foville's syndrome* following dorsal pontine injury includes lateral gaze palsy, ipsilateral facial palsy, and contralateral hemiparesis incurred by damage to descending corticospinal fibers. *Millard-*

 Gubler syndrome from ventral pontine injury is similar, except for the eye findings. There is lateral rectus weakness only, instead of gaze palsy, because the abducens fascicle is injured rather than the nucleus. Infarct, tumor, hemorrhage, vascular malformation, and multiple sclerosis are the most common etiologies of brainstem abducens palsy.

After leaving the ventral pons, the abducens nerve runs forward along the clivus to pierce the dura at the petrous apex, where it enters the cavernous sinus. Along its subarachnoid course it is susceptible to meningitis, tumor (meningioma, chordoma, carcinomatous meningitis), subarachnoid hemorrhage, trauma, and compression by aneurysm or dolichoectatic vessels. At the petrous apex, mastoiditis can produce deafness, pain, and ipsilateral abducens palsy (*Gradenigo's syndrome*). In the cavernous sinus, the nerve can be affected by carotid aneurysm, carotid cavernous fistula, tumor (pituitary adenoma, meningioma, nasopharyngeal carcinoma), herpes infection, and Tolosa-Hunt syndrome.

Unilateral or bilateral abducens palsy is a classic sign of raised intracranial pressure. The diagnosis can be confirmed if papilledema is observed on fundus examination. The mechanism is still debated but is probably related to rostral-caudal displacement of the brainstem. The same phenomenon accounts for abducens palsy from low intracranial pressure (e.g., after lumbar puncture, spinal anesthesia, or spontaneous dural cerebrospinal fluid leak).

Treatment of abducens palsy is aimed at prompt correction of the underlying cause. However, the cause remains obscure in many instances, despite diligent evaluation. As mentioned above for isolated trochlear or oculomotor palsy, most cases are assumed to represent microvascular infarcts because they often occur in the setting of diabetes or other vascular risk factors. Some cases may develop as a postinfectious mononeuritis (e.g., following a viral flu). Patching one eye or applying a temporary prism will provide relief of diplopia until the palsy resolves. If recovery is incomplete, eye muscle surgery can nearly always realign the eyes, at least in primary position. A patient with an abducens palsy that fails to improve should be reevaluated for an occult etiology (e.g., chordoma, carcinomatous meningitis, carotid cavernous fistula, myasthenia gravis).

Multiple Ocular Motor Nerve Palsies These should not be attributed to spontaneous microvascular events affecting more than one cranial nerve at a time. This remarkable coincidence does occur, especially in diabetic patients, but the diagnosis is made only in retrospect after exhausting all other diagnostic alternatives. Neuroimaging should focus on the cavernous sinus, superior orbital fissure, and orbital apex, where all three ocular motor nerves are in close proximity. In the diabetic or compromised host, fungal infection (*Aspergillus*, Mucorales, *Cryptococcus*) is a frequent cause of multiple nerve palsies. In the patient with systemic malignancy, carcinomatous meningitis is a likely diagnosis. Cytologic examination may be negative despite repeated sampling of the cerebrospinal fluid. The cancer-associated Lambert-Eaton myasthenic syndrome can also produce ophthalmoplegia. Giant cell (temporal) arteritis occasionally manifests as diplopia from ischemic palsies of extraocular muscles. Fisher syndrome, an ocular variant of Guillain-Barré, produces ophthalmoplegia with areflexia and ataxia. Often the ataxia is mild, and the reflexes are normal. Antiganglioside antibodies (GQ1b) can be detected in about 50% of cases.

Supranuclear Disorders of Gaze These are often mistaken for multiple ocular motor nerve palsies. For example, Wernicke's encephalopathy can produce nystagmus and a partial deficit of horizontal and vertical gaze that mimics a combined abducens and oculomotor nerve palsy. The disorder occurs in malnourished or alcoholic patients and can be reversed by thiamine. Infarct, hemorrhage, tumor, multiple sclerosis, encephalitis, vasculitis, and Whipple's disease are other important causes of supranuclear gaze palsy. Disorders of vertical gaze, especially downwards saccades, are an early feature of progressive supranuclear palsy. Smooth pursuit is affected later in the course of the disease. Parkinson's disease, Huntington's chorea, and olivopontocerebellar degeneration can also affect vertical gaze.

The *frontal eye field* of the cerebral cortex is involved in generation of saccades to the contralateral side. After hemispheric stroke, the eyes usually deviate towards the lesioned side because of the unopposed action of the frontal eye field in the normal hemisphere. With time, this deficit resolves. Seizures generally have the opposite effect: the eyes deviate conjugately away from the irritative focus. *Parietal lesions* disrupt smooth pursuit of targets moving toward the side of the lesion. Bilateral parietal lesions produce *Balint's syndrome*, characterized by impaired eye-hand coordination (optic ataxia), difficulty initiating voluntary eye movements (ocular apraxia), and visuospatial disorientation (simultanagnosia).

Horizontal Gaze Descending cortical inputs mediating horizontal gaze ultimately converge at the level of the pons. Neurons in the paramedian pontine reticular formation are responsible for controlling conjugate gaze toward the same side. They project directly to the ipsilateral abducens nucleus. A lesion of either the paramedian pontine reticular formation or the abducens nucleus causes an ipsilateral conjugate gaze palsy. Lesions at either locus produce nearly identical clinical syndromes, with the following exception: vestibular stimulation (oculocephalic maneuver or caloric irrigation) will succeed in driving the eyes conjugately to the side in a patient with a lesion of the paramedian pontine reticular formation, but not in a patient with a lesion of the abducens nucleus.

INTERNUCLEAR OPHTHALMOPLEGIA This results from damage to the medial longitudinal fasciculus ascending from the abducens nucleus in the pons to the oculomotor nucleus in the midbrain (hence, "internuclear"). Damage to fibers carrying the conjugate signal from abducens interneurons to the contralateral medial rectus motoneurons results in a failure of adduction on attempted lateral gaze. For example, a patient with a left internuclear ophthalmoplegia will have slowed or absent adducting movements of the left eye (Fig. 29-19). A patient with bilateral injury to the medial longitudinal fasciculus will have bilateral internuclear ophthalmoplegia. Multiple sclerosis is the most common cause, although tumor, stroke, trauma, or any brainstem process may be responsible. *One-and-a-half syndrome* is due to a combined lesion of the medial longitudinal fasciculus and the abducens nucleus on the same side. The patient's only horizontal eye movement is abduction of the eye on the other side.

Vertical Gaze This is controlled at the level of the midbrain. The neuronal circuits affected in disorders of vertical gaze are not fully elucidated, but lesions of the rostral interstitial nucleus of the medial longitudinal fasciculus and the interstitial nucleus of Cajal cause supranuclear paresis of upgaze, downgaze, or all vertical eye movements. Distal basilar artery ischemia is the most common etiology. *Skew deviation* refers to a vertical misalignment of the eyes, usually constant in all positions of gaze. The finding has poor localizing value because skew deviation has been reported after lesions in widespread regions of the brainstem and cerebellum.

PARINAUD'S SYNDROME Also known as dorsal midbrain syndrome, this is a distinct supranuclear vertical gaze disorder from damage to the posterior commissure. It is a classic sign of hydrocephalus from aqueductal stenosis. Pineal region tumors, cysticercosis, and stroke also cause Parinaud's syndrome. Features include loss of upgaze (and sometimes downgaze), convergence-retraction nystagmus on attempted upgaze, downwards ocular deviation ("setting sun" sign), lid retraction (Collier's sign), skew deviation, pseudoabducens palsy, and light-near dissociation of the pupils.

Nystagmus This is a rhythmical oscillation of the eyes, occurring physiologically from vestibular and optokinetic stimulation or pathologically in a wide variety of diseases (Chap. 22). Abnormalities of the eyes or optic nerves, present at birth or acquired in childhood, can

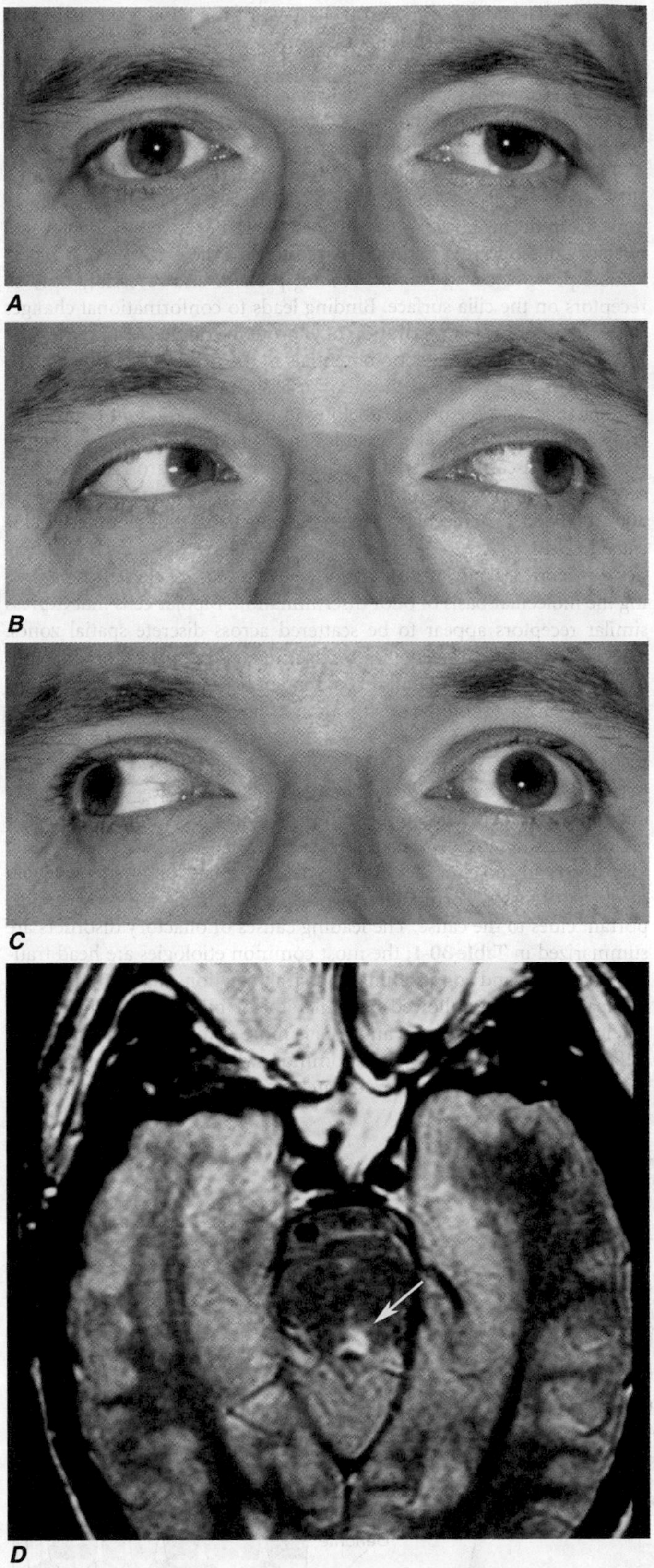

FIGURE 29-19 Left internuclear ophthalmoplegia (INO). ***A.*** In primary position of gaze the eyes appear normal. ***B.*** Horizontal gaze to the left is intact. ***C.*** On attempted horizontal gaze to the right, the left eye fails to adduct. In mildly affected patients the eye may adduct partially, or more slowly than normal. Nystagmus is usually present in the abducted eye. ***D.*** T2-weighted axial MRI image through the pons showing a demyelinating plaque in the left medial longitudinal fasciculus (*arrow*).

produce a complex, searching nystagmus with irregular pendular (sinusoidal) and jerk features. This nystagmus is commonly referred to as *congenital sensory nystagmus*. It is a poor term, because even in children with congenital lesions, the nystagmus does not appear until several months of age. *Congenital motor nystagmus*, which looks similar to congenital sensory nystagmus, develops in the absence of any abnormality of the sensory visual system. Visual acuity is also reduced in congenital motor nystagmus, probably by the nystagmus itself, but seldom below a level of 20/200.

JERK NYSTAGMUS This is characterized by a slow drift off the target, followed by a fast corrective saccade. By convention, the nystagmus is named after the quick phase. Jerk nystagmus can be downbeat, upbeat, horizontal (left or right), and torsional. The pattern of nystagmus may vary with gaze position. Some patients will be oblivious to their nystagmus. Others will complain of blurred vision, or a subjective, to-and-fro movement of the environment (oscillopsia) corresponding to their nystagmus. Fine nystagmus may be difficult to see upon gross examination of the eyes. Observation of nystagmoid movements of the optic disc on ophthalmoscopy is a sensitive way to detect subtle nystagmus.

GAZE-EVOKED NYSTAGMUS This is the most common form of jerk nystagmus. When the eyes are held eccentrically in the orbits, they have a natural tendency to drift back to primary position. The subject compensates by making a corrective saccade to maintain the deviated eye position. Many normal patients have mild gaze-evoked nystagmus. Exaggerated gaze-evoked nystagmus can be induced by drugs (sedatives, anticonvulsants, alcohol); muscle paresis; myasthenia gravis; demyelinating disease; and cerebellopontine angle, brainstem, and cerebellar lesions.

VESTIBULAR NYSTAGMUS *Vestibular nystagmus* results from dysfunction of the labyrinth (Ménière's disease), vestibular nerve, or vestibular nucleus in the brainstem. Peripheral vestibular nystagmus often occurs in discrete attacks, with symptoms of nausea and vertigo. There may be associated tinnitus and hearing loss. Sudden shifts in head position may provoke or exacerbate symptoms.

DOWNBEAT NYSTAGMUS *Downbeat nystagmus* occurs from lesions near the craniocervical junction (Chiari malformation, basilar invagination). It has also been reported in brainstem or cerebellar stroke, lithium or anticonvulsant intoxication, alcoholism, and multiple sclerosis. *Upbeat nystagmus* is associated with damage to the pontine tegmentum, from stroke, demyelination, or tumor.

Opsoclonus This rare, dramatic disorder of eye movements consists of bursts of consecutive saccades (saccadomania). When the saccades are confined to the horizontal plane, the term *ocular flutter* is preferred. It can occur from viral encephalitis, trauma, or a paraneoplastic effect of neuroblastoma, breast carcinoma, and other malignancies. It has also been reported as a benign, transient phenomenon in otherwise healthy patients.

FURTHER READINGS

Albert DM et al (eds): *Albert and Jakobiec's Principles and Practice of Ophthalmology*, 3d ed. Philadelphia, Saunders, 2007

Balcer LJ et al: Natalizumab reduces visual loss in patients with relapsing multiple sclerosis. Neurology 68:1299, 2007

Gariano RF, Gardner TW: Retinal angiogenesis in development and disease. Nature 438:960, 2005

Rosenfeld PJ et al: Ranibizumab for neovascular age-related macular degeneration. N Engl J Med 355:1419, 2006

Rutar T et al: Ophthalmic manifestations of infections caused by the USA300 clone of community-associated methicillin-resistant *Staphylococcus aureus*. Ophthalmology 113:1455, 2006

30 Disorders of Smell, Taste, and Hearing

Anil K. Lalwani

SMELL

The sense of smell determines the flavor and palatability of food and drink and serves, along with the trigeminal system, as a monitor of inhaled chemicals, including dangerous substances such as natural gas, smoke, and air pollutants. Olfactory dysfunction affects ~1% of people under age 60 and more than half of the population beyond this age.

DEFINITIONS

Smell is the perception of odor by the nose. *Taste* is the perception of salty, sweet, sour, or bitter by the tongue. Related sensations during eating such as somatic sensations of coolness, warmth, and irritation are mediated through the trigeminal, glossopharyngeal, and vagal afferents in the nose, oral cavity, tongue, pharynx, and larynx. *Flavor* is the complex interaction of taste, smell, and somatic sensation. Terms relating to disorders of smell include *anosmia*, an absence of the ability to smell; *hyposmia*, a decreased ability to smell; *hyperosmia*, an increased sensitivity to an odorant; *dysosmia*, distortion in the perception of an odor; *phantosmia*, perception of an odorant where none is present; and *agnosia*, inability to classify, contrast, or identify odor sensations verbally, even though the ability to distinguish between odorants or to recognize them may be normal. An odor stimulus is referred to as an *odorant*. Each category of smell dysfunction can be further subclassified as total (applying to all odorants) or partial (dysfunction of only select odorants).

PHYSIOLOGY OF SMELL

The *olfactory epithelium* is located in the superior part of the nasal cavities and is highly variable in its distribution between individuals. Over time the olfactory epithelium loses its homogeneity, as small areas undergo metaplasia producing islands of respiratory-like epithelium. This process is thought to be secondary to insults from environmental toxins, bacteria, and viruses. The primary sensory neuron in the olfactory epithelium is the bipolar cell. The dendritic process of the bipolar cell has a bulb-shaped vesicle that projects into the mucous layer and bears six to eight cilia containing odorant receptors. On average, each bipolar cell elaborates 56 cm^2 (9 $in.^2$) of surface area to receive olfactory stimuli. These primary sensory neurons are unique among sensory systems in that they are short-lived, regularly replaced, and regenerate and establish new central connections after injury. Basal stem cells, located on the basal surface of the olfactory epithelium, are the progenitors that differentiate into new bipolar cells (Fig. 30-1).

Between 50 and 200 unmyelinated axons of receptor cells form the fila of the olfactory nerve; they pass through the cribriform plate to terminate within spherical masses of neuropil, termed *glomeruli*, in the olfactory bulb. Olfactory ensheathing cells, which have features resembling glia of both the central and peripheral nervous systems, surround the axons along their course. The glomeruli are the focus of a high degree of convergence of information, since many more fibers enter than leave them. The main second-order neurons are mitral cells. The primary dendrite of each mitral cell extends into a single glomerulus. Axons of the mitral cells project along with the axons of adjacent tufted cells to the limbic system, including the anterior olfactory nucleus and the amygdala. Cognitive awareness of smell requires stimulation of the prepiriform cortex or amygdaloid nuclei.

A secondary site of olfactory chemosensation is located in the epithelium of the vomeronasal organ, a tubular structure that opens on the ventral aspect of the nasal septum. In humans, this structure is rudimentary and nonfunctional, without central projections. Sensory neurons located in the vomeronasal organ detect pheromones, nonvolatile chemical signals that in lower mammals trigger innate and stereotyped reproductive and social behaviors, as well as neuroendocrine changes.

The sensation of smell begins with introduction of an odorant to the cilia of the bipolar neuron. Most odorants are hydrophobic; as they move from the air phase of the nasal cavity to the aqueous phase of the olfactory mucous, they are transported toward the cilia by small water-soluble proteins called *odorant-binding proteins* and reversibly bind to receptors on the cilia surface. Binding leads to conformational changes in the receptor protein, activation of G protein–coupled second messengers, and generation of action potentials in the primary neurons. Intensity appears to be coded by the amount of firing in the afferent neurons.

Olfactory receptor proteins belong to the large family of G protein–coupled receptors that also includes rhodopsins; α- and β-adrenergic receptors; muscarinic acetylcholine receptors; and neurotransmitter receptors for dopamine, serotonin, and substance P. In humans, there are 300–1000 olfactory receptor genes belonging to 20 different families located in clusters at >25 different chromosomal locations. Each olfactory neuron expresses only one or, at most, a few receptor genes, thus providing the molecular basis of odor discrimination. Bipolar cells that express similar receptors appear to be scattered across discrete spatial zones. These similar cells converge on a select few glomeruli in the olfactory bulb. The result is a potential spatial map of how we receive odor stimuli, much like the tonotopic organization of how we perceive sound.

DISORDERS OF THE SENSE OF SMELL

These are caused by conditions that interfere with the access of the odorant to the olfactory neuroepithelium (transport loss), injure the receptor region (sensory loss), or damage central olfactory pathways (neural loss). Currently no clinical tests exist to differentiate these different types of olfactory losses. Fortunately, the history of the disease provides important clues to the cause. The leading causes of olfactory disorders are summarized in Table 30-1; the most common etiologies are head trauma in children and young adults, and viral infections in older adults.

Head trauma is followed by unilateral or bilateral impairment of smell in up to 15% of cases; anosmia is more common than hyposmia. Olfactory dysfunction is more common when trauma is associated with loss of consciousness, moderately severe head injury (grades II–

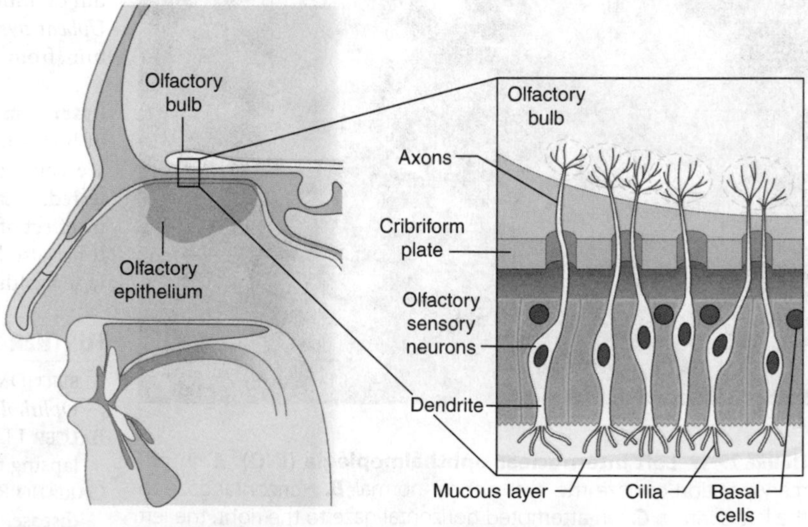

FIGURE 30-1 Olfaction. Olfactory sensory neurons (bipolar cells) are embedded in a small area of specialized epithelium in the dorsal posterior recess of the nasal cavity. These neurons project axons to the olfactory bulb of the brain, a small ovoid structure that rests on the cribriform plate of the ethmoid bone. Odorants bind to specific receptors on olfactory cilia and initiate a cascade of action potential events that lead to the production of action potentials in the sensory axons.

TABLE 30-1 CAUSES OF OLFACTORY DYSFUNCTION

Transport Losses	Neural Losses
Allergic rhinitis	AIDS
Bacterial rhinitis and sinusitis	Alcoholism
Congenital abnormalities	Alzheimer's disease
Nasal neoplasms	Cigarette smoke
Nasal polyps	Depression
Nasal septal deviation	Diabetes mellitus
Nasal surgery	Drugs/toxins
Viral infections	Huntington's chorea
Sensory Losses	Hypothyroidism
Drugs	Kallmann syndrome
Neoplasms	Malnutrition
Radiation therapy	Neoplasms
Toxin exposure	Neurosurgery
Viral infections	Parkinson's disease
	Trauma
	Vitamin B_{12} deficiency
	Zinc deficiency

V), and skull fracture. Frontal injuries and fractures disrupt the cribriform plate and olfactory axons that perforate it. Sometimes there is an associated cerebrospinal fluid (CSF) rhinorrhea resulting from a tearing of the dura overlying the cribriform plate and paranasal sinuses. Anosmia may also follow blows to the occiput. Once traumatic anosmia develops, it is usually permanent; only 10% of patients ever improve or recover. Perversion of the sense of smell may occur as a transient phase in the recovery process.

Viral infections can destroy the olfactory neuroepithelium, which is then replaced by respiratory epithelium. Parainfluenza virus type 3 appears to be especially detrimental to human olfaction. HIV infection is associated with subjective distortion of taste and smell, which may become more severe as the disease progresses. The loss of taste and smell may play an important role in the development and progression of HIV-associated wasting. Congenital anosmias are rare but important. Kallmann syndrome is an X-linked disorder characterized by congenital anosmia and hypogonadotropic hypogonadism resulting from a failure of migration from the olfactory placode of olfactory receptor neurons and neurons synthesizing gonadotropin-releasing hormone (Chap. 340). Anosmia can also occur in albinos. The receptor cells are present but are hypoplastic, lack cilia, and do not project above the surrounding supporting cells.

Meningiomas of the inferior frontal region are the most frequent neoplastic cause of anosmia; loss of smell may be the only neurologic abnormality. Rarely, anosmia can occur with gliomas of the frontal lobe. Occasionally, pituitary adenomas, craniopharyngiomas, suprasellar meningiomas, and aneurysms of the anterior part of the circle of Willis extend forward and damage olfactory structures. These tumors and hamartomas may also induce seizures with olfactory hallucinations, indicating involvement of the uncus of the temporal lobe.

Olfactory dysfunction is common in a variety of neurologic diseases, including Alzheimer's disease, Parkinson's disease, amyotrophic lateral sclerosis, and multiple sclerosis. In Alzheimer's and Parkinson's, olfactory loss may be the first clinical sign of the disease. In Parkinson's disease, bilateral olfactory deficits occur more commonly than the cardinal signs of the disorder such as tremor. In multiple sclerosis, olfactory loss is related to lesions visible by MRI, in olfactory processing areas in the temporal and frontal lobes.

Dysosmia, subjective distortions of olfactory perception, may occur with intranasal diseases that partially impair smell or during recovery from a neurogenic anosmia. Most dysosmic disorders consist of disagreeable odors, sometimes accompanied by distortions of taste. Dysosmia also can occur with depression.

APPROACH TO THE PATIENT: Disorders of the Sense of Smell

Unilateral anosmia is rarely a complaint and is only recognized by testing of smell in each nasal cavity separately. Bilateral anosmia, on the other hand, brings patients to medical attention. Anosmic patients usually complain of a loss of the sense of taste even though their taste thresholds may be within normal limits. In actuality, they are complaining of a loss of flavor detection, which is mainly an olfactory function. The physical examination should include a thorough inspection of the ears, upper respiratory tract, and head and neck. A neurologic examination emphasizing the cranial nerves and cerebellar and sensorimotor function is essential. Any signs of depression should be noted.

Sensory olfactory function can be assessed by several methods. The Odor Stix test uses a commercially available odor-producing magic marker–like pen held approximately 8–15 cm (3–6 in.) from the patient's nose. The 30-cm alcohol test uses a freshly opened isopropyl alcohol packet held ~30 cm (12 in.) from the patient's nose. There is a commercially available scratch-and-sniff card containing three odors available for gross testing of olfaction. A superior test is the University of Pennsylvania Smell Identification Test (UPSIT). This consists of a 40-item, forced choice, scratch-and-sniff paradigm. For example, one of the items reads, "This odor smells most like (a) chocolate, (b) banana, (c) onion, or (d) fruit punch." The test is highly reliable, is sensitive to age and sex differences, and provides an accurate quantitative determination of the olfactory deficit. The UPSIT, which is a forced-choice test, can also be used to identify malingerers who typically report fewer correct responses than would be expected by chance. The average score for total anosmics is slightly higher than that expected on the basis of chance because of the inclusion of some odorants that act by trigeminal stimulation.

Olfactory threshold testing is another method of assessing olfactory function. Following assessment of sensory olfactory function, the detection threshold for an odorant such as methyl ethyl carbinol is established using graduated concentrations for each side of the nose. Nasal resistance can also be measured with anterior rhinomanometry for each side of the nose.

CT or MRI of the head is required to rule out paranasal sinusitis; neoplasms of the anterior cranial fossa, nasal cavity, or paranasal sinuses; or unsuspected fractures of the anterior cranial fossa. Bone abnormalities are best seen with CT. MRI is the most sensitive method to visualize olfactory bulbs, ventricles, and other soft tissue of the brain. Coronal CT is optimal for assessing cribriform plate, anterior cranial fossa, and sinus anatomy.

Biopsy of the olfactory epithelium is possible. However, given the widespread degeneration of the olfactory epithelium and intercalation of respiratory epithelium in the olfactory area of adults with no apparent olfactory dysfunction, biopsy results must be interpreted with caution.

℞ DISORDERS OF THE SENSE OF SMELL

Therapy for patients with transport olfactory losses due to allergic rhinitis, bacterial rhinitis and sinusitis, polyps, neoplasms, and structural abnormalities of the nasal cavities can be undertaken with a high likelihood for improvement. Allergy management; antibiotic therapy; topical and systemic glucocorticoid therapy; and surgery for nasal polyps, deviation of the nasal septum, and chronic hyperplastic sinusitis are frequently effective in restoring the sense of smell.

There is no proven treatment for sensorineural olfactory losses. Fortunately, spontaneous recovery often occurs. Zinc and vitamin therapy (especially with vitamin A) are advocated by some. Profound zinc deficiency can produce loss and distortion of the sense of smell but is not a clinically important problem except in very limited geographic areas (Chap. 71). The epithelial degeneration associated with vitamin A deficiency can cause anosmia, but in western societies the prevalence of vitamin A deficiency is low. Exposure to cigarette smoke and other airborne toxic chemicals can cause metaplasia of the olfactory epithelium, and spontaneous recovery can occur if the insult is removed. Counseling of patients is therefore helpful in such cases.

More than half of people over age 60 suffer from olfactory dysfunction. No effective treatment exists for presbyosmia, but patients are often reassured to learn that this problem is common in their age group. In addition, early recognition and counseling can help patients to compensate for the loss of smell. The incidence of natural gas–related accidents is disproportionately high in the elderly, perhaps due in part to the gradual loss of smell. Mercaptan, the pungent odor in natural gas, is an olfactory stimulant that does not activate taste receptors. Many elderly with olfactory dysfunction experience a decrease in flavor sensation and find it necessary to hyperflavor food, usually by increasing the amount of salt in their diet.

TASTE

Compared with disorders of smell, gustatory disorders are uncommon. Loss of olfactory sensitivity is often accompanied by complaints of loss of the sense of taste, usually with normal detection thresholds for taste.

DEFINITIONS

Disturbances of the sense of taste may be categorized as *total ageusia*, total absence of gustatory function or inability to detect the qualities of sweet, salt, bitter, or sour; *partial ageusia*, ability to detect some but not all of the qualitative gustatory sensations; *specific ageusia*, inability to detect the taste quality of certain substances; *total hypogeusia*, decreased sensitivity to all tastants; *partial hypogeusia*, decreased sensitivity to some tastants; and *dysgeusia* or *phantogeusia*, distortion in the perception of a tastant, i.e., the perception of the wrong quality when a tastant is presented or the perception of a taste when there has been no tastant ingested. Confusion between sour and bitter, and less commonly between salty and bitter, may represent a semantic misunderstanding or have a true pathophysiologic basis. It may be possible to differentiate between the loss of flavor recognition in patients with olfactory losses who complain of a loss of taste as well as smell by asking if they are able to taste sweetness in sodas, saltiness in potato chips, etc.

PHYSIOLOGY OF TASTE

The taste receptor cells are located in the taste buds, spherical groups of cells arranged in a pattern resembling the segments of a citrus fruit (Fig. 30-2). At the surface, the taste bud has a pore into which microvilli of the receptor cells project. Unlike the olfactory system, the receptor cell is not the primary neuron. Instead, gustatory afferent nerve fibers contact individual taste receptor cells. The papillae lie along the lateral margin and dorsum of the tongue; at the junction of the dorsum and the base of the tongue; and in the palate, epiglottis, larynx, and esophagus.

Tastants gain access to the receptor cells through the taste pore. Four classes of taste have been traditionally recognized: sweet, salt, sour, and bitter, and more recently "umami" (monosodium glutamate, disodium gluanylate, disodium inosinate). Tastants enter the taste pore in a solution and initiate transduction by either activating receptors coupled to G-proteins or by directly activating ion channels on the microvillae within the taste bud. Individual gustatory afferent fibers almost always respond to a number of different chemicals. As with olfaction and other sensory systems, intensity appears to be encoded by the quantity of neural activity.

The sense of taste is mediated through the facial, glossopharyngeal, and vagal nerves. The chorda tympani branch of the facial nerve subserves taste from the anterior two-thirds of the tongue. The posterior third of the tongue is supplied by the lingual branch of the glossopharyngeal nerve. Afferents from the palate travel with the greater superficial petrosal nerve to the geniculate ganglion and then via the facial nerve to the brainstem. The internal branch of the superior laryngeal nerve of the vagus nerve contains the taste afferents from the larynx, including the epiglottis and esophagus.

The central connections of the nerves terminate in the brainstem in the nucleus of the tractus solitarius. The central pathway from the nucleus of the tractus solitarius projects to the ipsilateral parabrachial nuclei of the pons. Two divergent pathways project from the parabrachial nuclei. One ascends to the gustatory relay in the dorsal thalamus, synapses, and continues to the cortex of the insula. There is also evidence for a direct pathway from the parabrachial nuclei to the cortex. (Olfaction and gustation appear to be unique among sensory systems in that at least some fibers bypass the thalamus.) The other pathway from the parabrachial nuclei goes to the ventral forebrain, including the lateral hypothalamus, substantia innominata, central nucleus of the amygdala, and the stria terminalis.

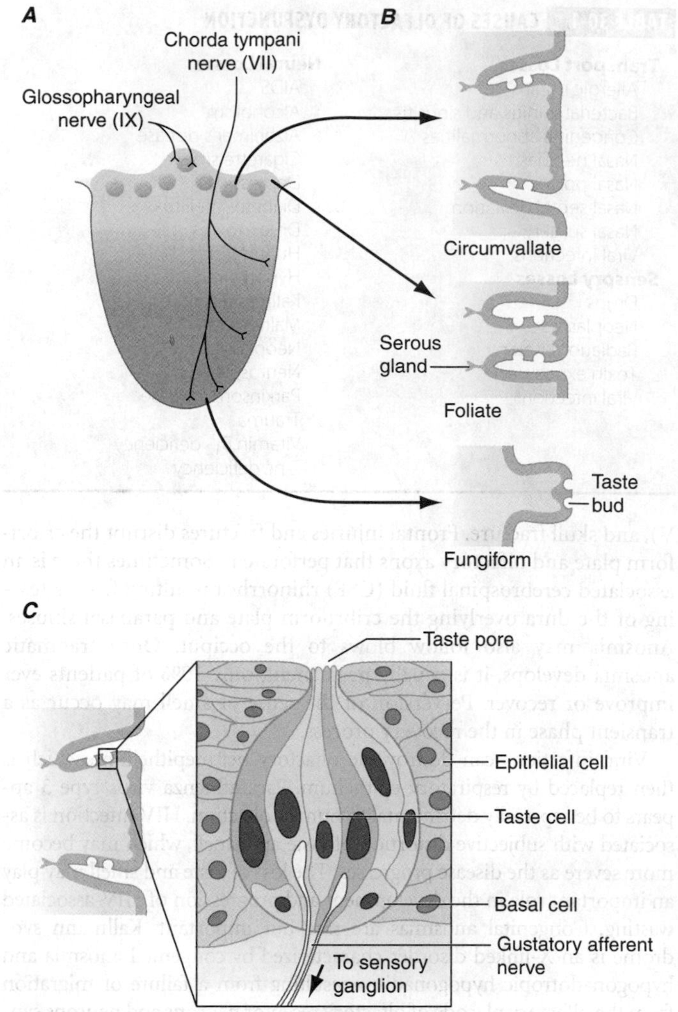

FIGURE 30-2 Taste. *A.* The taste buds of the anterior two-thirds of the tongue are innervated by the gustatory fibers that travel in a branch of the facial nerve (VII) called the chorda tympani. The taste buds of the posterior third of the tongue are innervated by gustatory fibers that travel in the lingual branch of the glossopharyngeal nerve (IX). *[Adapted from ER Kandel et al (eds): Principles of Neural Science, 4th ed, New York, McGraw-Hill, 2000; with permission.]* ***B.*** The main types of taste papillae are shown in schematic cross sections. Each type predominates in specific areas of the tongue, as indicated by the arrows from ***A. C.*** Each taste bud contains 50–150 taste cells that extend from the base of the taste bud to the taste pore, where the apical microvilli of taste cells have contact with tastants dissolved in saliva and taste pore mucus. Access of tastants to the basolateral regions of these cells is generally prevented by tight junctions between taste cells. Taste cells are short-lived cells that are replaced from stem cells at the base of the taste bud. Three types of taste cells in each taste bud (light cells, dark cells, and intermediate cells) may represent different stages of differentiation or different cell lineages. Taste stimuli, detected at the apical end of the taste cell, induce action potentials that cause the release of neurotransmitter at synapses formed at the base of the taste cell with gustatory fibers that transmit signals to the brain.

DISORDERS OF THE SENSE OF TASTE

Disorders of the sense of taste are caused by conditions that interfere with the access of the tastant to the receptor cells in the taste bud (transport loss), injure receptor cells (sensory loss), or damage gustatory afferent nerves and central gustatory pathways (neural loss) (Table 30-2). *Transport gustatory losses* result from xerostomia due to many causes, including Sjögren's syndrome, radiation therapy, heavy-metal intoxication, and bacterial colonization of the taste pore. *Sensory gustatory losses* are caused by inflammatory and degenerative diseases in the oral cavity; a vast number of drugs, particularly those that interfere with cell turnover such as antithyroid and antineoplastic agents;

TABLE 30-2 CAUSES OF GUSTATORY DYSFUNCTION

Transport Gustatory Losses	Neural Gustatory Losses
Drugs	Diabetes mellitus
Heavy-metal intoxication	Hypothyroidism
Radiation therapy	Oral neoplasms
Sjögren's syndrome	Oral surgery
Xerostomia	Radiation therapy
Sensory Gustatory Losses	Renal disease
Aging	Stroke and other CNS disorders
Candidiasis	Trauma
Drugs (antithyroid and antineoplastic)	Upper respiratory tract infections
Endocrine disorders	
Oral neoplasms	
Pemphigus	
Radiation therapy	
Viral infections (especially with herpes viruses)	

radiation therapy to the oral cavity and pharynx; viral infections; endocrine disorders; neoplasms; and aging. *Neural gustatory losses* occur with neoplasms, trauma, and surgical procedures in which the gustatory afferents are injured. Taste buds degenerate when their gustatory afferents are transected but remain when their somatosensory afferents are severed. Patients with renal disease have increased thresholds for sweet and sour tastes, which resolves with dialysis.

A side effect of medication is the single most common cause of taste dysfunction in clinical practice. Xerostomia, regardless of the etiology, can be associated with taste dysfunction. It is associated with poor oral clearance and poor dental hygiene and can adversely affect the oral mucosa, all leading to dysgeusia. However, severe salivary gland failure does not necessarily lead to taste complaints. Xerostomia, the use of antibiotics or glucocorticoids, or immunodeficiency can lead to overgrowth of *Candida*; overgrowth alone, without thrush or overt signs of infection, can be associated with bad taste or hypogeusia. When taste dysfunction occurs in a patient at risk for fungal overgrowth, a trial of nystatin or other antifungal medication is warranted.

Upper respiratory infections and head trauma can lead to both smell and taste dysfunction; taste is more likely to improve than smell. The mechanism of taste disturbance in these situations is not well understood. Trauma to the chorda tympani branch of the facial nerve during middle ear surgery or third molar extractions is relatively common and can cause dysgeusia. Bilateral chorda tympani injuries are usually associated with hypogeusia, whereas unilateral lesions produce only limited symptoms.

As noted above, aging itself may be associated with reduced taste sensitivity. The taste dysfunction may be limited to a single compound and may be mild.

APPROACH TO THE PATIENT: Disorders of the Sense of Taste

Patients who complain of loss of taste should be evaluated for both gustatory and olfactory function. Clinical assessment of taste is not as well developed or standardized as that of smell. The first step is to perform suprathreshold whole-mouth taste testing for quality, intensity, and pleasantness perception of four taste qualities: sweet, salty, sour, and bitter. Most commonly used reagents for taste testing are sucrose, citric acid or hydrochloric acid, caffeine or quinine (sulfate or hydrochloride), and sodium chloride. The taste stimuli should be freshly prepared and have similar viscosity. For quantification, detection thresholds are obtained by applying graduated dilutions to the tongue quadrants or by whole-mouth sips. Electric taste testing (*electrogustometry*) is used clinically to identify taste deficits in specific quadrants of the tongue. Regional gustatory testing may also be performed to assess for the possibility of loss localized to one or several receptor fields as a result of a peripheral or central lesion. The history of the disease and localization studies provide important clues to the causes of the taste disturbance. For example, absence of taste on the anterior two-thirds of the tongue associated with a facial paralysis indicates that the lesion is proximal to the juncture of the chorda tympani branch with the facial nerve in the mastoid.

Rx DISORDERS OF THE SENSE OF TASTE

Treatment of gustatory disorders is limited. No effective therapies exist for the sensorineural disorders of taste. Altered taste due to surgical stretch injury of the chorda tympani nerve usually improves within 3–4 months, while dysfunction is usually permanent with transection of the nerve. Taste dysfunction following trauma may resolve spontaneously without intervention and is more likely to do so than posttraumatic smell dysfunction. Idiopathic alterations of taste sensitivity usually remain stable or worsen; zinc and vitamin therapy are of unproven value. Directed therapy to address factors that affect taste perception can be of value. Xerostomia can be treated with artificial saliva, providing some benefit to patients with a disturbed salivary milieu. Oral pilocarpine may be beneficial for a variety of forms of xerostomia. Appropriate treatment of bacterial and fungal infections of the oral cavity can be of great help in improving taste function. Taste disturbance related to drugs can often be resolved by changing the prescribed medication.

HEARING

Hearing loss is one of the most common sensory disorders in humans and can present at any age. Nearly 10% of the adult population has some hearing loss, and one-third of individuals >65 years have a hearing loss of sufficient magnitude to require a hearing aid.

PHYSIOLOGY OF HEARING

(Fig. 30-3) The function of the external and middle ear is to amplify sound to facilitate mechanotransduction by hair cells in the inner ear. Sound waves enter the external auditory canal and set the tympanic membrane in motion, which in turn moves the malleus, incus, and stapes of the middle ear. Movement of the footplate of the stapes causes pressure changes in the fluid-filled inner ear eliciting a traveling wave in the basilar membrane of the cochlea. The tympanic membrane and the ossicular chain in the middle ear serve as an impedance-matching mechanism, improving the efficiency of energy transfer from air to the fluid-filled inner ear.

Stereocilia of the hair cells of the organ of Corti, which rests on the basilar membrane, are in contact with the tectorial membrane and are deformed by the traveling wave. A point of maximal displacement of the basilar membrane is determined by the frequency of the stimulating tone. High-frequency tones cause maximal displacement of the basilar membrane near the base of the cochlea. As the frequency of the stimulating tone decreases, the point of maximal displacement moves toward the apex of the cochlea.

The inner and outer hair cells of the organ of Corti have different innervation patterns, but both are mechanoreceptors. The afferent innervation relates principally to the inner hair cells, and the efferent innervation relates principally to outer hair cells. The motility of the outer hair cells alters the micromechanics of the inner hair cells, creating a cochlear amplifier, which explains the exquisite sensitivity and frequency selectivity of the cochlea.

Beginning in the cochlea, the frequency specificity is maintained at each point of the central auditory pathway: dorsal and ventral cochlear nuclei, trapezoid body, superior olivary complex, lateral lemniscus, inferior colliculus, medial geniculate body, and auditory cortex. At low frequencies, individual auditory nerve fibers can respond more or less synchronously with the stimulating tone. At higher frequencies, phase-locking occurs so that neurons alternate in response to particular phases of the cycle of the sound wave. Intensity is encoded by the amount of neural activity in individual neurons, the number of neurons that are active, and the specific neurons that are activated.

GENETIC CAUSES OF HEARING LOSS

More than half of childhood hearing impairment is thought to be hereditary; hereditary hearing impairment (HHI) can also manifest later in life. HHI may be classified as either nonsyndromic, when hearing loss is the only clinical abnormality, or syndromic, when hearing loss is associated with anomalies in other organ systems. Near-

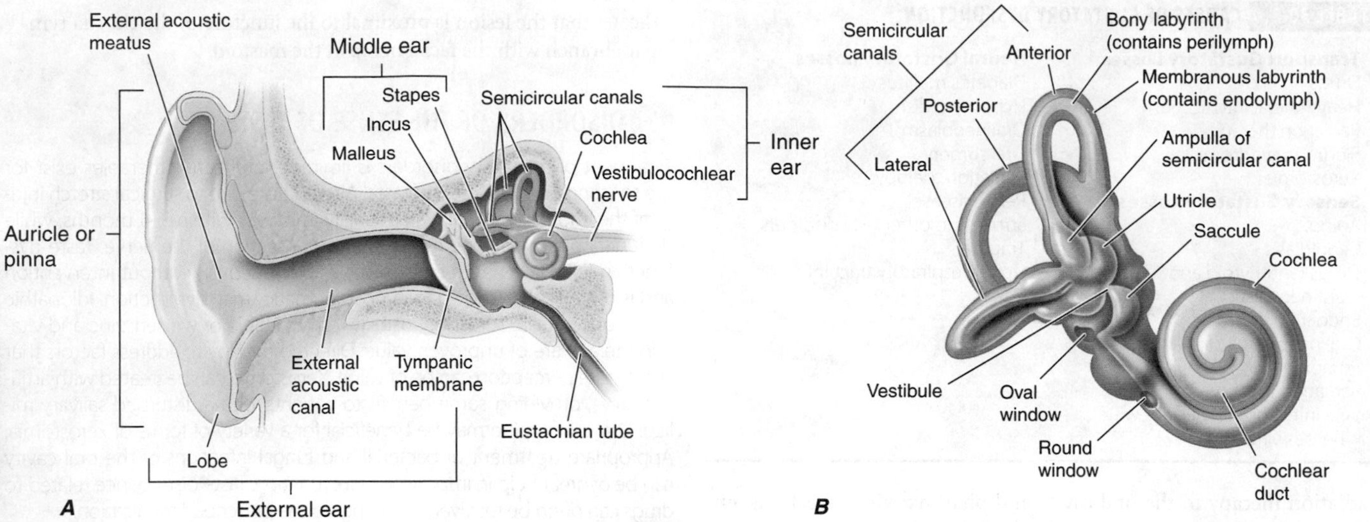

FIGURE 30-3 Ear anatomy. ***A.*** Drawing of modified coronal section through external ear and temporal bone, with structures of the middle and inner ear demonstrated. ***B.*** High-resolution view of inner ear.

ly two-thirds of HHIs are nonsyndromic, and the remaining one-third are syndromic. Between 70 and 80% of nonsyndromic HHI is inherited in an autosomal recessive manner and designated DFNB; another 15–20% is autosomal dominant (DFNA). Less than 5% is X-linked or maternally inherited via the mitochondria.

Nearly 100 loci harboring genes for nonsyndromic HHI have been mapped, with equal numbers of dominant and recessive modes of inheritance; numerous genes have now been cloned (Table 30-3). The hearing genes fall into the categories of structural proteins (MYH9, MYO7A, MYO15, TECTA, DIAPH1), transcription factors (POU3F4, POU4F3), ion channels (KCNQ4, SLC26A4), and gap junction proteins (GJB2, GJB3, GJB6). Several of these genes, including connexin 26 (GJB2), TECTA, and TMC1, cause both autosomal dominant and recessive forms of nonsyndromic HHI. In general, the hearing loss associated with dominant genes has its onset in adolescence or adulthood and varies in severity, whereas the hearing loss associated with recessive inheritance is congenital and profound. Connexin 26 is particularly important because it is associated with nearly 20% of cases of childhood deafness. Two frame-shift mutations, 35delG and 167delT, account for >50% of the cases; however, screening for these two mutations alone is insufficient to diagnose GJB2-related recessive deafness. The 167delT mutation is highly prevalent in Ashkenazi Jews; ~1 in 1765 individuals in this population are homozygous and affected. The hearing loss can also vary among the members of the same family, suggesting that other genes or factors influence the auditory phenotype.

The contribution of genetics to presbycusis (see below) is also becoming better understood. In addition to GJB2, several other nonsyndromic genes are associated with hearing loss that progresses with age. Sensitivity to aminoglycoside ototoxicity can be maternally transmitted through a mitochondrial mutation. Susceptibility to noise-induced hearing loss may also be genetically determined.

There are >400 syndromic forms of hearing loss. These include Usher syndrome (retinitis pigmentosa and hearing loss), Waardenburg syndrome (pigmentary abnormality and hearing loss), Pendred syndrome (thyroid organification defect and hearing loss), Alport syndrome (renal disease and hearing loss), Jervell and Lange-Nielsen syndrome (prolonged QT interval and hearing loss), neurofibromatosis type 2 (bilateral acoustic schwannoma), and mitochondrial disorders [mitochondrial encephalopathy, lactic acidosis, and stroke-like episodes (MELAS); myoclonic epilepsy and ragged red fibers (MERRF); progressive external ophthalmoplegia (PEO)] (Table 30-4).

DISORDERS OF THE SENSE OF HEARING

Hearing loss can result from disorders of the auricle, external auditory canal, middle ear, inner ear, or central auditory pathways (Fig. 30-4). *In general, lesions in the auricle, external auditory canal, or middle ear*

TABLE 30-3 HEREDITARY HEARING IMPAIRMENT GENES

Designation	Gene	Function
Autosomal Dominant		
	CRYM	Thyroid hormone binding protein
DFNA1	*DIAPH1*	Cytoskeletal protein
DFNA2	*GJB3 (Cx31)*	Gap junctions
DFNA2	*KCNQ4*	Potassium channel
DFNA3	*GJB2 (Cx26)*	Gap junctions
DFNA3	*GJB6 (Cx30)*	Gap junctions
DFNA4	*MYH14*	Class II nonmuscle myosin
DFNA5	*DFNA5*	Unknown
DFNA6/14/38	*WFS*	Transmembrane protein
DFNA8/12	*TECTA*	Tectorial membrane protein
DFNA9	*COCH*	Unknown
DFNA10	*EYA4*	Developmental gene
DFNA11	*MYO7A*	Cytoskeletal protein
DFNA13	*COL11A2*	Cytoskeletal protein
DFNA15	*POU4F3*	Transcription factor
DFNA17	*MYH9*	Cytoskeletal protein
DFNA20/26	*ACTG1*	Cytoskeletal protein
DFNA22	*MYO6*	Unconventional myosin
DFNA28	*TFCP2L3*	Transcription factor
DFNA36	*TMC1*	Transmembrane protein
DFNA48	*MYO1A*	Unconventional myosin
Autosomal Recessive		
	SLC26A5 (Prestin)	Motor protein
DFNB1	*GJB2 (CX26)*	Gap junction
	GJB6(CX30)	Gap junction
DFNB2	*MYO7A*	Cytoskeletal protein
DFNB3	*MYO15*	Cytoskeletal protein
DFNB4	*PDS(SLC26A4)*	Chloride/iodide transporter
DFNB6	*TMIE*	Transmembrane protein
DFNB7/B11	*TMC1*	Transmembrane protein
DFNB9	*OTOF*	Trafficking of membrane vesicles
DFNB8/10	*TMPRSS3*	Transmembrane serine protease
DFNB12	*CDH23*	Intercellular adherence protein
DFNB16	*STRC*	Stereocilia protein
DFNB18	*USH1C*	Unknown
DFNB21	*TECTA*	Tectorial membrane protein
DFNB22	*OTOA*	Gel attachement to nonsensory cell
DFNB23	*PCDH15*	Morphogenesis and cohesion
DFNB28	*TRIOBP*	Cytoskeletal-organizing protein
DFNB29	*CLDN14*	Tight junctions
DFNB30	*MYO3A*	Hybrid motor-signaling myosin
DFNB31	*WHRN*	PDZ domain–containing protein
DFNB36	*ESPN*	Ca-insensitive actin-bundling protein
DFNB37	*MYO6*	Unconventional myosin
DFNB67	*TMHS*	Unknown function; tetraspan protein

TABLE 30-4 SYNDROMIC HEREDITARY HEARING IMPAIRMENT GENES

Syndrome	Gene	Function
Alport syndrome	*COL4A3-5*	Cytoskeletal protein
BOR syndrome	*EYA1*	Developmental gene
	SIX1	Developmental gene
Jervell and Lange-Nielsen syndrome	*KVLQT1*	Delayed rectifier K^+ channel
	KCNE1	Delayed rectifier K^+ channel
Norrie disease	*Norrin*	Cell-cell interactions
Pendred syndrome	*SLC26A4*	Chloride/iodide transporter
Treacher Collins	*TCOF1*	Nucleolar-cytoplasmic transport
Usher syndrome	*MYO7A*	Cytoskeletal protein
	USH1C	Unknown
	CDH23	Intercellular adherence protein
	PCDH15	Cell adhesion molecule
	SANS	Harmonin associated protein
	USH2A	Cell adhesion molecule
	VLGR1	G protein–coupled receptor
	USH3	Unknown
WS type I, III	*PAX3*	Transcription factor
WS type II	*MITF*	Transcription factor
	SLUG	Transcription factor
WS type IV	*EDNRB*	Endothelin-B receptor
	EDN3	Endothelin-B receptor ligand
	SOX10	Transcription factor

Note: BOR, branchio-oto-renal syndrome; WS, Waardenburg syndrome.

cause conductive hearing losses, whereas lesions in the inner ear or eighth nerve cause sensorineural hearing losses.

Conductive Hearing Loss This results from obstruction of the external auditory canal by cerumen, debris, and foreign bodies; swelling of the lining of the canal; atresia or neoplasms of the canal; perforations of the tympanic membrane; disruption of the ossicular chain, as occurs with necrosis of the long process of the incus in trauma or infection; otosclerosis; or fluid, scarring, or neoplasms in the middle ear. Rarely, inner-ear malformations may present as conductive hearing loss beginning in adulthood.

Cholesteatoma, stratified squamous epithelium in the middle ear or mastoid, occurs frequently in adults. This is a benign, slowly growing lesion that destroys bone and normal ear tissue. Theories of pathogenesis include traumatic implantation and invasion, immigration and invasion through a perforation, and metaplasia following chronic infection and irritation. On examination, there is often a perforation of the tympanic membrane filled with cheesy white squamous debris. A chronically draining ear that fails to respond to appropriate antibiotic therapy should raise suspicion of a cholesteatoma. Conductive hearing loss secondary to ossicular erosion is common. Surgery is required to remove this destructive process.

Conductive hearing loss with a normal ear canal and intact tympanic membrane suggests ossicular pathology. Fixation of the stapes from *otosclerosis* is a common cause of low-frequency conductive hearing loss. It occurs equally in men and women and is inherited as an autosomal dominant trait with incomplete penetrance. Hearing impairment usually presents between the late teens to the forties. In women, the otosclerotic process is accelerated during pregnancy, and the hearing loss is often first noticeable at this time. A hearing aid or a simple outpatient surgical procedure (stapedectomy) can provide adequate auditory rehabilitation. Extension of otosclerosis beyond the stapes footplate to involve the cochlea (cochlear otosclerosis) can lead to mixed or sensorineural hearing loss. Fluoride therapy to prevent hearing loss from cochlear otosclerosis is of uncertain value.

Eustachian tube dysfunction is extremely common in adults and may predispose to acute otitis media (AOM) or serous otitis media (SOM). Trauma, AOM, or chronic otitis media are the usual factors

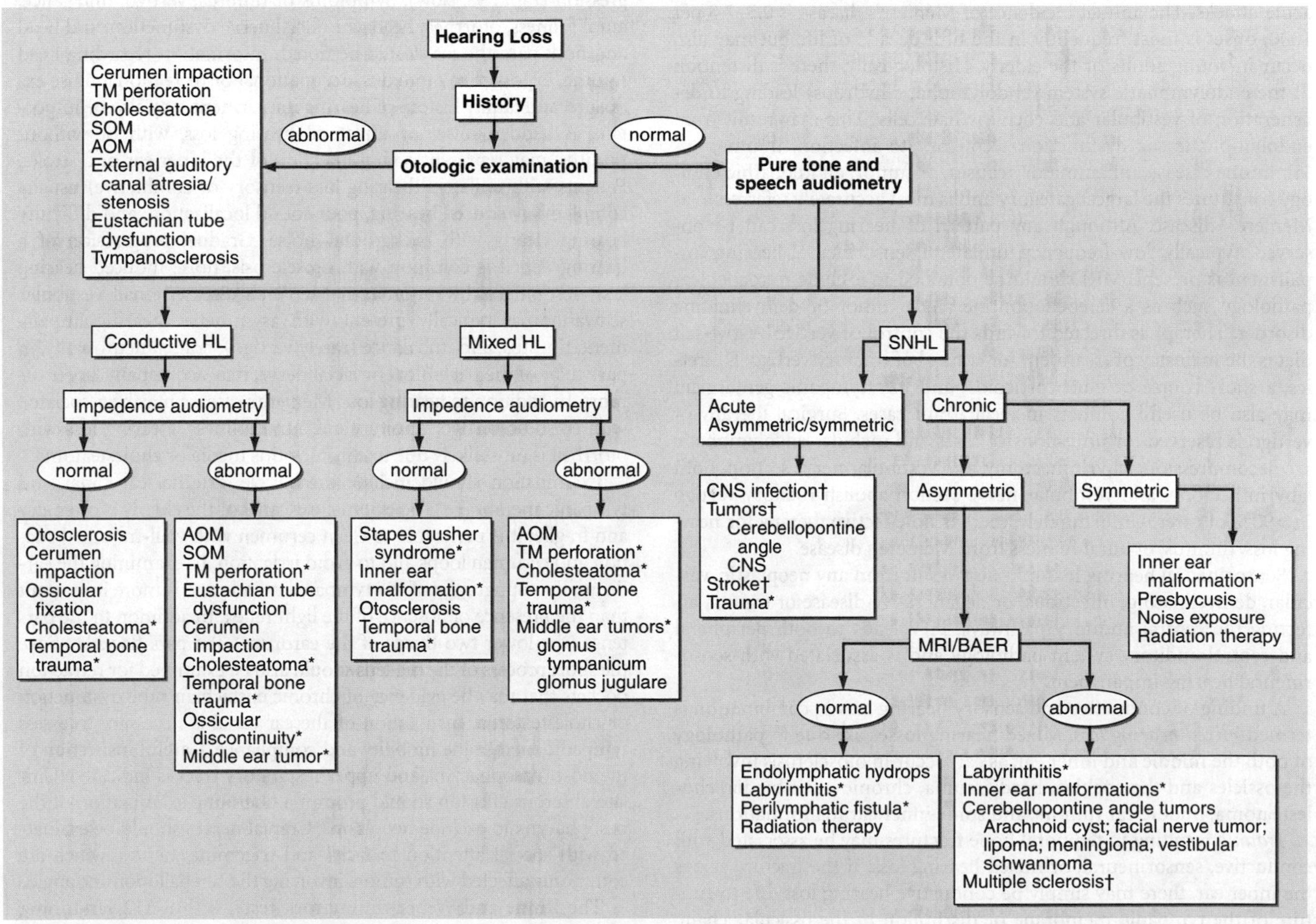

FIGURE 30-4 An algorithm for the approach to hearing loss. HL, hearing loss; SNHL, sensorineural hearing loss; TM, tympanic membrane; SOM, serous otitis media; AOM, acute otitis media; *, CT scan of temporal bone; †, MRI scan.

responsible for tympanic membrane perforation. While small perforations often heal spontaneously, larger defects usually require surgical intervention. Tympanoplasty is highly effective (>90%) in the repair of tympanic membrane perforations. Otoscopy is usually sufficient to diagnose AOM, SOM, chronic otitis media, cerumen impaction, tympanic membrane perforation, and eustachian tube dysfunction.

Sensorineural Hearing Loss Damage to the hair cells of the organ of Corti may be caused by intense noise, viral infections, ototoxic drugs (e.g., salicylates, quinine and its synthetic analogues, aminoglycoside antibiotics, loop diuretics such as furosemide and ethacrynic acid, and cancer chemotherapeutic agents such as cisplatin), fractures of the temporal bone, meningitis, cochlear otosclerosis (see above), Ménière's disease, and aging. Congenital malformations of the inner ear may be the cause of hearing loss in some adults. Genetic predisposition alone or in concert with environmental exposures may also be responsible.

Presbycusis (age-associated hearing loss) is the most common cause of sensorineural hearing loss in adults. In the early stages, it is characterized by symmetric, gentle to sharply sloping high-frequency hearing loss. With progression, the hearing loss involves all frequencies. More importantly, the hearing impairment is associated with significant loss in clarity. There is a loss of discrimination for phonemes, recruitment (abnormal growth of loudness), and particular difficulty in understanding speech in noisy environments. Hearing aids may provide limited rehabilitation once the word recognition score deteriorates below 50%. Cochlear implants are the treatment of choice when hearing aids prove inadequate, even when hearing loss is incomplete.

Ménière's disease is characterized by episodic vertigo, fluctuating sensorineural hearing loss, tinnitus, and aural fullness. Tinnitus and/or deafness may be absent during the initial attacks of vertigo, but invariably appear as the disease progresses and increase in severity during acute attacks. The annual incidence of Ménière's disease is 0.5–7.5 per 1000; onset is most frequently in the fifth decade of life but may also occur in young adults or the elderly. Histologically, there is distention of the endolymphatic system (endolymphatic hydrops) leading to degeneration of vestibular and cochlear hair cells. This may result from endolymphatic sac dysfunction secondary to infection, trauma, autoimmune disease, inflammatory causes, or tumor; an idiopathic etiology constitutes the largest category and is most accurately referred to as Ménière's disease. Although any pattern of hearing loss can be observed, typically, low-frequency, unilateral sensorineural hearing impairment is present. MRI should be obtained to exclude retrocochlear pathology such as a cerebellopontine angle tumor or demyelinating disorder. Therapy is directed towards the control of vertigo. A low-salt diet is the mainstay of treatment for control of rotatory vertigo. Diuretics, a short course of glucocorticoids, and intratympanic gentamicin may also be useful adjuncts in recalcitrant cases. Surgical therapy of vertigo is reserved for unresponsive cases and includes endolymphatic sac decompression, labyrinthectomy, and vestibular nerve section. Both labyrinthectomy and vestibular nerve section abolish rotatory vertigo in >90% of cases. Unfortunately, there is no effective therapy for hearing loss, tinnitus, or aural fullness from Ménière's disease.

Sensorineural hearing loss may also result from any neoplastic, vascular, demyelinating, infectious, or degenerative disease or trauma affecting the central auditory pathways. HIV leads to both peripheral and central auditory system pathology and is associated with sensorineural hearing impairment.

A finding of conductive and sensory hearing loss in combination is termed *mixed hearing loss*. Mixed hearing losses are due to pathology of both the middle and inner ear, as can occur in otosclerosis involving the ossicles and the cochlea, head trauma, chronic otitis media, cholesteatoma, middle ear tumors, and some inner ear malformations.

Trauma resulting in temporal bone fractures may be associated with conductive, sensorineural, or mixed hearing loss. If the fracture spares the inner ear, there may simply be conductive hearing loss due to rupture of the tympanic membrane or disruption of the ossicular chain. These abnormalities can be surgically corrected. Profound hearing loss and severe vertigo are associated with temporal bone fractures involving the inner ear. A perilymphatic fistula associated with leakage of inner-ear fluid into the middle ear can occur and may require surgical repair. An associated facial nerve injury is not uncommon. CT is best suited to assess fracture of the traumatized temporal bone, evaluate the ear canal, and determine the integrity of the ossicular chain and the involvement of the inner ear. CSF leaks that accompany temporal bone fractures are usually self-limited; the value of prophylactic antibiotics is uncertain.

Tinnitus is defined as the perception of a sound when there is no sound in the environment. It may have a buzzing, roaring, or ringing quality and may be pulsatile (synchronous with the heartbeat). Tinnitus is often associated with either a conductive or sensorineural hearing loss. The pathophysiology of tinnitus is not well understood. The cause of the tinnitus can usually be determined by finding the cause of the associated hearing loss. Tinnitus may be the first symptom of a serious condition such as a vestibular schwannoma. Pulsatile tinnitus requires evaluation of the vascular system of the head to exclude vascular tumors such as glomus jugulare tumors, aneurysms, and stenotic arterial lesions; it may also occur with SOM.

APPROACH TO THE PATIENT: Disorders of the Sense of Hearing

The goal in the evaluation of a patient with auditory complaints is to determine (1) the nature of the hearing impairment (conductive vs. sensorineural vs. mixed), (2) the severity of the impairment (mild, moderate, severe, profound), (3) the anatomy of the impairment (external ear, middle ear, inner ear, or central auditory pathway), and (4) the etiology. The history should elicit characteristics of the hearing loss, including the duration of deafness, unilateral vs. bilateral involvement, nature of onset (sudden vs. insidious), and rate of progression (rapid vs. slow). Symptoms of tinnitus, vertigo, imbalance, aural fullness, otorrhea, headache, facial nerve dysfunction, and head and neck paresthesias should be noted. Information regarding head trauma, exposure to ototoxins, occupational or recreational noise exposure, and family history of hearing impairment may also be important. A sudden onset of unilateral hearing loss, with or without tinnitus, may represent a viral infection of the inner ear or a stroke. Patients with unilateral hearing loss (sensory or conductive) usually complain of reduced hearing, poor sound localization, and difficulty hearing clearly with background noise. Gradual progression of a hearing deficit is common with otosclerosis, noise-induced hearing loss, vestibular schwannoma, or Ménière's disease. Small vestibular schwannomas typically present with asymmetric hearing impairment, tinnitus, and imbalance (rarely vertigo); cranial neuropathy, in particular of the trigeminal or facial nerve, may accompany larger tumors. In addition to hearing loss, Ménière's disease may be associated with episodic vertigo, tinnitus, and aural fullness. Hearing loss with otorrhea is most likely due to chronic otitis media or cholesteatoma.

Examination should include the auricle, external ear canal, and tympanic membrane. The external ear canal of the elderly is often dry and fragile; it is preferable to clean cerumen with wall-mounted suction and cerumen loops and to avoid irrigation. In examining the eardrum, the topography of the tympanic membrane is more important than the presence or absence of the light reflex. In addition to the pars tensa (the lower two-thirds of the eardrum), the pars flaccida above the short process of the malleus should also be examined for retraction pockets that may be evidence of chronic eustachian tube dysfunction or cholesteatoma. Insufflation of the ear canal is necessary to assess tympanic membrane mobility and compliance. Careful inspection of the nose, nasopharynx, and upper respiratory tract is indicated. Unilateral serous effusion should prompt a fiberoptic examination of the nasopharynx to exclude neoplasms. Cranial nerves should be evaluated with special attention to facial and trigeminal nerves, which are commonly affected with tumors involving the cerebellopontine angle.

The Rinne and Weber tuning fork tests, with a 512-Hz tuning fork, are used to screen for hearing loss, differentiate conductive from sensorineural hearing losses, and to confirm the findings of audiologic evaluation. Rinne's test compares the ability to hear by air conduction with the ability to hear by bone conduction. The tines of a vibrating tuning fork are held near the opening of the external auditory canal, and then the stem is placed on the mastoid process; for direct contact, it may be placed on teeth or dentures. The patient is asked to indicate whether the tone is louder by air conduction or bone conduction. Normally, and in the presence of sensorineural hearing loss, a tone is heard louder by air conduction than by bone conduction; however, with conductive hearing loss of ≥30 dB (see "Audiologic Assessment," below), the bone-conduction stimulus is perceived as louder than the air-conduction stimulus. For the Weber test, the stem of a vibrating tuning fork is placed on the head in the midline and the patient asked whether the tone is heard in both ears or better in one ear than in the other. With a unilateral conductive hearing loss, the tone is perceived in the affected ear. With a unilateral sensorineural hearing loss, the tone is perceived in the unaffected ear. A 5-dB difference in hearing between the two ears is required for lateralization.

LABORATORY ASSESSMENT OF HEARING

Audiologic Assessment The minimum audiologic assessment for hearing loss should include the measurement of pure tone air-conduction and bone-conduction thresholds, speech reception threshold, discrimination score, tympanometry, acoustic reflexes, and acoustic-reflex decay. This test battery provides a screening evaluation of the entire auditory system and allows one to determine whether further differentiation of a sensory (cochlear) from a neural (retrocochlear) hearing loss is indicated.

Pure tone audiometry assesses hearing acuity for pure tones. The test is administered by an audiologist and is performed in a sound-attenuated chamber. The pure tone stimulus is delivered with an audiometer, an electronic device that allows the presentation of specific frequencies (generally between 250 and 8000 Hz) at specific intensities. Air and bone conduction thresholds are established for each ear. Air conduction thresholds are determined by presenting the stimulus in air with the use of headphones. Bone conduction thresholds are determined by placing the stem of a vibrating tuning fork or an oscillator of an audiometer in contact with the head. In the presence of a hearing loss, broad-spectrum noise is presented to the nontest ear for *masking* purposes so that responses are based on perception from the ear under test.

The responses are measured in decibels. An *audiogram* is a plot of intensity in decibels of hearing threshold versus frequency. A decibel (dB) is equal to 20 times the logarithm of the ratio of the sound pressure required to achieve threshold in the patient to the sound pressure required to achieve threshold in a normal hearing person. Therefore, a change of 6 dB represents doubling of sound pressure, and a change of 20 dB represents a tenfold change in sound pressure. Loudness, which depends on the frequency, intensity, and duration of a sound, doubles with approximately each 10-dB increase in sound pressure level. Pitch, on the other hand, does not directly correlate with frequency. The perception of pitch changes slowly in the low and high frequencies. In the middle tones, which are important for human speech, pitch varies more rapidly with changes in frequency.

Pure tone audiometry establishes the presence and severity of hearing impairment, unilateral vs. bilateral involvement, and the type of hearing loss. Conductive hearing losses with a large mass component, as is often seen in middle-ear effusions, produce elevation of thresholds that predominate in the higher frequencies. Conductive hearing losses with a large stiffness component, as in fixation of the footplate of the stapes in early otosclerosis, produce threshold elevations in the lower frequencies. Often, the conductive hearing loss involves all frequencies, suggesting involvement of both stiffness and mass. In general, sensorineural hearing losses such as presbycusis affect higher frequencies more than lower frequencies. An exception is Ménière's disease, which is characteristically associated with low-frequency sensorineural hearing loss. Noise-induced hearing loss has an unusual pattern of hearing impairment in which the loss at 4000 Hz is greater than at higher frequencies. Vestibular schwannomas characteristically affect the higher frequencies, but any pattern of hearing loss can be observed.

Speech recognition requires greater synchronous neural firing than is necessary for appreciation of pure tones. *Speech audiometry* tests the clarity with which one hears. The *speech reception threshold* (SRT) is defined as the intensity at which speech is recognized as a meaningful symbol and is obtained by presenting two-syllable words with an equal accent on each syllable. The intensity at which the patient can repeat 50% of the words correctly is the SRT. Once the SRT is determined, discrimination or word recognition ability is tested by presenting one-syllable words at 25–40 dB above the SRT. The words are phonetically balanced in that the phonemes (speech sounds) occur in the list of words at the same frequency that they occur in ordinary conversational English. An individual with normal hearing or conductive hearing loss can repeat 88–100% of the phonetically balanced words correctly. Patients with a sensorineural hearing loss have variable loss of discrimination. As a general rule, neural lesions produce greater deficits in discrimination than do lesions in the inner ear. For example, in a patient with mild asymmetric sensorineural hearing loss, a clue to the diagnosis of vestibular schwannoma is the presence of a substantial deterioration in discrimination ability. Deterioration in discrimination ability at higher intensities above the SRT also suggests a lesion in the eighth nerve or central auditory pathways.

Tympanometry measures the impedance of the middle ear to sound and is useful in diagnosis of middle-ear effusions. A *tympanogram* is the graphic representation of change in impedance or compliance as the pressure in the ear canal is changed. Normally, the middle ear is most compliant at atmospheric pressure, and the compliance decreases as the pressure is increased or decreased; this pattern is seen with normal hearing or in the presence of sensorineural hearing loss. Compliance that does not change with change in pressure suggests middle-ear effusion. With a negative pressure in the middle ear, as with eustachian tube obstruction, the point of maximal compliance occurs with negative pressure in the ear canal. A tympanogram in which no point of maximal compliance can be obtained is most commonly seen with discontinuity of the ossicular chain. A reduction in the maximal compliance peak can be seen in otosclerosis.

During tympanometry, an intense tone elicits contraction of the stapedius muscle. The change in compliance of the middle ear with contraction of the stapedius muscle can be detected. The presence or absence of this *acoustic reflex* is important in the anatomic localization of facial nerve paralysis as well as hearing loss. Normal or elevated acoustic reflex thresholds in an individual with sensorineural hearing impairment suggests a cochlear hearing loss. Assessment of *acoustic reflex decay* helps differentiate sensory from neural hearing losses. In neural hearing loss, the reflex adapts or decays with time.

Otoacoustic emissions (OAE) can be measured with microphones inserted into the external auditory canal. The emissions may be spontaneous or evoked with sound stimulation. The presence of OAEs indicates that the outer hair cells of the organ of Corti are intact and can be used to assess auditory thresholds and to distinguish sensory from neural hearing losses.

Evoked Responses *Electrocochleography* measures the earliest evoked potentials generated in the cochlea and the auditory nerve. Receptor potentials recorded include the cochlear microphonic, generated by the outer hair cells of the organ of Corti, and the summating potential, generated by the inner hair cells in response to sound. The whole nerve action potential representing the composite firing of the first-order neurons can also be recorded during electrocochleography. Clinically, the test is useful in the diagnosis of Ménière's disease, where an elevation of the ratio of summating potential to action potential is seen.

Brainstem auditory evoked responses (BAERs) are useful in differentiating the site of sensorineural hearing loss. In response to sound, five distinct electrical potentials arising from different stations along the peripheral and central auditory pathway can be identified using computer averaging from scalp surface electrodes. BAERs are valuable in situations in which patients cannot or will not give reliable voluntary thresholds. They are also used to assess the integrity of the auditory nerve and brainstem in various clinical situations, including intraoperative monitoring and in determination of brain death.

The *vestibular-evoked myogenic potential (VEMP) test* elicits a vestibulocollic reflex whose afferent limb arises from acoustically sensitive cells in the saccule, with signals conducted via the inferior vestibular nerve. VEMP is a biphasic, short-latency response recorded from the tonically contracted sternocleidomastoid muscle in response to loud auditory clicks or tones. VEMPs may be diminished or absent in patients with early and late Ménière's disease, vestibular neuritis, benign paroxysmal positional vertigo, and vestibular schwannoma. On the other hand, the threshold for VEMPs may be lower in cases of superior canal dehiscence and perilymphatic fistula.

Imaging Studies The choice of radiologic tests is largely determined by whether the goal is to evaluate the bony anatomy of the external, middle, and inner ear or to image the auditory nerve and brain. Axial and coronal CT of the temporal bone with fine 1-mm cuts is ideal for determining the caliber of the external auditory canal, integrity of the ossicular chain, and presence of middle-ear or mastoid disease; it can also detect inner-ear malformations. CT is also ideal for the detection of bone erosion with chronic otitis media and cholesteatoma. MRI is superior to CT for imaging of retrocochlear pathology such as vestibular schwannoma, meningioma, other lesions of the cerebellopontine angle, demyelinating lesions of the brainstem, and brain tumors. Both CT and MRI are equally capable of identifying inner-ear malformations and assessing cochlear patency for preoperative evaluation of patients for cochlear implantation.

℞ DISORDERS OF THE SENSE OF HEARING

In general, conductive hearing losses are amenable to surgical correction, while sensorineural hearing losses are more difficult to manage. Atresia of the ear canal can be surgically repaired, often with significant improvement in hearing. Tympanic membrane perforations due to chronic otitis media or trauma can be repaired with an outpatient tympanoplasty. Likewise, conductive hearing loss associated with otosclerosis can be treated by stapedectomy, which is successful in 90–95% of cases. Tympanostomy tubes allow the prompt return of normal hearing in individuals with middle-ear effusions. Hearing aids are effective and well-tolerated in patients with conductive hearing losses.

Patients with mild, moderate, and severe sensorineural hearing losses are regularly rehabilitated with hearing aids of varying configuration and strength. Hearing aids have been improved to provide greater fidelity and have been miniaturized. The current generation of hearing aids can be placed entirely within the ear canal, thus reducing any stigma associated with their use. In general, the more severe the hearing impairment, the larger the hearing aid required for auditory rehabilitation. Digital hearing aids lend themselves to individual programming, and multiple and directional microphones at the ear level may be helpful in noisy surroundings. Since all hearing aids amplify noise as well as speech, the only absolute solution to the problem of noise is to place the microphone closer to the speaker than the noise source. This arrangement is not possible with a self-contained, cosmetically acceptable device.

In many situations, including lectures and the theater, hearing-impaired persons benefit from assistive devices that are based on the principle of having the speaker closer to the microphone than any source of noise. Assistive devices include infrared and frequency-modulated (FM) transmission as well as an electromagnetic loop around the room for transmission to the individual's hearing aid. Hearing aids with telecoils can also be used with properly equipped telephones in the same way.

In the event that the hearing aid provides inadequate rehabilitation, cochlear implants may be appropriate. Criteria for implantation include severe to profound hearing loss with word recognition score ≤30% under best aided conditions. Worldwide, >20,000 deaf individuals (including 4000 children) have received cochlear implants. Cochlear implants are neural prostheses that convert sound energy to electrical energy and can be used to stimulate the auditory division of the eighth nerve directly. In most cases of profound hearing impairment, the auditory hair cells are lost but the ganglionic cells of the auditory division of the eighth nerve are preserved. Cochlear implants consist of electrodes that are inserted into the cochlea through the round window, speech processors that extract acoustical elements of speech for conversion to electrical currents, and a means of transmitting the electrical energy through the skin. Patients with implants experience sound that helps with speech reading, allows open-set word recognition, and helps in modulating the person's own voice. Usually, within 3 months after implantation, adult patients can understand speech without visual cues. With the current generation of multichannel cochlear implants, nearly 75% of patients are able to converse on the telephone. For individuals who have had both eighth nerves destroyed by trauma or bilateral vestibular schwannomas (e.g., neurofibromatosis type 2), brainstem auditory implants placed near the cochlear nucleus may provide auditory rehabilitation.

Tinnitus often accompanies hearing loss. As for background noise, tinnitus can degrade speech comprehension in individuals with hearing impairment. Therapy for tinnitus is usually directed towards minimizing the appreciation of tinnitus. Relief of the tinnitus may be obtained by masking it with background music. Hearing aids are also helpful in tinnitus suppression, as are tinnitus maskers, devices that present a sound to the affected ear that is more pleasant to listen to than the tinnitus. The use of a tinnitus masker is often followed by several hours of inhibition of the tinnitus. Antidepressants have been shown to be beneficial in helping patients cope with tinnitus.

Hard-of-hearing individuals often benefit from a reduction in unnecessary noise (e.g., radio or television) to enhance the signal-to-noise ratio. Speech comprehension is aided by lip reading; therefore the impaired listener should be seated so that the face of the speaker is well-illuminated and easily seen. Although speech should be in a loud, clear voice, one should be aware that in sensorineural hearing losses in general and in hard-of-hearing elderly in particular, recruitment (abnormal perception of loud sounds) may be troublesome. Above all, optimal communication cannot take place without both parties giving it their full and undivided attention.

PREVENTION

Conductive hearing losses may be prevented by prompt antibiotic therapy of adequate duration for AOM and by ventilation of the middle ear with tympanostomy tubes in middle-ear effusions lasting ≥12 weeks. Loss of vestibular function and deafness due to aminoglycoside antibiotics can largely be prevented by careful monitoring of serum peak and trough levels.

Some 10 million Americans have noise-induced hearing loss, and 20 million are exposed to hazardous noise in their employment. Noise-induced hearing loss can be prevented by avoidance of exposure to loud noise or by regular use of ear plugs or fluid-filled ear muffs to attenuate intense sound. High-risk activities for noise-induced hearing loss include wood and metal working with electrical equipment and target practice and hunting with small firearms. All internal-combustion and electric engines, including snow and leaf blowers, snowmobiles, outboard motors, and chain saws, require protection of the user with hearing protectors. Virtually all noise-induced hearing loss is preventable through education, which should begin before the teenage years. Programs of industrial conservation of hearing are required when the exposure over an 8-h period averages 85 dB. Workers in such noisy environments can be protected with preemployment audiologic assessment, the mandatory use of hearing protectors, and annual audiologic assessments.

ACKNOWLEDGMENT

The author acknowledges the contributions of Dr. James B. Snow, Jr., to this chapter.

FURTHER READINGS

BENTON R: On the origin of smell: Odorant receptors in insects. Cell Mol Life Sci 63:1579, 2006

BREER H et al: The sense of smell: Multiple olfactory subsystems. Cell Mol Life Sci 63:1465, 2004

BRESLIN PA, HUANG L: Human taste: Peripheral anatomy, taste transduction, and coding. Adv Otorhinolaryngol 63:152, 2006

DULAC C: Sparse encoding of natural scents. Neuron 50:816, 2006

GATES GA, MILLS JH: Presbycusis. Lancet 366:1111, 2005

GUDZIOL V et al: Clinical significance of results from olfactory testing. Laryngoscope 116:1858, 2006

HECKMANN JG, LANG CJ: Neurological causes of taste disorders. Adv Otorhinolaryngol 63:255, 2006

LALWANI AK (ed): *Current Diagnosis and Treatment in Otolaryngology—Head & Neck Surgery*, 2d ed. New York, McGraw-Hill, 2007

RENNELS M, PICKERING LK: Sensorineural hearing loss in children. Lancet 365:2085, 2005

31 Pharyngitis, Sinusitis, Otitis, and Other Upper Respiratory Tract Infections

Michael A. Rubin, Ralph Gonzales, Merle A. Sande

Infections of the upper respiratory tract (URIs) have a tremendous impact on public health. They are among the most common reasons for visits to primary care providers, and, although the illnesses are typically mild, their high incidence and transmission rates place them among the leading causes of time lost from work or school. Even though the minority (~25%) of cases are caused by bacteria, URIs are the leading diagnoses for which antibiotics are prescribed on an outpatient basis in the United States. The enormous consumption of antibiotics for these illnesses has contributed to the rise in antibiotic resistance among common community-acquired pathogens such as *Streptococcus pneumoniae*—a trend that in itself has had an enormous influence on public health.

Although most URIs are caused by viruses, distinguishing patients with primary viral infection from those with primary bacterial infection is difficult. Signs and symptoms of bacterial and viral URIs are, in fact, indistinguishable. Because routine, rapid testing is neither available nor practical for most syndromes, acute infections are diagnosed largely on clinical grounds. Thus the judicious use of antibiotics in this setting is challenging.

NONSPECIFIC INFECTIONS OF THE UPPER RESPIRATORY TRACT

Nonspecific URIs are a broadly defined group of disorders that collectively constitute the leading cause of ambulatory care visits in the United States. By definition, nonspecific URIs have no prominent localizing features. They are identified by a variety of descriptive names, including *acute infective rhinitis, acute rhinopharyngitis/nasopharyngitis, acute coryza*, and *acute nasal catarrh*, as well as by the inclusive label *common cold*.

Etiology The large assortment of URI classifications reflects the wide variety of causative infectious agents and the varied manifestations of common pathogens. Nearly all nonspecific URIs are caused by viruses spanning multiple virus families and many antigenic types. For instance, there are at least 100 immunotypes of rhinovirus (Chap. 179), the most common cause of URI (~30–40% of cases); other causes include influenza virus (three immunotypes; Chap. 180) as well as parainfluenza virus (four immunotypes), coronavirus (at least three immunotypes), and adenovirus (47 immunotypes) (Chap. 179). Respiratory syncytial virus (RSV) also accounts for a small percentage of cases each year, as do some viruses not typically associated with URIs (e.g., enteroviruses, rubella virus, and varicella-zoster virus). Even with sophisticated diagnostic and culture techniques, a substantial proportion (25–30%) of cases have no assigned pathogen.

Clinical Manifestations The signs and symptoms of nonspecific URI are similar to those of other URIs but lack a pronounced localization to one particular anatomic location, such as the sinuses, pharynx, or lower airway. Nonspecific URI is commonly described as an acute, mild, and self-limited catarrhal syndrome, with a median duration of ~1 week. Signs and symptoms are diverse and frequently variable across patients. The principal signs and symptoms of nonspecific URI include rhinorrhea (with or without purulence), nasal congestion, cough, and sore throat. Other manifestations, such as fever, malaise, sneezing, and hoarseness, are more variable, with fever more common among infants and young children. Occasionally, clinical features reflect the underlying viral pathogen; myalgias and fatigue, for example, are sometimes seen with influenza and parainfluenza infections, while conjunctivitis may suggest infection with adenovirus or enterovirus. Findings on physical examination are frequently nonspecific and unimpressive. Between 0.5 and 2% of colds are complicated by secondary bacterial infections (e.g., rhinosinusitis, otitis media, and pneumonia), particularly in high-risk populations such as infants, elderly persons, and chronically ill patients. Secondary bacterial infections are usually associated with a prolonged course of illness, increased severity of illness, and localization of signs and symptoms. Purulent secretions from the nares or throat have often been used as an indication of sinusitis or pharyngitis. However, these secretions are also seen in nonspecific URI and, in the absence of other clinical features, are poor predictors of bacterial infection.

Rx UPPER RESPIRATORY INFECTIONS

Antibiotics have no role in the treatment of uncomplicated nonspecific URI. In the absence of clinical evidence of bacterial infection, treatment remains entirely symptom-based, with use of decongestants and nonsteroidal anti-inflammatory drugs. Other therapies directed at specific symptoms are often useful, including dextromethorphan for cough and lozenges with topical anesthetic for sore throat. Clinical trials of zinc, vitamin C, echinacea, and other alternative remedies have revealed no consistent benefit for the treatment of nonspecific URI.

INFECTIONS OF THE SINUS

Sinusitis refers to an inflammatory condition involving the four paired structures surrounding the nasal cavities. Although most cases of sinusitis involve more than one sinus, the maxillary sinus is most commonly involved; next in frequency are the ethmoid, frontal, and sphenoid sinuses. Each sinus is lined with a respiratory epithelium that produces mucus, which is transported out by ciliary action through the sinus ostium and into the nasal cavity. Normally, mucus does not accumulate in the sinuses, which remain sterile despite their adjacency to the bacterium-filled nasal passages. When the sinus ostia are obstructed, however, or when ciliary clearance is impaired or absent, the secretions can be retained, producing the typical signs and symptoms of sinusitis. The retained secretions may become infected with a variety of pathogens, including viruses, bacteria, and fungi. Sinusitis affects a tremendous proportion of the population, accounts for millions of visits to primary care physicians each year, and is the fifth leading diagnosis for which antibiotics are prescribed. It is typically classified by duration of illness (acute vs. chronic); by etiology (infectious vs. noninfectious); and, when infectious, by the offending pathogen type (viral, bacterial, or fungal).

ACUTE SINUSITIS

Acute sinusitis—defined as sinusitis of <4 weeks' duration—constitutes the vast majority of sinusitis cases. Most cases are diagnosed in the ambulatory care setting and occur primarily as a consequence of a preceding viral URI. Differentiating acute bacterial and viral sinusitis on clinical grounds is difficult. Therefore, it is perhaps unsurprising that antibiotics are prescribed frequently (in 85–98% of all cases) for this condition.

Etiology A number of infectious and noninfectious factors can contribute to acute obstruction of the sinus ostia or impairment of ciliary clearance, with consequent sinusitis. Noninfectious causes include allergic rhinitis (with either mucosal edema or polyp obstruction), barotrauma (e.g., from deep-sea diving or air travel), or chemical irritants. Illnesses such as nasal and sinus tumors (e.g., squamous cell carcinoma) or granulomatous diseases (e.g., Wegener's granulomatosis or rhinoscleroma) can also produce obstruction of the sinus ostia, while conditions leading to altered mucus content (e.g., cystic fibrosis) can cause sinusitis through impaired mucus clearance. In the hospital setting, nasotracheal intubation is a major risk factor for nosocomial sinusitis in intensive care units.

Acute infectious sinusitis can be caused by a variety of organisms, including viruses, bacteria, and fungi. Viral rhinosinusitis is far more common than bacterial sinusitis, although relatively few studies have sampled sinus aspirates for the presence of different viruses. In those studies that have done so, the viruses most commonly isolated—both alone and with bacteria—have been rhinovirus, parainfluenza virus, and influenza virus. Bacterial causes of sinusitis have been better described. Among community-acquired cases, *S. pneumoniae* and nontypable *Haemophilus influenzae* are the most common pathogens, accounting for 50–60% of cases.

Moraxella catarrhalis causes disease in a significant percentage (20%) of children but less often in adults. Other streptococcal species and *Staphylococcus aureus* cause only a small percentage of cases, although there is increasing concern about community strains of methicillin-resistant *S. aureus* (MRSA) as an emerging cause. Anaerobes are occasionally found in association with infections of the roots of premolar teeth that spread into the adjacent maxillary sinuses. The role of *Chlamydophila pneumoniae* and *Mycoplasma pneumoniae* in the pathogenesis of acute sinusitis is still unclear. Nosocomial cases are commonly associated with bacteria found in the hospital environment, including *S. aureus, Pseudomonas aeruginosa, Serratia marcescens, Klebsiella pneumoniae,* and *Enterobacter* species. Often, these infections are polymicrobial and involve organisms that are highly resistant to numerous antibiotics. Fungi are also established causes of sinusitis, although most acute cases are in immunocompromised patients and represent invasive, life-threatening infections. The best-known example is rhinocerebral mucormycosis caused by fungi of the order Mucorales, which includes *Rhizopus, Rhizomucor, Mucor, Absidia,* and *Cunninghamella.* These infections usually occur in diabetic patients with ketoacidosis but also develop in transplant recipients, patients with hematologic malignancies, and patients receiving chronic glucocorticoid or deferoxamine therapy. Other hyaline molds, such as *Aspergillus* and *Fusarium* species, are also occasional causes of this disease.

Clinical Manifestations Most cases of acute sinusitis present after or in conjunction with a viral URI, and it can be difficult to discriminate the clinical features of one from the other. A large proportion of patients with colds have sinus inflammation, although bacterial sinusitis complicates only 0.2–2% of these viral infections. Common presenting symptoms of sinusitis include nasal drainage and congestion, facial pain or pressure, and headache. Thick, purulent or discolored nasal discharge is often thought to indicate bacterial sinusitis but also occurs early in viral infections such as the common cold and is not specific to bacterial infection. Other nonspecific manifestations include cough, sneezing, and fever. Tooth pain, most often involving the upper molars, is associated with bacterial sinusitis, as is halitosis.

In acute sinusitis, sinus pain or pressure often localizes to the involved sinus (particularly the maxillary sinus) and can be worse when the patient bends over or is supine. Although rare, manifestations of advanced sphenoid or ethmoid sinus infection can be profound, including severe frontal or retroorbital pain radiating to the occiput, thrombosis of the cavernous sinus, and signs of orbital cellulitis. Acute focal sinusitis is uncommon but should be considered in the patient with severe symptoms over the maxillary sinus and fever, regardless of illness duration. Similarly, advanced frontal sinusitis can present with a condition known as *Pott's puffy tumor*, with soft tissue swelling and pitting edema over the frontal bone from a communicating subperiosteal abscess. Life-threatening complications include meningitis, epidural abscess, and cerebral abscess.

Patients with acute fungal sinusitis (such as mucormycosis) often present with symptoms related to pressure effects, particularly when the infection has spread to the orbits and cavernous sinus. Signs such as orbital swelling and cellulitis, proptosis, ptosis, and decreased extraocular movement are common, as is retroorbital or periorbital pain. Nasopharyngeal ulcerations, epistaxis, and headaches are also frequent, and involvement of cranial nerves V and VII has been described in more advanced cases. Bony erosion may be evident on examination. Oftentimes, the patient does not appear seriously ill despite the rapidly progressive nature of these infections.

Patients with acute nosocomial sinusitis are often critically ill and thus do not manifest the typical clinical features of sinus disease. This diagnosis should be suspected, however, when hospitalized patients who have appropriate risk factors (e.g., nasotracheal intubation) develop fever of unknown origin.

Diagnosis Distinguishing viral from bacterial sinusitis in the ambulatory setting is usually difficult, given the relatively low sensitivity and specificity of the common clinical features. One clinical feature that has been used to help guide diagnostic and therapeutic decision-making is illness duration. Because acute bacterial sinusitis is uncommon in patients whose symptoms have lasted <7 days, several authorities now recommend reserving this diagnosis for patients with "persistent" symptoms (i.e., symptoms lasting >7 days in adults or >10–14 days in children) accompanied by purulent nasal discharge (Table 31-1). Even among the patients who meet these criteria, only 40–50% have true bacterial sinusitis. The use of CT or sinus radiography is not recommended for routine cases, particularly early in the course of illness (i.e., at <7 days), given the high prevalence of similar abnormalities among cases of acute viral rhinosinusitis. In the evaluation of persistent, recurrent, or chronic sinusitis, CT of the sinuses is the radiographic study of choice.

The clinical history and/or setting can often identify cases of acute anaerobic bacterial sinusitis, acute fungal sinusitis, or sinusitis from noninfectious causes (e.g., allergic rhinosinusitis). In the case of an immunocompromised patient with acute fungal sinus infection, immediate examination by an otolaryngologist is required. Biopsy specimens from involved areas should be examined by a pathologist for evidence of fungal hyphal elements and tissue invasion. Cases of suspected acute nosocomial sinusitis should be confirmed by sinus CT. Because therapy should target the offending organism, a sinus aspirate should be obtained, if possible, for culture and susceptibility testing.

Rx ACUTE SINUSITIS

Most patients with a diagnosis of acute rhinosinusitis based on clinical grounds improve without antibiotic therapy. The preferred initial approach in patients with mild to moderate symptoms of short duration is therapy aimed at facilitating sinus drainage, such as oral and topical decongestants, nasal saline lavage, and—in patients with a history of chronic sinusitis or allergies—nasal glucocorticoids. Adult patients who do not improve after 7 days, children who do not improve after 10–14 days, and patients with more severe symptoms (regardless of duration) should be treated with antibiotics (Table 31-1). Empirical therapy should consist of the narrowest-spectrum agent active against the most common bacterial pathogens, including *S. pneumoniae* and *H. influenzae*—e.g., amoxicillin. No clinical trials support the use of broad-spectrum agents for routine cases of bacterial sinusitis, even in the current era of drug-resistant *S. pneumoniae*. Up to 10% of patients do not respond to initial antimicrobial therapy; sinus aspiration and/or lavage by an otolaryngologist should be considered in these cases. Antibiotic prophylaxis to prevent episodes of recurrent acute bacterial sinusitis is not recommended.

Surgical intervention and IV antibiotic administration are usually reserved for patients with severe disease or those with intracranial complications, such as abscess or orbital involvement. Immunocompromised patients with acute invasive fungal sinusitis usually require extensive surgical debridement and treatment with IV antifungal agents active against fungal hyphal forms, such as amphotericin B. Specific therapy should be individualized according to the fungal species and the individual patient's characteristics.

Treatment of nosocomial sinusitis should begin with broad-spectrum antibiotics to cover common pathogens such as *S. aureus* and gram-negative bacilli. Therapy should then be tailored to the results of culture and susceptibility testing of sinus aspirates.

CHRONIC SINUSITIS

Chronic sinusitis is characterized by symptoms of sinus inflammation lasting >12 weeks. This illness is most commonly associated with either bacteria or fungi, and clinical cure in most cases is very difficult. Many patients have undergone treatment with repeated courses of antibacterial agents and multiple sinus surgeries, increasing their risk of colonization with antibiotic-resistant pathogens and of surgical complications. Patients often suffer significant morbidity, sometimes over many years.

In *chronic bacterial sinusitis*, infection is thought to be due to the impairment of mucociliary clearance from repeated infections rather than to persistent bacterial infection. However, the pathogenesis of this condition is poorly understood. Although certain conditions (e.g., cystic fibrosis) can predispose patients to chronic bacterial sinusitis, most patients with this infection do not have obvious underlying conditions that result in the obstruction of sinus drainage, the impairment of ciliary action, or immune dysfunction. Patients experience constant nasal congestion and sinus pressure, with intermittent periods of greater severity,

TABLE 31-1 GUIDELINES FOR THE DIAGNOSIS AND TREATMENT OF ACUTE SINUSITIS

Age Group	Diagnostic Criteria	Treatment Recommendations[a]
Adults	Moderate symptoms (e.g., nasal purulence/ congestion or cough) for >7 d *or* Severe symptoms of any duration, including unilateral/focal facial swelling or tooth pain	*Initial therapy* Amoxicillin, 500 mg PO tid or 875 mg PO bid, *or* TMP-SMX, 1 DS tablet PO bid for 10–14 d *Exposure to antibiotics within 30 d or >30% prevalence of penicillin-resistant S. pneumoniae* Amoxicillin, 1000 mg PO tid, *or* Amoxicillin/clavulanate (extended release), 2000 mg PO bid, *or* Antipneumococcal fluoroquinolone (e.g., levofloxacin, 500 mg PO qd) *Recent treatment failure* Amoxicillin/clavulanate (extended release), 2000 mg PO bid, *or* Amoxicillin, 1500 mg bid, plus clindamycin, 300 mg PO qid, *or* Antipneumococcal fluoroquinolone (e.g., levofloxacin, 500 mg PO qd)
Children	Moderate symptoms (e.g., nasal purulence/congestion or cough) for >10–14 d *or* Severe symptoms of any duration, including fever (>102°F), unilateral/ focal facial swelling or pain	*Initial therapy* Amoxicillin, 45–90 mg/kg qd (up to 2 g) PO in divided doses (bid or tid), *or* Cefuroxime axetil, 30 mg/kg qd PO in divided doses (bid), *or* Cefdinir, 14 mg/kg PO qd *Exposure to antibiotics within 30 d, recent treatment failure, or >30% prevalence of penicillin-resistant S. pneumoniae* Amoxicillin, 90 mg/kg qd (up to 2 g) PO in divided doses (bid), plus clavulanate, 6.4 mg/kg qd PO in divided doses (bid) (extra-strength suspension), *or* Cefuroxime axetil, 30 mg/kg qd PO in divided doses (bid), *or* Cefdinir, 14 mg/kg PO qd

[a]Unless otherwise specified, the duration of therapy is generally 10 d, with appropriate follow-up.
Note: DS, double-strength; TMP-SMX, trimethoprim-sulfamethoxazole.
Sources: American Academy of Pediatrics Subcommittee on Management of Sinusitis and Committee on Quality Improvement, 2001; Hickner et al, 2001; Piccirillo, 2004; and Sinus and Allergy Health Partnership, 2004.

which may persist for years. CT can be helpful in determining the extent of disease and the response to therapy. The management team should include an otolaryngologist to conduct endoscopic examinations and obtain tissue samples for histologic examination and culture.

Chronic fungal sinusitis is a disease of immunocompetent hosts and is usually noninvasive, although slowly progressive invasive disease is sometimes seen. Noninvasive disease, which is typically associated with hyaline molds such as *Aspergillus* species and dematiaceous molds such as *Curvularia* or *Bipolaris* species, can present as a number of different scenarios. In mild, indolent disease, which usually occurs in the setting of repeated failures of antibacterial therapy, only nonspecific mucosal changes may be seen on sinus CT. Endoscopic surgery is usually curative in these patients, with no need for antifungal therapy. Another form of disease presents with long-standing, often unilateral symptoms and opacification of a single sinus on imaging studies as a result of a mycetoma (fungus ball) within the sinus. Treatment for this condition is also surgical, although systemic antifungal therapy may be warranted in the rare case where bony erosion occurs. A third form of disease, known as *allergic fungal sinusitis*, is seen in patients with a history of nasal polyposis and asthma, who often have had multiple sinus surgeries. Patients with this condition produce a thick, eosinophilic mucus with the consistency of peanut butter that contains sparse fungal hyphae on histologic examination. Patients often present with pansinusitis.

℞ CHRONIC SINUSITIS

Treatment of chronic bacterial sinusitis can be challenging and consists primarily of repeated culture-guided courses of antibiotics, sometimes for 3–4 weeks at a time; administration of intranasal glucocorticoids; and mechanical irrigation of the sinus with sterile saline solution. When this management approach fails, sinus surgery may be indicated and sometimes provides significant, albeit short-term, alleviation. Treatment of chronic fungal sinusitis consists of surgical removal of impacted mucus. Recurrence, unfortunately, is common.

INFECTIONS OF THE EAR AND MASTOID

Infections of the ear and associated structures can involve both the middle and external ear, including the skin, cartilage, periosteum, ear canal, and tympanic and mastoid cavities. Both viruses and bacteria are known causes of these infections, some of which result in significant morbidity if not treated appropriately.

INFECTIONS OF THE EXTERNAL EAR STRUCTURES

Infections involving the structures of the external ear are often difficult to differentiate from noninfectious inflammatory conditions with similar clinical manifestations. Clinicians should consider inflammatory disorders as a possible cause of external ear irritation, particularly in the absence of local or regional adenopathy. Aside from the more salient causes of inflammation such as trauma, insect bite, and overexposure to sunlight or extreme cold, the differential diagnosis should include less common conditions such as autoimmune disorders (e.g., lupus or relapsing polychondritis) and vasculitides (e.g., Wegener's granulomatosis).

Auricular Cellulitis Auricular cellulitis is an infection of the skin overlying the external ear and typically follows minor local trauma. It presents with the typical signs and symptoms of a skin/soft tissue infection, with tenderness, erythema, swelling, and warmth of the external ear (particularly the lobule) but without apparent involvement of the ear canal or inner structures. Treatment consists of warm compresses and oral antibiotics such as dicloxacillin that are active against typical skin and soft tissue pathogens (specifically, *S. aureus* and streptococci). IV antibiotics, such as a first-generation cephalosporin (e.g., cefazolin) or a penicillinase-resistant penicillin (e.g., nafcillin), are occasionally needed for more severe cases.

Perichondritis Perichondritis, an infection of the perichondrium of the auricular cartilage, typically follows local trauma (e.g., ear piercing, burns, or lacerations). Occasionally, when the infection spreads down to the cartilage of the pinna itself, patients may also have chondritis. The infection may closely resemble auricular cellulitis, with erythema, swelling, and extreme tenderness of the pinna, although the lobule is less often involved in perichondritis. The most common pathogens are *P. aeruginosa* and *S. aureus*, although other gram-negative and gram-positive organisms are occasionally involved. Treatment consists of systemic antibiotics active against both *P. aeruginosa* and *S. aureus*. An antipseudomonal penicillin (e.g., piperacillin) or a combination of a penicillinase-resistant penicillin plus an antipseudomonal quinolone (e.g., nafcillin plus ciprofloxacin) is typically used. Incision and drainage may be helpful for culture and for resolution of infection, which often takes weeks. When perichondritis fails to respond to adequate antimicrobial therapy, clinicians should consider a noninfectious inflammatory etiology; for example, relapsing polychondritis is often mistaken for infectious perichondritis.

Otitis Externa The term *otitis externa* refers to a collection of diseases involving primarily the auditory meatus. Otitis externa usually results from a combination of heat, retained moisture, and desquamation and maceration of the epithelium of the outer ear canal. The disease exists in several forms: localized, diffuse, chronic, and invasive. All forms are predominantly bacterial in origin, with *P. aeruginosa* and *S. aureus* the most common pathogens.

Acute localized otitis externa (*furunculosis*) can develop in the outer third of the ear canal, where skin overlies cartilage and hair follicles are numerous. As in furunculosis elsewhere on the body, *S. aureus* is the usual pathogen, and treatment typically consists of an oral antistaphylococcal penicillin (e.g., dicloxacillin), with incision and drainage in cases of abscess formation.

Acute diffuse otitis externa is also known as *swimmer's ear*, although it can develop in patients who have not recently been swimming. Heat, humidity, and the loss of protective cerumen lead to excessive moisture and elevation of the pH in the ear canal, which in turn lead to skin maceration and irritation. Infection may then occur; the predominant pathogen is *P. aeruginosa*, although other gram-negative and gram-positive organisms have been recovered from patients with this condition. The illness often starts with itching and progresses to severe pain, which is usually triggered by manipulation of the pinna or tragus. The onset of pain is generally accompanied by the development of an erythematous, swollen ear canal, often with scant white, clumpy discharge. Treatment consists of cleansing the canal to remove debris and to enhance the activity of topical therapeutic agents—usually hypertonic saline or mixtures of alcohol and acetic acid. Inflammation can also be decreased by adding glucocorticoids to the treatment regimen or by using Burow's solution (aluminum acetate in water). Antibiotics are most effective when given topically. Otic mixtures provide adequate pathogen coverage; these preparations usually combine neomycin with polymyxin, with or without glucocorticoids.

Chronic otitis externa is caused primarily by repeated local irritation, most commonly arising from persistent drainage from a chronic middle-ear infection. Other causes of repeated irritation, such as insertion of cotton swabs or other foreign objects into the ear canal, can lead to this condition, as can rare chronic infections such as syphilis, tuberculosis, or leprosy. Chronic otitis externa typically presents as erythematous, scaling dermatitis in which the predominant symptom is pruritus rather than pain; this condition must be differentiated from several others that produce a similar clinical picture, such as atopic dermatitis, seborrheic dermatitis, psoriasis, and dermatomycosis. Therapy consists of identifying and treating or removing the offending process, although successful resolution is frequently difficult.

Invasive otitis externa, also known as *malignant* or *necrotizing* otitis externa, is an aggressive and potentially life-threatening disease that occurs predominantly in elderly diabetic patients and other immunocompromised patients. The disease begins in the external canal, progresses slowly over weeks to months, and often is difficult to distinguish from a severe case of chronic otitis externa because of the presence of purulent otorrhea and an erythematous swollen ear and external canal. Severe, deep-seated otalgia is often noted and can help differentiate invasive from chronic otitis externa. The characteristic finding on examination is granulation tissue in the posteroinferior wall of the external canal, near the junction of bone and cartilage. If left unchecked, the infection can migrate to the base of the skull (resulting in skull-base osteomyelitis) and on to the meninges and brain, with a high associated mortality rate. Cranial nerve involvement is occasionally seen, with the facial nerve usually affected first and most often. Thrombosis of the sigmoid sinus can occur if the infection extends to that area. CT, which can reveal osseous erosion of the temporal bone and skull base, can be used to help determine the extent of disease, as can gallium and technetium-99 scintigraphy studies. *P. aeruginosa* is by far the most common pathogen, although *S. aureus*, *Staphylococcus epidermidis*, *Aspergillus*, *Actinomyces*, and some gram-negative bacteria have also been associated with this disease. In all cases, the external ear canal should be cleansed and a biopsy specimen of the granulation tissue within the canal (or of deeper tissues) should be obtained for culture of the offending organism. IV antibiotic therapy is directed specifically toward the recovered pathogen. For *P. aeruginosa*, the regimen typically includes an antipseudomonal penicillin or cephalosporin (e.g., piperacillin or ceftazidime) with an aminoglycoside. A fluoroquinolone antibiotic is frequently used in place of the aminoglycoside and can even be administered orally, given the excellent bioavailability of this drug class. In addition, antibiotic drops containing an agent active against *Pseudomonas* (e.g., ciprofloxacin) are usually prescribed and are combined with glucocorticoids to reduce inflammation. Cases of invasive *Pseudomonas* otitis externa recognized in the early stages can sometimes be treated with oral and otic fluoroquinolones alone, albeit with close follow-up. Extensive surgical debridement, once an important component of the treatment approach, is now rarely indicated.

INFECTIONS OF MIDDLE-EAR STRUCTURES

Otitis media is an inflammatory condition of the middle ear that results from dysfunction of the eustachian tube in association with a number of illnesses, including URIs and chronic rhinosinusitis. The inflammatory response to these conditions leads to the development of a sterile transudate within the middle-ear and mastoid cavities. Infection may occur if bacteria or viruses from the nasopharynx contaminate this fluid, producing an acute (or sometimes chronic) illness.

Acute Otitis Media Acute otitis media results when pathogens from the nasopharynx are introduced into the inflammatory fluid collected in the middle ear (e.g., by nose blowing during a URI). The proliferation of these pathogens in this space leads to the development of the typical signs and symptoms of acute middle-ear infection. The diagnosis of acute otitis media requires the demonstration of fluid in the middle ear (with tympanic membrane immobility) and the accompanying signs or symptoms of local or systemic illness (Table 31-2).

ETIOLOGY Acute otitis media typically follows a viral URI. The causative viruses (most commonly RSV, influenza virus, rhinovirus, and enterovirus) can themselves cause subsequent acute otitis media; more often, they predispose the patient to bacterial otitis media. Studies using tympanocentesis have consistently found *S. pneumoniae* to be the most important bacterial cause, isolated in up to 35% of cases. *H. influenzae* (nontypable strains) and *M. catarrhalis* are also common bacterial causes of acute otitis media, and concern is increasing about community strains of MRSA as an emerging etiologic agent. Viruses, such as those mentioned above, have been recovered either alone or with bacteria in 17–40% of cases.

CLINICAL MANIFESTATIONS Fluid in the middle ear is typically demonstrated or confirmed with pneumatic otoscopy. In the absence of fluid, the tympanic membrane moves visibly with the application of positive and negative pressure, but this movement is dampened when fluid is present. With bacterial infection, the tympanic membrane can also be erythematous, bulging, or retracted and occasionally can spontaneously perforate. The signs and symptoms accompanying infection can be local or systemic, including otalgia, otorrhea, diminished hearing, fever, or irritability. Erythema of the tympanic membrane is often evident but is nonspecific as it is frequently seen in association with inflammation of the upper respiratory mucosa (e.g., during examination of young children). Other signs and symptoms that are occasionally reported include vertigo, nystagmus, and tinnitus.

Rx ACUTE OTITIS MEDIA

There has been considerable debate on the usefulness of antibiotics for the treatment of acute otitis media. Although most cases resolve clinically 1 week after the onset of illness, antibiotics appear to be of some benefit. A higher proportion of treated than of untreated patients are free of illness 3–5 days after diagnosis. The difficulty of predicting which patients will benefit from antibiotic therapy has led to different approaches. In the Netherlands, for instance, physicians typically manage acute otitis media with initial observation, administering anti-inflammatory agents for aggressive pain management and reserving antibiotics for high-risk patients, patients with complicated disease, or patients who do not improve after 48–72 h. In contrast, many experts in the United States continue to recommend antibiotic therapy for children <6 months old in light of the higher

TABLE 31-2 GUIDELINES FOR THE DIAGNOSIS AND TREATMENT OF ACUTE OTITIS MEDIA

Illness Severity	Diagnostic Criteria	Treatment Recommendations
Mild to moderate	Fluid in the middle ear, evidenced by decreased tympanic membrane mobility, air/fluid level behind tympanic membrane, bulging tympanic membrane, purulent otorrhea *and* Acute onset of signs and symptoms of middle-ear inflammation, including fever, otalgia, decreased hearing, tinnitus, vertigo, erythematous tympanic membrane	*Initial therapy*[a] Observation alone (symptom relief only)[b] *or* Amoxicillin, 80–90 mg/kg qd (up to 2 g) PO in divided doses (bid or tid), *or* Cefdinir, 14 mg/kg qd PO in 1 dose or divided doses (bid), *or* Cefuroxime, 30 mg/kg qd PO in divided doses (bid), *or* Azithromycin, 10 mg/kg qd PO on day 1 followed by 5 mg/kg qd PO for 4 d *Exposure to antibiotics within 30 d or recent treatment failure*[a,c] Amoxicillin, 90 mg/kg qd (up to 2 g) PO in divided doses (bid), plus clavulanate, 6.4 mg/kg qd PO in divided doses (bid), *or* Ceftriaxone, 50 mg/kg IV/IM qd for 3 d, *or* Clindamycin, 30–40 mg/kg qd PO in divided doses (tid)
Severe	As above, with temperature ≥39.0°C *or* Moderate to severe otalgia	*Initial therapy*[a] Amoxicillin, 90 mg/kg qd (up to 2 g) PO in divided doses (bid), plus clavulanate, 6.4 mg/kg qd PO in divided doses (bid), *or* Ceftriaxone, 50 mg/kg IV/IM qd for 3 d *Exposure to antibiotics within 30 d or recent treatment failure*[a,c] Ceftriaxone, 50 mg/kg IV/IM qd for 3 d, *or* Clindamycin, 30–40 mg/kg qd PO in divided doses (tid), *or* Consider tympanocentesis with culture

[a]Duration (unless otherwise specified): 10 d for patients <6 years old and patients with severe disease; 5–7 d (with consideration of observation only in previously healthy individuals with mild disease) for patients ≥6 years old.

[b]Observation (deferring antibacterial treatment for 48–72 h and limiting management to symptom relief) is an option for mild to moderate disease in children 6 months to 2 years of age with an uncertain diagnosis and for children ≥2 years of age.

[c]Failure to improve and/or clinical worsening after 48–72 h of observation or treatment.

Sources: American Academy of Pediatrics Subcommittee on Management of Acute Otitis Media, 2004; Dowell et al, 1998.

frequency of secondary complications in this young and functionally immunocompromised population. However, observation without antimicrobial therapy is now generally considered a reasonable option in the United States for mild to moderate disease in children 6 months to 2 years of age with an uncertain diagnosis and for children ≥2 years of age (Table 31-2).

Given that most studies of the etiologic agents of acute otitis media consistently document similar pathogen profiles, therapy is generally empirical except in those few cases where tympanocentesis is warranted—e.g., cases in newborns, cases refractory to therapy, and cases in patients who are severely ill or immunodeficient. Despite resistance to penicillin and amoxicillin in roughly one-quarter of *S. pneumoniae* isolates, one-third of *H. influenzae* isolates, and nearly all *M. catarrhalis* isolates, outcome studies continue to find that amoxicillin is as successful as any other agent, and it remains the drug of first choice in recommendations from multiple sources (Table 31-2). Therapy for uncomplicated acute otitis media is typically administered for 5–7 days to patients ≥6 years old; longer courses (e.g., 10 days) should be reserved for children <6 years old and patients with severe disease, in whom short-course therapy may be inadequate.

A switch in regimen is recommended if there is no clinical improvement by the third day of therapy, given the possibility of infection with a β-lactamase-producing strain of *H. influenzae* or *M. catarrhalis* or with a strain of penicillin-resistant *S. pneumoniae.* Decongestants and antihistamines are frequently used as adjunctive agents to reduce congestion and relieve obstruction of the eustachian tube, but clinical trials have yielded no significant evidence of benefit with either class of agents.

Recurrent Acute Otitis Media Recurrent acute otitis media (more than three episodes within 6 months or four episodes within 12 months) is generally due to relapse or reinfection, although data indicate that the majority of early recurrences are new infections. In general, the same pathogens responsible for acute otitis media cause recurrent disease; even so, the recommended treatment consists of antibiotics active against β-lactamase-producing organisms. Antibiotic prophylaxis [e.g., with trimethoprim-sulfamethoxazole (TMP-SMX) or amoxicillin] can reduce recurrences in patients with recurrent acute otitis media by an average of one episode per year, but this benefit is small compared with the cost of the drug and the high likelihood of colonization with antibiotic-resistant pathogens. Other approaches, including placement of tympanostomy tubes, adenoidectomy, and tonsillectomy plus adenoidectomy, are of questionable overall value, given the relatively small benefit compared with the potential for complications.

Serous Otitis Media In serous otitis media (otitis media with effusion), fluid is present in the middle ear for an extended period and in the absence of signs and symptoms of infection. In general, acute effusions are self-limited; most resolve in 2–4 weeks. In some cases, however (in particular after an episode of acute otitis media), effusions can persist for months. These chronic effusions are often associated with a significant hearing loss in the affected ear. In younger children, persistent effusions and decreased hearing can be associated with impairment of language acquisition skills. The great majority of cases of otitis media with effusion resolve spontaneously within 3 months without antibiotic therapy. Antibiotic therapy or myringotomy with insertion of tympanostomy tubes is typically reserved for patients in whom bilateral effusion (1) has persisted for at least 3 months and (2) is associated with significant bilateral hearing loss. With this conservative approach and the application of strict diagnostic criteria for acute otitis media and otitis media with effusion, it is estimated that 6–8 million courses of antibiotics could be avoided each year in the United States.

Chronic Otitis Media Chronic suppurative otitis media is characterized by persistent or recurrent purulent otorrhea in the setting of tympanic membrane perforation. Usually, there is also some degree of conductive hearing loss. This condition can be categorized as active or inactive. Inactive disease is characterized by a central perforation of the tympanic membrane, which allows drainage of purulent fluid from the middle ear. When the perforation is more peripheral, squamous epithelium from the auditory canal may invade the middle ear through the perforation, forming a mass of keratinaceous debris (*cholesteatoma*) at the site of invasion. This mass can enlarge and has the potential to erode bone and promote further infection, which can lead to meningitis, brain abscess, or paralysis of cranial nerve VII. Treatment of chronic active otitis media is surgical; mastoidectomy, myringoplasty, and tympanoplasty can be performed as outpatient surgical procedures, with an overall success rate of ~80%. Chronic inactive otitis media is more difficult to cure, usually requiring repeated courses of topical antibiotic drops during periods of drainage. Systemic antibiotics may offer better cure rates, but their role in the treatment of this condition remains unclear.

Mastoiditis Acute mastoiditis was relatively common among children before the introduction of antibiotics. Because the mastoid air cells connect with the middle ear, the process of fluid collection and infection is usually the same in the mastoid as in the middle ear. Early and frequent treatment of acute otitis media is most likely the reason that

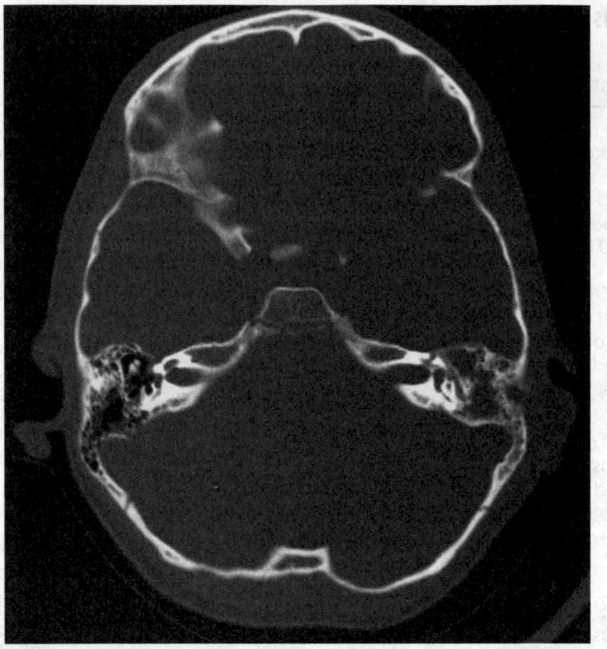

FIGURE 31-1 Acute mastoiditis. Axial CT image shows an acute fluid collection within the mastoid air cells on the left.

the incidence of acute mastoiditis has declined to only 1.2–2.0 cases per 100,000 person-years in countries with high prescribing rates for acute otitis media. In countries like the Netherlands, where antibiotics are used sparingly for acute otitis media, the incidence rate of acute mastoiditis is roughly twice that in countries like the United States. However, neighboring Denmark has a rate of acute mastoiditis similar to that in the Netherlands but an antibiotic-prescribing rate for acute otitis media more similar to that in the United States.

In typical acute mastoiditis, purulent exudate collects in the mastoid air cells (Fig. 31-1), producing pressure that may result in erosion of the surrounding bone and the formation of abscess-like cavities that are usually evident on CT. Patients typically present with pain, erythema, and swelling of the mastoid process along with displacement of the pinna, usually in conjunction with the typical signs and symptoms of acute middle-ear infection. Rarely, patients can develop severe complications if the infection tracks under the periosteum of the temporal bone to cause a subperiosteal abscess, erodes through the mastoid tip to cause a deep neck abscess, or extends posteriorly to cause septic thrombosis of the lateral sinus.

Purulent fluid should be cultured whenever possible to help guide antimicrobial therapy. Initial empirical therapy is usually directed against the typical organisms associated with acute otitis media, such as *S. pneumoniae*, *H. influenzae*, and *M. catarrhalis*. Some patients with more severe or prolonged courses of illness should be treated for infection with *S. aureus* and gram-negative bacilli (including *Pseudomonas*). Broad empirical therapy is usually narrowed once culture results become available. Most patients can be treated conservatively with IV antibiotics; surgery (cortical mastoidectomy) can be reserved for complicated cases and those in which conservative treatment has failed.

INFECTIONS OF THE PHARYNX AND ORAL CAVITY

Oropharyngeal infections range from mild, self-limited viral illnesses to serious, life-threatening bacterial infections. The most common presenting symptom is sore throat—one of the most frequent reasons for ambulatory care visits by both adults and children. Although sore throat is a symptom in many noninfectious illnesses as well, the overwhelming majority of patients with a new sore throat have acute pharyngitis of viral or bacterial etiology.

ACUTE PHARYNGITIS

Millions of visits to primary care providers each year are for sore throat; the majority of cases of acute pharyngitis are caused by typical respiratory viruses. The most important source of concern is infection with group A β-hemolytic *Streptococcus* (*S. pyogenes*), which is associated with acute glomerulonephritis and acute rheumatic fever. The risk of rheumatic fever can be reduced by timely penicillin therapy.

Etiology A wide variety of organisms cause acute pharyngitis. The relative importance of the different pathogens can only be estimated, since a significant proportion of cases (~30%) have no identified cause. Together, respiratory viruses are the most common identifiable cause of acute pharyngitis, with rhinoviruses and coronaviruses accounting for large proportions of cases (~20% and at least 5%, respectively). Influenza virus, parainfluenza virus, and adenovirus also account for a measurable share of cases, the latter as part of the more clinically severe syndrome of pharyngoconjunctival fever. Other important but less common viral causes include herpes simplex virus (HSV) types 1 and 2, coxsackievirus A, cytomegalovirus (CMV), and Epstein-Barr virus (EBV). Acute HIV infection can present as acute pharyngitis and should be considered in high-risk populations.

Acute bacterial pharyngitis is typically caused by *S. pyogenes*, which accounts for ~5–15% of all cases of acute pharyngitis in adults; rates vary with the season and with utilization of the health care system. Group A streptococcal pharyngitis is primarily a disease of children 5–15 years of age; it is uncommon among children <3 years old, as is rheumatic fever. Streptococci of groups C and G account for a minority of cases, although these serogroups are nonrheumatogenic. The remaining bacterial causes of acute pharyngitis are seen infrequently (<1% each) but should be considered in appropriate exposure groups because of the severity of illness if left untreated; these etiologic agents include *Neisseria gonorrhoeae*, *Corynebacterium diphtheriae*, *Corynebacterium ulcerans*, *Yersinia enterocolitica*, and *Treponema pallidum* (in secondary syphilis). Anaerobic bacteria can also cause acute pharyngitis (*Vincent's angina*) and can contribute to more serious polymicrobial infections, such as peritonsillar or retropharyngeal abscess (see below). Atypical organisms such as *M. pneumoniae* and *C. pneumoniae* have been recovered from patients with acute pharyngitis; whether these agents are commensals or causes of acute infection is debatable.

Clinical Manifestations Although the signs and symptoms accompanying acute pharyngitis are not reliable predictors of the etiologic agent, the clinical presentation occasionally suggests that one etiology is more likely than another. Acute pharyngitis due to respiratory viruses such as rhinovirus or coronavirus is usually not severe and is typically associated with a constellation of coryzal symptoms better characterized as nonspecific URI. Findings on physical examination are uncommon; fever is rare, and tender cervical adenopathy and pharyngeal exudates are not seen. In contrast, acute pharyngitis from influenza virus can be severe and is much more likely to be associated with fever as well as with myalgias, headache, and cough. The presentation of pharyngoconjunctival fever due to adenovirus infection is similar. Since pharyngeal exudate may be present on examination, this condition can be difficult to differentiate from streptococcal pharyngitis. However, adenoviral pharyngitis is distinguished by the presence of conjunctivitis in one-third to one-half of patients. Acute pharyngitis from primary HSV infection can also mimic streptococcal pharyngitis in some cases, with pharyngeal inflammation and exudate, but the presence of vesicles and shallow ulcers on the palate can help differentiate the two diseases. This HSV syndrome is distinct from pharyngitis caused by coxsackievirus (*herpangina*), which is associated with small vesicles that develop on the soft palate and uvula and then rupture to form shallow white ulcers. Acute exudative pharyngitis coupled with fever, fatigue, generalized lymphadenopathy, and (on occasion) splenomegaly is characteristic of infectious mononucleosis due to EBV or CMV. Acute primary infection with HIV is frequently associated with fever and acute pharyngitis as well as with myalgias, arthralgias, malaise, and occasionally a nonpruritic maculopapular rash, which later may be followed by lymphadenopathy and mucosal ulcerations without exudate.

The clinical features of acute pharyngitis caused by streptococci of groups A, C, and G are all similar, ranging from a relatively mild illness without many accompanying symptoms to clinically severe cases with profound pharyngeal pain, fever, chills, and abdominal pain. A hyperemic pharyngeal membrane with tonsillar hypertrophy and exudate is usually seen, along with tender anterior cervical adenopathy. Coryzal manifestations, including cough, are typically absent; when present, they suggest a viral etiology. Strains of *S. pyogenes* that generate erythrogenic toxin can also produce scarlet fever characterized by an erythematous rash and strawberry tongue. The other types of acute bacterial pharyngitis (e.g., gonococcal, diphtherial, and yersinial) often present as exudative pharyngitis with or without other clinical features. Their etiologies are often suggested only by the clinical history.

Diagnosis The primary goal of diagnostic testing is to separate acute streptococcal pharyngitis from pharyngitis of other etiologies (particularly viral) so that antibiotics can be prescribed more efficiently for patients to whom they may be beneficial. The most appropriate standard for the diagnosis of streptococcal pharyngitis, however, has not been definitively established. Throat swab culture is generally regarded as such. However, this method cannot distinguish between infection and colonization, and it takes 24–48 h to yield results that vary according to technique and culture conditions. Rapid antigen-detection tests offer good specificity (>90%) but lower sensitivity when implemented in routine practice. The sensitivity has also been shown to vary across the clinical spectrum of disease (65–90%). Several clinical prediction systems (Table 31-3) can increase the sensitivity of rapid antigen-detection tests to >90% in controlled settings. Since the sensitivities achieved in routine clinical practice are often lower, several medical and professional societies continue to recommend that all negative rapid antigen-detection tests in children be confirmed by a throat culture to limit transmission and complications of illness caused by group A streptococci. The Centers for Disease Control and Prevention, the Infectious Diseases Society of America, the American College of Physicians, and the American Academy of Family Physicians do not recommend backup culture when adults have negative results in a high-sensitivity, rapid antigen-detection test, however, given the lower prevalence and smaller benefit in this age group.

Cultures and rapid diagnostic tests for other causes of acute pharyngitis, such as influenza virus, adenovirus, HSV, EBV, CMV, and *M. pneumoniae*, are available in some locations and can be used when these infections are suspected. The diagnosis of acute EBV infection depends primarily on the detection of antibodies to the virus with a heterophile agglutination assay (monospot slide test) or enzyme-linked immunosorbent assay. Testing for HIV RNA or antigen (p24) should be performed when acute primary HIV infection is suspected. If other bacterial causes are suspected (particularly *N. gonorrhoeae*, *C. diphtheriae*, or *Y. enterocolitica*), specific cultures should be requested since these organisms may be missed on routine throat swab culture.

℞ PHARYNGITIS

Antibiotic treatment of pharyngitis due to *S. pyogenes* confers numerous benefits, including a decrease in the risk of rheumatic fever. The magnitude of this benefit is fairly small, however, since rheumatic fever is now a rare disease, even among untreated patients. When therapy is started within 48 h of illness onset, however, symptom duration is also decreased. An additional benefit of therapy is the potential to reduce the spread of streptococcal pharyngitis, particularly in areas of overcrowding or close contact. Antibiotic therapy for acute pharyngitis is therefore recommended in cases where *S. pyogenes* is confirmed as the etiologic agent by rapid antigen-detection test or throat swab culture. Otherwise, antibiotics should be given in routine cases only when another bacterial cause has been identified. Effective therapy for streptococcal pharyngitis consists of either a single dose of IM benzathine penicillin or a full 10-day course of oral penicillin

TABLE 31-3 GUIDELINES FOR THE DIAGNOSIS AND TREATMENT OF ACUTE PHARYNGITIS

Age Group	Diagnostic Criteria	Treatment Recommendations[a]
Adults	*Clinical suspicion of streptococcal pharyngitis* (e.g., fever, tonsillar swelling, exudate, enlarged/tender anterior cervical lymph nodes, absence of cough or coryza)[b] *with:* History of rheumatic fever *or* Documented household exposure *or* Positive rapid strep screen	Penicillin V, 500 mg PO tid, *or* Amoxicillin, 500 mg PO bid, *or* Erythromycin, 250 mg PO qid, *or* Benzathine penicillin G, single dose of 1.2 million units IM
Children	*Clinical suspicion of streptococcal pharyngitis* (e.g., tonsillar swelling, exudate, enlarged/tender anterior cervical lymph nodes, absence of coryza) *with:* History of rheumatic fever *or* Documented household exposure *or* Positive rapid strep screen *or* Positive throat culture (for patients with negative rapid strep screen)	Amoxicillin, 45 mg/kg qd PO in divided doses (bid or tid), *or* Penicillin VK, 50 mg/kg qd PO in divided doses (bid), *or* Cephalexin, 50 mg/kg qd PO in divided doses (qid), *or* Benzathine penicillin G, single dose of 25,000 units/kg IM

[a]Unless otherwise specified, the duration of therapy is generally 10 d, with appropriate follow-up.
[b]Some organizations support treating adults who have these symptoms and signs without administering a rapid streptococcal antigen test.
Sources: Cooper et al, 2001; Schwartz et al, 1998.

(Table 31-3). Erythromycin can be used in place of penicillin, although resistance to erythromycin among *S. pyogenes* strains in some parts of the world (particularly Europe) can prohibit the use of this drug. Newer (and more expensive) antibiotics are also active against streptococci but offer no greater efficacy than the above agents. Testing for cure is unnecessary and may reveal only chronic colonization. There is no evidence to support antibiotic treatment of group C or G streptococcal pharyngitis or of pharyngitis in which *Mycoplasma* or *Chlamydophila* has been recovered. Penicillin prophylaxis (benzathine penicillin G, 1.2 million units IM every 3–4 weeks) is indicated for patients at risk of recurrent rheumatic fever.

Treatment of viral pharyngitis is entirely symptom-based except in infection with influenza virus or HSV. For influenza, a number of therapeutic agents exist, including amantadine, rimantadine, and the two newer agents oseltamivir and zanamivir. All of these agents need to be started within 36–48 h of symptom onset to reduce illness duration meaningfully. Of these agents, only oseltamivir and zanamivir are active against both influenza A and influenza B and therefore can be used when local infection patterns are unknown. Oropharyngeal HSV infection sometimes responds to treatment with antiviral agents such as acyclovir, although these drugs are often reserved for immunosuppressed patients.

Complications Although rheumatic fever is the best-known complication of acute streptococcal pharyngitis, the risk of its following acute infection remains quite low. Other complications include acute glomerulonephritis and numerous suppurative conditions, such as peritonsillar abscess (*quinsy*), otitis media, mastoiditis, sinusitis, bacteremia, and pneumonia—all of which occur at low rates. Although antibiotic treatment of acute streptococcal pharyngitis can prevent the development of rheumatic fever, there is no evidence that it can prevent acute glomerulonephritis. Some evidence supports antibiotic use to prevent the suppurative complications of streptococcal pharyngitis, particularly peritonsillar abscess, which can also involve oral anaerobes such as *Fusobacterium*. Abscesses are usually accompanied by severe pharyngeal pain, dysphagia, fever, and dehydration; in addition, medial displacement of the tonsil and lateral displacement of the uvula are often evident on examination. Although early use of IV antibiotics (e.g., clindamycin; penicillin G with metronidazole) may obviate the need for surgical drainage in some cases, treatment typically involves needle aspiration or incision and drainage.

ORAL INFECTIONS

Aside from periodontal disease such as gingivitis, infections of the oral cavity most commonly involve HSV or *Candida* species. In addition to causing painful cold sores on the lips, HSV can infect the tongue and buccal mucosa, causing the formation of irritating vesicles. Although topical antiviral agents (e.g., acyclovir and penciclovir) can be used externally for cold sores, oral or IV acyclovir is often needed for primary infections, extensive oral infections, and infections in immunocompromised patients. Oropharyngeal candidiasis (*thrush*) is caused by a variety of *Candida* species, most often *C. albicans*. Thrush occurs predominantly in neonates, immunocompromised patients (especially those with AIDS), and recipients of prolonged antibiotic or glucocorticoid therapy. In addition to sore throat, patients often report a burning tongue, and physical examination reveals friable white or gray plaques on the gingiva, tongue, and oral mucosa. Treatment, which usually consists of an oral antifungal suspension (nystatin or clotrimazole) or oral fluconazole, is frequently successful. In the uncommon cases of fluconazole-refractory thrush that are seen in some patients with AIDS, other therapeutic options include oral formulations of itraconazole, amphotericin B, or voriconazole as well as the IV echinocandins (caspofungin, micafungin, and anidulafungin).

Vincent's angina, also known as *acute necrotizing ulcerative gingivitis* or *trench mouth*, is a unique and dramatic form of gingivitis characterized by painful, inflamed gingiva with ulcerations of the interdental papillae that bleed easily. Since oral anaerobes are the cause, patients typically have halitosis and frequently present with fever, malaise, and lymphadenopathy. Treatment consists of debridement and oral administration of penicillin plus metronidazole, with clindamycin alone as an alternative.

Ludwig's angina is a rapidly progressive, potentially fulminant cellulitis that involves the sublingual and submandibular spaces and that typically originates from an infected or recently extracted tooth, most commonly the lower second and third molars. Improved dental care has substantially reduced the incidence of this disorder. Infection in these areas leads to dysphagia, odynophagia, and "woody" edema in the sublingual region, forcing the tongue up and back with the potential for airway obstruction. Fever, dysarthria, and drooling may also be noted, and patients may speak in a "hot potato" voice. Intubation or tracheostomy may be necessary to secure the airway, as asphyxiation is the most common cause of death. Patients should be monitored closely and treated promptly with IV antibiotics directed against streptococci and oral anaerobes. Recommended agents include ampicillin/sulbactam and high-dose penicillin plus metronidazole.

Postanginal septicemia (*Lemierre's disease*) is a rare anaerobic oropharyngeal infection caused predominantly by *Fusobacterium necrophorum*. The illness typically starts as a sore throat (most commonly in adolescents and young adults), which may present as exudative tonsillitis or peritonsillar abscess. Infection of the deep pharyngeal tissue allows organisms to drain into the lateral pharyngeal space, which contains the carotid artery and internal jugular vein. Septic thrombophlebitis of the internal jugular vein can result, with associated pain, dysphagia, and neck swelling and stiffness. Sepsis usually occurs 3–10 days after the onset of sore throat and is often coupled with metastatic infection to the lung and other distant sites. Occasionally, the infection can extend along the carotid sheath and into the posterior mediastinum, resulting in mediastinitis, or it can erode into the carotid artery, with the early sign of repeated small bleeds into the mouth. The mortality rate from these invasive infections can be as high as 50%. Treatment consists of IV antibiotics (penicillin G or clindamycin) and surgical drainage of any purulent collections. The concomitant use of anticoagulants to prevent embolization remains controversial but is often advised.

INFECTIONS OF THE LARYNX AND EPIGLOTTIS

LARYNGITIS

Laryngitis is defined as any inflammatory process involving the larynx and can be caused by a variety of infectious and noninfectious processes. The vast majority of laryngitis cases seen in clinical practice in developed countries are acute. Acute laryngitis is a common syndrome caused predominantly by the same viruses responsible for many other URIs. In fact, most cases of acute laryngitis occur in the setting of a viral URI.

Etiology Nearly all major respiratory viruses have been implicated in acute viral laryngitis, including rhinovirus, influenza virus, parainfluenza virus, adenovirus, coxsackievirus, coronavirus, and RSV. Acute laryngitis can also be associated with acute bacterial respiratory infections, such as those caused by group A *Streptococcus* or *C. diphtheriae* (although diphtheria has been all but eliminated in the United States). Another bacterial pathogen thought to play a role (albeit unclear) in the pathogenesis of acute laryngitis is *M. catarrhalis*, which has been recovered on nasopharyngeal culture from a significant percentage of people with acute laryngitis. Chronic laryngitis of infectious etiology is much less common in developed than in developing countries. Laryngitis due to *Mycobacterium tuberculosis* is often difficult to distinguish from laryngeal cancer, in part because of the frequent absence of signs, symptoms, and radiographic findings typical of pulmonary disease. *Histoplasma* and *Blastomyces* may cause laryngitis, often as a complication of systemic infection. *Candida* species can cause laryngitis as well, often in association with thrush or esophagitis and particularly in immunosuppressed patients. Rare cases of chronic laryngitis are due to *Coccidioides* and *Cryptococcus*.

Clinical Manifestations Laryngitis is characterized by hoarseness and can also be associated with reduced vocal pitch or aphonia. As acute laryngitis is caused predominantly by respiratory viruses, these symptoms usually occur in association with other symptoms and signs of URI, including rhinorrhea, nasal congestion, cough, and sore throat. Direct laryngoscopy often reveals diffuse laryngeal erythema and edema, along with vascular engorgement of the vocal folds. In addition, chronic disease (e.g., tuberculous laryngitis) often includes mucosal nodules and ulcerations visible on laryngoscopy; these lesions are sometimes mistaken for laryngeal cancer.

℞ LARYNGITIS

Acute laryngitis is usually treated with humidification and voice rest alone. Antibiotics are not recommended except when group A *Streptococcus* is cultured, in which case penicillin is the drug of choice. The choice of therapy for chronic laryngitis depends on the pathogen, whose identification usually requires biopsy with culture. Patients with laryngeal tuberculosis are highly contagious because of the large number of organisms that are easily aerosolized. These patients should be managed in the same way as patients with active pulmonary disease.

CROUP

The term *croup* actually denotes a group of diseases collectively referred to as "croup syndrome," all of which are acute and predominantly viral respiratory illnesses characterized by marked swelling of the subglottic region of the larynx. Croup primarily affects children <6 years old. For a detailed discussion of this entity, the reader is referred to a text of pediatric medicine.

EPIGLOTTITIS

Acute epiglottitis (supraglottitis) is an acute, rapidly progressive cellulitis of the epiglottis and adjacent structures that can result in complete—and potentially fatal—airway obstruction in both children and adults. Before the widespread use of *H. influenzae* type b (Hib) vaccine, this entity was much more common among children, with a peak incidence at ~3.5 years of age. In some countries, mass vaccination against Hib has reduced the annual incidence of acute epiglottitis in children by >90%; in contrast, the annual incidence in adults has changed little since the introduction of Hib vaccine. Because of the danger of airway obstruction, acute epiglottitis constitutes a medical emergency, particularly in children, and prompt diagnosis and airway protection are of utmost importance.

Etiology After the introduction of the Hib vaccine in the mid-1980s, disease incidence among children in the United States declined dramatically. Nevertheless, lack of vaccination or vaccine failure has meant that many pediatric cases seen today are still due to Hib. In adults and (more recently) in children, a variety of other bacterial pathogens have been associated with epiglottitis, the most common

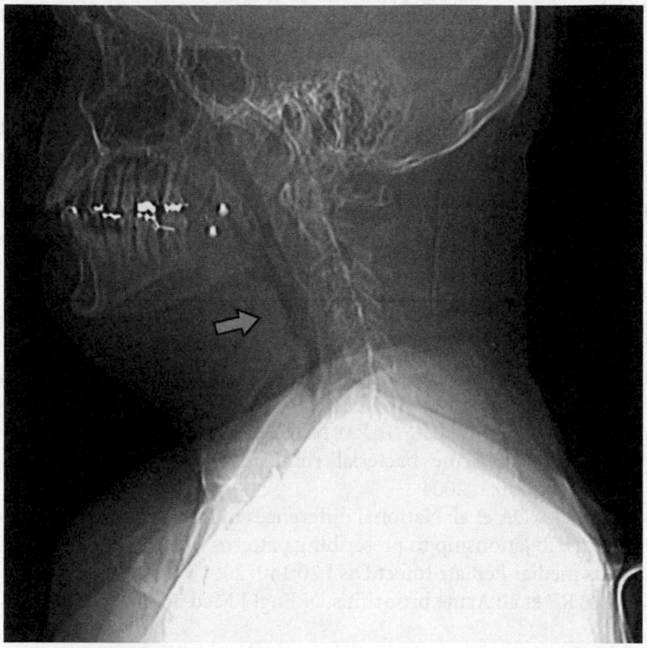

FIGURE 31-2 Acute epiglottitis. In this lateral soft tissue radiograph of the neck, the arrow indicates the enlarged edematous epiglottis (the "thumbprint sign").

being group A *Streptococcus*. Other pathogens seen less frequently include *S. pneumoniae*, *Haemophilus parainfluenzae*, and *S. aureus*. Viruses have not yet been established as causes of acute epiglottitis.

Clinical Manifestations and Diagnosis Epiglottitis typically presents more acutely in young children than in adolescents or adults. On presentation, most children have had symptoms for <24 h, including high fever, severe sore throat, tachycardia, systemic toxicity, and (in many cases) drooling while sitting forward. Symptoms and signs of respiratory obstruction may also be present and may progress rapidly. The somewhat milder illness in adolescents and adults often follows 1–2 days of severe sore throat and is commonly accompanied by dyspnea, drooling, and stridor. Physical examination of patients with acute epiglottitis may reveal moderate or severe respiratory distress, with inspiratory stridor and retractions of the chest wall. These findings *diminish* as the disease progresses and the patient tires. Conversely, oropharyngeal examination reveals injection that is much less severe than would be predicted from the symptoms—a finding that should alert the clinician to a cause of symptoms and obstruction that lies beyond the tonsils. The diagnosis is often made on clinical grounds, although direct fiberoptic laryngoscopy is frequently performed in a controlled environment (e.g., an operating room) in order to visualize and culture the typical edematous "cherry-red" epiglottis and to facilitate placement of an endotracheal tube. Direct visualization in an examination room (e.g., with a tongue blade and indirect laryngoscopy) is not recommended because of the risk of immediate laryngospasm and complete airway obstruction. Lateral neck radiographs and laboratory tests can assist in the diagnosis but may delay the critical securing of the airway and cause the patient to be moved or repositioned more than is necessary, thereby increasing the risk of further airway compromise. Neck radiographs typically reveal an enlarged edematous epiglottis (the "thumbprint sign," Fig. 31-2), usually with a dilated hypopharynx and normal subglottic structures. Laboratory tests characteristically document mild to moderate leukocytosis with a predominance of neutrophils. Blood cultures are positive in a significant proportion of cases.

℞ EPIGLOTTITIS

Security of the airway is always of primary concern in acute epiglottitis, even if the diagnosis is only suspected. Mere observation for signs of impending airway obstruction is not routinely recommended, particularly in children. Many adults have been managed with observation only since the illness is perceived to be milder in this age group, but some data suggest that this approach may be risky and probably should be reserved only for adult patients who have yet to develop dyspnea or stridor. Once the airway has been secured and specimens of blood and epiglottis tissue have been obtained for culture, treatment with IV antibiotics should be given to cover the most likely organisms, particularly *H. influenzae*. Because rates of ampicillin resistance in this organism have risen significantly in recent years, therapy with a β-lactam/β-lactamase inhibitor combination or a second- or third-generation cephalosporin is recommended. Typically, ampicillin/sulbactam, cefuroxime, cefotaxime, or ceftriaxone is given, with clindamycin and TMP-SMX reserved for patients allergic to β-lactams. Antibiotic therapy should be continued for 7–10 days and should be tailored, if necessary, to the organism recovered in culture. If the household contacts of a patient with *H. influenzae* epiglottitis include an unvaccinated child under the age of 4, all members of the household (including the patient) should receive prophylactic rifampin for 4 days to eradicate carriage of *H. influenzae*.

INFECTIONS OF THE DEEP NECK STRUCTURES

Deep neck infections are usually extensions of infection from other primary sites, most often within the pharynx or oral cavity. Many of these infections are life-threatening but are difficult to detect at early stages when they may be more easily managed. Three of the most clinically relevant spaces in the neck are the submandibular (and sublingual) space, the lateral pharyngeal (or parapharyngeal) space, and the retropharyngeal space. These spaces communicate with one another and with other important structures in the head, neck, and thorax, providing pathogens with easy access to areas including the mediastinum, carotid sheath, skull base, and meninges. Once infection reaches these sensitive areas, mortality rates can be as high as 20–50%.

Infection of the submandibular and/or sublingual space typically originates from an infected or recently extracted lower tooth. The result is the severe, life-threatening infection referred to as Ludwig's angina (see "Oral Infections," above). Infection of the lateral pharyngeal (or parapharyngeal) space is most often a complication of common infections of the oral cavity and upper respiratory tract, including tonsillitis, peritonsillar abscess, pharyngitis, mastoiditis, or periodontal infection. This space, located deep to the lateral wall of the pharynx, contains a number of sensitive structures, including the carotid artery, internal jugular vein, cervical sympathetic chain, and portions of cranial nerves IX through XII; at its distal end, it opens into the posterior mediastinum. Involvement of this space with infection can therefore be rapidly fatal. Examination may reveal some tonsillar displacement, trismus, and neck rigidity, but swelling of the lateral pharyngeal wall can easily be missed. The diagnosis can be confirmed by CT. Treatment consists of airway management, operative drainage of fluid collections, and at least 10 days of IV therapy with an antibiotic active against streptococci and oral anaerobes (e.g., ampicillin/sulbactam). A particularly severe form of this infection involving the components of the carotid sheath (postanginal septicemia, Lemierre's disease) is described above (see "Oral Infections"). Infection of the retropharyngeal space can also be extremely dangerous, as this space runs posterior to the pharynx from the skull base to the superior mediastinum. Infections in this space are more common among children <5 years old because of the presence of several small retropharyngeal lymph nodes that typically atrophy by the age of 4 years. Infection is usually a consequence of extension from another site of infection, most commonly acute pharyngitis. Other sources include otitis media, tonsillitis, dental infections, Ludwig's angina, and anterior extension of vertebral osteomyelitis. Retropharyngeal space infection can also follow penetrating trauma to the posterior pharynx (e.g., from an endoscopic procedure). Infections are commonly polymicrobial, involving a mixture of aerobes and anaerobes; group A β-hemolytic streptococci and *S. aureus* are the most common pathogens. *M. tuberculosis* was a frequent cause in the past but now is rarely involved in the United States.

Patients with retropharyngeal abscess typically present with sore throat, fever, dysphagia, and neck pain and are often drooling because of difficulty and pain with swallowing. Examination may reveal tender cervical adenopathy, neck swelling, and diffuse erythema and edema of the posterior pharynx as well as a bulge in the posterior pharyngeal wall that may not be obvious on routine inspection. A soft tissue mass is usually demonstrable by lateral neck radiography or CT. Because of the risk of airway obstruction, treatment begins with securing of the airway, which is followed by a combination of surgical drainage and IV antibiotic administration. Initial empirical therapy should cover streptococci, oral anaerobes, and *S. aureus*; ampicillin/sulbactam, clindamycin alone, or clindamycin plus ceftriaxone is usually effective. Complications result primarily from extension to other areas; for example, rupture into the posterior pharynx may lead to aspiration pneumonia and empyema. Extension may also occur to the lateral pharyngeal space and mediastinum, resulting in mediastinitis and pericarditis, or into nearby major blood vessels. All these events are associated with a high mortality rate.

FURTHER READINGS

AMERICAN ACADEMY OF PEDIATRICS SUBCOMMITTEE ON MANAGEMENT OF ACUTE OTITIS MEDIA: Diagnosis and management of acute otitis media. Pediatrics 113:1451, 2004

AMERICAN ACADEMY OF PEDIATRICS SUBCOMMITTEE ON MANAGEMENT OF SINUSITIS AND COMMITTEE ON QUALITY IMPROVEMENT: Clinical practice guideline: Management of sinusitis. Pediatrics 108:798, 2001

COOPER RJ et al: Principles of appropriate antibiotic use for acute pharyngitis in adults: Background. Ann Intern Med 134:509, 2001

DOWELL SF et al: Otitis media—principles of judicious use of antimicrobial agents. Pediatrics 101:165, 1998

GONZALES R et al: Principles of appropriate antibiotic use for treatment of nonspecific upper respiratory tract infections in adults: Background. Ann Intern Med 134:490, 2001

HICKNER JM et al: Principles of appropriate antibiotic use for acute rhinosinusitis in adults: Background. Ann Intern Med 134:498, 2001

PICCIRILLO JF: Acute bacterial sinusitis. N Engl J Med 351:902, 2004

RAFEI K et al: Airway infectious disease emergencies. Pediatr Clin North Am 53:215, 2006

SCHWARTZ B et al: Pharyngitis—principles of judicious use of antimicrobial agents. Pediatrics 101:171, 1998

SINUS AND ALLERGY HEALTH PARTNERSHIP: Antimicrobial treatment guidelines for acute bacterial rhinosinusitis. Otolaryngol Head Neck Surg 130:1, 2004

VAN ZUIJLEN DA et al: National differences in incidence of acute mastoiditis: Relationship to prescribing patterns of antibiotics for acute otitis media? Pediatr Infect Dis J 20:140, 2001

WENZEL RP et al: Acute bronchitis. N Engl J Med 355:2125, 2006

32 Oral Manifestations of Disease

Samuel C. Durso

As primary care physicians and consultants, internists are often asked to evaluate patients with disease of the oral soft tissues, teeth, and pharynx. Knowledge of the oral milieu and its unique structures is necessary to guide preventive services and recognize oral manifestations of local or systemic disease (**Chap. e7**). Furthermore, internists frequently collaborate with dentists in the care of patients who have a variety of medical conditions that affect oral health or who undergo dental procedures that increase their risk of medical complications.

DISEASES OF THE TEETH AND PERIODONTAL STRUCTURES

TOOTH AND PERIODONTAL STRUCTURE

Tooth formation begins during the sixth week of embryonic life and continues through the first 17 years of age. Tooth development begins in utero and continues until after the tooth erupts. Normally all 20 deciduous teeth have erupted by age 3 and have been shed by age 13. Permanent teeth, eventually totaling 32, begin to erupt by age 6 and have completely erupted by age 14, though third molars (wisdom teeth) may erupt later.

The erupted tooth consists of the visible crown covered with enamel and the root submerged below the gum line and covered with bonelike cementum. *Dentin*, a material that is denser than bone and exquisitely sensitive to pain, forms the majority of the tooth substance. Dentin surrounds a core of myxomatous *pulp* containing the vascular and nerve supply. The tooth is held firmly in the alveolar socket by the *periodontium*, supporting structures that consist of the gingivae, alveolar bone, cementum, and periodontal ligament. The periodontal ligament tenaciously binds the tooth's cementum to the alveolar bone. Above this ligament is a collar of attached gingiva just below the crown. A few millimeters of unattached or free gingiva (1–3 mm) overlap the base of the crown, forming a shallow sulcus along the gum-tooth margin.

Dental Caries, Pulpal and Periapical Disease, and Complications Dental caries begin asymptomatically as a destructive process of the hard surface of the tooth. *Streptococcus mutans*, principally, along with other bacteria colonize the organic buffering film on the tooth surface to produce *plaque*. If not removed by brushing or the natural cleaning action of saliva and oral soft tissues, bacterial acids demineralize the enamel. Fissures and pits on the occlusion surfaces are the most frequent sites of decay. Surfaces adjacent to tooth restorations and exposed roots are also vulnerable, particularly as teeth are retained in an aging population. Over time, dental caries extend to the underlying dentin, leading to cavitation of the enamel and ultimately penetration to the tooth pulp, producing *acute pulpitis*. At this early stage, when the pulp infection is limited, the tooth becomes sensitive to percussion and hot or cold, and pain resolves immediately when the irritating stimulus is removed. Should the infection spread throughout the pulp, *irreversible pulpitis* occurs, leading to pulp necrosis. At this late stage pain is severe and has a sharp or throbbing visceral quality that may be worse when the patient lies down. Once pulp necrosis is complete, pain may be constant or intermittent, but cold sensitivity is lost.

Treatment of caries involves removal of the softened and infected hard tissue; sealing the exposed dentin; and restoration of the tooth structure with silver amalgam, composite plastic, gold, or porcelain. Once irreversible pulpitis occurs, root canal therapy is necessary, and the contents of the pulp chamber and root canals are removed, followed by thorough cleaning, antisepsis, and filling with an inert material. Alternatively, the tooth may be extracted.

Pulpal infection, if it does not egress through the decayed enamel, leads to *periapical abscess* formation, which produces pain on chewing. If the infection is mild and chronic, a *periapical granuloma* or eventually a *periapical cyst* forms, either of which produces radiolucency at the root apex. When unchecked, a periapical abscess can erode into the alveolar bone producing osteomyelitis, penetrate and drain through the gingivae (parulis or gumboil), or track along deep fascial planes, producing a virulent cellulitis (Ludwig's angina) involving the submandibular space and floor of the mouth (Chap. 157). Elderly patients, those with diabetes mellitus, and patients taking glucocorticoids may experience little or no pain and fever as these complications develop.

Periodontal Disease Periodontal disease accounts for more tooth loss than caries, particularly in the elderly. Like dental caries, chronic infection of the gingiva and anchoring structures of the tooth begins with formation of bacterial plaque. The process begins invisibly above the gum line and in the gingival sulcus. Plaque, including mineralized plaque (calculus), is preventable by appropriate dental hygiene, including periodic professional cleaning. Left undisturbed, chronic inflammation ensues and produces a painless hyperemia of the free and attached gingivae (*gingivitis*) that typically bleeds with brushing. If ignored, severe *periodontitis* occurs, leading to deepening of the physiologic sulcus and destruction of the periodontal ligament. Pockets develop around the teeth and become filled with pus and debris. As the periodontium is destroyed, teeth loosen and exfoliate. Eventually there is resorption of the alveolar bone. A role for the chronic inflammation resulting from chronic periodontal disease in promoting coronary heart disease and stroke has been proposed. Epidemiologic studies demonstrate a moderate but significant association between chronic periodontal inflammation and atherogenesis, though a causal role remains unproven.

Acute and aggressive forms of periodontal disease are less common than the chronic forms described above. However, if the host is stressed or exposed to a new pathogen, rapidly progressive and destructive disease of the periodontal tissue can occur. A virulent example is *acute necrotizing ulcerative gingivitis* (ANUG), or *Vincent's infection*, characterized as "trench mouth" during World War I. Stress, poor oral hygiene, and tobacco and alcohol use are risk factors. The presentation includes sudden gingival inflammation, ulceration, bleeding, interdental gingival necrosis, and fetid halitosis. *Localized juvenile periodontitis*, seen in adolescents, is particularly destructive and appears to be associated with impaired neutrophil chemotaxis. *AIDS-related periodontitis* resembles ANUG in some patients or a more destructive form of adult chronic periodontitis in others. It may also produce a gangrene-like destructive process of the oral soft tissues and bone that resembles *noma*, seen in severely malnourished children in developing nations.

Prevention of Tooth Decay and Periodontal Infection Despite the reduced prevalence of dental caries and periodontal disease in the United States due in large part to water fluoridation and improved dental care, respectively, both diseases constitute a major public health problem worldwide and for certain groups. The internist should promote preventive dental care and hygiene as part of health maintenance. Special populations at high risk for dental caries and periodontal disease include those with xerostomia, diabetics, alcoholics, tobacco users, those with Down's syndrome, and those with gingival hyperplasia. Furthermore, patients lacking dental care access (low socioeconomic status) and those with reduced ability to provide self-care (e.g., nursing home residents, those with dementia or upper extremity disability) suffer at a disproportionate rate. It is important to provide counseling regarding regular dental hygiene and professional cleaning, use of fluoride-containing toothpaste, professional fluoride treatments, and use of electric toothbrushes for patients with limited dexterity and to give instruction to caregivers for those unable to perform self-care. Internists caring for international students studying in the United States should be aware of the high prevalence of dental decay in this population. Cost, fear of dental care, and language and cultural differences may create barriers that prevent some from seeking preventive dental services.

Developmental and Systemic Disease Affecting the Teeth and Periodontium Malocclusion is the most common developmental problem, which, in addition to a problem with cosmesis, can interfere with mastication unless corrected through orthodontic techniques. Impacted third molars are common and occasionally become infected. Acquired prognathism due to *acromegaly* may also lead to malocclusion, as may deformity of the maxilla and mandible due to *Paget's disease* of the bone. Delayed tooth eruption, receding chin, and a protruding tongue are occasional features of *cretinism* and *hypopituitarism*. Congenital syphilis produces tapering, notched (Hutchinson's) incisors and finely nodular (mulberry) molar crowns.

Enamel hypoplasia results in crown defects ranging from pits to deep fissures of primary or permanent teeth. Intrauterine infection (syphilis, rubella), vitamin deficiency (A, C, or D), disorders of calcium metabolism (malabsorption, vitamin D–resistant rickets, hypoparathyroidism), prematurity, high fever, or rare inherited defects (*amelogenesis imperfecta*) are all causes. Tetracycline, given in sufficiently high doses during the first 8 years, may produce enamel hypoplasia and discoloration. Exposure to endogenous pigments can discolor developing teeth: *erythroblastosis fetalis* (green or bluish-black), congenital liver disease (green or yellow-brown), and porphyria (red or brown that fluoresces with ultraviolet light). *Mottled enamel* occurs if excessive fluoride is ingested during development. Worn enamel is seen with age, bruxism, or excessive acid exposure (e.g., chronic gastric reflux or bulimia).

Premature tooth loss resulting from periodontitis is seen with cyclic neutropenia, Papillon-Lefèvre syndrome, Chédiak-Higashi syndrome, and leukemia. Rapid focal tooth loosening is most often due to infection, but rarer causes include histiocytosis X, Ewing's sarcoma, osteosarcoma, or Burkitt's lymphoma. Early loss of primary teeth is a feature of *hypophosphatasia*, a rare inborn error of metabolism.

Pregnancy may produce severe gingivitis and localized *pyogenic granulomas*. Severe periodontal disease occurs with Down's syndrome and diabetes mellitus. *Gingival hyperplasia* may be caused by phenytoin, calcium channel blockers (e.g., nifedipine), and cyclosporine. *Idiopathic familial gingival fibromatosis* and several syndrome-related disorders appear similar. Removal of the medication often reverses the drug-induced form, though surgery may be needed to control both. *Linear gingival erythema* is variably seen in patients with advanced HIV infection and probably represents immune deficiency and decreased neutrophil activity. Diffuse or focal gingival swelling may be a feature of early or late acute myelomonocytic leukemia (AML) as well as of other lymphoproliferative disorders. A rare, but pathognomonic, sign of Wegener's granulomatosis is a red-purplish, granular gingivitis (strawberry gums).

DISEASES OF THE ORAL MUCOSA

Infection Most oral mucosal diseases involve microorganisms (Table 32-1).

Pigmented Lesions See Table 32-2.

Dermatologic Diseases See Tables 32-1, 32-2, and 32-3 and Chaps. 52–56.

Diseases of the Tongue See Table 32-4.

HIV Disease and AIDS See Tables 32-1, 32-2, 32-3, and 32-5; Chap. 182; and Figs. 174-1 and 196-1.

Ulcers Ulceration is the most common oral mucosal lesion. Although there are many causes, the host and pattern of lesions, including the presence of systemic features, narrow the differential diagnosis (Table 32-1). Most acute ulcers are painful and self-limited. Recurrent aphthous ulcers and herpes simplex infection constitute the majority. Persistent and deep aphthous ulcers can be idiopathic or seen with HIV/AIDS. Aphthous lesions are often the presenting symptom in *Behçet's syndrome* (Chap. 320). Similar-appearing, though less painful, lesions may occur with Reiter's syndrome, and aphthous ulcers are occasionally present during phases of discoid or *systemic lupus erythematosus* (Chap. 316). Aphthous-like ulcers are seen in Crohn's disease (Chap. 289), but unlike the common aphthous variety, they may exhibit granulomatous inflammation histologically. Recurrent aphthae in some patients with *celiac disease* have been reported to remit with elimination of gluten.

Of major concern are chronic, relatively painless ulcers and mixed red/white patches (erythroplakia and leukoplakia) of more than 2 weeks' duration. Squamous cell carcinoma and premalignant dysplasia should be considered early and a diagnostic biopsy obtained. The importance is underscored because early-stage malignancy is vastly more treatable than late-stage disease. High-risk sites include the lower lip, floor of the mouth, ventral and lateral tongue, and soft palate–tonsillar pillar complex. Significant risk factors for oral cancer in Western countries include sun exposure (lower lip) and tobacco and alcohol use. In India and some other Asian countries, smokeless tobacco mixed with betel nut, slaked lime, and spices is a common cause of oral cancer. Less common etiologies include syphilis and Plummer-Vinson syndrome (iron deficiency).

Rarer causes of chronic oral ulcer such as tuberculosis, fungal infection, Wegener's granulomatosis, and midline granuloma may look identical to carcinoma. Making the correct diagnosis depends on recognizing other clinical features and biopsy of the lesion. The syphilitic chancre is typically painless and therefore easily missed. Regional lymphadenopathy is invariably present. Confirmation is achieved using appropriate bacterial and serologic tests.

TABLE 32-1 VESICULAR, BULLOUS, OR ULCERATIVE LESIONS OF THE ORAL MUCOSA

Condition	Usual Location	Clinical Features	Course
Viral Diseases			
Primary acute herpetic gingivostomatitis [herpes simplex virus (HSV) type 1, rarely type 2]	Lip and oral mucosa (buccal, gingival, lingual mucosa)	Labial vesicles that rupture and crust, and intraoral vesicles that quickly ulcerate; extremely painful; acute gingivitis, fever, malaise, foul odor, and cervical lymphadenopathy; occurs primarily in infants, children, and young adults	Heals spontaneously in 10–14 days. Unless secondarily infected, lesions lasting >3 weeks are not due to primary HSV infection.
Recurrent herpes labialis	Mucocutaneous junction of lip, perioral skin	Eruption of groups of vesicles that may coalesce, then rupture and crust; painful to pressure or spicy foods	Lasts about 1 week, but condition may be prolonged if secondarily infected. If severe, topical or oral antiviral may reduce healing time.
Recurrent intraoral herpes simplex	Palate and gingiva	Small vesicles on keratinized epithelium that rupture and coalesce; painful	Heals spontaneously in about 1 week. If severe, topical or oral antiviral may reduce healing time.
Chickenpox (varicella-zoster virus)	Gingiva and oral mucosa	Skin lesions may be accompanied by small vesicles on oral mucosa that rupture to form shallow ulcers; may coalesce to form large bullous lesions that ulcerate; mucosa may have generalized erythema	Lesions heal spontaneously within 2 weeks.
Herpes zoster (reactivation of varicella-zoster virus)	Cheek, tongue, gingiva, or palate	Unilateral vesicular eruptions and ulceration in linear pattern following sensory distribution of trigeminal nerve or one of its branches	Gradual healing without scarring unless secondarily infected; postherpetic neuralgia is common. Oral acyclovir, famcyclovir, or valacyclovir reduce healing time and postherpetic neuralgia
Infectious mononucleosis (Epstein-Barr virus)	Oral mucosa	Fatigue, sore throat, malaise, fever, and cervical lymphadenopathy; numerous small ulcers usually appear several days before lymphadenopathy; gingival bleeding and multiple petechiae at junction of hard and soft palates	Oral lesions disappear during convalescence; no treatment though glucocorticoids indicated if tonsillar swelling compromises airway
Herpangina (coxsackievirus A; also possibly coxsackie B and echovirus)	Oral mucosa, pharynx, tongue	Sudden onset of fever, sore throat, and oropharyngeal vesicles, usually in children under 4 years, during summer months; diffuse pharyngeal congestion and vesicles (1–2 mm), grayish-white surrounded by red areola; vesicles enlarge and ulcerate	Incubation period 2–9 days; fever for 1–4 days; recovery uneventful
Hand, foot, and mouth disease (coxsackievirus A16 most common)	Oral mucosa, pharynx, palms, and soles	Fever, malaise, headache with oropharyngeal vesicles that become painful, shallow ulcers; highly infectious; usually affects children under age 10	Incubation period 2–18 days; lesions heal spontaneously in 2–4 weeks
Primary HIV infection	Gingiva, palate, and pharynx	Acute gingivitis and oropharyngeal ulceration, associated with febrile illness resembling mononucleosis and including lymphadenopathy	Followed by HIV seroconversion, asymptomatic HIV infection, and usually ultimately by HIV disease
Bacterial or Fungal Diseases			
Acute necrotizing ulcerative gingivitis ("trench mouth," Vincent's infection)	Gingiva	Painful, bleeding gingiva characterized by necrosis and ulceration of gingival papillae and margins plus lymphadenopathy and foul odor	Debridement and diluted (1:3) peroxide lavage provide relief within 24 h; antibiotics in acutely ill patients; relapse may occur
Prenatal (congenital) syphilis	Palate, jaws, tongue, and teeth	Gummatous involvement of palate, jaws, and facial bones; Hutchinson's incisors, mulberry molars, glossitis, mucous patches, and fissures on corner of mouth	Tooth deformities in permanent dentition irreversible
Primary syphilis (chancre)	Lesion appears where organism enters body; may occur on lips, tongue, or tonsillar area	Small papule developing rapidly into a large, painless ulcer with indurated border; unilateral lymphadenopathy; chancre and lymph nodes containing spirochetes; serologic tests positive by third to fourth weeks	Healing of chancre in 1–2 months, followed by secondary syphilis in 6–8 weeks
Secondary syphilis	Oral mucosa frequently involved with mucous patches, primarily on palate, also at commissures of mouth	Maculopapular lesions of oral mucosa, 5–10 mm in diameter with central ulceration covered by grayish membrane; eruptions occurring on various mucosal surfaces and skin accompanied by fever, malaise, and sore throat	Lesions may persist from several weeks to a year
Tertiary syphilis	Palate and tongue	Gummatous infiltration of palate or tongue followed by ulceration and fibrosis; atrophy of tongue papillae produces characteristic bald tongue and glossitis	Gumma may destroy palate, causing complete perforation
Gonorrhea	Lesions may occur in mouth at site of inoculation or secondarily by hematogenous spread from a primary focus elsewhere	Most pharyngeal infection is asymptomatic; may produce burning or itching sensation; oropharynx and tonsils may be ulcerated and erythematous; saliva viscous and fetid	More difficult to eradicate than urogenital infection, though pharyngitis usually resolves with appropriate antimicrobial treatment

(continued)

TABLE 32-1 VESICULAR, BULLOUS, OR ULCERATIVE LESIONS OF THE ORAL MUCOSA (CONTINUED)

Condition	Usual Location	Clinical Features	Course
Tuberculosis	Tongue, tonsillar area, soft palate	A painless, solitary, 1–5 cm, irregular ulcer covered with a persistent exudate; ulcer has a firm undermined border	Autoinnoculation from pulmonary infection usual; lesions resolve with appropriate antimicrobial therapy
Cervicofacial actinomycosis	Swellings in region of face, neck, and floor of mouth	Infection may be associated with an extraction, jaw fracture, or eruption of molar tooth; in acute form resembles an acute pyogenic abscess, but contains yellow "sulfur granules" (gram-positive mycelia and their hyphae)	Typically swelling is hard and grows painlessly; multiple abscesses with draining tracks develop; penicillin first choice; surgery usually necessary
Histoplasmosis	Any area of the mouth, particularly tongue, gingiva, or palate	Nodular, verrucous, or granulomatous lesions; ulcers are indurated and painful; usual source hematogenous or pulmonary, but may be primary	Systemic antifungal therapy necessary to treat
Candidiasis (Table 32-3)			
Dermatologic Diseases			
Mucous membrane pemphigoid	Typically produces marked gingival erythema and ulceration; other areas of oral cavity, esophagus, and vagina may be affected	Painful, grayish-white collapsed vesicles or bullae of full-thickness epithelium with peripheral erythematous zone; gingival lesions desquamate, leaving ulcerated area	Protracted course with remissions and exacerbations; involvement of different sites occurs slowly; glucocorticoids may temporarily reduce symptoms but do not control the disease
Erythema multiforme minor and major (Stevens-Johnson syndrome)	Primarily the oral mucosa and the skin of hands and feet	Intraoral ruptured bullae surrounded by an inflammatory area; lips may show hemorrhagic crusts; the "iris," or "target," lesion on the skin is pathognomonic; patient may have severe signs of toxicity	Onset very rapid; usually idiopathic, but may be associated with trigger such as drug reaction; condition may last 3–6 weeks; mortality with EM major 5–15% if untreated
Pemphigus vulgaris	Oral mucosa and skin; sites of mechanical trauma (soft/hard palate, frenulum, lips, buccal mucosa)	Usually (>70%) presents with oral lesions; fragile, ruptured bullae and ulcerated oral areas; mostly in older adults	With repeated occurrence of bullae, toxicity may lead to cachexia, infection, and death within 2 years; often controllable with oral glucocorticoids
Lichen planus	Oral mucosa and skin	White striae in mouth; purplish nodules on skin at sites of friction; occasionally causes oral mucosal ulcers and erosive gingivitis	White striae alone usually asymptomatic; erosive lesions often difficult to treat, but may respond to glucocorticoids
Other Conditions			
Recurrent aphthous ulcers	Usually on nonkeratinized oral mucosa (buccal and labial mucosa, floor of mouth, soft palate, lateral and ventral tongue)	Single or clusters of painful ulcers with surrounding erythematous border; lesions may be 1–2 mm in diameter in crops (herpetiform), 1–5 mm (minor), or 5–15 mm (major)	Lesions heal in 1–2 weeks but may recur monthly or several times a year; protective barrier with orabase and topical steroids give symptomatic relief; systemic glucocorticoids may be needed in severe cases
Behçet's syndrome	Oral mucosa, eyes, genitalia, gut, and CNS	Multiple aphthous ulcers in mouth; inflammatory ocular changes, ulcerative lesions on genitalia; inflammatory bowel disease and CNS disease	Oral lesions often first manifestation; persist several weeks and heal without scarring
Traumatic ulcers	Anywhere on oral mucosa; dentures frequently responsible for ulcers in vestibule	Localized, discrete ulcerated lesions with red border; produced by accidental biting of mucosa, penetration by a foreign object, or chronic irritation by a denture	Lesions usually heal in 7–10 days when irritant is removed, unless secondarily infected
Squamous cell carcinoma	Any area in the mouth, most commonly on lower lip, tongue, and floor of mouth	Ulcer with elevated, indurated border; failure to heal, pain not prominent; lesions tend to arise in areas of erythro/leukoplakia or in smooth atrophic tongue	Invades and destroys underlying tissues; frequently metastasizes to regional lymph nodes
Acute myeloid leukemia (usually monocytic)	Gingiva	Gingival swelling and superficial ulceration followed by hyperplasia of gingiva with extensive necrosis and hemorrhage; deep ulcers may occur elsewhere on the mucosa complicated by secondary infection	Usually responds to systemic treatment of leukemia; occasionally requires local radiation therapy
Lymphoma	Gingiva, tongue, palate and tonsillar area	Elevated, ulcerated area that may proliferate rapidly, giving the appearance of traumatic inflammation	Fatal if untreated; may indicate underlying HIV infection
Chemical or thermal burns	Any area in mouth	White slough due to contact with corrosive agents (e.g., aspirin, hot cheese) applied locally; removal of slough leaves raw, painful surface	Lesion heals in several weeks if not secondarily infected

Note: CNS, central nervous system.

TABLE 32-2 PIGMENTED LESIONS OF THE ORAL MUCOSA

Condition	Usual Location	Clinical Features	Course
Oral melanotic macule	Any area of the mouth	Discrete or diffuse localized, brown to black macule	Remains indefinitely; no growth
Diffuse melanin pigmentation	Any area of the mouth	Diffuse pale to dark-brown pigmentation; may be physiologic ("racial") or due to smoking	Remains indefinitely
Nevi	Any area of the mouth	Discrete, localized, brown to black pigmentation	Remains indefinitely
Malignant melanoma	Any area of the mouth	Can be flat and diffuse, painless, brown to black, or can be raised and nodular	Expands and invades early; metastasis leads to death
Addison's disease	Any area of the mouth, but mostly buccal mucosa	Blotches or spots of bluish-black to dark-brown pigmentation occurring early in the disease, accompanied by diffuse pigmentation of skin; other symptoms of adrenal insufficiency	Condition controlled by adrenal steroid replacement
Peutz-Jeghers syndrome	Any area of the mouth	Dark-brown spots on lips, buccal mucosa, with characteristic distribution of pigment around lips, nose, eyes, and on hands; concomitant intestinal polyposis	Oral pigmented lesions remain indefinitely; gastrointestinal polyps may become malignant
Drug ingestion (neuroleptics, oral contraceptives, minocycline, zidovudine, quinine derivatives)	Any area of the mouth	Brown, black, or gray areas of pigmentation	Gradually disappears following cessation of drug
Amalgam tattoo	Gingiva and alveolar mucosa	Small blue-black pigmented areas associated with embedded amalgam particles in soft tissues; these may show up on radiographs as radiopaque particles in some cases	Remains indefinitely
Heavy metal pigmentation (bismuth, mercury, lead)	Gingival margin	Thin blue-black pigmented line along gingival margin; rarely seen except for children exposed to lead-based paint	Indicative of systemic absorption; no significance for oral health
Black hairy tongue	Dorsum of tongue	Elongation of filiform papillae of tongue, which become stained by coffee, tea, tobacco, or pigmented bacteria	Improves within 1–2 weeks with gentle brushing of tongue or discontinuation of antibiotic if due to bacterial overgrowth
Fordyce "spots"	Buccal and labial mucosa	Numerous small yellowish spots just beneath mucosal surface; no symptoms; due to hyperplasia of sebaceous glands	Benign; remains without apparent change
Kaposi's sarcoma	Palate most common, but may occur in any other site	Red or blue plaques of variable size and shape; often enlarge, become nodular and may ulcerate	Usually indicative of HIV infection or non-Hodgkin's lymphoma; rarely fatal, but may require treatment for comfort or cosmesis
Mucous retention cysts	Buccal and labial mucosa	Bluish-clear fluid-filled cyst due to extravasated mucous from injured minor salivary gland	Benign; painless unless traumatized; may be removed surgically

TABLE 32-3 WHITE LESIONS OF ORAL MUCOSA

Condition	Usual Location	Clinical Features	Course
Lichen planus	Buccal mucosa, tongue, gingiva, and lips; skin	Striae, white plaques, red areas, ulcers in mouth; purplish papules on skin; may be asymptomatic, sore, or painful; lichenoid drug reactions may look similar	Protracted; responds to topical glucocorticoids
White sponge nevus	Oral mucosa, vagina, anal mucosa	Painless white thickening of epithelium; adolescent/early adult onset; familial	Benign and permanent
Smoker's leukoplakia and smokeless tobacco lesions	Any area of oral mucosa, sometimes related to location of habit	White patch that may become firm, rough, or red-fissured and ulcerated; may become sore and painful but usually painless	May or may not resolve with cessation of habit; 2% develop squamous cell carcinoma; early biopsy essential
Erythroplakia with or without white patches	Floor of mouth common in men; tongue and buccal mucosa in women	Velvety, reddish plaque; occasionally mixed with white patches or smooth red areas	High risk of squamous cell cancer; early biopsy essential
Candidiasis	Any area in mouth	*Pseudomembranous type* ("thrush"): creamy white curdlike patches that reveal a raw, bleeding surface when scraped; found in sick infants, debilitated elderly patients receiving high doses of glucocorticoids or broad-spectrum antibiotics, or in patients with AIDS	Responds favorably to antifungal therapy and correction of predisposing causes where possible
		Erythematous type: flat, red, sometimes sore areas in same groups of patients	Course same as for pseudomembranous type
		Candidal leukoplakia: nonremovable white thickening of epithelium due to *Candida*	Responds to prolonged antifungal therapy
		Angular cheilitis: sore fissures at corner of mouth	Responds to topical antifungal therapy
Hairy leukoplakia	Usually lateral tongue, rarely elsewhere on oral mucosa	White areas ranging from small and flat to extensive accentuation of vertical folds; found in HIV carriers in all risk groups for AIDS	Due to EBV; responds to high dose acyclovir but recurs; rarely causes discomfort unless secondarily infected with *Candida*
Warts (papillomavirus)	Anywhere on skin and oral mucosa	Single or multiple papillary lesions, with thick, white keratinized surfaces containing many pointed projections; cauliflower lesions covered with normal-colored mucosa or multiple pink or pale bumps (focal epithelial hyperplasia)	Lesions grow rapidly and spread; consider squamous cell carcinoma and rule out with biopsy; excision or laser therapy; may regress in HIV infected patients on antiretroviral therapy

Note: EBV, Epstein-Barr virus.

TABLE 32-4 ALTERATIONS OF THE TONGUE

Type of Change	Clinical Features
Size or Morphology Changes	
Macroglossia	Enlarged tongue that may be part of a syndrome found in developmental conditions such as Down syndrome, Simpson-Golabi-Behmel syndrome, or Beckwith-Wiedemann syndrome may be due to tumor (hemangioma or lymphangioma), metabolic disease (such as primary amyloidosis), or endocrine disturbance (such as acromegaly or cretinism)
Fissured ("scrotal") tongue	Dorsal surface and sides of tongue covered by painless shallow or deep fissures that may collect debris and become irritated
Median rhomboid glossitis	Congenital abnormality of tongue with ovoid, denuded area in median posterior portion of the tongue; may be associated with candidiasis and may respond to antifungals
Color Changes	
"Geographic" tongue (benign migratory glossitis)	Asymptomatic inflammatory condition of the tongue, with rapid loss and regrowth of filiform papillae, leading to appearance of denuded red patches "wandering" across the surface of the tongue
Hairy tongue	Elongation of filiform papillae of the medial dorsal surface area due to failure of keratin layer of the papillae to desquamate normally; brownish-black coloration may be due to staining by tobacco, food, or chromogenic organisms
"Strawberry" and "raspberry" tongue	Appearance of tongue during scarlet fever due to the hypertrophy of fungiform papillae plus changes in the filiform papillae
"Bald" tongue	Atrophy may be associated with xerostomia, pernicious anemia, iron-deficiency anemia, pellagra, or syphilis; may be accompanied by painful burning sensation; may be an expression of erythmematous candidiasis and respond to antifungals

Disorders of mucosal fragility often produce painful oral ulcers that fail to heal within 2 weeks. *Mucous membrane pemphigoid* and *pemphigus vulgaris* are the major acquired disorders. While clinical features are often distinctive, immunohistochemical examination should be performed for diagnosis and to distinguish these entities from *lichen planus* and drug reactions.

Hematologic and Nutritional Disease Internists are more likely to encounter patients with acquired, rather than congenital, bleeding disorders. Bleeding after minor trauma should stop after 15 min and within an hour of tooth extraction if local pressure is applied. More prolonged bleeding, if not due to continued injury or rupture of a large vessel, should lead to investigation for a clotting abnormality. In addition to bleeding, petechiae and ecchymoses are prone to occur at the line of vibration between the soft and hard palates in patients with platelet dysfunction or thrombocytopenia.

All forms of leukemia, but particularly acute myelomonocytic leukemia, can produce gingival bleeding, ulcers, and gingival enlargement. Oral ulcers are a feature of agranulocytosis, and ulcers and mucositis are often severe complications of chemotherapy and radiation therapy for hematologic and other malignancies. Plummer-Vinson syndrome (iron deficiency, angular stomatitis, glossitis, and dysphagia) raises the risk of oral squamous cell cancer and esophageal cancer at the postcricoidal tissue web. Atrophic papillae and a red, burning tongue may occur with pernicious anemia. B group vitamin deficiencies produce many of these same symptoms as well as oral ulceration and cheilosis. Cheilosis may also be seen in iron deficiency. Swollen, bleeding gums, ulcers, and loosening of the teeth are a consequence of scurvy.

NONDENTAL CAUSES OF ORAL PAIN

Most but not all oral pain emanates from inflamed or injured tooth pulp or periodontal tissues. Nonodontogenic causes may be overlooked. In most instances toothache is predictable and proportional to the stimulus applied, and an identifiable condition (e.g., caries, abscess) is found. Local anesthesia eliminates pain originating from dental or periodontal structures, but not referred pains. The most common nondental origin is myofascial pain referred from muscles of mastication, which become tender and ache with increased use. Many sufferers exhibit bruxism (the grinding of teeth, often during sleep) that is secondary to stress and anxiety. *Temporomandibular disorder* is closely related. It predominantly affects females ages 15–45. Features include pain, limited mandibular movement, and temporomandibular joint sounds. The etiologies are complex, and malocclusion does not play the primary role once attributed to it. *Osteoarthritis* is a common cause of masticatory pain. Anti-inflammatory medication, jaw rest, soft foods, and heat provide relief. The temporomandibular joint is involved in 50% of patients with *rheumatoid arthritis* and is usually a late feature of severe disease. Bilateral preauricular pain, particularly in the morning, limits range of motion.

Migrainous neuralgia may be localized to the mouth. Episodes of pain and remission without identifiable cause and absence of relief with local anesthesia are important clues. *Trigeminal neuralgia* (*tic douloureaux*) may involve the entire branch or part of the mandibular or maxillary branches of the fifth cranial nerve and produce pain in one or a few teeth. Pain may occur spontaneously or may be triggered by touching the lip or gingiva, brushing the teeth, or chewing. *Glossopharyngeal neuralgia* produces similar acute neuropathic symptoms in the distribution of the ninth cranial nerve. Swallowing, sneezing, coughing, or pressure on the tragus of the ear triggers pain that is felt in the base of the tongue, pharynx, and soft palate and may be referred to the temporomandibular joint. *Neuritis* involving the maxillary and mandibular divisions of the trigeminal nerve (e.g., maxillary sinusitis, neuroma, and leukemic infiltrate) is distinguished from ordinary toothache by the neuropathic quality of the pain. Occasionally *phantom pain* follows tooth extraction.

TABLE 32-5 ORAL LESIONS ASSOCIATED WITH HIV INFECTION

Lesion Morphology	Etiologies
Papules, nodules, plaques	Candidiasis (hyperplastic and pseudomembranous)[a]
	Condyloma acuminatum (human papillomavirus infection)
	Squamous cell carcinoma (preinvasive and invasive)
	Non-Hodgkin's lymphoma[a]
	Hairy leukoplakia[a]
Ulcers	Recurrent aphthous ulcers[a]
	Angular cheilitis
	Squamous cell carcinoma
	Acute necrotizing ulcerative gingivitis[a]
	Necrotizing ulcerative periodontitis[a]
	Necrotizing ulcerative stomatitis
	Non-Hodgkin's lymphoma[a]
	Viral infection (herpes simplex, herpes zoster, cytomegalovirus)
	Mycobacterium tuberculosis, *Mycobacterium avium-intracellulare*
	Fungal infection (histoplasmosis, cryptococcosis, candidiasis, geotrichosis, aspergillosis)
	Bacterial infection (*Escherichia coli*, *Enterobacter cloacae*, *Klebsiella pneumoniae*, *Pseudomonas aeruginosa*)
	Drug reactions (single or multiple ulcers)
Pigmented lesions	Kaposi's sarcoma[a]
	Bacillary angiomatosis (skin and visceral lesions more common than oral)
	Zidovudine pigmentation (skin, nails, and occasionally oral mucosa)
	Addison's disease
Miscellaneous	Linear gingival erythema[a]

[a]Strongly associated with HIV infection.

Often the earliest symptom of Bell's palsy in the day or so before facial weakness develops is pain and hyperalgesia behind the ear and side of the face. Likewise, similar symptoms may precede visible lesions of herpes zoster infecting the seventh nerve (Ramsey-Hunt syndrome) or trigeminal nerve. *Postherpetic neuralgia* may follow either condition. *Coronary ischemia* may produce pain exclusively in the face and jaw and, like typical angina pectoris, is usually reproducible with increased myocardial demand. Aching in several upper molar or premolar teeth that is unrelieved by anesthetizing the teeth may point to *maxillary sinusitis*.

Giant cell arteritis is notorious for producing headache, but it may also produce facial pain or sore throat without headache. Jaw and tongue claudication with chewing or talking is relatively common. Tongue infarction is rare. Patients with subacute thyroiditis often experience pain referred to the face or jaw before the tender thyroid gland and transient hyperthyroidism are appreciated.

Burning mouth syndrome (glossodynia) is present in the absence of an identifiable cause (e.g., vitamin B_{12} deficiency, iron deficiency, Plummer-Vinson syndrome, diabetes mellitus, low-grade *Candida* infection, food sensitivity, or subtle xerostomia) and predominantly affects postmenopausal women. The etiology may be neuropathic. Clonazepam, alpha-lipoic acid and cognitive behavioral therapy have benefited some.

DISEASES OF THE SALIVARY GLANDS

Saliva is essential to oral health. Its major components, water and mucin, serve as a cleansing solvent and lubricating fluid. In addition, it contains antimicrobial factors (e.g., lysozyme, lactoperoxidase, secretory IgA), epidermal growth factor, minerals, and buffering systems. The major salivary glands secrete intermittently in response to autonomic stimulation, which is high during a meal but low otherwise. Hundreds of minor glands in the lips and cheeks secrete mucus continuously. Consequently, oral function becomes impaired when salivary function is reduced. Dry mouth (*xerostomia*) is perceived when salivary flow is reduced by 50%. The most common etiology is medication, especially drugs with anticholinergic properties, but also alpha and beta blockers, calcium channel blockers, and diuretics. Other causes include Sjögren's syndrome, chronic parotitis, salivary duct obstruction, diabetes mellitus, HIV/AIDS, and irradiation for head and neck cancer. Management involves eliminating or limiting drying medications, preventive dental care, and supplementing oral liquid. Sugarless mints or chewing gum may stimulate salivary secretion if dysfunction is mild. When sufficient exocrine tissue remains, pilocarpine or cevimeline has been shown to increase secretions. Commercial saliva substitutes or gels relieve dryness but must be supplemented with fluoride applications to prevent caries.

Sialolithiasis presents most often as painful swelling but in some instances as just swelling or pain. The obstructing stone produces spasm upon eating. Conservative therapy consists of local heat, massage, and hydration. Promotion of salivary secretion with mints or lemon drops may flush out small stones. Antibiotic treatment is necessary when bacterial infection in suspected. In adults, *acute bacterial parotitis* is typically unilateral and most commonly affects postoperative patients within the first 2 weeks of surgery. *Staphylococcus aureus* is the most common bacterial agent. Dehydration, advanced age, and chronic debilitating disease are major risks. Chronic bacterial sialadenitis results from lowered salivary secretion and recurrent bacterial infection. When suspected bacterial infection is not responsive to therapy, the differential diagnosis should be expanded to include benign and malignant neoplasms, lymphoproliferative disorders, Sjögren's syndrome, sarcoidosis, tuberculosis, lymphadenitis, actinomycosis, and Wegener's granulomatosis. Bilateral nontender parotid enlargement occurs with diabetes mellitus, cirrhosis, bulimia, HIV/AIDS, and drugs (e.g., iodide, propylthiouracil).

Pleomorphic adenoma comprises two-thirds of all salivary neoplasms. The parotid is the principal salivary gland affected, and the tumor presents as a firm, slow-growing mass. Though benign, recurrence is common if resection is incomplete. Malignant tumors such as mucoepidermoid carcinoma, adenoid cystic carcinoma, and adenocarcinoma tend to grow relatively fast, depending upon grade. They may ulcerate and invade nerves, producing numbness and facial paralysis. Neutron-beam radiation therapy is an effective treatment; 5-year survival is about 68% for malignant salivary gland tumors.

DENTAL CARE OF MEDICALLY COMPLEX PATIENTS

Routine dental care (e.g., extraction, scaling and cleaning, tooth restoration, and root canal) is remarkably safe. The most common concerns regarding care of dental patients with medical disease are fear of excessive bleeding for patients on anticoagulants, infection of the heart valves and prosthetic devices from hematogenous seeding of oral flora, and cardiovascular complications resulting from vasopressors used with local anesthetics during dental treatment. Experience confirms that the risks of any of these complications are very low.

Patients undergoing tooth extraction or alveolar and gingival surgery rarely experience uncontrolled bleeding when warfarin anticoagulation is maintained within the therapeutic range currently recommended for prevention of venous thrombosis, atrial fibrillation, or mechanical heart valve. Embolic complications and death, however, have been reported during subtherapeutic anticoagulation. Therapeutic anticoagulation should be confirmed before and continued through the procedure. Likewise, low-dose aspirin (e.g., 81–325 mg) can be safely continued.

Patients at high or moderate risk for bacterial endocarditis (Chap. 118) should maintain optimal oral hygiene, including flossing, and have regular professional cleaning. Prophylactic antibiotics are recommended for all at-risk patients who undergo dental and oral procedures likely to cause significant bleeding and bacteremia. Should unexpected bleeding occur, antibiotics given within 2 h following the procedure provide effective prophylaxis.

Hematogenous bacterial seeding from oral infection can undoubtedly produce late prosthetic joint infection and therefore requires removal of the infected tissue (e.g., drainage, extraction, root canal) and appropriate antibiotic therapy. However, evidence that late prosthetic joint infection occurs following routine dental procedures is lacking. For this reason, antibiotic prophylaxis is not recommended before dental surgery in patients with orthopedic pins, screws, and plates. It is, however, advised within the first 2 years after joint replacement for patients who have inflammatory arthropathies, immunosuppression, type 1 diabetes mellitus, previous prosthetic joint infection, hemophilia, or malnourishment.

Concern often arises regarding the use of vasoconstrictors in patients with hypertension and heart disease. Vasoconstrictors enhance the depth and duration of local anesthesia, thus reducing the anesthetic dose and potential toxicity. If intravascular injection is avoided, 2% lidocaine with 1:100,000 epinephrine (limited to a total of 0.036 mg epinephrine) can be used safely in those with controlled hypertension and stable coronary heart disease, arrhythmia, or congestive heart failure. Precaution should be taken with patients taking tricyclic antidepressants and nonselective beta blockers as these drugs may potentiate the effect of epinephrine.

Elective dental treatments should be postponed for at least 1 month after myocardial infarction, after which the risk of reinfarction is low provided the patient is medically stable (e.g., stable rhythm, stable angina, and free of heart failure). Patients who have suffered a stroke should have elective dental care deferred for 6 months. In both situations, effective stress reduction requires good pain control, including the use of the minimal amount of vasoconstrictor necessary to provide good hemostasis and local anesthesia.

Bisphosphonate therapy can be associated with *osteonecrosis* of the jaw. Most patients affected have received high dose aminobisphosphonate therapy for multiple myeloma or metastatic breast cancer and have undergone tooth extraction or dental surgery. Intra-oral lesions appear as exposed yellow-white hard bone involving the mandible or maxilla. Two-thirds are painful. Patients about to receive aminobisphosphonate therapy should receive preventive dental care that reduces the risk of infection and need for future dentoalveolar surgery.

HALITOSIS

Halitosis typically emanates from the oral cavity or nasal passages. Volatile sulfur compounds resulting from bacterial decay of food and cellular debris account for the malodor. Periodontal disease, caries, acute forms of gingivitis, poorly fitting dentures, oral abscess, and tongue coating are usual causes. Treatment includes correcting poor hygiene, treating infection, and tongue brushing. Xerostomia can produce and exacerbate halitosis. Pockets of decay in the tonsillar crypts, esophageal diverticulum, esophageal stasis (e.g., achalasia, stricture), sinusitis, and lung abscess account for some instances. A few systemic diseases produce distinctive odors: renal failure (ammoniacal), hepatic (fishy), and ketoacidosis (fruity). *Helicobacter pylori* gastritis can also produce ammoniac breath. If no odor is detectable, then pseudohalitosis or even halitophobia must be considered. These conditions represent varying degrees of psychiatric illness.

AGING AND ORAL HEALTH

While tooth loss and dental disease are not normal consequences of aging, a complex array of structural and functional changes occurs with age that can affect oral health. Subtle changes in tooth structure (e.g., diminished pulp space and volume, sclerosis of dentinal tubules, altered proportions of nerve and vascular pulp content) result in diminished or altered pain sensitivity, reduced reparative capacity, and increased tooth brittleness. In addition, age-associated fatty replacement of salivary acini may reduce physiologic reserve, thus increasing the risk of xerostomia.

Poor oral hygiene often results when vision fails or when patients lose manual dexterity and upper extremity flexibility. This is particularly common for nursing home residents and must be emphasized since regular oral cleaning and dental care has been shown to reduce the incidence of pneumonia. Other risks for dental decay include limited lifetime fluoride exposure and preference by some older adults for intensely sweet foods when taste and olfaction wane. These factors occur in an increasing proportion of persons over age 75 who retain teeth that have extensive restorations and exposed roots. Without assiduous care, decay can become quite advanced yet remain asymptomatic. Consequently, much or all of the tooth can be destroyed before the process is detected.

Periodontal disease, a leading cause of tooth loss, is indicated by loss of alveolar bone height. Over 90% of Americans have some degree of periodontal disease by age 50. Healthy adults who have not experienced significant alveolar bone loss by the sixth decade do not typically develop significant worsening with advancing age.

Complete edentulousness with advanced age, though less common than in previous decades, is still present in approximately 50% of Americans age ≥85. Speech, mastication, and facial contours are dramatically affected. Edentulousness may also worsen obstructive sleep apnea, particularly in those without symptoms while wearing dentures. Dentures can improve speech articulation and restore diminished facial contours. Mastication is restored less predictably, and those expecting dentures to improve oral intake are often disappointed. Dentures require periodic adjustment to accommodate inevitable remodeling that leads to a diminished volume of the alveolar ridge. Pain can result from friction or traumatic lesions produced by loose dentures. Poor fit and poor oral hygiene may permit candidiasis to develop. This may be asymptomatic or painful and is indicated by erythematous smooth or granular tissue conforming to an area covered by the appliance.

ACKNOWLEDGMENT
The author acknowledges the contribution to this chapter by the previous author, Dr. John S. Greenspan.

FURTHER READINGS

DURSO SC: Interaction with other health team members in caring for elderly patients. Dent Clin N Am 49:377, 2005

LITTLE JW et al (eds): *Dental Management of the Medically Compromised Patient*, 6th ed. St. Louis, Mosby, 2002

REGEZI JA, SCIUBBA JJ: *Oral Pathology: Clinical Pathologic Correlations*, 4th ed. Philadelphia, Saunders, 2002

SPAHR A et al: Periodontal infection and coronary heart disease. Role of periodontal bacteria and importance of total pathogen burden in the coronary event and periodontal disease (CORODONT) study. Arch Intern Med 166:554, 2006

WOO SB et al: Systematic Review: Bisphosphonates and osteonecrosis of the jaws. Ann Intern Med 144:753, 2006

SECTION 5 ALTERATIONS IN CIRCULATORY AND RESPIRATORY FUNCTIONS

33 Dyspnea and Pulmonary Edema

Richard M. Schwartzstein

DYSPNEA

The American Thoracic Society defines *dyspnea* as a "subjective experience of breathing discomfort that consists of qualitatively distinct sensations that vary in intensity. The experience derives from interactions among multiple physiological, psychological, social, and environmental factors, and may induce secondary physiological and behavioral responses." Dyspnea, a symptom, must be distinguished from the signs of increased work of breathing.

MECHANISMS OF DYSPNEA

Respiratory sensations are the consequence of interactions between the *efferent*, or outgoing, motor output from the brain to the ventilatory muscles (feed-forward) and the *afferent*, or incoming, sensory input from receptors throughout the body (feedback), as well as the integrative processing of this information that we infer must be occurring in the brain (Fig. 33-1). A given disease state may lead to dyspnea by one or more mechanisms, some of which may be operative under some circumstances but not others.

Motor Efferents Disorders of the ventilatory pump are associated with increased work of breathing or a sense of an increased effort to breathe. When the muscles are weak or fatigued, greater effort is required, even though the mechanics of the system are normal. The increased neural output from the motor cortex is thought to be sensed due to a corollary discharge that is sent to the sensory cortex at the same time that signals are sent to the ventilatory muscles.

Sensory Afferents Chemoreceptors in the carotid bodies and medulla are activated by hypoxemia, acute hypercapnia, and acidemia. Stimulation of these receptors, as well as others that lead to an increase in ventilation, produce a sensation of air hunger. Mechanoreceptors in the lungs, when stimulated by bronchospasm, lead to a sensation of chest tightness. J-receptors, sensitive to interstitial edema, and pulmonary vascular receptors, activated by acute changes in pulmonary artery pressure, appear to contribute to air hunger. Hyperinflation is associated with the sensation of an inability to get a deep breath or of an unsatisfying breath. It is not clear if this sensation arises from receptors in the lungs or chest wall, or if it is a variant of the sensation of air hunger. Metaboreceptors, located in skeletal muscle, are believed to be activated by changes in the local biochemical milieu of the tissue active during exercise and, when stimulated, contribute to the breathing discomfort.

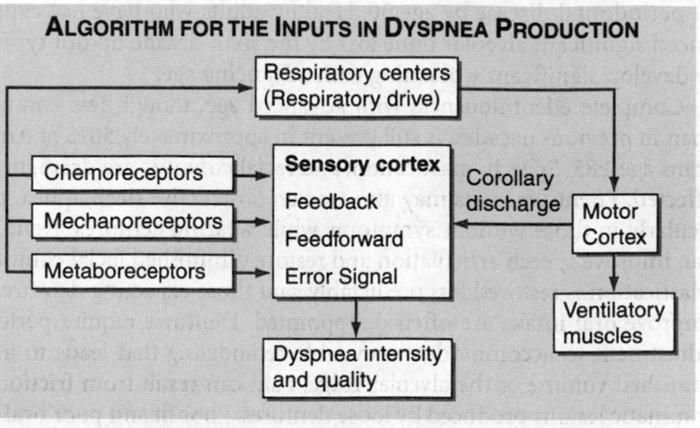

FIGURE 33-1 Hypothetical model for integration of sensory inputs in the production of dyspnea. Afferent information from the receptors throughout the respiratory system projects directly to the sensory cortex to contribute to primary qualitative sensory experiences and provide feedback on the action of the ventilatory pump. Afferents also project to the areas of the brain responsible for control of ventilation. The motor cortex, responding to input from the control centers, sends neural messages to the ventilatory muscles and a corollary discharge to the sensory cortex (feed-forward with respect to the instructions sent to the muscles). If the feed-forward and feedback messages do not match, an error signal is generated and the intensity of dyspnea increases. *(Adapted from Gillette and Schwartzstein.)*

Integration: Efferent-Reafferent Mismatch A discrepancy or mismatch between the feed-forward message to the ventilatory muscles and the feedback from receptors that monitor the response of the ventilatory pump increases the intensity of dyspnea. This is particularly important when there is a mechanical derangement of the ventilatory pump, such as in asthma or chronic obstructive pulmonary disease (COPD).

Anxiety Acute anxiety may increase the severity of dyspnea either by altering the interpretation of sensory data or by leading to patterns of breathing that heighten physiologic abnormalities in the respiratory system. In patients with expiratory flow limitation, for example, the increased respiratory rate that accompanies acute anxiety leads to hyperinflation, increased work of breathing, a sense of an increased effort to breathe, and a sense of an unsatisfying breath.

ASSESSING DYSPNEA

Quality of Sensation As with pain, dyspnea assessment begins with a determination of the quality of the discomfort (Table 33-1). Dyspnea questionnaires, or lists of phrases commonly used by patients, assist those who have difficulty describing their breathing sensations.

Sensory Intensity A modified Borg scale or visual analogue scale can be utilized to measure dyspnea at rest, immediately following exercise, or on recall of a reproducible physical task, e.g., climbing the stairs at home. An alternative approach is to inquire about the activities a patient can do, i.e., to gain a sense of the patient's disability. The Baseline Dyspnea Index and the Chronic Respiratory Disease Questionnaire are commonly used tools for this purpose.

TABLE 33-1 ASSOCIATION OF QUALITATIVE DESCRIPTORS AND PATHOPHYSIOLOGIC MECHANISMS OF SHORTNESS OF BREATH

Descriptor	Pathophysiology
Chest tightness or constriction	Bronchoconstriction, interstitial edema (asthma, myocardial ischemia)
Increased work or effort of breathing	Airway obstruction, neuromuscular disease (COPD, moderate to severe asthma, myopathy, kyphoscoliosis)
Air hunger, need to breathe, urge to breathe	Increased drive to breathe (CHF, pulmonary embolism, moderate to severe airflow obstruction)
Cannot get a deep breath, unsatisfying breath	Hyperinflation (asthma, COPD) and restricted tidal volume (pulmonary fibrosis, chest wall restriction)
Heavy breathing, rapid breathing, breathing more	Deconditioning

Note: CHF, congestive heart failure; COPD, chronic obstructive pulmonary disease.
Source: From Schwartzstein and Feller-Kopman.

Affective Dimension For a sensation to be reported as a symptom, it must be perceived as unpleasant and interpreted as abnormal. We are still in the early stages of learning the best ways to assess the affective dimension of dyspnea. Some therapies for dyspnea, such as pulmonary rehabilitation, may reduce breathing discomfort, in part, by altering this dimension.

DIFFERENTIAL DIAGNOSIS

Dyspnea is the consequence of deviations from normal function in the cardiopulmonary systems. Alterations in the respiratory system can be considered in the context of the controller (stimulation of breathing); the ventilatory pump (the bones and muscles that form the chest wall, the airways, and the pleura); and the gas exchanger (the alveoli, pulmonary vasculature, and surrounding lung parenchyma). Similarly, alterations in the cardiovascular system can be grouped into three categories: conditions associated with high, normal, and low cardiac output (Fig. 33-2).

Respiratory System Dyspnea • ***CONTROLLER*** Acute hypoxemia and hypercapnia are associated with increased activity in the controller. Stimulation of pulmonary receptors, as occurs in acute bronchospasm, interstitial edema, and pulmonary embolism, also leads to hyperventilation and air hunger, as well as a sense of chest tightness in the case of asthma. High altitude, high progesterone states such as pregnancy, and drugs such as aspirin stimulate the controller and can cause dyspnea even when the respiratory system is normal.

VENTILATORY PUMP Disorders of the airways (e.g., asthma, emphysema, chronic bronchitis, bronchiectasis) lead to increased airway resis-

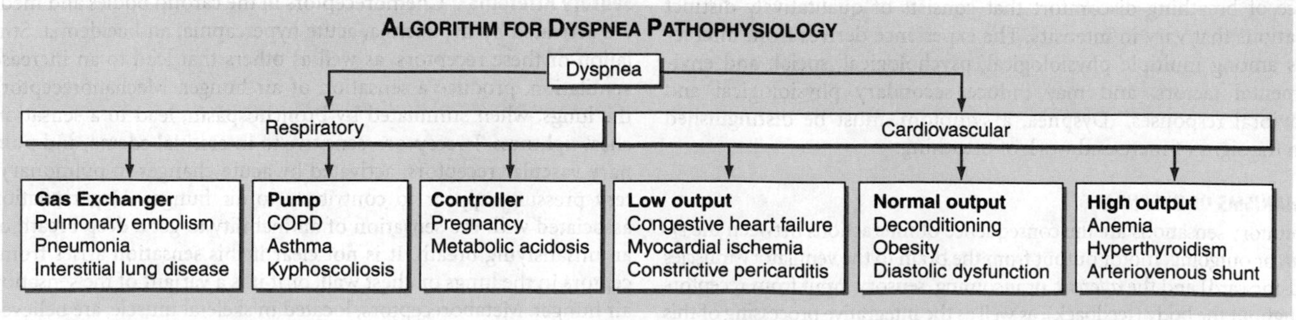

FIGURE 33-2 Pathophysiology of dyspnea. When confronted with a patient with shortness of breath of unclear cause, it is useful to begin the analysis with a consideration of the broad pathophysiologic categories that explain the vast majority of cases. COPD, chronic obstructive pulmonary disease. *(Adapted from Schwartzstein and Feller-Kopman.)*

tance and work of breathing. Hyperinflation further increases the work of breathing and can produce a sense of an inability to get a deep breath. Conditions that stiffen the chest wall, such as kyphoscoliosis, or that weaken ventilatory muscles, such as myasthenia gravis or the Guillain-Barré syndrome, are also associated with an increased effort to breathe. Large pleural effusions may contribute to dyspnea, both by increasing the work of breathing and by stimulating pulmonary receptors if there is associated atelectasis.

GAS EXCHANGER Pneumonia, pulmonary edema, and aspiration all interfere with gas exchange. Pulmonary vascular and interstitial lung disease and pulmonary vascular congestion may produce dyspnea by direct stimulation of pulmonary receptors. In these cases, relief of hypoxemia typically has only a small impact on the intensity of dyspnea.

Cardiovascular System Dyspnea • ***HIGH CARDIAC OUTPUT*** Mild to moderate anemia is associated with breathing discomfort during exercise. Left-to-right intracardiac shunts may lead to high cardiac output and dyspnea, although in their later stages these conditions may be complicated by the development of pulmonary hypertension, which contributes to dyspnea. The breathlessness associated with obesity is probably due to multiple mechanisms, including high cardiac output and impaired ventilatory pump function.

NORMAL CARDIAC OUTPUT Cardiovascular deconditioning is characterized by early development of anaerobic metabolism and stimulation of chemoreceptors and metaboreceptors. Diastolic dysfunction—due to hypertension, aortic stenosis, or hypertrophic cardiomyopathy—is an increasingly frequent recognized cause of exercise-induced breathlessness. Pericardial disease, e.g., constrictive pericarditis, is a relatively rare cause of chronic dyspnea.

LOW CARDIAC OUTPUT Diseases of the myocardium resulting from coronary artery disease and nonischemic cardiomyopathies result in a greater left ventricular end-diastolic volume and an elevation of the left ventricular end-diastolic as well as pulmonary capillary pressures. Pulmonary receptors are stimulated by the elevated vascular pressures and resultant interstitial edema, causing dyspnea.

APPROACH TO THE PATIENT: Dyspnea

(Fig. 33-3) In obtaining a *history*, the patient should be asked to describe in his/her own words what the discomfort feels like, as well as the effect of position, infections, and environmental stimuli on the dyspnea. Orthopnea is a common indicator of congestive heart failure, mechanical impairment of the diaphragm associated with obesity, or asthma triggered by esophageal reflux. Nocturnal dyspnea suggests congestive heart failure or asthma. Acute, intermittent episodes of dyspnea are more likely to reflect episodes of myocardial ischemia, bronchospasm, or pulmonary embolism, while chronic persistent dyspnea is typical of COPD and interstitial lung disease. Risk factors for occupational lung disease and for coronary artery disease should be solicited. Left atrial myxoma or hepatopulmonary syndrome should be considered when the patient complains of *platypnea*, defined as dyspnea in the upright position with relief in the supine position.

The *physical examination* should begin during the interview of the patient. Inability of the patient to speak in full sentences before stopping to get a deep breath suggests a condition that leads to stimulation of the controller or an impairment of the ventilatory pump with reduced vital capacity. Evidence for increased work of breathing (supraclavicular retractions, use of accessory muscles of ventilation, and the tripod position, characterized by sitting with one's hands braced on the knees) is indicative of disorders of the ventilatory pump, most commonly increased airway resistance or stiff lungs and chest wall. When measuring the vital signs, an accurate assessment of the respiratory rate should be obtained and examination for a pulsus paradoxus carried out (Chap. 232); if it is >10 mm Hg, consider the presence of COPD. During the general examination, signs of anemia (pale conjunctivae), cyanosis, and cirrhosis (spider angiomata, gynecomastia) should be sought. Examination of the chest should focus on symmetry of movement; percussion (dullness indicative of pleural effusion, hyper-resonance a sign of emphysema); and auscultation (wheezes, rales, rhonchi, prolonged expiratory phase, diminished breath sounds, which are clues to disorders of the airways, and interstitial edema or fibrosis). The cardiac examination should focus on signs of elevated right heart pressures (jugular venous distention, edema, accentuated pulmonic component to the second heart sound); left ventricular dysfunction (S3 and S4 gallops); and valvular disease (murmurs). When examining the abdomen with the patient in the supine position, it should be noted whether there is paradoxical movement of the abdomen (inward motion during inspiration), a sign of diaphragmatic weakness. Clubbing of the digits may be an indication of interstitial pulmonary fibrosis, and the presence of joint swelling or deformation as well as changes consistent with Raynaud's disease may be indicative of a collagen-vascular process that can be associated with pulmonary disease.

Patients with exertional dyspnea should be asked to walk under observation in order to reproduce the symptoms. The patient should be examined for new findings that were not present at rest and for oxygen saturation. A "picture" of the patient while symptomatic may be worth thousands of dollars in laboratory tests.

Following the history and physical examination, a *chest radiograph* should be obtained. The lung volumes should be assessed (hyperinflation indicates obstructive lung disease, low lung volumes suggest interstitial edema or fibrosis, diaphragmatic dysfunction, or impaired chest wall motion). The pulmonary parenchyma should be examined for evidence of interstitial disease and emphysema. Prominent pulmonary vasculature in the upper zones indicates pulmonary venous hypertension, while enlarged central pulmonary arteries suggest pulmonary artery hypertension. An enlarged cardiac silhouette suggests a dilated cardiomyopathy or valvular disease. Bilateral pleural effusions are typical of congestive heart failure and some forms of collagen vascular disease. Unilateral effusions raise the specter of carcinoma and pulmonary embolism but may also occur in heart failure. *Computed tomography* (CT) *of the chest* is generally reserved for further evaluation of the lung parenchyma (interstitial lung disease) and possible pulmonary embolism.

Laboratory studies should include an electrocardiogram to look for evidence of ventricular hypertrophy and prior myocardial infarction. Echocardiography is indicated in patients in whom systolic dysfunction, pulmonary hypertension, or valvular heart disease is suspected.

Distinguishing Cardiovascular from Respiratory System Dyspnea If a patient has evidence of both pulmonary and cardiac disease, a cardiopulmonary exercise test should be carried out to determine which system is responsible for the exercise limitation. If, at peak exercise, the patient achieves predicted maximal ventilation, demonstrates an increase in dead space or hypoxemia (oxygen saturation below 90%), or develops bronchospasm, the respiratory system is probably the cause of the problem. Alternatively, if the heart rate is >85% of the predicted maximum, if anaerobic threshold occurs early, if the blood pressure becomes excessively high or drops during exercise, if the O_2 pulse (O_2 consumption/heart rate, an indicator of stroke volume) falls, or if there are ischemic changes on the electrocardiogram, an abnormality of the cardiovascular system is likely the explanation for the breathing discomfort.

Rx DYSPNEA

The first goal is to correct the underlying problem responsible for the symptom. If this is not possible, one attempts to lessen the intensity of the symptom and its effect on the patient's quality of life. Supplemental O_2 should be administered if the resting O_2 saturation is ≤90% or if the pa-

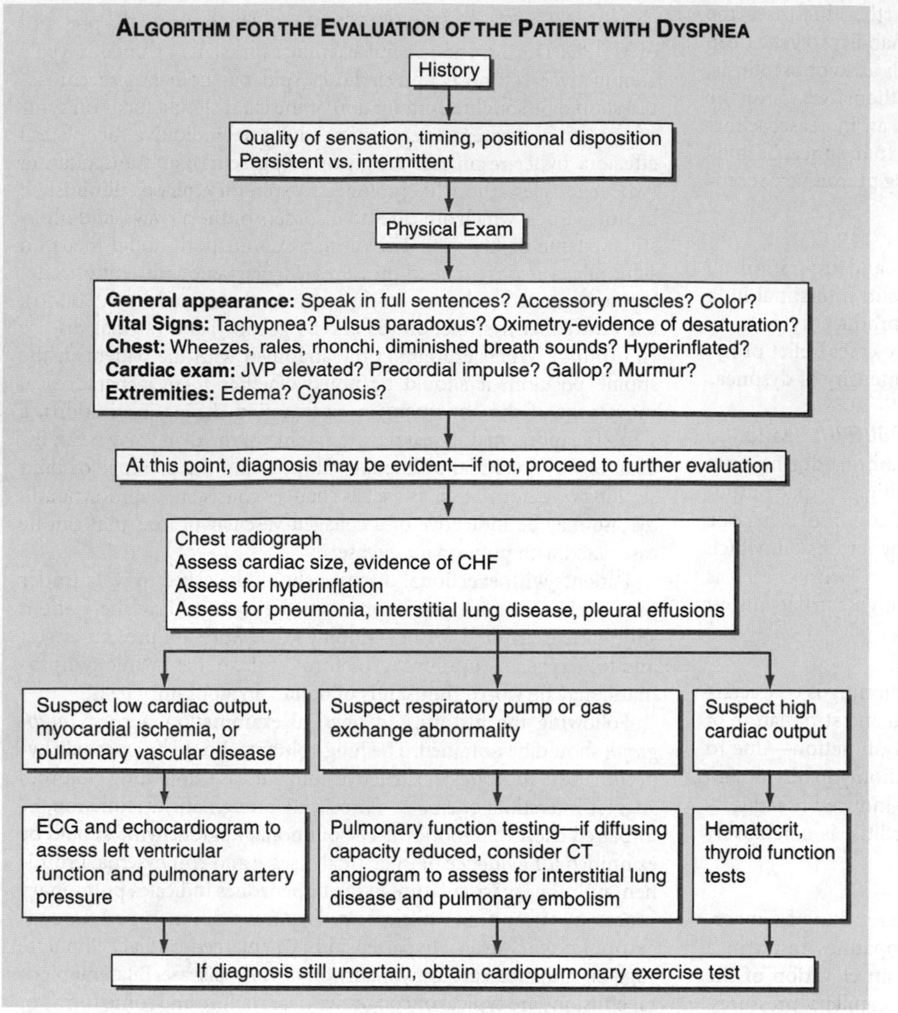
ALGORITHM FOR THE EVALUATION OF THE PATIENT WITH DYSPNEA
History
Quality of sensation, timing, positional disposition
Persistent vs. intermittent
Physical Exam
General appearance: Speak in full sentences? Accessory muscles? Color?
Vital Signs: Tachypnea? Pulsus paradoxus? Oximetry-evidence of desaturation?
Chest: Wheezes, rales, rhonchi, diminished breath sounds? Hyperinflated?
Cardiac exam: JVP elevated? Precordial impulse? Gallop? Murmur?
Extremities: Edema? Cyanosis?
At this point, diagnosis may be evident—if not, proceed to further evaluation
Chest radiograph
Assess cardiac size, evidence of CHF
Assess for hyperinflation
Assess for pneumonia, interstitial lung disease, pleural effusions
Suspect low cardiac output, myocardial ischemia, or pulmonary vascular disease
Suspect respiratory pump or gas exchange abnormality
Suspect high cardiac output
ECG and echocardiogram to assess left ventricular function and pulmonary artery pressure
Pulmonary function testing—if diffusing capacity reduced, consider CT angiogram to assess for interstitial lung disease and pulmonary embolism
Hematocrit, thyroid function tests
If diagnosis still uncertain, obtain cardiopulmonary exercise test

FIGURE 33-3 An algorithm for the evaluation of the patient with dyspnea. JVP, jugular venous pulse; CHF, congestive heart failure; ECG, electrocardiogram; CT, computed tomography. *(Adapted from Schwartzstein and Feller-Kopman.)*

tient's saturation drops to these levels with activity. For patients with COPD, pulmonary rehabilitation programs have demonstrated positive effects on dyspnea, exercise capacity, and rates of hospitalization. Studies of anxiolytics and antidepressants have not demonstrated consistent benefit. Experimental interventions—e.g., cold air on the face, chest wall vibration, and inhaled furosemide—to modulate the afferent information from receptors throughout the respiratory system are being studied.

PULMONARY EDEMA

MECHANISMS OF FLUID ACCUMULATION

The extent to which fluid accumulates in the interstitium of the lung depends on the balance of hydrostatic and oncotic forces within the pulmonary capillaries and in the surrounding tissue. Hydrostatic pressure favors movement of fluid from the capillary into the interstitium. The oncotic pressure, which is determined by the protein concentration in the blood, favors movement of fluid into the vessel. Albumin, the primary protein in the plasma, may be low in conditions such as cirrhosis and nephrotic syndrome. While hypoalbuminemia favors movement of fluid into the tissue for any given hydrostatic pressure in the capillary, it is usually not sufficient by itself to cause interstitial edema. In a healthy individual, the tight junctions of the capillary endothelium are impermeable to proteins, and the lymphatics in the tissue carry away the small amounts of protein that may leak out; together these factors result in an oncotic force that maintains fluid in the capillary. Disruption of the endothelial barrier, however, allows protein to escape the capillary bed and enhances the movement of fluid into the tissue of the lung.

Cardiogenic Pulmonary Edema (See also Chap. 266) Cardiac abnormalities that lead to an increase in pulmonary venous pressure shift the balance of forces between the capillary and the interstitium. Hydrostatic pressure is increased and fluid exits the capillary at an increased rate, resulting in interstitial and, in more severe cases, alveolar edema. The development of pleural effusions may further compromise respiratory system function and contribute to breathing discomfort.

Early signs of pulmonary edema include exertional dyspnea and orthopnea. Chest radiographs show peribronchial thickening, prominent vascular markings in the upper lung zones, and Kerley B lines. As the pulmonary edema worsens, alveoli fill with fluid; the chest radiograph shows patchy alveolar filling, typically in a perihilar distribution, which then progresses to diffuse alveolar infiltrates. Increasing airway edema is associated with rhonchi and wheezes.

Noncardiogenic Pulmonary Edema By definition, hydrostatic pressures are normal in noncardiogenic pulmonary edema. Lung water increases due to damage of the pulmonary capillary lining with leakage of proteins and other macromolecules into the tissue; fluid follows the protein as oncotic forces are shifted from the vessel to the surrounding lung tissue. This process is associated with dysfunction of the surfactant lining the alveoli, increased surface forces, and a propensity for the alveoli to collapse at low lung volumes. Physiologically, noncardiogenic pulmonary edema is characterized by intrapulmonary shunt with hypoxemia and decreased pulmonary compliance. Pathologically, hyaline membranes are evident in the alveoli, and inflammation leading to pulmonary fibrosis may be seen. Clinically, the picture ranges from mild dyspnea to respiratory failure. Auscultation of the lungs may be relatively normal despite chest radiographs that show diffuse alveolar infiltrates. CT scans demonstrate that the distribution of alveolar edema is more heterogeneous than was once thought.

It is useful to categorize the causes of noncardiogenic pulmonary edema in terms of whether the injury to the lung is likely to result from direct, indirect, or pulmonary vascular causes (Table 33-2). Direct inju-

TABLE 33-2 COMMON CAUSES OF NONCARDIOGENIC PULMONARY EDEMA

Direct Injury to Lung
Chest trauma, pulmonary contusion
Aspiration
Smoke inhalation
Pneumonia
Oxygen toxicity
Pulmonary embolism, reperfusion
Hematogenous Injury to Lung
Sepsis
Pancreatitis
Nonthoracic trauma
Leukoagglutination reactions
Multiple transfusions
Intravenous drug use, e.g., heroin
Cardiopulmonary bypass
Possible Lung Injury Plus Elevated Hydrostatic Pressures
High altitude pulmonary edema
Neurogenic pulmonary edema
Reexpansion pulmonary edema

ries are mediated via the airways (e.g. aspiration) or as the consequence of blunt chest trauma. Indirect injury is the consequence of mediators that reach the lung via the blood stream. The third category includes conditions that may be the consequence of acute changes in pulmonary vascular pressures, possibly the result of sudden autonomic discharge in the case of neurogenic and high-altitude pulmonary edema, or sudden swings of pleural pressure, as well as transient damage to the pulmonary capillaries in the case of reexpansion pulmonary edema.

Distinguishing Cardiogenic from Noncardiogenic Pulmonary Edema The *history* is essential for assessing the likelihood of underlying cardiac disease as well as for identification of one of the conditions associated with noncardiogenic pulmonary edema. The *physical examination* in cardiogenic pulmonary edema is notable for evidence of increased intracardiac pressures (S3 gallop, elevated jugular venous pulse, peripheral edema), and rales and/or wheezes on auscultation of the chest. In contrast, the physical examination in noncardiogenic pulmonary edema is dominated by the findings of the precipitating condition; pulmonary findings may be relatively normal in the early stages. The *chest radiograph* in cardiogenic pulmonary edema typically shows an enlarged cardiac silhouette, vascular redistribution, interstitial thickening, and perihilar alveolar infiltrates; pleural effusions are common. In noncardiogenic pulmonary edema, heart size is normal, alveolar infiltrates are distributed more uniformly throughout the lungs, and pleural effusions are uncommon. Finally, the *hypoxemia* of cardiogenic pulmonary edema is due largely to ventilation-perfusion mismatch and responds to the administration of supplemental oxygen. In contrast, hypoxemia in noncardiogenic pulmonary edema is due primarily to intrapulmonary shunting and typically persists despite high concentrations of inhaled O_2.

FURTHER READINGS

ABIDOV A et al: Prognostic significance of dyspnea in patients referred for cardiac stress testing. N Engl J Med 353:1889, 2005

Dyspnea mechanisms, assessment, and management: A consensus statement. Am Rev Resp Crit Care Med 159:321, 1999

GILLETTE MA, SCHWARTZSTEIN RM: Mechanisms of dyspnea, in *Supportive Care in Respiratory Disease*, SH Ahmedzai and MF Muer (eds). Oxford, U.K., Oxford University Press, 2005

MAHLER DA et al. Descriptors of breathlessness in cardiorespiratory diseases. Am J Respir Crit Care Med 154:1357, 1996

———, O'DONNELL DE (eds): *Dyspnea: Mechanisms, Measurement, and Management*. New York, Marcel Dekker, 2005

SCHWARTZSTEIN RM. The language of dyspnea, in *Dyspnea: Mechanisms, Measurement, and Management*, DA Mahler and DE O'Donnell (eds). New York, Marcel Dekker, 2005

———, FELLER-KOPMAN D. Shortness of breath, in *Primary Care Cardiology*, 2d ed, E Braunwald and L Goldman (eds). Philadelphia: WB Saunders, 2003

34 Cough and Hemoptysis

Steven E. Weinberger, David A. Lipson

COUGH

Cough is an explosive expiration that provides a normal protective mechanism for clearing the tracheobronchial tree of secretions and foreign material. When excessive or bothersome, it is also one of the most common symptoms for which patients seek medical attention. Reasons for this include discomfort from the cough itself, interference with normal lifestyle, and concern for the cause of the cough, especially fear of cancer.

MECHANISM

Coughing may be initiated either voluntarily or reflexively. As a defensive reflex it has both afferent and efferent pathways. The *afferent limb* includes receptors within the sensory distribution of the trigeminal, glossopharyngeal, superior laryngeal, and vagus nerves. The *efferent limb* includes the recurrent laryngeal nerve and the spinal nerves. The cough starts with a deep inspiration followed by glottic closure, relaxation of the diaphragm, and muscle contraction against a closed glottis. The resulting markedly positive intrathoracic pressure causes narrowing of the trachea. Once the glottis opens, the large pressure differential between the airways and the atmosphere coupled with tracheal narrowing produces rapid flow rates through the trachea. The shearing forces that develop aid in the elimination of mucus and foreign materials.

ETIOLOGY

Cough can be initiated by a variety of irritant triggers either from an exogenous source (smoke, dust, fumes, foreign bodies) or from an endogenous origin (upper airway secretions, gastric contents). These stimuli may affect receptors in the upper airway (especially the pharynx and larynx) or in the lower respiratory tract, following access to the tracheobronchial tree by inhalation or aspiration. When cough is triggered by upper airway secretions (as with postnasal drip) or gastric contents (as with gastroesophageal reflux), the initiating factor can go unrecognized and the cough may persist. Additionally, prolonged exposure to such irritants may initiate airway inflammation, which can itself precipitate cough and sensitize the airway to other irritants. Cough associated with gastroesophageal reflux is due only in part to irritation of upper airway receptors or to aspiration of gastric contents, as a vagally mediated reflex mechanism secondary to acid in the distal esophagus may also contribute.

Any disorder resulting in inflammation, constriction, infiltration, or compression of airways can be associated with cough. Inflammation commonly results from airway infections, ranging from viral or bacterial bronchitis to bronchiectasis. In viral bronchitis, airway inflammation sometimes persists long after resolution of the typical acute symptoms, thereby producing a prolonged cough that may last for weeks. Pertussis infection is also a possible cause of persistent cough in adults; however, diagnosis is generally made on clinical grounds (Chap. 142). Asthma is a common cause of cough. Although the clinical setting commonly suggests when a cough is secondary to asthma, some patients present with cough in the absence of wheezing or dyspnea, thus making the diagnosis more subtle ("cough variant asthma"). A neoplasm infiltrating the airway wall, such as bronchogenic carcinoma or a carcinoid tumor, is commonly associated with cough. Airway infiltration with granulomas may also trigger a cough, as seen with endobronchial sarcoidosis or tuberculosis. Compression of airways results from extrinsic masses such as lymph nodes or mediastinal tumors, or rarely from an aortic aneurysm.

Examples of parenchymal lung disease potentially producing cough include interstitial lung disease, pneumonia, and lung abscess. Congestive heart failure may be associated with cough, probably as a consequence of interstitial as well as peribronchial edema. A nonproductive cough complicates the use of angiotensin-converting enzyme (ACE) inhibitors in 5–20% of patients taking these agents. Onset is usually within 1 week of starting the drug but can be delayed up to 6 months. Although the mechanism is not known with certainty, it may relate to accumulation of bradykinin or substance P, both of which are degraded by ACE. In contrast, angiotensin II receptor antagonists do not seem to increase cough, likely because these drugs do not significantly increase bradykinin levels.

The most common causes of cough can be categorized according to the duration of the cough. Acute cough (<3 weeks) is most often due to upper respiratory infection (especially the common cold, acute bacterial sinusitis, and pertussis), but more serious disorders, such as pneumonia, pulmonary embolus, and congestive heart failure, can also present in this fashion. Subacute cough (between 3 and 8 weeks) is commonly post-infectious, resulting from persistent airway inflammation and/or postnasal drip following viral infection, pertussis, or infection with *Mycoplasma* or *Chlamydia.* In the patient with subacute cough that is not clearly post-infectious, the varied causes of chronic cough should be considered. Chronic cough (>8 weeks) in a smoker raises the possibilities of chronic obstructive lung disease or bronchogenic carcinoma. In a nonsmoker who has a normal chest radiograph and is not taking an ACE inhibitor, the most common causes of chronic cough are postnasal drip (sometimes termed the *upper airway cough syndrome*), asthma, and gastroesophageal reflux. Eosinophilic bronchitis in the absence of asthma has also been recognized as a potential cause of chronic cough.

APPROACH TO THE PATIENT: Cough

A detailed *history* frequently provides the most valuable clues for the etiology of the cough. Particularly important questions include:

1. Is the cough acute, subacute, or chronic?
2. At its onset, were there associated symptoms suggestive of a respiratory infection?
3. Is it seasonal or associated with wheezing?
4. Is it associated with symptoms suggestive of postnasal drip (nasal discharge, frequent throat clearing, a "tickle in the throat") or gastroesophageal reflux (heartburn or sensation of regurgitation)? However, the absence of such suggestive symptoms does not exclude either of these diagnoses.
5. Is it associated with fever or sputum? If sputum is present, what is its character?
6. Does the patient have any associated diseases or risk factors for disease (e.g., cigarette smoking, risk factors for infection with HIV, environmental exposures)?
7. Is the patient taking an ACE inhibitor?

The general *physical examination* may point to a systemic or nonpulmonary cause of cough, such as heart failure or primary nonpulmonary neoplasm. Examination of the oropharynx may provide suggestive evidence for postnasal drip, including oropharyngeal mucus or erythema, or a "cobblestone" appearance to the mucosa. Auscultation of the chest may demonstrate inspiratory stridor (indicative of upper airway disease), rhonchi or expiratory wheezing (indicative of lower airway disease), or inspiratory crackles (suggestive of a process involving the pulmonary parenchyma, such as interstitial lung disease, pneumonia, or pulmonary edema).

Chest radiography may be particularly helpful in suggesting or confirming the cause of the cough. Important potential findings include the presence of an intrathoracic mass lesion, localized pulmonary parenchymal opacification, or diffuse interstitial or alveolar disease. An area of honeycombing or cyst formation may suggest bronchiectasis, while symmetric bilateral hilar adenopathy may suggest sarcoidosis.

Pulmonary function testing (Chap. 246) is useful for assessing the functional abnormalities that accompany certain disorders producing cough. Measurement of forced expiratory flow rates can demonstrate reversible airflow obstruction characteristic of asthma. When asthma is considered but flow rates are normal, bronchoprovocation testing with methacholine or cold-air inhalation can demonstrate hyperreactivity of the airways to a bronchoconstrictive stimulus. Measurement of lung volumes and diffusing capacity is useful primarily for demonstration of a restrictive pattern, often seen with any of the diffuse interstitial lung diseases.

If *sputum* is produced, gross and microscopic examination may provide useful information. Purulent sputum suggests chronic bronchitis, bronchiectasis, pneumonia, or lung abscess. Blood in the sputum may be seen in the same disorders, but its presence also raises the question of an endobronchial tumor. Greater than 3% eosinophils seen on staining of induced sputum in a patient without asthma suggests the possibility of eosinophilic bronchitis. Gram and acid-fast stains and cultures may demonstrate a particular infectious pathogen, while sputum cytology may provide a diagnosis of a pulmonary malignancy.

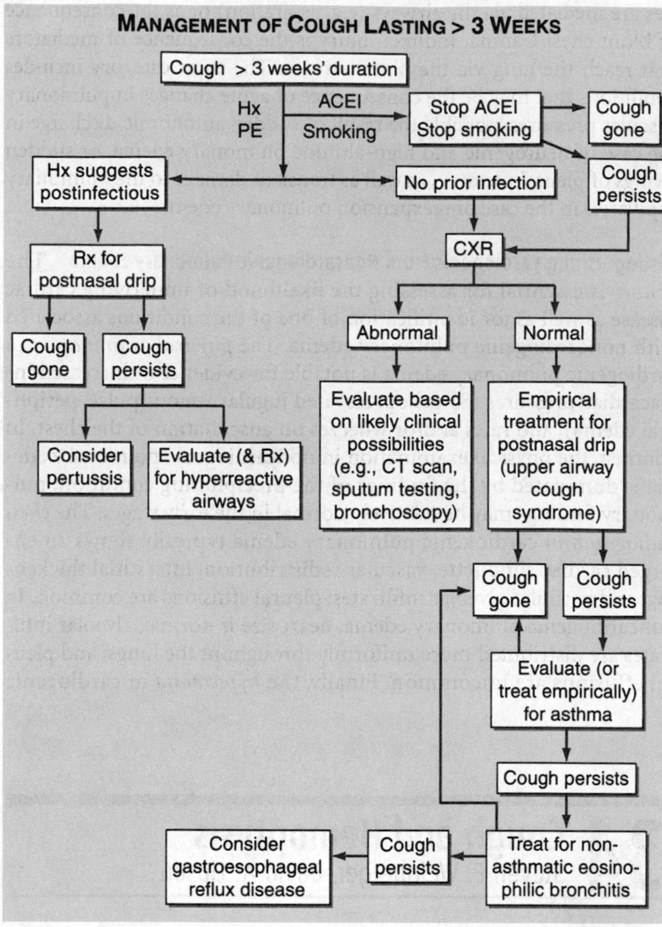

FIGURE 34-1 Algorithm for management of cough lasting >3 weeks. Cough between 3 and 8 weeks is considered subacute; cough >8 weeks is considered chronic. Hx, history; PE, physical examination; ACEI, angiotensin-converting enzyme inhibitor; Rx, treat; CXR, chest x-ray.

More specialized studies are helpful in specific circumstances. *Fiberoptic bronchoscopy* is the procedure of choice for visualizing an endobronchial tumor and collecting cytologic and histologic specimens. Inspection of the tracheobronchial mucosa can demonstrate endobronchial granulomas often seen in sarcoidosis, and endobronchial biopsy of such lesions or transbronchial biopsy of the lung interstitium can confirm the diagnosis. Inspection of the airway mucosa by bronchoscopy may also demonstrate the characteristic appearance of endobronchial Kaposi's sarcoma in patients with AIDS. *High-resolution computed tomography* (HRCT) can confirm the presence of interstitial lung disease and frequently suggests a diagnosis based on the specific abnormal pattern. It is the procedure of choice for demonstrating dilated airways and confirming the diagnosis of bronchiectasis.

A diagnostic algorithm for evaluation of subacute and chronic cough is presented in Fig. 34-1.

COMPLICATIONS

Common complications of coughing include chest and abdominal wall soreness, urinary incontinence, and exhaustion. On occasion, paroxysms of coughing may precipitate syncope (cough syncope; Chap. 21), consequent to markedly positive intrathoracic and alveolar pressures, diminished venous return, and decreased cardiac output. Although cough fractures of the ribs may occur in otherwise normal patients, their occurrence should at least raise the possibility of pathologic fractures, which are seen with multiple myeloma, osteoporosis, and osteolytic metastases.

Rx COUGH

Definitive treatment of cough depends on determining the underlying cause and then initiating specific therapy. Elimination of an exogenous inciting agent (cigarette smoke, ACE inhibitors) or an endogenous trigger (postnasal drip, gastroesophageal reflux) is usually effective when such a precipitant can be identified. Other important management considerations are treatment of specific respiratory tract infections, bronchodilators for potentially reversible airflow obstruction, inhaled glucocorticoids for eosinophilic bronchitis, chest physiotherapy and other methods to enhance clearance of secretions in patients with bronchiectasis, and treatment of endobronchial tumors or interstitial lung disease when such therapy is available and appropriate. In patients with chronic, unexplained cough, an empirical approach to treatment is often used for both diagnostic and therapeutic purposes, starting with an antihistamine-decongestant combination, nasal glucocorticoids, or nasal ipratropium spray to treat unrecognized postnasal drip. If ineffective, this may be followed sequentially by empirical treatment for asthma, nonasthmatic eosinophilic bronchitis, and gastroesophageal reflux.

Symptomatic or nonspecific therapy of cough should be considered when: (1) the cause of the cough is not known or specific treatment is not possible, and (2) the cough performs no useful function or causes marked discomfort or sleep disturbance. An irritative, nonproductive cough may be suppressed by an antitussive agent, which increases the latency or threshold of the cough center. Such agents include codeine (15 mg qid) or nonnarcotics such as dextromethorphan (15 mg qid). These drugs provide symptomatic relief by interrupting prolonged, self-perpetuating paroxysms. However, a cough productive of significant quantities of sputum should usually not be suppressed, since retention of sputum in the tracheobronchial tree may interfere with the distribution of alveolar ventilation and the ability of the lung to resist infection.

HEMOPTYSIS

Hemoptysis is defined as the expectoration of blood from the respiratory tract, a spectrum that varies from blood-streaking of sputum to coughing up large amounts of pure blood. *Massive hemoptysis* is variably defined as the expectoration of >100–600 mL over a 24-h period, although the patient's estimation of the amount of blood is notoriously unreliable. Expectoration of even relatively small amounts of blood is a frightening symptom and may be a marker for potentially serious disease, such as bronchogenic carcinoma. Massive hemoptysis, on the other hand, can represent an acutely life-threatening problem. Blood can fill the airways and the alveolar spaces, not only seriously disturbing gas exchange but potentially causing asphyxiation.

ETIOLOGY

Because blood originating from the nasopharynx or the gastrointestinal tract can mimic blood coming from the lower respiratory tract, it is important to determine initially that the blood is not coming from one of these alternative sites. Clues that the blood is originating from the gastrointestinal tract include a dark red appearance and an acidic pH, in contrast to the typical bright red appearance and alkaline pH of true hemoptysis.

An etiologic classification of hemoptysis can be based on the site of origin within the lungs (Table 34-1). The most common site of bleeding is the tracheobronchial tree, which can be affected by inflammation (acute or chronic bronchitis, bronchiectasis) or by neoplasm (bronchogenic carcinoma, endobronchial metastatic carcinoma, or bronchial carcinoid tumor). The bronchial arteries, which originate either from the aorta or from intercostal arteries and are therefore part of the high-pressure systemic circulation, are the source of bleeding in bronchitis or bronchiectasis or with endobronchial tumors. Blood originating from the pulmonary parenchyma can be either from a localized source, such as an infection (pneumonia, lung abscess, tuberculosis), or from a process diffusely affecting the parenchyma (as with a coagulopathy or with an autoimmune process such as Goodpasture's syndrome). Disorders primarily affecting the pulmonary vasculature include pulmonary embolic disease and those conditions associated with elevated pulmonary venous and capillary pressures, such as mitral stenosis or left ventricular failure.

TABLE 34-1 DIFFERENTIAL DIAGNOSIS OF HEMOPTYSIS

Source other than the lower respiratory tract
Upper airway (nasopharyngeal) bleeding
Gastrointestinal bleeding
Tracheobronchial source
Neoplasm (bronchogenic carcinoma, endobronchial metastatic tumor, Kaposi's sarcoma, bronchial carcinoid)
Bronchitis (acute or chronic)
Bronchiectasis
Broncholithiasis
Airway trauma
Foreign body
Pulmonary parenchymal source
Lung abscess
Pneumonia
Tuberculosis
Mycetoma ("fungus ball")
Goodpasture's syndrome
Idiopathic pulmonary hemosiderosis
Wegener's granulomatosis
Lupus pneumonitis
Lung contusion
Primary vascular source
Arteriovenous malformation
Pulmonary embolism
Elevated pulmonary venous pressure (esp. mitral stenosis)
Pulmonary artery rupture secondary to balloon-tip pulmonary artery catheter manipulation
Miscellaneous/rare causes
Pulmonary endometriosis (catamenial hemoptysis)
Systemic coagulopathy or use of anticoagulants or thrombolytic agents

Adapted from SE Weinberger: *Principles of Pulmonary Medicine*, 4th ed. Philadelphia, Saunders, 2004, with permission.

Although the relative frequency of the different etiologies of hemoptysis varies from series to series, most recent studies indicate that bronchitis and bronchogenic carcinoma are the two most common causes in the United States. Despite the lower frequency of tuberculosis and bronchiectasis seen in recent compared to older series, these two disorders still represent the most common causes of massive hemoptysis in several series, especially worldwide. Even after extensive evaluation, a sizable proportion of patients (up to 30% in some series) have no identifiable etiology for their hemoptysis. These patients are classified as having idiopathic or cryptogenic hemoptysis, and subtle airway or parenchymal disease is presumably responsible for the bleeding.

APPROACH TO THE PATIENT: Hemoptysis

The *history* is extremely valuable. Hemoptysis that is described as blood-streaking of mucopurulent or purulent sputum often suggests bronchitis. Chronic production of sputum with a recent change in quantity or appearance favors an acute exacerbation of chronic bronchitis. Fever or chills accompanying blood-streaked purulent sputum suggests pneumonia, whereas a putrid smell to the sputum raises the possibility of lung abscess. When sputum production has been chronic and copious, the diagnosis of bronchiectasis should be considered. Hemoptysis following the acute onset of pleuritic chest pain and dyspnea is suggestive of pulmonary embolism.

A history of previous or coexisting disorders should be sought, such as renal disease (seen with Goodpasture's syndrome or Wegener's granulomatosis), lupus erythematosus (with associated pulmonary hemorrhage from lupus pneumonitis), or a previous malignancy (either recurrent lung cancer or endobronchial metastasis from a nonpulmonary primary tumor) or treatment for malignancy (with recent chemotherapy or a bone marrow transplant). In a patient with AIDS, endobronchial or pulmonary parenchymal Kaposi's sarcoma should be considered. Risk factors for bronchogenic carcinoma, particularly smoking and asbestos exposure, should be sought. Patients should be questioned about previous bleeding disorders, treatment with anticoagulants, or use of drugs that can be associated with thrombocytopenia.

The *physical examination* may also provide helpful clues to the diagnosis. For example, examination of the lungs may demonstrate a pleural friction rub (pulmonary embolism), localized or diffuse crackles (parenchymal bleeding or an underlying parenchymal process associated with bleeding), evidence of airflow obstruction (chronic bronchitis), or prominent rhonchi, with or without wheezing or crackles (bronchiectasis). Cardiac examination may demonstrate findings of pulmonary arterial hypertension, mitral stenosis, or heart failure. Skin and mucosal examination may reveal Kaposi's sarcoma, arteriovenous malformations of Osler-Rendu-Weber disease, or lesions suggestive of systemic lupus erythematosus.

Diagnostic evaluation of hemoptysis starts with a chest radiograph (often followed by a CT scan) to look for a mass lesion, findings suggestive of bronchiectasis (Chap. 252), or focal or diffuse parenchymal disease (representing either focal or diffuse bleeding or a focal area of pneumonitis). Additional initial screening evaluation often includes a complete blood count, a coagulation profile, and assessment for renal disease with a urinalysis and measurement of blood urea nitrogen and creatinine levels. When sputum is present, examination by Gram and acid-fast stains (along with the corresponding cultures) is indicated.

Fiberoptic bronchoscopy is particularly useful for localizing the site of bleeding and for visualization of endobronchial lesions. When bleeding is massive, rigid bronchoscopy is often preferable to fiberoptic bronchoscopy because of better airway control and greater suction capability. In patients with suspected bronchiectasis, HRCT is the diagnostic procedure of choice.

A diagnostic algorithm for evaluation of nonmassive hemoptysis is presented in Fig. 34-2.

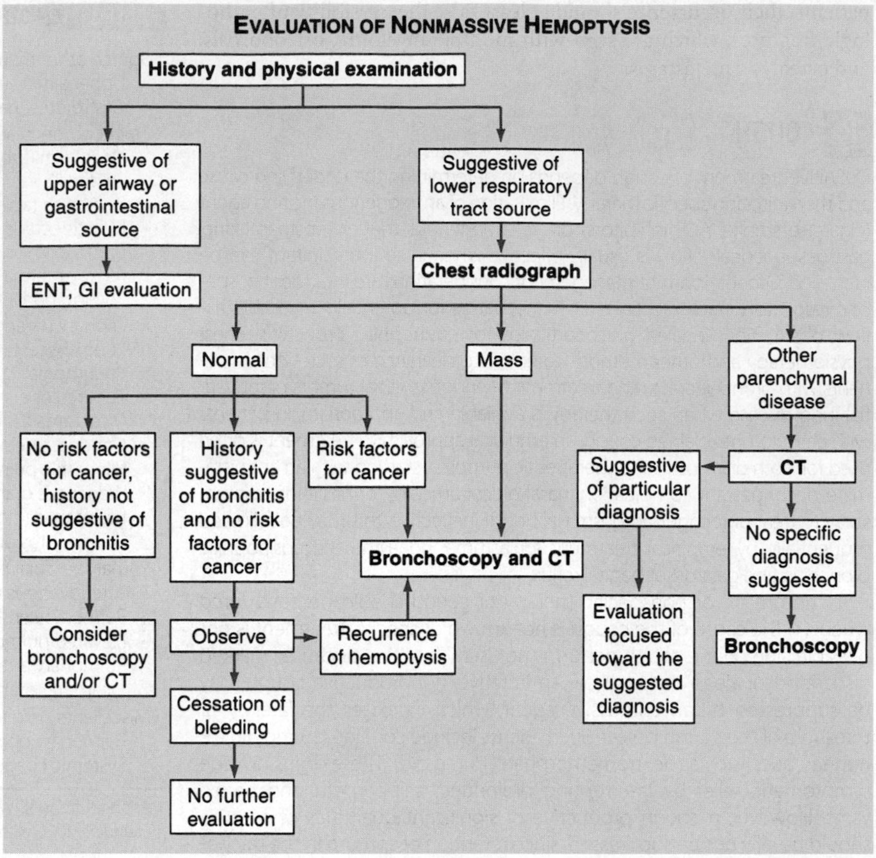

FIGURE 34-2 An algorithm for the evaluation of nonmassive hemoptysis. ENT, ear, nose, and throat; GI, gastrointestinal; CT, computed tomography.

℞ HEMOPTYSIS

The rapidity of bleeding and its effect on gas exchange determine the urgency of management. When the bleeding is confined to either blood-streaking of sputum or production of small amounts of pure blood, gas exchange is usually preserved; establishing a diagnosis is the first priority. When hemoptysis is massive, maintaining adequate gas exchange, preventing blood from spilling into unaffected areas of lung, and avoiding asphyxiation are the highest priorities. Keeping the patient at rest and partially suppressing cough may help the bleeding to subside. If the origin of the blood is known and is limited to one lung, the bleeding lung should be placed in the dependent position, so that blood is not aspirated into the unaffected lung.

With massive bleeding, the need to control the airway and maintain adequate gas exchange may necessitate endotracheal intubation and mechanical ventilation. In patients in danger of flooding the lung contralateral to the side of hemorrhage despite proper positioning, isolation of the right and left mainstem bronchi from each other can be achieved by selectively intubating the nonbleeding lung (often with bronchoscopic guidance) or by using specially designed double-lumen endotracheal tubes. Another option involves inserting a balloon catheter through a bronchoscope by direct visualization and inflating the balloon to occlude the bronchus leading to the bleeding site. This technique not only prevents aspiration of blood into unaffected areas but also may promote tamponade of the bleeding site and cessation of bleeding.

Other available techniques for control of significant bleeding include laser phototherapy, electrocautery, bronchial artery embolization, and surgical resection of the involved area of lung. With bleeding from an endobronchial tumor, argon plasma coagulation or the neodymium:yttrium-aluminum-garnet (Nd:YAG) laser can often achieve at least temporary hemostasis by coagulating the bleeding site. Electrocautery, which uses an electric current for thermal destruction of tissue, can be used similarly for management of bleeding from an endobronchial tumor. Bronchial artery embolization involves an arteriographic procedure in which a vessel proximal to the bleeding site is cannulated, and a material such as Gelfoam is injected to occlude the bleeding vessel. Surgical resection is a therapeutic option either for the emergent therapy of life-threatening hemoptysis that fails to respond to other measures or for the elective but definitive management of localized disease subject to recurrent bleeding.

FURTHER READINGS

AMERICAN COLLEGE OF CHEST PHYSICIANS: Diagnosis and management of cough: ACCP evidence-based clinical practice guidelines. Chest 129:1S, 2006

GIBSON PG et al: Eosinophilic bronchitis: Clinical manifestations and implications for treatment. Thorax 57:178, 2002

HAQUE RA et al: Chronic idiopathic cough. A discrete clinical entity? Chest 127:1710, 2005

IRWIN RS, MADISON JM: The diagnosis and treatment of cough. N Engl J Med 343:1715, 2000

———, ———: The persistently troublesome cough. Am J Respir Crit Care Med 165:1469, 2002

JEAN-BAPTISTE E: Clinical assessment and management of massive hemoptysis. Crit Care Med 28:1642, 2000

KHALIL A et al: Role of MDCT in identification of the bleeding site and the vessels causing hemoptysis. AJR Am J Roentgenol 188:W117, 2007

35 Hypoxia and Cyanosis

Eugene Braunwald

HYPOXIA

The fundamental task of the cardiorespiratory system is to deliver O_2 (and substrates) to the cells and to remove CO_2 (and other metabolic products) from them. Proper maintenance of this function depends on intact cardiovascular and respiratory systems, an adequate number of red blood cells and hemoglobin, and a supply of inspired gas containing adequate O_2.

EFFECTS

Decreased O_2 availability to cells results in an inhibition of the respiratory chain and increased anaerobic glycolysis. This switch from aerobic to anaerobic metabolism, Pasteur's effect, maintains some, albeit markedly reduced, adenosine triphosphate (ATP) production. In severe hypoxia, when ATP production is inadequate to meet the energy requirements of ionic and osmotic equilibrium, cell membrane depolarization leads to uncontrolled Ca^{2+} influx and activation of Ca^{2+}-dependent phospholipases and proteases. These events, in turn, cause cell swelling and ultimately cell necrosis.

The adaptations to hypoxia are mediated, in part, by the upregulation of genes encoding a variety of proteins, including glycolytic enzymes such as phosphoglycerate kinase and phosphofructokinase, as well as the glucose transporters Glut-1 and Glut-2; and by growth factors, such as vascular endothelial growth factor (VEGF) and erythropoietin, which enhance erythrocyte production.

During hypoxia systemic arterioles dilate, at least in part, by opening of K_{ATP} channels in vascular smooth-muscle cells due to the hypoxia-induced reduction in ATP concentration. By contrast, in pulmonary vascular smooth-muscle cells, inhibition of K^+ channels causes depolarization which, in turn, activates voltage-gated Ca^{2+} channels raising the cytosolic $[Ca^{2+}]$ and causing smooth-muscle cell contraction. Hypoxia-induced pulmonary arterial constriction shunts blood away from poorly ventilated toward better-ventilated portions of the lung; however, it also increases pulmonary vascular resistance and right ventricular afterload.

Effects on the Central Nervous System Changes in the central nervous system, particularly the higher centers, are especially important consequences of hypoxia. Acute hypoxia causes impaired judgment, motor incoordination, and a clinical picture resembling acute alcoholism. High-altitude illness is characterized by headache secondary to cerebral vasodilatation, and by gastrointestinal symptoms, dizziness, insomnia, and fatigue, or somnolence. Pulmonary arterial and sometimes venous constriction cause capillary leakage and high-altitude pulmonary edema (HAPE) (Chap. 33), which intensifies hypoxia and can initiate a vicious circle. Rarely, high-altitude cerebral edema (HACE) develops. This is manifest by severe headache and papilledema and can cause coma. As hypoxia becomes more severe, the centers of the brainstem are affected, and death usually results from respiratory failure.

CAUSES OF HYPOXIA

Respiratory Hypoxia When hypoxia occurs consequent to respiratory failure, Pa_{O_2} declines, and when respiratory failure is persistent, the hemoglobin-oxygen (Hb-O_2) dissociation curve (see Fig. 99-2) is displaced to the right, with greater quantities of O_2 released at any level of tissue P_{O_2}. Arterial hypoxemia, i.e., a reduction of O_2 saturation of arterial blood (Sa_{O_2}), and consequent cyanosis are likely to be more marked when such depression of Pa_{O_2} results from pulmonary disease than when the depression occurs as the result of a decline in the fraction of oxygen in inspired air (FI_{O_2}). In this latter situation, Pa_{CO_2} falls secondary to anoxia-induced hyperventilation and the Hb-O_2 dissociation curve is displaced to the left, limiting the decline in Sa_{O_2} at any level of Pa_{O_2}.

The most common cause of respiratory hypoxia is *ventilation-perfusion mismatch* resulting from perfusion of poorly ventilated alveoli. Respiratory hypoxemia may also be caused by *hypoventilation*, and it is then associated with an elevation of Pa_{CO_2} (Chap. 246). These two forms of respiratory hypoxia are usually correctable by inspiring 100% O_2 for several minutes. A third cause is shunting of blood across the lung from the pulmonary arterial to the venous bed (*intrapulmonary right-to-left shunting*) by perfusion of nonventilated portions of the lung, as in pulmonary atelectasis or through pulmonary arteriovenous connections. The low Pa_{O_2} in this situation is correctable only in part by an FI_{O_2} of 100%.

Hypoxia Secondary to High Altitude As one ascends rapidly to 3000 m (~10,000 ft), the reduction of the O_2 content of inspired air (FI_{O_2}) leads to a decrease in alveolar P_{O_2} to about 60 mmHg, and a condition termed *high-altitude illness* develops (see above). At higher altitudes, arterial saturation declines rapidly and symptoms become more serious; and at 5000 m, unacclimatized individuals usually cease to be able to function normally.

Hypoxia Secondary to Right-to-Left Extrapulmonary Shunting From a physiologic viewpoint, this cause of hypoxia resembles intrapulmonary right-to-left shunting but is caused by congenital cardiac malformations such as tetralogy of Fallot, transposition of the great arteries, and Eisenmenger's syndrome (Chap. 229). As in pulmonary right-to-left shunting, the Pa_{O_2} cannot be restored to normal with inspiration of 100% O_2.

Anemic Hypoxia A reduction in hemoglobin concentration of the blood is attended by a corresponding decline in the O_2-carrying capacity of the blood. Although the Pa_{O_2} is normal in anemic hypoxia, the absolute quantity of O_2 transported per unit volume of blood is diminished. As the anemic blood passes through the capillaries and the usual quantity of O_2 is removed from it, the P_{O_2} and saturation in the venous blood decline to a greater degree than normal.

Carbon Monoxide (CO) Intoxication (See also **Chap. e34**) Hemoglobin that is combined with CO (carboxyhemoglobin, COHb) is unavailable for O_2 transport. In addition, the presence of COHb shifts the Hb-O_2 dissociation curve to the left (see Fig. 99-2) so that O_2 is unloaded only at lower tensions, contributing further to tissue hypoxia.

Circulatory Hypoxia As in anemic hypoxia, the Pa_{O_2} is usually normal, but venous and tissue P_{O_2} values are reduced as a consequence of reduced tissue perfusion and greater tissue O_2 extraction. This pathophysiology leads to an increased arterial–mixed venous O_2 difference, or $(a - \bar{v})$ gradient. Generalized circulatory hypoxia occurs in heart failure (Chap. 227) and in most forms of shock (Chap. 264).

Specific Organ Hypoxia Localized circulatory hypoxia may occur consequent to decreased perfusion secondary to organic arterial obstruction, as in localized atherosclerosis in any vascular bed, or as a consequence of vasoconstriction, as observed in Raynaud's phenomenon (Chap. 243). Localized hypoxia may also result from venous obstruction and the resultant expansion of interstitial fluid causing arterial compression and, thereby, reduction of arterial inflow. Edema, which increases the distance through which O_2 must diffuse before it reaches cells, can also cause localized hypoxia. In an attempt to maintain adequate perfusion to more vital organs in patients with reduced cardiac output secondary to heart failure or hypovolemic shock, vasoconstriction may reduce perfusion in the limbs and skin, causing hypoxia of these regions.

Increased O_2 Requirements If the O_2 consumption of tissues is elevated without a corresponding increase in perfusion, tissue hypoxia ensues and the P_{O_2} in venous blood declines. Ordinarily, the clinical picture of patients with hypoxia due to an elevated metabolic rate, as in fever or thyrotoxicosis, is quite different from that in other types of hypoxia; the skin is warm and flushed owing to increased cutaneous blood flow that dissipates the excessive heat produced, and cyanosis is usually absent.

Exercise is a classic example of increased tissue O_2 requirements. These increased demands are normally met by several mechanisms operating simultaneously: (1) increasing the cardiac output and ventilation and, thus, O_2 delivery to the tissues; (2) preferentially directing the blood to the exercising muscles by changing vascular resistances in the circulatory beds of exercising tissues, directly and/or reflexly; (3) increasing O_2 extraction from the delivered blood and widening the arteriovenous O_2 difference; and (4) reducing the pH of the tissues and capillary blood, shifting the Hb-O_2 curve to the right (see Fig. 99-2) and unloading more O_2 from hemoglobin. If the capacity of these mechanisms is exceeded, then hypoxia, especially of the exercising muscles, will result.

Improper Oxygen Utilization Cyanide (**Chap. e35**) and several other similarly acting poisons cause cellular hypoxia. The tissues are unable to utilize O_2, and as a consequence, the venous blood tends to have a high O_2 tension. This condition has been termed *histotoxic hypoxia*.

ADAPTATION TO HYPOXIA

An important component of the respiratory response to hypoxia originates in special chemosensitive cells in the carotid and aortic bodies and in the respiratory center in the brainstem. The stimulation of these cells by hypoxia increases ventilation, with a loss of CO_2, and can lead to respiratory alkalosis. When combined with the metabolic acidosis resulting from the production of lactic acid, the serum bicarbonate level declines (Chap. 48).

With the reduction of Pa_{O_2}, cerebrovascular resistance decreases and cerebral blood flow increases in an attempt to maintain O_2 delivery to the brain. However, when the reduction of Pa_{O_2} is accompanied by hyperventilation and a reduction of Pa_{CO_2}, cerebrovascular resistance rises, cerebral blood flow falls, and hypoxia is intensified.

The diffuse, systemic vasodilation that occurs in generalized hypoxia raises the cardiac output. In patients with underlying heart disease, the requirements of peripheral tissues for an increase of cardiac output with hypoxia may precipitate congestive heart failure. In patients with ischemic heart disease, a reduced Pa_{O_2} may intensify myocardial ischemia and further impair left ventricular function.

One of the important mechanisms of compensation for chronic hypoxia is an increase in the hemoglobin concentration and in the number of red blood cells in the circulating blood, i.e., the development of polycythemia secondary to erythropoietin production (Chap. 103). In persons with chronic hypoxemia secondary to prolonged residence at a high altitude (>13,000 ft, 4200 m), a condition termed *chronic mountain sickness* develops. It is characterized by a blunted respiratory drive, reduced ventilation, erythrocytosis, cyanosis, weakness, right ventricular enlargement secondary to pulmonary hypertension, and even stupor.

CYANOSIS

Cyanosis refers to a bluish color of the skin and mucous membranes resulting from an increased quantity of reduced hemoglobin, or of hemoglobin derivatives, in the small blood vessels of those areas. It is usually most marked in the lips, nail beds, ears, and malar eminences. Cyanosis, especially if developed recently, is more commonly detected by a family member than the patient. The florid skin characteristic of polycythemia vera (Chap. 103) must be distinguished from the true cyanosis discussed here. A cherry-colored flush, rather than cyanosis, is caused by COHb (**Chap. e35**).

The degree of cyanosis is modified by the color of the cutaneous pigment and the thickness of the skin, as well as by the state of the cutaneous capillaries. The accurate clinical detection of the presence and degree of cyanosis is difficult, as proved by oximetric studies. In some instances, central cyanosis can be detected reliably when the Sa_{O_2} has fallen to 85%; in others, particularly in dark-skinned persons, it may not be detected until it has declined to 75%. In the latter case, examination of the mucous membranes in the oral cavity and the conjunctivae rather than examination of the skin is more helpful in the detection of cyanosis.

The increase in the quantity of reduced hemoglobin in the mucocutaneous vessels that produces cyanosis may be brought about either by an increase in the quantity of venous blood as a result of dilation of the venules and venous ends of the capillaries or by a reduction in the Sa_{O_2} in the capillary blood. In general, cyanosis becomes apparent when the concentration of reduced hemoglobin in capillary blood exceeds 40 g/L (4 g/dL).

It is the *absolute*, rather than the *relative*, quantity of reduced hemoglobin that is important in producing cyanosis. Thus, in a patient with severe anemia, the *relative* quantity of reduced hemoglobin in the venous blood may be very large when considered in relation to the total quantity of hemoglobin in the blood. However, since the concentration of the latter is markedly reduced, the *absolute* quantity of reduced hemoglobin may still be small, and, therefore, patients with severe anemia and even *marked* arterial desaturation may not display cyanosis. Conversely, the higher the total hemoglobin content, the greater is the tendency toward cyanosis; thus, patients with marked polycythemia tend to be cyanotic at higher levels of Sa_{O_2} than patients with normal hematocrit values. Likewise, local passive congestion, which causes an increase in the total quantity of reduced hemoglobin in the vessels in a given area, may cause cyanosis. Cyanosis is also observed when nonfunctional hemoglobin, such as methemoglobin or sulfhemoglobin (Chap. 99), is present in blood.

Cyanosis may be subdivided into central and peripheral types. In the *central* type, the Sa_{O_2} is reduced or an abnormal hemoglobin derivative is present, and the mucous membranes and skin are both affected. *Peripheral* cyanosis is due to a slowing of blood flow and abnormally great extraction of O_2 from normally saturated arterial blood. It results from vasoconstriction and diminished peripheral blood flow, such as occurs in cold exposure, shock, congestive failure, and peripheral vascular disease. Often in these conditions, the mucous membranes of the oral cavity or those beneath the tongue may be spared. Clinical differentiation between central and peripheral cyanosis may not always be simple, and in conditions such as cardiogenic shock with pulmonary edema there may be a mixture of both types.

DIFFERENTIAL DIAGNOSIS

Central Cyanosis (Table 35-1) Decreased Sa_{O_2} results from a marked reduction in the Pa_{O_2}. This reduction may be brought about by a decline in the FI_{O_2} without sufficient compensatory alveolar hyperventilation to maintain alveolar P_{O_2}. Cyanosis usually becomes manifest in an ascent to an altitude of 4000 m (13,000 ft).

Seriously *impaired pulmonary function*, through perfusion of unventilated or poorly ventilated areas of the lung or alveolar hypoventilation, is a common cause of central cyanosis (Chap. 246). This condition may occur acutely, as in extensive pneumonia or pulmonary edema, or chronically with chronic pulmonary diseases (e.g., emphysema). In the latter situation, secondary polycythemia is generally present and clubbing of the fingers (see below) may occur. Another cause of reduced

TABLE 35-1 CAUSES OF CYANOSIS

Central Cyanosis
Decreased arterial oxygen saturation
Decreased atmospheric pressure—high altitude
Impaired pulmonary function
Alveolar hypoventilation
Uneven relationships between pulmonary ventilation and perfusion (perfusion of hypoventilated alveoli)
Impaired oxygen diffusion
Anatomic shunts
Certain types of congenital heart disease
Pulmonary arteriovenous fistulas
Multiple small intrapulmonary shunts
Hemoglobin with low affinity for oxygen
Hemoglobin abnormalities
Methemoglobinemia—hereditary, acquired
Sulfhemoglobinema—acquired
Carboxyhemoglobinemia (not true cyanosis)
Peripheral Cyanosis
Reduced cardiac output
Cold exposure
Redistribution of blood flow from extremities
Arterial obstruction
Venous obstruction

Sa_{O_2} is *shunting of systemic venous blood into the arterial circuit.* Certain forms of congenital heart disease are associated with cyanosis on this basis (see above and Chap. 229).

Pulmonary arteriovenous fistulae may be congenital or acquired, solitary or multiple, microscopic or massive. The severity of cyanosis produced by these fistulae depends on their size and number. They occur with some frequency in hereditary hemorrhagic telangiectasia. Sa_{O_2} reduction and cyanosis may also occur in some patients with cirrhosis, presumably as a consequence of pulmonary arteriovenous fistulae or portal vein–pulmonary vein anastomoses.

In patients with cardiac or pulmonary right-to-left shunts, the presence and severity of cyanosis depend on the size of the shunt relative to the systemic flow as well as on the Hb-O_2 saturation of the venous blood. With increased extraction of O_2 from the blood by the exercising muscles, the venous blood returning to the right side of the heart is more unsaturated than at rest, and shunting of this blood intensifies the cyanosis. Secondary polycythemia occurs frequently in patients with arterial O_2 unsaturation and contributes to the cyanosis.

Cyanosis can be caused by small quantities of circulating methemoglobin and by even smaller quantities of sulfhemoglobin (Chap. 99). Although they are uncommon causes of cyanosis, these abnormal oxyhemoglobin derivatives should be sought by spectroscopy when cyanosis is not readily explained by malfunction of the circulatory or respiratory systems. Generally, digital clubbing does not occur with them.

Peripheral Cyanosis Probably the most common cause of peripheral cyanosis is the normal vasoconstriction resulting from exposure to cold air or water. When cardiac output is reduced, cutaneous vasoconstriction occurs as a compensatory mechanism so that blood is diverted from the skin to more vital areas such as the central nervous system and heart, and cyanosis of the extremities may result even though the arterial blood is normally saturated.

Arterial obstruction to an extremity, as with an embolus, or arteriolar constriction, as in cold-induced vasospasm (Raynaud's phenomenon, Chap. 243), generally results in pallor and coldness, and there may be associated cyanosis. Venous obstruction, as in thrombophlebitis, dilates the subpapillary venous plexuses and thereby intensifies cyanosis.

APPROACH TO THE PATIENT: Cyanosis

Certain features are important in arriving at the cause of cyanosis:

1. It is important to ascertain the time of onset of cyanosis. Cyanosis present since birth or infancy is usually due to congenital heart disease.
2. Central and peripheral cyanosis must be differentiated. Evidence of disorders of the respiratory or cardiovascular systems are helpful. Massage or gentle warming of a cyanotic extremity will increase peripheral blood flow and abolish peripheral, but not central, cyanosis.
3. The presence or absence of clubbing of the digits (see below) should be ascertained. The combination of cyanosis and clubbing is frequent in patients with congenital heart disease and right-to-left shunting, and is seen occasionally in patients with pulmonary disease such as lung abscess or pulmonary arteriovenous fistulae. In contrast, peripheral cyanosis or acutely developing central cyanosis is *not* associated with clubbed digits.
4. Pa_{O_2} and Sa_{O_2} should be determined, and in patients with cyanosis in whom the mechanism is obscure, spectroscopic examination of the blood performed to look for abnormal types of hemoglobin (critical in the differential diagnosis of cyanosis).

CLUBBING

The selective bullous enlargement of the distal segments of the fingers and toes due to proliferation of connective tissue, particularly on the dorsal surface, is termed *clubbing*; there is also increased sponginess of the soft tissue at the base of the nail. Clubbing may be hereditary, idiopathic, or acquired and associated with a variety of disorders, including cyanotic congenital heart disease (see above), infective endocarditis, and a variety of pulmonary conditions (among them primary and metastatic lung cancer, bronchiectasis, lung abscess, cystic fibrosis, and mesothelioma), as well as with some gastrointestinal diseases (including inflammatory bowel disease and hepatic cirrhosis). In some instances it is occupational, e.g., in jackhammer operators.

Clubbing in patients with primary and metastatic lung cancer, mesothelioma, bronchiectasis, and hepatic cirrhosis may be associated with *hypertrophic osteoarthropathy*. In this condition, the subperiosteal formation of new bone in the distal diaphyses of the long bones of the extremities causes pain and symmetric arthritis-like changes in the shoulders, knees, ankles, wrists, and elbows. The diagnosis of hypertrophic osteoarthropathy may be confirmed by bone radiographs. Although the mechanism of clubbing is unclear, it appears to be secondary to a humoral substance that causes dilation of the vessels of the fingertip.

FURTHER READINGS

FAWCETT RS et al: Nail abnormalities: Clues to systemic disease. Am Fam Physician 69:1417, 2004

GIORDANO FJ: Oxygen, oxidative stress, hypoxia, and heart failure. J Clin Invest 115:500, 2005

GRIFFEY RT et al: Cyanosis. J Emerg Med 18:369, 2000

HACKETT PH, ROACH RC: Current concepts: High altitude illness. N Engl J Med 345:107, 2001

LEVY MM: Pathophysiology of oxygen delivery in respiratory failure. Chest 128(Suppl 2):547S, 2005

MICHIELS C: Physiological and pathological responses to hypoxia. Am J Pathol 164:1875, 2004

TSAI BM et al: Hypoxic pulmonary vasoconstriction in cardiothoracic surgery: Basic mechanisms to potential therapies. Ann Thorac Surg 78:360, 2004

36 Edema

Eugene Braunwald, Joseph Loscalzo

Edema is defined as a clinically apparent increase in the interstitial fluid volume, which may expand by several liters before the abnormality is evident. Therefore, a weight gain of several kilograms usually precedes overt manifestations of edema, and a similar weight loss from diuresis can be induced in a slightly edematous patient before "dry weight" is achieved. *Anasarca* refers to gross, generalized edema. *Ascites* (Chap. 44) and *hydrothorax* refer to accumulation of excess fluid in the peritoneal and pleural cavities, respectively, and are considered to be special forms of edema.

Depending on its cause and mechanism, edema may be localized or have a generalized distribution; it is recognized in its generalized form by puffiness of the face, which is most readily apparent in the periorbital areas, and by the persistence of an indentation of the skin following pressure; this is known as "pitting" edema. In its more subtle form, edema may be detected by noting that after the stethoscope is removed from the chest wall, the rim of the bell leaves an indentation on the skin of the chest for a few minutes. When the ring on a finger fits more snugly than in the past or when a patient complains of difficulty in putting on shoes, particularly in the evening, edema may be present.

PATHOGENESIS

About one-third of total-body water is confined to the extracellular space. Approximately 75% of the latter, in turn, is interstitial fluid and the remainder is the plasma.

Starling Forces The forces that regulate the disposition of fluid between these two components of the extracellular compartment are frequently referred to as the *Starling forces*. The hydrostatic pressure within the vascular system and the colloid oncotic pressure in the interstitial fluid tend to promote movement of fluid from the vascular to the extravascular space. On the other hand, the colloid oncotic pressure contributed by plasma proteins and the hydrostatic pressure within the interstitial fluid, referred to as the *tissue tension*, promote the movement of fluid into the vascular compartment.

As a consequence of these forces, there is a movement of water and diffusible solutes from the vascular space at the arteriolar end of the capillaries. Fluid is returned from the interstitial space into the vascular system at the venous end of the capillaries and by way of the lymphatics. Unless these channels are obstructed, lymph flow rises with increases in net movement of fluid from the vascular compartment to the interstitium. These flows are usually balanced so that a steady state exists in the sizes of the intravascular and interstitial compartments, and, yet, a large exchange between them occurs. However, should either the hydrostatic or oncotic pressure gradient be altered significantly, a further net movement of fluid between the two components of the extracellular space will take place. The development of edema, then, depends on one or more alterations in the Starling forces so that there is increased flow of fluid from the vascular system into the interstitium or into a body cavity.

Edema due to an increase in capillary pressure may result from an elevation of venous pressure due to obstruction to venous and/or lymphatic drainage. An increase in capillary pressure may be generalized, as occurs in congestive heart failure (see below). The Starling forces may also be imbalanced when the colloid oncotic pressure of the plasma is reduced, owing to any factor that may induce hypoalbuminemia, such as severe malnutrition, liver disease, loss of protein into the urine or into the gastrointestinal tract, or a severe catabolic state. Edema may be localized to one extremity when venous pressure is elevated due to unilateral thrombophlebitis (see below).

Capillary Damage Edema may also result from damage to the capillary endothelium, which increases its permeability and permits the transfer of protein into the interstitial compartment. Injury to the capillary wall can result from drugs, viral or bacterial agents, and thermal or mechanical trauma. Increased capillary permeability may also be a consequence of a hypersensitivity reaction and is characteristic of immune injury. Damage to the capillary endothelium is presumably responsible for inflammatory edema, which is usually nonpitting, localized, and accompanied by other signs of inflammation—redness, heat, and tenderness.

Reduction of Effective Arterial Volume In many forms of edema, the effective arterial blood volume, a parameter that represents the filling of the arterial tree, is reduced. Underfilling of the arterial tree may be caused by a reduction of cardiac output and/or systemic vascular resistance. As a consequence of underfilling, a series of physiologic responses designed to restore the effective arterial volume to normal are set into motion. A key element of these responses is the retention of salt and, therefore, of water, ultimately leading to edema.

Renal Factors and the Renin-Angiotensin-Aldosterone (RAA) System (See also Chap. 336) In the final analysis, renal retention of Na^+ is central to the development of generalized edema. The diminished renal blood flow characteristic of states in which the effective arterial blood volume is reduced is translated by the renal juxtaglomerular cells (specialized myoepithelial cells surrounding the afferent arteriole) into a signal for increased renin release (Chap. 336). Renin is an enzyme with a molecular mass of about 40,000 Da that acts on its substrate, angiotensinogen, an α_2-globulin synthesized by the liver, to release angiotensin I, a decapeptide, which is broken down to angiotensin II (AII), an octapeptide. AII has generalized vasoconstrictor properties; it is especially active on the efferent arterioles. This efferent arteriolar constriction reduces the hydrostatic pressure in the peritubular capillaries, while the increased filtration fraction raises the colloid osmotic pressure in these vessels, thereby enhancing salt and water reabsorption in the proximal tubule as well as in the ascending limb of the loop of Henle.

The RAA system has long been recognized as a hormonal system; however, it also operates locally. Intrarenally produced AII contributes to glomerular efferent arteriolar constriction, and this "tubuloglomerular feedback" causes salt and water retention. These renal effects of AII are mediated by activation of AII type 1 receptors, which can be blocked by specific antagonists [angiotensin receptor blockers (ARBs)].

The mechanisms responsible for the increased release of renin when renal blood flow is reduced include: (1) a baroreceptor response in which reduced renal perfusion results in incomplete filling of the renal arterioles and diminished stretch of the juxtaglomerular cells, a signal that increases the elaboration and/or release of renin; (2) reduced glomerular filtration, which lowers the NaCl load reaching the distal renal tubules and the macula densa, cells in the distal convoluted tubules that act as chemoreceptors and that signal the neighboring juxtaglomerular cells to secrete renin; and (3) activation of the β-adrenergic receptors in the juxtaglomerular cells by the sympathetic nervous system and by circulating catecholamines, which also stimulates renin release. These three mechanisms generally act in concert to enhance Na^+ retention and, thereby, contribute to the formation of edema.

AII that enters the systemic circulation stimulates the production of aldosterone by the zona glomerulosa of the adrenal cortex. Aldosterone, in turn, enhances Na^+ reabsorption (and K^+ excretion) by the collecting tubule. In patients with heart failure, not only is aldosterone secretion elevated but the biologic half-life of aldosterone is prolonged, which increases further the plasma level of the hormone. A depression of hepatic blood flow, especially during exercise, is responsible for reduced hepatic catabolism of aldosterone. The activation of the RAA system is most striking in the early phase of acute, severe heart failure and is less intense in patients with chronic, stable, compensated heart failure.

Increased quantities of aldosterone are secreted in heart failure and in other edematous states, and blockade of the action of aldosterone by spironolactone (an aldosterone antagonist) or amiloride (a blocker of epithelial Na^+ channels) often induces a moderate diuresis in edematous states. Yet, persistently augmented levels of aldosterone (or other mineralocorticoids) alone do not always promote accumulation of edema, as witnessed by the lack of striking fluid retention in most instances of primary aldosteronism (Chap. 336). Furthermore, although normal individuals retain some NaCl and water with the administration of potent mineralocorticoids, such as deoxycorticosterone acetate or fludrocortisone, this accumulation is self-limiting, despite continued exposure to the steroid, a phenomenon known as *mineralocorticoid escape*. The failure of normal individuals who receive large doses of mineralocorticoids to accumulate large quantities of extracellular fluid and to develop edema is probably a consequence of an increase in glomerular filtration rate (pressure natriuresis) and the action of natriuretic substance(s) (see below). The continued secretion of aldosterone may be more important in the accumulation of fluid in edematous states because patients with edema secondary to heart failure, nephrotic syndrome, and hepatic cirrhosis are generally unable to repair the deficit in effective arterial blood volume. As a consequence, they do not develop pressure natriuresis.

Arginine Vasopressin (AVP) (See also Chap. 334) The secretion of AVP occurs in response to increased intracellular osmolar concentration, and by stimulating V_2 receptors, AVP increases the reabsorption of free water in the renal distal tubule and collecting duct, thereby increasing total-body water. Circulating AVP is elevated in many patients with heart failure secondary to a nonosmotic stimulus associated with decreased effective arterial volume. Such patients fail to show the normal reduction of AVP with a reduction of osmolality, contributing to edema formation and hyponatremia.

Endothelin This potent peptide vasoconstrictor is released by endothelial cells; its concentration is elevated in heart failure and contributes to renal vasoconstriction, Na^+ retention, and edema in heart failure.

Natriuretic Peptides Atrial distention and/or a Na^+ load cause release into the circulation of atrial natriuretic peptide (ANP), a polypeptide; a high-molecular-weight precursor of ANP is stored in secretory granules within atrial myocytes. Release of ANP causes (1) excretion of sodium and water by augmenting glomerular filtration rate, inhibiting sodium reabsorption in the proximal tubule, and inhibiting release of renin and aldosterone; and (2) arteriolar and venous dilation by antagonizing the vasoconstrictor actions of AII, AVP, and sympathetic stimulation. Thus, ANP has the capacity to oppose Na^+ retention and arterial pressure elevation in hypervolemic states.

The closely related brain natriuretic peptide (BNP) is stored primarily in ventricular myocardium and is released when ventricular diastolic pressure rises. Its actions are similar to those of ANP. Circulating levels of ANP and BNP are elevated in congestive heart failure and in cirrhosis with ascites, but obviously not sufficiently to prevent edema formation. In addition, in edematous states there is abnormal resistance to the actions of natriuretic peptides.

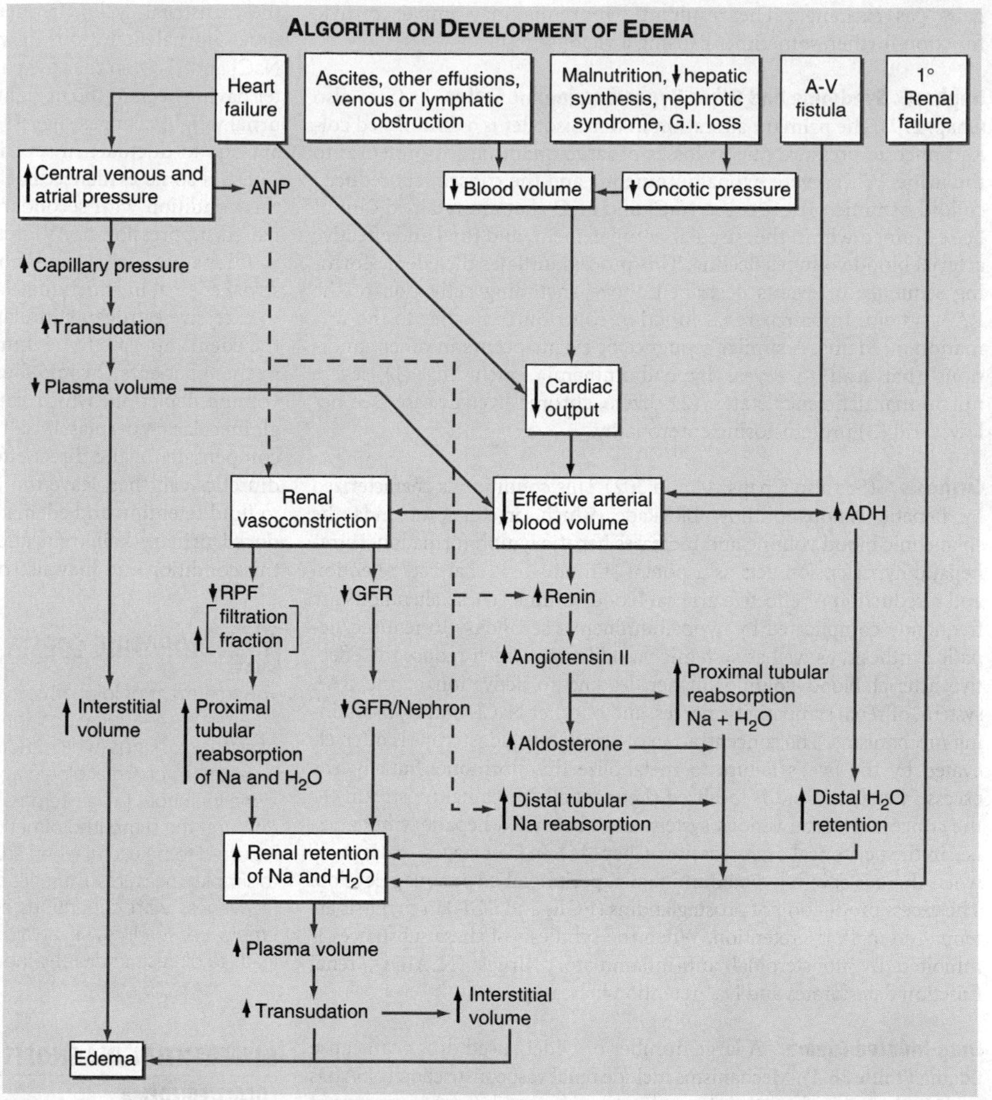

FIGURE 36-1 Sequence of events leading to the formation and retention of salt and water and the development of edema. ANP, atrial natriuretic peptide; RPF, renal plasma flow; GFR, glomerular filtration rate; ADH, antidiuretic hormone. Inhibitory influences are shown by broken lines.

CLINICAL CAUSES OF EDEMA

Obstruction of Venous (and Lymphatic) Drainage of a Limb In this condition the hydrostatic pressure in the capillary bed upstream (proximal) to the obstruction increases so that an abnormal quantity of fluid is transferred from the vascular to the interstitial space. Since the alternative route (i.e., the lymphatic channels) may also be obstructed or maximally filled, an increased volume of interstitial fluid in the limb develops, i.e., there is trapping of fluid in the extremity. Tissue tension rises in the affected limb until it counterbalances the primary alterations in the Starling forces, at which time no further fluid accumulates. The net effect is a local increase in the volume of interstitial fluid, causing local edema. The displacement of fluid into a limb may occur at the expense of the blood volume in the remainder of the body, thereby reducing effective arterial blood volume and leading to the retention of NaCl and H_2O until the deficit in plasma volume has been corrected. This same sequence occurs in ascites and hydrothorax, in which fluid is trapped or accumulates in the cavitary space, depleting the intravascular volume and leading to secondary salt and fluid retention.

Congestive Heart Failure (See also Chap. 227) In this disorder the impaired systolic emptying of the ventricle(s) and/or the impairment of ventricular relaxation promotes an accumulation of blood in the venous circulation at the expense of the effective arterial volume, and the aforementioned sequence of events (Fig. 36-1) is initiated. In mild heart failure, a small increment of total blood volume may repair the deficit of arterial volume and establish a new steady state. Through the operation of Starling's law of the heart, an increase in ventricular diastolic volume promotes a more forceful contraction and may thereby restore the cardiac output. However, if the cardiac disorder is more severe, fluid retention continues, and the increment in blood volume accumulates in the venous circulation. With reduction in cardiac output, a decrease in baroreflex-mediated inhibition of the vasomotor center activates renal vasoconstrictor nerves and the RAA system, causing Na^+ and H_2O retention.

Incomplete ventricular emptying (systolic heart failure) and/or inadequate ventricular relaxation (diastolic heart failure) both lead to an elevation of ventricular diastolic pressure. If the impairment of cardiac function primarily involves the right ventricle, pressures in the systemic veins and capillaries rise, augmenting the transudation of fluid into the interstitial space and enhancing the likelihood of peripheral edema. The elevated systemic venous pressure is transmitted to the thoracic duct with consequent reduction of lymph drainage, further increasing the accumulation of edema.

If the impairment of cardiac function (incomplete ventricular emptying and/or inadequate relaxation) involves the left ventricle primarily, then pulmonary venous and capillary pressures rise. Pulmonary artery pressure rises and this, in turn, interferes with the emptying of the right ventricle, leading to an elevation of right ventricular diastolic and of central and systemic venous pressures, thereby enhancing the likelihood of the formation of peripheral edema. The elevation of pulmonary capillary pressure may cause pulmonary edema, which impairs gas exchange. The resultant hypoxemia may impair cardiac function further, sometimes causing a vicious circle.

Nephrotic Syndrome and Other Hypoalbuminemic States (See also Chap. 277) The primary alteration in this disorder is a diminished colloid oncotic pressure due to losses of large quantities of protein into the urine. With severe hypoalbuminemia and the consequent reduced colloid osmotic pressure, the NaCl and H_2O that are retained cannot be restrained within the vascular compartment, and total and effective arterial blood volumes decline. This process initiates the edema-forming sequence of events described above, including activation of the RAA system. Impaired renal function contributes further to the formation of edema. A similar sequence of events occurs in other conditions that lead to *severe* hypoalbuminemia, including (1) severe nutritional deficiency states; (2) severe, chronic liver disease (see below); and (3) protein-losing enteropathy.

Cirrhosis (See also Chaps. 44 and 302) This condition is characterized by hepatic venous outflow blockade, which, in turn, expands the splanchnic blood volume and increases hepatic lymph formation. Intrahepatic hypertension acts as a potent stimulus for renal Na^+ retention and a reduction of effective arterial blood volume. These alterations are frequently complicated by hypoalbuminemia secondary to reduced hepatic synthesis, as well as systemic vasodilation, which reduce the effective arterial blood volume further, leading to activation of the RAA system, of renal sympathetic nerves, and of other NaCl- and H_2O-retaining mechanisms. The concentration of circulating aldosterone is often elevated by the liver's failure to metabolize this hormone. Initially, the excess interstitial fluid is localized preferentially proximal (upstream) to the congested portal venous system and obstructed hepatic lymphatics, i.e., in the peritoneal cavity (ascites, Chap. 44). In later stages, particularly when there is severe hypoalbuminemia, peripheral edema may develop. The excess production of prostaglandins (PGE_2 and PGI_2) in cirrhosis attenuates renal Na^+ retention. When the synthesis of these substances is inhibited by nonsteroidal anti-inflammatory drugs (NSAIDs), renal function deteriorates and Na^+ retention increases.

Drug-Induced Edema A large number of widely used drugs can cause edema (Table 36-1). Mechanisms include renal vasoconstriction (NSAIDs and cyclosporine), arteriolar dilatation (vasodilators), augmented renal Na^+ reabsorption (steroid hormones), and capillary damage (interleukin 2).

Idiopathic Edema This syndrome, which occurs almost exclusively in women, is characterized by periodic episodes of edema (unrelated to the menstrual cycle), frequently accompanied by abdominal distention. Diurnal alterations in weight occur with orthostatic retention of NaCl and H_2O, so that the patient may weigh several pounds more after having been in the upright posture for several hours. Such large diurnal weight changes suggest an increase in capillary permeability that appears to fluctuate in severity and to be aggravated by hot weather. There is some evidence that a reduction in plasma volume occurs in this condition with secondary activation of the RAA system and impaired suppression of AVP release.

Idiopathic edema should be distinguished from cyclical or premenstrual edema, in which the NaCl and H_2O retention may be secondary to excessive estrogen stimulation. There are also some cases in which the edema appears to be diuretic-induced. It has been postulated that in these patients chronic diuretic administration leads to mild blood volume depletion, which causes chronic hyperreninemia and juxtaglomerular hyperplasia. Salt-retaining mechanisms appear to overcompensate for the direct effects of the diuretics. *Acute* withdrawal of diuretics can then leave the Na^+-retaining forces unopposed, leading to fluid retention and edema. Decreased dopaminergic activity and reduced urinary kallikrein and kinin excretion have been reported in this condition and may also be of pathogenetic importance.

TABLE 36-1 DRUGS ASSOCIATED WITH EDEMA FORMATION

Nonsteroidal anti-inflammatory drugs
Antihypertensive agents
Direct arterial/arteriolar vasodilators
Hydralazine
Clonidine
Methyldopa
Guanethidine
Minoxidil
Calcium channel antagonists
α-Adrenergic antagonists
Thiazolidinediones
Steroid hormones
Glucocorticoids
Anabolic steroids
Estrogens
Progestins
Cyclosporine
Growth hormone
Immunotherapies
Interleukin 2
OKT3 monoclonal antibody

Source: From Chertow.

Rx IDIOPATHIC EDEMA

The treatment of idiopathic cyclic edema includes a reduction in NaCl intake, rest in the supine position for several hours each day, and the wearing of elastic stockings (which should be put on before arising in the morning). A variety of pharmacologic agents, including angiotensin-converting enzyme inhibitors, progesterone, the dopamine receptor agonist bromocriptine, and the sympathomimetic amine dextroamphetamine, have all been reported to be useful when administered to patients who do not respond to simpler measures. Diuretics may be helpful initially but may lose their effectiveness with continuous administration; accordingly, they should be employed sparingly, if at all. Discontinuation of diuretics paradoxically leads to diuresis in diuretic-induced edema, described above.

DIFFERENTIAL DIAGNOSIS

LOCALIZED EDEMA

(See also Chap. 243) Edema originating from inflammation or hypersensitivity is usually readily identified. Localized edema due to venous or lymphatic obstruction may be caused by thrombophlebitis, chronic lymphangitis, resection of regional lymph nodes, filariasis, etc. Lymphedema is particularly intractable because restriction of lymphatic flow results in increased protein concentration in the interstitial fluid, a circumstance that aggravates retention of fluid.

GENERALIZED EDEMA

The differences among the three major causes of generalized edema are shown in Table 36-2.

The great majority of patients with generalized edema suffer from advanced cardiac, renal, hepatic, or nutritional disorders. Consequently, the differential diagnosis of generalized edema should be directed toward identifying or excluding these several conditions.

Edema of Heart Failure (See also Chap. 227) The presence of heart disease, as manifested by cardiac enlargement and a gallop rhythm, together with evidence of cardiac failure, such as dyspnea, basilar rales, venous distention, and hepatomegaly, usually indicate that edema results from heart failure. Noninvasive tests, such as echocardiography, may be helpful in establishing the diagnosis of heart disease. The edema of heart failure typically occurs in the dependent portions of the body.

Edema of the Nephrotic Syndrome (See also Chap. 277) Marked proteinuria (>3.5 g/d), hypoalbuminemia (<35 g/L), and, in some instances, hypercholesterolemia are present. This syndrome may occur during the course of a variety of kidney diseases, which include glo-

TABLE 36-2 PRINCIPAL CAUSES OF GENERALIZED EDEMA: HISTORY, PHYSICAL EXAMINATION, AND LABORATORY FINDINGS

Organ System	History	Physical Examination	Laboratory Findings
Cardiac	Dyspnea with exertion prominent—often associated with orthopnea—or paroxysmal nocturnal dyspnea	Elevated jugular venous pressure, ventricular (S_3) gallop; occasionally with displaced or dyskinetic apical pulse; peripheral cyanosis, cool extremities, small pulse pressure when severe	Elevated urea nitrogen-to-creatinine ratio common; elevated uric acid; serum sodium often diminished; liver enzymes occasionally elevated with hepatic congestion
Hepatic	Dyspnea infrequent, except if associated with significant degree of ascites; most often a history of ethanol abuse	Frequently associated with ascites; jugular venous pressure normal or low; blood pressure lower than in renal or cardiac disease; one or more additional signs of chronic liver disease (jaundice, palmar erythema, Dupuytren's contracture, spider angiomata, male gynecomastia; asterixis and other signs of encephalopathy) may be present	If severe, reductions in serum albumin, cholesterol, other hepatic proteins (transferrin, fibrinogen); liver enzymes elevated, depending on the cause and acuity of liver injury; tendency toward hypokalemia, respiratory alkalosis; macrocytosis from folate deficiency
Renal	Usually chronic: may be associated with uremic signs and symptoms, including decreased appetite, altered (metallic or fishy) taste, altered sleep pattern, difficulty concentrating, restless legs or myoclonus; dyspnea can be present, but generally less prominent than in heart failure	Blood pressure may be elevated; hypertensive or diabetic retinopathy in selected cases; nitrogenous fetor; periorbital edema may predominate; pericardial friction rub in advanced cases with uremia	Albuminuria, hypoalbuminemia; sometimes, elevation of serum creatinine and urea nitrogen; hyperkalemia, metabolic acidosis, hyperphosphatemia, hypocalcemia, anemia (usually normocytic)

Source: From Chertow.

merulonephritis, diabetic glomerulosclerosis, and hypersensitivity reactions. A history of previous renal disease may or may not be elicited.

Edema of Acute Glomerulonephritis and Other Forms of Renal Failure (See also Chap. 277) The edema occurring during the acute phases of glomerulonephritis is characteristically associated with hematuria, proteinuria, and hypertension. Although some evidence supports the view that the fluid retention is due to increased capillary permeability, in most instances the edema results from primary retention of NaCl and H_2O by the kidneys owing to renal insufficiency. This state differs from congestive heart failure in that it is characterized by a normal (or sometimes even increased) cardiac output and a normal arterial–mixed venous oxygen difference. Patients with edema due to renal failure commonly have evidence of arterial hypertension as well as pulmonary congestion on chest roentgenograms even without cardiac enlargement, but they may not develop orthopnea. Patients with *chronic* renal failure may also develop edema due to primary renal retention of NaCl and H_2O.

Edema of Cirrhosis (See also Chap. 302) Ascites and biochemical and clinical evidence of hepatic disease (collateral venous channels, jaundice, and spider angiomas) characterize edema of hepatic origin. The ascites (Chap. 44) is frequently refractory to treatment because it collects as a result of a combination of obstruction of hepatic lymphatic drainage, portal hypertension, and hypoalbuminemia. A sizable accumulation of ascitic fluid may increase intraabdominal pressure and impede venous return from the lower extremities; hence, it tends to promote accumulation of edema in this region as well.

Edema of Nutritional Origin A diet grossly deficient in protein over a prolonged period may produce hypoproteinemia and edema. The latter may be intensified by the development of beriberi heart disease, also of nutritional origin, in which multiple peripheral arteriovenous fistulae result in reduced effective systemic perfusion and effective arterial blood volume, thereby enhancing edema formation (Chap. 71). Edema may actually become intensified when famished subjects are first provided with an adequate diet. The ingestion of more food may increase the quantity of NaCl ingested, which is then retained along with H_2O. So-called refeeding edema may also be linked to increased release of insulin, which directly increases tubular Na^+ reabsorption. In addition to hypoalbuminemia, hypokalemia and caloric deficits may be involved in the edema of starvation.

Other Causes of Edema These include hypothyroidism, in which the edema (myxedema) is located typically in the pretibial region and which may also be associated with periorbital puffiness; exogenous hyperadrenocortism; pregnancy; and administration of estrogens and vasodilators, particularly dihydropyridines such as nifedipine.

DISTRIBUTION OF EDEMA

The distribution of edema is an important guide to its cause. Thus, edema limited to one leg or to one or both arms is usually the result of venous and/or lymphatic obstruction. Edema resulting from hypoproteinemia characteristically is generalized, but it is especially evident in the very soft tissues of the eyelids and face and tends to be most pronounced in the morning because of the recumbent posture assumed during the night. Less common causes of facial edema include trichinosis, allergic reactions, and myxedema. Edema associated with heart failure, by contrast, tends to be more extensive in the legs and to be accentuated in the evening, a feature also determined largely by posture. When patients with heart failure have been confined to bed, edema may be most prominent in the presacral region. Paralysis reduces lymphatic and venous drainage on the affected side and may be responsible for unilateral edema.

ADDITIONAL FACTORS IN DIAGNOSIS

The color, thickness, and sensitivity of the skin are significant. Local tenderness and warmth suggest inflammation. Local cyanosis may signify venous obstruction. In individuals who have had repeated episodes of prolonged edema, the skin over the involved areas may be thickened, indurated, and often red.

Estimation of the venous pressure is of importance in evaluating edema. Ordinarily, a significant generalized increase in venous pressure can be recognized by the level at which cervical veins collapse (Chap. 220). In patients with obstruction of the superior vena cava, edema is confined to the face, neck, and upper extremities, in which the venous pressure is elevated compared with that in the lower extremities. Severe heart failure may cause ascites that may be distinguished from the ascites caused by hepatic cirrhosis by the jugular venous pressure, which is usually elevated in heart failure and normal in cirrhosis.

Determination of the concentration of serum albumin aids importantly in identifying those patients in whom edema is due, at least in part, to diminished intravascular colloid oncotic pressure. The presence of proteinuria also affords useful clues. The absence of proteinuria excludes nephrotic syndrome but cannot exclude nonproteinuric causes of renal failure. Slight to moderate proteinuria is the rule in patients with heart failure.

APPROACH TO THE PATIENT: Edema

An important first question is whether the edema is localized or generalized. If it is localized, those local phenomena that may be responsible should be considered. If the edema is generalized, it should be determined, first, if there is serious hypoalbuminemia, e.g., serum albumin <25 g/L. If so, the history, physical examination, urinalysis, and other laboratory data will help evaluate the question of cirrhosis, severe malnutrition, or the nephrotic syndrome as the underlying disorder. If hypoalbuminemia is not present, it should be determined if there is evidence of congestive heart failure of a severity to promote generalized edema. Finally, it should be determined whether the patient has an adequate urine output, or if there is significant oliguria or anuria. These abnormalities are discussed in Chaps. 45, 273, and 274.

FURTHER READINGS

ABASSI ZA et al: Control of extracellular fluid volume and the pathophysiology of edema formation, in *The Kidney*, 7th ed, BM Brenner (ed). Philadelphia, Saunders, 2004, pp 777–856

CHERTOW GM: Approach to the patient with edema, in *Cardiology for the Primary Care Physician*, 2d ed, E Braunwald, L Goldman (eds). Philadelphia, Saunders, 2003, pp 117–128

DISKIN CJ et al: Edema, oncotic pressure, and free entropy: Novel considerations for treatment of edema through attention to thermodynamics. Nephron 78:131, 1998

MCCULLOUGH JC: Renal disorders and heart disease, in *Braunwald's Heart Disease*, 7th ed, D Zipes et al (eds). Philadelphia, Saunders, 2005

O'BRIEN JG et al: Treatment of edema. Am Fam Physician 71:2111, 2005

STREETEN DH: Idiopathic edema. Pathogenesis, clinical features, and treatment. Endocrinol Metab Clin North Am 24:531, 1995

37 Palpitations

Joseph Loscalzo

Palpitations are extremely common among patients who present to their caregiver and can best be defined as an intermittent "thumping," "pounding," or "fluttering" sensation in the chest. This sensation can be either intermittent or sustained, and either regular or irregular. Most patients interpret palpitations as an unusual awareness of the heart beat and become especially concerned when they sense that they have had "skipped" or "missing" heart beats. Palpitations are often noted when the patient is quietly resting, during which time other stimuli are minimal. Palpitations that are positional may reflect a structural process within (e.g., atrial myxoma) or adjacent to (e.g., mediastinal mass) the heart.

Palpitations are brought about by cardiac (43%), psychiatric (31%), miscellaneous (10%), and unknown (16%) causes, according to one large series. Cardiac causes include premature atrial and ventricular contractions, supraventricular and ventricular arrhythmias, mitral valve prolapse, aortic regurgitation, and atrial myxoma. Intermittent palpitations are commonly caused by premature atrial or ventricular contractions: the postextrasystolic beat is sensed by the patient owing to the increase in ventricular end-diastolic dimension following the pause in the cardiac cycle and the increased strength of contraction (*postextrasystolic potentiation*) of that beat. Regular, sustained palpitations can be caused by regular supraventricular and ventricular tachycardias (Chap. 226). Irregular, sustained palpitations can be caused by atrial fibrillation.

It is important to note that most arrhythmias are not associated with palpitations. In those that are, it is often useful either to ask the patient to "tap out" the rhythm of the palpitations or to take his or her pulse while palpitations are occurring. In general, hyperdynamic cardiovascular states caused by catecholaminergic stimulation from exercise, stress, or pheochromocytoma can lead to palpitations. In addition, the enlarged ventricle of aortic regurgitation and accompanying hyperdynamic precordium frequently lead to the sensation of palpitations. Other factors that enhance the strength of myocardial contraction, including tobacco, caffeine, aminophylline, atropine, thyroxine, cocaine, and amphetamines, can cause palpitations.

Psychiatric causes of palpitations include panic attack or disorder, anxiety states, and somatization, alone or in combination. Patients with psychiatric causes for palpitations more commonly report a longer duration of the sensation (>15 min) and other accompanying symptoms than do patients with other causes. Among the miscellaneous causes of palpitations are included thyrotoxicosis, drugs (see above) and ethanol, spontaneous skeletal muscle contractions of the chest wall, pheochromocytoma, and systemic mastocytosis.

APPROACH TO THE PATIENT: Palpitations

The principal goal in assessing patients with palpitations is to determine if the symptom is caused by a life-threatening arrhythmia. Patients with preexisting coronary artery disease (CAD) or risk factors for CAD are at greatest risk for ventricular arrhythmias as a cause for palpitations. In addition, the association of palpitations with other symptoms suggesting hemodynamic compromise, including syncope or lightheadedness, supports this diagnosis. Palpitations caused by sustained tachyarrhythmias in patients with CAD can be accompanied by angina pectoris or dyspnea. In patients with ventricular dysfunction (systolic or diastolic), aortic stenosis, hypertrophic cardiomyopathy, or mitral stenosis, with or without CAD, palpitations can be accompanied by dyspnea from increased left atrial and pulmonary capillary wedge pressure.

Key features of the physical examination that will help confirm or refute the presence of an arrhythmia as a cause for the palpitations and its adverse hemodynamic consequences include measurement of the vital signs, assessment of the jugular venous pressure and pulse, and auscultation of the chest and precordium. A resting electrocardiogram can be used to document the arrhythmia. If exertion is known to induce the arrhythmia and accompanying palpitations, exercise electrocardiography can be used to make the diagnosis. If the arrhythmia is sufficiently infrequent, other methods must be used, including continuous electrocardiographic (Holter) monitoring; telephonic monitoring, through which the patient can transmit an electrocardiographic tracing during a sensed episode; and loop recordings (external or implantable), which can capture the electrocardiographic event for later review.

Most patients with palpitations do not have serious arrhythmias or underlying structural heart disease. Occasional benign atrial or ventricular premature contractions can often be managed with beta blocker therapy if sufficiently troubling to the patient. Palpitations incited by alcohol, tobacco, or illicit drugs need to be managed by abstention, while those caused by pharmacologic agents should be addressed by considering alternative therapies. Psychiatric causes of palpitations may benefit from cognitive or pharmacotherapies. The physician should note that palpitations are at the very least bothersome and, on occasion, frightening to the patient. Once serious causes for the symptom have been excluded, the patient should be reassured the palpitations will not adversely affect his or her prognosis.

ACKNOWLEDGMENT

Dr. Thomas Lee authored this chapter in previous editions. Some of the material from the 16th edition have been carried forward.

FURTHER READINGS

ABBOTT AV: Diagnostic approach to palpitations. Am Fam Physician 71:743, 2005

PICKETT CC, ZIMETBAUM PJ: Palpitations: A proper evaluation and approach to effective medical therapy. Curr Cardiol Rep 7:362, 2005

WEBER BE, KAPOOR WN: Evaluation and outcomes of patients with palpitations. Am J Med 100:138, 1996

SECTION 6 ALTERATIONS IN GASTROINTESTINAL FUNCTION

38 Dysphagia

Raj K. Goyal

Dysphagia is defined as a sensation of "sticking" or obstruction of the passage of food through the mouth, pharynx, or esophagus. However, it is often used as an umbrella term to include other symptoms related to swallowing difficulty. *Aphagia* signifies complete esophageal obstruction, which is usually due to bolus impaction and represents a medical emergency. *Difficulty in initiating a swallow* occurs in disorders of the voluntary phase of swallowing. However, once initiated, swallowing is completed normally. *Odynophagia* means painful swallowing. Frequently, odynophagia and dysphagia occur together. *Globus pharyngeus* is the sensation of a lump lodged in the throat. However, no difficulty is encountered when swallowing is performed. *Misdirection of food*, resulting in nasal regurgitation and laryngeal and pulmonary aspiration during swallowing, is characteristic of oropharyngeal dysphagia. *Phagophobia*, meaning fear of swallowing, and *refusal to swallow* may occur in hysteria, rabies, tetanus, and pharyngeal paralysis due to fear of aspiration. Painful inflammatory lesions that cause odynophagia may also cause refusal to swallow. Some patients may feel the food as it goes down the esophagus. This esophageal sensitivity is not associated with either food sticking or obstruction.

PHYSIOLOGY OF SWALLOWING

The process of swallowing begins with a voluntary (oral) phase that includes a preparatory phase during which a food bolus suitable for swallowing is prepared and a transfer phase during which the bolus is pushed into the pharynx by contraction of the tongue. The bolus then activates oropharyngeal sensory receptors that initiate the deglutition reflex. The deglutition reflex is centrally mediated and involves a complex series of events. It serves both to propel food through the pharynx and the esophagus and to prevent its entry into the airway. When the bolus is propelled backward by the tongue, the larynx moves forward and the upper esophageal sphincter (UES) opens. As the bolus moves into the pharynx, contraction of the superior pharyngeal constrictor against the contracted soft palate initiates a peristaltic contraction that proceeds rapidly downward to move the bolus through the pharynx and the esophagus. The lower esophageal sphincter (LES) opens as the food enters the esophagus and remains open until the peristaltic contraction has swept the bolus into the stomach. Peristaltic contraction in response to a swallow is called *primary peristalsis*. It involves inhibition followed by sequential contraction of muscles along the entire swallowing passage. The inhibition that precedes the peristaltic contraction is called *deglutitive inhibition*. Local distention of the esophagus from residual food activates *secondary peristalsis*.

Muscles of the oral cavity, pharynx, UES, and cervical esophagus are striated and are directly innervated by the lower motor neurons carried in the cranial nerves. Oral cavity muscles are innervated by the Vth and the VIIth cranial nerves and the tongue muscles by the XIIth cranial nerve. Pharyngeal muscles are innervated by the IXth and the Xth cranial nerves.

The UES consists of constrictor and dilator muscles. The constrictor muscles include the cricopharyngeus and inferior pharyngeal constrictor muscles. The dilator muscles include a number of suprahyoid muscles including the geniohyoid muscle. The constrictor muscles are innervated by the Xth cranial nerves and the dilator muscles are innervated by the XIIth and also the Vth and the VIIth cranial nerves. The UES remains closed owing to the elastic properties of its wall and to neurogenic tonic contraction of the cricopharyngeus muscle. Inhibition of the vagal excitatory activity in the central nervous system relaxes the cricopharyngeus, and contraction of the dilator muscles opens the UES by causing upward and forward displacement of the larynx.

The neuromuscular apparatus for peristalsis is different in cervical and thoracic parts of the esophagus. The cervical esophagus, like the pharyngeal muscles, is composed of striated muscles and is innervated by lower motor neurons in the vagus (Xth cranial) nerve. Peristalsis in the cervical esophagus is due to sequential activation of the vagal motor neurons in the nucleus ambiguus.

In contrast, the thoracic esophagus and LES are composed of smooth-muscle fibers and are innervated by excitatory and inhibitory neurons within the esophageal myenteric plexus. Neurotransmitters of the excitatory nerves are acetylcholine and substance P, and of the inhibitory nerves are vasoactive intestinal peptide (VIP) and nitric oxide. Separate groups of parasympathetic preganglionic nerve fibers in the Xth cranial nerve arising from its dorsal motor nucleus project onto the inhibitory and excitatory postganglionic myenteric neurons. Patterned activation of inhibitory followed by excitatory vagal pathways is responsible for peristalsis, which consists of a sequence of inhibition (deglutitive inhibition) followed by contraction. The LES relaxes, with deglutitive inhibition, at the onset of esophageal peristalsis.

The LES is closed at rest because of its intrinsic myogenic tone, influenced by excitatory and inhibitory nerves. The function of the LES is supplemented by the striated muscle of the diaphragmatic crura, which surrounds the LES and acts as an external LES.

PATHOPHYSIOLOGY OF DYSPHAGIA

Based on anatomic site of involvement, dysphagia may be divided into oral, pharyngeal, and esophageal dysphagia. Normal transport of an ingested bolus through the swallowing passage depends on the size of the ingested bolus and size of the lumen, the force of peristaltic contraction, and deglutitive inhibition, including normal relaxation of UES and LES during swallowing. Dysphagia caused by a large bolus or a narrow lumen is called *mechanical dysphagia*, whereas dysphagia due to weakness of peristaltic contractions or to impaired deglutitive inhibition causing nonperistaltic contractions and impaired sphincter relaxation is called *motor dysphagia*.

Oral and Pharyngeal (Oropharyngeal) Dysphagia Oral-phase dysphagia is associated with poor bolus formation and control, so that food may either drool out of the mouth or overstay in the mouth or the patient may experience difficulty in initiating the swallowing reflex. Poor bolus control may also lead to premature spillage of food into the pharynx and aspiration into the unguarded larynx and/or nasal cavity. Pharyngeal-phase dysphagia is associated with stasis of food in the pharynx due to poor pharyngeal propulsion and obstruction at the UES. Pharyngeal stasis leads to nasal regurgitation and laryngeal aspiration during or after a swallow. Nasal regurgitation and laryngeal aspiration during the process of swallowing are hallmarks of oropharyngeal dysphagia.

Oropharyngeal dysphagia may be due to mechanical causes, including a variety of developmental abnormalities, head and neck tumors, radiation therapy, and inflammatory processes (Table 38-1).

TABLE 38-1 OROPHARYNGEAL DYSPHAGIA

Oropharyngeal Mechanical Dysphagia

- I. Wall defects
  - A. Congenital
    - 1. Cleft lip, cleft palate
    - 2. Laryngeal clefts
  - B. Post surgical
- II. Intrinsic narrowing
  - A. Inflammatory
    - 1. Viral (herpes simplex, varicella-zoster, cytomegalovirus)
    - 2. Bacterial (peritonsillar abscess)
    - 3. Fungal *(Candida)*
    - 4. Mucocutaneous bullous diseases
    - 5. Caustic, chemical, thermal injury
  - B. Web
    - 1. Plummer-Vinson syndrome
  - C. Strictures
    - 1. Congenital microganthia
    - 2. Caustic ingestion
    - 3. Post-radiation
  - D. Tumors
    - 1. Benign
    - 2. Malignant
- III. Extrinsic compression
  - A. Retropharyngeal abscess, mass
  - B. Zenker's diverticulum
  - C. Thyroid disorders
  - D. Vertebral osteophytes

Oropharyngeal Motor Dysphagia

- I. Diseases of cerebral cortex and brainstem
  - A. With altered consciousness or dementia
    - 1. Dementias including Alzheimer's disease
    - 2. Altered consciousness, metabolic encephalopathy, encephalitis, meningitis, cerebrovascular accident, brain injury
  - B. With normal cognitive functions
    - 1. Brain injury
    - 2. Cerebral palsy
    - 3. Rabies, tetanus, neurosyphilis
    - 4. Cerebrovascular disease
    - 5. Parkinson's disease and other extrapyramidal lesions
    - 6. Multiple sclerosis (bulbar and pseudobulbar palsy)
    - 7. Amyotrophic lateral sclerosis (motor neuron disease)
    - 8. Poliomyelitis and post-poliomyelitis syndrome
- II. Diseases of cranial nerves (V, VII, IX, X, XII)
  - A. Basilar meningitis (chronic inflammatory, neoplastic)
  - B. Nerve injury
  - C. Neuropathy (Guillain-Barré syndrome, familial dysautonomia, sarcoid, diabetic and other causes)
- III. Neuromuscular
  - A. Myasthenia gravis
  - B. Eaton-Lambert syndrome
  - C. Botulinum toxin
  - D. Aminoglycoside and other drugs
- IV. Muscle disorders
  - A. Myositis (polymyositis, dermatomyositis, sarcoidosis)
  - B. Metabolic myopathy (mitochondrial myopathy, thyroid myopathy)
  - C. Primary myopathies (myotonic dystrophy, oculopharyngeal myopathy)

Oropharyngeal motor dysphagia results from impairment of the voluntary effort required in bolus preparation or neuromuscular disorders affecting bolus preparation, initiation of the swallowing reflex, timely passage of food through the pharynx, and prevention of entry of food into the nasal and the laryngeal opening. Paralysis of the suprahyoid muscles leads to loss of opening of the UES and severe dysphagia. Because each side of the pharynx is innervated by ipsilateral nerves, a unilateral lesion of motor neurons leads to unilateral pharyngeal paralysis.

Neuromuscular disorders causing dysphagia are listed in Table 38-1. They include a variety of cortical and suprabulbar disorders, lesions of the cranial nerves in their nuclei in the brain stem or their course to the muscles, defects of neurotransmission at the motor end plates, and muscular diseases. Some of these disorders also involve laryngeal muscles and vocal cords, causing hoarseness.

Since the oropharyngeal phase of swallowing lasts no more than a second, rapid-sequence videofluoroscopy is necessary to permit detection and analysis of abnormalities of oral and pharyngeal function. However, such studies can only be performed in a fully conscious and cooperative patient. A videofluoroscopic swallowing study (VFSS) using barium of different consistencies may reveal difficulties in the oral phase of swallowing. The pharynx is examined to detect stasis of barium in the valleculae and pyriform sinuses and regurgitation of barium into the nose and tracheobronchial tree. Pharyngeal contraction waves and opening of UES with a swallow are carefully monitored. Manometric studies may demonstrate reduced amplitude of pharyngeal contractions and reduced UES pressure without further fall in pressure on swallowing (see Fig. 286-3). General treatment consists of maneuvers to reduce pharyngeal stasis and to enhance airway protection under the direction of a trained swallow therapist. Feeding by a naso-gastric tube or an endoscopically placed gastrostomy tube may be necessary for nutritional support; however, these maneuvers do not provide protection against aspiration of salivary secretions. Gastrostomy tube feeding may actually increase gastroesophageal reflux and lead to more aspiration. Jejunostomy tube feeding may lessen reflux.

Dysphagia resulting from a cerebrovascular accident usually improves with time, although often not completely. Patients with myasthenia gravis (Chap. 381) and polymyositis (Chap. 383) may respond to treatment of the primary disease. Cricopharyngeal myotomy is usually not helpful. Extensive operative procedures to prevent aspiration are rarely needed. Death is often due to pulmonary complications.

A cricopharyngeal bar results from failure of the cricopharyngeus to relax but with normal activity of the suprahyoid muscles on swallowing. Barium swallow shows a prominent projection on the posterior wall of the pharynx at the level of the lower part of the cricoid cartilage (see Fig. 286-1). A transient cricopharyngeal bar is seen in up to 5% of individuals without dysphagia undergoing upper gastrointestinal studies; it can be produced in normal individuals during a Valsalva maneuver. A persistent cricopharyngeal bar may be caused by fibrosis in the cricopharyngeus. Cricopharyngeal myotomy may be helpful in severely symptomatic case with functional evidence of obstruction by the cricopharyngeus muscle, but is contraindicated in the presence of gastroesophageal reflux because it may lead to pharyngeal and pulmonary aspiration. Globus pharyngeus mainly occurs in individuals with emotional disorders, particularly in women. Results of barium studies and manometry are normal. Treatment consists primarily of reassurance. Some patients with globus pharyngeus have associated reflux esophagitis, and they may respond to treatment of the esophagitis.

Esophageal Dysphagia In an adult, the esophageal lumen can distend up to 4 cm in diameter. When the esophagus cannot dilate beyond 2.5 cm in diameter, dysphagia to normal solid food can occur. Dysphagia is always present when the esophagus cannot distend beyond 1.3 cm. Circumferential lesions produce dysphagia more consistently than do lesions that involve only a portion of circumferences of the esophageal wall, as uninvolved segments retain their distensibility. The esophageal causes of mechanical dysphagia are listed in Table 38-2. Common causes include carcinoma, peptic and other benign strictures, and lower esophageal ring. Esophageal motor dysphagia may result from abnormalities in peristalsis and deglutitive inhibition due to diseases of the esophageal striated or smooth muscle.

Diseases of the striated muscle often also involve the cervical part of the esophagus, in addition to affecting the oropharyngeal muscles. Clinical manifestations of the cervical esophageal involvement are usually overshadowed by those of the oropharyngeal dysphagia.

Diseases of the smooth-muscle segment involve the thoracic part of the esophagus and the LES. Dysphagia occurs when the peristaltic contractions are weak or absent or when the contractions are nonperistaltic. Loss of peristalsis may be associated with failure of LES relaxation. Weakness of contractile power occurs due to muscle weakness, as in scleroderma or impaired cholinergic effect. Nonperistaltic contractions and failure of LES relaxation occur due to impaired inhibitory innervation. In diffuse esophageal spasm (DES), inhibitory innervation only to the esophageal body is impaired, whereas in achalasia inhibitory innervation to both the esophageal body and LES is impaired. Dysphagia due to esophageal muscle

TABLE 38-2 ESOPHAGEAL DYSPHAGIA

Esophageal Mechanical Dysphagia

I. Wall defects
  A. Congenital
  B. Tracheoesophageal fistula
II. Intrinsic narrowing
  A. Inflammatory esophagitis
    1. Viral (herpes simplex, varicella-zoster, cytomegalovirus)
    2. Bacterial
    3. Fungal *(Candida)*
    4. Mucocutaneous bullous diseases
    5. Caustic, chemical, thermal injury
    6. Eosinophilic esophagitis
  B. Webs and rings
    1. Esophageal (congenital, inflammatory)
    2. Lower esophageal mucosal ring (Schatzki's ring)
    3. Eosinophilic esophagitis
    4. Host-versus-graft disease, mucocutaneous disorders
  C. Benign strictures
    1. Peptic
    2. Caustic
    3. Pill-induced
    4. Inflammatory (Crohn's disease, *Candida*, mucocutaneous lesions)
    5. Ischemic
    6. Postoperative
    7. Post-radiation
    8. Congenital
  D. Tumors
    1. Benign
    2. Malignant
III. Extrinsic compression
  A. Vascular compression (dysphagia lusoria, aberrant right subclavian artery, right-sided aorta, left atrial enlargement, aortic aneurysm)
  B. Posterior mediastinal mass
  C. Postvagotomy hematoma and fibrosis

Esophageal Motor Dysphagia

I. Disorders of cervical esophagus
  (see oropharyngeal motor disorders, Table 38-1)
II. Disorders of thoracic esophagus
  A. Diseases of smooth muscle or excitatory nerves
    1. Weak muscle contraction or LES tone
      a. Idiopathic
      b. Scleroderma and related collagen vascular diseases
      c. Hollow visceral myopathy
      d. Myotonic dystrophy
      e. Metabolic neuromyopathy (amyloid, alcohol?, diabetes?)
      f. Drugs: anticholinergics, smooth muscle relaxants
    2. Enhanced muscle contraction
      a. Hypertensive peristalsis (nutcracker esophagus)
      b. Hypertensive LES, hypercontracting LES
  B. Disorders of inhibitory innervation
    1. Diffuse esophageal spasm
    2. Achalasia
      a. Primary
      b. Secondary (Chagas' disease, carcinoma, lymphoma, neuropathic intestinal pseudo-obstruction syndrome)
    3. Contractile (muscular) lower esophageal ring

Note: LES, lower esophageal sphincter.

weakness is often associated with symptoms of gastroesophageal reflux disease (GERD). Dysphagia due to loss of the inhibitory innervation is typically not associated with GERD but may be associated with chest pain.

The causes of esophageal motor dysphagia are also listed in Table 38-2; they include scleroderma of the esophagus, achalasia, DES, and other motor disorders.

APPROACH TO THE PATIENT: Dysphagia

Figure 38-1 shows an algorithm of approach to a patient with dysphagia.

HISTORY The history can provide a presumptive diagnosis in >80% of patients. The site of dysphagia described by the patient helps to determine the site of esophageal obstruction; the lesion is at or below the perceived location of dysphagia.

Associated symptoms provide important diagnostic clues. Nasal regurgitation and tracheobronchial aspiration with swallowing are hallmarks of pharyngeal paralysis or a tracheoesophageal fistula. Tracheobronchial aspiration unrelated to swallowing may be due to achalasia, Zenker's diverticulum, or gastroesophageal reflux.

Association of laryngeal symptoms and dysphagia occurs in various neuromuscular disorders. The presence of hoarseness may be an important diagnostic clue. When hoarseness precedes dysphagia, the primary lesion is usually in the larynx; hoarseness following dysphagia may suggest involvement of the recurrent laryngeal nerve by extension of esophageal carcinoma. Sometimes hoarseness may be due to laryngitis secondary to gastroesophageal reflux. Hiccups may rarely occur with a lesion in the distal portion of the esophagus. Unilateral wheezing with dysphagia may indicate a mediastinal mass involving the esophagus and a large bronchus.

The type of food causing dysphagia provides useful information. Difficulty only with solids implies mechanical dysphagia with a lumen that is not severely narrowed. In advanced obstruction, dysphagia occurs with liquids as well as solids. In contrast, motor dysphagia due to achalasia and DES is equally affected by solids and liquids from the very onset. Patients with scleroderma have dysphagia to solids that is unrelated to posture and to liquids while recumbent but not upright. When peptic stricture develops in patients with scleroderma, dysphagia becomes more persistent.

The duration and course of dysphagia are helpful in diagnosis. Transient dysphagia may be due to an inflammatory process. Progressive dysphagia lasting a few weeks to a few months is suggestive of carcinoma of the esophagus. Episodic dysphagia to solids lasting several years indicates a benign disease characteristic of a lower esophageal ring.

Severe weight loss that is out of proportion to the degree of dysphagia is highly suggestive of carcinoma.

Chest pain with dysphagia occurs in DES and related motor disorders. Chest pain resembling DES may occur in esophageal obstruction due to a large bolus. A prolonged history of heartburn and reflux preceding dysphagia indicates peptic stricture. A history of prolonged nasogastric intubation, ingestion of caustic agents, ingestion of pills without water, previous radiation therapy, or associated mucocutaneous diseases may provide the cause of esophageal stricture. If odynophagia is present, candidal, herpes, or pill-induced esophagitis should be suspected.

In patients with AIDS or other immunocompromised states, esophagitis due to opportunistic infections such as *Candida*, herpes simplex virus, or cytomegalovirus and to tumors such as Kaposi's sarcoma and lymphoma should be considered.

PHYSICAL EXAMINATION Physical examination is important in oral and pharyngeal motor dysphagia. Signs of bulbar or pseudobulbar palsy, including dysarthria, dysphonia, ptosis, tongue atrophy, and hyperactive jaw jerk, in addition to evidence of generalized neuromuscular disease, should be sought. The neck should be examined for thyromegaly or a spinal abnormality. A careful inspection of the mouth and pharynx should disclose lesions that may interfere with passage of food. Pulmonary complications such as acute or chronic aspiration pneumonia may be present.

Physical examination is often unrevealing in esophageal dysphagia. Changes in the skin and extremities may suggest a diagnosis of scleroderma and other collagen vascular diseases or mucocutaneous diseases such as pemphigoid or epidermolysis bullosa, which may involve the esophagus. Cancer spread to lymph nodes and liver may be evident.

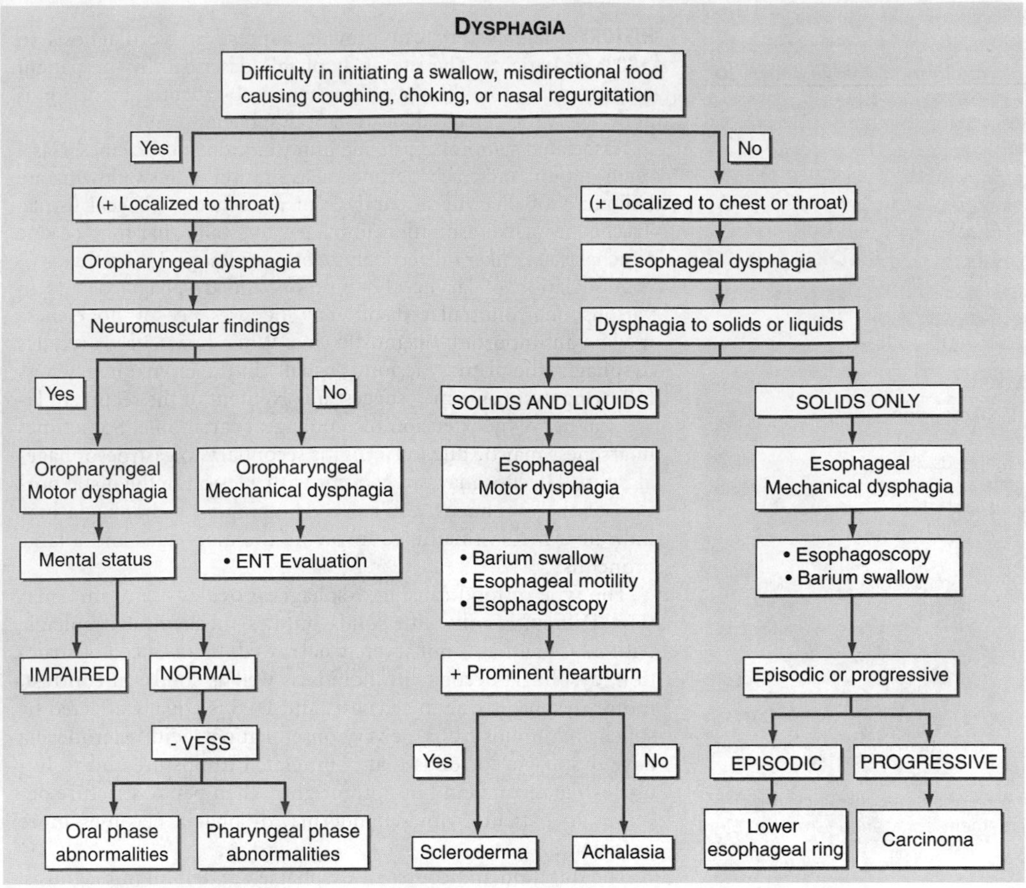

FIGURE 38-1 Approach to the patient with dysphagia. ENT, ear, nose, and throat; VFSS, videofluoroscopic swallowing study.

DIAGNOSTIC PROCEDURES Dysphagia is usually a symptom of organic disease rather than a functional complaint. If oral or pharyngeal dysphagia is suspected, VFSS by both a radiologist and a swallow therapist is the procedure of choice. Videoendoscopy is currently performed only in specialized centers. Otolaryngoscopic and neurologic evaluation are also usually required.

If esophageal mechanical dysphagia is suspected on clinical history, barium swallow and esophagogastroscopy with or without mucosal biopsies are the diagnostic procedures of choice. In some cases, CT examination and endoscopic ultrasound may be useful. For motor esophageal dysphagia, barium swallow, esophageal manometry, esophageal pH, and impedance testing are useful diagnostic tests. Esophagogastroscopy is also often performed in patients with motor dysphagia to exclude an associated structural abnormality (Chap. 286).

FURTHER READINGS

MASSEY B, SHAKER R: Oral pharyngeal and upper esophageal sphincter motility disorders. *http://www.nature.com/gimo/index.html*

MCCULLOUGH TM, JAFFE D: Head and neck disorders causing dysphagia. *http://www.nature.com/gimo/index.html*

PATERSON WG et al: Esophageal motility disorders. *http://www.nature.com/gimo/index.html*

39 Nausea, Vomiting, and Indigestion

William L. Hasler

Nausea is the subjective feeling of a need to vomit. *Vomiting* (emesis) is the oral expulsion of gastrointestinal contents resulting from contractions of gut and thoracoabdominal wall musculature. Vomiting is contrasted with *regurgitation*, the effortless passage of gastric contents into the mouth. *Rumination* is the repeated regurgitation of stomach contents, which may be rechewed and reswallowed. In contrast to vomiting, these phenomena often exhibit volitional control. *Indigestion* is a nonspecific term that encompasses a variety of upper abdominal complaints including nausea, vomiting, heartburn, regurgitation, and dyspepsia (the presence of symptoms thought to originate in the gastroduodenal region). Some individuals with dyspepsia report predominantly epigastric burning, gnawing discomfort, or pain. Others with dyspepsia experience a constellation of symptoms including postprandial fullness, early satiety (an inability to complete a meal due to premature fullness), bloating, eructation (belching), and anorexia.

NAUSEA AND VOMITING

MECHANISMS

Vomiting is coordinated by the brain stem and is effected by neuromuscular responses in the gut, pharynx, and thoracoabdominal wall. The mechanisms underlying nausea are poorly understood but likely involve the cerebral cortex, as nausea requires conscious perception. This is supported by electroencephalographic studies showing activation of temporofrontal cortical regions during nausea.

Coordination of Emesis Several brain stem nuclei—including the nucleus tractus solitarius, dorsal vagal and phrenic nuclei, medullary nuclei that regulate respiration, and nuclei that control pharyngeal, facial, and tongue movements—coordinate the initiation of emesis. Neurotransmitters involved in this coordination are uncertain; however, roles for neurokinin NK_1, serotonin 5-HT_3, and vasopressin pathways are postulated.

Somatic and visceral muscles exhibit stereotypic responses during emesis. Inspiratory thoracic and abdominal wall muscles contract, producing high intrathoracic and intraabdominal pressures that facilitate expulsion of gastric contents. The gastric cardia herniates across the diaphragm and the larynx moves upward to promote oral propulsion of the vomitus. Under normal conditions, distally migrating gut contractions are regulated by an electrical phenomenon, the slow wave, which cycles at 3 cycles/min in the stomach and 11 cycles/min in the duodenum. With emesis, there is slow-wave abolition and initiation of orally propagating spike activity, which evokes retrograde contractions that assist in oral expulsion of intestinal contents.

Activators of Emesis Emetic stimuli act at several sites. Emesis provoked by unpleasant thoughts or smells originates in the cerebral cortex, whereas cranial nerves mediate vomiting after gag reflex activation. Motion sickness and inner ear disorders act on the labyrinthine apparatus, whereas gastric irritants and cytotoxic agents such as cisplatin stimulate gastroduodenal vagal afferent nerves. Nongastric visceral afferents are activated by intestinal and colonic obstruction and mesenteric ischemia. The area postrema, a medullary nucleus, responds to bloodborne emetic stimuli and is termed the *chemoreceptor trigger zone.* Many emetogenic drugs act on the area postrema, as do bacterial toxins and metabolic factors produced during uremia, hypoxia, and ketoacidosis.

Neurotransmitters that mediate induction of vomiting are selective for these anatomic sites. Labyrinthine disorders stimulate vestibular cholinergic muscarinic M_1 and histaminergic H_1 receptors, whereas gastroduodenal vagal afferent stimuli activate serotonin 5-HT_3 receptors. The area postrema is richly served by nerve fibers acting on 5-HT_3, M_1, H_1, and dopamine D_2 receptor subtypes. Transmitter mediators in the cerebral cortex are poorly understood, although cortical cannabinoid CB_1 pathways have been characterized. Optimal pharmacologic management of vomiting requires understanding of these pathways.

TABLE 39-1 CAUSES OF NAUSEA AND VOMITING

Intraperitoneal	Extraperitoneal	Medications/Metabolic Disorders
Obstructing disorders	Cardiopulmonary disease	Drugs
Pyloric obstruction	Cardiomyopathy	Cancer chemotherapy
Small bowel obstruction	Myocardial infarction	Antibiotics
Colonic obstruction	Labyrinthine disease	Cardiac antiarrhythmics
Superior mesenteric artery syndrome	Motion sickness	Digoxin
Enteric infections	Labyrinthitis	Oral hypoglycemics
Viral	Malignancy	Oral contraceptives
Bacterial	Intracerebral disorders	Endocrine/metabolic disease
Inflammatory diseases	Malignancy	Pregnancy
Cholecystitis	Hemorrhage	Uremia
Pancreatitis	Abscess	Ketoacidosis
Appendicitis	Hydrocephalus	Thyroid and parathyroid disease
Hepatitis	Psychiatric illness	Adrenal insufficiency
Altered sensorimotor function	Anorexia and bulimia nervosa	Toxins
Gastroparesis	Depression	Liver failure
Intestinal pseudoobstruction	Postoperative vomiting	Ethanol
Functional dyspepsia		
Gastroesophageal reflux		
Chronic idiopathic nausea		
Functional vomiting		
Cyclic vomiting syndrome		
Biliary colic		
Abdominal irradiation		

DIFFERENTIAL DIAGNOSIS

Nausea and vomiting are caused by conditions within and outside the gut as well as by drugs and circulating toxins (Table 39-1).

Intraperitoneal Disorders Visceral obstruction and inflammation of hollow and solid viscera may produce vomiting as the main symptom. Gastric obstruction results from ulcer disease and malignancy, while small-bowel and colonic obstruction occur because of adhesions, benign or malignant tumors, volvulus, intussusception, or inflammatory diseases such as Crohn's disease. The superior mesenteric artery syndrome, occurring after weight loss or prolonged bed rest, results when the duodenum is compressed by the overlying superior mesenteric artery. Abdominal irradiation impairs intestinal contractile function and induces strictures. Biliary colic causes nausea via action on visceral afferent nerves. Vomiting with pancreatitis, cholecystitis, and appendicitis is due to localized visceral irritation and induction of ileus. Enteric infections with viruses or bacteria such as *Staphylococcus aureus* and *Bacillus cereus* are common causes of acute vomiting, especially in children. Opportunistic infections such as cytomegalovirus or herpes simplex virus induce emesis in immunocompromised individuals.

Disordered gut sensorimotor function also commonly causes nausea and vomiting. *Gastroparesis* is defined as a delay in emptying of food from the stomach and occurs after vagotomy, with pancreatic adenocarcinoma, with mesenteric vascular insufficiency, or in systemic diseases such as diabetes, scleroderma, and amyloidosis. Idiopathic gastroparesis occurring in the absence of systemic illness may follow a viral prodrome, suggesting an infectious etiology. Intestinal pseudoobstruction is characterized by disrupted intestinal and colonic motor activity and leads to retention of food residue and secretions, bacterial overgrowth, nutrient malabsorption, and symptoms of nausea, vomiting, bloating, pain, and altered defecation. *Intestinal pseudoobstruction* may be idiopathic or inherited as a familial visceral myopathy or neuropathy, or it may result from systemic disease or as a paraneoplastic complication of a malignancy such as small cell lung carcinoma. Patients with gastroesophageal reflux may report nausea and vomiting, as do some individuals with functional dyspepsia and irritable bowel syndrome.

Three other functional disorders without organic abnormalities have been characterized in adults. *Chronic idiopathic nausea* is defined as nausea without vomiting occurring several times weekly, whereas *functional vomiting* is defined as one or more vomiting episodes weekly in the absence of an eating disorder or psychiatric disease. *Cyclic vomiting syndrome* is a rare disorder of unknown etiology that produces periodic discrete episodes of relentless nausea and vomiting. The syndrome shows a strong association with migraine headaches, suggesting that some cases may be migraine variants. Cyclic vomiting is most common in children, although adult cases have been described in association with rapid gastric emptying and with chronic cannabis use.

Extraperitoneal Disorders Myocardial infarction and congestive heart failure are cardiac causes of nausea and vomiting. Postoperative emesis occurs after 25% of surgeries, most commonly laparotomy and orthopedic surgery, and is more prevalent in women. Increased intracranial pressure from tumors, bleeding, abscess, or obstruction to cerebrospinal fluid outflow produces prominent vomiting with or without nausea. Motion sickness, labyrinthitis, and Ménière's disease evoke symptoms via labyrinthine pathways. Patients with psychiatric illnesses including anorexia nervosa, bulimia nervosa, anxiety, and depression may report significant nausea that may be associated with delayed gastric emptying.

Medications and Metabolic Disorders Drugs evoke vomiting by action on the stomach (analgesics, erythromycin) or area postrema (digoxin, opiates, anti-Parkinsonian drugs). Emetogenic agents include antibiotics, cardiac antiarrhythmics, antihypertensives, oral hypoglycemics, and contraceptives. Cancer chemotherapy causes vomiting that is acute (within hours of administration), delayed (after 1 or more days), or anticipatory. Acute emesis resulting from highly emetogenic agents such as cisplatin is mediated by 5-HT_3 pathways, whereas delayed emesis is 5-HT_3-independent. Anticipatory nausea often responds better to anxiolytic therapy than to antiemetics.

Several metabolic disorders elicit nausea and vomiting. Pregnancy is the most prevalent endocrinologic cause of nausea, occurring in 70% of women in the first trimester. Hyperemesis gravidarum is a severe form of nausea of pregnancy which can produce significant fluid loss and electrolyte disturbances. Uremia, ketoacidosis, and adrenal insufficiency, as well as parathyroid and thyroid disease, are other metabolic causes of emesis.

Circulating toxins evoke symptoms via effects on the area postrema. Endogenous toxins are generated in fulminant liver failure, whereas exogenous enterotoxins may be produced by enteric bacterial infection. Ethanol intoxication is a common toxic etiology of nausea and vomiting.

APPROACH TO THE PATIENT: Nausea and Vomiting

HISTORY AND PHYSICAL EXAMINATION The history helps define the etiology of unexplained nausea and vomiting. Drugs, toxins, and gastrointestinal infections commonly cause acute symptoms, whereas established illnesses evoke chronic complaints. Pyloric obstruction and gastroparesis produce vomiting within 1 h of eating, whereas emesis from intestinal obstruction occurs later. In severe cases of gastroparesis, the vomitus may contain food residue ingested hours or days previously. Hematemesis raises suspicion of an ulcer, malignancy, or Mallory-Weiss tear, whereas feculent emesis is noted with distal intestinal or colonic obstruction. Bilious vomiting excludes gastric obstruction, while emesis of undigested food is consistent with a Zenker's diverticulum or achalasia. Relief of abdominal pain by emesis characterizes small-bowel obstruction, whereas vomiting has no effect on pancreatitis or cholecystitis pain. Pronounced weight loss raises concern about malignancy or obstruction. Fevers suggest inflammation; an intracranial source is considered if there are headaches or visual field changes. Vertigo or tinnitus indicates labyrinthine disease.

The physical examination complements information obtained in the history. Demonstration of orthostatic hypotension and reduced skin turgor indicate intravascular fluid loss. Pulmonary abnormalities raise concern for aspiration of vomitus. Abdominal auscultation may reveal absent bowel sounds with ileus. High-pitched rushes suggest bowel obstruction, while a succussion splash upon abrupt lateral movement of the patient is found with gastroparesis or pyloric obstruction. Tenderness or involuntary guarding raises suspicion of inflammation, whereas fecal blood suggests mucosal injury from ulcer, ischemia, or tumor. Neurologic etiologies present with papilledema, visual field loss, or focal neural abnormalities. Neoplasm is suggested by palpation of masses or adenopathy.

DIAGNOSTIC TESTING For intractable symptoms or an elusive diagnosis, selected diagnostic tests can direct clinical management. Electrolyte replenishment is indicated for hypokalemia or metabolic alkalosis. Detection of iron-deficiency anemia mandates a search for mucosal injury. Pancreaticobiliary disease is indicated by abnormal pancreatic enzymes or liver biochemistries, whereas endocrinologic, rheumatologic, or paraneoplastic etiologies are suggested by specific hormone or serologic testing. If luminal obstruction is suspected, supine and upright abdominal radiographs may show intestinal air-fluid levels with reduced colonic air. Ileus is characterized by diffusely dilated air-filled bowel loops.

Anatomic studies may be indicated if initial testing is nondiagnostic. Upper endoscopy detects ulcers or malignancy, while small-bowel barium radiography diagnoses partial small-bowel obstruction. Colonoscopy or contrast enema radiography can detect colonic obstruction. Abdominal ultrasound or computed tomography (CT) defines intraperitoneal inflammatory processes, while CT or magnetic resonance imaging (MRI) of the head can delineate intracranial disease. Mesenteric angiography or MRI is useful when ischemia is considered.

Gastrointestinal motility testing may detect a motor disorder that contributes to symptoms when anatomic abnormalities are absent. Gastroparesis commonly is diagnosed using gastric scintigraphy, by which emptying of a radiolabeled meal is measured. Isotopic breath tests and telemetry capsule methods also have been validated. Electrogastrography, a noninvasive test of gastric slow-wave activity using cutaneous electrodes placed over the stomach, has been proposed as an alternate means of diagnosing gastroparesis. The diagnosis of intestinal pseudoobstruction often is suggested by abnormal barium transit and luminal dilation on small-bowel contrast radiography. Small-intestinal manometry can confirm the diagnosis and further characterize the motor abnormality as neuropathic or myopathic based on contractile patterns. Such investigation can obviate the need for open intestinal biopsy to evaluate for smooth muscle or neuronal degeneration.

Rx NAUSEA AND VOMITING

GENERAL PRINCIPLES Therapy of vomiting is tailored to correction of medically or surgically remediable abnormalities if possible. Hospitalization is considered for severe dehydration especially if oral fluid replenishment cannot be sustained. Once oral intake is tolerated, nutrients are restarted with liquids that are low in fat, as lipids delay gastric emptying. Foods high in indigestible residues are avoided as these also prolong gastric retention.

ANTIEMETIC MEDICATIONS The most commonly used antiemetic agents act on sites within the central nervous system (**Table 39-2**). Antihistamines such as meclizine and dimenhydrinate and anticholinergic drugs like scopolamine act on labyrinthine-activated pathways and are useful in motion sickness and inner ear disorders. Dopamine D_2 antagonists treat emesis evoked by area postrema stimuli and are useful for medication, toxic, and metabolic etiologies. Dopamine antagonists freely cross the blood-brain barrier and cause anxiety, dystonic reactions, hyperprolactinemic effects (galactorrhea and sexual dysfunction), and irreversible tardive dyskinesia.

Other drug classes exhibit antiemetic properties. Serotonin 5-HT_3 antagonists such as ondansetron and granisetron exhibit utility in postoperative vomiting, after radiation therapy, and in the prevention of cancer chemotherapy–induced emesis. The usefulness of 5-HT_3 antagonists for other causes of emesis is less well established. Low-dose tricyclic antidepressant agents provide symptomatic benefit in patients with chronic idiopathic nausea and functional vomiting as well as in diabetic patients with nausea and vomiting whose disease is of long standing.

GASTROINTESTINAL MOTOR STIMULANTS Drugs that stimulate gastric emptying are indicated for gastroparesis (Table 39-2). Metoclopramide, a combined 5-HT_4 agonist and D_2 antagonist, exhibits efficacy in gastroparesis, but antidopaminergic side effects limit its use in 25% of patients. Erythromycin, a macrolide antibiotic, increases gastroduodenal motility by action on receptors for motilin, an endogenous stimulant of fasting motor activity. Intravenous erythromycin is useful for inpatients with refractory gastroparesis; however, oral forms also have some utility. Domperidone, a D_2 antagonist not available in the United States, exhibits prokinetic and antiemetic effects but does not cross into most other brain regions; thus, anxiety and dystonic reactions are rare. The main side effects of domperidone relate to induction of hyperprolactinemia via effects on pituitary regions served by a porous blood-brain barrier. The 5-HT_4 agonist tegaserod potently stimulates gastric emptying in patients with gastroparesis; however, its effects on symptoms of gastric retention are unproven.

Patients with refractory upper gut motility disorders pose significant challenges. Liquid suspensions of prokinetic drugs may be beneficial, as liquids empty from the stomach more rapidly than pills. Metoclopramide can be administered subcutaneously in patients unresponsive to oral drugs. Intestinal pseudoobstruction may respond to the somatostatin analogue octreotide, which induces propagative small intestinal motor complexes. Pyloric injections of botulinum toxin are reported in uncontrolled studies to benefit patients with gastroparesis. Placement of a feeding jejunostomy reduces hospitalizations and improves overall health in some patients with gastroparesis who do not respond to drug therapy. Surgical options are limited for refractory cases, but postvagotomy gastroparesis may improve with near-total resection of the stomach. Implanted gastric electrical stimulators may reduce symptoms, enhance nutrition, improve quality of life, and decrease health care expenditures in patients with medication-refractory gastroparesis.

SELECTED CLINICAL SETTINGS Cancer chemotherapeutic agents such as cisplatin are intensely emetogenic (Chap. 77). Given prophylactically, 5-HT_3 antagonists prevent chemotherapy-induced acute vomiting in most cases (Table 39-2). Optimal antiemetic effects often are obtained with a 5-HT_3 antagonist combined with a glucocorticoid. High-dose metoclopramide also exhibits efficacy in chemotherapy-evoked emesis, while benzodiazepines such as lorazepam are useful in reducing anticipatory nausea and vomiting. Therapy of delayed emesis 1–5 days after chemotherapy is less successful. Neurokinin NK_1 antagonists (e.g., aprepitant) exhibit antiemetic and antinausea effects during both the acute and delayed periods after chemotherapy. Cannabinoids such as tetrahydrocannabinol, long advocated for cancer-associated emesis, produce significant side effects and exhibit no

TABLE 39-2 TREATMENT OF NAUSEA AND VOMITING

Treatment	Mechanism	Examples	Clinical Indications
Antiemetic agents	Antihistaminergic	Dimenhydrinate, meclizine	Motion sickness, inner ear disease
	Anticholinergic	Scopolamine	Motion sickness, inner ear disease
	Antidopaminergic	Prochlorperazine, thiethylperazine	Medication-, toxin-, or metabolic-induced emesis
	5-HT_3 antagonist	Ondansetron, granisetron	Chemotherapy- and radiation-induced emesis, postoperative emesis
	NK_1 antagonist	Aprepitant	Chemotherapy-induced nausea and vomiting
	Tricyclic antidepressant	Amitriptyline, nortriptyline	Chronic idiopathic nausea, functional vomiting, cyclic vomiting syndrome
Prokinetic agents	5-HT_4 agonist and antidopaminergic	Metoclopramide	Gastroparesis
	Motilin agonist	Erythromycin	Gastroparesis, ?intestinal pseudoobstruction
	Peripheral antidopaminergic	Domperidone	Gastroparesis
	5-HT_4 agonist	Tegaserod	?Gastroparesis, ?intestinal pseudoobstruction
	Somatostatin analogue	Octreotide	Intestinal pseudoobstruction
Special settings	Benzodiazepines	Lorazepam	Anticipatory nausea and vomiting with chemotherapy
	Glucocorticoids	Methylprednisolone, dexamethasone	Chemotherapy-induced emesis
	Cannabinoids	Tetrahydrocannabinol	?Chemotherapy-induced emesis

more efficacy than antidopaminergic agents. Most current drug regimens produce greater reductions in vomiting than in nausea.

The clinician should exercise caution in managing the pregnant patient with nausea. Studies of the teratogenic effects of available antiemetic agents provide conflicting results. Few controlled trials have been performed in nausea of pregnancy, although antihistamines such as meclizine and antidopaminergics such as prochlorperazine demonstrate efficacy greater than placebo. Some obstetricians offer alternative therapies such as pyridoxine, acupressure, or ginger.

Controlling emesis in cyclic vomiting syndrome is a challenge. In many individuals, prophylactic treatment with tricyclic antidepressants, cyproheptadine, or β-adrenoceptor antagonists can reduce the frequency of attacks. Intravenous 5-HT_3 antagonists combined with the sedating effects of a benzodiazepine such as lorazepam are a mainstay of treatment of acute symptom flares. Small studies report benefits with antimigraine therapies, including the serotonin 5-HT_1 agonist sumatriptan as well as certain newer anticonvulsant drugs.

INDIGESTION

MECHANISMS

The most common causes of indigestion are gastroesophageal acid reflux and functional dyspepsia. Other cases are a consequence of a more serious organic illness.

Gastroesophageal Acid Reflux Acid reflux can result from a variety of physiologic defects. Reduced lower esophageal sphincter (LES) tone is an important cause of reflux in scleroderma and pregnancy; it may also be a factor in patients without other systemic conditions. Many individuals exhibit frequent transient LES relaxations during which acid bathes the esophagus. Overeating and aerophagia can transiently override the barrier function of the LES, whereas impaired esophageal body motility and reduced salivary secretion prolong acid exposure. The role of hiatal hernias is controversial—although most reflux patients exhibit hiatal hernias, most individuals with hiatal hernias do not have excess heartburn.

Gastric Motor Dysfunction Disturbed gastric motility is purported to cause acid reflux in some cases of indigestion. Delayed gastric emptying is also found in 25–50% of functional dyspeptics. The relation of these defects to symptom induction is uncertain; many studies show poor correlation between symptom severity and the degree of motor dysfunction. Impaired gastric fundus relaxation after eating may underlie selected dyspeptic symptoms like bloating, nausea, and early satiety.

Visceral Afferent Hypersensitivity Disturbed gastric sensory function is proposed as a pathogenic factor in functional dyspepsia. Visceral afferent hypersensitivity was first demonstrated in patients with irritable bowel syndrome who had heightened perception of rectal balloon inflation without changes in rectal compliance. Similarly, dyspeptic patients experience discomfort with fundic distention to lower pressures than healthy controls. Some patients with heartburn exhibit normal esophageal acid exposure. These individuals with functional heartburn are believed to have heightened perception of normal esophageal pH.

Other Factors *Helicobacter pylori* has a clear etiologic role in peptic ulcer disease, but ulcers cause a minority of cases of dyspepsia. Infection with *H. pylori* is considered to be a minor factor in the genesis of functional dyspepsia. In contrast, functional dyspepsia is associated with a reduced sense of physical and mental well-being and is exacerbated by stress, suggesting an important role for psychological factors. Analgesics cause dyspepsia, while nitrates, calcium channel blockers, theophylline, and progesterone promote acid reflux. Other exogenous stimuli that induce acid reflux include ethanol, tobacco, and caffeine via LES relaxation. Genetic factors may contribute to development of acid reflux.

DIFFERENTIAL DIAGNOSIS

Gastroesophageal Reflux Disease Gastroesophageal reflux disease (GERD) is prevalent in Western society. Heartburn is reported once monthly by 40% of Americans and daily by 7–10%. Most cases of heartburn occur because of excess acid reflux; however, approximately 10% of patients with functional heartburn exhibit normal degrees of esophageal acid exposure.

Functional Dyspepsia Nearly 25% of the populace has dyspeptic symptoms at least six times yearly, but only 10–20% of these individuals present to physicians. Functional dyspepsia, the cause of symptoms in 60% of dyspeptic patients, is defined as ≥3 months of bothersome postprandial fullness, early satiety, epigastric pain, or epigastric burning with symptom onset at least 6 months before diagnosis in the absence of organic cause. Most patients follow a benign course, but a small number with *H. pylori* infection or on nonsteroidal anti-inflammatory drugs (NSAIDs) progress to ulcer formation. As with idiopathic gastroparesis, some cases of functional dyspepsia result from prior gastrointestinal infection.

Ulcer Disease In most cases of GERD, there is no destruction of the esophagus. However, 5% of patients develop esophageal ulcers, and some form strictures. Symptoms do not reliably distinguish nonerosive from erosive or ulcerative esophagitis. Some 15–25% of cases of dyspepsia stem from ulcers of the stomach or duodenum. The most common causes of ulcer disease are gastric infection with *H. pylori* and use of NSAIDs. Other rare causes of gastroduodenal ulcer include Crohn's disease (Chap. 289) and Zollinger-Ellison syndrome (Chap. 287), a condition resulting from gastrin overproduction by an endocrine tumor.

Malignancy Dyspeptic patients often seek care because of fear of cancer. However, <2% of cases result from gastroesophageal malignancy. Esophageal squamous cell carcinoma occurs most often in those with histories of tobacco or ethanol intake. Other risk factors include prior caustic ingestion, achalasia, and the hereditary disorder tylosis. Esophageal adenocarcinoma usually complicates long-standing acid reflux. Between 8 and 20% of GERD patients exhibit intestinal metaplasia of the esophagus, termed *Barrett's metaplasia*. This condition predisposes to esophageal adenocarcinoma (Chap. 87). Gastric malignancies include adenocarcinoma, which is prevalent in certain Asian societies, and lymphoma.

Other Causes Alkaline reflux esophagitis produces GERD-like symptoms in patients who have had surgery for peptic ulcer disease. Opportunistic fungal or viral esophageal infections may produce heartburn or chest discomfort but more often cause odynophagia. Other causes of esophageal inflammation include eosinophilic esophagitis and pill esophagitis. Biliary colic is in the differential diagnosis of dyspepsia, but most patients with true biliary colic report discrete episodes of right upper quadrant or epigastric pain rather than chronic burning discomfort, nausea, and bloating. Intestinal lactase deficiency produces gas, bloating, discomfort, and diarrhea after lactose ingestion. Lactase deficiency occurs in 15–25% of Caucasians of northern European descent but is more common in African Americans and Asians. Intolerance of other carbohydrates (e.g., fructose, sorbitol) produces similar symptoms. Small-intestinal bacterial overgrowth may produce dyspepsia, often with bowel dysfunction, distention, and malabsorption. Pancreatic disease (chronic pancreatitis and malignancy), hepatocellular carcinoma, celiac disease, Ménétrier's disease, infiltrative diseases (sarcoidosis and eosinophilic gastroenteritis), mesenteric ischemia, thyroid and parathyroid disease, and abdominal wall strain cause dyspepsia. Extraperitoneal etiologies of indigestion include congestive heart failure and tuberculosis.

APPROACH TO THE PATIENT: Indigestion

HISTORY AND PHYSICAL EXAMINATION Care of the patient with indigestion requires a thorough interview. GERD classically produces heartburn, a substernal warmth in the epigastrium that moves toward the neck. Heartburn often is exacerbated by meals and may awaken the patient. Associated symptoms include regurgitation of acid and water brash, the reflex release of salty salivary secretions into the mouth. Atypical symptoms include pharyngitis, asthma, cough, bronchitis, hoarseness, and chest pain that mimics angina. Some patients with acid reflux on esophageal pH testing do not report heartburn and note abdominal pain or other symptoms.

Some individuals with dyspepsia report a predominance of epigastric pain or burning that is intermittent and not generalized or localized to other regions. Others experience a postprandial distress syndrome characterized by fullness occurring after normal-sized meals and early satiety that prevents completion of regular meals several times weekly, with associated bloating, belching, or nausea. Functional dyspepsia overlaps with other functional bowel disorders such as irritable bowel syndrome.

The physical exam with GERD and functional dyspepsia usually is normal. In atypical GERD, pharyngeal erythema and wheezing may be noted. Poor dentition may be seen with prolonged acid regurgitation. Functional dyspeptics may exhibit epigastric tenderness or abdominal distention.

Discrimination between functional and organic causes of indigestion mandates exclusion of selected historic and examination features. Odynophagia suggests esophageal infection, while dysphagia is worrisome for a benign or malignant esophageal blockage. Other alarming features include unexplained weight loss, recurrent vomiting, occult or gross gastrointestinal bleeding, jaundice, a palpable mass or adenopathy, and a family history of gastrointestinal malignancy.

DIAGNOSTIC TESTING As indigestion is prevalent and because most cases result from GERD or functional dyspepsia, a general principle is to perform only limited and directed diagnostic testing of selected individuals.

TABLE 39-3 ALARM SYMPTOMS IN GERD

Odynophagia
Unexplained weight loss
Recurrent vomiting
Occult or gross gastrointestinal bleeding
Jaundice
Palpable mass or adenopathy
Family history of gastrointestinal malignancy

Once alarm factors are excluded (Table 39-3), patients with typical GERD do not need further evaluation and are treated empirically. Upper endoscopy is indicated to exclude mucosal injury in cases with atypical symptoms, symptoms unresponsive to acid suppressing drugs, or alarm factors. For heartburn >5 years in duration, especially in patients >50 years old, endoscopy is recommended to screen for Barrett's metaplasia. However, the clinical benefits and cost-effectiveness of this approach have not been validated in controlled studies. Ambulatory esophageal pH testing using a catheter method or an implanted esophageal capsule device is considered for drug-refractory symptoms and atypical symptoms like unexplained chest pain. Esophageal manometry most commonly is ordered when surgical treatment of GERD is considered. A low LES pressure may predict failure of drug therapy and helps select patients who may require surgery. Demonstration of disordered esophageal body peristalsis may affect the decision to operate or modify the type of operation chosen. Manometry with provocative testing may clarify the diagnosis in patients with atypical symptoms. Blind perfusion of saline and then acid into the esophagus, known as the *Bernstein test*, can delineate whether unexplained chest discomfort results from acid reflux.

Upper endoscopy is performed as the initial diagnostic test in patients with unexplained dyspepsia who are >55 years old or have alarm factors because of the elevated risks of malignancy and ulcer in these groups. The management approach to patients <55 years old without alarm factors is dependent on the prevalence of *H. pylori* infection in the local population. For individuals who reside in regions with low *H. pylori* prevalence (<10%), a 4-week trial of a potent acid-suppressing medication such as a proton pump inhibitor is recommended. If this fails, a "test and treat" approach is most commonly applied. *H. pylori* status is determined with urea breath testing, stool antigen measurement, or blood serology testing. Those who are *H. pylori* positive are given therapy to eradicate the infection. If symptoms resolve on either of these regimens, no further intervention is required. For patients in areas with high *H. pylori* prevalence (>10%), an initial test and treat approach is advocated, with a subsequent trial of an acid-suppressing regimen offered for those who fail *H. pylori* treatment or for those who are negative for the infection. In each of these patient subsets, upper endoscopy is reserved for those who fail to respond to therapy.

Further testing is indicated if other factors are present. If bleeding is reported, a blood count is obtained to exclude anemia. Thyroid chemistries or calcium levels screen for metabolic disease, whereas specific serologies may suggest celiac disease. For suspected pancreaticobiliary causes, pancreatic and liver chemistries are obtained. If abnormalities are found, abdominal ultrasound or CT may give important information. Gastric emptying scintigraphy is considered to exclude gastroparesis in patients whose dyspeptic symptoms resemble postprandial distress when drug treatment fails. Gastric scintigraphy also assesses for gastroparesis in patients with GERD, especially if surgical intervention is being considered. Breath testing after carbohydrate ingestion may detect lactase deficiency, intolerance to other dietary carbohydrates, or small-intestinal bacterial overgrowth.

℞ INDIGESTION

GENERAL PRINCIPLES For mild indigestion, reassurance that a careful evaluation revealed no serious organic disease may be the only intervention needed. Drugs that cause acid reflux or dyspepsia should be stopped if possible. Patients with GERD should limit ethanol, caffeine, chocolate, and tobacco use because of their effects on the LES. Other measures in GERD include ingesting a low-fat diet, avoiding snacks before bedtime, and elevating the head of the bed.

Specific therapies for organic disease should be offered when possible. Surgery is appropriate in disorders like biliary colic, while diet changes are indicated for lactase deficiency or celiac disease. Some illnesses such as peptic ulcer disease may be cured by specific medical regimens. However, as most indigestion is caused by GERD or functional dyspepsia, medications that reduce gastric acid, stimulate motility, or blunt gastric sensitivity are indicated.

ACID-SUPPRESSING OR NEUTRALIZING MEDICATIONS Drugs that reduce or neutralize gastric acid are most often prescribed for GERD. Histamine H_2 antagonists such as cimetidine, ranitidine, famotidine, and nizatidine are useful in mild to moderate GERD. For severe symptoms or many cases of erosive or ulcerative esophagitis, proton pump inhibitors such as omeprazole, lansoprazole, rabeprazole, pantoprazole, or esomeprazole are needed. These drugs, which inhibit gastric H^+, K^+-ATPase activity, are more potent than H_2 antagonists. Acid suppressants may be taken continuously or on demand depending on symptom severity. Many patients initially started on a proton pump inhibitor can be stepped down to an H_2 antagonist. Combination therapy with a proton pump inhibitor and an H_2 antagonist has been proposed for some refractory cases.

Acid-suppressing drugs are also effective in appropriately selected patients with functional dyspepsia. Meta-analysis of eight controlled trials calculated a risk ratio of 0.86, with a 95% confidence interval of 0.78–0.95, favoring proton pump inhibitor therapy over placebo. The benefits of less potent acid reducing therapies such as H_2 antagonists are unproven.

Liquid antacids are useful for short-term control of mild GERD but are less effective for severe disease unless given at high doses that elicit side effects (diarrhea and constipation with magnesium- and aluminum-containing agents, respectively). Alginic acid in combination with antacids may form a floating barrier to acid reflux in individuals with upright symptoms. Sucralfate is a salt of aluminum hydroxide and sucrose octasulfate that buffers acid and binds pepsin and bile salts. Its efficacy in GERD is felt to be comparable to that of H_2 antagonists.

***HELICOBACTER PYLORI* ERADICATION** *H. pylori* eradication is clearly indicated only for peptic ulcer and mucosa-associated lymphoid tissue gastric lymphoma. The utility of eradication therapy in functional dyspepsia is less well established, but <15% of cases relate to this infection. Meta-analysis of 13 controlled trials calculated a risk ratio of 0.91, with a 95% confidence interval of 0.87–0.96, favoring *H. pylori* eradication therapy over placebo. Several drug combinations show efficacy in eliminating the infection (Chap. 287); most include 10–14 days of a proton pump inhibitor or bismuth subsalicylate in concert with two antibiotics. *H. pylori* infection is associated with reduced prevalence of GERD, especially in the elderly. However, eradication of the infection does not worsen GERD symptoms. To date, no consensus recommendations regarding *H. pylori* eradication in GERD patients have been offered.

GASTROINTESTINAL MOTOR STIMULANTS Motor stimulants (also known as prokinetics) such as metoclopramide, erythromycin, domperidone, and tegaserod have limited utility in GERD. The γ-aminobutyric acid B (GABA-B) agonist baclofen reduces esophageal acid exposure by inhibiting transient LES relaxations; the clinical benefits of this drug are yet to be defined in large trials. Several studies have evaluated the effectiveness of motor-stimulating drugs in functional dyspepsia; however, convincing evidence of their benefits has not been found. Some clinicians suggest that patients with symptoms resembling postprandial distress may respond preferentially to prokinetic drugs.

OTHER OPTIONS Antireflux surgery (fundoplication) is offered to GERD patients who are young and may require lifelong therapy, have typical heartburn and regurgitation, and are responsive to proton pump inhibitors. Individuals who may respond less well to operative therapy include those with atypical symptoms, those with poor response to proton pump inhibitors, and those who have esophageal motor disturbances. Fundoplications are performed laparoscopically when possible and include the Nissen and Toupet procedures in which the proximal stomach is partly or completely wrapped around the distal esophagus to increase LES pressure. Dysphagia, gas-bloat syndrome, and gastroparesis may be long-term complications of these procedures. Endoscopic therapies for increasing the barrier function of the gastroesophageal junction, including radiofrequency energy delivery, suturing, biopolymer implantation, and gastroplication, have been investigated in patients with refractory GERD with variable results and some adverse consequences.

Some patients with functional heartburn and functional dyspepsia refractory to standard therapies may respond to low-dose tricyclic antidepressants. Their mechanism of action is unknown but may involve blunting of visceral pain processing in the brain. Gas and bloating are among the most troubling symptoms in some patients with indigestion and can be difficult to treat. Dietary exclusion of gas-producing foods such as legumes and use of simethicone or activated charcoal provide symptom benefits in some patients. Therapies that modify gut flora, including antibiotics and probiotic preparations containing active bacterial cultures, are useful for cases of bacterial overgrowth and functional lower gastrointestinal disorders, but their utility in functional dyspepsia is unproven. Psychological treatments may be offered for refractory functional dyspepsia, but no convincing data suggest their efficacy.

FURTHER READINGS

ABELL TL et al: Treatment of gastroparesis: A multidisciplinary clinical review. Neurogastroenterol Motil 18:263, 2006

DEVAULT KR, CASTELL DO: American College of Gastroenterology. Updated guidelines for the diagnosis and treatment of gastroesophageal reflux disease. Am J Gastroenterol 100:190, 2005

GALMICHE JP et al: Functional esophageal disorders. Gastroenterology 130:1459, 2006

HASLER WL, CHEY WD: Nausea and vomiting. Gastroenterology 125:1860, 2003

KAHRILAS PJ, LEE TJ: Pathophysiology of gastroesophageal reflux disease. Thor Surg Clin 15:323, 2005

PARKMAN HP et al: American Gastroenterological Association technical review on the diagnosis and treatment of gastroparesis. Gastroenterology 127:1592, 2004

SCHWARTZBERG LS: Chemotherapy-induced nausea and vomiting: Clinician and patient perspectives. J Support Oncol 5(suppl 1):5, 2007

TACK J et al: Functional gastroduodenal disorders. Gastroenterology 130:1466, 2006

TALLEY NJ et al: American Gastroenterological Association technical review on the evaluation of dyspepsia. Gastroenterology 129:1756, 2005

TALLEY NJ et al: Guidelines for the management of dyspepsia. Am J Gastroenterol 100:2324, 2005

40 Diarrhea and Constipation

Michael Camilleri, Joseph A. Murray

Diarrhea and constipation are exceedingly common and together exact an enormous toll in terms of mortality, morbidity, social inconvenience, loss of work productivity, and consumption of medical resources. Worldwide, >1 billion individuals suffer one or more episodes of acute diarrhea each year. Among the 100 million persons affected annually by acute diarrhea in the United States, nearly half must restrict activities, 10% consult physicians, ~250,000 require hospitalization, and ~5000 die (primarily the elderly). The annual economic burden to society may exceed $20 billion. Acute infectious diarrhea remains one of the most common causes of mortality in developing countries, particularly among children, accounting for 2–3 million deaths per year. Constipation, by contrast, is rarely associated with mortality and is exceedingly common in developed countries, leading to frequent self-medication and, in a third of those, to medical consultation. Population statistics on chronic diarrhea and constipation are more uncertain, perhaps due to variable definitions and reporting, but the frequency of these conditions is also high. United States population surveys put prevalence rates for chronic diarrhea at 2–7% and for chronic constipation at 12–19%, with women being affected twice as often as men. Diarrhea and constipation are among the most common patient complaints faced by internists and primary care physicians, and they account for nearly 50% of referrals to gastroenterologists.

Although diarrhea and constipation may present as mere nuisance symptoms at one extreme, they can be severe or life-threatening at the other. Even mild symptoms may signal a serious underlying gastrointestinal lesion, such as colorectal cancer, or systemic disorder, such as thyroid disease. Given the heterogeneous causes and potential severity of these common complaints, it is imperative for clinicians to appreciate the pathophysiology, etiologic classification, diagnostic strategies, and principles of management of diarrhea and constipation, so that rational and cost-effective care can be delivered.

NORMAL PHYSIOLOGY

While the primary function of the small intestine is the digestion and assimilation of nutrients from food, the small intestine and colon together perform important functions that regulate the secretion and absorption of water and electrolytes, the storage and subsequent transport of intraluminal contents aborally, and the salvage of some nutrients after bacterial metabolism of carbohydrate that are not absorbed in the small intestine. The main motor functions are summarized in Table 40-1. Alterations in fluid and electrolyte handling contribute significantly to diarrhea. Alterations in motor and sensory functions of the colon result in highly prevalent syndromes such as irritable bowel syndrome (IBS), chronic diarrhea, and chronic constipation.

NEURAL CONTROL

The small intestine and colon have intrinsic and extrinsic innervation. The *intrinsic innervation*, also called the enteric nervous system, comprises myenteric, submucosal, and mucosal neuronal layers. The function of these layers is modulated by interneurons through the actions of neurotransmitter amines or peptides, including acetylcholine, vasoactive intestinal peptide (VIP), opioids, norepinephrine, serotonin, ATP, and nitric oxide. The myenteric plexus regulates smooth-muscle function, and the submucosal plexus affects secretion, absorption, and mucosal blood flow.

The *extrinsic innervations* of the small intestine and colon are part of the autonomic nervous system and also modulate motor and secretory functions. The parasympathetic nerves convey visceral sensory and excitatory pathways to the colon. Parasympathetic fibers via the vagus nerve reach the small intestine and proximal colon along the branches of the superior mesenteric artery. The distal colon is supplied by sacral parasympathetic nerves (S_{2-4}) via the pelvic plexus; these fibers course through the wall of the colon as ascending intracolonic fibers as far as, and in some instances including, the proximal colon. The chief excitatory neurotransmitters controlling motor function are acetylcholine and the tachykinins, such as substance P. The sympathetic nerve supply modulates motor functions and reaches the small intestine and colon alongside their arterial vessels. Sympathetic input to the gut is generally excitatory to sphincters and inhibitory to nonsphincteric muscle. Visceral afferents convey sensation from the gut to the central nervous system; initially, they course along sympathetic fibers, but as they approach the spinal cord they separate, have cell bodies in the dorsal root ganglion, and enter the dorsal horn of the spinal cord. Afferent signals are conveyed to the brain along the lateral spinothalamic tract and the nociceptive dorsal column pathway and are then projected beyond the thalamus and brainstem to the insula and cerebral cortex to be perceived. Other afferent fibers synapse in the prevertebral ganglia and reflexly modulate intestinal motility.

TABLE 40-1 NORMAL GASTROINTESTINAL MOTILITY: FUNCTIONS AT DIFFERENT ANATOMIC LEVELS

Stomach and small bowel
Synchronized MMCs in fasting
Accommodation, trituration, mixing, transit
Stomach ~3 h
Small bowel ~3 h
Ileal reservoir empties boluses
Colon: irregular mixing, fermentation, absorption, transit
Ascending, transverse: reservoirs
Descending: conduit
Sigmoid/rectum: volitional reservoir

Note: MMC, migrating motor complex.

INTESTINAL FLUID ABSORPTION AND SECRETION

On an average day, 9 L of fluid enter the gastrointestinal (GI) tract; ~1 L of residual fluid reaches the colon; the stool excretion of fluid constitutes about 0.2 L/d. The colon has a large capacitance and functional reserve and may recover up to four times its usual volume of 0.8 L/d, provided the rate of flow permits reabsorption to occur. Thus, the colon can partially compensate for excess fluid delivery to the colon because of intestinal absorptive or secretory disorders.

In the colon, sodium absorption is predominantly electrogenic, and uptake takes place at the apical membrane; it is compensated for by the export functions of the basolateral sodium pump. A variety of neural and non-neural mediators regulate colonic fluid and electrolyte balance, including cholinergic, adrenergic, and serotonergic mediators. Angiotensin and aldosterone also influence colonic absorption, reflecting the common embryologic development of the distal colonic epithelium and the renal tubules.

SMALL-INTESTINAL MOTILITY

During fasting, the motility of the small intestine is characterized by a cyclical event called the migrating motor complex (MMC), which serves to clear nondigestible residue from the small intestine (the intestinal "housekeeper"). This organized, propagated series of contractions lasts on average 4 min, occurs every 60–90 min, and usually involves the entire small intestine. After food ingestion, the small intestine produces irregular, mixing contractions of relatively low amplitude, except in the distal ileum where more powerful contractions occur intermittently and empty the ileum by bolus transfers.

ILEOCOLONIC STORAGE AND SALVAGE

The distal ileum acts as a reservoir, emptying intermittently by bolus movements. This action allows time for salvage of fluids, electrolytes, and nutrients. Segmentation by haustra compartmentalizes the colon and facilitates mixing, retention of residue, and formation of solid stools. There is increased appreciation of the intimate interaction between the colonic function and the luminal ecology. The resident bacteria in the colon are necessary for the digestion of unabsorbed carbohydrates that reach the colon even in health, thereby providing a vital source of nutrients to the mucosa. Normal colonic flora also keeps pathogens at bay by a variety of mechanisms. In health, the ascending and transverse regions of colon function as reservoirs (average transit, 15 h), and the descending colon acts as a conduit (average transit, 3 h). The colon is efficient at conserving sodium and water, a function that is particularly important in sodium-depleted patients in whom the small intestine alone is unable to maintain sodium balance. Diarrhea or constipation may result from alteration in the reservoir function of the proximal colon or the propulsive function of the left colon. Constipation may also result from disturbances of the rectal or sigmoid reservoir, typically as a result of dysfunction of the pelvic floor or the coordination of defecation.

COLONIC MOTILITY AND TONE

The small intestinal MMC only rarely continues into the colon. However, short duration or phasic contractions mix colonic contents, and high-amplitude (>75 mmHg) propagated contractions (HAPCs) are sometimes associated with mass movements through the colon and normally occur approximately five times per day, usually on awakening in the morning and postprandially. Increased frequency of HAPCs may result in diarrhea or urgency. The predominant phasic contractions in the colon are irregular and nonpropagated and serve a "mixing" function.

Colonic tone refers to the background contractility upon which phasic contractile activity (typically contractions lasting <15 s) is superimposed. It is an important cofactor in the colon's capacitance (volume accommodation) and sensation.

COLONIC MOTILITY AFTER MEAL INGESTION

After meal ingestion, colonic phasic and tonic contractility increase for a period of ~2 h. The initial phase (~10 min) is mediated by the vagus nerve in response to mechanical distention of the stomach. The subsequent response of the colon requires caloric stimulation and is mediated at least in part by hormones, e.g., gastrin and serotonin.

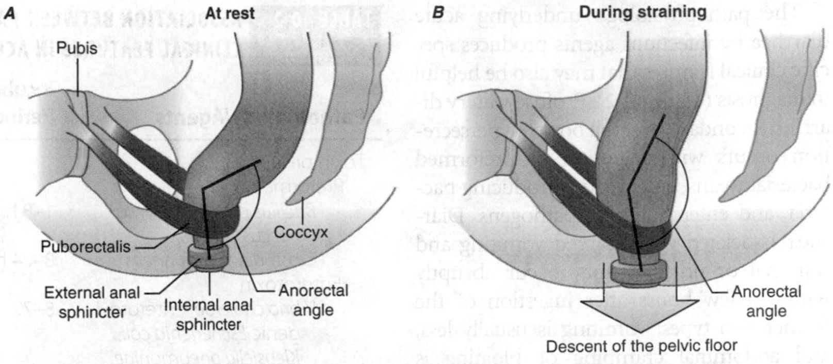

FIGURE 40-1 Sagittal view of the anorectum (*A*) at rest and (*B*) during straining to defecate. Continence is maintained by normal rectal sensation and tonic contraction of the internal anal sphincter and the puborectalis muscle, which wraps around the anorectum, maintaining an anorectal angle between 80° and 110°. During defecation, the pelvic floor muscles (including the puborectalis) relax, allowing the anorectal angle to straighten by at least 15°, and the perineum descends by 1.0–3.5 cm. The external anal sphincter also relaxes and reduces pressure on the anal canal. *(Reproduced with permission from Lembo and Camilleri.)*

DEFECATION

Tonic contraction of the puborectalis muscle, which forms a sling around the rectoanal junction, is important to maintain continence; during defecation, sacral parasympathetic nerves relax this muscle, facilitating the straightening of the rectoanal angle (Fig. 40-1). Distention of the rectum results in transient relaxation of the internal anal sphincter via intrinsic and reflex sympathetic innervation. As sigmoid and rectal contractions increase the pressure within the rectum, the rectosigmoid angle opens by >15°. Voluntary relaxation of the external anal sphincter (striated muscle innervated by the pudendal nerve) in response to the sensation produced by distention permits the evacuation of feces; this evacuation process can be augmented by an increase in intra-abdominal pressure created by the Valsalva maneuver. Defecation can also be delayed voluntarily by contraction of the external anal sphincter.

DIARRHEA

DEFINITION

Diarrhea is loosely defined as passage of abnormally liquid or unformed stools at an increased frequency. For adults on a typical Western diet, stool weight >200 g/d can generally be considered diarrheal. Diarrhea may be further defined as *acute* if <2 weeks, *persistent* if 2–4 weeks, and *chronic* if >4 weeks in duration.

Two common conditions, usually associated with the passage of stool totaling <200 g/d, must be distinguished from diarrhea, as diagnostic and therapeutic algorithms differ. *Pseudodiarrhea*, or the frequent passage of small volumes of stool, is often associated with rectal urgency and accompanies IBS or proctitis. *Fecal incontinence* is the involuntary discharge of rectal contents and is most often caused by neuromuscular disorders or structural anorectal problems. Diarrhea and urgency, especially if severe, may aggravate or cause incontinence. Pseudodiarrhea and fecal incontinence occur at prevalence rates comparable to or higher than that of chronic diarrhea and should always be considered in patients complaining of "diarrhea." Overflow diarrhea may occur in nursing home patients due to fecal impaction that is readily detectable by rectal examination. A careful history and physical examination generally allow these conditions to be discriminated from true diarrhea.

ACUTE DIARRHEA

More than 90% of cases of acute diarrhea are caused by infectious agents; these cases are often accompanied by vomiting, fever, and abdominal pain. The remaining 10% or so are caused by medications, toxic ingestions, ischemia, and other conditions.

Infectious Agents Most infectious diarrheas are acquired by fecal-oral transmission or, more commonly, via ingestion of food or water contaminated with pathogens from human or animal feces. In the immunocompetent person, the resident fecal microflora, containing >500 taxonomically distinct species, are rarely the source of diarrhea and may actually play a role in suppressing the growth of ingested pathogens. Disturbances of flora by antibiotics can lead to diarrhea by reducing the digestive function or by allowing the overgrowth of pathogens, such as *Clostridium difficile* (Chap. 123). Acute infection or injury occurs when the ingested agent overwhelms the host's mucosal immune and nonimmune (gastric acid, digestive enzymes, mucus secretion, peristalsis, and suppressive resident flora) defenses. Established clinical associations with specific enteropathogens may offer diagnostic clues.

In the United States, five high-risk groups are recognized:

1. *Travelers.* Nearly 40% of tourists to endemic regions of Latin America, Africa, and Asia develop so-called traveler's diarrhea, most commonly due to enterotoxigenic or enteroaggregative *Escherichia coli* as well as to *Campylobacter*, *Shigella*, *Aeromonas*, norovirus, *Coronavirus* and *Salmonella.* Visitors to Russia (especially St. Petersburg) may have increased risk of *Giardia*-associated diarrhea; visitors to Nepal may acquire *Cyclospora*. Campers, backpackers, and swimmers in wilderness areas may become infected with *Giardia*. Cruise ships may be affected by outbreaks of gastroenteritis caused by agents such as Norwalk virus.
2. *Consumers of certain foods.* Diarrhea closely following food consumption at a picnic, banquet, or restaurant may suggest infection with *Salmonella*, *Campylobacter*, or *Shigella* from chicken; enterohemorrhagic *E. coli* (O157:H7) from undercooked hamburger; *Bacillus cereus* from fried rice; *Staphylococcus aureus* or *Salmonella* from mayonnaise or creams; *Salmonella* from eggs; and *Vibrio* species, *Salmonella*, or acute hepatitis A from seafood, especially if raw.
3. *Immunodeficient persons.* Individuals at risk for diarrhea include those with either primary immunodeficiency (e.g., IgA deficiency, common variable hypogammaglobulinemia, chronic granulomatous disease) or the much more common secondary immunodeficiency states (e.g., AIDS, senescence, pharmacologic suppression). Common enteric pathogens often cause a more severe and protracted diarrheal illness, and, particularly in persons with AIDS, opportunistic infections, such as by *Mycobacterium* species, certain viruses (cytomegalovirus, adenovirus, and herpes simplex), and protozoa (*Cryptosporidium*, *Isospora belli*, Microsporida, and *Blastocystis hominis*) may also play a role (Chap. 182). In patients with AIDS, agents transmitted venereally per rectum (e.g., *Neisseria gonorrhoeae*, *Treponema pallidum*, *Chlamydia*) may contribute to proctocolitis. Persons with hemochromatosis are especially prone to invasive, even fatal, enteric infections with *Vibrio* species and *Yersinia* infections and should avoid raw fish.
4. *Daycare attendees and their family members.* Infections with *Shigella*, *Giardia*, *Cryptosporidium*, rotavirus, and other agents are very common and should be considered.
5. *Institutionalized persons.* Infectious diarrhea is one of the most frequent categories of nosocomial infections in many hospitals and long-term care facilities; the causes are a variety of microorganisms but most commonly *C. difficile.*

The pathophysiology underlying acute diarrhea by infectious agents produces specific clinical features that may also be helpful in diagnosis (Table 40-2). Profuse watery diarrhea secondary to small bowel hypersecretion occurs with ingestion of preformed bacterial toxins, enterotoxin-producing bacteria, and enteroadherent pathogens. Diarrhea associated with marked vomiting and minimal or no fever may occur abruptly within a few hours after ingestion of the former two types; vomiting is usually less, and abdominal cramping or bloating is greater; fever is higher with the latter. Cytotoxin-producing and invasive microorganisms all cause high fever and abdominal pain. Invasive bacteria and *Entamoeba histolytica* often cause bloody diarrhea (referred to as *dysentery*). *Yersinia* invades the terminal ileal and proximal colon mucosa and may cause especially severe abdominal pain with tenderness mimicking acute appendicitis.

Finally, infectious diarrhea may be associated with systemic manifestations. Reiter's syndrome (arthritis, urethritis, and conjunctivitis) may accompany or follow infections by *Salmonella*, *Campylobacter*, *Shigella*, and *Yersinia*. Yersiniosis may also lead to an autoimmune-type thyroiditis, pericarditis, and glomerulonephritis. Both enterohemorrhagic *E. coli* (O157:H7) and *Shigella* can lead to the *hemolytic-uremic syndrome* with an attendant high mortality rate. The syndrome of postinfectious IBS has now been recognized as a complication of infectious diarrhea. Acute diarrhea can also be a major symptom of several systemic infections including *viral hepatitis*, *listeriosis*, *legionellosis*, and *toxic shock syndrome*.

TABLE 40-2 ASSOCIATION BETWEEN PATHOBIOLOGY OF CAUSATIVE AGENTS AND CLINICAL FEATURES IN ACUTE INFECTIOUS DIARRHEA

Pathobiology/Agents	Incubation Period	Vomiting	Abdominal Pain	Fever	Diarrhea
Toxin producers					
Preformed toxin					
Bacillus cereus, *Staphylococcus aureus*,	1–8 h	3–4+	1–2+	0–1+	3–4+, watery
Clostridium perfringens	8–24 h				
Enterotoxin					
Vibrio cholerae, enterotoxigenic *Escherichia coli*, *Klebsiella pneumoniae*, *Aeromonas* species	8–72 h	2–4+	1–2+	0–1+	3–4+, watery
Enteroadherent					
Enteropathogenic and enteroadherent *E. coli*, *Giardia* organisms, cryptosporidiosis, helminths	1–8 d	0–1+	1–3+	0–2+	1–2+, watery, mushy
Cytotoxin-producers					
Clostridium difficile	1–3 d	0–1+	3–4+	1–2+	1–3+, usually watery, occasionally bloody
Hemorrhagic *E. coli*	12–72 h	0–1+	3–4+	1–2+	1–3+, initially watery, quickly bloody
Invasive organisms					
Minimal inflammation					
Rotavirus and Norwalk agent	1–3 d	1–3+	2–3+	3–4+	1–3+, watery
Variable inflammation					
Salmonella, *Campylobacter*, and *Aeromonas* species, *Vibrio parahaemolyticus*, *Yersinia*	12 h–11 d	0–3+	2–4+	3–4+	1–4+, watery or bloody
Severe inflammation					
Shigella species, enteroinvasive *E. coli*, *Entamoeba histolytica*	12 h–8 d	0–1+	3–4+	3–4+	1–2+, bloody

Source: Adapted from DW Powell, in T Yamada (ed): *Textbook of Gastroenterology and Hepatology*, 4th ed. Philadelphia, Lippincott Williams & Wilkins, 2003; and DR Syndman, in SL Gorbach (ed): *Infectious Diarrhea*. London, Blackwell, 1986.

Other Causes Side effects from medications are probably the most common noninfectious cause of acute diarrhea, and etiology may be suggested by a temporal association between use and symptom onset. Although innumerable medications may produce diarrhea, some of the more frequently incriminated include antibiotics, cardiac antidysrhythmics, antihypertensives, nonsteroidal anti-inflammatory drugs (NSAIDs), certain antidepressants, chemotherapeutic agents, bronchodilators, antacids, and laxatives. Occlusive or nonocclusive *ischemic colitis* typically occurs in persons >50 years; often presents as acute lower abdominal pain preceding watery, then bloody diarrhea; and generally results in acute inflammatory changes in the sigmoid or left colon while sparing the rectum. Acute diarrhea may accompany colonic *diverticulitis* and *graft-versus-host disease*. Acute diarrhea, often associated with systemic compromise, can follow ingestion of toxins including organophosphate insecticides, amanita and other mushrooms, arsenic, and preformed environmental toxins in seafood, such as ciguatera and scombroid. Conditions causing chronic diarrhea can also be confused with acute diarrhea early in their course. This confusion may occur with inflammatory bowel disease (IBD) and some of the other inflammatory chronic diarrheas that may have an abrupt rather than insidious onset and exhibit features that mimic infection.

APPROACH TO THE PATIENT: Acute Diarrhea

The decision to evaluate acute diarrhea depends on its severity and duration and on various host factors (Fig. 40-2). Most episodes of acute diarrhea are mild and self-limited and do not justify the cost and potential morbidity of diagnostic or pharmacologic interventions. Indications for evaluation include profuse diarrhea with dehydration, grossly bloody stools, fever ≥ 38.5° C, duration > 48 h without improvement, recent antibiotic use, new community outbreaks, associated severe abdominal pain in patients >50 years, and elderly (≥70 years) or immunocompromised patients. In some cases of moderately severe febrile diarrhea associated with fecal leukocytes (or increased fecal levels of the leukocyte proteins) or with gross blood, a diagnostic evaluation might be avoided in favor of an empirical antibiotic trial (see below).

The cornerstone of diagnosis in those suspected of severe acute infectious diarrhea is microbiologic analysis of the stool. Workup includes cultures for bacterial and viral pathogens, direct inspection for ova and parasites, and immunoassays for certain bacterial toxins (*C. difficile*), viral antigens (rotavirus), and protozoal antigens (*Giardia*, *E. histolytica*). The aforementioned clinical and epidemiologic associations may assist in focusing the evaluation. If a particular pathogen or set of possible pathogens is so implicated, then either the whole panel of routine studies may not be necessary or, in some instances, special cultures may be appropriate as for enterohemorrhagic and other types of *E. coli*, *Vibrio* species, and *Yersinia*. Molecular diagnosis of pathogens in stool can be made by identification of unique DNA sequences; and evolving microarray technologies could lead to a more rapid, sensitive, specific, and cost-effective diagnostic approach in the future.

Persistent diarrhea is commonly due to *Giardia* (Chap. 202), but additional causative organisms that should be considered include *C. difficile* (especially if antibiotics had been administered), *E. his-*

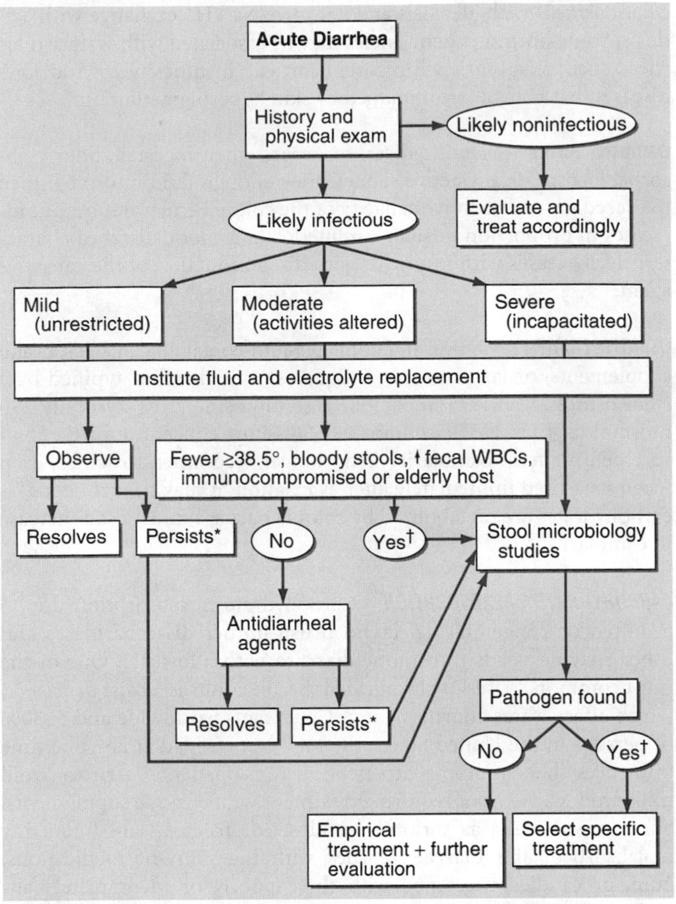

FIGURE 40-2 Algorithm for the management of acute diarrhea. Consider empirical Rx before evaluation with (*) metronidazole and with (†) quinolone. WBCs, white blood cells.

tolytica, *Cryptosporidium*, *Campylobacter*, and others. If stool studies are unrevealing, then flexible sigmoidoscopy with biopsies and upper endoscopy with duodenal aspirates and biopsies may be indicated. Brainerd diarrhea is an increasingly recognized entity characterized by an abrupt-onset diarrhea that persists for at least 4 weeks, but may last 1–3 years, and is thought to be of infectious origin. It may be associated with subtle inflammation of the distal small intestine or proximal colon.

Structural examination by sigmoidoscopy, colonoscopy, or abdominal CT scanning (or other imaging approaches) may be appropriate in patients with uncharacterized persistent diarrhea to exclude IBD, or as an initial approach in patients with suspected noninfectious acute diarrhea such as might be caused by ischemic colitis, diverticulitis, or partial bowel obstruction.

℞ ACUTE DIARRHEA

Fluid and electrolyte replacement are of central importance to all forms of acute diarrhea. Fluid replacement alone may suffice for mild cases. Oral sugar-electrolyte solutions (sport drinks or designed formulations) should be instituted promptly with severe diarrhea to limit dehydration, which is the major cause of death. Profoundly dehydrated patients, especially infants and the elderly, require IV rehydration.

In moderately severe nonfebrile and nonbloody diarrhea, antimotility and antisecretory agents such as loperamide can be useful adjuncts to control symptoms. Such agents should be avoided with febrile dysentery, which may be exacerbated or prolonged by them. Bismuth subsalicylate may reduce symptoms of vomiting and diarrhea but should not be used to treat immunocompromised patients or those with renal impairment because of the risk of bismuth encephalopathy.

Judicious use of antibiotics is appropriate in selected instances of acute diarrhea and may reduce its severity and duration (Fig. 40-2). Many physicians treat moderately to severely ill patients with febrile dysentery empirically without diagnostic evaluation using a quinolone, such as ciprofloxacin (500 mg bid for 3–5 d). Empirical treatment can also be considered for suspected giardiasis with metronidazole (250 mg qid for 7 d). Selection of antibiotics and dosage regimens are otherwise dictated by specific pathogens, geographic patterns of resistance, and conditions found (Chaps. 122, 143, and 146–152). Antibiotic coverage is indicated whether or not a causative organism is discovered in patients who are immunocompromised, have mechanical heart valves or recent vascular grafts, or are elderly. Antibiotic prophylaxis is indicated for certain patients traveling to high-risk countries in whom the likelihood or seriousness of acquired diarrhea would be especially high, including those with immunocompromise, IBD, hemochromatosis, or gastric achlorhydria. Use of trimethoprim/sulfamethoxazole, ciprofloxacin, or rifaximin may reduce bacterial diarrhea in such travelers by 90%, though rifaximin may not be suitable for invasive disease. Finally, physicians should be vigilant to identify if an outbreak of diarrheal illness is occurring and to alert the public health authorities promptly. This may reduce the ultimate size of the affected population.

CHRONIC DIARRHEA

Diarrhea lasting >4 weeks warrants evaluation to exclude serious underlying pathology. In contrast to acute diarrhea, most of the causes of chronic diarrhea are noninfectious. The classification of chronic diarrhea by pathophysiologic mechanism facilitates a rational approach to management, though many diseases cause diarrhea by more than one mechanism (Table 40-3).

Secretory Causes Secretory diarrheas are due to derangements in fluid and electrolyte transport across the enterocolonic mucosa. They are characterized clinically by watery, large-volume fecal outputs that are typically painless and persist with fasting. Because there is no malab-

TABLE 40-3 MAJOR CAUSES OF CHRONIC DIARRHEA ACCORDING TO PREDOMINANT PATHOPHYSIOLOGIC MECHANISM

Secretory causes Exogenous stimulant laxatives Chronic ethanol ingestion Other drugs and toxins Endogenous laxatives (dihydroxy bile acids) Idiopathic secretory diarrhea Certain bacterial infections Bowel resection, disease, or fistula (↓ absorption) Partial bowel obstruction or fecal impaction Hormone-producing tumors (carcinoid, VIPoma, medullary cancer of thyroid, mastocytosis, gastrinoma, colorectal villous adenoma) Addison's disease Congenital electrolyte absorption defects **Osmotic causes** Osmotic laxatives (Mg^{2+}, PO_4^{-3}, SO_4^{-2}) Lactase and other disaccharide deficiencies Nonabsorbable carbohydrates (sorbitol, lactulose, polyethylene glycol) **Steatorrheal causes** Intraluminal maldigestion (pancreatic exocrine insufficiency, bacterial overgrowth, bariatric surgery, liver disease) Mucosal malabsorption (celiac sprue, Whipple's disease, infections, abetalipoproteinemia, ischemia) Post-mucosal obstruction (1° or 2° lymphatic obstruction)	**Inflammatory causes** Idiopathic inflammatory bowel disease (Crohn's, chronic ulcerative colitis) Lymphocytic and collagenous colitis Immune-related mucosal disease (1° or 2° immunodeficiencies, food allergy, eosinophilic gastroenteritis, graft-vs-host disease) Infections (invasive bacteria, viruses, and parasites, Brainerd diarrhea) Radiation injury Gastrointestinal malignancies **Dysmotile causes** Irritable bowel syndrome (including post-infectious IBS) Visceral neuromyopathies Hyperthyroidism Drugs (prokinetic agents) Postvagotomy **Factitial causes** Munchausen Eating disorders **Iatrogenic causes** Cholecystectomy Ileal resection Bariatric surgery Vagotomy, fundoplication

sorbed solute, stool osmolality is accounted for by normal endogenous electrolytes with no fecal osmotic gap.

MEDICATIONS Side effects from regular ingestion of drugs and toxins are the most common secretory causes of chronic diarrhea. Hundreds of prescription and over-the-counter medications (see "Other Causes of Acute Diarrhea," above) may produce unwanted diarrhea. Surreptitious or habitual use of stimulant laxatives [e.g., senna, cascara, bisacodyl, ricinoleic acid (castor oil)] must also be considered. Chronic ethanol consumption may cause a secretory-type diarrhea due to enterocyte injury with impaired sodium and water absorption as well as rapid transit and other alterations. Inadvertent ingestion of certain environmental toxins (e.g., arsenic) may lead to chronic rather than acute forms of diarrhea. Certain bacterial infections may occasionally persist and be associated with a secretory-type diarrhea.

BOWEL RESECTION, MUCOSAL DISEASE, OR ENTEROCOLIC FISTULA These conditions may result in a secretory-type diarrhea because of inadequate surface for reabsorption of secreted fluids and electrolytes. Unlike other secretory diarrheas, this subset of conditions tends to worsen with eating. With disease (e.g., Crohn's ileitis) or resection of <100 cm of terminal ileum, dihydroxy bile acids may escape absorption and stimulate colonic secretion (cholorrheic diarrhea). This mechanism may contribute to so-called *idiopathic secretory diarrhea,* in which bile acids are functionally malabsorbed from a normal-appearing terminal ileum. Partial bowel obstruction, ostomy stricture, or fecal impaction may paradoxically lead to increased fecal output due to fluid hypersecretion.

HORMONES Although uncommon, the classic examples of secretory diarrhea are those mediated by hormones. *Metastatic gastrointestinal carcinoid tumors* or, rarely, *primary bronchial carcinoids* may produce watery diarrhea alone or as part of the carcinoid syndrome that comprises episodic flushing, wheezing, dyspnea, and right-sided valvular heart disease. Diarrhea is due to the release into the circulation of potent intestinal secretagogues including serotonin, histamine, prostaglandins, and various kinins. Pellagra-like skin lesions may rarely occur as the result of serotonin overproduction with niacin depletion. *Gastrinoma,* one of the most common neuroendocrine tumors, most typically presents with refractory peptic ulcers, but diarrhea occurs in up to one-third of cases and may be the only clinical manifestation in 10%. While other secretagogues released with gastrin may play a role, the diarrhea most often results from fat maldigestion owing to pancreatic enzyme inactivation by low intraduodenal pH. The watery diarrhea hypokalemia achlorhydria syndrome, also called *pancreatic cholera,* is due to a non-β cell pancreatic adenoma, referred to as a *VIPoma,* that secretes VIP and a host of other peptide hormones including pancreatic polypeptide, secretin, gastrin, gastrin-inhibitory polypeptide (also called glucose-dependent insulinotropic peptide), neurotensin, calcitonin, and prostaglandins. The secretory diarrhea is often massive with stool volumes >3 L/d; daily volumes as high as 20 L have been reported. Life-threatening dehydration; neuromuscular dysfunction from associated hypokalemia, hypomagnesemia, or hypercalcemia; flushing; and hyperglycemia may accompany a VIPoma. *Medullary carcinoma of the thyroid* may present with watery diarrhea caused by calcitonin, other secretory peptides, or prostaglandins. This tumor occurs sporadically or, in 25–50% of cases, as a feature of multiple endocrine neoplasia type 2a with pheochromocytomas and hyperparathyroidism. Prominent diarrhea is often associated with metastatic disease and poor prognosis. *Systemic mastocytosis,* which may be associated with the skin lesion urticaria pigmentosa, may cause diarrhea that is either secretory, and mediated by histamine, or inflammatory due to intestinal infiltration by mast cells. Large *colorectal villous adenomas* may rarely be associated with a secretory diarrhea that may cause hypokalemia, can be inhibited by NSAIDs, and is apparently mediated by prostaglandins.

CONGENITAL DEFECTS IN ION ABSORPTION Rarely, defects in specific carriers associated with ion absorption cause watery diarrhea from birth, and these disorders include defective Cl^-/HCO_3^- exchange (*congenital chloridorrhea*) with alkalosis and defective Na^+/H^+ exchange with acidosis. Some hormone deficiencies may be associated with watery diarrhea, such as occurs with adrenocortical insufficiency (Addison's disease) that may be accompanied by skin hyperpigmentation.

Osmotic Causes Osmotic diarrhea occurs when ingested, poorly absorbable, osmotically active solutes draw enough fluid into the lumen to exceed the reabsorptive capacity of the colon. Fecal water output increases in proportion to such a solute load. Osmotic diarrhea characteristically ceases with fasting or with discontinuation of the causative agent.

OSMOTIC LAXATIVES Ingestion of magnesium-containing antacids, health supplements, or laxatives may induce osmotic diarrhea typified by a stool osmotic gap (>50 mosmol/L): serum osmolarity (typically 290 mosmol/kg)[2 × (fecal sodium + potassium concentration)]. Measurement of fecal osmolarity is no longer recommended since, even when measured immediately after evacuation, it may be erroneous, as carbohydrates are metabolized by colonic bacteria, causing an increase in osmolarity.

CARBOHYDRATE MALABSORPTION Carbohydrate malabsorption due to acquired or congenital defects in brush-border disaccharidases and other enzymes leads to osmotic diarrhea with a low pH. One of the most common causes of chronic diarrhea in adults is *lactase deficiency,* which affects three-fourths of non-Caucasians worldwide and 5–30% of persons in the United States; the total lactose load at any one time influences the symptoms experienced. Most patients learn to avoid milk products without requiring treatment with enzyme supplements. Some sugars, such as sorbitol, lactulose, or fructose, are frequently malabsorbed, and diarrhea ensues with ingestion of medications, gum, or candies sweetened with these poorly or incompletely absorbed sugars.

Steatorrheal Causes Fat malabsorption may lead to greasy, foul-smelling, difficult-to-flush diarrhea often associated with weight loss and nutritional deficiencies due to concomitant malabsorption of amino acids and vitamins. Increased fecal output is caused by the osmotic effects of fatty acids, especially after bacterial hydroxylation, and, to a lesser extent, by the neutral fat. Quantitatively, steatorrhea is defined as stool fat exceeding the normal 7 g/d; rapid-transit diarrhea may result in fecal fat up to 14 g/d; daily fecal fat averages 15–25 g with small intestinal diseases and is often >32 g with pancreatic exocrine insufficiency. Intraluminal maldigestion, mucosal malabsorption, or lymphatic obstruction may produce steatorrhea.

INTRALUMINAL MALDIGESTION This condition most commonly results from pancreatic exocrine insufficiency, which occurs when >90% of pancreatic secretory function is lost. *Chronic pancreatitis,* usually a sequel of ethanol abuse, most frequently causes pancreatic insufficiency. Other causes include *cystic fibrosis, pancreatic duct obstruction,* and rarely, *somatostatinoma.* Bacterial overgrowth in the small intestine may deconjugate bile acids and alter micelle formation, impairing fat digestion; it occurs with stasis from a blind-loop, small bowel diverticulum or dysmotility and is especially likely in the elderly. Finally, cirrhosis or biliary obstruction may lead to mild steatorrhea due to deficient intraluminal bile acid concentration.

MUCOSAL MALABSORPTION Mucosal malabsorption occurs from a variety of enteropathies, but most commonly from *celiac disease.* This gluten-sensitive enteropathy affects all ages and is characterized by villous atrophy and crypt hyperplasia in the proximal small bowel and can present with fatty diarrhea associated with multiple nutritional deficiencies of varying severity. Celiac disease is much more frequent than previously thought; it affects ~1% of the population, frequently presents without steatorrhea, can mimic IBS, and has many other GI and extraintestinal manifestations. *Tropical sprue* may produce a similar histologic and clinical syndrome but occurs in residents of or travelers to tropical climates; abrupt onset and response to antibiotics suggest an infectious etiology. *Whipple's disease,* due to the bacillus *Tropheryma whipplei* and histiocytic infiltration of the small-bowel mucosa, is a less common cause of steatorrhea that most typically occurs in young or middle-aged men; it is frequently associated with arthralgias, fever, lymphadenopathy, and extreme fatigue and may affect the central nervous system and endocardium. A similar clinical and histologic picture results from *Mycobacterium avium-intracellulare* infection in patients with AIDS. *Abetalipoproteinemia* is a rare defect of chylomicron formation and fat malabsorption in children, associated with acanthocytic erythrocytes, ataxia, and retinitis pigmentosa. Several other conditions may cause mucosal malabsorption including infections, especially with protozoa such as *Giardia,* numerous medications (e.g., colchicine, cholestyramine, neomycin), and chronic ischemia.

POSTMUCOSAL LYMPHATIC OBSTRUCTION The pathophysiology of this condition, which is due to the rare *congenital intestinal lymphangiectasia* or to *acquired lymphatic obstruction* secondary to trauma, tumor, or infection, leads to the unique constellation of fat malabsorption with enteric losses of protein (often causing edema) and lymphocytopenia. Carbohydrate and amino acid absorption are preserved.

Inflammatory Causes Inflammatory diarrheas are generally accompanied by pain, fever, bleeding, or other manifestations of inflammation. The mechanism of diarrhea may not only be exudation but, depending on lesion site, may include fat malabsorption, disrupted fluid/electrolyte absorption, and hypersecretion or hypermotility from release of cytokines and other inflammatory mediators. The unifying feature on stool analysis is the presence of leukocytes or leukocyte-derived proteins such as calprotectin. With severe inflammation, exudative protein loss can lead to anasarca (generalized edema). Any middle-aged or older person with chronic inflammatory-type diarrhea, especially with blood, should be carefully evaluated to exclude a colorectal tumor.

IDIOPATHIC INFLAMMATORY BOWEL DISEASE The illnesses in this category, which include *Crohn's disease* and *chronic ulcerative colitis,* are among the most common organic causes of chronic diarrhea in adults and range in severity from mild to fulminant and life-threatening. They may be associated with uveitis, polyarthralgias, cholestatic liver disease (primary sclerosing cholangitis), and skin lesions (erythema nodosum, pyoderma gangrenosum). *Microscopic colitis,* including both lymphocytic and *collagenous colitis,* is an increasingly recognized cause of chronic watery diarrhea, especially in middle-aged women and those on NSAIDS; biopsy of a normal-appearing colon is required for histologic diagnosis. It may coexist with symptoms suggesting IBS or with celiac sprue. It typically responds well to anti-inflammatory drugs (e.g., bismuth), to the opioid agonist loperamide, or to budesonide.

PRIMARY OR SECONDARY FORMS OF IMMUNODEFICIENCY Immunodeficiency may lead to prolonged infectious diarrhea. With common variable *hypogammaglobulinemia,* diarrhea is particularly prevalent and often the result of giardiasis.

EOSINOPHILIC GASTROENTERITIS Eosinophil infiltration of the mucosa, muscularis, or serosa at any level of the GI tract may cause diarrhea, pain, vomiting, or ascites. Affected patients often have an atopic history, Charcot-Leyden crystals due to extruded eosinophil contents may be seen on microscopic inspection of stool, and peripheral eosinophilia is present in 50–75% of patients. While hypersensitivity to certain foods occurs in adults, true food allergy causing chronic diarrhea is rare.

OTHER CAUSES Chronic inflammatory diarrhea may be caused by *radiation enterocolitis, chronic graft-versus-host disease, Behçet's syndrome,* and *Cronkite-Canada syndrome,* among others.

Dysmotility Causes Rapid transit may accompany many diarrheas as a secondary or contributing phenomenon, but primary dysmotility is an unusual etiology of true diarrhea. Stool features often suggest a secretory diarrhea, but mild steatorrhea of up to 14 g of fat per day can be produced by maldigestion from rapid transit alone. *Hyperthyroidism, carcinoid syndrome,* and certain drugs (e.g., prostaglandins, prokinetic agents) may produce hypermotility with resultant diarrhea. Primary visceral neuromyopathies or idiopathic acquired intestinal pseudoobstruction may lead to stasis with secondary bacterial overgrowth causing diarrhea. *Diabetic diarrhea,* often accompanied by peripheral and generalized autonomic neuropathies, may occur in part because of intestinal dysmotility.

The exceedingly common *irritable bowel syndrome* (10% point prevalence, 1–2% per year incidence) is characterized by disturbed intestinal and colonic motor and sensory responses to various stimuli. Symptoms of stool frequency typically cease at night, alternate with periods of constipation, are accompanied by abdominal pain relieved with defecation, and rarely result in weight loss or true diarrhea.

Factitial Causes Factitial diarrhea accounts for up to 15% of unexplained diarrheas referred to tertiary care centers. Either as a form of *Munchausen syndrome* (deception or self-injury for secondary gain) or *eating disorders,* some patients covertly self-administer laxatives alone or in combination with other medications (e.g., diuretics) or surreptitiously add water or urine to stool sent for analysis. Such patients are typically women, often with histories of psychiatric illness and disproportionately from careers in health care. Hypotension and hypokalemia are common co-presenting features. The evaluation of such patients may be difficult: contamination of the stool with water or urine is suggested by very low or high stool osmolarity, respectively. Such patients often deny this possibility when confronted, but they do benefit from psychiatric counseling when they acknowledge their behavior.

APPROACH TO THE PATIENT: Chronic Diarrhea

The laboratory tools available to evaluate the very common problem of chronic diarrhea are extensive, and many are costly and invasive. As such, the diagnostic evaluation must be rationally directed by a careful history and physical examination (Fig. 40-3*A*). When this strategy is unrevealing, simple triage tests are often warranted to direct the choice of more complex investigations (Fig. 40-3*B*). The history, physical examination (Table 40-4), and routine blood studies should attempt to characterize the mechanism of diarrhea, identify diagnostically helpful associations, and assess the patient's fluid/electrolyte and nutritional status. Patients should be questioned about the onset, duration, pattern, aggravating (especially diet) and relieving factors, and stool characteristics of their diarrhea. The presence or absence of fecal incontinence, fever, weight loss, pain, certain exposures (travel, medications, contacts with diarrhea), and common extraintestinal manifestations (skin changes, arthralgias, oral aphthous ulcers) should be noted. A family history of IBD or sprue may indicate those possibilities. Physical findings may offer clues such as a thyroid mass, wheezing, heart murmurs, edema, hepatomegaly, abdominal masses, lymphadenopathy, mucocutaneous abnormalities, perianal fistulae, or anal sphincter laxity. Peripheral blood leukocytosis, elevated sedimentation rate, or C-reactive protein suggests inflammation; anemia reflects blood loss or nutritional deficiencies; or eosinophilia may occur with parasitoses, neoplasia, collagen-vascular disease, allergy, or eosinophilic gastroenteritis. Blood chemistries may demonstrate electrolyte, hepatic, or other metabolic disturbances. Measuring tissue transglutaminase antibodies may help detect celiac disease.

A therapeutic trial is often appropriate, definitive, and highly cost effective when a specific diagnosis is suggested on the initial physician encounter. For example, chronic watery diarrhea, which ceases with fasting in an otherwise healthy young adult, may justify a trial of a lactose-restricted diet; bloating and diarrhea persisting since a mountain backpacking trip may warrant a trial of metronidazole for likely giardiasis; and postprandial diarrhea persisting

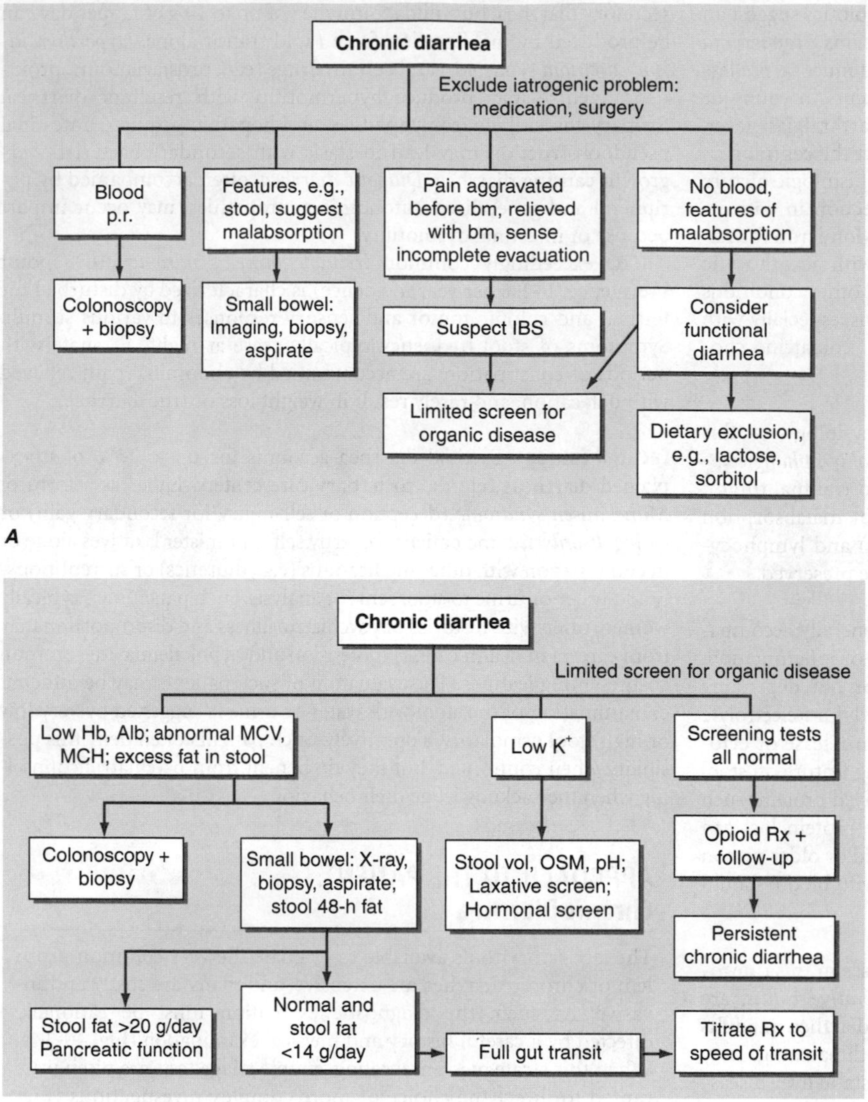

FIGURE 40-3 Chronic diarrhea. ***A.*** Initial management based on accompanying symptoms or features. ***B.*** Evaluation based on findings from a limited age appropriate screen for organic disease. p.r., per rectum; bm, bowel movement; IBS, irritable bowel syndrome; Hb, hemoglobin; Alb, albumin; MCV, mean corpuscular volume; MCH, mean corpuscular hemoglobin; OSM, osmolality. *(Reprinted from M Camilleri: Clin Gastroenterol Hepatol. 2:198, 2004.)*

since an ileal resection might be due to bile acid malabsorption and be treated with cholestyramine before further evaluation. Persistent symptoms require additional investigation.

Certain diagnoses may be suggested on the initial encounter, e.g., idiopathic IBD; however, additional focused evaluations may be necessary to confirm the diagnosis and characterize the severity or extent of disease so that treatment can be best guided. Patients suspected of having IBS should be initially evaluated with flexible sigmoidoscopy with colorectal biopsies; those with normal findings might be reassured and, as indicated, treated empirically with antispasmodics, antidiarrheals, bulk agents, anxiolytics, or antidepressants. Any patient who presents with chronic diarrhea and hematochezia should be evaluated with stool microbiologic studies and colonoscopy.

In an estimated two-thirds of cases, the cause for chronic diarrhea remains unclear after the initial encounter, and further testing is required. Quantitative stool collection and analyses can yield important objective data that may establish a diagnosis or characterize the type of diarrhea as a triage for focused additional studies (Fig. 40-3*B*). If stool weight is >200 g/d, additional stool analyses should be performed that might include electrolyte concentration, pH, occult blood testing, leukocyte inspection (or leukocyte protein assay), fat quantitation, and laxative screens.

For secretory diarrheas (watery, normal osmotic gap), possible medication-related side effects or surreptitious laxative use should be reconsidered. Microbiologic studies should be done including fecal bacterial cultures (including media for *Aeromonas* and *Pleisiomonas*), inspection for ova and parasites, and *Giardia* antigen assay (the most sensitive test for giardiasis). Small-bowel bacterial overgrowth can be excluded by intestinal aspirates with quantitative cultures or with glucose or lactulose breath tests involving measurement of breath hydrogen, methane, or other metabolite (e.g., $^{14}CO_2$). However, interpretation of these breath tests may be confounded by disturbances of intestinal transit. When suggested by history or other findings, screens for peptide hormones should be pursued (e.g., serum gastrin, VIP, calcitonin, and thyroid hormone/thyroid-stimulating hormone, or urinary 5-hydroxyindolacetic acid and histamine). Upper endoscopy and colonoscopy with biopsies and small-bowel barium x-rays are helpful to rule out structural or occult inflammatory disease.

Further evaluation of osmotic diarrhea should include tests for lactose intolerance and magnesium ingestion, the two most common causes. Low fecal pH suggests carbohydrate malabsorption; lactose malabsorption can be confirmed by lactose breath testing or by a therapeutic trial with lactose exclusion and observation of the effect of lactose challenge (e.g., a liter of milk). Lactase determination on small-bowel biopsy is generally not available. If fecal magnesium or laxative levels are elevated, then inadvertent or surreptitious ingestion should be considered and psychiatric help should be sought.

For those with proven fatty diarrhea, endoscopy with small-bowel biopsy (including aspiration for *Giardia* and quantitative cultures) should be performed; if this procedure is unrevealing, a small-bowel radiograph is often an appropriate next step. If small-bowel studies are negative or if pancreatic disease is suspected, pancreatic exocrine insufficiency should be excluded with direct tests, such as the secretin-cholecystokinin stimulation test or a variation that could be performed endoscopically. In general, indirect tests such as assay of fecal chymotrypsin activity or a bentiromide test have fallen out of favor because of low sensitivity and specificity.

TABLE 40-4 PHYSICAL EXAMINATION IN PATIENTS WITH CHRONIC DIARRHEA

1. Are there general features to suggest malabsorption or inflammatory bowel disease (IBD) such as anemia, dermatitis herpetiformis, edema, or clubbing?
2. Are there features to suggest underlying autonomic neuropathy or collagen-vascular disease in the pupils, orthostasis, skin, hands, or joints?
3. Is there an abdominal mass or tenderness?
4. Are there any abnormalities of rectal mucosa, rectal defects, or altered anal sphincter functions?
5. Are there any mucocutaneous manifestations of systemic disease such as dermatitis herpetiformis (celiac disease), erythema nodosum (ulcerative colitis), flushing (carcinoid), or oral ulcers for IBD or celiac disease?

Chronic inflammatory-type diarrheas should be suspected by the presence of blood or leukocytes in the stool. Such findings warrant stool cultures, inspection for ova and parasites, *C. difficile* toxin assay, colonoscopy with biopsies, and, if indicated, small-bowel contrast studies.

℞ CHRONIC DIARRHEA

Treatment of chronic diarrhea depends on the specific etiology and may be curative, suppressive, or empirical. If the cause can be eradicated, treatment is curative as with resection of a colorectal cancer, antibiotic administration for Whipple's disease, or discontinuation of a drug. For many chronic conditions, diarrhea can be controlled by suppression of the underlying mechanism. Examples include elimination of dietary lactose for lactase deficiency or gluten for celiac sprue, use of glucocorticoids or other anti-inflammatory agents for idiopathic IBDs, adsorptive agents such as cholestyramine for ileal bile acid malabsorption, proton pump inhibitors such as omeprazole for the gastric hypersecretion of gastrinomas, somatostatin analogues such as octreotide for malignant carcinoid syndrome, prostaglandin inhibitors such as indomethacin for medullary carcinoma of the thyroid, and pancreatic enzyme replacement for pancreatic insufficiency. When the specific cause or mechanism of chronic diarrhea evades diagnosis, empirical therapy may be beneficial. Mild opiates, such as diphenoxylate or loperamide, are often helpful in mild or moderate watery diarrhea. For those with more severe diarrhea, codeine or tincture of opium may be beneficial. Such antimotility agents should be avoided with IBD, as toxic megacolon may be precipitated. Clonidine, an α_2-adrenergic agonist, may allow control of diabetic diarrhea. For all patients with chronic diarrhea, fluid and electrolyte repletion is an important component of management (see "Acute Diarrhea," above). Replacement of fat-soluble vitamins may also be necessary in patients with chronic steatorrhea.

CONSTIPATION

DEFINITION

Constipation is a common complaint in clinical practice and usually refers to persistent, difficult, infrequent, or seemingly incomplete defecation. Because of the wide range of normal bowel habits, constipation is difficult to define precisely. Most persons have at least three bowel movements per week; however, low stool frequency alone is not the sole criterion for the diagnosis of constipation. Many constipated patients have a normal frequency of defecation but complain of excessive straining, hard stools, lower abdominal fullness, or a sense of incomplete evacuation. The individual patient's symptoms must be analyzed in detail to ascertain what is meant by "constipation" or "difficulty" with defecation.

Stool form and consistency are well correlated with the time elapsed from the preceding defecation. Hard, pellety stools occur with slow transit, while loose watery stools are associated with rapid transit. Both small pellety or very large stools are more difficult to expel than normal stools.

The perception of hard stools or excessive straining is more difficult to assess objectively, and the need for enemas or digital disimpaction is a clinically useful way to corroborate the patient's perceptions of difficult defecation.

Psychosocial or cultural factors may also be important. A person whose parents attached great importance to daily defecation will become greatly concerned when he or she misses a daily bowel movement; some children withhold stool to gain attention or because of fear of pain from anal irritation; and some adults habitually ignore or delay the call to have a bowel movement.

CAUSES

Pathophysiologically, chronic constipation generally results from inadequate fiber or fluid intake or from disordered colonic transit or anorectal function. These result from neurogastroenterologic disturbance, certain drugs, advancing age, or in association with a large number of systemic diseases that affect the gastrointestinal tract (Table 40-5). Constipation of recent onset may be a symptom of significant organic disease such as tumor or stricture. In *idiopathic constipation*, a subset of patients exhibit delayed emptying of the ascending and transverse colon with prolongation of transit (often in the proximal colon) and a reduced frequency of propulsive HAPCs. *Outlet obstruction to defecation* (also called *evacuation disorders*) may cause delayed colonic transit, which is usually corrected by biofeedback retraining of the disordered defecation. Constipation of any cause may be exacerbated by hospitalization or chronic illnesses that lead to physical or mental impairment and result in inactivity or physical immobility.

TABLE 40-5 CAUSES OF CONSTIPATION IN ADULTS

Types of Constipation and Causes	Examples
Recent onset	
Colonic obstruction	Neoplasm; stricture: ischemic, diverticular, inflammatory
Anal sphincter spasm	Anal fissure, painful hemorrhoids
Medications	
Chronic	
Irritable bowel syndrome	Constipation-predominant, alternating
Medications	Ca^{2+} blockers, antidepressants
Colonic pseudo-obstruction	Slow-transit constipation, megacolon (rare Hirschsprung's, Chagas)
Disorders of rectal evacuation	Pelvic floor dysfunction; anismus; descending perineum syndrome; rectal mucosal prolapse; rectocele
Endocrinopathies	Hypothyroidism, hypercalcemia, pregnancy
Psychiatric disorders	Depression, eating disorders, drugs
Neurologic disease	Parkinsonism, multiple sclerosis, spinal cord injury
Generalized muscle disease	Progressive systemic sclerosis

APPROACH TO THE PATIENT: Constipation

A careful history should explore the patient's symptoms and confirm whether he or she is indeed constipated based on frequency (e.g., fewer than three bowel movements per week), consistency (lumpy/hard), excessive straining, prolonged defecation time, or need to support the perineum or digitate the anorectum. In the vast majority of cases (probably >90%), there is no underlying cause (e.g., cancer, depression, or hypothyroidism), and constipation responds to ample hydration, exercise, and supplementation of dietary fiber (15–25 g/d). A good diet and medication history and attention to psychosocial issues are key. Physical examination and, particularly, a rectal examination should exclude fecal impaction and most of the important diseases that present with constipation and possibly indicate features suggesting an evacuation disorder (e.g., high anal sphincter tone).

The presence of weight loss, rectal bleeding, or anemia with constipation mandates either flexible sigmoidoscopy plus barium enema or colonoscopy alone, particularly in patients >40 years, to exclude structural diseases such as cancer or strictures. Colonoscopy alone is most cost effective in this setting since it provides an opportunity to biopsy mucosal lesions, perform polypectomy, or dilate strictures. Barium enema has advantages over colonoscopy in the patient with isolated constipation, since it is less costly and identifies colonic dilatation and all significant mucosal lesions or strictures that are likely to present with constipation. Melanosis coli, or pigmentation of the colon mucosa, indicates the use of anthraquinone laxatives such as cascara or senna; however, this is usually apparent from a careful history. An unexpected disorder such as megacolon or cathartic colon may also be detected by colonic radiographs. Measurement of serum calcium, potassium, and thyroid-stimulating hormone levels will identify rare patients with metabolic disorders.

Patients with more troublesome constipation may not respond to fiber alone and may be helped by a bowel training regimen: tak-

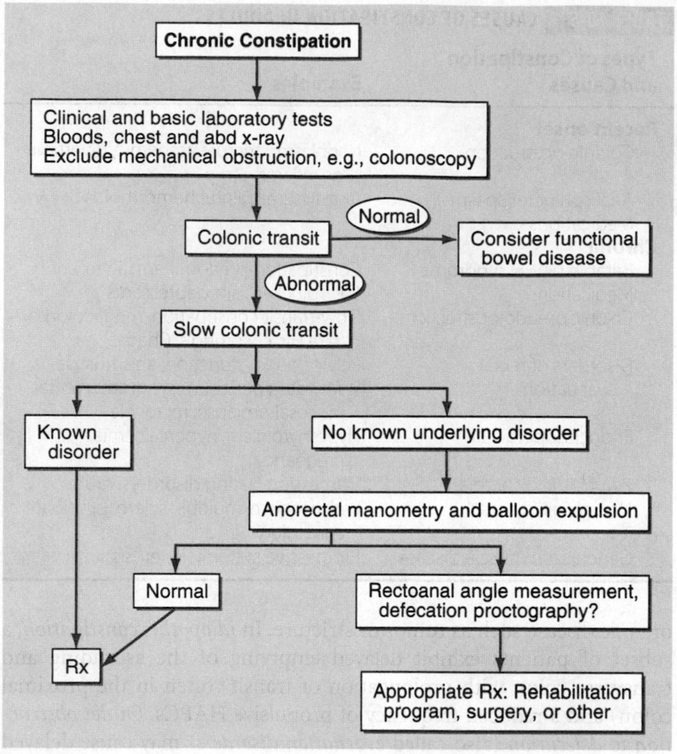

FIGURE 40-4 Algorithm for the management of constipation.

ing an osmotic laxative (lactulose, sorbitol, polyethylene glycol) and evacuating with enema or glycerine suppository as needed. After breakfast, a distraction-free 15–20 min on the toilet without straining is encouraged. Excessive straining may lead to development of hemorrhoids, and, if there is weakness of the pelvic floor or injury to the pudendal nerve, may result in obstructed defecation from descending perineum syndrome several years later. Those few who do not benefit from the simple measures delineated above or require long-term treatment with potent laxatives with the attendant risk of developing laxative abuse syndrome are assumed to have severe or intractable constipation and should have further investigation (Fig. 40-4). Novel agents that induce secretion (e.g., lubiprostone, a chloride channel activator) are also available.

INVESTIGATION OF SEVERE CONSTIPATION

A small minority (probably <5%) of patients have severe or "intractable" constipation. These are the patients most likely to be seen by gastroenterologists or in referral centers. Further observation of the patient may occasionally reveal a previously unrecognized cause, such as an evacuation disorder, laxative abuse, malingering, or psychological disorder. In these patients, evaluations of the physiologic function of the colon and pelvic floor and of psychological status aid in the rational choice of treatment. Even among these highly selected patients with severe constipation, a cause can be identified in only about two-thirds of tertiary referral patients (see below).

Measurement of Colonic Transit Radiopaque marker transit tests are easy, repeatable, generally safe, inexpensive, reliable, and highly applicable in evaluating constipated patients in clinical practice. Several validated methods are very simple. For example, radiopaque markers are ingested; an abdominal flat film taken 5 days later should indicate passage of 80% of the markers out of the colon without the use of laxatives or enemas. This test does not provide useful information about the transit profile of the stomach and small bowel.

Radioscintigraphy with a delayed-release capsule containing radiolabeled particles has been used to noninvasively characterize normal, accelerated, or delayed colonic function over 24–48 h with low radiation exposure. This approach simultaneously assesses gastric, small bowel (which may be important in ~20% of patients with delayed colonic transit since they reflect a more generalized GI motility disorder), and colonic transit. The disadvantages are the greater cost and the need for specific materials prepared in a nuclear medicine laboratory.

Anorectal and Pelvic Floor Tests Pelvic floor dysfunction is suggested by the inability to evacuate the rectum, a feeling of persistent rectal fullness, rectal pain, the need to extract stool from the rectum digitally, application of pressure on the posterior wall of the vagina, support of the perineum during straining, and excessive straining. These significant symptoms should be contrasted with the sense of incomplete rectal evacuation, which is common in IBS.

Formal psychological evaluation may identify eating disorders, "control issues," depression, or post-trauma stress disorders that may respond to cognitive or other intervention and may be important in restoring quality of life to patients who might present with chronic constipation.

A simple clinical test in the office to document a nonrelaxing puborectalis muscle is to have the patient strain to expel the index finger during a digital rectal examination. Motion of the puborectalis posteriorly during straining indicates proper coordination of the pelvic floor muscles.

Measurement of perineal descent is relatively easy to gauge clinically by placing the patient in the left decubitus position and watching the perineum to detect inadequate descent (<1.5 cm, a sign of pelvic floor dysfunction) or perineal ballooning during straining relative to bony landmarks (>4 cm, suggesting excessive perineal descent).

A useful overall test of evacuation is the balloon expulsion test. A balloon-tipped urinary catheter is placed and inflated with 50 mL of water. Normally, a patient can expel it while seated on a toilet or in the left lateral decubitus position. In the lateral position, the weight needed to facilitate expulsion of the balloon is determined; normally expulsion occurs with <200 g added.

Anorectal manometry when used in the evaluation of patients with severe constipation may find an excessively high resting (>80 mmHg) or squeeze anal sphincter tone, suggesting anismus (anal sphincter spasm). This test also identifies rare syndromes, such as adult Hirschsprung's disease, by the absence of the rectoanal inhibitory reflex.

Defecography (a dynamic barium enema including lateral views obtained during barium expulsion) reveals "soft abnormalities" in many patients; the most relevant findings are the measured changes in rectoanal angle, anatomic defects of the rectum such as internal mucosal prolapse, and enteroceles or rectoceles. Surgically remediable conditions are identified in only a few patients. These include severe, whole-thickness intussusception with complete outlet obstruction due to funnel-shaped plugging at the anal canal or an extremely large rectocele that fills preferentially during attempts at defecation instead of expulsion of the barium through the anus. In summary, defecography requires an interested and experienced radiologist, and abnormalities are not pathognomonic for pelvic floor dysfunction. The most common cause of outlet obstruction is failure of the puborectalis muscle to relax; this is not identified by defecography but requires a dynamic study such as proctography. MRI is being developed as an alternative and provides more information about the structure and function of the pelvic floor, distal colorectum, and anal sphincters.

Dynamic imaging studies such as proctography during defecation or scintigraphic expulsion of artificial stool help measure perineal descent and the rectoanal angle during rest, squeezing, and straining, and scintigraphic expulsion quantitates the amount of "artificial stool" emptied. Lack of straightening of the rectoanal angle by at least 15° during defecation confirms pelvic floor dysfunction.

Neurologic testing (electromyography) is more helpful in the evaluation of patients with incontinence than of those with symptoms suggesting obstructed defecation. The absence of neurologic signs in the lower extremities suggests that any documented denervation of the puborectalis results from pelvic (e.g., obstetric) injury or from stretching of the pudendal nerve by chronic, long-standing straining. Constipation is common among patients with spinal cord injuries, neurologic diseases such as Parkinson's disease, multiple sclerosis, and diabetic neuropathy.

Spinal-evoked responses during electrical rectal stimulation or stimulation of external anal sphincter contraction by applying magnetic stimulation over the lumbosacral cord identify patients with limited sacral neuropathies with sufficient residual nerve conduction to attempt biofeedback training.

In summary, a balloon expulsion test is an important screening test for anorectal dysfunction. If positive, an anatomic evaluation of the rectum or anal sphincters and an assessment of pelvic floor relaxation are the tools for evaluating patients in whom obstructed defecation is suspected.

℞ CONSTIPATION

After the cause of constipation is characterized, a treatment decision can be made. Slow-transit constipation requires aggressive medical or surgical treatment; anismus or pelvic floor dysfunction usually responds to biofeedback management (Fig. 40-4). However, only ~60% of patients with severe constipation are found to have such a physiologic disorder (half with colonic transit delay and half with evacuation disorder). Patients with spinal cord injuries or other neurologic disorders require a dedicated bowel regime that often includes rectal stimulation, enema therapy, and carefully timed laxative therapy.

Patients with slow-transit constipation are treated with bulk, osmotic, prokinetic, secretory, and stimulant laxatives including fiber, psyllium, milk of magnesia, lactulose, polyethylene glycol (colonic lavage solution), lubiprostone, and bisacodyl. Newer treatment aimed at enhancing motility and secretion may have application in circumstances such as constipation-predominant IBS in females or severe constipation. If a 3- to 6-month trial of medical therapy fails and patients continue to have documented slow-transit constipation unassociated with obstructed defecation, the patients should be considered for laparoscopic colectomy with ileorectostomy; however, this should not be undertaken if there is continued evidence of an evacuation disorder or a generalized GI dysmotility. Referral to a specialized center for further tests of colonic motor function is warranted. The decision to resort to surgery is facilitated in the presence of megacolon and megarectum. The complications after surgery include small-bowel obstruction (11%) and fecal soiling, particularly at night during the first postoperative year. Frequency of defecation is 3–8 per day during the first year, dropping to 1–3 per day from the second year after surgery.

Patients who have a combined (evacuation and transit/motility) disorder should pursue pelvic floor retraining (biofeedback and muscle relaxation), psychological counseling, and dietetic advice first, followed by colectomy and ileorectosomy if colonic transit studies do not normalize and symptoms are intractable despite biofeedback and optimized medical therapy. In patients with pelvic floor dysfunction alone, biofeedback training has a 70–80% success rate, measured by the acquisition of comfortable stool habits. Attempts to manage pelvic floor dysfunction with operations (internal anal sphincter or puborectalis muscle division) have achieved only mediocre success and have been largely abandoned.

FURTHER READINGS

BARTLETT JG: Narrative review: The new epidemic of *Clostridium difficile*-associated enteric disease. Ann Intern Med 145:758, 2006

CAMILLERI M: Chronic diarrhea: A review on pathophysiology and management for the clinical gastroenterologist. Clin Gastroenterol Hepatol 2:198, 2004

FARRELL RJ, KELLY CP: Celiac sprue. N Engl J Med 346:180, 2002

GADEWAR S, FASANO A: Current concepts in the evaluation, diagnosis and management of acute infectious diarrhea. Curr Opin Pharmacol 5:559, 2005

LEMBO A, CAMILLERI M: Chronic constipation. N Engl J Med 349:1360, 2003

MUSHER DM, MUSHER BL: Contagious acute gastrointestinal infections. N Engl J Med 351:2417, 2004

WALD A: Constipation in the primary care setting: Current concepts and misconceptions. Am J Med 119:736, 2006

WALD A: Clinical practice. Fecal incontinence in adults. N Engl J Med 356:1648, 2007

41 Weight Loss

Carol M. Reife

Significant unintentional weight loss in a previously healthy individual is often a harbinger of underlying systemic disease. During the routine medical examination, changes in weight should always be assessed; loss of 5% of body weight over 6–12 months should prompt further evaluation.

PHYSIOLOGY OF WEIGHT REGULATION

The normal individual maintains body weight at a remarkably stable "set point," given the wide variation in daily caloric intake and level of activity. Because of the physiologic importance of maintaining energy stores, voluntary weight loss is difficult to achieve and sustain.

Appetite and metabolism are regulated by an intricate network of neural and hormonal factors. The hypothalamic feeding and satiety centers play a central role in these processes (Chap. 74). Neuropeptides such as corticotropin-releasing hormone (CRH), α-melanocyte-stimulating hormone (α-MSH), and cocaine- and amphetamine-related transcript (CART) induce anorexia by acting centrally on satiety centers. The gastrointestinal peptides ghrelin, glucagon, somatostatin, and cholecystokinin signal satiety and thus decrease food intake. Hypoglycemia suppresses insulin, reducing glucose utilization and inhibiting the satiety center.

Leptin is produced by adipose tissue, and it plays a central role in the long-term maintenance of weight homeostasis by acting on the hypothalamus to decrease food intake and increase energy expenditure (Chap. 74). Leptin suppresses expression of hypothalamic neuropeptide Y, a potent appetite stimulatory peptide, and it increases the expression of α-MSH, which acts through the MC4R melanocortin receptor to decrease appetite. Thus, leptin activates a series of downstream neural pathways that alter food-seeking behavior and metabolism. Leptin deficiency, which occurs in conjunction with the loss of adipose tissue, stimulates appetite and induces adaptive responses including inhibition of hypothalamic thyrotropin-releasing hormone (TRH) and gonadotropin-releasing hormone (GnRH).

A variety of cytokines, including tumor necrosis factor α (TNF-α), interleukin (IL) 6 (IL-6), IL-1, interferon γ (IFN-γ), ciliary neurotrophic factor (CNTF), and leukemia inhibitory factor (LIF), can induce cachexia (Chap. 17). In addition to causing anorexia, these factors may stimulate fever, depress myocardial function, modulate immune and inflammatory responses, and induce a variety of specific metabolic alterations. TNF-α, for example, preferentially mobilizes fat but spares skeletal muscle. Levels of these cytokines may be increased in patients with cancer, sepsis, chronic inflammatory conditions, AIDS, or congestive heart failure.

Weight loss occurs when energy expenditure exceeds calories available for energy utilization (Chap. 72). In most individuals, approximately half of food energy is utilized for basal processes such as maintenance of body temperature. In a 70-kg person, basal activity consumes ~1800 kcal/d. About 40% of caloric intake is used for physical activity, although athletes may use >50% during vigorous exercise. About 10% of caloric intake is used for dietary thermogenesis, the energy expended for digestion, absorption, and metabolism of food.

Mechanisms of weight loss include decreased food intake, malabsorption, loss of calories, and increased energy requirements (Fig. 41-1). Changes in weight may involve loss of tissue mass or body fluid content. A deficit of 3500 kcal generally correlates with the loss of 0.45 kg (1 lb) of body fat, but one must also consider water weight [1 kg/L (2.2 lb/L)] gained or lost. Weight loss that persists over weeks to months reflects the loss of tissue mass.

Food intake may be influenced by a wide variety of visual, olfactory, and gustatory stimuli as well as by genetic, psychological, and social fac-

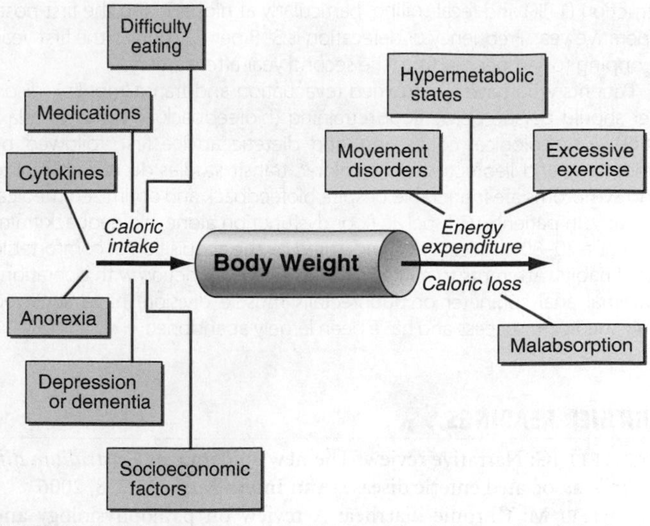

FIGURE 41-1 Energy balance and pathophysiology of weight loss.

tors. Absorption may be impaired because of pancreatic insufficiency, cholestasis, celiac sprue, intestinal tumors, radiation injury, inflammatory bowel disease, infection, or medication effect. These disease processes may be manifest as changes in stool frequency and consistency. Calories may also be lost due to vomiting or diarrhea, glucosuria in diabetes mellitus, or fistulous drainage. Resting energy expenditure decreases with age and can be affected by thyroid status. Beginning at about age 60, body weight declines by an average of 0.5% per year. Body composition is also affected by aging; adipose tissue increases and lean muscle mass decreases with age.

SIGNIFICANCE OF WEIGHT LOSS

Unintentional weight loss, especially in the elderly, is relatively common and is associated with increased morbidity and mortality rates, even after comorbid conditions have been taken into account. Prospective studies indicate that significant involuntary weight loss is associated with a mortality rate of 25% over the next 18 months. Retrospective studies of significant weight loss in the elderly document mortality rates of 9–38% over a 2- to 3-year period.

Cancer patients with weight loss have decreased performance status, impaired responses to chemotherapy, and reduced median survival (Chap. 77). Marked weight loss also predisposes to infection. Patients undergoing elective surgery, who have lost >4.5 kg (>10 lb) in 6 months, have higher surgical mortality rates. Vitamin and nutrient deficiencies may also accompany significant weight loss (Chap. 71).

CAUSES OF WEIGHT LOSS

The list of possible causes of weight loss is extensive (Table 41-1). In the elderly, the most common causes of weight loss are depression, cancer, and benign gastrointestinal disease. Lung and gastrointestinal cancer are the most common malignancies in patients presenting with weight loss. In younger individuals, diabetes mellitus, hyperthyroidism, psychiatric disturbances including eating disorders, and infection, especially with HIV, should be considered.

The cause of involuntary weight loss is rarely occult. Careful history and physical examination, in association with directed diagnostic testing, will identify the cause of weight loss in 75% of patients. The etiology of weight loss may not be found in the remaining patients, despite extensive testing. Patients with negative evaluations tend to have lower mortality rates than those found to have organic disease.

Patients with medical causes of weight loss usually have signs or symptoms that suggest involvement of a particular organ system. Gastrointestinal tumors, including those of the pancreas and liver, may affect food intake early in the course of illness, causing weight loss before other symptoms are apparent. Lung cancer may present with post-obstructive pneumonia, dyspnea, or cough and hemoptysis; however, it may be silent and should be considered even in those without a history of cigarette smoking. Depression and isolation can cause profound weight loss, especially in the elderly. Chronic pulmonary disease and congestive heart failure can produce anorexia, and they also increase resting energy expenditure. Weight loss may be the presenting sign of infectious diseases such as HIV infection, tuberculosis, endocarditis, and fungal or parasitic infections. Hyperthyroidism or pheochromocytoma increases metabolism. Elderly patients with apathetic hyperthyroidism may present with weight loss and weakness, with few other manifestations of thyrotoxicosis. New-onset diabetes mellitus is often accompanied by weight loss, reflecting glucosuria and loss of the anabolic actions of insulin. Adrenal insufficiency may be suggested by increased pigmentation, hyponatremia, and hyperkalemia.

TABLE 41-1 CAUSES OF WEIGHT LOSS

Cancer	Medications
Endocrine and metabolic	Antibiotics
Hyperthyroidism	Nonsteroidal anti-inflammatory drugs
Diabetes mellitus	Serotonin reuptake inhibitors
Pheochromocytoma	Metformin
Adrenal insufficiency	Levodopa
Gastrointestinal disorders	ACE inhibitors
Malabsorption	Other drugs
Obstruction	Disorders of the mouth and teeth
Pernicious anemia	Age-related factors
Cardiac disorders	Physiologic changes
Chronic ischemia	Decreased taste and smell
Chronic congestive heart failure	Functional disabilities
Respiratory disorders	Neurologic
Emphysema	Stroke
Chronic obstructive pulmonary disease	Parkinson's disease
Renal insufficiency	Neuromuscular disorders
Rheumatologic disease	Dementia
Infections	Social
HIV	Isolation
Tuberculosis	Economic hardship
Parasitic infection	Psychiatric and behavioral
Subacute bacterial endocarditis	Depression
	Anxiety
	Bereavement
	Alcoholism
	Eating disorders
	Increased activity or exercise
	Idiopathic

APPROACH TO THE PATIENT: Weight Loss

Before extensive evaluation is undertaken, it is important to confirm weight loss and to determine the time interval over which it has occurred. Almost half of patients who claim significant weight loss have no actual change when body weight is measured objectively. In the absence of documentation, changes in belt notch position or the fit of clothing may be confirmatory. Not infrequently, patients who have actually sustained significant weight loss are unaware that it has occurred. Routine documentation of weight during office visits is therefore important.

The review of systems should focus on signs or symptoms that are associated with disorders that commonly cause weight loss. These include fever, pain, shortness of breath or cough, palpitations, and evidence of neurologic disease. Gastrointestinal isturbances, including difficulty eating, dysphagia, anorexia, nausea, and change in bowel habits, should be sought. Travel history, use of cigarettes and alcohol, and all medications should be reviewed, and patients should be questioned about previous illness or surgery as well as diseases in family members. Risk factors for HIV infection should be assessed. Signs of depression, evidence of dementia, and social factors, including financial issues that might affect food intake, should be considered.

Physical examination should begin with weight determination and documentation of vital signs. The skin should be examined for pallor, jaundice, turgor, scars from prior surgery, and stigmata of systemic disease. The search for oral thrush or dental disease, thyroid gland enlargement, adenopathy, and respiratory or cardiac abnormalities and a detailed examination of the abdomen often lead to clues for further evaluation. Rectal examination, including prostate examination, should be performed in men; and all women should have a pelvic examination, even if they have had a hysterectomy. Neurologic examination should include mental status assessment and screening for depression.

Laboratory testing should confirm or exclude possible diagnoses elicited from the history and physical examination (Table 41-2). An initial phase of testing should include a complete blood count with differential, serum chemistry tests including glucose, electrolytes, renal and liver tests, calcium, thyroid-stimulating hormone (TSH), urinalysis, and chest x-ray. Patients at risk for HIV infection should have HIV antibody testing. In all cases, recommended cancer screening tests appropriate for the gender and age group, such as mammograms and colonoscopies, should be updated (Chap. 78).

TABLE 41-2 SCREENING TESTS FOR EVALUATION OF INVOLUNTARY WEIGHT LOSS

Initial testing	Additional testing
CBC	HIV test
Electrolytes, calcium, glucose	Upper and/or lower gastrointestinal endoscopy
Renal and liver function tests	Abdominal CT scan or MRI
Urinalysis	Chest CT scan
TSH	
Chest x-ray	
Recommended cancer screening	

If gastrointestinal signs or symptoms are present, upper and/or lower endoscopy and abdominal imaging with either CT or MRI have a relatively high yield, consistent with the high prevalence of gastrointestinal disorders in patients with weight loss. If an etiology of weight loss is not found, careful clinical follow-up, rather than persistent undirected testing, is reasonable.

FURTHER READINGS

ALIBHAI S: An approach to the management of unintentional weight loss in elderly people. CMAJ 172:773, 2005

BOURAS EP, LANGE SM: Rational approach to patients with unintentional weight loss. Mayo Clinic Proc 76:923, 2001

HERNANDEZ JL, MATORRAS JA: Involuntary weight loss without specific symptoms: A clinical prediction score for malignant neoplasm. Q J Med 96: 649, 2003

INUI A: Cancer anorexia-cachexia syndrome: Current issues in research and management. Cancer J Clinicians 52:72, 2002

NORA E, RAMAN A: Hypermetabolism, cachexia and wasting. Curr Opin Endocrinol Diabetes 12: 326, 2005

SCHWARTZ MW: Brain pathways controlling food intake and body weight. Exp Biol Med 226:978, 2001

STRASSER F, BRUERA ED: Update on anorexia and cachexia. Hematol Oncol Clin North Am 16:589, 2002

WALLACE JI: Involuntary weight loss in elderly outpatients: Recognition, etiologies, and treatment. Clin Geriatr Med 13:717, 1997

42 Gastrointestinal Bleeding

Loren Laine

Bleeding from the gastrointestinal (GI) tract may present in five ways. *Hematemesis* is vomitus of red blood or "coffee-grounds" material. *Melena* is black, tarry, foul-smelling stool. *Hematochezia* is the passage of bright red or maroon blood from the rectum. *Occult GI bleeding* (GIB) may be identified in the absence of overt bleeding by a fecal occult blood test or the presence of iron deficiency. Finally, patients may present only with *symptoms of blood loss or anemia* such as lightheadedness, syncope, angina, or dyspnea.

SOURCES OF GASTROINTESTINAL BLEEDING

Upper Gastrointestinal Sources of Bleeding (Table 42-1) The annual incidence of hospital admissions for upper GIB (UGIB) in the United States and Europe is ~0.1%, with a mortality rate of ~5–10%. Patients rarely die from exsanguination; rather, they die due to decompensation from other underlying illnesses. The mortality rate for patients <60 years in the absence of major concurrent illness is <1%. Independent predictors of rebleeding and death in patients hospitalized with UGIB include increasing age, comorbidities, and hemodynamic compromise (tachycardia or hypotension).

Peptic ulcers are the most common cause of UGIB, accounting for up to ~50% of cases; an increasing proportion is due to nonsteroidal anti-inflammatory drugs (NSAIDs), with the prevalence of *Helicobacter pylori* decreasing. Mallory-Weiss tears account for ~5–10 or 15% of cases. The proportion of patients bleeding from varices varies widely from ~5 to 30%, depending on the population. Hemorrhagic or erosive gastropathy (e.g., due to NSAIDs or alcohol) and erosive esophagitis often cause mild UGIB, but major bleeding is rare.

PEPTIC ULCERS In addition to clinical features, characteristics of an ulcer at endoscopy provide important prognostic information. One-third of patients with active bleeding or a nonbleeding visible vessel have further bleeding that requires urgent surgery if they are treated conservatively. These patients clearly benefit from endoscopic therapy with bipolar electrocoagulation, heater probe, injection therapy (e.g., absolute alcohol, 1:10,000 epinephrine), and/or clips with reductions in bleeding, hospital stay, mortality rate, and costs. In contrast, patients with clean-based ulcers have rates of recurrent bleeding approaching zero. If there is no other reason for hospitalization, such patients may be discharged on the first hospital day, following stabilization. Patients without clean-based ulcers should usually remain in the hospital for 3 days, as most episodes of recurrent bleeding occur within 3 days.

Randomized controlled trials document that a high-dose constant-infusion IV proton pump inhibitor (PPI) (e.g., omeprazole 80-mg bolus and 8-mg/h infusion), designed to sustain intragastric pH > 6 and enhance clot stability, decreases further bleeding (but not mortality), in patients with high-risk ulcers (active bleeding, nonbleeding visible vessel, adherent clot), even after appropriate endoscopic therapy. Institution of therapy at presentation in all patients with UGIB does not significantly improve outcomes such as further bleeding, transfusions, or mortality as compared to initiating therapy only when high-risk ulcers are identified at the time of endoscopy.

One-third of patients with a bleeding ulcer will rebleed within the next 1–2 years. Prevention of recurrent bleeding focuses on the three main factors in ulcer pathogenesis, *H. pylori*, NSAIDs, and acid. Eradi-

TABLE 42-1 SOURCES OF BLEEDING IN PATIENTS HOSPITALIZED FOR UPPER GI BLEEDING IN YEARS 2000–2002

Sources of Bleeding	Proportion of Patients, %
Ulcers	31–59
Varices	7–20
Mallory-Weiss tears	4–8
Gastroduodenal erosions	2–7
Erosive esophagitis	1–13
Neoplasm	2–7
Vascular ectasias	0–6
No source identified	8–14

Source: Data from M Van Leerdam et al: Am J Gastroenterol 98:1494, 2003; DM Jensen et al: Gastrointest Endosc 57:AB147, 2003; KC Thomopoulos et al: Eur J Gastroenterol Hepatol 16:177, 2004; F Di Fiore et al: Eur J Gastroenterol Hepatol 17:641, 2005.

cation of *H. pylori* in patients with bleeding ulcers decreases rates of rebleeding to <5%. If a bleeding ulcer develops in a patient taking NSAIDs, the NSAIDs should be discontinued, if possible. If NSAIDs must be continued, initial treatment should be with a PPI. Long-term preventive strategies to decrease NSAID-associated ulcers include use of a cyclooxygenase 2 (COX-2) selective inhibitor (coxib) or addition of GI co-therapy to a traditional NSAID. PPIs and misoprostol are effective co-therapies, but PPIs are more commonly used due to less frequent dosing (once daily) and fewer side effects (e.g., diarrhea). However, either PPI co-therapy alone or use of a coxib alone is associated with an annual rebleeding rate of ~10% in high-risk patients (i.e., a recent bleeding ulcer). Combination of a coxib and PPI provides a further significant decrease in ulcers and recurrent bleeding and should be employed in very high-risk patients. Patients with bleeding ulcers unrelated to *H. pylori* or NSAIDs should remain on full-dose antisecretory therapy indefinitely. Peptic ulcers are discussed in Chap. 287.

MALLORY-WEISS TEARS The classic history is vomiting, retching, or coughing preceding hematemesis, especially in an alcoholic patient. Bleeding from these tears, which are usually on the gastric side of the gastroesophageal junction, stops spontaneously in 80–90% of patients and recurs in only 0–7%. Endoscopic therapy is indicated for actively bleeding Mallory-Weiss tears. Angiographic therapy with embolization and operative therapy with oversewing of the tear are rarely required. Mallory-Weiss tears are discussed in Chap. 286.

ESOPHAGEAL VARICES Patients with variceal hemorrhage have poorer outcomes than patients with other sources of UGIB. Endoscopic therapy for acute bleeding and repeated sessions of endoscopic therapy to eradicate esophageal varices significantly reduce rebleeding and mortality. Ligation is the endoscopic therapy of choice for esophageal varices because it has less rebleeding, a lower mortality rate, fewer local complications, and requires fewer treatment sessions to achieve variceal eradication than sclerotherapy.

Octreotide (50-μg bolus and 50-μg/h IV infusion for 2–5 days) further helps in the control of acute bleeding when used in combination with endoscopic therapy. Other vasoactive agents such as somatostatin and terlipressin, available outside the United States, are also effective. Antibiotic therapy (e.g., quinolones) is also recommended for patients with cirrhosis presenting with UGIB, as antibiotics decrease bacterial infections and mortality in this population. Over the long term, treatment with nonselective beta blockers decreases recurrent bleeding from esophageal varices. Chronic therapy with beta blockers plus endoscopic ligation is recommended for prevention of recurrent esophageal variceal bleeding.

In patients who have persistent or recurrent bleeding despite endoscopic and medical therapy, more invasive therapy is warranted. Transjugular intrahepatic portosystemic shunt (TIPS) decreases rebleeding more effectively than endoscopic therapy, although hepatic encephalopathy is more common and the mortality rates are comparable. Most patients with TIPS have shunt stenosis within 1–2 years and require reintervention to maintain shunt patency, although the use of coated stents appears to markedly decrease shunt dysfunction, at least in the first year. A randomized comparison of TIPS and distal splenorenal shunt in Child-Pugh class A or B cirrhotic patients with refractory variceal bleeding revealed no significant difference in rebleeding, encephalopathy, or survival, but a much higher rate of reintervention with TIPS (82% vs. 11%). Therefore, TIPS is most appropriate in patients with more severe liver disease and those in whom transplant is anticipated. Patients with milder, well-compensated cirrhosis should require fewer re-interventions with decompressive surgery, although the higher initial risks of surgery must also be considered.

Portal hypertension is also responsible for bleeding from gastric varices, varices in the small and large intestine, and portal hypertensive gastropathy and enterocolopathy.

HEMORRHAGIC AND EROSIVE GASTROPATHY ("GASTRITIS") Hemorrhagic and erosive gastropathy, often labeled gastritis, refers to endoscopically visualized subepithelial hemorrhages and erosions. These are mucosal lesions and thus do not cause major bleeding. They develop in various clinical settings, the most important of which are NSAID use, alcohol intake, and stress. Half of patients who chronically ingest NSAIDs have erosions (15–30% have ulcers), while up to 20% of actively drinking alcoholic patients with symptoms of UGIB have evidence of subepithelial hemorrhages or erosions.

Stress-related gastric mucosal injury occurs only in extremely sick patients: those who have experienced serious trauma, major surgery, burns covering more than one-third of the body surface area, major intracranial disease, and severe medical illness (i.e., ventilator dependence, coagulopathy). Significant bleeding probably does not develop unless ulceration occurs. The mortality rate in these patients is quite high because of their serious underlying illnesses.

The incidence of bleeding from stress-related gastric mucosal injury or ulceration has decreased dramatically in recent years, most likely due to better care of critically ill patients. Pharmacologic prophylaxis for bleeding may be considered in the high-risk patients mentioned above. Multiple trials document the efficacy of intravenous H_2-receptor antagonist therapy, which is more effective than sucralfate but not superior to a PPI immediate-release suspension given via nasogastric tube. Prophylactic therapy decreases bleeding but does not lower the mortality rate.

OTHER CAUSES Other, less frequent causes of UGIB include erosive duodenitis, neoplasms, aortoenteric fistulas, vascular lesions [including hereditary hemorrhagic telangiectasias (Osler-Weber-Rendu) and gastric antral vascular ectasia ("watermelon stomach")], Dieulafoy's lesion (in which an aberrant vessel in the mucosa bleeds from a pinpoint mucosal defect), prolapse gastropathy (prolapse of proximal stomach into esophagus with retching, especially in alcoholics), and hemobilia and hemosuccus pancreaticus (bleeding from the bile duct or pancreatic duct).

Small-Intestinal Sources of Bleeding Small-intestinal sources of bleeding (bleeding from sites beyond the reach of the standard upper endoscope) are difficult to diagnose and are responsible for the majority of cases of obscure GIB. Fortunately, small-intestinal bleeding is uncommon. The most common causes are vascular ectasias and tumors (e.g., adenocarcinoma, leiomyoma, lymphoma, benign polyps, carcinoid, metastases, and lipoma). Other less common causes include Crohn's disease, infection, ischemia, vasculitis, small-bowel varices, diverticula, Meckel's diverticulum, duplication cysts, and intussusception. NSAIDs induce small-intestinal erosions and ulcers and may be a relatively common cause of chronic, obscure GIB; coxibs induce less small-intestinal injury than traditional NSAIDs.

Meckel's diverticulum is the most common cause of significant lower GIB (LGIB) in children, decreasing in frequency as a cause of bleeding with age. In adults <40–50 years, small-bowel tumors often account for obscure GIB; in patients >50–60 years, vascular ectasias are usually responsible.

Vascular ectasias should be treated with endoscopic therapy if possible. Surgical therapy can be used for vascular ectasias isolated to a segment of the small intestine when endoscopic therapy is unsuccessful. Although estrogen/progesterone compounds have been used for vascular ectasias, a double-blind trial found no benefit in prevention of recurrent bleeding. Isolated lesions, such as tumors, diverticula, or duplications, are generally treated with surgical resection.

Colonic Sources of Bleeding The incidence of hospitalizations for LGIB is about one-fifth that for UGIB. Hemorrhoids are probably the most common cause of LGIB; anal fissures also cause minor bleeding and pain. If these local anal processes, which rarely require hospitalization, are excluded, the most common causes of LGIB in adults are diverticula, vascular ectasias (especially in the proximal colon of patients >70 years), neoplasms (primarily adenocarcinoma), and colitis—most commonly infectious or idiopathic inflammatory bowel disease, but occasionally ischemic or radiation-induced. Uncommon causes include post-polypectomy bleeding, solitary rectal ulcer

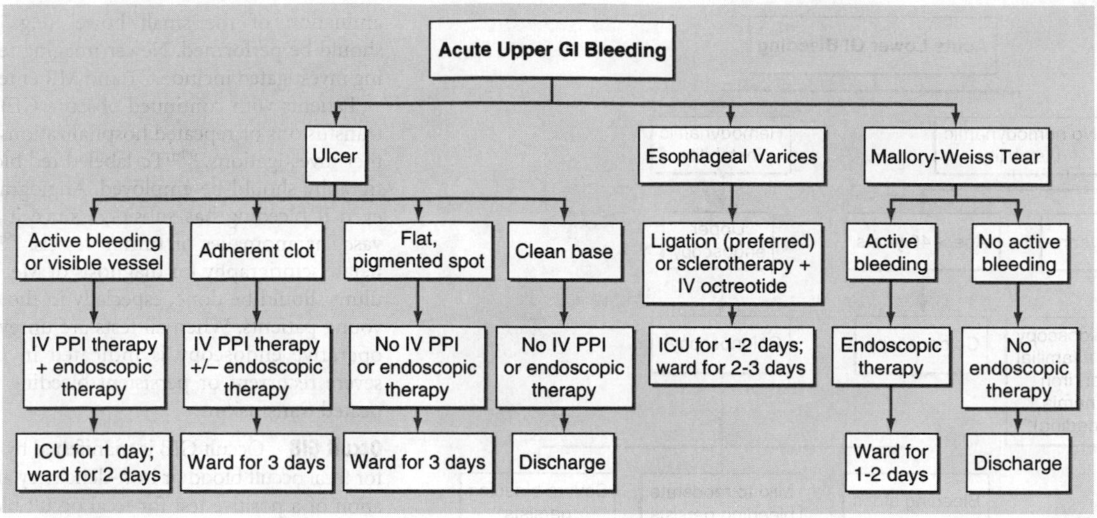

FIGURE 42-1 Suggested algorithm for patients with acute upper gastrointestinal bleeding. Recommendations on level of care and time of discharge assume patient is stabilized without further bleeding or other concomitant medical problems. PPI, proton pump inhibitor; ICU, intensive care unit.

syndrome, NSAID-induced ulcers or colitis, trauma, varices (most commonly rectal), lymphoid nodular hyperplasia, vasculitis, and aortocolic fistulas. In children and adolescents, the most common colonic causes of significant GIB are inflammatory bowel disease and juvenile polyps.

Diverticular bleeding is abrupt in onset, usually painless, sometimes massive, and often from the right colon; minor and occult bleeding is not characteristic. Clinical reports suggest that bleeding colonic diverticula stop bleeding spontaneously in ~80% of patients and rebleed in about 20–25% of patients. Intraarterial vasopressin or embolization by superselective technique should stop bleeding in a majority of patients. If bleeding persists or recurs, segmental surgical resection is indicated.

Bleeding from right colonic vascular ectasias in the elderly may be overt or occult; it tends to be chronic and only occasionally is hemodynamically significant. Endoscopic hemostatic therapy may be useful in the treatment of vascular ectasias, as well as discrete bleeding ulcers and post-polypectomy bleeding, while endoscopic polypectomy, if possible, is used for bleeding colonic polyps. Surgical therapy is generally required for major, persistent, or recurrent bleeding from the wide variety of colonic sources of GIB that cannot be treated medically, angiographically, or endoscopically.

APPROACH TO THE PATIENT: Gastrointestinal Bleeding

Measurement of the heart rate and blood pressure is the best way to assess a patient with GIB. Clinically significant bleeding leads to postural changes in heart rate or blood pressure, tachycardia, and, finally, recumbent hypotension. In contrast, the hemoglobin does not fall immediately with acute GIB, due to proportionate reductions in plasma and red cell volumes (i.e., "people bleed whole blood"). Thus, hemoglobin may be normal or only minimally decreased at the initial presentation of a severe bleeding episode. As extravascular fluid enters the vascular space to restore volume, the hemoglobin falls, but this process may take up to 72 h. Patients with slow, chronic GIB may have very low hemoglobin values despite normal blood pressure and heart rate. With the development of iron-deficiency anemia, the mean corpuscular volume will be low and red blood cell distribution width will be increased.

DIFFERENTIATION OF UPPER FROM LOWER GIB Hematemesis indicates an upper GI source of bleeding (above the ligament of Treitz). Melena indicates that blood has been present in the GI tract for at least 14 h. Thus, the more proximal the bleeding site, the more likely melena will occur. Hematochezia usually represents a lower GI source of bleeding, although an upper GI lesion may bleed so briskly that blood does not remain in the bowel long enough for melena to develop. When hematochezia is the presenting symptom of UGIB, it is associated with hemodynamic instability and dropping hemoglobin. Bleeding lesions of the small bowel may present as melena or hematochezia. Other clues to UGIB include hyperactive bowel sounds and an elevated blood urea nitrogen level (due to volume depletion and blood proteins absorbed in the small intestine).

A nonbloody nasogastric aspirate may be seen in up to 18% of patients with UGIB—usually from a duodenal source. Even a bile-stained appearance does not exclude a bleeding postpyloric lesion since reports of bile in the aspirate are incorrect in ~50% of cases. Testing of aspirates that are not grossly bloody for occult blood is not useful.

DIAGNOSTIC EVALUATION OF THE PATIENT WITH GIB **Upper GIB** (Fig. 42-1) History and physical examination are not usually diagnostic of the source of GIB. Upper endoscopy is the test of choice in patients with UGIB and should be performed urgently in patients with hemodynamic instability (hypotension, tachycardia, or postural changes in heart rate or blood pressure). Early endoscopy is also beneficial in cases of milder bleeding for management decisions. Patients with major bleeding and high-risk endoscopic findings (e.g., varices, ulcers with active bleeding or a visible vessel) benefit from endoscopic hemostatic therapy, while patients with low-risk lesions (e.g., clean-based ulcers, nonbleeding Mallory-Weiss tears, erosive or hemorrhagic gastropathy) who have stable vital signs and hemoglobin, and no other medical problems, can be discharged home.

Lower GIB (Fig. 42-2) Patients with hematochezia and hemodynamic instability should have upper endoscopy to rule out an upper GI source before evaluation of the lower GI tract. Patients with presumed LGIB may undergo early sigmoidoscopy for the detection of obvious, low-lying lesions. However, the procedure is difficult with brisk bleeding, and it is usually not possible to identify the area of bleeding. Sigmoidoscopy is useful primarily in patients <40 years with minor bleeding.

Colonoscopy after an oral lavage solution is the procedure of choice in patients admitted with LGIB unless bleeding is too massive or unless sigmoidoscopy has disclosed an obvious actively bleeding lesion. ^{99m}Tc-labeled red cell scan allows repeated imaging for up to 24 h and may identify the general location of bleeding. However, radionuclide scans should be interpreted with caution

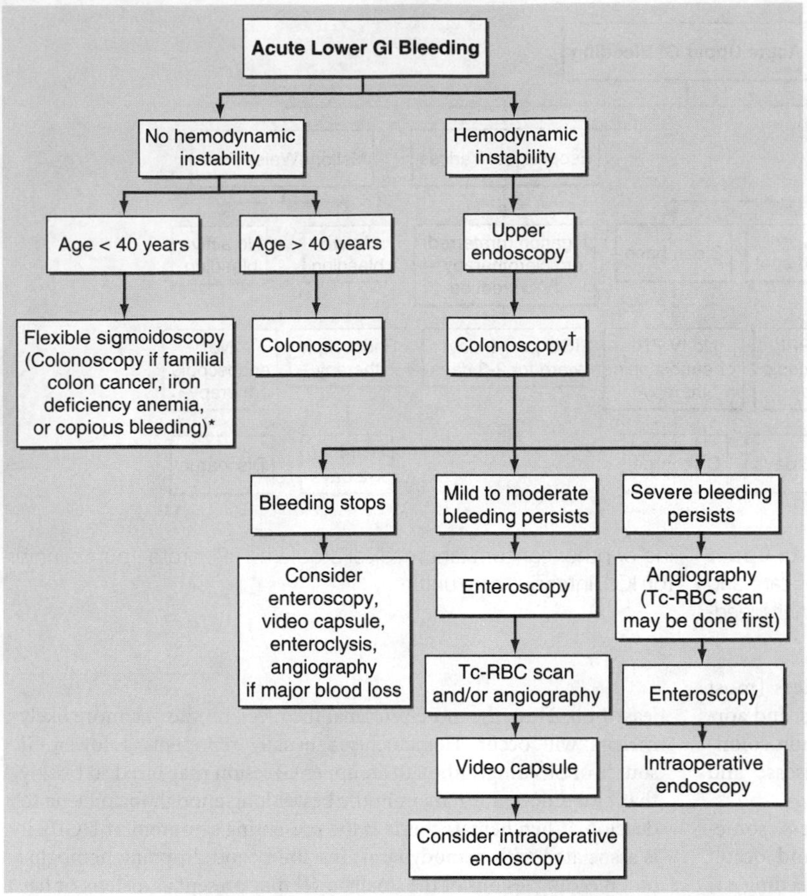

FIGURE 42-2 Suggested algorithm for patients with acute lower gastrointestinal bleeding. Sequential recommendations under "Hemodynamic instability" assume a test is found to be nondiagnostic before next test is performed. *Some suggest colonoscopy for any degree of rectal bleeding in patients <40 years as well. †If massive bleeding does not allow time for colonic lavage, proceed to angiography. Tc-RBC, ^{99m}technetium-labeled red blood cell.

because results, especially from later images, are highly variable. In active LGIB, angiography can detect the site of bleeding (extravasation of contrast into the gut) and permits treatment with intraarterial infusion of vasopressin or embolization. Even after bleeding has stopped, angiography may identify lesions with abnormal vasculature, such as vascular ectasias or tumors.

GIB of Obscure Origin Obscure GIB is defined as persistent or recurrent bleeding for which no source has been identified by routine endoscopic and contrast x-ray studies; it may be overt (e.g., melena, hematochezia) or occult. Push enteroscopy, with a specially designed enteroscope or a pediatric colonoscope to inspect the entire duodenum and part of the jejunum, is generally the next step. Push enteroscopy may identify probable bleeding sites in 20–40% of patients with obscure GIB. Video capsule endoscopy, which allows endoscopic examination of the entire small intestine, increases diagnostic yield in obscure GIB: a systematic review of 14 trials comparing push enteroscopy to capsule revealed "clinically significant findings" in 26% and 56% of patients, respectively. However, lack of control of the capsule prevents its manipulation and full visualization of the intestine; in addition, tissue cannot be sampled and therapy cannot be applied. A new endoscopic technique, double-balloon enteroscopy, allows the endoscopist to potentially examine and provide therapy to much or all of the small intestine. If enteroscopy and video capsule endoscopy are negative or unavailable, a specialized radiographic examination of the small bowel (e.g., enteroclysis) should be performed. Newer imaging techniques being investigated include CT and MR enterography.

Patients with continued obscure GIB who require transfusions or repeated hospitalizations warrant further investigations. ^{99m}Tc-labeled red blood cell scintigraphy should be employed. Angiography is useful even if bleeding has subsided, since it may disclose vascular anomalies or tumor vessels. ^{99m}Tc-pertechnetate scintigraphy for diagnosis of Meckel's diverticulum should be done, especially in the evaluation of young patients. When all tests are unrevealing, intraoperative endoscopy is indicated in patients with severe recurrent or persistent bleeding requiring repeated transfusions.

Occult GIB Occult GIB is manifested by a positive test for fecal occult blood or iron-deficiency anemia. Evaluation of a positive test for fecal occult blood generally should begin with colonoscopy, particularly in patients >40 years. If evaluation of the colon is negative, many perform upper endoscopy only if iron-deficiency anemia or upper GI symptoms are present, while others recommend upper endoscopy in all patients since up to 25–40% of these patients may have some abnormality noted on upper endoscopy. If standard endoscopic tests are unrevealing, enteroscopy, video capsule endoscopy, and/or enteroclysis may be considered in patients with iron-deficiency anemia.

FURTHER READINGS

CHAN FK et al: Proton pump inhibitor plus a COX-2 inhibitor for the prevention of recurrent ulcer bleeding in patients with arthritis: A double blinded, randomized trial. Gastroenterology 130:A-105, 2006

CIPOLLETTA L et al: Outpatient management for low-risk nonvariceal upper GI bleeding: A randomized controlled trial. Gastrointest Endosc 55:1, 2002

CONRAD SA et al: Randomized, double-blind comparison of immediate-release omeprazole oral suspension versus intravenous cimetidine for the prevention of upper gastrointestinal bleeding in critically ill patients. Crit Care Med 33:760, 2005

D'AMICO G et al: Pharmacological treatment of portal hypertension: An evidence-based approach. Semin Liver Dis 19:475, 1999

HENDERSON JM et al: Distal splenorenal shunt versus transjugular intrahepatic portal systematic shunt for variceal bleeding: A randomized trial. Gastroenterology 130:1643, 2006

LAINE L, COOK D: Endoscopic ligation compared with sclerotherapy for treatment of esophageal variceal bleeding: A meta-analysis. Ann Intern Med 123:280, 1995

LAU JYW et al: Effect of intravenous omeprazole on recurrent bleeding after endoscopic treatment of bleeding peptic ulcers. N Engl J Med 343:310, 2000

MARMO R et al: Dual therapy versus monotherapy in endoscopic treatment of high-risk bleeding ulcers: A meta-analysis of controlled trials. Am J Gastroenterol 102:279, 2007

ROCKALL TA et al: Risk assessment after acute upper gastrointestinal haemorrhage. Gut 38:316, 1996

TRIESTER SL et al. A meta-analysis of the yield of capsule endoscopy compared to other diagnostic modalities in patients with obscure gastrointestinal bleeding. Am J Gastroenterol 100:2407, 2005

43 Jaundice

Daniel S. Pratt, Marshall M. Kaplan

Jaundice, or icterus, is a yellowish discoloration of tissue resulting from the deposition of bilirubin. Tissue deposition of bilirubin occurs only in the presence of serum hyperbilirubinemia and is a sign of either liver disease or, less often, a hemolytic disorder. The degree of serum bilirubin elevation can be estimated by physical examination. Slight increases in serum bilirubin are best detected by examining the sclerae, which have a particular affinity for bilirubin due to their high elastin content. The presence of scleral icterus indicates a serum bilirubin of at least 51 μmol/L (3.0 mg/dL). The ability to detect scleral icterus is made more difficult if the examining room has fluorescent lighting. If the examiner suspects scleral icterus, a second place to examine is underneath the tongue. As serum bilirubin levels rise, the skin will eventually become yellow in light-skinned patients and even green if the process is long-standing; the green color is produced by oxidation of bilirubin to biliverdin.

The differential diagnosis for yellowing of the skin is limited. In addition to jaundice, it includes carotenoderma, the use of the drug quinacrine, and excessive exposure to phenols. Carotenoderma is the yellow color imparted to the skin by the presence of carotene; it occurs in healthy individuals who ingest excessive amounts of vegetables and fruits that contain carotene, such as carrots, leafy vegetables, squash, peaches, and oranges. Unlike jaundice, where the yellow coloration of the skin is uniformly distributed over the body, in carotenoderma the pigment is concentrated on the palms, soles, forehead, and nasolabial folds. Carotenoderma can be distinguished from jaundice by the sparing of the sclerae. Quinacrine causes a yellow discoloration of the skin in 4–37% of patients treated with it. Unlike carotene, quinacrine can cause discoloration of the sclerae.

Another sensitive indicator of increased serum bilirubin is darkening of the urine, which is due to the renal excretion of conjugated bilirubin. Patients often describe their urine as tea or cola colored. Bilirubinuria indicates an elevation of the direct serum bilirubin fraction and therefore the presence of liver disease.

Increased serum bilirubin levels occur when an imbalance exists between bilirubin production and clearance. A logical evaluation of the patient who is jaundiced requires an understanding of bilirubin production and metabolism.

PRODUCTION AND METABOLISM OF BILIRUBIN

(See also Chap. 297) Bilirubin, a tetrapyrrole pigment, is a breakdown product of heme (ferroprotoporphyrin IX). About 70–80% of the 250–300 mg of bilirubin produced each day is derived from the breakdown of hemoglobin in senescent red blood cells. The remainder comes from prematurely destroyed erythroid cells in bone marrow and from the turnover of hemoproteins such as myoglobin and cytochromes found in tissues throughout the body.

The formation of bilirubin occurs in reticuloendothelial cells, primarily in the spleen and liver. The first reaction, catalyzed by the microsomal enzyme heme oxygenase, oxidatively cleaves the α bridge of the porphyrin group and opens the heme ring. The end products of this reaction are biliverdin, carbon monoxide, and iron. The second reaction, catalyzed by the cytosolic enzyme biliverdin reductase, reduces the central methylene bridge of biliverdin and converts it to bilirubin. Bilirubin formed in the reticuloendothelial cells is virtually insoluble in water. This is due to tight internal hydrogen bonding between the water-soluble moieties of bilirubin, proprionic acid carboxyl groups of one dipyrrolic half of the molecule with the imino and lactam groups of the opposite half. This configuration blocks solvent access to the polar residues of bilirubin and places the hydrophobic residues on the outside. To be transported in blood, bilirubin must be solubilized. This is accomplished by its reversible, noncovalent binding to albumin. Unconjugated bilirubin bound to albumin is transported to the liver, where it, but not the albumin, is taken up by hepatocytes via a process that at least partly involves carrier-mediated membrane transport. No specific bilirubin transporter has yet been identified (Chap. 297, Fig. 297-1).

After entering the hepatocyte, unconjugated bilirubin is bound to the cytosolic protein ligandin, or glutathione S-transferase B. Whereas ligandin was initially thought to be a transport protein, responsible for delivering unconjugated bilirubin from the plasma membrane to the endoplasmic reticulum, it now appears that its role may in fact be to reduce bilirubin efflux back into the plasma. Studies suggest that unconjugated bilirubin may well rapidly diffuse unaided through the aqueous cytosol between membranes. In the endoplasmic reticulum, bilirubin is solubilized by conjugation to glucuronic acid, a process that disrupts the internal hydrogen bonds and yields bilirubin monoglucuronide and diglucuronide. The conjugation of glucuronic acid to bilirubin is catalyzed by bilirubin uridine diphosphate-glucuronosyl transferase (UDPGT). The now hydrophilic bilirubin conjugates diffuse from the endoplasmic reticulum to the canalicular membrane, where bilirubin monoglucuronide and diglucuronide are actively transported into canalicular bile by an energy-dependent mechanism involving the multiple drug resistance protein 2.

The conjugated bilirubin excreted into bile drains into the duodenum and passes unchanged through the proximal small bowel. Conjugated bilirubin is not taken up by the intestinal mucosa. When the conjugated bilirubin reaches the distal ileum and colon, it is hydrolyzed to unconjugated bilirubin by bacterial β-glucuronidases. The unconjugated bilirubin is reduced by normal gut bacteria to form a group of colorless tetrapyrroles called urobilinogens. About 80–90% of these products are excreted in feces, either unchanged or oxidized to orange derivatives called urobilins. The remaining 10–20% of the urobilinogens are passively absorbed, enter the portal venous blood, and are reexcreted by the liver. A small fraction (usually <3 mg/dL) escapes hepatic uptake, filters across the renal glomerulus, and is excreted in urine.

MEASUREMENT OF SERUM BILIRUBIN

The terms direct- and indirect-reacting bilirubin are based on the original van den Bergh reaction. This assay, or a variation of it, is still used in most clinical chemistry laboratories to determine the serum bilirubin level. In this assay, bilirubin is exposed to diazotized sulfanilic acid, splitting into two relatively stable dipyrrylmethene azopigments that absorb maximally at 540 nm, allowing for photometric analysis. The direct fraction is that which reacts with diazotized sulfanilic acid in the absence of an accelerator substance such as alcohol. The direct fraction provides an approximate determination of the conjugated bilirubin in serum. The total serum bilirubin is the amount that reacts after the addition of alcohol. The indirect fraction is the difference between the total and the direct bilirubin and provides an estimate of the unconjugated bilirubin in serum.

With the van den Bergh method, the normal serum bilirubin concentration usually is 17 μmol/L (<1 mg/dL). Up to 30%, or 5.1 μmol/L (0.3 mg/dL), of the total may be direct-reacting (conjugated) bilirubin. Total serum bilirubin concentrations are between 3.4 and 15.4 μmol/L (0.2 and 0.9 mg/dL) in 95% of a normal population.

Several new techniques, although less convenient to perform, have added considerably to our understanding of bilirubin metabolism. First, they demonstrate that in normal persons or those with Gilbert's syndrome, almost 100% of the serum bilirubin is unconjugated; <3% is monoconjugated bilirubin. Second, in jaundiced patients with hepatobiliary disease, the total serum bilirubin concentration measured by these new, more accurate methods is lower than the values found with diazo methods. This suggests that there are diazo-positive compounds distinct from bilirubin in the serum of patients with hepatobiliary disease. Third, these studies indicate that in jaundiced patients with hepatobiliary disease, monoglucuronides of bilirubin predominate over the diglucuronides. Fourth, part of the direct-reacting bilirubin fraction includes conjugated bilirubin that is covalently linked to albumin. This albumin-linked bilirubin fraction (*delta fraction,* or *biliprotein*) represents an important fraction of total serum bilirubin in patients with cholestasis and hepatobiliary disorders. Albumin-bound conjugated bilirubin is formed in serum when hepatic excretion of bilirubin glucuronides is impaired and the glucuronides are present in serum in increasing amounts. By virtue of its tight binding to albumin, the clearance rate of albumin-bound bilirubin from serum approximates the half-life of albumin, 12–14 days, rather than the short half-life of bilirubin, about 4 h.

The prolonged half-life of albumin-bound conjugated bilirubin explains two previously unexplained enigmas in jaundiced patients with liver disease: (1) that some patients with conjugated hyperbilirubinemia do not exhibit bilirubinuria during the recovery phase of their disease because the bilirubin is covalently bound to albumin and therefore not filtered by the renal glomeruli, and (2) that the elevated serum bilirubin level declines more slowly than expected in some patients who otherwise appear to be recovering satisfactorily. Late in the recovery phase of hepatobiliary disorders, all the conjugated bilirubin may be in the albumin-linked form. Its value in serum falls slowly because of the long half-life of albumin.

MEASUREMENT OF URINE BILIRUBIN
Unconjugated bilirubin is always bound to albumin in the serum, is not filtered by the kidney, and is not found in the urine. Conjugated bilirubin is filtered at the glomerulus and the majority is reabsorbed by the proximal tubules; a small fraction is excreted in the urine. Any bilirubin found in the urine is conjugated bilirubin. The presence of bilirubinuria implies the presence of liver disease. A urine dipstick test (Ictotest) gives the same information as fractionation of the serum bilirubin. This test is very accurate. A false-negative test is possible in patients with prolonged cholestasis due to the predominance of conjugated bilirubin covalently bound to albumin.

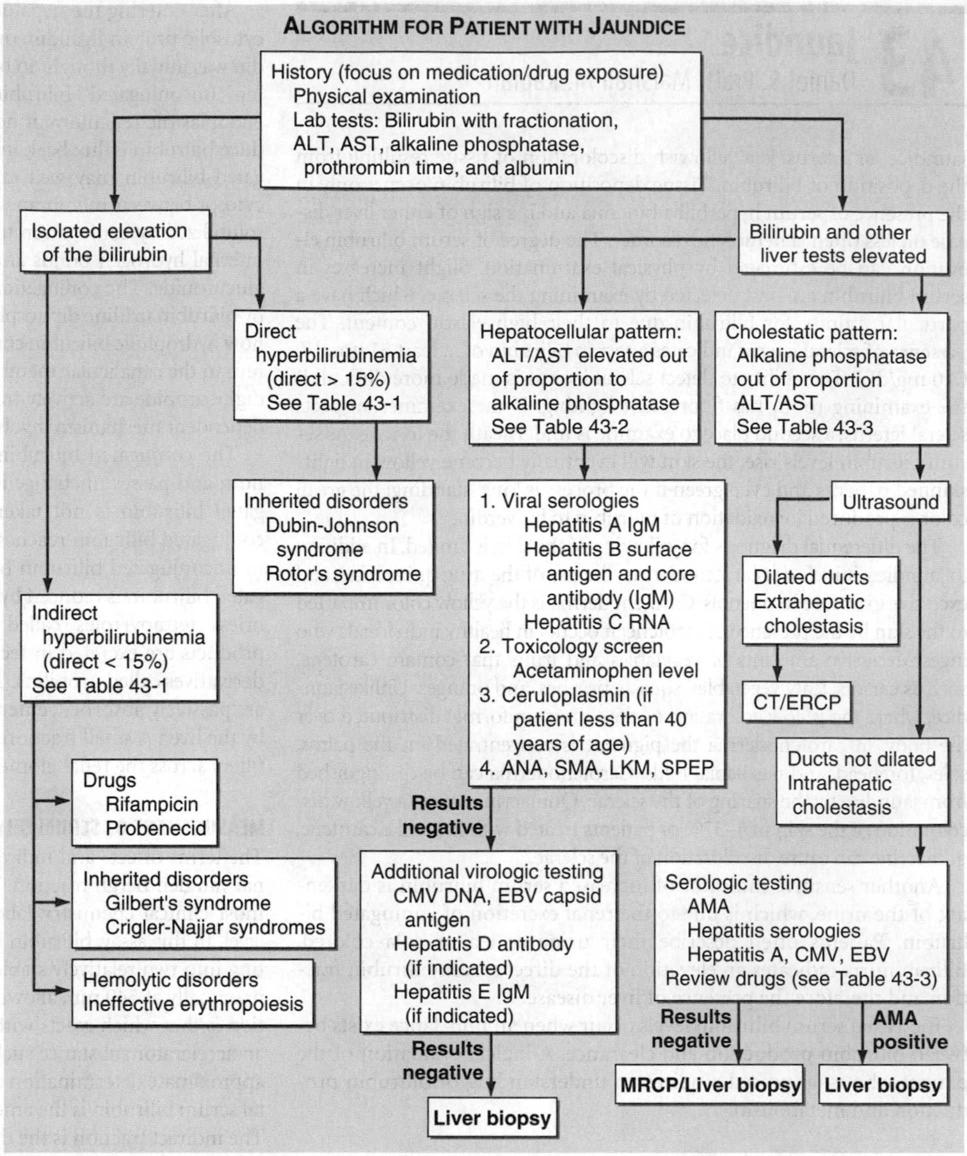

FIGURE 43-1 Evaluation of the patient with jaundice. MRCP, magnetic resonance cholangiopancreatography; ALT, alanine aminotransferase; AST, aspartate aminotransferase; SMA, smooth-muscle antibody; AMA, antimitochondrial antibody; LKM, liver-kidney microsomal antibody; SPEP, serum protein electrophoresis; CMV, cytomegalovirus; EBV, Epstein-Barr virus.

APPROACH TO THE PATIENT: Bilirubin

The bilirubin present in serum represents a balance between input from production of bilirubin and hepatic/biliary removal of the pigment. Hyperbilirubinemia may result from (1) overproduction of bilirubin; (2) impaired uptake, conjugation, or excretion of bilirubin; or (3) regurgitation of unconjugated or conjugated bilirubin from damaged hepatocytes or bile ducts. An increase in unconjugated bilirubin in serum results from either overproduction, impairment of uptake, or conjugation of bilirubin. An increase in conjugated bilirubin is due to decreased excretion into the bile ductules or backward leakage of the pigment. The initial steps in evaluating the patient with jaundice are to determine (1) whether the hyperbilirubinemia is predominantly conjugated or unconjugated in nature, and (2) whether other biochemical liver tests are abnormal. The thoughtful interpretation of limited data will allow for a rational evaluation of the patient (Fig. 43-1). This discussion will focus solely on the evaluation of the adult patient with jaundice.

ISOLATED ELEVATION OF SERUM BILIRUBIN **Unconjugated Hyperbilirubinemia** The differential diagnosis of an isolated unconjugated hyperbilirubinemia is limited (Table 43-1). The critical determination is whether the patient is suffering from a hemolytic process resulting in an overproduction of bilirubin (hemolytic disorders and ineffective erythropoiesis) or from impaired hepatic uptake/conjugation of bilirubin (drug effect or genetic disorders).

Hemolytic disorders that cause excessive heme production may be either inherited or acquired. Inherited disorders include spherocytosis, sickle cell anemia, thalassemia, and deficiency of red cell enzymes such as pyruvate kinase and glucose-6-phosphate dehydrogenase. In these conditions, the serum bilirubin rarely exceeds 86 μmol/L (5 mg/dL). Higher levels may occur when there is coexistent renal or hepatocellular dysfunction or in acute hemolysis such as a sickle cell crisis. In evaluating jaundice in patients with chronic hemolysis, it is important to remember the high incidence of pigmented (calcium bilirubinate) gallstones found in these patients, which increases the likelihood of choledocholithiasis as an alternative explanation for hyperbilirubinemia.

Acquired hemolytic disorders include microangiopathic hemolytic anemia (e.g., hemolytic-uremic syndrome), paroxysmal nocturnal hemoglobinuria, spur cell anemia, and immune hemolysis. Ineffective erythropoiesis occurs in cobalamin, folate, and iron deficiencies.

In the absence of hemolysis, the physician should consider a problem with the hepatic uptake or conjugation of bilirubin. Certain drugs, including rifampicin and probenecid, may cause unconjugated hyperbilirubinemia by diminishing hepatic uptake of

TABLE 43-1 CAUSES OF ISOLATED HYPERBILIRUBINEMIA

I. Indirect hyperbilirubinemia
- A. Hemolytic disorders
  - 1. Inherited
    - a. Spherocytosis, elliptocytosis
      Glucose-6-phosphate dehydrogenase and pyruvate kinase deficiencies
    - b. Sickle cell anemia
  - 2. Acquired
    - a. Microangiopathic hemolytic anemias
    - b. Paroxysmal nocturnal hemoglobinuria
    - c. Spur cell anemia
    - d. Immune hemolysis
- B. Ineffective erythropoiesis
  - 1. Cobalamin, folate, thalassemia, and severe iron deficiencies
- C. Drugs
  - 1. Rifampicin, probenecid, ribavirin
- D. Inherited conditions
  - 1. Crigler-Najjar types I and II
  - 2. Gilbert's syndrome

II. Direct hyperbilirubinemia
- A. Inherited conditions
  - 1. Dubin-Johnson syndrome
  - 2. Rotor's syndrome

bilirubin. Impaired bilirubin conjugation occurs in three genetic conditions: Crigler-Najjar syndrome, types I and II, and Gilbert's syndrome. *Crigler-Najjar type I* is an exceptionally rare condition found in neonates and characterized by severe jaundice [bilirubin > 342 μmol/L (>20 mg/dL)] and neurologic impairment due to kernicterus, frequently leading to death in infancy or childhood. These patients have a complete absence of bilirubin UDPGT activity, usually due to mutations in the critical 3′ domain of the *UDPGT* gene, and are totally unable to conjugate, hence cannot excrete bilirubin. The only effective treatment is orthotopic liver transplantation. Use of gene therapy and allogeneic hepatocyte infusion are experimental approaches of future promise for this devastating disease.

Crigler-Najjar type II is somewhat more common than type I. Patients live into adulthood with serum bilirubin levels that range from 103–428 μmol/L (6–25 mg/dL). In these patients, mutations in the bilirubin *UDPGT* gene cause reduced but not completely absent activity of the enzyme. Bilirubin *UDPGT* activity can be induced by the administration of phenobarbital, which can reduce serum bilirubin levels in these patients. Despite marked jaundice, these patients usually survive into adulthood, although they may be susceptible to kernicterus under the stress of intercurrent illness or surgery.

Gilbert's syndrome is also marked by the impaired conjugation of bilirubin due to reduced bilirubin UDPGT activity. Patients with Gilbert's syndrome have a mild unconjugated hyperbilirubinemia with serum levels almost always <103 μmol/L (6 mg/dL). The serum levels may fluctuate, and jaundice is often identified only during periods of fasting. One molecular defect that has been identified in patients with Gilbert's syndrome is in the TATAA element in the 5′ promoter region of the bilirubin *UDPGT* gene upstream of exon 1. This defect alone is not necessarily sufficient for producing the clinical syndrome of Gilbert's as there are patients who are homozygous for this defect yet do not have the levels of hyperbilirubinemia typically seen in Gilbert's syndrome. An enhancer polymorphism that lowers transcriptional activity has recently been identified. The decrease in transcription caused by both mutations together may be critical for producing the syndrome. Unlike both Crigler-Najjar syndromes, Gilbert's syndrome is very common. The reported incidence is 3–7% of the population with males predominating over females by a ratio of 2–7:1.

Conjugated Hyperbilirubinemia Elevated conjugated hyperbilirubinemia is found in two rare inherited conditions: *Dubin-Johnson syndrome* and *Rotor's syndrome* (Table 43-1). Patients with both conditions present with asymptomatic jaundice, typically in the second generation of life. The defect in Dubin-Johnson syndrome is mutations in the gene for multiple drug resistance protein 2. These patients have altered excretion of bilirubin into the bile ducts. Rotor's syndrome seems to be a problem with the hepatic storage of bilirubin. Differentiating between these syndromes is possible, but clinically unnecessary, due to their benign nature.

ELEVATION OF SERUM BILIRUBIN WITH OTHER LIVER TEST ABNORMALITIES The remainder of this chapter will focus on the evaluation of the patient with a conjugated hyperbilirubinemia in the setting of other liver test abnormalities. This group of patients can be divided into those with a primary hepatocellular process and those with intra- or extrahepatic cholestasis. Being able to make this differentiation will guide the physician's evaluation (Fig. 43-1). This differentiation is made on the basis of the history and physical examination as well as the pattern of liver test abnormalities.

History A complete medical history is perhaps the single most important part of the evaluation of the patient with unexplained jaundice. Important considerations include the use of or exposure to any chemical or medication, either physician-prescribed, over-the-counter, complementary or alternative medicines such as herbal and vitamin preparations, or other drugs such as anabolic steroids. The patient should be carefully questioned about possible parenteral exposures, including transfusions, IV and intranasal drug use, tattoos, and sexual activity. Other important questions include recent travel history, exposure to people with jaundice, exposure to possibly contaminated foods, occupational exposure to hepatotoxins, alcohol consumption, the duration of jaundice, and the presence of any accompanying symptoms such as arthralgias, myalgias, rash, anorexia, weight loss, abdominal pain, fever, pruritus, and changes in the urine and stool. While none of these latter symptoms are specific for any one condition, they can suggest a particular diagnosis. A history of arthralgias and myalgias predating jaundice suggests hepatitis, either viral or drug-related. Jaundice associated with the sudden onset of severe right upper quadrant pain and shaking chills suggests choledocholithiasis and ascending cholangitis.

Physical Examination The general assessment should include assessment of the patient's nutritional status. Temporal and proximal muscle wasting suggests long-standing diseases such as pancreatic cancer or cirrhosis. Stigmata of chronic liver disease, including spider nevi, palmar erythema, gynecomastia, caput medusae, Dupuytren's contractures, parotid gland enlargement, and testicular atrophy are commonly seen in advanced alcoholic (Laennec's) cirrhosis and occasionally in other types of cirrhosis. An enlarged left supraclavicular node (Virchow's node) or periumbilical nodule (Sister Mary Joseph's nodule) suggests an abdominal malignancy. Jugular venous distention, a sign of right-sided heart failure, suggests hepatic congestion. Right pleural effusion, in the absence of clinically apparent ascites, may be seen in advanced cirrhosis.

The abdominal examination should focus on the size and consistency of the liver, whether the spleen is palpable and hence enlarged, and whether there is ascites present. Patients with cirrhosis may have an enlarged left lobe of the liver, which is felt below the xiphoid, and an enlarged spleen. A grossly enlarged nodular liver or an obvious abdominal mass suggests malignancy. An enlarged tender liver could be viral or alcoholic hepatitis, an infiltrative process such as amyloid, or, less often, an acutely congested liver secondary to right-sided heart failure. Severe right upper quadrant tenderness with respiratory arrest on inspiration (Murphy's sign) suggests cholecystitis or, occasionally, ascending cholangitis. Ascites in the presence of jaundice suggests either cirrhosis or malignancy with peritoneal spread.

Laboratory Tests When the physician encounters a patient with unexplained jaundice, there is a battery of tests that are helpful in the initial evaluation. These include total and direct serum bilirubin with fractionation, aminotransferases, alkaline phosphatase, albumin, and prothrombin time tests. Enzyme tests [alanine aminotransferase (ALT), aspartate aminotransferase (AST), and alkaline phosphatase] are helpful in differentiating between a hepatocellular process and a cholestatic process (Table 296-1; Fig. 43-1), a critical step in determining what additional workup is indicated. Patients with a hepatocellular process generally have a disproportionate rise in the aminotransferases compared to the alkaline phosphatase. Patients with a cholestatic process have a disproportionate rise in the alkaline phosphatase compared to the aminotransferases. The bilirubin can be prominently elevated in both hepatocellular and cholestatic conditions and therefore is not necessarily helpful in differentiating between the two.

In addition to the enzyme tests, all jaundiced patients should have additional blood tests, specifically an albumin level and a prothrombin time, to assess liver function. A low albumin suggests a chronic process such as cirrhosis or cancer. A normal albumin is suggestive of a more acute process such as viral hepatitis or choledocholithiasis. An elevated prothrombin time indicates either vitamin K deficiency due to prolonged jaundice and malabsorption of vitamin K or significant hepatocellular dysfunction. The failure of the prothrombin time to correct with parenteral administration of vitamin K indicates severe hepatocellular injury.

The results of the bilirubin, enzyme tests, albumin, and prothrombin time tests will usually indicate whether a jaundiced patient has a hepatocellular or a cholestatic disease, as well as some indication of the duration and severity of the disease. The causes and evaluation of hepatocellular and cholestatic diseases are quite different.

Hepatocellular Conditions Hepatocellular diseases that can cause jaundice include viral hepatitis, drug or environmental toxicity, alcohol, and end-stage cirrhosis from any cause (Table 43-2). Wilson's disease, once believed to occur primarily in young adults, should be considered in all adults if no other cause of jaundice is found. Autoimmune hepatitis is typically seen in young to middle-aged women but may affect men and women of any age. Alcoholic hepatitis can be differentiated from viral and toxin-related hepatitis by the pattern of the aminotransferases. Patients with alcoholic hepatitis typically have an AST:ALT ratio of at least 2:1. The AST rarely exceeds 300 U/L. Patients with acute viral hepatitis and toxin-related injury severe enough to produce jaundice typically have aminotransferases > 500 U/L, with the ALT greater than or equal to the AST. The degree of aminotransferase elevation can occasionally help in differentiating between hepatocellular and cholestatic processes. While ALT and AST values less than 8 times normal may be seen in either hepatocellular or cholestatic liver disease, values 25 times normal or higher are seen primarily in acute hepatocellular diseases. Patients with jaundice from cirrhosis can have normal or only slight elevations of the aminotransferases.

When the physician determines that the patient has a hepatocellular disease, appropriate testing for acute viral hepatitis includes a hepatitis A IgM antibody, a hepatitis B surface antigen and core IgM antibody, and a hepatitis C viral RNA test. It can take many weeks for the hepatitis C antibody to become detectable, making it an unreliable test if acute hepatitis C is suspected. Depending on circumstances, studies for hepatitis D, E, Epstein-Barr virus (EBV), and cytomegalovirus (CMV) may be indicated. Ceruloplasmin is the initial screening test for Wilson's disease. Testing for autoimmune hepatitis usually includes an antinuclear antibody and measurement of specific immunoglobulins.

Drug-induced hepatocellular injury can be classified either as predictable or unpredictable. Predictable drug reactions are dose-dependent and affect all patients who ingest a toxic dose of the drug in question. The classic example is acetaminophen hepatotoxicity. Unpredictable or idiosyncratic drug reactions are not dose-dependent and occur in a minority of patients. A great number of drugs can cause idiosyncratic hepatic injury. Environmental toxins are also an important cause of hepatocellular injury. Examples include industrial chemicals such as vinyl chloride, herbal preparations containing pyrrolizidine alkaloids (Jamaica bush tea) and Kava Kava, and the mushrooms *Amanita phalloides* or *A. verna* that contain highly hepatotoxic amatoxins.

Cholestatic Conditions When the pattern of the liver tests suggests a cholestatic disorder, the next step is to determine whether it is intra- or extrahepatic cholestasis (Fig. 43-1). Distinguishing intrahepatic

TABLE 43-2 HEPATOCELLULAR CONDITIONS THAT MAY PRODUCE JAUNDICE

Viral hepatitis
Hepatitis A, B, C, D, and E
Epstein-Barr virus
Cytomegalovirus
Herpes simplex
Alcohol
Drug toxicity
Predictable, dose-dependent, e.g., acetaminophen
Unpredictable, idosyncratic, e.g., isoniazid
Environmental toxins
Vinyl chloride
Jamaica bush tea—pyrrolizidine alkaloids
Kava Kava
Wild mushrooms—*Amanita phalloides* or *A. verna*
Wilson's disease
Autoimmune hepatitis

from extrahepatic cholestasis may be difficult. History, physical examination, and laboratory tests are often not helpful. The next appropriate test is an ultrasound. The ultrasound is inexpensive, does not expose the patient to ionizing radiation, and can detect dilation of the intra- and extrahepatic biliary tree with a high degree of sensitivity and specificity. The absence of biliary dilatation suggests intrahepatic cholestasis, while the presence of biliary dilatation indicates extrahepatic cholestasis. False-negative results occur in patients with partial obstruction of the common bile duct or in patients with cirrhosis or primary sclerosing cholangitis (PSC) where scarring prevents the intrahepatic ducts from dilating.

Although ultrasonography may indicate extrahepatic cholestasis, it rarely identifies the site or cause of obstruction. The distal common bile duct is a particularly difficult area to visualize by ultrasound because of overlying bowel gas. Appropriate next tests include CT, magnetic resonance cholangiography (MRCP), and endoscopic retrograde cholangiopancreatography (ERCP). CT scanning and MRCP are better than ultrasonography for assessing the head of the pancreas and for identifying choledocholithiasis in the distal common bile duct, particularly when the ducts are not dilated. ERCP is the "gold standard" for identifying choledocholithiasis. It is performed by introducing a side-viewing endoscope perorally into the duodenum. The ampulla of Vater is visualized and a catheter is advanced through the ampulla. Injection of dye allows for the visualization of the common bile duct and the pancreatic duct. The success rate for cannulation of the common bile duct ranges from 80–95%, depending on the operator's experience. Beyond its diagnostic capabilities, ERCP allows for therapeutic interventions, including the removal of common bile duct stones and the placement of stents. In patients in whom ERCP is unsuccessful and there is a high likelihood of the need for a therapeutic intervention, transhepatic cholangiography can provide the same information and allow for intervention. MRCP is a now widely available, noninvasive technique for imaging the bile and pancreatic ducts; it has replaced ERCP as the initial diagnostic test in cases where the need for intervention is felt to be small.

In patients with apparent *intrahepatic cholestasis*, the diagnosis is often made by serologic testing in combination with percutaneous liver biopsy. The list of possible causes of intrahepatic cholestasis is long and varied (Table 43-3). A number of conditions that typically cause a hepatocellular pattern of injury can also present as a cholestatic variant. Both hepatitis B and C can cause a cholestatic hepatitis (fibrosing cholestatic hepatitis). This disease variant has been reported in patients who have undergone solid organ transplantation. Hepatitis A, alcoholic hepatitis, EBV, and CMV may also present as cholestatic liver disease.

Drugs may cause intrahepatic cholestasis, a variant of drug-induced hepatitis. Drug-induced cholestasis is usually reversible after eliminating the offending drug, although it may take many

TABLE 43-3 CHOLESTATIC CONDITIONS THAT MAY PRODUCE JAUNDICE

I. Intrahepatic
- A. Viral hepatitis
  - 1. Fibrosing cholestatic hepatitis—hepatitis B and C
  - 2. Hepatitis A, Epstein-Barr virus, cytomegalovirus
- B. Alcoholic hepatitis
- C. Drug toxicity
  - 1. Pure cholestasis—anabolic and contraceptive steroids
  - 2. Cholestatic hepatitis—chlorpromazine, erythromycin estolate
  - 3. Chronic cholestasis—chlorpromazine and prochlorperazine
- D. Primary biliary cirrhosis
- E. Primary sclerosing cholangitis
- F. Vanishing bile duct syndrome
  - 1. Chronic rejection of liver transplants
  - 2. Sarcoidosis
  - 3. Drugs
- G. Inherited
  - 1. Progressive familial intrahepatic cholestasis
  - 2. Benign recurrent cholestasis
- H. Cholestasis of pregnancy
- I. Total parenteral nutrition
- J. Nonhepatobiliary sepsis
- K. Benign postoperative cholestasis
- L. Paraneoplastic syndrome
- M. Venoocclusive disease
- N. Graft-versus-host disease
- O. Infiltrative disease
  - 1. TB
  - 2. Lymphoma
  - 3. Amyloid

II. Extrahepatic
- A. Malignant
  - 1. Cholangiocarcinoma
  - 2. Pancreatic cancer
  - 3. Gallbladder cancer
  - 4. Ampullary cancer
  - 5. Malignant involvement of the porta hepatis lymph nodes
- B. Benign
  - 1. Choledocholithiasis
  - 2. Postoperative biliary structures
  - 3. Primary sclerosing cholangitis
  - 4. Chronic pancreatitis
  - 5. AIDS cholangiopathy
  - 6. Mirizzi syndrome
  - 7. Parasitic disease (ascariasis)

months for cholestasis to resolve. Drugs most commonly associated with cholestasis are the anabolic and contraceptive steroids. Cholestatic hepatitis has been reported with chlorpromazine, imipramine, tolbutamide, sulindac, cimetidine, and erythromycin estolate. It also occurs in patients taking trimethoprim, sulfamethoxazole, and penicillin-based antibiotics such as ampicillin, dicloxacillin, and clavulinic acid. Rarely, cholestasis may be chronic and associated with progressive fibrosis despite early discontinuation of the drug. Chronic cholestasis has been associated with chlorpromazine and prochlorperazine.

Primary biliary cirrhosis is an autoimmune disease predominantly of middle-aged women in which there is a progressive destruction of interlobular bile ducts. The diagnosis is made by the presence of the antimitochondrial antibody that is found in 95% of patients. *Primary sclerosing cholangitis* is characterized by the destruction and fibrosis of larger bile ducts. The disease may involve only the intrahepatic ducts and present as intrahepatic cholestasis. However, in 95% of patients with PSC, both intra- and extrahepatic ducts are involved. The diagnosis of PSC is made by imaging the biliary tree. The pathognomonic findings are multiple strictures of bile ducts with dilatations proximal to the strictures. Approximately 75% of patients with PSC have inflammatory bowel disease.

The *vanishing bile duct syndrome* and *adult bile ductopenia* are rare conditions in which there are a decreased number of bile ducts seen in liver biopsy specimens. The histologic picture is similar to that found in primary biliary cirrhosis. This picture is seen in patients who develop chronic rejection after liver transplantation and in those who develop graft-versus-host disease after bone marrow transplantation. Vanishing bile duct syndrome also occurs in rare cases of sarcoidosis, in patients taking certain drugs including chlorpromazine, and idiopathically.

There are also familial forms of intrahepatic cholestasis. The familial intrahepatic cholestatic syndromes include *progressive familial intrahepatic cholestasis* (PFIC) *types 1–3*, and *benign recurrent cholestasis* (BRC). PFIC1 and BRC are autosomal recessive diseases that result from mutations in the *ATP8B1* gene that encodes a protein belonging to the subfamily of P-type ATPases; the exact function of this protein remains poorly defined. While PFIC1 is a progressive condition that manifests in childhood, BRC presents later than PFIC1 and is marked by recurrent episodes of jaundice and pruritus; the episodes are self-limited but can be debilitating. PFIC2 is caused by mutations in the *ABCB11* gene, which encodes the bile salt export pump, and PFIC3 is caused by mutations in the multidrug-resistant P-glycoprotein 3. *Cholestasis of pregnancy* occurs in the second and third trimesters and resolves after delivery. Its cause is unknown, but the condition is probably inherited and cholestasis can be triggered by estrogen administration.

Other causes of intrahepatic cholestasis include total parenteral nutrition (TPN), nonhepatobiliary sepsis, benign postoperative cholestasis, and a paraneoplastic syndrome associated with a number of different malignancies, including Hodgkin's disease, medullary thyroid cancer, renal cell cancer, renal sarcoma, T cell lymphoma, prostate cancer, and several gastrointestinal malignancies. The term *Stauffer's syndrome* has been used for intrahepatic cholestasis specifically associated with renal cell cancer. In patients developing cholestasis in the intensive care unit, the major considerations should be sepsis, shock liver, and TPN jaundice. Jaundice occurring after bone marrow transplantation is most likely due to venoocclusive disease or graft-versus-host disease.

Causes of *extrahepatic cholestasis* can be split into malignant and benign (Table 43-3). Malignant causes include pancreatic, gallbladder, ampullary, and cholangiocarcinoma. The latter is most commonly associated with PSC and is exceptionally difficult to diagnose because its appearance is often identical to that of PSC. Pancreatic and gallbladder tumors, as well as cholangiocarcinoma, are rarely resectable and have poor prognoses. Ampullary carcinoma has the highest surgical cure rate of all the tumors that present as painless jaundice. Hilar lymphadenopathy due to metastases from other cancers may cause obstruction of the extrahepatic biliary tree.

Choledocholithiasis is the most common cause of extrahepatic cholestasis. The clinical presentation can range from mild right upper quadrant discomfort with only minimal elevations of the enzyme tests to ascending cholangitis with jaundice, sepsis, and circulatory collapse. PSC may occur with clinically important strictures limited to the extrahepatic biliary tree. In cases where there is a dominant stricture, patients can be effectively managed with serial endoscopic dilatations. Chronic pancreatitis rarely causes strictures of the distal common bile duct, where it passes through the head of the pancreas. AIDS cholangiopathy is a condition, usually due to infection of the bile duct epithelium with CMV or cryptosporidia, which has a cholangiographic appearance similar to that of PSC. These patients usually present with greatly elevated serum alkaline phosphatase levels (mean, 800 IU/L), but the bilirubin is often near normal. These patients do not typically present with jaundice.

SUMMARY

The goal of this chapter is not to provide an encyclopedic review of all of the conditions that can cause jaundice. Rather, it is intended to provide a framework that helps a physician to evaluate the patient with jaundice in a logical way (Fig. 43-1).

Simply stated, the initial step is to obtain appropriate blood tests to determine if the patient has an isolated elevation of serum bilirubin. If so, is the bilirubin elevation due to an increased unconjugated or conjugated fraction? If the hyperbilirubinemia is accompanied by other liver test abnormalities, is the disorder hepatocellular or cholestatic? If cholestatic, is it intra- or extrahepatic? All of these questions can be answered with a thoughtful history, physical examination, and interpretation of laboratory and radiologic tests and procedures.

FURTHER READINGS

BOSMA PJ: Inherited disorders of bilirubin metabolism. J Hepatol 38:107, 2003

FERENCI P: Wilson's disease. Clin Gastroenterol Hepatol 3:726, 2005

FOX IJ et al: Treatment of the Crigler-Najjar syndrome type I with hepatocyte transplantation. N Engl J Med 338:1422, 1998

GLASOVA H, BEUERS U: Extrahepatic manifestations of cholestasis. J Gastroenterol Hepatol 9:938, 2002

PRATT DS, KAPLAN MM: Laboratory tests, in *Schiff's Diseases of the Liver*, 9th ed, ER Schiff et al (eds). Philadelphia, Lippincott Williams & Wilkins, 2003

TRAUNER M et al: Molecular pathogenesis of cholestasis. N Engl J Med 339:1217, 1998

44 Abdominal Swelling and Ascites

Robert M. Glickman, Roshini Rajapaksa

ABDOMINAL SWELLING

Abdominal swelling or distention is a common problem in clinical medicine and may be the initial manifestation of a systemic disease or of otherwise unsuspected abdominal disease. *Subjective* abdominal enlargement, often described as a sensation of fullness or bloating, is usually transient and is often related to a functional gastrointestinal disorder when it is not accompanied by objective physical findings of increased abdominal girth or local swelling. *Obesity* and lumbar lordosis, which may be associated with prominence of the abdomen, may usually be distinguished from true increases in the volume of the peritoneal cavity by history and careful physical examination.

CLINICAL HISTORY

Abdominal swelling may first be noticed by the patient because of a progressive increase in belt or clothing size, the appearance of abdominal or inguinal hernias, or the development of a localized swelling. Often, considerable abdominal enlargement has gone unnoticed for weeks or months, either because of coexistent obesity or because the ascites formation has been insidious, without pain or localizing symptoms. Progressive abdominal distention may be associated with a sensation of "pulling" or "stretching" of the flanks or groins and vague low back pain. Localized pain usually results from involvement of an abdominal organ (e.g., a passively congested liver, large spleen, or colonic tumor). Pain is uncommon in cirrhosis with ascites, and when it is present, pancreatitis, hepatocellular carcinoma, or peritonitis should be considered. Tense ascites or abdominal tumors may produce increased intraabdominal pressure, resulting in indigestion and heartburn due to gastroesophageal reflux or dyspnea, abdominal wall hernias (inguinal and umbilical), orthopnea, and tachypnea from elevation of the diaphragm. A coexistent pleural effusion, more commonly on the right, presumably due to leakage of ascitic fluid through lymphatic channels in the diaphragm, may also contribute to respiratory embarrassment. A large pleural effusion, obscuring most of the lung, is known as a *hepatic hydrothorax*. The patient with diffuse abdominal swelling should be questioned about increased alcohol intake, a prior episode of jaundice or hematuria, or a change in bowel habits. Such historic information may provide the clues that will lead one to suspect an occult cirrhosis, a colonic tumor with peritoneal seeding, congestive heart failure, or nephrosis.

PHYSICAL EXAMINATION

A carefully executed general physical examination can yield valuable clues concerning the etiology of abdominal swelling. Thus palmar erythema and spider angiomas suggest an underlying cirrhosis, while supraclavicular adenopathy (Virchow's node) should raise the question of an underlying gastrointestinal malignancy.

Inspection of the abdomen is important. By noting the abdominal contour, one may be able to distinguish localized from generalized swelling. The tensely distended abdomen with tightly stretched skin, bulging flanks, and everted umbilicus is characteristic of ascites. A prominent abdominal venous pattern with the direction of flow away from the umbilicus is often a reflection of portal hypertension; venous collaterals with flow from the lower part of the abdomen toward the umbilicus suggest obstruction of the inferior vena cava; flow downward toward the umbilicus suggests superior vena cava obstruction. "Doming" of the abdomen with visible ridges from underlying intestinal loops is usually due to intestinal obstruction or distention. An epigastric mass, with evident peristalsis proceeding from left to right, usually indicates underlying pyloric obstruction. A liver with metastatic deposits may be visible as a nodular right upper quadrant mass moving with respiration.

Auscultation may reveal the high-pitched, rushing sounds of early intestinal obstruction or a succussion sound due to increased fluid and gas in a dilated hollow viscus. Careful auscultation over an enlarged liver occasionally reveals a harsh bruit signifying a vascular tumor (especially a hepatocellular carcinoma) or alcoholic hepatitis, or the leathery friction rub of a surface nodule. A venous hum at the umbilicus may signify portal hypertension and an increased collateral blood flow around the liver. A fluid wave and flank dullness that shifts with change in position of the patient are important signs that indicate the presence of peritoneal fluid, although a minimum of 1500 mL of fluid is usually required to produce these findings. In obese patients, small amounts of fluid may be difficult to demonstrate and often can only be detected by ultrasound examination of the abdomen, which can detect as little as 100 mL of fluid. Careful percussion should serve to distinguish generalized abdominal enlargement from localized swelling due to an enlarged uterus, ovarian cyst, or distended bladder. Percussion can also outline an abnormally small or large liver. Loss of normal liver dullness may result from massive hepatic necrosis; it also may be a clue to free gas in the peritoneal cavity, as from perforation of a hollow viscus.

Palpation is often difficult with massive ascites, and ballottement of overlying fluid may be the only method of palpating the liver or spleen. A slightly enlarged spleen in association with ascites may be the only evidence of an occult cirrhosis. When there is evidence of portal hypertension, a soft liver suggests that obstruction to portal flow is extrahepatic; a firm liver suggests cirrhosis as the likely cause of the portal hypertension. A very hard or nodular liver is a clue that the liver is infiltrated with tumor, and when accompanied by ascites, it suggests that the latter is due to peritoneal seeding. The presence of a hard periumbilical nodule (Sister Mary Joseph's nodule) suggests metastatic disease from a pelvic or gastrointestinal primary tumor. A pulsatile liver and ascites may be found in tricuspid insufficiency.

An attempt should be made to determine whether a mass is solid or cystic, smooth or irregular, and whether it moves with respiration. The liver, spleen, and gallbladder should descend with respiration unless they are fixed by adhesions or extension of tumor beyond the organ. A fixed mass not descending with respiration may indicate that it is retroperitoneal. Tenderness, especially if localized, may indicate an inflammatory process such as an abscess; it also may be due to stretching of the visceral peritoneum or tumor necrosis. Rectal and pelvic examinations are mandatory; they may reveal otherwise undetected masses due to tumor or infection.

Radiographic and laboratory examinations are essential for confirming or extending the impressions gained on physical examination. Upright and recumbent films of the abdomen may demonstrate the dilated loops of intestine with fluid levels characteristic of intestinal obstruction or the diffuse abdominal haziness and loss of psoas margins suggestive of ascites. Ultrasonography is often of value in detecting ascites, determining the presence of a mass, or evaluating the size of the liver and

TABLE 44-1 CHARACTERISTICS OF ASCITIC FLUID IN VARIOUS DISEASE STATES

Condition	Gross Appearance	Protein, g/L	Serum-Ascites Albumin Gradient, g/dL	Cell Count: Red Blood Cells, >10,000/μL	Cell Count: White Blood Cells, per μL	Other Tests
Cirrhosis	Straw-colored or bile-stained	<25 (95%)	>1.1	1%	<250 (90%)[a]; predominantly mesothelial	
Neoplasm	Straw-colored, hemorrhagic, mucinous, or chylous	>25 (75%)	<1.1	20%	>1000 (50%); variable cell types	Cytology, cell block, peritoneal biopsy
Tuberculous peritonitis	Clear, turbid, hemorrhagic, chylous	>25 (50%)	<1.1	7%	>1000 (70%); usually >70% lymphocytes	Peritoneal biopsy, stain and culture for acid-fast bacilli
Pyogenic peritonitis	Turbid or purulent	If purulent, >25	<1.1	Unusual	Predominantly polymorphonuclear leukocytes	Positive Gram's stain, culture
Congestive heart failure	Straw-colored	Variable, 15–53	>1.1	10%	<1000 (90%); usually mesothelial, mononuclear	
Nephrosis	Straw-colored or chylous	<25 (100%)	<1.1	Unusual	<250; mesothelial, mononuclear	If chylous, ether extraction, Sudan staining
Pancreatic ascites (pancreatitis, pseudocyst)	Turbid, hemorrhagic, or chylous	Variable, often >25	<1.1	Variable, may be blood-stained	Variable	Increased amylase in ascitic fluid and serum

[a]Because the conditions of examining fluid and selecting patients were not identical in each series, the percentage figures (in parentheses) should be taken as an indication of the order of magnitude rather than as the precise incidence of any abnormal finding.

spleen. CT scanning provides similar information and is often necessary to visualize the retroperitoneum, pancreas, and lymph nodes. A plain film of the abdomen may reveal the distended colon of otherwise unsuspected ulcerative colitis and give valuable information as to the size of the liver and spleen. An irregular and elevated right side of the diaphragm may be a clue to a liver abscess or hepatocellular carcinoma. Studies of the gastrointestinal tract with barium or other contrast media are usually necessary in the search for a primary tumor.

Laboratory abnormalities that are highly suggestive of cirrhosis as the cause of ascites include unexplained thrombocytopenia, decreased albumin, and a prolonged prothrombin time.

ASCITES

The evaluation of a patient with ascites requires that the cause of the ascites be established. In most cases ascites appears as part of a well-recognized illness, i.e., cirrhosis, congestive heart failure, nephrosis, or disseminated carcinomatosis. In these situations, the physician should determine that the development of ascites is indeed a consequence of the basic underlying disease and not due to the presence of a separate or related disease process. This distinction is necessary even when the cause of ascites seems obvious. For example, when the patient with compensated cirrhosis and minimal ascites develops progressive ascites that is increasingly difficult to control with sodium restriction or diuretics, the temptation is to attribute the worsening of the clinical picture to progressive liver disease. However, an occult hepatocellular carcinoma, portal vein thrombosis, spontaneous bacterial peritonitis, alcoholic hepatitis, viral infection, or even tuberculosis may be responsible for the decompensation. The disappointingly low success in diagnosing tuberculous peritonitis or hepatocellular carcinoma in the patient with cirrhosis and ascites reflects the too-low index of suspicion for the development of such superimposed conditions. Similarly, the patient with congestive heart failure may develop ascites from a disseminated carcinoma with peritoneal seeding. It is important to note, however, that while there are many different causes of ascites, in the United States >80% of cases are due to cirrhosis. Risk factors for the development of cirrhosis include alcoholism, viral hepatitis, nonalcoholic steatohepatitis, and a family history of liver disease.

Diagnostic paracentesis (50–100 mL) should be part of the routine evaluation of the patient with ascites, and does not routinely require the prior administration of platelets or fresh-frozen plasma unless disseminated intravascular coagulation is suspected. The fluid should be examined for its gross appearance; protein content, albumin level, cell count, and differential cell count should be determined; and Gram's and acid-fast stains and culture should be performed. Cytologic and cell-block examination may disclose an otherwise unsuspected carcinoma. A serum ascites–albumin gradient (SAAG) should be calculated to determine if the fluid has the features of a transudate or an exudate. The gradient correlates directly with portal pressure. A gradient >1.1 g/dL (high gradient) is characteristic of uncomplicated cirrhotic ascites and differentiates ascites due to portal hypertension from ascites not due to portal hypertension >97% of the time. Other etiologies of high-gradient ascites include alcoholic hepatitis, congestive heart failure, hepatic metastases, constrictive pericarditis, and Budd-Chiari syndrome. A gradient <1.1 g/dL (low gradient) suggests that the ascites is not due to portal hypertension with >97% accuracy and mandates a search for other causes such as peritoneal carcinomatosis, tuberculous peritonitis, pancreatitis, serositis, pyogenic peritonitis, and nephrotic syndrome (Table 44-1). Table 44-1 presents some of the disease states that produce high-SAAG and low-SAAG ascites. Although there is variability of the ascitic fluid in any given disease state, some features are sufficiently characteristic to suggest certain diagnostic possibilities. For example, blood-stained fluid with >25 g/L protein is unusual in uncomplicated cirrhosis but is consistent with tuberculous peritonitis or neoplasm. Cloudy fluid with a predominance of polymorphonuclear cells (>250/μL) and a positive Gram's stain are characteristic of bacterial peritonitis, which requires antibiotic therapy; if most cells are lymphocytes, tuberculosis should be suspected. The complete examination of each fluid is most important, for occasionally only one finding may be abnormal. For example, if the fluid is a typical transudate but contains >250 white blood cells per microliter, the finding should be recognized as atypical for cirrhosis and should warrant a search for tumor or infection. This is especially true in the evaluation of cirrhotic ascites where occult peritoneal infection may be present with only minor elevations in the white blood cell count of the peritoneal fluid (300–500/μL). Since Gram's stain of the fluid may be negative in a high proportion of such cases, careful culture of the peritoneal fluid is mandatory. Bedside inoculation of blood culture flasks with ascitic fluid results in a dramatically increased incidence of positive cultures when bacterial infection is present (90 vs. 40% positivity with conventional cultures done by the laboratory). Direct visualization of the peritoneum (laparoscopy) may disclose peritoneal deposits of tumor, tuberculosis, or metastatic disease of the liver. Biopsies are taken under direct vision, often adding to the diagnostic accuracy of the procedure.

Chylous ascites refers to a turbid, milky, or creamy peritoneal fluid due to the presence of thoracic or intestinal lymph. Such a fluid shows Sudan-staining fat globules microscopically and an increased triglyceride content by chemical examination. Opaque milky fluid usually has a triglyceride concentration of >11.3 mmol/L (>1000 mg/dL), but a triglyceride concentration of >2.3 mmol/L (>200 mg/dL) is sufficient for the diagnosis. A turbid fluid due to leukocytes or tumor cells may be confused with chylous fluid (pseudochylous), and it is often helpful to carry out alkalinization and ether extraction of the specimen. Alkali tend to dissolve cellular proteins and thereby reduce turbidity; ether extraction leads to clearing if the turbidity of the fluid is due to lipid. Chylous ascites is most often the result of lymphatic disruption or obstruction from cirrhosis, tumor, trauma, tuberculosis, filariasis (Chap. 211), or congenital abnormalities. It may also be seen in the nephrotic syndrome.

Rarely, ascitic fluid may be *mucinous* in character, suggesting either pseudomyxoma peritonei (Chap. 291) or rarely a colloid carcinoma of the stomach or colon with peritoneal implants.

On occasion, ascites may develop as a seemingly isolated finding in the absence of a clinically evident underlying disease. Then, a careful analysis of ascitic fluid may indicate the direction the evaluation should take. A useful framework for the workup starts with an analysis of whether the fluid is classified as a high (transudate) or low (exudate) gradient fluid. *High-gradient (transudative) ascites* of unclear etiology is most often due to occult cirrhosis, right-sided venous hypertension raising hepatic sinusoidal pressure, Budd-Chiari syndrome, or massive hepatic metastases. Cirrhosis with well-preserved liver function (normal albumin) resulting in ascites is invariably associated with significant portal hypertension (Chap. 301). Evaluation should include liver function tests and a hepatic imaging procedure (i.e., CT or ultrasound) to detect nodular changes in the liver suggesting portal hypertension. On occasion, a wedged hepatic venous pressure can be useful to document portal hypertension. Finally, if clinically indicated, a liver biopsy will confirm the diagnosis of cirrhosis and perhaps suggest its etiology. Other etiologies may result in hepatic venous congestion and resultant ascites. Right-sided cardiac valvular disease and particularly constrictive pericarditis should raise a high index of suspicion and may require cardiac imaging and cardiac catheterization for definitive diagnosis. Hepatic vein thrombosis is evaluated by visualizing the hepatic veins with imaging techniques (Doppler ultrasound, angiography, CT scans, MRI) to demonstrate obliteration, thrombosis, or obstruction by tumor. Uncommonly, transudative ascites may be associated with benign tumors of the ovary, particularly fibroma (Meigs' syndrome) with ascites and hydrothorax.

Low-gradient (exudative) ascites should initiate an evaluation for primary peritoneal processes, most importantly infection and tumor. Tuberculous peritonitis (Table 44-1) is best diagnosed by peritoneal biopsy, either percutaneously or via laparoscopy. Histologic examination invariably shows granulomata that may contain acid-fast bacilli. Since cultures of peritoneal fluid and biopsies for tuberculosis may require 6 weeks, characteristic histology with appropriate stains allows antituberculosis therapy to be started promptly. Similarly, the diagnosis of peritoneal seeding by tumor can usually be made by cytologic analysis of peritoneal fluid or by peritoneal biopsy if cytology is negative. Appropriate diagnostic studies can then be undertaken to determine the nature and site of the primary tumor. Pancreatic ascites (Table 44-1) is invariably associated with an extravasation of pancreatic fluid from the pancreatic ductal system, most commonly from a leaking pseudocyst. Ultrasound or CT examination of the pancreas followed by visualization of the pancreatic duct by direct cannulation [viz., endoscopic retrograde cholangiopancreatography (ERCP)] usually discloses the site of leakage and permits resective surgery to be carried out.

An analysis of the physiologic and metabolic factors involved in the production of ascites (detailed in Chap. 301), coupled with a complete evaluation of the nature of the ascitic fluid, invariably discloses the etiology of the ascites and permits appropriate therapy to be instituted.

ACKNOWLEDGMENT

Dr. Kurt J. Isselbacher was the co-author of this chapter in previous editions.

FURTHER READINGS

LIPSKY MS, STERNBACH MR: Evaluation and initial management of patients with ascites. Am Fam Physician 54:1327, 1996

MCHUTCHISON JG: Differential diagnosis of ascites. Semin Liver Dis 17:191, 1997

PARSONS SL et al: Malignant ascites. Br J Surg 83:6, 1996

PINTO PC et al: Large volume paracentesis in nonedematous patients with tense ascites: Its effect on intravascular volume. Hepatology 8:207, 1988

RUNYON BA: Management of adult patients with ascites due to cirrhosis. Hepatology 39:841, 2004

SECTION 7 ALTERATIONS IN RENAL AND URINARY TRACT FUNCTION

45 Azotemia and Urinary Abnormalities

Bradley M. Denker, Barry M. Brenner

Normal kidney functions occur through numerous cellular processes to maintain body homeostasis. Disturbances in any of these functions can lead to a constellation of abnormalities that may be detrimental to survival. The clinical manifestations of these disorders will depend upon the pathophysiology of the renal injury and will often be initially identified as a complex of symptoms, abnormal physical findings, and laboratory changes that together make possible the identification of specific syndromes. These renal syndromes (Table 45-1) may arise as the consequence of a systemic illness or can occur as a primary renal disease. Nephrologic syndromes usually consist of several elements that reflect the underlying pathologic processes. The duration and severity of the disease will affect these findings and typically include one or more of the following: (1) disturbances in urine volume (oliguria, anuria, polyuria); (2) abnormalities of urine sediment [red blood cells (RBC); white blood cells, casts, and crystals]; (3) abnormal excretion of serum proteins (proteinuria); (4) reduction in glomerular filtration rate (GFR) (azotemia); (5) presence of hypertension and/or expanded total body fluid volume (edema); (6) electrolyte abnormalities; or (7) in some syndromes, fever/pain. The combination of these findings should permit identification of one of the major nephrologic syndromes (Table 45-1) and will allow differential diagnoses to be narrowed and the appropriate diagnostic evaluation and therapeutic course to be determined. Each of these syndromes and their associated diseases are discussed in more detail in subsequent chapters. This chapter will focus on several aspects of renal abnormalities that are critically important to distinguishing among these processes: (1) reduction in GFR leading to azotemia, (2) alterations of the urinary sediment and/or protein excretion, and (3) abnormalities of urinary volume.

TABLE 45-1 INITIAL CLINICAL AND LABORATORY DATA BASE FOR DEFINING MAJOR SYNDROMES IN NEPHROLOGY

Syndromes	Important Clues to Diagnosis	Findings That Are Common	Location of Discussion of Disease-Causing Syndrome
Acute or rapidly progressive renal failure	Anuria Oliguria Documented recent decline in GFR	Hypertension, hematuria Proteinuria, pyuria Casts, edema	Chaps. 273, 277, 279, 283
Acute nephritis	Hematuria, RBC casts Azotemia, oliguria Edema, hypertension	Proteinuria Pyuria Circulatory congestion	Chap. 277
Chronic renal failure	Azotemia for >3 months Prolonged symptoms or signs of uremia Symptoms or signs of renal osteodystrophy Kidneys reduced in size bilaterally Broad casts in urinary sediment	Proteinuria Casts Polyuria, nocturia Edema, hypertension Electrolyte disorders	Chaps. 272, 274
Nephrotic syndrome	Proteinuria >3.5 g per 1.73 m^2 per 24 h Hypoalbuminemia Edema Hyperlipidemia	Casts Lipiduria	Chap. 277
Asymptomatic urinary abnormalities	Hematuria Proteinuria (below nephrotic range) Sterile pyuria, casts		Chap. 277
Urinary tract infection/pyelonephritis	Bacteriuria >10^5 colonies per milliliter Other infectious agent documented in urine Pyuria, leukocyte casts Frequency, urgency Bladder tenderness, flank tenderness	Hematuria Mild azotemia Mild proteinuria Fever	Chap. 282
Renal tubule defects	Electrolyte disorders Polyuria, nocturia Renal calcification Large kidneys Renal transport defects	Hematuria "Tubular" proteinuria (<1 g/24 h) Enuresis	Chaps. 278, 279
Hypertension	Systolic/diastolic hypertension	Proteinuria Casts Azotemia	Chaps. 241, 280
Nephrolithiasis	Previous history of stone passage or removal Previous history of stone seen by x-ray Renal colic	Hematuria Pyuria Frequency, urgency	Chap. 281
Urinary tract obstruction	Azotemia, oliguria, anuria Polyuria, nocturia, urinary retention Slowing of urinary stream Large prostate, large kidneys Flank tenderness, full bladder after voiding	Hematuria Pyuria Enuresis, dysuria	Chap. 283

Note: GFR; glomerular filtration rate; RBC, red blood cell.

AZOTEMIA

ASSESSMENT OF GLOMERULAR FILTRATION RATE

Monitoring the GFR is important in both the hospital and outpatient settings, and several different methodologies are available (discussed below). In most acute clinical circumstances a measured GFR is not available, and the serum creatinine level is used to estimate the GFR in order to supply appropriate doses of renally excreted drugs and to follow short-term changes in GFR. Serum creatinine is the most widely used marker for GFR, and the GFR is related directly to the urine creatinine excretion and inversely to the serum creatinine (U_{Cr}/P_{Cr}). The creatinine clearance is calculated from these measurements for a defined time period (usually 24 h) and is expressed in mL/min. Based upon this relationship and some important caveats (discussed below), the GFR will fall in roughly inverse proportion to the rise in P_{Cr}. Failure to account for GFR reductions in drug dosing can lead to significant morbidity and mortality from drug toxicities (e.g., digoxin, aminoglycosides). In the outpatient setting, the serum creatinine is often used as a surrogate for GFR (although much less accurate; see below). In patients with chronic progressive renal disease there is an approximately linear relationship between $1/P_{Cr}$ and time. The slope of this line will remain constant for an individual patient, and when values are obtained that do not fall on this line, an investigation for a superimposed acute process (e.g., volume depletion, drug reaction) should be initiated. It should be emphasized that the signs and symptoms of uremia will develop at significantly different levels of serum creatinine depending upon the patient (size, age, and sex), the underlying renal disease, existence of concurrent diseases, and true GFR. In general, patients do not develop symptomatic uremia until renal insufficiency is usually quite severe (GFR < 15 mL/min).

A reduced GFR leads to retention of nitrogenous waste products (azotemia) such as urea and creatinine. Azotemia may result from reduced renal perfusion, intrinsic renal disease, or postrenal processes (ureteral obstruction; see below and Fig. 45-1). Precise determination of GFR is problematic as both commonly measured indices (urea and creatinine) have characteristics that affect their accuracy as markers of clearance. Urea clearance may significantly underestimate GFR because of tubule urea reabsorption. Creatinine is derived from muscle metabolism of creatine, and its generation varies little from day to day. Creatinine is useful for estimating GFR because it is a small, freely filtered solute. However, serum creatinine levels can increase acutely from dietary ingestion of cooked meat, and creatinine can be secreted into the proximal tubule through an organic cation pathway, leading to overestimation of the GFR. There are many clinical settings where a creatinine clearance is not available, and decisions concerning drug dosing must be made based on the serum creatinine. Two formulas are widely used to estimate GFR: (1) Cockcroft-Gault, which accounts for age and muscle mass (this value should be multiplied by 0.85 for women, since a lower fraction of the body weight is composed of muscle):

$$\text{Creatinine clearance (mL/min)} = \frac{(140 - \text{age}) \times \text{lean body weight (kg)}}{\text{plasma creatinine (mg/dL)} \times 72}$$

and (2) MDRD (modification of diet in renal disease):

$$\text{GFR (mL/min per 1.73 m}^2) = 186.3 \times P_{Cr}\ (e^{-1.154}) \times \text{age}\ (e^{-0.203}) \times (0.742 \text{ if female}) \times (1.21 \text{ if black}).$$

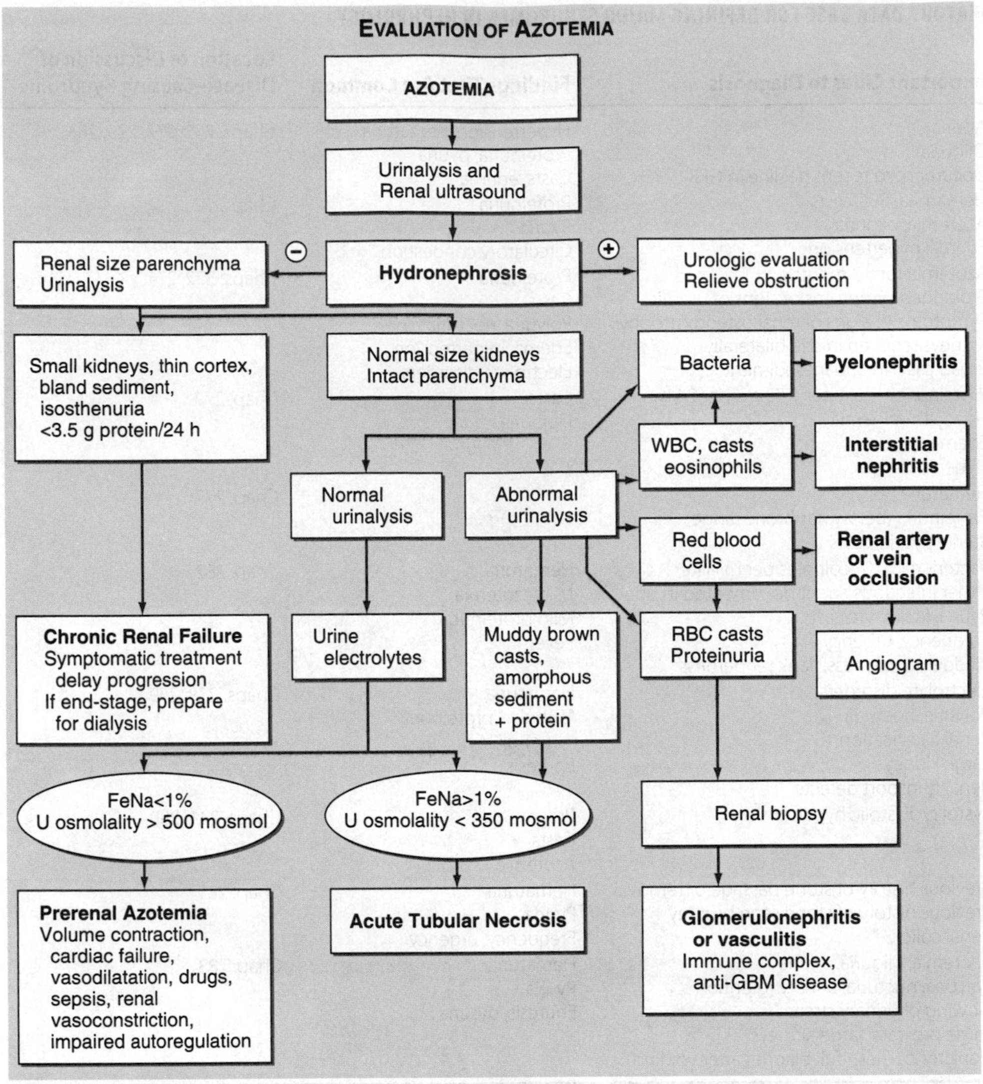

FIGURE 45-1 Approach to the patient with azotemia. WBC, white blood cell; RBC, red blood cell; GBM, glomerular basement membrane.

Although more cumbersome than Cockcroft-Gault, the MDRD equation is felt to be more accurate, and numerous websites are available for making the calculation (*www.kidney.org/professionals/kdoqi/gfr_calculator.cfm*).

The gradual loss of muscle from chronic illness, chronic use of glucocorticoids, or malnutrition can mask significant changes in GFR with small or imperceptible changes in serum creatinine concentration. More accurate determinations of GFR are available using inulin clearance or radionuclide-labeled markers such as ^{125}I-iothalamate or EDTA. These methods are highly accurate due to precise quantitation and the absence of any renal reabsorption/secretion and should be used to follow GFR in patients in whom creatinine is not likely to be a reliable indicator (patients with decreased muscle mass secondary to age, malnutrition, concurrent illnesses). (See also Table 274-2.) Cystatin C is a member of the cystatin superfamily of cysteine protease inhibitors and is produced at a relatively constant rate from all nucleated cells. Cystatin C production is not affected by diet or nutritional status and may provide a more sensitive indicator of GFR than the plasma creatinine concentration. However, it remains to be validated in many clinical settings.

APPROACH TO THE PATIENT: Azotemia

Once it has been established that GFR is reduced, the physician must decide if this represents acute or chronic renal injury. The clinical situation, history, and laboratory data often make this an easy distinction. However, the laboratory abnormalities characteristic of chronic renal failure, including anemia, hypocalcemia, and hyperphosphatemia, are often also present in patients presenting with acute renal failure. Radiographic evidence of renal osteodystrophy (Chap. 274) would be seen only in chronic renal failure but is a very late finding, and these patients are usually on dialysis. The urinalysis and renal ultrasound can occasionally facilitate distinguishing acute from chronic renal failure. An approach to the evaluation of azotemic patients is shown in Fig. 45-1. Patients with advanced chronic renal insufficiency often have some proteinuria, nonconcentrated urine (isosthenuria; isoosmotic with plasma), and small kidneys on ultrasound, characterized by increased echogenicity and cortical thinning. Treatment should be directed toward slowing the progression of renal disease and providing symptomatic relief for edema, acidosis, anemia, and hyperphosphatemia, as discussed in Chap. 274. Acute renal failure (Chap. 273) can result from processes affecting renal blood flow (prerenal azotemia), intrinsic renal diseases (affecting small vessels, glomeruli, or tubules), or postrenal processes (obstruction to urine flow in ureters, bladder, or urethra) (Chap. 283).

Prerenal Failure Decreased renal perfusion accounts for 40–80% of acute renal failure and, if appropriately treated, is readily reversible. The etiologies of prerenal azotemia include any cause of decreased circulating blood volume (gastrointestinal hemorrhage, burns, diarrhea, diuretics), volume sequestration (pancreatitis, peritonitis, rhabdomyolysis), or decreased effective arterial volume (cardiogenic shock, sepsis). Renal perfusion can also be affected by reductions in cardiac output from peripheral vasodilatation (sepsis, drugs) or profound renal vasoconstriction [severe heart failure, hepatorenal syndrome, drugs such as nonsteroidal anti-inflammatory drugs (NSAIDs)]. True, or "effective," arterial hypovolemia leads to a fall in mean arterial pressure, which in turn triggers a series of neural and humoral responses that include activation of the sympathetic nervous and renin-angiotensin-aldosterone systems and ADH release. GFR is maintained by prostaglandin-mediated relaxation of afferent arterioles and angiotensin II–mediated constriction of efferent arterioles. Once the mean arterial pressure falls below 80 mmHg, there is a steep decline in GFR.

Blockade of prostaglandin production by NSAIDs can result in severe vasoconstriction and acute renal failure. Angiotensin-converting enzyme (ACE) inhibitors decrease efferent arteriolar tone and in turn decrease glomerular capillary perfusion pressure. Patients on NSAIDs and/or ACE inhibitors are most susceptible to hemodynamically mediated acute renal failure when blood volume is reduced for any reason. Patients with bilateral renal artery stenosis (or stenosis in a solitary kidney) are dependent upon efferent arteriolar vasoconstriction for maintenance of glomerular filtration pressure and are particularly susceptible to precipitous decline in GFR when given ACE inhibitors.

Prolonged renal hypoperfusion can lead to acute tubular necrosis (ATN; an intrinsic renal disease discussed below). The urinalysis and urinary electrolytes can be useful in distinguishing prerenal azotemia from ATN (Table 45-2). The urine of patients with prerenal azotemia can be predicted from the stimulatory actions of norepinephrine, angiotensin II, ADH, and low tubule fluid flow rate on salt and water reabsorption. In prerenal conditions, the tubules are intact leading to a concentrated urine (>500 mosm), avid Na retention (urine Na concentration < 20 m*M*/L; fractional excretion of Na < 1%), and $U_{Cr}/P_{Cr} > 40$ (Table 45-2). The prerenal urine sediment is usually normal or has occasional hyaline and granular casts, while the sediment of ATN is usually filled with cellular debris and dark (muddy brown) granular casts.

Postrenal Azotemia Urinary tract obstruction accounts for <5% of cases of acute renal failure, but it is usually reversible and must be ruled out early in the evaluation (Fig. 45-1). Since a single kidney is capable of adequate clearance, acute renal failure from obstruction requires obstruction at the urethra or bladder outlet, bilateral ureteral obstruction, or unilateral obstruction in a patient with a single functioning kidney. Obstruction is usually diagnosed by the presence of ureteral and renal pelvic dilatation on renal ultrasound. However, early in the course of obstruction or if the ureters are unable to dilate (such as encasement by pelvic tumors or periureteral), the ultrasound examination may be negative. **The specific urologic conditions that cause obstruction are discussed in Chap. 283.**

Intrinsic Renal Disease When prerenal and postrenal azotemia have been excluded as etiologies of renal failure, an intrinsic parenchymal renal disease is present. Intrinsic renal disease can arise from processes involving large renal vessels, intrarenal microvasculature and glomeruli, or tubulointerstitium. Ischemic and toxic ATN account for ~90% of acute intrinsic renal failure. As outlined in Fig. 45-1, the clinical setting and urinalysis are helpful in separating the possible etiologies of acute intrinsic renal failure. Prerenal azotemia and ATN are part of a spectrum of renal hypoperfusion; evidence of structural tubule injury is present in ATN, whereas prompt reversibility occurs with prerenal azotemia upon restoration of adequate renal perfusion. Thus, ATN can often be distinguished from prerenal azotemia by urinalysis and urine electrolyte composition (Table 45-2 and Fig. 45-1). Ischemic ATN is observed most frequently in patients who have undergone major surgery, trauma, severe hypovolemia, overwhelming sepsis, or extensive burns. Nephrotoxic ATN complicates the administration of many common medications, usually by inducing a combination of intrarenal vasoconstriction, direct tubule toxicity, and/or tubule obstruction. The kidney is vulnerable to toxic injury by virtue of its rich blood supply (25% of cardiac output) and its ability to concentrate and metabolize toxins. A diligent search for hypotension and nephrotoxins will usually uncover the specific etiology of ATN.

TABLE 45-2 LABORATORY FINDINGS IN ACUTE RENAL FAILURE

Index	Prerenal Azotemia	Oliguric Acute Renal Failure
BUN/P_{Cr} Ratio	>20:1	10–15:1
Urine sodium (U_{Na}), meq/L	<20	>40
Urine osmolality, mosmol/L H_2O	>500	<350
Fractional excretion of sodium	<1%	>2%
$FE_{Na} = \dfrac{U_{Na} \times P_{Cr} \times 100}{P_{Na} \times U_{Cr}}$		
Urine/plasma creatinine (U_{Cr}/P_{Cr})	>40	<20

Note: BUN, Blood urea nitrogen; P_{Cr}, plasma creatinine; U_{Na}, urine sodium concentration; P_{Na}, plasma sodium concentration; U_{Cr}, urine creatinine concentration.

Discontinuation of nephrotoxins and stabilizing blood pressure will often suffice without the need for dialysis while the tubules recover. **An extensive list of potential drugs and toxins implicated in ATN can be found in Chap. 273.**

Processes that involve the tubules and interstitium can lead to acute renal failure. These include drug-induced interstitial nephritis (especially antibiotics, NSAIDs, and diuretics), severe infections (both bacterial and viral), systemic diseases (e.g., systemic lupus erythematosus), or infiltrative disorders (e.g., sarcoid, lymphoma, or leukemia). A list of drugs associated with allergic interstitial nephritis can be found in Chap. 279. The urinalysis usually shows mild to moderate proteinuria, hematuria, and pyuria (~75% of cases) and occasionally white blood cell casts. The finding of RBC casts in interstitial nephritis has been reported but should prompt a search for glomerular diseases (Fig. 45-1). Occasionally renal biopsy will be needed to distinguish among these possibilities. The finding of eosinophils in the urine is suggestive of allergic interstitial nephritis or atheroembolic renal disease and is optimally observed by using a Hansel stain. The absence of eosinophiluria, however, does not exclude these possible etiologies.

Occlusion of large renal vessels including arteries and veins is an uncommon cause of acute renal failure. A significant reduction in GFR by this mechanism suggests bilateral processes or a unilateral process in a patient with a single functioning kidney. Renal arteries can be occluded with atheroemboli, thromboemboli, in situ thrombosis, aortic dissection, or vasculitis. Atheroembolic renal failure can occur spontaneously but is most often associated with recent aortic instrumentation. The emboli are cholesterol-rich and lodge in medium and small renal arteries, leading to an eosinophil-rich inflammatory reaction. Patients with atheroembolic acute renal failure often have a normal urinalysis, but the urine may contain eosinophils and casts. The diagnosis can be confirmed by renal biopsy, but this is often unnecessary when other stigmata of atheroemboli are present (livedo reticularis, distal peripheral infarcts, eosinophilia). Renal artery thrombosis may lead to mild proteinuria and hematuria, whereas renal vein thrombosis typically induces heavy proteinuria and hematuria. **These vascular complications often require angiography for confirmation and are discussed in Chap. 280.**

Diseases of glomeruli (glomerulonephritis or vasculitis) and the renal microvasculature (hemolytic uremic syndromes, thrombotic thrombocytopenic purpura, or malignant hypertension) usually present with various combinations of glomerular injury: proteinuria, hematuria, reduced GFR, and alterations of Na excretion leading to hypertension, edema, and circulatory congestion (acute nephritic syndrome). These findings may occur as primary renal diseases or as renal manifestations of systemic diseases. The clinical setting and other laboratory data will help distinguish primary renal from systemic diseases. The finding of RBC casts in the urine is an indication for early renal biopsy (Fig. 45-1) as the pathologic pattern has important implications for diagnosis, prognosis, and treatment. Hematuria without RBC casts can also be an indication of glomerular disease, and this evaluation is summarized in Fig. 45-2. **A detailed discussion of glomerulonephritis and diseases of the microvasculature can be found in Chap. 277.**

Oliguria and Anuria *Oliguria* refers to a 24-h urine output of <500 mL, and *anuria* is the complete absence of urine formation (<50 mL). Anuria can be caused by total urinary tract obstruction, total renal artery or vein occlusion, and shock (manifested by severe hypotension and intense renal vasoconstriction). Cortical necrosis, ATN, and rapidly progressive glomerulonephritis can occasionally cause anuria. Oliguria can accompany any cause of acute renal failure and carries a more serious prognosis for renal recovery in all conditions except prerenal azotemia. *Nonoliguria* refers to urine output >500 mL/d in patients with acute or chronic azotemia. With nonoliguric ATN, disturbances of potassium and hydrogen balance are less severe than in oliguric patients, and recovery to normal renal function is usually more rapid.

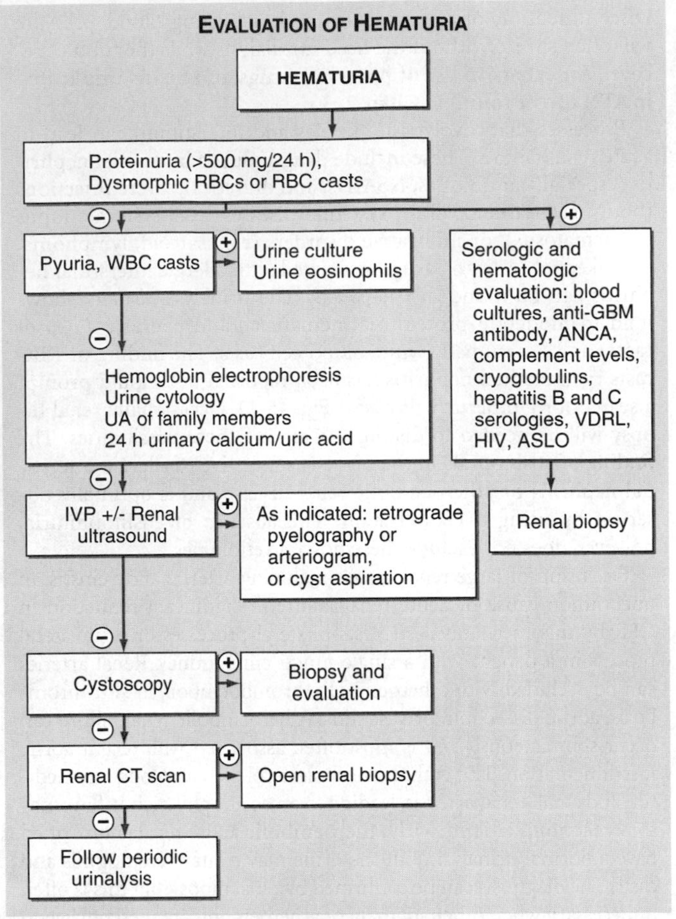

FIGURE 45-2 Approach to the patient with hematuria. RBC, red blood cell; WBC, white blood cell; GBM, glomerular basement membrane; ANCA, antineutrophil cytoplasmic antibody; VDRL, venereal disease research laboratory; ASLO, antistreptolysin O; UA, urinalysis; IVP, intravenous pyelography; CT, computed tomography.

ABNORMALITIES OF THE URINE

PROTEINURIA

The evaluation of proteinuria is shown schematically in Fig. 45-3 and is typically initiated after detection of proteinuria by dipstick examination. The dipstick measurement detects mostly albumin and gives false-positive results when pH > 7.0 and the urine is very concentrated or contaminated with blood. A very dilute urine may obscure significant proteinuria on dipstick examination, and proteinuria that is not predominantly albumin will be missed. This is particularly important for the detection of Bence-Jones proteins in the urine of patients with multiple myeloma. Tests to measure total urine concentration accurately rely on precipitation with sulfosalicylic or trichloracetic acids. Currently, ultrasensitive dipsticks are available to measure microalbuminuria (30–300 mg/d), an early marker of glomerular disease that has been shown to predict glomerular injury in early diabetic nephropathy (Fig. 45-3).

The magnitude of proteinuria and the protein composition of the urine depend upon the mechanism of renal injury leading to protein losses. Both charge and size selectivity normally prevent virtually all plasma albumin, globulins, and other large-molecular-weight proteins from crossing the glomerular wall. However, if this barrier is disrupted, there can be leakage of plasma proteins into the urine (glomerular proteinuria; Fig. 45-3). Smaller proteins (<20 kDa) are freely filtered but are readily reabsorbed by the proximal tubule. Normal individuals excrete <150 mg/d of total protein and <30 mg/d of albumin. The remainder of the protein in the urine is secreted by the tubules (Tamm-Horsfall, IgA, and urokinase) or represents small amounts of filtered β_2-microglobulin, apoproteins, enzymes, and peptide hormones. Another mechanism of proteinuria occurs when there is excessive production of an abnormal protein that exceeds the capacity of the tubule for reabsorption. This most commonly occurs with plasma cell dyscrasias such as multiple myeloma, amyloidosis, and lymphomas that are associated with monoclonal production of immunoglobulin light chains.

The normal glomerular endothelial cell forms a barrier composed of pores of ~100 nm that hold back blood cells but offer little impediment to passage of most proteins. The glomerular basement membrane traps most large proteins (>100 kDa), while the foot processes of epithelial cells (podocytes) cover the urinary side of the glomerular basement membrane and produce a series of narrow channels (slit diaphragms) to normally allow molecular passage of small solutes and water but not proteins. Some glomerular diseases, such as minimal change disease, cause fusion of glomerular epithelial cell foot processes, resulting in predominantly "selective" (Fig. 45-3) loss of albumin. Other glomerular diseases can present with disruption of the basement membrane and slit diaphragms (e.g., by immune complex deposition), resulting in losses of albumin and other plasma proteins. The fusion of foot processes causes increased pressure across the capillary basement membrane, resulting in areas with larger pore sizes. The combination of increased pressure and larger pores results in significant proteinuria ("nonselective"; Fig. 45-3).

When the total daily excretion of protein is >3.5 g, there is often associated hypoalbuminemia, hyperlipidemia, and edema (nephrotic syndrome; Fig. 45-3). However, total daily urinary protein excretion >3.5 g can occur without the other features of the nephrotic syndrome in a variety of other renal diseases (Fig. 45-3). Plasma cell dyscrasias (multiple myeloma) can be associated with large amounts of excreted light chains in the urine, which may not be detected by dipstick (which detects mostly albumin). The light chains produced from these disorders are filtered by the glomerulus and overwhelm the reabsorptive capacity of the proximal tubule. A sulfosalicylic acid precipitate that is out of proportion to the dipstick estimate is suggestive of light chains (Bence Jones protein), and light chains typically redissolve upon warming of the precipitate. Renal failure from these disorders occurs through a variety of mechanisms including tubule obstruction (cast nephropathy) and light chain deposition.

Hypoalbuminemia in nephrotic syndrome occurs through excessive urinary losses and increased proximal tubule catabolism of filtered albumin. Hepatic rates of albumin synthesis are increased although not to levels sufficient to prevent hypoalbuminemia. Edema forms from renal sodium retention and from reduced plasma oncotic pressure, which favors fluid movement from capillaries to interstitium. The mechanisms designed to correct the decrease in effective intravascular volume contribute to edema formation in some patients. These mechanisms include activation of the renin-angiotensin system, antidiuretic hormone, and the sympathetic nervous system, all of which promote excessive renal salt and water reabsorption.

The severity of edema correlates with the degree of hypoalbuminemia and is modified by other factors such as heart disease or peripheral vascular disease. The diminished plasma oncotic pressure and urinary losses of regulatory proteins appear to stimulate hepatic lipoprotein synthesis. The resulting hyperlipidemia results in lipid bodies (fatty casts, oval fat bodies) in the urine. Other proteins are lost in the urine, leading to a variety of metabolic disturbances. These include thyroxine-binding globulin, cholecalciferol-binding protein, transferrin, and metal-binding proteins. A hypercoagulable state frequently accompanies severe nephrotic syndrome due to urinary losses of antithrombin III, reduced serum levels of proteins S and C, hyperfibrinogenemia, and enhanced platelet aggregation. Some patients develop severe IgG deficiency with resulting defects in immunity. Many diseases (some listed in Fig. 45-3) and drugs can cause the nephrotic syndrome, and a complete list can be found in Chap. 277.

HEMATURIA, PYURIA, AND CASTS

Isolated hematuria without proteinuria, other cells, or casts is often indicative of bleeding from the urinary tract. Normal red blood cell excretion is up to 2 million RBCs per day. Hematuria is defined as two to five RBCs per high-power field (HPF) and can be detected by dipstick. Common causes of isolated hematuria include stones, neoplasms, tuberculosis, trauma, and prostatitis. Gross hematuria with blood clots is

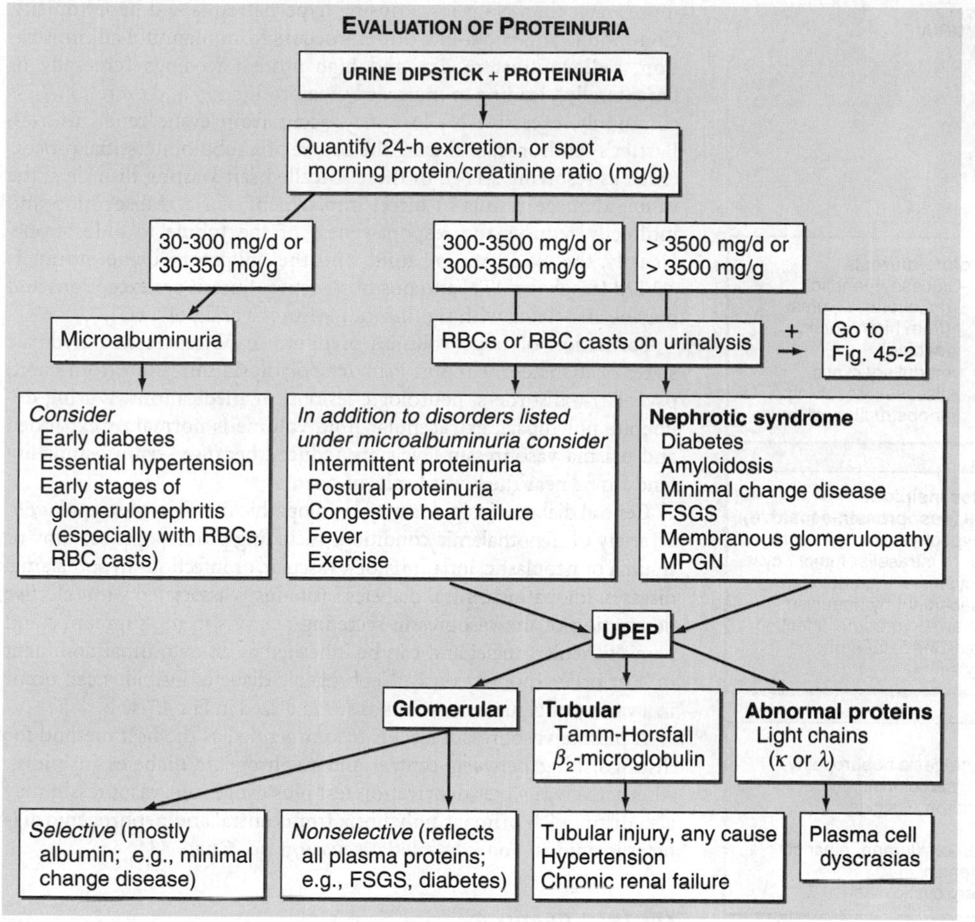

FIGURE 45-3 Approach to the patient with proteinuria. Investigation of proteinuria is often initiated by a positive dipstick on routine urinalysis. Conventional dipsticks detect predominantly albumin and cannot detect urinary albumin levels of 30–300 mg/d. However, more exact determination of proteinuria should employ a 24-h urine collection or a spot morning protein/creatinine ratio (mg/g). The pattern of proteinuria on UPEP (urine protein electrophoresis) can be classified as "glomerular," "tubular," or "abnormal" depending upon the origin of the urine proteins. Glomerular proteinuria is due to abnormal glomerular permeability. "Tubular proteins" such as Tamm-Horsfall are normally produced by the renal tubule and shed into the urine. Abnormal circulating proteins such as kappa or lambda light chains are readily filtered because of their small size. RBC, red blood cell; FSGS, focal segmental glomerulosclerosis; MPGN, membranoproliferative glomerulonephritis.

almost never indicative of glomerular bleeding; rather, it suggests a postrenal source in the urinary collecting system. Evaluation of patients presenting with microscopic hematuria is outlined in Fig. 45-2. A single urinalysis with hematuria is common and can result from menstruation, viral illness, allergy, exercise, or mild trauma. Annual urinalysis of servicemen over a 10-year period showed an incidence of 38%. However, persistent or significant hematuria (>three RBCs/HPF on three urinalyses, or a single urinalysis with >100 RBCs, or gross hematuria) identified significant renal or urologic lesions in 9.1%. Even patients who are chronically anticoagulated should be investigated as outlined in Fig. 45-2. The suspicion for urogenital neoplasms in patients with isolated painless hematuria (nondysmorphic RBCs) increases with age. Neoplasms are rare in the pediatric population, and isolated hematuria is more likely to be "idiopathic" or associated with a congenital anomaly. Hematuria with pyuria and bacteriuria is typical of infection and should be treated with antibiotics after appropriate cultures. Acute cystitis or urethritis in women can cause gross hematuria. Hypercalciuria and hyperuricosuria are also risk factors for unexplained isolated hematuria in both children and adults. In some of these patients (50–60%), reducing calcium and uric acid excretion through dietary interventions can eliminate the microscopic hematuria.

Isolated microscopic hematuria can be a manifestation of glomerular diseases. The RBCs of glomerular origin are often dysmorphic when examined by phase-contrast microscopy. Irregular shapes of RBCs may also occur due to pH and osmolarity changes produced along the distal nephron. There is, however, significant observer variability in detecting dysmorphic RBCs. The most common etiologies of isolated glomerular hematuria are IgA nephropathy, hereditary nephritis, and thin basement membrane disease. IgA nephropathy and hereditary nephritis can lead to episodic gross hematuria. A family history of renal failure is often present in patients with hereditary nephritis, and patients with thin basement membrane disease often have other family members with microscopic hematuria. A renal biopsy is needed for the definitive diagnosis of these disorders, which are discussed in more detail in Chap. 277. Hematuria with dysmorphic RBCs, RBC casts, and protein excretion >500 mg/d is virtually diagnostic of glomerulonephritis. RBC casts form as RBCs that enter the tubule fluid become trapped in a cylindrical mold of gelled Tamm-Horsfall protein. Even in the absence of azotemia, these patients should undergo serologic evaluation and renal biopsy as outlined in Fig. 45-2.

Isolated pyuria is unusual since inflammatory reactions in the kidney or collecting system are also associated with hematuria. The presence of bacteria suggests infection, and white blood cell casts with bacteria are indicative of pyelonephritis. White blood cells and/or white blood cell casts may also be seen in tubulointerstitial processes such as interstitial nephritis, systemic lupus erythematosus, and transplant rejection. In chronic renal diseases, degenerated cellular casts called *waxy casts* can be seen in the urine. *Broad casts* are thought to arise in the dilated tubules of enlarged nephrons that have undergone compensatory hypertrophy in response to reduced renal mass (i.e., chronic renal failure). A mixture of broad casts typically seen with chronic renal failure together with cellular casts and RBCs may be seen in smoldering processes such as chronic glomerulonephritis.

ABNORMALITIES OF URINE VOLUME

The volume of urine produced varies depending upon the fluid intake, renal function, and physiologic demands of the individual. See "Azotemia," above, for discussion of decreased (oliguria) or absent urine production (anuria). **The physiology of water formation and renal water conservation are discussed in Chap. 272.**

POLYURIA

By history, it is often difficult for patients to distinguish urinary frequency (often of small volumes) from polyuria (>3 L/d), and a 24-h urine collection is needed for evaluation (Fig. 45-4). Polyuria results from two potential mechanisms: (1) excretion of nonabsorbable solutes (such as glucose) or (2) excretion of water (usually from a defect in ADH production or renal responsiveness). To distinguish a solute diuresis from a water diuresis and to determine if the diuresis is appropriate for the clinical circumstances, a urine osmolality is measured.

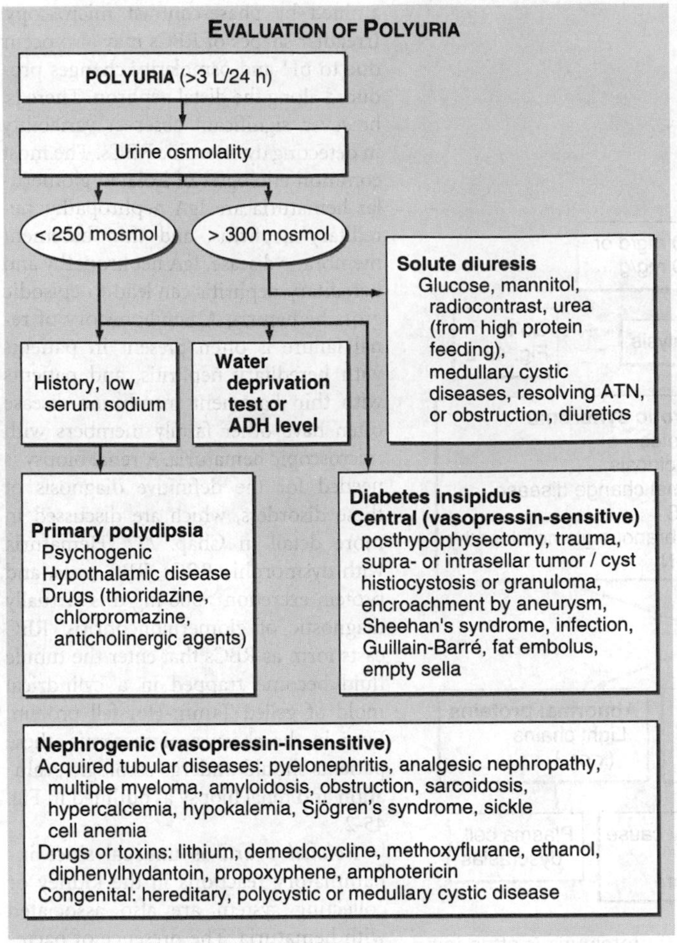

FIGURE 45-4 Approach to the patient with polyuria. ATN, acute tubular necrosis; ADH, antidiuretic hormone.

The average person excretes between 600 and 800 mosmol of solutes per day, primarily as urea and electrolytes. If the urine output is >3 L/d and the urine is dilute (<250 mosmol/L), then total mosmol excretion is normal and a water diuresis is present. This circumstance could arise from polydipsia, inadequate secretion of vasopressin (central diabetes insipidus), or failure of renal tubules to respond to vasopressin (nephrogenic diabetes insipidus). If the urine volume is >3 L/d and urine osmolality is >300 mosmol/L, then a solute diuresis is clearly present and a search for the responsible solute(s) is mandatory.

Excessive filtration of a poorly reabsorbed solute such as glucose, mannitol, or urea can depress reabsorption of NaCl and water in the proximal tubule and lead to enhanced excretion in the urine. Poorly controlled diabetes mellitus with glucosuria is the most common cause of a solute diuresis, leading to volume depletion and serum hypertonicity. Since the urine Na concentration is less than that of blood, more water than Na is lost, causing hypernatremia and hypertonicity. Common iatrogenic solute diuresis occurs from mannitol administration, radiocontrast media, and high-protein feedings (enterally or parenterally), leading to increased urea production and excretion. Less commonly, excessive Na loss may occur from cystic renal diseases, Bartter's syndrome, or during the course of a tubulointerstitial process (such as resolving ATN). In these so-called salt-wasting disorders, the tubule damage results in direct impairment of Na reabsorption and indirectly reduces the responsiveness of the tubule to aldosterone. Usually, the Na losses are mild, and the obligatory urine output is <2 L/d (resolving ATN and postobstructive diuresis are exceptions and may be associated with significant natriuresis and polyuria).

Formation of large volumes of dilute urine represent polydipsic states or diabetes insipidus. Primary polydipsia can result from habit, psychiatric disorders, neurologic lesions, or medications. During deliberate polydipsia, extracellular fluid volume is normal or expanded and plasma vasopressin levels are reduced because serum osmolality tends to be near the lower limits of normal.

Central diabetes insipidus may be idiopathic in origin or secondary to a variety of hypothalamic conditions including posthypophysectomy or trauma or neoplastic, inflammatory, vascular, or infectious hypothalamic diseases. Idiopathic central diabetes insipidus is associated with selective destruction of the vasopressin-secreting neurons in the supraoptic and paraventricular nuclei and can be inherited as an autosomal dominant trait or occur spontaneously. Nephrogenic diabetes insipidus can occur in a variety of clinical situations as summarized in Fig. 45-4.

A plasma vasopressin level is recommended as the best method for distinguishing between central and nephrogenic diabetes insipidus. Alternatively, a water deprivation test plus exogenous vasopressin may also distinguish primary polydipsia from central and nephrogenic diabetes insipidus. For a detailed discussion, see Chap. 334.

FURTHER READINGS

ANDERSON S et al: Renal and systemic manifestations of glomerular disease, in *Brenner & Rector's The Kidney*, 7th ed, BM Brenner (ed). Philadelphia, Saunders, 2004, pp 1927–1954

BERL T, VERBALIS J: Pathophysiology of water metabolism, in *Brenner & Rector's The Kidney*, 7th ed, BM Brenner (ed). Philadelphia, Saunders, 2004, pp 857–920

KASISKE BL, KEANE WF: Laboratory assessment of renal disease: Clearance, urinalysis and renal biopsy, in *Brenner & Rector's The Kidney*, 7th ed, BM Brenner (ed). Philadelphia, Saunders, 2004, pp 1107–1150

KHADRA MH et al: A prospective analysis of 1,930 patients with hematuria to evaluate current diagnostic practice. J Urol 163:524, 2000

RODRIGO E et al: Measurement of renal function in pre-ESRD patients. Kidney Int Suppl 80:11, 2002

SASAKI S: Nephrogenic diabetes insipidus: Update of genetic and clinical aspects. Nephrol Dial Transplant 19:1351, 2004

SHRIER RW et al: Acute renal failure: Definitions, diagnosis, pathogenesis and therapy. J Clin Invest 114:5, 2004

46 Fluid and Electrolyte Disturbances

Gary G. Singer, Barry M. Brenner

SODIUM AND WATER

Composition of Body Fluids Water is the most abundant constituent in the body, comprising approximately 50% of body weight in women and 60% in men. This difference is attributable to differences in the relative proportions of adipose tissue in men and women. Total body water is distributed in two major compartments: 55–75% is intracellular [intracellular fluid (ICF)], and 25–45% is extracellular [extracellular fluid (ECF)]. The ECF is further subdivided into intravascular (plasma water) and extravascular (interstitial) spaces in a ratio of 1:3.

The solute or particle concentration of a fluid is known as its *osmolality* and is expressed as milliosmoles per kilogram of water (mosmol/kg). Water crosses cell membranes to achieve osmotic equilibrium (ECF osmolality = ICF osmolality). The extracellular and intracellular solutes or osmoles are markedly different due to disparities in permeability and the presence of transporters and active pumps. The major ECF particles are Na^+ and its accompanying anions Cl^- and HCO_3^-, whereas K^+ and organic phosphate esters (ATP, creatine phosphate, and phospholipids) are the predominant ICF osmoles. Solutes that are restricted to the ECF or the ICF determine the *effective osmolality* (or *tonicity*) of that compartment. Since Na^+ is largely restricted to the extracellular compartment, total body Na^+ content is a reflection of ECF volume. Likewise, K^+ and its attendant anions are predominantly limited to the ICF and are necessary for normal cell function. Therefore, the number of intracellular particles is relatively constant, and a change in ICF osmolality is usually due to a change in ICF water content. However, in certain situations, brain cells can vary the number of intracellular solutes in order to defend against large water shifts. This process of *osmotic adaptation* is important in the defense of cell volume and occurs in chronic hyponatremia and hypernatremia. This response is mediated initially by transcellular shifts of K^+ and Na^+, followed by synthesis, import, or export of organic solutes (so-called osmolytes) such as inositol, betaine, and glutamine. During chronic hyponatremia, brain cells lose solutes, thereby defending cell volume and diminishing neurologic symptoms. The converse occurs during chronic hypernatremia. Certain solutes, such as urea, do not contribute to water shift across cell membranes and are known as *ineffective osmoles.*

Fluid movement between the intravascular and interstitial spaces occurs across the capillary wall and is determined by the Starling forces—capillary hydraulic pressure and colloid osmotic pressure. The transcapillary hydraulic pressure gradient exceeds the corresponding oncotic pressure gradient, thereby favoring the movement of plasma ultrafiltrate into the extravascular space. The return of fluid into the intravascular compartment occurs via lymphatic flow.

Water Balance (See also Chap. 272) The normal plasma osmolality is 275–290 mosmol/kg and is kept within a narrow range by mechanisms capable of sensing a 1–2% change in tonicity. To maintain a steady state, water intake must equal water excretion. Disorders of water homeostasis result in hypo- or hypernatremia. Normal individuals have an obligate water loss consisting of urine, stool, and evaporation from the skin and respiratory tract. Gastrointestinal excretion is usually a minor component of total water output, except in patients with vomiting, diarrhea, or high enterostomy output states. Evaporative or insensitive water losses are important in the regulation of core body temperature. Obligatory renal water loss is mandated by the minimum solute excretion required to maintain a steady state. Normally, about 600 mosmols must be excreted per day, and since the maximal urine osmolality is 1200 mosmol/kg, a minimum urine output of 500 mL/d is required for neutral solute balance.

WATER INTAKE The primary stimulus for water ingestion is *thirst*, mediated either by an increase in effective osmolality or a decrease in ECF volume or blood pressure. *Osmoreceptors*, located in the anterolateral hypothalamus, are stimulated by a rise in tonicity. Ineffective osmoles, such as urea and glucose, do not play a role in stimulating thirst. The average osmotic threshold for thirst is approximately 295 mosmol/kg and varies among individuals. Under normal circumstances, daily water intake exceeds physiologic requirements.

WATER EXCRETION In contrast to the ingestion of water, its excretion is tightly regulated by physiologic factors. The principal determinant of renal water excretion is *arginine vasopressin* (AVP; formerly antidiuretic hormone), a polypeptide synthesized in the supraoptic and paraventricular nuclei of the hypothalamus and secreted by the posterior pituitary gland. The binding of AVP to V_2 receptors on the basolateral membrane of principal cells in the collecting duct activates adenylyl cyclase and initiates a sequence of events that leads to the insertion of water channels into the luminal membrane. These water channels that are specifically activated by AVP are encoded by the *aquaporin-2* gene (Chap. 334). The net effect is passive water reabsorption along an osmotic gradient from the lumen of the collecting duct to the hypertonic medullary interstitium. The major stimulus for AVP secretion is hypertonicity. Since the major ECF solutes are Na^+ salts, effective osmolality is primarily determined by the plasma Na^+ concentration. An increase or decrease in tonicity is sensed by hypothalamic osmoreceptors as a decrease or increase in cell volume, respectively, leading to enhancement or suppression of AVP secretion. The osmotic threshold for AVP release is 280–290 mosmol/kg, and the system is sufficiently sensitive that plasma osmolality varies by no more than 1–2%.

Nonosmotic factors that regulate AVP secretion include *effective circulating (arterial) volume*, nausea, pain, stress, hypoglycemia, pregnancy, and numerous drugs. The hemodynamic response is mediated by baroreceptors in the carotid sinus. The sensitivity of these receptors is significantly lower than that of the osmoreceptors. In fact, depletion of blood volume sufficient to result in a decreased mean arterial pressure is necessary to stimulate AVP release, whereas small changes in effective circulating volume have little effect.

To maintain homeostasis and a normal plasma Na^+ concentration, the ingestion of solute-free water must eventually lead to the loss of the same volume of electrolyte-free water. Three steps are required for the kidney to excrete a water load: (1) filtration and delivery of water (and electrolytes) to the diluting sites of the nephron; (2) active reabsorption of Na^+ and Cl^- without water in the thick ascending limb of the loop of Henle (TALH) and, to a lesser extent, in the distal nephron; and (3) maintenance of a dilute urine due to impermeability of the collecting duct to water in the absence of AVP. Abnormalities of any of these steps can result in impaired free water excretion, and eventual hyponatremia.

Sodium Balance Sodium is actively pumped out of cells by the Na^+, K^+-ATPase pump. As a result, 85–90% of all Na^+ is extracellular, and the ECF volume is a reflection of total body Na^+ content. Normal volume regulatory mechanisms ensure that Na^+ loss balances Na^+ gain. If this does not occur, conditions of Na^+ excess or deficit ensue and are manifest as edematous or hypovolemic states, respectively. It is important to distinguish between disorders of osmoregulation and disorders of volume regulation since water and Na^+ balance are regulated independently. Changes in Na^+ concentration generally reflect disturbed water homeostasis, whereas alterations in Na^+ content are manifest as ECF volume contraction or expansion and imply abnormal Na^+ balance.

SODIUM INTAKE Individuals eating a typical western diet consume approximately 150 mmol of NaCl daily. This normally exceeds basal requirements. As noted above, sodium is the principal extracellular cation. Therefore, dietary intake of Na^+ results in ECF volume expansion, which in turn promotes enhanced renal Na^+ excretion to maintain steady state Na^+ balance.

SODIUM EXCRETION (See also Chap. 272) The regulation of Na^+ excretion is multifactorial and is the major determinant of Na^+ balance. A Na^+ deficit or excess is manifest as a decreased or increased effective circulating volume, respectively. Changes in effective circulating volume tend to lead to parallel changes in glomerular filtration rate (GFR). However, tubule Na^+ reabsorption, and not GFR, is the major regulatory mechanism controlling Na^+ excretion. Almost two-thirds of filtered Na^+ is reabsorbed in the proximal convoluted tubule; this process is electroneutral and isoosmotic. Further reabsorption (25–30%) occurs in the TALH via the apical *Na^+-K^+-$2Cl^-$ co-transporter;* this is an active process and is also electroneutral. Distal convoluted tubule reabsorption of Na^+ (5%) is mediated by the *thiazide-sensitive Na^+-Cl^- co-transporter*. Final Na^+ reabsorption occurs in the cortical and medullary collecting ducts, the amount excreted being reasonably equivalent to the amount ingested per day.

HYPOVOLEMIA

Etiology True volume depletion, or hypovolemia, generally refers to a state of combined salt and water loss exceeding intake, leading to ECF volume contraction. The loss of Na^+ may be renal or extrarenal (Table 46-1).

RENAL Many conditions are associated with excessive urinary NaCl and water losses, including diuretics. Pharmacologic diuretics inhibit specific pathways of Na^+ reabsorption along the nephron with a consequent increase in urinary Na^+ excretion. Enhanced filtration of nonreabsorbed solutes, such as glucose or urea, can also impair tubular reabsorption of Na^+ and water, leading to an osmotic or solute diuresis. This often occurs in poorly controlled diabetes mellitus and in patients receiving high-protein hyperalimentation. Mannitol is a diuretic

TABLE 46-1 CAUSES OF HYPOVOLEMIA

I. ECF volume contracted
  A. Extrarenal Na^+ loss
    1. Gastrointestinal (vomiting, nasogastric suction, drainage, fistula, diarrhea)
    2. Skin/respiratory (insensible losses, sweat, burns)
    3. Hemorrhage
  B. Renal Na^+ and water loss
    1. Diuretics
    2. Osmotic diuresis
    3. Hypoaldosteronism
    4. Salt-wasting nephropathies
  C. Renal water loss
    1. Diabetes insipidus (central or nephrogenic)
II. ECF volume normal or expanded
  A. Decreased cardiac output
    1. Myocardial, valvular, or pericardial disease
  B. Redistribution
    1. Hypoalbuminemia (hepatic cirrhosis, nephrotic syndrome)
    2. Capillary leak (acute pancreatitis, ischemic bowel, rhabdomyolysis)
  C. Increased venous capacitance
    1. Sepsis

Note: ECF, extracellular fluid.

that produces an osmotic diuresis because the renal tubule is impermeable to mannitol. Many tubule and interstitial renal disorders are associated with Na^+ wasting. Excessive renal losses of Na^+ and water may also occur during the diuretic phase of acute tubular necrosis (Chap. 273) and following the relief of bilateral urinary tract obstruction. Finally, mineralocorticoid deficiency (hypoaldosteronism) causes salt wasting in the presence of normal intrinsic renal function.

Massive renal water excretion can also lead to hypovolemia. The ECF volume contraction is usually less severe since two-thirds of the volume lost is intracellular. Conditions associated with excessive urinary water loss include *central diabetes insipidus* (CDI) and *nephrogenic diabetes insipidus* (NDI). These two disorders are due to impaired secretion of and renal unresponsiveness to AVP, respectively, and are discussed below.

EXTRARENAL Nonrenal causes of hypovolemia include fluid loss from the gastrointestinal tract, skin, and respiratory system and third-space accumulations (burns, pancreatitis, peritonitis). Approximately 9 L of fluid enters the gastrointestinal tract daily, 2 L by ingestion and 7 L by secretion. Almost 98% of this volume is reabsorbed so that fecal fluid loss is only 100–200 mL/d. Impaired gastrointestinal reabsorption or enhanced secretion leads to volume depletion. Since gastric secretions have a low pH (high H^+ concentration) and biliary, pancreatic, and intestinal secretions are alkaline (high HCO_3^- concentration), vomiting and diarrhea are often accompanied by metabolic alkalosis and acidosis, respectively.

Water evaporation from the skin and respiratory tract contributes to thermoregulation. These *insensible losses* amount to 500 mL/d. During febrile illnesses, prolonged heat exposure, exercise, or increased salt and water loss from skin, in the form of sweat, can be significant and lead to volume depletion. The Na^+ concentration of sweat is normally 20–50 mmol/L and decreases with profuse sweating due to the action of aldosterone. Since sweat is hypotonic, the loss of water exceeds that of Na^+. The water deficit is minimized by enhanced thirst. Nevertheless, ongoing Na^+ loss is manifest as hypovolemia. Enhanced evaporative water loss from the respiratory tract may be associated with hyperventilation, especially in mechanically ventilated febrile patients.

Certain conditions lead to fluid sequestration in a *third space*. This compartment is extracellular but is not in equilibrium with either the ECF or the ICF. The fluid is effectively lost from the ECF and can result in hypovolemia. Examples include the bowel lumen in gastrointestinal obstruction, subcutaneous tissues in severe burns, retroperitoneal space in acute pancreatitis, and peritoneal cavity in peritonitis. Finally, severe hemorrhage from any source can result in volume depletion.

Pathophysiology ECF volume contraction is manifest as a decreased plasma volume and hypotension. Hypotension is due to decreased venous return (preload) and diminished cardiac output; it triggers baroreceptors in the carotid sinus and aortic arch and leads to activation of the sympathetic nervous system and the renin-angiotensin system. The net effect is to maintain mean arterial pressure and cerebral and coronary perfusion. In contrast to the cardiovascular response, the renal response is aimed at restoring the ECF volume by decreasing the GFR and filtered load of Na^+ and, most importantly, by promoting tubular reabsorption of Na^+. Increased sympathetic tone increases proximal tubular Na^+ reabsorption and decreases GFR by causing preferential afferent arteriolar vasoconstriction. Sodium is also reabsorbed in the proximal convoluted tubule in response to increased angiotensin II and altered peritubular capillary hemodynamics (decreased hydraulic and increased oncotic pressure). Enhanced reabsorption of Na^+ by the collecting duct is an important component of the renal adaptation to ECF volume contraction. This occurs in response to increased *aldosterone* and AVP secretion and suppressed *atrial natriuretic peptide* secretion.

Clinical Features A careful history is often helpful in determining the etiology of ECF volume contraction (e.g., vomiting, diarrhea, polyuria, diaphoresis). Most symptoms are nonspecific and secondary to electrolyte imbalances and tissue hypoperfusion and include fatigue, weakness, muscle cramps, thirst, and postural dizziness. More severe degrees of volume contraction can lead to end-organ ischemia manifest as oliguria, cyanosis, abdominal and chest pain, and confusion or obtundation. Diminished skin turgor and dry oral mucous membranes are poor markers of decreased interstitial fluid. Signs of intravascular volume contraction include decreased jugular venous pressure, postural hypotension, and postural tachycardia. Larger and more acute fluid losses lead to hypovolemic shock, manifest as hypotension, tachycardia, peripheral vasoconstriction, and hypoperfusion—cyanosis, cold and clammy extremities, oliguria, and altered mental status.

Diagnosis A thorough history and physical examination are generally sufficient to diagnose the etiology of hypovolemia. Laboratory data usually confirm and support the clinical diagnosis. The blood urea nitrogen (BUN) and plasma creatinine concentrations tend to be elevated, reflecting a decreased GFR. Normally, the BUN:creatinine ratio is about 10:1. However, in *prerenal azotemia*, hypovolemia leads to increased urea reabsorption, a proportionately greater elevation in BUN than plasma creatinine, and a BUN:creatinine ratio of 20:1 or higher. An increased BUN (relative to creatinine) may also be due to increased urea production that occurs with hyperalimentation (high-protein), glucocorticoid therapy, and gastrointestinal bleeding.

The appropriate response to hypovolemia is enhanced renal Na^+ and water reabsorption, which is reflected in the urine composition. Therefore, the urine Na^+ concentration should usually be <20 mmol/L except in conditions associated with impaired Na^+ reabsorption, as in acute tubular necrosis (Chap. 273). Another exception is hypovolemia due to vomiting, since the associated metabolic alkalosis and increased filtered HCO_3^- impair proximal Na^+ reabsorption. In this case, the urine Cl^- is low (<20 mmol/L). The urine osmolality and specific gravity in hypovolemic subjects are generally >450 mosmol/kg and 1.015, respectively, reflecting the presence of enhanced AVP secretion. However, in hypovolemia due to diabetes insipidus, urine osmolality and specific gravity are indicative of inappropriately dilute urine.

℞ HYPOVOLEMIA

The therapeutic goals are to restore normovolemia with fluid similar in composition to that lost and to replace ongoing losses. Symptoms and signs, including weight loss, can help estimate the degree of volume contraction and should also be monitored to assess response to treatment. Mild volume contraction can usually be corrected via the oral route. More severe hypovolemia requires intravenous therapy. Isotonic or normal saline (0.9% NaCl or 154 mmol/L Na^+) is the solution of choice in normonatremic and most hyponatremic individuals and should be administered initially in patients with hypotension or shock. Hypernatremia reflects a proportionally greater deficit of water than Na^+, and its correction will therefore require a hypotonic solution such as half-normal saline (0.45% NaCl or 77 mmol/L Na^+) or 5% dextrose in water. Patients with significant hemorrhage, anemia, or intravascular volume depletion may require blood transfusion or colloid-containing solutions (albumin, dextran). Hypokalemia may be present initially or may ensue as a result of increased urinary K^+ excretion; it should be corrected by adding appropriate amounts of KCl to replacement solutions.

HYPONATREMIA

Etiology A plasma Na^+ concentration <135 mmol/L usually reflects a hypotonic state. However, plasma osmolality may be normal or increased in some cases of hyponatremia. Isotonic or slightly hypotonic hyponatremia may complicate transurethral resection of the prostate or bladder because large volumes of isoosmotic (mannitol) or hypoosmotic (sorbitol or glycine) bladder irrigation solution can be absorbed and result in a dilutional hyponatremia. The metabolism of sorbitol and glycine to CO_2 and water may lead to hypotonicity if the accumulated fluid and solutes are not rapidly excreted. Hypertonic hyponatremia is usually due to hyperglycemia or, occasionally, intravenous administration of mannitol. Relative insulin deficiency causes myocytes to become impermeable to glucose. Therefore, during poorly controlled diabetes mellitus, glucose is an effective osmole and draws water from muscle cells, resulting in hyponatremia. Plasma Na^+ concentration falls by 1.4 mmol/L for every 100 mg/dL rise in the plasma glucose concentration.

Most causes of hyponatremia are associated with a low plasma osmolality (Table 46-2). In general, hypotonic hyponatremia is due either to a primary water gain (and secondary Na^+ loss) or a primary Na^+ loss (and secondary water gain). In the absence of water intake or hypotonic fluid replacement, hyponatremia is usually associated with hypovolemic shock due to a profound sodium deficit and transcellular water shift. Contraction of the ECF volume stimulates thirst and AVP secretion. The increased water ingestion and impaired renal excretion result in hyponatremia. It is important to note that *diuretic-induced hyponatremia* is almost always due to thiazide diuretics. Loop diuretics decrease the tonicity of the medullary interstitium and impair maximal urinary concentrating capacity. This limits the ability of AVP to promote water retention. In contrast, thiazide diuretics lead to Na^+ and K^+ depletion and AVP-mediated water retention. Hyponatremia can also occur by a process of *desalination*. This occurs when the urine tonicity (the sum of the concentrations of Na^+ and K^+) exceeds that of administered intravenous fluids (including isotonic saline). This accounts for some cases of acute postoperative hyponatremia and cerebral salt wasting after neurosurgery.

Hyponatremia in the setting of ECF volume expansion is usually associated with edematous states, such as congestive heart failure, hepatic cirrhosis, and the nephrotic syndrome. These disorders all have in common a decreased effective circulating arterial volume, leading to increased thirst and increased AVP levels. Additional factors impairing the excretion of solute-free water include a reduced GFR, decreased delivery of ultrafiltrate to the diluting site (due to increased proximal fractional reabsorption of Na^+ and water), and diuretic therapy. The degree of hyponatremia often correlates with the severity of the underlying condition and is an important prognostic factor. Oliguric acute and chronic renal failure may be associated with hyponatremia if water intake exceeds the ability to excrete equivalent volumes.

TABLE 46-2 CAUSES OF HYPONATREMIA

I. Pseudohyponatremia
- A. Normal plasma osmolality
  1. Hyperlipidemia
  2. Hyperproteinemia
  3. Posttransurethral resection of prostate/bladder tumor
- B. Increased plasma osmolality
  1. Hyperglycemia
  2. Mannitol

II. Hypoosmolal hyponatremia
- A. Primary Na^+ loss (secondary water gain)
  1. Integumentary loss: sweating, burns
  2. Gastrointestinal loss: vomiting, tube drainage, fistula, obstruction, diarrhea
  3. Renal loss: diuretics, osmotic diuresis, hypoaldosteronism, salt-wasting nephropathy, postobstructive diuresis, nonoliguric acute tubular necrosis
- B. Primary water gain (secondary Na^+ loss)
  1. Primary polydipsia
  2. Decreased solute intake (e.g., beer potomania)
  3. AVP release due to pain, nausea, drugs
  4. Syndrome of inappropriate AVP secretion
  5. Glucocorticoid deficiency
  6. Hypothyroidism
  7. Chronic renal insufficiency
- C. Primary Na^+ gain (exceeded by secondary water gain)
  1. Heart failure
  2. Hepatic cirrhosis
  3. Nephrotic syndrome

Hyponatremia in the absence of ECF volume contraction, decreased effective circulating arterial volume, or renal insufficiency is usually due to increased AVP secretion resulting in impaired water excretion. Ingestion or administration of water is also required since high levels of AVP alone are usually insufficient to produce hyponatremia. This disorder, commonly termed the *syndrome of inappropriate antidiuretic hormone secretion* (SIADH), is the most common cause of normovolemic hyponatremia and is due to the nonphysiologic release of AVP from the posterior pituitary or an ectopic source (Chap. 334). Renal free-water excretion is impaired while the regulation of Na^+ balance is unaffected. The most common causes of SIADH include neuropsychiatric and pulmonary diseases, malignant tumors, major surgery (postoperative pain), and pharmacologic agents. Severe pain and nausea are physiologic stimuli of AVP secretion; these stimuli are inappropriate in the absence of hypovolemia or hyperosmolality. The pattern of AVP secretion can be used to classify SIADH into four subtypes: (1) erratic autonomous AVP secretion (ectopic production); (2) normal regulation of AVP release around a lower osmolality set point or *reset osmostat* (cachexia, malnutrition); (3) normal AVP response to hypertonicity with failure to suppress completely at low osmolality (incomplete pituitary stalk section); and (4) normal AVP secretion with increased sensitivity to its actions or secretion of some other antidiuretic factor (rare). Patients with the nephrogenic syndrome of inappropriate antidiuresis have clinical and laboratory features consistent with SIADH but undetectable levels of AVP. It is hypothesized that this disorder is due to gain of function mutations in the V2 receptor.

Hormonal excess or deficiency may cause hyponatremia. Adrenal insufficiency (Chap. 336) and hypothyroidism (Chap. 335) may present with hyponatremia and should not be confused with SIADH. Although decreased mineralocorticoids may contribute to the hyponatremia of adrenal insufficiency, it is the cortisol deficiency that leads to hypersecretion of AVP both indirectly (secondary to volume depletion) and directly (cosecreted with corticotropin-releasing factor). The mechanisms by which hypothyroidism leads to hyponatremia include decreased cardiac output and GFR and increased AVP secretion in response to hemodynamic stimuli.

Finally, hyponatremia may occur in the absence of AVP or renal failure if the kidney is unable to excrete the dietary water load. In psychogenic or primary polydipsia, compulsive water consumption may overwhelm the normally large renal excretory capacity of 12 L/d (Chap. 334). These patients often have psychiatric illnesses and may be taking medications, such as phenothiazines, that enhance the sensation of thirst by causing a dry mouth. The maximal urine output is a function of the minimum urine osmolality achievable and the mandatory solute excretion. Metabolism of a normal diet generates about 600 mosmol/d, and the minimum urine osmolality in humans is 50 mosmol/kg. Therefore, the maximum daily urine output will be about 12 L ($600 \div 50 = 12$). A solute excretion rate of greater than ~750 mosmol/d is, by definition, an *osmotic diuresis*. A low-protein diet may yield as few as 250 mosmol/d, which translates into a maximal urine output of 5 L/d at a minimum urine tonicity of 50 mosmol/kg. Beer drinkers typically have a poor dietary intake of protein and electrolytes and consume large volumes (of beer), which may exceed the renal excretory capacity and result in hyponatremia. This phenomenon is referred to as *beer potomania*.

Clinical Features The clinical manifestations of hyponatremia are related to osmotic water shift leading to increased ICF volume, specifically brain cell swelling or cerebral edema. Therefore the symptoms are primarily neurologic, and their severity is dependent on the rapidity of on-

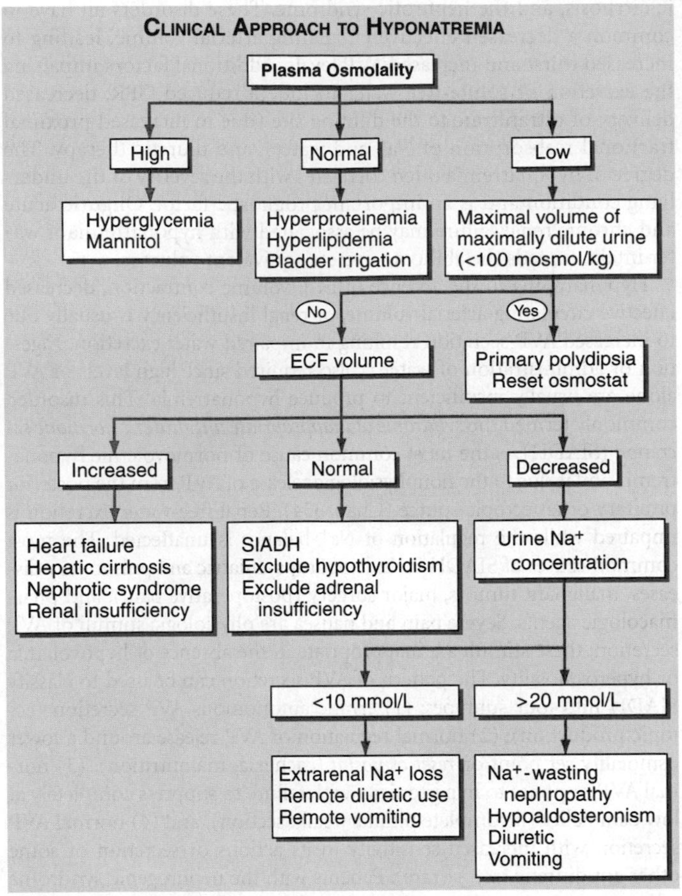

FIGURE 46-1 Algorithm depicting clinical approach to hyponatremia. ECF, extracellular fluid; SIADH, syndrome of inappropriate antidiuretic hormone secretion.

set and absolute decrease in plasma Na^+ concentration. Patients may be asymptomatic or complain of nausea and malaise. As the plasma Na^+ concentration falls, the symptoms progress to include headache, lethargy, confusion, and obtundation. Stupor, seizures, and coma do not usually occur unless the plasma Na^+ concentration falls acutely below 120 mmol/L or decreases rapidly. As described above, adaptive mechanisms designed to protect cell volume occur in chronic hyponatremia. Loss of Na^+ and K^+, followed by organic osmolytes, from brain cells decreases brain swelling due to secondary transcellular water shifts (from ICF to ECF). The net effect is to minimize cerebral edema and its symptoms.

Diagnosis (Fig. 46-1) Hyponatremia is not a disease but a manifestation of a variety of disorders. The underlying cause can often be ascertained from an accurate history and physical examination, including an assessment of ECF volume status and effective circulating arterial volume. The differential diagnosis of hyponatremia, an expanded ECF volume, and decreased effective circulating volume includes congestive heart failure, hepatic cirrhosis, and the nephrotic syndrome. Hypothyroidism and adrenal insufficiency tend to present with a near-normal ECF volume and decreased effective circulating arterial volume. All of these diseases have characteristic signs and symptoms. Patients with SIADH are usually euvolemic.

Four laboratory findings often provide useful information and can narrow the differential diagnosis of hyponatremia: (1) the plasma osmolality, (2) the urine osmolality, (3) the urine Na^+ concentration, and (4) the urine K^+ concentration. Since ECF tonicity is determined primarily by the Na^+ concentration, most patients with hyponatremia have a decreased plasma osmolality. The appropriate renal response to hypoosmolality is to excrete the maximum volume of dilute urine, i.e., urine osmolality and specific gravity of <100 mosmol/kg and 1.003, respectively. This occurs in patients with primary polydipsia. If this is not present, it suggests impaired free-water excretion due to the action of AVP on the kidney. The secretion of AVP may be a physiologic response to hemodynamic stimuli or it may be inappropriate in the presence of hyponatremia and euvolemia. Since Na^+ is the major ECF cation and is largely restricted to this compartment, ECF volume contraction represents a deficit in total body Na^+ content. Therefore, volume depletion in patients with normal underlying renal function results in enhanced tubule Na^+ reabsorption and a urine Na^+ concentration <20 mmol/L. The finding of a urine Na^+ concentration >20 mmol/L in hypovolemic hyponatremia implies a salt-wasting nephropathy, diuretic therapy, hypoaldosteronism, or occasionally vomiting. Both the urine osmolality and the urine Na^+ concentration can be followed serially when assessing response to therapy.

SIADH is characterized by hypoosmotic hyponatremia in the setting of an inappropriately concentrated urine (urine osmolality >100 mosmol/kg). Patients are typically normovolemic and have normal Na^+ balance. They tend to be mildly volume-expanded secondary to water retention and have a urine Na^+ excretion rate equal to intake (urine Na^+ concentration usually >40 mmol/L). By definition, they have normal renal, adrenal, and thyroid function and usually have normal K^+ and acid-base balance. SIADH is often associated with hypouricemia due to the uricosuric state induced by volume expansion. In contrast, hypovolemic patients tend to be hyperuricemic secondary to increased proximal urate reabsorption.

Rx HYPONATREMIA

The goals of therapy are twofold: (1) to raise the plasma Na^+ concentration by restricting water intake and promoting water loss and (2) to correct the underlying disorder. Mild asymptomatic hyponatremia is generally of little clinical significance and requires no treatment. The management of asymptomatic hyponatremia associated with ECF volume contraction should include Na^+ repletion, generally in the form of isotonic saline. The direct effect of the administered NaCl on the plasma Na^+ concentration is trivial. However, restoration of euvolemia removes the hemodynamic stimulus for AVP release, allowing the excess free water to be excreted. The hyponatremia associated with edematous states tends to reflect the severity of the underlying disease and is usually asymptomatic. These patients have increased total body water that exceeds the increase in total body Na^+ content. Treatment should include restriction of Na^+ and water intake, correction of hypokalemia, and promotion of water loss in excess of Na^+. The latter may require the use of loop diuretics with replacement of a proportion of the urinary Na^+ loss to ensure net free-water excretion. Dietary water restriction should be less than the urine output. Correction of the K^+ deficit may raise the plasma Na^+ concentration by favoring a shift of Na^+ out of cells as K^+ moves in. Water restriction is also a component of the therapeutic approach to hyponatremia associated with primary polydipsia, renal failure, and SIADH (Chap. 334). The recent development of nonpeptide vasopressin antagonists has introduced a new selective treatment for euvolemic and hypervolemic hyponatremia.

The rate of correction of hyponatremia depends on the absence or presence of neurologic dysfunction. This, in turn, is related to the rapidity of onset and magnitude of the fall in plasma Na^+ concentration. In asymptomatic patients, the plasma Na^+ concentration should be raised by no more than 0.5–1.0 mmol/L per h and by less than 10–12 mmol/L over the first 24 h. Acute or severe hyponatremia (plasma Na^+ concentration <110–115 mmol/L) tends to present with altered mental status and/or seizures and requires more rapid correction. Severe symptomatic hyponatremia should be treated with hypertonic saline, and the plasma Na^+ concentration should be raised by 1–2 mmol/L per hour for the first 3–4 h or until the seizures subside. Once again, the plasma Na^+ concentration should probably be raised by no more than 12 mmol/L during the first 24 h. The quantity of Na^+ required to increase the plasma Na^+ concentration by a given amount can be estimated by multiplying the deficit in plasma Na^+ concentration by the total body water.

Under normal conditions, total body water is 50 or 60% of lean body weight in women or men, respectively. Therefore, to raise the plasma Na^+ concentration from 105 to 115 mmol/L in a 70-kg man requires 420 mmol $[(115 - 105) \times 70 \times 0.6]$ of Na^+. The risk of correcting hyponatremia too rapidly is the development of the *osmotic demyelination syndrome* (ODS). This is a neurologic disorder characterized by flaccid paralysis, dysarthria, and dysphagia. The diagnosis is usually suspected clinically and can be confirmed by appropriate neuroimaging studies. There is no specific treatment for the disorder, which is associated with significant morbidity and mortality. Patients with chronic hyponatremia are most susceptible to the development of

ODS, since their brain cell volume has returned to near normal as a result of the osmotic adaptive mechanisms described above. Therefore, administration of hypertonic saline to these individuals can cause sudden osmotic shrinkage of brain cells. In addition to rapid or overcorrection of hyponatremia, risk factors for ODS include prior cerebral anoxic injury, hypokalemia, and malnutrition, especially secondary to alcoholism. Water restriction in primary polydipsia and intravenous saline therapy in ECF volume–contracted patients may also lead to overly rapid correction of hyponatremia as a result of AVP suppression and a brisk water diuresis. This can be prevented by administration of water or use of an AVP analogue to slow down the rate of free water excretion. **For further discussion, see Chap. 334.**

HYPERNATREMIA

Etiology Hypernatremia is defined as a plasma Na^+ concentration >145 mmol/L. Since Na^+ and its accompanying anions are the major effective ECF osmoles, hypernatremia is a state of hyperosmolality. As a result of the fixed number of ICF particles, maintenance of osmotic equilibrium in hypernatremia results in ICF volume contraction. Hypernatremia may be due to primary Na^+ gain or water deficit. The two components of an appropriate response to hypernatremia are increased water intake stimulated by thirst and the excretion of the minimum volume of maximally concentrated urine reflecting AVP secretion in response to an osmotic stimulus.

In practice, the majority of cases of hypernatremia result from the loss of water. Since water is distributed between the ICF and the ECF in a 2:1 ratio, a given amount of solute-free water loss will result in a twofold greater reduction in the ICF compartment than the ECF compartment. For example, consider three scenarios: the loss of 1 L of water, isotonic NaCl, or half-isotonic NaCl. If 1 L of water is lost, the ICF volume will decrease by 667 mL, whereas the ECF volume will fall by only 333 mL. Due to the fact that Na^+ is largely restricted to the ECF, this compartment will decrease by 1 L if the fluid lost is isoosmotic. One liter of half-isotonic NaCl is equivalent to 500 mL of water (one-third ECF, two-thirds ICF) plus 500 mL of isotonic saline (all ECF). Therefore, the loss of 1 L of half-isotonic saline decreases the ECF and ICF volumes by 667 mL and 333 mL, respectively.

The degree of hyperosmolality is typically mild unless the thirst mechanism is abnormal or access to water is limited. The latter occurs in infants, the physically handicapped, and patients with impaired mental status; in the postoperative state; and in intubated patients in the intensive care unit. On rare occasions, impaired thirst may be due to *primary hypodipsia*. This usually occurs as a result of damage to the hypothalamic osmoreceptors that control thirst and tends to be associated with abnormal osmotic regulation of AVP secretion. Primary hypodipsia may be due to a variety of pathologic changes, including granulomatous disease, vascular occlusion, and tumors. A subset of hypodipsic hypernatremia, referred to as *essential hypernatremia*, does not respond to forced water intake. This appears to be due to a specific osmoreceptor defect resulting in nonosmotic regulation of AVP release. Thus, the hemodynamic effects of water loading lead to AVP suppression and excretion of dilute urine.

The source of free water loss is either renal or extrarenal. Nonrenal loss of water may be due to evaporation from the skin and respiratory tract (insensible losses) or loss from the gastrointestinal tract. Insensible losses are increased with fever, exercise, heat exposure, and severe burns and in mechanically ventilated patients. Furthermore, the Na^+ concentration of sweat decreases with profuse perspiration, thereby increasing solute-free water loss. Diarrhea is the most common gastrointestinal cause of hypernatremia. Specifically, osmotic diarrheas (induced by lactulose, sorbitol, or malabsorption of carbohydrate) and viral gastroenteritides result in water loss exceeding that of Na^+ and K^+. In contrast, secretory diarrheas (e.g., cholera, carcinoid, VIPoma) have a fecal osmolality (twice the sum of the concentrations of Na^+ and K^+) similar to that of plasma and present with ECF volume contraction and a normal plasma Na^+ concentration or hyponatremia.

Renal water loss is the most common cause of hypernatremia and is due to drug-induced or osmotic diuresis or diabetes insipidus (Chap. 334). Loop diuretics interfere with the countercurrent mechanism and produce an isoosmotic solute diuresis. This results in a decreased medullary interstitial tonicity and impaired renal concentrating ability. The presence of non-reabsorbed organic solutes in the tubule lumen impairs the osmotic reabsorption of water. This leads to water loss in excess of Na^+ and K^+, known as an osmotic diuresis. The most frequent cause of an osmotic diuresis is hyperglycemia and glucosuria in poorly controlled diabetes mellitus. Intravenous administration of mannitol and increased endogenous production of urea (high-protein diet) can also result in an osmotic diuresis.

Hypernatremia secondary to nonosmotic urinary water loss is usually due to: (1) Central diabetes insipidus (CDI) characterized by impaired AVP secretion, or (2) NDI resulting from end-organ (renal) resistance to the actions of AVP. The most common cause of CDI is destruction of the neurohypophysis. This may occur as a result of trauma, neurosurgery, granulomatous disease, neoplasms, vascular accidents, or infection. In many cases, CDI is idiopathic and may occasionally be hereditary. The familial form of the disease is inherited in an autosomal dominant fashion and has been attributed to mutations in the propressophysin (AVP precursor) gene. Nephrogenic diabetes insipidus (NDI) may be either inherited or acquired. Congenital NDI is an X-linked recessive trait due to mutations in the V_2 receptor gene. Mutations in the autosomal *aquaporin-2* gene may also result in NDI. The *aquaporin-2* gene encodes the water channel protein whose membrane insertion is stimulated by AVP. The causes of sporadic NDI are numerous and include drugs (especially lithium), hypercalcemia, hypokalemia, and conditions that impair medullary hypertonicity (e.g., papillary necrosis or osmotic diuresis). Pregnant women, in the second or third trimester, may develop NDI as a result of excessive elaboration of vasopressinase by the placenta.

Finally, although infrequent, a primary Na^+ gain may cause hypernatremia. For example, inadvertent administration of hypertonic NaCl or $NaHCO_3$ or replacing sugar with salt in infant formula can produce this complication.

Clinical Features As a consequence of hypertonicity, water shifts out of cells, leading to a contracted ICF volume. A decreased brain cell volume is associated with an increased risk of subarachnoid or intracerebral hemorrhage. Hence, the major symptoms of hypernatremia are neurologic and include altered mental status, weakness, neuromuscular irritability, focal neurologic deficits, and occasionally coma or seizures. Patients may also complain of polyuria or thirst. For unknown reasons, patients with polydipsia from CDI tend to prefer ice-cold water. The signs and symptoms of volume depletion are often present in patients with a history of excessive sweating, diarrhea, or an osmotic diuresis. As with hyponatremia, the severity of the clinical manifestations is related to the acuity and magnitude of the rise in plasma Na^+ concentration. Chronic hypernatremia is generally less symptomatic as a result of adaptive mechanisms designed to defend cell volume. Brain cells initially take up Na^+ and K^+ salts, later followed by accumulation of organic osmolytes such as inositol. This serves to restore the brain ICF volume toward normal.

Diagnosis (Fig. 46-2) A complete history and physical examination will often provide clues as to the underlying cause of hypernatremia. Relevant symptoms and signs include the absence or presence of thirst, diaphoresis, diarrhea, polyuria, and the features of ECF volume contraction. The history should include a list of current and recent medications, and the physical examination is incomplete without a thorough mental status and neurologic assessment. Measurement of urine volume and osmolality are essential in the evaluation of hyperosmolality. The appropriate renal response to hypernatremia is the excretion of the minimum volume (500 mL/d) of maximally concentrated urine (urine osmolality >800 mosmol/kg). These findings suggest extrarenal or remote renal water loss or administration of hypertonic Na^+ salt solutions. The presence of a primary Na^+ excess can be confirmed by the presence of ECF volume expansion and natriuresis (urine Na^+ concentration usually >100 mmol/L).

Many causes of hypernatremia are associated with polyuria and a submaximal urine osmolality. The product of the urine volume and osmolality, i.e., the solute excretion rate, is helpful in determining the

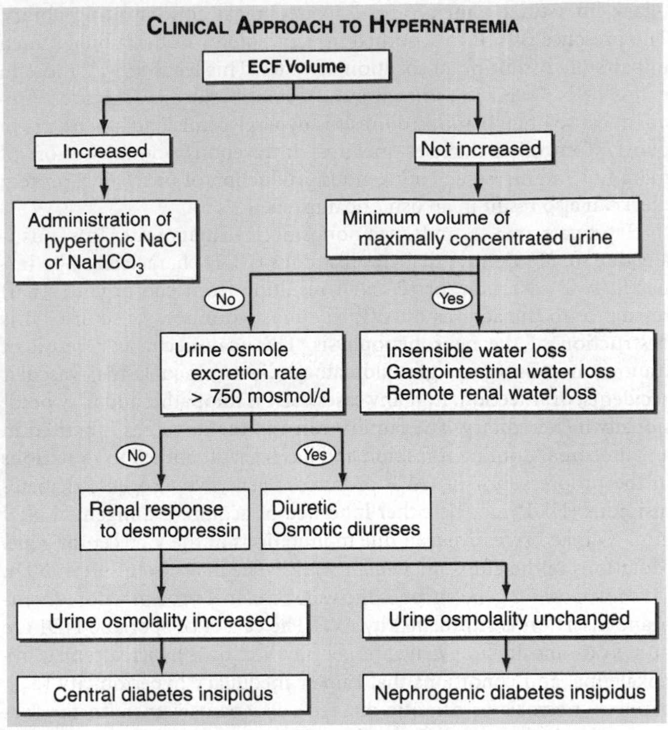

FIGURE 46-2 Algorithm depicting clinical approach to hypernatremia.

basis of the polyuria (see above). To maintain a steady state, total solute excretion must equal solute production. As stated above, individuals eating a normal diet generate ~600 mosmol/d. Therefore, daily solute excretion in excess of 750 mosmol defines an osmotic diuresis. This can be confirmed by measuring the urine glucose and urea. In general, both CDI and NDI present with polyuria and hypotonic urine (urine osmolality <250 mosmol/kg). The degree of hypernatremia is usually mild unless there is an associated thirst abnormality. The clinical history, physical examination, and pertinent laboratory data can often rule out causes of acquired NDI. CDI and NDI can generally be distinguished by administering the AVP analogue desmopressin (10 μg intranasally) after careful water restriction. The urine osmolality should increase by at least 50% in CDI and will not change in NDI. Unfortunately, the diagnosis may sometimes be difficult due to partial defects in AVP secretion and action.

℞ HYPERNATREMIA

The therapeutic goals are to stop ongoing water loss by treating the underlying cause and to correct the water deficit. The ECF volume should be restored in hypovolemic patients. The quantity of water required to correct the deficit can be calculated from the following equation:

$$\text{Water deficit} = \frac{\text{Plasma Na}^{+}\text{ concentration} - 140}{140} \times \text{Total body water}$$

In hypernatremia due to water loss, total body water is approximately 50 and 40% of lean body weight in men and women, respectively. For example, a 50-kg woman with a plasma Na^+ concentration of 160 mmol/L has an estimated free-water deficit of 2.9 L {[(160 – 140) ÷ 140] × (0.4 × 50)}. As in hyponatremia, rapid correction of hypernatremia is potentially dangerous. In this case, a sudden decrease in osmolality could potentially cause a rapid shift of water into cells that have undergone osmotic adaptation. This would result in swollen brain cells and increase the risk of seizures or permanent neurologic damage. Therefore, the water deficit should be corrected slowly over at least 48–72 h. When calculating the rate of water replacement, ongoing losses should be taken into account, and the plasma Na^+ concentration should be lowered by 0.5 mmol/L per h and by no more than 12 mmol/L over the first 24 h.

The safest route of administration of water is by mouth or via a nasogastric tube (or other feeding tube). Alternatively, 5% dextrose in water or half-isotonic saline can be given intravenously. The appropriate treatment of CDI consists of administering desmopressin intranasally (Chap. 334). Other options for decreasing urine output include a low-salt diet in combination with low-dose thiazide diuretic therapy. In some patients with partial CDI, drugs that either stimulate AVP secretion or enhance its action on the kidney have been useful. These include chlorpropamide, clofibrate, carbamazepine, and nonsteroidal anti-inflammatory drugs (NSAIDs). The concentrating defect in NDI may be reversible by treating the underlying disorder or eliminating the offending drug. Symptomatic polyuria due to NDI can be treated with a low-Na^+ diet and thiazide diuretics, as described above. This induces mild volume depletion, which leads to enhanced proximal reabsorption of salt and water and decreased delivery to the site of action of AVP, the collecting duct. By impairing renal prostaglandin synthesis, NSAIDs potentiate AVP action and thereby increase urine osmolality and decrease urine volume. Amiloride may be useful in patients with NDI who need to be on lithium. The nephrotoxicity of lithium requires the drug to be taken up into collecting duct cells via the amiloride-sensitive Na^+ channel.

POTASSIUM

Potassium Balance Potassium is the major intracellular cation. The normal plasma K^+ concentration is 3.5–5.0 mmol/L, whereas that inside cells is about 150 mmol/L. Therefore, the amount of K^+ in the ECF (30–70 mmol) constitutes <2% of the total body K^+ content (2500–4500 mmol). The ratio of ICF to ECF K^+ concentration (normally 38:1) is the principal result of the resting membrane potential and is crucial for normal neuromuscular function. The basolateral Na^+, K^+-ATPase pump actively transports K^+ in and Na^+ out of the cell in a 2:3 ratio, and the passive outward diffusion of K^+ is quantitatively the most important factor that generates the resting membrane potential. The activity of the electrogenic Na^+, K^+-ATPase pump may be stimulated as a result of an increased intracellular Na^+ concentration and inhibited in the setting of digoxin toxicity or chronic illness such as heart failure or renal failure.

The K^+ intake of individuals on an average western diet is 40–120 mmol/d, or approximately 1 mmol/kg per day, 90% of which is absorbed by the gastrointestinal tract. Maintenance of the steady state necessitates matching K^+ ingestion with excretion. Initially, extrarenal adaptive mechanisms, followed later by urinary excretion, prevent a doubling of the plasma K^+ concentration that would occur if the dietary K^+ load remained in the ECF compartment. Immediately following a meal, most of the absorbed K^+ enters cells as a result of the initial elevation in the plasma K^+ concentration and facilitated by insulin release and basal catecholamine levels. Eventually, however, the excess K^+ is excreted in the urine (see below). The regulation of gastrointestinal K^+ handling is not well understood. The amount of K^+ lost in the stool can increase from 10 to 50% or 60% (of dietary intake) in chronic renal insufficiency. In addition, colonic secretion of K^+ is stimulated in patients with large volumes of diarrhea, resulting in potentially severe K^+ depletion.

Potassium Excretion (See also Chap. 272) Renal excretion is the major route of elimination of dietary and other sources of excess K^+. The filtered load of K^+ (GFR × plasma K^+ concentration = 180 L/d × 4 mmol/L = 720 mmol/d) is ten- to twentyfold greater than the ECF K^+ content. Some 90% of filtered K^+ is reabsorbed by the proximal convoluted tubule and loop of Henle. Proximally, K^+ is reabsorbed passively with Na^+ and water, whereas the luminal Na^+-K^+-$2Cl^-$ co-transporter mediates K^+ uptake in the thick ascending limb of the loop of Henle. Therefore, K^+ delivery to the distal nephron [distal convoluted tubule and cortical collecting duct (CCD)] approximates dietary intake. Net distal K^+ secretion or reabsorption occurs in the setting of K^+ excess or depletion, respectively. The cell responsible for K^+ secretion in the late distal convoluted tubule (or connecting tubule) and CCD is the principal cell. Virtually all regulation of renal K^+ excretion and total body K^+ balance occurs in the distal nephron. Potassium secretion is regulated by two physiologic stimuli—aldosterone and hyperkalemia. Aldosterone is secreted by the zona glomerulosa cells of the adrenal cortex in response to high renin and angiotensin II or hyperkalemia. The plasma K^+ concentration, independent of

TABLE 46-3 CAUSES OF HYPOKALEMIA

I. Decreased intake
  A. Starvation
  B. Clay ingestion
II. Redistribution into cells
  A. Acid-base
    1. Metabolic alkalosis
  B. Hormonal
    1. Insulin
    2. β_2-Adrenergic agonists (endogenous or exogenous)
    3. α-Adrenergic antagonists
  C. Anabolic state
    1. Vitamin B_{12} or folic acid (red blood cell production)
    2. Granulocyte-macrophage colony stimulating factor (white blood cell production)
    3. Total parenteral nutrition
  D. Other
    1. Pseudohypokalemia
    2. Hypothermia
    3. Hypokalemic periodic paralysis
    4. Barium toxicity
III. Increased loss
  A. Nonrenal
    1. Gastrointestinal loss (diarrhea)
    2. Integumentary loss (sweat)
  B. Renal
    1. Increased distal flow: diuretics, osmotic diuresis, salt-wasting nephropathies
    2. Increased secretion of potassium
      a. Mineralocorticoid excess: primary hyperaldosteronism, secondary hyperaldosteronism (malignant hypertension, renin-secreting tumors, renal artery stenosis, hypovolemia), apparent mineralocorticoid excess (licorice, chewing tobacco, carbenoxolone), congenital adrenal hyperplasia, Cushing's syndrome, Bartter's syndrome
      b. Distal delivery of non-reabsorbed anions: vomiting, nasogastric suction, proximal (type 2) renal tubular acidosis, diabetic ketoacidosis, glue-sniffing (toluene abuse), penicillin derivatives
      c. Other: amphotericin B, Liddle's syndrome, hypomagnesemia

aldosterone, can directly affect K^+ secretion. In addition to the K^+ concentration in the lumen of the CCD, renal K^+ loss depends on the urine flow rate, a function of daily solute excretion (see above). Since excretion is equal to the product of concentration and volume, increased distal flow rate can significantly enhance urinary K^+ output. Finally, in severe K^+ depletion, secretion of K^+ is reduced and reabsorption in the cortical and medullary collecting ducts is upregulated.

HYPOKALEMIA

Etiology (Table 46-3) Hypokalemia, defined as a plasma K^+ concentration <3.5 mmol/L, may result from one (or more) of the following: decreased net intake, shift into cells, increased net loss. Diminished intake is seldom the sole cause of K^+ depletion since urinary excretion can be effectively decreased to <15 mmol/d as a result of net K^+ reabsorption in the distal nephron. With the exception of the urban poor and certain cultural groups, the amount of K^+ in the diet almost always exceeds that excreted in the urine. However, dietary K^+ restriction may exacerbate the hypokalemia secondary to increased gastrointestinal or renal loss. An unusual cause of decreased K^+ intake is ingestion of clay (geophagia), which binds dietary K^+ and iron. This custom was previously common among African Americans in the American South.

REDISTRIBUTION INTO CELLS Movement of K^+ into cells may transiently decrease the plasma K^+ concentration without altering total body K^+ content. For any given cause, the magnitude of the change is relatively small, often <1 mmol/L. However, a combination of factors may lead to a significant fall in the plasma K^+ concentration and may amplify the hypokalemia due to K^+ wasting. Metabolic alkalosis is often associated with hypokalemia. This occurs as a result of K^+ redistribution as well as excessive renal K^+ loss. Treatment of diabetic ketoacidosis with insulin may lead to hypokalemia due to stimulation of the Na^+-H^+ antiporter and (secondarily) the Na^+, K^+-ATPase pump. Furthermore, uncontrolled hyperglycemia often leads to K^+ depletion from an osmotic diuresis (see below). Stress-induced catecholamine release and administration of β_2-adrenergic agonists directly induce cellular uptake of K^+ and promote insulin secretion by pancreatic islet β cells. *Hypokalemic periodic paralysis* is a rare condition characterized by recurrent episodic weakness or paralysis (Chap. 382). Since K^+ is the major ICF cation, anabolic states can potentially result in hypokalemia due to a K^+ shift into cells. This may occur following rapid cell growth seen in patients with pernicious anemia treated with vitamin B_{12} or with neutropenia after treatment with granulocyte-macrophage colony stimulating factor. Massive transfusion with thawed washed red blood cells (RBCs) could cause hypokalemia since frozen RBCs lose up to half of their K^+ during storage.

NONRENAL LOSS OF POTASSIUM Excessive sweating may result in K^+ depletion from increased integumentary and renal K^+ loss. Hyperaldosteronism, secondary to ECF volume contraction, enhances K^+ excretion in the urine (Chap. 336). Normally, K^+ lost in the stool amounts to 5–10 mmol/d in a volume of 100–200 mL. Hypokalemia subsequent to increased gastrointestinal loss can occur in patients with profuse diarrhea (usually secretory), villous adenomas, VIPomas, or laxative abuse. However, the loss of gastric secretions does not account for the moderate to severe K^+ depletion often associated with vomiting or nasogastric suction. Since the K^+ concentration of gastric fluid is 5–10 mmol/L, it would take 30–80 L of vomitus to achieve a K^+ deficit of 300–400 mmol typically seen in these patients. In fact, the hypokalemia is primarily due to increased renal K^+ excretion. Loss of gastric contents results in volume depletion and metabolic alkalosis, both of which promote kaliuresis. Hypovolemia stimulates aldosterone release, which augments K^+ secretion by the principal cells. In addition, the filtered load of HCO_3^- exceeds the reabsorptive capacity of the proximal convoluted tubule, thereby increasing distal delivery of $NaHCO_3$, which enhances the electrochemical gradient favoring K^+ loss in the urine.

RENAL LOSS OF POTASSIUM (See also Chap. 336) In general, most cases of chronic hypokalemia are due to renal K^+ wasting. This may be due to factors that increase the K^+ concentration in the lumen of the CCD or augment distal flow rate. Mineralocorticoid excess commonly results in hypokalemia. *Primary hyperaldosteronism* is due to dysregulated aldosterone secretion by an adrenal adenoma (Conn's syndrome) or carcinoma or to adrenocortical hyperplasia. In a rare subset of patients, the disorder is familial (autosomal dominant) and aldosterone levels can be suppressed by administering low doses of exogenous glucocorticoid. The molecular defect responsible for *glucocorticoid-remediable hyperaldosteronism* is a rearranged gene (due to a chromosomal crossover), containing the 5′-regulatory region of the 11β-hydroxylase gene and the coding sequence of the aldosterone synthase gene. Consequently, mineralocorticoid is synthesized in the zona fasciculata and regulated by corticotropin. A number of conditions associated with hyperreninemia result in secondary hyperaldosteronism and renal K^+ wasting. High renin levels are commonly seen in both renovascular and malignant hypertension. Renin-secreting tumors of the juxtaglomerular apparatus are a rare cause of hypokalemia. Other tumors that have been reported to produce renin include renal cell carcinoma, ovarian carcinoma, and Wilms' tumor. Hyperreninemia may also occur secondary to decreased effective circulating arterial volume.

In the absence of elevated renin or aldosterone levels, enhanced distal nephron secretion of K^+ may result from increased production of nonaldosterone mineralocorticoids in *congenital adrenal hyperplasia.* Glucocorticoid-stimulated kaliuresis does not normally occur due to the conversion of cortisol to cortisone by 11β-hydroxysteroid dehydrogenase (11β-HSDH). Therefore, 11β-HSDH deficiency or suppression allows cortisol to bind to the aldosterone receptor and leads to the *syndrome of apparent mineralocorticoid excess.* Drugs that inhibit the activity of 11β-HSDH include glycyrrhetinic acid, present in licorice, chewing tobacco, and carbenoxolone. The presentation of Cushing's syndrome may include hypokalemia if the capacity of 11β-HSDH to inactivate cortisol is overwhelmed by persistently elevated glucocorticoid levels.

Liddle's syndrome is a rare familial (autosomal dominant) disease characterized by hypertension, hypokalemic metabolic alkalosis, renal

K^+ wasting, and suppressed renin and aldosterone secretion. Increased distal delivery of Na^+ with a nonreabsorbable anion (not Cl^-) enhances K^+ secretion. Classically, this is seen with *proximal (type 2) renal tubular acidosis* (RTA) and vomiting, associated with bicarbonaturia. Diabetic ketoacidosis and toluene abuse (glue sniffing) can lead to increased delivery of β-hydroxybutyrate and hippurate, respectively, to the CCD and to renal K^+ loss. High doses of penicillin derivatives administered to volume-depleted patients may likewise promote renal K^+ secretion as well as an osmotic diuresis. *Classic distal (type 1) RTA* is associated with hypokalemia due to increased renal K^+ loss, the mechanism of which is uncertain. Amphotericin B causes hypokalemia due to increased distal nephron permeability to Na^+ and K^+ and to renal K^+ wasting.

Bartter's syndrome is a disorder characterized by hypokalemia, metabolic alkalosis, hyperreninemic hyperaldosteronism secondary to ECF volume contraction, and juxtaglomerular apparatus hyperplasia. Finally, diuretic use and abuse are common causes of K^+ depletion. Carbonic anhydrase inhibitors, loop diuretics, and thiazides are all kaliuretic. The degree of hypokalemia tends to be greater with long-acting agents and is dose-dependent. Increased renal K^+ excretion is due primarily to increased distal solute delivery and secondary hyperaldosteronism (due to volume depletion). See also Chap. 278.

Clinical Features The clinical manifestations of K^+ depletion vary greatly between individual patients, and their severity depends on the degree of hypokalemia. Symptoms seldom occur unless the plasma K^+ concentration is <3 mmol/L. Fatigue, myalgia, and muscular weakness of the lower extremities are common complaints and are due to a lower (more negative) resting membrane potential. More severe hypokalemia may lead to progressive weakness, hypoventilation (due to respiratory muscle involvement), and eventually complete paralysis. Impaired muscle metabolism and the blunted hyperemic response to exercise associated with profound K^+ depletion increase the risk of rhabdomyolysis. Smooth-muscle function may also be affected and manifest as paralytic ileus.

The electrocardiographic changes of hypokalemia (Fig. 221-16) are due to delayed ventricular repolarization and do not correlate well with the plasma K^+ concentration. Early changes include flattening or inversion of the T wave, a prominent U wave, ST-segment depression, and a prolonged QU interval. Severe K^+ depletion may result in a prolonged PR interval, decreased voltage and widening of the QRS complex, and an increased risk of ventricular arrhythmias, especially in patients with myocardial ischemia or left ventricular hypertrophy. Hypokalemia may also predispose to digitalis toxicity. Hypokalemia is often associated with acid-base disturbances related to the underlying disorder. In addition, K^+ depletion results in intracellular acidification and an increase in net acid excretion or new HCO_3^- production. This is a consequence of enhanced proximal HCO_3^- reabsorption, increased renal ammoniagenesis, and increased distal H^+ secretion. This contributes to the generation of metabolic alkalosis frequently present in hypokalemic patients. NDI (see above) is not uncommonly seen in K^+ depletion and is manifest as polydipsia and polyuria. Glucose intolerance may also occur with hypokalemia and has been attributed to either impaired insulin secretion or peripheral insulin resistance.

Diagnosis (Fig. 46-3) In most cases, the etiology of K^+ depletion can be determined by a careful history. Diuretic and laxative abuse as well as surreptitious vomiting may be difficult to identify but should be excluded. Rarely, patients with a marked leukocytosis (e.g., acute myeloid leukemia) and normokalemia may have a low measured plasma K^+ concentration due to white blood cell uptake of K^+ at room temperature. This *pseudohypokalemia* can be avoided by storing the blood sample on ice or rapidly separating the plasma (or serum) from the cells.

After eliminating decreased intake and intracellular shift as potential causes of hypokalemia, examination of the renal response can help to clarify the source of K^+ loss. The appropriate response to K^+ depletion is to excrete <15 mmol/d of K^+ in the urine, due to increased reabsorption and decreased distal secretion. Hypokalemia with minimal renal K^+ excretion suggests that K^+ was lost via the skin or gastrointestinal tract or that there is a remote history of vomiting or diuretic use. As described above, renal K^+ wasting may be due to factors that either increase the K^+ concentration in the CCD or increase the distal flow rate (or both). The ECF volume status, blood pressure, and associated acid-base disorder may help to differentiate the causes of excessive renal K^+ loss. A rapid and simple test designed to evaluate the driving force for net K^+ secretion is the *transtubular K^+ concentration gradient* (TTKG). The TTKG is the ratio of the K^+ concentration in the lumen of the CCD ($[K^+]_{CCD}$) to that in peritubular capillaries or plasma ($[K^+]_P$). The validity of this measurement depends on three assumptions: (1) few solutes are reabsorbed in the medullary collecting duct (MCD), (2) K^+ is neither secreted nor reabsorbed in the MCD, and (3) the osmolality of the fluid in the terminal CCD is known. Significant reabsorption or secretion of K^+ in the MCD seldom occurs, except in profound K^+ depletion or excess, respectively. When AVP is acting ($OSM_U \geq OSM_P$), the osmolality in the terminal CCD is the same as that of plasma, and the K^+ concentration in the lumen of the distal nephron can be estimated by dividing the urine K^+ concentration ($[K^+]_U$) by the ratio of the urine to plasma osmolality (OSM_U/OSM_P):

$$[K^+]_{CCD} = [K^+]_U \div (OSM_U/OSM_P)\text{TTKG}$$
$$= [K^+]_{CCD}/[K^+]_P = [K^+]_U \div (OSM_U/OSM_P)/[K^+]_P$$

Hypokalemia with a TTKG greater than 4 suggests renal K^+ loss due to increased distal K^+ secretion. Plasma renin and aldosterone levels are often helpful in differentiating the various causes of hyperaldosteronism. Bicarbonaturia and the presence of other non-reabsorbed anions also increase the TTKG and lead to renal K^+-wasting.

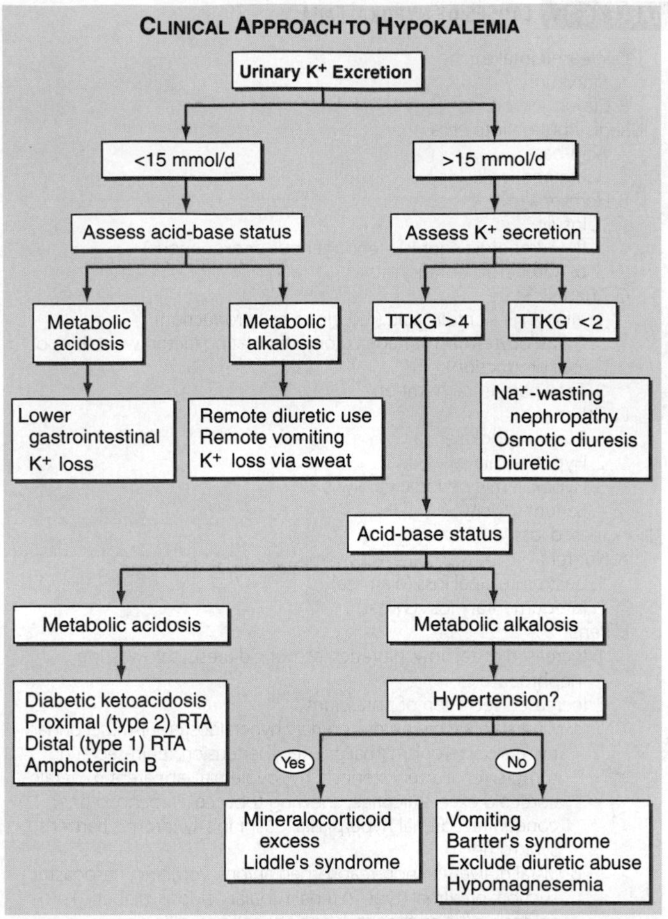

FIGURE 46-3 Algorithm depicting clinical approach to hypokalemia. TTKG, transtubular K^+ concentration gradient; RTA, renal tubular acidosis.

℞ HYPOKALEMIA

The therapeutic goals are to correct the K^+ deficit and to minimize ongoing losses. With the exception of periodic paralysis, hypokalemia resulting from transcellular shifts rarely requires intravenous K^+ supplementation, which can lead to rebound hyperkalemia. It is generally safer to correct hypokalemia via the oral route. The degree of K^+ depletion does not correlate well with the plasma K^+ concentration. A decrement of 1 mmol/L in the plasma K^+ concentration (from 4.0 to 3.0 mmol/L) may represent a total body K^+ deficit of 200–400 mmol, and patients with plasma levels under 3.0 mmol/L often require in excess of 600 mmol of K^+ to correct the deficit. Furthermore, factors promoting K^+ shift out of cells (e.g., insulin deficiency in diabetic ketoacidosis) may result in underestimation of the K^+ deficit. Therefore, the plasma K^+ concentration should be monitored frequently when assessing the response to treatment. Potassium chloride is usually the preparation of choice and will promote more rapid correction of hypokalemia and metabolic alkalosis. Potassium bicarbonate and citrate (metabolized to HCO_3^-) tend to alkalinize the patient and would be more appropriate for hypokalemia associated with chronic diarrhea or RTA.

Patients with severe hypokalemia or those unable to take anything by mouth require intravenous replacement therapy with KCl. The maximum concentration of administered K^+ should be no more than 40 mmol/L via a peripheral vein or 60 mmol/L via a central vein. The rate of infusion should not exceed 20 mmol/h unless paralysis or malignant ventricular arrhythmias are present. Ideally, KCl should be mixed in normal saline since dextrose solutions may initially exacerbate hypokalemia due to insulin-mediated movement of K^+ into cells. Rapid intravenous administration of K^+ should be used judiciously and requires close observation of the clinical manifestations of hypokalemia (electrocardiogram and neuromuscular examination).

HYPERKALEMIA

Etiology Hyperkalemia, defined as a plasma K^+ concentration >5.0 mmol/L, occurs as a result of either K^+ release from cells or decreased renal loss. Increased K^+ intake is rarely the sole cause of hyperkalemia since the phenomenon of *potassium adaptation* ensures rapid K^+ excretion in response to increases in dietary consumption. Iatrogenic hyperkalemia may result from overzealous parenteral K^+ replacement or in patients with renal insufficiency. *Pseudohyperkalemia* represents an artificially elevated plasma K^+ concentration due to K^+ movement out of cells immediately prior to or following venipuncture. Contributing factors include prolonged use of a tourniquet with or without repeated fist clenching, hemolysis, and marked leukocytosis or thrombocytosis. The latter two result in an elevated serum K^+ concentration due to release of intracellular K^+ following clot formation. Pseudohyperkalemia should be suspected in an otherwise asymptomatic patient with no obvious underlying cause. If proper venipuncture technique is used and a plasma (not serum) K^+ concentration is measured, it should be normal. Intravascular hemolysis, tumor lysis syndrome, and rhabdomyolysis all lead to K^+ release from cells as a result of tissue breakdown.

Metabolic acidoses, with the exception of those due to the accumulation of organic anions, can be associated with mild hyperkalemia resulting from intracellular buffering of H^+ (see above). Insulin deficiency and hypertonicity (e.g., hyperglycemia) promote K^+ shift from the ICF to the ECF. The severity of exercise-induced hyperkalemia is related to the degree of exertion. It is due to release of K^+ from muscles and is usually rapidly reversible, often associated with rebound hypokalemia. Treatment with beta blockers rarely causes hyperkalemia but may contribute to the elevation in plasma K^+ concentration seen with other conditions. *Hyperkalemic periodic paralysis* (Chap. 382) is a rare autosomal dominant disorder characterized by episodic weakness or paralysis, precipitated by stimuli that normally lead to mild hyperkalemia (e.g., exercise). The genetic defect appears to be a single amino acid substitution due to a mutation in the gene for the skeletal muscle Na^+ channel. Hyperkalemia may occur with severe digitalis toxicity due to inhibition of the Na^+,K^+-ATPase pump. Depolarizing muscle relaxants such as succinylcholine can increase the plasma K^+ concentration, especially in patients with massive trauma, burns, or neuromuscular disease.

Chronic hyperkalemia is virtually always associated with decreased renal K^+ excretion due to either impaired secretion or diminished distal solute delivery (Table 46-4). The latter is seldom the only cause of impaired K^+ excretion but may significantly contribute to hyperkalemia in protein-malnourished (low urea excretion) and ECF volume–contracted (decreased distal NaCl delivery) patients. Decreased K^+ secretion by the principal cells results from either impaired Na^+ reabsorption or increased Cl^- reabsorption.

TABLE 46-4 CAUSES OF HYPERKALEMIA

I. Renal failure
II. Decreased distal flow (i.e., decreased effective circulating arterial volume)
III. Decreased K^+ secretion
  A. Impaired Na^+ reabsorption
    1. Primary hypoaldosteronism: adrenal insufficiency, adrenal enzyme deficiency (21-hydroxylase, 3β-hydroxysteroid dehydrogenase, corticosterone methyl oxidase)
    2. Secondary hypoaldosteronism: hyporeninemia, drugs (ACE inhibitors, NSAIDs, heparin)
    3. Resistance to aldosterone: pseudohypoaldosteronism, tubulo-interstitial disease, drugs (K^+-sparing diuretics, trimethoprim, pentamidine)
  B. Enhanced Cl^- reabsorption (chloride shunt)
    1. Gordon's syndrome
    2. Cyclosporine

Note: ACE, angiotensin-converting enzyme; NSAIDs, nonsteroidal anti-inflammatory drugs.

Hyporeninemic hypoaldosteronism is a syndrome characterized by euvolemia or ECF volume expansion and suppressed renin and aldosterone levels (Chaps. 336 and 338). This disorder is commonly seen in mild renal insufficiency, diabetic nephropathy, or chronic tubulointerstitial disease. Patients frequently have an impaired kaliuretic response to exogenous mineralocorticoid administration, suggesting that enhanced distal Cl^- reabsorption (electroneutral Na^+ reabsorption) may account for many of the findings of hyporeninemic hypoaldosteronism. NSAIDs inhibit renin secretion and the synthesis of vasodilatory renal prostaglandins. The resultant decrease in GFR and K^+ secretion is often manifest as hyperkalemia. As a rule, the degree of hyperkalemia due to hypoaldosteronism is mild in the absence of increased K^+ intake or renal dysfunction.

Angiotensin-converting enzyme (ACE) inhibitors block the conversion of angiotensin I to angiotensin II. Angiotensin receptor antagonists directly inhibit the actions of angiotensin II on AT1 angiotensin II receptors. The actions of both of these classes of drugs result in impaired aldosterone release. Patients at increased risk of ACE inhibitor or angiotensin receptor antagonist–induced hyperkalemia include those with diabetes mellitus, renal insufficiency, decreased effective circulating arterial volume, bilateral renal artery stenosis, or concurrent use of K^+-sparing diuretics or NSAIDs.

Decreased aldosterone synthesis may be due to *primary adrenal insufficiency* (Addison's disease) or congenital adrenal enzyme deficiency (Chap. 336). Heparin (including low-molecular-weight heparin) inhibits production of aldosterone by the cells of the zona glomerulosa and can lead to severe hyperkalemia in a subset of patients with underlying renal disease, diabetes mellitus, or those receiving K^+-sparing diuretics, ACE inhibitors, or NSAIDs. *Pseudohypoaldosteronism* is a rare familial disorder characterized by hyperkalemia, metabolic acidosis, renal Na^+ wasting, hypotension, high renin and aldosterone levels, and end-organ resistance to aldosterone. The gene encoding the mineralocorticoid receptor is normal in these patients, and the electrolyte abnormalities can be reversed with supra-pharmacologic doses of an exogenous mineralocorticoid (e.g., 9α-fludrocortisone) or an inhibitor of 11β-HSDH (e.g., carbenoxolone). The kaliuretic response to aldosterone is impaired by K^+-sparing diuretics. Spironolactone is a competitive mineralocorticoid antagonist, whereas amiloride and triamterene block the apical Na^+ channel of the principal cell. Two other drugs that impair K^+ secretion by blocking distal nephron Na^+ reabsorption are trimethoprim and pentamidine. These antimicrobial agents may contribute to the hyperkalemia often seen in patients infected with HIV who are being treated for *Pneumocystis carinii* pneumonia.

Hyperkalemia frequently complicates acute oliguric renal failure due to increased K^+ release from cells (acidosis, catabolism) and decreased excretion. Increased distal flow rate and K^+ secretion per nephron compensate for decreased renal mass in chronic renal insufficiency. However, these adaptive mechanisms eventually fail to maintain K^+ balance when the GFR falls below 10–15 mL/min or oliguria ensues. Otherwise asymptomatic urinary tract obstruction is an often overlooked cause of hyperkalemia. Other nephropathies associated with impaired K^+ excretion include drug-induced interstitial nephritis, lupus nephritis, sickle cell disease, and diabetic nephropathy.

Gordon's syndrome is a rare condition characterized by hyperkalemia, metabolic acidosis, and a normal GFR. These patients are usually volume-expanded with suppressed renin and aldosterone levels as well as refractory to the kaliuretic effect of exogenous mineralocorticoids. It has been suggested that these findings could all be accounted for by increased distal Cl^- reabsorption (electroneutral Na^+ reabsorption), also referred to as a *Cl^- shunt.* A similar mechanism may be partially responsible for the hyperkalemia associated with cyclosporine nephrotoxicity. *Hyperkalemic distal (type 4) RTA* may be due to either hypoaldosteronism or a Cl^- shunt (aldosterone-resistant).

Clinical Features Since the resting membrane potential is related to the ratio of the ICF to ECF K^+ concentration, hyperkalemia partially depolarizes the cell membrane. Prolonged depolarization impairs membrane excitability and is manifest as weakness, which may progress to flaccid paralysis and hypoventilation if the respiratory muscles are involved. Hyperkalemia also inhibits renal ammoniagenesis and reabsorption of NH_4^+ in the TALH. Thus, net acid excretion is impaired and results in metabolic acidosis, which may further exacerbate the hyperkalemia due to K^+ movement out of cells.

The most serious effect of hyperkalemia is cardiac toxicity, which does not correlate well with the plasma K^+ concentration. The earliest electrocardiographic changes include increased T-wave amplitude, or peaked T waves. More severe degrees of hyperkalemia result in a prolonged PR interval and QRS duration, atrioventricular conduction delay, and loss of P waves. Progressive widening of the QRS complex and merging with the T wave produces a sine wave pattern. The terminal event is usually ventricular fibrillation or asystole.

Diagnosis (Fig. 46-4) With rare exceptions, chronic hyperkalemia is always due to impaired K^+ excretion. If the etiology is not readily apparent and the patient is asymptomatic, pseudohyperkalemia should be excluded, as described above. Oliguric acute renal failure and severe chronic renal insufficiency should also be ruled out. The history should focus on medications that impair K^+ handling and potential sources of K^+ intake. Evaluation of the ECF compartment, effective circulating volume, and urine output are essential components of the physical examination. The severity of hyperkalemia is determined by the symptoms, plasma K^+ concentration, and electrocardiographic abnormalities.

The appropriate renal response to hyperkalemia is to excrete at least 200 mmol of K^+ daily. In most cases, diminished renal K^+ loss is due to impaired K^+ secretion, which can be assessed by measuring the transtubular K^+ concentration gradient (TTKG). A TTKG <10 implies a decreased driving force for K^+ secretion due to either hypoaldosteronism or resistance to the renal effects of mineralocorticoid. This can be determined by evaluating the kaliuretic response to administration of mineralocorticoid (e.g., 9α-fludrocortisone). Primary adrenal insufficiency can be differentiated from hyporeninemic hypoaldosteronism by examining the renin-aldosterone axis. Renin and aldosterone levels should be measured in the supine and upright positions following 3 days of Na^+ restriction (Na^+ intake <10 mmol/d) in combination with a loop diuretic to induce mild volume contraction. Aldosterone-resistant hyperkalemia can result from the various causes of impaired distal Na^+ reabsorption or from a Cl^- shunt. The former leads to salt wasting, ECF volume contraction, and high renin and aldosterone levels. In contrast, enhanced distal Cl^- reabsorption is associated with volume expansion and suppressed renin and aldosterone secretion. As mentioned above, hypoaldosteronism seldom causes severe hyperkalemia in the absence of increased dietary K^+ intake, renal insufficiency, transcellular K^+ shifts, or antikaliuretic drugs.

℞ HYPERKALEMIA

The approach to therapy depends on the degree of hyperkalemia as determined by the plasma K^+ concentration, associated muscular weakness, and changes on the electrocardiogram. Potentially fatal hyperkalemia rarely occurs unless the plasma K^+ concentration exceeds 7.5 mmol/L and is usually associated with profound weakness and absent P waves, QRS widening, or ventricular arrhythmias on the electrocardiogram.

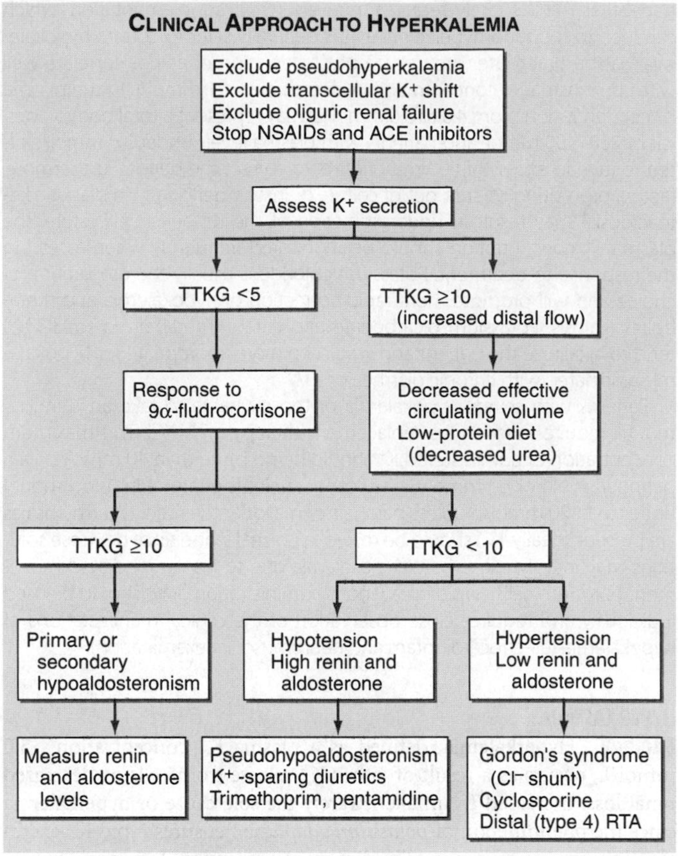

FIGURE 46-4 Algorithm depicting clinical approach to hyperkalemia. NSAID, nonsteroidal anti-inflammatory drug; ACE, angiotensin-converting enzyme; RTA, renal tubular acidosis; TTKG, transtubular K^+ concentration gradient.

Severe hyperkalemia requires emergent treatment directed at minimizing membrane depolarization, shifting K^+ into cells, and promoting K^+ loss. In addition, exogenous K^+ intake and antikaliuretic drugs should be discontinued. Administration of calcium gluconate decreases membrane excitability. The usual dose is 10 mL of a 10% solution infused over 2–3 min. The effect begins within minutes but is short-lived (30–60 min), and the dose can be repeated if no change in the electrocardiogram is seen after 5–10 min. Insulin causes K^+ to shift into cells by mechanisms described previously and will temporarily lower the plasma K^+ concentration. Although glucose alone will stimulate insulin release from normal pancreatic β cells, a more rapid response generally occurs when exogenous insulin is administered (with glucose to prevent hypoglycemia). A commonly recommended combination is 10–20 units of regular insulin and 25–50 g of glucose. Obviously, hyperglycemic patients should not be given glucose. If effective, the plasma K^+ concentration will fall by 0.5–1.5 mmol/L in 15–30 min, and the effect will last for several hours. Alkali therapy with intravenous $NaHCO_3$ can also shift K^+ into cells. This is safest when administered as an isotonic solution of 3 ampules per liter (134 mmol/L $NaHCO_3$) and ideally should be reserved for severe hyperkalemia associated with metabolic acidosis. Patients with end-stage renal disease seldom respond to this intervention and may not tolerate the Na^+ load and resultant volume expansion. When administered parenterally or in nebulized form, β_2-adrenergic agonists promote cellular uptake of K^+ (see above). The onset of action is 30 min, lowering the plasma K^+ concentration by 0.5 to 1.5 mmol/L, and the effect lasts 2–4 h.

Removal of K^+ can be achieved using diuretics, cation-exchange resin, or dialysis. Loop and thiazide diuretics, often in combination, may enhance K^+ excretion if renal function is adequate. Sodium polystyrene sulfonate is a cation-exchange resin that promotes the exchange of Na^+ for K^+ in the gastrointestinal tract. Each gram binds 1 mmol of K^+ and releases 2–3 mmol of Na^+. When given by mouth, the usual dose is 25–50 g mixed with 100 mL of 20% sorbitol to prevent constipation. This will generally lower the plasma K^+ concentration by 0.5–1.0 mmol/L within 1–2 h and last for 4–6 h. Sodium polystyrene sulfonate can also be administered as a retention enema consisting of 50 g of resin and 50 mL of 70% sorbitol mixed in 150 mL of tap water. The sorbitol should be omitted from the enema in postoperative patients due to the increased incidence of sorbitol-induced colonic necrosis, especially following renal transplantation. The most rapid and effective way of lowering the plasma K^+ concentration is hemodialysis. This should be reserved for patients with renal failure and those with severe life-threatening hyperkalemia unresponsive to more conservative measures. Peritoneal dialysis also removes K^+ but is only 15–20% as effective as hemodialysis. Finally, the underlying cause of the hyperkalemia should be treated. This may involve dietary modification, correction of metabolic acidosis, cautious volume expansion, and administration of exogenous mineralocorticoid.

FURTHER READINGS

ADROGUE HJ, MADIAS NE: Hypernatremia. N Engl J Med 342:1493, 2000

———: Hyponatremia. N Engl J Med 342:1581, 2000

BERL T, VERBALIS J: Pathophysiology of water metabolism, in *Brenner & Rector's The Kidney*, 7th ed, BM Brenner (ed). Philadelphia, Saunders, 2004

COHN JN et al: New guidelines for potassium replacement in clinical practice: A contemporary review by the National Council on Potassium in Clinical Practice. Arch Intern Med 160:2429, 2000

GOLDSZMIDT MA, ILIESCU EA: DDAVP to prevent rapid correction in hyponatremia. Clin Nephrol 53:226, 2000

GREENBERG A, VERBALIS JG: Vasopressin receptor antagonists. Kidney Int 69:2124, 2006

GROSS P: Treatment of severe hyponatremia. Kidney Int 60:2417, 2001

HARRIGAN MR: Cerebral salt wasting syndrome. Crit Care Clin 17:125, 2001

MOUNT DB: Disorders of potassium balance, in *Brenner & Rector's The Kidney*, 7th ed, BM Brenner (ed). Philadelphia, Saunders, 2004

NIELSEN S et al: Aquaporins in the kidney: From molecules to medicine. Physiol Rev 82:205, 2002

WARNOCK DG: Genetic forms of renal potassium and magnesium wasting. Am J Med 112:235, 2002

47 Hypercalcemia and Hypocalcemia

Sundeep Khosla

The calcium ion plays a critical role in normal cellular function and signaling, regulating diverse physiologic processes such as neuromuscular signaling, cardiac contractility, hormone secretion, and blood coagulation. Thus, extracellular calcium concentrations are maintained within an exquisitely narrow range through a series of feedback mechanisms that involve parathyroid hormone (PTH) and the active vitamin D metabolite 1,25-dihydroxyvitmin D [1,25(OH)$_2$D]. These feedback mechanisms are orchestrated by integrating signals between the parathyroid glands, kidney, intestine, and bone (Fig. 47-1) (Chap. 346).

Disorders of serum calcium concentration are relatively common and often serve as a harbinger of underlying disease. This chapter provides a brief summary of the approach to patients with altered serum calcium levels. See Chap. 347 for a detailed discussion of this topic.

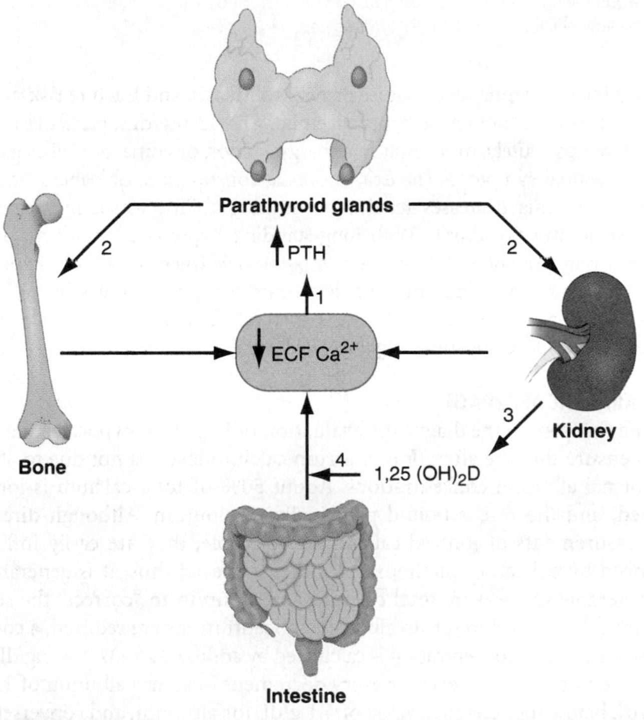

FIGURE 47-1 Feedback mechanisms maintaining extracellular calcium concentrations within a narrow, physiologic range [8.9–10.1 mg/dL (2.2–2.5 mM)]. A decrease in extracellular (ECF) calcium (Ca^{2+}) triggers an increase in parathyroid hormone (PTH) secretion (1) via activation of the calcium sensor receptor on parathyroid cells. PTH, in turn, results in increased tubular reabsorption of calcium by the kidney (2) and resorption of calcium from bone (2) and also stimulates renal 1,25(OH)$_2$D production (3). 1,25(OH)$_2$D, in turn, acts principally on the intestine to increase calcium absorption (4). Collectively, these homeostatic mechanisms serve to restore serum calcium levels to normal.

HYPERCALCEMIA

ETIOLOGY

The causes of hypercalcemia can be understood and classified based on derangements in the normal feedback mechanisms that regulate serum calcium (Table 47-1). Excess PTH production, which is not appropriately suppressed by increased serum calcium concentrations, occurs in primary neoplastic disorders of the parathyroid glands (parathyroid adenomas, hyperplasia, or, rarely, carcinoma) that are associated with increased parathyroid cell mass and impaired feedback inhibition by calcium. Inappropriate PTH secretion for the ambient level of serum calcium also occurs with heterozygous inactivating calcium sensor receptor (CaSR) mutations, which impair extracellular calcium sensing by the parathyroid glands and the kidneys, resulting in familial hypocalciuric hypercalcemia (FHH). Although PTH secretion by tumors is extremely rare, many solid tumors produce PTH-related peptide (PTHrP), which shares homology with PTH in the first 13 amino acids and binds the PTH receptor, thus mimicking effects of PTH on bone and the kidney. In PTHrP-mediated hypercalcemia of malignancy, PTH levels are suppressed by the high serum calcium levels. Hypercalcemia associated with granulomatous disease (e.g., sarcoidosis) or lymphomas is caused by enhanced conversion of 25(OH)D to the potent 1,25(OH)$_2$D. In these disorders, 1,25(OH)$_2$D enhances intestinal calcium absorption, resulting in hypercalcemia and suppressed PTH. Disorders that directly increase calcium mobilization from bone, such as hyperthyroidism or osteolytic metastases, also lead to hypercalcemia with suppressed PTH secretion, as does exogenous calcium overload, as in milk-alkali syndrome, or total parenteral nutrition with excessive calcium supplementation.

CLINICAL MANIFESTATIONS

Mild hypercalcemia (up to 11–11.5 mg/dL) is usually asymptomatic and recognized only on routine calcium measurements. Some patients may complain of vague neuropsychiatric symptoms, including trouble concentrating, personality changes, or depression. Other presenting symptoms

TABLE 47-1 CAUSES OF HYPERCALCEMIA

Excessive PTH production
Primary hyperparathyroidism (adenoma, hyperplasia, rarely carcinoma)
Tertiary hyperparathyroidism (long-term stimulation of PTH secretion in renal insufficiency)
Ectopic PTH secretion (very rare)
Inactivating mutations in the CaSR (FHH)
Alterations in CaSR function (lithium therapy)
Hypercalcemia of malignancy
Overproduction of PTHrP (many solid tumors)
Lytic skeletal metastases (breast, myeloma)
Excessive $1,25(OH)_2D$ production
Granulomatous diseases (sarcoidosis, tuberculosis, silicosis)
Lymphomas
Vitamin D intoxication
Primary increase in bone resorption
Hyperthyroidism
Immobilization
Excessive calcium intake
Milk-alkali syndrome
Total parenteral nutrition
Other causes
Endocrine disorders (adrenal insufficiency, pheochromocytoma, VIPoma)
Medications (thiazides, vitamin A, antiestrogens)

Note: CaSR, calcium sensor receptor; FHH, familial hypocalciuric hypercalcemia; PTH, parathyroid hormone; PTHrP, PTH-related peptide.

may include peptic ulcer disease or nephrolithiasis, and fracture risk may be increased. More severe hypercalcemia (>12–13 mg/dL), particularly if it develops acutely, may result in lethargy, stupor, or coma, as well as gastrointestinal symptoms (nausea, anorexia, constipation, or pancreatitis). Hypercalcemia decreases renal concentrating ability, which may cause polyuria and polydipsia. With long-standing hyperparathyroidism, patients may present with bone pain or pathologic fractures. Finally, hypercalcemia can result in significant electrocardiographic changes, including bradycardia, AV block, and short QT interval; changes in serum calcium can be monitored by following the QT interval (Fig. 221-16).

DIAGNOSTIC APPROACH

The first step in the diagnostic evaluation of hyper- or hypocalcemia is to ensure that the alteration in serum calcium levels is not due to abnormal albumin concentrations. About 50% of total calcium is ionized, and the rest is bound principally to albumin. Although direct measurements of ionized calcium are possible, they are easily influenced by collection methods and other artifacts; thus, it is generally preferable to measure total calcium and albumin to "correct" the serum calcium. When serum albumin concentrations are reduced, a corrected calcium concentration is calculated by adding 0.2 m*M* (0.8 mg/dL) to the total calcium level for every decrement in serum albumin of 1.0 g/dL below the reference value of 4.1 g/dL for albumin, and conversely for elevations in serum albumin.

A detailed history may provide important clues regarding the etiology of the hypercalcemia (Table 47-1). Chronic hypercalcemia is most commonly caused by primary hyperparathyroidism, as opposed to the second most common etiology of hypercalcemia, an underlying malignancy. The history should include medication use, previous neck surgery, and systemic symptoms suggestive of sarcoidosis or lymphoma.

Once true hypercalcemia is established, the second most important laboratory test in the diagnostic evaluation is a PTH level using a two-site assay for the intact hormone. Increases in PTH are often accompanied by hypophosphatemia. In addition, serum creatinine should be measured to assess renal function; hypercalcemia may impair renal function, and renal clearance of PTH may be altered depending on the fragments detected by the assay. If the PTH level is increased (or "inappropriately normal") in the setting of an elevated calcium and low phosphorus, the diagnosis is almost always primary hyperparathyroidism. Since individuals with familial hypocalciuric hypercalcemia (FHH) may also present with mildly elevated PTH levels and hypercalcemia, this diagnosis should be considered and excluded because parathyroid surgery is ineffective in this condition. A calcium/creatinine clearance ratio (calculated as urine calcium/serum calcium divided by urine creatinine/serum creatinine) of <0.01 is suggestive of FHH, particularly when there is a family history of mild, asymptomatic hypercalcemia. Ectopic PTH secretion is extremely rare.

A suppressed PTH level in the face of hypercalcemia is consistent with non-parathyroid-mediated hypercalcemia, most often due to underlying malignancy. Although a tumor that causes hypercalcemia is generally overt, a PTHrP level may be needed to establish the diagnosis of hypercalcemia of malignancy. Serum $1,25(OH)_2D$ levels are increased in granulomatous disorders, and clinical evaluation in combination with laboratory testing will generally provide a diagnosis for the various disorders listed in Table 47-1.

℞ HYPERCALCEMIA

Mild, asymptomatic hypercalcemia does not require immediate therapy, and management should be dictated by the underlying diagnosis. By contrast, significant, symptomatic hypercalcemia usually requires therapeutic intervention independent of the etiology of hypercalcemia. Initial therapy of significant hypercalcemia begins with volume expansion since hypercalcemia invariably leads to dehydration; 4–6 L of intravenous saline may be required over the first 24 h, keeping in mind that underlying comorbidities (e.g., congestive heart failure) may require the use of loop diuretics to enhance sodium and calcium excretion. However, loop diuretics should not be initiated until the volume status has been restored to normal. If there is increased calcium mobilization from bone (as in malignancy or severe hyperparathyroidism), drugs that inhibit bone resorption should be considered. Zoledronic acid (e.g., 4 mg intravenously over ~30 min), pamidronate (e.g., 60–90 mg intravenously over 2–4 h), and etidronate (e.g., 7.5 mg/kg per day for 3–7 consecutive days) are approved by the U.S. Food and Drug Administration for the treatment of hypercalcemia of malignancy in adults. Onset of action is within 1–3 days, with normalization of serum calcium levels occurring in 60–90% of patients. Bisphosphonate infusions may need to be repeated if hypercalcemia relapses. Because of their effectiveness, bisphosphonates have replaced calcitonin or plicamycin, which are rarely used in current practice for the management of hypercalcemia. In rare instances, dialysis may be necessary. Finally, while intravenous phosphate chelates calcium and decreases serum calcium levels, this therapy can be toxic because calcium-phosphate complexes may deposit in tissues and cause extensive organ damage.

In patients with $1,25(OH)_2D$-mediated hypercalcemia, glucocorticoids are the preferred therapy, as they decrease $1,25(OH)_2D$ production. Intravenous hydrocortisone (100–300 mg daily) or oral prednisone (40–60 mg daily) for 3–7 days are used most often. Other drugs, such as ketoconazole, chloroquine, and hydroxychloroquine, may also decrease $1,25(OH)_2D$ production and are used occasionally.

HYPOCALCEMIA

ETIOLOGY

The causes of hypocalcemia can be differentiated according to whether serum PTH levels are low (hypoparathyroidism) or high (secondary hyperparathyroidism). Although there are many potential causes of hypocalcemia, impaired PTH or vitamin D production are the most common etiologies (Table 47-2) (Chap. 347). Because PTH is the main defense against hypocalcemia, disorders associated with deficient PTH production or secretion may be associated with profound, life-threatening hypocalcemia. In adults, hypoparathyroidism most commonly results from inadvertent damage to all four glands during thyroid or parathyroid gland surgery. Hypoparathyroidism is a cardinal feature of autoimmune endocrinopathies (Chap. 345); rarely, it may be associated with infiltrative diseases such as sarcoidosis. Impaired PTH secretion may be secondary to magnesium deficiency or to activating mutations in the CaSR, which suppress PTH, leading to effects that are opposite to those that occur in FHH.

Vitamin D deficiency, impaired $1,25(OH)_2D$ production (primarily secondary to renal insufficiency), or, rarely, vitamin D resistance also cause hypocalcemia. However, the degree of hypocalcemia in these disorders is generally not as severe as that seen with hypoparathyroidism because the parathyroids are capable of mounting a compensatory increase in PTH secretion. Hypocalcemia may also occur in conditions associated with severe tissue injury such as burns, rhabdomyolysis, tumor lysis, or pancreatitis. The cause of hypocalcemia in these settings

TABLE 47-2 CAUSES OF HYPOCALCEMIA

Low Parathyroid Hormone Levels (Hypoparathyroidism)
Parathyroid agenesis
Isolated
DiGeorge syndrome
Parathyroid destruction
Surgical
Radiation
Infiltration by metastases or systemic diseases
Autoimmune
Reduced parathyroid function
Hypomagnesemia
Activating CaSR mutations
High Parathyroid Hormone Levels (Secondary Hyperparathyroidism)
Vitamin D deficiency or impaired $1,25(OH)_2D$ production/action
Nutritional vitamin D deficiency (poor intake or absorption)
Renal insufficiency with impaired $1,25(OH)_2D$ production
Vitamin D resistance, including receptor defects
Parathyroid hormone resistance syndromes
PTH receptor mutations
Pseudohypoparathyroidism (G protein mutations)
Drugs
Calcium chelators
Inhibitors of bone resorption (bisphosphonates, plicamycin)
Altered vitamin D metabolism (phenytoin, ketoconazole)
Miscellaneous causes
Acute pancreatitis
Acute rhabdomyolysis
Hungry bone syndrome after parathyroidectomy
Osteoblastic metastases with marked stimulation of bone formation (prostate cancer)

Note: CaSR, calcium sensor receptor; PTH, parathyroid hormone.

may include a combination of low albumin, hyperphosphatemia, tissue deposition of calcium, and impaired PTH secretion.

CLINICAL MANIFESTATIONS

Patients with hypocalcemia may be asymptomatic if the decreases in serum calcium are relatively mild and chronic, or they may present with life-threatening complications. Moderate to severe hypocalcemia is associated with paresthesias, usually of the fingers, toes, and circumoral regions, and is caused by increased neuromuscular irritability. On physical examination, a Chvostek's sign (twitching of the circumoral muscles in response to gentle tapping of the facial nerve just anterior to the ear) may be elicited, although it is also present in ~10% of normal individuals. Carpal spasm may be induced by inflation of a blood pressure cuff to 20 mmHg above the patient's systolic blood pressure for 3 min (Trousseau's sign). Severe hypocalcemia can induce seizures, carpopedal spasm, bronchospasm, laryngospasm, and prolongation of the QT interval.

DIAGNOSTIC APPROACH

In addition to measuring serum calcium, it is useful to determine albumin, phosphorus, and magnesium levels. As for the evaluation of hypercalcemia, determining the PTH level is central to the evaluation of hypocalcemia. A suppressed (or "inappropriately low") PTH level in the setting of hypocalcemia establishes absent or reduced PTH secretion (hypoparathyroidism) as the cause of the hypocalcemia. Further history will often elicit the underlying cause (i.e., parathyroid agenesis vs. destruction). By contrast, an elevated PTH level (secondary hyperparathyroidism) should direct attention to the vitamin D axis as the cause of the hypocalcemia. Nutritional vitamin D deficiency is best assessed by obtaining serum 25-hydroxyvitamin D levels, which reflect vitamin D stores. In the setting of renal insufficiency or suspected vitamin D resistance, serum $1,25(OH)_2D$ levels are informative.

℞ HYPOCALCEMIA

The approach to treatment depends on the severity of the hypocalcemia, the rapidity with which it develops, and the accompanying complications (e.g., seizures, laryngospasm). Acute, symptomatic hypocalcemia is initially managed with calcium gluconate, 10 mL 10% wt/vol (90 mg or 2.2 mmol) intravenously, diluted in 50 mL of 5% dextrose or 0.9% sodium chloride, given intravenously over 5 min. Continuing hypocalcemia often requires a constant intravenous infusion (typically 10 ampuls of calcium gluconate or 900 mg of calcium in 1 L of 5% dextrose or 0.9% sodium chloride administered over 24 h). Accompanying hypomagnesemia, if present, should be treated with appropriate magnesium supplementation.

Chronic hypocalcemia due to hypoparathyroidism is treated with calcium supplements (1000–1500 mg/d elemental calcium in divided doses) and either vitamin D_2 or D_3 (25,000–100,000 U daily) or calcitriol [$1,25(OH)_2D$, 0.25–2 μg/d]. Other vitamin D metabolites (dihydrotachysterol, alfacalcidiol) are now used less frequently. Vitamin D deficiency, however, is best treated using vitamin D supplementation, with the dose depending on the severity of the deficit and the underlying cause. Thus, nutritional vitamin D deficiency generally responds to relatively low doses of vitamin D (50,000 U, 2–3 times per week for several months), while vitamin D deficiency due to malabsorption may require much higher doses (100,000 U/d or more). The treatment goal is to bring serum calcium into the low normal range and to avoid hypercalciuria, which may lead to nephrolithiasis.

FURTHER READINGS

BILEZIKIAN JP, SILVERBERG SJ: Asymptomatic primary hyperparathyroidism. N Engl J Med 350:1746, 2004

FARFORD B et al: Nonsurgical management of primary hyperparathyroidism. Mayo Clin Proc 82(3):351, 2007

FINKELSTEIN JS, POTTS JT JR: Medical management of hypercalcemia, in *Endocrinology*, 5th ed, LJ DeGroot, JL Jameson (eds). Philadelphia, Elsevier, 2006

KIFOR O et al: Activating antibodies to the calcium-sensing receptor in two patients with autoimmune hypoparathyroidism. J Clin Endocrinol Metab 89:548, 2004

MARX SJ: Hyperparathyroid and hypoparathyroid disorders. N Engl J Med 343:1863, 2000

STEWART AF: Hypercalcemia associated with cancer. N Engl J Med 352:373, 2005

THAKKER RV: Genetics of endocrine and metabolic disorders: parathyroid. Rev Endocr Metab Disord 5:37, 2004

48 Acidosis and Alkalosis

Thomas D. DuBose, Jr.

NORMAL ACID-BASE HOMEOSTASIS

Systemic arterial pH is maintained between 7.35 and 7.45 by extracellular and intracellular chemical buffering together with respiratory and renal regulatory mechanisms. The control of arterial CO_2 tension (Pa_{CO_2}) by the central nervous system and respiratory systems and the control of the plasma bicarbonate by the kidneys stabilize the arterial pH by excretion or retention of acid or alkali. The metabolic and respiratory components that regulate systemic pH are described by the Henderson-Hasselbalch equation:

$$pH = 6.1 + \log \frac{HCO_3^-}{Pa_{CO_2} \times 0.0301}$$

Under most circumstances, CO_2 production and excretion are matched, and the usual steady-state Pa_{CO_2} is maintained at 40 mmHg.

Underexcretion of CO_2 produces hypercapnia, and overexcretion causes hypocapnia. Nevertheless, production and excretion are again matched at a new steady-state Pa_{CO_2}. Therefore, the Pa_{CO_2} is regulated primarily by neural respiratory factors (Chap. 258) and is not subject to regulation by the rate of CO_2 production. Hypercapnia is usually the result of hypoventilation rather than of increased CO_2 production. Increases or decreases in Pa_{CO_2} represent derangements of neural respiratory control or are due to compensatory changes in response to a primary alteration in the plasma [HCO_3^-].

The kidneys regulate plasma [HCO_3^-] through three main processes: (1) "reabsorption" of filtered HCO_3^-, (2) formation of titratable acid, and (3) excretion of NH_4^+ in the urine. The kidney filters ~4000 mmol of HCO_3^- per day. To reabsorb the filtered load of HCO_3^-, the renal tubules must therefore secrete 4000 mmol of hydrogen ions. Between 80 and 90% of HCO_3^- is reabsorbed in the proximal tubule. The distal nephron reabsorbs the remainder and secretes protons, as generated from metabolism, to defend systemic pH. While this quantity of protons, 40–60 mmol/d, is small, it must be secreted to prevent chronic positive H^+ balance and metabolic acidosis. This quantity of secreted protons is represented in the urine as titratable acid and NH_4^+. Metabolic acidosis in the face of normal renal function increases NH_4^+ production and excretion. NH_4^+ production and excretion are impaired in chronic renal failure, hyperkalemia, and renal tubular acidosis.

In sum, these regulatory responses, including chemical buffering, the regulation of Pa_{CO_2} by the respiratory system, and the regulation of [HCO_3^-] by the kidneys, act in concert to maintain a systemic arterial pH between 7.35 and 7.45.

TABLE 48-1 PREDICTION OF COMPENSATORY RESPONSES ON SIMPLE ACID-BASE DISTURBANCES AND PATTERN OF CHANGES

Disorder	Prediction of Compensation	Range of Values pH	HCO_3^-	Pa_{CO_2}
Metabolic acidosis	$Pa_{CO_2} = (1.5 \times HCO_3^-) + 8 \pm 2$ *or* Pa_{CO_2} will ↓ 1.25 mmHg per mmol/L ↓ in [HCO_3^-] *or* Pa_{CO_2} = [HCO_3^-] + 15	Low	Low	Low
Metabolic alkalosis	Pa_{CO_2} will ↑ 0.75 mmHg per mmol/L ↑ in [HCO_3^-] *or* Pa_{CO_2} will ↑ 6 mmHg per 10 mmol/L ↑ in [HCO_3^-] *or* Pa_{CO_2} = [HCO_3^-] + 15	High	High	High
Respiratory alkalosis		High	Low	Low
Acute	[HCO_3^-] will ↓ 0.2 mmol/L per mmHg ↓ in Pa_{CO_2}			
Chronic	[HCO_3^-] will ↓ 0.4 mmol/L per mmHg ↓ in Pa_{CO_2}			
Respiratory acidosis		Low	High	High
Acute	[HCO_3^-] will ↑ 0.1 mmol/L per mmHg ↑ in Pa_{CO_2}			
Chronic	[HCO_3^-] will ↑ 0.4 mmol/L per mmHg ↑ in Pa_{CO_2}			

DIAGNOSIS OF GENERAL TYPES OF DISTURBANCES

The most common clinical disturbances are simple acid-base disorders, i.e., metabolic acidosis or alkalosis or respiratory acidosis or alkalosis. Since compensation is not complete, the pH is abnormal in simple disturbances. More complicated clinical situations can give rise to mixed acid-base disturbances.

SIMPLE ACID-BASE DISORDERS

Primary respiratory disturbances (primary changes in Pa_{CO_2}) invoke compensatory metabolic responses (secondary changes in [HCO_3^-]), and primary metabolic disturbances elicit predictable compensatory respiratory responses. Physiologic compensation can be predicted from the relationships displayed in Table 48-1. Metabolic acidosis due to an increase in endogenous acids (e.g., ketoacidosis) lowers extracellular fluid [HCO_3^-] and decreases extracellular pH. This stimulates the medullary chemoreceptors to increase ventilation and to return the ratio of [HCO_3^-] to Pa_{CO_2}, and thus pH, toward normal, although not to normal. The degree of respiratory compensation expected in a simple form of metabolic acidosis can be predicted from the relationship: $Pa_{CO_2} = (1.5 \times [HCO_3^-]) + 8 \pm 2$, i.e., the Pa_{CO_2} is expected to decrease 1.25 mmHg for each mmol per liter decrease in [HCO_3^-]. Thus, a patient with metabolic acidosis and [HCO_3^-] of 12 mmol/L would be expected to have a Pa_{CO_2} between 24 and 28 mmHg. Values for Pa_{CO_2} <24 or >28 mmHg define a mixed disturbance (metabolic acidosis and respiratory alkalosis or metabolic alkalosis and respiratory acidosis, respectively). Another way to judge the appropriateness of the response in [HCO_3^-] or Pa_{CO_2} is to use an acid-base nomogram (Fig. 48-1). While the shaded areas of the nomogram show the 95% confidence limits for normal compensation in simple disturbances, finding acid-base values within the shaded area does not necessarily rule out a mixed disturbance. Imposition of one disorder over another may result in values lying within the area of a third. Thus, the nomogram, while convenient, is not a substitute for the equations in Table 48-1.

MIXED ACID-BASE DISORDERS

Mixed acid-base disorders—defined as independently coexisting disorders, not merely compensatory responses—are often seen in patients in critical care units and can lead to dangerous extremes of pH (Table 48-2). A patient with diabetic ketoacidosis (metabolic acidosis) may develop an independent respiratory problem leading to respiratory acidosis or alkalosis. Patients with underlying pulmonary disease may not respond to metabolic acidosis with an appropriate ventilatory response because of insufficient respiratory reserve. Such imposition of respiratory acidosis on metabolic acidosis can lead to severe acidemia and a poor outcome. When metabolic acidosis and metabolic alkalosis coexist in the same patient, the pH may be normal or near normal. When the pH is normal, an elevated anion gap (AG; see below) denotes the presence of a metabolic acidosis. A discrepancy in the ΔAG (prevailing minus nor-

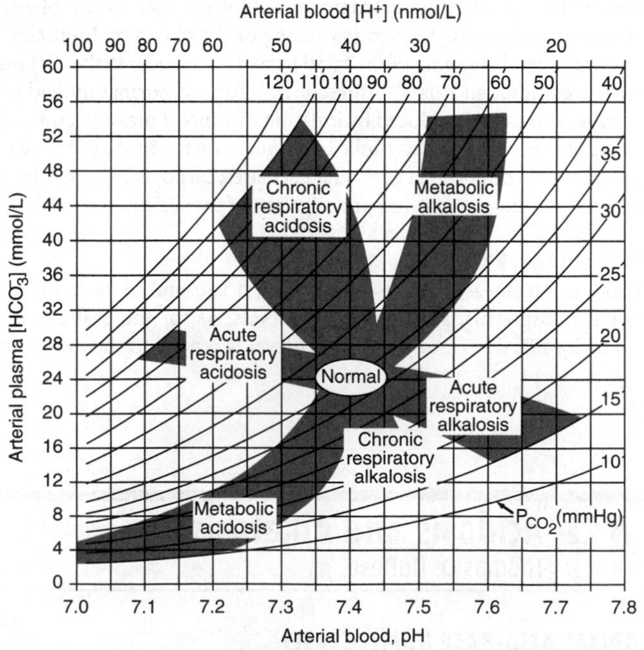

FIGURE 48-1 Acid-base nomogram. Shown are the 90% confidence limits (range of values) of the normal respiratory and metabolic compensations for primary acid-base disturbances. *(From DuBose, used with permission.)*

TABLE 48-2 EXAMPLES OF MIXED ACID-BASE DISORDERS

Mixed Metabolic and Respiratory
Metabolic acidosis – respiratory alkalosis Key: High- or normal-AG metabolic acidosis; prevailing Pa_{CO_2} *below* predicted value (Table 48-1) Example: Na^+, 140; K^+, 4.0; Cl^-, 106; HCO_3^-, 14; AG, 20; Pa_{CO_2}, 24; pH, 7.39 (lactic acidosis, sepsis in ICU)
Metabolic acidosis – respiratory acidosis Key: High- or normal-AG metabolic acidosis; prevailing Pa_{CO_2} *above* predicted value (Table 48-1) Example: Na^+, 140; K^+, 4.0; Cl^-, 102; HCO_3^-, 18; AG, 20; Pa_{CO_2}, 38; pH, 7.30 (severe pneumonia, pulmonary edema)
Metabolic alkalosis – respiratory alkalosis Key: Pa_{CO_2} does not increase as predicted; pH higher than expected Example: Na^+, 140; K^+, 4.0; Cl^-, 91; HCO_3^-, 33; AG, 16; Pa_{CO_2}, 38; pH, 7.55 (liver disease and diuretics)
Metabolic alkalosis – respiratory acidosis Key: Pa_{CO_2} higher than predicted; pH normal Example: Na^+, 140; K^+, 3.5; Cl^-, 88; HCO_3^-, 42; AG, 10; Pa_{CO_2}, 67; pH, 7.42 (COPD on diuretics)
Mixed Metabolic Disorders
Metabolic acidosis – metabolic alkalosis Key: Only detectable with high-AG acidosis; $\Delta AG >> \Delta HCO_3^-$ Example: Na^+, 140; K^+, 3.0; Cl^-, 95; HCO_3^-, 25; AG, 20; Pa_{CO_2}, 40; pH, 7.42 (uremia with vomiting)
Metabolic acidosis – metabolic acidosis Key: Mixed high-AG – normal-AG acidosis; ΔHCO_3^- accounted for by combined change in ΔAG and ΔCl^- Example: Na^+, 135; K^+, 3.0; Cl^-, 110; HCO_3^-, 10; AG, 15; Pa_{CO_2}, 25; pH, 7.20 (diarrhea and lactic acidosis, toluene toxicity, treatment of diabetic ketoacidosis)

Note: AG, anion gap; ICU, intensive care unit; COPD, chronic obstructive pulmonary disease.

mal AG) and the ΔHCO_3^- (normal minus prevailing HCO_3^-) indicates the presence of a mixed high-gap acidosis—metabolic alkalosis (see example below). A diabetic patient with ketoacidosis may have renal dysfunction resulting in simultaneous metabolic acidosis. Patients who have ingested an overdose of drug combinations such as sedatives and salicylates may have mixed disturbances as a result of the acid-base response to the individual drugs (metabolic acidosis mixed with respiratory acidosis or respiratory alkalosis, respectively). Even more complex are triple acid-base disturbances. For example, patients with metabolic acidosis due to alcoholic ketoacidosis may develop metabolic alkalosis due to vomiting and superimposed respiratory alkalosis due to the hyperventilation of hepatic dysfunction or alcohol withdrawal.

APPROACH TO THE PATIENT: Acid-Base Disorders

A stepwise approach to the diagnosis of acid-base disorders follows (Table 48-3). Care should be taken when measuring blood gases to obtain the arterial blood sample without using excessive heparin. Blood for electrolytes and arterial blood gases should be drawn simultaneously prior to therapy, since an increase in $[HCO_3^-]$ occurs with metabolic alkalosis and respiratory acidosis. Conversely, a decrease in $[HCO_3^-]$ occurs in metabolic acidosis and respiratory alkalosis. In the determination of arterial blood gases by the clinical laboratory, both pH and Pa_{CO_2} are measured, and the $[HCO_3^-]$ is calculated from the Henderson-Hasselbalch equation. This calculated value should be compared with the measured $[HCO_3^-]$ (total CO_2) on the electrolyte panel. These two values should agree within 2 mmol/L. If they do not, the values may not have been drawn simultaneously, a laboratory error may be present, or an error could have been made in calculating the $[HCO_3^-]$. After verifying the blood acid-base values, one can then identify the precise acid-base disorder.

TABLE 48-3 STEPS IN ACID-BASE DIAGNOSIS

1. Obtain arterial blood gas (ABG) and electrolytes simultaneously.
2. Compare $[HCO_3^-]$ on ABG and electrolytes to verify accuracy.
3. Calculate anion gap (AG).
4. Know four causes of high-AG acidosis (ketoacidosis, lactic acid acidosis, renal failure, and toxins).
5. Know two causes of hyperchloremic or nongap acidosis (bicarbonate loss from GI tract, renal tubular acidosis).
6. Estimate compensatory response (Table 48-1).
7. Compare ΔAG and ΔHCO_3^-.
8. Compare change in $[Cl^-]$ with change in $[Na^+]$.

CALCULATE THE ANION GAP All evaluations of acid-base disorders should include a simple calculation of the AG; it represents those unmeasured anions in plasma (normally 10 to 12 mmol/L) and is calculated as follows: $AG = Na^+ - (Cl^- + HCO_3^-)$. The unmeasured anions include anionic proteins, phosphate, sulfate, and organic anions. When acid anions, such as acetoacetate and lactate, accumulate in extracellular fluid, the AG increases, causing a high-AG acidosis. An increase in the AG is most often due to an increase in unmeasured anions and less commonly is due to a decrease in unmeasured cations (calcium, magnesium, potassium). In addition, the AG may increase with an increase in anionic albumin, because of either increased albumin concentration or alkalosis, which alters albumin charge. A decrease in the AG can be due to (1) an increase in unmeasured cations; (2) the addition to the blood of abnormal cations, such as lithium (lithium intoxication) or cationic immunoglobulins (plasma cell dyscrasias); (3) a reduction in the major plasma anion albumin concentration (nephrotic syndrome); (4) a decrease in the effective anionic charge on albumin by acidosis; or (5) hyperviscosity and severe hyperlipidemia, which can lead to an underestimation of sodium and chloride concentrations. A fall in serum albumin by 1 g/dL from the normal value (4.5 g/dL) decreases the anion gap by 2.5 meq/L. Know the common causes of a high-AG acidosis (Table 48-3).

In the face of a normal serum albumin, a high AG is usually due to non-chloride-containing acids that contain inorganic (phosphate, sulfate), organic (ketoacids, lactate, uremic organic anions), exogenous (salicylate or ingested toxins with organic acid production), or unidentified anions. The high AG is significant even if an additional acid-base disorder is superimposed to modify the $[HCO_3^-]$ independently. Simultaneous metabolic acidosis of the high-AG variety plus either chronic respiratory acidosis or metabolic alkalosis represents such a situation in which $[HCO_3^-]$ may be normal or even high (Table 48-2). Compare the change in $[HCO_3^-]$ (ΔHCO_3^-) and the change in the AG (ΔAG).

Similarly, normal values for $[HCO_3^-]$, Pa_{CO_2}, and pH do not ensure the absence of an acid-base disturbance. For instance, an alcoholic who has been vomiting may develop a metabolic alkalosis with a pH of 7.55, Pa_{CO_2} of 48 mmHg, $[HCO_3^-]$ of 40 mmol/L, $[Na^+]$ of 135, $[Cl^-]$ of 80, and $[K^+]$ of 2.8. If such a patient were then to develop a superimposed alcoholic ketoacidosis with a β-hydroxybutyrate concentration of 15 m*M*, arterial pH would fall to 7.40, $[HCO_3^-]$ to 25 mmol/L, and the Pa_{CO_2} to 40 mmHg. Although these blood gases are normal, the AG is elevated at 30 mmol/L, indicating a mixed metabolic alkalosis and metabolic acidosis. A mixture of high-gap acidosis and metabolic alkalosis is recognized easily by comparing the differences (Δ values) in the normal to prevailing patient values. In this example, the ΔHCO_3^- is 0 (25 – 25 mmol/L) but the ΔAG is 20 (30 – 10 mmol/L). Therefore, 20 mmol/L is unaccounted for in the Δ/Δ value (ΔAG to ΔHCO_3^-).

METABOLIC ACIDOSIS

Metabolic acidosis can occur because of an increase in endogenous acid production (such as lactate and ketoacids), loss of bicarbonate (as in diarrhea), or accumulation of endogenous acids (as in renal failure). Metabolic acidosis has profound effects on the respiratory, cardiac, and

TABLE 48-4 CAUSES OF HIGH-ANION-GAP METABOLIC ACIDOSIS

Lactic acidosis	Toxins
Ketoacidosis	Ethylene glycol
Diabetic	Methanol
Alcoholic	Salicylates
Starvation	Propylene glycol
	Pyroglutamic acid
	Renal failure (acute and chronic)

nervous systems. The fall in blood pH is accompanied by a characteristic increase in ventilation, especially the tidal volume (Kussmaul respiration). Intrinsic cardiac contractility may be depressed, but inotropic function can be normal because of catecholamine release. Both peripheral arterial vasodilation and central venoconstriction can be present; the decrease in central and pulmonary vascular compliance predisposes to pulmonary edema with even minimal volume overload. Central nervous system function is depressed, with headache, lethargy, stupor, and, in some cases, even coma. Glucose intolerance may also occur.

There are two major categories of clinical metabolic acidosis: high-AG and normal-AG, or hyperchloremic acidosis (Table 48-3 and Table 48-4).

Rx METABOLIC ACIDOSIS

Treatment of metabolic acidosis with alkali should be reserved for severe acidemia except when the patient has no "potential HCO_3^-" in plasma. Potential [HCO_3^-] can be estimated from the increment (Δ) in the AG (ΔAG = patient's AG – 10). It must be determined if the acid anion in plasma is metabolizable (i.e., β-hydroxybutyrate, acetoacetate, and lactate) or nonmetabolizable (anions that accumulate in chronic renal failure and after toxin ingestion). The latter requires return of renal function to replenish the [HCO_3^-] deficit, a slow and often unpredictable process. Consequently, patients with a normal AG acidosis (hyperchloremic acidosis), a slightly elevated AG (mixed hyperchloremic and AG acidosis), or an AG attributable to a nonmetabolizable anion in the face of renal failure should receive alkali therapy, either PO ($NaHCO_3$ or Shohl's solution) or IV ($NaHCO_3$), in an amount necessary to slowly increase the plasma [HCO_3^-] into the 20–22 mmol/L range.

Controversy exists, however, in regard to the use of alkali in patients with a pure AG acidosis owing to accumulation of a metabolizable organic acid anion (ketoacidosis or lactic acidosis). In general, severe acidosis (pH < 7.20) warrants the IV administration of 50–100 meq of $NaHCO_3$, over 30–45 min, during the initial 1–2 h of therapy. Provision of such modest quantities of alkali in this situation seems to provide an added measure of safety, but it is essential to monitor plasma electrolytes during the course of therapy, since the [K^+] may decline as pH rises. The goal is to increase the [HCO_3^-] to 10 meq/L and the pH to 7.15, not to increase these values to normal.

HIGH-ANION-GAP ACIDOSES

APPROACH TO THE PATIENT: High-Anion-Gap Acidoses

There are four principal causes of a high-AG acidosis: (1) lactic acidosis, (2) ketoacidosis, (3) ingested toxins, and (4) acute and chronic renal failure (Table 48-4). Initial screening to differentiate the high-AG acidoses should include (1) a probe of the history for evidence of drug and toxin ingestion and measurement of arterial blood gas to detect coexistent respiratory alkalosis (salicylates); (2) determination of whether diabetes mellitus is present (diabetic ketoacidosis); (3) a search for evidence of alcoholism or increased levels of β-hydroxybutyrate (alcoholic ketoacidosis); (4) observation for clinical signs of uremia and determination of the blood urea nitrogen (BUN) and creatinine (uremic acidosis); (5) inspection of the urine for oxalate crystals (ethylene glycol); and (6) recognition of the numerous clinical settings in which lactate levels may be increased (hypotension, shock, cardiac failure, leukemia, cancer, and drug or toxin ingestion).

Lactic Acidosis An increase in plasma L-lactate may be secondary to poor tissue perfusion (type A)—circulatory insufficiency (shock, cardiac failure), severe anemia, mitochondrial enzyme defects, and inhibitors (carbon monoxide, cyanide)—or to aerobic disorders (type B)—malignancies, nucleoside analogue reverse transcriptase inhibitors in HIV, diabetes mellitus, renal or hepatic failure, thiamine deficiency, severe infections (cholera, malaria), seizures, or drugs/toxins (biguanides, ethanol, methanol, propylene glycol, isoniazid, and fructose). Propylene glycol may be used as a vehicle for IV medications including lorazepam, and toxicity has been reported in several settings. Unrecognized bowel ischemia or infarction in a patient with severe atherosclerosis or cardiac decompensation receiving vasopressors is a common cause of lactic acidosis. Pyroglutamic acidemia has been reported in critically ill patients receiving acetaminophen, which is associated with depletion of glutathione. D-Lactic acid acidosis, which may be associated with jejunoileal bypass, short bowel syndrome, or intestinal obstruction, is due to formation of D-lactate by gut bacteria.

APPROACH TO THE PATIENT: Lactic Acid Acidosis

The underlying condition that disrupts lactate metabolism must first be corrected; tissue perfusion must be restored when inadequate. Vasoconstrictors should be avoided, if possible, since they may worsen tissue perfusion. Alkali therapy is generally advocated for acute, severe acidemia (pH < 7.15) to improve cardiac function and lactate utilization. However, $NaHCO_3$ therapy may paradoxically depress cardiac performance and exacerbate acidosis by enhancing lactate production (HCO_3^- stimulates phosphofructokinase). While the use of alkali in moderate lactic acidosis is controversial, it is generally agreed that attempts to return the pH or [HCO_3^-] to normal by administration of exogenous $NaHCO_3$ are deleterious. A reasonable approach is to infuse sufficient $NaHCO_3$ to raise the arterial pH to no more than 7.2 over 30–40 min.

$NaHCO_3$ therapy can cause fluid overload and hypertension because the amount required can be massive when accumulation of lactic acid is relentless. Fluid administration is poorly tolerated because of central venoconstriction, especially in the oliguric patient. When the underlying cause of the lactic acidosis can be remedied, blood lactate will be converted to HCO_3^- and may result in an overshoot alkalosis.

Ketoacidosis • ***DIABETIC KETOACIDOSIS (DKA)*** This condition is caused by increased fatty acid metabolism and the accumulation of ketoacids (acetoacetate and β-hydroxybutyrate). DKA usually occurs in insulin-dependent diabetes mellitus in association with cessation of insulin or an intercurrent illness, such as an infection, gastroenteritis, pancreatitis, or myocardial infarction, which increases insulin requirements temporarily and acutely. The accumulation of ketoacids accounts for the increment in the AG and is accompanied most often by hyperglycemia [glucose > 17 mmol/L (300 mg/dL)]. The relationship between the ΔAG and ΔHCO_3^- is ~1:1 in DKA but may decrease in the well-hydrated patient with preservation of renal function. Ketoacid excretion in the urine reduces the anion gap in this situation. It should be noted that since insulin prevents production of ketones, bicarbonate therapy is rarely needed except with extreme acidemia (pH < 7.1), and then in only limited amounts. Patients with DKA are typically volume depleted and require fluid resuscitation with isotonic saline. Volume overexpansion is not uncommon, however, after IV fluid administration, and contributes to the development of a hyperchloremic acidosis during treatment of DKA because volume expansion increases urinary ketoacid anion excretion (loss of potential bicarbonate). The mainstay for treatment of this condition is IV regular insulin and is described in Chap. 338 in more detail.

ALCOHOLIC KETOACIDOSIS (AKA) Chronic alcoholics can develop ketoacidosis when alcohol consumption is abruptly curtailed and nutrition is poor. AKA is usually associated with binge drinking, vomiting, abdominal pain, starvation, and volume depletion. The glucose concentration is variable, and acidosis may be severe because of elevated ketones, predominantly β-hydroxybutyrate. Hypoperfusion may enhance lactic acid production, chronic respiratory alkalosis may accompany liver disease, and metabolic alkalosis can result from vomiting (refer to the relationship between ΔAG and ΔHCO_3^-). Thus, mixed acid-base disorders are common in AKA. As the circulation is restored by administration of isotonic saline, the preferential accumulation of β-hydroxybutyrate is then shifted to acetoacetate. This explains the common clinical observation of an increasingly positive nitroprusside reaction as the patient improves. The nitroprusside ketone reaction (Acetest) can detect acetoacetic acid but not β-hydroxybutyrate, so that the degree of ketosis and ketonuria can not only change with therapy, but can be underestimated initially. Patients with AKA usually present with relatively normal renal function, as opposed to DKA where renal function is often compromised because of volume depletion (osmotic diuresis) or diabetic nephropathy. The AKA patient with normal renal function may excrete relatively large quantities of ketoacids in the urine, therefore, and may have a relatively normal AG and a discrepancy in the $\Delta AG/\Delta HCO_3^-$ relationship. Typically, insulin levels are low, and concentrations of triglyceride, cortisol, glucagon, and growth hormone are increased.

Rx ALCOHOLIC KETOACIDOSIS

Extracellular fluid deficits almost always accompany AKA and should be repleted by IV administration of saline and glucose (5% dextrose in 0.9% NaCl). Hypophosphatemia, hypokalemia, and hypomagnesemia may coexist and should be corrected. Hypophosphatemia usually emerges 12–24 h after admission, may be exacerbated by glucose infusion, and, if severe, may induce rhabdomyolysis. Upper gastrointestinal hemorrhage, pancreatitis, and pneumonia may accompany this disorder.

Drug- and Toxin-Induced Acidosis • ***SALICYLATES*** (See also **Chap. e34**) Salicylate intoxication in adults usually causes respiratory alkalosis or a mixture of high-AG metabolic acidosis and respiratory alkalosis. Only a portion of the AG is due to salicylates. Lactic acid production is also often increased.

Rx SALICYLATE-INDUCED ACIDOSIS

Vigorous gastric lavage with isotonic saline (not $NaHCO_3$) should be initiated immediately followed by administration of activated charcoal per NG tube. In the acidotic patient, to facilitate removal of salicylate, intravenous $NaHCO_3$ is administered in amounts adequate to alkalinize the urine and to maintain urine output (urine pH > 7.5). While this form of therapy is straightforward in acidotic patients, a coexisting respiratory alkalosis may make this approach hazardous. Alkalemic patients should not receive $NaHCO_3^-$. Acetazolamide may be administered in the face of alkalemia, when an alkaline diuresis cannot be achieved, or to ameliorate volume overload associated with $NaHCO_3^-$ administration, but this drug can cause systemic metabolic acidosis if HCO_3^- is not replaced. Hypokalemia should be anticipated with an alkaline diuresis and should be treated promptly and aggressively. Glucose-containing fluids should be administered because of the danger of hypoglycemia. Excessive insensible fluid losses may cause severe volume depletion and hypernatremia. If renal failure prevents rapid clearance of salicylate, hemodialysis can be performed against a bicarbonate dialysate.

ALCOHOLS Under most physiologic conditions, sodium, urea, and glucose generate the osmotic pressure of blood. Plasma osmolality is calculated according to the following expression: $P_{osm} = 2Na^+ + Glu + BUN$ (all in mmol/L), or, using conventional laboratory values in which glucose and BUN are expressed in milligrams per deciliter: $P_{osm} = 2Na^+ + Glu/18 + BUN/2.8$. The calculated and determined osmolality should agree within 10–15 mmol/kg H_2O. When the measured osmolality exceeds the calculated osmolality by >15–20 mmol/kg H_2O, one of two circumstances prevails. Either the serum sodium is spuriously low, as with hyperlipidemia or hyperproteinemia (pseudohyponatremia), or osmolytes other than sodium salts, glucose, or urea have accumulated in plasma. Examples include mannitol, radiocontrast media, isopropyl alcohol, ethylene glycol, propylene glycol, ethanol, methanol, and acetone. In this situation, the difference between the calculated osmolality and the measured osmolality (*osmolar gap*) is proportional to the concentration of the unmeasured solute. With an appropriate clinical history and index of suspicion, identification of an osmolar gap is helpful in identifying the presence of poison-associated AG acidosis. Three alcohols may cause fatal intoxications: ethylene glycol, methanol, and isopropyl alcohol. All cause an elevated osmolal gap, but only the first two cause a high-AG acidosis.

ETHYLENE GLYCOL (See also **Chap. e34**) Ingestion of ethylene glycol (commonly used in antifreeze) leads to a metabolic acidosis and severe damage to the central nervous system, heart, lungs, and kidneys. The increased AG and osmolar gap are attributable to ethylene glycol and its metabolites, oxalic acid, glycolic acid, and other organic acids. Lactic acid production increases secondary to inhibition of the tricarboxylic acid cycle and altered intracellular redox state. Diagnosis is facilitated by recognizing oxalate crystals in the urine, the presence of an osmolar gap in serum, and a high-AG acidosis. If antifreeze containing a fluorescent dye is ingested, a Wood's lamp applied to the urine may be revealing. Treatment should not be delayed while awaiting measurement of ethylene glycol levels in this setting.

Rx ETHYLENE GLYCOL–INDUCED ACIDOSIS

This includes the prompt institution of a saline or osmotic diuresis, thiamine and pyridoxine supplements, fomepizole or ethanol, and hemodialysis. The IV administration of the alcohol dehydrogenase inhibitor fomepizole (4-methylpyrazole; 7 mg/kg as a loading dose) or ethanol IV to achieve a level of 22 mmol/L (100 mg/dL) serves to lessen toxicity because they compete with ethylene glycol for metabolism by alcohol dehydrogenase. Fomepizole, although expensive, offers the advantages of a predictable decline in ethylene glycol levels without excessive obtundation during ethyl alcohol infusion.

METHANOL (See also **Chap. e34**) The ingestion of methanol (wood alcohol) causes metabolic acidosis, and its metabolites formaldehyde and formic acid cause severe optic nerve and central nervous system damage. Lactic acid, ketoacids, and other unidentified organic acids may contribute to the acidosis. Due to its low molecular weight (32 Da), an osmolar gap is usually present.

Rx METHANOL-INDUCED ACIDOSIS

This is similar to that for ethylene glycol intoxication, including general supportive measures, fomepizole or ethanol administration, and hemodialysis.

ISOPROPYL ALCOHOL Ingested isopropanol is absorbed rapidly and may be fatal when as little as 150 mL of rubbing alcohol, solvent, or de-icer is consumed. A plasma level >400 mg/dL is life threatening. Isopropyl alcohol differs from ethylene glycol and methanol in that the parent compound, not the metabolites, causes toxicity, and acidosis is not present because acetone is rapidly excreted.

Rx ISOPROPYL ALCOHOL TOXICITY

Isopropanol alcohol toxicity is treated by watchful waiting and supportive therapy; IV fluids, pressors, ventilatory support if needed, and occasionally hemodialysis for prolonged coma or levels >400 mg/dL.

Renal Failure (See also Chaps. 273 and 274) The hyperchloremic acidosis of moderate renal insufficiency is eventually converted to the high-AG acidosis of advanced renal failure. Poor filtration and reabsorption of organic anions contribute to the pathogenesis. As renal disease progresses, the number of functioning nephrons eventually becomes insufficient to keep pace with net acid production. Uremic acidosis is characterized, therefore, by a reduced rate of NH_4^+ production and excretion, primarily due to decreased renal mass. [HCO_3^-] rarely falls to <15 mmol/L, and the AG is rarely >20 mmol/L. The acid retained in chronic renal disease is buffered by alkaline salts from bone. Despite significant retention of acid (up to 20 mmol/d), the serum [HCO_3^-] does not decrease further, indicating participation of buffers

TABLE 48-5 CAUSES OF NON-ANION-GAP ACIDOSIS

I. Gastrointestinal bicarbonate loss
  A. Diarrhea
  B. External pancreatic or small-bowel drainage
  C. Ureterosigmoidostomy, jejunal loop, ileal loop
  D. Drugs
    1. Calcium chloride (acidifying agent)
    2. Magnesium sulfate (diarrhea)
    3. Cholestyramine (bile acid diarrhea)
II. Renal acidosis
  A. Hypokalemia
    1. Proximal RTA (type 2)
    2. Distal (classic) RTA (type 1)
  B. Hyperkalemia
    1. Generalized distal nephron dysfunction (type 4 RTA)
      a. Mineralocorticoid deficiency
      b. Mineralocorticoid resistance (autosomal dominant PHA I)
      c. Voltage defect (autosomal dominant PHA I and PHA II)
      d. Tubulointerstitial disease
III. Drug-induced hyperkalemia (with renal insufficiency)
  A. Potassium-sparing diuretics (amiloride, triamterene, spironolactone)
  B. Trimethoprim
  C. Pentamidine
  D. ACE-Is and ARBs
  E. Nonsteroidal anti-inflammatory drugs
  F. Cyclosporine and tacrolimus
IV. Other
  A. Acid loads (ammonium chloride, hyperalimentation)
  B. Loss of potential bicarbonate: ketosis with ketone excretion
  C. Expansion acidosis (rapid saline administration)
  D. Hippurate
  E. Cation exchange resins

Note: RTA, renal tubular acidosis; ACE-I, angiotensin-converting enzyme inhibitors; ARB, angiotensin receptor blocker; PHA, pseudohypoaldosteronism.

outside the extracellular compartment. Chronic metabolic acidosis results in significant loss of bone mass due to reduction in bone calcium carbonate. Chronic acidosis also increases urinary calcium excretion, proportional to cumulative acid retention.

℞ RENAL FAILURE

Because of the association of renal failure acidosis with muscle catabolism and bone disease, both uremic acidosis and the hyperchloremic acidosis of renal failure require oral alkali replacement to maintain the [HCO_3^-] between 20 and 24 mmol/L. This can be accomplished with relatively modest amounts of alkali (1.0–1.5 mmol/kg body weight per day). Sodium citrate (Shohl's solution) or $NaHCO_3$ tablets (650-mg tablets contain 7.8 meq) are equally effective alkalinizing salts. Citrate enhances the absorption of aluminum from the gastrointestinal tract and should never be given together with aluminum-containing antacids because of the risk of aluminum intoxication. When hyperkalemia is present, furosemide (60–80 mg/d) should be added.

HYPERCHLOREMIC (NONGAP) METABOLIC ACIDOSES

Alkali can be lost from the gastrointestinal tract in diarrhea or from the kidneys (renal tubular acidosis, RTA). In these disorders (Table 48-5), reciprocal changes in [Cl^-] and [HCO_3^-] result in a normal AG. In pure hyperchloremic acidosis, therefore, the increase in [Cl^-] above the normal value approximates the decrease in [HCO_3^-]. The absence of such a relationship suggests a mixed disturbance.

APPROACH TO THE PATIENT: Hyperchloremic Metabolic Acidoses

In diarrhea, stools contain a higher [HCO_3^-] and decomposed HCO_3^- than plasma so that metabolic acidosis develops along with volume depletion. Instead of an acid urine pH (as anticipated with systemic acidosis), urine pH is usually around 6 because metabolic acidosis and hypokalemia increase renal synthesis and excretion of NH_4^+, thus providing a urinary buffer that increases urine pH. Metabolic acidosis due to gastrointestinal losses with a high urine pH can be differentiated from RTA (Chap. 278) because urinary NH_4^+ excretion is typically low in RTA and high with diarrhea. Urinary NH_4^+ levels can be estimated by calculating the urine anion gap (UAG): UAG = $[Na^+ + K^+]_u - [Cl^-]_u$. When $[Cl^-]_u > [Na^+ + K^+]$, the urine gap is negative by definition. This indicates that the urine ammonium level is appropriately increased, suggesting an extrarenal cause of the acidosis. Conversely, when the urine anion gap is positive, the urine ammonium level is low, suggesting a renal cause of the acidosis.

Loss of functioning renal parenchyma by progressive renal disease leads to hyperchloremic acidosis when the glomerular filtration rate (GFR) is between 20 and 50 mL/min and to uremic acidosis with a high AG when the GFR falls to <20 mL/min. Such a progression occurs commonly with tubulointerstitial forms of renal disease, but hyperchloremic metabolic acidosis can persist with advanced glomerular disease. In advanced renal failure, ammoniagenesis is reduced in proportion to the loss of functional renal mass, and ammonium accumulation and trapping in the outer medullary collecting tubule may also be impaired. Because of adaptive increases in K^+ secretion by the collecting duct and colon, the acidosis of chronic renal insufficiency is typically normokalemic.

Proximal RTA (type 2 RTA) (Chap. 278) is most often due to generalized proximal tubular dysfunction manifested by glycosuria, generalized aminoaciduria, and phosphaturia (Fanconi syndrome). With a low plasma [HCO_3^-], the urine pH is acid (pH < 5.5). The fractional excretion of [HCO_3^-] may exceed 10–15% when the serum HCO_3^- > 20 mmol/L. Since HCO_3^- is not reabsorbed normally in the proximal tubule, therapy with $NaHCO_3$ will enhance renal potassium wasting and hypokalemia.

The typical findings in acquired or inherited forms of classic distal RTA (type 1 RTA) include hypokalemia, hyperchloremic acidosis, low urinary NH_4^+ excretion (positive UAG, low urine [NH_4^+]), and inappropriately high urine pH (pH > 5.5). Such patients are unable to acidify the urine below a pH of 5.5. Most patients have hypocitraturia and hypercalciuria, so nephrolithiasis, nephrocalcinosis, and bone disease are common. In generalized distal nephron dysfunction (type 4 RTA), hyperkalemia is disproportionate to the reduction in GFR because of coexisting dysfunction of potassium and acid secretion. Urinary ammonium excretion is invariably depressed, and renal function may be compromised, for example, due to diabetic nephropathy, amyloidosis, or tubulointerstitial disease.

Hyporeninemic hypoaldosteronism typically causes hyperchloremic metabolic acidosis, most commonly in older adults with diabetes mellitus or tubulointerstitial disease and renal insufficiency. Patients usually have mild to moderate renal insufficiency (GRF, 20–50 mL/min) and acidosis, with elevation in serum [K^+] (5.2–6.0 mmol/L), concurrent hypertension, and congestive heart failure. Both the metabolic acidosis and the hyperkalemia are out of proportion to impairment in GFR. Nonsteroidal anti-inflammatory drugs, trimethoprim, pentamidine, and angiotensin-converting enzyme (ACE) inhibitors can also cause hyperkalemia with hyperchloremic metabolic acidosis in patients with renal insufficiency (Table 48-5). **See Chap. 278 for the pathophysiology, diagnosis, and treatment of RTA.**

METABOLIC ALKALOSIS

Metabolic alkalosis is manifested by an elevated arterial pH, an increase in the serum [HCO_3^-], and an increase in Pa_{CO_2} as a result of compensatory alveolar hypoventilation (Table 48-1). It is often accompanied by hypochloremia and hypokalemia. The arterial pH establishes the diagnosis, since it is increased in metabolic alkalosis and decreased or normal in respiratory acidosis. Metabolic alkalosis frequently occurs in association with other disorders such as respiratory acidosis or alkalosis or metabolic acidosis.

PATHOGENESIS

Metabolic alkalosis occurs as a result of net gain of [HCO_3^-] or loss of nonvolatile acid (usually HCl by vomiting) from the extracellular fluid. Since it is unusual for alkali to be added to the body, the disorder involves a generative stage, in which the loss of acid usually causes alkalosis, and a maintenance stage, in which the kidneys fail to compensate by excreting HCO_3^-.

Under normal circumstances, the kidneys have an impressive capacity to excrete HCO_3^-. Continuation of metabolic alkalosis represents a failure of the kidneys to eliminate HCO_3^- in the usual manner. For HCO_3^- to be added to the extracellular fluid, it must be administered exogenously or synthesized endogenously, in part or entirely by the kidneys. The kidneys will retain, rather than excrete, the excess alkali and maintain the alkalosis if (1) volume deficiency, chloride deficiency, and K^+ deficiency exist in combination with a reduced GFR, which augments distal tubule H^+ secretion; or (2) hypokalemia exists because of autonomous hyperaldosteronism. In the first example, alkalosis is corrected by administration of NaCl and KCl, whereas in the latter it is necessary to repair the alkalosis by pharmacologic or surgical intervention, not with saline administration.

DIFFERENTIAL DIAGNOSIS

To establish the cause of metabolic alkalosis (Table 48-6), it is necessary to assess the status of the extracellular fluid volume (ECFV), the recumbent and upright blood pressure, the serum [K^+], and the renin-aldosterone system. For example, the presence of chronic hypertension and chronic hypokalemia in an alkalotic patient suggests either mineralocorticoid excess or that the hypertensive patient is receiving diuretics. Low plasma renin activity and normal urine [Na^+] and [Cl^-] in a patient who is not taking diuretics indicate a primary mineralocorticoid excess syndrome. The combination of hypokalemia and alkalosis in a normotensive, nonedematous patient can be due to Bartter's or Gitelman's syndrome, magnesium deficiency, vomiting, exogenous alkali, or diuretic ingestion. Determination of urine electrolytes (especially the urine [Cl^-]) and screening of the urine for diuretics may be helpful. If the urine is alkaline, with an elevated [Na^+] and [K^+] but low [Cl^-], the diagnosis is usually either vomiting (overt or surreptitious) or alkali ingestion. If the urine is relatively acid and has low concentrations of Na^+, K^+, and Cl^-, the most likely possibilities are prior vomiting, the posthypercapnic state, or prior diuretic ingestion. If, on the other hand, neither the urine sodium, potassium, nor chloride concentrations are depressed, magnesium deficiency, Bartter's or Gitelman's syndrome, or current diuretic ingestion should be considered. Bartter's syndrome is distinguished from Gitelman's syndrome because of hypocalciuria and hypomagnesemia in the latter disorder. The genetic and molecular basis of these two disorders has been elucidated recently (Chap. 278).

TABLE 48-6 CAUSES OF METABOLIC ALKALOSIS

I. Exogenous HCO_3^- loads
  A. Acute alkali administration
  B. Milk-alkali syndrome
II. Effective ECFV contraction, normotension, K^+ deficiency, and secondary hyperreninemic hyperaldosteronism
  A. Gastrointestinal origin
    1. Vomiting
    2. Gastric aspiration
    3. Congenital chloridorrhea
    4. Villous adenoma
  B. Renal origin
    1. Diuretics
    2. Posthypercapnic state
    3. Hypercalcemia/hypoparathyroidism
    4. Recovery from lactic acidosis or ketoacidosis
    5. Nonreabsorbable anions including penicillin, carbenicillin
    6. Mg^{2+} deficiency
    7. K^+ depletion
    8. Bartter's syndrome (loss of function mutations in TALH)
    9. Gitelman's syndrome (loss of function mutation in Na^+-Cl^- cotransporter in DCT)
III. ECFV expansion, hypertension, K^+ deficiency, and mineralocorticoid excess
  A. High renin
    1. Renal artery stenosis
    2. Accelerated hypertension
    3. Renin-secreting tumor
    4. Estrogen therapy
  B. Low renin
    1. Primary aldosteronism
      a. Adenoma
      b. Hyperplasia
      c. Carcinoma
    2. Adrenal enzyme defects
      a. 11 β-Hydroxylase deficiency
      b. 17 α-Hydroxylase deficiency
    3. Cushing's syndrome or disease
    4. Other
      a. Licorice
      b. Carbenoxolone
      c. Chewer's tobacco
IV. Gain-of-function mutation of renal sodium channel with ECFV expansion, hypertension, K^+ deficiency, and hyporeninemic-hypoaldosteronism
  A. Liddle's syndrome

Note: ECFV, extracellular fluid volume; TALH, thick ascending limb of Henle's loop; DCT, distal convoluted tubule.

Alkali Administration Chronic administration of alkali to individuals with normal renal function rarely, if ever, causes alkalosis. However, in patients with coexistent hemodynamic disturbances, alkalosis can develop because the normal capacity to excrete HCO_3^- may be exceeded or there may be enhanced reabsorption of HCO_3^-. Such patients include those who receive HCO_3^- (PO or IV), acetate loads (parenteral hyperalimentation solutions), citrate loads (transfusions), or antacids plus cation-exchange resins (aluminum hydroxide and sodium polystyrene sulfonate).

METABOLIC ALKALOSIS ASSOCIATED WITH ECFV CONTRACTION, K^+ DEPLETION, AND SECONDARY HYPERRENINEMIC HYPERALDOSTERONISM

Gastrointestinal Origin Gastrointestinal loss of H^+ from vomiting or gastric aspiration results in retention of HCO_3^-. The loss of fluid and NaCl in vomitus or nasogastric suction results in contraction of the ECFV and an increase in the secretion of renin and aldosterone. Volume contraction through a reduction in GFR results in an enhanced capacity of the renal tubule to reabsorb HCO_3^-. During active vomiting, however, the filtered load of bicarbonate is acutely increased to the point that the reabsorptive capacity of the proximal tubule for HCO_3^- is exceeded. The excess $NaHCO_3$ issuing out of the proximal tubule reaches the distal tubule, where H^+ secretion is enhanced by an aldosterone and the delivery of the poorly reabsorbed anion, HCO_3^-. Correction of the contracted ECFV with NaCl and repair of K^+ deficits corrects the acid-base disorder, and chloride deficiency.

Renal Origin • ***DIURETICS*** (See also Chap. 227) Drugs that induce chloruresis, such as thiazides and loop diuretics (furosemide, bumetanide, torsemide, and ethacrynic acid), acutely diminish the ECFV without altering the total body bicarbonate content. The serum [HCO_3^-] increases because the reduced ECFV "contracts" the [HCO_3^-] in the plasma (contraction alkalosis). The chronic administration of diuretics tends to generate an alkalosis by increasing distal salt delivery, so that K^+ and H^+ secretion are stimulated. The alkalosis is maintained by persistence of the contraction of the ECFV, secondary hyperaldosteronism, K^+ deficiency, and the direct effect of the diuretic (as long as diuretic administration continues). Repair of the alkalosis is achieved by providing isotonic saline to correct the ECFV deficit.

SOLUTE LOSING DISORDERS: BARTTER'S SYNDROME AND GITELMAN'S SYNDROME See Chap. 278.

NONREABSORBABLE ANIONS AND MAGNESIUM DEFICIENCY Administration of large quantities of nonreabsorbable anions, such as penicillin or carbenicillin, can enhance distal acidification and K^+ secretion by increasing the transepithelial potential difference (lumen negative). Mg^{2+} deficiency results in hypokalemic alkalosis by enhancing distal acidification through stimulation of renin and hence aldosterone secretion.

POTASSIUM DEPLETION Chronic K^+ depletion may cause metabolic alkalosis by increasing urinary acid excretion. Both NH_4^+ production and absorption are enhanced and HCO_3^- reabsorption is stimulated.

Chronic K^+ deficiency upregulates the renal H^+, K^+-ATPase to increase K^+ absorption at the expense of enhanced H^+ secretion. Alkalosis associated with severe K^+ depletion is resistant to salt administration, but repair of the K^+ deficiency corrects the alkalosis.

AFTER TREATMENT OF LACTIC ACIDOSIS OR KETOACIDOSIS When an underlying stimulus for the generation of lactic acid or ketoacid is removed rapidly, as with repair of circulatory insufficiency or with insulin therapy, the lactate or ketones are metabolized to yield an equivalent amount of HCO_3^-. Other sources of new HCO_3^- are additive with the original amount generated by organic anion metabolism to create a surfeit of HCO_3^-. Such sources include (1) new HCO_3^- added to the blood by the kidneys as a result of enhanced acid excretion during the preexisting period of acidosis, and (2) alkali therapy during the treatment phase of the acidosis. Acidosis-induced contraction of the ECFV and K^+ deficiency act to sustain the alkalosis.

POSTHYPERCAPNIA Prolonged CO_2 retention with chronic respiratory acidosis enhances renal HCO_3^- absorption and the generation of new HCO_3^- (increased net acid excretion). If the Pa_{CO_2} is returned to normal, metabolic alkalosis results from the persistently elevated $[HCO_3^-]$. Alkalosis develops if the elevated Pa_{CO_2} is abruptly returned toward normal by a change in mechanically controlled ventilation. Associated ECFV contraction does not allow complete repair of the alkalosis by correction of the Pa_{CO_2} alone, and alkalosis persists until Cl^- supplementation is provided.

METABOLIC ALKALOSIS ASSOCIATED WITH ECFV EXPANSION, HYPERTENSION, AND HYPERALDOSTERONISM
Increased aldosterone levels may be the result of autonomous primary adrenal overproduction or of secondary aldosterone release due to renal overproduction of renin. Mineralocorticoid excess increases net acid excretion and may result in metabolic alkalosis, which may be worsened by associated K^+ deficiency. ECFV expansion from salt retention causes hypertension. The kaliuresis persists because of mineralocorticoid excess and distal Na^+ absorption causing enhanced K^+ excretion, continued K^+ depletion with polydipsia, inability to concentrate the urine, and polyuria.

Liddle's syndrome (Chap. 278) results from increased activity of the collecting duct Na^+ channel (ENaC) and is a rare inherited disorder associated with hypertension due to volume expansion manifested as hypokalemic alkalosis and normal aldosterone levels.

Symptoms With metabolic alkalosis, changes in central and peripheral nervous system function are similar to those of hypocalcemia (Chap. 346); symptoms include mental confusion, obtundation, and a predisposition to seizures, paresthesia, muscular cramping, tetany, aggravation of arrhythmias, and hypoxemia in chronic obstructive pulmonary disease. Related electrolyte abnormalities include hypokalemia and hypophosphatemia.

Rx METABOLIC ALKALOSIS

This is primarily directed at correcting the underlying stimulus for HCO_3^- generation. If primary aldosteronism, renal artery stenosis, or Cushing's syndrome is present, correction of the underlying cause will reverse the alkalosis. $[H^+]$ loss by the stomach or kidneys can be mitigated by the use of proton pump inhibitors or the discontinuation of diuretics. The second aspect of treatment is to remove the factors that sustain the inappropriate increase in HCO_3^- reabsorption, such as ECFV contraction or K^+ deficiency. Although K^+ deficits should be repaired, NaCl therapy is usually sufficient to reverse the alkalosis if ECFV contraction is present, as indicated by a low urine $[Cl^-]$.

If associated conditions preclude infusion of saline, renal HCO_3^- loss can be accelerated by administration of acetazolamide, a carbonic anhydrase inhibitor, which is usually effective in patients with adequate renal function but can worsen K^+ losses. Dilute hydrochloric acid (0.1 *N* HCl) is also effective but can cause hemolysis, and must be delivered centrally and slowly. Hemodialysis against a dialysate low in $[HCO_3^-]$ and high in $[Cl^-]$ can be effective when renal function is impaired.

TABLE 48-7 RESPIRATORY ACID-BASE DISORDERS

I. Alkalosis	II. Acidosis
A. Central nervous system stimulation	A. Central
1. Pain	1. Drugs (anesthetics, morphine, sedatives)
2. Anxiety, psychosis	2. Stroke
3. Fever	3. Infection
4. Cerebrovascular accident	B. Airway
5. Meningitis, encephalitis	1. Obstruction
6. Tumor	2. Asthma
7. Trauma	C. Parenchyma
B. Hypoxemia or tissue hypoxia	1. Emphysema
1. High altitude, ↓Pa_{CO_2}	2. Pneumoconiosis
2. Pneumonia, pulmonary edema	3. Bronchitis
3. Aspiration	4. Adult respiratory distress syndrome
4. Severe anemia	5. Barotrauma
C. Drugs or hormones	D. Neuromuscular
1. Pregnancy, progesterone	1. Poliomyelitis
2. Salicylates	2. Kyphoscoliosis
3. Cardiac failure	3. Myasthenia
D. Stimulation of chest receptors	4. Muscular dystrophies
1. Hemothorax	E. Miscellaneous
2. Flail chest	1. Obesity
3. Cardiac failure	2. Hypoventilation
4. Pulmonary embolism	3. Permissive hypercapnia
E. Miscellaneous	
1. Septicemia	
2. Hepatic failure	
3. Mechanical hyperventilation	
4. Heat exposure	
5. Recovery from metabolic acidosis	

RESPIRATORY ACIDOSIS

Respiratory acidosis can be due to severe pulmonary disease, respiratory muscle fatigue, or abnormalities in ventilatory control and is recognized by an increase in Pa_{CO_2} and decrease in pH (Table 48-7). In acute respiratory acidosis, there is an immediate compensatory elevation (due to cellular buffering mechanisms) in HCO_3^-, which increases 1 mmol/L for every 10-mmHg increase in Pa_{CO_2}. In chronic respiratory acidosis (>24 h), renal adaptation increases the $[HCO_3^-]$ by 4 mmol/L for every 10-mmHg increase in Pa_{CO_2}. The serum HCO_3^- usually does not increase above 38 mmol/L.

The clinical features vary according to the severity and duration of the respiratory acidosis, the underlying disease, and whether there is accompanying hypoxemia. A rapid increase in Pa_{CO_2} may cause anxiety, dyspnea, confusion, psychosis, and hallucinations and may progress to coma. Lesser degrees of dysfunction in chronic hypercapnia include sleep disturbances, loss of memory, daytime somnolence, personality changes, impairment of coordination, and motor disturbances such as tremor, myoclonic jerks, and asterixis. Headaches and other signs that mimic raised intracranial pressure, such as papilledema, abnormal reflexes, and focal muscle weakness, are due to vasoconstriction secondary to loss of the vasodilator effects of CO_2.

Depression of the respiratory center by a variety of drugs, injury, or disease can produce respiratory acidosis. This may occur acutely with general anesthetics, sedatives, and head trauma or chronically with sedatives, alcohol, intracranial tumors, and the syndromes of sleep-disordered breathing, including the primary alveolar and obesity-hypoventilation syndromes (Chaps. 258 and 259). Abnormalities or disease in the motor neurons, neuromuscular junction, and skeletal muscle can cause hypoventilation via respiratory muscle fatigue. Mechanical ventilation, when not properly adjusted and supervised, may result in respiratory acidosis, particularly if CO_2 production suddenly rises (because of fever, agitation, sepsis, or overfeeding) or alveolar ventilation falls because of worsening pulmonary function. High levels of positive end-expiratory pressure in the presence of reduced cardiac output may cause hypercapnia as a result of large increases in alveolar dead space (Chap. 246). Permissive hypercapnia is being used with increasing frequency because of studies suggesting lower mortality rates than with conventional mechanical ventilation, especially with severe central nervous system or heart disease. The potential beneficial effects of permissive hypercapnia may be mitigated by correction of the acidemia by administration of $NaHCO_3$.

Acute hypercapnia follows sudden occlusion of the upper airway or generalized bronchospasm as in severe asthma, anaphylaxis, inhalational burn, or toxin injury. Chronic hypercapnia and respiratory acidosis occur in end-stage obstructive lung disease. Restrictive disorders involving both the chest wall and the lungs can cause respiratory acidosis because the high metabolic cost of respiration causes ventilatory muscle fatigue. Advanced stages of intrapulmonary and extrapulmonary restrictive defects present as chronic respiratory acidosis.

The diagnosis of respiratory acidosis requires, by definition, the measurement of Pa_{CO_2} and arterial pH. A detailed history and physical examination often indicate the cause. Pulmonary function studies (Chap. 246), including spirometry, diffusion capacity for carbon monoxide, lung volumes, and arterial Pa_{CO_2} and O_2 saturation, usually make it possible to determine if respiratory acidosis is secondary to lung disease. The workup for nonpulmonary causes should include a detailed drug history, measurement of hematocrit, and assessment of upper airway, chest wall, pleura, and neuromuscular function.

℞ RESPIRATORY ACIDOSIS

The management of respiratory acidosis depends on its severity and rate of onset. Acute respiratory acidosis can be life threatening, and measures to reverse the underlying cause should be undertaken simultaneously with restoration of adequate alveolar ventilation. This may necessitate tracheal intubation and assisted mechanical ventilation. Oxygen administration should be titrated carefully in patients with severe obstructive pulmonary disease and chronic CO_2 retention who are breathing spontaneously (Chap. 254). When oxygen is used injudiciously, these patients may experience progression of the respiratory acidosis. Aggressive and rapid correction of hypercapnia should be avoided, because the falling Pa_{CO_2} may provoke the same complications noted with acute respiratory alkalosis (i.e., cardiac arrhythmias, reduced cerebral perfusion, and seizures). The Pa_{CO_2} should be lowered gradually in chronic respiratory acidosis, aiming to restore the Pa_{CO_2} to baseline levels and to provide sufficient Cl^- and K^+ to enhance the renal excretion of HCO_3^-.

Chronic respiratory acidosis is frequently difficult to correct, but measures aimed at improving lung function (Chap. 254) can help some patients and forestall further deterioration in most.

RESPIRATORY ALKALOSIS

Alveolar hyperventilation decreases Pa_{CO_2} and increases the HCO_3^-/Pa_{CO_2} ratio, thus increasing pH (Table 48-7). Nonbicarbonate cellular buffers respond by consuming HCO_3^-. Hypocapnia develops when a sufficiently strong ventilatory stimulus causes CO_2 output in the lungs to exceed its metabolic production by tissues. Plasma pH and $[HCO_3^-]$ appear to vary proportionately with Pa_{CO_2} over a range from 40–15 mmHg. The relationship between arterial $[H^+]$ concentration and Pa_{CO_2} is ~0.7 mmol/L per mmHg (or 0.01 pH unit/mmHg), and that for plasma $[HCO_3^-]$ is 0.2 mmol/L per mmHg. Hypocapnia sustained for >2–6 h is further compensated by a decrease in renal ammonium and titratable acid excretion and a reduction in filtered HCO_3^- reabsorption. Full renal adaptation to respiratory alkalosis may take several days and requires normal volume status and renal function. The kidneys appear to respond directly to the lowered Pa_{CO_2} rather than to alkalosis per se. In chronic respiratory alkalosis a 1-mmHg fall in Pa_{CO_2} causes a 0.4- to 0.5-mmol/L drop in $[HCO_3^-]$ and a 0.3-mmol/L fall (or 0.003 rise in pH) in $[H^+]$.

The effects of respiratory alkalosis vary according to duration and severity but are primarily those of the underlying disease. Reduced cerebral blood flow as a consequence of a rapid decline in Pa_{CO_2} may cause dizziness, mental confusion, and seizures, even in the absence of hypoxemia. The cardiovascular effects of acute hypocapnia in the conscious human are generally minimal, but in the anesthetized or mechanically ventilated patient, cardiac output and blood pressure may fall because of the depressant effects of anesthesia and positive-pressure ventilation on heart rate, systemic resistance, and venous return. Cardiac arrhythmias may occur in patients with heart disease as a result of changes in oxygen unloading by blood from a left shift in the hemoglobin-oxygen dissociation curve (Bohr effect). Acute respiratory alkalosis causes intracellular shifts of Na^+, K^+, and PO_4^- and reduces free $[Ca^{2+}]$ by increasing the protein-bound fraction. Hypocapnia-induced hypokalemia is usually minor.

Chronic respiratory alkalosis is the most common acid-base disturbance in critically ill patients and, when severe, portends a poor prognosis. Many cardiopulmonary disorders manifest respiratory alkalosis in their early to intermediate stages, and the finding of normocapnia and hypoxemia in a patient with hyperventilation may herald the onset of rapid respiratory failure and should prompt an assessment to determine if the patient is becoming fatigued. Respiratory alkalosis is common during mechanical ventilation.

The hyperventilation syndrome may be disabling. Paresthesia, circumoral numbness, chest wall tightness or pain, dizziness, inability to take an adequate breath, and, rarely, tetany may themselves be sufficiently stressful to perpetuate the disorder. Arterial blood-gas analysis demonstrates an acute or chronic respiratory alkalosis, often with hypocapnia in the range of 15–30 mmHg and no hypoxemia. Central nervous system diseases or injury can produce several patterns of hyperventilation and sustained Pa_{CO_2} levels of 20–30 mmHg. Hyperthyroidism, high caloric loads, and exercise raise the basal metabolic rate, but ventilation usually rises in proportion so that arterial blood gases are unchanged and respiratory alkalosis does not develop. Salicylates are the most common cause of drug-induced respiratory alkalosis as a result of direct stimulation of the medullary chemoreceptor (**Chap. e34**). The methylxanthines, theophylline, and aminophylline stimulate ventilation and increase the ventilatory response to CO_2. Progesterone increases ventilation and lowers arterial Pa_{CO_2} by as much as 5–10 mmHg. Therefore, chronic respiratory alkalosis is a common feature of pregnancy. Respiratory alkalosis is also prominent in liver failure, and the severity correlates with the degree of hepatic insufficiency. Respiratory alkalosis is often an early finding in gram-negative septicemia, before fever, hypoxemia, or hypotension develops.

The diagnosis of respiratory alkalosis depends on measurement of arterial pH and Pa_{CO_2}. The plasma $[K^+]$ is often reduced and the $[Cl^-]$ increased. In the acute phase, respiratory alkalosis is not associated with increased renal HCO_3^- excretion, but within hours net acid excretion is reduced. In general, the HCO_3^- concentration falls by 2.0 mmol/L for each 10-mmHg decrease in Pa_{CO_2}. Chronic hypocapnia reduces the serum $[HCO_3^-]$ by 4.0 mmol/L for each 10-mmHg decrease in Pa_{CO_2}. It is unusual to observe a plasma $HCO_3^- < 12$ mmol/L as a result of a pure respiratory alkalosis.

When a diagnosis of respiratory alkalosis is made, its cause should be investigated. The diagnosis of hyperventilation syndrome is made by exclusion. In difficult cases, it may be important to rule out other conditions such as pulmonary embolism, coronary artery disease, and hyperthyroidism.

℞ RESPIRATORY ALKALOSIS

The management of respiratory alkalosis is directed toward alleviation of the underlying disorder. If respiratory alkalosis complicates ventilator management, changes in dead space, tidal volume, and frequency can minimize the hypocapnia. Patients with the hyperventilation syndrome may benefit from reassurance, rebreathing from a paper bag during symptomatic attacks, and attention to underlying psychological stress. Antidepressants and sedatives are not recommended. β-Adrenergic blockers may ameliorate peripheral manifestations of the hyperadrenergic state.

FURTHER READINGS

DuBose TD Jr: Acid-base disorders, in *Brenner and Rector's The Kidney*, 8th ed, BM Brenner (ed). Philadelphia, Saunders, 2007, in press

———, Alpern RJ: Renal tubular acidosis, in *The Metabolic and Molecular Bases of Inherited Disease*, 8th ed, CR Scriver et al (eds). New York, McGraw-Hill, 2001

Galla JH: Metabolic alkalosis, in *Acid-Base and Electrolyte Disorders—A Companion to Brenner and Rector's The Kidney*, TD DuBose, LL Hamm (eds). Philadelphia, Saunders, 2002, pp 109–128

296 LASKI ME, WESSON DE: Lactic acidosis, in *Acid-Base and Electrolyte Disorders—A Companion to Brenner and Rector's The Kidney*, TD DuBose, LL Hamm (eds). Philadelphia, Saunders, 2002, pp 83–107
MADIAS NE: Respiratory alkalosis, in *Acid-Base and Electrolyte Disorders—A Companion to Brenner and Rector's The Kidney*, TD DuBose, LL Hamm (eds). Philadelphia, Saunders, 2002, pp 147–164
WESSON DE et al: Clinical syndromes of metabolic alkalosis, in *The Kidney: Physiology and Pathophysiology*, 3d ed, DW Seldin, G Giebisch (eds). Philadelphia, Lippincott Williams and Wilkins, 2000, pp 2055–2072

SECTION 8 ALTERATIONS IN SEXUAL FUNCTION AND REPRODUCTION

49 Sexual Dysfunction

Kevin T. McVary

Male sexual dysfunction affects 10–25% of middle-aged and elderly men. Female sexual dysfunction occurs with a similar frequency. Demographic changes, the popularity of newer treatments, and greater awareness of sexual dysfunction by patients and society have led to increased diagnosis and associated health care expenditures for the management of this common disorder. Because many patients are reluctant to initiate discussion of their sex lives, the physician should address this topic directly to elicit a history of sexual dysfunction.

MALE SEXUAL DYSFUNCTION

PHYSIOLOGY OF MALE SEXUAL RESPONSE

Normal male sexual function requires (1) an intact libido, (2) the ability to achieve and maintain penile erection, (3) ejaculation, and (4) detumescence. *Libido* refers to sexual desire and is influenced by a variety of visual, olfactory, tactile, auditory, imaginative, and hormonal stimuli. Sex steroids, particularly testosterone, act to increase libido. Libido can be diminished by hormonal or psychiatric disorders or by medications.

Penile tumescence leading to erection depends on the increased flow of blood into the lacunar network accompanied by the complete relaxation of the arteries and corporal smooth muscle. The microarchitecture of the corpora is composed of a mass of smooth muscle (trabecula) which contains a network of endothelial-lined vessels (lacunar spaces). Subsequent compression of the trabecular smooth muscle against the fibroelastic tunica albuginea causes a passive closure of the emissary veins and accumulation of blood in the corpora. In the presence of a full erection and a competent valve mechanism, the corpora become noncompressible cylinders from which blood does not escape.

The central nervous system (CNS) exerts an important influence by either stimulating or antagonizing spinal pathways that mediate erectile function and ejaculation. The erectile response is mediated by a combination of central (psychogenic) and peripheral (reflexogenic) innervation. Sensory nerves that originate from receptors in the penile skin and glans converge to form the dorsal nerve of the penis, which travels to the S2-S4 dorsal root ganglia via the pudendal nerve. Parasympathetic nerve fibers to the penis arise from neurons in the intermediolateral columns of S2-S4 sacral spinal segments. Sympathetic innervation originates from the T-11 to the L-2 spinal segments and descends through the hypogastric plexus.

Neural input to smooth-muscle tone is crucial to the initiation and maintenance of an erection. There is also an intricate interaction between the corporal smooth muscle cell and its overlying endothelial cell lining (Fig. 49-1*A*). Nitric oxide, which induces vascular relaxation, promotes erection and is opposed by endothelin-1 (ET-1) and Rho kinase, which mediate vascular contraction. Nitric oxide is synthesized from L-arginine by nitric oxide synthase and is released from the nonadrenergic, noncholinergic (NANC) autonomic nerve supply to act postjunctionally on smooth-muscle cells. Nitric oxide increases the production of cyclic 3′,5′-guanosine monophosphate (cyclic GMP), which induces relaxation of the smooth muscle (Fig. 49-1*B*). Cyclic GMP is gradually broken down by phosphodiesterase type 5 (PDE-5). Inhibitors of PDE-5, such as the oral medications sildenafil, vardenifil, and tadalafil maintain erections by reducing the breakdown of cyclic GMP. However, if nitric oxide is not produced at some level, PDE-5 inhibitors are ineffective, as these drugs facilitate, but do not initiate, the initial enzyme cascade. In addition to nitric oxide, vasoactive prostaglandins (PGE_1, $PGF_{2\alpha}$) are synthesized within the cavernosal tissue and increase cyclic AMP levels, also leading to relaxation of cavernosal smooth-muscle cells.

Ejaculation is stimulated by the sympathetic nervous system, which results in contraction of the epididymis, vas deferens, seminal vesicles,

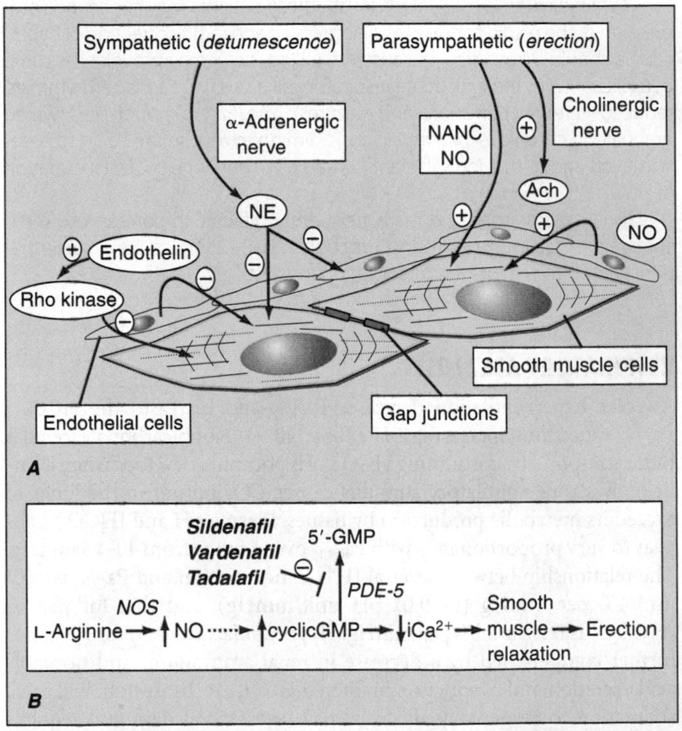

FIGURE 49-1 Pathways that control erection and detumescence. ***A.*** Erection is mediated by cholinergic parasympathetic pathways, and nonadrenergic, noncholinergic (NANC) pathways, which release nitric oxide (NO). Endothelial cells also release NO, which induces vascular smooth-muscle cell relaxation, allowing enhanced blood flow, and leading to erection. Detumescence is mediated by sympathetic pathways that release norepinephrine and stimulate α-adrenergic pathways, leading to contraction of vascular smooth-muscle cells. Endothelin, released from endothelial cells, also induces contraction. Rho kinase activation via endothelin activity (among others) also contributes to detumescence by alteration of calcium signaling. ***B.*** Biochemical pathways of NO synthesis and action. Sildenafil, vardenafil, and tadalafil enhance erectile function by inhibiting phosphodiesterase type 5 (PDE-5), thereby maintaining high levels of cyclic 3′,5′-guanosine monophosphate (cyclic GMP). NOS, nitric oxide synthase; iCa^{2+}, intracellular calcium.

and prostate, causing seminal fluid to enter the urethra. Seminal fluid emission is followed by rhythmic contractions of the bulbocavernosus and ischiocavernosus muscles, leading to ejaculation. *Premature ejaculation* is usually related to anxiety or a learned behavior and is amenable to behavioral therapy or treatment with medications such as selective serotonin reuptake inhibitors (SSRIs). *Retrograde ejaculation* results when the internal urethral sphincter does not close; it may occur in men with diabetes or after surgery involving the bladder neck.

Detumescence is mediated by norepinephrine from the sympathetic nerves, endothelin from the vascular surface, and smooth-muscle contraction induced by postsynaptic α-adrenergic receptors and activation of Rho kinase. These events increase venous outflow and restore the flaccid state. Venous leak can cause premature detumescence and is caused by insufficient relaxation of the corporal smooth muscle rather than a specific anatomic defect. *Priapism* refers to a persistent and painful erection and may be associated with sickle cell anemia, hypercoagulable states, spinal cord injury, or injection of vasodilator agents into the penis.

ERECTILE DYSFUNCTION

Epidemiology Erectile dysfunction (ED) is not considered a normal part of the aging process. Nonetheless, it is associated with certain physiologic and psychological changes related to age. In the Massachusetts Male Aging Study (MMAS), a community-based survey of men between the ages of 40 and 70, 52% of responders reported some degree of ED. Complete ED occurred in 10% of respondents, moderate ED occurred in 25%, and minimal ED in 17%. The incidence of moderate or severe ED more than doubled between the ages of 40 and 70. In the National Health and Social Life Survey (NHSLS), which was a nationally representative sample of men and women ages 18–59, 10% of men reported being unable to maintain an erection (corresponding to the proportion of men in the MMAS reporting severe ED). Incidence was highest among men in the 50–59 age group (21%) and among men who were poor (14%), divorced (14%), and less educated (13%).

The incidence of ED is also higher among men with certain medical disorders such as diabetes mellitus, obesity, lower urinary tract symptoms secondary to benign prostatic hyperplasia (BPH), heart disease, hypertension, and decreased HDL levels. Smoking is a significant risk factor in the development of ED. Medications used to treat diabetes or cardiovascular disease are additional risk factors (see below). There is a higher incidence of ED among men who have undergone radiation or surgery for prostate cancer and in those with a lower spinal cord injury. Psychological causes of ED include depression, anger, or stress from unemployment or other causes.

Pathophysiology ED may result from three basic mechanisms: (1) failure to initiate (psychogenic, endocrinologic, or neurogenic); (2) failure to fill (arteriogenic); or (3) failure to store adequate blood volume within the lacunar network (venoocclusive dysfunction). These categories are not mutually exclusive, and multiple factors contribute to ED in many patients. For example, diminished filling pressure can lead secondarily to venous leak. Psychogenic factor frequently coexist with other etiologic factors and should be considered in all cases. Diabetic, atherosclerotic, and drug-related causes account for >80% of cases of ED in older men.

VASCULOGENIC The most frequent organic cause of ED is a disturbance of blood flow to and from the penis. Atherosclerotic or traumatic arterial disease can decrease flow to the lacunar spaces, resulting in decreased rigidity and an increased time to full erection. Excessive outflow through the veins, despite adequate inflow, may also contribute to ED. Structural alterations to the fibroelastic components of the corpora may cause a loss of compliance and an inability to compress the tunical veins. This condition may result from aging, increased cross-linking of collagen fibers induced by nonenzymatic glycosylation, hypoxia, or altered synthesis of collagen associated with hypercholesterolemia.

NEUROGENIC Disorders that affect the sacral spinal cord or the autonomic fibers to the penis preclude nervous system relaxation of penile smooth muscle, thus leading to ED. In patients with spinal cord injury, the degree of ED depends on the completeness and level of the lesion. Patients with incomplete lesions or injuries to the upper part of the spinal cord are more likely to retain erectile capabilities than those with complete lesions or injuries to the lower part. Although 75% of patients with spinal cord injuries have some erectile capability, only 25% have erections sufficient for penetration. Other neurologic disorders commonly associated with ED include multiple sclerosis and peripheral neuropathy. The latter is often due to either diabetes or alcoholism. Pelvic surgery may cause ED through disruption of the autonomic nerve supply.

ENDOCRINOLOGIC Androgens increase libido, but their exact role in erectile function remains unclear. Individuals with castrate levels of testosterone can achieve erections from visual or sexual stimuli. Nonetheless, normal levels of testosterone appear to be important for erectile function, particularly in older males. Androgen replacement therapy can improve depressed erectile function when it is secondary to hypogonadism; however, it is not useful for ED when endogenous testosterone levels are normal. Increased prolactin may decrease libido by suppressing gonadotropin-releasing hormone (GnRH), and it also leads to decreased testosterone levels. Treatment of hyperprolactinemia with dopamine agonists can restore libido and testosterone.

DIABETIC ED occurs in 35–75% of men with diabetes mellitus. Pathologic mechanisms are primarily related to diabetes-associated vascular and neurologic complications. Diabetic macrovascular complications are mainly related to age, whereas microvascular complications correlate with the duration of diabetes and the degree of glycemic control (Chap. 338). Individuals with diabetes also have reduced amounts of nitric oxide synthase in both endothelial and neural tissues.

PSYCHOGENIC Two mechanisms contribute to the inhibition of erections in psychogenic ED. First, psychogenic stimuli to the sacral cord may inhibit reflexogenic responses, thereby blocking activation of vasodilator outflow to the penis. Second, excess sympathetic stimulation in an anxious man may increase penile smooth-muscle tone. The most common causes of psychogenic ED are performance anxiety, depression, relationship conflict, loss of attraction, sexual inhibition, conflicts over sexual preference, sexual abuse in childhood, and fear of pregnancy or sexually transmitted disease. Almost all patients with ED, even when it has a clear-cut organic basis, develop a psychogenic component as a reaction to ED.

MEDICATION-RELATED Medication-induced ED (Table 49-1) is estimated to occur in 25% of men seen in general medical outpatient clinics. Among the antihypertensive agents, the thiazide diuretics and beta blockers have been implicated most frequently. Calcium channel blockers and angiotensin-converting enzyme inhibitors are less frequently cited. These drugs may act directly at the corporal level (e.g., calcium channel blockers) or indirectly by reducing pelvic blood pressure, which is important in the development of penile rigidity. α Adrenergic blockers are less likely to cause ED. Estrogens, GnRH agonists, H_2 antagonists, and spironolactone cause ED by suppressing gonadotropin production or by blocking androgen action. Antidepressant and antipsychotic agents—particularly neuroleptics, tricyclics, and SSRIs—are associated with erectile, ejaculatory, orgasmic, and sexual desire difficulties.

Although many medications can cause ED, patients frequently have concomitant risk factors that confound the clinical picture. If there is a strong association between the institution of a drug and the onset of ED, alternative medications should be considered. Otherwise, it is often practical to treat the ED without attempting multiple changes in medications, as it may be difficult to establish a causal role for the drug.

APPROACH TO THE PATIENT: Erectile Dysfunction

A good physician-patient relationship helps to unravel the possible causes of ED, many of which require discussion of personal and some-

TABLE 49-1 DRUGS ASSOCIATED WITH ERECTILE DYSFUNCTION

Classification	Drugs
Diuretics	Thiazides Spironolactone
Antihypertensives	Calcium channel blockers Methyldopa Clonidine Reserpine β-Blockers Guanethidine
Cardiac/anti-hyperlipidemics	Digoxin Gemfibrozil Clofibrate
Antidepressants	Selective serotonin reuptake inhibitors Tricyclic antidepressants Lithium Monoamine oxidase inhibitors
Tranquilizers	Butyrophenones Phenothiazines
H_2 antagonists	Ranitidine Cimetidine
Hormones	Progesterone Estrogens Corticosteroids GnRH agonists 5α-Reductase inhibitors Cyproterone acetate
Cytotoxic agents	Cyclophosphamide Methotrexate Roferon-A
Anticholinergics	Disopyramide Anticonvulsants
Recreational	Ethanol Cocaine Marijuana

times embarrassing topics. For this reason, a primary care provider is often ideally suited to initiate the evaluation. A complete medical and sexual history should be taken in an effort to assess whether the cause of ED is organic, psychogenic, or multifactorial (Fig. 49-2). Initial questions should focus on the onset of symptoms, the presence and duration of partial erections, and the progression of ED. A history of nocturnal or early morning erections is useful for distinguishing physiologic from psychogenic ED. Nocturnal erections occur during rapid eye movement (REM) sleep and require intact neurologic and circulatory systems. Organic causes of ED are generally characterized by a gradual and persistent change in rigidity or the inability to sustain nocturnal, coital, or self-stimulated erections. The patient should be questioned about the presence of penile curvature or pain with coitus. It is also important to address libido, as decreased sexual drive and ED are sometimes the earliest signs of endocrine abnormalities (e.g., increased prolactin, decreased testosterone levels). It is useful to ask whether the problem is confined to coitus with one or other partners; ED arises not uncommonly in association with new or extramarital sexual relationships. Situational ED, as opposed to consistent ED, suggests psychogenic causes. Ejaculation is much less commonly affected than erection, but questions should be asked about whether ejaculation is normal, premature, delayed, or absent. Relevant risk factors should be identified, such as diabetes mellitus, coronary artery disease (CAD), or neurologic disorders. The patient's surgical history should be explored with an emphasis on bowel, bladder, prostate, or vascular procedures. A complete drug history is also important. Social changes that may precipitate ED are also crucial to the evaluation, including health worries, spousal death, divorce, relationship difficulties, and financial concerns.

Because ED commonly involves a host of endothelial cell risk factors, men with ED report higher rates of overt and silent myocardial infarction. As such, ED in an otherwise asymptomatic male warrants consideration of other vascular disorders including CAD.

The physical examination is an essential element in the assessment of ED. Signs of hypertension as well as evidence of thyroid,

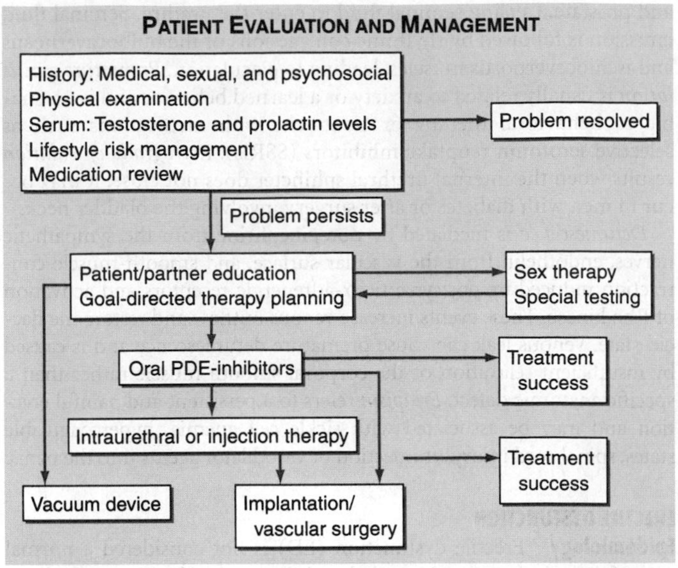

FIGURE 49-2 Algorithm for the evaluation and management of patients with ED.

hepatic, hematologic, cardiovascular, or renal diseases should be sought. An assessment should be made of the endocrine and vascular systems, the external genitalia, and the prostate gland. The penis should be carefully palpated along the corpora to detect fibrotic plaques. Reduced testicular size and loss of secondary sexual characteristics are suggestive of hypogonadism. Neurologic examination should include assessment of anal sphincter tone, the bulbocavernosus reflex, and testing for peripheral neuropathy.

Although hyperprolactinemia is uncommon, a serum prolactin level should be measured, as decreased libido and/or erectile dysfunction may be the presenting symptoms of a prolactinoma or other mass lesions of the sella (Chap. 333). The serum testosterone level should be measured and, if low, gonadotropins should be measured to determine whether hypogonadism is primary (testicular) or secondary (hypothalamic-pituitary) in origin (Chap. 340). If not performed recently, serum chemistries, CBC, and lipid profiles may be of value, as they can yield evidence of anemia, diabetes, hyperlipidemia, or other systemic diseases associated with ED. Determination of serum prostate specific antigen (PSA) should be conducted according to recommended clinical guidelines (Chap. 91).

Additional diagnostic testing is rarely necessary in the evaluation of ED. However, in selected patients, specialized testing may provide insight into pathologic mechanisms of ED and aid in the selection of treatment options. Optional specialized testing includes: (1) studies of nocturnal penile tumescence and rigidity; (2) vascular testing (in-office injection of vasoactive substances, penile Doppler ultrasound, penile angiography, dynamic infusion cavernosography/cavernosometry); (3) neurologic testing (biothesiometry-graded vibratory perception; somatosensory evoked potentials); and (4) psychological diagnostic tests. The information potentially gained from these procedures must be balanced against their invasiveness and cost.

℞ MALE SEXUAL DYSFUNCTION

PATIENT EDUCATION Patient and partner education is essential in the treatment of ED. In goal-directed therapy, education facilitates understanding of the disease, results of the tests, and selection of treatment. Discussion of treatment options helps to clarify how treatment is best offered and stratify first- and second-line therapies. Patients with high-risk lifestyle issues, such as smoking, alcohol abuse, or recreational drug use, should be counseled on the role these factors play in the development of ED.

ORAL AGENTS Sildenafil, tadalafil, and vardenifil are the only approved and effective oral agents for the treatment of ED. These three medications have markedly improved the management of ED because they are effective for the treatment of a broad range of causes, including psychogenic, diabetic, vasculogenic, postradical prostatectomy (nerve-sparing procedures), and spinal cord injury. They belong to a class of medications that are selective and potent inhibitors of PDE-5, the predominant phosphodiesterase isoform found in the penis. They are administered in graduated doses and enhance erections after sexual stimulation. The onset of action is approximately 60–120 min, depending on the medication used and other factors such as recent food intake. Reduced initial doses should be considered for patients who are elderly, taking concomitant alpha blockers, have renal insufficiency, or are taking medications that inhibit the CYP3A4 metabolic pathway in the liver (e.g., erythromycin, cimetidine, ketoconazole, and, possibly, itraconazole and mibefradil), as they may increase the serum concentration of the PDE-5 inhibitors or promote hypotension. Testosterone supplementation combined with a PDE-5 inhibitor may be beneficial in improving erectile function in hypogonadal men with erectile dysfunction who are unresponsive to PDE-5 inhibitors alone. These drugs do not affect ejaculation, orgasm, or sexual drive. Side effects associated with PDE-5 inhibitors include headaches (19%), facial flushing (9%), dyspepsia (6%), and nasal congestion (4%). Approximately 7% of men using sildenafil may experience transient altered color vision (blue halo effect), while 6% of men taking tadalafil may experience loin pain. PDE-5 inhibitors are contraindicated in men receiving nitrate therapy for cardiovascular disease, including agents delivered by oral, sublingual, transnasal, or topical routes. These agents can potentiate its hypotensive effect and may result in profound shock. Likewise, amyl/butyl nitrate "poppers" may have a fatal synergistic effect on blood pressure. PDE-5 inhibitors should also be avoided in patients with congestive heart failure and cardiomyopathy because of the risk of vascular collapse. Because sexual activity leads to an increase in physiologic expenditure [5–6 metabolic equivalents (METS)], physicians have been advised to exercise caution in prescribing any drug for sexual activity to those with active coronary disease, heart failure, borderline hypotension, or hypovolemia, and to those on complex antihypertensive regimens.

Although the PDE-5 inhibitors share a common mechanism of action, there are a few differences among the three agents. Having been on the market the longest, sildenafil has the most robust data confirming its activity, safety, and tolerability. It has recently been released for use in pulmonary hypertension as well as ED. Tadalafil is unique in its longer half-life. All three drugs are effective for patients with ED of all ages, severities, and etiologies. While there are pharmacokinetic and pharmacodynamic differences among these agents, clinically relevant differences are not clear.

ANDROGEN THERAPY Testosterone replacement is used to treat both primary and secondary causes of hypogonadism (Chap. 340). Androgen supplementation in the setting of normal testosterone is rarely efficacious and is discouraged. Methods of androgen replacement include transdermal patches and gels, parenteral administration of long-acting testosterone esters (enanthate and cypionate), and oral preparations (17 α-alkylated derivatives) (Chap. 340). Transdermal delivery of testosterone using patches or gels (50–100 mg/d) more closely mimics physiologic testosterone levels, but it is unclear whether this translates into improved sexual function. The administration of 200–300 mg intramuscularly every 2–3 weeks provides another option but is far from an ideal physiologic replacement. Oral androgen preparations have the potential for hepatotoxicity and should be avoided. Testosterone therapy is contraindicated in men with androgen-sensitive cancers (e.g., prostate) and may be inappropriate for men with bladder neck obstruction. It is generally advisable to measure PSA before giving androgen. Hepatic function should be tested before and during testosterone therapy.

VACUUM CONSTRICTION DEVICES Vacuum constriction devices (VCD) are a well-established, noninvasive therapy. They are a reasonable treatment alternative for select patients who cannot take sildenafil or do not desire other interventions. VCD draw venous blood into the penis and use a constriction ring to restrict venous return and maintain tumescence. Adverse events with VCD include pain, numbness, bruising, and altered ejaculation. Additionally, many patients complain that the devices are cumbersome and that the induced erections have a nonphysiologic appearance and feel.

INTRAURETHRAL ALPROSTADIL If a patient fails to respond to oral agents, a reasonable next choice is intraurethral or self-injection of vasoactive substances. Intraurethral prostaglandin E_1 (alprostadil), in the form of a semisolid pellet (doses of 125–1000 μg), is delivered with an applicator. Approximately 65% of men receiving intraurethral alprostadil respond with an erection when tested in the office, but only 50% of those achieve successful coitus at home. Intraurethral insertion is associated with a markedly reduced incidence of priapism in comparison to intracavernosal injection.

INTRACAVERNOSAL SELF-INJECTION Injection of synthetic formulations of alprostadil is effective in 70–80% of patients with ED, but discontinuation rates are high because of the invasive nature of administration. Doses range between 1 and 40 μg. Injection therapy is contraindicated in men with a history of hypersensitivity to the drug and in men at risk for priapism (hypercoagulable states, sickle cell disease). Side effects include local adverse events, prolonged erections, pain, and fibrosis with chronic use. Various combinations of alprostadil, phentolamine, and/or papaverine are sometimes used.

SURGERY A less frequently used form of therapy for ED involves the surgical implantation of a semirigid or inflatable penile prosthesis. These surgical treatments are invasive, associated with potential complications, and generally reserved for treatment of refractory ED. Despite their high cost and invasiveness, penile prostheses are associated with high rates of patient and partner satisfaction.

SEX THERAPY A course of sex therapy may be useful for addressing specific interpersonal factors that may affect sexual functioning. Sex therapy generally consists of in-session discussion and at-home exercises specific to the person and the relationship. It is preferable if therapy includes both partners, provided the patient is involved in an ongoing relationship.

FEMALE SEXUAL DYSFUNCTION

Female sexual dysfunction (FSD) has traditionally included disorders of desire, arousal, pain, and muted orgasm. The associated risk factors for FSD are similar to those in males: cardiovascular disease, endocrine disorders, hypertension, neurologic disorders, and smoking (Table 49-2).

EPIDEMIOLOGY

Epidemiologic data are limited, but the available estimates suggest that as many as 43% of women complain of at least one sexual problem. Despite the recent interest in organic causes of FSD, desire and arousal phase disorders (including lubrication complaints) remain the most common presenting problems when surveyed in a community-based population.

PHYSIOLOGY OF THE FEMALE SEXUAL RESPONSE

The female sexual response requires the presence of estrogens. A role for androgens is also likely but less well-established. In the CNS, estrogens and androgens work synergistically to enhance sexual arousal and response. A number of studies report enhanced libido in women during preovulatory phases of the menstrual cycle, suggesting that hormones involved in the ovulatory surge (e.g., estrogens) increase desire.

Sexual motivation is heavily influenced by context, including the environment and partner factors. Once sufficient sexual desire is reached, sexual arousal is mediated by the central and autonomic nervous systems. Cerebral sympathetic outflow is thought to increase desire, while peripheral parasympathetic activity results in clitoral vasocongestion and vaginal secretion (lubrication).

The neurotransmitters for clitoral corporal engorgement are similar to those in the male, with a prominent role for neural, smooth muscle,

TABLE 49-2 RISK FACTORS FOR FEMALE SEXUAL DYSFUNCTION

Neurologic disease: stroke, spinal cord injury, Parkinsonism
Trauma, genital surgery, radiation
Endocrinopathies: diabetes, hyperprolactinemia
Liver and/or renal failure
Cardiovascular disease
Psychological factors and interpersonal relationship disorders: sexual abuse, life stressors
Medications
Antiandrogens: cimetidine, spironolactone
Antidepressants, alcohol, hypnotics, sedatives
Antiestrogens or GnRH antagonists
Antihistamines, sympathomimetic amines
Antihypertensives: diuretics, calcium channel blockers
Alkylating agents
Anticholinergics

and endothelial released nitric oxide (NO). A fine network of vaginal nerves and arterioles promote a vaginal transudate. The major transmitters of this complex vaginal response are not certain, but roles for NO and vasointestinal polypeptide (VIP) are suspected. Investigators studying the normal female sexual response have challenged the long-held construct of a linear and unmitigated relationship between initial desire, arousal, vasocongestion, lubrication, and eventual orgasm. Caregivers should consider a paradigm of a positive emotional and physical outcome with one, many, or no orgasmic peak and release.

Although there are the obvious anatomic differences as well as variation in the density of vascular and neural beds in males and females, the primary effectors of sexual response are strikingly similar. Intact sensation is important for arousal. Thus, reduced levels of sexual functioning are more common in women with peripheral neuropathies (e.g., diabetes). Vaginal lubrication is a transudate of serum that results from the increased pelvic blood flow associated with arousal. Vascular insufficiency from a variety of causes may compromise adequate lubrication and result in dyspareunia. Cavernosal and arteriole smooth-muscle relaxation occurs via increased nitric oxide synthase (NOS) activity and produces engorgement in the clitoris and surrounding vestibule. Orgasm requires an intact sympathetic outflow tract; hence, orgasmic disorders are common in female patients with spinal cord injuries.

APPROACH TO THE PATIENT: Female Sexual Dysfunction

Many women do not volunteer information concerning their sexual response. Open-ended questions in a supportive atmosphere are helpful for initiating a discussion of sexual fitness in women who are reluctant to discuss such issues. Once a complaint has been voiced, a comprehensive evaluation should be performed, including a medical history, psychosocial history, physical examination, and limited laboratory testing.

The history should include the usual medical, surgical, obstetric, psychological, gynecologic, sexual, and social information. Past experiences, intimacy, knowledge, and partner availability should also be ascertained. Medical disorders that may impact sexual health should be delineated. These include diabetes, cardiovascular disease, gynecologic conditions, obstetric history, depression, anxiety disorders, and neurologic disease. Medications should be reviewed as they may impact arousal, libido, and orgasm. The need for counseling and life stresses should be identified. The physical examination should assess the genitalia, including clitoris. Pelvic floor examination may identify prolapse or other disorders. Laboratory studies are needed, especially if menopausal status is uncertain. Estradiol, FSH, and LH are usually obtained, and dehydroepiandrosterone (DHEA) should be considered as it reflects adrenal androgen secretion. A complete blood count, liver function assessment, and lipid studies may be useful, if not otherwise obtained. Complicated diagnostic evaluation, such as clitoral Doppler ultrasonography and biothesiometry, require expensive equipment and are of uncertain utility. It is important for the patient to identify which symptoms are most distressing.

The evaluation of FSD previously occurred mainly in a psychosocial context. However, inconsistencies between diagnostic categories based on only psychosocial considerations, and the emerging recognition of organic etiologies, has led to a new classification of FSD. This diagnostic scheme is based on four components that are not mutually exclusive: (1) *Hypoactive sexual desire*—the persistent or recurrent lack of sexual thoughts and/or receptivity to sexual activity, which causes personal distress. Hypoactive sexual desire may result from endocrine failure or may be associated with psychological or emotional disorders, (2) *Sexual arousal disorder*—the persistent or recurrent inability to attain or maintain sexual excitement, which causes personal distress, (3) *Orgasmic disorder*—the persistent or recurrent loss of orgasmic potential after sufficient sexual stimulation and arousal, which causes personal distress, (4) *Sexual pain disorder*—persistent or recurrent genital pain associated with noncoital sexual stimulation, which causes personal distress. This newer classification emphasizes "personal distress" as a requirement for dysfunction and provides clinicians with an organized framework for evaluation prior to or in conjunction with more traditional counseling methods.

℞ FEMALE SEXUAL DYSFUNCTION

GENERAL An open discussion with the patient is important as couples may need to be educated about normal anatomy and physiologic responses, including role of orgasm in sexual encounters. Physiologic changes associated with aging and/or disease should be explained. Couples may need to be reminded that clitoral stimulation rather than coital intromission may be more beneficial.

Behavioral modification and nonpharmacologic therapies should be a first step. Patient and partner counseling may improve communication and relationship strains. Lifestyle changes involving known risk factors can be an important part of the treatment process. Emphasis on maximizing physical health and avoiding lifestyles (e.g., smoking, alcohol abuse) and medications likely to produce FSD is important (Table 49-2). The use of topical lubricants may address complaints of dyspareunia and dryness. Contributing medications, such as antidepressants, may need to be altered, including the use of medications with less impact on sexual function, dose reduction, medication switching, or drug holidays.

HORMONAL THERAPY In postmenopausal women, estrogen replacement therapy may be helpful in treating vaginal atrophy, decreasing coital pain, and improving clitoral sensitivity (Chap. 342). Estrogen replacement in the form of local cream is the preferred method, as it avoids systemic side effects. Androgen levels in women decline substantially before menopause. However, low levels of testosterone or DHEA are not effective predictors of a positive therapeutic outcome with androgen therapy. The widespread use of exogenous androgens is not supported by the literature except in select circumstances (premature ovarian failure or menopausal states) and in secondary arousal disorders.

ORAL AGENTS The efficacy of PDE-5 inhibitors in FDS has been a marked disappointment given the proposed role of nitric oxide-dependent physiology in the normal female sexual response. The use of PDE-5 inhibitors for FSD should be discouraged pending proof that it is effective.

CLITORAL VACUUM DEVICE In patients with arousal and orgasmic difficulties, the option of using a clitoral vacuum device may be explored. This handheld battery-operated device has a small soft plastic cup that applies a vacuum over the stimulated clitoris. This causes increased cavernosal blood flow, engorgement, and vaginal lubrication.

FURTHER READINGS

ARAUJO AB et al: Changes in sexual function in middle-aged and older men: Longitudinal data from the Massachusetts male aging study. J Am Geriatr Soc 52:1502, 2004

BASSON R: Recent advances in women's sexual function and dysfunction. Menopause 11:714, 2004

BHASIN S et al: Sexual dysfunction in men and women with endocrine disorders. Lancet 369(9561):597, 2007

BURNETT AL: Erectile dysfunction. J Urol 175:S25, 2006

DAVIS SR et al: Endocrine aspects of female sexual dysfunction. J Sex Med 1:82, 2004

DOGGRELL SA: Comparison of clinical trials with sildenafil, vardenafil, and tadalafil in erectile dysfunction. Expert Opin Pharmacother 6:75, 2005

PAULS RN et al: Female sexual dysfunction: principles of diagnosis and therapy. Obstet Gynecol Surv 60:196, 2005

REES PM et al: Sexual function in men and women with neurological disorders. Lancet 369(9560):512, 2007

50 Hirsutism and Virilization

David A. Ehrmann

Hirsutism, defined as excessive male-pattern hair growth, affects approximately 10% of women. It usually represents a variation of normal hair growth, but rarely it is a harbinger of a serious underlying condition. Hirsutism is often idiopathic but may be caused by conditions associated with androgen excess, such as polycystic ovarian syndrome (PCOS) or congenital adrenal hyperplasia (CAH) (Table 50-1). Cutaneous manifestations commonly associated with hirsutism include acne and male-pattern balding (androgenic alopecia). *Virilization* refers to a condition in which androgen levels are sufficiently high to cause additional signs and symptoms such as deepening of the voice, breast atrophy, increased muscle bulk, clitoromegaly, and increased libido; virilization is an ominous sign that suggests the possibility of an ovarian or adrenal neoplasm.

HAIR FOLLICLE GROWTH AND DIFFERENTIATION

Hair can be categorized as either *vellus* (fine, soft, and not pigmented) or *terminal* (long, coarse, and pigmented). The number of hair follicles does not change over an individual's lifetime, but the follicle size and type of hair can change in response to numerous factors, particularly androgens. Androgens are necessary for terminal hair and sebaceous gland development and mediate differentiation of pilosebaceous units (PSUs) into either a terminal hair follicle or a sebaceous gland. In the former case, androgens transform the vellus hair into a terminal hair; in the latter, the sebaceous component proliferates and the hair remains vellus.

There are three phases in the cycle of hair growth: (1) *anagen* (growth phase), (2) *catagen* (involution phase), and (3) *telogen* (rest phase). Depending on the body site, hormonal regulation may play an important role in the hair growth cycle. For example, the eyebrows, eyelashes, and vellus hairs are androgen-insensitive, whereas the axillary and pubic areas are sensitive to low levels of androgens. Hair growth on the face, chest, upper abdomen, and back requires greater levels of androgens and is therefore more characteristic of the pattern typically seen in men. Androgen excess in women leads to increased hair growth in most androgen-sensitive sites except in the scalp region, where hair loss occurs because androgens cause scalp hairs to spend less time in the anagen phase.

Although androgen excess underlies most cases of hirsutism, there is only a modest correlation between androgen levels and the quantity of hair growth. This is due to the fact that hair growth from the follicle also depends on local growth factors, and there is variability in end-organ sensitivity. Genetic factors and ethnic background also influence hair growth. In general, dark-haired individuals tend to be more hirsute than blonde or fair individuals. Asians and Native Americans have relatively sparse hair in regions sensitive to high androgen levels, whereas people of Mediterranean descent are more hirsute.

TABLE 50-1 CAUSES OF HIRSUTISM

Gonadal hyperandrogenism
Ovarian hyperandrogenism
Polycystic ovary syndrome/functional ovarian hyperandrogenism
Ovarian steroidogenic blocks
Syndromes of extreme insulin resistance
Ovarian neoplasms
Adrenal hyperandrogenism
Premature adrenarche
Functional adrenal hyperandrogenism
Congenital adrenal hyperplasia (nonclassic and classic)
Abnormal cortisol action/metabolism
Adrenal neoplasms
Other endocrine disorders
Cushing's syndrome
Hyperprolactinemia
Acromegaly
Peripheral androgen overproduction
Obesity
Idiopathic
Pregnancy-related hyperandrogenism
Hyperreactio luteinalis
Thecoma of pregnancy
Drugs
Androgens
Oral contraceptives containing androgenic progestins
Minoxidil
Phenytoin
Diazoxide
Cyclosporine
True hermaphroditism

CLINICAL ASSESSMENT

Historic elements relevant to the assessment of hirsutism include the age of onset and rate of progression of hair growth and associated symptoms or signs (e.g., acne). Depending on the cause, excess hair growth is typically first noted during the second and third decades. The growth is usually slow but progressive. Sudden development and rapid progression of hirsutism suggest the possibility of an androgen-secreting neoplasm, in which case virilization also may be present.

The age of onset of menstrual cycles (menarche) and the pattern of the menstrual cycle should be ascertained; irregular cycles from the time of menarche onward are more likely to result from ovarian rather than adrenal androgen excess. Associated symptoms such as galactorrhea should prompt evaluation for hyperprolactinemia (Chap. 333) and possibly hypothyroidism (Chap. 335). Hypertension, striae, easy bruising, centripetal weight gain, and weakness suggest hypercortisolism (Cushing's syndrome; Chap. 336). Rarely, patients with growth hormone excess (i.e., acromegaly) will present with hirsutism. Use of medications such as phenytoin, minoxidil, or cyclosporine may be associated with androgen-independent excess hair growth (i.e., hypertrichosis). A family history of infertility and/or hirsutism may indicate disorders such as nonclassic CAH (Chap. 336).

Physical examination should include measurement of height, weight, and calculation of body mass index (BMI). A BMI >25 kg/m^2 is indicative of excess weight for height, and values >30 kg/m^2 are often seen in association with hirsutism. Notation should be made of blood pressure, as adrenal causes may be associated with hypertension. Cutaneous signs sometimes associated with androgen excess and insulin resistance include acanthosis nigricans and skin tags.

An objective clinical assessment of hair distribution and quantity is central to the evaluation in any woman presenting with hirsutism. This assessment permits the distinction between hirsutism and hypertrichosis and provides a baseline reference point to gauge the response to treatment. A simple and commonly used method to grade hair growth is the modified scale of Ferriman and Gallwey (Fig. 50-1), where each of nine androgen-sensitive sites is graded from 0 to 4. Approximately 95% of Caucasian women have a score below 8 on this scale; thus, it is normal for most women to have some hair growth in androgen-sensitive sites. Scores above 8 suggest excess androgen-mediated hair growth, a finding that should be assessed further by hormonal evaluation (see below). In racial/ethnic groups that are less likely to manifest hirsutism (e.g., Asian women), additional cutaneous evidence of androgen excess should be sought, including pustular acne or thinning hair.

HORMONAL EVALUATION

Androgens are secreted by the ovaries and adrenal glands in response to their respective tropic hormones, luteinizing hormone (LH) and adrenocorticotropic hormone (ACTH). The principal circulating steroids involved in the etiology of hirsutism are testosterone, androstenedione, and dehydroepiandrosterone (DHEA) and its sulfated form (DHEAS). The ovaries and adrenal glands normally contribute about equally to testosterone production. Approximately half of the total testosterone originates from direct glandular secretion, and the remainder is derived from the peripheral conversion of androstenedione and DHEA (Chap. 340).

Although it is the most important circulating androgen, testosterone is, in effect, the penultimate androgen in mediating hirsutism;

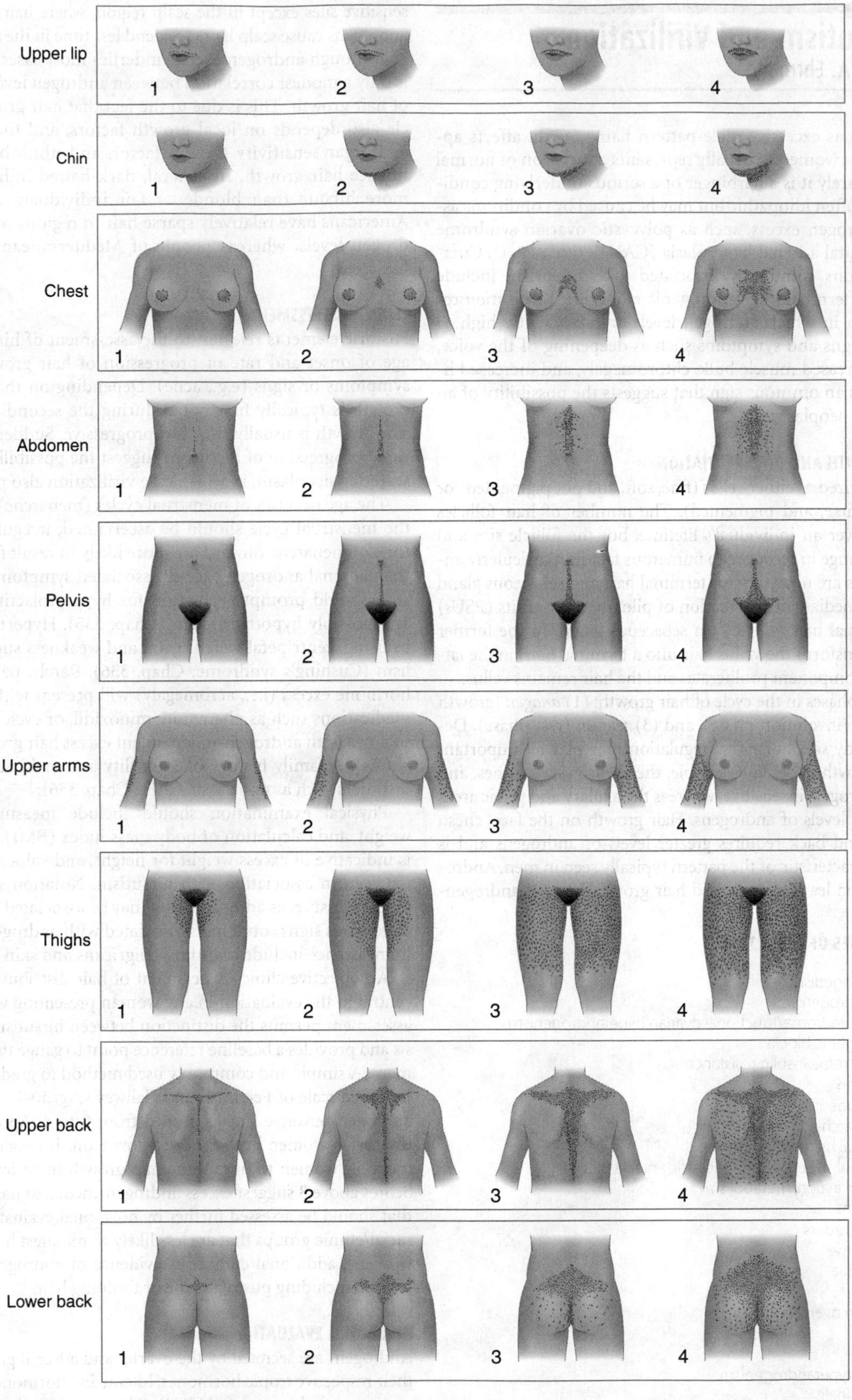

FIGURE 50-1 Hirsutism scoring scale of Ferriman and Gallwey. The nine body areas possessing androgen-sensitive areas are graded from 0 (no terminal hair) to 4 (frankly virile) to obtain a total score. A normal hirsutism score is less than 8. [*Modified from DA Ehrmann et al: Hyperandrogenism, hirsutism, and polycystic ovary syndrome, in LJ DeGroot and JL Jameson (eds), Endocrinology, 5th ed. Philadelphia, Saunders, 2006; with permission.*]

it is converted to the more potent dihydrotestosterone (DHT) by the enzyme 5α-reductase, which is located in the PSU. DHT has a higher affinity for, and slower dissociation from, the androgen receptor. The local production of DHT allows it to serve as the primary mediator of androgen action at the level of the pilosebaceous unit. There are two isoenzymes of 5α-reductase: type 2 is found in the prostate gland and in hair follicles, whereas type 1 is found primarily in sebaceous glands.

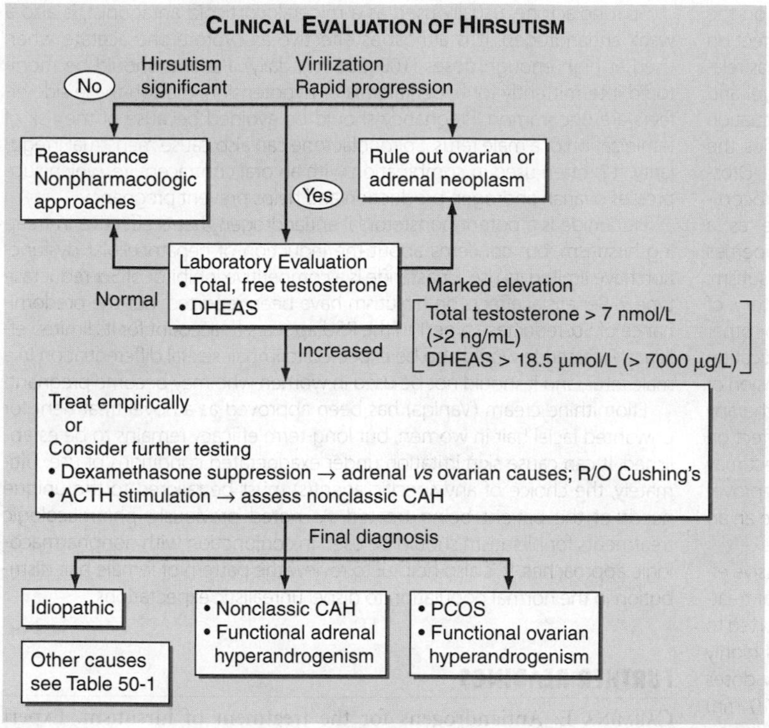

FIGURE 50-2 Algorithm for the evaluation and differential diagnosis of hirsutism. ACTH, adrenocorticotropic hormone; CAH, congenital adrenal hyperplasia; DHEAS, sulfated form of dehydroepiandrosterone; PCOS, polycystic ovarian syndrome.

One approach to testing for hyperandrogenemia is depicted in Fig. 50-2. In addition to measuring blood levels of testosterone and DHEAS, it is also important to measure the level of free (or unbound) testosterone. The fraction of testosterone that is not bound to its carrier protein, sex-hormone binding globulin (SHBG), is biologically available for conversion to DHT and for binding to androgen receptors. Hyperinsulinemia and/or androgen excess decrease hepatic production of SHBG, resulting in levels of total testosterone within the high-normal range, whereas the unbound hormone is more substantially elevated. Although there is a decline in ovarian testosterone production after menopause, ovarian estrogen production decreases to an even greater extent, and the concentration of SHBG is reduced. Consequently, there is an increase in the relative proportion of unbound testosterone, and it may exacerbate hirsutism after menopause.

A baseline plasma total testosterone level >12 nmol/L (>3.5 ng/mL) usually indicates a virilizing tumor, whereas a level >7 nmol/L (>2 ng/mL) is suggestive. A basal DHEAS level >18.5 µmol/L (>7000 µg/L) suggests an adrenal tumor. Although DHEAS has been proposed as a "marker" of predominant adrenal androgen excess, it is not unusual to find modest elevations in DHEAS among women with PCOS. Computed tomography (CT) or magnetic resonance imaging (MRI) should be used to localize an adrenal mass, and ultrasound will usually suffice to identify an ovarian mass if clinical evaluation and hormonal levels suggest these possibilities.

PCOS is the most common cause of ovarian androgen excess (Chap. 341). However, the increased ratio of LH to follicle-stimulating hormone that is characteristic of carefully studied patients with PCOS is not seen in up to half of these women due to the pulsatility of gonadotropins. If performed, ultrasound shows enlarged ovaries and increased stroma in many women with PCOS. However, polycystic ovaries may also be found in women without clinical or laboratory features of PCOS. Therefore, polycystic ovaries are a relatively insensitive and nonspecific finding for the diagnosis of ovarian hyperandrogenism. Although not usually necessary, gonadotropin-releasing hormone agonist testing can be used to make a specific diagnosis of ovarian hyperandrogenism. A peak 17-hydroxyprogesterone level ≥7.8 nmol/L (≥2.6 µg/L), after the administration of 100 µg nafarelin (or 10 µg/kg leuprolide) subcutaneously, is virtually diagnostic of ovarian hyperandrogenism.

Because adrenal androgens are readily suppressed by low doses of glucocorticoids, the dexamethasone androgen-suppression test may broadly distinguish ovarian from adrenal androgen overproduction. A blood sample is obtained before and after administering dexamethasone (0.5 mg orally every 6 h for 4 days). An adrenal source is suggested by suppression of unbound testosterone into the normal range; incomplete suppression suggests ovarian androgen excess. An overnight 1-mg dexamethasone suppression test, with measurement of 8:00 A.M. serum cortisol, is useful when there is clinical suspicion of Cushing's syndrome (Chap. 336).

Nonclassic CAH is most commonly due to 21-hydroxylase deficiency but can also be caused by autosomal recessive defects in other steroidogenic enzymes necessary for adrenal corticosteroid synthesis (Chap. 336). Because of the enzyme defect, the adrenal gland cannot secrete glucocorticoids efficiently (especially cortisol). This results in diminished negative feedback inhibition of ACTH, leading to compensatory adrenal hyperplasia and the accumulation of steroid precursors that are subsequently converted to androgen. Deficiency of 21-hydroxylase can be reliably excluded by determining a morning 17-hydroxyprogesterone level <6 nmol/L (<2 µg/L) (drawn in the follicular phase). Alternatively, 21-hydroxylase deficiency can be diagnosed by measurement of 17-hydroxyprogesterone 1 h after administration of 250 µg of synthetic ACTH (cosyntropin) intravenously.

℞ HIRSUTISM

Treatment of hirsutism may be accomplished pharmacologically or by mechanical means of hair removal. Nonpharmacologic treatments should be considered in all patients, either as the only treatment or as an adjunct to drug therapy.

Nonpharmacologic treatments include (1) bleaching; (2) depilatory (removal from the skin surface) such as shaving and chemical treatments; or (3) epilatory (removal of the hair including the root) such as plucking, waxing, electrolysis, and laser therapy. Despite perceptions to the contrary, shaving does not increase the rate or density of hair growth. Chemical depilatory treatments may be useful for mild hirsutism that affects only limited skin areas, though they can cause skin irritation. Wax treatment removes hair temporarily but is uncomfortable. Electrolysis is effective for more permanent hair removal, particularly in the hands of a skilled electrologist. Laser phototherapy appears to be efficacious for hair removal. It delays hair regrowth and causes permanent hair removal in most patients. The long-term effects and complications associated with laser treatment are still being evaluated.

Pharmacologic therapy is directed at interrupting one or more of the steps in the pathway of androgen synthesis and action: (1) suppression of adrenal and/or ovarian androgen production; (2) enhancement of androgen-binding to plasma-binding proteins, particularly SHBG; (3) impairment of the peripheral conversion of androgen precursors to active androgen; and (4) inhibition of androgen action at the target tissue level. Attenuation of hair growth is typically not evident until 4–6 months after initiation of medical treatment and, in most cases, leads to only a modest reduction in hair growth.

Combination estrogen-progestin therapy, in the form of an oral contraceptive, is usually the first-line endocrine treatment for hirsutism and acne, after cosmetic and dermatologic management. The estrogenic component of most oral contraceptives currently in use is either ethinyl estradiol or mestranol. The suppression of LH leads to reduced production of ovarian androgens. The reduced androgen levels also result in a dose-related increase in SHBG, thereby lowering the fraction of unbound plasma testosterone. Combination therapy has also been demonstrated to decrease DHEAS, perhaps by reducing ACTH levels. Estrogens also have a direct, dose-dependent suppressive effect on sebaceous cell function.

The choice of a specific oral contraceptive should be predicated on the progestational component, as progestins vary in their suppressive effect on SHBG levels and in their androgenic potential. Ethynodiol diacetate has relatively low androgenic potential, whereas progestins such as norgestrel and levonorgestrel are particularly androgenic, as judged from their attenuation of the estrogen-induced increase in SHBG. Norgestimate exemplifies the newer generation of progestins that are virtually nonandrogenic. Drospirenone, an analogue of spironolactone that has both antimineralocorticoid and antiandrogenic activities, has been approved for use as a progestational agent in combination with ethinyl estradiol. Its properties suggest that it should be the preferred choice for the treatment of hirsutism.

Oral contraceptives are contraindicated in women with a history of thromboembolic disease or in women with increased risk of breast or other estrogen-dependent cancers (Chap. 342). There is a relative contraindication to the use of oral contraceptives in smokers or in those with hypertension or a history of migraine headaches. In most trials, estrogen-progestin therapy alone improves the extent of acne by a maximum of 50–70%. The effect on hair growth may not be evident for 6 months, and the maximum effect may require 9–12 months owing to the length of the hair growth cycle. Improvements in hirsutism are typically in the range of 20%, but there may be an arrest of further progression of hair growth.

Adrenal androgens are more sensitive than cortisol to the suppressive effects of glucocorticoids. Therefore, glucocorticoids are the mainstay of treatment in patients with CAH. Although glucocorticoids have been reported to restore ovulatory function in some women with PCOS, this effect is highly variable. Because of side effects from excessive glucocorticoids, low doses should be used. Dexamethasone (0.2–0.5 mg) or prednisone (5–10 mg) should be taken at bedtime to achieve maximal suppression by inhibiting the nocturnal surge of ACTH.

Cyproterone acetate is the prototypic antiandrogen. It acts mainly by competitive inhibition of the binding of testosterone and DHT to the androgen receptor. In addition, it may enhance the metabolic clearance of testosterone by inducing hepatic enzymes. Although not available for use in the United States, cyproterone acetate is widely used in Canada, Mexico, and Europe. Cyproterone (50–100 mg) is given on days 1–15 and ethinyl estradiol (50 μg) is given on days 5–26 of the menstrual cycle. Side effects include irregular uterine bleeding, nausea, headache, fatigue, weight gain, and decreased libido.

Spironolactone, usually used as a mineralocorticoid antagonist, is also a weak antiandrogen. It is almost as effective as cyproterone acetate when used at high enough doses (100–200 mg daily). Patients should be monitored intermittently for hyperkalemia or hypotension, though these side effects are uncommon. Pregnancy should be avoided because of the risk of feminization of a male fetus. Spironolactone can also cause menstrual irregularity. It is often used in combination with an oral contraceptive, which suppresses ovarian androgen production and helps prevent pregnancy.

Flutamide is a potent nonsteroidal antiandrogen that is effective in treating hirsutism, but concerns about the induction of hepatocellular dysfunction have limited its use. Finasteride is a competitive inhibitor of 5α-reductase type 2. Beneficial effects on hirsutism have been reported, but the predominance of 5α-reductase type 1 in the PSU appears to account for its limited efficacy. Finasteride would also be expected to impair sexual differentiation in a male fetus, and it should not be used in women who may become pregnant.

Eflornithine cream (Vaniqa) has been approved as a novel treatment for unwanted facial hair in women, but long-term efficacy remains to be established. It can cause skin irritation under exaggerated conditions of use. Ultimately, the choice of any specific agent(s) must be tailored to the unique needs of the patient being treated. As noted previously, pharmacologic treatments for hirsutism should be used in conjunction with nonpharmacologic approaches. It is also helpful to review the pattern of female hair distribution in the normal population to dispel unrealistic expectations.

FURTHER READINGS

CARMINA E: Antiandrogens for the treatment of hirsutism. Expert Opin Investig Drugs 11:357, 2002

EHRMANN DA: Polycystic ovary syndrome. N Engl J Med 352:1223, 2005

HORDINSKY M et al: Hair loss and hirsutism in the elderly. Clin Geriatr Med 18:121, 2002

LANIGAN SW: Management of unwanted hair in females. Clin Exp Dermatol 26:644, 2001

ROSENFIELD RL: Clinical practice. Hirsutism. N Engl J Med 353:2578, 2005

SANCHEZ LA et al: Laser hair reduction in the hirsute patient: A critical assessment. Hum Reprod Update 8:169, 2002

51 Menstrual Disorders and Pelvic Pain

Janet E. Hall

Menstrual dysfunction can signal an underlying abnormality that may have long-term health consequences. Although frequent or prolonged bleeding usually prompts a woman to seek medical attention, infrequent or absent bleeding may seem less troubling, and the patient may not bring it to the attention of the physician. Thus, a focused menstrual history is a critical part of every female patient encounter. Pelvic pain is a common complaint that may relate to an abnormality of the reproductive organs but may also be of gastrointestinal, urinary tract, or musculoskeletal origin. Depending on its cause, pelvic pain may require urgent surgical attention.

MENSTRUAL DISORDERS

DEFINITION AND PREVALENCE

Amenorrhea refers to the absence of menstrual periods. Amenorrhea is classified as *primary* if menstrual bleeding has never occurred in the absence of hormonal treatment or *secondary* if menstrual periods are absent for 3–6 months. *Oligoamenorrhea* is defined as a cycle length >35 days or <10 menses per year. Both the frequency and amount of vaginal bleeding are irregular in oligoamenorrhea. It is often associated with anovulation, which can also occur with intermenstrual intervals of <24 days or vaginal bleeding for >7 days. Frequent or heavy irregular bleeding is termed *dysfunctional uterine bleeding* if anatomic uterine lesions or a bleeding diathesis have been excluded.

Primary Amenorrhea This is a rare disorder occurring in <1% of the female population. However, between 3 and 5% of women experience at least 3 months of secondary amenorrhea in a given year. There is no evidence that race or ethnicity influence the prevalence of amenorrhea. However, because of the importance of adequate nutrition for normal reproductive function, both the age at menarche and the prevalence of secondary amenorrhea vary significantly in different parts of the world.

The absence of menses by age 16 has been used traditionally to define primary amenorrhea. However, other factors such as growth, secondary sexual characteristics, the presence of cyclic pelvic pain, and the secular trend to an earlier age of menarche, particularly in African-American girls, also influence the age at which primary amenorrhea should be investigated. Thus, an evaluation for amenorrhea should be initiated by age 15 or 16 in the presence of normal growth and secondary sexual characteristics; age 13 in the absence of secondary sexual characteristics or if height is less than the third percentile; age 12 or 13 in the presence of breast development and cyclic pelvic pain; or within 2 years of breast development if menarche has not occurred.

Secondary Amenorrhea or Oligoamenorrhea Anovulation and irregular cycles are relatively common for 2–4 years after menarche and for 1–2 years before the final menstrual period. In the intervening years, menstrual cycle length is ~28 days, with an intermenstrual interval normally ranging between 25 and 35 days. Cycle-to-cycle variability in an individual woman who is consistently ovulating is generally +/– 2 days. Pregnancy is the most common cause of amenorrhea and should be excluded early in any evaluation of menstrual irregularity. However, many women will occasionally miss a single period. Three or more months of secondary amenorrhea should prompt an evaluation, as should a history of intermenstrual intervals of >35 or <21 days, or bleeding that persists for >7 days.

DIAGNOSIS

Evaluation of menstrual dysfunction depends on understanding the interrelationships between the four critical components of the reproductive tract: (1) the hypothalamus, (2) the pituitary, (3) the ovaries, and (4) the uterus and outflow tract (Fig. 51-1; Chap. 341). This system is maintained by complex negative and positive feedback loops involving the ovarian steroids (estradiol and progesterone) and peptides (inhibin B and inhibin A) and the hypothalamic [gonadotropin-releasing hormone (GnRH)] and pituitary [follicle-stimulating hormone (FSH) and luteinizing hormone (LH)] components of this system (Fig. 51-1).

Disorders of menstrual function can be thought of in two main categories: disorders of the uterus and outflow tract and disorders of ovulation. Many of the conditions that cause primary amenorrhea are congenital but go unrecognized until the time of normal puberty (e.g., genetic, chromosomal, and anatomic abnormalities). All causes of secondary amenorrhea can also cause primary amenorrhea.

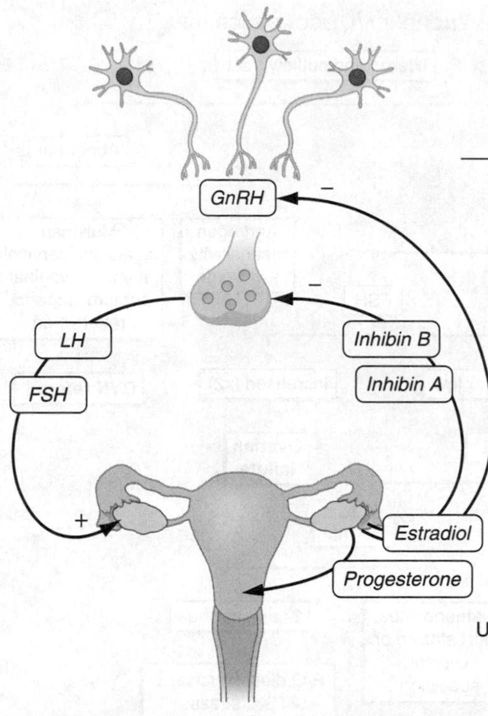

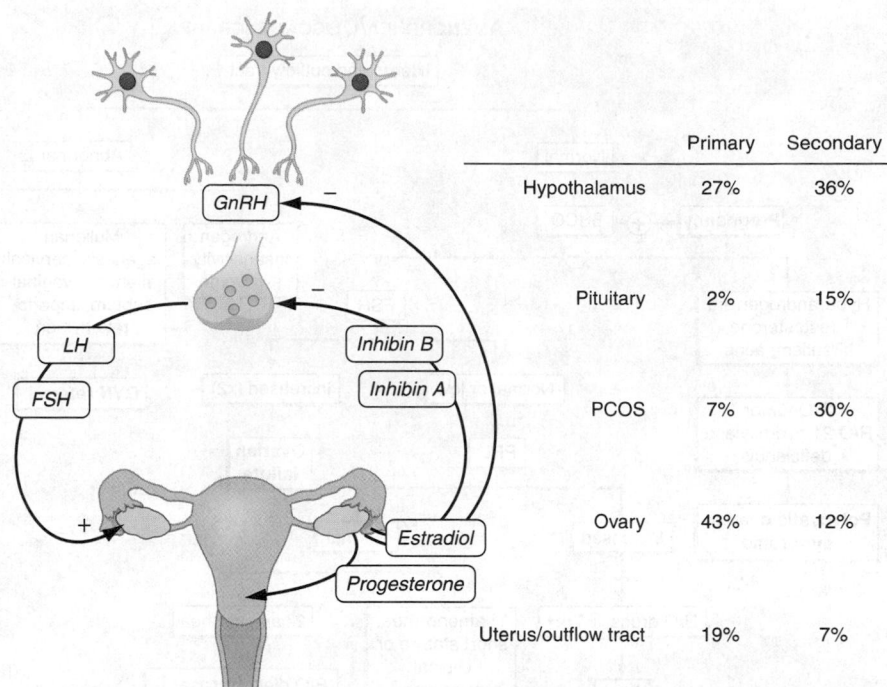

	Primary	Secondary
Hypothalamus	27%	36%
Pituitary	2%	15%
PCOS	7%	30%
Ovary	43%	12%
Uterus/outflow tract	19%	7%

FIGURE 51-1 Role of the hypothalamic-pituitary-gonadal axis in the etiology of amenorrhea. Gonadotropin-releasing hormone (GnRH) secretion from the hypothalamus stimulates follicle-stimulating hormone (FSH) and luteinizing hormone (LH) secretion from the pituitary to induce ovarian folliculogenesis and steroidogenesis. Ovarian secretion of estradiol and progesterone controls the shedding of the endometrium, resulting in menses and, in combination with the inhibins, provides feedback regulation of the hypothalamus and pituitary to control secretion of FSH and LH. The prevalence of amenorrhea resulting from abnormalities at each level of the reproductive system (hypothalamus, pituitary, ovary, uterus, and outflow tract) varies depending on whether amenorrhea is primary or secondary. PCOS, polycystic ovarian syndrome.

Disorders of the Uterus or Outflow Tract Abnormalities of the uterus and outflow tract typically present as primary amenorrhea. In patients with normal pubertal development and a blind vagina, the differential diagnosis includes *obstruction* by a transverse vaginal septum or imperforate hymen; *müllerian agenesis* (Mayer-Rokitansky-Kuster-Hauser syndrome), which has been associated with mutations in the *WNT4* gene; and *androgen insensitivity syndrome* (AIS), which is an X-linked recessive disorder that accounts for ~10% of all cases of primary amenorrhea (Chap. 340). Patients with AIS have a 46, XY karyotype, but because of the lack of androgen receptor responsiveness, they have severe underandrogenization and female external genitalia. The absence of pubic and axillary hair distinguishes them clinically from patients with müllerian agenesis. *Asherman syndrome* presents as secondary amenorrhea or hypomenorrhea and results from partial or complete obliteration of the uterine cavity by adhesions that prevent normal growth and shedding of the endometrium. Curettage performed for pregnancy complications accounts for >90% of cases; genital tuberculosis is an important cause in endemic regions.

℞ DISORDERS OF UTERUS OR OUTFLOW TRACT

Obstruction of the outflow tract requires surgical correction. The risk of endometriosis is increased with this condition, perhaps because of retrograde menstrual flow. *Müllerian agenesis* may also require surgical intervention, although vaginal dilatation is adequate in some patients. Because ovarian function is normal, assisted reproductive techniques can be used with a surrogate carrier. *Androgen resistance syndrome* requires gonadectomy because there is risk of gonadoblastoma in the dysgenetic gonads. Whether this should be performed in early childhood or after completion of breast development is controversial. Estrogen replacement is indicated after gonadectomy, and vaginal dilatation may be required to allow sexual intercourse.

Disorders of Ovulation Once uterus and outflow tract abnormalities have been excluded, all other causes of amenorrhea involve disorders of ovulation. The differential diagnosis is based on the results of initial tests including a pregnancy test, gonadotropins, and assessment of hyperandrogenism (Fig. 51-2).

HYPOGONADOTROPIC HYPOGONADISM Low estrogen levels in combination with normal or low levels of LH and FSH are seen with anatomic, genetic, or functional abnormalities that interfere with hypothalamic GnRH secretion or normal pituitary responsiveness to GnRH. Although relatively uncommon, tumors and infiltrative diseases should be considered in the differential diagnosis of hypogonadotropic hypogonadism (Chap. 333). These disorders may present with primary or secondary amenorrhea. They may occur in association with other features suggestive of hypothalamic or pituitary dysfunction such as short stature, diabetes insipidus, galactorrhea, or headache. Hypogonadotropic hypogonadism may also be seen following cranial irradiation. In the postpartum period, it may be due to pituitary necrosis (Sheehan syndrome) or lymphocytic hypophysitis. Because reproductive dysfunction is commonly associated with hyperprolactinemia, either from neuroanatomic lesions or medications, prolactin should be measured in all patients with hypogonadotropic hypogonadism (Chap. 333).

Isolated hypogonadotropic hypogonadism (IHH) is more common in men than women and is often associated with anosmia. IHH generally presents with primary amenorrhea. A number of genetic causes of IHH have been identified (Chaps. 340 and 341).

Functional hypothalamic amenorrhea (HA) is caused by a mismatch between energy expenditure and energy intake. Leptin secretion may play a key role in transducing the signals from the periphery to the hypothalamus in HA. The hypothalamic-pituitary-adrenal axis may also play a role. The diagnosis of HA can generally be made on the basis of a careful history, physical examination, and the demonstration of low levels of gonadotropins and normal prolactin levels. Eating disorders and chronic disease must be specifically excluded (Chap. 76). An atypical history, headache, signs of other hypothalamic dysfunction, or hyper-

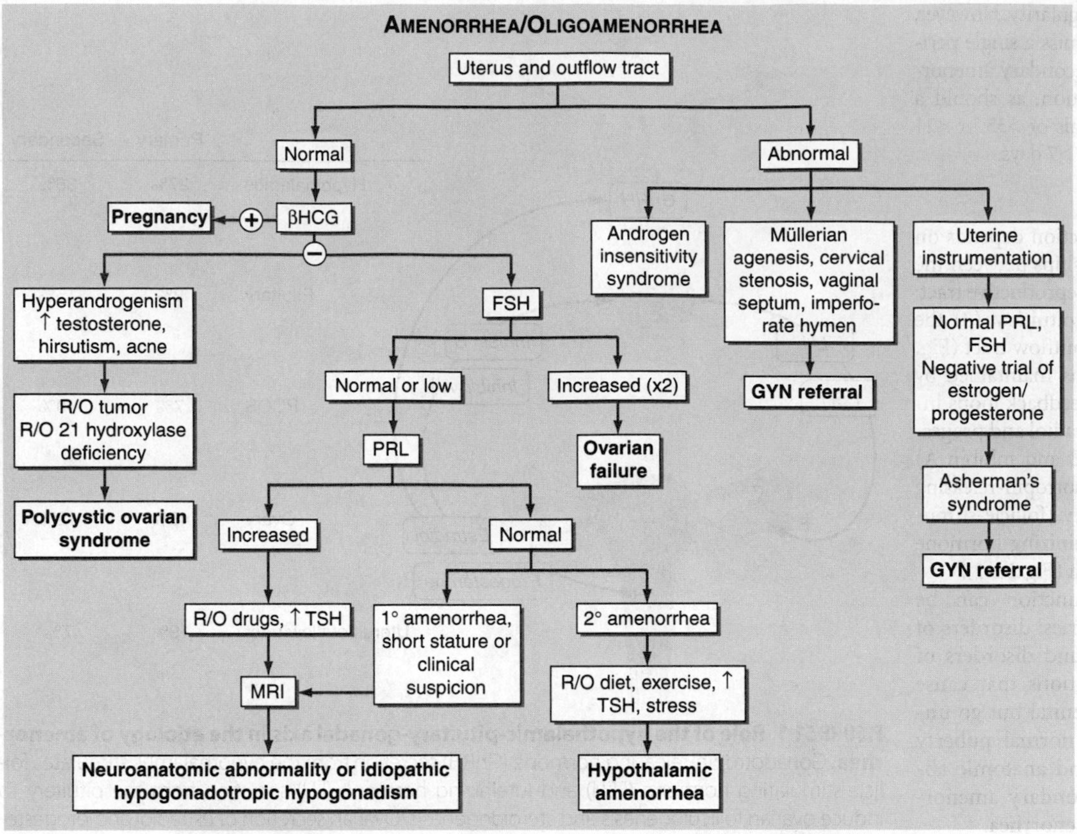

FIGURE 51-2 Algorithm for evaluation of amenorrhea. β-hCG, human chorionic gonadotropin; PRL, prolactin; FSH, follicle-stimulating hormone; TSH, thyroid-stimulating hormone.

prolactinemia, even if mild, necessitates cranial imaging with CT or MRI to exclude a neuroanatomic cause.

HYPERGONADOTROPIC HYPOGONADISM Ovarian failure is considered premature when it occurs in women younger than age 40. Ovarian failure is associated with the loss of negative-feedback restraint on the hypothalamus and pituitary, resulting in increased FSH and LH levels. FSH is a better marker of ovarian failure as its levels are less variable than LH. As with natural menopause, premature ovarian failure (POF) may wax and wane, and serial measurements may be necessary to establish the diagnosis.

Once the diagnosis of POF has been established, further evaluation is indicated because of other health problems that may be associated with POF. For example, POF is seen in association with a variety of chromosomal abnormalities including Turner syndrome, autoimmune polyglandular failure syndromes, radio- and chemotherapy, and galactosemia. In the majority of cases, however, a cause is not determined. The recognition that early ovarian failure occurs in premutation carriers of the fragile X syndrome is important because of increased risk of severe mental retardation in male children with *FMR1* mutations.

Hypergonadotropic hypogonadism occurs rarely in other disorders, such as mutations in the FSH or LH receptors. Aromatase deficiency and 17α-hydroxylase deficiency are associated with elevated gonadotropins with hyperandrogenism and hypertension, respectively. Gonadotropin-secreting tumors in women of reproductive age generally present with high, rather than low, estrogen levels and cause ovarian hyperstimulation or dysfunctional bleeding.

Rx AMENORRHEA CAUSED BY OVULATORY DISORDERS

Amenorrhea is almost always associated with chronically low levels of estrogen, whether it is caused by hypogonadotropic hypogonadism or ovarian failure. Development of secondary sexual characteristics requires gradual titration of estradiol replacement with eventual addition of a progestin. Symptoms of hypoestrogenism can be treated with hormone replacement therapy or oral contraceptive pills. Patients with hypogonadotropic hypogonadism who are interested in fertility require treatment with pulsatile GnRH or exogenous FSH and LH, whereas patients with ovarian failure can consider oocyte donation, which has a high chance of success in this population.

POLYCYSTIC OVARIAN SYNDROME (PCOS) This is diagnosed based on the presence of clinical or biochemical evidence of hyperandrogenism in association with amenorrhea or oligomenorrhea. Symptoms generally begin shortly after menarche and are slowly progressive. Lean patients with PCOS generally have high LH levels in the presence of normal to low levels of FSH and estradiol. The LH/FSH abnormality is less pronounced in obese patients in whom insulin resistance is a more prominent feature. Most patients also have a polycystic ovarian morphology on ultrasound, although there is controversy as to whether this morphology in combination with hyperandrogenism is sufficient for the diagnosis of PCOS.

Rx POLYCYSTIC OVARIAN SYNDROME

The major abnormality in patients with PCOS is the failure of regular, predictable ovulation. Thus, these patients are at risk for the development of dysfunctional bleeding and endometrial hyperplasia associated with unopposed estrogen exposure. Endometrial protection can be achieved with the use of oral contraceptives or progestins (medroxyprogesterone acetate, 5–10 mg, or prometrium, 200 mg daily for 10–14 days of each month). Oral contraceptives are also useful for management of hyperandrogenic symptoms, as is spironolactone, which functions as a weak androgen receptor antagonist. Management of the associated metabolic syndrome may be appropriate for some patients (Chap. 236). For patients interested in fertility, weight control is a critical first step. Clomiphene citrate is highly effective as first-line treatment, with or without the addition of metformin. Exogenous gonadotropins can be used by experienced practitioners.

PELVIC PAIN

The mechanisms causing pelvic pain are similar to those causing abdominal pain (Chap. 14) and include inflammation of the parietal peritoneum, obstruction of hollow viscera, vascular disturbances, and pain originating in the abdominal wall. Pelvic pain may reflect pelvic disease per se but may also reflect extrapelvic disorders that refer pain to the pel-

TABLE 51-1 CAUSES OF PELVIC PAIN		
	Acute	**Chronic**
Cyclic pelvic pain		Premenstrual symptoms Mittelschmerz Dysmenorrhea Endometriosis
Noncyclic pelvic pain	Pelvic inflammatory disease Ruptured or hemorrhagic ovarian cyst or ovarian torsion Ectopic pregnancy Endometritis Acute growth or degeneration of uterine myoma	Pelvic congestion syndrome Adhesions and retroversion of the uterus Pelvic malignancy Vulvodynia History of sexual abuse

vis. In up to 60% of cases, pelvic pain can be attributed to gastrointestinal problems including appendicitis, cholecystitis, infections, intestinal obstruction, diverticulitis, or inflammatory bowel disease. Urinary tract and musculoskeletal disorders are also common causes of pelvic pain.

APPROACH TO THE PATIENT: Pelvic Pain

A thorough history including the type, location, radiation, and status with respect to increasing or decreasing severity can help to identify the cause of acute pelvic pain. Specific associations with vaginal bleeding, sexual activity, defecation, urination, movement, or eating should be specifically sought. A careful menstrual history is essential to assess the possibility of pregnancy. Determination of whether the pain is acute versus chronic and cyclic versus noncyclic will direct further investigation (Table 51-1). However, disorders that cause cyclic pain may occasionally cause noncyclic pain, and the converse is also true.

ACUTE PELVIC PAIN

Pelvic inflammatory disease most commonly presents with bilateral lower abdominal pain. It is generally of recent onset and is exacerbated by intercourse or jarring movements. Fever is present in about half of patients; abnormal uterine bleeding occurs in about one-third. New vaginal discharge, urethritis, and chills may be present but are less specific signs. *Adnexal pathology* can present acutely and may be due to rupture, bleeding or torsion of cysts, or, much less commonly, neoplasms of the ovary, fallopian tubes, or paraovarian areas. Fever may be present with ovarian torsion. *Ectopic pregnancy* is associated with right or left sided lower abdominal pain, vaginal bleeding and menstrual cycle abnormalities, with clinical signs generally appearing 6–8 weeks after the last normal menstrual period. Orthostatic signs and fever may be present. Risk factors include the presence of known tubal disease, previous ectopic pregnancies, or a history of infertility, DES exposure of the mother in utero, or a history of pelvic infections. *Uterine pathology* includes endometritis and, less frequently, degenerating leiomyomas (fibroids). Endometritis is often associated with vaginal bleeding and systemic signs of infection. It occurs in the setting of sexually transmitted infections, uterine instrumentation, or postpartum infection.

A sensitive pregnancy test, complete blood count with differential, urinalysis, tests for chlamydial and gonococcal infections, and abdominal ultrasound aid in making the diagnosis and directing further management.

Rx ACUTE PELVIC PAIN

Treatment of acute pelvic pain depends on the suspected etiology but may require surgical or gynecologic intervention. Conservative management is an important consideration for ovarian cysts, if torsion is not suspected, to avoid unnecessary pelvic surgery and the subsequent risk of infertility due to adhesions. The majority of unruptured ectopic pregnancies are now treated with methotrexate, which is effective in 84–96% of cases. However, surgical treatment may be required.

CHRONIC PELVIC PAIN

Some women experience discomfort at the time of ovulation (*mittelschmerz*). Pain can be quite intense but is generally of short duration. The mechanism is thought to involve rapid expansion of the dominant follicle, although it may also be caused by peritoneal irritation by follicular fluid released at the time of ovulation. Many women experience premenstrual symptoms such as breast discomfort, food cravings, and abdominal bloating or discomfort. These moliminal symptoms are a good predictor of ovulation, although their absence is less helpful.

Dysmenorrhea *Dysmenorrhea* refers to the crampy lower abdominal discomfort that begins with the onset of menstrual bleeding and gradually decreases over the next 12–72 h. It may be associated with nausea, diarrhea, fatigue, and headache and occurs in 60–93% of adolescents, beginning with the establishment of regular ovulatory cycles. Its prevalence decreases after pregnancy and with the use of oral contraceptives.

Primary dysmenorrhea results from increased stores of prostaglandin precursors, which are generated by sequential stimulation of the uterus by estrogen and progesterone. During menstruation these precursors are converted to prostaglandins, which cause intense uterine contractions, decreased blood flow, and increased peripheral nerve hypersensitivity, resulting in pain.

Secondary dysmenorrhea is caused by underlying pelvic pathology. *Endometriosis* results from the presence of endometrial glands and stroma outside of the uterus. These deposits of ectopic endometrium respond to hormonal stimulation and cause dysmenorrhea, which generally precedes menstruation by several days. Endometriosis may also be associated with painful intercourse, painful bowel movements, and tender nodules in the uterosacral ligament. Fibrosis and adhesions can produce lateral displacement of the cervix. The CA125 level may be increased, but it has low negative predictive value. Definitive diagnosis requires laparoscopy. Symptomatology does not always predict the extent of endometriosis. Other secondary causes of dysmenorrhea include adenomyosis, a condition caused by the presence of ectopic endometrial glands and stroma within the myometrium. Cervical stenosis may result from trauma, infection, or surgery.

Rx DYSMENORRHEA

Local application of heat; use of vitamins B_1, B_6, and E and magnesium; acupuncture; yoga; and exercise are of some benefit for the treatment of dysmenorrhea. However, nonsteroidal anti-inflammatory drugs (NSAIDs) are the most effective treatment and provide >80% sustained response rates. Ibuprofen, naproxen, ketoprofen, mefanamic acid, and nimesulide are all superior to placebo. Treatment should be started a day before expected menses and is generally continued for 2–3 days. Oral contraceptives also reduce symptoms of dysmenorrhea. Failure of response to NSAIDs and oral contraceptives is suggestive of a pelvic disorder, such as endometriosis, and diagnostic laparoscopy should be considered to guide further treatment.

FURTHER READINGS

Dawood MY: Primary dysmenorrhea: Advances in pathogenesis and management. Obstet Gynecol 108:428, 2006

Genazzani AD et al: Diagnostic and therapeutic approach to hypothalamic amenorrhea. Ann NY Acad Sci 1092:103, 2006

Hall JE: Neuroendocrine control of the menstrual cycle, in *Yen and Jaffe's Reproductive Endocrinology*, 5th ed. JF Strauss, RL Barbieri (eds). Philadelphia, Elsevier, 2004, pp 195–211

Latthe P et al: Factors predisposing women to chronic pelvic pain: Systematic review. BMJ 332(7544):749, 2006

Pittock ST et al: Mayer-Rokitansky-Kuster-Hauser anomaly and its associated malformations. Am J Med Genet A 135:314, 2005

Wittenberger MD et al: The FMR1 premutation and reproduction. Fertil Steril 87:456, 2007

52 Approach to the Patient with a Skin Disorder

Thomas J. Lawley, Kim B. Yancey

The challenge of examining the skin lies in distinguishing normal from abnormal, significant findings from trivial ones, and in integrating pertinent signs and symptoms into an appropriate differential diagnosis. The fact that the largest organ in the body is visible is both an advantage and a disadvantage to those who examine it. It is advantageous because no special instrumentation is necessary and because the skin can be biopsied with little morbidity. However, the casual observer can be misled by a variety of stimuli and overlook important, subtle signs of skin or systemic disease. For instance, the sometimes minor differences in color and shape that distinguish a melanoma (Fig. 52-1) from a benign nevomelanocytic nevus (Fig. 52-2) can be difficult to recognize. To aid in the interpretation of skin lesions, a variety of descriptive terms have been developed to characterize cutaneous lesions (Tables 52-1, 52-2, and 52-3 as well as Fig. 52-3) and to formulate a differential diagnosis (Table 52-4). For instance, the finding of scaling papules (present in patients with psoriasis or atopic dermatitis) places the patient in a different diagnostic category than would hemorrhagic papules, which may indicate vasculitis or sepsis (Figs. 52-4 and 52-5, respectively). It is also important to differentiate primary from secondary skin lesions. If the examiner focuses on linear erosions overlying an area of erythema and scaling, he or she may incorrectly assume that the erosion is the primary lesion and the redness and scale are secondary, while the correct interpretation would be that the patient has a pruritic eczematous dermatitis with erosions caused by scratching.

APPROACH TO THE PATIENT: Skin Disorder

In examining the skin it is usually advisable to assess the patient before taking an extensive history. This way, the entire cutaneous surface is sure to be evaluated, and objective findings can be integrated with relevant historic data. Four basic features of a skin lesion must be noted and considered during a physical examination: the distribution of the eruption, the types of primary and secondary lesions, the shape of individual lesions, and the arrangement of the lesions. An ideal skin examination includes evaluation of the skin, hair, and

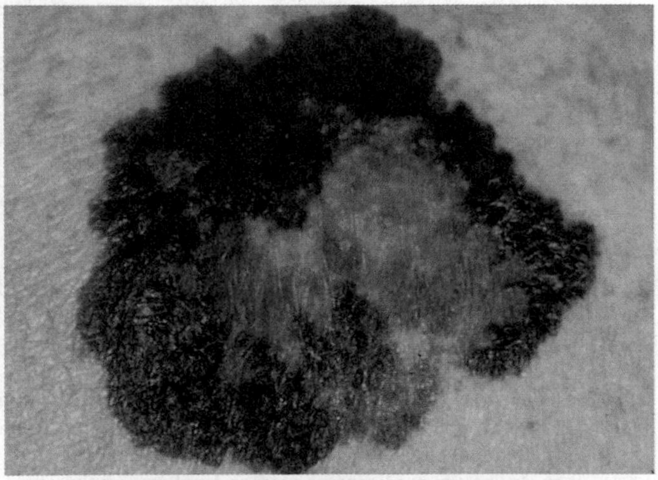

FIGURE 52-1 Superficial spreading melanoma. This is the most common type of melanoma. Such lesions usually demonstrate asymmetry, border irregularity, color variegation (black, blue, brown, pink, and white), a diameter >6 mm, and a history of change (e.g., an increase in size or development of associated symptoms such as pruritus or pain).

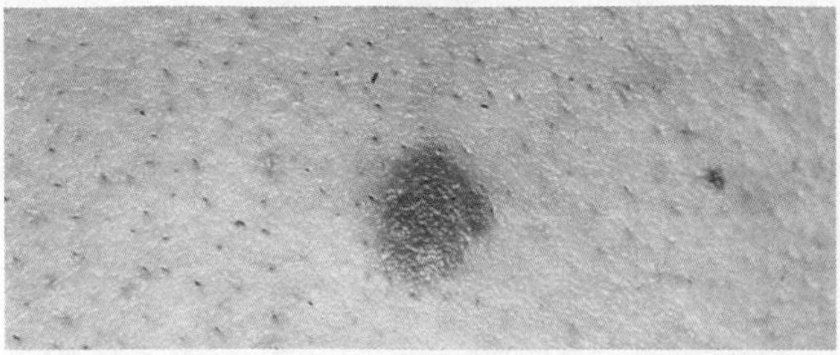

FIGURE 52-2 Nevomelanocytic nevus. Nevi are benign proliferations of nevomelanocytes characterized by regularly shaped hyperpigmented macules or papules of a uniform color.

TABLE 52-1 DESCRIPTION OF PRIMARY SKIN LESIONS

Macule: A flat, colored lesion, <2 cm in diameter, not raised above the surface of the surrounding skin. A "freckle," or ephelid, is a prototype pigmented macule.
Patch: A large (>2 cm) flat lesion with a color different from the surrounding skin. This differs from a macule only in size.
Papule: A small, solid lesion, <0.5 cm in diameter, raised above the surface of the surrounding skin and hence palpable (e.g., a closed comedone, or whitehead, in acne).
Nodule: A larger (0.5–5.0 cm), firm lesion raised above the surface of the surrounding skin. This differs from a papule only in size (e.g., a dermal nevomelanocytic nevus).
Tumor: A solid, raised growth >5 cm in diameter.
Plaque: A large (>1 cm), flat-topped, raised lesion; edges may either be distinct (e.g., in psoriasis) or gradually blend with surrounding skin (e.g., in eczematous dermatitis).
Vesicle: A small, fluid-filled lesion, <0.5 cm in diameter, raised above the plane of surrounding skin. Fluid is often visible, and the lesions are translucent [e.g., vesicles in allergic contact dermatitis caused by *Toxicodendron* (poison ivy)].
Pustule: A vesicle filled with leukocytes. Note: The presence of pustules does not necessarily signify the existence of an infection.
Bulla: A fluid-filled, raised, often translucent lesion >0.5 cm in diameter.
Wheal: A raised, erythematous, edematous papule or plaque, usually representing short-lived vasodilatation and vasopermeability.
Telangiectasia: A dilated, superficial blood vessel.

TABLE 52-2 DESCRIPTION OF SECONDARY SKIN LESIONS

Lichenification: A distinctive thickening of the skin that is characterized by accentuated skin-fold markings.
Scale: Excessive accumulation of stratum corneum.
Crust: Dried exudate of body fluids that may be either yellow (i.e., serous crust) or red (i.e., hemorrhagic crust).
Erosion: Loss of epidermis without an associated loss of dermis.
Ulcer: Loss of epidermis and at least a portion of the underlying dermis.
Excoriation: Linear, angular erosions that may be covered by crust and are caused by scratching.
Atrophy: An acquired loss of substance. In the skin, this may appear as a depression with intact epidermis (i.e., loss of dermal or subcutaneous tissue) or as sites of shiny, delicate, wrinkled lesions (i.e., epidermal atrophy).
Scar: A change in the skin secondary to trauma or inflammation. Sites may be erythematous, hypopigmented, or hyperpigmented depending on their age or character. Sites on hair-bearing areas may be characterized by destruction of hair follicles.

TABLE 52-3 COMMON DERMATOLOGIC TERMS

Alopecia: Hair loss; it may be partial or complete.
Annular: Ring-shaped lesions.
Cyst: A soft, raised, encapsulated lesion filled with semisolid or liquid contents.
Herpetiform: Grouped lesions.
Lichenoid: Violaceous to purple, polygonal lesions that resemble those seen in lichen planus.
Milia: Small, firm, white papules filled with keratin.
Morbilliform: Generalized, small erythematous macules and/or papules that resemble lesions seen in measles.
Nummular: Coin-shaped lesions.
Poikiloderma: Skin that displays variegated pigmentation, atrophy, and telangiectases.
Polycyclic: A configuration of skin lesions formed from coalescing rings or incomplete rings.
Pruritus: A sensation that elicits the desire to scratch. Pruritus is often the predominant symptom of inflammatory skin diseases (e.g., atopic dermatitis, allergic contact dermatitis); it is also commonly associated with xerosis and aged skin. Systemic conditions that can be associated with pruritus include chronic renal disease, cholestasis, pregnancy, malignancy, thyroid disease, polycythemia vera, and delusions of parasitosis.

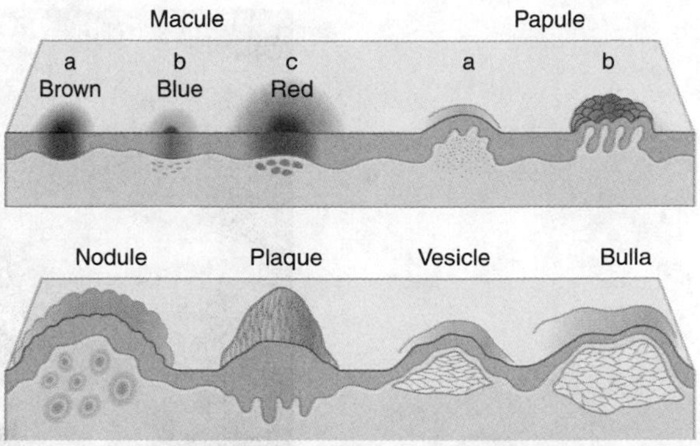

FIGURE 52-3 A schematic representation of several common primary skin lesions (see Table 52-1).

nails as well as the mucous membranes of the mouth, eyes, nose, nasopharynx, and anogenital region. In the initial examination it is important that the patient be disrobed as completely as possible. This will minimize chances of missing important individual skin

TABLE 52-4 SELECTED COMMON DERMATOLOGIC CONDITIONS

Diagnosis	Common Distribution	Usual Morphology
Acne vulgaris	Face, upper back	Open and closed comedones, erythematous papules, pustules, cysts
Rosacea	Blush area of cheeks, nose, forehead, chin	Erythema, telangiectases, papules, pustules
Seborrheic dermatitis	Scalp, eyebrows, perinasal areas	Erythema with greasy yellow-brown scale
Atopic dermatitis	Antecubital and popliteal fossae; may be widespread	Patches and plaques of erythema, scaling, and lichenification; pruritus
Stasis dermatitis	Ankles, lower legs	Patches of erythema and scaling on background of hyperpigmentation associated with signs of venous insufficiency
Dyshidrotic eczema	Palms, soles, sides of fingers and toes	Deep vesicles
Allergic contact dermatitis	Anywhere	Localized erythema, vesicles, scale, and pruritus (e.g., fingers, earlobes—nickel; dorsal aspect of foot—shoe; exposed surfaces—poison ivy)
Psoriasis	Elbows, knees, scalp, lower back, fingernails (may be generalized)	Papules and plaques covered with silvery scale; nails have pits
Lichen planus	Wrists, ankles, mouth (may be widespread)	Violaceous flat-topped papules and plaques
Keratosis pilaris	Extensor surfaces of arms and thighs, buttocks	Keratotic follicular papules with surrounding erythema
Melasma	Forehead, cheeks, temples, upper lip	Tan to brown patches
Vitiligo	Periorificial, trunk, extensor surfaces of extremities, flexor wrists, axillae	Chalk-white macules
Actinic keratosis	Sun-exposed areas	Skin-colored or red-brown macule or papule with dry, rough, adherent scale
Basal cell carcinoma	Face	Papule with pearly, telangiectatic border on sun-damaged skin
Squamous cell carcinoma	Face, especially lower lip, ears	Indurated and possibly hyperkeratotic lesions often showing ulceration and/or crusting
Seborrheic keratosis	Trunk, face	Brown plaques with adherent, greasy scale; "stuck on" appearance
Folliculitis	Any hair-bearing area	Follicular pustules
Impetigo	Anywhere	Papules, vesicles, pustules, often with honey-colored crusts
Herpes simplex	Lips, genitalia	Grouped vesicles progressing to crusted erosions
Herpes zoster	Dermatomal, usually trunk but may be anywhere	Vesicles limited to a dermatome (often painful)
Varicella	Face, trunk, relative sparing of extremities	Lesions arise in crops and quickly progress from erythematous macules to papules to vesicles to pustules to crusted sites
Pityriasis rosea	Trunk (Christmas tree pattern); herald patch followed by multiple smaller lesions	Symmetric erythematous patches with a collarette of scale
Tinea versicolor	Chest, back, abdomen, proximal extremities	Scaly hyper- or hypopigmented macules
Candidiasis	Groin, beneath breasts, vagina, oral cavity	Erythematous macerated areas with satellite pustules; white, friable patches on mucous membranes
Dermatophytosis	Feet, groin, beard, or scalp	Varies with site, (e.g., tinea corporis—scaly annular patch)
Scabies	Groin, axillae, between fingers and toes, beneath breasts	Excoriated papules, burrows, pruritus
Insect bites	Anywhere	Erythematous papules with central puncta
Cherry angioma	Trunk	Red, blood-filled papules
Keloid	Anywhere (site of previous injury)	Firm tumor, pink, purple, or brown
Dermatofibroma	Anywhere	Firm red to brown nodule that shows dimpling of overlying skin with lateral compression
Acrochordons (skin tags)	Groin, axilla, neck	Fleshy papules
Urticaria	Anywhere	Wheals, sometimes with surrounding flare; pruritus
Transient acantholytic dermatosis	Trunk, especially anterior chest	Erythematous papules
Xerosis	Extensor extremities, especially legs	Dry, erythematous, scaling patches; pruritus

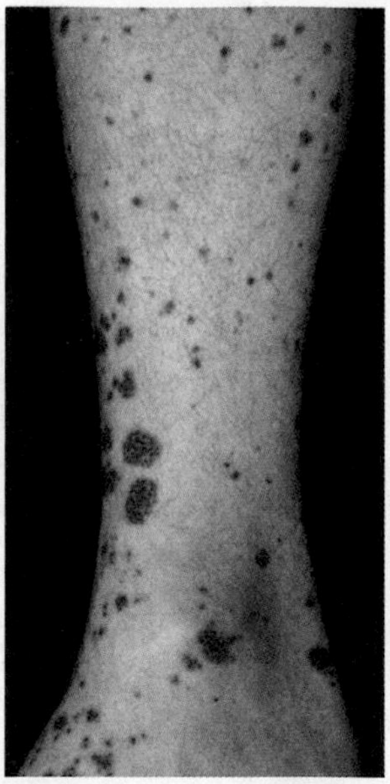

FIGURE 52-4 Necrotizing vasculitis. Palpable purpuric papules on the lower legs are seen in this patient with cutaneous small vessel vasculitis. *(Courtesy of Robert Swerlick, MD; with permission.)*

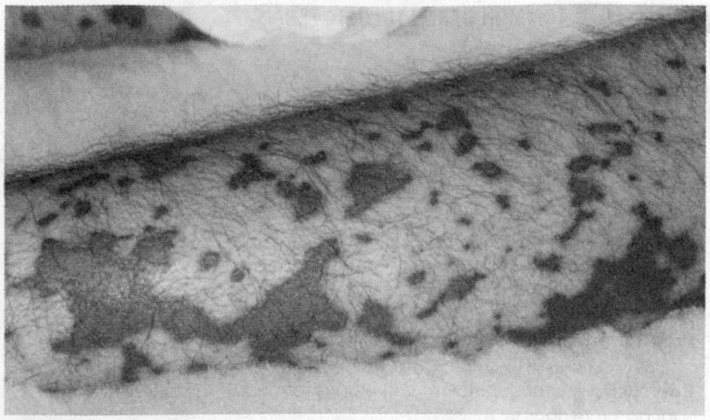

FIGURE 52-5 Meningococcemia. An example of fulminant meningococcemia with extensive angular purpuric patches. *(Courtesy of Stephen E. Gellis, MD; with permission.)*

lesions and make it possible to assess the distribution of the eruption accurately. The patient should first be viewed from a distance of about 1.5–2 m (4–6 ft) so that the general character of the skin and the distribution of lesions can be evaluated. Indeed, distribution of lesions often correlates highly with diagnosis (Fig. 52-6). For example, a hospitalized patient with a generalized erythematous exanthem is more likely to have a drug eruption than is a patient with a similar rash limited to the sun-exposed portions of the face. Once the distribution of the lesions has been established, the nature of the primary lesion must be determined. Thus, when lesions are distributed on elbows, knees, and scalp, the most likely possibility based solely on distribution is psoriasis or dermatitis herpetiformis (Figs. 52-7 and 52-8, respectively). The primary lesion in psoriasis is a scaly papule that soon forms erythematous plaques covered with a white scale, whereas that of dermatitis herpetiformis is an urticarial papule that quickly becomes a small vesicle. In this manner, identification of the primary lesion directs the examiner toward the proper diagnosis. Secondary changes in skin can also be quite helpful. For example, scale represents excessive epidermis, while crust is the result of a discontinuous epithelial cell layer. Palpation of skin lesions can also yield insight into the character of an eruption. Thus, red papules on the lower extremities that blanch with pressure can be a manifestation of many different diseases, but hemorrhagic red papules that do not blanch with pressure indicate palpable purpura characteristic of necrotizing vasculitis (Fig. 52-4).

The shape of lesions is also an important feature. Flat, round, erythematous papules and plaques are common in many cutaneous diseases. However, target-shaped lesions that consist in part of erythematous plaques are specific for erythema multiforme (Fig. 52-9). In the same way, the arrangement of individual lesions is important. Erythematous papules and vesicles can occur in many conditions, but their arrangement in a specific linear array suggests an external etiology such as allergic contact (Fig. 52-10) or primary irritant dermatitis. In contrast, lesions with a generalized arrangement are common and suggest a systemic etiology.

As in other branches of medicine, a complete history should be obtained to emphasize the following features:

1. Evolution of lesions
   a. Site of onset
   b. Manner in which the eruption progressed or spread

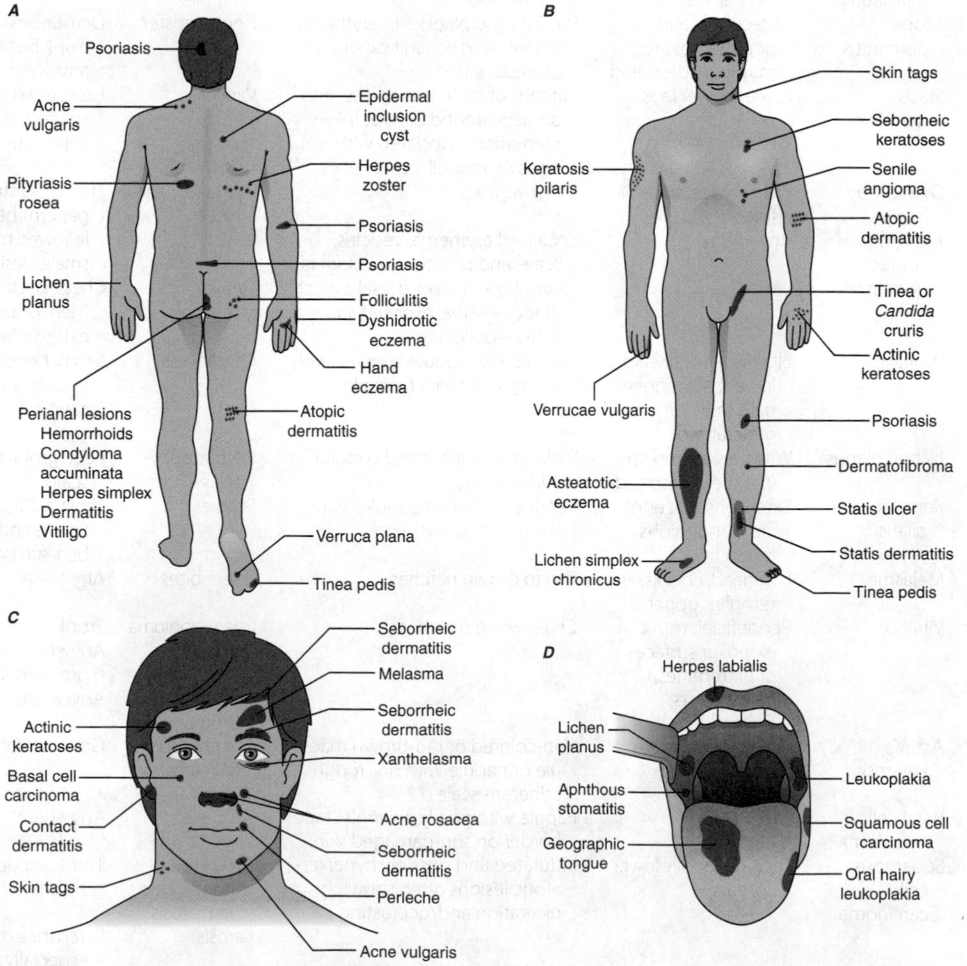

FIGURE 52-6 ***A–D.*** **The distribution of some common dermatologic diseases and lesions.**

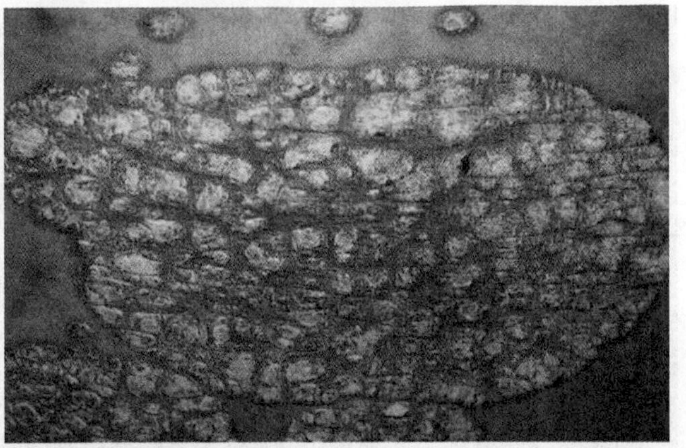

FIGURE 52-7 Psoriasis. This papulosquamous skin disease is characterized by small and large erythematous papules and plaques with overlying adherent silvery scale.

   c. Duration
   d. Periods of resolution or improvement in chronic eruptions
2. Symptoms associated with the eruption
   a. Itching, burning, pain, numbness
   b. What, if anything, has relieved symptoms
   c. Time of day when symptoms are most severe
3. Current or recent medications (prescribed as well as over-the-counter)
4. Associated systemic symptoms (e.g., malaise, fever, arthralgias)
5. Ongoing or previous illnesses
6. History of allergies
7. Presence of photosensitivity
8. Review of systems
9. Family history (particularly relevant for patients with melanoma, atopy, psoriasis, or acne)
10. Social, sexual, or travel history as relevant to the patient

DIAGNOSTIC TECHNIQUES

Many skin diseases can be diagnosed on gross clinical appearance, but sometimes relatively simple diagnostic procedures can yield valuable information. In most instances, they can be performed at the bedside with a minimum of equipment.

Skin Biopsy A skin biopsy is a straightforward minor surgical procedure; however, it is important to biopsy a lesion that is most likely to yield diagnostic findings. This decision may require expertise in skin diseases and knowledge of superficial anatomic structures in selected areas of the body. In this procedure, a small area of skin is anesthetized with 1% lidocaine with or without epinephrine. The skin lesion in question can be excised or saucerized with a scalpel or removed by punch biopsy. In the latter technique, a punch is pressed against the surface of the skin and rotated with downward pressure until it penetrates to the subcutaneous tissue. The circular biopsy is then lifted with forceps, and the bottom is cut with iris scissors. Biopsy sites may or may not need suture closure, depending on size and location.

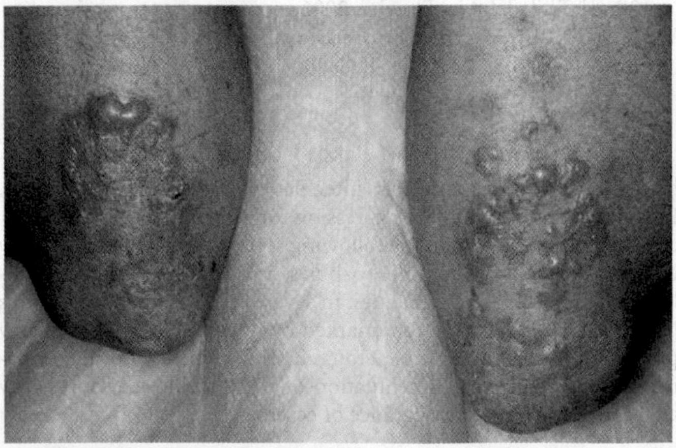

FIGURE 52-8 Dermatitis herpetiformis. This disorder typically displays pruritic, grouped papulovesicles on elbows, knees, buttocks, and posterior scalp. Vesicles are often excoriated due to associated pruritus.

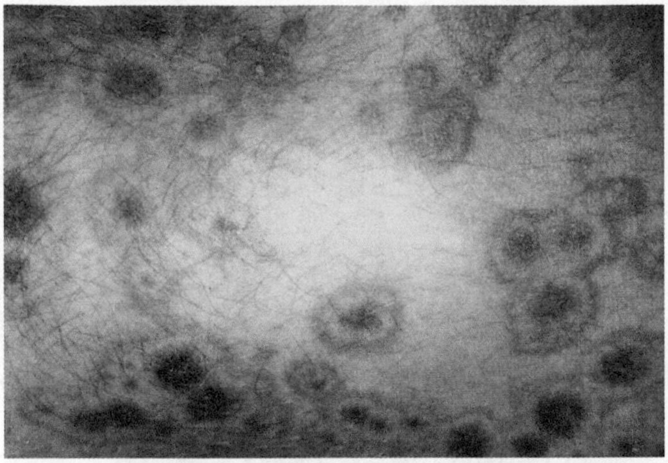

FIGURE 52-9 Erythema multiforme. This eruption is characterized by multiple erythematous plaques with a target or iris morphology. It usually represents a hypersensitivity reaction to drugs (e.g., sulfonylamides) or infections (e.g., HSV). *(Courtesy of the Yale Resident's Slide Collection; with permission.)*

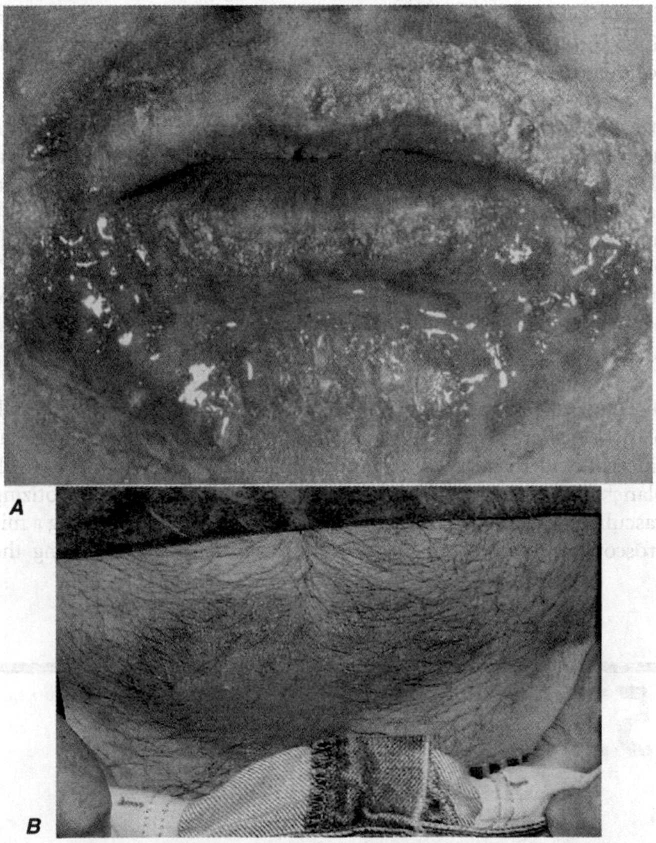

FIGURE 52-10 Allergic contact dermatitis (ACD). ***A.*** An example of ACD in its acute phase, with sharply demarcated, weeping, eczematous plaques in a perioral distribution. ***B.*** ACD in its chronic phase demonstrating an erythematous, lichenified, weeping plaque on skin chronically exposed to nickel in a metal snap. *(B, Courtesy of Robert Swerlick, MD; with permission.)*

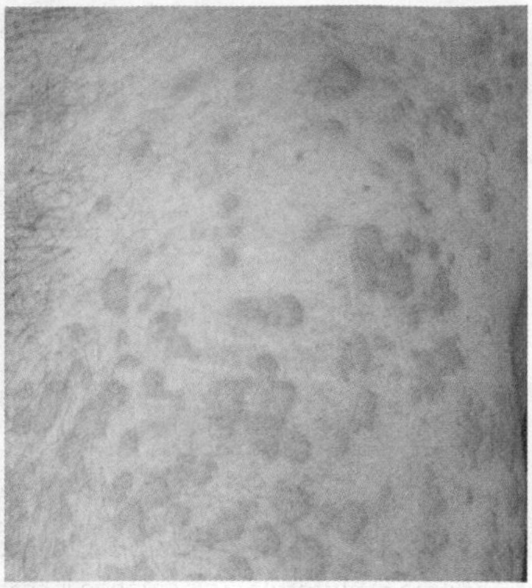

FIGURE 52-11 Urticaria. Discrete and confluent, edematous, erythematous papules and plaques are characteristic of this whealing eruption.

KOH Preparation A potassium hydroxide (KOH) preparation is performed on scaling skin lesions where a fungal infection is suspected. The edge of such a lesion is scraped gently with a no. 15 scalpel blade, and the removed scale is collected on a glass microscope slide then treated with 1 to 2 drops of a solution of 10–20% KOH. KOH dissolves keratin and allows easier visualization of fungal elements. Brief heating of the slide accelerates dissolution of keratin. When the preparation is viewed under the microscope, the refractile hyphae will be seen more easily when the light intensity is reduced and the condenser is lowered. This technique can be utilized to identify hyphae in dermatophyte infections, pseudohyphae and budding yeast in *Candida* infections (see Fig. 196-1), and "spaghetti and meatballs" yeast forms in tinea versicolor. The same sampling technique can be used to obtain scale for culture of selected pathogenic organisms.

Tzanck Smear A Tzanck smear is a cytologic technique most often used in the diagnosis of herpesvirus infections [herpes simplex virus (HSV) or varicella zoster virus (VZV)] (see Figs. 173-1 and 173-3). An early vesicle, not a pustule or crusted lesion, is unroofed, and the base of the lesion is scraped gently with a scalpel blade. The material is placed on a glass slide, air-dried, and stained with Giemsa or Wright's stain. Multinucleated epithelial giant cells suggest the presence of HSV or VZV; culture or immunofluorescence testing must be performed to identify the specific virus.

Diascopy Diascopy is designed to assess whether a skin lesion will blanch with pressure as, for example, in determining whether a red lesion is hemorrhagic or simply blood-filled. Urticaria (Fig. 52-11) will blanch with pressure, whereas a purpuric lesion caused by necrotizing vasculitis (Fig. 52-4) will not. Diascopy is performed by pressing a microscope slide or magnifying lens against a lesion and noting the amount of blanching that occurs. Granulomas often have an opaque to transparent, brown-pink "apple jelly" appearance on diascopy.

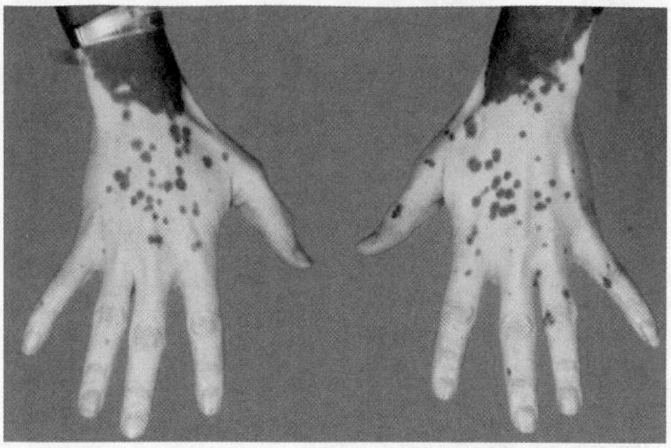

FIGURE 52-12 Vitiligo. Characteristic lesions display an acral distribution and striking depigmentation as a result of loss of melanocytes.

Wood's Light A Wood's lamp generates 360-nm ultraviolet (or "black") light that can be used to aid the evaluation of certain skin disorders. For example, a Wood's lamp will cause erythrasma (a superficial, intertriginous infection caused by *Corynebacterium minutissimum*) to show a characteristic coral pink color, and wounds colonized by *Pseudomonas* to appear pale blue. Tinea capitis caused by certain dermatophytes such as *Microsporum canis* or *M. audouini* exhibits a yellow fluorescence. Pigmented lesions of the epidermis such as freckles are accentuated, while dermal pigment such as postinflammatory hyperpigmentation fades under a Wood's light. Vitiligo (Fig. 52-12) appears totally white under a Wood's lamp, and previously unsuspected areas of involvement often become apparent. A Wood's lamp may also aid in the demonstration of tinea versicolor and in recognition of ash leaf spots in patients with tuberous sclerosis.

Patch Tests Patch testing is designed to document sensitivity to a specific antigen. In this procedure, a battery of suspected allergens is applied to the patient's back under occlusive dressings and allowed to remain in contact with the skin for 48 h. The dressings are removed, and the area is examined for evidence of delayed hypersensitivity reactions (e.g., erythema, edema, or papulovesicles). This test is best performed by physicians with special expertise in patch testing and is often helpful in the evaluation of patients with chronic dermatitis.

FURTHER READINGS

DERMATOLOGY LEXICON PROJECT: *www.futurehealth.rochester.edu/dlp2/*

JAMES WD et al: *Andrews' Diseases of the Skin: Clinical Dermatology*, 10th ed. Philadelphia, Elsevier, 2006

WOLFF K et al (eds): *Fitzpatrick's Dermatology in General Medicine*, 7th ed. New York, McGraw-Hill, 2008

53 Eczema, Psoriasis, Cutaneous Infections, Acne, and Other Common Skin Disorders

Calvin O. McCall, Thomas J. Lawley

ECZEMA AND DERMATITIS

Eczema is a type of dermatitis and these terms are often used synonymously (atopic eczema or atopic dermatitis). Eczema is a reaction pattern that presents with variable clinical findings and the common histologic finding of spongiosis (intercellular edema of the epidermis). Eczema is the final common expression for a number of disorders, including those discussed in the following sections. Primary lesions may include erythematous macules, papules, and vesicles, which can coalesce to form patches and plaques. In severe eczema, secondary lesions from infection or excoriation, marked by weeping and crusting, may predominate. In chronic eczematous conditions, lichenification (cutaneous hypertrophy and accentuation of normal skin markings) may alter the characteristic appearance of eczema.

ATOPIC DERMATITIS

Atopic dermatitis (AD) is the cutaneous expression of the atopic state, characterized by a family history of asthma, allergic rhinitis, or ecze-

TABLE 53-1 CLINICAL FEATURES OF ATOPIC DERMATITIS

1. Pruritus and scratching
2. Course marked by exacerbations and remissions
3. Lesions typical of eczematous dermatitis
4. Personal or family history of atopy (asthma, allergic rhinitis, food allergies, or eczema)
5. Clinical course lasting longer than 6 weeks
6. Lichenification of skin

ma. The prevalence of AD is increasing worldwide. Some of its features are shown in Table 53-1.

The etiology of AD is only partially defined, but there is a clear genetic predisposition. When both parents are affected by AD, >80% of their children manifest the disease. When only one parent is affected, the prevalence drops to slightly over 50%. Patients with AD may display a variety of immunoregulatory abnormalities including increased IgE synthesis, increased serum IgE, and impaired delayed-type hypersensitivity reactions.

The clinical presentation often varies with age. Half of patients with AD present within the first year of life, and 80% present by 5 years of age. About 80% ultimately coexpress allergic rhinitis or asthma. The infantile pattern is characterized by weeping inflammatory patches and crusted plaques on the face, neck, and extensor surfaces. The childhood and adolescent pattern is marked by dermatitis of flexural skin, particularly in the antecubital and popliteal fossae (Fig. 53-1). AD may resolve spontaneously, but over half of all individuals affected as children will have dermatitis in adult life. The distribution of lesions may be similar to those seen in childhood; however, adults frequently have localized disease, manifesting as lichen simplex chronicus or hand eczema (see below). In patients with localized disease, AD may be suspected because of a typical personal history, family history, or the presence of cutaneous stigmata of AD such as perioral pallor, an extra fold of skin beneath the lower eyelid (Dennie's line), increased palmar skin markings, and an increased incidence of cutaneous infections, particularly with *Staphylococcus aureus*. Regardless of other manifestations, pruritus is a prominent characteristic of AD in all age groups and is exacerbated by dry skin. Many of the cutaneous findings in affected patients, such as lichenification, are secondary to rubbing and scratching.

℞ ATOPIC DERMATITIS

Therapy of AD should include avoidance of cutaneous irritants, adequate moisturizing through the application of emollients, judicious use of topical anti-inflammatory agents, and prompt treatment of secondary infection. Patients should be instructed to bathe no more often than daily using warm or cool water, and to use only mild bath soap. Immediately after bathing while the skin is still moist, a topical anti-inflammatory agent in a cream or ointment base should be applied to areas of dermatitis, and all other skin areas should be lubricated with a moisturizer. Approximately 30 g of a topical agent is required to cover the entire body surface of an average adult.

Low- to midpotency topical glucocorticoids are employed in most treatment regimens for AD. Skin atrophy and the potential for systemic absorption are constant concerns, especially with more potent agents. Low-potency topical glucocorticoids or non-glucocorticoid anti-inflammatory agents should be selected for use on the face and intertriginous areas to minimize the risk of skin atrophy. Two non-glucocorticoid anti-inflammatory agents are now available, tacrolimus ointment and pimecrolimus cream. These agents are macrolide immunosuppressants that are approved by the U.S. Food and Drug Administration (FDA) for topical use in AD. Reports of broader effectiveness appear in the literature. These agents do not cause skin atrophy, nor do they suppress the hypothalamic-pituitary-adrenal axis. Recently, however, concerns have emerged regarding the potential for lymphomas in patients treated with these agents. Thus, caution should be exercised when considering these agents. Currently, they are also more costly than topical glucocorticoids.

Secondary infection of eczematous skin may lead to exacerbation of AD. Crusted and weeping skin lesions may be infected with *S. aureus*. When secondary infection is suspected, eczematous lesions should be cultured and patients treated with systemic antibiotics active against *S. aureus*. The initial use of penicillinase-resistant penicillins or cephalosporins is preferable. Dicloxacillin or cephalexin (250 mg qid for 7–10 days) is generally adequate; however, antibiotic selection must be directed by culture results and clinical response. More than 50% of *S. aureus* (SA) isolates are now methacillin resistant (MR) in some communities—community acquired MRSA (CA-MRSA). Current recommendations for the treatment of CA-MRSA infection in adults include trimethoprim/sulfamethoxazole (1–2 double strength bid), minocycline (100 mg bid), doxycycline (100 mg bid), or clindamycin (300–450 mg qid). Duration of therapy should be 7–10 days. Inducible resistance may limit clindamycin's usefulness. The latter can be detected by the double-disc diffusion test, which should be ordered if the isolate is erythromycin-resistant and clindamycin-sensitive. As an adjunct, the use of triclosan-containing antibacterial washes and intermittent nasal mupirocin may be useful.

Control of pruritus is essential for treatment, since AD often represents "an itch that rashes." Antihistamines are most often used to control pruritus, and mild sedation may be responsible for their antipruritic action. Sedation may also limit their usefulness; however, when used at bedtime, sedating antihistamines may improve the patient's sleep. Unlike their effects in urticaria, nonsedating antihistamines and selective H_2 blockers are of little use in controlling the pruritus of AD.

Treatment with systemic glucocorticoids should be limited to severe exacerbations unresponsive to topical therapy. In the patient with chronic AD, therapy with systemic glucocorticoids will generally clear the skin only briefly, and cessation of the systemic therapy will invariably be accompanied by return, if not worsening, of the dermatitis. Patients who do not respond to conventional therapies should be considered for patch testing to rule out allergic contact dermatitis. The role of dietary allergens in atopic dermatitis is controversial, and there is little evidence they play any role outside of infancy. Immunotherapy with aeroallergens has not proven useful in AD.

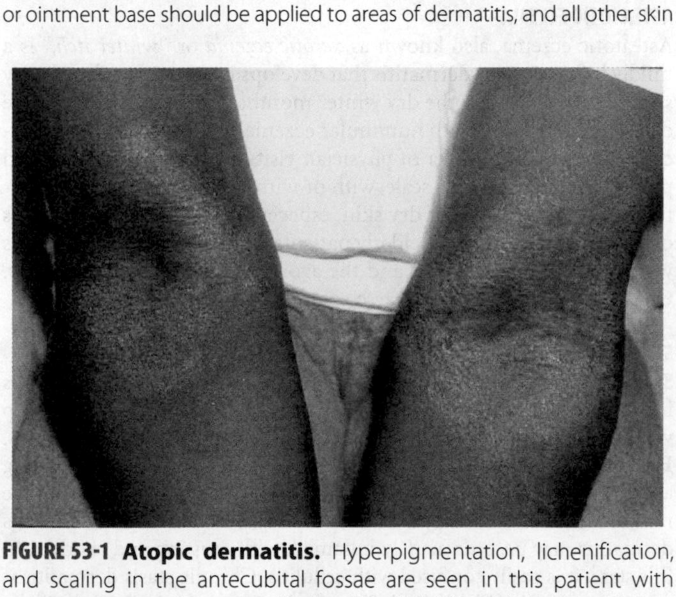

FIGURE 53-1 Atopic dermatitis. Hyperpigmentation, lichenification, and scaling in the antecubital fossae are seen in this patient with atopic dermatitis. (*Courtesy of Robert Swerlick, MD; with permission.*)

LICHEN SIMPLEX CHRONICUS

Lichen simplex chronicus may represent the end stage of a variety of pruritic and eczematous disorders, including atopic dermatitis. It consists of a circumscribed plaque or plaques of lichenified skin (thickening of the skin and accentuation of normal skin markings) due to chronic scratching or rubbing. Common areas involved include the posterior nuchal region, dorsum of the feet, and ankles. Treatment of lichen simplex chronicus centers on breaking the cycle of chronic itching and scratching. High-potency topical glucocorticoids are helpful in most cases, but in recalcitrant cases, application of topical glucocorticoids under occlusion, or intralesional injection of glucocorticoids may be required. Oral antihistamines such as hydroxyzine (10–25 mg every 6 h) or tricyclic antidepressants with antihistaminic activity, such as doxepin (10–25 mg at bedtime), are useful primarily due to their sedating action. Higher doses of these agents may be required, but sedation can become bothersome. Patients need to be counseled regarding driving or operating heavy equipment after taking these medications.

CONTACT DERMATITIS

Contact dermatitis is an inflammatory process in skin caused by an exogenous agent or agents that directly or indirectly injure the skin. This injury may be caused by an inherent characteristic of a compound—irritant contact dermatitis (ICD). An example of ICD would be dermatitis induced by a concentrated acid or base. Agents that cause allergic contact dermatitis (ACD) induce an antigen-specific immune response (poison ivy dermatitis). The clinical lesions of contact dermatitis may be acute (wet and edematous) or chronic (dry, thickened, and scaly), depending on the persistence of the insult (see Fig. 52-10).

Irritant Contact Dermatitis ICD is generally well demarcated and often localized to areas of thin skin (eyelids, intertriginous areas) or to areas where the irritant was occluded. Lesions may range from minimal skin erythema to areas of marked edema, vesicles, and ulcers. Chronic low-grade irritant dermatitis is the most common type of ICD, and the most common area of involvement is the hands (see below). The most common irritants encountered are chronic wet work, soaps, and detergents. Treatment should be directed to avoidance of irritants and use of protective gloves or clothing.

Allergic Contact Dermatitis ACD is a manifestation of delayed-type hypersensitivity mediated by memory T lymphocytes in the skin. The most common cause of ACD is exposure to plants, especially to members of the family Anacardiaceae, including the genus *Toxicodendron*. Poison ivy, poison oak, and poison sumac are members of this genus and cause an allergic reaction marked by erythema, vesiculation, and severe pruritus. The eruption is often linear or angular, corresponding to areas where plants have touched the skin. The sensitizing antigen common to these plants is urushiol, an oleoresin containing the active ingredient pentadecylcatechol. The oleoresin may adhere to skin, clothing, tools, and pets, and contaminated articles may cause dermatitis even after prolonged storage. Blister fluid does not contain urushiol and is not capable of inducing skin eruption in exposed subjects.

℞ CONTACT DERMATITIS

If contact dermatitis is suspected and an offending agent is identified and removed, the eruption will resolve. Usually, treatment with high-potency topical glucocorticoids is enough to relieve symptoms while the dermatitis runs its course. For those patients who require systemic therapy, daily oral prednisone beginning at 1 mg/kg, but usually ≤60 mg/d, is sufficient. It should be tapered over 2–3 weeks, and each daily dose given in the morning with food.

Identification of a contact allergen can be a difficult and time-consuming task. Patients with dermatitis unresponsive to conventional therapy or with an unusual and patterned distribution should be suspected of having ACD. They should be questioned carefully regarding occupational exposures and topical medications. Common sensitizers include preservatives in topical preparations, nickel sulfate, potassium dichromate, thimerosal, neomycin sulfate, fragrances, formaldehyde, and rubber-curing agents. Patch testing is helpful in identifying these agents but should not be attempted on patients with widespread active dermatitis or on those taking systemic glucocorticoids.

HAND ECZEMA

Hand eczema is a very common, chronic skin disorder in which both exogenous and endogenous factors play important roles. It may be associated with other cutaneous disorders such as atopic dermatitis, and contact with various agents may be involved. It represents a large proportion of occupation-associated skin disease. Chronic, excessive exposure to water and detergents, harsh chemicals, or allergens may initiate or aggravate this disorder. It may present with dryness and cracking of the skin of the hands as well as with variable amounts of erythema and edema. Often, the dermatitis will begin under rings where water and irritants are trapped. Dyshidrotic eczema, a variant of hand eczema, presents with multiple, intensely pruritic, small papules and vesicles occurring on the thenar and hypothenar eminences and the sides of the fingers (Fig. 53-2). Lesions tend to occur in crops that slowly form crusts and heal.

The evaluation of a patient with hand eczema should include an assessment of potential occupation-associated exposures. The history should be directed to identifying possible irritant or allergen exposures.

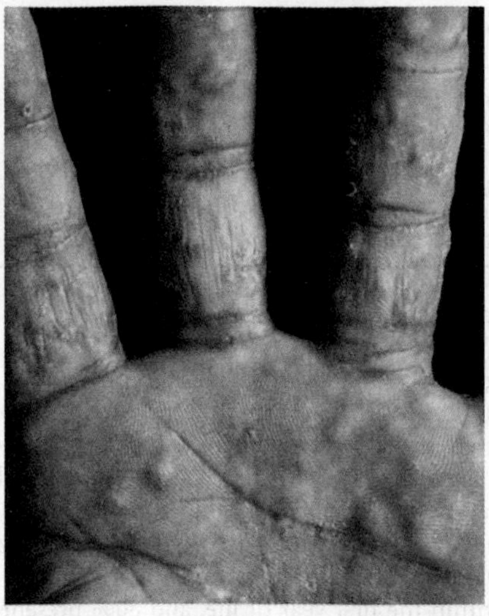

FIGURE 53-2 Dyshidrotic eczema. This example is characterized by deep-seated vesicles and scaling on palms and lateral fingers, and the disease is often associated with an atopic diathesis.

℞ HAND ECZEMA

Therapy of hand dermatitis is directed toward avoidance of irritants, identification of possible contact allergens, treatment of coexistent infection, and application of topical glucocorticoids. Whenever possible, the hands should be protected by gloves, preferably vinyl. The use of rubber gloves (latex) to protect dermatitic skin is sometimes associated with the development of hypersensitivity reactions to components of the gloves. Patients can be treated with cool moist compresses, followed by application of a mid- to high-potency topical glucocorticoid in a cream or ointment base. As with atopic dermatitis, treatment of secondary infection is essential for good control. Additionally, patients with hand dermatitis should be examined for dermatophyte infection by KOH preparation and culture (see below).

NUMMULAR ECZEMA

Nummular eczema is characterized by circular or oval "coinlike" lesions, beginning as small edematous papules that become crusted and scaly. The etiology of nummular eczema is unknown, but dry skin is a contributing factor. Common locations are the trunk or the extensor surfaces of the extremities, particularly on the pretibial areas or dorsum of the hands. It occurs more frequently in men and is most commonly seen in middle age. The treatment of nummular eczema is similar to that for atopic dermatitis.

ASTEATOTIC ECZEMA

Asteatotic eczema, also known as *xerotic eczema* or *"winter itch,"* is a mildly inflammatory dermatitis that develops in areas of extremely dry skin, especially during the dry winter months. Clinically, there may be considerable overlap with nummular eczema. This form of eczema accounts for a large number of physician visits because of the associated pruritus. Fine cracks and scale, with or without erythema, characteristically develop in areas of dry skin, especially on the anterior surfaces of the lower extremities in elderly patients. Asteatotic eczema responds well to topical moisturizers and the avoidance of cutaneous irritants. Overbathing and the use of harsh soaps exacerbate asteatotic eczema.

STASIS DERMATITIS AND STASIS ULCERATION

Stasis dermatitis develops on the lower extremities secondary to venous incompetence and chronic edema. Patients may give a history of deep venous thrombosis, have evidence of vein removal, or varicose veins. Early findings in stasis dermatitis consist of mild erythema and scaling associated with pruritus. The typical initial site of involvement is the medial aspect of the ankle, often over a distended vein (Fig. 53-3). Stasis dermatitis may become acutely inflamed, with crusting and exudate. In this state, it is easily confused with cellulitis. Chronic stasis dermatitis is often associated with dermal fibrosis that is recognized clinically as

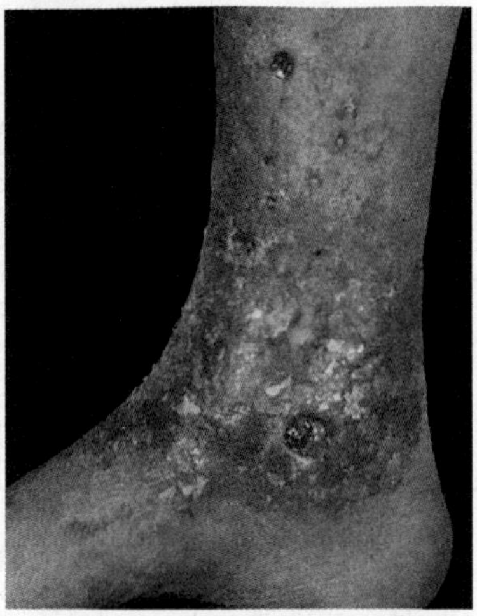

FIGURE 53-3 Stasis dermatitis. An example of stasis dermatitis showing erythematous, scaly, and oozing patches over the lower leg. Several stasis ulcers are also seen in this patient.

brawny edema of the skin. As the disorder progresses, the dermatitis becomes progressively pigmented, due to chronic erythrocyte extravasation leading to cutaneous hemosiderin deposition. Stasis dermatitis may be complicated by secondary infection and contact dermatitis. Severe stasis dermatitis may precede the development of stasis ulcers.

℞ STASIS DERMATITIS AND STASIS ULCERATION

Patients with stasis dermatitis and stasis ulceration benefit greatly from leg elevation and the routine use of compression stockings with a gradient of at least 30–40 mmHg. Stockings providing less compression, such as antiembolism hose, are poor substitutes. Use of emollients and/or midpotency topical glucocorticoids and avoidance of irritants are also helpful in treating stasis dermatitis. Protecting the legs from injury, including scratching, and control of chronic edema are essential to prevent ulcers. Diuretics may be required to adequately control chronic edema.

Stasis ulcers are difficult to treat, and resolution is slow. It is extremely important to elevate the affected limb as much as possible. The ulcer should be kept clear of necrotic material by gentle debridement and covered with a semipermeable dressing and a compression dressing or compression stocking. Glucocorticoids should not be applied to ulcers, since they may retard healing; however, they may be applied to the surrounding skin to control itching, scratching, and additional trauma. Secondarily infected lesions should be treated with appropriate oral antibiotics, but it should be noted that all ulcers will become colonized with bacteria, and the purpose of antibiotic therapy should not be to clear all bacterial growth. Care must be taken to exclude treatable causes of leg ulcers (hypercoagulation, vasculitis) before beginning the chronic management outlined above.

SEBORRHEIC DERMATITIS

Seborrheic dermatitis is a common, chronic disorder, characterized by greasy scales overlying erythematous patches or plaques. Induration and scale are generally less prominent than in psoriasis, but clinical overlap exists between these diseases—"sebopsoriasis." The most common location is in the scalp where it may be recognized as severe dandruff. On the face, seborrheic dermatitis affects the eyebrows, eyelids, glabella, and nasolabial folds (Fig. 53-4). Scaling of the external auditory canal is common in seborrheic dermatitis. Additionally, the postauricular areas often become macerated and tender. Seborrheic dermatitis may also develop in the central chest, axilla, groin, submammary folds, and gluteal cleft. Rarely, it may cause a widespread generalized dermatitis. Pruritus is variable.

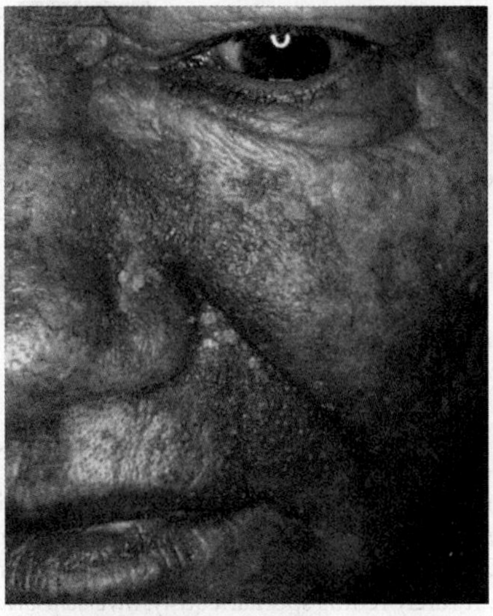

FIGURE 53-4 Seborrheic dermatitis. Central facial erythema with overlying greasy, yellowish scale is seen in this patient. (*Courtesy of Jean Bolognia, MD; with permission.*)

Seborrheic dermatitis may be evident within the first few weeks of life, and within this context it occurs in the scalp ("cradle cap"), face, or groin. It is rarely seen in children beyond infancy but becomes evident again during adult life. Although it is frequently seen in patients with Parkinson's disease, in those who have had cerebrovascular accidents, and in those with HIV infection, the overwhelming majority of individuals with seborrheic dermatitis have no underlying disorder.

℞ SEBORRHEIC DERMATITIS

Treatment with low-potency topical glucocorticoids in conjunction with a topical antifungal agent, such as ketoconazole cream or ciclopirox cream, is often effective. The scalp and beard areas may benefit from anti-dandruff shampoos, which should be left in place 3–5 min before rinsing. High-potency topical glucocorticoid solutions (betamethasone or clobetasol) are effective for control of severe scalp involvement. High potency glucocorticoids should not be used on the face since this is often associated with steroid-induced rosacea or atrophy. Tacrolimus and pimecrolimus are alternatives to topical glucocorticoids, especially when seborrheic dermatitis involves eyelids, although they are not FDA-approved for these indications.

PAPULOSQUAMOUS DISORDERS (Table 53-2)

PSORIASIS

Psoriasis is one of the most common dermatologic diseases, affecting up to 1% of the world's population. It is a chronic inflammatory skin disor-

TABLE 53-2 PAPULOSQUAMOUS DISORDERS

	Clinical Features	Other Notable Features	Histologic Features
Psoriasis	Sharply demarcated, erythematous plaques with mica-like scale; predominantly elbows, knees, and scalp; atypical forms may localize to intertriginous areas; eruptive forms may be associated with infection	May be aggravated by certain drugs, infection; severe forms seen associated with HIV	Acanthosis, vascular proliferation
Lichen planus	Purple polygonal papules marked by severe pruritus; lacy white markings, especially associated with mucous membrane lesions	Certain drugs may induce: thiazides, antimalarial drugs	Interface dermatitis
Pityriasis rosea	Rash often preceded by herald patch; oval to round plaques with trailing scale; most often affects the trunk, and eruption lines up in skin folds giving a "fir tree"-like appearance; generally spares palms and soles	Variable pruritus; self-limited resolving in 2–8 weeks; may be imitated by secondary syphilis	Pathologic features often nonspecific
Dermatophytosis	Polymorphous appearance depending on dermatophyte, body site, and host response; sharply defined to ill-demarcated scaly plaques with or without inflammation; may be associated with hair loss	KOH preparation may show branching hyphae; culture helpful	Hyphae and neutrophils in stratum corneum

der clinically characterized by erythematous, sharply demarcated papules and rounded plaques, covered by silvery micaceous scale. The skin lesions of psoriasis are variably pruritic. Traumatized areas often develop lesions of psoriasis (Koebner or isomorphic phenomenon). Additionally, other external factors may exacerbate psoriasis including infections, stress, and medications (lithium, beta blockers, and antimalarials).

The most common variety of psoriasis is called *plaque-type*. Patients with plaque-type psoriasis will have stable, slowly enlarging plaques, which remain basically unchanged for long periods of time. The most commonly involved areas are the elbows, knees, gluteal cleft, and the scalp. Involvement tends to be symmetric. Plaque psoriasis generally develops slowly and runs an indolent course. It rarely remits spontaneously. *Inverse psoriasis* affects the intertriginous regions including the axilla, groin, submammary region, and navel; it also tends to affect the scalp, palms, and soles. The individual lesions are sharply demarcated plaques (see Fig. 52-7), but they may be moist and without scale due to their location.

Guttate psoriasis (eruptive psoriasis) is most common in children and young adults. It develops acutely in individuals without psoriasis or in those with chronic plaque psoriasis. Patients present with many small erythematous, scaling papules, frequently after upper respiratory tract infection with β-hemolytic streptococci. The differential diagnosis should include pityriasis rosea and secondary syphilis.

Pustular psoriasis is another variant. Patients may have disease localized to the palms and soles, or the disease may be generalized. Regardless of the extent of disease, the skin is erythematous with pustules and variable scale. Localized to the palms and soles, it is easily confused with eczema. When generalized, episodes are characterized by fever (39°–40°C) lasting several days, an accompanying generalized eruption of sterile pustules, and a background of intense erythema; patients may become erythrodermic. Episodes of fever and pustules are recurrent. Local irritants, pregnancy, medications, infections, and systemic glucocorticoid withdrawal can precipitate this form of psoriasis. Oral retinoids are the treatment of choice in nonpregnant patients.

About half of all patients with psoriasis have fingernail involvement, appearing as punctate pitting, onycholysis, nail thickening, or subungual hyperkeratosis. About 5–10% of patients with psoriasis have associated arthralgias, and these are most often found in patients with fingernail involvement. Although some have the coincident occurrence of classic rheumatoid arthritis (Chap. 314), many have psoriatic arthritis that falls into one of three types: (1) asymmetric inflammatory arthritis most commonly involving the distal and proximal interphalangeal joints and less commonly the knees, hips, ankles, and wrists; (2) a seronegative rheumatoid arthritis–like disease; a significant portion of these patients go on to develop a severe destructive arthritis; or (3) disease limited to the spine (psoriatic spondylitis).

The etiology of psoriasis is still poorly understood, but there is clearly a genetic component to the disease. Over 50% of patients with psoriasis report a positive family history. Psoriatic lesions demonstrate infiltrates of activated T cells that are thought to elaborate cytokines responsible for keratinocyte hyperproliferation, which results in the characteristic clinical findings. Agents inhibiting T cell activation, clonal expansion, or release of proinflammatory cytokines are often effective for the treatment of severe psoriasis (see below).

TABLE 53-3 FDA-APPROVED SYSTEMIC THERAPY FOR PSORIASIS

Agent	Medication Class	Administration		Adverse Events (Selected)
		Route	Frequency	
Methotrexate	Antimetabolite	Oral	Weekly	Hepatotoxicity, pulmonary toxicity, pancytopenia, potential for increased malignancies, ulcerative stomatitis, nausea, diarrhea, teratogenicity
Acitretin	Retinoid	Oral	Daily	Teratogenicity, osteophyte formation, hyperlipidemia, flare of inflammatory bowel disease, hepatoxicity, depression
Cyclosporine	Calcineurin inhibitor	Oral	Twice daily	Renal dysfunction, hypertension, hyperkalemia, hyperuricemia, hypomagnesemia, hyperlipidemia, increased risk of malignancies

℞ PSORIASIS

Treatment of psoriasis depends on the type, location, and extent of disease. All patients should be instructed to avoid excess drying or irritation of their skin and to maintain adequate cutaneous hydration. Most patients with localized, plaque-type psoriasis can be managed with midpotency topical glucocorticoids, although their long-term use is often accompanied by loss of effectiveness (tachyphylaxis) and atrophy of the skin. A topical vitamin D analogue (calcipotriene) and a retinoid (tazarotene) are also efficacious in the treatment of limited psoriasis and have largely replaced other topical agents such as coal tar, salicylic acid, and anthralin.

Ultraviolet light, natural or artificial, is an effective therapy for many patients with widespread psoriasis. Ultraviolet B (UV-B) light, narrowband UV-B, and ultraviolet A (UV-A) spectrum with either oral or topical psoralens (PUVA) are also extremely effective. The long-term use of UV light may be associated with an increased incidence of non-melanoma and melanoma skin cancer. UV light therapy is contraindicated in patients receiving cyclosporine and should be used with great care in all immunocompromised patients due to an increased risk of developing skin cancers.

Various systemic agents can be used for severe, widespread psoriatic disease **(Table 53-3)**. Oral glucocorticoids should not be used for the treatment of psoriasis due to the potential for developing life-threatening pustular psoriasis when therapy is discontinued. Methotrexate is an effective agent, especially in patients with psoriatic arthritis. The synthetic retinoid, acitretin, is useful, especially when immunosuppression must be avoided; however, teratogenicity limits its use.

The evidence implicating psoriasis as a T cell–mediated disorder has directed therapeutic efforts to immunoregulation. Cyclosporine and other immunosuppressive agents can be very effective in the treatment of psoriasis, and much attention is currently directed toward the development of biologic agents with more selective immunosuppressive properties and better safety profiles **(Table 53-4)**. Experience with these agents is limited and information regarding combination therapy and adverse events continues to emerge. Use of TNF-α inhibitors may worsen congestive heart failure (CHF), and they should be used with caution in those at risk of or known to have CHF. Further, none of the immunosuppressive agents used in the treatment of psoriasis should be initiated if the patient has a severe infection; patients on such therapy should be routinely screened for tuberculosis. Malignancies, including a risk or history of certain malignancies, may limit the use of these systemic agents.

LICHEN PLANUS

Lichen planus (LP) is a papulosquamous disorder that may affect the skin, scalp, nails, and mucous membranes. The primary cutaneous lesions are pruritic, polygonal, flat-topped, violaceous papules. Close examination of the surface of these papules often reveals a network of gray lines (Wickham's striae). The skin lesions may occur anywhere but have a predilection for the wrists, shins, lower back, and genitalia **(Fig. 53-5)**. Involvement of the scalp, lichen planopilaris, may lead to scarring alopecia, and nail involvement may lead to permanent deformity or loss of fingernails and toenails. LP commonly involves mucous membranes, particularly the buccal mucosa, where it can present a spectrum of disease from a mild, white, reticulate eruption of the mucosa, to a severe, erosive stomatitis. Erosive stomatitis may persist for years and may be linked to an increased risk of oral squamous cell carcinoma. Cutaneous eruptions clinically resembling LP have been observed after administration of numerous drugs, including thiazide diuretics, gold, antimalarials, penicillamine, and phenothiazines, and in patients with skin lesions of chronic graft-versus-host disease. Additionally, LP may be associated with hepatitis C infection. The course of LP is variable, but most patients have spontaneous remissions 6 months to 2 years after the onset of disease. Topical glucocorticoids are the mainstay of therapy.

TABLE 53-4 BIOLOGICS APPROVED FOR PSORIASIS OR PSORIATIC ARTHRITIS

Agent	Mechanism of Action	Indication	Administration		Warnings
			Route	Frequency	
Alefacept	Anti-CD-2	Ps	IM	Once weekly × 12 weeks; may repeat	Lymphopenia, potential for increased malignancies, serious infections
Etanercept	Anti TNF-α	Ps, PsA	SC	Once or twice weekly	Serious infections, neurologic events, hematologic events, potential for increased malignancies
Efalizumab	Anti CD-11a	Ps	SC	Once weekly	Serious infections, potential for increased malignancies, thrombocytopenia, hemolytic anemia, psoriasis worsening
Adalimumab	Anti TNF-α	PsA	SC	Every other week	Serious infections, neurologic events, potential for increased malignancies, hypersensitivity reactions, hematologic events
Infliximab	Anti TNF-α	PsA	IV	Initial infusion followed by infusions at week 2, 6, then every 8 weeks	Serious infections, hepatotoxicity, hematologic events, hypersensitivity reactions, neurologic events, potential for increased malignancies

Ps, psoriasis; PsA, psoriatic arthritis; IM, intramuscular; SC, subcutaneous; TNF, tumor necrosis factor.

PITYRIASIS ROSEA

Pityriasis rosea (PR) is a papulosquamous eruption of unknown etiology occurring more commonly in the spring and fall. Its first manifestation is the development of a 2- to 6-cm annular lesion (the herald patch). This is followed in a few days to a few weeks by the appearance of many smaller annular or papular lesions with a predilection to occur on the trunk (Fig. 53-6). The lesions are generally oval, with their long axis parallel to the skin-fold lines. Individual lesions may range in color from red to brown and have a trailing scale. PR shares many clinical features with the eruption of secondary syphilis, but palm and sole lesions are extremely rare in PR and common in secondary syphilis. The eruption tends to be moderately pruritic and lasts 3–8 weeks. Treatment is directed at alleviating pruritus and consists of oral antihistamines, midpotency topical glucocorticoids, and, in some cases, the use of UV-B phototherapy.

CUTANEOUS INFECTIONS (Table 53-5)

IMPETIGO, ECTHYMA, AND FURUNCULOSIS

Impetigo is a common superficial bacterial infection of skin caused most often by *S. aureus* (Chap. 129), and in some cases by group A β-hemolytic streptococci (Chap. 130). The primary lesion is a superficial pustule that ruptures and forms a characteristic yellow-brown honey-colored crust (Chap. 130). Lesions may occur on normal skin—primary infection—or in areas already affected by another skin disease—secondary infection. Lesions caused by staphylococci may be tense, clear bullae, and this less common form of the disease is called *bullous impetigo*. Blisters are caused by the production of exfoliative toxin by *S. aureus* phage type II. This is the same toxin responsible for staphylococcal scalded-skin syndrome (SSSS), often resulting in dramatic loss of the superficial epidermis due to blistering. SSSS is much more common in children than in adults; however, it should be considered along with toxic epidermal necrolysis and severe drug eruptions in patients with widespread blistering of the skin. *Ecthyma* is a variant of impetigo that causes punched-out ulcerative lesions. It may result from neglected or inadequately treated impetigo. Treatment of both ecthyma and impetigo involves gentle debridement of adherent crusts, which is facilitated by the use of soaks and topical antibiotics, in conjunction with appropriate oral antibiotics. *Furunculosis* is also caused by *S. aureus*, and this disorder has gained prominence in the last decade because of CA-MRSA. A furuncle, or boil, is a painful, erythematous, nodule that can occur on any cutaneous surface. The lesions may be solitary but are most often multiple. Patients frequently believe they have been bitten by spiders or insects. Family members or close contacts may also be affected. Furuncles can rupture and drain spontaneously or may need incision and drainage, which may be adequate therapy for small solitary furuncles without cellulitis or systemic symptoms. Whenever possible, lesional material should be sent for culture. Current recommendations for methicillin-sensitive infections are β-lactam antibiotics. Therapy for CA-MRSA was discussed previously (see "Atopic Dermatitis"). Warm compresses and nasal mupirocin are helpful therapeutic additions. Severe infections may require IV antibiotics.

ERYSIPELAS AND CELLULITIS

See Chap. 119

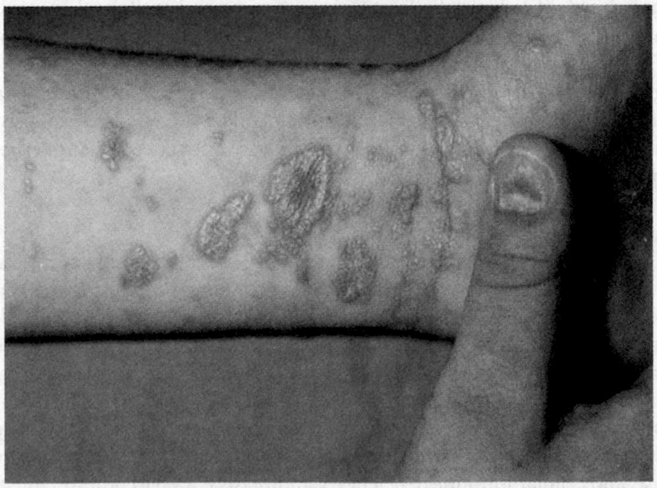

FIGURE 53-5 Lichen planus. An example of lichen planus showing multiple flat-topped, violaceous papules and plaques. Nail dystrophy as seen in this patient's thumbnail may also be a feature. (*Courtesy of Robert Swerlick, MD; with permission.*)

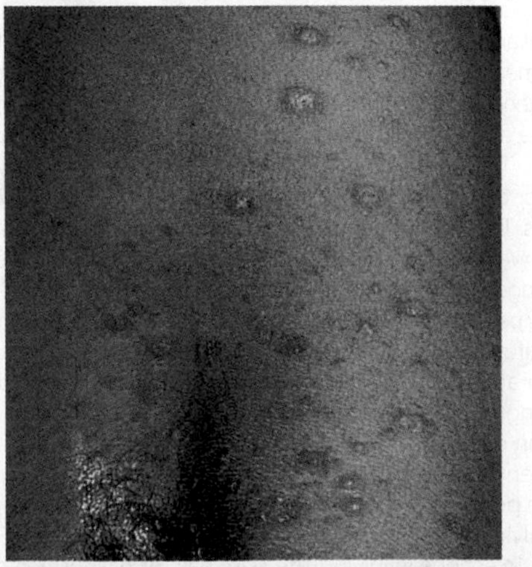

FIGURE 53-6 Pityriasis rosea. In this patient with pityriasis rosea, multiple round to oval erythematous patches with fine central scale are distributed along the skin tension lines on the trunk.

TABLE 53-5 COMMON SKIN INFECTIONS

	Clinical Features	Etiologic Agent	Treatment
Impetigo	Honey-colored crusted papules, plaques, or bullae	Group A Streptococcus and *Staphylococcus aureus*	Systemic or topical antistaphylococcal antibiotics
Dermatophytosis	Inflammatory or noninflammatory annular scaly plaques; may have hair loss; groin involvement spares scrotum; hyphae on KOH preparation	*Trichophyton, Epidermophyton,* or *Microsporum* sp.	Topical azoles, systemic griseofulvin, terbinafine, or azoles
Candidiasis	Inflammatory papules and plaques with satellite pustules, frequently in intertriginous areas; may involve scrotum; pseudohyphae on KOH preparation	*Candida albicans* and other *Candida* species	Topical nystatin or azoles; systemic azoles for resistant disease
Tinea versicolor	Hyperpigmented or hypopigmented scaly patches on the trunk; characteristic mixture of hyphae and spores on KOH preparation ("spaghetti and meatballs")	*Malassezia furfur*	Topical selenium sulfide lotion or azoles

DERMATOPHYTOSIS

Dermatophytes are fungi that infect skin, hair, and nails and include members of the genera *Trichophyton*, *Microsporum*, and *Epidermophyton*. Tinea corporis, or infection of the relatively hairless skin of the body (glabrous skin), may have a variable appearance depending on the extent of the associated inflammatory reaction (see Fig. 52-11). Typical infections have an annular appearance that patients refer to as "ringworm." Deep inflammatory nodules or granulomas occur in some infections—especially in those infections inappropriately treated with mid- to high-potency topical glucocorticoids. Involvement of the groin (tinea cruris) is more common in males than females. It presents as a scaling, erythematous eruption sparing the scrotum. Infection of the foot (tinea pedis) is the most common dermatophyte infection and is often chronic; it is characterized by variable erythema, edema, scaling, pruritus, and occasionally vesiculation. Involvement may be widespread or localized but generally involves the web space between the fourth and fifth toes. Infection of the nails (tinea unguium or onychomycosis) occurs in many patients with tinea pedis and is characterized by opacified, thickened nails and subungual debris. The distal-lateral variant is most common. Proximal subungual onychomycosis may be a marker for HIV infection or other immunocompromised states. Dermatophyte infection of the scalp (tinea capitis) has returned in epidemic proportions, particularly affecting inner-city children, but it also affects adults. The predominant organism is *T. tonsurans*, which can produce a relatively noninflammatory infection with mild scale and hair loss that is diffuse or localized. *T. tonsurans* can also cause a markedly inflammatory dermatosis with edema and nodules. This latter presentation is a kerion.

The diagnosis of tinea can be made from skin scrapings, nail scrapings, or hair by culture or direct microscopic examination with potassium hydroxide (KOH). Nail clippings may be sent for histologic examination with periodic acid Schiff (PAS) stain.

℞ DERMATOPHYTOSIS

Both topical and systemic therapies may be used to treat dermatophyte infections. Treatment depends on the site involved and the type of infection. Topical therapy is generally effective for uncomplicated tinea corporis, tinea cruris, and limited tinea pedis. It is not effective as a monotherapy for tinea capitis or onychomycosis. Topical imidazoles, triazoles, and allylamines may be effective therapies for dermatophyte infections, but nystatin is not active against dermatophytes. Topicals are generally applied twice daily, and treatment should continue 1 week beyond clinical resolution of the infection. Tinea pedis often requires longer treatment courses and frequently relapses. Oral antifungal agents may be required for recalcitrant tinea pedis or tinea corporis.

Oral antifungal agents are required for dermatophyte infections involving the hair and nails and for other infections unresponsive to topical therapy. A fungal etiology should be confirmed by direct microscopic examination or by culture prior to prescribing oral antifungal agents. All of the oral agents may cause hepatotoxicity and should not be used in women who are pregnant or breast-feeding.

Griseofulvin is the only oral agent approved in the United States for dermatophyte infections involving the skin, hair, or nails. When griseofulvin is used, a daily dose of 500 mg microsized or 375 mg ultramicrosized griseofulvin administered with a fatty meal is an adequate dose for most dermatophyte infections. Higher doses are required for some cases of tinea pedis and tinea capitis. The usual adult dose of griseofulvin for tinea capitis is 1 g microsized or 0.5 g ultramicrosized given daily. Markedly inflammatory tinea capitis may result in scarring and hair loss, and systemic or topical glucocorticoids may be helpful in preventing these sequelae. The duration of therapy may be 2 weeks for uncomplicated tinea corporis, 8–12 weeks for tinea capitis, or as long as 6–18 months for nail infections. Due to high relapse rates, griseofulvin is seldom used for nail infections. Common side effects of griseofulvin include gastrointestinal distress, headache, and urticaria.

Oral itraconazole and terbinafine are approved for onychomycosis. Itraconazole is given as either continuous daily therapy (200 mg/d) or pulses (200 mg bid for 1 week per month) administered with food. Fingernails require 2 months of continuous therapy or two pulses. Toenails require 3 months of continuous therapy or three pulses. Itraconazole has the potential for serious interactions with other drugs requiring the P450 enzyme system for metabolism. Terbinafine (250 mg/d) is also effective for onychomycosis. Therapy with terbinafine is continued for 6 weeks for fingernail infections and 12 weeks for toenail infections. Terbinafine has fewer drug-drug interactions, but caution should be used when patients are on multiple medications.

TINEA VERSICOLOR

Tinea versicolor is caused by a non-dermatophyte, dimorphic fungus, *Malassezia furfur*, a normal inhabitant of the skin. The expression of infection is promoted by heat and humidity. The typical lesions consist of oval scaly macules, papules, and patches concentrated on the chest, shoulders, and back but only rarely on the face or distal extremities. On dark skin, they often appear as hypopigmented areas, while on light skin, they are slightly erythematous or hyperpigmented. A KOH preparation from scaling lesions will demonstrate a confluence of short hyphae and round spores ("spaghetti and meatballs"). Lotions or shampoos containing sulfur, salicylic acid, or selenium sulfide will clear the infection if used daily for 1–2 weeks and then weekly thereafter. These preparations are irritating if left on the skin for more than 10 min; thus, they should be washed off completely. Treatment with some oral antifungal agents is also effective, but they do not provide lasting results, and they are not FDA-approved for this indication. Ketoconazole has been used as a single 400-mg dose; the patient waits 1 h, exercises to the point of sweating, then lets the skin dry. Itraconazole and fluconazole have also been used at various doses and frequencies. Griseofulvin is not effective, and terbenifine is not reliably effective for tinea versicolor.

CANDIDIASIS

Candidiasis is a fungal infection caused by a related group of yeasts, whose manifestations may be localized to the skin, or rarely, may be systemic and life-threatening. The causative organism is usually *Candida albicans*, but may also be *C. tropicalis*, *C. parapsilosis*, or *C. krusei*. These organisms are normal saprophytic inhabitants of the gastrointestinal tract but may overgrow (usually due to broad-spectrum antibiotic therapy) and cause disease at a number of cutaneous sites. Other predisposing factors include diabetes mellitus, chronic intertrigo, oral contraceptive use, and cellular immune deficiency. Candidiasis is a very common infection in HIV-infected individuals (Chap. 182). The oral cavity is commonly involved. Lesions may occur on the tongue or buccal mucosa (thrush) and appear as white plaques (see Fig. 52-12). Microscopic examination of scrapings demonstrate both pseudohyphae and yeast forms. Fissured, macerated lesions at the corners of the mouth (perlèche) are often seen in individuals with poorly fitting dentures and may also be associated with candidal infection. Additionally, candidal infections have an affinity for sites that are chronically wet and macerated, including the skin around nails (onycholysis and paronychia) and in intertriginous areas. Intertriginous lesions are characteristically edematous, erythematous, and scaly, with scattered "satellite pustules." In males, there is often involvement of the penis and scrotum as well as the inner aspect of the thighs. In contrast to dermatophyte infections, candidal infections are frequently painful and accompanied by a marked inflammatory response. Diagnosis of candidal infection is based upon the clinical pattern and demonstration of yeast on KOH preparation or culture.

℞ CANDIDIASIS

Treatment involves removing any predisposing factors such as antibiotic therapy or chronic wetness and the use of appropriate topical or systemic antifungal agents. Effective topicals include nystatin or azoles (miconazole, clotrimazole, econazole, or ketoconazole). The associated inflammatory response accompanying candidal infection on glabrous skin can be treated with a mild glucocorticoid lotion or cream (2.5% hydrocortisone). Systemic therapy is usually reserved for immunosuppressed patients or individuals with chronic or recurrent disease who fail to respond to appropriate topical therapy. Oral agents approved for the treatment of candidiasis include itraconazole and fluconazole. Oral nystatin is only effective for candidiasis of the gastrointestinal tract. Griseofulvin and terbenifine are not effective.

WARTS

Warts are cutaneous neoplasms caused by papilloma viruses. More than 100 different human papilloma viruses (HPV) have been described. A typical wart, verruca vulgaris, is sessile, dome-shaped, and usually about a centimeter in diameter. Its surface is hyperkeratotic consisting of many small filamentous projections. The HPV that cause typical verruca vulgaris also cause typical plantar warts, flat warts (or verruca plana), and filiform warts. Plantar warts are endophytic and are covered by thick keratin. Paring of the wart will generally demonstrate a central core of keratinized debris and punctate bleeding points. Filiform warts are most commonly seen on the face, neck, and skin folds and present as papillomatous lesions on a narrow base. Flat warts are only slightly elevated and have a velvety, nonverrucous surface. They have a propensity for the face, arms, and legs and are often spread by shaving.

Genital warts begin as small papillomas that may grow to form large fungating lesions. In women, they may involve either the labia, perineum, or perianal skin. Additionally, the mucosa of the vagina, urethra, and anus can be involved, as well as the cervical epithelium. In men, the lesions often occur initially in the coronal sulcus but may be seen on the shaft of the penis, the scrotum, perianal skin, or in the urethra.

Appreciable evidence has accumulated that suggests HPV plays a role in the development of neoplasia of the uterine cervix and anogenital skin (Chap. 93). HPV types 16 and 18 have been most intensely studied and are the major risk factors for intraepithelial neoplasia and squamous cell carcinoma of the cervix, anus, vulva, and penis. The risk is higher in patients immunosuppressed after solid organ transplantation and in those infected with HIV. Recent evidence also implicates other types. Histologic examination of biopsies from affected sites may reveal changes associated with typical warts and/or features typical of intraepidermal carcinoma (Bowen's disease). Squamous cell carcinomas associated with HPV infections have also been observed in extragenital skin (Chap. 83). This is most commonly seen in patients immunosuppressed after organ transplantation. Patients on long-term immunosuppression should be monitored for the development of squamous cell carcinoma and other cutaneous malignancies.

℞ WARTS

Treatment of warts, other than anogenital warts, should be tempered by the observation that a majority of warts in normal individuals resolve spontaneously within 1–2 years. There are many modalities available to treat warts, but no single therapy is universally effective. Factors that influence the choice of therapy include the location of the wart, extent of disease, the age and immunologic status of the patient, and the patient's desire for therapy. Perhaps the most useful and convenient method for treating warts in almost any location is cryotherapy with liquid nitrogen. Equally effective for non-genital warts, but requiring much more patient compliance, is the use of keratolytic agents such as salicylic acid plasters or solutions. For genital warts, in-office application of a podophyllin solution is moderately effective but may be associated with marked local reactions. Prescription preparations of dilute, purified podophyllin are available for home use. Topical imiquimod, a potent inducer of local cytokine release, has also been approved for use in genital warts. Conventional and laser surgical procedures may be required for recalcitrant warts. Recurrence of warts appears to be common to all these modalities. A highly effective vaccine for selected types of HPV has been recently approved by the FDA, and its use will likely reduce the incidence of anogenital and cervical carcinoma.

HERPES SIMPLEX

See Chap. 172

HERPES ZOSTER

See Chap. 173

ACNE

ACNE VULGARIS

Acne vulgaris is a self-limited disorder primarily of teenagers and young adults, although perhaps 10–20% of adults may continue to experience some form of the disorder. The permissive factor for the expression of the disease in adolescence is the increase in sebum production by sebaceous glands after puberty. Small cysts, called *comedones*, form in hair follicles due to blockage of the follicular orifice by retention of keratinous material and sebum. The activity of bacteria (*Proprionobacterium acnes*) within the comedones releases free fatty acids from sebum, causes inflammation within the cyst, and results in rupture of the cyst wall. An inflammatory foreign-body reaction develops as result of extrusion of oily and keratinous debris from the cyst.

The clinical hallmark of acne vulgaris is the comedone, which may be closed (whitehead) or open (blackhead). Closed comedones appear as 1- to 2-mm pebbly white papules, which are accentuated when the skin is stretched. They are the precursors of inflammatory lesions of acne vulgaris. The contents of closed comedones are not easily expressed. Open comedones, which rarely result in inflammatory acne lesions, have a large dilated follicular orifice and are filled with easily expressible oxidized, darkened, oily debris. Comedones are usually accompanied by inflammatory lesions: papules, pustules, or nodules.

The earliest lesions seen in adolescence are generally mildly inflamed or noninflammatory comedones on the forehead. Subsequently, more typical inflammatory lesions develop on the cheeks, nose, and chin (Fig. 53-7). The most common location for acne is the face, but involvement of the chest and back is common. Most disease remains mild and does not lead to scarring. A small number of patients develop large inflam-

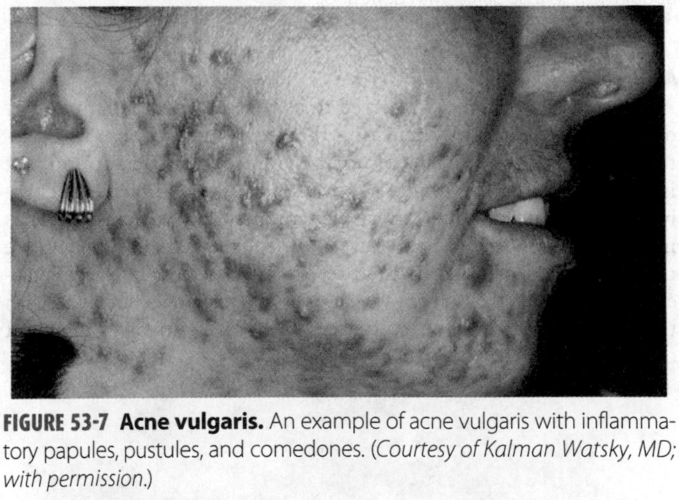

FIGURE 53-7 Acne vulgaris. An example of acne vulgaris with inflammatory papules, pustules, and comedones. (*Courtesy of Kalman Watsky, MD; with permission.*)

matory cysts and nodules, which may drain and result in significant scarring. Regardless of the severity, acne may affect a patient's quality of life. If adequately treated, this may be a transient effect. In the case of severe, scarring acne, the effects can be permanent and profound. Early therapeutic intervention in severe acne is essential.

Exogenous and endogenous factors can alter the expression of acne vulgaris. Friction and trauma (from headbands or chin straps of athletic helmets), application of comedogenic topical agents (cosmetics or hair preparations), or chronic topical exposure to certain industrial compounds may elicit or aggravate acne. Glucocorticoids, topical or systemic, may also elicit acne. Other systemic medications such as oral contraceptive pills, lithium, isoniazid, androgenic steroids, halogens, phenytoin, and phenobarbital may produce acneiform eruptions or aggravate preexisting acne. Genetic factors and polycystic ovary disease may also play a role.

℞ ACNE VULGARIS

Treatment of acne vulgaris is directed toward elimination of comedones by normalization of follicular keratinization, decreasing sebaceous gland activity, decreasing the population of *P. acnes*, and decreasing inflammation. Minimal to moderate, pauci-inflammatory disease may respond adequately to local therapy alone. Although areas affected with acne should be kept clean, overly vigorous scrubbing may aggravate acne due to mechanical rupture of comedones. Topical agents such as retinoic acid, benzoyl peroxide, or salicylic acid may alter the pattern of epidermal desquamation, preventing the formation of comedones and aiding in the resolution of preexisting cysts. Topical antibacterial agents such as azelaic acid, topical erythromycin (with or without zinc), or clindamycin are also useful adjuncts to therapy.

Patients with moderate to severe acne with a prominent inflammatory component will benefit from the addition of systemic therapy, such as tetracycline in doses of 250–500 mg bid, or doxycycline, 100 mg bid. Minocycline may also be useful. Such antibiotics appear to have an anti-inflammatory effect independent of their antibacterial effect. Female patients who do not respond to oral antibiotics may benefit from hormonal therapy. Women placed on oral contraceptives containing ethinyl estradiol and norgestimate have demonstrated improvement in their acne when compared to a placebo control.

Patients with severe nodulocystic acne unresponsive to the therapies discussed above may benefit from treatment with the synthetic retinoid, isotretinoin. Its dose is based on the patient's weight, and it is given once daily for 5 months. Results are excellent in appropriately selected patients. Its use is highly regulated due to its potential for severe adverse events, primarily teratogenicity. Additionally, patients receiving this medication develop extremely dry skin, cheilitis, and must be followed for development of hypertriglyceridemia. Recently there have also been concerns that it is associated with severe depression in some patients. The latter has not been proved. At present, prescribers must enroll in a program designed to prevent pregnancy and adverse events while patients are taking isotretinoin. These measures are imposed to ensure that all prescribers are familiar with the risks of isotretinoin; that all female patients have two negative pregnancy tests prior to initiating therapy and a negative pregnancy test prior to each refill; and that all patients have been warned about the risks associated with isotretinoin.

ACNE ROSACEA

Acne rosacea, commonly referred to as rosacea, is an inflammatory disorder predominantly affecting the central face. Those most often affected are Caucasians of northern European background, but it is seen in patients with dark skin also. It is seen almost exclusively in adults, only rarely affecting patients <30 years. Rosacea is more common in women, but those most severely affected are men. It is characterized by the presence of erythema, telangiectases, and superficial pustules (Fig. 53-8), but is not associated with the presence of comedones. Rosacea only rarely involves the chest or back.

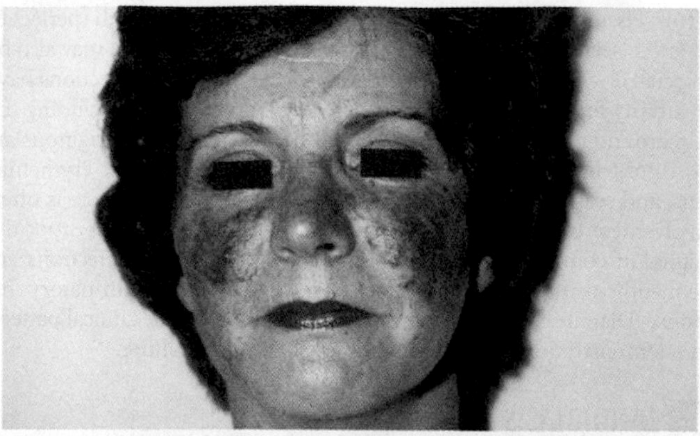

FIGURE 53-8 Acne rosacea. Prominent facial erythema, telangiectasia, scattered papules, and small pustules are seen in this patient with acne rosacea. (*Courtesy of Robert Swerlick, MD; with permission.*)

There is a relationship between the tendency for facial flushing and the subsequent development of acne rosacea. Often, individuals with rosacea initially demonstrate a pronounced flushing reaction. This may be in response to heat, emotional stimuli, alcohol, hot drinks, or spicy foods. As the disease progresses, the flush persists longer and longer and may eventually become permanent. Papules, pustules, and telangiectases can become superimposed on the persistent flush. Rosacea of very long standing may lead to connective tissue overgrowth, particularly of the nose (rhinophyma). Rosacea may also be complicated by various inflammatory disorders of the eye, including keratitis, blepharitis, iritis, and recurrent chalazion. These ocular problems are potentially sight-threatening and warrant ophthalmologic evaluation.

℞ ACNE ROSACEA

Acne rosacea can be treated topically or systemically. Mild disease often responds to topical metronidazole or sodium sulfacetamide. More severe disease requires oral tetracyclines: tetracycline 250–500 mg bid, doxycycline 100 mg bid, or minocycline 50–100 mg bid. Residual telangiectasia may respond to laser therapy. Topical glucocorticoids, especially potent agents, should be avoided since chronic use of these preparations may elicit rosacea. Topical therapy of the skin is not effective treatment for ocular disease.

SKIN DISEASES AND SMALLPOX VACCINATION

Given the potential threat of a bioterrorism attack with smallpox, vaccinations against smallpox are available to the general public, although they are not recommended. Because of a higher incidence of adverse events associated with smallpox vaccination in patients with a history of certain skin diseases, including atopic dermatitis, eczema, and psoriasis, such vaccination is contraindicated in patients with these conditions in the absence of a bioterrorism attack and a real or potential exposure to smallpox. In the case of such exposure, the risk of smallpox infection outweighs the risk of adverse events from the vaccine (Chap. 214).

FURTHER READINGS

James WD et al: *Andrews' Diseases of the Skin Clinical Dermatology*, 10th ed. Philadelphia, Saunders-Elsevier, 2006

Wolff K, Johnson RA: *Fitzpatrick's Color Atlas and Synopsis of Clinical Dermatology*, 5th ed. New York, McGraw-Hill, 2005

Wolff K et al (eds): *Fitzpatrick's Dermatology in General Medicine*, 7th ed. New York, McGraw-Hill, 2008

Wolverton SE (ed): *Comprehensive Dermatologic Drug Therapy*. Philadelphia, Saunders, 2001

54 Skin Manifestations of Internal Disease

Jean L. Bolognia, Irwin M. Braverman

It is now a generally accepted concept in medicine that the skin can show signs of internal disease. Therefore, in textbooks of medicine one finds a chapter describing in detail the major systemic disorders that can be identified by cutaneous signs. The underlying assumption of such a chapter is that the clinician has been able to identify the disorder in the patient and needs only to read about it in the textbook. In reality, concise differential diagnoses and the identification of these disorders are actually difficult for the nondermatologist because he or she is not well versed in the recognition of cutaneous lesions or their spectrum of presentations. Therefore, the authors of this chapter have decided to cover this particular topic of cutaneous medicine not by discussing individual disorders but by describing and discussing the various presenting clinical signs and symptoms that indicate the presence of these disorders. Concise differential diagnoses will be generated in which the significant diseases will be briefly discussed and distinguished from the more common disorders that have no significance for internal diseases. The latter disorders are reviewed in table form and always need to be excluded when considering the former. For a detailed description of individual diseases, the reader should consult a dermatologic text.

PAPULOSQUAMOUS SKIN LESIONS

(Table 54-1) When an eruption is characterized by elevated lesions, papules (<1 cm), or plaques (>1 cm), in association with scale, it is referred to as a *papulosquamous lesion*. The most common papulosquamous diseases—*psoriasis*, *tinea*, *pityriasis rosea*, and *lichen planus*—are primary cutaneous disorders (Chap. 53). When psoriatic lesions are accompanied by arthritis, the possibility of psoriatic arthritis or *Reiter's disease* should be considered. A history of oral ulcers, conjunctivitis, uveitis, and/or urethritis points to the latter diagnosis. Lithium, beta blockers, HIV or streptococcal infections, and a rapid taper of systemic glucocorticoids are known to exacerbate psoriasis.

Whenever the diagnosis of pityriasis rosea or lichen planus is made, it is important to review the patient's medications because the eruption can be treated by simply discontinuing the offending agent. Pityriasis rosea–like drug eruptions are seen most commonly with beta blockers, angiotensin-converting enzyme (ACE) inhibitors, gold, and metronidazole, while the drugs that can produce a lichenoid eruption include thiazides, antimalarials, gold, quinidine, phenothiazines, sulfonylureas, and ACE inhibitors. In some populations, there is a higher prevalence of hepatitis C viral infection in patients with lichen planus. Lichen planus–like lesions are also observed in chronic graft-versus-host disease.

TABLE 54-1 SELECTED CAUSES OF PAPULOSQUAMOUS SKIN LESIONS

1. Primary cutaneous disorders
   - a. Psoriasis[a]
   - b. Tinea[a]
   - c. Pityriasis rosea[a]
   - d. Lichen planus[a]
   - e. Parapsoriasis
   - f. Bowen's disease (squamous cell carcinoma in situ)[b]
2. Drugs
3. Systemic diseases
   - a. Lupus erythematosus[c]
   - b. Cutaneous T cell lymphoma
   - c. Secondary syphilis
   - d. Reiter's disease
   - e. Sarcoidosis[d]

[a]Discussed in detail in Chap. 53.
[b]Associated with chronic sun exposure and exposure to arsenic.
[c]See also Red Lesions in "Papulonodular Skin Lesions."
[d]See also Red-Brown Lesions in "Papulonodular Skin Lesions."

In its early stages, *cutaneous T cell lymphoma* (CTCL) may be confused with eczema or psoriasis, but it often fails to respond to the appropriate therapy for those inflammatory diseases. CTCL can develop within lesions of large-plaque parapsoriasis and is suggested by an increase in the thickness of the lesions. The diagnosis of CTCL is established by skin biopsy in which collections of atypical T lymphocytes are found in the epidermis and dermis. As the disease progresses, cutaneous tumors and lymph node involvement may appear.

In *secondary syphilis* there are scattered red-brown papules with thin scale. The eruption often involves the palms and soles and can resemble pityriasis rosea. Associated findings are helpful in making the diagnosis and include annular plaques on the face, nonscarring alopecia, condyloma lata (broad-based and moist), and mucous patches as well as lymphadenopathy, malaise, fever, headache, and myalgias. The interval between the primary chancre and the secondary stage is usually 4–8 weeks, and spontaneous resolution without appropriate therapy is seen.

ERYTHRODERMA

(Table 54-2) *Erythroderma* is the term used when the majority of the skin surface is erythematous (red in color). There may be associated scale, erosions, or pustules as well as shedding of the hair and nails. Potential systemic manifestations include fever, chills, hypothermia, reactive lymphadenopathy, peripheral edema, hypoalbuminemia, and high-output cardiac failure. The major etiologies of erythroderma are (1) cutaneous diseases such as psoriasis and dermatitis (Table 54-3); (2) drugs; (3) systemic diseases, most commonly CTCL; and (4) idiopathic. In the first three groups, the location and description of the initial lesions, prior to the development of the erythroderma, aid in the diagnosis. For example, a history of red scaly plaques on the elbows and knees would point to psoriasis. It is also important to examine the skin carefully for a migration of the erythema and associated secondary changes such as pustules or erosions. Migratory waves of erythema studded with superficial pustules are seen in *pustular psoriasis*.

Drug-induced erythroderma (exfoliative dermatitis) may begin as an exanthematous (morbilliform) eruption (Chap. 56) or may arise as diffuse erythema. A number of drugs can produce an erythroderma, including penicillins, sulfonamides, carbamazepine, phenytoin, gold, allopurinol, and zalcitabine. Fever and peripheral eosinophilia often accompany the eruption, and there may also be facial swelling, hepatitis, and allergic interstitial nephritis; this constellation is frequently referred to as *drug reaction with eosinophilia and systemic symptoms* (DRESS). In addition, reactions to anticonvulsants can lead to a pseudolymphoma syndrome (with adenopathy and circulating atypical lymphocytes), while reactions to allopurinol may be accompanied by gastrointestinal bleeding.

The most common malignancy that is associated with erythroderma is CTCL; in some series, up to 25% of the cases of erythroderma were due to CTCL. The patient may progress from isolated plaques and tumors, but more commonly the erythroderma is present throughout the course of the disease (Sézary syndrome). In the Sézary syndrome, there are circulating atypical T lymphocytes, pruritus, and lymphadenopathy. In cases of erythroderma where there is no apparent cause (idiopathic), longitudinal follow-up is mandatory to monitor for the possible development of CTCL. There have been isolated case reports of erythroderma secondary to some solid tumors—lung, liver, prostate, thyroid, and colon—but it is usually in a late stage of the disease.

TABLE 54-2 CAUSES OF ERYTHRODERMA

1. Primary cutaneous disorders
   - a. Psoriasis[a]
   - b. Dermatitis [atopic, contact >> seborrheic or stasis (with autosensitization)][a]
   - c. Pityriasis rubra pilaris
2. Drugs
3. Systemic diseases
   - a. Cutaneous T cell lymphoma
   - b. Lymphoma
4. Idiopathic

[a]Discussed in detail in Chap. 53.

TABLE 54-3 ERYTHRODERMA (PRIMARY CUTANEOUS DISORDERS)

	Initial Lesions	Location of Initial Lesions	Other Findings	Diagnostic Aids	Treatment
Psoriasis[a]	Pink-red, silvery scale, sharply demarcated	Elbows, knees, scalp, presacral area	Nail dystrophy, arthritis, pustules	Skin biopsy	Topical glucocorticoids, vitamin D; UV-B (narrowband); oral retinoid and/or PUVA; MTX, cyclosporine, anti-TNF agents
Dermatitis[a]					
Atopic	Acute: Erythema, fine scale, crust, indistinct borders Chronic: Lichenification (increased skin markings)	Antecubital and popliteal fossae, neck, hands	Pruritus Family history of atopy, including asthma, allergic rhinitis or conjunctivitis, and atopic dermatitis Exclude secondary infection with *S. aureus* Exclude superimposed irritant or allergic contact dermatitis	Skin biopsy	Topical glucocorticoids, tacrolimus, pimecrolimus, tar, and antipruritics; oral antihistamines; open wet dressings; UV-B ± UV-A; PUVA; oral/IM glucocorticoids; MTX; cyclosporine Topical or oral antibiotics
Contact	Local: Erythema, crusting, vesicles, and bullae	Depends on offending agent	Irritant—onset often within hours Allergic—delayed-type hypersensitivity; lag time of 48 h	Patch testing	Remove irritant or allergen; topical glucocorticoids; oral antihistamines; oral/IM glucocorticoids
	Systemic: Erythema, fine scale, crust	Generalized	Patient has history of allergic contact dermatitis to topical agent and then receives systemic medication that is structurally related, e.g., ethylenediamine (topical), aminophylline (IV)	Patch testing	Same as local
Seborrheic (rare)	Pink-red, greasy scale	Scalp, nasolabial folds, eyebrows, intertriginous zones	Flares with stress, HIV infection Associated with Parkinson's disease	Skin biopsy	Topical glucocorticoids and imidazoles
Stasis (with autosensitization)	Erythema, crusting, excoriations	Lower extremities	Pruritus, lower extremity edema History of venous ulcers, thrombophlebitis, and/or cellulitis Exclude cellulitis Exclude superimposed contact dermatitis, e.g., topical neomycin	Skin biopsy	Topical glucocorticoids; open wet dressings; leg elevation; pressure stockings
Pityriasis rubra pilaris	Orange-red, perifollicular papules	Generalized, but characteristic "skip" areas of normal skin	Wax-like keratoderma Exclude cutaneous T cell lymphoma	Skin biopsy	Isotretinoin or acitretin; methotrexate

[a]Discussed in detail in Chap. 53.

Note: PUVA, psoralens + ultraviolet A irradiation; UV-B, ultraviolet B; UV-A, ultraviolet A; MTX, methotrexate; TNF, tumor necrosis factor.

ALOPECIA

(Table 54-4) The two major forms of alopecia are scarring and nonscarring. In *scarring alopecia* there are associated fibrosis, inflammation, and loss of hair follicles. A smooth scalp with a decreased number of follicular openings is usually observed clinically, but in some cases the changes are seen only in biopsy specimens from the affected areas. In *nonscarring alopecia* the hair shafts are gone, but the hair follicles are preserved, explaining the reversible nature of nonscarring alopecia.

The most common causes of nonscarring alopecia include *telogen effluvium*, *androgenetic alopecia*, *alopecia areata*, *tinea capitis*, and some cases of *traumatic alopecia* (Table 54-5). In women with androgenetic alopecia, an elevation in circulating levels of androgens may be seen as a result of ovarian or adrenal gland dysfunction. When there are signs of virilization, such as a deepened voice and enlarged clitoris, the possibility of an ovarian or adrenal gland tumor should be considered.

Exposure to various drugs can also cause diffuse hair loss, usually by inducing a telogen effluvium. An exception is the anagen effluvium observed with antimitotic agents such as daunorubicin. Alopecia is a side effect of the following drugs: warfarin, heparin, propylthiouracil, carbimazole, vitamin A, isotretinoin, acitretin, lithium, beta blockers, colchicine, and amphetamines. Fortunately, spontaneous regrowth usually follows discontinuation of the offending agent.

Less commonly, nonscarring alopecia is associated with *lupus erythematosus* and *secondary syphilis.* In systemic lupus there are two forms of alopecia—one is scarring secondary to discoid lesions (see below) and the other is nonscarring. The latter form may be diffuse and involve the entire

TABLE 54-4 CAUSES OF ALOPECIA

I. Nonscarring alopecia
   A. Primary cutaneous disorders
      1. Telogen effluvium
      2. Androgenetic alopecia
      3. Alopecia areata
      4. Tinea capitis
      5. Traumatic alopecia[a]
   B. Drugs
   C. Systemic diseases
      1. Lupus erythematosus
      2. Secondary syphilis
      3. Hypothyroidism
      4. Hyperthyroidism
      5. Hypopituitarism
      6. Deficiencies of protein, iron, biotin, and zinc
II. Scarring alopecia
   A. Primary cutaneous disorders
      1. Cutaneous lupus (chronic discoid)
      2. Lichen planus
      3. Folliculitis decalvans
      4. Linear scleroderma (morphea)
      5. Central centrifugal cicatricial alopecia
   B. Systemic diseases
      1. Lupus erythematosus
      2. Sarcoidosis
      3. Cutaneous metastases

[a]Most patients with trichotillomania, pressure-induced alopecia.

TABLE 54-5 NONSCARRING ALOPECIA (PRIMARY CUTANEOUS DISORDERS)

	Clinical Characteristics	Pathogenesis	Treatment
Telogen effluvium	Diffuse shedding of normal hairs Follows either major stress (high fever, severe infection) or change in hormones (post partum) Reversible without treatment	Stress causes the normally asynchronous growth cycles of individual hairs to become synchronous; therefore, large numbers of growing (anagen) hairs simultaneously enter the dying (telogen) phase	Observation; discontinue any drugs that have alopecia as a side effect; must exclude underlying metabolic causes, e.g., hypothyroidism, hyperthyroidism
Androgenetic alopecia (male pattern; female pattern)	Miniaturization of hairs along the midline of the scalp Recession of the anterior scalp line in men and some women	Increased sensitivity of affected hairs to the effects of testosterone Increased levels of circulating androgens (ovarian or adrenal source in women)	If no evidence of hyperandrogen state, then topical minoxidil; finasteride[a]; hair transplant
Alopecia areata	Well-circumscribed, circular areas of hair loss, 2–5 cm in diameter In extensive cases, coalescence of lesions and/or involvement of other hair-bearing surfaces of the body Pitting of the nails	The germinative zones of the hair follicles are surrounded by T lymphocytes Occasional associated diseases: hyperthyroidism, hypothyroidism, vitiligo, Down syndrome	Topical anthralin; intralesional glucocorticoids; topical contact sensitizers
Tinea	Varies from scaling with minimal hair loss to discrete patches with "black dots" (broken hairs) to boggy plaque with pustules (kerion)	Invasion of hairs by dermatophytes, most commonly *Trichophyton tonsurans*	Oral griseofulvin or terbinafine plus 2.5% selenium sulfide or ketoconazole shampoo; examine family members
Traumatic alopecia[b]	Broken hairs Irregular outline	Traction with curlers, rubber bands, braiding Exposure to heat or chemicals (e.g., hair straighteners) Mechanical pulling (trichotillomania)	Discontinuation of offending hair style or chemical treatments; trichotillomania may require hair clipping and observation of shaved hairs or biopsy for diagnosis, possibly followed by psychotherapy

[a]To date, FDA-approved for men.

[b]May also be scarring.

scalp, or it may be localized to the frontal scalp, eventually resulting in multiple short hairs ("lupus hairs"). Scattered, poorly circumscribed patches of alopecia with a "moth-eaten" appearance are a manifestation of the secondary stage of syphilis. Diffuse thinning of the hair is also associated with hypothyroidism and hyperthyroidism (Table 54-4).

Scarring alopecia is more frequently the result of a primary cutaneous disorder such as *lichen planus, folliculitis decalvans, chronic cutaneous (discoid) lupus*, or *linear scleroderma* (*morphea*) than it is a sign of systemic disease. Although the scarring lesions of *discoid lupus* can be seen in patients with systemic lupus, in the majority of cases the disease process is limited to the skin. Less common causes of scarring alopecia include *sarcoidosis* (see "Papulonodular Skin Lesions," below) and *cutaneous metastases*.

In the early phases of discoid lupus, lichen planus, and folliculitis decalvans, there are circumscribed areas of alopecia. Fibrosis and subsequent loss of follicles are observed primarily in the center of the individual lesions, while the inflammatory process is most prominent at the periphery. The areas of active inflammation in discoid lupus are erythematous with scale, whereas the areas of previous inflammation are often hypopigmented with a rim of hyperpigmentation. In lichen planus the peripheral perifollicular macules are usually violet-colored. Complete examination of the skin and oral mucosa combined with a biopsy and direct immunofluorescence microscopy will aid in distinguishing these two entities. The peripheral active lesions in folliculitis decalvans are follicular pustules; these patients can develop a reactive arthritis.

FIGURATE SKIN LESIONS

(Table 54-6) In *figurate eruptions*, the lesions form rings and arcs that are usually erythematous but can be skin-colored to brown. Most commonly, they are due to primary cutaneous diseases such as *tinea, urticaria, erythema annulare centrifugum*, and *granuloma annulare* (Chaps. 53 and 55). An underlying systemic illness is found in a second, less common group of migratory annular erythemas. It includes *erythema gyratum repens, erythema migrans, erythema marginatum*, and *necrolytic migratory erythema*.

In erythema gyratum repens, one sees numerous mobile concentric arcs and wavefronts that resemble the grain in wood. A search for an underlying malignancy is mandatory in a patient with this eruption. Erythema migrans is the cutaneous manifestation of Lyme disease, which is caused by the spirochete *Borrelia burgdorferi*. In the initial stage (3–30 days after tick bite), a single annular lesion is usually seen, which can expand to ≥10 cm in diameter. Within several days, approximately half the patients develop multiple smaller erythematous lesions at sites distant from the bite. Associated symptoms include fever, headache, photophobia, myalgias, arthralgias, and malar rash. Erythema marginatum is seen in patients with rheumatic fever, primarily on the trunk. Lesions are pink-red in color, flat to mildly elevated, and transient.

There are additional cutaneous diseases that present as annular eruptions but lack an obvious migratory component. Examples include *CTCL, subacute cutaneous lupus, secondary syphilis*, and *sarcoidosis* (see "Papulonodular Skin Lesions," below).

ACNE

(Table 54-7) In addition to *acne vulgaris* and *acne rosacea*, the two major forms of acne (Chap. 53), there are drugs and systemic diseases that can lead to acneiform eruptions (Table 54-7).

TABLE 54-6 CAUSES OF FIGURATE SKIN LESIONS

I. Primary cutaneous disorders
  A. Tinea
  B. Urticaria (≥90% of cases)
  C. Erythema annulare centrifugum
  D. Granuloma annulare
  E. Psoriasis
II. Systemic diseases
  A. Migratory
    1. Erythema migrans
    2. Urticaria (≤10% of cases)
    3. Erythema gyratum repens
    4. Erythema marginatum
    5. Pustular psoriasis
    6. Necrolytic migratory erythema (glucagonoma syndrome)[a]
  B. Nonmigratory
    1. Sarcoidosis
    2. Subacute lupus erythematosus
    3. Secondary syphilis
    4. Cutaneous T cell lymphoma (e.g., mycosis fungoides)

[a]Migratory erythema with erosions; favors lower extremities and girdle area.

TABLE 54-7 CAUSES OF ACNEIFORM ERUPTIONS

I. Primary cutaneous disorders
  A. Acne vulgaris
  B. Acne rosacea
II. Drugs, e.g., anabolic steroids, glucocorticoids, lithium, iodides, EGFR[a] inhibitors
III. Systemic diseases
  A. Increased androgen production
    1. Adrenal origin, e.g., Cushing's disease, 21-hydroxylase deficiency
    2. Ovarian origin, e.g., polycystic ovary syndrome
  B. Cryptococcosis, disseminated
  C. Dimorphic fungi
  D. Behçet's disease

[a]EGFR, epidermal growth factor receptor.

Patients with the *carcinoid syndrome* have episodes of flushing of the head, neck, and sometimes the trunk. Resultant skin changes of the face, in particular telangiectasias, may mimic the clinical appearance of acne rosacea.

PUSTULAR LESIONS

Acneiform eruptions (see "Acne," above) and *folliculitis* represent the most common pustular dermatoses. An important consideration in the evaluation of follicular pustules is a determination of the associated pathogen, e.g., normal flora, *Staphylococcus aureus*, *Pseudomonas aeruginosa* ("hot tub" folliculitis), *Malassezia*, dermatophytes (Majocchi's granuloma). Noninfectious forms of folliculitis include HIV-associated eosinophilic folliculitis and folliculitis secondary to drugs such as glucocorticoids and lithium. Administration of high-dose systemic glucocorticoids can result in a widespread eruption of follicular pustules on the trunk, characterized by lesions in the same stage of development. With regard to underlying systemic diseases, nonfollicular-based pustules are a characteristic component of pustular psoriasis and can be seen in septic emboli of bacterial or fungal origin (see "Purpura," below).

TELANGIECTASIAS

(Table 54-8) In order to distinguish the various types of telangiectasias, it is important to examine the shape and configuration of the dilated blood vessels. *Linear telangiectasias* are seen on the face of patients with *actinically damaged skin* and *acne rosacea,* and they are found on the legs of patients with *venous hypertension* and *essential telangiectasia*. Patients with an unusual form of *mastocytosis* (telangiectasia macularis eruptiva perstans) and the *carcinoid syndrome* (see "Acne," above) also have linear telangiectasias. Lastly, linear telangiectasias are found in areas of cutaneous inflammation. For example, lesions of discoid lupus frequently have telangiectasias within them.

TABLE 54-8 CAUSES OF TELANGIECTASIAS

I. Primary cutaneous disorders	
A. Linear	B. Poikiloderma
1. Acne rosacea	1. Ionizing radiation[a]
2. Actinically damaged skin	2. Poikiloderma vasculare atrophicans
3. Venous hypertension	C. Spider angioma
4. Essential telangiectasia	1. Idiopathic
5. Within basal cell carcinomas	2. Pregnancy
II. Systemic diseases	
A. Linear	D. Periungual
1. Carcinoid	1. Lupus erythematosus
2. Ataxia-telangiectasia	2. Scleroderma
3. Mastocytosis	3. Dermatomyositis
B. Poikiloderma	4. Hereditary hemorrhagic telangiectasia
1. Dermatomyositis	E. Papular
2. Cutaneous T cell lymphoma	1. Hereditary hemorrhagic telangiectasia
3. Xeroderma pigmentosum	F. Spider angioma
C. Mat	1. Cirrhosis
1. Scleroderma	

[a]Becoming less common.

Poikiloderma is a term used to describe a patch of skin with (1) reticulated hypo- and hyperpigmentation, (2) wrinkling secondary to epidermal atrophy, and (3) telangiectasias. Poikiloderma does not imply a single disease entity—although becoming less common, it is seen in skin damaged by *ionizing radiation* as well as in patients with autoimmune connective tissue diseases, primarily *dermatomyositis* (DM), and rare genodermatoses (e.g., Kindler syndrome).

In *scleroderma*, the dilated blood vessels have a unique configuration and are known as *mat telangiectasias*. The lesions are broad macules that usually measure 2–7 mm in diameter but occasionally are larger. Mats have a polygonal or oval shape, and their erythematous color may be uniform or the result of delicate telangiectasias. The most common locations for mat telangiectasias are the face, oral mucosa, and hands—peripheral sites that are prone to intermittent ischemia. The CREST (*c*alcinosis cutis, *R*aynaud's phenomenon, *e*sophageal dysmotility, *s*clerodactyly, and *t*elangiectasia) variant of scleroderma (Chap. 316) is associated with a chronic course and anticentromere antibodies. Mat telangiectasias are an important clue to the diagnosis of the CREST syndrome as well as systemic scleroderma, for they may be the only cutaneous finding.

Periungual telangiectasias are pathognomonic signs of the three major autoimmune connective tissue diseases—*lupus erythematosus*, *scleroderma*, and *DM*. They are easily visualized by the naked eye and occur in at least two-thirds of these patients. In both DM and lupus there is associated nailfold erythema, and in DM the erythema is often accompanied by "ragged" cuticles and fingertip tenderness. Under 10× magnification, the blood vessels in the nailfolds of lupus patients are tortuous and resemble "glomeruli," whereas in scleroderma and DM there is a loss of capillary loops and those that remain are markedly dilated.

In *hereditary hemorrhagic telangiectasia* (Osler-Rendu-Weber disease), the lesions usually appear during adulthood and are most commonly seen on the mucous membranes, face, and distal extremities, including under the nails. They represent arteriovenous (AV) malformations of the dermal microvasculature, are dark red in color, and are usually slightly elevated. When the skin is stretched over an individual lesion, an eccentric punctum with radiating legs is seen. Although the degree of systemic involvement varies in this autosomal dominant disease (due to mutations in either the endoglin or activin receptor–like kinase gene), the major symptoms are recurrent epistaxis and gastrointestinal bleeding. The fact that these mucosal telangiectasias are actually AV communications helps to explain their tendency to bleed.

HYPOPIGMENTATION

(Table 54-9) Disorders of hypopigmentation are often classified as either diffuse or localized. The classic example of *diffuse hypopigmentation* is *oculocutaneous albinism* (OCA). The most common forms are due to mutations in the tyrosinase gene (type I) or the *P* gene (type II); patients with type IA OCA have a total lack of enzyme activity. At birth, different forms of OCA can appear similar—white hair, gray-blue eyes, and pink-white skin. However, the patients with no tyrosinase activity maintain this phenotype, whereas those with decreased activity will acquire some pigmentation of the eyes, hair, and skin as they age. The degree of pigment formation is also a function of racial background, and the pigmentary dilution is readily apparent when patients are compared to their first-degree relatives. The ocular findings in OCA correlate with the degree of hypopigmentation and include decreased visual acuity, nystagmus, photophobia, and a lack of normal binocular vision.

The differential diagnosis of *localized hypomelanosis* includes the following primary cutaneous disorders: *idiopathic guttate hypomelanosis, postinflammatory hypopigmentation, tinea (pityriasis) versicolor, vitiligo, chemical leukoderma, nevus depigmentosus* (see below), and *piebaldism* (Table 54-9). In this group of diseases, the areas of involvement are macules or patches with a decrease or absence of pigmentation. Patients with vitiligo also have an increased incidence of several autoimmune disorders, including hypothyroidism, Graves' disease, pernicious anemia, Addison's disease, uveitis, alopecia areata, chronic mucocutaneous candidiasis, and the polyglandular autoimmune syndromes (types I and II). Diseases of the thyroid gland are the most frequently associated disorders, occurring in up to 30% of patients with

TABLE 54-9 CAUSES OF HYPOPIGMENTATION

I. Primary cutaneous disorders
  A. Diffuse
  1. Generalized vitiligo[a]
  B. Localized
    1. Idiopathic guttate hypomelanosis
    2. Postinflammatory
    3. Tinea (pityriasis) versicolor
    4. Vitiligo
    5. Chemical leukoderma
    6. Nevus depigmentosus
    7. Piebaldism
II. Systemic diseases
  A. Diffuse
    1. Oculocutaneous albinism[b]
      a. Hermansky-Pudlak syndrome[c]
      b. Chédiak-Higashi syndrome[d]
    2. Phenylketonuria
    3. Homocystinuria
  B. Localized
    1. Vogt-Koyanagi-Harada
    2. Scleroderma
    3. Melanoma-associated leukoderma
    4. Tuberous sclerosis
    5. Hypomelanosis of Ito/mosaicism
    6. Incontinentia pigmenti (stage IV)
    7. Sarcoidosis
    8. Tuberculoid and indeterminate leprosy
    9. Cutaneous T cell lymphoma
    10. Onchocerciasis

[a]Absence of melanocytes.
[b]Normal number of melanocytes.
[c]Platelet storage defect and restrictive lung disease secondary to deposits of ceroid-like material; one form due to mutations in β subunit of adaptor protein.
[d]Giant lysosomal granules and recurrent infections.

vitiligo. Circulating autoantibodies are often found, and the most common ones are antithyroglobulin, antimicrosomal, and antithyroid-stimulating hormone receptor antibodies.

There are four systemic diseases that should be considered in a patient with skin findings suggestive of vitiligo—*Vogt-Koyanagi-Harada syndrome*, *scleroderma*, *onchocerciasis*, and *melanoma-associated leukoderma*. A history of aseptic meningitis, nontraumatic uveitis, tinnitus, hearing loss, and/or dysacusis points to the diagnosis of the Vogt-Koyanagi-Harada syndrome. In these patients, the face and scalp are the most common locations of pigment loss. The vitiligo-like leukoderma seen in patients with scleroderma has a clinical resemblance to idiopathic vitiligo that has begun to repigment as a result of treatment; that is, perifollicular macules of normal pigmentation are seen within areas of depigmentation. The basis of this leukoderma is unknown; there is no evidence of inflammation in areas of involvement, but it can resolve if the underlying connective tissue disease becomes inactive. In contrast to idiopathic vitiligo, melanoma-associated leukoderma often begins on the trunk, and its appearance should prompt a search for metastatic disease. It is also seen in patients undergoing immunotherapy for melanoma, with cytotoxic T lymphocytes presumably recognizing cell surface antigens common to melanoma cells and melanocytes.

There are two systemic disorders (neurocristopathies) that may have the cutaneous findings of piebaldism (Table 54-10). They are *Shah-Waardenburg syndrome* and *Waardenburg syndrome*. A possible explanation for both disorders is an abnormal embryonic migration or survival of two neural crest–derived elements, one of them being melanocytes and the other myenteric ganglion cells (leading to Hirschsprung disease in Shah-Waardenburg syndrome) or auditory nerve cells (Waardenburg syndrome). The latter syndrome is characterized by congenital sensorineural hearing loss, dystopia canthorum (lateral displacement of the inner canthi but normal interpupillary distance), heterochromic irises, and a broad nasal root, in addition to the piebaldism. Patients with Waardenburg syndrome have been shown to have mutations in three genes including two (*PAX-3* and *MITF*) that encode DNA-binding proteins, while patients with Hirschsprung disease plus white spotting have mutations in one of three genes—endothelin 3, endothelin B receptor, and *SOX-10*.

In *tuberous sclerosis*, the earliest cutaneous sign is an ash leaf spot. These lesions are often present at birth and are usually multiple; however, detection may require Wood's lamp examination, especially in fair-skinned individuals. The pigment within them is reduced but not absent. The average size is 1–3 cm, and the common shapes are polygonal and lance-ovate. Examination of the patient for additional cutaneous signs such as multiple angiofibromas of the face (adenoma sebaceum), ungual and gingival fibromas, fibrous plaques of the forehead, and connective tissue nevi (shagreen patches) is recommended. It is important to remember that an ash leaf spot on the scalp will result in *poliosis*, which is a circumscribed patch of gray-white hair. Internal manifestations include seizures, mental retardation, central nervous system (CNS) and retinal hamartomas, renal angiomyolipomas, and cardiac rhabdomyomas. The latter can be detected in up to 60% of children (<18 years) with tuberous sclerosis by echocardiography.

Nevus depigmentosus is a stable, well-circumscribed hypomelanosis that is present at birth. There is usually a single oval or rectangular lesion, but occasionally the nevus has a segmental or whorled pattern (also referred to as *linear nevoid hypopigmentation*). It is important to distinguish this more common entity from ash leaf spots of tuberous sclerosis, especially when there are multiple lesions. In *hypomelanosis of Ito*, swirls and streaks of hypopigmentation run parallel to one another in a pattern that resembles a marble cake. Lesions may progress or regress with time, and in up to a third of patients, associated abnormalities are found involving the musculoskeletal system (asymmetry), the CNS (seizures and mental retardation), and the eyes (strabismus and hypertelorism). Chromosomal mosaicism has been detected in these patients, lending support to the hypothesis that the pattern is the result of the migration of two clones of primordial melanocytes, each with a different pigment potential.

Localized areas of decreased pigmentation are commonly seen as a result of cutaneous inflammation (Table 54-10) and have been observed in the skin overlying active lesions of sarcoidosis (see "Papulonodular Skin Lesions," below) as well as in CTCL. Cutaneous infections also present as disorders of hypopigmentation, and in *tuberculoid leprosy* there are a few asymmetric patches of hypomelanosis that have associated anesthesia, anhidrosis, and alopecia. Biopsy specimens of the palpable border show dermal granulomas that contain rare, if any, *Mycobacterium leprae* organisms.

HYPERPIGMENTATION

(Table 54-11) Disorders of hyperpigmentation are also divided into two groups—localized and diffuse. The localized forms are due to an epidermal alteration, a proliferation of melanocytes, or an increase in pigment production. Both seborrheic keratoses and acanthosis nigricans belong to the first group. *Seborrheic keratoses* are common lesions, but in one rare clinical setting they are a sign of systemic disease, and that setting is the sudden appearance of multiple lesions, often with an inflammatory base and in association with acrochordons (skin tags) and acanthosis nigricans. This is termed the *sign of Leser-Trélat* and alerts the clinician to search for an internal malignancy. *Acanthosis nigricans* can also be a reflection of an internal malignancy, most commonly of the gastrointestinal tract, and it appears as velvety hyperpigmentation, primarily in flexural areas. In the majority of patients, acanthosis nigricans is associated with obesity and insulin resistance, but it may be a reflection of an endocrinopathy such as acromegaly, Cushing's syndrome, polycystic ovary syndrome, or insulin-resistant diabetes mellitus (type A, type B, and lipoatrophic forms).

A proliferation of melanocytes results in the following pigmented lesions: *lentigo*, *melanocytic nevus*, and *melanoma* (Chap. 83). In an adult, the majority of lentigines are related to sun exposure, which explains their distribution. However, in the Peutz-Jeghers and LEOPARD [*l*entigines; *E*CG abnormalities, primarily conduction defects; *o*cular hypertelorism; *p*ulmonary stenosis and subaortic valvular stenosis; *a*bnormal genitalia (cryptorchidism, hypospadias); *r*etardation of growth; and *d*eafness (sensorineural)] syndromes, lentigines do serve

TABLE 54-10 HYPOPIGMENTATION (PRIMARY CUTANEOUS DISORDERS, LOCALIZED)

	Clinical Characteristics	Wood's Lamp Examination (UV-A; Peak = 365 nm)	Skin Biopsy Specimen	Pathogenesis	Treatment
Idiopathic guttate hypomelanosis	Common; acquired; 1–4 mm in diameter Shins and extensor forearms	Less enhancement than vitiligo	Abrupt decrease in epidermal melanin content	Possible somatic mutations as a reflection of aging; UV exposure	None
Postinflammatory hypopigmentation	Can develop within active lesions, as in subacute lupus, or after the lesion fades, as in dermatitis	Depends on particular disease Usually less enhancement than in vitiligo	Type of inflammatory infiltrate depends on specific disease	Block in transfer of melanin from melanocytes to keratinocytes could be secondary to edema or decrease in contact time Destruction of melanocytes if inflammatory cells attack basal layer	Treat underlying inflammatory disease
Tinea (pityriasis) versicolor	Common disorder Upper trunk and neck Shawl-like distribution Young adults Macules have fine white scale when scratched	Golden fluorescence	Hyphae and budding yeast in stratum corneum	Invasion of stratum corneum by the yeast *Malassezia* Yeast is lipophilic and produces C_9 and C_{11} dicarboxylic acids, which in vitro inhibit tyrosinase	Selenium sulfide 2.5%; topical imidazoles; oral imidazoles or triazoles
Vitiligo	Acquired; progressive Symmetric areas of complete pigment loss Periorificial—around mouth, nose, eyes, nipples, umbilicus, anus Other areas—flexor wrists, extensor distal extremities Segmental form is less common—unilateral, dermatomal-like	More apparent Chalk-white	Absence of melanocytes Mild inflammation	Possible autoimmune phenomenon that results in destruction of melanocytes—cellular and/or humoral Alternative hypothesis is self-destruction of melanocytes and circulating antibodies or cytotoxic T cells as a secondary phenomenon	Topical glucocorticoids; topical calcineurin inhibitors; UV-B; PUVA; transplants; depigmentation if widespread
Chemical leukoderma	Similar appearance to vitiligo Often begins on hands Satellite lesions in areas not exposed to chemicals	More apparent Chalk-white	Decreased number or absence of melanocytes	Exposure to chemicals that selectively destroy melanocytes, in particular phenols and catechols (germicides; adhesives) Release of cellular antigens and activation of circulating lymphocytes may explain satellite phenomenon	Avoid exposure to offending agent, then treat as vitiligo
Piebaldism	Autosomal dominant Congenital, stable White forelock Areas of hypomelanosis contain normally pigmented and hyperpigmented macules of various sizes Symmetric involvement of central forehead, ventral trunk, and mid regions of upper and lower extremities	Enhancement of leukoderma and hyperpigmented macules	Hypomelanotic areas—few to no melanocytes	Defect in migration of melanoblasts from neural crest to ventral skin or failure of melanoblasts to survive or differentiate in these areas Mutations within the *c-kit* proto-oncogene that encodes the tyrosine kinase receptor for stem cell growth factor	None; occasionally transplants

***Note:** PUVA, psoralens +ultraviolet A irradiation; UV-B, ultraviolet B.*

as a clue to systemic disease. In *LEOPARD syndrome*, hundreds of lentigines develop during childhood and are scattered over the entire surface of the body. The lentigines in patients with *Peutz-Jeghers syndrome* are located primarily around the nose and mouth, on the hands and feet, and within the oral cavity. While the pigmented macules on the face may fade with age, the oral lesions persist. However, similar intraoral lesions are also seen in Addison's disease and as a normal finding in darkly pigmented individuals. Patients with this autosomal dominant syndrome (due to mutations in a novel serine threonine kinase gene) have multiple benign polyps of the gastrointestinal tract, testicular tumors, and an increased risk of developing gastrointestinal (primarily colon), pancreatic, and gynecologic cancers.

In the Carney complex, numerous lentigines are also seen, but in association with cardiac myxomas. This autosomal dominant disorder is also known as the *LAMB* (*l*entigines, *a*trial myxomas, *m*ucocutaneous myxomas, and *b*lue nevi) *syndrome* or *NAME* [*n*evi, *a*trial myxoma, *m*yxoid neurofibroma, and *e*phelides (freckles)] *syndrome.* These patients can also have evidence of endocrine overactivity in the form of Cushing's syndrome, acromegaly, or sexual precocity.

The third type of localized hyperpigmentation is due to a local increase in pigment production, and it includes *ephelides* and café au lait macules (CALM). The latter are most commonly associated with two disorders—neurofibromatosis (NF) and McCune-Albright syndrome. *CALM* are flat, uniformly brown in color (usually two shades darker than uninvolved skin), and can vary in size from 0.5–12 cm. Approximately 80–90% of adult patients with *type I NF* will have six or more CALM measuring ≥1.5 cm in diameter. Additional findings are discussed in the section on neurofibromas (see "Papulonodular Skin Le-

TABLE 54-11 CAUSES OF HYPERPIGMENTATION

I. Primary cutaneous disorders
A. Localized
1. Epidermal alteration
a. Seborrheic keratosis
b. Acanthosis nigricans (obesity)
c. Pigmented actinic keratosis
2. Proliferation of melanocytes
a. Lentigo
b. Nevus
c. Melanoma
3. Increased pigment production
a. Ephelides (freckles)
b. Café au lait macule
c. Postinflammatory hyperpigmentation
B. Localized and diffuse
1. Drugs
II. Systemic diseases
A. Localized
1. Epidermal alteration
a. Seborrheic keratoses (sign of Leser-Trélat)
b. Acanthosis nigricans (endocrine disorders, paraneoplastic)
2. Proliferation of melanocytes
a. Lentigines (Peutz-Jeghers and LEOPARD syndromes; xeroderma pigmentosum)
b. Nevi [Carney complex (LAMB and NAME syndromes)][a]
3. Increased pigment production
a. Café au lait macules (neurofibromatosis, McCune-Albright syndrome[b])
b. Urticaria pigmentosa[c]
4. Dermal pigmentation
a. Incontinentia pigmenti (stage III)
b. Dyskeratosis congenita
B. Diffuse
1. Endocrinopathies
a. Addison's disease
b. Nelson syndrome
c. Ectopic ACTH syndrome
2. Metabolic
a. Porphyria cutanea tarda
b. Hemochromatosis
c. Vitamin B_{12}, folate deficiency
d. Pellagra
e. Malabsorption, Whipple's disease
3. Melanosis secondary to metastatic melanoma
4. Autoimmune
a. Biliary cirrhosis
b. Scleroderma
c. POEMS syndrome
d. Eosinophilia-myalgia syndrome[d]
5. Drugs and metals

[a] Also lentigines.
[b] Polyostotic fibrous dysplasia.
[c] See also "Papulonodular Skin Lesions."
[d] Late 1980s.

sions," below). In comparison with NF, the CALM in patients with *McCune-Albright syndrome* [polyostotic fibrous dysplasia with precocious puberty in females due to mosaicism for an activating mutation in a G protein ($G_s\alpha$) gene] are usually larger, more irregular in outline, and tend to respect the midline. CALM have also been associated with pulmonary stenosis (Watson syndrome), tuberous sclerosis, the LEOPARD syndrome, and multiple endocrine neoplasia (MEN), but a few such lesions can be found in normal individuals.

In incontinentia pigmenti, dyskeratosis congenita, and bleomycin pigmentation, the areas of localized hyperpigmentation form a pattern—swirled in the first, reticulated in the second, and flagellate in the third. In *dyskeratosis congenita*, atrophic reticulated hyperpigmentation is seen on the neck, trunk, and thighs and is accompanied by nail dystrophy, pancytopenia, and leukoplakia of the oral and anal mucosae. The latter often develops into squamous cell carcinoma. In addition to the flagellate pigmentation (linear streaks) on the trunk, patients receiving bleomycin often have hyperpigmentation overlying the elbows, knees, and small joints of the hand.

Localized hyperpigmentation is seen as a side effect of several other *systemic medications*, including those that produce fixed drug reactions [nonsteroidal anti-inflammatory drugs (NSAIDs), sulfonamides, barbiturates, and tetracyclines] and those that can complex with melanin (antimalarials) or iron (minocycline). Fixed drug eruptions recur in the exact same location as circular areas of erythema that can become bullous and then resolve as brown macules. The eruption usually appears within hours of administration of the offending agent, and common locations include the genitalia, extremities, and perioral region. Chloroquine and hydroxychloroquine produce gray-brown to blue-black discoloration of the shins, hard palate, and face, while blue macules (often misdiagnosed as bruises) can be seen on the lower extremities and in sites of inflammation with prolonged minocycline administration. Estrogen in oral contraceptives can induce melasma—symmetric brown patches on the face, especially the cheeks, upper lip, and forehead. Similar changes are seen in pregnancy and in patients receiving phenytoin.

In the diffuse forms of hyperpigmentation, the darkening of the skin may be of equal intensity over the entire body or may be accentuated in sun-exposed areas. The causes of diffuse hyperpigmentation can be divided into four major groups—endocrine, metabolic, autoimmune, and drugs. The endocrinopathies that frequently have associated hyperpigmentation include *Addison's disease*, *Nelson syndrome*, and *ectopic ACTH syndrome*. In these diseases, the increased pigmentation is diffuse but is accentuated in the palmar creases, sites of friction, scars, and the oral mucosa. An overproduction of the pituitary hormones α-MSH (melanocyte-stimulating hormone) and ACTH can lead to an increase in melanocyte activity. These peptides are products of the proopiomelanocortin gene and exhibit homology; e.g., α-MSH and ACTH share 13 amino acids. A minority of the patients with Cushing's disease or hyperthyroidism have generalized hyperpigmentation.

The metabolic causes of hyperpigmentation include *porphyria cutanea tarda* (PCT), *hemochromatosis*, *vitamin B_{12} deficiency*, *folic acid deficiency*, *pellagra*, *malabsorption*, and *Whipple's disease*. In patients with PCT (see "Vesicles/Bullae," below), the skin darkening is seen in sun-exposed areas and is a reflection of the photoreactive properties of porphyrins. The increased level of iron in the skin of patients with hemochromatosis stimulates melanin pigment production and leads to the classic bronze color. Patients with pellagra have a brown discoloration of the skin, especially in sun-exposed areas, as a result of nicotinic acid (niacin) deficiency. In the areas of increased pigmentation, there is a thin varnish-like scale. These changes are also seen in patients who are vitamin B_6 deficient, have functioning carcinoid tumors (increased consumption of niacin), or take isoniazid. Approximately 50% of the patients with Whipple's disease have an associated generalized hyperpigmentation in association with diarrhea, weight loss, arthritis, and lymphadenopathy. A diffuse slate-blue color is seen in patients with melanosis secondary to metastatic melanoma. Although there is a debate as to whether the color is due to single-cell metastases in the dermis or to a widespread deposition of melanin resulting from the high concentration of circulating melanin precursors, there is more evidence to support the latter.

Of the autoimmune diseases associated with diffuse hyperpigmentation, *biliary cirrhosis* and *scleroderma* are the most common, and occasionally both disorders are seen in the same patient. The skin is dark brown in color, especially in sun-exposed areas. In biliary cirrhosis the hyperpigmentation is accompanied by pruritus, jaundice, and xanthomas, whereas in scleroderma it is accompanied by sclerosis of the extremities, face, and, less commonly, the trunk. Additional clues to the diagnosis of scleroderma are telangiectasias, calcinosis cutis, Raynaud's phenomenon, and distal ulcerations (see "Telangiectasias," above). The differential diagnosis of cutaneous sclerosis with hyperpigmentation includes the POEMS [*p*olyneuropathy; *o*rganomegaly (liver, spleen, lymph nodes); *e*ndocrinopathies (impotence, gynecomastia); *M*-protein; and *s*kin changes] syndrome. The skin changes include hyperpigmentation, skin thickening, hypertrichosis, and angiomas.

Diffuse hyperpigmentation that is due to drugs or metals can result from one of several mechanisms—induction of melanin pigment formation, complexing of the drug or its metabolites to melanin, and deposits of the drug in the dermis. Busulfan, cyclophosphamide, 5-fluorouracil, and inorganic arsenic induce pigment production. Complexes containing melanin or hemosiderin plus the drug or its metabolites are seen in patients receiving chlorpromazine and minocycline. The sun-exposed skin as well as the conjunctivae of patients on long-term, high-dose chlorpromazine can become blue-gray in color. Patients taking minocycline may develop a diffuse blue-gray, muddy appearance in sun-exposed areas in addition to pigmentation of the mucous membranes, teeth, nails, bones, and thyroid. Administration of amiodarone can result in both a phototoxic eruption (exaggerated sunburn) and/or a brown or blue-gray discoloration of sun-exposed skin. Biopsy specimens of the latter show yellow-brown granules in dermal macrophages, which represent intralysosomal accumulations of lipids, amiodarone, and its metabolites. Actual deposits of a particular drug or metal in the skin are seen with silver (argyria), where the skin appears blue-gray in color; gold (chrysiasis), where the skin has a brown to blue-gray color; and clofazimine, where the skin appears reddish brown. The associated hyperpigmentation is accentuated in sun-exposed areas, and discoloration of the eye is seen with gold (sclerae) and clofazimine (conjunctivae).

VESICLES/BULLAE

(Table 54-12) Depending on their size, cutaneous blisters are referred to as *vesicles* (<0.5 cm) or *bullae* (>0.5 cm). The primary blistering disorders include *pemphigus vulgaris, pemphigus foliaceus, pemphigus erythematosus, paraneoplastic pemphigus, bullous pemphigoid, gestational pemphigoid, cicatricial pemphigoid, epidermolysis bullosa acquisita, linear IgA bullous dermatosis*, and *dermatitis herpetiformis* (Chap. 55).

Vesicles and bullae are also seen in *contact dermatitis*, both allergic and irritant forms (Chap. 53). When there is a linear arrangement of vesicular lesions, an exogenous cause should be suspected. Bullous disease secondary to the ingestion of drugs can take one of several forms, including phototoxic eruptions, isolated bullae, Stevens-Johnson syndrome (SJS), and toxic epidermal necrolysis (TEN) (Chap. 56). Clinically, phototoxic eruptions resemble an exaggerated sunburn with diffuse erythema and bullae in sun-exposed areas. The most commonly associated drugs are doxycycline, sulfonamides, thiazides, NSAIDs, and psoralens. The development of a phototoxic eruption is dependent on the doses of both the drug and ultraviolet (UV)-A irradiation.

Toxic epidermal necrolysis is characterized by bullae that arise on widespread areas of erythema and then slough. This results in large areas of denuded skin. The associated morbidity, such as sepsis, and mortality are relatively high and are a function of the extent of epidermal necrosis. In addition, these patients may also have involvement of the mucous membranes and intestinal tract. Drugs are the primary cause of TEN, and the most common offenders are phenytoin, barbiturates, carbamazepine, sulfonamides, penicillins, and NSAIDs. Severe acute graft-versus-host disease (grade 4) can also resemble TEN.

In *erythema multiforme* (EM), the primary lesions are pink-red macules and edematous papules, the centers of which may become vesicular. The clue to the diagnosis of EM, as opposed to a morbilliform exanthem, is the development of a "dusky" violet color or petechiae in the center of the lesions. Target or iris lesions are also characteristic of EM and arise as a result of active centers and borders in combination with centrifugal spread. However, iris lesions need not be present to make the diagnosis of EM.

EM has been subdivided into two major groups: (1) EM minor due to herpes simplex virus (HSV); and (2) EM major due to HSV, *Mycoplasma pneumoniae*, or rarely drugs. Involvement of the mucous membranes (oral, nasal, ocular, and genital) is seen more commonly in the latter form. Hemorrhagic crusts of the lips are characteristic of EM major and SJS as well as herpes simplex, pemphigus vulgaris, and paraneoplastic pemphigus. Fever, malaise, myalgias, sore throat, and cough may precede or accompany the eruption. The lesions of EM usually resolve over 3–6 weeks but may be recurrent, especially when due to HSV. In addition to HSV (in which lesions appear 7–12 days after the viral eruption), EM can also follow vaccinations, radiation therapy, and exposure to environmental toxins.

Induction of SJS is most often due to drugs, especially sulfonamides, phenytoin, barbiturates, penicillins, and carbamazepine. Widespread dusky macules and significant mucosal involvement are characteristic of SJS, and the cutaneous lesions may or may not develop epidermal detachment. If the latter occurs, by definition, it is limited to <10% of the body surface area (BSA). Greater involvement leads to the diagnosis of SJS/TEN overlap (10–30% BSA) or TEN (>30% BSA).

In addition to primary blistering disorders and hypersensitivity reactions, bacterial and viral infections can lead to vesicles and bullae. The most common infectious agents are HSV (Chap. 172), varicella-zoster virus (Chap. 173), and *S. aureus* (Chap. 129).

Staphylococcal scalded-skin syndrome (SSSS) and *bullous impetigo* are two blistering disorders associated with staphylococcal (phage group II) infection. In SSSS, the initial findings are redness and tenderness of the central face, neck, trunk, and intertriginous zones. This is followed by short-lived flaccid bullae and a slough or exfoliation of the superficial epidermis. Crusted areas then develop, characteristically around the mouth. SSSS is distinguished from TEN by the following features: younger age group (primarily infants), more superficial site of blister formation, no oral lesions, shorter course, less morbidity and mortality, and an association with staphylococcal exfoliative toxin ("exfoliatin"), not drugs. A rapid diagnosis of SSSS versus TEN can be made by a frozen section of the blister roof or exfoliative cytology of the blister contents. In SSSS the site of staphylococcal infection is usually extracutaneous (conjunctivitis, rhinorrhea, otitis media, pharyngitis, tonsillitis), and the cutaneous lesions are sterile, whereas in bullous impetigo the skin lesions are the site of infection. Impetigo is more localized than SSSS and usually presents with honey-colored crusts. Occasionally, superficial purulent blisters also form. *Cutaneous emboli* from gram-negative infections may present as isolated bullae, but the base of the lesion is purpuric or necrotic, and it may develop into an ulcer (see "Purpura," below).

TABLE 54-12 CAUSES OF VESICLES/BULLAE

- I. Primary cutaneous diseases
  - A. Primary blistering diseases (autoimmune)
    1. Pemphigus[a]
    2. Bullous pemphigoid[b]
    3. Gestational pemphigoid[b]
    4. Cicatricial pemphigoid[b]
    5. Dermatitis herpetiformis[b,c]
    6. Linear IgA bullous dermatosis[b]
    7. Epidermolysis bullosa acquisita[b,d]
  - B. Secondary blistering diseases
    1. Contact dermatitis[a]
    2. Erythema multiforme[a,b]
    3. Stevens-Johnson syndrome
    4. Toxic epidermal necrolysis[b]
  - C. Infections
    1. Varicella/zoster virus[a,e]
    2. Herpes simplex virus[a,e]
    3. Enteroviruses, e.g., hand-foot-and-mouth disease
    4. Staphylococcal scalded-skin syndrome[a,f]
    5. Bullous impetigo[a]
- II. Systemic diseases
  - A. Autoimmune
    1. Paraneoplastic pemphigus[a]
  - B. Infections
    1. Cutaneous emboli[b]
  - C. Metabolic
    1. Diabetic bullae[a,b]
    2. Porphyria cutanea tarda[b]
    3. Porphyria variegata[b]
    4. Pseudoporphyria[b]
    5. Bullous dermatosis of hemodialysis[b]
  - D. Ischemia
    1. Coma bullae

[a]Intraepidermal.
[b]Subepidermal.
[c]Associated with gluten enteropathy.
[d]Associated with inflammatory bowel disease.
[e]Also systemic.
[f]In adults, associated with renal failure and immunocompromised state.

Several metabolic disorders are associated with blister formation, including diabetes mellitus, renal failure, and porphyria. Local hypoxia secondary to decreased cutaneous blood flow can also produce blisters, which explains the presence of bullae over pressure points in comatose patients (coma bullae). In *diabetes mellitus*, tense bullae with clear viscous fluid arise on normal skin. The lesions can be as large as 6 cm in diameter and are located on the distal extremities. There are several types of porphyria, but the most common form with cutaneous findings is *PCT*. In sun-exposed areas (primarily the face and hands), the skin is very fragile, and trauma leads to erosions and tense vesicles. These lesions then heal with scarring and formation of milia; the latter are firm, 1- to 2-mm white or yellow papules that represent epidermoid inclusion cysts. Associated findings can include hypertrichosis of the lateral malar region (men) or face (women) and, in sun-exposed areas, hyperpigmentation and firm sclerotic plaques. An elevated level of urinary uroporphyrins confirms the diagnosis and is due to a decrease in uroporphyrinogen decarboxylase activity. Precipitating agents include alcohol, iron, chlorinated hydrocarbons, hepatitis C infection, and hepatomas.

The differential diagnosis of PCT includes (1) *porphyria variegata*—the skin signs of PCT plus the systemic findings of acute intermittent porphyria; it has a diagnostic plasma porphyrin fluorescence emission at 626 nm; (2) *drug-induced* pseudoporphyria—the clinical and histologic findings are similar to PCT, but porphyrins are normal; etiologic agents include naproxen, furosemide, tetracycline, and nalidixic acid; (3) *bullous dermatosis of hemodialysis*—the same appearance as PCT, but porphyrins are usually normal or occasionally borderline elevated; patients have chronic renal failure and are on hemodialysis; (4) PCT associated with hepatomas, hepatic carcinomas, and hemodialysis; and (5) *epidermolysis bullosa acquisita* (Chap. 55).

EXANTHEMS

(Table 54-13) Exanthems are characterized by an acute generalized eruption. The two most common presentations are erythematous macules and papules (morbilliform) and confluent blanching erythema (scarlatiniform). *Morbilliform* eruptions are usually due to either drugs or viral infections. For example, up to 5% of the patients receiving penicillins, sulfonamides, phenytoin, or gold will develop a maculopapular eruption. Accompanying signs may include pruritus, fever, eosinophilia, and transient lymphadenopathy. Similar maculopapular eruptions are seen in the classic childhood viral exanthems, including (1) *rubeola* (measles)—a prodrome of coryza, cough, and conjunctivitis followed by Koplik's spots on the buccal mucosa; the eruption begins behind the ears, at the hairline, and on the forehead and then spreads down the body, often becoming confluent; (2) *rubella*—the eruption begins on the forehead and face and then spreads down the body; it resolves in the same order and is associated with retroauricular and suboccipital lymphadenopathy; and (3) *erythema infectiosum* (fifth disease)—erythema of the cheeks is followed by a reticulated pattern on extremities; it is secondary to a parvovirus B19 infection, and an associated arthritis is seen in adults.

TABLE 54-13 CAUSES OF EXANTHEMS

I. Morbilliform
  A. Drugs
  B. Viral
    1. Rubeola (measles)
    2. Rubella
    3. Erythema infectiosum
    4. Epstein-Barr virus, echovirus, coxsackievirus, CMV,[a] and adenovirus
    5. Early HIV (plus mucosal ulcerations)
  C. Bacterial
    1. Typhoid fever
    2. Early secondary syphilis
    3. Early *Rickettsia*
    4. Early meningococcemia
  D. Acute graft-versus-host disease
  E. Kawasaki disease
II. Scarlatiniform
  A. Scarlet fever
  B. Toxic shock syndrome
  C. Kawasaki disease
  D. Early staphylococcal scalded-skin syndrome

[a]CMV, cytomegalovirus.

Both measles and rubella are seen in unvaccinated young adults, and an atypical form of measles is seen in adults immunized with either killed measles vaccine or killed vaccine followed in time by live vaccine. In contrast to classic measles, the eruption of atypical measles begins on the palms, soles, wrists, and knuckles, and the lesions may become purpuric. The patient with atypical measles can have pulmonary involvement and be quite ill. Rubelliform and roseoliform eruptions are also associated with *Epstein-Barr virus* (5–15% of patients), *echovirus, coxsackievirus, cytomegalovirus*, and *adenovirus* infections. Detection of specific IgM antibodies or fourfold elevations in IgG antibodies allows the proper diagnosis. Occasionally, a maculopapular drug eruption is a reflection of an underlying viral infection. For example, about 95% of the patients with infectious mononucleosis who are given ampicillin will develop a rash.

Of note, early in the course of infections with *Rickettsia* and meningococcus, prior to the development of purpura, the lesions may be erythematous macules and papules. This is also the case in chickenpox prior to the development of vesicles. Maculopapular eruptions are associated with early *HIV infection*, early secondary *syphilis, typhoid fever*, and *acute graft-versus-host disease*. In the last, lesions frequently begin on the palms and soles; the macular rose spots of typhoid fever involve primarily the anterior trunk.

The prototypic *scarlatiniform* eruption is seen in *scarlet fever* and is due to an erythrotoxin produced by group A β-hemolytic streptococcal infections, most commonly pharyngitis. This eruption is characterized by diffuse erythema, which begins on the neck and upper trunk, and red follicular puncta. Additional findings include a white strawberry tongue (white coating with red papillae) followed by a red strawberry tongue (red tongue with red papillae); petechiae of the palate; a facial flush with circumoral pallor; linear petechiae in the antecubital fossae; and desquamation of the involved skin, palms, and soles 5–20 days after onset of the eruption. A similar desquamation of the palms and soles is seen in toxic shock syndrome (TSS), Kawasaki's disease, and after severe febrile illnesses. Certain strains of staphylococci also produce an erythrotoxin that leads to the same clinical findings as in streptococcal scarlet fever, except that the anti-streptolysin O or -DNase B titers are not elevated.

In *toxic shock syndrome*, staphylococcal (phage group I) infections produce an exotoxin (TSST-1) that causes the fever and rash, as well as enterotoxins. Initially, the majority of cases were reported in menstruating women who were using tampons. However, other sites of infection, including wounds and vaginitis, can lead to TSS. The diagnosis of TSS is based on clinical criteria (Chap. 129), and three of these involve mucocutaneous sites (diffuse erythema of the skin, desquamation of the palms and soles 1–2 weeks after onset of illness, and involvement of the mucous membranes). The latter is characterized as hyperemia of the vagina, oropharynx, or conjunctivae. Similar systemic findings have been described in *streptococcal toxic shock–like syndrome* (Chap. 130), and although an exanthem is seen less often than in TSS due to a staphylococcal infection, the underlying infection is often in the soft tissue.

The cutaneous eruption in *Kawasaki's disease* (mucocutaneous lymph node syndrome) (Chap. 319) is polymorphous, but the two most common forms are morbilliform and scarlatiniform. Additional mucocutaneous findings include bilateral conjunctival injection; erythema and edema of the hands and feet followed by desquamation; and diffuse erythema of the oropharynx, red strawberry tongue, and erosions with crusting on the lips. This clinical picture can resemble TSS and scarlet fever, but clues to the diagnosis of Kawasaki's disease are cervical lymphadenopathy, lip erosions, and thrombocytosis. The most serious associated systemic finding in this disease is coronary aneurysm secondary to arteritis. Aneurysms may lead to sudden death, primarily within the first 30 days of the illness. Scarlatiniform eruptions are also seen in the early phase of SSSS (see "Vesicles/Bullae," above) and as reactions to drugs.

URTICARIA

(Table 54-14) *Urticaria* (hives) are transient lesions that are composed of a central wheal surrounded by an erythematous halo. Individual lesions are round, oval, or figurate and are often pruritic. Acute and chronic urticaria has a wide variety of allergic etiologies and reflect edema in the dermis. Urticarial lesions can also be seen in patients with mastocytosis (urticaria pigmentosa), hyperthyroidism, and systemic-onset juvenile idiopathic arthritis (Still's disease). In both juvenile- and adult-onset Still's disease, the lesions coincide with the fever spike, are transient, and are due to dermal infiltrates of neutrophils.

The common *physical urticarias* include dermographism, solar urticaria, cold urticaria, and cholinergic urticaria. Patients with *dermographism* exhibit linear wheals following minor pressure or scratching of the skin. It is a common disorder, affecting ~5% of the population. *Solar urticaria* characteristically occurs within minutes of sun exposure and is a skin sign of one systemic disease—erythropoietic protoporphyria. In addition to the urticaria, these patients have subtle pitted scarring of the nose and hands. *Cold urticaria* is precipitated by exposure to the cold, and therefore exposed areas are usually affected. In some patients, the disease is associated with abnormal circulating proteins—more commonly cryoglobulins and less commonly cryofibrinogens or cold agglutinins. Additional systemic symptoms include wheezing and syncope, thus explaining the need for these patients to avoid swimming in cold water. *Cholinergic urticaria* is precipitated by heat, exercise, or emotion and is characterized by small wheals with relatively large flares. It is occasionally associated with wheezing.

Whereas urticarias are the result of dermal edema, subcutaneous edema leads to the clinical picture of *angioedema*. Sites of involvement include the eyelids, lips, tongue, larynx, and gastrointestinal tract as well as the subcutaneous tissue. Angioedema occurs alone or in combination with urticaria, including urticarial vasculitis and the physical urticarias. Both acquired and hereditary (autosomal dominant) forms of angioedema occur (Chap. 311), and in the latter, urticaria is rarely, if ever, seen.

Urticarial vasculitis is an immune complex disease that may be confused with simple urticaria. In contrast to simple urticaria, individual lesions tend to last longer than 24 h and usually develop central petechiae that can be observed even after the urticarial phase has resolved. The patient may also complain of burning rather than pruritus. On biopsy, there is a leukocytoclastic vasculitis of the small blood vessels. Although many cases of urticarial vasculitis are idiopathic in origin, it can be a reflection of an underlying systemic illness such as lupus erythematosus, Sjögren's syndrome, or hereditary complement deficiency. There is a spectrum of urticarial vasculitis that ranges from purely cutaneous to multisystem involvement. The most common systemic signs and symptoms are arthralgias and/or arthritis, nephritis, and crampy abdominal pain, with asthma and chronic obstructive lung disease seen less often. Hypocomplementemia occurs in one- to two-thirds of patients, even in the idiopathic cases. Urticarial vasculitis can also be seen in patients with *hepatitis B* and *hepatitis C* infections, *serum sickness*, and *serum sickness–like illnesses*.

TABLE 54-14 CAUSES OF URTICARIA AND ANGIOEDEMA

I. Primary cutaneous disorders
A. Acute and chronic urticaria[a]
B. Physical urticaria
1. Dermatographism
2. Solar urticaria[b]
3. Cold urticaria[b]
4. Cholinergic urticaria[b]
C. Angioedema (hereditary and acquired)[b]
II. Systemic diseases
A. Urticarial vasculitis
B. Hepatitis B or C infection
C. Serum sickness
D. Angioedema (hereditary and acquired)

[a]A small minority develop anaphylaxis.
[b]Also systemic.

PAPULONODULAR SKIN LESIONS

(Table 54-15) In the *papulonodular diseases*, the lesions are elevated above the surface of the skin and may coalesce to form plaques. The location, consistency, and color of the lesions are the keys to their diagnosis; this section is organized on the basis of color.

WHITE LESIONS

In *calcinosis cutis* there are firm white to white-yellow papules with an irregular surface. When the contents are expressed, a chalky white material is seen. *Dystrophic calcification* is seen at sites of previous inflammation or damage to the skin. It develops in acne scars as well as on the distal extremities of patients with scleroderma and in the subcutaneous tissue and intermuscular fascial planes in DM. The latter is more extensive and is more commonly seen in children. An elevated calcium phosphate product, most commonly due to secondary hyperparathyroidism in the setting of renal failure, can lead to nodules of *metastatic calcinosis cutis*, which tend to be subcutaneous and periarticular. These patients can also develop calcification of muscular arteries and subsequent ischemic necrosis (calciphylaxis).

SKIN-COLORED LESIONS

There are several types of skin-colored lesions, including epidermoid inclusion cysts, lipomas, rheumatoid nodules, neurofibromas, angiofibromas, neuromas, and adnexal tumors such as tricholemmomas. Both *epidermoid inclusion cysts* and *lipomas* are very common mobile subcutaneous nodules—the former are rubbery and drain cheeselike material (sebum and keratin) if incised. Lipomas are firm and somewhat lobulated on palpation. When extensive facial epidermoid inclusion cysts develop during childhood or there is a family history of such lesions, the patient should be examined for other signs of Gardner syndrome, including osteomas and desmoid tumors. *Rheumatoid nodules* are firm, 0.5- to 4-cm nodules that tend to localize around pressure points, especially the elbows. They are seen in ~20% of patients with rheumatoid arthritis and 6% of patients with Still's disease. Biopsies of the nodules show palisading granulomas. Similar lesions that are smaller and shorter-lived are seen in rheumatic fever.

Neurofibromas (benign Schwann cell tumors) are soft papules or nodules that exhibit the "button-hole" sign, that is, they invaginate into the skin with pressure in a manner similar to a hernia. Single lesions are seen in normal individuals, but multiple neurofibromas, usually in combination with six or more CALM measuring >1.5 cm (see "Hyperpigmentation," above), axillary freckling, and multiple Lisch nodules, are seen in von Recklinghausen's disease (NF type I; Chap. 375). In some patients the neurofibromas are localized and unilateral due to somatic mosaicism.

Angiofibromas are firm, pink to skin-colored papules that measure from 3 mm to a few centimeters in diameter. When multiple lesions are located on the central cheeks (adenoma sebaceum), the patient has tuberous sclerosis or MEN syndrome, type 1. The former is an autosomal disorder due to mutations in two different genes, and the associated findings are discussed in the section on ash leaf spots as well as in Chap. 375.

Neuromas (benign proliferations of nerve fibers) are also firm, skin-colored papules. They are more commonly found at sites of amputation and as rudimentary supernumerary digits. However, when there are multiple neuromas on the eyelids, lips, distal tongue, and/or oral mucosa, the patient should be investigated for other signs of the MEN syndrome, type 2b. Associated findings include marfanoid habitus, protuberant lips, intestinal ganglioneuromas, and medullary thyroid carcinoma (>75% of patients; Chap. 345).

Adnexal tumors are derived from pluripotent cells of the epidermis that can differentiate toward hair, sebaceous, apocrine, or eccrine glands or remain undifferentiated. *Basal cell carcinomas* (BCCs) are examples of adnexal tumors that have little or no evidence of differentiation. Clinically, they are translucent papules with rolled borders, telangiectasias, and central erosion. BCCs commonly arise in sun-damaged skin of the head and neck as well as the upper trunk. When a patient has multiple BCCs, especially prior to age 30, the possibility of the nevoid basal cell carcinoma syndrome should be raised. It is inherited as an autosomal

TABLE 54-15 PAPULONODULAR SKIN LESIONS ACCORDING TO COLOR GROUPS

I. White
- A. Calcinosis cutis

II. Skin-colored
- A. Rheumatoid nodules
- B. Neurofibromas (von Recklinghausen's disease)
- C. Angiofibromas (tuberous sclerosis, MEN syndrome, type 1)
- D. Neuromas (MEN syndrome, type 2b)
- E. Adnexal tumors
  1. Basal cell carcinomas (nevoid basal cell carcinoma syndrome)
  2. Tricholemmomas (Cowden disease)
- F. Osteomas (Gardner syndrome)
- G. Primary cutaneous disorders
  1. Epidermal inclusion cysts
  2. Lipomas

III. Pink/translucent[a]
- A. Amyloidosis
- B. Papular mucinosis

IV. Yellow
- A. Xanthomas
- B. Tophi
- C. Necrobiosis lipoidica
- D. Pseudoxanthoma elasticum
- E. Sebaceous adenomas (Torre syndrome)

V. Red[a]
- A. Papules
  1. Angiokeratomas (Fabry disease)
  2. Bacillary angiomatosis (primarily in AIDS)
- B. Papules/plaques
  1. Cutaneous lupus
  2. Lymphoma cutis
  3. Leukemia cutis
- C. Nodules
  1. Panniculitis
  2. Cutaneous polyarteritis nodosa
  3. Systemic vasculitis
- D. Primary cutaneous disorders
  1. Arthropod bites
  2. Cherry hemangiomas
  3. Infections, e.g., erysipelas, sporotrichosis
  4. Polymorphous light eruption
  5. Lymphocytoma cutis (pseudolymphoma)

VI. Red-brown[a]
- A. Sarcoidosis
- B. Sweet's syndrome
- C. Urticaria pigmentosa
- D. Erythema elevatum diutinum (chronic leukocytoclastic vasculitis)
- E. Lupus vulgaris

VII. Blue[a]
- A. Venous malformations (blue rubber bleb syndrome)
- B. Primary cutaneous disorders
  1. Venous lake
  2. Blue nevus

VIII. Violaceous
- A. Lupus pernio (sarcoidosis)
- B. Lymphoma cutis
- C. Cutaneous lupus

IX. Purple
- A. Kaposi's sarcoma
- B. Angiosarcoma
- C. Palpable purpura

X. Brown-black[b]

XI. Any color
- A. Metastases

[a]May have darker hue in more darkly pigmented individuals.
[b]See also "Hyperpigmentation."
Note: MEN, multiple endocrine neoplasia.

dominant trait and is associated with jaw cysts, palmar and plantar pits, frontal bossing, medulloblastomas, and calcification of the falx cerebri and diaphragma sellae. *Tricholemmomas* are also skin-colored adnexal tumors but differentiate toward hair follicles and can have a wartlike appearance. The presence of multiple tricholemmomas on the face and cobblestoning of the oral mucosa points to the diagnosis of Cowden disease (multiple hamartoma syndrome) due to mutations in the *PTEN* gene. Internal organ involvement (in decreasing order of frequency) includes fibrocystic disease and carcinoma of the breast, adenomas and carcinomas of the thyroid, and gastrointestinal polyposis. Keratoses of the palms, soles, and dorsal aspect of the hands are also seen.

PINK LESIONS

The cutaneous lesions associated with primary systemic *amyloidosis* are often pink in color and translucent. Common locations are the face, especially the periorbital and perioral regions, and flexural areas. On biopsy, homogeneous deposits of amyloid are seen in the dermis and in the walls of blood vessels; the latter lead to an increase in vessel wall fragility. As a result, petechiae and purpura develop in clinically normal skin as well as in lesional skin following minor trauma, hence the term *pinch purpura*. Amyloid deposits are also seen in the striated muscle of the tongue and result in macroglossia.

Even though specific mucocutaneous lesions are rarely seen in secondary amyloidosis and are present in only ~30% of the patients with primary amyloidosis, a rapid diagnosis of systemic amyloidosis can be made by an examination of abdominal subcutaneous fat. By special staining, deposits are seen around blood vessels or individual fat cells in 40–50% of patients. There are also three forms of amyloidosis that are limited to the skin and that should not be construed as cutaneous lesions of systemic amyloidosis. They are macular amyloidosis (upper back), lichenoid amyloidosis (usually lower extremities), and nodular amyloidosis. In macular and lichenoid amyloidosis, the deposits are composed of altered epidermal keratin. Recently, macular and lichenoid amyloidosis have been associated with MEN syndrome, type 2a.

Patients with *multicentric reticulohistiocytosis* also have pink-colored papules and nodules on the face and mucous membranes as well as on the extensor surface of the hands and forearms. They have a polyarthritis that can mimic rheumatoid arthritis clinically. On histologic examination, the papules have characteristic giant cells that are not seen in biopsies of rheumatoid nodules. Pink to skin-colored papules that are firm, 2–5 mm in diameter, and often in a linear arrangement are seen in patients with *papular mucinosis*. This disease is also referred to as *generalized lichen myxedematosus* or *scleromyxedema*. The latter name comes from the brawny induration of the face and extremities that may accompany the papular eruption. Biopsy specimens of the papules show localized mucin deposition, and serum protein electrophoresis and/or immunofixation electrophoresis demonstrates a monoclonal spike of IgG, usually with a λ light chain.

YELLOW LESIONS

Several systemic disorders are characterized by yellow-colored cutaneous papules or plaques—hyperlipidemia (xanthomas), gout (tophi), diabetes (necrobiosis lipoidica), pseudoxanthoma elasticum, and Torre syndrome (sebaceous tumors). Eruptive xanthomas are the most common form of *xanthomas* and are associated with hypertriglyceridemia (types I, III, IV, and V). Crops of yellow papules with erythematous halos occur primarily on the extensor surfaces of the extremities and the buttocks, and they spontaneously involute with a fall in serum triglycerides. Increased β-lipoproteins (primarily types II and III) result in one or more of the following types of xanthoma: xanthelasma, tendon xanthomas, and plane xanthomas. Xanthelasma are found on the eyelids, whereas tendon xanthomas are frequently associated with the Achilles and extensor finger tendons; plane xanthomas are flat and favor the palmar creases, face, upper trunk, and scars. Tuberous xanthomas are frequently associated with hypertriglyceridemia, but they are also seen in patients with hypercholesterolemia (type II) and are found most frequently over the large joints or hand. Biopsy specimens of xanthomas show collections of lipid-containing macrophages (foam cells).

Patients with several disorders, including biliary cirrhosis, can have a secondary form of hyperlipidemia with associated tuberous and planar xanthomas. However, patients with myeloma have *normolipemic flat xanthomas*. This latter form of xanthoma may be ≥12 cm in diameter and is most frequently seen on the upper trunk or side of the neck. It is important to note that the most common setting for eruptive xanthomas is uncontrolled diabetes mellitus. The least specific sign for hyperlipidemia is xanthelasma, because at least 50% of the patients with this finding have normal lipid profiles.

In *tophaceous gout* there are deposits of monosodium urate in the skin around the joints, particularly those of the hands and feet. Additional sites of *tophi* formation include the helix of the ear and the olecranon and prepatellar bursae. The lesions are firm, yellow in color, and occasionally discharge a chalky material. Their size varies from 1 mm to 7 cm, and the diagnosis can be established by polarization of the aspirated contents of a lesion. Lesions of *necrobiosis lipoidica* are found primarily on the shins (90%), and patients can have diabetes mellitus or develop it subsequently. Characteristic findings include a central yellow color, atrophy (transparency), telangiectasias, and an erythematous border. Ulcerations can also develop within the plaques. Biopsy specimens show necrobiosis of collagen, granulomatous inflammation, and obliterative endarteritis.

In *pseudoxanthoma elasticum* (PXE) there is an abnormal deposition of calcium on the elastic fibers of the skin, eye, and blood vessels. In the skin, the flexural areas such as the neck, axillae, antecubital fossae, and inguinal area are the primary sites of involvement. Yellow papules coalesce to form reticulated plaques that have an appearance similar to that of plucked chicken skin. In severely affected skin, hanging, redundant folds develop. Biopsy specimens of involved skin show swollen and irregularly clumped elastic fibers with deposits of calcium. In the eye, the calcium deposits in Bruch's membrane lead to angioid streaks and choroiditis; in the arteries of the heart, kidney, gastrointestinal tract, and extremities, the deposits lead to angina, hypertension, gastrointestinal bleeding, and claudication, respectively. Long-term administration of D-penicillamine can lead to PXE-like skin changes as well as elastic fiber alterations in internal organs.

Adnexal tumors that have differentiated toward sebaceous glands include sebaceous adenoma, sebaceous carcinoma, and sebaceous hyperplasia. Except for sebaceous hyperplasia, which is commonly seen on the face, these tumors are fairly rare. Patients with Torre syndrome have one or more *sebaceous adenoma(s)*, and they can also have sebaceous carcinomas and sebaceous hyperplasia as well as keratoacanthomas. The internal manifestations of Torre syndrome include *multiple* carcinomas of the gastrointestinal tract (primarily colon) as well as cancers of the larynx, genitourinary tract, and endometrium.

RED LESIONS

Cutaneous lesions that are red in color have a wide variety of etiologies; in an attempt to simplify their identification, they will be subdivided into papules, papules/plaques, and subcutaneous nodules. Common red papules include *arthropod bites* and *cherry hemangiomas*; the latter are small, bright-red, dome-shaped papules that represent benign proliferation of capillaries. In patients with AIDS, the development of multiple red hemangioma-like lesions points to bacillary angiomatosis, and biopsy specimens show clusters of bacilli that stain positive with the Warthin-Starry stain; the pathogens have been identified as *Bartonella henselae* and *B. quintana*. Disseminated visceral disease is seen primarily in immunocompromised hosts but can occur in immunocompetent individuals.

Multiple *angiokeratomas* are seen in Fabry disease, an X-linked recessive lysosomal storage disease that is due to a deficiency of α-galactosidase A. The lesions are red to red-blue in color and can be quite small in size (1–3 mm), with the most common location being the lower trunk. Associated findings include chronic renal failure, peripheral neuropathy, and corneal opacities (cornea verticillata). Electron photomicrographs of angiokeratomas and clinically normal skin demonstrate lamellar lipid deposits in fibroblasts, pericytes, and endothelial cells that are diagnostic of this disease. Widespread acute eruptions of erythematous papules are discussed in the section on exanthems.

There are several infectious diseases that present as erythematous papules or nodules in a lymphocutaneous or sporotrichoid pattern, i.e., in a linear arrangement along the lymphatic channels. The two most common etiologies are *Sporothrix schenckii* (sporotrichosis) and *M. marinum* (mycobacteria other than tuberculosis; atypical mycobacteria). The organisms are introduced as a result of trauma, and a primary inoculation site is often seen in addition to the lymphatic nodules. Additional causes include *Nocardia*, *Leishmania*, and other dimorphic fungi; culture of lesional tissue will aid in the diagnosis.

The diseases that are characterized by erythematous plaques with scale are reviewed in the papulosquamous section, and the various forms of dermatitis are discussed in the section on erythroderma. Additional disorders in the differential diagnosis of red papules/plaques include *erysipelas*, *polymorphous light eruption* (PMLE), *cutaneous lymphoid hyperplasia* (lymphocytoma cutis), *cutaneous lupus*, *lymphoma cutis*, and *leukemia cutis*. The first three diseases represent primary cutaneous disorders. PMLE is characterized by erythematous papules and plaques in a primarily sun-exposed distribution—dorsum of the hand, extensor forearm, and upper trunk. Lesions follow exposure to UV-B and/or UV-A, and in northern latitudes PMLE is most severe in the late spring and early summer. A process referred to as "hardening" occurs with continued UV exposure, and the eruption fades, but in temperate climates it will recur in the spring. PMLE must be differentiated from cutaneous lupus, and this is accomplished by histologic examination and direct immunofluorescence of the lesions. Cutaneous lymphoid hyperplasia (pseudolymphoma) is a *benign* polyclonal proliferation of lymphocytes in the skin that presents as infiltrated pink-red to red-purple papules and plaques; it must be distinguished from lymphoma cutis.

Several types of red plaques are seen in patients with systemic *lupus*, including (1) erythematous urticarial plaques across the cheeks and nose in the classic butterfly rash; (2) erythematous discoid lesions with fine or "carpet-tack" scale, telangiectasias, central hypopigmentation, peripheral hyperpigmentation, follicular plugging, and atrophy located on the face, scalp, external ears, arms, and upper trunk; and (3) psoriasiform or annular lesions of subacute lupus with hypopigmented centers located primarily on the extensor arms and upper trunk. Additional cutaneous findings include (1) a violaceous flush on the face and V of the neck; (2) urticarial vasculitis (see "Urticaria," above); (3) lupus panniculitis (see below); (4) diffuse alopecia; (5) alopecia secondary to discoid lesions; (6) periungual telangiectasias and erythema; (7) EM-like lesions that may become bullous; and (8) distal ulcerations secondary to Raynaud's phenomenon, vasculitis, or livedoid vasculopathy. Patients with only discoid lesions usually have the form of lupus that is limited to the skin. However, 2–10% of these patients eventually develop systemic lupus. Direct immunofluorescence of involved skin shows deposits of IgG or IgM and C3 in a granular distribution along the dermal-epidermal junction.

In *lymphoma cutis* there is a proliferation of malignant lymphocytes or histiocytes in the skin, and the clinical appearance resembles that of cutaneous lymphoid hyperplasia—infiltrated pink-red to red-purple papules and plaques. Lymphoma cutis can occur anywhere on the surface of the skin, whereas the sites of predilection for lymphocytomas include the malar ridge, tip of the nose, and earlobes. Patients with non-Hodgkin lymphomas have specific cutaneous lesions more often than those with Hodgkin disease, and occasionally, the skin nodules precede the development of extracutaneous non-Hodgkin lymphoma or represent the only site of involvement (e.g., primary cutaneous B cell lymphoma). Arcuate lesions are sometimes seen in lymphoma and lymphocytoma cutis as well as in CTCL. *Adult T cell leukemia/lymphoma* that develops in association with HTLV-1 infection is characterized by cutaneous plaques, hypercalcemia, and circulating CD25+ lymphocytes. *Leukemia cutis* has the same appearance as lymphoma cutis, and specific lesions are seen more commonly in monocytic leukemias than in lymphocytic or granulocytic leukemias. Cutaneous chloromas (granulocytic sarcomas) may precede the appearance of circulating blasts in acute myelogeneous leukemia and, as such, represent a form of aleukemic leukemia cutis.

Common causes of erythematous subcutaneous nodules include inflamed epidermoid inclusion cysts, acne cysts, and furuncles. *Panniculitis*, an inflammation of the fat, also presents as subcutaneous nodules and is frequently a sign of systemic disease. There are several forms of panniculitis, including erythema nodosum, erythema induratum/nodular vasculitis, lupus profundus, lipodermatosclerosis, α_1-antitrypsin deficiency, factitial, and fat necrosis secondary to pancreatic disease. Except for erythema nodosum, these lesions may break down and ulcerate or heal with a scar. The shin is the most common location for the nodules of erythema nodosum, whereas the calf is the most common location for lesions of erythema induratum. In erythema nodosum the nodules are initially red but then develop a blue color as they resolve. Patients with erythema nodosum but no underlying systemic illness can still have fever, malaise, leukocytosis, arthralgias, and/or arthritis. However, the possibility of an underlying illness should be excluded, and the most common associations are streptococcal infections, upper respiratory viral infections, sarcoidosis, and inflammatory bowel disease in addition to drugs (oral contraceptives, sulfonamides, penicillins, bromides, iodides). Less common associations include bacterial gastroenteritis (*Yersinia, Salmonella*) and coccidioidomycosis followed by tuberculosis, histoplasmosis, brucellosis, and infections with *Chlamydophila pneumoniae* or *Chlamydia trachomatis, M. pneumoniae,* or hepatitis B virus.

Erythema induratum and nodular vasculitis share a similar histology and were thought to represent the clinical spectrum of a single entity; subsequently they have been separated, with the latter usually idiopathic and the former associated with the presence of *M. tuberculosis* DNA by polymerase chain reaction (PCR) within skin lesions. The lesions of lupus profundus are found primarily on the upper arms and buttocks (sites of abundant fat) and are seen in both the cutaneous and systemic forms of lupus. The overlying skin may be normal, erythematous, or have the changes of discoid lupus. The subcutaneous fat necrosis that is associated with pancreatic disease is presumably secondary to circulating lipases and is seen in patients with pancreatic carcinoma as well as in patients with acute and chronic pancreatitis. In this disorder there may be an associated arthritis, fever, and inflammation of visceral fat. Histologic examination of deep incisional biopsy specimens will aid in the diagnosis of the particular type of panniculitis.

Subcutaneous erythematous nodules are also seen in *cutaneous polyarteritis nodosa* (PAN) and as a manifestation of *systemic vasculitis,* e.g., systemic PAN, allergic granulomatosis, or Wegener's granulomatosis (Chap. 319). Cutaneous PAN presents with painful subcutaneous nodules and ulcers within a red-purple, netlike pattern of livedo reticularis. The latter is due to slowed blood flow through the superficial horizontal venous plexus. The majority of lesions are found on the lower extremity, and while arthralgias and myalgias may accompany cutaneous PAN, there is no evidence of systemic involvement. In both the cutaneous and systemic forms of vasculitis, skin biopsy specimens of the associated nodules will show the changes characteristic of a vasculitis; the size of the vessel involved will depend on the particular disease.

RED-BROWN LESIONS

The cutaneous lesions in *sarcoidosis* (Chap. 322) are classically red to red-brown in color, and with diascopy (pressure with a glass slide) a yellow-brown residual color is observed that is secondary to the granulomatous infiltrate. The waxy papules and plaques may be found anywhere on the skin, but the face is the most common location. Usually there are no surface changes, but occasionally the lesions will have scale. Biopsy specimens of the papules show "naked" granulomas in the dermis, i.e., granulomas surrounded by a minimal number of lymphocytes. Other cutaneous findings in sarcoidosis include annular lesions with an atrophic or scaly center, papules within scars, hypopigmented macules and papules, alopecia, acquired ichthyosis, erythema nodosum, and lupus pernio (see below).

The differential diagnosis of sarcoidosis includes foreign-body granulomas produced by chemicals such as beryllium and zirconium, late secondary syphilis, and *lupus vulgaris.* Lupus vulgaris is a form of cutaneous tuberculosis that is seen in previously infected and sensitized individuals. There is often underlying active tuberculosis elsewhere, usually in the lungs or lymph nodes. At least 90% of the lesions occur in the head and neck area and are red-brown plaques with a yellow-brown color on diascopy. Secondary scarring and squamous cell carcinomas can develop within the plaques. Cultures or PCR analysis of the lesions should be done because it is rare for the acid-fast stain to show bacilli within the dermal granulomas.

Sweet's syndrome is characterized by red to red-brown plaques and nodules that are frequently painful and occur primarily on the head, neck, and upper extremities. The patients also have fever, neutrophilia, and a dense dermal infiltrate of neutrophils in the lesions. In ~10% of the patients there is an associated malignancy, most commonly acute myelogenous leukemia. Sweet's syndrome has also been reported with lymphoma, myeloma, myelodysplastic syndromes, and solid tumors (primarily of the genitourinary tract) as well as drugs (e.g., *all-trans*-retinoic acid). The differential diagnosis includes neutrophilic eccrine hidradenitis and atypical forms of pyoderma gangrenosum. Extracutaneous sites of involvement include joints, muscles, eye, kidney (proteinuria, occasionally glomerulonephritis), and lung (neutrophilic infiltrates). The idiopathic form of Sweet's syndrome is seen more often in women, following a respiratory tract infection.

A generalized distribution of red-brown macules and papules is seen in the form of mastocytosis known as *urticaria pigmentosa* (Chap. 311). Each lesion represents a collection of mast cells in the dermis, with hyperpigmentation of the overlying epidermis. Stimuli such as rubbing cause these mast cells to degranulate, and this leads to the formation of localized urticaria (Darier's sign). Additional symptoms can result from mast cell degranulation and include headache, flushing, diarrhea, and pruritus. Mast cells also infiltrate various organs such as the liver, spleen, and gastrointestinal tract, and accumulations of mast cells in the bones may produce either osteosclerotic or osteolytic lesions on radiographs. In the majority of these patients, however, the internal involvement remains indolent. A subtype of chronic cutaneous small-vessel vasculitis, *erythema elevatum diutinum* (EED), also presents with papules that are red-brown in color. The papules coalesce into plaques on the extensor surfaces of knees, elbows, and the small joints of the hand. Flares of EED have been associated with streptococcal infections.

BLUE LESIONS

Lesions that are blue in color are the result of either vascular ectasias and tumors or melanin pigment in the dermis. *Venous lakes* (ectasias) are compressible dark-blue lesions that are found commonly in the head and neck region. *Venous malformations* are also compressible blue papulonodules and plaques that can occur anywhere on the body, including the oral mucosa. When there are multiple rather than single congenital lesions, the patient may have the blue rubber bleb syndrome or Mafucci's syndrome. Patients with the blue rubber bleb syndrome also have vascular anomalies of the gastrointestinal tract that may bleed, whereas patients with Mafucci's syndrome have associated dyschondroplasia and osteochondromas. *Blue nevi* (moles) are seen when there are collections of pigment-producing nevus cells in the dermis. These benign papular lesions are dome-shaped and occur most commonly on the dorsum of the hand or foot or in the head and neck region.

VIOLACEOUS LESIONS

Violaceous papules and plaques are seen in *lupus pernio, lymphoma cutis,* and *cutaneous lupus.* Lupus pernio is a particular type of sarcoidosis that involves the tip and alar rim of the nose as well as the earlobes, with lesions that are violaceous in color rather than red-brown. This form of sarcoidosis is associated with involvement of the upper respiratory tract. The plaques of lymphoma cutis and cutaneous lupus may be red or violaceous in color and were discussed above.

PURPLE LESIONS

Purple-colored papules and plaques are seen in vascular tumors, such as *Kaposi's sarcoma* (Chap. 182) and *angiosarcoma,* and when there is extravasation of red blood cells into the skin in association with inflammation, as in *palpable purpura* (see "Purpura," below). Patients with congenital or acquired AV fistulas and venous hypertension can develop purple papules on the lower extremities that can resemble Kaposi's sarcoma clinically and histologically; this condition is referred to as pseudo-Kaposi sarcoma (acral angiodermatitis). Angiosarcoma is found most commonly on the scalp and face of elderly patients or within areas of chronic lymphedema and presents as purple papules and plaques. In the head and neck region the tumor often extends beyond the clinically defined borders and may be accompanied by facial edema.

BROWN AND BLACK LESIONS

Brown- and black-colored papules are reviewed in "Hyperpigmentation," above.

CUTANEOUS METASTASES

These are discussed last because they can have a wide range of colors. Most commonly they present as either firm, skin-colored subcutaneous nodules or firm, red to red-brown papulonodules. The lesions of lymphoma cutis range from pink-red to plum in color, whereas metastatic melanoma can be pink, blue, or black in color. Cutaneous metastases develop from hematogenous or lymphatic spread and are most often due to the following primary carcinomas: in men, lung, colon, melanoma, and oral cavity; and in women, breast, melanoma, and lung. These metastatic lesions may be the initial presentation of the carcinoma, especially when the primary site is the lung, kidney, or ovary.

PURPURA

(Table 54-16) *Purpura* are seen when there is an extravasation of red blood cells into the dermis and, as a result, the lesions do not blanch with pressure. This is in contrast to those erythematous or violet-colored lesions that are due to localized vasodilatation—they do blanch with pressure. Purpura (≥3 mm) and petechiae (≤2 mm) are divided into two major groups, palpable and nonpalpable. The most frequent causes of *nonpalpable* petechiae and purpura are primary cutaneous disorders such as *trauma*, *solar (actinic) purpura*, and *capillaritis*. Less common causes are *steroid purpura* and *livedoid vasculopathy* (see "Ulcers," below). Solar purpura are seen primarily on the extensor forearms, while steroid purpura secondary topotent topical glucocorticoids or endogenous or exogenous Cushing's syndrome can be more widespread. In both cases there is alteration of the supporting connective tissue that surrounds the dermal blood vessels. In contrast, the petechiae that result from capillaritis are found primarily on the lower extremities. In capillaritis there is an extravasation of erythrocytes as a result of perivascular lymphocytic inflammation. The petechiae are bright red, 1–2 mm in size, and scattered within annular or coin-shaped yellow-brown macules. The yellow-brown color is caused by hemosiderin deposits within the dermis.

TABLE 54-16 CAUSES OF PURPURA

I. Primary cutaneous disorders
A. Nonpalpable
1. Trauma
2. Solar purpura
3. Steroid purpura
4. Capillaritis
5. Livedoid vasculopathy[a]
II. Systemic diseases
A. Nonpalpable
1. Clotting disturbances
a. Thrombocytopenia (including ITP)
b. Abnormal platelet function
c. Clotting factor defects
2. Vascular fragility
a. Amyloidosis
b. Ehlers-Danlos syndrome
c. Scurvy
3. Thrombi
a. Disseminated intravascular coagulation
b. Monoclonal cryoglobulinemia
c. Heparin-induced thrombocytopenia and thrombosis
d. Thrombotic thrombocytopenic purpura
e. Warfarin reaction
4. Emboli
a. Cholesterol
b. Fat
5. Possible immune complex
a. Gardner-Diamond syndrome (autoerythrocyte sensitivity)
b. Waldenström's hypergammaglobulinemic purpura
B. Palpable
1. Vasculitis
a. Cutaneous small-vessel vasculitis
b. Polyarteritis nodosa
2. Emboli[b]
a. Acute meningococcemia
b. Disseminated gonococcal infection
c. Rocky Mountain spotted fever
d. Ecthyma gangrenosum

[a]Also associated with systemic diseases.
[b]Bacterial, fungal, or parasitic.
Note: ITP, idiopathic thrombocytopenic purpura.

Systemic causes of nonpalpable purpura fall into several categories, and those secondary to clotting disturbances and vascular fragility will be discussed first. The former group includes *thrombocytopenia* (Chap. 109), *abnormal platelet function* as is seen in uremia, and *clotting factor defects*. The initial site of presentation for thrombocytopenia-induced petechiae is the distal lower extremity. Capillary fragility leads to nonpalpable purpura in patients with systemic *amyloidosis* (see "Papulonodular Skin Lesions," above), disorders of collagen production such as *Ehlers-Danlos syndrome*, and *scurvy*. In scurvy there are flattened corkscrew hairs with surrounding hemorrhage on the lower extremities, in addition to gingivitis. Vitamin C is a cofactor for lysyl hydroxylase, an enzyme involved in the posttranslational modification of procollagen that is necessary for cross-link formation.

In contrast to the previous group of disorders, the purpura seen in the following group of diseases are associated with thrombi formation within vessels. It is important to note that these thrombi are demonstrable in skin biopsy specimens. This group of disorders includes disseminated intravascular coagulation (DIC), monoclonal cryoglobulinemia, thrombotic thrombocytopenic purpura, and reactions to warfarin and heparin (heparin-induced thrombocytopenia and thrombosis). DIC is triggered by several types of infection (gram-negative, gram-positive, viral, and rickettsial) as well as by tissue injury and neoplasms. Widespread purpura and hemorrhagic infarcts of the distal extremities are seen. Similar lesions are found in purpura fulminans, which is a form of DIC associated with fever and hypotension that occurs more commonly in children following an infectious illness such as varicella, scarlet fever, or an upper respiratory tract infection. In both disorders, hemorrhagic bullae can develop in involved skin.

Monoclonal cryoglobulinemia is associated with multiple myeloma, Waldenström's macroglobulinemia, lymphocytic leukemia, and lymphoma. Purpura, primarily of the lower extremities, and hemorrhagic infarcts of the fingers and toes are seen in these patients. Exacerbations of disease activity can follow cold exposure or an increase in serum viscosity. Biopsy specimens show precipitates of the cryoglobulin within dermal vessels. Similar deposits have been found in the lung, brain, and renal glomeruli. Patients with *thrombotic thrombocytopenic purpura* can also have hemorrhagic infarcts as a result of intravascular thromboses. Additional signs include thrombocytopenic purpura, fever, and microangiopathic hemolytic anemia (Chap. 101).

Administration of *warfarin* can result in painful areas of erythema that become purpuric and then necrotic with an adherent black eschar; the condition is referred to as warfarin-induced necrosis. This reaction is seen more often in women and in areas with abundant subcutaneous fat—breasts, abdomen, buttocks, thighs, and calves. The erythema and purpura develop between the third and tenth day of therapy, most likely as a result of a transient imbalance in the levels of anticoagulant and procoagulant vitamin K–dependent factors. Continued therapy does not exacerbate preexisting lesions, and patients with an inherited or acquired deficiency of protein C are at increased risk for this particular reaction as well as for purpura fulminans.

Purpura secondary to *cholesterol emboli* are usually seen on the lower extremities of patients with atherosclerotic vascular disease. They often follow anticoagulant therapy or an invasive vascular procedure such as an arteriogram but also occur spontaneously from disintegration of atheromatous plaques. Associated findings include livedo reticularis, gangrene, cyanosis, and ischemic ulcerations. Multiple step sections of the biopsy specimen may be necessary to demonstrate the cholesterol clefts within the vessels. Petechiae are also an important sign of *fat embolism* and occur primarily on the upper body 2–3 days after a major injury. By using special fixatives, the emboli can be demonstrated in biopsy specimens of the petechiae. Emboli of tumor or thrombus are seen in patients with atrial myxomas and marantic endocarditis.

In the *Gardner-Diamond syndrome* (autoerythrocyte sensitivity), female patients develop large ecchymoses within areas of painful, warm erythema. Intradermal injections of autologous erythrocytes or phosphatidyl serine derived from the red cell membrane can reproduce the lesions in some patients; however, there are instances where a reaction is seen at an injection site of the forearm but not in the midback region. The latter has led some observers to view Gardner-Diamond syndrome as a cutaneous manifestation of severe emotional stress. More recently, the possibility of platelet dysfunction (as assessed via aggregation studies) has been raised. *Waldenström's hypergammaglobulinemic purpura* is a chronic disorder characterized by petechiae on the lower extremities. There are circulating complexes of IgG–anti-IgG molecules, and exacerbations are associated with prolonged standing or walking.

Palpable purpura are further subdivided into vasculitic and embolic. In the group of vasculitic disorders, cutaneous small-vessel vasculitis, also known as *leukocytoclastic vasculitis* (LCV), is the one most commonly associated with palpable purpura (Chap. 319). Underlying etiologies include drugs (e.g., antibiotics), infections (e.g., hepatitis C virus), and autoimmune connective tissue diseases. *Henoch-Schönlein purpura* is a subtype of acute LCV that is seen primarily in children and adolescents following an upper respiratory infection. The majority of lesions are found on the lower extremities and buttocks. Systemic manifestations include fever, arthralgias (primarily of the knees and ankles), abdominal pain, gastrointestinal bleeding, and nephritis. Direct immunofluorescence examination shows deposits of IgA within dermal blood vessel walls. In *polyarteritis nodosa*, specific cutaneous lesions result from a vasculitis of arterial vessels or there may be an associated LCV. The arteritis leads to ischemia of the skin, and this explains the irregular outline of the purpura (see below).

Several types of infectious emboli can give rise to palpable purpura. These embolic lesions are usually *irregular* in outline as opposed to the lesions of LCV, which are *circular* in outline. The irregular outline is indicative of a cutaneous infarct, and the size corresponds to the area of skin that received its blood supply from that particular arteriole or artery. The palpable purpura in LCV are circular because the erythrocytes simply diffuse out evenly from the postcapillary venules as a result of inflammation. Infectious emboli are most commonly due to gram-negative cocci (meningococcus, gonococcus), gram-negative rods (Enterobacteriaceae), and gram-positive cocci (*Staphylococcus*). Additional causes include *Rickettsia* and, in immunocompromised patients, *Candida* and opportunistic fungi.

The embolic lesions in *acute meningococcemia* are found primarily on the trunk, lower extremities, and sites of pressure, and a gunmetal-gray color often develops within them. Their size varies from 1 mm to several centimeters, and the organisms can be cultured from the lesions. Associated findings include a preceding upper respiratory tract infection, fever, meningitis, DIC, and, in some patients, a deficiency of the terminal components of complement. In *disseminated gonococcal infection* (arthritis-dermatitis syndrome), a small number of papules and vesicopustules with central purpura or hemorrhagic necrosis are found on the distal extremities. Additional symptoms include arthralgias, tenosynovitis, and fever. To establish the diagnosis, a Gram stain of these lesions should be performed. *Rocky Mountain spotted fever* is a tick-borne disease that is caused by *R. rickettsii*. A several-day history of fever, chills, severe headache, and photophobia precedes the onset of the cutaneous eruption. The initial lesions are erythematous macules and papules on the wrists, ankles, palms, and soles. With time, the lesions spread centripetally and become purpuric.

Lesions of *ecthyma gangrenosum* begin as edematous, erythematous papules or plaques and then develop central purpura and necrosis. Bullae formation also occurs in these lesions, and they are frequently found in the girdle region. The organism that is classically associated with ecthyma gangrenosum is *Pseudomonas aeruginosa*, but other gram-negative rods such as *Klebsiella*, *Escherichia coli*, and *Serratia* can produce similar lesions. In immunocompromised hosts, the list of potential pathogens is expanded to include *Candida* and opportunistic fungi.

ULCERS

The approach to the patient with a cutaneous ulcer is outlined in Table 54-17. Peripheral vascular diseases of the extremities are reviewed in Chap. 243, as is Raynaud's phenomenon.

TABLE 54-17 CAUSES OF CUTANEOUS ULCERS

I. Primary cutaneous disorders
- A. Peripheral vascular disease (Chap. 243)
  1. Venous
  2. Arterial
- B. Livedoid vasculopathy[a]
- C. Squamous cell carcinoma, e.g., within scars
- D. Infections, e.g., ecthyma caused by *Streptococcus* (Chap. 130)

II. Systemic diseases
- A. Lower legs
  1. Cutaneous small-vessel vasculitis[b]
  2. Hemoglobinopathies (Chap. 99)
  3. Cryoglobulinemia,[b] cryofibrinogenemia
  4. Cholesterol emboli[b]
  5. Necrobiosis lipoidica[c]
  6. Antiphospholipid syndrome (Chap. 110)
  7. Neuropathic[d] (Chap. 338)
  8. Panniculitis
- B. Hands and feet
  1. Raynaud's phenomenon (Chap. 243)
- C. Generalized
  1. Pyoderma gangrenosum
  2. Calciphylaxis (Chap. 347)
  3. Infections, e.g., dimorphic fungi, chronic herpes simplex
  4. Lymphoma
- D. Mucosal
  1. Behçet's syndrome (Chap. 320)
  2. Erythema multiforme major, Stevens-Johnson syndrome, TEN
  3. Primary blistering disorders (Chap. 55)
  4. Lupus erythematosus
  5. Inflammatory bowel disease

[a]Also associated with systemic diseases.
[b]Reviewed in section on Purpura.
[c]Reviewed in section on Papulonodular Skin Lesions.
[d]Favors plantar surface of the foot.
Note: TEN, toxic epidermal necrolysis.

Livedoid vasculopathy (livedoid vasculitis; atrophie blanche) represents a combination of a vasculopathy plus intravascular thrombosis. Purpuric lesions and livedo reticularis are found in association with *painful* ulcerations of the lower extremities. These ulcers are often slow to heal, but when they do, irregularly shaped white scars are formed. The majority of cases are secondary to venous hypertension, but possible underlying illnesses include cryofibrinogenemia and disorders of hypercoagulability, e.g., the antiphospholipid syndrome (Chaps. 111 and 313).

In *pyoderma gangrenosum*, the border of the ulcers has a characteristic appearance of an undermined necrotic violaceous edge and a peripheral erythematous halo. The ulcers often begin as pustules that then expand rather rapidly to a size as large as 20 cm. Although these lesions are most commonly found on the lower extremities, they can arise anywhere on the surface of the body, including sites of trauma (pathergy). An estimated 30–50% of cases are idiopathic, and the most common associated disorders are ulcerative colitis and Crohn's disease. Less commonly, pyoderma gangrenosum is associated with seropositive rheumatoid arthritis, acute and chronic myelogenous leukemia, hairy cell leukemia, and myelofibrosis. Additional findings in these patients, even those with idiopathic disease, are cutaneous anergy and a monoclonal gammopathy, usually IgA. Because the histology of pyoderma gangrenosum may be nonspecific (dermal infiltrate of neutrophils when in untreated state), the diagnosis is usually made clinically and includes excluding less common causes of similar-appearing ulcers such as necrotizing vasculitis, Meleney's ulcer (synergistic infection at a site of trauma or surgery), dimorphic fungi, cutaneous amebiasis, spider bites, and factitial. In the myeloproliferative disorders, the ulcers may be more superficial with a pustulobullous border, and these lesions provide a connection between classic pyoderma gangrenosum and acute febrile neutrophilic dermatosis (Sweet's syndrome).

FEVER AND RASH

The major considerations in a patient with a fever and a rash are inflammatory diseases versus infectious diseases. In the hospital setting, the most common scenario is a patient who has a drug rash plus a fever secondary to an underlying infection. However, it should be emphasized that a drug reaction can lead to both a cutaneous eruption and a fever ("drug fever"), especially in the setting of DRESS. Additional inflammatory diseases that are often associated with a fever include pustular psoriasis, erythroderma, and Sweet's syndrome. Lyme disease, secondary syphilis, and viral and bacterial exanthems (see "Exanthems," above) are examples of infectious diseases that produce a rash and a fever. Lastly, it is important to determine whether or not the cutaneous lesions represent septic emboli (see "Purpura," above). Such lesions usually have evidence of ischemia in the form of purpura, necrosis, or impending necrosis (gunmetal-gray color). In the patient with thrombocytopenia, however, purpura can be seen in inflammatory reactions such as morbilliform drug eruptions and infectious lesions.

FURTHER READINGS

BOLOGNIA JL et al: *Dermatology*, 2d ed. Philadelphia, Mosby, 2007

BRAVERMAN IM: *Skin Signs of Systemic Disease*, 3d ed. Philadelphia, Saunders, 1998

CALLEN JP et al: *Dermatological Signs of Internal Disease*, 3d ed. Philadelphia, Saunders, 2003

MCKEE PH et al: *Pathology of the Skin*, 3d ed. London, Elsevier, 2005

SPITZ JL: *Genodermatoses: A Clinical Guide to Genetic Skin Disorders*, 2d ed. Lippincott Williams & Wilkins, 2004

55 Immunologically Mediated Skin Diseases

Kim B. Yancey, Thomas J. Lawley

A number of immunologically mediated skin diseases and immunologically mediated systemic disorders with cutaneous manifestations are now recognized as distinct entities with consistent clinical, histologic, and immunopathologic findings. Many of these disorders are due to autoimmune mechanisms. Clinically, they are characterized by morbidity (pain, pruritus, disfigurement) and in some instances by mortality (largely due to loss of epidermal barrier function and/or secondary infection). The major features of the more common immunologically mediated skin diseases are summarized in this chapter (Table 55-1), as are the systemic disorders with cutaneous manifestations.

AUTOIMMUNE CUTANEOUS DISEASES

PEMPHIGUS VULGARIS

Pemphigus refers to a group of autoantibody-mediated intraepidermal blistering diseases characterized by loss of cohesion between epidermal cells (a process termed *acantholysis*). Manual pressure to the skin of these patients may elicit the separation of the epidermis (Nikolsky's sign). This finding, while characteristic of pemphigus, is not specific to this group of disorders and is also seen in toxic epidermal necrolysis, Stevens-Johnson syndrome, and a few other skin diseases.

Pemphigus vulgaris (PV) is a mucocutaneous blistering disease that predominates in patients >40 years. PV typically begins on mucosal surfaces; it often progresses to a mucocutaneous disease in which fragile, flaccid blisters rupture to produce extensive denudation of the skin (Fig. 55-1). PV typically involves the mouth, scalp, face, neck, axilla, groin, and trunk. PV may be associated with severe skin pain; some patients experience pruritus as well. Lesions usually heal without scarring, except at sites complicated by secondary infection or mechanically induced dermal wounds. Postinflammatory

TABLE 55-1 IMMUNOLOGICALLY MEDIATED BLISTERING DISEASES

Disease	Clinical	Histology	Immunopathology	Autoantigens[a]
Pemphigus foliaceus	Crusts and shallow erosions on scalp, central face, upper chest, and back	Acantholytic blister formed in superficial layer of epidermis	Cell surface deposits of IgG on keratinocytes	Dsg1
Pemphigus vulgaris	Flaccid blisters, denuded skin, oromucosal lesions	Acantholytic blister formed in suprabasal layer of epidermis	Cell surface deposits of IgG on keratinocytes	Dsg3 (plus Dsg1 in patients with skin involvement)
Paraneoplastic pemphigus	Painful stomatitis with papulosquamous or lichenoid eruptions that progress to blisters	Acantholysis, keratinocyte necrosis and vacuolar interface dermatitis	Cell surface deposits of IgG and C3 on keratinocytes and (variably) similar immunoreactants in epidermal BMZ	Plakin protein family members and desmosomal cadherins (see text for details)
Bullous pemphigoid	Large tense blisters on flexor surfaces and trunk	Subepidermal blister with eosinophil-rich infiltrate	Linear band of IgG and/or C3 in epidermal BMZ	BPAG1, BPAG2
Pemphigoid gestationis	Pruritic, urticarial plaques, rimmed by vesicles and bullae on the trunk and extremities	Teardrop-shaped, subepidermal blisters in dermal papillae; eosinophil-rich infiltrate	Linear band of C3 in epidermal BMZ	BPAG2 (plus BPAG1 in some patients)
Linear IgA disease	Pruritic small papules on extensor surfaces; occasionally larger, arciform blisters	Subepidermal blister with neutrophil-rich infiltrate	Linear band of IgA in epidermal BMZ	BPAG2 (see text for specific details)
Cicatricial pemphigoid	Erosive and/or blistering lesions of mucous membranes and possibly the skin; scarring of some sites	Subepidermal blister that may or may not include a leukocytic infiltrate	Linear band of IgG, IgA, and/or C3 in epidermal BMZ	BPAG2, laminin 5, or others
Epidermolysis bullosa acquisita	Blisters, erosions, scars, and milia on sites exposed to trauma; widespread, inflammatory, tense blisters may be seen initially	Subepidermal blister that may or may not include a leukocytic infiltrate	Linear band of IgG and/or C3 in epidermal BMZ	Type VII collagen
Dermatitis herpetiformis	Extremely pruritic small papules and vesicles on elbows, knees, buttocks, and posterior neck	Subepidermal blister with neutrophils in dermal papillae	Granular deposits of IgA in dermal papillae	Epidermal transglutaminase

[a]Autoantigens bound by these patients' autoantibodies are defined as follows: Dsg1, desmoglein 1; Dsg3, desmoglein 3; BPAG1, bullous pemphigoid antigen 1; BPAG2, bullous pemphigoid antigen 2.

Note: BMZ, basement membrane zone.

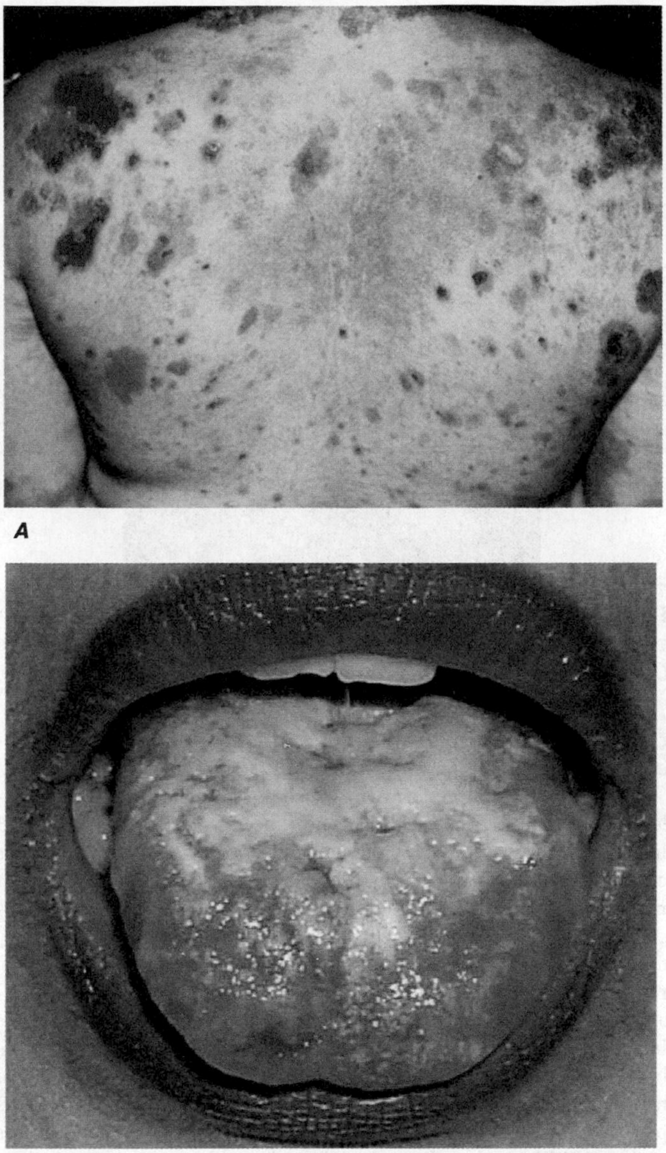

FIGURE 55-1 Pemphigus vulgaris. ***A.*** Pemphigus vulgaris demonstrating flaccid bullae that are easily ruptured, resulting in multiple erosions and crusted plaques. ***B.*** Pemphigus vulgaris almost invariably involves the oral mucosa and may present with erosions involving the gingiva, buccal mucosa, palate, posterior pharynx, or the tongue. (***B,*** *Courtesy of Robert Swerlick, MD; with permission.*)

hyperpigmentation is usually present at sites of healed lesions for some time.

Biopsies of early lesions demonstrate intraepidermal vesicle formation secondary to loss of cohesion between epidermal cells (i.e., acantholytic blisters). Blister cavities contain acantholytic epidermal cells, which appear as round homogeneous cells containing hyperchromatic nuclei. Basal keratinocytes remain attached to the epidermal basement membrane, hence blister formation is within the suprabasal portion of the epidermis. Lesional skin may contain focal collections of intraepidermal eosinophils within blister cavities; dermal alterations are slight, often limited to an eosinophil-predominant leukocytic infiltrate. Direct immunofluorescence microscopy of lesional or intact patient skin shows deposits of IgG on the surface of keratinocytes; deposits of complement components are typically found in lesional but not uninvolved skin. Deposits of IgG on keratinocytes are derived from circulating autoantibodies directed against cell-surface autoantigens. Such circulating autoantibodies can be demonstrated in 80–90% of PV patients by indirect immunofluorescence microscopy; monkey esophagus is the optimal substrate for these studies. Patients with PV have IgG autoantibodies directed against *desmogleins* (Dsgs), transmembrane desmosomal glycoproteins that belong to the cadherin family of calcium-dependent adhesion molecules. Such autoantibodies can be precisely quantitated by enzyme-linked immunosorbent assay (ELISA). Patients with early PV (i.e., mucosal disease) have only IgG autoantibodies directed against Dsg3; patients with advanced PV (i.e., mucocutaneous disease) have IgG autoantibodies directed against both Dsg3 and Dsg1. Experimental studies have shown that autoantibodies from patients with PV are pathogenic (i.e., responsible for blister formation) and that their titer correlates with disease activity. Recent studies have shown that the anti-Dsg autoantibody profile in these patients' sera as well as the tissue distribution of Dsg3 and Dsg1 determine the site of blister formation in patients with pemphigus. Coexpression of Dsg3 and Dsg1 by epidermal cells protects against pathogenic IgG directed against either cadherin but not pathogenic autoantibodies directed against both.

PV can be life-threatening. Prior to the availability of glucocorticoids, the mortality ranged from 60–90%; the current mortality is ~5%. Common causes of morbidity and mortality are infection and complications of treatment with glucocorticoids. Bad prognostic factors include advanced age, widespread involvement, and the requirement for high doses of glucocorticoids (with or without other immunosuppressive agents) for control of disease. The course of PV in individual patients is variable and difficult to predict. Some patients achieve remission, while others may require long-term treatment or succumb to complications of their disease or its treatment. The mainstay of treatment is systemic glucocorticoids. Patients with moderate to severe PV are usually started on prednisone, 1 mg/kg per day. If new lesions continue to appear after 1–2 weeks of treatment, the dose may need to be increased. Many regimens combine an immunosuppressive agent with systemic glucocorticoids for control of PV. The most frequently used are azathioprine (2–2.5 mg/kg per day), mycophenolate mofetil (20–35 mg/kg per day), or cyclophosphamide (1–2 mg/kg per day). Patients with severe, treatment-resistant disease may derive benefit from plasmapheresis [six high-volume exchanges (i.e., 2–3 liters per exchange) over ~2 weeks], IV immunoglobulin (2 g/kg over 3–5 days every 6–8 weeks), or rituximab (375 mg/m^2 per week × 4). It is important to bring severe or progressive disease under control quickly to lessen the severity and/or duration of this disorder.

PEMPHIGUS FOLIACEUS

Pemphigus foliaceus (PF) is distinguished from PV by several features. In PF, acantholytic blisters are located high within the epidermis, usually just beneath the stratum corneum. Hence PF is a more superficial blistering disease than PV. The distribution of lesions in the two disorders is much the same, except that in PF mucous membranes are almost always spared. Patients with PF rarely demonstrate intact blisters but rather exhibit shallow erosions associated with erythema, scale, and crust formation. Mild cases of PF resemble severe seborrheic dermatitis; severe PF may cause extensive exfoliation. Sun exposure (ultraviolet irradiation) may be an aggravating factor. *Fogo selvagem* (FS), an endemic form of PF thought to develop as a consequence of environmental stimuli (e.g., insect bites), is found in south central rural Brazil as well as selected sites in Latin America and Tunisia.

Patients with PF have immunopathologic features in common with PV. Specifically, direct immunofluorescence microscopy of perilesional skin demonstrates IgG on the surface of keratinocytes. Similarly, patients with PF have circulating IgG autoantibodies directed against the surface of keratinocytes. Guinea pig esophagus is the optimal substrate for indirect immunofluorescence microscopy studies of sera from patients with PF. In PF, autoantibodies are directed against Dsg1, a 160-kDa desmosomal cadherin. As noted for PV, the autoantibody profile in patients with PF (i.e., anti-Dsg1 IgG) and the tissue distribution of this autoantigen (i.e., expression in oral mucosa that is compensated by coexpression of Dsg3) is thought to account for the distribution of lesions in this disease.

Although pemphigus has been associated with several autoimmune diseases, its association with thymoma and/or myasthenia gravis is particularly notable. To date, >30 cases of thymoma and/or myasthenia gravis have been reported in association with pemphigus, usually with PF. Patients may also develop pemphigus as a consequence of drug exposure; drug-induced pemphigus usually resembles PF rather than PV. Drugs containing a thiol group in their chemical structure (e.g., penicillamine, captopril, enalapril) are most commonly associated with drug-induced pemphigus. Nonthiol drugs linked to pemphigus include penicillins, cephalosporins, and piroxicam. It has been suggested that thiol- and nonthiol-containing drugs induce pemphigus via biochemical and immunologic mechanisms, respectively. Hence, the better prognosis upon drug withdrawal in cases of pemphigus induced by thiol-containing medications. Some cases of drug-induced pemphigus are durable and require treatment with systemic glucocorticoids and/or immunosuppressive agents.

PF is generally a less severe disease than PV and carries a better prognosis. Localized disease can sometimes be treated with topical or intralesional glucocorticoids; more active cases can usually be controlled with systemic glucocorticoids. Patients with severe, treatment-resistant disease may require more aggressive interventions as described above for patients with severe PV.

PARANEOPLASTIC PEMPHIGUS

Paraneoplastic pemphigus (PNP) is an autoimmune acantholytic mucocutaneous disease associated with an occult or confirmed neoplasm. Patients with PNP typically show painful mucosal erosive lesions in association with papulosquamous and/or lichenoid eruptions that often progress to blisters. Palm and sole involvement is common in these patients and raises the possibility that prior reports of neoplasia-associated erythema multiforme actually may have represented unrecognized cases of PNP. Biopsies of lesional skin from these patients show varying combinations of acantholysis, keratinocyte necrosis, and vacuolar-interface dermatitis. Direct immunofluorescence microscopy of patient skin shows deposits of IgG and complement on the surface of keratinocytes and (variably) similar immunoreactants in the epidermal basement membrane zone. Patients with PNP have IgG autoantibodies against cytoplasmic proteins that are members of the plakin family (e.g., desmoplakins I and II, bullous pemphigoid antigen 1, envoplakin, periplakin, and plectin) and cell-surface proteins that are members of the cadherin family (e.g., Dsg3 and Dsg1). Passive transfer studies have shown that autoantibodies from patients with PNP are pathogenic.

The predominant neoplasms associated with PNP are non-Hodgkin's lymphoma, chronic lymphocytic leukemia, thymoma, spindle cell tumors, Waldenström's macroglobulinemia, and Castleman's disease; the latter is particularly common among children with PNP. In addition to severe skin lesions, many patients with PNP develop life-threatening bronchiolitis obliterans. PNP is generally resistant to conventional therapies (i.e., those used to treat PV); rare patients may improve (or even remit) following ablation or removal of underlying neoplasms.

BULLOUS PEMPHIGOID

Bullous pemphigoid (BP) is a polymorphic autoimmune subepidermal blistering disease usually seen in the elderly. Initial lesions may consist of urticarial plaques; most patients eventually display tense blisters on either normal-appearing or erythematous skin (Fig. 55-2). The lesions are usually distributed over the lower abdomen, groin, and flexor surface of the extremities; oral mucosal lesions are found in some patients. Pruritus may be nonexistent or severe. As lesions evolve, tense blisters tend to rupture and be replaced by erosions with or without surmounting crust. Nontraumatized blisters heal without scarring. The major histocompatibility complex class II allele HLA-DQβ1*0301 is prevalent in patients with BP. Despite isolated reports, several studies have shown that patients with BP do not have an increased incidence of malignancy in comparison with appropriately age- and gender-matched controls.

Biopsies of early lesional skin demonstrate subepidermal blisters and histologic features that roughly correlate with the clinical character of the particular lesion under study. Lesions on normal-appearing skin generally show a sparse perivascular leukocytic infiltrate with some eosinophils; conversely, biopsies of inflammatory lesions typically show an eosinophil-rich infiltrate at sites of vesicle formation and in perivascular areas. In addition to eosinophils, cell-rich lesions also contain mononuclear cells and neutrophils. It is not possible to distinguish BP from other subepidermal blistering diseases by routine histologic techniques alone.

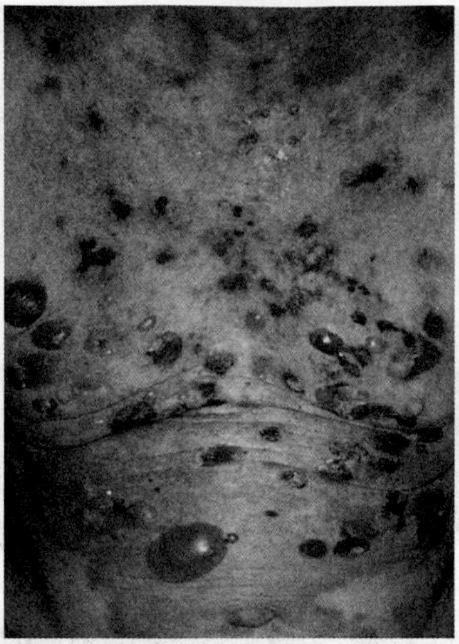

FIGURE 55-2 Bullous pemphigoid with tense vesicles and bullae on erythematous, urticarial bases. *(Courtesy of the Yale Resident's Slide Collection; with permission.)*

Direct immunofluorescence microscopy of normal-appearing perilesional skin from patients with BP shows linear deposits of IgG and/or C3 in the epidermal basement membrane. The sera of ~70% of these patients contain circulating IgG autoantibodies that bind the epidermal basement membrane of normal human skin in indirect immunofluorescence microscopy. IgG from an even higher percentage of patients shows reactivity to the epidermal side of 1 *M* NaCl split skin [an alternative immunofluorescence microscopy test substrate used to distinguish circulating IgG anti-basement membrane autoantibodies in patients with BP from those in patients with similar, yet different, subepidermal blistering diseases (see below)]. In BP, circulating autoantibodies recognize 230- and 180-kDa hemidesmosome-associated proteins in basal keratinocytes [i.e., bullous pemphigoid antigen (BPAG)1 and BPAG2, respectively]. Autoantibodies against BPAG2 are thought to deposit in situ, activate complement, produce dermal mast cell degranulation, and generate granulocyte-rich infiltrates that cause tissue damage and blister formation.

BP may persist for months to years, with exacerbations or remissions. Although extensive involvement may result in widespread erosions and compromise cutaneous integrity, the mortality rate is relatively low. Nonetheless, deaths may occur in elderly and/or debilitated patients. The mainstay of treatment is systemic glucocorticoids. Patients with local or minimal disease can sometimes be controlled with topical glucocorticoids alone; patients with more extensive lesions generally respond to systemic glucocorticoids either alone or in combination with immunosuppressive agents. Patients will usually respond to prednisone, 0.75–1 mg/kg per day. In some instances, azathioprine (2–2.5 mg/kg per day), mycophenolate mofetil (20–35 mg/kg per day), or cyclophosphamide (1–2 mg/kg per day) are necessary adjuncts.

PEMPHIGOID GESTATIONIS

Pemphigoid gestationis (PG), also known as *herpes gestationis*, is a rare, nonviral, subepidermal blistering disease of pregnancy and the puerperium. PG may begin during any trimester of pregnancy or present shortly after delivery. Lesions are usually distributed over the abdomen, trunk, and extremities; mucous membrane lesions are rare. Skin lesions in these patients may be quite polymorphic and consist of erythematous urticarial papules and plaques, vesiculopapules, and/or frank bullae. Lesions are almost always very pruritic. Severe exacerbations of PG frequently occur after delivery, typically within 24–48 h. PG tends to recur in subsequent pregnancies, often beginning earlier during such gestations. Brief flare-ups of disease may occur with resumption of menses and may develop in patients later exposed to oral contraceptives. Occasionally, infants of affected mothers demonstrate transient skin lesions.

Biopsies of early lesional skin show teardrop-shaped subepidermal vesicles forming in dermal papillae in association with an eosinophil-rich leukocytic infiltrate. Differentiation of PG from other subepidermal bullous diseases by light microscopy is difficult. However, direct immunofluorescence microscopy of perilesional skin from PG patients reveals the immunopathologic hallmark of this disorder—linear deposits of C3 in epidermal basement membrane. These deposits develop as a consequence of complement activation produced by low titer IgG anti-basement membrane autoantibodies directed against BPAG2, the same hemidesmosome-associated protein that is targeted by autoantibodies in patients with BP—a subepidermal bullous disease that resembles PG clinically, histologically, and immunopathologically.

The goals of therapy in patients with PG are to prevent the development of new lesions, relieve intense pruritus, and care for erosions at sites of blister formation. Many patients require treatment with moderate doses of daily glucocorticoids (i.e., 20–40 mg prednisone) at some point in their course. Mild cases (or brief flare-ups) may be controlled by vigorous use of potent topical glucocorticoids. Infants born of mothers with PG appear to be at increased risk of being slightly premature or "small for dates." Current evidence suggests that there is no difference in the incidence of uncomplicated live births in PG patients treated with systemic glucocorticoids and in those managed more conservatively. If systemic glucocorticoids are administered, newborns are at risk for development of reversible adrenal insufficiency.

DERMATITIS HERPETIFORMIS

Dermatitis herpetiformis (DH) is an intensely pruritic, papulovesicular skin disease characterized by lesions symmetrically distributed over extensor surfaces (i.e., elbows, knees, buttocks, back, scalp, and posterior neck) (see Fig. 52-8). Primary lesions in this disorder consist of papules, papulovesicles, or urticarial plaques. Because pruritus is prominent, patients may present with excoriations and crusted papules but no observable primary lesions. Patients sometimes report that their pruritus has a distinctive burning or stinging component; the onset of such local symptoms reliably heralds the development of distinct clinical lesions 12–24 h later. Almost all DH patients have an associated, usually subclinical, gluten-sensitive enteropathy (Chap. 288), and >90% express the HLA-B8/DRw3 and HLA-DQw2 haplotypes. DH may present at any age, including childhood; onset in the second to fourth decades is most common. The disease is typically chronic.

Biopsy of early lesional skin reveals neutrophil-rich infiltrates within dermal papillae. Neutrophils, fibrin, edema, and microvesicle formation at these sites are characteristic of early disease. Older lesions may demonstrate nonspecific features of a subepidermal bulla or an excoriated papule. Because the clinical and histologic features of this disease can be variable and resemble other subepidermal blistering disorders, the diagnosis is confirmed by direct immunofluorescence microscopy of normal-appearing perilesional skin. Such studies demonstrate granular deposits of IgA (with or without complement components) in the papillary dermis and along the epidermal basement membrane zone. IgA deposits in the skin are unaffected by control of disease with medication; however, these immunoreactants may diminish in intensity or disappear in patients maintained for long periods on a strict gluten-free diet (see below). Patients with DH have granular deposits of IgA in their epidermal basement membrane zone and should be distinguished from individuals with linear IgA deposits at this site (see below).

Although most DH patients do not report overt gastrointestinal symptoms or have laboratory evidence of malabsorption, biopsies of small bowel usually reveal blunting of intestinal villi and a lymphocytic infiltrate in the lamina propria. As is true for patients with celiac disease, this gastrointestinal abnormality can be reversed by a gluten-free diet. Moreover, if maintained, this diet alone may control the skin disease and eventuate in clearance of IgA deposits from these patients' epidermal basement membrane zone. Subsequent gluten exposure in such patients alters the morphology of their small bowel, elicits a flare-up of their skin disease, and is associated with the reappearance of IgA in their epidermal basement membrane zone. As in patients with celiac disease, dietary gluten sensitivity in patients with DH is associated with IgA anti-endomysial autoantibodies that target tissue transglutaminase. Recent studies suggest that patients with DH also have high-avidity IgA autoantibodies against epidermal transglutaminase 3 and that the latter is co-localized with granular deposits of IgA in the papillary dermis of DH patients. Patients with DH also have an increased incidence of thyroid abnormalities, achlorhydria, atrophic gastritis, and antigastric parietal cell autoantibodies. These associations likely relate to the high frequency of the HLA-B8/DRw3 haplotype in these patients, since this marker is commonly linked to autoimmune disorders. The mainstay of treatment of DH is dapsone, a sulfone. Patients respond rapidly (24–48 h) to dapsone (50–200 mg/d) but require careful pretreatment evaluation and close follow-up to ensure that complications are avoided or controlled. All patients on >100 mg/d dapsone will have some hemolysis and methemoglobinemia. These are expected pharmacologic side effects of this agent. Gluten restriction can control DH and lessen dapsone requirements; this diet must rigidly exclude gluten to be of maximal benefit. Many months of dietary restriction may be necessary before a beneficial result is achieved. Good dietary counseling by a trained dietitian is essential.

LINEAR IgA DISEASE

Linear IgA disease, once considered a variant form of dermatitis herpetiformis, is actually a separate and distinct entity. Clinically, these patients may resemble individuals with DH, BP, or other subepidermal blistering diseases. Lesions typically consist of papulovesicles, bullae, and/or urticarial plaques predominantly on central or flexural sites. Oral mucosal involvement occurs in some patients. Severe pruritus resembles that seen in patients with DH. Patients with linear IgA disease do not have an increased frequency of the HLA-B8/DRw3 haplotype or an associated enteropathy and hence are not candidates for treatment with a gluten-free diet.

The histologic alterations in early lesions may be virtually indistinguishable from those in DH. However, direct immunofluorescence microscopy of normal-appearing perilesional skin reveals linear deposits of IgA (and often C3) in the epidermal basement membrane zone. Most patients with linear IgA disease demonstrate circulating IgA anti-basement membrane autoantibodies directed against neoepitopes in the proteolytically processed extracellular domain of BPAG2. These patients generally respond to treatment with dapsone, 50–200 mg/d.

EPIDERMOLYSIS BULLOSA ACQUISITA

EBA is a rare, noninherited, polymorphic, chronic, subepidermal blistering disease. (The inherited form is discussed in Chap. 357.) Patients with classic or noninflammatory EBA have blisters on noninflamed skin, atrophic scars, milia, nail dystrophy, and oral lesions. Because lesions generally occur at sites exposed to minor trauma, classic EBA is considered to be a mechanobullous disease. Other patients with EBA have widespread inflammatory, scarring, and bullous lesions that resemble severe BP. Inflammatory EBA may evolve into the classic, noninflammatory form of this disease. Rare patients present with lesions that predominate on mucous membranes. The HLA-DR2 haplotype is found with increased frequency in EBA patients. Recent studies suggest that EBA is often associated with inflammatory bowel disease (especially Crohn's disease).

The histology of lesional skin varies depending on the character of the lesion being studied. Noninflammatory bullae show subepidermal blisters with a sparse leukocytic infiltrate and resemble those in patients with porphyria cutanea tarda. Inflammatory lesions consist of neutrophil-rich subepidermal blisters. EBA patients have continuous deposits of IgG (and frequently C3 as well as other complement components) in a linear pattern within the epidermal basement membrane zone. Ultrastructurally, these immunoreactants are found in the sublamina densa region in association with anchoring fibrils. Approximately 50% of EBA patients have demonstrable circulating IgG anti-basement membrane autoantibodies directed against type VII collagen—the collagen species that comprises anchoring fibrils. Such IgG autoantibodies bind the dermal side of 1 *M* NaCl split skin (in contrast to IgG autoantibodies in patients with BP). Recent studies have shown that passive transfer of experimental or patient IgG directed against type VII collagen can produce lesions in mice that clinically, histologically, and immunopathologically resemble those seen in patients with inflammatory EBA.

Treatment of EBA is generally unsatisfactory. Some patients with inflammatory EBA may respond to systemic glucocorticoids, either alone or in combination with immunosuppressive agents. Other patients (especially those with neutrophil-rich inflammatory lesions) may respond to dapsone. The chronic, noninflammatory form of this disease is largely resistant to treatment, although some patients may respond to cyclosporine, azathioprine, or IV immunoglobulin (IVIg).

CICATRICIAL PEMPHIGOID

Cicatricial pemphigoid (CP) is a rare, acquired, subepithelial immunobullous disease characterized by erosive lesions of mucous membranes and skin that result in scarring of at least some sites of involvement. Common sites of involvement include the oral mucosa (especially the gingiva) and conjunctiva; other sites that may be affected include the nasopharyngeal, laryngeal, esophageal, and anogenital mucosa. Skin lesions (present in about one-third of patients) tend to predominate on the scalp, face, and upper trunk and generally consist of a few scattered erosions or tense blisters on an erythematous or urticarial base. CP is typically a chronic and progressive disorder. Serious complications may arise as a consequence of ocular, laryngeal, esophageal, or anogenital lesions. Erosive conjunctivitis may result in shortened fornices, symblepharа, ankyloblepharon, entropion, corneal opacities, and (in severe cases) blindness. Similarly, erosive lesions of the larynx may cause hoarseness, pain, and tissue loss that, if unrecognized and untreated, may eventuate in complete destruction of the airway. Esophageal lesions may result in stenosis and/or strictures that may place patients at risk for aspiration. Strictures may also complicate anogenital involvement.

Biopsies of lesional tissue generally demonstrate subepithelial vesiculobullae and a mononuclear leukocytic infiltrate. Neutrophils and eosinophils may be seen in biopsies of early lesions; older lesions may demonstrate a scant leukocytic infiltrate and fibrosis. Direct immunofluorescence microscopy of perilesional tissue typically demonstrates deposits of IgG, IgA, and/or C3 in the epidermal basement membrane of these patients. Because many of these patients show no evidence of circulating anti-basement membrane autoantibodies, testing of perilesional skin is important diagnostically. Although CP was once thought to be a single nosologic entity, it is now largely regarded as a disease phenotype that may develop as a consequence of an autoimmune reaction against a variety of different molecules in epidermal basement membrane (e.g., BPAG2, laminin 5, type VII collagen, and other antigens yet to be completely defined). Recent studies suggest that CP patients with anti-laminin 5 autoantibodies have an increased relative risk for cancer. Treatment of CP is largely dependent upon sites of involvement. Due to potentially severe complications, patients with ocular, laryngeal, esophageal, and/or anogenital involvement require aggressive systemic treatment with dapsone, prednisone, or the latter in combination with another immunosuppressive agent (e.g., azathioprine, mycophenolate mofetil, or cyclophosphamide) or IVIg. Less threatening forms of the disease may be managed with topical or intralesional glucocorticoids.

AUTOIMMUNE SYSTEMIC DISEASES WITH PROMINENT CUTANEOUS FEATURES

DERMATOMYOSITIS

The cutaneous manifestations of dermatomyositis (Chap. 383) are often distinctive but at times may resemble those of systemic lupus erythematosus (SLE) (Chap. 313), scleroderma (Chap. 316), or other overlapping connective tissue diseases (Chap. 316). The extent and severity of cutaneous disease may or may not correlate with the extent and severity of the myositis. The cutaneous manifestations of dermatomyositis are similar whether the disease appears in children or the elderly, except that calcification of subcutaneous tissue is a common late sequela in childhood dermatomyositis.

The cutaneous signs of dermatomyositis may precede or follow the development of myositis by weeks to years. Cases lacking muscle involvement (i.e., dermatomyositis sine myositis) have also been reported. The most common manifestation is a purple-red discoloration of the upper eyelids, sometimes associated with scaling ("heliotrope" erythema; Fig. 55-3) and periorbital edema. Erythema on the cheeks and nose in a "butterfly" distribution may resemble the malar eruption of SLE. Erythematous or violaceous scaling patches are common on the upper anterior chest, posterior neck, scalp, and the extensor surfaces of the arms, legs, and hands. Erythema and scaling may be particularly prominent over the elbows, knees, and the dorsal interphalangeal joints. Approximately one-third of patients have violaceous, flat-topped papules over the dorsal interphalangeal joints that are pathognomonic of dermatomyositis (Gottron's sign or Gottron's papules; Fig. 55-4). These lesions can be contrasted with the erythema and scaling on the dorsum of the fingers in some patients with SLE, which spares the skin over the interphalangeal joints. Periungual telangiectasia may be prominent. Lacy or reticulated erythema may be associated with fine scaling on the extensor surfaces of the thighs and upper arms. Other patients, particularly those with longstanding disease, develop areas of hypopigmentation, hyperpigmentation, mild atrophy, and telangiectasia known as *poikiloderma*. Poikiloderma is rare in both SLE and scleroderma and thus can serve as a clinical sign that distinguishes dermatomyositis from these two diseases. Cutaneous changes may be similar in scleroderma and dermatomyositis and may include thickening and binding down of the skin of the hands (sclerodac-

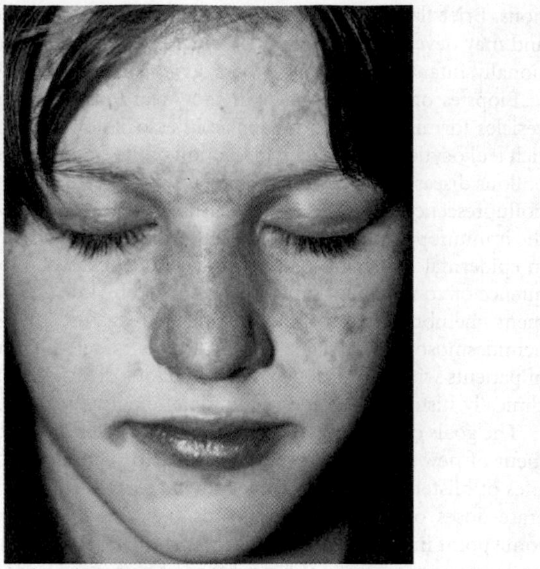

FIGURE 55-3 Dermatomyositis. Periorbital violaceous erythema characterizes the classic heliotrope rash. (*Courtesy of James Krell, MD; with permission.*)

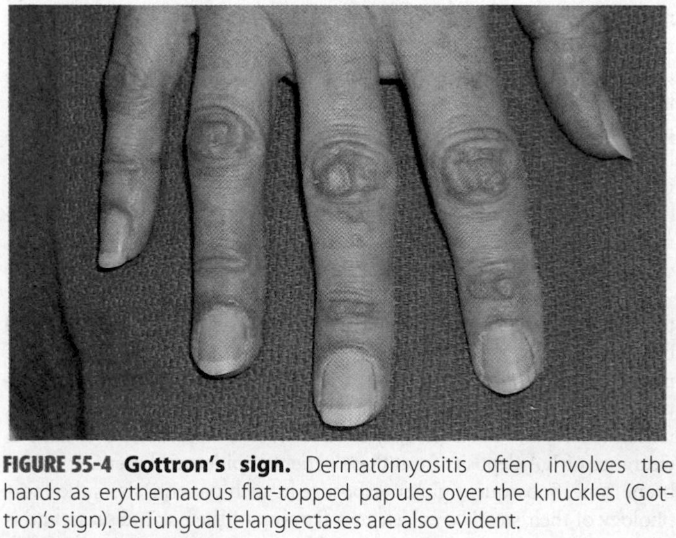

FIGURE 55-4 Gottron's sign. Dermatomyositis often involves the hands as erythematous flat-topped papules over the knuckles (Gottron's sign). Periungual telangiectases are also evident.

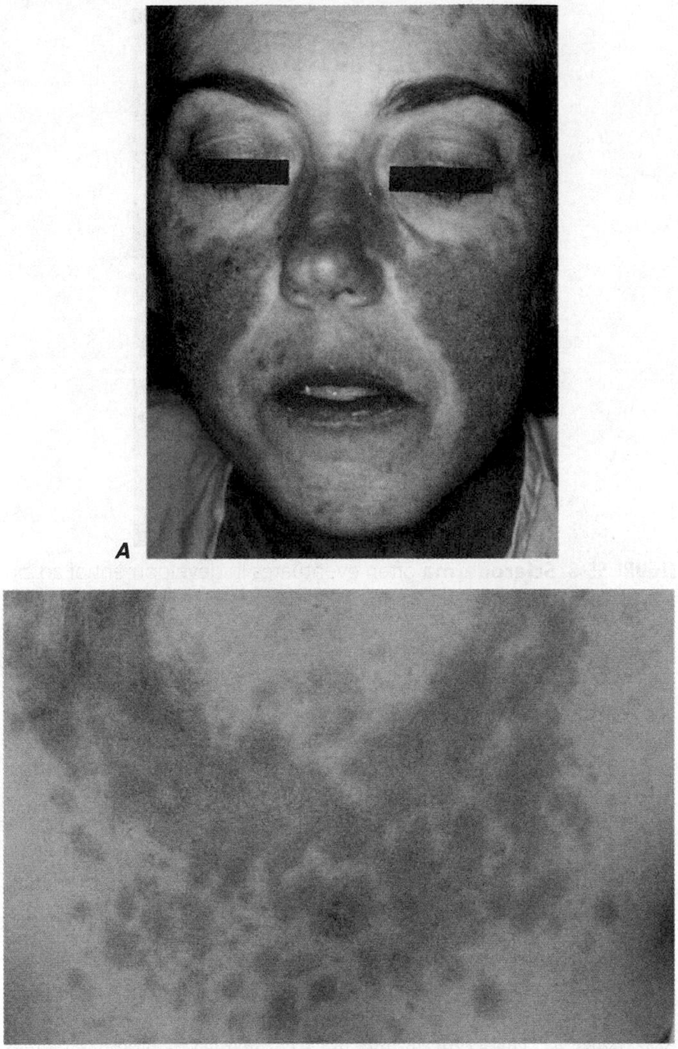

FIGURE 55-5 ***A.*** **Acute cutaneous lupus erythematosus** showing prominent, scaly, malar erythema. Involvement of other sun-exposed sites is also common. ***B.*** **Acute cutaneous LE** on the upper chest demonstrating brightly erythematous and slightly edematous papules and plaques. (***B,*** *Courtesy of Robert Swerlick, MD; with permission.*)

tyly) as well as Raynaud's phenomenon. However, the presence of severe muscle disease, Gottron's papules, heliotrope erythema, and poikiloderma serve to distinguish patients with dermatomyositis. Skin biopsy of erythematous, scaling lesions of dermatomyositis may reveal only mild nonspecific inflammation but sometimes may show changes indistinguishable from those found in SLE, including epidermal atrophy, hydropic degeneration of basal keratinocytes, edema of the upper dermis, and a mild mononuclear cell infiltrate. Direct immunofluorescence microscopy of lesional skin is usually negative, although granular deposits of immunoglobulin(s) and complement in the epidermal basement membrane zone have been described in some patients. Treatment should be directed at the systemic disease. Topical glucocorticoids are sometimes useful; patients should avoid exposure to ultraviolet irradiation and use photoprotective measures such as broad-spectrum sunscreens.

LUPUS ERYTHEMATOSUS

The cutaneous manifestations of lupus erythematosus (LE) (Chap. 313) can be divided into acute, subacute, and chronic types. *Acute cutaneous LE* is characterized by erythema of the nose and malar eminences in a "butterfly" distribution (Fig. 55-5). The erythema is often sudden in onset, accompanied by edema and fine scale, and correlated with systemic involvement. Patients may have widespread involvement of the face as well as erythema and scaling of the extensor surfaces of the extremities and upper chest. These acute lesions, while sometimes evanescent, usually last for days and are often associated with exacerbations of systemic disease. Skin biopsy of acute lesions may show only a sparse dermal infiltrate of mononuclear cells and dermal edema. In some instances, cellular infiltrates around blood vessels and hair follicles are notable, as is hydropic degeneration of basal cells of the epidermis. Direct immunofluorescence microscopy of lesional skin frequently reveals deposits of immunoglobulin(s) and complement in the epidermal basement membrane zone. Treatment is aimed at control of systemic disease; photoprotection in this, as well as in other forms of LE, is very important.

Subacute cutaneous lupus erythematosus (SCLE) is characterized by a widespread photosensitive, nonscarring eruption. Most of these patients have SLE in which renal and central nervous system involvement is mild or absent. SCLE may present as a papulosquamous eruption that resembles psoriasis or annular lesions that resemble those seen in erythema multiforme. In the papulosquamous form, discrete erythematous papules arise on the back, chest, shoulders, extensor surfaces of the arms, and the dorsum of the hands; lesions are uncommon on the face, flexor surfaces of the arms, and below the waist. These slightly scaling papules tend to merge into large plaques, some with a reticulate appearance. The annular form involves the same areas and presents with erythematous papules that evolve into oval, circular, or polycyclic lesions. The lesions of SCLE are more widespread but have less tendency for scarring than do lesions of discoid LE. Skin biopsy reveals a dense mononuclear cell infiltrate around hair follicles and blood vessels in the superficial dermis, combined with hydropic degeneration of basal cells in the epidermis. Direct immunofluorescence microscopy of lesional skin reveals deposits of immunoglobulin(s) in the epidermal basement membrane zone in about half these cases. A particulate pattern of IgG deposition throughout the epidermis has recently been associated with SCLE. Most SCLE patients have anti-Ro autoantibodies. Local therapy alone is usually unsuccessful. Most patients require treatment with aminoquinoline antimalarials. Low-dose therapy with oral glucocorticoids is sometimes necessary. Photoprotective measures against both ultraviolet B and A wavelengths are very important.

Discoid lupus erythematosus (DLE, also called *chronic cutaneous LE*) is characterized by discrete lesions, most often found on the face, scalp, and/or external ears. The lesions are erythematous papules or plaques with a thick, adherent scale that occludes hair follicles (follicular plugging). When the scale is removed, its underside shows small excrescences that correlate with the openings of hair follicles (so called "carpet tacking"), a finding relatively specific for DLE. Long-standing lesions develop central atrophy, scarring, and hypopigmentation but frequently have erythematous, sometimes raised borders (Fig. 55-6). These lesions persist for years and tend to expand slowly. Only 5–10% of patients with DLE meet the American Rheumatism Association criteria for SLE. However, typical discoid lesions are frequently seen in patients with SLE. Biopsy of DLE lesions shows hyperkeratosis, follicular plugging, atrophy of the epidermis, hydropic degeneration of basal keratinocytes, and a mononuclear cell infiltrate adjacent to epidermal, adnexal, and microvascular basement membranes. Direct immunofluorescence microscopy demonstrates immunoglobulin(s) and complement deposits at the basement membrane zone in ~90% of cases. Treatment is focused on control of local cutaneous disease and consists mainly of photoprotection and topical or intralesional glucocorticoids. If local therapy is ineffective, use of aminoquinoline antimalarials may be indicated.

SCLERODERMA AND MORPHEA

The skin changes of scleroderma (Chap. 316) usually begin on the hands, feet, and face, with episodes of recurrent nonpitting edema. Sclerosis of the skin begins distally on the fingers (sclerodactyly) and spreads proximally, usually accompanied by resorption of bone of the fingertips, which may have punched out ulcers, stellate scars, or areas of hemorrhage (Fig. 55-7). The fingers may actually shrink in size and become sausage-shaped, and since the fingernails are usually unaffected, the nails may curve over the end of the fingertips. Periungual telangiectases are usually present, but periungual erythema is rare. In advanced cases, the extremities show contractures and calcinosis cutis. Facial involvement includes a smooth, unwrinkled brow, taut skin over the nose,

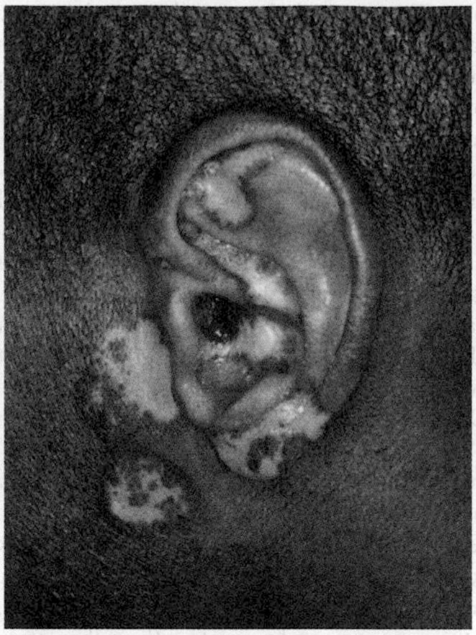

FIGURE 55-6 Discoid lupus erythematosus. Violaceous, hyperpigmented, atrophic plaques, often with evidence of follicular plugging, which may result in scarring, are characteristic of discoid lupus erythematosus (also called chronic cutaneous lupus erythematosus).

shrinkage of tissue around the mouth, and perioral radial furrowing (Fig. 55-8). Matlike telangiectases are often present, particularly on the face and hands. Involved skin feels indurated, smooth, and bound to underlying structures; hyperpigmentation and hypopigmentation are also often present. Raynaud's phenomenon, i.e., cold-induced blanching, cyanosis, and reactive hyperemia, is present in almost all patients and can precede development of scleroderma by many years. The combination of calcinosis cutis, Raynaud's phenomenon, esophageal dysmotility, sclerodactyly, and telangiectasia has been termed the *CREST syndrome*. Anticentromere antibodies have been reported in a very high percentage of patients with the CREST syndrome but in only a small minority of patients with scleroderma. Skin biopsy reveals thickening of the dermis and homogenization of collagen bundles. Direct immunofluorescence microscopy of lesional skin is usually negative.

Morphea is characterized by localized thickening and sclerosis of skin, usually affecting young adults or children. Morphea begins as erythematous or flesh-colored plaques that become sclerotic, develop central hypopigmentation, and demonstrate an erythematous border. In most cases, patients have one or a few lesions, and the disease is termed *localized morphea*. In some patients, widespread cutaneous lesions may occur, without systemic involvement. This form is called *generalized morphea*. Most patients with morphea do not have autoantibodies. Skin

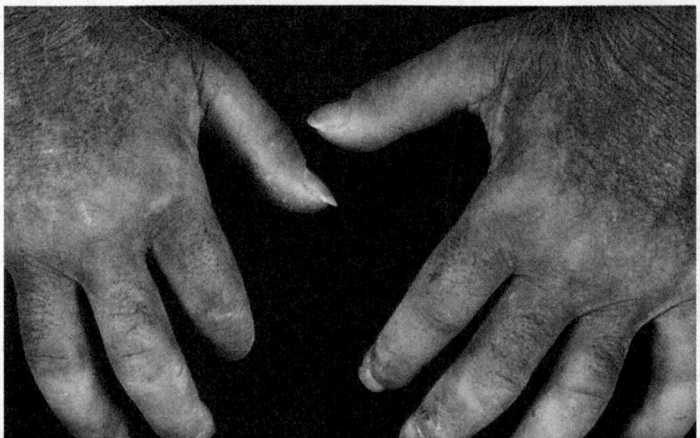

FIGURE 55-7 Scleroderma showing acral sclerosis and focal digital ulcers.

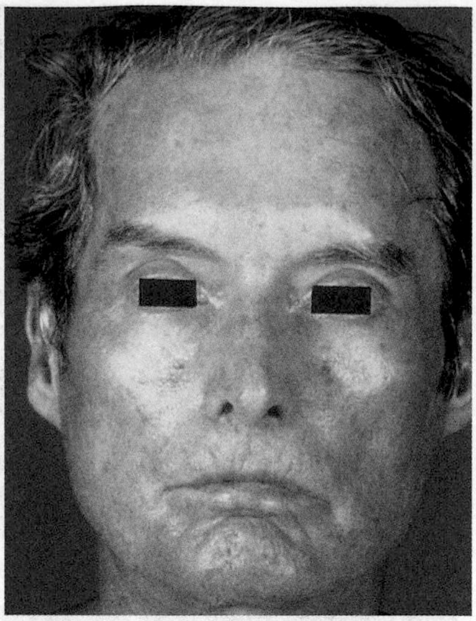

FIGURE 55-8 Scleroderma often eventuates in development of an expressionless, mask-like facies.

biopsy of morphea is indistinguishable from that of scleroderma. Linear scleroderma is a limited form of disease that presents in a linear, band-like distribution and tends to involve deep as well as superficial layers of skin. Scleroderma and morphea are usually quite resistant to therapy. For this reason, physical therapy to prevent joint contractures and to maintain function is employed and is often helpful.

Diffuse fasciitis with eosinophilia is a clinical entity that can sometimes be confused with scleroderma. There is usually the sudden onset of swelling, induration, and erythema of the extremities frequently following significant physical exertion. The proximal portions of extremities (arms, forearms, thighs, legs) are more often involved than are the hands and feet. While the skin is indurated, it is usually not bound down as in scleroderma; contractures may occur early secondary to fascial involvement. The latter may also cause muscle groups to be separated and veins to appear depressed. These skin findings are accompanied by peripheral blood eosinophilia, increased erythrocyte sedimentation rate, and sometimes hypergammaglobulinemia. Deep biopsy of affected areas of skin reveals inflammation and thickening of the deep fascia overlying muscle. An inflammatory infiltrate composed of eosinophils and mononuclear cells is usually found. Patients with eosinophilic fasciitis appear to be at increased risk to develop bone marrow failure or other hematologic abnormalities. While the ultimate course of eosinophilic fasciitis is uncertain, many patients respond favorably to treatment with prednisone in doses ranging from 40–60 mg/d.

The *eosinophilia-myalgia syndrome*, a disorder reported in epidemic numbers in 1989 and linked to ingestion of L-tryptophan manufactured by a single company in Japan, is a multisystem disorder characterized by debilitating myalgias and absolute eosinophilia in association with varying combinations of arthralgias, pulmonary symptoms, and peripheral edema. In a later phase (i.e., 3–6 months after initial symptoms), these patients often develop localized sclerodermatous skin changes, weight loss, and/or neuropathy (Chap. 316). The precise cause of this syndrome, which may resemble other sclerotic skin conditions, is unknown. However, the implicated lots of L-tryptophan contained the contaminant 1,1-ethylidene bis[tryptophan]. This contaminant may be pathogenic or a marker for another substance that provokes the disorder.

FURTHER READINGS

ANHALT GJ: Paraneoplastic pemphigus. J Investig Dermatol Symp Proc 9:29, 2004

BRAVERMAN IM: Connective tissue diseases, in *Skin Signs of Systemic Disease*, 3d ed. Philadelphia, Saunders, 1998

MUTASIM DF et al: Immunobullous diseases. J Am Acad Dermatol 52:1029, 2005

PAYNE AS et al: Desmosomes and disease: Pemphigus and bullous impetigo. Curr Opin Cell Biol 16:536, 2004

SCHMIDT E, ZILLIKENS D: Autoimmune and inherited subepidermal blistering diseases: Advances in the clinic and the laboratory. Adv Dermatol 16:113, 2000

SONTHEIMER RD: Skin manifestations of systemic autoimmune connective tissue disease: Diagnostics and therapeutics. Best Pract Res Clin Rheumatol 18:429, 2004

UDEY MC, STANLEY JR: Pemphigus—diseases of antidesmosomal autoimmunity. JAMA 282:572, 1999

YANCEY KB, EGAN CA: Pemphigoid: Clinical, histologic, immunopathologic, and therapeutic considerations. JAMA 284:350, 2000

56 Cutaneous Drug Reactions

Jean-Claude Roujeau, Robert S. Stern, Bruce U. Wintroub

Cutaneous reactions are among the most frequent adverse reactions to drugs. Every physician will see patients suffering from them. Most are benign, but a few can be life-threatening. Prompt recognition of severe reactions, drug withdrawal, and appropriate therapeutic interventions can minimize toxicity. This chapter focuses on adverse cutaneous reactions to drugs other than topical agents; it covers their incidence, patterns, and pathogenesis and provides some practical guidelines on treatment, assessment of causality, and future utilization of drugs.

USE OF PRESCRIPTION DRUGS IN THE UNITED STATES

In the United States more than 3 billion prescriptions for over 60,000 drug products, which include more than 2000 different active agents, are dispensed annually. Hospital inpatients alone annually receive about 120 million courses of drug therapy, and half of adult Americans receive prescription drugs on a regular outpatient basis. Many additional patients use over-the-counter medicines that may cause adverse cutaneous reactions.

INCIDENCE OF CUTANEOUS REACTIONS

Several large cohort studies established that acute cutaneous reaction to drugs affected about 3% of hospital inpatients. Reactions usually occur a few days to 4 weeks after initiation of therapy.

Many drugs of common use are associated with a 1–2% rate of "rashes" during premarketing clinical trials. The risk is often higher when medications are used in general unselected populations. The rate may reach 3–7% for amoxicillin, sulfamethoxazole, and many anticonvulsants (Table 56-1). It may be even higher with anti-HIV agents.

In addition to acute eruptions, a variety of skin diseases can be induced or exacerbated by prolonged utilization of drugs, e.g., pruritus, pigmentation, nail or hair disorders, psoriasis, and pemphigus. These chronic drug reactions are not frequent, but neither their incidence nor their impact on public health has been evaluated.

In a series of 48,005 inpatients over a 20-year period, morbilliform rash (91%) and urticaria (6%) were the most frequent skin reactions. Severe reactions are actually too rare to be detected in such cohorts. Their incidence has been estimated to be in the range of 1 in 10,000 to 1 in 1 million users. Even though they are rare, severe cutaneous reactions to drugs have an important impact on health and on the risk-versus-benefit evaluation of medicines because of significant mortality and sequelae.

Some populations are at increased risks of drug reactions: patients with collagen vascular diseases, bone marrow graft recipients, and those with acute Epstein-Barr virus infection. It has also been established that HIV infection increases the risk of drug allergy (Chap. 182). This was true for many drugs but has been evaluated mainly with sulfamethoxazole. Up to 40% of HIV-infected patients had skin reactions when treated with high doses, and about 15% reacted to the same dosage that induced 3–5% eruptions in non-HIV-infected populations. How HIV promotes allergy to certain medications has not yet been explained.

TABLE 56-1 CUTANEOUS REACTIONS TO DRUGS RECEIVED BY AT LEAST 1000 PATIENTS (BCDSP)[a]

Drug	Reactions, No.	Recipients, No.	Rate, %	95% Confidence Interval
Amoxicillin	63	1225	5.1	3.9–6.4
Ampicillin	215	4763	4.5	3.9–5.1
Co-trimoxazole	46	1235	3.7	2.7–4.8
Semisynthetic penicillins	41	1436	2.9	2.0–3.7
Red blood cells	67	3386	2.0	1.5–2.4
Penicillin G	68	4204	1.6	1.2–2.0
Cephalosporins	27	1781	1.5	0.9–2.1
Gentamicin	13	1277	1.0	0.5–1.6

[a]BCDSP, Boston Collaborative Drug Surveillance Program.
Source: Adapted from Bigby.

PATHOGENESIS OF DRUG REACTIONS

Untoward cutaneous responses to drugs can arise as a result of immunologic or nonimmunologic mechanisms. A variety of adverse reactions result from mechanisms that do not involve an immunologic process. Drug reactions are a public health problem because of their frequent occurrence, occasional severity, and impact on the use of medications. The skin is among the organs most often affected by adverse drug reactions. The list of conditions that can be triggered by medications includes nearly all dermatologic diseases. Many of these adverse reactions result from mechanisms that do not involve an immunologic process. Obvious examples are pigmentary changes related to accumulation in the dermis of amiodarone, antimalarials, minocycline, quinolones, alteration of hair follicules by cytostatics, and lipodystrophy associated with metabolic effects of anti-HIV medications. These side effects are mostly toxic, predictable, and often can be avoided at least in part by simple preventive measures.

IMMUNOLOGIC DRUG REACTIONS

For most acute drug eruptions, benign or severe, accumulated data suggest an immunologic basis. In the last 10 years drug-specific T cell clones were derived from the blood lymphocytes or from skin lesions of patients with a variety of drug allergies. Since these clones had been obtained after several stimulations in vitro with the drug, their relevance to explain the original manifestations of allergy can be questioned. Regardless, these T cell clones brought definite evidence that drugs can be recognized as antigens by human T cells, and that these T cells play a role in drug allergy. Specific clones were obtained with penicillin G, amoxicillin, cephalosporins, sulfamethoxazole, phenobarbital, carbamazepine, lamotrigine, i.e., many of the medications that are frequently a cause of drug eruptions. Both CD4 and CD8 clones were often obtained, whatever the clinical type of eruption.

Some clones produced a T_H0 profile of cytokines (simultaneous release of IL-4 and IFN-γ). A T_H2 orientation was frequent in CD4+ clones while CD8+ clones were usually T_H1 and often cytotoxic. Drug presentation to T cell was MHC-restricted, usually as expected by HLA class II for CD4+ cells and by HLA class I for CD8. But there were also less classic situations like HLA class II restricted cytotoxic CD4 clones. With many drugs, an original observation was that the drug could be presented to the TCR and activate a specific clone without prior processing by the antigen-presenting cell and through a noncovalent binding to the MHC or its embedded peptide. Actually, some specific TCR could recognize sulfamethoxazole presented either in covalent or noncovalent bound form, but the former was the exception and the latter the rule. Since the noncovalent binding is reminiscent of the pharmacologic interaction between a drug and its receptor, the denomination of pharmoco-immune (p-i) concept has been proposed.

Once a drug has induced an immune response, the final phenotype of the reaction probably depends on the nature of effectors: cytotoxic (CD8+) T cells in blistering reactions, chemokines for reactions mediated by neutrophils or eosinophils, and collaboration with B cells for production of specific antibodies for urticarial reactions.

Immediate Reactions Immediate reactions depend on the release of mediators of inflammation by tissue mast cells or circulating basophilic leukocytes. These mediators include histamine, leukotrienes, prostaglandins, platelet-activating factor, enzymes, and proteoglycans. Drugs can trigger mediator release either directly ("anaphylactoid" reaction) or through IgE-specific antibodies. These reactions are usually manifest in the skin and gastrointestinal, respiratory, and cardiovascular systems (Chap. 311). Primary symptoms and signs include pruritus, urticaria, nausea, vomiting, cramps, bronchospasm, and laryngeal edema—and, occasionally, anaphylactic shock with hypotension and death. They occur within minutes of drug exposure. Nonsteroidal anti-inflammatory drugs (NSAIDs), including aspirin, and radiocontrast media are frequent causes of pharmacologically mediated anaphylactoid reactions, which can occur on first exposure. Penicillins and myorelaxants used in general anesthesia are the most frequent causes of IgE-dependent reactions to drugs, which require prior sensitization. Release of mediators is triggered when polyvalent drug protein conjugates cross-link IgE molecules fixed to sensitized cells. Certain routes of administration favor different clinical patterns (e.g., gastrointestinal effects from oral route, circulatory effects from intravenous route).

Immune Complex–Dependent Reactions Because the use of nonhuman sera is now uncommon, this mechanism is rarely relevant to adverse reactions seen today. Serum sickness is produced by tissue deposition of circulating immune complexes with consumption of complement. It is characterized by fever, arthritis, nephritis, neuritis, edema, and an urticarial, papular, or purpuric rash (Chap. 319). It was first described following administration of foreign sera; it may now occur with monoclonal antibodies. In classic serum sickness, symptoms develop 6 days or more after exposure to a drug, the latent period representing the time needed to synthesize antibody. Cephalosporin administration in febrile children may be associated with a clinically similar "serum sickness–like" reaction. The real mechanism of this reaction is unknown but is unrelated to complement activation.

Cutaneous or systemic vasculitis, a relatively rare cutaneous complication of drugs, may also be a result of immune complex deposition (Chap. 319).

Delayed Hypersensitivity Delayed hypersensitivity mechanisms directed by drug-specific T cells are probably the most important mechanisms in the etiology of the most common drug eruptions—morbilliform exanthems—and also of rare and severe forms such as hypersensitivity syndrome, acute generalized exanthematous pustulosis (AGEP), Stevens-Johnson syndrome (SJS), and toxic epidermal necrolysis (TEN). Drug-specific T cells have been detected in these types of drug eruptions.

Contrary to what has been believed for years, the antigen is more often the native drug itself than its metabolites. It remains to better understand why the stimulation of T cells by medications leads to reactions that are clinically so diverse. Some answers were provided by the study of effector cells obtained at the site of skin lesions. Drug-specific cytotoxic T cells have been detected in the skin lesions of fixed drug eruptions and of TEN. In TEN, blisters that result from accumulation of interstitial fluid under the necrotic epidermis contain T lymphocytes that are able to kill autologous lymphocytes and keratinocytes in a drug-specific, HLA-restricted, and perforin/granzyme-mediated pathway.

Drug-specific clones producing CXCL8, a neutrophil-attracting chemokine, were obtained from skin tests of patients with AGEP, a neutrophil-mediated drug reaction.

One may therefore assume that the final pattern of drug eruptions results both from the nature of effectors—cytotoxic T cells in blistering reactions, chemokines in reactions mediated by neutrophils or eosinophils—and from the intensity of stimulation and response.

Genetic Factors and Cutaneous Drug Reactions Specific genetically determined defects in the ability of an individual to detoxify toxic reactive drug metabolites predispose such individuals to the development of drug toxicity. It has also been suspected that a slow acetylator phenotype increases the risk of rash from sulfonamides. However, in two large prospective cohorts of HIV-infected patients treated with sulfonamides, no association of drug eruption with acetylation genotype was found.

Recent literature shows that genetic factors may be important predictors of severe drug reactions. Hypersensitivity to the anti-HIV medication abacavir was strongly associated with HLA B*5701. In Taiwan, within a homogeneous Han Chinese population, a 100% association was observed between SJS or TEN related to carbamazepine and HLA B*1502. In the same population, another 100% association was found between SJS, TEN, or hypersensitivity syndrome/drug reaction with eosinophilia and systemic symptoms (DRESS) related to allopurinol and HLA B*5801. These observations have important theoretical implications. By pointing to HLA genes, they strongly support a key role for immune mechanisms. However, the strong associations found in Taiwan have not been observed in other countries with more heterogenous populations. Therefore, widespread practical applications of these findings are not yet possible.

CLINICAL PRESENTATION OF CUTANEOUS DRUG REACTIONS

NONIMMUNE CUTANEOUS REACTIONS

Exacerbation or Induction of Dermatologic Diseases A variety of agents can exacerbate preexisting diseases or sometimes induce a disease that may or may not disappear after withdrawal of the inducing medication. For example, NSAIDs, lithium, beta blockers, and angiotensin-converting enzyme (ACE) inhibitors can exacerbate plaque psoriasis, while antimalarials can worsen pustular psoriasis. Acne may be induced by glucocorticoids, androgens, and lithium. Minocycline and thiazide diuretics may exacerbate subacute systemic lupus erythematosus, and pemphigus can be induced by D-penicillamine, captopril, and other ACE inhibitors. The hypothesis that a drug may be responsible should always be considered, especially in cases with atypical clinical presentation, unusual age of onset, or unexpected evolution.

Photosensitivity Eruptions Photosensitivity eruptions are usually most marked in sun-exposed areas but may extend to sun-protected areas. The mechanism is almost always phototoxicity. Phototoxic reactions resemble sunburn and can occur with first exposure to a drug. Their severity depends on the tissue level of the drug, its efficiency as a photosensitizer, and the extent of exposure to the activating wavelengths of ultraviolet light (Chap. 57).

Common orally administered photosensitizing drugs include many fluoroquinolones and cycline antibiotics. Other drugs less frequently encountered are chlorpromazine, thiazides, and several NSAIDs (ibuprofen, naproxen, piroxicam). Because UV-A and visible light, which trigger these reactions, are not easily absorbed by nonopaque sunscreens and are transmitted through window glass, photosensitivity reactions may be difficult to block.

Photosensitivity reactions abate with removal of either the drug or ultraviolet radiation, use of high-potency sunscreens that block UV-A light, and treating the reaction as one would a sunburn. Rarely, individuals develop persistent reactivity to light, necessitating long-term avoidance of sun exposure.

Pigmentation Changes Drugs, either systemic or topical, may cause a variety of pigmentary changes in the skin. Oral contraceptives may induce melasma. Long-term minocycline or pefloxacin may cause blue-gray pigmentation, while amiodarone causes a more purple coloration. Long-term high-dose phenothiazine results in gray-brown pigmentation of sun-exposed areas. Numerous cancer chemotherapeutic agents may be associated with pigmentation, e.g., bleomycin, busulfan, daunorubicin, cyclophosphamide, hydroxyurea, and methotrexate. Pigmentation changes may also occur in mucous membranes (busulfan), nails (zidovudine), hair, and teeth.

Warfarin Necrosis of Skin This rare reaction usually occurs between the third and tenth days of therapy with warfarin derivatives, usually in women. The more common sites are breasts, thighs, and buttocks. Lesions are sharply demarcated, erythematous, indurated, and purpuric and may resolve or progress to form large, irregular, hemorrhagic bullae with eventual necrosis and slow-healing eschar formation.

Development of the syndrome is unrelated to drug dose, and the course is not altered by discontinuation of the drug after onset of the eruption. Warfarin reactions are associated with protein C deficiency. Warfarin anticoagulation in heterozygotes for protein C deficiency causes a precipitous fall in circulating levels of protein C, permitting hypercoagulability and thrombosis in the cutaneous microvasculature, with consequent areas of necrosis. Similar reactions have been associated with heparin. Heparin-induced necrosis may have clinically similar features but is probably due to heparin-induced platelet aggregation with subsequent occlusion of blood vessels.

Warfarin-induced cutaneous necrosis is treated with vitamin K and heparin. Treatment with protein C concentrates may also be helpful.

Drug-Induced Hair Disorders • ***DRUG-INDUCED HAIR LOSS*** Medications may affect hair follicles at two different phases of their cycle. *Anagen effluvium* occurs within days of drug administration, whereas in *telogen effluvium*, the delay is 2–4 months. Both present as diffuse nonscarring alopecia most often reversible after discontinuation of the responsible agent.

The prevalence and severity of alopecia depend on the drug as well as on individual predisposition. A considerable number of drugs have been reported to induce hair loss. These include antineoplastic agents (alkylating agents, bleomycin, vinca alkaloids, platinum compounds), anticonvulsants (carbamazepine, valproate), antihypertensive drugs (beta blockers), antidepressants, antithyroid drugs, interferons (IFNs), oral contraceptives, and hypolipidemics.

HIRSUTISM Hirsutism is an excessive growth of coarse hair with masculine characteristics in a female, most often on the lateral aspects of face and back. Hirsutism results from androgenic stimulation of hormone-sensitive hair follicles.

Anabolic steroids, oral contraceptives of the nonsteroid progesterone type, testosterone, and corticotropin can induce hirsutism.

HYPERTRICHOSIS Hypertrichosis differs from hirsutism by being located mainly on the forehead and temporal regions. It is usually reversible. Drugs responsible for hypertrichosis include anti-inflammatory drugs, glucocorticoids, vasodilators (diazoxide, minoxidil), diuretics (acetazolamide), anticonvulsants (phenytoin), immunosuppressive agents, psoralens, and zidovudine.

Changes in hair color or structure are uncommon adverse effects from medications. Hair discoloration may occur with chloroquine, IFN-α, chemotherapeutic agents, and tyrosine kinase inhibitors. Changes in hair structure have been observed in patients given EGFR inhibitors.

Drug-Induced Nail Disorders These usually involve several or all 20 nails and need months to resolve after withdrawal of the offending agent. The pathogenesis is most often toxic. Drug-induced nail changes include Beau's line (transversal depression of the nail plate), onycholysis (detachment of the distal part of the nail plate), onychomadesis (detachment of the proximal part of the nail plate), pigmentation, and paronychia (inflammation of periungual skin).

ONYCHOLYSIS Onycholysis may occur as a consequence of phototoxic reactions, particularly with tetracyclines, fluoroquinolones, phenothiazines, and psoralens, as well as in persons taking NSAIDs, captopril, retinoids, sodium valproate, and many chemotherapeutic agents such as anthracyclines or taxanes including paclitaxel and docetaxel. The risk of onycholysis in patients receiving cytotoxic drugs can be increased by exposure to sunlight.

ONYCHOMADESIS Onychomadesis is caused by temporary arrest of nail matrix mitotic activity. Common drugs reported to induce onychomadesis include carbamazepine, lithium, retinoids, and chemotherapeutic agents such as cyclophosphamide and vincristine.

PARONYCHIA Paronychia and multiple pyogenic granuloma with progressive and painful periungual abscess of fingers and toes are a side effect of systemic retinoids, lamivudine, indinavir, and anti-EGFR monoclonal antibodies (cetuximab, gefitinib).

NAIL DISCOLORATION Some drugs, including anthracyclines, taxanes, fluorouracil, and zidovudine, may induce nail bed hyperpigmentation through melanocyte stimulation. It appears to be reversible and dose-dependent.

Pruritus Pruritus is a common symptom of most drug eruptions, but it may also occur without skin lesions as the only manifestation of drug intolerance. Severe pruritus may occur in up to 50% of African patients treated with antimalarials and lead to poor compliance. It is much rarer in Caucasians.

IMMUNE CUTANEOUS REACTIONS: BENIGN

Maculopapular Eruptions Morbilliform or maculopapular eruptions are the most common of all drug-induced reactions, often start on the trunk or areas of pressure or trauma, and consist of erythematous macules and papules that are frequently symmetric and may become confluent. Involvement of mucous membranes is unusual, with the exception of scaly lips; the eruption may be associated with moderate to severe pruritus and fever. Diagnosis is rarely assisted by laboratory testing. Skin biopsy is useless because it shows normal skin or very mild and nonspecific changes. A viral exanthem is the principal differential diagnostic consideration, especially in children. Absence of enanthems, absence of symptoms in ears, nose, and throat and upper respiratory tract, and polymorphism of the skin lesions support a drug rather than a viral eruption.

Maculopapular reactions usually develop within 1 week of initiation of therapy and last less than 2 weeks. Occasionally these eruptions may decrease or fade with continued use of the responsible drug. Since the eruption may also worsen, the suspect drug should be discontinued unless it is essential. Oral antihistamines, emollients, and soothing baths may help relieve pruritus. Short courses of potent topical glucocorticoids can reduce inflammation and symptoms. Systemic glucocorticoid treatment is rarely indicated.

Urticaria/Angioedema *Urticaria* is the second most frequent type of cutaneous reaction to drugs. However, "drug allergy" explains no more than 10–20% of acute urticaria cases. It is a skin reaction characterized by pruritic, red wheals of varying size. Individual lesions rarely last more than 24 h. Deep edematous dermal and subcutaneous tissues are known as *angioedema*. Angioedema may involve mucous membranes. Urticaria and angioedema may be part of a life-threatening anaphylactic reaction.

Drug-induced urticaria may be caused by three mechanisms: an IgE-dependent mechanism, circulating immune complexes (serum sickness), and nonimmunologic activation of effector pathways. IgE-dependent urticarial reactions usually occur within 36 h of drug exposure but can occur within minutes. Immune complex–induced urticaria associated with serum sickness usually occurs 6–12 days after first exposure. In this syndrome, the urticarial eruption may be accompanied by fever, hematuria, arthralgias, hepatic dysfunction, and neurologic symptoms.

Certain drugs, such as NSAIDs, ACE inhibitors, angiotensin II antagonists, and radiographic dyes, may induce urticarial reactions, angioedema, and anaphylaxis in the absence of drug-specific antibody. Although ACE inhibitors, aspirin, penicillin, and blood products are the most frequent causes of urticarial eruptions, urticaria has been observed in association with nearly all drugs. Drugs may also cause chronic urticaria, which lasts more than 6 weeks. Aspirin frequently exacerbates this problem.

The treatment of urticaria or angioedema depends on the severity of the reaction and the rate at which it is evolving. In severe cases, with respiratory or cardiovascular compromise, epinephrine is the mainstay of therapy, but its effect is reduced in patients using beta blockers. Treatment with systemic glucocorticoids, sometimes administered IV, is helpful. In addition to drug withdrawal, for patients with only cutaneous symptoms and without symptoms of angioedema or anaphylaxis, oral antihistamines are usually sufficient.

Fixed Drug Eruptions These reactions are characterized by one or more sharply demarcated, erythematous lesions, sometimes leading to a blister. Hyperpigmentation results after resolution of the acute inflammation. With rechallenge, the lesion recurs in the same (i.e., fixed) location. Lesions often involve the lips, hands, legs, face, genitalia, and oral mucosa and cause a burning sensation. Most patients have multiple lesions. Fixed drug eruptions have been associated with phenolphthalein, sulfonamides, cyclines, dipyrone, NSAIDs, and barbiturates. Patch testing has been used in Europe to help establish the etiology.

IMMUNE CUTANEOUS REACTIONS: SEVERE

Vasculitis Cutaneous necrotizing vasculitis often presents as palpable purpuric lesions that may be generalized or limited to the lower extremities or other dependent areas (Chap. 319). Urticarial lesions, ulcers, and hemorrhagic blisters also occur. Vasculitis may involve other organs, including the liver, kidney, brain, and joints. Drugs are an infrequent cause of vasculitis. Infection and collagen vascular disease are responsible for the majority of cases.

Propylthiouracil induces a cutaneous vasculitis that is accompanied by leukopenia and splenomegaly. Direct immunofluorescent changes in these lesions suggest immune-complex deposition. Drugs implicated in vasculitis include allopurinol, thiazides, sulfonamides, other antimicrobials, and several NSAIDs. The presence of eosinophils in the perivascular infiltrate of skin biopsy may indicate a higher probability of a drug etiology.

Pustular Eruptions AGEP is a rare reaction pattern, often associated with exposure to drugs. Usually beginning on the face or intertriginous areas, small nonfollicular pustules overlying erythematous and edematous skin may coalesce and lead to superficial ulceration. Differentiating this eruption from TEN in its initial stages may be difficult. A skin biopsy is important and shows scattered pustules in the upper part of the epidermis instead of the full-thickness necrosis that characterizes TEN. Fever is present with elevated neutrophil counts, and sepsis is often suspected. Acute pustular psoriasis is the principal differential diagnostic consideration. AGEP often begins within a few days of initiating drug treatment, most notably antibiotics. For other associated drugs, diltiazem, chloroquine, hydroxychloroquine or terbinafine, AGEP begins later: 7–14 days after initiation of treatment.

Hypersensitivity Syndrome Initially described with phenytoin, hypersensitivity syndrome—a multiorgan drug-induced reaction—is also known as *DRESS* and *drug-induced hypersensitivity syndrome* (*DIHS*). It presents as a widespread erythematous eruption that may become purpuric or lichenoid and is accompanied by many of the following features: fever, facial and periorbital edema, tender generalized lymphadenopathy, leukocytosis (often with atypical lymphocytes and eosinophils), hepatitis, and sometimes nephritis or pneumonitis. The cutaneous reaction usually begins 2–8 weeks after the drug is started and lasts longer than mild eruptions after drug cessation. Symptoms may persist for several weeks, especially hepatitis. The eruption recurs with rechallenge, and cross-reactions among aromatic anticonvulsants, including phenytoin, carbamazepine, and barbiturates, are frequent. Other drugs causing this syndrome include lamotrigine, minocycline, dapsone, allopurinol, and sulfonamides, as well as abacavir and zalcitabine in HIV-infected patients. Reactivation of herpes viruses, especially of herpes virus 6, has been reported to be frequent in this syndrome. The role of virus infection is still unclear; it may contribute to long-lasting manifestations such as hepatitis or encephalitis. Mortality as high as 10% has been reported. In life-threatening situations such as pneumonitis or nephritis, systemic glucocorticoids (prednisone, 0.5–1.0 mg/kg) seem to reduce symptoms. Topical high-potency glucocorticoids may also be helpful. In all cases, rapid withdrawal of the suspected drug is required.

Stevens-Johnson Syndrome and Toxic Epidermal Necrolysis *SJS* and *TEN* are terms that, most believe, describe the same usually drug-induced disorder, which is characterized by blisters and epidermal detachment resulting from epidermal necrosis in the absence of substantial dermal inflammation. The term *SJS* is now used to describe cases with blisters developing on dusky or purpuric macules in which total body surface area blistering and eventual detachment is <10%. The term *SJS/TEN* is used to describe cases with 10–30% detachment, and *TEN* is used to describe cases with >30% detachment. Erythema multiforme major is now considered by most to be different from SJS, characterized by typical "target" lesions and resulting from a reaction to infection, most commonly from herpes simplex virus.

Patients with SJS, SJS/TEN, or TEN initially present with acute symptoms, painful skin lesions, fever >39°C (102.2°F), sore throat, and visual impairment resulting from mucous membrane and ocular lesions. Intestinal and pulmonary involvements are associated with a poor prognosis, as are a greater extent of epidermal detachment and older age. About 10% and 30% of SJS- and TEN-affected persons die from their disease, respectively. Drugs that most commonly cause SJS or TEN are anti-infectious sulfonamides, nevirapine, allopurinol, lamotrigine, aromatic anticonvulsants, and oxicam NSAIDs. At this time SJS or TEN have no treatment of proven efficacy. The best results come from early diagnosis, immediate discontinuation of any suspected drug, and supportive therapy, paying close attention to ocular complications, often in burn units or intensive care units.

DRUGS OF SPECIAL INTEREST

ALLOPURINOL

Together with sulfonamides and antiepileptics, allopurinol is one of the "usual suspects" that induce frequently mild maculopapular eruptions (in at least 3% of users) and may also cause more severe reactions including hypersensitivity/DRESS and SJS/TEN. Because of increasing utilization it is one of the most frequent causes of life-threatening reactions.

ANTI-HIV MEDICATIONS

In clinical trials, combinations of highly active antiretroviral treatments were frequently associated with ≥10% "drug eruptions." Two drugs, nevirapine and abacavir, have been associated with specific risks.

Nevirapine has both a high risk of maculopapular eruptions and a very high risk (about 1 in 1000) of SJS or TEN. Progressive escalation of daily doses has been shown to decrease the risk of mild eruption but does not abrogate the risk of severe reactions.

Abacavir is associated with a 4–5% risk of a hypersensitivity reaction, which is remarkable because of the association of symptoms suggesting a type I reaction (dyspnea, diarrhea, low blood pressure, shock on rechallenge) and signs of delayed hypersensitivity (rash, late onset, hepatitis). The risk is lower in patients of African ancestry and strongly correlated with HLAB*5701.

PENICILLIN

The utilization rate of penicillin has decreased markedly since it has been the subject of many investigations and a model for "drug allergy." Incidence of cutaneous reactions is about 1%. About 85% of cutaneous reactions to penicillin are morbilliform, and about 10% are urticaria or angioedema. Anaphylaxis and serum sickness appear to be due to IgE antibodies in serum.

Delayed reactions, mainly maculopapular eruptions, are much more common with aminopenicillins, involving 4–7% of users. The question of cross-reactivity between β-lactam antibiotics and preventing the risk of anaphylaxis is discussed below ("Management of a Patient with a Drug Eruption").

NONSTEROIDAL ANTI-INFLAMMATORY DRUGS

Most NSAIDs, including aspirin, cause immediate allergy-like symptoms in susceptible individuals. Approximately 1% of persons experience urticaria or angioedema, and about half as many (0.5%) experience rhinosinusitis and asthma.

Urticaria/angioedema may be delayed up to 24 h and may occur at any age. The rhinosinusitis-asthma syndrome generally develops within 1 h of drug administration. Recurrences are frequent and can be complicated by nasal and sinus infection, polyposis, bloody discharge, and nasal eosinophilia. In many individuals with this syndrome, asthma that can be life-threatening eventually ensues whenever NSAIDs are subsequently ingested. Proof of the association of symptoms and NSAID use requires either clear-cut history of symptoms following drug ingestion or an oral challenge. That procedure must be conducted only in a hospital setting by experienced personnel. Cross-reactivity between NSAIDs that inhibit cyclooxygenase (COX) 1 is common, while reactivity to COX-2 inhibitors is less frequent. The reaction is pharmacologic, and patients who are sensitive to NSAIDs cannot be identified by assessment of IgE antibody to aspirin, lymphocyte sensitization, or in vitro immunologic testing.

Other reactions can also occur with NSAIDs, including phototoxicity with many agents, a pattern of pseudoporphyria being often related to naproxen, hypersensitivity/DRESS (oxicam derivatives, COX-2 inhibitors), and SJS or TEN (phenylbutazone, oxicam derivatives, diclofenac).

RADIOCONTRAST MEDIA

Large numbers of patients are exposed to radiocontrast agents. High-osmolality radiocontrast media were about five times more likely to induce urticaria (1%) or anaphylaxis than were newer low-osmolality media. Severe reactions are rare with either type of contrast media. About one-third of those with mild reactions to previous exposure re-react on re-exposure. In most cases, these reactions are probably not immunologic. Pretreatment with prednisone and diphenhydramine reduces reaction rates. Persons with a reaction to a high-osmolality contrast media should be given low-osmolality media if later contrast studies are required.

ANTICONVULSANTS

Along with sulfonamide antibiotics, phenobarbital, phenytoin, and carbamazepine among the older anticonvulsants, and lamotrigine among the newer, are associated with many types of severe reactions and a high incidence of less severe reactions, particularly in children. These drugs have among the highest risk of SJS, TEN, and hypersensitivity syndrome in immunologically normal patients. The aromatic anticonvulsants can induce a pseudolymphoma syndrome and induce gingival hyperplasia.

SULFONAMIDES

Antibacterial sulfonamides have a rather high risk of causing cutaneous eruptions and are among the drugs most frequently implicated in SJS and TEN. The combination of sulfamethoxazole and trimethoprim frequently induces adverse cutaneous reactions in patients with AIDS (Chap. 182). Desensitization is often successful in AIDS patients with morbilliform eruptions but is not recommended in AIDS patients who manifested erythroderma or a bullous reaction in response to their earlier sulfonamide exposure.

Reaction rates are much lower with nonantibiotic sulfonamides, including diuretics or antidiabetic agents. Cross-reactivity between antibiotic and nonantibiotic sulfonamides is, at most, infrequent.

VANCOMYCIN

Vancomycin causes two unusual but recognizable cutaneous reactions: linear IgA bullous dermatosis (a transient blistering eruption) and *red man syndrome*. Red man syndrome occurs during rapid IV infusion of vancomycin. This is thought to be a histamine-related anaphylactoid reaction characterized by flushing, diffuse maculopapular eruption, hypotension, and, in rare cases, cardiac arrest.

AGENTS USED IN CANCER CHEMOTHERAPY

Since many agents used in cancer chemotherapy inhibit cell division, rapidly proliferating elements of the skin, including hair, mucous membranes, and appendages, are sensitive to their effects. As a result, stomatitis and alopecia are among the most frequent dose-dependent side effects of chemotherapy. Various nail abnormalities have been described: onycholysis, dystrophy, Beau's lines, white lines, and pigmentation. Sterile cellulitis and phlebitis and ulceration of pressure areas occur with many of these agents. Also reported is acral erythema, which begins with dysesthesia followed by redness and a painful edematous eruption of the palms and soles; it is caused by cytarabine, doxorubicin, methotrexate, and 5-fluorouracil. Urticaria, angioedema, and exfoliative dermatitis also have been seen, as has local and diffuse hyperpigmentation.

Hypersensitivity to carboplatin or cisplatin is not rare (with an incidence of 10–20%) among patients receiving multiple treatments with these drugs. It is probably IgE mediated. Moderate to severe reactions including respiratory distress and hypotension are also observed in 10–20% of patients receiving paclitaxel regardless of premedication with glucocorticoids and histamine H(1) and H(2) antagonists.

GLUCOCORTICOIDS

Both systemic and topical glucocorticoids cause a variety of skin changes, including acneiform eruptions, atrophy, striae, and other stigmata of Cushing's syndrome, and in sufficiently high doses can retard wound healing. Patients using glucocorticoids are at higher risk for bacterial, yeast, and fungal skin infections that may be misinterpreted as drug eruptions but are instead drug side effects. Allergy to glucocorticoids may also occur either as contact dermatitis to topical formulations or as systemic reactions, including anaphylaxis.

BIOLOGIC THERAPIES

These include cytokines and monoclonal antibodies.

Injection-site reactions are the most frequent adverse event. The severity varies from mild redness to deep inflammation and necrosis. In most cases the treatment can be continued and the severity of reactions will decrease with time.

Like all foreign proteins, monoclonal antibodies may induce urticaria, angioedema, anaphylactic reactions, and serum sickness.

Alopecia is a common complication of IFN-α. A nonspecific highly pruritic "dermatitis" is frequent in patients receiving IFN and ribavirin for hepatitis C.

Induction or exacerbation of various immune-mediated disorders, especially lupus erythematosus, has been reported with many biologicals (interleukin 2, IFN-α, anti–tumor necrosis factor α).

Granulocyte colony-stimulating factor may induce various neutrophilic dermatoses, including Sweet's syndrome and pyoderma gangrenosum, and can exacerbate psoriasis.

Cetuximab is a member of a new family of antineoplastic agents that inhibit the EGF receptor. These molecules induce acneiform eruptions after a mean interval of 10 days in a majority of patients. The severity of the eruption was shown to correlate with a better anticancer effect. Systemic antibiotics and topical anti-acne treatments are helpful.

Although not usually classified as adverse drug reactions, skin infections and skin cancer could become a major concern with long-term use of immune-modifying biologicals.

ANTIMALARIAL AGENTS

Antimalarial agents are used as therapy for several skin diseases, including the skin manifestations of lupus and polymorphous light eruption, but they can also induce cutaneous reactions. The most frequent is pruritus, which occurs in up to 50% of African patients receiving chloroquine and may be severe enough to lead to discontinuation of treatment.

Pigmentation disturbances, including black pigmentation of the face, mucous membranes, and pretibial and subungual areas, occur

TABLE 56-2 CLINICAL AND LABORATORY FINDINGS ASSOCIATED WITH MORE SERIOUS DRUG-INDUCED CUTANEOUS CLINICAL FINDINGS

Cutaneous
- Confluent erythema
- Facial edema or central facial involvement
- Skin pain
- Palpable purpura
- Skin necrosis
- Blisters or epidermal detachment
- Positive Nikolsky's sign
- Mucous membrane erosions
- Urticaria
- Swelling of tongue

General
- High fever [temperature >40°C (>104°F)]
- Enlarged lymph nodes
- Arthralgias or arthritis
- Shortness of breath, wheezing, hypotension

Laboratory results
- Eosinophil count >1000/μL
- Lymphocytosis with atypical lymphocytes
- Abnormal liver function tests

Source: Adapted from Roujeau and Stern.

with antimalarials. Quinacrine (mepacrine) causes generalized, cutaneous yellow discoloration. Less frequent reactions include pustular eruptions (AGEP) and hypersensitivity/DRESS.

MANAGEMENT OF A PATIENT WITH A DRUG ERUPTION

There are four main questions to be answered when seeing an eruption:

1. Is it a severe eruption or the onset of a form that may become severe?
2. Is it a drug reaction?
3. Which drug(s) are suspected, and which should be withdrawn?
4. What is recommended for future use of drugs?

EARLY DIAGNOSIS OF SEVERE ERUPTIONS

Many patients who experience a severe skin reaction complain that the diagnosis has been delayed, sometimes for several days. Initially, most eruptions look nonspecific. Of special importance is the rapid recognition of reactions that may become serious or life-threatening. Table 56-2 lists clinical and laboratory features that, if present, suggest the reaction may be serious. Table 56-3 provides key features of the most serious adverse cutaneous reactions. Intensity of symptoms and rapid progression of signs should raise the suspicion of a severe eruption. Any doubt should lead to consultation with a dermatologist and/or referral of the patient to a specialized center.

CONFIRMATION OF DRUG REACTION

The probability of drug etiology varies with the pattern of the reaction. Only fixed drug eruptions are always drug-induced. Maculopapular eruptions are usually viral in children and drug-induced in adults. Among severe reactions, attribution to drugs varies from 10–20% for anaphylaxis and vasculitis to 70–90% for AGEP, DRESS, SJS, or TEN. Skin biopsy helps in characterizing the reaction but does not indicate drug causality. Blood counts and liver and renal function tests are important for evaluating organ involvement. The association of mild elevation of liver enzymes and high eosinophil count is frequent but not specific for a drug reaction. Blood tests that could identify an alternative cause, antinuclear antibody tests, and serology or polymerase chain reaction for infections may be of great importance for final assessment of etiology.

WHICH DRUG(S) TO SUSPECT AND WITHDRAW

Most cases of drug eruptions occur during the first course of treatment with a new medication, after a delay that varies with the type of reaction. A notable exception is IgE-mediated urticaria and anaphylaxis that need presensitization and develop a few minutes to a few hours after rechallenge. Characteristic time lags between onset of treatment and reaction are 4–14 days for maculopapular eruptions, 7–21 days for SJS/TEN, and 14–48 days for DRESS. Medications introduced for the first time in the relevant time frame are prime suspects. Two other important elements to suspect causality at this stage are (1) previous experience with the drug in the population and (2) alternative etiologic candidates.

TABLE 56-3 CLINICAL FEATURES OF SELECTED SEVERE CUTANEOUS REACTIONS OFTEN INDUCED BY DRUGS

Diagnosis	Mucosal Lesions	Typical Skin Lesions	Frequent Signs and Symptoms	Alternative Causes Not Related to Drugs
Stevens-Johnson syndrome	Erosions usually at ≥two sites	Small blisters on dusky purpuric macules or atypical targets; rare areas of confluence; detachment ≤10% of body surface area	Most cases involve fever	10–20% cause not determined
Toxic epidermal necrolysis[a]	Erosions usually at ≥two sites	Individual lesions like those seen in Stevens-Johnson syndrome; confluent erythema; outer layer of epidermis separates readily from basal layer with lateral pressure; large sheet of necrotic epidermis; total detachment of >30% of body surface area	Nearly all cases involve fever, "acute skin failure," leukopenia	10–20% cause not determined
Hypersensitivity syndrome	Infrequent	Severe exanthematous rash (may become purpuric), exfoliative dermatitis	30–50% of cases involve fever, lymphadenopathy, hepatitis, nephritis, carditis, eosinophilia, atypical lymphocytes	Cutaneous lymphoma
Acute generalized exanthematous pustulosis	About 20% erosions mouth, tongue	Initially nonfollicular small pustules overlying edematous erythema, sometimes leading to superficial ulcers	Fever, burning, pruritus, facial swelling, leukocytosis, hypocalcemia	Infection
Serum sickness or reactions resembling serum sickness	Absent	Morbilliform lesions, sometimes with urticaria	Fever, arthralgias	Infection
Anticoagulant-induced necrosis	Infrequent	Erythema then purpura and necrosis, especially of fatty areas	Pain in affected areas	Disseminated intravascular coagulopathy, septicemia
Angioedema	Often involved	Urticaria or swelling of central part of face	Respiratory distress, cardiovascular collapse	Insect stings, foods

[a]Overlap of Stevens-Johnson syndrome and toxic epidermal necrolysis with features of both and attachment of 10 to 30% of body surface area may occur.

Source: Adapted from Roujeau and Stern.

The decision to continue or discontinue any medication will depend on the severity of the reaction, the severity of the primary disease, degree of suspicion of causality, and feasibility of an alternative safer treatment. In many instances when a decision of "treating through" an eruption has been made, the rash disappears in a few days. This was seen in patients with AIDS treated for opportunistic infections with antibacterial sulfonamides. The decision to treat through an eruption should, however, remain the exception and withdrawal of every suspect drug the general rule. On the other hand, drugs that are not suspected and are important for the patient, e.g., antidiabetic or antihypertensive agents, generally should not be withdrawn. This approach prevents reluctance to future utilization of these agents.

RECOMMENDATION FOR FUTURE USE OF DRUGS

The aims are (1) to prevent the recurrence of the drug eruption and (2) not to compromise future treatments by contraindicating otherwise useful medications.

Begin with thorough assessment of drug causality. Drug causality is evaluated based on timing of the reaction, evaluation of other possible causes, effect of drug withdrawal or continuation, and knowledge of medications that have been associated with the observed reaction. Combination of these criteria leads to considering the causality as definite, probable, possible, or unlikely.

A drug with "unlikely" causality or that has been continued when the reaction improved or reintroduced without a reaction can be administered safely.

A drug with a "definite" or "probable" causality should be contraindicated, and a warning card given to the patient.

A drug with a "possible" causality may be submitted to further investigations depending on the expected need for future treatment.

The usefulness of drug tests is still debated. Many in vitro tests have been developed. They include lymphocyte proliferation assays, measuring the production of cytokines by patient lymphocytes in presence of medication, lymphocyte toxicity tests, and basophil degranulation assays. The predictive value of these tests has not been validated in any large series of affected patients, and these tests are research and not clinical tools.

In patients with history suggesting immediate IgE-mediated reactions to penicillin, skin testing with major and minor determinants of penicillins or cephalosporins has proved useful for identifying patients at risk of anaphylactic reactions to these agents. However, skin tests themselves carry a small risk of anaphylaxis. Negative skin tests do not totally rule out IgE-mediated reactivity, but the risk of anaphylaxis in response to penicillin administration in patients with negative skin tests is about 1% while about two-thirds of patients with a positive skin test experience an allergic response on rechallenge.

For patients with late drug reactions, the clinical usefulness of skin tests is more questionable. At least one of a combination of several tests (prick, patch, and intradermal) is positive in 50–70% of patients with a reaction "definitely" attributed to a single medication. This low sensitivity probably contributes to the fact that readministration of drugs that had been tested negative resulted in up to 17% eruptions.

CROSS-SENSITIVITY

Because of the possibility of cross-sensitivity among chemically related drugs, many physicians recommend avoidance of not only the medication that induced the reaction but also all drugs of the same group.

There are two types of cross-sensitivity. Reactions that depend on a pharmacologic interaction may recur with all drugs that target the same pathway, whether structurally similar or not. This is the case with angioedema caused by NSAIDs and ACE inhibitors. In this situation, the risk of recurrence varies from drug to drug in a particular class; however, avoidance of all drugs in the class is usually recommended. The other cross-sensitivity manifests in the risk that structurally related drugs are cross-recognized by the immune system. This is a real problem with aromatic antiepileptics (barbiturates, phenytoin, carbamazepine), with up to 50% reaction to a second drug in patients who reacted to one. For other drugs, in vitro as well as in vivo data have suggested that cross-reactivity existed only between compounds with very similar chemical structures. Sulfamethoxazole-specific lymphocytes may occasionally recognize a few other antibacterial sulfonamides but not diuretics, antidiabetic drugs, or anti-COX2 NSAIDs with a sulfonamide group.

Recent data suggest that although the risk of a drug eruption to another drug was increased in persons with a prior reaction, "cross-sensitivity" was probably not the explanation. As an example, persons with a history of an allergic-like reaction to penicillin were at higher risk to develop a reaction to antibacterial sulfonamides than to cephalosporin.

These data suggest that the list of drugs to avoid after a drug reaction should be limited to the causative one(s) and to a few very similar medications.

Because of growing evidence that some severe cutaneous reactions to drugs are associated with HLA genes, it is probably wise to recommend that first-degree family members of patients with severe cutaneous reactions also should avoid these causative medications.

Desensitization can be considered in those with history of reaction to a medication that must be used again. Efficacy of such procedures has been demonstrated in cases of immediate reaction to penicillin and positive skin tests, anaphylactic reactions to platinum chemotherapy, and delayed reactions to sulfonamides in patients with AIDS. Various protocols are available, including oral and parenteral approaches. Oral desensitization appears to have a lower risk of serious anaphylactic reactions. However, desensitization carries the risk of anaphylaxis regardless of how it is performed. After desensitization, many patients experience non-life-threatening reactions during therapy with the culprit drug.

REPORTING

Any severe reaction to drugs should be notified to a regulatory agency or to pharmaceutical companies. Because severe reactions are too rare to be detected in premarketing clinical trials, spontaneous reports are of critical importance for early detection of unexpected life-threatening events. To be useful, the report should contain enough details to permit ascertainment of severity and drug causality. This permits recognition of similar cases that may be reported from several different sources.

FURTHER READINGS

AUQUIER-DUNANT A et al: Severe cutaneous adverse reactions. Correlations between clinical patterns and causes of erythema multiforme majus, Stevens-Johnson syndrome, and toxic epidermal necrolysis: Results of an international prospective study. Arch Dermatol 138:1019, 2002

BAHRAMI S et al: Tissue eosinophilia as an indicator of drug-induced cutaneous small-vessel vasculitis. Arch Dermatol 142:155, 2006

BIGBY M: Rates of cutaneous reactions to drugs. Arch Dermatol 137:765, 2001

BREATHNACH SM: Adverse cutaneous reactions to drugs. Clin Med 2:15, 2002

ELIASZEWICZ M et al: Prospective evaluation of risk factors of cutaneous drug reactions to sulfonamides in patients with AIDS. J Am Acad Dermatol 47:40, 2002

HUNG SI et al: HLAB*5801 allele as a genetic marker for severe cutaneous reactions caused by allopurinol. Proc Natl Acad Sci USA 102:4134, 2005

LEE CW et al: Rapid inpatient/outpatient desensitization for chemotherapy hypersensitivity: Standard protocol effective in 57 patients for 255 courses. Gynecol Oncol 99:393, 2005

MESSAAD D et al: Drug provocation tests in patients with a history suggesting an immediate drug hypersensitivity reaction. Ann Intern Med 140:130, 2004

PICHLER WJ: Delayed drug hypersensitivity reactions. Ann Intern Med 139:683, 2003

ROUJEAU JC: Immune mechanisms in drug allergy. Allergology Internat J 55:27, 2006

ROUJEAU JC, STERN RS: Severe adverse cutaneous reactions to drugs. N Engl J Med 331:1272, 1994

WYATT AJ et al: Cutaneous reactions to chemotherapy and their management. Am J Clin Dermatol 7:45, 2006

57 Photosensitivity and Other Reactions to Light

David R. Bickers

SOLAR RADIATION

Sunlight is the most visible and obvious source of comfort in the environment. The sun provides the beneficial effects of warmth and vitamin D synthesis; however, acute and chronic sun exposure also have pathologic consequences. Few effects of sun exposure beyond those affecting the skin have been identified, but cutaneous exposure to sunlight is the major cause of human skin cancer and can exert immunosuppressive effects as well.

The sun's energy reaching the earth's surface is limited to components of the ultraviolet (UV), the visible, and portions of the infrared spectra. The cutoff at the short end of the UV is at ~290 nm; this is due primarily to stratospheric ozone formed by highly energetic ionizing radiation, thereby preventing penetration to the earth's surface of the shorter, more energetic, potentially more harmful wavelengths of solar radiation. Indeed, concern about destruction of the ozone layer by chlorofluorocarbons released into the atmosphere has led to international agreements to reduce production of these chemicals.

Measurements of solar flux indicate that there is a twentyfold regional variation in the amount of energy at 300 nm that reaches the earth's surface. This variability relates to seasonal effects; the path of sunlight transmission through ozone and air; the altitude (4% increase for each 300 m of elevation); the latitude (increasing intensity with decreasing latitude); and the amount of cloud cover, fog, and pollution.

The major components of the photobiologic action spectrum capable of affecting human skin include the UV and visible wavelengths between 290 and 700 nm. In addition, the wavelengths beyond 700 nm in the infrared spectrum primarily emit heat and under certain circumstances may exacerbate the pathologic effects of energy in the UV and visible spectra.

The UV spectrum reaching the earth represents <10% of total incident solar energy and is arbitrarily divided into two major segments, UV-B and UV-A, comprising the wavelengths from 290–400 nm. UV-B consists of wavelengths between 290 and 320 nm. This portion of the photobiologic action spectrum is the most efficient in producing redness or erythema in human skin and hence is sometimes known as the "sunburn spectrum." UV-A represents those wavelengths between 320 and 400 nm and is ~1000-fold less efficient in producing skin redness than is UV-B.

The wavelengths between 400 and 700 nm are visible to the human eye. The photon energy in the visible spectrum is not capable of damaging human skin in the absence of a photosensitizing chemical. Without the absorption of energy by a molecule there can be no photosensitivity. Thus the *absorption spectrum* of a molecule is defined as the range of wavelengths absorbed by it, whereas the *action spectrum* for an effect of incident radiation is defined as the range of wavelengths that evoke the response.

Photosensitivity occurs when a photon-absorbing chemical (chromophore) present in the skin absorbs incident energy, becomes excited, and transfers the absorbed energy to various structures or to oxygen.

UV RADIATION (UVR) AND SKIN STRUCTURE AND FUNCTION

Skin consists of two major compartments: the outer epidermis, a stratified squamous epithelium, and the underlying dermis rich in matrix proteins such as collagen and elastin. Both of these compartments are susceptible to damage from sun exposure. The epidermis and the dermis contain several chromophores capable of absorbing incident solar energy including nucleic acids, proteins, and lipids. The outermost epidermal layer, the stratum corneum, is a major absorber of UV-B, and <10% of incident UV-B wavelengths penetrate through the epidermis to the dermis. Approximately 3% of radiation below 300 nm, 20% of radiation below 360 nm, and 33% of short visible radiation reaches the basal cell layer in untanned human skin. In contrast, UV-A readily penetrates to the dermis and is capable of altering structural and matrix proteins that contribute to photoaging of chronically sun-exposed skin, particularly in individuals of light complexion.

Molecular Targets for UVR-Induced Skin Effects Epidermal DNA, predominantly in keratinocytes and in Langerhans cells (LCs), which are dendritic antigen-presenting cells, absorbs UV-B and undergoes structural changes including the formation of cyclobutane dimers and 6,4-photoproducts. These structural changes are potentially mutagenic and can be repaired by mechanisms that result in their recognition and excision and the reestablishment of normal base sequences. The efficient repair of these structural aberrations is crucial, since individuals with defective DNA repair are at high risk for the development of cutaneous cancer. For example, patients with xeroderma pigmentosum (XP), an autosomal recessive disorder, are characterized by variably deficient repair of UV-induced photoproducts, and their skin phenotype often manifests the dry, leathery appearance of prematurely photoaged skin as well as basal cell and squamous cell carcinomas and melanoma in the first two decades of life. Studies in mice using knockout gene technology have verified the importance of functional genes regulating these repair pathways in preventing the development of UV-induced cancer. Furthermore, incorporation of a bacterial DNA repair enzyme, T4N5 endonuclease, into liposomes in a product applied to skin of patients with XP selectively removes cyclobutane pyrimidine dimers and reduces the degree of solar damage and skin cancer. DNA damage in LCs may contribute to the known immunosuppressive effects of UV-B (see "Immunologic Effects," below).

Cutaneous Optics and Chromophores Chromophores are endogenous or exogenous chemical components that can absorb physical energy. Endogenous chromophores are of two types: (1) chemicals that are normal components of skin, including nucleic acids, proteins, lipids, and 7-dehydrocholesterol, the precursor of vitamin D; and (2) chemicals, such as porphyrins, synthesized elsewhere in the body that circulate in the bloodstream and diffuse into the skin. Normally, only trace amounts of porphyrins are present in the skin, but in selected diseases known as the porphyrias (Chap. 352), increased amounts are released into the circulation from the bone marrow and the liver and are transported to the skin, where they absorb incident energy both in the Soret band, around 400 nm (short visible), and to a lesser extent in the red portion of the visible spectrum (580–660 nm). This results in the generation of reactive oxygen species that can mediate structural damage to the skin, manifest as erythema, edema, urticaria, or blister formation.

Acute Effects of Sun Exposure The acute effects of skin exposure to sunlight include sunburn and vitamin D synthesis. Molecular targets for UVR in addition to DNA include molecular oxygen leading to the generation of reactive oxygen species (ROS), cell membranes, and urocanic acid.

SUNBURN This painful skin condition is caused predominantly by UV-B. Generally speaking, an individual's ability to tolerate sunlight is inversely proportional to the degree of melanin pigmentation. Melanin, a complex tyrosine polymer, is synthesized in specialized epidermal dendritic cells known as melanocytes and is packaged into *melanosomes* that are transferred via dendritic process into *keratinocytes*, thereby providing photoprotection and simultaneously darkening the skin. Sun-induced melanogenesis is a consequence of increased tyrosinase activity in melanocytes that in turn is a consequence of a human gene, the melanocortin1 receptor (*MC1R*), that accounts for the wide variation in human skin and hair color. Human *MC1R* encodes a 317-amino-acid G-coupled receptor (melanocortin receptor) that binds α-melanocyte-stimulating hormone. This leads to increased intracellular cyclic AMP and protein kinase A, followed by increased transcription of microphthalmia transcription factor

TABLE 57-1 SKIN TYPE AND SUNBURN SENSITIVITY (FITZPATRICK CLASSIFICATION)

Type	Description
I	Always burn, never tan
II	Always burn, sometimes tan
III	Sometimes burn, sometimes tan
IV	Sometimes burn, always tan
V	Never burn, sometimes tan
VI	Never burn, always tan

(MITF) that regulates melanogenesis. *MC1R* mutations account for population differences in skin color, ability to tan, and cancer susceptibility. The Fitzpatrick classification of human skin is a function of the efficiency of the epidermal-melanin unit and can usually be ascertained by asking an individual two questions: (1) Do you burn after sun exposure? and (2) Do you tan after sun exposure? The answers to these questions permit division of the population into six skin types varying from type I (always burn, never tan) to type VI (never burn, always tan) (Table 57-1).

Sunburn is due to vasodilatation of dermal blood vessels. There is a lag in time between skin exposure to sunlight and the development of visible redness (usually 4–12 h), suggesting that an epidermal chromophore causes delayed production and/or release of vasoactive mediator(s), or cytokines, that diffuse to the dermal vasculature to evoke vasodilatation.

The action spectrum for sunburn erythema includes the UV-B and UV-A. Photons in the UV-B are at least 1000-fold more efficient than photons in the UV-A in evoking the response. However, UV-A may contribute to sunburn erythema at midday when much more UV-A than UV-B is present in the solar spectrum. UV-induced activation of nuclear factor-κB (NF-κB)-dependent gene transactivation can augment release of several proinflammatory cytokines including interleukin (IL) 1B, 1L-6, IL-8, vascular endothelial growth factor, prostaglandin E_2, and tumor necrosis factor α. Local accumulation of these cytokines occurs in sunburned skin, providing chemotactic factors that attract neutrophils and macrophages. It is of interest that nonsteroidal anti-inflammatory drugs (NSAIDs) can reduce sunburn erythema, perhaps by blocking I-κB kinase 2, the enzyme essential for nuclear translocation of cytosolic NF-κB.

VITAMIN D PHOTOCHEMISTRY Cutaneous exposure to UV-B causes photolysis of epidermal 7-dehydrocholesterol converting it to pre-vitamin D_3, which then undergoes a temperature-dependent isomerization to form the stable hormone vitamin D_3. This compound then diffuses to the dermal vasculature and circulates systemically where it is converted to the functional hormone 1,25-dihydroxyvitamin $D_3[1,25(OH)_2D_3]$. Vitamin D metabolites from the circulation or those produced in the skin itself can augment epidermal differentiation signaling. Controversy exists regarding the importance of sun exposure in vitamin D homeostasis. At present, it is important to emphasize that the use of sunscreens does not substantially diminish vitamin D levels. Since aging also substantially decreases the ability of human skin to photocatalytically produce vitamin D_3, the widespread use of sunscreens that filter out UV-B has led to concern that vitamin D deficiency may become a significant clinical problem in the elderly.

Chronic Effects of Sun Exposure: Nonmalignant The clinical features of photodamaged sun-exposed skin consist of wrinkling, blotchiness, and telangiectasia and a roughened, irregular, "weather-beaten" leathery appearance. Whether this photoaging represents accelerated chronologic aging or a separate and distinct process is not clear.

Within chronically sun-exposed epidermis, there is thickening (acanthosis) and morphologic heterogeneity within the basal cell layer. Higher but irregular melanosome content may be present in some keratinocytes, indicating prolonged residence of the cells in the basal cell layer. These structural changes may help to explain the leathery texture and the blotchy discoloration of sun-damaged skin.

UV-A is important in the pathogenesis of photoaging in human skin, and ROS are likely involved. The dermis and its connective tissue matrix are the major site for sun-associated chronic damage, manifest as solar elastosis, a massive increase in thickened irregular masses of abnormal elastic fibers. Collagen fibers are also abnormally clumped in the deeper dermis of sun-damaged skin. The chromophore(s), the action spectra, and the specific biochemical events orchestrating these changes are only partially understood, although UV-A seems to be primarily involved. Chronologically aged, sun-protected skin and photoaged skin share important molecular features including connective tissue damage and elevated matrix metalloproteinases (MMPs). MMPs are enzymes involved in the degradation of the extracellular matrix, and UV-A induces MMP-1 and MMP-3 mRNA expression, leading to enhanced collagen breakdown. In addition, UV-A reduces type I procollagen mRNA expression.

Chronic Effects of Sun Exposure: Malignant One of the major known consequences of chronic skin exposure to sunlight is nonmelanoma skin cancer. The two types of nonmelanoma skin cancer are *basal cell carcinoma* (BCC) and *squamous cell carcinoma* (SCC; Chap. 83). There are three major steps for cancer induction: initiation, promotion, and progression. Exposure of human skin to sunlight results in *initiation*, a step whereby structural (mutagenic) changes in DNA evoke an irreversible alteration in the target cell (*keratinocyte*) that begins the tumorigenic process. Exposure to a tumor initiator such as UV-B is believed to be a necessary but not sufficient step in the malignant process, since initiated skin cells not exposed to tumor promoters do not generally develop tumors. The second stage in tumor development is *promotion*, a multistep process whereby chronic exposure to sunlight evokes epigenetic changes that culminate in the clonal expansion of initiated cells and cause the development, over many years, of premalignant growths known as *actinic keratoses*, a minority of which may progress to form skin cancer. Based on extensive studies it seems clear that UV-B is a *complete carcinogen*, meaning that it can act as both a tumor initiator and a promoter.

The third and final step in the malignant process is *malignant conversion* of benign precursors into malignant lesions, a process thought to require additional genetic alterations in already transformed cells. Skin carcinogenesis is thought to be caused by the accumulation of mutations in the tumor-suppressor gene *p53* as a result of UV-induced DNA damage. Indeed both human and murine UV-induced skin cancers have unique *p53* mutations (C → T and CC → TT transitions) that are present in the majority of these lesions. Studies have shown that sunscreens can substantially reduce the frequency of these signature mutations in *p53* and can dramatically inhibit the induction of tumors. The *p53* mutations are present in sun-exposed normal human skin, in actinic keratoses, and in nonmelanoma skin cancers including BCC and SCC.

BCCs also manifest mutations in the tumor-suppressor gene known as *patched*, which results in activation of hedgehog signaling, and enhanced activity of *smoothened*, which in turn causes downstream activation of transcription factors that augment cell proliferation. Thus, these tumors can manifest mutations in both p53 and in *patched*.

Sun exposure causes nonmelanoma cancers and melanoma of the skin, although the evidence is far more direct for its role in nonmelanoma (BCC and SCC) than in melanoma. Approximately 80% of nonmelanoma skin cancers develop on exposed body areas, including the face, the neck, and the hands. Major risk factors include male sex, childhood sun exposures, older age, fair skin, and residence at latitudes closer to the equator. Whites of darker complexions (e.g., Hispanics) have one-tenth the risk of developing such cancers compared to fair-skinned individuals. Blacks are at substantially reduced risk for all forms of skin cancer. More than 1.3 million individuals in the United States develop nonmelanoma skin cancer annually, and the lifetime risk for a fair-skinned individual to develop such a neoplasm is estimated at ~15%. A consensus exists that the incidence of nonmelanoma skin cancer in the population is increasing at the rate of 2–3% per year, for unknown reasons. One potential explanation is the widespread use of indoor tanning. It is estimated that 30 million people tan indoors in the United States annually, including >2 million adolescents.

The relationship of sun exposure to melanoma development is less clear-cut, but suggestive evidence supports an association. The strongest risk factors for melanoma include positive family history for melanoma, multiple dysplastic nevi, and prior melanoma. Melanomas occasionally develop by the teenage years, indicating that the latent period for tumor growth is less than that of nonmelanoma skin cancer. Melanomas are among the most rapidly increasing of all human malignancies (Chap. 83). Epidemiologic studies of immigrant populations of similar ethnic stock indicate that individuals born in one area or who migrate to the same locale before age 10 have higher age-specific melanoma rates than individuals arriving later. It is thus reasonable to conclude that life in a sunny climate from birth or early childhood increases the risk of melanoma. In general, risk does not correlate with cumulative sun exposure but may relate to the duration and extent of exposure in childhood. Epidemiologic studies have shown that indoor tanning is a risk factor for melanoma.

Meta-analysis of 17 case-control studies in patients with melanoma concluded that the protective effect of sunscreens against this type of tumor could not be substantiated, but this is likely due to failure to control for confounding factors such as sunscreen stability and frequency of application. Since no prospective studies are available to address this issue, it seems reasonable to recommend that patients at risk for melanoma utilize photoprotection such as sun avoidance, high sun protective factor (SPF) sunscreens, and protective clothing.

Immunologic Effects Exposure to solar radiation causes local (inhibition of immune responses to antigens applied at the irradiated site) and systemic (inhibition of immune responses to antigens applied at remote unirradiated sites) immunosuppression. The action spectrum for UV-induced immunosuppression closely mimics the absorption spectrum of DNA. Pyrimidine dimers in LCs may inhibit antigen presentation. The absorption spectrum of epidermal urocanic acid closely mimics the action spectrum for UV-B-induced immunosuppression. *Trans-cis* isomerization of urocanic acid in the stratum corneum leads to its systemic absorption and consequent immunosuppressive effects. Furthermore administration of modest doses of UV-B to human skin reduces the degree of allergic sensitization to the potent contact allergen, dinitrochlorobenzene. This is associated with ROS-induced depletion of epidermal LCs.

Higher doses of UV-radiation evoke diminished immunologic responses to antigens introduced either epicutaneously or intracutaneously at sites distant from the irradiated site. These suppressed responses are also associated with the induction of antigen-specific suppressor T lymphocytes and may be mediated by as yet undefined factors that are released from epidermal cells at the irradiated site. One important consequence of chronic sun exposure and the concomitant immunosuppression is enhanced risk of skin cancer. Perhaps the most graphic demonstration of the role of immunosuppression in enhancing the risk of nonmelanoma skin cancer has come from studies of patients receiving organ transplantation who are on chronic immunosuppressive antirejection drug regimens. More than 50% of transplant patients develop BCCs and SCCs, and these cancers are the most common malignancy arising in immunosuppressed solid-organ transplant recipients. Human papilloma viruses (HPVs) may also play a role in the increased risk of SCCs in these patients since tumors display an HPV DNA carriage rate of almost 80%. These patients require close periodic monitoring and rigorous photoprotection using sunscreens, protective clothing, and sun avoidance.

PHOTOSENSITIVITY DISEASES

The diagnosis of photosensitivity requires a careful history to define the duration of the signs and symptoms, the length of time between exposure to sunlight and the development of subjective complaints, and visible changes in the skin. The age of onset can also be a helpful clue; for example, the acute photosensitivity of erythropoietic protoporphyria almost always begins in childhood, whereas the chronic photosensitivity of porphyria cutanea tarda (PCT) typically begins in the fourth and fifth decades. A history of exposure to topical and systemic drugs and chemicals may provide important clues. Many classes of drugs can cause photosensitivity on the basis of either phototoxicity or photoallergy. Fragrances such as musk ambrette that were previously present in numerous cosmetic products are also potent photosensitizers.

TABLE 57-2 CLASSIFICATION OF PHOTOSENSITIVITY DISEASES

Type	Disease
Genetic	Erythropoietic porphyria
	Erythropoietic protoporphyria
	Porphyria cutanea tarda—familial
	Variegate porphyria
	Hepatoerythropoietic porphyria
	Albinism
	Xeroderma pigmentosum
	Rothmund-Thompson disease
	Bloom syndrome
	Cockayne's disease
	Kindler syndrome
	Phenylketonuria
Metabolic	Porphyria cutanea tarda—sporadic
	Hartnup disease
	Kwashiorkor
	Pellagra
	Carcinoid syndrome
Phototoxic	
Internal	Drugs
External	Drugs, plants, food
Photoallergic	
Immediate	Solar urticaria
Delayed	Drug photoallergy
	Persistent light reaction/chronic actinic dermatitis
Neoplastic and degenerative	Photoaging
	Actinic keratosis
	Melanoma and nonmelanoma skin cancer
Idiopathic	Polymorphous light eruption
	Hydroa aestivale
	Actinic prurigo
Photoaggravated	Lupus erythematosus
	Systemic
	Subacute cutaneous
	Discoid
	Dermatomyositis
	Herpes simplex
	Lichen planus actinicus
	Acne vulgaris (aestivale)

Examination of the skin may also offer important clues. Anatomic areas that are naturally protected from direct sunlight such as the hairy scalp, the upper eyelids, the retroauricular areas, and the infranasal and submental regions may be spared, whereas exposed areas show characteristic features of the pathologic process. These anatomic localization patterns are often helpful, but not infallible, in making the diagnosis. For example, airborne contact sensitizers that are blown onto the skin may produce dermatitis that can be difficult to distinguish from photosensitivity, despite the fact that such material may trigger skin reactivity in areas shielded from direct sunlight.

Many dermatologic conditions may be caused or aggravated by sunlight (Table 57-2). The role of light in evoking these responses may be dependent on genetic abnormalities ranging from well-described defects in DNA repair that occur in XP to the inherited abnormalities in heme synthesis that characterize the porphyrias. In certain photosensitivity diseases, the chromophore has been identified, whereas in the majority, the energy-absorbing agent is unknown.

Polymorphous Light Eruption After sunburn, the most common type of photosensitivity disease is *polymorphous light eruption* (PLE), the mechanism of which is unknown. Many affected individuals never seek medical attention because the condition is often transient, becoming manifest each spring with initial sun exposure but then subsiding spontaneously with continuing exposure, a phenomenon known as "hardening." The major manifestations of PLE include pruritic (often intensely so) erythematous papules that may coalesce into plaques in a patchy distribution on exposed areas of the trunk and forearms. The face is usually less seriously involved.

The diagnosis can be confirmed by skin biopsy and by performing phototest procedures in which skin is exposed to multiple erythema doses of UV-A and UV-B. The action spectrum for PLE is usually within these portions of the solar spectrum.

Treatment of this PLE includes the use of sunscreens and the induction of hardening by the cautious administration of artificial UV-B (broad-band or narrow-band) and/or UV-A radiation for 2–3 weeks prior to initial sun exposure.

Phototoxicity and Photoallergy These photosensitivity disorders are related to the topical or systemic administration of drugs and other chemicals. Both reactions require the absorption of energy by a drug or chemical resulting in the production of an excited-state photosensitizer that can transfer its absorbed energy to a bystander molecule or to molecular oxygen, thereby generating tissue-destructive chemical species, including ROS.

Phototoxicity is a nonimmunologic reaction caused by drugs and chemicals, a few of which are listed in Table 57-3. The usual clinical manifestations include erythema resembling a sunburn reaction that quickly desquamates, or "peels," within several days. In addition, edema, vesicles, and bullae may occur.

Photoallergy is much less common and is distinct in that this is an immunopathologic process. The excited-state photosensitizer may create highly unstable haptenic free radicals that bind covalently to macromolecules to form a functional antigen capable of evoking a delayed hypersensitivity response. Some of the drugs and chemicals that produce photoallergy are listed in Table 57-4. The clinical manifestations typically differ from those of phototoxicity in that an intensely pruritic eczematous dermatitis tends to predominate and evolves into lichenified, thickened, "leathery" changes in sun-exposed areas. A small subset (perhaps 5–10%) of patients with photoallergy may develop a persistent exquisite hypersensitivity to light even when the offending drug or chemical is identified and eliminated, a condition known as *persistent light reaction*.

A very uncommon type of persistent photosensitivity is known as *chronic actinic dermatitis*. These patients are typically elderly men with a long history of preexisting allergic contact dermatitis or photosensitivity. They are usually exquisitely sensitive to UV-B, UV-A, and visible wavelengths.

Diagnostic confirmation of phototoxicity and photoallergy can often be obtained using phototest procedures. In patients with suspected phototoxicity, determining the minimal erythema dose (MED) while the patient is exposed to a suspected agent and then repeating the MED after discontinuation of the agent may provide a clue to the causative drug or chemical. Photopatch testing can be performed to confirm the diagnosis of photoallergy. This is a simple variant of ordinary patch testing in which a series of known photoallergens is applied to the skin in duplicate and one set is irradiated with a suberythema dose of UV-A. Development of eczematous changes at sites exposed to sensitizer and light is a positive result. The characteristic abnormality in patients with persistent light reaction is a diminished threshold to erythema evoked by UV-B. Patients with chronic actinic dermatitis usually manifest a broad spectrum of UV hyperresponsiveness and require meticulous photoprotection including avoiding sun exposure, high (>30) SPF sunscreens, and in severe cases systemic immunosuppression, preferably with azathioprine (1–2 mg/kg per day).

TABLE 57-3 PHOTOTOXIC DRUGS

	Topical	Systemic
Amiodarone		+
Dacarbazine		+
Fluoroquinolones		+
5-Fluorouracil	+	+
Furosemide		+
Nalidixic acid		+
Phenothiazines		+
Psoralens	+	+
Retinoids	+/–	+
Sulfonamides		+
Sulfonylureas		+
Tetracyclines		+
Thiazides		+
Vinblastine		+

TABLE 57-4 PHOTOALLERGIC DRUGS

	Topical	Systemic
6-Methylcoumarin	+	
Aminobenzoic acid and esters	+	
Bithionol	+	
Chlorpromazine		+
Diclofenac		+
Fluoroquinolones		+
Halogenated salicylanilides	+	
Hypericin (St John's Wort)	+	+
Musk ambrette	+	
Piroxicam		+
Promethazine		+
Sulfonamides		+
Sulfonylureas		+

The management of drug photosensitivity involves first and foremost the elimination of exposure to the chemical agents responsible for the reaction and minimization of sun exposure. The acute symptoms of phototoxicity may be ameliorated by cool, moist compresses, topical glucocorticoids, and systemically administered NSAIDs. In severely affected individuals, a rapidly tapered course of systemic glucocorticoids may be useful. Judicious use of analgesics may be necessary.

Photoallergic reactions require a similar management approach. Furthermore, patients with persistent light reaction and chronic actinic dermatitis must be meticulously protected against light exposure. In selected patients in whom chronic systemic high-dose glucocorticoids pose unacceptable risks, it may be necessary to employ immunosuppressive drugs such as azathioprine, cyclophosphamide, cyclosporine, or mycophenolate mofetil.

Porphyria The porphyrias (Chap. 352) are a group of diseases that have in common inherited or acquired derangements in the synthesis of heme. Heme is an iron-chelated tetrapyrrole or porphyrin, and the nonmetal chelated porphyrins are potent photosensitizers that absorb light intensely in both the short (400–410 nm) and the long (580–650 nm) portions of the visible spectrum.

Heme cannot be reutilized and must be continuously synthesized, and the two body compartments with the largest capacity for its production are the bone marrow and the liver. Accordingly, the porphyrias originate in one or the other of these organs, with the end result of excessive endogenous production of potent photosensitizing porphyrins. The porphyrins circulate in the bloodstream and diffuse into the skin, where they absorb solar energy, become photoexcited, generate ROS, and evoke cutaneous photosensitivity. The mechanism of porphyrin photosensitization is known to be photodynamic, or oxygen-dependent, and is mediated by ROS such as singlet oxygen and superoxide anions.

Porphyria cutanea tarda is the most common type of human porphyria and is associated with decreased activity of the enzyme uroporphyrinogen decarboxylase associated with a number of gene mutations. There are two basic types of PCT: (1) the sporadic or acquired type, generally seen in individuals ingesting ethanol or receiving estrogens; and (2) the inherited type, in which there is autosomal dominant transmission of deficient enzyme activity. Both forms are associated with increased hepatic iron stores.

In both types of PCT, the predominant feature is a chronic photosensitivity characterized by increased fragility of sun-exposed skin, particularly areas subject to repeated trauma such as the dorsa of the hands, the forearms, the face, and the ears. The predominant skin lesions are vesicles and bullae that rupture, producing moist erosions, often with a hemorrhagic base, that heal slowly with crusting and purplish discoloration of the affected skin. Hypertrichosis, mottled pigmentary change, and scleroderma-like induration are associated features. Biochemical confirmation of the diagnosis can be obtained by measurement of urinary porphyrin excretion, plasma porphyrin assay, and by assay of erythrocyte and/or hepatic uroporphyrinogen decarboxylase. Multiple mutations of the uroporphyrinogen decarboxylase gene have been identified in human populations, including exon skipping and base substitutions. Some patients with PCT have associated mutations in the *HFE* gene linked to hemochromatosis. This could contribute to the iron overload seen in PCT, although iron status as measured by serum ferritin, iron levels, and transferrin saturation is no different from that in PCT patients without *HFE* mutations. Prior hepatitis C virus infection appears to be an independent risk factor for PCT.

Treatment of PCT consists of repeated phlebotomies to diminish the excessive hepatic iron stores and/or intermittent low doses of the antimalarial drugs chloroquine and hydroxychloroquine. Long-term remission of the disease can be achieved if the patient eliminates exposure to porphyrinogenic agents.

Erythropoietic protoporphyria originates in the bone marrow and is due to a decrease in the mitochondrial enzyme ferrochelatase secondary to numerous gene mutations. The major clinical features include an acute photosensitivity characterized by subjective burning and stinging of exposed skin that often develops during or just after exposure. There may be associated skin swelling and, after repeated episodes, a waxlike scarring.

The diagnosis is confirmed by demonstration of elevated levels of free erythrocyte protoporphyrin. Detection of increased plasma protoporphyrin helps to differentiate lead poisoning and iron-deficiency anemia, in both of which elevated erythrocyte protoporphyrin levels occur in the absence of cutaneous photosensitivity and of elevated plasma protoporphyrin levels.

Treatment consists of reducing sun exposure and the oral administration of the carotenoid β-carotene, which is an effective scavenger of free radicals. This drug increases tolerance to sun exposure in many affected individuals, although it has no effect on deficient ferrochelatase.

An algorithm for managing patients with photosensitivity is illustrated in Fig. 57-1.

PHOTOPROTECTION

Since photosensitivity of the skin results from exposure to sunlight, it follows that absolute avoidance of the sun would eliminate these disorders. Unfortunately, contemporary life-styles make this an impractical alternative for most individuals, and this has led to a search for better approaches to photoprotection.

Natural photoprotection is provided by structural proteins in the epidermis, particularly keratins and melanin. The amount of melanin and its distribution in cells is genetically regulated, and individuals of darker complexion (skin types IV–VI) are at decreased risk for the development of acute sunburn and cutaneous malignancy.

Other forms of photoprotection include clothing and sunscreens. Clothing constructed of tightly woven sun-protective fabrics, irrespective of color, affords substantial protection. Wide-brimmed hats, long sleeves, and trousers all reduce direct exposure. Sunscreens are now considered to be over-the-counter drugs and category I ingredients are recognized by the U.S. Food and Drug Administration (FDA) as monographed and safe and effective. These are listed in Table 57-5. Sunscreens are rated for their photoprotective effect by their SPF. The SPF is simply a ratio of the time required to produce sunburn erythema with and without sunscreen application. The monograph stipulates that sunscreens must be rated on a scale ranging from minimal (SPF ≮2 and ≯12) to moderate (SPF ≮12 and ≯30) to high (SPF ≥30, labeled as 30+). No SPF number >30 can be placed on the label.

In addition to light absorption, a critical determinant of the sustained photoprotective effect of sunscreens is their water-resistance.

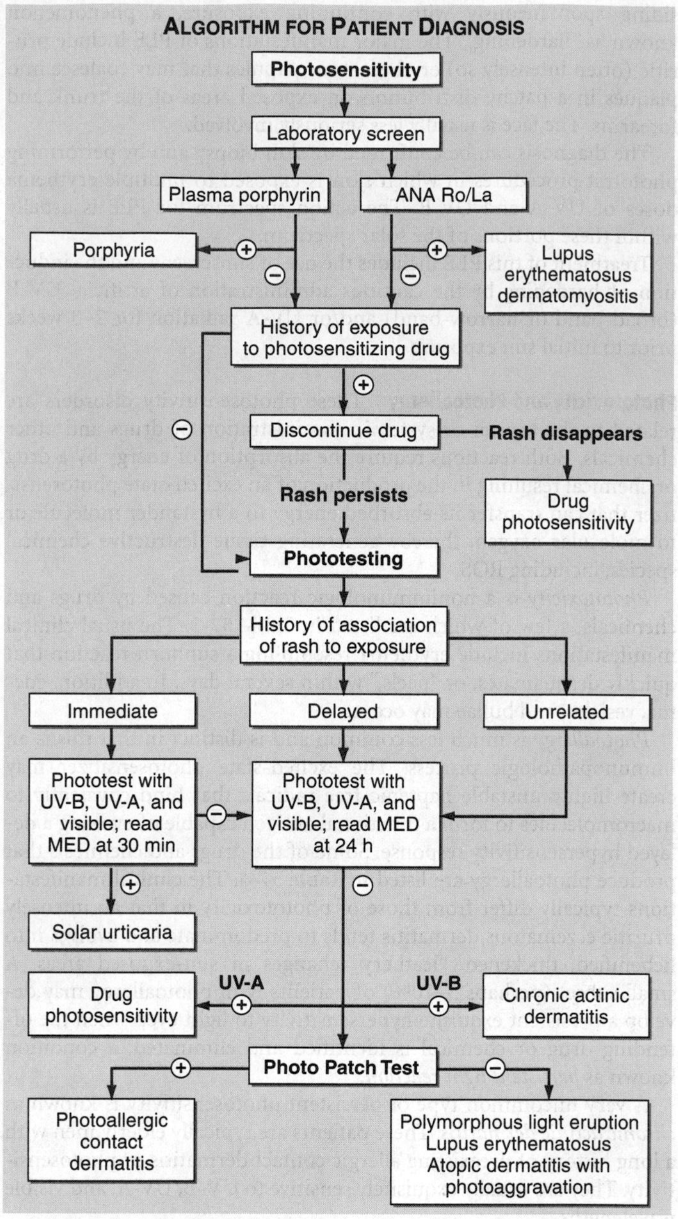

FIGURE 57-1 An algorithm for the diagnosis of a patient with photosensitivity.

TABLE 57-5 FDA CATEGORY 1 MONOGRAPHED SUNSCREEN INGREDIENTS[a]

Ingredients	Maximum Concentration, %
p-Aminobenzoic acid (PABA)	15
Avobenzone	3
Cinoxate	3
Dioxybenzone (benzophenone-8)	3
Ecamsule[b]	15
Homosalate	15
Menthyl anthranilate	5
Octocrylene	10
Octyl methoxycinnamate	7.5
Octyl salicylate	5
Oxybenzone (benzophenone-3)	6
Padimate O (octyl dimethyl PABA)	8
Phenylbenzimidazole sulfonic acid	4
Sulisobenzone (benzophenone-4)	10
Titanium dioxide	25
Trolamine salicylate	12
Zinc oxide	25

[a]FDA, U.S. Food and Drug Administration.
[b]Recently approved by the FDA.

The FDA monograph has also defined strict testing criteria for sunscreens making this claim.

Some degree of photoprotection can also be achieved by limiting the time of exposure during the day. Since the majority of an individual's total lifetime sun exposure may occur by the age of 18, it is important to educate parents and young children about the hazards of sunlight. Simply eliminating exposure at midday will substantially reduce lifetime UV-B exposure.

PHOTOTHERAPY AND PHOTOCHEMOTHERAPY

UV can also be used therapeutically. The administration of UV-B alone or in combination with topically applied agents can induce remissions of psoriasis and atopic dermatitis.

Photochemotherapy in which topically applied or systemically administered psoralens are combined with UV-A (PUVA) is also effective in treating psoriasis and in the early stages of cutaneous T cell lymphoma and vitiligo. Psoralens are tricyclic furocoumarins that, when intercalated into DNA and exposed to UV-A, form adducts with pyrimidine bases and eventually form DNA cross-links. These structural changes are thought to decrease DNA synthesis and relate to the improvement that occurs in psoriasis. The reason that PUVA photochemotherapy is effective in cutaneous T cell lymphoma is not clear.

In addition to its effects on DNA, PUVA photochemotherapy also stimulates epidermal thickening and melanin synthesis; the latter provides the rationale for its use in the depigmenting disease vitiligo. Oral 8-methoxypsoralen and UV-A appear to be most effective in this regard, but as many as 100 treatments extending over 12–18 months may be required to promote satisfactory repigmentation.

Not surprisingly the major side effects of long-term UV-B phototherapy and PUVA photochemotherapy mimic those seen in individuals with chronic sun exposure and include skin dryness, actinic keratoses, and an increased risk of skin cancer. Despite these risks, the therapeutic index of these modalities continues to be excellent.

FURTHER READINGS

LIM HW et al: Sunlight, tanning booths, and vitamin D. J Am Acad Dermatol 52:868, 2005

MILLER AJ, MIHM MC JR: Melanoma. N Engl J Med 355:51, 2006

MORISON WL: Photosensitivity. N Engl J Med 350:111, 2004

SCHADE N et al: Ultraviolet B radiation–induced immunosuppression: Molecular mechanisms and cellular alterations. Photochem Photobiol Sci 3:699, 2005

WONG TH, REES JL: The relation between melanocortin I receptor variation and generation of phenotypic diversity in the cutaneous response to ultraviolet radiation. Peptides 26:1965, 2005

SECTION 10 HEMATOLOGIC ALTERATIONS

58 Anemia and Polycythemia

John W. Adamson, Dan L. Longo

HEMATOPOIESIS AND THE PHYSIOLOGIC BASIS OF RED CELL PRODUCTION

Hematopoiesis is the process by which the formed elements of the blood are produced. The process is regulated through a series of steps beginning with the pluripotent hematopoietic stem cell. Stem cells are capable of producing red cells, all classes of granulocytes, monocytes, platelets, and the cells of the immune system. The precise molecular mechanism—either intrinsic to the stem cell itself, or through the action of extrinsic factors—by which the stem cell becomes committed to a given lineage is not fully defined. However, experiments in mice suggest that erythroid cells come from a common erythroid/megakaryocyte progenitor that does not develop in the absence of expression of the GATA-1 and FOG-1 (friend of GATA-1) transcription factors (Chap. 68). Following lineage commitment, hematopoietic progenitor and precursor cells come increasingly under the regulatory influence of growth factors and hormones. For red cell production, erythropoietin (EPO) is the regulatory hormone. EPO is required for the maintenance of committed erythroid progenitor cells that, in the absence of the hormone, undergo programmed cell death (*apoptosis*). The regulated process of red cell production is *erythropoiesis*, and its key elements are illustrated in Fig. 58-1.

In the bone marrow, the first morphologically recognizable erythroid precursor is the pronormoblast. This cell can undergo 4–5 cell divisions that result in the production of 16–32 mature red cells. With increased EPO production, or the administration of EPO as a drug, early progenitor cell numbers are amplified and, in turn, give rise to increased numbers of erythrocytes. The regulation of EPO production itself is linked to O_2 availability.

In mammals, O_2 is transported to tissues bound to the hemoglobin contained within circulating red cells. The mature red cell is 8 μm in diameter, anucleate, discoid in shape, and extremely pliable in order to traverse the microcirculation successfully; its membrane integrity is maintained by the intracellular generation of ATP. Normal red cell production results in the daily replacement of 0.8–1% of all circulating red cells in the body, since the average red cell lives 100–120 days. The organ responsible for red cell production is called the *erythron*. The erythron is a dynamic organ made up of a rapidly proliferating pool of marrow erythroid precursor cells and a large mass of mature circulating red blood cells. The size of the red cell mass reflects the balance of red cell production and destruction. The physiologic basis of red cell production and destruction provides an understanding of the mechanisms that can lead to anemia.

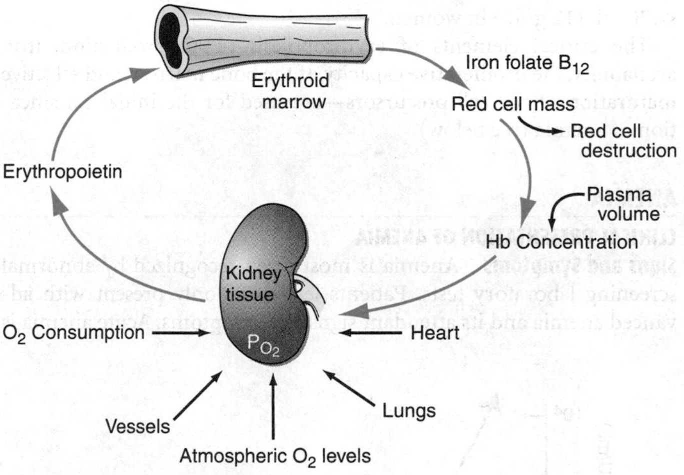

FIGURE 58-1 The physiologic regulation of red cell production by tissue oxygen tension. Hb, hemoglobin.

The physiologic regulator of red cell production, the glycoprotein hormone EPO, is produced and released by peritubular capillary lining cells within the kidney. These cells are highly specialized epithelial-like cells. A small amount of EPO is produced by hepatocytes. The fundamental stimulus for EPO production is the availability of O_2 for tissue metabolic needs. Impaired O_2 delivery to the kidney can result from a decreased red cell mass (*anemia*), impaired O_2 loading of the hemoglobin molecule or a high O_2 affinity mutant hemoglobin (*hypoxemia*), or, rarely, impaired blood flow to the kidney (renal artery stenosis). EPO governs the day-to-day production of red cells, and ambient levels of the hormone can be measured in the plasma by sensitive immunoassays—the normal level being 10–25 U/L. When the hemoglobin concentration falls below 100–120 g/L (10–12 g/dL), plasma EPO levels increase in proportion to the severity of the anemia (Fig. 58-2). In circulation, EPO has a half-clearance time of 6–9 h. EPO acts by binding to specific receptors on the surface of marrow erythroid precursors, inducing them to proliferate and to mature. With EPO stimulation, red cell production can increase four- to fivefold within a 1- to 2-week period but only in the presence of adequate nutrients, especially iron. The functional capacity of the erythron, therefore, requires normal renal production of EPO, a functioning erythroid marrow, and an adequate supply of substrates for hemoglobin synthesis. A defect in any of these key components can lead to anemia. Generally, anemia is recognized in the laboratory when a patient's hemoglobin level or hematocrit is reduced below an expected value (the normal range). The likelihood and severity of anemia are defined based on the deviation of the patient's hemoglobin/hematocrit from values expected for age- and sex-matched normal subjects. The hemoglobin concentration in adults has a Gaussian distribution. The mean hematocrit value for adult males is 47% (± SD 7) and that for adult females is 42% (± 5). Any single hematocrit or hemoglobin value carries with it a likelihood of associated anemia. Thus, a hematocrit of ≤39% in an adult male or <35% in an adult female has only about a 25% chance of being normal. Suspected low hemoglobin or hematocrit values are more easily interpreted if previous values for the same patient are known for comparison. The World Health Organization (WHO) defines anemia as a hemoglobin level < 130 g/L (13 g/dL) in men and <120 g/L (12 g/dL) in women.

The critical elements of erythropoiesis—EPO production, iron availability, the proliferative capacity of the bone marrow, and effective maturation of red cell precursors—are used for the initial classification of anemia (see below).

ANEMIA

CLINICAL PRESENTATION OF ANEMIA

Signs and Symptoms Anemia is most often recognized by abnormal screening laboratory tests. Patients less commonly present with advanced anemia and its attendant signs and symptoms. Acute anemia is nearly always due to blood loss or hemolysis. If blood loss is mild, enhanced O_2 delivery is achieved through changes in the O_2-hemoglobin dissociation curve mediated by a decreased pH or increased CO_2 (*Bohr effect*). With acute blood loss, hypovolemia dominates the clinical picture and the hematocrit and hemoglobin levels do not reflect the volume of blood lost. Signs of vascular instability appear with acute losses of 10–15% of the total blood volume. In such patients, the issue is not anemia but hypotension and decreased organ perfusion. When >30% of the blood volume is lost suddenly, patients are unable to compensate with the usual mechanisms of vascular contraction and changes in regional blood flow. The patient prefers to remain supine and will show postural hypotension and tachycardia. If the volume of blood lost is >40% (i.e., >2 L in the average-sized adult), signs of hypovolemic shock including confusion, dyspnea, diaphoresis, hypotension, and tachycardia appear (Chap. 101). Such patients have significant deficits in vital organ perfusion and require immediate volume replacement.

With acute hemolytic disease, the signs and symptoms depend on the mechanism that leads to red cell destruction. Intravascular hemolysis with release of free hemoglobin may be associated with acute back pain, free hemoglobin in the plasma and urine, and renal failure. Symptoms associated with more chronic or progressive anemia depend on the age of the patient and the adequacy of blood supply to critical organs. Symptoms associated with moderate anemia include fatigue, loss of stamina, breathlessness, and tachycardia (particularly with physical exertion). However, because of the intrinsic compensatory mechanisms that govern the O_2-hemoglobin dissociation curve, the gradual onset of anemia—particularly in young patients—may not be associated with signs or symptoms until the anemia is severe [hemoglobin <70–80 g/L (7–8 g/dL)]. When anemia develops over a period of days or weeks, the total blood volume is normal to slightly increased and changes in cardiac output and regional blood flow help compensate for the overall loss in O_2-carrying capacity. Changes in the position of the O_2-hemoglobin dissociation curve account for some of the compensatory response to anemia. With chronic anemia, intracellular levels of 2,3-bisphosphoglycerate rise, shifting the dissociation curve to the right and facilitating O_2 unloading. This compensatory mechanism can only maintain normal tissue O_2 delivery in the face of a 20–30 g/L (2–3 g/dL) deficit in hemoglobin concentration. Finally, further protection of O_2 delivery to vital organs is achieved by the shunting of blood away from organs that are relatively rich in blood supply, particularly the kidney, gut, and skin.

Certain disorders are commonly associated with anemia. Chronic inflammatory states (e.g., infection, rheumatoid arthritis) are associated with mild to moderate anemia, whereas lymphoproliferative disorders, such as chronic lymphocytic leukemia and certain other B cell neoplasms, may be associated with autoimmune hemolysis.

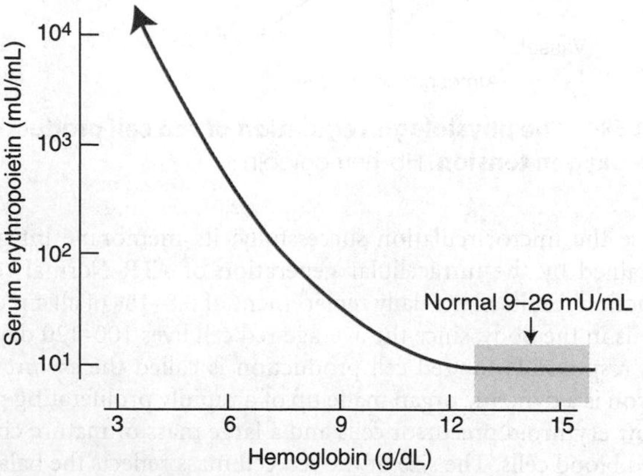

FIGURE 58-2 Erythropoietin levels in response to anemia. When the hemoglobin level falls to 120 g/L (12 g/dL), plasma erythropoietin levels increase logarithmically. In the presence of renal disease or chronic inflammation, EPO levels are typically lower than expected for a particular level of anemia. As individuals age, the level of EPO needed to sustain normal hemoglobin levels appears to increase. (*From Hillman et al.*)

APPROACH TO THE PATIENT: Anemia

The evaluation of the patient with anemia requires a careful history and physical examination. Nutritional history related to drugs or alcohol intake and family history of anemia should always be assessed. Certain geographic backgrounds and ethnic origins are associated with an increased likelihood of an inherited disorder of the hemoglobin molecule or intermediary metabolism. Glucose-6-phosphate dehydrogenase (G6PD) deficiency and certain hemoglobinopathies are seen more commonly in those of Middle Eastern or African origin, including African Americans who have a high frequency of G6PD deficiency. Other information that may be useful includes exposure to certain toxic agents or drugs and symptoms related to other disorders commonly associated with anemia. These include symptoms and signs such as bleeding, fatigue, malaise, fever, weight loss, night sweats, and other systemic symptoms. Clues to the mechanisms of anemia may be provided on physical examination by findings of infection, blood in the stool, lymphadenopathy, splenomegaly, or petechiae. Splenomegaly and lymphade-

TABLE 58-1 LABORATORY TESTS IN ANEMIA DIAGNOSIS

I. Complete blood count (CBC)
- A. Red blood cell count
  - 1. Hemoglobin
  - 2. Hematocrit
  - 3. Reticulocyte count
- B. Red blood cell indices
  - 1. Mean cell volume (MCV)
  - 2. Mean cell hemoglobin (MCH)
  - 3. Mean cell hemoglobin concentration (MCHC)
  - 4. Red cell distribution width (RDW)
- C. White blood cell count
  - 1. Cell differential
  - 2. Nuclear segmentation of neutrophils
- D. Platelet count
- E. Cell morphology
  - 1. Cell size
  - 2. Hemoglobin content
  - 3. Anisocytosis
  - 4. Poikilocytosis
  - 5. Polychromasia

II. Iron supply studies
- A. Serum iron
- B. Total iron-binding capacity
- C. Serum ferritin

III. Marrow examination
- A. Aspirate
  - 1. M/E ratio[a]
  - 2. Cell morphology
  - 3. Iron stain
- B. Biopsy
  - 1. Cellularity
  - 2. Morphology

[a]M/E ratio, ratio of myeloid to erythroid precursors.

nopathy suggest an underlying lymphoproliferative disease, while petechiae suggest platelet dysfunction. Past laboratory measurements may be helpful to determine a time of onset.

In the anemic patient, physical examination may demonstrate a forceful heartbeat, strong peripheral pulses, and a systolic "flow" murmur. The skin and mucous membranes may be pale if the hemoglobin is <80–100 g/L (8–10 g/dL). This part of the physical examination should focus on areas where vessels are close to the surface such as the mucous membranes, nail beds, and palmar creases. If the palmar creases are lighter in color than the surrounding skin when the hand is hyperextended, the hemoglobin level is usually <80 g/L (8 g/dL).

LABORATORY EVALUATION Table 58-1 lists the tests used in the initial workup of anemia. A routine complete blood count (CBC) is required as part of the evaluation and includes the hemoglobin, hematocrit, and red cell indices: the mean cell volume (MCV) in femtoliters, mean cell hemoglobin (MCH) in picograms per cell, and mean concentration of hemoglobin per volume of red cells (MCHC) in grams per liter (non-SI: grams per deciliter). The red cell indices are calculated as shown in Table 58-2, and the normal variations in the hemoglobin and hematocrit with age are shown in Table 58-3. A number of physiologic factors affect the CBC including age, sex, pregnancy, smoking, and altitude. High-normal hemoglobin values may be seen in men and women who live at altitude or smoke heavily. Hemoglobin elevations due to smoking reflect normal compensation due to the displacement of O_2 by CO in hemoglobin binding. Other important information is provided by the reticulocyte count and measurements of iron supply including *serum iron*, *total iron-binding capacity* (TIBC; an indirect measure of the transferrin level), and *serum ferritin*. Marked alterations in the red cell indices usually reflect disorders of maturation or iron deficiency. A careful evaluation of the peripheral blood smear is important, and clinical laboratories often provide a description of both the red and white cells, a white cell differential count, and the platelet count. In patients with severe anemia and abnormalities in red blood cell morphology and/or low reticulocyte counts, a bone marrow aspirate or biopsy may be important to assist in the diagnosis. Other tests of value in the diagnosis of specific anemias are discussed in chapters on specific disease states.

TABLE 58-2 RED BLOOD CELL INDICES

Index	Normal Value
Mean cell volume (MCV) = (hematocrit × 10)/(red cell count × 10^6)	90 ± 8 fL
Mean cell hemoglobin (MCH) = (hemoglobin × 10)/(red cell count × 10^6)	30 ± 3 pg
Mean cell hemoglobin concentration = (hemoglobin × 10)/hematocrit, or MCH/MCV	33 ± 2%

TABLE 58-3 CHANGES IN NORMAL HEMOGLOBIN/HEMATOCRIT VALUES WITH AGE AND PREGNANCY

Age/Sex	Hemoglobin g/dL	Hematocrit %
At birth	17	52
Childhood	12	36
Adolescence	13	40
Adult man	16 (±2)	47 (±6)
Adult woman (menstruating)	13 (±2)	40 (±6)
Adult woman (postmenopausal)	14 (±2)	42 (±6)
During pregnancy	12 (±2)	37 (±6)

Source: From Hillman et al.

The components of the CBC also help in the classification of anemia. *Microcytosis* is reflected by a lower than normal MCV (<80), whereas high values (>100) reflect *macrocytosis*. The MCH and MCHC reflect defects in hemoglobin synthesis (*hypochromia*). Automated cell counters describe the red cell volume distribution width (RDW). The MCV (representing the peak of the distribution curve) is insensitive to the appearance of small populations of macrocytes or microcytes. An experienced laboratory technician will be able to identify minor populations of large or small cells or hypochromic cells before the red cell indices change.

Peripheral Blood Smear The peripheral blood smear provides important information about defects in red cell production. As a complement to the red cell indices, the blood smear also reveals variations in cell size (*anisocytosis*) and shape (*poikilocytosis*). The degree of anisocytosis usually correlates with increases in the RDW or the range of cell sizes. Poikilocytosis suggests a defect in the maturation of red cell precursors in the bone marrow or fragmentation of circulating red cells. The blood smear may also reveal *polychromasia*—red cells that are slightly larger than normal and grayish blue in color on the Wright-Giemsa stain. These cells are reticulocytes that have been prematurely released from the bone marrow, and their color represents residual amounts of ribosomal RNA. These cells appear in circulation in response to EPO stimulation or to architectural damage of the bone marrow (fibrosis, infiltration of the marrow by malignant cells, etc.) that results in their disordered release from the marrow. The appearance of nucleated red cells, Howell-Jolly bodies, target cells, sickle cells, and others may provide clues to specific disorders (Figs. 58-3 to 58-11).

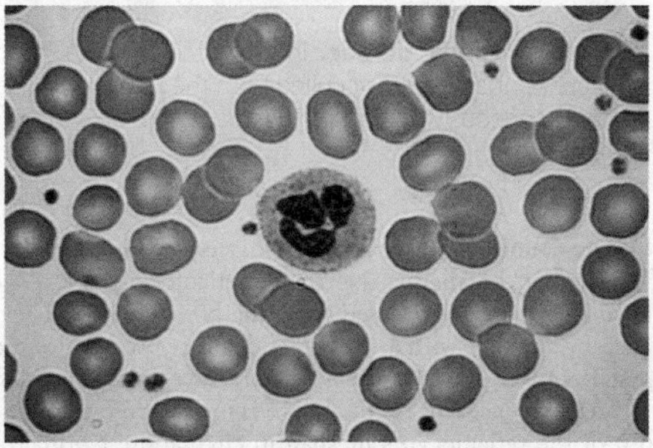

FIGURE 58-3 Normal blood smear (Wright's stain). High-power field showing normal red cells, a neutrophil, and a few platelets. (*From Hillman et al.*)

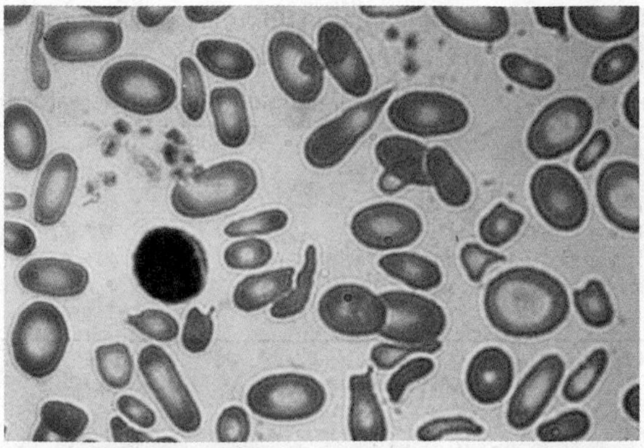

FIGURE 58-4 Severe iron-deficiency anemia. Microcytic and hypochromic red cells smaller than the nucleus of a lymphocyte associated with marked variation in size (anisocytosis) and shape (poikilocytosis). (*From Hillman et al.*)

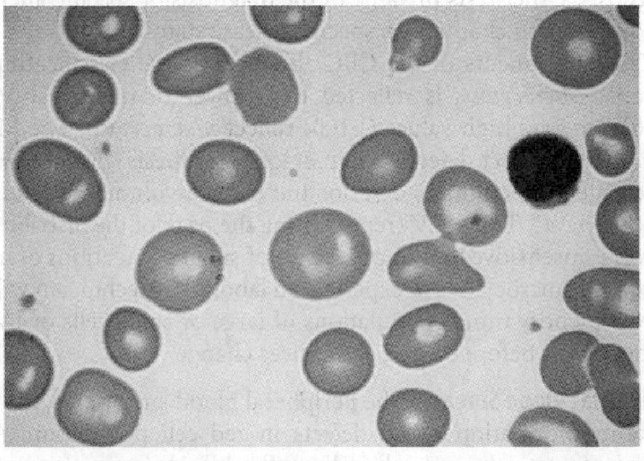

FIGURE 58-5 Macrocytosis. Red cells are larger than a small lymphocyte and well hemoglobinized. Often macrocytes are oval-shaped (macroovalocytes).

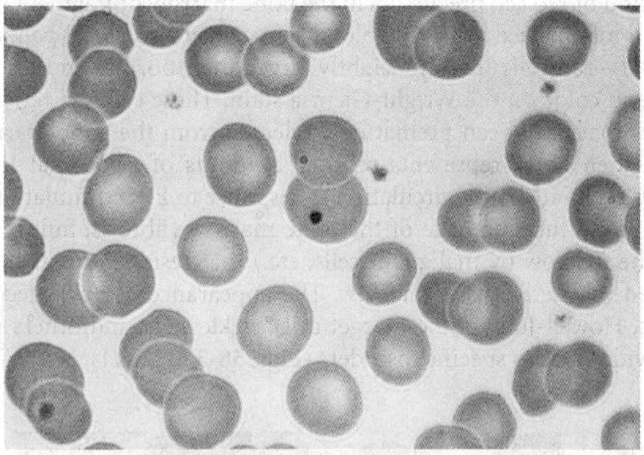

FIGURE 58-6 Howell-Jolly bodies. In the absence of a functional spleen, nuclear remnants are not culled from the red cells and remain as small homogeneously staining blue inclusions on Wright stain. (*From Hillman et al.*)

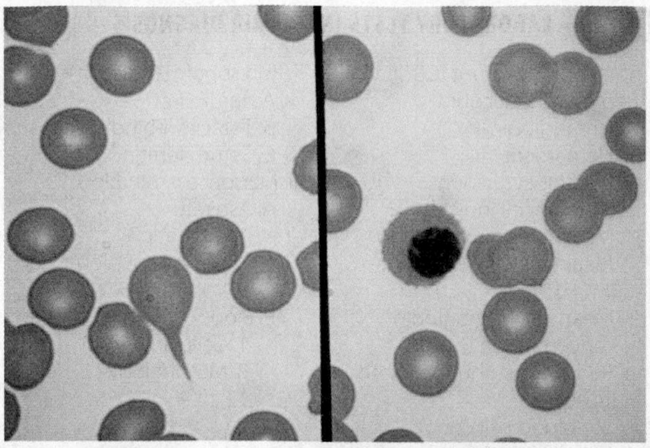

FIGURE 58-7 Red cell changes in myelofibrosis. The left panel shows a teardrop-shaped cell. The right panel shows a nucleated red cell. These forms are seen in myelofibrosis with extramedullary hematopoiesis.

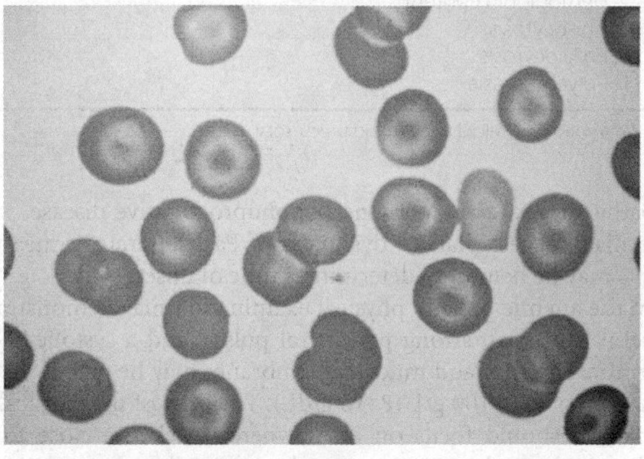

FIGURE 58-8 Target cells. Target cells have a bull's-eye appearance and are seen in thalassemia and in liver disease. (*From Hillman et al.*)

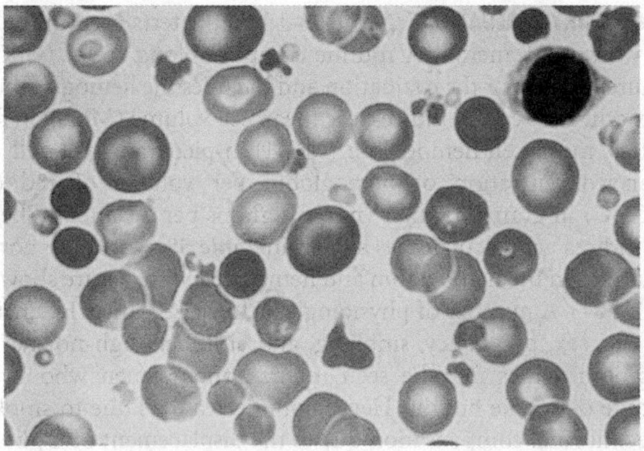

FIGURE 58-9 Red cell fragmentation. Red cells may become fragmented in the presence of foreign bodies in the circulation such as mechanical heart valves or in the setting of thermal injury. (*From Hillman et al.*)

Reticulocyte Count An accurate reticulocyte count is key to the initial classification of anemia. Normally, reticulocytes are red cells that have been recently released from the bone marrow. They are identified by staining with a supravital dye that precipitates the ribosomal RNA (Fig. 58-12). These precipitates appear as blue or black punctate spots. This residual RNA is metabolized over the first 24–36 h of the reticulocyte's lifespan in circulation. Normally, the reticulocyte count ranges from 1–2% and reflects the daily replacement of 0.8–1.0% of the circulating red cell population. A reticulocyte count provides a reliable measure of red cell production.

In the initial classification of anemia, the patient's reticulocyte count is compared with the expected reticulocyte response. In general, if the EPO and erythroid marrow responses to moderate anemia [hemoglobin < 100 g/L (10 g/dL)] are intact, the red cell production rate increases to two to three times normal within 10 days following the onset of anemia. In the face of established anemia, a reticulocyte response less than two to three times normal indicates an inadequate marrow response.

In order to use the reticulocyte count to estimate marrow response, two corrections are necessary. The first correction adjusts

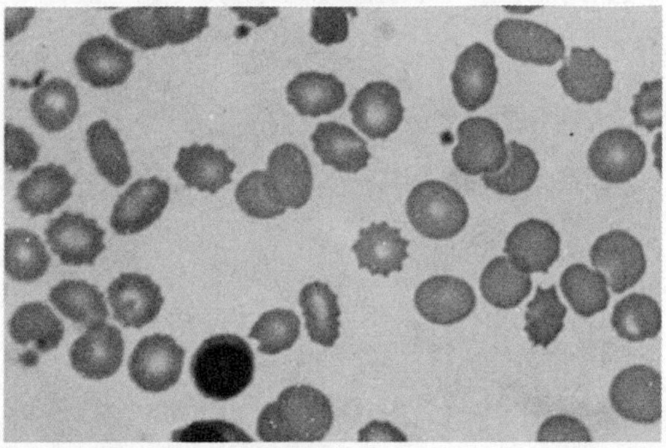

FIGURE 58-10 Uremia. The red cells in uremia may acquire numerous, regularly spaced, small spiny projections. Such cells, called burr cells or echinocytes, are readily distinguishable from irregularly spiculated acanthocytes shown in Fig. 58-11.

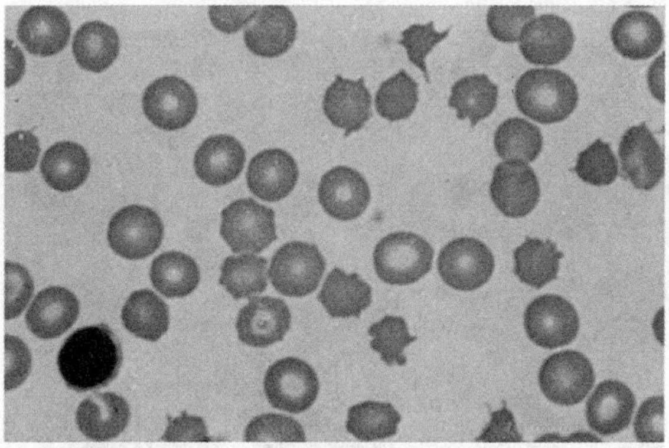

FIGURE 58-11 Spur cells. Spur cells are recognized as distorted red cells containing several irregularly distributed thornlike projections. Cells with this morphologic abnormality are also called acanthocytes. (*From Hillman et al.*)

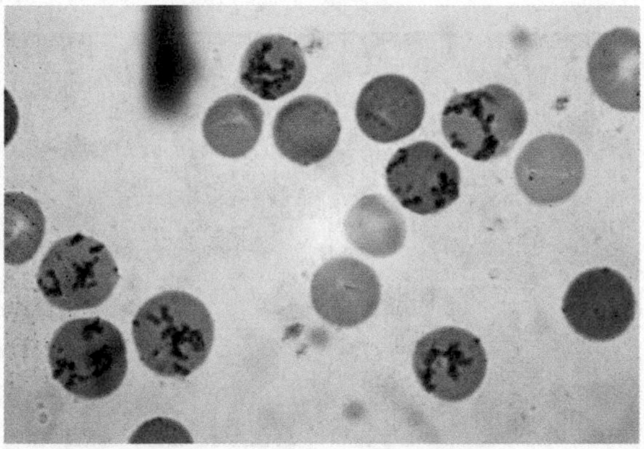

FIGURE 58-12 Reticulocytes. Methylene blue stain demonstrates residual RNA in newly made red cells. (*From Hillman et al.*)

the reticulocyte count based on the reduced number of circulating red cells. With anemia, the percentage of reticulocytes may be increased while the absolute number is unchanged. To correct for this effect, the reticulocyte percentage is multiplied by the ratio of the patient's hemoglobin or hematocrit to the expected hemoglobin/hematocrit for the age and gender of the patient (Table 58-4). This provides an estimate of the reticulocyte count corrected for anemia. In order to convert the corrected reticulocyte count to an index of marrow production, a further correction is required, depending on whether some of the reticulocytes in circulation have been released from the marrow prematurely. For this second correction, the peripheral blood smear is examined to see if there are polychromatophilic macrocytes present. These cells, representing

TABLE 58-4 CALCULATION OF RETICULOCYTE PRODUCTION INDEX

Correction #1 for anemia:
This correction produces the corrected reticulocyte count
In a person whose reticulocyte count is 9%, hemoglobin 7.5 g/dL, hematocrit 23%, the absolute reticulocyte count = 9 × (7.5/15) [or × (23/45)]= 4.5%

Correction #2 for longer life of prematurely released reticulocytes in the blood:
This correction produces the reticulocyte production index
In a person whose reticulocyte count is 9%, hemoglobin 7.5 gm/dL, hematocrit 23%, the reticulocyte production index

$$= 9 \times \frac{(7.5/15)(\text{hemoglobin correction})}{2\ (\text{maturation time correction})} = 2.25$$

prematurely released reticulocytes, are referred to as "shift" cells, and the relationship between the degree of shift and the necessary shift correction factor is shown in **Fig. 58-13**. The correction is necessary because these prematurely released cells survive as reticulocytes in circulation for >1 day, thereby providing a falsely high estimate of daily red cell production. If polychromasia is increased, the reticulocyte count, already corrected for anemia, should be divided again by a factor of 2 to account for the prolonged reticulocyte maturation time. The second correction factor varies from 1–3 depending on the severity of anemia. In general, a correction of 2 is commonly used. An appropriate correction is shown in Table 58-4. If polychromatophilic cells are not seen on the blood smear, the second correction is not required. The now doubly corrected reticulocyte count is the *reticulocyte production index*, and it provides an estimate of marrow production relative to normal.

Premature release of reticulocytes is normally due to increased EPO stimulation. However, if the integrity of the bone marrow release process is lost through tumor infiltration, fibrosis, or other disorders, the appearance of nucleated red cells or polychromatophilic macrocytes should still invoke the second reticulocyte correction. The shift correction should always be applied to a patient with anemia and a very high reticulocyte count to provide a true index of effective red cell production. Patients with severe chronic hemolytic anemia may increase red cell production as much as six- to sevenfold. This measure alone, therefore, confirms the fact that the patient has an appropriate EPO response, a normally functioning bone marrow, and sufficient iron available to meet the de-

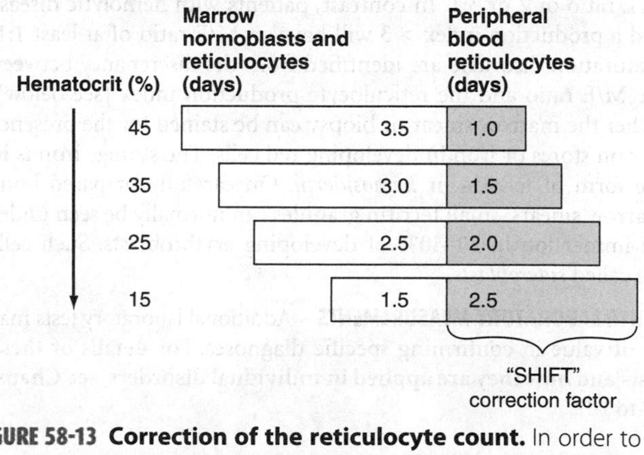

FIGURE 58-13 Correction of the reticulocyte count. In order to use the reticulocyte count as an indicator of effective red cell production, the reticulocyte number must be corrected based on the level of anemia and the circulating life span of the reticulocytes. Erythroid cells take ~4.5 days to mature. At normal hematocrit levels, they are released to the circulation with ~1 day left as reticulocytes. However, with different levels of anemia, erythroid cells are released from the marrow prematurely. Most patients come to clinical attention with hematocrits in the mid-20s and thus a correction factor of 2 is commonly used because the observed reticulocytes will live for 2 days in the circulation before losing their RNA.

TABLE 58-5 NORMAL MARROW RESPONSE TO ANEMIA

Hematocrit	Production Index	Reticulocytes (incl corrections)	Marrow M:E Ratio
45	1	1	3:1
35	2.0–3.0	4.8%/3.8/2.5	2:1–1:1
25	3.0–5.0	14%/8/4.0	1:1–1:2
15	3.0–5.0	30%/10/4.0	1:1–1:2

mands for new red cell formation. Table 58-5 demonstrates the normal marrow response to anemia. If the reticulocyte production index is <2 in the face of established anemia, a defect in erythroid marrow proliferation or maturation must be present.

Tests of Iron Supply and Storage The laboratory measurements that reflect the availability of iron for hemoglobin synthesis include the serum iron, the TIBC, and the percent transferrin saturation. The percent transferrin saturation is derived by dividing the serum iron level (× 100) by the TIBC. The normal serum iron ranges from 9–27 μmol/L (50–150 μg/dL), while the normal TIBC is 54–64 μmol/L (300–360 μg/dL); the normal transferrin saturation ranges from 25–50%. A diurnal variation in the serum iron leads to a variation in the percent transferrin saturation. The serum ferritin is used to evaluate total-body iron stores. Adult males have serum ferritin levels that average ~100 μg/L, corresponding to iron stores of ~1 g. Adult females have lower serum ferritin levels averaging 30 μg/L, reflecting lower iron stores (300 mg). A serum ferritin level of 10–15 μg/L represents depletion of body iron stores. However, ferritin is also an acute-phase reactant and, in the presence of acute or chronic inflammation, may rise severalfold above baseline levels. As a rule, a serum ferritin > 200 μg/L means there is at least some iron in tissue stores.

Bone Marrow Examination A bone marrow aspirate and smear or a needle biopsy may be useful in the evaluation of some patients with anemia. In patients with hypoproliferative anemia and normal iron status, a bone marrow is indicated. Marrow examination can diagnose primary marrow disorders such as myelofibrosis, a red cell maturation defect, or an infiltrative disease (Figs. 58-14 to 58-16). The increase or decrease of one cell lineage (myeloid vs. erythroid) compared to another is obtained by a differential count of nucleated cells in a bone marrow smear [the myeloid/erythroid (M/E) ratio]. A patient with a hypoproliferative anemia (see below) and a reticulocyte production index < 2 will demonstrate an M/E ratio of 2 or 3:1. In contrast, patients with hemolytic disease and a production index > 3 will have an M/E ratio of at least 1:1. Maturation disorders are identified from the discrepancy between the M/E ratio and the reticulocyte production index (see below). Either the marrow smear or biopsy can be stained for the presence of iron stores or iron in developing red cells. The storage iron is in the form of ferritin or *hemosiderin*. On carefully prepared bone marrow smears, small ferritin granules can normally be seen under oil immersion in 20–40% of developing erythroblasts. Such cells are called *sideroblasts*.

OTHER LABORATORY MEASUREMENTS Additional laboratory tests may be of value in confirming specific diagnoses. For details of these tests and how they are applied in individual disorders, see Chaps. 98 to 102.

DEFINITION AND CLASSIFICATION OF ANEMIA

Initial Classification of Anemia The functional classification of anemia has three major categories. These are: (1) marrow production defects (*hypoproliferation*), (2) red cell maturation defects (*ineffective erythropoiesis*), and (3) decreased red cell survival (*blood loss/hemolysis*). The classification is shown in Fig. 58-17. A hypoproliferative anemia is typically seen with a low reticulocyte production index together with little or no change in red cell morphology (a normocytic, normochromic anemia) (Chap. 98). Maturation disorders typically have a slight to moderately elevated reticulocyte production index that is accompanied by either macrocytic (Chap. 100) or microcytic (Chaps. 98, 99) red cell indices. Increased red blood cell destruction secondary to hemolysis results in an increase in the reticulocyte production index to at least three times normal (Chap. 101), provided sufficient iron is available. Hemorrhagic anemia does not typically result in production indices of more than 2.0–2.5 times normal because of the limitations placed on expansion of the erythroid marrow by iron availability.

In the first branch point of the classification of anemia, a reticulocyte production index > 2.5 indicates that hemolysis is most likely. A reticulocyte production index < 2 indicates either a hypoproliferative anemia or maturation disorder. The latter two possibilities can often

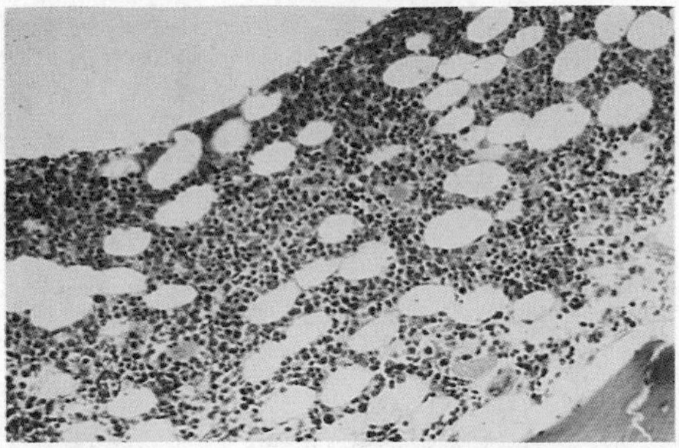

FIGURE 58-14 Normal bone marrow. This is a low-power view of a section of a normal bone marrow biopsy stained with hematoxylin and eosin (H&E). Note that the nucleated cellular elements account for ~40–50% and the fat (clear areas) accounts for ~50–60% of the area. (*From Hillman et al.*)

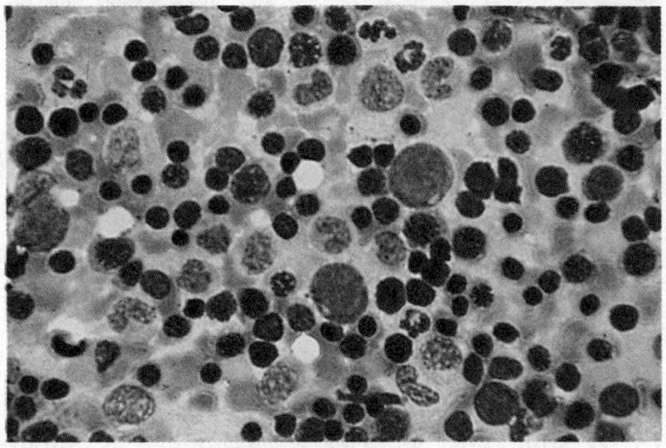

FIGURE 58-15 Erythroid hyperplasia. This marrow shows an increase in the fraction of cells in the erythroid lineage as might be seen when a normal marrow compensates for acute blood loss or hemolysis. The M/E ratio is about 1:1. (*From Hillman et al.*)

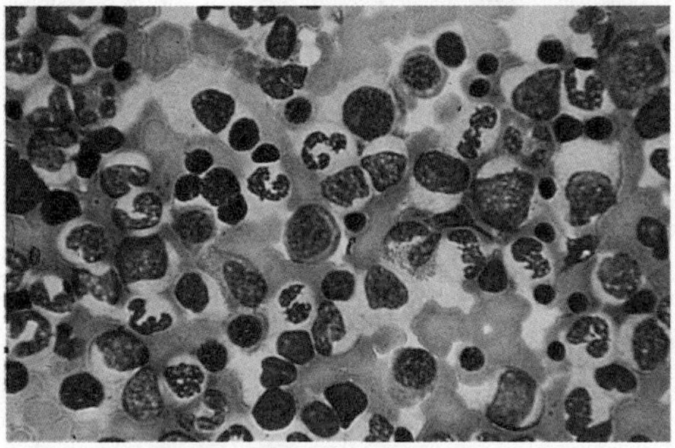

FIGURE 58-16 Myeloid hyperplasia. This marrow shows an increase in the fraction of cells in the myeloid or granulocytic lineage as might be seen in a normal marrow responding to infection. The M/E ratio is >3:1. (*From Hillman et al.*)

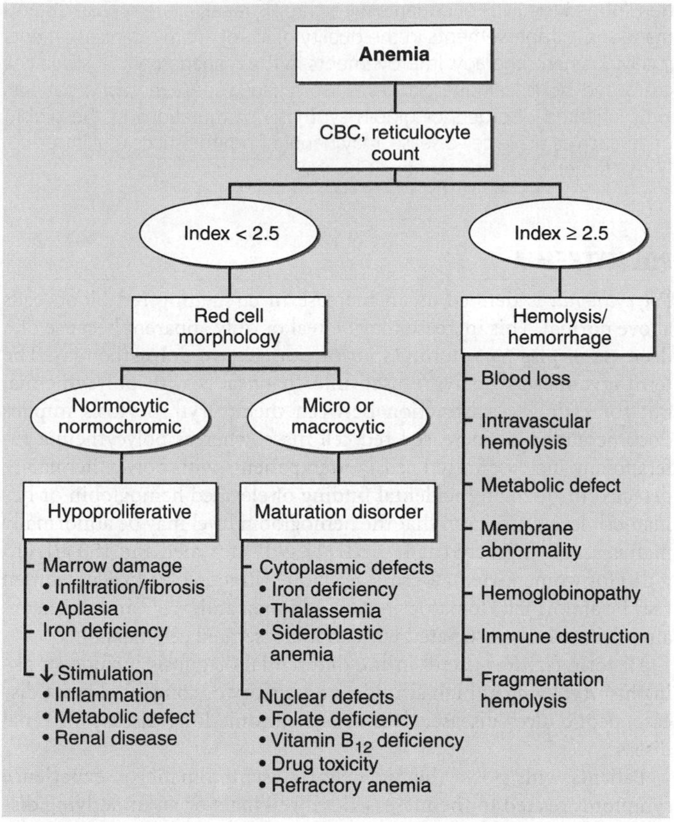

FIGURE 58-17 The physiologic classification of anemia. CBC, complete blood count.

be distinguished by the red cell indices, by examination of the peripheral blood smear, or by a marrow examination. If the red cell indices are normal, the anemia is almost certainly hypoproliferative in nature. Maturation disorders are characterized by ineffective red cell production and a low reticulocyte production index. Bizarre red cell shapes—macrocytes or hypochromic microcytes—are seen on the peripheral blood smear. With a hypoproliferative anemia, no erythroid hyperplasia is noted in the marrow, whereas patients with ineffective red cell production have erythroid hyperplasia and an M/E ratio < 1:1.

Hypoproliferative Anemias At least 75% of all cases of anemia are hypoproliferative in nature. A hypoproliferative anemia reflects absolute or relative marrow failure in which the erythroid marrow has not proliferated appropriately for the degree of anemia. The majority of hypoproliferative anemias are due to mild to moderate iron deficiency or inflammation. A hypoproliferative anemia can result from marrow damage, iron deficiency, or inadequate EPO stimulation. The last may reflect impaired renal function, suppression of EPO production by inflammatory cytokines such as interleukin 1, or reduced tissue needs for O_2 from metabolic disease such as hypothyroidism. Only occasionally is the marrow unable to produce red cells at a normal rate, and this is most prevalent in patients with renal failure. With diabetes mellitus or myeloma, the EPO deficiency may be more marked than would be predicted by the degree of renal insufficiency. In general, hypoproliferative anemias are characterized by normocytic, normochromic red cells, although microcytic, hypochromic cells may be observed with mild iron deficiency or long-standing chronic inflammatory disease. The key laboratory tests in distinguishing between the various forms of hypoproliferative anemia include the serum iron and iron-binding capacity, evaluation of renal and thyroid function, a marrow biopsy or aspirate to detect marrow damage or infiltrative disease, and serum ferritin to assess iron stores. Occasionally, an iron stain of the marrow will be needed to determine the pattern of iron distribution. Patients with the anemia of acute or chronic inflammation show a distinctive pattern of serum iron (low), TIBC (normal or low), percent transferrin saturation (low), and serum ferritin (normal or high). These changes in iron values are brought about by hepcidin, the iron regulatory hormone that is increased in inflammation (Chap. 98). A distinct pattern of results is noted in mild to moderate iron deficiency (low serum iron, high TIBC, low percent transferrin saturation, low serum ferritin) (Chap. 98). Marrow damage by drugs, such as the antiretrovirals used to treat HIV infection, infiltrative disease such as leukemia or lymphoma, or marrow aplasia can usually be diagnosed from the peripheral blood and bone marrow morphology. With infiltrative disease or fibrosis, a marrow biopsy is required.

Maturation Disorders The presence of anemia with an inappropriately low reticulocyte production index, macro- or microcytosis on smear, and abnormal red cell indices suggests a maturation disorder. Maturation disorders are divided into two categories: nuclear maturation defects, associated with macrocytosis and abnormal marrow development, and cytoplasmic maturation defects, associated with microcytosis and hypochromia usually from defects in hemoglobin synthesis. The inappropriately low reticulocyte production index is a reflection of the ineffective erythropoiesis that results from the destruction within the marrow of developing erythroblasts. Bone marrow examination shows erythroid hyperplasia.

Nuclear maturation defects result from vitamin B_{12} or folic acid deficiency, drug damage, or myelodysplasia. Drugs that interfere with cellular DNA metabolism, such as methotrexate or alkylating agents, can produce a nuclear maturation defect. Alcohol, alone, is also capable of producing macrocytosis and a variable degree of anemia, but this is usually associated with folic acid deficiency. Measurements of folic acid and vitamin B_{12} are key not only in identifying the specific vitamin deficiency but also because they reflect different pathogenetic mechanisms.

Cytoplasmic maturation defects result from severe iron deficiency or abnormalities in globin or heme synthesis. Iron deficiency occupies an unusual position in the classification of anemia. If the iron-deficiency anemia is mild to moderate, erythroid marrow proliferation is decreased and the anemia is classified as hypoproliferative. However, if the anemia is severe and prolonged, the erythroid marrow will become hyperplastic despite the inadequate iron supply, and the anemia will be classified as ineffective erythropoiesis with a cytoplasmic maturation defect. In either case, an inappropriately low reticulocyte production index, microcytosis, and a classic pattern of iron values make the diagnosis clear and easily distinguish iron deficiency from other cytoplasmic maturation defects such as the thalassemias. Defects in heme synthesis, in contrast to globin synthesis, are less common and may be acquired or inherited (Chap. 352). Acquired abnormalities are usually associated with myelodysplasia, may lead to either a macro- or microcytic anemia, and are frequently associated with mitochondrial iron loading. In these cases, iron is taken up by the mitochondria of the developing erythroid cell but not incorporated into heme. The iron-encrusted mitochondria surround the nucleus of the erythroid cell, forming a ring. Based on the distinctive finding of so-called ringed sideroblasts on the marrow iron stain, patients are diagnosed as having a sideroblastic anemia—almost always reflecting myelodysplasia. Again, studies of iron parameters are helpful in the differential diagnosis and management of these patients.

Blood Loss/Hemolytic Anemia In contrast to anemias associated with an inappropriately low reticulocyte production index, hemolysis is associated with red cell production indices ≥2.5 times normal. The stimulated erythropoiesis is reflected in the blood smear by the appearance of increased numbers of polychromatophilic macrocytes. A marrow examination is rarely indicated if the reticulocyte production index is increased appropriately. The red cell indices are typically normocytic or slightly macrocytic, reflecting the increased number of reticulocytes. Acute blood loss is not associated with an increased reticulocyte production index because of the time required to increase EPO production and, subsequently, marrow proliferation. Subacute blood loss may be associated with modest reticulocytosis. Anemia from chronic blood loss presents more often as iron deficiency than with the picture of increased red cell production.

The evaluation of blood loss anemia is usually not difficult. Most problems arise when a patient presents with an increased red cell production index from an episode of acute blood loss that went unrecognized. The cause of the anemia and increased red cell production may not be obvious. The confirmation of a recovering state may require observations over a period of 2–3 weeks, during which the hemoglobin concentration will be seen to rise and the reticulocyte production index fall.

Hemolytic disease, while dramatic, is among the least common forms of anemia. The ability to sustain a high reticulocyte production index reflects the ability of the erythroid marrow to compensate for hemolysis and, in the case of extravascular hemolysis, the efficient recycling of iron from the destroyed red cells to support red cell production. With intravascular hemolysis, such as paroxysmal nocturnal hemoglobinuria, the loss of iron may limit the marrow response. The level of response depends on the severity of the anemia and the nature of the underlying disease process.

Hemoglobinopathies, such as sickle cell disease and the thalassemias, present a mixed picture. The reticulocyte index may be high but is inappropriately low for the degree of marrow erythroid hyperplasia (Chap. 99).

Hemolytic anemias present in different ways. Some appear suddenly as an acute, self-limited episode of intravascular or extravascular hemolysis, a presentation pattern often seen in patients with autoimmune hemolysis or with inherited defects of the Embden-Meyerhof pathway or the glutathione reductase pathway. Patients with inherited disorders of the hemoglobin molecule or red cell membrane generally have a lifelong clinical history typical of the disease process. Those with chronic hemolytic disease, such as hereditary spherocytosis, may actually present not with anemia but with a complication stemming from the prolonged increase in red cell destruction such as symptomatic bilirubin gallstones or splenomegaly. Patients with chronic hemolysis are also susceptible to aplastic crises if an infectious process interrupts red cell production.

The differential diagnosis of an acute or chronic hemolytic event requires the careful integration of family history, the pattern of clinical presentation and—whether the disease is congenital or acquired—by a careful examination of the peripheral blood smear. Precise diagnosis may require more specialized laboratory tests, such as hemoglobin electrophoresis or a screen for red cell enzymes. Acquired defects in red cell survival are often immunologically mediated and require a direct or indirect antiglobulin test or a cold agglutinin titer to detect the presence of hemolytic antibodies or complement-mediated red cell destruction.

Rx ANEMIA

An overriding principle is to initiate treatment of mild to moderate anemia only when a specific diagnosis is made. Rarely, in the acute setting, anemia may be so severe that red cell transfusions are required before a specific diagnosis is made. Whether the anemia is of acute or gradual onset, the selection of the appropriate treatment is determined by the documented cause(s) of the anemia. Often, the cause of the anemia may be multifactorial. For example, a patient with severe rheumatoid arthritis who has been taking anti-inflammatory drugs may have a hypoproliferative anemia associated with chronic inflammation as well as chronic blood loss associated with intermittent gastrointestinal bleeding. In every circumstance, it is important to evaluate the patient's iron status fully before and during the treatment of any anemia. **Transfusion is discussed in Chap. 107; iron therapy is discussed in Chap. 98; treatment of megaloblastic anemia is discussed in Chap. 100; treatment of other entities is discussed in their respective chapters (sickle cell anemia, Chap. 99; hemolytic anemias, Chap. 101; aplastic anemia and myelodysplasia, Chap. 102).**

Therapeutic options for the treatment of anemias have expanded dramatically during the past 25 years. Blood component therapy is available and safe. Recombinant EPO as an adjunct to anemia management has transformed the lives of patients with chronic renal failure on dialysis and made some improvements in the quality of life of anemic cancer patients receiving chemotherapy. Improvements in the management of sickle cell crises and sickle cell anemia have also taken place. Eventually, patients with inherited disorders of globin synthesis or mutations in the globin gene, such as sickle cell disease, may benefit from the successful introduction of targeted genetic therapy (Chap. 65).

POLYCYTHEMIA

Polycythemia is defined as an increase in circulating red blood cells above normal. This increase may be real or only apparent because of a decrease in plasma volume (spurious or relative polycythemia). The term *erythrocytosis* may be used interchangeably with polycythemia, but some draw a distinction between them; erythrocytosis implies documentation of increased red cell mass, whereas polycythemia refers to any increase in red cells. Often patients with polycythemia are detected through an incidental finding of elevated hemoglobin or hematocrit levels. Concern that the hemoglobin level may be abnormally high is usually triggered at 170 g/L (17 g/dL) for men and 150 g/L (15 g/dL) for women. Hematocrit levels >50% in men or >45% in women may be abnormal. Hematocrits >60% in men and >55% in women are almost invariably associated with an increased red cell mass.

Historic features useful in the differential diagnosis include smoking history; living at high altitude; or a history of congenital heart disease, peptic ulcer disease, sleep apnea, chronic lung disease, or renal disease.

Patients with polycythemia may be asymptomatic or experience symptoms related to the increased red cell mass or an underlying disease process that leads to increased red cell production. The dominant symptoms from increased red cell mass are related to hyperviscosity and thrombosis (both venous and arterial), because the blood viscosity increases logarithmically at hematocrits >55%. Manifestations range from digital ischemia to Budd-Chiari syndrome with hepatic vein thrombosis. Abdominal thromboses are particularly common. Neurologic symptoms such as vertigo, tinnitus, headache, and visual disturbances may occur. Hypertension is often present. Patients with *polycythemia vera* may have aquagenic pruritus and symptoms related to hepatosplenomegaly. Patients may have easy bruising, epistaxis, or bleeding from the gastrointestinal tract. Patients with hypoxemia may develop cyanosis on minimal exertion or have headache, impaired mental acuity, and fatigue.

The physical examination usually reveals a ruddy complexion. Splenomegaly favors polycythemia vera as the diagnosis (Chap. 103). The presence of cyanosis or evidence of a right-to-left shunt suggests congenital heart disease presenting in the adult, particularly tetralogy of Fallot or Eisenmenger syndrome (Chap. 229). Increased blood viscosity raises pulmonary artery pressure; hypoxemia can lead to increased pulmonary vascular resistance. Together these factors can produce cor pulmonale.

Polycythemia can be spurious (related to a decrease in plasma volume; Gaisbock's syndrome), primary, or secondary in origin. The secondary causes are all associated with increases in EPO levels: either a physiologically adapted appropriate elevation based on tissue hypoxia (lung disease, high altitude, CO poisoning, high-affinity hemoglobinopathy) or an abnormal overproduction (renal cysts, renal artery stenosis, tumors with ectopic EPO production). A rare familial form of polycythemia is associated with normal EPO levels but hyperresponsive EPO receptors due to mutations.

APPROACH TO THE PATIENT: Polycythemia

As shown in Fig. 58-18, the first step is to document the presence of an increased red cell mass using the principle of isotope dilution by administering ^{51}Cr-labeled autologous red blood cells to the patient and sampling blood radioactivity over a 2-h period. If the red

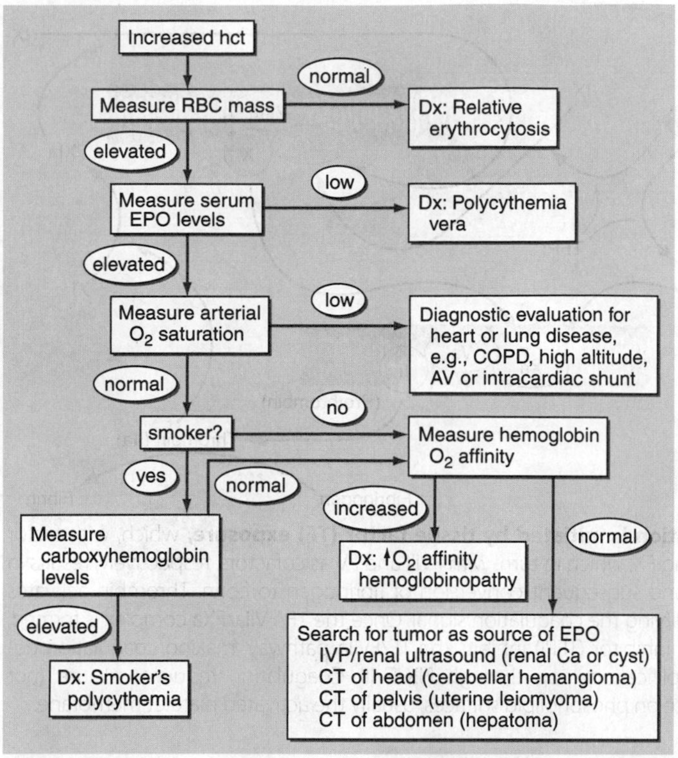

FIGURE 58-18 An approach to diagnosing patients with polycythemia. RBC, red blood cell; EPO, erythropoietin; COPD, chronic obstructive pulmonary disease; AV, atrioventricular; IVP, intravenous pyelogram; hct, hematocrit.

cell mass is normal (<36 mL/kg in men, <32 mL/kg in women), the patient has spurious polycythemia. If the red cell mass is increased (>36 mL/kg in men, >32 mL/kg in women), serum EPO levels should be measured. If EPO levels are low or unmeasurable, the patient most likely has polycythemia vera. Ancillary tests that support this diagnosis include elevated white blood cell count, increased absolute basophil count, and thrombocytosis. A mutation in *JAK-2* (Val617Phe), a key member of the cytokine intracellular signaling pathway, can be found in 70–95% of patients with polycythemia vera.

If serum EPO levels are elevated, one attempts to distinguish whether the elevation is a physiologic response to hypoxia or is related to autonomous production. Patients with low arterial O_2 saturation (<92%) should be further evaluated for the presence of heart or lung disease, if they are not living at high altitude. Patients with normal O_2 saturation who are smokers may have elevated EPO levels because of CO displacement of O_2. If carboxyhemoglobin (COHb) levels are high, the diagnosis is smoker's polycythemia. Such patients should be urged to stop smoking. Those who cannot stop smoking require phlebotomy to control their polycythemia. Patients with normal O_2 saturation who do not smoke either have an abnormal hemoglobin that does not deliver O_2 to the tissues (evaluated by finding elevated O_2-hemoglobin affinity) or have a source of EPO production that is not responding to the normal feedback inhibition. Further workup is dictated by the differential diagnosis of EPO-producing neoplasms. Hepatoma, uterine leiomyoma, and renal cancer or cysts are all detectable with abdominopelvic CT scans. Cerebellar hemangiomas may produce EPO, but they nearly always present with localizing neurologic signs and symptoms rather than polycythemia-related symptoms.

ACKNOWLEDGMENT

Dr. Robert S. Hillman wrote this chapter in the 14th edition, and elements of his chapter were retained here.

FURTHER READINGS

HILLMAN RS et al: *Hematology in Clinical Practice*, 4th ed. New York, McGraw-Hill, 2005

59 Bleeding and Thrombosis

Barbara A. Konkle

The human hemostatic system provides a natural balance between procoagulant and anticoagulant forces. The procoagulant forces include platelet adhesion and aggregation and fibrin clot formation; anticoagulant forces include the natural inhibitors of coagulation and fibrinolysis. Under normal circumstances, hemostasis is regulated to promote blood flow; however, it is also prepared to clot blood rapidly to arrest blood flow and prevent exsanguination. After bleeding is successfully halted, the system remodels the damaged vessel to restore normal blood flow. The major components of the hemostatic system, which function in concert, are (1) platelets and other formed elements of blood, such as monocytes and red cells; (2) plasma proteins (the coagulation and fibrinolytic factors and inhibitors); and (3) the vessel wall itself.

STEPS OF NORMAL HEMOSTASIS

PLATELET PLUG FORMATION

On vascular injury, platelets adhere to the site of injury, usually the denuded vascular intimal surface. Platelet adhesion is mediated primarily by von Willebrand factor (vWF), a large multimeric protein present in both plasma and in the extracellular matrix of the subendothelial vessel wall, which serves as the primary "molecular glue," providing sufficient strength to withstand the high levels of shear stress that would tend to detach them with the flow of blood. Platelet adhesion is also facilitated by direct binding to subendothelial collagen through specific platelet membrane collagen receptors.

Platelet adhesion results in subsequent platelet activation and aggregation. This process is enhanced and amplified by humoral mediators in plasma (e.g., epinephrine, thrombin); mediators released from activated platelets (e.g., adenosine diphosphate, serotonin); and vessel wall extracellular matrix constituents that come in contact with adherent platelets (e.g., collagen, vWF). Activated platelets undergo the release reaction, during which they secrete contents that further promote aggregation and inhibit the naturally anticoagulant endothelial cell factors. During platelet aggregation (platelet-platelet interaction), additional platelets are recruited from the circulation to the site of vascular injury, leading to the formation of an occlusive platelet thrombus. The platelet plug is anchored and stabilized by the developing fibrin mesh.

The platelet glycoprotein (Gp) IIb/IIIa ($\alpha_{IIb}\beta_3$) complex is the most abundant receptor on the platelet surface. Platelet activation converts the normally inactive GpIIb/IIIa receptor into an active receptor, enabling binding to fibrinogen and vWF. Because the surface of each platelet has about 50,000 GpIIb/IIIa fibrinogen binding sites, numerous activated platelets recruited to the site of vascular injury can rapidly form an occlusive aggregate by means of a dense network of intercellular fibrinogen bridges. Since this receptor is the key mediator of platelet aggregation, it has become an effective target for antiplatelet therapy.

FIBRIN CLOT FORMATION

Plasma coagulation proteins (*clotting factors*) normally circulate in plasma in their inactive forms. The sequence of coagulation protein reactions that culminate in the formation of fibrin was originally described as a *waterfall* or a *cascade*. Two pathways of blood coagulation have been described in the past: the so-called extrinsic, or tissue factor, pathway and the so-called intrinsic, or contact activation, pathway. We now know that coagulation is normally initiated through tissue factor (TF) exposure and activation through the classic *extrinsic pathway*, but with critically important amplification through elements of the classic *intrinsic pathway*, as illustrated in Fig. 59-1. These reactions take place on phospholipid surfaces, usually the activated platelet surface. Coagulation testing in the laboratory can reflect other influences due to the artificial nature of the in vitro systems used (see below).

The immediate trigger for coagulation is vascular damage that exposes blood to TF that is constitutively expressed on the surfaces of subendothelial cellular components of the vessel wall, such as smooth-muscle cells and fibroblasts. TF is also present in circulating microparticles, presumably shed from cells including monocytes and platelets. TF binds the serine protease factor VIIa; the complex activates factor X to factor Xa. Alternatively, the complex can indirectly activate factor X by initially converting factor IX to factor IXa, which then activates factor X. The participation of factor XI in hemostasis is not dependent on its activation by factor XIIa but rather on its positive feedback activation by thrombin. Thus, factor XIa functions in the propagation and amplification, rather than in the initiation, of the coagulation cascade.

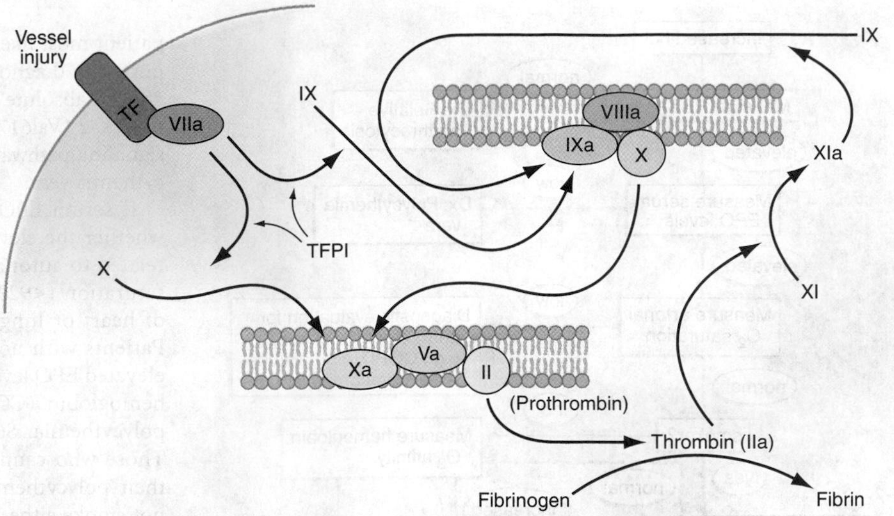

FIGURE 59-1 Coagulation is initiated by tissue factor (TF) exposure, which, with factor (F)VIIa, activates FIX and FX, which in turn, with FVIII and FV as cofactors, respectively, results in thrombin formation and subsequent conversion of fibrinogen to fibrin. Thrombin activates FXI, FVIII, and FV, amplifying the coagulation signal. Once the TF/FVIIa/FXa complex is formed, tissue factor pathway inhibitor (TFPI) inhibits the TF/FVIIa pathway, making coagulation dependent on the amplification loop through FIX/FVIII. Coagulation requires calcium (not shown) and takes place on phospholipid surfaces, usually the activated platelet membrane.

Factor Xa, which can be formed through the actions of either the tissue factor/factor VIIa complex or factor IXa (with factor VIIIa as a cofactor), converts prothrombin to thrombin, the pivotal protease of the coagulation system. The essential cofactor for this reaction is factor Va. Like the homologous factor VIIIa, factor Va is produced by thrombin-induced limited proteolysis of factor V. Thrombin is a multifunctional enzyme that converts soluble plasma fibrinogen to an insoluble fibrin matrix. Fibrin polymerization involves an orderly process of intermolecular associations (Fig. 59-2). Thrombin also activates factor XIII (fibrin-stabilizing factor) to factor XIIIa, which covalently cross-links and thereby stabilizes the fibrin clot.

The assembly of the clotting factors on activated cell membrane surfaces greatly accelerates their reaction rates and also serves to localize blood clotting to sites of vascular injury. The critical cell membrane components, acidic phospholipids, are not normally exposed on resting cell membrane surfaces. However, when platelets, monocytes, and endothelial cells are activated by vascular injury or inflammatory stimuli, the procoagulant head groups of the membrane anionic phospholipids become translocated to the surfaces of these cells or released as part of microparticles, making them available to support and promote the plasma coagulation reactions.

ANTITHROMBOTIC MECHANISMS

Several physiologic antithrombotic mechanisms act in concert to prevent clotting under normal circumstances. These mechanisms operate to preserve blood fluidity and limit blood clotting to specific focal sites of vascular injury. Endothelial cells have many antithrombotic effects. They produce prostacyclin, nitric oxide, and ectoADPase/CD39, which act to inhibit platelet binding, secretion, and aggregation. Endothelial cells produce anticoagulant factors including heparan proteoglycans, antithrombin, TF pathway inhibitor, and thrombomodulin. They also activate fibrinolytic mechanisms through the production of tissue plasminogen activator 1, urokinase, plasminogen activator inhibitor, and annexin-2. The sites of action of the major physiologic antithrombotic pathways are shown in Fig. 59-3.

Antithrombin (or antithrombin III) is the major plasma protease inhibitor of thrombin and the other clotting factors in coagulation. Antithrombin neutralizes thrombin and other activated coagulation factors by forming a complex between the active site of the enzyme and the reactive center of antithrombin. The rate of formation of these inactivating complexes increases by a factor of several thousand in the presence of heparin. Antithrombin inactivation of thrombin and other activated clotting factors occurs physiologically on vascular surfaces, where glycosaminoglycans, including heparan sulfates, are present to catalyze these reactions. Inherited quantitative or qualitative deficiencies of antithrombin lead to a lifelong predisposition to venous thromboembolism.

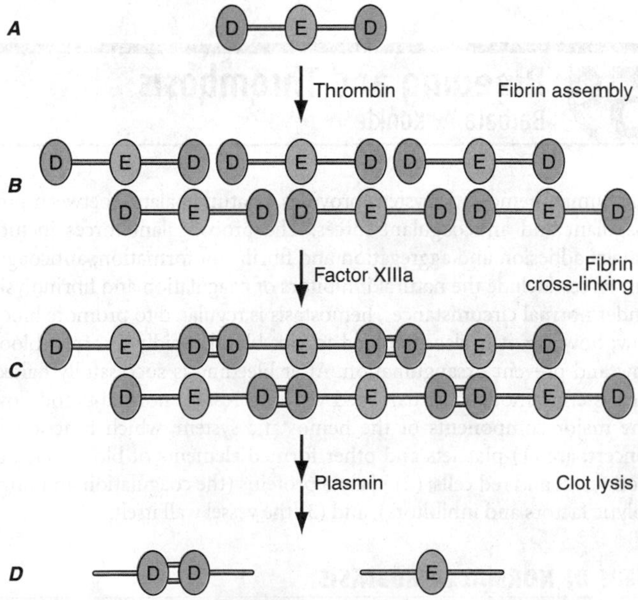

FIGURE 59-2 Fibrin formation and dissolution. *A.* Fibrinogen is a trinodular structure consisting of 2 D domains and 1 E domain. Thrombin activation results in an ordered lateral assembly of protofibrils ***(B)*** with noncovalent associations. FXIIIa cross-links the D domains on adjacent molecules ***(C)***. Fibrin and fibrinogen (not shown) lysis by plasmin occurs at discrete sites and results in intermediary fibrin(ogen) degradation products (not shown). D-Dimers are the product of complete lysis of fibrin, maintaining the cross-linked D domains.

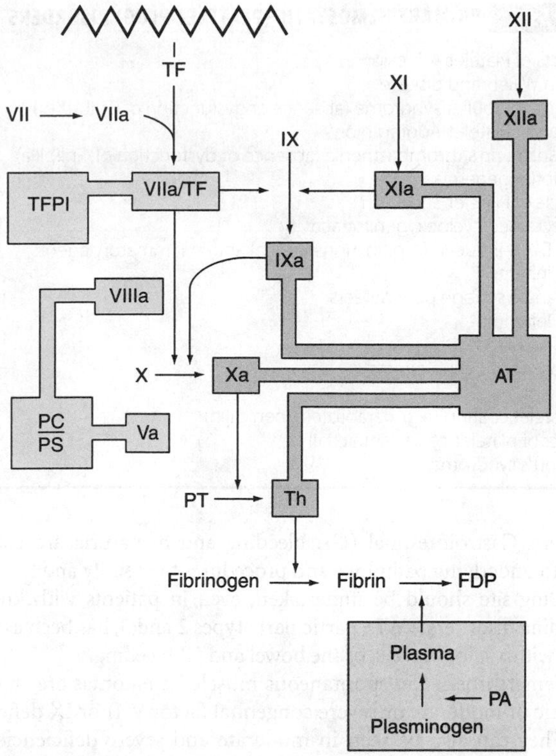

FIGURE 59-3 Sites of action of the four major physiologic antithrombotic pathways: antithrombin (AT); protein C/S (PC/PS); tissue factor pathway inhibitor (TFPI); and the fibrinolytic system, consisting of plasminogen, plasminogen activator (PA), and plasmin. PT, prothrombin; Th, thrombin; FDP, fibrin(ogen) degradation products. *[Modified from BA Konkle, AI Schafer, in DP Zipes et al (eds): Braunwald's Heart Disease, 7th ed. Philadelphia, Saunders, 2005.]*

Protein C is a plasma glycoprotein that becomes an anticoagulant when it is activated by thrombin. The thrombin-induced activation of protein C occurs physiologically on thrombomodulin, a transmembrane proteoglycan binding site for thrombin on endothelial cell surfaces. The binding of protein C to its receptor on endothelial cells places it in proximity to the thrombin-thrombomodulin complex, therefore enhancing its activation efficiency. Activated protein C acts as an anticoagulant by cleaving and inactivating activated factors V and VIII. This reaction is accelerated by a cofactor, protein S, which, like protein C, is a glycoprotein that undergoes vitamin K–dependent posttranslational modification. Quantitative or qualitative deficiencies of protein C or protein S, or resistance to the action of activated protein C by a specific mutation at its target cleavage site in factor Va (Factor V Leiden), lead to hypercoagulable states.

Tissue factor pathway inhibitor (TFPI) is a plasma protease inhibitor that regulates the TF-induced extrinsic pathway of coagulation. TFPI inhibits the TF/FVIIa/FXa complex, essentially turning off the TF/FVIIa initiation of coagulation, which then becomes dependent on the "amplification loop" via FXI and FVIII activation by thrombin. TFPI is bound to lipoprotein and can also be released by heparin from endothelial cells, where it is bound to glycosaminoglycans, and from platelets. The heparin-mediated release of TFPI may play a role in the anticoagulant effects of unfractionated and low-molecular-weight heparins.

THE FIBRINOLYTIC SYSTEM

Any thrombin that escapes the inhibitory effects of the physiologic anticoagulant systems is available to convert fibrinogen to fibrin. In response, the endogenous fibrinolytic system is then activated to dispose of intravascular fibrin and thereby maintain or reestablish the patency of the circulation. Just as thrombin is the key protease enzyme of the coagulation system, plasmin is the major protease enzyme of the fibrinolytic system, acting to digest fibrin to fibrin degradation products. The general scheme of fibrinolysis is shown in Fig. 59-4.

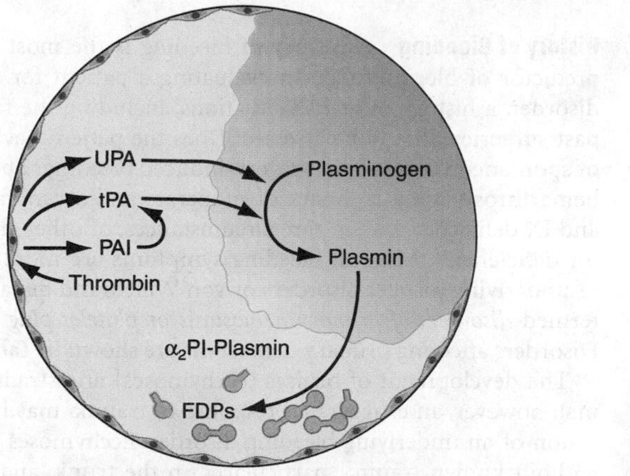

FIGURE 59-4 A schematic diagram of the fibrinolytic system. Tissue plasminogen activator (tPA) is released from endothelial cells, binds the fibrin clot, and activates plasminogen to plasmin. Excess fibrin is degraded by plasmin to distinct degradation products (FDPs). Any free plasmin is complexed with α_2-antiplasmin (α_2PI).

The plasminogen activators, tissue type plasminogen activator (tPA) and the urokinase type plasminogen activator (uPA), cleave the Arg560-Val561 bond of plasminogen to generate the active enzyme plasmin. The lysine-binding sites of plasmin (and plasminogen) permit it to bind to fibrin, so that physiologic fibrinolysis is "fibrin specific." Both plasminogen (through its lysine-binding sites) and tPA possess specific affinity for fibrin and thereby bind selectively to clots. The assembly of a ternary complex, consisting of fibrin, plasminogen, and tPA, promotes the localized interaction between plasminogen and tPA and greatly accelerates the rate of plasminogen activation to plasmin. Moreover, partial degradation of fibrin by plasmin exposes new plasminogen and tPA binding sites in carboxy-terminus lysine residues of fibrin fragments to enhance these reactions further. This creates a highly efficient mechanism to generate plasmin focally on the fibrin clot, which then becomes plasmin's substrate for digestion to fibrin degradation products.

Plasmin cleaves fibrin at distinct sites of the fibrin molecule leading to the generation of characteristic fibrin fragments during the process of fibrinolysis (Fig. 59-2). The sites of plasmin cleavage of fibrin are the same as those in fibrinogen. However, when plasmin acts on covalently cross-linked fibrin, D-dimers are released; hence, D-dimers can be measured in plasma as a relatively specific test of fibrin (rather than fibrinogen) degradation. D-Dimer assays can be used as sensitive markers of blood clot formation, and some have been validated for clinical use to exclude the diagnosis of deep venous thrombosis (DVT) and pulmonary embolism in selected populations.

Physiologic regulation of fibrinolysis occurs primarily at two levels: (1) plasminogen activator inhibitors (PAIs), specifically PAI1 and PAI2, inhibit the physiologic plasminogen activators; and (2) α_2 antiplasmin inhibits plasmin. PAI1 is the primary inhibitor of tPA and uPA in plasma. α_2 antiplasmin is the main inhibitor of plasmin in human plasma, inactivating any nonfibrin clot–associated plasmin.

APPROACH TO THE PATIENT: Bleeding and Thrombosis

CLINICAL PRESENTATION Disorders of hemostasis may be either inherited or acquired. A detailed personal and family history is key in determining the chronicity of symptoms and the likelihood of the disorder being inherited and it provides clues to underlying conditions that have contributed to the bleeding or thrombotic state. In addition, the history can give clues as to the etiology by determining (1) the bleeding (mucosal and/or joint) or thrombosis (arterial and/or venous) site, and (2) whether an underlying bleeding or clotting tendency was enhanced by another medical condition or the introduction of medications or dietary supplements.

History of Bleeding A history of bleeding is the most important predictor of bleeding risk. In evaluating a patient for a bleeding disorder, a history of at-risk situations, including the response to past surgeries, should be assessed. Does the patient have a history of spontaneous or trauma/surgery-induced bleeding? Spontaneous hemarthroses are a hallmark of moderate and severe factors VIII and IX deficiency and, in rare circumstances, of other clotting factor deficiencies. Mucosal bleeding symptoms are more suggestive of underlying platelet disorders or von Willebrand disease (vWD), termed *disorders of primary hemostasis or platelet plug formation*. Disorders affecting primary hemostasis are shown in Table 59-1.

The development of bruises (ecchymoses) after trauma is normal; however, an exaggerated response to trauma may be an indication of an underlying bleeding disorder. Ecchymoses presenting without known trauma, particularly on the trunk, and especially large ecchymoses, >2 in. in diameter, may be a sign of an underlying bleeding disorder. The introduction of medications or nutritional supplements with platelet inhibitory activity often enhance bruising and bleeding in a patient with an underlying bleeding disorder. Easy bruising can also be a sign of medical conditions in which there is no identifiable coagulopathy; instead, the conditions are caused by an abnormality of blood vessels or their supporting tissues. In Ehlers-Danlos syndrome there may be posttraumatic bleeding and a history of joint hyperextensibility. Cushing's syndrome, chronic steroid use, and aging result in changes in skin and subcutaneous tissue, and subcutaneous bleeding occurs in response to minor trauma. The latter has been termed *senile purpura*.

Epistaxis is a common symptom, particularly in children and in dry climates, and may not reflect an underlying bleeding disorder. However, it is the most common symptom in hereditary hemorrhagic telangiectasia and in boys with vWD. Clues that epistaxis is a symptom of an underlying bleeding disorder include lack of seasonal variation and bleeding that requires medical evaluation or treatment, including cauterization. Bleeding with eruption of primary teeth is seen in children with more severe bleeding disorders, such as moderate and severe hemophilia. It is uncommon in children with mild bleeding disorders. Patients with disorders of primary hemostasis (platelet adhesion) do have increased bleeding after dental cleanings and other procedures that involve gum manipulation.

Menorrhagia is defined quantitatively as a loss of >80 cc of blood per cycle, based on blood loss required to produce iron-deficiency anemia. A complaint of heavy menses is subjective and has a poor correlation with excessive blood loss. Predictors of menorrhagia include bleeding resulting in iron-deficiency anemia or a need for blood transfusion, excessive pad or tampon use, menses lasting longer than 8 days, passage of clots, bleeding through protection, or flooding at night. Menorrhagia is a common symptom in women with underlying bleeding disorders and is reported in the majority of women with vWD and factor XI deficiency and in symptomatic carriers of hemophilia A. Women with underlying bleeding disorders are more likely to have other bleeding symptoms, including bleeding after dental extractions, postoperative bleeding, and postpartum bleeding, and are much more likely to have menorrhagia beginning at menarche than women with menorrhagia due to other causes.

Postpartum hemorrhage is a common symptom in women with underlying bleeding disorders. This occurs most commonly in the first 48 h after delivery, but it may also be manifest by prolonged or excessive bleeding after discharge from the hospital. Women with a history of postpartum hemorrhage have a high risk of recurrence with subsequent pregnancies. Rupture of ovarian cysts with intra-abdominal hemorrhage has also been reported in women with underlying bleeding disorders.

Tonsillectomy is a major hemostatic challenge, as intact hemostatic mechanisms are essential to prevent excessive bleeding from the tonsillar bed. Bleeding may occur early after surgery or after approximately 7 days postoperatively, with loss of the eschar at the operative site. Similar delayed bleeding is seen after colonic polyp resection by cautery. Gastrointestinal (GI) bleeding and hematuria are usually due to underlying pathology and procedures to identify and treat the bleeding site should be undertaken, even in patients with known bleeding disorders. vWD, particularly types 2 and 3, has been associated with angiodysplasia of the bowel and GI bleeding.

TABLE 59-1 PRIMARY HEMOSTATIC (PLATELET PLUG) DISORDERS

Defects of Platelet Adhesion
von Willebrand disease
Bernard-Soulier syndrome (absence of dysfunction of GpIb-IX-V)
Defects of Platelet Aggregation
Glanzmann's thrombasthenia (absence or dysfunction of GpIIbIIIa)
Afibrinogenemia
Defects of Platelet Secretion
Decreased cyclooxygenase activity
Drug-induced (aspirin, nonsteroidal anti-inflammatory agents)
Inherited
Granule storage pool defects
Inherited
Acquired
Nonspecific drug effects
Uremia
Platelet coating (e.g., paraprotein, penicillin)
Defect of platelet coagulant activity
Scott's syndrome

Hemarthroses and spontaneous muscle hematomas are characteristic of moderate or severe congenital factor VIII or IX deficiency. They can also be seen in moderate and severe deficiencies of fibrinogen, prothrombin, and of factors V, VII, and X. Spontaneous hemarthroses occur rarely in other bleeding disorders except for severe vWD, with associated FVIII levels <5%. Muscle and soft tissue bleeds are also common in acquired FVIII deficiency. Bleeding into a joint results in severe pain and swelling, as well as loss of function, but is rarely associated with discoloration from bruising around the joint. Life-threatening sites of bleeding include bleeding into the oropharynx, where bleeding can obstruct the airway, into the central nervous system, and into the retroperitoneum. Central nervous system bleeding is the major cause of bleeding-related deaths in patients with severe congenital factor deficiencies.

Prohemorrhagic Effects of Medications and Dietary Supplements Aspirin and other nonsteroidal anti-inflammatory drugs (NSAIDs) that inhibit cyclooxygenase 1 impair primary hemostasis and may exacerbate bleeding from another cause or even unmask a previously occult mild bleeding disorder such as vWD. All NSAIDs, however, can precipitate gastrointestinal bleeding, which may be more severe in patients with underlying bleeding disorders. The aspirin effect on platelet function as assessed by aggregometry can persist for up to 7 days, although it has frequently returned to normal by 3 days after the last dose. The effect of other NSAIDs is shorter, as the inhibitor effect is reversed when the drug is removed.

Many herbal supplements can impair hemostatic function (Table 59-2). Some have been more convincingly associated with a bleeding risk than others. Fish oil or concentrated omega 3 fatty acid supplements impair platelet activation. They alter platelet biochemistry to produce more PGI3, a more potent platelet inhibitor than prostacyclin (PGI2), and more thromboxane A3, a less potent platelet activator than thromboxane A2. In fact, diets naturally rich in omega 3 fatty acids can result in a prolonged bleeding time and abnormal platelet aggregation studies, but the actual associated bleeding risk is unclear. Vitamin E appears to inhibit protein kinase C–mediated platelet aggregation and nitric oxide production. In patients with unexplained bruising or bleeding, it is prudent to review any new medications or supplements and discontinue those that may be associated with bleeding.

Underlying Systemic Diseases That Cause or Exacerbate a Bleeding Tendency Acquired bleeding disorders are commonly secondary to, or associated with, systemic disease. The clinical evaluation of a patient with a bleeding tendency must therefore include a thorough

TABLE 59-2 HERBAL SUPPLEMENTS ASSOCIATED WITH INCREASED BLEEDING

Herbs with Potential Anti-Platelet Activity
- Ginkgo (*Ginkgo biloba L.*)
- Garlic (*Allium sativum*)
- Bilberry (*Vaccinium myrtillus*)
- Ginger (*Gingiber officinale*)
- Dong quai (*Angelica sinensis*)
- Feverfew (*Tanacetum parthenium*)
- Asian Ginseng (*Panax ginseng*)
- American Ginseng (*Panax quinquefolius*)
- Siberian ginseng/eleuthero (*Eleutherococcus senticosus*)
- Tumeric (*Circuma longa*)
- Meadowsweet (*Filipendula ulmaria*)
- Willow (*Salix* spp.)

Coumarin-Containing Herbs
- Motherworth (*Leonurus cardiaca*)
- Chamomile (*Matricaria recutita, Chamaemelum mobile*)
- Horse chestnut (*Aesculus hippocastanum*)
- Red clover (*Trifolium pratense*)
- Fenugreek (*Trigonella foenum-graecum*)

assessment for evidence of underlying disease. Bruising or mucosal bleeding may be the presenting complaint in liver disease, severe renal impairment, hypothyroidism, paraproteinemias or amyloidosis, and conditions causing bone marrow failure. All coagulation factors are synthesized in the liver and hepatic failure results in combined factor deficiencies. This is often compounded by thrombocytopenia from splenomegaly due to portal hypertension. Coagulation factors II, VII, IX, X and proteins C, S, and Z are dependent on vitamin K for posttranslational modification. Although Vitamin K is required in both procoagulant and anticoagulant processes, the phenotype of vitamin K deficiency or the warfarin effect on coagulation is bleeding.

The normal blood platelet count is 150,000–450,000/μL. Thrombocytopenia results from decreased production, increased destruction, and/or sequestration. Although the bleeding risk varies somewhat by the reason for the thrombocytopenia, bleeding rarely occurs in isolated thrombocytopenia at counts <50,000/μL and usually not until <10,000–20,000/μL. Coexisting coagulopathies, as seen in liver failure or disseminated coagulation; infection; platelet-inhibitory drugs; and underlying medical conditions can all increase the risk of bleeding in the thrombocytopenic patient. Most procedures can be performed in patients with a platelet count of 50,000/μL. The level needed for major surgery will depend on the type of surgery and the patients' underlying medical state, although a count of approximately 80,000/μL is likely sufficient.

History of Thrombosis The risk of thrombosis, like that of bleeding, is influenced by both genetic and environmental influences. The major risk factor for arterial thrombosis is atherosclerosis, while those for venous thrombosis are immobility, surgery, underlying medical conditions such as malignancy, medications such as hormonal therapy, obesity, and genetic predispositions. Factors that increase risks for venous and both venous and arterial thromboses are shown in Table 59-3.

The most important point in a history related to venous thrombosis is whether the thrombotic event was idiopathic (meaning there was no clear precipitating factor) or was a precipitated event. In patients without underlying malignancy, having an idiopathic event is the strongest predictor of recurrence of venous thromboembolism. In patients who have a vague history of thrombosis, a history of being treated with warfarin suggests a past DVT. Age is an important risk factor for venous thrombosis; the risk of DVT increases per decade, with an approximate incidence of 1/100,000 per year in early childhood to 1/200 per year among octogenarians. Family history is helpful in determining if there is a genetic predisposition and how strong that predisposition appears to be.

A genetic thrombophilia that confers a relatively small increased risk, such as being a heterozygote for the prothrombin G20210A or factor V Leiden mutation, may be a relatively minor determinant of

TABLE 59-3 RISK FACTORS FOR THROMBOSIS

Venous	Venous and Arterial
Inherited	Inherited
Factor V Leiden	Homocystinuria
Prothrombin G20210A	Dysfibrinogenemia
Antithrombin deficiency	
Protein C deficiency	Mixed (inherited and acquired)
Protein S deficiency	Hyperhomocysteinemia
Elevated FVIII	
	Acquired
Acquired	Malignancy
Age	Antiphospholipid antibody syndrome
Previous thrombosis	Hormonal therapy
Immobilization	Polycythemia vera
Major surgery	Essential thrombocythemia
Pregnancy & puerperium	Paroxysmal nocturnal hemoglobinuria
Hospitalization	Thrombotic thrombocytopenic purpura
Obesity	
Infection	Heparin-induced thrombocytopenia
APC resistance, nongenetic	Disseminated intravascular coagulation
Unknown[a]	
Elevated factor II, IX, XI	
Elevated TAFI levels	
Low levels of TFPI	

[a]Unknown whether risk is inherited or acquired.
Note: APC, activated protein C; TAFI, thrombin-activatable fibrinolysis inhibitor; TFPI, tissue factor pathway inhibitor.

risk in an elderly individual undergoing a high risk surgical procedure. As shown in Fig. 59-5, a thrombotic event often has more than one contributing factor. Predisposing factors must be carefully assessed to determine the risk of recurrent thrombosis, and with consideration of the patient's bleeding risk, determine the length of anticoagulation. Similar consideration should be given to determining the need to test the patient and family members for genetic thrombophilias.

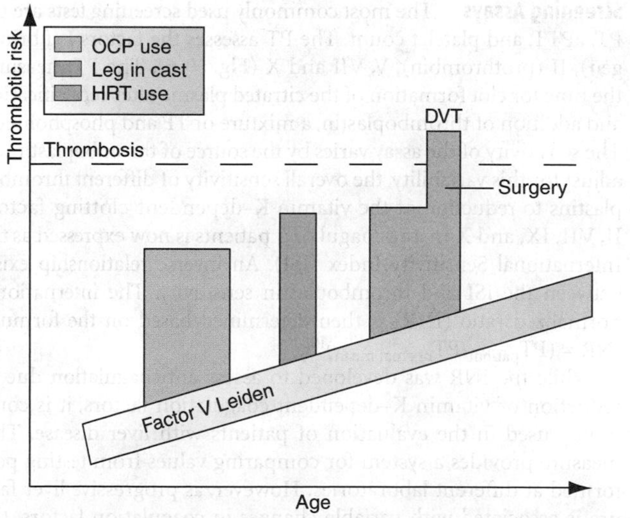

FIGURE 59-5 Thrombotic risk over time. Shown schematically is an individual's thrombotic risk over time. An underlying Factor V Leiden mutation provides a "theoretically" constant increased risk. The thrombotic risk increases with age and, intermittently, with oral contraceptive (OCP) or hormone replacement (HRT) use; other events may increase the risk further. At some point the cumulative risk may increase to the threshold for thrombosis and result in deep venous thrombosis (DVT). Note: The magnitude and duration of risk portrayed in the figure is meant for example only and may not precisely reflect the relative risk determined by clinical study. *[From BA Konkle, A Schafer, in DP Zipes et al (eds): Braunwald's Heart Disease, 7th ed. Philadelphia, Saunders, 2005; modified with permission from FR Rosendaal: Venous thrombosis: A multicausal disease. Lancet 353:1167, 1999.]*

LABORATORY EVALUATION Careful history taking and clinical examination are essential components in the assessment of bleeding and thrombotic risk. The use of laboratory tests of coagulation complement, but cannot substitute for, clinical assessment. No test provides a global assessment of hemostasis. The bleeding time has been used to assess bleeding risk; however, it does not predict bleeding risk with surgery and is not recommended for this indication. The PFA-100, an instrument that measures platelet-dependent coagulation under flow conditions, is more sensitive and specific for platelet disorders and vWD than the bleeding time; however, it is not sensitive enough to rule out underlying mild bleeding disorders. Also, it has not been evaluated prospectively to determine its utility in predicting bleeding risk, although such studies are underway.

For routine preoperative and preprocedure testing, an abnormal prothrombin time (PT) may detect liver disease or vitamin K deficiency that had not been previously appreciated. Studies have not confirmed the usefulness of an activated partial thromboplastin time (aPTT) in preoperative evaluations in patients with a negative bleeding history. The primary use of coagulation testing should be to confirm the presence and type of bleeding disorder in a patient with a suspicious clinical history.

Because of the nature of coagulation assays, proper sample acquisition and handling is critical to obtaining valid results. In patients with abnormal coagulation assays who have no bleeding history, repeat studies with attention to these factors frequently results in normal values. Most coagulation assays are performed in sodium citrate anticoagulated plasma that is recalcified for the assay. Because the anticoagulant is in liquid solution and needs to be added to blood in proportion to the plasma volume, incorrectly filled or inadequately mixed blood collection tubes will give erroneous results. Vacutainer tubes should be filled to >90% of the recommended fill, which is usually denoted by a line on the tube. An elevated hematocrit (>55%) can result in a false value due to a decreased plasma to anticoagulant ratio.

Screening Assays The most commonly used screening tests are the PT, aPTT, and platelet count. The PT assesses the factors I (fibrinogen), II (prothrombin), V, VII and X (Fig. 59-6). The PT measures the time for clot formation of the citrated plasma after recalcification and addition of thromboplastin, a mixture of TF and phospholipids. The sensitivity of the assay varies by the source of thromboplastin. To adjust for this variability, the overall sensitivity of different thromboplastins to reduction of the vitamin K–dependent clotting factors II, VII, IX, and X in anticoagulated patients is now expressed as the International Sensitivity Index (ISI). An inverse relationship exists between the ISI and thromboplastin sensitivity. The international normalized ratio (INR) is then determined based on the formula: $INR = (PT_{patient}/PT_{normal\ mean})^{ISI}$.

While the INR was developed to assess anticoagulation due to reduction of vitamin K–dependent coagulation factors, it is commonly used in the evaluation of patients with liver disease. This measure provides a system for comparing values from testing performed at different laboratories. However, as progressive liver failure is associated with variable changes in coagulation factors, the degree of prolongation of either the PT or the INR only roughly predicts the bleeding risk. Thrombin generation has been shown to be normal in many patients with mild to moderate liver dysfunction. As the PT only measures one aspect of hemostasis affected by liver dysfunction, we likely overestimate the bleeding risk of a mildly elevated INR in this setting.

The aPTT assesses the intrinsic and common coagulation pathways, factors XI, IX, VIII, X, V, II, fibrinogen, and also prekallikrein, high molecular weight kininogen and factor XII (Fig. 59-6). The aPTT reagent contains phospholipids derived from either animal or vegetable sources that function as a platelet substitute in the coagulation pathways and includes an activator of the intrinsic coagulation system, such as ellagic acid or the particulate activators kaolin, celite, or micronized silica.

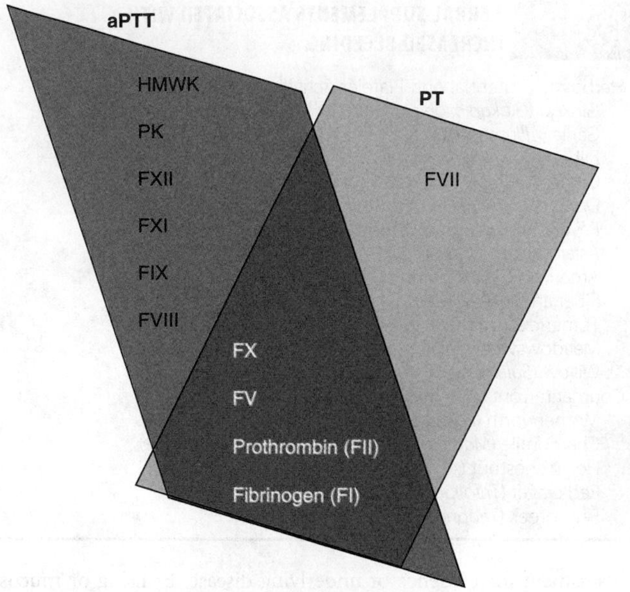

FIGURE 59-6 Coagulation factor activity tested in the activated partial thromboplastin time (aPTT) in red and prothrombin time (PT) in green, or both. HMWK, high-molecular-weight kininogen; PK, prekallikrein; F, factor.

The phospholipid composition of aPTT reagents varies, which influences the sensitivity of individual reagents to clotting factor deficiencies and to inhibitors such as heparin and lupus anticoagulants. Thus, aPTT results will vary from one laboratory to another, and the normal range in the laboratory where the testing occurs should be used in the interpretation. Local laboratories can relate their aPTT values to therapeutic heparin anticoagulation by correlating aPTT values with direct measurements of heparin activity (anti-Xa or protamine titration assays) in samples from heparinized patients, although correlation between these assays is often poor. The aPTT reagent will vary in sensitivity to individual factor deficiencies and usually becomes prolonged with individual factor deficiencies of 30–50%. The relationship between defects in secondary hemostasis (fibrin formation) and coagulation test abnormalities is shown in Table 59-4.

Mixing Studies Mixing studies are used to evaluate a prolonged aPTT or, less commonly PT, to distinguish between a factor deficiency and an inhibitor. In this assay, normal plasma and patient plasma are mixed in a 50:50 ratio, and the aPTT or PT is determined immediately and after incubation at 37°C for varying times, typically 30, 60, and/or 120 min. With isolated factor deficiencies, the aPTT will correct with mixing and stay corrected with incubation. With aPTT prolongation due to a lupus anticoagulant, the mixing and incubation will show no correction. In acquired neutralizing factor antibodies, such as an acquired factor VIII inhibitor, the initial assay may or may not correct immediately after mixing but will prolong or remain prolonged with incubation at 37°C. Failure to correct with mixing can also be due to the presence of other inhibitors or interfering substances such as heparin, fibrin split products, and paraproteins.

Specific Factor Assays Decisions to proceed with specific clotting factor assays will be influenced by the clinical situation and the results of coagulation screening tests. Precise diagnosis and effective management of inherited and acquired coagulation deficiencies necessitate quantitation of the relevant factors. When bleeding is severe, specific assays are often urgently required to guide appropriate therapy. Individual factor assays are usually performed as modifications of the mixing study, where the patient's plasma is

TABLE 59-4 HEMOSTATIC DISORDERS AND COAGULATION TEST ABNORMALITIES

Prolonged activated partial thromboplastin time (aPTT)
- No clinical bleeding – ↓ factors XII, high-molecular-weight kininogen, protein kinase
- Variable, but usually mild, bleeding – ↓ factor XI, mild ↓ FVIII and FIX
- Frequent, severe bleeding – severe deficiencies of FVIII and FIX
- Heparin

Prolonged prothrombin time (PT)
- Factor VII deficiency
- Vitamin K deficiency – early
- Warfarin anticoagulation

Prolonged aPTT and PT
- Factor II, V or X deficiency
- Vitamin K deficiency – late
- Direct thrombin inhibitors

Prolonged thrombin time
- Heparin or heparin-like inhibitors
- Mild or no bleeding – dysfibrinogenemia
- Frequent, severe bleeding – afibrinogenemia

Prolonged PT and/or aPTT not correct with mixing with normal plasma
- Bleeding – specific factor inhibitor
- No symptoms, or clotting and/or pregnancy loss – lupus anticoagulant
- Disseminated intravascular coagulation
- Heparin or direct thrombin inhibitor

Abnormal clot solubility
- Factor XIII deficiency
- Inhibitors or defective cross-linking

Rapid clot lysis
- Deficiency of α_2-antiplasmin or plasminogen activator inhibitor 1
- Treatment with fibrinolytic therapy

mixed with plasma deficient in the factor being studied. This will correct all factor deficiencies to >50%, thus making prolongation of clot formation due to a factor deficiency dependent on the factor missing from the added plasma.

Testing for Antiphospholipid Antibodies Antibodies to phospholipids (cardiolipin) or phospholipid-binding proteins (β_2-microglobulin and others) are detected by ELISA. When these antibodies interfere with phospholipid-dependent coagulation tests, they are termed *lupus anticoagulants.* The aPTT has variable sensitivity to lupus anticoagulants, depending in part on the aPTT reagents used. An assay utilizing a sensitive reagent has been termed an *LA-PTT*. The dilute Russell Viper Venom test (dRVVT) and the tissue thromboplastin time (TTI) are modifications of standard tests with the phospholipid reagent decreased, thus increasing the sensitivity to antibodies that interfere with the phospholipid component. The tests, however, are not specific for lupus anticoagulants, as factor deficiencies or other inhibitors also result in prolongation. Documentation of a lupus anticoagulant requires not only prolongation of a phospholipid-dependent coagulation test but also lack of correction when mixed with normal plasma and correction with the addition of activated platelet membranes or certain phospholipids, e.g., hexagonal phase.

Other Coagulation Tests The thrombin time and the reptilase time measure fibrinogen conversion to fibrin and are prolonged when the fibrinogen level is low (usually <80–100 mg/dL); qualitatively abnormal, as seen in inherited or acquired dysfibrinogenemias; or when fibrin/fibrinogen degradation products interfere. The thrombin time, but not the reptilase time, is prolonged in the presence of heparin. Measurement of anti-factor Xa plasma inhibitory activity is a test frequently used to assess low-molecular-weight heparin (LMWH) activity or as a direct measurement of unfractionated heparin (UFH) activity. Heparin in the patient sample inhibits the enzymatic conversion of an Xa-specific chromogenic substrate to colored product by factor Xa. Standard curves are created using multiple concentrations of UFH and LMWH and are used to calculate the concentration of anti-Xa activity in the patient plasma.

Laboratory Testing for Thrombophilia Laboratory assays to detect thrombophilic states include molecular diagnostic, immunologic and functional assays. These assays vary in their sensitivity and specificity for the condition being tested. Furthermore, acute thrombosis, acute illnesses, inflammatory conditions, pregnancy, and medications affect levels of many coagulation factors and their inhibitors. Antithrombin is decreased by heparin and in the setting of acute thrombosis. Protein C and S levels may be increased in the setting of acute thrombosis and are decreased by warfarin. Antiphospholipid antibodies are frequently transiently positive in acute illness. As thrombophilia evaluations are usually performed to assess the need to extend anticoagulation, testing should be performed in a steady state, remote from the acute event. In most instances warfarin anticoagulation can be stopped after the initial 3–6 months of treatment, and testing is performed at least 3 weeks later. Furthermore, sensitive markers of coagulation activation, notably the D-dimer assay and the thrombin generation test, hold promise as predictors, when elevated, of recurrent thrombosis when measured at least 1 month from discontinuation of warfarin, although further study is needed to better support this application.

Measures of Platelet Function The bleeding time has been used to assess bleeding risk; however, it has not been found to predict bleeding risk with surgery, and it is not recommended for use for this indication. The PFA-100 and similar instruments that measure platelet-dependent coagulation under flow conditions are generally more sensitive and specific for platelet disorders and vWD than the bleeding time; however, data are insufficient to support their use to predict bleeding risk or monitor response to therapy. When they are used in the evaluation of a patient with bleeding symptoms, abnormal results, as with the bleeding time, require specific testing, such as vWF assays and/or platelet aggregation studies. Since all of these "screening" assays may miss patients with mild bleeding disorders, further studies are needed to define their role in hemostasis testing.

For classic platelet aggregometry, various agonists are added to the patient's platelet-rich plasma, and platelet agglutination and aggregation are observed. Tests of platelet secretion in response to agonists can also be measured. These tests are affected by many factors, including numerous medications, and the association between minor defects in aggregation or secretion in these assays and bleeding risk is not clearly established.

ACKNOWLEDGMENT
Robert I. Handin, MD, contributed this chapter in the 16th edition and some material from that chapter have been retained here.

FURTHER READINGS

BAUER KA: Management of thrombophilia. J Thromb Haemost 1:1429, 2003

BOCKENSTEDT PL: Laboratory methods in hemostasis, in *Thrombosis and Hemorrhage*, 3d ed, J Loscalzo, AI Schafer (eds). Philadelphia, Lippincott Williams & Wilkins, 2003, pp 363–423

COLMAN RW et al: Overview of hemostasis, in *Hemostasis and Thrombosis,* 5th ed, RW Colman et al (eds). Philadelphia, Lippincott Williams & Wilkins, 2006, pp 3–16

HEIT JA: The epidemiology of venous thromboembolism in the community: Implications for prevention and management. J Thromb Thrombol 21:23, 2006

KONKLE BA: Clinical approach to the bleeding patient, in *Hemostasis and Thrombosis,* 5th ed, RW Colman et al (eds). Philadelphia, Lippincott Williams & Wilkins, 2006, pp 1147–1158

ORTEL TL: The antiphospholipid syndrome: What are we really measuring? How do we measure it? And how do we treat it? J Thromb Thrombol 21:79, 2006

ROBERTS HR et al: A cell-based model of thrombin generation. Sem Thromb Hemost 32(Suppl 1):32, 2006

60 Enlargement of Lymph Nodes and Spleen

Patrick H. Henry, Dan L. Longo

This chapter is intended to serve as a guide to the evaluation of patients who present with enlargement of the lymph nodes (*lymphadenopathy*) or the spleen (*splenomegaly*). Lymphadenopathy is a rather common clinical finding in primary care settings, whereas palpable splenomegaly is less so.

LYMPHADENOPATHY

Lymphadenopathy may be an incidental finding in patients being examined for various reasons, or it may be a presenting sign or symptom of the patient's illness. The physician must eventually decide whether the lymphadenopathy is a normal finding or one that requires further study, up to and including biopsy. Soft, flat, submandibular nodes (<1 cm) are often palpable in healthy children and young adults, and healthy adults may have palpable inguinal nodes of up to 2 cm, which are considered normal. Further evaluation of these normal nodes is not warranted. In contrast, if the physician believes the node(s) to be abnormal, then pursuit of a more precise diagnosis is needed.

APPROACH TO THE PATIENT: Lymphadenopathy

Lymphadenopathy may be a primary or secondary manifestation of numerous disorders, as shown in Table 60-1. Many of these disorders are infrequent causes of lymphadenopathy. In primary care practice, more than two-thirds of patients with lymphadenopathy have nonspecific causes or upper respiratory illnesses (viral or bacterial), and <1% have a malignancy. In one study, 84% of patients referred for evaluation of lymphadenopathy had a "benign" diagnosis. The remaining 16% had a malignancy (lymphoma or metastatic adenocarcinoma). Of the patients with benign lymphadenopathy, 63% had a nonspecific or reactive etiology (no causative agent found), and the remainder had a specific cause demonstrated, most commonly infectious mononucleosis, toxoplasmosis, or tuberculosis. Thus, the vast majority of patients with lymphadenopathy will have a nonspecific etiology requiring few diagnostic tests.

CLINICAL ASSESSMENT The physician will be aided in the pursuit of an explanation for the lymphadenopathy by a careful medical history, physical examination, selected laboratory tests, and perhaps an excisional lymph node biopsy.

The *medical history* should reveal the setting in which lymphadenopathy is occurring. Symptoms such as sore throat, cough, fever, night sweats, fatigue, weight loss, or pain in the nodes should be sought. The patient's age, sex, occupation, exposure to pets, sexual behavior, and use of drugs such as diphenylhydantoin are other important historic points. For example, children and young adults usually have benign (i.e., nonmalignant) disorders, such as viral or bacterial upper respiratory infections, infectious mononucleosis, toxoplasmosis, and, in some countries, tuberculosis, which account for the observed lymphadenopathy. In contrast, after age 50 the incidence of malignant disorders increases and that of benign disorders decreases.

The *physical examination* can provide useful clues such as the extent of lymphadenopathy (localized or generalized), size of nodes, texture, presence or absence of nodal tenderness, signs of inflammation over the node, skin lesions, and splenomegaly. A thorough ear, nose, and throat (ENT) examination is indicated in adult patients with cervical adenopathy and a history of tobacco use. Localized or regional adenopathy implies involvement of a single anatomic area. Generalized adenopathy has been defined as involvement of three or more noncontiguous lymph node areas. Many of the causes of lymphadenopathy (Table 60-1) can produce localized *or* generalized adenopathy, so this distinction is of limited utility in the differential diagnosis. Nevertheless, generalized lymphadenopathy is frequently associated with nonmalignant disorders such as infectious mononucleosis [Epstein-Barr virus (EBV) or cytomegalovirus (CMV)], toxoplasmosis, AIDS, other viral infections, systemic lupus erythematosus (SLE), and mixed connective tissue disease. Acute and chronic lymphocytic leukemias and malignant lymphomas also produce generalized adenopathy in adults.

The site of localized or regional adenopathy may provide a useful clue about the cause. Occipital adenopathy often reflects an infection of the scalp, and preauricular adenopathy accompanies conjunctival infections and cat-scratch disease. The most frequent site of regional adenopathy is the neck, and most of the causes are benign—upper respiratory infections, oral and dental lesions, infectious mononucleosis, other viral illnesses. The chief malignant causes include metastatic cancer from head and neck, breast, lung, and thyroid primaries. Enlargement of supraclavicular and scalene

TABLE 60-1 DISEASES ASSOCIATED WITH LYMPHADENOPATHY

1. Infectious diseases
   a. Viral—infectious mononucleosis syndromes (EBV, CMV), infectious hepatitis, herpes simplex, herpesvirus-6, varicella-zoster virus, rubella, measles, adenovirus, HIV, epidemic keratoconjunctivitis, vaccinia, herpesvirus-8
   b. Bacterial—streptococci, staphylococci, cat-scratch disease, brucellosis, tularemia, plague, chancroid, melioidosis, glanders, tuberculosis, atypical mycobacterial infection, primary and secondary syphilis, diphtheria, leprosy
   c. Fungal—histoplasmosis, coccidioidomycosis, paracoccidioidomycosis
   d. Chlamydial—lymphogranuloma venereum, trachoma
   e. Parasitic—toxoplasmosis, leishmaniasis, trypanosomiasis, filariasis
   f. Rickettsial—scrub typhus, rickettsialpox, Q fever
2. Immunologic diseases
   a. Rheumatoid arthritis
   b. Juvenile rheumatoid arthritis
   c. Mixed connective tissue disease
   d. Systemic lupus erythematosus
   e. Dermatomyositis
   f. Sjögren's syndrome
   g. Serum sickness
   h. Drug hypersensitivity—diphenylhydantoin, hydralazine, allopurinol, primidone, gold, carbamazepine, etc.
   i. Angioimmunoblastic lymphadenopathy
   j. Primary biliary cirrhosis
   k. Graft-vs.-host disease
   l. Silicone-associated
   m. Autoimmune lymphoproliferative syndrome
3. Malignant diseases
   a. Hematologic—Hodgkin's disease, non-Hodgkin's lymphomas, acute or chronic lymphocytic leukemia, hairy cell leukemia, malignant histiocytosis, amyloidosis
   b. Metastatic—from numerous primary sites
4. Lipid storage diseases—Gaucher's, Niemann-Pick, Fabry, Tangier
5. Endocrine diseases—hyperthyroidism
6. Other disorders
   a. Castleman's disease (giant lymph node hyperplasia)
   b. Sarcoidosis
   c. Dermatopathic lymphadenitis
   d. Lymphomatoid granulomatosis
   e. Histiocytic necrotizing lymphadenitis (Kikuchi's disease)
   f. Sinus histiocytosis with massive lymphadenopathy (Rosai-Dorfman disease)
   g. Mucocutaneous lymph node syndrome (Kawasaki's disease)
   h. Histiocytosis X
   i. Familial mediterranean fever
   j. Severe hypertriglyceridemia
   k. Vascular transformation of sinuses
   l. Inflammatory pseudotumor of lymph node
   m. Congestive heart failure

Note: EBV, Epstein-Barr virus; CMV, cytomegalovirus.

nodes is always abnormal. Because these nodes drain regions of the lung and retroperitoneal space, they can reflect lymphomas, other cancers, or infectious processes arising in these areas. Virchow's node is an enlarged left supraclavicular node infiltrated with metastatic cancer from a gastrointestinal primary. Metastases to supraclavicular nodes also occur from lung, breast, testis, or ovarian cancers. Tuberculosis, sarcoidosis, and toxoplasmosis are nonneoplastic causes of supraclavicular adenopathy. Axillary adenopathy is usually due to injuries or localized infections of the ipsilateral upper extremity. Malignant causes include melanoma or lymphoma and, in women, breast cancer. Inguinal lymphadenopathy is usually secondary to infections or trauma of the lower extremities and may accompany sexually transmitted diseases such as lymphogranuloma venereum, primary syphilis, genital herpes, or chancroid. These nodes may also be involved by lymphomas and metastatic cancer from primary lesions of the rectum, genitalia, or lower extremities (melanoma).

The size and texture of the lymph node(s) and the presence of pain are useful parameters in evaluating a patient with lymphadenopathy. Nodes $<1.0\ cm^2$ in area (1.0 cm × 1.0 cm or less) are almost always secondary to benign, nonspecific reactive causes. In one retrospective analysis of younger patients (9–25 years) who had a lymph node biopsy, a maximum diameter of >2 cm served as one discriminant for predicting that the biopsy would reveal malignant or granulomatous disease. Another study showed that a lymph node size of $2.25\ cm^2$ (1.5 cm × 1.5 cm) was the best size limit for distinguishing malignant or granulomatous lymphadenopathy from other causes of lymphadenopathy. Patients with node(s) $\leq 1.0\ cm^2$ should be observed after excluding infectious mononucleosis and/or toxoplasmosis unless there are symptoms and signs of an underlying systemic illness.

The texture of lymph nodes may be described as soft, firm, rubbery, hard, discrete, matted, tender, movable, or fixed. Tenderness is found when the capsule is stretched during rapid enlargement, usually secondary to an inflammatory process. Some malignant diseases such as acute leukemia may produce rapid enlargement and pain in the nodes. Nodes involved by lymphoma tend to be large, discrete, symmetric, rubbery, firm, mobile, and nontender. Nodes containing metastatic cancer are often hard, nontender, and nonmovable because of fixation to surrounding tissues. The coexistence of splenomegaly in the patient with lymphadenopathy implies a systemic illness such as infectious mononucleosis, lymphoma, acute or chronic leukemia, SLE, sarcoidosis, toxoplasmosis, cat-scratch disease, or other less common hematologic disorders. The patient's story should provide helpful clues about the underlying systemic illness.

Nonsuperficial presentations (thoracic or abdominal) of adenopathy are usually detected as the result of a symptom-directed diagnostic workup. Thoracic adenopathy may be detected by routine chest radiography or during the workup for superficial adenopathy. It may also be found because the patient complains of a cough or wheezing from airway compression; hoarseness from recurrent laryngeal nerve involvement; dysphagia from esophageal compression; or swelling of the neck, face, or arms secondary to compression of the superior vena cava or subclavian vein. The differential diagnosis of mediastinal and hilar adenopathy includes primary lung disorders and systemic illnesses that characteristically involve mediastinal or hilar nodes. In the young, mediastinal adenopathy is associated with infectious mononucleosis and sarcoidosis. In endemic regions, histoplasmosis can cause unilateral paratracheal lymph node involvement that mimics lymphoma. Tuberculosis can also cause unilateral adenopathy. In older patients, the differential diagnosis includes primary lung cancer (especially among smokers), lymphomas, metastatic carcinoma (usually lung), tuberculosis, fungal infection, and sarcoidosis.

Enlarged intraabdominal or retroperitoneal nodes are usually malignant. Although tuberculosis may present as mesenteric lymphadenitis, these masses usually contain lymphomas or, in young men, germ cell tumors.

LABORATORY INVESTIGATION The laboratory investigation of patients with lymphadenopathy must be tailored to elucidate the etiology suspected from the patient's history and physical findings. One study from a family practice clinic evaluated 249 younger patients with "enlarged lymph nodes, not infected" or "lymphadenitis." No laboratory studies were obtained in 51%. When studies were performed, the most common were a complete blood count (CBC) (33%), throat culture (16%), chest x-ray (12%), or monospot test (10%). Only eight patients (3%) had a node biopsy, and half of those were normal or reactive. The CBC can provide useful data for the diagnosis of acute or chronic leukemias, EBV or CMV mononucleosis, lymphoma with a leukemic component, pyogenic infections, or immune cytopenias in illnesses such as SLE. Serologic studies may demonstrate antibodies specific to components of EBV, CMV, HIV, and other viruses; *Toxoplasma gondii*; *Brucella*; etc. If SLE is suspected, then antinuclear and anti-DNA antibody studies are warranted.

The chest x-ray is usually negative, but the presence of a pulmonary infiltrate or mediastinal lymphadenopathy would suggest tuberculosis, histoplasmosis, sarcoidosis, lymphoma, primary lung cancer, or metastatic cancer and demands further investigation.

A variety of imaging techniques (CT, MRI, ultrasound, color Doppler ultrasonography) have been employed to differentiate benign from malignant lymph nodes, especially in patients with head and neck cancer. CT and MRI are comparably accurate (65–90%) in the diagnosis of metastases to cervical lymph nodes. Ultrasonography has been used to determine the long (L) axis, short (S) axis, and a ratio of long to short axis in cervical nodes. An L/S ratio of <2.0 has a sensitivity and a specificity of 95% for distinguishing benign and malignant nodes in patients with head and neck cancer. This ratio has greater specificity and sensitivity than palpation or measurement of either the long or the short axis alone.

The indications for lymph node biopsy are imprecise, yet it is a valuable diagnostic tool. The decision to biopsy may be made early in a patient's evaluation or delayed for up to 2 weeks. Prompt biopsy should occur if the patient's history and physical findings suggest a malignancy; examples include a solitary, hard, nontender cervical node in an older patient who is a chronic user of tobacco; supraclavicular adenopathy; and solitary or generalized adenopathy that is firm, movable, and suggestive of lymphoma. If a primary head and neck cancer is suspected as the basis of a solitary, hard cervical node, then a careful ENT examination should be performed. Any mucosal lesion that is suspicious for a primary neoplastic process should be biopsied first. If no mucosal lesion is detected, an excisional biopsy of the largest node should be performed. Fine-needle aspiration should not be performed as the first diagnostic procedure. Most diagnoses require more tissue than such aspiration can provide, and it often delays a definitive diagnosis. Fine-needle aspiration should be reserved for thyroid nodules and for confirmation of relapse in patients whose primary diagnosis is known. If the primary physician is uncertain about whether to proceed to biopsy, consultation with a hematologist or medical oncologist should be helpful. In primary care practices, <5% of lymphadenopathy patients will require a biopsy. That percentage will be considerably larger in referral practices, i.e., hematology, oncology, or ENT.

Two groups have reported algorithms that they claim will identify more precisely those lymphadenopathy patients who should have a biopsy. Both reports were retrospective analyses in referral practices. The first study involved patients 9–25 years of age who had a node biopsy performed. Three variables were identified that predicted those young patients with peripheral lymphadenopathy who should undergo biopsy; lymph node size >2 cm in diameter and abnormal chest x-ray had positive predictive values, whereas recent ENT symptoms had negative predictive values. The second study evaluated 220 lymphadenopathy patients in a hematology unit and identified five variables [lymph node size, location (supraclavicular or nonsupraclavicular), age (>40 years or <40 years), texture (nonhard or hard), and tenderness] that were utilized in a mathematical model to identify those patients requiring a biopsy. Positive predictive value was found for age >40 years, supraclavicular location, node size >2.25 cm^2, hard texture, and lack of pain or tenderness. Negative predictive value was evident for age <40 years, node size <1.0 cm^2, nonhard texture, and tender or painful nodes. Ninety-one percent of those who required biopsy were correctly classified by this model. Since both of these studies were retrospective analyses and one was limited to young patients, it is not known how useful these models would be if applied prospectively in a primary care setting.

Most lymphadenopathy patients do not require a biopsy, and at least half require no laboratory studies. If the patient's history and physical findings point to a benign cause for lymphadenopathy, then careful follow-up at a 2- to 4-week interval can be employed. The patient should be instructed to return for reevaluation if the node(s) increase in size. Antibiotics are not indicated for lymphadenopathy unless strong evidence of a bacterial infection is present. Glucocorticoids should not be used to treat lymphadenopathy because their lympholytic effect obscures some diagnoses (lymphoma, leukemia, Castleman's disease) and they contribute to delayed healing or activation of underlying infections. An exception to this statement is the life-threatening pharyngeal obstruction by enlarged lymphoid tissue in Waldeyer's ring that is occasionally seen in infectious mononucleosis.

SPLENOMEGALY

STRUCTURE AND FUNCTION OF THE SPLEEN

The spleen is a reticuloendothelial organ that has its embryologic origin in the dorsal mesogastrium at about 5 weeks' gestation. It arises in a series of hillocks, migrates to its normal adult location in the left upper quadrant (LUQ), and is attached to the stomach via the gastrolienal ligament and to the kidney via the lienorenal ligament. When the hillocks fail to unify into a single tissue mass, accessory spleens may develop in around 20% of persons. The function of the spleen has been elusive. Galen believed it was the source of "black bile" or melancholia, and the word *hypochondria* (literally, beneath the ribs) and the idiom "to vent one's spleen" attest to the beliefs that the spleen had an important influence on the psyche and emotions. In humans its normal physiologic roles seem to be the following:

1. Maintenance of quality control over erythrocytes in the red pulp by removal of senescent and defective red blood cells. The spleen accomplishes this function through a unique organization of its parenchyma and vasculature (Fig. 60-1).
2. Synthesis of antibodies in the white pulp.
3. The removal of antibody-coated bacteria and antibody-coated blood cells from the circulation.

An increase in these normal functions may result in splenomegaly.

The spleen is composed of *red pulp* and *white pulp*, which are Malpighi's terms for the red blood–filled sinuses and reticuloendothelial cell–lined cords and the white lymphoid follicles arrayed within the red pulp matrix. The spleen is in the portal circulation. The reason for this is unknown but may relate to the fact that lower blood pressure allows less rapid flow and minimizes damage to normal erythrocytes. Blood flows into the spleen at a rate of about 150 mL/min through the splenic artery, which ultimately ramifies into central arterioles. Some blood goes from the arterioles to capillaries and then to splenic veins and out of the spleen, but the majority of blood from central arterioles flows into the macrophage-lined sinuses and cords. The blood entering the sinuses reenters the circulation through the splenic venules, but the blood entering the cords is subjected to an inspection of sorts.

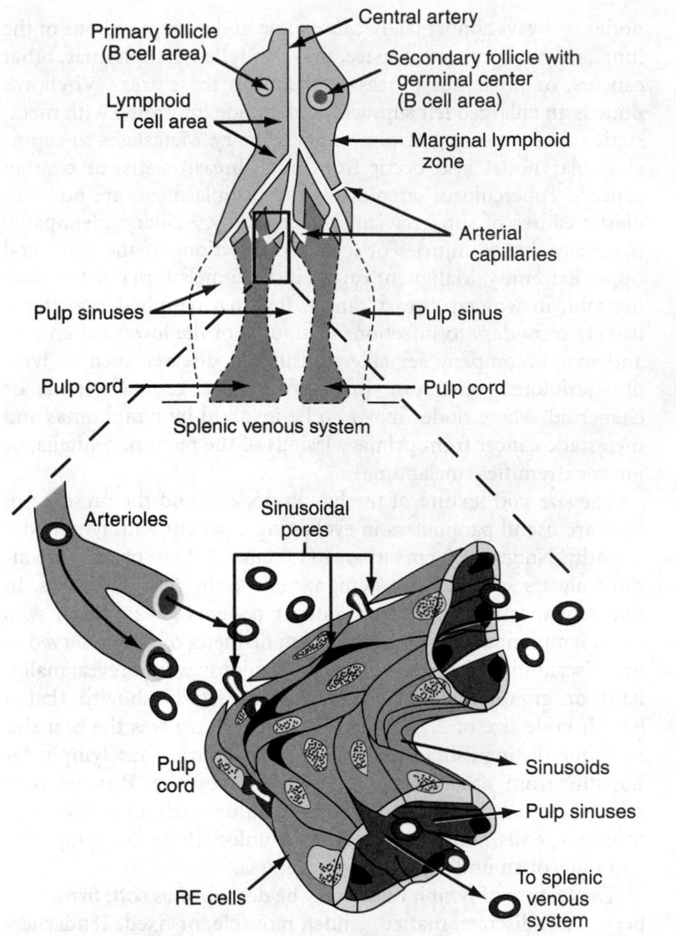

FIGURE 60-1 Schematic spleen structure. The spleen comprises many units of red and white pulp centered around small branches of the splenic artery, called *central arteries*. White pulp is lymphoid in nature and contains B cell follicles, a marginal zone around the follicles, and T cell–rich areas sheathing arterioles. The red pulp areas include pulp sinuses and pulp cords. The cords are dead ends. In order to regain access to the circulation, red blood cells must traverse tiny openings in the sinusoidal lining. Stiff, damaged, or old red cells cannot enter the sinuses. *(Top portion of figure from CA Janeway et al: Immunobiology, 5th ed., New York, Garland, 2001; bottom portion of figure from RS Hillman, KA Ault: Hematology in Clinical Practice, 4th ed. New York, McGraw-Hill, 2005.)*

In order to return to the circulation, the blood cells in the cords must squeeze through slits in the cord lining to enter the sinuses that lead to the venules. Old and damaged erythrocytes are less deformable and are retained in the cords, where they are destroyed and their components recycled. Red cell inclusion bodies such as parasites (Chap. 203 and **e18**), nuclear residua (Howell-Jolly bodies, Fig. 58-6), or denatured hemoglobin (Heinz bodies) are pinched off in the process of passing through the slits, a process called *pitting*. The culling of dead and damaged cells and the pitting of cells with inclusions appear to occur without significant delay since the blood transit time through the spleen is only slightly slower than in other organs.

The spleen is also capable of assisting the host in adapting to its hostile environment. It has at least three adaptive functions: (1) clearance of bacteria and particulates from the blood, (2) the generation of immune responses to certain pathogens, and (3) the generation of cellular components of the blood under circumstances in which the marrow is unable to meet the needs (i.e., extramedullary hematopoiesis). The latter adaptation is a recapitulation of the blood-forming function the spleen plays during gestation. In some animals, the spleen also serves a role in the vascular adaptation to stress because it stores red blood cells (often hemoconcentrated to higher hematocrits than normal) under normal circumstances and contracts under the influence of β-adrenergic stimulation to provide the animal with an autotransfusion and improved oxygen-carrying capacity. However, the normal human spleen does not sequester or store red blood cells and does not contract in response to sympathetic stimuli. The normal human spleen contains approximately one-third of the total body platelets and a significant number of marginated neutrophils. These sequestered cells are available when needed to respond to bleeding or infection.

APPROACH TO THE PATIENT: Splenomegaly

CLINICAL ASSESSMENT The most common *symptoms* produced by diseases involving the spleen are pain and a heavy sensation in the LUQ. Massive splenomegaly may cause early satiety. Pain may result from acute swelling of the spleen with stretching of the capsule, infarction, or inflammation of the capsule. For many years it was believed that splenic infarction was clinically silent, which at times is true. However, Soma Weiss, in his classic 1942 report of the self-observations by a Harvard medical student on the clinical course of subacute bacterial endocarditis, documented that severe LUQ and pleuritic chest pain may accompany thromboembolic occlusion of splenic blood flow. Vascular occlusion, with infarction and pain, is commonly seen in children with sickle cell crises. Rupture of the spleen, from either trauma or infiltrative disease that breaks the capsule, may result in intraperitoneal bleeding, shock, and death. The rupture itself may be painless.

A palpable spleen is the major *physical sign* produced by diseases affecting the spleen and suggests enlargement of the organ. The normal spleen is said to weigh <250 g, decreases in size with age, normally lies entirely within the rib cage, has a maximum cephalocaudad diameter of 13 cm by ultrasonography or maximum length of 12 cm and/or width of 7 cm by radionuclide scan, and is usually not palpable. However, a palpable spleen was found in 3% of 2200 asymptomatic, male, freshman college students. Follow-up at 3 years revealed that 30% of those students still had a palpable spleen without any increase in disease prevalence. Ten-year follow-up found no evidence for lymphoid malignancies. Furthermore, in some tropical countries (e.g., New Guinea) the incidence of splenomegaly may reach 60%. Thus, the presence of a palpable spleen does not always equate with presence of disease. Even when disease is present, splenomegaly may not reflect the primary disease but rather a reaction to it. For example, in patients with Hodgkin's disease, only two-thirds of the palpable spleens show involvement by the cancer.

Physical examination of the spleen utilizes primarily the techniques of palpation and percussion. Inspection may reveal fullness in the LUQ that descends on inspiration, a finding associated with a massively enlarged spleen. Auscultation may reveal a venous hum or friction rub.

Palpation can be accomplished by bimanual palpation, ballotment, and palpation from above (Middleton maneuver). For bimanual palpation, which is at least as reliable as the other techniques, the patient is supine with flexed knees. The examiner's left hand is placed on the lower rib cage and pulls the skin toward the costal margin, allowing the fingertips of the right hand to feel the tip of the spleen as it descends while the patient inspires slowly, smoothly, and deeply. Palpation is begun with the right hand in the left lower quadrant with gradual movement toward the left costal margin, thereby identifying the lower edge of a massively enlarged spleen. When the spleen tip is felt, the finding is recorded as centimeters below the left costal margin at some arbitrary point, i.e., 10–15 cm, from the midpoint of the umbilicus or the xiphisternal junction. This allows other examiners to compare findings or the initial examiner to determine changes in size over time. Bimanual palpation in the right lateral decubitus position adds nothing to the supine examination.

Percussion for splenic dullness is accomplished with any of three techniques described by Nixon, Castell, or Barkun:

1. *Nixon's method*: The patient is placed on the right side so that the spleen lies above the colon and stomach. Percussion begins at the lower level of pulmonary resonance in the posterior axillary line and proceeds diagonally along a perpendicular line toward the lower midanterior costal margin. The upper border of dullness is normally 6–8 cm above the costal margin. Dullness >8 cm in an adult is presumed to indicate splenic enlargement.
2. *Castell's method*: With the patient supine, percussion in the lowest intercostal space in the anterior axillary line (8th or 9th) produces a resonant note if the spleen is normal in size. This is true during expiration or full inspiration. A dull percussion note on full inspiration suggests splenomegaly.
3. *Percussion of Traube's semilunar space*: The borders of Traube's space are the sixth rib superiorly, the left midaxillary line laterally, and the left costal margin inferiorly. The patient is supine with the left arm slightly abducted. During normal breathing, this space is percussed from medial to lateral margins, yielding a normal resonant sound. A dull percussion note suggests splenomegaly.

Studies comparing methods of percussion and palpation with a standard of ultrasonography or scintigraphy have revealed sensitivity of 56–71% for palpation and 59–82% for percussion. Reproducibility among examiners is better for palpation than percussion. Both techniques are less reliable in obese patients or patients who have just eaten. Thus, the physical examination techniques of palpation and percussion are imprecise at best. It has been suggested that the examiner perform percussion first and, if positive, proceed to palpation; if the spleen is palpable, then one can be reasonably confident that splenomegaly exists. However, not all LUQ masses are enlarged spleens; gastric or colon tumors and pancreatic or renal cysts or tumors can mimic splenomegaly.

The presence of an enlarged spleen can be more precisely determined, if necessary, by liver-spleen radionuclide scan, CT, MRI, or ultrasonography. The latter technique is the current procedure of choice for routine assessment of spleen size (normal = a maximum cephalocaudad diameter of 13 cm) because it has high sensitivity and specificity and is safe, noninvasive, quick, mobile, and less costly. Nuclear medicine scans are accurate, sensitive, and reliable but are costly, require greater time to generate data, and utilize immobile equipment. They have the advantage of demonstrating accessory splenic tissue. CT and MRI provide accurate determination of spleen size, but the equipment is immobile and the procedures are expensive. MRI appears to offer no advantage over CT. Changes in spleen structure such as mass lesions, infarcts, inhomogeneous infiltrates, and cysts are more readily assessed by CT, MRI, or ultrasonography. None of these techniques is very reliable in the detection of patchy infiltration (e.g., Hodgkin's disease).

DIFFERENTIAL DIAGNOSIS Many of the diseases associated with splenomegaly are listed in Table 60-2. They are grouped according to the presumed basic mechanisms responsible for organ enlargement:

1. Hyperplasia or hypertrophy related to a particular splenic function such as reticuloendothelial hyperplasia (work hypertrophy) in diseases such as hereditary spherocytosis or thalassemia syndromes that require removal of large numbers of defective red blood cells; immune hyperplasia in response to systemic infection (infectious mononucleosis, subacute bacterial endocarditis) or to immunologic diseases (immune thrombocytopenia, SLE, Felty's syndrome).
2. Passive congestion due to decreased blood flow from the spleen in conditions that produce portal hypertension (cirrhosis, Budd-Chiari syndrome, congestive heart failure).
3. Infiltrative diseases of the spleen (lymphomas, metastatic cancer, amyloidosis, Gaucher's disease, myeloproliferative disorders with extramedullary hematopoiesis).

TABLE 60-2 DISEASES ASSOCIATED WITH SPLENOMEGALY GROUPED BY PATHOGENIC MECHANISM

Enlargement Due to Increased Demand for Splenic Function	Enlargement Due to Abnormal Splenic or Portal Blood Flow
Reticuloendothelial system hyperplasia (for removal of defective erythrocytes)	Cirrhosis
Spherocytosis	Hepatic vein obstruction
Early sickle cell anemia	Portal vein obstruction, intrahepatic or extrahepatic
Ovalocytosis	Cavernous transformation of the portal vein
Thalassemia major	Splenic vein obstruction
Hemoglobinopathies	Splenic artery aneurysm
Paroxysmal nocturnal hemoglobinuria	Hepatic schistosomiasis
Pernicious anemia	Congestive heart failure
Immune hyperplasia	Hepatic echinococcosis
Response to infection (viral, bacterial, fungal, parasitic)	Portal hypertension (any cause including the above): "Banti's disease"
Infectious mononucleosis	
AIDS	**Infiltration of the Spleen**
Viral hepatitis	
Cytomegalovirus	*Intracellular or extracellular depositions*
Subacute bacterial endocarditis	Amyloidosis
Bacterial septicemia	Gaucher's disease
Congenital syphilis	Niemann-Pick disease
Splenic abscess	Tangier disease
Tuberculosis	Hurler's syndrome and other mucopolysaccharidoses
Histoplasmosis	Hyperlipidemias
Malaria	*Benign and malignant cellular infiltrations*
Leishmaniasis	Leukemias (acute, chronic, lymphoid, myeloid, monocytic)
Trypanosomiasis	Lymphomas
Ehrlichiosis	Hodgkin's disease
Disordered immunoregulation	Myeloproliferative syndromes (e.g., polycythemia vera, essential thrombocytosis)
Rheumatoid arthritis (Felty's syndrome)	Angiosarcomas
Systemic lupus erythematosus	Metastatic tumors (melanoma is most common)
Collagen vascular diseases	Eosinophilic granuloma
Serum sickness	Histiocytosis X
Immune hemolytic anemias	Hamartomas
Immune thrombocytopenias	Hemangiomas, fibromas, lymphangiomas
Immune neutropenias	Splenic cysts
Drug reactions	
Angioimmunoblastic lymphadenopathy	**Unknown Etiology**
Sarcoidosis	
Thyrotoxicosis (benign lymphoid hypertrophy)	Idiopathic splenomegaly
Interleukin 2 therapy	Berylliosis
Extramedullary hematopoiesis	Iron-deficiency anemia
Myelofibrosis	
Marrow damage by toxins, radiation, strontium	
Marrow infiltration by tumors, leukemias, Gaucher's disease	

The differential diagnostic possibilities are much fewer when the spleen is "massively enlarged," palpable more than 8 cm below the left costal margin or its drained weight is ≥1000 g (Table 60-3). The vast majority of such patients will have non-Hodgkin's lymphoma, chronic lymphocytic leukemia, hairy cell leukemia, chronic myelogenous leukemia, myelofibrosis with myeloid metaplasia, or polycythemia vera.

LABORATORY ASSESSMENT The major laboratory abnormalities accompanying splenomegaly are determined by the underlying systemic illness. Erythrocyte counts may be normal, decreased (thalassemia major syndromes, SLE, cirrhosis with portal hypertension), or increased (polycythemia vera). Granulocyte counts may be normal, decreased (Felty's syndrome, congestive splenomegaly, leukemias), or increased (infections or inflammatory disease, myeloproliferative disorders). Similarly, the platelet count may be normal, decreased when there is enhanced sequestration or destruction of platelets in an enlarged spleen (congestive splenomegaly, Gaucher's disease, immune thrombocytopenia), or increased in the myeloproliferative disorders such as polycythemia vera.

The CBC may reveal cytopenia of one or more blood cell types, which should suggest *hypersplenism.* This condition is characterized by splenomegaly, cytopenia(s), normal or hyperplastic bone marrow, and a response to splenectomy. The latter characteristic is less precise because reversal of cytopenia, particularly granulocytopenia, is sometimes not sustained after splenectomy. The cytopenias result from increased destruction of the cellular elements secondary to reduced flow of blood through enlarged and congested cords (congestive splenomegaly) or to immune-mediated mechanisms. In hypersplenism, various cell types usually have normal morphology on the peripheral blood smear, although the red cells may be spherocytic due to loss of surface area during their longer transit through the enlarged spleen. The increased marrow production of red cells should be reflected as an increased reticulocyte production index, although the value may be less than expected due to increased sequestration of reticulocytes in the spleen.

The need for additional laboratory studies is dictated by the differential diagnosis of the underlying illness of which splenomegaly is a manifestation.

TABLE 60-3 DISEASES ASSOCIATED WITH MASSIVE SPLENOMEGALY[a]

Chronic myelogenous leukemia	Gaucher's disease
Lymphomas	Chronic lymphocytic leukemia
Hairy cell leukemia	Sarcoidosis
Myelofibrosis with myeloid metaplasia	Autoimmune hemolytic anemia
Polycythemia vera	Diffuse splenic hemangiomatosis

[a]The spleen extends greater than 8 cm below left costal margin and/or weighs more than 1000 g.

SPLENECTOMY

Splenectomy is infrequently performed for diagnostic purposes, especially in the absence of clinical illness or other diagnostic tests that suggest underlying disease. More often splenectomy is performed for symptom control in patients with massive splenomegaly, for disease control in patients with traumatic splenic rupture, or for correction of cytopenias in patients with hypersplenism or immune-mediated destruction of one or more cellular blood elements. Splenectomy is necessary for staging of patients with Hodgkin's disease only in those with clinical stage I or II disease in whom radiation therapy alone is contemplated as the treatment. Noninvasive staging of the spleen in Hodgkin's disease is not a sufficiently reliable basis for treatment decisions because one-third of normal-sized spleens will be involved with Hodgkin's disease and one-third of enlarged spleens will be tumor-free. Although splenectomy in chronic myelogenous leukemia does not affect the natural history of disease, removal of the massive spleen usually makes patients significantly more comfortable and simplifies their management by significantly reducing transfusion requirements. Splenectomy is an effective secondary or tertiary treatment for two chronic B cell leukemias, hairy cell leukemia and prolymphocytic leukemia, and for the very rare splenic mantle cell or marginal zone lymphoma. Splenectomy in these diseases may be associated with significant tumor regression in bone marrow and other sites of disease.

Similar regressions of systemic disease have been noted after splenic irradiation in some types of lymphoid tumors, especially chronic lymphocytic leukemia and prolymphocytic leukemia. This has been termed the *abscopal effect*. Such systemic tumor responses to local therapy directed at the spleen suggest that some hormone or growth factor produced by the spleen may affect tumor cell proliferation, but this conjecture is not yet substantiated. A common therapeutic indication for splenectomy is traumatic or iatrogenic splenic rupture. In a fraction of patients with splenic rupture, peritoneal seeding of splenic fragments can lead to *splenosis*—the presence of multiple rests of spleen tissue not connected to the portal circulation. This ectopic spleen tissue may cause pain or gastrointestinal obstruction, as in endometriosis. A large number of hematologic, immunologic, and congestive causes of splenomegaly can lead to destruction of one or more cellular blood elements. In the majority of such cases, splenectomy can correct the cytopenias, particularly anemia and thrombocytopenia. In a large series of patients seen in two tertiary care centers, the indication for splenectomy was diagnostic in 10% of patients, therapeutic in 44%, staging for Hodgkin's disease in 20%, and incidental to another procedure in 26%. Perhaps the only contraindication to splenectomy is the presence of marrow failure, in which the enlarged spleen is the only source of hematopoietic tissue.

The absence of the spleen has minimal long-term effects on the hematologic profile. In the immediate postsplenectomy period, leukocytosis (up to 25,000/μL) and thrombocytosis (up to 1×10^6/μL) may develop, but within 2–3 weeks, blood cell counts and survival of each cell lineage are usually normal. The chronic manifestations of splenectomy are marked variation in size and shape of erythrocytes (anisocytosis, poikilocytosis) and the presence of Howell-Jolly bodies (nuclear remnants), Heinz bodies (denatured hemoglobin), basophilic stippling, and an occasional nucleated erythrocyte in the peripheral blood. When such erythrocyte abnormalities appear in a patient whose spleen has not been removed, one should suspect splenic infiltration by tumor that has interfered with its normal culling and pitting function.

The most serious consequence of splenectomy is increased susceptibility to bacterial infections, particularly those with capsules such as *Streptococcus pneumoniae*, *Haemophilus influenzae*, and some gram-negative enteric organisms. Patients under age 20 years are particularly susceptible to overwhelming sepsis with *S. pneumoniae*, and the overall actuarial risk of sepsis in patients who have had their spleens removed is about 7% in 10 years. The case-fatality rate for pneumococcal sepsis in splenectomized patients is 50–80%. About 25% of patients without spleens will develop a serious infection at some time in their life. The frequency is highest within the first 3 years after splenectomy. About 15% of the infections are polymicrobial, and lung, skin, and blood are the most common sites. No increased risk of viral infection has been noted in patients who have no spleen. The susceptibility to bacterial infections relates to the inability to remove opsonized bacteria from the bloodstream and a defect in making antibodies to T cell–independent antigens such as the polysaccharide components of bacterial capsules. Pneumococcal vaccine (23-valent polysaccharide vaccine) should be administered to all patients 2 weeks before elective splenectomy. The Advisory Committee on Immunization Practices recommends that even splenectomized patients receive pneumococcal vaccine with a repeat vaccination 5 years later. Efficacy has not been proven in this setting, and the recommendation discounts the possibility that administration of the vaccine may actually lower the titer of specific pneumococcal antibodies. A more effective pneumococcal conjugate vaccine that involves T cells in the response is now available (Prevenar, 7-valent). The vaccine to *Neisseria meningitidis* should also be given to patients in whom elective splenectomy is planned. Although efficacy data for *Haemophilus influenzae* type b vaccine are not available for older children or adults, it may be given to patients who have had a splenectomy.

Splenectomized patients should be educated to consider any unexplained fever as a medical emergency. Prompt medical attention with evaluation and treatment of suspected bacteremia may be life-saving. Routine chemoprophylaxis with oral penicillin can result in the emergence of drug-resistant strains and is not recommended.

In addition to an increased susceptibility to bacterial infections, splenectomized patients are also more susceptible to the parasitic disease babesiosis. The splenectomized patient should avoid areas where the parasite *Babesia* is endemic (e.g., Cape Cod, MA).

Surgical removal of the spleen is an obvious cause of hyposplenism. Patients with sickle cell disease often suffer from autosplenectomy as a result of splenic destruction by the numerous infarcts associated with sickle cell crises during childhood. Indeed, the presence of a palpable spleen in a patient with sickle cell disease after age 5 suggests a coexisting hemoglobinopathy, e.g., thalassemia or hemoglobin C. In addition, patients who receive splenic irradiation for a neoplastic or autoimmune disease are also functionally hyposplenic. The term *hyposplenism* is preferred to *asplenism* in referring to the physiologic consequences of splenectomy because asplenia is a rare, specific, and fatal congenital abnormality in which there is a failure of the left side of the coelomic cavity (which includes the splenic anlagen) to develop normally. Infants with asplenia have no spleens, but that is the least of their problems. The right side of the developing embryo is duplicated on the left so there is liver where the spleen should be, there are two right lungs, and the heart comprises two right atria and two right ventricles.

FURTHER READINGS

BARKUN AN et al: The bedside assessment of splenic enlargement. Am J Med 91:512, 1991

GRAVES SA et al: Does this patient have splenomegaly? JAMA 270:2218, 1993

KRAUS MD et al: The spleen as a diagnostic specimen: A review of ten years' experience at two tertiary care institutions. Cancer 91:2001, 2001

MCINTYRE OR, EBAUGH FG JR: Palpable spleens: Ten year follow-up. Ann Intern Med 90:130, 1979

PANGALIS GA et al: Clinical approach to lymphadenopathy. Semin Oncol 20:570, 1993

Recommended Adult Immunization Schedule—United States, October 2005–September 2006. MMWR 54(40):Q1, 2005

WILLIAMSON HA JR: Lymphadenopathy in a family practice: A descriptive study of 240 cases. J Fam Pract 20:449, 1985

61 Disorders of Granulocytes and Monocytes

Steven M. Holland, John I. Gallin

Leukocytes, the major cells comprising inflammatory and immune responses, include neutrophils, T and B lymphocytes, natural killer (NK) cells, monocytes, eosinophils, and basophils. These cells have specific functions, such as antibody production by B lymphocytes or destruction of bacteria by neutrophils, but in no single infectious disease is the exact role of the cell types completely established. Thus, whereas neutrophils are classically thought to be critical to host defense against bacteria, they may also play important roles in defense against viral infections.

The blood delivers leukocytes to the various tissues from the bone marrow, where they are produced. Normal blood leukocyte counts are $4.3–10.8 \times 10^9$/L, with neutrophils representing 45–74% of the cells, bands 0–4%, lymphocytes 16–45%, monocytes 4–10%, eosinophils 0–7%, and basophils 0–2%. Variation among individuals and among different ethnic groups can be substantial with lower leukocyte numbers for certain African-American ethnic groups. The various leukocytes are derived from a common stem cell in the bone marrow. Three-

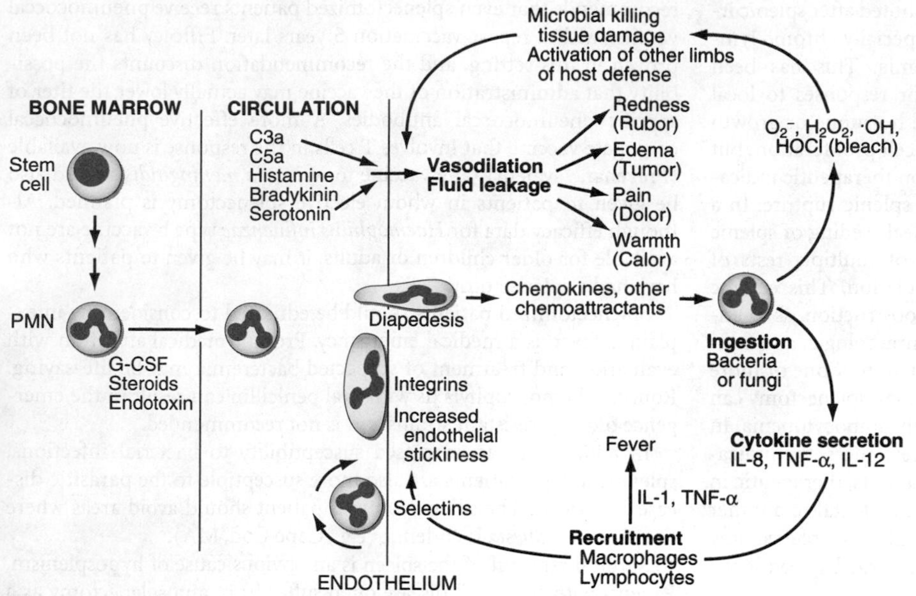

FIGURE 61-1 Schematic events in neutrophil production, recruitment, and inflammation. The four cardinal signs of inflammation (rubor, tumor, calor, dolor) are indicated, as are the interactions of neutrophils with other cells and cytokines. PMN, polymorphonuclear leukocytes; G-CSF, granulocyte colony-stimulating factor; IL, interleukin; TNF-α, tumor necrosis factor α.

fourths of the nucleated cells of bone marrow are committed to the production of leukocytes. Leukocyte maturation in the marrow is under the regulatory control of a number of different factors, known as colony-stimulating factors (CSFs) and interleukins (ILs). Because an alteration in the number and type of leukocytes is often associated with disease processes, total white blood count (WBC) (cells per μL) and differential counts are informative. This chapter focuses on neutrophils, monocytes, and eosinophils. Lymphocytes and basophils are discussed in Chaps. 308 and 311, respectively.

NEUTROPHILS

MATURATION

Important events in neutrophil life are summarized in Fig. 61-1. In normal humans, neutrophils are produced only in the bone marrow. The minimum number of stem cells necessary to support hematopoiesis is estimated to be 400–500 at any one time. Human blood monocytes, tissue macrophages, and stromal cells produce CSFs, hormones required for the growth of monocytes and neutrophils in the bone marrow. The hematopoietic system not only produces enough neutrophils (~1.3×10^{11} cells per 80-kg person per day) to carry out physiologic functions but also has a large reserve stored in the marrow, which can be mobilized in response to inflammation or infection. An increase in the number of blood neutrophils is called *neutrophilia*, and the presence of immature cells is termed a *shift to the left*. A decrease in the number of blood neutrophils is called *neutropenia*.

Neutrophils and monocytes evolve from pluripotent stem cells under the influence of cytokines and CSFs (Fig. 61-2). The proliferation phase through the metamyelocyte takes about 1 week, while the maturation phase from metamyelocyte to mature neutrophil takes another week. The myeloblast is the first recognizable precursor cell and is followed by the *promyelocyte*. The promyelocyte evolves when the classic lysosomal granules, called the *primary*, or *azurophil, granules* are produced. The primary granules contain hydrolases, elastase, myeloperoxidase, cathepsin G, cationic proteins, and bactericidal/permeability-increasing protein, which is important for killing gram-negative bacteria. Azurophil granules also contain *defensins*, a family of cysteine-rich polypeptides with broad antimicrobial activity against bacteria, fungi, and certain enveloped viruses. The promyelocyte divides to produce the *myelocyte*, a cell responsible for the synthesis of the *specific*, or *secondary, granules*, which contain unique (specific) constituents such as lactoferrin, vitamin B_{12}–binding protein, membrane components of the reduced nicotinamide-adenine dinucleotide phosphate (NADPH) oxidase required for hydrogen peroxide production, histaminase, and receptors for certain chemoattractants and adherence-promoting factors (CR3) as well as receptors for the basement membrane component, laminin. The secondary granules do not contain acid hydrolases and therefore are not classic lysosomes. Packaging of secondary granule contents during myelopoiesis is controlled by CCAAT/enhancer binding protein-ε. Secondary granule contents are readily released extracellularly, and their mobilization is important in modulating inflammation. During the final stages of maturation, no cell division occurs, and the cell passes through the metamyelocyte stage and then to the band neutrophil with a sausage-shaped nucleus (Fig. 61-3). As the band cell matures, the nucleus assumes a lobulated configuration. The nucleus of neutrophils normally contains up to four segments (Fig. 61-4). Excessive segmentation (more than five nuclear lobes) may be a manifestation of folate or vitamin B_{12} deficiency (see Fig. 100-4) and the congenital neutropenia syndrome of warts, hypogammaglobulinemia, infections, and myelokathexis (WHIM) described below. The Pelger-Hüet anomaly (Fig. 61-5), an infrequent dominant benign inherited trait, results in neutrophils with distinctive bilobed nuclei that must be distinguished from band forms. Acquired

Cell	Stage	Surface Markers[a]	Characteristics
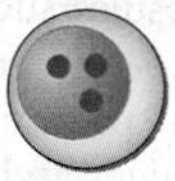	MYELOBLAST	CD33, CD13, CD15	Prominent nucleoli
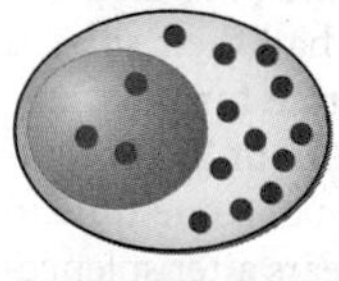	PROMYELOCYTE	CD33, CD13, CD15	Large cell Primary granules appear
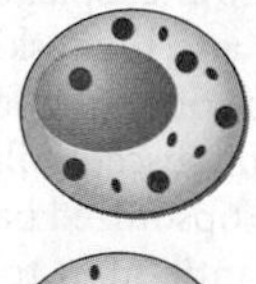	MYELOCYTE	CD33, CD13, CD15, CD14, CD11b	Secondary granules appear
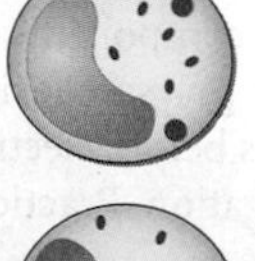	METAMYELOCYTE	CD33, CD13, CD15, CD14, CD11b	Kidney bean–shaped nucleus
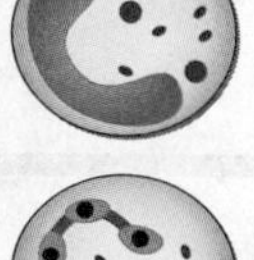	BAND FORM	CD33, CD13, CD15, CD14, CD11b CD10, CD16	Condensed, band–shaped nucleus
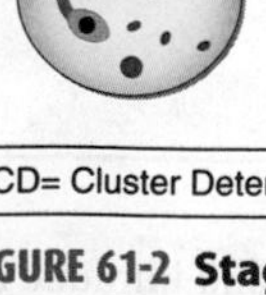	NEUTROPHIL	CD33, CD13, CD15, CD14, CD11b CD10, CD16	Condensed, multilobed nucleus

[a]CD= Cluster Determinant; ● Nucleolus; ● Primary granule; • Secondary granule.

FIGURE 61-2 Stages of neutrophil development shown schematically. G-CSF (granulocyte colony-stimulating factor) and GM-CSF (granulocyte-macrophage colony-stimulating factor) are critical to this process. Identifying cellular characteristics and specific cell-surface markers are listed for each maturational stage.

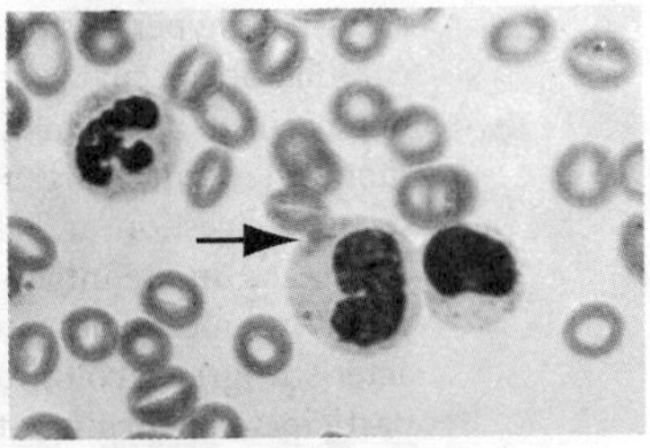

FIGURE 61-3 Neutrophil band with Döhle body. The neutrophil with a sausage-shaped nucleus in the center of the field is a band form. Döhle bodies are discrete, blue-staining nongranular areas found in the periphery of the cytoplasm of the neutrophil in infections and other toxic states. They represent aggregates of rough endoplasmic reticulum.

bilobed nuclei, pseudo Pelger-Huet anomaly, can occur with acute infections or in myelodysplastic syndromes. The physiologic role of the normal multilobed nucleus of neutrophils is unknown, but it may allow great deformation of neutrophils during migration into tissues at sites of inflammation.

In severe acute bacterial infection, prominent neutrophil cytoplasmic granules, called *toxic granulations*, are occasionally seen. Toxic granulations are immature or abnormally staining azurophil granules. Cytoplasmic inclusions, also called *Döhle bodies* (Fig. 61-3), can be seen during infection and are fragments of ribosome-rich endoplasmic reticulum. Large neutrophil vacuoles are often present in acute bacterial infection and probably represent pinocytosed (internalized) membrane.

Neutrophils are heterogeneous in function. Monoclonal antibodies have been developed that recognize only a subset of mature neutrophils. The meaning of neutrophil heterogeneity is not known.

The morphology of eosinophils and basophils is shown in Fig. 61-6.

MARROW RELEASE AND CIRCULATING COMPARTMENTS

Specific signals, including IL-1, tumor necrosis factor α (TNF-α), the CSFs, complement fragments, and chemokines, mobilize leukocytes from the bone marrow and deliver them to the blood in an unstimulated state. Under normal conditions, ~90% of the neutrophil pool is in the bone marrow, 2–3% in the circulation, and the remainder in the tissues (Fig. 61-7).

The circulating pool exists in two dynamic compartments: one freely flowing and one marginated. The freely flowing pool is about one-half the neutrophils in the basal state and is composed of those cells that are in the blood and not in contact with the endothelium. Marginated leukocytes are those that are in close physical contact with the endothelium (Fig. 61-8). In the pulmonary circulation, where an extensive capillary bed (~1000 capillaries per alveolus) exists, margination occurs because the capillaries are about the same size as a mature neutrophil. Therefore, neutrophil fluidity and deformability are necessary to make the transit through the pulmonary bed. Increased neutrophil rigidity and decreased deformability lead to augmented neutrophil trapping and margination in the lung. In contrast, in the systemic postcapillary venules, margination is mediated by the interaction of specific cell-surface molecules called *selectins*. Selectins are glycoproteins expressed on neutrophils and endothelial cells, among others, that cause a low-affinity interaction, resulting in "rolling" of the neutrophil along the endothelial surface. On neutrophils, the molecule L-selectin [cluster determinant (CD) 62L] binds to glycosylated proteins on endothelial cells [e.g., glycosylation-dependent cell adhesion molecule (GlyCAM1) and CD34]. Glycoproteins on neutrophils, most importantly sialyl-Lewis^x (SLe^x, CD15s), are targets for binding of selectins expressed on endothelial cells [E-selectin (CD62E) and P-selectin (CD62P)] and other leukocytes. In response to chemotactic stimuli from injured tissues (e.g., complement product C5a, leukotriene B_4, IL-8) or bacterial products [e.g., *N*-formylmethionylleucylphenylalanine (f-metleuphe)], neutrophil adhesiveness increases, and the cells "stick" to the endothelium through *integrins*. The integrins are leukocyte glycoproteins that exist as complexes of a common CD18 β chain with CD11a (LFA-1), CD11b (called Mac-1, CR3, or the C3bi receptor), and CD11c (called p150, 95 or CR4). CD11a/CD18 and CD11b/CD18 bind to specific endothelial receptors [intercellular adhesion molecules (ICAM) 1 and 2].

On cell stimulation, L-selectin is shed from neutrophils, and E-selectin increases in the blood, presumably because it is shed from endothelial cells; receptors for chemoattractants and opsonins are mobilized; and the phagocytes orient toward the chemoattractant source in the extravascular space, increase their motile activity (chemokinesis), and migrate directionally (chemotaxis) into tissues. The process of migration into tissues is called *diapedesis* and involves the crawling of neutrophils between postcapillary endothelial cells that open junctions between ad-

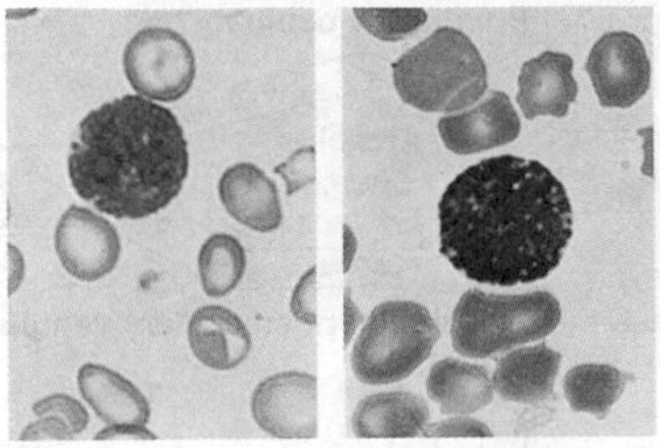

FIGURE 61-6 Normal eosinophil and basophil. The eosinophil contains large, bright orange granules and usually a bilobed nucleus. The basophil contains large purple-black granules that fill the cell and obscure the nucleus.

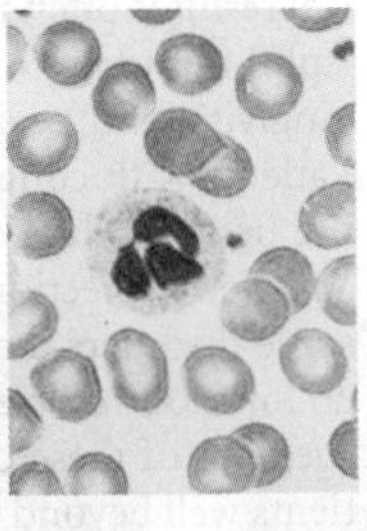

FIGURE 61-4 Normal granulocyte. The normal granulocyte has a segmented nucleus with heavy, clumped chromatin; fine neutrophilic granules are dispersed throughout the cytoplasm.

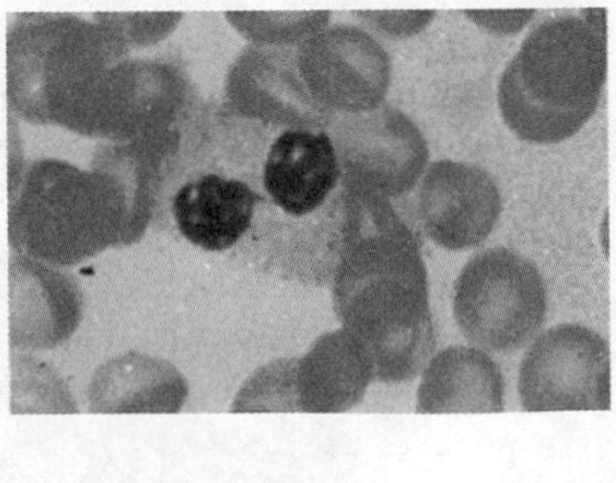

FIGURE 61-5 Pelger-Hüet anomaly. In this benign disorder, the majority of granulocytes are bilobed. The nucleus frequently has a spectacle-like, or "pince-nez," configuration.

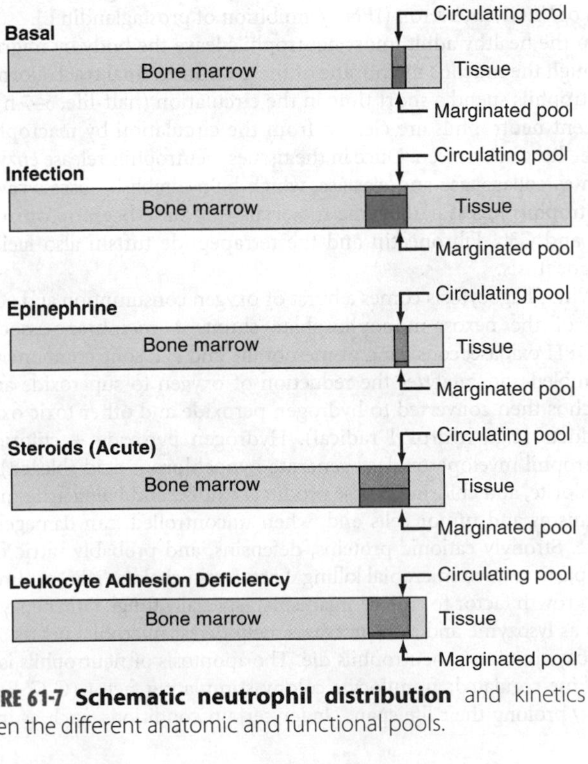

FIGURE 61-7 Schematic neutrophil distribution and kinetics between the different anatomic and functional pools.

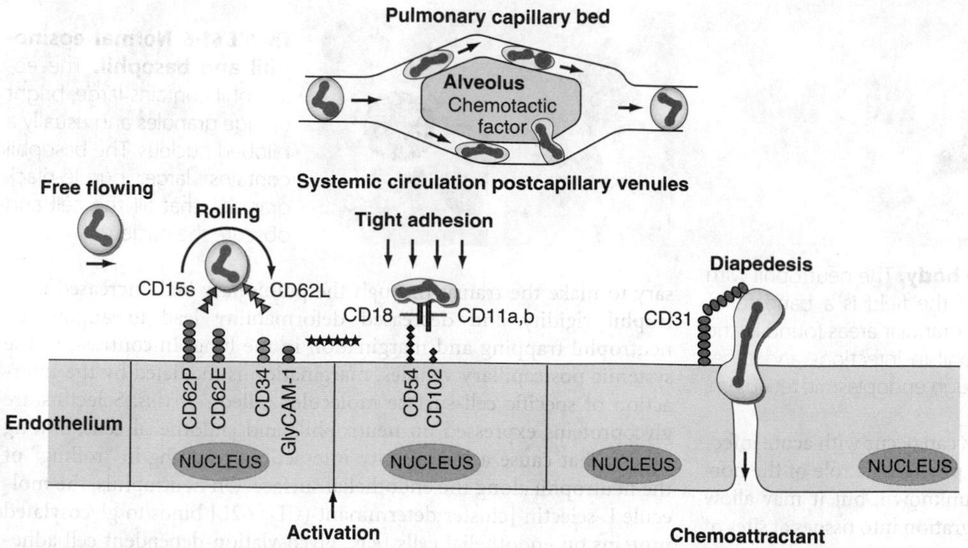

FIGURE 61-8 Neutrophil travel through the pulmonary capillaries is dependent on neutrophil deformability. Neutrophil rigidity (e.g., caused by C5a) enhances pulmonary trapping and response to pulmonary pathogens in a way that is not so dependent on cell-surface receptors. Intraalveolar chemotactic factors, such as those caused by certain bacteria (e.g., *Streptococcus pneumoniae*) lead to diapedesis of neutrophils from the pulmonary capillaries into the alveolar space. Neutrophil interaction with the endothelium of the systemic postcapillary venules is dependent on molecules of attachment. The neutrophil "rolls" along the endothelium using selectins: neutrophil CD15s (sialyl-Lewis^{x}) binds to CD62E (E-selectin) and CD62P (P-selectin) on endothelial cells; CD62L (L-selectin) on neutrophils binds to CD34 and other molecules (e.g., GlyCAM-1) expressed on endothelium. Chemokines or other activation factors stimulate integrin-mediated "tight adhesion": CD11a/CD18 (LFA-1) and CD11b/CD18 (Mac-1, CR3) bind to CD54 (ICAM-1) and CD102 (ICAM-2) on the endothelium. Diapedesis occurs between endothelial cells: CD31 (PECAM-1) expressed by the emigrating neutrophil interacts with CD31 expressed at the endothelial cell-cell junction.

jacent cells to permit leukocyte passage. Diapedesis involves platelet/endothelial cell adhesion molecule (PECAM) 1 (CD31), which is expressed on both the emigrating leukocyte and the endothelial cells. The endothelial responses (increased blood flow from increased vasodilation and permeability) are mediated by anaphylatoxins (e.g., C3a and C5a) as well as vasodilators such as histamine, bradykinin, serotonin, nitric oxide, vascular endothelial growth factor (VEGF), and prostaglandins E and I. Cytokines regulate some of these processes [e.g., TNF-α induction of VEGF, interferon (IFN) γ inhibition of prostaglandin E].

In the healthy adult, most neutrophils leave the body by migration through the mucous membrane of the gastrointestinal tract. Normally, neutrophils spend a short time in the circulation (half-life, 6–7 h). Senescent neutrophils are cleared from the circulation by macrophages in the lung and spleen. Once in the tissues, neutrophils release enzymes, such as collagenase and elastase, which help establish abscess cavities. Neutrophils ingest pathogenic materials that have been opsonized by IgG and C3b. Fibronectin and the tetrapeptide tuftsin also facilitate phagocytosis.

With phagocytosis comes a burst of oxygen consumption and activation of the hexose-monophosphate shunt. A membrane-associated NADPH oxidase, consisting of membrane and cytosolic components, is assembled and catalyzes the reduction of oxygen to superoxide anion, which is then converted to hydrogen peroxide and other toxic oxygen products (e.g., hydroxyl radical). Hydrogen peroxide + chloride + neutrophil myeloperoxidase generate hypochlorous acid (bleach), hypochlorite, and chlorine. These products oxidize and halogenate microorganisms and tumor cells and, when uncontrolled, can damage host tissue. Strongly cationic proteins, defensins, and probably nitric oxide also participate in microbial killing. Lactoferrin chelates iron, an important growth factor for microorganisms, especially fungi. Other enzymes, such as lysozyme and acid proteases, help digest microbial debris. After 1–4 days in tissues, neutrophils die. The apoptosis of neutrophils is also cytokine-regulated; granulocyte colony-stimulating factor (G-CSF) and IFN-γ prolong their life span. Under certain conditions, such as in delayed-type hypersensitivity, monocyte accumulation occurs within 6–12 h of initiation of inflammation. Neutrophils, monocytes, microorganisms in various states of digestion, and altered local tissue cells make up the inflammatory exudate, pus. Myeloperoxidase confers the characteristic green color to pus and may participate in turning off the inflammatory process by inactivating chemoattractants and immobilizing phagocytic cells.

Neutrophils respond to certain cytokines [IFN-γ, granulocyte-macrophage colony-stimulating factor (GM-CSF), IL-8] and produce cytokines and chemotactic signals [TNF-α, IL-8, macrophage inflammatory protein (MIP) 1] that modulate the inflammatory response. In the presence of fibrinogen, f-met leu phe or leukotriene B_4 induces IL-8 production by neutrophils, providing autocrine amplification of inflammation. *Chemokines* (*chemo*attractant cyto*kines*) are small proteins produced by many different cell types, including endothelial cells, fibroblasts, epithelial cells, neutrophils, and monocytes, that regulate neutrophil, monocyte, eosinophil, and lymphocyte recruitment and activation. Chemokines transduce their signals through heterotrimeric G protein–linked receptors that have seven cell membrane–spanning domains, the same type of cell-surface receptor that mediates the response to the classic chemoattractants f-metleuphe and C5a. Four major groups of chemokines are recognized based on the cysteine structure near the N terminus: C, CC, CXC, and CXXXC. The CXC cytokines such as IL-8 mainly attract neutrophils; CC chemokines such as MIP-1 attract lymphocytes, monocytes, eosinophils, and basophils; the C chemokine lymphotactin is T cell tropic; the CXXXC chemokine fractalkine attracts neutrophils, monocytes, and T cells. These molecules and their receptors not only regulate the trafficking and activation of inflammatory cells, but specific chemokine receptors serve as co-receptors for HIV infection (Chap. 182) and have a role in atherogenesis.

NEUTROPHIL ABNORMALITIES

A defect in the neutrophil life cycle can lead to dysfunction and compromised host defenses. Inflammation is often depressed, and the clinical result is often recurrent with severe bacterial and fungal infections. Aphthous ulcers of mucous membranes (gray ulcers without pus) and gingivitis and periodontal disease suggest a phagocytic cell disorder. Patients with congenital phagocyte defects can have infections within the first few days of life. Skin, ear, upper and lower respiratory tract, and bone infections are common. Sepsis and meningitis are rare. In some disorders the frequency of infection is variable, and patients can go for months or even years without major infection. Aggressive management of these congenital diseases has extended the life span of patients well beyond 30 years.

Neutropenia The consequences of absent neutrophils are dramatic. Susceptibility to infectious diseases increases sharply when neutrophil counts fall below 1000 cells/μL. When the absolute neutrophil count (ANC; band forms and mature neutrophils combined) falls to <500 cells/μL, control of endogenous microbial flora (e.g., mouth, gut) is impaired; when the ANC is <200/μL, the inflammatory process is absent. Neutropenia can be due to depressed production, increased peripheral destruction, or excessive peripheral pooling. A falling neutrophil count or a significant decrease in the number of neutrophils below steady-state levels, together with a failure to increase neutrophil counts in the setting of infection or other challenge, requires investigation. Acute neutropenia, such as that caused by cancer chemotherapy, is more likely to be associated with increased risk of infection than neutropenia of long duration (months to years) that reverses in response to infection or carefully controlled administration of endotoxin (see "Laboratory Diagnosis," below).

Some causes of inherited and acquired neutropenia are listed in Table 61-1. The most common neutropenias are iatrogenic, resulting from the use of cytotoxic or immunosuppressive therapies for malignancy or control of autoimmune disorders. These drugs cause neutropenia because they result in decreased production of rapidly growing progenitor (stem) cells of the marrow. Certain antibiotics such as chloramphenicol, trimethoprim-sulfamethoxazole, flucytosine, vidarabine, and the antiretroviral drug zidovudine may cause neutropenia by inhibiting proliferation of myeloid precursors. The marrow suppression is generally dose-related and dependent on continued administration of the drug. Recombinant human G-CSF usually reverses this form of neutropenia.

Another important mechanism for iatrogenic neutropenia is the effect of drugs that serve as immune haptens and sensitize neutrophils or neutrophil precursors to immune-mediated peripheral destruction. This form of drug-induced neutropenia can be seen within 7 days of exposure to the drug; with previous drug exposure, resulting in preexisting antibodies, neutropenia may occur a few hours after administration of the drug. Although any drug can cause this form of neutropenia, the most frequent causes are commonly used antibiotics, such as sulfa-containing compounds, penicillins, and cephalosporins. Fever and eosinophilia may also be associated with drug reactions, but often these signs are not present. Drug-induced neutropenia can be severe, but discontinuation of the sensitizing drug is sufficient for recovery, which is usually seen within 5–7 days and is complete by 10 days. Readministration of the sensitizing drug should be avoided, since abrupt neutropenia will often result. For this reason, diagnostic challenge should be avoided.

Autoimmune neutropenias caused by circulating antineutrophil antibodies are another form of acquired neutropenia that results in increased destruction of neutrophils. Acquired neutropenia may also be seen with viral infections, including infection with HIV. Acquired neutropenia may be cyclic in nature, occurring at intervals of several weeks. Acquired cyclic or stable neutropenia may be associated with an expansion of large granular lymphocytes (LGLs), which may be T cells, NK cells, or NK-like cells. Patients with LGL lymphocytosis may have moderate blood and bone marrow lymphocytosis, neutropenia, polyclonal hypergammaglobulinemia, splenomegaly, rheumatoid arthritis, and absence of lymphadenopathy. Such patients may have a chronic and relatively stable course. Recurrent bacterial infections are frequent. Benign and malignant forms of this syndrome occur. In some patients, a spontaneous regression has occurred even after 11 years, suggesting an immunoregulatory defect as the basis for at least one form of the disorder. Glucocorticoids, cyclosporine, IFN-α, and nucleosides such as 2-chlorodeoxyadenosine each have induced remission.

Hereditary Neutropenias Hereditary neutropenias are rare and may manifest in early childhood as a profound constant neutropenia or agranulocytosis. Congenital forms of neutropenia include Kostmann's syndrome (neutrophil count <100/μL), which is often fatal due to mutations in the anti-apoptosis gene HAX-1; severe chronic neutropenia (neutrophil count of 300–1500/μL) due to mutations in neutrophil elastase; hereditary cyclic neutropenia, or, more appropriately, cyclic hematopoiesis, also due to mutations in neutrophil elastase; the cartilage-hair hypoplasia syndrome due to mutations in the mitochondrial RNA-processing endoribonuclease RMRP; Shwachman-Diamond syndrome associated with pancreatic insufficiency due to mutations in the Shwachman-Bodian-Diamond syndrome gene *SBDS*; the WHIM [warts, *h*ypogammaglobulinemia, *i*nfections, *m*yelokathexis (retention of WBCs in the marrow)] syndrome, characterized by neutrophil hypersegmentation and bone marrow myeloid arrest due to mutations in the chemokine receptor CXCR4; and neutropenias associated with other immune defects, such as X-linked agammaglobulinemia, Wiskott-Aldrich syndrome, and CD40 ligand deficiency. Mutations in the G-CSF receptor can develop in severe congenital neutropenia and are linked to leukemia.

Maternal factors can be associated with neutropenia in the newborn. Transplacental transfer of IgG directed against antigens on fetal neutrophils can result in peripheral destruction. Drugs (e.g., thiazides) ingested during pregnancy can cause neutropenia in the newborn by either depressed production or peripheral destruction.

In Felty's syndrome—the triad of rheumatoid arthritis, splenomegaly, and neutropenia (Chap. 314)—spleen-produced antibodies can shorten neutrophil life span, while LGLs can attack marrow neutrophil precursors. Splenectomy may increase neutrophil count in Felty's syndrome and lower serum neutrophil-binding IgG. Some Felty's syndrome patients also have neutropenia associated with an increased number of LGLs. Splenomegaly with peripheral trapping and destruction of neutrophils is also seen in lysosomal storage diseases and in portal hypertension.

Neutrophilia Neutrophilia results from increased neutrophil production, increased marrow release, or defective margination (Table 61-2). The most important acute cause of neutrophilia is infection.

TABLE 61-1 CAUSES OF NEUTROPENIA

Decreased Production
Drug-induced—alkylating agents (nitrogen mustard, busulfan, chlorambucil, cyclophosphamide); antimetabolites (methotrexate, 6-mercaptopurine, 5-flucytosine); noncytotoxic agents [antibiotics (chloramphenicol, penicillins, sulfonamides), phenothiazines, tranquilizers (meprobamate), anticonvulsants (carbamazepine), antipsychotics (clozapine), certain diuretics, anti-inflammatory agents, antithyroid drugs, many others]
Hematologic diseases—idiopathic, cyclic neutropenia, Chédiak-Higashi syndrome, aplastic anemia, infantile genetic disorders (see text)
Tumor invasion, myelofibrosis
Nutritional deficiency—vitamin B_{12}, folate (especially alcoholics)
Infection—tuberculosis, typhoid fever, brucellosis, tularemia, measles, infectious mononucleosis, malaria, viral hepatitis, leishmaniasis, AIDS
Peripheral Destruction
Antineutrophil antibodies and/or splenic or lung trapping
Autoimmune disorders—Felty's syndrome, rheumatoid arthritis, lupus erythematosus
Drugs as haptens—aminopyrine, α-methyldopa, phenylbutazone, mercurial diuretics, some phenothiazines
Wegener's granulomatosis
Peripheral Pooling (Transient Neutropenia)
Overwhelming bacterial infection (acute endotoxemia)
Hemodialysis
Cardiopulmonary bypass

TABLE 61-2 CAUSES OF NEUTROPHILIA

Increased Production
Idiopathic
Drug-induced—glucocorticoids, G-CSF
Infection—bacterial, fungal, sometimes viral
Inflammation—thermal injury, tissue necrosis, myocardial and pulmonary infarction, hypersensitivity states, collagen vascular diseases
Myeloproliferative diseases—myelocytic leukemia, myeloid metaplasia, polycythemia vera
Increased Marrow Release
Glucocorticoids
Acute infection (endotoxin)
Inflammation—thermal injury
Decreased or Defective Margination
Drugs—epinephrine, glucocorticoids, nonsteroidal anti-inflammatory agents
Stress, excitement, vigorous exercise
Leukocyte adhesion deficiency type 1 (integrin β chain, CD18); leukocyte adhesion deficiency type 2 (selectin ligand, CD15s, sialyl-Lewis[x])
Miscellaneous
Metabolic disorders—ketoacidosis, acute renal failure, eclampsia, acute poisoning
Drugs—lithium
Other—metastatic carcinoma, acute hemorrhage or hemolysis

TABLE 61-3 TYPES OF GRANULOCYTE AND MONOCYTE DISORDERS

Function	Cause of Indicated Dysfunction: Drug-Induced	Acquired	Inherited
Adherence-aggregation	Aspirin, colchicine, alcohol, glucocorticoids, ibuprofen, piroxicam	Neonatal state, hemodialysis	Leukocyte adhesion deficiency types 1 and 2
Deformability		Leukemia, neonatal state, diabetes mellitus, immature neutrophils	
Chemokinesis-chemotaxis	Glucocorticoids (high dose), auranofin, colchicine (weak effect), phenylbutazone, naproxen, indomethacin, interleukin 2	Thermal injury, malignancy, malnutrition, periodontal disease, neonatal state, systemic lupus erythematosus, rheumatoid arthritis, diabetes mellitus, sepsis, influenza virus infection, herpes simplex virus infection, acrodermatitis enteropathica, AIDS	Chédiak-Higashi syndrome, neutrophil-specific granule deficiency, hyper IgE–recurrent infection (Job's) syndrome (in some patients), Down syndrome, α-mannosidase deficiency, severe combined immunodeficiency, Wiskott-Aldrich syndrome
Microbicidal activity	Colchicine, cyclophosphamide, glucocorticoids (high dose), TNF-α blocking antibodies	Leukemia, aplastic anemia, certain neutropenias, tuftsin deficiency, thermal injury, sepsis, neonatal state, diabetes mellitus, malnutrition, AIDS	Chédiak-Higashi syndrome, neutrophil-specific granule deficiency, chronic granulomatous disease, defects in IFN-γ/IL-12 axis

Neutrophilia from acute infection represents both increased production and increased marrow release. Increased production is also associated with chronic inflammation and certain myeloproliferative diseases. Increased marrow release and mobilization of the marginated leukocyte pool are induced by glucocorticoids. Release of epinephrine, as with vigorous exercise, excitement, or stress, will demarginate neutrophils in the spleen and lungs and double the neutrophil count in minutes. Cigarette smoking can increase neutrophil counts into the abnormal range. Leukocytosis with cell counts of 10,000–25,000/μL occurs in response to infection and other forms of acute inflammation and results from both release of the marginated pool and mobilization of marrow reserves. Persistent neutrophilia with cell counts of ≥30,000–50,000/μL is called a *leukemoid reaction*, a term often used to distinguish this degree of neutrophilia from leukemia. In a leukemoid reaction, the circulating neutrophils are usually mature and not clonally derived.

Abnormal Neutrophil Function Inherited and acquired abnormalities of phagocyte function are listed in Table 61-3. The resulting diseases are best considered in terms of the functional defects of adherence, chemotaxis, and microbicidal activity. The distinguishing features of the important inherited disorders of phagocyte function are shown in Table 61-4.

DISORDERS OF ADHESION Two main types of leukocyte adhesion deficiency (LAD) have been described, LAD 1 and LAD 2. Both are autosomal recessive traits and result in the inability of neutrophils to exit the circulation to sites of infection, leading to leukocytosis and increased susceptibility to infection (Fig. 61-8). Patients with LAD 1 have mutations in CD18, the common component of the integrins LFA-1, Mac-1, and p150,95, leading to a defect in tight adhesion between neutrophils and the endothelium. The heterodimer formed by CD18/CD11b (Mac-1) is also the receptor for the complement-derived opsonin C3bi (CR3). The *CD18* gene is located on distal chromosome 21q. The severity of the defect determines the severity of clinical disease. Complete lack of expression of the leukocyte integrins results in a severe phenotype in which inflammatory stimuli do not increase the expression of leukocyte integrins on neutrophils or activated T and B cells. Neutrophils (and monocytes) from patients with LAD 1 adhere poorly to endothelial cells and protein-coated surfaces and exhibit defective spreading, aggregation, and chemotaxis. Patients with LAD 1 have recurrent bacterial infections involving the skin, oral and genital mucosa, and respiratory and intestinal tracts; persistent leukocytosis (neutrophil counts of 15,000–20,000/μL) because cells do not marginate; and, in severe cases, a history of delayed separation of the umbilical stump. Infections, especially of the skin, may become necrotic with progressively enlarging borders, slow healing, and development of dysplastic scars. The most common bacteria are *Staphylococcus aureus* and enteric gram-negative bacteria. LAD 2 is caused by an abnormality of fucosylation of SLe^x (CD15s), the ligand on neutrophils that interacts with selectins on endothelial cells and is responsible for neutrophil rolling along the endothelium. Infection susceptibility in LAD 2 appears to be less severe than in LAD 1. LAD 2 is also known as *congenital disorder of glycosylation IIc* (CDGIIc).

DISORDERS OF NEUTROPHIL GRANULES The most common neutrophil defect is myeloperoxidase deficiency, a primary granule defect inherited as an autosomal recessive trait; the incidence is ~1 in 2000 persons. Isolated myeloperoxidase deficiency is not associated with clinically compromised defenses, presumably because other defense systems such as hydrogen peroxide generation are amplified. Microbicidal activity of neutrophils is delayed but not absent. Myeloperoxidase deficiency may make other acquired host defense defects more serious. An acquired form of myeloperoxidase deficiency occurs in myelomonocytic leukemia and acute myeloid leukemia.

Chédiak-Higashi syndrome (CHS) is a rare disease with autosomal recessive inheritance due to defects in the lysosomal transport protein LYST, encoded by the gene *CHS1* at 1q42. This protein is required for normal packaging and disbursement of granules. Neutrophils (and all cells containing lysosomes) from patients with CHS characteristically have large granules (Fig. 61-9) making it a systemic disease. Patients with CHS have nystagmus, partial oculocutaneous albinism, and an increased number of infections resulting from many bacterial agents. Some CHS patients develop an "accelerated phase" in childhood with a hemophagocytic syndrome and an aggressive lymphoma requiring bone marrow transplantation. CHS neutrophils and monocytes have impaired chemotaxis and abnormal rates of microbial killing due to slow rates of fusion of the lysosomal granules with phagosomes. NK cell function is also impaired. CHS patients may develop a severe disabling peripheral neuropathy in adulthood that can lead to bed confinement.

Specific granule deficiency is a rare autosomal recessive disease in which the production of secondary granules and their contents, as well as the primary granule component defensins, is defective. The defect in bacterial killing leads to severe bacterial infections. One type of specific granule deficiency is due to a mutation in the CCAAT/enhancer binding protein-ε, a regulator of expression of granule components.

CHRONIC GRANULOMATOUS DISEASE Chronic granulomatous disease (CGD) is a group of disorders of granulocyte and monocyte oxidative metabolism. Although CGD is rare, with an incidence of 1 in 200,000 individuals, it is an important model of defective neutrophil oxidative metabolism. Most often CGD is inherited as an X-linked recessive trait; 30% of patients inherit the disease in an autosomal recessive pattern.

TABLE 61-4 INHERITED DISORDERS OF PHAGOCYTE FUNCTION: DIFFERENTIAL FEATURES

Clinical Manifestations	Cellular or Molecular Defects	Diagnosis
Chronic Granulomatous Diseases (70% X-linked, 30% Autosomal Recessive)		
Severe infections of skin, ears, lungs, liver, and bone with catalase-positive microorganisms such as *S. aureus*, *Burkholderia cepacia*, *Aspergillus* spp., *Chromobacterium violaceum*; often hard to culture organism; excessive inflammation with granulomas, frequent lymph node suppuration; granulomas can obstruct GI or GU tracts; gingivitis, aphthous ulcers, seborrheic dermatitis	No respiratory burst due to the lack of one of four NADPH oxidase subunits in neutrophils, monocytes, and eosinophils	NBT or DHR test; no superoxide and H_2O_2 production by neutrophils; immunoblot for NADPH oxidase components; genetic detection
Chédiak-Higashi Syndrome (Autosomal Recessive)		
Recurrent pyogenic infections, especially with *S. aureus*; many patients get lymphoma-like illness during adolescence; periodontal disease; partial oculocutaneous albinism, nystagmus, progressive peripheral neuropathy, mental retardation in some patients	Reduced chemotaxis and phagolysosome fusion, increased respiratory burst activity, defective egress from marrow, abnormal skin window; defect in LYST	Giant primary granules in neutrophils and other granule-bearing cells (Wright's stain); genetic detection
Specific Granule Deficiency (Autosomal Recessive)		
Recurrent infections of skin, ears, and sinopulmonary tract; delayed wound healing; decreased inflammation; bleeding diathesis	Abnormal chemotaxis, impaired respiratory burst and bacterial killing, failure to upregulate chemotactic and adhesion receptors with stimulation, defect in transcription of granule proteins; defect in C/EBPε	Lack of secondary (specific) granules in neutrophils (Wright's stain), no neutrophil-specific granule contents (i.e., lactoferrin), no defensins, platelet α granule abnormality; genetic detection
Myeloperoxidase Deficiency (Autosomal Recessive)		
Clinically normal except in patients with underlying disease such as diabetes mellitus; then candidiasis or other fungal infections	No myeloperoxidase due to pre- and post-translational defects	No peroxidase in neutrophils; genetic detection
Leukocyte Adhesion Deficiency		
Type 1: Delayed separation of umbilical cord, sustained neutrophilia, recurrent infections of skin and mucosa, gingivitis, periodontal disease	Impaired phagocyte adherence, aggregation, spreading, chemotaxis, phagocytosis of C3bi-coated particles; defective production of CD18 subunit common to leukocyte integrins	Reduced phagocyte surface expression of the CD18-containing integrins with monoclonal antibodies against LFA-1 (CD18/CD11a), Mac-1 or CR3 (CD18/CD11b), p150,95 (CD18/CD11c); genetic detection
Type 2: Mental retardation, short stature, Bombay (hh) blood phenotype, recurrent infections, neutrophilia	Impaired phagocyte rolling along endothelium	Reduced phagocyte surface expression of Sialyl-Lewis^X, with monoclonal antibodies against CD15s; genetic detection
Phagocyte Activation Defects (X-linked and Autosomal Recessive)		
NEMO deficiency: mild hypohidrotic ectodermal dysplasia; broad based immune defect: pyogenic and encapsulated bacteria, viruses, *Pneumocystis*, mycobacteria; X-linked	Impaired phagocyte activiation by IL-1, IL-18, TLR, CD40, TNF-α leading to problems with inflammation and antibody production	Poor in vitro response to endotoxin; lack of NF-κB activation; genetic detection
IRAK4 deficiency: susceptibility to pyogenic bacteria such as staphylococci, streptococci, clostridia; resistant to mycobacteria; autosomal recessive	Impaired phagocyte activation by endotoxin through TLR and other pathways; TNF-α signaling preserved	Poor in vitro response to endotoxin; lack of NF-κB activation by endotoxin; genetic detection
Hyper IgE–Recurrent Infection Syndrome (Autosomal Dominant) (Job's Syndrome)		
Eczematoid or pruritic dermatitis, "cold" skin abscesses, recurrent pneumonias with *S. aureus* with bronchopleural fistulae and cyst formation, mild eosinophilia, mucocutaneous candidiasis, characteristic facies, restrictive lung disease, scoliosis, delayed primary dental deciduation	Reduced chemotaxis in some patients, reduced suppressor T cell activity	Clinical features, involving lungs, skeleton, and immune system; serum IgE > 2000 IU/mL
Mycobacteria Susceptibility (Autosomal Dominant and Recessive Forms)		
Severe local or disseminated infections with bacille Calmette-Guérin (BCG), nontuberculous mycobacteria, salmonella, histoplasmosis, poor granuloma formation	Inability to kill intracellular organisms due to low IFN-γ production; mutations in IFN-γ receptors, IL-12 receptor, IL-12 p40, STAT-1, NEMO	Low or very high levels of IFN-γ receptor 1; functional assays of cytokine production and response; genetic detection

Abbreviations: GI, gastrointestinal; GU, genitourinary; NADPH, nicotinamide-adenine dinucleotide phosphate, NBT, nitroblue tetrazolium (dye test), DHR, dihydrorhodamine (oxidation test); LYST, lysosomal transport protein; C/EBPε, CCAAT/enhancer binding protein-ε; NEMO, NF-κB essential modulator; TLR, Toll-like receptor; IL, interleukin; TNF, tumor necrosis factor; IRAK4, IL-1 receptor–associated kinase protein-ε, NEMO 4; IFN, interferon.

Mutations in the genes for the four proteins that assemble at the plasma membrane account for all patients with CGD. Two proteins (a 91-kDa protein, abnormal in X-linked CGD, and a 22-kDa protein, absent in one form of autosomal recessive CGD) form the heterodimer cytochrome b-558 in the plasma membrane. Two other proteins (47 and 67 kDa, abnormal in the other autosomal recessive forms of CGD) are cytoplasmic in origin and interact with the cytochrome after cell activation to form NADPH oxidase, required for hydrogen peroxide production. Leukocytes from patients with CGD have severely diminished hydrogen peroxide production. The genes involved in each of the defects have been

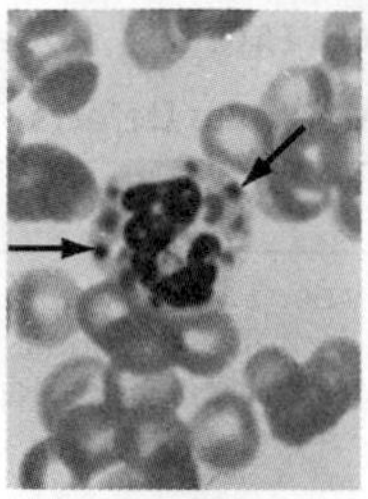

FIGURE 61-9 Chédiak-Higashi syndrome. The granulocytes contain huge cytoplasmic granules formed from aggregation and fusion of azurophilic and specific granules. Large abnormal granules are found in other granule-containing cells throughout the body.

cloned and sequenced and the chromosome locations identified. Patients with CGD characteristically have increased numbers of infections due to catalase-positive microorganisms (organisms that destroy their own hydrogen peroxide). When patients with CGD become infected, they often have extensive inflammatory reactions, and lymph node suppuration is common despite the administration of appropriate antibiotics. Aphthous ulcers and chronic inflammation of the nares are often present. Granulomas are frequent and can obstruct the gastrointestinal or genitourinary tracts. The excessive inflammation probably reflects failure to inhibit the synthesis or degradation of chemoattractants and antigens, leading to persistent neutrophil accumulation. Impaired killing of intracellular microorganisms by macrophages may lead to persistent cell-mediated immune activation and granuloma formation. Autoimmune complications such as immune thrombocytopenic purpura and juvenile rheumatoid arthritis are also increased in CGD. In addition, discoid lupus is more common in X-linked carriers.

DISORDERS OF PHAGOCYTE ACTIVATION Phagocytes depend on cell-surface stimulation to induce signals that evoke multiple levels of the inflammatory response, including cytokine synthesis, chemotaxis, and antigen presentation. Mutations affecting the major pathway that signals through NF-κB have been noted in patients with a variety of infection susceptibility syndromes. If the defects are at a very late stage of signal transduction, in the protein critical for NF-κB activation known as the NF-κB essential modulator (NEMO), then affected males develop ectodermal dysplasia and severe immune deficiency with susceptibility to bacteria, fungi, mycobacteria, and viruses. If the defect in NF-κB activation is closer to the signaling source, in the IL-1 receptor–associated kinase 4 (IRAK4), then children have a marked susceptibility to pyogenic infections early in life but develop resistance to infection later.

MONONUCLEAR PHAGOCYTES

The mononuclear phagocyte system is composed of monoblasts, promonocytes, and monocytes, in addition to the structurally diverse tissue macrophages that make up what was previously referred to as the reticuloendothelial system. Macrophages are long-lived phagocytic cells capable of many of the functions of neutrophils. They are also secretory cells that participate in many immunologic and inflammatory processes distinct from neutrophils. Monocytes leave the circulation by diapedesis more slowly than neutrophils and have a half-life in the blood of 12–24 h.

After blood monocytes arrive in the tissues, they differentiate into macrophages ("big eaters") with specialized functions suited for specific anatomic locations. Macrophages are particularly abundant in capillary walls of the lung, spleen, liver, and bone marrow, where they function to remove microorganisms and other noxious elements from the blood. Alveolar macrophages, liver Kupffer cells, splenic macrophages, peritoneal macrophages, bone marrow macrophages, lymphatic macrophages, brain microglial cells, and dendritic macrophages all have specialized functions. Macrophage-secreted products include lysozyme, neutral proteases, acid hydrolases, arginase, complement components, enzyme inhibitors (plasmin, α_2-macroglobulin), binding proteins (transferrin, fibronectin, transcobalamin II), nucleosides, and cytokines (TNF-α; IL-1, -8, -12, -18). IL-1 (Chaps. 17 and 308) has many functions, including initiating fever in the hypothalamus, mobilizing leukocytes from the bone marrow, and activating lymphocytes and neutrophils. TNF-α is a pyrogen that duplicates many of the actions of IL-1 and plays an important role in the pathogenesis of gram-negative shock (Chap. 265). TNF-α stimulates production of hydrogen peroxide and related toxic oxygen species by macrophages and neutrophils. In addition, TNF-α induces catabolic changes that contribute to the profound wasting (cachexia) associated with many chronic diseases.

Other macrophage-secreted products include reactive oxygen and nitrogen metabolites, bioactive lipids (arachidonic acid metabolites and platelet-activating factors), chemokines, CSFs, and factors stimulating fibroblast and vessel proliferation. Macrophages help regulate the replication of lymphocytes and participate in the killing of tumors, viruses, and certain bacteria (*Mycobacterium tuberculosis* and *Listeria monocytogenes*). Macrophages are key effector cells in the elimination of intracellular microorganisms. Their ability to fuse to form giant cells that coalesce into granulomas in response to some inflammatory stimuli is important in the elimination of intracellular microbes and is under the control of IFN-γ. Nitric oxide induced by IFN-γ is an important effector against intracellular parasites, including tuberculosis and *Leishmania*.

Macrophages play an important role in the immune response (Chap. 308). They process and present antigen to lymphocytes and secrete cytokines that modulate and direct lymphocyte development and function. Macrophages participate in autoimmune phenomena by removing immune complexes and other substances from the circulation. Polymorphisms in macrophage receptors for immunoglobulin (FcγRII) determine susceptibility to some infections and autoimmune diseases. In wound healing, they dispose of senescent cells, and they contribute to atheroma development. Macrophage elastase mediates development of emphysema from cigarette smoking.

DISORDERS OF THE MONONUCLEAR PHAGOCYTE SYSTEM

Many disorders of neutrophils extend to mononuclear phagocytes. Thus, drugs that suppress neutrophil production in the bone marrow can cause monocytopenia. Transient monocytopenia occurs after stress or glucocorticoid administration. Monocytosis is associated with tuberculosis, brucellosis, subacute bacterial endocarditis, Rocky Mountain spotted fever, malaria, and visceral leishmaniasis (kala azar). Monocytosis also occurs with malignancies, leukemias, myeloproliferative syndromes, hemolytic anemias, chronic idiopathic neutropenias, and granulomatous diseases such as sarcoidosis, regional enteritis, and some collagen vascular diseases. Patients with LAD, hyperimmunoglobulin E–recurrent infection (Job's) syndrome, CHS, and CGD all have defects in the mononuclear phagocyte system.

Monocyte cytokine production or response is impaired in some patients with disseminated nontuberculous mycobacterial infection who are not infected with HIV. Genetic defects in the pathways regulated by IFN-γ and IL-12 lead to impaired killing of intracellular bacteria, mycobacteria, salmonellae, and certain viruses (Fig. 61-10).

Certain viral infections impair mononuclear phagocyte function. For example, influenza virus infection causes abnormal monocyte chemotaxis. Mononuclear phagocytes can be infected by HIV using CCR5, the chemokine receptor that acts as a co-receptor with CD4 for HIV. T lymphocytes produce IFN-γ, which induces FcR expression and phagocytosis and stimulates hydrogen peroxide production by mononuclear phagocytes and neutrophils. In certain diseases, such as AIDS, IFN-γ production may be deficient, while in other diseases, such as T cell lymphomas, excessive release of IFN-γ may be associated with erythrophagocytosis by splenic macrophages.

Autoinflammatory diseases are characterized by abnormal cytokine regulation leading to excess inflammation in the absence of infection. These diseases can mimic infectious or immunodeficient syndromes. Gain-of-function mutations in the TNF-α receptor cause TNF-α receptor–associated periodic syndrome (TRAPS), which is characterized by recurrent fever in the absence of infection, due to persistent stimulation of the TNF-α receptor (Chap. 323). Diseases with abnormal IL-1 regulation leading to fever include familial Mediterranean fever due to mutations in *pyrin*. Mutations in *cold-induced autoinflammatory syndrome 1* lead to neonatal onset multisystem autoinflammatory disease, familial

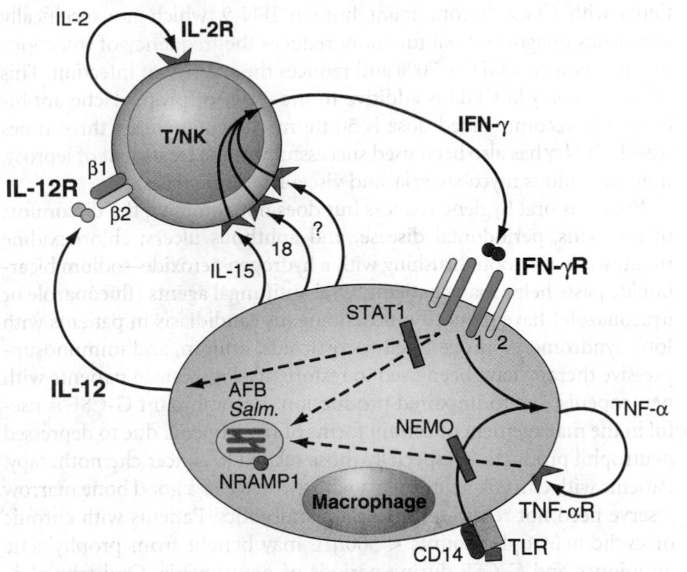

FIGURE 61-10 Lymphocyte-macrophage interactions underlying resistance to mycobacteria and other intracellular parasites such as *Salmonella*. Mycobacteria infect macrophages, leading to the production of IL-12, which activates T or NK cells through its receptor, leading to production of IL-2 and IFN-γ. IFN-γ acts through its receptor on macrophages to upregulate TNF-α and IL-12 and kill intracellular parasites. Mutant forms of the cytokines and receptors shown in large type have been found in severe cases of nontuberculous mycobacterial infection and salmonellosis.

cold urticaria, and Muckle-Wells syndrome. Pyoderma gangrenosum, acne, and sterile pyogenic arthritis is caused by mutations in CD2BP1. In contrast to these syndromes of overexpression of proinflammatory cytokines, blockade of TNF-α by the antagonists infliximab, etanercept, and adalimumab has been associated with severe infections due to tuberculosis, nontuberculous mycobacteria, and fungi (Chap. 323).

Monocytopenia occurs with acute infections, with stress, and after treatment with glucocorticoids. Monocytopenia also occurs in aplastic anemia, hairy cell leukemia, acute myeloid leukemia, and as a direct result of myelotoxic drugs.

EOSINOPHILS

Eosinophils and neutrophils share similar morphology, many lysosomal constituents, phagocytic capacity, and oxidative metabolism. Eosinophils express a specific chemoattractant receptor and respond to a specific chemokine, eotaxin. Little is known about the role of eosinophils. Eosinophils are much longer lived than neutrophils, and unlike neutrophils, tissue eosinophils can recirculate. During most infections, eosinophils are not important. However, in invasive helminthic infections, such as hookworm, schistosomiasis, strongyloidiasis, toxocariasis, trichinosis, filariasis, echinococcosis, and cysticercosis, the eosinophil plays a central role in host defense. Eosinophils are associated with bronchial asthma, cutaneous allergic reactions, and other hypersensitivity states.

The distinctive feature of the red-staining (Wright's stain) eosinophil granule is its crystalline core consisting of an arginine-rich protein (major basic protein) with histaminase activity, important in host defense against parasites. Eosinophil granules also contain a unique eosinophil peroxidase that catalyzes the oxidation of many substances by hydrogen peroxide and may facilitate killing of microorganisms.

Eosinophil peroxidase, in the presence of hydrogen peroxide and halide, initiates mast cell secretion in vitro and thereby promotes inflammation. Eosinophils contain cationic proteins, some of which bind to heparin and reduce its anticoagulant activity. Eosinophil-derived neurotoxin and eosinophil cationic protein are ribonucleases that can kill respiratory syncytial virus. Eosinophil cytoplasm contains Charcot-Leyden crystal protein, a hexagonal bipyramidal crystal first observed in a patient with leukemia and then in sputum of patients with asthma; this protein is lysophospholipase and may function to detoxify certain lysophospholipids.

Several factors enhance the eosinophil's function in host defense. T cell–derived factors enhance the ability of eosinophils to kill parasites. Mast cell–derived eosinophil chemotactic factor of anaphylaxis (ECFa) increases the number of eosinophil complement receptors and enhances eosinophil killing of parasites. Eosinophil CSFs (e.g., IL-5) produced by macrophages increase eosinophil production in the bone marrow and activate eosinophils to kill parasites.

EOSINOPHILIA

Eosinophilia is the presence of >500 eosinophils per μL of blood and is common in many settings besides parasite infection. Significant tissue eosinophilia can occur without an elevated blood count. A common cause of eosinophilia is allergic reaction to drugs (iodides, aspirin, sulfonamides, nitrofurantoin, penicillins, and cephalosporins). Allergies such as hay fever, asthma, eczema, serum sickness, allergic vasculitis, and pemphigus are associated with eosinophilia. Eosinophilia also occurs in collagen vascular diseases (e.g., rheumatoid arthritis, eosinophilic fasciitis, allergic angiitis, and periarteritis nodosa) and malignancies (e.g., Hodgkin's disease; mycosis fungoides; chronic myeloid leukemia; and cancer of the lung, stomach, pancreas, ovary, or uterus), as well as in Job's syndrome and CGD. Eosinophilia is commonly present in the helminthic infections. IL-5 is the dominant eosinophil growth factor. Therapeutic administration of the cytokines IL-2 and GM-CSF frequently leads to transient eosinophilia. The most dramatic hypereosinophilic syndromes are Loeffler's syndrome, tropical pulmonary eosinophilia, Loeffler's endocarditis, eosinophilic leukemia, and idiopathic hypereosinophilic syndrome (50,000–100,000/μL).

The idiopathic hypereosinophilic syndrome represents a heterogeneous group of disorders with the common feature of prolonged eosinophilia of unknown cause and organ system dysfunction, including the heart, central nervous system, kidneys, lungs, gastrointestinal tract, and skin. The bone marrow is involved in all affected individuals, but the most severe complications involve the heart and central nervous system. Clinical manifestations and organ dysfunction are highly variable. Eosinophils are found in the involved tissues and likely cause tissue damage by local deposition of toxic eosinophil proteins such as eosinophil cationic protein and major basic protein. In the heart, the pathologic changes lead to thrombosis, endocardial fibrosis, and restrictive endomyocardiopathy. The damage to tissues in other organ systems is similar. Some cases are due to mutations involving the platelet-derived growth factor receptor, and these are extremely sensitive to the tyrosine kinase inhibitor imatinib. Glucocorticoids, hydroxyurea, and IFN-α each have been used successfully, as have therapeutic antibodies against IL-5. Cardiovascular complications are managed aggressively.

The *eosinophilia-myalgia syndrome* is a multisystem disease, with prominent cutaneous, hematologic, and visceral manifestations, that frequently evolves into a chronic course and can occasionally be fatal. The syndrome is characterized by eosinophilia (eosinophil count >1000/μL) and generalized disabling myalgias without other recognized causes. Eosinophilic fasciitis, pneumonitis, and myocarditis; neuropathy culminating in respiratory failure; and encephalopathy may occur. The disease is caused by ingesting contaminants in L-tryptophan–containing products. Eosinophils, lymphocytes, macrophages, and fibroblasts accumulate in the affected tissues, but their role in pathogenesis is unclear. Activation of eosinophils and fibroblasts and the deposition of eosinophil-derived toxic proteins in affected tissues may contribute. IL-5 and transforming growth factor β have been implicated as potential mediators. Treatment is withdrawal of products containing L-tryptophan and the administration of glucocorticoids. Most patients recover fully, remain stable, or show slow recovery, but the disease can be fatal in up to 5% of patients.

EOSINOPENIA

Eosinopenia occurs with stress, such as acute bacterial infection, and after treatment with glucocorticoids. The mechanism of eosinopenia of acute bacterial infection is unknown but is independent of endogenous glucocorticoids, since it occurs in animals after total adrenalectomy. There is no known adverse effect of eosinopenia.

HYPERIMMUNOGLOBULIN E–RECURRENT INFECTION SYNDROME

The hyperimmunoglobulin E–recurrent infection syndrome, or Job's syndrome, is a rare multisystem disease in which the immune system, bone, teeth, lung, and skin are affected. Abnormal chemotaxis is a variable feature. The molecular basis for this syndrome is still not known, but some cases show clear autosomal dominant transmission with linkage to 4q. Patients with this syndrome have characteristic facies with broad nose, kyphoscoliosis and osteoporosis, and eczema. The primary teeth erupt normally but do not deciduate, often requiring extraction. Patients develop recurrent sinopulmonary and cutaneous infections that tend to be much less inflamed than appropriate for the degree of infection and have been referred to as "cold abscesses." A high degree of suspicion is required to diagnose infections in these patients, who may appear well despite extensive disease. The cold abscesses have been considered a reflection of too few phagocytes arriving too late, perhaps due to a lymphocyte factor inhibiting chemotaxis. However, the chemotactic defect in these patients is variable, and the fundamental basis for the impaired defenses is complex and poorly defined.

LABORATORY DIAGNOSIS AND MANAGEMENT

Initial studies of WBC and differential and often a bone marrow examination may be followed by assessment of bone marrow reserves (steroid challenge test), marginated circulating pool of cells (epinephrine challenge test), and marginating ability (endotoxin challenge test) (Fig. 61-7). In vivo assessment of inflammation is possible with a Rebuck skin window test or an in vivo skin blister assay, which measures the ability of leukocytes and inflammatory mediators to accumulate locally in the skin. In vitro tests of phagocyte aggregation, adherence, chemotaxis, phagocytosis, degranulation, and microbicidal activity (for *S. aureus*) may help pinpoint cellular or humoral lesions. Deficiencies of oxidative metabolism are detected with either the nitroblue tetrazolium (NBT) dye test or the dihydrorhodamine (DHR) oxidation test. These tests are based on the ability of products of oxidative metabolism to alter the oxidation states of reporter molecules so that they can be detected microscopically (NBT) or by flow cytometry (DHR). Qualitative studies of superoxide and hydrogen peroxide production may further define neutrophil oxidative function.

Patients with leukopenias or leukocyte dysfunction often have delayed inflammatory responses. Therefore, clinical manifestations may be minimal despite overwhelming infection, and unusual infections must always be suspected. Early signs of infection demand prompt, aggressive culturing for microorganisms, use of antibiotics, and surgical drainage of abscesses. Prolonged courses of antibiotics are often required. In patients with CGD, prophylactic antibiotics (trimethoprim-sulfamethoxazole) and antifungals (itraconazole) markedly diminish the frequency of life-threatening infections. Short courses of glucocorticoids may relieve gastrointestinal or genitourinary tract obstruction by granulomas in patients with CGD. Recombinant human IFN-γ, which nonspecifically stimulates phagocytic cell function, reduces the frequency of infections in patients with CGD by 70% and reduces the severity of infection. This effect of IFN-γ in CGD is additive to the effect of prophylactic antibiotics. The recommended dose is 50 μg/m^2 subcutaneously three times weekly. IFN-γ has also been used successfully in the treatment of leprosy, nontuberculous mycobacteria, and visceral leishmaniasis.

Rigorous oral hygiene reduces but does not eliminate the discomfort of gingivitis, periodontal disease, and aphthous ulcers; chlorhexidine mouthwash and tooth brushing with a hydrogen peroxide–sodium bicarbonate paste helps many patients. Oral antifungal agents (fluconazole or itraconazole) have reduced mucocutaneous candidiasis in patients with Job's syndrome. Androgens, glucocorticoids, lithium, and immunosuppressive therapy have been used to restore myelopoiesis in patients with neutropenia due to impaired production. Recombinant G-CSF is useful in the management of certain forms of neutropenia due to depressed neutrophil production, especially those related to cancer chemotherapy. Patients with chronic neutropenia with evidence of a good bone marrow reserve need not receive prophylactic antibiotics. Patients with chronic or cyclic neutrophil counts < 500/μL may benefit from prophylactic antibiotics and G-CSF during periods of neutropenia. Oral trimethoprim-sulfamethoxazole (160/800 mg) twice daily can prevent infection. Increased numbers of fungal infections are not seen in patients with CGD on this regimen. Oral quinolones such as levofloxacin and ciprofloxacin are alternatives.

In the setting of cytotoxic chemotherapy with severe, persistent neutropenia, trimethoprim-sulfamethoxazole prevents *Pneumocystis jiroveci* pneumonia. These patients, and patients with phagocytic cell dysfunction, should avoid heavy exposure to airborne soil, dust, or decaying matter (mulch, manure), which are often rich in *Nocardia* and the spores of *Aspergillus* and other fungi. Restriction of activities or social contact has no proven role in reducing risk of infection.

Cure of some congenital phagocyte defects is possible by bone marrow transplantation (Chap. 108). However, complications of bone marrow transplantation are still serious, and with rigorous medical care many patients with phagocytic disorders can go for years without a life-threatening infection. The identification of specific gene defects in patients with LAD 1, CGD, and other immunodeficiencies has led to gene therapy trials in a number of genetic white cell disorders.

FURTHER READINGS

HORWITZ MS et al: Neutrophil elastase in cyclic and severe congenital neutropenia. Blood 109:1817, 2007

KLION AD et al: Approaches to the treatment of hypereosinophilic syndromes: A workshop summary report. J Allergy Clin Immunol 117:1292, 2006

NATHAN C: Neutrophils and immunity: Challenges and opportunities. Nat Rev Immunol 6:173, 2006

PUEL A et al: Heritable defects of the human TLR signalling pathways. J Endotoxin Res 11:220, 2005

ROSENZWEIG SD, HOLLAND SM: Phagocyte immunodeficiencies and their infections. J Allergy Clin Immunol 113:620, 2004

SEGAL BH et al: Genetic, biochemical, and clinical features of chronic granulomatous disease. Medicine (Baltimore) 79:170, 2000

62 Principles of Human Genetics

J. Larry Jameson, Peter Kopp

IMPACT OF GENETICS ON MEDICAL PRACTICE

The beginning of the new millennium was marked by the announcement that the vast majority of the human genome had been sequenced. This milestone in the exploration of the human genome was preceded by numerous conceptual and technological advances. They include, among others, the elucidation of the DNA double-helix structure, the discovery of restriction enzymes and the polymerase chain reaction (PCR), the development and automatization of DNA sequencing, and the generation of genetic and physical maps by the Human Genome Project (HGP). The consequences of this wealth of knowledge for the practice of medicine are profound. To date, the most significant impact of genetics has been to enhance our understanding of disease etiology and pathogenesis. However, genetics is rapidly playing a more prominent role in the diagnosis, prevention, and treatment of disease (Chap. 64). Genetic approaches have proven invaluable for the detection of infectious pathogens and are used clinically to identify agents that are difficult to culture such as mycobacteria, viruses, and parasites. In many cases, molecular genetics has improved the feasibility and accuracy of diagnostic testing and is beginning to open new avenues for therapy, including gene and cellular therapy (Chaps. 65 and 67). Molecular genetics has already significantly changed the treatment of human disease. Peptide hormones, growth factors, cytokines, and vaccines can now be produced in large amounts using recombinant DNA technology. Targeted modification of these peptides provides the practitioner with improved therapeutic tools, as illustrated by genetically modified insulin analogues with more favorable kinetics. There is hope that a better understanding of the genetic basis of human disease will also have an increasing impact on disease prevention.

Genetics has traditionally been viewed through the window of relatively rare single-gene diseases. Taken together, these disorders account for ~10% of pediatric admissions and childhood mortality. It is, however, increasingly apparent that virtually every medical condition, maybe with the exception of simple trauma, has a genetic component. As is often evident from a patient's family history, many common disorders such as hypertension, heart disease, asthma, diabetes mellitus, and mental illnesses are significantly influenced by the genetic background. These polygenic or multifactorial (complex) disorders involve the contributions of many different genes, as well as environmental factors, that can modify disease risk (Chap. 64). A major current challenge is to elucidate the genetic components that contribute to the pathogenesis of complex disorders. The recent publication of a comprehensive catalogue of human single-nucleotide polymorphism (SNP) haplotypes, the HapMap Project, provides an essential resource for genome-wide association studies (see below).

Cancer has a genetic basis since it results from acquired somatic mutations in genes controlling growth, apoptosis, and cellular differentiation (Chap. 79). In addition, the development of many cancers is associated with a hereditary predisposition. The prevalence of genetic diseases, combined with their severity and chronic nature, imposes a great financial, social, and emotional burden on society.

Genetics has historically focused on chromosomal and metabolic disorders, reflecting the long-standing availability of techniques to diagnose these conditions. For example, conditions such as trisomy 21 (Down syndrome) or monosomy X (Turner syndrome) can be diagnosed using cytogenetics (Chap. 63). Likewise, many metabolic disorders (e.g., phenylketonuria, familial hypercholesterolemia) are diagnosed using biochemical analyses. Recent advances in DNA diagnostics have extended the field of genetics to include virtually all medical specialties. In cardiology, for example, the molecular basis of inherited cardiomyopathies and ion channel defects that predispose to arrhythmias is being defined (Chaps. 226 and 231). In neurology, genetics has unmasked the pathophysiology of a startling number of neurodegenerative disorders (Chap. 360). Hematology has evolved dramatically, from its incipient genetic descriptions of hemoglobinopathies to the current understanding of the molecular basis of red cell membrane defects, clotting disorders, and thrombotic disorders (Chaps. 99 and 110).

New concepts derived from genetic studies can sometimes clarify the pathogenesis of disorders that were previously opaque. For example, although many different genetic defects can cause peripheral neuropathies, disruption of the normal folding of the myelin sheaths is frequently a common final pathway (Chap. 379). Several genetic causes of obesity appear to converge on a physiologic pathway that involves products of the proopiomelanocortin polypeptide and the MC4R receptor, thus identifying a key mechanism for appetite control (Chap. 74). A similar phenomenon is emerging for genetically distinct forms of Alzheimer's disease, several of which lead to the formation of neurofibrillary tangles (Chap. 365). The identification of defective genes often leads to the detection of cellular pathways involved in key physiologic processes. Examples include identification of the cystic fibrosis conductance regulator (*CFTR*) gene; the Duchenne muscular dystrophy (*DMD*) gene, which encodes dystrophin; and the fibroblast growth factor receptor-3 (*FGFR3*) gene, which is responsible for achondroplastic dwarfism. Similarly, transgenic (over)expression, and targeted gene "knock-out" and "knock-in" models help to unravel the physiologic function of genes.

The astounding rate at which new genetic information is being generated creates a major challenge for physicians, health care providers, and basic investigators. The terminology and techniques used for discovery evolve continuously. Much genetic information presently resides in computer databases or is being published in basic science journals. Databases provide easy access to the expanding information about the human genome, genetic disease, and genetic testing (Table 62-1). For example, several thousand monogenic disorders are summarized in a large, continuously evolving compendium, referred to as the *Online Mendelian Inheritance in Man* (OMIM) catalogue (Table 62-1). The ongoing refinement of bioinformatics is simplifying the access to this seemingly daunting onslaught of new information.

CHROMOSOMES AND DNA REPLICATION

Organization of DNA into Chromosomes • *SIZE OF THE HUMAN GENOME*

The human genome is divided into 23 different chromosomes, including 22 autosomes (numbered 1–22) and the X and Y sex chromosomes. Adult cells are *diploid*, meaning they contain two homologous sets of 22 autosomes and a pair of sex chromosomes. Females have two X chromosomes (XX), whereas males have one X and one Y chromosome (XY). As a consequence of meiosis, germ cells (sperm or oocytes) are haploid and contain one set of 22 autosomes and one of the sex chromosomes. At the time of fertilization, the diploid genome is reconstituted by pairing of the homologous chromosomes from the mother and father. With each cell division (mitosis), chromosomes are replicated, paired, segregated, and divided into two daughter cells (Chap. 63).

The human genome is estimated to contain ~30,000–40,000 genes, a smaller number than initially predicted, that are divided among the 23 chromosomes. A *gene* is a functional unit that is regulated by transcription (see below) and encodes a RNA product, which is most commonly, but not always, translated into a protein that exerts activity within or outside the cell. Historically, genes were identified because they conferred specific traits that are transmitted from one generation to the next. Increasingly, they are characterized based on expression in

TABLE 62-1 SELECTED DATABASES RELEVANT FOR GENOMICS AND GENETIC DISORDERS

Site	URL	Comment
National Center for Biotechnology Information (NCBI)	*http://www.ncbi.nlm.nih.gov/*	Molecular biology information, public databases, computational biology. Software for analyzing genome data. Extensive links to other databases, genome resources, and tutorials
National Human Genome Research Institute	*http://www.genome.gov/*	Web links providing information about the human genome sequence, genomes of other organisms, and genomic research
Ensembl Genome browser	*http://www.ensembl.org/*	Maps and sequence information of eukaryotic genomes
Online Mendelian Inheritance in Man	*http://www.ncbi.nlm.nih.gov/omim/*	Online compendium of Mendelian disorders and human genes causing genetic disorders
Office of Biotechnology Activities National Institutes of Health	*www4.od.nih.gov/oba/*	Information about recombinant DNA and gene transfer
		Medical, ethical, legal, and social issues raised by genetic testing
		Medical, ethical, legal, and social issues raised by xenotransplantation
American College of Medical Genetics	*http://www.acmg.net/*	Extensive links to other databases relevant for the diagnosis, treatment, and prevention of genetic disease
Cancer Genome Anatomy Project (CGAP)	*http://cgap.nci.nih.gov/*	Information about gene expression profiles of normal, precancer, and cancer cells
GenLink	*http://www.genlink.wustl.edu*	Multimedia database resource for human genetics and telomere research
GeneTests	*http://www.genetests.org/*	International directory of genetic testing laboratories and prenatal diagnosis clinics
		Reviews and educational materials
Genomes Online Database (GOLD)	*http://www.genomesonline.org/*	Information on published and unpublished genomes
HUGO Gene Nomenclature	*http://www.gene.ucl.ac.uk/nomenclature*	Gene names and symbols
MITOMAP, a human mitochondrial genome database	*http://www.mitomap.org/*	A compendium of polymorphisms and mutations of the human mitochondrial DNA
Mitochondrial disorders	*http://www.neuro.wustl.edu/neuromuscular/mitosyn.html*	Overview on clinical syndromes associated with mtDNA mutations
DNA repeat sequences & disease	*http://www.neuro.wustl.edu/neuromuscular/mother/dnarep.htm*	Overview on clinical syndromes associated with DNA repeats
Online Mendelian Inheritance in Animals (OMIA)	*http://omia.angis.org.au/*	Online compendium of Mendelian disorders in animals
The Jackson Laboratory	*http://www.jax.org/*	Information about murine models and the mouse genome
International HapMap Project	*http://www.hapmap.org/*	Catalogue of haplotypes in different ethnic groups relevant for association studies and pharmacogenomics
Nuclear Receptor Signaling Atlas	*http://nursa.org*	Atlas of nuclear receptors, coregulators, and ligands
Dolan DNA Learning Center, Cold Spring Harbor Laboratories	*http://www.dnalc.org/*	Educational material about selected genetic disorders, DNA, eugenics, and genetic origin
The Online Metabolic and Molecular Bases of Inherited Disease (OMMBID)	*http://genetics.accessmedicine.com*	Online version of the comprehensive text on The Metabolic and Molecular Bases of Inherited Disease, 8e

Note: Databases are evolving constantly. Pertinent information may be found by using links listed in the few selected databases. Instructions for the use of genome-related databases have been published [Nat Genet 32(Suppl):1–79, 2002].

various tissues. The number of genes greatly underestimates the complexity of genetic expression, as single genes can generate multiple spliced mRNA products, which are translated into proteins that are subject to complex posttranslational modification, such as phosphorylation. *Proteomics,* the study of the proteome using technologies of large-scale protein separation and identification, is an emerging field focused on protein variation and function. Similarly, the field of *metabolomics* aims at determining the composition and modifications of the *metabolome,* the complement of low-molecular-weight molecules, many of which participate in various metabolic functions. These analyses, which are heavily dependent on bioinformatics, reveal that physiologic or pathologic alterations have myriad effects on the proteome and the metabolome and emphasize that these processes involve *modular networks* rather than *linear pathways.*

Human DNA consists of ~3 billion base pairs (bp) of DNA per haploid genome. DNA length is normally measured in units of 1000 bp (kilobases, kb) or 1,000,000 bp (megabases, Mb). Not all DNA encodes genes. In fact, genes account for only ~10–15% of DNA. Much of the remaining DNA consists of highly repetitive sequences, the function of which is poorly understood. These repetitive DNA regions, along with nonrepetitive sequences that do not encode genes, may serve a structural role in the packaging of DNA into chromatin, i.e., DNA bound to histone proteins, and chromosomes (Fig. 62-1). If only 10% of DNA is expressed and there are 30,000 genes, the average gene would be ~10 kb in length. Although many genes are about this size, the range is quite broad. For example, some genes are only a few hundred bp, whereas others, such as the *DMD* gene, are extraordinarily large (2 Mb).

STRUCTURE OF DNA Each gene is composed of a linear polymer of DNA. DNA is a double-stranded helix composed of four different bases: adenine (A), thymidine (T), guanine (G), and cytosine (C). Adenine is paired to thymidine, and guanine is paired to cytosine, by hydrogen bond interactions that span the double helix. DNA has several remarkable features that make it ideal for the transmission of genetic information. It is relatively stable, at least in comparison to RNA or proteins. The double-stranded nature of DNA and its feature of strict base-pair complementarity permit faithful replication during cell division. As described below, complementarity also allows the transmission of genetic information from DNA → RNA → protein (Fig. 62-2). Messenger RNA (mRNA) is encoded by the so-called sense or coding strand of the DNA double helix and is translated into proteins by ribosomes.

The presence of four different bases provides surprising genetic diversity. In the protein-coding regions of genes, the DNA bases are arranged into codons, a triplet of bases that specifies a particular amino acid. It is possible to arrange the four bases into 64 different triplet codons (4^3). Each codon specifies 1 of the 20 different amino acids, or a regulatory signal, such as initiation and stop of translation. Because there are more codons than amino acids, the genetic code is degenerate; that is, most amino acids can be specified by several different codons. By arranging the codons in different combinations and in various lengths, it is possible to generate the tremendous diversity of primary protein structure.

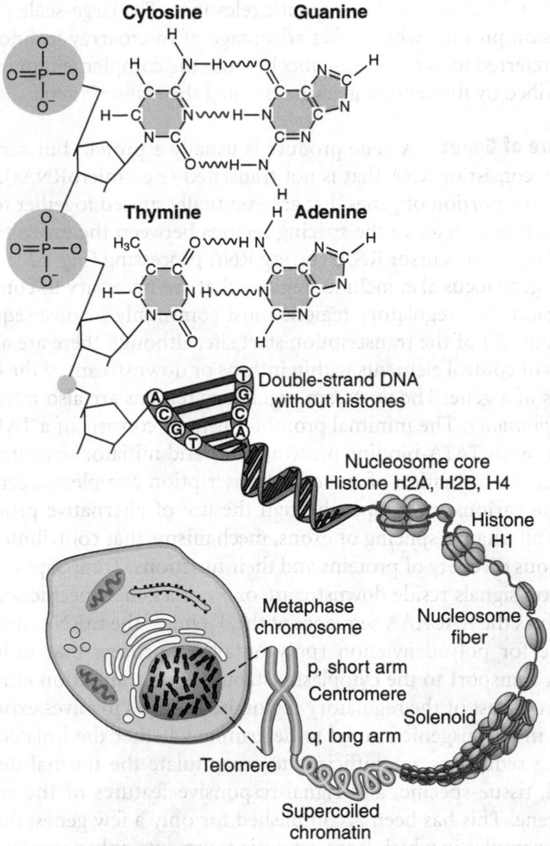

FIGURE 62-1 Structure of chromatin and chromosomes. Chromatin is composed of double-strand DNA that is wrapped around histone and nonhistone proteins forming nucleosomes. The nucleosomes are further organized into solenoid structures. Chromosomes assume their characteristic structure, with short (p) and long (q) arms at the metaphase stage of the cell cycle.

Replication of DNA and Mitosis Genetic information in DNA is transmitted to daughter cells under two different circumstances: (1) somatic cells divide by mitosis, allowing the diploid ($2n$) genome to replicate itself completely in conjunction with cell division; and (2) germ cells (sperm and ova) undergo meiosis, a process that enables the reduction of the diploid ($2n$) set of chromosomes to the haploid state ($1n$) (Chap. 63).

Prior to mitosis, cells exit the resting, or G_0 state, and enter the cell cycle (Chap. 80). After traversing a critical checkpoint in G_1, cells undergo DNA synthesis (S phase), during which the DNA in each chromosome is replicated, yielding two pairs of sister chromatids ($2n \rightarrow 4n$). The process of DNA synthesis requires stringent fidelity in order to avoid transmitting errors to subsequent generations of cells. Genetic abnormalities of DNA mismatch/repair include xeroderma pigmentosum, Bloom syndrome, ataxia telangiectasia, and hereditary nonpolyposis colon cancer (HNPCC), among others. Many of these disorders strongly predispose to neoplasia because of the rapid acquisition of additional mutations (Chap. 79). After completion of DNA synthesis, cells enter G_2 and progress through a second checkpoint before entering mitosis. At this stage, the chromosomes condense and are aligned along the equatorial plate at metaphase. The two identical sister chromatids, held together at the centromere, divide and migrate to opposite poles of the cell (see Fig. 63-3). After formation of a nuclear membrane around the two separated sets of chromatids, the cell divides and two daughter cells are formed, thus restoring the diploid ($2n$) state.

Assortment and Segregation of Genes during Meiosis Meiosis occurs only in germ cells of the gonads. It shares certain features with mitosis but involves two distinct steps of cell division that reduce the chromosome number to the haploid state. In addition, there is active recombination that generates genetic diversity. During the first cell division, two sister chromatids ($2n \rightarrow 4n$) are formed for each chromosome pair and there is an exchange of DNA between homologous paternal and maternal chromosomes. This process involves the formation of *chiasmata*, structures that correspond to the DNA segments that cross over between the maternal and paternal homologues (Fig. 62-3). Usually there is at least one crossover on each chromosomal arm; recombination occurs more frequently in female meiosis than in male meiosis. Subsequently, the chromosomes segregate randomly. Because there are 23 chromosomes, there exist 2^{23} (>8 million) possible combinations of chromosomes. Together with the genetic exchanges that occur during recombination, chromosomal segregation generates tremendous diversity, and each gamete is genetically unique. The process of recom-

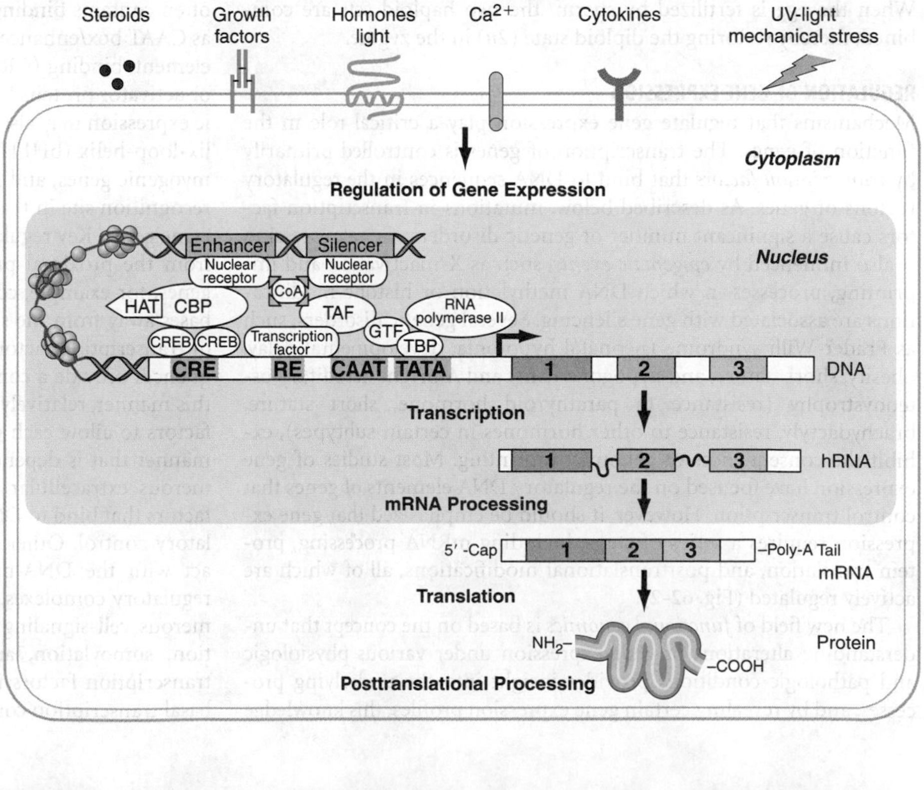

FIGURE 62-2 Flow of genetic information. Multiple extracellular signals activate intracellular signal cascades that result in altered regulation of gene expression through the interaction of transcription factors with regulatory regions of genes. RNA polymerase transcribes DNA into RNA that is processed to mRNA by excision of intronic sequences. The mRNA is translated into a polypeptide chain to form the mature protein after undergoing posttranslational processing. HAT, histone acetyl transferase; CBP, CREB-binding protein; CREB, cyclic AMP response element–binding protein; CRE, cyclic AMP responsive element; CoA, Co activator; TAF, TBP-associated factors; GTF, general transcription factors; TBP, TATA-binding protein; TATA, TATA box; RE, response element; NH_2, aminoterminus; COOH, carboxyterminus.

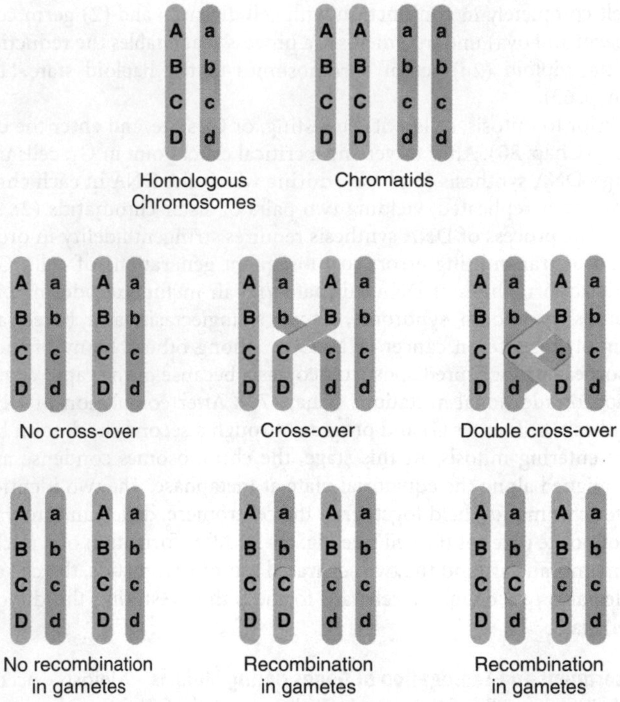

FIGURE 62-3 Crossing-over and genetic recombination. During chiasma formation, either of the two sister chromatids on one chromosome pairs with one of the chromatids of the homologous chromosome. Genetic recombination occurs through crossing-over and results in recombinant and nonrecombinant chromosome segments in the gametes. Together with the random segregation of the maternal and paternal chromosomes, recombination contributes to genetic diversity and forms the basis of the concept of linkage.

bination, and the independent segregation of chromosomes, provide the foundation for performing linkage analyses, whereby one attempts to correlate the inheritance of certain chromosomal regions (or linked genes) with the presence of a disease or genetic trait (see below).

After the first meiotic division, which results in two daughter cells ($2n$), the two chromatids of each chromosome separate during a second meiotic division to yield four gametes with a haploid state ($1n$). When the egg is fertilized by sperm, the two haploid sets are combined, thereby restoring the diploid state ($2n$) in the zygote.

REGULATION OF GENE EXPRESSION

Mechanisms that regulate gene expression play a critical role in the function of genes. The transcription of genes is controlled primarily by *transcription factors* that bind to DNA sequences in the regulatory regions of genes. As described below, mutations in transcription factors cause a significant number of genetic disorders. Gene expression is also influenced by *epigenetic events*, such as X-inactivation and imprinting, processes in which DNA methylation or histone modifications are associated with gene silencing. Several genetic disorders, such as Prader-Willi syndrome (neonatal hypotonia, developmental delay, obesity, short stature, and hypogonadism) and Albright hereditary osteodystrophy (resistance to parathyroid hormone, short stature, brachydactyly, resistance to other hormones in certain subtypes), exhibit the consequences of genomic imprinting. Most studies of gene expression have focused on the regulatory DNA elements of genes that control transcription. However, it should be emphasized that gene expression requires a series of steps, including mRNA processing, protein translation, and posttranslational modifications, all of which are actively regulated (Fig. 62-2).

The new field of *functional genomics* is based on the concept that understanding alterations of gene expression under various physiologic and pathologic conditions provides insight into the underlying processes, and by revealing certain gene expression profiles, this knowledge may be of diagnostic and therapeutic relevance. The large-scale study of expression profiles, which takes advantage of microarray technologies, is also referred to as *transcriptomics* because the complement of mRNAs transcribed by the cellular genome is called the *transcriptome.*

Structure of Genes A gene product is usually a protein but can occasionally consist of RNA that is not translated (e.g., microRNAs). *Exons* refer to the portion of genes that are eventually spliced together to form mRNA. *Introns* refer to the spacing regions between the exons that are spliced out of precursor RNAs during RNA processing (Fig. 62-2).

The gene locus also includes regions that are necessary to control its expression. The regulatory regions most commonly involve sequences upstream (5′) of the transcription start site, although there are also examples of control elements within introns or downstream of the coding regions of a gene. The upstream regulatory regions are also referred to as the *promoter*. The minimal promoter usually consists of a TATA box (which binds TATA-binding protein, TBP) and initiator sequences that enhance the formation of an active transcription complex. A gene may generate various transcripts through the use of alternative promoters and/or alternative splicing of exons, mechanisms that contribute to the enormous diversity of proteins and their functions. Transcriptional termination signals reside downstream, or 3′, of a gene. Specific sequences, such as the AAUAAA sequence at the 3′ end of the mRNA, designate the site for polyadenylation (poly-A tail), a process that influences mRNA transport to the cytoplasm, stability, and translation efficiency. A rigorous test of the regulatory region boundaries involves expressing a gene in a transgenic animal to determine whether the isolated DNA flanking sequences are sufficient to recapitulate the normal developmental, tissue-specific, and signal-responsive features of the endogenous gene. This has been accomplished for only a few genes; there are many examples in which large genomic fragments only partially reconstitute normal gene regulation in vivo, implying the presence of distant regulatory sequences. Genome-wide analyses of selected transcription factor binding sites, such as for the estrogen receptor, reveal that the majority of regulatory sites are very distant from the transcription start sites of genes. A detailed understanding of mechanisms that regulate genes is also relevant for gene therapy strategies that require normal gene regulation (Chap. 65).

The number of DNA sequences and transcription factors that regulate transcription is much greater than originally anticipated. Most genes contain at least 15–20 discrete regulatory elements within 300 bp of the transcription start site. This densely packed promoter region often contains binding sites for ubiquitous transcription factors such as CAAT box/enhancer binding protein (C/EBP), cyclic AMP response element–binding (CREB) protein, selective promoter factor 1 (Sp-1), or activator protein 1 (AP-1). However, factors involved in cell-specific expression may also bind to these sequences. For example, basic helix-loop-helix (bHLH) proteins bind to E-boxes in the promoters of myogenic genes, and steroidogenic factor 1 (SF-1) binds to a specific recognition site in the regulatory region of multiple steroidogenic enzyme genes. Key regulatory elements may also reside at a large distance from the proximal promoter. The globin and the immunoglobulin genes, for example, contain *locus control regions* that are several kilobases away from the structural sequences of the gene. Specific groups of transcription factors that bind to these promoter and enhancer sequences provide a combinatorial code for regulating transcription. In this manner, relatively ubiquitous factors interact with more restricted factors to allow each gene to be expressed and regulated in a unique manner that is dependent on developmental state, cell type, and numerous extracellular stimuli. As described below, the transcription factors that bind to DNA actually represent only the first level of regulatory control. Other proteins—*coactivators* and *co-repressors*—interact with the DNA-binding transcription factors to generate large regulatory complexes. These complexes are subject to control by numerous cell-signaling pathways, including phosphorylation, acetylation, sumoylation, and ubiquitinylation. Ultimately, the recruited transcription factors interact with, and stabilize, components of the basal transcription complex that assembles at the site of the TATA box

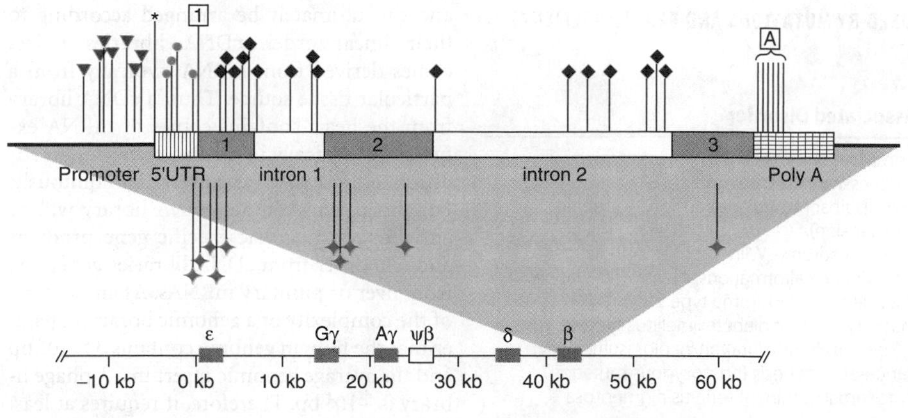

FIGURE 62-4 Point mutations causing β-thalassemia as example of allelic heterogeneity. The β-globin gene is located in the globin gene cluster. Point mutations can be located in the promoter, the CAP site, the 5′-untranslated region, the initiation codon, each of the three exons, the introns, or the polyadenylation signal. Many mutations introduce missense or nonsense mutations, whereas others cause defective RNA splicing. Not shown here are deletion mutations of the β-globin gene or larger deletions of the globin locus that can also result in thalassemia. ▼, Promoter mutations; *, CAP site; •, 5′UTR; 1, Initiation codon; ♦, Defective RNA processing; ✦, Missense and nonsense mutations; A, Poly A signal.

and initiator region. This basal transcription factor complex consists of >30 different proteins. Gene transcription occurs when RNA polymerase begins to synthesize RNA from the DNA template.

Mutations can occur in all domains of a gene (Fig. 62-4). A point mutation occurring within the coding region leads to an amino acid substitution if the codon is altered. Point mutations that introduce a premature stop codon result in a truncated protein. Large deletions may affect a portion of a gene or an entire gene, whereas small deletions and insertions alter the reading frame if they do not represent a multiple of three bases. These "frameshift" mutations lead to an entirely altered carboxy terminus. Mutations occurring in regulatory or intronic regions may result in altered expression or splicing of genes. Examples are shown in Fig. 62-5.

Transcriptional Activation and Repression Every gene is controlled uniquely, whether in its spatial or temporal pattern of expression or in its response to extracellular signals. It is estimated that transcription factors account for ~30% of expressed genes. A growing number of identified genetic diseases involve transcription factors (Table 62-2). The MODY (maturity-onset diabetes of the young) disorders are representative of this group of diseases; mutations in several different islet cell–specific transcription factors cause various forms of MODY (Chap. 338).

Transcriptional activation can be divided into three main mechanisms:

1. Events that alter chromatin structure can enhance the access of transcription factors to DNA. For example, histone acetylation generally opens chromatin structure and is correlated with transcriptional activation.
2. Posttranslational modifications of transcription factors, such as phosphorylation, can induce the assembly of active transcription complexes. As an example, phosphorylation of CREB protein on serine 133 induces a conformational change that allows the recruitment of CREB-binding protein (CBP), a factor that integrates the actions of many transcription factors, including proteins, with histone acetyltransferase activity.
3. Transcriptional activators can displace a repressor protein. This mechanism is particularly common during development when the pattern of transcription factor expression changes dynamically.

Of course, these mechanisms are not mutually exclusive, and most genes are activated by some combination of these events.

Suppression of gene expression is as important as gene activation in the control of cell differentiation and function. Some mechanisms of repression are the corollary of activation. For example, repression is often associated with histone deacetylation or protein dephosphorylation. For nuclear hormone receptors, transcriptional silencing involves the recruitment of repression complexes that contain histone deacetylase activity. Aberrant expression of repressor proteins is sometimes associated with neoplasia. The t(15;17) chromosomal translocation that occurs in promyelocytic leukemia fuses the *PML* gene to a portion of the retinoic acid receptor α (*RAR α*) gene (Table 62-2). This event causes unregulated transcriptional repression in a manner that precludes normal cellular differentiation. The addition of the RAR ligand, retinoic acid, activates the receptor, thereby relieving repression and allowing cells to differentiate and ultimately undergo apoptosis. This mechanism has therapeutic importance as the addition of retinoic acid to treatment regimens induces a higher remission rate in patients with promyelocytic leukemia (Chap. 104). Methylation of promoter regions is frequently found in neoplasms and silences gene expression.

CLONING AND SEQUENCING DNA

A description of recombinant DNA techniques, the methodology used for the manipulation, analysis, and characterization of DNA segments, is beyond the scope of this chapter. As these methods are wide-

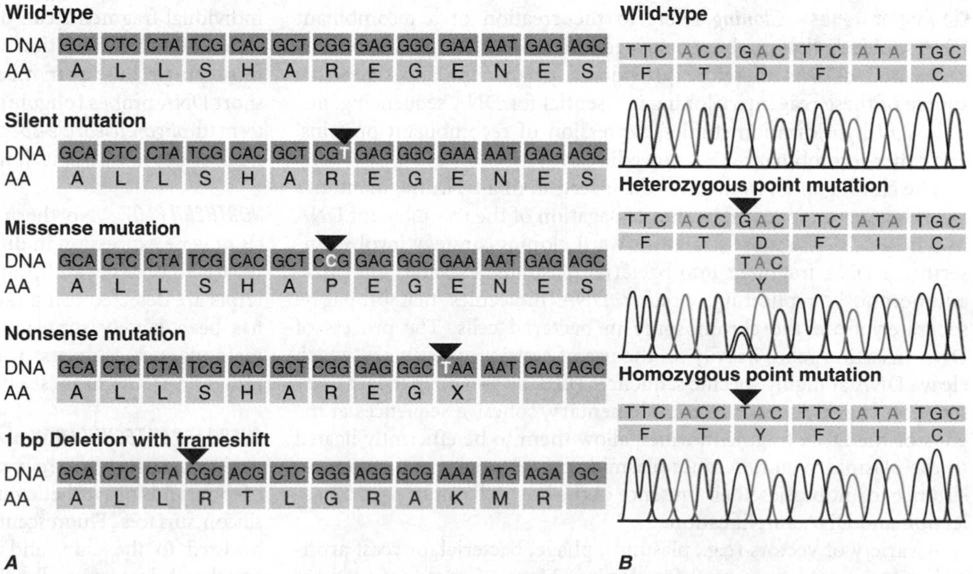

FIGURE 62-5 ***A.*** Examples of mutations. The coding strand is shown with the encoded amino acid sequence. ***B.*** Chromatograms of sequence analyses after amplification of genomic DNA by polymerase chain reaction.

TABLE 62-2 SELECTED EXAMPLES OF DISEASES CAUSED BY MUTATIONS AND REARRANGEMENTS IN TRANSCRIPTION FACTOR CLASSES

Transcription Factor Class	Example	Associated Disorder
Nuclear receptors	Androgen receptor	Complete or partial androgen insensitivity (recessive missense mutations) Spinobulbar muscular atrophy (CAG repeat expansion)
Zinc finger proteins	WT1	WAGR syndrome: Wilm's tumor, aniridia, genitourinary malformations, mental retardation
Basic helix-loop-helix	MITF	Waardenburg syndrome type 2A
Homeobox	IPF1	Maturity onset of diabetes mellitus type 4 (heterozygous mutation/haploinsufficiency) Pancreatic agenesis (homozygous mutation)
Leucine zipper	Retina leucine zipper (NRL)	Autosomal dominant retinitis pigmentosa
High mobility group (HMG) proteins	SRY	Sex-reversal
Forkhead	HNF4α, HNF1α, HNF1β	Maturity-onset of diabetes mellitus types 1, 3, 5
Paired box	PAX3	Waardenburg syndrome types 1 and 3
T-box	TBX5	Holt-Oram syndrome (thumb anomalies, atrial or ventricular septum defects, phocomelia)
Cell cycle control proteins	P53	Li-Fraumeni syndrome, other cancers
Coactivators	CREB binding protein (CBP)	Rubinstein-Taybi syndrome
General transcription factors	TATA-binding protein (TBP)	Spinocerebellar ataxia 17 (CAG expansion)
Transcription elongation factor	VHL	Von Hippel–Lindau syndrome (renal cell carcinoma, pheochromocytoma, pancreatic tumors, hemangioblastomas) Autosomal dominant inheritance, somatic inactivation of second allele (Knudson two-hit model)
Runt	CBFA2	Familial thrombocytopenia with propensity to acute myelogenous leukemia
Chimeric proteins due to translocations	PML—RAR	Acute promyelocytic leukemia t(15;17)(q22;q11.2-q12) translocation

Note: Selected abbreviations include: SRY, sex determining region Y; HNF, hepatocyte nuclear factor; CREB (cAMP responsive element binding) binding protein; VHL, Von Hippel–Lindau; PML, promyelocytic leukemia; RAR, retinoic acid receptor.

ly used in genetics and molecular diagnostics, however, it is useful to review briefly some of the fundamental principles of cloning and DNA sequencing.

Cloning of Genes *Cloning* refers to the creation of a recombinant DNA molecule that can be propagated indefinitely. The ability to clone genes and cDNAs therefore provides a permanent and renewable source of these reagents. Cloning is essential for DNA sequencing, nucleic acid hybridization studies, expression of recombinant proteins, and other recombinant DNA procedures.

The cloning of DNA involves the insertion of a DNA fragment into a cloning vector, followed by the propagation of the recombinant DNA in a host cell. The most straightforward cloning strategy involves inserting a DNA fragment into bacterial plasmids. Plasmids are small, autonomously replicating, circular DNA molecules that propagate separately from the chromosome in bacterial cells. The process of DNA insertion relies heavily on the use of restriction enzymes, which cleave DNA at highly specific sequences (usually 4–6 bp in length). Restriction enzymes generate complementary, cohesive sequences at the ends of the DNA fragment, which allow them to be efficiently ligated to the plasmid vector. Because plasmids contain genes that confer resistance to antibiotics, their presence in the host cell can be used for selection and DNA amplification.

A variety of vectors (e.g., plasmids, phage, bacterial, or yeast artificial chromosomes) are used for cloning. Many of these are used for creating *libraries*, a term that refers to a collection of DNA clones. A genomic library represents an array of clones derived from genomic DNA. These overlapping DNA fragments represent the entire genome and can ultimately be arranged according to their linear order. cDNA libraries reflect clones derived from mRNA, typically from a particular tissue source. Thus, a cDNA library from the heart contains copies of mRNA expressed specifically in cardiac myocytes, in addition to those that are expressed ubiquitously. For this reason, a heart cDNA library will be enriched with cardiac-specific gene products and will differ from cDNA libraries generated from liver or pituitary mRNAs. As an example of the complexity of a genomic library, consider that the human genome contains 3×10^9 bp and the average genomic insert in a λ phage library is ~10^4 bp. Therefore, it requires at least 3×10^5 clones to represent all genomic DNA. Specific clones are isolated from the several hundred thousand clones by using DNA hybridization.

With completion of the HGP, all human genes have been cloned and sequenced. As a result, many of these cloning procedures are now unnecessary or greatly facilitated by the extensive information concerning DNA markers and the sequence of DNA (see below).

Nucleic Acid Hybridization Nucleic acid *hybridization* is a fundamental principle in molecular biology that takes advantage of the fact that the two complementary strands of nucleic acids bind, or *hybridize*, to one another with very high specificity. The goal of hybridization is to detect specific nucleic acid (DNA or RNA) sequences in a complex background of other sequences. This technique is used for Southern blotting, Northern blotting, and for screening libraries (see above). Further adaptation of hybridization techniques has led to the development of microarray DNA chips.

SOUTHERN BLOT Southern blotting is used to analyze whether genes have been deleted or rearranged. It is also used to detect restriction fragment length polymorphisms (RFLPs). Genomic DNA is digested with restriction endonucleases and separated by gel electrophoresis. Individual fragments can then be transferred to a membrane and detected after hybridization with specific radioactive DNA probes. Because single base-pair mismatches can disrupt the hybridization of short DNA probes (oligonucleotides), a variation of the Southern blot, termed *oligonucleotide-specific hybridization* (OSH), uses short oligonucleotides to distinguish normal from mutant genes.

NORTHERN BLOT Northern blots are used to analyze patterns and levels of gene expression in different tissues. In a Northern blot, mRNA is separated on a gel and transferred to a membrane, and specific transcripts are detected using radiolabeled DNA as a probe. This technique has been largely supplanted by more sensitive and comprehensive methods such as reverse transcriptase (RT)–PCR and gene expression arrays on DNA chips (see below).

MICROARRAY TECHNOLOGY A comprehensive approach to genome-scale studies consists of *microarrays*, or *DNA chips*. These microarrays consist of thousands of synthetic nucleic acid sequences aligned on thin glass or silicon surfaces. Fluorescently labeled test sample DNA or RNA is hybridized to the chip, and a computerized scanner detects sequence matches. Microarrays allow the detection of variations in DNA sequence and are used for mutational analysis and genotyping. Alternatively, the expression pattern of large numbers of mRNA transcripts can be determined by hybridization of RNA samples to cDNA or genomic microarrays. This method has tremendous potential in the era of functional genomics and permits comprehensive analyses of gene expression profiles. As one example, microarrays can be used to develop genetic fingerprints of different types of malignancies, providing information useful for classification, pathophysiology, prognosis, and treatment.

The Polymerase Chain Reaction The PCR, introduced in 1985, has revolutionized the way DNA analyses are performed and has become a cornerstone of molecular biology and genetic analysis. In essence, PCR provides a rapid way of amplifying specific DNA fragments in vitro. Exquisite specificity is conferred by the use of PCR primers, which are designed for a given DNA sequence. The geometric amplification of the DNA after multiple cycles yields remarkable sensitivity. As a result, PCR can be used to amplify DNA from very small samples, including single cells. These properties also allow DNA amplification from a variety of tissue sources including blood samples, biopsies, surgical or autopsy specimens, or cells from hair or saliva. PCR can also be used to study mRNA. In this case, the enzyme RT is first used to convert the RNA to DNA, which can then be amplified by PCR. This procedure, commonly known as *RT-PCR*, is useful as a quantitative measure of gene expression.

PCR provides a key component of molecular diagnostics. It provides a strategy for the rapid amplification of DNA (or mRNA) to search for mutations by a wide array of techniques, including DNA sequencing. PCR is also used for the amplification of highly polymorphic di- or trinucleotide repeat sequences or the genotyping of SNPs, which allow various polymorphic alleles to be traced in genetic linkage or association studies. PCR is increasingly used to diagnose various microbial pathogens.

DNA Sequencing DNA sequencing is now an automated procedure. Although many protocols exist, the most commonly used strategy currently uses the capillary electrophoresis-based Sanger method in which dideoxynucleotides are used to randomly terminate DNA polymerization at each of the four bases (A,G,T,C). After separating the array of terminated DNA fragments using high-resolution gel or capillary electrophoresis, it is possible to deduce the DNA sequence by examining the progression of fragment lengths generated in each of the four nucleotide reactions. The use of fluorescently labeled dideoxynucleotides allows automated detection of the different bases and direct computer analysis of the DNA sequence (Fig. 62-5). Significant efforts are underway to develop faster, more cost-effective DNA sequencing technologies. These include the use of pyrosequencing chemistries; whole-genome sequencing using solid-phase sequencing; mass spectrometry; detection of fluorescently labeled bases in flow cytometry; direct reading of the DNA sequence by scanning, tunneling, or atomic force microscopy; and sequence analysis using DNA chips.

TRANSGENIC MICE AS MODELS OF GENETIC DISEASE

Several organisms have been studied extensively as genetic models, including *Mus musculus* (mouse), *Drosophila melanogaster* (fruit fly), *Caenorhabditis elegans* (nematode), *Saccharomyces cerevisiae* (baker's yeast), and *Escherichia coli* (colonic bacterium). The ability to use these evolutionarily distant organisms as genetic models that are relevant to human physiology reflects a surprising conservation of genetic pathways and gene function. Transgenic mouse models have been particularly valuable, because many human and mouse genes exhibit similar structure and function, and because manipulation of the mouse genome is relatively straightforward compared to those of other mammalian species.

Transgenic strategies in mice can be divided into two main approaches: (1) expression of a gene by random insertion into the genome, and (2) deletion or targeted mutagenesis of a gene by homologous recombination with the native endogenous gene (knock-out, knock-in) (Fig. 62-6; Table 62-3). Transgenic mice are generated by pronuclear injection of foreign DNA into fertilized mouse oocytes and subsequent transfer into the oviduct of pseudopregnant foster mothers.

Transgenic expression of genes can be useful for studying disorders that are sensitive to gene dosage. Overexpression of *PMP22*, for example, mimics a common duplication of this gene in type IA Charcot-Marie-Tooth disease (Chap. 379). Duplication of the *PMP22* gene results in high levels of expression of peripheral myelin protein 22, and this dosage effect is responsible for the demyelinating neuropathy. Expression of the Y chromosome–specific gene, *SRY*, in XX females demonstrates that *SRY* is sufficient to induce the formation of testes. This finding confirms the pathogenic role of *SRY* translocations to the X chromosome in sex-reversed XX females. Huntington disease is an autosomal dominant disorder caused by expansion of a CAG trinucleotide repeat that encodes a polyglutamine tract. Targeted deletion of the Huntington disease (*HD*) gene does not induce the neurologic disorder. On the other hand, transgenic expression of the entire gene or of the first exon containing the sequence encoding the expanded polyglutamine repeat is sufficient to cause many features of the neurologic disorder, indicating a gain-of-function property for the expanded polyglutamine-containing protein. Transgenic strategies can also be used as a precursor to gene therapy. Expression of dystrophin, the pro-

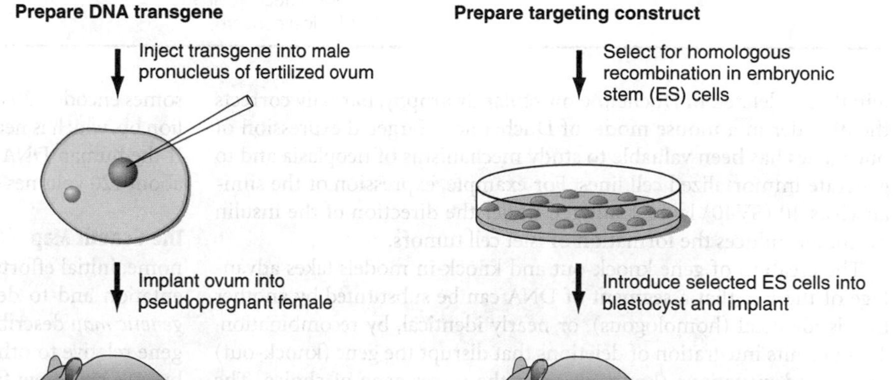

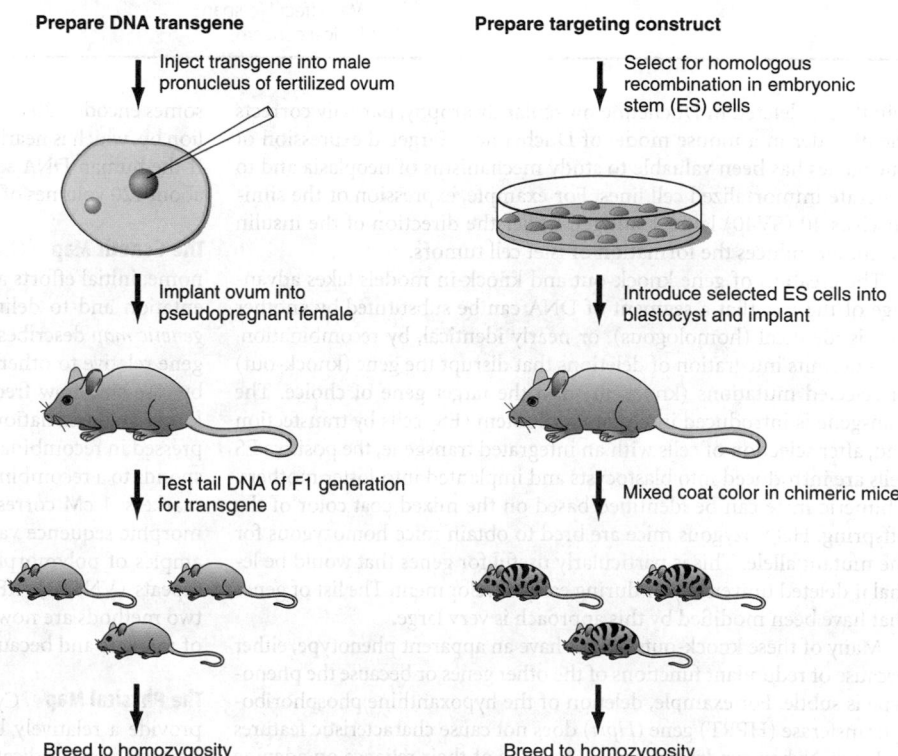

FIGURE 62-6 Transgenic mouse models. *Left.* Transgenic mice are generated by pronuclear injection of foreign DNA into fertilized mouse oocytes and subsequent transfer into the oviduct of pseudopregnant foster mothers. ***Right.*** For targeted mutagenesis (gene knock-out/knock-in), embryonic stem (ES) cells are transfected with the targeted (mutagenized) transgene. The transgene undergoes homologous recombination with the wild-type gene. After selection, positive ES cells are introduced into blastocysts and implanted into foster mothers. Chimeric mice can be identified based on the mixed coat color of the offspring. Heterozygous mice are bred to obtain mice homozygous for the mutant allele.

TABLE 62-3 GENETICALLY MODIFIED ANIMALS

Commonly Used Description	Technical Principle	Remarks
Transgenic	Pronuclear injection of transgene	Commonly used Genomic DNA or cDNA constructs Random integration of transgene Variable copy numbers of transgene Variable expression in each individual founder Gain-of-function models due to overexpression using tissue-specific promoters Loss-of-function models using anti-sense and dominant negative transgenes Inducible expression possible (Tetracycline, ecdysone) Applicable to several species
(Targeted) Knock-out	Substitution of functional gene with inactive gene by homologous recombination in embryonic stem cells	Predominantly used in mice Tissue-specific knock-out possible (Cre/lox) Absence of phenotype possible due to redundancy
(Targeted) Knock-in	Introduction of subtle mutation(s) into gene by substitution of endogenous gene with gene carrying a specific mutation. Homologous recombination in embryonic stem cells	Predominantly used in mice Can accurately model human disease
Forward genetics	Mutations created randomly by ENU (*N*-ethyl-*N*-nitrourea)	Selection of phenotype followed by genetic characterization Useful for identifying novel genes
Congenic strains	Mating of an inbred *donor* strain with a disease phenotype with an inbred *recipient* strain in order to define the genomic region responsible for the disorder	Useful for mapping disease-causing genes
Cloning	Introduction of nucleus into enucleated eggs (nuclear transfer)	Successful in several mammalian species including sheep (Dolly), mice, cows, monkeys Cloning of genetically identical individuals May affect life-span Ethical concerns

tein that is deleted in Duchenne muscular dystrophy, partially corrects the disorder in a mouse model of Duchenne's. Targeted expression of oncogenes has been valuable to study mechanisms of neoplasia and to generate immortalized cell lines. For example, expression of the simian virus 40 (SV40) large T antigen under the direction of the insulin promoter induces the formation of islet cell tumors.

The creation of gene knock-out and knock-in models takes advantage of the fact that a segment of DNA can be substituted by another that is identical (homologous), or nearly identical, by recombination. This permits integration of deletions that disrupt the gene (knock-out) or selected mutations (knock-in) into the target gene of choice. The transgene is introduced into embryonic stem (ES) cells by transfection and, after selection of cells with an integrated transgene, the positive ES cells are introduced into blastocysts and implanted into foster mothers. Chimeric mice can be identified based on the mixed coat color of the offspring. Heterozygous mice are bred to obtain mice homozygous for the mutant allele. This is particularly useful for genes that would be lethal if deleted universally or during early development. The list of genes that have been modified by this approach is very large.

Many of these knock-outs do not have an apparent phenotype, either because of redundant functions of the other genes or because the phenotype is subtle. For example, deletion of the hypoxanthine phosphoribosyltransferase (HPRT) gene (*Hprt*) does not cause characteristic features of Lesch-Nyhan syndrome in mice because of their reliance on adenine phosphoribosyltransferase (APRT) in the purine salvage pathway. Deletion of the retinoblastoma (*Rb*) gene encoding p105 does not lead to retinoblastoma or other tumors that characterize the human syndrome. However, mice with combinatorial deletion of several Rb-related proteins exhibit features similar to the human disorder. These examples underscore the fact that the functions of genes, and their interactions with genetic background and the environment, are not necessarily identical in mice and humans. On the other hand, the deletion of many genes provides a remarkably faithful model of human disorders. In addition to clarifying pathophysiology, these models facilitate the development of therapies, both genetic and pharmaceutical.

Many variations of these basic approaches now exist that allow genes to be expressed or deleted in specific cell types, at different times during development, or at varying levels. Consequently, transgenic technology has emerged as a powerful strategy for defining the physiologic effects of deleting or overexpressing a gene, as well as providing unique genetic models for dissecting pathophysiology or testing therapies. In addition to transgenic animal models, naturally occurring mutations in mice and other species continue to provide fundamental insights into human disease. A compendium of natural and transgenic animal models is provided in continuously evolving databases (Table 62-1).

IMPLICATIONS OF THE HUMAN GENOME PROJECT

The HGP was initiated in the mid-1980s as an ambitious effort to characterize the human genome, culminating in a complete DNA sequence. The initial main goals were (1) creation of genetic maps, (2) development of physical maps, and (3) determination of the complete human DNA sequence. Some analogies help in appreciating the scope of the HGP. The 23 pairs of human chromosomes encode ~30,000–40,000 genes. The total length of DNA is ~3 billion bp, which is nearly 1000-fold greater than that of the *E. coli* genome. If the human DNA sequence were printed out, it would correspond to about 120 volumes of *Harrison's Principles of Internal Medicine*.

The Genetic Map Given the size and complexity of the human genome, initial efforts aimed at developing genetic maps to provide orientation and to delimit where a gene of interest may be located. A *genetic map* describes the order of genes and defines the position of a gene relative to other loci on the same chromosome. It is constructed by assessing how frequently two markers are inherited together (i.e., *linked*) by association studies. Distances of the genetic map are expressed in recombination units, or centiMorgans (cM). One cM corresponds to a recombination frequency of 1% between two polymorphic markers; 1 cM corresponds to ~1 Mb of DNA (Fig. 62-3). Any polymorphic sequence variation can be useful for mapping purposes. Examples of polymorphic markers include variable number of tandem repeats (VNTRs), RFLPs, microsatellite repeats, and SNPs; the latter two methods are now used predominantly because of the high density of markers and because they are amenable to automated procedures.

The Physical Map Cytogenetics and chromosomal banding techniques provide a relatively low-resolution microscopic view of genetic loci. Physical maps indicate the position of a locus or gene in absolute values. Sequence-tagged sites (STSs) are used as a standard unit for physical mapping and serve as sequence-specific landmarks for arranging overlapping cloned fragments in the same order as they occur in the genome. These overlapping clones allow the characterization of contiguous DNA sequences, commonly referred to as *contigs*. This approach led to high-resolution physical maps by cloning the whole genome into overlapping fragments and has been essential for the identification of disease-causing genes by positional cloning.

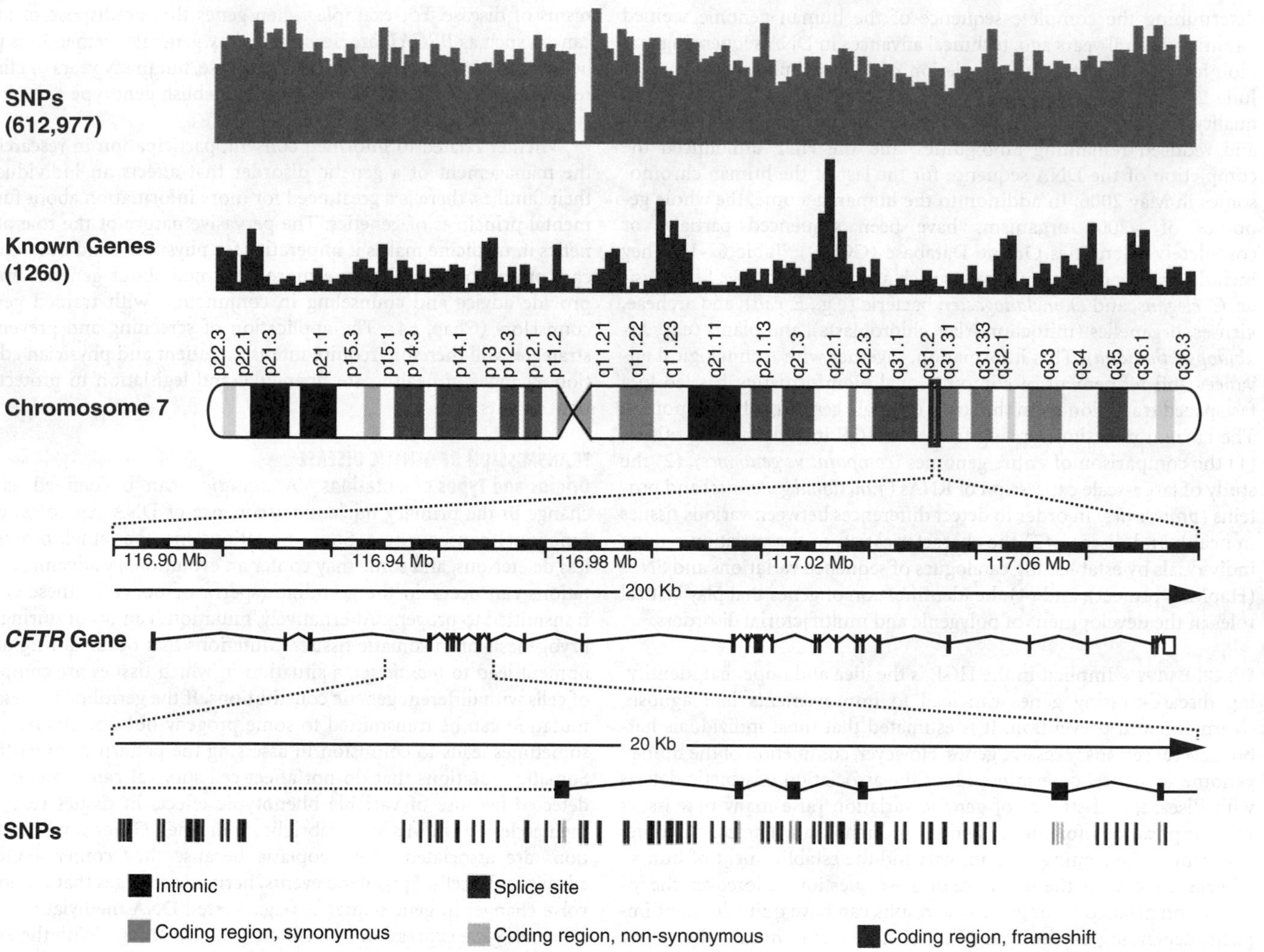

FIGURE 62-7 Chromosome 7 is shown with the density of single nucleotide polymorphisms (SNPs) and genes above. A 200-kb region in 7q31.2 containing the *CFTR* gene is shown below. The *CFTR* gene contains 27 exons. More than 1420 mutations in this gene have been found in patients with cystic fibrosis. A 20-kb region encompassing exons 4–9 is shown in further amplified in order to illustrate the SNPs in this region.

Recent insights into the structure of the normal human genome show that certain blocks of DNA sequences, often containing numerous genes, can be duplicated one or several times. This *copy number variation* (CNV), which tends to vary in a specific manner among different populations, is associated with hot spots of chromosomal rearrangements and is thought to play an important role in normal human variation and in genetic disease.

The identification of the ~10 million SNPs estimated to occur in the human genome has generated a catalogue of common genetic variants that occur in human beings from distinct ethnic backgrounds (Fig. 62-7). SNPs that are in close proximity are inherited together, i.e., they are linked, and are referred to as *haplotypes*, hence the name HapMap (Fig. 62-8). The HapMap describes the nature and location of these SNP haplotypes and how they are distributed among individuals within and among populations. The HapMap information is greatly facilitating genome-wide association studies designed to elucidate the complex interactions among multiple genes and lifestyle factors in multifactorial disorders (see below). Moreover, haplotype analyses may become useful to assess variations in responses to medications (*pharmacogenomics*) and environmental factors, as well as the prediction of disease predisposition.

The Human DNA Sequence The complete DNA sequence of each chromosome provides the highest resolution physical map. The primary focus of the HGP was to obtain DNA sequence for the entire human genome as well as model organisms. Although the prospect of

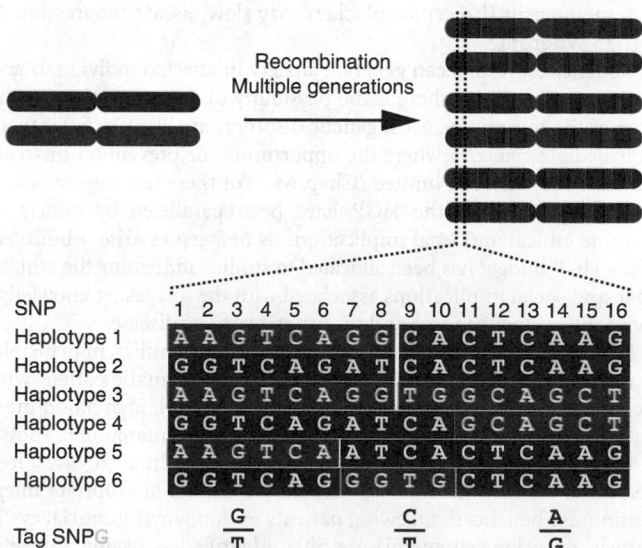

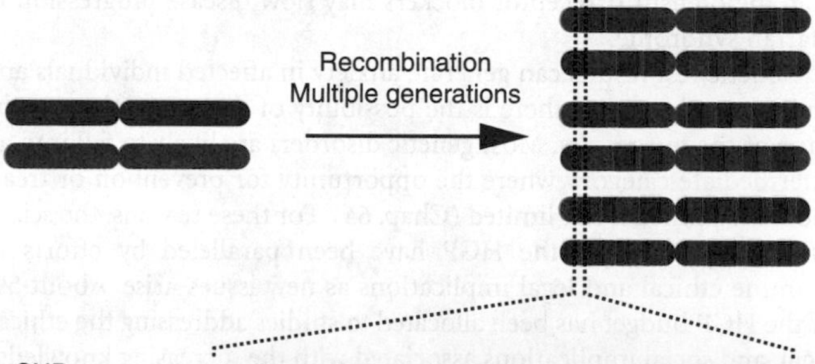

FIGURE 62-8 The origin of haplotypes is due to repeated recombination events occurring in multiple generations. Over time, this leads to distinct haplotypes. These haplotype blocks can often be characterized by genotyping selected Tag single nucleotide polymorphisms, an approach that now facilitates performing genome-wide association studies.

determining the complete sequence of the human genome seemed daunting several years ago, technical advances in DNA sequencing and bioinformatics led to the completion of a draft human sequence in June 2000, well in advance of the original goal year of 2003. High-quality reference sequences, completed in 2003, further closed gaps and reduced remaining ambiguities, and the HGP announced the completion of the DNA sequence for the last of the human chromosomes in May 2006. In addition to the human genome, the whole genomes of >2000 organisms have been sequenced partially or completely [Genomes Online Database (GOLD); Table 62-1]. They include, among others, eukaryotes such as man and mouse; *S. cerevisiae*, *C. elegans*, and *D. melanogaster*; bacteria (e.g., *E. coli*); and archeae, viruses, organelles (mitochondriae, chloroplasts), and plants (e.g., *Arabidopsis thaliana*). This information, together with technological advances and refinement of computational bioinformatics, has led to a fast-paced transition from the study of single genes to whole genomes. The current directions arising from the HGP include, among others, (1) the comparison of entire genomes (*comparative genomics*), (2) the study of large-scale expression of RNAs (*functional genomics)* and proteins *(proteomics*) in order to detect differences between various tissues in health and disease, (3) the characterization of the variation among individuals by establishing catalogues of sequence variations and SNPs (HapMap project), and (4) the identification of genes that play critical roles in the development of polygenic and multifactorial disorders.

Ethical Issues Implicit in the HGP is the idea and hope that identifying disease-causing genes can lead to improvements in diagnosis, treatment, and prevention. It is estimated that most individuals harbor several serious recessive genes. However, completion of the human genome sequence, determination of the association of genetic defects with disease, and studies of genetic variation raise many new issues with implications for the individual and mankind. The controversies concerning the cloning of mammals and the establishment of human ES cells underscore the relevance of these questions. Moreover, the information gleaned from genotypic results can have quite different impacts, depending on the availability of strategies to modify the course of disease. For example, the identification of mutations that cause multiple endocrine neoplasia (MEN) type 2 or hemochromatosis allows specific interventions for affected family members. On the other hand, at present, the identification of an Alzheimer or Huntington disease gene does not alter therapy and outcomes. In addition, the progress in this area is unpredictable, as underscored by the finding that angiotensin II receptor blockers may slow disease progression in Marfan syndrome.

Genetic test results can generate anxiety in affected individuals and family members, and there is the possibility of discrimination on the basis of the test results. Most genetic disorders are likely to fall into an intermediate category where the opportunity for prevention or treatment is significant but limited (Chap. 64). For these reasons, the scientific components of the HGP have been paralleled by efforts to examine ethical and legal implications as new issues arise. About 5% of the HGP budget has been allocated to studies addressing the ethical, legal, and social implications associated with the increasing knowledge about the human genome and the genetic basis of disease.

Many issues raised by the genome project are familiar, in principle, to medical practitioners. For example, an asymptomatic patient with increased low-density lipoprotein (LDL) cholesterol, high blood pressure, or a strong family history of early myocardial infarction is known to be at increased risk of coronary heart disease. In such cases, it is clear that the identification of risk factors and an appropriate intervention are beneficial. Likewise, patients with phenylketonuria, cystic fibrosis, or sickle cell anemia are often identified as having a genetic disease early in life. These precedents can be helpful for adapting policies that relate to genetic information. We can anticipate similar efforts, whether based on genotypes or other markers of genetic predisposition, to be applied to many disorders. One confounding aspect of the rapid expansion of information is that our ability to make clinical decisions often lags behind initial insights into genetic mechanisms of disease. For example, when genes that predispose to breast cancer, such as *BRCA1*, are described, they generate tremendous public interest in the potential to predict disease, but many years of clinical research are still required to rigorously establish genotype and phenotype correlations.

Whether related to informed consent, participation in research, or the management of a genetic disorder that affects an individual or their families, there is a great need for more information about fundamental principles of genetics. The pervasive nature of the role of genetics in medicine makes it imperative for physicians and other health care professionals to become more informed about genetics and to provide advice and counseling in conjunction with trained genetic counselors (Chap. 64). The application of screening and prevention strategies will therefore require intensive patient and physician education, changes in health care financing, and legislation to protect patient's rights.

TRANSMISSION OF GENETIC DISEASE

Origins and Types of Mutations A *mutation* can be defined as any change in the primary nucleotide sequence of DNA regardless of its functional consequences. Some mutations may be lethal, others are less deleterious, and some may confer an evolutionary advantage. Mutations can occur in the germline (sperm or oocytes); these can be transmitted to progeny. Alternatively, mutations can occur during embryogenesis or in somatic tissues. Mutations that occur during development lead to *mosaicism*, a situation in which tissues are composed of cells with different genetic constitutions. If the germline is mosaic, a mutation can be transmitted to some progeny but not others, which sometimes leads to confusion in assessing the pattern of inheritance. Somatic mutations that do not affect cell survival can sometimes be detected because of variable phenotypic effects in tissues (e.g., pigmented lesions in McCune-Albright syndrome). Other somatic mutations are associated with neoplasia because they confer a growth advantage to cells. Epigenetic events, heritable changes that do not involve changes in gene sequence (e.g., altered DNA methylation), may influence gene expression or facilitate genetic damage. With the exception of triplet nucleotide repeats, which can expand (see below), mutations are usually stable.

Mutations are structurally diverse—they can involve the entire genome, as in triploidy (one extra set of chromosomes), or gross numerical or structural alterations in chromosomes or individual genes (Chap. 63). Large deletions may affect a portion of a gene or an entire gene, or, if several genes are involved, they may lead to a *contiguous gene syndrome*. Unequal crossing-over between homologous genes can result in fusion gene mutations, as illustrated by color blindness (Chap. 29). Mutations involving single nucleotides are referred to as *point mutations* (Fig. 62-5). Substitutions are called *transitions* if a purine is replaced by another purine base (A ↔ G) or if a pyrimidine is replaced by another pyrimidine (C ↔ T). Changes from a purine to a pyrimidine, or vice versa, are referred to as *transversions*. If the DNA sequence change occurs in a coding region and alters an amino acid, it is called a *missense mutation*. Depending on the functional consequences of such a missense mutation, amino acid substitutions in different regions of the protein can lead to distinct phenotypes. *Polymorphisms* are sequence variations that have a frequency of at least 1%. Usually, they do not result in a perceptible phenotype. Often they consist of single base-pair substitutions that do not alter the protein coding sequence because of the degenerate nature of the genetic code (synonymous polymorphism), although it is possible that some might alter mRNA stability, translation, or the amino acid sequence (nonsynonymous polymorphism) (Fig. 62-7). These types of base substitutions are encountered frequently during genetic testing and must be distinguished from true mutations that alter protein expression or function. Small nucleotide deletions or insertions cause a shift of the codon reading frame (*frameshift*). Most commonly, reading frame alterations result in an abnormal protein segment of variable length before termination of translation occurs at a stop codon (*nonsense mutation*) (Fig. 62-5). Mutations in intronic sequences or in exon junctions may destroy or create splice donor or splice acceptor sites. Mutations may also be found in the regulatory sequences of genes, resulting in reduced gene transcription.

MUTATION RATES As noted before, mutations represent an important cause of genetic diversity as well as disease. Mutation rates are difficult to determine in humans because many mutations are silent and because testing is often not adequate to detect the phenotypic consequences. Mutation rates vary in different genes but are estimated to occur at a rate of $\sim 10^{-10}$/bp per cell division. Germline mutation rates (as opposed to somatic mutations) are relevant in the transmission of genetic disease. Because the population of oocytes is established very early in development, only ~20 cell divisions are required for completed oogenesis, whereas spermatogenesis involves ~30 divisions by the time of puberty and 20 cell divisions each year thereafter. Consequently, the probability of acquiring new point mutations is much greater in the male germline than the female germline, in which rates of aneuploidy are increased (Chap. 63). Thus, the incidence of new point mutations in spermatogonia increases with paternal age (e.g., achondrodysplasia, Marfan syndrome, neurofibromatosis). It is estimated that about 1 in 10 sperm carries a new deleterious mutation. The rates for new mutations are calculated most readily for autosomal dominant and X-linked disorders and are $\sim 10^{-5}$–10^{-6}/locus per generation. Because most monogenic diseases are relatively rare, new mutations account for a significant fraction of cases. This is important in the context of genetic counseling, as a new mutation can be transmitted to the affected individual but does not necessarily imply that the parents are at risk to transmit the disease to other children. An exception to this is when the new mutation occurs early in germline development, leading to *gonadal mosaicism*.

UNEQUAL CROSSING-OVER Normally, DNA recombination in germ cells occurs with remarkable fidelity to maintain the precise junction sites for the exchanged DNA sequences (Fig. 62-3). However, mispairing of homologous sequences leads to unequal crossover, with gene duplication on one of the chromosomes and gene deletion on the other chromosome. A significant fraction of growth hormone (*GH*) gene deletions, for example, involve unequal crossing-over (Chap. 333). The *GH* gene is a member of a large gene cluster that includes a growth hormone variant gene as well as several structurally related chorionic somatomammotropin genes and pseudogenes (highly homologous but functionally inactive relatives of a normal gene). Because such gene clusters contain multiple homologous DNA sequences arranged in tandem, they are particularly prone to undergo recombination and, consequently, gene duplication or deletion. On the other hand, duplication of the *PMP22* gene because of unequal crossing-over results in increased gene dosage and type IA Charcot-Marie-Tooth disease. Unequal crossing-over resulting in deletion of *PMP22* causes a distinct neuropathy called *hereditary liability to pressure palsy* (Chap. 379).

Glucocorticoid-remediable aldosteronism (GRA) is caused by a rearrangement involving the genes that encode aldosterone synthase (*CYP11B2*) and steroid 11β-hydroxylase (*CYP11B1*), normally arranged in tandem on chromosome 8q. These two genes are 95% identical, predisposing to gene duplication and deletion by unequal crossing-over. The rearranged gene product contains the regulatory regions of 11β-hydroxylase fused to the coding sequence of aldosterone synthetase. Consequently, the latter enzyme is expressed in the adrenocorticotropic hormone (ACTH)-dependent zona fasciculata of the adrenal gland, resulting in overproduction of mineralocorticoids and hypertension (Chap. 336).

Gene conversion refers to a nonreciprocal exchange of homologous genetic information; it is probably more common than generally recognized. In human genetics, gene conversion has been used to explain how an internal portion of a gene is replaced by a homologous segment copied from another allele or locus; these genetic alterations may range from a few nucleotides to a few thousand nucleotides. As a result of gene conversion, it is possible for short DNA segments of two chromosomes to be identical, even though these sequences are distinct in the parents. A practical consequence of this phenomenon is that nucleotide substitutions can occur during gene conversion between related genes, often altering the function of the gene. In disease states, gene conversion often involves intergenic exchange of DNA between a gene and a related pseudogene. For example, the 21-hydroxylase gene (*CYP21A2*) is adjacent to a nonfunctional pseudogene (*CYP21A1P*). Many of the nucleotide substitutions that are found in the *CYP21A2* gene in patients with congenital adrenal hyperplasia correspond to sequences that are present in the *CYP21A1P* pseudogene, suggesting gene conversion as a mechanism of mutagenesis. In addition, mitotic gene conversion has been suggested as a mechanism to explain revertant mosaicism in which an inherited mutation is "corrected" in certain cells. For example, patients with autosomal recessive generalized atrophic benign epidermolysis bullosa have acquired reverse mutations in one of the two mutated *COL17A1* alleles, leading to clinically unaffected patches of skin.

INSERTIONS AND DELETIONS Though many instances of insertions and deletions occur as a consequence of unequal crossing-over, there is also evidence for internal duplication, inversion, or deletion of DNA sequences. The fact that certain deletions or insertions appear to occur repeatedly as independent events suggests that specific regions within the DNA sequence predispose to these errors. For example, certain regions of the *DMD* gene appear to be hot spots for deletions. Some regions within the human genome are rearrangement hot spots and lead to CNVs (see above).

ERRORS IN DNA REPAIR Because mutations caused by defects in DNA repair accumulate as somatic cells divide, these types of mutations are particularly important in the context of neoplastic disorders (Chap. 80). Several genetic disorders involving DNA repair enzymes underscore their importance. Patients with xeroderma pigmentosum have defects in DNA damage recognition or in the nucleotide excision and repair pathway (Chap. 83). Exposed skin is dry and pigmented and is extraordinarily sensitive to the mutagenic effects of ultraviolet irradiation. More than 10 different genes have been shown to cause the different forms of xeroderma pigmentosum. This finding is consistent with the earlier classification of this disease into different complementation groups in which normal function is rescued by the fusion of cells derived from two different forms of xeroderma pigmentosum.

Ataxia telangiectasia causes large telangiectatic lesions of the face, cerebellar ataxia, immunologic defects, and hypersensitivity to ionizing radiation (Chap. 368). The discovery of the ataxia telangiectasia mutated (*ATM*) gene reveals that it is homologous to genes involved in DNA repair and control of cell cycle checkpoints. Mutations in the *ATM* gene give rise to defects in meiosis as well as increasing susceptibility to damage from ionizing radiation. Fanconi's anemia is also associated with an increased risk of multiple acquired genetic abnormalities. It is characterized by diverse congenital anomalies and a strong predisposition to develop aplastic anemia and acute myelogenous leukemia (Chap. 104). Cells from these patients are susceptible to chromosomal breaks caused by a defect in genetic recombination. At least eight different complementation groups have been identified, and several loci and genes associated with Fanconi's anemia have been mapped or cloned. HNPCC (Lynch syndrome) is characterized by autosomal dominant transmission of colon cancer, young age (<50 years) of presentation, predisposition to lesions in the proximal large bowel, and associated malignancies such as uterine cancer and ovarian cancer. HNPCC is caused by mutations in one of several different mismatch repair (MMR) genes including MutS homologue 2 (*MSH2*), MutL homologue 1 (*MLH1*), and *MSH6* (Chap. 87). These enzymes are involved in the detection of nucleotide mismatches and in the recognition of slipped-strand trinucleotide repeats. Germline mutations in these genes lead to microsatellite instability and a high mutation rate in colon cancer. Genetic screening tests for this disorder are now being used for families considered to be at risk (Chap. 64). Recognition of HNPCC allows early screening with colonoscopy and the implementation of prevention strategies using nonsteroidal anti-inflammatory drugs.

DIPYRIMIDINE AND CPG SEQUENCES Certain DNA sequences are particularly susceptible to mutagenesis. Successive pyrimidine residues (e.g., T-T or C-C) are subject to the formation of ultraviolet light–induced photoadducts. If these pyrimidine dimers are not repaired by the nucleotide excision repair pathway, mutations will be introduced after DNA synthesis. The dinucleotide C-G, or CpG, is also a hot spot for a specific type of mutation. In this case, methylation of the cytosine is associated with an enhanced rate of deamination to uracil, which is then replaced with thymine. This C → T transition (or G → A on the opposite strand) accounts for at least one-third of point mutations associated with polymorphisms and mutations. Many of the *MSH2* mutations in HNPCC, for example, involve CpG sequences. In addition to the fact that certain types of mutations (C → T or G → A) are relatively common, the nature of the genetic code also results in overrepresentation of certain amino acid substitutions.

UNSTABLE DNA SEQUENCES *Trinucleotide repeats* may be unstable and expand beyond a critical number. Mechanistically, the expansion is thought to be caused by unequal recombination and slipped mispairing. A premutation represents a small increase in trinucleotide copy number. In subsequent generations, the expanded repeat may increase further in length and result in an increasingly severe phenotype, a process called *dynamic mutation* (see below for discussion of anticipation). Trinucleotide expansion was first recognized as a cause of the fragile X syndrome, one of the most common causes of mental retardation. Other disorders arising from a similar mechanism include Huntington disease (Chap. 365), X-linked spinobulbar muscular atrophy (Chap. 369), and myotonic dystrophy (Chap. 382). Malignant cells are also characterized by genetic instability, indicating a breakdown in mechanisms that regulate DNA repair and the cell cycle.

Functional Consequences of Mutations Functionally, mutations can be broadly classified as gain-of-function and loss-of-function mutations. Gain-of-function mutations are typically dominant, i.e., they result in phenotypic alterations when a single allele is affected. Inactivating mutations are usually recessive, and an affected individual is homozygous or compound heterozygous (e.g., carrying two different mutant alleles of the same gene) for the disease-causing mutations. Alternatively, mutation in a single allele can result in ***haploinsufficiency***, a situation in which one normal allele is not sufficient to maintain a normal phenotype. Haploinsufficiency is a commonly observed mechanism in diseases associated with mutations in transcription factors (Table 62-2). Remarkably, the clinical features among patients with an identical mutation in a transcription factor often vary significantly. One mechanism underlying this variability consists in the influence of modifying genes. Haploinsufficiency can also affect the expression of rate-limiting enzymes. For example, haploinsufficiency in enzymes involved in heme synthesis can cause porphyrias (Chap. 352).

An increase in dosage of a gene product may also result in disease, as illustrated by the duplication of the *DAX1* gene in dosage-sensitive sex-reversal (Chap. 343). Mutation in a single allele can also result in loss of function due to a dominant-negative effect. In this case, the mutated allele interferes with the function of the normal gene product by one of several different mechanisms: (1) a mutant protein may interfere with the function of a multimeric protein complex, as illustrated by mutations in type 1 collagen (*COL1A1*, *COL1A2*) genes in osteogenesis imperfecta (Chap. 357); (2) a mutant protein may occupy binding sites on proteins or promoter response elements, as illustrated by thyroid hormone resistance, a disorder in which inactivated thyroid hormone receptor binds to target genes and functions as an antagonist of normal receptors (Chap. 335); or (3) a mutant protein can be cytotoxic as in α_1 antitrypsin deficiency (Chap. 254) or autosomal dominant neurohypophyseal diabetes insipidus (Chap. 334), in which the abnormally folded proteins are trapped within the endoplasmic reticulum and ultimately cause cellular damage.

Genotype and Phenotype • ***ALLELES, GENOTYPES, AND HAPLOTYPES*** An observed trait is referred to as a *phenotype*; the genetic information defining the phenotype is called the *genotype*. Alternative forms of a gene or a genetic marker are referred to as *alleles*. Alleles may be polymorphic variants of nucleic acids that have no apparent effect on gene expression or function. In other instances, these variants may have subtle effects on gene expression, thereby conferring the adaptive advantages associated with genetic diversity. On the other hand, allelic variants may reflect mutations in a gene that clearly alter its function. The common Glu6Val (E6V) sickle cell mutation in the β-*globin* gene and the ΔF508 deletion of phenylalanine (F) in the *CFTR* gene are examples of allelic variants of these genes that result in disease. Because each individual has two copies of each chromosome (one inherited from the mother and one inherited from the father), he or she can have only two alleles at a given locus. However, there can be many different alleles in the population. The normal or common allele is usually referred to as *wild type*. When alleles at a given locus are identical, the individual is *homozygous*. Inheriting identical copies of a mutant allele occurs in many autosomal recessive disorders, particularly in circumstances of consanguinity. If the alleles are different on the maternal and the paternal copy of the gene, the individual is *heterozygous* at this locus (Fig. 62-5). If two different mutant alleles are inherited at a given locus, the individual is said to be a *compound heterozygote*. *Hemizygous* is used to describe males with a mutation in an X chromosomal gene or a female with a loss of one X chromosomal locus.

Genotypes describe the specific alleles at a particular locus. For example, there are three common alleles (E2, E3, E4) of the apolipoprotein E (*APOE*) gene. The genotype of an individual can therefore be described as *APOE3/4* or *APOE4/4* or any other variant. These designations indicate which alleles are present on the two chromosomes in the *APOE* gene at locus 19q13.2. In other cases, the genotype might be assigned arbitrary numbers (e.g., 1/2) or letters (e.g., B/b) to distinguish different alleles.

A *haplotype* refers to a group of alleles that are closely linked together at a genomic locus (Fig. 62-8). Haplotypes are useful for tracking the transmission of genomic segments within families and for detecting evidence of genetic recombination, if the crossover event occurs between the alleles (Fig. 62-3). As an example, various alleles at the histocompatibility locus antigen (HLA) on chromosome 6p are used to establish haplotypes associated with certain disease states. For example, 21-hydroxylase deficiency, complement deficiency, and hemochromatosis are each associated with specific HLA haplotypes. It is now recognized that these genes lie in close vicinity to the HLA locus, which explains why HLA associations were identified even before the disease genes were cloned and localized. In other cases, specific HLA associations with diseases such as ankylosing spondylitis (HLA-B27) or type 1 diabetes mellitus (HLA-DR4) reflect the role of specific HLA allelic variants in susceptibility to these autoimmune diseases. The recent characterization of common SNP haplotypes in four populations from different parts of the world through the HapMap project is providing a novel tool for association studies designed to detect genes involved in the pathogenesis of complex disorders (Table 62-1). The presence or absence of certain haplotypes may also become relevant for the customized choice of medical therapies (pharmacogenomics) or for preventative strategies.

ALLELIC HETEROGENEITY *Allelic heterogeneity* refers to the fact that different mutations in the same genetic locus can cause an identical or similar phenotype. For example, many different mutations of the β-globin locus can cause β-thalassemia (Table 62-4) (Fig. 62-4). In essence, allelic heterogeneity reflects the fact that many different mutations are capable of altering protein structure and function. For this reason, maps of inactivating mutations in genes usually show a near-random distribution. Exceptions include: (1) a founder effect, in which a particular mutation that does not affect reproductive capacity can be traced to a single individual; (2) "hot spots" for mutations, in which the nature of the DNA sequence predisposes to a recurring mutation; and (3) localization of mutations to certain domains that are particularly critical for protein function. Allelic heterogeneity creates a practical problem for genetic testing because one must often examine the entire genetic locus for mutations, as these can differ in each pa-

TABLE 62-4 SELECTED EXAMPLES OF LOCUS HETEROGENEITY AND PHENOTYPIC HETEROGENEITY

Phenotypic Heterogeneity

Gene, Protein	Phenotype	Inheritance	OMIM
LMNA, Lamin A/C	Emery–Dreifuss muscular dystrophy (AD)	AD	181350
	Familial partial lipodystrophy Dunnigan	AD	151660
	Hutchinson-Gilford progeria	AD	176670
	Atypical Werner syndrome	AD	150330
	Dilated cardiomyopathy	AD	115200
	Early-onset atrial fibrillation	AD	607554
	Emery–Dreifuss muscular dystrophy (AR)	AR	604929
	Limb-girdle muscular dystrophy type 1B	AR	159001
	Charcot-Marie-Tooth type 2B1	AR	605588
KRAS	Noonan syndrome	AD	163950
	Cardio-facio-cutaneous syndrome	AD	115150

Locus Heterogeneity

Phenotype	Gene	Chromosomal Location	Protein
Familial hypertrophic cardiomyopathy			
Genes encoding sarcomeric proteins	*MYH7*	14q12	Myosin heavy chain beta
	TNNT2	1q2	Troponin-T2
	TPM1	15q22.1	Tropomyosin alpha
	MYBPC3	11p11q	Myosin binding protein C
	TNNI3	19q13.4	Troponin 1
	MYL2	12q23-24.3	Myosin light chain 2
	MYL3	3p	Myosin light chain 3
	TTN	2q24.3	Cardiac titin
	ACTC	15q11	Cardiac alpha actin
	MYH6	14q1	Myosin heavy chain alpha
	MYLK2	20q13.3	Myosin light-peptide kinase
	CAV3	3p25	Caveolin 3
Genes encoding nonsarcomeric proteins	*MTT1*	Mitochondrial	tRNA isoleucine
	MTTG	Mitochondrial	tRNA glycine
	PRKAG2	7q35-q36	AMP-activated protein kinase γ2 subunit
	DMPK	19q13.2-13.3	Myotonin protein kinase (myotonic dystrophy)
	FRDA	9q13	Frataxin (Friedreich ataxia)
Polycystic kidney disease	*PKD1*	16p13.3-13.12	Polycystin 1 (AD)
	PKD2	4q21.-23	Polycystin 2 (AD)
	PKHD1	6p21.1-p12	Fibrocystin (AR)
Noonan syndrome	PTPN11	12q24.1	Protein-tyrosine phosphatase 2c
	KRAS	12p12.1	KRAS

Note: AD, autosomal dominant; AR, autosomal recessive.

tient. For example, there are >1400 reported mutations in the *CFTR* gene (Fig. 62-7). The mutational analysis initially focuses on a panel of mutations that are particularly frequent (often taking the ethnic background of the patient into account), but a negative result does not exclude the presence of a mutation elsewhere in the gene. One should also be aware that mutational analyses generally focus on the coding region of a gene without considering regulatory and intronic regions. Because disease-causing mutations may be located outside the coding regions, negative results should be interpreted with caution.

PHENOTYPIC HETEROGENEITY *Phenotypic heterogeneity* occurs when more than one phenotype is caused by allelic mutations (e.g., different mutations in the same gene) (Table 62-4). For example, laminopathies are monogenic multisystem disorders that result from mutations in the *LMNA* gene, which encodes the nuclear lamins A and C. Twelve autosomal dominant and four autosomal recessive disorders are caused by mutations in the *LMNA* gene. They include several forms of lipodystrophies, Emery-Dreifuss muscular dystrophy, progeria syndromes, a form of neuronal Charcot-Marie-Tooth disease (type 2B1), and a group of overlapping syndromes. Remarkably, hierarchical cluster analysis has revealed that the phenotypes vary depending on the position of the mutation. Similarly, identical mutations in the *FGFR2* gene can result in very distinct phenotypes: Crouzon syndrome (craniofacial synostosis), or Pfeiffer syndrome (acrocephalopolysyndactyly).

LOCUS OR NONALLELIC HETEROGENEITY AND PHENOCOPIES *Nonallelic or locus heterogeneity* refers to the situation in which a similar disease phenotype results from mutations at different genetic loci. This often occurs when more than one gene product produces different subunits of an interacting complex or when different genes are involved in the same genetic cascade or physiologic pathway. For example, osteogenesis imperfecta can arise from mutations in two different procollagen genes (*COL1A1* or *COL1A2*) that are located on different chromosomes (Chap. 357). The effects of inactivating mutations in these two genes are similar because the protein products comprise different subunits of the helical collagen fiber. Similarly, muscular dystrophy syndromes can be caused by mutations in various genes, consistent with the fact that it can be transmitted in an X-linked (Duchenne or Becker), autosomal dominant (limb-girdle muscular dystrophy type 1), or autosomal recessive (limb-girdle muscular dystrophy type 2) manner (Chap. 382). Mutations in the X-linked *DMD* gene, which encodes dystrophin, are the most common cause of muscular dystrophy. This feature reflects the large size of the gene as well as the fact that the phenotype is expressed in hemizygous males because they have only a single copy of the X chromosome. Dystrophin is associated with a large protein complex linked to the membrane-associated cytoskeleton in muscle. Mutations in several different components of this protein complex can also cause muscular dystrophy syndromes. Although the phenotypic features of some of these disorders are distinct, the phenotypic spectrum caused by mutations in different genes overlaps, thereby leading to nonallelic heterogeneity. It should be noted that mutations in dystrophin also cause allelic heterogeneity. For example, mutations in the *DMD* gene can cause either Duchenne or the less severe Becker muscular dystrophy, depending on the severity of the protein defect.

Recognition of nonallelic heterogeneity is important for several reasons: (1) the ability to identify disease loci in linkage studies is reduced by including patients with similar phenotypes but different genetic disorders; (2) genetic testing is more complex because several different genes need to be considered along with the possibility of different mutations in each of the candidate genes; and (3) novel information is gained about how genes or proteins interact, providing unique insights into molecular physiology.

Phenocopies refer to circumstances in which nongenetic conditions mimic a genetic disorder. For example, features of toxin- or drug-induced neurologic syndromes can resemble those seen in Huntington disease, and vascular causes of dementia share phenotypic features with familial forms of Alzheimer dementia (Chap. 365). Children born with activating mutations of the thyroid-stimulating hormone receptor (TSH-R) exhibit goiter and thyrotoxicosis similar to that seen in neonatal Graves' disease, which is caused by the transfer of maternal autoantibodies to the fetus (Chap. 335). As in nonallelic heterogeneity, the presence of phenocopies has the potential to confound linkage studies and genetic testing. Patient history and subtle differences in phenotype can often provide clues that distinguish these disorders from related genetic conditions.

VARIABLE EXPRESSIVITY AND INCOMPLETE PENETRANCE The same genetic mutation may be associated with a phenotypic spectrum in different affected individuals, thereby illustrating the phenomenon of *variable expressivity*. This may include different manifestations of a disorder variably involving different organs (e.g., MEN), the severity of the disorder (e.g., cystic fibrosis), or the age of disease onset (e.g., Alzheimer dementia). MEN-1 illustrates several of these features. Families with this autosomal dominant disorder develop tumors of the parathyroid gland, endocrine pancreas, and the pituitary gland (Chap. 345). However, the pattern of tumors in the different glands, the age at which tumors develop, and the types of hormones produced vary among affected individuals, even within a given family. In this example, the phenotypic variability arises, in part, because of the requirement for a second mutation in the normal copy of the *MEN1* gene, as well as the large array of different cell types that are susceptible to the effects of *MEN1* gene mutations. In part, variable expression reflects the influence of modifier genes, or genetic background, on the effects of a particular mutation. Even in identical twins, in whom the genetic constitution is essentially the same, one can occasionally see variable expression of a genetic disease.

Interactions with the environment can also influence the course of a disease. For example, the manifestations and severity of hemochromatosis can be influenced by iron intake (Chap. 351), and the course of phenylketonuria is affected by exposure to phenylalanine in the diet (Chap. 358). Other metabolic disorders, such as hyperlipidemias and porphyria, also fall into this category. Many mechanisms, including genetic effects and environmental influences, can therefore lead to variable expressivity. In genetic counseling, it is particularly important to recognize this variability, as one cannot always predict the course of disease, even when the mutation is known.

Penetrance refers to the proportion of individuals with a mutant genotype that express the phenotype. If all carriers of a mutant express the phenotype, penetrance is complete, whereas it is said to be *incomplete* or *reduced* if some individuals do not have any features of the phenotype. Dominant conditions with incomplete penetrance are characterized by skipping of generations with unaffected carriers transmitting the mutant gene. For example, hypertrophic obstructive cardiomyopathy (HCM) caused by mutations in the *myosin-binding protein C* gene is a dominant disorder with clinical features in only a subset of patients who carry the mutation (Chap. 231). Patients who have the mutation but no evidence of the disease can still transmit the disorder to subsequent generations. In many conditions with postnatal onset, the proportion of gene carriers who are affected varies with age. Thus, when describing penetrance, one has to specify age. For example, for disorders such as Huntington disease or familial amyotrophic lateral sclerosis, which present late in life, the rate of penetrance is influenced by the age at which the clinical assessment is performed. *Imprinting* can also modify the penetrance of a disease (see below). For example, in patients with Albright hereditary osteodystrophy, mutations in the Gsα subunit (*GNAS1* gene) are expressed clinically only in individuals who inherit the mutation from their mother (Chap. 347).

SEX-INFLUENCED PHENOTYPES Certain mutations affect males and females quite differently. In some instances, this is because the gene resides on the X or Y sex chromosomes (X-linked disorders and Y-linked disorders). As a result, the phenotype of mutated X-linked genes will be expressed fully in males but variably in heterozygous females, depending on the degree of X-inactivation and the function of the gene. For example, most heterozygous female carriers of factor VIII deficiency (hemophilia A) are asymptomatic because sufficient factor VIII is produced to prevent a defect in coagulation (Chap. 110). On the other hand, some females heterozygous for the X-linked lipid storage defect caused by α-galactosidase A deficiency (Fabry disease) experience mild manifestations of painful neuropathy, as well as other features of the disease (Chap. 355). Because only males have a Y chromosome, mutations in genes such as *SRY*, which causes male-to-female sex-reversal, or *DAZ* (deleted in azoospermia), which causes abnormalities of spermatogenesis, are unique to males (Chap. 343).

Other diseases are expressed in a sex-limited manner because of the differential function of the gene product in males and females. Activating mutations in the luteinizing hormone receptor cause dominant male-limited precocious puberty in boys (Chap. 340). The phenotype is unique to males because activation of the receptor induces testosterone production in the testis, whereas it is functionally silent in the immature ovary. Biallelic inactivating mutations of the follicle-stimulating hormone (FSH) receptor cause primary ovarian failure in females because the follicles do not develop in the absence of FSH action. In contrast, affected males have a more subtle phenotype, because testosterone production is preserved (allowing sexual maturation) and spermatogenesis is only partially impaired (Chap. 340). In congenital adrenal hyperplasia, most commonly caused by 21-hydroxylase deficiency, cortisol production is impaired and ACTH stimulation of the adrenal gland leads to increased production of androgenic precursors (Chap. 336). In females, the increased androgen level causes ambiguous genitalia, which can be recognized at the time of birth. In males, the diagnosis may be made on the basis of adrenal insufficiency at birth, because the increased adrenal androgen level does not alter sexual differentiation, or later in childhood, because of the development of precocious puberty. Hemochromatosis is more common in males than in females, presumably because of differences in dietary iron intake and losses associated with menstruation and pregnancy in females (Chap. 351).

Chromosomal Disorders Chromosomal or cytogenetic disorders are caused by numerical or structural aberrations in chromosomes. Deviations in chromosome number are common causes of abortions, developmental disorders, and malformations. *Contiguous gene syndromes*, i.e., large deletions affecting several genes, have been useful for identifying the location of new disease-causing genes. Because of the variable size of gene deletions in different patients, a systematic comparison of phenotypes and locations of deletion breakpoints allows positions of particular genes to be mapped within the critical genomic region. For discussion of disorders of chromosome number and structure, see Chap. 63.

Monogenic Mendelian Disorders Monogenic human diseases are frequently referred to as *Mendelian disorders* because they obey the principles of genetic transmission originally set forth in Gregor Mendel's classic work. The continuously updated OMIM catalogue lists several thousand of these disorders and provides information about the clinical phenotype, molecular basis, allelic variants, and pertinent animal models (Table 62-1). The mode of inheritance for a given phenotypic trait or disease is determined by pedigree analysis. All affected and unaffected individuals in the family are recorded in a pedigree using standard symbols (Fig. 62-9). The principles of allelic segregation, and the transmission of alleles from parents to children, are illustrated in Fig. 62-10. One dominant (A) allele and one recessive (a) allele can display three Mendelian modes of inheritance: autosomal dominant, autosomal recessive, and X-chromosomal. About 65% of human monogenic disorders are autosomal dominant, 25% are autosomal recessive, and 5% are X-linked. Genetic testing is now available for many of these disorders and plays an increasingly important role in clinical medicine (Chap. 64).

AUTOSOMAL DOMINANT DISORDERS Autosomal dominant disorders assume particular relevance because mutations in a single allele are sufficient to cause the disease. In contrast to recessive disorders, in which disease pathogenesis is relatively straightforward because there is loss of gene function, dominant disorders can be caused by various disease mechanisms, many of which are unique to the function of the genetic pathway involved.

In autosomal dominant disorders, individuals are affected in successive generations; the disease does not occur in the offspring of unaffected individuals. Males and females are affected with equal frequency because the defective gene resides on one of the 22 autosomes (Fig. 62-11A). Autosomal dominant mutations alter one of the two alleles at a given locus. Because the alleles segregate randomly at meiosis, the probability that an offspring will be affected is 50%. Unless there is a new germline mutation, an affected individual has an af-

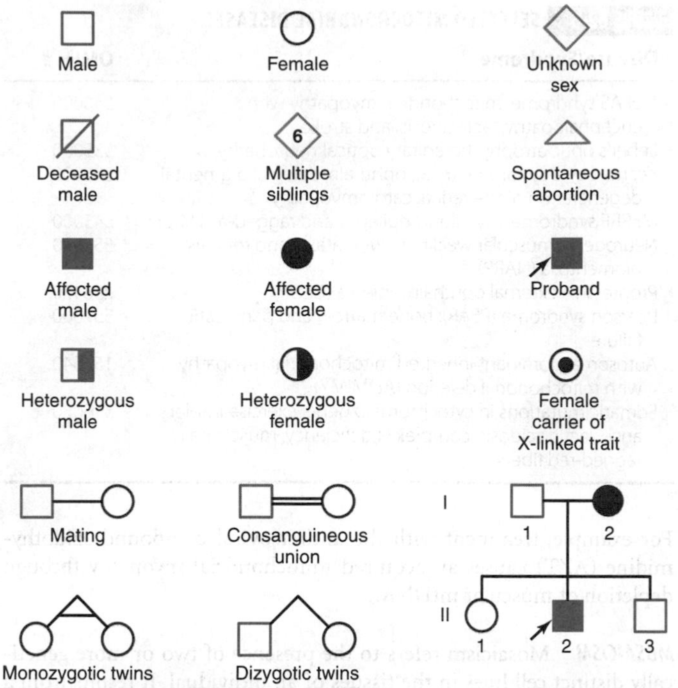

FIGURE 62-9 Standard pedigree symbols.

fected parent. Children with a normal genotype do not transmit the disorder. Due to differences in penetrance or expressivity (see above), the clinical manifestations of autosomal dominant disorders may be variable. Because of these variations, it is sometimes challenging to determine the pattern of inheritance.

It should be recognized, however, that some individuals acquire a mutated gene from an unaffected parent. De novo germline mutations occur more frequently during later cell divisions in gametogenesis, which explains why siblings are rarely affected. As noted before, new germline mutations occur more frequently in fathers of advanced age. For example, the average age of fathers with new germline mutations that cause Marfan's syndrome is ~37 years, whereas fathers who transmit the disease by inheritance have an average age of ~30 years.

AUTOSOMAL RECESSIVE DISORDERS In recessive disorders, the mutated alleles result in a complete or partial loss of function. They frequently involve enzymes in metabolic pathways, receptors, or proteins in signaling cascades. In an autosomal recessive disease, the affected individual, who can be of either sex, is a homozygote or compound heterozygote for a single-gene defect. With a few important exceptions, autosomal recessive diseases are rare and often occur in the context of parental consanguinity. The relatively high frequency of certain recessive disorders, such as sickle cell anemia, cystic fibrosis, and thalassemia, is partially explained by a selective biologic advantage for the heterozygous state (see below). Though heterozygous carriers of a defective allele are usually clinically normal, they may display subtle differences in phenotype that only become apparent with more precise

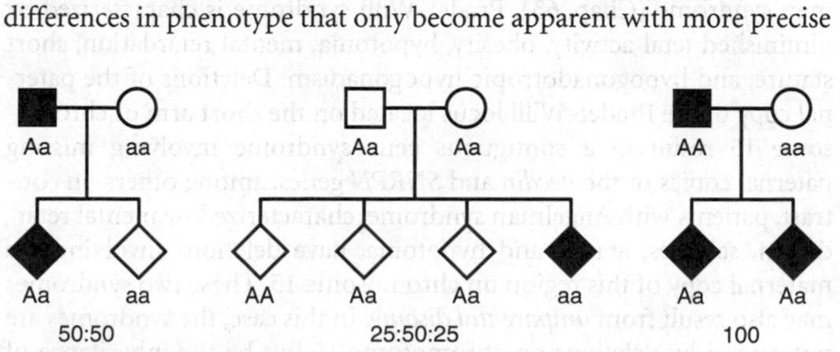

FIGURE 62-10 Segregation of alleles. Segregation of genotypes in the offspring of parents with one dominant (A) and one recessive (a) allele. The distribution of the parental alleles to their offspring depends on the combination present in the parents. Filled symbols = affected individuals.

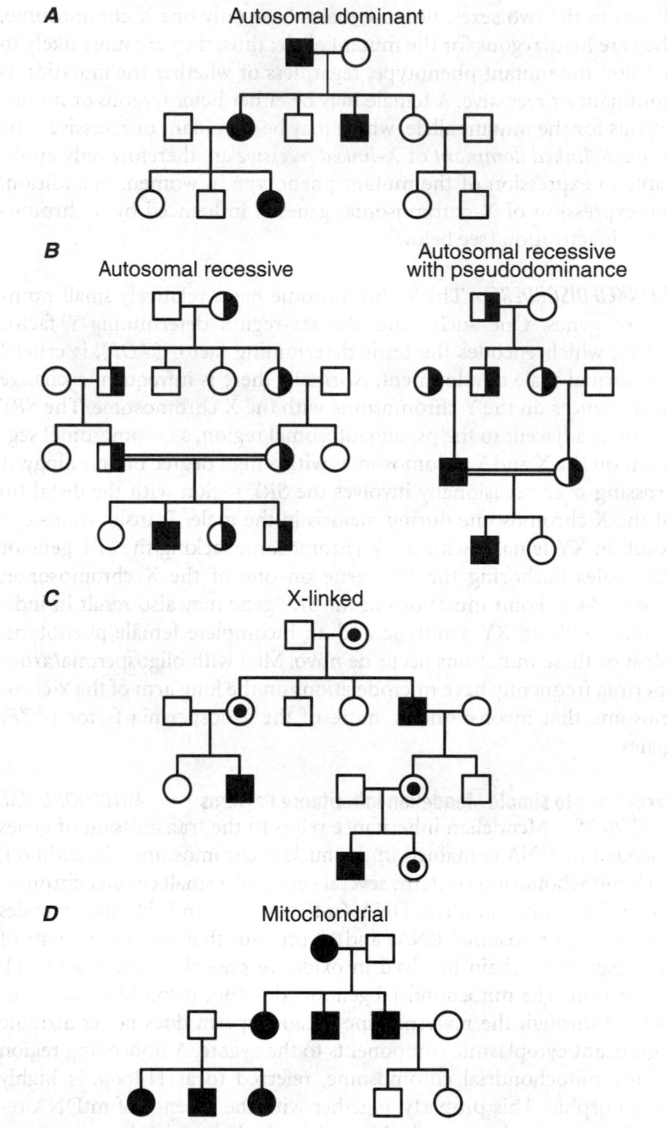

FIGURE 62-11 Dominant, recessive, X-linked, and mitochondrial (matrilinear) inheritance.

testing or in the context of certain environmental influences. In sickle cell anemia, for example, heterozygotes are normally asymptomatic. However, in situations of dehydration or diminished oxygen pressure, sickle cell crises can also occur in heterozygotes (Chap. 99).

In most instances, an affected individual is the offspring of heterozygous parents. In this situation, there is a 25% chance that the offspring will have a normal genotype, a 50% probability of a heterozygous state, and a 25% risk of homozygosity for the recessive alleles (Figs. 62-10, 62-11*B*). In the case of one unaffected heterozygous and one affected homozygous parent, the probability of disease increases to 50% for each child. In this instance, the pedigree analysis mimics an autosomal dominant mode of inheritance (*pseudodominance*). In contrast to autosomal dominant disorders, new mutations in recessive alleles are rarely manifest because they usually result in an asymptomatic carrier state.

X-LINKED DISORDERS Males have only one X chromosome; consequently, a daughter always inherits her father's X chromosome in addition to one of her mother's two X chromosomes. A son inherits the Y chromosome from his father and one maternal X chromosome. Thus, the characteristic features of X-linked inheritance are (1) the absence of father-to-son transmission, and (2) the fact that all daughters of an affected male are obligate carriers of the mutant allele (Fig. 62-11*C*). The risk of developing disease due to a mutant X-chromosomal gene differs in the two sexes. Because males have only one X chromosome, they are hemizygous for the mutant allele; thus, they are more likely to develop the mutant phenotype, regardless of whether the mutation is dominant or recessive. A female may be either heterozygous or homozygous for the mutant allele, which may be dominant or recessive. The terms *X-linked dominant* or *X-linked recessive* are therefore only applicable to expression of the mutant phenotype in women. In addition, the expression of X-chromosomal genes is influenced by X chromosome inactivation (see below).

Y-LINKED DISORDERS The Y chromosome has a relatively small number of genes. One such gene, the sex-region determining Y factor (*SRY*), which encodes the testis-determining factor (*TDF*), is crucial for normal male development. Normally there is infrequent exchange of sequences on the Y chromosome with the X chromosome. The *SRY* region is adjacent to the pseudoautosomal region, a chromosomal segment on the X and Y chromosomes with a high degree of homology. A crossing-over occasionally involves the *SRY* region with the distal tip of the X chromosome during meiosis in the male. Translocations can result in XY females with the Y chromosome lacking the *SRY* gene or XX males harboring the *SRY* gene on one of the X chromosomes (Chap. 343). Point mutations in the *SRY* gene may also result in individuals with an XY genotype and an incomplete female phenotype. Most of these mutations occur de novo. Men with oligospermia/azoospermia frequently have microdeletions on the long arm of the Y chromosome that involve one or more of the azoospermia factor (*AZF*) genes.

Exceptions to Simple Mendelian Inheritance Patterns • ***MITOCHONDRIAL DISORDERS*** Mendelian inheritance refers to the transmission of genes encoded by DNA contained in the nuclear chromosomes. In addition, each mitochondrion contains several copies of a small circular chromosome. The mitochondrial DNA (mtDNA) is ~16.5 kb and encodes transfer and ribosomal RNAs and 13 proteins that are components of the respiratory chain involved in oxidative phosphorylation and ATP generation. The mitochondrial genome does not recombine and is inherited through the maternal line because sperm does not contribute significant cytoplasmic components to the zygote. A noncoding region of the mitochondrial chromosome, referred to as D-loop, is highly polymorphic. This property, together with the absence of mtDNA recombination, makes it a valuable tool for studies tracing human migration and evolution, and it is also used for specific forensic applications.

Inherited mitochondrial disorders are transmitted in a matrilineal fashion; all children from an affected mother will inherit the disease, but it will not be transmitted from an affected father to his children (Fig. 62-11*D*). Alterations in the mtDNA affecting enzymes required for oxidative phosphorylation lead to reduction of ATP supply, generation of free radicals, and induction of apoptosis. Several syndromic disorders arising from mutations in the mitochondrial genome are known in humans and they affect both protein-coding and tRNA genes (Table 62-1 and Table 62-5). The broad clinical spectrum often involves (cardio)myopathies and encephalopathies because of the high dependence of these tissues on oxidative phosphorylation. The age of onset and the clinical course are highly variable because of the unusual mechanisms of mtDNA transmission, which replicates independently from nuclear DNA. During cell replication, the proportion of wild-type and mutant mitochondria can drift among different cells and tissues. The resulting heterogeneity in the proportion of mitochondria with and without a mutation is referred to as *heteroplasmia* and underlies the phenotypic variability that is characteristic of mitochondrial diseases.

Acquired somatic mutations in mitochondria are thought to be involved in several age-dependent degenerative disorders affecting predominantly muscle and the peripheral and central nervous system (e.g., Alzheimer's and Parkinson's disease). Establishing that a mtDNA alteration is causal for a clinical phenotype is challenging because of the high degree of polymorphism in mtDNA and the phenotypic variability characteristic of these disorders. Certain pharmacologic treatments may have an impact on mitochondria and/or their function.

TABLE 62-5 SELECTED MITOCHONDRIAL DISEASES

Disease/Syndrome	OMIM #
MELAS syndrome: mitochondrial myopathy with encephalopathy, lactacidosis, and stroke	540000
Leber's optic atrophy: hereditary optical neuropathy	535000
Kearns-Sayre syndrome (KSS): ophthalmoplegia, pigmental degeneration of the retina, cardiomyopathy	530000
MERRF syndrome: myoclonic epilepsy and ragged-red fibers	545000
Neurogenic muscular weakness with ataxia and retinitis pigmentosa (NARP)	551500
Progressive external ophthalmoplegia (CEOP)	258470
Pearson syndrome (PEAR): bone marrow and pancreatic failure	557000
Autosomal dominant inherited mitochondrial myopathy with mitochondrial deletion (ADMIMY)	157640
Somatic mutations in cytochrome *b* gene: exercise intolerance, lactic acidosis, complex III deficiency, muscle pain, ragged-red fibers	516020

For example, treatment with the antiretroviral compound azidothymidine (AZT) causes an acquired mitochondrial myopathy through depletion of muscular mtDNA.

MOSAICISM Mosaicism refers to the presence of two or more genetically distinct cell lines in the tissues of an individual. It results from a mutation that occurs during embryonic, fetal, or extrauterine development. The developmental stage at which the mutation arises will determine whether germ cells and/or somatic cells are involved. Chromosomal mosaicism results from non-disjunction at an early embryonic mitotic division, leading to the persistence of more than one cell line, as exemplified by some patients with Turner syndrome (Chap. 343). Somatic mosaicism is characterized by a patchy distribution of genetically altered somatic cells. The McCune-Albright syndrome, for example, is caused by activating mutations in the stimulatory G protein α ($G_s\alpha$) that occur early in development (Chap. 347). The clinical phenotype varies depending on the tissue distribution of the mutation; manifestations include ovarian cysts that secrete sex steroids and cause precocious puberty, polyostotic fibrous dysplasia, café-au-lait skin pigmentation, growth hormone–secreting pituitary adenomas, and hypersecreting autonomous thyroid nodules (Chap. 341).

X-INACTIVATION, IMPRINTING, AND UNIPARENTAL DISOMY According to traditional Mendelian principles, the parental origin of a mutant gene is irrelevant for the expression of the phenotype. There are, however, important exceptions to this rule. *X-inactivation* prevents the expression of most genes on one of the two X-chromosomes in every cell of a female. Gene inactivation also occurs on selected chromosomal regions of autosomes. This phenomenon, referred to as *genomic imprinting*, leads to inheritable preferential expression of one of the parental alleles. It is of pathophysiologic importance in disorders where the transmission of disease is dependent on the sex of the transmitting parent and, thus, plays an important role in the expression of certain genetic disorders. Two classic examples are the Prader-Willi syndrome and Angelman syndrome (Chap. 63). Prader-Willi syndrome is characterized by diminished fetal activity, obesity, hypotonia, mental retardation, short stature, and hypogonadotropic hypogonadism. Deletions of the paternal copy of the Prader-Willi locus located on the short arm of chromosome 15 result in a contiguous gene syndrome involving missing paternal copies of the *necdin* and *SNRPN* genes, among others. In contrast, patients with Angelman syndrome, characterized by mental retardation, seizures, ataxia, and hypotonia, have deletions involving the maternal copy of this region on chromosome 15. These two syndromes may also result from *uniparental disomy*. In this case, the syndromes are not caused by deletions on chromosome 15 but by the inheritance of either two maternal chromosomes (Prader-Willi syndrome) or two paternal chromosomes (Angelman syndrome).

Imprinting and the related phenomenon of allelic exclusion may be more common than currently documented, as it is difficult to examine

TABLE 62-6 SELECTED TRINUCLEOTIDE REPEAT DISORDERS

Disease	Locus	Repeat	Triplet Length (Normal/Disease)	Inheritance	Gene Product
X-chromosomal spinobulbar muscular atrophy (SBMA)	Xq11-q12	CAG	11–34/40–62	XR	Androgen receptor
Fragile X-syndrome (FRAXA)	Xq27.3	CGG	6–50/200–300	XR	FMR-1 protein
Fragile X-syndrome (FRAXE)	Xq28	GCC	6–25/>200	XR	FMR-2 protein
Dystrophia myotonica (DM)	19q13.2-q13.3	CTG	5–30/200–1000	AD, variable penetrance	Myotonin protein kinase
Huntington disease (HD)	4p16.3	CAG	6–34/37–180	AD	Huntingtin
Spinocerebellar ataxia type 1 (SCA1)	6p21.3-21.2	CAG	6–39/40–88	AD	Ataxin 1
Spinocerebellar ataxia type 2 (SCA2)	12q24.1	CAG	15–31/34–400	AD	Ataxin 2
Spinocerebellar ataxia type 3 (SCA3); Machado Joseph disease (MD)	14q21	CAG	13–36/55–86	AD	Ataxin 3
Spinocerebellar ataxia type 6 (SCA6, CACNAIA)	19p13.1-13.2	CAG	4–16/20–33	AD	Alpha 1A voltage-dependent L-type calcium channel
Spinocerebellar ataxia type 7 (SCA7)	3p21.1-p12	CAG	4–19/37 to >300	AD	Ataxin 7
Spinocerebellar ataxia type 12 (SCA12)	5q31	CAG	6–26/66–78	AD	Protein phosphatase 2A
Dentorubral pallidoluysiane atrophy (DRPLA)	12p	CAG	7–23/49–75	AD	Atrophin 1
Friedreich ataxia (FRDA1)	9q13-21	GAA	7–22/200–900	AR	Frataxin

Note: AD, autosomal dominant; AR, autosomal recessive; XR, X-linked recessive.

levels of mRNA expression from the maternal and paternal alleles in specific tissues or in individual cells. Genomic imprinting, or uniparental disomy, is involved in the pathogenesis of several other disorders and malignancies (Chap. 63). For example, hydatidiform moles contain a normal number of diploid chromosomes, but they are all of paternal origin. The opposite situation occurs in ovarian teratomata, with 46 chromosomes of maternal origin. Expression of the imprinted gene for insulin-like growth factor II (IGF-II) is involved in the pathogenesis of the cancer-predisposing Beckwith-Wiedemann syndrome (BWS) (Chap. 79). These children show somatic overgrowth with organomegalies and hemihypertrophy, and they have an increased risk of embryonal malignancies such as Wilm's tumor. Normally, only the paternally derived copy of the *IGF-II* gene is active and the maternal copy is inactive. Imprinting of the *IGF-II* gene is regulated by *H19*, which encodes an RNA transcript that is not translated into protein. Disruption or lack of *H19* methylation leads to a relaxation of *IGF-II* imprinting and expression of both alleles.

Meiotically and mitotically heritable changes in gene expression not associated with DNA sequence alterations are referred to as *epigenetic effects*. These changes involve DNA methylation, histone modifications, and RNA-mediated silencing, resulting in gene repression without a change in the coding sequence. Epigenetic alterations are increasingly recognized to play a role in human diseases such as cancer, mental retardation, hematologic disorders, and possibly in aging. For example, de novo methylation of CpG islands, regions of >500 bp in size with a GC content >55% in promoter regions that are normally unmethylated, is a hallmark of human cancers. Inhibitors of enzymes controlling epigenetic modifications such as histone deacetylases and DNA methyltransferases reverse gene silencing and represent a promising new group of antineoplastic agents.

SOMATIC MUTATIONS Cancer can be defined as a genetic disease at the cellular level (Chap. 79). Cancers are monoclonal in origin, indicating that they have arisen from a single precursor cell with one or several mutations in genes controlling growth (proliferation or apoptosis) and/or differentiation. These acquired somatic mutations are restricted to the tumor and its metastases and are not found in the surrounding normal tissue. The molecular alterations include dominant gain-of-function mutations in oncogenes, recessive loss-of-function mutations in tumor-suppressor genes and DNA repair genes, gene amplification, and chromosome rearrangements. Rarely, a single mutation in certain genes may be sufficient to transform a normal cell into a malignant cell. In most cancers, however, the development of a malignant phenotype requires several genetic alterations for the gradual progression from a normal cell to a cancerous cell, a phenomenon termed *multistep carcinogenesis* (Chaps. 79, 80). Most human tumors express telomerase, an enzyme formed of a protein and an RNA component, which adds telomere repeats at the ends of chromosomes during replication. This mechanism impedes shortening of the telomers, which is associated with senescence in normal cells, and is associated with enhanced replicative capacity in cancer cells. Telomerase inhibitors may provide a novel strategy for treating advanced human cancers.

In many cancer syndromes, there is an inherited *predisposition* to tumor formation. In these instances, a germline mutation is inherited in an autosomal dominant fashion inactivating one allele of an autosomal tumor-suppressor gene. If the second allele is inactivated by a somatic mutation or by epigenetic silencing in a given cell, this will lead to neoplastic growth (Knudson two-hit model). Thus, the defective allele in the germline is transmitted in a dominant mode, though tumorigenesis results from a biallelic loss of the tumor-suppressor gene in an affected tissue. The classic example to illustrate this phenomenon is retinoblastoma, which can occur as a sporadic or hereditary tumor. In sporadic retinoblastoma, both copies of the retinoblastoma (*RB*) gene are inactivated through two somatic events. In hereditary retinoblastoma, one mutated or deleted *RB* allele is inherited in an autosomal dominant manner and the second allele is inactivated by a subsequent somatic mutation. This two-hit model applies to other inherited cancer syndromes such as MEN-1 (Chap. 345) and neurofibromatosis type 2 (Chap. 374).

NUCLEOTIDE REPEAT EXPANSION DISORDERS Several diseases are associated with an increase in the number of nucleotide repeats above a certain threshold (Table 62-6). The repeats are sometimes located within the coding region of the genes, as in Huntington disease or the X-linked form of spinal and bulbar muscular atrophy (SBMA, Kennedy syndrome). In other instances, the repeats probably alter gene regulatory sequences. If an expansion is present, the DNA fragment is unstable and tends to expand further during cell division. The length of the nucleotide repeat often correlates with the severity of the disease. When repeat length increases from one generation to the next, disease manifestations may worsen or be observed at an earlier age; this phenomenon is referred to as *anticipation*. In Huntington disease, for example, there is a correlation between age of onset and length of the triplet codon expansion (Chap. 360). Anticipation has also been documented in other diseases caused by dynamic mutations in trinucleotide repeats (Table 62-6). The repeat number may also vary in a tissue-specific manner. In myotonic dystrophy, the CTG repeat may be tenfold greater in muscle tissue than in lymphocytes (Chap. 382).

Complex Genetic Disorders The expression of many common diseases such as cardiovascular disease, hypertension, diabetes, asthma, psychiatric disorders, and certain cancers is determined by a combination of ge-

TABLE 62-7 GENES AND LOCI INVOLVED IN MONO- AND POLYGENIC FORMS OF DIABETES

Disorder	Genes or Susceptibility Locus	Chromosomal Location	Other Factors
Monogenic forms of diabetes			
MODY 1	HNF4α (hepatocyte nuclear factor 4α)	20q12-q13.1	AD inheritance
MODY 1	GCK (glucokinase)	7p15-p13	
MODY 1	HNF1α (hepatocyte nuclear factor 1α)	12q24.2	
MODY 1	IPF1 (insulin receptor substrate)	13q12.1	
MODY 5 (renal cysts, diabetes)	HNF1β (hepatocyte nuclear factor 1β)	17cen-q21.3	
MODY 6	NeuroD1 (neurogenic differention factor 1)	2q32	
Diabetes mellitus type 2; loci and genes linked and/or associated with susceptibility for diabetes mellitus type 2	Genes and loci identified by linkage/association studies		
	CPN10 (Calpain-10)	2q37.3	Diet
	HNF4α (hepatocyte nuclear factor 4α)	20q12-q13.1	Energy expenditure
	PTPN1 (protein-tyrosine phosphatase)	20q13.1-q13.2	Obesity
	PKLR (liver pyruvate kinase)	1q21	
	CASQ1 (calsequestrin 1)	1q21	
	APM1 (adiponectin)	3q27	
	TCF7L2 (transcription factor 7-like 2)	10q25.3	
	1q21-23	1q21-23	
	2q	2q	
	3q22-27	3q22-27	
	8p21-23	8p21-23	
	11q	11q	
	12q24	12q24	
	15	15	
	18p11	18p11	
	20q	20q	
	20p	20p	
	Selected candidate genes with possible contribution		
	PPARγ (Peroxisome proliferator receptor γ)	3p25	
	KCNJ11(ATP-sensitive K channel Kir6.2)	11p15.1	
	ABCC8 (ATP-binding cassette, subfamily c, member 8)	11p15.1	
	Insulin VNTR	11p15	
	IRS-1 (insulin receptor substrate)	2q36	
	PGC1α (PPAR γ coactivatory α)	4p15.1	
	ENPP1 (ectonucleotide pyrophosphatase/phosphodiesterase 1)	6q22-23	

Note: MODY, maturity onset diabetes of the young; AD, autosomal dominant; VNTR, variable number of tandem repeats.

netic background, environmental factors, and lifestyle. A trait is called *polygenic* if multiple genes contribute to the phenotype or *multifactorial* if multiple genes are assumed to interact with environmental factors. Genetic models for these complex traits need to account for genetic heterogeneity and interactions with other genes and the environment. Complex genetic traits may be influenced by modifying genes that are not linked to the main gene involved in the pathogenesis of the trait. This type of gene-gene interaction, or *epistasis*, plays an important role in polygenic traits that require the simultaneous presence of variations in multiple genes to result in a pathologic phenotype.

Type 2 diabetes mellitus provides a paradigm for considering a multifactorial disorder, as genetic, nutritional, and lifestyle factors are intimately interrelated in disease pathogenesis (Table 62-7) (Chap. 338). The identification of genetic variations and environmental factors that either predispose to or protect against disease is essential for predicting disease risk, designing preventive strategies, and developing novel therapeutic approaches. The study of rare monogenic diseases may provide insight into some of genetic and molecular mechanisms important in the pathogenesis of complex diseases. For example, the identification of the hepatocyte nuclear factor α (HNFα) in maturity-onset of diabetes type 4 defined it as a *candidate gene* in the pathogenesis of diabetes mellitus type 2 (Tables 62-2 and 62-8). Genome scans have identified various loci that may be associated with susceptibility to development of diabetes mellitus in certain populations. Efforts to identify susceptibility genes require very large sample sizes, and positive results may depend on ethnicity, ascertainment criteria, and statistical analysis. Association studies analyzing the potential influence of (biologically functional) SNPs and SNP haplotypes on a particular phenotype are a promising approach for the detection of involved genes.

Linkage and Association Studies There are two primary strategies for mapping genes that cause or increase susceptibility to human disease: (1) classic linkage can be performed based on a known genetic model or, when the model is unknown, by studying pairs of affected relatives; or (2) disease genes can be mapped using allelic association studies (Table 62-8).

GENETIC LINKAGE *Genetic linkage* refers to the fact that genes are physically connected, or linked, to one another along the chromosomes. Two fundamental principles are essential for understanding the concept of linkage: (1) when two genes are close together on a chromosome, they are usually transmitted together, unless a recombination event separates them (Figs. 62-3, 62-8); and (2) the odds of a crossover, or recombination event, between two linked genes is proportional to the distance that separates them. Thus, genes that are further apart are more likely to undergo a recombination event than genes that are very close together. The detection of chromosomal loci that segregate with a disease by linkage can be used to identify the gene responsible for the disease (*positional cloning)* and to predict the odds of disease gene transmission in genetic counseling.

Polymorphisms are essential for linkage studies because they provide a means to distinguish the maternal and paternal chromosomes in an individual. On average, 1 out of every 1000 bp varies from one person to the next. Although this degree of variation seems low (99.9% identical), it means that >3 million sequence differences exist between any two unrelated individuals and the probability that the sequence at such loci will differ on the two homologous chromosomes is high (often >70–90%). These sequence variations include VNTRs, short tandem repeats (STRs), and SNPs. Most STRs, also called *polymorphic microsatellite markers*, consist of di-, tri-, or tetranucleotide repeats that can be measured readily using PCR (Fig. 62-12). Characterization of SNPs, using DNA chips, provides an important new tool for comprehensive analyses of genetic variation, linkage, and association studies. Although these sequence variations usually have no apparent functional consequences, they provide much of the basis for variation in genetic traits.

TABLE 62-8 GENETIC APPROACHES FOR IDENTIFYING DISEASE GENES

Method	Indications and Advantages	Limitations
Linkage Studies		
Classical linkage analysis (parametric methods)	Analysis of monogenic traits Suitable for genome scan Control population not required Useful for multifactorial disorders in isolated populations	Difficult to collect large informative pedigrees Difficult to obtain sufficient statistical power for complex traits
Allele-sharing methods (nonparametric methods) Affected sib and relative pair analyses Sib pair analysis	Suitable for identification of susceptibility genes in polygenic and multifactorial disorders Suitable for genome scan Control population not required if allele frequencies are known Statistical power can be increased by including parents and relatives	Difficult to collect sufficient number of subjects Difficult to obtain sufficient statistical power for complex traits Reduced power compared to classical linkage, but not sensitive to specification of genetic mode
Association Studies		
Case-control studies Linkage disequilibrium Transmission disequilibrium test (TDT) Whole-genome association studies	Suitable for identification of susceptibility genes in polygenic and multifactorial disorders Suitable for testing specific allelic variants of known candidate loci Facilitated by HapMap data, making whole-genome studies more feasible Does not necessarily need relatives	Requires large sample size and matched control population False-positive results in the absence of suitable control population Candidate gene approach does not permit to detect novel genes and pathways Whole-genome association studies very expensive

In order to identify a chromosomal locus that segregates with a disease, it is necessary to characterize polymorphic DNA markers from affected and unaffected individuals of one or several pedigrees. One can then assess whether certain marker alleles cosegregate with the disease. Markers that are closest to the disease gene are less likely to undergo recombination events and therefore receive a higher linkage score. Linkage is expressed as a lod (logarithm of odds) score—the ratio of the probability that the disease and marker loci are linked rather than unlinked. Lod scores of +3 (1000:1) are generally accepted as supporting linkage, whereas a score of –2 is consistent with the absence of linkage.

An example of the use of linkage analysis is shown in Fig. 62-12. In this case, the gene for the autosomal dominant disorder MEN-1 is known to be located on chromosome 11q13. Using positional cloning, the *MEN1* gene was identified and shown to encode menin, a tumor suppressor. Affected individuals inherit a mutant form of the *MEN1* gene, predisposing them to certain types of tumors (parathyroid, pituitary, pancreatic islet) (Chap. 345). In the tissues that develop a tumor, a "second hit" occurs in the normal copy of the *MEN1* gene. This somatic mutation may be a point mutation, a microdeletion, or loss of a chromosomal fragment (detected as loss of heterozygosity, LOH). Within a given family, linkage to the *MEN1* gene locus can be assessed without necessarily knowing

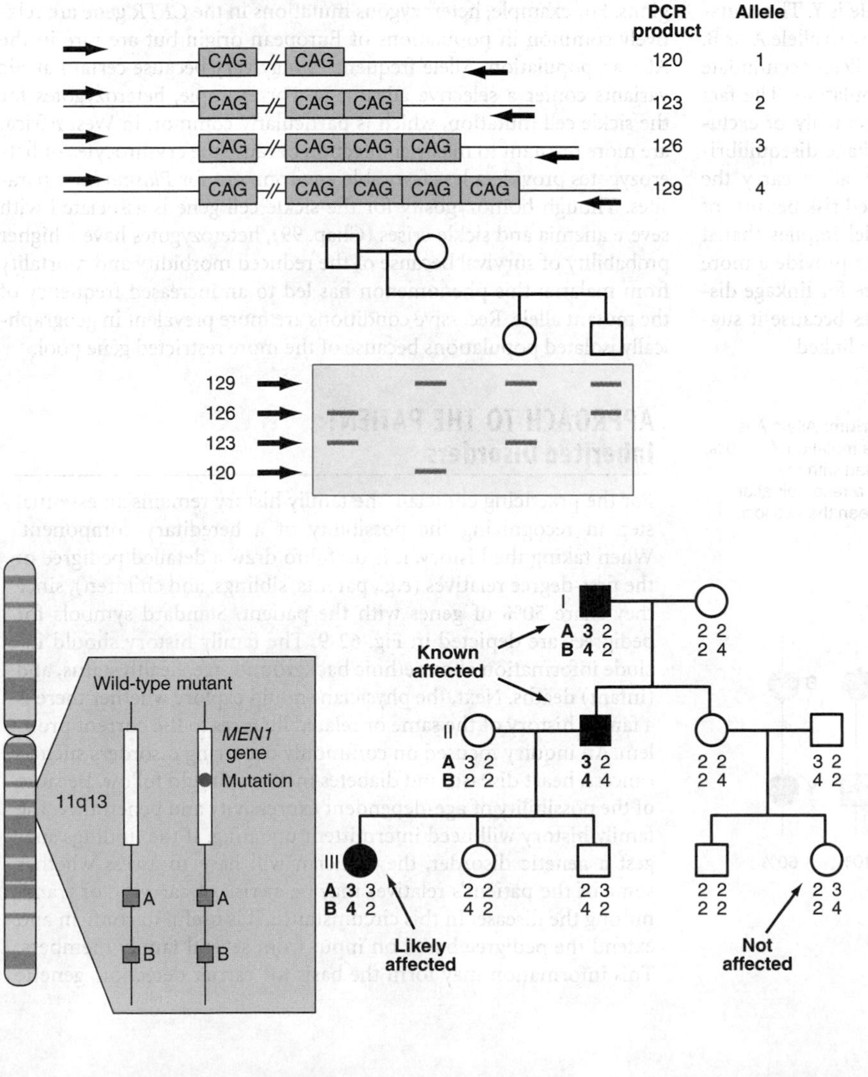

FIGURE 62-12 CAG repeat length and linkage analysis in multiple endocrine neoplasia (MEN) type 1. *Upper panel.* Detection of different alleles using polymorphic microsatellite markers. The example depicts a CAG trinucleotide repeat. PCR with primers flanking the polymorphic region results in products of variable length, depending on the number of CAG repeats. After characterization of the alleles in the parents, transmission of the paternal and maternal alleles can be determined. ***Lower panel.*** Genotype analysis using microsatellite markers in a family with MEN-1. Two microsatellite markers, A and B, are located in close proximity to the *MEN1* gene on chromosome 11q13. For each individual, the A and B alleles have been determined. Based on this analysis, the genotype A3,B4 is linked to the disease because it occurs in the two affected individuals I-1 and II-1 but not in unaffected siblings. Because the disease allele is linked to A3,B4 within the affected family, it is likely that the individual III-1 is a carrier of the mutated *MEN1* gene. Although III-5 also has the A3,B4 genotype, she has inherited the allele from her unaffected father (II-4), who is not related to the original family. The A3,B4 genotype is only associated with MEN-1 in the original family, but not in the general population. Therefore, individual III-5 is not at risk for developing the disease.

the specific mutation in the *MEN1* gene. Using polymorphic STRs that are close to the *MEN1* gene, one can assess transmission of the different *MEN1* alleles and compare this pattern to development of the disorder to determine which allele is associated with risk of MEN-1. In the pedigree shown, the affected grandfather in generation I carries alleles 3 and 4 on the chromosome with the mutated *MEN1* gene and alleles 2 and 2 on his other chromosome 11. Consistent with linkage of the 3/4 genotype to the *MEN1* locus, his son in generation II is affected, whereas his daughter (who inherits the 2/2 genotype from her father) is unaffected. In the third generation, transmission of the 3/4 genotype indicates risk of developing MEN-1, assuming that no genetic recombination between the 3/4 alleles and the *MEN1* gene has occurred. After a specific mutation in the *MEN1* gene is identified within a family, it is possible to track transmission of the mutation itself, thereby eliminating uncertainty caused by recombination.

ALLELIC ASSOCIATION, LINKAGE DISEQUILIBRIUM, AND HAPLOTYPES *Allelic association* refers to a situation in which the frequency of an allele is significantly increased or decreased in individuals affected by a particular disease in comparison to controls. Linkage and association differ in several aspects. Genetic linkage is demonstrable in families or sibships. Association studies, on the other hand, compare a population of affected individuals with a control population. Association studies can be performed as case-control studies that include unrelated affected individuals and matched controls, or as family-based studies that compare the frequencies of alleles transmitted or not transmitted to affected children.

Allelic association studies are particularly useful for identifying susceptibility genes in complex diseases. When alleles at two loci occur more frequently in combination than would be predicted (based on known allele frequencies and recombination fractions), they are said to be in *linkage disequilibrium*. In Fig. 62-13, a mutation, Z, has occurred at a susceptibility locus where the normal allele is Y. The mutation is in close proximity to a genetic polymorphism with allele A or B. With time, the chromosomes carrying the A and Z alleles accumulate and represent 10% of the chromosomes in the population. The fact that the disease susceptibility gene, Z, is found preferentially, or exclusively, in association with the A allele illustrates linkage disequilibrium. Though not all chromosomes carrying the A allele carry the disease gene, the A allele is associated with an increased risk because of its possible association with the Z allele. This model implies that it may be possible in the future to identify Z directly to provide a more accurate prediction of disease susceptibility. Evidence for linkage disequilibrium can be helpful in mapping disease genes because it suggests that the two loci, in this case A and Z, are tightly linked.

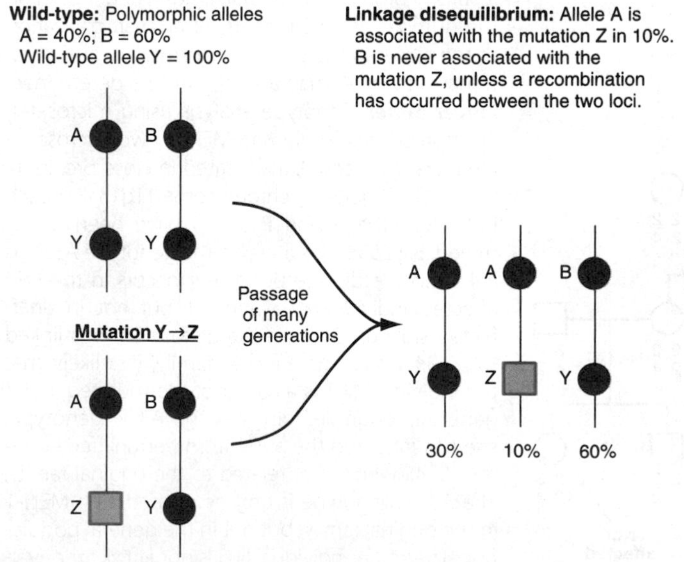

FIGURE 62-13 Linkage disequilibrium.

Detecting the genetic factors contributing to the pathogenesis of common complex disorders remains a great challenge. In many instances, these are low-penetrance alleles, i.e., variations that individually only have a subtle effect on disease development, and they can only be identified by unbiased genome-wide association studies. Most variants are in noncoding or regulatory sequences but do not alter protein structure. The analysis of complex disorders is further complicated by ethnic differences in disease prevalence, differences in allele frequencies in known susceptibility genes among different populations, locus and allelic heterogeneity, gene-gene and gene-environment interactions, and the possibility of phenocopies. The HapMap Project is now making genome-wide association studies for the characterization of complex disorders more realistic. Adjacent SNPs are inherited together as blocks, and these blocks can be identified by genotyping selected marker SNPs, so-called *Tag SNPs*, thereby reducing cost and workload (Fig. 62-8). The availability of this information permits the characterization of a limited number of SNPs to identify the set of haplotypes present in an individual, e.g., in cases and controls. This, in turn, permits genome-wide association studies by searching for associations of certain haplotypes with a disease phenotype of interest, an essential step for unraveling the genetic factors contributing to complex disorders.

POPULATION GENETICS In population genetics, the focus changes from alterations in an individual's genome to the distribution pattern of different genotypes in the population. In a case where there are only two alleles, A and a, the frequency of the genotypes will be $p^2 + 2pq + q^2 = 1$, with p^2 corresponding to the frequency of AA, $2pq$ to the frequency of Aa, and q^2 to aa. When the frequency of an allele is known, the frequency of the genotype can be calculated. Alternatively, one can determine an allele frequency, if the genotype frequency has been determined.

Allele frequencies vary among ethnic groups and geographical regions. For example, heterozygous mutations in the *CFTR* gene are relatively common in populations of European origin but are rare in the African population. Allele frequencies may vary because certain allelic variants confer a selective advantage. For example, heterozygotes for the sickle cell mutation, which is particularly common in West Africa, are more resistant to malarial infection because the erythrocytes of heterozygotes provide a less favorable environment for *Plasmodium* parasites. Though homozygosity for the sickle cell gene is associated with severe anemia and sickle crises (Chap. 99), heterozygotes have a higher probability of survival because of the reduced morbidity and mortality from malaria; this phenomenon has led to an increased frequency of the mutant allele. Recessive conditions are more prevalent in geographically isolated populations because of the more restricted gene pool.

APPROACH TO THE PATIENT: Inherited Disorders

For the practicing clinician, the family history remains an essential step in recognizing the possibility of a hereditary component. When taking the history, it is useful to draw a detailed pedigree of the first-degree relatives (e.g., parents, siblings, and children), since they share 50% of genes with the patient. Standard symbols for pedigrees are depicted in Fig. 62-9. The family history should include information about ethnic background, age, health status, and (infant) deaths. Next, the physician should explore whether there is a family history of the same or related illnesses to the current problem. An inquiry focused on commonly occurring disorders such as cancers, heart disease, and diabetes mellitus should follow. Because of the possibility of age-dependent expressivity and penetrance, the family history will need intermittent updating. If the findings suggest a genetic disorder, the clinician will have to assess whether some of the patient's relatives may be at risk of carrying or transmitting the disease. In this circumstance, it is useful to confirm and extend the pedigree based on input from several family members. This information may form the basis for carrier detection, genetic counseling, early intervention, and prevention of a disease in relatives of the index patient (Chap. 64).

In instances where a diagnosis at the molecular level may be relevant, the physician will have to identify an appropriate laboratory that can perform the test. Genetic testing is becoming more readily available through commercial laboratories. For uncommon disorders, the test may only be performed in a specialized research laboratory. Approved laboratories offering testing for inherited disorders can be identified in continuously updated on-line resources (GeneTests; Table 62-1). If genetic testing is considered, the patient and the family should be informed about the potential implications of positive results, including psychological distress and the possibility of discrimination. The patient or caretakers should be informed about the meaning of a negative result, technical limitations, and the possibility of false-negative and inconclusive results. For these reasons, genetic testing should only be performed after obtaining *informed consent*. Published ethical guidelines address the specific aspects that should be considered when testing children and adolescents. Genetic testing should usually be limited to situations in which the results may have an impact on the medical management.

IDENTIFYING THE DISEASE-CAUSING GENE *Genomic medicine* aims to enhance the quality of medical care through the use of genotypic analysis (DNA testing) to identify genetic predisposition to disease, to select more specific pharmacotherapy, and to design individualized medical care based on genotype. Genotype can be deduced by analysis of protein (e.g., hemoglobin, apoprotein E), mRNA, or DNA. However, technological advances have made DNA analysis particularly useful because it can be readily applied to all but the largest genes (Fig. 62-14).

DNA testing is performed by mutational analysis or linkage studies in individuals at risk for a genetic disorder known to be present in a family. Mass screening programs require tests of high sensitivity and specificity to be cost-effective. Prerequisites for the success of genetic screening programs include the following: that the disorder is potentially serious; that it can be influenced at a presymptomatic stage by changes in behavior, diet, and/or pharmaceutical manipulations; and that the screening does not result in any harm or discrimination. Screening in Jewish populations for the autosomal recessive neurodegenerative storage disease Tay-Sachs has reduced the number of affected individuals. In contrast, screening for sickle cell trait/disease in African Americans has led to unanticipated problems of discrimination by health insurers and employers. Mass screening programs harbor additional potential problems. For example, screening for the most common genetic alteration in cystic fibrosis, the ΔF508 mutation with a frequency of ~70% in northern Europe, is feasible and seems to be effective. One has to keep in mind, however, that there is pronounced allelic heterogeneity and that the disease can be caused by >1400 other mutations. The search for these less common mutations would substantially increase costs but not the effectiveness of the screening program as a whole. Occupational screening programs aim to detect individuals with increased risk for certain professional activities (e.g., α_1 antitrypsin deficiency and smoke or dust exposure).

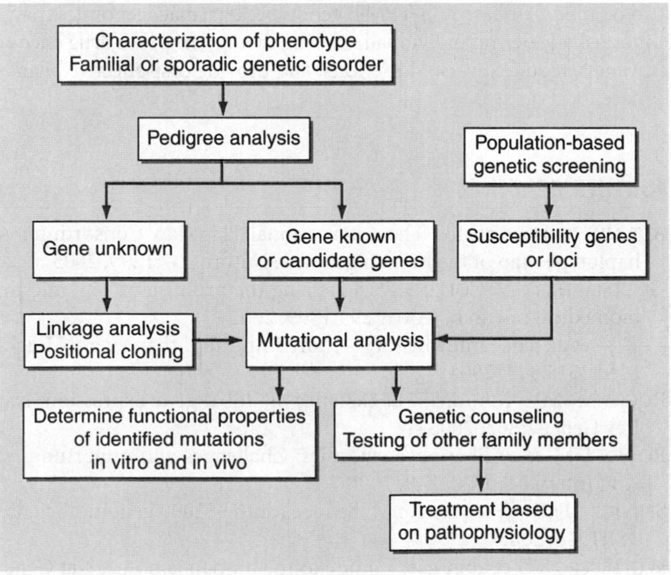

FIGURE 62-14 Approach to genetic disease.

Mutational Analyses DNA sequence analysis is increasingly used as a diagnostic tool and has significantly enhanced diagnostic accuracy. It is used for determining carrier status and for prenatal testing in monogenic disorders (Chap. 64). Numerous techniques are available for the detection of mutations (Table 62-9). In a very broad sense, one can distinguish between techniques that allow for screening the absence or presence of known mutations (screening mode) or techniques that definitively characterize mutations. Analyses of large alterations in the genome are possible using classic methods such as cytogenetics, fluorescent in situ hybridization (FISH), and Southern blotting (Chap. 63), as well as more sensitive novel techniques that search for multiple single exon deletions or duplications.

More discrete sequence alterations rely heavily on the use of the PCR, which allows rapid gene amplification and analysis. Moreover, PCR makes it possible to perform genetic testing and mutational analysis with small amounts of DNA extracted from leukocytes or even from single cells, buccal cells, or hair roots. Screening for point mutations can be performed by numerous methods (Table 62-9); most are based on the recognition of mismatches between nucleic acid duplexes, electrophoretic separation of single- or double-stranded DNA, or sequencing of DNA fragments amplified by PCR. DNA sequencing can be performed directly on PCR products or on fragments cloned into plasmid vectors amplified in bacterial host cells.

RT-PCR may be useful to detect absent or reduced levels of mRNA expression due to a mutated allele. Protein truncation tests (PTT) can be used to detect the broad array of mutations that result in premature termination of a polypeptide during its synthesis. The isolated cDNA is transcribed and translated in vitro, and the proteins are analyzed by gel electrophoresis. Comparison of electrophoretic mobility with the wild-type protein allows detection of truncated mutants.

The majority of traditional diagnostic methods are gel-based. Novel technologies for the analysis of mutations, genotyping, large-scale sequencing, and mRNA expression profiles are in rapid development. DNA chip technologies allow hybridization of DNA or RNA to hundreds of thousands of probes simultaneously. Microarrays are being used clinically for mutational analysis of several human disease genes, as well as for the identification of viral sequence variations. Together with the knowledge gained from the HGP, these technologies provide the foundation to expand from a focus on single genes to analyses at the scale of the genome. Faster and cheaper sequencing technologies are under development, and it has been anticipated that sequencing the whole genome of an individual for a cost of ≤$1000 will become a reality within this decade. The availability of comprehensive individual sequence information is expected to have a significant impact on medical care and preventative strategies, but it also raises ethical and legal concerns how such information may be used by insurers and employers.

A general algorithm for the approach to mutational analysis is outlined in Fig. 62-14. The importance of a detailed clinical phenotype cannot be overemphasized. This is the step where one should also consider the possibility of genetic heterogeneity and phenocopies. If obvious candidate genes are suggested by the phenotype, they can be analyzed directly. After identification of a mutation, it is essential to demonstrate that it segregates with the phenotype. The functional characterization of novel mutations is labor inten-

TABLE 62-9 METHODS USED FOR THE DETECTION OF MUTATIONS

Method	Principle	Type of Mutation Detected
Commonly Used Techniques		
Cytogenetic analysis	Unique visual appearance of various chromosomes	Numerical or structural abnormalities in chromosomes
Fluorescent in situ hybridization (FISH)	Hybridization to chromosomes with fluorescently labeled probes	Numerical or structural abnormalities in chromosomes
Southern blot	Hybridization with genomic probe or cDNA probe after digestion of high molecular DNA	Large deletion, insertion, rearrangement, expansions of triplet repeat, amplification
Polymerase chain reaction (PCR)	Amplification of DNA segment	Expansion of triplet repeats, variable number of tandem repeats (VNTR), gene rearrangements, translocations; prepare DNA for other mutation methods
Reverse transcriptase PCR (RT-PCR)	Reverse transcription, amplification of DNA segment → absence or reduction of mRNA transcription	Analyze expressed mRNA (cDNA) sequence; detect loss of expression
DNA sequencing	Direct sequencing of PCR products Sequencing of DNA segments cloned into plasmid vectors	Point mutations, small deletions and insertions
Restriction fragment polymorphism (RFLP)	Detection of altered restriction pattern of genomic DNA (Southern blot) or PCR products	Point mutations, small deletions and insertions
Other Techniques		
Single-strand conformational polymorphism (SSCP)	PCR of DNA segment: Mutations result in conformational change and altered mobility	Point mutations, small deletions and insertions
Denaturing gradient gel electrophoresis (DGGE)	PCR of DNA segment: Mutations result in conformational change and altered mobility	Point mutations, small deletions and insertions
RNAse cleavage	Cleavage of mismatch between mutated and wild-type sequence	Point mutations, small deletions and insertions
Oligonucleotide specific hybridization (OSH)	Hybridization of PCR products to wild-type or mutated oligonucleotides immobilized on chips or slides	Point mutations, small deletions and insertions
Microarrays	Hybridization of PCR products to wild-type or mutated oligonucleotides	Point mutations, small deletions and insertions Genotyping of SNPs
Protein truncation test (PTT)	Transcription/translation of cDNA isolated from tissue sample	Mutations leading to premature truncations
Pyrosequencing	Clonal amplification of single DNA fragments on microparticles followed by massive parallel sequencing	Sequencing of whole genomes of microorganisms, resequencing of amplicons
Multiplex ligation-dependent probe amplification (MLPA)	Quantification of PCR-generated amplicons reflecting the number of copies of a specific DNA sequence	Copy number variations

sive and may require analyses in vitro or in transgenic models in order to document the relevance of the genetic alteration.

Prenatal diagnosis of numerous genetic diseases in instances with a high risk for certain disorders is now possible by direct DNA analysis. *Amniocentesis* involves the removal of a small amount of amniotic fluid, usually at 16 weeks of gestation. Cells can be collected and submitted for karyotype analyses, FISH, and mutational analysis of selected genes. The main indications for amniocentesis include advanced maternal age above age 35, abnormal serum triple marker test (α-fetoprotein, β human chorionic gonadotropin, pregnancy-associated plasma protein A, or unconjugated estriol), a family history of chromosomal abnormalities, or a Mendelian disorder amenable to genetic testing. Prenatal diagnosis can also be performed by *chorionic villus sampling* (CVS), in which a small amount of the chorion is removed by a transcervical or transabdominal biopsy. Chromosomes and DNA obtained from these cells can be submitted for cytogenetic and mutational analyses. CVS can be performed earlier in gestation (weeks 9–12) than amniocentesis, an aspect that may be of relevance when termination of pregnancy is a consideration. Later in pregnancy, beginning at about 18 weeks of gestation, percutaneous umbilical blood sampling (PUBS) permits collection of fetal blood for lymphocyte culture and analysis. In combination with in vitro fertilization (IVF) techniques, it is even possible to perform genetic diagnoses in a single cell removed from the four- to eight-cell embryo or to analyze the first polar body from an oocyte. Preconceptual diagnosis thereby avoids therapeutic abortions but is extremely costly and labor intensive. Lastly, it has to be emphasized that excluding a specific disorder by any of these approaches is never equivalent to the assurance of having a normal child.

Mutations in certain cancer susceptibility genes, such as *BRCA1* and *BRCA2*, may identify individuals with an increased risk for the development of malignancies and result in risk-reducing interventions. The detection of mutations is an important diagnostic and prognostic tool in leukemias and lymphomas. The demonstration of the presence or absence of mutations and polymorphisms is also relevant for the rapidly evolving field of pharmacogenomics, including the identification of differences in drug treatment response or metabolism as a function of genetic background. For example, the thiopurine drugs 6-mercaptopurine and azathioprine are commonly used cytotoxic and immunosuppressive agents. They are metabolized by thiopurine methyltransferase (TPMT), an enzyme with variable activity associated with genetic polymorphisms in 10% of Caucasians and complete deficiency in about 1/300 individuals. Patients with intermediate or deficient TPMT activity are at risk for excessive toxicity, including fatal myelosuppression. Characterization of these polymorphisms allows mercaptopurine doses to be modified based on TPMT genotype. Pharmacogenomics may increasingly permit individualized drug therapy, improve drug effectiveness, reduce adverse side effects, and provide cost-effective pharmaceutical care.

FURTHER READINGS

ALTSHULER D et al: for The International HapMap Consortium: A haplotype map of the human genome. Nature 437:1299, 2005

GUTTMACHER AE, COLLINS FS: Realizing the promise of genomics in biomedical research. JAMA 294:1399, 2005

——— et al: The family history—more important than ever. N Engl J Med 351:2333, 2004

ROCKMAN MV, KRUGLYAK L: Genetics of global gene expression. Nat Rev Genet 7:862, 2006

RODEN DM et al: Pharmacogenomics: Challenges and opportunities. Ann Intern Med 145:749, 2006

SERVICE RF: Gene sequencing. The race for the $1000 genome. Science 311:1544, 2006

WOLFSBERG TG et al: A user's guide to the human genome. Nat Genet 35(Suppl 1): 2003

63 Chromosome Disorders

Terry Hassold, Stuart Schwartz

In humans, the normal diploid number of chromosomes is 46, consisting of 22 pairs of autosomal chromosomes (numbered 1–22 in decreasing size) and one pair of sex chromosomes (XX in females and XY in males). The genome is estimated to contain between 30,000 and 40,000 genes. Even the smallest autosome contains between 200 and 300 genes. Not surprisingly, duplications or deletions of chromosomes, or even small chromosome segments, have profound consequences on normal gene expression, leading to severe developmental and physiologic abnormalities.

Deviations in number or structure of the 46 human chromosomes are astonishingly common, despite severe deleterious consequences. Chromosomal disorders occur in an estimated 10–25% of all pregnancies. They are the leading cause of fetal loss and, among pregnancies surviving to term, the leading known cause of birth defects and mental retardation.

In recent years, the practice of cytogenetics has shifted from conventional cytogenetic methodology to a union of cytogenetic and molecular techniques. Formerly the province of research laboratories, fluorescence in situ hybridization (FISH) and related molecular cytogenetic technologies have been incorporated into everyday practice in clinical laboratories. As a result, there is an increased appreciation of the importance of "subtle" constitutional cytogenetic abnormalities, such as microdeletions and imprinting disorders, as well as previously recognized translocations and disorders of chromosome number.

VISUALIZING CHROMOSOMES

CONVENTIONAL CYTOGENETIC ANALYSIS

In theory, chromosome preparations can be obtained from any actively dividing tissue by causing the cells to arrest in metaphase, the stage of the cell cycle when chromosomes are maximally condensed. In practice, only a small number of tissues are used for routine chromosome analysis: amniocytes or chorionic villi for prenatal testing and blood, bone marrow, or skin fibroblasts for postnatal studies. Samples of blood, bone marrow, and chorionic villi can be processed using short-term culture techniques that yield results in 1–3 days. Analysis of other tissue types typically involves long-term cell culture, requiring 1–3 weeks of processing before cytogenetic analysis is possible.

Cells are isolated at metaphase or prometaphase and treated chemically or enzymatically to reveal chromosome "bands" (Fig. 63-1). Analysis of the number of chromosomes in the cell and the distribution of bands on individual chromosomes allow the identification of numerical or structural abnormalities. This strategy is useful for characterizing the normal chromosome complement and determining the incidence and types of major chromosome abnormalities.

Each human chromosome contains two specialized structures: a centromere and two telomeres. The centromere, or primary constriction, divides the chromosome into short (p) and long (q) arms and is responsible for the segregation of chromosomes during cell division. The telomeres, or chromosome ends, "cap" the p and q arms and are important for allowing DNA replication at the ends of the chromosomes. Prior to DNA replication, each chromosome consists of a single chromatid copy of the DNA double helix. After DNA replication and continuing until the time of cell division (including metaphase, when chromosomes are typically visualized), each chromosome consists of two identical sister chromatids (Fig. 63-1).

MOLECULAR CYTOGENETICS

The introduction of FISH methodologies in the late 1980s revolutionized the field of cytogenetics. In principle, FISH is similar to other DNA-DNA hybridization methodologies. The probe is labeled with a hapten, such as biotin or digoxigenin, to allow detection with a fluorophore (e.g., FITC or rhodamine). After the hybridization step, the specimen is counter-stained and the preparations are visualized with a fluorescence microscope.

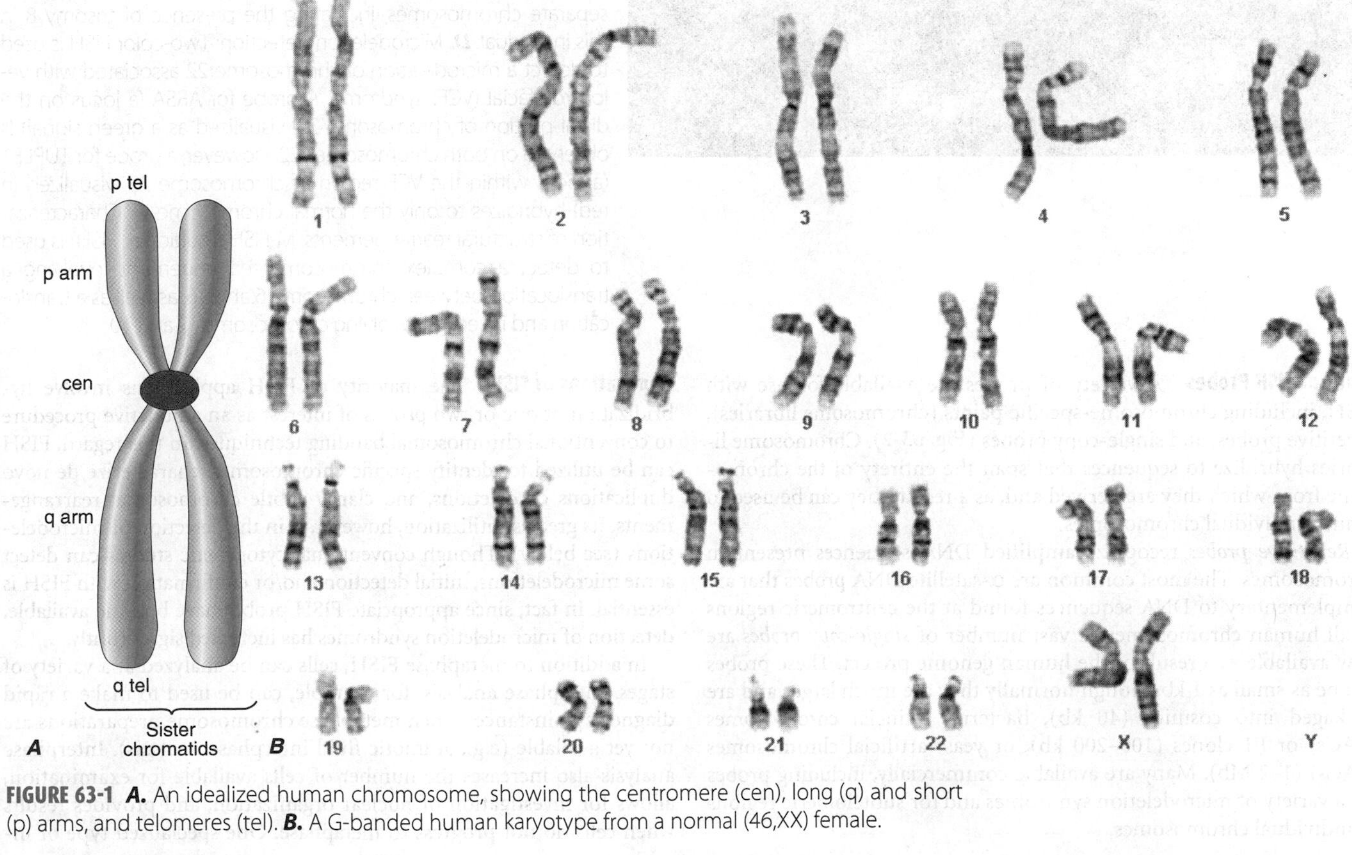

FIGURE 63-1 ***A.*** An idealized human chromosome, showing the centromere (cen), long (q) and short (p) arms, and telomeres (tel). ***B.*** A G-banded human karyotype from a normal (46,XX) female.

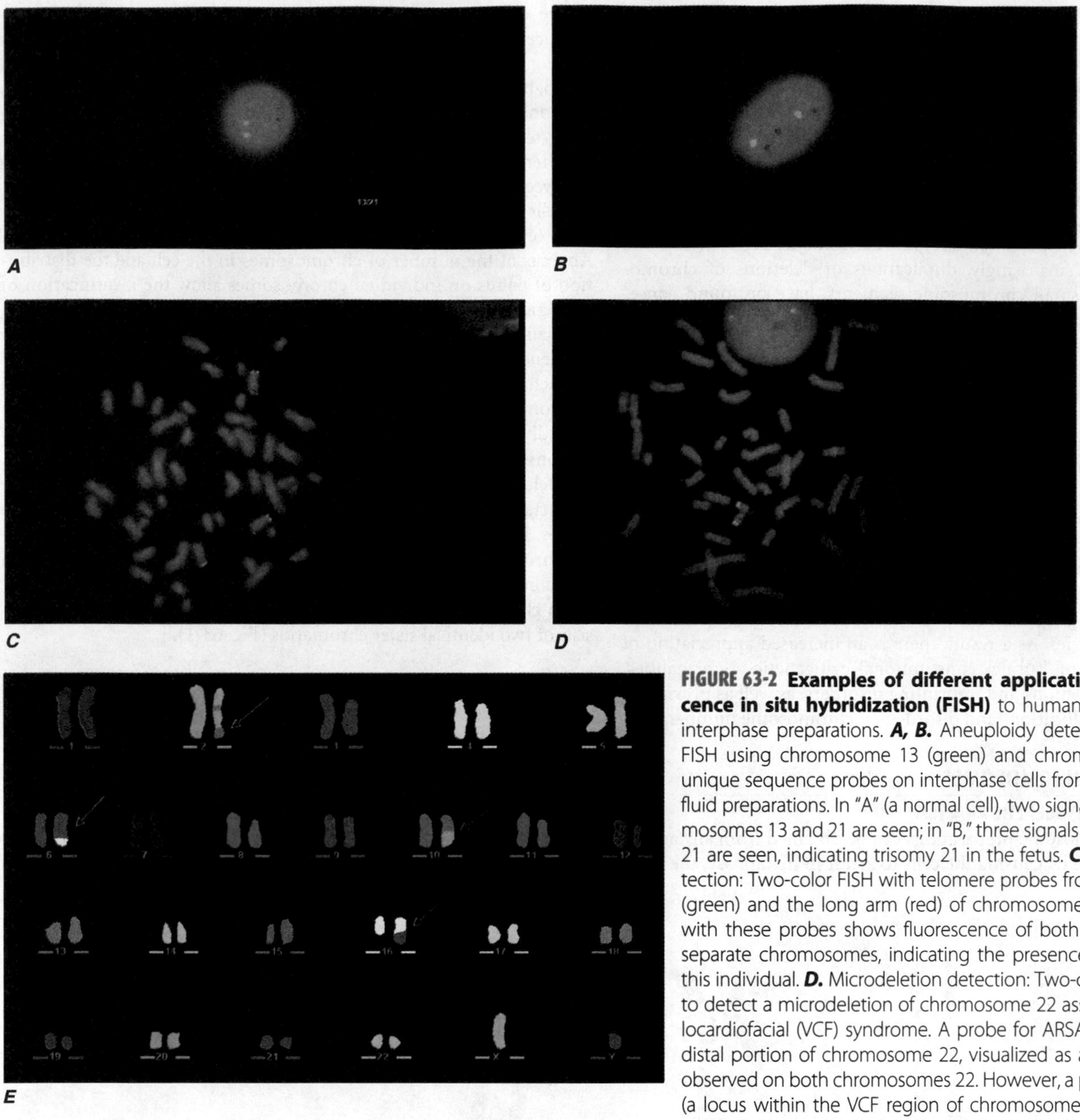

FIGURE 63-2 Examples of different applications of fluorescence in situ hybridization (FISH) to human metaphase and interphase preparations. ***A, B.*** Aneuploidy detection: Interphase FISH using chromosome 13 (green) and chromosome 21 (red) unique sequence probes on interphase cells from direct amniotic fluid preparations. In "A" (a normal cell), two signals for both chromosomes 13 and 21 are seen; in "B," three signals for chromosome 21 are seen, indicating trisomy 21 in the fetus. ***C.*** Aneuploidy detection: Two-color FISH with telomere probes from the short arm (green) and the long arm (red) of chromosome 8. Hybridization with these probes shows fluorescence of both probes to three separate chromosomes, indicating the presence of trisomy 8 in this individual. ***D.*** Microdeletion detection: Two-color FISH is used to detect a microdeletion of chromosome 22 associated with velocardiofacial (VCF) syndrome. A probe for ARSA (a locus on the distal portion of chromosome 22, visualized as a green signal) is observed on both chromosomes 22. However, a probe for TUPLE1 (a locus within the VCF region of chromosome 22, visualized in red) hybridizes to only the normal chromosome. ***E.*** Characterization of structural rearrangements: M-FISH (multicolor FISH) is used to detect a complex chromosome rearrangement involving a translocation between chromosome 6 and 16, as well as a translocation and inversion involving chromosomes 2 and 10.

Types of FISH Probes A variety of probes are available for use with FISH, including chromosome-specific paints (chromosome libraries), repetitive probes, and single-copy probes (Fig. 63-2). Chromosome libraries hybridize to sequences that span the entirety of the chromosome from which they are derived and, as a result, they can be used to "paint" individual chromosomes.

Repetitive probes recognize amplified DNA sequences present in chromosomes. The most common are α-satellite DNA probes that are complementary to DNA sequences found at the centromeric regions of all human chromosomes. A vast number of *single-copy probes* are now available as a result of the human genome project. These probes can be as small as 1 kb, though normally they are much larger and are packaged into cosmids (40 kb), bacterial artificial chromosomes (BACs) or P1 clones (100–200 kb), or yeast artificial chromosomes (YACs) (1–2 Mb). Many are available commercially, including probes for a variety of microdeletion syndromes and for subtelomeric regions of individual chromosomes.

Applications of FISH The majority of FISH applications involve hybridization of one or two probes of interest as an adjunctive procedure to conventional chromosomal banding techniques. In this regard, FISH can be utilized to identify specific chromosomes, characterize de novo duplications or deletions, and clarify subtle chromosomal rearrangements. Its greatest utilization, however, is in the detection of microdeletions (see below). Though conventional cytogenetic studies can detect some microdeletions, initial detection and/or confirmation with FISH is essential. In fact, since appropriate FISH probes have become available, detection of microdeletion syndromes has increased significantly.

In addition to metaphase FISH, cells can be analyzed at a variety of stages. Interphase analysis, for example, can be used to make a rapid diagnosis in instances when metaphase chromosome preparations are not yet available (e.g., amniotic fluid interphase analysis). Interphase analysis also increases the number of cells available for examination, allows for investigation of nuclear organization, and provides results when cells do not progress to metaphase. One specialized type of interphase analysis involves the application of FISH to paraffin-embedded sections, thereby preserving the architecture of the tissue.

The use of interphase FISH has increased recently, especially for analyses of amniocentesis samples. These studies are performed on uncultured amniotic fluid, typically using DNA probes specific for the chromosomes most commonly identified in trisomies (chromosomes 13, 18, 21, and the X and Y). These studies can be performed rapidly (24–72 h) and will ascertain about 60% of the abnormalities detected prenatally. Another area in which interphase analysis is routinely utilized is cancer cytogenetics (Chap. 79). Many site-specific translocations are associated with specific types of malignancies. For example, there are probes available for both the Abelson (Abl) oncogene and breakpoint cluster region (bcr) involved in chronic myelogenous leukemia (CML); these probes are labeled in red and green, respectively; the fusion of these genes in CML combines the fluorescent colors and appears as a yellow hybridization signal.

In addition to standard metaphase and interphase FISH analyses, a number of enhanced techniques have been developed for specific types of analysis, including multicolor FISH techniques, reverse painting, comparative genomic hybridization, and fiber FISH. *Spectral karyotyping* (SKY) and multicolor FISH (m-FISH) techniques use combinatorially labeled probes that create a unique color for individual chromosomes. This technology is useful in the identification of unknown chromosome material (such as markers of duplications) but is most commonly used with the complex rearrangements seen in cancer specimens.

Fiber FISH is a technique in which chromosomes are mechanically stretched, using a variety of different methods. It provides a higher resolution of analysis than conventional FISH.

Comparative genomic hybridization (CGH) is a method that can be used only when DNA is available from a specimen of interest. The entire DNA specimen from the sample of interest is labeled in one color (e.g., green), and the normal control DNA specimen is indicated by another color (e.g., red). These are mixed in equal amounts and hybridized to normal metaphase chromosomes. The red-to-green ratio is analyzed by a computer program, which determines where the DNA of interest may have gains or losses of material. This technique is useful in the analysis of tumors, particularly in those cases where cytogenetic analysis is not possible.

An extension of CGH promises to yield another major advance for examining human chromosomes. Specifically, the development of CGH "arrays" uses protocols that are similar to standard CGH, except that test DNA is hybridized to DNAs that are spread on arrays, rather than hybridized to normal chromosomes. Depending on the type of array (most are constructed utilizing either BACs or oligonucleotides), the resolution can be up to 150 kb, far greater than for standard chromosome analysis. This technology has been used to study cryptic chromosomal imbalances in patients with mental retardation and multiple congenital anomalies, as well as in prenatal diagnosis. It has also been used to detect microdeletions and microduplications in cancer and in previously unidentified genomic disorders. Although this technology is still in development, its use is anticipated to increase in the near term.

INDICATIONS FOR CYTOGENETIC ANALYSIS

Primary indications for karyotypic analysis vary according to the developmental stage/age of the conceptus/individual under investigation. One especially important application is in prenatal diagnosis (particularly for pregnancies involving older women), assaying for chromosomal abnormalities in either chorionic villi of first-trimester fetuses or amniotic fluid of second-trimester fetuses. Tissue specimens from spontaneously aborted fetuses or stillbirths can also be examined for chromosome abnormalities. Interphase cytogenetics (using FISH) is increasingly being used to study individual blastomeres of preimplantation embryos (with in vitro fertilization–derived pregnancies). This makes it possible to detect aneuploid or structurally unbalanced embryos or, in the case of sex-linked disorders, to identify male conceptuses; such embryos would not be used to initiate pregnancies.

Among infants and children, peripheral blood is examined, most often in individuals with specific phenotypic abnormalities. For example, karyotypic analysis can be used for the confirmation or exclusion of a specific chromosomal syndrome (e.g., trisomy 21); in patients with unexplained psychomotor retardation with or without dysmorphic features; in cases of monogenic disorders associated with mental retardation and/or dysmorphic features; and with abnormalities of sexual differentiation and development.

In adults, peripheral blood can be examined in patients with infertility or recurrent miscarriages, since chromosome abnormalities can lead to meiotic arrest or to genetically unbalanced gametes. An important branch of cytogenetics is concerned with analyses of bone marrow, unstimulated peripheral blood, and lymph nodes of tumors, as chromosomal abnormalities are a common correlate of leukemia, lymphoma, and solid tumors (Chap. 79).

CYTOGENETIC TESTING IN PRENATAL DIAGNOSIS

The vast majority of prenatal diagnostic studies are performed to rule out a chromosomal abnormality, but cells may also be propagated for biochemical studies or molecular analyses of DNA. Three procedures are used to obtain samples for prenatal diagnosis: amniocentesis, chorionic villus sampling (CVS), and fetal blood sampling. Amniocentesis is the most common procedure and is routinely performed at 15–17 weeks of gestation. On some occasions, early amniocentesis at 12–14 weeks is performed to expedite results, although less fluid is obtained at this time. Early amniocentesis carries a greater risk of spontaneous abortion or fetal injury but provides results at an earlier stage of pregnancy.

The vast majority of amniocenteses are performed in the context of advanced maternal age, the best-known correlate of trisomy (see below). Additional reasons for amniocentesis referral include an abnormal "triple- or quad-marker assay" and/or detection of ultrasound abnormalities. In this assay, levels of human chorionic gonadotropin, α-fetoprotein, and unconjugated estriol (and, in the quad assay, inhibin) in the maternal serum are quantified and used to adjust the maternal age-predicted risk of a trisomy 21 or trisomy 18 fetus. Specific ultrasound abnormalities, when detected at midtrimester, can also be associated with chromosomal defects. When a nonspecific ultrasound abnormality is present, the estimated risk of a chromosomal defect is ~16%. Associations of chromosomal abnormalities and specific types of abnormal ultrasound findings are listed in Table 63-1.

CVS is the second most common procedure for genetic prenatal diagnosis. Because this procedure is routinely performed at about 10–12 weeks of gestation, it allows for an earlier detection of abnormalities and a safer pregnancy termination, if desired. CVS is a relatively safe procedure (spontaneous abortions, <0.5–1%). Because there is an increased association of limb defects when the procedure is performed earlier (<10 weeks of gestation), CVS is applicable during a narrow time frame of gestation. CVS involves the use of a catheter inserted transvaginally; ~25 mg of villi are aspirated from the chorion frondosum (the fetal portion of the placenta). By adding colchicine directly to the rapidly dividing cytotrophoblasts, results can be obtained within 24–48 h. Findings from these procedures should be confirmed

TABLE 63-1 FREQUENCY OF CHROMOSOME ABNORMALITIES, IDENTIFIED ON THE BASIS OF ABNORMAL ULTRASOUND FINDINGS

	Chromosomal Abnormalities (Frequency)	
Ultrasound Finding	**Average, %**	**Range in Different Studies, %**
Abnormal ultrasound (nonspecific)	16	13–35
Omphalocele	39	26–54
Cystic hygroma	68	46–78
Congenital heart disease	30	8–40
Choroid plexus cyst	5	4–10

by analyses of cultured mesenchymal cells, as they are more reliably derived from the fetus.

Percutaneous umbilical blood sampling (PUBS) is a method for obtaining fetal blood during the second and third trimesters of pregnancy. PUBS is usually performed when ultrasound abnormalities are detected late in the second trimester. PUBS is also used when cytogenetic results from amniocentesis need clarification, such as in the detection of mosaicism.

CHROMOSOME ABNORMALITIES

CHROMOSOMES IN CELL DIVISION

To understand the etiology of chromosome abnormalities, it is important to review the movement of chromosomes during cell division. In somatic tissues, chromosomes are replicated during the S-phase of the cell cycle, so that each replicated chromosome consists of two identical sister chromatids. When the cell enters mitosis, each of the 46 chromosomes align on the metaphase plate, with the centromeres co-oriented toward opposite spindle poles (Fig. 63-3). At anaphase the sister chromatids separate, with each of the daughter cells receiving one sister chromatid from each of the 46 chromosomes.

Chromosome segregation is more complicated in germ cell division, since the number of chromosomes must be reduced from 46 to 23 in the mature sperm and eggs. This is accomplished by two rounds of division—meiosis I and meiosis II (Fig. 63-3). In meiosis I, homologous chromosomes pair and exchange genetic material, then align on the metaphase plate, and finally separate from one another. Thus, by the end of meiosis I, only 23 of the original 46 chromosomes are represented in each of the two daughter cells. Meiosis II quickly follows meiosis I and is essentially a "haploid mitosis," involving separation of the sister chromatids in each of the 23 chromosomes.

Although the fundamentals of meiosis are the same in males and females, there are important distinctions, particularly in the timing of meiotic divisions. In males, meiosis begins with puberty and continues throughout the individual's lifetime. In females, meiosis begins prenatally, with oocytes proceeding through the first stages of meiosis I but arresting at mid-prophase. At the time of birth, the first meiotic division is suspended in oocytes. Only after ovulation many years later do oocytes complete meiosis I and proceed to the metaphase stage of meiosis II; if fertilized, the oocyte then completes the second meiotic division. Thus, in females, the first meiotic division takes at least 10–15 years and as many as 40–45 years to complete. Maternal age–related increases in the incidence of trisomy are likely the consequence of this protracted process of cell division.

INCIDENCE AND TYPES OF CHROMOSOME ABNORMALITIES

Errors in meiosis, or in early cleavage divisions, occur with extraordinary frequency. At least 10–25% of all pregnancies, for example, involve chromosomally abnormal conceptions. A large proportion of these terminate in the earliest stages of pregnancy, many of which go unrecognized. Nevertheless, even among clinically recognized pregnancies, nearly 10% of fetuses are chromosomally unbalanced. For the three types of clinically recognized pregnancies—spontaneous abortions, stillbirths, and livebirths—the frequencies of different chromosomal abnormalities are summarized in Table 63-2. The most common abnormalities are numerical, involving fetuses with additional (trisomy) or missing (monosomy) chromosomes, or those with one (triploidy) or two (tetraploidy) additional sets of chromosomes. Structural chromosome abnormalities are much less common, although several of the most important clinical chromosomal disorders involve structural rearrangements (see below).

By far the most common abnormality is trisomy, which is identified in ~25% of spontaneous abortions and 0.3% of newborns. Trisomies for all chromosomes have now been identified in embryos or fetuses, but there is considerable variation in frequency for various chromosomes. For example, trisomy 16 is extraordinarily common, accounting for about one-third of all trisomies in spontaneous abortions, whereas trisomies 1, 5, 11, and 19 have been identified less often. Available evidence suggests two reasons for this variation: (1) some chromosomes (e.g., chromosome 16) are more likely to segregate abnormally or undergo nondisjunction during meiosis than are others; and (2) the potential for development varies widely among different trisomic conditions, with some being eliminated very early in gestation, others surviving to the time of clinical pregnancy recognition, and some (e.g., trisomies 13, 18, and 21 and sex chromosome trisomies) being compatible with survival to term.

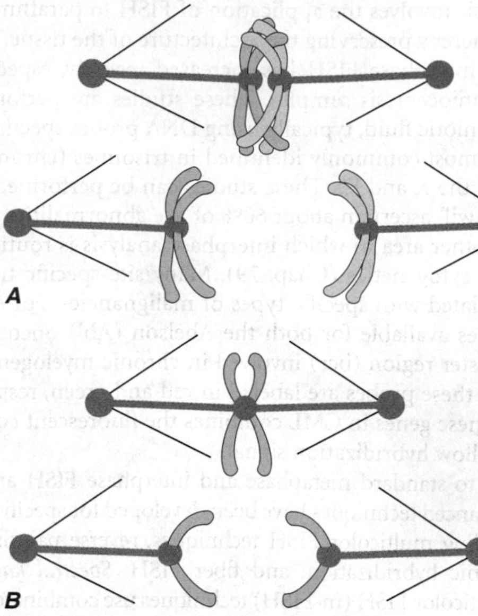

FIGURE 63-3 Chromosome segregation in meiosis. ***A.*** In meiosis I, each of the 23 pairs of chromosomes finds its "partner," or homologue, and exchanges genetic material (recombines) with it. At metaphase, each homologous pair aligns on the equatorial plate; at anaphase, each member of the homologous pair segregates from its partner. Thus, at the end of meiosis I, each daughter cell contains 23 chromosomes, with each chromosome consisting of two sister chromatids. ***B.*** In meiosis II, each chromosome aligns on the metaphase plate, and at anaphase, each of the two sister chromatids divides from the other. Thus, at the end of meiosis II, each daughter cell (e.g., the oocyte or spermatocyte) contains 23 chromosomes, with each chromosome consisting of one sister chromatid. In mitosis, the chromosomes behave exactly as they do in meiosis II, except that somatically dividing cells contain 46 chromosomes, not the 23 that are present in the meiosis II cell.

TABLE 63-2 FREQUENCY AND DISTRIBUTION OF CHROMOSOME ABNORMALITIES IN DIFFERENT TYPES OF CLINICALLY RECOGNIZABLE PREGNANCIES

	Frequency of Abnormality			
Chromosome Abnormality	**Spontaneous Abortion**	**Stillbirth**	**Livebirth**	**Probability of Surviving to Term, %**
Trisomy, all	25.1	4.0	0.3	5
+13, 18, 21	4.5	2.7	0.14	15
+16	7.5	—	—	0
Sex chromosome monosomy (45,X)	8.7	0.1	0.01	1
Triploidy	6.4	0.2	—	0
Tetraploidy	2.4	—	—	0
Structural abnormality	2.0	0.8	0.3	45
Total abnormalities	50.0	5.1	0.6	5

CHROMOSOMAL SYNDROMES

While most chromosomally abnormal conceptions perish in utero, several conditions are compatible with survival to term. The best-characterized of these are numerical abnormalities, involving loss or gain of individual chromosomes, and abnormalities resulting from unbalanced translocations. FISH and other molecular studies have led to the identification of two "new" types of chromosome abnormalities, commonly referred to as *microdeletion syndromes* and *imprinting syndromes.*

NUMERICAL ABNORMALITIES

Virtually all types of numerical abnormalities are eliminated prenatally, so that only those involving small, gene-poor autosomes or the sex chromosomes are identified with any frequency among live-borns. Clinically, the most important of these is trisomy 21, the most frequent cause of Down syndrome. Depending on the maternal age structure of the population and the utilization of prenatal testing, the incidence of trisomy 21 ranges from 1/600 to 1/1000 live births, making it the most common chromosome abnormality in live-born individuals. Like most trisomies, the incidence of trisomy 21 is highly correlated with maternal age, increasing from about 1/1500 live births for women 20 years of age to 1/30 for women ≥45 years.

In addition to trisomy 21, only two other autosomal trisomies, 13 and 18, occur with any frequency in livebirths. Incidence rates for trisomies 13 and 18 in livebirths are 1/20,000 and 1/10,000, respectively. Unlike trisomy 21, which is associated with near-normal life expectancy, both trisomies 13 and 18 are associated with death in infancy, typically occurring during the first year of life.

Three sex chromosome trisomies—the 47,XXX, 47,XXY (Klinefelter syndrome), and 47,XYY conditions—are quite common, with each occurring in about 1/2000 newborns. Of all the trisomic conditions, these three have the fewest phenotypic complications. In fact, with the exception of infertility in Klinefelter syndrome (Chap. 343), it is likely that most individuals with such trisomic conditions would go undetected. The additional Y chromosome in the 47,XYY condition is small and contains only a few genes. Most Y-linked genes are involved in testicular development or spermatogenesis. Thus, dosage imbalance of Y-linked genes has relatively little effect on other developmental processes. The 47,XYY genotype is associated with increased height. Its role in antisocial behavior, postulated initially because of an increased prevalence among some penalized populations, is unclear.

For the 47,XXX and 47,XXY conditions, the situation is different—the X chromosome contains >1000 genes, many of them essential for normal development. How, then, are 47,XXX and 47,XXY individuals spared from the catastrophic consequences of dosage imbalance? The answer lies in the biology of X chromosome gene expression. In normal females, one of the chromosomes undergoes *X inactivation* in somatic cells. The inactivation of the paternal or maternal X chromosome occurs randomly in each somatic cell and thereby serves as a mechanism of dosage compensation, ensuring that males and females have equal expression of most X-linked genes. The inactivation process occurs at the blastocyst stage of development; prior to this, both X chromosomes are active. In addition, not all X-linked genes are inactivated. Some genes on the X chromosome "escape" the inactivating mechanism and are expressed from both X chromosomes. In disorders such as Klinefelter syndrome, some genes may be expressed from both X chromosomes, resulting in its phenotypic features.

As a rule, monosomic conditions are incompatible with fetal development and, consequently, autosomal monosomies are only rarely identified in spontaneous abortions and are not found among live-born individuals. In fact, the only monosomy compatible with live birth is the 45,X condition, which causes Turner syndrome. The 45,X chromosome constitution occurs with surprisingly high frequency, present in at least 1–2% of all pregnancies. More than 99% of all 45,X conceptions are spontaneously aborted. Thus, live-born individuals with a 45,X chromosome constitution represent a rare group of survivors. The 45,X phenotype is mild, presumably because the second copy of many X chromosomal genes is normally inactivated. Nonetheless, Turner syndrome causes gonadal dysgenesis, resulting in infertility and failure to undergo secondary sexual development, along with a number of other phenotypic features (Chap. 343). Several other structural abnormalities of the X chromosome such as deletions, isochromosome X, or ring chromosomes can cause Turner syndrome. Mosaicism, including 45,X/45,XX, 45X/45,XXX, 45,X/45,XY, and others, also occurs (see below) and contributes to the phenotypic spectrum in Turner syndrome.

TABLE 63-3 STUDIES OF THE PARENT AND MEIOTIC/MITOTIC STAGE OF ORIGIN OF HUMAN TRISOMIES AND SEX CHROMOSOME MONOSOMY

	Origin, %				
	Paternal		Maternal		
	I	II	I	II	Mitotic
Trisomy					
2	28	—	54	13	6
7	—	—	17	26	57
15	—	15	76	9	—
16	—	1	96	3	—
18	—	—	33	56	11
21	3	5	67	22	2
22	3	—	94	3	—
XXY	46	—	38	14	3
XXX	—	6	60	16	18
Monosomy					
X[a]	80		20		

[a]Results pertain to nonmosaic 45,X individuals.

Because numerical abnormalities originate in meiosis (Table 63-3), affected individuals have missing or extra chromosomes in all cells. In a small proportion of cases, a mitotic nondisjunctional event occurs at an early stage in an individual with an initially normal chromosome constitution. Alternatively, a "normalizing" mitotic nondisjunctional event may result in a normal chromosome complement in some cells of an embryo. In either case, the embryo is a mosaic, with some cells bearing a normal chromosome constitution and others an aneuploid number of chromosomes. The phenotypic consequences are difficult to predict because they depend on the timing of nondisjunction and the distribution of normal and abnormal cells in different tissues. Nevertheless, mosaicism may lead to clinical abnormalities indistinguishable from those of nonmosaic individuals; for example, nearly 5% of all cases of Down syndrome involve individuals with mosaic trisomy 21, and about 15% of individuals with Turner syndrome are mosaic for various sex chromosomal constitutions as described above.

The Origin and Etiology of Numerical Abnormalities Over the past decade, a number of studies have used DNA polymorphisms to investigate the origin of different types of chromosome abnormalities (Fig. 63-4). The most thoroughly investigated types have been numerical abnormalities (Table 63-3). Sex chromosome monosomy usually results from loss of the paternal sex chromosome, regardless of whether the conception is live-born or spontaneously aborted.

Trisomies show remarkable variation in parental origin. For example, paternal nondisjunction is responsible for nearly 50% of 47,XXY but only 5–10% of cases of trisomies 13, 14, 15, 21, and 22; it is rarely, if ever, the source of the additional chromosome in trisomy 16. Similarly, there is considerable variability in the meiotic stage of origin. For example, all cases of trisomy 16 may be due to meiosis I errors, whereas for trisomy 21, one-third of cases are associated with meiosis II errors, and for trisomy 18, the majority of cases are apparently due to meiosis II nondisjunction. In spite of this variation in parental and meiotic origin, nondisjunction at maternal meiosis I appears to be the most common source of trisomy.

Maternal Age and Trisomy The association between increasing maternal age and trisomy is the most important etiologic factor in con-

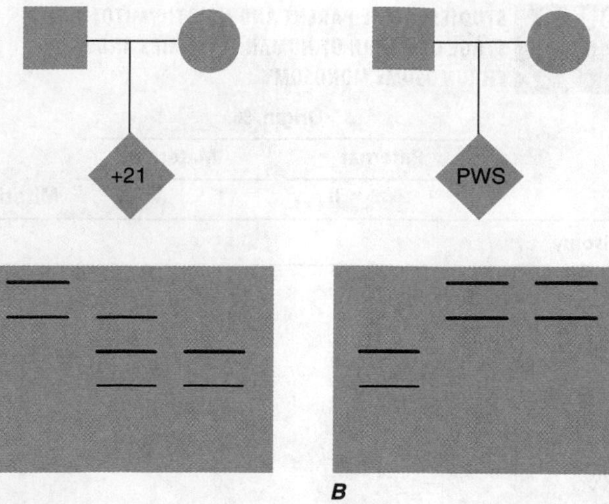

FIGURE 63-4 Use of DNA technology to determine the origin of chromosome abnormalities. ***A.*** Analysis of a chromosome 21–specific DNA polymorphism demonstrates that the trisomic individual received two chromosomes 21 from his mother and one from his father; thus, the extra chromosome 21 resulted from an error in oogenesis. ***B.*** Inheritance of a chromosome 15–specific DNA polymorphism in an individual with Prader-Willi syndrome (PWS). The affected individual has received two maternal, but no paternal, chromosomes 15; thus, the individual is said to have maternal uniparental disomy 15, a common cause of PWS.

genital chromosomal disorders. Among women under the age of 25, ~2% of all clinically recognized pregnancies are trisomic; by the age of 36, however, this figure increases to 10% and by the age of 42, to >33% (Fig. 63-5). This association between maternal age and trisomy is exerted without respect to race, geography, or socioeconomic factors and likely affects segregation of all chromosomes.

Despite the importance of increasing age, little is known about the mechanism by which aging leads to abnormal chromosomal segregation. As noted above, it is thought to originate in maternal meiosis I owing to the protracted time to completion (often ≥40 years) in females, and recent studies suggest that it may be associated with alterations in meiotic crossing-over. In trisomy 21, for example, crossover patterns appear to be similarly abnormal in younger and older mothers of trisomic conceptions. Thus, it has been suggested that two distinct steps, or "hits," may be involved in maternal age–related nondisjunction. The first hit, which is age independent, involves the establishment of a "vulnerable" crossover configuration in the fetal oocyte; the second hit, which is age dependent, involves abnormal processing of the vulnerable bivalent structure at metaphase I. If this model is correct, it suggests that the nondisjunctional process is the same in younger and older women, but it occurs more frequently with aging, possibly because of age-dependent degradation of meiotic proteins.

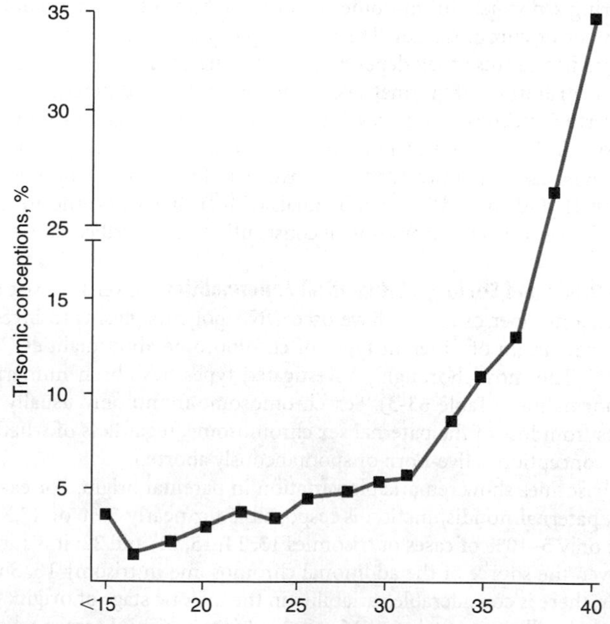

FIGURE 63-5 Estimated maternal age–adjusted rates of trisomy among all clinically recognized pregnancies (e.g., spontaneous abortions, stillbirths, and livebirths). Among women in their forties, over 25% of all pregnancies are estimated to involve a trisomic conception; the vast majority of these spontaneously abort, with only trisomies 13, 18, and 21 and sex chromosome trisomies surviving to term with any appreciable frequency.

STRUCTURAL CHROMOSOME ABNORMALITIES

Structural rearrangements involve breakage and reunion of chromosomes. Although less common than numerical abnormalities, they present additional challenges from a genetic counseling standpoint. This is because structural abnormalities, unlike numerical abnormalities, can be present in "balanced" form in clinically normal individuals but transmitted in "unbalanced" form to progeny, thereby resulting in a hereditary form of chromosome abnormality.

Rearrangements may involve exchanges of material between different chromosomes (translocations) or loss, gain, or rearrangements of individual chromosomes (e.g., deletions, duplications, inversions, rings, or isochromosomes). Of particular clinical importance are *translocations*, which involve two basic types: Robertsonian and reciprocal. Robertsonian rearrangements are a special class of translocation, in which the long arms of two acrocentric chromosomes (chromosomes 13, 14, 15, 21, and 22) join together, generating a fusion chromosome that contains virtually all of the genetic material of the original two chromosomes. If the Robertsonian translocation is present in unbalanced form, a monosomic or trisomic conception ensues. For example, ~3% of Down syndrome cases are attributable to unbalanced Robertsonian translocations, most often involving chromosomes 14 and 21. In this instance, the affected individual has 46 chromosomes, including one structurally normal chromosome 14, two structurally normal chromosomes 21, and one fusion 14/21 chromosome. This effect leads to a normal diploid dosage for chromosome 14 and to a triplication of chromosome 21, thus resulting in Down syndrome. Similarly, a small proportion of individuals with trisomy 13 syndrome are clinically affected because of an unbalanced Robertsonian translocation.

Reciprocal translocations involve mutual exchanges between any two chromosomes. In this circumstance, the phenotypic consequences associated with unbalanced translocations depend on the location of the breakpoints, which dictate the amount of material that has been "exchanged" between the two chromosomes. Because most reciprocal translocations involve unique sets of breakpoints, it is difficult to predict the phenotypic consequences in any one situation. In general, severity is determined by the amount of excess or missing chromosome material in individuals with unbalanced translocations.

In addition to rearrangements between chromosomes, there are several examples of intrachromosome structural abnormalities. The most common and deleterious of these involve loss of chromosome material due to deletions. The two best-characterized deletion syndromes, Wolf-Hirschhorn syndrome and cri-du-chat syndrome, result from loss of relatively small chromosomal segments on chromosomes 4p and 5p, respectively. Nonetheless, each is associated with multiple congenital anomalies, developmental delays, profound retardation, and reduced lifespan.

Microdeletion Syndromes The term *contiguous gene syndrome* refers to genetic disorders that mimic a combination of single-gene disorders. They result from the deletion of a small number of tightly clustered genes. Because some are too small to be detected cytogenetically, they are termed *microdeletions*. The application of molecular tech-

TABLE 63-4 SOME COMMONLY IDENTIFIED MICRODELETION AND MICRODUPLICATION SYNDROMES

Syndrome	Cytogenetic Location	Principal Features	Imprinting Effects
Langer-Giedion syndrome	8q24.1 (del)	Sparse hair, bulbous nose, variable mental retardation	No
WAGR complex	11p13 (del)	Wilms' tumor, aniridia, genitourinary disorders, mental retardation	No
Beckwith-Wiedemann syndrome	11p15 (dup)	Macrosomia, macroglossia, omphalocoele	Yes, occasionally associated with "paternal uniparental disomy" (see text)
Retinoblastoma	13q14.11 (del)	Retinoblastoma due to homozygous loss of functional RB allele	No obvious effect, although abnormal RB allele more likely to be paternal
Prader-Willi syndrome	15q11-13 (del)	Obesity, hypogonadism, mental retardation	Yes, prototypic imprinting disorder (see text)
Angelman syndrome	15q11-13 (del)	Ataxic gait	With Prader-Willi syndrome, prototypic imprinting disorder (see text)
α-Thalassemia and mental retardation	16p13.3 (del)	α-Thalassemia and mental retardation, due to deletion of distal 16p, including α-globin locus	No
Smith-Magenis syndrome	17p11.2 (del)	Brachycephaly, midface hypoplasia, mental retardation	No
Miller-Dieker syndrome	17p13 (del)	Dysmorphic facies, lissencephaly	No
Charcot-Marie-Tooth syndrome type 1A	17p11.2 (dup)	Progressive neuropathy due to microduplication	No
DiGeorge syndrome/ velocardiofacial syndrome	22q11 (del)	Abnormalities of third and fourth branchial arches	No

niques has led to the identification of at least 18 of these microdeletion syndromes (Table 63-4). Some of the more common ones include the Wilms' tumor–aniridia complex (WAGR), Miller Dieker syndrome (MDS), and velocardiofacial (VCF) syndrome. WAGR is characterized by mental retardation and involvement of multiple organs, including kidney (Wilm's tumor), eye (aniridia), and the genitourinary system. The cytogenetic abnormality involves a deletion of a part of the short arm of chromosome 11 (11p13), which typically is detectable on well-banded chromosome preparations. In MDS, a disorder characterized by mental retardation, dysmorphic faces, and lissencephaly, the deletion involves chromosome 17 (17p13). Using FISH, 17p deletions have been detected in >90% of patients with MDS as well as in 20% of cases of isolated lissencephaly.

Deletions involving the long arm of chromosome 22 (22q11) are the most common microdeletions identified to date, present in ~1/3000 newborns. VCF syndrome, the most commonly associated syndrome, consists of learning disabilities or mild mental retardation, palatal defects, a hypoplastic aloe nasi and long nose, and congenital heart defects (conotruncal defect). Some individuals with 22q11 deletion are more severely affected and present with DiGeorge syndrome, which involves abnormalities in the development of the third and fourth branchial arches leading to thymic hypoplasia, parathyroid hypoplasia, and conotruncal heart defects. In ~30% of these cases, a deletion at 22q11 can be detected with high-resolution banding; by combing conventional cytogenetics, FISH, and molecular detection techniques (i.e., Southern blotting or polymerase chain reaction analyses), these rates improve to >90%. Additional studies have demonstrated a surprisingly high frequency of 22q11 deletions in individuals with nonsyndromic conotruncal defects. Approximately 10% of individuals with a 22q11 deletion inherited it from a parent with a similar deletion.

Smith-Magenis syndrome involves a microdeletion localized to the proximal region of the short arm of chromosome 17 (17p11.2). Affected individuals have mental retardation, dysmorphic facial features, delayed speech, peripheral neuropathy, and behavior abnormalities. Most of these deletions can be detected with cytogenetic analysis, although FISH is available to confirm these findings. In contrast, William syndrome, a chromosome 7 (7q11.23) microdeletion, cannot be diagnosed with standard or high-resolution analysis; it is only detectable utilizing FISH or other molecular methods. William syndrome involves a deletion of the elastin gene and is characterized by mental retardation, dysmorphic features, a gregarious personality, premature aging, and congenital heart disease (usually supravalvular aortic stenosis).

In addition to microdeletion syndromes, there is now at least one well-described microduplication syndrome, Charcot-Marie-Tooth type 1A (CMT1A). This is a nerve conduction disease previously thought to be transmitted as a simple autosomal dominant disorder. Recent molecular studies have demonstrated that affected individuals are heterozygous for duplication of a small region of chromosome 17 (17p11.2–12). Although it is not yet clear why increased gene dosage would result in CMT1A, the inheritance pattern is explained by the fact that one-half of the offspring of affected individuals inherit the duplication-carrying chromosome.

IMPRINTING DISORDERS

Two other microdeletion syndromes, Prader-Willi syndrome (PWS) and Angelman syndrome (AS), exhibit parent-of-origin, or "imprinting," effects. For many years, it has been known that cytogenetically detectable deletions of chromosome 15 occur in a proportion of patients with PWS, as well as in those with AS. This seemed curious, as the clinical manifestations of the two syndromes are very dissimilar. PWS is characterized by obesity, hypogonadism, and mild to moderate mental retardation, whereas AS is associated with microcephaly, ataxic gait, seizures, inappropriate laughter, and severe mental retardation. New insight into the pathogenesis of these disorders has been provided by the recognition that parental origin of the deletion determines which phenotype ensues: if the deletion is paternal, the result is PWS, whereas if the deletion is maternal, the result is AS (Fig. 63-2).

This scenario is complicated further by the recognition that not all individuals with PWS or AS carry the chromosome 15 deletion. For such individuals, the parental origin of the chromosome 15 region is again the important determinant. In PWS, for example, nondeletion patients invariably have two maternal and no paternal chromosomes 15 [maternal uniparental disomy (UPD)], whereas for some nondeletion AS patients the reverse is true (paternal UPD). This indicates that at least some genes on chromosome 15 are differently expressed, depending on which parent contributed the chromosome. Additionally, this means that normal fetal development requires the presence of one maternal and one paternal copy of chromosome 15.

Approximately 70% of PWS cases are due to paternal deletions of 15q11-q13, whereas 25% are due to maternal UPD, and about 5% are caused by mutations in a chromosome 15 imprinting center. In AS, 75% of cases are due to maternal deletions, and only 2% are due to paternal UPD. The remaining cases are presumably caused by imprinting mutations (5%), or mutations in the *UBE3A* gene, which is associated with AS. The UPD cases are mostly caused by meiotic nondisjunction resulting in trisomy 15, subsequently followed by a normalizing mitotic nondisjunction event ("trisomy rescue") resulting in two normal chromosomes 15, both from the same parent. *UBE3A* is the only maternally imprinted gene known in the critical region of chromosome 15. However, several paternally imprinted genes, or expressed-sequence tags (ESTs), have been identified, including *ZNF127*, *IPW*, *SNRPN*, *SNURF*, *PAR1*, and *PAR5*.

Chromosomal regions that behave in the manner observed in PWS and AS are said to be *imprinted*. This phenomenon is involved in differential expression of certain genes on different chromosomes. Chromosome 11 is one of these with an imprinted region, since it is known that a small proportion of individuals with the Beckwith-Wiedemann overgrowth syndrome have two paternal but no maternal copies of this chromosome.

ACQUIRED CHROMOSOME ABNORMALITIES IN CANCER

In addition to the constitutional cytogenetic chromosomal abnormalities that are present at birth, somatic chromosomal changes can be acquired later in life and are often associated with malignant conditions. As with constitutional abnormalities, somatic changes can include the net loss of chromosomal material (due to a deletion or loss of a chromosome), net gain of material (duplication or gain of a chromosome), and relocation of DNA sequences (translocation). Cytogenetic changes have been particularly well studied in (1) leukemias, e.g., Philadelphia chromosome translocation in CML [t(9;22)(q34.1;q11.2)]; and (2) lymphomas, e.g., translocations of *MYC* in Burkitt's [t(8;14)(q24; q32)]. These and other translocations are useful for diagnosis, classification, and prognosis. Analyses of cytogenetic changes are also useful in certain solid tumors. For example, a complex karyotype with Wilms' tumor, diploidy in medulloblastoma, and Her-2/neu amplification in breast cancer are poor prognostic signs. For detailed discussion of cancer genetics, see Chap. 79.

FURTHER READINGS

Dave BJ, Sanger WG: Role of cytogenetics and molecular cytogenetics in the diagnosis of genetic imbalances. Semin Pediatr Neurol 14(1):2, 2007

Jiang F, Katz RL: Use of interphase fluorescence in situ hybridization as a powerful diagnostic tool in cytology. Diagn Mol Pathol 11:47, 2002

Lee C et al: Multicolor fluorescence in situ hybridization in clinical cytogenetic diagnostics. Curr Opin Pediatr 13:550, 2002

Menten B et al: Emerging patterns of cryptic chromosomal imbalance in patients with idiopathic mental retardation and multiple congenital anomalies: A new series of 140 patients and review of published reports. J Med Genet 43:625, 2006

Nasmyth K: Segregating sister genomes: The molecular biology of chromosome separation. Science 297:559, 2002

Rickman L et al: Prenatal detection of unbalanced chromosomal rearrangements by array CGH. J Med Genet 43: 353, 2006

Rimoin DL et al (eds): *Emery and Rimoin's Principles and Practice of Medical Genetics*, 4th ed. Philadelphia, Churchill Livingstone, 2001

Sharp AJ et al: Discovery of previously unidentified genomic disorders from the duplication architecture of the human genome. Nat Genet 38:1038, 2006

64 The Practice of Genetics in Clinical Medicine

Susan Miesfeldt, J. Larry Jameson

IMPLICATIONS OF MOLECULAR GENETICS FOR INTERNAL MEDICINE

The field of medical genetics has traditionally focused on chromosomal abnormalities (Chap. 63) and Mendelian disorders (Chap. 62). However, there is genetic susceptibility to many common adult-onset diseases, including atherosclerosis, cardiac disorders, asthma, hypertension, autoimmune diseases, diabetes mellitus, macular degeneration, Alzheimer's disease, psychiatric disorders, and many forms of cancer. Genetic contributions to these common disorders involve more than the ultimate expression of an illness; these genes can also influence the severity of infirmity, effect of treatment, and progression of disease.

The primary care clinician is now faced with the role of recognizing and counseling patients at risk for a number of genetically influenced illnesses. Among the greater than 20,000 genes in the human genome, it is estimated that each of us harbors several potentially deleterious mutations. Fortunately, many of these alterations are recessive and clinically silent. An even greater number, however, represent genetic variants that alter disease susceptibility, severity, or response to therapy.

Genetic medicine is changing the way diseases are classified, enhancing our understanding of pathophysiology, providing practical information concerning drug metabolism and therapeutic responses, and allowing for individualized screening and health care management programs. In view of these changes, the physician must integrate personal medical history, family history, and diagnostic molecular testing into the overall care of individual patients and their families. Surveys indicate that patients still turn to their primary care internist for guidance about genetic disorders, even though they may be seeing other specialists. The internist has an important role in educating patients about the indications, benefits, risks, and limitations of genetic testing in the management of a number of diverse diseases. This is a difficult task, as scientific advances in genetic medicine have outpaced the translation of these discoveries into standards of clinical care.

COMMON ADULT-ONSET GENETIC DISORDERS

MULTIFACTORIAL INHERITANCE

The risk for many adult-onset disorders reflects the combined effects of genetic factors at multiple loci that may function independently or in combination with other genes or environmental factors. Our understanding of the genetic basis of these disorders is incomplete, despite the clear recognition of genetic susceptibility. In type 2 diabetes mellitus, for example, the concordance rate in monozygotic twins ranges between 50 and 90%. Diabetes or impaired glucose tolerance occurs in 40% of siblings and in 30% of the offspring of an affected individual. Despite the fact that diabetes affects 5% of the population and exhibits a high degree of heritability, only a few genetic mutations (most of which are rare) that might account for the familial nature of the disease have been identified. They include certain mitochondrial DNA disorders (Chap. 62), mutations in a cascade of genes that control pancreatic islet cell development and function (*HNF4α, HNF1α, IPF1, TCF7L2, glucokinase*), insulin receptor mutations, and others (Chap. 338). Superimposed on this genetic background are environmental influences such as diet, exercise, pregnancy, and medications.

Identifying susceptibility genes associated with multifactorial adult-onset disorders is a formidable task. Nonetheless, a reasonable goal for these types of diseases is to identify genes that increase (or decrease) disease risk by a factor of two or more. For common diseases such as diabetes or heart disease, this level of risk has important implications for health. In much the same way that cholesterol is currently used as a biochemical marker of cardiovascular risk, we can anticipate the development of genetic panels with similar predictive power. The advent of DNA-sequencing chips represents an important technical advance that promises to make large-scale testing more feasible (Chap. 62). Whether to perform a genetic test for a particular inherited adult-onset disorder, such as hemochromatosis, multiple endocrine neoplasia (MEN) type 1, prolonged QT syndrome, or Huntington disease, is a complex decision; it depends on the clinical features of the disorder, the desires of the patient and family, and whether the results of genetic testing will alter medical decision-making or treatment (see below).

Population Screening Mass genetic screening programs require tests of high enough sensitivity and specificity to be cost-effective. An effective screening program should fulfill the following criteria: that the tested disorder is prevalent and serious; that it can be influenced presymptomatically through lifestyle changes, screening, or medications;

and that identification of risk does not result in undue discrimination or harm. Screening individuals of Jewish descent for the autosomal recessive neurodegenerative disorder Tay-Sachs disease has resulted in a dramatic decline in the incidence of this syndrome in the United States. On the other hand, screening for sickle cell disease or trait in the African-American population has sometimes resulted in insurance and employment discrimination.

Mass screening for complex genetic disorders can result in potential problems. For example, cystic fibrosis is most commonly associated with alterations in ΔF508. This variant accounts for 30–80% of mutant alleles depending on the ethnic group. Nevertheless, cystic fibrosis is associated with pronounced genetic heterogeneity with more than 1000 disease-related mutations. The American College of Medical Genetics recommends a panel of 23 alleles, including the ΔF508 allele, for routine diagnostic and carrier testing. Analysis for the less common cystic fibrosis–associated mutations would greatly impact the cost of testing without significantly influencing the effectiveness of mass screening. Nevertheless, the individual who carries one of the less common cystic fibrosis–associated alterations will not benefit if testing is limited to a routine panel.

Occupational health screening programs hold promise but also raise concerns about employment discrimination. These concerns were brought to light in 2001 when it was discovered that a railroad company was testing its employees, without consent, for a rare genetic condition that results in susceptibility to carpal tunnel syndrome. The Equal Employment Opportunity Commission argued that the tests were unlawful under the Americans with Disabilities Act.

THE FAMILY HISTORY

When two or more first-degree relatives are affected with asthma, cardiovascular disease, type 2 diabetes, breast cancer, colon cancer, or melanoma, the relative risk ranges from two- to fivefold, underscoring the importance of family history for these prevalent disorders. Pending further advances in genetic testing, the key to assessing the inherited risk for common adult-onset diseases rests in the collection and interpretation of a detailed personal and family medical history in conjunction with a directed physical examination. For example, a history of multiple family members with early-onset coronary artery disease, glucose intolerance, and hypertension should suggest increased risk for genetic, and perhaps environmental, predisposition to metabolic syndrome (Chap. 236). Individual patients with this family history should be monitored for the possible development of hypertension, diabetes, and hyperlipidemia. They should be counseled about the importance of avoiding additional risk factors such as obesity and cigarette smoking.

Family history should be recorded in the form of a pedigree. At a minimum, pedigrees should convey health-related data on all first-degree relatives and selected second-degree relatives, including grandparents. When pedigrees appear to suggest an inherited disease, they should be extended to include additional family members. The determination of risk for an asymptomatic individual will vary depending on the size of the pedigree, the number of unaffected relatives, and the types of diagnoses, as well as the ages of disease onset within the family. For example, a woman with two first-degree relatives with breast cancer is at greater risk for a Mendelian disorder if she has a total of three female first-degree relatives than if she has a total of ten female first-degree relatives. Additional variables that should be documented in the pedigree include the presence or absence of nonhereditary risk factors among those affected with diseases, and the finding of multiple diseases in an individual patient. For instance, a woman with a history of both colon cancer and endometrial cancer is at risk for hereditary nonpolyposis colon cancer (HNPCC) regardless of her family history.

When assessing the personal and family history, the physician should be alert to a younger age of disease onset than is usually seen in the general population. A 30-year-old with acute myocardial infarction should be considered at risk for a hereditary trait, even if there is no family history of premature coronary artery disease (Chap. 235). The absence of the nonhereditary risk factors typically associated with a disease also raises the prospect of genetic causation. A personal or family history of deep-vein thrombosis, in the absence of known environmental or medical risk factors, suggests a hereditary thrombotic disorder (Chap. 111). The physical examination also may provide important clues about the risk for a specific inherited disorder. A patient presenting with xanthomas at a young age should prompt consideration of familial hypercholesterolemia. Some adult-onset disease-causing mutations are more prevalent in certain ethnic groups. For instance, >2% of the Ashkenazi population carry one of three specific mutations in the *BRCA1* or *BRCA2* genes. The prevalence of the factor V Leiden allele ranges from 3 to 7% in Caucasians but is much lower in Africans or Asians.

Recall of family history is often inaccurate. This is especially so when the history is remote and families become more dispersed geographically. It can be helpful to ask patients to fill out family history forms before or after their visits, as this provides them with an opportunity to contact relatives. Attempts should be made to confirm the illnesses reported in the family history before making important and, in certain circumstances, irreversible management decisions. This process is often labor intensive and ideally involves interviews of additional family members or reviewing medical records, autopsy reports, and death certificates.

Although many inherited disorders will be suggested by the clustering of relatives with the same or related conditions, it is important to note that *disease penetrance* is incomplete for most multifactorial genetic disorders. As a result, the pedigree obtained in such families may not exhibit a clear Mendelian inheritance pattern, as not all family members carrying the disease-associated alleles will manifest a clinical disorder. Furthermore, genes associated with some of these disorders often exhibit *variable expression* of disease. For example, the breast cancer–associated gene *BRCA1* can predispose to several different malignancies in the same family, including cancers of the breast, ovary, and prostate (Chap. 79). For common diseases such as breast cancer, some family members without the disease-causing mutation may also develop breast cancer, representing another confounding variable in the pedigree analysis.

Some of the aforementioned features of the family history are illustrated in Fig. 64-1. In this example, the proband, a 36-year-old woman (IV-1), has a strong history of breast and ovarian cancer on the paternal side of her family. The early age of onset, as well as the co-occurrence of breast and ovarian cancer in this family, suggests the

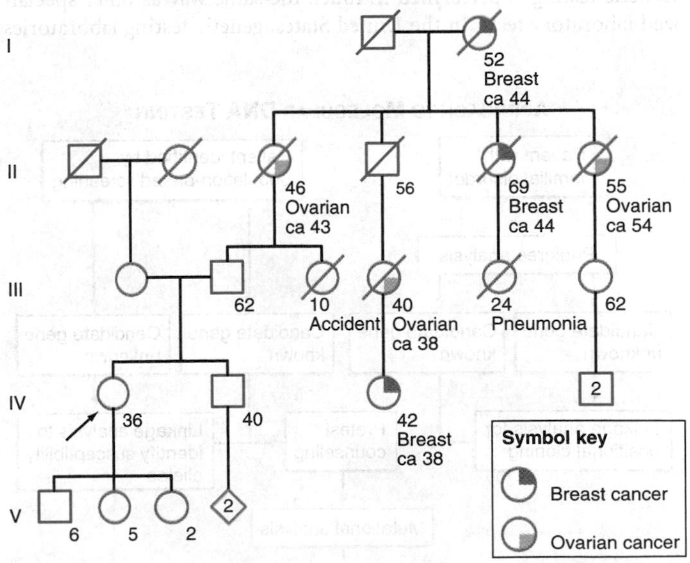

FIGURE 64-1 A 36-year-old woman (*arrow*) seeks consultation because of her family history of cancer. The patient expresses concern that the multiple cancers in her relatives imply an inherited predisposition to develop cancer. The family history is recorded and records of the patient's relatives confirm the reported diagnoses.

possibility of an inherited mutation in *BRCA1* or *BRCA2*. It is unclear though—without genetic testing—whether her father inherited such a mutation and transmitted it to her. After appropriate genetic counseling of the proband and her family, one approach to DNA analysis in this family is to test the cancer-affected 42-year-old living cousin for the presence of a *BRCA1* or *BRCA2* mutation. If a mutation is found, then it is possible to test for this particular alteration in the proband and other family members, if they so desire. In the example shown, if the proband's father has the *BRCA1* mutation, there is a 50:50 probability that the mutation was transmitted to her, and genetic testing can be used to establish the absence or presence of this alteration.

GENETIC TESTING FOR ADULT-ONSET DISORDERS

A critical first step before initiating genetic testing is to ensure that the correct clinical diagnosis has been made, whether based on family history, characteristic physical findings, or biochemical testing. Careful clinical assessment can define the *phenotype*, thereby preventing unnecessary testing and directing testing toward the most probable candidate genes (Fig. 64-2). For patients identified by population-based screening (e.g., diabetes, hypercholesterolemia), testing might involve known candidate genes, or genome-wide linkage studies (HapMap) of the population could be used as part of a research study to identify susceptibility alleles. For patients with a strong family history (e.g., breast cancer, hemochromatosis), testing often includes known candidate genes, or traditional linkage analyses within pedigrees can identify disease-causing genes. Once candidate genes are known, mutational analyses can be performed after pretest genetic counseling (see below).

Many disorders exhibit the feature of *locus heterogeneity*, which refers to the fact that mutations in different genes can cause phenotypically similar disorders. For example, osteogenesis imperfecta (Chap. 357), long QT syndrome (Chap. 226), muscular dystrophy (Chap. 382), homocystinuria (Chap. 358), retinitis pigmentosa (Chap. 29), and hereditary predisposition to colon cancer (Chap. 87) or breast cancer (Chap. 86) can each be caused by mutations in distinct genes. The pattern of disease transmission, clinical course, and treatment may differ significantly, depending on the specific gene affected. In these cases, the choice of which genes to test is often determined by unique clinical and family history features, the relative prevalence of mutations in various genes, or test availability.

METHODOLOGIC APPROACHES TO GENETIC TESTING

Genetic testing is performed in much the same way as other specialized laboratory tests. In the United States, genetic testing laboratories are CLIA (Clinical Laboratory Improvement Act) approved to ensure that they meet quality and proficiency standards. A useful source for various genetic tests is *www.genetests.org*.

DNA testing is most commonly performed by DNA sequence analysis for mutations, although genotype can also be deduced through the study of RNA or protein (e.g., apoprotein E, hemoglobin, immunohistochemistry). The determination of DNA sequence alterations relies heavily on the use of polymerase chain reaction (PCR), which allows rapid amplification and analysis of the gene of interest. In addition, PCR enables genetic testing on minimal amounts of DNA extracted from a wide range of tissue sources including leukocytes, fibroblasts, epithelial cells in saliva or hair, and archival tissues. Amplified DNA can be analyzed directly by DNA sequencing or it can be hybridized to DNA chips or blots to detect the presence of normal and mutant DNA sequences. Direct DNA sequencing is increasingly used for prenatal diagnosis as well as for determination of hereditary disease susceptibility. Analyses of large alterations in the genome are possible using cytogenetics, fluorescent in situ hybridization (FISH), or Southern blotting (Chap. 63).

Protein truncation tests (PTTs) are used to detect mutations that result in the premature termination of a polypeptide occurring during protein synthesis. In this assay, the isolated complementary DNA (cDNA) is transcribed and translated in vitro, and the protein is analyzed by gel electrophoresis. The truncated (mutant) gene product is readily identified as its electrophoretic mobility differs from that of the normal protein. This test is used most commonly for analyses of large genes with significant genetic heterogeneity such as *DMD*, *APC*, and the *BRCA* genes.

Like all laboratory tests, there are limitations to the accuracy and interpretation of genetic tests. In addition to technical errors, genetic tests are sometimes designed to detect only the most common mutations. In this case, a negative result must be qualified by the possibility that the individual may have a mutation that is not included in the test. In addition, a negative result does not mean that there is not a mutation in some other gene that causes a similar inherited disorder.

In addition to molecular testing for established disease, genetic testing for susceptibility to chronic disease is being increasingly integrated into the practice of medicine. In most cases, however, the discovery of disease-associated genes has greatly outpaced studies that assess clinical outcomes and the impact of interventions. Until such evidence-based studies are available, predictive molecular testing must be approached with caution and should be offered only to patients who have been adequately counseled and have provided informed consent. In the majority of cases, genetic testing should be offered only to individuals with a suggestive personal or family medical history or in the context of a clinical trial.

Predictive genetic testing falls into two distinct categories. *Presymptomatic testing* applies to diseases where a specific genetic alteration is associated with a near 100% likelihood of developing disease. In contrast, *predisposition testing* predicts a risk for disease that is less than 100%. For example, presymptomatic testing is available for those at risk for Huntington's disease, whereas predisposition testing is considered for those at risk for hereditary breast cancer. It is important to note that, for the majority of adult-onset, multifactorial genetic disorders, testing is purely predictive. Test results cannot reveal with confidence whether, when, or how the disease will manifest itself. For example, not everyone with the apolipoprotein E allele (ε4) will develop Alzheimer's disease, and individuals without this genetic marker can still develop the disorder (Chap. 365).

Molecular analysis is generally more informative if testing is initiated in a symptomatic family member, since the identification of a mutation can direct the testing of other at-risk family members (whether they are symptomatic or not). In the absence of additional familial or environmental risk factors, individuals who test negative for the mutation found in the affected family member can be informed that they are at general population risk for that particular disease. Furthermore, they can be reassured that they are not at risk for passing on the mutation to their children. On the other hand, asymptomatic family members who test positive for the known mutation must be informed that they are at increased risk for disease development and for transmitting the alteration to their children.

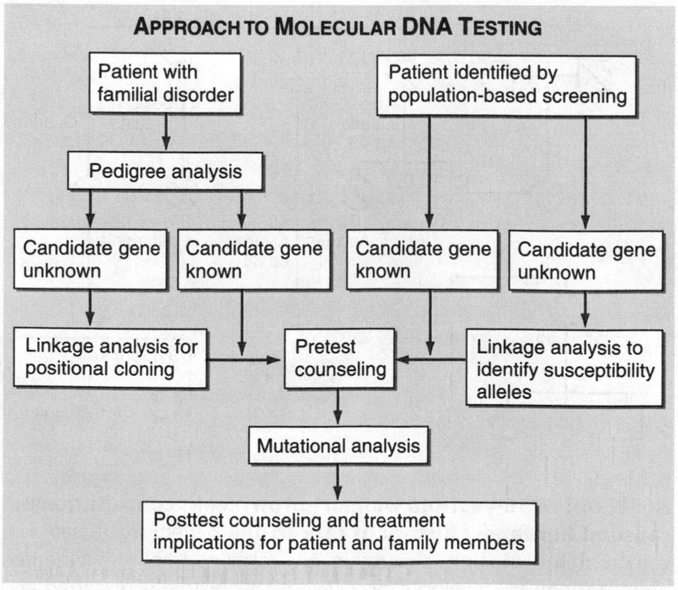

FIGURE 64-2 Approach to identifying a disease-causing gene.

Clinicians providing pretest counseling and education should assess the patient's ability to cope with test results. Individuals who demonstrate signs and symptoms of emotional distress should have their psychosocial needs addressed before proceeding with molecular testing. Generally, genetic testing should not be offered at a time of personal crisis or acute illness within the family. Patients will derive more benefit from test results if they are emotionally able to comprehend and absorb the information. It is important to assess patients' preconceived notions of their personal likelihood of disease in preparing pretest educational strategies. Often, patients harbor unwarranted fear or denial of their likelihood of genetic risk.

Genetic testing has the potential of affecting the way individual family members relate to one another, both negatively and positively. As a result, patients addressing the option of molecular testing must consider how test results might impact their relationships with relatives, partners, spouses, and friends. In families with a known genetic mutation, those who test positive must consider the impact of their carrier status on their present and future lifestyles; those who test negative may manifest *survivor guilt.* Family members are likely to differ in their emotional and social responses to the same information. Counseling should also address the potential consequences of test results on relationships with a spouse or child. Parents who are found to have a disease-associated mutation often express considerable anxiety and despair as they address the issue of risk to their children.

When a condition does not manifest until adulthood, clinicians will be faced with the question of whether at-risk children should be offered molecular testing and, if so, at what age. Although the matter is debated, several professional organizations have cautioned that genetic testing for adult-onset disorders should not be offered to children. Many of these conditions are not preventable; consequently, such information can pose significant psychosocial risk to the child. In addition, there is concern that testing during childhood violates a child's right to make an informed decision regarding testing upon reaching adulthood. On the other hand, testing should be offered in childhood for disorders that may manifest early in life, especially when management options are available. For example, children at risk for familial adenomatous polyposis (FAP), associated with alterations in the *APC* gene, may develop polyps as early as their teens, and progression to an invasive cancer can occur by their twenties. Likewise, children at risk for MEN type 2, which is caused by mutations in the *RET* proto-oncogene, may develop medullary thyroid cancer early in childhood, and the issue of prophylactic thyroidectomy should be addressed with the parents of children with documented mutations (Chap. 345).

INFORMED CONSENT

When the issue of testing is addressed, patients should be strongly encouraged to involve other relatives in the decision-making process, as molecular diagnostics will likely have an impact on the entire family. Informed consent for molecular testing begins with detailed education and counseling (Fig. 64-3). The patient must fully understand the risks, benefits, and limitations of undergoing the analysis. Informed consent should include a written document, drafted clearly and concisely in a language and format that is comprehensible to the patient, who should be made aware of the disposition of test results. Informed consent should also include a discussion of the mechanics of testing. Most molecular testing for hereditary disease involves DNA-based analysis of peripheral blood. In the majority of circumstances, test results should be given only to the individual, in person, and with a support person in the room.

Because molecular testing of an asymptomatic individual often allows prediction of future risk, the patient should understand any potential long-term medical, psychological, and social implications of this decision. In the United States, legislation affecting this area is still evolving, and it is important to explore with the patient the potential impact that test results may have on employment and future health, as well as disability and life insurance coverage.

Patients should understand that alternatives to molecular analysis remain available if they decide not to proceed with this option. They should also be notified that testing is available in the future if they are not currently prepared to undergo analysis. The option of DNA banking should be presented so that samples are readily available for future use by family members, if needed.

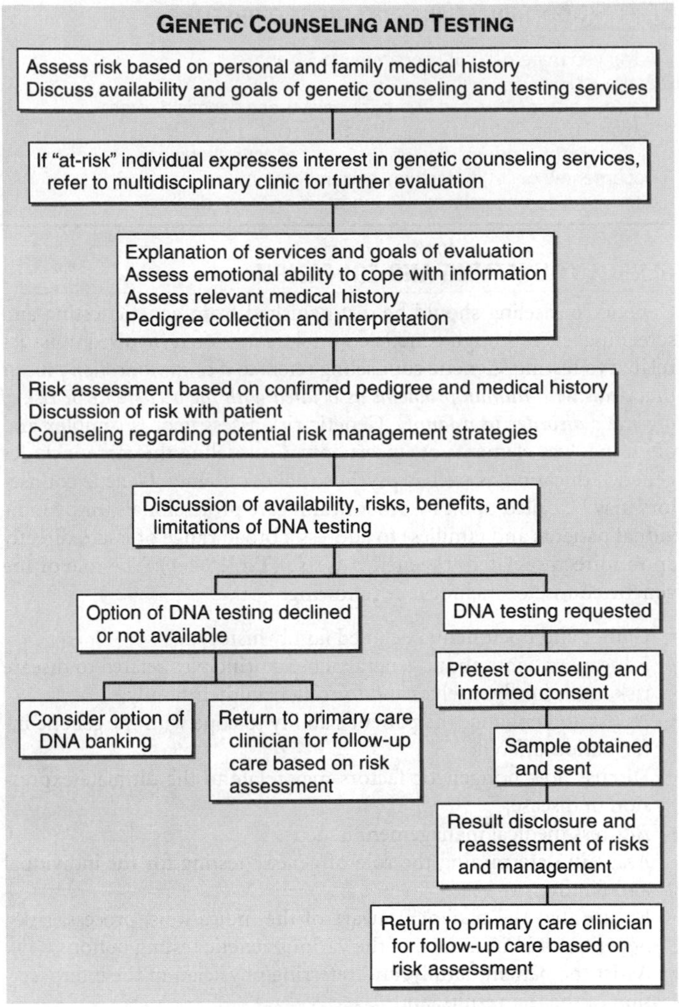
GENETIC COUNSELING AND TESTING
Assess risk based on personal and family medical history
Discuss availability and goals of genetic counseling and testing services
If "at-risk" individual expresses interest in genetic counseling services, refer to multidisciplinary clinic for further evaluation
Explanation of services and goals of evaluation
Assess emotional ability to cope with information
Assess relevant medical history
Pedigree collection and interpretation
Risk assessment based on confirmed pedigree and medical history
Discussion of risk with patient
Counseling regarding potential risk management strategies
Discussion of availability, risks, benefits, and limitations of DNA testing
Option of DNA testing declined or not available
DNA testing requested
Pretest counseling and informed consent
Consider option of DNA banking
Return to primary care clinician for follow-up care based on risk assessment
Sample obtained and sent
Result disclosure and reassessment of risks and management
Return to primary care clinician for follow-up care based on risk assessment

FIGURE 64-3 Algorithm for genetic counseling in association with genetic testing.

FOLLOW-UP CARE AFTER TESTING

Depending on the nature of the genetic disorder, posttest interventions may include (1) cautious surveillance and appropriate health care screening, (2) specific medical interventions, (3) chemoprevention, (4) risk avoidance, and (5) referral to support services. For example, patients with known pathologic mutations in *BRCA1* or *BRCA2* are offered intensive screening as well as the option of prophylactic mastectomy and oophorectomy. In addition, such women may be eligible for preventive treatment with tamoxifen, or enrollment in a chemoprevention clinical trial. In contrast, those at known risk for Huntington's disease are offered continued follow-up and supportive services, including physical and occupational therapy, and social services or support groups, as indicated. Specific interventions will change as translational research continues to enhance our understanding of these genetic diseases and as more is learned about the functions of the gene products involved.

Individuals who test negative for a mutation in a disease-associated gene identified in an affected family member must be reminded that they may still be at risk for the disease. This is of particular importance for common diseases such as diabetes mellitus, cancer, and coronary artery disease. For example, a woman who finds that she does not carry the disease-associated mutation in *BRCA2* previously discovered in her family must be reminded that she still requires the same breast cancer screening recommended for the general population.

TABLE 64-1 INDICATIONS FOR GENETIC COUNSELING

Advanced maternal (>35) or paternal (>50) age
Consanguinity
Previous history of a child with birth defects or a genetic disorder
Personal or family history suggestive of a genetic disorder
High-risk ethnic groups; known carriers of genetic alterations
Documented genetic alteration in a family member
Ultrasound or prenatal testing suggesting a genetic disorder

GENETIC COUNSELING AND EDUCATION

Genetic counseling should be distinguished from genetic testing and screening, even though genetic counselors are often involved in issues related to testing. Genetic counseling refers to *a communication process that deals with human problems associated with the occurrence or risk of a genetic disorder in a family*. Genetic risk assessment is complex and often involves elements of uncertainty. Counseling therefore includes genetic education as well as psychosocial counseling. Genetic counselors may be called upon by other health care professionals (or by individual patients and families) to address a broad range of issues directly and indirectly related to genetic disease (Table 64-1). The role of the genetic counselor includes the following:

- Gather and document a detailed family history;
- Educate patients about general genetic principles related to disease risk, both for themselves and for others in their family;
- Assess and enhance the patient's ability to cope with the genetic information offered;
- Discuss how nongenetic factors may relate to the ultimate expression of disease;
- Address medical management issues;
- Assist in determining the role of genetic testing for the individual and family;
- Ensure that the patient is aware of the indications, process, risks, benefits, and limitations of the various genetic testing options;
- Assist the patient, family, and referring physician in the interpretation of the test results; and
- Refer the patient and other at-risk family members for additional medical and support services, if necessary.

The complexity of genetic counseling and the broad scope of genetic diseases have led to the development of specialized, multidisciplinary clinics designed to provide broad-based support and medical care for those at risk and their family members. Such specialty clinics are well established in the areas of cancer and neurodegenerative disorders. The multidisciplinary teams are often composed of medical geneticists, specialist physicians, genetic counselors, nurses, psychologists, social workers, and biomedical ethicists who work together to consider difficult diagnostic, treatment, and testing decisions. Such a format also provides primary care physicians with invaluable support and assistance as they follow and treat at-risk patients.

The approach to genetic counseling has important ethical, social, and financial implications. Philosophies related to genetic counseling vary widely by country and center. In North American centers, for example, counseling is generally offered in a nondirective manner, wherein patients learn to understand how their values factor into a particular medical decision. Nondirective counseling is particularly appropriate when there are no data demonstrating a clear benefit associated with a particular intervention or when an intervention is considered experimental. For example, nondirective genetic counseling is employed when a person is deciding whether to undergo genetic testing for Huntington's disease (Chap. 365). At this time, there is no clear benefit (in terms of medical outcome) to an at-risk individual undergoing genetic testing for this disease, as its course cannot be altered by therapeutic interventions. However, testing can have an important impact on this individual's perception of the future and his or her interpersonal relationships and plans for reproduction. Therefore, the decision to pursue testing rests on the individual's belief system and values. On the other hand, a more directive approach is appropriate when a condition can be treated. In a family with FAP, colon cancer screening and prophylactic colectomy should be recommended for known *APC* mutation carriers. The counselor and clinician following this family must ensure that the at-risk family members have access to the resources necessary to adhere to these recommendations.

Genetic education is central to an individual's ability to make an informed decision regarding testing options and treatment. Although genetic counselors represent one source of genetic education, other health care providers also need to contribute to patient education. Patients at risk for genetic disease should understand fundamental medical genetic principles and terminology relevant to their situation. This includes the concept of genes, how they are transmitted, and how they confer hereditary disease risk. An adequate knowledge of patterns of inheritance will allow patients to understand the probability of disease risk for themselves and other family members. It is also important to impart the concepts of disease penetrance and expression. For most complex adult-onset genetic disorders, asymptomatic patients should be advised that a positive test result does not always translate into future disease development. In addition, the role of nongenetic factors, such as environmental exposures, must be discussed in the context of multifactorial disease risk and disease prevention. Finally, patients should understand the natural history of the disease as well as the potential options for intervention, including screening, prevention, and—in certain circumstances—pharmacologic treatment or prophylactic surgery.

THERAPEUTIC INTERVENTIONS BASED ON GENETIC RISK FOR DISEASE

Specific treatments are now available for an increasing number of genetic disorders, whether identified through population-based screening or directed testing (Table 64-2). Although the strategies for therapeutic interventions are best developed for childhood hereditary metabolic diseases, these principles are making their way into the diagnosis and

TABLE 64-2 EXAMPLES OF GENETIC TESTING AND POSSIBLE INTERVENTIONS

Genetic Disorder	Inheritance	Genes	Interventions
Oncologic			
Hereditary nonpolyposis colon cancer	AD	*MSH2, MLH1, MSH6, PMS1, PMS2, TGFBR2*	Early endoscopic screening
Familial adenomatous polyposis	AD	*APC*	Early endoscopic screening Nonsteroidal anti-inflammatory drugs Colectomy
Familial breast and ovarian cancer	AD	*BRCA1, BRCA2*	Estrogen receptor antagonists Early screening by exams and mammography Consideration of prophylactic surgery
Familial melanoma	AD	*CDKN2A*	Avoidance of UV light Screening and biopsies
Basal cell nevus syndrome	AD	*PTCH*	Avoidance of UV light Screening and biopsies

(continued)

TABLE 64-2 EXAMPLES OF GENETIC TESTING AND POSSIBLE INTERVENTIONS (CONTINUED)

Genetic Disorder	Inheritance	Genes	Interventions
Hematologic			
Factor V Leiden	AD	*F5*	Avoidance of thrombogenic risk factors and oral contraceptives
Hemophilia A	XL	*F8C*	Factor VIII replacement
Hemophilia B	XL	*F9*	Factor IX replacement Possible gene therapy
Glucose 6-PO4 dehydrogenase deficiency	XL	*G6PD*	Avoidance of oxidant drugs
Cardiovascular			
Hypertrophic cardiomyopathy	AD	*MYH7, MYBPC3, TMSA, TNNT2, TPM1*	Echocardiographic screening Early pharmacologic intervention Myomectomy
Long QT syndrome	AD	*KCNQ1, SCN5A, HERG, MiRP1, KCNE1, KCNE2*	Electrocardiographic screening Early pharmacologic intervention Implantable cardioverter defibrillator devices
Marfan syndrome	AD	*FBN1*	Echocardiographic screening Prophylactic beta blockers
Gastrointestinal			
Familial Mediterranean fever	AR	*MEFV*	Colchicine treatment
Hemochromatosis	AR	*HFE*	Phlebotomy
Pulmonary			
α_1 Antitrypsin deficiency	AR	*PI*	Avoidance of smoking Avoidance of occupational and environmental toxins
Primary pulmonary hypertension	AD	*BMPR2*	Treatment with pulmonary vasodilators
Renal			
Polycystic kidney disease	AD	*PKHD1, PKHD2*	Prevention of hypertension Prevention of urinary tract infections Kidney transplantation
Nephrogenic diabetes insipidus	XL, AR	*AVPR2, AQP2*	Fluid replacement Thiazides, amiloride
Endocrine			
Neurohypophyseal diabetes insipidus	AD	*AVP*	Replace vasopressin
Maturity-onset diabetes of the young	AD	Multiple genes	Screen and treat for diabetes
Familial hypocalciuric hypercalcemia	AD	*CASR*	Avoidance of parathyroidectomy
Kallmann syndrome	XL	*KAL*	Induction of puberty with hormone replacement
Multiple endocrine neoplasia type 2	AD	*RET*	Prophylactic thyroidectomy Screening for pheochromocytoma and hyperparathyroidism
21-hydroxylase deficiency	AR	*CYP21*	Glucocorticoid and mineralocorticoid treatment
Neurologic			
Malignant hyperthermia	AD	*RYR1*	Avoidance of precipitating anesthetics
Hyperkalemic periodic paralysis	AD	*SCN4A*	Acetazolamide
Adrenoleukodystrophy	XL	*ABCD1*	Possible bone marrow transplant for severe childhood CNS form
Duchenne and Becker muscular dystrophy	XL	*DMD*	Corticosteroids Possible future myoblast transfer
Familial Parkinson disease	AD	*SNCA, PARK2*	Amantadine, anticholinergics, levodopa, monoamine oxidase B inhibitors
Wilson disease	AR	*ATP7B*	Zinc, trientene

Abbreviations: AD, autosomal dominant; AR, autosomal recessive; CNS, central nervous system; XL, X-linked.

management of adult-onset disorders. Hereditary hemochromatosis illustrates many of the issues raised by the availability of genetic screening in the adult population. For instance, it is relatively common (approximately 1 in 200 individuals of northern European descent are homozygous), and its complications are potentially preventable through phlebotomy (Chap. 351). The identification of the *HFE* gene, mutations of which are associated with this syndrome, has sparked interest in the use of DNA-based testing for presymptomatic diagnosis of the disorder. However, up to one-third of individuals who are homozygous for the *HFE* mutation do not have evidence of iron overload. Consequently, in the absence of a positive family history, current recommendations include phenotypic screening for evidence of iron overload followed by genetic testing. Whether genetic screening for hemochromatosis will someday be coupled to assessment of phenotypic expression awaits further studies. In contrast to the issue of population screening, it is important to test and counsel other family members when the diagnosis of hemochromatosis has been made in a proband. Testing allows the physician to exclude family members who are not at risk. It also permits presymptomatic detection of iron overload and the institution of treatment (phlebotomy) before the development of organ damage.

Preventive measures and therapeutic interventions are not restricted to metabolic disorders. Identification of familial forms of long QT syndrome, associated with ventricular arrhythmias, allows early electrocardiographic testing and the use of prophylactic antiarrhythmic therapy, overdrive pacemakers, or defibrillators (Chap. 226). Individuals with familial hypertrophic cardiomyopathy can be screened by ultrasound, treated with beta blockers or other drugs, and counseled about the importance of avoiding strenuous exercise and dehydration (Chap. 231). Likewise, individuals with Marfan syndrome can be treated with beta blockers and monitored for the development of aortic aneurysms (Chap. 242). Individuals with α_1 antitrypsin deficiency can be strongly counseled to avoid cigarette smoking and exposure to environmental pulmonary and hepatotoxins. Various host genes influence the pathogenesis of certain infectious diseases in humans, including HIV (Chap. 182). The factor V Leiden allele increases risk of thrombosis (Chap. 59). Approximately 3% of the worldwide population is heterozygous for this mutation. Moreover, it is found in up to 25% of patients with recurrent deep-vein thrombosis or pulmonary embolism. Women who are heterozygous or homozygous for this allele should therefore avoid the use of oral contraceptives and receive heparin prophylaxis after surgery or trauma.

The field of pharmacogenomics seeks to identify genes that alter drug metabolism or confer susceptibility to toxic drug reactions. Pharmacogenomics permits individualized drug therapy, resulting in improved treatment outcomes, reduced toxicities, and more cost-effective pharmaceutical care. Examples include succinylcholine sensitivity, thiopurine methyltransferase (TPMT) deficiency, malignant hyperthermia, dihydropyrimidine dehydrogenase deficiency, the porphyrias, and glucose-6-phosphase dehydrogenase (G6PD) deficiency.

As noted above, the identification of genes that increase the risk of specific types of neoplasia is rapidly changing the management of many cancers. Identifying family members with mutations that predispose to FAP or hereditary nonpolyposis colon cancer (HNPCC) can lead to recommendations of early cancer screening or prophylactic surgery (Chap. 87). Similar principles apply to familial forms of melanoma, basal cell carcinoma, and cancers of the breast, ovary, and thyroid gland. It should be recognized, however, that most cancers harbor several distinct genetic abnormalities by the time they acquire invasive or metastatic potential (Chaps. 79 and 80). Consequently, the major impact of genetic testing in these cases is to allow more intensive clinical screening, as it remains very challenging to predict disease penetrance, expression, or clinical course.

Although genetic diagnosis of these and other disorders is only beginning to be used in the clinical setting, predictive testing holds the promise of allowing earlier and more targeted interventions that can reduce morbidity and mortality. We can expect the availability of genetic tests to expand. A critical challenge for physicians and other health care providers is to keep pace with these advances in genetic medicine and to implement testing judiciously.

FURTHER READINGS

CLAYTON EW: Ethical, legal, and social implications of genomic medicine. N Engl J Med 349:562, 2003

COLLINS FS, WATSON JD: Genetic discrimination: Time to act. Science 302:745, 2003

ENSENAUER RE: Genetic testing: Practical, ethical, and counseling considerations. Mayo Clin Proc 80:63, 2005

GUTTMACHER AE, COLLINS FS: Genomic medicine—a primer. N Engl J Med 347:1512, 2002

HARPER PS: *Practical Genetic Counselling*, 5th ed. Oxford, Butterworth Heinmann, 1998

MCCANDLESS SE et al: The burden of genetic disease on inpatient care in a children's hospital. Am J Hum Genet 74:121, 2004

WOLFBERG AJ: Genes on the web—Direct-to-consumer marketing of genetic testing. N Engl J Med 355:543, 2006

65 Gene Therapy in Clinical Medicine

Katherine A. High

Gene transfer is a novel area of therapeutics in which the active agent is a nucleic acid sequence rather than a protein or small molecule. Because delivery of naked DNA or RNA to a cell is an inefficient process, most gene transfer is carried out using a vector, or gene delivery vehicle. These vehicles have generally been engineered from viruses by deleting some or all of the viral genome and replacing it with the therapeutic gene of interest under the control of a suitable promoter (Table 65-1). Gene transfer strategies can be described in terms of three essential elements: (1) a vector, (2) a gene to be delivered, and

TABLE 65-1 CHARACTERISTICS OF GENE DELIVERY VEHICLES

	Viral Vectors							
Features	**Retroviral**	**Lentiviral**	**Adenoviral**	**AAV**	**Human Foamy Virus**	**HSV-1**	**SV-40**	**Alpha-Viruses**
Viral genome	RNA	RNA	DNA	DNA	RNA	DNA	DNA	RNA
Cell division requirement	Yes	G1 phase	No	No	No	No	No	No
Packaging limitation	8 kb	8 kb	8–30 kb	5 kb	8.5 kb	40–150 kb	5 kb	5 kb
Immune responses to vector	Few	Few	Extensive	Few	Few	Few in recombinant virus	Few	Few
Genome integration	Yes	Yes	Poor	Poor	Yes	No	Poor	No
Long-term expression	Yes	Yes	No	Yes	Yes	No	No	No
Main advantages	Persistent gene transfer in dividing cells	Persistent gene transfer in transduced tissues	Highly effective in transducing various tissues	Elicits few inflammatory responses, nonpathogenic	Persistent gene expression in both dividing and nondividing cells	Large packaging capacity with persistent gene transfer	Wide host cell range; lack of immunogenicity	Limited immune responses against the vector
Main disadvantages	Theoretical risk of insertional mutagenesis (occurred in 3 cases)	Might induce oncogenesis in some cases	Viral capsid elicits strong immune responses	Limited packaging capacity	In need of a stable packaging system	Residual cytotoxicity with neuron specificity	Limited packaging capacity	Transduced gene expression is transient

Note: AAV, adeno-associated virus; HSV, herpes simplex virus; SV, sarcoma virus.

(3) a relevant target cell to which the DNA or RNA is delivered. The series of steps in which the donated DNA enters the target cell and begins expression is referred to as *transduction*. Gene delivery can take place in vivo, in which the vector is directly injected into the patient or, in the case of hematopoietic and some other target cells, ex vivo, with removal of the target cells from the patient, followed by return of the modified autologous cells after gene transfer in the laboratory. The latter approach offers opportunities to integrate gene transfer techniques with cellular therapies (Chap. 67).

Gene transfer technology is still under development and protocols are experimental. Gene therapy is one of the most complex therapeutic modalities yet attempted, and each new disease represents a therapeutic problem for which dosing, safety, and efficacy must be defined. Nonetheless, gene transfer remains one of the most powerful concepts in modern molecular medicine and has the potential to address a host of diseases for which there are currently no cures or, in some cases, no available treatment. Over 5000 subjects have been enrolled in gene transfer studies, and serious adverse events have been rare. Gene therapies are being developed for a wide variety of disease entities (Fig. 65-1).

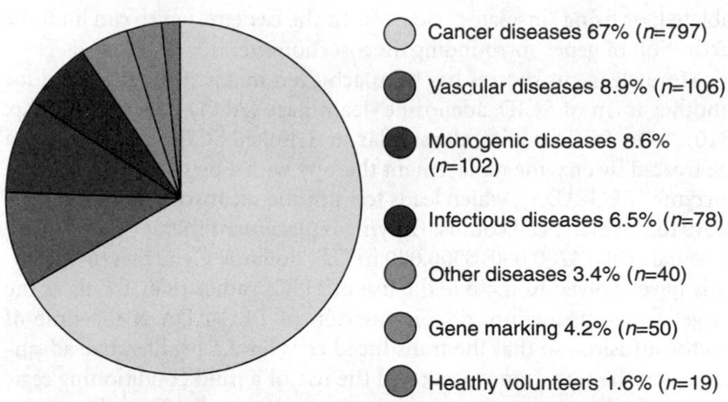

FIGURE 65-1 Indications in gene therapy clinical trials. The chart divides clinical gene transfer studies by disease classification. A majority of trials have addressed cancer, with monogenic disorders and cardiovascular diseases the next largest categories. *(Reproduced with permission from J Gene Med. New Jersey, Wiley, 2006.)*

GENE TRANSFER FOR GENETIC DISEASE

Gene transfer strategies for genetic disease generally involve gene addition therapy. This approach most commonly involves transfer of the missing gene to a physiologically relevant target cell. However, other strategies are possible, including supplying a gene that achieves a similar biologic effect through an alternative pathway (e.g., factor VIIa for hemophilia A); supplying an antisense oligonucleotide to splice out a mutant exon if the sequence is not critical to the function of the protein (as has been done with the dystrophin gene in Duchenne muscular dystrophy); or downregulating a harmful response through an siRNA. Two distinct strategies are used to achieve long-term gene expression: one is to transduce stem cells with an integrating vector, so that all progeny cells will carry the donated gene; the other is to transduce long-lived cells, such as skeletal muscle or neural cells. In the case of long-lived cells, integration into the target cell genome is unnecessary, provided the donated DNA can be stabilized in an episomal form.

Immunodeficiency Disorders: Proof of Principle Early attempts to provide gene replacement into hematopoietic stem cells (HSCs) were stymied by the relatively low transduction efficiency of retroviral vectors, which require dividing target cells for integration. Because HSCs are normally quiescent, they are a formidable transduction target. However, identification of cytokines that induced cell division without promoting differentiation of stem cells, along with technical improvements in the isolation and transduction of HSCs, led to modest but real gains in transduction efficiency.

The first convincing therapeutic effect from gene transfer occurred with X-linked severe combined immunodeficiency disease (SCID), which results from mutations in the gene (*IL2RG*) encoding the γc subunit of a cytokine receptor required for normal development of T and NK cells (Chap. 310). Affected infants present in the first few months of life with overwhelming infections and/or failure to thrive. In this disorder, it was recognized that the transduced cells, even if few in number, would have a proliferative advantage compared to the nontransduced cells, which lack receptors for the cytokines required for lymphocyte development and maturation. Complete reconstitution of the immune system, including documented responses to standard childhood vaccinations, clearing of infections, and remarkable gains in growth occurred in most of the treated children. However, two developed a syndrome similar to T cell acute lymphocytic leukemia, with splenomegaly, rising white counts, and the emergence of a single clone of T cells. In these children, the retroviral vector had integrated within a gene, *LMO-2* (LIM only-2), which encodes a component of a transcription factor complex involved in hematopoietic development. Insertion of the retroviral long terminal repeat is thought to increase the expression of *LMO-2*.

The X-linked SCID studies were a watershed event in the evolution of gene therapy. They demonstrated conclusively that gene therapy could cure disease; of the 16 infants eventually treated in these trials, 15 achieved correction of the immunodeficiency disorder. Unfortunately, 3 later developed a leukemia-like disorder, but 12 are alive and free of complications at time periods ranging up to 7 years after initial treatment. These studies also demonstrated that insertional mutagenesis leading to cancer was more than a hypothetical possibility. As a result of the experience in these trials, all protocols using integrating vectors in hematopoietic cells must include a plan for monitoring sites of insertion and clonal proliferation. Strategies to overcome this complication have included employing a "suicide" gene cassette in the vector, so that errant clones can be quickly

	Non-Viral Vectors			
Features	**Transposon/ Transposase System**	**Liposomes**	**Naked DNA**	**Site-Specific Integrase**
Viral genome	N/A	N/A	N/A	N/A
Cell division requirement	No	No	No	No
Packaging limitation	Undetermined, probably large	Undetermined, probably large	Undetermined, probably large	Undetermined, probably large
Immune responses to vector	No	No	No	No
Genome integration	Yes	No	No	Yes
Long-term expression	Yes	No	No	Undetermined
Main advantages	Transfects many cell types with long-term gene expression	Transfects many cell types. Large holding capacity to enable a high number of base pairs	Efficient in gene transfer; limited immunogenicity	Specific integration site
Main disadvantages	Early stage in development	Expensive to produce	Transient and low-level expression	Early stage in development

ablated; or using "insulator" elements in the cassette, which can limit the activation of genes surrounding the insertion site.

More clear-cut success has been achieved in a gene therapy trial for another form of SCID, adenosine deaminase (ADA) deficiency (Chap. 310). ADA-SCID is clinically similar to X-linked SCID, although it can be treated by enzyme replacement therapy with a pegylated form of the enzyme (PEG-ADA), which leads to immune reconstitution but not always to normal T cell counts. Enzyme replacement therapy is expensive (annual costs: $200,000–$300,000 in U.S. dollars). Gene therapy protocols have evolved to include the use of HSCs rather than T cells as the target for transduction; discontinuation of PEG-ADA at the time of vector infusion, so that the transduced cells have a proliferative advantage over the non-transduced; and the use of a mild conditioning regimen to facilitate engraftment of the transduced cells. There have been no complications in the six children treated on this protocol, with a median follow-up of >4 years. Based on current data, the efficacy of gene transfer for ADA-SCID is convincing, but longer term follow-up will be required to determine whether this approach is sufficiently safe to be routinely recommended as an alternative to PEG-ADA.

Other diseases likely to be amenable to transduction of HSCs include Wiskott-Aldrich syndrome (trials underway), chronic granulomatous disease, sickle cell disease, and thalassemia.

Long-Term Expression in Genetic Disease: In Vivo Gene Transfer with Recombinant Adeno-Associated Viral (AAV) Vectors Recombinant AAV vectors have emerged as attractive gene delivery vehicles for genetic disease. Engineered from a small replication-defective DNA virus, they are devoid of viral coding sequences and trigger very little immune response in experimental animals. They are capable of transducing nondividing target cells, and the donated DNA is stabilized primarily in an episomal form, thus minimizing risks associated with insertional mutagenesis. Because the vector has a tropism for certain long-lived cell types, such as skeletal muscle, the central nervous system (CNS), and hepatocytes, long-term expression can be achieved even in the absence of integration.

Clinical trials using recombinant AAV vectors are now ongoing for muscular dystrophies, α_1-antitrypsin deficiency, lipoprotein lipase deficiency, hemophilia B, and a form of congenital blindness called Leber's congenital amaurosis. Hemophilia is often considered a promising disease model for gene transfer, as the gene product does not require precise regulation of expression and biologically active clotting factors can be synthesized in a variety of tissue types, permitting latitude in choice of target tissue. Moreover, raising circulating factor levels from <1% (levels seen in those severely affected) into the range of 5% greatly improves the phenotype of the disease. Preclinical studies with recombinant AAV vectors infused into skeletal muscle or liver have resulted in long-term (>5 years) expression of factor VIII or factor IX in the hemophilic dog model. Administration to skeletal muscle of an AAV vector expressing factor IX in patients with hemophilia was safe and resulted in long-term expression as measured by muscle biopsy, but circulating levels never rose >1% for sustained periods, and a large number of IM injections (>80–100) was required to access a large muscle mass. Intravascular vector delivery has been employed to access large areas of skeletal muscle in animal models of hemophilia and will likely be tested in upcoming trials. Administration of an AAV vector expressing factor IX to the liver in humans with hemophilia resulted in therapeutic circulating levels at the highest dose tested, but expression at these levels (>5%) lasted for only 6–10 weeks before declining to baseline (<1%). A memory T cell response to viral capsid, present in humans but not in other animal species (which are not natural hosts for the virus), may be a contributing factor in the loss of expression. Fortunately, triggering of the memory T cell response appears tissue-specific, and it is possible that introduction of the vector into immunoprivileged sites, such as the CNS (e.g., for Parkinson's disease) or the retina, will avoid this complication.

Leber's congenital amaurosis (LCA) is a form of retinal degenerative disease, characterized by severe early-onset blindness. This disease, not currently treatable, is caused by mutations in several different genes; ~15% of cases of LCA are due to a mutation in a gene, *RPE65*, encoding a retinal pigment epithelial protein. In dogs with a null mutation in *RPE65*, sight has been restored after subretinal injection of an AAV vector expressing *RPE65*. Transgene expression appears to be stable, with the first animals treated >5 years ago continuing to manifest electrophysiologic and behavioral evidence of visual function. As is the case for X-linked SCID, gene transfer must occur relatively early in life to achieve correction of the genetic disease, although the exact limitations imposed by age await clinical studies. AAV-RPE65 trials have now been approved in both the United States and Great Britain. Other inherited retinal degenerative disorders may also be amenable to correction by gene transfer, as are certain complex acquired disorders such as age-related macular degeneration, which affects several million people worldwide. The neovascularization that occurs in age-related macular degeneration can be inhibited by expression of vascular endothelial growth factor (VEGF) inhibitors such as angiostatin, or through the use of RNAi-mediated knockdown of VEGF. Early-phase trials of siRNAs that target VEGF RNA are underway, but these require repeated intravitreal injection of the siRNAs; an AAV vector–mediated approach might allow long-term knockdown of VEGF.

GENE THERAPY FOR CANCER

The majority of clinical gene transfer experience has been in subjects with cancer (Fig. 65-1). As a general rule, a feature that distinguishes gene therapies from conventional cancer therapeutics is that the former are less toxic, in some cases because they are delivered locally (e.g., intratumoral injections), and in other cases because they are targeted specifically to elements of the tumor (immunotherapies, antiangiogenic approaches).

Cancer gene therapies can be divided into local and systemic approaches (Table 65-2). Some of the earliest cancer gene therapy trials focused on local delivery of a prodrug or a suicide gene that would increase sensitivity of tumor cells to cytotoxic drugs. A frequently used strategy has been intratumoral injection of an adenoviral vector expressing the thymidine kinase (*TK*) gene. Cells that take up and express the *TK* gene can be killed after the administration of ganciclovir, which is phosphorylated to a toxic nucleoside by *TK*. Because cell division is required for the toxic nucleoside to affect cell viability, this strategy was initially used in aggressive brain tumors (glioblastoma multiforme) where the cycling tumor cells were affected but the nondividing normal neurons were not. More recently, this approach has been explored for locally recurrent prostate, breast, and colon tumors, among others.

Another local approach uses adenoviral-mediated expression of the tumor suppressor p53, which is mutated in a wide variety of cancers. This strategy has shown complete and partial responses in squamous cell carcinoma of the head and neck, esophageal cancer, and non-small cell lung cancer after direct intratumoral injection of the vector. Response rates (~15%) are comparable to those of other single agents. The use of oncolytic viruses that selectively replicate in tumor cells but not in normal cells has also shown promise in squamous cell carcinoma of the head and neck and in other solid tumors. This approach is based on the observation that deletion of certain viral genes abolishes their ability to replicate in normal cells but not in tumor cells. An advantage of this strategy is that the replicating vector can proliferate and spread within the tumor, facilitating eventual tumor clearance. However, physical limitations to viral spread, including fibrosis, intermixed normal cells, basement membranes, and necrotic areas within the tu-

TABLE 65-2 GENE THERAPY STRATEGIES IN CANCER

- Local/regional approaches
  - Suicide gene/prodrug
  - Suppressor oncogene
  - Oncolytic virus
- Systemic response
  - Chemoprotection
  - Immunomodulation
  - Anti-angiogenesis

mor, may reduce clinical efficacy. Oncolytic viruses are licensed and available in some countries, but not in the United States.

Because metastatic disease rather than uncontrolled growth of the primary tumor is the source of mortality for most cancers, there has been considerable interest in developing systemic gene therapy approaches. One strategy has been to promote more efficient recognition of tumor cells by the immune system. Approaches have included transduction of tumor cells with immune-enhancing genes encoding cytokines, chemokines, or co-stimulatory molecules. Sustained clinical responses provide evidence that the transduced cells can act as a vaccine. In a related approach, patient lymphocytes have been transduced with genes encoding a T cell receptor–like molecule, with a tumor antigen–binding domain fused to an intracellular signaling domain to allow T cell activation, thereby converting normal lymphocytes into cells capable of recognizing and destroying tumor cells. A third immunotherapy approach relies on ex vivo manipulation of dendritic cells to enhance the presentation of tumor antigens. These immunologic approaches may be of particular value in treating minimal residual disease after other anticancer modalities.

Gene transfer strategies have also been developed for inhibiting tumor angiogenesis. These have included constitutive expression of angiogenesis inhibitors such as angiostatin and endostatin; use of siRNA to reduce levels of VEGF or VEGF receptor; and combined approaches in which autologous T cells are genetically modified to recognize antigens specific to tumor vasculature. These studies are still in early-phase testing.

Another novel systemic approach is the use of gene transfer to protect normal cells from the toxicities of chemotherapy. The most extensively studied of these approaches has been transduction of hematopoietic cells with genes encoding resistance to chemotherapeutic agents, including the multidrug resistance gene *MDRI* or the gene encoding O^6-methylguanine DNA methyltransferase (*MGMT*). Ex vivo transduction of hematopoietic cells, followed by autologous transplantation, is being investigated as a strategy for allowing administration of higher doses of chemotherapy than would otherwise be tolerated.

GENE THERAPY FOR VASCULAR DISEASE

The third major category addressed by gene transfer studies is cardiovascular disease. The most extensive experience has been in trials designed to increase blood flow to either skeletal (critical limb ischemia) or cardiac muscle (angina/myocardial ischemia). Initial treatment options for both of these groups include mechanical revascularization or medical management, but a subset of patients are not candidates for, or fail, these approaches. These patients have formed the first cohorts for evaluation of gene transfer to achieve therapeutic angiogenesis. The major transgene used has been VEGF, attractive because of its specificity for endothelial cells; other transgenes have included fibroblast growth factor (FGF) and hypoxia-inducible factor 1, α subunit (HIF-1α). The design of most of the trials has included direct IM (or myocardial) injection of either a plasmid or an adenoviral vector expressing the transgene. Both of these vectors are likely to result in only short-term expression of VEGF. This strategy may be adequate, however, as there is no need for continued transgene expression once the new vessels have formed. Direct injection favors local expression, which should help to avoid systemic effects such as retinal neovascularization or new vessel formation in a nascent tumor. Initial trials of adeno-VEGF or plasmid-VEGF injection have resulted in improvement over baseline in terms of frequency of claudication/angina or amounts of nitroglycerin consumption. Study designs including placebo control groups and more objective endpoints (exercise duration at 3 or 6 months, rest and stress cardiac perfusion scans, and regional wall motion assessed by nonfluoroscopic electroanatomic mapping) continue to suggest a beneficial effect of gene transfer, although definitive conclusions will require larger studies. Continuing areas of investigation include choice of the optimal vector (adenoviral vs. plasmid), the optimal transgene (VEGF, HIF-1α, FGF, etc.), the optimal method of delivery in cardiac indications (intracoronary vs. direct myocardial), ideal objective endpoints, and whether concurrent administration of cytokines to mobilize endothelial progenitor cells will augment the therapeutic effect.

TABLE 65-3 TAKING HISTORY FROM SUBJECTS ENROLLED IN GENE TRANSFER STUDIES

Elements of History for Subjects Enrolled in Gene Transfer Trials

1. What vector was administered? Is it predominantly integrating [retroviral, lentiviral, herpesvirus (latency and reactivation)], or non-integrating (plasmid, adenoviral, AAV)?
2. What was the route of administration of the vector?
3. What was the target tissue?
4. What gene was transferred in? A disease-related gene? A marker?
5. Were there any adverse events noted after gene transfer?

Screening Questions for Long-Term Follow-Up in Gene Transfer Subjects[a]

1. Has a new malignancy been diagnosed?
2. Has a new neurologic/ophthalmologic disorder, or exacerbation of a pre-existing disorder, been diagnosed?
3. Has a new autoimmune or rheumatologic disorder been diagnosed?
4. Has a new hematologic disorder been diagnosed?

[a]Factors influencing long-term risk include: integration of the vector into the genome; vector persistence without integration; and transgene-specific effects.

OTHER DISEASES

The power and versatility of gene transfer approaches are such that there are few serious disease entities for which gene transfer therapies are *not* under development. Besides those already discussed, other areas of interest include gene therapies for HIV and for neurodegenerative disorders. The latter include studies in patients with Parkinson's disease, where AAV vectors expressing enzymes required for enhanced production of dopamine, or of the inhibitory neurotransmitter γ-aminobutyric acid, have been introduced into affected areas of the brain (striatum, subthalamic nucleus) by stereotactic neurosurgery. In Alzheimer's disease, an ex vivo approach in which autologous fibroblasts are transduced with a retroviral vector expressing nerve growth factor, then reimplanted into the basal forebrain, has slowed the rate of cognitive decline in a small Phase I study.

SUMMARY

The development of new classes of therapeutics typically takes two to three decades; monoclonal antibodies and recombinant proteins are recent examples. Gene therapeutics, which entered clinical testing in the early 1990s, are well along in the course of development, and are likely to become increasingly important as a therapeutic modality in the twenty-first century. A central question to be addressed is the long-term safety of gene transfer, and regulatory agencies have mandated a 15-year follow-up for subjects enrolled in gene therapy trials (Table 65-3). Realization of the therapeutic benefits of the Human Genome Project, and of new discoveries such as RNAi, will depend on continued progress in gene transfer technology.

ACKNOWLEDGMENT

I would like to thank Valder Arruda, MD, PhD, for his review of the manuscript.

FURTHER READINGS

HACEIN-BEY-ABINA S et al: LMO2-associated clonal T cell proliferation in two patients after gene therapy for SCID-XI. Science 302:415, 2003

LIN E, NEMUNAITIS J: Oncolytic viral therapies. Cancer Gene Ther 11:643, 2004

MANNO CS et al: Successful transduction of liver in hemophilia by AAV-Factor IX and limitations imposed by the host immune response. Nat Med 12:342, 2006

SADELAIN M et al: Targeting tumours with genetically enhanced T lymphocytes. Nat Rev Cancer 3:35, 2003

SHAH PB, LOSORDO DW: Non-viral vectors for gene therapy: Clinical trials in cardiovascular disease. Adv Genet 54:339, 2005

SKARLATOS SI: New programs for gene- and cell-based therapies at NHLBI. Clin Pharmacol Ther 82:334, 2007

Gene Therapy Clinical Trials Worldwide. J Gene Med, New Jersey, Wiley, 2006 *www.abedia.com/wiley/indications.php*

66 Stem Cell Biology

Minoru S. H. Ko

Stem cell biology is a relatively new field that explores the characteristics and possible clinical applications of the different types of pluripotential cells that serve as the progenitors of more differentiated cell types. In addition to potential therapeutic applications (Chap. 67), patient-derived stem cells can also provide disease models and a means to test drug effectiveness.

IDENTIFICATION, ISOLATION, AND DERIVATION OF STEM CELLS

Resident Stem Cells The definition of stem cells remains elusive. Stem cells were originally postulated as *unspecified* or *undifferentiated* cells that provide a source of renewal of skin, intestine, and blood cells throughout the lifespan. These *resident stem cells* are now identified in a variety of organs, i.e., epithelia of the skin and digestive system, bone marrow, blood vessels, brain, skeletal muscle, liver, testis, and pancreas, based on their specific locations, morphology, and biochemical markers.

Isolated Stem Cells Unequivocal identification of stem cells requires the separation and purification of cells, usually based on a combination of specific cell-surface markers. These *isolated stem cells*, e.g., hematopoietic stem (HS) cells, can be studied in detail and used in clinical applications, such as bone marrow transplantation (Chap. 68). However, the lack of specific cell-surface markers for other types of stem cells has made it difficult to isolate them in large quantities. This challenge has been partially addressed in animal models by genetically marking different cell types with green fluorescence protein driven by cell-specific promoters. Alternatively, putative stem cells have been isolated from a variety of tissues as side population (SP) cells using fluorescence-activated cell sorting after staining with Hoechst 33342 dye. However, the SP phenotype should be used with caution as it may not be function for stem cells.

Cultured Stem Cells It is desirable to culture and expand stem cells in vitro to obtain a sufficient quantity for analysis and potential therapeutic use. Although the derivation of stem cells in vitro has been a major obstacle in stem cell biology, the number and types of *cultured stem cells* have increased progressively (Table 66-1). The cultured stem cells derived from resident stem cells are often called *adult stem cells* to indicate their adult origins and to distinguish them from *embryonic stem* (ES) and *embryonic germ* (EG) *cells*. However, considering the presence of embryo-derived tissue-specific stem cells, e.g., trophoblast stem (TS) cells, and the possible derivation of similar cells from embryo/fetus, e.g., neural stem (NS) cells, it is more appropriate to use the term, *tissue stem cells*.

Successful derivation of cultured stem cells (both embryonic and tissue stem cells) often requires the identification of necessary growth factors and culture conditions, mimicking the microenvironment or *niche* of the resident stem cells. For example, the derivation of mouse TS cells, once considered impossible, became possible by using FGF4, a ligand known to be expressed by cells adjacent to the developing trophoblast in vivo. Therefore, it may be possible to culture other resident stem cells (e.g., intestinal stem cells) or isolated stem cells (e.g., HS cells) by studying the factors that constitute their normal niche.

SELF-RENEWAL AND PROLIFERATION OF STEM CELLS

Symmetric and Asymmetric Cell Division The most widely accepted stem cell definition is a cell with a unique capacity to produce unaltered daughter cells (*self-renewal*) and to generate specialized cell types (*potency*). Self-renewal can be achieved in two ways. *Asymmetric cell division* produces one daughter cell that is identical to the parental cell and one daughter cell that is different from the parental cell and is a progenitor or differentiated cell. Asymmetric cell division does not increase the number of stem cells. *Symmetric cell division* produces two identical daughter cells. For stem cells to proliferate in vitro, they must divide symmetrically. Self-renewal alone cannot define stem cells, because any established cell line, e.g., HeLa cells or NIH3T3 cells, proliferate by symmetric cell division.

Unlimited Expansion In Vitro Resident stem cells are often quiescent and divide infrequently. However, once the stem cells are successfully cultured in vitro, they often acquire the capacity to divide continuously and the ability to proliferate beyond the normal limit of passages typical of primary cultured cells (sometimes called *immortality*). These features are primarily seen in ES cells, but have also been demonstrated for NS cells, MS cells, MAPCs, maGSCs (adult-derived tissue stem cells), and USSCs (newborn-derived tissue stem cells), thereby enhancing the potential of these cells for therapeutic use (Table 66-1).

Stability of Genotype and Phenotype The capacity to actively proliferate is associated with the potential accumulation of chromosomal abnormalities and mutations. Mouse ES cells have been extensively used to produce gene-targeted animals and are known to maintain their euploid karyotype and genome integrity. In contrast, human ES cells appear to be more susceptible to mutations after long-term culture. Another limitation is the possible formation of tumors after transplanting actively dividing stem cells. Mouse ES cells can form teratomas when injected into immunosuppressed animals.

POTENCY AND DIFFERENTIATION OF STEM CELLS

Developmental Potency The term *potency* is used to indicate a cell's ability to differentiate into specialized cell types. The current lack of knowledge about the molecular nature of potency requires the experimental manipulation of stem cells to demonstrate their potency. For example, in vivo testing can be done by injecting stem cells into mouse blastocysts or immunosuppressed adult mice and determining how many different cell types are formed from the injected cells. In vitro testing can be done by differentiating cells in various culture conditions to determine how many different cell types are formed from the cells. The in vivo assays are not applicable to human stem cells. The formal demonstration of self-renewal and potency is performed by demonstrating that a single cell possesses such abilities in vitro (*clonality*). Cultured stem cells are tentatively grouped according to their potency (Fig. 66-1).

From Totipotency to Unipotency *Totipotent cells* can form an entire organism autonomously. Only a fertilized egg (zygote) possesses this feature. *Pluripotent cells* (e.g., ES cells) can form almost all the body's cell lineages (endoderm, mesoderm, and ectoderm), including germ cells. *Multipotent cells* (e.g., HS cells) can form multiple cell lineages but cannot form all of the body's cell lineages. *Oligopotent cells* (e.g., NS cells) can form more than one cell lineage but are more restricted than multipotent cells. Oligopotent cells are sometimes called *progenitor cells* or *precursor cells*; however, these terms are often more strictly used to define partially differentiated or lineage-committed cells (e.g., myeloid progenitor cells) that can divide into different cell types but lack self-renewing capacity. *Unipotent cells* or *monopotent cells*, e.g., spermatogonial stem (SS) cells, can form a single differentiated cell lineage. Terminally differentiated cells, such as fibroblast cells, also have a capacity to proliferate (which may be called self-renewal) but maintain the same cell type (e.g., no potency to form another cell type) and are not, therefore, considered unipotent cells.

Nuclear Reprogramming Development naturally progresses from totipotent fertilized eggs to pluripotent epiblast cells, to multipotent cells, and finally to terminally differentiated cells. According to Wad-

TABLE 66-1 TYPES OF CULTURED STEM CELLS

Name	Source, Derivation, Maintenance, and Properties
Embryonic stem cells (ES, ESC)	ES cells can be derived by culturing blastocysts or immuno-surgically isolated inner cell mass (ICM) from blastocysts on a feeder layer of MEFs with LIF (m) or without LIF (h). ES cells are to originate from the epiblast (m, h). ES cells grow as tightly adherent multicellular colonies with a population doubling time of ~12 h (m), maintain a stable euploid karyotype even after extensive culture and manipulation, can differentiate into a variety of cell types in vitro, and can contribute to all cell types, including functional sperm and oocytes, when injected into a blastocyst (m). ES cells form relatively flat, compact colonies with the population doubling time of 35–40 h (h).
Embryonic germ cells (EG, EGC)	EG cells can be derived by culturing primordial germ cells (PGCs) from embryos at E8.5–E12.5 on a feeder layer of MEFs with FGF2 and LIF (m). EG cells can be derived by culturing gonadal tissues from 5–11 week post-fertilization embryo/fetus on a feeder layer of MEFs with FGF2, forskolin, and LIF (h). EG cells show essentially the same pluripotency as ES cells when injected into mouse blastocysts (m). The only known difference is the imprinting status of some genes (e.g., Igf2r): Imprinting is normally erased during germline development, and thus, the imprinting status of in EG cells is different from that of ES cells.
Trophoblast stem cells (TS, TSC)	TS cells can be derived by culturing trophectoderm cells of E3.5 blastocysts, extraembryonic ectoderm of E6.5 embryos, and chorionic ectoderm of E7.5 embryos on a feeder layer of MEFs with FGF4 (m). TS cells can differentiate into trophoblast giant cells in vitro (m). TS can contribute exclusively to all trophoblast subtypes when injected into blastocysts (m).
Extraembryonic endoderm cells (XEN)	XEN cells can be derived by culturing the ICM in non-ES cell culture condition (m). XEN cells can contribute only to the parietal endoderm lineage when injected into a blastocyst (m).
Embryonic carcinoma cells (EC)	EC cells can be derived from teratocarcinoma—a type of cancer that most commonly develops in the testes. EC cells rarely show pluripotency in vitro, but they can contribute to all cell types when injected into blastocysts. EC cells often have an aneuploid karyotype and other genome alterations.
Mesenchymal stem cells (MS, MSC)	MS cells can be derived from bone marrow, muscle, adipose tissue, peripheral blood, and umbilical cord blood (m, h). MS cells can differentiate into mesenchymal cell types, including adipocytes, osteocytes, chondrocytes, and myocytes (m, h).
Multipotent adult stem cells (MAPC)	MAPCs can be derived by culturing bone marrow mononuclear cells, after depleting CD45$^+$ and GlyA$^+$ cells, with FCS, EGF, and PDGF-BB (h). MAPCs are very rare cells that are present within MSC cultures from postnatal bone marrow (m, h). MAPCs can also be isolated from postnatal muscle and brain (m). MAPCs can be cultured for >120 population doublings. MAPCs can differentiate into all tissues in vivo when injected into a mouse blastocyst, and can differentiate into various cell lineages of mesodermal, ectodermal, and endodermal origin in vitro (m).
Spermatogonial stem cells (SS, SSC)	SS cells can be derived by culturing newborn testis on STS-feeder cells with GDNF (m). SS cells can reconstitute long-term spermatogenesis after transplantation into recipient testes and restore fertility.
Germline stem cells (GS, GSC)	GS cells can be derived from neonatal testis (m). GS cells can differentiate into three germlayers in vitro and contribute to a variety of tissues, including germline, when injected into blastocysts.
Multipotent adult germline stem cells (maGSC)	maGSC can be derived from adult testis (m). maGSC can differentiate into three germlayers in vitro and can contribution to a variety of tissues, including germline, when injected into blastocysts.
Neural stem cells (NS, NSC)	NS cells can be derived from fetal and adult brain (subventricular zone, ventricular zone, and hippocampus) and cultured as a heterogeneous cell population of monolayer or floating cell clusters called *neurospheres*. NS cells can differentiate into neuron and glia in vivo and in vitro. Recently, the culture of pure population of symmetrically dividing adherent NS cells became possible in the presence of FGF2 and EGF.
Unrestricted somatic stem cells (USSC)	USSCs are rare cells derived from newborn cord blood (h). USSCs can be derived by culturing the mononuclear fraction of cord blood in the presence of 30% FCS and 10^{-7} *M* dexamethasone. USSCs can differentiate into a variety of cell types in vitro and can contribute a variety of cells types in in vivo transplantation experiments in rat, mouse, and sheep (h). USSCs are CD45$^-$ adherent cells and can be expanded to 10^{15} cells without losing pluripotency (h).

Note: m, mouse; h, human; FGF, fibroblast growth factor; FCS, fetal calf serum; EGF, epidermal growth factor; PDGF, platelet-derived growth factor; GDNF, glial cell line–derived neurotrophic factor; LIF, leukemia inhibitory factor; MEF, mouse embryonic fibroblast.

dington's epigenetic landscape, this is analogous to a ball moving down a slope. The reversal of the terminally differentiated cells to totipotent or pluripotent cells (called *nuclear reprogramming*) can thus be seen as an uphill gradient that never occurs in normal conditions. However, nuclear reprogramming has been achieved using *nuclear transplantation*, or *nuclear transfer* (NT), procedures (often called "cloning"), where the nucleus of a differentiated cell is transferred into an enucleated oocyte. Although this is an error-prone procedure and the success rate is very low, live animals have been produced using adult somatic cells as donors in sheep, mouse, and other mammals. In mice, it has been demonstrated that ES cells derived from blastocysts made by somatic cell NT are indistinguishable from normal ES cells. NT can potentially be used to produce *patient-specific ES cells* carrying a genome identical to that of the patient. However, the successful implementation of this procedure has not been reported in humans. Setting aside technical and ethical issues, the limited supply of human oocytes will be a major problem for clinical applications of NT. Alternatively, successful nuclear reprogramming of somatic cells by fusing them with ES cells has been demonstrated in mouse and human. However, it is not yet clear how ES-derived DNA can be removed from hybrid cells. More direct nuclear reprogramming of somatic cells by transfecting specific genes or by exposing the cells to ES cell extracts is the subject of current research.

Stem Cell Plasticity or Transdifferentiation The prevailing paradigm in developmental biology is that once cells are differentiated, their phenotypes are stable. However, a number of reports have shown that tissue stem cells, which are thought to be lineage-committed multipotent cells, possess the capacity to differentiate into cell types outside their lineage restrictions (called *transdifferentiation*). For example, HS cells may be converted into neurons as well as germ cells. This feature may provide a means to use tissue stem cells derived directly from a patient for therapeutic purposes, thereby eliminating the need to use embryonic stem cells or elaborate procedures such as nuclear reprogramming a patient's somatic cells. However, more strict criteria and rigorous validation are required to establish tissue stem cell plasticity. For example, observations of transdifferentiation may reflect cell fusion, contamination with progenitor cells from other cell lineages, or persistence of pluripotent embryonic cells in adult organs. Therefore, the assignment of potency to each cultured stem cell in Fig. 66-1 should be taken with caution. Whether transdifferentiation exists and can be used for therapeutic purposes remains to be determined conclusively.

Directed Differentiation of Stem Cells Pluripotent stem cells (e.g., ES cells) can differentiate into multiple cell types, but in culture they normally differentiate into heterogeneous cell populations in a stochastic manner. However, for therapeutic uses, it is desirable to direct stem cells into specific cell types (e.g., insulin-secreting beta cells). This is an active area of stem cell research, and protocols are being developed to achieve this goal. In any of these directed cell differentiation systems, the cell phenotype must be evaluated critically. Interestingly, it has been reported that mouse ES cells can differentiate in vitro into oocytes as well as sperm, which are capable of fertilizing an oocyte to produce live offspring.

Stage / Potency	Preimplantation	Embryonic, fetal	Postnatal	Adult
Totipotent	Zygote^{m,h}			
Pluripotent	ES^{m,h}	EG^{m,h}	GS^{m} USSC^{h} MAPC^{m,h}	EC^{m,h} maGSC^{m} MAPC^{m,h}
Multipotent				MS^{m,h}
Oligopotent	TS^{m}			NS^{m,h}
Unipotent	XEN^{m}			SSC^{m}
Terminally differentiated cells				

FIGURE 66-1 Potency and source developmental stage of cultured stem cells. For abbreviations of stem cells, see Table 66-1. Note that stem cells are often abbreviated with or without "cells," e.g., ES cells or ESCs for embryonic stem cells. m, mouse; h, human.

MOLECULAR CHARACTERIZATION OF STEM CELLS

Genomics and Proteomics In addition to standard molecular biological approaches, genomics and proteomics have been extensively applied to the analysis of stem cells. For example, DNA microarray analyses have revealed the expression levels of essentially all genes and identified specific markers for some stem cells. Similarly, the protein profiles of stem cells have been assessed by using mass spectrophotometry. These methodologies are beginning to provide a novel means to characterize and classify various stem cells and the molecular mechanisms that give them their unique characteristics.

Stemness This term has been used to designate the essential molecular characteristics of stem cells. It is also used to indicate common genetic programs shared among ES cells and tissue stem cells (HS and NS cells). A number of common genes, such as stress-response genes, have been identified, but the lack of commonality among different studies raises concerns about the validity of this concept.

Pivotal Genes Involved in ES Cell Regulation Recent work has begun to identify genes involved in the regulation of stem cell function. For example, three genes—*Pou5f1* (Oct3/4), *Nanog,* and *Sox2*—govern key gene regulatory pathways/networks for the maintenance of self-renewal and pluripotency of mouse and human ES cells. Similarly, it has been shown that the interaction and balance among three transcription factors—*Pou5f1, Cdx2,* and *Gata6*—determine the fate of mouse ES cells: upregulation of *Cdx2* differentiates ES cells into trophoblast cells, whereas upregulation of *Gata6* differentiates ES cells into primitive endoderm. These types of analyses should provide molecular clues about the function of stem cells and lead to a more effective means to manipulate stem cells for future therapeutic use.

FURTHER READINGS

CERVERA RP, STOJKOVIC M: Human embryonic stem cell derivation and nuclear transfer: Impact on regenerative therapeutics and drug discovery. Clin Pharmacol Ther 82(3):310, 2007

DEPARTMENT OF HEALTH AND HUMAN SERVICES: Regenerative Medicine 2006. August 2006. *http://stemcells.nih.gov/info/scireport*

KO MSH, MCLAREN A: Epigenetics of germ cells, stem cells, and early embryos. Dev Cell 10:161, 2006

LANZA R et al (eds): *Handbook of Stem Cells,* vols 1 and 2. London, Elsevier Academic Press, 2004

MARSHAK DR et al (eds): *Stem Cell Biology,* New York, Cold Spring Harbor Laboratory Press, 2001

ODORICO J et al (eds): *Human Embryonic Stem Cells.* New York, BIOS Scientific Publishers, 2005

67 Applications of Stem Cell Biology in Clinical Medicine

John A. Kessler

Organ damage and the resultant inflammatory responses initiate a series of repair processes, including stem cell proliferation, migration, and differentiation, often in combination with angiogenesis and remodeling of the extracellular matrix. Endogenous stem cells in tissues such as liver and skin have a remarkable ability to regenerate the organs, whereas heart and brain have a much more limited capability for self-repair. Under rare circumstances, circulating stem cells may contribute to regenerative responses by migrating into a tissue and differentiating into organ-specific cell types. The goal of stem cell therapies is to promote cell replacement in organs that are damaged beyond their ability for self-repair.

SOURCES OF STEM CELLS FOR TISSUE REPAIR

Different types of stem cells include embryonic stem (ES) cells, umbilical cord blood stem cells, organ-specific somatic stem cells (e.g., neural stem cells for treatment of the brain), and somatic stem cells capable of generating cell types specific for the target rather than the donor organ (e.g., bone marrow mesenchymal stem cells for cardiac repair) (Chap. 66). ES cells self-renew endlessly so that a single cell line with carefully characterized traits can generate large numbers of cells that can be immunologically matched with potential transplant recipients. However, little is currently known about the mechanisms that govern differentiation of these cells or processes that limit their unbridled proliferation. Human ES cells are difficult to culture and grow slowly. ES cells tend to develop abnormal karyotypes and have the potential to form teratomas if they are not committed to the desired cell types before transplantation. The study of human ES cells has been controversial, and their use in clinical applications would be unacceptable to some patients and physicians despite their enormous potential. Somatic cell nuclear transfer ("therapeutic cloning") represents an alternative method for creating ES cell lines that are genetically identical to the patient. It may also be possible to derive pluripotent stem cells from spermatogonia in the adult human testis, providing another strategy for obtaining genetically identical stem cells.

Umbilical cord blood stem/progenitor cells are associated with less graft-versus-host disease compared to marrow stem cells. They have less HLA restriction than adult marrow stem cells, and they are less likely to be contaminated with herpesvirus. However, it is unclear how many different cell types these cells can generate, and methods for differentiating them into nonhematopoietic phenotypes are largely lacking. The quantity of cells from any single source can also be limiting.

Organ-specific multipotent stem cells are already somewhat specialized and may be easier to induce into desired cell types. These cells could potentially be obtained from the patient and amplified in culture, thereby circumventing the problems associated with immune rejection. Multipotent stem cells are relatively easy to harvest from bone marrow (Chap. 68) but are more difficult to isolate from other tissues, such as heart and brain. Substantial efforts have therefore been devoted to obtaining more pluripotent stem cell populations, such as bone marrow mesenchymal stem cells (MSCs) or adipose stem cells, for use in regenerative strategies. Tissue culture evidence suggests that these stem cell populations are able to generate a variety of cell types, including myocytes, chondrocytes, tendon cells, osteoblasts, cardiomyocytes, adipocytes, hepatocytes, and neurons, through a process known as transdifferentiation. However, it is unclear how effectively these differentiated cells integrate into organs, survive, and function after transplantation in vivo. Early studies of bone marrow–derived stem cells transplanted into heart, liver, and other organs suggested that the cells had differentiated into organ-specific cell types. Subsequent studies, however, revealed that the stem cells had fused with cells resident in the organs. Further studies will be necessary to determine whether transdifferentiation of MSCs or other stem cell populations occurs at a high enough frequency to be useful for stem cell replacement therapy.

Regardless of the source of the stem cells used in regenerative strategies, a number of generic problems must be overcome for the development of successful clinical applications. These include development of methods for reliably generating large numbers of specific cell types, minimizing the risk of tumor formation or proliferation of inappropriate cell types, ensuring the viability and function of the engrafted cells, overcoming immune rejection when autografts are not used, and facilitating revascularization of the regenerated tissue. Each organ system will also pose tissue-specific problems for stem cell therapies.

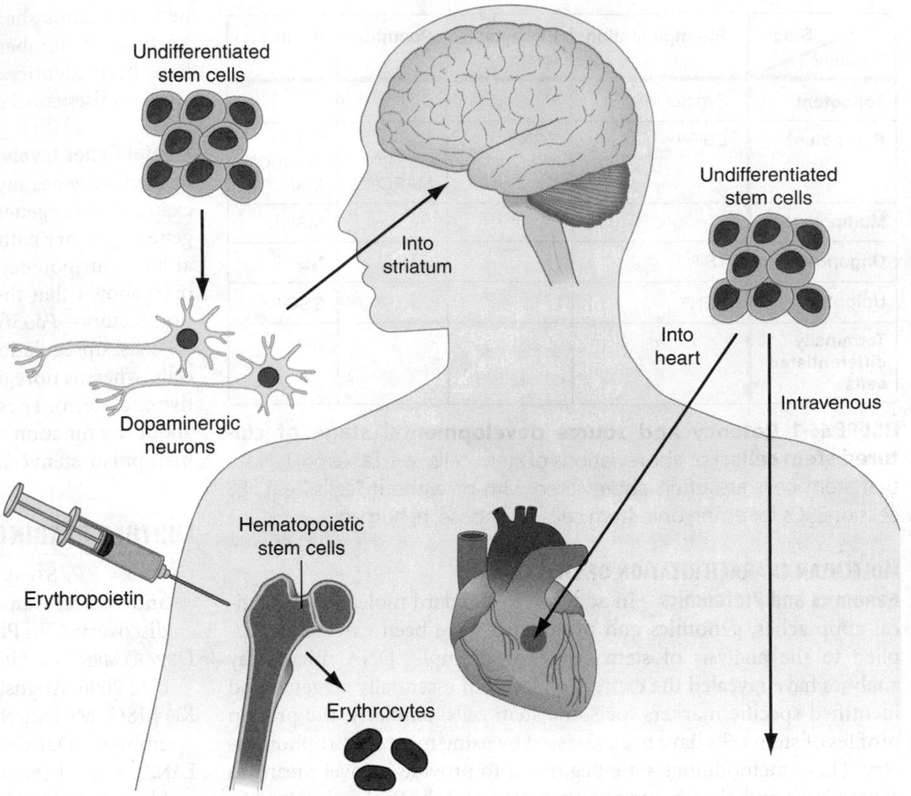

FIGURE 67-1 Strategies for transplantation of stem cells. 1. Undifferentiated or partially differentiated stem cells may be injected directly in the target organ or intravenously. 2. Stem cells may be differentiated ex vivo prior to injection into the target organ. 3. Growth factors or other drugs may be injected to stimulate endogenous stem cell populations.

STRATEGIES FOR STEM CELL REPLACEMENT

Stem cell transplantation is not a new concept and it is already part of established medical practice. Hematopoietic stem cells (HSCs) (Chap. 68) are responsible for the long-term repopulation of all blood elements in bone marrow transplant recipients. HSC transplantation is now the gold standard against which other stem cell transplantation therapies will be measured. Transplantation of differentiated cells is also a clinical reality, as donated organs (e.g., liver, kidney) and tissues (i.e., cornea, eye, skin) are often used to replace damaged tissues. However, the clinical need for transplantable tissues and organs far outweighs the available supply, and organ transplantation has limited potential for some tissues such as the brain. Stem cells offer the possibility of a renewable source of cell replacement for virtually all organs.

At least three different therapeutic concepts for cell replacement have been considered (Fig. 67-1): (1) injection of stem cells directly into the damaged organ or into the circulation, allowing them to "home" into the damaged tissue; (2) in vitro differentiation of stem cells followed by transplantation into a damaged organ—e.g., pancreatic islet cells could be generated from stem cells prior to transplantation into patients with diabetes, whereas cardiomyocytes could be generated to treat ischemic heart disease; and (3) stimulation of endogenous stem cells to facilitate repair—e.g., administration of appropriate growth factors to amplify numbers of endogenous stem/progenitor cells or direct them to differentiate into the desired cell types. In addition to these strategies for cell replacement, the ex vivo or in situ generation of tissues provides an alternative means of tissue engineering (Chap. 69). Stem cells are also excellent vehicles for cellular gene therapy (Chap. 65).

DISEASE-SPECIFIC STEM CELL APPROACHES

ISCHEMIC HEART DISEASE AND CARDIOMYOCYTE REGENERATION

Because of the high prevalence of ischemic heart disease, extensive efforts have been devoted to cell replacement of cardiomyocytes. Historically, the adult heart has been viewed as a terminally differentiated organ without the capacity for regeneration. However, the heart has the ability to achieve low levels of cardiomyocyte regeneration as well as revascularization. This regeneration is likely accomplished by cardiac stem cells resident in the heart, and possibly by cells originating in the bone marrow. If such cells could be characterized, isolated, and amplified ex vivo, they might provide an ideal source of stem cells for therapeutic use. For effective myocardial repair, cells must be delivered either systemically or locally, and the cells must survive, engraft, and differentiate into functional cardiomyocytes that couple mechanically and electrically with the recipient myocardium. The optimal method for cell delivery is not yet clear, and various experimental studies have employed intramyocardial, transendocardial, intravenous, and intracoronary injections. In experimental myocardial infarction, functional improvements have been achieved after transplantation of a variety of different cell types, including ES cells, bone marrow stem cells, endothelial stem cells, and adipose stem cells. Bone marrow stem cells in particular have been examined in clinical trials of human ischemic heart disease. These have largely been small, nonrandomized studies that typically combine cell treatment with conventional therapies. Although the fate of the cells and mechanisms by which they altered cardiac function are open questions, these studies have shown small but measurable improvement in cardiac function and, in some cases, reduction in infarct size. The preponderance of evidence suggests that the functional benefits are not derived from direct generation of cardiomyocytes but rather from indirect effects of the stem cells on resident cells. This may reflect the release of soluble growth factors, induction of angiogenesis, or some other mechanism.

DIABETES MELLITUS

The success of islet cell and pancreas transplantation provides proof of concept for a cell-based approach for type I diabetes. However, the demand for donor pancreata far exceeds the number available, and maintenance of long-term graft survival remains a problem. The search for a renewable source of stem cells capable of regenerating pancreatic islets has therefore been intensive.

Pancreatic β cell turnover occurs in the normal pancreas, although the source of the new β cells is controversial. Attempts to promote endogenous regenerative processes have not yet been successful, but this remains a potentially viable approach. A number of different cell types are candidates for use in stem cell replacement, including ES cells, hepatic progenitor cells, pancreatic ductal progenitor cells, and bone marrow stem cells. Successful therapy will depend on developing a source of cells that can be amplified and have the ability to synthesize, store, and release insulin when it is required, primarily in response to changes in the glucose level. The proliferative capacity of the replacement cells must be tightly regulated to avoid excessive expansion of β cell numbers with the consequent development of hyperinsulinemia/hypoglycemia, and the cells must avoid immune rejection. Although ES cells can be differentiated into cells that produce insulin, these cells have relatively low insulin content and a high rate of apoptosis, and they generally lack the capacity to normalize blood glucose in diabetic animals. Thus, ES cells have not yet been useful for the large-scale production of differentiated islet cells.

During embryogenesis, the pancreas, liver, and gastrointestinal tract are all derived from the anterior endoderm, and transdifferentiation of the pancreas to liver and vice versa has been observed in certain pathologic conditions. Multipotential stem cells also reside within gastric glands and intestinal crypts. Thus, hepatic, pancreatic, and/or gastrointestinal precursor cells may be candidates for cell-based therapy of diabetes.

NERVOUS SYSTEM

Neural cells have been differentiated from a variety of stem cell populations. Human ES cells can be induced to generate neural stem cells, and these cells can give rise to neurons, oligodendroglia, and astrocytes. These neural stem cells have been transplanted into the rodent brain with formation of appropriate cell types and no tumor formation. Multipotent stem cells present in the adult brain can also generate all of the major neural cell types, but highly invasive procedures would be necessary to obtain autologous cells. Fetal neural stem cells derived from miscarriages or abortuses are an alternative, and a clinical trial of fetal neural stem cells in Batten disease is commencing. Transdifferentiation of bone marrow and adipose stem cells into neural stem cells, and vice versa, has been reported, and clinical trials of such cells have begun for a number of neurologic disorders. Clinical trials of a conditionally immortalized human cell line and of human umbilical cord blood cells in stroke are also planned. Neurologic disorders that have already been targeted for stem cell therapies include spinal cord injury, amyotrophic lateral sclerosis, stroke, traumatic brain injury, Batten disease, and Parkinson's disease. In Parkinson's disease, the major motor features result from the loss of a single cell population, dopaminergic neurons within the substantia nigra pars compacta. Two clinical trials of fetal nigral transplantation failed to meet their primary endpoint and were complicated by the development of dyskinesia. Transplantation of stem cell–derived dopamine-producing cells offers a number of potential advantages over fetal transplants, including the ability of stem cells to migrate and disperse within tissue, the potential for engineering regulatable release of dopamine, and the ability to engineer cells to produce factors that will enhance cell survival. Nevertheless, the experience with fetal transplants points out the difficulties that may be encountered.

At least some of the neurologic dysfunction after spinal cord injury reflects demyelination, and both ES cells and marrow-derived stem cells are able to facilitate remyelination after experimental spinal cord injury. Clinical trials of marrow-derived stem cells have already begun, and this may be the first disease targeted for the clinical use of ES cells. Marrow-derived stem cells are also being used in the treatment of stroke, traumatic brain injury, and amyotrophic lateral sclerosis (ALS), where possible benefits are more likely to be indirect trophic effects or remyelination rather than neuron replacement. At present, no population of transplanted stem cells has been shown to generate neurons that extend axons over long distances to form synaptic connections (such as would be necessary for replacement of upper motor neurons in ALS, stroke, or other disorders).

LIVER

Transplantation is currently the only successful treatment for end-stage liver diseases, but this approach is limited by the shortage of liver grafts. Clinical trials of hepatocyte transplantation demonstrate that it can potentially substitute for organ transplantation, but the paucity of available cells also limits this strategy. Potential sources of stem cells include endogenous liver stem cells (such as oval cells), ES cells, bone marrow cells, and umbilical cord blood cells. Although a series of studies in humans as well as animals suggested that transplanted bone marrow stem cells can generate hepatocytes, this phenomenon largely reflects the fusion of the transplanted cells with endogenous liver cells, giving the erroneous appearance of new hepatocytes. ES cells have been differentiated into hepatocytes and transplanted in animal models of liver failure without formation of teratomas.

OTHER ORGAN SYSTEMS AND THE FUTURE

The use of stem cells in regenerative medicine has been studied for many other organ systems and cell types, including skin, eye, cartilage, bone, kidney, lung, endometrium, vascular endothelium, smooth muscle, striated muscle, and others. In fact, the potential for stem cell regeneration of damaged organs and tissues is virtually limitless. However, numerous obstacles must be overcome before stem cell therapies can become a widespread clinical reality. Only HSCs have been adequately characterized by surface markers to allow unambiguous identification, a prerequisite for reliable clinical applications. The pathways for differentiating stem cells into specific cellular phenotypes are still unknown, the migration of transplanted cells is uncontrolled, and the response of the cells to the environment of diseased organs is unpredictable. Future strategies may employ the coadministration of scaffolding, artificial extracellular matrix, and/or growth factors to orchestrate differentiation of stem cells and their organization into appropriate constituents of the organ. Imaging techniques are needed to visualize stem cells in vivo after transplantation into humans. Fortunately, stem cells can be engineered before transplantation to contain contrast agents that may make this feasible. The potential for tumor formation and the problems associated with immune rejection are significant impediments. Many strategies for cell replacement already include vasoactive endothelial growth factor (VEGF) coadministration to foster vascularization, which is required for survival and function of the transplant. Some stem cells have been engineered to have an inducible suicide gene so that the cells can be eradicated in the event of tumor formation or some other complication. The potential for stem cell therapies to revolutionize medical care is extraordinary, and disorders such as myocardial infarction, diabetes, Parkinson's disease and many others are attractive targets. However, such stem cell–based therapies are at a very early stage of development, and perfection of techniques for clinical transplantation of predictable, well-characterized cells will be a difficult and lengthy undertaking.

ETHICAL ISSUES

Stem cell therapies raise contentious ethical issues that must be addressed in parallel with the scientific and medical opportunities. Our society has great diversity in religious beliefs, concepts of individual rights, tolerance for uncertainty and risk, and boundaries for how scientific interventions should be used to alter the outcome of disease. In the United States, the federal government has authorized research using human ES lines in existence before August 2001 but has restricted the use of federal funds for developing new human ES lines. However, these existing lines develop abnormalities with time in culture and are contaminated with mouse proteins. These findings have sparked renewed debate about the need to develop new human ES cell lines.

In considering ethical issues associated with the use of stem cells, it is helpful to draw from experience with other scientific advances, such as organ transplantation, recombinant DNA technology, implantation of mechanical devices, neuroscience and cognitive research, in vitro fertilization, and prenatal genetic testing. From these and other precedents, we learn the importance of understanding and testing fundamental biology in the laboratory setting and in animal models before applying new techniques in carefully controlled clinical trials. When these trials occur, they must include full informed consent and have careful oversight by external review groups.

Ultimately, medical interventions will be scientifically feasible but ethically or socially unacceptable to some members of a society. Stem cell research raises questions about the definition of human life, and it has raised deep fears about our ability to balance issues of justice and safety with the needs of critically ill patients. Health care providers and experts with backgrounds in ethics, law, and sociology must help guard against the premature or inappropriate application stem cell therapies, and the inappropriate use of vulnerable population groups. On the other hand, these therapies offer important new strategies for the treatment of otherwise irreversible disorders. An open dialogue between the scientific community, physicians, patients, and their advocates, lawmakers, and the lay population is important to raise and address ethical issues and to balance the benefits and risks associated with stem cell transfer.

ACKNOWLEDGMENTS

The author acknowledges the contributions of David Bodine, J. Larry Jameson, and Ron McKay to this chapter in the 16th edition.

FURTHER READINGS

COMMITTEE ON THE BIOLOGICAL AND BIOMEDICAL APPLICATIONS OF STEM CELL RESEARCH et al: Stem Cells and the Future of Regenerative Medicine. Washington, D.C., National Academies Press, 2002

HOLLAND S et al: The Human Embryonic Stem Cell Debate: Science, Ethics and Public Policy. Cambridge, MA, MIT Press, 2001

LANZA R et al (eds): Essentials of Stem Cell Biology. San Diego, Elsevier Academic Press, 2006

MIMEAULT M et al: Stem cells: A revolution in therapeutics-recent advances in stem cell biology and their therapeutic applications in regenerative medicine and cancer therapies. Clin Pharmacol Ther 82(3):252, 2007

NATIONAL INSTITUTES OF HEALTH: Stem cell information page. URL: *http://stemcells.nih.gov/index.asp.*

PUCEAT M, BALLIS A: Embryonic stem cells: From bench to bedside. Clin Pharmacol Ther 82(3):337, 2007

SUGARMAN J: Ethics and stem cell therapeutics for cardiovascular disease. Prog Cardiovasc Dis 50(1):1, 2007

VATS A et al: Stem cells. Lancet 366:592, 2005

68 Hematopoietic Stem Cells

David T. Scadden, Dan L. Longo

All of the cell types in the peripheral blood and some cells in every tissue of the body are derived from hematopoietic (*hemo*: blood; *poiesis*: creation) stem cells. If the hematopoietic stem cell is damaged and can no longer function (e.g., due to the nuclear accident at Chernobyl), a person would survive 2–4 weeks in the absence of extraordinary support measures. With the clinical use of hematopoietic stem cells, tens of thousands of lives are saved each year (Chap. 108). Stem cells produce tens of billions of blood cells daily from a stem cell pool that is estimated to be only in the hundreds of thousands. How stem cells do this, how they persist for many decades despite the production demands, and how they may be better used in clinical care are important issues in medicine.

The study of blood cell production has become a paradigm for how other tissues may be organized and regulated. Basic research in hematopoiesis that includes defining stepwise molecular changes accompanying functional changes in maturing cells, aggregating cells into functional subgroups, and demonstrating hematopoietic stem cell regulation by a specialized microenvironment are concepts worked out in hematology, but they offer models for other tissues. Moreover, these concepts may not be restricted to normal tissue function but extend to malignancy. Stem cells are rare cells among a heterogeneous population of cell types, and their behavior is assessed mainly in experimental animal models involving reconstitution of hematopoiesis. Thus, much of what we know about stem cells is imprecise and based on inferences from genetically manipulated animals.

CARDINAL FUNCTIONS OF HEMATOPOIETIC STEM CELLS

All stem cell types have two cardinal functions: self-renewal and differentiation (Fig. 68-1). Stem cells exist to generate, maintain, and repair tissues. They function successfully if they can replace a wide variety of shorter-lived mature cells over prolonged periods. The process of self-renewal (see below) assures that a stem cell population can be sustained over time. Without self-renewal, the stem cell pool could exhaust over time and tissue maintenance would not be possible. The process of differentiation provides the effectors of tissue function: mature cells. Without proper differentiation, the integrity of tissue function would be compromised and organ failure would ensue.

In the blood, mature cells have variable average life spans, ranging from 7 h for mature neutrophils to a few months for red blood cells to many years for memory lymphocytes. However, the stem cell pool is the central, durable source of all blood and immune cells, maintaining a capacity to produce a broad range of cells from a single cell source and yet keeping itself vigorous over decades of life. As an individual stem cell divides, it has the capacity to accomplish one of three division outcomes: two stem cells, two cells destined for differentiation, or one stem cell and one differentiating cell. The former two outcomes are the result of symmetric cell division, whereas the latter indicates a different outcome for the two daughter cells—an event termed *asymmetric cell division.* The relative balance for these types of outcomes may change during development and under particular kinds of demands on the stem cell pool.

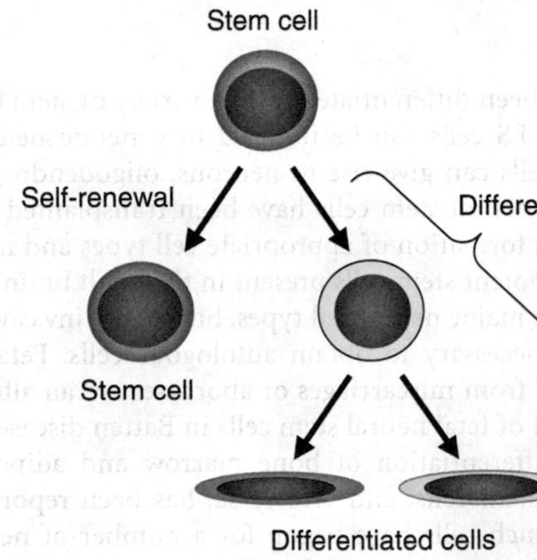

FIGURE 68-1 Signature characteristics of the stem cell. Stem cells have two essential features: the capacity to differentiate into a variety of mature cell types and the capacity for self-renewal. Intrinsic factors associated with self-renewal include expression of Bmi-1, Gfi-1, PTEN, STAT5, Tel/Atv6, p21, p18, MCL-1, Mel-18, RAE28, and HoxB4. Extrinsic signals for self-renewal include Notch, Wnt, SHH, and Tie2/Ang-1. Based mainly on murine studies, hematopoietic stem cells express the following cell surface molecules: CD34, Thy-1 (CD90), c-Kit receptor (CD117), CD133, CD164, and c-Mpl (CD110, also known as the thrombopoietin receptor).

DEVELOPMENTAL BIOLOGY OF HEMATOPOIETIC STEM CELLS

During development, blood cells are produced at different sites. Initially, the yolk sac provides oxygen-carrying red blood cells, and then several sites of intraembryonic blood cell production become involved. These intraembryonic sites engage in sequential order, moving from the genital ridge at a site where the aorta, gonadal tissue, and mesonephros are emerging to the fetal liver and then, in the second trimester, to the bone marrow and spleen. As the location of stem cells changes, the relative abundance of cells they produce also changes, progressively increasing in the complexity of cell types from those simply carrying oxygen to platelets supporting a more complex vasculature to the cells of innate immunity and finally to the cells of adaptive immunity. Stem cell proliferation remains high, even in the bone marrow, until shortly after birth, when it appears to dramatically decline. The cells in the bone marrow are thought to arrive by the bloodborne transit of cells from the fetal liver after calcification of the long bones has begun. The presence of stem cells in the circulation is not unique to a time window in development. Rather, hematopoietic stem cells appear to circulate throughout life. The time that cells spend freely circulating appears to be brief (measured in minutes in the mouse), but the cells that do circulate are functional and can be used for transplantation. The number of stem cells that circulate can be increased in a number of ways to facilitate harvest and transfer to the same or a different host.

MOBILITY OF HEMATOPOIETIC STEM CELLS

Cells entering and exiting the bone marrow do so through a series of molecular interactions. Circulating stem cells (through CD162 and CD44) engage the lectins P- and E-selectin on the endothelial surface to slow the movement of the cells to a rolling phenotype. Stem cell integrins are then activated and accomplish firm adhesion between the stem cell and vessel wall, with a particularly important role for stem cell VCAM-1 engaging endothelial VLA-4. The chemokine CXCL12 (SDF1) interacting with stem cell CXCR4 receptors also appears to be important in the process of stem cells getting from the circulation to where they engraft in the bone marrow. This is particularly true in the developmental move from fetal liver to bone marrow; however, the role for this molecule in adults appears to be more related to retention of stem cells in the bone marrow rather the process of getting them there. Interrupting that retention process through either specific molecular blockers of the CXCR4/CXCL12 interaction, cleavage of CXCL12, or downregulation of the receptor can all result in the release of stem cells into the circulation. This process is an increasingly important aspect of recovering stem cells for therapeutic use as it has permitted the harvesting process to be done by leukapheresis rather than bone marrow punctures in the operating room. Refining our knowledge of how stem cells get into and out of the bone marrow may improve our ability to obtain stem cells and make them more efficient at finding their way to the specific sites for blood cell production, the so-called stem cell niche.

HEMATOPOIETIC STEM CELL MICROENVIRONMENT

The concept of a specialized microenvironment, or stem cell niche, was first proposed to explain why cells derived from the bone marrow of one animal could be used in transplantation and again be found in the bone marrow of the recipient. This niche is more than just a housing site for stem cells, however. It is an anatomic location where regulatory signals are provided that allow the stem cells to thrive, to expand if needed, and to provide varying amounts of descendant daughter cells. In addition, unregulated growth of stem cells may be problematic based on their undifferentiated state and self-renewal capacity. Thus, the niche must also regulate the number of stem cells produced. In this manner, the niche has the dual functions of serving as a site of nurture but imposing limits for stem cells: in effect, acting as both a nest and a cage.

The niche for blood stem cells changes with each of the sites of blood production during development, but for most of human life it is located in the bone marrow. Within the bone marrow, at least two niche sites have been proposed: on trabecular bone surfaces and in the perivascular space. Stem cells may be found in both places by histologic analysis, and functional regulation has been shown at the bone surface. Specifically, bone-forming mesenchymal cells, osteoblasts, participate in hematopoietic stem cell function, affecting their location, proliferation, and number. The basis for this interaction is through a number of molecules mediating location, such as the chemokine CXCL12 (SDF1) and N-cadherin, through proliferation signals mediated by angiopoietin 1, and signaling to modulate self-renewal or survival by factors such as Notch ligands, kit ligand, and Wnts. Other bone components, such as the extracellular matrix glycoprotein, osteopontin, and the high ionic calcium found at trabecular surfaces, contribute to the unique microenvironment, or stem cell niche, on trabecular bone. This physiology has practical applications. First, medications altering niche components may have an effect on stem cell function. This has now been shown for a number of compounds, and some are being clinically tested. Second, it is now possible to assess whether the niche participates in disease states and to examine whether targeting the niche with medications may alter the outcome of certain diseases.

EXCESS CAPACITY OF HEMATOPOIETIC STEM CELLS

In the absence of disease, one never runs out of hematopoietic stem cells. Indeed, serial transplantation studies in mice suggest that sufficient stem cells are present to reconstitute several animals in succession, with each animal having normal blood cell production. The fact that allogeneic stem cell transplant recipients also never run out of blood cells in their life span, which can extend for decades, argues that even the limiting numbers of stem cells provided to them are sufficient. How stem cells respond to different conditions to increase or decrease their mature cell production remains poorly understood. Clearly, negative feedback mechanisms affect the level of production of most of the cells, leading to the normal tightly regulated blood cell counts. However, many of the regulatory mechanisms that govern production of more mature progenitor cells do not apply or apply differently to stem cells. Similarly, most of the molecules shown to be able to change the size of the stem cell pool have little effect on more mature blood cells. For example, the growth factor erythropoietin, which stimulates red blood cell production from more mature precursor cells, has no effect on stem cells. Similarly, granulocyte colony-stimulating factor drives the rapid proliferation of granulocyte precursors but does not affect cell cycling of stem cells. Rather, it changes the location of stem cells by indirect means, altering molecules such as CXCL12 that tether stem cells to their niche. Molecules shown to be important for altering the proliferation of stem cells, such as the cyclin-dependent kinase inhibitor p21Cip1, have little or no effect on progenitor proliferation. Hematopoietic stem cells have governing mechanisms that are distinct from the cells they generate.

HEMATOPOIETIC STEM CELL DIFFERENTIATION

Hematopoietic stem cells sit at the base of a branching hierarchy of cells culminating in the many mature cell types that compose the blood and immune system (Fig. 68-2). The maturation steps leading to terminally differentiated and functional blood cells take place both as a consequence of intrinsic changes in gene expression and niche-directed and cytokine-directed changes in the cells. Our knowledge of the details remains incomplete (see *http://stemcell.princeton.edu/* for a comprehensive listing of gene expression in stem cells). As stem cells mature to progenitors, precursors, and, finally, mature effector cells, they undergo a series of functional changes. These include the obvious acquisition of functions defining mature blood cells, such as phagocytic capacity or hemoglobinization. They also include the progressive loss of plasticity, i.e., the ability to become other cell types. For example, the myeloid progenitor can make all cells in the myeloid series but none in the lymphoid series. As common myeloid progenitors mature, they become precursors for either monocytes and granulocytes or erythrocytes and megakaryocytes, but not both. Some amount of reversibility of this process may exist early in the differentiation cascade, but that is lost beyond a distinct stage. As cells differentiate, they may also lose proliferative capacity (Fig. 68-3). Mature granulocytes are incapable of proliferation and only increase in number by increased production from precursors. Lymphoid cells retain the capacity to proliferate but have linked their proliferation to the recognition of particular proteins or peptides by specific antigen receptors on their surface. In most tissues the proliferative cell population is a more immature progenitor population. In general, cells within the highly proliferative progenitor cell compartment are also relatively short-lived, making their way through the differentiation process in a defined molecular program involving the sequential activation of particular sets

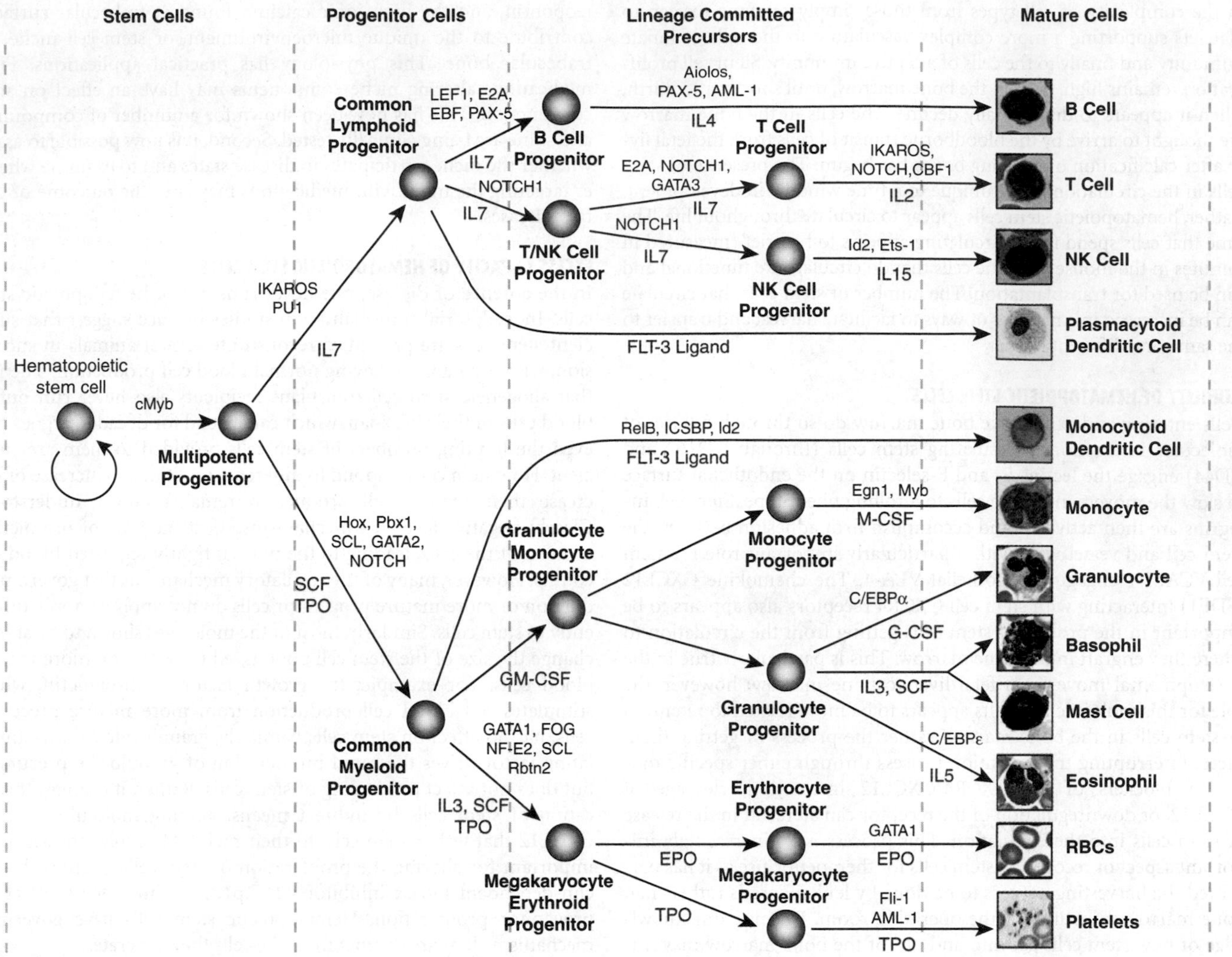

FIGURE 68-2 Hierarchy of hematopoietic differentiation. *Stem cells* are multipotent cells that are the source of all descendant cells and have the capacity to provide either long-term (measured in years) or short-term (measured in months) cell production. *Progenitor cells* have a more limited spectrum of cells they can produce and are generally a short-lived, highly proliferative population also known as transient amplifying cells. *Precursor cells* are cells committed to a single blood cell lineage but with a continued ability to proliferate; they do not have all the features of a fully mature cell. *Mature cells* are the terminally differentiated product of the differentiation process and are the effector cells of specific activities of the blood and immune system. Progress through the pathways is mediated by alterations in gene expression. The regulation of the differentiation by soluble factors and cell-cell communications within the bone marrow niche are still being defined. The transcription factors that characterize particular cell transitions are illustrated on the arrows; the soluble factors that contribute to the differentiation process are in blue. SCF, stem cell factor; EPO, erythropoietin; TPO, thrombopoietin.

of genes. For any particular cell type, the differentiation program is difficult to speed up. The time it takes for hematopoietic progenitors to become mature cells is ~10–14 days in humans, evident clinically by the interval between cytotoxic chemotherapy and blood count recovery in patients.

SELF-RENEWAL

The hematopoietic stem cell must balance its three potential fates: apoptosis, self-renewal, and differentiation. The proliferation of cells is generally not associated with the ability to undergo a self-renewing division except among memory T and B cells and among stem cells. Self-renewal capacity gives way to differentiation as the only option after cell division when cells leave the stem cell compartment, until they have the opportunity to become memory lymphocytes. In addition to this self-renewing capacity, stem cells have an additional feature characterizing their proliferation machinery. Stem cells in most mature adult tissues are deeply quiescent. In the hematopoietic system, stem cells are also highly cytokine-resistant, remaining dormant even when cytokines drive bone marrow progenitors to proliferation rates measured in hours, not days. Stem cells, in contrast, are thought to divide at intervals measured in months to years, at least as estimated in nonhuman primates. This deep quiescence is difficult to overcome in vitro, limiting the ability to effectively expand human hematopoietic stem cells. The process may be controlled by particularly high levels of expression of cyclin-dependent kinase inhibitors that restrict entry of stem cells into cell cycle, blocking the G1-S transition. Modifying the levels of molecules such as p21Cip1 and p18INK4c in the laboratory has resulted in increased stem cell proliferation and number in mice and in some limited human cell studies. Exogenous signals from the niche also appear to enforce quiescence, including the activation of the tyrosine kinase receptor Tie2 on stem cells by angiopoietin 1 on osteoblasts.

The regulation of stem cell proliferation also appears to change with age. In mice, the cyclin-dependent kinase inhibitor p16INK4a accumulates in stem cells in older animals and is associated with a change in five different stem cell functions, including cell cycling. Lowering expression of p16INK4a in older animals improves stem cell cycling and capacity to reconstitute hematopoiesis in adoptive hosts, making them similar to younger animals. Mature cell numbers are unaffected. Therefore, molecular events governing the specific functions of stem cells are being gradually made clear and offer the potential of new ap-

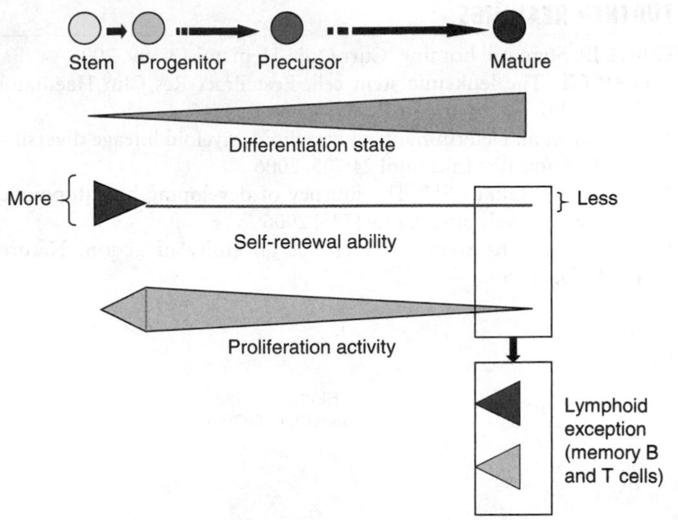

FIGURE 68-3 Relative function of cells in the hematopoietic hierarchy. The boxes represent distinct functional features of cells in the myeloid (*upper box*) versus lymphoid (*lower box*) lineages.

proaches to changing stem cell function for therapy. One critical stem cell function that remains poorly defined is the molecular regulation of self-renewal.

For medicine, self-renewal is perhaps the most important function of stem cells because it is critical in regulating the number of stem cells. Stem cell number is a key limiting parameter for both autologous and allogeneic stem cell transplantation. Were we to have the ability to use fewer stem cells or expand limited numbers of stem cells ex vivo, it might be possible to reduce the morbidity and expense of stem cell harvests and enable use of other stem cell sources. Specifically, umbilical cord blood is a rich source of stem cells. However, the volume of cord blood units is extremely small, and therefore the total number of hematopoietic stem cells that can be obtained is generally only sufficient to transplant an individual of <40 kg. This limitation restricts what would otherwise be an extremely promising source of stem cells. Two features of cord blood stem cells are particularly important. (1) They are derived from a diversity of individuals that far exceeds the adult donor pool and therefore can overcome the majority of immunologic cross-matching obstacles. (2) Cord blood stem cells have a large number of T cells associated with them, but (paradoxically) they appear to be associated with a lower incidence of graft-versus-host disease when compared with similarly mismatched stem cells from other sources. If stem cell expansion by self-renewal could be achieved, the number of cells available might be sufficient for use in larger adults. An alternative approach to this problem is to improve the efficiency of engraftment of donor stem cells. Graft engineering is exploring methods of adding cell components that may enhance engraftment. Furthermore, at least some data suggest that depletion of host NK (natural killer) cells may lower the number of stem cells necessary to reconstitute hematopoiesis.

Some limited understanding of self-renewal exists and, intriguingly, implicates gene products that are associated with the chromatin state, a high-order organization of chromosomal DNA that influences transcription. These include members of the polycomb family, a group of zinc finger–containing transcriptional regulators that interact with the chromatin structure, contributing to the accessibility of groups of genes for transcription. Certain members, including Bmi-1 and Gfi-1, are important in enabling hematopoietic stem cell self-renewal through modification of cell cycle regulators such as the cyclin-dependent kinase inhibitors. In the absence of either of these genes, hematopoietic stem cells decline in number and function. In contrast, dysregulation of *Bmi-1* has been associated with leukemia; it may promote leukemic stem cell self-renewal when it is overexpressed. Other transcription regulators have also been associated with self-renewal, particularly homeobox, or "hox," genes. These transcription factors are named for their ability to govern large numbers of genes, including those determining body patterning in invertebrates. HoxB4 is capable of inducing extensive self-renewal of stem cells through its DNA-binding motif. Other members of the hox family of genes have been noted to affect normal stem cells, but they are also associated with leukemia. External signals that may influence the relative self-renewal versus differentiation outcomes of stem cell cycling include the Notch ligands and specific Wnt ligands. Intracellular signal transducing intermediates are also implicated in regulating self-renewal but, interestingly, are not usually associated with the pathways activated by Notch or Wnt receptors. They include PTEN, an inhibitor of the AKT pathway, and STAT5, both of which are usually downstream of activated growth factor receptors and necessary for normal stem cell functions, including self-renewal, at least in mouse models. The connections between these molecules remain to be defined, and their role in physiologic regulation of stem cell self-renewal is still poorly understood.

CANCER IS SIMILAR TO AN ORGAN WITH SELF-RENEWING CAPACITY

The relationship of stem cells to cancer is an important evolving dimension of adult stem cell biology. Cancer may share principles of organization with normal tissues. Cancer might have the same hierarchical organization of cells with a base of stemlike cells capable of the signature stem-cell features, self-renewal and differentiation. These stemlike cells might be the basis for perpetuation of the tumor and represent a slowly dividing, rare population with distinct regulatory mechanisms, including a relationship with a specialized microenvironment. A subpopulation of self-renewing cells in cancer has been defined. A more sophisticated understanding of the stem-cell organization of cancers may lead to improved strategies for attacking the many common and difficult-to-treat types of malignancies that have been relatively refractory to interventions aimed at dividing cells.

Does the concept of cancer stem cells provide insight into the cellular origin of cancer? The fact that some cells within a cancer have stem cell–like properties does not necessarily mean that the cancer arose in the stem cell itself. Rather, more mature cells could have acquired the self-renewal characteristics of stem cells. Any single genetic event is unlikely to be sufficient to enable full transformation of a normal cell to a frankly malignant one. Rather, cancer is a multistep process, and for the multiple steps to accumulate, the cell of origin must be able to persist for prolonged periods. It must also be able to generate large numbers of daughter cells. The normal stem cell has these properties and, by virtue of its having intrinsic self-renewal capability, may be more readily converted to a malignant phenotype. This hypothesis has been tested experimentally in the hematopoietic system. Taking advantage of the cell-surface markers that distinguish hematopoietic cells of varying maturity, stem cells, progenitors, precursors, and mature cells can be isolated. Powerful transforming gene constructs were placed in these cells, and it was found that the cell with the greatest potential to produce a malignancy was indeed the stem cell. This does not prove that stem cells give rise to all tumors, but it does suggest that stem cells may be susceptible to malignant conversion and may be the population of greatest interest in developing strategies to protect against, monitor, or treat nascent malignancy.

WHAT ELSE CAN HEMATOPOIETIC STEM CELLS DO?

Some experimental data have suggested that hematopoietic stem cells or other cells mobilized into the circulation by the same factors that mobilize hematopoietic stem cells are capable of playing a role in healing the vascular and tissue damage associated with stroke and myocardial infarction. These data are controversial, and the applicability of a stem-cell approach to nonhematopoietic conditions remains experimental. However, the application of the evolving knowledge of hematopoietic stem cell biology may lead to wide-ranging clinical uses.

The stem cell therefore represents a true dual-edged sword. It has tremendous healing capacity and is essential for life. Uncontrolled, it can threaten the life it maintains. Understanding how stem cells function, the signals that modify their behavior, and the tissue niches that modulate stem cell responses to injury and disease are critical for more effectively developing stem cell–based medicine. That aspect of medicine will include the use of the stem cells and the use of drugs to target stem cells to enhance repair of damaged tissues. It will also include the careful balance of interventions to control stem cells where they may be dysfunctional or malignant.

FURTHER READINGS

CHUTE JP: Stem cell homing. Curr Opin Hematol 13:399, 2006

JORDAN CT: The leukemic stem cell. Best Pract Res Clin Haematol 20:13, 2007

LAIOSA CV et al: Determinants of lymphoid-myeloid lineage diversification. Annu Rev Immunol 24:705, 2006

MIKKOLA HK, ORKIN SH: The journey of developing hematopoietic stem cells. Development 133:3733, 2006

SCADDEN DT: The stem cell niche as an entity of action. Nature 441:1075, 2006

69 Tissue Engineering

Jennifer Anderson, Joseph P. Vacanti

The origins of tissue engineering date to the sixteenth century when complex skin flaps were used to replace the nose. Modern tissue engineering combines the disciplines of materials sciences and life sciences to replace a diseased or damaged organ with a living, functional substitute. The most common tissue engineering approach combines cells and matrices to produce a living structure (Fig. 69-1). These strategies also include the use of scaffolding, cells, and growth factors to shape new tissues. The term *regenerative medicine* has emerged as a concept inclusive of tissue engineering and stem cell therapy (Chap. 67).

CELLULAR COMPONENTS OF TISSUE ENGINEERING

The foundation of tissue engineering is the combination of a three-dimensional scaffold with live and functional cells. Cells used in tissue engineering should be easily accessible and capable of proliferation while maintaining their differentiated function. There are three possible sources for cells: autologous, allogenic, and xenogenic. *Autologous cells* are isolated directly from the patient. They have the advantage of avoiding immune-mediated rejection. However, a potential limitation is that they may not be available or able to proliferate to the required tissue mass. *Allogenic cells* are harvested from a donor other than the patient. They have the advantage of being more readily available, but the immune system must be modulated to avoid rejection. *Xenogenic cells*, or those from a different species, may also be used but also risk immune rejection or transmission of animal pathogens.

Although cells such as fibroblasts and smooth-muscle cells proliferate rapidly, other cells proliferate slowly or lose their tissue-specific function when cultured, thereby limiting their use. In addition, cellular characteristics may depend on their location within the body. For example, the cell-to-cell interactions and function of endothelial cells in the pulmonary microvasculature are different from those in the blood-brain barrier. The microenvironment of the cell, including the presence of other cell types, soluble factors, and the presence of physical or mechanical forces may also alter the function of a transplanted cell.

Stem cells provide a promising cell source because they are capable of rapid proliferation and they can be induced to differentiate into multiple cell lineages (Chaps. 66 and 67). Human embryonic stem cells are capable of differentiating into endoderm, mesoderm, or ectoderm tissue types. Multipotent adult stem cells have been found in multiple mature tissues including the bone marrow, brain, heart, and liver. In addition to being able to differentiate into numerous lineages, adult stem cells generate a relatively muted immune response.

SCAFFOLDS

A scaffold provides a three-dimensional framework to support the tissue or organ-specific cells. The scaffold not only provides mechanical support, but it must also supply critical nutrients and transport metabolites to and from the developing tissue. Important scaffold properties vary depending on the tissue but typically include specific

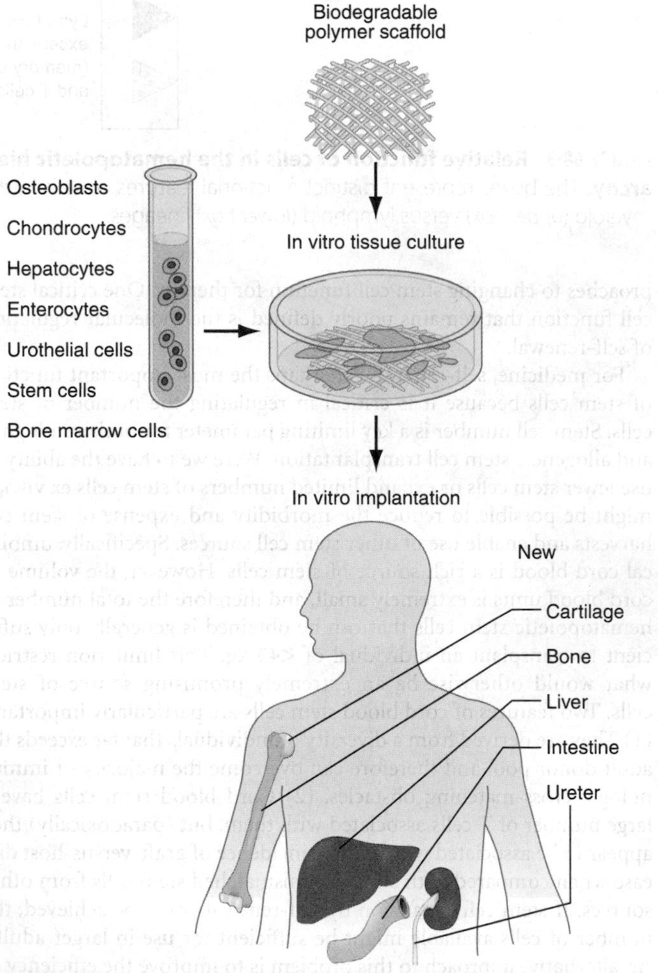

FIGURE 69-1 Schematic of basic principles of tissue engineering. *[From Langer R, Vacanti J: Tissue engineering. Science 260:1993 (Fig. 1), with permission.]*

biomechanical properties, porosity, biocompatibility, and appropriate surface characteristics for cell adhesion and differentiation.

Scaffolds can be natural materials or synthetic polymers and are typically biodegradable. Natural materials such as collagen and alginates are biocompatible. However, it is difficult to control their mechanical properties, and they may generate an immune reaction. Synthetic polymers such as polyglycolic acid and polyethylene, on the other hand, can be tailored to provide more acceptable mechanical properties but are associated with a strong inflammatory response. Nonbiodegradable synthetic polymers such as polytetrafluoroethylene and polyethylene provide well-defined mechanical and structural properties. However, their long-term presence in the body can lead to a chronic inflammatory response, which results in poor tissue quality. Polylactic acid and polyglycolic acid are examples of biodegradable polymers. Although the degradation of these materials can be partially

TABLE 69-1 FDA-APPROVED TISSUE-ENGINEERED PRODUCTS

Name of Product	Brief Description
Alloderm (LifeCell)	Acellular dermal matrix for tissue repair
Apligraf (Organogenesis)	Living skin equivalent approved for the treatment of venous leg ulcers and diabetic foot ulcers
Carticel (Genzyme Biosurgery)	Autologous chondrocytes approved for cartilage repair
Dermagraft (Smith and Nephew)	Living skin equivalent approved for full-thickness diabetic foot ulcers
Durasis (Cook Surgical Products)	Porcine small-intestine submucosa for replacement of dura mater
Epicel (Genzyme Biosurgery)	Living skin equivalent approved for burn patients
OrCel (Ortec)	Living skin equivalent approved for burn patients
Surgisis (Cook Surgical Products)	Porcine small-intestine submucosa for dermal wounds and reinforcement of weakened tissue

controlled, nonuniform degradation and varying degradation rates in different anatomic locations represent challenges.

The surface properties of the materials used for the scaffold are important for adhesion, migration, and cell differentiation. Ongoing research is focused on tethering growth factors or peptide sequences to the surface of the scaffold to improve adhesion and migration.

BIOREACTORS

Initially, cells used in tissue engineering were cultured in static conditions. Improvements in bioreactor technology more closely approximate physiologic parameters for tissue growth. By modulating rates of flow and mixing, the transfer of nutrients, gases, metabolites, and regulatory molecules can be maximized. Mechanical stimuli can also impact the newly forming tissue. For example, tissue-engineered blood vessels exposed to shear stress in a pulsatile flow bioreactor have greater burst strength and collagen content than those not exposed to shear stress.

TISSUE ENGINEERING SUCCESSES

Several tissue-engineered skin substitutes have been approved by the U.S. Food and Drug Administration (FDA) and in use for >10 years (Table 69-1). One of these products uses neonatal dermal fibroblasts isolated from human foreskins cultured on a scaffold of polylactide coglycolide. The polymer scaffold gradually degrades in the presence of water. A bilayer skin substitute has also been developed: dermal fibroblasts are cultured in a collagen solution and then coated with several layers of keratinocytes. Cartilage tissue engineering is also showing promise; autologous chondrocytes from a healthy portion of the patient's joint are expanded in culture and then implanted into the site of injury. Other scaffold-based products are based on processed animal submucosa or dura. In addition to these FDA-approved products, numerous tissue-engineered products are currently in clinical trials (Table 69-2). Engineered tissues being actively investigated include bone, mandible, teeth, cartilage, skin, cornea, bladder, urethra, small-diameter blood vessels, and the pulmonary artery.

CHALLENGES TO TISSUE ENGINEERING

The greatest success in tissue engineering to date has been in tissues such as skin and cartilage where the requirements for nutrients and oxygen are relatively low. Due to oxygen diffusion limitations, the maximal thickness of an engineered tissue is 150–200 μm if there is not an intrinsic capillary network. Strategies used to overcome this limitation include transplantation of the tissue directly into the patient's vasculature or trying to induce angiogenesis by incorporating growth factors such as vascular endothelial cell growth factor into the scaffold. A more recent approach involves the creation of an intrinsic network of vascular channels immediately adjacent to the engineered tissue. A combination of microelectro mechanical systems (MEMS) fabrication technology and computational models of fractal branching allows the construction of an intrinsic microvascular network scaffold within a biocompatible polymer. This preformed capillary-like network can be seeded with cells and ultimately sustains the growth and function of complex three-dimensional tissues.

Immune rejection of allogenic cells is another major obstacle. The use of immunosuppressive drugs is not considered an optimal solution to this problem. One potential solution is to develop "universal donor" cells by masking the histocompatibility proteins on the cell surface.

Off-the-shelf availability will need to be addressed for tissue engineering products to be used widely. Ideally, products should be reproducible and available at a wide variety of hospitals, including those without sophisticated facilities for cell culture and cell proliferation.

TABLE 69-2 TISSUE-ENGINEERING PRODUCTS IN CLINICAL TRIALS

TRC (Aastrom)	Autologous adult bone marrow cells for bone grafting
LiverX2000 (Algenix)	Extracorporeal liver assist device
Encapsulated proliferated islet (Amcyte)	Encapsulated islet cells
Myocell (Bioheart)	Encapsulated cells for myocardial infarction
BioSeed-C, BioSeed-Oral Bone (Biotissue Technologies)	Autologous tissue repair for bone and cartilage
E-matrix (Encelle)	Repair or regeneration of diseased or damaged tissue
MarkII (Excorp)	Extracorporeal liver assist device
ICX-PRO, ICX-TRC (Intercytex)	Wound repair and hair regeneration
HuCNS-SC (Stem Cell Inc)	Human central nervous system stem cells
NT-501 (Neurotech SA)	Encapsulated cell technology for long-term delivery of therapeutic factors to retina
Procord (Proneuron)	Autologous activated macrophage therapy for patients with acute complete spinal cord injury
ChondroCelect (Tigenix)	Autologous chondrocyte implantation
Spheramine (Titan Pharmaceutical)	Retinal pigment epithelial cells in microcarriers to provide continuous source of dopamine in the brain
ELAD (Vigagen)	Extracorporeal liver assist device

FURTHER READINGS

AHSAN T, NEREM RM: Bioengineered tissues: The science, the technology, and the industry. Orthod Craniofacial Res 8:134, 2005

LAVIK E, LANGER R: Tissue engineering: Current state and perspectives. Appl Microbiol Biotechnol 65:1, 2004

LYSAGHT MJ, HAZLEHURST AL: Tissue engineering: The end of the beginning. Tissue Engineering 10:12, 2004

SHEIH SJ, VACANTI JP: State-of-the-art tissue engineering: From tissue engineering to organ building. Surgery 137:1, 2005

YOW KH et al: Tissue engineering of vascular conduits. Br J Surg 93(6):652, 2006

70 Nutritional Requirements and Dietary Assessment

Johanna Dwyer

Nutrients are substances that must be supplied by the diet because they are not synthesized in the body in sufficient amounts. Nutrient requirements for groups of healthy persons have been determined experimentally. For good health we require energy-providing nutrients (protein, fat, and carbohydrate), vitamins, minerals, and water. Specific nutrient requirements include 9 essential amino acids, several fatty acids, 4 fat-soluble vitamins, 10 water-soluble vitamins, and choline. Several inorganic substances, including 4 minerals, 7 trace minerals, 3 electrolytes, and the ultratrace elements, also must be supplied in the diet.

The required amounts of the essential nutrients differ by age and physiologic state. Conditionally essential nutrients are not required in the diet but must be supplied to individuals who do not synthesize them in adequate amounts, such as those with genetic defects, those having pathologic states with nutritional implications, and developmentally immature infants. Many organic phytochemicals and zoochemicals present in foods have health effects. For example, dietary fiber has beneficial effects on gastrointestinal function. Other bioactive food constituents or contaminants such as lead may have negative health effects.

ESSENTIAL NUTRIENT REQUIREMENTS

ENERGY

For weight to remain stable, energy intake must match energy output. The major components of energy output are resting energy expenditure (REE) and physical activity; minor sources include the energy cost of metabolizing food (thermic effect of food or specific dynamic action) and shivering thermogenesis (e.g., cold-induced thermogenesis). The average energy intake is about 2800 kcal/d for American men and about 1800 kcal/d for American women, although these estimates vary with body size and activity level. Formulas for estimating REE are useful for assessing the energy needs of an individual whose weight is stable. Thus, for males, $REE = 900 + 10w$, and for females, $REE = 700 + 7w$, where w is weight in kilograms. The calculated REE is then adjusted for physical activity level by multiplying by 1.2 for sedentary, 1.4 for moderately active, or 1.8 for very active individuals. The final figure provides a rough estimate of total caloric needs in a state of energy balance. Formulas to provide more precise estimates of energy requirements are provided by the Food and Nutrition Board, Institute of Medicine, National Academy of Sciences in recent reports on dietary reference intakes. For further discussion of energy balance in health and disease, see Chap. 72.

PROTEIN

Dietary protein consists of both essential and other amino acids that are required for protein synthesis. The nine essential amino acids are histidine, isoleucine, leucine, lysine, methionine/cystine, phenylalanine/tyrosine, threonine, tryptophan, and valine. All amino acids can be used for energy, and certain amino acids (e.g., alanine) can also be used for gluconeogenesis. When energy intake is inadequate, protein intake must be increased, since ingested amino acids are diverted into pathways of glucose synthesis and oxidation. In extreme energy deprivation, protein-calorie malnutrition may ensue (Chap. 72).

For adults, the recommended dietary allowance (RDA) for protein is about 0.6 g/kg desirable body weight per day, assuming that energy needs are met and that the protein is of relatively high biologic value. Current recommendations for a healthy diet call for at least 10–14% of calories from protein. Biologic value tends to be highest for animal proteins, followed by proteins from legumes (beans), cereals (rice, wheat, corn), and roots. Combinations of plant proteins that complement one another in biologic value or combinations of animal and plant proteins can increase biologic value and lower total protein requirements.

Protein needs increase during growth, pregnancy, lactation, and rehabilitation after malnutrition. Tolerance to normal amounts of dietary protein is decreased in renal insufficiency and liver failure, precipitating encephalopathy in patients with cirrhosis of the liver.

FAT AND CARBOHYDRATE

Fats are a concentrated source of energy and constitute on average 34% of calories in U.S. diets. For optimal health, saturated fat and trans-fat should be limited to <10% of calories, and polyunsaturated fats to <10% of calories, with monounsaturated fats constituting the remainder of fat intake. At least 55% of total calories should be derived from carbohydrates. The brain requires about 100 g/d of glucose for fuel; other tissues use about 50 g/d. Some tissues (e.g., brain and red blood cells) rely on glucose supplied either exogenously or from muscle proteolysis. Over time, some adaptations in carbohydrate needs are possible in other tissues during hypocaloric states (Chap. 339).

WATER

For adults, 1.0–1.5 mL water per kcal of energy expenditure is sufficient under usual conditions to allow for normal variations in physical activity, sweating, and solute load of the diet. Water losses include 50–100 mL/d in the feces, 500–1000 mL/d by evaporation or exhalation, and, depending on the renal solute load, ≥1000 mL/d in the urine. If external losses increase, intakes must increase accordingly to avoid underhydration. Fever increases water losses by approximately 200 mL/d per °C; diarrheal losses vary but may be as great as 5 L/d with severe diarrhea. Heavy sweating and vomiting also increase water losses. When renal function is normal and solute intakes are adequate, the kidneys can adjust to increased water intake by excreting up to 18 L/d of excess water (Chap. 334). However, obligatory urine outputs can compromise hydration status when there is inadequate intake or when losses increase in disease or kidney damage.

Infants have high requirements for water because of their large ratio of surface area to volume, the limited capacity of the immature kidney to handle high renal solute loads, and their inability to communicate their thirst. During pregnancy, 30 mL/d additional water is needed. During lactation, milk production increases water requirements by approximately 1000 mL/d, or 1 mL for each mL of milk produced. Special attention must be paid to the water needs of the elderly, who have reduced total body water and blunted thirst sensation, and may be taking diuretics.

OTHER NUTRIENTS

See Chap. 71 for a detailed description of vitamins and trace minerals.

DIETARY REFERENCE INTAKES AND RECOMMENDED DIETARY ALLOWANCES

Fortunately, human life and well-being can be maintained within a fairly wide range for most nutrients. However, the capacity for adaptation is not infinite—too much of a nutrient, as well as too little, may have adverse effects on health. Therefore, quantitative benchmark recommendations on nutrient intakes have been developed to guide clinical practice. These estimates are collectively referred to as the *dietary reference intakes* (DRIs). The DRIs supplant but include the *recommended dietary allowances* (RDAs), the single reference values used in the United States since 1989. DRIs include the *estimated average requirement* (EAR) of a nutrient, as well as three other reference values used for dietary planning for individuals: the RDA, or, if it cannot be established, the *adequate intake* (AI), and the tolerable *upper level* (UL). The current DRIs for vitamins and elements are provided in Tables 70-1 and 70-2, respectively.

TABLE 70-1 DIETARY REFERENCE INTAKES: RECOMMENDED INTAKES FOR INDIVIDUALS—VITAMINS

Life-Stage Group	Vitamin, μg/d: A[a]	C	D[b,c]	E[d]	K	Thiamine, mg/d	Riboflavin, mg/d	Niacin, mg/d[e]	Vitamin B_6, mg/d	Folate, μg/d[f]	Vitamin B_{12}, μg/d	Pantothenic Acid, mg/d	Biotin, μg/d	Choline, mg/d[g]
Infants														
0–6 mo	400	40	5	4	2.0	0.2	0.3	2	0.1	65	0.4	1.7	5	125
7–12 mo	500	50	5	5	2.5	0.3	0.4	4	0.3	80	0.5	1.8	6	150
Children														
1–3 y	**300**	**15**	5	**6**	30	**0.5**	**0.5**	**6**	**0.5**	**150**	**0.9**	2	8	200
4–8 y	**400**	**25**	5	**7**	55	**0.6**	**0.6**	**8**	**0.6**	**200**	**1.2**	3	12	250
Males														
9–13 y	**600**	**45**	5	**11**	60	**0.9**	**0.9**	**12**	**1.0**	**300**	**1.8**	4	20	375
14–18 y	**900**	**75**	5	**15**	75	**1.2**	**1.3**	**16**	**1.3**	**400**	**2.4**	5	25	550
19–30 y	**900**	**90**	5	**15**	120	**1.2**	**1.3**	**16**	**1.3**	**400**	**2.4**	5	30	550
31–50 y	**900**	**90**	5	**15**	120	**1.2**	**1.3**	**16**	**1.3**	**400**	**2.4**	5	30	550
51–70 y	**900**	**90**	10	**15**	120	**1.2**	**1.3**	**16**	**1.7**	**400**	**2.4**[h]	5	30	550
>70 y	**900**	**90**	15	**15**	120	**1.2**	**1.3**	**16**	**1.7**	**400**	**2.4**[h]	5	30	550
Females														
9–13 y	**600**	**45**	5	**11**	60	**0.9**	**0.9**	**12**	**1.0**	**300**	**1.8**	4	20	375
14–18 y	**700**	**65**	5	**15**	75	**1.0**	**1.0**	**14**	**1.2**	**400**[i]	**2.4**	5	25	400
19–30 y	**700**	**75**	5	**15**	90	**1.1**	**1.1**	**14**	**1.3**	**400**[i]	**2.4**	5	30	425
31–50 y	**700**	**75**	5	**15**	90	**1.1**	**1.1**	**14**	**1.3**	**400**[i]	**2.4**	5	30	425
51–70 y	**700**	**75**	10	**15**	90	**1.1**	**1.1**	**14**	**1.5**	**400**	**2.4**[h]	5	30	425
>70 y	**700**	**75**	15	**15**	90	**1.1**	**1.1**	**14**	**1.5**	**400**	**2.4**[h]	5	30	425
Pregnancy														
≤18 y	**750**	**80**	5	**15**	75	**1.4**	**1.4**	**18**	**1.6**	**600**[j]	**2.6**	6	30	450
19–30 y	**770**	**85**	5	**15**	90	**1.4**	**1.4**	**18**	**1.9**	**600**[j]	**2.6**	6	30	450
31–50 y	**770**	**85**	5	**15**	90	**1.4**	**1.4**	**18**	**1.9**	**600**[j]	**2.6**	6	30	450
Lactation														
≤18 y	**1200**	**115**	5	**19**	75	**1.4**	**1.6**	**17**	**2.0**	**500**	**2.8**	7	35	550
19–30 y	**1300**	**120**	5	**19**	90	**1.4**	**1.6**	**17**	**2.0**	**500**	**2.8**	7	35	550
31–50 y	**1300**	**120**	5	**19**	90	**1.4**	**1.6**	**17**	**2.0**	**500**	**2.8**	7	35	550

Note: This table presents recommended dietary allowances (RDAs) in **bold type** and adequate intakes (AIs) in ordinary type. RDAs and AIs may both be used as goals for individual intake. RDAs are set to meet the needs of almost all individuals (97 to 98%) in a group. For healthy breastfed infants, the AI is the mean intake. The AI for other life stage and gender groups is believed to cover needs of all individuals in the group, but lack of data or uncertainty in the data prevent being able to specify with confidence the percentage of individuals covered by this intake.

[a]As retinol activity equivalents (RAEs). 1 RAE = 1 μg retinol, 12 μg β-carotene, 24 μg α-carotene, or 24 μg β-cryptoxanthin. To calculate RAEs from retinol equivalents (REs) of provitamin A carotenoids in foods, divide the REs by 2. For preformed vitamin A in foods or supplements and for provitamin A carotenoids in supplements, 1 RE = 1 RAE.

[b]As calciferol. 1 μg calciferol = 40 IU vitamin D.

[c]In the absence of adequate exposure to sunlight.

[d]As α-tocopherol. α-Tocopherol includes *RRR*-α-tocopherol, the only form of α-tocopherol that occurs naturally in foods, and the *2R*-stereoisomeric forms of α-tocopherol (*RRR-*, *RSR-*, *RRS-*, and *RSS*-α-tocopherol) that occur in fortified foods and supplements. It does not include the *2S*-stereoisomeric forms of α-tocopherol (*SRR-*, *SSR-*, *SRS-*, and *SSS*-α-tocopherol), also found in fortified foods and supplements.

[e]As niacin equivalents (NE). 1 mg of niacin = 60 mg of tryptophan; 0–6 months = preformed niacin (not NE).

[f]As dietary folate equivalents (DFEs). 1 DFE = 1 μg food folate = 0.6 μg of folic acid from fortified food or as a supplement consumed with food = 0.5 μg of a supplement taken on an empty stomach.

[g]Although AIs have been set for choline, there are few data to assess whether a dietary supply of choline is needed at all stages of the life cycle, and it may be that the choline requirement can be met by endogenous synthesis at some of these stages.

[h]Because 10 to 30% of older people may malabsorb food-bound B_{12}, it is advisable for those >50 years to meet their RDA mainly by consuming foods fortified with B_{12} or a supplement containing B_{12}.

[i]In view of evidence linking inadequate folate intake with neural tube defects in the fetus, it is recommended that all women capable of becoming pregnant consume 400 μg from supplements or fortified foods in addition to intake of food folate from a varied diet.

[j]It is assumed that women will continue consuming 400 μg from supplements or fortified food until their pregnancy is confirmed and they enter prenatal care, which ordinarily occurs after the end of the periconceptional period—the critical time for formation of the neural tube.

Source: Food and Nutrition Board, Institute of Medicine—National Academy of Sciences Dietary Reference Intakes, 2000, 2002, reprinted with permission. Courtesy of the National Academy Press, Washington, DC. *http://www.nap.edu*

ESTIMATED AVERAGE REQUIREMENT

When florid manifestations of the classic dietary deficiency diseases such as rickets, scurvy, xerophthalmia, and protein-calorie malnutrition were common, nutrient adequacy was inferred from the absence of their clinical signs. Later, it was determined that biochemical and other changes were evident long before the clinical deficiency became apparent. Consequently, criteria of nutrient adequacy are now based on biologic markers when they are available. Priority is given to sensitive biochemical, physiologic, or behavioral tests that reflect early changes in regulatory processes or maintenance of body stores of nutrients. Current definitions focus on the amount of a nutrient that minimizes the risk of chronic degenerative diseases.

The EAR is the amount of a nutrient estimated to be adequate for half of the healthy individuals of a specific age and sex. The types of evidence and criteria used to establish nutrient requirements vary by nutrient, age, and physiologic group. The EAR is not useful clinically for estimating nutrient adequacy in individuals because it is a median requirement for a group; 50% of individuals in a group fall below the requirement and 50% fall above it. Thus, a person with a usual intake at the EAR has a 50% risk of an inadequate intake. For these reasons, other standards, described below, are more useful for clinical purposes.

RECOMMENDED DIETARY ALLOWANCES

The RDA is the nutrient-intake goal for planning diets of individuals; it is used in the MyPyramid food guide of the U.S. Department of Agriculture (USDA), therapeutic diets, and descriptions of the nutritional content of processed foods and dietary supplements. The nutrient content in a food is stated by weight or as a percentage of the daily value (DV), a variant of the RDA that, for an adult, represents the highest RDA for an adult consuming 2000 kcal/d.

The RDA is the average daily dietary intake level that meets the nutrient requirements of nearly all healthy persons of a specific sex, age, life stage, or physiologic condition (such as pregnancy or lactation).

The RDA is defined statistically as 2 standard deviations (SD) above the EAR to ensure that the needs of most individuals are met.

The risk of dietary inadequacy increases as intake falls further below the RDA. However, the RDA is an overly generous criterion for evaluating nutrient adequacy. For example, by definition the RDA exceeds the actual requirements of all but about 2 to 3% of the population. Therefore, many people whose intake falls below the RDA may still be getting enough of the nutrient.

ADEQUATE INTAKE

It is not possible to set an RDA for some nutrients that do not have an established EAR. In this circumstance, the AI is based on observed, or experimentally determined, approximations of nutrient intakes in healthy people. In the DRIs established to date, AIs rather than RDAs are proposed for infants up to age 1 year, as well as for calcium, chromium, vitamin D, fluoride, manganese, pantothenic acid, biotin, choline, sodium, chloride, potassium, and water for persons of all ages.

TOLERABLE UPPER LEVELS OF NUTRIENT INTAKE

Healthy individuals derive no established benefit from consuming nutrient levels above the RDA or AI. Excessive nutrient intake can disturb body functions and cause acute, progressive, or permanent disabilities. The tolerable UL is the highest level of chronic nutrient intake (usually daily) that is unlikely to pose a risk of adverse health effects for most of the population. Data on the adverse effects of large amounts of many nutrients are unavailable or too limited to establish a UL. Therefore, the lack of a UL does *not* mean that the risk of adverse effects from high intake is nonexistent. Individual nutrients in foods that most people eat rarely reach levels that exceed the UL. However, nutritional supplements provide more concentrated amounts of nutrients per dose and, as a result, pose a greater potential risk of toxicity. Nutrient supplements are labeled with "Supplement Facts" that express the amount of nutrient in absolute units or as the percent of the DV provided per recommended serving size. Total nutrient consumption, including both food and supplements, should not exceed RDA levels.

FACTORS ALTERING NUTRIENT NEEDS

The DRIs are affected by age, sex, rate of growth, pregnancy, lactation, physical activity, composition of diet, coexisting diseases, and drugs. When only slight differences exist between the requirements for nutrient sufficiency and excess, dietary planning becomes more difficult.

PHYSIOLOGIC FACTORS

Growth, strenuous physical activity, pregnancy, and lactation increase needs for energy and several essential nutrients, including water. Energy needs rise during pregnancy, due to the demands of fetal growth, and during lactation, because of the increased energy required for milk production. Energy needs decrease with loss of lean body mass, the major determinant of REE. Because both health and physical activity tend to decline with age, energy needs in older persons, especially those over 70, tend to be less than those of younger persons.

DIETARY COMPOSITION

Dietary composition affects the biologic availability and utilization of nutrients. For example, the absorption of iron may be impaired by high amounts of calcium or lead; non-heme iron uptake may be impaired by the lack of ascorbic acid and amino acids in the meal. Protein utilization by the body may be decreased when essential amino acids are not present in sufficient amounts. Animal foods, such as

TABLE 70-2 DIETARY REFERENCE INTAKES: RECOMMENDED INTAKES FOR INDIVIDUALS—ELEMENTS

Life-Stage Group	Calcium, mg/d	Chromium, µg/d	Copper, µg/d	Fluoride, mg/d	Iodine, µg/d	Iron, mg/d	Magnesium, mg/d	Manganese, mg/d	Molybdenum, µg/d	Phosphorus mg/d	Selenium, µg/d	Zinc, mg/d
Infants												
0–6 mo	210	0.2	200	0.01	110	0.27	30	0.003	2	100	15	2
7–12 mo	270	5.5	220	0.5	130	**11**	75	0.6	3	275	20	**3**
Children												
1–3 y	500	11	**340**	0.7	**90**	**7**	**80**	1.2	**17**	**460**	**20**	**3**
4–8 y	800	15	**440**	1	**90**	**10**	**130**	1.5	**22**	**500**	**30**	**5**
Males												
9–13 y	1300	25	**700**	2	**120**	**8**	**240**	1.9	**34**	**1250**	**40**	**8**
14–18 y	1300	35	**890**	3	**150**	**11**	**410**	2.2	**43**	**1250**	**55**	**11**
19–30 y	1000	35	**900**	4	**150**	**8**	**400**	2.3	**45**	**700**	**55**	**11**
31–50 y	1000	35	**900**	4	**150**	**8**	**420**	2.3	**45**	**700**	**55**	**11**
51–70 y	1200	30	**900**	4	**150**	**8**	**420**	2.3	**45**	**700**	**55**	**11**
>70 y	1200	30	**900**	4	**150**	**8**	**420**	2.3	**45**	**700**	**55**	**11**
Females												
9–13 y	1300	21	**700**	2	**120**	**8**	**240**	1.6	**34**	**1250**	**40**	**8**
14–18 y	1300	24	**890**	3	**150**	**15**	**360**	1.6	**43**	**1250**	**55**	**9**
19–30 y	1000	25	**900**	3	**150**	**18**	**310**	1.8	**45**	**700**	**55**	**8**
31–50 y	1000	25	**900**	3	**150**	**18**	**320**	1.8	**45**	**700**	**55**	**8**
51–70 y	1200	20	**900**	3	**150**	**8**	**320**	1.8	**45**	**700**	**55**	**8**
>70 y	1200	20	**900**	3	**150**	**8**	**320**	1.8	**45**	**700**	**55**	**8**
Pregnancy												
≤18 y	1300	29	**1000**	3	**220**	**27**	**400**	2.0	**50**	**1250**	**60**	**12**
19–30 y	1000	30	**1000**	3	**220**	**27**	**350**	2.0	**50**	**700**	**60**	**11**
31–50 y	1000	30	**1000**	3	**220**	**27**	**360**	2.0	**50**	**700**	**60**	**11**
Lactation												
≤18 y	1300	44	**1300**	3	**290**	**10**	**360**	2.6	**50**	**1250**	**70**	**13**
19–30 y	1000	45	**1300**	3	**290**	**9**	**310**	2.6	**50**	**700**	**70**	**12**
31–50 y	1000	45	**1300**	3	**290**	**9**	**320**	2.6	**50**	**700**	**70**	**12**

Note: This table presents recommended dietary allowances (RDAs) in **bold type** and adequate intakes (AIs) in ordinary type. RDAs and AIs may both be used as goals for individual intake. RDAs are set to meet the needs of almost all individuals (97 to 98%) in a group. For healthy breastfed infants, the AI is the mean intake. The AI for other life stage and gender groups is believed to cover needs of all individuals in the group, but lack of data or uncertainty in the data prevent being able to specify with confidence the percentage of individuals covered by this intake.

Source: Food and Nutrition Board, Institute of Medicine—National Academy of Sciences Dietary Reference Intakes, 2000, 2002, reprinted with permission. Courtesy of the National Academy Press, Washington, DC. *http://www.nap.edu*

milk, eggs, and meat, have high biologic values with most of the needed amino acids present in adequate amounts. Plant proteins in corn (maize), soy, and wheat have lower biologic values and must be combined with other plant or animal proteins to achieve optimal utilization by the body.

ROUTE OF ADMINISTRATION

The RDAs apply only to oral intakes. When nutrients are administered parenterally, similar values can sometimes be used for amino acids, carbohydrates, fats, sodium, chloride, potassium, and most of the vitamins, since their intestinal absorption is nearly 100%. However, the oral bioavailability of most mineral elements may be only half that obtained by parenteral administration. For some nutrients that are not readily stored in the body, or cannot be stored in large amounts, timing of administration may also be important. For example, amino acids cannot be used for protein synthesis if they are not supplied together; instead they will be used for energy production.

DISEASE

Specific dietary deficiency diseases include protein-calorie malnutrition; iron, iodine, and vitamin A deficiency; megaloblastic anemia due to vitamin B_{12} or folic acid deficiency; vitamin D–deficiency rickets; scurvy due to lack of ascorbic acid; beriberi due to lack of thiamine; and pellagra due to lack of niacin and protein (Chaps. 71 and 72). Each deficiency disease is characterized by imbalances at the cellular level between the supply of nutrients or energy and the body's nutritional needs for growth, maintenance, and other functions. Imbalances in nutrient intakes are recognized as risk factors for certain chronic degenerative diseases, such as saturated and trans-fat and cholesterol in coronary artery disease; sodium in hypertension; obesity in hormone-dependent endometrial and breast cancers; and ethanol in alcoholism. However, the etiology and pathogenesis of these disorders are multifactorial, and diet is only one of many risk factors. Osteoporosis, for example, is associated with calcium deficiency as well as risk factors related to environment (e.g., smoking, sedentary lifestyle), physiology (e.g., estrogen deficiency), genetic determinants (e.g., defects in collagen metabolism), and drug use (chronic steroids) (Chap. 348).

DIETARY ASSESSMENT

In clinical situations, nutritional assessment is an iterative process that involves (1) screening for malnutrition; (2) assessing food and dietary supplement intake, and establishing the absence or presence of malnutrition and its possible causes; and (3) planning for the most appropriate nutritional therapy. Some disease states affect the bioavailability, requirements, utilization, or excretion of specific nutrients. In these circumstances, specific measurements of various nutrients may be required to ensure adequate replacement (Chap. 72).

Most health care facilities have a nutrition screening process in place for identifying possible malnutrition after hospital admission. Nutritional screening is required by the Joint Commission on Accreditation of Healthcare Organizations (JCAHO), but there are no universally recognized or validated standards. The factors that are usually assessed include abnormal weight for height or body mass index (e.g., BMI <18.5 or >25); reported weight change (involuntary loss or gain of >5 kg in the past 6 months) (Chap. 41); diagnoses with known nutritional implications (metabolic disease, any disease affecting the gastrointestinal tract, alcoholism, and others); present therapeutic dietary prescription; chronic poor appetite; presence of chewing and swallowing problems or major food intolerances; need for assistance with preparing or shopping for food, eating, or other aspects of self care; and social isolation. Reassessment of nutrition status should occur periodically in hospitalized patients—at least once every week.

A more complete dietary assessment is indicated for patients who exhibit a high risk of malnutrition based on nutrition screening. The type of assessment varies with the clinical setting, severity of the patient's illness, and stability of his or her condition.

ACUTE CARE SETTINGS

Acute care settings, anorexia, various diseases, test procedures, and medications can compromise dietary intake. Under such circumstances, the goal is to identify and avoid inadequate intake and ensure appropriate alimentation. Dietary assessment focuses on what patients are currently eating, whether they are able and willing to eat, and whether they experience any problems with eating. Dietary intake assessment is based on information from observed intakes; medical record; history; clinical examination; and anthropometric, biochemical, and functional status. The objective is to gather enough information to establish the likelihood of malnutrition due to poor dietary intake or other causes and to assess whether nutritional therapy is indicated.

Simple observations may suffice to suggest inadequate oral intake. These include dietitians' and nurses' notes, the amount of food eaten on trays, frequent tests and procedures that are likely to cause meals to be skipped, nutritionally inadequate diet orders such as clear liquids or full liquids for more than a few days, fever, gastrointestinal distress, vomiting, diarrhea, a comatose state, and diseases or treatments that involve any part of the alimentary tract. Acutely ill patients with diet-related diseases such as diabetes require assessment because an inappropriate diet may exacerbate these conditions and adversely affect other therapies. Abnormal biochemical values [serum albumin levels <35 g/L (<3.5 mg/dL); serum cholesterol levels <3.9 mmol/L (<150 mg/dL)] are nonspecific but may also indicate a need for further nutritional assessment.

Most therapeutic diets offered in hospitals are calculated to meet individual nutrient requirements and the RDA. However, there are exceptions including clear liquids, some full liquid diets, and test diets, which are inadequate for several nutrients and should not be used, if possible, for more than 24 h. As much as half of the food served to hospitalized patients is not eaten, so it cannot be assumed that the intakes of hospitalized patients are adequate. Dietary assessment should compare how much and what food the patient has consumed with the diet that has been provided. Major deviations in intakes of energy, protein, fluids, or other nutrients of special concern for the patient's illness should be noted and corrected.

Nutritional monitoring is especially important for patients who are very ill and who have extended lengths of stay. Patients who are fed by special enteral and parenteral routes also require special nutritional assessment and monitoring by physicians with training in nutrition support and/or dietitians with certification in nutrition support (Chap. 73).

AMBULATORY SETTINGS

The aim of dietary assessment in the outpatient setting is to determine whether the patient's usual diet is a health risk in itself or if it contributes to existing chronic disease-related problems. Dietary assessment also provides the basis for planning a diet that fulfills therapeutic goals while ensuring patient adherence. The outpatient dietary assessment should review the adequacy of present and usual food intakes, including vitamin and mineral supplements, medications, and alcohol, as all of these may affect the patient's nutritional status. The assessment should focus on the dietary constituents that are most likely to be involved or compromised by a specific diagnosis, as well as any comorbidities that are present. More than one day's intake should be reviewed to provide a better representation of the usual diet.

There are many ways to assess the adequacy of the patient's habitual diet. These include a food guide, a food exchange list, a diet history, or a food frequency questionnaire. A commonly used food guide for healthy persons is the USDA's food pyramid, which is useful as a basis for identifying inadequate intakes of essential nutrients, as well as likely excesses in fat, saturated fat, sodium, sugar, and alcohol (Table 70-3). The guide is available online (*www.MyPyramid.gov*) and can be tailored to the needs of persons of different ages and life stages by varying the number of servings. The process of reviewing the guide with patients helps to identify food groups eaten in excess of recommendations or in insufficient quantities and helps them to transition to healthier dietary patterns. For those prescribed therapeutic diets, assessment against prescriptions stated as food exchange lists may be useful. These include, for example, the American Diabetes Association food exchange lists for diabetes, or the American Dietetic Association food exchange lists for renal disease.

TABLE 70-3 MY PYRAMID: THE USDA FOOD GUIDE PYRAMID FOR HEALTHY PERSONS

Servings and Examples of Standard Portion Sizes	Lower: 1600 kcal	Moderate: 2200 kcal	Higher: 2800 kcal
Fruits, cups	1.5	2	2.5
Vegetables, cups	2	3	3.5
Grains, oz eq (1 slice bread, 1 cup ready to eat cereal, 0.5 cup cooked rice, pasta, cooked cereal)	5	7	10
Meat and beans, oz eq (1 oz lean meat, poultry, or fish; 1 egg, 1 Tbsp. peanut butter, 0.25 cup cooked dry beans, or 0.5 oz nuts or seeds)	5	6	7
Milk, cups (1 cup milk or yogurt, 1.5 oz natural or 2 oz processed cheese)	3	3	3
Oils, tsp	5	6	8
Discretionary calorie allowance, kcal (remaining calories after accounting for all of the above)	132	290	426

Abbreviation: oz eq, ounce equivalent.
Source: Data from United States Department of Agriculture. *http://www.MyPyramid.com*

NUTRITIONAL STATUS ASSESSMENT

Full nutritional status assessment is reserved for seriously ill patients and those at very high nutritional risk when the cause of malnutrition is still uncertain after initial clinical evaluation and dietary assessment. It involves multiple dimensions, including documentation of dietary intake, anthropometric measurements, biochemical measurements of blood and urine, clinical examination, health history, and functional status. For further discussion of nutritional assessment, see Chap. 72.

GLOBAL CONSIDERATIONS

New nutrient-based terminologies with dietary reference intakes have been developed not only in North America, but in the United Kingdom and Europe, and by the World Health Organization/Food and Agricultural Organization of the United Nations (WHO/FAO). These different standards have many similarities in their basic concepts, definitions, and levels of nutrients recommended, but there are some differences, owing to assumptions made, functional criteria chosen, the timeliness of the evidence reviewed, and expert judgment.

FURTHER READINGS

Gibson RS: *Principles of Nutritional Assessment*, 2d ed. Oxford University Press, London, 2005

Murphy SP et al: Multivitamin-multimineral supplements' effect on total nutrient intake. Am J Clin Nutr 85(1): 280S, 2007

Shils ME et al (eds): *Modern Nutrition in Health and Disease*, 10th ed. Philadelphia, Lippincott Williams and Wilkins, 2005

71 Vitamin and Trace Mineral Deficiency and Excess

Robert M. Russell, Paolo M. Suter

Vitamins and trace minerals are required constituents of the human diet since they are either inadequately synthesized or not synthesized in the human body. Only small amounts of these substances are needed for carrying out essential biochemical reactions (e.g., acting as coenzymes or prosthetic groups). Overt vitamin or trace mineral deficiencies are rare in Western countries due to a plentiful, varied, and inexpensive food supply; however, multiple nutrient deficiencies may appear together in persons who are chronically ill or alcoholic. Moreover, subclinical vitamin and trace mineral deficiencies, as diagnosed by laboratory testing, are quite common in the normal population—especially in the geriatric age group.

Famine, emergency-affected and displaced populations, and refugees are at increased risk for protein-energy malnutrition and classic micronutrient deficiencies (vitamin A, iron, iodine), as well as for thiamine (beriberi), riboflavin, vitamin C (scurvy), and niacin (pellagra) overt deficiencies.

Body stores of vitamins and minerals vary tremendously. For example, vitamin B_{12} and vitamin A stores are large, and an adult may not become deficient for 1 or more years after being on a depleted diet. However, folate and thiamine may become depleted within weeks when eating a deficient diet. Therapeutic modalities can deplete essential nutrients from the body; for example, hemodialysis removes water-soluble vitamins, which must be replaced by supplementation.

There are several roles for vitamins and trace minerals in diseases: (1) deficiencies of vitamins and minerals may be caused by disease states such as malabsorption; (2) both deficiency and excess of vitamins and minerals can cause disease in and of themselves (e.g., vitamin A intoxication and liver disease); and (3) vitamins and minerals in high doses may be used as drugs (e.g., niacin for hypercholesterolemia). The hematologic-related vitamins and minerals (Chaps. 98, 100) are considered only briefly in this chapter, as are the bone-related vitamins and minerals (vitamin D, calcium, phosphorus; Chap. 346), since they are covered elsewhere (Tables 71-1, 71-2, and Fig. 71-1).

VITAMINS

THIAMINE (VITAMIN B_1)

Thiamine was the first B vitamin to be identified and is therefore also referred to as vitamin B_1. Thiamine functions in the decarboxylation of α-ketoacids, such as pyruvate α-ketoglutarate, and branched-chain amino acids and thus is a source of energy generation. In addition, thiamine pyrophosphate acts as a coenzyme for a transketolase reaction that mediates the conversion of hexose and pentose phosphates. It has also been postulated that thiamine plays a role in peripheral nerve conduction, although the exact chemical reactions underlying this function are unknown.

Food Sources The median intake of thiamine in the United States from food alone is 2 mg/d. Primary food sources for thiamine include yeast, organ meat, pork, legumes, beef, whole grains, and nuts. Milled rice or grains contain little thiamine, if any. Thiamine deficiency is therefore more common in cultures that rely heavily on a rice-based diet. Tea, coffee (regular and decaffeinated), raw fish, and shellfish contain thiaminases, which can destroy the vitamin. Thus, drinking large amounts of tea or coffee can theoretically lower thiamine body stores.

Deficiency Most dietary deficiency of thiamine worldwide is the result of poor dietary intake. In Western countries, the primary causes of thiamine deficiency are alcoholism and chronic illness, such as cancer. Alcohol interferes directly with the absorption of thiamine and with the synthesis of thiamine pyrophosphate. Thiamine should always be replenished when refeeding a patient with alcoholism, as carbohydrate repletion without adequate thiamine can precipitate acute thiamine deficiency. Other at-risk populations are women with prolonged hyperemesis gravidarum and anorexia, patients with an overall poor nutritional status on parenteral glucose, and patients on chronic diuretic therapy due to increased urinary thiamine losses. Maternal thiamine deficiency can lead to infantile beriberi in breast-fed children. Thiamine deficiency should also be considered in the setting of motor vehicle accidents associated with head injury.

Thiamine deficiency in its early stage induces anorexia and nonspecific symptoms (e.g., irritability, decrease in short-term memory). Prolonged thiamine deficiency causes beriberi, which is classically categorized as wet or dry, although there is considerable overlap. In either

TABLE 71-1 PRINCIPAL CLINICAL FINDINGS OF VITAMIN MALNUTRITION

Nutrient	Clinical Finding	Dietary Level per Day Associated with Overt Deficiency in Adults	Contributing Factors to Deficiency
Thiamine	Beriberi: neuropathy, muscle weakness and wasting, cardiomegaly, edema, ophthalmoplegia, confabulation	<0.3 mg/1000 kcal	Alcoholism, chronic diuretic use, hyperemesis
Riboflavin	Magenta tongue, angular stomatitis, seborrhea, cheilosis	<0.6 mg	—
Niacin	Pellagra: pigmented rash of sun-exposed areas, bright red tongue, diarrhea, apathy, memory loss, disorientation	<9.0 niacin equivalents	Alcoholism, vitamin B_6 deficiency, riboflavin deficiency, tryptophan deficiency
Vitamin B_6	Seborrhea, glossitis convulsions, neuropathy, depression, confusion, microcytic anemia	<0.2 mg	Alcoholism, isoniazid
Folate	Megaloblastic anemia, atrophic glossitis, depression, ↑ homocysteine	<100 μg/d	Alcoholism, sulfasalazine, pyrimethamine, triamterene
Vitamin B_{12}	Megaloblastic anemia, loss of vibratory and position sense, abnormal gait, dementia, impotence, loss of bladder and bowel control, ↑ homocysteine, ↑ methylmalonic acid	<1.0 μg/d	Gastric atrophy (pernicious anemia), terminal ileal disease, strict vegetarianism, acid reducing drugs (e.g., H_2 blockers)
Vitamin C	Scurvy: petechiae, ecchymosis, coiled hairs, inflamed and bleeding gums, joint effusion, poor wound healing, fatigue	<10 mg/d	Smoking, alcoholism
Vitamin A	Xerophthalmia, nightblindness, Bitot's spots, follicular hyperkeratosis, impaired embryonic development, immune dysfunction	<300 μg/d	Fat malabsorption, infection, measles, alcoholism, protein-energy malnutrition
Vitamin D	Rickets: skeletal deformation, rachitic rosary, bowed legs; osteomalacia	<2.0 μg/d	Aging, lack of sunlight exposure, fat malabsorption, deeply pigmented skin
Vitamin E	Peripheral neuropathy, spinocerebellar ataxia, skeletal muscle atrophy, retinopathy	Not described unless underlying contributing factor is present	Occurs only with fat malabsorption, or genetic abnormalities of vitamin E metabolism/transport
Vitamin K	Elevated prothrombin time, bleeding	<10 μg/d	Fat malabsorption, liver disease, antibiotic use

form of beriberi, patients may complain of pain and paresthesia. *Wet beriberi* presents primarily with cardiovascular symptoms, due to impaired myocardial energy metabolism and dysautonomia, and can occur after 3 months of a thiamine-deficient diet. Patients present with an enlarged heart, tachycardia, high-output congestive heart failure, peripheral edema, and peripheral neuritis. Patients with *dry beriberi* present with a symmetric peripheral neuropathy of the motor and sensory systems with diminished reflexes. The neuropathy affects the legs most markedly, and patients have difficulty rising from a squatting position.

Alcoholic patients with chronic thiamine deficiency may also have central nervous system (CNS) manifestations known as *Wernicke's encephalopathy*, consisting of horizontal nystagmus, ophthalmoplegia (due to weakness of one or more extraocular muscles), cerebellar ataxia, and mental impairment (Chap. 387). When there is an additional loss of memory and a confabulatory psychosis, the syndrome is known as *Wernicke-Korsakoff syndrome*. Despite the typical clinical picture and history, Wernicke-Korsakoff syndrome is underdiagnosed.

The laboratory diagnosis of thiamine deficiency is usually made by a functional enzymatic assay of transketolase activity measured before and after the addition of thiamine pyrophosphate. A >25% stimulation by the addition of thiamine pyrophosphate (an activity coefficient of 1.25) is taken as abnormal. Thiamine or the phosphorylated esters of thiamine in serum or blood can also be measured by high-performance liquid chromatography (HPLC) to detect deficiency.

℞ THIAMINE DEFICIENCY

In acute thiamine deficiency with either cardiovascular or neurologic signs, 100 mg/d of thiamine should be given parenterally for 7 days, followed by 10 mg/d orally until there is complete recovery. Cardiovascular improvement occurs within 24 h, and ophthalmoplegic improvement occurs within 24 h. Other manifestations gradually clear, although psychosis in Wernicke-Korsakoff syndrome may be permanent or persist for several months.

Toxicity Although anaphylaxis has been reported after high doses of thiamine, no adverse effects have been recorded from either food or supplements at high doses. Thiamine supplements may be bought over the counter in doses of up to 50 mg/d.

RIBOFLAVIN (VITAMIN B_2)

Riboflavin is important for the metabolism of fat, carbohydrate, and protein, reflecting its role as a respiratory coenzyme and an electron donor. Enzymes that contain flavin adenine dinucleotide (FAD) or flavin-mononucleotide (FMN) as prosthetic groups are known as *flavoenzymes* (e.g., succinic acid dehydrogenase, monoamine oxidase, glutathione reductase). FAD is a cofactor for methyltetrahydrofolate reductase and therefore modulates homocysteine metabolism. The vitamin also plays a role in drug and steroid metabolism, including detoxification reactions.

Although much is known about the chemical and enzymatic reactions of riboflavin, the clinical manifestations of riboflavin deficiency are nonspecific and similar to those of other B vitamin deficiencies. Riboflavin deficiency is manifested principally by lesions of the mucocutaneous surfaces of the mouth and skin (Table 71-1). In addition to the mucocutaneous lesions, corneal vascularization, anemia, and personality changes have been described with riboflavin deficiency.

Deficiency and Excess Riboflavin deficiency is almost always due to dietary deficiency. Milk, other dairy products, and enriched breads and cereals are the most important dietary sources of riboflavin in the United States, although lean meat, fish, eggs, broccoli, and legumes are also good sources. Riboflavin is extremely sensitive to light, and milk should be stored in containers that protect against photodegradation. Laboratory diagnosis of riboflavin deficiency can be made by measurement of red blood cell or urinary riboflavin concentrations or by measurement of erythrocyte glutathione reductase activity, with and without added FAD. Because the capacity of the gastrointestinal tract to absorb riboflavin is limited (~20 mg if given in one oral dose), riboflavin toxicity has not been described.

NIACIN (VITAMIN B_3)

The term *niacin* refers to nicotinic acid and nicotinamide and their biologically active derivatives. Nicotinic acid and nicotinamide serve as precursors of two coenzymes, nicotinamide adenine dinucleotide (NAD) and NAD phosphate (NADP), which are important in numerous oxidation and reduction reactions in the body. In addition, NAD and NADP are active in adenine diphosphate–ribose transfer reactions involved in DNA repair and calcium mobilization.

Metabolism and Requirements Nicotinic acid and nicotinamide are absorbed well from the stomach and small intestine. Niacin bioavailability is high from beans, milk, meat, and eggs; bioavailability from cereal grains is lower. Since flour is enriched with the "free" niacin (i.e., non-coenzyme form), bioavailability is excellent. Median intakes of niacin in the United States considerably exceed the recommended dietary allowance (RDA).

The amino acid tryptophan can be converted to niacin with an efficiency of 60:1 by weight. Thus, the RDA for niacin is expressed in niacin equivalents. A lower conversion of tryptophan to niacin occurs in vitamin B_6 and/or riboflavin deficiencies, or in the presence of isoniazid. The urinary excretion products of niacin include 2-pyridone and 2-methyl nicotinamide, measurements of which are used in diagnosis of niacin deficiency.

Deficiency Niacin deficiency causes *pellagra*, which is mostly found among people eating corn-based diets in parts of China, Africa, and India. Pellagra in North America is found mainly among alcoholics; in patients with congenital defects of intestinal and kidney absorption of tryptophan (Hartnup disease; Chap. 358); and in patients with carcinoid syndrome (Chap. 344), where there is increased conversion of tryptophan to serotonin. In the setting of famine or population displacement, the occurrence of pellagra results from the absolute lack of niacin but also the deficiency of micronutrients required for the conversion of tryptophan to niacin (e.g., iron, riboflavin, and pyridoxine). The early symptoms of pellagra include loss of appetite, generalized weakness and irritability, abdominal pain, and vomiting. Bright red glossitis then ensues, followed by a characteristic skin rash that is pigmented and scaling, particularly in skin areas exposed to sunlight. This rash is known as *Casal's necklace* because it forms a ring around the neck; it is seen in advanced cases. Vaginitis and esophagitis may also occur. Diarrhea (in part due to proctitis and in part due to malabsorption), depression, seizures, and dementia are also part of the pellagra syndrome—the four *D*s: *d*ermatitis, *d*iarrhea, and *d*ementia leading to *d*eath.

℞ PELLAGRA

Treatment of pellagra consists of oral supplementation of 100–200 mg of nicotinamide or nicotinic acid three times daily for 5 days. High doses of nicotinic acid (2 g/d in a time-release form) are used for the treatment of elevated cholesterol and triglyceride levels and/or low high-density lipoprotein (HDL) cholesterol level (Chap. 350).

Toxicity Prostaglandin-mediated flushing due to binding of the vitamin to a G protein–coupled receptor has been observed at daily doses as low as 50 mg of niacin when taken as a supplement or as therapy for dyslipidemia. There is no evidence of toxicity from niacin derived from food sources. Flushing always starts in the face and may be accompanied by skin dryness, itching, paresthesia, and headache. Premedication with aspirin may alleviate these symptoms. Flushing is subject to tachyphylaxis and often improves with time. Nausea, vomiting, and abdominal pain also occur at similar doses of niacin. Hepatic toxicity is the most serious toxic reaction due to niacin and may present as jaundice with elevated aspartate aminotransferase (AST) and alanine aminotransferase (ALT) levels. A few cases of fulminant hepatitis requiring liver transplantation have been reported at doses of

TABLE 71-2 DEFICIENCIES AND TOXICITIES OF METALS

Element	Deficiency	Toxicity	Tolerable Upper (Dietary) Intake Level
Boron	No biologic function determined	Developmental defects, male sterility, testicular atrophy	20 mg/d (extrapolated from animal data)
Calcium	Reduced bone mass, osteoporosis	Renal insufficiency (milk-alkalai syndrome), nephrolithiasis, impaired iron absorption	2500 mg/d (milk-alkalai)
Copper	Anemia, growth retardation, defective keratinization and pigmentation of hair, hypothermia, degenerative changes in aortic elastin, osteopenia, mental deterioration	Nausea, vomiting, diarrhea, hepatic failure, tremor, mental deterioration, hemolytic anemia, renal dysfunction	10 mg/d (liver toxicity)
Chromium	Impaired glucose tolerance	Occupational: renal failure, dermatitis, pulmonary cancer	ND
Fluoride	↑ Dental caries	Dental and skeletal fluorosis, osteosclerosis	10 mg/d (fluorosis)
Iodine	Thyroid enlargement, ↓ T_4, cretinism	Thyroid dysfunction, acne-like eruptions	1100 μg/d (thyroid dysfunction)
Iron	Muscle abnormalities, kilonychia, pica, anemia, ↓ work performance, impaired cognitive development, premature labor, ↑ perinatal maternal mortality	Gastrointestinal effects (nausea, vomiting, diarrhea, constipation), iron overload with organ damage, acute systemic toxicity	45 mg/d of elemental iron (GI side effects)
Manganese	Impaired growth and skeletal development, reproduction, lipid and carbohydrate metabolism; upper body rash	General: Neurotoxicity, Parkinson-like symptoms Occupational: Encephalitis-like syndrome, Parkinson-like syndrome, psychosis, pneumoconiosis	11 mg/d (neurotoxicity)
Molybdenum	Severe neurologic abnormalities	Reproductive and fetal abnormalities	2 mg/d extrapolated from animal data
Selenium	Cardiomyopathy, heart failure, striated muscle degeneration	General: Alopecia, nausea, vomiting, abnormal nails, emotional lability, peripheral neuropathy, lassitude, garlic odor to breath, dermatitis Occupational: Lung and nasal carcinomas, liver necrosis, pulmonary inflammation	400 μg/d (hair, nail changes)
Phosphorous	Rickets (osteomalacia), proximal muscle weakness, rhabdomyolysis, paresthesia, ataxia, seizure, confusion, heart failure, hemolysis, acidosis	Hyperphosphatemia	4000 mg/d
Zinc	Growth retardation, ↓ taste and smell, alopecia, dermatitis, diarrhea, immune dysfunction, failure to thrive, gonadal atrophy, congenital malformations	General: Reduced copper absorption, gastritis, sweating, fever, nausea, vomiting Occupational: Respiratory distress, pulmonary fibrosis	40 mg/d (impaired copper metabolism)

Note: ND, not determined; GI, gastrointestinal.

3–9 g/d. Other toxic reactions include glucose intolerance, hyperuricemia, macular edema, and macular cysts. The upper limit for daily niacin intake has been set at 35 mg. However, this upper limit does not pertain to the therapeutic use of niacin.

PYRIDOXINE (VITAMIN B_6)

Vitamin B_6 refers to a family of compounds including pyridoxine, pyridoxal, pyridoxamine, and their 5′-phosphate derivatives. 5′-Pyridoxal phosphate (PLP) is a cofactor for more than 100 enzymes involved in amino acid metabolism. Vitamin B_6 is also involved in heme and neurotransmitter synthesis and in the metabolism of glycogen, lipids, steroids, sphingoid bases, and several vitamins, including the conversion of tryptophan to niacin.

Dietary Sources Plants contain vitamin B_6 in the form of pyridoxine, whereas animal tissues contain PLP and pyridoxamine phosphate. The vitamin B_6 contained in plants is less bioavailable than that from animal tissues. Rich food sources of vitamin B_6 include legumes, nuts, wheat bran, and meat, although it is present in all food groups.

Deficiency Symptoms of vitamin B_6 deficiency include epithelial changes, as seen frequently with other B vitamin deficiencies. In addition, severe vitamin B_6 deficiency can lead to peripheral neuropathy, abnormal electroencephalograms, and personality changes including depression and confusion. In infants, diarrhea, seizures, and anemia have been reported. Microcytic, hypochromic anemia is due to diminished hemoglobin synthesis, since the first enzyme involved in heme biosynthesis (aminolevulinate synthase) requires PLP as a cofactor (Chap. 98). In some case reports, platelet dysfunction has also been reported. Since vitamin B_6 is necessary for the conversion of homocysteine to cystathionine, it is possible that chronic low-grade vitamin B_6 deficiency may result in hyperhomocysteinemia and increased risk of cardiovascular disease (Chaps. 235, 358). Independent of homocysteine, low levels of circulating vitamin B_6 have also been associated with inflammation and elevated C-reactive protein levels.

Vitamin	Active derivative or cofactor form	Principal function
Thiamine (B_1) 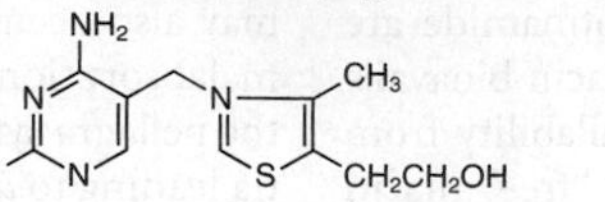	Thiamine pyrophosphate	Coenzyme for cleavage of carbon-carbon bonds; amino acid and carbohydrate metabolism
Riboflavin (B_2) 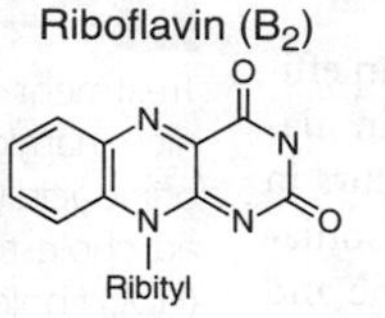	Flavin mononucleotide (FMN) and flavin adenine dinucleotide (FAD)	Cofactor for oxidation, reduction reactions, and covalently attached prosthetic groups for some enzymes
Niacin 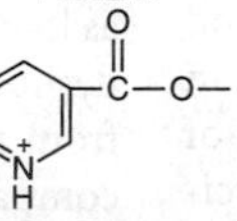	Nicotinamide adenine dinucleotide phosphate (NADP) and nicotinamide adenine dinucleotide (NAD)	Coenzymes for oxidation and reduction reactions
Vitamin B_6 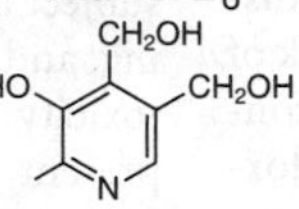	Pyridoxal phosphate	Cofactor for enzymes of amino acid metabolism
Folate 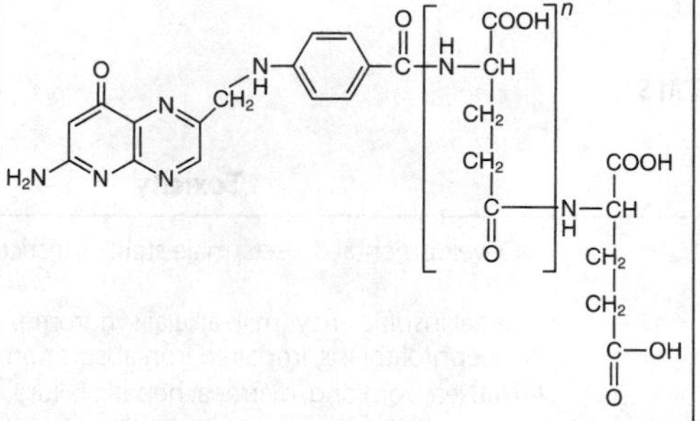	Polyglutamate forms of (5, 6, 7, 8) tetrahydrofolate with carbon unit attachments	Coenzyme for one carbon transfer in nucleic acid and amino acid metabolism
Vitamin B_{12} 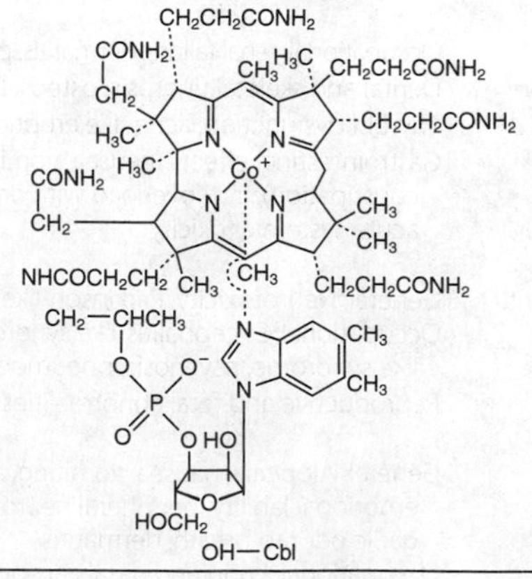	Methylcobalamine Adenosylcobalamin	Coenzyme for methionine synthase and L-methylmalonyl-CoA mutase

FIGURE 71-1 The structures and principal functions of vitamins associated with human disorders.

Certain medications such as isoniazid, L-dopa, penicillamine, and cycloserine interact with PLP due to a reaction with carbonyl groups. Pyridoxine should be given concurrently with isoniazid to avoid neuropathy. The increased ratio of AST (or SGOT) to ALT (or SGPT) seen in alcoholic liver disease reflects the relative vitamin B_6 dependence of ALT. Vitamin B_6 dependency syndromes that require pharmacologic doses of vitamin B_6 are rare; they include cystathionine β-synthase deficiency, pyridoxine-responsive (primarily sideroblastic) anemias, and gyrate atrophy with chorioretinal degeneration due to decreased activity of the mitochondrial enzyme ornithine aminotransferase. In these situations, 100–200 mg/d of oral vitamin B_6 is required for treatment.

High doses of vitamin B_6 have been used to treat carpal tunnel syndrome, premenstrual syndrome, schizophrenia, autism, and diabetic neuropathy but have not been found to be effective.

Vitamin	Active derivative or cofactor form	Principal function
Vitamin C 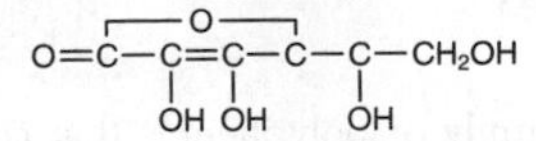	Ascorbic acid and dehydrascorbic acid	Participation as a redox ion in many biological oxidation and hydrogen transfer reactions
Vitamin A 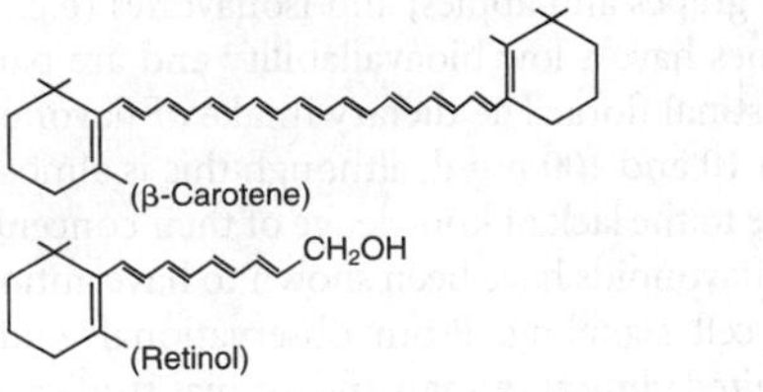	Retinol, retinaldehyde, and retinoic acid	Formation of rhodopsin (vision) and glycoproteins (epithelial cell function); also regulates gene transcription
Vitamin D 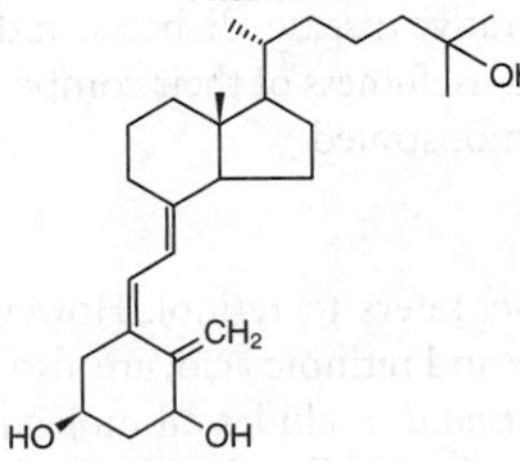	1, 25-Dihydroxyvitamin D	Maintenance of blood calcium and phosphorous levels; antiproliferative hormone
Vitamin E 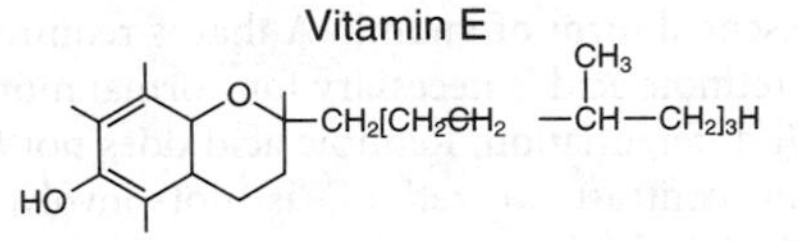	Tocopherols and tocotrienols	Antioxidants
Vitamin K 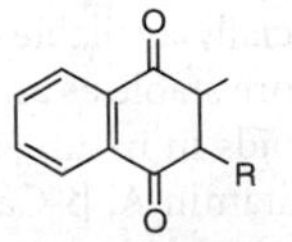	Vitamin K hydroquinone	Cofactor for posttranslation carboxylation of many proteins including essential clotting factors

FIGURE 71-1 (***Continued***) **The structures and principal functions of vitamins** associated with human disorders.

The laboratory diagnosis of vitamin B_6 deficiency is generally made on the basis of low plasma PLP values (<20 nmol/L). Treatment of vitamin B_6 deficiency is 50 mg/d; higher doses of 100–200 mg/d are given if vitamin B_6 deficiency is related to medication use. Vitamin B_6 should not be given with L-dopa, since the vitamin interferes with the action of this drug.

Toxicity The safe upper limit for vitamin B_6 has been set at 100 mg/d, although no adverse effects have been associated with high intakes of vitamin B_6 from food sources only. When toxicity occurs, it causes a severe sensory neuropathy, leaving patients unable to walk. Some cases of photosensitivity and dermatitis have also been reported.

FOLATE, VITAMIN B_{12}

See Chap. 100.

VITAMIN C

Both ascorbic acid and its oxidized product dehydroascorbic acid are biologically active. Actions of vitamin C include antioxidant activity, promotion of nonheme iron absorption, carnitine biosynthesis, the conversion of dopamine to norepinephrine, and the synthesis of many peptide hormones. Vitamin C is also important for connective tissue metabolism and cross-linking (proline hydroxylation), and it is a component of many drug-metabolizing enzyme systems, particularly the mixed-function oxidase systems.

Absorption and Dietary Sources Almost complete absorption of vitamin C occurs if <100 mg is administered in a single dose; however, only 50% or less is absorbed at doses >1 g. Enhanced degradation and fecal and urinary excretion of vitamin C occur at higher intake levels.

Good dietary sources of vitamin C include citrus fruits, green vegetables (especially broccoli), tomatoes, and potatoes. Consumption of five servings of fruits and vegetables a day provides vitamin C in excess of the RDA, 90 mg/d for males and 75 mg/d for females. In addition, approximately 40% of the U.S. population consumes vitamin C as a dietary supplement in which "natural forms" of vitamin C are no more bioavailable than synthetic forms. Smoking, hemodialysis, pregnancy, and stress (e.g., infection, trauma) appear to increase vitamin C requirements.

Deficiency Vitamin C deficiency causes scurvy. In the United States, this is seen primarily among the poor and elderly, in alcoholics who consume <10 mg/d of vitamin C, and also in individuals consuming macrobiotic diets. In addition to generalized fatigue, symptoms of scurvy primarily reflect impaired formation of mature connective tissue and include bleeding into skin (petechiae, ecchymoses, perifollicular hemorrhages); inflamed and bleeding gums; and manifestations of bleeding into joints, the peritoneal cavity, pericardium, and the adrenal glands. In children, vitamin C deficiency may cause impaired bone growth. Laboratory diagnosis of vitamin C deficiency is made on the basis of low plasma or leukocyte levels.

Administration of vitamin C (200 mg/d) improves the symptoms of scurvy within a matter of several days. High-dose vitamin C supplementation (e.g., 1–2 g/d) might slightly decrease the symptoms and duration of upper respiratory tract infections. Vitamin C supplementation has also been reported to be useful in Chédiak-Higashi syndrome (Chap. 61) and osteogenesis imperfecta (Chap. 357). Diets high in vitamin C have been claimed to lower the incidence of certain cancers, particularly esophageal and gastric cancers. If proved, this effect may be due to the fact that vitamin C can prevent the conversion of nitrites and secondary amines to carcinogenic nitrosamines. However, one intervention study from China did not show vitamin C to be protective.

Toxicity Taking >2 g of vitamin C in a single dose may result in abdominal pain, diarrhea, and nausea. Since vitamin C may be metabolized to oxalate, it is feared that chronic, high-dose vitamin C supplementation could result in an increased prevalence of kidney stones. However, this has not been borne out in several trials, except in patients with preexisting renal disease. Thus, it is reasonable to advise patients with a past history of kidney stones to not take large doses of vitamin C. There is also an unproven but possible risk that chronic high doses of vitamin C could promote iron overload in patients taking supplemental iron. High doses of vitamin C can induce hemolysis in patients with glucose-6-phosphate dehydrogenase deficiency, and doses >1 g/d can cause false-negative guaiac reactions as well as interfere with tests for urinary glucose.

BIOTIN

Biotin is a water-soluble vitamin that plays a role in gene expression, gluconeogenesis, and fatty acid synthesis and serves as a CO_2 carrier on the surface of both cytosolic and mitochondrial carboxylase enzymes. The vitamin also functions in the catabolism of specific amino acids (e.g., leucine). Excellent food sources of biotin include organ meat such as liver or kidney, soy, beans, yeast, and egg yolks; however, egg white contains the protein avidin, which strongly binds the vitamin and reduces its bioavailability.

Biotin deficiency due to low dietary intake is rare; rather, deficiency is due to inborn errors of metabolism. Biotin deficiency has been induced by experimental feeding of egg white diets and in patients with short bowels who received biotin-free parenteral nutrition. In the adult, biotin deficiency results in mental changes (depression, hallucinations), paresthesia, anorexia, and nausea. A scaling, seborrheic, and erythematous rash may occur around the eyes, nose, and mouth as well as on the extremities. In infants, biotin deficiency presents as hypotonia, lethargy, and apathy. In addition, the infant may develop alopecia and a characteristic rash that includes the ears. The laboratory diagnosis of biotin deficiency can be established based on a decreased urinary concentration or an increased urinary excretion of 3-hydroxyisovaleric acid after a leucine challenge. Treatment requires pharmacologic doses of biotin, using up to 10 mg/d. No toxicity is known.

PANTOTHENIC ACID (VITAMIN B_5)

Pantothenic acid is a component of coenzyme A and phosphopantetheine, which are involved in fatty acid metabolism and the synthesis of cholesterol, steroid hormones, and all compounds formed from isoprenoid units. In addition, pantothenic acid is involved in the acetylation of proteins. The vitamin is excreted in the urine, and the laboratory diagnosis of deficiency is made on the basis of low urinary vitamin levels.

The vitamin is ubiquitous in the food supply. Liver, yeast, egg yolks, whole grains, and vegetables are particularly good sources. Human pantothenic acid deficiency has been demonstrated only in experimental feeding of diets low in pantothenic acid or by giving a specific pantothenic acid antagonist. The symptoms of pantothenic acid deficiency are nonspecific and include gastrointestinal disturbance, depression, muscle cramps, paresthesia, ataxia, and hypoglycemia. Pantothenic acid deficiency is believed to have caused the burning feet syndrome seen in prisoners of war during World War II. No toxicity of this vitamin has been reported.

CHOLINE

Choline is a precursor for acetylcholine, phospholipids, and betaine. Choline is necessary for the structural integrity of cell membranes, cholinergic neurotransmission, lipid and cholesterol metabolism, methyl-group metabolism, and transmembrane signaling. Recently, a recommended adequate intake was set at 550 mg/d for adult males and 425 mg/d for adult females, although certain genetic polymorphisms can increase an individual's requirement for choline. Choline is thought to be a "conditionally essential" nutrient, in that de novo synthesis occurs in the liver and is less than the vitamin's utilization only under certain stress conditions (e.g., alcoholic liver disease). The dietary requirement of choline depends on the status of other methyl-group donors (folate, vitamin B_{12}, and methionine) and thus varies widely. Choline is widely distributed in food (e.g., egg yolk, wheat germ, organ meat, milk) in the form of lecithin (phosphatidylcholine). Choline deficiency has occurred in patients receiving parenteral nutrition devoid of choline. Deficiency results in fatty liver, elevated transaminase levels, and skeletal muscle damage with high creatine phosphokinase values. The diagnosis of choline deficiency is currently made on the basis of low plasma levels, although nonspecific conditions (e.g., heavy exercise) may suppress plasma levels.

Toxicity from choline results in hypotension, cholinergic sweating, diarrhea, salivation, and a fishy body odor. The upper limit for choline has been set at 3.5 g/d. Therapeutically, choline has been suggested for patients with dementia and for patients at high risk of cardiovascular disease, due to its ability to lower cholesterol and homocysteine levels. However, such benefits have yet to be documented. Choline- and betaine-restricted diets are of therapeutic value in trimethylaminuria (fish odor syndrome).

FLAVONOIDS

Flavonoids constitute a large family of polyphenols that contribute to the aroma, taste, and color of fruits and vegetables. Major groups of dietary flavonoids include anthocyanidins in berries; catechins in green tea and chocolate; flavonols (e.g., quercitin) in broccoli, kale, leeks, onion, and the skins of grapes and apples; and isoflavones (e.g., genistein) in legumes. Isoflavones have a low bioavailability and are partially metabolized by the intestinal flora. The dietary intake of flavonoids is estimated to be between 10 and 100 mg/d, although this is almost certainly an underestimate due to the lack of knowledge of their concentrations in many foods. Several flavonoids have been shown to have antioxidant activity and to affect cell signaling. From observational epidemiologic studies and from limited clinical human and animal studies, flavonoids have been postulated to play a role in the prevention of several chronic diseases, including neurodegenerative disease, diabetes, and osteoporosis. The ultimate importance and usefulness of their compounds against human disease have yet to be demonstrated.

VITAMIN A

Vitamin A, in the strictest sense, refers to retinol. However, the oxidized metabolites, retinaldehyde and retinoic acid, are also biologically active compounds. The term *retinoids* includes all molecules (including synthetic molecules) that are chemically related to retinol. Retinaldehyde (11-*cis*) is the essential form of vitamin A that is required for normal vision, whereas retinoic acid is necessary for normal morphogenesis, growth, and cell differentiation. Retinoic acid does not function in vision and, in contrast to retinol, is not involved in reproduction. Vitamin A also plays a role in iron utilization, humoral immunity, T cell–mediated immunity, natural killer cell activity, and phagocytosis. Vitamin A is commercially available in esterified forms (e.g., acetate, palmitate) since it is more stable as an ester.

There are more than 600 carotenoids in nature, and approximately 50 of these can be metabolized to vitamin A. β-Carotene is the most prevalent carotenoid in the food supply that has provitamin A activity. In humans, significant fractions of carotenoids are absorbed intact and are stored in liver and fat. It is now estimated that 12 μg or greater of dietary β-carotene is equivalent to 1 μg of retinol, whereas 24 μg or greater of other dietary provitamin A carotenoids (e.g., cryptoxanthin, α-carotene) is equivalent to 1 μg of retinol.

Metabolism The liver contains approximately 90% of the vitamin A reserves and secretes vitamin A in the form of retinol, which is bound to retinol-binding protein. Once this has occurred, the retinol-binding protein complex interacts with a second protein, transthyretin. This trimolecular complex functions to prevent vitamin A from being filtered by the kidney glomerulus, to protect the body against the toxicity of retinol and to allow retinol to be taken up by specific cell-surface receptors that recognize retinol-binding protein. A certain amount of vitamin A enters peripheral cells even if it is not bound to retinol-binding protein. After retinol is internalized by the cell, it becomes bound to a series of cellular retinol-binding proteins, which function as sequestering and transporting agents as well as co-ligands for enzymatic reactions. Certain cells also contain retinoic acid–binding proteins, which have sequestering functions but also shuttle retinoic acid to the nucleus and enable its metabolism.

Retinoic acid is a ligand for certain nuclear receptors that act as transcription factors. Two families of receptors (RAR and RXR receptors) are active in retinoid-mediated gene transcription. Retinoid receptors regulate transcription by binding as dimeric complexes to specific DNA sites, the retinoic acid response elements, in target genes (Chap. 332). The receptors can either stimulate or repress gene expression in response to their ligands. RAR binds all-*trans* retinoic acid and 9-*cis* retinoic acid, whereas RXR binds only 9-*cis* retinoic acid.

The retinoid receptors play an important role in controlling cell proliferation and differentiation. Retinoic acid is useful in the treatment of promyelocytic leukemia (Chap. 104) and is also used in the treatment of cystic acne because it inhibits keratinization, decreases sebum secretion, and possibly alters the inflammatory reaction (Chap. 53). RXRs dimerize with other nuclear receptors to function as coregulators of genes responsive to retinoids, thyroid hormone, and calcitriol. RXR agonists induce insulin sensitivity experimentally, perhaps because RXR is a cofactor for the peroxisome-proliferator-activated receptors (PPARs), which are targets for the thiazolidinedione drugs such as rosiglitazone and troglitazone (Chap. 338).

Dietary Sources The retinol activity equivalent (RAE) is used to express the vitamin A value of food. One RAE is defined as 1 μg of retinol (0.003491 mmol), 12 μg of β-carotene, and 24 μg of other provitamin A carotenoids. In older literature, vitamin A was often expressed in international units (IU), with 1 RAE being equal to 3.33 IU of retinol and 20 IU of β-carotene, but these units are no longer in current scientific use.

Liver, fish, and eggs are excellent food sources for preformed vitamin A; vegetable sources of provitamin A carotenoids include dark green and deeply colored fruits and vegetables. Moderate cooking of vegetables enhances carotenoid release for uptake in the gut. Carotenoid absorption is also aided by some fat in a meal. Infants are particularly susceptible to vitamin A deficiency because neither breast nor cow's milk supplies enough vitamin A to prevent deficiency. In developing countries, chronic dietary deficit is the main cause of vitamin A deficiency and is exacerbated by infection. In early childhood, low vitamin A status results from inadequate intakes of animal food sources and edible oils, both of which are expensive, coupled with seasonal unavailability of vegetables and fruits, and lack of marketed fortified food products. Concurrent zinc deficiency can interfere with the mobilization of vitamin A from liver stores. Alcohol interferes with the conversion of retinol to retinaldehyde in the eye by competing for alcohol (retinol) dehydrogenase. Drugs that interfere with the absorption of vitamin A include mineral oil, neomycin, and cholestyramine.

Deficiency Vitamin A deficiency is endemic where diets are chronically poor, especially in Southern Asia, Sub-Saharan Africa, some areas of Latin America, and the Western Pacific, including parts of China. Vitamin A status is usually assessed by measuring serum retinol [normal range, 1.05–3.50 μmol/L (30–100 μg/dL)] or blood spot retinol or by tests of dark adaptation. Stable isotopic or invasive liver biopsy methods exist to estimate total body stores of vitamin A. Based on deficient serum retinol [<0.70 μmol/L (20 μg/dL)], there are more than 125 million preschool-age children with vitamin A deficiency, among whom ~4 million have an ocular manifestation of deficiency termed *xerophthalmia*. This condition includes milder stages of night blindness and conjunctival xerosis (dryness) with Bitot's spots (white patches of keratinized epithelium appearing on the sclera) as well as rare, potentially blinding corneal ulceration and necrosis. Keratomalacia (softening of the cornea) leads to corneal scarring that blinds at least a quarter of a million children each year and is associated with a fatality rate of 4–25%. However, vitamin A deficiency at any stage poses an increased risk of mortality from diarrhea, dysentery, measles, malaria, and respiratory disease. Vitamin A deficiency can compromise barrier and innate and acquired immune defenses to infection. Vitamin A supplementation can markedly reduce risk of child mortality (23–34%, on average) where deficiency is widely prevalent. About 10% of pregnant women in undernourished settings also develop night blindness, assessed by history, during the latter half of pregnancy and this moderate vitamin A deficiency is associated with an increased risk of maternal infection and mortality.

Rx VITAMIN A DEFICIENCY

Any stage of xerophthalmia should be treated with 60 mg of vitamin A in oily solution, usually contained in a soft-gel capsule. The same dose is repeated 1 and 14 days later. Doses should be reduced by half for patients 6–11 months of age. Mothers with night blindness or Bitot's spots should be given vitamin A orally, either 3 mg daily or 7.5 mg twice a week for 3 months. These regimens are efficacious, and they are less expensive and more widely available than injectable water-miscible vitamin A. A common approach to prevention is to supplement young children living in high-risk areas with 60 mg every 4–6 months, with a half-dose given to infants 6–11 months of age.

Uncomplicated vitamin A deficiency rarely occurs in industrialized countries. One high-risk group, extremely low-birth-weight infants (<1000 g), is likely to be vitamin A–deficient and should be supplemented with 1500 μg (or RAE) of vitamin A, three times a week for 4 weeks. Severe measles in any society can lead to secondary vitamin A deficiency. Children hospitalized with measles should receive two 60-mg doses of vitamin A on two consecutive days. Vitamin A deficiency most often occurs in patients with malabsorptive diseases (e.g., celiac sprue, short-bowel syndrome), who have abnormal dark adaptation or symptoms of night blindness without other ocular changes. Typically, such patients are treated for 1 month with 15 mg/d of a water-miscible preparation of vitamin A. This is followed by a lower maintenance dose with the exact amount determined by monitoring serum retinol.

There are no specific deficiency signs or symptoms that result from carotenoid deficiency. It was postulated that β-carotene would be an effective chemopreventive agent for cancer because numerous epidemiologic studies had shown that diets high in β-carotene were associated with lower incidences of cancers of the respiratory and digestive systems. However, intervention studies in smokers found that treatment with high doses of β-carotene actually resulted in more lung cancers than did treatment with placebo. Non–provitamin A carotenoids, such as lutein and zeaxanthin, have been suggested to protect against macular degeneration. The non–provitamin A carotenoid lycopene has been proposed to protect against prostate cancer. However, the effectiveness of these agents has not been proven by intervention studies, and the mechanisms underlying these purported biologic actions are unknown.

Toxicity Acute toxicity of vitamin A was first noted in Arctic explorers who ate polar bear liver and has also been seen after administration of 150 mg in adults or 100 mg in children. Acute toxicity is manifested by increased intracranial pressure, vertigo, diplopia, bulging fontanels in children, seizures, and exfoliative dermatitis; it may result in death. In children being treated for vitamin A deficiency according to the protocols outlined above, transient bulging of fontanels occurs in 2% of infants, and transient nausea, vomiting, and headache occur in 5% of preschoolers. Chronic vitamin A intoxication is largely a concern in industrialized countries and has been seen in normal adults who ingest 15 mg/d and children who ingest 6 mg/d of vitamin A over a period of several months. Manifestations include dry skin, cheilosis, glossitis, vomiting, alopecia, bone demineralization and pain, hypercalcemia, lymph node enlargement, hyperlipidemia, amenorrhea, and features of pseudotumor cerebri with increased intracranial pressure and papilledema. Liver fibrosis with portal hypertension and bone demineralization may result from chronic vitamin A intoxication. When vitamin A is provided in excess to pregnant women, congenital malformations have included spontaneous abortions, craniofacial abnormalities, and valvular heart disease. In pregnancy, the daily dose of vitamin A should not exceed 3 mg. Commercially available retinoid derivatives are also toxic, including 13-*cis*-retinoic acid, which has been associated with birth defects. As a result, contraception should be continued for a least 1 year, and possibly longer, in women who have taken 13-*cis* retinoic acid.

High doses of carotenoids do not result in toxic symptoms but should be avoided in smokers due to an increased risk of lung cancer. Carotenemia, which is characterized by a yellowing of the skin (creases of the palms and soles) but not the sclerae, may be present after ingestion of >30 mg of β-carotene daily. Hypothyroid patients are particularly susceptible to the development of carotenemia due to impaired breakdown of carotene to vitamin A. Reduction of carotenes from the diet results in the disappearance of skin yellowing and carotenemia over a period of 30–60 days.

VITAMIN D

See Chap. 346, Fig. 71-1, and Table 71-1.

VITAMIN E

Vitamin E is a collective name for all stereoisomers of tocopherols and tocotrienols, although only the 2R tocopherols meet human requirements. Vitamin E acts as a chain-breaking antioxidant and is an efficient pyroxyl radical scavenger, which protects low-density lipoproteins (LDLs) and polyunsaturated fats in membranes from oxidation. A network of other antioxidants (e.g., vitamin C, glutathione) and enzymes maintains vitamin E in a reduced state. Vitamin E also inhibits prostaglandin synthesis and the activities of protein kinase C and phospholipase A_2.

Absorption and Metabolism After absorption, vitamin E is taken up from chylomicrons by the liver, and a hepatic α tocopherol transport protein mediates intracellular vitamin E transport and incorporation into very low-density lipoprotein (VLDL). The transport protein has particular affinity for the RRR isomeric form of α tocopherol; thus this natural isomer has the most biologic activity.

Requirement Vitamin E is widely distributed in the food supply and is particularly high in sunflower oil, safflower oil, and wheat germ oil; γ tocotrienols are notably present in soybean and corn oils. Vitamin E is also found in meats, nuts, and cereal grains, and small amounts are present in fruits and vegetables. Vitamin E pills containing doses of 50–1000 mg are ingested by a large fraction of the U.S. population. The RDA for vitamin E is 15 mg/d (34.9 μmol or 22.5 IU) for all adults. Diets high in polyunsaturated fats may necessitate a slightly higher requirement for vitamin E.

Dietary deficiency of vitamin E does not exist. Vitamin E deficiency is seen in only severe and prolonged malabsorptive diseases, such as celiac disease, or after small-intestinal resection. Children with cystic fibrosis or prolonged cholestasis may develop vitamin E deficiency characterized by areflexia and hemolytic anemia. Children with abetalipoproteinemia cannot absorb or transport vitamin E and become deficient quite rapidly. A familial form of isolated vitamin E deficiency also exists; it is due to a defect in the α tocopherol transport protein. Vitamin E deficiency causes axonal degeneration of the large myelinated axons and results in posterior column and spinocerebellar symptoms. Peripheral neuropathy is initially characterized by areflexia, with progression to an ataxic gait, and by decreased vibration and position sensations. Ophthalmoplegia, skeletal myopathy, and pigmented retinopathy may also be features of vitamin E deficiency. Either vitamin E or selenium deficiency in the host has been shown to increase certain viral mutations and, therefore, virulence. The laboratory diagnosis of vitamin E deficiency is made on the basis of low blood levels of α tocopherol (<5 μg/mL, or <0.8 mg of α tocopherol per gram of total lipids).

℞ VITAMIN E DEFICIENCY

Symptomatic vitamin E deficiency should be treated with 800–1200 mg of α tocopherol per day. Patients with abetalipoproteinemia may need as much as 5000–7000 mg/d. Children with symptomatic vitamin E deficiency should be treated with 400 mg/d orally of water-miscible esters; alternatively, 2 mg/kg per d may be administered intramuscularly. Vitamin E in high doses may protect against oxygen-induced retrolental fibroplasia and bronchopulmonary dysplasia, as well as intraventricular hemorrhage of prematurity. Vitamin E has been suggested to increase sexual performance, to treat intermittent claudication, and to slow the aging process, but evidence for these properties is lacking. When given in combination with other antioxidants, vitamin E may help to prevent macular degeneration. High doses (60–800 mg/d) of vitamin E have been shown in controlled trials to improve parameters of immune function and to reduce colds in nursing home residents, but intervention studies using vitamin E to prevent cardiovascular disease or cancer have not shown efficacy and, at doses >400 mg/d, may even increase all-cause mortality.

Toxicity All forms of vitamin E are absorbed and could contribute to toxicity. High doses of vitamin E (>800 mg/d) may reduce platelet aggregation and interfere with vitamin K metabolism and are therefore contraindicated in patients taking warfarin. Nausea, flatulence, and diarrhea have been reported at doses >1 g/d.

VITAMIN K

There are two natural forms of vitamin K: vitamin K_1, also known as *phylloquinone*, from vegetable and animal sources, and vitamin K_2, or *menaquinone*, which is synthesized by bacterial flora and found in hepatic tissue. Phylloquinone can be converted to menaquinone in some organs.

Vitamin K is required for the posttranslational carboxylation of glutamic acid, which is necessary for calcium binding to γ-carboxylated proteins such as prothrombin (factor II); factors VII, IX, and X; protein C; protein S; and proteins found in bone (osteocalcin) and vascular smooth muscle (e.g., matrix Gla protein). However, the importance of vitamin K for bone mineralization and prevention of vascular calcification is not known. Warfarin-type drugs inhibit γ-carboxylation by preventing the conversion of vitamin K to its active hydroquinone form.

Dietary Sources Vitamin K is found in green leafy vegetables such as kale and spinach, and appreciable amounts are also present in margarine and liver. Vitamin K is present in vegetable oils and is particularly rich in olive, canola, and soybean oils. The average daily intake by Americans is estimated to be approximately 100 μg/d.

Deficiency The symptoms of vitamin K deficiency are due to hemorrhage, and newborns are particularly susceptible because of low fat stores, low breast milk levels of vitamin K, sterility of the infantile intestinal tract, liver immaturity, and poor placental transport. Intracranial bleeding, as well as gastrointestinal and skin bleeding, can occur in vitamin K–deficient infants 1–7 days after birth. Thus, vitamin K (1 mg IM) is given prophylactically at the time of delivery.

Vitamin K deficiency in adults may be seen in patients with chronic small-intestinal disease (e.g., celiac disease, Crohn's disease), in those with obstructed biliary tracts, or after small-bowel resection. Broad-spectrum antibiotic treatment can precipitate vitamin K deficiency by reducing gut bacteria, which synthesize menaquinones, and by inhibiting the metabolism of vitamin K. In patients with warfarin therapy, the antiobesity drug orlistat can lead to INR changes due to vitamin K malabsorption. The diagnosis of vitamin K deficiency is usually made on the basis of an elevated prothrombin time or reduced clotting factors, although vitamin K may also be measured directly by HPLC. Vitamin K deficiency is treated using a parenteral dose of 10 mg. For patients with chronic malabsorption, 1–2 mg/d of vitamin K should be given orally, or 1–2 mg/week can be taken parenterally. Patients with liver disease may have an elevated prothrombin time because of liver cell destruction as well as vitamin K deficiency. If an elevated prothrombin time does not improve on vitamin K therapy, it can be deduced that it is not the result of vitamin K deficiency.

Toxicity Toxicity from dietary phylloquinones and menaquinones has not been described. High doses of vitamin K can impair the actions of oral anticoagulants.

MINERALS

Table 71-2.

CALCIUM

See Chap. 346.

ZINC

Zinc is an integral component of many metalloenzymes in the body; it is involved in the synthesis and stabilization of proteins, DNA, and

RNA and plays a structural role in ribosomes and membranes. Zinc is necessary for the binding of steroid hormone receptors and several other transcription factors to DNA. Zinc is absolutely required for normal spermatogenesis, fetal growth, and embryonic development.

Absorption The absorption of zinc from the diet is inhibited by dietary phytate, fiber, oxalate, iron, and copper, as well as by certain drugs including penicillamine, sodium valproate, and ethambutol. Meat, shellfish, nuts, and legumes are good sources of bioavailable zinc, whereas zinc in grains and legumes is less available for absorption.

Deficiency Mild zinc deficiency has been described in many diseases, including diabetes mellitus, HIV/AIDS, cirrhosis, alcoholism, inflammatory bowel disease, malabsorption syndromes, and sickle cell disease. In these diseases, mild chronic zinc deficiency can cause stunted growth in children, decreased taste sensation (hypogeusia), and impaired immune function. Severe chronic zinc deficiency has been described as a cause of hypogonadism and dwarfism in several Middle Eastern countries. In these children, hypopigmented hair is also part of the syndrome. Acrodermatitis enteropathica is a rare autosomal recessive disorder characterized by abnormalities in zinc absorption. Clinical manifestations include diarrhea, alopecia, muscle wasting, depression, irritability, and a rash involving the extremities, face, and perineum. The rash is characterized by vesicular and pustular crusting with scaling and erythema. Occasional patients with Wilson's disease have developed zinc deficiency as a consequence of penicillamine therapy (Chap. 354).

The diagnosis of zinc deficiency is usually made by a serum zinc level of <12 μmol/L (<70 μg/dL). Pregnancy and birth control pills may cause a slight depression in serum zinc levels, and hypoalbuminemia from any cause can result in hypozincemia. In acute stress situations, zinc may be redistributed from serum into tissues. Zinc deficiency may be treated with 60 mg elemental zinc, orally twice a day. Zinc gluconate lozenges (13 mg elemental zinc every 2 h while awake) have been reported to reduce the duration and symptoms of the common cold in adults, but studies are conflicting.

Zinc deficiency is prevalent in many developing countries and usually coexists with other micronutrient deficiencies (especially iron). Zinc (20 mg/d) may be an effective adjunctive therapeutic strategy for diarrheal disease in children.

Toxicity Acute zinc toxicity after oral ingestion causes nausea, vomiting, and fever. Zinc fumes from welding may also be toxic and cause fever, respiratory distress, excessive salivation, sweating, and headache. Chronic large doses of zinc may depress immune function and cause hypochromic anemia as a result of copper deficiency.

COPPER

Copper is an integral part of numerous enzyme systems including amine oxidases, ferroxidase (ceruloplasmin), cytochrome-*c* oxidase, superoxide dismutase, and dopamine hydroxylase. Copper is also a component of ferroprotein, a transport protein involved in the basolateral transfer of iron during absorption from the enterocyte. As such, copper plays a role in iron metabolism, melanin synthesis, energy production, neurotransmitter synthesis, and CNS function; the synthesis and cross-linking of elastin and collagen; and the scavenging of superoxide radicals. Dietary sources of copper include shellfish, liver, nuts, legumes, bran, and organ meats.

Deficiency Dietary copper deficiency is relatively rare, although it has been described in premature infants who are fed milk diets and in infants with malabsorption (Table 71-2). Copper-deficiency anemia has been reported in patients with malabsorptive diseases and nephrotic syndrome and in patients treated for Wilson's disease with chronic high doses of oral zinc, which can interfere with copper absorption. Menkes kinky hair syndrome is an X-linked metabolic disturbance of copper metabolism characterized by mental retardation, hypocupremia, and decreased circulating ceruloplasmin (Chap. 357). It is caused by mutations in the copper-transporting *ATP7A* gene. Children with this disease often die within 5 years because of dissecting aneurysms or cardiac rupture. Aceruloplasminemia is a rare autosomal recessive disease characterized by tissue iron overload, mental deterioration, microcytic anemia, and low serum iron and copper concentrations.

The diagnosis of copper deficiency is usually made on the basis of low serum levels of copper (<65 μg/dL) and low ceruloplasmin levels (<20 mg/dL). Serum levels of copper may be elevated in pregnancy or stress conditions since ceruloplasmin is an acute-phase reactant and 90% of circulating copper is bound to ceruloplasmin.

Toxicity Copper toxicity is usually accidental (Table 71-2). In severe cases, kidney failure, liver failure, and coma may ensue. In Wilson's disease, mutations in the copper-transporting *ATP7B* gene lead to accumulation of copper in the liver and brain, with low blood levels due to decreased ceruloplasmin (Chap. 354).

SELENIUM

Selenium, in the form of selenocysteine, is a component of the enzyme glutathione peroxidase, which serves to protect proteins, cell membranes, lipids, and nucleic acids from oxidant molecules. As such, selenium is being actively studied as a chemopreventive agent against certain cancers, such as prostate. Selenocysteine is also found in the deiodinase enzymes, which mediate the deiodination of thyroxine to triiodothyronine (Chap. 335). Rich dietary sources of selenium include seafood, muscle meat, and cereals, although the selenium content of cereal is determined by the soil concentration. Countries with low soil concentrations include parts of Scandinavia, China, and New Zealand. *Keshan disease* is an endemic cardiomyopathy found in children and young women residing in regions of China where dietary intake of selenium is low (<20 μg/d). Concomitant deficiencies of iodine and selenium may worsen the clinical manifestations of cretinism. Chronic ingestion of high amounts of selenium leads to selenosis characterized by hair and nail brittleness and loss, garlic breath odor, skin rash, myopathy, irritability, and other abnormalities of the nervous system.

CHROMIUM

Chromium potentiates the action of insulin in patients with impaired glucose tolerance, presumably by increasing insulin receptor–mediated signaling, although its usefulness in treating type II diabetes is uncertain. In addition, improvement in blood lipid profiles has been reported in some patients. The usefulness of chromium supplements in muscle building is not substantiated. Rich food sources of chromium include yeast, meat, and grain products. Chromium in the trivalent state is found in supplements and is largely nontoxic; however, chromium-6 is a product of stainless steel welding and is a known pulmonary carcinogen, as well as a cause of liver, kidney, and CNS damage.

MAGNESIUM

See Chap. 346.

FLUORIDE, MANGANESE, AND ULTRATRACE ELEMENTS

An essential function for fluoride in humans has not been described, although it is useful for the maintenance of structure in teeth and bone. Adult fluorosis results in mottled and pitted defects in tooth enamel as well as brittle bone (skeletal fluorosis).

Manganese and molybdenum deficiencies have been reported in patients with rare genetic abnormalities and in a few patients receiving prolonged total parenteral nutrition. Several manganese-specific enzymes have been identified (e.g., manganese superoxide dismutase). Deficiencies of manganese have been reported to result in bone demineralization, poor growth, ataxia, disturbances in carbohydrate and lipid metabolism, and convulsions.

Ultratrace elements are defined as those needed in amounts <1 mg/d. Essentiality has not been established for most ultratrace elements, although selenium, chromium, and iodine are clearly essential (Chap. 335). *Molybdenum* is necessary for the activity of sulfite and xanthine oxidase, and molybdenum deficiency may result in skeletal and brain lesions.

FURTHER READINGS

BONAA KH et al: Homocysteine lowering and cardiovascular events after acute myocardial infarction. N Engl J Med 354:1578, 2006

DAY E et al: Thiamine for Wernicke-Korsakoff Syndrome in people at risk from alcohol abuse. Cochrane Database Syst Rev CD004033, 2004

LICHTENSTEIN AH, RUSSELL RM: Essential nutrients in a healthy diet: Food or supplements? JAMA 294:1, 2005

MILLER ER et al: Meta-analysis: High-dosage vitamin E supplementation may increase all-cause mortality. Ann Intern Med 142:37, 2005

MORRIS MC et al: Dietary folate and vitamin B12 intake and cognitive decline among community-dwelling older persons. Arch Neurol 62:641, 2005

MURPHY SP et al: Multivitamin-multimineral supplements' effect on total nutrient intake. Am J Clin Nutr 85(1):280S, 2007

PENNISTON KL, TANUMIHARDJO: The acute and chronic toxic effects of vitamin A. Am J Clin Nutr 83:191, 2006

PRENTICE RL: Clinical trials and observational studies to assess the chronic disease benefits and risks of multivitamin-multimineral supplements. Am J Clin Nutr 85(1):308S, 2007

TOUVIER M et al: Dual association of beta-carotene with risk of tobacco-related cancers in a cohort of French women. J Natl Cancer Inst 97:1338, 2005

VERMEER C et al: Beyond deficiency: Potential benefits of increased intakes of vitamin K for bone and vascular health. Eur J Nutr 43:325, 2004

72 Malnutrition and Nutritional Assessment

Douglas C. Heimburger

Malnutrition can arise from primary or secondary causes, with the former resulting from inadequate or poor-quality food intake and the latter from diseases that alter food intake or nutrient requirements, metabolism, or absorption. Primary malnutrition occurs mainly in developing countries and under conditions of war or famine. Secondary malnutrition, the main form encountered in industrialized countries, was largely unrecognized until the early 1970s, when it became appreciated that persons with adequate food supplies can become malnourished as a result of acute or chronic diseases that alter nutrient intake or metabolism. Various studies have shown that protein-energy malnutrition (PEM) affects one-third to one-half of patients on general medical and surgical wards in teaching hospitals. The consistent finding that nutritional status influences patient prognosis underscores the importance of preventing, detecting, and treating malnutrition.

PROTEIN-ENERGY MALNUTRITION

The two major types of PEM are *marasmus* and *kwashiorkor*. These conditions are compared in Table 72-1. Marasmus and kwashiorkor can occur singly or in combination, as *marasmic kwashiorkor*. Kwashiorkor can occur rapidly, whereas marasmus is the end result of a gradual wasting process that passes through stages of underweight, then mild, moderate, and severe cachexia.

MARASMUS

The end stage of cachexia, marasmus is a state in which virtually all available body fat stores have been exhausted due to starvation. Conditions that produce marasmus in developed countries tend to be chronic and indolent, such as cancer, chronic pulmonary disease, and anorexia nervosa. Marasmus is easy to detect because of the patient's starved appearance. The diagnosis is based on severe fat and muscle wastage resulting from prolonged calorie deficiency. Diminished skin-fold thickness reflects the loss of fat reserves; reduced arm muscle circumference with temporal and interosseous muscle wasting reflects the catabolism of protein throughout the body, including vital organs such as the heart, liver, and kidneys.

The laboratory findings in marasmus are relatively unremarkable. The creatinine-height index (the 24-h urinary creatinine excretion compared with normal values based on height) is low, reflecting the loss of muscle mass. Occasionally, the serum albumin level is reduced, but it stays above 2.8 g/dL in uncomplicated cases. Despite a morbid appearance, immunocompetence, wound healing, and the ability to handle short-term stress are reasonably well preserved in most patients with marasmus.

Marasmus is a chronic, fairly well-adapted form of starvation rather than an acute illness; it should be treated cautiously, in an attempt to reverse the downward trend gradually. Although nutritional support is necessary, overly aggressive repletion can result in severe, even life-threatening metabolic imbalances such as hypophosphatemia and cardiorespiratory failure. When possible, oral or enteral nutritional support is preferred; treatment started slowly allows readaptation of metabolic and intestinal functions (Chap. 73).

KWASHIORKOR

In contrast to marasmus, kwashiorkor in developed countries occurs mainly in connection with acute, life-threatening illnesses such as trauma and sepsis, and chronic illnesses that involve acute-phase in-

TABLE 72-1 COMPARISON OF MARASMUS AND KWASHIORKOR

	Marasmus	Kwashiorkor[a]
Clinical setting	↓ Energy intake	↓ Protein intake during stress state
Time course to develop	Months or years	Weeks
Clinical features	Starved appearance Weight <80% standard for height Triceps skinfold <3 mm Mid-arm muscle circumference <15 cm	Well-nourished appearance Easy hair pluckability[b] Edema
Laboratory findings	Creatinine-height index <60% standard	Serum albumin <2.8 g/dL Total iron-binding capacity <200 μg/dL Lymphocytes <1500/μL Anergy
Clinical course	Reasonably preserved responsiveness to short-term stress	Infections Poor wound healing, decubitus ulcers, skin breakdown
Mortality	Low unless related to underlying disease	High
Diagnostic criteria	Triceps skinfold <3 mm Mid-arm muscle circumference <15 cm	Serum albumin <2.8 g/dL At least one of the following: Poor wound healing, decubitus ulcers, or skin breakdown Easy hair pluckability[b] Edema

[a]The findings used to diagnose kwashiorkor must be unexplained by other causes.

[b]Tested by *firmly* pulling a lock of hair from the top (not the sides or back), grasping with the thumb and forefinger. An average of three or more hairs removed easily and painlessly is considered abnormal hair pluckability.

flammatory responses. The physiologic stress produced by these illnesses increases protein and energy requirements at a time when intake is often limited. A classic scenario for kwashiorkor is the acutely stressed patient who receives only 5% dextrose solutions for periods as brief as 2 weeks. Although the etiologic mechanisms are not clear, the protein-sparing response normally seen in starvation is blocked by the stressed state and by carbohydrate infusion.

In its early stages, the physical findings of kwashiorkor are few and subtle. Fat reserves and muscle mass are initially unaffected, giving the deceptive appearance of adequate nutrition. Signs that support the diagnosis of kwashiorkor include easy hair pluckability, edema, skin breakdown, and poor wound healing. The major *sine qua non* is severe reduction of levels of serum proteins such as albumin (<2.8 g/dL) and transferrin (<150 mg/dL) or iron-binding capacity (<200 μg/dL). Cellular immune function is depressed, reflected by lymphopenia (<1500 lymphocytes/μL in adults and older children) and lack of response to skin test antigens (anergy).

The prognosis of adult patients with full-blown kwashiorkor is not good, even with aggressive nutritional support. Surgical wounds often dehisce (fail to heal), pressure sores develop, gastroparesis and diarrhea can occur with enteral feeding, the risk of gastrointestinal bleeding from stress ulcers is increased, host defenses are compromised, and death from overwhelming infection may occur despite antibiotic therapy. Unlike treatment in marasmus, aggressive nutritional support is indicated to restore better metabolic balance rapidly (Chap. 73). Although kwashiorkor in children is less foreboding, perhaps because a lesser degree of stress is required to precipitate the disorder, it is still a serious condition.

MARASMIC KWASHIORKOR

Marasmic kwashiorkor, the combined form of PEM, develops when the cachectic or marasmic patient experiences acute stress such as surgery, trauma, or sepsis, superimposing kwashiorkor onto chronic starvation. An extremely serious, life-threatening situation can occur because of the high risk of infection and other complications. It is important to determine the major component of PEM so that the appropriate nutritional plan can be developed. If kwashiorkor predominates, the need for vigorous nutritional therapy is urgent; if marasmus predominates, feeding should be more cautious.

PHYSIOLOGIC CHARACTERISTICS OF HYPOMETABOLIC AND HYPERMETABOLIC STATES

The metabolic characteristics and nutritional needs of hypermetabolic patients who are stressed from injury, infection, or chronic inflammatory illness differ from those of hypometabolic patients who are unstressed but chronically starved. In both cases, nutritional support is important, but misjudgments in selecting the appropriate approach may have disastrous consequences.

The hypometabolic patient is typified by the relatively unstressed but mildly catabolic and chronically starved individual who, with time, will develop marasmus. The hypermetabolic patient stressed from injury or infection is catabolic (experiencing rapid breakdown of body mass) and is at high risk for developing kwashiorkor, if nutritional needs are not met and/or the illness does not resolve quickly. As summarized in Table 72-2, the two states are distinguished by differing perturbations of metabolic rate, rates of protein breakdown (proteolysis), and rates of gluconeogenesis. These differences are mediated by proinflammatory cytokines and counterregulatory hormones—tumor necrosis factor, interleukins 1 and 6, C-reactive protein, catecholamines (epinephrine and norepinephrine), glucagon, and cortisol—that are relatively reduced in hypometabolic patients and increased in hypermetabolic patients. Although insulin levels are also elevated in stressed patients, insulin resistance in the target tissues prevents insulin-mediated anabolic actions.

METABOLIC RATE

In starvation and semistarvation, the resting metabolic rate falls between 10% and 30% as an adaptive response to energy restriction, slowing the rate of weight loss. By contrast, resting metabolic rate rises

TABLE 72-2 PHYSIOLOGIC CHARACTERISTICS OF HYPOMETABOLIC AND HYPERMETABOLIC STATES

Physiologic Characteristics	Hypometabolic, Nonstressed Patient (Cachectic, Marasmic)	Hypermetabolic, Stressed Patient (Kwashiorkor Risk[a])
Cytokines, catecholamines, glucagon, cortisol, insulin	↓	↑
Metabolic rate, O_2 consumption	↓	↑
Proteolysis, gluconeogenesis	↓	↑
Ureagenesis, urea excretion	↓	↑
Fat catabolism, fatty acid utilization	↑	↑
Adaptation to starvation	Normal	Abnormal

[a]These changes characterize the stressed, kwashiorkor-risk patient seen in developed countries; they differ in some respects from the characteristics of primary kwashiorkor seen in developing countries.

in the presence of physiologic stress in proportion to the degree of the insult. It may increase by about 10% after elective surgery, 20–30% after bone fractures, 30–60% with severe infections such as peritonitis or gram-negative septicemia, and as much as 110% after major burns.

If the metabolic rate (energy requirement) is not matched by energy intake, weight loss results—slowly in hypometabolism and quickly in hypermetabolism. Losses of up to 10% of body weight are unlikely to be detrimental; however, losses greater than this in acutely ill hypermetabolic patients may be associated with rapid deterioration in body function.

PROTEIN CATABOLISM

The rate of endogenous protein breakdown (catabolism) to supply energy needs normally falls during uncomplicated energy deprivation. After about 10 days of total starvation, the unstressed individual loses about 12–18 g/d protein (equivalent to approximately 2 oz of muscle tissue or 2–3 g of nitrogen). By contrast, in injury and sepsis, protein breakdown accelerates in proportion to the degree of stress, to 30–60 g/d after elective surgery, 60–90 g/d with infection, 100–130 g/d with severe sepsis or skeletal trauma, and >175 g/d with major burns or head injuries. These losses are reflected by proportional increases in the excretion of urea nitrogen, the major byproduct of protein breakdown.

GLUCONEOGENESIS

The major aim of protein catabolism during a state of starvation is to provide the glucogenic amino acids (especially alanine and glutamine) that serve as substrates for endogenous glucose production (gluconeogenesis) in the liver. In the hypometabolic/starved state, protein breakdown for gluconeogenesis is minimized, especially as ketones derived from fatty acids become the substrate preferred by certain tissues. In the hypermetabolic/stress state, gluconeogenesis increases dramatically and in proportion to the degree of the insult, to increase the supply of glucose (the major fuel of reparation). Glucose is the only fuel that can be utilized by hypoxic tissues (anaerobic glycolysis), white blood cells, and newly generated fibroblasts. Infusions of glucose partially offset a negative energy balance but do not significantly suppress the high rates of gluconeogenesis in the catabolic patient. Hence, adequate supplies of protein are needed to replace the amino acids utilized for this metabolic response.

In summary, the hypometabolic patient is adapted to starvation and conserves body mass by reducing the metabolic rate and using fat as the primary fuel (rather than glucose and its precursor amino acids). The hypermetabolic patient also uses fat as a fuel but rapidly breaks down body protein to produce glucose, causing loss of muscle and organ tissue and endangering vital body functions.

MICRONUTRIENT MALNUTRITION

The same illnesses and reductions in nutrient intake that lead to PEM often produce deficiencies of vitamins and minerals as well (Chap. 71).

Deficiencies of nutrients that are stored in small amounts (such as the water-soluble vitamins) are lost through external secretions, such as zinc in diarrhea fluid or burn exudate, and are probably more common than generally recognized.

Deficiencies of vitamin C, folic acid, and zinc are reasonably common in sick patients. Signs of scurvy such as corkscrew hairs on the lower extremities are frequently found in chronically ill and/or alcoholic patients. The diagnosis can be confirmed with plasma vitamin C levels. Folic acid intakes and blood levels are often less than optimal, even among healthy persons; when illness, alcoholism, poverty, or poor dentition is present, deficiencies are common. Low blood zinc levels are prevalent in patients with malabsorption syndromes such as inflammatory bowel disease. Patients with zinc deficiency often exhibit poor wound healing, pressure ulcer formation, and impaired immunity. Thiamine deficiency is a common complication of alcoholism, but its manifestations are often prevented by therapeutic doses of thiamine in patients treated for alcohol abuse.

Patients with low plasma vitamin C levels usually respond to the doses found in multivitamin preparations, but patients with deficiencies should be supplemented with 250–500 mg/d. Folic acid is absent from some oral multivitamin preparations; patients with deficiencies should be supplemented with about 1 mg/d. Patients with zinc deficiencies resulting from large external losses sometimes require oral daily supplementation with 220 mg of zinc sulfate one to three times daily. For these reasons, laboratory assessments of the micronutrient status of patients at high risk are desirable.

Hypophosphatemia develops in hospitalized patients with remarkable frequency and generally results from rapid intracellular shifts of phosphate in cachectic or alcoholic patients receiving intravenous glucose (Chap. 46). The adverse clinical sequelae are numerous; some, such as acute cardiopulmonary failure, can be life-threatening.

NUTRITIONAL ASSESSMENT

Because interactions between illness and nutrition are complex, many physical and laboratory findings reflect both underlying disease and nutritional status. Therefore, the nutritional evaluation of a patient requires an integration of the history, physical examination, anthropometrics, and laboratory studies. This approach helps both to detect nutritional problems and to avoid concluding that isolated findings indicate nutritional problems when they do not. For example, hypoalbuminemia caused by an underlying illness does not necessarily indicate malnutrition.

NUTRITIONAL HISTORY

A nutritional history is directed toward identifying underlying mechanisms that put patients at risk for nutritional depletion or excess. These mechanisms include inadequate intake, impaired absorption, decreased utilization, increased losses, and increased requirements of nutrients.

Individuals with the characteristics listed in Table 72-3 are at particular risk for nutritional deficiencies.

PHYSICAL EXAMINATION

Physical findings that suggest vitamin, mineral, and protein-energy deficiencies and excesses are outlined in Table 72-4. Most of the physical findings are not specific for individual nutrient deficiencies, and they must be integrated with the historic, anthropometric, and laboratory findings. For example, the finding of follicular hyperkeratosis on the back of the arms is a fairly common, normal finding. On the other hand, if it is widespread in a person who consumes little fruit and vegetables and smokes regularly (increasing ascorbic acid requirements), vitamin C deficiency is likely. Similarly, easily pluckable hair may be a consequence of chemotherapy, but in a hospitalized patient who has poorly healing surgical wounds and hypoalbuminemia, it suggests kwashiorkor.

TABLE 72-3 THE HIGH-RISK PATIENT

Underweight (body mass index <18.5) and/or recent loss of ≥10% of usual body weight
Poor intake: anorexia, food avoidance (e.g., psychiatric condition), or NPO status for more than about 5 days
Protracted nutrient losses: malabsorption, enteric fistulae, draining abscesses or wounds, renal dialysis
Hypermetabolic states: sepsis, protracted fever, extensive trauma or burns
Alcohol abuse or use of drugs with antinutrient or catabolic properties: steroids, antimetabolites (e.g., methotrexate), immunosuppressants, antitumor agents
Impoverishment, isolation, advanced age

ANTHROPOMETRICS

Anthropometric measurements provide information on body muscle mass and fat reserves. The most practical and commonly used measurements are body weight, height, triceps skinfold (TSF), and mid-arm muscle circumference (MAMC). Body weight is one of the most useful nutritional parameters to follow in patients who are acutely or chronically ill. Unintentional weight loss during illness often reflects loss of lean body mass (muscle and organ tissue), especially if it is rapid and not caused by diuresis. This can be an ominous sign since it indicates use of vital body protein stores as a metabolic fuel. The reference standard for normal body weight, body mass index (BMI, or weight in kilograms divided by height, in meters, squared), is discussed in Chap 75. BMIs <18.5 are considered underweight, 18.5–24.9 are normal, 25–29.9 are overweight, and ≥30 are obese.

Measurement of skinfold thickness is useful for estimating body fat stores, because about 50% of body fat is normally located in the subcutaneous region. Skinfold thicknesses can also permit discrimination of fat mass from muscle mass. The TSF is a convenient site that is generally representative of the body's overall fat level. A thickness of <3 mm suggests virtually complete exhaustion of fat stores. The MAMC, often used to estimate skeletal muscle mass, is calculated as follows:

$$\text{MAMC (cm)} = \text{upper arm circumference (cm)} - [0.314 \times \text{TSF (mm)}]$$

LABORATORY STUDIES

A number of laboratory tests used routinely in clinical medicine can yield valuable information about a patient's nutritional status if a slightly different approach to their interpretation is used. For example, abnormally low serum albumin levels, total iron-binding capacity, and anergy may have a distinct explanation, but collectively they may represent kwashiorkor. In the clinical setting of a hypermetabolic, acutely ill patient who is edematous and has easily pluckable hair and inadequate protein intake, the diagnosis of kwashiorkor is clear-cut. Commonly used laboratory tests for assessing nutritional status are outlined in Table 72-5. The table also provides tips to help avoid assigning nutritional significance to tests that may be abnormal for nonnutritional reasons.

Assessment of Circulating (Visceral) Proteins The serum proteins most used to assess nutritional status include albumin, total iron-binding capacity (or transferrin), thyroxine-binding prealbumin (or transthyretin), and retinol-binding protein. Because they have differing synthesis rates and half-lives—the half-life of serum albumin is about 21 days whereas those of prealbumin and retinol-binding protein are about 2 days and 12 h, respectively—some of these proteins reflect changes in nutritional status more quickly than others. However, rapid fluctuations can also make shorter-half-life proteins less reliable.

Levels of circulating proteins are influenced by their rates of synthesis and catabolism, "third spacing" (loss into interstitial spaces), and, in some cases, external loss. Although an adequate intake of calories and protein is necessary to achieve optimal circulating protein levels, serum protein levels generally do not reflect protein intake. For example, a drop in the serum level of albumin or transferrin often accompanies significant physiologic stress (e.g., from infection

TABLE 72-4 PHYSICAL FINDINGS OF NUTRITIONAL DEFICIENCIES

Clinical Findings	Possible Deficiency[a]	Possible Excess
Hair, Nails		
Corkscrew hairs and unemerged coiled hairs	Vitamin C	
Easily pluckable hair	Protein	
Flag sign (transverse depigmentation of hair)	Protein	
Sparse hair	Protein, biotin, zinc	Vitamin A
Transverse ridging of nails	Protein	
Skin		
Cellophane appearance	Protein	
Cracking (flaky paint or crazy pavement dermatosis)	Protein	
Follicular hyperkeratosis	Vitamins A, C	
Petechiae (especially perifollicular)	Vitamin C	
Purpura	Vitamins C, K	
Pigmentation, scaling of sun-exposed areas	Niacin	
Poor wound healing, decubitus ulcers	Protein, vitamin C, zinc	
Scaling	Vitamin A, essential fatty acids, biotin	Vitamin A
Yellow pigmentation sparing sclerae (benign)	Zinc (hyperpigmented)	Carotene
Eyes		
Night blindness	Vitamin A	
Papilledema		Vitamin A
Perioral		
Angular stomatitis	Riboflavin, pyridoxine, niacin	
Cheilosis (dry, cracking, ulcerated lips)	Riboflavin, pyridoxine, niacin	
Oral		
Atrophic lingual papillae (slick tongue)	Riboflavin, niacin, folate, vitamin B_{12}, protein, iron	
Glossitis (scarlet, raw tongue)	Riboflavin, niacin, pyridoxine, folate, vitamin B_{12}	
Hypogeusesthesia, hyposmia	Zinc	
Swollen, retracted, bleeding gums (if teeth present)	Vitamin C	
Bones, Joints		
Beading of ribs, epiphyseal swelling, bowlegs	Vitamin D	
Tenderness, subperiosteal hemorrhage in children	Vitamin C	
Neurologic		
Confabulation, disorientation	Thiamine (Korsakoff psychosis)	
Drowsiness, lethargy, vomiting		Vitamin A
Dementia	Niacin, vitamin B_{12}, folate	
Headache		Vitamin A
Ophthalmoplegia	Thiamine, phosphorus	
Peripheral neuropathy (e.g., weakness, paresthesias, ataxia, foot drop, and decreased tendon reflexes, fine tactile sense, vibratory sense, and position sense)	Thiamine, pyridoxine, vitamin B_{12}	Pyridoxine
Tetany	Calcium, magnesium	
Other		
Edema	Protein, thiamine	
Heart failure	Thiamine ("wet" beriberi), phosphorus	
Hepatomegaly	Protein	Vitamin A
Parotid enlargement	Protein (consider also bulimia)	
Sudden heart failure, death	Vitamin C	

[a]In this table, "protein deficiency" is used to signify kwashiorkor.

or injury) and is not necessarily an indication of malnutrition or poor intake. A low serum albumin level in a burned patient with both hypermetabolism and increased dermal losses of protein may not indicate malnutrition. On the other hand, adequate nutritional support of the patient's calorie and protein needs is critical for returning circulating proteins to normal levels as stress resolves. Thus low values by themselves do not define malnutrition, but they often point to increased risk of malnutrition because of the hypermetabolic stress state. As long as significant physiologic stress persists, serum protein levels remain low, even with aggressive nutritional support. However, if the levels do not rise after the underlying illness improves, the patient's protein and calorie needs should be reassessed to ensure that intake is sufficient.

Assessment of Vitamin and Mineral Status The use of laboratory tests to confirm suspected micronutrient deficiencies is desirable because the physical findings for these are often equivocal or nonspecific. Low blood micronutrient levels can predate more serious clinical manifestations and may also indicate drug-nutrient interactions.

ESTIMATING ENERGY AND PROTEIN REQUIREMENTS

A patient's basal energy expenditures (BEE, measured in kilocalories per day) can be estimated from height, weight, age, and gender using the Harris-Benedict equations:

$$\text{Men: BEE} = 66.47 + 13.75W + 5.00H - 6.76A$$

$$\text{Women: BEE} = 655.10 + 9.56W + 1.85H - 4.68A$$

where W is weight in kg; H is height in cm, and A is age in years. After solving these equations, total energy requirements are estimated by multiplying the BEE by a factor that accounts for the stress of illness. Multiplying by 1.1–1.4 yields a range 10–40% above basal that estimates the 24-h energy expenditure of the majority of patients. The lower value (1.1) is used for patients without evidence of significant physiologic stress; the higher value (1.4) is appropriate for patients with marked stress such as sepsis or trauma. The result is used as a 24-h energy goal for feeding.

When it is important to have a more accurate assessment of energy expenditure, it can be measured at the bedside using indirect calorimetry. This technique is useful in patients who are believed to be hypermetabolic from sepsis or trauma and whose body weights cannot be obtained accurately. Indirect calorimetry can also be useful in patients having difficulty weaning from a ventilator, as their energy needs should not be exceeded to avoid excessive CO_2 production. Patients at the extremes of weight (e.g., obese persons) and/or age are good candidates as well, because the Harris-Benedict equations were developed from measurements in adults with roughly normal body weights.

Because urea is a major byproduct of protein catabolism, the amount of urea nitrogen excreted each day can be used to estimate the rate of protein catabolism and to determine if protein intake is adequate to offset it. Total protein loss and protein balance can be calculated from the urinary urea nitrogen (UUN) as follows:

$$\text{Protein catabolic rate (g/d)} = [\text{24-h UUN (g)} + 4] \times 6.25 \text{ (g protein/g nitrogen)}$$

The value of 4 g added to the UUN represents a liberal estimate of the unmeasured nitrogen lost in the urine (e.g., creatinine and uric acid), sweat, hair, skin, and feces. When protein intake is low (e.g., less

TABLE 72-5 LABORATORY TESTS FOR NUTRITIONAL ASSESSMENT

Test (Normal Values)	Nutritional Use	Causes of Normal Value Despite Malnutrition	Other Causes of Abnormal Value
Serum albumin (3.5–5.5 g/dL)	2.8–3.5: Compromised protein status <2.8: Possible kwashiorkor Increasing value reflects positive protein balance	Dehydration Infusion of albumin, fresh frozen plasma, or whole blood	**Low** Common: Infection and other stress, especially with poor protein intake Burns, trauma Congestive heart failure Fluid overload Severe liver disease Uncommon: Nephrotic syndrome Zinc deficiency Bacterial stasis/overgrowth of small intestine
Serum prealbumin, also called transthyretin (20–40 mg/dL; lower in prepubertal children)	10–15 mg/dL: Mild protein depletion 5–10 mg/dL: Moderate protein depletion <5 mg/dL: Severe protein depletion Increasing value reflects positive protein balance	Chronic renal failure	Similar to serum albumin
Serum total iron binding capacity (TIBC) 240–450 μg/dL	<200: Compromised protein status, possible kwashiorkor Increasing value reflects positive protein balance More labile than albumin	Iron deficiency	**Low** Similar to serum albumin **High** Iron deficiency
Prothrombin time 12.0–15.5 sec	Prolongation: vitamin K deficiency		**Prolonged** Anticoagulant therapy (warfarin) Severe liver disease
Serum creatinine 0.6–1.6 mg/dL	<0.6: Muscle wasting due to prolonged energy deficit Reflects muscle mass		**High** Despite muscle wasting: Renal failure Severe dehydration
24-h urinary creatinine 500–1200 mg/d (standardized for height and sex)	Low value: muscle wasting due to prolonged energy deficit	>24-h collection Decreasing serum creatinine	**Low** Incomplete urine collection Increasing serum creatinine Neuromuscular wasting
24-h urinary urea nitrogen (UUN) <5 g/d (depends on level of protein intake)	Determine level of catabolism (as long as protein intake is ≥10 g below calculated protein loss or <20 g total, but at least 100 g carbohydrate is provided) 5–10 g/d = mild catabolism or normal fed state 10–15 g/d = moderate catabolism >15 g/d = severe catabolism Estimate protein balance Protein balance = protein intake – protein loss where protein loss (protein catabolic rate) = [24-h UUN (g) + 4] × 6.25 Adjustments required in burn patients and others with large nonurinary nitrogen losses and in patients with fluctuating BUN levels (e.g., renal failure)		
Blood urea nitrogen (BUN) 8–23 mg/dL	<8: Possibly inadequate protein intake 12–23: Possibly adequate protein intake >23: Possibly excessive protein intake If serum creatinine is normal, use BUN If serum creatinine is elevated, use BUN/creatinine ratio (normal range is essentially the same as for BUN)		**Low** Severe liver disease Anabolic state Syndrome of inappropriate antidiuretic hormone **High** Despite poor protein intake: Renal failure (use BUN/creatinine ratio) Congestive heart failure Gastrointestinal hemorrhage

than about 20 g/d), the equation indicates both the patient's protein requirement and the severity of the catabolic state (Table 72-5). More substantial protein intakes can raise the UUN because some of the ingested (or infused) protein is catabolized and converted to UUN. Thus at lower protein intakes the equation is useful for estimating *requirements*, and at higher protein intakes it is useful for assessing protein *balance*.

$$\text{Protein balance (g/d)} = \text{Protein intake} - \text{Protein catabolic rate}$$

FURTHER READINGS

American Society for Parenteral and Enteral Nutrition: *The science and practice of nutrition support: A case-based core curriculum*. Dubuque, Kendall/Hunt, 2001. Available online at: *www.nutritioncare.org*

Baker H: Nutrition in the elderly: Hypovitaminosis and its implications. Geriatrics 62(8):22, 2007

Chapman IM: Nutritional disorders in the elderly. Med Clin North Am 90(5):887, 2006

Heimburger DC, Ard JD (eds): *Handbook of Clinical Nutrition*, 4th ed. Philadelphia, Mosby Elsevier, 2006

Shils ME et al (eds): *Modern Nutrition in Health and Disease*, 10th ed. Baltimore, Lippincott Williams & Wilkins, 2005

73 Enteral and Parenteral Nutrition Therapy

Bruce R. Bistrian, David F. Driscoll

The ability to provide specialized nutritional support (SNS) represents a major advance in medical therapy. Nutritional support, via either enteral or parenteral routes, is used in two main settings: (1) to provide adequate nutritional intake during the recuperative phase of illness or injury, when the patient's ability to ingest or absorb nutrients is impaired, and (2) to support the patient during the systemic response to inflammation, injury, or infection during an extended critical illness. SNS is also used in patients with permanent loss of intestinal length or function. In addition, an increasing number of elderly patients living in nursing homes and chronic care facilities receive enteral feeding, usually as a consequence of inadequate nutritional intake.

Enteral refers to feeding via a tube placed into the gut to deliver liquid formulas containing all essential nutrients. *Parenteral* refers to the infusion of complete nutrient solutions into the bloodstream via a peripheral vein or, more commonly, by central venous access to meet nutritional needs. Enteral feeding is generally the preferred route because of benefits derived from maintaining the digestive, absorptive, and immunologic barrier functions of the gastrointestinal tract. Small-bore pliable tubes have largely replaced large-bore rubber tubes, making placement easier and more acceptable to patients. Infusion pumps have also improved the delivery of nutrient solutions.

For short-term use, enteral tubes can be placed via the nose into the stomach, duodenum, or jejunum. For long-term use, these sites can be accessed through the abdominal wall using endoscopic, radiologic, or surgical procedures. Intestinal tolerance of tube feeding may be limited during acute illness by gastric retention or diarrhea. Parenteral feeding has greater risk of infection, reflecting the need for venous access, and a greater propensity for inducing hyperglycemia. However, these risks can generally be managed successfully by SNS teams. For the postoperative patient with preexisting malnutrition, or in trauma patients who were previously well nourished, SNS is strikingly cost-effective. In the most critically ill patient in the intensive care unit, SNS can dramatically enhance survival. Although enteral nutrition (EN) can be provided by most health care teams caring for hospitalized patients, safe and effective parenteral nutrition (PN) usually requires specialized teams.

APPROACH TO THE PATIENT: Requirements for Specialized Nutritional Support

INDICATIONS FOR SPECIALIZED NUTRITIONAL SUPPORT Although at least 15–20% of patients in acute care hospitals have evidence of significant malnutrition, only a small fraction will benefit from SNS. For others, wasting is an inevitable component of a terminal disease and the course of the disease will not be altered by SNS. The decision to use SNS should be based on the likelihood that preventing protein-calorie malnutrition (PCM) will increase the likelihood of recovery, reduce infection rates, improve healing, or otherwise shorten the hospital stay. In the case of the elderly or chronically ill patient for whom full recovery is not anticipated, the decision to feed is usually based on whether SNS will extend the duration and quality of life. The decision-making process used to decide when to use SNS is depicted in Fig. 73-1.

The first step in deciding to administer SNS is to consider the nutritional implications of the disease process. Is the condition or its treatment likely to impair food intake and absorption for a prolonged period of time? For example, a well-nourished individual can tolerate approximately 7 days of starvation while experiencing a systemic response to inflammation (SRI). The second step is to determine if the patient is already significantly malnourished to the degree that critical functions such as wound healing, immune function, or ventilatory function are impaired (Chap. 72). An unintentional weight loss of >10% during the previous 6 months or a weight/height <90% of standard, when associated with physiologic impairment, represents significant PCM. Weight loss >20% of usual or <80% of standard reflects severe PCM. The presence or absence of SRI should be noted, since inflammation, injury, and infection increase the rate of lean tissue loss. SRI also has pathophysiologic effects that influence nutritional responses such as fluid retention and hyperglycemia, as well as impairment of anabolic responses to nutritional support.

Once it is determined that a patient is already or at risk of becoming malnourished, the next step is to decide whether SNS will impact positively on the patient's response to disease. In the end stages of many chronic illnesses with accompanying PCM, particularly those due to cancer or terminal neurologic disorders, nutrition may not reverse the PCM or improve quality of life. While the provision of food and water is part of basic medical care, nutrition delivered by tube or catheter, either enterally or parenterally, is associated with risk and discomfort. Thus, SNS should be recommended only when potential benefits exceed risks, and should be undertaken with the consent of the patient. Like other life support measures, enteral or parenteral therapy is difficult to withdraw once started. Initiating nutrition support may be appropriate before a final prognosis can be determined, but this should not preclude its subsequent withdrawal. If preventing or treating PCM with SNS is appropriate, nutritional requirements and the method of delivery should be determined. The optimal route depends on the degree of gut function and somewhat on the available technical resources.

The timing of nutritional support is based on evaluation of the preexisting nutritional status, the presence and extent of SRI, and the anticipated clinical course. SRI is identified by the standard clinical signs of leukocytosis, tachycardia, tachypnea, and/or temperature elevation or depression. Although the degree of hypoalbuminemia provides an estimate of SRI severity, normal serum albumin levels will not be restored by adequate nutritional support until the SRI remits, even though nutritional benefits can be achieved by adequate feeding.

The SRI can be graded as severe, moderate, or mild. Examples of severe SRI include sepsis or other inflammatory conditions like pancreatitis requiring ICU care, multiple trauma with an Injury Severity Score > 20–25 or APACHE II > 25, closed head injury with a Glasgow Coma Scale < 8, or major third-degree burns of >40% of body surface area. Moderate SRI includes less severe infections, injuries, or inflammatory conditions like pneumonia, major surgery, acute hepatic or renal insufficiency, and exacerbations of ulcerative colitis or regional enteritis requiring hospitalization. PCM should also be defined as severe, moderate, or minimal as assessed by weight/height, percent recent weight loss, and body mass index. The body mass index in relation to nutritional status is listed in Table 73-1. A patient with a severe SRI requires early feeding within the first several days of care because the condition is likely to produce inadequate spontaneous intake over the next 7 days. A moderate SRI, as commonly seen during a postoperative period without oral intake that exceeds 5 days, benefits from adequate feeding by day 5–7 if the patient was initially well nourished. If severely malnourished, candidates for elective major surgery benefit from preoperative nutritional repletion for 5–7 days. However, this is not often possible. Thus, early postoperative feeding is indicated. Patients with a moderate SRI and moderate PCM also benefit from earlier feeding within the first several days.

EFFICACY OF SNS IN DIFFERENT DISEASE STATES Efficacy studies have shown that malnourished patients undergoing major thoracoabdominal surgery benefit from SNS. Critical illness requiring ICU care including major burns, major trauma, severe sepsis, closed

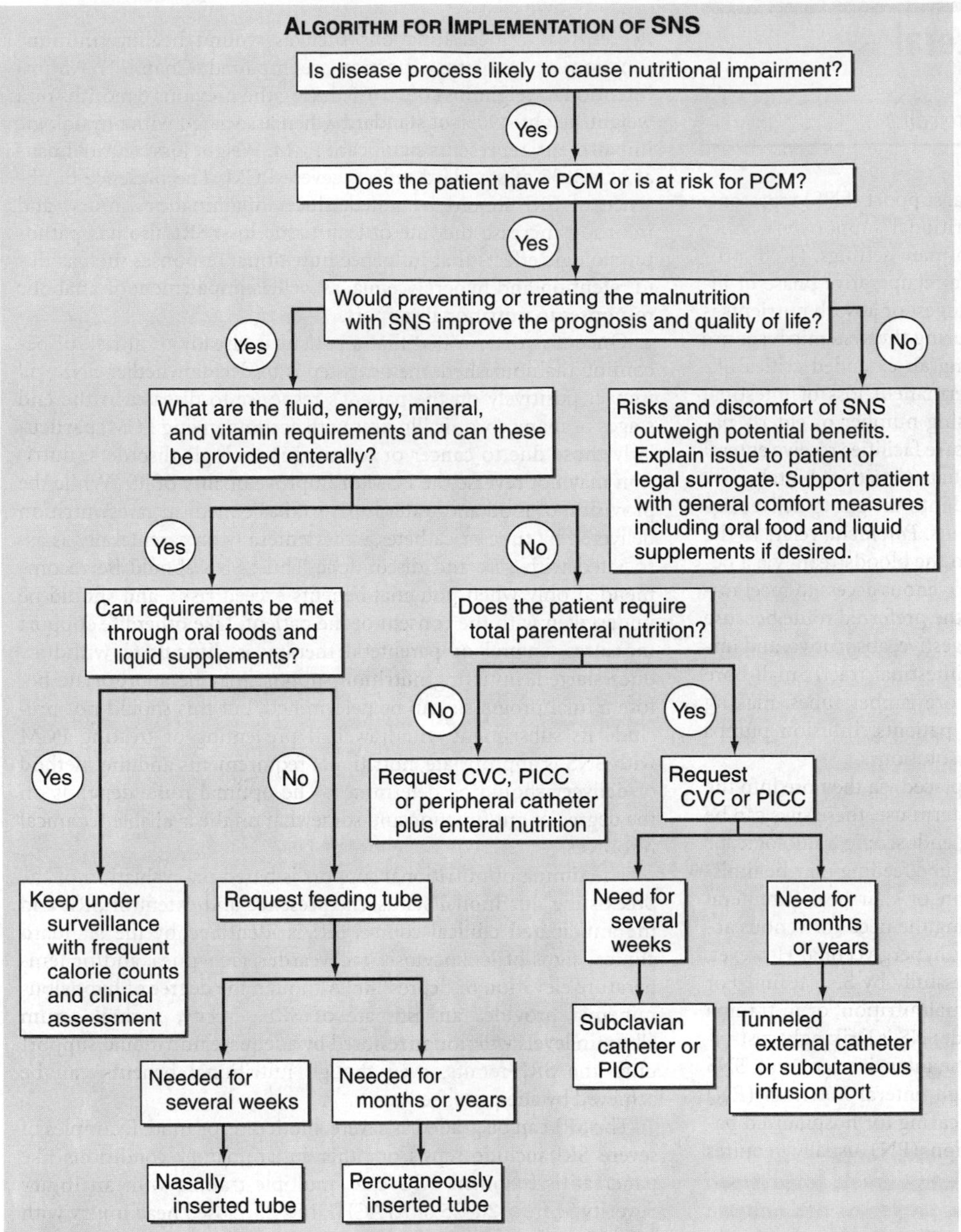
ALGORITHM FOR IMPLEMENTATION OF SNS
Is disease process likely to cause nutritional impairment?
Yes
Does the patient have PCM or is at risk for PCM?
Yes
Would preventing or treating the malnutrition with SNS improve the prognosis and quality of life?
Yes
No
What are the fluid, energy, mineral, and vitamin requirements and can these be provided enterally?
Risks and discomfort of SNS outweigh potential benefits. Explain issue to patient or legal surrogate. Support patient with general comfort measures including oral food and liquid supplements if desired.
Yes
No
Can requirements be met through oral foods and liquid supplements?
Does the patient require total parenteral nutrition?
Yes
No
No
Yes
Request CVC, PICC or peripheral catheter plus enteral nutrition
Request CVC or PICC
Keep under surveillance with frequent calorie counts and clinical assessment
Request feeding tube
Need for several weeks
Need for months or years
Subclavian catheter or PICC
Tunneled external catheter or subcutaneous infusion port
Needed for several weeks
Needed for months or years
Nasally inserted tube
Percutaneously inserted tube

FIGURE 73-1 Decision-making for the implementation of specialized nutrition support (SNS). CVC, central venous catheter; PICC, peripherally inserted central catheter. *(Adapted from previous chapter by Lyn Howard, MD.)*

head injury, and severe pancreatitis [positive CT scan and Acute Physiology and Chronic Health Evaluation II (APACHE II) > 10] all benefit by early SNS, as indicated by reduced mortality and morbidity. In critical illness, initiation of SNS within 24 h of injury or ICU admission is associated with a ~50% reduction in mortality. Patients with nitrogen accumulation disorders of renal and hepatic failure have a likelihood of PCM of >50% and at least a moderate SRI. Improvements in morbidity, including infection rates, encephalopathy, liver or renal function, and length of hospital stay have been found with SNS. Inflammatory bowel disease—including Crohn's disease particularly, and, to a lesser degree, ulcerative colitis—often produce PCM. In the outpatient setting, SNS in Crohn's disease can improve nutritional status, quality of life, and the likelihood of remission. With pulmonary disease in the critically ill, SNS improves ventilatory status, and in acute lung injury the use of omega 3 fats as a component of SNS improves gas exchange and respiratory dynamics and reduces the need for mechanical ventilation. Low body weight in chronic obstructive pulmonary disease is associated with diminished pulmonary status and exercise capacity and higher mortality rates. However, there is little convincing evidence that SNS as caloric supplementation improves nutrition or pulmonary function. PCM is also common in the course of cancer and HIV disease, although less so in the latter with the advent of highly active antiretroviral therapy. When PCM develops as a consequence of SRI in these conditions, there is limited likelihood of substantial efficacy or benefit from SNS. However, when PCM develops as a consequence of gastrointestinal dysfunction, SNS can be effective. Although no randomized trials have been performed for SNS provided for hyperemesis gravidarum, there is considerable clinical evidence that it improves pregnancy outcomes.

RISKS AND BENEFITS OF SPECIALIZED NUTRITION SUPPORT The risks are determined primarily by patient factors such as state of alertness, swallowing competence, the route of delivery, underlying conditions, and the experience of the supervising clinical team. The safest and least costly approach is to avoid SNS by close attention to oral food intake, by adding an oral liquid supplement, or in certain chronic conditions by using medications to stimulate appetite. Nutrient intake monitoring by frequent calorie counts or oral formula selection is best performed by a nutritionist.

Enteral tube feeding is often required in patients with anorexia, impaired swallowing, or bowel disease. The bowel and its associated digestive organs derive 70% of their required nutrients directly from food in the lumen. Arginine, glutamine, short-chain fatty acids, long-chain omega 3 fatty acids, and nucleotides available in some specialty enteral formulas are particularly important for maintaining immunity. Enteral feeding also supports gut function by stimulating splanchnic blood flow, neuronal activity, IgA antibody release, and secretion of gastrointestinal hormones that stimulate gut trophic activity. These factors

TABLE 73-1 BODY MASS INDEX (BMI) AND NUTRITIONAL STATUS

BMI	Nutritional Status
>30 kg/m^2	Obese
>25–30 kg/m^2	Overweight
20–25 kg/m^2	Normal
<18.5 kg/m^2	Moderate malnutrition
<16 kg/m^2	Severe malnutrition
<13 kg/m^2	Lethal in males
<11 kg/m^2	Lethal in females

From D Driscoll, B Bistrian: Parenteral and enteral nutrition in the intensive care unit, in *Intensive Care Medicine*, R Irwin, J Rippe (eds). Lippincott Williams & Wilkins, Philadelphia, 2003.

support the gut as an immunologic barrier against enteric pathogens. For these reasons, some luminal nutrition should be provided, even when PN is required to provide most of the nutritional support. The combination of some enteral feeding either by mouth or by enteral tube with parenteral feeding often shortens the transition to full enteral feeding, which can generally be used when >50% of requirements can be met enterally. Substantial nutritional benefit can be achieved by providing ~50% of energy needs for periods of up to 10 days, if protein and other essential nutrient requirements are met. For longer periods of time, it may be preferable to provide 75–80% of energy needs, rather than full feeding, if this improves gastrointestinal tolerance, glycemic control, and avoidance of excess fluid administration.

In the past, bowel rest through PN was the cornerstone of treatment for many severe gastrointestinal disorders. However, the value of providing even minimal amounts of EN is now widely accepted. The development of protocols to facilitate more widespread use of EN include initiation within 24 h of ICU admission; aggressive use of the head-upright position; postpyloric and nasojejunal feeding tubes; prokinetic agents; more rapid increases in feeding rates; tolerance of higher gastric residuals; and nurse-administered algorithms. PN alone is generally necessary only for severe gut dysfunction due to prolonged ileus, obstruction, or severe hemorrhagic pancreatitis. In the critically ill, feeding adequately by PN beginning within the first 24 h of care improves mortality and is more effective than delayed EN. Early feeding of the critically ill in the ICU is associated with a 50% reduction in mortality, but there is also a 50% increase in infection risk. Much of the increase in morbidity related to PN and EN is due to hyperglycemia, which can be significantly reduced by insulin therapy. The level of glycemia necessary to accomplish this goal, whether <110 mg/dL or only <150 mg/dL, is not yet defined.

Although PN was initially relatively expensive, its components are often less expensive than specialty enteral formulas. Percutaneous placement of a central venous catheter into the subclavian or internal jugular vein with advancement into the superior vena cava can be accomplished at the bedside by trained personnel using sterile techniques. Peripherally inserted central catheters can also be placed within the lumen in the central vein, but this technique is usually more appropriate for non-ICU patients. The subclavian or internal jugular lines can be changed over a wire, but this carries a greater risk of pneumothorax or serious vascular damage. The peripherally inserted catheters are subject to position-related flow, and the catheter cannot be changed over a wire. Inserting a nasogastric tube is a bedside procedure, but many critically ill patients have impaired gastric emptying that increases the risk of aspiration pneumonia. This risk can be reduced by feeding directly into the jejunum beyond the ligament of Treitz. This usually requires fluoroscopic guidance or endoscopic placement. In patients who have planned laparotomies or other conditions likely to require a prolonged need for SNS, it is advantageous to place a jejunal feeding tube at the time of surgery.

Although most SNS is delivered in hospitals, some patients require it on a long-term basis. If they have a safe environment and a willingness to learn the self-care techniques, SNS can be administered at home. The clinical outcomes of patients with severe intestinal disorders treated with home PN or EN are summarized in Table 73-2. PN infused at home is usually cycled overnight to give greater daytime freedom. Other important considerations in determining the appropriateness of home PN or EN are that the patient's prognosis is longer than several months and that the therapy benefits quality of life.

DISEASE-SPECIFIC NUTRITIONAL SUPPORT SNS is basically a support therapy and is primary therapy only for the treatment or prevention of malnutrition. Certain conditions require modification of nutritional support because of organ or system impairment. For instance, in nitrogen accumulation disorders, protein intake may need to be reduced. However, in renal disease, except for brief periods of several days, protein intakes should approach requirement levels of at least 0.8 g/kg or higher up to 1.2 g/kg as long as the

TABLE 73-2 SUMMARY OF OUTCOMES FOR PATIENTS ON HOME PARENTERAL AND ENTERAL NUTRITION (HPEN)

				Therapy Status, % at 1 year[b]			Rehabilitation[c] Status, % in 1st year			Complications[d] per Patient-Year	
Diagnosis	Number in Group	Age in Years	% Survival[a] on Therapy	Full Oral Nutrition	Continued on HPEN Rx	Died	C	P	M	HPEN	NonHPEN
Home Parenteral Nutrition											
Crohn's disease	562	36	96	70	25	2	60	38	2	0.9	1.1
Ischemic bowel disease	331	49	87	27	48	19	53	41	6	1.4	1.1
Motility disorder	299	45	87	31	44	21	49	39	12	1.3	1.1
Congenital bowel defect	172	5	94	42	47	9	63	27	11	2.1	1.0
Hyperemesis gravidarum	112	28	100	100	0	0	83	16	1	1.5	3.5
Chronic pancreatitis	156	42	90	82	10	5	60	38	2	1.2	2.5
Radiation enteritis	145	58	87	28	49	22	42	49	9	0.8	1.1
Chronic adhesive obstructions	120	53	83	47	34	13	23	68	10	1.7	1.4
Cystic fibrosis	51	17	50	38	13	36	24	66	16	0.8	3.7
Cancer	2122	44	20	26	8	63	29	57	14	1.1	3.3
AIDS	280	33	10	13	6	73	8	63	29	1.6	3.3
Home Enteral Nutrition											
Neurologic disorders of swallowing	1134	65	55	19	25	48	5	24	71	0.3	0.9
Cancer	1644	61	30	30	6	59	21	59	21	0.4	2.7

[a]Survival rates on therapy are values at 1 year, calculated by the life table method. This will differ from the percentage listed as died under Therapy Status, since all patients with known end points are considered in this latter measure. The ratio of observed versus expected deaths is equivalent to a Standard Mortality Ratio.

[b]Not shown are those patients who were back in hospital or who had changed therapy type by 12 months.

[c]Rehabilitation is designated complete (C), partial (P), or minimal (M), relative to the patient's ability to sustain normal age-related activity.

[d]Complications refer only to those complications that resulted in rehospitalization.

Source: Derived from North American HPEN Registry.

Table taken from previous chapter by Lyn Howard, MD.

blood urea nitrogen does not exceed 100 mg/dL. If this is not possible, then dialysis or hemofiltration should be considered to allow better feeding. In hepatic failure, intakes of 1.2–1.4 g/kg up to the optimal 1.5 g/kg should be attempted, as long as encephalopathy due to protein intolerance is not encountered. In the presence of protein intolerance, formulas containing 33–50% branched-chain amino acids are available at the 1.2–1.4-g/kg level. Cardiac patients, and many severely stressed patients, often benefit from fluid and sodium restriction to levels of 1000 mL of total parenteral nutrition (TPN) formula and 5–20 meq of sodium per day. In patients with severe chronic PCM characterized by severe weight loss and tissue wasting, TPN must be instituted gradually because of the profound antinatriuresis, antidiuresis, and intracellular accumulation of potassium, magnesium, and phosphorus. This is usually accomplished by limiting fluid intakes initially to about 1000 mL containing modest carbohydrate content of 10–20% dextrose, low sodium, and ample potassium, magnesium, and phosphorus, with careful assessment of fluid and electrolyte status. Protein need not be restricted.

THE DESIGN OF INDIVIDUAL REGIMENS

FLUID REQUIREMENTS

The normal daily requirement for fluid is 30 mL/kg of body weight from all sources (IV infusions, per tube, or oral intake), plus any replacement of abnormal losses such as an osmotic diuresis, nasogastric drainage, wound output, or diarrheal/ostomy losses. Electrolyte and mineral losses can be estimated or measured and also need to be replaced (Table 73-3). Fluid restriction may be necessary in patients with fluid overload, and fluid inputs can be limited to 1200 mL/d if urine is the only significant fluid output. When severe fluid overload occurs, the optimal PN solution for central venous administration is a concentrated 1-L solution of 7% crystalline amino acids (70 g) and 21% dextrose (210 g), which provides an amount of nitrogen and glucose that is effective at protein-sparing.

Patients requiring PN or EN in the acute care setting generally have some element of associated hormonal adaptations (e.g., increased secretion of antidiuretic hormone, aldosterone, insulin, glucagon, or cortisol) that cause fluid retention and hyperglycemia. Weight gain in the critically ill, whether receiving SNS or not, is invariably the consequence of fluid retention, since lean tissue accretion is minimal in the acute phase of illness. Because excess fluid removal can be difficult, limiting fluid intake to allow for balanced intake and output is more effective.

ENERGY REQUIREMENTS

Total energy expenditure comprises resting energy expenditure (two-thirds) plus activity energy expenditure (one-third) (Chap. 72). Resting energy expenditure includes the calories necessary for basal metabolism at bed rest. Activity energy expenditure represents one-fourth to one-third of the total, and the thermal effect of feeding is about 10% of the total energy expenditure. For normally nourished healthy individuals, the total energy expenditure is about 30–35 kcal/kg. Although critical illness increases resting energy expenditure, only in initially well-nourished individuals with the highest systemic inflammatory response, such as that from severe multiple trauma, burns, closed head injury, or sepsis, do total energy expenditures reach 40–45 kcal/kg. The chronically ill patient with lean tissue loss has reduced basal energy expenditure, and inactivity which results in a total energy expenditure of about 20–25 kcal/kg. About 95% of such patients need <30 kcal/kg to achieve energy balance. Because providing about 50% of measured energy expenditure as SNS is at least equally efficacious for the first 10 days of critical illness, actual measurement of energy expenditure is not generally necessary in the early period of SNS. However, in patients who remain critically ill beyond several weeks, in the severely malnourished for whom estimates of energy expenditure are unreliable, or in those who are difficult to wean from ventilators, it is reasonable to actually measure energy expenditure and to aim for energy balance with SNS.

Insulin resistance is associated with increased gluconeogenesis and reduced glucose utilization, predisposing a patient to hyperglycemia. This is aggravated in patients receiving exogenous carbohydrate from SNS. Normalization of blood glucose levels by insulin infusion in critically ill patients receiving SNS reduces morbidity and mortality. In mild or moderately malnourished patients, a reasonable goal is to provide metabolic support to improve protein synthesis and maintain metabolic homeostasis. Hypocaloric nutrition providing only about 1000 kcal/d and 70 g protein for up to 10 days requires less fluid and reduces the likelihood of poor glycemic control. Energy content can be advanced to 20–25 kcal/kg with 1.5 g protein/kg as conditions permit and definitely during the second week of SNS. Patients with multiple trauma, closed head injury, and severe burns often have much higher energy expenditures, but there is little evidence that providing more than 30 kcal/kg has additional benefit, and it risks hyperglycemia.

Generally, because glucose is an essential tissue fuel, glucose and amino acids are provided parenterally until the level of resting energy expenditure is reached. At this point, adding fat becomes beneficial, since more parenteral glucose stimulates de novo lipogenesis by the liver—an energy-inefficient process. Polyunsaturated long-chain triglycerides are the chief ingredient in most parenteral fat emulsions and the majority of the fat in enteral feeding formulas. These vegetable oil–based emulsions provide essential fatty acids. Enteral feeding formulas have fat content that ranges from 3% of calories up to as much as 50% of calories, while parenteral fat comes in separate containers as 10, 20, and 30% emulsions that can be infused separately or mixed by the pharmacy under controlled conditions as all-in-one or total nutrient admixture with glucose, amino acids, lipid, electrolytes, vitamins, and minerals. Although parenteral fat is required at only about 3% of energy requirements to meet essential fatty acid requirements, when provided as an all-in-one mixture of carbohydrate, fat, and protein, 2–3% fat in the TPN mixtures, representing about 20–30% of calories as fat, is provided to ensure emulsion stability. If given separately, parenteral fat should not be provided at rates exceeding 0.11 g/kg body weight per h or about 100 g over 12 h—equivalent to 1 L of 10% parenteral fat and 500 mL of 20% parenteral fat.

Medium-chain triglycerides, which contain saturated fatty acids with chain lengths of 6, 8, 10, or 12 carbons, are provided in a number of enteral feeding formulas because they are absorbed preferentially. Fish oil contains polyunsaturated fatty acids of the omega 3 family, which have been shown to improve immune function and reduce the inflammatory response. Parenteral emulsions containing medium-chain triglycerides, olive oil, and fish oil are available in Europe and Japan but not yet in the United States.

Carbohydrates are provided as hydrous glucose providing 3.4 kcal/g in PN formulas. In enteral formulas, glucose is the carbohydrate source in so-called monomeric diets. These diets provide protein as amino acids and fat in minimal amounts (3%) to meet essential fatty acid requirements. Monomeric formulas are designed to optimize absorption in the seriously compromised gut. These formulas, like the im-

TABLE 73-3 ENTERIC FLUID VOLUMES AND THEIR ELECTROLYTE CONTENT[a]

	L/d	Na	K	Cl	HCO_3	H
Oral intake	2–3					
Enteric secretions						
Saliva	1–2	15	30	15	50	—
Gastric juice	1.5–2	50–70	5–15	90–120	0	70–100
Bile	0.5–1.5	120–150	5–15	80–120	30–50	—
Pancreatic	0.5–1	100–140	10	70–100	60–110	—
Small intestine	1–2	80–140	10–20	80–120	20–40	—

[a]All in mEq/L.

Source: Adapted from previous chapter by Lyn Howard, MD, in *Harrison's Principles of Internal Medicine*.

mune-enhancing diets, are quite expensive. In polymeric diets, the carbohydrate source is usually an osmotically less active polysaccharide, protein is usually soy or casein protein, and fat is present in amounts from 25 to 50%. Such formulas are usually well tolerated by patients with normal intestinal length, and some are acceptable for oral consumption.

PROTEIN OR AMINO ACID REQUIREMENTS

Although the recommended dietary allowance for protein is 0.8 g/kg per d, maximal rates of repletion occur with 1.5 g/kg in the malnourished. In the severely catabolic patient, this higher level minimizes protein loss. In patients requiring SNS in the acute care setting, at least 1 g/kg is recommended, with greater amounts up to 1.5 g/kg as volume, renal, and hepatic tolerances allow. The standard parenteral and enteral formulas contain protein of high biologic value and meet the requirements for the eight essential amino acids. In protein-intolerant conditions such as renal and hepatic failure, modified amino acid formulas should be considered. In hepatic failure, higher branched-chain amino acid–enriched formulas appear to improve outcomes. Conditionally essential amino acids like arginine and glutamine may also have some benefit in supplemental amounts.

Protein (nitrogen) balance provides a measure of feeding efficacy of PN or EN. It is calculated as protein intake/6.25 because proteins are on average 16% nitrogen (N), minus the 24-h urine urea N (UUN) plus 4 g N, which reflects other N losses. In the critically ill, a mild negative balance of 2–4 g N/d is usually achievable with a similarly mild positive balance in the recuperating patient. Each g N represents approximately 30 g lean tissue.

MINERAL AND VITAMIN REQUIREMENTS

Parenteral electrolyte, vitamin, and trace mineral requirements are summarized in Tables 73-4, 73-5, and 73-6. Electrolyte modifications are necessary with substantial gastrointestinal losses from nasogastric drainage or intestinal losses from fistulas, diarrhea or ostomy outputs. Such losses also imply extra calcium, magnesium, and zinc losses. Excessive urine or potassium losses with amphotericin, or magnesium losses with cisplatin or in renal failure, necessitate adjustments in sodium, potassium, magnesium, phosphorus, and acid-base balance. Vitamin and trace element requirements are met by the daily provision of a complete parenteral vitamin supplement and trace elements for PN, and with the provision of adequate amounts of enteral feeding formulas that contain these micronutrients.

PARENTERAL NUTRITION

INFUSION TECHNIQUE AND PATIENT MONITORING

Parenteral feeding through a peripheral vein is limited by osmolality and volume constraints. Solutions that contain more than 3% amino acids and 5% glucose (290 kcal/L) are poorly tolerated peripherally. Parenteral fat (20%) can be given to increase the calories delivered. The total volume required to provide a marginal protein intake of 60 g and 1680 total kcal is 2.5 L. However, the risk of significant morbidity and mortality from incompatibilities of calcium and phosphate salts is greatest in these low-osmolality, low-glucose regimens. Parenteral feeding via a peripheral vein is generally intended as a supplement to oral feeding and is not optimal for the critically ill. Peripheral parenteral nutrition may benefit from small amounts of heparin at 1000 U/L and co-infusion with parenteral fat to reduce osmolality, but volume constraints still limit the value of this therapy. Peripherally inserted central catheters (PICCs) can be used for the short term to provide concentrated glucose parenteral solutions of 20–25% dextrose and 4–7% amino acids, while avoiding some of the complications of catheter placement via a large central vein. With PICC lines, however, flow can be position-related, and the lines cannot be exchanged over a wire for infection monitoring. For these reasons, in the critically ill, centrally placed catheters are preferred. The subclavian approach is best tolerated by the patient and is the easiest to dress. The jugular approach is less likely to lead to a pneumothorax. The femoral approach is discouraged because of the greater risk of catheter infection. For long-term feeding in the home, tunneled catheters and implanted ports reduce infection risk and are more acceptable to patients. However, tunneled catheters require placement in the operating room.

Catheters are made of silastic, polyurethane, or polyvinyl chloride. Silastic catheters are less thrombogenic and are best for tunneled catheters. Polyurethane is best for temporary catheters. Dressing changes with dry gauze at regular intervals should be performed by nurses skilled in catheter care to avoid infection. Chlorhexidine solution is more effective than alcohol or iodine compounds. Appropriate monitoring for patients receiving PN is summarized in Table 73-7.

TABLE 73-4 USUAL DAILY ELECTROLYTE ADDITIONS TO PARENTERAL NUTRITION

Electrolyte	Parenteral Equivalent of RDA	Usual Intake
Sodium		1–2 meq/kg + replacement, but can be as low as 5–40 meq/d
Potassium		40–100 meq/d + replacement of unusual losses
Chloride		As needed for acid-base balance, but usually 2:1 to 1:1 with acetate
Acetate		As needed for acid-base balance
Calcium	10 meq	10–20 meq/d
Magnesium	10 meq	8–16 meq/d
Phosphorus	30 mmol	20–40 mmol

TABLE 73-5 PARENTERAL MULTIVITAMIN REQUIREMENTS FOR ADULTS

Vitamin	Recently Revised Value
Vitamin A	3300 IU
Thiamin (B_1)	6 mg
Riboflavin (B_2)	3.6 mg
Niacin (B_3)	40 mg
Folic acid	600 μg
Pantothenic acid	15 mg
Pyridoxine (B_6)	6 mg
Cyanocobalamin (B_{12})	5 μg
Biotin	60 μg
Ascorbic acid (C)	200 mg
Vitamin D	200 IU
Vitamin E	10 IU
Vitamin K[a]	150 μg

[a]A product is available that does not contain vitamin K. Vitamin K supplementation is recommended at 2–4 mg/week in patients not receiving oral anticoagulation therapy if using this product.

TABLE 73-6 PARENTERAL TRACE METAL SUPPLEMENTATION FOR ADULTS[a]

Trace Mineral	Intake
Zinc	2.5–4 mg/d, an additional 10–15 mg/d per L of stool or ileostomy output
Copper	0.5–1.5 mg/d, possibility of retention in biliary tract obstruction
Manganese	0.1–0.3 mg/d, possibility of retention in biliary tract obstruction
Chromium	10–15 μg/d
Selenium	20–100 μg/d, necessary for long-term PN, optional for short-term TPN
Molybdenum	20–120 μg/d, necessary for long-term PN, optional for short-term PN
Iodine	75–150 μg/d, necessary for long-term PN, optional for short-term PN

[a]Commercial products are available that have the first four, first five, and all seven of these metals in recommended amounts.

Note: PN, parenteral nutrition; TPN, total parenteral nutrition.

TABLE 73-7 MONITORING THE PATIENT ON PARENTERAL NUTRITION

Clinical Data Monitored Daily	
General sense of well-being	
Strength as evidenced in getting out of bed, walking, resistance exercise as appropriate	
Vital signs including temperature, blood pressure, pulse, and respiratory rate	
Fluid balance: weight at least several times weekly, fluid intake (parenteral and enteral) vs fluid output (urine, stool, gastric drainage, wound, ostomy)	
Parenteral nutrition delivery equipment: tubing, pump, filter, catheter, dressing	
Nutrient solution composition	
Laboratory Daily	
Finger-stick glucose	Three times daily until stable
Blood glucose, Na, K, Cl, HCO_3, BUN	Daily until stable and fully advanced, then twice weekly
Serum creatinine, albumin, PO_4, Ca, Mg, Hb/Hct, WBC	Baseline, then twice weekly
INR	Baseline, then weekly
Micronutrient tests	As indicated

Note: Hb, hemoglobin; Hct, hematocrit; INR, international normalized ratio; WBC, white blood cell count.
Source: Adapted from chapter by Lyn Howard, MD, in HPIM, 16e.

COMPLICATIONS

Mechanical The insertion of a central venous catheter should be performed by trained and experienced personnel using aseptic techniques to limit the major common complications of pneumothorax and inadvertent arterial puncture or injury. Catheter position should be radiographically confirmed to be in the superior vena cava distal to the junction with the jugular or subclavian vein and not directly against the vessel wall. Thrombosis related to the catheter may occur at the site of entry into the vein and extend to encase the catheter. Catheter infection predisposes to thrombosis, as does the systemic inflammatory response. The addition of 6000 U of heparin in the daily parenteral formula in hospitalized patients with temporary catheters reduces the risk of fibrin sheath formation and catheter infection. Temporary catheters that develop a thrombus should be removed and, based on clinical findings, treated with anticoagulants. Thrombolytic therapy can be considered for patients with permanent catheters depending on the ease of replacement and presence of alternate, reasonably acceptable venous access sites. Low-dose warfarin therapy of 1 mg/d reduces the risk of thrombosis in permanent catheters used for home PN, but full anticoagulation may be required in patients who have recurrent thrombosis related to permanent catheters. A recent U.S. Food and Drug Administration mandate to reformulate parenteral multivitamins to include vitamin K at a dose of 150 μg daily may affect the efficacy of low-dose warfarin therapy. There is a "no vitamin K" version available for patients receiving this therapy. Catheters can become mechanically occluded and may also become occluded by fibrin at the tip, or by fat, minerals, or drugs intraluminally. These occlusions can be managed with low-dose alteplase for fibrin, with indwelling 70% alcohol for fat, with 0.1 *N* hydrochloric acid for mineral precipitates, and with either 0.1 *N* hydrochloric acid or 0.1 *N* sodium hydroxide for drugs, depending on their pH.

Metabolic The most common problems related to PN are fluid overload and hyperglycemia (Table 73-8). Hypertonic dextrose stimulates a much higher insulin level than meal feeding. Because insulin is a potent antinatriuretic and antidiuretic hormone, hyperinsulinemia leads to sodium and fluid retention. In the absence of gastrointestinal losses or renal dysfunction, net fluid retention is likely when total fluid intake exceeds 2000 mL/d. Close monitoring of body weight, as well as fluid intake and output, is necessary to prevent this complication. In the absence of significant renal impairment, the sodium content of the urine is likely to be <10 meq/L. Providing sodium in limited amounts of 40 meq/d and the use of both glucose and fat in the PN mixture to lower total glucose and sodium will help reduce fluid retention. The elevated insulin also increases the intracellular transport of potassium, magnesium, and phosphorus, which can precipitate a dangerous refeeding syndrome if the total glucose content of the PN solution is advanced too quickly in severely malnourished patients. It is generally best to start PN with <200 g glucose/d to assess glucose tolerance. Regular insulin can be added to the PN formula to establish glycemic control, and the insulin doses can be increased proportionately as the glucose is advanced. As a general rule, patients with insulin-dependent diabetes require about twice their usual home insulin doses when they are receiving TPN at 20–25 kcal/kg, largely as a consequence of parenteral glucose administration and some loss of insulin to the TPN container. As a rough estimate, the amount of insulin can be provided in a similar proportion to the amount of calories provided as TPN relative to full feeding, and the insulin can be placed in the TPN formula. Subcutaneous regular insulin can be provided to improve glucose control as assessed by measurements of blood glucose every 6 h. About two-

TABLE 73-8 SELECTED METABOLIC DISTURBANCES AND THEIR CORRECTION

Disturbance	Cause	Corrective Action with PN
Hyponatremia	Increased total body water or decreased total body sodium	Decrease free water or increase sodium
Hypernatremia	Occurs commonly with excessive isotonic or hypertonic fluid followed by diuretic administration with free water clearance; can also occur with dehydration and normal total body sodium	Increase free water to produce net positive fluid balance maintaining sodium and chloride balance
Hypokalemia	Inadequate intake relative to need	Use supplements
	Excessive diuresis, tubular dysfunction	Use supplements
	Magnesium deficiency	Increase PN magnesium
	Metabolic alkalosis	Correct alkalosis
	Hyperinsulinemia	Maintain constant PN, increase potassium
Hyperkalemia	Excessive provision	Reduce supplements
	Metabolic acidosis	Evaluate alkalosis, treat with PN acetate salt and decrease potassium
	Renal deterioration	Evaluate patient and adjust PN as indicated
Hypocalcemia	Reciprocal response to phosphorus repletion	Increase calcium
	Critical illness effect	Increase calcium
	Severe malabsorption	Supplement calcium
Hypercalcemia	Excessive administration or pathologic (cancer, hyperparathyroidism)	Reduce or eliminate calcium
Hypomagnesemia	Increased requirements due to diuretic use, alcoholism, malabsorption, malnutrition	Supplement magnesium
	Critical illness	Supplement magnesium
Hypophosphatemia	Inadequate intake relative to needs related to malnutrition, alcohol use	Supplement phosphorus
	Increased calcium intake	Use supplements
Hyperphosphatemia	Excessive administration or worsening renal function	Reduce phosphorus
Azotemia	Excessive amino acid infusion or worsening renal function	Reduce amino acid level but consider renal replacement therapy if cannot provide 1 g protein per kg for prolonged periods

Note: PN, parenteral nutrition.

thirds of the total 24-h amount can be added to the next day's order, with subcutaneous insulin supplements as needed. Advances in TPN concentration should be made when reasonable glucose control is established, and the insulin dose adjusted proportionately to the calories added as glucose and amino acids. These are general rules, and they are conservative. Given the adverse clinical impact of hyperglycemia, it may be necessary to use continuous insulin therapy as a separate infusion with a standard protocol to initially establish control. Once established, this insulin dose can be added to the PN formula. Acid-base imbalance is also common during PN therapy. Amino acid formulas are buffered, but critically ill patients are prone to metabolic acidosis, often due to renal tubular impairment. The use of sodium and potassium acetate salts in the PN formula may address this problem. Bicarbonate salts should not be used because they are incompatible with TPN formulations. Nasogastric drainage produces a hypochloremic alkalosis that can be managed by attention to chloride balance. Occasionally, hydrochloric acid may be required for a more rapid response or when diuretic therapy limits the ability to provide substantial sodium chloride. Up to 100 meq/L and up to 150 meq of hydrochloric acid per day may be placed in a fat-free PN formula.

Infectious Infections of the central access catheter rarely occur in the first 72 h. Fever during this period is usually from infection elsewhere or another cause. Fever that develops during PN can be addressed by checking the catheter site and, if the site looks clean, exchanging the catheter over a wire with cultures taken through the catheter and at the catheter tip. If these cultures are negative, as they are most of the time, the new catheter can continue to be used. If a culture is positive for a relatively nonpathogenic bacteria like *Staphylococcus epidermidis*, consider a second exchange over a wire with repeat cultures or replace the catheter depending on the clinical circumstances. If cultures are positive for more pathogenic bacteria, or for fungi like *Candida albicans*, it is generally best to replace the catheter at a new site. Whether antibiotic treatment is required is a clinical decision, but *C. albicans* grown from the blood culture in a patient receiving PN should always be treated because the consequences of failure to treat can be dire.

Catheter infections can be minimized by dedicating the feeding catheter to PN, without blood sampling or medication administration. Central catheter infections are a serious complication with an attributed mortality of 12–25%. Infections in central venous catheters dedicated to feeding should occur less frequently than 3 per 1000 catheter-days. Home PN catheters that become infected may be treated through the catheter without removal of the catheter, particularly if the offending organism is *S. epidermidis*. Clearing of the biofilm and fibrin sheath by local treatment of the catheter with indwelling alteplase may increase the likelihood of eradication. Antibiotic lock therapy with high concentrations of antibiotic, with or without heparin in addition to systemic therapy, may improve efficacy. Sepsis with hypotension should precipitate catheter removal in either the temporary or permanent PN setting.

ENTERAL NUTRITION

TUBE PLACEMENT AND PATIENT MONITORING

The types of enteral feeding tubes, methods of insertion, their clinical uses, and potential complications are outlined in Table 73-9. The different types of enteral formulas are listed in Table 73-10. Patients receiving EN are at risk for many of the same metabolic complications as those who receive PN and should be monitored in the same manner. EN can be a source of similar problems, but not to the same degree, because the insulin response to EN is about half of that seen with PN. Enteral feeding formulas have fixed electrolyte compositions that are generally modest in sodium and somewhat higher in potassium content. Acid-base disturbances can be addressed to a more limited extent with EN. Acetate salts can be added to the formula to treat chronic metabolic acidosis. Calcium chloride can be added to treat mild chronic metabolic alkalosis. Medications and other additives to enteral feeding formulas can clog the tubes (e.g., calcium chloride may interact with casein-based formulas to produce insoluble calcium caseinate products) and may reduce the efficacy of some drugs (e.g., phenytoin). Since small-bore tubes are easily displaced, tube position should be checked at intervals by aspirating and measuring the pH of the gut fluid (<4 in the stomach, >6 in the jejunum).

COMPLICATIONS

Aspiration The debilitated patient with poor gastric emptying and impairment of swallowing and cough is at risk for aspiration; this is particularly true for those who are mechanically ventilated. Tracheal suctioning induces coughing and gastric regurgitation, and cuffs on endotracheal or tracheostomy tubes seldom protect against aspiration. Preventive measures include elevating the head of the bed to 30 degrees,

TABLE 73-9 ENTERAL FEEDING TUBES

Type/Insertion Technique	Clinical Uses	Potential Complications
Nasogastric Tube		
External measurement: nostril, ear, xiphisternum; tube stiffened by ice water or stylet; position verified by injecting air and auscultating, or by x-ray	Short-term clinical situation (weeks) or longer periods with intermittent insertion; bolus feeding simpler, but continuous drip with pump better tolerated	Aspiration; ulceration of nasal and esophageal tissues, leading to stricture
Nasoduodenal Tube		
External measurement: nostril, ear, anterior superior iliac spine; tube stiffened by stylet and passed through pylorus under fluoroscopy or with endoscopic loop	Short-term clinical situations where gastric emptying impaired or proximal leak suspected; requires continuous drip with pump	Spontaneous pulling back into stomach (position verified by aspirating content, pH > 6); diarrhea common, fiber-containing formulas may help
Gastrostomy Tube		
Percutaneous placement endoscopically, radiologically, or surgically; after tract established, can be converted to a gastric "button"	Long-term clinical situations, swallowing disorders, or impaired small-bowel absorption requiring continuous drip	Aspiration; irritation around tube exit site; peritoneal leak; balloon migration and obstruction of pylorus
Jejunostomy Tube		
Percutaneous placement endoscopically or radiologically via pylorus or endoscopically or surgically directly into the jejunum	Long-term clinical situations where gastric emptying impaired; requires continuous drip with pump; direct endoscopic placement (PEJ) is the most comfortable for patient	Clogging or displacement of tube; jejunal fistula if large-bore tube used; diarrhea from dumping; irritation of surgical anchoring suture
Combined Gastrojejunostomy Tube		
Percutaneous placement endoscopically, radiologically, or surgically; intragastric arm for continuous or intermittent gastric suction; jejunal arm for enteral feeding	Used for patients with impaired gastric emptying and at high risk for aspiration or patients with acute pancreatitis or proximal leaks	Clogging: especially of small bore jejunal tube

Note: All small tubes are at risk for clogging, especially if used for crushed medications. In long-term enteral patients, gastrostomy and jejunostomy tubes can be exchanged for a low-profile "button" once the tract is established.
Source: Adapted from chapter in *Harrison's Principles of Internal Medicine*, 16e, by Lyn Howard, MD.

TABLE 73-10 ENTERAL FORMULAS

Composition Characteristics	Clinical Indications
Standard Enteral Formula	
1. Complete dietary products (+)[a]	Suitable for most patients requiring tube feeding; some can be used orally
a. Caloric density 1 kcal/mL	
b. Protein ~14% cals, caseinates, soy, lactalbumin	
c. CHO ~60% cals, hydrolyzed corn starch, maltodextrin, sucrose	
d. Fat ~30% cals, corn, soy, safflower oils	
e. Recommended daily intake of all minerals and vitamins in >1500 kcal/d	
f. Osmolality (mosmol/kg): ~300	
Modified Enteral Formulas	
1. Caloric density 1.5–2 kcal/mL (+)	Fluid-restricted patients
2. a. High protein ~20–25% protein (+)	Critically ill patients
b. Hydrolyzed protein to small peptides (+)	Impaired absorption
c. ↑ Arginine, glutamine, nucleotides, ω3 fat (+++)	Immune-enhancing diets
d. ↑ Branched-chain amino acids, ↓ aromatic amino acids (+++)	Liver failure patients intolerant of 0.8 g/kg protein
e. Low protein of high biologic value	Renal failure patient for brief periods if critically ill
3. a. Low fat, partial MCT substitution (+)	Fat malabsorption
b. ↑ Fat >40% cals (++)	Pulmonary failure with CO_2 retention on standard formula, limited utility
c. ↑ Fat from MUFA (++)	Improvement in glycemic index control in diabetes
d. ↑ Fat from ω3 and ↓ ω6 linoleic acid (+++)	Improved ventilation in ARDS
4. Fiber provided as soy polysaccharide (+)	Improved laxation

Cost: + inexpensive; ++ moderately expensive; +++ very expensive.

Note: ARDS, acute respiratory distress syndrome; CHO, carbohydrate; MCT, medium-chain triglyceride; MUFA, monounsaturated fatty acids; ω3 or ω6, polyunsaturated fat with first double bond at carbon 3 (fish oils) or carbon 6 (vegetable oils).

Source: Adapted from chapter in *Harrison's Principles of Internal Medicine*, 16e, by Lyn Howard, MD.

using nurse-directed algorithms for formula advancement, combining enteral with parenteral feeding, and using post–ligament of Treitz feeding. Tube feeding should not be discontinued for gastric residuals of <300 mL unless there are other signs of gastrointestinal intolerance such as nausea, vomiting, or abdominal distention. Continuous feeding using pumps is better tolerated intragastrically and is essential for feeding into the jejunum. For small-bowel feeding, residuals are not assessed but abdominal pain and distention should be monitored.

Diarrhea Enteral feeding often leads to diarrhea, especially if bowel function is compromised by disease or drugs, particularly broad-spectrum antibiotics. Diarrhea may be controlled by the use of a continuous drip, with a fiber-containing formula, or by adding an antidiarrheal agent to the formula. However, *Clostridium difficile*, which is a common cause of diarrhea in patients being tube fed, should be ruled out before using antidiarrheal agents. H2 blockers may also assist in reducing the net fluid presented to the colon. Diarrhea associated with enteral feeding does not necessarily imply inadequate absorption of nutrients other than water and electrolytes. Amino acids and glucose are particularly well absorbed in the upper small bowel except in the most diseased or shortest bowel. Since luminal nutrients exert trophic effects on the gut mucosa, it is often appropriate to persist with tube feeding, despite the diarrhea, even when this necessitates supplemental parenteral fluid support.

ACKNOWLEDGMENT

The authors acknowledge the contributions of Lyn Howard, MD, the author in earlier editions of HPIM, to material in this chapter.

FURTHER READINGS

AUGUST D et al: Evidence-based approach to optimal management of HPEN access. J Parenter Enteral Nutr 30:S5, 2006

BISTRIAN B, MCCOWEN K: Nutritional support in the adult intensive care unit: Key controversies. Crit Care Med 34:1525, 2006

CENTERS FOR DISEASE CONTROL AND PREVENTION: Reduction in central line–associated bloodstream infections among patients in intensive care units—Pennsylvania, April 2001–March 2005. MMWR 54:1013, 2005

DEBAVEYE Y, VAN DEN BERGHE G: Risks and benefits of nutritional support during critical illness. Annu Rev Nutr 26:513, 2006

KORETZ RL et al: Does enteral nutrition affect clinical outcome? A systematic review of the randomized trials. Am J Gastroenterol 102(2):412, 2007

MILNE A et al: Meta-analysis: Protein and energy supplementation in older people. Ann Intern Med 144:37, 2006

PLANK LD, HILL GL: Energy balance in critical illness. Proc Nutr Soc 62:545, 2003

SIMPSON F, DOIG GS: Parenteral vs. enteral nutrition in the critically ill patient: A meta-analysis of trials using the intention to treat principle. Intensive Care Med 31:12, 2005

VAN DEN BERGHE G et al: Intensive insulin therapy in the critically ill patients. N Engl J Med 345:1359, 2001

74 Biology of Obesity

Jeffrey S. Flier, Eleftheria Maratos-Flier

In a world where food supplies are intermittent, the ability to store energy in excess of what is required for immediate use is essential for survival. Fat cells, residing within widely distributed adipose tissue depots, are adapted to store excess energy efficiently as triglyceride and, when needed, to release stored energy as free fatty acids for use at other sites. This physiologic system, orchestrated through endocrine and neural pathways, permits humans to survive starvation for as long as several months. However, in the presence of nutritional abundance and a sedentary lifestyle, and influenced importantly by genetic endowment, this system increases adipose energy stores and produces adverse health consequences.

DEFINITION AND MEASUREMENT

Obesity is a state of excess adipose tissue mass. Although often viewed as equivalent to increased body weight, this need not be the case—lean but very muscular individuals may be overweight by numerical standards without having increased adiposity. Body weights are distributed continuously in populations, so that choice of a medically meaningful distinction between lean and obese is somewhat arbitrary. Obesity is therefore more effectively defined by assessing its linkage to morbidity or mortality.

Although not a direct measure of adiposity, the most widely used method to gauge obesity is the *body mass index* (BMI), which is equal to weight/height^2 (in kg/m^2) **(Fig. 74-1)**. Other approaches to quantifying obesity include anthropometry (skin-fold thickness), densitometry (underwater weighing), CT or MRI, and electrical impedance. Using data from the Metropolitan Life Tables, BMIs for the midpoint of all heights and frames among both men and women range from 19–26 kg/m^2; at a similar BMI, women have more body fat than men. Based on data of substantial morbidity, a BMI of 30 is most commonly used as a threshold for obesity in both men and women. Large-scale epidemiologic studies suggest that all-cause, metabolic, cancer, and cardiovascular morbidity begin to rise (albeit at a slow rate) when BMIs are ≥ 25, suggesting that the cut-off for obesity should be low-

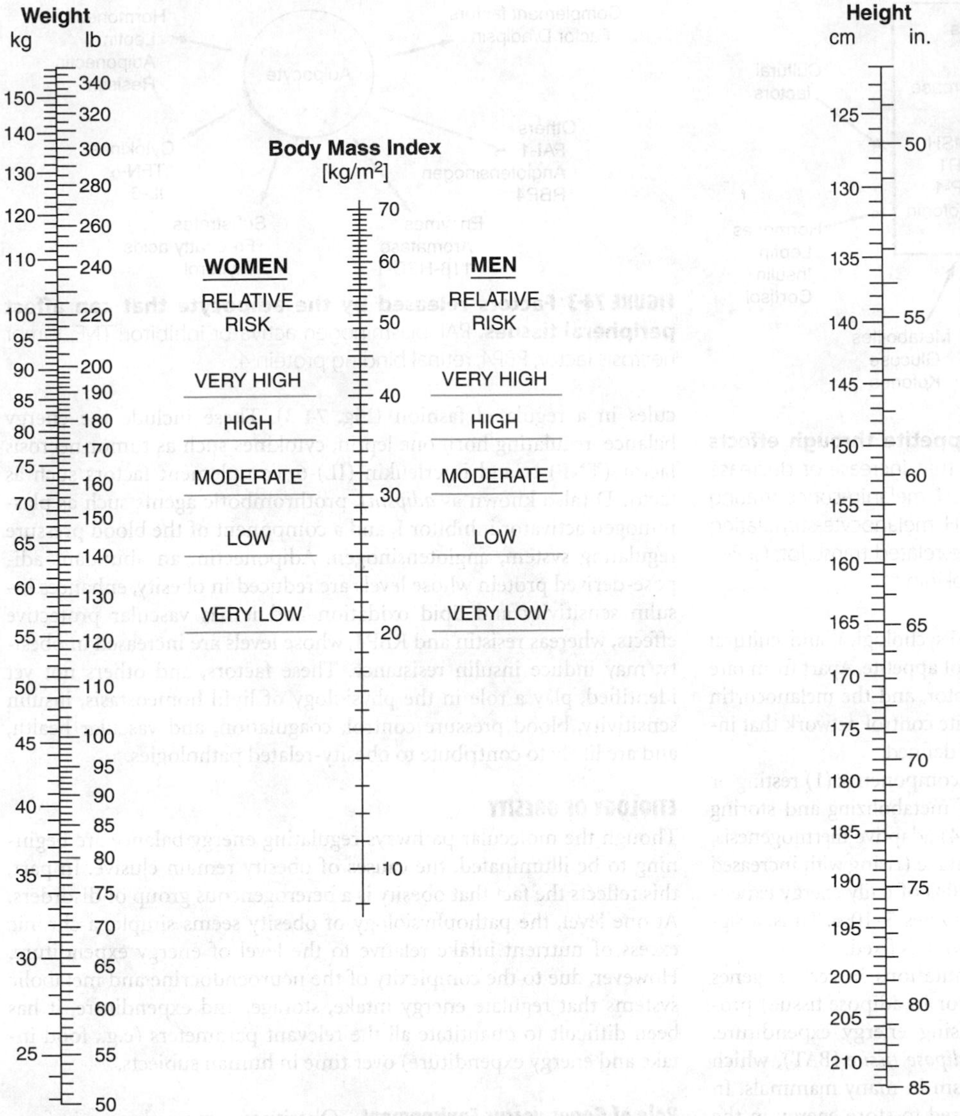

FIGURE 74-1 Nomogram for determining body mass index. To use this nomogram, place a ruler or other straight edge between the body weight (without clothes) in kilograms or pounds located on the left-hand line and the height (without shoes) in centimeters or inches located on the right-hand line. The body mass index is read from the middle of the scale and is in metric units. *(Copyright 1979, George A. Bray, M.D.; used with permission.)*

ered. Most authorities use the term *overweight* (rather than obese) to describe individuals with BMIs between 25 and 30. A BMI between 25 and 30 should be viewed as medically significant and worthy of therapeutic intervention, especially in the presence of risk factors that are influenced by adiposity, such as hypertension and glucose intolerance.

The distribution of adipose tissue in different anatomic depots also has substantial implications for morbidity. Specifically, intraabdominal and abdominal subcutaneous fat have more significance than subcutaneous fat present in the buttocks and lower extremities. This distinction is most easily made clinically by determining the waist-to-hip ratio, with a ratio >0.9 in women and >1.0 in men being abnormal. Many of the most important complications of obesity, such as insulin resistance, diabetes, hypertension, hyperlipidemia, and hyperandrogenism in women, are linked more strongly to intraabdominal and/or upper body fat than to overall adiposity (Chap. 236). The mechanism underlying this association is unknown but may relate to the fact that intraabdominal adipocytes are more lipolytically active than those from other depots. Release of free fatty acids into the portal circulation has adverse metabolic actions, especially on the liver. Whether adipokines and cytokines secreted by visceral adipocytes play an additional role in systemic complications of obesity is an area of active investigation.

PREVALENCE

Data from the National Health and Nutrition Examination Surveys (NHANES) show that the percent of the American adult population with obesity (BMI > 30) has increased from 14.5% (between 1976 and 1980) to 30.5% (between 1999 and 2000). As many as 64% of U.S. adults ≥20 years of age were overweight (defined as BMI > 25) between the years of 1999 and 2000. Extreme obesity (BMI ≥40) has also increased and affects 4.7% of the population. The increasing prevalence of medically significant obesity raises great concern. Obesity is more common among women and in the poor; the prevalence in children is also rising at a worrisome rate.

PHYSIOLOGIC REGULATION OF ENERGY BALANCE

Substantial evidence suggests that body weight is regulated by both endocrine and neural components that ultimately influence the effector arms of energy intake and expenditure. This complex regulatory system is necessary because even small imbalances between energy intake and expenditure will ultimately have large effects on body weight. For example, a 0.3% positive imbalance over 30 years would result in a 9-kg (20-lb) weight gain. This exquisite regulation of energy balance cannot be monitored easily by calorie-counting in relation to physical activity. Rather, body weight regulation or dysregulation depends on a complex interplay of hormonal and neural signals. Alterations in stable weight by forced overfeeding or food deprivation induce physiologic changes that resist these perturbations: with weight loss, appetite increases and energy expenditure falls; with overfeeding, appetite falls and energy expenditure increases. This latter compensatory mechanism frequently fails, however, permitting obesity to develop when food is abundant and physical activity is limited. A major regulator of these adaptive responses is the adipocyte-derived hormone leptin, which acts through brain circuits (predominantly in the hypothalamus) to influence appetite, energy expenditure, and neuroendocrine function (see below).

Appetite is influenced by many factors that are integrated by the brain, most importantly within the hypothalamus (Fig. 74-2). Signals that impinge on the hypothalamic center include neural afferents, hormones, and metabolites. Vagal inputs are particularly important, bringing information from viscera, such as gut distention. Hormonal signals include leptin, insulin, cortisol, and gut peptides. Among the latter are ghrelin, which is made in the stomach and stimulates feeding, and peptide YY (PYY) and cholecystokinin, which are made in the small intestine and signal to the brain through direct action on hypothalamic control centers and/or via the vagus nerve. Metabolites, including glucose, can influence appetite, as seen by the effect of hypoglycemia to induce hunger; however, glucose is not normally a major regulator of appetite. These diverse hormonal, metabolic, and neural signals act by influencing the expression and release of various hypothalamic peptides [e.g., neuropeptide Y (NPY), Agouti-related peptide (AgRP), α-melanocyte-stimulating hormone (α-MSH), and melanin-concentrating hormone (MCH)] that are integrated with serotonergic, catecholaminergic, endocannabinoid,

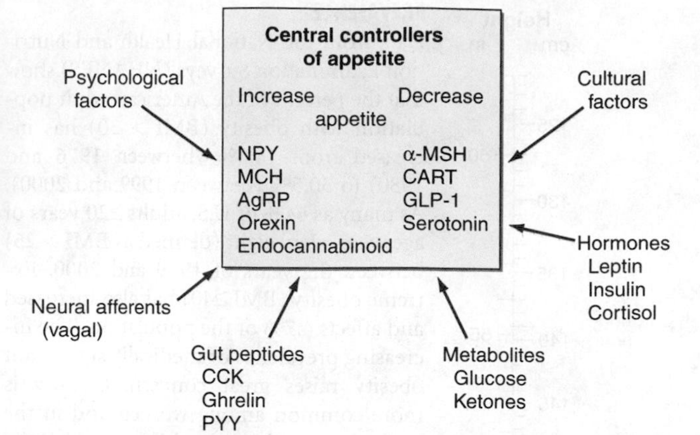

FIGURE 74-2 The factors that regulate appetite through effects on central neural circuits. Some factors that increase or decrease appetite are listed. NPY, neuropeptide Y; MCH, melanin-concentrating hormone; AgRP, Agouti-related peptide; MSH, melanocyte-stimulating hormone; CART, cocaine- and amphetamine-related transcript; GLP-1, glucagon-related peptide-1; CCK, cholecystokinin.

and opioid signaling pathways (see below). Psychological and cultural factors also play a role in the final expression of appetite. Apart from rare genetic syndromes involving leptin, its receptor, and the melanocortin system, specific defects in this complex appetite control network that influence common cases of obesity are not well defined.

Energy expenditure includes the following components: (1) resting or basal metabolic rate; (2) the energy cost of metabolizing and storing food; (3) the thermic effect of exercise; and (4) adaptive thermogenesis, which varies in response to chronic caloric intake (rising with increased intake). Basal metabolic rate accounts for ~70% of daily energy expenditure, whereas active physical activity contributes 5–10%. Thus, a significant component of daily energy consumption is fixed.

Genetic models in mice indicate that mutations in certain genes (e.g., targeted deletion of the insulin receptor in adipose tissue) protect against obesity, apparently by increasing energy expenditure. Adaptive thermogenesis occurs in *brown adipose tissue* (BAT), which plays an important role in energy metabolism in many mammals. In contrast to white adipose tissue, which is used to store energy in the form of lipids, BAT expends stored energy as heat. A mitochondrial *uncoupling protein* (UCP-1) in BAT dissipates the hydrogen ion gradient in the oxidative respiration chain and releases energy as heat. The metabolic activity of BAT is increased by a central action of leptin, acting through the sympathetic nervous system, which heavily innervates this tissue. In rodents, BAT deficiency causes obesity and diabetes; stimulation of BAT with a specific adrenergic agonist (β_3 agonist) protects against diabetes and obesity. Although BAT exists in humans (especially neonates), its physiologic role is not yet established. Homologues of UCP-1 (UCP-2 and -3) may mediate uncoupled mitochondrial respiration in other tissues.

THE ADIPOCYTE AND ADIPOSE TISSUE

Adipose tissue is composed of the lipid-storing adipose cell and a stromal/vascular compartment in which cells including preadipocytes and macrophages reside. Adipose mass increases by enlargement of adipose cells through lipid deposition, as well as by an increase in the number of adipocytes. Obese adipose tissue is also characterized by increased numbers of infiltrating macrophages. The process by which adipose cells are derived from a mesenchymal preadipocyte involves an orchestrated series of differentiation steps mediated by a cascade of specific transcription factors. One of the key transcription factors is *peroxisome proliferator-activated receptor* γ (PPARγ), a nuclear receptor that binds the thiazolidinedione class of insulin-sensitizing drugs used in the treatment of type 2 diabetes (Chap. 338).

Although the adipocyte has generally been regarded as a storage depot for fat, it is also an endocrine cell that releases numerous mole-

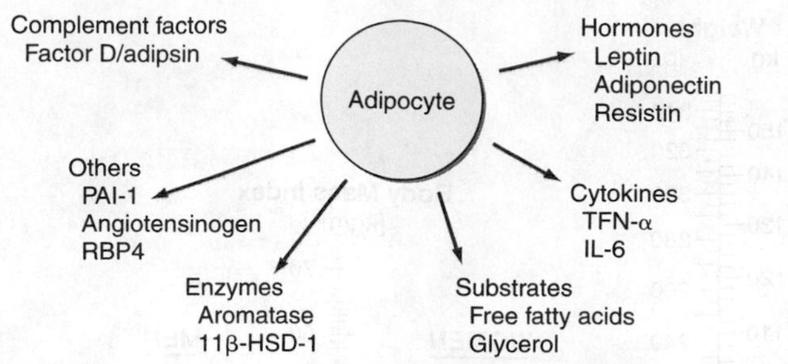

FIGURE 74-3 Factors released by the adipocyte that can affect peripheral tissues. PAI, plasminogen activator inhibitor; TNF, tumor necrosis factor; RBP4, retinal binding protein 4.

cules in a regulated fashion (Fig. 74-3). These include the energy balance–regulating hormone leptin, cytokines such as tumor necrosis factor (TNF) α and interleukin (IL)-6, complement factors such as factor D (also known as *adipsin*), prothrombotic agents such as plasminogen activator inhibitor I, and a component of the blood pressure regulating system, angiotensinogen. Adiponectin, an abundant adipose-derived protein whose levels are reduced in obesity, enhances insulin sensitivity and lipid oxidation and it has vascular protective effects, whereas resistin and RBP4, whose levels are increased in obesity, may induce insulin resistance. These factors, and others not yet identified, play a role in the physiology of lipid homeostasis, insulin sensitivity, blood pressure control, coagulation, and vascular health, and are likely to contribute to obesity-related pathologies.

ETIOLOGY OF OBESITY

Though the molecular pathways regulating energy balance are beginning to be illuminated, the causes of obesity remain elusive. In part, this reflects the fact that obesity is a heterogeneous group of disorders. At one level, the pathophysiology of obesity seems simple: a chronic excess of nutrient intake relative to the level of energy expenditure. However, due to the complexity of the neuroendocrine and metabolic systems that regulate energy intake, storage, and expenditure, it has been difficult to quantitate all the relevant parameters (e.g., food intake and energy expenditure) over time in human subjects.

Role of Genes versus Environment Obesity is commonly seen in families, and the heritability of body weight is similar to that for height. Inheritance is usually not Mendelian, however, and it is difficult to distinguish the role of genes and environmental factors. Adoptees more closely resemble their biologic than adoptive parents with respect to obesity, providing strong support for genetic influences. Likewise, identical twins have very similar BMIs whether reared together or apart, and their BMIs are much more strongly correlated than those of dizygotic twins. These genetic effects appear to relate to both energy intake and expenditure.

Whatever the role of genes, it is clear that the environment plays a key role in obesity, as evidenced by the fact that famine prevents obesity in even the most obesity-prone individual. In addition, the recent increase in the prevalence of obesity in the United States is far too rapid to be due to changes in the gene pool. Undoubtedly, genes influence the susceptibility to obesity in response to specific diets and availability of nutrition. Cultural factors are also important—these relate to both availability and composition of the diet and to changes in the level of physical activity. In industrial societies, obesity is more common among poor women, whereas in underdeveloped countries, wealthier women are more often obese. In children, obesity correlates to some degree with time spent watching television. Although the role of diet composition in obesity continues to generate controversy, it appears that high-fat diets may promote obesity, especially when combined with diets rich in simple (as opposed to complex) carbohydrates.

Additional environmental factors may contribute to the increasing obesity prevalence. Both epidemiologic correlations and experimental data suggest that sleep deprivation leads to increased obesity. Less well

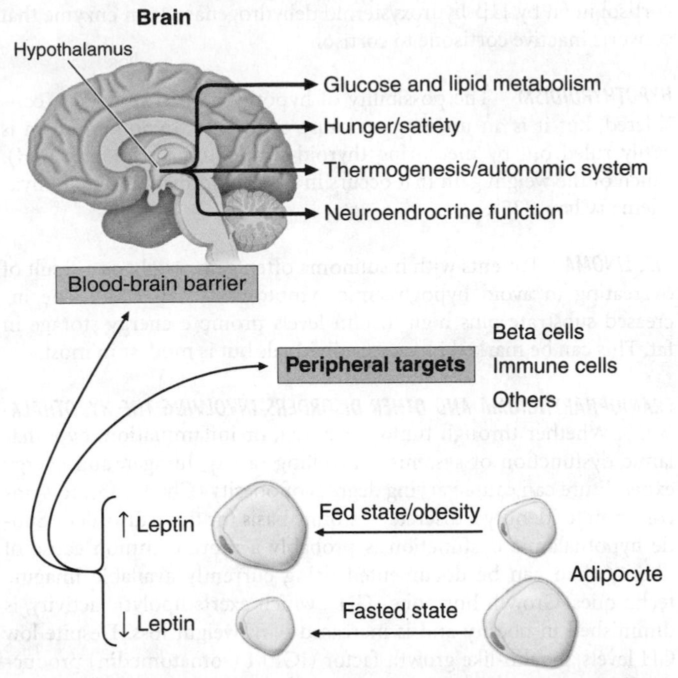

FIGURE 74-4 The physiologic system regulated by leptin. Rising or falling leptin levels act through the hypothalamus to influence appetite, energy expenditure, and neuroendocrine function and through peripheral sites to influence systems such as the immune system.

supported in humans are potential changes in gut flora with capacity to alter energy balance and a possible role for obesigenic viral infections.

Specific Genetic Syndromes For many years obesity in rodents has been known to be caused by a number of distinct mutations distributed through the genome. Most of these single-gene mutations cause both hyperphagia and diminished energy expenditure, suggesting a physiologic link between these two parameters of energy homeostasis. Identification of the *ob* gene mutation in genetically obese (ob/ob) mice represented a major breakthrough in the field. The ob/ob mouse develops severe obesity, insulin resistance, and hyperphagia, as well as efficient metabolism (e.g., it gets fat even when ingesting the same number of calories as lean litter mates). The product of the *ob* gene is the peptide leptin, a name derived from the Greek root *leptos*, meaning thin. Leptin is secreted by adipose cells and acts primarily through the hypothalamus. Its level of production provides an index of adipose energy stores (Fig. 74-4). High leptin levels decrease food intake and increase energy expenditure. Another mouse mutant, db/db, which is resistant to leptin, has a mutation in the leptin receptor and develops a similar syndrome. The *OB* gene is present in humans and expressed in fat. Several families with morbid, early-onset obesity caused by inactivating mutations in either leptin or the leptin receptor have been described, thus demonstrating the biologic relevance of leptin in humans. The obesity in these individuals begins shortly after birth, is severe, and is accompanied by neuroendocrine abnormalities. The most prominent of these is hypogonadotropic hypogonadism, which is reversed by leptin replacement. Central hypothyroidism and growth retardation are seen in the mouse model, but their occurrence in leptin-deficient humans is less clear. To date, there is no evidence to suggest that mutations or polymorphisms in the leptin or leptin receptor genes play a prominent role in common forms of obesity.

Mutations in several other genes cause severe obesity in humans (Table 74-1); each of these syndromes is rare. Mutations in the gene encoding proopiomelanocortin (POMC) cause severe obesity through failure to synthesize α-MSH, a key neuropeptide that inhibits appetite in the hypothalamus. The absence of POMC also causes secondary adrenal insufficiency due to absence of adrenocorticotropic hormone (ACTH), as well as pale skin and red hair due to absence of α-MSH. Proenzyme convertase 1 (PC-1) mutations are thought to cause obesity by preventing synthesis of α-MSH from its precursor peptide, POMC. α-MSH binds to the type 4 melanocortin receptor (MC4R), a key hypothalamic receptor that inhibits eating. Heterozygous loss-of-function mutations of this receptor account for as much as 5% of severe obesity. These five genetic defects define a pathway through which leptin (by stimulating POMC and increasing α-MSH) restricts food intake and limits weight (Fig. 74-5).

In addition to these human obesity genes, studies in rodents reveal several other molecular candidates for hypothalamic mediators of human obesity or leanness. The *tub* gene encodes a hypothalamic peptide of unknown function; mutation of this gene causes late-onset obesity. The *fat* gene encodes carboxypeptidase E, a peptide-processing enzyme; mutation of this gene is thought to cause obesity by disrupting production of one or more neuropeptides. AgRP is coexpressed with NPY in arcuate nucleus neurons. AgRP antagonizes α-MSH action at MC4 receptors, and its overexpression induces obesity. In contrast, a mouse deficient in the peptide MCH, whose administration causes feeding, is lean.

A number of complex human syndromes with defined inheritance are associated with obesity (Table 74-2). Although specific genes are undefined at present, their identification will likely enhance our understanding of more common forms of human obesity. In the Prader-Willi syndrome, obesity coexists with short stature, mental retardation, hypogonadotropic hypogonadism, hypotonia, small hands and feet, fish-shaped mouth, and hyperphagia. Most patients have a chromosome 15 deletion, and reduced expression of the signaling protein necdin may be an important cause of defective hypothalamic neural development in this disorder (Chap. 63). Bardet-Biedl syndrome

TABLE 74-1 SOME OBESITY GENES IN HUMANS AND MICE

Gene	Gene Product	Mechanism of Obesity	In Human	In Rodent
Lep (ob)	Leptin, a fat-derived hormone	Mutation prevents leptin from delivering satiety signal; brain perceives starvation	Yes	Yes
LepR (db)	Leptin receptor	Same as above	Yes	Yes
POMC	Proopiomelanocortin, a precursor of several hormones and neuropeptides	Mutation prevents synthesis of melanocyte-stimulating hormone (MSH), a satiety signal	Yes	Yes
MC4R	Type 4 receptor for MSH	Mutation prevents reception of satiety signal from MSH	Yes	Yes
AgRP	Agouti-related peptide, a neuropeptide expressed in the hypothalamus	Overexpression inhibits signal through MC4R	No	Yes
PC-1	Prohormone convertase 1, a processing enzyme	Mutation prevents synthesis of neuropeptide, probably MSH	Yes	No
Fat	Carboxypeptidase E, a processing enzyme	Same as above	No	Yes
Tub	Tub, a hypothalamic protein of unknown function	Hypothalamic dysfunction	No	Yes
TrkB	TrkB, a neurotrophin receptor	Hyperphagia due to uncharacterized hypothalamic defect	Yes	Yes

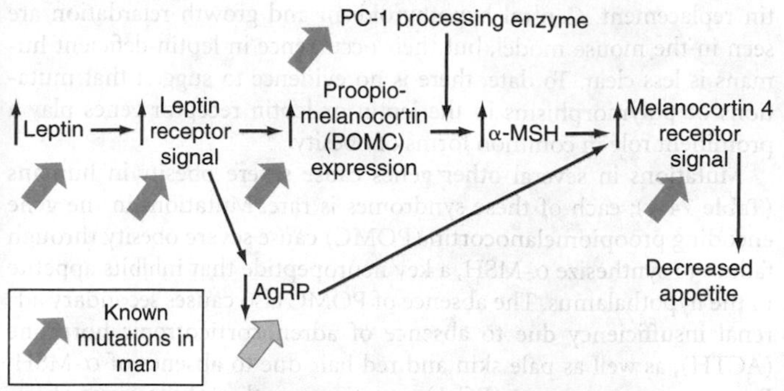

FIGURE 74-5 A central pathway through which leptin acts to regulate appetite and body weight. Leptin signals through proopiomelanocortin (POMC) neurons in the hypothalamus to induce increased production of α-melanocyte-stimulating hormone (α-MSH), requiring the processing enzyme PC-1 (proenzyme convertase 1). α-MSH acts as an agonist on melanocortin-4 receptors to inhibit appetite, and the neuropeptide AgRp (Agouti-related peptide) acts as an antagonist of this receptor. Mutations that cause obesity in humans are indicated by the solid green arrows.

(BBS) is a genetically heterogeneous disorder characterized by obesity, mental retardation, retinitis pigmentosa, renal and cardiac malformations, polydactyly, and hypogonadotropic hypogonadism. At least eight genetic loci have been identified, and BBS may involve defects in ciliary function.

Other Specific Syndromes Associated with Obesity • ***CUSHING'S SYNDROME*** Although obese patients commonly have central obesity, hypertension, and glucose intolerance, they lack other specific stigmata of Cushing's syndrome (Chap. 336). Nonetheless, a potential diagnosis of Cushing's syndrome is often entertained. Cortisol production and urinary metabolites (17OH steroids) may be increased in simple obesity. Unlike in Cushing's syndrome, however, cortisol levels in blood and urine in the basal state and in response to corticotropin-releasing hormone (CRH) or ACTH are normal; the overnight 1-mg dexamethasone suppression test is normal in 90%, with the remainder being normal on a standard 2-day low-dose dexamethasone suppression test. Obesity may be associated with excessive local reactivation of cortisol in fat by 11β-hydroxysteroid dehydrogenase 1, an enzyme that converts inactive cortisone to cortisol.

HYPOTHYROIDISM The possibility of hypothyroidism should be considered, but it is an uncommon cause of obesity; hypothyroidism is easily ruled out by measuring thyroid-stimulating hormone (TSH). Much of the weight gain that occurs in hypothyroidism is due to myxedema (Chap. 335).

INSULINOMA Patients with insulinoma often gain weight as a result of overeating to avoid hypoglycemic symptoms (Chap. 339). The increased substrate plus high insulin levels promote energy storage in fat. This can be marked in some individuals but is modest in most.

CRANIOPHARYNGIOMA AND OTHER DISORDERS INVOLVING THE HYPOTHALAMUS Whether through tumors, trauma, or inflammation, hypothalamic dysfunction of systems controlling satiety, hunger, and energy expenditure can cause varying degrees of obesity (Chap. 333). It is uncommon to identify a discrete anatomic basis for these disorders. Subtle hypothalamic dysfunction is probably a more common cause of obesity than can be documented using currently available imaging techniques. Growth hormone (GH), which exerts lipolytic activity, is diminished in obesity and is increased with weight loss. Despite low GH levels, insulin-like growth factor (IGF) I (somatomedin) production is normal, suggesting that GH suppression is a compensatory response to increased nutritional supply.

Pathogenesis of Common Obesity Obesity can result from increased energy intake, decreased energy expenditure, or a combination of the two. Thus, identifying the etiology of obesity should involve measurements of both parameters. However, it is nearly impossible to perform direct and accurate measurements of energy intake in free-living individuals, and the obese, in particular, often underreport intake. Measurements of chronic energy expenditure have only recently become available using doubly labeled water or metabolic chamber/rooms. In subjects at stable weight and body composition, energy intake equals expenditure. Consequently, these techniques allow assessment of energy intake in free-living individuals. The level of energy expenditure differs in established obesity, during periods of weight gain or loss, and in the pre- or postobese state. Studies that fail to take note of this phenomenon are not easily interpreted.

TABLE 74-2 A COMPARISON OF SYNDROMES OF OBESITY—HYPOGONADISM AND MENTAL RETARDATION

	Syndrome				
Feature	**Prader-Willi**	**Laurence-Moon-Biedl**	**Ahlstrom**	**Cohen**	**Carpenter**
Inheritance	Sporadic; two-thirds have defect	Autosomal recessive	Autosomal recessive	Probably autosomal recessive	Autosomal recessive
Stature	Short	Normal; infrequently short	Normal; infrequently short	Short or tall	Normal
Obesity	Generalized Moderate to severe Onset 1–3 yrs	Generalized Early onset, 1–2 yrs	Truncal Early onset, 2–5 yrs	Truncal Mid-childhood, age 5	Truncal, gluteal
Craniofacies	Narrow bifrontal diameter Almond-shaped eyes Strabismus V-shaped mouth High-arched palate	Not distinctive	Not distinctive	High nasal bridge Arched palate Open mouth Short philtrum	Acrocephaly Flat nasal bridge High-arched palate
Limbs	Small hands and feet Hypotonia	Polydactyly	No abnormalities	Hypotonia Narrow hands and feet	Polydactyly Syndactyly Genu valgum
Reproductive status	1° Hypogonadism	1° Hypogonadism	Hypogonadism in males but not in females	Normal gonadal function or hypogonadotrophic hypogonadism	2° Hypogonadism
Other features	Enamel hypoplasia Hyperphagia Temper tantrums Nasal speech			Dysplastic ears Delayed puberty	
Mental retardation	Mild to moderate		Normal intelligence	Mild	Slight

There is continued interest in the concept of a body weight "set point." This idea is supported by physiologic mechanisms centered around a sensing system in adipose tissue that reflects fat stores and a receptor, or "adipostat," that is in the hypothalamic centers. When fat stores are depleted, the adipostat signal is low, and the hypothalamus responds by stimulating hunger and decreasing energy expenditure to conserve energy. Conversely, when fat stores are abundant, the signal is increased, and the hypothalamus responds by decreasing hunger and increasing energy expenditure. The recent discovery of the *ob* gene, and its product leptin, and the *db* gene, whose product is the leptin receptor, provides important elements of a molecular basis for this physiologic concept (see above).

What Is the Status of Food Intake in Obesity? (Do the Obese Eat More Than the Lean?) This question has stimulated much debate, due in part to the methodologic difficulties inherent in determining food intake. Many obese individuals believe that they eat small quantities of food, and this claim has often been supported by the results of food intake questionnaires. However, it is now established that average energy expenditure increases as individuals get more obese, due primarily to the fact that metabolically active lean tissue mass increases with obesity. Given the laws of thermodynamics, the obese person must therefore eat more than the average lean person to maintain their increased weight. It may be the case, however, that a subset of individuals who are predisposed to obesity have the capacity to become obese initially without an absolute increase in caloric consumption.

What Is the State of Energy Expenditure in Obesity? The average total daily energy expenditure is higher in obese than lean individuals when measured at stable weight. However, energy expenditure falls as weight is lost, due in part to loss of lean body mass and to decreased sympathetic nerve activity. When reduced to near-normal weight and maintained there for a while, (some) obese individuals have lower energy expenditure than (some) lean individuals. There is also a tendency for those who will develop obesity as infants or children to have lower resting energy expenditure rates than those who remain lean.

The physiologic basis for variable rates of energy expenditure (at a given body weight and level of energy intake) is essentially unknown. A mutation in the human β_3-adrenergic receptor may be associated with increased risk of obesity and/or insulin resistance in certain (but not all) populations. Homologues of the BAT uncoupling protein, named UCP-2 and UCP-3, have been identified in both rodents and humans. UCP-2 is expressed widely, whereas UCP-3 is primarily expressed in skeletal muscle. These proteins may play a role in disordered energy balance.

One newly described component of thermogenesis, called *nonexercise activity thermogenesis* (NEAT), has been linked to obesity. It is the thermogenesis that accompanies physical activities other than volitional exercise, such as the activities of daily living, fidgeting, spontaneous muscle contraction, and maintaining posture. NEAT accounts for about two-thirds of the increased daily energy expenditure induced by overfeeding. The wide variation in fat storage seen in overfed individuals is predicted by the degree to which NEAT is induced. The molecular basis for NEAT and its regulation is unknown.

Leptin in Typical Obesity The vast majority of obese persons have increased leptin levels but do not have mutations of either leptin or its receptor. They appear, therefore, to have a form of functional "leptin resistance." Data suggesting that some individuals produce less leptin per unit fat mass than others or have a form of relative leptin deficiency that predisposes to obesity are at present contradictory and unsettled. The mechanism for leptin resistance, and whether it can be overcome by raising leptin levels, is not yet established. Some data suggest that leptin may not effectively cross the blood-brain barrier as levels rise. It is also apparent from animal studies that leptin signaling inhibitors, such as SOCS3 and PTP1b, are involved in the leptin-resistant state.

PATHOLOGIC CONSEQUENCES OF OBESITY

(See also Chap. 75) Obesity has major adverse effects on health. Obesity is associated with an increase in mortality, with a 50–100% increased risk of death from all causes compared to normal-weight individuals, mostly due to cardiovascular causes. Obesity and overweight together are the second leading cause of preventable death in the United States, accounting for 300,000 deaths per year. Mortality rates rise as obesity increases, particularly when obesity is associated with increased intraabdominal fat (see above). Life expectancy of a moderately obese individual could be shortened by 2–5 years, and a 20- to 30-year-old male with a BMI > 45 may lose 13 years of life. It is also apparent that the degree to which obesity affects particular organ systems is influenced by susceptibility genes that vary in the population.

Insulin Resistance and Type 2 Diabetes Mellitus Hyperinsulinemia and insulin resistance are pervasive features of obesity, increasing with weight gain and diminishing with weight loss (Chap. 236). Insulin resistance is more strongly linked to intraabdominal fat than to fat in other depots. The molecular link between obesity and insulin resistance in tissues such as fat, muscle, and liver has been sought for many years. Major factors under investigation include: (1) insulin itself, by inducing receptor downregulation; (2) free fatty acids, known to be increased and capable of impairing insulin action; (3) intracellular lipid accumulation; and (4) various circulating peptides produced by adipocytes, including the cytokines TNF-α and IL-6, RBP4, and the "adipokines" adiponectin and resistin, which are produced by adipocytes, have altered expression in obese adipocytes, and are capable of modifying insulin action. Despite nearly universal insulin resistance, most obese individuals do not develop diabetes, suggesting that the onset of diabetes requires an interaction between obesity-induced insulin resistance and other factors that predispose to diabetes, such as impaired insulin secretion (Chap. 338). Obesity, however, is a major risk factor for diabetes, and as many as 80% of patients with type 2 diabetes mellitus are obese. Weight loss and exercise, even of modest degree, are associated with increased insulin sensitivity and often improve glucose control in diabetes.

Reproductive Disorders Disorders that affect the reproductive axis are associated with obesity in both men and women. Male hypogonadism is associated with increased adipose tissue, often distributed in a pattern more typical of females. In men >160% ideal body weight, plasma testosterone and sex hormone–binding globulin (SHBG) are often reduced, and estrogen levels (derived from conversion of adrenal androgens in adipose tissue) are increased (Chap. 340). Gynecomastia may be seen. However, masculinization, libido, potency, and spermatogenesis are preserved in most of these individuals. Free testosterone may be decreased in morbidly obese men whose weight is >200% ideal body weight.

Obesity has long been associated with menstrual abnormalities in women, particularly in women with upper body obesity (Chap. 341). Common findings are increased androgen production, decreased SHBG, and increased peripheral conversion of androgen to estrogen. Most obese women with oligomenorrhea have the polycystic ovarian syndrome (PCOS), with its associated anovulation and ovarian hyperandrogenism; 40% of women with PCOS are obese. Most nonobese women with PCOS are also insulin-resistant, suggesting that insulin resistance, hyperinsulinemia, or the combination of the two are causative or contribute to the ovarian pathophysiology in PCOS in both obese and lean individuals. In obese women with PCOS, weight loss or treatment with insulin-sensitizing drugs often restores normal menses. The increased conversion of androstenedione to estrogen, which occurs to a greater degree in women with lower body obesity, may contribute to the increased incidence of uterine cancer in postmenopausal women with obesity.

Cardiovascular Disease The Framingham Study revealed that obesity was an independent risk factor for the 26-year incidence of cardiovascular disease in men and women [including coronary disease, stroke, and congestive heart failure (CHF)]. The waist/hip ratio may be the best predictor of these risks. When the additional effects of hypertension and glucose intolerance associated with obesity are included, the adverse impact of obesity is even more evident. The effect of obesity on cardiovascular mortality in women may be seen at BMIs as low as 25. Obesity, especially abdominal obesity, is associated with an atherogenic lipid profile; with increased low-density lipoprotein (LDL) cholesterol, very low density lipoprotein, and triglyceride; and with decreased high-density lipoprotein cholesterol and decreased levels of the vascular protective adipokine adiponectin (Chap. 350). Obesity is also associated with hypertension. Measurement of blood pressure in the obese requires use of a larger cuff size to avoid artifactual increases. Obesity-induced hypertension is associated with increased peripheral resistance and cardiac output, increased sympathetic nervous system tone, increased salt sensitivity, and insulin-mediated salt retention; it is often responsive to modest weight loss.

Pulmonary Disease Obesity may be associated with a number of pulmonary abnormalities. These include reduced chest wall compliance, increased work of breathing, increased minute ventilation due to increased metabolic rate, and decreased functional residual capacity and expiratory reserve volume (Chap. 246). Severe obesity may be associated with obstructive sleep apnea and the "obesity hypoventilation syndrome" with attenuated hypoxic and hypercapnic ventilatory responses (Chap. 258). Sleep apnea can be obstructive (most common), central, or mixed and is associated with hypertension. Weight loss (10–20 kg) can bring substantial improvement, as can major weight loss following gastric bypass or restrictive surgery. Continuous positive airway pressure has been used with some success.

Gallstones Obesity is associated with enhanced biliary secretion of cholesterol, supersaturation of bile, and a higher incidence of gallstones, particularly cholesterol gallstones (Chap. 305). A person 50% above ideal body weight has about a sixfold increased incidence of symptomatic gallstones. Paradoxically, fasting increases supersaturation of bile by decreasing the phospholipid component. Fasting-induced cholecystitis is a complication of extreme diets.

Cancer Obesity in males is associated with higher mortality from cancer, including cancer of the esophagus, colon, rectum, pancreas, liver, and prostate; obesity in females is associated with higher mortality from cancer of the gallbladder, bile ducts, breasts, endometrium, cervix, and ovaries. Some of the latter may be due to increased rates of conversion of androstenedione to estrone in adipose tissue of obese individuals. It was recently estimated that obesity accounts for 14% of cancer deaths in men and 20% in women in the United States.

Bone, Joint, and Cutaneous Disease Obesity is associated with an increased risk of osteoarthritis, no doubt partly due to the trauma of added weight bearing and joint malalignment. The prevalence of gout may also be increased (Chap. 327). Among the skin problems associated with obesity is acanthosis nigricans, manifested by darkening and thickening of the skin folds on the neck, elbows, and dorsal interphalangeal spaces. Acanthosis reflects the severity of underlying insulin resistance and diminishes with weight loss. Friability of skin may be increased, especially in skin folds, enhancing the risk of fungal and yeast infections. Finally, venous stasis is increased in the obese.

FURTHER READINGS

FAROOQI IS, O'RAHILLY S: Genetics of obesity. Philos Trans R Soc Lond B Biol Sci 361:1095, 2006

FLIER JS: Obesity wars: Molecular progress confronts an expanding epidemic. Cell 116:337, 2004

KERSHAW EE, FLIER JS: Adipose tissue as an endocrine organ. J Clin Endocrinol Metab 89:2548, 2004

MORTON GJ et al: Central nervous system control of food intake and body weight. Nature 443:289, 2006

MURPHY KG et al: Gut peptides in the regulation of food intake and energy homeostasis. Endocr Rev 27:719, 2006

OGDEN CL et al: The epidemiology of obesity. Gastroenterology 132(6):2087, 2007

OGDEN CL et al: Prevalence of overweight and obesity in the United States, 1999–2004. JAMA 295:1549, 2006

75 Evaluation and Management of Obesity

Robert F. Kushner

Over 66% of U.S. adults are currently categorized as overweight or obese, and the prevalence of obesity is increasing rapidly throughout most of the industrialized world. Based on statistics from the World Health Organization, overweight and obesity may soon replace more traditional public health concerns such as undernutrition and infectious diseases as the most significant contributors to ill health. Children and adolescents are also becoming more obese, indicating that the current trends will accelerate over time. Obesity is associated with an increased risk of multiple health problems, including hypertension, type 2 diabetes, dyslipidemia, degenerative joint disease, and some malignancies. Thus, it is important for physicians to routinely identify, evaluate, and treat patients for obesity and associated comorbid conditions.

EVALUATION

The U.S. Preventive Services Task Force recommends that physicians screen all adult patients for obesity and offer intensive counseling and behavioral interventions to promote sustained weight loss. This recommendation is consistent with previously released guidelines from the National Heart, Lung, and Blood Institute (NHLBI) and a number of medical societies. The five main steps in the evaluation of obesity are described below and include (1) focused obesity-related history, (2) physical examination to determine the degree and type of obesity, (3) comorbid conditions, (4) fitness level, and (5) the patient's readiness to adopt lifestyle changes.

The Obesity-Focused History Information from the history should address the following six questions:

- What factors contribute to the patient's obesity?
- How is the obesity affecting the patient's health?
- What is the patient's level of risk from obesity?
- What are the patient's goals and expectations?
- Is the patient motivated to begin a weight management program?
- What kind of help does the patient need?

Although the vast majority of obesity can be attributed to behavioral features that affect diet and physical activity patterns, the history may suggest secondary causes that merit further evaluation. Disorders to consider include polycystic ovarian syndrome, hypothyroidism, Cushing's syndrome, and hypothalamic disease. Drug-induced weight gain should also to be considered. Common causes include antidiabetes agents (insulin, sulfonylureas, thiazolidinediones); steroid hormones; psychotropic agents; mood stabilizers (lithium); antidepressants (tricyclics, monoamine oxidase inhibitors, paraxetine, mirtazapine); and antiepileptic drugs (valproate, gabapentin, carbamazapine). Other medications such as nonsteroidal anti-inflammatory drugs and calcium-channel blockers may cause peripheral edema, but they do not increase body fat.

The patient's current diet and physical activity patterns may reveal factors that contribute to the development of obesity in addition to identifying behaviors to target for treatment. This type of historical information is best obtained by using a questionnaire in combination with an interview.

TABLE 75-1 BODY MASS INDEX (BMI) TABLE

BMI	19	20	21	22	23	24	25	26	27	28	29	30	31	32	33	34	35
Height, inches	Body Weight, pounds																
58	91	96	100	105	110	115	119	124	129	134	138	143	148	153	158	162	167
59	94	99	104	109	114	119	124	128	133	138	143	148	153	158	163	168	173
60	97	102	107	112	118	123	128	133	138	143	148	153	158	163	168	174	179
61	100	106	111	116	122	127	132	137	143	148	153	158	164	169	174	180	185
62	104	109	115	120	126	131	136	142	147	153	158	164	169	175	180	186	191
63	107	113	118	124	130	135	141	146	152	158	163	169	175	180	186	191	197
64	110	116	122	128	134	140	145	151	157	163	169	174	180	186	192	197	204
65	114	120	126	132	138	144	150	156	162	168	174	180	186	192	198	204	210
66	118	124	130	136	142	148	155	161	167	173	179	186	192	198	204	210	216
67	121	127	134	140	146	153	159	166	172	178	185	191	198	204	211	217	223
68	125	131	138	144	151	158	164	171	177	184	190	197	203	210	216	223	230
69	128	135	142	149	155	162	169	176	182	189	196	203	209	216	223	230	236
70	132	139	146	153	160	167	174	181	188	195	202	209	216	222	229	236	243
71	136	143	150	157	165	172	179	186	193	200	208	215	222	229	236	243	250
72	140	147	154	162	169	177	184	191	199	206	213	221	228	235	242	250	258
73	144	151	159	166	174	182	189	197	204	212	219	227	235	242	250	257	265
74	148	155	163	171	179	186	194	202	210	218	225	233	241	249	256	264	272
75	152	160	168	176	184	192	200	208	216	224	232	240	248	256	264	272	279
76	156	164	172	180	189	197	205	213	221	230	238	246	254	263	271	279	287

BMI	36	37	38	39	40	41	42	43	44	45	46	47	48	49	50	51	52	53	54
58	172	177	181	186	191	196	201	205	210	215	220	224	229	234	239	244	248	253	258
59	178	183	188	193	198	203	208	212	217	222	227	232	237	242	247	252	257	262	267
60	184	189	194	199	204	209	215	220	225	230	235	240	245	250	255	261	266	271	276
61	190	195	201	206	211	217	222	227	232	238	243	248	254	259	264	269	275	280	285
62	196	202	207	213	218	224	229	235	240	246	251	256	262	267	273	278	284	289	295
63	203	208	214	220	225	231	237	242	248	254	259	265	270	278	282	287	293	299	304
64	209	215	221	227	232	238	244	250	256	262	267	273	279	285	291	296	302	308	314
65	216	222	228	234	240	246	252	258	264	270	276	282	288	294	300	306	312	318	324
66	223	229	235	241	247	253	260	266	272	278	284	291	297	303	309	315	322	328	334
67	230	236	242	249	255	261	268	274	280	287	293	299	306	312	319	325	331	338	344
68	236	243	249	256	262	269	276	282	289	295	302	308	315	322	328	335	341	348	354
69	243	250	257	263	270	277	284	291	297	304	311	318	324	331	338	345	351	358	365
70	250	257	264	271	278	285	292	299	306	313	320	327	334	341	348	355	362	369	376
71	257	265	272	279	286	293	301	308	315	322	329	338	343	351	358	365	372	379	386
72	265	272	279	287	294	302	309	316	324	331	338	346	353	361	368	375	383	390	397
73	272	280	288	295	302	310	318	325	333	340	348	355	363	371	378	386	393	401	408
74	280	287	295	303	311	319	326	334	342	350	358	365	373	381	389	396	404	412	420
75	287	295	303	311	319	327	335	343	351	359	367	375	383	391	399	407	415	423	431
76	295	304	312	320	328	336	344	353	361	369	377	385	394	402	410	418	426	435	443

BMI and Waist Circumference Three key anthropometric measurements are important to evaluate the degree of obesity—weight, height, and waist circumference. The body mass index (BMI), calculated as weight (kg)/height $(m)^2$, or as weight (lbs)/height $(inches)^2 \times 703$, is used to classify weight status and risk of disease (Tables 75-1 and 75-2). BMI is used since it provides an estimate of body fat and is related to risk of disease. Lower BMI thresholds for overweight and obesity have been proposed for the Asia-Pacific region since this population appears to be at-risk at lower body weights for glucose and lipid abnormalities.

Excess abdominal fat, assessed by measurement of waist circumference or waist-to-hip ratio, is independently associated with higher risk for diabetes mellitus and cardiovascular disease. Measurement of the waist circumference is a surrogate for visceral adipose tissue and should be performed in the horizontal plane above the iliac crest. Cut points that define higher risk for men and women based on ethnicity have been proposed by the International Diabetes Federation (Table 75-3).

TABLE 75-2 CLASSIFICATION OF WEIGHT STATUS AND RISK OF DISEASE

	BMI (kg/m^2)	Obesity Class	Risk of Disease
Underweight	<18.5		
Healthy weight	18.5–24.9		
Overweight	25.0–29.9		Increased
Obesity	30.0–34.9	I	High
Obesity	35.0–39.9	II	Very high
Extreme Obesity	≥40	III	Extremely high

Source: Adapted from National Institutes of Health, National Heart, Lung, and Blood Institute: *Clinical Guidelines on the Identification, Evaluation, and Treatment of Overweight and Obesity in Adults.* U.S. Department of Health and Human Services, Public Health Service, 1998.

TABLE 75-3 ETHNIC-SPECIFIC VALUES FOR WAIST CIRCUMFERENCE

Ethnic Group	Waist Circumference
Europeans	
Men	>94 cm (37 in)
Women	>80 cm (31.5 in)
South Asians and Chinese	
Men	>90 cm (35 in)
Women	>80 cm (31.5 in)
Japanese	
Men	>85 cm (33.5 in)
Women	>90 cm (35 in)
Ethnic south and central Americans	Use south Asian recommendations until more specific data are available.
Sub-Saharan Africans	Use European data until more specific data are available.
Eastern Mediterranean and Middle East (Arab) populations	Use European data until more specific data are available.

Source: From KGMM Alberti et al for the IDF Epidemiology Task Force Consensus Group: The metabolic syndrome—a new worldwide definition. Lancet 366:1059, 2005.

Physical Fitness Several prospective studies have demonstrated that physical fitness, reported by questionnaire or measured by a maximal treadmill exercise test, is an important predictor of all-cause mortality independent of BMI and body composition. These observations highlight the importance of taking an exercise history during examination as well as emphasizing physical activity as a treatment approach.

Obesity-Associated Comorbid Conditions The evaluation of comorbid conditions should be based on presentation of symptoms, risk factors, and index of suspicion. All patients should have a fasting lipid panel (total, LDL, and HDL cholesterol and triglyceride levels) and blood glucose measured at presentation along with blood pressure determination. Symptoms and diseases that are directly or indirectly related to obesity are listed in Table 75-4. Although individuals vary, the number and severity of organ-specific comorbid conditions usually rise with increasing levels of obesity. Patients at very high absolute risk include the following: established coronary heart disease; presence of other atherosclerotic diseases such as peripheral arterial disease, abdominal aortic aneurysm, and symptomatic carotid artery disease; type 2 diabetes; and sleep apnea.

Assessing the Patient's Readiness to Change An attempt to initiate lifestyle changes when the patient is not ready usually leads to frustration and may hamper future weight-loss efforts. Assessment includes patient motivation and support, stressful life events, psychiatric status, time availability and constraints, and appropriateness of goals and expectations. Readiness can be viewed as the balance of two opposing forces: (1) motivation, or the patient's desire to change; and (2) resistance, or the patient's resistance to change.

A helpful method to begin a readiness assessment is to "anchor" the patient's interest and confidence to change on a numerical scale. Using this technique, the patient is asked to rate his or her level of interest and confidence on a scale from 0 to 10, with 0 being not so important (or confident) and 10 being very important (or confident) to lose weight at this time. This exercise helps to establish readiness to change and also serves as a basis for further dialogue.

℞ OBESITY

THE GOAL OF THERAPY The primary goal of treatment is to improve obesity-related comorbid conditions and reduce the risk of developing future comorbidities. Information obtained from the history, physical examination, and diagnostic tests is used to determine risk and develop a treatment plan (Fig. 75-1). The decision of how aggressively to treat the patient, and which modalities to use, is determined by the patient's risk status, expectations, and available resources. Therapy for obesity always begins with lifestyle management and may include pharmacotherapy or surgery, depending on BMI risk category (Table 75-5). Setting an initial weight-loss goal of 10% over 6 months is a realistic target.

LIFESTYLE MANAGEMENT Obesity care involves attention to three essential elements of lifestyle: dietary habits, physical activity, and behavior modification. Because obesity is fundamentally a disease of energy imbalance, all patients must learn how and when energy is consumed (diet), how and when energy is expended (physical activity), and how to incorporate this information into their daily life (behavior therapy). Lifestyle management has been shown to result in a modest (typically 3–5 kg) weight loss compared to no treatment or usual care.

Diet Therapy The primary focus of diet therapy is to reduce overall calorie consumption. The NHLBI guidelines recommend initiating treatment with a calorie deficit of 500–1000 kcal/d compared to the patient's habitual diet. This reduction is consistent with a goal of losing approximately 1–2 lb per week. This calorie deficit can be accomplished by suggesting substitutions or alternatives to the diet. Examples include choosing smaller portion sizes, eating more fruits and vegetables, consuming more whole-grain cereals, selecting leaner cuts of meat and skimmed dairy products, reducing fried foods and other added fats and oils, and drinking water instead of caloric beverages. It is important that the dietary counseling remains patient-centered and that the goals are practical, realistic, and achievable.

The macronutrient composition of the diet will vary depending on the patient's preference and medical condition. The 2005 U.S. Department of Agriculture Dietary Guidelines for Americans (Chap. 70), which focus on health promotion and risk reduction, can be applied to treatment of the overweight or obese patient. The recommendations include maintaining a diet rich in whole grains, fruits, vegetables, and dietary fiber; consuming two servings (8 oz) of fish high in omega 3 fatty acids per week; decreasing sodium to <2300 mg/d; consuming 3 cups of milk (or equivalent low-fat or fat-free dairy products) per day; limiting cholesterol to <300 mg/d; and keeping total fat between 20 and 35% of daily calories and saturated fats to <10% of daily calories. Application of these guidelines to specific calorie goals can be found on the website *www.mypyramid.gov*. The revised Dietary Reference Intakes for Macronutrients released by the Institute of Medicine recommends 45–65% of calories from carbohydrates, 20–35% from fat, and 10–35% from protein. The guidelines also recommend daily fiber intake of 38 g (men) and 25 g (women) for persons over 50 years of age and 30 g (men) and 21 g (women) for those under 50.

TABLE 75-4 OBESITY-RELATED ORGAN SYSTEMS REVIEW

Cardiovascular	**Respiratory**
Hypertension	Dyspnea
Congestive heart failure	Obstructive sleep apnea
Cor pulmonale	Hypoventilation syndrome
Varicose veins	Pickwickian syndrome
Pulmonary embolism	Asthma
Coronary artery disease	**Gastrointestinal**
Endocrine	Gastroesophageal reflux disease
Metabolic syndrome	Nonalcoholic fatty liver disease
Type 2 diabetes	Cholelithiasis
Dyslipidemia	Hernias
Polycystic ovarian syndrome	Colon cancer
Musculoskeletal	**Genitourinary**
Hyperuricemia and gout	Urinary stress incontinence
Immobility	Obesity-related glomerulopathy
Osteoarthritis (knees and hips)	Hypogonadism (male)
Low back pain	Breast and uterine cancer
Carpal tunnel syndrome	Pregnancy complications
Psychological	**Neurologic**
Depression/low self-esteem	Stroke
Body image disturbance	Idiopathic intracranial hypertension
Social stigmatization	Meralgia paresthetica
Integument	Dementia
Striae distensae	
Stasis pigmentation of legs	
Lymphedema	
Cellulitis	
Intertrigo, carbuncles	
Acanthosis nigricans	
Acrochordon (skin tags)	
Hidradenitis suppurativa	

Since portion control is one of the most difficult strategies for patients to manage, the use of pre-prepared products, such as meal replacements, is a simple and convenient suggestion. Examples include frozen entrees, canned beverages and bars. Use of meal replacements in the diet has been shown to result in a 7–8% weight loss.

A current area of controversy is the use of low-carbohydrate, high-protein diets for weight loss. These diets are based on the concept that carbohydrates are the primary cause of obesity and lead to insulin resistance. Most low-carbohydrate diets (e.g., South Beach, Zone, and Sugar Busters!) recommend a carbohydrate level of approximately 40–46% of energy. The Atkins diet contains 5–15% carbohydrate, depending on the phase of the diet. Several randomized, controlled trials of these low-carbohydrate diets have demonstrated greater weight loss at 6 months with improvement in coronary heart disease risk factors, including an increase in HDL cholesterol and a decrease in triglyceride levels. Weight loss between groups did not remain statistically significant at 1 year; however, low-carbohydrate diets appear to be at least as effective as low-fat diets in inducing weight loss for up to 1 year.

Another dietary approach to consider is the concept of energy density, which refers to the number of calories (energy) a food contains per unit of weight. People tend to ingest a constant volume of food, regardless of caloric or macronutrient content. Adding water or fiber to a food decreases its energy density by increasing weight without affecting caloric content. Examples of foods with low-energy density include soups, fruits, vegetables, oatmeal, and lean meats. Dry foods and high-fat foods such as pret-

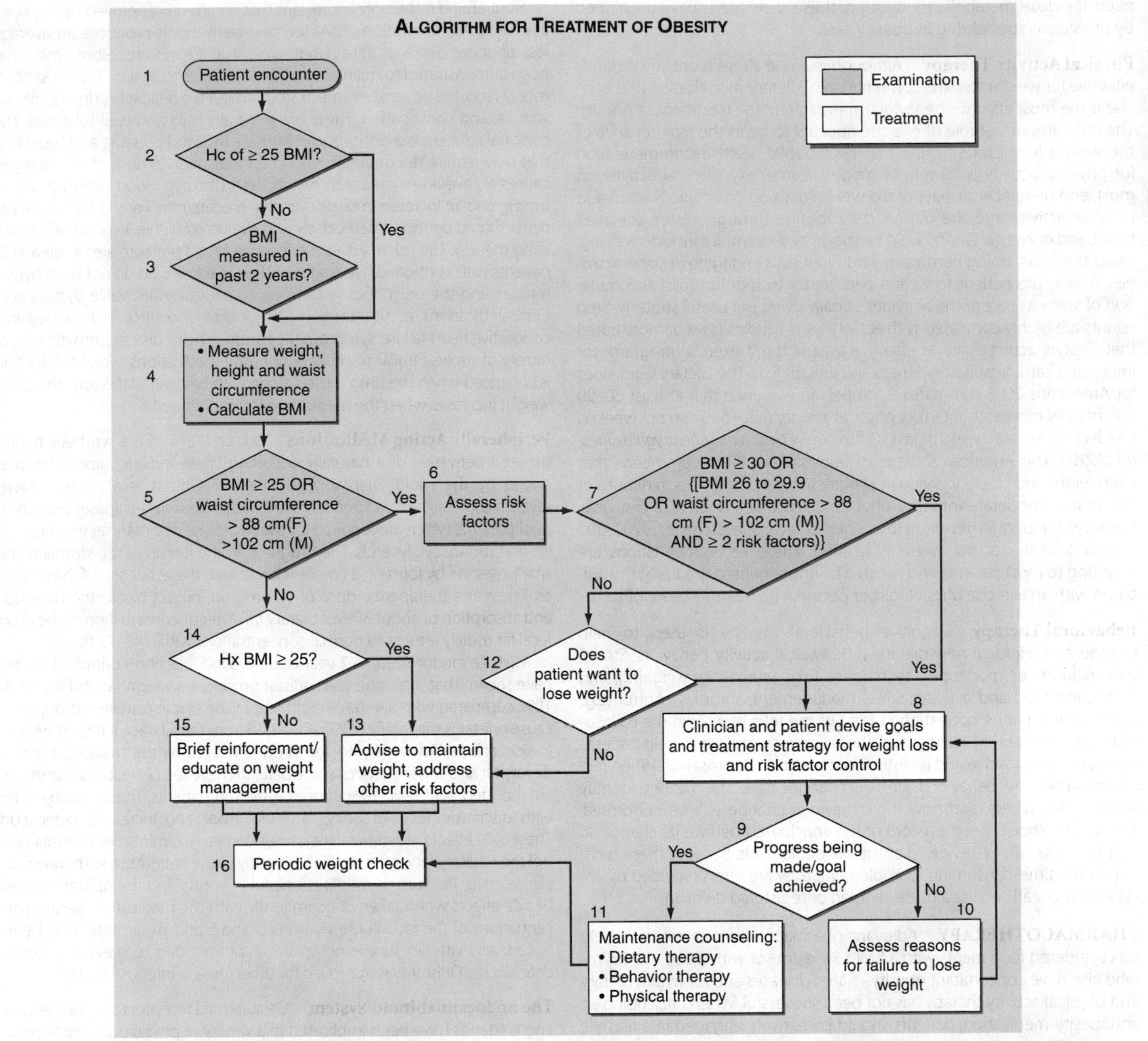
ALGORITHM FOR TREATMENT OF OBESITY
Examination
Treatment
1 Patient encounter
2 Hc of ≥ 25 BMI?
No
Yes
3 BMI measured in past 2 years?
4 • Measure weight, height and waist circumference
• Calculate BMI
5 BMI ≥ 25 OR waist circumference > 88 cm(F) >102 cm (M)
Yes
6 Assess risk factors
7 BMI ≥ 30 OR {[BMI 26 to 29.9 OR waist circumference > 88 cm (F) > 102 cm (M)] AND ≥ 2 risk factors)}
Yes
No
No
14 Hx BMI ≥ 25?
Yes
12 Does patient want to lose weight?
Yes
No
No
15 Brief reinforcement/ educate on weight management
13 Advise to maintain weight, address other risk factors
8 Clinician and patient devise goals and treatment strategy for weight loss and risk factor control
9 Progress being made/goal achieved?
Yes
No
16 Periodic weight check
11 Maintenance counseling:
• Dietary therapy
• Behavior therapy
• Physical therapy
10 Assess reasons for failure to lose weight

FIGURE 75-1 Treatment algorithm. This algorithm applies only to the assessment for overweight and obesity and subsequent decisions on that assessment. It does not reflect any initial overall assessment for other conditions that the physician may wish to perform. Ht, height; Hx, history; Wt, weight. *(From National, Heart, Lung, and Blood Institute: Clinical guidelines on the identification, evaluation, and treatment of overweight and obesity in adults: The evidence report. Washington, DC, US Department of Health and Human Services, 1998.)*

zels, cheese, egg yolks, potato chips, and red meat have a high-energy density. Diets containing low-energy dense foods have been shown to control hunger and result in decreased caloric intake and weight loss.

Occasionally, very-low-calorie diets (VLCDs) are prescribed as a form of aggressive dietary therapy. The primary purpose of a VLCD is to promote a rapid and significant (13–23 kg) short-term weight loss over a 3–6 month period. These propriety formulas typically supply ≤800 kcal, 50–80 g protein, and 100% of the recommended daily intake for vitamins and minerals. According to a review by the National Task Force on the Prevention and Treatment of Obesity, indications for initiating a VLCD include well-motivated individuals who are moderately to severely obese (BMI >30), have failed at more conservative approaches to weight loss, and have a medical condition that would be immediately improved with rapid weight loss. These conditions include poorly controlled type 2 diabetes, hypertriglyceridemia, obstructive sleep apnea, and symptomatic peripheral edema. The risk for gallstone formation increases exponentially at rates of weight loss >1.5 kg/week (3.3 lb/week). Prophylaxis against gallstone formation with ursodeoxycholic acid, 600 mg/d, is effective in reducing this risk. Because of the

TABLE 75-5 A GUIDE TO SELECTING TREATMENT

	BMI Category				
Treatment	**25–26.9**	**27–29.9**	**30–35**	**35–39.9**	**≥40**
Diet, exercise, behavior therapy	With comorbidities	With comorbidities	+	+	+
Pharmacotherapy		With comorbidities	+	+	+
Surgery				With comorbidities	+

Source: From National Heart, Lung, and Blood Institute, North American Association for the Study of Obesity (2000).

need for close metabolic monitoring, these diets are usually prescribed by physicians specializing in obesity care.

Physical Activity Therapy Although exercise alone is only moderately effective for weight loss, the combination of dietary modification and exercise is the most effective behavioral approach for the treatment of obesity. The most important role of exercise appears to be in the maintenance of the weight loss. Currently, the *minimum* public health recommendation for physical activity is 30 min of moderate intensity physical activity on most, and preferably all, days of the week. Focusing on simple ways to add physical activity into the normal daily routine through leisure activities, travel, and domestic work should be suggested. Examples include walking, using the stairs, doing home and yard work, and engaging in sport activities. Asking the patient to wear a pedometer to monitor total accumulation of steps as part of the activities of daily living is a useful strategy. Step counts are highly correlated with activity level. Studies have demonstrated that lifestyle activities are as effective as structured exercise programs for improving cardiorespiratory fitness and weight loss. The Dietary Guidelines for Americans 2005 summarizes compelling evidence that at least 60–90 min of daily moderate-intensity physical activity (420–630 min per week) is needed to sustain weight loss (*http://www.health.gov/dietaryguidelines/dga2005/*). The American College of Sports Medicine recommends that overweight and obese individuals progressively increase to a minimum of 150 min of moderate intensity physical activity per week as a first goal. However, for long-term weight loss, a higher level of exercise (e.g., 200–300 min or ≥2000 kcal per week) is needed. These recommendations are daunting to most patients and need to be implemented gradually. Consultation with an exercise physiologist or personal trainer may be helpful.

Behavioral Therapy Cognitive behavioral therapy is used to help change and reinforce new dietary and physical activity behaviors. Strategies include self-monitoring techniques (e.g., journaling, weighing, and measuring food and activity); stress management; stimulus control (e.g., using smaller plates, not eating in front of the television or in the car); social support; problem solving; and cognitive restructuring to help patients develop more positive and realistic thoughts about themselves. When recommending any behavioral lifestyle change, have the patient identify what, when, where, and how the behavioral change will be performed. The patient should keep a record of the anticipated behavioral change so that progress can be reviewed at the next office visit. Because these techniques are time-consuming to implement, they are often provided by ancillary office staff such as a nurse clinician or registered dietitian.

PHARMACOTHERAPY Adjuvant pharmacologic treatments should be considered for patients with a BMI >30 kg/m^2 or with a BMI >27 kg/m^2 who also have concomitant obesity-related diseases and for whom dietary and physical activity therapy has not been successful. When prescribing an antiobesity medication, patients should be actively engaged in a lifestyle program that provides the strategies and skills needed to effectively use the drug since this support increases total weight loss.

There are several potential targets of pharmacologic therapy for obesity. The most thoroughly explored treatment is suppression of appetite via centrally active medications that alter monoamine neurotransmitters. A second strategy is to reduce the absorption of selective macronutrients from the gastrointestinal (GI) tract, such as fat. These two mechanisms form the basis for all currently prescribed antiobesity agents. A third target, selective blocking of the endocannabinoid system, has recently been identified.

Centrally Acting Anorexiant Medications Appetite-suppressing drugs, or anorexiants, affect satiety—the absence of hunger after eating—and hunger—a biologic sensation that initiates eating. By increasing satiety and decreasing hunger, these agents help patients reduce caloric intake without a sense of deprivation. The target site for the actions of anorexiants is the ventromedial and lateral hypothalamic regions in the central nervous system (Chap. 74). Their biological effect on appetite regulation is produced by augmenting the neurotransmission of three monoamines: norepinephrine; serotonin [5-hydroxytryptamine (5-HT)]; and, to a lesser degree, dopamine. The classic sympathomimetic adrenergic agents (benzphetamine, phendimetrazine, diethylpropion, mazindol, and phentermine) function by stimulating norepinephrine release or by blocking its reuptake. In contrast, sibutramine (Meridia) functions as a serotonin and norepinephrine reuptake inhibitor. Unlike other previously used anorexiants, sibutramine is not pharmacologically related to amphetamine and has no addictive potential.

Sibutramine is the only anorexiant that is currently approved by the Food and Drug Administration (FDA) for long-term use. It produces an average loss of about 5–9% of initial body weight at 12 months. Sibutramine has been demonstrated to maintain weight loss for up to 2 years. The most commonly reported adverse events of sibutramine are headache, dry mouth, insomnia, and constipation. These are generally mild and well-tolerated. The principal concern is a dose-related increase in blood pressure and heart rate that may require discontinuation of the medication. A dose of 10–15 mg/d causes an average increase in systolic and diastolic blood pressure of 2–4 mmHg and an increase in heart rate of 4–6 beats/min. For this reason, all patients should be monitored closely and evaluated within 1 month after initiating therapy. The risk of adverse effects on blood pressure are no greater in patients with controlled hypertension than in those who do not have hypertension, and the drug does not appear to cause cardiac valve dysfunction. Contraindications to sibutramine use include uncontrolled hypertension, congestive heart failure, symptomatic coronary heart disease, arrhythmias, or history of stroke. Similar to other antiobesity medications, weight reduction is enhanced when the drug is used along with behavioral therapy, and body weight increases when the medication is discontinued.

Peripherally Acting Medications Orlistat (Xenical) is a synthetic hydrogenated derivative of a naturally occurring lipase inhibitor, lipostatin, produced by the mold *Streptomyces toxytricini*. Orlistat is a potent, slowly reversible inhibitor of pancreatic, gastric, and carboxylester lipases and phospholipase A2, which are required for the hydrolysis of dietary fat into fatty acids and monoacylglycerols. The drug acts in the lumen of the stomach and small intestine by forming a covalent bond with the active site of these lipases. Taken at a therapeutic dose of 120 mg tid, orlistat blocks the digestion and absorption of about 30% of dietary fat. After discontinuation of the drug, fecal fat usually returns to normal concentrations within 48–72 h.

Multiple randomized, 1–2 year double-blind, placebo-controlled studies have shown that after one year, orlistat produces a weight loss of about 9–10%, compared with a 4–6% weight loss in the placebo-treated groups. Because orlistat is minimally (<1%) absorbed from the GI tract, it has no systemic side effects. Tolerability to the drug is related to the malabsorption of dietary fat and subsequent passage of fat in the feces. GI tract adverse effects are reported in at least 10% of orlistat-treated patients. These include flatus with discharge, fecal urgency, fatty/oily stool, and increased defecation. These side effects are generally experienced early, diminish as patients control their dietary fat intake, and infrequently cause patients to withdraw from clinical trials. Psyllium mucilloid is helpful in controlling the orlistat-induced GI side effects when taken concomitantly with the medication. Serum concentrations of the fat-soluble vitamins D and E and β-carotene may be reduced, and vitamin supplements are recommended to prevent potential deficiencies. Orlistat was approved for other-the-counter use in 2007.

The Endocannabinoid System Cannabinoid receptors and their endogenous ligands have been implicated in a variety of physiologic functions, including feeding, modulation of pain, emotional behavior, and peripheral lipid metabolism. Cannabis and its main ingredient, Δ^9-tetrahydrocannabinol (THC), is an exogenous cannabinoid compound. Two endocannabinoids have been identified, anandamide and 2-arachidonyl glyceride. Two cannabinoid receptors have been identified: CB_1 (abundant in the brain) and CB_2 (present in immune cells). The brain endocannabinoid system is thought to control food intake through reinforcing motivation to find and consume foods with high incentive value and to regulate actions of other mediators of appetite. The first selective cannabinoid CB_1 receptor antagonist, rimonabant, was discovered in 1994. The medication antagonizes the orexigenic effect of THC and suppresses appetite when given alone in animal models. Several large prospective, randomized controlled trials have demonstrated the effectiveness of rimonabant as a weight-loss agent. Taken as a 20 mg dose, subjects lost an average of 6.5 kg (14.32 lb) compared to 1.5 kg (3.3 lb) for placebo at 1 year. Concomitant improvements were seen in waist circumference and cardiovascular risk factors. The most common reported side effects include depression, anxiety, and nausea. FDA approval of Rimonabant is still pending.

SURGERY Bariatric surgery can be considered for patients with severe obesity (BMI ≥40 kg/m^2) or those with moderate obesity (BMI ≥35 kg/m^2) associated with a serious medical condition. Surgical weight loss functions by reducing caloric intake and, depending on the procedure, macronutrient absorption.

Weight-loss surgeries fall into one of two categories: restrictive and restrictive-malabsorptive (**Fig. 75-2**). Restrictive surgeries limit the amount of food the stomach can hold and slow the rate of gastric emptying. The vertical

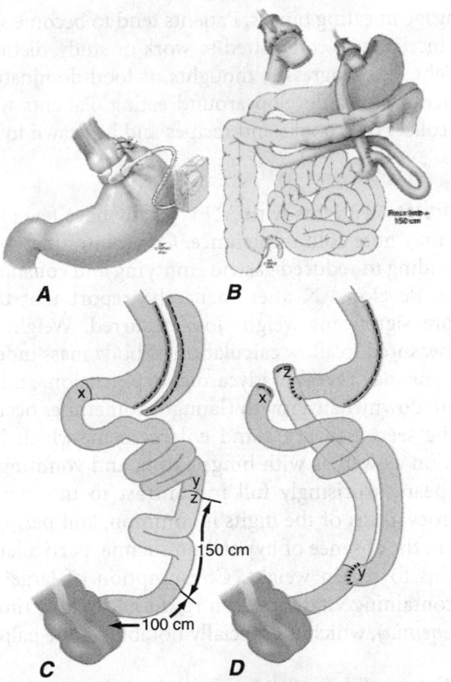

FIGURE 75-2 Bariatric surgical procedures. Examples of operative interventions used for surgical manipulation of the gastrointestinal tract. ***A.*** Laparoscopic gastric band (LAGB). ***B.*** The Roux-en-Y gastric bypass. ***C.*** Biliopancreatic diversion with duodenal switch. ***D.*** Biliopancreatic diversion. *(From ML Kendrick, GF Dakin. Surgical approaches to obesity. Mayo Clin Proc 815:518, 2006; with permission.)*

banded gastroplasty (VBG) is the prototype of this category but is currently performed on a very limited basis due to lack of effectiveness in long-term trials. Laparoscopic adjustable silicone gastric banding (LASGB) has replaced the VBG as the most commonly performed restrictive operation. The first banding device, the lap-band, was approved for use in the United States in 2001. In contrast to previous devices, the diameter of this band is adjustable by way of its connection to a reservoir that is implanted under the skin. Injection or removal of saline into the reservoir tightens or loosens the band's internal diameter, thus changing the size of the gastric opening.

The three restrictive-malabsorptive bypass procedures combine the elements of gastric restriction and selective malabsorption. These procedures include Roux-en-Y gastric bypass (RYGB), biliopancreatic diversion (BPD), and biliopancreatic diversion with duodenal switch (BPDDS) (Fig. 75-2). RYGB is the most commonly performed and accepted bypass procedure. It may be performed with an open incision or laparoscopically.

Although no recent randomized controlled trials compare weight loss after surgical and nonsurgical interventions, data from meta-analyses and large databases, primarily obtained from observational studies, suggest that bariatric surgery is the most effective weight-loss therapy for those with clinically severe obesity. These procedures generally produce a 30–35% average total body weight loss that is maintained in nearly 60% of patients at 5 years. In general, mean weight loss is greater after the combined restrictive-malabsorptive procedures compared to the restrictive procedures. An abundance of data supports the positive impact of bariatric surgery on obesity-related morbid conditions, including diabetes mellitus, hypertension, obstructive sleep apnea, dyslipidemia, and nonalcoholic fatty liver disease.

Surgical mortality from bariatric surgery is generally <1% but varies with the procedure, patient's age and comorbid conditions, and experience of the surgical team. The most common surgical complications include stomal stenosis or marginal ulcers (occurring in 5–15% of patients) that present as prolonged nausea and vomiting after eating or inability to advance the diet to solid foods. These complications are typically treated by endoscopic balloon dilatation and acid suppression therapy, respectively. For patients who undergo LASGB, there are no intestinal absorptive abnormalities other than mechanical reduction in gastric size and outflow. Therefore, selective deficiencies occur uncommonly unless eating habits become unbalanced. In contrast, the restrictive-malabsorptive procedures increase risk for micronutrient deficiencies of vitamin B_{12}, iron, folate, calcium, and vitamin D. Patients with restrictive-malabsorptive procedures require lifelong supplementation with these micronutrients.

FURTHER READINGS

BRAY GA, GREENWAY FL: Pharmacologic treatment of the overweight patient. Pharmacol Rev 59:151, 2007

BRAY GA, RYAN DH: Drug treatment of the overweight patient. Gastroenterology 132(6):2239, 2007

BUCHWALD H et al: Bariatric surgery: A systematic review and meta-analysis. JAMA 292:1724, 2004

DEMARIA EJ: Bariatric surgery for morbid obesity. N Engl J Med 356:2176, 2007

HASLAM DW, JAMES WPT: Obesity. Lancet 366:1197, 2005

KUSHNER RF: Roadmaps for clinical practice: Case studies in disease prevention and health promotion—assessment and management of adult obesity: A primer for physicians. Chicago, American Medical Association, 2003. (Available online at *www.ama-assn.org/ama/pub/category/10931.html*)

MCTIGUE KM et al: Screening and interventions for obesity in adults: Summary of the evidence for the U.S. Preventive Services Task Force. Ann Intern Med 139:933, 2003. (Appendix tables available at *www.annals.org*)

NATIONAL HEART, LUNG, AND BLOOD INSTITUTE, NORTH AMERICAN ASSOCIATION FOR THE STUDY OF OBESITY: Practical guide: Identification, evaluation, and treatment of overweight and obesity in adults. Bethesda, MD, National Institutes of Health pub number 00-4084, Oct. 2000. Available online: *http://www.nhlbi.nih.gov/guidelines/obesity/practgde.htm*

PADWAL R et al: Long-term pharmacotherapy for overweight and obesity: A systematic review and meta-analysis of randomized controlled trials. Int J Obesity 27:1437, 2003

WADDEN TA et al: Lifestyle modification for the management of obesity. Gastroenterology 132(6):2226, 2007

76 Eating Disorders

B. Timothy Walsh

Anorexia nervosa and bulimia nervosa are characterized by severe disturbances of eating behavior. The salient feature of *anorexia nervosa* (AN) is a refusal to maintain a minimally normal body weight. *Bulimia nervosa* (BN) is characterized by recurrent episodes of binge eating followed by abnormal compensatory behaviors, such as self-induced vomiting. AN and BN are distinct clinical syndromes but share certain features in common. Both disorders occur primarily among previously healthy young women who become overly concerned with body shape and weight. Many patients with BN have past histories of anorexia nervosa, and many patients with AN engage in binge eating and purging behavior. In the current diagnostic system, the critical distinction between AN and BN depends on body weight: patients with AN are, by definition, significantly underweight, whereas patients with BN have body weights in the normal range or above.

Binge eating disorder (BED) is a more recently described syndrome characterized by repeated episodes of binge eating, similar to those of BN, in the absence of inappropriate compensatory behavior. Patients with BED are typically middle-aged men or women with significant obesity. They have an increased frequency of anxiety and depression compared to similarly obese patients without BED. It is not established that patients with BED are at increased risk for medical complications or that they require specific treatment interventions.

EPIDEMIOLOGY

Among women, the lifetime prevalence of the full syndrome of AN is approximately 1%. AN is much less common in males. AN is more prevalent in cultures where food is plentiful and in which being thin is associated with attractiveness. Individuals who pursue interests that place a premium on thinness, such as ballet and modeling, are at greater risk. The incidence of AN has increased in recent decades.

ETIOLOGY

The etiology of AN is unknown but appears to involve a combination of psychological, biologic, and cultural risk factors. Risk factors, such as sexual or physical abuse and a family history of mood disturbance, are best viewed as nonspecific risk factors that increase vulnerability to a range of psychiatric disorders, including AN.

Patients who develop AN are inclined to be more obsessional and perfectionist than their peers. The disorder often begins as a diet not distinguishable at the outset from those undertaken by many adolescents and young women. As weight loss progresses, the fear of gaining weight grows; dieting becomes stricter; and psychological, behavioral, and medical aberrations increase. Eating disorders, including AN, may develop among individuals with type 1 diabetes mellitus and are associated with poorer glycemic control and an increased frequency of complications (Chap. 338).

Numerous physiologic disturbances, including abnormalities in a variety of neurotransmitter systems, have been described in AN (see below). It is difficult to distinguish neurochemical, metabolic, and hormonal changes that may have a role in the initiation or perpetuation of the syndrome from those that are secondary to the disorder. The resolution of most of these abnormalities with weight restoration argues against an etiologic role.

Genetic factors contribute to the risk of development of AN, as its incidence is greater in families with one affected member and the concordance in monozygotic twins is greater than in dizygotic twins. However, specific genes have not been identified.

CLINICAL FEATURES

AN typically begins in mid to late adolescence, sometimes in association with a stressful life event such as leaving home for school (Table 76-1). The disorder occasionally develops in early puberty, before menarche, but seldom begins after age 40. Despite being underweight, patients with AN are irrationally afraid of gaining weight, often out of a concern that weight gain will get "out of control." They also exhibit a distortion of body image, which may express itself in several ways. For example, despite being emaciated, patients with AN may believe that their body as a whole, or some part of their body, is too fat. Further weight loss is viewed by the patient as a fulfilling accomplishment, while weight gain is seen as a personal failure. Patients with AN rarely complain of hunger or fatigue and often exercise extensively. Despite the denial of hunger, one-quarter to one-half of patients with AN engage in eating binges. Patients tend to become socially withdrawn and increasingly committed to work or study, dieting, and exercise. As weight loss progresses, thoughts of food dominate mental life and idiosyncratic rules develop around eating. Patients with AN may obsessively collect cookbooks and recipes and be drawn to food-related occupations.

Physical Features Patients with AN typically have few physical complaints but may note cold intolerance. Gastrointestinal motility is diminished, leading to reduced gastric emptying and constipation. Some women who develop AN after menarche report that their menses ceased before significant weight loss occurred. Weight and height should be measured to allow calculation of body mass index (BMI; kg/m^2). Vital signs may reveal bradycardia, hypotension, and mild hypothermia. Soft, downy hair growth (lanugo) sometimes occurs, and alopecia may be seen. Salivary gland enlargement, which is associated with starvation as well as with binge eating and vomiting, may make the face appear surprisingly full in contrast to the marked general wasting. Acrocyanosis of the digits is common, and peripheral edema can be seen in the absence of hypoalbuminemia, particularly when the patient begins to regain weight. Consumption of large amounts of vegetables containing vitamin A can result in a yellow tint to the skin (*hypercarotenemia*), which is especially notable on the palms.

Laboratory Abnormalities Mild normochromic, normocytic anemia is frequent, as is mild to moderate leukopenia, with a disproportionate reduction of polymorphonuclear leukocytes. Dehydration may result in slightly increased levels of blood urea nitrogen and creatinine. Serum transaminase levels may increase, especially during the early phases of refeeding. The level of serum proteins is usually normal. Blood sugar is often low and serum cholesterol may be moderately elevated. Hypokalemic alkalosis suggests self-induced vomiting or the use

TABLE 76-1 COMMON CHARACTERISTICS OF ANOREXIA NERVOSA AND BULIMIA NERVOSA

	Anorexia Nervosa[a]	Bulimia Nervosa
Clinical Characteristics		
Onset	Mid-adolescence	Late adolescence/early adulthood
Female:male	10:1	10:1
Lifetime prevalence in women	1%	1–3%
Weight	Markedly decreased	Usually normal
Menstruation	Absent	Usually normal
Binge eating	25–50%	Required for diagnosis
Mortality	~5% per decade	Low
Physical and Laboratory Findings[a]		
Skin/extremities	Lanugo Acrocyanosis Edema	
Cardiovascular	Bradycardia Hypotension	
Gastrointestinal	Salivary gland enlargement Slow gastric emptying Constipation Elevated liver enzymes	Salivary gland enlargement Dental erosion
Hematopoietic	Normochromic, normocytic anemia Leukopenia	
Fluid/Electrolyte	Increased BUN, creatinine Hypokalemia	Hypokalemia Hypochloremia Alkalosis
Endocrine	Hypoglycemia Low estrogen or testosterone Low LH and FSH Low-normal thyroxine Normal TSH Increased cortisol	
Bone	Osteopenia	

[a]Patients with the binge-eating/purging subtype of anorexia nervosa may also exhibit the physical and laboratory findings associated with bulimia nervosa.

Abbreviations: BUN, blood urea nitrogen; LH, luteinizing hormone; FSH, follicle stimulating hormone; TSH, thyroid stimulating hormone.

of diuretics. Hyponatremia is common and may result from excess fluid intake and disturbances in the secretion of antidiuretic hormone.

Endocrine Abnormalities The regulation of virtually every endocrine system is altered in AN, but the most striking changes occur in the reproductive system. Amenorrhea is hypothalamic in origin and reflects diminished production of gonadotropin-releasing hormone (GnRH). When exogenous GnRH is administered in a pulsatile manner, pituitary responses of luteinizing hormone (LH) and follicle-stimulating hormone (FSH) are normalized, indicating the absence of a primary pituitary abnormality. The resulting gonadotropin deficiency causes low plasma estrogen in women and reduced testosterone in men. The hypothalamic GnRH pulse generator is exquisitely sensitive, particularly in women, to body weight, stress, and exercise, each of which may contribute to *hypothalamic amenorrhea* in AN (Chap. 341).

Serum leptin levels are markedly reduced in AN as a result of undernutrition and decreased body fat mass. The reduction in leptin appears to be the primary factor responsible for the disturbances of the hypothalamic-pituitary-gonadal axis, and to be an important mediator of the other neuroendocrine abnormalities characteristic of AN (Chap. 74).

Serum cortisol and 24-h urine free cortisol levels are generally elevated but without characteristic clinical signs of cortisol excess. Thyroid function tests resemble the pattern seen in euthyroid sick syndrome (Chap. 335). Thyroxine (T_4) and free T_4 levels are usually in the low-normal range, triiodothyronine (T_3) levels are reduced, and reverse T_3 (rT_3) is elevated. The level of thyroid-stimulating hormone (TSH) is normal or partially suppressed. Growth hormone is increased, but insulin-like growth factor 1 (IGF-1), which is produced mainly by the liver, is reduced, as in other conditions of starvation. Diminished bone density is routinely observed in AN and reflects the effects of multiple nutritional deficiencies, reduced gonadal steroids, and increased cortisol. The degree of bone density reduction is proportional to the length of the illness, and patients are at risk for the development of symptomatic fractures. The occurrence of AN during adolescence may lead to the premature cessation of linear bone growth and a failure to achieve expected adult height.

Cardiac Abnormalities Cardiac output is reduced, and congestive heart failure occurs rarely during rapid refeeding. The electrocardiogram usually shows sinus bradycardia, reduced QRS voltage, and nonspecific ST-T-wave abnormalities. Some patients develop a prolonged QT_c interval, which may predispose to serious arrhythmias, particularly when electrolyte abnormalities also are present.

DIAGNOSIS

The diagnosis of AN is based on the presence of characteristic behavioral, psychological, and physical attributes (Table 76-2). Widely accepted diagnostic criteria are provided by the American Psychiatric Association's *Diagnostic and Statistical Manual of Mental Disorders* (DSM-IV). These criteria include weight <85% of that expected for age and height, which is roughly equivalent to a BMI of 18.5 kg/m^2 for adult women. This weight criterion is somewhat arbitrary, so that a patient who meets all other diagnostic criteria but weighs between 85 and 90% of expected would still merit the diagnosis of AN. The current diagnostic criteria require that women with AN not have spontaneous menses, but occasional patients with the characteristics and complications of AN describe regular menstruation. Two mutually exclusive subtypes of AN are specified in DSM-IV. Patients whose weight loss is maintained primarily by caloric restriction, perhaps augmented by excessive exercise, are considered to have the "restricting" subtype of AN. The "binge eating/purging" subtype is characterized by binge eating and self-induced vomiting and/or laxative abuse. Patients with the binge/purge subtype are more prone to develop electrolyte imbalances, are more emotionally labile, and are more likely to have other problems with impulse control, such as drug abuse.

The diagnosis of AN can usually be made confidently in a patient with a history of weight loss accomplished by restrictive dieting and excessive exercise, accompanied by a marked reluctance to gain weight. Patients with AN often deny that they have a serious problem and may be brought to medical attention by concerned family or friends. In atypical presentations, other causes of significant weight loss in previously healthy young people should be considered, including inflammatory bowel disease, gastric outlet obstruction, diabetes mellitus, central nervous system (CNS) tumors, or neoplasm (Chap. 41).

TABLE 76-2 DIAGNOSTIC FEATURES OF ANOREXIA NERVOSA

Refusal to maintain body weight at or above a minimally normal weight for age and height. (This includes a failure to achieve weight gain expected during a period of growth leading to an abnormally low body weight.)

Intense fear of weight gain or becoming fat.

Distortion of body image (e.g., feeling fat despite an objectively low weight or minimizing the seriousness of low weight).

Amenorrhea. (This criterion is met if menstrual periods occur only following hormone—e.g., estrogen—administration.)

PROGNOSIS

The course and outcome of AN are highly variable. One-quarter to one-half of patients eventually recover fully, with few psychological or physical sequelae. However, many patients have persistent difficulties with weight maintenance, depression, and eating disturbances, including BN. The development of obesity following AN is rare. The long-term mortality of AN is among the highest associated with any psychiatric disorder. Approximately 5% of patients die per decade of follow-up, primarily due to the physical effects of chronic starvation or by suicide.

Virtually all of the physiologic abnormalities associated with AN are observed in other forms of starvation and markedly improve or disappear with weight gain. A worrisome exception is the reduction in bone mass, which may not recover fully, particularly when AN occurs during adolescence when peak bone mass is normally achieved.

Rx ANOREXIA NERVOSA

Because of the profound physiologic and psychological effects of starvation, there is a broad consensus that weight restoration to at least 90% of predicted weight is the primary goal in the treatment of AN. Unfortunately, because most patients resist this goal, the management of AN is often accompanied by frustration for the patient, the family, and the physician. Patients typically exaggerate their food intake and minimize their symptoms. Some patients resort to subterfuge to make their weights appear higher, for example, by water-loading before they are weighed. In attempting to engage the patient in treatment, it may be useful for the physician to elicit the patient's physical concerns (e.g., about osteoporosis, weakness, or fertility) and, provide education about the importance of normalizing nutritional status in order to address those concerns. The physician should reassure the patient that weight gain will not be permitted to get "out of control" but simultaneously emphasize that weight restoration is medically and psychologically imperative.

The intensity of the initial treatment, including the need for hospitalization, is determined by the patient's current weight, the rapidity of recent weight loss, and the severity of medical and psychological complications (**Fig. 76-1**). Hospitalization should be strongly considered for patients weighing <75% of expected, even if the results of routine blood studies are within normal limits. Acute medical problems, such as severe electrolyte imbalances, should be identified and addressed. Nutritional restoration can almost always be successfully accomplished by oral feeding, and parenteral methods are rarely required. For severely underweight patients, sufficient calories (approximately 1200–1800 kcal/d) should be provided initially in divided meals as food or liquid supplements to maintain weight and to permit stabilization of fluid and electrolyte balance. Calories can then be gradually increased to achieve a weight gain of 1–2 kg (2–4 lb) per week, typically requiring an intake of 3000–4000 kcal/d. Meals must be supervised, ideally by personnel who are firm regarding the necessity of food consumption, empathic regarding the challenges entailed, and reassuring about the patient's eventual recovery. Patients have great psychological difficulty complying with the need for increased caloric consumption, and the assistance of psychiatrists or psychologists experienced in the treatment of AN is usually necessary.

Less severely affected patients may be treated in a partial hospitalization program where medical and psychiatric supervision is available and

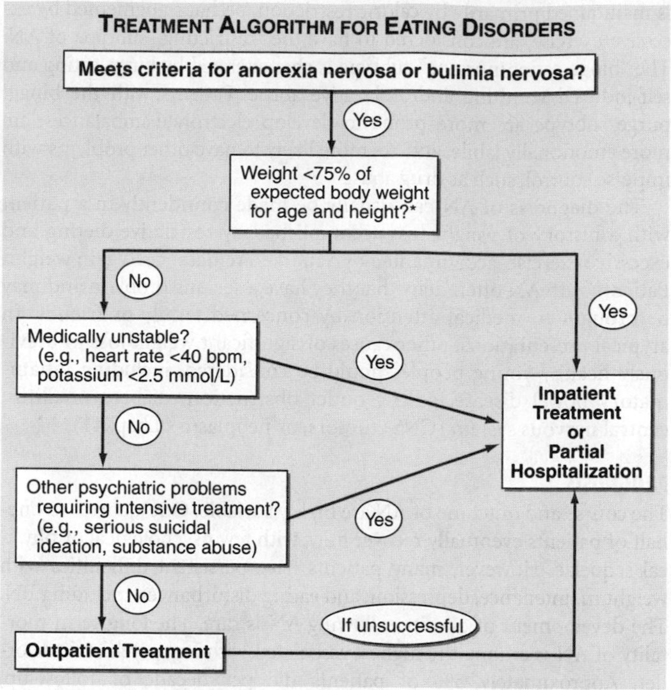

FIGURE 76-1 An algorithm for basic treatment decisions regarding patients with anorexia nervosa or bulimia nervosa. Based on the American Psychiatric Association's practice guidelines for the treatment of patients with eating disorders. *Although outpatient management may be considered for patients with anorexia nervosa weighing more than 75% of expected, there should be a low threshold for using more intensive interventions if the weight loss has been rapid or if current weight is <80% of expected.

several meals can be monitored each day. Outpatient treatment may suffice for mildly ill patients. Weight must be monitored at frequent intervals, and explicit goals agreed on for weight gain, with the understanding that more intensive treatment will be required if the level of care initially employed is not successful. For younger patients, the active involvement of the family in treatment is crucial regardless of the treatment venue.

Psychiatric treatment focuses primarily on two issues. First, patients require much emotional support during the period of weight gain. Patients often intellectually agree with the need to gain weight, but strenuously resist increases in caloric intake, and often surreptitiously discard food that is provided. Second, patients must learn to base their self-esteem not on the achievement of an inappropriately low weight, but on the development of satisfying personal relationships and the attainment of reasonable academic and occupational goals. While this is often possible, some patients with AN develop other serious emotional and behavioral symptoms such as depression, self-mutilation, obsessive-compulsive behavior, and suicidal ideation. These symptoms may require additional therapeutic interventions, in the form of psychotherapy, medication, or hospitalization.

Medical complications occasionally occur during refeeding. Especially in the early stages of treatment, severely malnourished patients may develop a "refeeding syndrome" characterized by hypophosphatemia, hypomagnesemia, and cardiovascular instability. Acute gastric dilatation has been described when refeeding is rapid. As in other forms of malnutrition, fluid retention and peripheral edema may occur, but they generally do not require specific treatment in the absence of cardiac, renal, or hepatic dysfunction. Transient modest elevations in serum liver enzyme levels occasionally occur. Multivitamins should be given, and an adequate intake of vitamin D (400 IU/d) and calcium (1500 mg/d) should be provided to minimize bone loss.

No psychotropic medications are of established value in the treatment of AN; tricyclic antidepressants are contraindicated when there is prolongation of the QT_C interval. The alterations of cortisol and thyroid hormone metabolism do not require specific treatment and are corrected by weight gain. Estrogen treatment appears to have minimal impact on bone density in underweight patients, and the small benefit of bisphosphonate treatment appears to be outweighed by the potential risks of such agents in young women.

BULIMIA NERVOSA

EPIDEMIOLOGY

In women, the full syndrome of BN occurs with a lifetime prevalence of 1–3%. Variants of the disorder, such as occasional binge eating or purging, are much more common and occur in 5–10% of young women. The frequency of BN among men is less than one-tenth of that among women. The prevalence of BN increased dramatically in the early 1970s and 1980s but may have leveled off or declined somewhat in recent years.

ETIOLOGY

As with AN, the etiology of BN is likely to be multifactorial. Patients who develop BN describe a higher-than-expected prevalence of childhood and parental obesity, suggesting that a predisposition toward obesity may increase vulnerability to this eating disorder. The marked increase in the number of cases of BN during the past 25 years and the rarity of BN in underdeveloped countries suggest that cultural factors are important. Several biologic abnormalities in patients with BN may perpetuate this disorder once it has begun. These include abnormalities of CNS serotonergic function, which is involved in eating behavior, and disruption of peripheral satiety mechanisms, including the release of cholecystokinin (CCK) from the small intestine.

CLINICAL FEATURES

The typical patient presenting for treatment of BN is a woman of normal weight in her mid-twenties who reports binge eating and purging 5–10 times a week for 5–10 years (Table 76-3). The disorder usually begins in late adolescence or early adulthood during or following a diet, often in association with depressed mood. The self-imposed caloric restriction leads to increased hunger and to overeating. In an attempt to avoid weight gain, the patient induces vomiting, takes laxatives or diuretics, or engages in some other form of compensatory behavior. During binges, patients with this disorder tend to consume large amounts of sweet foods with a high fat content, such as dessert items. The most frequent compensatory behaviors are self-induced vomiting and laxative abuse, but a wide variety of techniques have been described, including the omission of insulin injections by individuals with type 1 diabetes mellitus. Initially, patients may experience a sense of satisfaction that appealing food can be eaten without weight gain. However, as the disorder progresses, patients perceive diminished control over eating. Binges increase in size and frequency and are provoked by a variety of stimuli, such as transient depression, anxiety, or a sense that too much food has been consumed in a normal meal. Between binges, patients restrict caloric intake, which increases hunger and sets the stage for the next binge. Typically, patients with BN are ashamed of their behavior and endeavor to keep their disorder hidden from family and friends. Like patients with AN, those with BN place an unusual emphasis on weight and shape as a basis for their self-esteem. Many patients with BN have mild symptoms of depression. Some patients exhibit serious mood and behavioral disturbances, such as suicide attempts, sexual promiscuity, and drug and alcohol abuse. Although vomiting may be

TABLE 76-3 DIAGNOSTIC FEATURES OF BULIMIA NERVOSA

Recurrent episodes of binge eating, which is characterized by the consumption of a large amount of food in a short period of time and a feeling that the eating is out of control.
Recurrent inappropriate behavior to compensate for the binge eating, such as self-induced vomiting.
The occurrence of both the binge eating and the inappropriate compensatory behavior at least twice weekly, on average, for 3 months.
Overconcern with body shape and weight.

Note: If the diagnostic criteria for anorexia nervosa are simultaneously met, only the diagnosis of anorexia nervosa is given.

triggered initially by manual stimulation of the gag reflex, most patients with BN develop the ability to induce vomiting at will. Rarely, patients resort to the regular use of syrup of ipecac. Laxatives and diuretics are frequently taken in impressive quantities, such as 30 or 60 laxative pills on a single occasion. The resulting fluid loss produces dehydration and a feeling of emptiness but has little impact on caloric balance.

The physical abnormalities associated with BN primarily result from the purging behavior. Painless bilateral salivary gland hypertrophy (sialadenosis) may be noted. A scar or callus on the dorsum of the hand may develop due to repeated trauma from the teeth among patients who manually stimulate the gag reflex. Recurrent vomiting and the exposure of the lingual surfaces of the teeth to stomach acid lead to loss of dental enamel and eventually to chipping and erosion of the front teeth. Laboratory abnormalities are surprisingly infrequent, but hypokalemia, hypochloremia, and hyponatremia are observed occasionally. Repeated vomiting may lead to alkalosis, whereas repeated laxative abuse may produce a mild metabolic acidosis. Serum amylase may be slightly elevated due to an increase in the salivary isoenzyme.

Serious physical complications resulting from BN are rare. Oligomenorrhea and amenorrhea are more frequent than among women without eating disorders. Arrhythmias occasionally occur secondary to electrolyte disturbances. Tearing of the esophagus and rupture of the stomach have been reported and constitute life-threatening events. Some patients who chronically abuse laxatives or diuretics develop transient peripheral edema when this behavior ceases, presumably due to high levels of aldosterone secondary to persistent fluid and electrolyte depletion.

DIAGNOSIS

The critical diagnostic features of BN are repeated episodes of binge eating followed by inappropriate and abnormal behaviors aimed at avoiding weight gain (Table 76-3). The diagnosis of BN requires a candid history from the patient detailing frequent, large eating binges followed by the purposeful use of inappropriate mechanisms to avoid weight gain. Most patients with BN who present for treatment are distressed by their inability to control their eating behavior but are able to provide such details if queried in a supportive and nonjudgmental fashion.

As in AN, there are two subtypes of BN. Patients with the "purging" subtype utilize compensatory behaviors that directly rid the body of calories or fluids (e.g., self-induced vomiting, laxative, or diuretic abuse), whereas those with the "nonpurging" subtype attempt to compensate for binges by fasting or by excessive exercise. Patients with the nonpurging subtype tend to be heavier and are less prone to fluid and electrolyte disturbances.

PROGNOSIS

The prognosis of BN is much more favorable than that of AN. Mortality is low, and full recovery occurs in approximately 50% of patients within 10 years. Approximately 25% of patients have persistent symptoms of BN over many years. Few patients progress from BN to AN.

℞ BULIMIA NERVOSA

BN can usually be treated on an outpatient basis (Fig. 76-1). Cognitive behavioral therapy (CBT) is a short-term (4–6 months) psychological treatment that focuses on the intense concern with shape and weight, the persistent dieting, and the binge eating and purging that characterize this disorder. Patients are directed to monitor the circumstances, thoughts, and emotions associated with binge/purge episodes, to eat regularly, and to challenge their assumptions linking weight to self-esteem. CBT produces symptomatic remission in 25–50% of patients.

Numerous double-blind, placebo-controlled trials have documented that antidepressant medications are useful in the treatment of BN but are probably somewhat less effective than CBT. Although efficacy has been established for virtually all chemical classes of antidepressants, only the selective serotonin reuptake inhibitor fluoxetine (Prozac) has been approved for use in BN by the U.S. Food and Drug Administration. Antidepressant medications are helpful even for patients with BN who are not depressed, and the dose of fluoxetine recommended for BN (60 mg/d) is higher than that typically used to treat depression. These observations suggest that different mechanisms may underlie the utility of these medications in BN and in depression.

A subset of patients does not respond to CBT, antidepressant medication, or their combination. More intensive forms of treatment, including hospitalization, may be required.

FURTHER READINGS

American Psychiatric Association: Practice guidelines for the treatment of patients with eating disorders, third edition. Am J Psychiatry, 2006

Chan JL, Mantzoros CS: Role of leptin in energy-deprivation states: Normal human physiology and clinical implications for hypothalamic amenorrhoea and anorexia nervosa. Lancet 366:74, 2005

Katzman DK: Medical complications in adolescents with anorexia: A review of the literature. Int J Eat Disord 37(Suppl):S52, 2005

Keski-Rahkonen A et al: Epidemiology and course of anorexia nervosa in the community. Am J Psychiatry 164(8):1259, 2007

Klein DA, Walsh BT: Eating disorders: Clinical features and pathophysiology. Physiol Behav 81:359, 2004

Mehler PS: Clinical practice. Bulimia nervosa. N Engl J Med 349:875, 2003

Sysko R, Walsh BT: A critical evaluation of the efficacy of self-help interventions for the treatment of bulimia nervosa and binge-eating disorder. Int J Eat Disord Oct 5 2007, epub ahead of print

Yager J, Andersen AE: Clinical practice. Anorexia nervosa. N Engl J Med 353:1481, 2005

SECTION 1 NEOPLASTIC DISORDERS

77 Approach to the Patient with Cancer

Dan L. Longo

The application of current treatment techniques (surgery, radiation therapy, chemotherapy, and biological therapy) results in the cure of nearly two of three patients diagnosed with cancer. Nevertheless, patients experience the diagnosis of cancer as one of the most traumatic and revolutionary events that has ever happened to them. Independent of prognosis, the diagnosis brings with it a change in a person's self-image and in his or her role in the home and workplace. The prognosis of a person who has just been found to have pancreatic cancer is the same as the prognosis of the person with aortic stenosis who develops the first symptoms of congestive heart failure (median survival, ~8 months). However, the patient with heart disease may remain functional and maintain a self-image as a fully intact person with just a malfunctioning part, a diseased organ ("a bum ticker"). By contrast, the patient with pancreatic cancer has a completely altered self-image and is viewed differently by family and anyone who knows the diagnosis. He or she is being attacked and invaded by a disease that could be anywhere in the body. Every ache or pain takes on desperate significance. Cancer is an exception to the coordinated interaction among cells and organs. In general, the cells of a multicellular organism are programmed for collaboration. Many diseases occur because the specialized cells fail to perform their assigned task. Cancer takes this malfunction one step further. Not only is there a failure of the cancer cell to maintain its specialized function, but it also strikes out on its own; the cancer cell competes to survive using natural mutability and natural selection to seek advantage over normal cells in a recapitulation of evolution. One consequence of the traitorous behavior of cancer cells is that the patient feels betrayed by his or her body. The cancer patient feels that he or she, and not just a body part, is diseased.

THE MAGNITUDE OF THE PROBLEM

No nationwide cancer registry exists; therefore, the incidence of cancer is estimated on the basis of the National Cancer Institute's Surveillance, Epidemiology, and End Results (SEER) database, which tabulates cancer incidence and death figures from nine sites, accounting for about 10% of the U.S. population, and from population data from the U.S. Census Bureau. In 2007, 1.445 million new cases of invasive cancer (766,860 men, 678,060 women) were diagnosed and 559,650 persons (289,550 men, 270,100 women) died from cancer. The percent distribution of new cancer cases and cancer deaths by site for men and women are shown in Table 77-1. Cancer incidence has been declining by about 2% each year since 1992.

The most significant risk factor for cancer overall is age; two-thirds of all cases were in those over age 65. Cancer incidence increases as the third, fourth, or fifth power of age in different sites. For the interval between birth and age 39, 1 in 72 men and 1 in 51 women will develop cancer; for the interval between ages 40 and 59, 1 in 12 men and 1 in 11 women will develop cancer; and for the interval between ages 60 and 79, 1 in 3 men and 1 in 5 women will develop cancer. Overall, men have a 45% risk of developing cancer at some time during their lives; women have a 37% lifetime risk.

Cancer is the second leading cause of death behind heart disease. Deaths from heart disease have declined 45% in the United States since 1950 and continue to decline. Cancer has overtaken heart disease as the number one cause of death in persons under age 85 years (Fig. 77-1). After a 70-year period of increases, cancer deaths began to decline in 1997 (Fig. 77-2). The five leading causes of cancer deaths are shown for various populations in Table 77-2. Along with the decrease in incidence has come an increase in survival for cancer patients. The 5-year survival for white patients was 39% in 1960–1963 and 68% in 1996–2002. Cancers are more often deadly in blacks; the 5-year survival was 57% for the 1996–2002 interval. Incidence and mortality vary among racial and ethnic groups (Table 77-3). The basis for these differences is unclear.

CANCER AROUND THE WORLD

In 2002, 11 million new cancer cases and 7 million cancer deaths were estimated worldwide. When broken down by region of the world, ~45% of cases were in Asia, 26% in Europe, 14.5% in North America, 7.1% in Central/South America, 6% in Africa, and 1% in Australia/New Zealand (Fig. 77-3). Lung cancer is the most common cancer and the most common cause of cancer death in the world. Its incidence is highly variable, affecting only 2 per 100,000 African women but as many as 61 per 100,000 North American men. Breast cancer is the second most common cancer worldwide; however, it ranks fifth as a cause of death behind lung, stomach, liver, and colorectal cancer. Among the eight most common forms of cancer, lung (2-fold), breast (3-fold), prostate (2.5-fold), and colorectal (3-fold) cancers are more common in more developed countries than in less developed countries. By contrast, liver (2-fold), cervical (2-fold), and esophageal (2- to 3-fold) cancers are more common in less developed

TABLE 77-1 DISTRIBUTION OF CANCER INCIDENCE AND DEATHS FOR 2007

	Male			Female	
Sites	**%**	**Number**	**Sites**	**%**	**Number**
Cancer Incidence					
Prostate	29	218,890	Breast	26	178,480
Lung	15	114,760	Lung	15	98,620
Colorectal	10	79,130	Colorectal	11	74,630
Bladder	7	50,040	Endometrial	6	39,080
Lymphoma	4	34,200	Lymphoma	4	28,990
Melanoma	4	33,910	Melanoma	4	26,030
Kidney	4	31,590	Thyroid	4	25,480
Leukemia	3	24,800	Ovary	3	22,430
Oral cavity	3	24,180	Kidney	3	19,600
Pancreas	2	18,830	Leukemia	3	19,440
All others	18	136,530	All others	21	145,280
All sites	100	776,860	All sites	100	678,060
Cancer Deaths					
Lung	31	89,510	Lung	26	70,880
Prostate	9	27,050	Breast	15	40,460
Colorectal	9	26,000	Colorectal	10	26,180
Pancreas	6	16,840	Pancreas	6	16,530
Leukemia	4	12,320	Ovary	6	15,280
Liver	4	11,280	Leukemia	4	9470
Esophagus	4	10,900	Lymphoma	3	9060
Bladder	3	9630	Endometrial	3	7400
Lymphoma	3	9600	CNS	2	5590
Kidney	3	8080	Liver	2	5500
All others	24	68,340	All others	23	63,750
All sites	100	289,550	All sites	100	270,100

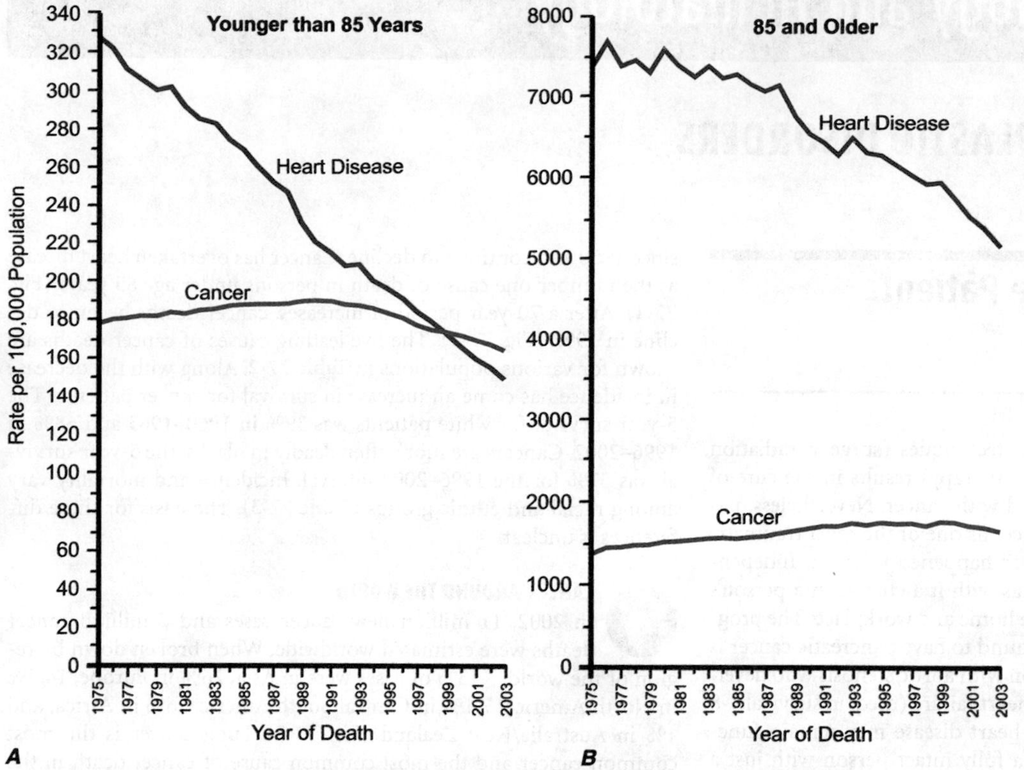

FIGURE 77-1 Death rates for heart disease and cancer among people younger and older than age 85. ***A.*** In people younger than 85 years, cancer has overtaken heart disease as the largest cause of death. ***B.*** In people over 85 years, heart disease is by far the major cause of death. *(From Jemal et al.)*

countries. Stomach cancer incidence is similar in more and less developed countries but is much more common in Asia than North America or Africa. The most common cancers in Africa are cervical, breast, and liver cancers. It has been estimated that nine modifiable risk factors are responsible for more than one-third of cancers worldwide. These include smoking, alcohol consumption, obesity, physical inactivity, low fruit and vegetable consumption, unsafe sex, air pollution, indoor smoke from household fuels, and contaminated injections.

PATIENT MANAGEMENT

Important information is obtained from every portion of the routine history and physical examination. The duration of symptoms may reveal the chronicity of disease. The past medical history may alert the physician to the presence of underlying diseases that may affect the choice of therapy or the side effects of treatment. The social history may reveal occupational exposure to carcinogens or habits, such as smoking or alcohol consumption, that may influence the course of disease and its treatment. The family history may suggest an underlying familial cancer predisposition and point out the need to begin surveillance or other preventive therapy for unaffected siblings of the patient. The review of systems may suggest early symptoms of metastatic disease or a paraneoplastic syndrome.

DIAGNOSIS

The diagnosis of cancer relies most heavily on invasive tissue biopsy and should never be made without obtaining tissue; no noninvasive diagnostic test is sufficient to define a disease process as cancer. Although in rare clinical settings (e.g., thyroid nodules) fine-needle aspiration is an acceptable diagnostic procedure, the diagnosis generally depends on obtaining adequate tissue to permit careful evaluation of the histology of the tumor, its grade, and its invasiveness and to yield further molecular diagnostic information, such as the expression of cell-surface markers or intracellular proteins that typify a particular cancer, or the presence of a molecular marker, such as the t(8;14) translocation of Burkitt's lymphoma. Increasing evidence links the expression of certain genes with the prognosis and response to therapy (Chaps. 79, 80).

Occasionally a patient will present with a metastatic disease process that is defined as cancer on biopsy but has no apparent primary site of disease. Efforts should be made to define the primary site based on age, sex, sites of involvement, histology and tumor markers, and personal and family history. Particular attention should be focused on ruling out the most treatable causes (Chap. 95).

Once the diagnosis of cancer is made, the management of the patient is best undertaken as a multidisciplinary collaboration among the primary care physician, medical oncologists, surgical oncologists, radiation oncologists, oncology nurse specialists, pharmacists, social workers, rehabilitation medicine specialists, and a number of other consulting professionals working closely with each other and with the patient and family.

DEFINING THE EXTENT OF DISEASE AND THE PROGNOSIS

The first priority in patient management after the diagnosis of cancer is established and shared with the patient is to determine the extent of disease. The curability of a tumor usually is inversely proportional to the tumor burden. Ideally, the tumor will be diagnosed before symptoms develop or as a consequence of screening efforts (Chap. 78). A very high proportion of such patients can be cured. However, most patients with cancer present with symptoms related to the cancer, caused either by mass effects of the tumor or by alterations associated with the production of cytokines or hormones by the tumor.

For most cancers, the extent of disease is evaluated by a variety of noninvasive and invasive diagnostic tests and procedures. This process is called *staging*. There are two types. *Clinical staging* is based on physical examination, radiographs, isotopic scans, CT scans, and other imaging procedures; *pathologic staging* takes into account information obtained during a surgical procedure, which might include intraoperative palpation, resection of regional lymph nodes and/or tissue adjacent to the tumor, and inspection and biopsy of organs commonly involved in disease spread. Pathologic staging includes histologic examination of all tissues removed during the surgical procedure. Surgical procedures performed may include a simple lymph node biopsy or more extensive procedures such as thoracotomy, mediastinoscopy, or laparotomy. Surgical staging may occur in a separate procedure or may be done at the time of definitive surgical resection of the primary tumor.

Knowledge of the predilection of particular tumors for spread to adjacent or distant organs helps direct the staging evaluation.

Information obtained from staging is used to define the extent of disease either as localized, as exhibiting spread outside of the organ of origin to regional but not distant sites, or as metastatic to distant sites. The most widely used system of staging is the TNM (tumor, node, metastasis) system codified by the International Union Against Cancer and the American Joint Committee on Cancer (AJCC). The TNM classification is an anatomically based system that categorizes the tumor on the basis of the size of the primary tumor lesion (T1–4, where a higher number indicates a tumor of larger size), the presence of nodal involvement (usually N0 and N1 for the absence and presence, respectively, of involved nodes, although some tumors have more elaborate

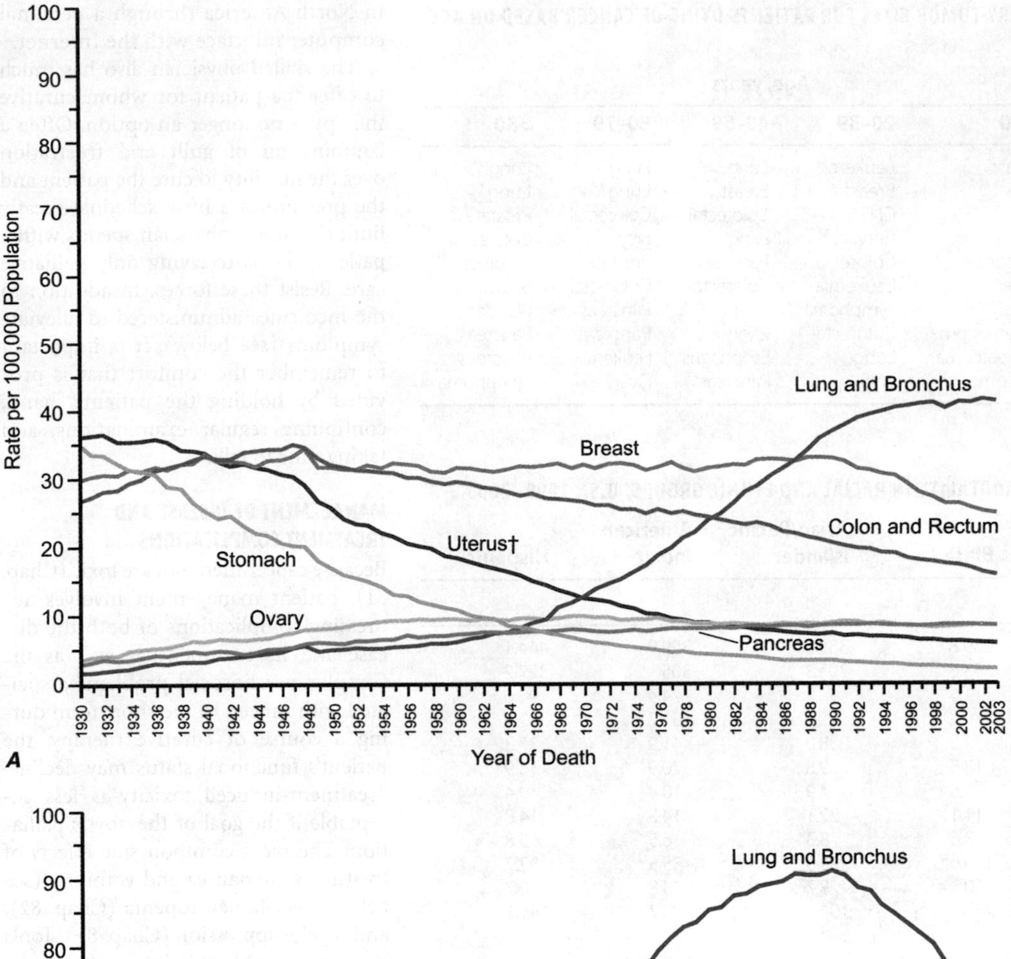

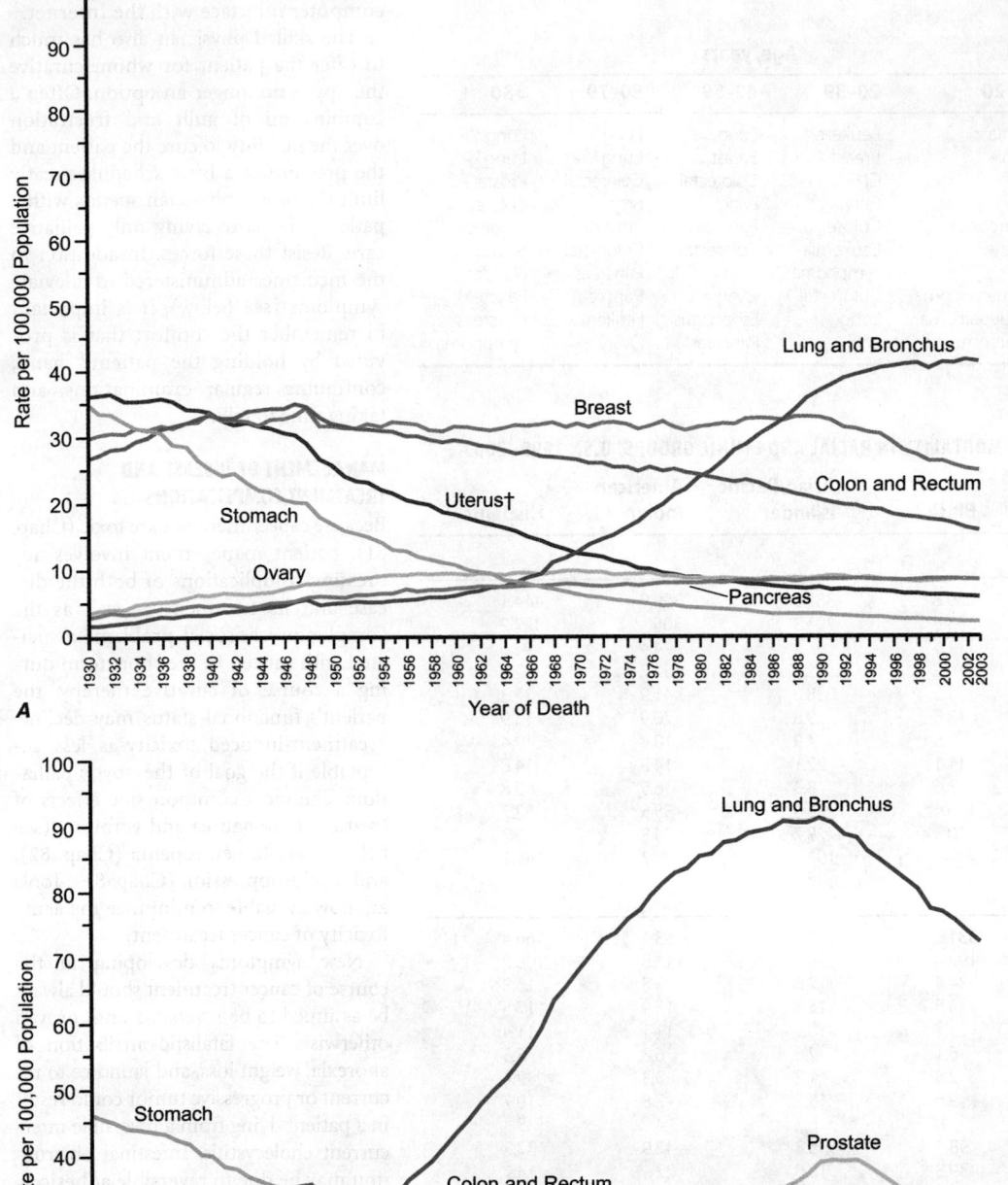

FIGURE 77-2 Sixty-year trend in cancer death rates for (*A*) women and (*B*) men, by site in the United States, 1930–2003. Rates are per 100,000 age-adjusted to the 2000 U.S. standard population. (*From Jemal et al.*)

systems of nodal grading), and the presence of metastatic disease (M0 and M1 for the absence and presence, respectively, of metastases). The various permutations of T, N, and M scores (sometimes including tumor histologic grade G) are then broken into stages, usually designated by the roman numerals I through IV. Tumor burden increases and curability decreases with increasing stage. Other anatomic staging systems are used for some tumors, e.g., the Dukes classification for colorectal cancers, the International Federation of Gynecologists and Obstetricians (FIGO) classification for gynecologic cancers, and the Ann Arbor classification for Hodgkin's disease.[1]

Certain tumors cannot be grouped on the basis of anatomic considerations. For example, hematopoietic tumors such as leukemia, myeloma, and lymphoma are often disseminated at presentation and do not spread like solid tumors. For these tumors, other prognostic factors have been identified (Chaps. 104–106).

In addition to tumor burden, a second major determinant of treatment outcome is the physiologic reserve of the patient. Patients who are bedridden before developing cancer are likely to fare worse, stage for stage, than fully active patients. Physiologic reserve is a determinant of how a patient is likely to cope with the physiologic stresses imposed by the cancer and its treatment. This factor is difficult to assess directly. Instead, surrogate markers for physiologic reserve are used, such as the patient's age or Karnofsky performance status (Table 77-4). Older patients and those with a Karnofsky performance status <70 have a poor prognosis unless the poor performance is a reversible consequence of the tumor.

Increasingly, biologic features of the tumor are being related to prognosis. The expression of particular oncogenes, drug-resistance genes, apoptosis-related genes, and genes involved in metastasis are being found to influence response to therapy and prognosis. The presence of selected cytogenetic abnormalities may influence survival. Tumors with higher growth fractions, as assessed by expression of proliferation-related markers such as proliferating cell nuclear antigen (PCNA), behave more aggressively than tumors with lower growth fractions. Information obtained from studying the tumor itself will increasingly be used to influence treatment decisions. Host genes involved in drug metabolism can influence the safety and efficacy of particular treatments.

MAKING A TREATMENT PLAN

From information on the extent of disease and the prognosis and in conjunction with the patient's wishes, it is determined whether the treatment approach should be curative or palliative in intent. Cooperation among the various professionals involved in cancer treat-

[1]The AJCC *Manual for Staging Cancer*, 5th edition, can be obtained from the AJCC at 55 East Erie Street, Chicago, IL, 60611.

TABLE 77-2 THE FIVE LEADING PRIMARY TUMOR SITES FOR PATIENTS DYING OF CANCER BASED ON AGE AND SEX IN 2004

Rank		All Ages	Under 20	Age, years 20–39	40–59	60–79	>80
1	M	Lung	Leukemia	Leukemia	Lung	Lung	Lung
	F	Lung	Leukemia	Breast	Breast	Lung	Lung
2	M	Prostate	CNS	CNS	Colorectal	Colorectal	Prostate
	F	Breast	CNS	Cervix	Lung	Breast	Colorectal
3	M	Colorectal	Bone sarcoma	Colorectal	Pancreas	Prostate	Colorectal
	F	Colorectal	Endocrine	Leukemia	Colorectal	Colorectal	Breast
4	M	Pancreas	Endocrine	Lymphoma	Liver	Pancreas	Bladder
	F	Pancreas	Soft tissue sarcoma	Colorectal	Ovary	Pancreas	Pancreas
5	M	Leukemia	Soft tissue sarcoma	Lung	Esophagus	Leukemia	Pancreas
	F	Ovary	Bone sarcoma	CNS	Pancreas	Ovary	Lymphoma

Note: M, male; F, female.

TABLE 77-3 CANCER INCIDENCE AND MORTALITY IN RACIAL AND ETHNIC GROUPS, U.S., 1999–2003

Site		White	Black	Asian/Pacific Islander	American Indian	Hispanic
Incidence per 100,000 Population						
All	M	555	639.8	385.5	359.9	444.1
	F	421.1	383.8	303.3	305	327.2
Breast		130.8	111.5	91.2	74.4	92.6
Colorectal	M	63.7	70.2	52.6	52.7	52.4
	F	45.9	53.5	38.0	41.9	37.3
Kidney	M	18	18.5	9.8	20.9	16.9
	F	9.3	9.5	4.9	10	9.4
Liver	M	7.2	11.1	22.1	14.5	14.8
	F	2.7	3.6	8.3	6.5	5.8
Lung	M	88.8	110.6	56.6	55.5	52.7
	F	56.2	50.3	28.7	33.8	26.7
Prostate		156	243	104	70.7	141.1
Deaths per 100,000 Population						
All	M	239.2	331	144.9	153.4	166.4
	F	163.4	192.4	98.8	111.6	108.8
Breast		25.4	34.4	12.6	13.8	16.3
Colorectal	M	23.7	33.6	15.3	15.9	17.5
	F	16.4	23.7	10.5	11.1	11.4
Kidney	M	6.2	6.1	2.6	6.8	5.5
	F	2.8	2.8	1.2	3.3	2.4
Liver	M	6.3	9.6	15.5	7.8	10.7
	F	2.8	3.8	6.7	4	5
Lung	M	73.8	98.4	38.8	42.9	37.2
	F	42	39.8	18.8	27	14.7
Prostate		26.7	65.1	11.8	18	22.1

Note: M, male; F, female.

in North America through a personal computer interface with the Internet.[2]

The skilled physician also has much to offer the patient for whom curative therapy is no longer an option. Often a combination of guilt and frustration over the inability to cure the patient and the pressure of a busy schedule greatly limit the time a physician spends with a patient who is receiving only palliative care. Resist these forces. In addition to the medicines administered to alleviate symptoms (see below), it is important to remember the comfort that is provided by holding the patient's hand, continuing regular examinations, and taking time to talk.

MANAGEMENT OF DISEASE AND TREATMENT COMPLICATIONS

Because cancer therapies are toxic (Chap. 81), patient management involves addressing complications of both the disease and its treatment as well as the complex psychosocial problems associated with cancer. In the short term during a course of curative therapy, the patient's functional status may decline. Treatment-induced toxicity is less acceptable if the goal of therapy is palliation. The most common side effects of treatment are nausea and vomiting (see below), febrile neutropenia (Chap. 82), and myelosuppression (Chap. 81). Tools are now available to minimize the acute toxicity of cancer treatment.

New symptoms developing in the course of cancer treatment should always be assumed to be reversible until proven otherwise. The fatalistic attribution of anorexia, weight loss, and jaundice to recurrent or progressive tumor could result in a patient dying from a reversible intercurrent cholecystitis. Intestinal obstruction may be due to reversible adhesions rather than progressive tumor. Systemic infections, sometimes with unusual pathogens, may be a consequence of the immunosuppression associated with cancer therapy. Some drugs used to treat cancer or its complications (e.g., nausea) may produce central nervous system symptoms that look like metastatic disease or may mimic paraneoplastic syndromes such as the syndrome of inappropriate antidiuretic hormone. A definitive diagnosis should be pursued and may even require a repeat biopsy.

A critical component of cancer management is assessing the response to treatment. In addition to a careful physical examination in which all sites of disease are physically measured and recorded in a flow chart by date, response assessment usually requires periodic repeating of imaging

ment is of the utmost importance in treatment planning. For some cancers, chemotherapy or chemotherapy plus radiation therapy delivered before the use of definitive surgical treatment (so-called neoadjuvant therapy) may improve the outcome, as seems to be the case for locally advanced breast cancer and head and neck cancers. In certain settings in which combined modality therapy is intended, coordination among the medical oncologist, radiation oncologist, and surgeon is crucial to achieving optimal results. Sometimes the chemotherapy and radiation therapy need to be delivered sequentially, and other times concurrently. Surgical procedures may precede or follow other treatment approaches. It is best for the treatment plan either to follow a standard protocol precisely or else to be part of an ongoing clinical research protocol evaluating new treatments. Ad hoc modifications of standard protocols are likely to compromise treatment results.

The choice of treatment approaches was formerly dominated by the local culture in both the university and the practice settings. However, it is now possible to gain access electronically to standard treatment protocols and to every approved clinical research study

[2]The National Cancer Institute maintains a database called PDQ (Physician Data Query) that is accessible on the Internet under the name CancerNet at *wwwicic.nci.nih.gov/health.htm*. Information can be obtained through a facsimile machine using CancerFax by dialing 301-402-5874. Patient information is also provided by the National Cancer Institute in at least three formats: on the Internet via CancerNet at *wwwicic.nci.nih.gov/patient.htm*, through the CancerFax number listed above, or by calling 1-800-4-CANCER. The quality control for the information provided through these services is rigorous.

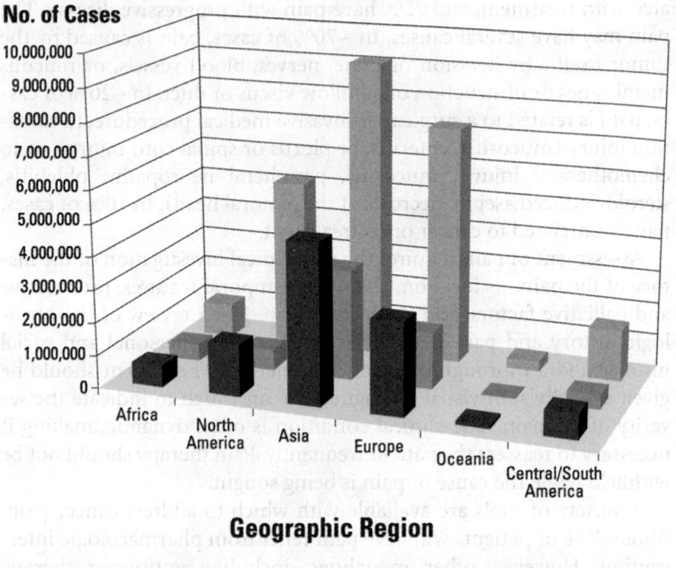

FIGURE 77-3 Worldwide overall annual cancer incidence, mortality and 5-year prevalence for the period of 1993–2001. (*From Kamangar et al.*)

TABLE 77-4 KARNOFSKY PERFORMANCE INDEX

Performance Status	Functional Capability of the Patient
100	Normal; no complaints; no evidence of disease
90	Able to carry on normal activity; minor signs or symptoms of disease
80	Normal activity with effort; some signs or symptoms of disease
70	Cares for self; unable to carry on normal activity or do active work
60	Requires occasional assistance but is able to care for most needs
50	Requires considerable assistance and frequent medical care
40	Disabled; requires special care and assistance
30	Severely disabled; hospitalization is indicated although death is not imminent
20	Very sick; hospitalization necessary; active supportive treatment is necessary
10	Moribund, fatal processes progressing rapidly
0	Dead

tests that were abnormal at the time of staging. If imaging tests have become normal, repeat biopsy of previously involved tissue is performed to document complete response by pathologic criteria. Biopsies are not usually required if there is macroscopic residual disease. A *complete response* is defined as disappearance of all evidence of disease, and a *partial response* as >50% reduction in the sum of the products of the perpendicular diameters of all measurable lesions. The determination of partial response may also be based on a 30% decrease in the sums of the longest diameters of lesions (Response Evaluation Criteria in Solid Tumors, or RECIST, criteria). *Progressive disease* is defined as the appearance of any new lesion or an increase of >25% in the sum of the products of the perpendicular diameters of all measurable lesions (or an increase of 20% in the sums of the longest diameters by RECIST). Tumor shrinkage or growth that does not meet any of these criteria is considered *stable disease.* Some sites of involvement (e.g., bone) or patterns of involvement (e.g., lymphangitic lung or diffuse pulmonary infiltrates) are considered unmeasurable. No response is complete without biopsy documentation of their resolution, but partial responses may exclude their assessment unless clear objective progression has occurred.

Tumor markers may be useful in patient management in certain tumors. Response to therapy may be difficult to gauge with certainty. However, some tumors produce or elicit the production of markers that can be measured in the serum or urine and, in a particular patient, rising and falling levels of the marker are usually associated with increasing or decreasing tumor burden, respectively. Some clinically useful tumor markers are shown in **Table 77-5**. Tumor markers are not in themselves specific enough to permit a diagnosis of malignancy to be made, but once a malignancy has been diagnosed and shown to be associated with elevated levels of a tumor marker, the marker can be used to assess response to treatment.

The recognition and treatment of depression are important components of management. The incidence of depression in cancer patients is ~25% overall and may be greater in patients with greater debility. This diagnosis is likely in a patient with a depressed mood (dysphoria) and/or a loss of interest in pleasure (anhedonia) for at least 2 weeks. In addition, three or more of the following symptoms are usually present: appetite change, sleep problems, psychomotor retardation or agitation, fatigue, feelings of guilt or worthlessness, inability to concentrate, and suicidal ideation. Patients with these symptoms should receive therapy. Medical therapy with a serotonin reuptake inhibitor such as fluoxetine (10–20 mg/d), sertraline (50–150 mg/d), or paroxetine (10–20 mg/d) or a tricyclic antidepressant such as amitriptyline (50–100 mg/d) or desipramine

TABLE 77-5 TUMOR MARKERS

Tumor Markers	Cancer	Non-Neoplastic Conditions
Hormones		
Human chorionic gonadotropin	Gestational trophoblastic disease, gonadal germ cell tumor	Pregnancy
Calcitonin	Medullary cancer of the thyroid	
Catecholamines	Pheochromocytoma	
Oncofetal Antigens		
Alphafetoprotein	Hepatocellular carcinoma, gonadal germ cell tumor	Cirrhosis, hepatitis
Carcinoembryonic antigen	Adenocarcinomas of the colon, pancreas, lung, breast, ovary	Pancreatitis, hepatitis, inflammatory bowel disease, smoking
Enzymes		
Prostatic acid phosphatase	Prostate cancer	Prostatitis, prostatic hypertrophy
Neuron-specific enolase	Small cell cancer of the lung, neuroblastoma	
Lactate dehydrogenase	Lymphoma, Ewing's sarcoma	Hepatitis, hemolytic anemia, many others
Tumor-Associated Proteins		
Prostate-specific antigen	Prostate cancer	Prostatitis, prostatic hypertrophy
Monoclonal immunoglobulin	Myeloma	Infection, MGUS[a]
CA-125	Ovarian cancer, some lymphomas	Menstruation, peritonitis, pregnancy
CA 19-9	Colon, pancreatic, breast cancer	Pancreatitis, ulcerative colitis
CD30	Hodgkin's disease, anaplastic large cell lymphoma	—
CD25	Hairy cell leukemia, adult T cell leukemia/lymphoma	—

[a]MGUS, monoclonal gammopathy of uncertain significance.

(75–150 mg/d) should be tried, allowing 4–6 weeks for response. Effective therapy should be continued at least 6 months after resolution of symptoms. If therapy is unsuccessful, other classes of antidepressants may be used. In addition to medication, psychosocial interventions such as support groups, psychotherapy, and guided imagery may be of benefit.

Many patients opt for unproven or unsound approaches to treatment when it appears that conventional medicine is unlikely to be curative. Those seeking such alternatives are often well educated and may be early in the course of their disease. Unsound approaches are usually hawked on the basis of unsubstantiated anecdotes and not only cannot help the patient but may be harmful. Physicians should strive to keep communications open and nonjudgmental, so that patients are more likely to discuss with the physician what they are actually doing. The appearance of unexpected toxicity may be an indication that a supplemental therapy is being taken.[3]

LONG-TERM FOLLOW-UP/LATE COMPLICATIONS

At the completion of treatment, sites originally involved with tumor are reassessed, usually by radiography or imaging techniques, and any persistent abnormality is biopsied. If disease persists, the multidisciplinary team discusses a new salvage treatment plan. If the patient has been rendered disease-free by the original treatment, the patient is followed regularly for disease recurrence. The optimal guidelines for follow-up care are not known. For many years, a routine practice has been to follow the patient monthly for 6–12 months, then every other month for a year, every 3 months for a year, every 4 months for a year, every 6 months for a year, and then annually. At each visit, a battery of laboratory and radiographic and imaging tests were obtained on the assumption that it is best to detect recurrent disease before it becomes symptomatic. However, where follow-up procedures have been examined, this assumption has been found to be untrue. Studies of breast cancer, melanoma, lung cancer, colon cancer, and lymphoma have all failed to support the notion that asymptomatic relapses are more readily cured by salvage therapy than symptomatic relapses. In view of the enormous cost of a full battery of diagnostic tests and their manifest lack of impact on survival, new guidelines are emerging for less frequent follow-up visits, during which the history and physical examination are the major investigations performed.

As time passes, the likelihood of recurrence of the primary cancer diminishes. For many types of cancer, survival for 5 years without recurrence is tantamount to cure. However, important medical problems can occur in patients treated for cancer and must be examined (**Chap. e13**). Some problems emerge as a consequence of the disease and some as a consequence of the treatment. An understanding of these disease- and treatment-related problems may help in their detection and management.

Despite these concerns, most patients who are cured of cancer return to normal lives.

SUPPORTIVE CARE

In many ways, the success of cancer therapy depends on the success of the supportive care. Failure to control the symptoms of cancer and its treatment may lead patients to abandon curative therapy. Of equal importance, supportive care is a major determinant of quality of life. Even when life cannot be prolonged, the physician must strive to preserve its quality. Quality-of-life measurements have become common endpoints of clinical research studies. Furthermore, palliative care has been shown to be cost-effective when approached in an organized fashion. A credo for oncology could be to cure sometimes, to extend life often, and to comfort always.

Pain Pain occurs with variable frequency in the cancer patient: 25–50% of patients present with pain at diagnosis, 33% have pain associated with treatment, and 75% have pain with progressive disease. The pain may have several causes. In ~70% of cases, pain is caused by the tumor itself—by invasion of bone, nerves, blood vessels, or mucous membranes or obstruction of a hollow viscus or duct. In ~20% of cases, pain is related to a surgical or invasive medical procedure, to radiation injury (mucositis, enteritis, or plexus or spinal cord injury), or to chemotherapy injury (mucositis, peripheral neuropathy, phlebitis, steroid-induced aseptic necrosis of the femoral head). In 10% of cases, pain is unrelated to cancer or its treatment.

Assessment of pain requires the methodical investigation of the history of the pain, its location, character, temporal features, provocative and palliative factors, and intensity (Chap. 12); a review of the oncologic history and past medical history as well as personal and social history; and a thorough physical examination. The patient should be given a 10-division visual analogue scale on which to indicate the severity of the pain. The clinical condition is often dynamic, making it necessary to reassess the patient frequently. Pain therapy should not be withheld while the cause of pain is being sought.

A variety of tools are available with which to address cancer pain. About 85% of patients will have pain relief from pharmacologic intervention. However, other modalities, including antitumor therapy (such as surgical relief of obstruction, radiation therapy, and strontium-89 or samarium-153 treatment for bone pain), neurostimulatory techniques, regional analgesia, or neuroablative procedures are effective in an additional 12% or so. Thus, very few patients will have inadequate pain relief if appropriate measures are taken. **A specific approach to pain relief is detailed in Chap. 11.**

Nausea Emesis in the cancer patient is usually caused by chemotherapy (Chap. 81). Its severity can be predicted from the drugs used to treat the cancer. Three forms of emesis are recognized on the basis of their timing with regard to the noxious insult. *Acute emesis*, the most common variety, occurs within 24 h of treatment. *Delayed emesis* occurs 1–7 days after treatment; it is rare, but, when present, usually follows cisplatin administration. *Anticipatory emesis* occurs before administration of chemotherapy and represents a conditioned response to visual and olfactory stimuli previously associated with chemotherapy delivery.

Acute emesis is the best understood form. Stimuli that activate signals in the chemoreceptor trigger zone in the medulla, the cerebral cortex, and peripherally in the intestinal tract lead to stimulation of the vomiting center in the medulla, the motor center responsible for coordinating the secretory and muscle contraction activity that leads to emesis. Diverse receptor types participate in the process, including dopamine, serotonin, histamine, opioid, and acetylcholine receptors. The serotonin receptor antagonists ondansetron and granisetron are the most effective drugs against highly emetogenic agents, but they are expensive.

As with the analgesia ladder, emesis therapy should be tailored to the situation. For mildly and moderately emetogenic agents, prochlorperazine, 5–10 mg PO or 25 mg PR, is effective. Its efficacy may be enhanced by administering the drug before the chemotherapy is delivered. Dexamethasone, 10–20 mg IV, is also effective and may enhance the efficacy of prochlorperazine. For highly emetogenic agents such as cisplatin, mechlorethamine, dacarbazine, and streptozocin, combinations of agents work best and administration should begin 6–24 h before treatment. Ondansetron, 8 mg PO every 6 h the day before therapy and IV on the day of therapy, plus dexamethasone, 20 mg IV before treatment, is an effective regimen. Addition of oral aprepitant (a substance P/neurokinin 1 receptor antagonist) to this regimen (125 mg on day 1, 80 mg on days 2 and 3) further decreases the risk of both acute and delayed vomiting. Like pain, emesis is easier to prevent than to alleviate.

Delayed emesis may be related to bowel inflammation from the therapy and can be controlled with oral dexamethasone and oral metoclopramide, a dopamine receptor antagonist that also blocks serotonin receptors at high dosages. The best strategy for preventing anticipatory emesis is to control emesis in the early cycles of therapy to prevent the conditioning from taking place. If this is unsuccessful, pro-

---

[3]Information about unsound methods may be obtained from the National Council Against Health Fraud, Box 1276, Loma Linda, CA 92354, or from the Center for Medical Consumers and Health Care Information, 237 Thompson Street, New York, NY 10012.

phylactic antiemetics the day before treatment may help. Experimental studies are evaluating behavior modification.

Effusions Fluid may accumulate abnormally in the pleural cavity, pericardium, or peritoneum. Asymptomatic malignant effusions may not require treatment. Symptomatic effusions occurring in tumors responsive to systemic therapy usually do not require local treatment but respond to the treatment for the underlying tumor. Symptomatic effusions occurring in tumors unresponsive to systemic therapy may require local treatment in patients with a life expectancy of at least 6 months.

Pleural effusions due to tumors may or may not contain malignant cells. Lung cancer, breast cancer, and lymphomas account for ~75% of malignant pleural effusions. Their exudative nature is usually gauged by an effusion/serum protein ratio of ≥0.5 or an effusion/serum lactate dehydrogenase ratio of ≥0.6. When the condition is symptomatic, thoracentesis is usually performed first. In most cases, symptomatic improvement occurs for <1 month. Chest tube drainage is required if symptoms recur within 2 weeks. Fluid is aspirated until the flow rate is <100 mL in 24 h. Then either 60 units of bleomycin or 1 g of doxycycline is infused into the chest tube in 50 mL of 5% dextrose in water; the tube is clamped; the patient is rotated on four sides, spending 15 min in each position; and, after 1–2 h, the tube is again attached to suction for another 24 h. The tube is then disconnected from suction and allowed to drain by gravity. If <100 mL drains over the next 24 h, the chest tube is pulled, and a radiograph taken 24 h later. If the chest tube continues to drain fluid at an unacceptably high rate, sclerosis can be repeated. Bleomycin may be somewhat more effective than doxycycline but is very expensive. Doxycycline is usually the drug of first choice. If neither doxycycline nor bleomycin is effective, talc can be used.

Symptomatic pericardial effusions are usually treated by creating a pericardial window or by stripping the pericardium. If the patient's condition does not permit a surgical procedure, sclerosis can be attempted with doxycycline and/or bleomycin.

Malignant ascites is usually treated with repeated paracentesis of small volumes of fluid. If the underlying malignancy is unresponsive to systemic therapy, peritoneovenous shunts may be inserted. Despite the fear of disseminating tumor cells into the circulation, widespread metastases are an unusual complication. The major complications are occlusion, leakage, and fluid overload. Patients with severe liver disease may develop disseminated intravascular coagulation.

Nutrition Cancer and its treatment may lead to a decrease in nutrient intake of sufficient magnitude to cause weight loss and alteration of intermediary metabolism. The prevalence of this problem is difficult to estimate because of variations in the definition of cancer cachexia, but most patients with advanced cancer experience weight loss and decreased appetite. A variety of both tumor-derived factors (e.g., bombesin, adrenocorticotropic hormone) and host-derived factors (e.g., tumor necrosis factor, interleukins 1 and 6, growth hormone) contribute to the altered metabolism, and a vicious cycle is established in which protein catabolism, glucose intolerance, and lipolysis cannot be reversed by the provision of calories.

It remains controversial how to assess nutritional status and when and how to intervene. Efforts to make the assessment objective have included the use of a prognostic nutritional index based on albumin levels, triceps skin fold thickness, transferrin levels, and delayed-type hypersensitivity skin testing. However, a simpler approach has been to define the threshold for nutritional intervention as >10% unexplained body weight loss, serum transferrin level <1500 mg/L (150 mg/dL), and serum albumin <34 g/L (3.4 g/dL).

The decision is important, because it appears that cancer therapy is substantially more toxic and less effective in the face of malnutrition. Nevertheless, it remains unclear whether nutritional intervention can alter the natural history. Unless some pathology is affecting the absorptive function of the gastrointestinal tract, enteral nutrition provided orally or by tube feeding is preferred over parenteral supplementation. However, the risks associated with the tube may outweigh the benefits. Megestrol acetate, a progestational agent, has been advocated as a pharmacologic intervention to improve nutritional status. Research in this area may provide more tools in the future as cytokine-mediated mechanisms are further elucidated.

Psychosocial Support The psychosocial needs of patients vary with their situation. Patients undergoing treatment experience fear, anxiety, and depression. Self-image is often seriously compromised by deforming surgery and loss of hair. Women who receive cosmetic advice that enables them to look better also feel better. Loss of control over how one spends time can contribute to the sense of vulnerability. Juggling the demands of work and family with the demands of treatment may create enormous stresses. Sexual dysfunction is highly prevalent and needs to be discussed openly with the patient. An empathetic health care team is sensitive to the individual patient's needs and permits negotiation where such flexibility will not adversely affect the course of treatment.

Cancer survivors have other sets of difficulties. Patients may have fears associated with the termination of a treatment they associate with their continued survival. Adjustments are required to physical losses and handicaps, real and perceived. Patients may be preoccupied with minor physical problems. They perceive a decline in their job mobility and view themselves as less desirable workers. They may be victims of job and/or insurance discrimination. Patients may experience difficulty reentering their normal past life. They may feel guilty for having survived and may carry a sense of vulnerability to colds and other illnesses. Perhaps the most pervasive and threatening concern is the ever-present fear of relapse (the Damocles syndrome).

Patients in whom therapy has been unsuccessful have other problems related to the end of life.

Death and Dying The most common causes of death in patients with cancer are infection (leading to circulatory failure), respiratory failure, hepatic failure, and renal failure. Intestinal blockage may lead to inanition and starvation. Central nervous system disease may lead to seizures, coma, and central hypoventilation. About 70% of patients develop dyspnea preterminally. However, many months usually pass between the diagnosis of cancer and the occurrence of these complications, and during this period the patient is severely affected by the possibility of death. The path of unsuccessful cancer treatment usually occurs in three phases. First, there is optimism at the hope of cure; when the tumor recurs, there is the acknowledgment of an incurable disease, and the goal of palliative therapy is embraced in the hope of being able to live with disease; finally, at the disclosure of imminent death, another adjustment in outlook takes place. The patient imagines the worst in preparation for the end of life and may go through stages of adjustment to the diagnosis. These stages include denial, isolation, anger, bargaining, depression, acceptance, and hope. Of course, patients do not all progress through all the stages or proceed through them in the same order or at the same rate. Nevertheless, developing an understanding of how the patient has been affected by the diagnosis and is coping with it is an important goal of patient management.

It is best to speak frankly with the patient and the family regarding the likely course of disease. These discussions can be difficult for the physician as well as for the patient and family. The critical features of the interaction are to reassure the patient and family that everything that can be done to provide comfort will be done. They will not be abandoned. Many patients prefer to be cared for in their homes or in a hospice setting rather than a hospital. The American College of Physicians has published a book called *Home Care Guide for Cancer: How to Care for Family and Friends at Home* that teaches an approach to successful problem-solving in home care. With appropriate planning, it should be possible to provide the patient with the necessary medical care as well as the psychological and spiritual support that will prevent the isolation and depersonalization that can attend in-hospital death.

The care of dying patients may take a toll on the physician. A "burnout" syndrome has been described that is characterized by fatigue, disengagement from patients and colleagues, and a loss of self-fulfillment. Efforts at stress reduction, maintenance of a balanced life, and setting realistic goals may combat this disorder.

End-of-Life Decisions Unfortunately, a smooth transition in treatment goals from curative to palliative may not be possible in all cases because of the occurrence of serious treatment-related complications or rapid disease progression. Vigorous and invasive medical support for a reversible disease or treatment complication is assumed to be justified. However, if the reversibility of the condition is in doubt, the patient's wishes determine the level of medical care. These wishes should be elicited before the terminal phase of illness and reviewed periodically. Information about advance directives can be obtained from the American Association of Retired Persons, 601 E Street, NW, Washington, DC 20049, 202-434-2277 or Choice in Dying, 250 West 57th Street, New York, NY 10107, 212-366-5540. **A full discussion of end-of-life management is in Chap. 11.**

78 Prevention and Early Detection of Cancer

Otis W. Brawley, Barnett S. Kramer

Improved understanding of carcinogenesis has allowed cancer prevention and early detection (also known as cancer control) to expand beyond the identification and avoidance of carcinogens. Specific interventions to prevent cancer in those at risk, and more sensitive and specific screening for early detection of cancer are the goals.

Carcinogenesis is not simply an event but a process, a continuum of discrete cellular changes over time resulting in more autonomous cellular processes. Prevention concerns the identification and manipulation of the genetic, biologic, and environmental factors in the causal pathway of cancer.

EDUCATION AND HEALTHFUL HABITS

Public education on the avoidance of identified risk factors for cancer and encouraging healthy habits contributes to cancer prevention and control. The physician is a powerful messenger in this education campaign. The patient-physician encounter provides an opportunity to teach patients about the hazards of smoking, the features of a healthy lifestyle (including diet and exercise), use of proven cancer screening methods, and sun avoidance.

Smoking Cessation Tobacco smoking is the most modifiable risk factor for cardiovascular disease, pulmonary disease, and cancer. Smokers have a 33% lifetime risk of dying prematurely from a tobacco-related cancer, cardiovascular, or pulmonary disease. Tobacco use causes more deaths from cardiovascular disease than from cancer. Lung cancer and cancers of the larynx, oropharynx, esophagus, kidney, bladder, pancreas, and stomach are all tobacco-related.

The degree of smoke exposure, meaning the number of cigarettes smoked per day as well as the level of inhalation of cigarette smoke, is correlated with risk of lung cancer mortality. Light- and low-tar cigarettes are not safer because smokers tend to inhale them more frequently and deeply.

Those who stop smoking have a 30–50% lower 10-year lung cancer mortality rate compared to those who continue smoking, despite the fact that some carcinogen-induced gene mutations persist for years after smoking cessation. Smoking cessation and avoidance have the potential to save more lives than any other public health activity.

FURTHER READINGS

GRUNBERG SM, HESKETH PJ: Control of chemotherapy-induced emesis. N Engl J Med 329:1790, 1993

JEMAL A et al: Cancer statistics, 2007. CA Cancer J Clin 57:43, 2007

KAMANGAR F et al: Patterns of cancer incidence, mortality, and prevalence across five continents: Defining priorities to reduce cancer disparities in different geographic regions of the world. J Clin Oncol 24:2137, 2006

LEVY MH: Pharmacologic treatment of cancer pain. N Engl J Med 335:1124, 1996

THERASSE P et al: New guidelines to evaluate response to treatment in solid tumors. J Natl Cancer Inst 92:205, 2000

U.S. DEPARTMENT OF HEALTH AND HUMAN SERVICES: *Clinical Practice Guideline Number 9, Management of Cancer Pain.* U.S. Department of Health and Human Services, Agency for Health Care Policy and Research publication no. 94-0592, 1994

WALSH D et al: The symptoms of advanced cancer: Relationship to age, gender, and performance status in 1000 patients. Support Care Cancer 8:175, 2000

The risk of tobacco smoke is not limited to the smoker. Environmental tobacco smoke, known as second hand or passive smoke, causes lung cancer and other cardiopulmonary diseases in nonsmokers.

Tobacco prevention is a pediatric issue. Over 80% of adult American smokers began smoking before the age of 18. Nearly 20% of Americans aged 12–18 have smoked a cigarette in the past month. Counseling of adolescents and young adults is critical to prevent smoking. A physician's simple advice to not start smoking or to quit smoking can be of benefit. Physicians should query patients on tobacco use on every office visit, record the answer with the vital signs, and ask smokers if they would like assistance in quitting.

Current approaches to smoking cessation recognize that smoking is an addiction (Chap. 390). The smoker who is quitting goes through a process with identifiable stages that include contemplation of quitting, an action phase in which the smoker quits, and a maintenance phase. Smokers who quit completely are more likely to be successful than those who gradually reduce the number of cigarettes smoked or change to lower tar or nicotine cigarettes. More than 90% of the Americans who have successfully quit smoking did so on their own without participation in an organized cessation program, but cessation programs are helpful for some smokers. The Community Intervention Trial for Smoking Cessation (COMMIT) was a 4-year program; it demonstrated that light smokers (<25 cigarettes per day) were more likely to benefit from simple cessation messages and cessation programs. Quit rates were 30.6% in the intervention group and 27.5% in the control group. The COMMIT interventions were not successful in heavy smokers (>25 cigarettes per day). Heavy smokers may need an intensive broad-based cessation program that includes counseling, behavioral strategies, and pharmacologic adjuncts, such as nicotine replacement (gum, patches, sprays, lozenges, and inhalers) and bupropion.

Cigar smoking has increased in the past decade. The health risks of cigars are similar to those of cigarettes. Smoking one or two cigars daily doubles the risk for oral and esophageal cancers; three or four cigars daily increases the risk of oral cancers more than eightfold and esophageal cancer fourfold. The risks of occasional use are unknown.

Smokeless tobacco is the fastest growing part of the tobacco industry and represents a substantial health risk. Chewing tobacco is a carcinogen linked to dental caries, gingivitis, oral leukoplakia, and oral cancer. The systemic effects of smokeless tobacco may increase risks for other cancers. Esophageal cancer is linked to carcinogens in tobacco being dissolved in saliva, swallowed, and coming into contact with the esophagus.

Physical Activity Physical activity is associated with a decreased risk of colon and breast cancer. A variety of mechanisms have been proposed. However, such studies are prone to confounding factors such as recall bias, association of exercise with other health-related practices, and effects of preclinical cancers on exercise habits (reverse causality). Recommending adults to engage in at least 30 min of vigorous activity for ≥3 days a week is good health advice, though its effects on cancer incidence are unproven.

Diet Modification International epidemiologic studies suggest that diets high in fat are associated with increased risk for cancers of the breast, colon, prostate, and endometrium. These cancers have their highest incidence and mortalities in western culture where fat comprises an average of 40–45% of the total calories consumed. In populations at low risk for these cancers, fat accounts for <20% of dietary calories.

Despite correlations, dietary fat has not been proven to cause cancer. Case-control and cohort epidemiologic studies give conflicting results. In addition, diet is a highly complex exposure to many nutrients and chemicals. Low-fat diets are associated with many dietary changes beyond simple subtraction of fat. Other lifestyle changes are also associated with adherence to a low-fat diet. The Women's Intervention Nutrition Study (WINS) evaluated the effects of low-fat diet on breast cancer recurrence in previously treated postmenopausal breast cancer patients. Breast cancer patients, mean age 62 years, were randomly assigned to a standard diet (40% fat) or a low-fat diet (26% fat). At 5 years, breast cancer had recurred in 9.8% of women in the low-fat diet group compared to 12.4% of women on the standard diet.

In observational studies, dietary fiber lowers the risk of colonic polyps and invasive cancer of the colon. However, cancer protective effects of increasing fiber and lowering dietary fat have not been proven in the context of a prospective clinical trial. The putative protective mechanisms are complex and speculative. Fiber binds oxidized bile acids and generates soluble fiber products, such as butyrate, that may have differentiating properties. Fiber does not increase bowel transit times. High-fiber diets could lower the risk of breast and prostate cancer by absorbing and inactivating dietary estrogenic and androgenic cancer promoters. However, two large prospective cohort studies of >100,000 health professionals showed no association between fruit and vegetable intake and risk of cancer.

The Polyp Prevention Trial randomly assigned 2000 elderly persons, who had polyps removed, to a low-fat, high-fiber diet versus routine diet for 4 years. No differences were noted in polyp formation.

The U.S. National Institutes of Health Women's Health Initiative, launched in 1994, is a long-term clinical trial enrolling >100,000 women aged 45–69. It placed women in 22 intervention groups. Participants received calcium/vitamin D supplementation, hormone-replacement therapy, and counseling to increase exercise, eat a low-fat diet, and cease smoking. The study showed that while dietary fat intake was significantly lower in the diet intervention group, invasive breast cancers were not reduced over an 8-year follow-up period compared to the control group. The difference in dietary fat averaged ~10% between the two groups. Scientific evidence does not currently establish the anticarcinogenic value of vitamin, mineral, or nutritional supplements in amounts greater than those provided by a balanced diet. However, consuming at least five servings of fruits and vegetables a day decreases dietary fat and increases fiber; such a diet may lower the risk of cardiovascular disease even if it does not influence cancer.

Energy Balance Risk of cancer increases as body mass index increases over 25 kg/m^2. Obesity increases risks for cancers of the colon, breast (female postmenopausal), endometrium, kidney (renal cell), and esophagus, although causality is not established.

Relative risks of colon cancer are increased in obesity by 1.5–2.0 for men and 1.2–1.5 for women. Obese postmenopausal women have a 30–50% increased risk of breast cancer. A hypothesis for the association is that adipose tissue serves as a depot for aromatase that facilitates estrogen production. Adiposity is also associated with poorer survival and increased risk of recurrence after treatment.

Sun Avoidance Nonmelanoma skin cancers (basal cell and squamous cell) are induced by cumulative exposure to ultraviolet (UV) radiation. Intermittent acute sun exposure and sun damage have been linked to melanoma. Sunburns, especially in childhood and adolescence, are associated with increased risk of melanoma in adulthood. Reduction of sun exposure through use of protective clothing and changing patterns of outdoor activities can reduce skin cancer risk. Sunscreens decrease the risk of actinic keratoses, the precursor to squamous cell skin cancer, but melanoma risk may be increased. Sunscreens prevent burning, but they may encourage more prolonged exposure to the sun and may not filter out wavelengths of energy that cause melanoma.

Educational interventions to help individuals accurately assess their risk of developing skin cancer have some impact. Self examination for skin pigment characteristics associated with melanoma, such as freckling, may be useful in identifying people at high risk. Those who recognize themselves as being at risk tend to be more compliant with sun-avoidance recommendations. Risk factors for melanoma include a propensity to sunburn, a large number of benign melanocytic nevi, and atypical nevi.

CANCER CHEMOPREVENTION

Chemoprevention involves the use of specific natural or synthetic chemical agents to reverse, suppress, or prevent carcinogenesis before the development of invasive malignancy.

Cancer develops through an accumulation of genetic and epigenetic changes that are potential points of intervention to prevent cancer. The initial changes are termed *initiation*. The alteration can be inherited or acquired through the action of physical, infectious, or chemical carcinogens. Like most human diseases, cancer arises from an interaction between genetics and environmental exposures (Table 78-1). Influences that cause the initiated cell to progress through the carcinogenic process and change

TABLE 78-1 SUSPECTED CARCINOGENS

Carcinogens[a]	Associated Cancer or Neoplasm
Alkylating agents	Acute myeloid leukemia, bladder cancer
Androgens	Prostate cancer
Aromatic amines (dyes)	Bladder cancer
Arsenic	Cancer of the lung, skin
Asbestos	Cancer of the lung, pleura, peritoneum
Benzene	Acute myelocytic leukemia
Chromium	Lung cancer
Diethylstilbestrol (prenatal)	Vaginal cancer (clear cell)
Epstein-Barr virus	Burkitt's lymphoma, nasal T cell lymphoma
Estrogens	Cancer of the endometrium, liver, breast
Ethyl alcohol	Cancer of the liver, esophagus, head and neck
Helicobacter pylori	Gastric cancer, gastric MALT lymphoma
Hepatitis B or C virus	Liver cancer
Human immunodeficiency virus	Non-Hodgkin's lymphoma, Kaposi's sarcoma, squamous cell carcinomas (especially of the urogenital tract)
Human papilloma virus	Cervix cancer, head and neck cancer
Human T cell lymphotropic virus type I (HTLV-I)	Adult T cell leukemia/lymphoma
Immunosuppressive agents (azathioprine, cyclosporine, glucocorticoids)	Non-Hodgkin's lymphoma
Nitrogen mustard gas	Cancer of the lung, head and neck, nasal sinuses
Nickel dust	Cancer of the lung, nasal sinuses
Phenacetin	Cancer of the renal pelvis and bladder
Polycyclic hydrocarbons	Cancer of the lung, skin (especially squamous cell carcinoma of scrotal skin)
Schistosomiasis	Bladder cancer (squamous cell)
Sunlight (ultraviolet)	Skin cancer (squamous cell and melanoma)
Tobacco (including smokeless)	Cancer of the upper aerodigestive tract, bladder
Vinyl chloride	Liver cancer (angiosarcoma)

[a]Agents that are thought to act as cancer initiators and/or promoters.

phenotypically are termed *promoters*. Promoters include hormones such as androgens, linked to prostate cancer, and estrogen, linked to breast and endometrial cancer. The distinction between an initiator and promoter is sometimes arbitrary; some components of cigarette smoke are "complete carcinogens," acting as both initiators and promoters. Cancer can be prevented or controlled through interference with the factors that cause cancer initiation, promotion, or progression. Compounds of interest in chemoprevention often have antimutagenic, antioxidant, anti-inflammatory, antiproliferative, or pro-apoptotic activity (or a combination).

Chemoprevention of Cancers of the Upper Aerodigestive Tract Smoking causes diffuse epithelial injury in the head, neck, esophagus, and lung. Patients cured of squamous cell cancers of the lung, esophagus, head, and neck are at risk (as high as 5% per year) of developing second cancers of the upper aerodigestive tract. Cessation of cigarette smoking does not markedly decrease the cured cancer patient's risk of second malignancy, even though it does lower the cancer risk in those who have never developed a malignancy. Smoking cessation may halt the early stages of the carcinogenic process (such as metaplasia), but it may have no effect on late stages of carcinogenesis. This "field carcinogenesis" hypothesis for upper aerodigestive tract cancer has made "cured" patients an important population for chemoprevention of second malignancies.

Oral leukoplakia, a premalignant lesion commonly found in smokers, has been used as an intermediate marker allowing demonstration of chemopreventive activity in smaller shorter duration, randomized, placebo-controlled trials. Response was associated with upregulation of retinoic acid receptor-β (RAR-β). Therapy with high, relatively toxic doses of isoretinoin (13-*cis*-retinoic acid) causes regression of oral leukoplakia. However, the lesions recur when the therapy is withdrawn, suggesting the need for chronic administration. More tolerable doses of isoretinoin have not proven beneficial in the prevention of head and neck cancer. Isoretinoin also failed to prevent second malignancies in patients cured of early-stage non-small cell lung cancer; mortality rates were actually increased in current smokers.

Premalignant lesions in the oropharyngeal area have also responded to retinol, α-tocopherol (vitamin E), and selenium. Further study to define the activity of these drugs is ongoing.

Several large-scale trials have assessed agents in the chemoprevention of lung cancer in patients at high risk. In the α-tocopherol/β-carotene (ATBC) Lung Cancer Prevention Trial participants were male smokers, age 50–69 at entry. Participants had smoked an average of one pack of cigarettes per day for 35.9 years. Participants received α-tocopherol, β-carotene, and/or placebo in a randomized, 2 × 2 factorial design. After median follow-up of 6.1 years, lung cancer incidence and mortality were statistically significantly increased in those receiving β-carotene. α-Tocopherol had no effect on lung cancer mortality, and no evidence suggested interaction between the two drugs. Patients receiving α-tocopherol had a higher incidence of hemorrhagic stroke.

The β-Carotene and Retinol Efficacy Trial (CARET) involved 17,000 American smokers and workers with asbestos exposure. Entrants were randomly assigned to one of four arms and received β-carotene, retinol, and/or placebo in a 2 × 2 factorial design. This trial also demonstrated harm from β-carotene: a lung cancer rate of 5 per 1000 subjects per year for those taking placebo and of 6 per 1000 subjects per year for those taking β-carotene.

The ATBC and CARET results demonstrate the importance of testing chemoprevention hypotheses thoroughly before their widespread implementation as the results contradict a number of observational studies. In the ATBC trial, those taking α-tocopherol had a one-third reduction in the incidence of prostate cancer, compared to those not taking α-tocopherol. The Physicians' Health Trial showed no change in the risk of lung cancer for those taking β-carotene; fewer of its participants were smokers than those in the ATBC and CARET studies.

Chemoprevention of Colon Cancer Many of the current colon cancer prevention trials are based on the premise that most colorectal cancers develop from adenomatous polyps. These trials use adenoma recurrence or disappearance as a surrogate endpoint for colon cancer prevention. Early clinical trial results suggest that nonsteroidal anti-inflammatory drugs (NSAIDs), such as piroxicam, sulindac, and aspirin, may prevent adenoma formation or cause regression of adenomatous polyps. The mechanism of action of NSAIDs is unknown, but they are presumed to work through the cyclooxygenase pathway. In the Physicians' Health Trial, aspirin had no effect on colon cancer incidence, although the 6-year assessment period may not have been long enough to evaluate this endpoint definitively. A number of studies suggest that NSAID use is associated with a lower risk of adenomatous polyps and invasive cancer. However, prospective trials have not shown that NSAIDs prevent colon cancer.

Cyclooxygenase-2 (COX-2) inhibitors may be even more effective. In a placebo-controlled trial, high-dose celecoxib reduced the recurrence of colorectal polyps in patients with familial adenomatous polyposis. The effect on colon cancer occurrence is unknown. Trials for prevention of sporadic colorectal cancers with COX-2 inhibitors were initiated but have been complicated by the association of these drugs with cardiovascular disease.

Epidemiologic studies suggest that diets high in calcium lower colon cancer risk. Calcium binds bile and fatty acids, which cause proliferation of colonic epithelium. It is hypothesized that calcium reduces intraluminal exposure to these compounds. Calcium supplementation decreases the risk of adenomatous polyp recurrence by ~20%. Trials of calcium with cancer-incidence endpoints are underway.

The Women's Health Initiative demonstrated that postmenopausal women taking premarin plus progestin have a 44% lower risk of colorectal cancer compared to women taking placebo. Of >16,600 women randomized and followed for a median of 5.6 years, 43 invasive colorectal cancers occurred in the hormone group and 72 in the placebo group. The positive effect on colon cancer is mitigated by the modest increase in cardiovascular and breast cancer risks associated with combined estrogen plus progestin therapy. Colorectal cancers diagnosed in women taking estrogen and progestin were in more advanced stage than those in women taking placebo.

A case-control study suggested that statins decrease the incidence of colorectal cancer. However, a meta-analysis of statin use showed no protective effect of statins on overall cancer incidence or death.

Chemoprevention of Breast Cancer Hormonal manipulation is being tested in the primary prevention of breast cancer. Tamoxifen is an antiestrogen with partial estrogen agonistic activity in some tissues, such as endometrium and bone. One of its actions is to upregulate transforming growth factor β, which decreases breast cell proliferation. In randomized placebo-controlled trials to assess tamoxifen as adjuvant therapy for breast cancer, tamoxifen reduced the number of new breast cancers in the opposite breast by more than a third. In a randomized placebo-controlled prevention trial involving >13,000 women at high risk, tamoxifen decreased the risk of developing breast cancer by 49% (from 43.4 to 22.0 per 1000 women) after a median follow-up of nearly 6 years. The International Breast Cancer Intervention Study (IBIS-I) trial had similar findings. In both studies tamoxifen also reduced bone fractures; a small increase in risk of endometrial cancer, stroke, pulmonary emboli, and deep vein thrombosis was noted. Tamoxifen has been approved by the U.S. Food and Drug Administration for reduction of breast cancer in women at high risk for the disease (1.66% risk at 5 years based on the Gail risk model: *http://www.nci.nih.gov/cancertopics/pdq/genetics/breast-and-ovarian/healthprofessional#Section_66*).

A trial comparing tamoxifen with another selective estrogen receptor modulator, raloxifene, showed that raloxifene is comparable to tamoxifen in cancer prevention. Raloxifene is associated with more noninvasive breast cancer than tamoxifen; the drugs are similar in risks of other cancers, fractures, ischemic heart disease, and stroke. Because the aromatase inhibitors are even more effective than tamoxifen in adjuvant breast cancer therapy, it is hoped that they also are more effective in breast cancer prevention. However, no data are available on this point.

Chemoprevention of Prostate Cancer Finasteride is a 5-α-reductase inhibitor. It inhibits conversion of testosterone to dihydrotestosterone

(DHT), a potent stimulator of prostate cell proliferation. The Prostate Cancer Prevention Trial randomly assigned men ≥55 years at average risk of prostate cancer to finasteride or placebo. After 7 years of therapy, the incidence of prostate cancer was 18.4% in the finasteride arm and 24.8% in the placebo arm, a statistically significant difference. However, the finasteride group had more patients with tumors of Gleason score 7 and higher compared to the placebo arm (6.4% vs 5.1%). The clinical significance of this finding, if any, is unknown.

Selenium is being tested as a prostate cancer preventive based on laboratory studies, epidemiologic data, and a small randomized skin cancer prevention trial that showed a significantly decreased number of prostate cancers in men taking selenium. In the placebo group, 16 prostate cancers were diagnosed versus 4 in the treatment group among the 843 men who began the study with a serum prostate specific antigen level <4 ng/mL.

The ATBC study cited above showed in secondary analysis that the risk of prostate cancer was reduced 33% in men taking α-tocopherol (99 cases in those on the drug; 151 cases on placebo). A prospective randomized trial to assess these drugs is ongoing.

Vaccines and Cancer Prevention A number of infectious agents cause cancer. Hepatitis B and C are linked to liver cancer, some human papilloma virus (HPV) strains are linked to cervical and head and neck cancer, and *Helicobacter pylori* is associated with gastric cancer and lymphoma. Vaccines to protect against these agents may reduce the risk of their associated cancers.

The hepatitis B vaccine is effective in preventing hepatitis and hepatomas due to chronic hepatitis B infection. Public health officials are encouraging widespread administration of the hepatitis B vaccine, especially in Asia, where the disease is epidemic.

A four-valent HPV vaccine (Gardasil) is 100% effective at preventing infection with any of the four component strains (6, 11, 16, 18). The vaccine is recommended for girls and women ages 9–26 years. Reduction in these HPV types could prevent >70% of the cervical cancers worldwide.

SURGICAL PREVENTION OF CANCER

Some organs in some individuals are at such high risk of developing cancer that surgical removal of the organ at risk is recommended. Women with severe cervical dysplasia are treated with conization and occasionally even hysterectomy. Colectomy is used to prevent colon cancer in patients with familial polyposis or ulcerative colitis.

Prophylactic bilateral mastectomy is chosen for breast cancer prevention among women with genetic predisposition to breast cancer. In a prospective series of 139 women with *BRCA1* and *BRCA2* mutations, 76 chose to undergo prophylactic mastectomy and 63 chose close surveillance. At 3 years, no cases of breast cancer had been diagnosed in those opting for surgery, but eight in the surveillance group had developed breast cancer. A larger retrospective cohort study reported that prophylactic mastectomy could reduce risk of breast cancer by 90%. The effect of the procedure on mortality is unknown. Observational studies are prone to a variety of biases associated with the choice to undergo prophylactic surgery; thus, such studies can give an overestimate of the magnitude of benefit.

Surgery is also used to manage hormonal cancers. Orchiectomy is an effective method of androgen deprivation in prostate cancer, and oophorectomy is effective in hormone-dependent breast cancer.

CANCER SCREENING

Screening is a means of detecting disease early in asymptomatic individuals, with the goal of decreasing morbidity and mortality. While screening can potentially save lives and has been shown to do so in cervical, colon, and probably breast cancer, it is also subject to a number of biases that can suggest a benefit when actually there is none. Biases can even mask net harm. Early detection does not in itself confer benefit. To be of value, screening must detect disease earlier, and treatment of earlier disease must yield a better outcome than treatment at the onset of symptoms. Cause-specific mortality, rather than survival after diagnosis, is the preferred endpoint (see below).

Because screening is done on asymptomatic, healthy persons, it should offer substantial likelihood of benefit that outweighs harm. Screening tests and their appropriate use should be carefully evaluated before their use is widely encouraged in screening programs, as a matter of public policy.

Screening examinations, tests, or procedures are usually not diagnostic of cancer but instead indicate that a cancer may be present. The diagnosis is then made following a workup that includes a biopsy and pathologic confirmation.

A number of genes have been identified that predispose for a disease, and many more will be identified in the near future. Testing for these genes can define a high-risk population. The ability to predict the development of a particular cancer may some day present therapeutic options as well as ethical dilemmas. It may eventually allow for early intervention to prevent a cancer or limit its severity. People at high risk may be ideal candidates for chemoprevention and screening; however, efficacy of these interventions in the high-risk population should be investigated. Currently, persons at high risk for a particular cancer can engage in intensive screening. While this course is clinically prudent, it is not known if it saves lives in these populations.

The Accuracy of Screening A screening test's accuracy or ability to discriminate disease is described by four indices: sensitivity, specificity, positive predictive value, and negative predictive value (Table 78-2). *Sensitivity*, also called the true positive rate, is the proportion of persons with the disease testing positive in the screen (i.e., the ability of the test to detect disease when it is present). *Specificity*, or 1-false positive rate, is the proportion of persons who do not have the disease and test negative in the screening test (i.e., the ability of a test to correctly identify that the disease is not present). The *positive predictive value* is the proportion of persons that test positive who actually have the disease. Similarly, *negative predictive value* is the proportion testing negative who do not have the disease. The sensitivity and specificity of a test are relatively independent of the underlying prevalence (or risk) of the disease in the population screened, but the predictive values depend strongly on the prevalence of the disease.

Screening is most beneficial, efficient, and economical when the target disease is common in the population being screened. To be valuable, the screening test should have a high specificity; sensitivity need not be very high.

Potential Biases of Screening Tests The common biases of screening are lead time, length-biased sampling, and selection. These biases can

TABLE 78-2 ASSESSMENT OF THE VALUE OF A DIAGNOSTIC TEST[a]

	Condition Present	Condition Absent
Positive test	*a*	*b*
Negative test	*c*	*d*

a = true positive
b = false positive
c = false negative
d = true negative

Sensitivity	The proportion of persons with the condition who test positive: $a/(a + c)$
Specificity	The proportion of persons without the condition who test negative: $d/(b + d)$
Positive predictive value (PPV)	The proportion of persons with a positive test who have the condition: $a/(a + b)$
Negative predictive value	The proportion of persons with a negative test who do not have the condition: $d/(c + d)$

Prevalence, sensitivity, and specificity determine PPV

$$\text{PPV} = \frac{\text{prevalence} \times \text{sensitivity}}{(\text{prevalence} \times \text{sensitivity}) + (1 - \text{prevalence})(1 - \text{specificity})}$$

[a]For diseases of low prevalence, such as cancer, poor specificity has a dramatic adverse effect on PPV such that only a small fraction of positive tests are true positives.

TABLE 78-3 SCREENING RECOMMENDATIONS FOR ASYMPTOMATIC NORMAL-RISK SUBJECTS[a]

Test or Procedure	USPSTF	ACS	CTFPHC
Sigmoidoscopy	Fair evidence to recommend	≥50, every 5 years	Fair evidence to consider
Fecal occult blood testing	≥50, good evidence for every 1–2 years	≥50, every year	Good evidence, age ≥50
Colonoscopy	No direct evidence	≥50, every 10 years	No direct evidence
Digital rectal examination	No recommendation	No recommendation	No recommendation
Prostate-specific antigen	Insufficient evidence to recommend	M: ≥50, every year	Recommendation against
Pap test	F: 18–65, every 1–3 years	F: with uterine cervix, beginning 3 years after first intercourse or by age 21. Yearly for standard Pap; every 2 years with liquid test.	Fair evidence to include in examination of sexually active women
Pelvic examination	No recommendation, advise adnexal palpation during exam for other reasons	F: 18–40, every 1–3 years with Pap test; >40, every year	Not considered
Breast self-examination	No recommendation	≥20, monthly	Fair evidence to exclude
Breast clinical examination	Insufficient evidence as a stand-alone without mammography	F: 20–40, every 3 years; >40, yearly	F: 50–69, every 1–2 years
Mammography	F: 40–75, every 1–2 years (fair evidence)	F: ≥40, every year	F: 50–69, every 1–2 years
Complete skin examination	Insufficient evidence for or against	Periodic exam	Poor evidence to include or exclude

[a]Summary of the screening procedures recommended for the general population by U.S. Preventive Services Task Force (USPSTF), the American Cancer Society (ACS), and the Canadian Task Force on Prevention Health Care (CTFPHC). These recommendations refer to asymptomatic persons who have no risk factors, other than age or gender, for the targeted condition.

Note: F, female; M, male.

make a screening test seem beneficial when actually it is not (or even causes net harm). Whether beneficial or not, screening can create the false impression of an epidemic by increasing the number of cancers diagnosed. It can also produce a shift in proportion of patients diagnosed at an early stage that improves survival statistics without reducing mortality (i.e., the number of deaths from a given cancer relative to the number of those at risk for the cancer). In such a case, the *apparent* duration of survival (measured from date of diagnosis) increases without lives being saved or life expectancy changed.

Lead-time bias occurs when a test does not influence the natural history of the disease; the patient is merely diagnosed at an earlier date. When lead-time bias occurs, survival *appears* increased, but life is not really prolonged. The screening test only prolongs the time the subject is aware of the disease and spends as a patient.

Length-biased sampling occurs when slow-growing, less aggressive cancers are detected during screening. Cancers diagnosed due to the onset of symptoms between scheduled screenings are on average more aggressive, and treatment outcomes are not as favorable. An extreme form of length bias sampling is termed *overdiagnosis*, the detection of "pseudo disease." The reservoir of some undetected slow-growing tumors is large. Many of these tumors fulfill the histologic criteria of cancer but will never become clinically significant or cause death. This problem is compounded by the fact that the most common cancers appear most frequently at ages when competing causes of death are more frequent.

Selection bias must be considered in assessing the results of any screening effort. The population most likely to seek screening may differ from the general population to which the screening test might be applied. The individuals screened may have volunteered because of a particular risk factor not found in the general population, such as a strong family history. In general, volunteers for studies are more health conscious and likely to have a better prognosis or lower mortality rate, irrespective of the screening result. This is termed the *healthy volunteer effect.*

Potential Drawbacks of Screening Risks associated with screening include harm caused by the screening intervention itself, harm due to the further investigation of persons with positive tests (both true and false positives), and harm from the treatment of persons with a true-positive result, even if life is extended by treatment. The diagnosis and treatment of cancers that would never have caused medical problems can lead to the harm of unnecessary treatment and give patients the anxiety of a cancer diagnosis. The psychosocial impact of cancer screening can also be substantial when applied to the entire population.

Assessment of Screening Tests Good clinical trial design can offset some biases of screening and demonstrate the relative risks and benefits of a screening test. A randomized, controlled screening trial with cause-specific mortality as the endpoint provides the strongest support for a screening intervention. Overall survival should also be reported to detect an adverse effect of screening and treatment on other disease outcomes (e.g., cardiovascular disease). In a randomized trial, two like populations are randomly established. One is given the medical standard of care (which may be no screening at all) and the other receives the screening intervention being assessed. The two populations are compared over time. Efficacy for the population studied is established when the group receiving the screening test has a better cause-specific mortality rate than the control group. Studies showing a reduction in the incidence of advanced-stage disease, an improved survival, or a stage shift are weaker (and possibly misleading) evidence of benefit. These latter criteria are necessary but not sufficient to establish the value of a screening test.

Although a randomized, controlled screening trial provides the strongest evidence to support a screening test, it is not perfect. Unless the trial is population-based, it does not remove the question of generalizability to the target population. Screening trials generally involve thousands of persons and last for years. Less definitive study designs are therefore often used to estimate the effectiveness of screening practices. After a randomized controlled clinical trial, in descending order of strength, evidence may be derived from the findings of internally controlled trials using intervention allocation methods other than randomization (e.g., allocation by birth date, date of clinic visit); the findings of cohort or case-control analytic observational studies; the results of multiple time series study with or without the intervention; the opinions of respected authorities based on clinical experience, descriptive studies, or consensus reports of experts (the weakest form of evidence because even experts can be misled by biases).

Screening for Specific Cancers Widespread screening for cervical, colon, and likely breast cancer is beneficial for certain age groups. A number of organizations have considered whether or not to endorse routine use of certain screening tests. Because these groups have not used the same criteria to judge whether a screening test should be endorsed, they have arrived at different recommendations. The U.S. Preventive Services Task Force (USPSTF), the Canadian Task Force on Preventive Health Care, and the American Cancer Society (ACS) publish screening guidelines (Table 78-3). Special surveillance of those at high risk for a specific cancer because of a family history or a genetic risk factor may be prudent, but few studies have assessed the influence on mortality.

BREAST CANCER Breast self-examination, clinical breast examination by a care giver, and mammography have been advocated as useful screening tools. Only screening mammography alone and screening mammography with clinical examination have been evaluated in randomized controlled trials. MRI is being assessed and is more accurate than mammography in women at high risk due to genetic predisposition or in women with very dense breast tissue.

A number of trials have suggested that annual or biennial screening with mammography or mammography plus clinical breast examination in normal-risk women over the age of 50 decreases breast cancer mortality. Each trial has been criticized for design flaws. In most trials, breast cancer mortality rate is decreased by 20–30%. Experts disagree on whether average-risk women age 40–49 should receive regular screening (Table 78-3). The significance of the screening effect in women aged 40–49 depends on the statistical test used. An analysis of eight large randomized trials showed no benefit from mammography screening for women aged 40–49 when assessed 5–7 years after trial entry. However, a small benefit emerged 10–12 years after study entry. What proportion of this benefit is due to screening after these women turned 50 is not known. In randomized screening studies of women aged 50–69, the mortality decline begins about 5 years after initiation of screening. Nearly half of women aged 40–49 screened annually will have false-positive mammograms necessitating further evaluation, often including biopsy. The risk of false-positive testing should be discussed with the patient.

No study of breast self-examination has shown it to decrease mortality; however, it is recommended as prudent by many organizations. A substantial fraction of breast cancers are first detected by patients. Self-examination leads to increased biopsy rate without reducing breast cancer mortality.

Genetic screening for *BRCA1* and *BRCA2* mutations and other markers of breast cancer risk has identified a group of women at high risk for breast cancer. Unfortunately when to begin and the optimal frequency of screening have not been defined. Mammography is less sensitive at detecting breast cancers in women carrying *BRCA1* and *-2* mutations, possibly because such cancers occur in younger women, in whom mammography is known to be less sensitive. MRI screening may be more effective.

CERVICAL CANCER Screening with Papanicolaou smears decreases cervical cancer mortality. The cervical cancer mortality rate has fallen substantially since the widespread use of the Pap smear. Most screening guidelines recommend regular Pap testing for all women who are or have been sexually active for 3 years or have reached the age of 21. With the onset of sexual activity comes the risk of sexual transmission of HPV, the most common etiologic factor for cervical cancer. The recommended interval for Pap screening varies from 1–3 years. At age 30, women who have had three normal test results in a row may get screened every 2–3 years. An upper age limit at which screening ceases to be effective is not known, but women ≥70 years with no abnormal results in the previous 10 years may choose to stop screening.

COLORECTAL CANCER Fecal occult blood testing (FOBT), digital rectal examination (DRE), rigid and flexible sigmoidoscopy, radiographic barium contrast studies, and colonoscopy have been considered for colorectal cancer screening. Annual FOBT could reduce colorectal cancer mortality by a third. The sensitivity for fecal occult blood is increased if specimens are re-hydrated before testing, but at the cost of lower specificity. The false-positive rate for rehydrated FOBT is high; 1–5% of persons tested have a positive test. Only 2–10% of those with occult blood in the stool have cancer and 20–30% have adenomas. The high false-positive rate of FOBT dramatically increases the number of colonoscopies performed.

Two case-control studies suggest that regular screening of those >50 years with sigmoidoscopy decreases mortality. This type of study is prone to selection biases. A quarter to a third of polyps can be discovered with the rigid sigmoidoscope; half are found with a 35-cm flexible scope and two-thirds to three-quarters are found with a 60-cm scope. Diagnosis of adenomatous polyps by sigmoidoscopy should lead to evaluation of the entire colon with colonoscopy and/or barium enema. The most efficient interval for screening sigmoidoscopy is unknown, but 5 years is often recommended. Case-control studies suggest that intervals of up to 15 years may confer benefit.

One-time colonoscopy detects ~25% more advanced lesions (polyps > 10 mm, villous adenomas, adenomatous polyps with high-grade dysplasia, invasive cancer) than one-time FOBT with sigmoidoscopy. Colonoscopy is well suited to screening subjects at high risk, such as those with ulcerative colitis or family predisposition. Perforation rates are 3/1000 for colonoscopy and 1/1000 for sigmoidoscopy. Debate continues on whether colonoscopy is too expensive and invasive for widespread use as a screening tool in standard-risk populations. DRE and barium enema are both insensitive as screening tools.

LUNG CANCER Chest x-ray and sputum cytology have been evaluated in randomized lung cancer screening trials. No reduction in lung cancer mortality has been seen, although all the controlled trials have had low statistical power. Even screening of high-risk subjects (smokers) has not proven beneficial. Spiral CT can diagnose lung cancers at early stages; however, false-positive rates are high. Spiral CT screening increases the number of lesions detected and increases the number of diagnostic and therapeutic procedures. However, its capacity to save lives is unproven.

OVARIAN CANCER Adnexal palpation, transvaginal ultrasound, and serum CA-125 assay have been considered for ovarian cancer screening. These tests alone and in combination do not have sufficiently high sensitivity or specificity to be recommended for routine screening of ovarian cancer. The risks and costs associated with the high number of false-positive results is an impediment to routine use of these modalities for screening. Most expert panels have concluded that routine screening for ovarian cancer is not indicated for standard-risk women or those with single affected family members, but might be worthwhile in families with genetic ovarian cancer syndromes.

PROSTATE CANCER The most common prostate cancer screening modalities are DRE and serum prostate-specific antigen (PSA) assay. Newer serum tests, such as measurement of bound to free serum PSA, have yet to be fully evaluated. An emphasis on PSA screening has caused prostate cancer to become the most common non-skin cancer diagnosed in American males. This disease is prone to lead-time bias, length bias, and overdiagnosis, and substantial debate rages among experts as to whether it is effective. Some experts are concerned that prostate cancer screening, more than screening for other cancers, may cause net harm. Prostate cancer screening clearly detects many asymptomatic cancers, but the ability to distinguish tumors that are lethal but still curable from those that pose little or no threat to health is limited. Men over age 50 have a high prevalence of indolent, clinically insignificant prostate cancers. No trial has yet demonstrated the benefit of prostate cancer screening and treatment.

The placebo arm of the Prostate Cancer Prevention Trial showed that rigorous screening of low-risk men for 7 years leads to the diagnosis of prostate cancer in >12% of patients. In addition, 15% of men who had normal DRE and PSA levels after 7 years were found to have prostate cancer on biopsy despite the normal screening tests. Thus, screening missed more disease than it found and >27% of normal-risk men in their late 60s were found to have prostate cancer.

The effectiveness of treatments for low-stage prostate cancer are under study. However, both surgery and radiation therapy may cause significant morbidity, such as impotence and urinary incontinence. Comparison of radical prostatectomy to "watchful waiting" in clinically diagnosed (not screen-detected) prostate cancers showed a small decrease in prostate cancer death rate in the surgery arm. One life was saved for every 18–20 men treated with radical prostatectomy. Urinary incontinence and sexual impotence were more common in the surgery arm. One current screening recommendation is that men over age 50 be offered screening and allowed to make a choice after being informed of potential risks and benefits (Table 78-3). A man should have a life expectancy of at least 10 years to be eligible for screening. The USPSTF has found insufficient evidence to recommend prostate cancer screening.

ENDOMETRIAL CANCER Transvaginal ultrasound and endometrial sampling have been advocated as screening tests for endometrial cancer. Benefit from routine screening has not been shown. Transvaginal ultrasound and endometrial sampling are indicated for workup of vaginal bleeding in postmenopausal women but are not considered as screening tests in symptomatic women.

SKIN CANCER Visual examination of all skin surfaces by the patient or by a health care provider is used in screening for basal and squamous cell cancers and melanoma. No prospective randomized study has been performed to look for a mortality decrease. Observational epidemiologic evidence from Scotland and Australia suggests that screening programs have caused a stage shift in melanomas diagnosed. Screening may reinforce sun avoidance and other skin cancer prevention behaviors.

FURTHER READINGS

BACH PB et al: Computed tomography screening and lung cancer outcomes. JAMA 297:953, 2007

BARRETT-CONNOR E et al: Effects of raloxifene on cardiovascular events and breast cancer in postmenopausal women. N Engl J Med 355:125, 2006

FISHER B et al: Tamoxifen for prevention of breast cancer: report of the National Surgical Adjuvant Breast and Bowel Project P-1 Study. J Natl Cancer Inst 90:1371, 1998

FREEDLAND SJ, PARTIN AW: Prostate-specific antigen: Update 2006. Urology 67:458, 2006

HUMPHREY LL et al: Breast cancer screening: A summary of the evidence for the U.S. Preventive Services Task Force. Ann Intern Med 137:347, 2002

PRENTICE RL et al: Low-fat dietary pattern and risk of invasive breast cancer. The Women's Health Initiative randomized controlled dietary modification trial. JAMA 295:629, 2006

WINAWER SJ et al: Guidelines for colonoscopy surveillance after polypectomy: A consensus update by the Multi-Society Task Force on Colorectal Cancer and the American Cancer Society. Gastroenterology 130:1872, 2006

WEBSITES

The Canadian Taskforce on Preventive Health Care
http://www.ctfphc.org/
The National Cancer Institute Cancernet
http://cancernet.nci.nih.gov/

79 Cancer Genetics

Pat J. Morin, Jeffrey M. Trent, Francis S. Collins, Bert Vogelstein

CANCER IS A GENETIC DISEASE

Cancer arises through a series of somatic alterations in DNA that result in unrestrained cellular proliferation. Most of these alterations involve actual sequence changes in DNA (i.e., mutations). They may arise as a consequence of random replication errors, exposure to carcinogens (e.g., radiation), or faulty DNA repair processes. While most cancers arise sporadically, familial clustering of cancers occurs in certain families that carry a germline mutation in a cancer gene.

HISTORICAL PERSPECTIVE

The idea that cancer progression is driven by sequential somatic mutations in specific genes has only gained general acceptance in the past 25 years. Before the advent of the microscope, cancer was believed to be composed of aggregates of mucus or other noncellular matter. By the middle of the nineteenth century, it became clear that tumors were masses of cells and that these cells arose from the normal cells of the tissue in which the cancer originated. However, the molecular basis for the uncontrolled proliferation of cancer cells was to remain a mystery for another century. During that time, a number of theories for the origin of cancer were postulated. The great biochemist Otto Warburg proposed the combustion theory of cancer, which stipulated that cancer was due to abnormal oxygen metabolism: while normal cells required oxygen, cancer cells could survive in its absence. In addition, some believed that all cancers were caused by viruses, and that cancer was in fact a contagious disease.

In the end, observations of cancer occurring in chimney sweeps, studies of x-rays, and the overwhelming data demonstrating cigarette smoke as a causative agent in lung cancer, together with Ames's work on chemical mutagenesis, were sufficient to convince many that cancer originated through changes in DNA. Although the viral theory of cancer did not prove to be generally accurate, the study of retroviruses led to the discovery of the first human *oncogenes* in the mid to late 1970s. Soon after, the study of families with genetic predisposition to cancer was instrumental in the discovery of *tumor-suppressor genes*. The field that studies the type of mutations, as well as the consequence of these mutations in tumor cells, is now known as *cancer genetics*.

THE CLONAL ORIGIN AND MULTISTEP NATURE OF CANCER

Nearly all cancers originate from a single cell; this clonal origin is a critical discriminating feature between neoplasia and hyperplasia. Multiple cumulative mutational events are invariably required for the progression from normal to fully malignant phenotype. The process can be seen as Darwinian microevolution in which, at each successive step, the mutated cells gain a growth advantage resulting in an increased representation relative to their neighbors (Fig. 79-1). It is believed that five to ten accumulated mutations are necessary for a cell to progress from the normal to the fully malignant phenotype.

We are beginning to understand the precise nature of the genetic alterations responsible for some malignancies and to get a sense of the order in which they occur. The best studied example is colon cancer, in which analyses of DNA from tissues extending from normal colon epithelium through adenoma to carcinoma have identified some of the genes mutated in the process (Fig. 79-2). Similar progression models are being elucidated for other malignancies.

GENERAL CLASSES OF CANCER GENES

There are two major classes of cancer genes. The first class comprises genes that directly affect cell growth either positively (*oncogenes*) or

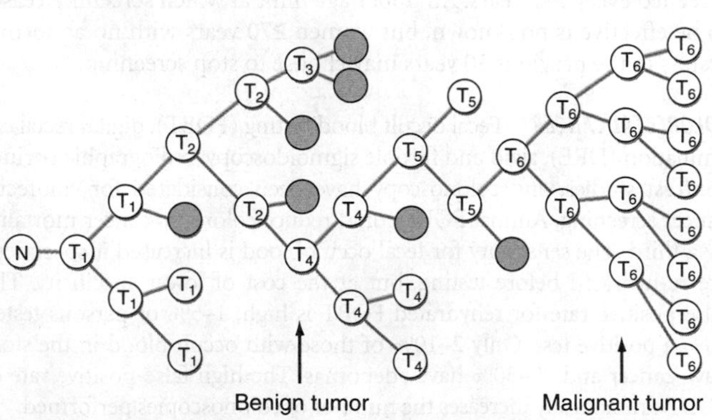

FIGURE 79-1 Multistep clonal development of malignancy. In this diagram a series of five cumulative mutations (T1, T2, T4, T5, T6), each with a modest growth advantage acting alone, eventually results in a malignant tumor. Note that not all such alterations result in progression; for example, the T3 clone is a dead end. The actual number of cumulative mutations necessary to transform from the normal to the malignant state is unknown in most tumors. (*After P Nowell, Science 194:23, 1976, with permission.*)

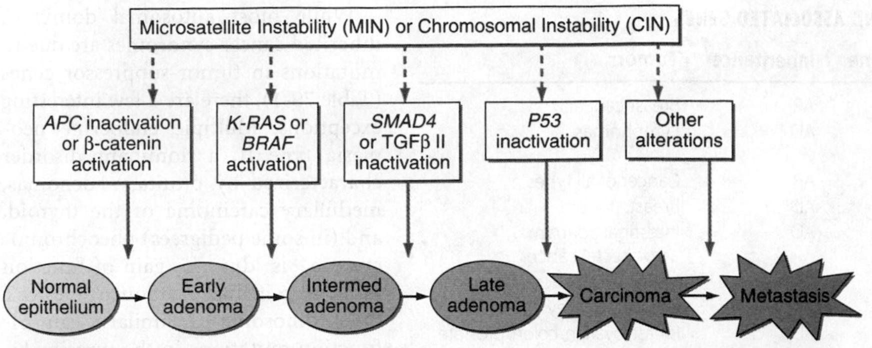

FIGURE 79-2 Progressive somatic mutational steps in the development of colon carcinoma. The accumulation of alterations in a number of different genes results in the progression from normal epithelium through adenoma to full-blown carcinoma. Genetic instability (microsatellite or chromosomal) accelerates the progression by increasing the likelihood of mutation at each step. Patients with familial polyposis are already one step into this pathway, since they inherit a germline alteration of the *APC* gene. TGF, transforming growth factor.

negatively (*tumor-suppressor genes*). These genes exert their effects on tumor growth through their ability to control cell division (cell birth) or cell death (apoptosis). Oncogenes are tightly regulated in normal cells. In cancer cells, oncogenes acquire mutations that relieve this control and lead to increased activity of the gene product. This mutational event typically occurs in a single allele of the oncogene and acts in a dominant fashion. In contrast, the normal function of tumor-suppressor genes is to restrain cell growth, and this function is lost in cancer. Because of the diploid nature of mammalian cells, both alleles must be inactivated to completely lose the function of a tumor-suppressor gene, leading to a recessive mechanism at the cellular level. From these ideas and studies on the inherited form of retinoblastoma, Knudson and others formulated the *two-hit hypothesis*, which in its modern version states that both copies of a tumor-suppressor gene must be inactivated in cancer.

The second class of cancer genes, the *caretakers*, does not directly affect cell growth but rather affects the ability of the cell to maintain the integrity of its genome. Cells with deficiency in these genes have an increased rate of mutations in all the genes, including oncogenes and tumor-suppressor genes. This "mutator" phenotype was first hypothesized by Loeb to explain how the multiple mutational events required for tumorigenesis can occur in the lifetime of an individual. A mutation phenotype has now been observed in cancer at both the nucleotide sequence and chromosomal levels.

MECHANISMS OF TUMOR-SUPPRESSOR INACTIVATION

The two major types of somatic lesions observed in tumor-suppressor genes during tumor development are *point mutations* and *large deletions.* Point mutations in the coding region of tumor-suppressor genes will frequently lead to truncated protein products or otherwise nonfunctional proteins. Similarly, deletions lead to the loss of a functional product and sometimes encompass the entire gene or even the entire chromosome arm, leading to loss of heterozygosity (LOH) in the tumor DNA compared to the corresponding normal tissue DNA (Fig. 79-3). LOH in tumor DNA is considered a hallmark for the presence of a tumor-suppressor gene at a particular locus, and LOH studies have been useful in the positional cloning of many tumor-suppressor genes. Gene silencing, which occurs in conjunction with hypermethylation of the promoter, is another mechanism of tumor-suppressor gene inactivation. Silencing is an epigenetic change rather than a sequence alteration.

FAMILIAL CANCER SYNDROMES

A small fraction of cancers occur in patients with a genetic predisposition. In these families, the affected individuals have a predisposing loss-of-function mutation in one allele of a tumor-suppressor gene or caretaker gene. The tumors in these patients show a loss of the remaining normal allele as a result of somatic events (point mutations or deletions), in agreement with the Knudson hypothesis (Fig. 79-3). Thus, most cells of an individual with an inherited loss-of-function mutation in a tumor-suppressor gene are functionally normal, and only the rare cells that develop a mutation in the remaining normal allele will exhibit uncontrolled growth. The normal function of tumor suppressors is to restrain growth, to promote differentiation (gatekeeper genes), or to preserve genome integrity (caretaker genes).

Roughly 100 syndromes of familial cancer have been reported, although many are rare. The majority are inherited as autosomal dominant traits, although some of those associated with DNA repair abnormalities (xeroderma pigmentosum, Fanconi's anemia, ataxia telangiectasia) are autosomal recessive. Table 79-1 shows a number of cancer predisposition syndromes and the responsible genes. The current paradigm states that the genes mutated in familial syndromes can also be targets for somatic mutations in sporadic (noninherited) tumors. The study of cancer syndromes has thus provided invaluable insights into the mechanisms of progression for many tumor types. This section examines the case of inherited colon cancer in detail, but the same general lessons can be applied to all the cancer syndromes listed in Table 79-1.

Familial adenomatous polyposis (FAP) is a dominantly inherited colon cancer syndrome due to germline mutations in the adenomatous polyposis coli (*APC*) tumor-suppressor gene on chromosome 5. Patients with this syndrome develop hundreds to thousands of adenomas in the colon. Each of these adenomas has lost the normal remaining allele of *APC* but has not yet accumulated the required additional mutations to generate fully malignant cells (Fig. 79-2). However, out of these thousands of benign adenomas, several will invariably acquire further abnormalities and a subset will even develop into fully malignant cancers. *APC* is thus considered to be a gatekeeper for colon tumorigenesis; Fig. 79-4 shows germline and somatic mutations found

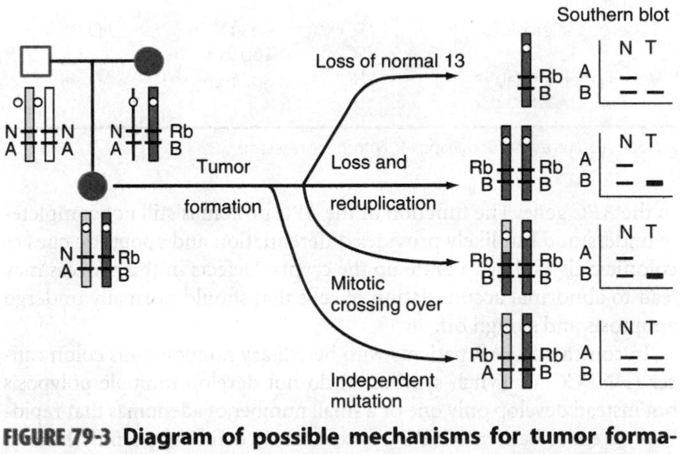

FIGURE 79-3 Diagram of possible mechanisms for tumor formation in an individual with hereditary (familial) retinoblastoma. On the left is shown the pedigree of an affected individual who has inherited the abnormal (Rb) allele from her affected mother. The four chromosomes of her two parents are drawn to indicate their origin. Just below the retinoblastoma locus a polymorphic marker is also analyzed in this family. The patient is AB at this locus, like her mother, whereas her father is AA. Thus the B allele must be on the chromosome carrying the retinoblastoma disease gene. Tumor formation results when the normal allele (N), which this patient inherited from her father, is inactivated. On the right are shown four possible ways in which this could occur. In each case, the resulting chromosome 13 arrangement is shown, as well as the results of a Southern blot comparing normal tissue with tumor tissue. Note that in the first three situations the normal allele (A) has been lost in the tumor tissue, which is referred to as loss of heterozygosity (LOH). (*From TD Gelehrter and FS Collins, in Principles of Medical Genetics, Baltimore, Williams and Wilkins, 1990, with permission.*)

TABLE 79-1 CANCER PREDISPOSITION SYNDROMES AND ASSOCIATED GENES

Syndrome	Gene	Chromosome	Inheritance	Tumors
Ataxia telangiectasia	*ATM*	11q22-q23	AR	Breast cancer
Autoimmune lymphoproliferative syndrome	*FAS* *FASL*	10q24 1q23	AD	Lymphomas
Bloom syndrome	*BLM*	15q26.1	AR	Cancer of all types
Cowden syndrome	*PTEN*	10q23	AD	Breast, thyroid
Familial adenomatous polyposis	*APC*	5q21	AD	Intestinal adenoma, colorectal cancer
Familial melanoma	*p16INK4*	9p21	AD	Melanoma, pancreatic cancer
Familial Wilms tumor	*WT1*	11p13	AD	Pediatric kidney cancer
Hereditary breast/ovarian cancer	*BRCA1* *BRCA2*	17q21 13q12.3	AD	Breast, ovarian, colon, prostate
Hereditary diffuse gastric cancer	*CDH1*	16q22	AD	Stomach cancers
Hereditary multiple exostoses	*EXT1* *EXT2*	8q24 11p11-12	AD	Exostoses, chondrosarcoma
Hereditary prostate cancer	*HPC1*	1q24-25	AD	Prostate carcinoma
Hereditary retinoblastoma	*RB1*	13q14.2	AD	Retinoblastoma, osteosarcoma
Hereditary nonpolyposis colon cancer (HNPCC)	*MSH2* *MLH1* *MSH6* *PMS2*	2p16 3p21.3 2p16 7p22	AD	Colon, endometrial, ovarian, stomach, small bowel, ureter carcinoma
Hereditary papillary renal carcinoma	*MET*	7q31	AD	Papillary renal tumor
Juvenile polyposis	*SMAD4*	18q21	AD	Gastrointestinal, pancreatic cancers
Li-Fraumeni	*TP53*	17p13.1	AD	Sarcoma, breast cancer
Multiple endocrine neoplasia type 1	*MEN1*	11q13	AD	Parathyroid, endocrine, pancreas, and pituitary
Multiple endocrine neoplasia type 2a	*RET*	10q11.2	AD	Medullary thyroid carcinoma, pheochromocytoma
Neurofibromatosis type 1	*NF1*	17q11.2	AD	Neurofibroma, neurofibrosarcoma, brain tumor
Neurofibromatosis type 2	*NF2*	22q12.2	AD	Vestibular schwannoma, meningioma, spine
Nevoid basal cell carcinoma syndrome (Gorlin's syndrome)	*PTCH*	9q22.3	AD	Basal cell carcinoma, medulloblastoma, jaw cysts
Tuberous sclerosis	*TSC1* *TSC2*	9q34 16p13.3	AD	Angiofibroma, renal angiomyolipoma
Von Hippel–Lindau	*VHL*	3p25-26	AD	Kidney, cerebellum, pheochromocytoma

Note: AD, autosomal dominant; AR, autosomal recessive.

in the *APC* gene. The function of the APC protein is still not completely understood but likely provides differentiation and apoptotic cues to colonic cells as they migrate up the crypts. Defects in this process may lead to abnormal accumulation of cells that should normally undergo apoptosis and slough off.

In contrast to FAP, patients with hereditary nonpolyposis colon cancer (HNPCC, or Lynch syndrome) do not develop multiple polyposis but instead develop only one or a small number of adenomas that rapidly progress to cancer. HNPCC is commonly defined by family history, with at least three individuals over at least two generations developing colon or endometrial cancer, and with at least one individual diagnosed before the age of 50. Most HNPCC is due to mutations in one of four DNA mismatch repair genes (Table 79-1), which are components of a repair system that is normally responsible for correcting errors in freshly replicated DNA. Germline mutations in *MSH2* and *MLH1* account for >60% of HNPCC cases, while mutations in *MSH6* and *PMS2* are much less frequent. When a somatic mutation inactivates the remaining wild-type allele of a mismatch repair gene, the cell develops a hypermutable phenotype characterized by profound genomic instability, especially for the short repeated sequences called *microsatellites*. This microsatellite instability (MIN) favors the development of cancer by increasing the rate of mutations in many genes, including oncogenes and tumor-suppressor genes (Fig. 79-2). These genes can thus be considered caretakers. Figure 79-5 shows an example of the instability in allele sizes for dinucleotide repeats in the cancers of HNPCC patients.

While most autosomal dominant inherited cancer syndromes are due to mutations in tumor-suppressor genes (Table 79-1), there are a few interesting exceptions. Multiple endocrine neoplasia type II, a dominant disorder characterized by pituitary adenomas, medullary carcinoma of the thyroid, and (in some pedigrees) pheochromocytoma, is due to gain-of-function mutations in the protooncogene *RET* on chromosome 10. Similarly, gain-of-function mutations in the tyrosine kinase domain of the *MET* oncogene lead to hereditary papillary renal carcinoma. Interestingly, loss-of-function mutations in the *RET* gene cause a completely different disease, Hirschsprung's disease [aganglionic megacolon (Chaps. 291 and 345)].

Although the Mendelian forms of cancer have taught us much about the mechanisms of growth control, most forms of cancer do not follow simple patterns of inheritance. In many instances (e.g., lung cancer), a strong environmental contribution is at work. Even in such circumstances, however, some individuals may be more genetically susceptible to developing cancer, given the appropriate exposure, due to the presence of modifier alleles.

GENETIC TESTING FOR FAMILIAL CANCER

The discovery of cancer susceptibility genes raises the possibility of DNA testing to predict the risk of cancer in individuals of affected families. An algorithm for cancer risk assessment and decision-making in high-risk families using genetic testing is shown in Fig. 79-6. Once a mutation is discovered in a family, subsequent testing of asymptomatic family members can be crucial in patient management. A negative gene test in these individuals can prevent years of anxiety in the knowledge that their cancer risk is no higher than that of the general population. On the other hand, a positive test may lead to alteration of clinical management, such as increased frequency of cancer screening and, when feasible and appropriate, prophylactic surgery. Potential negative consequences of a positive test result include psychological distress (anxiety, depression) and discrimination (insurance, employment). Testing should therefore not be conducted without counseling before and after disclosure of the test result. In addition, the decision to test should depend on whether effective interventions exist for the particular type of cancer to be tested. Despite these caveats, genetic cancer testing for some cancer syndromes already appears to have greater benefits than risks, and many companies now offer testing for various genes associated with the predisposition to breast cancer (*BRCA1* and *BRCA2*), melanoma (*p16INK4*), and colon cancer (*APC* and the HNPCC genes).

Because of the inherent problems of genetic testing such as cost, specificity, and sensitivity, it is not yet appropriate to offer these tests to the general population. However, testing may be appropriate in some subpopulations with a known increased risk, even without a defined family history. For example, two mutations in the breast cancer susceptibility gene *BRCA1*, 185delAG and 5382insC, exhibit a sufficiently high frequency in the Ashkenazi Jewish population that genetic testing of an individual of this ethnic group may be warranted.

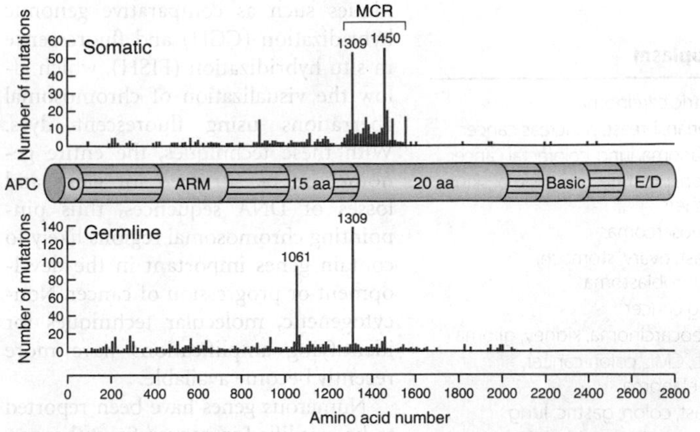

FIGURE 79-4 Germline and somatic mutations in the tumor-suppressor gene *APC*. *APC* encodes a 2843-amino-acid protein with 6 major domains: an oligomerization region (O), armadillo repeats (ARM), 15-amino-acid repeats (15 AA), 20-amino-acid repeats (20 AA), a basic region, and a domain involved in binding EB1 and the *Drosophila* discs large homologue (E/D). Shown are the positions within the *APC* gene of a total of 650 somatic and 826 germline mutations (from the APC database at *http://p53.free.fr*). The vast majority of these mutations result in the truncation of the APC protein. Germline mutations are found to be relatively evenly distributed up to codon 1600 except for 2 mutation hotspots at amino acids 1061 and 1309, which together account for one-third of the mutations found in familial adenomatous polyposis (FAP) families. Somatic *APC* mutations in colon tumors cluster in an area of the gene known as the *mutation cluster region* (MCR). The location of the MCR suggests that the 20-amino-acid domain plays a crucial role in tumor suppression. Note that loss of the second functional *APC* allele in tumors from FAP families often occurs through loss of heterozygosity.

It is important that genetic test results be communicated to families by trained genetic counselors. To ensure that the families clearly understand its advantages and disadvantages and the impact it may have on their management and psyche, genetic testing should never be done before counseling. Significant expertise is needed to communicate the results of genetic testing to families. For example, one common mistake is to misinterpret the result of negative genetic tests. For many cancer predisposition genes, the sensitivity of genetic testing is only ≤70% (i.e., of 100 kindreds tested, disease-causing mutations can be identified in only 70). Therefore, such testing should in general begin with an affected member of the kindred (the youngest family member still alive who has had the cancer of interest). If a mutation is not identified in this individual, then the test should be reported as noninformative (Fig. 79-6) rather than negative (because it is possible that the mutation in this individual is not detectable by standard genetic assays for purely technical reasons). On the other hand, if a mutation can be identified in this individual, then testing of other family members can be performed, and the sensitivity of such subsequent tests will be 100% (because the mutation in the family is in this case known to be detectable by the assay methods used).

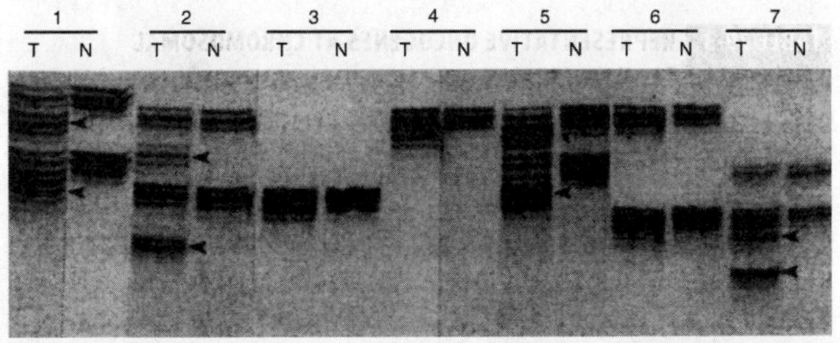

FIGURE 79-5 Demonstration of microsatellite instability in normal and tumor tissue from hereditary nonpolyposis colon cancer (HNPCC) patients. In each case the lane marked T contains DNA from a tumor, and the lane marked N contains DNA from normal tissue of the same patient. The marker (*D2S123*, located on chromosome 2) is a microsatellite composed of a tandem repeat of the dinucleotide CA, which varies in length from chromosome to chromosome. Normally, however, the length of the repeat is stable in somatic tissues. In this example, a polymerase chain reaction analysis has been applied to genomic DNA, and new alleles for the marker are apparent in tumors 1, 2, 5, and 7. Because the tumor tissue is defective in DNA mismatch repair, clonal abnormalities in copying of the CA repeat have arisen. Errors are also occurring in functional genes, eventually resulting in the malignant phenotype. (*From LA Aaltonen et al, Clues to the pathogenesis of familial colorectal cancer. Science 260:812, 1993, with permission; Copyright 1993 AAAS.*)

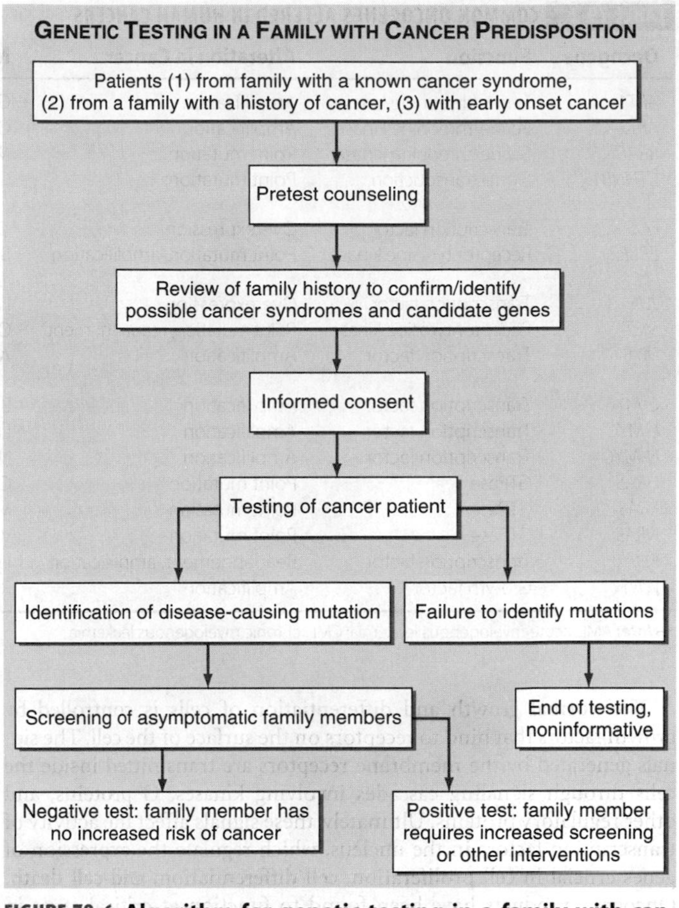

FIGURE 79-6 Algorithm for genetic testing in a family with cancer predisposition. The key step is the identification of a mutation in a cancer patient, which allows testing of asymptomatic family members. Asymptomatic family members who test positive may require increased screening or surgery, whereas others are at no greater risk for cancer than the general population.

ONCOGENES IN HUMAN CANCER

Oncogenes of the kind found in human cancers were initially discovered through their presence in the genome of retroviruses capable of causing cancers in chickens, mice, and rats. The cellular homologues of these viral genes are often targets of mutation or aberrant regulation in human cancer. Whereas many oncogenes were discovered because of their presence in retroviruses, other oncogenes, particularly those involved in translocations characteristic of particular leukemias and lymphomas, were isolated through genomic approaches. Investigators cloned the sequences surrounding the chromosomal translocations observed cytogenetically and then deduced the nature of the genes that were the targets of these translocations (see below). Some of these were oncogenes known from retroviruses [like *ABL*, involved in chronic myelogenous leukemia (CML)], while others were new (like *BCL2*, involved in B cell lymphoma). In the normal cellular environment, protooncogenes have crucial roles in cell proliferation and differentiation. Table 79-2 is a partial list of oncogenes known to be involved in human cancer.

TABLE 79-2 COMMON ONCOGENES ALTERED IN HUMAN CANCERS

Oncogene	Function	Alteration in Cancer	Neoplasm
AKT1	Serine/threonine kinase	Amplification	Gastric carcinoma
AKT2	Serine/threonine kinase	Amplification	Ovarian, breast, pancreas cancer
BRAF	Serine/threonine kinase	Point mutation	Melanoma, lung, colorectal cancer
CTNNB1	Signal transduction	Point mutation	Colon, prostate, melanoma, skin, others
FOS	Transcription factor	Overexpression	Osteosarcomas
ERBB2	Receptor tyrosine kinase	Point mutation, amplification	Breast, ovary, stomach, neuroblastoma
JUN	Transcription factor	Overexpression	Lung cancer
MET	Receptor tyrosine kinase	Point mutation, rearrangement	Osteocarcinoma, kidney, glioma
MYB	Transcription factor	Amplification	AML, CML, colon cancer, melanoma
C-MYC	Transcription factor	Amplification	Breast, colon, gastric, lung
L-MYC	Transcription factor	Amplification	Lung carcinoma, bladder
N-MYC	Transcription factor	Amplification	Neuroblastoma, lung cancer
HRAS	GTPase	Point mutation	Colon, lung, pancreas
KRAS	GTPase	Point mutation	Melanoma, colorectal cancer, AML
NRAS	GTPase	Point mutation	Various carcinomas, melanoma
REL	Transcription factor	Rearrangement, amplification	Lymphomas
WNT1	Growth factor	Amplification	Retinoblastoma

Note: AML, acute myelogenous leukemia; CML, chronic myelogenous leukemia.

The normal growth and differentiation of cells is controlled by growth factors that bind to receptors on the surface of the cell. The signals generated by the membrane receptors are transmitted inside the cells through signaling cascades involving kinases, G proteins, and other regulatory proteins. Ultimately, these signals affect the activity of transcription factors in the nucleus, which regulate the expression of genes crucial in cell proliferation, cell differentiation, and cell death. Oncogene products have been found to function at critical steps in these pathways (Chap. 80), and inappropriate activation of these pathways can lead to tumorigenesis.

MECHANISMS OF ONCOGENE ACTIVATION

Mechanisms that upregulate (or activate) cellular oncogenes fall into three broad categories: point mutation, DNA amplification, and chromosomal rearrangement.

Point Mutation Point mutation is a common mechanism of oncogene activation. For example, mutations in one of the *RAS* genes (*HRAS*, *KRAS*, or *NRAS*) are present in up to 85% of pancreatic cancers and 50% of colon cancers but are relatively uncommon in other cancer types. Remarkably—and in contrast to the diversity of mutations found in tumor-suppressor genes (Fig. 79-4)—most of the activated *RAS* genes contain point mutations in codons 12, 13, or 61 (which convey resistance to GAP, a protein that interacts with RAS and inactivates it through substitution of the GTP cofactor with GDP). The restricted pattern of mutation compared to tumor-suppressor genes reflects the fact that gain-of-function mutations of oncogenes are more difficult to attain than simple inactivation. Indeed, inactivation of a gene can be attained through the introduction of a stop codon anywhere in the coding sequence, whereas activations require precise substitutions at residues that normally downregulate the activity of the encoded protein. The specificity of oncogene mutations provides specific diagnostic opportunities, as it is much simpler to find mutations at specified positions than it is when mutations can be scattered throughout the gene (as in tumor-suppressor genes).

DNA Amplification The second mechanism for activation of oncogenes is DNA sequence amplification, leading to overexpression of the gene product. This increase in DNA copy number may cause cytologically recognizable chromosome alterations referred to as *homogeneous staining regions* (HSRs), if integrated within chromosomes, or *double minutes* (dmins), if extrachromosomal in nature. The recognition of DNA amplification is accomplished through various cytogenetic techniques such as comparative genomic hybridization (CGH) and fluorescence in situ hybridization (FISH), which allow the visualization of chromosomal aberrations using fluorescent dyes. With these techniques, the entire genome can be surveyed for gains and losses of DNA sequences, thus pinpointing chromosomal regions likely to contain genes important in the development or progression of cancer. Noncytogenetic, molecular techniques for identifying amplifications have more recently become available.

Numerous genes have been reported to be amplified in cancer. Several genes, including *NMYC* and *LMYC*, were identified through their presence within the amplified DNA sequences of a tumor and had homology to known oncogenes. Because the region amplified often extends to hundreds of thousands of base pairs, more than one oncogene may be amplified in some cancers (particularly sarcomas). Genes simultaneously amplified in many cases include *MDM2*, *GLI*, *CDK4*, and *SAS*. Demonstration of amplification of a cellular gene is often a predictor of poor prognosis. For example, *ERBB2/HER2* and *NMYC* are often amplified in aggressive breast cancers and neuroblastoma, respectively.

Chromosomal Rearrangement Chromosomal alterations provide important clues to the genetic changes in cancer. The chromosomal alterations in human solid tumors such as carcinomas are heterogeneous and complex and likely reflect selection for the loss of tumor-suppressor genes on the involved chromosome. In contrast, the chromosome alterations in myeloid and lymphoid tumors are often simple translocations, i.e., reciprocal transfers of chromosome arms from one chromosome to another. Consequently, many detailed and informative chromosome analyses have been performed on hematopoietic cancers. The breakpoints of recurring chromosome abnormalities usually occur at the site of cellular oncogenes. Table 79-3 lists representative examples of recurring chromosome alterations in malignancy and the

TABLE 79-3 REPRESENTATIVE ONCOGENES AT CHROMOSOMAL TRANSLOCATIONS

Gene (Chromosome)	Translocation	Malignancy
ABL (9q34.1)–BCR (22q11)	(9;22)(q34;q11)	Chronic myelogenous leukemia
ATF1 (12q13)–EWS (22q12)	(12;22)(q13;q12)	Malignant melanoma of soft parts (MMSP)
BCL1 (11q13.3)–IgH (14q32)	(11;14)(q13;q32)	Mantle cell lymphoma
BCL2 (18q21.3)–IgH (14q32)	(14;18)(q32;q21)	Follicular lymphoma
FLI1 (11q24)–EWS (22q12)	(11;22)(q24;q12)	Ewing's sarcoma
LCK (1p34)–TCRB (7q35)	(1;7)(p34;q35)	T cell acute lymphocytic leukemia (ALL)
MYC (8q24)–IgH (14q32)	(8;14)(q24;q32)	Burkitt's lymphoma, B cell ALL
WT1 (11p13)–EWS (22q12)	(11;22)(p13;q12)	Desmoplastic small round cell tumor (DSRCT)
PAX3 (2q35)–FKHR/ALV(13q14)	(2;13)(q35;q14)	Alveolar rhabdomyosarcoma
PAX7 (1p36)–KHR/ALV(13q14)	(1;13)(p36;q14)	Alveolar rhabdomyosarcoma
RET (10q11.2)	(10;17)(q11.2;q23)	Papillary thyroid carcinomas

Source: From R Hesketh: *The Oncogene and Tumour Suppressor Gene Facts Book*, 2d ed. San Diego, Academic Press, 1997; with permission.

associated gene(s) rearranged or deregulated by the chromosomal rearrangement. Translocations are particularly common in lymphoid tumors, probably because these cell types normally rearrange their DNA to generate antigen receptors. Indeed, antigen receptor genes are commonly involved in the translocations, implying that an imperfect regulation of receptor gene rearrangement may be involved in the pathogenesis. An example is Burkitt's lymphoma, a B cell tumor characterized by a reciprocal translocation between chromosomes 8 and 14. Molecular analysis of Burkitt's lymphomas demonstrated that the breakpoints occurred within or near the *MYC* locus on chromosome 8 and within the immunoglobulin heavy chain locus on chromosome 14, resulting in the transcriptional activation of *MYC*. Enhancer activation by translocation, although not universal, appears to play an important role in malignant progression. In addition to transcription factors and signal transduction molecules, translocation may result in the overexpression of cell cycle regulatory proteins such as cyclins and of proteins that regulate cell death such as bcl-2.

The first reproducible chromosome abnormality detected in human malignancy was the Philadelphia chromosome detected in CML. This cytogenetic abnormality is generated by reciprocal translocation involving the *ABL* oncogene, a tyrosine kinase on chromosome 9, being placed in proximity to the *BCR* (breakpoint cluster region) on chromosome 22. Figure 79-7 illustrates the generation of the translocation and its protein product. The consequence of expression of the *BCR-ABL* gene product is the activation of signal transduction pathways leading to cell growth independent of normal external signals. Imatinib, a drug that specifically blocks the activity of *BCR-ABL* has shown remarkable efficacy with little toxicity in patients with CML. Knowledge of genetic alterations in cancer can lead to mechanism-based design and development of cancer drugs.

CHROMOSOMAL INSTABILITY IN SOLID TUMORS

Solid tumors are generally highly aneuploid, containing an abnormal number of chromosomes; these chromosomes also exhibit structural alterations such as translocations, deletions, and amplifications. Again, colon cancer has proven to be a particularly useful model for the study of chromosomal instability (CIN). As described above, some familial cases are characterized by the presence of MIN. Interestingly, MIN and CIN appear to be mutually exclusive in colon cancer, suggesting that they represent alternative mechanisms for the generation of a mutator phenotype in this cancer (Fig. 79-2). Other cancer types rarely exhibit MIN but almost always exhibit CIN. Normal cells possess several cell cycle checkpoints, often defined as quality-control requirements that have to be met before subsequent events are allowed to take place. The spindle checkpoint, which ensures proper chromosome attachment to the mitotic spindle before allowing the sister chromatids to separate, has been shown to be deficient in certain cancers. The genes that, when mutated, may cause CIN have in general not yet been identified, although a few candidates mutated in a small number of tumors have been discovered. The identification of the cause of CIN in tumors will likely be a formidable task, considering that several hundred genes are thought to control the mitotic checkpoint and other cellular processes assuring proper chromosome segregation. Regardless of the mechanisms underlying CIN, the measurement of the number of chromosomal alterations present in tumors is now possible with both cytogenetic and molecular techniques, and several studies have shown that this information can be useful for prognostic purposes.

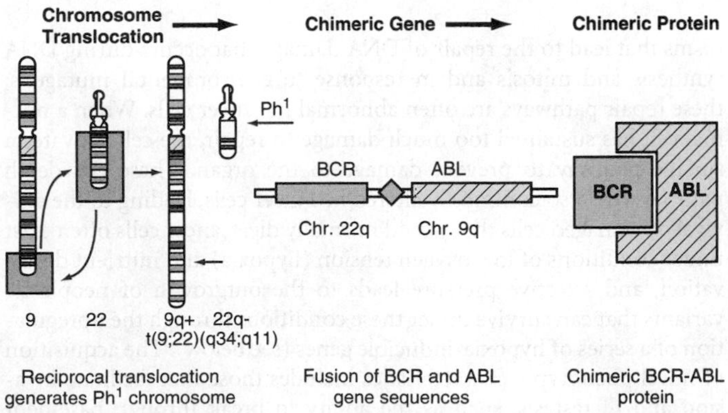

FIGURE 79-7 Specific translocation seen in chronic myelogenous leukemia (CML). The Philadelphia chromosome (Ph) is derived from a reciprocal translocation between chromosomes 9 and 22 with the breakpoint joining the sequences of the *ABL* oncogene with the *BCR* gene. The fusion of these DNA sequences allows the generation of an entirely novel fusion protein with modified function. (*Courtesy of ER Fearon and KR Cho; with permission.*)

VIRUSES IN HUMAN CANCER

Certain human malignancies are associated with viruses. Examples include Burkitt's lymphoma (Epstein-Barr virus), hepatocellular carcinoma (hepatitis virus), cervical cancer [human papillomavirus (HPV)], and T cell leukemia (retroviruses). The mechanisms of action of these viruses are varied but always involve activation of growth-promoting pathways or inhibition of tumor-suppressor products in the infected cells. For example, HPV proteins E6 and E7 bind and inactivate cellular tumor suppressors p53 and pRB, respectively. Viruses are not sufficient for cancer development but constitute one alteration in the multistep process of cancer.

EPIGENETIC REGULATION OF GENE EXPRESSION IN CANCER

An *epigenetic modification* refers to a change in the genome, heritable by cell progeny, that does not involve a change in the DNA sequence. The inactivation of the second X chromosome in female cells is an example of an epigenetic mechanism that prevents gene expression from the inactivated chromosome. During embryologic development, regions of chromosomes from one parent are silenced and gene expression proceeds from the chromosome of the other parent. For most genes, expression occurs from both alleles or randomly from one allele or the other. The preferential expression of a particular gene exclusively from the allele contributed by one parent is called *parental imprinting* and is thought to be regulated by covalent modifications of chromatin protein and DNA (often methylation) of the silenced allele.

The role of epigenetic control mechanisms in the development of human cancer is unclear. However, a general decrease in the level of DNA methylation has been noted as a common change in cancer. In addition, numerous genes, including some tumor-suppressor genes, appear to become hypermethylated and silenced during tumorigenesis. *VHL* and *p16INK4* are well-studied examples of tumor-suppressor genes that are silenced through methylation in human cancers. Overall, epigenetic mechanisms may be responsible for reprogramming the expression of a large number of genes in cancer and, together with the mutation of specific genes, are likely to be crucial in the development of human malignancies.

GENE EXPRESSION AND MUTATIONAL PROFILING IN CANCER

The tumorigenesis process, driven by alterations in tumor suppressors, oncogenes, and epigenetic regulation, is accompanied by changes in gene expression. The advent of powerful new techniques such as microarrays and serial analysis of gene expression (SAGE) has allowed the study of gene expression in neoplastic cells on a scale never before accomplished. Indeed, it is now possible to identify expression levels of thousands of genes expressed in normal and cancer tissues. Figure 79-8 shows a typical cDNA array experiment examining gene expression in cancer. This global knowledge of gene expression allows the identification of differentially expressed genes and, in principle, the understanding of the complex molecular circuitry regulating normal and neoplastic behaviors. Such studies have led to molecular profiling of tumors, which has suggested general methods for distinguishing tumors of various biologic behaviors (molecular classification), elucidating pathways relevant to the development of tumors, and identifying molecular targets for the detection and therapy of cancer. The first practical applications of this technology have suggested that global

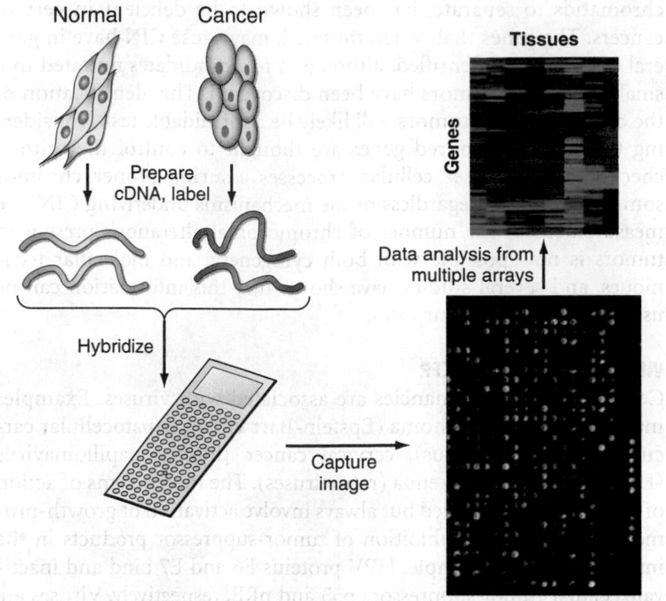

FIGURE 79-8 A cDNA array experiment. RNA is prepared from cells, reverse transcribed to cDNA, and labeled with fluorescent dyes (typically green for normal cells and red for cancer cells). The fluorescent probes are mixed and hybridized to the cDNA array. Each spot on the array is a cDNA fragment that represents a different gene. The image is then captured with a fluorescence camera; red spots indicate higher expression in tumor compared with reference while green spots represent the opposite. Yellow signals indicate equal expression levels in normal and tumor specimens. After clustering analysis of multiple arrays, the results are typically represented graphically using Treeview software, which shows, for each sample, a color-coded representation of gene expression for every gene on the array.

gene expression profiling can provide prognostic information not evident from other clinical or laboratory tests. The National Cancer Institute, in conjunction with the National Center for Biotechnology Information, has undertaken the Cancer Genome Anatomy Project (CGAP) (*http://cgap.nci.nih.gov/*) to collect data on gene expression in normal and malignant tissues and make it available on the Internet.

In addition, with the completion of the Human Genome Project and advances in sequencing technologies, large-scale mutational profiling of the cancer genome has become possible. Hundreds of genes from a given pathway (MAPK pathway, for example) or from a gene family can be systematically sequenced in a large number of cancers in order to identify genes that are crucial to human oncogenesis. This approach has been used to identify several novel targets in various cancers. For example, *B-RAF* mutations were identified in a large fraction of melanomas and *PIK3CA* mutations were identified in large fractions of colon, breast, and hepatocellular cancers. Most recently, this approach has been applied to an unbiased set of genes including about two-thirds of all those known to encode proteins. Hundreds of genes not previously implicated in cancers were shown to be altered in breast and colorectal cancers.

THE FUTURE

A revolution in cancer genetics has occurred in the past 25 years. Identification of cancer genes has led to a better understanding of the tumorigenesis process and has had important repercussions on all fields of biology. In spite of these spectacular advances, however, there has been little overall improvement in cancer death rates. It is hoped that, as the molecular mechanisms of cancer initiation and development continue to be elucidated, novel therapies based on pathophysiology rather than empiricism will emerge. Time will tell whether these strategies will rely on novel combinations or dosing schedules of conventional drugs or will be based on new approaches such as those involving gene therapy or immunotherapy. In addition, a better understanding of the molecular pathways and genetic alterations in cancer cells may lead to the development of sensitive strategies for early detection of cancer.

FURTHER READINGS

GARBER JE, OFFIT K: Hereditary cancer predisposition syndromes. J Clin Oncol 23:276, 2005

GOLUB TR et al: Molecular classification of cancer: Class discovery and class prediction by gene expression monitoring. Science 286:531, 1999

JALLEPALLI PV, LENGAUER C: Chromosome segregation and cancer: Cutting through the mystery. Nat Rev Cancer 1:109, 2001

LOEB LA: Mutator phenotype may be required for multistage carcinogenesis. Cancer Res 51:3075, 1991

MUNGER K: Disruption of oncogene/tumor suppressor networks during human carcinogenesis. Cancer Invest 20:71, 2002

PARSONS DW et al: Colorectal cancer: Mutations in a signaling pathway. Nature 436:792, 2005

STRAUSBERG RL et al: In silico analysis of cancer through the Cancer Genome Anatomy Project. Trends Cell Biol 11:S66, 2001

VOGELSTEIN B, KINZLER KW: The multistep nature of cancer. Trends Genet 9:138, 1993

80 Cancer Cell Biology and Angiogenesis

Robert G. Fenton, Dan L. Longo

Two characteristic features define a cancer: unregulated cell growth and tissue invasion/metastasis. Unregulated cell growth without invasion is a feature of *benign neoplasms*, or new growths. Cancer is a synonym for *malignant neoplasm*. Cancers of epithelial tissues are called *carcinomas*; cancers of nonepithelial (mesenchymal) tissues are called *sarcomas*. Cancers arising from hematopoietic or lymphoid cells are called *leukemias* or *lymphomas*.

Cancer is a genetic disease. The malignant phenotype often requires mutations in several different genes that regulate cell proliferation, survival, DNA repair, motility, invasion, and angiogenesis (Table 80-1). Cancer-causing mutations often activate signal transduction pathways leading to aberrant cell proliferation and perturbations of tissue-specific differentiation programs. The normal cell has protective mechanisms that lead to the repair of DNA damage that occurs during DNA synthesis and mitosis and in response to environmental mutagens; these repair pathways are often abnormal in cancer cells. When a normal cell has sustained too much damage to repair, the cell activates a suicide pathway to prevent damage to the organ. These cell death pathways are also commonly altered in cancer cells, leading to the survival of damaged cells that would normally die. Cancer cells often exist under conditions of low oxygen tension (hypoxia) and nutrient deprivation, and selective pressure leads to the outgrowth of neoplastic variants that can survive under these conditions through the upregulation of a series of hypoxia-inducible genes (see below). The acquisition of novel phenotypic characteristics includes those that facilitate invasion and metastasis, such as the ability to break through basement membranes, migrate through the extracellular matrix and into the vascular compartment, and generate new blood vessels to support colonization in remote sites. The accumulation of genetic lesions may lead through an identifiable progression of altered phenotypes as is noted in colon cancer: hyperplasia → adenoma → dysplasia → carcinoma in situ → invasive carcinoma. Premalignant changes have also been identified in prostate, breast, and pancreatic cancers.

TABLE 80-1 PHENOTYPIC CHARACTERISTICS OF MALIGNANT CELLS
Deregulated cell proliferation: Loss of negative regulators (suppressor oncogenes, i.e., Rb, p53), and increased positive regulators (oncogenes, i.e., *Ras, Myc*). Leads to aberrant cell cycle control and includes loss of normal checkpoint responses.
Failure to differentiate: Arrest at a stage prior to terminal differentiation. May retain stem cell properties. (Frequently observed in leukemias due to transcriptional repression of developmental programs by the gene products of chromosomal translocations.)
Loss of normal apoptosis pathways: Inactivation of p53, increases in Bcl-2 family members. This defect enhances the survival of cells with oncogenic mutations and genetic instability and allows clonal expansion and diversification within the tumor without activation of physiologic cell death pathways.
Genetic instability: Defects in DNA repair pathways leading to either single or oligo-nucleotide mutations, (as in microsatellite instability, MIN) or more commonly chromosomal instability (CIN) leading to aneuploidy. Caused by loss of function of p53, BRCA1/2, mismatch repair genes, and others.
Loss of replicative senescence: Normal cells stop dividing after 25–50 population doublings. Arrest is mediated by the Rb, $p16^{INK4a}$, and p53 pathways. Further replication leads to telomere loss, with crisis. Surviving cells often harbor gross chromosomal abnormalities.
Increased angiogenesis: Due to increased gene expression of proangiogenic factors (VEGF, FGF, IL-8) by tumor or stromal cells, or loss of negative regulators (endostatin, tumstatin, thrombospondin).
Invasion: Loss of cell-cell contacts (gap junctions, cadherens) and increased production of matrix metalloproteinases (MMPs). Often takes the form of epithelial-to-mesenchymal transition (EMT) with anchored epithelial cells becoming more like motile fibroblasts.
Metastasis: Spread of tumor cells to lymph nodes or distant tissue sites. Limited by the ability of tumor cells to survive in a foreign environment.
Evasion of the immune system: Downregulation of MHC class I and II molecules; induction of T cell tolerance; inhibition of normal dendritic cell and/or T cell function; antigenic loss variants and clonal heterogeneity.

Note: VEGF, vascular endothelial growth factor; FGF, fibroblast growth factor; IL, interleukin.

CANCER CELL BIOLOGY

The treatment of most human cancers with conventional cytoreductive agents has been unsuccessful due to the Gompertzian-like growth kinetics of solid tumors (i.e., tumor growth is exponential in small tumors, with increasing doubling times as tumors expand; since conventional chemotherapeutic agents target proliferating cells, noncycling cells in large tumors are relatively resistant). Genetic instability is inherent in most cancer cells and predisposes to the development of intrinsic and acquired drug resistance. Thus, although tumors arise from a single cell (i.e., they are clonal), large tumors become very heterogeneous with multiple related subclones, some of which will be resistant to specific therapies, leading to the selection of progressively more resistant tumors as treatment progresses. Since a 1-cm tumor often contains 10^9 cells, and patients typically present to their physicians with 10^{10}–10^{11} tumor cells, the obstacle to curative treatment becomes more understandable. Rationally designed, target-based therapeutic agents, directed against the specific molecular derangements that distinguish malignant from nonmalignant cells, have become possible with advances in the understanding of oncogene and tumor-suppressor pathways. This chapter describes the convergence of scientific, pharmacologic, and medical knowledge that has led to the targeted therapy of cancer.

THERAPEUTIC APPROACHES TO CELL CYCLE ABNORMALITIES IN CANCER

The mechanism of cell division is substantially the same in all dividing cells and has been conserved throughout evolution. The process assures that the cell accurately duplicates its contents, especially its chromosomes. The cell cycle is divided into four phases. During M-phase, the replicated chromosomes are separated and packaged into two new nuclei by mitosis and the cytoplasm is divided between the two daughter cells by cytokinesis. The other three phases of the cell cycle are called *interphase*: G_1 (gap 1), during which the cell determines its readiness to commit to DNA synthesis; S (DNA synthesis), during which the genetic material is replicated and no re-replication is permitted; and G_2 (gap 2), during which the fidelity of DNA replication is assessed and errors are corrected.

Deregulation of the molecular mechanisms controlling cell cycle progression is a hallmark of cancer. Progression from one phase of the cell cycle to the next is controlled by the orderly activation of cyclin-dependent kinases (CDKs) that are regulated by signaling events that couple a cell's physiologic response to its extracellular milieu. In normal cells, specific molecular signals, called *checkpoints*, prevent progression into the next phase of the cell cycle until all requisite physiologic processes are complete. Cancer cells often have defective cell cycle checkpoints. The transition through G_1 into S-phase is a critical regulator of cell proliferation, and the phosphorylation state of the retinoblastoma tumor-suppressor protein (pRB) at the restriction point in late G_1 determines whether a cell will enter S-phase. The complex of CDK4 or CDK6 with D type cyclins forms a G_1-specific kinase whose activity is regulated by growth factors, nutrients, and cell-cell and cell-matrix interactions. Subsequent formation of an active CDK2/cyclin E complex results in full phosphorylation of pRB, relieving its inhibitory effects on the S-phase-regulating transcription factor E2F/DP1, and permitting the activation of genes required for S-phase (such as dihydrofolate reductase, thymidine kinase, ribonucleotide reductase, and DNA polymerase). The activity of CDK/cyclin complexes can be blocked by CDK-inhibitors including $p21^{Cip1/Waf1}$, $p16^{Ink4a}$, and $p27^{Kip1}$, which block S-phase progression by preventing the phosphorylation of pRB.

Genetic lesions that render the retinoblastoma pathway nonfunctional are thought to occur in all human cancers. Loss of function of pRB as guardian of the G_1 restriction point enables cancer cells to enter a mitotic cycle without the normal input from external signals. Current therapeutic efforts to reverse the derangements of the retinoblastoma pathway have taken two main approaches. All kinases require the binding of ATP (and substrate) to the enzyme active site, followed by transfer of the γ-phosphate to serine, threonine, or tyrosine residues of the substrate. Flavopiridol was the first relatively selective CDK inhibitor identified, with Ki or IC_{50}s in the 40- to 400-n*M* range. Although flavopiridol was initially thought to prevent tumor cell proliferation by inhibition of cell cycle CDKs, it is now clear that regulation of cellular transcription elongation by the CDK7/cyclin H and CDK9/cyclin T1 complexes may be the critical target of flavopiridol. Phase II clinical trials of flavopiridol are in progress; responses have been reported in chronic lymphocytic leukemia after a dosing schedule was defined to optimize the pharmacokinetics of the drug. Laboratory efforts are focused on the development of novel classes of CDK inhibitors capable of specifically targeting individual CDK/cyclin complexes. A second therapeutic endeavor to regain control of pRB function involves reversing the epigenetic silencing of $p16^{Ink4a}$ gene and is discussed below.

p53, the "guardian of the genome," is a sequence-specific transcription factor whose activity is regulated through tight control of p53 protein levels. Normally, levels of p53 are kept low by its association with the mdm2 oncogene product, which binds p53 and shuttles it out of the nucleus for proteolytic degradation. p53 levels are regulated by two checkpoint pathways that are activated in response to DNA damage or oncogene-induced cell proliferation (Fig. 80-1). The loss of p53 function abrogates these checkpoints and enables tumor cells to escape cell cycle arrest, senescence, or apoptosis despite accumulation of mutations and aberrant passage through the cell cycle.

Acquired mutation in p53 is the most common genetic alteration found in human cancer (>50%); germline mutation in p53 is the causative genetic lesion of the Li-Fraumeni familial cancer syndrome. In many tumors, one p53 allele on chromosome 17p is deleted and the other is mutated. The mutations often abrogate the DNA binding function of p53 that is required for its transcription factor activity and tumor-suppressor functions, and also result in high intracellular levels of p53 protein. Inactivation of the p53 pathway compromises cell cycle arrest, attenuates apoptosis induced by DNA damage or other stimuli, and predisposes cells to chromosome instability. This genomic instability greatly increases the probability that p53 null cells will acquire additional mutations and become malignant. *In summary, it is likely*

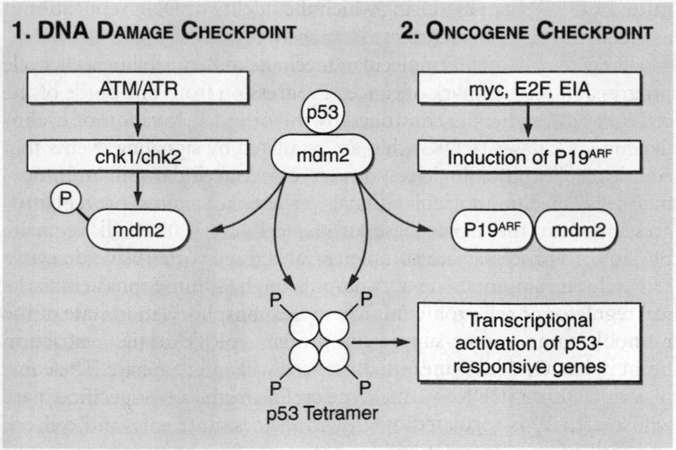

FIGURE 80-1 Induction of p53 by the DNA damage and oncogene checkpoints. In response to noxious stimuli, p53 and mdm2 are phosphorylated by the ataxia telangiectasia mutated (ATM) and related ATR serine/threonine kinases, as well as the immediated downstream checkpoint kinases, Chk1 and Chk2. This causes dissociation of p53 from mdm2, leading to increased p53 protein levels and transcription of genes leading to cell cycle arrest ($p21^{Cip1/Waf1}$) or apoptosis (e.g., the proapoptotic Bcl-2 family members Noxa and Puma). Inducers of p53 include hypoxia, DNA damage (caused by ultraviolet radiation, gamma irradiation, or chemotherapy), ribonucleotide depletion, and telomere shortening. A second mechanism of p53 induction is activated by oncogenes such as *Myc*, which promote aberrant G_1/S transition. This pathway is regulated by a second product of the Ink4a locus, $p19^{ARF}$, which is encoded by an *a*lternative *r*eading *f*rame of the same stretch of DNA that codes for $p16^{Ink4a}$. Levels of ARF are upregulated by *Myc* and E2F, and ARF binds to mdm2 and rescues p53 from its inhibitory effect. This *oncogene checkpoint* leads to the death or senescence (an irreversible arrest in G1 of the cell cycle) of renegade cells that attempt to enter S phase without appropriate physiologic signals. Senescent cells have been identified in patients whose premalignant lesions harbor activated oncogenes, for instance, dysplastic nevi that encode an activated form of BRAF (see below), demonstrating that induction of senescence is a protective mechanism that operates in humans to prevent the outgrowth of neoplastic cells.

that all human cancers have genetic alterations that inactivate the Rb and p53 tumor-suppressor pathways.

Tumors expressing mutant p53 are more resistant to radiation therapy and chemotherapy than tumors with wild-type p53. If the transcriptional functions of the mutant p53 could be reestablished in tumor cells, massive apoptosis might ensue, whereas normal cells would be protected because they express very low levels of wild-type p53. Investigators have screened chemical libraries for compounds that inhibit tumor cell growth in a mutant p53-dependent manner. One compound entered cells and induced mutant p53 to adopt an active conformation such that p53-dependent transcriptional activation was restored and apoptosis was selectively induced. This compound also had anti-tumor activity in murine xenograft models. Other investigators have identified a low-molecular-weight, cell-permeable compound that inhibits the apoptotic functions of wild-type p53 found in normal host cells. This compound protected mice from the toxic effects of radiation therapy and chemotherapy, including bone marrow suppression, gastrointestinal dysfunction, and hair loss. Taken together, these approaches provide proof of principle for the pharmacologic manipulation of p53 function (mutant or wild-type) that could greatly enhance therapeutic efficacy while decreasing toxicity.

Knowledge of the molecular events governing cell cycle regulation has led to the development of viruses that replicate selectively in tumor cells with defined genetic lesions. Such "oncolytic" viruses include adenoviruses designed to replicate in tumor cells that lack functional p53 or have defects in the pRB pathway. The former group includes an adenovirus mutant in which the viral p55 protein (which binds and inhibits p53) was deleted; this virus selectively replicates in tumor cells lacking p53 function. This virus has shown efficacy in phase II clinical trials of head and neck tumors, especially when combined with 5-fluorouracil and cisplatin (50% partial or complete response). The complexities of virus-host interactions (i.e., immune response against replicating virus) will require further refinements of this novel technology before the clinical utility of this approach can be fully realized.

TELOMERASE

DNA polymerase is unable to replicate the tips of chromosomes, resulting in the loss of DNA at the specialized ends of chromosomes (called *telomeres*) with each replication cycle. At birth, human telomeres are 15- to 20-kb pairs long and are composed of tandem repeats of a six-nucleotide sequence (TTAGGG) that associate with specialized telomere-binding proteins to form a T-loop structure that protects the ends of chromosomes from being mistakenly recognized as damaged. The loss of telomeric repeats with each cell division cycle causes gradual telomere shortening, leading to growth arrest (called *replicative senescence*) when one or more critically short telomeres triggers a p53-regulated DNA-damage checkpoint response. Cells can bypass this growth arrest if pRB and p53 are nonfunctional, but cell death ensues when the unprotected ends of chromosomes precipitate chromosome fusions or other catastrophic DNA rearrangements (termed *crisis*). *The ability to bypass telomere-based growth limitations is thought to be a critical step in the evolution of most malignancies.* This occurs by the reactivation of telomerase expression in cancer cells. Telomerase is an enzyme that adds TTAGGG repeats onto the 3′ ends of chromosomes. It contains a catalytic subunit with reverse transcriptase activity (hTERT) and an RNA component that provides the template for telomere extension. Most normal somatic cells do not express sufficient telomerase to prevent telomere attrition with each cell division. Exceptions include stem cells (such as those found in hematopoietic tissues, gut and skin epithelium, and germ cells) that require extensive cell division to maintain tissue homeostasis. More than 90% of human cancers express high levels of telomerase that prevent telomere exhaustion and allow indefinite cell proliferation. In vitro experiments indicate that inhibition of telomerase activity leads to tumor cell apoptosis. Major efforts are underway to develop methods to inhibit telomerase activity in cancer cells. The reverse transcriptase activity of telomerase is a prime target for small-molecule pharmaceuticals. The protein component of telomerase (hTERT) can act as a tumor-associated antigen recognized by antigen-specific cytotoxic T lymphocytes (CTL) that lyse human melanoma, prostate, lung, breast, and colon cancer cells in vitro. Clinical trials of telomerase vaccines are underway.

SIGNAL TRANSDUCTION PATHWAYS AS THERAPEUTIC TARGETS IN CANCER CELLS

Since the discovery that the v-*src* oncogene has protein tyrosine kinase activity, the central role of tyrosine phosphorylation in cellular responses to growth factors has become apparent. Many tyrosine kinases act at the apex of signaling pathways and are transmembrane proteins (receptor tyrosine kinases, RTK) or are associated with structures at the plasma membrane (*Src*-, Janus-, and *Fak*-family kinases). RTKs are transmembrane glycoproteins that undergo dimerization upon ligand binding, with activation of their cytoplasmic tyrosine kinase domains by proximity-induced trans-phosphorylation of the activation loop. Tyrosine residues of the receptor or adaptor proteins (such as IRS-1 or Shc) are phosphorylated and act as docking sites for proteins containing SH2 (Src-homology 2) or PTB (phosphotyrosine binding) domains, thus initiating multiple signal transduction pathways (Fig. 80-2). Normally, tyrosine kinase activity is short-lived and reversed by protein tyrosine phosphatases (PTP). However, in many human cancers, tyrosine kinases or components of their downstream pathways are activated by mutation, gene amplification, or chromosomal translocations. Because these pathways regulate proliferation, survival, migration, and angiogenesis, they have been identified as important targets for cancer therapeutics.

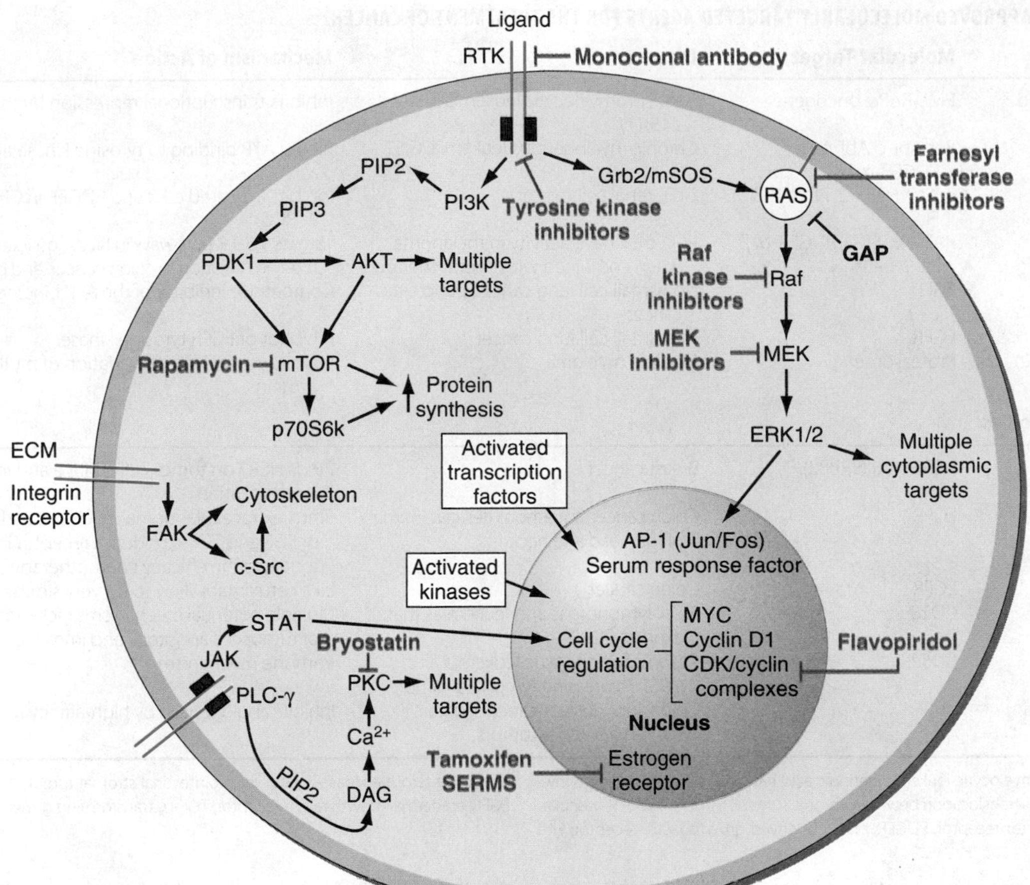

FIGURE 80-2 Therapeutic targeting of signal transduction pathways in cancer cells. Three major signal transduction pathways are activated by receptor tyrosine kinases (RTK). 1. The protooncogene Ras is activated by the Grb2/mSOS guanine nucleotide exchange factor, which induces an association with Raf and activation of downstream kinases (MEK and ERK1/2). 2. Activated PI3K phosphorylates the membrane lipid PIP_2 to generate PIP_3, which acts as a membrane-docking site for a number of cellular proteins including the serine/threonine kinases PDK1 and Akt. PDK1 has numerous cellular targets including Akt and mTOR. Akt phosphorylates target proteins that promote resistance to apoptosis and enhance cell cycle progression, while mTOR and its target p70S6K upregulate protein synthesis to potentiate cell growth. 3. Activation of PLC-γ leads the formation of diacylglycerol (DAG) and increased intracellular calcium, with activation of multiple isoforms of PKC and other enzymes regulated by the calcium/calmodulin system. Other important signaling pathways involve non-RTKs that are activated by cytokine or integrin receptors. Janus kinases (JAK) phosphorylate STAT (signal transducer and activator of transcription) transcription factors, which translocate to the nucleus and activate target genes. Integrin receptors mediate cellular interactions with the extracellular matrix (ECM), inducing activation of FAK (focal adhesion kinase) and c-Src, which activate multiple downstream pathways, including modulation of the cell cytoskeleton. Many activated kinases and transcription factors migrate into the nucleus where they regulate gene transcription, thus completing the path from extracellular signals, such as growth factors, to a change in cell phenotype, such as induction of differentiation or cell proliferation. The nuclear targets of these processes include transcription factors (e.g., Myc, AP-1, and serum response factor) and the cell cycle machinery (CDKs and cyclins). Inhibitors of many of these pathways have been developed for the treatment of human cancers. Examples of inhibitors that are currently being evaluated in clinical trials are shown in purple.

TARGETING Bcr-Abl WITH IMATINIB: PROOF OF PRINCIPLE

The protein product of the Philadelphia chromosome occurs in all patients with chronic myeloid leukemia (CML) and in ~30% of patients with adult acute lymphoid leukemia (ALL) and encodes the fusion protein Bcr-Abl. Although the c-*Abl* protooncogene is a nuclear protein whose kinase activity is tightly regulated as a part of the DNA damage response pathway (and actually induces growth arrest), the Bcr-Abl fusion protein is largely cytoplasmic with a constitutively activated tyrosine kinase domain. The deregulated tyrosine kinase activity of Bcr-Abl is required for its transforming activity. *The Abl tyrosine kinase inhibitor, imatinib mesylate (Gleevec), has validated the concept of a molecularly targeted approach to cancer treatment.*

Imatinib is a low-molecular-weight competitive inhibitor of the ATP binding site of Bcr-Abl, c-Abl, platelet-derived growth factor receptor (PDGFR), and c-Kit; hence it is not absolutely specific for the *Bcr-Abl* oncogene product (Table 80-2). Clinical studies have demonstrated remarkable activity of this agent in CML. In phase II studies of 532 chronic phase CML patients in whom interferon treatment had failed, 95% obtained a hematologic complete response, with only 9% relapse after a median follow-up of 18 months. With longer follow-up, 75% of patients treated with imatinib in chronic phase remain in remission after nearly 4 years. Imatinib was also active in CML blast crisis with a 52% response rate, although the responses were short-lived (78% relapse within 1 year). Relapse during treatment with imatinib was associated with reactivation of the tyrosine kinase either by amplification of the *Bcr-Abl* locus leading to increased levels of Bcr-Abl protein or, more commonly, by point mutations within the Bcr-Abl kinase domain that decreased imatinib binding without loss of Bcr-Abl kinase activity. These data constitute genetic proof that the target of imatinib is the Bcr-Abl tyrosine kinase, and that Bcr-Abl kinase activity is still required by imatinib-resistant cells. Two drugs have been developed (dasatinib and nilotinib) that are potent inhibitors against most imatinib resistant mutants; these compounds have demonstrated significant activity in patients with imatinib-resistant CML.

TABLE 80-2 FDA-APPROVED MOLECULARLY TARGETED AGENTS FOR THE TREATMENT OF CANCER

Drug	Molecular Target	Disease	Mechanism of Action
All-*trans* retinoic acid (ATRA)	PML-RARα oncogene	Acute promyelocytic leukemia M3 AML; t(15;17)	Inhibits transcriptional repression by the PML-RARα
Imatinib (Gleevec)	Bcr-Abl, c-Abl, c-Kit, PDGFR-α/β,	Chronic myelogenous leukemia; GIST	Blocks ATP binding to tyrosine kinase active site.
Sunitinib (Sutent)	c-Kit, VEGFR-2, PDGFR-β, Flt-3	GIST; renal cell cancer	Inhibits activated c-Kit and PDGFR in GIST; inhibits VEGFR in RCC.
Sorafinib (Nexavar)	RAF, VEGFR-2, PDGFR-α/β, Flt-3, c-Kit	RCC; may have activity in melanoma when combined with chemotherapy	Targets VEGFR pathways in RCC. Possible activity against BRAF in melanoma, colon cancer, and others.
Erlotinib (Tarceva)	EGFR	Non-small cell lung cancer; pancreatic cancer	Competitive inhibitor of the ATP binding site of the EGFR.
Gefitinb (Iressa)	EGFR	Non-small cell lung cancer	Inhibitor of EGFR tyrosine kinase.
Bortezomib (Velcade)	Proteasome	Multiple myeloma	Inhibits proteolytic degradation of multiple cellular proteins.
Monoclonal Antibodies			
Trastuzumab (Herceptin)	HER2/neu (ERBB2)	Breast cancer	Binds HER2 on tumor cell surface and induces receptor internalization.
Cetuximab (Erbitux)	EGFR	Colon cancer, squamous cell carcinoma of the head and neck	Binds extracellular domain of EGFR and blocks binding of EGF and TGF-α; induces receptor internalization. Potentiates the efficacy chemotherapy and radiotherapy.
Panitumomab (Vectibix)	EGFR	Colon cancer	Like cetuximab; likely to be very similar in clinical activity
Rituximab (Rituxan)	CD20	B cell lymphomas and leukemias that express CD20	Multiple potential mechanisms including direct induction of tumor cell apoptosis and immune mechanisms.
Alemtuzumab (Campath)	CD52	Chronic lymphocytic leukemia and CD52-expressing lymphoid tumors	Immune mechanisms
Bevacizumab (Avastin)	VEGF	Colon, lung, breast cancers; data pending in other tumors	Inhibits angiogenesis by high-affinity binding to VEGF.

Note: PML-RARα, promyelocytic leukemia–retinoic acid receptor-alpha; AML, acute myeloid leukemia; t(15;17), translocation between chromosomes 15 and 17; VEGFR, vascular endothelial growth factor receptor; PDGFR, platelet-derived growth factor receptor; Flt-3, fms-like tyrosine kinase-3; GIST, gastrointestinal stromal tumor; RCC, renal cell cancer; EGFR, epidermal growth factor receptor; TGF-α, transforming growth factor alpha.

Imatinib has also demonstrated targeted activity in other diseases, including gastrointestinal stromal tumors (GIST), rare mesenchymal tumors of the GI tract (stomach and small intestine). The pathogenic molecular event for most patients with this disease is mutation of the proto-oncogene *c-Kit*, leading to the constitutive activation of this receptor tyrosine kinase without the binding of its physiologic ligand, stem cell factor. About 10% of GISTs encode activating mutations of the PDGFRα instead of *c-Kit*. GISTs are thought to arise from or share a common stem cell with the interstitial cells of Cajal, which give rise to the myenteric plexus of the GI tract. Imatinib, which inhibits the c-Kit kinase domain, has demonstrated significant activity (>50% partial responses usually lasting 1–2 years) in this chemotherapy-refractory tumor. Resistance to imatinib develops due to secondary mutations in c-Kit, and many of these tumors are susceptible to treatment with the multitargeted TK inhibitor sunitinib that has activity against c-Kit as well as the PDGF and vascular endothelial growth factor (VEGF) receptors. Sunitinib is approved by the U.S. Food and Drug Administration for treatment of patients with imatinib-resistant GIST or who are intolerant of imatinib (Table 80-2). Interestingly, tumors with mutations in exon 11 of c-Kit's juxtamembrane region are particularly sensitive to imatinib, whereas those with exon 9 mutations (extracellular domain) respond better to sunitinib than imatinib. In the future, primary therapy for GIST may be determined by the specific molecular defect in c-Kit. Patients with chronic myelomonocytic leukemia (CMML, a myeloproliferative disorder) often harbor a Tel-PDGFR translocation that results in constitutive activation of the PDGFR kinase domain exclusively in the leukemic cells. Imatinib inhibits this kinase and has demonstrated significant activity in this disease. *These examples extend the proof of principle that targeting of signaling pathways in cancer cells can be highly efficacious with minimal toxicity, even when the drug does not have absolute target specificity.* Imatinib has become the paradigm of targeted drug development in other diseases.

TARGETING OTHER RECEPTOR TYROSINE KINASES

Epidermal growth factor receptor (EGFR) mutations define a novel subset of lung cancers. Clinical studies of two high-affinity competitive inhibitors of the ATP binding site in the EGFR kinase domain, gefitinib and erlotinib, have provided important insights into the pathogenesis of different subsets of patients with non-small cell lung cancer (NSCLC). Phase III studies led to FDA approval after ~10–20% of advanced-stage patients treated with single-agent gefitinib or erlotinib had objective tumor responses. Responders tended to have adenocarcinoma or bronchoalveolar histology (not squamous or large cell), and were never-smokers, women, and of Eastern Asian origin. DNA sequence analysis of the *EGFR* gene isolated from the tumors of responding patients (mostly nonsmokers) demonstrated that most had acquired mutations of the kinase domain that led to increased tyrosine kinase activity. Frequently, patients with mutated alleles also had evidence of *EGFR* gene amplification by fluorescence in situ hybridization (FISH). These tumors exhibited euploid chromosome content, in contrast to tumors from smokers, which were most often aneuploid and harbored mutations in the K-*Ras* oncogene. In fact, mutated K-*Ras*, which occurs to the exclusion of EGFR mutation, appears to define a subset of patients with low likelihood of response to EGFR inhibitors. Thus the model has been proposed that the pathogenesis of NSCLC in never-smokers occurs through a novel pathway that is dependent on activated EGFR, and that tumors are *addicted* to this oncogene, rendering them highly susceptible to its inhibition (see Fig. 80-7). No EGFR kinase domain mutations have yet been found in tumors other than NSCLC. *Thus, these studies define a novel oncogenic pathway for an important human cancer, and provide a mechanism to identify subsets of patients likely to respond to the targeted therapy.* The wild-type EGFR is expressed by many other human cancers, and in colon cancer and head and neck cancers, targeting of the EGFR with a monoclonal antibody (cetuximab) has demonstrated improved survival when combined with chemotherapy or radiation therapy.

HER2/*neu* is a target in human breast cancer. The gene encoding HER2/*neu*, a member of the EGFR family, is amplified in ~20% of breast cancers. Tumors that overexpress HER2/*neu* are less responsive to chemotherapy, and patients with these tumors have a reduced survival compared with patients with normal levels of HER2/*neu*. Trastuzumab (Herceptin) is a humanized monoclonal antibody that binds HER2/*neu* on the surface of tumor cells and induces internalization of the receptor, thereby reducing the level of surface expression. This leads to inhibition of cell cycle progression and renders cancer cells more susceptible to the induction of apoptosis. Phase III clinical trials demonstrated that combining trastuzumab with chemotherapy significantly improved response rates and overall survival in patients with metastatic HER2-positive disease, leading to FDA approval. In addition, five randomized trials demonstrated that the addition of trastuzumab to chemotherapy in the adjuvant setting for patients with HER2-positive disease reduces the risk of recurrence by nearly 50%. These studies emphasize the critical pathogenic role of HER2-overexpression in a subset of breast cancer patients.

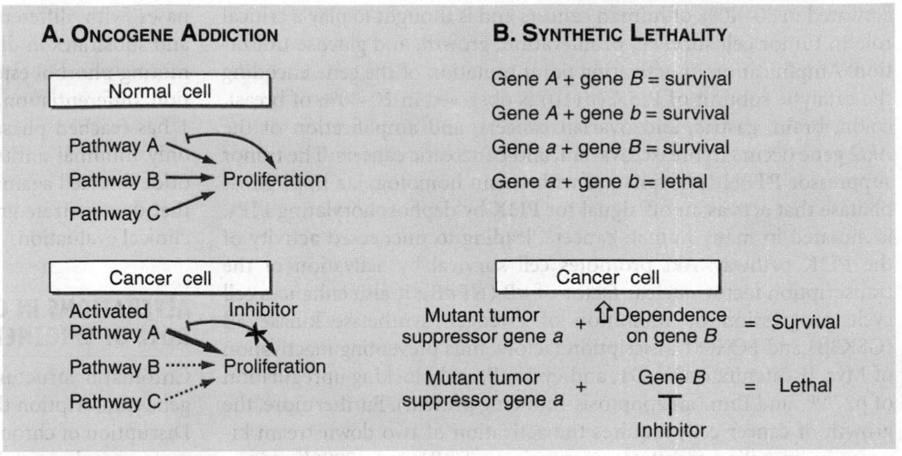

FIGURE 80-3 Oncogene addiction and synthetic lethality: keys to discovery of new anti-cancer drugs. Panel ***A.*** Normal cells receive environmental signals that activate signaling pathways (pathways A, B, and C) that together promote G1 to S phase transition and passage through the cell cycle. Inhibition of one pathway (such as pathway A by a targeted inhibitor) has no significant effect due to redundancy provided by pathways B and C. In cancer cells, oncogenic mutations lead over time to dependency on the activated pathway, with loss of significant input from pathways B and C. The dependency or addiction of the cancer cell to pathway A makes it highly vulnerable to inhibitors that target components of this pathway. Clinically relevant examples include Bcr-Abl (CML), amplified HER2/*neu* (breast cancer), overexpressed or mutated EGF receptors (lung cancer), and mutated *BRAF* (melanoma). Panel ***B.*** Genes are said to have a synthetic lethal relationship when mutation of either gene alone is tolerated by the cell, but mutation of both genes leads to lethality. Thus, in the example, mutant *gene a* and *gene b* have a synthetic lethal relationship, implying that the loss of one gene makes the cell dependent on the function of the other gene. In cancer cells, loss of function of a tumor-suppressor gene (wild-type designated *gene A;* mutant designated *gene a*) may render the cancer cells dependent on an alternative pathway of which *gene B* is a component. As shown in the figure, if an inhibitor of *gene B* can be identified, this can cause death of the cancer cell, without harming normal cells (which maintain wild-type function for *gene A*). High-throughput screens can now be performed using isogenic cell line pairs in which one cell line has a defined defect in a tumor-suppressor pathway. Compounds can be identified that selectively kill the mutant cell line; targets of these compounds have a synthetic lethal relationship to the tumor-suppressor pathway, and are potentially important targets for future therapeutics. Note that this approach allows discovery of drugs that indirectly target deleted tumor-suppressor genes and hence greatly expands the list of physiologically relevant cancer targets.

The PDGFR and its ligand, platelet-derived growth factor (PDGF), are overexpressed in many glioblastomas and in subsets of melanoma, ovarian, pancreatic, gastric, lung, and prostate cancers. Overexpression of the hepatocyte growth factor receptor c-MET has been observed in many human cancers and correlates with a poor prognosis, perhaps due to its role in invasion and metastasis. Small-molecule inhibitors of these RTKs are being developed for clinical use. As described below, the vascular endothelial growth factor receptor (VEGFR), TIE, and EPH RTK families have been identified as important therapeutic targets for inhibition of angiogenesis.

Signaling Pathways Downstream of RTKs: Ras and PI3K Several oncogene and tumor-suppressor gene products are components of signal transduction pathways that emanate from RTK activation (Fig. 80-2). The most extensively studied are the Ras/mitogen-activated protein (MAP) kinase pathway and the phosphatidylinositol-3-kinase (PI3K) pathway, both of which regulate multiple processes in cancer cells, including cell cycle progression, resistance to apoptotic signals, angiogenesis, and cell motility. The development of inhibitors of these pathways is an important avenue of anticancer drug development.

Mutation of the *Ras* protooncogene occurs in 20% of human cancers and results in loss of the response of oncogenic Ras to GTPase-activating proteins (GAPs). The constitutively activated, GTP-bound Ras activates downstream effectors including the MAP kinase and PI3K/Akt pathways. Cancers of the pancreas, colon, and lung and AML harbor frequent *Ras* mutations, with the K-*Ras* allele affected more commonly (85%) than N-*Ras* (15%); H-*Ras* mutations are uncommon in human cancers. In addition, *Ras* activity in tumor cells can be increased by other mechanisms, including upregulation of RTK activity and mutation of GAP proteins (e.g., *NF1* mutations in type I neurofibromatosis). Ras proteins localize to the inner plasma membrane and require posttranslational modifications, including addition of a farnesyl lipid moiety to the cysteine residue of the carboxy-terminal CAAX-box motif. Inhibition of RAS farnesylation by rationally designed farnesyltransferase inhibitors (FTIs) demonstrated encouraging efficacy in preclinical models, most of which utilized oncogenic forms of H-Ras. Despite this, clinical trials of FTIs in patients whose tumors harbor *Ras* mutations have been disappointing, although some activity has been seen in AML. Upon further study, it appears that in the presence of FTIs, lipid modification of the K- and N-Ras proteins occurs by addition of a distinct lipid (geranylgeranyl) through the action of geranylgeranyl transferase-I (GGT-I), which results in restoration of Ras function. Thus, while FTIs are likely to have antitumor activity in select human cancers, their mechanism of action appears to occur by inhibition of farnesylation of proteins other than Ras, perhaps RhoB or Rheb (an activator of mTOR). Oncologists anxiously await the development of bona fide Ras-targeted therapeutics.

Effector pathways downstream of Ras are also targets of anticancer drug efforts. Activation of the Raf serine/threonine kinase is induced by binding to Ras and leads to activation of the MAP kinase pathway (Fig. 80-2). Two-thirds of melanomas and 10% of colon cancers harbor activating mutations in the *BRAF* oncogene, leading to constitutive activation of the downstream MAP/ERK kinase (MEK) and extracellular signal-regulated kinases (ERK1/2). This results in the phosphorylation of ERK's cytoplasmic and nuclear targets and alters the pattern of normal cellular gene expression. Inhibitors of Raf kinases (e.g., sorafinib) have entered clinical trials; their activity against tumors expressing mutant *BRAF* have been disappointing as single agents, but they appear to increase the activity of chemotherapy in some cases. Sorafinib also has significant activity against VEGFRs, and this may account for its clinical activity observed in highly vascular renal cell cancers (see below). Cells harboring mutant *BRAF* are highly sensitive to MEK inhibition, providing another example of "oncogene addiction" (Fig. 80-3).

PI3K is a heterodimeric lipid kinase that catalyses the conversion of phosphatidylinositol bisphosphate (PIP_2) to phosphatidylinositol trisphosphate (PIP_3), which acts as a plasma membrane docking site for proteins that contain a pleckstrin homology (PH) domain. These include the serine/threonine kinases Akt and PDK1 that are key downstream effectors of PI3K action (Fig. 80-2). The PI3K pathway is activated in 30–40% of human cancers and is thought to play a critical role in tumor cell survival, proliferation, growth, and glucose utilization. Amplification or activating point mutation of the gene encoding the catalytic subunit of PI3K (p110) is observed in 20–30% of breast, colon, brain, gastric, and ovarian cancers, and amplification of the *Akt2* gene occurs in breast, ovarian, and pancreatic cancers. The tumor suppressor PTEN (phosphatase with tensin homology), a lipid phosphatase that acts as an off signal for PI3K by dephosphorylating PIP_3, is mutated in many human cancers, leading to unchecked activity of the PI3K pathway. Akt promotes cell survival by activation of the transcription factor nuclear factor of κB (NFκB); it also enhances cell cycle progression by inhibition of glycogen synthetase kinase 3β (GSK3β) and FOXO transcription factors, thus preventing inactivation of Myc, β-catenin, cyclin D1, and cyclin E, and blocking upregulation of $p27^{Kip1}$ and Bim (an apoptosis-inducing protein). Furthermore, the growth of cancer cells requires the activation of two downstream kinases, mammalian target of rapamycin (mTOR) and p70S6K, whose activities promote the translation of cellular mRNAs. Targeted interruption of the PI3K pathway is being attempted at multiple levels. Inhibitors of mTOR, including rapamycin and its more soluble ester derivative temsirolimus (tem), selectively kill human tumor cell lines with PTEN mutations and upregulated PI3K pathway activity. Early clinical data indicate that tem has activity in renal cell cancer, perhaps by blocking the translation of the transcription factor hypoxia-inducible factor (HIF)-1α mRNA, a mediator of cellular responses to hypoxia, which requires mTOR activity for efficient translation.

RTKs activate other signaling pathways. Activation of phospholipase C-γ(PLC) results in the hydrolysis of PIP_2 into diacylglycerol (DAG) and IP_3. DAG together with calcium ion (Ca^{2+}) activates protein kinase C (PKC), a family of serine/threonine-specific protein kinases with different activation requirements, subcellular locations, and substrates in different cell types. PKC is the target of tumor-promoting phorbol esters, and its activation can modulate cell proliferation, differentiation, and tumorigenesis. The PKC inhibitor bryostatin 1 has reached phase II clinical trials and thus far has demonstrated only minimal antitumor activity. However, an antisense oligonucleotide directed against PKC and a number of small molecule inhibitors that demonstrate greater selectivity for PKC isoforms are undergoing clinical evaluation.

ALTERATIONS IN GENE TRANSCRIPTION IN CANCER CELLS: ROLE OF EPIGENETIC CHANGES

Chromatin structure regulates the hierarchical order of sequential gene transcription that governs differentiation and tissue homeostasis. Disruption of chromatin remodeling leads to aberrant gene expression and can induce proliferation of undifferentiated cells, leading to cancer. *Epigenetics* is defined as changes that alter the pattern of gene expression that persist across at least one cell division, but are not caused by changes in the DNA code. Epigenetic changes include alterations of chromatin structure mediated by methylation of cytosine residues in CpG dinucleotides, modification of histones by acetylation or methylation, or changes in higher-order chromosome structure (**Fig. 80-4**). The transcriptional regulatory regions of active genes often contain a high frequency of CpG dinucleotides (referred to as *CpG islands*), which under normal circumstances remain unmethylated. Expression of these genes is controlled by transient association with repressor or activator proteins that regulate transcriptional activation. However, hypermethylation of promoter regions is a common mechanism by which tumor-suppressor loci are epigenetically silenced in cancer cells.

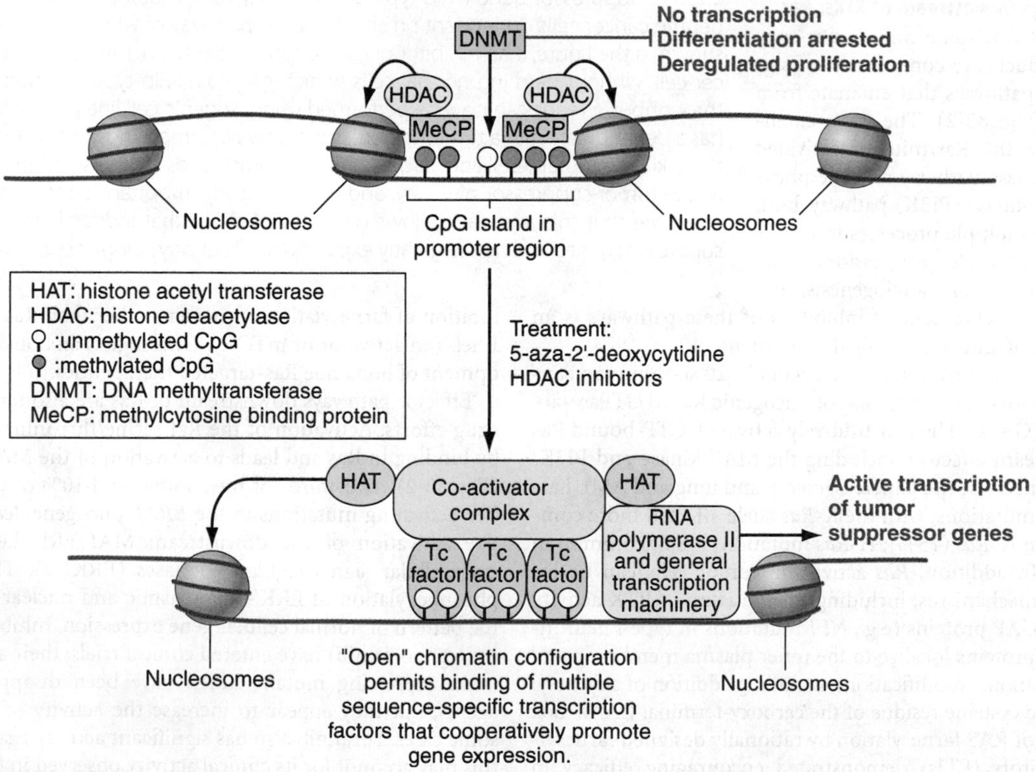

FIGURE 80-4 Epigenetic regulation of gene expression in cancer cells. Tumor-suppressor genes are often epigenetically silenced in cancer cells. In the upper portion, a CpG island within the promoter and enhancer regions of the gene has been methylated, resulting in the recruitment of methyl-cytosine binding proteins (MeCP) and complexes with histone deacetylase (HDAC) activity. Chromatin is in a condensed, nonpermissive conformation that inhibits transcription. Clinical trials are under way utilizing the combination of demethylating agents such as 5-aza-2′-deoxycytidine plus HDAC inhibitors, which together confer an open, permissive chromatin structure (*lower portion*). Transcription factors bind to specific DNA sequences in promoter regions and, through protein-protein interactions, recruit coactivator complexes containing histone acetyl transferase (HAT) activity. This enhances transcription initiation by RNA polymerase II and associated general transcription factors. The expression of the tumor-suppressor gene commences, with phenotypic changes that may include growth arrest, differentiation, or apoptosis.

Thus one allele may be inactivated by mutation or deletion (as occurs in loss of heterozygosity), while expression of the other allele is epigenetically silenced. The mechanisms that target suppressor oncogenes for this form of gene silencing are unknown.

Acetylation of the amino terminus of the core histones H3 and H4 induces an open chromatin conformation that promotes transcription initiation. Histone acetylases are components of coactivator complexes recruited to promoter/enhancer regions by sequence-specific transcription factors during the activation of genes (Fig. 80-4). Histone deacetylases (HDACs; at least 17 are encoded in the human genome) are recruited to genes by transcriptional repressors and prevent the initiation of gene transcription. Methylated cytosine residues in promoter regions become associated with methyl-cytosine–binding proteins that recruit protein complexes with HDAC activity. The balance between permissive and inhibitory chromatin structure is therefore largely determined by the activity of transcription factors in modulating the "histone code" and the methylation status of the genetic regulatory elements of genes.

The pattern of gene transcription is aberrant in all human cancers, and in many cases, epigenetic events are responsible. Unlike genetic events that alter DNA primary structure (e.g., deletions), epigenetic changes are potentially reversible and appear amenable to therapeutic intervention. In many human cancers, including pancreatic cancer and multiple myeloma, the $p16^{Ink4a}$ promoter is inactivated by methylation, thus permitting the unchecked activity of CDK4/cyclin D and rendering pRB nonfunctional. In sporadic forms of renal, breast, and colon cancer, the von Hippel–Lindau (*VHL*), breast cancer 1 (*BRCA1*), and serine/threonine kinase 11 (*STK11*) genes, respectively, are epigenetically silenced. Other targeted genes include the $p15^{Ink4b}$ CDK inhibitor, glutathione-S-transferase (which detoxifies reactive oxygen species), and the E-cadherin molecule (important for junction formation between epithelial cells). Epigenetic silencing can occur in premalignant lesions and can affect genes involved in DNA repair, thus predisposing to further genetic damage. Examples include MLH1 (mut L homologue) in hereditary nonpolyposis colon cancer (HNPCC, also called Lynch syndrome), which is critical for repair of mismatched bases that occur during DNA synthesis, and 0^6-methylguanine-DNA methyltransferase, which removes alkylated guanine adducts from DNA and is often silenced in colon, lung, and lymphoid tumors.

Many human leukemias have chromosomal translocations that code for novel fusion proteins with enzymatic activities that alter chromatin structure. The PML-RAR fusion protein, generated by the t(15;17) observed in most cases of acute promyelocytic leukemia (APL), binds to promoters containing retinoic acid response elements and recruits HDAC to these promoters, effectively inhibiting gene expression. This arrests differentiation at the promyelocyte stage and promotes tumor cell proliferation and survival. Treatment with pharmacologic doses of all-*trans* retinoic acid (ATRA), the ligand for RARα, results in the release of HDAC activity and the recruitment of coactivators, which overcomes the differentiation block. This induced differentiation of APL cells has greatly improved treatment of these patients and has provided a treatment paradigm for the reversal of epigenetic changes in cancer. However, for other leukemia-associated fusion proteins, such as AML-ETO and the MLL fusion proteins seen in AML and ALL, no ligand is known. Therefore, efforts are ongoing to determine the structural basis for interactions between translocation fusion proteins and chromatin remodeling proteins, and to use this information to rationally design small molecules that will disrupt specific protein-protein associations. Drugs that block the enzymatic activity of HDAC are being developed. A number of different chemical classes of HDAC inhibitors have demonstrated antitumor activity in clinical studies against cutaneous T cell lymphoma (e.g., vorinostat) and some solid tumors. HDAC inhibitors may target cancer cells via a number of mechanisms including upregulation of death receptors (DR4/5, FAS, and their ligands) and $p21^{Cip1/Waf1}$, as well as inhibition of cell cycle checkpoints.

Major therapeutic efforts are also under way to reverse the hypermethylation of CpG islands that characterizes many solid tumors. Drugs that induce DNA demethylation, such as 5-aza-2′-deoxycytidine, can lead to reexpression of silenced genes in cancer cells with restoration of function. However, 5-aza-2′-deoxycytidine has limited aqueous solubility and is myelosuppressive. Other inhibitors of DNA methyltransferases are in development. In ongoing clinical trials, inhibitors of DNA methylation are being combined with HDAC inhibitors. The hope is that by reversing coexisting epigenetic changes, the deregulated patterns of gene transcription in cancer cells will be at least partially reversed.

Aberrant signal transduction pathways activate a number of transcription factors that promote tumor cell proliferation and survival. These include signal transducer and activator of transcription (STAT)-3 and STAT5, NFκB, β-catenin (a component of the APC tumor-suppressor pathway), the heterodimer of c-Jun and Fos known as AP1, and c-Myc. The ability to target these transcription factors therapeutically does not currently exist. However, structural and molecular approaches may make it possible to identify small molecules that would inhibit protein-protein interactions needed for transcription factor dimerization or interaction with coactivator proteins. A small-molecule inhibitor has been developed that blocks the association of Myc with its partner Max, thereby inhibiting Myc-induced transformation. Many transcription factors are activated by phosphorylation, which can be prevented by tyrosine- or serine/threonine kinase inhibitors. The transcription factor NFκB is a heterodimer composed of p65 and p50 subunits that associate with an inhibitor, IκB, in the cell cytoplasm. In response to growth factor or cytokine signaling, a multi-subunit kinase called IKK (IκB-kinase) phosphorylates IκB and directs its degradation by the ubiquitin/proteasome system. NFκB, free of its inhibitor, translocates to the nucleus and activates target genes, many of which promote the survival of tumor cells. Novel drugs called *proteasome inhibitors* block the proteolysis of IκB, thereby preventing NFκB activation. For unexplained reasons, this is selectively toxic to tumor cells. Further studies have indicated that the antitumor effects of proteasome inhibitors are more complicated and involve the inhibition of the degradation of multiple cellular proteins. Proteasome inhibitors [bortezomib (Velcade)] have shown very significant activity in patients with multiple myeloma, including partial and complete remissions. Inhibitors of IKK are also in development, with the hope of more selectively blocking the degradation of IκB, thus "locking" NFκB in an inhibitory complex and rendering the cancer cell more susceptible to apoptosis-inducing agents.

Estrogen receptors (ERs) and androgen receptors, members of the steroid hormone family of nuclear receptors, are targets of inhibition by drugs used to treat breast and prostate cancers, respectively. Tamoxifen, a partial agonist and antagonist of ER function, can mediate tumor regression in metastatic breast cancer and can prevent disease recurrence in the adjuvant setting, saving thousands of lives each year. Tamoxifen binds to the ER and modulates its transcriptional activity, inhibiting activity in the breast but promoting activity in bone and uterine epithelium. Selective estrogen receptor modulators (SERMs) have been developed with the hope of a more beneficial modulation of ER activity, i.e., antiestrogenic activity in the breast, uterus, and ovary, but estrogenic for bone, brain, and cardiovascular tissues. Aromatase inhibitors, which block the conversion of androgens to estrogens in breast and subcutaneous fat tissues, have demonstrated improved clinical efficacy compared with tamoxifen and are often used as first-line therapy in patients with ER-positive disease (Chap. 86).

APOPTOSIS

Tissue homeostasis requires a balance between the death of aged, terminally differentiated cells and their renewal by proliferation of committed progenitors. Genetic damage to growth-regulating genes of stem cells could lead to catastrophic results for the host as a whole. However, genetic events causing activation of oncogenes or loss of tumor suppressors, which would be predicted to lead to unregulated cell proliferation, instead activate signal transduction pathways that block aberrant cell proliferation. These pathways can lead to programmed cell death (*apoptosis*) or irreversible growth arrest (*senescence*). Much as a pano-

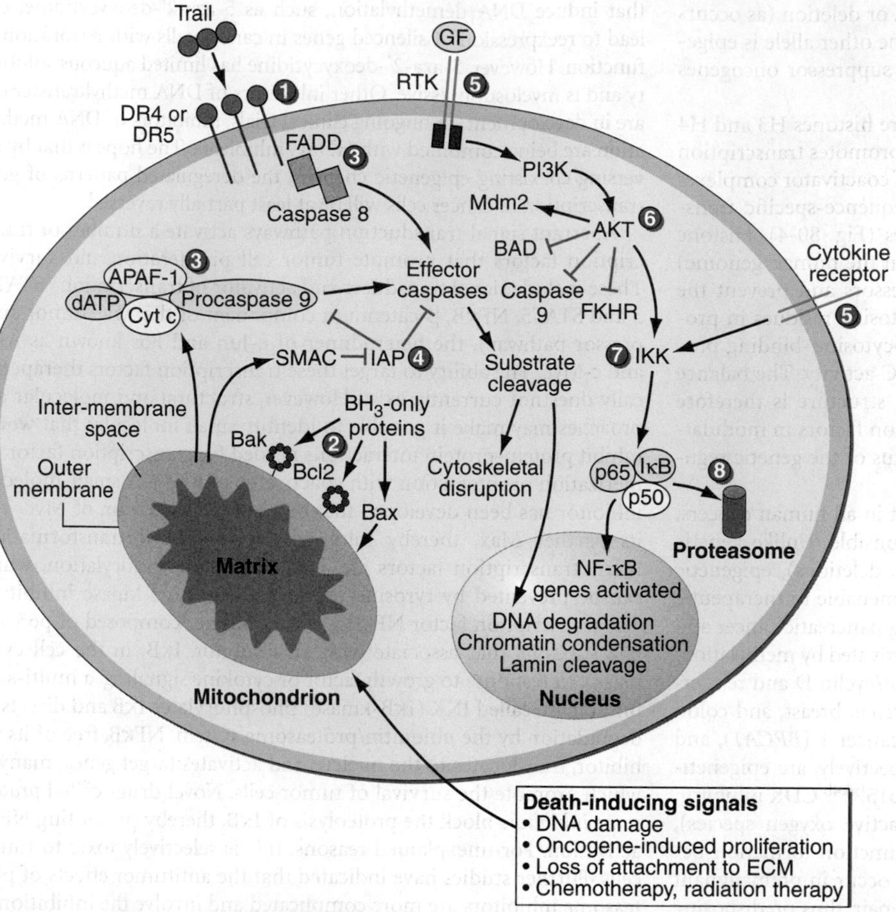

FIGURE 80-5 Therapeutic strategies to overcome aberrant survival pathways in cancer cells. ***1.*** The extrinsic pathway of apoptosis can be selectively induced in cancer cells by TRAIL (the ligand for death receptors 4 and 5) or by agonistic monoclonal antibodies. ***2.*** Inhibition of antiapoptotic Bcl-2 family members with antisense oligonucleotides or inhibitors of the BH_3-binding pocket will promote formation of Bak- or Bax-induced pores in the mitochondrial outer membrane. ***3.*** Epigenetic silencing of APAF-1, caspase-8, and other proteins can be overcome using demethylating agents and inhibitors of histone deacetylases. ***4.*** Inhibitor of apoptosis proteins (IAP) blocks activation of caspases; small-molecule inhibitors of IAP function (mimicking SMAC action) should lower the threshold for apoptosis. ***5.*** Signal transduction pathways originating with activation of receptor tyrosine kinase receptors (RTKs) or cytokine receptors promote survival of cancer cells by a number of mechanisms. Inhibiting receptor function with monoclonal antibodies, such as trastuzumab or cetuximab, or inhibiting kinase activity with small-molecular inhibitors can block the pathway. ***6.*** The Akt kinase phosphorylates many regulators of apoptosis to promote cell survival; inhibitors of Akt may render tumor cells more sensitive to apoptosis-inducing signals; however, the possibility of toxicity to normal cells may limit the therapeutic value of these agents. ***7*** and ***8.*** Activation of the transcription factor NFκB (composed of p65 and p50 subunits) occurs when its inhibitor, IκB, is phosphorylated by IκB-kinase (IKK), with subsequent degradation of IκB by the proteasome. Inhibition of IKK activity should selectively block the activation of NFκB target genes, many of which promote cell survival. Inhibitors of proteasome function are FDA approved and may work in part by preventing destruction of IκB, thus blocking NFκB nuclear localization. NFκB is unlikely to be the only target for proteasome inhibitors.

ply of intra- and extracellular signals impinge upon the core cell cycle machinery to regulate cell division, so too these signals are transmitted to a core enzymatic machinery that regulates cell death and survival.

Apoptosis is induced by two main pathways (Fig. 80-5). The extrinsic pathway of apoptosis is activated by cross-linking members of the tumor necrosis factor (TNF) receptor superfamily, such as CD95 (Fas) and death receptors DR4 and DR5, by their receptors, Fas ligand or TRAIL (TNF-related apoptosis-inducing ligand), respectively. This induces the association of FADD (Fas-associated death domain) and procaspase-8 to death domain motifs of the receptors. Caspase-8 is activated and then cleaves and activates effector caspases-3 and -7, which then target cellular constituents (including caspase-activated DNAse, cytoskeletal proteins, and a number of regulatory proteins), inducing the morphologic appearance characteristic of apoptosis. The intrinsic pathway of apoptosis is initiated by the release of cytochrome c and SMAC (second mitochondrial activator of caspases) from the mitochondrial intermembrane space in response to a variety of noxious stimuli, including DNA damage, loss of adherence to the extracellular matrix (ECM), oncogene-induced proliferation, and growth factor deprivation. Upon release into the cytoplasm, cytochrome c associates with dATP, procaspase-9, and the adaptor protein APAF-1, leading to the sequential activation of caspase-9 and effector caspases. SMAC binds to and blocks the function of inhibitor of apoptosis proteins (IAPs), negative regulators of caspase activation.

The release of apoptosis-inducing proteins from the mitochondria is regulated by pro- and antiapoptotic members of the Bcl-2 family. Antiapoptotic members (e.g., Bcl-2, Bcl-XL, and Mcl-1) associate with the mitochondrial outer membrane via their carboxy termini, exposing to the cytoplasm a hydrophobic binding pocket composed of Bcl-2 homology (BH) domains 1, 2, and 3 that is crucial for their activity. Perturbations of normal physiologic processes in specific cellular compartments lead to the activation of BH3-only proapoptotic family members (such as Bad, Bim, Bid, Puma, Noxa, and others) that can alter the conformation of the outer-membrane proteins Bax and Bak, which then oligomerize to form pores in the mitochondrial outer membrane resulting in cytochrome c release. If BH3-only proteins are sequestered by Bcl-2, Bcl-XL, or Mcl-1, pores do not form and apoptosis-inducing proteins are not released from the mitochondrion. The relative levels of expression of antiapoptotic Bcl-2 family members compared to the levels of proapoptotic BH3-only proteins at the mitochondrial membrane determines the activation state of the intrinsic pathway. The mitochondrion must therefore be recognized not only as an organelle with vital roles in intermediary metabolism and oxidative phosphorylation but also as a central regulatory structure of the apoptotic process.

The evolution of tumor cells to a more malignant phenotype requires the acquisition of genetic changes that subvert apoptosis pathways and promote cancer cell survival and resistance to anticancer therapies. However, because of their deranged physiology, cancer cells may be more vulnerable than normal cells to therapeutic interventions that target the apoptosis pathways that cancer cells are very dependent upon. For instance, overexpression of Bcl-2 as a result of the t(14;18) translocation contributes to follicular lymphoma. Upregulation of Bcl-2 expression is also observed in prostate, breast, and lung cancers and melanoma. Targeting of antiapoptotic Bcl-2 family members has been accomplished by the identification of several low-molecular-weight compounds that bind to the hydrophobic pockets of either Bcl-2 or Bcl-XL and block their ability to associate with death-inducing BH3-only proteins. These compounds inhibit the antiapoptotic activities of Bcl-2 and Bcl-XL at nanomolar concentrations and will soon be entering clinical trials, first as single agents and then in combination with cytotoxic agents.

Preclinical studies targeting death receptors DR4 and -5 have demonstrated that recombinant, soluble, human TRAIL or humanized monoclonal antibodies with agonist activity against DR4 or -5 can induce apoptosis of tumor cells while sparing normal cells. The mechanisms for this selectivity may include expression of decoy receptors or elevated levels of intracellular inhibitors (such as FLIP, which competes with caspase-8 for FADD) by normal cells but not tumor cells. Synergy has been shown between TRAIL-induced apoptosis and chemotherapeutic agents. For instance, some colon cancers encode mutated Bax protein as the result of mismatch repair (MMR) defects and are resistant to TRAIL. However, upregulation of Bak by chemotherapy restores the ability of TRAIL to activate the mitochondrial pathway of apoptosis. In early phase clinical trials, agonistic antibodies for DR4 and -5 and recombinant TRAIL trimers have led to the stabilization of tumor growth with a few cases of tumor shrinkage; however, studies have not yet shown that clinical activity correlates with activation of the extrinsic pathway of apoptosis.

Many of the signal transduction pathways perturbed in cancer promote tumor cell survival (Fig. 80-5). These include activation of the PI3K/Akt pathway, increased levels of the NFκB transcription factor, and epigenetic silencing of genes such as APAF-1 and caspase-8. Each of these pathways is a target for therapeutic agents that, in addition to affecting cancer cell proliferation or gene expression, may render cancer cells more susceptible to apoptosis, thus promoting synergy when combined with other chemotherapeutic agents.

Some tumor cells resist drug-induced apoptosis by expression of one or more members of the ABC family of ATP-dependent efflux pumps that mediate the multidrug resistance (MDR) phenotype. The prototype, P-glycoprotein (PGP), spans the plasma membrane 12 times and has two ATP-binding sites. Hydrophobic drugs (e.g., anthracyclines and vinca alkaloids) are recognized by PGP as they enter the cell and are pumped out. Numerous clinical studies have failed to demonstrate that drug resistance can be overcome using inhibitors of PGP. However, ABC transporters have different substrate specificities, and inhibition of a single family member may not be sufficient to overcome the MDR phenotype. A more rational targeting of specific transporters expressed by distinct tumor types may lead to increased efficacy.

METASTASIS: DETERMINING RISK AND DEVELOPING THERAPEUTIC STRATEGIES

The three major features of tissue invasion are cell adhesion to the basement membrane, local proteolysis of the membrane, and movement of the cell through the rent in the membrane and the ECM. Malignant cells that gain access to the circulation must then repeat those steps at a remote site, find a hospitable niche in a foreign tissue, and induce the growth of new blood vessels. There are currently few drugs that directly target the process of metastasis. Metalloproteinase inhibitors (see "Tumor Angiogenesis," below) represent an initial attempt to inhibit the migration of tumor cells into blood and lymphatic vessels. The rate-limiting step for metastasis is the ability for tumor cells to survive and expand in the novel microenvironment of the metastatic site, and multiple host-tumor interactions determine the ultimate outcome (Fig. 80-6).

The metastatic phenotype may be a characteristic of all cells constituting the primary tumor; however, it is likely that variants with metastatic potential arise due to genetic and epigenetic events that characterize tumor progression (Fig. 80-6). A number of candidate metastasis-suppressor genes have been identified. The loss of function of these genes enhances metastasis, and although the molecular mechanisms are in many cases uncertain, one common theme is an enhancing of the ability of the metastatic tumor cells to overcome the many apoptosis signals they encounter during the metastatic process. Gene expression profiling is being used to study the metastatic process with the goal of identifying signatures characteristic of primary tumors that have a high propensity to metastasize, leading to a more rational basis for the use of adjuvant chemotherapy.

Bone metastases are extremely painful, cause fractures of weight-bearing bones, can lead to hypercalcemia, and are a major cause of morbidity for cancer patients. Osteoclasts and their monocyte–derived precursors express the surface receptor RANK (receptor activator of NFκB), which is required for terminal differentiation and activation of osteoclasts. Osteo-

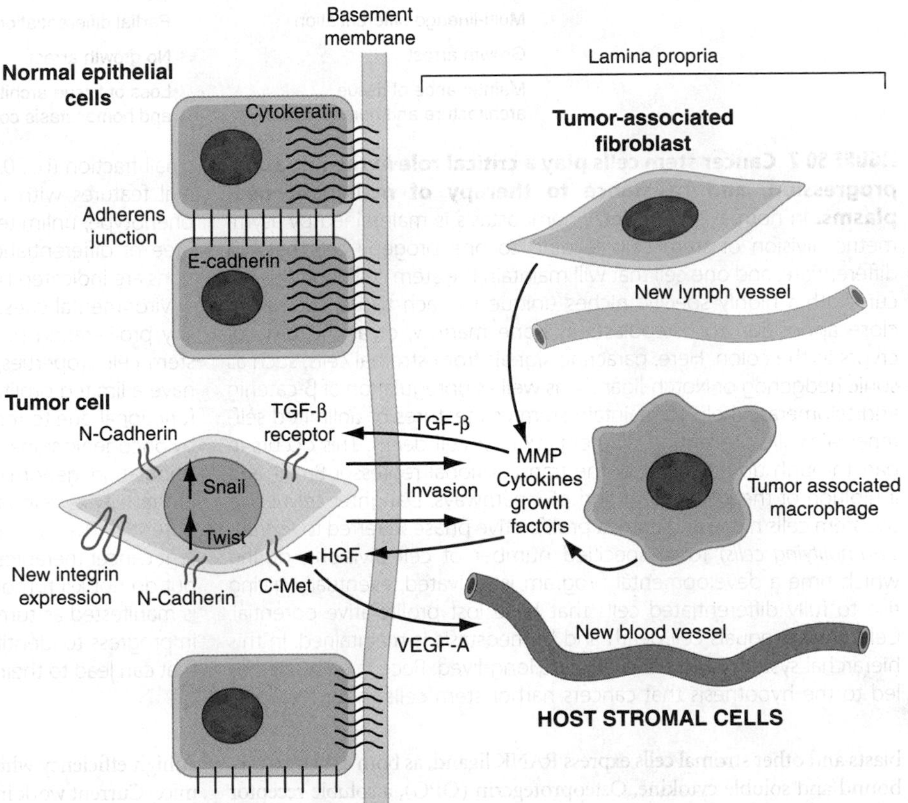

FIGURE 80-6 Oncogene signaling pathways are activated during tumor progression and promote metastatic potential. This figure shows a cancer cell that has undergone epithelial to mesenchymal transition (EMT) under the influence of several environmental signals. Critical components include activated transforming growth factor beta (TGF-β) and the hepatocyte growth factor (HGF)/c-Met pathways, as well as changes in the expression of adhesion molecules that mediate cell-cell and cell-extracellular matrix interactions. Important changes in gene expression are mediated by the Snail and Twist family of transcriptional repressors (whose expression is induced by the oncogenic pathways), leading to reduced expression of E-cadherin, a key component of adherens junctions between epithelial cells. This, in conjunction with upregulation of N-cadherin, a change in the pattern of expression of integrins (which mediate cell-extracellular matrix associations that are important for cell motility), and a switch in intermediate filament expression from cytokeratin to vimentin, results in the phenotypic change from adherent highly organized epithelial cells to motile and invasive cells with a fibroblast or mesenchymal morphology. EMT is thought to be an important step leading to metastasis in some human cancers. Host stromal cells, including tumor-associated fibroblasts and macrophages, play an important role in modulating tumor cell behavior through secretion of growth factors and proangiogenic cytokines, and matrix metalloproteinases that degrade the basement membrane. VEGF-A, -C, and -D are produced by tumor cells and stromal cells in response to hypoxia or oncogenic signals, and induce production of new blood vessels and lymphatic channels through which tumor cells metastasize to lymph nodes or tissues.

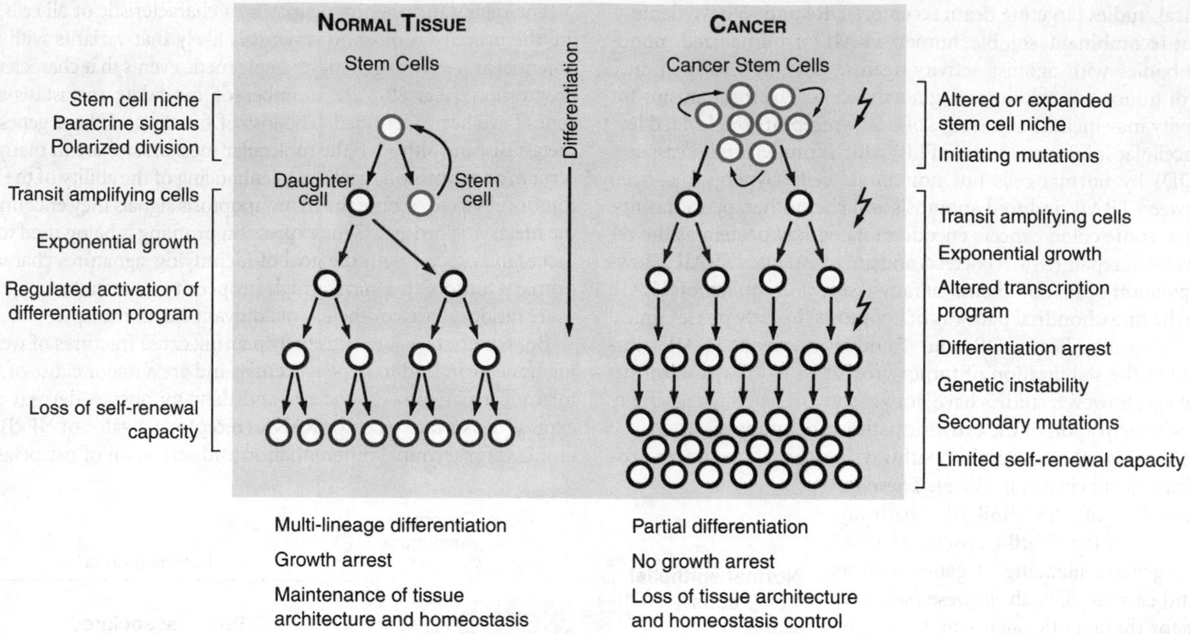

FIGURE 80-7 Cancer stem cells play a critical role in the initiation, progression, and resistance to therapy of malignant neoplasms. In normal tissues (***left***), homeostasis is maintained by asymmetric division of stem cells leading to one progeny cell that will differentiate, and one cell that will maintain the stem cell pool. This occurs within highly specific niches unique to each tissue, such as in close apposition to osteoblasts in bone marrow, or at the base of crypts in the colon. Here, paracrine signals from stromal cells, such as sonic hedgehog or Notch-ligands, as well as upregulation of β-catenin and telomerase, help to maintain stem cell features of unlimited self-renewal while preventing differentiation or cell death. This occurs in part through upregulation of the transcriptional repressor Bmi-1 and inhibition of the $p16^{Ink4a}$/Arf and p53 pathways. Daughter cells leave the stem cells niche and enter a proliferative phase (referred to as *transit-amplifying cells*) for a specified number of cell divisions, during which time a developmental program is activated, eventually giving rise to fully differentiated cells that have lost proliferative potential. Cell renewal equals cell death and homeostasis is maintained. In this hierarchal system, only stem cells are long-lived. Recent evidence has led to the hypothesis that cancers harbor stem cells that make up a small fraction (i.e., 0.001–1%) of all cancer cells. These cells share several features with normal stem cells, including an undifferentiated phenotype, unlimited self-renewal potential, a capacity for some degree of differentiation; however, due to initiating mutations (mutations are indicated by lightning bolts), they are no longer regulated by environmental cues. The cancer stem cell pool is expanded, and rapidly proliferating progeny, through additional mutations, may attain stem cell properties, although most of this population is thought to have a limited proliferative capacity. Differentiation programs are dysfunctional due to reprogramming of the pattern of gene transcription by oncogenic signaling pathways. Within the cancer transit-amplifying population, genomic instability generates aneuploidy and clonal heterogeneity as cells attain a fully malignant phenotype with metastatic potential. The cancer stem cell hypothesis has led to the idea that current cancer therapies may be effective at killing the bulk of tumor cells, but do not kill tumor stem cells, leading to a regrowth of tumors that is manifested as tumor recurrence or disease progression. Research is in progress to identify unique molecular features of cancer stem cells that can lead to their direct targeting by novel therapeutic agents.

blasts and other stromal cells express RANK ligand, as both a membrane-bound and soluble cytokine. Osteoprotegerin (OPG), a soluble receptor for RANK ligand produced by stromal cells, acts as a decoy receptor to inhibit RANK activation. The relative balance of RANK ligand and OPG determines the activation state of RANK on osteoclasts. Many tumors increase osteoclast activity by secretion of substances such as parathyroid hormone (PTH), PTH-related peptide, interleukin (IL)-1, or Mip1, that perturb the homeostatic balance of bone remodeling by increasing RANK signaling. One example is multiple myeloma, where tumor cell–stromal cell interactions activate osteoclasts and inhibit osteoblasts, leading to the development of multiple lytic bone lesions. Inhibition of RANK ligand by IV administration of recombinant OPG or the extracellular domain of RANK linked to an immunoglobulin Fc-receptor (RANK-Fc) can prevent further bone destruction. Bisphosphonates are also effective inhibitors of osteoclast function that are used in the treatment of cancer patients with bone metastases.

NEW CONCEPTS IN THE DEVELOPMENT OF CANCER THERAPEUTICS

CANCER STEM CELLS

It has long been recognized that only a small proportion of the cells within a tumor are capable of initiating colonies in vitro or of forming tumors at high efficiency when injected into immunocompromised NOD/SCID mice. Current work indicates that human acute and chronic myeloid leukemias (AML and CML) have a small population of cells (<1%) that have properties of stem cells, such as unlimited self-renewal and the capacity to cause leukemia when serially transplanted in mice. These cells have an undifferentiated phenotype ($Thy1^-CD34^+CD38^-$, and negative for other differentiation markers) and resemble normal stem cells in many ways, but are no longer under homeostatic control (Fig. 80-7). Solid tumors may also contain a population of stem cells. Cancer stem cells, like their normal counterparts, have unlimited proliferative capacity and paradoxically traverse the cell cycle at a very slow rate; cancer growth occurs largely due to expansion of the stem cell pool, the unregulated proliferation of the transit amplifying population, and failure of apoptosis pathways (Fig. 80-7). Slow cell cycle progression, plus high levels of expression of anti-apoptotic Bcl-2 family members and drug efflux pumps of the MDR family, render cancer stem cells less vulnerable to cancer chemotherapy or radiation therapy. Implicit in the cancer stem cell hypothesis is the idea that failure to cure most human cancers is due to the fact that current therapeutic agents do not kill the stem cells. If cancer stem cells can be identified and isolated, then aberrant signaling pathways that distinguish these cells from normal tissue stem cells can be identified and targeted. Oncologists eagerly await a new class of agent that may directly attack the cells that drive tumor growth.

ONCOGENE ADDICTION AND SYNTHETIC LETHALITY

The concepts of oncogene addiction and synthetic lethality have spurred new drug development targeting oncogene and tumor-suppressor pathways. As discussed earlier in this chapter and outlined in Fig. 80-3, cancer cells become physiologically dependent upon signaling pathways containing activated oncogenes; this can effect proliferation (i.e., mutated Ras, BRAF, overexpressed Myc, or activated tyrosine kinases), survival (overexpression of Bcl-2 or NFκB), cell metabolism (as occurs when HIF-1α and Akt increase dependence on glycolysis), and perhaps angiogenesis (production of VEGF, e.g., renal cell cancer). In such cases, targeted inhibition of the pathway can lead to specific killing of the cancer cells. However, targeting defects in tumor-suppressor genes has been much more difficult, since the target of the mutation is often deleted. However, identifying genes that have a synthetic lethal relationship to tumor-suppressor pathways may allow targeting of proteins required uniquely by the tumor cells (Fig. 80-3, panel *B*). Several examples of this have been identified. For instance, the von Hippel–Landau tumor-suppressor-protein is inactivated in 60% of renal cell cancers, leading to overexpression of HIF-1α and the subsequent activation of downstream genes that promote angiogenesis, proliferation, survival, and altered glucose metabolism. HIF-1α mRNA has a complex 5′-terminus that indirectly requires the activity of mTOR (via activation of p70S6K and inhibition of 4E-BP) for efficient protein translation. Inhibitors of mTOR block HIF-1α translation and have significant clinical activity in renal cell cancer. In this case, mTOR is synthetic lethal to VHL loss (Fig. 80-3), and its inhibition results in selective killing of cancer cells. Conceptually, this provides a framework for genetic screens to identify other synthetic lethal combinations involving known tumor-suppressor genes, and development of novel therapeutic agents to target dependent pathways.

In summary, our expanding knowledge of the genetic and molecular abnormalities in cancer cells, and their phenotypic correlates, has led to the development and FDA approval of a number of targeted pharmaceutical agents for the treatment of cancer (Table 80-2). This list will expand to include inhibitors of pathways currently under investigation and those yet to be discovered, yielding novel therapeutics with greater efficacy with less toxicity.

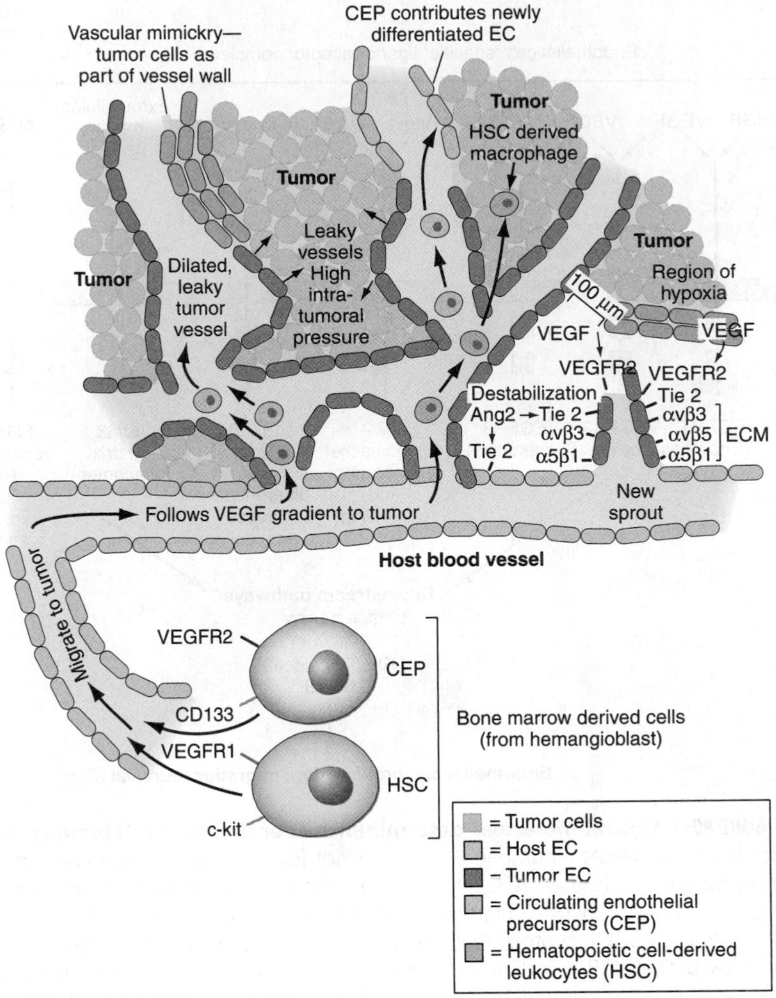

FIGURE 80-8 Tumor angiogenesis is a complex process involving many different cell types that must proliferate, migrate, invade, and differentiate in response to signals from the tumor microenvironment. Endothelial cells (ECs) sprout from host vessels in response to VEGF, bFGF, Ang2, and other proangiogenic stimuli. Sprouting is stimulated by VEGF/VEGFR2, Ang2/Tie-2, and integrin/extracellular matrix (ECM) interactions. Bone marrow–derived circulating endothelial precursors (CEPs) migrate to the tumor in response to VEGF and differentiate into ECs, while hematopoietic stem cells differentiate into leukocytes, including tumor-associated macrophages that secrete angiogenic growth factors and produce MMPs that remodel the ECM and release bound growth factors. Tumor cells themselves may directly form parts of vascular channels within tumors. The pattern of vessel formation is haphazard: vessels are tortuous, dilated, leaky, and branch in random ways. This leads to uneven blood flow within the tumor, with areas of acidosis and hypoxia (which stimulate release of angiogenic factors) and high intratumoral pressures that inhibit delivery of therapeutic agents.

TUMOR ANGIOGENESIS

The growth of primary and metastatic tumors to larger than a few millimeters requires the recruitment of neighboring blood vessels and vascular endothelial cells to support their metabolic requirements. The diffusion limit for oxygen in tissues is ~100 μm. A critical element in the growth of primary tumors and formation of metastatic sites is the *angiogenic switch*: the ability of the tumor to promote the formation of new capillaries from preexisting host vessels. The angiogenic switch is a phase in tumor development when the dynamic balance of pro- and antiangiogenic factors is tipped in favor of vessel formation by the effects of the tumor on its immediate environment. Stimuli for tumor angiogenesis include hypoxia, inflammation, and genetic lesions in oncogenes or tumor suppressors that alter tumor cell gene expression. Angiogenesis consists of several steps, including the stimulation of endothelial cells (ECs) by growth factors, the degradation of the ECM by proteases, proliferation of ECs and migration into the tumor, and the eventual formation of new capillary tubes.

Tumor blood vessels are not normal; they have chaotic architecture and blood flow. Due to an imbalance of angiogenic regulators such as VEGF and angiopoietins (see below), tumor vessels are tortuous and dilated with an uneven diameter, excessive branching, and shunting. Tumor blood flow is variable, with areas of hypoxia and acidosis leading to the selection of variants that are resistant to hypoxia-induced apoptosis (often due to the loss of p53 expression). Tumor vessel walls have numerous openings, widened interendothelial junctions, and discontinuous or absent basement membrane; this contributes to the high vascular permeability of these vessels and, together with lack of functional intratumoral lymphatics, causes interstitial hypertension within the tumor (which also interferes with the delivery of therapeutics to the tumor; Figs. 80-8, 80-9, and 80-10). Tumor blood vessels lack perivascular cells such as pericytes and smooth-muscle cells that normally regulate flow in response to tissue metabolic needs.

Unlike normal blood vessels, the vascular lining of tumor vessels is not a homogeneous layer of ECs but often consists of a mosaic of ECs and tumor cells; the concept of cancer cell–derived vascular channels, which may be lined by ECM secreted by the tumor cells, is referred to

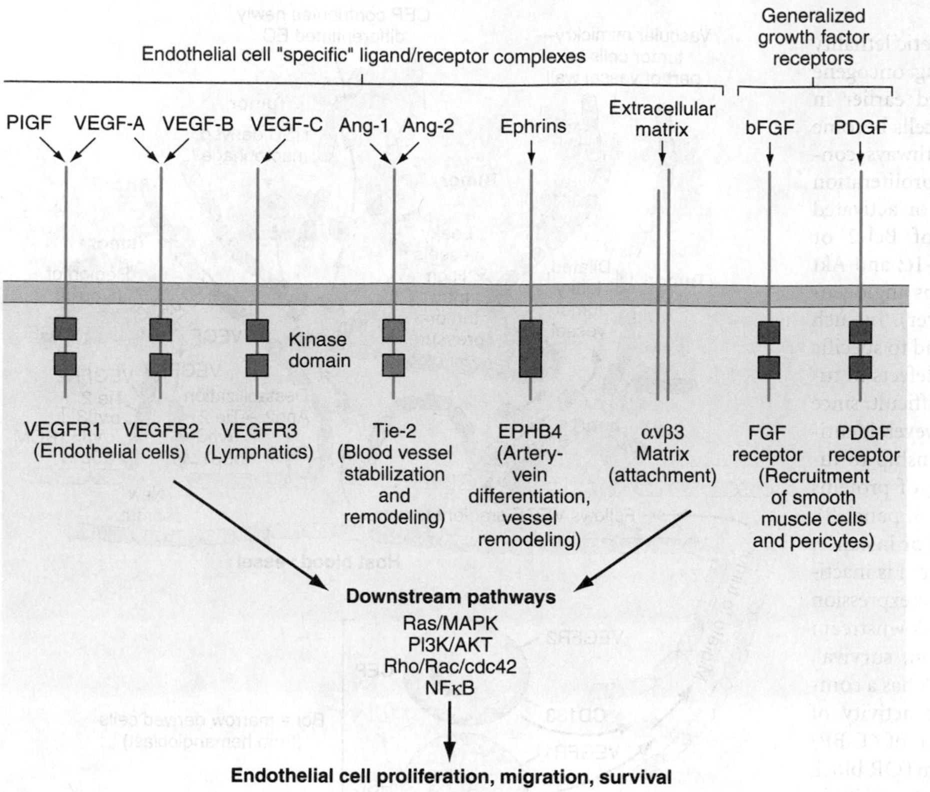

FIGURE 80-9 Critical molecular determinants of endothelial cell biology. Angiogenic endothelium expresses a number of receptors not found on resting endothelium. These include receptor tyrosine kinases (RTK) and integrins that bind to the extracellular matrix and mediate endothelial cells adhesion, migration, and invasion. Endothelial cells (ECs) also express RTK (i.e., the FGF and PDGF receptors) that are found on many other cell types. Critical functions mediated by activated RTK include proliferation, migration, and enhanced survival of endothelial cells, as well as regulation of the recruitment of perivascular cells and bloodborne circulating endothelial precursors and hematopoietic stem cells to the tumor. Intracellular signaling via EC-specific RTK utilizes molecular pathways that may be targets for future antiangiogenic therapies.

as *vascular mimickry*. It is unclear whether tumor cells actually form structural elements of vascular channels or represent tumor cells in transit into or out of the vessel. However, the former is supported by evidence that in some human colon cancers, tumor cells can comprise up to 15% of vessel walls. The ECs of angiogenic blood vessels are unlike quiescent ECs found in adult vessels, where only 0.01% of ECs are dividing. During tumor angiogenesis, ECs are highly proliferative and express a number of plasma membrane proteins that are characteristic of activated endothelium, including growth factor receptors and adhesion molecules such as integrins.

MECHANISMS OF TUMOR VESSEL FORMATION

Tumors utilize a number of mechanisms to promote their vascularization, and in each case they subvert normal angiogenic processes to suit this purpose (Fig. 80-8). Primary or metastatic tumor cells sometimes arise in proximity to host blood vessels and grow around these vessels, parasitizing nutrients by coopting the local blood supply. However, most tumor blood vessels arise by the process of *sprouting*, in which tumors secrete trophic angiogenic molecules, the most potent being VEGF, that induce the proliferation and migration of host ECs into the tumor. Sprouting in normal and pathogenic angiogenesis is regulated by three families of transmembrane RTKs expressed on ECs and their ligands (VEGFs, angiopoietins, ephrins; Fig. 80-9), which are produced by tumor cells, inflammatory cells, or stromal cells in the tumor microenvironment.

When tumor cells arise in or metastasize to an avascular area, they grow to a size limited by hypoxia and nutrient deprivation. Hypoxia, a key regulator of tumor angiogenesis, causes the transcriptional induction of the gene encoding VEGF by a process that involves stabilization of HIF-1α. Under normoxic conditions, HIF-1α levels are maintained at a low level by proteasome-mediated destruction regulated by a ubiquitin E3-ligase encoded by the VHL tumor-suppressor locus. However, under hypoxic conditions, HIF-1α is not hydroxylated and association with VHL does not occur; therefore HIF-1 levels increase, and target genes including VEGF, nitric oxide synthetase (NOS), and Ang2 are induced. Loss of the *VHL* genes, as occurs in familial and sporadic renal cell carcinomas, results in HIF-1α stabilization and induction of VEGF. Most tumors have hypoxic regions due to poor blood flow, and tumor cells in these areas stain positive for HIF-1α expression; in renal cancers with *VHL* deletion, all of the tumor cells express high levels of HIF-1α, and VEGF-induced angiogenesis leads to high microvascular density (hence the term *hypernephroma*).

VEGF and its receptors are required for *vasculogenesis* (the de novo formation of blood vessels from differentiating endothelial cells, as occurs during embryonic development) and angiogenesis under normal (wound healing, corpus luteum formation) and pathologic processes (tumor angiogenesis, inflammatory conditions such as rheumatoid arthritis). VEGF-A is a heparin-binding glycoprotein with at least four isoforms (splice variants) that regulates blood vessel formation by binding to the RTKs VEGFR1 and VEGFR2, which are expressed on all ECs in addition to a subset of hematopoietic cells (Fig. 80-8). VEGFR2 regulates EC proliferation, migration, and survival, while VEGFR1 may act as an antagonist of R1 in ECs but is probably also important for angioblast differentiation during embryogenesis. Tumor vessels appear to be more dependent on VEGFR signaling for growth and survival than normal ECs. While VEGF signaling is a critical initiator of angiogenesis, this is a complex process regulated by additional signaling pathways (Fig. 80-9). The angiopoietin, Ang1, produced by stromal cells, binds to the EC RTK Tie-2 and promotes the interaction of ECs with the ECM and perivascular cells, such as pericytes and smooth-muscle cells, to form tight, non-leaky vessels. PDGF and basic fibroblast growth factor (bFGF) help to recruit these perivascular cells. Ang1 is required for maintaining the quiescence and stability of mature blood vessels and prevents the vascular permeability normally induced by VEGF and inflammatory cytokines.

For tumor cell–derived VEGF to initiate sprouting from host vessels, the stability conferred by the Ang1/Tie2 pathway must be perturbed; this occurs by the secretion of Ang2 by ECs that are undergoing active remodeling. Ang2 binds to Tie2 and is a competitive inhibitor of Ang1 action: under the influence of Ang2, preexisting blood vessels become more responsive to remodeling signals, with less adherence of ECs to stroma and associated perivascular cells and more responsiveness to VEGF. Therefore, Ang2 is required at early stages of tumor angiogenesis for destabilizing the vasculature by making host ECs more sensitive to angiogenic signals. Since tumor ECs are blocked by Ang2, there is no stabilization by the Ang1/Tie2 interaction, and tumor blood vessels are leaky, hemorrhagic, and have poor association of ECs with underlying stroma. Sprouting tumor ECs express high levels of the transmembrane protein ephrin-B2 and its receptor, the RTK EPH whose signaling appears to work with the angiopoietins during vessel remodeling. During embryogenesis, EPH receptors are ex-

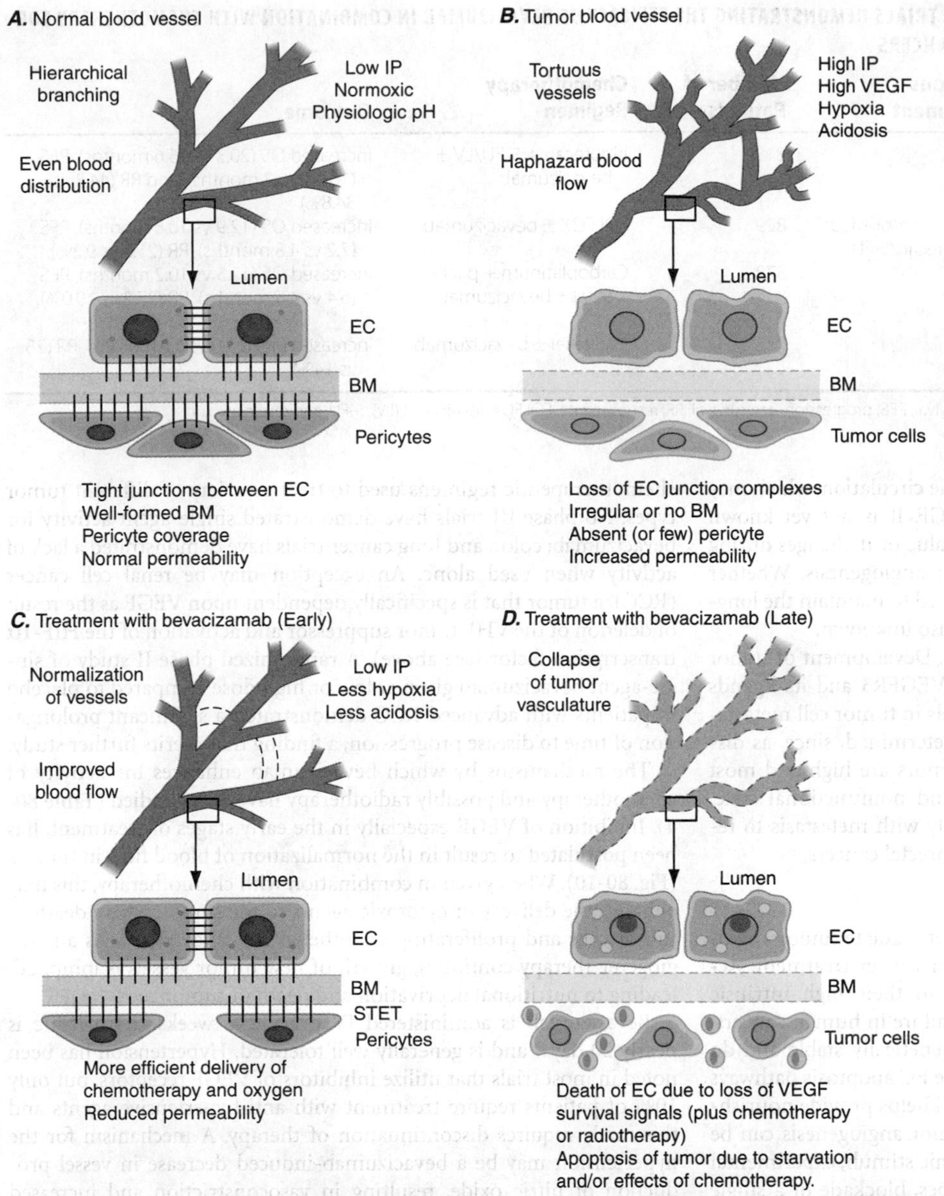

FIGURE 80-10 Normalization of tumor blood vessels due to inhibition of VEGF signaling. ***A.*** Blood vessels in normal tissues exhibit a regular hierarchical branching pattern that delivers blood to tissues in a spatially and temporally efficient manner to meet the metabolic needs of the tissue (top). At the microscopic level, tight junctions are maintained between endothelial cells (EC), which are adherent to a thick and evenly distributed basement membrane (BM). Pericytes form a surrounding layer that provides trophic signals to the EC and helps maintain proper vessel tone. Vascular permeability is regulated, interstitial fluid pressure is low, and oxygen tension and pH are physiologic. ***B.*** Tumors have abnormal vessels with tortuous branching and dilated, irregular interconnecting branches, causing uneven blood flow with areas of hypoxia and acidosis. This harsh environment selects genetic events that result in resistant tumor variants, such as the loss of p53. High levels of VEGF (secreted by tumor cells) disrupt gap junction communication, tight junctions, and adherens junctions between EC via src-mediated phosphorylation of proteins such as connexin 43, zonula occludens-1, VE-cadherin, and α/β-catenins. Tumor vessels have thin, irregular BM, and pericytes are sparse or absent. Together, these molecular abnormalities result in a vasculature that is permeable to serum macromolecules, leading to high tumor interstitial pressure, which can prevent the delivery of drugs to the tumor cells. This is made worse by the binding and activation of platelets at sites of exposed BM, with release of stored VEGF and microvessel clot formation, creating more abnormal blood flow and regions of hypoxia. ***C.*** In experimental systems, treatment with bevacizumab or blocking antibodies to VEGFR2 leads to changes in the tumor vasculature that has been termed *vessel normalization*. During the first week of treatment, abnormal vessels are eliminated or pruned (dotted lines), leaving a more normal branching pattern. ECs partially regain features such as cell-cell junctions, adherence to a more normal BM, and pericyte coverage. These changes lead to a decrease in vascular permeability, reduced interstitial pressure, and a transient increase in blood flow within the tumor. Note that in murine models, this normalization period lasts only for ~5–6 days. ***D.*** After continued anti-VEGF/VEGFR therapy (which is often combined with chemo- or radiotherapy), ECs die, leading to tumor cell death (either due to direct effects of the chemotherapy or lack of blood flow).

pressed on the endothelium of primordial venous vessels while the transmembrane ligand ephrin-B2 is expressed by cells of primordial arteries; the reciprocal expression may regulate differentiation and patterning of the vasculature.

A number of ubiquitously expressed host molecules play critical roles in normal and pathologic angiogenesis. Proangiogenic cytokines, chemokines, and growth factors secreted by stromal cells or inflammatory cells make important contributions to neovascularization, including bFGF, transforming growth factor-α (TGF-α), TNF-α, and IL-8. In contrast to normal endothelium, angiogenic endothelium overexpresses specific members of the integrin family of ECM-binding proteins that mediate EC adhesion, migration, and survival. Specifically, expression of integrins $\alpha_v\beta_3$, $\alpha_v\beta_5$, and $\alpha_5\beta_1$ mediate spreading and migration of ECs and are required for angiogenesis induced by VEGF and bFGF, which in turn can upregulate EC integrin expression. The $\alpha_v\beta_3$ integrin physically associates with VEGFR2 in the plasma membrane and promotes signal transduction from each receptor to promote EC proliferation (via focal adhesion kinase, src, PI3K, and other pathways) and survival (by inhibition of p53 and increasing the Bcl-2/Bax expression ratio). In addition, $\alpha_v\beta_3$ forms cell surface complexes with matrix metalloproteinases (MMPs), zinc-requiring proteases that cleave ECM proteins, leading to enhanced EC migration and the release of heparin-binding growth factors including VEGF and bFGF. EC adhesion molecules can be upregulated (i.e., by VEGF, TNF-α) or downregulated (by TGF-β); this, together with chaotic blood flow explains poor leukocyte-endothelial interactions in tumor blood vessels and may help tumor cells avoid immune surveillance.

Cells derived from hematopoietic progenitors in the host bone marrow contribute to tumor angiogenesis in a process linked to the secretion of VEGF and PlGF (placenta-derived growth factor) by tumor cells and their surrounding stroma. VEGF promotes the mobilization and recruitment of circulating endothelial cell precursors (CEPs) and hematopoietic stem cells (HSCs) to tumors where they co-localize and appear to cooperate in neovessel formation. CEPs express VEGFR2, while HSCs express VEGFR1, a receptor for VEGF and PlGF. Both CEPs and HSCs are derived from a common precursor, the hemangioblast. CEPs are thought to differentiate into ECs, whereas the role of HSC-derived cells (such as tumor-associated macrophages) may be to secrete angiogenic factors required for sprouting and stabilization of ECs (VEGF, bFGF, angiopoietins) and to activate MMPs, resulting in ECM remodeling and growth factor release. In mouse tumor models and in human cancers, increased numbers of CEPs and subsets of

TABLE 80-3 RANDOMIZED PHASE III CLINICAL TRIALS DEMONSTRATING THE EFFICACY OF BEVACIZUMAB IN COMBINATION WITH CHEMOTHERAPY FOR THE TREATMENT OF ADVANCED CANCERS

Tumor Type	Stage of Disease	Previous Treatment	Number of Patients	Chemotherapy Regimen	Outcome
Colon cancer	Metastatic	No	813	Irinotecan + 5-FU/LV ± bevacizumab	Increased OS (20.3 vs 15.6 months), PFS (10.6 vs 6.2 months), and RR (44.8 vs 34.8%)
Colon cancer	Metastatic	Second line; previous irinotecan/5-FU	829	FOLFOX ± bevacizumab	Increased OS (12.9 vs 10.8 months), PFS (7.2 vs 4.8 months), RR (21.8 vs 9.2%).
Non-small cell lung cancer (excluding squamous histology)	Metastatic	No	878	Carboplatinum + paclitaxel ± bevacizumab	Increased OS (12.5 vs 10.2 months), PFS (6.4 vs 4.5 months), RR (27.2 vs 10.0%).
Breast cancer	Recurrent or metastatic	No	722	Paclitaxel ± bevacizumab	Increased PFS (11.0 vs 6.2 months), RR (28 vs 14%).

Note: 5-FU, 5-fluorouracil; LV, leucovoran; OS, overall survival; PFS, progression-free survival; RR, response rate; FOLFOX, folinic acid (LV), 5-FU, and oxaliplatinum.

VEGFR-expressing HSCs can be detected in the circulation, which may correlate with increased levels of serum VEGF. It is not yet known whether levels of these cells have prognostic value or if changes during treatment correlate with inhibition of tumor angiogenesis. Whether CEPs and VEGFR1-expressing HSCs are required to maintain the long-term integrity of established tumor vessels is also unknown.

Lymphatic vessels also exist within tumors. Development of tumor lymphatics is associated with expression of VEGFR3 and its ligands VEGF-C and VEGF-D. The role of these vessels in tumor cell metastasis to regional lymph nodes remains to be determined, since, as discussed above, interstitial pressures within tumors are high and most lymphatic vessels may exit in a collapsed and nonfunctional state. However, VEGF-C levels correlate significantly with metastasis to regional lymph nodes in lung, prostate, and colorectal cancers,

ANTIANGIOGENIC THERAPY

Understanding the molecular mechanisms that regulate tumor angiogenesis may provide unique opportunities for cancer treatment. Acquired drug resistance of tumor cells due to their high intrinsic mutation rate is a major cause of treatment failure in human cancers. ECs comprising the tumor vasculature are genetically stable and do not share genetic changes with tumor cells; the EC apoptosis pathways are therefore intact. Each EC of a tumor vessel helps provide nourishment to many tumor cells, and although tumor angiogenesis can be driven by a number of exogenous proangiogenic stimuli, experimental data indicate that at least in some tumor types, blockade of a single growth factor (e.g., VEGF) may inhibit tumor-induced vascular growth. Angiogenesis inhibitors function by targeting the critical molecular pathways involved in EC proliferation, migration, and/or survival, many of which are unique to the activated endothelium in tumors. Inhibition of growth factor and adhesion-dependent signaling pathways can induce EC apoptosis with concomitant inhibition of tumor growth. Different types of tumors use distinct molecular mechanisms to activate the angiogenic switch. Therefore, it is doubtful that a single antiangiogenic strategy will suffice for all human cancers; rather, a number of agents will be needed, each responding to distinct programs of angiogenesis used by different human cancers.

Four randomized phase III clinical trials have demonstrated that the addition of bevacizumab (Avastin; a humanized monoclonal antibody that binds and inhibits VEGF) to chemotherapy results in significantly improved response rates, progression-free survival, and overall survival when compared to treatment with chemotherapy alone (Table 80-3). This effect was shown in the first-line treatment of patients with advanced colon, lung, and breast cancers, and in the second-line treatment of colon cancer. However, not all trials have been positive; in previously treated breast cancer, the addition of bevacizumab to capecitabine (an oral fluoropyrimidine) did not increase efficacy, and in previously untreated pancreatic cancer, bevacizumab did not enhance the efficacy of gemcitabine.

Several general principles have arisen from these studies. Bevacizumab appears to potentiate the effects of many different types of active chemotherapeutic regimens used to treat a variety of different tumor types. No phase III trials have demonstrated single-agent activity for bevacizumab; colon and lung cancer trials have demonstrated a lack of activity when used alone. An exception may be renal cell cancer (RCC), a tumor that is specifically dependent upon VEGF as the result of deletion of the VHL tumor suppressor and activation of the HIF-1α transcription factor (see above). A randomized phase II study of single-agent bevacizumab given at low or high dose compared to placebo in patients with advanced RCC demonstrated a significant prolongation of time to disease progression, a finding that merits further study.

The mechanisms by which bevacizumab enhances the activity of chemotherapy and possibly radiotherapy have been studied (Table 80-4). Inhibition of VEGF, especially in the early stages of treatment, has been postulated to result in the normalization of blood flow in tumors (Fig. 80-10). When given in combination with chemotherapy, this may enhance the delivery of cytotoxic agents to the tumor, where death of tumor cells and proliferating endothelial cells may result. As antiangiogenic therapy continues, growth of new tumor vessels is inhibited, leading to nutritional deprivation and death of tumor cells.

Bevacizumab is administered IV every 2–3 weeks (its half-life is nearly 20 days) and is generally well tolerated. Hypertension has been noted in most trials that utilize inhibitors of VEGF receptors, but only 10% of patients require treatment with anti-hypertensive agents and this rarely requires discontinuation of therapy. A mechanism for the hypertension may be a bevacizumab-induced decrease in vessel production of nitric oxide, resulting in vasoconstriction and increased blood pressure. Rare but serious side effects of bevacizumab include an increased risk of arterial thromboembolic events including stroke and myocardial infarction, usually in patients over the age of 65 with a history of cardiovascular disease. An increased risk of hemorrhage was noted in lung cancer patients with a squamous histology and large central tumors near the major mediastinal blood vessels. Cavitation of the

TABLE 80-4 MECHANISMS OF BEVACIZUMAB ACTION

1. Inhibition of VEGF-dependent signaling pathways required for the proliferation and survival of endothelial cells within the tumor vasculature. This may enhance the direct toxic effects of chemotherapy on tumor endothelial cells.
2. Inhibition of vascular permeability, decreasing interstitial pressure in tumors, and promoting delivery of therapeutic drugs and oxygen (a process termed *vessel normalization*).
3. Prevention of neoangiogenesis between cycles of chemotherapy, blocking tumor regrowth.
4. Inhibition of the recruitment of proangiogenic bone marrow–derived cells (including circulating endothelial precursors and monocytes) to the tumor vasculature.
5. Blocking potential direct effects of VEGF on tumors that have been reported to express VEGFR2, e.g., colon and pancreatic cancer cells.
6. Reversing the inhibitory activity of VEGF on dendritic cells, thereby promoting antitumor immunity.

Note: VEGF(R), vascular endothelial growth factor (receptor).

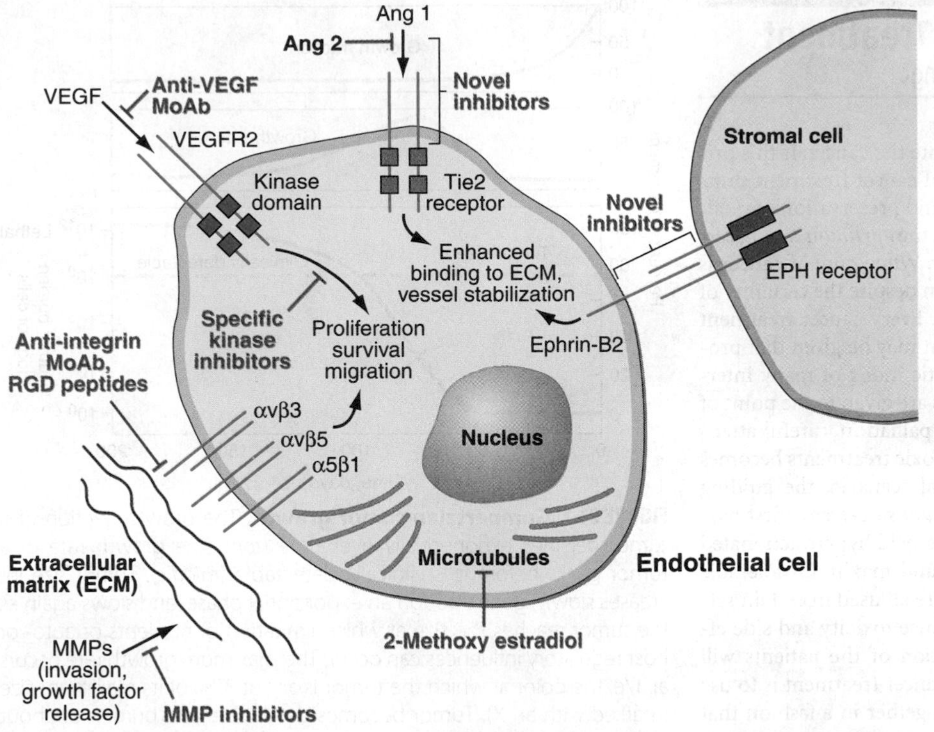

FIGURE 80-11 Knowledge of the molecular events governing tumor angiogenesis has led to a number of therapeutic strategies to block tumor blood vessel formation. The successful therapeutic targeting of VEGF is described in the text. Other endothelial cell–specific receptor tyrosine kinase pathways (e.g., angiopoietin/Tie2 and ephrin/EPH) are likely targets for the future. Ligation of the $\alpha_v\beta_3$ integrin is required for EC survival. Integrins are also required for EC migration and are important regulators of matrix metalloproteinase (MMP) activity, which modulates EC movement through the ECM as well as release of bound growth factors. Targeting of integrins includes development of blocking antibodies, small peptide inhibitors of integrin signaling, and arg-gly-asp-containing peptides that prevent integrin:ECM binding. Peptides derived from normal proteins by protealytic cleavage, including endostatin and tumstatin, inhibit angiogenesis by mechanisms that include interfering with integrin function. Signal transduction pathways that are dysregulated in tumor cells indirectly regulate EC function. Inhibition of EGF-family receptors, whose signaling activity is upregulated in a number of human cancers (e.g., breast, colon, and lung cancers), results in downregulation of VEGF and IL-8, while increasing expression of the antiangiogenic protein thrombospondin-1. The Ras/MAPK, PI3K/Akt, and Src kinase pathways constitute important anti-tumor targets that also regulate the proliferation and survival of tumor-derived EC. The discovery that EC from normal tissues express tissue-specific "vascular addressins" on their cell surface suggests that targeting specific EC subsets may be possible.

tumor with vessel rupture and massive hemoptysis lead to the exclusion of squamous cell cancers from treatment with bevacizumab. This potentially fatal side effect may actually reflect an increased activity of bevacizumab plus chemotherapy in squamous cell cancers. Other serious complications include bowel perforations that have been observed in 1–3% of patients (mainly those with colon and ovarian cancers).

Important questions remain concerning the clinical use of bevacizumab. Do patients develop resistance to this agent? Although patients with advanced colon, lung, and breast cancers benefit from treatment with bevacizumab-containing regiments, few patients are cured and most will relapse and die of their disease. While resistance of cancer cells to chemotherapeutic agents is expected, it is unclear to what extent the relapses reflect resistance to bevacizumab (if at all). Preclinical studies have demonstrated that inhibition of VEGF-mediated angiogenic pathways can select for tumor variants that utilize other angiogenic mechanisms, such as the secretion of the proangiogenic chemokine IL-8, which is a downstream mediator of the EGFR pathway. This has led to studies in which bevacizumab has been combined with cetuximab or erlotinib (inhibitors of EGFR signaling), and preliminary phase II studies have shown efficacy of these combinations in heavily pretreated patients with colon and lung cancers.

The bevacizumab experience suggests that inhibition of the VEGF pathway will be most efficacious when combined with agents that directly target tumor cells. This also appears to be the case in the development of small-molecule inhibitors (SMI) that target VEGF receptor tyrosine kinase activity but are also inhibitory to other kinases that are expressed by tumor cells and important for their proliferation and survival. Sunitinib, FDA approved for the treatment of GIST (see above and Table 80-2), has activity directed against mutant c-Kit receptors, but also targets VEGFR and PDGFR, and has shown significant antitumor activity against metastatic RCC, presumably on the basis of its antiantiogenic activity. Similarly, sorafenib, originally developed as a Raf kinase inhibitor but with potent activity against VEGF and PDGF receptors, increases progression-free survival in RCC. Thus, agents that target both angiogenesis and tumor-specific signaling pathways may have greater efficacy against a broad range of cancers. A caveat is that RCC and GIST are highly dependent upon single signaling pathways (VEGF and c-Kit, respectively) whereas most solid tumors use a panoply of interconnected proliferation and survival pathways that are redundant and likely to be less amenable to single-agent targeting.

The success in targeting tumor angiogenesis has led to enhanced enthusiasm for the development of drugs that target other aspects of the angiogenic process; some of these therapeutic approaches are outlined in Fig. 80-11.

FURTHER READINGS

Bild AH et al: Oncogenic pathway signatures in human cancers as a guide to targeted therapies. Nature 439:353, 2006

Dai Y, Grant S: Targeting multiple arms of the apoptotic regulatory machinery. Cancer Res 67:2908, 2007

Ferrara N, Kerbel RS: Angiogenesis as a therapeutic target. Nature 438:967, 2005

Finkel T et al: The common biology of cancer and ageing. Nature 448:767, 2007

Huber MA et al: Molecular requirements for epithelial-mesenchymal transition during tumor progression. Curr Opin Cell Biol 17:548, 2005

Kaelin Jr WG: The concept of synthetic lethality in the context of anticancer therapy. Nat Rev Cancer 5:686, 2005

Panares RL, Garcia AA: Bevacizumab in the management of solid tumors. Expert Rev Anticancer Ther 7:434, 2007

Sharma SV et al: Epidermal growth factor receptor mutations in lung cancer. Nat Rev Cancer 7:169, 2007

Sherbenou DW, Drucker BJ: Applying the discovery of the Philadelphia chromosome. J Clin Invest 117:2068, 2007

Vousden KH, Lane DP: p53 in health and disease. Nat Rev Mol Cell Biol 8:275, 2007

81 Principles of Cancer Treatment

Edward A. Sausville, Dan L. Longo

The goal of cancer treatment is first to eradicate the cancer. If this primary goal cannot be accomplished, the goal of cancer treatment shifts to palliation, the amelioration of symptoms, and preservation of quality of life while striving to extend life. The dictum *primum non nocere* is not the guiding principle of cancer therapy. When cure of cancer is possible, cancer treatments may be undertaken despite the certainty of severe and perhaps life-threatening toxicities. Every cancer treatment has the potential to cause harm, and treatment may be given that produces toxicity with no benefit. The therapeutic index of many interventions is quite narrow, and most treatments are given to the point of toxicity. Conversely, when the clinical goal is palliation, careful attention to minimizing the toxicity of potentially toxic treatments becomes a significant goal. Irrespective of the clinical scenario, the guiding principle of cancer treatment should be *primum succerrere*, "first hasten to help." Radical surgical procedures, large-field hyperfractionated radiation therapy, high-dose chemotherapy, and maximum tolerable doses of cytokines such as interleukin (IL) 2 are all used in certain settings where 100% of the patients will experience toxicity and side effects from the intervention and only a fraction of the patients will experience benefit. One of the challenges of cancer treatment is to use the various treatment modalities alone and together in a fashion that maximizes the chances for patient benefit.

Cancer treatments are divided into four main types: surgery, radiation therapy (including photodynamic therapy), chemotherapy (including hormonal therapy and molecularly targeted therapy), and biologic therapy (including immunotherapy and gene therapy). The modalities are often used in combination, and agents in one category can act by several mechanisms. For example, cancer chemotherapy agents can induce differentiation, and antibodies (a form of immunotherapy) can be used to deliver radiation therapy. Surgery and radiation therapy are considered local treatments, though their effects can influence the behavior of tumor at remote sites. Chemotherapy and biologic therapy are usually systemic treatments. *Oncology*, the study of tumors including treatment approaches, is a multidisciplinary effort with surgical-, radiotherapy-, and internal medicine–related areas of expertise. Treatments for patients with hematologic malignancies are often shared by hematologists and medical oncologists.

In many ways, cancer mimics an organ attempting to regulate its own growth. However, cancers have not set an appropriate limit on how much growth should be permitted. Normal organs and cancers share the property of having (1) a population of cells in cycle and actively renewing and (2) a population of cells not in cycle. In cancers, cells that are not dividing are heterogeneous; some have sustained too much genetic damage to replicate but have defects in their death pathways that permit their survival, some are starving for nutrients and oxygen, and some are out of cycle but poised to be recruited back into cycle and expand if needed (i.e., reversibly growth–arrested). Severely damaged and starving cells are unlikely to kill the patient. The problem is that the cells that are reversibly not in cycle are capable of replenishing tumor cells physically removed or damaged by radiation and chemotherapy. These include *cancer stem cells*, whose properties are being elucidated. The stem cell fraction may define new targets for therapies that will retard their ability to reenter the cell cycle.

Tumors follow a Gompertzian growth curve (Fig. 81-1); the growth fraction of a neoplasm starts at 100% with the first transformed cell and declines exponentially over time until at the time of diagnosis, with a tumor burden of 1–5 × 10^9 tumor cells, the growth fraction is usually 1–4%. Thus, peak growth rate occurs before the tumor is detectable. A key feature of a successful tumor is the ability to stimulate the development of a new supporting stroma through angiogenesis and production of proteases to allow invasion through basement membranes and normal tissue barriers (Chap. 80). Specific cellular mechanisms promote entry or withdrawal of tumor cells from the cell

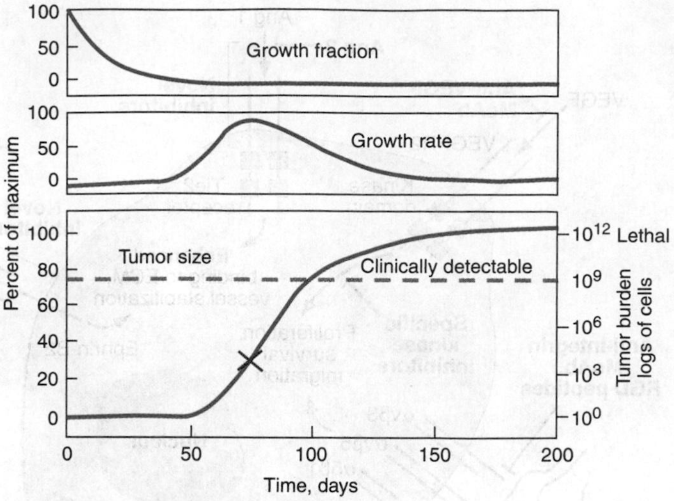

FIGURE 81-1 Gompertzian tumor growth. The growth fraction of a tumor declines exponentially over time (*top*). The growth rate of a tumor peaks before it is clinically detectable (*middle*). Tumor size increases slowly, goes through an exponential phase, and slows again as the tumor reaches the size at which limitation of nutrients or auto- or host regulatory influences can occur. The maximum growth rate occurs at 1/e, the point at which the tumor is about 37% of its maximum size (marked with an X). Tumor becomes detectable at a burden of about 10^9 (1 cm^3) cells and kills the patient at a tumor cell burden of about 10^{12} (1 kg). Efforts to treat the tumor and reduce its size can result in an increase in the growth fraction and an increase in growth rate.

cycle. For example, when a tumor recurs after surgery or chemotherapy, frequently its growth is accelerated and the growth fraction of the tumor is increased. This pattern is similar to that seen in regenerating organs. Partial resection of the liver results in the recruitment of cells into the cell cycle, and the resected liver volume is replaced. Similarly, chemotherapy-damaged bone marrow increases its growth to replace cells killed by chemotherapy. However, cancers do not recognize a limit on their expansion. Monoclonal gammopathy of uncertain significance may be an example of a clonal neoplasm with intrinsic features that stop its growth before a lethal tumor burden is reached. A fraction of patients with this disorder go on to develop fatal multiple myeloma, but probably this occurs because of the accumulation of additional genetic lesions. Elucidation of the mechanisms that regulate this "organ-like" behavior of tumors may provide additional clues to cancer control and treatment.

PRINCIPLES OF CANCER SURGERY

Surgery is used in cancer prevention, diagnosis, staging, treatment (for both localized and metastatic disease), palliation, and rehabilitation.

PROPHYLAXIS

Cancer can be prevented by surgery in people who have premalignant lesions resected (e.g., premalignant lesions of skin, colon, cervix) and in those who are at increased risk of cancer from either an underlying disease (colectomy in those with pancolonic involvement with ulcerative colitis), the presence of genetic lesions (colectomy for familial polyposis, thyroidectomy for multiple endocrine neoplasia type 2, bilateral mastectomy or oophorectomy for familial breast or ovarian cancer syndromes), or a developmental anomaly (orchiectomy in those with an undescended testis). In some cases, prophylactic surgery is more radical than the surgical procedures used to treat the cancer after it develops. The assessment of risk involves many factors and should be undertaken with care before advising a patient to undergo such a major procedure. For breast cancer prevention, many experts use a 20% risk of developing breast cancer over the next 5 years as a threshold. However, patient fears play a major role in defining candidates for cancer prevention surgery. Counseling and education may not be enough to allay the fears of someone who has lost close family members to a malignancy.

DIAGNOSIS

The underlying principle in cancer diagnosis is to obtain as much tissue as safely possible. Owing to tumor heterogeneity, pathologists are better able to make the diagnosis when they have more tissue to examine. In addition to light-microscopic inspection of a tumor for pattern of growth, degree of cellular atypia, invasiveness, and morphologic features that aid in the differential diagnosis, sufficient tissue is of value in searching for genetic abnormalities and protein expression patterns, such as hormone receptor expression in breast cancers, that may aid in differential diagnosis or provide information about prognosis or likely response to treatment. Histologically similar tumors may have very different gene expression patterns when assessed by such techniques as microarray analysis using gene chips, with important differences in response to treatment. Such testing requires that the tissue be handled properly (e.g., immunologic detection of proteins is more effective in fresh-frozen tissue rather than in formalin-fixed tissue). Coordination among the surgeon, pathologist, and primary care physician is essential to ensure that the amount of information learned from the biopsy material is maximized.

These goals are best met by an *excisional biopsy* in which the entire tumor mass is removed with a small margin of normal tissue surrounding it. If an excisional biopsy cannot be performed, *incisional biopsy* is the procedure of second choice. A wedge of tissue is removed, and an effort is made to include the majority of the cross-sectional diameter of the tumor in the biopsy to minimize sampling error. The biopsy techniques that involve cutting into tumor carry with them a risk of facilitating the spread of the tumor. *Core-needle biopsy* usually obtains considerably less tissue, but this procedure often provides enough information to plan a definitive surgical procedure. *Fine-needle aspiration* generally obtains only a suspension of cells from within a mass. This procedure is minimally invasive, and if positive for cancer it may allow inception of systemic treatment when metastatic disease is evident, or it can provide a basis for planning a more meticulous and extensive surgical procedure.

STAGING

As noted in Chap. 77, an important component of patient management is defining the extent of disease. Radiographic and other imaging tests can be helpful in defining the clinical stage; however, pathologic staging requires defining the extent of involvement by documenting the histologic presence of tumor in tissue biopsies obtained through a surgical procedure. Axillary lymph node sampling in breast cancer and lymph node sampling at laparotomy for lymphomas and testicular, colon, and other intraabdominal cancers may provide crucial information for treatment planning and may determine the extent and nature of primary cancer treatment.

TREATMENT

Surgery is the most effective means of treating cancer. Today about 40% of cancer patients are cured by surgery. Unfortunately, a large fraction of patients with solid tumors (perhaps 60%) have metastatic disease that is not accessible for removal. However, even when the disease is not curable by surgery alone, the removal of tumor can obtain important benefits, including local control of tumor, preservation of organ function, debulking that permits subsequent therapy to work better, and staging information on extent of involvement. Cancer surgery aiming for cure is usually planned to excise the tumor completely with an adequate margin of normal tissue (the margin varies with the tumor and the anatomy), touching the tumor as little as possible to prevent vascular and lymphatic spread, and minimizing operative risk. Extending the procedure to resect draining lymph nodes obtains prognostic information, but such resections alone generally do not improve survival.

Increasingly, laparoscopic approaches are being used to address primary abdominal and pelvic tumors. Lymph node spread may be assessed using the sentinel node approach, in which the first draining lymph node a spreading tumor would encounter is defined by injecting a dye into the tumor site at operation and then resecting the first node to turn blue. The sentinel node assessment is continuing to undergo clinical evaluation but appears to provide reliable information without the risks (lymphedema, lymphangiosarcoma) associated with resection of all the regional nodes. Advances in adjuvant chemotherapy and radiation therapy following surgery have permitted a substantial decrease in the extent of primary surgery necessary to obtain the best outcomes. Thus, lumpectomy with radiation therapy is as effective as modified radical mastectomy for breast cancer, and limb-sparing surgery followed by adjuvant radiation therapy and chemotherapy has replaced radical primary surgical procedures involving amputation and disarticulation for childhood rhabdomyosarcomas. More limited surgery is also being employed to spare organ function, as in larynx and bladder cancer. The magnitude of operations necessary to optimally control and cure cancer has also been diminished by technical advances; for example, the circular anastomotic stapler has allowed narrower (<2 cm) margins in colon cancer without compromise of local control rates, and many patients who would have had colostomies are able to maintain normal anatomy.

In some settings—e.g., bulky testicular cancer or stage III breast cancer—surgery is not the first treatment modality employed. After an initial diagnostic biopsy, chemotherapy and/or radiation therapy is delivered to reduce the size of the tumor and clinically control undetected metastatic disease. Such therapy is followed by a surgical procedure to remove residual masses; this is called *neoadjuvant therapy*. Because the sequence of treatment is critical to success and is different from the standard surgery-first approach, coordination among the surgical oncologist, radiation oncologist, and medical oncologist is crucial.

Surgery may be curative in a subset of patients with metastatic disease. Patients with lung metastases from osteosarcoma may be cured by resection of the lung lesions. In patients with colon cancer who have fewer than five liver metastases restricted to one lobe and no extrahepatic metastases, hepatic lobectomy may produce long-term disease-free survival in 25% of selected patients. Surgery can also be associated with systemic antitumor effects. In the setting of hormonally responsive tumors, oophorectomy and/or adrenalectomy may control estrogen production, and orchiectomy may reduce androgen production; both have effects on metastatic tumor growth. If resection of the primary lesion takes place in the presence of metastases, acceleration of metastatic growth may occur, perhaps based on the removal of a source of angiogenesis inhibitors and mass-related growth regulators in the tumor.

In selecting a surgeon or center for primary cancer treatment, consideration must be given to the volume of cancer surgeries undertaken by the site. Studies in a variety of cancers have shown that increased annual procedure volume appears to correlate with outcome. In addition, facilities with extensive support systems—e.g., for joint thoracic and abdominal surgical teams with cardiopulmonary bypass, if needed—may allow resection of certain tumors that would otherwise not be possible.

PALLIATION

Surgery is employed in a number of ways for supportive care: insertion of central venous catheters, control of pleural and pericardial effusions and ascites, caval interruption for recurrent pulmonary emboli, stabilization of cancer-weakened weight-bearing bones, and control of hemorrhage, among others. Surgical bypass of gastrointestinal, urinary tract, or biliary tree obstruction can alleviate symptoms and prolong survival. Surgical procedures may provide relief of otherwise intractable pain or reverse neurologic dysfunction (cord decompression). Splenectomy may relieve symptoms and reverse hypersplenism. Intrathecal or intrahepatic therapy relies on surgical placement of appropriate infusion portals. Surgery may correct other treatment-related toxicities such as adhesions or strictures.

REHABILITATION

Surgical procedures are also valuable in restoring a cancer patient to full health. Orthopedic procedures may be necessary to assure proper ambulation. Breast reconstruction can make an enormous impact on the patient's perception of successful therapy. Plastic and reconstructive surgery can correct the effects of disfiguring primary treatment.

PRINCIPLES OF RADIATION THERAPY

PHYSICAL PROPERTIES AND BIOLOGIC EFFECTS

Exposure to ionizing radiation is constant. Radiation comes from the sun and other cosmic sources, the ground, the air we breathe, the food we ingest, and from within our bodies. Radiation therapy uses radiation to treat cancer. Radiation is a physical form of treatment that damages any tissue in its path; its selectivity for cancer cells may be due to defects in a cancer cell's ability to repair sublethal DNA and other damage. Radiation causes breaks in DNA and generates free radicals from cell water that may damage cell membranes, proteins and organelles. Radiation damage is dependent on oxygen; hypoxic cells are more resistant. Augmentation of oxygen is the basis for radiation sensitization. Sulfhydryl compounds interfere with free radical generation and may act as radiation protectors.

Most radiation-induced cell damage is due to the formation of hydroxyl radicals:

$$\text{Ionizing radiation} + H_2O \rightarrow H_2O^+ + e^-$$

$$H_2O^+ + H_2O \rightarrow H_3O^+ + OH^{\cdot}$$

$$OH^{\cdot} \rightarrow \text{cell damage}$$

The dose-response curve for cells has both linear and exponential components. The linear component is from double-stranded DNA breaks produced by single hits. The exponential component represents breaks produced by multiple hits (Fig. 81-2). Plotting the fraction of surviving cells against doses of x-rays or gamma radiation, the curve has a shoulder that reflects the cell's repair of sublethal damage, followed by a linear portion reflecting greater cell kill with larger doses. The features that make a particular cell more sensitive or more resistant to the biologic effects of radiation are not completely defined.

Although radiation can interfere with many cellular processes, many experts feel that a cell must undergo a double-strand DNA break from radiation in order to be killed. The factors that influence tumor cell killing include the D_0 of the tumor (the dose required to deliver an average of one lethal hit to all the cells in a population), the D_q of the tumor (the threshold dose—a measure of the cell's ability to repair sublethal damage), hypoxia, tumor mass, growth fraction, and cell cycle time and phase (cells in late G_1 and S are more resistant). Rate of clinical response is not predictive; some cells do not die after radiation exposure until they attempt to replicate.

Therapeutic radiation is delivered in three ways: (1) *teletherapy*, with beams of radiation generated at a distance and aimed at the tumor within the patient; (2) *brachytherapy*, with encapsulated sources of radiation implanted directly into or adjacent to tumor tissues; and (3) *systemic therapy*, with radionuclides targeted in some fashion to a site of tumor. Teletherapy is the most commonly used form of radiation therapy.

Radiation from any source decreases in intensity as a function of the square of the distance from the source (inverse square law). Thus, if the radiation source is 5 cm above the skin surface and the tumor is 5 cm below the skin surface, the intensity of radiation in the tumor will be $5^2/10^2$, or 25% of the intensity at the skin. By contrast, if the radiation source is moved to 100 cm from the patient, the intensity of radiation in the tumor will be $100^2/105^2$, or 91% of the intensity at the skin. Teletherapy maintains intensity over a larger volume of target tissue by increasing the source-to-surface distance. In brachytherapy, the source-to-surface distance is small; thus, the effective treatment volume is small.

X-rays and gamma rays are the forms of radiation most commonly used to treat cancer. They are both electromagnetic, nonparticulate waves that cause the ejection of an orbital electron when absorbed. This orbital electron ejection is called *ionization*. X-rays are generated by linear accelerators; gamma rays are generated from decay of atomic nuclei in radioisotopes such as cobalt and radium. These waves behave biologically as packets of energy, called *photons*. Particulate forms of radiation are also used in certain circumstances. Electron beams have a very low tissue penetrance and are used to treat skin conditions such as mycosis fungoides. Neutron beams may be somewhat more effective than x-rays in treating salivary gland tumors. However, aside from these specialized uses, particulate forms of radiation such as neutrons, protons, and negative mesons, which should do more tissue damage because of their higher linear energy transfer and be less dependent on oxygen, have not yet found wide applicability to cancer treatment.

A number of parameters influence the damage done to tissue by radiation. Hypoxic cells are relatively resistant. Nondividing cells are more resistant than dividing cells. In addition to these biologic parameters, physical parameters of the radiation are also crucial. The energy of the radiation determines its ability to penetrate tissue. Low-energy orthovoltage beams (150–400 kV) scatter when they strike the body, much like light diffuses when it strikes particles in the air. Such beams result in more damage to adjacent normal tissues and less radiation delivered to the tumor. Megavoltage radiation (>1 MeV) has very low lateral scatter; this produces a skin-sparing effect, more homogeneous distribution of the radiation energy, and greater deposit of the energy

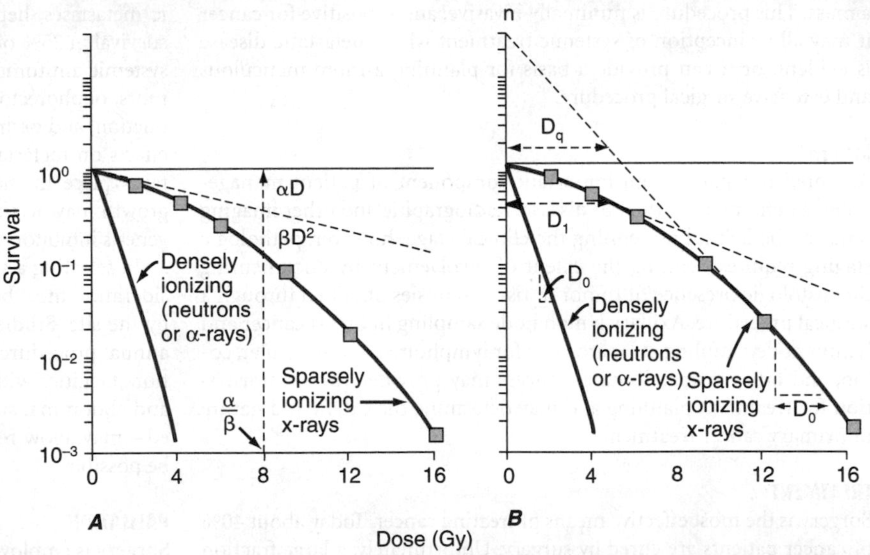

FIGURE 81-2 Shape of survival curve for mammalian cells exposed to radiation. The fraction of cells surviving is plotted on a logarithmic scale against dose on a linear scale. For alpha particles or low-energy neutrons (said to be densely ionizing), the dose-response curve is a straight line from the origin (i.e., survival is an exponential function of dose). The survival curve can be described by just one parameter, the slope. For x-rays or gamma rays (said to be sparsely ionizing), the dose-response curve has an initial linear slope, followed by a shoulder; at higher doses the curve tends to become straight again. ***A.*** The experimental data are fitted to a linear-quadratic function. There are two components of cell killing: one is proportional to dose (αD), while the other is proportional to the square of the dose (βD²). The dose at which the linear and quadratic components are equal is the ratio α/β. The linear-quadratic curve bends continuously but is a good fit to experimental data for the first few decades of survival. ***B.*** The curve is described by the initial slope (D_1), the final slope (D_0), and a parameter that represents the width of the shoulder, either *n* or D_q. *(From EJ Hall: Radiobiology for the Radiologist, 5th ed. Philadelphia, Lippincott Williams & Wilkins, 2000; with permission.)*

in the tumor, or *target volume*. The tissues that the beam passes through to get to the tumor are called the *transit volume*. The maximum dose in the target volume is often the cause of complications to tissues in the transit volume, and the minimum dose in the target volume influences the likelihood of tumor recurrence. Dose homogeneity in the target volume is the goal.

Radiation is quantitated on the basis of the amount of radiation absorbed in the patient; it is not based on the amount of radiation generated by the machine. The *rad* (radiation *a*bsorbed *d*ose) is defined as 100 erg of energy per gram of tissue. The International System (SI) unit for rad is the Gray (Gy); 1 Gy = 100 rad. Radiation dose is measured by placing detectors at the body surface or calculating the dose based on radiating phantoms that resemble human form and substance. Radiation dose has three determinants: total absorbed dose, number of fractions, and time. A frequent error is to omit the number of fractions and the duration of treatment. This is analogous to saying that a runner completed a race in 20 s; without knowing how far he or she ran, the result is difficult to interpret. The time could be very good for a 200-m race or very poor for a 100-m race. Thus, a typical course of radiation therapy should be described as 4500 cGy delivered to a particular target (e.g., mediastinum) over 5 weeks in 180-cGy fractions. Most curative radiation treatment programs are delivered once a day, 5 days a week in 150- to 200-cGy fractions.

Compounds that incorporate into DNA and alter its stereochemistry (e.g., halogenated pyrimidines, cisplatin) augment radiation effects. Hydroxyurea, another DNA synthesis inhibitor, also potentiates radiation effects. Compounds that deplete thiols (e.g., buthionine sulfoximine) can also augment radiation effects. Hypoxia is a major factor that interferes with radiation effects.

APPLICATION TO PATIENTS

Teletherapy Radiation therapy can be used alone or together with chemotherapy to produce cure of localized tumors and control of the primary site of disease in tumors that have disseminated. Therapy is planned based on the use of a simulator with the treatment field or fields designed to accommodate an individual patient's anatomic features. Individualized treatment planning employs lead shielding tailored to shape the field and limit the radiation exposure of normal tissue. Often the radiation is delivered from two or three different positions. Conformal three-dimensional treatment planning permits the delivery of higher doses of radiation to the target volume without increasing complications in the transit volume.

Radiation therapy is a component of curative therapy for a number of diseases, including breast cancer, Hodgkin's disease, head and neck cancer, prostate cancer, and gynecologic cancers. Radiation therapy can also palliate disease symptoms in a variety of settings: relief of bone pain from metastatic disease, control of brain metastases, reversal of spinal cord compression and superior vena caval obstruction, shrinkage of painful masses, and opening of threatened airways. In high-risk settings, radiation therapy can prevent the development of leptomeningeal disease and brain metastases in acute leukemia and lung cancer.

Brachytherapy Brachytherapy involves placing a sealed source of radiation into or adjacent to the tumor and withdrawing the radiation source after a period of time precisely calculated to deliver a chosen dose of radiation to the tumor. This approach is often used to treat brain tumors and cervical cancer. The difficulty with brachytherapy is the short range of radiation effects (the inverse square law) and the inability to shape the radiation to fit the target volume. Normal tissue may receive toxic exposure to the radiation, with attendant radiation enteritis or cystitis in cervix cancer or brain injury in brain tumors.

Radionuclides and Radioimmunotherapy Nuclear medicine physicians or radiation oncologists may administer radionuclides with therapeutic effects. Iodine 131 is used to treat thyroid cancer since iodine is naturally taken up preferentially by the thyroid; it emits gamma rays that destroy the normal thyroid as well as the tumor. Strontium 89 and samarium 153 are two radionuclides that are preferentially taken up in bone, particularly sites of new bone formation. Both are capable of controlling bone metastases and the pain associated with them, but the dose-limiting toxicity is myelosuppression.

Monoclonal antibodies and other ligands can be attached to radioisotopes by conjugation (for nonmetal isotopes) or by chelation (for metal isotopes), and the targeting moiety can result in the accumulation of the radionuclide preferentially in tumor. Iodine 131–labeled anti-CD20 and yttrium 90–labeled anti-CD20 are active in B cell lymphoma, and other labeled antibodies are being evaluated. Thyroid uptake of labeled iodine is blocked by cold iodine. Dose-limiting toxicity is myelosuppression.

Photodynamic Therapy Some chemical structures (porphyrins, phthalocyanines) are selectively taken up by cancer cells by mechanisms not fully defined. When light, usually delivered by a laser, is shone on cells containing these compounds, free radicals are generated and the cells die. Hematoporphyrins and light are being used with increasing frequency to treat skin cancer; ovarian cancer; and cancers of the lung, colon, rectum, and esophagus. Palliation of recurrent locally advanced disease can sometimes be dramatic and last many months.

TOXICITY

Though radiation therapy is most often administered to a local region, systemic effects, including fatigue, anorexia, nausea, and vomiting, may develop that are related in part to the volume of tissue irradiated, dose fractionation, radiation fields, and individual susceptibility. Bone is among the most radioresistant organs, radiation effects being manifested mainly in children through premature fusion of the epiphyseal growth plate. By contrast, the male testis, female ovary, and bone marrow are the most sensitive organs. Any bone marrow in a radiation field will be eradicated by therapeutic irradiation. Organs with less need for cell renewal, such as heart, skeletal muscle, and nerves, are more resistant to radiation effects. In radiation-resistant organs, the vascular endothelium is the most sensitive component. Organs with more self-renewal as a part of normal homeostasis, such as the hematopoietic system and mucosal lining of the intestinal tract, are more sensitive. Acute toxicities include mucositis, skin erythema (ulceration in severe cases), and bone marrow toxicity. Often these can be alleviated by interruption of treatment.

Chronic toxicities are more serious. Radiation of the head and neck region often produces thyroid failure. Cataracts and retinal damage can lead to blindness. Salivary glands stop making saliva, which leads to dental caries and poor dentition. Taste and smell can be affected. Mediastinal irradiation leads to a threefold increased risk of fatal myocardial infarction. Other late vascular effects include chronic constrictive pericarditis, lung fibrosis, viscus stricture, spinal cord transection, and radiation enteritis. A serious late toxicity is the development of second solid tumors in or adjacent to the radiation fields. Such tumors can develop in any organ or tissue and occur at a rate of about 1% per year beginning in the second decade after treatment. Some organs vary in susceptibility to radiation carcinogenesis. A woman who receives mantle field radiation therapy for Hodgkin's disease at age 25 has a 30% risk of developing breast cancer by age 55 years. This is comparable in magnitude to genetic breast cancer syndromes. Women treated after age 30 have little or no increased risk of breast cancer. No data suggest that a threshold dose of therapeutic radiation exists below which the incidence of second cancers is decreased. High rates of second tumors occur in people who receive as little as 1000 cGy.

PRINCIPLES OF CHEMOTHERAPY

Medical oncology is the subspecialty of internal medicine that cares for and designs treatment approaches to patients with cancer, in conjunction with surgical and radiation oncologists. The core skills of the medical oncologist include the use of drugs that may have a beneficial effect on the natural history of the patient's illness or favorably influence the patient's quality of life. In general, the curability of a tumor is inversely related to tumor volume and directly related to drug dose.

Chemotherapy agents may be used for the treatment of active, clinically apparent cancer. Table 81-1, *A* lists those tumors considered curable by conventionally available chemotherapeutic agents when used to address disseminated or metastatic cancers. If a tumor is localized to a single site, serious consideration of surgery or primary radiation therapy should be given, as these treatment modalities may be curative as local treatments. Chemotherapy may be employed after the failure of these modalities to eradicate a local tumor or as part of multimodality approaches to offer primary treatment to a clinically localized tumor. In this event, it can allow organ preservation when given with radiation, as in the larynx or other upper airway sites; or sensitize tumors to radiation when given, for example, to patients concurrently receiving radiation for lung or cervix cancer (Table 81-1, *B*). Chemotherapy can be administered as an adjuvant, i.e., in addition to surgery (Table 81-1, *C*) or radiation, after all clinically apparent disease has been removed. This use of chemotherapy may have curative potential in breast and colorectal neoplasms, as it attempts to eliminate clinically unapparent tumor that may have already disseminated. As noted above, small tumors frequently have high growth fractions and therefore may be intrinsically more susceptible to the action of antiproliferative agents. Chemotherapy is routinely used in "conventional" dose regimens. In general, these doses produce reversible acute side effects, primarily consisting of transient myelosuppression with or without gastrointestinal toxicity (usually nausea), which are readily managed. High-dose chemotherapy regimens are predicated on the observation that the dose-response curve for many anticancer agents is rather steep, and increased dose can produce markedly increased therapeutic effect, although at the cost of potentially life-threatening complications that require intensive support, usually in the form of hematopoietic stem cell support from the patient (*autologous*) or from donors matched for histocompatibility loci (*allogeneic*). High-dose regimens have definite curative potential in defined clinical settings (Table 81-1, *D*).

TABLE 81-1 CURABILITY OF CANCERS WITH CHEMOTHERAPY

A. Advanced cancers with possible cure
- Acute lymphoid and acute myeloid leukemia (pediatric/adult)
- Hodgkin's disease (pediatric/adult)
- Lymphomas—certain types (pediatric/adult)
- Germ cell neoplasms
  - Embryonal carcinoma
  - Teratocarcinoma
  - Seminoma or dysgerminoma
  - Choriocarcinoma
- Gestational trophoblastic neoplasia
- Pediatric neoplasms
  - Wilm's tumor
  - Embryonal rhabdomyosarcoma
  - Ewing's sarcoma
  - Peripheral neuroepithelioma
  - Neuroblastoma
- Small-cell lung carcinoma
- Ovarian carcinoma

B. Advanced cancers possibly cured by chemotherapy and radiation
- Squamous carcinoma (head and neck)
- Squamous carcinoma (anus)
- Breast carcinoma
- Carcinoma of the uterine cervix
- Non-small cell lung carcinoma (stage III)
- Small-cell lung carcinoma

C. Cancers possibly cured with chemotherapy as adjuvant to surgery
- Breast carcinoma
- Colorectal carcinoma[a]
- Osteogenic sarcoma
- Soft tissue sarcoma

D. Cancers possibly cured with "high-dose" chemotherapy with stem cell support
- Relapsed leukemias, lymphoid and myeloid
- Relapsed lymphomas, Hodgkin's and non-Hodgkin's
- Chronic myeloid leukemia
- Multiple myeloma

E. Cancers responsive with useful palliation, but not cure, by chemotherapy
- Bladder carcinoma
- Chronic myeloid leukemia
- Hairy cell leukemia
- Chronic lymphocytic leukemia
- Lymphoma—certain types
- Multiple myeloma
- Gastric carcinoma
- Cervix carcinoma
- Endometrial carcinoma
- Soft tissue sarcoma
- Head and neck cancer
- Adrenocortical carcinoma
- Islet-cell neoplasms
- Breast carcinoma
- Colorectal carcinoma
- Renal carcinoma

F. Tumor poorly responsive in advanced stages to chemotherapy
- Pancreatic carcinoma
- Biliary-tract neoplasms
- Thyroid carcinoma
- Carcinoma of the vulva
- Non-small cell lung carcinoma
- Prostate carcinoma
- Melanoma
- Hepatocellular carcinoma

[a]Rectum also receives radiation therapy.

Karnofsky was among the first to champion the evaluation of a chemotherapeutic agent's benefit by carefully quantitating its effect on tumor size and using these measurements to objectively decide the basis for further treatment of a particular patient or further clinical evaluation of a drug's potential. A partial response (PR) is defined conventionally as a decrease by at least 50% in a tumor's bidimensional area; a complete response (CR) connotes disappearance of all tumor; progression of disease signifies an increase in size of existing lesions by >25% from baseline or best response or development of new lesions; and "stable" disease fits into none of the above categories. Newer evaluation systems utilize unidimensional measurement, but the intent is similar in rigorously defining evidence for the activity of the agent in assessing its value to the patient.

If cure is not possible, chemotherapy may be undertaken with the goal of palliating some aspect of the tumor's effect on the host. Common tumors that may be meaningfully addressed with palliative intent are listed in Table 81-1, *E*. Usually, tumor-related symptoms may manifest as pain, weight loss, or some local symptom related to the tumor's effect on normal structures. Patients treated with palliative intent should be aware of their diagnosis and the limitations of the proposed treatments, have access to supportive care, and have suitable "performance status," according to assessment algorithms such as the one developed by Karnofsky or by the Eastern Cooperative Oncology Group (ECOG). ECOG performance status 0 (PS0) patients are without symptoms; PS1 patients are ambulatory but restricted in strenuous physical activity; PS2 patients are ambulatory but unable to work and are up and about 50% or more of the time; PS3 patients are capable of limited self-care and are up <50% of the time; PS4 patients are totally confined to bed or chair and incapable of self-care. Only PS0, PS1, and PS2 patients are generally considered suitable for palliative (noncurative) treatment. If there is curative potential, even poor-performance status patients may be treated, but their prognosis is usually inferior to that of good-performance patients treated with similar regimens.

An important perspective the primary care provider may bring to patients and their families facing incurable cancer is that, given the limited value of chemotherapeutic approaches at some point in the natural history, *palliative care* or *hospice-based* approaches, with meticulous and ongoing attention to symptom relief and with family, psychological, and spiritual support, should receive prominent attention as a valuable therapeutic plan (Chap. 11). Optimizing the quality of life rather than attempting to extend it becomes a valued intervention. Patients facing the impending progression of disease in a life-threatening way frequently choose to undertake toxic treatments of little to no potential value, and support provided by the primary caregiver in accessing palliative and hospice-based options can be critical in providing a basis for patients to make sensible choices.

CANCER DRUGS: OVERVIEW AND PRINCIPLES FOR USE

Cancer drug treatments are of four broad types. *Conventional chemotherapy agents* were historically derived by the empirical observation that these "small molecules" (generally with molecular weight <1500 Da) could cause major regression of experimental tumors growing in animals. These agents mainly target DNA structure or segregation of DNA as chromosomes in mitosis. *Targeted agents* refer to small molecules or "biologicals" (generally macromolecules such as antibodies or cytokines) designed and developed to interact with a defined molecular target important in either maintaining the malignant state or selectively expressed by the tumor cells. As described in Chapter 80, successful tumors have activated biochemical pathways that lead to uncontrolled proliferation through the action of, e.g., oncogene products, loss of cell cycle inhibitors, or loss of cell death regulation, and have acquired the capacity to replicate chromosomes indefinitely, invade, metastasize, and evade the immune system. Targeted therapies seek to capitalize on the biology behind the aberrant cellular behavior as a basis for therapeutic effects. *Hormonal therapies* (the first form of targeted therapy) capitalize on the biochemical pathways underlying estrogen and androgen function and action as a therapeutic basis for approaching patients with tumors of breast, prostate, uterus, and ovarian origin. *Biologic therapies* are often macromolecules that have a particular target (e.g., antigrowth factor or cytokine antibodies) or may have the capacity to orchestrate or regulate the host immune response to kill tumor cells. Thus, biologic therapies include not only antibodies but cytokines and gene therapies.

The usefulness of any drug is governed by the extent to which a given dose causes a useful result (therapeutic effect; in the case of anticancer agents, toxicity to tumor cells) as opposed to a toxic effect. The *therapeutic index* is the degree of separation between toxic and therapeutic doses. Really useful drugs have large therapeutic indices, and this usually occurs when the drug target is expressed in the disease-causing compartment as opposed to the normal compartment. Classically, selective toxicity of an agent for an organ is governed by the expression of an agent's target or by differential accumulation into or elimination from compartments where toxicity is experienced or ameliorated, respectively. Currently used chemotherapeutic agents have the unfortunate property that their targets are present in both normal and tumor tissues. Therefore, they have relatively narrow therapeutic indices.

Following demonstration of activity in animal models, conventional chemotherapeutic agents are further evaluated to define an optimal schedule of administration and arrive at a drug formulation designed for a given route and schedule. Safety testing in two species on an analogous schedule of administration defines the starting dose for a phase I trial in humans. This is established as a fraction, usually one-sixth to one-tenth, of the dose just causing easily reversible toxicity in the more sensitive animal species. Escalating doses of the drug are then given during the human phase I trial until reversible toxicity is observed. Dose-limiting toxicity (DLT) defines a dose that conveys greater toxicity than would be acceptable in routine practice, allowing definition of a lower maximal tolerated dose (MTD). The occurrence of toxicity is, if possible, correlated with plasma drug concentrations. The MTD or a dose just lower than the MTD is usually the dose suitable for phase II trials, where a fixed dose is administered to a relatively homogeneous set of patients with a particular tumor type in an effort to define whether the drug causes regression of tumors. An "active" agent conventionally has PR rates of at least 20–25% with reversible non-life-threatening side effects, and it may then be suitable for study in phase III trials to assess efficacy in comparison to standard or no therapy.

Response, defined as tumor shrinkage, is but the most immediate indicator of drug effect. To be clinically valuable, responses must translate into clinical benefit. This is conventionally established by a beneficial effect on overall survival, or at least an increased time to further progression of disease. Active efforts are being made to quantitate effects of anticancer agents on quality of life. Cancer drug clinical trials conventionally use a toxicity grading scale where grade I toxicities do not require treatment, grade II often require symptomatic treatment but are not life-threatening, grade III toxicities are potentially life-threatening if untreated, grade IV toxicities are actually life-threatening, and grade V toxicities are those that result in the patient's death.

Development of targeted agents should proceed quite differently. While Phase I–III trials are still conducted, molecular analysis of human tumors more precisely defines targets expressed in a patient's tumor and should allow patient selection to enrich all trial phases with patients potentially responsive to the agent by virtue of expressing the target in the tumor. Clinical trials may be designed that assess the behavior of the drug in relation to its target. Ideally, the plasma concentration that affects the drug target is known, so escalation to MTD may not be necessary. Rather, the correlation of host toxicity while achieving an "optimal biologic dose" becomes a more relevant endpoint for Phase I and early Phase II trials with targeted agents.

Valuable cancer drug treatment strategies using conventional chemotherapy agents, targeted agents, hormonal treatments, or biologicals have one of two valuable outcomes. They can induce cancer cell death, resulting in tumor shrinkage with corresponding improvement in patient survival, or increase the time until the disease progresses. Another potential outcome is to induce cancer cell *differentiation* or dormancy with loss of tumor cell replicative potential and reacquisition of phenotypic properties resembling normal cells. Blocking tumor cell differentiation may be a key feature in the pathogenesis of certain leukemias.

Cell death is a closely regulated process. *Necrosis* refers to cell death induced, for example, by physical damage with the hallmarks of cell swelling and membrane disruption. *Apoptosis*, or programmed cell death, refers to a highly ordered process whereby cells respond to defined stimuli by dying, and it recapitulates the necessary cell death observed during the ontogeny of the organism. *Anoikis* refers to the death of epithelial cells after removal from the normal milieu of substrate, particularly from cell-to-cell contact. Cancer chemotherapeutic agents can cause both necrosis and apoptosis. Apoptosis is characterized by chromatin condensation (giving rise to "apoptotic bodies"); cell shrinkage; and, in living animals, phagocytosis by surrounding stromal cells without evidence of inflammation. This process is regulated either by signal transduction systems that promote a cell's demise after a certain level of insult is achieved, or in response to specific cell-surface receptors that mediate cell death signals. Modulation of apoptosis by manipulation of signal transduction pathways has emerged as a basis for understanding the actions of drugs and designing new strategies to improve their use.

A general view of how cancer treatments work is that the interaction of a chemotherapeutic drug with its target induces a "cascade" of further signaling steps. These signals ultimately lead to cell death by triggering an "execution phase" where proteases, nucleases, and endogenous regulators of the cell death pathway are activated (Fig. 81-3).

Targeted agents differ from chemotherapy agents in that they do not indiscriminately cause macromolecular lesions but regulate the action of particular pathways. For example, the $p210^{bcr\text{-}abl}$ fusion protein tyrosine kinase drives chronic myeloid leukemia (CML), and HER-2/neu stimulates the proliferation of certain breast cancers. The tumor has been described as "addicted" to the function of these molecules in the sense that without the pathway's continued action, the tumor cell cannot survive. In this way, targeted agents may alter the "threshold" tumors have for undergoing apoptosis without actually creating any molecular lesions such as direct DNA strand breakage or altered membrane function.

While apoptotic mechanisms are important in regulating cellular proliferation and the behavior of tumor cells in vitro, in vivo it is unclear whether all of the actions of chemotherapeutic agents to cause cell death can be attributed to apoptotic mechanisms. However, changes in molecules that regulate apoptosis are correlated with clinical outcomes (e.g., *bcl2* overexpression in certain lymphomas conveys poor prognosis; pro-apoptotic bax expression is associated with a better outcome after chemotherapy for ovarian carcinoma). A better understanding of the relationship of cell death and cell survival mechanisms is needed.

Resistance to chemotherapy drugs has been postulated to arise either from cells not being in the appropriate phase of the cell cycle to allow drug lethality, or from decreased uptake, increased efflux, metabolism of the drug, or alteration of the target, e.g., by mutation or overexpression. Indeed, p170PGP (p170 P-glycoprotein; *mdr* gene product) was recognized from experiments with cells growing in tissue culture as mediating the efflux of chemotherapeutic agents in resistant cells. Certain neoplasms, particularly hematopoietic tumors, have an adverse prognosis if they express high levels of p170PGP, and modulation of this protein's function has been attempted by a variety of strategies.

Chemotherapeutic agents where drugs acting by different mechanisms were combined (e.g., an alkylating agent plus an antimetabolite plus a mitotic spindle blocker) proved to be more effective than single agents. Particular combinations were chosen to emphasize drugs whose individual toxicities to the host were, if possible, distinct. As agents emerge with novel mechanisms of action, combinations of drugs and targeted agents may maximize the chances of affecting critical pathways in the tumor.

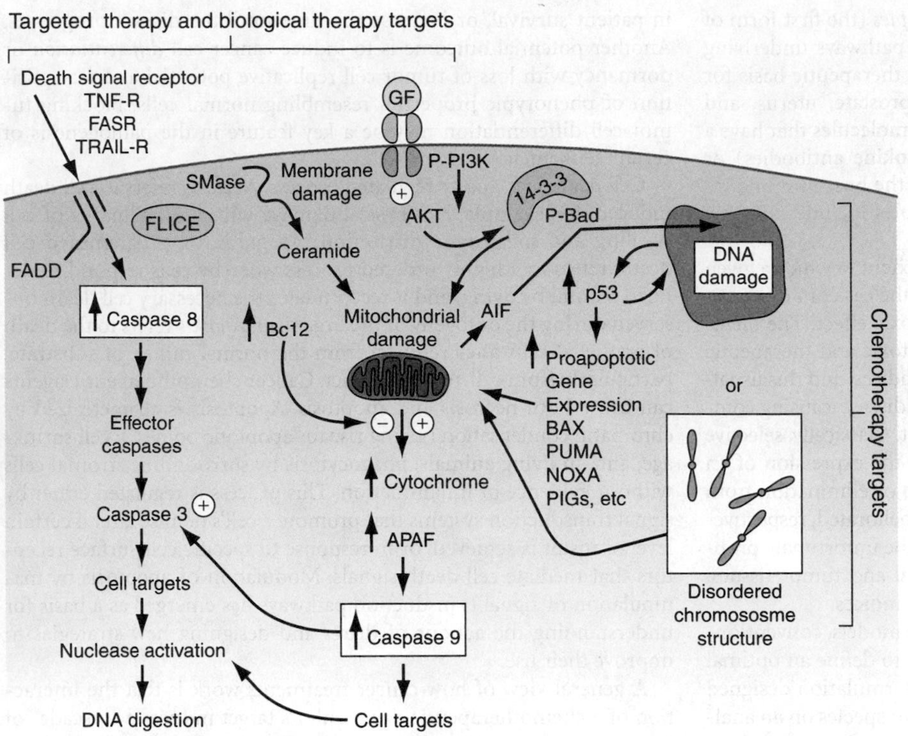

FIGURE 81-3 Integration of cell death responses. Cell death through an apoptotic mechanism requires active participation of the cell. In response to interruption of growth factor (GF) or propagation of certain cytokine death signals (e.g., tumor necrosis factor receptor, TNF-R), there is activation of "upstream" cysteine aspartyl proteases (caspases), which then directly digest cytoplasmic and nuclear proteins, resulting in activation of "downstream" caspases; these cause activation of nucleases, resulting in the characteristic DNA fragmentation that is a hallmark of apoptosis. Chemotherapy agents that create lesions in DNA or alter mitotic spindle function seem to activate aspects of this process by damage ultimately conveyed to the mitochondria, perhaps by activating the transcription of genes whose products can produce or modulate the toxicity of free radicals. In addition, membrane damage with activation of sphingomyelinases results in the production of ceramides that can have a direct action at mitochondria. The antiapoptotic protein bcl2 attenuates mitochondrial toxicity, while proapoptotic gene products such as bax antagonize the action of bcl2. Damaged mitochondria release cytochrome C and apoptosis-activating factor (APAF), which can directly activate caspase 9, resulting in propagation of a direct signal to other downstream caspases through protease activation. Apoptosis-inducing factor (AIF) is also released from the mitochondrion and then can translocate to the nucleus, bind to DNA, and generate free radicals to further damage DNA. An additional proapoptotic stimulus is the bad protein, which can heterodimerize with *bcl2* gene family members to antagonize apoptosis. Importantly, though, bad protein function can be retarded by its sequestration as phospho-bad through the 14-3-3 adapter proteins. The phosphorylation of bad is mediated by the action of the AKT kinase in a way that defines how growth factors that activate this kinase can retard apoptosis and promote cell survival.

CHEMOTHERAPEUTIC AGENTS USED FOR CANCER TREATMENT

Table 81-2 lists commonly used cancer chemotherapy agents and pertinent clinical aspects of their use. The drugs and schedules listed are examples that have proved tolerable and useful; the specific doses that may be used in a particular patient may vary somewhat with the particular treatment protocol, or plan, of treatment. Significant variation from these dose ranges should be carefully verified to avoid or anticipate toxicity. Not included in Table 81-2 are hormone receptor–directed agents, as the side effects are generally those expected from the interruption or augmentation of hormonal effect, and doses used in most cases are those that adequately saturate the intended hormone receptor. The drugs listed may be usefully grouped into three general categories: those affecting DNA, those affecting microtubules, and molecularly targeted agents.

Direct DNA-Interactive Agents DNA replication occurs during the synthesis or S-phase of the cell cycle, with chromosome segregation of the replicated DNA occurring in the M, or mitosis, phase. The G1 and G2 "gap phases" precede S and M, respectively. Historically, chemotherapeutic agents have been divided into "phase-nonspecific" agents, which can act in any phase of the cell cycle, and "phase-specific" agents, which require the cell to be at a particular cell cycle phase to cause greatest effect. Once the agent has acted, cells may progress to "checkpoints" in the cell cycle where the drug-related damage may be assessed and either repaired or allowed to initiate apoptosis. An important function of certain tumor-suppressor genes such as p53 may be to modulate checkpoint function.

FORMATION OF COVALENT DNA ADDUCTS Alkylating agents as a class are cell cycle phase-nonspecific agents. They break down, either spontaneously or after normal organ or tumor cell metabolism, to reactive intermediates that covalently modify bases in DNA. This leads to cross-linkage of DNA strands or the appearance of breaks in DNA as a result of repair efforts. "Broken" or cross-linked DNA is intrinsically unable to complete normal replication or cell division; in addition, it is a potent activator of cell cycle checkpoints and further activates cell-signaling pathways that can precipitate apoptosis. As a class, alkylating agents share similar toxicities: myelosuppression, alopecia, gonadal dysfunction, mucositis, and pulmonary fibrosis. They differ greatly in a spectrum of normal organ toxicities. As a class they share the capacity to cause "second" neoplasms, particularly leukemia, many years after use, particularly when used in low doses for protracted periods.

Cyclophosphamide is inactive unless metabolized by the liver to 4-hydroxy-cyclophosphamide, which decomposes into an alkylating species, as well as to chloroacetaldehyde and acrolein. The latter causes chemical cystitis; therefore, excellent hydration must be maintained while using cyclophosphamide. If severe, the cystitis may be effectively treated by mesna (2-mercaptoethanesulfonate). Liver disease impairs drug activation. Sporadic interstitial pneumonitis leading to pulmonary fibrosis can accompany the use of cyclophosphamide, and high doses used in conditioning regimens for bone marrow transplant can cause cardiac dysfunction. Ifosfamide is a cyclophosphamide analogue also activated in the liver, but more slowly, and it requires coadministration of mesna to prevent bladder injury. Central nervous system (CNS) effects, including somnolence, confusion, and psychosis, can follow ifosfamide use; the incidence appears related to low body surface area or the presence of nephrectomy.

Several alkylating agents are less commonly used. Nitrogen mustard (mechlorethamine) is the prototypic agent of this class, decomposing rapidly in aqueous solution to potentially yield a bifunctional carbonium ion. It must be administered shortly after preparation into a rapidly flowing intravenous line. It is a powerful vesicant, and infiltration may be symptomatically ameliorated by infiltration of the affected site with 1/6 *M* thiosulfate. Even without infiltration, aseptic thrombophlebitis is frequent. It can be used topically as a dilute solution in cutaneous lymphomas, with a notable incidence of hypersensitivity reactions. It causes moderate nausea after intravenous administration.

Chlorambucil causes predictable myelosuppression, azoospermia, nausea, and pulmonary side effects. Busulfan can cause profound

TABLE 81-2 COMMONLY USED CANCER CHEMOTHERAPY AGENTS

Drug	Examples of Usual Doses	Toxicity	Interactions, Issues
Direct DNA-Interacting Agents			
Alkylators			
Cyclophosphamide	400–2000 mg/m^2 IV 100 mg/m^2 PO qd	Marrow (relative platelet sparing) Cystitis Common alkylator[a] Cardiac (high dose)	Liver metabolism required to activate to phosphoramide mustard + acrolein Mesna protects against "high-dose" bladder damage
Mechlorethamine	6 mg/m^2 IV day 1 and day 8	Marrow Vesicant Nausea	Topical use in cutaneous lymphoma
Chlorambucil	1–3 mg/m^2 qd PO	Marrow Common alkylator[a]	
Melphalan	8 mg/m^2 qd × 5, PO	Marrow (delayed nadir) GI (high dose)	Decreased renal function delays clearance
Carmustine (BCNU)	200 mg/m^2 IV 150 mg/m^2 PO	Marrow (delayed nadir) GI, liver (high dose) Renal	
Lomustine (CCNU)	100–300 mg/m^2 PO	Marrow (delayed nadir)	
Ifosfamide	1.2 g/m^2 per day qd × 5 + mesna	Myelosuppressive Bladder Neurologic Metabolic acidosis Neuropathy	Isomeric analogue of cyclophosphamide More lipid soluble Greater activity vs testicular neoplasms and sarcomas Must use mesna
Procarbazine	100 mg/m^2 per day qd ×14	Marrow Nausea Neurologic Common alkylator[a]	Liver and tissue metabolism required Disulfiran-like effect with ethanol Acts as MAOI HBP after tyrosinase-rich foods
Dacarbazine (DTIC)	375 mg/m^2 IV day 1 and day 15	Marrow Nausea Flulike	Metabolic activation
Temozolomide	150–200 mg/m^2 qd × 5 q28d *or* 75 mg/m^2 qd × 6–7 weeks	Nausea/vomiting Headache/fatigue Constipation	Infrequent myelosuppression
Altretamine (formerly hexamethyl-melamine)	260 mg/m^2 per day qd ×14–21 as 4 divided oral doses	Nausea Neurologic (mood swing) Neuropathy Marrow (less)	Liver activation Barbiturates enhance/cimetidine diminishes
Cisplatin	20 mg/m^2 qd ×5 IV 1 q3–4 weeks *or* 100–200 mg/m^2 per dose IV q3–4 weeks	Nausea Neuropathy Auditory Marrow platelets > WBCs Renal Mg^{2+}, Ca^{2+}	Maintain high urine flow; osmotic diuresis, monitor intake/output K^+, Mg^{2+} Emetogenic—prophylaxis needed Full dose if CrCl > 60 mL/min and tolerate fluid push
Carboplatin	365 mg/m^2 IV q3–4 weeks as adjusted for CrCl	Marrow platelets > WBCs Nausea Renal (high dose)	Reduce dose according to CrCl: to AUC of 5–7 mg/mL per min [AUC = dose/(CrCl + 25)]
Oxaliplatin	130 mg/m^2 q3 weeks over 2 h *or* 85 mg/m^2 q2 weeks	Nausea Anemia	Acute reversible neurotoxicity; chronic sensory neurotox cumulative with dose; reversible laryngopharyngeal spasm
Antitumor antibiotics			
Bleomycin	15–25 mg/d qd ×5 IV bolus *or* continuous IV	Pulmonary Skin effects Raynaud's Hypersensitivity	Inactivate by bleomycin hydrolase (decreased in lung/skin) O_2 enhances pulmonary toxicity Cisplatin-induced decrease in CrCl may increase skin/lung toxicity Reduce dose if CrCl < 60 mL/min
Actinomycin D	10–15 μg/kg per day qd ×5 IV bolus	Marrow Nausea Mucositis Vesicant Alopecia	Radiation recall
Mitomycin C	6–10 mg/m^2 q6 weeks	Marrow Vesicant Hemolytic-uremic syndrome Lung CV—heart failure	Treat superficial bladder cancers by intravesical infusion Delayed marrow toxicity Cumulative marrow toxicity
Etoposide (VP16-213)	100–150 mg/m^2 IV qd ×3–5d *or* 50 mg/m^2 PO qd ×21d *or* up to 1500 mg/m^2 per dose (high dose with stem cell support)	Marrow (WBCs > platelet) Alopecia Hypotension Hypersensitivity (rapid IV) Nausea Mucositis (high dose)	Hepatic metabolism—renal 30% Reduce doses with renal failure Schedule-dependant (5 day better than 1 day) Late leukemogenic Accentuate antimetabolite action

(continued)

TABLE 81-2 COMMONLY USED CANCER CHEMOTHERAPY AGENTS (CONTINUED)

Drug	Examples of Usual Doses	Toxicity	Interactions, Issues
Topotecan	20 mg/m² IV q3–4 weeks over 30 min *or* 1.5–3 mg/m² q3–4 weeks over 24 h *or* 0.5 mg/m² per day over 21 days	Marrow Mucositis Nausea Mild alopecia	Reduce dose with renal failure No liver toxicity
Irinotecan (CPT II)	100–150 mg/m² IV over 90 min q3–4 weeks *or* 30 mg/m² per day over 120 h	Diarrhea: "early onset" with cramping, flushing, vomiting; "late onset" after several doses Marrow Alopecia Nausea Vomiting Pulmonary	Prodrug requires enzymatic clearance to active drug "SN 38" Early diarrhea likely due to biliary excretion Late diarrhea, use "high-dose" loperamide (2 mg q2–4 h)
Doxorubicin and daunorubicin	45–60 mg/m² dose q3–4 weeks *or* 10–30 mg/m² dose q week *or* continuous-infusion regimen	Marrow Mucositis Alopecia Cardiovascular acute/chronic Vesicant	Heparin aggregate; coadministration increases clearance Acetaminophen, BCNU increase liver toxicity Radiation recall
Idarubicin	10–15 mg/m² IV q 3 weeks *or* 10 mg/m² IV qd ×3	Marrow Cardiac (less than doxorubicin)	None established
Epirubicin	150 mg/m² IV q3 weeks	Marrow Cardiac	None established
Mitoxantrone	12 mg/m² qd ×3 *or* 12–14 mg/m² q3 weeks	Marrow Cardiac (less than doxorubicin) Vesicant (mild) Blue urine, sclerae, nails	Interacts with heparin Less alopecia, nausea than doxorubicin Radiation recall
Indirect DNA-Interacting Agents			
Antimetabolites			
Deoxycoformycin	4 mg/m² IV every other week	Nausea Immunosuppression Neurologic Renal	Excretes in urine Reduce dose for renal failure Inhibits adenosine deaminase
6-Mercaptopurine	75 mg/m² PO *or* up 500 mg/m² PO (high dose)	Marrow Liver Nausea	Variable bioavailability Metabolize by xanthine oxidase Decrease dose with allopurinol Increased toxicity with thiopurine methyltransferase deficiency
6-Thioguanine	2–3 mg/kg per day for up to 3–4 weeks	Marrow Liver Nausea	Variable bioavailability Increased toxicity with thiopurine methyltransferase deficiency
Azathioprine	1–5 mg/kg per day	Marrow Nausea Liver	Metabolizes to 6MP, therefore reduce dose with allopurinol Increased toxicity with thiopurine methyltransferase deficiency
2-Chlorodeoxyadenosine	0.09 mg/kg per day qd ×7 as continuous infusion	Marrow Renal Fever	Notable use in hairy cell leukemia
Hydroxyurea	20–50 mg/kg (lean body weight) PO qd *or* 1–3 g/d	Marrow Nausea Mucositis Skin changes Rare renal, liver, lung, CNS	Decrease dose with renal failure Augments antimetabolite effect
Methotrexate	15–30 mg PO or IM qd ×3–5 *or* 30 mg IV days 1 and 8 *or* 1.5–12 g/m² per day (with leucovorin)	Marrow Liver/lung Renal tubular Mucositis	Rescue with leucovorin Excreted in urine Decrease dose in renal failure NSAIDs increase renal toxicity
5-Fluorouracil	375 mg/m² IV qd ×5 *or* 600 mg/m² IV days 1 and 8	Marrow Mucositis Neurologic Skin changes	Toxicity enhanced by leucovorin Dihydropyrimidine dehydrogenase deficiency increases toxicity Metabolizes in tissues
Capecitabine	665 mg/m² bid continuous; 1250 mg/m² bid 2 weeks on/ 1 off; 829 mg/m² bid 2 weeks on/ 1 off + 60 mg/d leucovorin	Diarrhea Hand-foot syndrome	Prodrug of 5FU due to intratumoral metabolism
Cytosine arabinoside	100 mg/m² per day qd ×7 by continuous infusion *or* 1–3 g/m² dose IV bolus	Marrow Mucositis Neurologic (high dose) Conjunctivitis (high dose) Noncardiogenic pulmonary edema	Enhances activity of alkylating agents Metabolizes in tissues by deamination
Azacytidine	750 mg/m² per week *or* 150–200 mg/m² per day ×5–10 (bolus) or (continuous IV)	Marrow Nausea Liver Neurologic Myalgia	Use limited to leukemia Altered methylation of DNA alters gene expression

(continued)

TABLE 81-2 COMMONLY USED CANCER CHEMOTHERAPY AGENTS (CONTINUED)

Drug	Examples of Usual Doses	Toxicity	Interactions, Issues
Gemcitabine	1000 mg/m² IV weekly ×7	Marrow Nausea Hepatic Fever/"flu syndrome"	
Fludarabine phosphate	25 mg/m² IV qd ×5	Marrow Neurologic Lung	Dose reduction with renal failure Metabolized to F-ara converted to F-ara ATP in cells by deoxycytidine kinase
Asparaginase	25,000 IU/m² q3–4 weeks *or* 6000 IU/m² per day qod for 3–4 weeks *or* 1000–2000 IU/m² for 10–20 days	Protein synthesis Clotting factors Glucose Albumin Hypersensitivity CNS Pancreatitis Hepatic	Blocks methotrexate action
Pemetrexed	200 mg/m² q3 weeks	Anemia Neutropenia Thrombocytopenia	Supplement folate/B_{12} Caution in renal failure
Antimitotic agents			
Vincristine	1–1.4 mg/m² per week	Vesicant Marrow Neurologic GI: ileus/constipation; bladder hypotoxicity; SIADH Cardiovascular	Hepatic clearance Dose reduction for bilirubin >1.5 mg/dL Prophylactic bowel regimen
Vinblastine	6–8 mg/m² per week	Vesicant Marrow Neurologic (less common but similar spectrum to other vincas) Hypertension Raynaud's	Hepatic clearance Dose reduction as with vincristine
Vinorelbine	15–30 mg/m² per week	Vesicant Marrow Allergic/bronchospasm (immediate) Dyspnea/cough (subacute) Neurologic (less prominent but similar spectrum to other vincas)	Hepatic clearance
Paclitaxel	135–175 mg/m² per 24-h infusion *or* 175 mg/m² per 3-h infusion *or* 140 mg/m² per 96-h infusion *or* 250 mg/m² per 24-h infusion plus G-CSF	Hypersensitivity Marrow Mucositis Alopecia Sensory neuropathy CV conduction disturbance Nausea—infrequent	Premedicate with steroids, H_1 and H_2 blockers Hepatic clearance Dose reduction as with vincas
Docetaxel	100 mg/m² per 1-h infusion q3 weeks	Hypersensitivity Fluid retention syndrome Marrow Dermatologic Sensory neuropathy Nausea infrequent Some stomatitis	Premedicate with steroids, H_1 and H_2 blockers
Estramustine phosphate	14 mg/kg per day in 3–4 divided doses with water >2 h after meals Avoid Ca^{2+}-rich foods	Nausea Vomiting Diarrhea CHF Thrombosis Gynecomastia	
NAB-Paclitaxel (protein bound)	260 mg/m² q3 weeks	Neuropathy Anemia Neutropenia Thrombocytopenia	Caution in hepatic insufficiency
Molecularly Targeted Agents			
Imatinib	400 mg/d, continuous	Nausea Periorbital edema	Myelosuppression not frequent in solid tumor indications
Tretinoin	45 mg/m² per day until complete response + anthrocycline-based regimen in APL	Teratogenic Cutaneous	APL differentiation syndrome: pulmonary dysfunction/infiltrate, pleural/pericardial effusion, fever
Bexarotene	300–400 mg/m² per day, continuous	Hypercholesterolemia Hypertriglyceridemia Cutaneous Teratogenic	Central hypothyroidism

(continued)

TABLE 81-2 COMMONLY USED CANCER CHEMOTHERAPY AGENTS (CONTINUED)

Drug	Examples of Usual Doses	Toxicity	Interactions, Issues
Gemtuzumab ozogamicin	9 mg/m^2 over 2 h q2 weeks, usually followed by chemotherapy or marrow transplant	Neutropenia Thrombocytopenia Hepatic	Postinfusion syndrome: fever, chills, hypotension Rare hepatic venoocclusive disease Mucositis uncommon
Denileukin diftitox	9–18 μg/kg per day × 5 d q 3 wk	Nausea/vomiting Chills/fever Asthenia Hepatic	Acute hypersensitivity: hypotension, vasodilation, rash, chest tightness Vascular leak: hypotension, edema, hypoalbuminemia, thrombotic events (MI, DVT, CVA)
Gefitinib	250 mg PO per day	Rash Diarrhea	In U.S., only with prior documented benefit
Erlotinib	150 mg PO per day	Rash Diarrhea	1 h before, 2 h after meals
Dasatinib	70 mg PO bid	Liver changes Rash Neutropenia Thrombocytopenia	
Sorafenib	400 mg PO bid	Diarrhea Hand-foot syndrome Other rash	
Sunitinib	50 mg PO qd for 4 of 6 weeks	Fatigue Diarrhea Neutropenia	
Miscellaneous			
Arsenic trioxide	0.16 mg/kg per day up to 50 days in APL	↑QT_c Peripheral neuropathy Musculoskeletal pain Hyperglycemia	APL differentiation syndrome (see under tretinoin)

[a]Common alkylator: alopecia, pulmonary, infertility, plus teratogenesis.

Note: APL, acute promyelocytic leukemia; AUC, area under the curve; CHF, congestive heart failure; CNS, central nervous system; CrCl, creatinine clearance; CV, cardiovascular; CVA, cerebrovascular accident; DVT, deep venous thrombosis; G-CSF, granulocyte colony-stimulating factor; GI, gastrointestinal; HBP, high blood pressure; MAOI, monoamine oxidase inhibitors; MI, myocardial infarction; 6MP, 6-mercaptopurine; NSAIDs, nonsteroidal anti-inflammatory drugs; SIADH, syndrome of inappropriate antidiuretic hormone; WBCs, white blood cells.

myelosuppression, alopecia, and pulmonary toxicity but is relatively "lymphocyte sparing." Its routine use in treatment of CML has been curtailed in favor of imatinib (Gleevec)or dasatinib, but it is still employed in transplant preparation regimens. Melphalan shows variable oral bioavailability and undergoes extensive binding to albumin and α_1-acidic glycoprotein. Mucositis appears more prominently; however, it has prominent activity in multiple myeloma.

Nitrosoureas break down to carbamoylating species that not only cause a distinct pattern of DNA base pair–directed toxicity but also can covalently modify proteins. They share the feature of causing relatively delayed bone marrow toxicity, which can be cumulative and long-lasting. Streptozotocin is unique in that its glucose-like structure conveys specific toxicity to the islet cells of the pancreas (for whose derivative tumor types it is prominently indicated) as well as causing renal toxicity in the form of Fanconi syndrome, including amino aciduria, glycosuria, and renal tubular acidosis. Methyl CCNU (lomustine) causes direct glomerular as well as tubular damage, cumulatively related to dose and time of exposure.

Procarbazine is metabolized in the liver and possibly in tumor cells to yield a variety of free radical and alkylating species. In addition to myelosuppression, it causes hypnotic and other CNS effects, including vivid nightmares. It can cause a disulfiram-like syndrome on ingestion of ethanol. Altretamine (formerly hexamethylmelamine) and thiotepa can chemically give rise to alkylating species, although the nature of the DNA damage has not been well characterized in either case. Thiotepa can be used for intrathecal treatment of neoplastic meningitis. Dacarbazine (DTIC) is activated in the liver to yield the highly reactive methyl diazonium cation. It causes only modest myelosuppression 21–25 days after a dose but causes prominent nausea on day 1. Temozolomide is structurally related to dacarbazine but was designed to be activated by nonenzymatic hydrolysis in tumors and is bioavailable orally.

Cisplatin was discovered fortuitously by observing that bacteria present in electrolysis solutions could not divide. Only the *cis* diamine configuration is active as an antitumor agent. It is hypothesized that in the intracellular environment, a chloride is lost from each position, being replaced by a water molecule. The resulting positively charged species is an efficient bifunctional interactor with DNA, forming Pt-based cross-links. Cisplatin requires administration with adequate hydration, including forced diuresis with mannitol to prevent kidney damage; even with the use of hydration, gradual decrease in kidney function is common, along with noteworthy anemia. Hypomagnesemia frequently attends cisplatin use and can lead to hypocalcemia and tetany. Other common toxicities include neurotoxocity with stocking-and-glove sensorimotor neuropathy. Hearing loss occurs in 50% of patients treated with conventional doses. Cisplatin is intensely emetogenic, requiring prophylactic antiemetics. Myelosuppression is less evident than with other alkylating agents. Chronic vascular toxicity (Raynaud's phenomenon, coronary artery disease) is a more unusual toxicity. Carboplatin displays less nephro-, oto-, and neurotoxicity. However, myelosuppression is more frequent, and as the drug is exclusively cleared through the kidney, adjustment of dose for creatinine clearance must be accomplished through use of various dosing nomograms. Oxaliplatin is a platinum analog with noteworthy activity in colon cancers refractory to other treatments. It is prominently neurotoxic.

ANTITUMOR ANTIBIOTICS AND TOPOISOMERASE POISONS Antitumor antibiotics are substances produced by bacteria that in nature appear to provide a chemical defense against other hostile microorganisms. As a class they bind to DNA directly and can frequently undergo electron transfer reactions to generate free radicals in close proximity to DNA, leading to DNA damage in the form of single-strand breaks or cross-links. Topoisomerase poisons include natural products or semisynthetic species derived ultimately from plants, and they modify enzymes that regulate the capacity of DNA to unwind to allow normal replication or transcription. These include topoisomerase I, which creates single-strand breaks that then rejoin following the passage of the other DNA strand through the break. Topoisomerase II creates double-strand breaks through which another segment of DNA duplex passes before rejoining. DNA damage from these agents can occur in any cell cycle phase, but cells tend to arrest in S-phase or G_2 of the cell cycle in cells with p53 and Rb pathway lesions as the result of defective checkpoint mechanisms in cancer cells. Owing to the role of topoisomerase I in the procession of the replication fork, topoisomerase I poisons cause lethality if the topoisomerase I–induced lesions are made in S-phase.

Doxorubicin can intercalate into DNA, thereby altering DNA structure, replication, and topoisomerase II function. It can also undergo reduction reactions by accepting electrons into its quinone ring system, with the capacity to undergo reoxidation to form reactive oxygen radicals after reoxidation. It causes predictable myelosuppression, alopecia, nausea, and mucositis. In addition, it causes acute cardiotoxicity in the form of atrial and ventricular dysrhythmias, but these are rarely of clinical significance. In contrast, cumulative doses >550 mg/m^2 are associated with a 10% incidence of chronic cardiomyopathy. The incidence of cardiomyopathy appears to be related to schedule (peak serum concentration), with low dose, frequent treatment, or continuous infusions better tolerated than intermittent higher dose exposures. Cardiotoxicity has been related to iron-catalyzed oxidation and reduction of doxorubicin, and not to topoisomerase action. Cardiotoxicity is related to peak plasma dose; thus, lower doses and continuous infusions are less likely to cause heart damage. Doxorubicin's cardiotoxicity is increased when given together with trastuzumab (Herceptin), the anti-HER-2/neu antibody. Radiation recall or interaction with concomitantly administered radiation to cause local site complications is frequent. The drug is a powerful vesicant, with necrosis of tissue apparent 4–7 days after an extravasation; therefore it should be administered into a rapidly flowing intravenous line. Dexrazoxane is an antidote to doxorubicin-induced extravasation. Doxorubicin is metabolized by the liver, so doses must be reduced by 50–75% in the presence of liver dysfunction. Daunorubicin is closely related to doxorubicin and was actually introduced first into leukemia treatment, where it remains part of curative regimens and has been shown preferable to doxorubicin owing to less mucositis and colonic damage. Idarubicin is also used in acute myeloid leukemia treatment and may be preferable to daunorubicin in activity. Encapsulation of daunorubicin into a liposomal formulation has attenuated cardiac toxicity and antitumor activity in Kaposi's sarcoma and ovarian cancer.

Bleomycin refers to a mixture of glycopeptides that have the unique feature of forming complexes with Fe^{2+} while also bound to DNA. Oxidation of Fe^{2+} gives rise to superoxide and hydroxyl radicals. The drug causes little, if any, myelosuppression. The drug is cleared rapidly, but augmented skin and pulmonary toxicity in the presence of renal failure has led to the recommendation that doses be reduced by 50–75% in the face of a creatinine clearance <25 mL/min. Bleomycin is not a vesicant and can be administered intravenously, intramuscularly, or subcutaneously. Common side effects include fever and chills, facial flush, and Raynaud's phenomenon. Hypertension can follow rapid intravenous administration, and the incidence of anaphylaxis with early preparations of the drug has led to the practice of administering a test dose of 0.5–1 unit before the rest of the dose. The most feared complication of bleomycin treatment is pulmonary fibrosis, which increases in incidence at >300 cumulative units administered and is minimally responsive to treatment (e.g., glucocorticoids). The earliest indicator of an adverse effect is a decline in the DL_{CO}, although cessation of drug immediately upon documentation of a decrease in DL_{CO} may not prevent further decline in pulmonary function. Bleomycin is inactivated by a bleomycin hydrolase, whose concentration is diminished in skin and lung. Because bleomycin-dependent electron transport is dependent on O_2, bleomycin toxicity may become apparent after exposure to transient very high PI_{O2}. Thus, during surgical procedures, patients with prior exposure to bleomycin should be maintained on the lowest PI_{O2} consistent with maintaining adequate tissue oxygenation.

Mitomycin C undergoes reduction of its quinone function to generate a bifunctional DNA alkylating agent. It is a broadly active antineoplastic agent with a number of unpredictable toxicities, including delayed bronchospasm 12–14 h after dosing and a chronic pulmonary fibrosis syndrome more frequent at doses of 50–60 mg/m^2. Cardiomyopathy has been described, particularly in a setting of prior radiation therapy. A hemolytic/uremic syndrome carries an ultimate mortality rate of 25–50% and is poorly treated by conventional component support and exchange transfusion. Mitomycin is a notable vesicant and causes substantial nausea and vomiting. It can be used for intravesical instillation for curative treatment of superficial transitional bladder carcinomas and, with radiation therapy, for curative treatment of anal carcinoma.

Mitoxantrone is a synthetic compound that was designed to recapitulate features of doxorubicin but with less cardiotoxicity. It is quantitatively less cardiotoxic (comparing the ratio of cardiotoxic to therapeutically effective doses) but is still associated with a 10% incidence of cardiotoxicity at cumulative doses of >150 mg/m^2. It also causes alopecia. Cases of acute promyelocytic leukemia (APL) have arisen shortly after exposure of patients to mitoxantrone, particularly in the adjuvant treatment of breast cancer. While chemotherapy-associated leukemia is generally of the acute myeloid type, APL arising in the setting of prior mitoxantrone treatment had the typical t(15;17) chromosome translocation associated with APL, but the breakpoints of the translocation appeared to be at topoisomerase II sites that would be preferred sites of mitoxantrone action, clearly linking the action of the drug to the generation of the leukemia.

Etoposide was synthetically derived from the plant product podophyllotoxin; it binds directly to topoisomerase II and DNA in a reversible ternary complex. It stabilizes the covalent intermediate in the enzyme's action where the enzyme is covalently linked to DNA. This "alkali-labile" DNA bond was historically a first hint that an enzyme such as a topoisomerase might exist. The drug therefore causes a prominent G_2 arrest, reflecting the action of a DNA damage checkpoint. Prominent clinical effects include myelosuppression, nausea, and transient hypotension related to the speed of administration of the agent. Etoposide is a mild vesicant but is relatively free from other large-organ toxicities. When given at high doses or very frequently, topoisomerase II inhibitors may cause acute leukemia associated with chromosome 11q23 abnormalities in up to 1% of exposed patients.

Camptothecin was isolated from extracts of a Chinese tree and had notable antileukemia activity. Early clinical studies with the sodium salt of the hydrolyzed camptothecin lactone showed evidence of toxicity with little antitumor activity. Identification of topoisomerase I as the target of camptothecins and the need to preserve lactone structure allowed additional efforts to identify active members of this series. Topoisomerase I is responsible for unwinding the DNA strand by introducing single-strand breaks and allowing rotation of one strand about the other. In S-phase, topoisomerase I–induced breaks that are not promptly resealed lead to progress of the replication fork off the end of a DNA strand. The DNA damage is a potent signal for induction of apoptosis. Camptothecins promote the stabilization of the DNA linked to the enzyme in a so-called cleavable complex, analogous to the action of etoposide with topoisomerase II. Topotecan is a camptothecin derivative approved for use in gynecologic tumors and small cell lung cancer. Toxicity is limited to myelosuppression and mucositis. CPT-11, or irinotecan, is a camptothecin with evidence of activity in colon carcinoma. In addition to myelosuppression, it causes a secretory diarrhea related to the toxicity of a metabolite called SN-38. The diarrhea can be treated effectively with loperamide or octreotide.

Indirect Effectors of DNA Function: Antimetabolites A broad definition of antimetabolites would include compounds with structural similarity to precursors of purines or pyrimidines, or compounds that interfere with purine or pyrimidine synthesis. Antimetabolites can cause DNA damage indirectly, through misincorporation into DNA, abnormal timing or progression through DNA synthesis, or altered function of pyrimidine and purine biosynthetic enzymes. They tend to convey greatest toxicity to cells in S-phase, and the degree of toxicity increases with duration of exposure. Common toxic manifestations include stomatitis, diarrhea, and myelosuppression. Second malignancies are not associated with their use.

Methotrexate inhibits dihydrofolate reductase, which regenerates reduced folates from the oxidized folates produced when thymidine monophosphate is formed from deoxyuridine monophosphate. Without reduced folates, cells die a "thymine-less" death. N5-tetrahydrofolate or N5-formyltetrahydrofolate (leucovorin) can bypass this block and rescue cells from methotrexate, which is maintained in cells by polyglutamylation. The drug and other reduced folates are transported into cells by the folate carrier, and high concentrations of drug can bypass this carrier and allow diffusion of drug directly into cells. These properties have suggested the design of "high-dose" methotrexate regimens with leucovorin rescue of normal marrow and mucosa as part of curative approaches to osteosarcoma in the adjuvant setting and hematopoietic neoplasms of children and adults. Methotrexate is cleared by the kidney via both glomerular filtration and tubular secretion, and toxicity is augmented by renal dysfunction and drugs such as salicylates, probenecid, and nonsteroidal anti-inflammatory agents that undergo tubular secretion. With normal renal function, 15 mg/m^2 leucovorin will rescue 10^{-8} to 10^{-6} *M* methotrexate in three to four doses. However, with decreased creatinine clearance, doses of 50–100 mg/m^2 are continued until methotrexate levels are $<5 \times 10^{-8}$ *M*. In addition to bone marrow suppression and mucosal irritation, methotrexate can cause renal failure itself at high doses owing to crystallization in renal tubules; therefore, high-dose regimens require alkalinization of urine with increased flow by hydration. Methotrexate can be sequestered in third-space collections and leech back into the general circulation, causing prolonged myelosuppression. Less frequent adverse effects include reversible increases in transaminases and hypersensitivity-like pulmonary syndrome. Chronic low-dose methotrexate can cause hepatic fibrosis. When administered to the intrathecal space, methotrexate can cause chemical arachnoiditis and CNS dysfunction.

Pemetrexed is a novel folate-directed antimetabolite. It is "multitargeted" in that it inhibits the activity of several enzymes, including thymidylate synthetase, dihydrofolate reductase, and glycinamide ribonucleotide formyltransferase, thereby affecting the synthesis of both purine and pyrimidine nucleic acid precursors. To avoid significant toxicity to the normal tissues, patients receiving pemetrexed should also receive low-dose folate and vitamin B12 supplementation. Pemetrexed has notable activity against certain lung cancers and, in combination with cisplatin, also against mesotheliomas.

5-Fluorouracil (5FU) represents an early example of "rational" drug design in that it originated from the observation that tumor cells incorporate radiolabeled uracil more efficiently into DNA than normal cells, especially gut. 5FU is metabolized in cells to 5′FdUMP, which inhibits thymidylate synthetase (TS). In addition, misincorporation can lead to single-strand breaks, and RNA can aberrantly incorporate FUMP. 5FU is metabolized by dihydropyrimidine dehydrogenase, and deficiency of this enzyme can lead to excessive toxicity from 5FU. Oral bioavailability varies unreliably, but orally administered analogues of 5FU such as capecitabine have been developed that allow at least equivalent activity to many parenteral 5FU-based approaches to refractory cancers. Intravenous administration of 5FU leads to bone marrow suppression after short infusions but to stomatitis after prolonged infusions. Leucovorin augments the activity of 5FU by promoting formation of the ternary covalent complex of 5FU, the reduced folate, and TS. Less frequent toxicities include CNS dysfunction, with prominent cerebellar signs, and endothelial toxicity manifested by thrombosis, including pulmonary embolus and myocardial infarction.

Cytosine arabinoside (ara-C) is incorporated into DNA after formation of ara-CTP, resulting in S-phase–related toxicity. Continuous infusion schedules allow maximal efficiency, with uptake maximal at 5–7 μM. Ara-C can be administered intrathecally. Adverse effects include nausea, diarrhea, stomatitis, chemical conjunctivitis, and cerebellar ataxia. Gemcitabine is a cytosine derivative that is similar to ara-C in that it is incorporated into DNA after anabolism to the triphosphate, rendering DNA susceptible to breakage and repair synthesis, which differs from that in ara-C in that gemcitabine-induced lesions are very inefficiently removed. In contrast to ara-C, gemcitabine appears to have useful activity in a variety of solid tumors, with limited nonmyelosuppressive toxicities. 6-Thioguanine and 6-mercaptopurine (6MP) are used in the treatment of acute lymphoid leukemia. Although administered orally, they display variable bioavailability. 6MP is metabolized by xanthine oxidase and therefore requires dose reduction when used with allopurinol.

Fludarabine phosphate is a prodrug of F-adenine arabinoside (F-ara-A), which in turn was designed to diminish the susceptibility of ara-A to adenosine deaminase. F-ara-A is incorporated into DNA and can cause delayed cytotoxicity even in cells with low growth fraction, including chronic lymphocytic leukemia and follicular B cell lymphoma. CNS and peripheral nerve dysfunction and T cell depletion leading to opportunistic infections can occur in addition to myelosuppression. 2-Chlorodeoxyadenosine is a similar compound with activity in hairy cell leukemia. 2-Deoxycoformycin inhibits adenosine deaminase, with resulting increase in dATP levels. This causes inhibition of ribonucleotide reductase as well as augmented susceptibility to apoptosis, particularly in T cells. Renal failure and CNS dysfunction are notable toxicities in addition to immunosuppression. Hydroxyurea inhibits ribonucleotide reductase, resulting in S-phase block. It is orally bioavailable and useful for the acute management of myeloproliferative states.

Asparaginase is a bacterial enzyme that causes breakdown of extracellular asparagine required for protein synthesis in certain leukemic cells. This effectively stops tumor cell DNA synthesis, as DNA synthesis requires concurrent protein synthesis. The outcome of asparaginase action is therefore very similar to the result of the small-molecule antimetabolites. As asparaginase is a foreign protein, hypersensitivity reactions are common, as are effects on organs such as pancreas and liver that normally require continuing protein synthesis. This may result in decreased insulin secretion with hyperglycemia, with or without hyperamylasemia and clotting function abnormalities. Close monitoring of clotting functions should accompany use of asparaginase. Paradoxically, owing to depletion of rapidly turning over anticoagulant factors, thromboses particularly affecting the CNS may also be seen with asparaginase.

Mitotic Spindle Inhibitors Microtubules are cellular structures that form the mitotic spindle, and in interphase cells they are responsible for the cellular "scaffolding" along which various motile and secretory processes occur. Microtubules are composed of repeating noncovalent multimers of a heterodimer of α and subunits of the protein tubulin. Vincristine binds to the tubulin dimer with the result that microtubules are disaggregated. This results in the block of growing cells in M-phase; however, toxic effects in G_1 and S-phase are also evident. Vincristine is metabolized by the liver, and dose adjustment in the presence of hepatic dysfunction is required. It is a powerful vesicant, and infiltration can be treated by local heat and infiltration of hyaluronidase. At clinically used intravenous doses, neurotoxicity in the form of glove-and-stocking neuropathy is frequent. Acute neuropathic effects include jaw pain, paralytic ileus, urinary retention, and the syndrome of inappropriate antidiuretic hormone secretion. Myelosuppression is not seen. Vinblastine is similar to vincristine, except that it tends to be more myelotoxic, with more frequent thrombocytopenia and also mucositis and stomatitis. Vinorelbine is a vinca alkaloid that appears to have differences in resistance patterns in comparison to vincristine and vinblastine; it may be administered orally.

The taxanes include paclitaxel and docetaxel. These agents differ from the vinca alkaloids in that the taxanes stabilize microtubules against depolymerization. The "stabilized" microtubules function abnormally and are not able to undergo the normal dynamic changes of microtubule structure and function necessary for cell cycle completion. Taxanes are among the most broadly active antineoplastic agents for use in solid tumors, with evidence of activity in ovarian cancer, breast cancer, Kaposi's sarcoma, and lung tumors. They are administered intravenously, and paclitaxel requires use of a Cremophor-containing vehicle that can cause hypersensitivity reactions. Premedication with dexamethasone (20 mg orally or intravenously 12 and 6 h before treatment) and diphenhydramine (50 mg) and cimetidine (300 mg), both 30 min before treatment, decreases but does not eliminate the risk of hypersensitivity reactions to the paclitaxel vehicle. Docetaxel uses a polysorbate 80 formulation, which can cause fluid retention in addition to hypersensitivity reactions, and dexamethasone premedication with or without antihistamines is frequently used. A protein-bound formulation of paclitaxel (called *nab-paclitaxel*) has at least equivalent antineoplastic activity and decreased risk of hypersensitivity reactions. Paclitaxel may also cause hypersensitivity reactions, myelosuppression, neurotoxicity in the form of glove-and-stocking numbness, and paresthesia. Cardiac rhythm disturbances were observed in phase I and II trials, most commonly asymptomatic bradycardia but also, much more rarely, varying degrees of heart block. These have not emerged as clinically significant in the majority of patients. Docetaxel causes comparable degrees of myelosuppression and neuropathy. Hypersensitivity reactions, including bronchospasm, dyspnea, and hypotension, are less frequent but occur to some degree in up to 25% of patients. Fluid retention appears to result from a vascular leak syndrome that can aggravate preexisting effusions. Rash can complicate docetaxel administration, appearing prominently as a pruritic maculopapular rash affecting the forearms, but it has also been associated with fingernail ridging, breakdown, and skin discoloration. Stomatitis appears to be somewhat more frequent than with paclitaxel.

Estramustine was originally synthesized as a mustard derivative that might be useful in neoplasms that possessed estrogen receptors. However, no evidence of interaction with DNA was observed. Surprisingly, the drug caused metaphase arrest, and subsequent study revealed that it binds to microtubule-associated proteins, resulting in abnormal microtubule function. Estramustine binds to estramustine-binding proteins (EMBPs), which are notably present in prostate tumor tissue. The drug is used as an oral formulation in patients with prostate cancer. Gastrointestinal and cardiovascular adverse effects related to the estrogen moiety occur in up to 10% of patients, including worsened heart failure and thromboembolic phenomena. Gynecomastia and nipple tenderness can also occur.

Hormonal Agents The family of steroid hormone receptor–related molecules has emerged as prominent targets for small molecules useful in cancer treatment. When bound to their cognate ligands, these receptors can alter gene transcription and, in certain tissues, induce apoptosis. The pharmacologic effect is a mirror or parody of the normal effects of the agent acting in nontransformed tissue, although the effects on tumors are mediated by indirect effects in some cases.

Glucocorticoids are generally given in "pulsed" high doses in leukemias and lymphomas, where they induce apoptosis in tumor cells. Cushing's syndrome or inadvertent adrenal suppression on withdrawal from high-dose glucocorticoids can be significant complications, along with infections common in immunosuppressed patients, in particular *Pneumocystis* pneumonia, which classically appears a few days after completing a course of high-dose glucocorticoids.

Tamoxifen is a partial estrogen receptor antagonist; it has a tenfold greater antitumor activity in breast cancer patients whose tumors express estrogen receptors than in those who have low or no levels of expression. Side effects include a somewhat increased risk of estrogen-related cardiovascular complications, such as thromboembolic phenomena, and a small increased incidence of endometrial carcinoma, which appears after chronic use (usually >5 years). Progestational agents—including medroxyprogesterone acetate, androgens including fluoxymesterone (Halotestin), and, paradoxically, estrogens—have approximately the same degree of activity in primary hormonal treatment of breast cancers that have elevated expression of estrogen receptor protein. Estrogen is not used often owing to prominent cardiovascular and uterotropic activity.

Aromatase refers to a family of enzymes that catalyze the formation of estrogen in various tissues, including the ovary and peripheral adipose tissue and some tumor cells. Aromatase inhibitors are of two types, the irreversible steroid analogs such as exemestane and the reversible inhibitors such as anastrozole or letrozole. Anastrozole is superior to tamoxifen in the adjuvant treatment of breast cancer in postmenopausal patients with estrogen receptor–positive tumors. Letrozole treatment affords benefit following tamoxifen treatment. Adverse effects of aromatase inhibitors may include an increased risk of osteoporosis.

Prostate cancer is classically treated by androgen deprivation. Diethylstilbestrol (DES) acting as an estrogen at the level of the hypothalamus to downregulate hypothalamic luteinizing hormone (LH) production results in decreased elaboration of testosterone by the testicle. For this reason, orchiectomy is equally as effective as moderate-dose DES, inducing responses in 80% of previously untreated patients with prostate cancer but without the prominent cardiovascular side effects of DES, including thrombosis and exacerbation of coronary artery disease. In the event that orchiectomy is not accepted by the patient, testicular androgen suppression can also be effected by luteinizing hormone–releasing hormone (LHRH) agonists such as leuprolide and goserelin. These agents cause tonic stimulation of the LHRH receptor, with the loss of its normal pulsatile activation resulting in decreased output of LH by the anterior pituitary. Therefore, as primary hormonal manipulation in prostate cancer, one can choose orchiectomy or leuprolide, but not both. The addition of androgen receptor blockers, including flutamide or bicalutamide, is of uncertain additional benefit in extending overall response duration; the combined use of orchiectomy or leuprolide plus flutamide is referred to as *total androgen blockade*.

Tumors that respond to a primary hormonal manipulation may frequently respond to second and third hormonal manipulations. Thus, breast tumors that had previously responded to tamoxifen have, on relapse, notable response rates to withdrawal of tamoxifen itself or to subsequent addition of an aromatase inhibitor or progestin. Likewise, initial treatment of prostate cancers with leuprolide plus flutamide may be followed after disease progression by response to withdrawal of flutamide. These responses may result from the removal of antagonists from mutant steroid hormone receptors that have come to depend on the presence of the antagonist as a growth-promoting influence.

Additional strategies to treat refractory breast and prostate cancers that possess steroid hormone receptors may also address adrenal capacity to produce androgens and estrogens, even after orchiectomy or oophorectomy, respectively. Thus, aminoglutethimide or ketoconazole can be used to block adrenal synthesis by interfering with the enzymes of steroid hormone metabolism. Administration of these agents requires concomitant hydrocortisone replacement and additional glucocorticoid doses administered in the event of physiologic stress.

Humoral mechanisms can also result in complications of an underlying malignancy. Adrenocortical carcinomas can cause Cushing's syndrome as well as syndromes of androgen or estrogen excess. Mitotane can counteract these by decreasing synthesis of steroid hormones. Islet cell neoplasms can cause debilitating diarrhea, treated with the somatostatin analogue octreotide. Prolactin-secreting tumors can be effectively managed by the dopaminergic agonist bromocriptine.

TARGETED THERAPIES

A better understanding of cancer cell biology has suggested many new targets for cancer drug discovery and development. These include the products of oncogenes and tumor-suppressor genes, regulators of cell death pathways, mediators of cellular immortality such as telomerase, and molecules responsible for microenvironmental molding such as proteases or angiogenic factors. The essential difference in the development of agents that would target these processes is that the basis for discovery of the candidate drug is the a priori importance of the target in the biology of the tumor, rather than the initial detection of drug candidates based on the phenomenon of tumor cell regression in tissue culture or in animals. The following examples reflect the rapidly evolving clinical research activity in this area. Figure 81-4 summarizes how FDA-approved targeted agents act.

Hematopoietic Neoplasms Imatinib targets the ATP binding site of the p210$^{bcr\text{-}abl}$ protein tyrosine kinase that is formed as the result of the chromosome 9,22 translocation producing the Philadelphia chromosome in CML. Imatinib is superior to interferon plus chemotherapy in

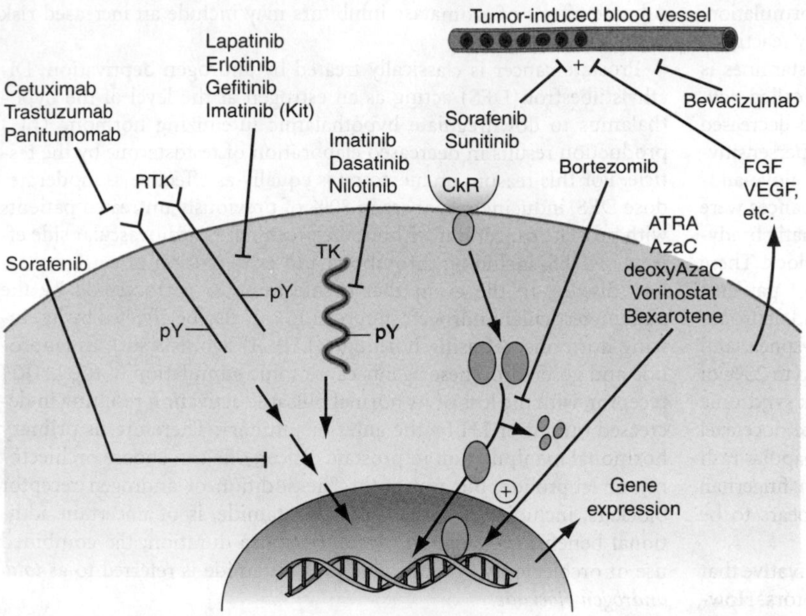

FIGURE 81-4 Site of action of targeted agents. Signals proceeding from growth factor–related receptor tyrosine kinases (RTKs) such as EGF-R, erbB2, or c-kit can be interrupted by lapatinib, erlotinib, gefitinib, and imatinib, acting at the ATP binding site; or by cetuximab, trastuzumab, or panitumomab. Tyrosine kinases (TKs) that are not directly stimulated by growth factors such as p210 bcr-abl or src can be inhibited by imatinib, dasatinib, or nilotinib. Signals projected downstream from growth factor receptors can be affected by the multitargeted kinase inhibitor sorafenib, acting on c-raf, and, upon arrival at the nucleus, affect gene expression, which can be affected by the targeted transcriptional modulators vorinostat (targeting histone deacetylase), azacytidine derivatives (targeting DNA methyltransferase), or retinoid receptor modulators all-*trans*-retinoic acid (ATRA) or bexarotene. Cytokine receptors (CkRs) are one stimulus for degradation of the inhibitory subunit of the NFκB transcription factor by the proteosome. Bortezomib inhibits this process and can prevent activation of NFκB-dependent genes, among other growth-related effects. Sorafenib and sunitinib, acting as inhibitors of VEGF receptors, can modulate tumor blood vessel function through their action on endothelial cells, while bevacizumab targets the same process by combining with VEGF itself.

the initial treatment of the chronic phase of this disorder. It has lesser activity in the blast phase of CML, where the cells may have acquired additional mutations in p210$^{bcr\text{-}abl}$ itself or other genetic lesions. Its side effects are relatively tolerable in most patients and include hepatic dysfunction, diarrhea, and fluid retention. Rarely, patients receiving imatinib have decreased cardiac function, which may persist after discontinuation of the drug. The quality of response to imatinib enters into the decision about when to refer patients with CML for consideration of transplant approaches. Nilotinib is a tyrosine protein kinase inhibitor with a similar spectrum of activity to imatinib, but with increased potency and perhaps better tolerance by certain patients. Dasatinib, another inhibitor of the p210$^{bcr\text{-}abl}$ oncoproteins, is active in certain mutant variants of p210$^{bcr\text{-}abl}$ that are refractory to imatinib and arise during therapy with imatinib or are present de novo. Dasatinib also has inhibitory action against kinases belonging to the src tyrosine protein kinase family; this activity may contribute to its effects in hematopoietic tumors and suggest a role in solid tumors where src kinases are active. Only the T315I mutant is resistant to dasatinib; a new class of inhibitors called aurora kinase inhibitors is in development to address this problem.

All-*trans*-retinoic acid (ATRA) targets the PML-retinoic acid receptor (RAR) α fusion protein, which is the result of the chromosome 15,17 translocation pathogenic for most forms of APL. Administered orally, it causes differentiation of the neoplastic promyelocytes to mature granulocytes and attenuates the rate of hemorrhagic complications. Adverse effects include headache with or without pseudotumor cerebri and gastrointestinal and cutaneous toxicities. Another active retinoid is the synthetic retinoid X receptor ligand bexarotene, which has activity in cutaneous T cell lymphoma.

Bortezomib is an inhibitor of the proteasome, the multi-subunit assembly of protease activities responsible for the selective degradation of proteins important in regulating activation of transcription factors, including NFκB and proteins regulating cell cycle progression. It has activity in multiple myeloma and certain lymphomas. Adverse effects include neuropathy, orthostatic hypotension with or without hyponatremia, and reversible thrombocytopenia.

Vorinostat is an inhibitor of histone deacetylases, responsible for maintaining the proper orientation of histones on DNA, with resulting capacity for transcriptional readiness. Acetylated histones allow entry of transcription factors and therefore increased expression of genes that are selectively repressed in tumors. The result can be differentiation with the emergence of a more normal cellular phenotype, or cell cycle arrest with expression of endogenous regulators of cell cycle progression. Vorinostat is approved for clinical use in cutaneous T cell lymphoma, with dramatic skin clearing and very few side effects.

DNA methyltransferase inhibitors including 5-azacytidine and 2′-deoxy-5-azacytidine can also increase transcription of genes "silenced" during the pathogenesis of a tumor by causing demethylation of the methylated cytosines that are acquired as an "epigenetic" (i.e., after the DNA is replicated) modification of DNA. These drugs were originally considered antimetabolites but have clinical value in myelodysplastic syndromes and certain leukemias when administered at low doses. Combinations of DNA methyltransferase inhibitors and histone deacetylase inhibitors may offer new approaches to reregulate chromatin function.

Targeted toxins utilize macromolecules such as antibodies or cytokines with high affinity for defined tumor cell surface molecules, such as a leukemia differentiation antigen, to which a therapeutic antibody can deliver a covalently linked potent cytotoxin (e.g., gemtuzumab ozogamicin, a drug linked to anti-CD33), or a growth factor such as IL-2 to deliver a toxin (in the form of diphtheria toxin in denileukin diftitox) to cells bearing the IL-2 receptor. The value of such targeted approaches is that in addition to maximizing the therapeutic index by differential expression of the target in tumor (as opposed to nonrenewable normal cells), selection of patients for clinical use can capitalize on assessing the target in the tumor.

Solid Tumors Small-molecule epidermal growth factor (EGF) antagonists act at the ATP binding site of the EGF receptor tyrosine kinase. In early clinical trials, gefitinib showed evidence of responses in a small fraction of patients with non-small cell lung cancer. Side effects were generally acceptable, consisting mostly of rash and diarrhea. Gefitinib was found to have antitumor activity mainly in the subset of patients with tumors containing activating mutations in the EGF receptor. Often patients who developed resistance to gefitinib have acquired additional mutations in the enzyme, similar to what was seen in imatinib-resistant CML. Erlotinib is another EGF receptor tyrosine kinase antagonist with somewhat superior activity to gefitinib in clinical trials in non-small cell lung cancer. Even patients with wild-type EGF receptors may benefit from erlotinib treatment. Lapitinib is a combined EGF receptor and erbB2 tyrosine kinase antagonist with activity in breast cancers refractory to anti-erbB2 antibodies.

In addition to the p210$^{bcr\text{-}abl}$ kinase, imatinib also has activity against the c-kit tyrosine kinase, activated in gastrointestinal stromal sarcoma, and the platelet derived growth factor receptor (PDGF-R), activated by translocation in certain sarcomas. Imatinib has found clinical utility in these neoplasms previously refractory to chemotherapeutic approaches.

TABLE 81-3 INDICATIONS FOR THE CLINICAL USE OF G-CSF OR GM-CSF

Preventive Uses
- With the first cycle of chemotherapy (so-called primary CSF administration)
  - Not needed on a routine basis
  - Use if the probability of febrile neutropenia is ≥20%
  - Use if patient has preexisting neutropenia or active infection
  - Age >65 treated for lymphoma with curative intent or other tumor treated by similar regimens
  - Poor performance status
  - Extensive prior chemotherapy
  - Dose-dense regimens in a clinical trial or with strong evidence of benefit
- With subsequent cycles if febrile neutropenia has previously occurred (so-called secondary CSF administration)
  - Not needed after short duration neutropenia without fever
  - Use if patient had febrile neutropenia in previous cycle
  - Use if prolonged neutropenia (even without fever) delays therapy

Therapeutic Uses
- Afebrile neutropenic patients
  - No evidence of benefit
- Febrile neutropenic patients
  - No evidence of benefit
  - May feel compelled to use in the face of clinical deterioration from sepsis, pneumonia, or fungal infection, but benefit unclear
- In bone marrow or peripheral blood stem cell transplantation
  - Use to mobilize stem cells from marrow
  - Use to hasten myeloid recovery
- In acute myeloid leukemia
  - G-CSF of minor or no benefit
  - GM-CSF of no benefit and may be harmful
- In myelodysplastic syndromes
  - Not routinely beneficial
  - Use intermittently in subset with neutropenia and recurrent infection

What Dose and Schedule Should Be Used?
- G-CSF: 5 μg/kg per day subcutaneously
- GM-CSF: 250 μg/m^2 per day subcutaneously
- Peg-filgrastim: one dose of 6 mg 24 h after chemotherapy

When Should Therapy Begin and End?
- When indicated, start 24–72 h after chemotherapy
- Continue until absolute neutrophil count is 10,000/μL
- Do not use concurrently with chemotherapy or radiation therapy

Note: G-CSF, granulocyte colony-stimulating factor; GM-CSF, granulocyte-macrophage colony-stimulating factor.
Source: From the American Society of Clinical Oncology.

"Multitargeted" kinase antagonists are small-molecule ATP site-directed antagonists that inhibit more than one protein kinase. Drugs of this type with prominent activity against the vascular endothelial growth factor receptor (VEGF-R) tyrosine kinase have activity in renal cell carcinoma. Sorafenib is a VEGF-R antagonist with activity against the *raf* serine-threonine protein kinase as well. Sunitinib has anti-VEGF-R as well as anti-PDGF-R and anti-c-kit activity. It causes prominent responses as well as stabilization of disease in renal cell cancers and gastrointestinal stromal tumors. Side effects for both agents are mostly acceptable, with fatigue and diarrhea encountered with both agents. The "hand-foot syndrome" with erythema and desquamation of the distal extremities, in some cases requiring dose modification, may be seen with sorafenib. Temsirolimus, an mTOR inhibitor, has activity in renal and breast cancer. It produces some hyperlipidemia (10%), myelosuppression (10%), and rare lung toxicity.

ACUTE COMPLICATIONS OF CANCER CHEMOTHERAPY

Myelosuppression The common cytotoxic chemotherapeutic agents almost invariably affect bone marrow function. Titration of this effect determines the MTD of the agent on a given schedule. The normal kinetics of blood cell turnover influence the sequence and sensitivity of each of the formed elements. Polymorphonuclear leukocytes (PMNs; $t_{1/2}$ = 6–8 h), platelets ($t_{1/2}$ = 5–7 days), and red blood cells (RBCs; $t_{1/2}$ = 120 days) respectively have most, less, and least susceptibility to usually administered cytotoxic agents. The nadir count of each cell type in response to classes of agents is characteristic. Maximal neutropenia occurs 6–14 days after conventional doses of anthracyclines, antifolates, and antimetabolites. Alkylating agents differ from each other in the timing of cytopenias. Nitrosoureas, DTIC, and procarbazine can display delayed marrow toxicity, first appearing 6 weeks after dosing.

Complications of myelosuppression result from the predictable sequelae of the missing cells' function. *Febrile neutropenia* refers to the clinical presentation of fever (one temperature ≥38.5°C or three readings ≥38°C but ≤38.5°C per 24 h) in a neutropenic patient with an uncontrolled neoplasm involving the bone marrow or, more usually, in a patient undergoing treatment with cytotoxic agents. Mortality from uncontrolled infection varies inversely with the neutrophil count. If the nadir neutrophil count is >1000/μL, there is little risk; if <500/μL, risk of death is markedly increased. Management of febrile neutropenia has conventionally included empirical coverage with antibiotics for the duration of neutropenia (Chap. 82). Selection of antibiotics is governed by the expected association of infections with certain underlying neoplasms; careful physical examination (with scrutiny of catheter sites, dentition, mucosal surfaces, and perirectal and genital orifices by gentle palpation); chest x-ray; and Gram stain and culture of blood, urine, and sputum (if any) to define a putative site of infection. In the absence of any originating site, a broadly acting β-lactam with anti-*Pseudomonas* activity, such as ceftazidime, is begun empirically. The addition of vancomycin to cover potential cutaneous sites of origin (until these are ruled out or shown to originate from methicillin-sensitive organisms) or metronidazole or imipenem for abdominal or other sites favoring anaerobes reflects modifications tailored to individual patient presentations. The coexistence of pulmonary compromise raises a distinct set of potential pathogens, including *Legionella*, *Pneumocystis*, and fungal agents that may require further diagnostic evaluations such as bronchoscopy with bronchoalveolar lavage. Febrile neutropenic patients can be stratified broadly into two prognostic groups. The first, with expected short duration of neutropenia and no evidence of hypotension or abdominal or other localizing symptoms, may be expected to do well even with oral regimens, e.g., ciprofloxacin or moxifloxacin, or amoxicillin plus clavulinic acid. A less favorable prognostic group are patients with expected prolonged neutropenia, evidence of sepsis, and end-organ compromise, particularly pneumonia. These patients clearly require tailoring of their antibiotic regimen to their underlying presentation, with frequent empirical addition of antifungal agents if fever persists for 7 days without identification of an adequately treated organism or site.

Transfusion of granulocytes has no role in the management of febrile neutropenia, owing to their exceedingly short half-life, mechanical fragility, and clinical syndromes of pulmonary compromise with leukostasis after their use. Instead, colony-stimulating factors (CSFs) are used to augment bone marrow production of PMNs. Early-acting factors such as IL-1, IL-3, and stem cell factor, have not been as useful clinically as late-acting, lineage-specific factors such as G-CSF (granulocyte colony-stimulating factor) or GM-CSF (granulocyte-macrophage colony-stimulating factor), erythropoietin (EPO), thrombopoietin, IL-6, and IL-11. CSFs may easily become overused in oncology practice. The settings in which their use has been proved effective are limited. G-CSF, GM-CSF, EPO, and IL-11 are currently approved for use. The American Society of Clinical Oncology has developed practice guidelines for the use of G-CSF and GM-CSF (Table 81-3).

Primary prophylaxis (i.e., shortly after completing chemotherapy to reduce the nadir) of G-CSF to patients receiving cytotoxic regimens is associated with a 20% incidence of febrile neutropenia. "Dose-dense" regimens, where cycling of chemotherapy is intended to be completed without delay of administered doses, may also benefit, but such patients should be on a clinical trial. Administration of G-CSF in these circumstances has reduced the incidence of febrile neutropenia in several studies by about 50%. Most patients, however, receive regimens that do not have such a high risk of expected febrile neutropenia, and therefore most patients initially should not receive G-CSF or GM-CSF. Special circumstances—such as a documented history of febrile neutropenia with the regimen in a particular patient or categories of patient at increased risk, such as patients > age 65 with aggressive lymphoma treated with curative chemotherapy regimens; extensive compromise of marrow by prior radiation or chemotherapy; or active, open wounds or deep-seated infection—may support primary treatment with G-CSF or GM-CSF. Administration of G-CSF or GM-CSF to afebrile neutropenic patients or to patients with low-risk febrile neutropenia is not recommended, and patients receiving concomitant chemoradiation treatment, particularly those with thoracic neoplasms, likewise are not generally recommended for treatment. In contrast, administration of G-CSF to high-risk patients with febrile neutropenia and evidence of organ compromise including sepsis syndrome, invasive fungal infection, concurrent hospitalization at the time fever develops, pneumonia, profound neutropenia ($<0.1 \times 10^9$/L), or age >65 years is reasonable.

Secondary prophylaxis refers to the administration of CSFs in patients who have experienced a neutropenic complication from a prior cycle of chemotherapy; dose reduction or delay may be a reasonably considered alternative. G-CSF or GM-CSF is conventionally started 24–72 h after completion of chemotherapy and continued until a PMN count of 10,000/μL is achieved, unless a "depot" preparation of G-CSF such as peg-filgrastim is used, where one dose is administered at least 14 days before the next scheduled administration of chemotherapy. Also, patients with myeloid leukemias undergoing induction therapy may have a slight reduction in the duration of neutropenia if G-CSF is commenced after completion of therapy and may be of particular value in elderly patients, but the influence on long-term outcome has not been defined. GM-CSF probably has a more restricted utility than G-CSF, with its use currently limited to patients after autologous bone marrow transplants, although proper head-to-head comparisons with G-CSF have not been conducted in most instances. GM-CSF may be associated with more systemic side effects.

Dangerous degrees of thrombocytopenia do not frequently complicate the management of patients with solid tumors receiving cytotoxic chemotherapy (with the possible exception of certain carboplatin-containing regimens), but they are frequent in patients with certain hematologic neoplasms where marrow is infiltrated with tumor. Severe bleeding related to thrombocytopenia occurs with increased frequency at platelet counts <20,000/μL and is very prevalent at counts <5000/μL.

The precise "trigger" point at which to transfuse patients is being evaluated in a randomized study. This issue is important not only because of the costs of frequent transfusion, but unnecessary platelet transfusions expose the patient to the risks of allosensitization and loss of value from subsequent transfusion owing to rapid platelet clearance, as well as the infectious and hypersensitivity risks inherent in any transfusion. Prophylactic transfusions to keep platelets >20,000/μL are reasonable in patients with leukemia who are stressed by fever or concomitant medical conditions (the threshold for transfusion is 10,000/μL in patients with solid tumors and no other bleeding diathesis or physiologic stressors such as fever or hypotension, a level that might also be reasonably considered for leukemia patients who are thrombocytopenic but not stressed or bleeding). In contrast, patients with myeloproliferative states may have functionally altered platelets despite normal platelet counts, and transfusion with normal donor platelets should be considered for evidence of bleeding in these patients. Careful review of medication lists to prevent exposure to nonsteroidal anti-inflammatory agents and maintenance of clotting factor levels adequate to support near-normal prothrombin and partial thromboplastin time tests are important in minimizing the risk of bleeding in the thrombocytopenic patient.

Certain cytokines in clinical investigation have shown an ability to increase platelets (e.g., IL-6, IL-1, thrombopoietin), but clinical benefit and safety are not yet proven. IL-11 (oprelvekin) is approved for use in the setting of expected thrombocytopenia, but its effects on platelet counts are small, and it is associated with side effects such as headache, fever, malaise, syncope, cardiac arrhythmias, and fluid retention.

Anemia associated with chemotherapy can be managed by transfusion of packed RBCs. Transfusion is not undertaken until the hemoglobin falls to <80 g/L (8 g/dL) or if compromise of end-organ function occurs or an underlying condition (e.g., coronary artery disease) calls for maintenance of hemoglobin >90 g/L (9 g/dL). Patients who are to receive therapy for >2 months on a "stable" regimen and who are likely to require continuing transfusions are also candidates for EPO to maintain hemoglobin of 90–100 g/L (9–10 g/dL). In the setting of adequate iron stores and serum EPO levels <100 ng/mL, EPO, 150 U three times a week, can produce a slow increase in hemoglobin over about 2 months of administration. Depot formulations can be administered less frequently. It is unclear whether higher hemoglobin levels, up to 110–120 g/L (11–12 g/dL), are associated with improved quality of life to a degree that justifies the more intensive EPO use. Efforts to achieve levels at or above 120 g/L (12 g/dL) have been associated with increased thromboses and mortality. EPO may rescue hypoxic cells from death and contribute to tumor radioresistance. This may be a disadvantage in cancer but a great advantage in the setting of heart attacks and strokes.

Nausea and Vomiting The most common side effect of chemotherapy administration is nausea, with or without vomiting. Nausea may be acute (within 24 h of chemotherapy), delayed (>24 h), or anticipatory of the receipt of chemotherapy. Patients may be likewise stratified for their risk of susceptibility to nausea and vomiting, with increased risk in young, female, heavily pretreated patients without a history of alcohol or drug use but with a history of motion or morning sickness. Antineoplastic agents vary in their capacity to cause nausea and vomiting. Highly emetogenic drugs (>90%) include mechlorethamine, streptozotocin, DTIC, cyclophosphamide at >1500 mg/m^2, and cisplatin; moderately emetogenic drugs (30–90% risk) include carboplatin, cytosine arabinoside (>1 mg/m^2), ifosfamide, conventional-dose cyclophosphamide, and anthracyclines; low-risk (10–30%) agents include fluorouracil, taxanes, etoposide, and bortezomib, with minimal risk (<10%) afforded by treatment with antibodies, bleomycin, busulfan, fludarabine, and vinca alkaloids. *Emesis* is a reflex caused by stimulation of the vomiting center in the medulla. Input to the vomiting center comes from the chemoreceptor trigger zone (CTZ) and afferents from the peripheral gastrointestinal tract, cerebral cortex, and heart. The different emesis "syndromes" require distinct management approaches. In addition, a conditioned reflex may contribute to anticipatory nausea arising after repeated cycles of chemotherapy. Accordingly, antiemesis agents differ in their locus and timing of action. Combining agents from different classes or the sequential use of different classes of agent is the cornerstone of successful management of chemotherapy-induced nausea and vomiting. Of great importance are the prophylactic administration of agents and such psychological techniques as the maintenance of a supportive milieu, counseling, and relaxation to augment the action of antiemetic agents.

Serotonin antagonists (5HT3) and neurokine (NK1) receptor antagonists are useful in "high-risk" chemotherapy regimens. The combination acts at both peripheral gastrointestinal as well as CNS sites that control nausea and vomiting. For example, the 5HT3 blocker dolasetron (Anzamet), 100 mg IV or p.o.; dexamethasone, 12 mg; and the NK1 antagonist aprepitant, 125 mg p.o., are combined on the day of administration of severely emetogenic regimens, with repetition of dexamethasone (8 mg) and aprepitant (80 mg) on days 2 and 3 for delayed nausea. Alternate 5HT3 antagonists include ondansetron (Zofran), given as 0.15 mg/kg intravenously for three doses just before and at 4 and 8 h after chemotherapy; palonosetron (Aloxi) at 0.25 mg over 30 s, 30 min prechemotherapy; and granisetron (Kytril,) given as a single dose of 0.01 mg/kg just before chemotherapy. Emesis from moderately emetic chemotherapy regimens may be prevented with a 5HT3 antagonist and dexamethasone alone for patients not receiving doxorubicin and cyclophosphamide combinations; the latter combination requires the 5HT3/dexamethasone/aprepitant on day 1 but aprepitant alone on days 2 and 3. Emesis from low-emetic-risk regimens may be prevented with 8 mg of dexamethasone alone, or with non-5HT3, non-NK1 antagonist approaches including the following.

Antidopaminergic phenothiazines act directly at the CTZ and include prochlorperazine (Compazine), 10 mg intramuscularly or intravenously, 10–25 mg orally or 25 mg per rectum every 4–6 h for up to four doses; and thiethylperazine (Torecan), 10 mg by potentially all the above routes every 6 h. Haloperidol (Haldol) is a butyrophenone dopamine antagonist given at 0.5–1.0 mg intramuscularly or orally every 8 h. Antihistamines such as diphenhydramine (Benadryl) have little intrinsic antiemetic capacity but are frequently given to prevent or treat dystonic reactions that can complicate use of the antidopaminergic agents. Lorazepam (Ativan) is a short-acting benzodiazepine that provides an anxiolytic effect to augment the effectiveness of a variety of agents when used at 1–2 mg intramuscularly, intravenously, or orally every 4–6 h. Metoclopramide (Reglan) acts on peripheral dopamine receptors to augment gastric emptying and is used in high doses for highly emetogenic regimens (1–2 mg/kg intravenously 30 min before chemotherapy and every 2 h for up to three additional doses as needed); intravenous doses of 10–20 mg every 4–6 h as needed or 50 mg orally 4 h before and 8 and 12 h after chemotherapy are used for moderately emetogenic regimens.

5-9-Tetrahydrocannabinol (Marinol) is a rather weak antiemetic compared to other available agents, but it may be useful for persisting nausea and is used orally at 10 mg every 3–4 h as needed.

Diarrhea Regimens that include fluorouracil infusions and/or irinotecan may produce severe diarrhea. Similar to the vomiting syndromes, chemotherapy-induced diarrhea may be immediate or can occur in a delayed fashion up to 48–72 h after the drugs. Careful attention to maintained hydration and electrolyte repletion, intravenously if necessary, along with antimotility treatments such as "high-dose" loperamide, commenced with 4 mg at the first occurrence of diarrhea, with 2 mg repeated every 2 h until 12 h without loose stools. Octreotide (100–150 μg), a somatostatin analog, or opiate-based preparations may be considered for patients not responding to loperamide.

Mucositis Irritation and inflammation of the mucous membranes particularly afflicting the oral and anal mucosa, but potentially involving the gastrointestinal tract, may accompany cytotoxic chemotherapy. Mucositis is due to damage to the proliferating cells at the base of the mucosal squamous epithelia or in the intestinal crypts. Topical therapies, including anesthetics and barrier-creating preparations, may provide symptomatic relief in mild cases. Palifermin or keratinocyte growth factor, a member of the fibroblast growth factor family, is effective in preventing severe mucositis in the setting of high-dose chemotherapy with stem cell transplantation for hematologic malignancies. It may also prevent mucositis from radiation.

Alopecia Chemotherapeutic agents vary widely in causing alopecia, with anthracyclines, alkylating agents, and topoisomerase inhibitors reliably causing near-total alopecia when given at therapeutic doses. Antimetabolites are more variably associated with alopecia. Psychological support and the use of cosmetic resources are to be encouraged, and "chemo caps" that reduce scalp temperature to decrease the degree of alopecia should be discouraged, particularly during treatment with curative intent of neoplasms such as leukemia or lymphoma, or in adjuvant breast cancer therapy. The richly vascularized scalp can certainly harbor micrometastatic or disseminated disease.

Gonadal Dysfunction and Pregnancy Cessation of ovulation and azoospermia reliably result from alkylating agent– and topoisomerase poison–containing regimens. The duration of these effects varies with age and sex. Males treated for Hodgkin's disease with mechlorethamine- and procarbazine-containing regimens are effectively sterile, whereas fertility usually returns after regimens that include cisplatin, vinblastine, or etoposide and after bleomycin for testicular cancer. Sperm banking before treatment may be considered to support patients likely to be sterilized by treatment. Females experience amenorrhea with anovulation after alkylating agent therapy; they are likely to recover normal menses if treatment is completed before age 30 but unlikely to recover menses after age 35. Even those who regain menses usually experience premature menopause. As the magnitude and extent of decreased fertility can be difficult to predict, patients should be counseled to maintain effective contraception, preferably by barrier means, during and after therapy. Resumption of efforts to conceive should be considered in the context of the patient's likely prognosis. Hormone replacement therapy should be undertaken in women who do not have a hormonally responsive tumor. For those patients who have had a hormone-sensitive tumor primarily treated by a local modality, conventional practice would counsel against hormone replacement, but this issue is under investigation.

Chemotherapy agents have variable effects on the success of pregnancy (Chap. 7). All agents tend to have increased risk of adverse outcomes when administered during the first trimester, and strategies to delay chemotherapy, if possible, until after this milestone should be considered if the pregnancy is to continue to term. Patients in their second or third trimester can be treated with most regimens for the common neoplasms afflicting women in their childbearing years, with the exception of antimetabolites, particularly antifolates, which have notable teratogenic or fetotoxic effects throughout pregnancy. The need for anticancer chemotherapy per se is infrequently a clear basis to recommend termination of a concurrent pregnancy, although each treatment strategy in this circumstance must be tailored to the individual needs of the patient. Chronic effects of cancer treatment are reviewed in **Chap. e13**.

BIOLOGIC THERAPY

The goal of biologic therapy is to manipulate the host-tumor interaction in favor of the host. Theoretically, biologic approaches should reflect a bell-shaped dose-response curve where the maximum biologic effect is less than the MTD. However, empirical trial and error has led to the discovery that a number of biologic treatment approaches may produce antitumor effects, but nearly all of them are most active at their MTD. As a class, biologic therapies may be distinguished from molecularly targeted agents in that many biologic therapies require an active response (e.g., reexpression of silenced genes, or antigen expression) on the part of the tumor cell or on the part of the host (e.g., immunologic effects) to allow therapeutic effect. This may be contrasted with the more narrowly defined antiproliferative or apoptotic response that is the ultimate goal of molecularly targeted agents discussed above. However, there is much commonality in the strategies to evaluate and use molecularly targeted and biologic therapies.

IMMUNE MEDIATORS OF ANTITUMOR EFFECTS

The very existence of a cancer in a person is testimony to the failure of the immune system to deal effectively with the cancer. Tumors have a variety of means of avoiding the immune system: (1) they are often only subtly different from their normal counterparts; (2) they are capable of downregulating their major histocompatibility complex antigens, effectively masking them from recognition by T cells; (3) they are inefficient at presenting antigens to the immune system; (4) they can cloak themselves in a protective shell of fibrin to minimize contact with surveillance mechanisms; and (5) they can produce a range of soluble molecules, including potential immune targets, that can distract the immune system from recognizing the tumor cell or can kill the immune effector cells. Some of the cell products initially polarize the immune response away from cellular immunity (shifting from T_H1 to T_H2 responses; Chap. 308) and ultimately lead to defects in T cells that prevent their activation and cytotoxic activity. Cancer treatment further suppresses host immunity. A variety of strategies are being tested to overcome these barriers.

Cell-Mediated Immunity The strongest evidence that the immune system can exert clinically meaningful antitumor effects comes from allogeneic bone marrow transplantation. Adoptively transferred T cells from the donor expand in the tumor-bearing host, recognize the tumor as being foreign, and can mediate impressive antitumor effects (graft-versus-tumor effects). Three types of experimental interventions are being developed to take advantage of the ability of T cells to kill tumor cells.

1. Allogeneic T cells are transferred to cancer-bearing hosts in three major settings: in the form of allogeneic bone marrow transplantation, as pure lymphocyte transfusions following bone marrow re-

covery after allogeneic bone marrow transplantation, and as pure lymphocyte transfusions following immunosuppressive (but not myeloablative) therapy (so-called minitransplants). In each of these settings, the effector cells are donor T cells that recognize the tumor as being foreign, probably through minor histocompatibility differences. The main risk of such therapy is the development of graft-versus-host disease because of the minimal difference between the cancer and the normal host cells. This approach has been highly effective in certain hematologic cancers.

2. Autologous T cells are removed from the tumor-bearing host, manipulated in several ways in vitro, and given back to the patient. The two major classes of autologous T cell manipulation are (a) to develop tumor antigen–specific T cells and expand them to large numbers over many weeks ex vivo before administration, and (b) to activate the cells with polyclonal stimulators such as anti-CD3 and anti-CD28 after a short period ex vivo and try to expand them in the host after adoptive transfer with stimulation by IL-2, for example. Short periods removed from the patient permit the cells to overcome the tumor-induced T cell defects, and such cells traffic and home to sites of disease better than cells that have been in culture for many weeks. Individual centers have successful experiences with one or the other approach but not both, and whether one is superior to the other is not known.
3. Tumor vaccines are aimed at boosting T cell immunity. The finding that mutant oncogenes that are expressed only intracellularly can be recognized as targets of T cell killing greatly expanded the possibilities for tumor vaccine development. No longer is it difficult to find something different about tumor cells. However, major difficulties remain in getting the tumor-specific peptides presented in a fashion to prime the T cells. Tumors themselves are very poor at presenting their own antigens to T cells at the first antigen exposure (*priming*). Priming is best accomplished by professional antigen-presenting cells (dendritic cells). Thus, a number of experimental strategies are aimed at priming host T cells against tumor-associated peptides. Vaccine adjuvants such as GM-CSF appear capable of attracting antigen-presenting cells to a skin site containing a tumor antigen. Such an approach has been documented to eradicate microscopic residual disease in follicular lymphoma and give rise to tumor-specific T cells. Purified antigen-presenting cells can be pulsed with tumor, its membranes, or particular tumor antigens and delivered as a vaccine. Tumor cells can be transfected with genes that attract antigen-presenting cells. Other ideas are also being tested. In a variation on the theme of adoptive transfer, the tumor vaccine may be given to the normal bone marrow and lymphoid cell donor of an allogeneic transplant so that the donor immune system has more cells capable of recognizing the tumor specifically. Vaccines against viruses that cause cancers are safe and effective. Hepatitis B vaccine prevents hepatocellular carcinoma and a tetravalent human papilloma virus vaccine prevents infection by virus types currently accounting for 70% of cervical cancer. These vaccines are ineffective at treating patients who have developed a virus-induced cancer. Investigational vaccines have shown preliminary evidence of activity against multiple myeloma, certain lymphomas, and melanomas.

Antibodies In general, antibodies are not very effective at killing cancer cells. Because the tumor seems to influence the host toward making antibodies rather than generating cellular immunity, it is inferred that antibodies are easier for the tumor to fend off. Many patients can be shown to have serum antibodies directed at their tumors, but these do not appear to influence disease progression. However, the ability to grow very large quantities of high-affinity antibody directed at a tumor by the hybridoma technique has led to the application of antibodies to the treatment of cancer.

Clinical antitumor efficacy has been obtained using antibodies where the antigen-combining regions are grafted onto human immunoglobulin gene products (chimerized or humanized), or derive de novo from mice bearing human immunoglobulin gene loci. Such humanized antibodies against the CD20 molecule expressed on B cell lymphomas (rituximab) and against the HER-2/neu receptor overexpressed on epithelial cancers, especially breast cancer (trastuzumab), have become reliable tools in the oncologist's armamentarium. Each used alone can cause tumor regression (rituximab more than trastuzumab), and both appear to potentiate the effects of combination chemotherapy given just after antibody administration. Antibodies to CD52 are active in chronic lymphoid leukemia and T cell malignancies. EGF-R–directed antibodies (such as cetuximab and panitumomab) have activity in colorectal cancer refractory to chemotherapy, particularly when utilized to augment the activity of an additional chemotherapy program, and in the primary treatment of head and neck cancers treated with radiation therapy. The mechanism of action is unclear. Direct effects on the tumor may mediate an antiproliferative effect as well as stimulate the participation of host mechanisms involving immune cell or complement-mediated response to tumor cell–bound antibody. Alternatively, the antibody may alter the release of paracrine factors promoting tumor cell survival.

The anti-VEGF antibody bevacizumab shows little evidence of antitumor effect when used alone, but when combined with chemotherapeutic agents it improves the magnitude of tumor shrinkage and time to disease progression in colorectal, lung, and breast cancer. The mechanism for the effect is unclear and may relate to the capacity of the antibody to alter delivery and tumor uptake of the active chemotherapeutic agent.

Side effects include infusion–related hypersensitivity reactions, usually limited to the first infusion, which can be managed with glucocorticoid and/or antihistamine prophylaxis. In addition, distinct syndromes have emerged with different antibodies. Anti-EGF-R antibodies produce an acneiform rash that poorly responds to steroid cream treatment. Trastuzumab (anti-HER-2) can inhibit cardiac function, particularly in those patients with prior exposure to anthracyclines. Bevacizumab has a number of side effects of medical significance, including hypertension, proteinuria, hemorrhage, and gastrointestinal perforations with or without prior surgeries.

Conjugation of antibodies to drugs and toxins is discussed above; conjugates of antibodies with isotopes, photodynamic agents, and other killing moieties may also be effective. Radioconjugates targeting CD20 on lymphomas have been approved for use [ibritumomab tiuxetan (Zevalin), using yttrium-90 or ^{131}I-tositumomab]. Other conjugates are associated with problems that have not yet been solved (e.g., antigenicity, instability, poor tumor penetration).

Cytokines There are >70 separate proteins and glycoproteins with biologic effects in humans: interferon (IFN) α, β, γ; IL-1 through -29 (so far); the tumor necrosis factor (TNF) family [including lymphotoxin, TNF-related apoptosis-inducing ligand (TRAIL), CD40 ligand, and others]; and the chemokine family. Only a fraction of these has been tested against cancer; only IFN-α and IL-2 are in routine clinical use.

About 20 different genes encode IFN-α, and their biologic effects are indistinguishable. Interferon induces the expression of many genes, inhibits protein synthesis, and exerts a number of different effects on diverse cellular processes. Its antitumor effects appear to be antagonized in vitro by thymidine, suggesting that de novo thymidylate synthesis is also affected. The two recombinant forms that are commercially available are IFN-α2a and -α2b. In general, interferon antitumor effects are dose-related, and IFN is most effective at its MTD. Interferon is not curative for any tumor but can induce partial responses in follicular lymphoma, hairy cell leukemia, CML, melanoma, and Kaposi's sarcoma. It has been used in the adjuvant setting in stage II melanoma, multiple myeloma, and follicular lymphoma, with uncertain effects on survival. It produces fever, fatigue, a flulike syndrome, malaise, myelosuppression, and depression and can induce clinically significant autoimmune disease.

IL-2 must exert its antitumor effects indirectly through augmentation of immune function. Its biologic activity is to promote the growth and activity of T cells and natural killer (NK) cells. High doses of IL-2 can produce tumor regression in certain patients with metastatic melanoma and renal cell cancer. About 2–5% of patients may experience complete remissions that are durable, unlike any other treatment for these tumors. IL-2 is associated with myriad clinical side effects: intravascular volume depletion, capillary leak syndrome, adult respiratory distress syndrome, hypotension, fever, chills, skin rash, and impaired renal and liver function. Patients may require blood pressure support and intensive care to manage the toxicity. However, once the agent is stopped, most of the toxicities reverse completely within 3–6 days.

GENE THERAPIES

No gene therapy has been approved for routine clinical use. Several strategies are under evaluation, including the use of viruses that cannot replicate to express genes that can allow the action of drugs or directly inhibit cancer cell growth, viruses that can actually replicate but only in the context of the tumor cell, or viruses that can express antigens in the context of the tumor and therefore provoke a host-mediated immune response. Key issues in the success of these approaches will be in defining safe viral vector systems that escape host immune function and effectively target the tumor or tumor cell milieu. Other gene therapy strategies would utilize therapeutic oligonucleotides to target the expression of genes important in the maintenance of tumor cell viability.

ACKNOWLEDGMENTS

Stephen M. Hahn, MD, and Eli Glatstein, MD, contributed a chapter on radiation therapy in the prior edition, and some of their material has been incorporated into this chapter.

FURTHER READINGS

American Society of Clinical Oncology: 2006 Update of recommendations for the use of white blood cell growth factors: An evidence-based clinical practice guideline. J Clin Oncol 24:3187, 2006

———: Guideline for antiemetics in oncology: Update 2006. J Clin Oncol 24:2932, 2006

Chabner BA, Longo DL (eds): *Cancer Chemotherapy and Biotherapy: Principles and Practice*, 4th ed. Philadelphia, Lippincott Williams & Wilkins, 2006

Folkman J: Angiogenesis: An organizing principle for drug discovery? Nat Rev Drug Discov 6:273, 2007

Krause DS, Van Etten RA: Tyrosine kinases as targets for cancer therapy. N Engl J Med 353:17, 2005

82 Infections in Patients with Cancer

Robert Finberg

Infections are a common cause of death and an even more common cause of morbidity in patients with a wide variety of neoplasms. Autopsy studies show that most deaths from acute leukemia and half of deaths from lymphoma are caused directly by infection. With more intensive chemotherapy, patients with solid tumors have also become more likely to die of infection. Fortunately, an evolving approach to prevention and treatment of infectious complications of cancer has decreased rates of infection-associated mortality and will probably continue to do so. This accomplishment has resulted from three major steps:

1. The concept of "early empirical" antibiotics reduced mortality rates among patients with leukemia and bacteremia from 84% in 1965 to 44% in 1972. With better availability (and early use) of broad-spectrum antibiotics, this figure has recently dropped to 20–36%.
2. "Empirical" antifungal therapy has lowered the incidence of disseminated fungal infection; in trial settings, mortality rates now range from 7 to 21%. An antifungal agent is administered—on the basis of likely fungal infection—to neutropenic patients who, after 4–7 days of antibiotic therapy, remain febrile but have no positive cultures.
3. Use of antibiotics for afebrile neutropenic patients as broad-spectrum prophylaxis against infections promises to decrease both mortality and morbidity even further.

A physical predisposition to infection in patients with cancer (Table 82-1) can be a result of the neoplasm's production of a break in the skin. For example, a squamous cell carcinoma may cause local invasion of the epidermis, which allows bacteria to gain access to the subcutaneous tissue and permits the development of cellulitis. The artificial closing of a normally patent orifice can also predispose to infection: Obstruction of a ureter by a tumor can cause urinary tract infection, and obstruction of the bile duct can cause cholangitis. Part of the host's normal defense against infection depends on the continuous emptying of a viscus; without emptying, a few bacteria present as a result of bacteremia or local transit can multiply and cause disease.

A similar problem can affect patients whose lymph node integrity has been disrupted by radical surgery, particularly patients who have had radical node dissections. A common clinical problem following radical mastectomy is the development of cellulitis (usually caused by

TABLE 82-1 DISRUPTION OF NORMAL BARRIERS THAT MAY PREDISPOSE TO INFECTIONS IN PATIENTS WITH CANCER

Type of Defense	Specific Lesion	Cells Involved	Organism	Cancer Association	Disease
Physical barrier	Breaks in skin	Skin epithelial cells	Staphylococci, streptococci	Head and neck, squamous cell carcinoma	Cellulitis, extensive skin infection
Emptying of fluid collections	Occlusion of orifices: ureters, bile duct, colon	Luminal epithelial cells	Gram-negative bacilli	Renal, ovarian, biliary tree, metastatic diseases of many cancers	Rapid, overwhelming bacteremia; urinary tract infection
Lymphatic function	Node dissection	Lymph nodes	Staphylococci, streptococci	Breast cancer surgery	Cellulitis
Splenic clearance of microorganisms	Splenectomy	Splenic reticuloendothelial cells	*Streptococcus pneumoniae*, *Haemophilus influenzae*, *Neisseria meningitidis*, *Babesia*, *Capnocytophaga canimorsus*	Hodgkin's disease, leukemia, idiopathic thrombocytopenic purpura	Rapid, overwhelming sepsis
Phagocytosis	Lack of granulocytes	Granulocytes (neutrophils)	Staphylococci, streptococci, enteric organisms, fungi	Hairy cell, acute myelocytic, and acute lymphocytic leukemias	Bacteremia
Humoral immunity	Lack of antibody	B cells	*S. pneumoniae*, *H. influenzae*, *N. meningitidis*	Chronic lymphocytic leukemia, multiple myeloma	Infections with encapsulated organisms, sinusitis, pneumonia
Cellular immunity	Lack of T cells	T cells and macrophages	*Mycobacterium tuberculosis*, *Listeria*, herpesviruses, fungi, other intracellular parasites	Hodgkin's disease, leukemia, T cell lymphoma	Infections with intracellular bacteria, fungi, parasites

TABLE 82-2 VACCINATION OF CANCER PATIENTS RECEIVING CHEMOTHERAPY

	Use in Indicated Patients		
Vaccine	**Intensive Chemotherapy**	**Hodgkin's Disease**	**Hematopoietic Stem Cell Transplantation**
Diphtheria-tetanus[a]	Primary series and boosters as necessary	No special recommendation	12, 14, and 24 months after transplantation
Poliomyelitis[b]	Complete primary series and boosters	No special recommendation	12, 14, and 24 months after transplantation
Haemophilus influenzae type b conjugate	Primary series and booster for children	Immunization before treatment and booster 3 months afterward	12, 14, and 24 months after transplantation
Hepatitis A	Not routinely recommended	Not routinely recommended	Not routinely recommended
Hepatitis B	Complete series	No special recommendation	12, 14, and 24 months after transplantation
23-Valent pneumococcal polysaccharide[c]	Every 5 years	Immunization before treatment and booster 3 months afterward	12 and 24 months after transplantation
4-Valent meningococcal conjugate[d]	Should be administered to splenectomized patients and patients living in endemic areas, including college students in dormitories	Should be administered to splenectomized patients and patients living in endemic areas, including college students in dormitories	Should be administered to splenectomized patients and patients living in endemic areas, including college students in dormitories
Influenza	Seasonal immunization	Seasonal immunization	Seasonal immunization
Measles/mumps/rubella	Contraindicated	Contraindicated during chemotherapy	After 24 months in patients without graft-versus-host disease
Varicella-zoster virus	Contraindicated[e]	Contraindicated	Contraindicated

[a]The Td (tetanus-diphtheria) combination is currently recommended for adults. Pertussis vaccines have not been recommended for people >6 years of age in the past. However, recent data indicate that the Tdap (tetanus–diphtheria–acellular pertussis) product is both safe and efficacious in adults.
[b]Live-virus vaccine is contraindicated; inactivated vaccine should be used.
[c]The seven-serotype pneumococcal conjugate vaccine is currently recommended only for children. It is anticipated that future vaccines will include more serotypes and will be recommended for adults.
[d]Currently licensed for people 11–55 years of age.
[e]Contact the manufacturer for more information on use in children with acute lymphocytic leukemia.

streptococci or staphylococci) because of lymphedema and/or inadequate lymph drainage. In most cases, this problem can be addressed by local measures designed to prevent fluid accumulation and breaks in the skin, but antibiotic prophylaxis has been necessary in refractory cases.

A life-threatening problem common to many cancer patients is the loss of the reticuloendothelial capacity to clear microorganisms after splenectomy. Splenectomy may be performed as part of the management of hairy cell leukemia, chronic lymphocytic leukemia (CLL), and chronic myelocytic leukemia (CML) and in Hodgkin's disease. Even after curative therapy for the underlying disease, the lack of a spleen predisposes such patients to rapidly fatal infections. The loss of the spleen through trauma similarly predisposes the normal host to overwhelming infection for life after splenectomy. The splenectomized patient should be counseled about the risks of infection with certain organisms, such as the protozoan *Babesia* (Chap. 204) and *Capnocytophaga canimorsus* (formerly dysgonic fermenter 2, or DF-2), a bacterium carried in the mouths of animals (Chaps. 140 and **e14**). Since encapsulated bacteria (*Streptococcus pneumoniae*, *Haemophilus influenzae*, and *Neisseria meningitidis*) are the organisms most commonly associated with postsplenectomy sepsis, splenectomized persons should be vaccinated (and revaccinated; Table 82-2 and Chap. 116) against the capsular polysaccharides of these organisms. Many clinicians recommend giving splenectomized patients a small supply of antibiotics effective against *S. pneumoniae*, *N. meningitidis*, and *H. influenzae* to avert rapid, overwhelming sepsis in the event that they cannot present for medical attention immediately after the onset of fever or other symptoms of bacterial infection. A few amoxicillin/clavulanic acid tablets are a reasonable choice for this purpose.

The level of suspicion of infections with certain organisms should depend on the type of cancer diagnosed (Table 82-3). Diagnosis of multiple myeloma or CLL should alert the clinician to the possibility of hypogammaglobulinemia. While immunoglobulin replacement therapy can be effective, in most cases prophylactic antibiotics are a cheaper, more convenient method of eliminating bacterial infections in CLL patients with hypogammaglobulinemia. Patients with acute lymphocytic leukemia (ALL), patients with non-Hodgkin's lymphoma, and all cancer patients treated with high-dose glucocorticoids (or glucocorticoid-containing chemotherapy regimens) should receive antibiotic prophylaxis for *Pneumocystis* infection (Table 82-3) for the duration of their chemotherapy. In addition to exhibiting susceptibility to certain infectious organisms, patients with cancer are likely to manifest their infections in characteristic ways.

TABLE 82-3 INFECTIONS ASSOCIATED WITH SPECIFIC TYPES OF CANCER

Cancer	Underlying Immune Abnormality	Organisms Causing Infection
Multiple myeloma	Hypogammaglobulinemia	*Streptococcus pneumoniae*, *Haemophilus influenzae*, *Neisseria meningitidis*
Chronic lymphocytic leukemia	Hypogammaglobulinemia	*S. pneumoniae*, *H. influenzae*, *N. meningitidis*
Acute myelocytic or lymphocytic leukemia	Granulocytopenia, skin and mucous-membrane lesions	Extracellular gram-positive and gram-negative bacteria, fungi
Hodgkin's disease	Abnormal T cell function	Intracellular pathogens (*Mycobacterium tuberculosis*, *Listeria*, *Salmonella*, *Cryptococcus*, *Mycobacterium avium*)
Non-Hodgkin's lymphoma and acute lymphocytic leukemia	Glucocorticoid chemotherapy, T and B cell dysfunction	*Pneumocystis*
Colon and rectal tumors	Local abnormalities[a]	*Streptococcus bovis* (bacteremia)
Hairy cell leukemia	Abnormal T cell function	Intracellular pathogens (*M. tuberculosis*, *Listeria*, *Cryptococcus*, *M. avium*)

[a]The reason for this association is not well defined.

SYSTEM-SPECIFIC SYNDROMES

SKIN-SPECIFIC SYNDROMES

Skin lesions are common in cancer patients, and the appearance of these lesions may permit the diagnosis of systemic bacterial or fungal

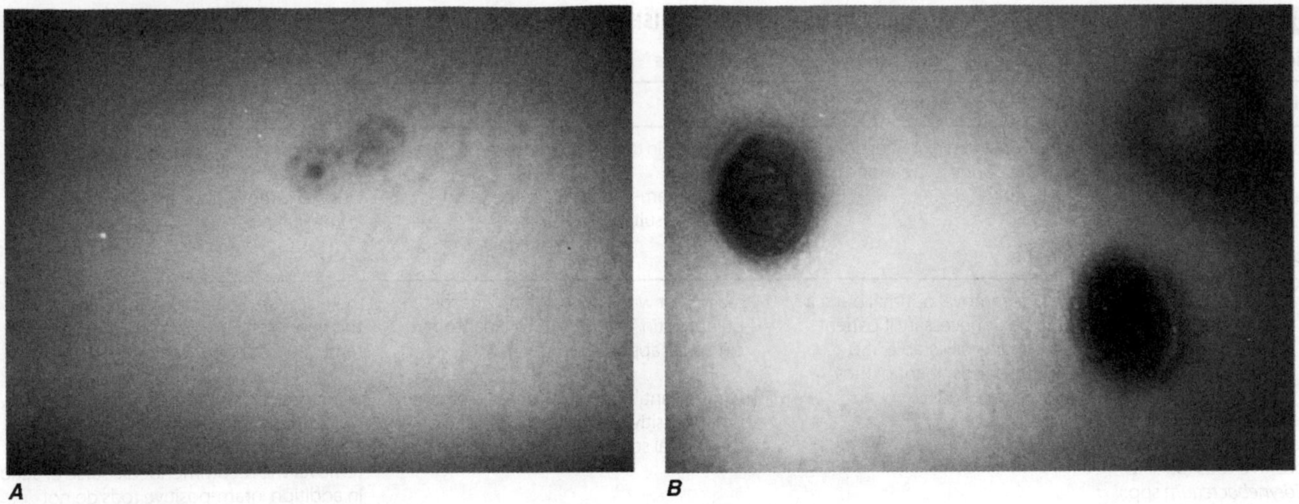

A B

FIGURE 82-1 ***A.*** **Papules related to** ***Escherichia coli*** bacteremia in a neutropenic patient with acute lymphocytic leukemia. ***B.*** The same lesion the following day.

infection. While cellulitis caused by skin organisms such as *Streptococcus* or *Staphylococcus* is common, neutropenic patients—i.e., those with <500 functional polymorphonuclear leukocytes (PMNs)/μL—and patients with impaired blood or lymphatic drainage may develop infections with unusual organisms. Innocent-looking macules or papules may be the first sign of bacterial or fungal sepsis in immunocompromised patients (Fig. 82-1). In the neutropenic host, a macule progresses rapidly to ecthyma gangrenosum, a usually painless, round, necrotic lesion consisting of a central black or gray-black eschar with surrounding erythema. Ecthyma gangrenosum, which is located in nonpressure areas (as distinguished from necrotic lesions associated with lack of circulation), is often associated with *Pseudomonas aeruginosa* bacteremia (Chap. 145) but may be caused by other bacteria.

Candidemia (Chap. 196) is also associated with a variety of skin conditions and commonly presents as a maculopapular rash. Punch biopsy of the skin may be the best method for diagnosis.

Cellulitis, an acute spreading inflammation of the skin, is most often caused by infection with group A *Streptococcus* or *Staphylococcus aureus*, virulent organisms normally found on the skin (Chap. 119). Although cellulitis tends to be circumscribed in normal hosts, it may spread rapidly in neutropenic patients. A tiny break in the skin may lead to spreading cellulitis, which is characterized by pain and erythema; in the affected patients, signs of infection (e.g., purulence) are often lacking. What might be a furuncle in a normal host may require amputation because of uncontrolled infection in a patient presenting with leukemia. A dramatic response to an infection that might be trivial in a normal host can mark the first sign of leukemia. Fortunately, granulocytopenic patients are likely to be infected with certain types of organisms (Table 82-4); thus the selection of an antibiotic regimen is

TABLE 82-4 ORGANISMS LIKELY TO CAUSE INFECTIONS IN GRANULOCYTOPENIC PATIENTS

Gram-positive cocci	*Enterobacter* spp.
Staphylococcus epidermidis	*Serratia* spp.
Staphylococcus aureus	*Acinetobacter* spp.[a]
Viridans *Streptococcus*	*Citrobacter* spp.
Enterococcus faecalis	Gram-positive bacilli
Streptococcus pneumoniae	Diphtheroids
Gram-negative bacilli	JK bacillus[a]
Escherichia coli	Fungi
Klebsiella spp.	*Candida* spp.
Pseudomonas aeruginosa	*Aspergillus* spp.
Non-*aeruginosa Pseudomonas* spp.[a]	

[a]Often associated with intravenous catheters.

somewhat easier than it might otherwise be (see "Antibacterial Therapy," below). It is essential to recognize cellulitis early and to treat it aggressively. Patients who are neutropenic or have previously received antibiotics for other reasons may develop cellulitis with unusual organisms (e.g., *Escherichia coli*, *Pseudomonas*, or fungi). Early treatment, even of innocent-looking lesions, is essential to prevent necrosis and loss of tissue. Debridement to prevent spread may sometimes be necessary early in the course of disease, but it can often be performed after chemotherapy, when the PMN count increases.

Sweet's syndrome, or *febrile neutrophilic dermatosis*, was originally described in women with elevated white blood cell (WBC) counts. The disease is characterized by the presence of leukocytes in the lower dermis, with edema of the papillary body. Ironically, this disease now is usually seen in neutropenic patients with cancer, most often in association with acute leukemia but also in association with a variety of other malignancies. Sweet's syndrome usually presents as red or bluish-red papules or nodules that may coalesce and form sharply bordered plaques. The edema may suggest vesicles, but on palpation the lesions are solid, and vesicles probably never arise in this disease. The lesions are most common on the face, neck, and arms. On the legs, they may be confused with erythema nodosum. The development of lesions is often accompanied by high fevers and an elevated erythrocyte sedimentation rate. Both the lesions and the temperature elevation respond dramatically to glucocorticoid administration. Treatment begins with high doses of glucocorticoids (60 mg/d of prednisone) followed by tapered doses over the next 2–3 weeks.

Data indicate that *erythema multiforme* with mucous membrane involvement is often associated with herpes simplex virus (HSV) infection and is distinct from Stevens-Johnson syndrome, which is associated with drugs and tends to have a more widespread distribution. Since cancer patients are both immunosuppressed (and therefore susceptible to herpes infections) and heavily treated with drugs (and therefore subject to Stevens-Johnson syndrome), both of these conditions are common in this population.

Cytokines, which are used as adjuvants or primary treatments for cancer, can themselves cause characteristic rashes, further complicating the differential diagnosis. This phenomenon is a particular problem in bone marrow transplant recipients (Chap. 126), who, in addition to having the usual chemotherapy-, antibiotic-, and cytokine-induced rashes, are plagued by graft-versus-host disease.

CATHETER-RELATED INFECTIONS

Because IV catheters are commonly used in cancer chemotherapy and are prone to infection (Chap. 125), they pose a major problem in the care of patients with cancer. Some catheter-associated infections can be treated with antibiotics, while in others the catheter must be re-

TABLE 82-5 APPROACH TO CATHETER INFECTIONS IN IMMUNOCOMPROMISED PATIENTS

Clinical Presentation	Catheter Removal	Antibiotics	Comments
Evidence of Infection, Negative Blood Cultures			
Exit-site erythema	Not necessary if infection responds to treatment	Usually begin treatment for gram-positive cocci.	Coagulase-negative staphylococci are most common.
Tunnel-site erythema	Required	Treat for gram-positive cocci pending culture results.	Failure to remove the catheter may lead to complications.
Blood Culture–Positive Infections			
Coagulase-negative staphylococci	Line removal optimal but may be unnecessary if patient is clinically stable and responds to antibiotics	Usually start with vancomycin. (Linezolid, quinupristin/dalfopristin, and daptomycin are all appropriate.)	If there are no contraindications to line removal, this course of action is optimal. If the line is removed, antibiotics may not be necessary.
Other gram-positive cocci (e.g., *Staphylococcus aureus, Enterococcus*); gram-positive rods (*Bacillus, Corynebacterium* spp.)	Recommended	Treat with antibiotics to which the organism is sensitive, with duration based on the clinical setting.	The incidence of metastatic infections following *S. aureus* infection and the difficulty of treating enterococcal infection make line removal the recommended course of action. In addition, gram-positive rods do not respond readily to antibiotics alone.
Gram-negative bacteria	Recommended	Use an agent to which the organism is shown to be sensitive.	Organisms like *Stenotrophomonas, Pseudomonas*, and *Burkholderia* are notoriously hard to treat.
Fungi	Recommended	—	Fungal infections of catheters are extremely difficult to treat.

moved (Table 82-5). If the patient has a "tunneled" catheter (which consists of an entrance site, a subcutaneous tunnel, and an exit site), a red streak over the subcutaneous part of the line (the tunnel) is grounds for immediate removal of the catheter. Failure to remove catheters under these circumstances may result in extensive cellulitis and tissue necrosis.

More common than tunnel infections are exit-site infections, often with erythema around the area where the line penetrates the skin. Most authorities (Chap. 129) recommend treatment (usually with vancomycin) for an exit-site infection caused by a coagulase-negative *Staphylococcus*. Treatment of coagulase-positive staphylococcal infection is associated with a poorer outcome, and it is advisable to remove the catheter if possible. Similarly, many clinicians remove catheters associated with infections due to *P. aeruginosa* and *Candida* species, since such infections are difficult to treat and bloodstream infections with these organisms are likely to be deadly. Catheter infections caused by *Burkholderia cepacia*, *Stenotrophomonas* spp., *Agrobacterium* spp., and *Acinetobacter baumannii* as well as *Pseudomonas* spp. other than *aeruginosa* are likely to be very difficult to eradicate with antibiotics alone. Similarly, isolation of *Bacillus*, *Corynebacterium*, and *Mycobacterium* spp. should prompt removal of the catheter.

GASTROINTESTINAL TRACT–SPECIFIC SYNDROMES

Upper Gastrointestinal Tract Disease • ***INFECTIONS OF THE MOUTH*** The oral cavity is rich in aerobic and anaerobic bacteria (Chap. 157) that normally live in a commensal relationship with the host. The antimetabolic effects of chemotherapy cause a breakdown of host defenses, leading to ulceration of the mouth and the potential for invasion by resident bacteria. Mouth ulcerations afflict most patients receiving chemotherapy and have been associated with viridans streptococcal bacteremia. The use of keratinocyte growth factor (palifermin) in a daily dose of 60 μg/kg for 3 days before chemotherapy and total-body irradiation is of proven value in preventing mucosal ulceration after stem cell transplantation. Fluconazole is clearly effective in the treatment of both local infections (thrush) and systemic infections (esophagitis) due to *Candida albicans*. Newer azoles (such as voriconazole) are similarly effective.

Noma (*cancrum oris*), commonly seen in malnourished children, is a penetrating disease of the soft and hard tissues of the mouth and adjacent sites, with resulting necrosis and gangrene. It has a counterpart in immunocompromised patients and is thought to be due to invasion of the tissues by *Bacteroides*, *Fusobacterium*, and other normal inhabitants of the mouth. Noma is associated with debility, poor oral hygiene, and immunosuppression.

Viruses, particularly HSV, are a prominent cause of morbidity in immunocompromised patients, in whom they are associated with severe mucositis. The use of acyclovir, either prophylactically or therapeutically, is of value.

ESOPHAGEAL INFECTIONS The differential diagnosis of esophagitis (usually presenting as substernal chest pain upon swallowing) includes herpes simplex and candidiasis, both of which are readily treatable.

Lower Gastrointestinal Tract Disease Hepatic candidiasis (Chap. 196) results from seeding of the liver (usually from a gastrointestinal source) in neutropenic patients. It is most common in patients being treated for acute leukemia and usually presents symptomatically around the time the neutropenia resolves. The characteristic picture is that of persistent fever unresponsive to antibiotics; abdominal pain and tenderness or nausea; and elevated serum levels of alkaline phosphatase in a patient with hematologic malignancy who has recently recovered from neutropenia. The diagnosis of this disease (which may present in an indolent manner and persist for several months) is based on the finding of yeasts or pseudohyphae in granulomatous lesions. Hepatic ultrasound or CT may reveal bull's-eye lesions. In some cases, MRI reveals small lesions not visible by other imaging modalities. The pathology (a granulomatous response) and the timing (with resolution of neutropenia and an elevation in granulocyte count) suggest that the host response to *Candida* is an important component of the manifestations of disease. In many cases, although organisms are visible, cultures of biopsied material may be negative. The designation *hepatosplenic candidiasis* or *hepatic candidiasis* is a misnomer because the disease often involves the kidneys and other tissues; the term *chronic disseminated candidiasis* may be more appropriate. Because of the risk of bleeding with liver biopsy, diagnosis is often based on imaging studies (MRI, CT). Amphotericin B is traditionally used for therapy (often for several months, until all manifestations of disease have disappeared), but fluconazole may be useful for outpatient therapy. The use of other antifungal agents and combination therapy is less well studied.

Typhlitis *Typhlitis* (also referred to as necrotizing colitis, neutropenic colitis, necrotizing enteropathy, ileocecal syndrome, and cecitis) is a clinical syndrome of fever and right-lower-quadrant tenderness in an immunosuppressed host. This syndrome is classically seen in neutropenic patients after chemotherapy with cytotoxic drugs. It may be more common among children than among adults and appears to be much more common among patients with acute myelocytic leukemia (AML) or ALL than among those with other types of cancer; a similar syndrome has been reported in patients infected with HIV type 1. Physical examination reveals right-lower-quadrant tenderness, with or without rebound tenderness. Associated diarrhea (often bloody) is common, and the diagnosis can be confirmed by the finding of a thickened cecal wall on CT, MRI, or ultrasonography. Plain films may reveal a right-lower-quadrant mass, but CT with contrast or MRI is a much more sensitive means of making the diagnosis. Although surgery is sometimes attempted to avoid perforation from ischemia, most cases resolve with medical therapy alone. The disease is sometimes associated with positive blood cultures (which usually yield aerobic gram-negative bacilli), and therapy is recommended for a broad spectrum of bacteria (particularly gram-negative bacilli, which are likely to be found in the bowel flora). Surgery is indicated in the case of perforation.

***Clostridium difficile*-Induced Diarrhea** Patients with cancer are predisposed to the development of *C. difficile* diarrhea (Chap. 123) as a consequence of chemotherapy alone. Thus, they may have positive toxin tests before receiving antibiotics. Obviously, such patients are also subject to *C. difficile*–induced diarrhea as a result of antibiotic pressure. *C. difficile* should always be considered as a possible cause of diarrhea in cancer patients who have received antibiotics.

CENTRAL NERVOUS SYSTEM–SPECIFIC SYNDROMES

Meningitis The presentation of meningitis in patients with lymphoma or CLL, patients receiving chemotherapy (particularly with glucocorticoids) for solid tumors, and patients who have received bone marrow transplants suggests a diagnosis of cryptococcal or listerial infection. As noted previously, splenectomized patients are susceptible to rapid, overwhelming infection with encapsulated bacteria (including *S. pneumoniae*, *H. influenzae*, and *N. meningitidis*). Similarly, patients who are antibody-deficient (such as patients with CLL, those who have received intensive chemotherapy, or those who have undergone bone marrow transplantation) are likely to have infections caused by these bacteria. Other cancer patients, however, because of their defective cellular immunity, are likely to be infected with other pathogens (Table 82-3).

Encephalitis The spectrum of disease resulting from viral encephalitis is expanded in immunocompromised patients. A predisposition to infections with intracellular organisms similar to those encountered in patients with AIDS (Chap. 182) is seen in cancer patients receiving (1) high-dose cytotoxic chemotherapy, (2) chemotherapy affecting T cell function (e.g., fludarabine), or (3) antibodies that eliminate T cells (e.g., anti-CD3) or cytokine activity. Infection with varicella-zoster virus (VZV) has been associated with encephalitis that may be caused by VZV-related vasculitis. Chronic viral infections may also be associated with dementia and encephalitic presentations, and a diagnosis of progressive multifocal leukoencephalopathy should be considered when a patient who has received chemotherapy presents with dementia (Table 82-6). Other abnormalities of the central nervous system (CNS) that may be confused with infection include normal-pressure hydrocephalus and vasculitis resulting from CNS irradiation. It may be possible to differentiate these conditions by MRI.

Brain Masses Mass lesions of the brain most often present as headache with or without fever or neurologic abnormalities. Infections associated with mass lesions may be caused by bacteria (particularly *Nocardia*), fungi (particularly *Cryptococcus* or *Aspergillus*), or parasites (*Toxoplasma*). Epstein-Barr virus (EBV)–associated lymphoproliferative disease may also present as single or multiple mass lesions of the brain. A biopsy may be required for a definitive diagnosis.

PULMONARY INFECTIONS

Pneumonia (Chap. 251) in immunocompromised patients may be difficult to diagnose because conventional methods of diagnosis depend on the presence of neutrophils. Bacterial pneumonia in neutropenic patients may present without purulent sputum—or, in fact, without any sputum at all—and may not produce physical findings suggestive of chest consolidation (rales or egophony).

In granulocytopenic patients with persistent or recurrent fever, the chest x-ray pattern may help to localize an infection and thus to determine which investigative tests and procedures should be undertaken and which therapeutic options should be considered (Table 82-7). The difficulties encountered in the management of pulmonary infiltrates relate in part to the difficulties of performing diagnostic procedures on the patients involved. When platelet counts can be increased to adequate levels by transfusion, microscopic and microbiologic evaluation of the fluid obtained by endoscopic bronchial lavage is often diagnostic. Lavage fluid should be cultured for *Mycoplasma*, *Chlamydophila*, *Legionella*, *Nocardia*, more common bacterial pathogens, and fungi. In addition, the possibility of *Pneumocystis* pneumonia should be considered, especially in patients with ALL or lymphoma who have not received prophylactic trimethoprim-sulfamethoxazole (TMP-SMX). The characteristics of the infiltrate may be helpful in decisions about further diagnostic and therapeutic maneuvers. Nodular infiltrates suggest fungal pneumonia (e.g., that caused by *Aspergillus* or *Mucor*). Such lesions may best be approached by visualized biopsy procedures.

Aspergillus spp. (Chap. 197) can colonize the skin and respiratory tract or cause fatal systemic illness. Although *Aspergillus* may cause aspergillomas in a previously existing cavity or may produce allergic bronchopulmonary aspergillosis, the major problem posed by this genus in neutropenic patients is invasive disease due to *A. fumigatus* or *A. flavus*. The organisms enter the host following colonization of the respiratory tract, with subsequent invasion of the blood vessels. The disease is likely to present as a thrombotic or embolic event because of the organisms' ability to invade blood vessels. The risk of infection with *Aspergillus* correlates directly with the duration of neutropenia. In prolonged neutropenia, positive surveillance cultures for colonization of the nasopharynx with *Aspergillus* may predict the development of disease.

TABLE 82-6 DIFFERENTIAL DIAGNOSIS OF CENTRAL NERVOUS SYSTEM INFECTIONS IN PATIENTS WITH CANCER

	Underlying Predisposition	
Findings on CT or MRI	**Prolonged Neutropenia**	**Defects in Cellular Immunity**[a]
Mass lesions	*Aspergillus* brain abscess *Nocardia* brain abscess *Cryptococcus* brain abscess	Toxoplasmosis EBV-LPD
Diffuse encephalitis	PML (J-C virus)	Infection with VZV, CMV, HSV, HHV-6, J-C virus (PML), *Listeria*

[a]High-dose glucocorticoid therapy, cytotoxic chemotherapy.

Abbreviations: CMV, cytomegalovirus; EBV-LPD, Epstein-Barr virus lymphoproliferative disease; HHV-6, human herpesvirus type 6; HSV, herpes simplex virus; PML, progressive multifocal leukoencephalopathy; VZV, varicella-zoster virus.

TABLE 82-7 DIFFERENTIAL DIAGNOSIS OF CHEST INFILTRATES IN IMMUNOCOMPROMISED PATIENTS

	Cause of Pneumonia	
Infiltrate	**Infectious**	**Noninfectious**
Localized	Bacteria, *Legionella*, mycobacteria	Local hemorrhage or embolism, tumor
Nodular	Fungi (e.g., *Aspergillus* or *Mucor*), *Nocardia*	Recurrent tumor
Diffuse	Viruses (especially CMV), *Chlamydophila*, *Pneumocystis*, *Toxoplasma gondii*, mycobacteria	Congestive heart failure, radiation pneumonitis, drug-induced lung injury, diffuse alveolar hemorrhage (described after BMT)

Abbreviations: BMT, bone marrow transplantation; CMV, cytomegalovirus.

Patients with *Aspergillus* infection often present with pleuritic chest pain and fever, which are sometimes accompanied by cough. Hemoptysis may be an ominous sign. Chest x-rays may reveal new focal infiltrates or nodules. Chest CT may reveal a characteristic halo consisting of a mass-like infiltrate surrounded by an area of low attenuation. The presence of a "crescent sign" on a chest x-ray or a chest CT scan, in which the mass progresses to central cavitation, is characteristic of invasive *Aspergillus* infection but may develop as the lesions are resolving.

In addition to causing pulmonary disease, *Aspergillus* may invade through the nose or palate, with deep sinus penetration. The appearance of a discolored area in the nasal passages or on the hard palate should prompt a search for invasive *Aspergillus*. This situation is likely to require surgical debridement. Catheter infections with *Aspergillus* usually require both removal of the catheter and antifungal therapy.

Diffuse interstitial infiltrates suggest viral, parasitic, or *Pneumocystis* pneumonia. If the patient has a diffuse interstitial pattern on chest x-ray, it may be reasonable to institute empirical treatment with TMP-SMX (for *Pneumocystis*) and a quinolone (for *Chlamydophila, Mycoplasma,* and *Legionella*) or an erythromycin derivative (e.g., azithromycin) while considering invasive diagnostic procedures. Noninvasive procedures, such as staining of sputum smears for *Pneumocystis*, serum cryptococcal antigen tests, and urine testing for *Legionella* antigen, may be helpful. In transplant recipients who are seropositive for cytomegalovirus (CMV), a determination of CMV load in the serum should be considered. Viral load studies (which allow physicians to quantitate viruses) have superseded simple measurement of serum IgG, which merely documents prior exposure to virus. Infections with viruses that cause only upper respiratory symptoms in immunocompetent hosts, such as respiratory syncytial virus (RSV), influenza viruses, and parainfluenza viruses, may be associated with fatal pneumonitis in immunocompromised hosts. An attempt at early diagnosis by nasopharyngeal aspiration should be considered so that appropriate treatment can be instituted.

Bleomycin is the most common cause of chemotherapy-induced lung disease. Other causes include alkylating agents (such as cyclophosphamide, chlorambucil, and melphalan), nitrosoureas [carmustine (BCNU), lomustine (CCNU), and methyl-CCNU], busulfan, procarbazine, methotrexate, and hydroxyurea. Both infectious and noninfectious (drug- and/or radiation-induced) pneumonitis can cause fever and abnormalities on chest x-ray; thus, the differential diagnosis of an infiltrate in a patient receiving chemotherapy encompasses a broad range of conditions (Table 82-7). Since the treatment of radiation pneumonitis (which may respond dramatically to glucocorticoids) or drug-induced pneumonitis is different from that of infectious pneumonia, a biopsy may be important in the diagnosis. Unfortunately, no definitive diagnosis can be made in ~30% of cases, even after bronchoscopy.

Open-lung biopsy is the "gold standard" of diagnostic techniques. Biopsy via a visualized thoracostomy can replace an open procedure in many cases. When a biopsy cannot be performed, empirical treatment can be undertaken with a quinolone or erythromycin (or an erythromycin derivative such as azithromycin) and TMP-SMX (in the case of diffuse infiltrates) or with amphotericin B or other antifungal agents (in the case of nodular infiltrates). The risks should be weighed carefully in these cases. If inappropriate drugs are administered, empirical treatment may prove toxic or ineffective; either of these outcomes may be riskier than biopsy.

CARDIOVASCULAR INFECTIONS

Patients with Hodgkin's disease are prone to persistent infections by *Salmonella*, sometimes (and particularly often in elderly patients) affecting a vascular site. The use of IV catheters deliberately lodged in the right atrium is associated with a high incidence of bacterial endocarditis, presumably related to valve damage followed by bacteremia. Nonbacterial thrombotic endocarditis has been described in association with a variety of malignancies (most often solid tumors) and may follow bone marrow transplantation as well. The presentation of an embolic event with a new cardiac murmur suggests this diagnosis. Blood cultures are negative in this disease of unknown pathogenesis.

ENDOCRINE SYNDROMES

Infections of the endocrine system have been described in immunocompromised patients. *Candida* infection of the thyroid may be difficult to diagnose during the neutropenic period. It can be defined by indium-labeled WBC scans or gallium scans after neutrophil counts increase. CMV infection can cause adrenalitis with or without resulting adrenal insufficiency. The presentation of a sudden endocrine anomaly in an immunocompromised patient may be a sign of infection in the involved end organ.

MUSCULOSKELETAL INFECTIONS

Infection that is a consequence of vascular compromise, resulting in gangrene, can occur when a tumor restricts the blood supply to muscles, bones, or joints. The process of diagnosis and treatment of such infection is similar to that in normal hosts, with the following caveats:

1. *In terms of diagnosis,* a lack of physical findings resulting from a lack of granulocytes in the granulocytopenic patient should make the clinician more aggressive in obtaining tissue rather than relying on physical signs.

2. *In terms of therapy,* aggressive debridement of infected tissues may be required, but it is usually difficult to operate on patients who have recently received chemotherapy, both because of a lack of platelets (which results in bleeding complications) and because of a lack of WBCs (which may lead to secondary infection). A blood culture positive for *Clostridium perfringens*—an organism commonly associated with gas gangrene—can have a number of meanings (Chap. 135). Bloodstream infections with intestinal organisms such as *Streptococcus bovis* and *C. perfringens* may arise spontaneously from lower gastrointestinal lesions (tumor or polyps); alternatively, these lesions may be harbingers of invasive disease. The clinical setting must be considered in order to define the appropriate treatment for each case.

RENAL AND URETERAL INFECTIONS

Infections of the urinary tract are common among patients whose ureteral excretion is compromised (Table 82-1). *Candida*, which has a predilection for the kidney, can invade either from the bloodstream or in a retrograde manner (via the ureters or bladder) in immunocompromised patients. The presence of "fungus balls" or persistent candiduria suggests invasive disease. Persistent funguria (with *Aspergillus* as well as *Candida*) should prompt a search for a nidus of infection in the kidney.

Certain viruses are typically seen only in immunosuppressed patients. BK virus (polyomavirus hominis 1) has been documented in the urine of bone marrow transplant recipients and, like adenovirus, may be associated with hemorrhagic cystitis. BK-induced cystitis usually remits with decreasing immunosuppression. Anecdotal reports have described the treatment of infections due to adenovirus and BK virus with cidofovir.

ABNORMALITIES THAT PREDISPOSE TO INFECTION (Table 82-1)

THE LYMPHOID SYSTEM

It is beyond the scope of this chapter to detail how all the immunologic abnormalities that result from cancer or from chemotherapy for cancer lead to infections. Disorders of the immune system are discussed in other sections of this book. As has been noted, patients with antibody deficiency are predisposed to overwhelming infection with encapsulated bacteria (including *S. pneumoniae, H. influenzae,* and *N. meningitidis*). Infections that result from the lack of a functional cellular immune system are described in Chap. 182. It is worth mentioning, however, that patients undergoing intensive chemotherapy for any form of cancer will have not only defects due to granulocytopenia but also lymphocyte dysfunction, which may be profound. Thus, these patients—especially those receiving glucocorticoid-containing regimens or drugs that inhibit T cell activation or cytokine induction—should be given prophylaxis for *Pneumocystis* pneumonia.

Initial studies in the 1960s revealed a dramatic increase in the incidence of infections (fatal and nonfatal) among cancer patients with a granulocyte count of <500/μL. More recent studies have cited a figure of 48.3 infections per 100 neutropenic patients (<1000 granulocytes/μL) with hematologic malignancies and solid tumors, or 46.3 infections per 1000 days at risk.

Neutropenic patients are unusually susceptible to infection with a wide variety of bacteria; thus, antibiotic therapy should be initiated promptly to cover likely pathogens if infection is suspected. Indeed, early initiation of antibacterial agents is mandatory to prevent deaths. These patients are susceptible to gram-positive and gram-negative organisms found commonly on the skin and in the bowel (Table 82-4). Because treatment with narrow-spectrum agents leads to infection with organisms not covered by the antibiotics used, the initial regimen should target pathogens likely to be initial causes of bacterial infection in neutropenic hosts (Fig. 82-2).

Rx INFECTIONS IN CANCER PATIENTS

ANTIBACTERIAL THERAPY Hundreds of antibacterial regimens have been tested for use in patients with cancer. The major risk of infection is related to the degree of neutropenia seen as a consequence of either the disease or the therapy. Many of the relevant studies involved small populations in which the outcomes were generally good, and most lacked the statistical power to detect differences among the regimens studied. Each febrile neutropenic patient should be approached as a unique problem, with particular attention given to previous infections and recent antibiotic exposures. Several general guidelines are useful in the initial treatment of neutropenic patients with fever (Fig. 82-2):

1. In the initial regimen, it is necessary to use antibiotics active against both gram-negative and gram-positive bacteria (Table 82-4).
2. An aminoglycoside or an antibiotic without good activity against gram-positive organisms (e.g., ciprofloxacin or aztreonam) alone is not adequate in this setting.
3. The agents used should reflect both the epidemiology and the antibiotic resistance pattern of the hospital.
4. If the pattern of resistance justifies its use, a single third-generation cephalosporin constitutes an appropriate initial regimen in many hospitals.
5. Most standard regimens are designed for patients who have not previously received prophylactic antibiotics. The development of fever in a patient who has received antibiotics affects the choice of subsequent therapy, which should target resistant organisms and organisms known to cause infections in patients being treated with the antibiotics already administered.
6. Randomized trials have indicated the safety of oral antibiotic regimens in the treatment of "low-risk" patients with fever and neutropenia. Outpatients who are expected to remain neutropenic for <10 days and who have no concurrent medical problems (such as hypotension, pulmonary compromise, or abdominal pain) can be classified as low risk and treated with a broad-spectrum oral regimen.
7. Several large-scale studies indicate that prophylaxis with a fluoroquinolone (ciprofloxacin or levofloxacin) decreases morbidity and mortality rates among afebrile patients who are anticipated to have neutropenia of long duration.

The initial antibacterial regimen should be refined on the basis of culture results (Fig. 82-2). Blood cultures are the most relevant on which to base therapy; surface cultures of skin and mucous membranes may be misleading. In the case of gram-positive bacteremia or another gram-positive infection, it is important that the antibiotic be optimal for the organism isolated. Although it is not desirable to leave the patient unprotected, the addition of more and more antibacterial agents to the regimen is not appropriate unless there is a clinical or microbiologic reason to do so. Planned progressive therapy (the serial, empirical addition of one drug after another without culture data) is not efficacious in most settings and may have unfortunate consequences. Simply adding another antibiotic for fear that a gram-negative infection is present is a dubious practice. The synergy exhibited by β-lactams and aminoglycosides against certain gram-negative organisms (especially *P. aeruginosa*) provides the rationale for using two antibiotics in this setting, but recent analyses suggest that efficacy is not enhanced by the addition of aminoglycosides, while toxicity may be increased. Mere "double coverage," with the addition of a quinolone or another antibiotic that is not likely to exhibit synergy, has not been shown to be of benefit and may cause additional toxicities and side effects. Cephalosporins can cause bone marrow suppression, and vancomycin is associated with neutropenia in some healthy individuals (Chap. 127). Furthermore, the addition of multiple cephalosporins may induce β-lactamase production by some organisms; cephalosporins and double β-lactam combinations should probably be avoided altogether in *Enterobacter* infections.

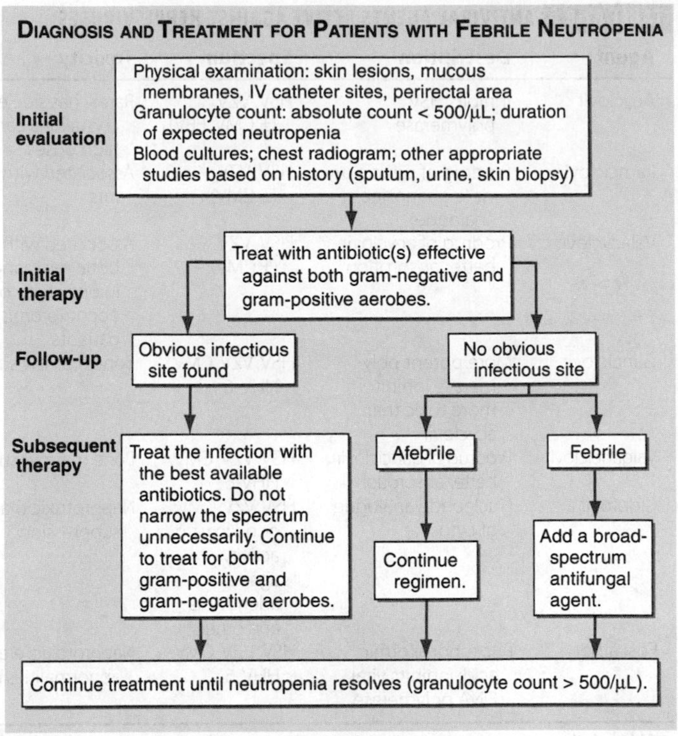

FIGURE 82-2 Algorithm for the diagnosis and treatment of febrile neutropenic patients.

ANTIFUNGAL THERAPY Fungal infections in cancer patients are most often associated with neutropenia. Neutropenic patients are predisposed to the development of invasive fungal infections, most commonly those due to *Candida* and *Aspergillus* species and occasionally those caused by *Fusarium*, *Trichosporon*, and *Bipolaris*. Cryptococcal infection, which is common among patients taking immunosuppressive agents, is uncommon among neutropenic patients receiving chemotherapy for AML. Invasive candidal disease is usually caused by *C. albicans* or *C. tropicalis* but can be caused by *C. krusei*, *C. parapsilosis*, and *C. glabrata*.

For decades it has been common clinical practice to add amphotericin B to antibacterial regimens if a neutropenic patient remains febrile despite 4–7 days of treatment with antibacterial agents. The rationale for the empirical addition of amphotericin B is that it is difficult to culture fungi before they cause disseminated disease and that mortality rates from disseminated fungal infections in granulocytopenic patients are high. Before the introduction of newer azoles into clinical practice, amphotericin B was the mainstay of antifungal therapy. The insolubility of amphotericin B has resulted in the marketing of several lipid formulations that are less toxic than the amphotericin B deoxycholate complex. However, because of the high cost of the lipid preparations, their use at many centers is reserved for patients who fail to respond to standard amphotericin B. Since the side effects of the formulations differ, unnecessary switching from one to another is not recommended.

Although fluconazole is efficacious in the treatment of infections due to many *Candida* spp., its use against serious fungal infections in immunocompromised patients is limited by its narrow spectrum: it has no activity against *Aspergillus* or against several non-*albicans Candida* spp. The release of newer broad-spectrum azoles (such as voriconazole and posaconazole) has provided another option for the treatment of *Aspergillus* infection (including CNS infection, in which amphotericin B has usually failed). In fact,

TABLE 82-8 ANTIVIRAL AGENTS ACTIVE AGAINST HERPESVIRUSES

Agent	Description	Spectrum	Toxicity	Other Issues
Acyclovir	Inhibits HSV polymerase	HSV, VZV (± CMV, EBV)	Rarely has side effects; crystalluria can occur at high doses	Long history of safety; original antiviral agent
Famciclovir	Prodrug of penciclovir (a guanosine analogue)	HSV, VZV (± CMV)	Associated with cancer in rats	Longer effective half-life than acyclovir
Valacyclovir	Prodrug of acyclovir; better absorption	HSV, VZV (± CMV)	Associated with thrombotic microangiopathy in one study of immunocompromised patients	Better oral absorption and longer effective half-life than acyclovir; can be given as a single daily dose for prophylaxis
Ganciclovir	More potent polymerase inhibitor; more toxic than acyclovir	HSV, VZV, CMV, HHV-6	Bone marrow suppression	Neutropenia may respond to G-CSF or GM-CSF
Valganciclovir	Prodrug of ganciclovir; better absorption	HSV, VZV, CMV, HHV-6	Bone marrow suppression	—
Cidofovir	Nucleotide analogue of cytosine	HSV, VZV, CMV; good in vitro activity against adenovirus and others	Nephrotoxic marrow suppression	Given IV once a week
Foscarnet	Phosphonoformic acid; inhibits viral DNA polymerase	HSV, VZV, CMV, HHV-6	Nephrotoxic; electrolyte abnormalities common	IV only

Abbreviations: ±, agent has some activity but not enough for the treatment of infections; CMV, cytomegalovirus; EBV, Epstein-Barr virus; G-CSF, granulocyte colony-stimulating factor; GM-CSF, granulocyte-macrophage colony-stimulating factor; HHV, human herpesvirus; HSV, herpes simplex virus; VZV, varicella-zoster virus.

experience indicates that these drugs may well supplant amphotericin B as the mainstay of treatment because of their lesser toxicity and better penetration into cerebrospinal fluid and other sites. Clinicians should be aware that the spectrum of each azole is somewhat different and that no drug can be assumed to be efficacious against all fungi. For example, while voriconazole is active against *Pseudallescheria boydii*, amphotericin B is not; however, voriconazole has no activity against *Mucor*. Recent studies suggest a role for posaconazole as a prophylactic agent in patients with prolonged neutropenia. **For a full discussion of antifungal therapy, see Chap. 191.**

Echinocandins (such as caspofungin) are useful in the treatment of infections caused by azole-resistant *Candida*. Studies in progress are assessing the use of these agents in combinations to determine whether treatment with multiple antifungal agents leads to better outcomes.

ANTIVIRAL THERAPY The availability of a variety of agents active against herpes-group viruses, including some new agents with a broader spectrum of activity, has heightened focus on the treatment of viral infections, which pose a major problem in cancer patients. Viral diseases caused by the herpes group are prominent. Serious (and sometimes fatal) infections due to HSV and CMV are well documented, and VZV infections may be fatal to patients receiving chemotherapy. The roles of human herpesvirus (HHV) 6, HHV-7, and HHV-8 (Kaposi's sarcoma herpesvirus) in cancer patients are being defined (Chap. 175). While clinical experience is most extensive with acyclovir, which can be used therapeutically or prophylactically, a number of derivative drugs offer advantages over this agent **(Table 82-8)**.

In addition to the herpes group, several respiratory viruses (especially RSV) may cause serious disease in cancer patients. While vaccination with influenza vaccine is recommended (see below), it may be ineffective in this patient population. The availability of antiviral drugs with activity against influenza viruses gives the clinician additional options for the treatment of these patients **(Table 82-9)**.

OTHER THERAPEUTIC MODALITIES Another way to address the problems of the febrile neutropenic patient is to replenish the neutrophil population. Although granulocyte transfusions are efficacious in the treatment of refractory gram-negative bacteremia, they do not have a documented role in prophylaxis. Because of the expense, the risk of leukoagglutinin reactions (which has probably been decreased by improved cell-separation procedures), and the risk of transmission of CMV from unscreened donors (which has been reduced by the use of filters), granulocyte transfusion is reserved for patients unresponsive to antibiotics. This modality is efficacious for documented gram-negative bacteremia refractory to antibiotics, particularly in situations where granulocyte numbers will be depressed for only a short period. The demonstrated usefulness of granulocyte colony-stimulating factor (G-CSF) in mobilizing neutrophils and advances in preservation techniques may make this option more useful than in the past.

A variety of cytokines, including G-CSF and granulocyte-macrophage colony-stimulating factor, enhance granulocyte recovery after chemotherapy and consequently shorten the period of maximal vulnerability to fatal infections. The role of these cytokines in routine practice is still a matter of some debate. Most authorities recommend their use only when neutropenia is both severe and prolonged. The cytokines themselves may have adverse effects, including fever, hypoxemia, and pleural effusions or serositis in other areas (Chap. 308). Since there is little evidence that their routine administration lessens the risk of death and since they are still expensive, the use of these cytokines has not become the standard of care in all centers. The role of other cytokines (such as macrophage colony-stimulating factor for monocytes or interferon-γ) in preventing or treating infections in granulocytopenic patients is under investigation.

TABLE 82-9 OTHER ANTIVIRAL AGENTS USEFUL IN THE TREATMENT OF INFECTIONS IN CANCER PATIENTS

Agent	Description	Spectrum	Toxicity	Other Issues
Amantadine, rimantadine	Interfere with uncoating	Influenza A only	5–10% fewer CNS effects with rimantadine	May be given prophylactically
Zanamivir	Neuraminidase inhibitor	Influenza A and B	Usually well tolerated	Inhalation only
Oseltamivir	Neuraminidase inhibitor	Influenza A and B	Usually well tolerated	PO dosing
Pleconaril	Blocks enterovirus binding and uncoating	90% of enteroviruses, 80% of rhinoviruses	Generally well tolerated	Decreases duration of meningitis; available for compassionate use only
Interferons	Cytokines with broad spectrum of activity	Used locally for warts, systemically for hepatitis	Fever, myalgias, bone marrow suppression	Not shown to be helpful in CMV infection; use limited by toxicity
Ribavirin	Purine analogue (precise mechanism of action unknown)	Broad theoretical spectrum; documented use against RSV, Lassa fever virus, and hepatitis viruses (with interferon)	IV form causes anemia	Given by aerosol for RSV infection (efficacy in doubt); approved for use in children with heart/lung disease

Abbreviations: CMV, cytomegalovirus; CNS, central nervous system; RSV, respiratory syncytial virus.

Once neutropenia has resolved, patients are not at increased risk of infection. However, depending on what drugs they receive, patients who continue on chemotherapeutic protocols remain at high risk for certain diseases. Any patient receiving more than a maintenance dose of glucocorticoids (including many treatment regimens for diffuse lymphoma) should also receive prophylactic TMP-SMX because of the risk of *Pneumocystis* infection; those with ALL should receive such prophylaxis for the duration of chemotherapy.

PREVENTION OF INFECTION IN CANCER PATIENTS

EFFECT OF THE ENVIRONMENT

Outbreaks of fatal *Aspergillus* infection have been associated with construction projects and materials in several hospitals. The association between spore counts and risk of infection suggests the need for a high-efficiency air-handling system in hospitals that care for large numbers of neutropenic patients. The use of laminar-flow rooms and prophylactic antibiotics has decreased the number of infectious episodes in severely neutropenic patients. However, because of the expense of such a program and the failure to show that it dramatically affects mortality rates, most centers do not routinely use laminar flow to care for neutropenic patients. Some centers use "reverse isolation," in which health care providers and visitors to a patient who is neutropenic wear gowns and gloves. Since most of the infections these patients develop are due to organisms that colonize the patients' own skin and bowel, the validity of such schemes is dubious, and limited clinical data do not support their use. Hand washing by all staff caring for neutropenic patients should be required to prevent the spread of resistant organisms.

The presence of large numbers of bacteria (particularly *P. aeruginosa*) in certain foods, especially fresh vegetables, has led some authorities to recommend a special "low-bacteria" diet. A diet consisting of cooked and canned food is satisfactory to most neutropenic patients and does not involve elaborate disinfection or sterilization protocols. However, there are no studies to support even this type of dietary restriction. Counseling of patients to avoid leftovers, deli foods, and unpasteurized dairy products is recommended.

PHYSICAL MEASURES

Although few studies address this issue, patients with cancer are predisposed to infections resulting from anatomic compromise (e.g., lymphedema resulting from node dissections after radical mastectomy). Surgeons who specialize in cancer surgery can provide specific guidelines for the care of such patients, and patients benefit from common-sense advice about how to prevent infections in vulnerable areas.

IMMUNOGLOBULIN REPLACEMENT

Many patients with multiple myeloma or CLL have immunoglobulin deficiencies as a result of their disease, and all allogeneic bone marrow transplant recipients are hypogammaglobinemic for a period after transplantation. However, current recommendations reserve intravenous immunoglobulin (IVIg) replacement therapy for those patients with severe (<400 mg/dL), prolonged hypogammaglobulinemia. Antibiotic prophylaxis has been shown to be cheaper and efficacious in preventing infections in most CLL patients with hypogammaglobulinemia. Routine use of IVIg replacement is not recommended.

SEXUAL PRACTICES

The use of condoms is recommended for severely immunocompromised patients. Any sexual practice that results in oral exposure to feces is not recommended. Neutropenic patients should be advised to avoid any practice that results in trauma, as even microscopic cuts may result in bacterial invasion and fatal sepsis.

ANTIBIOTIC PROPHYLAXIS

Several studies indicate that the use of oral fluoroquinolones prevents infection and decreases mortality rates among severely neutropenic patients. Fluconazole prevents *Candida* infections when given prophylactically to patients receiving bone marrow transplants. The use of broader-spectrum antifungal agents (e.g., posaconazole) appears to be more efficacious. Prophylaxis for *Pneumocystis* is mandatory for patients with ALL and for all cancer patients receiving glucocorticoid-containing chemotherapy regimens.

VACCINATION OF CANCER PATIENTS

In general, patients undergoing chemotherapy respond less well to vaccines than do normal hosts. Their greater need for vaccines thus leads to a dilemma in their management. Purified proteins and inactivated vaccines are almost never contraindicated and should be given to patients even during chemotherapy. For example, all adults should receive diphtheria-tetanus toxoid boosters at the indicated times as well as seasonal influenza vaccine. However, if possible, vaccination should not be undertaken concurrent with cytotoxic chemotherapy. If patients are expected to be receiving chemotherapy for several months and vaccination is indicated (for example, influenza vaccination in the fall), the vaccine should be given midcycle—as far apart in time as possible from the antimetabolic agents that will prevent an immune response. The meningococcal and pneumococcal polysaccharide vaccines should be given to patients before splenectomy, if possible. The *H. influenzae* type b conjugate vaccine should be administered to all splenectomized patients.

In general, live virus (or live bacterial) vaccines should not be given to patients during intensive chemotherapy because of the risk of disseminated infection. Recommendations on vaccination are summarized in Table 82-2.

FURTHER READINGS

BOHLIUS J et al: Granulopoiesis-stimulating factors to prevent adverse effects in the treatment of malignant lymphoma. Cochrane Database Syst Rev 3:CD003189, 2004

GAFTER-GVILI A et al: Antibiotic prophylaxis for bacterial infections in afebrile neutropenic patients following chemotherapy. Cochrane Database Syst Rev 4:CD004386, 2005

HALL K et al: Diagnosis and management of long-term central venous catheter infections. J Vasc Interv Radiol 15:327, 2004

PAUL M et al: Empirical antibiotic monotherapy for febrile neutropenia: Systematic review and meta-analysis of randomized controlled trials. J Antimicrob Chemother 57:176, 2006

ULLMANN AJ et al: Posaconazole or fluconazole for prophylaxis in severe graft-versus-host disease. N Engl J Med 356:335, 2007

83 Cancer of the Skin

Arthur J. Sober, Hensin Tsao, Carl V. Washington

MELANOMA

Pigmented lesions are among the most common findings on skin examination. The challenge is to distinguish cutaneous melanomas, which may be lethal, from the remainder, which with rare exceptions are benign. Examples of malignant and benign pigmented lesions are shown in Fig. 83-1.

EPIDEMIOLOGY

Melanomas originate from neural crest-derived melanocytes; pigment cells present normally in the epidermis and sometimes in the dermis. This tumor affects around 62,000 individuals per year in the United States, resulting in 7910 deaths. Melanoma is the fifth most common cancer in men (5% of cancers) and the sixth most common in women (4% of cancers). The tumor can affect adults of all ages, even young

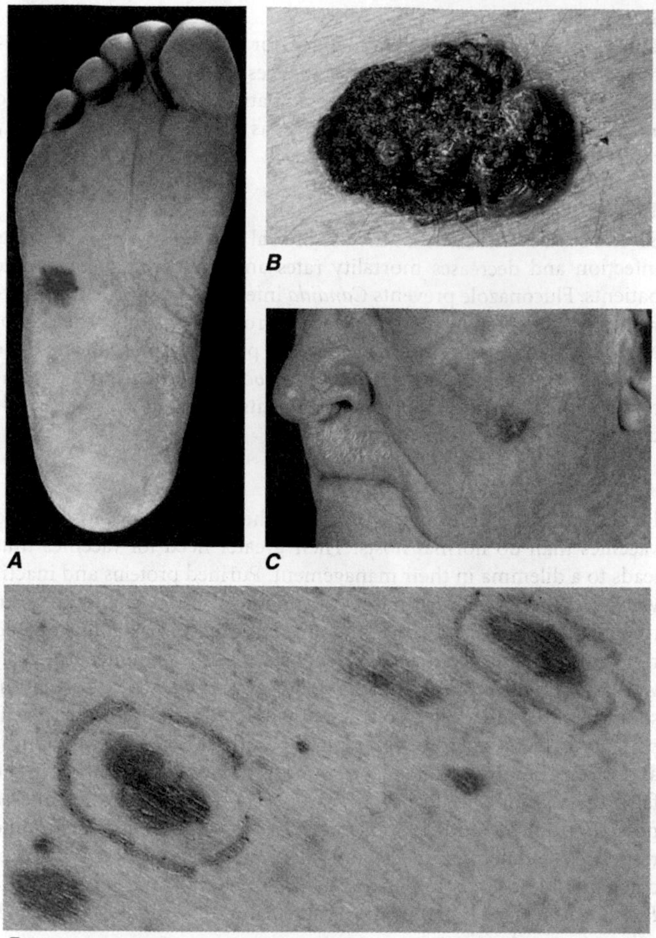

FIGURE 83-1 Atypical and malignant pigmented lesions. The most common melanoma is superficial spreading melanoma (not pictured). ***A.*** Acral lentiginous melanoma is the most common melanoma in blacks, Asians, and Hispanics and occurs as an enlarging hyperpigmented macule or plaque on the palms and soles. Lateral pigment diffusion is present. ***B.*** Nodular melanoma most commonly manifests itself as a rapidly growing, often ulcerated or crusted black nodule. ***C.*** Lentigo maligna melanoma occurs on sun-exposed skin as a large, hyperpigmented macule or plaque with irregular borders and variable pigmentation. ***D.*** Dysplastic nevi are irregularly pigmented and shaped nevomelanocytic lesions which may be associated with familial melanoma.

individuals (starting in the mid-teens); has distinct clinical features that make it detectable at a time when cure by surgical excision is possible; and is located on the skin surface, where it is visible. The incidence has increased dramatically (6% per year from 1973 to 1980, then 3% per year). Current lifetime risk ratio is 1:53 in males and 1:78 in females. The reason for this increase is uncertain but may involve increased recreational sun exposure, especially early in life. Individuals of similar ethnic background who immigrate after childhood to areas of high sun exposure (e.g., Israel and Australia) have lower melanoma rates than individuals of similar age who were either born in those countries or immigrated before age 10. The individuals most susceptible to development of melanoma are those with fair complexions, red or blond hair, blue eyes, and freckles and who tan poorly and sunburn easily. Other factors associated with increased risk include a family history of melanoma (~1 in 10 melanoma patients have a family member with melanoma), the presence of a clinically atypical mole (dysplastic nevus) or a giant congenital melanocytic nevus, the presence of a higher than average number of ordinary melanocytic nevi, and immunosuppression (Table 83-1). Individuals with 50 or more moles ≥2 mm in size have a 64-fold increased risk. About 30% of melanomas

TABLE 83-1 RISK FACTORS FOR CUTANEOUS MELANOMA

High risk (>50-fold increase in risk)
Persistently changing mole
Clinically atypical moles in patient with two family members with melanoma
Adulthood (vs. childhood)
>50 nevi ≥2 mm in diameter
Intermediate risk (~10-fold increase in risk)
Family history of melanoma
Sporadic clinically atypical moles
Congenital nevi (?)
White ethnicity (vs. black or East Asian ethnicity)
Personal history of prior melanoma
Low risk (2- to 4-fold increase in risk)
Immunosuppression
Sun sensitivity or excess exposure to sun

Source: Adapted from AR Rhodes et al: JAMA 258:3146, 1987.

arise in a nevus. Some individuals with multiple primary melanomas and/or a strong family history have heritable mutations in the *CDKN2A* gene. Melanoma is relatively rare in heavily pigmented peoples. Dark-skinned populations (such as those of India and Puerto Rico), blacks, and East Asians have rates 10–20 times lower than lighter-skinned whites. In keeping with the role of sun exposure, the incidence is inversely correlated with the latitude of residence; at any latitude, darker-skinned persons have the lowest incidence. Melanoma is rare in children under age 10.

CLINICAL CHARACTERISTICS

There are four types of cutaneous melanoma (Table 83-2). In three of these—*superficial spreading melanoma*, *lentigo maligna melanoma*, and *acral lentiginous melanoma*—the lesion has a period of superficial (so-called radial) growth during which it increases in size but does not penetrate deeply. It is during this period that the melanoma is most capable of being cured by surgical excision. The fourth type—*nodular melanoma*—does not have a recognizable radial growth phase and usually presents as a deeply invasive lesion, capable of early metastasis. When tumors begin to penetrate deeply into the skin, they are in the so-called vertical growth phase. Melanomas with a radial growth phase are characterized by irregular and sometimes notched borders, variation in pigment pattern, and variation in color. An increase in size or change in color is noted by the patient in 70% of early lesions. Bleeding, ulceration, and pain are late signs and are of little help in early recognition. Superficial spreading melanoma is the most frequent variant observed in the white population. Melanomas arising in dysplastic nevi (see below) are usually of this type. The back is the most common site for melanoma in men. In women, the back and the lower leg (from knee to ankle) are common sites. Nodular melanomas are dark brown-black to blue-black nodules. Lentigo maligna melanoma is usually confined to chronically sun-damaged, sun-exposed sites (face, neck, back of hands) in older individuals. Acral lentiginous melanoma occurs on the palms, soles, nail beds, and mucous membranes. While this type occurs in whites, it is most frequent (along with nodular melanoma) in blacks and East Asians.

A fifth type of melanoma, the *desmoplastic melanoma*, is recognized. This tumor type is associated with a fibrotic response to the tumor, neural invasion, and a higher tendency to local recurrence. Occasionally, melanomas can be amelanotic, in which case the diagnosis is established histologically after biopsy of a new or changing skin nodule or because of a suspicion of a basal cell carcinoma (see below).

PROGNOSTIC FACTORS

The most important prognostic factor is the stage at the time of presentation. Fortunately, most melanomas are diagnosed in clinical stages I and II. The revised American Joint Committee on Cancer (AJCC) staging system for melanoma is based on microscopic primary tumor depth (Breslow's thickness), presence of ulceration, evidence of nodal involvement, and presence of metastatic disease to internal sites (Table 83-3). Certain anatomic sites may affect the prognosis. The favorable

TABLE 83-2 CLINICAL FEATURES OF MALIGNANT MELANOMA

Type	Site	Average Age at Diagnosis, Years	Duration of Known Existence, Years	Color
Lentigo maligna melanoma	Sun-exposed surfaces, particularly malar region of cheek and temple	70	5–20[a] or longer	In flat portions, shades of brown and tan predominant, but whitish gray occasionally present; in nodules, shades of reddish brown, bluish gray, bluish black
Superficial spreading melanoma	Any site (more common on upper back and, in women, on lower legs)	40–50	1–7	Shades of brown mixed with bluish red (violaceous), bluish black, reddish brown, and often whitish pink, and the border of lesion is at least in part visibly and/or palpably elevated
Nodular melanoma	Any site	40–50	Months to less than 5 years	Reddish blue (purple) or bluish black; either uniform in color or mixed with brown or black
Acral lentiginous melanoma	Palm, sole, nail bed, mucous membrane	60	1–10	In flat portions, dark brown predominantly; in raised lesions (plaques) brown-black or blue-black predominantly

[a]During much of this time, the precursor stage, lentigo maligna, is confined to the epidermis.

Source: Adapted from AJ Sober, in *Pathophysiology of Dermatologic Diseases*, NA Soter, HP Baden (eds). New York, McGraw-Hill, 1984.

sites appear to be the forearm and leg (excluding feet), while unfavorable sites include scalp, hands, feet, and mucous membranes. In general, women with stage I or II disease have a better survival than men, perhaps in part because of earlier diagnosis; women frequently have melanomas on the lower leg, where self-recognition is more likely and prognosis is better. Older individuals, especially men over 60, have poorer prognoses. This finding has been explained in part by a tendency toward later diagnosis (and thus thicker tumors) in men and by a higher proportion in men of acral melanomas (palmar-plantar), which have a poorer prognosis. Melanoma may recur after many years. About 10–15% of first-time recurrences develop >5 years after treatment of the original lesion. The time to recurrence varies inversely with tumor thickness. An alternative prognostic scheme for clinical stages I and II melanoma, proposed by Clark, is based on the anatomic level of invasion in the skin. Level I is intraepidermal (in situ); level II penetrates the papillary dermis; level III spans the papillary dermis; level IV penetrates the reticular dermis; and level V penetrates into the subcutaneous fat. The 5-year survival for these stages averages 100, 95, 82, 71, and 49%, respectively.

TABLE 83-3 PROGNOSIS OF MELANOMA BY THICKNESS (BRESLOW) AND REVISED AJCC STAGES: 5-YEAR SURVIVAL RATES

AJCC Stage	Thickness, mm	Ulceration	Nodal Disease	Distant Metastases
0	In situ	N/A	No	No
IA	<1	No	No	No
IB	<1	Yes	No	No
	1.01–2.0	No	No	No
IIA	1.01–2.0	Yes	No	No
	2.01–4.0	No	No	No
IIB	2.01–4.0	Yes	No	No
	>4.0	No	No	No
IIC	>4.0	Yes	No	No
IIIA	Any	No	Yes	
			1 node w/microscopic disease	No
			2–3 nodes w/microscopic disease	No
IIIB	Any	Yes	1 node w/microscopic disease	No
	Any	Yes	2–3 nodes w/microscopic disease	No
	Any	No	1 node w/macroscopic disease	No
	Any	No	2–3 nodes w/macroscopic disease	No
	Any	Any	In transit or satellite disease w/out nodal disease	No
IIIC	Any	Yes	1 node w/macroscopic disease	No
		Yes	2–3 nodes w/macroscopic disease	No
		Any	≥4 metastatic or matted nodes, or in transit mets/ satellites or metastatic nodes	No
IV	Any	Any	Any	Yes

Note: AJCC, American Joint Commission for Cancer.

NATURAL HISTORY

Melanomas may spread by the lymphatic channels or the bloodstream. The earliest metastases are often to regional lymph nodes. Lymphadenectomy may control early regional disease. Liver, lung, bone, and brain are common sites of hematogenous spread, but unusual sites, such as the anterior chamber of the eye, may also be involved. Once metastatic disease is established, cure is unlikely.

MANAGEMENT

The entire cutaneous surface, including the scalp and mucous membranes, should be examined in each patient. Bright room illumination is important, and a 7× to 10× hand lens is helpful for evaluating variation in pigment pattern. A history of relevant risk factors should be elicited. Any suspicious lesions should be biopsied, evaluated by a specialist, or recorded by chart and/or photography for follow-up. Examination of the lymph nodes and palpation of the abdominal viscera are part of the staging examination for suspected melanoma. The patient should be advised to have other family members screened if either melanoma or clinically atypical moles (dysplastic nevi) are present. The detection of early melanoma in relatives has been reported.

Melanoma prevention is based on protection from the sun. Routine use of a broad spectrum UV-A/UV-B sunblock with sun protection factor ≥15, use of protective clothing, and avoiding intense midday ultraviolet exposure should be recommended. The patient should be educated in the clinical features of melanoma and advised to report any growth or other change in a pigmented lesion. Patient education brochures are available from the American Cancer Society, the American Academy of Dermatology, the National Cancer Institute, and the Skin Cancer Foundation. Self-examination at 6- to 8-week intervals may enhance the likelihood of detecting change. The importance of routine follow-up visits for melanoma patients and patients with clinically atypical moles (dysplastic nevi) should be emphasized, as these visits may facilitate early detection of new primary tumors.

Precursor Lesions Clinically atypical moles, also termed *dysplastic nevi*, occur in certain families affected by melanoma. In some families, melanomas occur nearly exclusively in

TABLE 83-4 CLINICAL FEATURES DISTINGUISHING ATYPICAL MOLES FROM BENIGN ACQUIRED NEVI

Clinical Feature	Clinically Atypical Moles	Benign Acquired Nevi
Color	Variable mixtures of tan, brown, black, or red/pink within a single nevus; nevi may look very different from each other	Uniformly tan or brown
Shape	Irregular borders; pigment may fade off into surrounding skin; macular portion at the edge of the nevus	Round; sharp, clear-cut borders between the nevus and the surrounding skin; may be flat or elevated
Size	Usually >6 mm in diameter; may be >10 mm; occasionally <6 mm	Usually <6 mm in diameter
Number	Often very many (>100), but occasionally may be only one	In a typical adult, 10 to 40 are scattered over the body; perhaps 15% of patients have no nevi
Location	Sun-exposed areas; the back is the most common site, but dysplastic nevi may also be seen on the scalp, breasts, and buttocks	Generally on the sun-exposed surfaces of the skin above the waist; the scalp, breasts, and buttocks are rarely involved

Source: Modified from RJ Friedman et al: CA—A Cancer J Clinicians 33(3):130, 1985.

the individuals with dysplastic nevi. In other families, the nevi may not be present in all individuals with an increased risk of melanoma. The melanomas may arise in clinically atypical moles or in normal skin (in the latter situation the moles act as markers of increased risk). Individuals with clinically atypical moles and a strong family history of melanoma have been reported to have a >50% lifetime risk for developing melanoma. Table 83-4 lists the features that are characteristic of clinically atypical moles and that differentiate them from benign acquired nevi. The number of clinically atypical moles may vary from one to several hundred. Clinically atypical moles usually differ from each other in appearance. The borders are often hazy and indistinct, and the pigment pattern is more highly varied than that in benign acquired nevi. Of the 90% of melanoma patients whose disease is regarded as sporadic (i.e., who lack a family history of melanoma), ~40% have clinically atypical moles, as compared with an estimated 5–10% of the population at large. Further studies to determine the background frequency of clinically atypical moles are required, once greater unanimity exists regarding their clinical and histopathologic features. The observation that sporadic melanomas can arise in association with a clinically atypical mole makes this the most important precursor for melanoma. Less frequent precursors include the giant congenital melanocytic nevus. Congenital melanocytic nevi are present at birth or appear in the neonatal period (tardive form). The *giant melanocytic nevus*, also called the bathing trunk, cape, or garment nevus, is a rare malformation that affects perhaps 1 in 30,000 to 1 in 100,000 individuals. These nevi are usually >20 cm in diameter and may cover more than half the body surface. Giant nevi often occur in association with multiple small congenital nevi. The borders are sharp, and hair may be present. The lesions are usually dark brown and may have darker and lighter areas. Pigment is haphazardly displayed. The surface is smooth to rugose or cerebriform and may vary from one portion of the lesion to another.

A lifetime risk of melanoma development of 6% has been estimated. The risk is greatest before age 5 and next greatest between ages 5 and 10. Early detection of melanoma is difficult in these lesions because of the deep dermal or subcutaneous origin of primary melanoma and because of the large and varied surface of the nevus. Prophylactic excision early in life can be accomplished by staged removal with coverage by split-thickness skin grafts. Surgery cannot remove all at-risk nevus cells as some may penetrate into the muscles or central nervous system below the nevus. At present there are no uniform management guidelines for giant congenital nevi. The *small- to medium-sized congenital melanocytic nevus*, which affects approximately 1% of persons, usually presents as a raised dark- to medium-brown lesion with a smooth or papillomatous surface. The border is sharp, and lesions may be oriented along lines of skin cleavage. Follicular hyper- and hypopigmentation may coexist in a salt-and-pepper configuration. The lesion may have an excess of thick, coarse hairs. The risk of melanoma developing in these lesions is not known but appears to be relatively small. The management of small- to medium-sized congenital melanocytic nevi remains controversial. Melanomas in small congenital melanocytic nevi appear to occur after puberty, unlike melanomas that arise in giant congenital nevi and tend to occur much earlier in life. Melanomas can also arise in benign dermal and compound moles. Overall, it has been estimated that for a 20-year-old individual, the lifetime risk of any selected mole transforming into melanoma by age 80 years is approximately 0.03% (1 in 3,164) for men and 0.009% (1 in 10,800) for women.

Differential Diagnosis The aim of differential diagnosis is to distinguish benign pigmented lesions from melanoma and its precursor. If melanoma is a consideration, then biopsy is appropriate. Some benign look-alikes may be removed in the process of trying to detect authentic melanoma. Table 83-5 summarizes the distinguishing features of benign lesions that may be confused with melanoma. Early detection of melanoma may be facilitated by applying the "ABCD rules": A—asymmetry, benign lesions are usually symmetrical; B—border irregularity, most nevi have clear-cut borders; C—color variegation, benign lesions usually have uniform light or dark pigment; D—diameter >6 mm (the size of a pencil eraser). Of these criteria, the weakest is diameter >6

TABLE 83-5 PIGMENTED LESIONS THAT MUST BE DISTINGUISHED FROM CUTANEOUS MELANOMA AND ITS PRECURSORS

Blue nevus	Gunmetal or cerulean blue, blue-gray. Stable over time. One-half occur on dorsa of hands and feet. Lesions are usually single, small, 3 mm to <1 cm. Must be distinguished from nodular melanoma.
Compound nevus	Round or oval shape, well-demarcated, smooth-bordered. May be dome-shaped or papillomatous; colors range from flesh colored to very dark brown, with individual nevi being relatively homogeneous in color.
Hemangioma	Dome-shaped reddish, purple, blue nodule. Compression with a glass microscope slide may result in blanching. Must be distinguished from nodular melanoma.
Junctional nevus	Flat to barely raised brown lesion. Sharp border. Fine pigmentary stippling visible, especially upon magnification.
Lentigo Juvenile Solar	Flat, uniformly medium or dark brown lesion with sharp border. Solar lentigines are acquired lesions on sites of chronic solar exposure (face and backs of hands). Lesions are 2 mm to ≥1 cm. Solar lentigines have reticulate pigmentation upon magnification.
Pigmented basal cell carcinoma	Papular border. May have central ulceration. Usually on a sun-exposed surface in an older patient. Patient usually has dark brown eyes and dark brown or black hair.
Pigmented dermatofibroma	Lesion is not well demarcated visually, is firm, and dimples downward when compressed laterally. Usually on extremities. Usually <6 mm.
Seborrheic keratosis	Rough, sharp-bordered lesions that feel waxy and "stuck on"; range in color from flesh to tan, to dark brown. Presence of keratin plugs in surface is helpful for discriminating especially dark lesions from melanoma.
Subungual hematoma	Maroon (red-brown) coloration. As lesion grows out from nail fold, a curving clear area is seen.
Tattoo (medical or traumatic)	In medical tattoo, lesions are small pigmentary dots, often blue or green, which make a regular pattern (rectangle). Traumatic tattoos are irregular, and pigmentation may appear black.

mm since a significant fraction of melanomas are now diagnosed with diameters <6 mm. In addition, the above features are less helpful in the recognition of nodular melanomas, which may be symmetrical and have uniform colors. "Different" has been substituted for "diameter" by some. Addition of an "E" for evolution has been proposed as other features may become more significant if the lesion is changing.

Biopsy Any pigmented cutaneous lesion that has changed in size or shape or has other features suggestive of malignant melanoma is a candidate for biopsy. The recommended technique is an excisional biopsy, as that facilitates pathologic assessment of the lesion, permits accurate measurement of thickness if the lesion is melanoma, and constitutes treatment if the lesion is benign. For large lesions or lesions on anatomic sites where excisional biopsy may not be feasible (such as the face, hands, or feet), an incisional biopsy through the most nodular or darkest area of the lesion is acceptable; this should include the vertical growth phase of the primary tumor, if present. Incisional biopsy does not appear to facilitate the spread of melanoma.

Staging Once the diagnosis of malignant melanoma has been confirmed, the tumor must be staged to determine prognosis and treatment. The history should probe for evidence of metastatic disease, such as malaise, weight loss, headaches, visual difficulty, or bone pain. The physical examination should be directed especially to the skin, regional draining lymph nodes, central nervous system, liver, and spleen. In the absence of signs or symptoms of metastasis, few laboratory or radiologic tests are indicated for staging purposes. No tests or scans are routinely indicated unless the history or physical examination suggests metastasis to a specific organ. Once signs of metastasis exist, favored sites of spread, such as the liver, lungs, bone, and brain, should be evaluated. Patients are classified into four stages (Table 83-3).

℞ MELANOMA

SURGICAL MANAGEMENT For a newly diagnosed cutaneous melanoma, wide surgical excision of the lesion with a margin of normal skin is necessary to remove all malignant cells and minimize possible local recurrence. The appropriate width of the margin is a source of controversy. A World Health Organization trial that prospectively randomized between 1- and 3-cm margins in 612 patients with thin malignant melanomas (≤2 mm thick) reported that the narrower margin resulted in higher rates of local recurrence but no difference in rates of nodal or distant metastases, disease-free survival, or overall survival. Another large randomized trial comparing 2- or 4-cm surgical margins for intermediate-thickness lesions (1–4 mm thick) also found no significant differences in overall survival. The following margins can be recommended for primary melanoma: in situ: 0.5 cm; invasive up to 1 mm thick: 1.0 cm; >1 mm: 2.0 cm. For lesions on the face, hands, and feet, strict adherence to these margins must give way to individual considerations about the constraints of surgery and minimization of morbidity. In all instances, however, inclusion of subcutaneous fat in the surgical specimen facilitates adequate thickness measurement and assessment of surgical margins by the pathologist.

Sentinel Node Biopsy Sentinel node biopsy (SLNB) has replaced elective regional nodal dissection for the evaluation of regional nodal status. The initial draining node(s) from the primary site is/are identified by injecting a blue dye and a radioisotope around the primary site. The initial draining node(s) is/are then identified by inspection of the nodal basin for the blue stained node and/or the node with high uptake of the radioisotope. The identified nodes are removed and subjected to careful histopathologic processing with serial section hematoxylin and eosin stains as well as immunohistochemical stains that identify melanocytes. Sentinel lymph node examination is a valuable staging tool, and in the instance of a negative biopsy, SLNB may obviate the need for complete nodal dissection. Patients with lesions <0.75 mm thick have an excellent prognosis and are not candidates for SLNB unless other high-risk features are present (ulceration, shave biopsy with base involved, etc.). At the other extreme, patients with lesions >4 mm thick have such a high risk for distant metastases that controlling nodal disease may not alter the ultimate clinical outcome. A subset of patients with lesions of intermediate thickness may have a survival benefit from regional node dissection. SLNB is of value in selecting patients who may benefit from adjuvant therapy. Survival benefit of SLNB remains to be proven.

ADJUVANT THERAPY FOR NODAL DISEASE For patients who are free of disease but at high risk for metastases, adjuvant therapy that complements surgery is needed to destroy occult micrometastases, prolong disease-free survival, and improve the cure rate. Many strategies have been tried unsuccessfully. However, adjuvant interferon (IFN) α2b may be capable of improving disease-free and overall survival in patients with nodal metastases (stage III disease). The U.S. Food and Drug Administration has approved a high-dose IFN adjuvant protocol consisting of 20 million units per square meter intravenously 5 days a week for 4 weeks followed by 10 million units per square meter subcutaneously three times a week for 11 months. In a large fraction of patients, these doses of IFN are associated with severe toxicity, including a flulike illness and decline in performance status. The toxicity in most patients reverses promptly with lower doses and when therapy is stopped.

TREATMENT OF METASTATIC DISEASE Melanoma can metastasize to any internal organ, the brain being a particularly common site. Metastatic melanoma is generally incurable, with survival in patients with visceral metastases generally <1 year. Thus, the goal of treatment is usually palliation. Patients with soft tissue and nodal metastases fare better than those with liver and brain metastases. Metastases limited to regional nodes (AJCC stage III disease) warrant a therapeutic lymph node dissection. Surgical excision of a single metastasis to the lung or to a surgically accessible brain site can prolong survival. Stereotactic radiosurgery has been successful in the treatment of isolated brain metastases. Radiation therapy can provide local palliation for recurrent tumors or metastases. Patients who have advanced regional disease limited to a limb may benefit from hyperthermic limb perfusion with melphalan. High complete response rates have been reported, and responses are associated with significant palliation of symptoms.

A number of drugs and biological therapies have demonstrated minimal antitumor activity (15–20% partial response rates) in metastatic melanoma, including dacarbazine (DTIC); the nitrosoureas carmustine (BCNU), lomustine (CCNU), and semustine (methyl-CCNU); platinum analogues such as cisplatin and carboplatin; vinca alkaloids such as vincristine, vinblastine, and vindesine; the taxanes paclitaxel and docetaxel; IFN-α; and interleukin 2 (IL-2). Although limited in efficacy, single-agent dacarbazine is still considered the standard treatment. Ongoing trials are attempting to define superior combinations. IL-2 produces response rates similar to those seen with cytotoxic agents; however, active doses usually cause greater toxicity than chemotherapy. Response rates of >50% have been observed with IL-2 for intracutaneous and subcutaneous disease.

Melanoma can express cell-surface antigens that may be recognized by host immune cells. These melanoma-associated antigens alone or in combination may make it possible to develop vaccination strategies against melanoma. Such strategies include the use of purified tumor proteins as immunogens and the use of genetically altered tumor cells to elicit a T cell response. Alternative experimental approaches include efforts to expand tumor-specific T cells (either obtained from the tumor as tumor-infiltrating lymphocytes or harvested from the peripheral blood after vaccination) in vitro and transfer them into patients in large numbers. In addition, monoclonal antibodies to tumor antigens are being evaluated. Agents directed against the cell cycle pathways are also currently in trial. All of these experimental approaches will need considerable further development before being applicable on a wide scale. Advances in treating metastatic disease may also prove applicable in the adjuvant setting.

The absence of curative therapy for patients with metastatic melanoma underscores the importance of early detection and prevention as strategies to decrease melanoma mortality. Patients with stage 4 melanoma are best treated by medical oncologists with expertise in treating patients with advanced disease. Clinical trials should be considered as an option for this patient group.

NONMELANOMA SKIN CANCER

Nonmelanoma skin cancer (NMSC) is the most common cancer in the United States, with an estimated annual incidence of >1.5 million

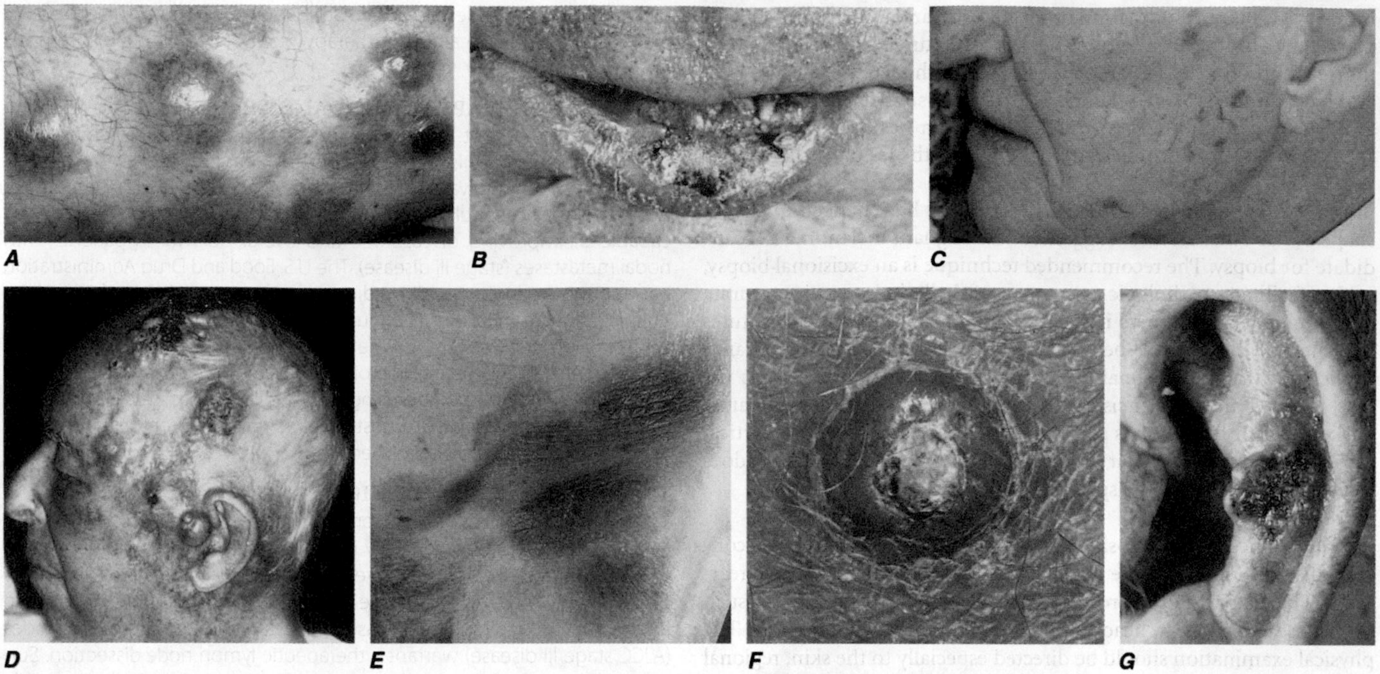

FIGURE 83-2 Cutaneous neoplasms. ***A.*** Non-Hodgkin's lymphoma involves the skin with typical violaceous, "plum-colored" nodules. ***B.*** Squamous cell carcinoma is seen here as a hyperkeratotic crusted and somewhat eroded plaque on the lower lip. Sun-exposed skin such as the head, neck, hands, and arms are other typical sites of involvement. ***C.*** Actinic keratoses consists of hyperkeratotic erythematous papules and patches on sun-exposed skin. They arise in middle-aged to older adults and have some potential for malignant transformation. ***D.*** Metastatic carcinoma to the skin is characterized by inflammatory, often ulcerated dermal nodules. ***E.*** Mycosis fungoides is a cutaneous T cell lymphoma, and plaque stage lesions are seen in this patient. ***F.*** Keratoacanthoma is a low-grade squamous cell carcinoma that presents as an exophytic nodule with central keratinous debris. ***G.*** This basal cell carcinoma shows central ulceration and a pearly, rolled, telangiectatic tumor border.

cases. Basal cell carcinomas (BCCs) account for 70–80% of NMSCs. Squamous cell carcinomas (SCCs), while representing only ~20% of NMSC, are more significant because of their ability to metastasize (Fig. 83-2); they account for most of the 2400 deaths annually. Incidence rates have risen dramatically over the past decade.

ETIOLOGY

The causes of BCC and SCC are multifactorial. Cumulative exposure to sunlight, principally the ultraviolet B (UV-B) spectrum, is the most significant factor. Emerging data suggest that ultraviolet A radiation may be more carcinogenic than previously believed. Other factors associated with a higher incidence of skin cancer are male sex, older age, Celtic descent, a fair complexion, a tendency to sunburn easily, and an outdoor occupation. The incidence of these tumors increases with decreasing latitude. Most tumors develop on sun-exposed areas of the head and neck. Tumors are more common on the left side of the body in the United States but on the right side in England, presumably owing to asymmetric exposure during driving. As the earth's ozone shield continues to thin, further increases in the incidence of skin cancer are anticipated. In certain geographic areas, exposure to arsenic in well water or from industrial sources may significantly increase the risk of BCC and SCC. Skin cancer in affected individuals may be seen with or without other cutaneous markers of chronic arsenism (e.g., arsenical keratoses). Less common is exposure to the cyclic aromatic hydrocarbons in tar, soot, or shale. The risk of lip or oral SCC is increased with cigarette smoking. Human papillomaviruses and UV radiation may act as cocarcinogens.

Host factors associated with a high risk of skin cancer include immunosuppression induced by disease or drugs. Transplant recipients receiving chronic immunosuppressive therapy are particularly prone to SCC. The frequency of skin cancer is proportional to the duration of immunosuppression and the extent of sun exposure both before and after transplantation. Skin cancer is not uncommon in patients infected with HIV, and it may be more aggressive in this setting. Other factors include ionizing radiation, thermal burn scars, and chronic ulcerations. Several heritable conditions are associated with skin cancer (e.g., albinism, xeroderma pigmentosum, and basal cell nevus syndrome). Mutations in the tumor suppressor *patch* gene have been implicated in the development of BCC.

CLINICAL PRESENTATION

NMSCs are often asymptomatic, but nonhealing ulceration, bleeding, or pain can occur in advanced lesions.

Basal Cell Carcinoma BCC is a malignancy arising from epidermal basal cells. The least invasive of BCC subtypes, *superficial BCC*, classically consists of truncal erythematous, scaling plaques that slowly enlarge. This BCC subtype may be confused with benign inflammatory dermatoses, especially nummular eczema and psoriasis. BCC can also present as a small, slow-growing pearly nodule, often with small telangiectatic vessels on its surface (*nodular BCC*). The occasional presence of melanin in this variant of nodular BCC (*pigmented BCC*) may lead to confusion clinically with melanoma. *Morpheaform (fibrosing) BCC* and *micronodular BCC*, the most invasive subtypes, manifest as solitary, flat or slightly depressed, indurated, whitish or yellowish plaques. Borders are typically indistinct, a feature associated with a greater potential for extensive subclinical spread.

Squamous Cell Carcinoma Primary *cutaneous SCC* is a malignant neoplasm of keratinizing epidermal cells. SCC can grow rapidly and metastasize. The clinical features of SCC vary widely. Commonly, SCC appears as an ulcerated erythematous nodule or superficial erosion on the skin or lower lip, but it may present as a verrucous papule or plaque. Overlying telangiectasias are uncommon. The margins of this tumor may be ill-defined, and fixation to underlying structures may occur. Cutaneous SCC may develop anywhere on the body but usually arises on sun-damaged skin. A related neoplasm, keratoacanthoma, typically appears as a dome-shaped papule with a central keratotic crater, expands rapidly, and commonly regresses without therapy. This lesion can be difficult to differentiate from SCC.

Actinic keratoses and *cheilitis*, both premalignant forms of SCC, present as hyperkeratotic papules on sun-exposed areas. The potential for malignant degeneration in untreated lesions ranges from 0.25 to 20%. *Bowen's disease*, an in situ form of SCC, presents as a scaling, erythematous plaque. Treatment of premalignant and in situ lesions reduces the subsequent risk of invasive disease.

NATURAL HISTORY

Basal Cell Carcinoma The natural history of BCC is that of a slowly enlarging, locally invasive neoplasm. The degree of local destruction and risk of recurrence vary with the size, duration, location, and histologic subtype of the tumor; presence of recurrent disease; and various patient characteristics. Location on the central face, ears, or scalp may portend a higher risk. Small nodular, pigmented, cystic, or superficial BCCs respond well to most treatments. Large lesions and micronodular and morpheaform subtypes may be more aggressive. The metastatic potential of BCC has been estimated to be 0.0028–0.1%. Persons with either BCC or SCC have an increased risk of developing subsequent skin cancers, estimated to be up to 40% in 5 years.

Squamous Cell Carcinoma The natural history of SCC depends on both tumor and host characteristics. Tumors arising on actinically damaged skin have a lower metastatic potential than those on protected surfaces. The metastatic frequency of cutaneous SCC, reported at 0.3–5.2%, occurs most frequently in regional draining lymph nodes. Tumors occurring on the lower lip and ear have metastatic potentials approaching 13 and 11%, respectively. The metastatic potential of SCC arising in scars, chronic ulcerations, and genital or mucosal surfaces is higher. The overall metastatic rate for recurrent tumors may approach 30%. Large, poorly differentiated, deep tumors, with perineural or lymphatic invasion, often behave aggressively. Multiple tumors with rapid growth and aggressive behavior can be a therapeutic challenge in immunosuppressed patients.

℞ NONMELANOMA SKIN CANCER

BASAL CELL CARCINOMA The most frequently employed treatment modalities for BCC include electrodesiccation and curettage (ED&C), excision, cryosurgery, radiation therapy, laser therapy, Mohs micrographic surgery (MMS), topical 5-fluorouracil, and topical immunomodulators. The mode of therapy chosen depends on tumor characteristics, patient age, medical status, preferences of the patient, and other factors. ED&C remains the method most commonly employed by dermatologists. This method is selected for low-risk tumors (e.g., a small primary tumor of a less aggressive subtype in a favorable location). Excision, which offers the advantage of histologic control, is usually selected for more aggressive tumors or those in high-risk locations or, in many instances, for aesthetic reasons. Cryosurgery employing liquid nitrogen may be used for certain low-risk tumors but requires specialized equipment (cryoprobes) to be effective for advanced neoplasms. Radiation therapy, while not used as often, offers an excellent chance for cure in many cases of BCC. It is useful in patients not considered surgical candidates and as a surgical adjunct in high-risk tumors. Younger patients may not be good candidates for radiation therapy because of the risks of long-term carcinogenesis and radiodermatitis. Despite rapidly advancing technology in laser development, their long-term efficacy in treating infiltrative or recurrent lesions is still unknown. On the other hand, MMS, a specialized type of surgical excision that permits the best histologic control and preservation of uninvolved tissue, is associated with cure rates >98%. It is the preferred modality for lesions that are recurrent, in a high-risk location, or large and ill-defined and where maximal tissue conservation is critical (e.g., the eyelids). Topical 5-fluorouracil therapy should be limited to superficial BCC. New topicals, the immunomodulators, show promise in their efficacy at treating superficial and even nodular BCCs. Imiquimod, a relatively well-tolerated cream, has successfully undergone phase III clinical trials. Intralesional chemotherapy (5-fluorouracil and INF) and photodynamic therapy (which employs selective activation of a photoactive drug by visible light) have been used successfully in patients with numerous tumors. A topical endonuclease (T4N5 liposome lotion) has been shown to repair DNA and may decrease the rate of NMSC in xeroderma pigmentosum.

TABLE 83-6 OTHER NONMELANOMA CUTANEOUS MALIGNANCIES

Tumor Type	Most Common Location	Recurrence Rate,[a] %	Metastatic Rate, %
Atypical fibroxanthoma	Head and neck	21	4
Merkel cell carcinoma	Head and neck	40	75
Dermatofibrosarcoma protuberans	Trunk	50	1
Sebaceous carcinoma	Eyelid	12	30
Microcystic adnexal carcinoma	Face	50	1 case
Porocarcinoma	Extremity	20	10
Eccrine carcinoma	Head and neck	36	11
Angiosarcoma	Head and neck	75	75

[a]Recurrence rates are the highest reported and were established prior to widespread use of Mohs micrographic surgery.

SQUAMOUS CELL CARCINOMA The therapy of cutaneous SCC should be based on an analysis of risk factors influencing the biologic behavior of the tumor. These include the size, location, and degree of histologic differentiation of the tumor as well as the age and physical condition of the patient. Surgical excision, MMS, and radiation therapy are standard methods of treatment. Cryosurgery and ED&C have been used successfully for premalignant lesions and small primary tumors. Metastases are treated with lymph node dissection, irradiation, or both. 13-*cis*-retinoic acid (1 mg orally every day) plus INF-α (3 million units subcutaneously or intramuscularly every day) may produce a partial response in most patients. Systemic chemotherapy combinations that include cisplatin may also be palliative in some patients.

PREVENTION

As the vast majority of skin cancers are related to chronic UV radiation exposure, patient and physician education could dramatically reduce their incidence. Emphasis should be placed on preventive measures beginning early in life. Patients must understand that damage from UV-B begins early, despite the fact that cancers develop years later. Regular use of sunscreens and protective clothing should be encouraged. Avoidance of tanning salons and midday (10 A.M.–2 P.M.) sun exposure is recommended. Precancerous and in situ lesions should be treated early. Early detection of small tumors affords simpler treatment modalities with higher cure rates and lower morbidity. In patients with a history of skin cancer, long-term follow-up for the detection of recurrence, metastasis, and new skin cancers should be emphasized. Chemoprophylaxis using synthetic retinoids is useful in controlling new lesions in some patients with multiple tumors.

OTHER NONMELANOMA CUTANEOUS MALIGNANCIES

Neoplasms of cutaneous adnexa and sarcomas of fibrous, mesenchymal, fatty, and vascular tissues make up 1–2% of NMSC (Table 83-6). Some can portend a poor prognosis such as *Merkel cell carcinoma*, which is a neural crest-derived, highly aggressive malignancy that exhibits a metastatic rate of 75% and a 5-year survival rate of 30–40%. Others, such as the human herpes virus 8-induced, HIV-related *Kaposi's sarcoma*, exhibit a more indolent course. The marked decrease in incidence of this tumor parallels the institution of the highly active antiretroviral therapy.

ACKNOWLEDGMENT

Katarina G. Chiller, MD, and Howard K. Koh, MD, contributed to this chapter in the 16th edition and material from that chapter is included here.

FURTHER READINGS

AMERICAN CANCER SOCIETY: Website at *www.cancer.org*

BALCH CM et al: Prognostic factors analysis of 17,600 melanoma patients: Validation of the American Joint Committee on Cancer melanoma staging system. J Clin Oncol 19:3622, 2001

BALCH CM et al: Final version of the AJCC staging system for cutaneous melanoma. J Clin Oncol 19:3635, 2001

DRAKE LA et al: Guidelines of care of basal cell carcinoma. J Am Acad Dermatol 26:117, 1992

——— et al: Guidelines of care for cutaneous squamous cell carcinoma. J Am Acad Dermatol 28:628, 1993

GEISSE JK et al: Imiquimod 5% cream for the treatment of superficial basal cell carcinoma: A double-blind, randomized, vehicle-controlled study. J Am Acad Dermatol 47:390, 2002

JOHNSON TM et al: Staging workup, sentinel node biopsy, and follow-up tests for melanoma: Update of current concepts, Arch Dermatol 140:107, 2004

MORTON DL et al: Sentinel-node biopsy on nodal observation in melanoma. N Engl J Med 355:1307, 2006

PETRELLA T et al: Single agent interleukin-2 in the treatment of metastatic melanoma: A systematic review. Cancer Treat Rev 2007 [epub ahead of print] PMID: 17562357

RIGEL DS et al: ABCDE: An evolving concept in the early diagnosis of melanoma. Arch Dermatol 141:1032, 2005

TSAO H et al: Management of cutaneous melanoma. N Engl J Med 351:998, 2004

84 Head and Neck Cancer

Everett E. Vokes

Epithelial carcinomas of the head and neck arise from the mucosal surfaces in the head and neck area and typically are squamous cell in origin. This category includes tumors of the paranasal sinuses, the oral cavity, and the nasopharynx, oropharynx, hypopharynx, and larynx. Tumors of the salivary glands differ from the more common carcinomas of the head and neck in etiology, histopathology, clinical presentation, and therapy. Thyroid malignancies are described in Chap. 335.

INCIDENCE AND EPIDEMIOLOGY

The number of new cases of head and neck cancers in the United States was 40,500 in 2006, accounting for about 3% of adult malignancies. The worldwide incidence exceeds half a million cases annually. In North America and Europe, the tumors usually arise from the oral cavity, oropharynx, or larynx, whereas nasopharyngeal cancer is more common in the Mediterranean countries and in the Far East.

ETIOLOGY AND GENETICS

Alcohol and tobacco use are the most common risk factors for head and neck cancer in the United States. Smokeless tobacco is an etiologic agent for oral cancers. Other potential carcinogens include marijuana and occupational exposures such as nickel refining, exposure to textile fibers, and woodworking.

Dietary factors may contribute. The incidence of head and neck cancer is highest in people with the lowest consumption of fruits and vegetables. Certain vitamins, including carotenoids, may be protective if included in a balanced diet. Supplements of retinoids such as *cis*-retinoic acid have not been shown to prevent head and neck cancers (or lung cancer) and may increase the risk in active smokers.

Some head and neck cancers may have a viral etiology. The DNA of human papillomavirus (HPV) has been detected in the tissue of oral and tonsil cancers, and may predispose to oral and tonsillar cancer in the absence of tobacco and alcohol use. These patients can present at a somewhat younger age. The incidence of HPV-related head and neck cancer may be increasing. Epstein-Barr virus (EBV) infection is associated with nasopharyngeal cancer. Nasopharyngeal cancer occurs endemically in some countries of the Mediterranean and Far East, where EBV antibody titers can be measured to screen high-risk populations. Nasopharyngeal cancer has also been associated with consumption of salted fish.

No specific risk factors or environmental carcinogens have been identified for salivary gland tumors.

HISTOPATHOLOGY, CARCINOGENESIS, AND MOLECULAR BIOLOGY

Squamous cell head and neck cancers can be divided into well-differentiated, moderately well-differentiated, and poorly differentiated categories. Poorly differentiated tumors have a worse prognosis than well-differentiated tumors. For nasopharyngeal cancers, the less common differentiated squamous cell carcinoma is distinguished from nonkeratinizing and undifferentiated carcinoma (lymphoepithelioma) that contains infiltrating lymphocytes.

Salivary gland tumors can arise from the major (parotid, submandibular, sublingual) or minor salivary glands (located in the submucosa of the upper aerodigestive tract). Most parotid tumors are benign, but half of submandibular and sublingual gland tumors and most minor salivary gland tumors are malignant. Malignant tumors include mucoepidermoid and adenoidcystic carcinomas and adenocarcinomas.

The mucosal surface of the entire pharynx is exposed to alcohol- and tobacco-related carcinogens and is at risk for the development of a premalignant or malignant lesion, such as erythroplakia or leukoplakia (hyperplasia, dysplasia), that can progress to invasive carcinoma. Alternatively, multiple synchronous or metachronous cancers can develop. In fact, over time patients with early-stage head and neck cancer are at greater risk of dying from a second malignancy than from a recurrence of the primary disease.

Second head and neck malignancies are usually not therapy-induced; they reflect the exposure of the upper aerodigestive mucosa to the same carcinogens that caused the first cancer. These second primaries develop in the head and neck area, the lung, or the esophagus. Rarely, patients can develop a radiation therapy–induced sarcoma after having undergone prior radiotherapy for a head and neck cancer.

Chromosomal deletions and other alterations, most frequently involving chromosomes 3p, 9p, 17p, and 13q, have been identified in both premalignant and malignant head and neck lesions, as have mutations in tumor suppressor genes, such as the p53 gene. Amplification of oncogenes is less common, but overexpression of PRAD-1/bcl-1 (cyclin D1), bcl-2, transforming growth factor β, and the epidermal growth factor receptor (EGFR) have been described. EGFR overexpression has been shown to be very common, and its extent seems to be of prognostic importance.

Resected tumor specimens with histopathologically negative margins ("complete resection") can have residual tumor cells with persistent p53 mutations at the margins. Thus, a tumor-specific p53 mutation can be detected in some phenotypically "normal" surgical margins, indicating residual disease. Patients with such submicroscopic marginal involvement may have a worse prognosis than patients with truly negative margins.

CLINICAL PRESENTATION AND DIFFERENTIAL DIAGNOSIS

Most head and neck cancers occur after age 50, although these cancers can appear in younger patients, including those without known risk factors. The manifestations vary according to the stage and primary site of the tumor. Patients with nonspecific signs and symptoms in the head and neck area should be evaluated with a thorough otolaryngologic exam, particularly if symptoms persist longer than 2–4 weeks.

Cancer of the nasopharynx typically does not cause early symptoms. However, on occasion it may cause unilateral serous otitis media due to obstruction of the eustachian tube, unilateral or bilateral nasal obstruction, or epistaxis. Advanced nasopharyngeal carcinoma causes neuropathies of the cranial nerves.

Carcinomas of the oral cavity present as nonhealing ulcers, changes in the fit of dentures, or painful lesions. Tumors of the tongue base or oropharynx can cause decreased tongue mobility and alterations in speech. Cancers of the oropharynx or hypopharynx rarely cause early symptoms, but they may cause sore throat and/or otalgia.

Hoarseness may be an early symptom of laryngeal cancer, and persistent hoarseness requires referral to a specialist for indirect laryngoscopy and/or radiographic studies. If a head and neck lesion treated initially with antibiotics does not resolve in a short period, further workup is indicated; to simply continue the antibiotic treatment may be to lose the chance of early diagnosis of a malignancy.

Advanced head and neck cancers in any location can cause severe pain, otalgia, airway obstruction, cranial neuropathies, trismus, odynophagia, dysphagia, decreased tongue mobility, fistulas, skin involvement, and massive cervical lymphadenopathy, which may be unilateral or bilateral. Some patients have enlarged lymph nodes even though no primary lesion can be detected by endoscopy or biopsy; these patients are considered to have carcinoma of unknown primary (Fig. 84-1). If the enlarged nodes are located in the upper neck and the tumor cells are of squamous cell histology, the malignancy probably arose from a mucosal surface in the head or neck. Tumor cells in supraclavicular lymph nodes may also arise from a primary site in the chest or abdomen.

The physical examination should include inspection of all visible mucosal surfaces and palpation of the floor of mouth and tongue and of the neck. In addition to tumors themselves, leukoplakia (a white mucosal patch) or erythroplakia (a red mucosal patch) may be observed; these "premalignant" lesions can represent hyperplasia, dysplasia, or carcinoma in situ. All visible or palpable lesions should be biopsied. Further examination should be performed by a specialist. Additional staging procedures include CT of the head and neck to identify the extent of the disease. Patients with lymph node involvement should have chest radiography and a bone scan to screen for distant metastases. The definitive staging procedure is an endoscopic examination under anesthesia, which may include laryngoscopy, esophagoscopy, and bronchoscopy; during this procedure, multiple biopsy samples are obtained to establish a primary diagnosis, define the extent of primary disease, and identify any additional premalignant lesions or second primaries.

Head and neck tumors are classified according to the TNM system of the American Joint Committee on Cancer. This classification varies according to the specific anatomic subsite (Tables 84-1 and 84-2). Distant metastases are found in <10% of patients at initial diagnosis, but in autopsy series, microscopic involvement of the lungs, bones, or liver is more common, particularly in patients with advanced neck lymph node disease. Modern imaging techniques may increase the number of patients with clinically detectable distant metastases in the future.

In patients with lymph node involvement and no visible primary, the diagnosis should be made by lymph node excision. If the results indicate squamous cell carcinoma, a panendoscopy should be performed, with biopsy of all suspicious-appearing areas and directed biopsies of common primary sites, such as the nasopharynx, tonsil, tongue base, and pyriform sinus.

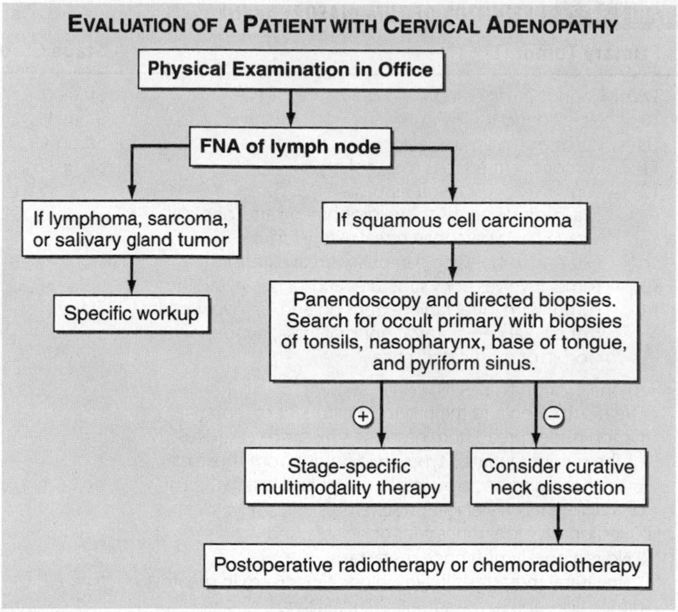

FIGURE 84-1 Evaluation of a patient with cervical adenopathy without a primary mucosal lesion; a diagnostic workup. FNA, fine-needle aspiration.

TABLE 84-1 TNM CLASSIFICATION FOR HEAD AND NECK CANCER (EXCEPT NASOPHARYNGEAL)

Primary Tumor Site

T Grade	Oropharynx	Hypopharynx
T1	0–2 cm	0–2 cm
T2	2.1–4 cm	>1 site, 2–4 cm
T3	>4 cm	>4 cm
T4a	Larynx, muscle of tongue, medial pterygoid, hard palate, mandible invasion	Thyroid/cricoid cartilage, hyoid bone, thyroid gland, esophagus, or central compartment soft tissue invasion
T4b	Lateral pterygoid muscle, pterygoid plates, lateral nasopharynx, or skull base or encases carotid artery invasion	Invasion of prevertebral fascia, encases carotid artery, or involves mediastinal structures

Regional Lymph Nodes (N)

NX	Regional lymph nodes cannot be assessed
N0	No regional lymph node metastasis
N1	Unilateral metastasis in lymph node(s), ≤6 cm in greatest dimension, above the supraclavicular fossa
N2	Bilateral metastasis in lymph node(s), ≤6 cm in greatest dimension, above the supraclavicular fossa
N3	Metastasis in a lymph node(s) >6 cm and/or to supraclavicular fossa N3a > 6 cm N3b Extension to the supraclavicular fossa
MX	Distant metastasis cannot be assessed
M0	No distant metastasis
M1	Distant metastasis

Stage Grouping

Stage 0	Tis	N0	M0
Stage I	T1	N0	M0
Stage II	T2	N0	M0
Stage III	T3	N0	M0
	T1	N1	M0
	T2	N1	M0
	T3	N1	M0
Stage IVA	T4a	N0	M0
	T4a	N1	M0
	T1	N2	M0
	T2	N2	M0
	T3	N2	M0
	T4a	N2	M0
Stage IVB	T4b	Any N	M0
	Any T	N3	M0
Stage IVC	Any T	Any N	M1

TABLE 84-2 DEFINITION OF TNM–NASOPHARYNX

Primary Tumor (T)		Stage Grouping			
TX	Cannot be assessed	Stage 0	Tis	N0	M0
T0	No evidence	Stage I	T1	N0	M0
Tis	Carcinoma in situ	Stage IIA	T2a	N0	M0
T1	Tumor confined to the nasopharynx	Stage IIB	T1	N1	M0
T2	Tumor extends to soft tissues		T2	N1	M0
	T2a Tumor extends to the oropharynx and/or nasal cavity w/o parapharyngeal extension		T2a	N1	M0
	T2b Any tumor with parapharyngeal extension		T2b	N1	M0
T3	Tumor involves bony structures and/or paranasal sinuses		T2b	N1	M0
T4	Tumor with intracranial extension and/or involvement of cranial nerves, infratemporal fossa, hypopharynx, orbit, or masticator space	Stage III	T1	N2	M0
			T2a	N2	M0
Regional Lymph Nodes (N)			T2b	N2	M0
The distribution and the prognostic impact of regional lymph node spread from nasopharynx cancer, particularly of the undifferentiated type, are different from those of other head and neck mucosal cancers and justify the use of a different N classification scheme.			T3	N0	M0
NX Regional lymph nodes cannot be assessed			T3	N1	M0
N0 No regional lymph node metastasis			T3	N2	M0
N1 Unilateral metastasis in lymph node(s), ≤6 cm in greatest dimension, above the supraclavicular fossa			T4	N0	M0
N2 Bilateral metastasis in lymph node(s), ≤6 cm in greatest dimension, above the supraclavicular fossa			T4	N1	M0
N3 Metastasis in lymph node(s), >6 cm and/or to supraclavicular fossa			T4	N2	M0
N3a Greater than 6 cm in dimension			Any T	N3	M0
N3b Extension to the supraclavicular fossa			Any T	Any N	M1

℞ HEAD AND NECK CANCER

Patients with head and neck cancer can be categorized into three clinical groups: those with localized disease, those with locally or regionally advanced disease, and those with recurrent and/or metastatic disease. Comorbidities associated with tobacco and alcohol abuse can affect treatment outcome and define long-term risks for patients who are cured of their disease.

LOCALIZED DISEASE Nearly one-third of patients have localized disease; that is, T1 or T2 (stage I or stage II) lesions without detectable lymph node involvement or distant metastases. These lesions are treated with curative intent by surgery or radiation therapy. The choice of modality differs according to anatomic location and institutional expertise. Radiation therapy is often preferred for laryngeal cancer to preserve voice function, and surgery is preferred for small lesions in the oral cavity to avoid the long-term complications of radiation, such as xerostomia and dental decay. Overall 5-year survival is 60–90%. Most recurrences occur within the first 2 years following diagnosis and are usually local.

LOCALLY OR REGIONALLY ADVANCED DISEASE Locally or regionally advanced disease—disease with a large primary tumor and/or lymph node metastases—is the stage of presentation for >50% of patients. Such patients can also be treated with curative intent, but not with surgery or radiation therapy alone. Combined modality therapy including surgery, radiation therapy, and chemotherapy is most successful. Concomitant chemotherapy and radiation therapy appears to be the most effective approach. It can be administered either as a primary treatment for patients with unresectable disease, to pursue an organ preserving approach, or in the postoperative setting for intermediate-stage resectable tumors.

Induction Chemotherapy In this strategy, patients receive chemotherapy [usually cisplatin and fluorouracil (5-FU)] before surgery and radiation therapy. Most patients who receive three cycles show tumor reduction, and the response is clinically "complete" in up to half. This "sequential" multimodality therapy allows for organ preservation in patients with laryngeal and hypopharyngeal cancer, and it has been shown to result in higher cure rates compared with radiotherapy alone when drug combinations including cisplatin, 5-FU, and a taxane are used.

Concomitant Chemoradiotherapy With the concomitant strategy, chemotherapy and radiation therapy are given simultaneously rather than sequentially. Because most patients with head and neck cancer develop recurrent disease in the head and neck area, this approach is aimed at killing radiation-resistant cancer cells with chemotherapy. In addition, chemotherapy can enhance cell killing by radiation therapy. Toxicity (especially mucositis, grade 3 or 4 in 70–80%) is increased with concomitant chemoradiotherapy. However, metaanalyses of randomized trials document an improvement in 5-year survival of 8% with concomitant chemotherapy and radiation therapy. Results seem even more favorable when more active combinations of drugs are used but have not yet been validated in randomized trials. Five-year survival is 34–50%. In addition, concomitant chemoradiotherapy produces better laryngectomy-free survival (organ preservation) than radiation therapy alone in patients with advanced larynx cancer. The use of radiation therapy together with cisplatin has produced markedly improved survival in patients with advanced nasopharyngeal cancer.

The success of concomitant chemoradiotherapy in patients with unresectable disease has led to the testing of a similar approach in patients with resected disease as a postoperative therapy. Concomitant chemoradiotherapy produces a significant improvement over postoperative radiation therapy alone for patients whose tumors demonstrate higher risk features, such as spread beyond nodes, involvement of multiple lymph nodes, or positive margins following surgery.

Monoclonal antibody to the EGFR (cetuximab) increases survival rates when administered during radiotherapy. EGFR blockade results in radiation sensitization and has milder side effects than traditional chemotherapy agents. The integration of cetuximab into current standard chemoradiotherapy regimens is under investigation.

RECURRENT AND/OR METASTATIC DISEASE Ten percent of patients present with metastatic disease, and over half of patients with locoregionally advanced disease have recurrence, 20% outside the head and neck region. Patients with recurrent and/or metastatic disease are, with few exceptions, treated with palliative intent. Some patients may require local or regional radiation therapy for pain control, but most are given chemotherapy. Response rates to chemotherapy average only 30–50%; the duration of response averages only 3 months, and the median survival time is 6–8 months. Therefore, chemotherapy provides transient symptomatic benefit. Drugs with single-agent activity in this setting include methotrexate, 5-FU, cisplatin, paclitaxel, and docetaxel. Combinations of cisplatin with 5-FU, carboplatin with 5-FU, and cisplatin or carboplatin with paclitaxel or docetaxel are frequently used

EGFR-directed therapies, including monoclonal antibodies (e.g., cetuximab) and tyrosine kinase inhibitors (TKI) of the EGFR signaling pathway (e.g., erlotinib or gefitinib) have single-agent activity of approximately 10%. Side effects are usually limited to an acneiform rash and diarrhea (for the TKIs). Their impact on survival times when combined with traditional agents or in combination with other novel agents such as antiangiogenic compounds is under investigation.

CHEMOPREVENTION

β-Carotene and *cis*-retinoic acid can lead to the regression of leukoplakia. However, *cis*-retinoic acid does not reduce the incidence of second primaries.

TREATMENT COMPLICATIONS

Complications from treatment of head and neck cancer are usually correlated to the extent of surgery and exposure of normal tissue structures to radiation. Currently, the extent of surgery has been limited or completely replaced by chemotherapy and radiation therapy as the primary approach. Acute complications of radiation include mucositis and dysphagia. Long-term complications include xerostomia, loss of taste, decreased tongue mobility, second malignancies, dysphagia, and neck fibrosis. The complications of chemotherapy vary with the regimen used but usually include myelosuppression, mucositis, nausea and vomiting, and nephrotoxicity (with cisplatin).

The mucosal side effects of therapy can lead to malnutrition and dehydration. Many centers address issues of dentition before starting treatment, and some place feeding tubes to assure control of hydration and nutrition intake. About 50% of patients develop hypothyroidism from the treatment; thus, thyroid function should be monitored.

SALIVARY GLAND TUMORS

Most benign salivary gland tumors are treated with surgical excision, and patients with invasive salivary gland tumors are treated with surgery and radiation therapy. Neutron radiation may be particularly effective. These tumors may recur regionally; adenoidcystic carcinoma has a tendency to recur along the nerve tracks. Distant metastases may occur as late as 10–20 years after the initial diagnosis. For metastatic disease, therapy is given with palliative intent, usually chemotherapy with doxorubicin and/or cisplatin.

FURTHER READINGS

ADELSTEIN DJ et al: An intergroup phase III comparison of standard radiation therapy and two schedules of concurrent chemoradiotherapy in patients with unresectable squamous cell head and neck cancer. J Clin Oncol 21:92, 2003

BERNIER J et al: Postoperative irradiation with or without concomitant chemotherapy for locally advanced head and neck cancer. N Engl J Med 350:1945, 2004

BONNER JA et al: Radiotherapy plus cetuximab for squamous-cell carcinoma of the head and neck. N Engl J Med 354:567, 2006

BROCKSTEIN B, VOKES EE: Concurrent chemoradiotherapy for head and neck cancer. Semin Oncol 31:786, 2004

COHEN EE et al: The expanding role of systemic therapy in head and neck cancer. J Clin Oncol 22:1743, 2004

FORASTIERE AA et al: Concurrent chemotherapy and radiotherapy for organ preservation in advanced laryngeal cancer. N Engl J Med 349:2091, 2003

PFISTER DG et al: American Society of Clinical Oncology clinical practice guideline for the use of larynx-preservation strategies in the treatment of laryngeal cancer. J Clin Oncol 24:3693, 2006

SEIWERT TY et al: The chemoradiation paradigm in head and neck cancer. Nat Clin Pract Oncol 4:145, 2007

SLEBOS RJ et al: Gene expression differences associated with human papillomavirus status in head and neck squamous cell carcinoma. Clin Cancer Res 12:701, 2006

VOKES E et al: Weekly carboplatin and paclitaxel followed by concomitant TFHX chemoradiotherapy: Curative and organ preserving therapy for advanced head and neck cancer. J Clin Oncol 21:320, 2003

85 Neoplasms of the Lung

John D. Minna, Joan H. Schiller

THE MAGNITUDE OF THE PROBLEM

In 2007, primary carcinoma of the lung affected 114,760 males and 98,620 females in the United States; 86% die within 5 years of diagnosis, making it the leading cause of cancer death in both men and women. The incidence of lung cancer peaks between ages 55 and 65 years. Lung cancer accounts for 29% of all cancer deaths (31% in men, 26% in women). Lung cancer is responsible for more deaths in the United States each year than breast cancer, colon cancer, and prostate cancer combined; more women die each year of lung cancer than of breast cancer. The age-adjusted lung cancer death rate in males is decreasing, but in females it is stable or still increasing. These death rates are related to smoking; smoking cessation efforts begun 40 years ago in men are largely responsible for the change in incidence and death rates. However, women started smoking in substantial numbers about 10–15 years later than men; smoking cessation efforts need to increase for women. The 5-year overall lung cancer survival rate (15%) has nearly doubled in the past 30 years. The improvement is due to advances in combined-modality treatment with surgery, radiotherapy, and chemotherapy. The International Agency for Research on Cancer estimates that there will be over 1.18 million deaths from lung cancer worldwide in 2007, which will rise to 10 million deaths per year by 2030. This represents one lung cancer case for every 3 million cigarettes smoked. Thus, primary carcinoma of the lung is a major health problem with a generally grim prognosis.

PATHOLOGY

The term *lung cancer* is used for tumors arising from the respiratory epithelium (bronchi, bronchioles, and alveoli). Mesotheliomas, lymphomas, and stromal tumors (sarcomas) are distinct from epithelial lung cancer. Four major cell types make up 88% of all primary lung neoplasms according to the World Health Organization classification (Table 85-1). These are *squamous* or *epidermoid carcinoma*, *small cell* (also called *oat cell*) *carcinoma*, *adenocarcinoma* (including bronchioloalveolar), and *large cell carcinoma*. The remainder include undifferentiated carcinomas, carcinoids, bronchial gland tumors (including adenoid cystic carcinomas and mucoepidermoid tumors), and rarer tumor types. The various cell types have different natural histories and responses to therapy, and thus a correct histologic diagnosis by an experienced pathologist is the first step to correct treatment. In the past 25 years, adenocarcinoma has replaced squamous cell carcinoma as the most frequent histologic subtype, and the incidence of small cell carcinoma is on the decline.

Major treatment decisions are made on the basis of whether a tumor is classified as a small cell lung carcinoma (SCLC) or as one of the non-small cell lung cancer (NSCLC) varieties (squamous, adenocarcinoma, large cell carcinoma, bronchioloalveolar carcinoma, and mixed ver-

TABLE 85-1 FREQUENCY, AGE-ADJUSTED INCIDENCE, AND SURVIVAL RATES FOR DIFFERENT HISTOLOGIC TYPES OF LUNG CANCER[a]

Histologic Type of Thoracic Malignancy	Frequency, %	Age-Adjusted Rate	5-Year Survival Rate (All Stages)
Adenocarcinoma (and all subtypes)	32	17	17
Bronchioloalveolar carcinoma	3	1.4	42
Squamous cell (epidermoid) carcinoma	29	15	15
Small cell carcinoma	18	9	5
Large cell carcinoma	9	5	11
Carcinoid	1.0	0.5	83
Mucoepidermoid carcinoma	0.1	<0.1	39
Adenoid cystic carcinoma	<0.1	<0.1	48
Sarcoma and other soft tissue tumors	0.1	0.1	30
All others and unspecified carcinomas	11.0	6	NA
Total	100	52	14

[a]Data on histology frequency and age-adjusted incidence rates per 100,000 U.S. population are from 60,514 cases of invasive lung cancer involving all races and both sexes obtained from the data for 1983–1987 of the Surveillance, Epidemiology, and End Results (SEER) Program of the National Cancer Institute; 5-year relative survival rates for all stages, all races, and both sexes are from the SEER data on 87,128 carcinomas, 1978–1986. NA, not available.

Source: Summarized from Travis et al: Cancer 75:191, 1995.

sions of these). The histologic distinctions between SCLC and NSCLC include the following: SCLC has scant cytoplasm, small hyperchromatic nuclei with fine chromatin pattern and indistinct nucleoli with diffuse sheets of cells, while NSCLC has abundant cytoplasm, pleomorphic nuclei with coarse chromatin pattern, prominent nucleoli, and glandular or squamous architecture. Among the molecular distinctions, SCLC displays neuroendocrine properties absent in NSCLCs, production of specific peptide hormones [such as adrenocorticotropic hormone (ACTH), arginine vasopressin (AVP), atrial natriuretic factor (ANF), gastrin-releasing peptide (GRP)] and differences in oncogene and tumor-suppressor gene changes (SCLCs have *RB* mutations in 90% and *p16* abnormalities in 10% but never have *KRAS* or *EGFR* mutations, while NSCLCs have *RB* mutations in only 20%, *p16* changes in 50%, *KRAS* mutations in 30%, and *EGFR* mutations in ~10%). Both types have frequent *p53* mutations (>70% in SCLC and >50% in NSCLC), 3p allele loss (>90% in both), telomerase expression (>90% in both), and tumor-acquired promoter methylation in multiple genes (>80% in both, often involving the same genes, including *RASSF1A*). SCLCs are initially very responsive to combination chemotherapy (>70% responses, with 30% complete responses) and to radiotherapy (>90% responses); however, most SCLCs ultimately relapse. By contrast, NSCLCs have objective tumor shrinkage following radiotherapy in 30–50% of cases and response to combination chemotherapy in 20–35% of cases. At presentation, SCLCs usually have already spread such that surgery is unlikely to be curative and, given their responsiveness to chemotherapy, are managed primarily by chemotherapy with or without radiotherapy. Chemotherapy clearly provides symptom relief and survival advantage. By contrast, NSCLCs that are clinically localized at the time of presentation may be cured with either surgery or radiotherapy. The beneficial role of chemotherapy in NSCLC is in palliation of symptoms and improving survival modestly.

Although it is important to differentiate whether a tumor is SCLC or NSCLC for both prognostic and therapeutic reasons, it is less important to identify the histologic subtypes of NSCLC. Stage for stage, the histology of NSCLC is not an important prognostic factor, and in the past the different subtypes of NSCLC were rarely treated differently. However, lung adenocarcinomas (often with bronchioloalveolar features) may be responsive to therapy aimed at the epidermal growth factor receptor (EGFR) (see below). In addition, patients with squamous cell carcinoma may not be appropriate candidates for antiangiogenic therapy due to an increased risk of bleeding (see below).

Eighty-five percent of patients with lung cancer of all histologic types are current or former cigarette smokers. Of the annual 213,380 new cases of lung cancer, ~50% develop in former smokers. With increased success in smoking cessation efforts, the number of former smokers will grow, and these individuals will be important candidates for early detection and chemoprevention efforts.

All histologic types of lung cancer are due to smoking. However, lung cancer can also occur in individuals who have never smoked. By far the most common form of lung cancer arising in lifetime nonsmokers, in women, and in young patients (<45 years) is adenocarcinoma. However, in nonsmokers with adenocarcinoma involving the lung, the possibility of other primary sites should be considered. Squamous and small cell cancers usually present as central masses with endobronchial growth, while adenocarcinomas and large cell cancers tend to present as peripheral nodules or masses, frequently with pleural involvement. Squamous and large cell cancers cavitate in 10–20% of cases. Bronchioloalveolar carcinoma (BAC) is a subtype of adenocarcinoma that grows along the alveoli without invasion and can present radiographically as a single mass; as a diffuse, multinodular lesion; as a fluffy infiltrate; and on screening CT scans as a "ground glass" opacity. The male to female ratio is 1:1, and while BAC can be associated with smoking, it is often found in nonsmokers. Histologically pure BAC is relatively rare. More common is adenocarcinoma with BAC features. BAC may present in a mucinous form, which tends to be multicentric, and a nonmucinous form, which tends to be solitary. Many of the EGFR mutations found in nonsmoking lung cancers occur in adenocarcinomas with BAC histologic features.

ETIOLOGY

Most lung cancers are caused by carcinogens and tumor promoters inhaled via cigarette smoking. The prevalence of smoking in the United States is 28% for males and 25% for females, age 18 years or older; 38% of high school seniors smoke. The relative risk of developing lung cancer is increased about thirteenfold by active smoking and about 1.5-fold by long-term passive exposure to cigarette smoke. Chronic obstructive pulmonary disease, which is also smoking-related, further increases the risk of developing lung cancer. The lung cancer death rate is related to the total amount (often expressed in "cigarette pack-years") of cigarettes smoked, such that the risk is increased 60- to 70-fold for a man smoking two packs a day for 20 years as compared with a nonsmoker. Conversely, the chance of developing lung cancer decreases with cessation of smoking but may never return to the nonsmoker level. The increase in lung cancer rate in women is also associated with a rise in cigarette smoking. Women have a higher relative risk per given exposure than men (~1.5-fold higher). This sex difference may be due to a greater susceptibility to tobacco carcinogens in women, although the data are controversial.

About 15% of lung cancers occur in individuals who have never smoked. The majority of these are found in women. The reason for this sex difference is not known but may be related to hormonal factors.

Efforts to get people to stop smoking are mandatory. However, smoking cessation is extremely difficult, because the smoking habit represents a powerful addiction to nicotine (Chap. 390). Smoking addiction is both biologic and psychosocial. Different methods are available to help motivated smokers give up the habit, including counseling, behavioral therapy, nicotine replacement (gum, patch, sublingual spray, inhaler), and antidepressants (such as bupropion). However, one year after starting such smoking cessation aids, the methods are successful in only 20–25% of individuals. Preventing people from starting to smoke is thus very important, and this primary prevention effort needs to be targeted to children since most cigarette smoking addiction occurs during the teenage years.

Radiation is another environmental cause of lung cancer. People exposed to high levels of radon or receiving thoracic radiation therapy have a higher than normal incidence of lung cancer, particularly if they smoke.

BIOLOGY AND MOLECULAR PATHOGENESIS

Molecular genetic studies have shown the acquisition by lung cancer cells of a number of genetic lesions, including activation of dominant oncogenes and inactivation of tumor-suppressor or recessive oncogenes (Chaps. 79 and 80). In fact, lung cancer cells may have to accumulate a large number (perhaps ≥20) of such lesions. A small subpopulation (perhaps <1%) of cells within a tumor are responsible for the full malignant behavior of the tumor;—these are referred to as *cancer stem cells*. As part of this concept, the large bulk of the cells in a cancer are "offspring" of these cancer stem cells and, while clonally related to the cancer stem cell subpopulation, by themselves cannot regenerate the full malignant phenotype such as metastatic disease and unlimited replicative potential. These cancer stem cells are very important to identify since successful treatment of the tumor will require eradication of this stem cell component. These cancer stem cells may be more resistant to chemotherapy than the bulk of the tumor. Features that distinguish cancer stem cells from the remaining tumor cells have not been defined and validated.

Activation of Dominant Oncogenes Changes in dominant oncogenes include point mutations in the coding regions of the *RAS* family of oncogenes (particularly in the *KRAS* gene in adenocarcinoma of the lung); mutations in the tyrosine kinase domain of the EGFR found in adenocarcinomas from nonsmokers (~10% in the United States with rates >50% in nonsmoking East Asian patients); occasional mutations in *BRAF* and *PIK3CA* or activation of the PIK3CA/AKT/mTor pathway; amplification, rearrangement, and/or loss of transcriptional control of *myc* family oncogenes (c-, N-, and L-*myc*; changes in c-*myc* are found in non-small cell cancers, while changes in all *myc* family members are found in SCLC); overexpression of bcl-2 and other antiapoptotic proteins; overexpression of other EGFR family members such as Her-2/neu, and ERBB3; and activated expression of the telomerase gene in >90% of lung cancers. Genome-wide approaches are identifying other amplified or mutated dominant oncogenes that could be important new therapeutic targets.

Inactivation of Tumor-Suppressor Genes A large number of tumor-suppressor genes (recessive oncogenes) have been identified that are inactivated during the pathogenesis of lung cancer. This usually occurs by a tumor-acquired inactivating mutation of one allele [seen, for example, in the *p53* and retinoblastoma (*RB*) tumor-suppressor gene] or tumor-acquired inactivation of expression by tumor-acquired promoter DNA methylation (seen, for example, in the case of the *p16* and *RASSF1A* tumor-suppressor genes), which is then coupled with physical loss of the other parental allele ("loss of heterozygosity"). This leaves the tumor cell with only the functionally inactive allele and thus loss of function of the growth-regulatory tumor-suppressor gene. Genome-wide approaches have identified many such genes involved in lung cancer pathogenesis, including *p53*, *RB*, *RASSF1A*, *SEMA3B*, *SEMA3F*, *FUS1*, *p16*, *LKB1*, *RARβ*, and *FHIT*. Several tumor-suppressor genes on chromosome 3p appear to be involved in nearly all lung cancers. Allelic loss for this region occurs very early in lung cancer pathogenesis, including in histologically normal smoking-damaged lung epithelium.

Autocrine Growth Factors The large number of genetic and epigenetic lesions shows that lung cancer, like other common epithelial malignancies, arises as a multistep process that is likely to involve both carcinogens causing mutation ("initiation") and tumor promoters. Prevention can be directed at both processes. Lung cancer cells produce many peptide hormones and express receptors for these hormones. They can promote tumor cell growth in an "autocrine" fashion.

Highly carcinogenic derivatives of nicotine are formed in cigarette smoke. Lung cancer cells of all histologic types (and the cells from which they are derived) express nicotinic acetylcholine receptors. Nicotine activates signaling pathways in tumor and normal cells that block apoptosis. Thus, nicotine itself could be directly involved in lung cancer pathogenesis both as a mutagen and tumor promoter.

Inherited Predisposition to Lung Cancer While an inherited predisposition to develop lung cancer is not common, several features suggest a potential for familial association. People with inherited mutations in *RB* (patients with retinoblastomas living to adulthood) and *p53* (Li-Fraumeni syndrome) genes may develop lung cancer. First-degree relatives of lung cancer probands have a two- to threefold excess risk of lung cancer or other cancers, many of which are not smoking-related. An as yet unidentified gene in chromosome region 6q23 was found to segregate in families at high risk of developing lung cancer of all histologic types. Finally, certain polymorphisms of the P450 enzyme system (which metabolizes carcinogens) or chromosome fragility (*mutagen sensitivity*) genotypes are associated with the development of lung cancer. The use of any of these inherited differences to identify persons at very high risk of developing lung cancer would be useful in early detection and prevention efforts.

Therapy Targeted at Molecular Abnormalities A detailed understanding of the molecular pathogenesis should be applicable to new methods of early diagnosis, prevention, and treatment of lung cancer. Two examples of this translation involve EGFR and vascular endothelial growth factor (VEGF). EGFR belongs to the ERBB (HER) family of protooncogenes, including EGFR (ERBB1), Her2/neu (ERBB2), HER3 (ERBB3), and HER4 (ERBB4), cell-surface receptors consisting of an extracellular ligand-binding domain, a transmembrane structure, and an intracellular tyrosine kinase (TK) domain. The binding of ligand to receptor activates receptor dimerization and TK autophosphorylation, initiating a cascade of intracellular events, leading to increased cell proliferation, angiogenesis, metastasis, and a decrease in apoptosis (Chap. 80). Overexpression of EGFR protein or amplification of the *EGFR* gene has been found in as many as 70% of NSCLCs.

Activating/oncogenic mutations (usually a missense or a small deletion mutation) in the TK domain of EGFR have been identified. These are found most commonly in women, East Asians, patients who have never smoked, and those with adenocarcinoma and BAC histology. This is also the group of patients who are most likely to have dramatic responses to drugs that inhibit TK activation [tyrosine kinase inhibitors (TKIs)]. EGFR mutations are almost never found in cancers other than lung cancer, nor in lung cancers that have *KRAS* mutations. These EGFR mutations, often associated with amplification of the *EGFR* gene, usually confer sensitivity of these lung cancers to EGFR TKIs (such as gefitinib or erlotinib), resulting in clinically beneficial tumor responses that unfortunately are still not permanent. In many cases the development of EGFR TKI resistance is associated with the development of another mutation in the *EGFR* gene (*T790M* mutation), or amplification of the *c-met* oncogene. However, other drugs with EGFR TKI activity are in development to which the lung cancers with these resistance mutations will respond as are drugs targeting c-met or its pathways.

The discovery of EGFR mutation/amplification driving lung cancer growth and the dramatic response of these tumors to oral EGFR TKI therapy has prompted a widespread search for other drugs "targeted" against oncogenic changes in lung cancer. An important example of another such target is VEGF, which, while not mutated, is inappropriately produced by lung cancers and stimulates tumor angiogenesis (Chap. 80). VEGF is often overexpressed in lung cancer, and the resulting increase in tumor microvessel density correlates with poor prognosis. A monoclonal antibody to the VEGF ligand, bevacizumab, has significant antitumor effects when used with chemotherapy in lung cancer (see below).

Molecular Profiles Predict Survival and Response Just as the presence of EGFR TK domain mutations and amplification is an excellent predictor of response to EGFR TKIs, molecular predictors of response to standard chemotherapy and other new targeted agents are being sought. Lung cancers can be molecularly typed at the time of diagnosis to yield information that predicts survival and defines agents to which the tumor is most likely to respond. One example is the identification of alterations in lung cancer DNA repair pathways that may predict resistance to chemotherapy. Patients whose tumors exhibit low activity of the excision-repair-cross complementation group 1 (ERCC1) proteins typically have a worse prognosis as they are unable to repair DNA adducts in the tumor. However, retrospective analysis shows that when treated with cisplatin, patients with tumors expressing low levels of ERCC1 activity appear to do better, as they are unable to repair DNA adducts caused by cisplatin, while patients with high ERCC1 activity actually do worse with cisplatin-based chemotherapy. Although these protein or gene expression "signatures" have yet to be validated in large prospective studies, it is possible that such information will allow future therapy to be tailored to the characteristics of each patient's tumor. Mass spectroscopy-based proteomic studies have identified unique protein patterns in the serum of patients, one of which allows for early diagnosis, while another can predict sensitivity or resistance to drugs. However, such methods have not been validated and may be difficult to implement in a patient care setting.

CLINICAL MANIFESTATIONS

Lung cancer gives rise to signs and symptoms caused by local tumor growth, invasion or obstruction of adjacent structures, growth in regional nodes through lymphatic spread, growth in distant metastatic sites after hematogenous dissemination, and remote effects of tumor products (paraneoplastic syndromes) (Chaps. 96 and 97).

Although 5–15% of patients with lung cancer are identified while they are asymptomatic, usually as a result of a routine chest radiograph or through the use of screening CT scans, most patients present with some sign or symptom. Central or endobronchial growth of the primary tumor may cause cough, hemoptysis, wheeze and stridor, dyspnea, and postobstructive pneumonitis (fever and productive cough). Peripheral growth of the primary tumor may cause pain from pleural or chest wall involvement, dyspnea on a restrictive basis, and symptoms of lung abscess resulting from tumor cavitation. Regional spread of tumor in the thorax (by contiguous growth or by metastasis to regional lymph nodes) may cause tracheal obstruction, esophageal compression with dysphagia, recurrent laryngeal nerve paralysis with hoarseness, phrenic nerve paralysis with elevation of the hemidiaphragm and dyspnea, and sympathetic nerve paralysis with Horner's syndrome (enophthalmos, ptosis, miosis, and ipsilateral loss of sweating). Malignant pleural effusion often leads to dyspnea. *Pancoast's* (or *superior sulcus tumor*) *syndrome* results from local extension of a tumor growing in the apex of the lung with involvement of the eighth cervical and first and second thoracic nerves, with shoulder pain that characteristically radiates in the ulnar distribution of the arm, often with radiologic destruction of the first and second ribs. Often Horner's syndrome and Pancoast's syndrome coexist. Other problems of regional spread include *superior vena cava syndrome* from vascular obstruction; pericardial and cardiac extension with resultant tamponade, arrhythmia, or cardiac failure; lymphatic obstruction with resultant pleural effusion; and lymphangitic spread through the lungs with hypoxemia and dyspnea. In addition, BAC can spread transbronchially, producing tumor growing along multiple alveolar surfaces with impairment of gas exchange, respiratory insufficiency, dyspnea, hypoxemia, and sputum production.

Extrathoracic metastatic disease is found at autopsy in >50% of patients with squamous carcinoma, 80% of patients with adenocarcinoma and large cell carcinoma, and >95% of patients with small cell cancer. Lung cancer metastases may occur in virtually every organ system. Common clinical problems related to metastatic lung cancer include brain metastases with headache, nausea, and neurologic deficits; bone metastases with pain and pathologic fractures; bone marrow invasion with cytopenias or leukoerythroblastosis; liver metastases causing liver dysfunction, biliary obstruction, anorexia, and pain; lymph node metastases in the supraclavicular region and occasionally in the axilla and groin; and spinal cord compression syndromes from epidural or bone metastases. Adrenal metastases are common but rarely cause adrenal insufficiency.

Paraneoplastic syndromes are common in patients with lung cancer and may be the presenting finding or first sign of recurrence. In addition, paraneoplastic syndromes may mimic metastatic disease and, unless detected, lead to inappropriate palliative rather than curative treatment. Often the paraneoplastic syndrome may be relieved with successful treatment of the tumor. In some cases, the pathophysiology of the paraneoplastic syndrome is known, particularly when a hormone with biologic activity is secreted by a tumor (Chap. 96). However, in many cases the pathophysiology is unknown. Systemic symptoms of anorexia, cachexia, weight loss (seen in 30% of patients), fever, and suppressed immunity are paraneoplastic syndromes of unknown etiology. *Endocrine syndromes* are seen in 12% of patients: hypercalcemia and hypophosphatemia resulting from the ectopic production by squamous tumors of parathyroid hormone (PTH) or, more commonly, PTH-related peptide; hyponatremia with the syndrome of inappropriate secretion of antidiuretic hormone or possibly atrial natriuretic factor by small cell cancer; and ectopic secretion of ACTH by small cell cancer. ACTH secretion usually results in additional electrolyte disturbances, especially hypokalemia, rather than the changes in body habitus that occur in Cushing's syndrome from a pituitary adenoma.

Skeletal–connective tissue syndromes include clubbing in 30% of cases (usually non-small cell carcinomas) and hypertrophic pulmonary osteoarthropathy in 1–10% of cases (usually adenocarcinomas), with periostitis and clubbing causing pain, tenderness, and swelling over the affected bones and a positive bone scan. *Neurologic-myopathic syndromes* are seen in only 1% of patients but are dramatic and include the myasthenic *Eaton-Lambert syndrome* and retinal blindness with small cell cancer, while peripheral neuropathies, subacute cerebellar degeneration, cortical degeneration, and polymyositis are seen with all lung cancer types. Many of these are caused by autoimmune responses such as the development of anti-voltage-gated calcium channel antibodies in the Eaton-Lambert syndrome (Chap. 97). Coagulation, thrombotic, or other hematologic manifestations occur in 1–8% of patients and include migratory venous thrombophlebitis (*Trousseau's syndrome*), nonbacterial thrombotic (marantic) endocarditis with arterial emboli, disseminated intravascular coagulation with hemorrhage, anemia, granulocytosis, and leukoerythroblastosis. Thrombotic disease complicating cancer is usually a poor prognostic sign. Cutaneous manifestations such as dermatomyositis and acanthosis nigricans are uncommon (1%), as are the renal manifestations of nephrotic syndrome or glomerulonephritis (≤1%).

DIAGNOSIS AND STAGING

SCREENING

Most patients with lung cancer present with advanced disease, raising the question of whether screening would detect these tumors at an earlier stage when they are theoretically more curable. The role of screening high-risk patients (for example current or former smokers >50 years of age) for early stage lung cancers is debated. Results from five randomized screening studies in the 1980s of chest x-rays with or without cytologic analysis of sputum did not show any impact on lung cancer–specific mortality from screening high-risk patients, although earlier-stage cancers were detected in the screened groups. These studies have been criticized for their design and statistical analyses, but they led to current recommendations not to use these tools to screen for lung cancer. However, low-dose, noncontrast, thin-slice, helical, or spiral CT has emerged as a possible new tool for lung cancer screening. Spiral CT is a scan in which only the pulmonary parenchyma is examined, thus negating the use of intravenous contrast and the necessity of a physician being present at the exam. The scan can usually be done quickly (within one breath) and involves low doses of radiation. In a nonrandomized study of current and former smokers from the Early Lung Cancer Action Project (ELCAP), low-dose CT was shown to be more sensitive than chest x-ray for detecting lung nodules and lung cancer in early stages. Survival from date of diagnosis is also long (10-year survival predicted to be 92% in screening-detected stage I NSCLC patients). Other nonrandomized CT screening studies of asymptomatic current or former smokers also found that early lung cancer cases were diagnosed more often with CT screening than predicted by standard incidence data. However, no decline in the number of advanced lung cancer cases or deaths from lung cancer was noted in the screened group. Thus, spiral CT appears to diagnose more lung cancer without improving lung cancer mortality. Concerns include the influence of lead-time bias, length-time bias, and over-diagnosis (cancers so slow-growing that they are unlikely to cause the death of the patient). Over-diagnosis is a well-established problem in prostate cancer screening, but it is surprising that some lung cancers are not fatal. However, many of the small adenocarcinomas found as "ground glass" opacities on screening CT appear to have such long doubling times (>400 days) that they may never harm the patient. While CT screening will detect lung cancer in 1–4% of the patients screened over a 5-year period, it also detects a substantial number of false-positive lung lesions (ranging from 25 to 75% in different series) that need follow-up and evaluation. The appropriate management of these small lesions is undefined. Unnecessary treatment of these patients may include thoracotomy and lung resection, thus adding to the cost, mortality, and morbidity of treatment. A large, randomized trial of CT screening for lung cancer (National Lung Cancer Screening Trial) involving ~55,000 individuals has completed accrual and will provide definitive data in the next several years on whether screening reduces lung cancer mortality. Until these results become available, routine CT screening for lung cancer cannot be recommended for any risk group. For those patients who want to be screened, physicians need to discuss the possible benefits and risks of such screening, including the risk of false-positive scans that could result in multiple follow-up CTs and possible biopsies for a malignancy that may not be life-threatening.

ESTABLISHING A DIAGNOSIS OF LUNG CANCER

Once signs, symptoms, or screening studies suggest lung cancer, a tissue diagnosis must be established. Tumor tissue can be obtained by a bronchial or transbronchial biopsy during fiberoptic bronchoscopy; by node biopsy during mediastinoscopy; from the operative specimen at the time of definitive surgical resection; by percutaneous biopsy of an enlarged lymph node, soft tissue mass, lytic bone lesion, bone marrow, or pleural lesion; by fine-needle aspiration of thoracic or extrathoracic tumor masses using CT guidance; or from an adequate cell block obtained from a malignant pleural effusion. In most cases, the pathologist should be able to make a definite diagnosis of epithelial malignancy and distinguish small cell from non-small cell lung cancer.

STAGING PATIENTS WITH LUNG CANCER

Lung cancer staging consists of two parts: first, a determination of the location of tumor (anatomic staging) and, second, an assessment of a patient's ability to withstand various antitumor treatments (physiologic staging). In a patient with NSCLC, *resectability* (whether the tumor can be entirely removed by a standard surgical procedure such as a lobectomy or pneumonectomy), which depends on the anatomic stage of the tumor, and *operability* (whether the patient can tolerate such a surgical procedure), which depends on the cardiopulmonary function of the patient, are determined.

Non-Small Cell Lung Cancer The TNM International Staging System should be used for cases of NSCLC, particularly in preparing patients for curative attempts with surgery or radiotherapy (Table 85-2). The various T (tumor size), N (regional node involvement), and M (presence or absence of distant metastasis) factors are combined to form different stage groups. At presentation, approximately one-third of patients have disease localized enough for a curative attempt with surgery or radiotherapy (patients with stage I or II disease and some with stage IIIA disease), one-third have distant metastatic disease (stage IV disease), and one-third have local or regional disease that may or may not be amenable to a curative attempt (some patients with stage IIIA disease and others with stage IIIB disease) (see below). This staging system provides useful prognostic information.

Small Cell Lung Cancer A simple two-stage system is used. In this system, *limited-stage disease* (seen in about 30% of all patients with SCLC) is defined as disease confined to one hemithorax and regional lymph nodes (including mediastinal, contralateral hilar, and usually ipsilateral supraclavicular nodes), while *extensive-stage disease* (seen in about 70% of patients) is defined as disease exceeding those boundaries. Clinical studies such as physical examination, x-rays, CT and bone scans, and bone marrow examination are used in staging. In part, the definition of limited-stage disease relates to whether the known tumor can be encompassed within a tolerable radiation therapy port. Thus, contralateral supraclavicular nodes, recurrent laryngeal nerve involvement, and superior vena caval obstruction can all be part of limited-stage disease. However, cardiac tamponade, malignant pleural effusion, and bilateral pulmonary parenchymal involvement generally qualify disease as extensive-stage because the organs within a curative radiation therapy port cannot safely tolerate curative radiation doses.

LUNG CANCER STAGING PROCEDURES

(Table 85-3) All patients with lung cancer should have a complete history and physical examination, with evaluation of all other medical problems, determination of performance status and history of weight loss, and a CT scan of the chest and abdomen with contrast. Positron emission tomography (PET) scans are sensitive in detecting both intrathoracic and metastatic disease. PET is useful in assessing the mediastinum and solitary pulmonary nodules. A standardized uptake value (SUV) of >2.5 is highly suspicious for malignancy. False negatives can be seen in diabetes, in slow-growing tumors such as BAC, in concurrent infection such as tuberculosis, and in lesions <8 mm. False positives can also be seen in infections and granulomatous disease. Thus, PET should never be used alone to diagnose lung cancer, mediastinal involvement, or metastases. Instead, its primary function is to help guide a mediastinal biopsy for staging purposes and to help identify sites of metastatic disease. Fiberoptic bronchoscopy obtains material for pathologic examination

TABLE 85-2 TUMOR, NODE, METASTASIS INTERNATIONAL STAGING SYSTEM FOR LUNG CANCER

		5-Year Survival Rate, %	
Stage	TNM Descriptors	Clinical Stage	Surgical-Pathologic Stage
IA	T1 N0 M0	61	67
IB	T2 N0 M0	38	57
IIA	T1 N1 M0	34	55
IIB	T2 N1 M0	24	39
IIB	T3 N0 M0	22	38
IIIA	T3 N1 M0	9	25
	T1–2–3 N2 M0	13	23
IIIB	T4 N0–1–2 M0	7	<5
	T1–2–3–4 N3 M0	3	<3
IV	Any T any N M1	1	<1

Tumor (T) Status Descriptor

T0	No evidence of a primary tumor
TX	Primary tumor cannot be assessed, or tumor proven by the presence of malignant cells in sputum or bronchial washings but not visualized by imaging or bronchoscopy
TIS	Carcinoma in situ
T1	Tumor <3 cm in greatest dimension, surrounded by lung or visceral pleura, without bronchoscopic evidence of invasion more proximal than lobar bronchus (i.e., not in main bronchus)
T2	Tumor with any of following: >3 cm in greatest dimension; involves main bronchus, ≥2 cm distal to the carina; invades visceral pleura; associated with atelectasis or obstructive pneumonitis extending to hilum but does not involve entire lung
T3	Tumor of any size that directly invades any of the following: chest wall (including superior sulcus tumors), diaphragm, mediastinal pleura, parietal pericardium; or tumor in main bronchus <2 cm distal to carina but without involvement of carina; or associated atelectasis or obstructive pneumonitis of entire lung
T4	Tumor of any size that invades any of the following: mediastinum, heart, great vessels, trachea, esophagus, vertebral body, carina; or tumor with a malignant pleural or pericardial effusion,[a] or with satellite tumor nodule(s) within the ipsilateral primary-tumor lobe of the lung.

Lymph Node (N) Involvement Descriptor

NX	Regional lymph nodes cannot be assessed
N0	No regional lymph node metastasis
N1	Metastasis to ipsilateral peribronchial and/or ipsilateral hilar lymph nodes, and intrapulmonary nodes involved by direct extension of the primary tumor
N2	Metastasis to ipsilateral mediastinal and/or subcarinal lymph node(s)
N3	Metastasis to contralateral mediastinal, contralateral hilar, ipsilateral or contralateral scalene, or supraclavicular lymph node(s)

Distant Metastasis (M) Descriptor

MX	Presence of distant metastasis cannot be assessed
M0	No distant metastasis
M1	Distant metastasis present[b]

[a]Most pleural effusions associated with lung cancer are due to tumor. However, in a few patients with multiple negative cytopathologic exams of a non-bloody, non-exudative pleural or pericardial effusion that clinical judgment dictates is not related to the tumor, the effusion should be excluded as a staging element and the patient's disease staged as T1, T2, or T3.

[b]Separate metastatic pulmonary tumor nodule(s) in the ipsilateral nonprimary tumor lobe(s) of the lung are classified as M1.

Source: Adapted from CF Mountain. Revisions in the International System for Staging of Lung Cancer. Chest 111:1710, 1997; with permission.

TABLE 85-3 PRETREATMENT STAGING PROCEDURES FOR PATIENTS WITH LUNG CANCER

All Patients
Complete history and physical examination
Determination of performance status and weight loss
Complete blood count with platelet determination
Measurement of serum electrolytes, glucose, and calcium; renal and liver function tests
Electrocardiogram
Skin test for tuberculosis
Chest x-ray
CT scan of chest and abdomen
CT or MRI scan of brain and radionuclide scan of bone if any finding suggests the presence of tumor metastasis in these organs
Fiberoptic bronchoscopy with washings, brushings, and biopsy of suspicious lesions unless medically contraindicated or if it would not alter therapy (e.g., very late stage patient)
X-rays of suspicious bony lesions detected by scan or symptom
Barium swallow radiographic examination if esophageal symptoms exist
Pulmonary function studies and arterial blood gas measurements if signs or symptoms of respiratory insufficiency are present
Biopsy of accessible lesions suspicious for cancer if a histologic diagnosis is not yet made or if treatment or staging decisions would be based on whether or not a lesion contained cancer
Patients with Non-small Cell Lung Cancer Who Have No Contraindication[a] to Curative Surgery or Radiotherapy with or without Chemotherapy
All the above procedures, plus the following:
PET scan to evaluate mediastinum and detect metastatic disease
Pulmonary function tests and arterial blood gas measurements
Coagulation tests
CT or MRI scan of brain if symptoms suggestive
Cardiopulmonary exercise testing if performance status or pulmonary function tests are borderline
If surgical resection is planned: surgical evaluation of the mediastinum at mediastinoscopy or at thoracotomy
If the patient is a poor surgical risk or a candidate for curative radiotherapy: transthoracic fine-needle aspiration biopsy or transbronchial forceps biopsy of peripheral lesions if material from routine fiberoptic bronchoscopy is negative
Patients Presenting with Small Cell or Advanced Non-small Cell Lung Cancer
For proven small cell lung cancer, all the procedures under "All Patients," plus the following:
CT or MRI scan of brain
Bone marrow aspiration and biopsy (if peripheral blood counts abnormal)
For non-small cell lung cancer or cancer of unknown histology, all the procedures under "All Patients," plus the following:
Fiberoptic bronchoscopy if indicated by hemoptysis, obstruction, pneumonitis, or no histologic diagnosis of cancer
Biopsy of accessible lesions suspicious for tumor to obtain a histologic diagnosis or if therapy would be altered by finding of tumor
Transthoracic fine-needle aspiration biopsy or transbronchial forceps biopsy of peripheral lesions if fiberoptic bronchoscopy is negative and no other material exists for a histologic diagnosis
Diagnostic and therapeutic thoracentesis if a pleural effusion is present

[a]Patients with non-small cell lung cancer and extrathoracic metastatic disease, malignant pleural effusion, or intrathoracic disease beyond the bounds of a tolerable radiotherapy port.

Note: CT, computed tomography; PET, positron emission tomography.

and information on tumor size, location, degree of bronchial obstruction (i.e., assesses resectability), and recurrence.

Chest radiographs and CT scans are needed to evaluate tumor size and nodal involvement; old radiographs are useful for comparison. CT scans of the thorax and upper abdomen are of use in the preoperative staging of NSCLC to detect mediastinal nodes and pleural extension and occult abdominal disease (e.g., liver, adrenal), and in planning curative radiation therapy. However, mediastinal nodal involvement should be documented histologically if the findings will influence therapeutic decisions. Thus, sampling of lymph nodes via mediastinoscopy or thoracotomy to establish the presence or absence of N2 or N3 nodal involvement is crucial in considering a curative surgical approach for patients with NSCLC with clinical stage I, II, or III disease, regardless of whether the PET is positive or negative. A preoperative mediastinoscopy may not need to be done in patients with normal-size nodes (by CT) that are PET-negative, as the discovery of micrometastases is unlikely to change the preoperative management of the disease, although lymph node sampling should be done intraoperatively. A standard nomenclature for referring to the location of lymph nodes involved with cancer has evolved (Fig. 85-1). Unless the CT-detected abnormalities are unequivocal, histology of suspicious extrathoracic lesions should be confirmed by procedures such as fine-needle aspiration if the patient would otherwise be considered for curative treatment. In SCLC, CT scans are used in the planning of chest radiation treatment and in the assessment of the response to chemotherapy and radiation therapy. Surgery or radiotherapy can make interpretation of conventional chest x-rays difficult; after treatment, CT scans can provide good evidence of tumor recurrence.

If signs or symptoms suggest involvement by tumor, brain CT or bone scans are performed, as well as radiography of any suspicious bony lesions. Any accessible lesions suspicious for cancer should be biopsied if involvement would influence treatment.

In patients presenting with a mass lesion on chest x-ray or CT scan and no obvious contraindications to a curative approach after the initial evaluation, the mediastinum must be investigated. Approaches vary among centers and include performing chest CT scan and mediastinoscopy (for right-sided tumors) or mediastinotomy (for left-sided lesions) on all patients and proceeding directly to thoracotomy for staging of the mediastinum. Patients who present with disease that is confined to the chest but not resectable, and who thus are candidates for neoadjuvant chemotherapy plus surgery or for curative radiotherapy with or without chemotherapy, should have additional tests done as indicated to evaluate specific symptoms. In patients presenting with NSCLC that is not curable, all the general staging procedures are done, plus fiberoptic bronchoscopy as indicated to evaluate hemoptysis, obstruction, or pneumonitis, as well as thoracentesis with cytologic examination (and chest tube drainage as indicated) if fluid is present. As a rule, a radiographic finding of an isolated lesion (such as an enlarged adrenal gland) should be confirmed as cancer by fine-needle aspiration before a curative attempt is rejected.

STAGING OF SMALL CELL LUNG CANCER

Pretreatment staging for patients with SCLC includes the initial general lung cancer evaluation with chest and abdominal CT scans (because of the high frequency of hepatic and adrenal involvement) as well as fiberoptic bronchoscopy with washings and biopsies to determine the tumor extent before therapy; brain CT scan (10% of patients have metastases); and radionuclide scans (bone) if symptoms or other findings suggest disease involvement in these areas. Bone marrow biopsies and aspirations are rarely performed given the low incidence of isolated bone marrow metastases. Chest and abdominal CT scans are very useful to evaluate and follow tumor response to therapy, and chest CT scans are helpful in planning chest radiotherapy ports.

If signs or symptoms of spinal cord compression or leptomeningitis develop at any time in lung cancer patients with disease of any histologic type, a spinal CT scan or MRI scan and examination of the cerebrospinal fluid cytology are performed. If malignant cells are detected, radiotherapy to the site of compression and intrathecal chemotherapy (usually with methotrexate) are given. In addition, a brain CT or MRI scan is performed to search for brain metastases, which often are associated with spinal cord or leptomeningeal metastases.

RESECTABILITY AND OPERABILITY

In patients with NSCLC, the following are major contraindications to curative surgery or radiotherapy alone: extrathoracic metastases; superior vena cava syndrome; vocal cord and, in most cases, phrenic nerve paralysis; malignant pleural effusion; cardiac tamponade; tumor within 2 cm of the carina (not curable by surgery but potentially curable by radiotherapy); metastasis to the contralateral lung; bilateral

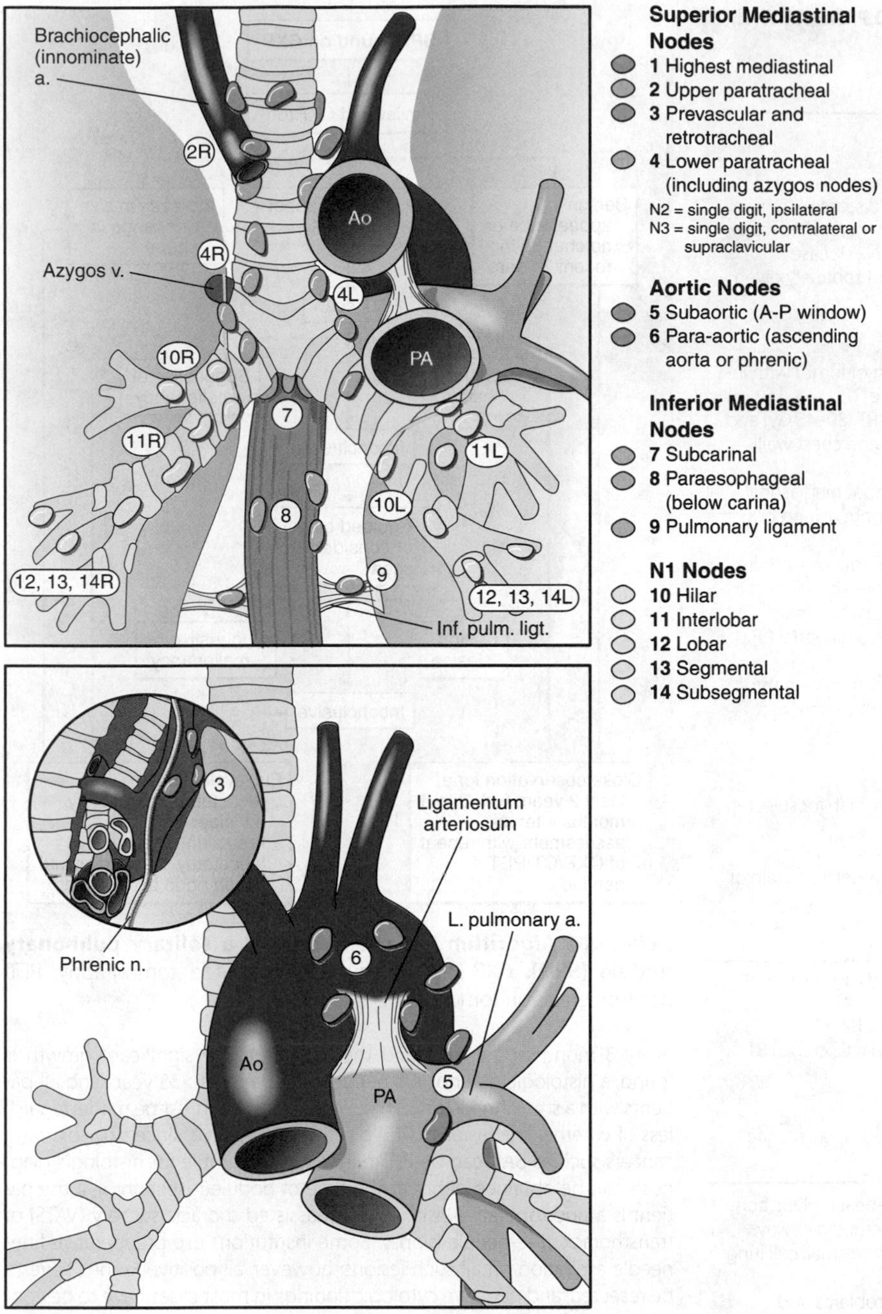

FIGURE 85-1 Regional lymph node stations for lung cancer staging. *(Used by permission from CF Mountain, C Dresler: Chest 111:1718, 1997.)*

endobronchial tumor (potentially curable by radiotherapy); metastasis to the supraclavicular lymph nodes; contralateral mediastinal node metastases (potentially curable by radiotherapy); and involvement of the main pulmonary artery. Pleural effusions are generally considered malignant regardless of whether they are cytology positive, particularly if they are exudative, bloody, and have no other probable etiology. Most patients with SCLC have unresectable disease; however, if clinical findings suggest the potential for resection (most common with peripheral lesions), that option should be considered.

PHYSIOLOGIC STAGING

Patients with lung cancer often have cardiopulmonary and other problems related to chronic obstructive pulmonary disease as well as other medical problems. To improve their preoperative condition, correctable problems (e.g., anemia, electrolyte and fluid disorders, infections, and arrhythmias) should be addressed, smoking stopped, and appropriate chest physical therapy instituted. Since it is not always possible to predict whether a lobectomy or pneumonectomy will be required until the time of operation, a conservative approach is to restrict resectional surgery to patients who could potentially tolerate a pneumonectomy. In addition to nonambulatory performance status, a myocardial infarction within the past 3 months is a contraindication to thoracic surgery because 20% of patients will die of reinfarction. An infarction in the past 6 months is a relative contraindication. Other major contraindications include uncontrolled major arrhythmias, an FEV_1 (forced expiratory volume in 1 s) <1 L, CO_2 retention (resting P_{CO_2} >45 mmHg), DL_{CO} <40%, and severe pulmonary hypertension. Recommending surgery when the FEV_1 is 1.1–2.0 L or <80% predicted requires careful judgment, while an FEV_1 >2.5 L or >80% predicted usually permits a pneumonectomy. In patients with borderline lung function but a resectable tumor, cardiopulmonary exercise testing could be performed as part of the physiologic evaluation. This test allows an estimate of the maximal oxygen consumption ($\dot{V}_{O_2}$max). A $\dot{V}_{O_2}$max <15 mL/kg per min predicts for high risk of postoperative complications.

℞ LUNG CANCER

The overall treatment approach to patients with lung cancer is shown in **Table 85-4**. Patients should be encouraged to stop smoking, particularly if they will be undergoing surgery or radiation therapy. Those who do fare better than those who continue to smoke.

MANAGEMENT OF OCCULT AND STAGE 0 CARCINOMAS In the uncommon situation where malignant cells are identified in a sputum or bronchial washing specimen but the chest radiograph appears normal (TX tumor stage), the lesion must be localized. More than 90% can be localized by meticulous examination of the bronchial tree with a fiberoptic bronchoscope under general anesthesia and collection of a series of differential brushings and biopsies. Often, carcinoma in situ or multicentric lesions are found in these patients. Current recommendations are for the most conservative surgical resection, allowing removal of the cancer and conservation of lung parenchyma, even if the bronchial margins are positive for carcinoma in situ. The 5-year overall survival rate for these occult cancers is ~60%. Close follow-up of these patients is indicated because of the high incidence of second primary lung cancers (5% per patient per year). One approach to in situ or multicentric lesions uses systemically administered hematoporphyrin (which localizes to tumors and sensitizes them to light) followed by bronchoscopic phototherapy.

SOLITARY PULMONARY NODULE AND "GROUND GLASS" OPACITY Occasionally, when an x-ray or CT scan is done for another purpose, a patient will present with an incidental finding of an asymptomatic, solitary pulmonary nodule (SPN, defined as an x-ray density completely surrounded by normal aerated lung, with circumscribed margins, of any shape, usually 1–6 cm in greatest diameter). A decision to resect or follow the nodule must be made. Nodules of this size discovered in CT screening for lung cancer would also be of the size requiring a biopsy for tissue. Approximately 35% of all such lesions in adults are malignant, most being primary lung cancer, while <1% are malignant in nonsmokers <35 years of age. A complete history, including a smoking history, physical examination, routine laboratory tests, chest CT scan, fiberoptic bronchoscopy, and old chest x-rays or CT scans are obtained if available.

TABLE 85-4 SUMMARY OF TREATMENT APPROACH TO PATIENTS WITH LUNG CANCER

Non-Small Cell Lung Cancer
Stages IA, IB, IIA, IIB, and some IIIA:
Surgical resection for stages IA, IB, IIA, and IIB
Surgical resection with complete-mediastinal lymph node dissection and consideration of neoadjuvant CRx for stage IIIA disease with "minimal N2 involvement" (discovered at thoracotomy or mediastinoscopy)
Consider postoperative RT for patients found to have N2 disease
Stage IB: discussion of risk/benefits of adjuvant CRx; not routinely given
Stage II: Adjuvant CRx
Curative potential RT for "nonoperable" patients
Stage IIIA with selected types of stage T3 tumors:
Tumors with chest wall invasion (T3): en bloc resection of tumor with involved chest wall and consideration of postoperative RT
Superior sulcus (Pancoast's) (T3) tumors: preoperative RT (30–45 Gy) and CRx followed by en bloc resection of involved lung and chest wall with postoperative RT
Proximal airway involvement (<2 cm from carina) without mediastinal nodes: sleeve resection if possible preserving distal normal lung or pneumonectomy
Stages IIIA "advanced, bulky, clinically evident N2 disease" (discovered preoperatively) and IIIB disease that can be included in a tolerable RT port:
Curative potential concurrent RT + CRx if performance status and general medical condition are reasonable; otherwise, sequential CRx followed by RT, or RT alone
Stage IIIB disease with carinal invasion (T4) but without N2 involvement:
Consider pneumonectomy with tracheal sleeve resection with direct reanastomosis to contralateral mainstem bronchus
Stage IV and more advanced IIIB disease:
RT to symptomatic local sites
CRx for ambulatory patients; consider CRx and bevacizumab for selected patients
Chest tube drainage of large malignant pleural effusions
Consider resection of primary tumor and metastasis for isolated brain or adrenal metastases
Small Cell Lung Cancer
Limited stage (good performance status): combination CRx + concurrent chest RT
Extensive stage (good performance status): combination CRx
Complete tumor responders (all stages): consider prophylactic cranial RT
Poor-performance-status patients (all stages):
Modified-dose combination CRx
Palliative RT
All Patients
RT for brain metastases, spinal cord compression, weight-bearing lytic bony lesions, symptomatic local lesions (nerve paralyses, obstructed airway, hemoptysis, intrathoracic large venous obstruction, in non-small cell lung cancer and in small cell cancer not responding to CRx)
Appropriate diagnosis and treatment of other medical problems and supportive care during CRx
Encouragement to stop smoking
Entrance into clinical trial, if eligible

Abbreviations: CRx, chemotherapy; RT, radiotherapy.

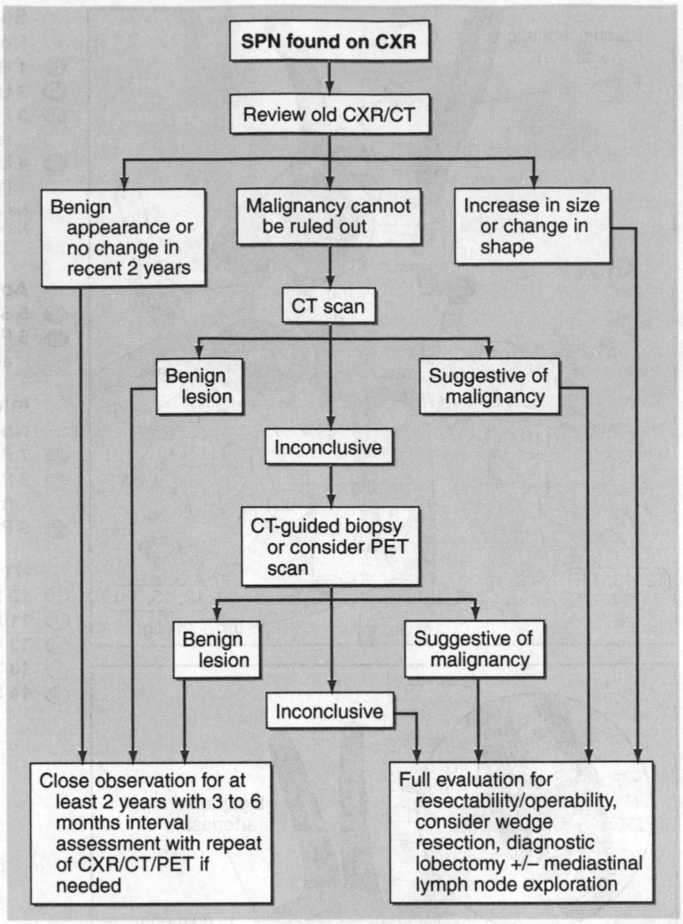

FIGURE 85-2 Algorithm for evaluation of a solitary pulmonary nodule (SPN). CXR, chest x-ray; CT, computed tomography; PET, positron emission tomography.

PET scans are useful in detecting lung cancers >7–8 mm in diameter. If no diagnosis is immediately apparent, the following risk factors would all argue strongly in favor of proceeding with resection to establish a histologic diagnosis: a history of cigarette smoking; age ≥35 years; a relatively large lesion; lack of calcification; chest symptoms; associated atelectasis, pneumonitis, or adenopathy; growth of the lesion revealed by comparison with old x-rays/CT scans; or a positive PET scan. At present, only two radiographic criteria are reliable predictors of the benign nature of an SPN: lack of growth over a period >2 years and certain characteristic patterns of calcification. Calcification alone does not exclude malignancy. However, a dense central nidus, multiple punctate foci, and "bull's eye" (granuloma) and "popcorn ball" (hamartoma) calcifications are all highly suggestive of a benign lesion. An algorithm for evaluating an SPN is shown in Fig. 85-2.

When old x-rays are not available, the PET scan is negative, and the characteristic calcification patterns are absent, the following approach is reasonable. Nonsmoking patients <35 years can be followed with serial CT every 3 months for 1 year and then yearly; if any significant growth is found, a histologic diagnosis is needed. For patients >35 years and all patients with a smoking history, a histologic diagnosis must be made, regardless of whether the lesion is PET positive or negative, since slow-growing cancers such as BAC can be PET negative. The sample for histologic diagnosis can be obtained either at the time of nodule resection or, if the patient is a poor operative risk, via video-assisted thoracic surgery (VATS) or transthoracic fine-needle biopsy. Some institutions use preoperative fine-needle aspiration on all such lesions; however, all positive lesions have to be resected, and negative cytologic findings in most cases have to be confirmed by histology on a resected specimen. Much has been made of sparing patients an operation; however, the high probability of finding a malignancy (particularly in smokers >35 years) and the excellent chance for surgical cure when the tumor is small both suggest an aggressive approach to these lesions.

Since the advent of screening CTs, small "ground-glass" opacities ("GGOs") have often been observed, particularly as the increased sensitivity of CTs enables detection of smaller lesions. Many of these GGOs, when biopsied, are found to be BAC. Some of the GGOs are semiopaque and referred to as "partial" GGOs, which are often more slowly growing, with atypical adenomatous hyperplasia histology, a lesion of unclear prognostic significance. By contrast, "solid" GGOs have a faster growth rate and usually are typical adenocarcinomas histologically.

NON-SMALL CELL LUNG CANCER NSCLC Stages I and II

Surgery In patients with NSCLC stages IA, IB, IIA and IIB (Table 85-2) who can tolerate operation, the treatment of choice is pulmonary resection. If a complete resection is possible, the 5-year survival rate for N0 disease is about 60–80%, depending on the size of the tumor. The 5-year survival drops to about 50% when N1 (hilar node involvement) disease is present.

The extent of resection is a matter of surgical judgment based on findings at exploration. Clinical trials have shown that lobectomy is superior to wedge resection in reducing the rate of local recurrence. Pneumonectomy is reserved for patients with tumors involving multiple lobes or very central tumors and should only be performed in patients with excellent pulmonary reserve. In addition, patients undergoing a right-sided pneumonectomy after induction chemotherapy and radiation therapy (see below) have a high mortality rate and should be carefully selected before surgery. Wedge resection and segmentectomy (potentially by VATS) are reserved for patients with poor pulmonary reserve and small peripheral lesions.

Radiotherapy with Curative Intent Patients with stage I or II disease who refuse surgery or are not candidates for pulmonary resection should be considered for radiation therapy with curative intent. The decision to administer high-dose radiotherapy is based on the extent of disease and the volume of the chest that requires irradiation. Patients with distant metastases, malignant pleural effusion, or cardiac involvement are not considered candidates for curative radiation treatment. The long-term survival for patients with all stages of lung cancer who receive radiation with curative intent is about 20%. In addition to being potentially curative, radiotherapy may increase the quality and length of life by controlling the primary tumor and preventing symptoms related to local recurrence in the lung.

Treatment with curative intent usually involves midplane doses of 60–64 Gy, while palliative thoracic radiation (see below) involves delivery of 30–45 Gy. The major dose-limiting concern is the amount of lung parenchyma and other organs in the thorax that are included in the treatment plan, including the spinal cord, heart, and esophagus. In patients with a major degree of underlying pulmonary disease, the treatment plan may have to be compromised because of the deleterious effects of radiation on pulmonary function.

The most common side effect of curative thoracic radiation is esophagitis. Other side effects include fatigue, radiation myelitis (rare), and radiation pneumonitis, which can sometimes progress to pulmonary fibrosis. The risk of radiation pneumonitis is proportional to the radiation dose and the volume of lung in the field. The full clinical syndrome (dyspnea, fever, and radiographic infiltrate corresponding to the treatment port) occurs in 5% of cases and is treated with glucocorticoids. Acute radiation esophagitis occurs during treatment but is usually self-limited, unlike spinal cord injury, which may be permanent and should be avoided by careful treatment planning. Brachytherapy (local radiotherapy delivered by placing radioactive "seeds" in a catheter in the tumor bed) provides a way to give a high local dose while sparing surrounding normal tissue.

NSCLC Stage IA Patients with resected stage IA NSCLC receive no other therapy but are at a high risk of recurrence (~2–3% annually) or developing a second primary lung cancer. Thus, it is reasonable to follow these patients with CT scans for the first 5 years and consider entering them onto early detection and chemoprevention studies.

Adjuvant Chemotherapy for NSCLC Stages IB and II A meta-analysis of more than 4300 patients showed a trend toward improved survival of ~5% at 5 years with cisplatin-based adjuvant therapy (p = .08). Subsequently, three randomized studies demonstrated no significant survival advantage despite the addition of more "modern" postoperative adjuvant chemotherapy regimens. However, since then at least three additional randomized trials and two meta-analyses showed a survival benefit in response to postoperative adjuvant-based therapy (**Table 85-5**). Consequently, adjuvant chemotherapy is now routinely recommended in NSCLC patients with a good performance status and stage IIA or IIB disease, though the beneficial effects are modest.

TABLE 85-5 RANDOMIZED STUDIES OF ADJUVANT CHEMOTHERAPY IN NSCLC

Study	Treatment	Number of Patients	5-Year Survival (%)	Median Survival	Hazard Ratio (95% CI)	*p* Value
ECOG 3590 (II–IIIA)	Surgery → RT vs. Surgery + post-op concurrent RT + cis/etoposide	242 246	39% 33%	39 months vs. 38 months	0.93 (0.74–1.18)	0.56
ALPI (I–IIIA)	Surgery alone vs. Surgery + post-op mitomycin/vindesine/cisplatin	603 606	51% 43%	NR	0.96 (0.8–1.1)	0.59
Big Lung Trial (I–IIIB)	Surgery alone vs. Surgery + post-op chemotherapy[a]	189 192		33 months 34 months	1.02 (0.77–1.35)	0.90
IALT IB–IIIA	Surgery alone vs. Surgery + post-op Cis + VP16/vinca	405 361	40% 44.5%	NR	0.86 (0.76–0.98)	<0.03
UFT IA–IB	Surgery alone vs. Surgery + post-op UFT	488 469	85% 88%	—	0.71 (0.52–0.98)	0.04
CALGB IB (ASCO 06)	Surgery alone vs. Surgery + post-op carbo/paclitaxel	172 172	57% 59%	78 months 95 months	0.80 (0.60–1.07)	0.10
NCI-C IB–II	Surgery alone vs. Surgery + post-op Cis/vinorelbine	241 241	54% 69%	73 months 94 months	0.69 (0.52–0.91)	0.04
ANITA IB, II, IIIA	Surgery alone vs. Surgery + post-op Cis/vinorelbine	433 407	43% 51%	44 months 66 months	0.79 (50–88.5)	0.017

[a]Chemotherapy allowed: mitomycin, cisplatin, ifosfamide; mitomycin, vinblastine, cisplatin; cisplatin, vindesine; cisplatin, vinorelbine.

Note: RT, radiation therapy; NR, not reported; UFT, tegafur and uracil.

The role of adjuvant chemotherapy for stage IB disease is undefined. Subset analysis of all the randomized studies showed no benefit in patients with stage IB. In addition, one clinical trial focusing solely on IB disease and using carboplatin and paclitaxel (one of the most commonly used regimens for advanced disease) found a hazard ratio of 0.80 (20% reduction in death with adjuvant chemotherapy) that was not statistically significant. Thus, patients with stage IB NSCLC are not routinely given adjuvant therapy.

Adjuvant Radiotherapy for NSCLC Stages I–II After apparent complete resection, postoperative adjuvant radiation therapy does not improve survival and may actually be detrimental to survival in N0 and N1 disease.

Superior Sulcus or Pancoast Tumors Non-small cell carcinomas of the superior pulmonary sulcus producing *Pancoast's syndrome* appear to behave differently than lung cancers at other sites and are usually treated with combined radiotherapy and surgery. Patients with these carcinomas should have the usual preoperative staging procedures, including mediastinoscopy and CT and PET scans, to determine tumor extent and a neurologic examination (and sometimes nerve conduction studies) to document involvement or impingement of nerves in the region. If mediastinoscopy is negative, curative approaches may be used in treating Pancoast's syndrome despite its apparent locally invasive nature. The best results reported thus employed concurrent preoperative irradiation [30 Gy in 10 treatments] and cisplatin and etoposide, followed by an en bloc resection of the tumor and involved chest wall 3–6 weeks later; 65% of thoracotomy specimens showed either a complete response or minimal residual microscopic disease on pathologic evaluation. The 2-year survival rate was 55% for all eligible patients and 70% for patients who had a complete resection.

NSCLC with T3, N0 Disease (Stage IIB) The subset of T3, N0 disease (which does not present as Pancoast tumor) was initially considered stage III disease. However, it has a different natural history and treatment strategy than stage III N2 disease and is now considered as stage IIB. Patients with peripheral chest wall invasion should have resection of the involved ribs and underlying lung. Chest wall defects are then repaired with chest wall musculature or Marlex mesh and methylmethacrylate. Five-year survival rates as high as 35–50% have been found, and adjuvant chemotherapy is usually recommended.

NSCLC Stage III Treatment of locally advanced NSCLC is one of the most controversial issues in the management of lung cancer. Treatment options include a local therapy (surgery or radiation therapy) combined with systemic chemotherapy to control micrometastases. Interpretation of the results of clinical trials involving patients with locally advanced disease has been clouded by a number of issues, including changing diagnostic techniques, different staging systems, and heterogeneous patient populations with tumors that range from nonbulky stage IIIA (clinical N1 nodes with N2 nodes discovered only at the time of surgery, despite a negative mediastinoscopy) to bulky N2 nodes (enlarged adenopathy clearly visible on chest x-rays or multiple nodal level involvement) to clearly inoperable stage IIIB disease. Thus, a team approach involving pulmonary medicine, thoracic surgery, and medical and radiation oncology is essential for the management of these patients.

NSCLC Stage IIIA ***Nonbulky IIIA*** Surgery for N2 disease is a controversial area in the management of lung cancer. Patients with N2 disease can be divided into "minimal" disease (involvement of only one node with microscopic foci, usually discovered at thoracotomy or mediastinoscopy) and the more common "advanced" bulky disease, clinically obvious on CT scans and discovered preoperatively. Patients who have an incidental finding of N2 disease at the time of resection should receive adjuvant chemotherapy.

Bulky IIIA No evidence suggests that patients with "bulky," multilevel ipsilateral mediastinal nodes (N2) have improved survival with surgery and either pre- or postoperative chemotherapy compared to treatment with chemotherapy plus radiation therapy. This important issue was addressed in the multicenter randomized Intergroup 0139 Trial involving patients with pathologically staged N2 disease who received 45 Gy of induction radiation therapy plus two cycles of cisplatin and etoposide to "debulk" tumors. The patients were then randomly assigned to surgical resection of any residual tumor or to boost radiation therapy plus an additional two cycles of chemotherapy. Although a significant improvement in progression-free survival was observed at 5 years for those patients randomized to surgical resection (22% vs. 11%; $p = .017$), the difference in 5-year overall survival while favoring surgery (22% vs. 11%; $p = .10$) was not significant. This is important since treatment-related mortality was greater in the surgery arm (8% vs. 2%), with the majority of deaths occurring in patients undergoing pneumonectomy. Patients who had persistent N2 disease following neoadjuvant chemotherapy did particularly poorly, leading some oncologists to conclude that surgery for bulky IIIA disease should only be conducted in patients who have clearing of their mediastinal nodes following neoadjuvant therapy. The main role of neoadjuvant chemotherapy is to control micrometastatic disease, and if this macroscopically evident disease is not sensitive to chemotherapy, it is unlikely that the microscopic disease will be controlled. Thus, surgical removal of the primary tumor after such chemotherapy is probably fruitless. Likewise, neoadjuvant chemotherapy generally should not be used to render inoperable disease operable. One exception to this approach is T4, N0 or T4, N1 (stage IIIB, see below) disease for which preoperative chemotherapy may provide enough tumor debulking to allow otherwise unresectable disease to be resected. Chemotherapy may allow chest wall resection for direct extension of tumor, tracheal sleeve pneumonectomy, and sleeve lobectomy for lesions near the carina.

Bulky NSCLC Stage IIIA and Dry IIIB (IIIB without a Pleural Effusion) The presence of pathologically involved N2 nodes should be confirmed histologically because enlarged nodes detected by CT will be negative for cancer in ~30% of patients. Chemotherapy plus radiation therapy is the treatment of choice for patients with bulky stage IIIA or IIIB disease without pleural effusion (referred to as "dry IIIB"). Randomized studies demonstrate an improvement in median and long-term survival with chemotherapy followed by radiation therapy, compared with radiation therapy alone. Subsequent randomized trials have shown that administering chemotherapy and radiation therapy concurrently results in improved survival compared to sequential chemotherapy and radiation therapy, albeit with more side effects, such as fatigue, esophagitis, and neutropenia. Frequently, an additional two to three cycles of chemotherapy are also given. However, it is not clear whether these additional cycles should be administered before or after the chemoradiation, what the optimal drugs are, or whether doses should be attenuated during the radiation but given more frequently. (Lower doses of drugs may "sensitize" the tumor to radiation therapy but may not by themselves remove other microscopic disease.)

DISSEMINATED NON-SMALL CELL LUNG CANCER **Symptomatic Management of Metastatic Disease** Patients who present with or progress to metastatic NSCLC have a poor prognosis, as do patients with pleural effusions. Untreated, the median survival of both of these patient groups is roughly 4–6 months. They are often treated in the same way. Standard medical management, the judicious use of pain medications, the appropriate use of radiotherapy, and outpatient chemotherapy form the cornerstone of this management.

Palliative Radiation Therapy Patients whose primary tumor is causing urgent severe symptoms such as bronchial obstruction with pneumonitis, hemoptysis, upper airway or superior vena cava obstruction, brain or spinal cord compression, or painful bony metastases should have radiotherapy to the primary tumor to relieve these symptoms. Usually, radiation therapy is given as a course of 30–40 Gy over 2–4 weeks for palliative purposes. Radiation therapy provides relief of intrathoracic symptoms: hemoptysis, 84%; superior vena cava syndrome, 80%; dyspnea, 60%; cough, 60%; atelectasis, 23%; and vocal cord paralysis, 6%. Cardiac tamponade (treated with pericardiocentesis and radiation therapy to the heart), painful bony metastases (with relief in 66%), brain or spinal cord compression, and brachial plexus involvement may also be palliated with radiotherapy.

Brain metastases are often isolated sites of relapse in patients with adenocarcinoma of the lung otherwise controlled by surgery or radiotherapy. These are usually treated with radiation therapy and, in highly selected cases, with surgical resection. Usually, in addition to radiotherapy for brain metastases and cord compression, dexamethasone (25–100 mg/d in four divided doses) is also given and then rapidly tapered to the lowest dosage that relieves symptoms. Because of the high frequency of brain metastases, the use of prophylactic cranial irradiation (PCI, given to the whole brain before metastatic disease becomes manifest) has been considered. However, PCI is of no proven value. Screening asymptomatic patients with head CT scans to find such lesions before such metastases become clinically evident is also not proven beneficial.

Pleural effusions are common and are usually treated with thoracentesis. If they recur and are symptomatic, a pleurex catheter or chest tube drainage followed by pleurodesis with a sclerosing agent such as intrapleural talc, bleomycin, or tetracycline can be used. These sclerosing agents may be administered through the chest tube, or, in the case of talc, via thorascopic insufflation. In the former case, the chest cavity is completely drained. Xylocaine 1% is instilled (15 mL), followed by 50 mL normal saline. Then the sclerosing agent is dissolved in 100 mL normal saline, and this solution is injected through the chest tube. The chest tube is clamped for 4 h if tolerated, and the patient is rotated onto different sides to distribute the sclerosing agent. The chest tube is removed 24–48 h later, after drainage has become slight (usually <100 mL/24 h). While sclerosing agents have been widely used, an indwelling pleurex catheter is equivalent to chest tube drainage and better tolerated by patients. In this situation, the pleurex catheter is tunneled under the skin and can remain in place for weeks. The patient periodically drains the catheter into a specially designed bag, as needed.

Symptomatic endobronchial lesions that recur after surgery or radiotherapy or develop in patients with severely compromised pulmonary function are difficult to treat with conventional therapy. Neodymium-YAG (yttrium-aluminum-garnet) laser therapy administered through a flexible fiberoptic bronchoscope (usually under general anesthesia) can provide palliation in 80–90% of such patients even when the tumor has relapsed after radiotherapy. Local radiotherapy delivered by brachytherapy, photodynamic therapy using a photosensitizing agent, and endobronchial stents are other measures that can relieve airway obstruction from recurrent tumor.

Chemotherapy Chemotherapy palliates symptoms, improves the quality of life, and improves survival in newly diagnosed patients with stage IV NSCLC, particularly in patients with good performance status. Whereas the median survival for untreated patients is roughly 4–6 months, and 1-year survival is 5–10%, with combination chemotherapy the median survival is 8–10 months, 1-year survival is 30–35%, and 2-year survival 10–15%. Combination chemotherapy produces an objective tumor response in 20–30% of patients, although the response is complete in <5%. In addition, economic analysis has found chemotherapy to be cost-effective palliation for stage IV NSCLC. However, the use of chemotherapy for NSCLC requires clinical experience and careful judgment to balance potential benefits and toxicities for these patients.

Chemotherapy for previously untreated, good-performance-status patients typically consists of two drugs ("doublets"). Traditionally, one of the two drugs has been either cisplatin or carboplatin, and the other drug is a taxane (paclitaxel or docetaxel), gemcitabine, or a vinca alkaloid such as vinorelbine. No major difference in outcome has been observed between the standard chemotherapy doublets, although they differ in terms of schedule, side effects, and cost. Cytotoxic chemotherapy for first-line chemotherapy is typically administered for four to six cycles; no benefit has been shown for continuing the same chemotherapy beyond that point. After four to six cycles, chemotherapy is usually stopped and the patient observed closely for tumor progression, at which point second-line chemotherapy may be started if the patient's performance status remains good. Nausea with typical first-line regimens is usually mild, particularly when 5-HT3 serotonin antagonists are used as antiemetics. Hair loss depends on the choice of regimen and should be discussed with the patient. All regimens cause myelosuppression, but the incidence of neutropenic fevers, bleeding episodes, or anemia requiring transfusions is low. Growth-factor support is rarely needed. Elderly patients without significant comorbid conditions benefit from and tolerate chemotherapy much the same as their younger counterparts. However, patients with a poorer performance status seem to obtain less benefit.

Docetaxel and pemetrexed are second-line agents for patients who have progressive disease on first-line chemotherapy and still have a good performance status. Docetaxel improves progression-free survival and overall survival compared to best supportive care, and pemetrexed has roughly the same efficacy as docetaxel, but with fewer side effects.

VEGF Targeted Therapy Bevacizumab, a monoclonal antibody to VEGF, improves response rate, progression-free survival, and overall survival of patients with advanced disease when combined with chemotherapy (paclitaxel/carboplatin). Median, 1-year, and 2-year survival in response to chemotherapy plus bevacizumab was 12.3 months, 51%, and 23%, compared, respectively, to 10.3 months, 44%, and 15% with chemotherapy alone (hazard ratio 0.79, $p = 0.003$). A 1-year survival of >50% and a 2-year survival of >20% represents a significant improvement in long-term prognosis. The dose of bevacizumab administered on this trial was 15 mg/kg IV every 3 weeks. Bevacizumab side effects include bleeding, hypertension, and proteinuria, and the hemorrhagic side effects make this agent risky to use. Patients with squamous cancer cannot receive bevacizumab because of their tendency toward serious hemorrhagic side effects. Patients with brain metastases, hemoptysis, and bleeding disorders or who need anticoagulation are also not eligible to receive the agent. Despite these restrictions and careful patient selection, significant bleeding is noted in about 4% of patients.

EGFR Targeted Therapy Erlotinib is an oral inhibitor of the EGFR kinase that is used in second- and third-line therapy of NSCLC. Clinical responses have been seen in a large fraction of the small subset of patients with tumors bearing mutations in the EGFR. Prolonged survival with EGFR TKI treatment has also been observed in some patients whose tumors have amplification of the *EGFR* gene or overexpression of the receptor. Side effects of erlotinib differ from chemotherapy side effects of hair loss, nausea, and neutropenia, but they include acneiform skin rash and diarrhea. For patients whose tumors respond to EGFR TKI therapy, substantial clinical benefit is seen.

SMALL CELL LUNG CANCER SCLC is a chemotherapy-sensitive disease. Patients with limited stage disease have high response rates (60–80%) and a 10–30% complete response rate. The response rates in patients with extensive disease are somewhat lower (50%) and almost always partial responses. Tumor regressions usually occur quickly, within the first two cycles of treatment, and provide rapid palliation of tumor-related symptoms.

Chemotherapy significantly prolongs survival. Untreated, patients with limited-stage SCLC have a median survival of 12 weeks; the median survival with chemotherapy is 18 months, and long-term (>3 year) survival is 30–40%. The median survival of extensive-stage patients is 9 months; <5% of patients survive 2 years. Thus, although initially responsive, most patients with SCLC relapse, presumably due to the emergence of chemotherapy resistance.

Chemotherapy The chemotherapy combination most widely used for SCLC is etoposide plus cisplatin or carboplatin, given every 3 weeks on an outpatient basis for four to six cycles. Increased dose intensity of chemotherapy adds toxicity without clear survival benefit. Appropriate supportive care (antiemetics, fluid support with cisplatin, monitoring of blood counts and blood chemistries, monitoring for signs of bleeding or infection, and, as required, use of hematopoietins) and adjustment of chemotherapy doses on the basis of nadir granulocyte counts are essential.

The prognosis of patients who relapse is poor. Patients who relapse >3 months since the completion of their initial chemotherapy (so-called chemosensitive disease) have a median survival of 4–5 months; patients who do not respond to initial chemotherapy or relapse within 3 months (chemorefractory disease) have a median survival of only 2–3 months. Patients with chemosensitive disease may be retreated with their initial regimen. Topotecan has modest activity as second-line therapy, or patients can be entered onto clinical trials testing new agents.

Considerations for Therapy of SCLC Limited-Stage Disease ***Combined-Modality Chemoradiotherapy*** Radiation therapy to the thorax is associated with a small but significant improvement in long-term survival for patients with limited-stage SCLC (5% at 3 years). Chemotherapy given concurrently with thoracic radiation is more effective than sequential chemoradiation but is associated with significantly more esophagitis and hematologic toxicity. In one randomized study, twice-daily hyperfractionated radiation was compared with a once-daily schedule; both were administered concurrently with four cycles of cisplatin and etoposide. Survival was significantly higher with the twice-daily regimen (median survival 23 months compared with 19 months; 5-year survival 26% compared with 16%), but the twice-daily regimen gave more grade 3 esophagitis and pulmonary toxicity. Patients should be carefully selected for concurrent chemoradiation therapy based on good performance status and pulmonary reserve.

PCI significantly decreases the development of brain metastases (which occur in about two-thirds of patients who do not receive PCI) and results in a small survival benefit (~5%) in patients who have obtained a complete response to induction chemotherapy. Deficits in cognitive ability following PCI are uncommon and often difficult to sort out from effects of chemotherapy or normal aging.

Radiation Therapy for Palliation Palliative radiation therapy is an important component of the management of SCLC patients. Cranial radiation often decreases the signs and symptoms of brain metastases. In the case of symptomatic, progressive lesions in the chest or at other critical sites, if radiotherapy has not yet been given to these areas, it may be administered in full doses (e.g., 40 Gy to the chest tumor mass).

Surgery Although surgical resection is not routinely recommended for SCLC, occasional patients meet the usual requirements for resectability (stage I or II disease with negative mediastinal nodes). Often this histologic diagnosis is made in some patients only on review of the resected surgical specimen. However, when such SCLC patients are discovered, they should receive standard SCLC chemotherapy. Retrospective series have reported high cure rates if postoperative chemotherapy is used, although it is unclear what the outcome would be with chemoradiation therapy alone, given the relatively low bulk disease of these patients.

LUNG CANCER PREVENTION

Deterring children from taking up smoking and helping young adults stop is likely to be the most effective lung cancer prevention. Smoking cessation programs are successful in 5–20% of volunteers; the poor efficacy is due to the addictive nature of nicotine use, which is as strong as addiction to heroin.

Chemoprevention is an experimental approach to reduce lung cancer risk; no benefit has yet been shown for chemoprevention. Two putative chemoprevention agents, vitamin E and β-carotene, actually increased the risk of lung cancer in heavy smokers.

BENIGN LUNG NEOPLASMS

The benign neoplasms of the lung, representing <5% of all primary tumors, include bronchial adenomas and hamartomas (90% of such lesions) and a group of very uncommon benign neoplasms (epithelial tumors such as bronchial papillomas, fibroepithelial polyps; mesenchymal tumors such as chondromas, fibromas, lipomas, hemangiomas, leiomyomas, pseudolymphomas; tumors of mixed origin such as teratomas; and other diseases such as endometriosis). The diagnostic and primary-treatment approach (surgery) is basically the same for all these neoplasms. They can present as central masses causing airway obstruction, cough, hemoptysis, and pneumonitis. The masses may or may not be visible on radiographs but are usually accessible to fiberoptic bronchoscopy. Alternatively, they can present without symptoms as SPNs and are evaluated accordingly. In all cases, the extent of surgery must be determined at operation, and a conservative procedure with appropriate reconstructions is usually performed.

BRONCHIAL ADENOMAS

Bronchial adenomas (80% are central) are slow-growing endobronchial lesions; they represent 50% of all benign pulmonary neoplasms. About 80–90% are carcinoids, 10–15% are adenocystic tumors (or cylindromas), and 2–3% are mucoepidermoid tumors. Adenomas present in patients 15–60 years old (average age 45) as endobronchial lesions and are often symptomatic for several years. Patients may have a chronic cough, recurrent hemoptysis, or obstruction with atelectasis, lobar collapse, or pneumonitis and abscess formation.

Bronchial adenomas of all types, because of their endobronchial and often central location, are usually visible by fiberoptic bronchoscopy. Because they are hypervascular, they can bleed profusely after bronchoscopic biopsy, and this problem should be anticipated. Bronchial adenomas must be considered as potentially malignant, thus requiring removal for symptom relief and because they can be locally invasive or recurrent, potentially can metastasize, and may produce paraneoplastic syndromes. Surgical excision is the primary treatment for all types of bronchial adenomas. The extent of surgery is determined at operation and should be as conservative as possible. Often bronchotomy with local excision, sleeve resection, segmental resection, or lobectomy is sufficient. Five-year survival rate after surgical resection is 95%, decreasing to 70% if regional nodes are involved. The treatment of metastatic pulmonary carcinoids is unclear because they can either be indolent or behave more like SCLC (Chap. 344). Assessment of the tempo and histology of the disease in the individual patient is necessary to determine if and when chemotherapy or radiotherapy is indicated.

CARCINOID AND OTHER NEUROENDOCRINE LUNG TUMORS

Neuroendocrine lung tumors represent a spectrum of pathologic entities, including typical carcinoid, atypical carcinoid, and large cell neuroendocrine cancer, as well as SCLC. SCLC and large cell neuroendocrine cancer are high-grade neuroendocrine tumors and in general should be treated as described for SCLC. By contrast, typical carcinoid and atypical carcinoids are low- and intermediate-grade tumors with different treatment approaches and in general are resistant to chemotherapy (Chap. 44). Carcinoids, like SCLCs, may secrete other hormones, such as ACTH or AVP, and can cause paraneoplastic syndromes that resolve on resection. Uncommonly, bronchial carcinoid metastases (usually to the liver) may produce the carcinoid syndrome, with cutaneous flush, bronchoconstriction, diarrhea, and cardiac valvular lesions, which SCLC does not do. Carcinoid tumors that have an unusually aggressive histologic appearance (referred to as *atypical carcinoids*) metastasize in 70% of cases to regional nodes, liver, or bone, compared with only a 5% rate of metastasis for carcinoids with typical histology. Large cell neuroendocrine cancer is a high-grade NSCLC with neuroendocrine features. These tumors are characterized by histologic features similar to small cell cancer, but they are formed by larger cells. The prognosis for patients with large cell neuroendocrine cancer is significantly worse than that for patients with atypical carcinoid and classic large cell cancer. Five-year survival is 21% for patients with large cell neuroendocrine cancer, 65% for atypical carcinoid, and 90% for typical carcinoid.

THYMOMAS

See **Chap. e12.**

HAMARTOMAS

Pulmonary hamartomas have a peak incidence at age 60 and are more frequent in men than in women. Histologically, they contain normal pulmonary tissue components (smooth muscle and collagen) in a disorganized fashion. They are usually peripheral, clinically silent, and benign in their behavior. Unless the radiographic findings are pathognomonic for hamartoma, with "popcorn" calcification, the lesions usually have to be resected for diagnosis, particularly if the patient is a smoker. VATS may minimize the surgical complications.

METASTATIC PULMONARY TUMORS

The lung is a frequent site of metastases from primary cancers outside the lung. Usually such metastatic disease is incurable. However, two special situations should be borne in mind. The first is the development of an SPN or a mass on chest x-ray in a patient known to have an extrathoracic neoplasm. This nodule may represent a metastasis or a new primary lung cancer. Because the natural history of lung cancer is often worse than that of other primary tumors, a single pulmonary nodule in a patient with a known extrathoracic tumor is approached as though the nodule is a primary lung cancer, particularly if the patient is >35 years and a smoker. If a vigorous search for other sites of active cancer proves negative, the nodule is surgically resected. Second, in some cases multiple metastatic pulmonary nodules can be resected with curative intent. This tactic is usually recommended if, after careful staging, it is found that (1) the patient can tolerate the contemplated pulmonary resection, (2) the primary tumor has been definitively and successfully treated (disease-free for >1 year), and (3) all known metastatic disease can be encompassed by the projected pulmonary resection. Patients with uncontrolled primary tumors and other extrapulmonary metastases are not considered. Primary tumors whose pulmonary metastases have been successfully resected for cure include osteogenic and soft tissue sarcomas; colon, rectal, uterine, cervix, and corpus tumors; head and neck, breast, testis, and salivary gland cancer; melanoma; and bladder and kidney tumors. Five-year survival rates of 20–30% have been found in selected series, and dramatic results have been achieved in patients with osteogenic sarcomas, where resection of pulmonary metastases (sometimes requiring several thoracotomies) is a standard curative treatment approach.

FURTHER READINGS

Black C et al: Population screening for lung cancer using computed tomography: Is there evidence of clinical effectiveness? A systematic review of the literature. Thorax 62:131, 2007

Eberhardt W et al: Chemoradiation paradigm for the treatment of lung cancer. Nat Clin Pract Oncol 3:188, 2006

Hayes DN et al: Gene expression profiling reveals reproducible human lung adenocarcinoma subtypes in multiple independent patient cohorts. J Clin Oncol 24:5079, 2006

Sato M et al: Molecular genetics of lung cancer and translation to the clinic. J Thorac Oncol 2:327, 2007

Stinnett S et al: Role of chemotherapy for palliation in the lung cancer patient. J Support Oncol 5:19, 2007

Subramanian J, Govindan R: Lung cancer in never smokers: A review. J Clin Oncol 25:561, 2007

Sun S et al: Of molecules and cancer stem cells: Novel therapeutic strategies for lung cancer. J Clin Invest 117, 2007

Wright G et al: Surgery for non-small cell lung cancer: Systematic review and meta-analysis of randomised controlled trials. Thorax 61:597, 2006

86 Breast Cancer

Marc E. Lippman

Breast cancer is a malignant proliferation of epithelial cells lining the ducts or lobules of the breast. In the year 2007, about 180,510 cases of invasive breast cancer and 40,910 deaths occurred in the United States. Epithelial malignancies of the breast are the most common cause of cancer in women (excluding skin cancer), accounting for about one-third of all cancer in women. As a result of improved treatment and earlier detection, mortality from breast cancer has begun to decrease substantially in the United States. This chapter will not consider rare malignancies presenting in the breast, such as sarcomas and lymphomas, but will focus on the epithelial cancers. Human breast cancer is a clonal disease; a single transformed cell—the product of a series of somatic (acquired) or germline mutations—is eventually able to express full malignant potential. Thus, breast cancer may exist for a long period as either a noninvasive disease or an invasive but nonmetastatic disease. These facts have significant clinical ramifications.

GENETIC CONSIDERATIONS Not more than 10% of human breast cancers can be linked directly to germline mutations. Several genes have been implicated in familial cases. The Li-Fraumeni syndrome is characterized by inherited mutations in the p53 tumor-suppressor gene, which lead to an increased incidence of breast cancer, osteogenic sarcomas, and other malignancies. Inherited mutations in *PTEN* have also been reported in breast cancer.

Another tumor-suppressor gene, *BRCA-1*, has been identified at the chromosomal locus 17q21; this gene encodes a zinc finger protein, and the product therefore may function as a transcription factor. The gene appears to be involved in gene repair. Women who inherit a mutated allele of this gene from either parent have at least a 60–80% lifetime chance of developing breast cancer and about a 33% chance of developing ovarian cancer. The risk is higher among women born after 1940, presumably due to promotional effects of hormonal factors. Men who carry a mutant allele of the gene have an increased incidence of prostate cancer and breast cancer. A fourth gene, termed *BRCA-2*, which has been localized to chromosome 13q12, is also associated with an increased incidence of breast cancer in men and women.

Germline mutations in *BRCA-1* and *BRCA-2* can be readily detected; patients with these mutations can be counseled appropriately. All women with strong family histories for breast cancer should be referred to genetic screening programs, particularly women of Ashkenazi Jewish descent who have a high likelihood of a specific *BRCA-1* mutation (deletion of adenine and guanine at position 185).

Even more important than the role these genes play in inherited forms of breast cancer may be their role in sporadic breast cancer. The p53 mutation is present in nearly 40% of human breast cancers as an acquired defect. Acquired mutations in *PTEN* occur in about 10% of the cases. *BRCA-1* mutation in sporadic primary breast cancer has not been reported. However, decreased expression of *BRCA-1* mRNA (possibly via gene methylation) and abnormal cellular location of the *BRCA-1* protein have been found in some breast cancers. Loss of heterozygosity of *BRCA-1* and *BRCA-2* suggests that tumor-suppressor activity may be inactivated in sporadic cases of human breast cancer. Finally, increased expression of a dominant oncogene plays a role in about a quarter of human breast cancer cases. The product of this gene, a member of the epidermal growth factor receptor superfamily, is called *erbB2* (HER-2, neu) and is overexpressed in these breast cancers due to gene amplification; this overexpression can contribute to transformation of human breast epithelium and is the target of effective systemic therapy in adjuvant and metastatic disease settings.

EPIDEMIOLOGY

Breast cancer is a hormone-dependent disease. Women without functioning ovaries who never receive estrogen-replacement therapy do not develop breast cancer. The female:male ratio is about 150:1. For most epithelial malignancies, a log-log plot of incidence versus age shows a single-component straight-line increase with every year of life. A similar plot for breast cancer shows two components: a straight-line increase with age but with a decrease in slope beginning at the age of menopause. The three dates in a woman's life that have a major impact on breast cancer incidence are age at menarche, age at first full-term pregnancy, and age at menopause. Women who experience menarche at age 16 have only 50–60% of the breast cancer risk of a woman having menarche at age 12; the lower risk persists throughout life. Similarly, menopause occurring 10 years before the median age of menopause (52 years), whether natural or surgically induced, reduces lifetime breast cancer risk by about 35%. Women who have a first full-term pregnancy by age 18 have a 30–40% lower risk of breast cancer compared with nulliparous women. Thus, length of menstrual life—particularly the fraction occurring before first full-term pregnancy—is a substantial component of the total risk of breast cancer. These three factors (menarche, age of first full-term pregnancy, and menopause) can account for 70–80% of the variation in breast cancer frequency in different countries. A meta-analysis has shown that duration of maternal nursing correlates with substantial risk reduction independent of either parity or age at first full-term pregnancy.

International variation in incidence has provided some of the most important clues on hormonal carcinogenesis. A woman living to age 80 in North America has one chance in nine of developing invasive breast cancer. Asian women have one-fifth to one-tenth the risk of breast cancer of women in North America or Western Europe. Asian women have substantially lower concentrations of estrogens and progesterone. These differences cannot be explained on a genetic basis because Asian women living in a western environment have sex steroid hormone concentrations and risks identical to those of their western counterparts. These migrant women and more notably their daughters also differ markedly in height and weight from Asian women in Asia; height and weight are critical regulators of age of menarche and have substantial effects on plasma concentrations of estrogens.

The role of diet in breast cancer etiology is controversial. While there are associative links between total caloric and fat intake and breast cancer risk, the exact role of fat in the diet is unproven. Increased caloric intake contributes to breast cancer risk in multiple ways: earlier menarche, later age at menopause, and increased postmenopausal estrogen concentrations reflecting enhanced aromatase activities in fatty tissues. Moderate alcohol intake also increases the risk by an unknown mechanism. Folic acid supplementation appears to modify risk in women who use alcohol but is not additionally protective in abstainers. Recommendations favoring abstinence from alcohol must be weighed against other social pressures and the possible cardioprotective effect of moderate alcohol intake.

Understanding the potential role of exogenous hormones in breast cancer is of extraordinary importance because millions of American women regularly use oral contraceptives and postmenopausal hormone replacement therapy. The most credible meta-analyses of oral contraceptive use suggest that these agents cause little if any increased risk of breast cancer. By contrast, oral contraceptives offer a substantial protective effect against ovarian epithelial tumors and endometrial cancers. Far more controversial are the data surrounding HRT in postmenopausal women. Data from the Women's Health Initiative (WHI) trial showed in a prospectively randomized design that conjugated equine estrogens plus progestins increased the risk of breast cancer and adverse cardiovascular events but with decreases in bone fractures and colorectal cancer. On balance there were more negative events with HRT. A parallel WHI trial with >12,000 women enrolled testing conjugated estrogens alone (in women who have had hysterectomies) showed no significant increase in breast cancer incidence. A meta-analysis of nonrandomized HRT studies suggests that most of the previously attributed benefit of HRT can be accounted for by higher socioeconomic status among users, which is presumably associated with better access to health care and healthier behaviors. Certain potential benefits of HRT, such as a putative protective effect on cognition with age, were not assessed in WHI. HRT is an area of rapid reevaluation, but it would appear (at least from breast cancer and cardiovascular disease vantage points) that there are serious concerns about long-term HRT use. HRT in women previously diagnosed with breast cancer increases recurrence rates.

In addition to the other factors, radiation is a risk factor in younger women. Women who have been exposed before age 30 to radiation in the form of multiple fluoroscopies (200–300 cGy) or treatment for Hodgkin's disease (>3600 cGy) have a substantial increase in risk of breast cancer, whereas radiation exposure after age 30 appears to have a minimal carcinogenic effect on the breast.

EVALUATION OF BREAST MASSES IN MEN AND WOMEN

Because the breasts are a common site of potentially fatal malignancy in women and because they frequently provide clues to underlying systemic diseases in both men and women, examination of the breast is an essential part of the physical examination. Unfortunately, internists frequently do not examine breasts in men, and, in women, they are apt to defer this evaluation to gynecologists. Because of the plausible association between early detection and improved outcome, it is the duty of every physician to distinguish breast abnormalities at the earliest possible stage and to institute a diagnostic workup. Women should be trained in breast self-examination (BSE). Although breast cancer in men is unusual, unilateral lesions should be evaluated in the same manner as in women, with the recognition that gynecomastia in men can sometimes begin unilaterally and is often asymmetric.

Virtually all breast cancer is diagnosed by biopsy of a nodule detected either on a mammogram or by palpation. Algorithms have been developed to enhance the likelihood of diagnosing breast cancer and reduce the frequency of unnecessary biopsy (Fig. 86-1).

THE PALPABLE BREAST MASS

Women should be strongly encouraged to examine their breasts monthly. A potentially flawed study from China has suggested that BSE does not alter survival, but given its safety, the procedure should still be encouraged. At worst, this practice increases the likelihood of detecting a mass at a smaller size when it can be treated with more limited surgery. Breast examination by the physician should be performed in good light so as to see retractions and other skin changes. The nipple and areolae should be inspected, and an attempt should be made to elicit nipple discharge. All regional lymph node groups should be examined, and any lesions should be measured. Physical examination alone cannot exclude malignancy. Lesions with certain features are more likely to be cancerous (hard, irregular, tethered or fixed, or painless lesions). A negative mammogram in the presence of a persistent lump in the breast does not exclude malignancy. Palpable lesions require additional diagnostic procedures including biopsy.

In premenopausal women, lesions that are either equivocal or nonsuspicious on physical examination should be reexamined in 2–4 weeks, during the follicular phase of the menstrual cycle. Days 5–7 of the cycle are the best time for breast examination. A dominant mass in a postmenopausal woman or a dominant mass that persists through a menstrual cycle in a premenopausal woman should be aspirated by fine-needle biopsy or referred to a surgeon. If nonbloody fluid is aspirated, the diagnosis (cyst) and therapy have been accomplished together. Solid lesions that are persistent, recurrent, complex, or bloody cysts require mammography and biopsy, although in selected patients the so-called triple diagnostic techniques (palpation, mammography, aspiration) can be used to avoid biopsy (Figs. 86-1, 86-2, and 86-3). Ultrasound can be used in place of fine-needle aspiration to distinguish cysts from solid lesions. Not all solid masses are detected by ultrasound; thus, a palpable mass that is not visualized on ultrasound must be presumed to be solid.

Several points are essential in pursuing these management decision trees. First, risk-factor analysis is not part of the decision structure. No constellation of risk factors, by their presence or absence, can be used to exclude biopsy. Second, fine-needle aspiration should be used only in centers that have proven skill in obtaining such specimens and ana-

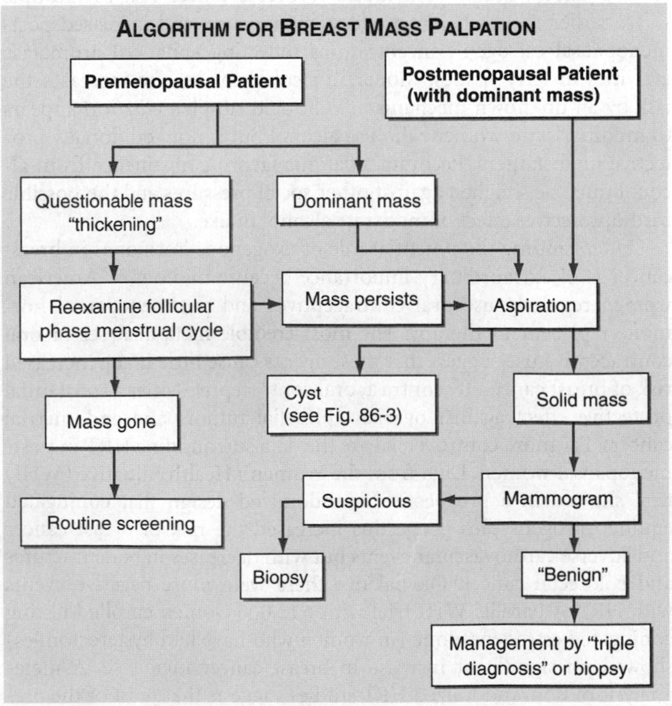

FIGURE 86-1 Approach to a palpable breast mass.

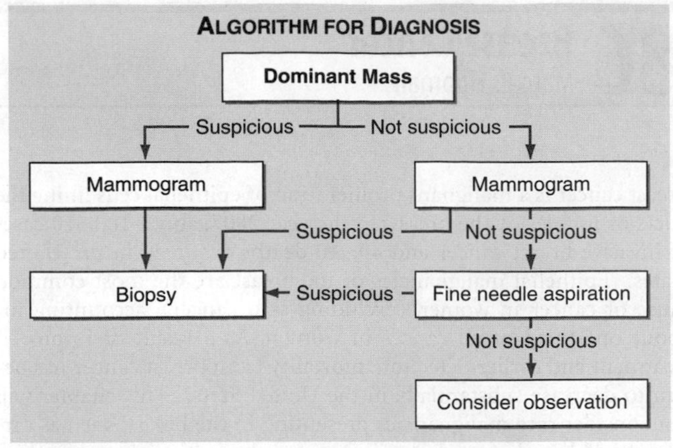

FIGURE 86-2 The "triple diagnosis" technique.

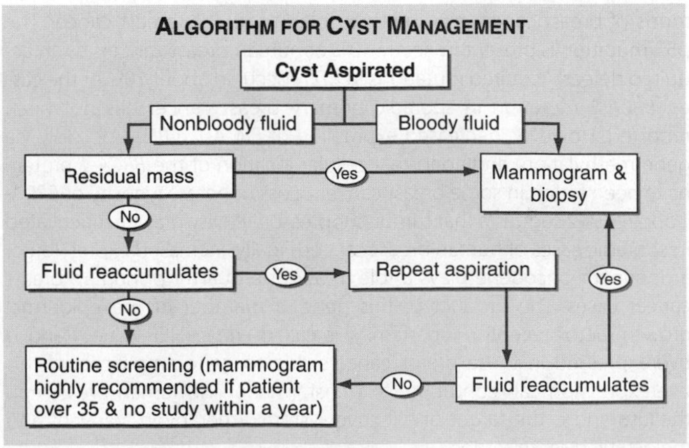

FIGURE 86-3 Management of a breast cyst.

lyzing them. The likelihood of cancer is low in the setting of a "triple negative" (benign-feeling lump, negative mammogram, and negative fine-needle aspiration), but it is not zero. The patient and physician must be aware of a 1% risk of false negatives. Third, additional technologies such as MRI, ultrasound, and sestamibi imaging cannot be used to exclude the need for biopsy, although in unusual circumstances they may provoke a biopsy.

THE ABNORMAL MAMMOGRAM

Diagnostic mammography should not be confused with *screening mammography*, which is performed after a palpable abnormality has been detected. Diagnostic mammography is aimed at evaluating the rest of the breast before biopsy is performed or occasionally is part of the triple-test strategy to exclude immediate biopsy.

Subtle abnormalities that are first detected by screening mammography should be evaluated carefully by compression or magnified views. These abnormalities include clustered microcalcifications, densities (especially if spiculated), and new or enlarging architectural distortion. For some nonpalpable lesions, ultrasound may be helpful either to identify cysts or to guide biopsy. If there is no palpable lesion and detailed mammographic studies are unequivocally benign, the patient should have routine follow-up appropriate to the patient's age.

If a nonpalpable mammographic lesion has a low index of suspicion, mammographic follow-up in 3–6 months is reasonable. Workup of indeterminate and suspicious lesions has been rendered more complex by the advent of stereotactic biopsies. Morrow and colleagues have suggested that these procedures are indicated for lesions that require biopsy but are likely to be benign—that is, for cases in which the procedure probably will eliminate additional surgery. When a lesion is more probably malignant, open biopsy should be performed with a needle localization technique. Others have proposed more widespread use of stereotactic core biopsies for nonpalpable lesions on economic grounds and because diagnosis leads to earlier treatment planning. However, stereotactic diagnosis of a malignant lesion does not eliminate the need for definitive surgical procedures, particularly if breast conservation is attempted. For example, after a breast biopsy with needle localization (i.e., local excision) of a stereotactically diagnosed malignancy, reexcision may still be necessary to achieve negative margins. To some extent, these issues are decided on the basis of referral pattern and the availability of the resources for stereotactic core biopsies. A reasonable approach is shown in Fig. 86-4.

BREAST MASSES IN THE PREGNANT OR LACTATING WOMAN

During pregnancy, the breast grows under the influence of estrogen, progesterone, prolactin, and human placental lactogen. Lactation is suppressed by progesterone, which blocks the effects of prolactin. After delivery, lactation is promoted by the fall in progesterone levels, which leaves the effects of prolactin unopposed. The development of a dominant mass during pregnancy or lactation should never be attributed to hormonal changes. A dominant mass must be treated with the same concern in a pregnant woman as any other. Breast cancer develops in 1 in every 3000–4000 pregnancies. Stage for stage, breast cancer in pregnant patients is no different from premenopausal breast cancer in nonpregnant patients. However, pregnant women often have more advanced disease because the significance of a breast mass was not fully considered and/or because of endogenous hormone stimulation. Persistent lumps in the breast of pregnant or lactating women *cannot* be attributed to benign changes based on physical findings; such patients should be promptly referred for diagnostic evaluation.

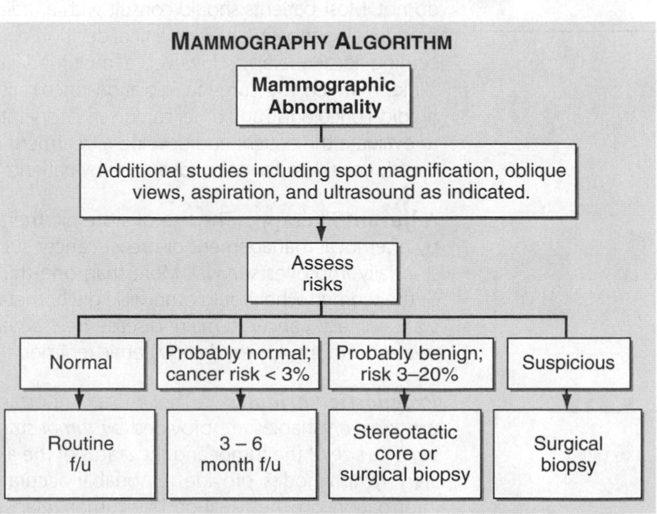

FIGURE 86-4 Approaches to abnormalities detected by mammogram. f/u, follow-up.

BENIGN BREAST MASSES

Only about 1 in every 5–10 breast biopsies leads to a diagnosis of cancer, although the rate of positive biopsies varies in different countries and clinical settings. (These differences may be related to interpretation, medicolegal considerations, and availability of mammograms.) The vast majority of benign breast masses are due to "fibrocystic" disease, a descriptive term for small fluid-filled cysts and modest epithelial cell and fibrous tissue hyperplasia. However, fibrocystic disease is a histologic, not a clinical, diagnosis, and women who have had a biopsy with benign findings are at greater risk of developing breast cancer than those who have not had a biopsy. The subset of women with ductal or lobular cell proliferation (about 30% of patients), particularly the small fraction (3%) with atypical hyperplasia, have a fourfold greater risk of developing breast cancer than unbiopsied women, and the increase in the risk is about ninefold for women in this category who also have an affected first-degree relative. Thus, careful follow-up of these patients is required. By contrast, patients with a benign biopsy without atypical hyperplasia are at little risk and may be followed routinely.

SCREENING

Breast cancer is virtually unique among the epithelial tumors in adults in that screening (in the form of annual mammography) improves survival. Meta-analysis examining outcomes from every randomized trial of mammography conclusively shows a 25–30% reduction in the chance of dying from breast cancer with annual screening after age 50; the data for women between ages 40 and 50 are almost as positive. While controversy continues to surround the assessment of screening mammography, the preponderance of data strongly supports the benefits of screening mammography. New analyses of older randomized studies have suggested that screening may not work. While the design defects in some older studies cannot be retrospectively corrected, most experts, including panels of the American Society of Clinical Oncology and the American Cancer Society, continue to believe that screening conveys substantial benefit. Furthermore, the profound drop in breast cancer mortality seen over the past decade is unlikely to be solely attributable to improvements in therapy. It seems prudent to recommend annual mammography for women past the age of 40. Although no randomized study of BSE has ever shown any improvement in survival, its major benefit is identification of tumors appropriate for conservative local therapy. Better mammographic technology, including digitized mammography, routine use of magnified views, and greater skill in mammographic interpretation, combined with newer diagnostic techniques (MRI, magnetic resonance spectroscopy, positron emission tomography, etc.) may make it possible to identify breast cancers even more reliably and earlier. Screening by any technique other than mammography is not indicated; however, younger women who are *BRCA-1* or *BRCA-2* carriers may benefit from MRI screening where the higher sensitivity may outweigh the loss of specificity.

STAGING

Correct staging of breast cancer patients is of extraordinary importance. Not only does it permit an accurate prognosis, but in many cases therapeutic decision-making is based largely on the TNM (primary tumor, regional nodes, metastasis) classification (Table 86-1). Comparison with historic series should be undertaken with caution, as the staging has changed several times in the past 20 years. The current staging is complex and results in significant changes in outcome by stage as compared with prior staging systems.

℞ BREAST CANCER

PRIMARY BREAST CANCER Breast-conserving treatments, consisting of the removal of the primary tumor by some form of lumpectomy with or without irradiating the breast, result in a survival that is as good as (or slightly superior to) that after extensive surgical procedures, such as mastectomy or modified radical mastectomy, with or without further irradiation. Postlumpectomy breast irradiation greatly reduces the risk of recurrence in the breast. While breast conservation is associated with a possibility of recurrence in the breast, 10-year survival is at least as good as that after more radical surgery. Postoperative radiation to regional nodes following mastectomy is also associated with an improvement in survival. Since radiation therapy can also reduce the rate of local or regional recurrence, it should be strongly considered following mastectomy for women with high-risk primary tumors (i.e., T2 in size, positive margins, positive nodes). At present, nearly one-third of women in the United States are managed by lumpectomy. Breast-conserving surgery is not suitable for all patients: it is not generally suitable for tumors >5 cm (or for smaller tumors if the breast is small), for tumors involving the nipple areola complex, for tumors with extensive intraductal disease involving multiple quadrants of the breast, for women with a history of collagen-vascular disease, and for women who either do not have the motivation for breast conservation or do not have convenient access to radiation therapy. However, these groups probably do not account for more than one-third of patients who are treated with mastectomy. Thus, a great many women still undergo mastectomy who could safely avoid this procedure and probably would if appropriately counseled.

An extensive intraductal component is a predictor of recurrence in the breast, and so are several clinical variables. Both axillary lymph node involvement and involvement of vascular or lymphatic channels by metastatic tumor in the breast are associated with a higher risk of relapse in the breast but are not contraindications to breast-conserving treatment. When these patients are excluded, and when lumpectomy with negative tumor margins is achieved, breast conservation is associated with a recurrence rate in the breast of substantially <10%. The survival of patients who have recurrence in the breast is somewhat worse than that of women who do not. Thus, recurrence in the breast is a negative prognostic variable for long-term survival. However, recurrence in the breast is not the *cause* of distant metastasis. If recurrence in the breast caused metastatic disease, then women treated with lumpectomy, who have a higher rate of recurrence in the breast, should have poorer survival than women treated with mastectomy, and they do not. Most patients should consult with a radiation oncologist before making a final decision concerning local therapy. However, a multimodality clinic in which the surgeon, radiation oncologist, medical oncologist, and other caregivers cooperate to evaluate the patient and develop a treatment is usually considered a major advantage by patients.

TABLE 86-1 STAGING OF BREAST CANCER

Primary Tumor (T)	
T0	No evidence of primary tumor
TIS	Carcinoma in situ
T1	Tumor ≤2 cm
T1a	Tumor >0.1 cm but ≤0.5 cm
T1b	Tumor >0.5 but ≤1 cm
T1c	Tumor >1 cm but ≤2 cm
T2	Tumor >2 cm but ≤5 cm
T3	Tumor >5 cm
T4	Extension to chest wall, inflammation, satellite lesions, ulcerations
Regional Lymph Nodes (N)	
PN0(i-)	No regional lymph node metastasis histologically, negative IHC
PN0(i+)	No regional lymph node metastasis histologically, positive IHC, no IHC cluster greater than 0.2 mm
PN0(mol-)	No regional lymph node metastasis histologically, negative molecular findings (RT-PCR)[a]
PN0(mol+)	No regional lymph node metastasis histologically, positive molecular findings (RT-PCR)[a]
PN1	Metastasis in one to three axillary lymph nodes, or in internal mammary nodes with microscopic disease detected by sentinal lymph node dissection but not clinically apparent
PN1mi	Micrometastasis (>0.2mm, none >2.0 mm)
PN1a	Metastasis in one to three axillary lymph nodes
PN1b	Metastasis in internal mammary nodes with microscopic disease detected by sentinel lymph node dissection but not *clinically apparent*[b]
PN1c	Metastasis in one to three axillary lymph nodes and in internal mammary lymph nodes with microscopic disease detected by sentinel lymph node dissection but not clinically apparent.[b] (If associated with greater than three positive axillary lymph nodes, the internal mammary nodes are classified as pN3b to reflect increased tumor burden.)
pN2	Metastasis in four to nine axillary lymph nodes, or in clinically apparent internal mammary lymph nodes in the *absence* of axillary lymph node metastasis
pN3	Metastasis in ten or more axillary lymph nodes, or in infraclavicular lymph nodes, or in clinically apparent[c] ipsilateral internal mammary lymph nodes in the *presence* of 1 or more positive axillary lymph nodes; or in more than 3 axillary lymph nodes with clinically negative microscopic metastasis in internal mammary lymph nodes; or in ipsilateral SCLNs
Distant Metastasis (M)	
M0	No distant metastasis
M1	Distant metastasis (includes spread to ipsilateral supraclavicular nodes)

Stage Grouping

Stage 0	TIS	N0	M0
Stage I	T1	N0	M0
Stage IIA	T0	N1	M0
	T1	N1	M0
	T2	N0	M0
Stage IIB	T2	N1	M0
	T3	N0	M0
Stage IIIA	T0	N2	M0
	T1	N2	M0
	T2	N2	M0
	T3	N1, N2	M0
Stage IIIB	T4	Any N	M0
	Any T	N3	M0
Stage IIIC	Any T	N3	M0
Stage IV	Any T	Any N	M1

[a]RT-PCR, reverse transcriptase/polymerase chain reaction.
[b]Clinically apparent is defined as detected by imaging studies (excluding lymphoscintigraphy) or by clinical examination.
[c]T1 includes T1mic.
Source: Used with permission of the American Joint Committee on Cancer (AJCC), Chicago, Illinois. The original source for this material is the AJCC Cancer Staging Manual, Sixth Edition (2002) published by Springer-New York, www.springeronline.com.

Adjuvant Therapy The use of systemic therapy after local management of breast cancer substantially improves survival. More than one-third of the women who would otherwise die of metastatic breast cancer remain disease-free when treated with the appropriate systemic regimen.

Prognostic Variables The most important prognostic variables are provided by *tumor staging*. The size of the tumor and the status of the axillary lymph nodes provide reasonably accurate information on the likelihood of tumor relapse. The relation of pathologic stage to 5-year survival is shown in Table 86-2. For most women, the need for adjuvant therapy can be readily defined

TABLE 86-2 5-YEAR SURVIVAL RATE FOR BREAST CANCER BY STAGE

Stage	5-Year Survival, %
0	99
I	92
IIA	82
IIB	65
IIIA	47
IIIB	44
IV	14

Source: Modified from data of the National Cancer Institute—Surveillance, Epidemiology, and End Results (SEER).

on this basis alone. In the absence of lymph node involvement, involvement of microvessels (either capillaries or lymphatic channels) in tumors is nearly equivalent to lymph node involvement. The greatest controversy concerns women with intermediate prognoses. *There is rarely justification for adjuvant chemotherapy in most women with tumors <1 cm in size whose axillary lymph nodes are negative.* Detection of breast cancer cells either in the circulation or bone marrow is associated with an increased relapse rate. The most exciting development in this area is the use of gene expression arrays to analyze patterns of tumor gene expression. Several groups have independently defined gene sets that reliably predict disease-free and overall survival far more accurately than any single prognostic variable. Their value is now being assessed in prospective randomized trials. In addition, gene sets capable of predicting responses to endocrine therapy and specific chemotherapeutic drugs have also been described.

Estrogen and progesterone receptor status are of prognostic significance. Tumors that lack either or both of these receptors are more likely to recur than tumors that have them.

Several *measures of tumor growth rate* correlate with early relapse. S-phase analysis using flow cytometry is the most accurate measure. Indirect S-phase assessments using antigens associated with the cell cycle, such as PCNA (Ki67), are also valuable. Tumors with a high proportion (more than the median) of cells in S phase pose a greater risk of relapse; chemotherapy offers the greatest survival benefit for these tumors. Assessment of DNA content in the form of ploidy is of modest value, with nondiploid tumors having a somewhat worse prognosis.

Histologic classification of the tumor has also been used as a prognostic factor. Tumors with a poor nuclear grade have a higher risk of recurrence than tumors with a good nuclear grade. Semiquantitative measures such as the Elston score improve the reproducibility of this measurement.

Molecular changes in the tumor are also useful. Tumors that overexpress *erbB2* (HER-2/neu) or have a mutated p53 gene have a worse prognosis. Particular interest has centered on *erbB2* overexpression as measured by histochemistry or by fluorescence in situ hybridization. Tumors that overexpress *erbB2* are more likely to respond to higher doses of doxorubicin-containing regimens and predict those tumors that will respond to HER-2/neu antibodies (trastuzumab) (herceptin) and a Her-2/neu kinase inhibitor.

To grow, tumors must generate a neovasculature (Chap. 80). The presence of more microvessels in a tumor, particularly when localized in so-called "hot spots," is associated with a worse prognosis. This may assume even greater significance in light of blood vessel–targeting therapies such as bevacizumab (avastin).

Other variables that have also been used to evaluate prognosis include proteins associated with invasiveness, such as type IV collagenase, cathepsin D, plasminogen activator, plasminogen activator receptor, and the metastasis-suppressor gene *nm23*. None of these has been widely accepted as a prognostic variable for therapeutic decision-making. One problem in interpreting these prognostic variables is that most of them have not been examined in a study using a large cohort of patients.

Adjuvant Regimens Adjuvant therapy is the use of systemic therapies in patients whose known disease has received local therapy but who are at risk of relapse. Selection of appropriate adjuvant chemotherapy or hormone therapy is highly controversial in some situations. Meta-analyses have helped to define broad limits for therapy but do not help in choosing optimal regimens or in choosing a regimen for certain subgroups of patients. A summary of recommendations is shown in Table 86-3. In general, premenopausal women for whom any form of adjuvant systemic therapy is indicated should receive multidrug chemotherapy. The antiestrogen tamoxifen improves survival in premenopausal patients with positive estrogen receptors and should be added following completion of chemotherapy. Prophylactic castration may also be associated with a substantial survival benefit (primarily in estrogen receptor–positive patients) but is not widely used in this country.

Data on postmenopausal women are also controversial. The impact of adjuvant chemotherapy is quantitatively less clear-cut than in premenopausal patients, although survival advantages have been shown. The first decision is whether chemotherapy or endocrine therapy should be used. While adjuvant tamoxifen improves survival regardless of axillary lymph node status, the improvement in survival is modest for patients in whom multiple lymph nodes are involved. For this reason, it has been usual to give chemotherapy to postmenopausal patients who have no medical contraindications and who have more than one positive lymph node; tamoxifen is commonly given simultaneously or subsequently. For postmenopausal women for whom systemic therapy is warranted but who have a more favorable prognosis, tamoxifen may be used as a single agent. Large clinical trials have shown superiority for aromatase inhibitors over tamoxifen alone in the adjuvant setting. Unfortunately the optimal plan is unclear. Tamoxifen for 5 years followed by an aromatase inhibitor, the reverse strategy, or even switching to an aromatase inhibitor after 2–3 years of tamoxifen has been shown to be better than tamoxifen alone. No valid information currently permits selection among the three clinically approved aromatase inhibitors. Large clinical trials currently underway will help address these questions.

Most comparisons of adjuvant chemotherapy regimens show little difference among them, although small advantages for doxorubicin-containing regimens are usually seen.

One approach—so-called neoadjuvant chemotherapy—involves the administration of adjuvant therapy before definitive surgery and radiation

TABLE 86-3 SUGGESTED APPROACHES TO ADJUVANT THERAPY

Age Group	Lymph Node Status[a]	Endocrine Receptor (ER) Status	Tumor	Recommendation
Premenopausal	Positive	Any	Any	Multidrug chemotherapy + tamoxifen if ER-positive + trastuzumab in HER-2/neu positive tumors
Premenopausal	Negative	Any	>2 cm, or 1–2 cm with other poor prognostic variables	Multidrug chemotherapy + tamoxifen if ER-positive + trastuzumab in HER-2/neu positive tumors
Postmenopausal	Positive	Negative	Any	Multidrug chemotherapy + trastuzumab in HER-2/neu positive tumors
Postmenopausal	Positive	Positive	Any	Aromatase inhibitors and tamoxifen with or without chemotherapy + trastuzumab in HER-2/neu positive tumors
Postmenopausal	Negative	Positive	>2 cm, or 1–2 cm with other poor prognostic variables	Aromatase inhibitors and tamoxifen + trastuzumab in HER-2/neu positive tumors
Postmenopausal	Negative	Negative	>2 cm, or 1–2 cm with other poor prognostic variables	Consider multidrug chemotherapy + trastuzumab in HER-2/neu positive tumors

[a]As determined by pathologic examination.

therapy. Because the objective response rates of patients with breast cancer to systemic therapy in this setting exceed 75%, many patients will be "downstaged" and may become candidates for breast-conserving therapy. However, overall survival has not been improved using this approach.

Other adjuvant treatments under investigation include the use of taxanes, such as paclitaxel and docetaxel, and therapy based on alternative kinetic and biologic models. In such approaches, high doses of single agents are used separately in relatively dose-intensive cycling regimens. Node-positive patients treated with doxorubicin-cyclophosphamide for four cycles followed by four cycles of a taxane have a substantial improvement in survival as compared with women receiving doxorubicin-cyclophosphamide alone, particularly in women with estrogen receptor–negative tumors. In addition, administration of the same drug combinations at the same dose but at more frequent intervals (q2 weeks with cytokine support as compared with the standard q3 weeks) is even more effective. Among the 25% of women whose tumors overexpress HER-2/neu, addition of trastuzumab given concurrently with a taxane and then for a year after chemotherapy produces significant improvement in survival. Though longer follow-up will be important, this is now the standard care for most women with HER-2/neu positive breast cancers. Cardiotoxicity, immediate and long-term, remains a concern, and further efforts to exploit nonanthracycline-containing regimens are being pursued. Very-high-dose therapy with stem cell transplantation in the adjuvant setting has not proved superior to standard dose therapy and should not be routinely used.

SYSTEMIC THERAPY OF METASTATIC DISEASE Nearly half of patients treated for apparently localized breast cancer develop metastatic disease. Although a small number of these patients enjoy long remissions when treated with combinations of systemic and local therapy, most eventually succumb to metastatic disease. Soft tissue, bony, and visceral (lung and liver) metastases each account for approximately one-third of sites of initial relapses. However, by the time of death, most patients will have bony involvement. Recurrences can appear at any time after primary therapy. Half of all initial cancer recurrences occur >5 years after initial therapy.

Because the diagnosis of metastatic disease alters the outlook for the patient so drastically, it should rarely be made without biopsy. Every oncologist has seen patients with tuberculosis, gallstones, sarcoidosis, or other nonmalignant diseases misdiagnosed and treated as though they had metastatic breast cancer or even second malignancies such as multiple myeloma thought to be recurrent breast cancer. This is a catastrophic mistake and justifies biopsy for virtually every patient at the time of initial suspicion of metastatic disease.

The choice of therapy requires consideration of local therapy needs, the overall medical condition of the patient, and the hormone receptor status of the tumor, as well as clinical judgment. Because therapy of systemic disease is palliative, the potential toxicities of therapies should be balanced against the response rates. Several variables influence the response to systemic therapy. For example, the presence of estrogen and progesterone receptors is a strong indication for endocrine therapy. On the other hand, patients with short disease-free intervals, rapidly progressive visceral disease, lymphangitic pulmonary disease, or intracranial disease are unlikely to respond to endocrine therapy.

In many cases, systemic therapy can be withheld while the patient is managed with appropriate local therapy. Radiation therapy and occasionally surgery are effective at relieving the symptoms of metastatic disease, particularly when bony sites are involved. Many patients with bone-only or bone-dominant disease have a relatively indolent course. Under such circumstances, systemic chemotherapy has a modest effect, whereas radiation therapy may be effective for long periods. Other systemic treatments, such as strontium 89 and/or bisphosphonates, may provide a palliative benefit without inducing objective responses. Most patients with metastatic disease and certainly all who have bone involvement should receive concurrent bisphosphonates. Since the goal of therapy is to maintain well-being for as long as possible, emphasis should be placed on avoiding the most hazardous complications of metastatic disease, including pathologic fracture of the axial skeleton and spinal cord compression. New back pain in patients with cancer should be explored aggressively on an emergent basis; to wait for neurologic symptoms is a potentially catastrophic error. Metastatic involvement of endocrine organs can cause profound dysfunction, including adrenal insufficiency and hypopituitarism. Similarly, obstruction of the biliary tree or other impaired organ function may be better managed with a local therapy than with a systemic approach.

TABLE 86-4 ENDOCRINE THERAPIES FOR BREAST CANCER

Therapy	Comments
Castration	For premenopausal women
Surgical	
LHRH agonists	
Antiestrogens	
Tamoxifen	Useful in pre- and postmenopausal women
"Pure" antiestrogens	Responses in tamoxifen-resistant and aromatase inhibitor resistant patients
Surgical adrenalectomy	Rarely employed second-line choice
Aromatase inhibitors	Low toxicity; now first choice for metastatic disease
High-dose progestogens	Common fourth-line choice after AIs, tamoxifen and fulvestrant
Hypophysectomy	Rarely used
Additive androgens or estrogens	Plausible fourth-line therapies; potentially toxic

Note: LHRH, luteinizing hormone–releasing hormone.

Endocrine Therapy Normal breast tissue is estrogen-dependent. Both primary and metastatic breast cancer may retain this phenotype. The best means of ascertaining whether a breast cancer is hormone-dependent is through analysis of estrogen and progesterone receptor levels on the tumor. Tumors that are positive for the estrogen receptor and negative for the progesterone receptor have a response rate of ~30%. Tumors that have both receptors have a response rate approaching 70%. If neither receptor is present, the objective response rates are <10%. Receptor analyses provide information as to the correct ordering of endocrine therapies as opposed to chemotherapy. Because of their lack of toxicity and because some patients whose receptor analyses are reported as negative respond to endocrine therapy, an endocrine treatment should be attempted in virtually every patient with metastatic breast cancer. Potential endocrine therapies are summarized in Table 86-4. The choice of endocrine therapy is usually determined by toxicity profile and availability. In most patients, the initial endocrine therapy should be an aromatase inhibitor rather than tamoxifen. For the subset of women who are ER positive but also HER-2/neu positive, response rates to aromatase inhibitors are very substantially higher than to tamoxifen. Newer "pure" antiestrogens that are free of agonistic effects are also in clinical trial. Cases in which tumors shrink in response to tamoxifen withdrawal (as well as withdrawal of pharmacologic doses of estrogens) have been reported. Endogenous estrogen formation may be blocked by analogues of luteinizing hormone–releasing hormone in premenopausal women. Additive endocrine therapies, including treatment with progestogens, estrogens, and androgens, may also be tried in patients who respond to initial endocrine therapy; the mechanism of action of these latter therapies is unknown. Patients who respond to one endocrine therapy have at least a 50% chance of responding to a second endocrine therapy. It is not uncommon for patients to respond to two or three sequential endocrine therapies; however, combination endocrine therapies do not appear to be superior to individual agents, and combinations of chemotherapy with endocrine therapy are not useful. The median survival of patients with metastatic disease is approximately 2 years, and many patients, particularly older persons and those with hormone-dependent disease, may respond to endocrine therapy for 3–5 years or longer.

Chemotherapy Unlike many other epithelial malignancies, breast cancer responds to multiple chemotherapeutic agents, including anthracyclines, alkylating agents, taxanes, and antimetabolites. Multiple combinations of these agents have been found to improve response rates somewhat, but they have had little effect on duration of response or survival. The choice among multidrug combinations frequently depends on whether adjuvant chemotherapy was administered and, if so, what type. While patients treated with adjuvant regimens such as cyclophosphamide, methotrexate, and fluorouracil (CMF regimens) may subsequently respond to the same combination in the metastatic disease setting, most oncologists use drugs to which the patients have not been previously exposed. Once patients have progressed after combination drug therapy, it is most common to treat them with single agents. Given the significant toxicity of most drugs, the use of a single effective agent will minimize toxicity by sparing the patient exposure to drugs that would be of little value. No method to select the drugs most efficacious for a given patient has been demonstrated to be useful.

Most oncologists use either an anthracycline or paclitaxel following failure with the initial regimen. However, the choice has to be balanced with individual needs. One randomized study has suggested docetaxel may be superior to paclitaxel. A nanoparticle formulation of paclitaxel (abraxane) has also shown promise.

The use of a humanized antibody to *erbB2* [trastuzumab (Herceptin)] combined with paclitaxel can improve response rate and survival for women whose metastatic tumors overexpress *erbB2*. The magnitude of the survival extension is modest in patients with metastatic disease. Similarly, the use of bevacizumab (avastin) has improved the response rate and response duration to paclitaxel. Objective responses in previously treated patients may also be seen with gemcitabine, capecitabine, navelbine, and oral etoposide.

High-Dose Chemotherapy Including Autologous Bone Marrow Transplantation Autologous bone marrow transplantation combined with high doses of single agents can produce objective responses even in heavily pretreated patients. However, such responses are rarely durable and do not alter the clinical course for most patients with advanced metastatic disease.

STAGE III BREAST CANCER Between 10 and 25% of patients present with so-called locally advanced, or stage III, breast cancer at diagnosis. Many of these cancers are technically operable, whereas others, particularly cancers with chest wall involvement, inflammatory breast cancers, or cancers with large matted axillary lymph nodes, cannot be managed with surgery initially. Although no randomized trials have proved the efficacy of neoadjuvant chemotherapy, this approach has gained widespread use. More than 90% of patients with locally advanced breast cancer show a partial or better response to multidrug chemotherapy regimens that include an anthracycline. Early administration of this treatment reduces the bulk of the disease and frequently makes the patient a suitable candidate for salvage surgery and/or radiation therapy. These patients should be managed in multimodality clinics to coordinate surgery, radiation therapy, and systemic chemotherapy. Such approaches produce long-term disease-free survival in about 30–50% of patients.

BREAST CANCER PREVENTION Women who have one breast cancer are at risk of developing a contralateral breast cancer at a rate of approximately 0.5% per year. When adjuvant tamoxifen is administered to these patients, the rate of development of contralateral breast cancers is reduced. In other tissues of the body, tamoxifen has estrogen-like effects that are beneficial: preservation of bone mineral density and long-term lowering of cholesterol. However, tamoxifen has estrogen-like effects on the uterus, leading to an increased risk of uterine cancer (0.75% incidence after 5 years on tamoxifen). Tamoxifen also increases the risk of cataract formation. The Breast Cancer Prevention Trial (BCPT) revealed a >49% reduction in breast cancer among women with a risk of at least 1.66% taking the drug for 5 years. Raloxifene has shown similar breast cancer prevention potency but may have different effects on bone and heart. The two agents have been compared in a prospective randomized prevention trial (the STAR trial). The agents are approximately equivalent in preventing breast cancer with fewer thromboembolic events and endometrial cancers with raloxifene; however, raloxifene did not reduce noninvasive cancers as effectively as tamoxifen, so no clear winner has emerged.

NONINVASIVE BREAST CANCER Breast cancer develops as a series of molecular changes in the epithelial cells that lead to ever more malignant behavior. Increased use of mammography has led to more frequent diagnosis of noninvasive breast cancer. These lesions fall into two groups: ductal carcinoma in situ (DCIS) and lobular carcinoma in situ (lobular neoplasia). The management of both entities is controversial.

Ductal Carcinoma In Situ (DCIS) Proliferation of cytologically malignant breast epithelial cells within the ducts is termed *DCIS*. Atypical hyperplasia may be difficult to differentiate from DCIS. At least one-third of patients with untreated DCIS develop invasive breast cancer within 5 years. For many years, the standard treatment for this disease was mastectomy. However, treatment of this condition by lumpectomy and radiation therapy gives survival that is as good as the survival for invasive breast cancer treated by mastectomy. In one randomized trial, the combination of wide excision plus irradiation for DCIS caused a substantial reduction in the local recurrence rate as compared with wide excision alone with negative margins, though survival was identical in the two arms. No studies have compared either of these regimens to mastectomy. Addition of tamoxifen to any DCIS surgical/radiation therapy regimen further improves local control. Data for aromatase inhibitors in this setting are not available.

Several prognostic features may help to identify patients at high risk for local recurrence after either lumpectomy alone or lumpectomy with radiation therapy. These include extensive disease; age <40; and cytologic features such as necrosis, poor nuclear grade, and comedo subtype with overexpression of *erbB2*. Some data suggest that adequate excision with careful determination of pathologically clear margins is associated with a low recurrence rate. When surgery is combined with radiation therapy, recurrence (which is usually in the same quadrant) occurs with a frequency of ≤10%. Given the fact that half of these recurrences will be invasive, about 5% of the initial cohort will eventually develop invasive breast cancer. A reasonable expectation of mortality for these patients is about 1%, a figure that approximates the mortality rate for DCIS managed by mastectomy. Although this train of reasoning has not formally been proved valid, it is reasonable to recommend that patients who desire breast preservation, and in whom DCIS appears to be reasonably localized, be managed by adequate surgery with meticulous pathologic evaluation, followed by breast irradiation and tamoxifen. For patients with localized DCIS, axillary lymph node dissection is unnecessary. More controversial is the question of what management is optimal when there is any degree of invasion. Because of a significant likelihood (10–15%) of axillary lymph node involvement even when the primary lesion shows only microscopic invasion, it is prudent to do at least a level 1 and 2 axillary lymph node dissection for all patients with any degree of invasion; sentinel node biopsy may be substituted. Further management is dictated by the presence of nodal spread.

Lobular Neoplasia Proliferation of cytologically malignant cells within the lobules is termed *lobular neoplasia*. Nearly 30% of patients who have had adequate local excision of the lesion develop breast cancer (usually infiltrating ductal carcinoma) over the next 15–20 years. Ipsilateral and contralateral cancers are equally common. Therefore, lobular neoplasia may be a premalignant lesion that suggests an elevated risk of subsequent breast cancer, rather than a form of malignancy itself, and aggressive local management seems unreasonable. Most patients should be treated with tamoxifen for 5 years and followed with careful annual mammography and semiannual physical examinations. Additional molecular analysis of these lesions may make it possible to discriminate between patients who are at risk of further progression and require additional therapy and those in whom simple follow-up is adequate.

MALE BREAST CANCER Breast cancer is about 1/150th as frequent in men as in women; 1720 men developed breast cancer in 2006. It usually presents as a unilateral lump in the breast and is frequently not diagnosed promptly. Given the small amount of soft tissue and the unexpected nature of the problem, locally advanced presentations are somewhat more common. When male breast cancer is matched to female breast cancer by age and stage, its overall prognosis is identical. Although gynecomastia may initially be unilateral or asymmetric, any unilateral mass in a man over the age of 40 should receive a careful workup including biopsy. On the other hand, bilateral symmetric breast development rarely represents breast cancer and is almost invariably due to endocrine disease or a drug effect. It should be kept in mind, nevertheless, that the risk of cancer is much greater in men with gynecomastia; in such men, gross asymmetry of the breasts should arouse suspicion of cancer. Male breast cancer is best managed by mastectomy and axillary lymph node dissection (modified radical mastectomy). Patients with locally advanced disease or positive nodes should also be treated with irradiation. Approximately 90% of male breast cancers contain estrogen receptors, and approximately 60% of cases with metastatic disease respond to endocrine therapy. No randomized studies have evaluated adjuvant therapy for male breast cancer. Two historic experiences suggest that the disease responds well to adjuvant systemic therapy, and, if not medically contraindicated, the same criteria for the use of adjuvant therapy in women should be applied to men.

The sites of relapse and spectrum of response to chemotherapeutic drugs are virtually identical for breast cancers in either sex.

FOLLOW-UP OF BREAST CANCER PATIENTS

Despite the availability of sophisticated and expensive imaging techniques and a wide range of serum tumor marker tests, survival is not

TABLE 86-5 BREAST CANCER SURVEILLANCE GUIDELINES

Test	Frequency
Recommended	
History; eliciting symptoms; physical examination	q3–6 months × 3 years; q6–12 months × 2 years; then annually
Breast self-examination	Monthly
Mammography	Annually
Pelvic examination	Annually
Patient education about symptoms of recurrence	Ongoing
Coordination of care	Ongoing
Not Recommended	
Complete blood count	
Serum chemistry studies	
Chest radiographs	
Bone scans	
Ultrasound examination of the liver	
Computed tomography of chest, abdomen, or pelvis	
Tumor marker CA 15-3, CA 27-29	
Tumor marker CEA	

Source: *Recommended Breast Cancer Surveillance Guidelines,* ASCO Education Book, Fall, 1997.

influenced by early diagnosis of relapse. Surveillance guidelines are given in Table 86-5.

FURTHER READINGS

BREAST INTERNATIONAL GROUP (BIG) 1-98 COLLABORATIVE GROUP: A comparison of letrozole and tamoxifen in postmenopausal women with early breast cancer. N Engl J Med 353:2747, 2005

CITRON ML et al: Randomized trial of dose-dense versus conventionally scheduled and sequential versus concurrent combination chemotherapy as postoperative adjuvant treatment of node-positive primary breast cancer: First report of intergroup trial C9741/cancer and leukemia group B trial 9741. J Clin Oncol 21:1431, 2003

CLEATOR S et al: Triple-negative breast cancer: Therapeutic options. Lancet Oncol 8:235, 2007

EARLY BREAST CANCER TRIALISTS' COLLABORATIVE GROUP: Effects of chemotherapy and hormonal therapy for early breast cancer on recurrence and 15-year survival: An overview of the randomised trials. Lancet 365:1687, 2005

———: Effects of radiotherapy and of differences in the extent of surgery for early breast cancer on local recurrence and 15-year survival: An overview of the randomised trials. Lancet 366:2087, 2005

GIORDANO S et al: Breast cancer in men. Ann Intern Med 137:678, 2002

INGLE JN et al: Fulvestrant in women with advanced breast cancer after progression on prior aromatase inhibitor therapy: North central cancer treatment group trial N0032. J Clin Oncol 24:1052, 2006

JAKESZ R et al: Switching of postmenopausal women with endocrine-responsive early breast cancer to anastrozole after 2 years' adjuvant tamoxifen: Combined results of ABCSG trial 8 and ARNO 95 trial. Lancet 366:455, 2005

PARTRIDGE A, SCHAPIRA L: Pregnancy and breast cancer. Oncology 19:693, 2005

ROMOND EH et al: Trastuzumab plus adjuvant chemotherapy for operable HER2-positive breast cancer. N Engl J Med 353:1673, 2005

SANTEN RJ, MANSEL R: Benign breast disorders. N Engl J Med 353:275, 2005

SHAPIRO CL, WINER EL (eds): Late effects of treatment and survivorship issues in early-stage breast cancer. Sem Oncol 30:729, 2003

87 Gastrointestinal Tract Cancer

Robert J. Mayer

The gastrointestinal tract is the second most common noncutaneous site for cancer and the second major cause of cancer-related mortality in the United States.

ESOPHAGEAL CANCER

INCIDENCE AND ETIOLOGY

Cancer of the esophagus is a relatively uncommon but extremely lethal malignancy. The diagnosis was made in 15,560 Americans in 2007 and led to 13,940 deaths. Worldwide, the incidence of esophageal cancer varies strikingly. It occurs frequently within a geographic region extending from the southern shore of the Caspian Sea on the west to northern China on the east and encompassing parts of Iran, Central Asia, Afghanistan, Siberia, and Mongolia. High-incidence "pockets" of the disease are also present in such disparate locations as Finland, Iceland, Curaçao, southeastern Africa, and northwestern France. In North America and western Europe, the disease is more common in blacks than whites and in males than females; it appears most often after age 50 and seems to be associated with a lower socioeconomic status.

A variety of causative factors have been implicated in the development of the disease (Table 87-1). In the United States, esophageal cancer cases are either squamous cell carcinomas or adenocarcinomas. The etiology of squamous cell esophageal cancer is related to excess alcohol consumption and/or cigarette smoking. The relative risk increases with the amount of tobacco smoked or alcohol consumed, with these factors acting synergistically. The consumption of whiskey is linked to a higher incidence than the consumption of wine or beer. Squamous cell esophageal carcinoma has also been associated with the ingestion of nitrites, smoked opiates, and fungal toxins in pickled vegetables, as well as mucosal damage caused by such physical insults as long-term exposure to extremely hot tea, the ingestion of lye, radiation-induced strictures, and chronic achalasia. The presence of an esophageal web in association with glossitis and iron deficiency (i.e., Plummer-Vinson or Paterson-Kelly syndrome) and congenital hyperkeratosis and pitting of the palms and soles (i.e., tylosis palmaris et plantaris) have each been linked with squamous cell esophageal cancer, as have dietary deficiencies of molybdenum, zinc, and vitamin A.

TABLE 87-1 SOME ETIOLOGIC FACTORS BELIEVED TO BE ASSOCIATED WITH ESOPHAGEAL CANCER

- Excess alcohol consumption
- Cigarette smoking
- Other ingested carcinogens
  - Nitrates (converted to nitrites)
  - Smoked opiates
  - Fungal toxins in pickled vegetables
- Mucosal damage from physical agents
  - Hot tea
  - Lye ingestion
  - Radiation-induced strictures
  - Chronic achalasia
- Host susceptibility
  - Esophageal web with glossitis and iron deficiency (i.e., Plummer-Vinson or Paterson-Kelly syndrome)
  - Congenital hyperkeratosis and pitting of the palms and soles (i.e., tylosis palmaris et plantaris)
- ? Dietary deficiencies molybdenum, zinc, vitamin A
- ? Celiac sprue
- Chronic gastric reflux (i.e., Barrett's esophagus) for adenocarcinoma

For unclear reasons, the incidence of squamous cell esophageal cancer has decreased somewhat in both the black and white population in the United States over the past 30 years, while the rate of adenocarcinoma has risen dramatically, particularly in white males. Adenocarcinomas arise in the distal esophagus in the presence of chronic gastric reflux and gastric metaplasia of the epithelium (Barrett's esophagus), which is more common in obese persons. Adenocarcinomas arise within dysplastic columnar epithelium in the distal esophagus. Even before frank neoplasia is detectable, aneuploidy and p53 mutations are found in the dysplastic epithelium. These adenocarcinomas behave clinically like gastric adenocarcinoma and now account for >60% of esophageal cancers.

CLINICAL FEATURES

About 10% of esophageal cancers occur in the upper third of the esophagus (cervical esophagus), 35% in the middle third, and 55% in the lower third. Squamous cell carcinomas and adenocarcinomas cannot be distinguished radiographically or endoscopically.

Progressive dysphagia and weight loss of short duration are the initial symptoms in the vast majority of patients. Dysphagia initially occurs with solid foods and gradually progresses to include semisolids and liquids. By the time these symptoms develop, the disease is usually incurable, since difficulty in swallowing does not occur until >60% of the esophageal circumference is infiltrated with cancer. Dysphagia may be associated with pain on swallowing (odynophagia), pain radiating to the chest and/or back, regurgitation or vomiting, and aspiration pneumonia. The disease most commonly spreads to adjacent and supraclavicular lymph nodes, liver, lungs, pleura, and bone. Tracheoesophageal fistulas may develop as the disease advances, leading to severe suffering. As with other squamous cell carcinomas, hypercalcemia may occur in the absence of osseous metastases, probably from parathormone-related peptide secreted by tumor cells (Chap. 96).

DIAGNOSIS

Attempts at endoscopic and cytologic screening for carcinoma in patients with Barrett's esophagus, while effective as a means of detecting high-grade dysplasia, have not yet been shown to improve the prognosis in individuals found to have a carcinoma. Routine contrast radiographs effectively identify esophageal lesions large enough to cause symptoms. In contrast to benign esophageal leiomyomas, which result in esophageal narrowing with preservation of a normal mucosal pattern, esophageal carcinomas show ragged, ulcerating changes in the mucosa in association with deeper infiltration, producing a picture resembling achalasia. Smaller, potentially resectable tumors are often poorly visualized despite technically adequate esophagograms. Because of this, esophagoscopy should be performed in all patients suspected of having an esophageal abnormality, to visualize the tumor and to obtain histopathologic confirmation of the diagnosis. Because the population of persons at risk for squamous cell carcinoma of the esophagus (i.e., smokers and drinkers) also has a high rate of cancers of the lung and the head and neck region, endoscopic inspection of the larynx, trachea, and bronchi should also be done. A thorough examination of the fundus of the stomach (by retroflexing the endoscope) is imperative as well. Endoscopic biopsies of esophageal tumors fail to recover malignant tissue in one-third of cases because the biopsy forceps cannot penetrate deeply enough through normal mucosa pushed in front of the carcinoma. Cytologic examination of tumor brushings complements standard biopsies and should be performed routinely. The extent of tumor spread to the mediastinum and para-aortic lymph nodes should be assessed by CT scans of the chest and abdomen and by endoscopic ultrasound. Positron emission tomography scanning provides a useful assessment of resectability, offering accurate information regarding spread to mediastinal lymph nodes.

℞ ESOPHAGEAL CANCER

The prognosis for patients with esophageal carcinoma is poor. Fewer than 5% of patients survive 5 years after the diagnosis; thus, management focuses on symptom control. Surgical resection of all gross tumor (i.e., total resection) is feasible in only 45% of cases, with residual tumor cells frequently present at the resection margins. Such esophagectomies have been associated with a postoperative mortality rate of 5–10% due to anastomotic fistulas, subphrenic abscesses, and respiratory complications. About 20% of patients who survive a total resection live 5 years. The efficacy of primary radiation therapy (5500–6000 cGy) for squamous cell carcinomas is similar to that of radical surgery, sparing patients perioperative morbidity but often resulting in less satisfactory palliation of obstructive symptoms. The evaluation of chemotherapeutic agents in patients with esophageal carcinoma has been hampered by ambiguity in the definition of "response" and the debilitated physical condition of many treated individuals. Nonetheless, significant reductions in the size of measurable tumor masses have been reported in 15–25% of patients given single-agent treatment and in 30–60% of patients treated with drug combinations that include cisplatin. Combination chemotherapy and radiation therapy as the initial therapeutic approach, either alone or followed by an attempt at operative resection, seems to be beneficial. When administered along with radiation therapy, chemotherapy produces a better survival outcome than radiation therapy alone. The use of preoperative chemotherapy and radiation therapy followed by esophageal resection appears to prolong survival as compared with controls in small, randomized trials, and some reports suggest that no additional benefit accrues when surgery is added if significant shrinkage of tumor has been achieved by the chemoradiation combination.

For the incurable, surgically unresectable patient with esophageal cancer, dysphagia, malnutrition, and the management of tracheoesophageal fistulas are major issues. Approaches to palliation include repeated endoscopic dilatation, the surgical placement of a gastrostomy or jejunostomy for hydration and feeding, and endoscopic placement of an expansive metal stent to bypass the tumor. Endoscopic fulguration of the obstructing tumor with lasers is the most promising of these techniques.

TUMORS OF THE STOMACH

GASTRIC ADENOCARCINOMA

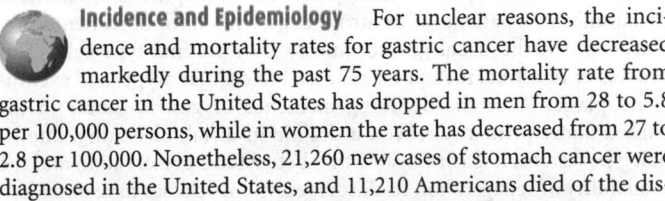

Incidence and Epidemiology For unclear reasons, the incidence and mortality rates for gastric cancer have decreased markedly during the past 75 years. The mortality rate from gastric cancer in the United States has dropped in men from 28 to 5.8 per 100,000 persons, while in women the rate has decreased from 27 to 2.8 per 100,000. Nonetheless, 21,260 new cases of stomach cancer were diagnosed in the United States, and 11,210 Americans died of the disease in 2007. Gastric cancer incidence has decreased worldwide but remains high in Japan, China, Chile, and Ireland.

The risk of gastric cancer is greater among lower socioeconomic classes. Migrants from high- to low-incidence nations maintain their susceptibility to gastric cancer, while the risk for their offspring approximates that of the new homeland. These findings suggest that an environmental exposure, probably beginning early in life, is related to the development of gastric cancer, with dietary carcinogens considered the most likely factor(s).

Pathology About 85% of stomach cancers are adenocarcinomas, with 15% due to lymphomas and gastrointestinal stromal tumors (GIST) and leiomyosarcomas. Gastric adenocarcinomas may be subdivided into two categories: a *diffuse type*, in which cell cohesion is absent, so that individual cells infiltrate and thicken the stomach wall without forming a discrete mass; and an *intestinal type*, characterized by cohesive neoplastic cells that form glandlike tubular structures. The diffuse carcinomas occur more often in younger patients, develop throughout the stomach (including the cardia), result in a loss of distensibility of the gastric wall (so-called linitis plastica, or "leather bottle" appearance), and carry a poorer prognosis. Intestinal-type lesions are frequently ulcerative, more commonly appear in the antrum and lesser curvature of the stomach, and are often preceded by a prolonged precancerous process. While the incidence of diffuse carcinomas is similar in most populations, the intestinal type tends to predominate in the high-risk geographic regions and is less likely to be found in areas where the frequency of gastric cancer is declining. Thus, different etiologic factor(s) may be involved in these

TABLE 87-2 NITRATE-CONVERTING BACTERIA AS A FACTOR IN THE CAUSATION OF GASTRIC CARCINOMA[a]

Exogenous sources of nitrate-converting bacteria:
Bacterially contaminated food (common in lower socioeconomic classes, who have a higher incidence of the disease; diminished by improved food preservation and refrigeration)
? *Helicobacter pylori* infection
Endogenous factors favoring growth of nitrate-converting bacteria in the stomach:
Decreased gastric acidity
Prior gastric surgery (antrectomy) (15- to 20-year latency period)
Atrophic gastritis and/or pernicious anemia
? Prolonged exposure to histamine H_2-receptor antagonists

[a]Hypothesis: Dietary nitrates are converted to carcinogenic nitrites by bacteria.

two subtypes. In the United States, ~30% of gastric cancers originate in the distal stomach, ~20% arise in the midportion of the stomach, and ~37% originate in the proximal third of the stomach. The remaining 13% involve the entire stomach.

Etiology The long-term ingestion of high concentrations of nitrates in dried, smoked, and salted foods appears to be associated with a higher risk. The nitrates are thought to be converted to carcinogenic nitrites by bacteria (Table 87-2). Such bacteria may be introduced exogenously through the ingestion of partially decayed foods, which are consumed in abundance worldwide by the lower socioeconomic classes. Bacteria such as *Helicobacter pylori* may also contribute to this effect by causing chronic gastritis, loss of gastric acidity, and bacterial growth in the stomach. The effect of *H. pylori* eradication on the subsequent risk for gastric cancer in high-incidence areas is under investigation. Loss of acidity may occur when acid-producing cells of the gastric antrum have been removed surgically to control benign peptic ulcer disease or when achlorhydria, atrophic gastritis, and even pernicious anemia develop in the elderly. Serial endoscopic examinations of the stomach in patients with atrophic gastritis have documented replacement of the usual gastric mucosa by intestinal-type cells. This process of intestinal metaplasia may lead to cellular atypia and eventual neoplasia. Since the declining incidence of gastric cancer in the United States primarily reflects a decline in distal, ulcerating, intestinal-type lesions, it is conceivable that better food preservation and the availability of refrigeration to all socioeconomic classes have decreased the dietary ingestion of exogenous bacteria. *H. pylori* has not been associated with the diffuse, more proximal form of gastric carcinoma.

Several additional etiologic factors have been associated with gastric carcinoma. Gastric ulcers and adenomatous polyps have occasionally been linked, but data on a cause-and-effect relationship are unconvincing. The inadequate clinical distinction between benign gastric ulcers and small ulcerating carcinomas may, in part, account for this presumed association. The presence of extreme hypertrophy of gastric rugal folds (i.e., Ménétrier's disease), giving the impression of polypoid lesions, has been associated with a striking frequency of malignant transformation; such hypertrophy, however, does not represent the presence of true adenomatous polyps. Individuals with blood group A have a higher incidence of gastric cancer than persons with blood group O; this observation may be related to differences in the mucous secretion, leading to altered mucosal protection from carcinogens. A germline mutation in the E-cadherin gene, inherited in an autosomal dominant pattern and coding for a cell adhesion protein, has been linked to a high incidence of occult gastric cancers in young asymptomatic carriers. Duodenal ulcers are not associated with gastric cancer.

Clinical Features Gastric cancers, when superficial and surgically curable, usually produce no symptoms. As the tumor becomes more extensive, patients may complain of an insidious upper abdominal discomfort varying in intensity from a vague, postprandial fullness to a severe, steady pain. Anorexia, often with slight nausea, is very common but is not the usual presenting complaint. Weight loss may eventually be observed, and nausea and vomiting are particularly prominent with tumors of the pylorus; dysphagia and early satiety may be the major symptoms caused by diffuse lesions originating in the cardia. There are no early physical signs. A palpable abdominal mass indicates long-standing growth and predicts regional extension.

Gastric carcinomas spread by direct extension through the gastric wall to the perigastric tissues, occasionally adhering to adjacent organs such as the pancreas, colon, or liver. The disease also spreads via lymphatics or by seeding of peritoneal surfaces. Metastases to intraabdominal and supraclavicular lymph nodes occur frequently, as do metastatic nodules to the ovary (Krukenberg's tumor), periumbilical region ("Sister Mary Joseph node"), or peritoneal cul-de-sac (Blumer's shelf palpable on rectal or vaginal examination); malignant ascites may also develop. The liver is the most common site for hematogenous spread of tumor.

The presence of iron-deficiency anemia in men and of occult blood in the stool in both sexes mandates a search for an occult gastrointestinal tract lesion. A careful assessment is of particular importance in patients with atrophic gastritis or pernicious anemia. Unusual clinical features associated with gastric adenocarcinomas include migratory thrombophlebitis, microangiopathic hemolytic anemia, and acanthosis nigricans.

Diagnosis A double-contrast radiographic examination is the simplest diagnostic procedure for the evaluation of a patient with epigastric complaints. The use of double-contrast techniques helps to detect small lesions by improving mucosal detail. The stomach should be distended at some time during every radiographic examination, since decreased distensibility may be the only indication of a diffuse infiltrative carcinoma. Although gastric ulcers can be detected fairly early, distinguishing benign from malignant lesions radiographically is difficult. The anatomic location of an ulcer is not in itself an indication of the presence or absence of a cancer.

Gastric ulcers that appear benign by radiography present special problems. Some physicians believe that gastroscopy is not mandatory if the radiographic features are typically benign, if complete healing can be visualized by x-ray within 6 weeks, and if a follow-up contrast radiograph obtained several months later shows a normal appearance. However, we recommend gastroscopic biopsy and brush cytology for all patients with a gastric ulcer in order to exclude a malignancy. Malignant gastric ulcers must be recognized before they penetrate into surrounding tissues, because the rate of cure of early lesions limited to the mucosa or submucosa is >80%. Since gastric carcinomas are difficult to distinguish clinically or radiographically from gastric lymphomas, endoscopic biopsies should be made as deeply as possible, due to the submucosal location of lymphoid tumors.

The staging system for gastric carcinoma is shown in Table 87-3.

Rx GASTRIC ADENOCARCINOMA

Complete surgical removal of the tumor with resection of adjacent lymph nodes offers the only chance for cure. However, this is possible in less than a third of patients. A subtotal gastrectomy is the treatment of choice for patients with distal carcinomas, while total or near-total gastrectomies are required for more proximal tumors. The inclusion of extended lymph node dissection in these procedures appears to confer an added risk for complications without enhancing survival. The prognosis following complete surgical resection depends on the degree of tumor penetration into the stomach wall and is adversely influenced by regional lymph node involvement, vascular invasion, and abnormal DNA content (i.e., aneuploidy), characteristics found in the vast majority of American patients. As a result, the probability of survival after 5 years for the 25–30% of patients able to undergo complete resection is ~20% for distal tumors and <10% for proximal tumors, with recurrences continuing for at least 8 years after surgery. In the absence of ascites or extensive hepatic or peritoneal metastases, even patients whose disease is believed to be incurable by surgery should be offered resection of the primary lesion. Reduction of tumor bulk is the best form of palliation and may enhance the probability of benefit from subsequent therapy.

TABLE 87-3 STAGING SYSTEM FOR GASTRIC CARCINOMA

Stage	TNM	Features	Data from ACS	
			No. of Cases, %	5-Year Survival, %
0	TisN0M0	Node negative; limited to mucosa	1	90
IA	T1N0M0	Node negative; invasion of lamina propria or submucosa	7	59
IB	T2N0M0	Node negative; invasion of muscularis propria	10	44
II	T1N2M0 T2N1M0 T3N0M0	Node positive; invasion beyond mucosa but within wall *or* Node negative; extension through wall	17	29
IIIA	T2N2M0 T3N1-2M0	Node positive; invasion of muscularis propria or through wall	21	15
IIIB	T4N0-1M0	Node negative; adherence to surrounding tissue	14	9
IV	T4N2M0 T1-4N0-2M1	Node positive; adherence to surrounding tissue *or* Distant metastases	30	3

Note: ACS, American Cancer Society.

Gastric adenocarcinoma is a relatively radioresistant tumor, and adequate control of the primary tumor requires doses of external beam irradiation that exceed the tolerance of surrounding structures, such as bowel mucosa and spinal cord. As a result, the major role of radiation therapy in patients has been palliation of pain. Radiation therapy alone after a complete resection does not prolong survival. In the setting of surgically unresectable disease limited to the epigastrium, patients treated with 3500–4000 cGy did not live longer than similar patients not receiving radiotherapy; however, survival was prolonged slightly when 5-fluorouracil (5-FU) was given in combination with radiation therapy. In this clinical setting, the 5-FU may be functioning as a radiosensitizer.

The administration of combinations of cytotoxic drugs to patients with advanced gastric carcinoma has been associated with partial responses in 30–50% of cases; responders appear to benefit from treatment. Such drug combinations have generally included cisplatin combined with either epirubicin and infusional 5-FU or with irinotecan. Despite this encouraging response rate, complete remissions are uncommon, the partial responses are transient, and the overall influence of multidrug therapy on survival has been unclear. The use of adjuvant chemotherapy alone following the complete resection of a gastric cancer has only minimally improved survival. However, combination chemotherapy administered before and after surgery (*perioperative treatment*) as well as postoperative chemotherapy combined with radiation therapy reduces the recurrence rate and prolongs survival.

PRIMARY GASTRIC LYMPHOMA

Primary lymphoma of the stomach is relatively uncommon, accounting for <15% of gastric malignancies and ~2% of all lymphomas. The stomach is, however, the most frequent extranodal site for lymphoma, and gastric lymphoma has increased in frequency during the past 30 years. The disease is difficult to distinguish clinically from gastric adenocarcinoma; both tumors are most often detected during the sixth decade of life; present with epigastric pain, early satiety, and generalized fatigue; and are usually characterized by ulcerations with a ragged, thickened mucosal pattern demonstrated by contrast radiographs. The diagnosis of lymphoma of the stomach may occasionally be made through cytologic brushings of the gastric mucosa but usually requires a biopsy at gastroscopy or laparotomy. Failure of gastroscopic biopsies to detect lymphoma in a given case should not be interpreted as being conclusive, since superficial biopsies may miss the deeper lymphoid infiltrate. The macroscopic pathology of gastric lymphoma may also mimic adenocarcinoma, consisting of either a bulky ulcerated lesion localized in the corpus or antrum or a diffuse process spreading throughout the entire gastric submucosa and even extending into the duodenum. Microscopically, the vast majority of gastric lymphoid tumors are non-Hodgkin's lymphomas of B cell origin; Hodgkin's disease involving the stomach is extremely uncommon. Histologically, these tumors may range from well-differentiated, superficial processes [mucosa-associated lymphoid tissue (MALT)] to high-grade, large-cell lymphomas. Like gastric adenocarcinoma, infection with *H. pylori* increases the risk for gastric lymphoma in general and MALT lymphomas in particular. Gastric lymphomas spread initially to regional lymph nodes (often to Waldeyer's ring) and may then disseminate. Gastric lymphomas are staged like other lymphomas (Chap. 105).

℞ PRIMARY GASTRIC LYMPHOMA

Primary gastric lymphoma is a far more treatable disease than adenocarcinoma of the stomach, a fact that underscores the need for making the correct diagnosis. Antibiotic treatment to eradicate *H. pylori* infection has led to regression of about 75% of gastric MALT lymphomas and should be considered before surgery, radiation therapy, or chemotherapy are undertaken in patients having such tumors. A lack of response to such antimicrobial treatment has been linked to a specific chromosomal abnormality, i.e., t(11;18). Responding patients should undergo periodic endoscopic surveillance because it remains unclear whether the neoplastic clone is eliminated or merely suppressed, although the response to antimicrobial treatment is quite durable. Subtotal gastrectomy, usually followed by combination chemotherapy, has led to 5-year survival rates of 40–60% in patients with localized high-grade lymphomas. The need for a major surgical procedure has been questioned, particularly in patients with preoperative radiographic evidence of nodal involvement, for whom chemotherapy [CHOP (cyclophosphamide, doxorubicin, vincristine, and prednisone)] plus rituximab is effective therapy. A role for radiation therapy is not defined because most recurrences develop at distant sites.

GASTRIC (NONLYMPHOID) SARCOMA

Leiomyosarcomas and GISTs make up 1–3% of gastric neoplasms. They most frequently involve the anterior and posterior walls of the gastric fundus and often ulcerate and bleed. Even those lesions that appear benign on histologic examination may behave in a malignant fashion. These tumors rarely invade adjacent viscera and characteristically do not metastasize to lymph nodes, but they may spread to the liver and lungs. The treatment of choice is surgical resection. Combination chemotherapy should be reserved for patients with metastatic disease. All such tumors should be analyzed for a mutation in the c-*kit* receptor. GISTs are unresponsive to conventional chemotherapy; ~50% of patients experience objective response and prolonged survival when treated with imatinib mesylate (Gleevec) (400–800 mg PO daily), a selective inhibitor of the c-*kit* tyrosine kinase. Many patients with GIST whose tumors have become refractory to imatinib subsequently benefit from sunitinib (Sutent), another inhibitor of the c-*kit* tyrosine kinase.

COLORECTAL CANCER

INCIDENCE

Cancer of the large bowel is second only to lung cancer as a cause of cancer death in the United States: 153,760 new cases occurred in 2007, and 52,180 deaths were due to colorectal cancer. The incidence rate has remained relatively unchanged during the past 30 years, while the mortality rate has decreased, particularly in females. Colorectal cancer generally occurs in persons ≥50 years.

POLYPS AND MOLECULAR PATHOGENESIS

Most colorectal cancers, regardless of etiology, arise from adenomatous polyps. A polyp is a grossly visible protrusion from the mucosal surface and may be classified pathologically as a nonneoplastic hamartoma (*juvenile polyp*), a hyperplastic mucosal proliferation (*hyperplastic polyp*), or an adenomatous polyp. Only adenomas are clearly premalignant, and only a minority of such lesions becomes cancer. Adenomatous polyps may be found in the colons of ~30% of middle-aged and ~50% of elderly people; however, <1% of polyps ever become malignant. Most polyps produce no symptoms and remain clinically undetected. Occult blood in the stool is found in <5% of patients with polyps.

A number of molecular changes are noted in adenomatous polyps, dysplastic lesions, and polyps containing microscopic foci of tumor cells (carcinoma in situ), which are thought to reflect a multistep process in the evolution of normal colonic mucosa to life-threatening invasive carcinoma. These developmental steps toward carcinogenesis include, but are not restricted to, point mutations in the K-*ras* protooncogene; hypomethylation of DNA, leading to gene activation; loss of DNA (*allelic loss*) at the site of a tumor-suppressor gene [the adenomatous polyposis coli (*APC*) gene] on the long arm of chromosome 5 (5q21); allelic loss at the site of a tumor-suppressor gene located on chromosome 18q [the deleted in colorectal cancer (*DCC*) gene]; and allelic loss at chromosome 17p, associated with mutations in the p53 tumor-suppressor gene (see Fig. 79-2). Thus, the altered proliferative pattern of the colonic mucosa, which results in progression to a polyp and then to carcinoma, may involve the mutational activation of an oncogene followed by and coupled with the loss of genes that normally suppress tumorigenesis. It remains uncertain whether the genetic aberrations always occur in a defined order. Based on this model, however, cancer is believed to develop only in those polyps in which most (if not all) of these mutational events take place.

Clinically, the probability of an adenomatous polyp becoming a cancer depends on the gross appearance of the lesion, its histologic features, and its size. Adenomatous polyps may be pedunculated (stalked) or sessile (flat-based). Cancers develop more frequently in sessile polyps. Histologically, adenomatous polyps may be tubular, villous (i.e., papillary), or tubulovillous. Villous adenomas, most of which are sessile, become malignant more than three times as often as tubular adenomas. The likelihood that any polypoid lesion in the large bowel contains invasive cancer is related to the size of the polyp, being negligible (<2%) in lesions <1.5 cm, intermediate (2–10%) in lesions 1.5–2.5 cm in size, and substantial (10%) in lesions >2.5 cm.

Following the detection of an adenomatous polyp, the entire large bowel should be visualized endoscopically or radiographically, since synchronous lesions are noted in about one-third of cases. Colonoscopy should then be repeated periodically, even in the absence of a previously documented malignancy, since such patients have a 30–50% probability of developing another adenoma and are at a higher-than-average risk for developing a colorectal carcinoma. Adenomatous polyps are thought to require >5 years of growth before becoming clinically significant; colonoscopy need not be carried out more frequently than every 3 years.

ETIOLOGY AND RISK FACTORS

Risk factors for the development of colorectal cancer are listed in Table 87-4.

Diet The etiology for most cases of large-bowel cancer appears to be related to environmental factors. The disease occurs more often in upper socioeconomic populations who live in urban areas. Mortality from colorectal cancer is directly correlated with per capita consumption of calories, meat protein, and dietary fat and oil as well as elevations in the serum cholesterol concentration and mortality from coronary artery disease. Geographic variations in incidence are unrelated to genetic differences, since migrant groups tend to assume the large-bowel cancer incidence rates of their adopted countries. Furthermore, population groups such as Mormons and Seventh Day Adventists, whose lifestyle and dietary habits differ somewhat from those of their neighbors, have significantly lower-than-expected incidence and mortality rates for colorectal cancer. Colorectal cancer has increased in Japan since that nation has adopted a more "western" diet. At least three hypotheses have been proposed to explain the relationship to diet, none of which is fully satisfactory.

TABLE 87-4 RISK FACTORS FOR THE DEVELOPMENT OF COLORECTAL CANCER

Diet: Animal fat
Hereditary syndromes (autosomal dominant inheritance)
Polyposis coli
Nonpolyposis syndrome (Lynch syndrome)
Inflammatory bowel disease
Streptococcus bovis bacteremia
Ureterosigmoidostomy
? Tobacco use

ANIMAL FATS One hypothesis is that the ingestion of animal fats found in red meats and processed meat leads to an increased proportion of anaerobes in the gut microflora, resulting in the conversion of normal bile acids into carcinogens. This provocative hypothesis is supported by several reports of increased amounts of fecal anaerobes in the stools of patients with colorectal cancer. Diets high in animal (but not vegetable) fats are also associated with high serum cholesterol, which is also associated with enhanced risk for the development of colorectal adenomas and carcinomas.

INSULIN RESISTANCE The large number of calories in "western" diets coupled with physical inactivity has been associated with a higher prevalence of obesity. Obese persons develop insulin resistance with increased circulating levels of insulin, leading to higher circulating concentrations of insulin-like growth factor type I (IGF-I). This growth factor appears to stimulate proliferation of the intestinal mucosa.

FIBER Contrary to prior beliefs, the results of randomized trials and case-controlled studies have failed to show any value for dietary fiber or diets high in fruits and vegetables in preventing the recurrence of colorectal adenomas or the development of colorectal cancer. The weight of epidemiologic evidence, however, implicates diet as being the major etiologic factor for colorectal cancer, particularly diets high in animal fat and in calories.

HEREDITARY FACTORS AND SYNDROMES

Up to 25% of patients with colorectal cancer have a family history of the disease, suggesting a hereditary predisposition. Inherited large-bowel cancers can be divided into two main groups: the well-studied but uncommon polyposis syndromes and the more common nonpolyposis syndromes (Table 87-5).

Polyposis Coli Polyposis coli (familial polyposis of the colon) is a rare condition characterized by the appearance of thousands of adenomatous polyps throughout the large bowel. It is transmitted as an autosomal dominant trait; the occasional patient with no family history probably developed the condition due to a spontaneous mutation. Polyposis coli is associated with a deletion in the long arm of chromosome 5 [including the *APC* (adenomatous polyposis coli) gene] in both neoplastic (somatic mutation) and normal (germline mutation) cells. The loss of this genetic material (i.e., allelic loss) results in the absence of tumor-suppressor genes whose protein products would normally inhibit neoplastic growth. The presence of soft tissue and bony tumors, congenital hypertrophy of the retinal pigment epithelium, mesenteric desmoid tumors, and ampullary cancers in addition to the colonic polyps characterizes a subset of polyposis coli known as *Gardner's syndrome.* The appearance of malignant tumors of the central nervous system accompanying polyposis coli defines *Turcot's syndrome.* The colonic polyps in all these conditions are rarely present before puberty but are generally evident in affected individuals by age 25. If the polyposis is not treated surgically, colorectal cancer will develop in almost all patients before age 40. Polyposis coli results from a defect in the colonic mucosa, leading to an abnormal proliferative pattern

TABLE 87-5 HEREDITABLE (AUTOSOMAL DOMINANT) GASTROINTESTINAL POLYPOSIS SYNDROMES

Syndrome	Distribution of Polyps	Histologic Type	Malignant Potential	Associated Lesions
Familial adenomatous polyposis	Large intestine	Adenoma	Common	None
Gardner's syndrome	Large and small intestines	Adenoma	Common	Osteomas, fibromas, lipomas, epidermoid cysts, ampullary cancers, congenital hypertrophy of retinal pigment epithelium
Turcot's syndrome	Large intestine	Adenoma	Common	Brain tumors
Nonpolyposis syndrome (Lynch syndrome)	Large intestine (often proximal)	Adenoma	Common	Endometrial and ovarian tumors
Peutz-Jeghers syndrome	Small and large intestines, stomach	Hamartoma	Rare	Mucocutaneous pigmentation; tumors of the ovary, breast, pancreas, endometrium
Juvenile polyposis	Large and small intestines, stomach	Hamartoma, rarely progressing to adenoma	Rare	Various congenital abnormalities

and impaired DNA repair mechanisms. Once the multiple polyps are detected, patients should undergo a total colectomy. The ileoanal anastomotic technique allows removal of the entire bowel while retaining the anal sphincter. Medical therapy with nonsteroidal anti-inflammatory drugs (NSAIDs) such as sulindac and cyclooxygenase-2 inhibitors such as celecoxib can decrease the number and size of polyps in patients with polyposis coli; however, this effect on polyps is only temporary, and NSAIDs are not proven to reduce the risk of cancer. Colectomy remains the primary therapy/prevention. The offspring of patients with polyposis coli, who often are prepubertal when the diagnosis is made in the parent, have a 50% risk for developing this premalignant disorder and should be carefully screened by annual flexible sigmoidoscopy until age 35. Proctosigmoidoscopy is a sufficient screening procedure because polyps tend to be evenly distributed from cecum to anus, making more-invasive and expensive techniques such as colonoscopy or barium enema unnecessary. Testing for occult blood in the stool is an inadequate screening maneuver. An alternative method for identifying carriers is testing DNA from peripheral blood mononuclear cells for the presence of a mutated *APC* gene. The detection of such a germline mutation can lead to a definitive diagnosis before the development of polyps.

Hereditary Nonpolyposis Colon Cancer Hereditary nonpolyposis colon cancer (HNPCC), also known as *Lynch syndrome*, is another autosomal dominant trait. It is characterized by the presence of three or more relatives with histologically documented colorectal cancer, one of whom is a first-degree relative of the other two; one or more cases of colorectal cancer diagnosed before age 50 in the family; and colorectal cancer involving at least two generations. In contrast to polyposis coli, HNPCC is associated with an unusually high frequency of cancer arising in the proximal large bowel. The median age for the appearance of an adenocarcinoma is <50 years, 10–15 years younger than the median age for the general population. Despite having a poorly differentiated histologic appearance, the proximal colon tumors in HNPCC have a better prognosis than sporadic tumors from patients of similar age. Families with HNPCC often include individuals with multiple primary cancers; the association of colorectal cancer with either ovarian or endometrial carcinomas is especially strong in women. It has been recommended that members of such families undergo biennial colonoscopy beginning at age 25 years, with intermittent pelvic ultrasonography and endometrial biopsy for afflicted women; such a screening strategy has not yet been validated. HNPCC is associated with germline mutations of several genes, particularly *hMSH2* on chromosome 2 and *hMLH1* on chromosome 3. These mutations lead to errors in DNA replication and are thought to result in DNA instability because of defective repair of DNA mismatches, resulting in abnormal cell growth and tumor development. Testing tumor cells through molecular analysis of DNA or immunohistochemical staining of paraffin-fixed tissue for "microsatellite instability" (sequence changes reflecting defective mismatch repair) in patients under age 50 with colorectal cancer and a positive family history for colorectal or endometrial cancer may identify probands with HNPCC.

INFLAMMATORY BOWEL DISEASE

(Chap. 289) Large-bowel cancer is increased in incidence in patients with long-standing inflammatory bowel disease (IBD). Cancers develop more commonly in patients with ulcerative colitis than in those with granulomatous colitis, but this impression may result in part from the occasional difficulty of differentiating these two conditions. The risk of colorectal cancer in a patient with IBD is relatively small during the initial 10 years of the disease, but then it appears to increase at a rate of ~0.5–1% per year. Cancer may develop in 8–30% of patients after 25 years. The risk is higher in younger patients with pancolitis.

Cancer surveillance in patients with IBD is unsatisfactory. Symptoms such as bloody diarrhea, abdominal cramping, and obstruction, which may signal the appearance of a tumor, are similar to the complaints caused by a flare-up of the underlying disease. In patients with a history of IBD lasting ≥15 years who continue to experience exacerbations, the surgical removal of the colon can significantly reduce the risk for cancer and also eliminate the target organ for the underlying chronic gastrointestinal disorder. The value of such surveillance techniques as colonoscopy with mucosal biopsies and brushings for less-symptomatic individuals with chronic IBD is uncertain. The lack of uniformity regarding the pathologic criteria that characterize dysplasia and the absence of data that such surveillance reduces the development of lethal cancers have made this costly practice an area of controversy.

OTHER HIGH-RISK CONDITIONS

***Streptococcus bovis* Bacteremia** For unknown reasons, individuals who develop endocarditis or septicemia from this fecal bacterium have a high incidence of occult colorectal tumors and, possibly, upper gastrointestinal cancers as well. Endoscopic or radiographic screening appears advisable.

Tobacco Use Cigarette smoking is linked to the development of colorectal adenomas, particularly after >35 years of tobacco use. No biologic explanation for this association has yet been proposed.

PRIMARY PREVENTION

Several orally administered compounds have been assessed as possible inhibitors of colon cancer. The most effective class of chemopreventive agents is aspirin and other NSAIDs, which are thought to suppress cell proliferation by inhibiting prostaglandin synthesis. Regular aspirin use reduces the risk of colon adenomas and carcinomas as well as death from large-bowel cancer; such use also appears to diminish the likelihood for developing additional premalignant adenomas following treatment for a prior colon carcinoma. This effect of aspirin on colon carcinogenesis increases with the duration and dosage of drug use. Oral folic acid supplements and oral calcium supplements reduce the risk of adenomatous polyps and colorectal cancers in case-controlled studies. Antioxidant vitamins such as ascorbic acid, tocopherols, and β-carotene are ineffective at reducing the incidence of subsequent adenomas in patients who have undergone the removal of a colon adenoma. Estrogen-replacement therapy has been associated with a reduction in the risk of colorectal cancer in women, conceivably by an effect on bile acid synthesis and composition or by decreasing synthesis of IGF-I.

The otherwise unexplained reduction in colorectal cancer mortality in women may be a result of the widespread use of estrogen replacement in postmenopausal individuals.

SCREENING

The rationale for colorectal cancer screening programs is that earlier detection of localized, superficial cancers in asymptomatic individuals will increase the surgical cure rate. Such screening programs are important for individuals having a family history of the disease in first-degree relatives. The relative risk for developing colorectal cancer increases to 1.75 in such individuals and may be even higher if the relative was afflicted before age 60. The prior use of proctosigmoidoscopy as a screening tool was based on the observation that 60% of early lesions are located in the rectosigmoid. For unexplained reasons, however, the proportion of large-bowel cancers arising in the rectum has been decreasing during the past several decades, with a corresponding increase in the proportion of cancers in the more proximal descending colon. As such, the potential for rigid proctosigmoidoscopy to detect a sufficient number of occult neoplasms to make the procedure cost-effective has been questioned. Flexible, fiberoptic sigmoidoscopes permit trained operators to visualize the colon for up to 60 cm, which enhances the capability for cancer detection. However, this technique still leaves the proximal half of the large bowel unscreened.

Most programs directed at the early detection of colorectal cancers have focused on digital rectal examinations and fecal occult blood testing. The digital examination should be part of any routine physical evaluation in adults older than age 40, serving as a screening test for prostate cancer in men, a component of the pelvic examination in women, and an inexpensive maneuver for the detection of masses in the rectum. The development of the Hemoccult test has greatly facilitated the detection of occult fecal blood. Unfortunately, even when performed optimally, the Hemoccult test has major limitations as a screening technique. About 50% of patients with documented colorectal cancers have a negative fecal Hemoccult test, consistent with the intermittent bleeding pattern of these tumors. When random cohorts of asymptomatic persons have been tested, 2–4% have Hemoccult-positive stools. Colorectal cancers have been found in <10% of these "test-positive" cases, with benign polyps being detected in an additional 20–30%. Thus, a colorectal neoplasm will not be found in most asymptomatic individuals with occult blood in their stool. Nonetheless, persons found to have Hemoccult-positive stool routinely undergo further medical evaluation, including sigmoidoscopy, barium enema, and/or colonoscopy—procedures that are not only uncomfortable and expensive but also associated with a small risk for significant complications. The added cost of these studies would appear justifiable if the small number of patients found to have occult neoplasms because of Hemoccult screening could be shown to have an improved prognosis and prolonged survival. Prospectively controlled trials showed a statistically significant reduction in mortality from colorectal cancer for individuals undergoing annual screening. However, this benefit only emerged after >13 years of follow-up and was extremely expensive to achieve, since all positive tests (most of which were false-positive) were followed by colonoscopy. Moreover, these colonoscopic examinations quite likely provided the opportunity for cancer prevention through the removal of potentially premalignant adenomatous polyps since the eventual development of cancer was reduced by 20% in the cohort undergoing annual screening.

Screening techniques for large-bowel cancer in asymptomatic persons remain unsatisfactory. Compliance with any screening strategy within the general population is poor. At present, the American Cancer Society suggests fecal Hemoccult screening annually and flexible sigmoidoscopy every 5 years beginning at age 50 for asymptomatic individuals having no colorectal cancer risk factors. The American Cancer Society has also endorsed a "total colon examination" (i.e., colonoscopy or double-contrast barium enema) every 10 years as an alternative to Hemoccult testing with periodic flexible sigmoidoscopy. Colonoscopy has been shown to be superior to double-contrast barium enema and also to have a higher sensitivity for detecting villous or dysplastic adenomas or cancers than the strategy employing occult fecal blood testing and flexible sigmoidoscopy. Whether colonoscopy performed every 10 years beginning after age 50 will prove to be cost-effective and whether it may be supplanted as a screening maneuver by sophisticated radiographic techniques ("virtual colonoscopy") remains unclear. More effective techniques for screening are needed, perhaps taking advantage of the molecular changes that have been described in these tumors. Analysis of fecal DNA for multiple mutations associated with colorectal cancer is being tested.

CLINICAL FEATURES

Presenting Symptoms Symptoms vary with the anatomic location of the tumor. Since stool is relatively liquid as it passes through the ileocecal valve into the right colon, cancers arising in the cecum and ascending colon may become quite large without resulting in any obstructive symptoms or noticeable alterations in bowel habits. Lesions of the right colon commonly ulcerate, leading to chronic, insidious blood loss without a change in the appearance of the stool. Consequently, patients with tumors of the ascending colon often present with symptoms such as fatigue, palpitations, and even angina pectoris and are found to have a hypochromic, microcytic anemia indicative of iron deficiency. Since the cancer may bleed intermittently, a random fecal occult blood test may be negative. As a result, the unexplained presence of iron-deficiency anemia in any adult (with the possible exception of a premenopausal, multiparous woman) mandates a thorough endoscopic and/or radiographic visualization of the entire large bowel (Fig. 87-1).

Since stool becomes more formed as it passes into the transverse and descending colon, tumors arising there tend to impede the passage of stool, resulting in the development of abdominal cramping, occasional obstruction, and even perforation. Radiographs of the abdomen often reveal characteristic annular, constricting lesions ("apple-core" or "napkin-ring") (Fig. 87-2).

Cancers arising in the rectosigmoid are often associated with hematochezia, tenesmus, and narrowing of the caliber of stool; anemia is an infrequent finding. While these symptoms may lead patients and their physicians to suspect the presence of hemorrhoids, the development of rectal bleeding and/or altered bowel habits demands a prompt digital rectal examination and proctosigmoidoscopy.

Staging, Prognostic Factors, and Patterns of Spread The prognosis for individuals having colorectal cancer is related to the depth of tumor penetration into the bowel wall and the presence of both regional

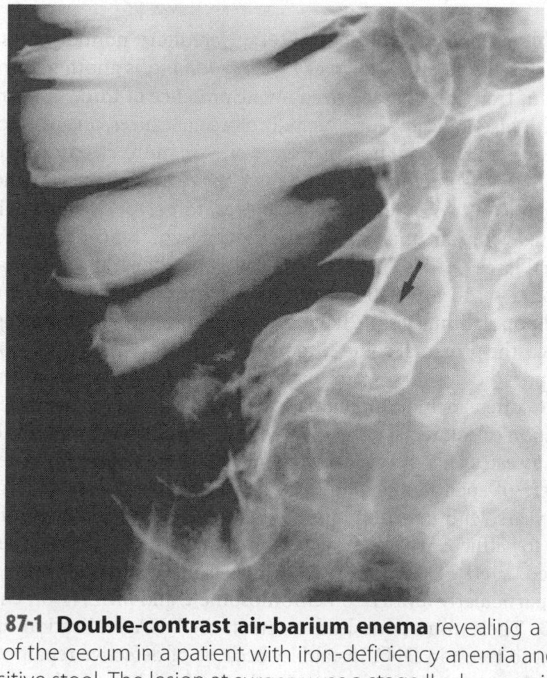

FIGURE 87-1 Double-contrast air-barium enema revealing a sessile tumor of the cecum in a patient with iron-deficiency anemia and guaiac-positive stool. The lesion at surgery was a stage II adenocarcinoma.

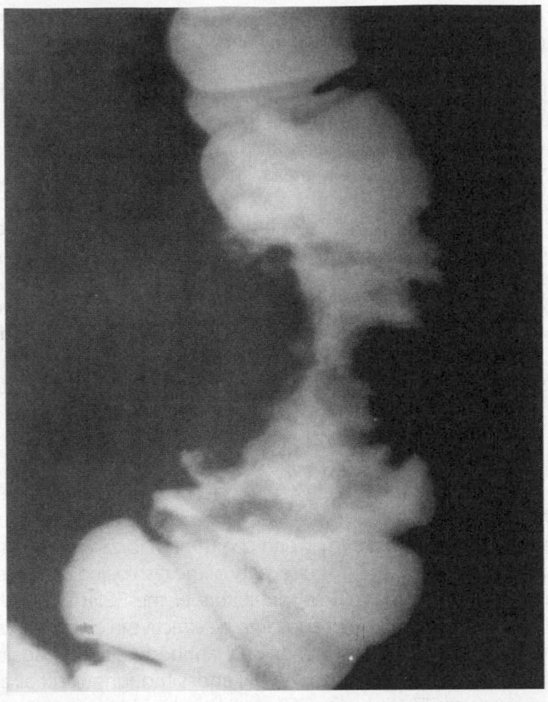

FIGURE 87-2 Annular, constricting adenocarcinoma of the descending colon. This radiographic appearance is referred to as an "apple-core" lesion and is always highly suggestive of malignancy.

lymph node involvement and distant metastases. These variables are incorporated into the staging system introduced by Dukes and applied to a TNM classification method, in which T represents the depth of tumor penetration, N the presence of lymph node involvement, and M the presence or absence of distant metastases (Fig. 87-3). Superficial lesions that do not involve regional lymph nodes and do not penetrate through the submucosa (T_1) or the muscularis (T_2) are designated as *stage I* ($T_{1-2}N_0M_0$) disease; tumors that penetrate through the muscularis but have not spread to lymph nodes are *stage II* disease ($T_3N_0M_0$); regional lymph node involvement defines *stage III* ($T_xN_1M_0$) disease; and metastatic spread to sites such as liver, lung, or bone indicates *stage IV* ($T_xN_xM_1$) disease. Unless gross evidence of metastatic disease is present, disease stage cannot be determined accurately before surgical resection and pathologic analysis of the operative specimens. It is not clear whether the detection of nodal metastases by special immunohistochemical molecular techniques has the same prognostic implications as disease detected by routine light microscopy.

Most recurrences after a surgical resection of a large-bowel cancer occur within the first 4 years, making 5-year survival a fairly reliable indicator of cure. The likelihood for 5-year survival in patients with colorectal cancer is stage-related (Fig. 87-3). That likelihood has improved during the past several decades when similar surgical stages have been compared. The most plausible explanation for this improvement is more thorough intraoperative and pathologic staging. In particular, more exacting attention to pathologic detail has revealed that the prognosis following the resection of a colorectal cancer is not related merely to the presence or absence of regional lymph node involvement. Prognosis may be more precisely gauged by the number of involved lymph nodes (one to three lymph nodes versus four or more lymph nodes). A minimum of 12 sampled lymph nodes is thought necessary to accurately define tumor stage. Other predictors of a poor prognosis after a total surgical resection include tumor penetration through the bowel wall into pericolic fat, poorly differentiated histology, perforation and/or tumor adherence to adjacent organs (increasing the risk for an anatomically adjacent recurrence), and venous invasion by tumor (Table 87-6). Regardless of the clinicopathologic stage, a preoperative elevation of the plasma carcinoembryonic antigen (CEA) level predicts eventual tumor recurrence. The presence of aneuploidy and specific chromosomal deletions, such as allelic loss in chromosome 18q (involving the *DCC* gene) in tumor cells, appears to predict a higher risk for metastatic spread, particularly in patients with stage II ($T_3N_0M_0$) disease. Conversely, the detection of microsatellite instability in tumor tissue indicates a more favorable outcome. In contrast to most other cancers, the prognosis in colorectal cancer is not influenced by the size of the primary lesion when adjusted for nodal involvement and histologic differentiation.

Cancers of the large bowel generally spread to regional lymph nodes or to the liver via the portal venous circulation. The liver represents the most frequent visceral site of metastasis; it is the initial site of distant spread in one-third of recurring colorectal cancers and is involved in more than two-thirds of such patients at the time of death. In general, colorectal cancer rarely spreads to the lungs, supraclavicular lymph nodes, bone, or brain without prior spread to the liver. A major exception to this rule occurs in patients having primary tumors in the distal rectum, from which tumor cells may spread through the paravertebral venous plexus, escaping the portal venous system and thereby reaching the lungs or supraclavicular lymph nodes without hepatic involvement. The median survival after the detection of distant metastases has ranged in the past from 6–9 months (hepatomegaly, abnormal liver chemistries) to 24–30 months (small liver nodule initially identified by elevated CEA level and subsequent CT scan), but effective systemic therapy is improving the prognosis.

℞ COLORECTAL CANCER

Total resection of tumor is the optimal treatment when a malignant lesion is detected in the large bowel. An evaluation for the presence of metastatic disease, including a thorough physical examination, chest radiograph, biochemical assessment of liver function, and measurement of the plasma CEA level, should be performed before surgery. When possible, a colonoscopy of the entire large bowel should be performed to identify synchronous neo-

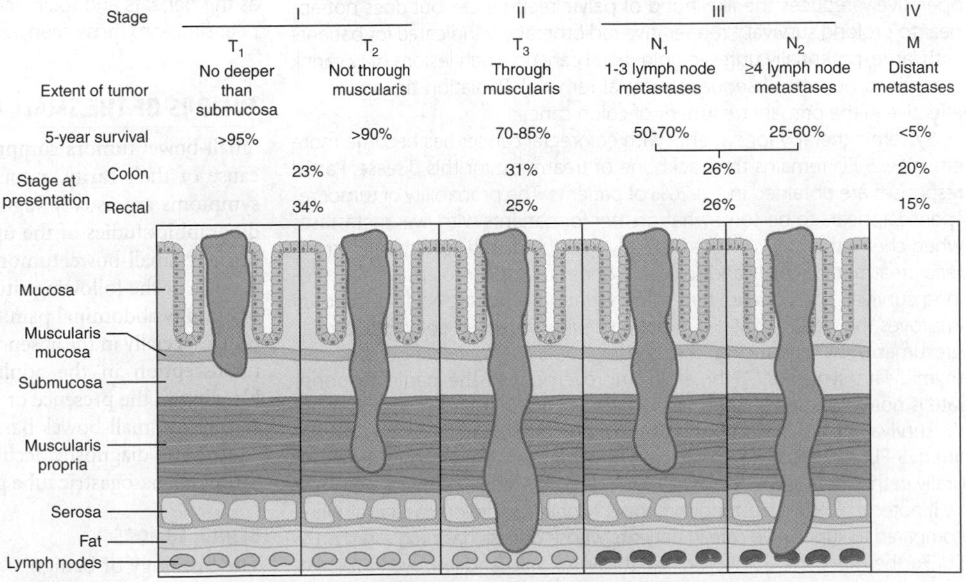

FIGURE 87-3 Staging and prognosis for patients with colorectal cancer.

TABLE 87-6 PREDICTORS OF POOR OUTCOME FOLLOWING TOTAL SURGICAL RESECTION OF COLORECTAL CANCER

Tumor spread to regional lymph nodes
Number of regional lymph nodes involved
Tumor penetration through the bowel wall
Poorly differentiated histology
Perforation
Tumor adherence to adjacent organs
Venous invasion
Preoperative elevation of CEA titer (>5.0 ng/mL)
Aneuploidy
Specific chromosomal deletion (e.g., allelic loss on chromosome 18q)

Note: CEA, carcinoembryonic antigen.

plasms and/or polyps. The detection of metastases should not preclude surgery in patients with tumor-related symptoms such as gastrointestinal bleeding or obstruction, but it often prompts the use of a less radical operative procedure. At the time of laparotomy, the entire peritoneal cavity should be examined, with thorough inspection of the liver, pelvis, and hemidiaphragm and careful palpation of the full length of the large bowel. Following recovery from a complete resection, patients should be observed carefully for 5 years by semiannual physical examinations and yearly blood chemistry measurements. If a complete colonoscopy was not performed preoperatively, it should be carried out within the first several postoperative months. Some authorities favor measuring plasma CEA levels at 3-month intervals because of the sensitivity of this test as a marker for otherwise undetectable tumor recurrence. Subsequent endoscopic or radiographic surveillance of the large bowel, probably at triennial intervals, is indicated, since patients who have been cured of one colorectal cancer have a 3–5% probability of developing an additional bowel cancer during their lifetime and a >15% risk for the development of adenomatous polyps. Anastomotic ("suture-line") recurrences are infrequent in colorectal cancer patients provided the surgical resection margins are adequate and free of tumor. The value of periodic CT scans of the abdomen, assessing for an early, asymptomatic indication of tumor recurrence, is an area of uncertainty, with some experts recommending the test be performed annually for the first three postoperative years.

Radiation therapy to the pelvis is recommended for patients with rectal cancer because it reduces the 20–25% probability of regional recurrences following complete surgical resection of stage II or III tumors, especially if they have penetrated through the serosa. This alarmingly high rate of local disease recurrence is believed to be due to the fact that the contained anatomic space within the pelvis limits the extent of the resection and because the rich lymphatic network of the pelvic side wall immediately adjacent to the rectum facilitates the early spread of malignant cells into surgically inaccessible tissue. The use of sharp rather than blunt dissection of rectal cancers (*total mesorectal excision*) appears to reduce the likelihood of local disease recurrence to ~10%. Radiation therapy, either pre- or postoperatively, reduces the likelihood of pelvic recurrences but does not appear to prolong survival. Preoperative radiotherapy is indicated for patients with large, potentially unresectable rectal cancers; such lesions may shrink enough to permit subsequent surgical removal. Radiation therapy is not effective in the primary treatment of colon cancer.

Systemic therapy for patients with colorectal cancer has become more effective. 5-FU remains the backbone of treatment for this disease. Partial responses are obtained in 15–20% of patients. The probability of tumor response appears to be somewhat greater for patients with liver metastases when chemotherapy is infused directly into the hepatic artery, but intraarterial treatment is costly and toxic and does not appear to appreciably prolong survival. The concomitant administration of folinic acid (leucovorin) improves the efficacy of 5-FU in patients with advanced colorectal cancer, presumably by enhancing the binding of 5-FU to its target enzyme, thymidylate synthase. A threefold improvement in the partial response rate is noted when folinic acid is combined with 5-FU; however, the effect on survival is marginal, and the optimal dose schedule remains to be defined. 5-FU is generally administered intravenously but may also be given orally in the form of capecitabine with seemingly similar efficacy.

Irinotecan (CPT-11), a topoisomerase 1 inhibitor, prolongs survival when compared to supportive care in patients whose disease has progressed on 5-FU. Furthermore, the addition of irinotecan to 5-FU and leucovorin (LV) improves response rates and survival of patients with metastatic disease. The *FOLFIRI regimen* is as follows: irinotecan, 180 mg/m^2 as a 90-min infusion day 1; LV, 400 mg/m^2 as a 2-h infusion during irinotecan, immediately followed by 5-FU bolus, 400 mg/m^2 and 46-h continuous infusion of 2.4–3 g/m^2 every 2 weeks. Diarrhea is the major side effect from irinotecan. Oxaliplatin, a platinum analogue, also improves the response rate when added to 5-FU and LV as initial treatment of patients with metastatic disease. The *FOLFOX regimen* is the following: 2-h infusion of LV (400 mg/m^2 per day) followed by a 5-FU bolus (400 mg/m^2 per day) and 22-h infusion (1200 mg/m^2) every 2 weeks, together with oxaliplatin, 85 mg/m^2 as a 2-h infusion on day 1. Oxaliplatin frequently causes a dose-dependent sensory neuropathy that usually resolves following the cessation of therapy. FOLFIRI and FOLFOX are equal in efficacy.

Monoclonal antibodies are also effective in patients with advanced colorectal cancer. Cetuximab (Erbitux) and panitumumab (Vectibix) are directed against the epidermal growth factor receptor (EGFR), a transmembrane glycoprotein involved in signaling pathways affecting growth and proliferation of tumor cells. Both cetuximab and panitumumab, when given alone, have been shown to benefit a small proportion of previously treated patients, and cetuximab appears to have therapeutic synergy with such chemotherapeutic agents as irinotecan, even in patients previously resistant to this drug; this suggests that cetuximab can reverse cellular resistance to cytotoxic chemotherapy. The use of both cetuximab and panitumumab can lead to an acne-like rash with the development and severity of the rash being correlated with the likelihood of antitumor efficacy. Inhibitors of the EGFR tyrosine kinase such as erlotinib (Tarceva) do not appear to be effective in colorectal cancer.

Bevacizumab (Avastin) is a monoclonal antibody directed against the vascular endothelial growth factor (VEGF) and is thought to act as an anti-angiogenesis agent. The addition of bevacizumab to irinotecan-containing combinations and to FOLFOX improves the outcome observed with the chemotherapy alone. The use of bevacizumab can lead to hypertension, proteinuria, and an increased likelihood of thromboembolic events.

Patients with solitary hepatic metastases without clinical or radiographic evidence of additional tumor involvement should be considered for partial liver resection, because such procedures are associated with 5-year survival rates of 25–30% when performed on selected individuals by experienced surgeons.

The administration of 5-FU and LV for 6 months after resection of tumor in patients with stage III disease leads to a 40% decrease in recurrence rates and 30% improvement in survival. The likelihood of recurrence has been further reduced when oxaliplatin has been combined with 5-FU and LV (e.g. FOLFOX); unexpectedly, the addition of irinotecan to 5-FU and LV did not enhance outcome. Patients with stage II tumors do not appear to benefit from adjuvant therapy. In rectal cancer, the delivery of preoperative or postoperative combined modality therapy (5-FU plus radiation therapy) reduces the risk of recurrence and increases the chance of cure for patients with stages II and III tumors, with the preoperative approach being better tolerated. The 5-FU acts as a radiosensitizer when delivered together with radiation therapy. Life-extending adjuvant therapy is used in only about half of patients over age 65 years. This age bias is completely inappropriate as the benefits and tolerance of adjuvant therapy in patients age 65+ appear similar to those seen in younger individuals.

TUMORS OF THE SMALL INTESTINE

Small-bowel tumors comprise <3% of gastrointestinal neoplasms. Because of their rarity, a correct diagnosis is often delayed. Abdominal symptoms are usually vague and poorly defined, and conventional radiographic studies of the upper and lower intestinal tract often appear normal. Small-bowel tumors should be considered in the differential diagnosis in the following situations: (1) recurrent, unexplained episodes of crampy abdominal pain; (2) intermittent bouts of intestinal obstruction, especially in the absence of IBD or prior abdominal surgery; (3) intussusception in the adult; and (4) evidence of chronic intestinal bleeding in the presence of negative conventional contrast radiographs. A careful small-bowel barium study is the diagnostic procedure of choice; the diagnostic accuracy may be improved by infusing barium through a nasogastric tube placed into the duodenum (enteroclysis).

BENIGN TUMORS

The histology of benign small-bowel tumors is difficult to predict on clinical and radiologic grounds alone. The symptomatology of benign tumors is not distinctive, with pain, obstruction, and hemorrhage being the most frequent symptoms. These tumors are usually discovered during the fifth and sixth decades of life, more often in the distal rather than the proximal small intestine. The most common benign tumors are adenomas, leiomyomas, lipomas, and angiomas.

Adenomas These tumors include those of the islet cells and Brunner's glands as well as polypoid adenomas. *Islet cell adenomas* are occasionally located outside the pancreas; the associated syndromes are discussed in Chap. 344. *Brunner's gland adenomas* are not truly neoplastic but represent a hypertrophy or hyperplasia of submucosal duodenal glands. These appear as small nodules in the duodenal mucosa that secrete a highly viscous alkaline mucus. Most often, this is an incidental radiographic finding not associated with any specific clinical disorder.

Polypoid Adenomas About 25% of benign small-bowel tumors are polypoid adenomas (Table 87-5). They may present as single polypoid lesions or, less commonly, as papillary villous adenomas. As in the colon, the sessile or papillary form of the tumor is sometimes associated with a coexisting carcinoma. Occasionally, patients with Gardner's syndrome develop premalignant adenomas in the small bowel; such lesions are generally in the duodenum. Multiple polypoid tumors may occur throughout the small bowel (and occasionally the stomach and colorectum) in the Peutz-Jeghers syndrome. The polyps are usually hamartomas (juvenile polyps) having a low potential for malignant degeneration. Mucocutaneous melanin deposits as well as tumors of the ovary, breast, pancreas, and endometrium are also associated with this autosomal dominant condition.

Leiomyomas These neoplasms arise from smooth-muscle components of the intestine and are usually intramural, affecting the overlying mucosa. Ulceration of the mucosa may cause gastrointestinal hemorrhage of varying severity. Cramping or intermittent abdominal pain is frequently encountered.

Lipomas These tumors occur with greatest frequency in the distal ileum and at the ileocecal valve. They have a characteristic radiolucent appearance, are usually intramural and asymptomatic, but on occasion cause bleeding.

Angiomas While not true neoplasms, these lesions are important because they frequently cause intestinal bleeding. They may take the form of telangiectasia or hemangiomas. Multiple intestinal telangiectasias occur in a nonhereditary form confined to the gastrointestinal tract or as part of the hereditary Osler-Rendu-Weber syndrome. Vascular tumors may also take the form of isolated hemangiomas, most commonly in the jejunum. Angiography, especially during bleeding, is the best procedure for evaluating these lesions.

MALIGNANT TUMORS

While rare, small-bowel malignancies occur in patients with long-standing regional enteritis and celiac sprue as well as in individuals with AIDS. Malignant tumors of the small bowel are frequently associated with fever, weight loss, anorexia, bleeding, and a palpable abdominal mass. After ampullary carcinomas (many of which arise from biliary or pancreatic ducts), the most frequently occurring small-bowel malignancies are adenocarcinomas, lymphomas, carcinoid tumors, and leiomyosarcomas.

Adenocarcinomas The most common primary cancers of the small bowel are adenocarcinomas, accounting for ~50% of malignant tumors. These cancers occur most often in the distal duodenum and proximal jejunum, where they tend to ulcerate and cause hemorrhage or obstruction. Radiologically, they may be confused with chronic duodenal ulcer disease or with Crohn's disease if the patient has long-standing regional enteritis. The diagnosis is best made by endoscopy and biopsy under direct vision. Surgical resection is the treatment of choice.

Lymphomas Lymphoma in the small bowel may be primary or secondary. A diagnosis of a primary intestinal lymphoma requires histologic confirmation in a clinical setting in which palpable adenopathy and hepatosplenomegaly are absent and no evidence of lymphoma is seen on chest radiograph, CT scan, or peripheral blood smear or on bone marrow aspiration and biopsy. Symptoms referable to the small bowel are present, usually accompanied by an anatomically discernible lesion. Secondary lymphoma of the small bowel consists of involvement of the intestine by a lymphoid malignancy extending from involved retroperitoneal or mesenteric lymph nodes (Chap. 105).

Primary intestinal lymphoma accounts for ~20% of malignancies of the small bowel. These neoplasms are non-Hodgkin's lymphomas; they usually have a diffuse, large-cell histology and are of T cell origin. Intestinal lymphoma involves the ileum, jejunum, and duodenum, in decreasing frequency, a pattern that mirrors the relative amount of normal lymphoid cells in these anatomic areas. The risk of small-bowel lymphoma is increased in patients with a prior history of malabsorptive conditions (e.g., celiac sprue), regional enteritis, and depressed immune function due to congenital immunodeficiency syndromes, prior organ transplantation, autoimmune disorders, or AIDS.

The development of localized or nodular masses that narrow the lumen results in periumbilical pain (made worse by eating) as well as weight loss, vomiting, and occasional intestinal obstruction. The diagnosis of small-bowel lymphoma may be suspected from the appearance on contrast radiographs of patterns such as infiltration and thickening of mucosal folds, mucosal nodules, areas of irregular ulceration, or stasis of contrast material. The diagnosis can be confirmed by surgical exploration and resection of involved segments. Intestinal lymphoma can occasionally be diagnosed by peroral intestinal mucosal biopsy, but since the disease mainly involves the lamina propria, full-thickness surgical biopsies are usually required.

Resection of the tumor constitutes the initial treatment modality. While postoperative radiation therapy has been given to some patients following a total resection, most authorities favor short-term (three cycles) systemic treatment with combination chemotherapy. The frequent presence of widespread intraabdominal disease at the time of diagnosis and the occasional multicentricity of the tumor often make a total resection impossible. The probability of sustained remission or cure is ~75% in patients with localized disease but is ~25% in individuals with unresectable lymphoma. In patients whose tumors are not resected, chemotherapy may lead to bowel perforation.

A unique form of small-bowel lymphoma, diffusely involving the entire intestine, was first described in oriental Jews and Arabs and is referred to as *immunoproliferative small intestinal disease* (IPSID), *Mediterranean lymphoma*, or *α-heavy chain disease*. This is a B cell tumor. The typical presentation includes chronic diarrhea and steatorrhea associated with vomiting and abdominal cramps; clubbing of the digits may be observed. A curious feature in many patients with IPSID is the presence in the blood and intestinal secretions of an abnormal IgA that contains a shortened α-heavy chain and is devoid of light chains. It is suspected that the abnormal α chains are produced by plasma cells infiltrating the small bowel. The clinical course of patients with IPSID is generally one of exacerbations and remissions, with death frequently resulting from either progressive malnutrition and wasting or the development of an aggressive lymphoma. The use of oral antibiotics such as tetracycline appears to be beneficial in the early phases of the disorder, suggesting a possible infectious etiology. Combination chemotherapy has been administered during later stages of the disease, with variable results. Results are better when antibiotics and chemotherapy are combined.

Carcinoid Tumors Carcinoid tumors arise from argentaffin cells of the crypts of Lieberkühn and are found from the distal duodenum to the ascending colon, areas embryologically derived from the midgut. More than 50% of intestinal carcinoids are found in the distal ileum, with most congregating close to the ileocecal valve. Most intestinal carcinoids are asymptomatic and of low malignant potential, but invasion and metastases may occur, leading to the carcinoid syndrome (Chap. 344).

Leiomyosarcomas Leiomyosarcomas often are >5 cm in diameter and may be palpable on abdominal examination. Bleeding, obstruction, and perforation are common. Such tumors should be analyzed for the expression of mutant *c-kit* receptor (defining GIST), and in the presence of metastatic disease, justifying treatment with imatinib mesylate (Gleevec) or, in imatinib refractory patients, sunitinib (Sutent).

CANCERS OF THE ANUS

Cancers of the anus account for 1–2% of the malignant tumors of the large bowel. Most such lesions arise in the anal canal, the anatomic area extending from the anorectal ring to a zone approximately halfway between the pectinate (or dentate) line and the anal verge. Carcinomas arising proximal to the pectinate line (i.e., in the transitional zone between the glandular mucosa of the rectum and the squamous epithelium of the distal anus) are known as *basaloid, cuboidal*, or *cloacogenic* tumors; about one-third of anal cancers have this histologic pattern. Malignancies arising distal to the pectinate line have squamous histology, ulcerate more frequently, and constitute ~55% of anal cancers. The prognosis for patients with basaloid and squamous cell cancers of the anus is identical when corrected for tumor size and the presence or absence of nodal spread.

The development of anal cancer is associated with infection by human papillomavirus, the same organism etiologically linked to cervical cancer. The virus is sexually transmitted. The infection may lead to anal warts (condyloma accuminata), which may progress to anal intraepithelial neoplasia and on to squamous cell carcinoma. The risk for anal cancer is increased among homosexual males, presumably related to anal intercourse. Anal cancer risk is increased in both men and women with AIDS, possibly because their immunosuppressed state permits more severe papillomavirus infection. Anal cancers occur most commonly in middle-aged persons and are more frequent in women than men. At diagnosis, patients may experience bleeding, pain, sensation of a perianal mass, and pruritus.

Radical surgery (abdominal-perineal resection with lymph node sampling and a permanent colostomy) was once the treatment of choice for this tumor type. The 5-year survival rate after such a procedure was 55–70% in the absence of spread to regional lymph nodes and <20% if nodal involvement was present. An alternative therapeutic approach combining external beam radiation therapy with concomitant chemotherapy has resulted in biopsy-proven disappearance of all tumor in >80% of patients whose initial lesion was <3 cm in size. Tumor recurrences develop in <10% of these patients, meaning that ~70% of patients with anal cancers can be cured with nonoperative treatment. Surgery should be reserved for the minority of individuals who are found to have residual tumor after being managed initially with radiation therapy combined with chemotherapy.

FURTHER READINGS

CRUMP W et al: Lymphoma of the gastrointestinal tract. Semin Oncol 26:324, 1999

DEMETRI GD et al: Efficacy and safety of imatinib mesylate in advanced gastrointestinal stromal tumors. N Engl J Med 347:472, 2002

ENZINGER PC, MAYER RJ: Esophageal cancer. N Engl J Med 349:2241, 2003

HOHENBERGER P, GRETSCHEL S: Gastric cancer. Lancet 362:305, 2003

LYNCH HT, DE LA CHAPELLE A: Hereditary colorectal cancer. N Engl J Med 348:919, 2003

MEYERHARDT JA, MAYER RJ: Systemic therapy for colorectal cancer. N Engl J Med 352:476, 2005

ROSTRUM A et al: Nonsteroidal anti-inflammatory drugs and cyclooxygenase-2 inhibitors for primary prevention of colorectal cancer: A systematic review prepared for the US Preventive Services Task Force. Ann Intern Med 146:376, 2007

RYAN DP et al: Carcinoma of the anal canal. N Engl J Med 342:792, 2000

SPECHLER SJ: Barrett's esophagus. N Engl J Med 346:836, 2002

UEMURA N et al: *Helicobacter pylori* infection and the development of gastric cancer. N Engl J Med 345:784, 2001

WALSH JME, TERDIMAN JP: Colorectal cancer screening. JAMA 289:1288, 2003

WEITZ J et al: Colorectal cancer. Lancet 365:153, 2005

WOLAN BM et al: Adjuvant treatment of colorectal cancer. CA Cancer Clin J 57:168, 2007

88 Tumors of the Liver and Biliary Tree

Brian I. Carr

HEPATOCELLULAR CARCINOMA

INCIDENCE

Hepatocellular carcinoma (HCC) is one of the most common malignancies worldwide. The annual global incidence is about 1 million cases, with a male to female ratio of about 4:1. The incidence rate equals the death rate. In the United States, 19,160 new cases and 16,780 deaths were noted in 2007. The death rate in males in low-incidence countries such as the United States is 1.9 per 100,000 per year; in intermediate-incidence areas such as Austria and South Africa, annual death rates range from 5.1–20.0 per 100,000; and in high-incidence areas such as in Asia (China and Korea), death rates are as high as 23.1–150 per 100,000 per year (Table 88-1). The incidence of HCC in the United States is around 3 per 100,000 persons, with significant sex, ethnic, and geographic variations. These numbers are rapidly increasing and may be an underestimate. Around 4 million persons in the United States are chronic carriers of hepatitis C virus (HCV). About 10% of them, or 400,000, are likely to develop cirrhosis. Around 5% or 20,000 of these may develop HCC annually. Add to this the two other common predisposing factors—hepatitis B virus (HBV) and chronic alcohol consumption—and 60,000 new HCC cases annually seem possible. Future advances in HCC survival will likely depend on immunization strategies for HBV and HCV and earlier diagnosis by screening of patients at risk of HCC development.

TABLE 88-1 AGE-ADJUSTED INCIDENCE RATES FOR HEPATOCELLULAR CARCINOMA

	Persons per 100,000 per Year	
Country	**Male**	**Female**
Argentina	6.0	2.5
Brazil, Recife	9.2	8.3
Brazil, Sao Paulo	3.8	2.6
Mozambique	112.9	30.8
South Africa, Cape: Black	26.3	8.4
South Africa, Cape: White	1.2	0.6
Senegal	25.6	9.0
Nigeria	15.4	3.2
Gambia	33.1	12.6
Burma	25.5	8.8
Japan	7.2	2.2
Korea	13.8	3.2
China, Shanghai	34.4	11.6
India, Bombay	4.9	2.5
India, Madras	2.1	0.7
Great Britain	1.6	0.8
France	6.9	1.2
Italy, Varese	7.1	2.7
Norway	1.8	1.1
Spain, Navarra	7.9	4.7

EPIDEMIOLOGY

Endemic hot spots occur in areas of China and sub-Saharan Africa, which are associated with both high endemic hepatitis B carrier rates and mycotoxin contamination of foodstuffs, stored grains, drinking water, and soil. Environmental factors are important; Japanese in Japan have a higher incidence than those living in Hawaii, who in turn have a higher incidence than those living in California.

ETIOLOGIC FACTORS

Chemical Carcinogens Probably the best-studied and most potent ubiquitous natural chemical carcinogen is a product of the *Aspergillus* fungus, called aflatoxin B_1. This mold and aflatoxin product can be found in stored grains in hot, humid places, where peanuts and rice are stored in unrefrigerated conditions. Aflatoxin contamination of foodstuffs correlates well with incidence rates in Africa and to some extent in China. In endemic areas of China, even farm animals such as ducks have HCC. The most potent carcinogens appear to be natural products of plants, fungi, and bacteria, such as bush trees containing pyrrolizidine alkaloids as well as tannic acid and safrole. Pollutants such as pesticides and insecticides are known rodent carcinogens.

Hepatitis Both case-control and cohort studies have shown a strong association between chronic hepatitis B carrier rates and increased incidence of HCC. In Taiwanese male postal carriers who were hepatitis B surface antigen (HBsAg)-positive, a 98-fold greater risk for HCC was found compared to HBsAg-negative individuals. The incidence of HCC in Alaskan natives is markedly increased related to a high prevalence of HBV infection. HBV-based HCC may arise from rounds of hepatic destruction with subsequent proliferation and not necessarily from frank cirrhosis. The increase in Japanese HCC incidence rates in the past three decades is thought to be from hepatitis C. A large-scale intervention study sponsored by the World Health Organization (WHO) is currently underway in Asia involving HBV vaccination of the newborn. HCC in African blacks is not associated with severe cirrhosis but is poorly differentiated and very aggressive. Despite uniform HBV carrier rates among the South African Bantu, there is a ninefold difference in HCC incidence between Mozambicans living along the coast and inland. These differences are attributed to the additional exposure to dietary aflatoxin B_1 and other carcinogenic mycotoxins. A typical interval between HCV-associated transfusion and subsequent HCC is ~30 years. HCV-associated HCC patients tend to have more frequent and advanced cirrhosis, but in HBV-associated HCC, only half the patients have cirrhosis; the remainder have chronic active hepatitis (Chap. 300).

Other Etiologic Conditions The 75–85% association of HCC with underlying cirrhosis has long been recognized, more typically with macronodular cirrhosis in Southeast Asia but also with micronodular cirrhosis (alcohol) in Europe and the United States (Chap. 302). It is still not clear whether cirrhosis itself is a predisposing factor to the development of HCC or whether the underlying causes of the cirrhosis are actually the carcinogenic factors. However, ~20 % of U.S. patients with HCC do not have underlying cirrhosis. Several underlying conditions are associated with an increased risk for cirrhosis-associated HCC (Table 88-2), including hepatitis, alcohol abuse, autoimmune chronic active hepatitis, cryptogenic cirrhosis, and nonalcoholic steatohepatitis (NASH). A less common association is with primary biliary cirrhosis and several metabolic diseases, including hemochromatosis, Wilson's disease, α_1-antitrypsin deficiency, tyrosinemia, porphyria cutanea tarda, glycogenesis types 1 and 3, citrullinemia, and orotic aciduria. The etiology of HCC in those 20% of patients who have no cirrhosis is unclear, and their HCC natural history not well-defined.

TABLE 88-2 RISK FACTORS FOR HEPATOCELLULAR CARCINOMA

Common	Unusual
Cirrhosis from any cause	Primary biliary cirrhosis
Hepatitis B or C chronic infection	Hemochromatosis
Ethanol chronic consumption	α_1 Antitrypsin deficiency
Nonalcoholic steatohepatitis (NASH)	Glycogen storage diseases
Aflatoxin B_1 or other mycotoxins	Citrullinemia
	Porphyria cutanea tarda
	Hereditary tyrosinemia
	Wilson's disease

CLINICAL FEATURES

Symptoms in HCC patients include abdominal pain, weight loss, weakness, abdominal fullness and swelling, jaundice, and nausea (Table 88-3). Presenting signs and symptoms differ somewhat between high- and low-incidence areas. The most common symptom is abdominal pain in high-risk areas, especially in South African blacks; by contrast, only 40–50% of Chinese and Japanese patients present with abdominal pain. Abdominal swelling may occur as a consequence of ascites due to the underlying chronic liver disease or may be due to a rapidly expanding tumor. Occasionally, central necrosis or acute hemorrhage into the peritoneal cavity leads to death. In countries with an active surveillance program, HCC tends to be identified at an earlier stage when symptoms may be due only to the underlying disease. Jaundice is usually due to obstruction of the intrahepatic ducts by the underlying liver disease. Hematemesis may occur due to esophageal varices from the underlying portal hypertension. Bone pain is seen in 3–12% of patients, but necropsies show bone metastases in ~20% of patients. Patients may be asymptomatic.

Physical Signs Hepatomegaly is the most common physical sign, occurring in 50–90% of patients. Abdominal bruits are noted in 6–25%, and ascites occurs in 30–60% of patients. Ascites should be examined

TABLE 88-3 HEPATOCELLULAR CARCINOMA: CLINICAL PRESENTATION AT THE UNIVERSITY OF PITTSBURGH LIVER CANCER CENTER ($n = 547$)

	Number of Patients (%)
Symptom	
No symptom	129 (24)
Abdominal pain	219 (40)
Other (workup of anemia and various diseases)	64 (12)
Routine physical exam finding, elevated LFTs	129 (24)
Weight loss	112 (20)
Appetite loss	59 (11)
Weakness/malaise	83 (15)
Jaundice	30 (5)
Routine CT scan screening of known cirrhosis	92 (17)
Cirrhosis symptoms (ankle swelling, abdominal bloating, increased girth, pruritus, GI bleed)	98 (18)
Diarrhea	7 (1)
Tumor rupture	1
Patient characteristics	
Mean age (years)	56 ± 13
Male: Female	3:1
Ethnicity	
Caucasian	72%
Middle Eastern	10%
Asian	13%
African American	5%
Cirrhosis	81%
No cirrhosis	19%
Tumor characteristics	
Hepatic tumor numbers	
1	20%
2	25%
3 or more	65%
Portal vein invasion	75%
Unilobar	25%
Bilobar	75%

Note: LFTs, liver function tests; GI, gastrointestinal.

by cytology. Splenomegaly is mainly due to portal hypertension. Weight loss and muscle wasting are common, particularly with rapidly growing or large tumors. Fever is found in 10–50% of patients, from unclear cause. The signs of chronic liver disease may be present, including jaundice, dilated abdominal veins, palmar erythema, gynecomastia, testicular atrophy, and peripheral edema. Budd-Chiari syndrome can occur due to HCC invasion of the hepatic veins; it should be suspected in patients with tense ascites and a large tender liver (Chap. 302).

Paraneoplastic Syndromes Most paraneoplastic syndromes in HCC are biochemical abnormalities without associated clinical consequences. They include hypoglycemia (also caused by end-stage liver failure), erythrocytosis, hypercalcemia, hypercholesterolemia, dysfibrinogenemia, carcinoid syndrome, increased thyroxin-binding globulin, changes in secondary sex characteristics (gynecomastia, testicular atrophy, and precocious puberty), and porphyria cutanea tarda. Mild hypoglycemia occurs in rapidly growing HCC as part of terminal illness, and profound hypoglycemia may occur, although the cause is unclear. Erythrocytosis occurs in 3–12% of patients, and hypercholesterolemia in 10–40%. A high percentage of patients have thrombocytopenia or leukopenia not caused by cancer infiltration of bone marrow, as in other tumor types.

STAGING

Although the TNM (primary *t*umor, regional *n*odes, *m*etastasis) staging system set up by the American Joint Commission for Cancers (AJCC) is sometimes used, the newer Cancer of the Liver Italian Program (CLIP) system is now popular as it takes cirrhosis into account, as does the Okuda system (Table 88-4). Other staging systems have been proposed and a consensus is needed. The best prognosis is stage I, solitary tumor <2 cm in diameter without vascular invasion. Adverse prognostic features include ascites, vascular invasion, and lymph node spread. Vascular invasion, in particular, has profound effects on prognosis and may be microscopic or macroscopic (visible on CT). Most large tumors have microscopic vascular invasion, so full staging can usually be made only after surgical resection. Stage III disease contains a mixture of lymph node–positive and –negative tumors. Stage III patients with positive lymph node disease have a poor prognosis, and few patients survive 1 year. The prognosis of stage IV is poor after either resection or transplantation, and 1-year survival is rare. A working staging system based entirely on clinical grounds that incorporates the contribution of the underlying liver disease was originally developed by Okuda et al. (Table 88-4). Patients with Okuda stage III have a dire prognosis, because they usually cannot be curatively resected and the condition of their liver typically precludes chemotherapy.

TABLE 88-4 CLIP AND OKUDA STAGING SYSTEMS FOR HEPATOCELLULAR CARCINOMA

CLIP Classification

	Points		
Variables	**0**	**1**	**2**
i. Tumor number	Single	Multiple	—
Hepatic replacement by tumor (%)[a]	<50	<50	>50
ii. Child-Pugh score	A	B	C
iii. α-Fetoprotein level (ng/mL)	<400	≥400	—
iv. Portal vein thrombosis (CT)	No	Yes	—

CLIP stages (score = sum of points): CLIP 0, 0 points; CLIP 1, 1 point; CLIP 2, 2 points; CLIP 3, 3 points.

Okuda Classification

Tumor Size[a]		Ascites		Albumin (g/L)		Bilirubin (mg/dL)	
≥50% (+)	<50 (–)	+ (+)	– (–)	≤3 (+)	>3 (–)	≥3 (+)	<3 (–)

Okuda stages: stage 1, all (–); stage 2, 1 or 2 (+); stage 3, 3 or 4 (+).

[a]Extent of liver occupied by tumor.
Note: CLIP, Cancer of the Liver Italian Program.

APPROACH TO THE PATIENT: Hepatocellular Carcinoma

History and Physical The history is important in evaluating putative predisposing factors, including a history of hepatitis or jaundice, blood transfusion, or use of intravenous drugs. A family history of HCC or hepatitis should be sought, and a detailed social history taken to include job descriptions for industrial exposure to possible carcinogenic drugs as well as contraceptive hormones. Physical examination should include assessing stigmata of underlying liver disease such as jaundice, ascites, peripheral edema, spider nevi, palmar erythema, and weight loss. Evaluation of the abdomen for hepatic size, masses or ascites, hepatic nodularity and tenderness, and splenomegaly is needed, as is assessment of overall clinical performance status and psychosocial evaluation.

Serologic Assays α-Fetoprotein (AFP) is a serum tumor marker in HCC; however, it is only increased in about half of U.S. patients. The other widely used assay is that for des-γ-carboxy prothrombin (DCP), a protein induced by vitamin K absence (PIVKA-2). This protein is increased in as many as 80% of HCC patients but may also be elevated in patients with vitamin K deficiency; it is always elevated after use of warfarin. It may predict for portal vein invasion. In a patient presenting with either a new hepatic mass or other indications of recent hepatic decompensation, carcinoembryonic antigen (CEA), vitamin B_{12}, AFP, ferritin, PIVKA-2, and antimitochondrial Ab should be measured, and standard liver function tests should be performed, including prothrombin time (PT), partial thromboplastin time (PTT), albumin, transaminases, γ-glutamyl transpeptidase, and alkaline phosphatase. Decreases in platelet count and white blood cell count may reflect portal hypertension and associated hypersplenism. Hepatitis A, B, and C serology should be measured. If HBV or HCV serology is positive, quantitative measurements of HBV DNA or HCV RNA are needed.

Radiology An ultrasound examination of the liver is an excellent screening tool. The two characteristic vascular abnormalities are hypervascularity of the tumor mass (neovascularization or abnormal tumor-feeding arterial vessels) and thrombosis by tumor invasion of otherwise normal portal veins. To determine tumor size and extent and the presence of portal vein invasion accurately, a helical/triphasic CT scan of the abdomen and pelvis with fast contrast bolus technique should be performed to detect the vascular lesions typical of HCC. Portal vein invasion is normally detected as an obstruction and expansion of the vessel. A chest CT is used to exclude metastases. MRI can also provide detailed information, especially with the newer contrast agents. Ethiodol (Lipiodol) is an ethiodized oil emulsion retained by liver tumors that can be delivered by hepatic artery injection (5–15 mL) for CT imaging 1 week later. For small tumors, ethiodol injection is very helpful before biopsy because its histologic presence constitutes proof that the needle biopsied the mass under suspicion. A prospective comparison of triphasic CT, gadolinium-enhanced MRI, ultrasound, and fluorodeoxyglucose positron emission tomography (FDG-PET) scans demonstrated similar results for CT, MRI, and ultrasound; PET imaging was unsuccessful.

Pathologic Diagnosis Histologic proof of the presence of HCC is obtained through a core liver biopsy of the mass under ultrasound guidance as well as random biopsy of the underlying liver. Bleeding risk is increased compared to other cancers because (1) the tumors are hypervascular, and (2) patients often have thrombocytopenia and decreased clotting factors. Bleeding risk is further increased in the presence of ascites. Tracking of tumor has been an uncommon problem. Fine-needle aspirates may provide sufficient material for diagnosis of cancer, but core biopsies are preferred. Tissue architecture must be examined to distinguish between HCC and metastatic adenocarcinoma; laparoscopic approaches can also be used. For patients suspected of having portal vein involvement, a core biopsy of the portal vein may be performed safely. If positive, this is regarded as an exclusion criterion for transplantation for HCC.

SCREENING HIGH-RISK POPULATIONS

Screening has not been shown to save lives. Prospective studies in high-risk populations showed that ultrasound was more sensitive than AFP elevations. An Italian study in patients with cirrhosis identified a yearly HCC incidence of 3% but showed no increase in the rate of detection of potentially curable tumors with aggressive screening. Prevention strategies including universal vaccination against hepatitis viruses are more likely to be effective than screening efforts. Despite absence of formal guidelines, most practitioners obtain 6-monthly AFP levels and perform CT (or ultrasound) when following high-risk patients (HBV carriers, HCV cirrhosis, family history of HCC).

Rx HEPATOCELLULAR CARCINOMA

Most HCC patients have two liver diseases, cirrhosis and HCC, each of which is an independent cause of death. The presence of cirrhosis usually places constraints on resection surgery, ablative therapies, and chemotherapy. Thus patient assessment and treatment planning have to take the severity of the nonmalignant liver disease into account. The clinical management choices for HCC can be complex (Fig. 88-1). The natural history of HCC is highly variable. Patients presenting with advanced tumors (vascular invasion, symptoms, extrahepatic spread) have a median survival of ~4 months, with or without treatment. Treatment results from the literature are difficult to interpret. Survival is not always a measure of the efficacy of therapy because of the adverse effects on survival of the underlying liver disease. A multidisciplinary team, including a hepatologist, interventional radiologist, surgical oncologist, transplant surgeon, and medical oncologist, is important for the comprehensive management of HCC patients.

STAGES I AND II HCC Early-stage tumors are successfully treated using various techniques, including surgical resection, local ablation (thermal or radiofrequency), and local injection therapies (ethanol or acetic acid). Because the majority of patients with HCC suffer from a field defect in the cirrhotic liver, they are at risk for subsequent multiple primary liver tumors. Many will also have significant underlying liver disease and may not tolerate major surgical loss of hepatic parenchyma; they may be eligible for orthotopic liver transplant (OLTX) in the future. An important principle in treating early-stage HCC is to use liver-sparing treatments and to focus on treatment of both the tumor and the cirrhosis.

Surgical Excision The risk of major hepatectomy is high (5–10% mortality) due to the underlying liver disease and the potential for liver failure. Preoperative portal vein occlusion can sometimes be performed to cause atrophy of the HCC-involved lobe and compensatory hypertrophy of the noninvolved liver, permitting safer resection. Intraoperative ultrasound is useful for planning the surgical approach. In cirrhotic patients, any major liver surgery can result in liver failure. The Child-Pugh classification of liver failure (Chap. 295) is a reliable prognosticator for tolerance of hepatic surgery, and only Child A patients should be considered for surgical resection. Child B and C patients with stages I and II HCC should be referred for OLTX if appropriate, as should patients with ascites or a recent history of variceal bleeding. Although open surgical excision is the most reliable, the patient may be better served with a laparoscopic approach to resection, using RFA or percutaneous ethanol injection (PEI). No adequate comparisons of these different techniques have been undertaken, and the choice of treatment is usually based on physician skill.

Local Ablation Strategies Radiofrequency ablation (RFA) uses heat to ablate tumors. The maximum size of the probe arrays allows for a 7-cm zone of necrosis, which would be adequate for a 3- to 4-cm tumor. The heat reliably kills cells within the zone of necrosis. Treatment of tumors close to the main portal pedicles can lead to bile duct injury and obstruction. This limits the tumors that are anatomically suited for this technique. RFA can be performed percutaneously with CT or ultrasound guidance, or by laparoscopy with ultrasound guidance.

Local Injection Therapy Numerous agents have been used for local injection into tumors, most commonly, ethanol (PEI). The relatively soft HCC within the hard background of cirrhotic liver allows for injection of large volumes of ethanol into the tumor without diffusion into the hepatic parenchyma or leakage out of the liver. PEI causes direct destruction of cancer cells, but it is not selective for cancer cells and will destroy normal cells in the vicinity. It usually requires multiple injections (average of three), in contrast to one for RFA. The maximum size of tumor reliably treated is 3 cm, even with multiple injections.

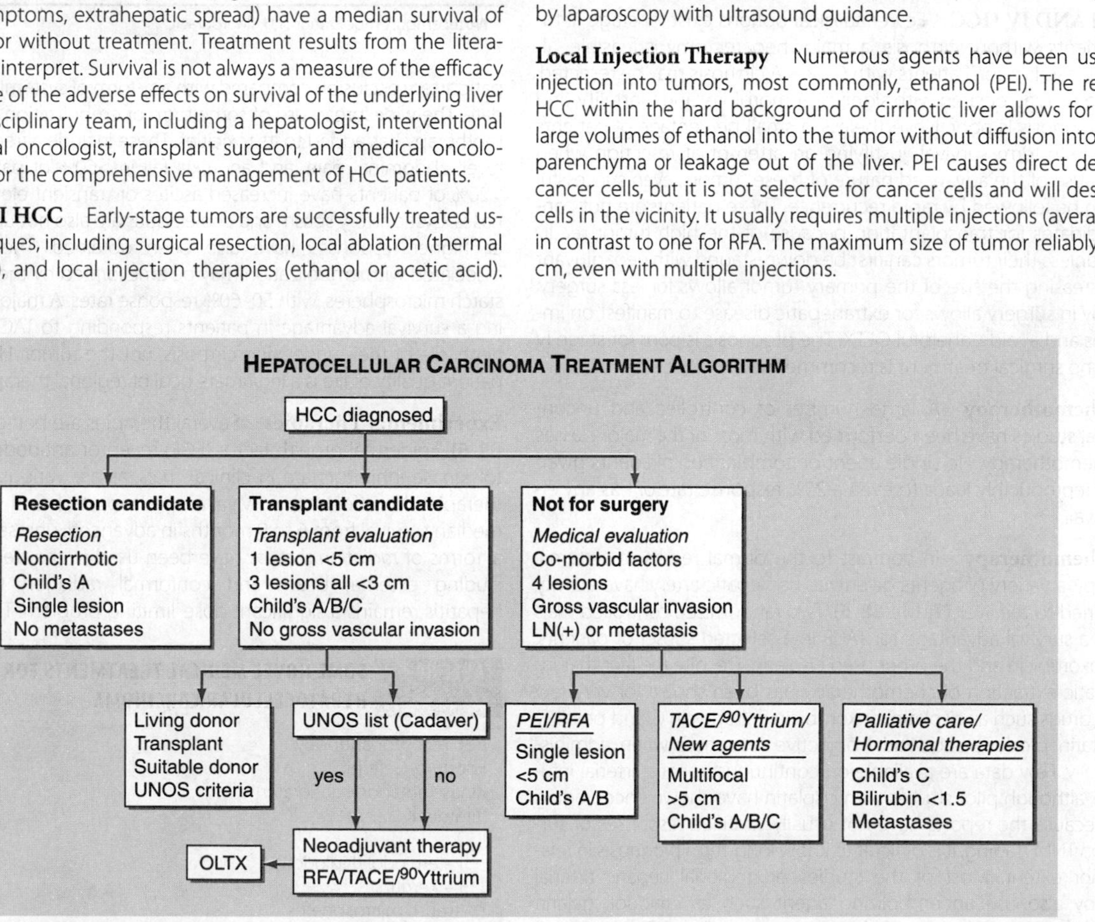

FIGURE 88-1 Treatment approach to patients with hepatocellular carcinoma. The initial clinical evaluation is aimed at assessing the extent of the tumor and the underlying functional compromise of the liver by cirrhosis. Patients are classified as having resectable disease, unresectable disease, or as transplantation candidates. Abbreviations: OLTX, orthotopic liver transplantation; TACE, transarterial chemoembolization; PEI, percutaneous ethanol injection; RFA, radiofrequency ablation; LN, lymph node. Child's A/B/C refers to the Child-Pugh classification of liver failure.

Liver Transplantation A viable option for stages I and II tumors in the setting of cirrhosis is OLTX, with survival approaching that for noncancer cases. OLTX for patients with a single lesion ≤ 5 cm or three or fewer nodules, each ≤ 3 cm (Milan criteria), resulted in excellent tumor-free survival (≥70% at 5 years). For advanced HCC, OLTX has been abandoned due to high tumor recurrence rates. Priority scoring for OLTX previously led to HCC patients waiting too long for their OLTX, resulting in some tumors becoming too advanced during the patient's wait for a donated liver. A variety of therapies were used as a "bridge" to OLTX, including RFA, PEI, and transarterial chemoembolization (TACE). These pretransplant treatments allow patients to remain on the waiting list longer, giving them greater opportunities to be transplanted. What remains unclear is whether this translates into prolonged survival after transplant. Further, it is not known whether patients who have had their tumor(s) treated preoperatively follow the recurrence pattern predicted by their tumor status at the time of transplant (i.e., post local ablative therapy), or if they follow the course set by their tumor parameters present before such treatment. The United Network for Organ Sharing (UNOS) point system for priority scoring of OLTX recipients now includes additional points for patients with HCC. The success of living related donor liver transplantation programs has also led to patients receiving transplantation earlier for HCC and often with greater than minimal tumors.

Adjuvant Therapy The role of adjuvant chemotherapy for patients after resection or OLTX remains unclear. No clear advantage in disease-free or overall survival has been found for either adjuvant or neoadjuvant approaches, though a meta-analysis of several trials revealed a significant improvement in disease-free and overall survival. Analysis of postoperative adjuvant systemic chemotherapy trials demonstrated no disease-free or overall survival advantage, but single studies of TACE and neoadjuvant ^{131}I-ethiodol have shown enhanced survival after resection.

STAGES III AND IV HCC Fewer surgical options exist for stage III tumors. In patients without cirrhosis, a major hepatectomy is feasible, although prognosis is poor. Patients with Child's A cirrhosis may be resected, but a lobectomy is associated with significant morbidity and mortality, and long-term prognosis is poor. Nevertheless, a small percentage of patients will achieve long-term survival, justifying an attempt at resection when feasible. Because of the advanced nature of these tumors, even successful resection can be followed by rapid recurrence. These patients are not considered candidates for transplantation because of the high tumor recurrence rates, unless their tumors can first be down-staged with neoadjuvant therapy. Decreasing the size of the primary tumor allows for less surgery, and the delay in surgery allows for extrahepatic disease to manifest on imaging studies and avoid unhelpful OLTX. The prognosis is poor for stage IV tumors, and no surgical treatment is recommended.

Systemic Chemotherapy A large number of controlled and uncontrolled clinical studies have been performed with most of the major classes of cancer chemotherapy. No single agent or combination of agents given systemically reproducibly leads to even a 25% response rate or has any effect on survival.

Regional Chemotherapy In contrast to the dismal results of systemic chemotherapy, a variety of agents given via the hepatic artery have activity in HCC confined to the liver **(Table 88-5)**. Two randomized controlled trials have shown a survival advantage for TACE in a selected subset of patients. One used doxorubicin and the other used cisplatin. Despite the fact that increased hepatic extraction of chemotherapy has been shown for very few drugs, some drugs such as cisplatin, doxorubicin, mitomycin C, and possibly neocarzinostatin produce substantial objective responses when administered regionally. Few data are available on continuous hepatic arterial infusion for HCC, although pilot studies with cisplatin have shown encouraging responses. Because the reports have not usually stratified responses or survival based on TNM staging, it is difficult to know long-term prognosis in relation to tumor extent. Most of the studies on regional hepatic arterial chemotherapy also use an embolizing agent such as ethiodol, gelatin sponge particles (Gelfoam), starch (Spherex), or microspheres. Two products are composed of microspheres of defined size ranges—Embospheres (Biospheres) and Contour SE—using particles of 40–120, 100–300, 300–500, and 500–1000 μm in size. The optimal diameter of the particles for TACE has yet to be defined. Consistently higher objective response rates appear to be reported for arterial administration of drugs together with some form of hepatic artery occlusion compared with any form of systemic chemotherapy to date. The widespread use of some form of embolization in addition to chemotherapy has added to its toxicities. These include a frequent but transient fever, abdominal pain, and anorexia (all in >60% of patients). In addition, >20% of patients have increased ascites or transient elevation of transaminases. Cystic artery spasm and cholecystitis are also not uncommon. However, higher responses have also been obtained. The hepatic toxicities associated with embolization may be ameliorated by the use of degradable starch microspheres, with 50–60% response rates. A major problem in showing a survival advantage in patients responding to TACE is that many patients die of their underlying cirrhosis, not the tumor. However, improving patient quality of life is a legitimate goal of regional therapies.

TABLE 88-5 SOME RANDOMIZED CLINICAL TRIALS INVOLVING TRANSHEPATIC ARTERY CHEMOEMBOLIZATION (TACE) FOR HEPATOCELLULAR CARCINOMA

Author	Year	Agents 1	Agents 2	Survival Effect
Kawaii	1992	Doxorubicin + embo	Embo	No
Chang	1994	Cisplatin + embo	Embo	No
Hatanaka	1995	Cisplatin, doxorubicin + embo	Same + ethiodol	No
Uchino	1993	Cisplatin, doxorubicin + oral FU	Same + tamoxifen	No
Lin	1988	Embo	Embo + IV FU	No
Yoshikawa	1994	Epirubicin + ethiodol (Lipiodol)	Epirubicin	No
Pelletier	1990	Doxorubicin + Gelfoam	None	No
Trinchet	1995	Cisplatin + Gelfoam	None	No
Bruix	1998	Coils and Gelfoam	None	No
Pelletier	1998	Cisplatin + ethiodol	None	No
Trinchet	1995	Cisplatin + Gelfoam	None	No
Pelletier	1998	Cisplatin + ethiodol	None	No
Lo	2002	Cisplatin + ethiodol	None	Yes
Llovet	2002	Doxorubicin + ethiodol	None	Yes

Note: embo, embolization; FU, fluorouracil.

Experimental Therapies Several therapies are being evaluated **(Table 88-6)**. Epidermal growth factor (EGF) receptor antibodies and EGF receptor kinase inhibitors are in clinical trials, as are various anti-angiogenesis therapies. No effects on survival are yet reported. Oral sorafenib increases median survival from 6 to 9 months in advanced, unresectable HCC. Several forms of *radiation therapy* have been used in the treatment of HCC, including external beam and conformal radiation therapy. Radiation hepatitis remains a significant dose-limiting problem. The pure beta emit-

TABLE 88-6 SOME NOVEL MEDICAL TREATMENTS FOR HEPATOCELLULAR CARCINOMA

EGF receptor antibody
Erlotinib, Gefitinib
Kinase antagonists, Sorafenib
Vitamin K
IL-2
^{131}I – ethiodol (Lipiodol)
^{131}I – Ferritin
^{90}Yttrium microspheres
^{166}Holmium
Three-dimensional conformal radiation
Proton beam high-dose radiotherapy
Anti-angiogenesis strategies, Bevacizumab

Note: EGF, epidermal growth factor; IL, interleukin.

ter ^{90}yttrium attached to either glass or resin microspheres has been assessed in phase II trials of HCC and has encouraging survival effects with minimal toxicities. Randomized trials have yet to be performed. Vitamin K has been assessed in clinical trials at high dosage for its HCC-inhibitory actions. This idea is based on the characteristic biochemical defect in HCC of elevated plasma levels of immature prothrombin (DCP or PIVKA-2), due to a defect in the activity of prothrombin carboxylase, a vitamin K–dependent enzyme. Two vitamin K randomized controlled trials from Japan show decreased tumor occurrence. Patient participation in clinical trials aimed at assessing new therapies is encouraged.

SUMMARY

Most Common Modes of Patient Presentation

1. A patient with known history of hepatitis, jaundice, or cirrhosis, with an abnormality on ultrasound or CT scan, or rising AFP or DCP (PIVKA-2)
2. A patient with an abnormal liver function test as part of a routine examination
3. Radiologic workup for liver transplant for cirrhosis
4. Symptoms of HCC including cachexia, abdominal pain, or fever.

History and Physical Examination

1. Clinical jaundice, asthenia, itching (scratches), tremors, or disorientation
2. Hepatomegaly, splenomegaly, ascites, peripheral edema, skin signs of liver failure.

Clinical Evaluation

1. Blood tests: full blood count (splenomegaly), liver function tests, ammonia levels, electrolytes, α-fetoprotein and DCP (PIVKA-2), Ca^{2+} and Mg^{2+}; hepatitis B and C serology (and quantitative HBV DNA or HCV RNA, if either is positive); neurotensin (specific for fibrolamellar HCC)
2. Triphasic dynamic helical (spiral) CT scan of liver (if inadequate, then follow with an MRI); chest CT scan; upper and lower gastrointestinal endoscopy (for varices, bleeding, ulcers); and brain scan (only if symptoms suggest)
3. A core biopsy: of the tumor and separately of the underlying liver.

Therapy (See also Fig. 88-1)

1. HCC < 2 cm: RFA ablation, PEI, or resection
2. HCC > 2 cm, no vascular invasion: liver resection, RFA, or OLTX
3. Multiple unilobar tumors or tumor with vascular invasion: TACE
4. Bilobar tumors, no vascular invasion: TACE with OLTX for patients whose tumors have a response
5. Extrahepatic HCC or elevated bilirubin: Phase I and II studies.

OTHER PRIMARY LIVER TUMORS

FIBROLAMELLAR HCC (FL-HCC)

This rarer variant of HCC has a different biology than adult-type HCC. None of the known HCC causative factors seem important here. It is typically a disease of younger adults, often teenagers and predominantly females. It is AFP negative, but patients typically have elevated blood neurotensin levels, normal liver function tests, and no cirrhosis. Radiology is similar for HCC, except that characteristic adult-type portal vein invasion is less common. Although it is often multifocal in the liver, and therefore not resectable, metastases are common, especially to lungs and locoregional lymph nodes, but survival is often much better than with adult-type HCC. Resectable tumors are associated with 5-year survival of ≥50%. Patients often present with a huge liver or unexplained weight loss, fever, or elevated liver function tests on routine evaluations. These huge masses suggest slow growth. Surgical resection is the best management option, even for metastases, since these tumors respond much less well to chemotherapy than adult-type HCC. Although several series of OLTX for FL-HCC have been reported, the patients usually to die from tumor recurrences, with a 2- to 5-year lag compared with OLTX for adult-type HCC. Anecdotal responses to gemcitabine plus cisplatin-TACE are reported.

EPITHELIOID HEMANGIOENDOTHELIOMA (EHE)

This rare vascular tumor of adults is also usually multifocal and can also be associated with prolonged survival, even in the presence of metastases, which are commonly in the lung. There is usually no underlying cirrhosis. Histologically, these tumors are usually of borderline malignancy and express factor VIII antigen, confirming their endothelial origin. OLTX may be associated with prolonged survival.

CHOLANGIOCARCINOMA (CCC)

CCC typically refers to mucin-producing adenocarcinomas (different from HCC) that arise from the bile ducts. They are grouped by their anatomic site of origin as intrahepatic, hilar (central, ~65% of CCCs), and peripheral (or distal, ~30% of CCCs). They arise on the basis of cirrhosis less frequently than HCC, excepting primary biliary cirrhosis. Nodular tumors arising at the bifurcation of the common bile duct are called *Klatskin tumors* and are often associated with a collapsed gallbladder, a finding that mandates visualization of the entire biliary tree. The approach to management of central and peripheral CCC is quite different. The incidence seems to be increasing in the United States. Although most CCCs have no obvious cause, several predisposing factors have been identified, including primary sclerosing cholangitis, an autoimmune disease (10–20% of PSC patients), and liver fluke in Asians, especially *Opisthorchis viverrini* and *Clonorchis sinensis*. CCC seems also to be associated with any cause of chronic biliary inflammation and injury, with alcoholic liver disease, choledocholithiasis, choledochal cysts (10%), and Caroli's disease. CCC most typically presents as painless jaundice, often with pruritus or weight loss, and acholic stools. Diagnosis is made by biopsy, percutaneously for peripheral liver lesions or, more commonly, via endoscopic retrograde cholangiopancreatography (ERCP) under direct vision for central lesions. The tumors often stain positively for cytokeratins 7, 8, and 19 and negatively for cytokeratin 20. However, histology alone cannot usually distinguish CCC from metastases from primary tumors of the colon or pancreas. Serologic tumor markers appear to be nonspecific, but CEA, CA 19-9, and CA-125 are often elevated in CCC patients and are useful for following response to therapy. Radiologic evaluation typically starts with ultrasound, which is useful in visualizing dilated bile ducts, and then proceeds with either MRI or magnetic resonance cholangiopancreatography (MRCP) or helical CT scans. Invasive ERCP is then needed to define the biliary tree and obtain a biopsy or is needed therapeutically to decompress an obstructed biliary tree with internal stent placement. If that fails, then percutaneous biliary drainage will be needed, with the biliary drainage flowing into an external bag. Central tumors often invade the porta hepatis, and locoregional lymph node involvement by tumor is frequent.

℞ CHOLANGIOCARCINOMA

Hilar CCC is resectable in ~30% of patients and usually involves bile duct resection and lymphadenectomy. Typical survival is around 24 months, with recurrences being mainly in the operative bed but with ~30% in the lungs and liver. Distal CCC, which involves the main ducts, is normally treated by resection of the extrahepatic bile ducts, often with pancreaticoduodenectomy. Survival is similar. Due to the high rates of locoregional recurrences or positive surgical margins, many patients get treated with postoperative adjuvant radiotherapy. Its effect on survival has not been assessed. Intraluminal brachyradiotherapy has also shown some promise. However, photodynamic therapy enhanced survival in one study. In this technique, sodium porfimer is injected IV and then subjected to intraluminal red light laser photoactivation. OLTX has been assessed for treatment of unresectable CCC, but 5-year survival was previously ~20%, so enthusiasm waned. However, neoadjuvant radiotherapy with sensitizing chemotherapy has shown better survival rates for CCC treated by OLTX from one institution; confirmation is needed. Multiple chemotherapeutic agents have been assessed for activity and survival in unresectable CCC. Most have been inactive. However, both systemic and hepatic arterial gemcitabine have shown promising results. The combination of this drug with others and with radiotherapy is being explored.

GALLBLADDER CANCER (GB Ca)

GB Ca has an even worse prognosis than CCC, with typical survival ~6 months or less. Women are affected much more commonly than men (4:1), unlike in HCC or CCC, and GB Ca is more common than CCC. Most patients have a history of gallstones, but very few patients with gallstones develop GB Ca (~0.2%). It presents similarly to CCC and is often diagnosed unexpectedly during gallstone or cholecystitis surgery. Presentation is typically that of chronic cholecystitis, chronic right upper quadrant pain and weight loss. Useful but nonspecific serum markers include CEA and CA 19-9. CT scans or MRCP typically reveal a gallbladder mass. The mainstay of treatment is surgical, either simple or radical cholecystectomy for stages I or II disease, respectively. Survival is nearly 100% at 5 years for stage I, and ranges from 60–90% at 5 years for stage II. More advanced GB Ca has worse survival, and many are unresectable. Adjuvant radiotherapy, used in the presence of local lymph node disease, has not been shown to enhance survival. Similar to CCC, chemotherapy is not useful in advanced or metastatic GB Ca.

CARCINOMA OF THE AMPULLA OF VATER

This tumor arises within 2 cm of the distal end of the common bile duct, and is mainly (90%) an adenocarcinoma. Locoregional lymph nodes are commonly involved (50%), and the liver is the most frequent site for metastases. The commonest clinical presentation is jaundice, and many patients also have pruritus, weight loss, and epigastric pain. Initial evaluation is performed with an abdominal ultrasound to assess vascular involvement, biliary dilatation, and liver lesions. This is followed by a CT scan, or MRI and especially MRCP. The most effective therapy is resection by pylorus-sparing pancreaticoduodenectomy, an aggressive procedure resulting in better survival rates than local resection. Survival rates are ~25% at 5 years in operable patients with involved lymph nodes and ~50% in patients without involved nodes. Unlike CCC, ~80% of patients are thought to be resectable at diagnosis. Adjuvant chemotherapy or radiotherapy has not been shown to be useful in enhancing survival. For metastatic tumors, chemotherapy is currently experimental.

TUMORS METASTATIC TO THE LIVER

These are predominantly from colon, pancreas, and breast primary tumors but can originate from any organ primary. Ocular melanomas are prone to liver metastasis. Tumor spread to the liver normally carries a poor prognosis for that tumor type. Colorectal and breast hepatic metastases were previously treated with continuous hepatic arterial infusion chemotherapy. However, more effective systemic drugs for these cancers, especially the addition of oxaliplatin to colorectal cancer regimens, have reduced the use of hepatic artery infusion therapy. In a large randomized study of systemic versus infusional plus systemic chemotherapy for resected colorectal metastases to the liver, the patients receiving infusional therapy had no survival advantage, mainly due to extrahepatic tumor spread. ^{90}Yttrium resin beads are approved in the United States for treatment of colorectal hepatic metastases. The role of this modality, either alone or in combination with chemotherapy, is being evaluated in many centers. Palliation may be obtained from chemoembolization, PEI, or RFA.

BENIGN LIVER TUMORS

Three common benign tumors occur and all are found predominantly in women. They are *hemangiomas, adenomas,* and *focal nodular hyperplasia* (FNH). FNH is typically benign, and usually no treatment is needed. Hemangiomas are the commonest and are entirely benign. Treatment is unnecessary unless their expansion causes symptoms. Adenomas are associated with contraceptive hormone use. They can cause pain and can bleed or rupture, causing acute problems. Their main interest for the physician is a low potential for malignant change and a 30% risk of bleeding. For this reason, considerable effort has gone into differentiating these three entities radiologically. Upon discovery of a liver mass, patients are usually advised to stop taking sex steroids, since adenoma regression may then occasionally occur. Adenomas can often be large masses ranging from 8–15 cm. Due to their size and definite, but low, malignant potential and potential for bleeding, adenomas are typically resected. The most useful diagnostic differentiating tool is a triphasic CT scan performed with HCC fast bolus protocol for arterial-phase imaging, together with subsequent delayed venous-phase imaging. Adenomas usually do not appear on the basis of cirrhosis, although both adenomas and HCCs are intensely vascular on the CT arterial phase and both can exhibit hemorrhage (40% of adenomas). However, adenomas have smooth, well-defined edges and enhance homogeneously, especially in the portal venous phase on delayed images, when HCCs no longer enhance. FNHs exhibit a characteristic central scar that is hypovascular on the arterial-phase and hypervascular on the delayed-phase CT images. MRI is even more sensitive in depicting the characteristic central scar of FNH.

FURTHER READINGS

FURUKAWA H et al: Living-donor liver transplantation for hepatocellular carcinoma. J Hepatobiliary Pancreat Surg 13:393, 2006

GOIN JE et al: Treatment of unresectable hepatocellular carcinoma with intrahepatic yttrium 90 microspheres. J Vasc Interv Radiol 16:161, 2005

LLOVET JM et al: A molecular signature to discriminate dysplastic nodules from early hepatocellular carcinoma. Gastroenterology 131:1758, 2006

PARIKH S, HYMAN D: Hepatocellular cancer: A guide for the internist. Am J Med 120:194, 2007

STEEL JL et al: Clinically meaningful changes in health-related quality of life in patients with hepatobiliary cancer. Ann Oncol 17:304, 2006

THORGEIRSSON S et al: Molecular prognostication of liver cancer: End of the beginning. J Hepatol 44:798, 2006

89 Pancreatic Cancer

Yu Jo Chua, David Cunningham

Over 90% of pancreatic cancers are ductal adenocarcinomas of the exocrine pancreas. These tumors occur twice as frequently in the pancreatic head compared to the rest of the organ, and tend to be aggressive, often presenting when locally inoperable or after distal metastases have occurred. Patients with pancreatic cancer have a poor prognosis, with a 5-year survival of only 5%. The discussion of pancreatic cancer here will be limited to ductal adenocarcinomas. Other types of pancreatic neoplasms include islet cell tumors and neuroendocrine tumors (Chap. 344).

INCIDENCE AND ETIOLOGY

Epidemiology The lifetime risk of being diagnosed with pancreatic cancer in the United States is 1.27%. In the United States, it is estimated that approximately 37,170 people will be diagnosed with pancreatic cancer in 2007. Consistent with its associated poor prognosis, 33,370 are expected to die from this disease in the same year, making it the fourth leading cause of cancer-related death. The median age of diagnosis of pancreatic cancer is 72 years, with the peak incidence of diagnosis between the ages of 65 and 84; it is rarely diagnosed in those below the age of 50. The incidence is slightly higher in men than women, and it is also higher in African Americans than in Caucasians.

Etiology Cigarette smoking, obesity, and nonhereditary chronic pancreatitis appear to be risk factors for the development of pancreatic cancer. With smoking, the risk seems to increase with the number of cigarettes consumed and decreases with smoking cessation. Less clear, and sometimes conflicting associations, have been observed for other environmental factors such as diet, coffee and alcohol consumption, previous partial gastrectomy or cholecystectomy, and *Helicobacter pylori*. An epidemiologic association between diabetes mellitus and pancreatic cancer has also been demonstrated; however, it is uncertain if diabetes is a precedent of, or consequence of, pancreatic cancer.

GENETIC CONSIDERATIONS Five to 10% of patients with pancreatic cancer also have an affected first-degree relative, suggesting that in some cases genetic factors are involved. These patients seem to present earlier than sporadic cases. The risk of pancreatic cancer is increased in certain syndromes, whether directly or indirectly, such as hereditary chronic pancreatitis, Peutz-Jeghers syndrome, Von Hippel-Lindau syndrome, familial atypical multiple-mole melanoma syndrome, ataxia-telangiectasia, Gardner's syndrome [a variant of familial adenomatous polyposis (FAP)] and Lynch syndrome II, a subtype of hereditary nonpolyposis colorectal cancer (HNPCC). Heavy smokers who also have homozygous deletions of the gene for glutathione-S transferase T1 (GSTT1), a carcinogen metabolizing enzyme, may be at particular risk. Activating mutations in the K-*ras* oncogene are found in nearly all pancreatic cancer. Loss-of-function mutations in several tumor suppressor genes occur in this disease, including p53, *CDKN2A* gene (also called multiple tumor suppressor-1 gene, leading in many cases to loss of function of p16), *DPC4*, and *BRCA2*. A feature almost unique to pancreatic cancer is the combination of K-*ras* and *CDKN2A* mutations.

CLINICAL FEATURES

Presenting Features Common presenting features of pancreatic cancer include pain (present in >80% of patients with locally advanced or metastatic disease), obstructive jaundice, weight loss, and anorexia. Patients with jaundice may also have pruritus, pale stools, and dark urine; they often have tumors in the pancreatic head, and tend to be diagnosed earlier and with earlier stage disease. Other symptoms tend to be more insidious, so that in the absence of jaundice, the interval between onset and diagnosis can be prolonged. Pain, for example, is often more of a problem in patients with lesions in the body or tail of the pancreas where the primary tumor is more likely to become quite large or to invade adjacent structures (such as the splanchnic nerves) before becoming manifest; these patients frequently have inoperable disease. When present, pain is often felt as a dull ache in the upper abdomen and may radiate to the back, and characteristically may improve upon leaning forward. It may initially be intermittent, and may worsen with meals. These patients may suffer from marked weight loss, which may result from a combination of anorexia, early satiety, malabsorption or diarrhea/steatorrhea. Other less common presenting features include the diagnosis of glucose intolerance (particularly within 2 years of cancer diagnosis), previous pancreatitis, migratory superficial thrombophlebitis (Trousseau's syndrome), gastrointestinal hemorrhage from varices, and splenomegaly.

Physical Findings Patients with early disease may not have any significant abnormalities detectable on physical examination. Jaundice may be a presenting feature in some; in these patients a palpable, nontender gallbladder (Courvoisier's sign) may be palpated under the right costal margin. Patients with more advanced disease may have an abdominal mass, hepatomegaly, splenomegaly, or ascites. The left supraclavicular lymph node (Virchow's node) may be involved with tumor, or widespread peritoneal disease may be palpable on rectal examination in the pouch of Douglas.

DIAGNOSTIC PROCEDURES

Imaging Studies (Fig. 89-1) Ultrasound is often used as an initial investigation for patients with jaundice, or with less-specific symptoms such as upper abdominal discomfort, and is able to assess the biliary tract, gall bladder, pancreas, and liver. Computed tomography (CT) scanning is preferable to ultrasound even though it is more costly, as it is less operator-dependent, more reproducible, and less susceptible to interference from intestinal gas. The sensitivity and specificity of CT is markedly improved by the use of pancreatic protocol scanning on modern multislice scanners. CT may show a pancreatic mass, dilatation of the biliary system or pancreatic duct, or distal spread to the liver, regional lymph nodes, or peritoneum (and/or associated ascites). When helical CT is combined with the use of intravenous contrast, it may also help determine resectability by providing information on the involvement of important vascular structures such as the celiac axis, superior mesenteric or portal vessels. Endoscopic retrograde cholangiopancreatography (ERCP) is also widely used in the diagnosis of pancreatic cancer, particularly when CT and ultrasound fail to show a mass lesion, and may reveal either stricture or obstruction in either the pancreatic or common bile duct. ERCP can also be used to obtain brushings of a stricture for cytology or for placing stents in order to relieve obstructive jaundice. Endoscopic ultrasound (EUS) may be useful in the diagnosis of small lesions (<2–3 cm in diameter) and, in some cases, for local staging as well as evaluating invasion of major vascular structures. EUS-guided fine-needle aspiration may also be used to obtain cytology for confirming the diagnosis, particularly in patients with potentially operable disease (see below). While magnetic resonance imaging (MRI) does not offer any advantages over CT in the routine evaluation of patients with possible pancreatic cancer, magnetic resonance cholangiopancreatography (MRCP) may be better than CT for defining the anatomy of the pancreatic duct and biliary tree, being able to image the ducts both above and below a stricture. The sensitivity of MRCP is comparable to ERCP, but does not require contrast administration to the ductal system, so that there is less associated morbidity. MRCP may be useful when cannulation of the pancreatic duct by ERCP has been unsuccessful or may be difficult, such as when normal anatomy is changed by surgery. Positron-emission tomography with ^{18}F-fluoro-2deoxyglucose (FDG-PET) may be useful for excluding occult distal metastasis in patients with localized disease who are being worked up for surgery or in patients with unresectable localized disease being considered for chemoradiotherapy.

Tissue Diagnosis and Cytology Patients with disease that is potentially curable by surgery, and in whom a highly suspicious lesion is seen on imaging, are often taken directly to surgery without prior tissue confirmation of cancer. This is because of theoretical concerns that a percutaneous fine-needle aspiration may result in dissemination of cancer intraperitoneally or along the track of the biopsy needle. In addition, negative cytology may not be sufficient evidence to avoid surgery, particularly with small lesions. EUS-guided fine-needle aspiration is increasingly being used, even in patients with potentially resectable disease, as there is less risk of intraperitoneal spread of cancer. Other methods of obtaining specimens for cytological analysis include sampling of pancreatic juices or brushings of ductal lesions obtained by ERCP.

Serum Markers The most widely used serum marker in pancreatic cancer is cancer-associated antigen 19-9 (CA 19-9). It has a reported sensitivity and specificity of about 80–90%, and is suggestive, rather than confirmatory, of the diagnosis of pancreatic cancer. Serum levels of CA 19-9 can be elevated in patients with jaundice without pancreatic cancer present. The level of CA 19-9 may have prognostic implications, with very high levels sometimes found in patients with inoperable disease. In advanced disease, patients treated with chemotherapy who had high pretreatment levels of CA 19-9 have also been found to have a worse survival, whereas those patients whose levels of marker fell with treatment had a better outcome. In patients with cancers with elevated CA 19-9, serial evaluation of this marker is useful for monitoring re-

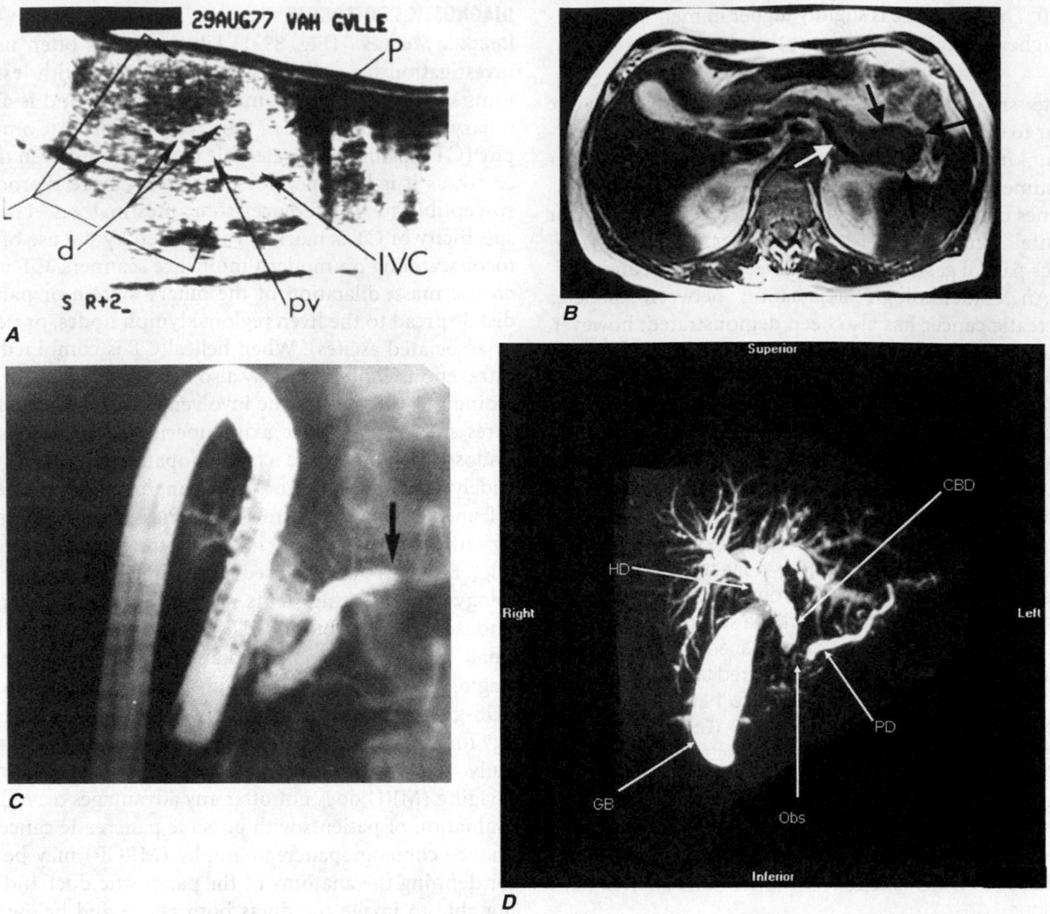

FIGURE 89-1 Carcinoma of the pancreas. ***A.*** Sonogram showing pancreatic carcinoma (P), dilated intrahepatic bile ducts (d), dilated portal vein (pv), and inferior vena cava (IVC). ***B.*** Computed tomography scan showing pancreatic carcinoma (*dark arrows*). ***C.*** Endoscopic retrograde showing abrupt cutoff of the duct of Wirsung (*arrow*). ***D.*** Magnetic resonance cholangiopancreatography showing obstruction (Obs) in the pancreatic duct (PD). The gallbladder (GB), hepatic duct (HD), and common bile duct (CBD) are labeled.

sponses to treatment. In patients with completely resected tumors, follow-up with CA 19-9 is useful for detecting recurrence.

Staging In pancreatic cancer, which has a poor prognosis, the value of detailed clinical staging is limited. The most clinically relevant distinction to make is between patients with disease that may be resected with curative intent, and those with advanced disease in whom treatment is palliative (Table 89-1).

Surveillance in High-Risk Individuals Routine screening for pancreatic cancer is not recommended due to a high false-positive rate of the available tests. However, screening may be reasonable in certain high-risk individuals, such as those with strong family histories, although the optimal timing, frequency, and method of screening is unknown.

TABLE 89-1 STAGING OF PANCREATIC CARCINOMA

	Stage Grouping	TNM Staging^a
Localized resectable	I	T1–2 N0 M0
	II	T3 N0 M0 or T1–3 N1 M0
Locally advanced	III	T4 N(any) M0
Metastatic	IV	T(any) N(any) M1

^{a}TNM, tumor, nodes, metastasis.

Note: T1, tumor limited to pancreas, ≤2 cm; T2, tumor limited to pancreas, >2 cm; T3, tumor extends beyond the pancreas but without involvement of celiac axis or superior mesenteric artery; T4, tumor involves celiac axis or the superior mesenteric artery (unresectable primary tumor); N0, no regional lymph node metastasis (regional lymph nodes are the peripancreatic lymph nodes, including the lymph nodes along the hepatic artery, celiac axis and pyloric/splenic regions); N1, regional lymph node metastasis; M0, no distal metastasis; M1, distal metastasis.

Source: Modified from Greene, Page; with permission.

One recommendation is to commence screening at the age of 35 in patients with hereditary pancreatitis, or 10 years before the age of the youngest diagnosis of pancreatic cancer in those with a significant family history using spiral CT, followed by EUS when CT results have been indeterminate.

℞ PANCREATIC CANCER

Symptoms and the associated impaired performance status are significant issues in the management of patients with pancreatic cancer, as they can have a marked negative impact on the ability to safely deliver chemotherapy or perform curative surgery. For example, patients with malabsorption secondary to pancreatic insufficiency may be treated with pancreatic enzyme supplementation. Indeed effective symptom management is as important a therapeutic goal as survival prolongation.

ADVANCED PANCREATIC CANCER These patients have metastatic or locally advanced inoperable disease and are the majority with newly diagnosed disease. Debulking surgery or partial resections have no role, as these procedures are associated with the same risks as a curative resection but are unlikely to improve survival. Many patients may, however, benefit from endoscopic biliary or duodenal stenting, and some patients from nerve plexus blocks or ablation. Less frequently, intestinal bypass surgery is required.

The deoxycytidine analogue gemcitabine, given as a single agent (gemcitabine 1000 mg/m^2 weekly for 7 weeks followed by 1 week rest, then weekly for 3 weeks every 4 weeks thereafter), has been the preferred treatment for these patients since it was shown to yield clinical benefit (a composite parameter for evaluating symptomatic benefit of treatment used in some trials of this disease) and improved survival compared to 5-fluorouracil. The median survival observed with single-agent gemcitabine in randomized trials is about 6 months, with a 12-month survival of approximately 18%. Furthermore, two randomized trials have shown improved survival from the addition of either the oral fluoropyrimidine, capecitabine (gemcitabine 1000 mg/m^2 days 1, 8, and 15 plus capecitabine 1660 mg/m^2 days 1–21, repeated every 28 days), or the tyrosine kinase inhibitor of the epidermal growth factor receptor (EGFR), erlotinib (standard gemcitabine plus erlotinib 100 mg daily). The survival improvement observed with both of these combinations appears similar, and the addition of capecitabine to gemcitabine in this regimen does not appear to increase the toxicity above single-agent gemcitabine. Either combination should, therefore, be considered as options for treating these patients. Second-line treatment options in pancreatic cancer are limited although there may be an emerging role for oxaliplatin-based chemotherapy; fit patients who have failed first-line treatment should be offered entry into clinical trials. On-going clinical trials are evaluating the potential benefits of incorporating other novel targeted agents into the treatment of pancreatic cancer, usually together with gemcitabine.

In patients with locally advanced unresectable disease, external beam chemoradiotherapy may be useful, either as initial treatment or as consolidation after induction chemotherapy.

OPERABLE DISEASE Complete surgical resection in patients with localized disease (stage I or II disease), with distal metastases excluded by prior CT scan of the abdomen and pelvis, and CT of the chest or chest x-ray, is potentially curative. However, such surgery is only possible in 10–15% of patients, many of whom will suffer from recurrences of their disease. Indeed, the 5-year survival reported in randomized trials with surgery alone is approximately 10%, although modern series have improved on these results. Outcomes tend to be more favorable in patients with lymph node–negative disease, smaller tumors (less than 3 cm), negative resection margins and well-differentiated tumors. Despite a dismal long term outcome, these patients still have a better survival with surgery than with other palliative measures.

Surgery is usually preceded by laparoscopy in order to exclude peritoneal metastases not seen on other staging investigations. Pancreaticoduodenectomy, also known as the Whipple procedure, is the standard operation for cancers of the head or uncinate process of the pancreas. The procedure involves resection of the pancreatic head, duodenum, first 15 cm of the jejunum, common bile duct, and gallbladder, and a partial gastrectomy, with the pancreatic and biliary anastomosis placed 45 to 60 cm proximal to the gastrojejunostomy. Perioperative mortality rates have fallen to less than 5%, reflecting greater experience with the surgery and perioperative management of these patients. However, this type of surgery is highly specialized and should ideally only occur in dedicated centers with a high volume of these cases and specialized surgeons.

Adjuvant treatment for patients with curatively resected pancreatic cancer is controversial, with divergent treatment approaches preferred in the United States and in Europe, based on the results of different randomized trials conducted on both sides of the Atlantic. In the United States, fluoropyrimidine-based postoperative chemoradiotherapy followed by adjuvant chemotherapy is preferred. In Europe, because a large randomized trial (the European Study Group for Pancreatic Cancer 1 or ESPAC1 trial) showed a survival benefit for adjuvant chemotherapy with 5-fluorouracil (5FU) **(Fig. 89-2)**, this approach is more common practice.

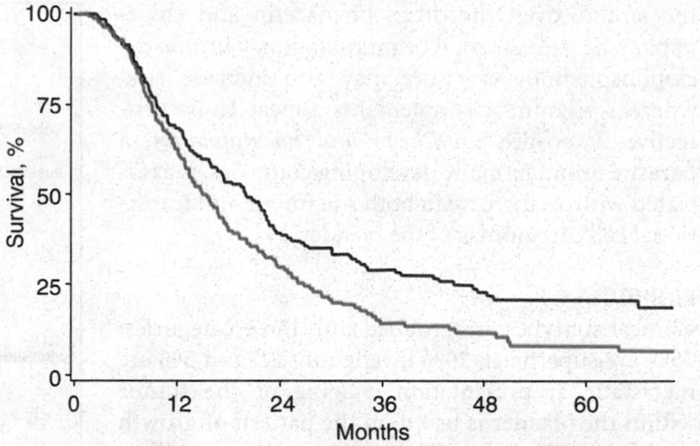

No. at Risk						
No CT —	142	89	41	18	11	7
CT —	147	99	56	38	22	11

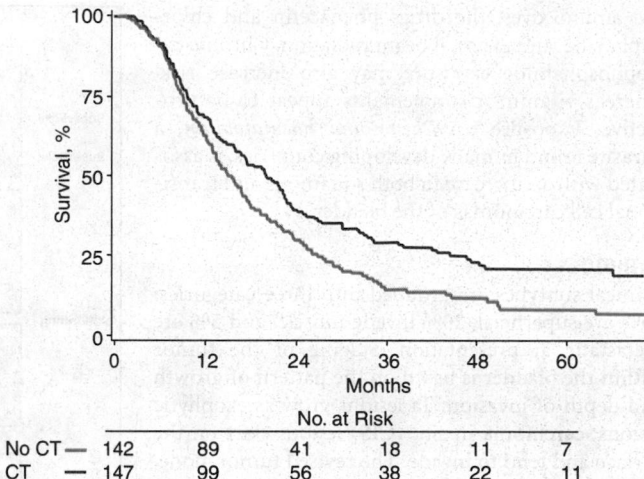

FIGURE 89-2 Survival by adjuvant chemotherapy. Kaplan-Meier estimates of survival from the European Study Group for Pancreatic Cancer 1 (ESPAC1) trial for the comparison of adjuvant chemotherapy versus no adjuvant chemotherapy (CT) in patients with resected pancreatic cancer (hazard ratio for death, 0.71; 95% confidence interval, 0.55 to 0.92; $p = .009$). *(Reprinted with permission from JP Neoptolemos, DD Stocken, H Friess, et al: A randomized trial of chemoradiotherapy and chemotherapy after resection of pancreatic cancer. N Engl J Med 350:1200–1210, 2004. Copyright 2004, Massachusetts Medical Society.)*

FURTHER READINGS

Alexakis N et al: Current standards of surgery for pancreatic cancer. Br J Surg 91:1410, 2004

Barugola G et al: The determinant factors of recurrence following resection for ductal pancreatic cancer. JOP 8(Suppl 1):132, 2007

Chua YJ, Cunningham D: Chemotherapy for advanced pancreatic cancer. Best Pract Res Clin Gastroenterol 20:327, 2006

DiMagno EP et al: AGA technical review on the epidemiology, diagnosis, and treatment of pancreatic ductal adenocarcinomas. American Gastroenterological Association. Gastroenterology 117:1464, 1999

Greene FL, Page DL (eds.): *Exocrine Pancreas, AJCC Cancer Staging Manual*, 6th ed, New York, Springer, pp 157–164, 2002

Neoptolemos JP et al: A randomized trial of chemoradiotherapy and chemotherapy after resection of pancreatic cancer. N Engl J Med 350:1200, 2004

Willett CG et al: Locally advanced pancreatic cancer. J Clin Oncol 23:4538, 2005

90 Bladder and Renal Cell Carcinomas

Howard I. Scher, Robert J. Motzer

BLADDER CANCER

A transitional cell epithelium lines the urinary tract from the renal pelvis to the ureter, urinary bladder, and the proximal two-thirds of the urethra. Cancers can occur at any point: 90% of malignancies develop in the bladder, 8% in the renal pelvis, and the remaining 2% in the ureter or urethra. Bladder cancer is the fourth most common cancer in men and the thirteenth in women, with an estimated 67,160 new cases and 13,750 deaths in the United States predicted for the year 2007. The almost 5:1 ratio of incidence to mortality reflects the higher frequency of the less lethal superficial variants compared to the more lethal invasive and metastatic variants. The incidence is three times higher in men than in women, and twofold higher in whites than blacks, with a median age at diagnosis of 65 years.

Once diagnosed, urothelial tumors exhibit polychronotropism—the tendency to recur over time and in new locations in the urothelial tract. As long as urothelium is present, continuous monitoring of the tract is required.

EPIDEMIOLOGY

Cigarette smoking is believed to contribute to up to 50% of the diagnosed urothelial cancers in men and up to 40% in women. The risk of developing a urothelial malignancy in male smokers is increased two- to fourfold relative to nonsmokers and continues for 10 years or longer after cessation. Other implicated agents include the aniline dyes, the drugs phenacetin and chlornaphazine, and external beam radiation. Chronic cyclophosphamide exposure may also increase risk, whereas vitamin A supplements appear to be protective. Exposure to *Schistosoma haematobium*, a parasite found in many developing countries, is associated with an increase in both squamous and transitional cell carcinomas of the bladder.

PATHOLOGY

Clinical subtypes are grouped into three categories: 75% are superficial, 20% invade muscle, and 5% are metastatic at presentation. Staging of the tumor within the bladder is based on the pattern of growth and depth of invasion: Ta lesions grow as exophytic lesions; carcinoma in situ (CIS) lesions start on the surface and tend to invade. The revised tumor, node, metastasis (TNM) staging system is illustrated in Fig. 90-1. About half of invasive tumors presented originally as superficial lesions that later progressed. Tumors are also rated by grade. Grade I lesions (highly differentiated tumors) rarely progress to a higher stage, whereas grade III tumors do.

More than 95% of urothelial tumors in the United States are transitional in origin. Pure squamous cancers with keratinization constitute 3%, adenocarcinomas 2%, and small cell tumors (with paraneoplastic syndromes) <1%. Adenocarcinomas develop primarily in the urachal remnant in the dome of the bladder or in the periurethral tissues; some assume a signet cell histology. Lymphomas and melanomas are rare. Of the transitional cell tumors, low-grade papillary lesions that grow on a central stalk are most common. These tumors are very friable, have a tendency to bleed, are at high risk for recurrence, and yet rarely progress to the more lethal invasive variety. In contrast, CIS is a high-grade tumor that is considered a precursor of the more lethal muscle-invasive disease.

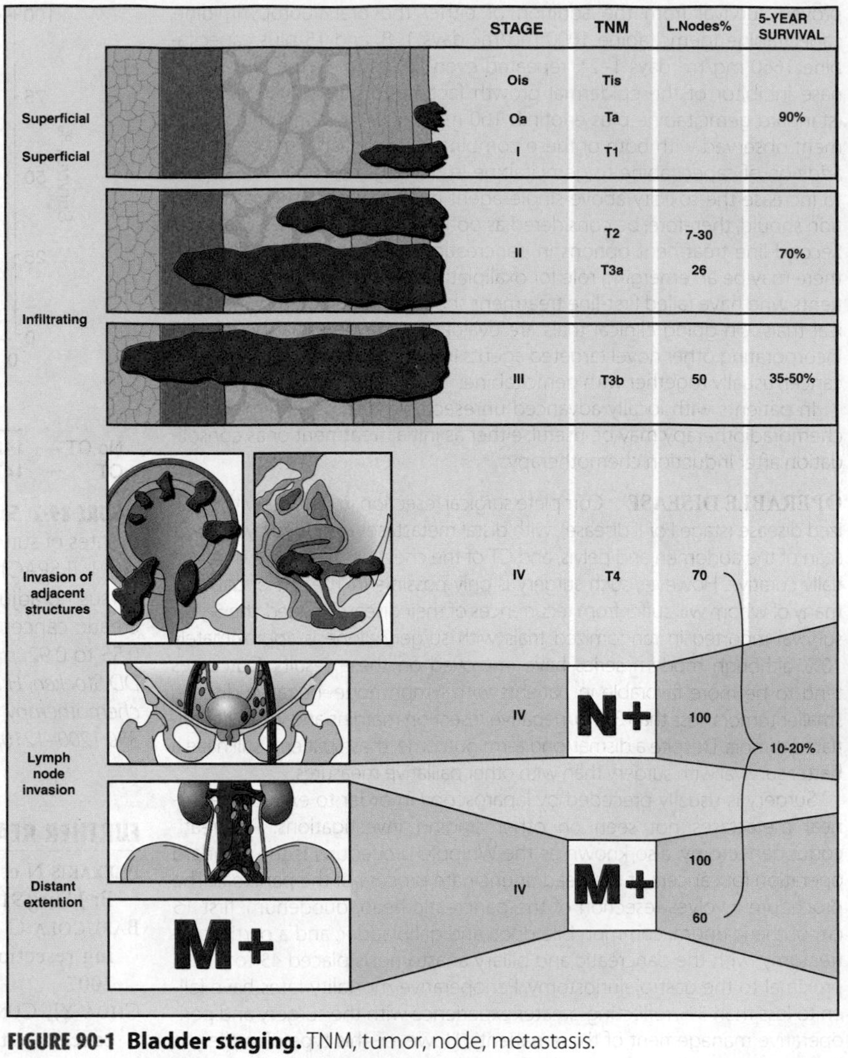

FIGURE 90-1 Bladder staging. TNM, tumor, node, metastasis.

PATHOGENESIS

The multicentric nature of the disease and high rate of recurrence has led to the hypothesis of a field defect in the urothelium that results in a predisposition to cancer. Molecular genetic analyses suggest that the superficial and invasive lesions develop along distinct molecular pathways in which primary tumorigenic aberrations precede secondary changes associated with progression to a more advanced stage. Low-grade papillary tumors that do not tend to invade or metastasize harbor constitutive activation of the receptor-tyrosine kinase-Ras signal transduction pathway and a high frequency of fibroblast growth factor receptor 3 (FGFR3) mutations. In contrast, CIS and invasive tumors have a higher frequency of *TP53* and *RB* gene alternations. Within all clinical stages, including Tis, T1, and T2 or greater lesions, tumors with alterations in *p53*, *p21*, and/or *RB* have a higher probability of recurrence, metastasis, and death from disease.

CLINICAL PRESENTATION, DIAGNOSIS, AND STAGING

Hematuria occurs in 80–90% of patients and often reflects exophytic tumors. The bladder is the most common source of gross hematuria (40%), but benign cystitis (22%) is a more common cause than bladder cancer (15%) (Chap. 45). Microscopic hematuria is more commonly of prostate origin (25%); only 2% of bladder cancers produce microscopic hematuria. Once hematuria is documented, a urinary cytology, visualization of the urothelial tract by CT or intravenous pyelogram, and cystoscopy are recommended if no other etiology is found. Screening asymptomatic individuals for hematuria increases the diagnosis of tumors at an early stage but has not been shown to prolong life. After hematuria, irritative symptoms are the next most common presentation, which may reflect in situ disease. Obstruction of the ureters may cause flank pain. Symptoms of metastatic disease are rarely the first presenting sign.

The endoscopic evaluation includes an examination under anesthesia to determine whether a palpable mass is present. A flexible endoscope is inserted into the bladder, and bladder barbotage is performed. The visual inspection includes mapping the location, size, and number of lesions, as well as a description of the growth pattern (solid vs. papillary). An intraoperative video is often recorded. All visible tumors should be resected, and a sample of the muscle underlying the tumor should be obtained to assess the depth of invasion. Normal-appearing areas are biopsied at random to ensure no field defect. A notation is made as to whether a tumor was completely or incompletely resected. Selective catheterization and visualization of the upper tracts should be performed if the cytology is positive and no disease is visible in the bladder. Ultrasonography, CT, and/or MRI may help to determine whether a tumor extends to perivesical fat (T3) and to document nodal spread. Distant metastases are assessed by CT of the chest and abdomen, MRI, or radionuclide imaging of the skeleton.

℞ BLADDER CANCER

Management depends on whether the tumor invades muscle and whether it has spread to the regional lymph nodes and beyond. The probability of spread increases with increasing T stage.

SUPERFICIAL DISEASE At a minimum, the management of a superficial tumor is complete endoscopic resection with or without intravesical therapy. The decision to recommend intravesical therapy depends on the histologic subtype, number of lesions, depth of invasion, presence or absence of CIS, and antecedent history. Recurrences develop in upward of 50% of cases, of which 5–20% progress to a more advanced stage. In general, solitary papillary lesions are managed by transurethral surgery alone. CIS and recurrent disease are treated by transurethral surgery followed by intravesical therapy.

Intravesical therapies are used in two general contexts: as an adjuvant to a complete endoscopic resection to prevent recurrence or, less commonly, to eliminate disease that cannot be controlled by endoscopic resection alone. Intravesical treatments are advised for patients with recurrent disease, >40% involvement of the bladder surface by tumor, diffuse CIS, or T1 disease. The standard intravesical therapy, based on randomized comparisons, is bacillus Calmette-Guerin (BCG) in six weekly instillations, followed by monthly maintenance administrations for ≥1 year. Other agents with activity include mitomycin-C, interferon (IFN), and gemcitabine. The side effects of intravesical therapies include dysuria, urinary frequency, and, depending on the drug, myelosuppression or contact dermatitis. Rarely, intravesical BCG may produce a systemic illness associated with granulomatous infections in multiple sites that requires antituberculin therapy.

Following the endoscopic resection, patients are monitored for recurrence at 3-month intervals during the first year. Recurrence may develop anywhere along the urothelial tract, including the renal pelvis, ureter, or urethra. A consequence of the "successful" treatment of tumors in the bladder is an increase in the frequency of extravesical recurrences (e.g., urethra or ureter). Those with persistent disease or new tumors are generally considered for a second course of BCG or for intravesical chemotherapy with valrubicin or gemcitabine. In some cases cystectomy is recommended, although the specific indications vary. Tumors in the ureter or renal pelvis are typically managed by resection during retrograde examination or, in some cases, by instillation through the renal pelvis. Tumors of the prostatic urethra may require cystectomy if the tumor cannot be resected completely.

INVASIVE DISEASE The treatment of a tumor that has invaded muscle can be separated into control of the primary tumor and, depending on the pathologic findings at surgery, systemic chemotherapy. Radical cystectomy is the standard, although in selected cases a bladder-sparing approach is used; this approach includes complete endoscopic resection; partial cystectomy; or a combination of resection, systemic chemotherapy, and external beam radiation therapy. In some countries, external beam radiation therapy is considered standard. In the United States, its role is limited to those patients deemed unfit for cystectomy, those with unresectable local disease, or as part of an experimental bladder-sparing approach.

Indications for cystectomy include muscle-invading tumors not suitable for segmental resection; low-stage tumors unsuitable for conservative management (e.g., due to multicentric and frequent recurrences resistant to intravesical instillations); high-grade tumors (T1G3) associated with CIS; and bladder symptoms, such as frequency or hemorrhage, that impair quality of life.

Radical cystectomy is major surgery that requires appropriate preoperative evaluation and management. The procedure involves removal of the bladder and pelvic lymph nodes and creation of a conduit or reservoir for urinary flow. Grossly abnormal lymph nodes are evaluated by frozen section. If metastases are confirmed, the procedure is often aborted. In males, radical cystectomy includes the removal of the prostate, seminal vesicles, and proximal urethra. Impotence is universal unless the nerves responsible for erectile function are preserved. In females, the procedure includes removal of the bladder, urethra, uterus, fallopian tubes, ovaries, anterior vaginal wall, and surrounding fascia.

Previously, urine flow was managed by directing the ureters to the abdominal wall, where it was collected in an external appliance. Currently, most patients receive either a continent cutaneous reservoir constructed from detubularized bowel or an orthotopic neobladder. Some 70% of men receive a neobladder. With a continent reservoir, 65–85% of men will be continent at night and 85–90% during the day. Cutaneous reservoirs are drained by intermittent catheterization; orthotopic neobladders are drained more naturally. Contraindications to a neobladder include renal insufficiency, an inability to self-catheterize, or an exophytic tumor or CIS in the urethra. Diffuse CIS in the bladder is a relative contraindication based on the risk of a urethral recurrence. Concurrent ulcerative colitis or Crohn's disease may hinder the use of resected bowel.

A partial cystectomy may be considered when the disease is limited to the dome of the bladder, a margin of at least 2 cm can be achieved, there is no CIS in other sites, and the bladder capacity is adequate after the tumor

TABLE 90-1 SURVIVAL FOLLOWING SURGERY FOR BLADDER CANCER

Pathologic Stage	5-Year Survival, %	10-Year Survival, %
T2,N0	89	87
T3a,N0	78	76
T3b,N0	62	61
T4,N0	50	45
Any T,N1	35	34

has been removed. This occurs in 5–10% of cases. Carcinomas in the ureter or in the renal pelvis are treated with nephroureterectomy with a bladder cuff to remove the tumor.

The probability of recurrence following surgery is predicted on the basis of pathologic stage, presence or absence of lymphatic or vascular invasion, and nodal spread. Among those whose cancers recur, the recurrence develops in a median of 1 year (range 0.04–11.1 years). Long-term outcomes vary by pathologic stage and histology (**Table 90-1**). The number of lymph nodes removed is also prognostic, whether or not the nodes contained tumor.

Chemotherapy (described below) has been shown to prolong the survival of patients with invasive disease, but only when combined with definitive treatment of the bladder by radical cystectomy or radiation therapy. Thus, for the majority of patients, chemotherapy alone is inadequate to clear the bladder of disease. Experimental studies are evaluating bladder preservation strategies by combining chemotherapy and radiation therapy in patients whose tumors were endoscopically removed.

METASTATIC DISEASE The primary goal of treatment for metastatic disease is to achieve complete remission with chemotherapy alone or with a combined-modality approach of chemotherapy followed by surgical resection of residual disease, as is done routinely for the treatment of germ cell tumors. One can define a goal in terms of cure or palliation on the basis of the probability of achieving a complete response to chemotherapy using prognostic factors, such as Karnofsky Performance Status (KPS) (<80%), and whether the pattern of spread is nodal or visceral (liver, lung, or bone). For those with zero, one, or two risk factors, the probability of complete remission is 38, 25, and 5%, respectively, and median survival is 33, 13.4, and 9.3 months, respectively. Patients who are functionally compromised or who have visceral disease or bone metastases rarely achieve long-term survival. The toxicities also vary as a function of risk, and treatment-related mortality rates are as high as 3–4% using some combinations in these poor-risk patient groups.

CHEMOTHERAPY A number of chemotherapeutic drugs have shown activity as single agents; cisplatin, paclitaxel, and gemcitabine are considered most active. Standard therapy consists of two-, three-, or four-drug combinations. Overall response rates of >50% have been reported using combinations such as methotrexate, vinblastine, doxorubicin, and cisplatin (M-VAC); cisplatin and paclitaxel (PT); gemcitabine and cisplatin (GC); or gemcitabine, paclitaxel, and cisplatin (GTC). M-VAC was considered standard, but the toxicities of neutropenia and fever, mucositis, diminished renal and auditory function, and peripheral neuropathy led to the development of alternative regimens. At present, GC is used more commonly than M-VAC, based on the results of a comparative trial of M-VAC versus GC that showed less neutropenia and fever, and less mucositis for the GC regimen. Anemia and thrombocytopenia were more common with GC. GTC is not more effective than GC.

Chemotherapy has also been evaluated in the neoadjuvant and adjuvant settings. In a randomized trial, patients receiving three cycles of neoadjuvant M-VAC followed by cystectomy had a significantly better median (6.2 years) and 5-year survival (57%) compared to cystectomy alone (median survival 3.8 years; 5-year survival 42%). Similar results were obtained in an international study of three cycles of cisplatin, methotrexate, and vinblastine (CMV) followed by either radical cystectomy or radiation therapy. The decision to administer adjuvant therapy is based on the risk of recurrence after cystectomy. Indications for adjuvant chemotherapy include the presence of nodal disease, extravesical tumor extension, or vascular invasion in the resected specimen. Another study of adjuvant therapy found that four cycles of CMV delayed recurrence, although an effect on survival was less clear. Additional trials are studying taxane- and gemcitabine-based combinations.

The management of bladder cancer is summarized in **Table 90-2**.

TABLE 90-2 MANAGEMENT OF BLADDER CANCER

Nature of Lesion	Management Approach
Superficial	Endoscopic removal, usually with intravesical therapy
Invasive disease	Cystectomy ± systemic chemotherapy (before or after surgery)
Metastatic disease	Curative or palliative chemotherapy (based on prognostic factors) ± surgery

CARCINOMA OF THE RENAL PELVIS AND URETER

About 2500 cases of renal pelvis and ureter cancer occur each year; nearly all are transitional cell carcinomas similar to bladder cancer in biology and appearance. This tumor is also associated with chronic phenacetin abuse and with Balkan nephropathy, a chronic interstitial nephritis endemic in Bulgaria, Greece, Bosnia-Herzegovina, and Romania.

The most common symptom is painless gross hematuria, and the disease is usually detected on intravenous pyelogram during the work-up for hematuria. Patterns of spread are like those in bladder cancer. For low-grade disease localized to the renal pelvis and ureter, nephroureterectomy (including excision of the distal ureter with a portion of the bladder) is associated with 5-year survival of 80–90%. More invasive or histologically poorly differentiated tumors are more likely to recur locally and to metastasize. Metastatic disease is treated with the chemotherapy used in bladder cancer, and the outcome is similar to that of metastatic transitional cell cancer of bladder origin.

RENAL CELL CARCINOMA

Renal cell carcinomas account for 90–95% of malignant neoplasms arising from the kidney. Notable features include resistance to cytotoxic agents, infrequent responses to biologic response modifiers such as interleukin (IL) 2, and a variable clinical course for patients with metastatic disease, including anecdotal reports of spontaneous regression.

EPIDEMIOLOGY

The incidence of renal cell carcinoma continues to rise and is now nearly 51,000 cases annually in the United States, resulting in 13,000 deaths. The male to female ratio is 2:1. Incidence peaks between the ages of 50–70, although this malignancy may be diagnosed at any age. Many environmental factors have been investigated as possible contributing causes; the strongest association is with cigarette smoking (accounting for 20–30% of cases). Risk is also increased for patients who have acquired cystic disease of the kidney associated with end-stage renal disease, and for those with tuberous sclerosis. Most cases are sporadic, although familial forms have been reported. One is associated with von Hippel-Lindau (VHL) syndrome, which predisposes to renal cell carcinomas, retinal hemangioma, hemangioblastoma of the spinal cord and cerebellum, and pheochromocytoma. Roughly 35% of individuals with VHL disease develop renal cell cancer. An increased incidence has also been reported for first-degree relatives.

PATHOLOGY AND GENETICS

Renal cell neoplasia represents a heterogeneous group of tumors with distinct histopathologic, genetic, and clinical features ranging from benign to high-grade malignant (Table 90-3). They are classified on the basis of morphology and histology. Categories include clear cell carcinoma (60% of cases), papillary tumors (5–15%), chromophobic tumors (5–10%), oncocytomas (5–10%), and collecting or Bellini duct tumors (<1%). Papillary tumors tend to be bilateral and multifocal. Chromophobic tumors have a more indolent clinical course, and oncocytomas are considered benign neoplasms. In contrast, Bellini duct carcinomas, which are thought to arise from the collecting ducts within the renal medulla, are very rare but very aggressive. They tend to affect younger patients.

TABLE 90-3 CLASSIFICATION OF EPITHELIAL NEOPLASMS ARISING FROM THE KIDNEY

Carcinoma Type	Growth Pattern	Cell of Origin	Cytogenetics
Clear cell	Acinar or sarcomatoid	Proximal tubule	3p–
Papillary	Papillary or sarcomatoid	Proximal tubule	+7, +17, –Y
Chromophobic	Solid, tubular, or sarcomatoid	Cortical collecting duct	Hypodiploid
Oncocytic	Tumor nests	Cortical collecting duct	Undetermined
Collecting duct	Papillary or sarcomatoid	Medullary collecting duct	Undetermined

Clear cell tumors, the predominant histology, are found in >80% of patients who develop metastases. Clear cell tumors arise from the epithelial cells of the proximal tubules and usually show chromosome 3p deletions. Deletions of 3p21–26 (where the *VHL* gene maps) are identified in patients with familial as well as sporadic tumors. *VHL* encodes a tumor-suppressor protein that is involved in regulating the transcription of vascular endothelial growth factor (VEGF), platelet-derived growth factor (PDGF), and a number of other hypoxia-inducible proteins. Inactivation of *VHL* leads to overexpression of these agonists of the VEGF and PDGF receptors, which promote tumor angiogenesis and tumor growth. Agents that inhibit proangiogenic growth factor activity show antitumor effects.

CLINICAL PRESENTATION

The presenting signs and symptoms include hematuria, abdominal pain, and a flank or abdominal mass. This classic triad occurs in 10–20% of patients. Other symptoms are fever, weight loss, anemia, and a varicocele (Table 90-4). The tumor can also be found incidentally on a radiograph. Widespread use of radiologic cross-sectional imaging procedures (CT, ultrasound, MRI) contributes to earlier detection, including incidental renal masses detected during evaluation for other medical conditions. The increasing number of incidentally discovered low-stage tumors has contributed to an improved 5-year survival for patients with renal cell carcinoma and increased use of nephron-sparing surgery (partial nephrectomy). A spectrum of paraneoplastic syndromes has been associated with these malignancies, including erythrocytosis, hypercalcemia, nonmetastatic hepatic dysfunction (Stauffer syndrome), and acquired dysfibrinogenemia. Erythrocytosis is noted at presentation in only about 3% of patients. Anemia, a sign of advanced disease, is more common.

The standard evaluation of patients with suspected renal cell tumors includes a CT scan of the abdomen and pelvis, chest radiograph, urine analysis, and urine cytology. If metastatic disease is suspected from the chest radiograph, a CT of the chest is warranted. MRI is useful in evaluating the inferior vena cava in cases of suspected tumor involvement or invasion by thrombus. In clinical practice, any solid

TABLE 90-4 SIGNS AND SYMPTOMS IN PATIENTS WITH RENAL CELL CANCER

Presenting Sign or Symptom	Incidence, %
Classic triad: hematuria, flank pain, flank mass	10–20
Hematuria	40
Flank pain	40
Palpable mass	25
Weight loss	33
Anemia	33
Fever	20
Hypertension	20
Abnormal liver function	15
Hypercalcemia	5
Erythrocytosis	3
Neuromyopathy	3
Amyloidosis	2
Increased erythrocyte sedimentation rate	55

renal masses should be considered malignant until proven otherwise; a definitive diagnosis is required. If no metastases are demonstrated, surgery is indicated, even if the renal vein is invaded. The differential diagnosis of a renal mass includes cysts, benign neoplasms (adenoma, angiomyolipoma, oncocytoma), inflammatory lesions (pyelonephritis or abscesses), and other primary or metastatic cancers. Other malignancies that may involve the kidney include transitional cell carcinoma of the renal pelvis, sarcoma, lymphoma, and Wilms' tumor. All of these are less common causes of renal masses than is renal cell cancer.

STAGING AND PROGNOSIS

Two staging systems used are the Robson classification and the American Joint Committee on Cancer (AJCC) staging system. According to the AJCC system, stage I tumors are <7 cm in greatest diameter and confined to the kidney, stage II tumors are ≥7 cm and confined to the kidney, stage III tumors extend through the renal capsule but are confined to Gerota's fascia (IIIa) or involve a single hilar lymph node (N1), and stage IV disease includes tumors that have invaded adjacent organs (excluding the adrenal gland) or involve multiple lymph nodes or distant metastases. The rate of 5-year survival varies by stage: >90% for stage I, 85% for stage II, 60% for stage III, and 10% for stage IV.

℞ RENAL CELL CARCINOMA

LOCALIZED TUMORS The standard management for stage I or II tumors and selected cases of stage III disease is radical nephrectomy. This procedure involves en bloc removal of Gerota's fascia and its contents, including the kidney, the ipsilateral adrenal gland, and adjacent hilar lymph nodes. The role of a regional lymphadenectomy is controversial. Extension into the renal vein or inferior vena cava (stage III disease) does not preclude resection even if cardiopulmonary bypass is required. If the tumor is resected, half of these patients have prolonged survival.

Nephron-sparing approaches via open or laparoscopic surgery may be appropriate for patients who have only one kidney, depending on the size and location of the lesion. A nephron-sparing approach can also be used for patients with bilateral tumors, accompanied by a radical nephrectomy on the opposite side. Partial nephrectomy techniques are being applied electively to resect small masses for patients with a normal contralateral kidney. Adjuvant therapy following this surgery does not improve outcome, even in cases with a poor prognosis.

ADVANCED DISEASE Surgery has a limited role for patients with metastatic disease. However, long-term survival may occur in patients who relapse after nephrectomy in a solitary site that can be removed. One indication for nephrectomy with metastases at initial presentation is to alleviate pain or hemorrhage of a primary tumor. Also, a cytoreductive nephrectomy before systemic treatment improves survival for carefully selected patients with stage IV tumors.

Metastatic renal cell carcinoma is highly refractory to chemotherapy and only infrequently responsive to cytokine therapy with IL-2 or IFN-α. IFN-α and IL-2 produce regressions in 10–20% of patients, but on occasion these responses are durable. IL-2 was approved on the observation of durable complete remission in a small proportion of cases.

The situation changed dramatically when two large-scale randomized trials established a role for antiangiogenic therapy in this disease as predicted by the genetic studies. These trials separately evaluated two orally administered antiangiogenic agents, sorafenib and sunitinib, that inhibited receptor tyrosine kinase signaling through the VEGF and PDGF receptors. Both showed efficacy as second-line treatment following progression during cytokine treatment, resulting in approval by regulatory authorities for the treatment of advanced renal cell carcinoma. A randomized phase 3 trial comparing sunitinib to IFN-α showed superior efficacy for sunitinib with an acceptable safety profile. The trial resulted in a change in the standard first-line treatment from IFN to sunitinib. Sunitinib is usually given orally at a dose of 50 mg/d for 4 weeks out of 6. Diarrhea is the main toxicity. Sorafenib is usually given orally at a dose of 400 mg bid. In addition to diarrhea, toxicities include rash, fatigue, and hand-foot syndrome. Temsirolimus, a mammalian target of rapamycin (mTOR) inhibitor, also has activity in previously treated patients. The usual dosage is 25 mg IV weekly.

The prognosis of metastatic renal cell carcinoma is variable. In one analysis, no prior nephrectomy, a KPS <80, low hemoglobin, high corrected calcium, and abnormal lactate dehydrogenase were poor prognostic factors. Patients with zero, one or two, and three or more factors had a median survival of 24, 12, and 5 months, respectively. These tumors may follow an unpredictable and protracted clinical course. It may be best to document progression before considering systemic treatment.

FURTHER READINGS

Black PC et al: Molecular markers of urothelial cancer and their use in the monitoring of superficial urothelial cancer. J Clin Oncol 24:5528, 2006

Brassell SA, Kamat AM: Contemporary intravesical treatment options for urothelial carcinoma of the bladder. J Natl Compr Canc Netw 4:1027, 2006

Cohen HT, McGovern FJ: Renal-cell carcinoma. N Engl J Med 353:2477, 2005

Huang WC et al: Chronic kidney disease after nephrectomy in patients with renal cortical tumours: A retrospective cohort study. Lancet Oncol 7:735, 2006

Mitra AP et al: Molecular pathways in invasive bladder cancer: New insights into mechanisms, progression, and target identification. J Clin Oncol 24:5552, 2006

Motzer RJ et al: Sunitinib in patients with metastatic renal cell carcinoma. JAMA 295:2516, 2006

Nelson EC et al: Renal cell carcinoma: Current status and emerging therapies. Cancer Treat Rev 33:299, 2007

Sugano K, Kakizoe T: Genetic alterations in bladder cancer and their clinical applications in molecular tumor staging. Nature Clin Pract 3:642, 2006

Winquist E et al: Neoadjuvant chemotherapy for transitional cell carcinoma of the bladder: A systematic review and meta-analysis. J Urol 171:561, 2004

91 Benign and Malignant Diseases of the Prostate

Howard I. Scher

Benign and malignant changes in the prostate increase with age. Autopsies of men in the eighth decade of life show hyperplastic changes in >90% and malignant changes in >70% of individuals. The high prevalence of these diseases among the elderly, who often have competing causes of morbidity and mortality, mandates a risk-adapted approach to diagnosis and treatment. This can be achieved by considering these diseases as a series of states. Each state represents a distinct clinical milestone for which intervention(s) may be recommended based on current symptoms or the risk of developing symptoms or death from disease within a given time frame (Fig. 91-1). For benign proliferative disorders, symptoms of urinary frequency, infection, and potential for obstruction are weighed against the side effects and complications of medical or surgical therapy. For prostate malignancies, the risks of developing the disease, symptoms, or death from cancer are balanced against the morbidities of the interventions recommended and preexisting comorbid conditions.

ANATOMY AND PATHOLOGY

The prostate is located in the pelvis and is surrounded by the rectum, the bladder, the periprostatic and dorsal vein complexes that are responsible for erectile function, and the urinary sphincter that is re-

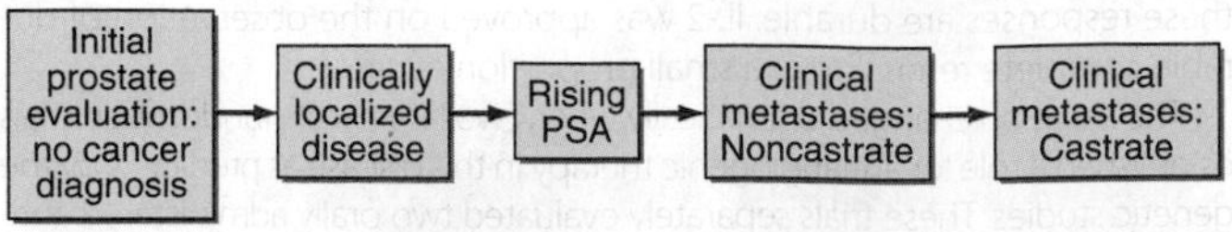

FIGURE 91-1 Clinical states of prostate cancer. PSA, prostate-specific antigen.

sponsible for passive urinary control. The prostate is composed of branching tubuloalveolar glands arranged in lobules and surrounded by a stroma. The acinal unit includes an epithelial compartment made up of epithelial, basal, and neuroendocrine cells and a stromal compartment that includes fibroblasts and smooth-muscle cells. The compartments are separated by a basement membrane. Prostate-specific antigen (PSA) and acid phosphatase are produced in the epithelial cells. Both prostate epithelial cells and stromal cells express androgen receptors and depend on androgens for growth. Testosterone, the major circulating androgen, is converted by the enzyme 5α-reductase to dihydrotestosterone in the gland.

The periurethral portion of the gland increases in size during puberty and after the age of 55 due to the growth of nonmalignant cells in the transition zone of the prostate that surrounds the urethra. Most cancers develop in the peripheral zone, and cancers in this location can often be palpated during a digital rectal examination (DRE).

PROSTATE CANCER

In 2007 in the United States, ~218,890 prostate cancer cases were diagnosed, and 27,050 men died from prostate cancer. The absolute number of prostate cancer deaths has decreased in the past 5 years; this has been attributed by some to the widespread use of PSA-based detection strategies. However, screening has not been shown to improve survival in prospective randomized trials. The paradox of management is that although the disease remains the second leading cause of cancer deaths in men, only 1 man in 8 with prostate cancer will die of his disease.

EPIDEMIOLOGY

Epidemiologic studies show that the risk of being diagnosed with prostate cancer increases by a factor of 2 if one first-degree relative is affected and by 4 if two or more are affected. Current estimates are that 40% of early-onset and 5–10% of all prostate cancers are hereditary. Prostate cancer affects ethnic groups differently. Matched for age, African-American males compared to white males have both a greater number of prostatic intraepithelial neoplasia (PIN) lesions, which are precursors to cancer, and larger tumors, possibly related to the higher levels of testosterone seen in African-American males. PIN, the precursor of cancer, is typically multifocal and highly unstable. Polymorphic variants of the androgen receptor gene, the cytochrome P450 C17 gene, and the steroid 5α-reductase type II (*SRD5A2*) gene have also been implicated in the variations in incidence.

The incidence of autopsy-detected cancers is similar around the world, while the incidence of clinical disease varies. Thus, environmental factors may play a role. High consumption of dietary fats, such as α-linoleic acid, or the polycyclic aromatic hydrocarbons that form when red meats are cooked is believed to increase risk. Similar to breast cancer in Asian women, the risk of prostate cancer in Asian men increases when they move to Western environments. Protective factors include consumption of the isoflavinoid genistein (which inhibits 5α-reductase), cruciferous vegetables that contain the isothiocyanate sulforaphane, retinoids such as lycopene (in tomatoes), and inhibitors of cholesterol biosynthesis (e.g., statin drugs). The antioxidants α-tocopherol (vitamin E) and selenium may also reduce risk.

The development of a prostate cancer is a multistep process. One early change is hypermethylation of the GSTP1 gene promoter, which leads to loss of function of a gene that detoxifies carcinogens. A role for inflammation has been suggested based on the finding that many prostate cancers occur adjacent to a lesion termed *PIA (proliferative-inflammatory atrophy)*. This also suggests a role for oxidative damage.

DIAGNOSIS AND TREATMENT BY CLINICAL STATE

The disease continuum—from the appearance of a preneoplastic and invasive lesion localized to the prostate, to a metastatic lesion that results in symptoms and, ultimately, mortality from prostate cancer—can span decades. Management at all points is centered on competing risks that are defined by considering the disease as a series of clinical states (Fig. 91-1). The states are defined operationally, on the basis of whether or not a cancer diagnosis has been established and, for those already diagnosed, whether or not metastases are detectable on imaging studies and the measured level of testosterone in the blood. With this approach, an individual resides in only one state and remains in that state until he has progressed. At each assessment, the decision to offer treatment and the specific form of treatment is based on the risk posed by the cancer, relative to competing causes of mortality that may be present in that individual. It follows that the more advanced the disease, the greater the need for treatment. For those without a cancer diagnosis, the decision to undergo testing to detect a cancer is based on the probability that a clinically significant cancer may be present. For those with a prostate cancer diagnosis, the clinical state model considers the probability of developing symptoms or dying from disease. Thus, a patient with localized prostate cancer who has had all cancer removed surgically remains in the state of localized disease as long as the PSA remains undetectable. The time within a state becomes a measure of the efficacy of an intervention, though the effect may not be assessable for years. As many men with active cancer are not at risk for developing metastases, symptoms, or death, the states model allows a distinction between *cure*—the elimination of all cancer cells, the primary therapeutic objective when treating most cancers—and *cancer control*, in which the tempo of the illness is altered and symptoms controlled until the patient dies of other causes. These can be equivalent therapeutically from a patient standpoint if the patient has not experienced symptoms of the disease or the treatment needed to control it. Even when a recurrence is documented, immediate therapy is not always necessary. Rather, as at the time of diagnosis, the need for intervention is based on the tempo of the illness as it unfolds in the individual, relative to the risk-to-benefit ratio of the therapy being considered.

NO CANCER DIAGNOSIS

Prevention Several agents are under investigation for their potential to reduce the risk of clinically significant prostate cancer. Finasteride, a 5α-reductase inhibitor, has been tested in men ages ≥55 years in the Prostate Cancer Prevention Trial, a double-blind, randomized multicenter trial. The prostate cancer detection rate was 18.4% (803 of 4364) in the finasteride group and 24.4% (1147 of 4692) in the placebo group. Early concerns that the cancers detected in the finasteride group were high-grade [37% (280 of 757 cancers) vs. 22% (237 of 1068 cancers) for the placebo group] have been shown to be an artifact of the reduced volume of the malignant epithelial cells in finasteride-treated patients. No effect on survival was detected. Vitamin E and selenium are also being tested as preventive agents (the SELECT study).

Physical Examination The need to pursue a diagnosis of prostate cancer is based on symptoms, an abnormal DRE, or an elevated serum PSA. The urologic history should focus on symptoms of outlet obstruction, continence, potency, or change in ejaculatory pattern.

The DRE focuses on prostate size and consistency and abnormalities within or beyond the gland. Many cancers occur in the peripheral zone and can be palpated on DRE. Carcinomas are characteristically hard, nodular, and irregular, while induration may be due to benign prostatic hypertrophy (BPH) or to calculi or tumor. Overall, 20–25% of men with an abnormal DRE have cancer.

Prostate-Specific Antigen PSA is a kallikrein-like serine protease that causes liquefaction of seminal coagulum. It is produced by both nonmalignant and malignant epithelial cells. PSA is prostate-specific, not prostate cancer–specific, and serum PSA increases may occur from prostatitis, BPH, and prostate cancer. The performance of a prostate biopsy can increase PSA levels up to tenfold for 8–10 weeks. The serum PSA level is not affected by DRE. PSA circulates in the blood as an inactive complex with the protease inhibitors α_1-antichymotrypsin and β_2-macroglobulin, and it has an estimated half-life in serum of 2–3 days. Levels should be undetectable if the prostate has been removed. Immunohistochemical staining for PSA can be used to establish a prostate cancer diagnosis.

PSA testing was approved in 1994 for early detection of prostate cancer, but there is controversy on its use. The American Cancer Society recommends that physicians offer PSA testing and a DRE on an annual basis for men over age 50 with an anticipated survival of >10 years; this includes men up to age 76 years. For African Americans and men with a family history of prostate cancer, testing is advised to begin at age 45. The American Urologic Association recommendations are similar, with a proviso that the risks and benefits of the performance of these tests are not defined. The National Comprehensive Cancer Network advises testing at age 40, tailoring additional testing to the age-specific median. The American College of Physicians recommends that physicians "describe the potential benefits and known harms of screening" and to "individualize the decision to screen." PSA values may fluctuate for no apparent reason; thus, an isolated abnormal value should be confirmed before proceeding with further testing.

The PSA criteria used to recommend a diagnostic prostate biopsy have evolved over time. The goal is to increase the sensitivity of the test for younger men more likely to die of the disease and to reduce the frequency of detecting cancers of low malignant potential in elderly men more likely to die of other causes. Age-specific reference ranges reduce the upper limit of normal for younger men and increase it for older men. Different thresholds alter the sensitivity and specificity of detection. The threshold for performance of a biopsy was 4.0 ng/mL, which has been reduced to 2.6 ng/mL for men <60 by many groups based on the finding that nearly half of the men with PSAs who reached this level increased to 4 within a relatively short (4-year) time frame, and that, once diagnosed, nearly one-third had spread beyond the confines of the gland. Most PSA is complexed to α_1-chymotrypsin (ACT); only a small percentage is "free." To improve diagnostic accuracy for men with a PSA between 4 and 10, the risk of cancer is under 10% if the free PSA is >25% but as high as 56% for those with a free PSA <10%. PSA density measurements were developed to correct for the contribution of BPH to the total PSA level. PSA density is calculated by dividing the serum PSA by the prostate weight estimated from transrectal ultrasound (TRUS). Values <0.10 ng/mL per cm^3 are consistent with BPH, while those >0.15 suggest cancer. *PSA velocity* is the rate of change in PSA levels over time and is expressed most commonly as the PSA doubling time. It is particularly useful for men with seemingly normal values that are rising. For men with a PSA above 4, rates of rise >0.75 ng/mL per year suggest cancer, while for those with lower PSA levels, rates above 0.5 ng/mL per year should be used to advise a biopsy. As an example, an increase from 2.5 to 3.2 in a 1-year period would warrant further testing. Free and complexed PSA measurements are used when levels are between 4 and 10 ng/mL to decide whether a biopsy is needed. The level of free PSA is lower in men with cancer. The ratios of free to total, complexed to total, and free to complexed PSA have also been used. In one series, specificity improved by 20% by defining normal ranges as free/total >0.15, complexed/total <0.70, and free/complexed >0.25.

PSA-based detection strategies have changed the clinical spectrum of the disease. Now, 95–99% of newly diagnosed cancers are clinically localized, 40% are not palpable, and of these, 70% are pathologically organ-confined. The downside of widespread PSA screening is the detection and treatment of cancers with such a low malignant potential that they would not have shortened survival or produced symptoms during the patient's lifetime. The side effects of treatment, including impotence, incontinence, and bowel dysfunction, are unacceptable for these patients. Formal clinical trials to assess the value of screening on prostate cancer morbidity and mortality are ongoing. Until the results of these studies are available, men are advised to make an informed decision about whether to undergo testing.

A diagnostic algorithm based on the DRE and PSA findings is illustrated in Fig. 91-2. In general, a biopsy is recommended if the DRE or PSA is abnormal. Twenty-five percent of men with a PSA >4 ng/mL

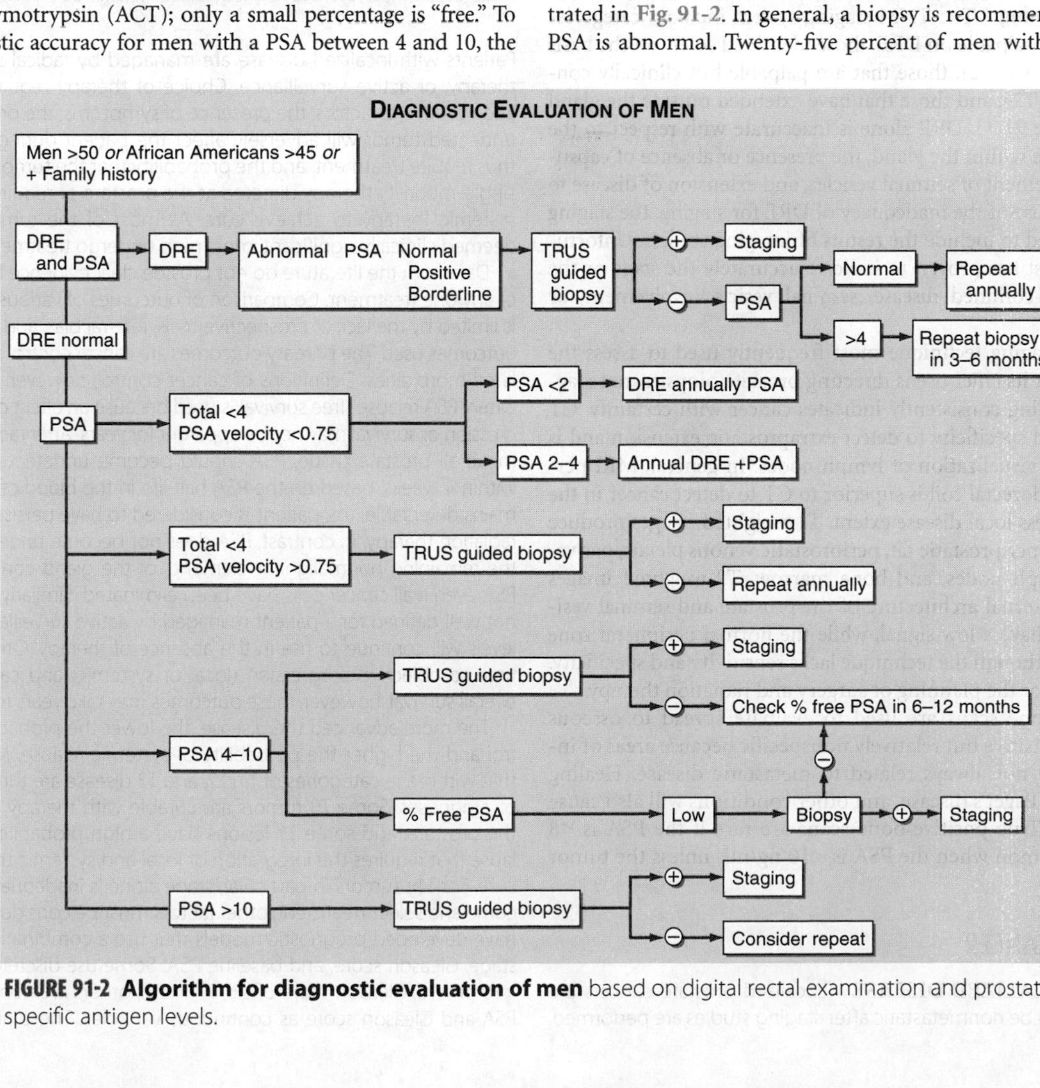

FIGURE 91-2 Algorithm for diagnostic evaluation of men based on digital rectal examination and prostate-specific antigen levels.

and an abnormal DRE have cancer, as do 17% of men with a PSA of 2.5–4.0 ng/mL and normal DRE.

Prostate Biopsy A diagnosis of cancer is established by a TRUS-guided needle biopsy. Direct visualization by ultrasound or MRI assures that all areas of the gland are sampled. A minimum of six separate cores, three from the right and three from the left, is advised, as is a separate biopsy of the transition zone if clinically indicated. More commonly, 12–14 cores are advised to increase the diagnostic yield. Patients with prostatitis should have a course of antibiotics before biopsy. Men with an abnormal PSA and negative biopsy are advised to undergo a repeat biopsy.

Each core of the biopsy is examined for the presence of cancer, and the amount of cancer is quantified based on the length of the tumor within the core and the percentage of the core involved.

Pathology The noninvasive proliferation of epithelial cells within ducts is termed *prostatic intraepithelial neoplasia.* PIN is a precursor of cancer, but not all PIN lesions develop into invasive cancers. Of the cancers identified, >95% are adenocarcinomas; the remainder are squamous or transitional cell tumors or, rarely, carcinosarcomas. Metastases to the prostate are rare, but in some cases colon cancers or transitional cell tumors of the bladder invade the gland by direct extension. When prostate cancer is diagnosed, a measure of histologic aggressiveness is assigned using the *Gleason grading system,* in which the dominant and secondary glandular histologic patterns are scored from 1 (well-differentiated) to 5 (undifferentiated) and summed to give a total score of 2–10 for each tumor. The most poorly differentiated area of tumor (i.e., the area with the highest histologic grade) often determines biologic behavior. The presence or absence of perineural invasion and extracapsular spread are also recorded.

Prostate Cancer Staging The TNM staging system includes categories for cancers that are palpable on DRE, those identified solely on the basis of an abnormal PSA (T1c), those that are palpable but clinically confined to the gland (T2), and those that have extended outside the gland (T3 and T4) (Table 91-1). DRE alone is inaccurate with respect to the extent of the disease within the gland, the presence or absence of capsular invasion, involvement of seminal vesicles, and extension of disease to lymph nodes. Because of the inadequacy of DRE for staging, the staging system was modified to include the results of imaging studies. Unfortunately, no single test has proven to indicate accurately the stage or the presence of organ-confined disease, seminal vesicle involvement, or lymph node spread.

TRUS is the imaging technique most frequently used to assess the primary tumor, but its chief use is directing prostate biopsies, not staging. No TRUS finding consistently indicates cancer with certainty. CT lacks sensitivity and specificity to detect extraprostatic extension and is inferior to MRI in visualization of lymph nodes. In general, MRI performed with an endorectal coil is superior to CT to detect cancer in the prostate and to assess local disease extent. T1-weighted images produce a high signal in the periprostatic fat, periprostatic venous plexus, perivesicular tissues, lymph nodes, and bone marrow. T2-weighted images demonstrate the internal architecture of the prostate and seminal vesicles. Most cancers have a low signal, while the normal peripheral zone has a high signal, although the technique lacks sensitivity and specificity. MRI is also useful for the planning of surgery and radiation therapy.

Radionuclide bone scans are used to evaluate spread to osseous sites. This test is sensitive but relatively nonspecific because areas of increased uptake are not always related to metastatic disease. Healing fractures, arthritis, Paget's disease, and other conditions will also cause abnormal uptake. True-positive bone scans are rare if the PSA is <8 ng/mL and uncommon when the PSA is <10 ng/mL unless the tumor is high-grade.

TABLE 91-1 COMPARISON OF CLINICAL STAGE BY THE TNM CLASSIFICATION SYSTEM AND THE WHITMORE-JEWETT STAGING SYSTEM

TNM Stage	Description	Whitmore-Jewett Stage	Description
T1a	Nonpalpable, with 5% or less of resected tissue with cancer	A1	Well differentiated tumor on few chips from one lobe
T1b	Nonpalpable, with >5% of resected tissue with cancer	A2	Involvement more diffuse
T1c	Nonpalpable, detected due to elevated serum PSA		
T2a	Palpable, half of one lobe or less	BIN	Palpable, < one lobe, surrounded by normal tissue
T2b	Palpable, > half of one lobe but not both lobes	B1	Palpable, < one lobe
T2c	Palpable, involves both lobes	B2	Palpable, one entire lobe or both lobes
T3a	Palpable, unilateral extra-capsular extension	C1	Palpable, outside capsule, not into seminal vesicles
T3b	Palpable, bilateral extra-capsular extension		
T3c	Tumor invades seminal vesicle(s)	C2	Palpable, seminal vesicle involved
M1	Distant metastases	D	Metastatic disease

Source: Adapted from FF Schroder et al: TNM classification of prostate cancer. Prostate (Suppl) 4:129, 1992; and American Joint Committee on Cancer, 1992.

℞ PROSTATE CANCER

CLINICALLY LOCALIZED DISEASE Localized prostate cancers are those that appear to be nonmetastatic after staging studies are performed. Patients with localized disease are managed by radical surgery, radiation therapy, or active surveillance. Choice of therapy requires the consideration of several factors: the presence of symptoms, the probability that the untreated tumor will adversely affect the patient during his lifetime and thus require treatment, and the probability that the tumor can be cured by single-modality therapy directed at the prostate or requires both local and systemic therapy to achieve cure. As most of the tumors detected are deemed clinically significant, most men undergo treatment.

Data from the literature do not provide clear evidence for the superiority of any one treatment. Comparison of outcomes of various forms of therapy is limited by the lack of prospective trials, referral bias, and differences in the outcomes used. The primary outcomes are cancer control and treatment-related morbidities. Definitions of cancer control, however, vary by modality. Often, PSA relapse–free survival is used because an effect on metastatic progression or survival may not be apparent for years. After radical surgery to remove all prostate tissue, PSA should become undetectable in the blood within 4 weeks, based on the PSA half-life in the blood of 3 days. If PSA remains detectable, the patient is considered to have persistent disease. After radiation therapy, in contrast, PSA does not become undetectable because the remaining nonmalignant elements of the gland continue to produce PSA even if all cancer cells have been eliminated. Similarly, cancer control is not well-defined for a patient managed by active surveillance because PSA levels will continue to rise in the absence of therapy. Other outcomes are time to objective progression (local or systemic) and cancer-specific and overall survival; however, these outcomes may take years to assess.

The more advanced the disease, the lower the probability of local control and the higher the probability of systemic relapse. More important is that within the categories of T1, T2, and T3 disease are tumors with a range of prognoses. Some T3 tumors are curable with therapy directed solely at the prostate, and some T1 lesions have a high probability of systemic relapse that requires the integration of local and systemic therapy to achieve cure. For T1c tumors in particular, stage alone is inadequate to predict outcome and select treatment; other factors must be considered. Many groups have developed prognostic models that use a combination of the initial T stage, Gleason score, and baseline PSA. Some use discrete cut points (PSA <10 or ≥10; Gleason score of ≤6, 7, or ≥8); others are nomograms that use PSA and Gleason score as continuous variables. These algorithms can be used to predict disease extent (organ-confined vs. non-organ-confined, node-negative or -positive) and the probability of success of treatment using a PSA-based definition specific to the local therapy under consideration. Specific nomograms have been developed for radical prostatectomy, external beam radiation therapy, and brachytherapy (seed implantation). These are being refined continually to incorporate other clinical parameters and biologic determinants. Surgical technique, radiation therapy delivery, and criteria for active surveillance continue to be refined and improved; the year of treatment affects outcomes independent of other factors. The improvements make treatment decisions a dynamic process.

The frequency of adverse events for the different treatment modalities varies with the modality used and the experience of the treating team. For example, following radical prostatectomy, incontinence rates range from 2 to 47% and impotence rates range from 25 to 89%. Part of the variability relates to how the complication is defined and whether the patient or physician is reporting the event. The time of the assessment is also important. After surgery, impotence is immediate but may reverse over time, while with radiation therapy impotence is not immediate but may develop over time. Of greatest concern to patients are the effects on continence, sexual potency, and bowel function.

Radical Prostatectomy The goal of radical prostatectomy is to excise the cancer completely with a clear margin, to maintain continence by preserving the external sphincter, and to preserve potency by preserving the autonomic nerves in the neurovascular bundle. Radical prostatectomy is advised for patients with a life expectancy of >10 years and is performed using a retropubic, perineal, or laparoscopic approach. Outcomes can be predicted using postoperative nomograms that consider pretreatment factors and the pathologic findings at surgery. PSA failure is defined as a value above 0.2 or 0.4 ng/mL, although the exact definition varies among series.

There is controversy over the definition of what constitutes "high risk" based on a predicted probability of success or failure. In these situations, nomograms and predictive models can only go so far. Exactly what probability of success or failure would lead a physician to recommend and a patient to seek alternative approaches is controversial. For example, it may be appropriate to recommend radical surgery for a younger patient with a low probability of cure.

Prostatectomy techniques continue to improve as the ability to determine whether the tumor is localized to the gland improves based on different biopsy algorithms and with imaging. The result is better case selection and better surgical planning, which in turn have led to more rapid recovery and higher rates of continence and potency. Factors associated with incontinence include older age and shorter urethra length. The specific surgical technique, open vs. laparoscopic vs. robotic, as well as the skill and experience of the surgeon are also factors for the preservation of neurovascular bundles and development of an anastomotic stricture. Surgical experience is also a factor. In a series treated at an academic center, 6% of patients had mild stress urinary incontinence (SUI) (requiring 1 pad/day), 2% moderate SUI (>1 pad/day), and 0.3% severe SUI (requiring an artificial urinary sphincter). At 1 year, 92% were completely continent. In contrast, the results in a Medicare population treated at multiple centers showed that at 3, 12, and 24 months following surgery, 58, 35, and 42% (respectively) wore pads in their underwear, and 24, 11, and 15% reported "a lot" of urine leakage.

Factors associated with recovery of erectile function include younger age, quality of erections before surgery, and the absence of damage to the neurovascular bundles. Erectile function returns in a median of 4–6 months if both bundles are preserved. Potency is reduced by half if at least one nerve bundle is sacrificed. In cases where cancer control requires the removal of both bundles, sural nerve grafts are being explored. Overall, with the availability of drugs such as sildenafil, intraurethral inserts of alprostadil, and intracavernosal injections of vasodilators, many patients recover satisfactory sexual function.

Neoadjuvant hormonal therapy has been explored in an attempt to improve the outcomes of surgery for high-risk patients. The results of several large trials testing 3 or 8 months of androgen depletion before surgery showed that serum PSA levels decreased by 96%, prostate volumes decreased by 34%, and margin positivity rates decreased from 41 to 17%. Unfortunately, hormones did not produce an improvement in PSA relapse–free survival. Thus, neoadjuvant hormonal therapy is not recommended.

Radiation Therapy Radiation therapy is given by external beam, by radioactive sources implanted into the gland, or by a combination.

External Beam Radiation Therapy Contemporary external beam radiation techniques now use three-dimensional conformal treatment plans with intensity-modulated radiation therapy (IMRT) to maximize the dose to the prostate and to minimize the exposure of the surrounding normal structures. The addition of IMRT has permitted further shaping of the dose, allowing the delivery of still higher doses to the prostate and a further reduction in normal tissue exposure. These advances have enabled the safe administration of doses >80 Gy, higher local control rates, and fewer side effects.

Cancer control after radiation therapy has been defined by various criteria, including a decline in PSA to <0.5 or 1 ng/mL, "nonrising" PSA values, and a negative biopsy of the prostate 2 years after completion of treatment. PSA relapse is defined as three consecutive rising PSA values from the nadir value, with the time to failure as a rise by 2 ng/mL or greater above the posttreatment nadir value.

Radiation dose is important. A PSA nadir of <1.0 ng/mL was observed in 90% of patients receiving 75.6 or 81.0 Gy vs. 76 and 56% of those receiving 70.2 Gy and 64.8 Gy, respectively. The positive biopsy rates at 2.5 years were 4% for those treated with 81 Gy vs. 27 and 36% for those receiving 75.6 or 70.2 Gy. The frequency of rectal complications relates directly to the volume of the anterior rectal wall receiving full-dose treatment.

Overall, radiation therapy is associated with a higher frequency of bowel complications (mainly diarrhea and proctitis) than surgery. Grade 3 rectal or urinary toxicities were seen in 2.1% of patients who received a median dose of 75.6 Gy. Grade 3 urethral strictures requiring dilatation developed in 1% of cases, all of whom had undergone a transurethral resection of the prostate (TURP). Pooled data show that the frequency of grade 3 and 4 toxicities is 6.9 and 3.5%, respectively, for patients who received >70 Gy. The frequency of erectile dysfunction is related to the quality of erections pretreatment, the dose administered, and the time of assessment. Postradiation erectile dysfunction is related to a disruption of the vascular supply and not the nerve fibers.

Neoadjuvant hormone therapy has also been studied in combination with radiation therapy. The aim is to decrease the size of the prostate and, consequently, to reduce the exposure of normal tissues to full-dose radiation, to increase local control rates, and to decrease the rate of systemic failure. Short-term hormone therapy can reduce toxicities and improve local control rates, but long-term treatment (2–3 years) is needed to prolong the time to PSA failure and lower the risk of metastatic disease. The impact on survival has been less clear.

Brachytherapy Brachytherapy is the direct implantation of radioactive sources into the prostate. It is based on the principle that the deposition of radiation energy in tissues decreases as a function of the square of the distance from the source (Chap. 81). The goal is to deliver intensive irradiation to the prostate, minimizing the exposure of the surrounding tissues. The current standard technique achieves a more homogeneous dose distribution by placing seeds according to a customized template based on CT and ultrasonographic assessment of the tumor and computer-optimized dosimetry. The implantation is performed transperineally, without an open procedure, with real-time imaging.

The improvements in brachytherapy techniques have resulted in fewer complications and a marked reduction in local failure rates. In a series of 197 patients followed for a median of 3 years, 5-year actuarial PSA relapse–free survival for patients with pretherapy PSA levels of 0–4, 4–10, and >10 ng/mL were 98, 90, and 89%, respectively. In a separate report of 201 patients who underwent posttreatment biopsies, 80% were negative, 17% were indeterminate, and 3% were positive. The results did not change with longer follow-up. Nevertheless, many physicians feel that implantation is best reserved for patients with good or intermediate prognostic features.

Brachytherapy is well tolerated, although most patients experience urinary frequency and urgency that can persist for several months. Incontinence has been seen in 2–4% of cases. Higher complication rates are observed in patients who have undergone a prior TURP or who have obstructive symptoms at baseline. Proctitis has been reported in <2% of patients.

Active Surveillance Active surveillance, described previously as *watchful waiting*, or *deferred therapy*, is a policy of monitoring the illness at fixed intervals with DREs, PSA measurements, and repeat biopsies of the prostate as indicated, but with no therapeutic intervention(s) until the tumor progresses. Progression can be based on PSA changes, local tumor growth, the development of symptoms, or metastatic disease. The practice evolved from studies of predominantly elderly men with well-differentiated tumors who demonstrated no clinically significant progression for protracted periods, during which a significant proportion died of intercurrent disease. In a structured literature review of patients treated by radical surgery, external beam radiation, or a deferred approach, the 10-year survival rates were 93% for radical prostatectomy, 74% for external beam radiation, and 84% for deferred treatment. Arguing against active surveillance are the results of a Swedish randomized trial of radical prostatectomy vs. active surveillance. With a median follow-up of 6.2 years, men treated by radical surgery had a lower risk of prostate cancer death relative to active surveillance patients (4.6% vs. 8.9%) and a lower risk of metastatic progression (hazard ratio 0.63).

Case selection is critical, and the criteria to select men who can safely choose active surveillance are under intense study. In a prostatectomy series, it was estimated that 10–15% of patients had "insignificant" cancers. Given the multifocality of the disease, a concern is the limited ability to predict pathologic findings on the basis of a needle biopsy, even when multiple cores are obtained. Nomograms to help predict which patients can safely be managed by active surveillance have been developed, and as their predictive accuracy improves, it can be anticipated that more patients will be candidates.

RISING PSA This state consists of patients in whom the sole manifestation of disease is a rising PSA after surgery and/or radiation therapy. By definition, patients have no evidence of disease on scan. For these patients the central issue is whether the rise in PSA results from persistent disease in the primary site, systemic disease, or both. In theory, disease in the primary site may still be curable by additional local treatment; external beam radiation for patients who had undergone surgery, prostatectomy for patients who had undergone radiation therapy.

The decision to recommend radiation therapy after prostatectomy is often made on the basis of the pathologic findings at surgery, as imaging studies such as CT and bone scan are typically uninformative. Some recommend a Prostascint scan: imaging with a radiolabeled antibody to prostate-specific membrane antigen (PSMA), which is highly expressed on prostate epithelial cells, to help with this distinction. Antibody localization to the prostatic fossa suggests local recurrence; localization to extrapelvic sites predicts failure of radiation therapy. Others recommend that a biopsy of the urethrovesical anastomosis be obtained before considering radiation. Factors that predict for response to salvage radiation therapy are a positive surgical margin, lower Gleason grade, long interval from surgery to PSA failure, slow PSA doubling time, and low (<0.5–1.0 ng/mL) PSA value at the time of radiation treatment. Radiation therapy is generally not recommended if the PSA was persistently elevated after surgery, which usually indicates that the disease had spread outside of the area of the prostate bed and is unlikely to be controlled with radiation therapy.

For patients with a rising PSA after radiation therapy, salvage prostatectomy can be considered if the disease was "curable" at the outset, if persistent disease has been documented by a biopsy of the prostate, and if no metastatic disease is seen on imaging studies. Unfortunately, case selection is poorly defined in most series, and morbidities are significant. As currently performed, virtually all patients are impotent after salvage radical prostatectomy, and ~45% have either total urinary incontinence or stress incontinence. Major bleeding, bladder neck contractures, and rectal injury are not uncommon.

In many cases, the rise in PSA after surgery or radiation therapy indicates subclinical metastatic disease. In these cases, the need for treatment depends, in part, on the estimated probability that the patient will show evidence of metastatic disease on a scan and in what time frame. That immediate therapy is not always required was shown in a series where patients received no systemic therapy until metastatic disease was documented. Overall, the median time to metastatic progression was 8 years, and 63% of the patients with rising PSA values remained free of metastases at 5 years. Factors associated with progression included the Gleason grade of the primary tumor, time to recurrence, and PSA doubling times. For those with Gleason grade ≥8 tumors, the probability of metastatic progression was 37, 51, and 71% at 3, 5, and 7 years, respectively. If the time to recurrence was <2 years and PSA doubling time was long (>10 months), the proportion with metastatic disease at the same time intervals was 23, 32, and 53%, vs. 47, 69, and 79% if the doubling time was short (<10 months). A difficulty with predicting the course of disease in the rising PSA state is that most patients receive some form of therapy before the development of metastases. Nevertheless, predictive models continue to be refined. PSA doubling times are prognostic for survival. In one series, all patients who succumbed to disease had PSA doubling times of 3 months or less. Most physicians advise treatment when PSA doubling times are 12 months or less.

METASTATIC DISEASE: NONCASTRATE *Metastatic disease noncastrate* refers to patients with metastases visible on an imaging study and noncastrate levels of testosterone. The patient may be newly diagnosed or have a recurrence after treatment for localized disease. Symptoms of metastatic disease include pain from osseous spread, although many patients are asymptomatic despite extensive spread. Less common are symptoms related to marrow compromise (myelophthisis), coagulopathy, or spinal cord compression.

Standard treatment for noncastrate metastatic disease is to deplete androgens by medical or surgical means. Over 90% of male hormones originate in the testes; <10% are synthesized in the adrenal gland. Surgical orchiectomy is the "gold standard" approach but is least acceptable to patients. Medical therapies can be divided into agents that lower testosterone levels and antiandrogens that bind to the androgen receptor but do not signal **(Fig. 91-3)**.

Testosterone-Lowering Agents Medical therapies that lower testosterone levels include the gonadotropin-releasing hormone (GnRH) analogues, estrogens, and progestational agents. Estrogens such as diethylstilbestrol have fallen out of favor due to the risk of vascular complications such as fluid retention, phlebitis, emboli, and stroke. GnRH analogues (leuprolide acetate and goserelin acetate) initially produce a rise in luteinizing hormone and follicle-stimulating hormone followed by a downregulation of receptors in the pituitary gland, which effects a chemical castration. They were approved on the basis of randomized comparisons showing an improved safety profile (specifically, reduced cardiovascular toxicities) relative to diethylstilbestrol, with equivalent potency. The initial rise in testosterone may result in a clinical flare of the disease. These agents are therefore contraindicated in men with significant obstructive symptoms, cancer-related pain, or spinal cord compromise.

Agents that lower testosterone are associated with an androgen-depletion syndrome that includes hot flushes, weakness, fatigue, impotence, loss of muscle mass, changes in personality, anemia, depression, and a reduction in bone density. The bone changes can be prevented by treatment with bisphosphonates along with vitamin D and calcium supplementation. GnRH analogues also lead to an alteration in body composition and to glucose intolerance. Many taking them develop the metabolic syndrome.

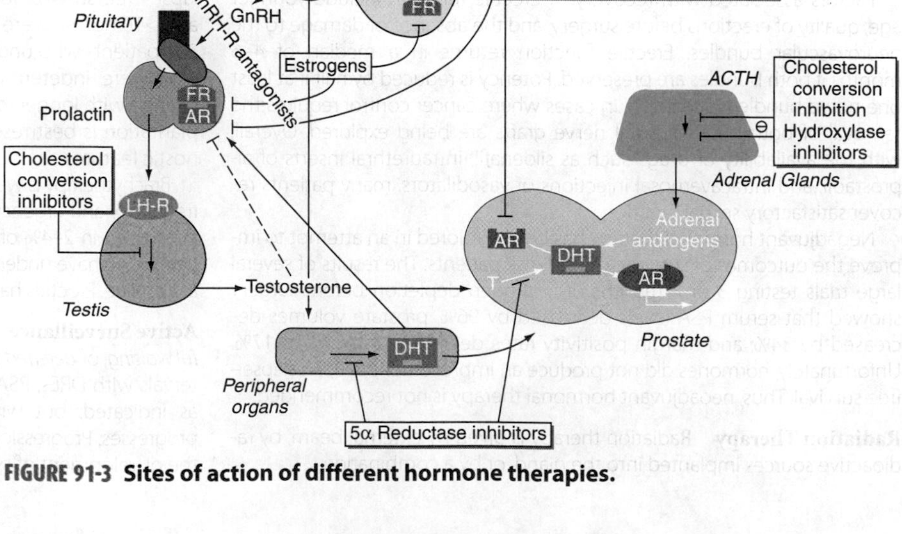

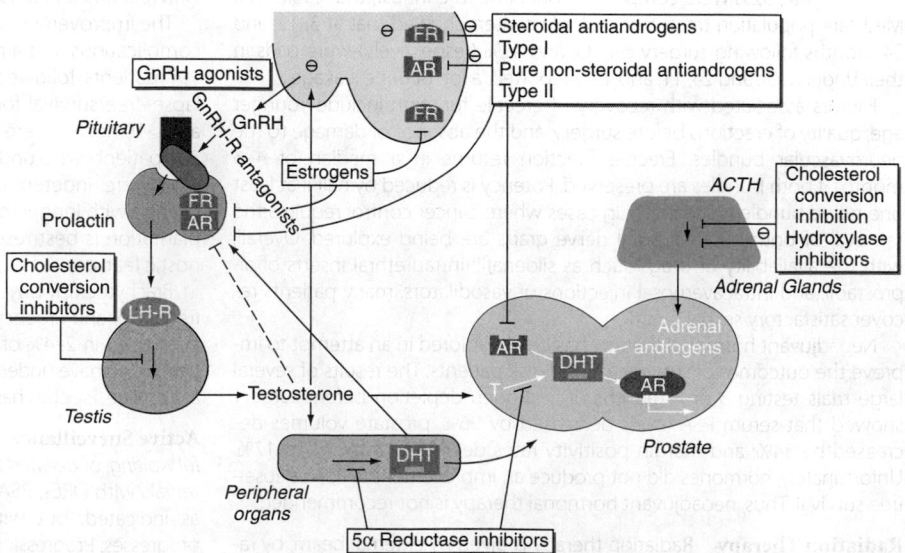

FIGURE 91-3 Sites of action of different hormone therapies.

Antiandrogens Nonsteroidal antiandrogens such as flutamide, bicalutamide, and nilutamide block the binding of androgens to the receptor. When an antiandrogen is given alone, testosterone levels remain the same or increase. Compared to testosterone-lowering therapies, antiandrogens cause fewer hot flashes, less of an effect on libido, less muscle wasting, fewer personality changes, and less bone loss. Gynecomastia remains a significant problem but can be alleviated in part by tamoxifen.

Antiandrogens were approved initially to block the flare that results from GnRH analogue administration. They have also been studied as monotherapy and as part of a combined androgen blockade (also called maximal androgen blockade). Most reported randomized trials suggest that the cancer-specific outcomes are inferior when antiandrogens are used alone. Bicalutamide, even at 150 mg (three times the recommended dose), was associated with a shorter time to progression and inferior survival compared to surgical castration for patients with established metastatic disease. Nevertheless, some men may accept the trade-off of a potentially inferior cancer outcome for an improved quality of life.

Combined androgen blockade—the administration of an antiandrogen plus a GnRH analogue or surgical orchiectomy—was designed to inhibit both testicular and adrenal androgens at the outset. Cumulative results of randomized comparisons involving thousands of patients showed no advantage for combining an antiandrogen with surgical orchiectomy, while separate analyses of trials combining an antiandrogen with a GnRH analogue have shown a modest (<10%) survival advantage. Meta-analysis of all combined androgen blockade trials concluded that the approach was not more effective. In practice, most patients treated with a GnRH analogue receive an antiandrogen for the first 2–4 weeks of treatment to protect against the flare.

Intermittent Hormone Therapy Another way to reduce the side effects of androgen depletion is to administer hormones on an intermittent basis. This was proposed as a way to prevent the selection of cells that are resistant to androgen depletion. The hypothesis is that by allowing endogenous testosterone levels to rise, the cells that survive androgen depletion will induce a normal differentiation pathway. In this way, the surviving cells that are allowed to proliferate in the presence of androgen will retain sensitivity to subsequent androgen depletion. Applied in the clinic, androgen depletion is continued for 2–6 months beyond the point of maximal response. Once treatment is stopped, endogenous testosterone levels increase, and the symptoms associated with hormone treatment abate. PSA levels also begin to rise, and at some level treatment is restarted. With this approach, multiple cycles of regression and proliferation have been documented in individual patients. It is unknown whether the intermittent approach increases, decreases, or does not change the overall duration of sensitivity to androgen depletion. The preliminary reports suggest that the approach is safe, but long-term data are needed to assess the course in men with low PSA levels. A trial to address this question is ongoing.

Outcomes of Androgen Depletion The antiprostate cancer effects of the various androgen depletion strategies are similar, and the clinical course is predictable: an initial response, then a period of stability in which tumor cells are dormant and not proliferating, followed after a variable period of time by a rise in PSA and regrowth that is visible on a scan as a castration-resistant lesion. Androgen depletion is not curative because cells that survive castration are present when the disease is first diagnosed. Considered by disease manifestation, PSA levels return to normal in 60–70% of patients, and measurable disease regression occurs in 50%; improvements in bone scan occur in 25% of cases, but the majority remains stable. Duration of survival is inversely proportional to disease extent at the time androgen depletion is first started.

An active question is whether hormones should be given in the adjuvant setting after surgery or radiation treatment of the primary tumor or at the time that a PSA recurrence is documented, or to wait until metastatic disease or symptoms of disease are manifest. Trials in support of early therapy have often been underpowered relative to the reported benefit or have been criticized on methodologic grounds. One trial, although it showed a survival benefit for patients treated with radiation therapy and 3 years of androgen depletion relative to radiation alone, was criticized for the poor outcomes of the control group. Another showing a survival benefit for patients with positive lymph nodes who were randomized to immediate medical or surgical castration compared to observation ($p = .02$) was criticized because the confidence intervals around the 5- and 8-year survival distributions for the two groups overlapped. A large randomized study comparing early to late hormone treatment (orchiectomy or GnRH analogue) in patients with locally advanced or asymptomatic metastatic disease showed that patients treated early were less likely to progress from M0 to M1 disease, to develop pain, and to die of prostate cancer. This trial was criticized because therapy was delayed "too long" in the late-treatment group. When patients treated by radical surgery, radiation therapy, or active surveillance were randomly assigned to receive bicalutamide, 150 mg, or placebo, hormone treatment produced a significant reduction in the proportion of patients who developed osseous metastases at 2 years (9% for bicalutamide; 13.8% for placebo). This result has not gained acceptance in part because too many "good-risk" patients were treated and because no effect on survival was demonstrated. These criticisms are valid; however, the net influence on survival from early hormone intervention is similar to that observed in patients with breast cancer, for which adjuvant hormonal therapy is routinely given.

METASTATIC DISEASE: CASTRATE Castration-resistant disease can manifest in many ways. For some it is a rise in PSA with no change in radiographs and no new symptoms. In others it is a rising PSA and progression in bone with or without symptoms of disease. Still others will show soft tissue disease with or without osseous metastases, and others have visceral spread. The prognosis, which is highly variable, can be predicted using nomograms designed for the castration-resistant disease state. The important point is that despite the failure of first-line hormone treatment, the majority of these tumors remain sensitive to second- and third-line hormonal treatments. Castration resistance does not indicate that the tumor is "hormone-refractory." The rising PSA is an indication of continued signaling through the androgen receptor axis.

The manifestations of disease in this patient group hinder the assessment of drugs and treatment standards because traditional measures of outcome such as tumor regression do not apply. Bone scans can be inaccurate for assessing changes in osseous disease, and no PSA-based outcome is a true surrogate for survival benefit. It is essential to define therapeutic objectives before initiating treatment, as there are defined standards of care for different disease manifestations. Therapeutic objectives need not be defined by survival only as useful endpoints also include relief of symptoms and delay of metastases or new symptoms of disease.

The management of patients with castrate metastatic disease requires first that the castrate status be documented. Patients receiving an antiandrogen alone, whose serum testosterone levels are elevated, should be treated first with a GnRH analogue or orchiectomy and observed for response. Patients on an antiandrogen in combination with a GnRH analogue should have the antiandrogen discontinued, as ~20% will respond to the selective discontinuation of the antiandrogen. Any withdrawal response occurs within weeks of stopping flutamide but may take 8–12 weeks with nilutamide and bicalutamide because of their long terminal half-lives. At the time of progression, a different antiandrogen can be given, as some tumors are not cross-resistant. An additional consideration in this setting is that significant androgen production persists in the adrenal gland and that one of the adaptive/selective changes, which occurs in the tumor itself, is the upregulation of adrenal synthetic enzymes, leading to autocrine signaling. High-dose ketoconazole, which inhibits adrenal androgen synthesis, is also often effective in these cases. Other hormones that may be active include estrogens, progestins, and glucocorticoids. Cytotoxic agents are considered when hormones are no longer effective, or the tempo of the illness suggests a more aggressive approach is needed.

Mitoxantrone was the first cytotoxic agent approved to provide palliation of pain secondary to castrate metastatic disease. The results established the important principle that systemic chemotherapy can provide palliation of pain in the absence of a survival benefit. In this trial, mitoxantrone-treated patients had a greater reduction in pain, less use of narcotics, and less fatigue. In 2004, docetaxel was established as the first-line standard cytotoxic drug for patients in this state, based on a trial showing that q3w docetaxel was superior to weekly therapy and to mitoxantrone. The results were confirmed in a second trial of estramustine/docetaxel vs. mitoxantrone. The addition of estramustine produced significant toxicity with no apparent improvement in survival and has been dropped from these regimens. Docetaxel and other microtubule targeted agents produce PSA declines in 50% of patients, measurable disease regression in 25%, and both an improvement in preexisting and prevention of future cancer-related pain.

Management of pain is a critical part of therapy. Optimal palliation requires assessing whether the symptoms and metastases are focal or diffuse and

TABLE 91-2 AUA SYMPTOM INDEX

	AUA Symptom Score (Circle 1 Number on Each Line)					
Questions to Be Answered	**Not at All**	**Less than 1 Time in 5**	**Less than Half the Time**	**About Half the Time**	**More than Half the time**	**Almost Always**
Over the past month, how often you have had a sensation of not emptying your bladder completely after you finished urinating?	0+	1	2	3	4	5
Over the past month, how often have you had to urinate again less than 2 h after you finished urinating?	0	1	2	3	4	5
Over the past month, how often have you found you stopped and started again several times when you urinated?	0	1	2	3	4	5
Over the past month, how often have you found it difficult to postpone urination?	0	1	2	3	4	5
Over the past month, how often have you had a weak urinary stream?	0	1	2	3	4	5
Over the past month, how often have you had to push or strain to begin urination?	0	1	2	3	4	5
Over the past month, how many times did you most typically get up to urinate from the time you went to bed at night until the time you got up in the morning?	(None)	(1 time)	(2 times)	(3 times)	(4 times)	(5 times)
Sum of 7 circled numbers (AUA Symptom Score): ____						

Note: AUA, American Urological Association.
Source: Barry MJ et al: J Urol 148:1549, 1992. Used with permission.

whether disease threatens the spinal cord, the cauda equina, or the base of the skull. Neurologic symptoms require emergency evaluation because loss of function may be permanent if not addressed quickly. Single sites of pain and areas of neurologic involvement are best treated with external beam radiation. As the disease is often diffuse, palliation at one site often is followed by the emergence of symptoms in a separate site that had not received radiation.

Given the bone-dominant pattern of prostate cancer spread, two bone-seeking radioisotopes, ^{89}Sr (Metastron) and ^{153}Sm-EDTMP (Quadramet), are approved for palliation of pain, although they have no effect on PSA or survival. Fewer patients treated with one of these isotopes developed new areas of pain or required additional radiation therapy compared to patients receiving external beam radiation therapy alone. Additionally, patients randomly assigned to a combination of ^{89}Sr and doxorubicin after induction chemotherapy had fewer skeletal events and longer survival than patients treated with doxorubicin alone. Confirmatory studies are ongoing. Addition of the bisphosphonate zoledronate to "standard therapy" in patients with castration-resistant disease resulted in fewer skeletal events relative to placebo. The skeletal events included microfractures, new pain, and need for radiation therapy. Bisphosphonates have a dual role: to protect against the bone loss associated with androgen depletion and to prevent skeletal events.

BENIGN DISEASE

SYMPTOMS

Benign proliferative disease may produce hesitancy, intermittent voiding, a diminished stream, incomplete emptying, and postvoid leakage. The severity of these symptoms can be quantitated with the self-administered American Urological Association Symptom Index (Table 91-2), although the degree of symptoms does not always relate to gland size. Resistance to urine flow reduces bladder compliance, leading to nocturia, urgency, and, ultimately, urinary retention. An episode of urinary retention may be precipitated by infection, tranquilizing drugs, antihistamines, and alcohol. Prostatitis often produces pain or induration. Typically, the symptoms remain stable over time and obstruction does not occur.

DIAGNOSTIC PROCEDURES AND TREATMENT

Asymptomatic patients do not require treatment regardless of the size of the gland, while those with an inability to urinate, gross hematuria, recurrent infection, or bladder stones may require surgery. In patients with symptoms, uroflowmetry can identify those with normal flow rates who are unlikely to benefit from surgery and those with high postvoid residuals who may need other interventions. Pressure-flow studies detect primary bladder dysfunction. Cystoscopy is recommended if hematuria is documented and to assess the urinary outflow tract before surgery. Imaging of the upper tracts is advised for patients with hematuria, a history of calculi, or prior urinary tract problems.

Medical therapies for BPH include 5α-reductase inhibitors and α-adrenergic blockers. Finasteride (10 mg/d PO) and other 5α-reductase inhibitors that block the conversion of testosterone to dihydrotestosterone decrease prostate size, increase urine flow rates, and improve symptoms. They also lower baseline PSA levels by 50%, an important consideration when using PSA to guide biopsy recommendations. α-Adrenergic blockers such as terazosin (1–10 mg PO at bedtime) act by relaxing the smooth muscle of the bladder neck and increasing peak urinary flow rates. No data show that these agents influence the progression of the disease.

Surgical approaches include TURP, transurethral incision, or removal of the gland via a retropubic, suprapubic, or perineal approach. Also utilized are TULIP (transurethral ultrasound-guided laser-induced prostatectomy), stents, and hyperthermia.

FURTHER READINGS

LOBLAW DA et al: Initial hormonal management of androgen-sensitive metastatic, recurrent or progressive prostate cancer: 2006 update of an American Society of Clinical Oncology practice guideline. J Clin Oncol 25:1596, 2007

LOEB S, CATALONA WJ: Prostate-specific antigen in clinical practice. Cancer Letters 249:30, 2007

NELSON WG et al: Prostate cancer. N Engl J Med 349:366, 2003

SCHER HI, HELLER G: Clinical states in prostate cancer: Toward a dynamic model of disease progression. Urology 55:323, 2000

TANNOCK IM et al: Docetaxel plus prednisone or mitoxantrone plus prednisone for advanced prostate cancer. N Engl J Med 351:1502, 2004

THOMPSON IM et al: The influence of finasteride on the development of prostate cancer. N Engl J Med 349:215, 2003

THORPE A, NEAL D: Benign prostatic hyperplasia. Lancet 366:1359, 2003

YAO SL, DIPAOLA RS: Evidence-based approach to prostate cancer follow-up. Semin Oncol 30:390, 2003

92 Testicular Cancer

Robert J. Motzer, George J. Bosl

Primary germ cell tumors (GCTs) of the testis, arising by the malignant transformation of primordial germ cells, constitute 95% of all testicular neoplasms. Infrequently, GCTs arise from an extragonadal site, including the mediastinum, retroperitoneum, and, very rarely, the pineal gland. This disease is notable for the young age of the afflicted patients, the totipotent capacity for differentiation of the tumor cells, and its curability; about 95% of newly diagnosed patients are cured. Experience in the management of GCTs leads to improved outcome.

INCIDENCE AND EPIDEMIOLOGY

In 2007, 7920 new cases of testicular GCT were diagnosed in the United States; the incidence is decreasing after having increased slowly over the past 40 years. The tumor occurs most frequently in men between the ages of 20 and 40. A testicular mass in a male ≥50 years should be regarded as a lymphoma until proved otherwise. GCT is at least four to five times more common in white than in African-American males, and a higher incidence has been observed in Scandinavia and New Zealand than in the United States.

ETIOLOGY AND GENETICS

Cryptorchidism is associated with a severalfold higher risk of GCT. Abdominal cryptorchid testes are at a higher risk than inguinal cryptorchid testes. Orchiopexy should be performed before puberty, if possible. Early orchiopexy reduces the risk of GCT and improves the ability to save the testis. An abdominal cryptorchid testis that cannot be brought into the scrotum should be removed. About 2% of men with GCTs of one testis will develop a primary tumor in the other testis. Testicular feminization syndromes increase the risk of testicular GCT, and Klinefelter's syndrome is associated with mediastinal GCT.

An isochromosome of the short arm of chromosome 12 [i(12p)] is pathognomonic for GCT of all histologic types. Excess 12p copy number, either in the form of i(12p) or as increased 12p on aberrantly banded marker chromosomes, occurs in nearly all GCTs, but the gene(s) on 12p involved in the pathogenesis are not yet defined.

CLINICAL PRESENTATION

A painless testicular mass is pathognomonic for a testicular malignancy. More commonly, patients present with testicular discomfort or swelling suggestive of epididymitis and/or orchitis. In this circumstance, a trial of antibiotics is reasonable. However, if symptoms persist or a residual abnormality remains, then testicular ultrasound examination is indicated.

Ultrasound of the testis is indicated whenever a testicular malignancy is considered and for persistent or painful testicular swelling. If a testicular mass is detected, a radical inguinal orchiectomy should be performed. Because the testis develops from the gonadal ridge, its blood supply and lymphatic drainage originate in the abdomen and descend with the testis into the scrotum. An inguinal approach is taken to avoid breaching anatomic barriers and permitting additional pathways of spread.

Back pain from retroperitoneal metastases is common and must be distinguished from musculoskeletal pain. Dyspnea from pulmonary metastases occurs infrequently. Patients with increased serum levels of human chorionic gonadotropin (hCG) may present with gynecomastia. A delay in diagnosis is associated with a more advanced stage and possibly worse survival.

The staging evaluation for GCT includes a determination of serum levels of fetoprotein (AFP), hCG, and lactate dehydrogenase (LDH). After orchiectomy, a chest radiograph and a CT scan of the abdomen and pelvis should be performed. A chest CT scan is required if pulmonary nodules or mediastinal or hilar disease is suspected. Stage I disease is limited to the testis, epididymis, or spermatic cord. Stage II disease is limited to retroperitoneal (regional) lymph nodes. Stage III disease is disease outside the retroperitoneum, involving supradiaphragmatic nodal sites or viscera. The staging may be "clinical"—defined solely by physical examination, blood marker evaluation, and radiographs—or "pathologic"—defined by an operative procedure.

The regional draining lymph nodes for the testis are in the retroperitoneum, and the vascular supply originates from the great vessels (for the right testis) or the renal vessels (for the left testis). As a result, the lymph nodes that are involved first by a right testicular tumor are the interaortocaval lymph nodes just below the renal vessels. For a left testicular tumor, the first involved lymph nodes are lateral to the aorta (para-aortic) and below the left renal vessels. In both cases, further nodal spread is inferior, contralateral, and, less commonly, above the renal hilum. Lymphatic involvement can extend cephalad to the retrocrural, posterior mediastinal, and supraclavicular lymph nodes. Treatment is determined by tumor histology (seminoma versus nonseminoma) and clinical stage (Table 92-1).

PATHOLOGY

GCTs are divided into nonseminoma and seminoma subtypes. Nonseminomatous GCTs are most frequent in the third decade of life and can display the full spectrum of embryonic and adult cellular differentiation. This entity comprises four histologies: embryonal carcinoma, teratoma, choriocarcinoma, and endodermal sinus (yolk sac) tumor. Choriocarcinoma, consisting of both cytotrophoblasts and syncytiophoblasts, represents malignant trophoblastic differentiation and is invariably associated with secretion of hCG. Endodermal sinus tumor is the malignant counterpart of the fetal yolk sac and is associated with secretion of AFP. Pure embryonal carcinoma may secrete AFP or hCG, or both; this pattern is biochemical evidence of differentiation. Teratoma is composed of somatic cell types derived from two or more germ layers (ectoderm, mesoderm, or endoderm). Each of these histologies may be present alone or in combination with others. Nonseminomatous GCTs tend to metastasize early to sites such as the retroperitoneal lymph nodes and lung parenchyma. One-third of patients present with disease limited to the testis (stage I), one-third with retroperitoneal metastases (stage II), and one-third with more extensive supradiaphragmatic nodal or visceral metastases (stage III).

Seminoma represents about 50% of all GCTs, has a median age in the fourth decade, and generally follows a more indolent clinical

TABLE 92-1 GERM CELL TUMOR STAGING AND TREATMENT

		Treatment	
Stage	**Extent of Disease**	**Seminoma**	**Nonseminoma**
IA	Testis only, no vascular/lymphatic invasion (T1)	Radiation therapy	RPLND or observation
IB	Testis only, with vascular/lymphatic invasion (T2), or extension through tunica albuginea (T2), or involvement of spermatic cord (T3) or scrotum (T4)	Radiation therapy	RPLND
IIA	Nodes < 2 cm	Radiation therapy	RPLND or chemotherapy often followed by RPLND
IIB	Nodes 2–5 cm	Radiation therapy	RPLND +/– adjuvant chemotherapy or chemotherapy followed by RPLND
IIC	Nodes > 5 cm	Chemotherapy	Chemotherapy, often followed by RPLND
III	Distant metastases	Chemotherapy	Chemotherapy, often followed by surgery (biopsy or resection)

Note: RPLND, retroperitoneal lymph node dissection.

course. Most patients (70%) present with stage I disease, about 20% with stage II disease, and 10% with stage III disease; lung or other visceral metastases are rare. Radiation therapy is the treatment of choice in patients with stage I disease and stage II disease where the nodes are <5 cm in maximum diameter. When a tumor contains both seminoma and nonseminoma components, patient management is directed by the more aggressive nonseminoma component.

TUMOR MARKERS

Careful monitoring of the serum tumor markers AFP and hCG is essential in the management of patients with GCT, as these markers are important for diagnosis, as prognostic indicators, in monitoring treatment response, and in the detection of early relapse. Approximately 70% of patients presenting with disseminated nonseminomatous GCT have increased serum concentrations of AFP and/or hCG. While hCG concentrations may be increased in patients with either nonseminoma or seminoma histology, the AFP concentration is increased only in patients with nonseminoma. The presence of an increased AFP level in a patient whose tumor shows only seminoma indicates that an occult nonseminomatous component exists and the patient should be treated for nonseminomatous GCT. LDH levels are not as specific as AFP or hCG but are increased in 50–60% patients with metastatic nonseminoma and in up to 80% of patients with advanced seminoma.

AFP, hCG, and LDH levels should be determined before and after orchiectomy. Increased serum AFP and hCG concentrations decay according to first-order kinetics; the half-life is 24–36 h for hCG and 5–7 days for AFP. AFP and hCG should be assayed serially during and after treatment. The reappearance of hCG and/or AFP or the failure of these markers to decline according to the predicted half-life is an indicator of persistent or recurrent tumor.

Rx TESTICULAR CANCER

STAGE I NONSEMINOMA If, after an orchiectomy (for clinical stage I disease), radiographs and physical examination show no evidence of disease and serum AFP and hCG concentrations are either normal or declining to normal according to the known half-life, patients may be managed by either a nerve-sparing retroperitoneal lymph node dissection (RPLND) or surveillance. The retroperitoneal lymph nodes are involved by GCT (pathologic stage II) in 20–50% of these patients. The choice of surveillance or RPLND is based on the pathology of the primary tumor. If the primary tumor shows no evidence for lymphatic or vascular invasion and is limited to the testis (T1), then either option is reasonable. If lymphatic or vascular invasion is present or the tumor extends into the tunica, spermatic cord, or scrotum (T2 through T4), then surveillance should not be offered. Either approach should cure >95% of patients.

RPLND is the standard operation for removal of the regional lymph nodes of the testis (retroperitoneal nodes). The operation removes the lymph nodes ipsilateral to the primary site and the nodal groups adjacent to the primary landing zone. The standard (modified bilateral) RPLND removes all node-bearing tissue down to the bifurcation of the great vessels, including the ipsilateral iliac nodes. The major long-term effect of this operation is retrograde ejaculation and infertility. Nerve-sparing RPLND, usually accomplished by identification and dissection of individual nerve fibers, may avoid injury to the sympathetic nerves responsible for ejaculation. Normal ejaculation is preserved in ~90% of patients. Patients with pathologic stage I disease are observed, and only the <10% who relapse require additional therapy. If retroperitoneal nodes are found to be involved at RPLND, then a decision regarding adjuvant chemotherapy is made on the basis of the extent of retroperitoneal disease (see below).

Surveillance is an option in the management of clinical stage I disease when no vascular/lymphatic invasion is found (T1). Only 20–30% of patients have pathologic stage II disease, implying that most RPLNDs in this situation are not therapeutic. Surveillance and RPLND lead to equivalent long-term survival rates. Patient compliance is essential if surveillance is to be successful. Patients must be carefully followed with periodic chest radiography, physical examination, CT scan of the abdomen, and serum tumor marker determinations. The median time to relapse is about 7 months, and late relapses (>2 years) are rare. The 70–80% of patients who do not relapse require no intervention after orchiectomy; treatment is reserved for those who do relapse. When the primary tumor is classified as T2 through T4 (extension beyond testis and epididymis or lymphatic/vascular invasion is identified), nerve-sparing RPLND is preferred. About 50% of these patients have pathologic stage II disease and are destined to relapse without the RPLND.

STAGE II NONSEMINOMA Patients with limited, ipsilateral retroperitoneal adenopathy (nodes usually ≤3 cm in largest diameter) and normal levels of AFP and hCG generally undergo a modified bilateral RPLND as primary management. Increased levels of either AFP or hCG or both imply metastatic disease outside the retroperitoneum; chemotherapy is used in this setting. The local recurrence rate after a properly performed RPLND is very low. Depending on the extent of disease, the postoperative management options include either surveillance or two cycles of adjuvant chemotherapy. Surveillance is the preferred approach for patients with resected "low-volume" metastases (tumor nodes ≤2 cm in diameter *and* <6 nodes involved) because the probability of relapse is one-third or less. For those who relapse, risk-directed chemotherapy is indicated (see below). Because relapse occurs in ≥50% of patients with "high-volume" metastases (>6 nodes involved, *or* any involved node >2 cm in largest diameter, *or* extranodal tumor extension), two cycles of adjuvant chemotherapy should be considered, as it results in cure in ≥98% of patients. Regimens consisting of etoposide (100 mg/m^2 daily on days 1–5) plus cisplatin (20 mg/m^2 daily on days 1–5) with or without bleomycin (30 units per day on days 2, 9, and 16) given at 3-week intervals are effective and well tolerated.

STAGES I AND II SEMINOMA Inguinal orchiectomy followed by retroperitoneal radiation therapy cures ~98% of patients with stage I seminoma. The dose of radiation therapy (2500–3000 cGy) is low and well tolerated, and the in-field recurrence rate is negligible. About 2% of patients relapse with supradiaphragmatic or systemic disease. Surveillance has been proposed as an option, and studies have shown that about 15% of patients relapse. The median time to relapse is 12–15 months, and late relapses (>5 years) may be more frequent than with nonseminoma. The relapse is usually treated with chemotherapy. Surveillance for clinical stage I seminoma is not recommended.

Nonbulky retroperitoneal disease (stage IIA and IIB) is also treated with radiation therapy. Prophylactic supradiaphragmatic fields are not used. Relapses in the anterior mediastinum are unusual. Approximately 90% of patients achieve relapse-free survival with retroperitoneal masses <5 cm in diameter. Because at least one-third of patients with bulkier disease relapse, initial chemotherapy is preferred for stage IIC disease.

CHEMOTHERAPY FOR ADVANCED GCT Regardless of histology, patients with stage IIC and stage III GCT are treated with chemotherapy. Combination chemotherapy programs based on cisplatin at doses of 100 mg/m^2 plus etoposide at doses of 500 mg/m^2 per cycle cure 70–80% of such patients, with or without bleomycin, depending on risk stratification (see below). A complete response (the complete disappearance of all clinical evidence of tumor on physical examination and radiography plus normal serum levels of AFP and hCG for ≥1 month) occurs after chemotherapy alone in ~60% of patients, and another 10–20% become disease-free with surgical resection of residual masses containing viable GCT. Lower doses of cisplatin result in inferior survival rates.

The toxicity of four cycles of the cisplatin/bleomycin/etoposide (BEP) regimen is substantial. Nausea, vomiting, and hair loss occur in most patients, although nausea and vomiting have been markedly ameliorated by modern antiemetic regimens. Myelosuppression is frequent, and symptomatic bleomycin pulmonary toxicity occurs in ~5% of patients. Treatment-induced mortality due to neutropenia with septicemia or bleomycin-induced pulmonary failure occurs in 1–3% of patients. Dose reductions for myelosuppression are rarely indicated. Long-term permanent toxicities include nephrotoxicity (reduced glomerular filtration and persistent magnesium wasting), ototoxicity, and peripheral neuropathy. When bleomycin is administered by weekly bolus injection, Raynaud's phenomenon appears in 5–10% of patients. Other evidence of small blood vessel damage is seen less often, including transient ischemic attacks and myocardial infarction.

RISK-DIRECTED CHEMOTHERAPY Because not all patients are cured and treatment may cause significant toxicities, patients are stratified into "good-risk" and "poor-risk" groups according to pretreatment clinical features. For good-risk patients, the goal is to achieve maximum efficacy with minimal toxicity. For poor-risk patients, the goal is to identify more effective therapy with tolerable toxicity.

TABLE 92-2 IGCCCG RISK CLASSIFICATION FOR ADVANCED GERM CELL TUMORS

Risk	Nonseminoma	Seminoma
Good	Gonadal or retroperitoneal primary site Absent nonpulmonary visceral metastases AFP < 1000 ng/mL Beta-hCG < 5000 mIU/mL LDH < 1.5 × upper limit or normal (ULN)	Any primary site Absent nonpulmonary visceral metastases Any LDH, hCG
Intermediate	Gonadal or retroperitoneal primary site Absent nonpulmonary visceral metastases AFP 1000–10,000 ng/mL Beta-hCG 5000–50,000 mIU/mL LDH 1.5–10 × ULN	Any primary site Presence of nonpulmonary visceral metastases Any LDH, hCG
Poor	Mediastinal primary site Presence of nonpulmonary visceral metastases AFP ≥ 10,000 ng/mL Beta-hCG > 50,000 mIU/mL LDH > 10 × ULN	No patients classified as poor prognosis

Note: AFP, α fetoprotein; hCG, human chorionic gonadotropin; LDH, lactate dehydrogenase.
Source: From International Germ Cell Cancer Consensus Group.

The International Germ Cell Cancer Consensus Group developed criteria to assign patients to three risk groups (good, intermediate, poor) **(Table 92-2)**. The marker cut-offs have been incorporated into the revised TNM (primary tumor, regional nodes, metastasis) staging of GCT. Hence, TNM stage groupings are now based on both anatomy (site and extent of disease) and biology (marker status and histology). Seminoma is either good or intermediate risk, based on the absence or presence of nonpulmonary visceral metastases. No poor-risk category exists for seminoma. Marker levels play no role in defining risk for seminoma. Nonseminomas have good-, intermediate-, and poor-risk categories based on the site of the primary tumor, the presence or absence of nonpulmonary visceral metastases, and marker levels.

For ~90% of patients with good-risk GCTs, four cycles of etoposide plus cisplatin (EP) or three cycles of BEP produce durable complete responses, with minimal acute and chronic toxicity. Pulmonary toxicity is absent when bleomycin is not used and is rare when therapy is limited to 9 weeks; myelosuppression with neutropenic fever is less frequent; and the treatment mortality rate is negligible. About 75% of intermediate-risk patients and 45% of poor-risk patients achieve durable complete remission with four cycles of BEP, and no regimen has proved superior. More effective therapy is needed.

POSTCHEMOTHERAPY SURGERY Resection of residual metastases after the completion of chemotherapy is an integral part of therapy. If the initial histology is nonseminoma and the marker values have normalized, all sites of residual disease should be resected. In general, residual retroperitoneal disease requires a modified bilateral RPLND. Thoracotomy (unilateral or bilateral) and neck dissection are less frequently required to remove residual mediastinal, pulmonary parenchymal, or cervical nodal disease. Viable tumor (seminoma, embryonal carcinoma, yolk sac tumor, or choriocarcinoma) will be present in 15%, mature teratoma in 40%, and necrotic debris and fibrosis in 45% of resected specimens. The frequency of teratoma or viable disease is highest in residual mediastinal tumors. If necrotic debris or mature teratoma is present, no further chemotherapy is necessary. If viable tumor is present but is completely excised, two additional cycles of chemotherapy are given.

If the initial histology is pure seminoma, mature teratoma is rarely present, and the most frequent finding is necrotic debris. For residual retroperitoneal disease, a complete RPLND is technically difficult owing to extensive postchemotherapy fibrosis. Observation is recommended when no radiographic abnormality exists on CT scan. Positive findings on a positron emission tomography (PET) scan correlate with viable seminoma in residua, and mandate surgical excision or biopsy.

SALVAGE CHEMOTHERAPY Of patients with advanced GCT, 20–30% fail to achieve a durable complete response to first-line chemotherapy. A combination of cisplatin, ifosfamide, and vinblastine (VeIP) will cure about 25% of patients as a second-line therapy. Substitution of paclitaxel for vinblastine may be more effective in this setting. Patients are more likely to achieve a durable complete response if they had a testicular primary tumor and relapsed from a prior complete remission to first-line cisplatin-containing chemotherapy. In contrast, if the patient failed to achieve a complete response or has a primary mediastinal nonseminoma, then standard-dose salvage therapy is rarely beneficial. Treatment options for such patients include dose-intensive treatment, experimental therapies, and surgical resection.

Chemotherapy consisting of dose-intensive, high-dose carboplatin (≥1500 mg/m^2) plus etoposide (≥1200 mg/m^2), with or without cyclophosphamide, or ifosfamide, with peripheral blood stem cell support, induces a complete response in 25–40% of patients who have progressed after ifosfamide-containing salvage chemotherapy. About one-half of the complete responses will be durable. High-dose therapy is the treatment of choice and standard of care for this patient population. Paclitaxel is also active in previously treated patients and shows promise in high-dose combination programs. Cure is still possible in some relapsed patients.

EXTRAGONADAL GCT AND MIDLINE CARCINOMA OF UNCERTAIN HISTOGENESIS

The prognosis and management of patients with extragonadal GCT depends on the tumor histology and site of origin. All patients with a diagnosis of extragonadal GCT should have a testicular ultrasound examination. Nearly all patients with retroperitoneal or mediastinal seminoma achieve a durable complete response to BEP or EP. The clinical features of patients with primary retroperitoneal nonseminoma GCT are similar to those of patients with a primary of testis origin, and careful evaluation will find evidence of a primary testicular GCT in about two-thirds of cases. In contrast, a primary mediastinal nonseminomatous GCT is associated with a poor prognosis; one-third of patients are cured with standard therapy (four cycles of BEP). Patients with newly diagnosed mediastinal nonseminoma are considered to have poor-risk disease and should be considered for clinical trials testing regimens of possibly greater efficacy. In addition, mediastinal nonseminoma is associated with hematologic disorders, including acute myelogenous leukemia, myelodysplastic syndrome, and essential thrombocytosis unrelated to previous chemotherapy. These hematologic disorders are very refractory to treatment. Nonseminoma of any primary site may change into other malignant histologies such as embryonal rhabdomyosarcoma or adenocarcinoma. This is called malignant transformation. i(12p) has been identified in the transformed cell type, indicating GCT clonal origin.

A group of patients with poorly differentiated tumors of unknown histogenesis, midline in distribution, and not associated with secretion of AFP or hCG has been described; a few (10–20%) are cured by standard cisplatin-containing chemotherapy. i(12p) is present in ~25% of such tumors (the fraction that are cisplatin-responsive), confirming their origin from primitive germ cells. This finding is also predictive of the response to cisplatin-based chemotherapy and resulting long-term survival. These tumors are heterogeneous; neuroepithelial tumors and lymphoma may also present in this fashion.

FERTILITY

Infertility is an important consequence of the treatment of GCTs. Preexisting infertility or impaired fertility is often present. Azoospermia and/or oligospermia are present at diagnosis in at least 50% of patients with testicular GCTs. Ejaculatory dysfunction is associated with RPLND, and germ cell damage may result from cisplatin-containing chemotherapy. Nerve-sparing techniques to preserve the retroperitoneal sympathetic nerves have made retrograde ejaculation less likely in the subgroups of patients who are candidates for this operation. Spermatogenesis does recur in some patients after chemotherapy. However, because of the significant risk of impaired reproductive capacity, semen analysis and cryopreservation of sperm in a sperm bank should be recommended to all patients before treatment.

BOSL GJ et al: Testicular germ-cell cancer. N Engl J Med 337:242, 1997

——— et al: Cancer of the testis, in *Cancer: Principles and Practice of Oncology*, 7th ed, VT DEVITA et al (eds). Philadelphia, Lippincott Williams & Wilkins, 2005, pp 1269–1294

CHAGANTI RSK, HOULDSWORTH J: Genetics and biology of human male germ cell tumors. Cancer Res 60:1475, 2000

INTERNATIONAL GERM CELL CANCER CONSENSUS GROUP: International Germ Cell Consensus Classification: A prognostic factor-based staging system for metastatic germ cell cancers. J Clin Oncol 15:594, 1997

KONDAGUNTA GV et al: Etoposide and cisplatin chemotherapy for metastatic good-risk germ cell tumors. J Clin Oncol 23: 9290, 2005

MOORE CJ et al: Management of difficult germ-cell tumors. Oncology 20:1565, 2006

MOTZER R et al: Sequential dose-intensive paclitaxel, ifosfamide, carboplatin, and etoposide salvage therapy for germ cell tumor patients. J Clin Oncol 18:1173, 2000

SONPAUDE G et al: Management of recurrent testicular germ cell tumors. Oncologist 12:51, 2007

93 Gynecologic Malignancies

Robert C. Young

OVARIAN CANCER

INCIDENCE AND EPIDEMIOLOGY

Ovarian cancer can develop from three distinctive cell types (germ cells, stromal cells, and epithelial cells), and each of these presents with distinctive features and outcomes and requires widely different management approaches. Epithelial ovarian cancer is the most common of the three and the leading cause of death from gynecologic cancer in the United States. In 2007, 22,430 new cases were diagnosed, and 15,280 women died from ovarian cancer. Epithelial ovarian cancer accounts for 5% of all cancer deaths in women in the United States; more women die of this disease than from cervical and endometrial cancer combined.

The age-specific incidence of the common epithelial type of ovarian cancer increases progressively and peaks in the eighth decade. Epithelial tumors, unlike germ cell and stromal tumors, are uncommon before the age of 40. Epidemiologic studies suggest higher incidences in women with a family history; in those who have been exposed to asbestos or talc; in industrialized nations; and in women with disordered ovarian function, including infertility, nulliparity, and frequent miscarriages. The use of ovulation-inducing drugs such as clomiphene has been implicated, but the studies have produced mixed results. Reduction in ovarian cancer risk is associated with pregnancy (each pregnancy reduces the ovarian cancer risk by about 10%), breast-feeding, and tubal ligation. Oral contraceptives reduce the risk of ovarian cancer in patients with a family history of cancer and in the general population. Many of these risk-reduction factors support the "incessant ovulation" hypothesis for ovarian cancer etiology, which implies that an aberrant repair process of the surface epithelium is central to ovarian cancer development. Estrogen replacement after menopause does not appear to increase the risk of ovarian cancer, although its use has declined substantially since the HRT trials demonstrated an increased cardiovascular risk.

Familial cases account for about 10% of all ovarian cancer. Compared to a lifetime risk of 1.6% in the general population, women with one affected first-degree relative have a 5% risk. In families with two or more affected first-degree relatives, the risk may exceed 50%. Two types of autosomal dominant familial cancers have been identified: (1) breast/ovarian cancer syndrome; and (2) the Lynch type II cancer family syndrome with nonpolyposis colorectal cancer, endometrial cancer, and ovarian cancer.

ETIOLOGY AND GENETICS

In women with hereditary breast/ovarian cancer, two susceptibility loci have been identified: *BRCA1*, located on chromosome 17q12-21, and *BRCA2*, on 13q12-13. Both are tumor-suppressor genes that produce nuclear proteins that interact with RAD 51, which effects genomic integrity. Both genes are large, and numerous mutations have been described; most are frameshift or nonsense mutations, and 86% produce truncated protein products. The implications of the many other mutations, including many missense mutations, are not known. The cumulative risk of ovarian cancer with critical mutations of *BRCA1* or *-2* is 25%. Mutated genes can be inherited from either parent, so a complete family history is required. Men in such families have an increased risk of prostate cancer.

The Lynch type II syndrome is associated with an increased risk of ovarian cancer. Affected women often present at a younger age (<50 years). The predisposition results from germline mutations of mismatch repair genes (*MSH2, MLH1, MLH6, PMS1*, and *PMS2*). Because the risk of both endometrial and ovarian cancer is high, intensified screening and prophylactic surgery are often considered.

CLINICAL PRESENTATION AND DIFFERENTIAL DIAGNOSIS

Seventy percent of patients with ovarian cancer are first diagnosed when the disease has already spread beyond the true pelvis. The occurrence of abdominal pain, bloating, and urinary symptoms usually indicates advanced disease. Localized ovarian cancer is generally asymptomatic. However, progressive enlargement of a localized ovarian tumor can produce urinary frequency or constipation. Rarely, torsion of an ovarian mass causes acute abdominal pain or a surgical abdomen. In contrast to cervical or endometrial cancer, vaginal bleeding or discharge is rarely seen with early ovarian cancer. The diagnosis of early disease usually occurs with palpation of an asymptomatic adnexal mass during routine pelvic examination or as an incidental finding at surgery. However, most ovarian enlargements discovered on physical examination, especially in premenopausal women, are benign functional cysts that characteristically resolve over one to three menstrual cycles. Adnexal masses in premenarchal or postmenopausal women are more likely to be pathologic. A solid, irregular, fixed pelvic mass is usually ovarian cancer. Ultrasound studies usually show complex cysts with solid elements. Other causes of adnexal masses include pedunculated uterine fibroids, endometriosis, benign ovarian neoplasms, and inflammatory lesions of the bowel.

Evaluation of patients with suspected ovarian cancer should include measurement of CA-125. Between 80 and 85% of patients with epithelial ovarian cancer have levels of CA-125 ≥ 35 U/mL. Other malignant tumors can also elevate CA-125 levels, including cancers of the endometrium, cervix, fallopian tubes, pancreas, breast, lung, and colon. Certain nonmalignant conditions that can produce moderate elevations of CA-125 levels include pregnancy, endometriosis, pelvic inflammatory disease, and uterine fibroids. About 1% of normal females have serum CA-125 levels >35 U/mL. However, in postmenopausal women with an asymptomatic pelvic mass and CA-125 levels ≥65 U/mL, the test has a sensitivity of 97% and a specificity of 78%.

SCREENING

In contrast to patients who present with advanced disease, patients with early ovarian cancers (stages I and II) are commonly curable with conventional therapy. Thus, effective screening procedures would improve the cure rate in this disease. Although pelvic examination and CA-125 can occasionally detect early disease, these are relatively insensitive screening procedures. Transvaginal sonography is often used, but significant false-positive results are noted, particularly in premenopausal women. Doppler flow imaging coupled with transvaginal ultrasound may improve accuracy and reduce the high rate of false positives.

TABLE 93-1 STAGING AND SURVIVAL IN GYNECOLOGIC MALIGNANCIES

Stage	Ovarian	5-Year Survival, %	Endometrial	5-Year Survival, %	Cervix	5-Year Survival, %
0	—		—		Carcinoma in situ	100
I	Confined to ovary	90	Confined to corpus	89	Confined to uterus	85
II	Confined to pelvis	70	Involves corpus and cervix	73	Invades beyond uterus but not to pelvic wall	65
III	Intraabdominal spread	25–50	Extends outside the uterus but not outside the true pelvis	52	Extends to pelvic wall and/or lower third of vagina, or hydronephrosis	35
IV	Spread outside abdomen	1–5	Extends outside the true pelvis or involves the bladder or rectum	17	Invades mucosa of bladder or rectum or extends beyond the true pelvis	7

CA-125 has significant limitations as a screening test. Half of women with stages I and II ovarian cancer have normal CA-125 levels. Attempts have been made to improve the sensitivity and specificity by combinations of procedures, commonly transvaginal ultrasound and CA-125. In a screening study of 22,000 women, 42 had a positive screen and 11 had ovarian cancer (seven with advanced disease). In addition, eight women with a negative screen developed ovarian cancer. Thus, the false-positive rate would lead to a large number of unnecessary (i.e., negative) laparotomies if each positive screen resulted in a surgical exploration. In the United Kingdom, a large collaborative screening trial is underway to prospectively compare various screening techniques with controls. Until the results of such trials are available, the National Institutes of Health Consensus Conference recommended against screening for ovarian cancer among the general population without known risk factors for the disease. Although no evidence shows that screening saves lives, many physicians use annual pelvic examinations, transvaginal ultrasound, and CA-125 to screen women with a family history of ovarian cancer, Lynch type II, or breast/ovarian cancer syndrome.

Proteomic technologies have been used to identify patterns of proteins associated with early disease. Preliminary studies identified all 50 stage I patients with a sensitivity of 100%, a specificity of 95%, and a positive predictive value of 94%. However, difficulty in consistency of replicate samples, variability of results from different spectroscopy equipment, and the tendency of the artificial intelligence algorithms to overfit the data have limited its utility. Most proteins identified to date have been acute phase reactants, and extensive fractionation is necessary to identify unique cancer-specific proteins.

PATHOLOGY

Common epithelial tumors comprise most (85%) of the ovarian neoplasms. These may be benign (50%), malignant (33%), or tumors of low malignant potential (16%) (i.e., tumors of borderline malignancy). Epithelial tumors of low malignant potential have the cytologic features of malignancy but do not invade the ovarian stroma. More than 75% of borderline malignancies present in early stage and generally occur in the fourth or fifth decade of life. They usually have 10-year survival of 80–90%.

There are five major subtypes of common epithelial tumors: serous (50%); mucinous (25%), endometrioid (15%); clear cell (5%); and Brenner tumors (1%), the latter derived from the urothelium. Benign common epithelial tumors are almost always serous or mucinous and develop in women ages 20–60. They are frequently large (20–30 cm), bilateral, and cystic. Malignant epithelial tumors are usually seen in women over 40.

Although most ovarian tumors are epithelial, two other ovarian tumor types, stromal and germ cell tumors, are distinct in their cell of origin, have different clinical presentations and natural histories, and require different management (see below).

Metastasis to the ovary can occur from breast, colon, gastric, and pancreatic cancers. The Krukenberg tumor was classically described as bilateral ovarian masses from metastatic mucin-secreting gastrointestinal cancers.

STAGING AND PROGNOSTIC FACTORS

Laparotomy is the primary procedure used to establish the diagnosis and provide accurate staging. Less-invasive studies may help define the extent of spread, including chest x-rays, abdominal CT or MRI scans, and abdominal and pelvic sonography. Symptoms of bladder or renal dysfunction are evaluated by cystoscopy or intravenous pyelography.

A careful staging laparotomy with a total abdominal hysterectomy and bilateral salpingo-oophorectomy will establish the stage and extent of disease and allow for the cytoreduction of tumor masses in patients with advanced disease. Proper laparotomy requires a vertical incision of sufficient length to ensure adequate examination of the abdominal contents. The presence, amount, and cytology of any ascitic fluid should be noted. The primary tumor should be evaluated for rupture, excrescences, or dense adherence. Careful visual and manual inspection of the diaphragm and peritoneal surfaces is required. A partial omentectomy should be performed and the paracolic gutters inspected. Pelvic lymph nodes as well as para-aortic nodes in the region of the renal hilus should be biopsied. Since this surgical procedure defines stage, establishes prognosis, and determines the necessity for subsequent therapy, it should be performed by a surgeon with special expertise in ovarian cancer staging. Studies have shown that patients operated upon by gynecologic oncologists were properly staged 97% of the time, compared to 52 and 35% of cases staged by obstetricians/gynecologists and general surgeons, respectively. After staging, ~23% of women have stage I disease (cancer confined to the ovary or ovaries), 13% have stage II (disease confined to the true pelvis), 47% have stage III (disease spread into but confined to the abdomen), and 16% have stage IV disease (spread outside the pelvis and abdomen). The 5-year survival correlates with stage of disease: stage I, 90–95%; stage II, 70–80%; stage III, 25–50%; and stage IV, 1–5% (Table 93-1).

Prognosis in ovarian cancer is dependent not only on stage but on the extent of residual disease and histologic grade. Patients presenting with advanced disease but left without significant residual disease after surgery have a median survival of 39 months, compared to 17 months for those with suboptimal tumor resection.

If initial surgery does not produce minimal residual disease, a second cytoreductive surgery has been used after the first three cycles of chemotherapy; in one trial it was associated with a 6-month improvement in median duration of survival. Another randomized trial where more aggressive debulking surgery was initially carried out was unable to confirm this benefit.

Prognosis of epithelial tumors is also highly influenced by histologic grade but less so by histologic type. Although grading systems differ among pathologists, all grading systems show a better prognosis for well- or moderately differentiated tumors than for poorly differentiated histologies. Estimated 5-year survivals for patients by tumor grade are: well-differentiated, 88%; moderately differentiated, 58%; poorly differentiated, 27%.

The prognostic significance of pre- and postoperative CA-125 levels is uncertain. CA-125 levels generally reflect volume of disease, and high levels usually indicate unresectability and a poorer survival. Postoperative levels, if elevated, usually indicate residual disease. The rate of decline of CA-125 levels during initial therapy or the absolute level after one to three cycles of chemotherapy correlates with prognosis but is not sufficiently accurate to guide individual treatment decisions. Even when the CA-125 level falls to normal after surgery or chemotherapy, "second-look" laparotomy identifies residual disease in 60% of women.

Genetic and biologic factors may influence prognosis. Increased tumor levels of p53 are associated with a poorer prognosis in advanced disease. Epidermal growth factor receptors in ovarian cancer are associated with a decrease in disease-free survival, but the increased expression of HER-2/neu has given conflicting prognostic results. HER-2/neu is overexpressed in 20% of ovarian cancers, and responses have been seen to trastuzumab in this subset of patients.

℞ OVARIAN CANCER

The selection of therapy for patients with epithelial ovarian cancer depends on the stage, extent of residual tumor, and histologic grade. In general, patients are considered in three separate treatment groups: (1) those with early (stages I and II) ovarian cancer and microscopic or no residual disease, (2) patients with advanced (stage III) disease but minimal residual tumor (<1 cm) after initial surgery, and (3) patients with bulky residual tumor and advanced (stage III or IV) disease.

Patients with stage I disease, no residual tumor, and well or moderately differentiated tumors need no adjuvant therapy after definitive surgery, and 5-year survival exceeds 95%. For all other patients with early disease and those stage I patients with poor prognosis histologic grade, adjuvant platinum-based therapy is warranted. Large prospective randomized trials have demonstrated that adjuvant therapy improves disease-free and overall survival by 8% (82% vs. 74%, $p = .008$).

For patients with advanced (stage III) disease but with limited or no residual disease after definitive cytoreductive surgery (about half of all stage III patients), the primary therapy is platinum-based combination chemotherapy. Approximately 70% of women respond to initial combination chemotherapy, and 40–50% have a complete regression of disease. Unfortunately, only about half of these patients are free of disease if surgically restaged. Although a variety of combinations are active, a randomized prospective trial of paclitaxel and cisplatin compared to paclitaxel and carboplatin in patients with optimally resected advanced disease demonstrated equivalent disease-free and overall survivals but with significantly reduced toxicity with the carboplatin combination. This regimen of paclitaxel, 175 mg/m^2 by 3-h infusion, and carboplatin, dosed to an AUC (area under the curve) of 7.5, is the preferred treatment choice for patients with previously untreated advanced-stage disease.

Three randomized trials using intraperitoneal (IP) chemotherapy have demonstrated improved disease-free and overall survival compared to the intravenous administration of the same drugs. However, the increased toxicity (neuropathy, nephropathy, and catheter complications) is significant, and only about 40% of patients were able to receive full courses of therapy. Furthermore, the optimal dose and schedule of IP therapy has not been established, nor have any of the IP regimens been prospectively compared to the standard intravenous carboplatin-paclitaxel regimen. The ultimate role of IP therapy in the treatment of advanced ovarian cancer is unresolved.

Patients with advanced disease (stages III and IV) and bulky residual tumor are generally treated with intravenous paclitaxel-platinum combination, and while the overall prognosis is poorer, 5-year survival may reach 15–20%.

Historically, patients who had an excellent initial response to chemotherapy and no clinical evidence of disease had a second-look laparotomy. The second-look surgical procedure itself does not prolong overall survival, and outside of clinical trials its routine use is no longer recommended. Maintenance therapy may extend progression-free survival but has not improved overall survival.

Patients with advanced disease whose disease recurs after initial treatment are usually not curable but may benefit significantly from limited surgery to relieve intestinal obstruction, localized radiation therapy to relieve pressure or pain from mass lesions or metastasis, or palliative chemotherapy. The selection of chemotherapy for palliation depends on the initial regimen and evidence of drug resistance. Patients who had a complete regression of disease lasting ≥6 months often respond to reinduction with the same agents; patients relapsing within the first 6 months of initial therapy rarely do. Progestational agents, tamoxifen, or aromatase inhibitors produce responses in 5–15% of patients and have minimal side effects. Agents with >15% response rates in patients relapsing after initial combination chemotherapy include gemcitabine, topotecan, liposomal doxorubicin, and bevicizumab.

Bevicizumab is a monoclonal antibody that targets the vascular endothelial growth factor. Initial trials produced a 17% overall response rate in heavily pretreated patients. However, hypertension, thrombosis, and bowel perforations have been reported in some trials.

Patients with tumors of low malignant potential, even with advanced-stage disease, have longer survivals (80–90%) when managed with surgery alone. Radiation and chemotherapy do not improve outcome.

OVARIAN GERM CELL TUMORS

Fewer than 5% of all ovarian tumors are germ cell in origin. They include teratoma, dysgerminoma, endodermal sinus tumor, and embryonal carcinoma. Germ cell tumors of the ovary generally occur in younger women (75% of ovarian malignancies in women <30), display an unusually aggressive natural history, and are commonly cured with less-extensive nonsterilizing surgery and chemotherapy. Women cured of these malignancies are able to conceive and have normal children.

These neoplasms can be divided into three major groups: (1) benign tumors (usually dermoid cysts); (2) malignant tumors that arise from dermoid cysts; and (3) primitive malignant germ cell tumors, including dysgerminoma, yolk sac tumors, immature teratomas, embryonal carcinomas, and choriocarcinoma.

Dermoid cysts are teratomatous cysts usually lined by epidermis and skin appendages. They often contain hair, and calcified bone or teeth can sometimes be seen on conventional pelvic x-ray. They are almost always curable by surgical resection. Approximately 1% of these tumors have malignant elements, usually squamous cell carcinoma.

Malignant germ cell tumors are usually large (median—16 cm). Bilateral disease is rare except in dysgerminoma (10–15% bilaterality). Abdominal or pelvic pain in young women is the usual presenting symptom. Serum human chorionic gonadotropin (β-hCG) and α fetoprotein levels are useful in the diagnosis and management of these patients. Before the advent of chemotherapy, extensive surgery was routine, but it has now been replaced by careful evaluation of extent of spread, followed by resection of bulky disease and preservation of one ovary, the uterus, and the cervix, if feasible. This allows many affected women to preserve fertility. After surgical staging, 60–75% of women have stage I disease and 25–30% have stage III disease. Stages II and IV are infrequent.

Most of the malignant germ cell tumors are managed with chemotherapy after surgery. Regimens similar to those used in testicular cancer, such as BEP (bleomycin, etoposide, and cisplatin), with three or four courses given at 21-day intervals, have produced 95% long-term survival in patients with disease stages I–III. This regimen is the treatment of choice for all malignant germ cell tumors except grade I, stage I immature teratoma, where surgery alone is adequate, and perhaps early-stage dysgerminoma, where surgery and radiation therapy are used.

Dysgerminoma is the ovarian counterpart of testicular seminoma. The tumor is very sensitive to radiation therapy. The 5-year disease-free survival is 100% in early-stage patients and 61% in stage III disease. Unfortunately, the use of radiation therapy makes many patients infertile. BEP chemotherapy is equally or more effective and does not cause infertility. In incompletely resected patients with dysgerminoma treated with BEP, the 2-year disease-free survival is 95% and infertility is not observed. Combination chemotherapy (BEP) has replaced postoperative radiation therapy as the treatment of choice in women with ovarian dysgerminoma.

OVARIAN STROMAL TUMORS

Stromal tumors make up <10% of ovarian tumors. They are named for the stromal tissue involved: granulosa, theca, Sertoli, Leydig, and collagen-producing stromal cells. The granulosa and theca cell stromal cell tumors occur most frequently in the first three decades of life. Granulosa cell tumors frequently produce estrogen and cause menstrual abnormalities, bleeding, and precocious puberty. Endometrial carcinoma can be seen in 5% of these women, perhaps related to the persistent hyperestrogenism. Sertoli and Leydig cell tumors, when functional, produce androgens with resultant virilization or hirsutism. Some 75% of these stromal cell tumors present in stage I and can be cured with total abdominal hysterectomy and bilateral salpingo-oophorectomy. Stromal tumors generally grow slowly, and recurrences can occur 5–10 years after initial surgery; serum markers such as estradiol, inhibin, and müllerian inhibitory substance may be useful in monitoring patients. Neither radiation therapy nor chemotherapy has been documented to be consistently effective, and surgical management remains the primary treatment.

Ovarian stromal and germ cell tumors are sometimes components of complex genetic syndromes. Peutz-Jeghers syndrome (mucocutaneous pigmentation and intestinal polyps) is associated with ovarian sex cord stromal tumors and Sertoli cell tumors in men. Patients with gonadal dysgenesis (46XY genotype or mosaic for Y-containing cell lines) develop gonadoblastomas, and women with nevoid basal cell carcinomas have an increased risk of ovarian fibromas.

CARCINOMA OF THE FALLOPIAN TUBE

The fallopian tube is a very rare site of cancer in the female genital tract, although its epithelial surface far exceeds that of the ovary, where epithelial cancer is 20 times more common. Approximately 300 new cases occur yearly; 90% are papillary serous adenocarcinomas, with the remainder being mixed mesodermal, endometrioid, and transitional cell tumors. *BRCA1* and *-2* mutations are found in 16% of cases. The gross and microscopic characteristics and the spread of tumor are similar to those of ovarian cancer but can be distinguished if the tumor arises from the endosalpinx, where the tubal epithelium shows a transition between benign and malignant, and the ovaries and endometrium are normal or minimally involved. The differential diagnosis includes primary or metastatic ovarian cancer, chronic salpingitis, tuberculous salpingitis, salpingitis isthmica nodosa, and cautery artifact.

Unlike patients with ovarian cancer, patients often present with early symptoms, usually postmenopausal vaginal bleeding, pain, and leukorrhea. Surgical staging is similar to that used for ovarian cancer, and prognosis is related to stage and extent of residual disease. Patients with stages I and II disease are generally treated with surgery alone or with surgery and pelvic radiation therapy, although radiation therapy does not clearly improve 5-year survival (5-year survival, stage I: 74% vs. 75%; stage II: 43% vs. 48%). Patients with stages III and IV disease are treated with the same chemotherapy regimens used in advanced ovarian cancer; 5-year survival is similar (stage III, 20%; stage IV, 5%).

UTERINE CANCER

INCIDENCE AND EPIDEMIOLOGY

Carcinoma of the endometrium is the most common female pelvic malignancy. Approximately 39,080 new cases are diagnosed yearly, although in most (75%), tumor is confined to the uterine corpus at diagnosis, and therefore most can be cured. The 7400 deaths yearly make uterine cancer only the eighth leading cause of cancer death in females. It is primarily a disease of postmenopausal women, although 25% of cases occur in women ages <50 and 5% ages <40. The disease is common in Eastern Europe and the United States and uncommon in Asia.

Proliferation of the endometrium is under the control of estrogen, and prolonged exposure to unopposed estrogen from either endogenous or exogenous sources plays a central etiologic role. Risk factors for endometrial cancer include obesity, low fertility index, early menarche, late menopause, and chronic anovulation. Granulosa cell tumors of the ovary that secrete estrogen may present with synchronous endometrial cancers. Chronic unapposed estrogen replacement increases the risk, and women taking tamoxifen for breast cancer treatment or prevention have a twofold increased risk.

The Lynch syndrome occurs in families with an autosomal dominant mutation of mismatch repair genes *MLH1*, *MSH2*, *MSH6*, and *PMS2*, which predispose to nonpolyposis colon cancer as well as endometrial and ovarian cancer. The estimated lifetime risk for endometrial cancer is 40–60%, with a mean age around 50 years. Unlike colorectal cancer, endometrial cancer risk is not lower in *MSH6* mutation carriers. Most women present with stage I disease, and the survival rate is generally good (5-year survival 88%). No unique endometrial screening strategies have been established for Lynch family gene carriers.

CLINICAL PRESENTATION

Endometrial carcinoma occurs most often in the sixth and seventh decades of life. Symptoms often include abnormal vaginal discharge (90%), abnormal postmenopausal bleeding (80%), and leukorrhea (10%). The risk of endometrial cancer associated with postmenopausal bleeding increases with advancing age (9% at age 50 vs. 60% at age 80). Evaluation of such patients should include a history and physical with pelvic examination followed by an endometrial biopsy or a fractional dilation and curettage. Outpatient procedures such as endometrial biopsy or aspiration curettage can be used but are definitive only when positive.

PATHOLOGY

Between 75 and 80% of all endometrial carcinomas are adenocarcinomas, and the prognosis depends on stage, histologic grade, and extent of myometrial invasion. Grade I tumors are highly differentiated adenocarcinomas, grade II tumors contain some solid areas, and grade III tumors are largely solid or undifferentiated. Adenocarcinoma with squamous differentiation is seen in 10% of patients; the most differentiated form is known as *adenoacanthoma*, and the poorly differentiated form is called *adenosquamous carcinoma*. Other less common pathologies include mucinous carcinoma (5%) and papillary serous carcinoma (<10%). This latter type has a natural history similar to ovarian carcinoma and should be managed in the same way. Rarer histologies include secretory (2%), ciliated, clear cell, and undifferentiated carcinomas.

STAGING

The staging of endometrial cancer requires surgery to establish the extent of disease and the depth of myometrial invasion. A total abdominal hysterectomy and bilateral salpingo-oophorectomy should be performed and peritoneal fluid sampled. Frozen sections of the uterine specimen are used to determine the histology and grade and depth of invasion. If indicated, pelvic and para-aortic lymphadenectomy is performed. After evaluation and staging, ~75% of patients are stage I, 13% are stage II, 9% are stage III, and 3% are stage IV. Five-year survival declines with advancing stage: stage I, 89%; stage II, 73%; stage III, 52%; and stage IV, 17% (Table 93-1).

Rx UTERINE CANCER

Patients with uncomplicated stage I endometrial carcinoma are effectively managed with total abdominal hysterectomy and bilateral salpingo-oophorectomy. Pre- or postoperative irradiation has been used, and although vaginal cuff recurrence is reduced, survival is not altered. In women with poor histologic grade, deep myometrial invasion, or extensive involvement of the lower uterine segment or cervix, intracavitary or external beam irradiation is warranted.

About 15% of women have endometrial carcinoma with extension to the cervix only (stage II), and management depends on the extent of cervical invasion. Superficial cervical invasion can be managed like stage I disease, but extensive cervical invasion requires radical hysterectomy or preoperative radiotherapy followed by extrafascial hysterectomy. Once disease is outside the uterus but still confined to the true pelvis (stage III), management generally includes surgery and irradiation. Patients who have involvement only of the ovary or fallopian tubes generally do well with such therapy (5-year survival of 80%). Other stage III patients with disease extending beyond the adnexa or those with serous carcinomas of the endometrium have a significantly poorer prognosis (5-year survival of 15%). Patients with positive para-aortic nodes (stage IIIC) or those with upper abdominal involvement (stage IV) have shown improved survival with platinum-based chemotherapy compared to whole-abdominal irradiation alone.

Patients with stage IV disease (outside the abdomen or invading the bladder or rectum) are treated palliatively with irradiation, surgery, and platinum-based chemotherapy. Progestational agents produce responses in ~10–20% of patients. Well-differentiated tumors respond most frequently, and response can be correlated with the level of progesterone receptor expression in the tumor. The commonly used progestational agents hydroxyprogesterone (Dilalutin), megestrol (Megace), and deoxyprogesterone (Provera) all produce similar response rates, and the antiestrogen tamoxifen (Nolvadex) produces responses in 10–25% of patients in a salvage setting.

Chemotherapy is not very successful in advanced endometrial carcinoma. The most active single agents with consistent response rates of ≥20% include cisplatin, carboplatin, doxorubicin, epirubicin, and paclitaxel. Combinations of drugs with or without progestational agents have generally produced response rates similar to single agents.

CERVIX CANCER

INCIDENCE AND EPIDEMIOLOGY

Carcinoma of the cervix was once the most common cause of cancer death in women, but over the past 40 years, the mortality rate has decreased by 50% due to widespread screening with the Pap smear. In 2007, ~11,150 new cases of invasive cervix cancer occurred, and >50,000 cases of carcinoma in situ were detected. There were 3670 deaths from the disease, and of those patients, ~85% had never had a Pap smear. Worldwide, cervical cancer is the third commonest cancer diagnosed, and it remains the major gynecologic cancer in underdeveloped countries. It is more common in lower socioeconomic groups, in women with early initial sexual activity and/or multiple sexual partners, and in smokers.

ETIOLOGY AND GENETICS

Venereal transmission of human papilloma virus (HPV) has an important etiologic role. Over 66 types of HPVs have been isolated, and many are associated with genital warts. Those types commonly associated with cervical carcinoma are 16, 18, 31, 33, 52, and 58, but 70% of cases are caused by HPV-16 and -18. These, along with many other types, are also associated with cervical intraepithelial neoplasia (CIN). The protein product of HPV-16, the E7 protein, binds and inactivates the tumor-suppressor gene Rb, and the E6 protein of HPV-18 has sequence homology to the SV40 large T antigen and the capacity to bind and inactivate the tumor-suppressor gene p53. E6 and E7 are both necessary and sufficient to cause cell transformation in vitro. These binding and inactivation events may explain the carcinogenic effects of the viruses (Chap. 178).

SCREENING AND PREVENTION

Vaccination against pathologic HPV appears to be an effective cervix cancer prevention strategy. Vaccines are made with inactivated virus-like particles that are noninfectious but highly immunogenic. The administration of a quadrivalent HPV vaccine against types 16, 18, 6, and 11 in a double-blind study of 2392 women completely prevented infection with the virus, and no cases of HPV-16–related CIN were seen in vaccinated women. This quadrivalent vaccine has been approved for use by the FDA for patients 9–26 years old and must be administered before HPV exposure to be effective. A second study with a bivalent vaccine (types 16 and 18) is underway. Both vaccines appear highly effective in preventing their particular HPV infections, and protection has persisted for at least 4.5 years after three injections over a 6-month period. Since not all oncogenic HPVs are targeted, patients will need to continue PAP smear surveillance.

Uncomplicated HPV infection in the lower genital tract can progress to CIN. This lesion precedes invasive cervical carcinoma and is classified as low-grade squamous intraepithelial lesion (SIL), high-grade SIL, and carcinoma in situ. Carcinoma in situ demonstrates cytologic evidence of neoplasia without invasion through the basement membrane and can persist unchanged for 10–20 years, but most of these eventually progress to invasive carcinoma.

The Pap smear is 90–95% accurate in detecting early lesions such as CIN but is less sensitive in detecting cancer when frankly invasive cancer or fungating masses are present. Inflammation, necrosis, and hemorrhage may produce false-positive smears, and colposcopic-directed biopsy is required when any lesion is visible on the cervix, regardless of Pap smear findings. The American Cancer Society recommends that women after onset of sexual activity, or >age 20, have two consecutive yearly smears. If negative, smears should be repeated every 3 years until age 65. The Pap smear can be reported as normal (includes benign, reactive, or reparative changes); atypical squamous cells of undetermined significance (ASCUS) or cannot exclude high-grade SIL (ASC-H); low- or high-grade CIN; or frankly malignant. Women with ASCUS, ASC-H, or low-grade CIN should have repeat smears in 3–6 months and be tested for HPV. Women with high-grade CIN or frankly malignant Pap smears should have colposcopic-directed cervical biopsy. Colposcopy is a technique using a binocular microscope and 3% acetic acid applied to the cervix in which abnormal areas appear white and can be biopsied directly. Cone biopsy is still required when endocervical tumor is suspected, colposcopy is inadequate, the biopsy shows microinvasive carcinoma, or when a discrepancy is noted between the Pap smear and the colposcopic findings. Cone biopsy alone is therapeutic for CIN in many patients, although a less radical electrocautery excision may be sufficient.

Approximately 70% of invasive cervix cancers are squamous cell tumors, 20–25% are adenocarcinomas, and 2–5% are adenosquamous with epithelial and glandular structures.

CLINICAL PRESENTATION AND STAGING

Patients with cervix cancer generally are asymptomatic, and the disease is detected on routine pelvic examination. Others present with abnormal bleeding or postcoital spotting that may increase to intermenstrual or prominent menstrual bleeding. Yellowish vaginal discharge, lumbosacral back pain, lower-extremity edema, and urinary symptoms may be present.

The staging of cervical carcinoma is clinical and generally completed with a pelvic examination under anesthesia with cystoscopy and proctoscopy. Chest x-rays, intravenous pyelograms, and CT are generally required, and MRI may be used to assess extracervical extension. Stage 0 is carcinoma in situ, stage I is disease confined to the cervix, stage II disease invades beyond the cervix but not to the pelvic wall or lower third of the vagina, stage III disease extends to the pelvic wall or lower third of the vagina or causes hydronephrosis, and stage IV is present when the tumor invades the mucosa of bladder or rectum or extends beyond the true pelvis (Fig. 93-1). Five-year survivals by stage are: stage I, 85%; stage II, 65%; stage III, 35%; and stage IV, 7% (Table 93-1).

Rx CERVIX CANCER

Carcinoma in situ (stage 0) can be managed successfully by cone biopsy or by abdominal hysterectomy. For stage I disease, results appear equivalent for either radical hysterectomy or radiation therapy. Patients with disease stages II–IV are primarily managed with external beam irradiation and intracavitary treatment or combined modality therapy. Retroperitoneal lymphadenectomy has no proven therapeutic role. Pelvic exenterations have become increasingly rare due to improved radiation control. However, they are sometimes performed for centrally recurrent or persistent disease.

In women with locally advanced disease (stages IIB–IVA), platinum-based chemotherapy given concomitantly with radiation therapy improves survival compared to radiation therapy alone. Cisplatin, 75 mg/m^2 over 4 h, followed by 5-fluorouracil (5-FU), 4 g given by 96-h infusion on days 1–5 of radiation therapy, is a common regimen. Two additional cycles of chemotherapy are given at 3-week intervals. Three randomized trials of platinum-based chemotherapy reduced the risk of recurrence by 30–50% across a wide spectrum of stages and presentations and were found to improve the survival rate in bulky stage I as well as locally advanced (stages IIB–IV) cervical cancer.

Chemotherapy has some palliative benefit in patients with unresectable advanced disease or recurrent disease. Active agents with ≥20% response rates include cisplatin, paclitaxel, vinorelbine, ifosfamide, and topotecan. The combination of topotecan and cisplatin has a modest survival advantage over cisplatin alone.

GESTATIONAL TROPHOBLASTIC NEOPLASIA

Gestational trophoblastic diseases are a group of related diseases that form a spectrum from benign hydatidiform mole to trophoblastic malignancy (placental-site trophoblastic tumor and choriocarcinoma). Malignant forms account for <1% of female gynecologic malignancies and can be cured with appropriate chemotherapy. Deaths from this disease have become rare in the United States.

EPIDEMIOLOGY

The incidence is about 1 per 1500 pregnancies in the United States and is nearly tenfold higher in Asia. Maternal age >45 years is a risk factor for hydatidiform mole as is a prior history of molar pregnancy. Choriocarcinoma occurs in ~1 in 25,000 pregnancies or 1 in 20,000 live births. Prior history of hydatidiform mole is a risk factor for choriocarcinoma. A woman with a previous molar pregnancy is 1000 times more likely to develop choriocarcinoma than a woman with a prior normal-term pregnancy.

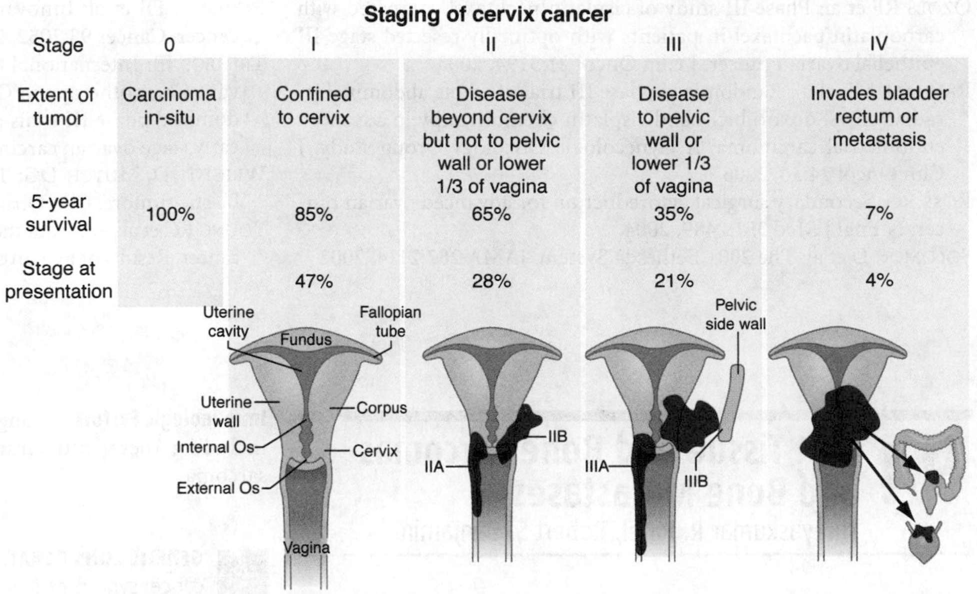

FIGURE 93-1 Anatomic display of the stages of cervix cancer defined by location, extent of tumor, frequency of presentation, and 5-year survival.

PATHOLOGY AND ETIOLOGY

The trophoblastic neoplasms have been divided by morphology into complete or partial hydatidiform mole, invasive mole, placental-site trophoblastomas, and choriocarcinomas. Hydatidiform moles contain clusters of villi with hydropic changes, hyperplasia of the trophoblast, and the absence of fetal vessels. Invasive moles differ only by invasion into the uterine myometrium. Placental-site trophoblastic tumors are predominately made up of cytotrophoblast cells arising from the placental implantation site. Choriocarcinomas consist of anaplastic trophoblastic tissue with both cytotrophoblastic and syncytiotrophoblastic elements and no identifiable villi.

Complete moles result from uniparental disomy in which loss of the maternal genes (23 autosomes plus X) occurs by unknown mechanisms and is followed by duplication of the paternal haploid genome (23 autosomes plus X). Uncommonly (5%), moles result from dispermic fertilization of an empty egg, resulting in either 46XY or 46XX genotype. Partial moles result from dispermic fertilization of an egg with retention of the maternal haploid set of chromosomes, resulting in diandric triploidy (Chap. 62).

CLINICAL PRESENTATION

Molar pregnancies are generally associated with first-trimester bleeding and excessive uterine size. About 45% of patients have ovarian theca-lutein cysts present on ultrasound. The β-hCG levels are generally markedly elevated. Fetal parts and heart sounds are not present. The diagnosis is generally made by the passage of grapelike clusters from the uterus, but ultrasound demonstration of the hydropic mole can be diagnostic. Patients suspected of a molar pregnancy require a chest film, careful pelvic examinations, and weekly serial monitoring of β-hCG levels.

℞ GESTATIONAL TROPHOBLASTIC NEOPLASIA

Patients with hydatidiform moles require suction curettage coupled with postevacuation monitoring of β-hCG levels. In most women (80%), the β-hCG titer progressively declines within 8–10 days of evacuation (serum half-life is 24–36 h). Patients should be monitored on a monthly basis and should not become pregnant for at least a year. Patients found to have invasive mole at curettage are generally treated with hysterectomy and chemotherapy. Approximately half of patients with choriocarcinoma develop the malignancy after a molar pregnancy, and the other half develop the malignancy after abortion, ectopic pregnancy, or occasionally after a normal full-term pregnancy.

Chemotherapy is used for gestational trophoblastic neoplasia and often as chemoprophylaxis after molar evacuation to reduce postmolar tumors. It is also used in hydatidiform mole if β-hCG levels rise or plateau or if metastases develop. Patients with invasive mole or choriocarcinoma require chemotherapy. Several regimens are effective for low-risk patients, including methotrexate at 30 mg/m^2 intramuscularly on a weekly basis until β-hCG titers are normal. However, methotrexate (1 mg/kg) every other day for four doses, followed by leukovorin (0.1 mg/kg) intravenously 24 h after methotrexate, is associated with a cure rate of ≥90% and low toxicity. Intermittent courses are continued until the β-hCG titer becomes undetectable for 3 consecutive weeks; then patients are monitored monthly for a year.

Patients with high-risk tumors (high β-hCG levels, disease presenting ≥4 months after antecedent pregnancy, brain or liver metastasis, or failure of single-agent methotrexate) are initially treated with combination chemotherapy. EMA-CO (a cyclic non-cross-resistant combination of etoposide, methotrexate, and dactinomycin alternating with cyclophosphamide and vincristine); cisplatin, bleomycin, and vinblastine; and cisplatin, etoposide, and bleomycin are effective regimens. EMA-CO is now the regimen of choice for patients with high-risk disease because of excellent survival rates (>80%) and less toxicity. The use of etoposide carries a 1.5% lifetime risk of acute myeloid leukemia (sixteenfold relative risk) and other solid tumors. As a result, etoposide-containing regimens should be reserved for patients with high-risk features. Patients with brain or liver metastases are usually treated with local irradiation to metastatic sites in conjunction with chemotherapy. Long-term studies of patients cured of trophoblastic disease have not demonstrated an increased risk of maternal complications or fetal abnormalities with subsequent pregnancies.

FURTHER READINGS

CHAMPION V et al: Quality of life in long-term survivors of ovarian germ cell tumors: A gynecologic oncology group study. Gynecol Oncol 105:687, 2007

KOUTSKY LA: A controlled trial of a human papilloma virus type 16 vaccine. N Engl J Med 347:1645, 2002

LINDOR NM et al: Recommendations for the care of individuals with an inherited predisposition to Lynch Syndrome. JAMA 296:1507, 2006

MODUGNO F: Ovarian Cancer and High Risk Women Symposium Presenters. Ovarian cancer and high-risk women: Implications for prevention, screening and early detection. Gynecol Oncol 91:15, 2003

OZOLS RF et al: Phase III study of cisplatin/paclitaxel compared with carboplatin/paclitaxel in patients with optimally resected stage III epithelial ovarian cancer. J Clin Oncol 21:3194, 2003

RANDALL ME et al: Randomized phase III trial of whole abdominal irradiation vs. doxorubicin and cisplatin chemotherapy in advanced endometrial carcinoma: A Gynecologic Oncology Group study. J Clin Oncol 24:36, 2006

ROSE PG: Secondary surgical cytoreduction for advanced ovarian cancer. N Engl J Med 351:2489, 2004

SOLOMON D et al: The 2001 Bethesda System. JAMA 287:2114, 2002

STEHMAN FB et al: Innovations in the treatment of invasive cervical cancer. Cancer 98:2052, 2003

TRIMBOS JB: International Collaborative Neoplasm Trial I and Adjuvant Chemotherapy in Ovarian Neoplasm Trial: Two parallel randomized phase III trials of adjuvant chemotherapy in patients with early stage ovarian carcinoma. J Natl Cancer Inst 95:105, 2003

WRIGHT JD, MUTCH DG: Treatment of high-risk gestational trophoblastic tumors. Clin Obstet Gynecol 46:593, 2003

YOUNG RC et al: Adjuvant therapy in stage I and stage II epithelial ovarian cancer. Results of two prospective trials. N Engl J Med 327:1021, 1990

94 Soft Tissue and Bone Sarcomas and Bone Metastases

Shreyaskumar R. Patel, Robert S. Benjamin

Sarcomas are rare (<1% of all malignancies) mesenchymal neoplasms that arise in bone and soft tissues. These tumors are usually of mesodermal origin, although a few are derived from neuroectoderm, and they are biologically distinct from the more common epithelial malignancies. Sarcomas affect all age groups; 15% are found in children <15 years and 40% occur after age 55. Sarcomas are one of the most common solid tumors of childhood and are the fifth most common cause of cancer deaths in children. Sarcomas may be divided into two groups, those derived from bone and those derived from soft tissues.

SOFT TISSUE SARCOMAS

Soft tissues include muscles, tendons, fat, fibrous tissue, synovial tissue, vessels, and nerves. Approximately 60% of soft tissue sarcomas arise in the extremities, with the lower extremities involved three times as often as the upper extremities. Thirty percent arise in the trunk, the retroperitoneum accounting for 40% of all trunk lesions. The remaining 10% arise in the head and neck.

INCIDENCE

Approximately 9220 new cases of soft tissue sarcomas occurred in the United States in 2007. The annual age-adjusted incidence is 3.0 per 100,000 population, but the incidence varies with age. Soft tissue sarcomas constitute 0.7% of all cancers in the general population and 6.5% of all cancers in children.

EPIDEMIOLOGY

Malignant transformation of a benign soft tissue tumor is extremely rare, with the exception that malignant peripheral nerve sheath tumors (neurofibrosarcoma, malignant schwannoma) can arise from neurofibromas in patients with neurofibromatosis. Several etiologic factors have been implicated in soft tissue sarcomas.

Environmental Factors Trauma or previous injury is rarely involved, but sarcomas can arise in scar tissue resulting from a prior operation, burn, fracture, or foreign body implantation. Chemical carcinogens such as polycyclic hydrocarbons, asbestos, and dioxin may be involved in the pathogenesis.

Iatrogenic Factors Sarcomas in bone or soft tissues occur in patients who are treated with radiation therapy. The tumor nearly always arises in the irradiated field. The risk increases with time.

Viruses Kaposi's sarcoma (KS) in patients with HIV type 1, classic KS, and KS in HIV-negative homosexual men is caused by human herpes virus (HHV) 8 (Chap. 175). No other sarcomas are associated with viruses.

Immunologic Factors Congenital or acquired immunodeficiency, including therapeutic immunosuppression, increases the risk of sarcoma.

GENETIC CONSIDERATIONS Li-Fraumeni syndrome is a familial cancer syndrome in which affected individuals have germ-line abnormalities of the tumor-suppressor gene p53 and an increased incidence of soft tissue sarcomas and other malignancies, including breast cancer, osteosarcoma, brain tumor, leukemia, and adrenal carcinoma (Chap. 79). Neurofibromatosis 1 (NF-1, peripheral form, von Recklinghausen's disease) is characterized by multiple neurofibromas and café au lait spots. Neurofibromas occasionally undergo malignant degeneration to become malignant peripheral nerve sheath tumors. The gene for NF-1 is located in the pericentromeric region of chromosome 17 and encodes neurofibromin, a tumor-suppressor protein with GTPase-activating activity that inhibits Ras function (Chap. 374). Germ-line mutation of the *Rb-1* locus (chromosome 13q14) in patients with inherited retinoblastoma is associated with the development of osteosarcoma in those who survive the retinoblastoma and of soft tissue sarcomas unrelated to radiation therapy. Other soft tissue tumors, including desmoid tumors, lipomas, leiomyomas, neuroblastomas, and paragangliomas, occasionally show a familial predisposition.

Ninety percent of synovial sarcomas contain a characteristic chromosomal translocation t(X;18)(p11;q11) involving a nuclear transcription factor on chromosome 18 called *SYT* and two breakpoints on X. Patients with translocations to the second X breakpoint (*SSX2*) may have longer survival than those with translocations involving *SSX1*.

Insulin-like growth factor (IGF) type 2 is produced by some sarcomas and may act as an autocrine growth factor and as a motility factor that promotes metastatic spread. IGF-2 stimulates growth through IGF-1 receptors, but its effects on motility are through different receptors. If secreted in large amounts, IGF-2 may produce hypoglycemia (Chaps. 96, 339).

CLASSIFICATION

Approximately 20 different groups of sarcomas are recognized on the basis of the pattern of differentiation toward normal tissue. For example, rhabdomyosarcoma shows evidence of skeletal muscle fibers with cross-striations; leiomyosarcomas contain interlacing fascicles of spindle cells resembling smooth muscle; and liposarcomas contain adipocytes. When precise characterization of the group is not possible, the tumors are called *unclassified sarcomas*. All of the primary bone sarcomas can also arise from soft tissues (e.g., extraskeletal osteosarcoma). The entity *malignant fibrous histiocytoma* includes many tumors previously classified as fibrosarcomas or as pleomorphic variants of other sarcomas and is characterized by a mixture of spindle (fibrous) cells and round (histiocytic) cells arranged in a storiform pattern with frequent giant cells and areas of pleomorphism.

For purposes of treatment, most soft tissue sarcomas can be considered together. However, some specific tumors have distinct features. For example, *liposarcoma* can have a spectrum of behaviors. Pleomorphic liposarcomas and dedifferentiated liposarcomas behave like other high-grade sarcomas; in contrast, well-differentiated liposarcomas (better termed *atypical lipomatous tumors*) lack metastatic potential, and myxoid liposarcomas metastasize infrequently but, when they do, have a predilection for unusual metastatic sites containing fat, such as the retroperitoneum, mediastinum, and subcutaneous tissue. Rhabdomyosarcomas, Ewing's sarcoma, and other small-cell sarcomas tend to be more aggressive and are more responsive to chemotherapy than other soft tissue sarcomas.

Gastrointestinal stromal cell tumors (GISTs), previously classified as gastrointestinal leiomyosarcomas, are now recognized as a distinct entity within soft tissue sarcomas. Its cell of origin resembles the interstitial cell of Cajal, which controls peristalsis. The majority of malignant GISTs have activating mutations of the *c-kit* gene that result in ligand-independent phosphorylation and activation of the KIT receptor tyrosine kinase, leading to tumorigenesis.

TABLE 94-1 AJCC STAGING SYSTEM FOR SARCOMAS

Histologic Grade (G)	Tumor Size (T)	Node Status (N)	Metastases (M)
Well differentiated (G1)	≤5 cm (T1)	Not involved (N0)	Absent (M0)
Moderately differentiated (G2)	>5 cm (T2)	Involved (N1)	Present (M1)
Poorly differentiated (G3)	Superficial fascial involvement (Ta)		
Undifferentiated (G4)	Deep fascial involvement (Tb)		

Disease Stage	5-Year Survival, %
Stage I	98.8
A: G1,2; T1a,b; N0; M0	
B: G1,2; T2a; N0; M0	
Stage II	81.8
A: G1,2; T2b; N0; M0	
B: G3,4; T1; N0; M0	
C: G3,4; T2a; N0; M0	
Stage III G3,4; T2b; N0; M0	51.7
Stage IV	<20
A: any G; any T; N1; M0	
B: any G; any T; any N; M1	

DIAGNOSIS

The most common presentation is an asymptomatic mass. Mechanical symptoms referable to pressure, traction, or entrapment of nerves or muscles may be present. All new and persistent or growing masses should be biopsied, either by a cutting needle (core-needle biopsy) or by a small incision, placed so that it can be encompassed in the subsequent excision without compromising a definitive resection. Lymph node metastases occur in 5%, except in synovial and epithelioid sarcomas, clear-cell sarcoma (melanoma of the soft parts), angiosarcoma, and rhabdomyosarcoma, where nodal spread may be seen in 17%. The pulmonary parenchyma is the most common site of metastases. Exceptions are GISTs, which metastasize to the liver; myxoid liposarcomas, which seek fatty tissue; and clear-cell sarcomas, which may metastasize to bones. Central nervous system metastases are rare, except in alveolar soft part sarcoma.

Radiographic Evaluation Imaging of the primary tumor is best with plain radiographs and MRI for tumors of the extremities or head and neck and by CT for tumors of the chest, abdomen, or retroperitoneal cavity. A radiograph and CT scan of the chest are important for the detection of lung metastases. Other imaging studies may be indicated, depending on the symptoms, signs, or histology.

STAGING AND PROGNOSIS

The histologic grade, relationship to fascial planes, and size of the primary tumor are the most important prognostic factors. The current American Joint Commission on Cancer (AJCC) staging system is shown in Table 94-1. Prognosis is related to the stage. Cure is common in the absence of metastatic disease, but a small number of patients with metastases can also be cured. Most patients with stage IV disease die within 12 months, but some patients may live with slowly progressive disease for many years.

Rx SOFT TISSUE SARCOMAS

AJCC stage I patients are adequately treated with surgery alone. Stage II patients are considered for adjuvant radiation therapy. Stage III patients may benefit from adjuvant chemotherapy. Stage IV patients are managed primarily with chemotherapy, with or without other modalities.

SURGERY Soft tissue sarcomas tend to grow along fascial planes, with the surrounding soft tissues compressed to form a pseudocapsule that gives the sarcoma the appearance of a well-encapsulated lesion. This is invariably deceptive because "shelling out," or marginal excision, of such lesions results in a 50–90% probability of local recurrence. Wide excision with a negative margin, incorporating the biopsy site, is the standard surgical procedure for local disease. The adjuvant use of radiation therapy and/or chemotherapy improves the local control rate and permits the use of limb-sparing surgery with a local control rate (85–90%) comparable to that achieved by radical excisions and amputations. Limb-sparing approaches are indicated except when negative margins are not obtainable, when the risks of radiation are prohibitive, or when neurovascular structures are involved so that resection will result in serious functional consequences to the limb.

RADIATION THERAPY External beam radiation therapy is an adjuvant to limb-sparing surgery for improved local control. Preoperative radiation therapy allows the use of smaller fields and smaller doses but results in a higher rate of wound complications. Postoperative radiation therapy must be given to larger fields, as the entire surgical bed must be encompassed, and in higher doses to compensate for hypoxia in the operated field. Brachytherapy or interstitial therapy, in which the radiation source is inserted into the tumor bed, is comparable in efficacy (except in low-grade lesions), less time-consuming, and less expensive.

ADJUVANT CHEMOTHERAPY Chemotherapy is the mainstay of treatment for Ewing's primitive neuroectodermal tumors (PNET) and rhabdomyosarcomas. Meta-analysis of 14 randomized trials revealed a significant improvement in local control and disease-free survival in favor of doxorubicin-based chemotherapy. Overall survival improvement was 4% for all sites and 7% for the extremity site. A chemotherapy regimen including an anthracycline and ifosfamide with growth factor support improved overall survival by 19% for high-risk (high-grade, ≥5 cm primary, or locally recurrent) extremity soft tissue sarcomas.

ADVANCED DISEASE Metastatic soft tissue sarcomas are largely incurable, but up to 20% of patients who achieve a complete response become long-term survivors. The therapeutic intent, therefore, is to produce a complete remission with chemotherapy (<10%) and/or surgery (30–40%). Surgical resection of metastases, whenever possible, is an integral part of the management. Some patients benefit from repeated surgical excision of metastases. The two most active chemotherapeutic agents are doxorubicin and ifosfamide. These drugs show a steep dose-response relationship in sarcomas. Gemcitabine with or without docetaxel has become an established second-line regimen and is particularly active in patients with leiomyosarcomas. Dacarbazine also has some modest activity. Taxanes have selective activity in angiosarcomas, and vincristine, etoposide, and irinotecan are effective in rhadomyosarcomas and Ewing's sarcomas. Imatinib mesylate targets the KIT tyrosine kinase activity and is standard therapy for advanced/metastatic GISTs.

BONE SARCOMAS

INCIDENCE AND EPIDEMIOLOGY

Bone sarcomas are rarer than soft tissue sarcomas; they accounted for only 0.2% of all new malignancies and 2370 new cases in the United

States in 2007. Several benign bone lesions have the potential for malignant transformation. Enchondromas and osteochondromas can transform into chondrosarcoma; fibrous dysplasia, bone infarcts, and Paget's disease of bone can transform into either malignant fibrous histiocytoma or osteosarcoma.

CLASSIFICATION

Benign Tumors The common benign bone tumors include enchondroma, osteochondroma, chondroblastoma, and chondromyxoid fibroma, of cartilage origin; osteoid osteoma and osteoblastoma, of bone origin; fibroma and desmoplastic fibroma, of fibrous tissue origin; hemangioma, of vascular origin; and giant cell tumor, of unknown origin.

Malignant Tumors The most common malignant tumors of bone are plasma cell tumors (Chap. 106). The four most common malignant nonhematopoietic bone tumors are osteosarcoma, chondrosarcoma, Ewing's sarcoma, and malignant fibrous histiocytoma. Rare malignant tumors include chordoma (of notochordal origin), malignant giant cell tumor and adamantinoma (of unknown origin), and hemangioendothelioma (of vascular origin).

Musculoskeletal Tumor Society Staging System Sarcomas of bone are staged according to the Musculoskeletal Tumor Society staging system based on grade and compartmental localization. A Roman numeral reflects the tumor grade: stage I is low-grade, stage II is high-grade, and stage III includes tumors of any grade that have lymph node or distant metastases. In addition, the tumor is given a letter reflecting its compartmental localization. Tumors designated A are intracompartmental (i.e., confined to the same soft tissue compartment as the initial tumor), and tumors designated B are extracompartmental (i.e., extending into the adjacent soft tissue compartment or into bone). The tumor node metastasis (TNM) staging system is shown in Table 94-2.

OSTEOSARCOMA

Osteosarcoma, accounting for almost 45% of all bone sarcomas, is a spindle cell neoplasm that produces osteoid (unmineralized bone) or bone. About 60% of all osteosarcomas occur in children and adolescents in the second decade of life, and about 10% occur in the third decade of life. Osteosarcomas in the fifth and sixth decades of life are frequently secondary to either radiation therapy or transformation in a preexisting benign condition, such as Paget's disease. Males are affected 1.5–2 times as often as females. Osteosarcoma has a predilection for metaphyses of long bones; the most common sites of involvement are the distal femur, proximal tibia, and proximal humerus. The classification of osteosarcoma is complex, but 75% of osteosarcomas fall in the "classic" category, which include osteoblastic, chondroblastic, and fibroblastic osteosarcomas. The remaining 25% are classified as "variants" on the basis of (1) clinical characteristics, as in the case of osteosarcoma of the jaw, postradiation osteosarcoma, or Paget's osteosarcoma; (2) morphologic characteristics, as in the case of telangiectatic osteosarcoma, small cell osteosarcoma, or epithelioid osteosarcoma; or (3) location, as in parosteal or periosteal osteosarcoma. Diagnosis usually requires a synthesis of clinical, radiologic, and pathologic features. Patients typically present with pain and swelling of the affected area. A plain radiograph reveals a destructive lesion with a moth-eaten appearance, a spiculated periosteal reaction (sunburst appearance), and a cuff of periosteal new bone formation at the margin of the soft tissue mass (Codman's triangle). A CT scan of the primary tumor is best for defining bone destruction and the pattern of calcification, whereas MRI is better for defining intramedullary and soft tissue extension. A chest radiograph and CT scan are used to detect lung metastases. Metastases to the bony skeleton should be imaged by a bone scan. Almost all osteosarcomas are hypervascular. Angiography is not helpful for diagnosis, but it is the most sensitive test for assessing the response to preoperative chemotherapy. Pathologic diagnosis is established either with a core-needle biopsy, where feasible, or with an open biopsy with an appropriately placed incision that does not compromise future limb-sparing resection. Most osteosarcomas are high-grade. The most important prognostic factor for long-term survival is response to chemotherapy. Preoperative chemotherapy followed by limb-sparing surgery (which can be accomplished in >80% of patients) followed by postoperative chemotherapy is standard management. The effective drugs are doxorubicin, ifosfamide, cisplatin, and high-dose methotrexate with leucovorin rescue. The various combinations of these agents that have been used have all been about equally successful. Long-term survival rates in extremity osteosarcoma range from 60 to 80%. Osteosarcoma is radioresistant; radiation therapy has no role in the routine management. Malignant fibrous histiocytoma is considered a part of the spectrum of osteosarcoma and is managed similarly.

TABLE 94-2 STAGING SYSTEM FOR BONE SARCOMAS

Primary tumor (T)	TX	Primary tumor cannot be assessed
	T0	No evidence of primary tumor
	T1	Tumor ≤8 cm in greatest dimension
	T2	Tumor >8 cm in greatest dimension
	T3	Discontinuous tumors in the primary bone site
Regional lymph nodes (N)	NX	Regional lymph nodes cannot be assessed
	N0	No regional lymph node metastasis
	N1	Regional lymph node metastasis
Distant metastasis (M)	MX	Distant metastasis cannot be assessed
	M0	No distant metastasis
	M1	Distant metastasis
	M1a	Lung
	M1b	Other distant sites
Histologic grade (G)	GX	Grade cannot be assessed
	G1	Well differentiated—low grade
	G2	Moderately differentiated—low grade
	G3	Poorly differentiated—high grade
	G4	Undifferentiated—high grade (Ewing's is always classed G4)

Stage Grouping

Stage IA	T1	N0	M0	G1,2 low grade
Stage IB	T2	N0	M0	G1,2 low grade
Stage IIA	T1	N0	M0	G3,4 high grade
Stage IIB	T2	N0	M0	G3,4 high grade
Stage III	T3	N0	M0	Any G
Stage IVA	Any T	N0	M1a	Any G
Stage IVB	Any T	N1	Any M	Any G
	Any T	Any N	M1b	Any G

CHONDROSARCOMA

Chondrosarcoma, which constitutes ~20–25% of all bone sarcomas, is a tumor of adulthood and old age with a peak incidence in the fourth to sixth decades of life. It has a predilection for the flat bones, especially the shoulder and pelvic girdles, but can also affect the diaphyseal portions of long bones. Chondrosarcomas can arise de novo or as a malignant transformation of an enchondroma or, rarely, of the cartilaginous cap of an osteochondroma. Chondrosarcomas have an indolent natural history and typically present as pain and swelling. Radiographically, the lesion may have a lobular appearance with mottled or punctate or annular calcification of the cartilaginous matrix. It is difficult to distinguish low-grade chondrosarcoma from benign lesions by x-ray or histologic examination. The diagnosis is therefore influenced by clinical history and physical examination. A new onset of pain, signs of inflammation, and progressive increase in the size of the mass suggest malignancy. The histologic classification is complex, but most tumors fall within the classic category. Like other bone sarcomas, high-grade chondrosarcomas spread to the lungs. Most chondrosarcomas are resistant to chemotherapy, and surgical resection of primary or recurrent tumors, including pulmonary metastases, is the mainstay of therapy. This rule does not hold for two histologic variants. Dedifferentiated chondrosarcoma has a high-grade osteosarcoma or a malignant fibrous histiocytoma component that responds to chemotherapy. Mesenchymal chondrosarcoma, a rare variant composed of a small cell element, also is responsive to systemic chemotherapy and is treated like Ewing's sarcoma.

EWING'S SARCOMA

Ewing's sarcoma, which constitutes ~10–15% of all bone sarcomas, is common in adolescence and has a peak incidence in the second decade of life. It typically involves the diaphyseal region of long bones and also has an affinity for flat bones. The plain radiograph may show a characteristic "onion peel" periosteal reaction with a generous soft tissue mass, which is better demonstrated by CT or MRI. This mass is composed of sheets of monotonous, small, round, blue cells and can be confused with lymphoma, embryonal rhabdomyosarcoma, and small-cell carcinoma. The presence of p30/32, the product of the *mic-2* gene (which maps to the pseudoautosomal region of the X and Y chromosomes) is a cell-surface marker for Ewing's sarcoma (and other members of a family of tumors called PNETs). Most PNETs arise in soft tissues; they include peripheral neuroepithelioma, Askin's tumor (chest wall), and esthesioneuroblastoma. Glycogen-filled cytoplasm detected by staining with periodic acid–Schiff is also characteristic of Ewing's sarcoma cells. The classic cytogenetic abnormality associated with this disease (and other PNETs) is a reciprocal translocation of the long arms of chromosomes 11 and 22, t(11;22), which creates a chimeric gene product of unknown function with components from the *fli-1* gene on chromosome 11 and *ews* on 22. This disease is very aggressive, and it is therefore considered a systemic disease. Common sites of metastases are lung, bones, and bone marrow. Systemic chemotherapy is the mainstay of therapy, often being used before surgery. Doxorubicin, cyclophosphamide or ifosfamide, etoposide, vincristine, and dactinomycin are active drugs. Local treatment for the primary tumor includes surgical resection, usually with limb salvage or radiation therapy. Patients with lesions below the elbow and below the mid-calf have a 5-year survival rate of 80% with effective treatment. Ewing's sarcoma is a curable tumor, even in the presence of obvious metastatic disease, especially in children <11 years old.

TUMORS METASTATIC TO BONE

Bone is a common site of metastasis for carcinomas of the prostate, breast, lung, kidney, bladder, and thyroid and for lymphomas and sarcomas. Prostate, breast, and lung primaries account for 80% of all bone metastases. Metastatic tumors of bone are more common than primary bone tumors. Tumors usually spread to bone hematogenously, but local invasion from soft tissue masses also occurs. In descending order of frequency, the sites most often involved are the vertebrae, proximal femur, pelvis, ribs, sternum, proximal humerus, and skull. Bone metastases may be asymptomatic or may produce pain, swelling, nerve root or spinal cord compression, pathologic fracture, or myelophthisis (replacement of the marrow). Symptoms of hypercalcemia may be noted in cases of bony destruction.

Pain is the most frequent symptom. It usually develops gradually over weeks, is usually localized, and often is more severe at night. When patients with back pain develop neurologic signs or symptoms, emergency evaluation for spinal cord compression is indicated (Chap. 270). Bone metastases exert a major adverse effect on quality of life in cancer patients.

Cancer in the bone may produce osteolysis, osteogenesis, or both. Osteolytic lesions result when the tumor produces substances that can directly elicit bone resorption (vitamin D–like steroids, prostaglandins, or parathyroid hormone–related peptide) or cytokines that can induce the formation of osteoclasts (interleukin 1 and tumor necrosis factor). Osteoblastic lesions result when the tumor produces cytokines that activate osteoblasts. In general, purely osteolytic lesions are best detected by plain radiography, but they may not be apparent until they are >1 cm. These lesions are more commonly associated with hypercalcemia and with the excretion of hydroxyproline-containing peptides indicative of matrix destruction. When osteoblastic activity is prominent, the lesions may be readily detected using radionuclide bone scanning (which is sensitive to new bone formation), and the radiographic appearance may show increased bone density or sclerosis. Osteoblastic lesions are associated with higher serum levels of alkaline phosphatase and, if extensive, may produce hypocalcemia. Although some tumors may produce mainly osteolytic lesions (e.g., kidney cancer) and others mainly osteoblastic lesions (e.g., prostate cancer), most metastatic lesions produce both types of lesion and may go through stages where one or the other predominates.

In older patients, particularly women, it may be necessary to distinguish metastatic disease of the spine from osteoporosis. In osteoporosis, the cortical bone may be preserved, whereas cortical bone destruction is usually noted with metastatic cancer.

Rx METASTATIC BONE DISEASE

Treatment of metastatic bone disease depends on the underlying malignancy and the symptoms. Some metastatic bone tumors are curable (lymphoma, Hodgkin's disease), and others are treated with palliative intent. Pain may be relieved by local radiation therapy. Hormonally responsive tumors are responsive to hormone inhibition (antiandrogens for prostate cancer, antiestrogens for breast cancer). Strontium 89 and samarium 153 are bone-seeking radionuclides that can exert antitumor effects and relieve symptoms. Bisphosphonates such as pamidronate may relieve pain and inhibit bone resorption, thereby maintaining bone mineral density and reducing risk of fractures in patients with osteolytic metastases from breast cancer and multiple myeloma. Careful monitoring of serum electrolytes and creatinine is recommended. Monthly administration prevents bone-related clinical events and may reduce the incidence of bone metastases in women with breast cancer. When the integrity of a weight-bearing bone is threatened by an expanding metastatic lesion that is refractory to radiation therapy, prophylactic internal fixation is indicated. Overall survival is related to the prognosis of the underlying tumor. Bone pain at the end of life is particularly common; an adequate pain relief regimen including sufficient amounts of narcotic analgesics is required. **The management of hypercalcemia is discussed in Chap. 347.**

FURTHER READINGS

BORDEN EC et al: Soft tissue sarcomas of adults: State of the translational science. Clin Cancer Res 9:1941, 2003

HELMAN LJ, MELTZER P: Mechanisms of sarcoma development. Nat Rev Cancer 3:685, 2003

MOCELLIN S et al: Adult soft tissue sarcomas: Conventional therapies and molecularly targeted approaches. Cancer Treat Rev 32:9, 2006

PISTERS PW et al: Evidence-based recommendations for local therapy for soft tissue sarcomas. J Clin Oncol 25:1003, 2007

SCURR M, JUDSON I: How to treat the Ewing's family of sarcomas in adult patients. Oncologist 11:65, 2006

VERWEIJ J et al: Progression-free survival in gastrointestinal stromal tumors with high-dose imatinib: Randomized trial. Lancet 364:1127, 2004

95 Carcinoma of Unknown Primary

Gauri R. Varadhachary, James L. Abbruzzese

Carcinoma of unknown primary (CUP) is a biopsy-proven (mainly epithelial) malignancy for which the anatomic site of origin remains unidentified after an intensive search. CUP is one of the 10 most frequently diagnosed cancers worldwide, accounting for approximately 3–5% of all cancer cases. Most investigators do not consider lymphomas, metastatic melanomas, and metastatic sarcomas that present without a known primary tumor to be CUP because these cancers have specific stage- and histology-based treatments that can guide management.

A standard workup for CUP includes a medical history; physical examination; and laboratory studies, including liver and renal function tests, hemogram, chest x-ray, CT scan of the abdomen and pelvis, mammography in women, and prostate-specific antigen (PSA) test in men. With the increasing availability of additional sophisticated imaging techniques and the emergence of targeted therapies that have been shown to be effective in several cancers, oncologists must decide on the extent of workup that is warranted. Specifically, they must consider how additional diagnostic procedures may affect the choice of therapy and the patient's survival and quality of life.

The reason tumors present as CUP remains unclear. One hypothesis is that the primary tumor either regresses after seeding the metastasis or remains so small that it is not detected. It is possible that CUP falls on the continuum of cancer presentation where the primary has been contained or eliminated by the natural body defenses. Alternatively, CUP may represent a specific malignant event that results in an increase in metastatic spread or survival relative to the primary. Whether the CUP metastases truly define a clone that is genetically and phenotypically unique to this diagnosis remains to be determined.

CUP BIOLOGY

No characteristics that are unique to CUP relative to metastases from known primaries have been identified. Abnormalities in chromosomes 1 and 12 and other complex abnormalities have been found. Aneuploidy has been described in 70% of CUP patients with metastatic adenocarcinoma or undifferentiated carcinoma. The overexpression of various genes, including *Ras*, *bcl-2* (40%), *her-2* (11%), and *p53* (26–53%), has been studied in CUP samples, but they seem to have no effect on response to therapy or survival. The extent of angiogenesis in CUP relative to that in metastases from known primaries has also been evaluated, but no consistent findings have emerged.

CLINICAL EVALUATION

Obtaining a thorough medical history from CUP patients is essential, paying particular attention to previous surgeries, removed lesions, and family medical history to assess potential hereditary cancers. Physical examination, including a digital rectal examination in men and breast and pelvic examinations in women, should be performed. Determining the patient's performance status, nutritional status, comorbid illnesses, and cancer-induced complications is essential since they may affect treatment planning.

Role of Serum Tumor Markers and Cytogenetics Most tumor markers, including CEA, CA-125, CA 19-9, and CA 15-3, when elevated, are nonspecific and not helpful in determining the primary tumor site. Men who present with adenocarcinoma and osteoblastic metastasis should undergo a PSA test. Patients with an elevated PSA should be treated as having prostate cancer. In patients with undifferentiated or poorly differentiated carcinoma (especially with a midline tumor), elevated β-human chorionic gonadotropin (βhCG) and α fetoprotein (AFP) levels suggest the possibility of an extragonadal germ cell (testicular) tumor. Cytogenetic studies had a larger role in the past, although interpretation of these older studies can be challenging. In our opinion, with the availability of immunohistochemical stains, cytogenetic analyses are indicated only occasionally. We reserve them for undifferentiated neoplasms with inconclusive immunohistochemical stains and those for which a high suspicion of lymphoma exists.

Role of Imaging Studies Chest x-rays are always obtained in CUP workups but are often negative, especially with low-volume disease. CT scans of the chest, abdomen, and pelvis can be used to help find the primary, evaluate the extent of disease, and select the most favorable biopsy site. Older studies suggested that the primary tumor site is detected in 20–35% of patients who undergo a CT scan of the abdomen and pelvis, although by current definition these patients would not be considered as having CUP. Older studies also suggest a latent primary tumor prevalence of 20%; with more sophisticated imaging, this prevalence is <10% today.

Mammography should be performed in all women who present with metastatic adenocarcinoma, especially in those with adenocarcinoma and isolated axillary adenopathy. MRI of the breast is a recognized follow-up modality in patients with suspected occult primary breast carcinoma (following negative mammography and sonography findings). The results of these imaging modalities can influence surgical management; a negative breast MRI result predicts a low tumor yield at mastectomy.

A conventional workup for a cervical CUP (neck lymphadenopathy with no known primary tumor) includes a CT scan or MRI and invasive studies, including indirect and direct laryngoscopy, bronchoscopy, and upper endoscopy. Ipsilateral (or bilateral) tonsillectomy (with histopathology) has been recommended for cervical CUP patients. [^{18}F]-fluorodeoxyglucose (FDG) positron emission tomography (PET) scans are useful in this patient population and may help guide the biopsy; determine the extent of disease; facilitate the appropriate treatment, including planning radiation fields; and help with disease surveillance. Several studies have evaluated the utility of PET in patients with cervical CUP. These trials have included a small number of patients; primary tumors were identified in ~21–30%.

The diagnostic contribution of PET to the evaluation of noncervical CUP is controversial. PET or PET-CT helps to detect primary tumor in 20–35% of patients. PET-CT can be helpful for patients who are candidates for surgical intervention for solitary metastatic disease because the presence of disease outside the primary site will affect surgical consolidation planning.

Invasive studies, including upper endoscopy, colonoscopy, and bronchoscopy, should be limited to symptomatic patients or those with laboratory or pathologic abnormalities suggesting that these techniques will result in a high tumor yield.

PATHOLOGIC DIAGNOSIS OF CUP

A detailed pathologic examination of the most accessible biopsied tissue specimen is mandatory in CUP cases. Pathologic evaluation typically consists of hematoxylin-and-eosin stains and immunohistochemical tests. Electron microscopy is rarely used currently, although it may be selectively useful when making treatment decisions.

Light Microscopy Evaluation Adequate tissue obtained by fine-needle aspiration or core-needle biopsy should first be stained with hematoxylin and eosin and subjected to light microscopic examination. On light microscopy, 60% of CUPs are found to be adenocarcinoma, and 5% are squamous cell carcinoma. The remaining 30% of lesions are diagnosed as poorly differentiated adenocarcinoma, poorly differentiated carcinoma, or poorly differentiated neoplasm. A small percentage of lesions are diagnosed as neuroendocrine cancers (2%), mixed tumors (adenosquamous, or sarcomatoid carcinomas), or undifferentiated neoplasm (Table 95-1).

Role of Immunohistochemical Analysis Immunohistochemical stains are peroxidase-labeled antibodies against specific tumor antigens that are used to define tumor lineage. The number of available immunohistochemical stains is ever-increasing. However, in CUP cases, more is not necessarily better, and immunohistochemical stains should be used in conjunction with the patient's clinical presentation and imaging studies to select the best therapy. Communication between the cli-

TABLE 95-1 MAJOR HISTOLOGIES IN CUP

Histology	Proportion, %
Well to moderately differentiated adenocarcinoma	60
Squamous cell cancer	5
Poorly differentiated adenocarcinoma, poorly differentiated carcinoma	30
Neuroendocrine	2
Undifferentiated malignancy	3

nician and pathologist is essential. No stain is 100% specific, and overinterpretation should be avoided. PSA and thyroglobulin tissue markers, which are positive in prostate and thyroid cancer, respectively, are the most specific of the current marker panel. However, these cancers rarely present as CUP, so the yield of these tests may be low. Fig. 95-1 delineates a simple algorithm for immunohistochemical staining in CUP cases. Table 95-2 lists additional tests that may be useful to further define the tumor lineage. A more comprehensive algorithm may improve the diagnostic accuracy but can make the process complex. With the use of immunohistochemical markers, electron microscopic analysis, which is time-consuming and expensive, is rarely needed.

There are 20 subtypes of cytokeratin (CK) intermediate filaments with different molecular weights and differential expression in various cell types and cancers. Monoclonal antibodies to specific CK subtypes have been used to help classify tumors according to their site of origin; commonly used CK stains in CUP are CK7 and CK20. CK7 is found in tumors of the lung, ovary, endometrium, and breast and not in those of the lower gastrointestinal tract, whereas CK20 is normally expressed in the gastrointestinal epithelium, urothelium, and Merkel's cells. CK20+/CK7– strongly suggest a primary tumor of the colon; 75–95% of colon tumors show this pattern of staining. CK20–/CK7+ suggests cancer of the lung, breast, ovary, endometrium, and pancreaticobiliary tract; some of these can also be CK20+. The nuclear CDX-2 transcription factor, which is the product of a homeobox gene necessary for intestinal organogenesis, is often used to aid in the diagnosis of gastrointestinal adenocarcinomas.

Thyroid transcription factor 1 (TTF-1) is a 38-kDa homeodomain-containing nuclear protein that plays a role in transcriptional activation during embryogenesis in the thyroid, diencephalon, and respiratory epithelium. TTF-1 nuclear staining is typically positive in lung and thyroid cancers. Approximately 68% of adenocarcinomas and 25% of squamous cell lung cancers stain positive for TTF-1, which helps differentiate a lung primary tumor from metastatic adenocarcinoma in a pleural effusion, the mediastinum, or the lung parenchyma.

Distinguishing pleural mesothelioma from lung adenocarcinoma can be challenging. Calretinin, Wilms' tumor gene-1 (WT-1), and mesothelin have been suggested as useful markers for mesothelioma.

Gross cystic disease fibrous protein-15, a 15-kDa monomer protein, is a marker of apocrine differentiation that is detected in 62–72% of breast carcinomas. UROIII, high-molecular-weight cytokeratin, thrombomodulin, and CK20 are the markers used to diagnose lesions of urothelial origin.

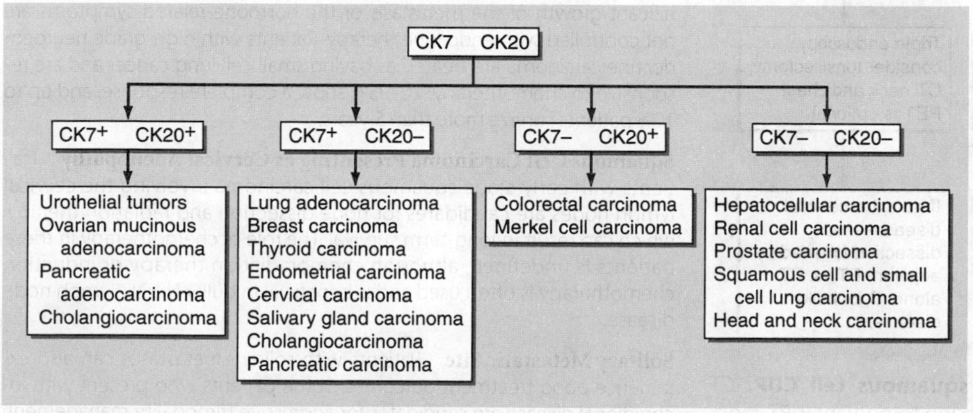

FIGURE 95-1 Approach to cytokeratin (CK7 and CK20) markers used in CUP.

TABLE 95-2 ADDITIONAL IMMUNOHISTOCHEMICAL STAINS USEFUL IN THE DIAGNOSIS OF CUP

Tissue Marker	Diagnosis
Estrogen and progesterone receptors	Breast cancer
BRST-1	Breast cancer
Gross cystic disease fibrous protein-15	Breast cancer
Thyroid transcription factor 1	Lung and thyroid cancer
Thyroglobulin	Thyroid cancer
Chromogranin, synaptophysin, neuron specific enolase	Neuroendocrine cancer
CDX-2	Gastrointestinal cancer
Calretinin, mesothelin	Mesothelioma
Leukocyte common antigen	Lymphoma
S-100, HMB-45	Melanoma
URO-III, thrombomodulin	Bladder cancer
α Fetoprotein	Hepatocellular cancer, germ cell cancer
β-Human chronic gonadotropin	Germ cell cancer
Prostate specific antigen	Prostate cancer

ROLE OF DNA MICROARRAY AND REVERSE TRANSCRIPTASE POLYMERASE CHAIN REACTION (RT-PCR) IN CUP

In the absence of a known primary, developing therapeutic strategies for CUP is challenging. The current diagnostic yield with imaging and immunochemistry is ~20–30% for CUP patients. The use of gene expression studies holds the promise of substantially increasing this yield. Gene expression profiles are most commonly generated using quantitative RT-PCR or DNA microarray.

Neural network programs have been used to develop predictive algorithms from the gene expression profiles. Typically, a training set of gene profiles from known cancers (preferably from metastatic sites) are used to train the software. The program can then be used to predict the origin of a test tumor, and presumably of true CUP. Comprehensive gene expression databases that have become available for common malignancies may also be useful in CUP. Investigators have used expression data from normal differentiated tissues to identify conserved expression profiles found in malignant tissue as a basis for predicting the tissue of origin. These approaches have been effective in blind testing against known primary cancers and their metastasis. However, because, by definition, the primary tumor site is not identifiable in CUP, validation of site prediction in this setting can be challenging, and any predictions currently must be supported by clinical and pathologic correlation. Prospective validation trials are currently evaluating the role of molecular studies in CUP.

Rx CARCINOMA OF UNKNOWN PRIMARY

GENERAL CONSIDERATIONS The treatment of CUP continues to evolve, albeit slowly. The median survival duration of most patients with disseminated CUP is ~6–10 months. Systemic chemotherapy is the primary treatment modality in most cases, but the careful integration of surgery, radiation therapy, and even periods of observation are important in the overall management of this condition (**Figs. 95-2** and **95-3**). Prognostic factors include performance status, site and number of metastases, response to chemotherapy, and serum lactate dehydrogenase (LDH) levels. Culine and colleagues developed a prognostic model using performance status and serum LDH levels, which allowed the assignment of patients into two subgroups with divergent outcomes. Future prospective trials using this prognostic model are warranted. Clinically, several CUP diagnoses fall into a favorable prog-

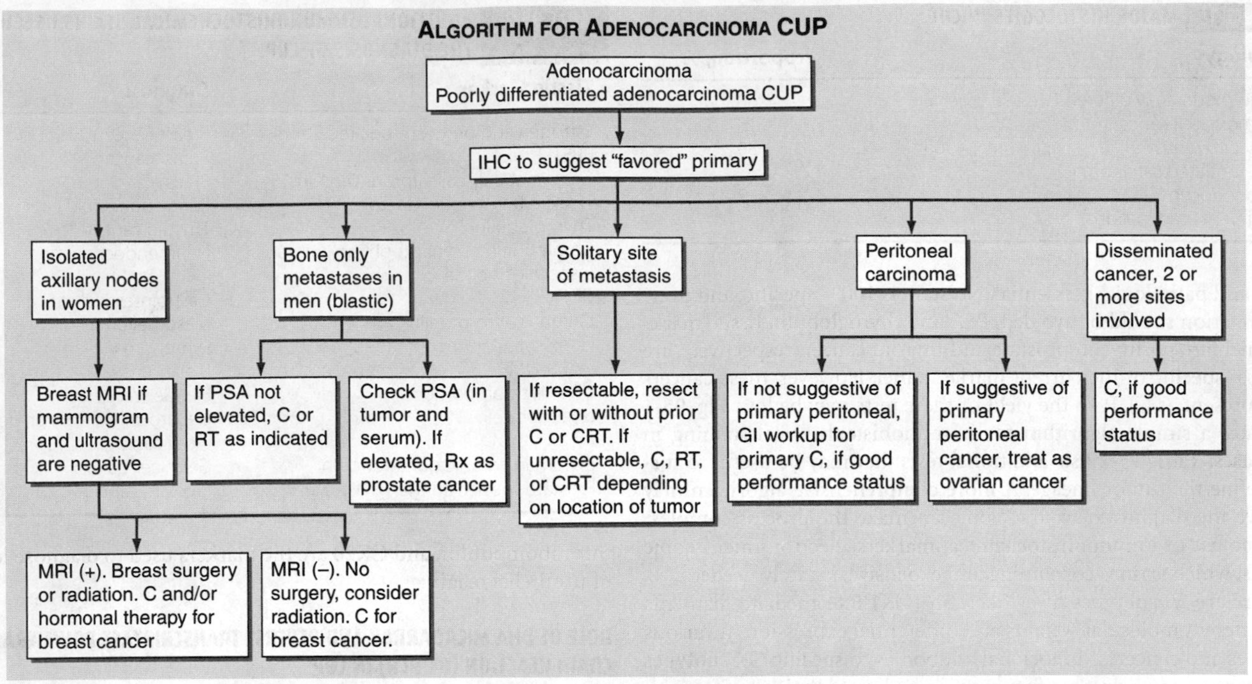

FIGURE 95-2 Treatment algorithm for adenocarcinoma and poorly differentiated adenocarcinoma CUP. C, chemotherapy; IHC, immunohistochemistry; GI, gastrointestinal; CRT, chemoradiation; RT, radiation; PSA, prostate-specific antigen; MRI, magnetic resonance imaging.

nostic subset. Others, including those with disseminated CUP, have a more unfavorable prognosis.

TREATMENT OF FAVORABLE SUBSETS OF CUP **Women with Isolated Axillary Adenopathy** Women with isolated axillary adenopathy with adenocarcinoma or carcinoma should be treated for stage II or III breast cancer. These patients should undergo a breast MRI if mammogram and ultrasound are negative. Radiation therapy to the ipsilateral breast is indicated if the breast MRI is positive. Chemotherapy and/or hormonal therapy is indicated based on patient's age (premenopausal or postmenopausal), nodal disease bulk, and hormone receptor status (Chap. 86).

Women with Peritoneal Carcinomatosis The term *primary peritoneal papillary serous carcinoma* (PPSC) has been used to describe CUP with carcinomatosis with the pathologic and laboratory (elevated CA-125 antigen) characteristics of ovarian cancer but no ovarian primary tumor identified on transvaginal sonography or laparotomy. Studies suggest that ovarian cancer and PPSC, which are both of mullerian origin, have similar gene expression profiles. Similar to patients with ovarian cancer, patients with PPSC are candidates for cytoreductive surgery, followed by adjuvant taxane and platinum-based chemotherapy. In one retrospective study of 258 women with peritoneal carcinomatosis who had undergone cytoreductive surgery and chemotherapy, 22% of patients had a complete response to chemotherapy; the median survival duration was 18 months (range 11–24 months).

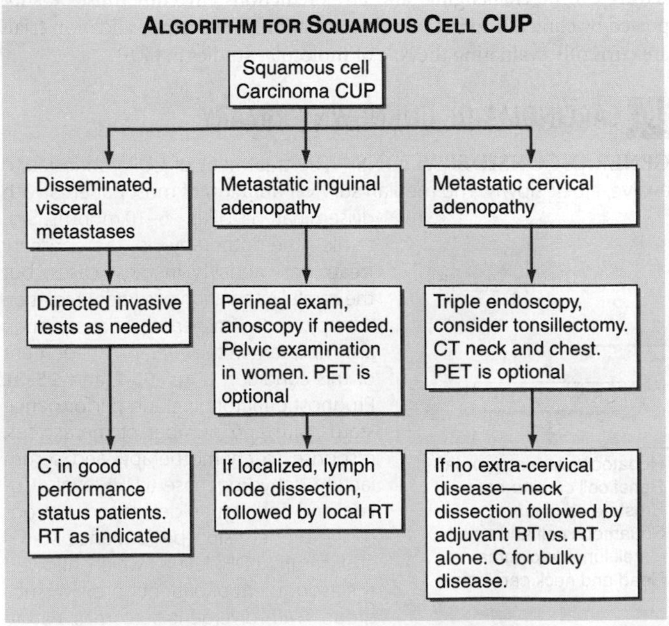

FIGURE 95-3 Treatment algorithm for squamous cell CUP. CT, computed tomography; PET, positron emission tomography; RT, radiation; C, chemotherapy.

Poorly Differentiated Carcinoma with Midline Adenopathy Men with poorly differentiated or undifferentiated carcinoma that presents as a midline adenopathy should be evaluated for extragonadal germ cell malignancy. They often experience a good response to treatment with platinum-based combination chemotherapy. Response rates of >50% have been noted, and 10–15% long-term survivors have been reported.

Neuroendocrine Carcinoma Low-grade neuroendocrine carcinoma often has an indolent course, and treatment decisions are based on symptoms and tumor bulk. Urine 5-HIAA and serum chromogranin may be elevated and can be followed as markers. Often the patient is treated with somatostatin analogues alone for hormone-related symptoms (diarrhea, flushing, nausea). Specific local therapies or systemic therapy would only be indicated if the patient is symptomatic with local pain secondary to significant growth of the metastasis or the hormone-related symptoms are not controlled with endocrine therapy. Patients with high-grade neuroendocrine carcinoma are treated as having small cell lung cancer and are responsive to chemotherapy; 20–25% show a complete response, and up to 10% patients survive more than 5 years.

Squamous Cell Carcinoma Presenting as Cervical Adenopathy Patients with early-stage squamous cell carcinoma involving the cervical lymph nodes are candidates for node dissection and radiation therapy, which can result in long-term survival. The role of chemotherapy in these patients is undefined, although chemoradiation therapy or induction chemotherapy is often used and is beneficial in bulky N2/N3 lymph node disease.

Solitary Metastatic Site Patients with solitary metastases can also experience good treatment outcomes. Some patients who present with locoregional disease are candidates for aggressive trimodality management; both prolonged disease-free interval and occasionally cure are possible.

Men with Blastic Skeletal Metastases and Elevated PSA Blastic bone-only metastasis is a rare presentation, and elevated serum PSA or tumor staining with PSA may provide confirmatory evidence of prostate cancer in these patients. Those with elevated levels are candidates for hormonal therapy for prostate cancer, although it is important to rule out other primary tumors (lung most common).

MANAGEMENT OF DISSEMINATED CUP Patients who present with liver, brain, and adrenal metastatic disease usually have a poor prognosis. Beside primary peritoneal carcinoma, carcinomatosis presenting as CUP in other settings is not uncommon. Gastric, appendicular, colon, pancreas, and cholangiocarcinoma are all possible primaries, and imaging, endoscopy, and pathologic data help in the evaluation.

Traditionally, platinum-based combination chemotherapy regimens have been used to treat patients with CUP. In a phase II study by Hainsworth and colleagues, 55 mostly chemotherapy-naive patients were treated with paclitaxel, carboplatin, and oral etoposide every 3 weeks. The overall response rate was 47%, with median overall survival duration of 13.4 months. Briasoulis and colleagues reported similar response rates and survival durations in 77 patients with CUP who had been treated with paclitaxel and carboplatin. In this study, patients with nodal or pleural disease and women with peritoneal carcinomatosis had higher response rates and overall survival durations of 13 and 15 months, respectively. Studies incorporating newer agents, including gemcitabine, irinotecan, and targeted agents, are showing higher response rates. In a phase II randomized trial by Culine and colleagues, 80 patients were randomly assigned to receive gemcitabine with cisplatin or irinotecan with cisplatin; 78 patients were assessible for efficacy and toxicity. Objective responses were observed in 21 patients (55%) in the gemcitabine and cisplatin arm and in 15 patients (38%) in the irinotecan and cisplatin arm. The median survival was 8 months for gemcitabine and cisplatin and 6 months for irinotecan and cisplatin.

The role of second-line chemotherapy in CUP is poorly defined. Gemcitabine as a single agent has shown a partial response rate of 8%, and 25% of patients had minor responses or stable disease, with improved symptoms. Combination chemotherapy as a second- and third-line treatment may result in a slightly improved response.

Combination targeted therapy is being evaluated. Hainsworth and colleagues studied the combination of bevacizumab and erlotinib in 51 patients; 25% were chemotherapy-naive and had advanced bone or liver metastases, while the rest had been previously treated with 1 or 2 chemotherapy regimens. Responses were noted in 4 patients (8%), and 30 patients (59%) experienced stable disease or a minor response. The median overall survival was 8.9 months, with 42% of patients alive at 1 year.

Historically, patients with CUP have been treated with "global" regimens that work for a variety of primary cancers. With incremental improved responses over the past decade in known cancer types, we anticipate overall better response rates with newer regimens for selected CUP patients. With a more robust immunohistochemical panel (directed approach) and new molecular data, one may be able to create a more tailored algorithm for CUP patients.

SUMMARY

Patients with CUP should undergo a directed diagnostic search for the primary tumor on the basis of clinical and pathologic data. Subsets of patients have prognostically favorable disease, as defined by clinical or histologic criteria, and may substantially benefit from aggressive treatment and expect prolonged survival. However, for most patients who present with advanced CUP, the prognosis remains poor, with early resistance to available cytotoxic therapy. Research into the metastatic phenotype will help us improve our understanding of CUP tumor biology. Whether the CUP clone is a distinct molecular genotype-phenotype that is different from metastases of known primary tumors remains to be elucidated. The identification of specific CUP-related molecular and biochemical targets may help exploit therapeutic targeted agents for this entity.

FURTHER READINGS

Abbruzzese JL et al: The biology of unknown primary tumors. Semin Oncol 20:238, 1993

Bugat R et al: Summary of the standards, options and recommendations for the management of patients with carcinoma of unknown primary site. Br J Cancer 89(Suppl 1):S59, 2003

Culine S et al: Cisplatin in combination with either gemcitabine or irinotecan in carcinomas of unknown primary site: Results of a randomized phase II study—trial for the French Study Group on Carcinomas of Unknown Primary (GEFCAPI 01). J Clin Oncol 21:3479, 2003

Dennis JL, Oien KA: Hunting the primary: novel strategies for defining the origin of tumours. J Pathol 205:236, 2005

Greco FA, Hainsworth JD: One-hour paclitaxel, carboplatin, and extended-schedule etoposide in the treatment of carcinoma of unknown primary site. Semin Oncol 24(6 Suppl 19):S19, 1997

Kende AI et al: Expression of cytokeratins 7 and 20 in carcinomas of the gastrointestinal tract. Histopathology 42:137, 2003

Lobins R, Floyd J: Small cell carcinoma of unknown primary. Semin Oncol 34:39, 2007.

Olson JA Jr et al: Magnetic resonance imaging facilitates breast conservation for occult breast cancer. Ann Surg Oncol 7:411, 2000

Rusthoven KE et al: The role of fluorodeoxyglucose positron emission tomography in cervical lymph node metastases from an unknown primary tumor. Cancer 101:2641, 2004

Varadhachary GR et al: Diagnostic strategies for unknown primary cancer. Cancer 100:1776, 2004

96 Paraneoplastic Syndromes: Endocrinologic/Hematologic

J. Larry Jameson, Bruce E. Johnson

In addition to local tissue invasion and metastasis, neoplastic cells can produce a variety of peptides that that can stimulate hormonal, hematologic, dermatologic, or neurologic responses. *Paraneoplastic syndromes* refer to the disorders that accompany benign or malignant tumors but are not directly related to mass effects or invasion. Tumors of neuroendocrine origin, such as small cell lung carcinoma (SCLC) and carcinoids, produce a wide array of peptide hormones and are common causes of paraneoplastic syndromes. However, almost every type of malignancy has the potential to produce hormones or cytokines, or to induce immunologic responses. Careful studies of the prevalence of paraneoplastic syndromes indicate that they are more common than is generally appreciated. The signs, symptoms, and metabolic alterations associated with paraneoplastic disorders may be overlooked in the context of a malignancy and its treatment. Consequently, atypical clinical manifestations in a patient with cancer should prompt consideration of a paraneoplastic syndrome. The most common endocrinologic and hematologic syndromes associated with underlying neoplasia will be discussed here.

ENDOCRINE PARANEOPLASTIC SYNDROMES

Etiology Hormones can be produced from eutopic or ectopic sources. *Eutopic* refers to the expression of a hormone from its normal tissue of origin, whereas *ectopic* refers to hormone production from an atypical tissue source. For example, adrenocorticotropic hormone (ACTH) is expressed eutopically by the corticotrope cells of the anterior pituitary but it can be expressed ectopically in SCLC. Many hormones are produced at low levels from a wide array of tissues, in addition to the classic endocrine source. Thus, ectopic expression is often a quantitative change rather than an absolute change in tissue expression. Nevertheless, the term *ectopic expression* is firmly entrenched and conveys the abnormal physiology associated with neoplastic hormone production. In addition to high levels of hormones, ectopic expression is typically characterized by abnormal regulation of hormone production (e.g., defective feedback control) and peptide processing (resulting in large, unprocessed precursors).

A diverse array of molecular mechanisms has been suggested to cause ectopic hormone production, but this process remains incompletely understood. In rare instances, genetic rearrangements explain aberrant hormone expression. For example, translocation of the *parathyroid hormone (PTH)* gene resulted in high levels of PTH expression in an ovarian carcinoma, presumably because the genetic rearrangement brings the *PTH* gene under the control of ovary-specific regulatory elements. A related phenomenon is well documented in many forms of leukemia and lymphoma, in which somatic genetic rearrangements confer a growth advantage and alter cellular differentiation and function (Chap. 105). Although genetic rearrangements may cause selected cases of ectopic hormone production, this mechanism is probably unusual, as many tumors are associated with excessive production of numerous peptides. It is likely that cellular dedifferentiation underlies most cases of ectopic hormone production. In support of this idea, many cancers are poorly differentiated histologically, and certain tumor products, such as human chorionic gonadotropin (hCG), parathyroid hormone–related protein (PTHrP), and α fetoprotein, are characteristic of gene expression at earlier developmental stages. On the other hand, the propensity of certain cancers to produce particular hormones (e.g., squamous cell carcinomas produce PTHrP) suggests that dedifferentiation is partial or that selective pathways are derepressed. These expression profiles are likely to be driven by alterations in transcriptional repression, changes in DNA methylation, or other factors that govern cell differentiation. Consistent with this idea, many solid tumors harbor poorly differentiated "cancer stem cells," a subpopulation of cells that are capable of initiating new tumors.

In SCLC, the pathway of differentiation has been defined. The neuroendocrine phenotype is dictated in part by the basic-helix-loop-helix (bHLH) transcription factor human achaete-scute homologue 1 (hASH-1), which is expressed at abnormally high levels in SCLC associated with ectopic ACTH. The activity of hASH-1 is inhibited by hairy enhancer of split 1 (HES-1) and by Notch proteins, which are also capable of inducing growth arrest. Thus, abnormal expression of these developmental transcription factors appears to provide a link between cell proliferation and differentiation.

Ectopic hormone production would only be an epiphenomenon associated with cancer if it did not result in clinical manifestations. Excessive and unregulated production of hormones such as ACTH, PTHrP, or vasopressin can lead to substantial morbidity and can complicate the cancer treatment plan. Moreover, the paraneoplastic endocrinopathies are sometimes the presenting feature of underlying malignancy and may prompt the search for an unrecognized tumor.

A large number of paraneoplastic endocrine syndromes have been described, linking overproduction of particular hormones with specific types of tumors. However, certain recurring syndromes emerge from this group (Table 96-1). The most common paraneoplastic endocrine syndromes include hypercalcemia from overproduction of PTHrP and other factors, hyponatremia from excess vasopressin, and Cushing's syndrome from ectopic ACTH.

TABLE 96-1 PARANEOPLASTIC SYNDROMES CAUSED BY ECTOPIC HORMONE PRODUCTION

Paraneoplastic Syndrome	Ectopic Hormone	Typical Tumor Types[a]
Common		
Hypercalcemia of malignancy	Parathyroid hormone-related protein (PTHrP)	Squamous cell (head and neck, lung, skin), breast, genitourinary, gastrointestinal
	1,25 dihydroxyvitamin D	Lymphomas
	Parathyroid hormone (PTH) (rare)	Lung, ovary
	Prostaglandin E2 (PGE2) (rare)	Renal, lung
Syndrome of inappropriate antidiuretic hormone secretion (SIADH)	Vasopressin	Lung (squamous, small cell), gastrointestinal, genitourinary, ovary
Cushing's syndrome	Adrenocorticotropic hormone (ACTH)	Lung (small cell, bronchial carcinoid, adenocarcinoma, squamous), thymus, pancreatic islet, medullary thyroid carcinoma
	Corticotropin-releasing hormone (CRH) (rare)	Pancreatic islet, carcinoid, lung, prostate
	Ectopic expression of gastric inhibitory peptide (GIP), luteinizing hormone (LH)/ human chorionic gonadotropin (hCG), other G protein–coupled receptors (rare)	Macronodular adrenal hyperplasia
Less Common		
Non-islet cell hypoglycemia	Insulin-like growth factor (IGF-II)	Mesenchymal tumors, sarcomas, adrenal, hepatic, gastrointestinal, kidney, prostate
	Insulin (rare)	Cervix (small cell carcinoma)
Male feminization	hCG[b]	Testis (embryonal, seminomas), germinomas, choriocarcinoma, lung, hepatic, pancreatic islet
Diarrhea or intestinal hypermotility	Calcitonin[c]	Lung, colon, breast, medullary thyroid carcinoma
	Vasoactive intestinal peptide (VIP)	Pancreas, pheochromocytoma, esophagus
Rare		
Oncogenic osteomalacia	Phosphatonin [fibroblast growth factor 23 (FGF23)]	Hemangiopericytomas, osteoblastomas, fibromas, sarcomas, giant cell tumors, prostate, lung
Acromegaly	Growth hormone–releasing hormone (GHRH)	Pancreatic islet, bronchial and other carcinoids
	Growth hormone (GH)	Lung, pancreatic islet
Hyperthyroidism	Thyroid-stimulating hormone (TSH)	Hydatidiform mole, embryonal tumors, struma ovarii
Hypertension	Renin	Juxtaglomerula tumors, kidney, lung, pancreas, ovary

[a]Only the most common tumor types are listed. For most ectopic hormone syndromes, an extensive list of tumors has been reported to produce one or more hormones.

[b]hCG is produced eutopically by trophoblastic tumors. Certain tumors produce disproportionate amounts of the hCG α or hCG β subunits. High levels of hCG rarely cause hyperthyroidism because of weak binding to the TSH receptor.

[c]Calcitonin is produced eutopically by medullary thyroid carcinoma and is used as a tumor marker.

HYPERCALCEMIA CAUSED BY ECTOPIC PRODUCTION OF PTHrP

(See also Chap. 347)

Etiology Humoral hypercalcemia of malignancy (HHM) occurs in up to 20% of patients with cancer. HHM is most common in cancers of the lung, head and neck, skin, esophagus, breast, genitourinary tract, and in multiple myeloma and lymphomas. Several distinct humoral causes of HHM occur, most commonly overproduction of PTHrP. In addition to acting as a circulating humoral factor, bone metastases (e.g., breast, multiple myeloma) may produce PTHrP, leading to local osteolysis and hypercalcemia.

PTHrP is structurally related to PTH and it binds to the PTH receptor, explaining the similar biochemical features of HHM and hyperparathyroidism. PTHrP plays a key role in skeletal development and regulates cellular proliferation and differentiation in other tissues including skin, bone marrow, breast, and hair follicles. The mechanism of PTHrP induction in malignancy is incompletely understood; however, tumor-bearing tissues commonly associated with HHM normally produce PTHrP during development or cell renewal. Mutations in certain oncogenes, such as *Ras*, can activate PTHrP expression. In adult T cell lymphoma, the transactivating Tax protein produced by human T-cell lymphotropic virus I (HTLV-I) stimulates PTHrP promoter activity. Metastatic lesions to bone are more likely to produce PTHrP than are metastases in other tissues, suggesting that bone produces factors that enhance PTHrP production, or that PTHrP-producing metastases have a selective growth advantage in bone. Thus, PTHrP production can be stimulated by mutations in oncogenes, by altered expression of viral or cellular transcription factors, and by local growth factors.

Another relatively common cause of HHM is excess production of 1,25-dihydroxyvitamin D. Like granulomatous disorders associated with hypercalcemia, lymphomas can produce an enzyme that converts 25-hydroxyvitamin D to the more active 1,25-dihydroxyvitamin D, leading to enhanced gastrointestinal calcium absorption. Other causes of HHM include tumor-mediated production of osteolytic cytokines and inflammatory mediators.

Clinical Manifestations The typical presentation of HHM is a patient with a known malignancy who is found to be hypercalcemic on routine laboratory tests. Less often, hypercalcemia is the initial presenting feature of malignancy. Particularly when calcium levels are markedly increased [>3.5 mmol/L (>14 mg/dL)], patients may experience fatigue, mental status changes, dehydration, or symptoms of nephrolithiasis.

Diagnosis Features that favor HHM, as opposed to primary hyperparathyroidism, include known malignancy, recent onset of hypercalcemia, and very high serum calcium levels. Like hyperparathyroidism, hypercalcemia caused by PTHrP is accompanied by hypercalciuria and hypophosphatemia. Measurement of PTH is useful to exclude primary hyperparathyroidism; the PTH level should be suppressed in HHM. An elevated PTHrP level confirms the diagnosis, and it is increased in ~80% of hypercalcemic patients with cancer. 1,25-Dihydroxyvitamin D levels may be increased in patients with lymphoma.

Rx HUMORAL HYPERCALCEMIA OF MALIGNANCY

The management of HHM begins with removal of excess calcium in the diet, medications, or IV solutions. Oral phosphorus (e.g., 250 mg Neutra-Phos 3–4 times daily) should be given until serum phosphorus is >1.0 mmol/L (>3 mg/dL). Saline rehydration is used to dilute serum calcium and promote calciuresis. Forced diuresis with furosemide or other loop diuretics can enhance calcium excretion but provides relatively little value except in life-threatening hypercalcemia. When used, loop diuretics should be administered only after complete rehydration and with careful monitoring of fluid balance. Bisphosphonates such as pamidronate (30–90 mg IV), zolendronate (4–8 mg IV), or etidronate (7.5 mg/kg per day PO for 3–7 consecutive days) can reduce serum calcium within 1–2 days and suppress calcium release for several weeks. Bisphosphonate infusions can be repeated or oral bisphosphonates can be used for chronic treatment. Dialysis should be considered in severe hypercalcemia when saline hydration and bisphosphonate treatments are not possible or are too slow in onset. Previously used agents, such as calcitonin and mithramycin, have little utility now that bisphosphonates are available. Calcitonin (2–8 U/kg SC every 6–12 h) should be considered when rapid correction of severe hypercalcemia is needed. Hypercalcemia associated with lymphomas, multiple myeloma, or leukemia may respond to glucocorticoid treatment (e.g., prednisone 40–100 mg PO in four divided doses).

ECTOPIC VASOPRESSIN: TUMOR-ASSOCIATED SIADH

(See also Chap. 46)

Etiology Vasopressin is an antidiuretic hormone normally produced by the posterior pituitary gland. Ectopic vasopressin production by tumors is a common cause of the syndrome of inappropriate antidiuretic hormone (SIADH), occurring in at least half of patients with SCLC. Compensatory mechanisms, such as decreased thirst, suppression of aldosterone, and production of atrial natriuretic peptide (ANP), may mitigate the development of hyponatremia in patients who produce excessive vasopressin. Tumors with neuroendocrine features, such as SCLC and carcinoids, are the most common sources of ectopic vasopressin production, but it also occurs in other forms of lung cancer and with central nervous system (CNS) lesions, head and neck cancer, and genitourinary, gastrointestinal, and ovarian cancers. The mechanism of activation of the vasopressin gene in these tumors is unknown but often involves concomitant expression of the adjacent oxytocin gene, suggesting derepression of this locus.

Clinical Manifestations Most patients with ectopic vasopressin secretion are asymptomatic and are identified because of the presence of hyponatremia on routine chemistry testing. Symptoms may include weakness, lethargy, nausea, confusion, depressed mental status, and seizures. The severity of symptoms reflects the rapidity of onset as well as the extent of hyponatremia. Hyponatremia usually develops slowly but may be exacerbated by the administration of IV fluids or the institution of new medications. Thirst is typically suppressed.

Diagnosis The diagnostic features of ectopic vasopressin production are the same as those of other causes of SIADH (Chaps. 46 and 334). Hyponatremia and reduced serum osmolality occur in the setting of an inappropriately normal or increased urine osmolality. Urine sodium excretion is normal or increased unless volume depletion is present. Other causes of hyponatremia should be excluded, including renal, adrenal, or thyroid insufficiency. Physiologic sources of vasopressin stimulation (CNS lesions, pulmonary disease, nausea), adaptive circulatory mechanisms (hypotension, heart failure, hepatic cirrhosis), and medications, including many chemotherapeutic agents, should also be considered as possible causes of hyponatremia. Vasopressin assay is not usually necessary to make the diagnosis.

Rx ECTOPIC VASOPRESSIN: TUMOR-ASSOCIATED SIADH

Most patients with ectopic vasopressin production develop hyponatremia over several weeks or months. The disorder should be corrected gradually unless mental status is altered or there is risk of seizures. Treatment of the underlying malignancy may reduce ectopic vasopressin production but this response is slow, if it occurs at all. Fluid restriction to less than urine output, plus insensible losses, is often sufficient to partially correct hyponatremia. However, strict monitoring of the amount and types of liquids consumed or administered intravenously is required for fluid restriction to be effective. Salt tablets or saline are not helpful unless volume depletion is also present. Demeclocycline (150–300 mg orally three to four times daily) can be used to inhibit vasopressin action on the renal distal tubule but its onset of action is relatively slow (1–2 weeks). Conivaptan, a nonpeptide V_2-receptor antagonist, can be administered either PO (20–120 mg bid) or IV (10–40 mg), and is particularly effective when used in combination with fluid restriction in euvolemic hyponatremia. Severe hyponatremia (Na <

115 meq/L) or mental status changes may require treatment with hypertonic (3%) or normal saline infusion together with furosemide, to enhance free water clearance. The rate of sodium correction should be slow (0.5–1 meq/L per h) to prevent rapid fluid shifts and the possible development of central pontine myelinolysis.

CUSHING'S SYNDROME CAUSED BY ECTOPIC ACTH PRODUCTION

(See also Chap. 336)

Etiology Ectopic ACTH production accounts for 10–20% of Cushing's syndrome. The syndrome is particularly common in neuroendocrine tumors. SCLC (>50%) is by far the most common cause of ectopic ACTH, followed by thymic carcinoid (15%), islet cell tumors (10%), bronchial carcinoid (10%), other carcinoids (5%), and pheochromocytomas (2%). Ectopic ACTH production is caused by increased expression of the proopiomelanocortin (POMC) gene, which encodes ACTH, along with melanocyte-stimulating hormone (MSH), β lipotropin, and several other peptides. In many tumors, there is abundant but aberrant expression of the POMC gene from an internal promoter, proximal to the third exon, which encodes ACTH. However, because this product lacks the signal sequence necessary for protein processing, it is not secreted. Increased production of ACTH arises instead from less abundant, but unregulated, POMC expression from the same promoter site used in the pituitary. However, because the tumors lack many of the enzymes needed to process the POMC polypeptide, it is typically released as multiple large, biologically inactive fragments along with relatively small amounts of fully processed, active ACTH.

Rarely, corticotropin-releasing hormone (CRH) is produced by pancreatic islet tumors, SCLC, medullary thyroid cancer, carcinoids, or prostate cancer. When levels are high enough, CRH can cause pituitary corticotrope hyperplasia and Cushing's syndrome. Tumors that produce CRH sometimes also produce ACTH, raising the possibility of a paracrine mechanism for ACTH production.

A distinct mechanism for ACTH-independent Cushing's syndrome involves ectopic expression of various G protein–coupled receptors in the adrenal nodules. Ectopic expression of the gastric inhibitory peptide (GIP) receptor is the best-characterized example of this mechanism. In this case, meals induce GIP secretion, which inappropriately stimulates adrenal growth and glucocorticoid production.

Clinical Manifestations The clinical features of hypercortisolemia are detected in only a small fraction of patients with documented ectopic ACTH production. Patients with ectopic ACTH syndrome generally exhibit less marked weight gain and centripetal fat redistribution, probably because the exposure to excess glucocorticoids is relatively short and because cachexia reduces the propensity for weight gain and fat deposition. The ectopic ACTH syndrome is associated with several clinical features that distinguish it from other causes of Cushing's syndrome (e.g., pituitary adenomas, adrenal adenomas, iatrogenic glucocorticoid excess). The metabolic manifestations of ectopic ACTH syndrome are dominated by fluid retention and hypertension, hypokalemia, metabolic alkalosis, glucose intolerance, and, often, steroid psychosis. The very high ACTH levels often cause increased pigmentation, and melanotrope-stimulating hormone (MSH) activity derived from the POMC precursor peptide is also increased. The extraordinarily high glucocorticoid levels in patients with ectopic sources of ACTH can lead to marked skin fragility and easy bruising. In addition, the high cortisol levels often overwhelm the renal 11β-hydroxysteroid dehydrogenase type II enzyme, which normally inactivates cortisol and prevents it from binding to renal mineralocorticoid receptors. Consequently, in addition to the excess mineralocorticoids produced by ACTH stimulation of the adrenal gland, high levels of cortisol exert activity through the mineralocorticoid receptor, leading to severe hypokalemia.

Diagnosis The diagnosis of ectopic ACTH syndrome is usually not difficult in the setting of a known malignancy. Urine free cortisol levels fluctuate but are typically greater than two to four times normal and the plasma ACTH level is usually >22 pmol/L (>100 pg/mL). A suppressed ACTH level excludes this diagnosis and indicates an ACTH-independent cause of Cushing's syndrome (e.g., adrenal or exogenous glucocorticoid). In contrast to pituitary sources of ACTH, most ectopic sources of ACTH do not respond to glucocorticoid suppression. Therefore, high-dose dexamethasone (8 mg PO) suppresses 8:00 A.M. serum cortisol (50% decrease from baseline) in ~80% of pituitary ACTH-producing adenomas but fails to suppress ectopic ACTH in ~90% of cases. Bronchial and other carcinoids are well-documented exceptions to these general guidelines, as these ectopic sources of ACTH may exhibit feedback regulation indistinguishable from pituitary adenomas, including suppression by high-dose dexamethasone, and ACTH responsiveness to adrenal blockade with metyrapone. If necessary, petrosal sinus catheterization can be used to evaluate a patient with ACTH-dependent Cushing's syndrome when the source of ACTH is unclear. After CRH stimulation, a 3:1 petrosal sinus:peripheral ACTH ratio strongly suggests a pituitary ACTH source. Imaging studies are also useful in the evaluation of suspected carcinoid lesions, allowing biopsy and characterization of hormone production using special stains.

Rx CUSHING'S SYNDROME CAUSED BY ECTOPIC ACTH PRODUCTION

The morbidity associated with the ectopic ACTH syndrome can be substantial. Patients may experience depression or personality changes because of extreme cortisol excess. Metabolic derangements including diabetes mellitus and hypokalemia can worsen fatigue. Poor wound healing and predisposition to infections can complicate the surgical management of tumors, and opportunistic infections, caused by organisms such as *Pneumocystis carinii* and mycoses, are often the cause of death in patients with ectopic ACTH production. Depending on prognosis and treatment plans for the underlying malignancy, measures to reduce cortisol levels are often indicated. Treatment of the underlying malignancy may reduce ACTH levels but is rarely sufficient to reduce cortisol levels to normal. Adrenalectomy is not practical for most of these patients but should be considered if the underlying tumor is not resectable and the prognosis is otherwise favorable (e.g., carcinoid). Medical therapy with ketoconazole (200–400 mg PO bid), metyrapone (250–500 mg PO every 6 h), mitotane (3–6 g PO in four divided doses, tapered to maintain low cortisol production), or other agents that block steroid synthesis or action is often the most practical strategy for managing the hypercortisolism associated with ectopic ACTH production (Chap. 333). Glucocorticoid replacement should be provided to avoid adrenal insufficiency. Unfortunately, many patients will eventually progress despite medical blockade.

TUMOR-INDUCED HYPOGLYCEMIA CAUSED BY EXCESS PRODUCTION OF IGF-II

(See also Chap. 339) Mesenchymal tumors, hemangiopericytomas, hepatocellular tumors, adrenal carcinomas, and a variety of other large tumors have been reported to produce excessive amounts of insulin-like growth factor type II (IGF-II) precursor, which binds weakly to insulin receptors and strongly to IGF-I receptors, leading to insulin-like actions. The gene encoding IGF-II resides on a chromosome 11p15 locus that is normally imprinted (that is, expression is exclusively from a single parental allele). Biallelic expression of the IGF-II gene occurs in a subset of tumors, suggesting loss of methylation and loss of imprinting as a mechanism for gene induction. In addition to increased IGF-II production, IGF-II bioavailability is increased due to complex alterations in circulating binding proteins. Increased IGF-II suppresses growth hormone (GH) and insulin, resulting in reduced IGF binding protein 3 (IGFBP-3), IGF-I, and acid-labile subunit (ALS). The reduction in ALS and IGFBP-3, which normally sequester IGF-II, causes it to be displaced to a small circulating complex that has greater access to insulin target tissues. For this reason, circulating IGF-II levels may not be markedly increased, despite causing hypoglycemia. In addition to IGF-II–mediated hypoglycemia, tumors may occupy enough of the liver to impair gluconeogenesis.

In most cases, the tumor causing hypoglycemia is clinically apparent and hypoglycemia develops in association with fasting. The diagnosis is made by documenting low serum glucose and suppressed insulin levels in association with symptoms of hypoglycemia. Serum IGF-II levels may not be increased (IGF-II assays may not detect IGF-II precursors). Increased IGF-II mRNA expression is found in most of these tumors. Any medications associated with hypoglycemia should be eliminated. Treatment of the underlying malignancy, if possible, may reduce the predisposition to hypoglycemia. Frequent meals and IV glucose, especially during sleep or fasting, are often necessary to prevent hypoglycemia. Glucagon, GH, and glucocorticoids have also been used to enhance glucose production.

HUMAN CHORIONIC GONADOTROPIN

hCG is composed of α and β subunits and can be produced as intact hormone, which is biologically active, or as uncombined biologically inert subunits. Ectopic production of intact hCG occurs most often in association with testicular embryonal tumors, germ cell tumors, extragonadal germinomas, lung cancer, hepatoma, and pancreatic islet tumors. Eutopic production of hCG occurs with trophoblastic malignancies. Low levels of hCG or its uncombined α or β subunits have been reported in a wide array of tumors. hCG α subunit production is particularly common in lung cancer and pancreatic islet cancer. In men, high hCG levels stimulate steroidogenesis and aromatase activity in testicular Leydig cells, resulting in increased estrogen production and the development of gynecomastia. Precocious puberty in boys or gynecomastia in men should prompt measurement of hCG and consideration of a testicular tumor or another source of ectopic hCG production. Most women are asymptomatic. hCG is easily measured. Treatment should be directed at the underlying malignancy.

ONCOGENIC OSTEOMALACIA

Hypophosphatemic oncogenic osteomalacia, also called tumor-induced osteomalacia (TIO), is characterized by markedly reduced serum phosphorus and renal phosphate wasting, leading to muscle weakness, bone pain, and osteomalacia. Serum calcium and PTH levels are normal and 1,25-dihydroxyvitamin D is low. Oncogenic osteomalacia is usually caused by benign mesenchymal tumors, such as hemangiopericytomas, fibromas, or giant cell tumors, often of the skeletal extremities or head. It has also been described in sarcomas and in patients with prostate and lung cancer. Resection of the tumor reverses the disorder, confirming its humoral basis. The circulating phosphaturic factor is called *phosphatonin*—a factor that inhibits renal tubular reabsorption of phosphate and renal conversion of 25-hydroxyvitamin D to 1,25-dihydroxyvitamin D. Phosphatonin has been identified as fibroblast growth factor 23 (FGF23). FGF23 levels are increased in some, but not all, patients with osteogenic osteomalacia. The disorder exhibits biochemical features similar to those seen with inactivating mutations in the *PHEX* gene, the cause of hereditary X-linked hypophosphatemia. The *PHEX* gene encodes a protease that activates FGF23. Treatment involves removal of the tumor, if possible, and supplementation with phosphate and vitamin D. Octreotide treatment reduces phosphate wasting in some patients with tumors that express somatostatin receptor subtype 2. Octreotide scans may also be useful to detect these tumors.

HEMATOLOGIC SYNDROMES

The elevation of granulocyte, platelet, and eosinophil counts in most patients with myeloproliferative disorders is caused by the proliferation of the myeloid elements due to the underlying disease rather than a paraneoplastic syndrome. The paraneoplastic hematologic syndromes in patients with solid tumors are less well characterized than the endocrine syndromes because the ectopic hormone(s) or cytokines responsible have not been identified in most of these tumors (Table 96-2). The extent of the paraneoplastic syndromes parallels the course of the cancer.

ERYTHROCYTOSIS

Ectopic production of erythropoietin by cancer cells causes most paraneoplastic erythrocytosis. The ectopically produced erythropoietin stimulates the production of red blood cells (RBC) in the bone marrow and raises the hematocrit. Other lymphokines and hormones produced by cancer cells may stimulate erythropoietin release but have not been proven to cause erythrocytosis.

TABLE 96-2 PARANEOPLASTIC HEMATOLOGIC SYNDROMES

Syndrome	Proteins	Cancers Typically Associated with Syndrome
Erythrocytosis	Erythropoietin	Renal cancers Hepatocarcinoma Cerebellar hemangioblastomas
Granulocytosis	G-CSF GM-CSF IL-6	Lung cancer Gastrointestinal cancer Ovarian cancer Genitourinary cancer Hodgkin's disease
Thrombocytosis	IL-6	Lung cancer Gastrointestinal cancer Breast cancer Ovarian cancer Lymphoma
Eosinophilia	IL-5	Lymphoma Leukemia Lung cancer
Thrombophlebitis	Unknown	Lung cancer Pancreatic cancer Gastrointestinal cancer Breast cancer Genitourinary cancer Ovarian cancer Prostate cancer Lymphoma

Note: G-CSF, granulocyte colony-stimulating factor; GM-CSF, granulocyte-macrophage CSF; IL, interleukin.

Most patients with erythrocytosis have an elevated hematocrit (>52% in men; >48% in women) that is detected on a routine blood count. Approximately 3% of patients with renal cell cancer, 10% of patients with hepatoma, and 15% of patients with cerebellar hemangioblastomas have erythrocytosis. In most cases the erythrocytosis is asymptomatic.

Patients with erythrocytosis due to a renal cell cancer, hepatoma, or CNS cancer should have measurement of red cell mass. If the red cell mass is elevated, the serum erythropoietin level should then be measured. Patients with an appropriate cancer, elevated erythropoietin levels, and no other explanation for erythrocytosis (e.g., hemoglobinopathy that causes increased O_2 affinity; Chap. 58) have the paraneoplastic syndrome.

℞ ERYTHROCYTOSIS

Successful resection of the cancer usually resolves the erythrocytosis. If the tumor cannot be resected or treated effectively with radiation therapy or chemotherapy, phlebotomy may control any symptoms related to erythrocytosis.

GRANULOCYTOSIS

Approximately 30% of patients with solid tumors have granulocytosis (granulocyte count > 8000/μL). In about half of patients with granulocytosis and cancer, the granulocytosis has an identifiable nonparaneoplastic etiology (infection, tumor necrosis, glucocorticoid administration, etc.). The other patients have proteins in urine and serum that stimulate the growth of bone marrow cells. Tumors and tumor cell lines from patients with lung, ovarian, and bladder cancers have been documented to produce granulocyte colony-stimulating factor (G-CSF), granulocyte-macrophage colony-stimulating factor (GM-CSF), and/or interleukin 6 (IL-6). However, the etiology of granulocytosis has not been characterized in most patients.

Patients with granulocytosis are nearly all asymptomatic, and the differential white blood cell count does not have a shift to immature forms of neutrophils. Granulocytosis occurs in 40% of patients with lung and gastrointestinal cancers, 20% of patients with breast cancer, 30% of patients with brain tumors and ovarian cancers, 20% of patients with Hodgkin's disease, and 10% of patients with renal cell carcinoma. Patients with advanced-stage disease are more likely to have granulocytosis than those with early-stage disease.

Paraneoplastic granulocytosis does not require treatment. The granulocytosis resolves when the underlying cancer is treated.

THROMBOCYTOSIS

Some 35% of patients with thrombocytosis (platelet count > 400,000/μL) have an underlying diagnosis of cancer. IL-6, a candidate molecule for the etiology of paraneoplastic thrombocytosis, stimulates the production of platelets in vitro and in vivo. Some patients with cancer and thrombocytosis have elevated levels of IL-6 in plasma. Another candidate molecule is thrombopoietin, a peptide hormone that stimulates megakaryocyte proliferation and platelet production. The etiology of thrombocytosis has not been established in most cases.

Patients with thrombocytosis are nearly all asymptomatic. Thrombocytosis is not clearly linked to thrombosis in patients with cancer. Thrombocytosis is present in 40% of patients with lung and gastrointestinal cancers, 20% of patients with breast, endometrial, and ovarian cancers, and 10% of patients with lymphoma. Patients with thrombocytosis are more likely to have advanced-stage disease and have a poorer prognosis than patients without thrombocytosis. Paraneoplastic thrombocytosis does not require treatment.

EOSINOPHILIA

Eosinophilia is present in ~1% of patients with cancer. Tumors and tumor cell lines from patients with lymphomas or leukemia may produce IL-5, which stimulates eosinophil growth. Activation of IL-5 transcription in lymphomas and leukemias may involve translocation of the long arm of chromosome 5, to which the genes for IL-5 and other cytokines map.

Patients with eosinophilia are typically asymptomatic. Eosinophilia is present in 10% of patients with lymphoma, 3% of patients with lung cancer, and occasional patients with cervical, gastrointestinal, renal, and breast cancer. Patients with markedly elevated eosinophil counts (>5000/μL) can develop shortness of breath and wheezing. A chest radiograph may reveal diffuse pulmonary infiltrates from eosinophil infiltration and activation in the lungs.

Rx EOSINOPHILIA

Definitive treatment is directed at the underlying malignancy: tumors should be resected or treated with radiation or chemotherapy. In most patients who develop shortness of breath related to eosinophilia, symptoms resolve with the use of oral or inhaled glucocorticoids.

THROMBOPHLEBITIS

Deep venous thrombosis and pulmonary embolism are the most common thrombotic conditions in patients with cancer. Migratory or recurrent thrombophlebitis may be the initial manifestation of cancer. Nearly 15% of patients who develop deep venous thrombosis or pulmonary embolism have a diagnosis of cancer (Chap. 111). The coexistence of peripheral venous thrombosis with visceral carcinoma, particularly pancreatic cancer, is called *Trousseau's syndrome.*

Pathogenesis Patients with cancer are predisposed to thromboembolism because they are often at bedrest or immobilized, and tumors may obstruct or slow blood flow. Chronic IV catheters also predispose to clotting. In addition, clotting may be promoted by release of procoagulants or cytokines from tumor cells or associated inflammatory cells, or by platelet adhesion or aggregation. The specific molecules that promote thromboembolism have not been identified.

In addition to cancer causing secondary thrombosis, primary thrombophilic diseases may be associated with cancer. For example, the antiphospholipid antibody syndrome is associated with a wide range of pathologic manifestations. About 20% of patients with this syndrome have cancers. Among patients with cancer and antiphospholipid antibodies, 35–45% develop thrombosis.

Clinical Manifestations Patients with cancer who develop deep venous thrombosis usually develop swelling or pain in the leg, and physical examination reveals tenderness, warmth, and redness. Patients who present with pulmonary embolism develop dyspnea, chest pain, and syncope, and physical examination shows tachycardia, cyanosis, and hypotension. Some 5% of patients with no history of cancer who have a diagnosis of deep venous thrombosis or pulmonary embolism will have a diagnosis of cancer within 1 year. The most common cancers associated with thromboembolic episodes include lung, pancreatic, gastrointestinal, breast, ovarian, and genitourinary cancers, lymphomas, and brain tumors. Patients with cancer who undergo surgical procedures requiring general anesthesia have a 20–30% risk of deep venous thrombosis.

Diagnosis The diagnosis of deep venous thrombosis in patients with cancer is made by impedance plethysmography or bilateral compression ultrasonography of the leg veins. Patients with a noncompressible venous segment have deep venous thrombosis. If compression ultrasonography is normal and a high clinical suspicion exists for deep venous thrombosis, venography should be done to look for a luminal filling defect. Elevation of D-dimer is not as predictive of deep venous thrombosis in patients with cancer as it is in patients without cancer.

Patients with symptoms and signs suggesting a pulmonary embolism should be evaluated with a chest radiograph, electrocardiogram, arterial blood gas analysis, and ventilation–perfusion scan. Patients with mismatched segmental perfusion defects have a pulmonary embolus. Patients with equivocal ventilation–perfusion findings should be evaluated as described above for deep venous thrombosis in their legs. If deep venous thrombosis is detected, they should be anticoagulated. If deep venous thrombosis is not detected, they should be considered for a pulmonary angiogram.

Patients without a diagnosis of cancer who present with an initial episode of thrombophlebitis or pulmonary embolus need no additional tests for cancer other than a careful history and physical examination. In light of the many possible primary sites, diagnostic testing in asymptomatic patients is wasteful. However, if the clot is refractory to standard treatment or is in an unusual site, or if the thrombophlebitis is migratory or recurrent, efforts to find an underlying cancer are indicated.

Rx THROMBOPHLEBITIS

Patients with cancer and a diagnosis of deep venous thrombosis or pulmonary embolism should be treated initially with IV unfractionated heparin or low-molecular-weight heparin for at least 5 days and warfarin started within 1 or 2 days. The warfarin dose should be adjusted so the international normalized ratio (INR) is 2–3. Patients with proximal deep venous thrombosis and a relative contraindication to heparin anticoagulation (hemorrhagic brain metastases or pericardial effusion) should be considered for placement of a filter in the inferior vena cava (Greenfield filter) to prevent pulmonary embolism. Warfarin should be administered for 3–6 months. An alternative approach is to use low-molecular-weight heparin for 6 months. Patients with cancer who undergo a major surgical procedure should be considered for heparin prophylaxis or pneumatic boots. Breast cancer patients undergoing chemotherapy and patients with implanted catheters should be considered for prophylaxis (1 mg/d warfarin).

Cutaneous paraneoplastic syndromes are discussed in Chap. 54. Neurologic paraneoplastic syndromes are discussed in Chap. 97.

FURTHER READINGS

AL-TOURAH AJ et al: Paraneoplastic erythropoietin-induced polycythemia associated with small lymphocytic lymphoma. J Clin Oncol 24:2388, 2006

DELELLIS RA, XIA L: Paraneoplastic endocrine syndromes: A review. Endocr Pathol 14:303, 2003

EMEL EA et al: Sensitivity of fibroblast growth factor 23 measurements in tumor-induced osteomalacia. J Clin Endocrinol Metab 91:2055, 2006

GABRILOVICH M et al: Paraneoplastic polymyositis associated with squamous cell carcinoma of the lung. Chest 129(6):1721, 2006

JAN DE BEUR SM: Tumor-induced osteomalacia. JAMA 294:1260, 2005

JONES PA, BAYLIN SB: The fundamental role of epigenetic events in cancer. Nat Rev Genet 3:415, 2002

STEWART AF: Clinical practice. Hypercalcemia associated with cancer. N Engl J Med 352:373, 2005

97 Paraneoplastic Neurologic Syndromes

Josep Dalmau, Myrna R. Rosenfeld

Paraneoplastic neurologic disorders (PNDs) are cancer-related syndromes that can affect any part of the nervous system (Table 97-1). They are remote effects of cancer, caused by mechanisms other than metastasis or by any of the complications of cancer such as coagulopathy, stroke, metabolic and nutritional conditions, infections, and side effects of cancer therapy. In 60% of patients the neurologic symptoms precede the cancer diagnosis. Overall, clinically disabling PNDs occur in 0.5–1% of all cancer patients, but they occur in 2–3% of patients with neuroblastoma or small cell lung cancer (SCLC), and in 30–50% of patients with thymoma or sclerotic myeloma.

PATHOGENESIS

Most PNDs are mediated by immune responses triggered by neuronal proteins (onconeuronal antigens) expressed by tumors. In PNDs of the central nervous system (CNS), many antibody-associated immune responses have been identified (Table 97-2). These antibodies usually react with the patient's tumor, and their detection in serum or cerebrospinal fluid (CSF) strongly predicts the presence of cancer. The target antigens are usually intracellular proteins with roles in neuronal development and function. Some of the antibodies react with epitopes located in critical protein domains, disrupting protein function and leading to neuronal apoptosis. In addition to onconeuronal antibodies, most PNDs of the CNS are associated with infiltrates of CD4+ and CD8+ T cells, microglial activation, gliosis, and variable neuronal loss. The infiltrating T cells are often in close contact with neurons undergoing degeneration, suggesting a primary pathogenic role. T cell–mediated cytotoxicity may contribute directly to cell death in these PNDs. Thus both humoral and cellular immune mechanisms participate in the pathogenesis of many PNDs. This complex immunopathogenesis may underlie the resistance of many of these conditions to therapy.

Neuronal cell-surface antigens can be the target of antibodies in some patients with paraneoplastic encephalitis. A few of these antigens have been identified, including the NR1/NR2 subunits of NMDA receptors (Fig. 97-1) and voltage-gated potassium channels (VGKC). These disorders are more responsive to immunotherapy than those associated with immune responses to intracellular antigens.

Only four of the antibodies listed in Table 97-2 have been shown to play a direct pathogenic role in PNDs; all produce distinctive disorders of the peripheral nervous system. These are: antibodies to P/Q-type voltage-gated calcium channels (VGCC) in patients with the Lambert-Eaton myasthenic syndrome (LEMS); antibodies to acetylcholine receptors in patients with myasthenia gravis; antibodies to VGKC in some patients with peripheral nerve hyperexcitability (neuromyotonia); and antibodies to ganglionic acetylcholine receptors in some patients with autonomic neuropathy. Common features of these four antibodies are that they target cell-surface molecules and that their passive transfer to animals reproduces the disorders. Plasma exchange or immunomodulation with intravenous immunoglobulin (IVIg) usually produces neurologic improvement. Each of these disorders can occur without cancer, and therefore detection of these antibodies does not predict the presence of cancer.

Other PNDs are likely immune-mediated, although their antigens are unknown. These include several syndromes of inflammatory neuropathies and myopathies. In addition, many patients with typical PND syndromes are antibody-negative.

For still other PNDs, the cause remains quite obscure. These include, among others, several neuropathies that occur in the terminal stages of cancer and a number of neuropathies associated with plasma cell dyscrasias or lymphoma without evidence of inflammatory infiltrates or deposits of immunoglobulin, cryoglobulin, or amyloid.

TABLE 97-1 PARANEOPLASTIC SYNDROMES OF THE NERVOUS SYSTEM

Syndromes of the brain, brainstem, and cerebellum
Focal encephalitis
Cortical encephalitis
Limbic encephalitis
Brainstem encephalitis
Cerebellar dysfunction
Autonomic dysfunction
Paraneoplastic cerebellar degeneration
Opsoclonus-myoclonus
Syndromes of the spinal cord
Subacute necrotizing myelopathy
Motor neuron dysfunction
Myelitis
Stiff-person syndrome
Syndromes of dorsal root ganglia
Sensory neuronopathy
Multiple levels of involvement
Encephalomyelitis,[a] sensory neuronopathy, autonomic dysfunction
Syndromes of peripheral nerve
Chronic and subacute sensorimotor peripheral neuropathy
Vasculitis of nerve and muscle
Neuropathy associated with malignant monoclonal gammopathies
Peripheral nerve hyperexcitability
Autonomic neuropathy
Syndromes of the neuromuscular junction
Lambert-Eaton myasthenic syndrome
Myasthenia gravis
Syndromes of the muscle
Polymyositis/dermatomyositis
Acute necrotizing myopathy
Syndromes affecting the visual system
Cancer-associated retinopathy (CAR)
Melanoma-associated retinopathy (MAR)
Uveitis (usually in association with encephalomyelitis)

[a]Includes cortical, limbic, or brainstem encephalitis, cerebellar dysfunction, myelitis.

APPROACH TO THE PATIENT: Paraneoplastic Neurologic Disorders

The diagnosis and management of PNDs may be difficult for several reasons. First, it is common for symptoms to appear before the presence of a tumor is known. Second, the neurologic syndrome can evolve in a rapidly progressive fashion, producing a severe and usually irreversible neurologic deficit in a short period of time. There is evidence that prompt tumor control improves the course of PNDs. Therefore, the major concern of the physician is to recognize a disorder promptly as paraneoplastic in order to identify and treat the tumor.

PND OF THE CENTRAL NERVOUS SYSTEM AND DORSAL ROOT GANGLIA

When symptoms involve brain, spinal cord, or dorsal root ganglia, the suspicion of PND is usually based on a combination of clinical, radiologic, and CSF findings. In these cases, a biopsy of the affected tissue is often difficult to obtain, and although useful to rule out other disorders (e.g., metastasis, infection), neuropathologic findings are

TABLE 97-2 PARANEOPLASTIC ANTINEURONAL ANTIBODIES, ASSOCIATED SYNDROMES AND CANCERS

Antibody	Syndrome	Associated Cancers
Anti-Hu (ANNA-1)	PEM (including cortical, limbic, brainstem encephalitis, cerebellar dysfunction, myelitis), PSN, autonomic dysfunction	SCLC, other neuroendocrine tumors
Anti-Yo (PCA-1)	PCD	Ovary and other gynecologic cancers, breast
Anti-Ri (ANNA-2)	PCD, brainstem encephalitis, opsoclonus-myoclonus	Breast, gynecological, SCLC
Anti-Tr	PCD	Hodgkin's lymphoma
Anti-Zic	PCD, encephalomyelitis	SCLC and other neuroendocrine tumors
Anti-CV_2/CRMP5	PEM, PCD, chorea, peripheral neuropathy, uveitis	SCLC, thymoma, other
Anti-Ma proteins[a]	Limbic, hypothalamic, brainstem encephalitis (infrequently PCD)	Germ-cell tumors of testis, lung cancer, other solid tumors
Anti-NR1/NR2 subunits of NMDA receptor	Encephalitis with prominent psychiatric symptoms, seizures, hypoventilation	Ovarian teratoma
Anti-amphiphysin	Stiff-person syndrome, PEM	Breast, SCLC
Anti-VGCC[b]	LEMS, PCD	SCLC, lymphoma
Anti-AChR[b]	MG	Thymoma
Anti-VGKC[b]	Peripheral nerve hyperexcitability (neuromyotonia), limbic encephalitis	Thymoma, SCLC, others
Anti-recoverin	Cancer-associated retinopathy (CAR)	SCLC and other
Anti-bipolar cells of the retina	Melanoma-associated retinopathy (MAR)	Melanoma

[a]Patients with antibodies to Ma2 are usually men with testicular cancer. Patients with additional antibodies to other Ma proteins are men or women with a variety of solid tumors.

[b]These antibodies can occur with or without a cancer association.

Note: PEM: paraneoplastic encephalomyelitis; PCD, paraneoplastic cerebellar degeneration; PSN, paraneoplastic sensory neuronopathy; LEMS, Lambert-Eaton myasthenic syndrome; MG, myasthenia gravis; VGCC, voltage-gated calcium channel; AChR, acetylcholine receptor; VGKC, voltage-gated potassium channel; SCLC, small-cell lung cancer; NMDA, *N*-methyl-D-aspartate.

not specific for PND. Furthermore, there are no specific radiologic or electrophysiologic tests that are diagnostic of PND. The presence of antineuronal antibodies (Table 97-2) may help in the diagnosis with the following caveats: (1) antibodies are detected in only 60–70% of PNDs of the CNS; (2) antibodies may be present in both the serum and CSF, but in some patients only the CSF is positive (especially with antibodies to Tr and Ma proteins); (3) antibodies (usually at low titer) are present in a variable proportion of cancer patients without PND; (4) there is an imperfect correlation between antibody titers and the course of the neurologic disorder; (5) several antibodies may associate with a similar syndrome, with the antibody specificity often correlating with the tumor type (e.g., cerebellar degeneration is associated with anti-Tr antibodies if the tumor is Hodgkin's disease but with anti-Yo antibodies if the tumor is ovarian or breast cancer); and (6) several antibodies may be present in the serum or CSF of the same patient (e.g., anti-Hu and anti-CV_2/CRMP5).

MRI and CSF studies are important to rule out neurologic complications due to the direct spread of cancer, particularly metastatic and leptomeningeal disease. In most PNDs the MRI findings are nonspecific. Paraneoplastic limbic encephalitis is usually associated with characteristic MRI abnormalities in the mesial temporal lobes (see below), but similar findings can occur with other disorders [e.g., nonparaneoplastic limbic encephalitis with antibodies to VGKC, human herpesvirus (HHV) 6 encephalitis] (Fig. 97-2). The CSF profile of patients with PND of the CNS or dorsal root ganglia typically consists of mild to moderate pleocytosis (<200 mononuclear cells, predominantly lymphocytes), an increase in the protein concentration, intrathecal synthesis of IgG, and a variable presence of oligoclonal bands.

PND OF NERVE AND MUSCLE If symptoms involve peripheral nerve, neuromuscular junction, or muscle, the diagnosis of a specific PND is usually established on clinical, electrophysiologic, and pathologic grounds. The clinical history, accompanying symptoms (e.g., anorexia, weight loss), and type of syndrome dictate the studies and degree of effort needed to demonstrate a neoplasm. For ex-

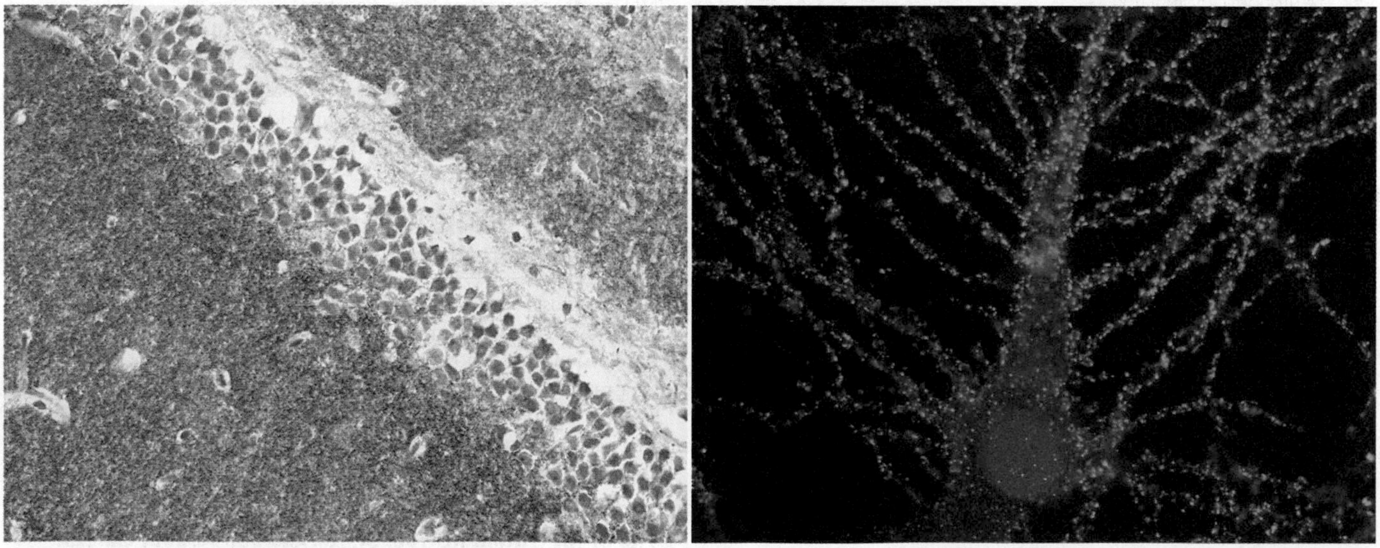

A B

FIGURE 97-1 Antibodies to NR1/NR2 subunits of the NMDA receptor in a patient with paraneoplastic encephalitis and ovarian teratoma. ***Panel A*** is a section of dentate gyrus of rat hippocampus immunolabeled (brown staining) with the patient's antibodies. The reactivity predominates in the molecular layer, which is highly enriched in dendritic processes. ***Panel B*** shows the antibody reactivity with cultures of rat hippocampal neurons; the intense green immunolabeling is due to the antibodies against the NR1/NR2 subunits of NMDA receptors.

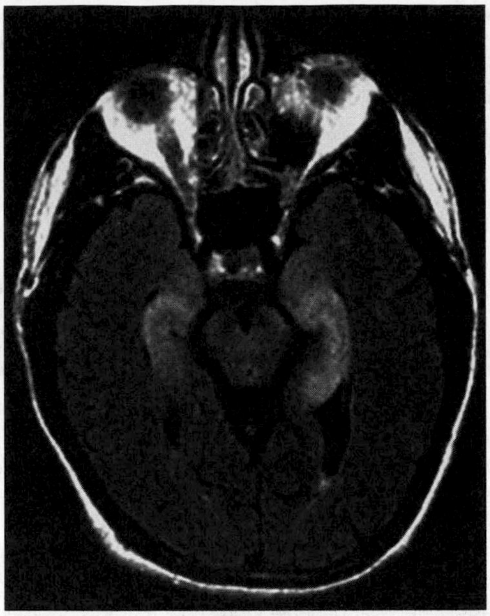

FIGURE 97-2 Fluid-attenuated inversion recovery sequence MRI of a patient with limbic encephalitis and voltage-gated potassium channel antibodies. Note the abnormal hyperintensity involving the medial aspect of the temporal lobes.

ample, the frequent association of LEMS with SCLC should lead to a chest and abdomen CT or body positron emission tomography (PET) scan and, if negative, periodic tumor screening for at least 3 years after the neurologic diagnosis. In contrast, the weak association of polymyositis with cancer calls into question the need for repeated cancer screenings in this situation. Serum and urine immunofixation studies should be considered in patients with peripheral neuropathy of unknown cause; detection of a monoclonal gammopathy suggests the need for additional studies to uncover a B cell or plasma cell malignancy. In paraneoplastic neuropathies, diagnostically useful antineuronal antibodies are limited to anti-CV_2/CRMP5 and anti-Hu.

For any type of PND, if antineuronal antibodies are negative, the diagnosis relies on the demonstration of cancer and the exclusion of other cancer-related or independent neurologic disorders. Body PET scans often uncover tumors undetected by other tests.

SPECIFIC PARANEOPLASTIC NEUROLOGIC SYNDROMES (Table 97-3)

PARANEOPLASTIC ENCEPHALOMYELITIS AND FOCAL ENCEPHALITIS

The term *encephalomyelitis* describes an inflammatory process with multifocal involvement of the nervous system, including brain, brainstem, cerebellum, and spinal cord. It is often associated with dorsal root ganglia and autonomic dysfunction. For any given patient, the clinical manifestations are determined by the area or areas predominantly involved, but pathology almost always reveals abnormalities (inflammatory infiltrates, neuronal loss, gliosis) beyond the symptomatic regions. Several clinicopathologic syndromes may occur alone or in combination: (1) *cortical encephalitis*, which may present as "epilepsia partialis continua"; (2) *limbic encephalitis*, characterized by confusion, depression, agitation, anxiety, severe short-term memory deficits, partial complex seizures, and dementia; the MRI usually shows unilateral or bilateral medial temporal lobe abnormalities, best seen with T2 and fluid-attenuated inversion recovery sequences, and occasionally enhancing with gadolinium; (3) *brainstem encephalitis*, resulting in eye movement disorders (nystagmus, opsoclonus, supranuclear or nuclear paresis), cranial nerve paresis, dysarthria, dysphagia, and central autonomic dysfunction; (4) *cerebellar gait and limb ataxia*; (5) *myelitis*, which may cause lower or upper motor neuron symptoms, myoclonus, muscle rigidity, and spasms; and (6) *autonomic dysfunction* as a result of involvement of the neuraxis at multiple levels, including hypothalamus, brainstem, and autonomic nerves (see autonomic neuropathy). Cardiac arrhythmias, postural hypotension, or central hypoventilation are frequent causes of death in patients with encephalomyelitis.

Paraneoplastic encephalomyelitis and focal encephalitis are usually associated with SCLC, but many other cancers have also been reported. Patients with SCLC and these syndromes usually have anti-Hu antibodies in serum and CSF. Anti-CV_2/CRMP5 antibodies occur less frequently; some of these patients may develop chorea or uveitis. Antibodies to Ma proteins are associated with limbic, hypothalamic and brainstem encephalitis and occasionally with cerebellar symptoms (Fig. 97-3); some patients develop hypersomnia, cataplexy, and severe hypokinesia. MRI abnormalities are frequent, including those described with limbic encephalitis and variable

TABLE 97-3 ANTIBODY-ASSOCIATED PARANEOPLASTIC AND NONPARANEOPLASTIC SYNDROMES[a]

	Antibodies		
	Paraneoplastic		
Syndrome	**Frequent**	**Infrequent**	**Nonparaneoplastic**
Limbic encephalitis	Ma2, Hu, CV_2/CRMP5, *anti-NR1/NR2 of NMDA receptor*	Tr, VGKC	VGKC
Cerebellar degeneration	Yo, Tr, P/Q VGCC, Hu, Zic, Ri, CV_2/CRMP5, Ma1-2	*mGluR1*; *MAZ*	Gliadin, GAD
Hypothalamic, brainstem encephalitis	Ma2, Hu	CV_2/CRMP5	
Encephalomyelitis	Hu, Zic	CV_2/CRMP5, Ri, amphiphysin	
Chorea	CV_2/CRMP5		
Opsoclonus-myoclonus	Ri	Hu, Ma2, Yo,	
Stiff-person syndrome	Amphiphysin	*Gephyrin*, Ri	GAD
PNH (neuromyotonia)	VGKC		VGKC
Myasthenia gravis	AChR		AChR, MuSK
LEMS	P/Q-type VGCC	*MysB*	P/Q-type VGCC
Sensory neuronopathy	Hu		
Axonal sensorimotor neuropathy	Hu, CV_2/CRMP5		Monoclonal gammopathy (M protein)[b]
Autonomic neuropathy	Hu	CV_2/CRMP5, ganglionic AChR	Ganglionic AChR
Predominant sensory demyelinating neuropathy		MAG, ganglioside antibodies: often present with Waldenström's macroglobulinemia	MAG, ganglioside antibodies, often present with MGUS
Paraneoplastic retinopathy	Recoverin (CAR), anti-bipolar cell antibodies (*MAR*), *anti-enolase*	*Tubby-like protein 1*, *PNR*	*Anti-enolase*

[a]Antibodies have been validated by more than one laboratory and/or the protein sequence of the target antigen is known.

[b]The M protein usually does not have specific antibody activity.

Note: *Italics* indicate that commercial testing for these antibodies is not available. PNH, peripheral nerve hyperexcitability; CAR, cancer-associated retinopathy; MAR, melanoma-associated retinopathy; PNR, photoreceptor-specific nuclear receptor; MGUS, monoclonal gammopathy of uncertain significance; VGKC, voltage-gated potassium channel; GAD, glutamic acid decarboxylase; AChR, acetylcholine receptor; LEMS, Lambert-Eaton myasthenic syndrome; VGCC, voltage-gated calcium channel; MAG, myelin-associated glycoprotein; NMDA, *N*-methyl-D-aspartate.

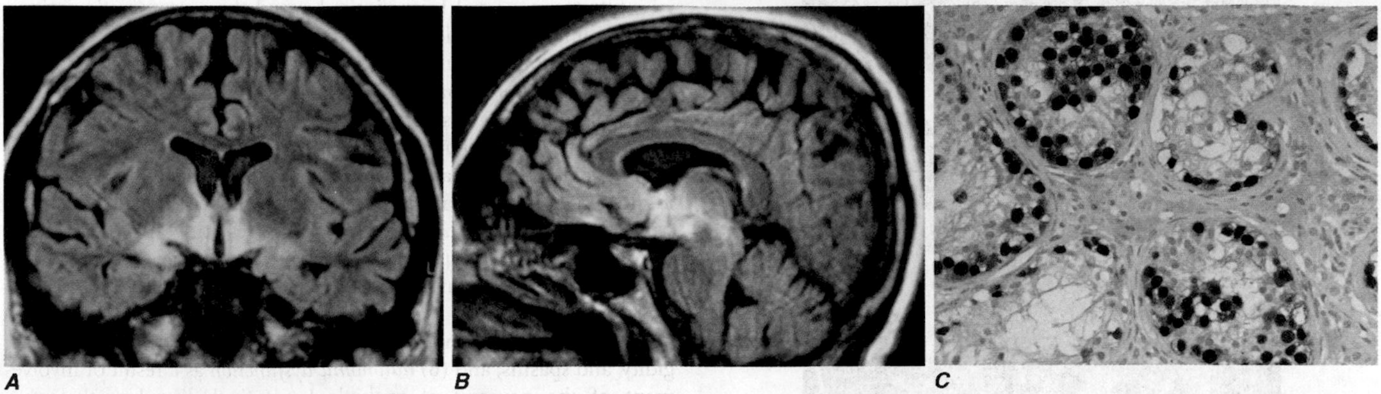

FIGURE 97-3 MRI and tumor of a patient with anti-Ma2-associated encephalitis. ***Panels A*** and ***B*** are fluid-attenuated inversion recovery MRI sequences showing abnormal hyperintensities in the medial temporal lobes, hypothalamus and upper brainstem. ***Panel C*** corresponds to a section of the patient's orchiectomy incubated with a specific marker (Oct4) of germ-cell tumors. The positive (brown) cells correspond to an intratubular germ-cell neoplasm.

involvement of the hypothalamus, basal ganglia, or upper brainstem. Antibodies to NR1/NR2 subunits of the NMDA receptor associate with a severe, potentially lethal, but treatment-responsive encephalitis. The affected patients are young women who develop combinations of psychiatric symptoms, seizures, dyskinesias, stupor and hypoventilation. The oncologic associations of these antibodies are shown in Table 97-2.

Rx ENCEPHALITIS AND ENCEPHALOMYELITIS

Most types of paraneoplastic encephalitis and encephalomyelitis respond poorly to treatment. Stabilization of symptoms or partial neurologic improvement may occasionally occur, particularly if there is a satisfactory response of the tumor to treatment. The roles of plasma exchange, IVIg, and immunosuppression have not been established. Approximately 30% of patients with anti-Ma2-associated encephalitis respond to treatment of the tumor (usually a germ-cell neoplasm of the testis) and immunotherapy. Two other syndromes that are responsive to treatment of the tumor and immunotherapy are the encephalitis that associates with antibodies to the NR1/NR2 subunits of NMDA receptors in patients with teratoma of the ovary, and the encephalitis that associates with VGKC antibodies in some patients with thymoma or SCLC.

PARANEOPLASTIC CEREBELLAR DEGENERATION

This disorder is often preceded by a prodrome that may include dizziness, oscillopsia, blurry or double vision, nausea, and vomiting. A few days or weeks later, dysarthria, gait and limb ataxia, and variable dysphagia can appear. The examination usually shows downbeating nystagmus and, rarely, opsoclonus. Brainstem dysfunction, upgoing toes, or a mild neuropathy may occur, but more often the symptoms and signs are restricted to the cerebellum. Early in the course, MRI studies are usually normal; later, the MRI typically reveals cerebellar atrophy. The disorder results from extensive degeneration of Purkinje cells, with variable involvement of other cerebellar cortical neurons, deep cerebellar nuclei, and spinocerebellar tracts. The tumors more frequently involved are SCLC, cancer of the breast and ovary, and Hodgkin's lymphoma.

Anti-Yo antibodies in patients with breast and gynecologic cancers and anti-Tr antibodies in patients with Hodgkin's lymphoma are the two paraneoplastic antibodies typically associated with prominent or pure cerebellar degeneration. Antibodies to P/Q-type VGCC occur in some patients with SCLC and cerebellar dysfunction; only some of these patients develop LEMS. Of note, a variable degree of cerebellar dysfunction can be associated with virtually any type of antibody-related PND of the CNS (Table 97-2).

Rx CEREBELLAR DEGENERATION

A number of single case reports have described neurologic improvement after tumor removal, plasma exchange, IVIg, cyclophosphamide, rituximab, or glucocorticoids. However, large series of patients with antibody-positive paraneoplastic cerebellar degeneration show that this disorder rarely improves with any treatment.

PARANEOPLASTIC OPSOCLONUS-MYOCLONUS SYNDROME

Opsoclonus is a disorder of eye movement characterized by involuntary, chaotic saccades that occur in all directions of gaze; it is frequently associated with myoclonus and ataxia. Opsoclonus-myoclonus may be cancer-related or idiopathic. When the cause is paraneoplastic, the tumors involved are usually cancer of the lung and breast in adults and neuroblastoma in children. The pathologic substrate of opsoclonus-myoclonus is unclear. Most SCLC patients do not have detectable antineuronal antibodies. A small subset of patients with ataxia, opsoclonus, and other eye movement disorders develop anti-Ri antibodies; in rare instances muscle rigidity, autonomic dysfunction, and dementia also occur. The tumor most frequently involved in anti-Ri-associated syndromes is breast cancer.

If the tumor is not successfully treated, the paraneoplastic opsoclonus-myoclonus syndrome in adults often progresses to encephalopathy, coma, and death. In addition to treating the tumor, symptoms may respond to immunotherapy (glucocorticoids, plasma exchange, and/or IVIg).

At least 50% of children with opsoclonus-myoclonus have an underlying neuroblastoma. Hypotonia, ataxia, behavioral changes, and irritability are frequent accompanying symptoms. Many patients harbor antibodies to neuronal cell surface antigens of unknown identity. Neurologic symptoms often improve with treatment of the tumor (including chemotherapy) and with glucocorticoids, adrenocorticotropic hormone (ACTH), plasma exchange, IVIg, and rituximab. Many patients are left with psychomotor retardation and behavioral and sleep problems.

PARANEOPLASTIC SYNDROMES OF THE SPINAL CORD

The number of reports of paraneoplastic spinal cord syndromes, such as *subacute motor neuronopathy* and *acute necrotizing myelopathy*, has decreased in recent years. This may represent a true decrease in incidence, due to improved and prompt oncologic interventions, or may be because of the identification of nonparaneoplastic etiologies.

Some patients with cancer develop *upper* or *lower motor neuron dysfunction* or both, resembling amyotrophic lateral sclerosis. It is unclear whether these disorders have a paraneoplastic etiology or simply coincide with the presence of cancer. There are isolated case reports of cancer patients with motor neuron dysfunction who had neurologic improvement after tumor treatment. A more than coincidental association occurs between lymphoma and motor neuron dysfunction. A search for lymphoma should be undertaken in patients with a motor neuron syndrome who are found to have a monoclonal protein in serum or CSF.

Paraneoplastic myelitis may present with upper or lower motor neuron symptoms, segmental myoclonus, and rigidity. This syndrome can appear as the presenting manifestation of encephalomyelitis and may be associated with SCLC and serum anti-Hu, anti-CV_2/CRMP5, or anti-amphiphysin antibodies.

Paraneoplastic myelopathy can also produce several syndromes characterized by prominent muscle stiffness and rigidity. The spectrum ranges from focal symptoms in one or several extremities (*stiff-limb syndrome* or *stiff-person syndrome*) to a disorder that also affects the brainstem (known as *encephalomyelitis with rigidity*) and likely has a different pathogenesis.

PARANEOPLASTIC STIFF-PERSON SYNDROME

This disorder is characterized by progressive muscle rigidity, stiffness, and painful spasms triggered by auditory, sensory, or emotional stimuli. Rigidity mainly involves the lower trunk and legs, but it can affect the upper extremities and neck. Symptoms improve with sleep and general anesthetics. Electrophysiologic studies demonstrate continuous motor unit activity. Antibodies associated with the stiff-person syndrome target proteins [glutamic acid decarboxylase (GAD), amphiphysin] involved in the function of inhibitory synapses utilizing γ-aminobutyric acid (GABA) or glycine as neurotransmitters. Paraneoplastic stiff-person syndrome and amphiphysin antibodies are often related to breast cancer. By contrast, antibodies to GAD may occur in some cancer patients but are much more frequently present in the nonparaneoplastic disorder.

Rx STIFF-PERSON SYNDROME

Optimal treatment of stiff-person syndrome requires therapy of the underlying tumor, glucocorticoids, and symptomatic use of drugs that enhance GABA-ergic transmission (diazepam, baclofen, sodium valproate, tiagabine, vigabatrin). A benefit of IVIg has been demonstrated for the nonparaneoplastic disorder but remains to be established for the paraneoplastic syndrome.

PARANEOPLASTIC SENSORY NEURONOPATHY OR DORSAL ROOT GANGLIONOPATHY

This syndrome is characterized by sensory deficits that may be symmetric or asymmetric, painful dysesthesias, radicular pain, and decreased or absent reflexes. All modalities of sensation and any part of the body including face and trunk can be involved. Specialized sensations such as taste and hearing can also be affected. Electrophysiologic studies show decreased or absent sensory nerve potentials with normal or near-normal motor conduction velocities. Symptoms result from an inflammatory, likely immune-mediated, process that targets the dorsal root ganglia, causing neuronal loss, proliferation of satellite cells, and secondary degeneration of the posterior columns of the spinal cord. The dorsal nerve roots, and less frequently the anterior nerve roots and peripheral nerves, may also be involved.

Rx SENSORY NEUROPATHY

This disorder often precedes or is associated with encephalomyelitis and autonomic dysfunction and has the same immunologic and oncologic associations, e.g., anti-Hu antibodies and SCLC. As with anti-Hu-associated encephalomyelitis, the therapeutic approach focuses on prompt treatment of the tumor. Glucocorticoids occasionally produce clinical stabilization or improvement. The benefit of IVIg and plasma exchange is not proved.

PARANEOPLASTIC PERIPHERAL NEUROPATHIES

These disorders may develop any time during the course of the neoplastic disease. Neuropathies occurring at late stages of cancer or lymphoma usually cause mild to moderate sensorimotor deficits due to axonal degeneration of unclear etiology. These neuropathies are often masked by concurrent neurotoxicity from chemotherapy and other cancer therapies. In contrast, the neuropathies that develop in the early stages of cancer often show a rapid progression, sometimes with a relapsing and remitting course, and evidence of inflammatory infiltrates and axonal loss or demyelination in biopsy studies. If demyelinating features predominate (Chap. 379), IVIg or glucocorticoids may improve symptoms. Occasionally anti-CV_2/CRMP5 antibodies are present; detection of anti-Hu suggests concurrent dorsal root ganglionitis.

Guillain-Barré syndrome and *brachial plexitis* have occasionally been reported in patients with lymphoma, but there is no clear evidence of a paraneoplastic association.

Malignant monoclonal gammopathies include: (1) multiple myeloma and sclerotic myeloma associated with IgG or IgA monoclonal proteins; and (2) Waldenström's macroglobulinemia, B cell lymphoma, and chronic B cell lymphocytic leukemia associated with IgM monoclonal proteins. These disorders may cause neuropathy by a variety of mechanisms, including compression of roots and plexuses by metastasis to vertebral bodies and pelvis, deposits of amyloid in peripheral nerves, and paraneoplastic mechanisms. The paraneoplastic variety has several distinctive features. Approximately half of patients with sclerotic myeloma develop a sensorimotor neuropathy with predominantly motor deficits, resembling a chronic inflammatory demyelinating neuropathy (Chap. 380); some patients develop elements of the POEMS syndrome (*p*olyneuropathy, *o*rganomegaly, *e*ndocrinopathy, *M* protein, *s*kin changes). Treatment of the plasmacytoma or sclerotic lesions usually improves the neuropathy. In contrast, the sensorimotor or sensory neuropathy associated with multiple myeloma rarely responds to treatment. Between 5 and 10% of patients with Waldenström's macroglobulinemia develop a distal symmetric sensorimotor neuropathy with predominant involvement of large sensory fibers. These patients may have IgM antibodies in their serum against myelin-associated glycoprotein and various gangliosides (Chap. 380). In addition to treating the Waldenström's macroglobulinemia, other therapies may improve the neuropathy, including plasma exchange, IVIg, chlorambucil, cyclophosphamide, fludarabine, or rituximab.

Vasculitis of the nerve and muscle causes a painful symmetric or asymmetric distal sensorimotor neuropathy with variable proximal weakness. It predominantly affects elderly men and is associated with an elevated erythrocyte sedimentation rate and increased CSF protein concentration. SCLC and lymphoma are the primary tumors involved. Pathology demonstrates axonal degeneration and T cell infiltrates involving the small vessels of the nerve and muscle. Immunosuppressants (glucocorticoids and cyclophosphamide) often result in neurologic improvement.

Peripheral nerve hyperexcitability (*neuromyotonia,* or *Isaacs' syndrome*) is characterized by spontaneous and continuous muscle fiber activity of peripheral nerve origin. Clinical features include cramps, muscle twitching (fasciculations or myokymia), stiffness, delayed muscle relaxation (pseudomyotonia), and spontaneous or evoked carpal or pedal spasms. The involved muscles may be hypertrophic, and some patients develop paresthesias and hyperhydrosis. CNS dysfunction, including mood changes, sleep disorder, or hallucinations, may occur. The electromyogram (EMG) shows fibrillations; fasciculations; and doublet, triplet, or multiplet single unit (myokymic) discharges that have a high intraburst frequency. An immune pathogenesis is suggested by the frequent presence of serum antibodies to VGKC. The disorder often occurs without cancer; if paraneoplastic, benign and malignant thymomas and SCLC are the usual tumors. Phenytoin, carbamazepine, and plasma exchange improve symptoms.

Paraneoplastic autonomic neuropathy usually develops as a component of other disorders, such as LEMS and encephalomyelitis. It may rarely occur as a pure or predominantly autonomic neuropathy with adrenergic or cholinergic dysfunction at the pre- or postganglionic levels. Patients can develop several life-threatening complications, such as gastrointestinal paresis with pseudoobstruction, cardiac dysrhythmias, and postural hypotension. Other symptoms include dry mouth, erectile dysfunction, anhidrosis, and sphincter dysfunction; abnormal pupillary responses may be found. The disorder has been reported to occur in association with several tumors, including SCLC, cancer of the pancreas or testis, carcinoid tumors, and lymphoma. Because autonomic symptoms can also be the presenting feature of encephalomyelitis, serum anti-Hu and anti-CV_2/CRMP5 antibodies should also be sought. Serum antibodies to ganglionic acetylcholine receptors have been reported in this syndrome, but they also occur without a cancer association. (See Chap. 370.)

LAMBERT-EATON MYASTHENIC SYNDROME

LEMS is discussed in Chap. 381.

MYASTHENIA GRAVIS

Myasthenia gravis is discussed in Chap. 381.

POLYMYOSITIS-DERMATOMYOSITIS

Polymyositis and dermatomyositis are discussed in detail in Chap. 383.

ACUTE NECROTIZING MYOPATHY

Patients with this syndrome develop myalgias and rapid progression of weakness involving the extremities and the pharyngeal and respiratory muscles, often resulting in death. Serum muscle enzymes are elevated, and muscle biopsy shows extensive necrosis with minimal or absent inflammation and sometimes deposits of complement. The disorder occurs as a paraneoplastic manifestation of a variety of cancers including SCLC and cancer of the gastrointestinal tract, breast, kidney, and prostate, among others. Glucocorticoids or treatment of the underlying tumor rarely control the disorder.

PARANEOPLASTIC VISUAL SYNDROMES

This group of disorders involves the retina and, less frequently, the uvea and optic nerves. The term *cancer-associated retinopathy* is used to describe paraneoplastic cone and rod dysfunction characterized by photosensitivity, progressive loss of vision and color perception, central or ring scotomas, night blindness, and attenuation of photopic and scotopic responses in the electroretinogram (ERG). The most commonly associated tumor is SCLC. Melanoma-associated retinopathy affects patients with metastatic cutaneous melanoma. Patients develop the acute onset of night blindness and shimmering, flickering, or pulsating photopsias that often progress to visual loss. The ERG demonstrates reduction in the b-wave amplitude. Paraneoplastic optic neuritis and uveitis are very uncommon and can develop in association with encephalomyelitis. Some patients with paraneoplastic uveitis harbor anti-CV_2/CRMP5 antibodies.

Some paraneoplastic retinopathies are associated with serum antibodies that specifically react with the subset of retinal cells undergoing degeneration, supporting an immune-mediated pathogenesis (Tables 97-2 and 97-3). Paraneoplastic retinopathies usually fail to improve with treatment, although rare responses to glucocorticoids, plasma exchange, and IVIg have been reported.

FURTHER READINGS

ANTOINE JC, CAMDESSANCHÉ JP: Peripheral nervous system involvement in patients with cancer. Lancet Neurol 6:75, 2007

BATALLER L et al: Autoimmune limbic encephalitis in 39 patients: Immunophenotypes and outcomes. J Neurol Neurosurg Psychiatry 78:381, 2007

DALMAU J et al: Paraneoplastic anti-*N*-methyl-D-aspartate receptor encephalitis associated with ovarian teratoma. Ann Neurol 61:25, 2007

MATHEW RM et al: Orchiectomy for suspected microscopic tumor in patients with anti-Ma2-associated encephalitis. Neurology 68:900, 2007

ROSENFELD MR, DALMAU J: Current therapies for neuromuscular manifestations of paraneoplastic syndromes. Curr Neurol Neurosci Rep 6:77, 2006

SECTION 2 HEMATOPOIETIC DISORDERS

98 Iron Deficiency and Other Hypoproliferative Anemias

John W. Adamson

Anemias associated with normocytic and normochromic red cells and an inappropriately low reticulocyte response (reticulocyte index <2.0–2.5) are *hypoproliferative anemias*. This category includes early iron deficiency (before hypochromic microcytic red cells develop), acute and chronic inflammation (including many malignancies), renal disease, hypometabolic states such as protein malnutrition and endocrine deficiencies, and anemias from marrow damage. Marrow damage states are discussed in Chap. 102.

Hypoproliferative anemias are the most common anemias, and anemia associated with acute and chronic inflammation is the most common of these. The anemia of inflammation, like iron deficiency, is related in part to abnormal iron metabolism. The anemias associated with renal disease, inflammation, cancer, and hypometabolic states are characterized by an abnormal erythropoietin response to the anemia.

IRON METABOLISM

Iron is a critical element in the function of all cells, although the amount of iron required by individual tissues varies during development. At the same time, the body must protect itself from free iron, which is highly toxic in that it participates in chemical reactions that generate free radicals such as singlet O_2 or OH^-. Consequently, elaborate mechanisms have evolved that allow iron to be made available for physiologic functions while at the same time conserving this element and handling it in such a way that toxicity is avoided.

The major role of iron in mammals is to carry O_2 as part of hemoglobin. O_2 is also bound by myoglobin in muscle. Iron is a critical element in iron-containing enzymes, including the cytochrome system in mitochondria. Iron distribution in the body is shown in Table 98-1. Without iron, cells lose their capacity for electron transport and energy metabolism. In erythroid cells, hemoglobin synthesis is impaired, resulting in anemia and reduced O_2 delivery to tissue.

THE IRON CYCLE IN HUMANS

Figure 98-1 outlines the major pathways of internal iron exchange in humans. Iron absorbed from the diet or released from stores circulates in the plasma bound to *transferrin*, the iron transport protein. Trans-

TABLE 98-1 BODY IRON DISTRIBUTION

	Iron Content, mg	
	Adult Male, 80 kg	Adult Female, 60 kg
Hemoglobin	2500	1700
Myoglobin/enzymes	500	300
Transferrin iron	3	3
Iron stores	600–1000	0–300

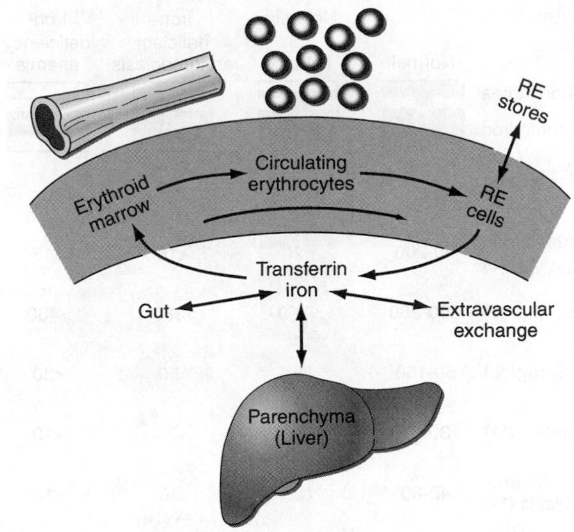

FIGURE 98-1 Internal iron exchange. Normally about 80% of iron passing through the plasma transferrin pool is recycled from broken-down red cells. Absorption of about 1 mg/d is required from the diet in men, 1.4 mg/d in women to maintain homeostasis. As long as transferrin saturation is maintained between 20–60% and erythropoiesis is not increased, iron stores are not required. However, in the event of blood loss, dietary iron deficiency, or inadequate iron absorption, up to 40 mg/d of iron can be mobilized from stores. RE, reticuloendothelial.

ferrin is a bilobed glycoprotein with two iron binding sites. Transferrin that carries iron exists in two forms—*monoferric* (one iron atom) or *diferric* (two iron atoms). The turnover (half-clearance time) of transferrin-bound iron is very rapid—typically 60–90 min. Because almost all of the iron transported by transferrin is delivered to the erythroid marrow, the clearance time of transferrin-bound iron from the circulation is affected most by the plasma iron level and the erythroid marrow activity. When erythropoiesis is markedly stimulated, the pool of erythroid cells requiring iron increases and the clearance time of iron from the circulation decreases. The half-clearance time of iron in the presence of iron deficiency is as short as 10–15 min. With suppression of erythropoiesis, the plasma iron level typically increases and the half-clearance time may be prolonged to several hours. Normally, the iron bound to transferrin turns over 10–20 times per day. Assuming a normal plasma iron level of 80–100 μg/dL, the amount of iron passing through the transferrin pool is 20–24 mg/d.

The iron-transferrin complex circulates in the plasma until it interacts with specific *transferrin receptors* on the surface of marrow erythroid cells. Diferric transferrin has the highest affinity for transferrin receptors; apotransferrin (transferrin not carrying iron) has very little affinity. While transferrin receptors are found on cells in many tissues within the body—and all cells at some time during development will display transferrin receptors—the cell having the greatest number of receptors (300,000 to 400,000/cell) is the developing erythroblast.

Once the iron-bearing transferrin interacts with its receptor, the complex is internalized via clathrin-coated pits and transported to an acidic endosome, where the iron is released at the low pH. The iron is then made available for heme synthesis while the transferrin-receptor complex is recycled to the surface of the cell, where the bulk of the transferrin is released back into circulation and the transferrin receptor reanchors into the cell membrane. At this point a certain amount of the transferrin receptor protein may be released into circulation and can be measured as soluble transferrin receptor protein. Within the erythroid cell, iron in excess of the amount needed for hemoglobin synthesis binds to a storage protein, *apoferritin*, forming *ferritin*. This mechanism of iron exchange also takes place in other cells of the body expressing transferrin receptors, especially liver parenchymal cells where the iron can be incorporated into heme-containing enzymes or stored. The iron incorporated into hemoglobin subsequently enters the circulation as new red cells are released from the bone marrow. The iron is then part of the red cell mass and will not become available for reutilization until the red cell dies.

In a normal individual, the average red cell life span is 120 days. Thus, 0.8–1.0% of red cells turn over each day. At the end of its life span, the red cell is recognized as senescent by the cells of the *reticuloendothelial (RE) system*, and the cell undergoes phagocytosis. Once within the RE cell, the hemoglobin from the ingested red cell is broken down, the globin and other proteins are returned to the amino acid pool, and the iron is shuttled back to the surface of the RE cell, where it is presented to circulating transferrin. It is the efficient and highly conserved recycling of iron from senescent red cells that supports steady state (and even mildly accelerated) erythropoiesis.

Since each milliliter of red cells contains 1 mg of elemental iron, the amount of iron needed to replace those red cells lost through senescence amounts to 16–20 mg/d (assuming an adult with a red cell mass of 2 L). Any additional iron required for daily red cell production comes from the diet. Normally, an adult male will need to absorb at least 1 mg of elemental iron daily to meet needs, while females in the childbearing years will need to absorb an average of 1.4 mg/d. However, to achieve a maximum proliferative erythroid marrow response to anemia, additional iron must be available. With markedly stimulated erythropoiesis, demands for iron are increased by as much as six- to eightfold. With extravascular hemolytic anemia, the rate of red cell destruction is increased, but the iron recovered from the red cells is efficiently reutilized for hemoglobin synthesis. In contrast, with intravascular hemolysis or blood loss anemia, the rate of red cell production is limited by the amount of iron that can be mobilized from stores. Typically, the rate of mobilization under these circumstances will not support red cell production more than 2.5 times normal. If the delivery of iron to the stimulated marrow is suboptimal, the marrow's proliferative response is blunted, and hemoglobin synthesis is impaired. The result is a hypoproliferative marrow accompanied by microcytic, hypochromic anemia.

While blood loss or hemolysis places a demand on the iron supply, conditions associated with inflammation interfere with iron release from stores and can result in a rapid decrease in the serum iron (see below).

NUTRITIONAL IRON BALANCE

The balance of iron in humans is tightly controlled and designed to conserve iron for reutilization. There is no regulated excretory pathway for iron, and the only mechanisms by which iron is lost from the body are blood loss (via gastrointestinal bleeding, menses, or other forms of bleeding) and the loss of epithelial cells from the skin, gut, and genitourinary tract. Normally, the only route by which iron comes into the body is via absorption from food or from medicinal iron taken orally. Iron may also enter the body through red-cell transfusions or injection of iron complexes. The margin between the amount of iron available for absorption and the requirement for iron in growing infants and the adult female is narrow; this accounts for the great prevalence of iron deficiency worldwide—currently estimated at one-half billion people.

The amount of iron required from the diet to replace losses averages about 10% of body iron content a year in men and 15% in women of childbearing age. Dietary iron content is closely related to total caloric intake (approximately 6 mg of elemental iron per 1000 calories). Iron bioavailability is affected by the nature of the foodstuff, with heme iron (e.g., red meat) being most readily absorbed. In the United States, the average iron intake in an adult male is 15 mg/d with 6% absorption; for the average female, the daily intake is 11 mg/d with 12% absorption. An individual with iron deficiency can increase iron absorption to about 20% of the iron present in a meat-containing diet but only 5–10% of the iron in a vegetarian diet. As a result, one-third of the female population in the United States has virtually no iron stores. Vegetarians are at an additional disadvantage because certain foodstuffs that include phytates and phosphates reduce iron absorption by about 50%. When ionizable iron salts are given together with food, the amount of iron absorbed is reduced. When the percentage of iron absorbed from individual food items is compared with the percentage for an equivalent amount of ferrous salt, iron in vegetables is only about one-twentieth as available, egg iron one-eighth, liver iron one-half, and heme iron one-half to two-thirds.

Infants, children, and adolescents may be unable to maintain normal iron balance because of the demands of body growth and lower dietary intake of iron. During the last two trimesters of pregnancy, daily iron requirements increase to 5–6 mg. That is the reason why iron supplements are strongly recommended for pregnant women in developed countries. Enthusiasm for supplementing foods such as bread and cereals with iron has waned in the face of concerns that the very prevalent hemochromatosis gene would result in an unacceptable risk of iron overload.

Iron absorption takes place largely in the proximal small intestine and is a carefully regulated process. For absorption, iron must be taken up by the luminal cell. That process is facilitated by the acidic contents of the stomach, which maintains the iron in solution. At the brush border of the absorptive cell, the ferric iron is converted to the ferrous form by a ferrireductase. Transport across the membrane is accomplished by divalent metal transporter 1 (DMT-1, also known as Nramp 2 or DCT-1). DMT-1 is a general cation transporter. Once inside the gut cell, iron may be stored as ferritin or transported through the cell to be released at the basolateral surface to plasma transferrin through the membrane-embedded iron exporter, ferroportin. The function of ferroportin is negatively regulated by hepcidin, the principal iron regulatory hormone. In the process of release, iron interacts with another ferroxidase, hephaestin, which oxidizes the iron to the ferric form for transferrin binding. Hephaestin is similar to ceruloplasmin, the copper-carrying protein.

Iron absorption is influenced by a number of physiologic states. Erythroid hyperplasia, for example, stimulates iron absorption, even in the face of normal or increased iron stores, and hepcidin levels are inappropriately low. The molecular mechanism underlying this relationship is not known. Thus, patients with anemias associated with high levels of ineffective erythropoiesis absorb excess amounts of dietary iron. Over time, this may lead to iron overload and tissue damage. In iron deficiency, hepcidin levels are low and iron is much more efficiently absorbed from a given diet; the contrary is true in states of secondary iron overload. The normal individual can reduce iron absorption in situations of excessive intake or medicinal iron intake; however, while the percentage of iron absorbed goes down, the absolute amount goes up. This accounts for the acute iron toxicity occasionally seen when children ingest large numbers of iron tablets. Under these circumstances, the amount of iron absorbed exceeds the transferrin binding capacity of the plasma, resulting in free iron that affects critical organs such as cardiac muscle cells.

IRON-DEFICIENCY ANEMIA

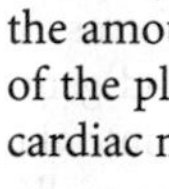

Iron deficiency is one of the most prevalent forms of malnutrition. Globally, 50% of anemia is attributable to iron deficiency and accounts for around 841,000 deaths annually worldwide. Africa and parts of Asia bear 71% of the global mortality burden; North America represents only 1.4% of the total morbidity and mortality associated with iron deficiency.

STAGES OF IRON DEFICIENCY

Iron-deficiency anemia is the condition in which there is anemia and clear evidence of iron lack. The progression to iron deficiency can be divided into three stages (Fig. 98-2). The first stage is *negative iron balance*, in which the demands for (or losses of) iron exceed the body's ability to absorb iron from the diet. This stage results from a number of physiologic mechanisms, including blood loss, pregnancy (in which the demands for red cell production by the fetus outstrip the mother's ability to provide iron), rapid growth spurts in the adolescent, or inadequate dietary iron intake. Blood loss in excess of 10–20 mL of red cells per day is greater than the amount of iron that the gut can absorb from a normal diet. Under these circumstances the iron deficit must be made up by mobilization of iron from RE storage sites. During this period, iron stores—reflected by the serum ferritin level or the appearance of stainable iron on bone marrow aspirations—decrease. As long as iron stores are present and can be mobilized, the serum iron, total iron-binding capacity (TIBC), and red cell protoporphyrin levels remain within normal limits. At this stage, red cell morphology and indices are normal.

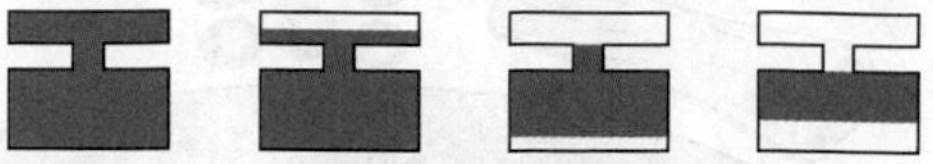

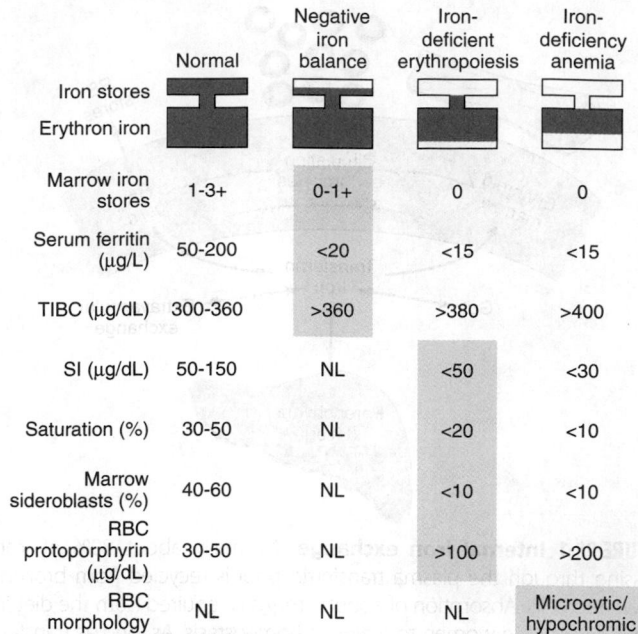

	Normal	Negative iron balance	Iron-deficient erythropoiesis	Iron-deficiency anemia
Marrow iron stores	1-3+	0-1+	0	0
Serum ferritin (μg/L)	50-200	<20	<15	<15
TIBC (μg/dL)	300-360	>360	>380	>400
SI (μg/dL)	50-150	NL	<50	<30
Saturation (%)	30-50	NL	<20	<10
Marrow sideroblasts (%)	40-60	NL	<10	<10
RBC protoporphyrin (μg/dL)	30-50	NL	>100	>200
RBC morphology	NL	NL	NL	Microcytic/ hypochromic

FIGURE 98-2 Laboratory studies in the evolution of iron deficiency. Measurements of marrow iron stores, serum ferritin, and total iron-binding capacity (TIBC) are sensitive to early iron-store depletion. Iron-deficient erythropoiesis is recognized from additional abnormalities in the serum iron (SI), percent transferrin saturation, the pattern of marrow sideroblasts, and the red cell protoporphyrin level. Patients with iron-deficiency anemia demonstrate all the same abnormalities plus hypochromic microcytic anemia. *(From Hillman and Finch, with permission.)*

When iron stores become depleted, the serum iron begins to fall. Gradually, the TIBC increases, as do red cell protoporphyrin levels. By definition, marrow iron stores are absent when the serum ferritin level is <15 μg/L. As long as the serum iron remains within the normal range, hemoglobin synthesis is unaffected despite the dwindling iron stores. Once the transferrin saturation falls to 15–20%, hemoglobin synthesis becomes impaired. This is a period of *iron-deficient erythropoiesis.* Careful evaluation of the peripheral blood smear reveals the first appearance of microcytic cells, and if the laboratory technology is available, one finds hypochromic reticulocytes in circulation. Gradually, the hemoglobin and hematocrit begin to fall, reflecting *iron-deficiency anemia.* The transferrin saturation at this point is 10–15%.

When moderate anemia is present (hemoglobin 10–13 g/dL), the bone marrow remains hypoproliferative. With more severe anemia (hemoglobin 7–8 g/dL), hypochromia and microcytosis become more prominent, target cells and misshapen red cells (poikilocytes) appear on the blood smear as cigar- or pencil-shaped forms, and the erythroid marrow becomes increasingly ineffective. Consequently, with severe prolonged iron-deficiency anemia, erythroid hyperplasia of the marrow develops, rather than hypoproliferation.

CAUSES OF IRON DEFICIENCY

Conditions that increase demand for iron, increase iron loss, or decrease iron intake or absorption can produce iron deficiency (Table 98-2).

CLINICAL PRESENTATION OF IRON DEFICIENCY

Certain clinical conditions carry an increased likelihood of iron deficiency. Pregnancy, adolescence, periods of rapid growth, and an intermittent history of blood loss of any kind should alert the clinician to possible iron deficiency. A cardinal rule is that the appearance of iron deficiency in an adult male means gastrointestinal blood loss until

TABLE 98-2 CAUSES OF IRON DEFICIENCY

Increased demand for iron and/or hematopoiesis
rapid growth in infancy or adolescence
pregnancy
erythropoietin therapy
Increased iron loss
chronic blood loss
menses
acute blood loss
blood donation
phlebotomy as treatment for polycythemia vera
Decreased iron intake or absorption
inadequate diet
malabsorption from disease (sprue, Crohn's disease)
malabsorption from surgery (post-gastrectomy)
acute or chronic inflammation

proven otherwise. Signs related to iron deficiency depend on the severity and chronicity of the anemia in addition to the usual signs of anemia—fatigue, pallor, and reduced exercise capacity. *Cheilosis* (fissures at the corners of the mouth) and *koilonychia* (spooning of the fingernails) are signs of advanced tissue iron deficiency. The diagnosis of iron deficiency is typically based on laboratory results.

LABORATORY IRON STUDIES

Serum Iron and Total Iron-Binding Capacity The serum iron level represents the amount of circulating iron bound to transferrin. The TIBC is an indirect measure of the circulating transferrin. The normal range for the serum iron is 50–150 μg/dL; the normal range for TIBC is 300–360 μg/dL. Transferrin saturation, which is normally 25–50%, is obtained by the following formula: serum iron × 100 ÷ TIBC. Iron-deficiency states are associated with saturation levels below 18%. In evaluating the serum iron, the clinician should be aware that there is a diurnal variation in the value. A transferrin saturation >50% indicates that a disproportionate amount of the iron bound to transferrin is being delivered to nonerythroid tissues. If this persists for an extended time, tissue iron overload may occur.

Serum Ferritin Free iron is toxic to cells, and the body has established an elaborate set of protective mechanisms to bind iron in various tissue compartments. Within cells, iron is stored complexed to protein as ferritin or hemosiderin. Apoferritin binds to free ferrous iron and stores it in the ferric state. As ferritin accumulates within cells of the RE system, protein aggregates are formed as hemosiderin. Iron in ferritin or hemosiderin can be extracted for release by the RE cells, although hemosiderin is less readily available. Under steady-state conditions, the serum ferritin level correlates with total body iron stores; thus, the serum ferritin level is the most convenient laboratory test to estimate iron stores. The normal value for ferritin varies according to the age and gender of the individual (Fig. 98-3). Adult males have serum ferritin values averaging about 100 μg/L, while adult females have levels averaging 30 μg/L. As iron stores are depleted, the serum ferritin falls to <15 μg/L. Such levels are diagnostic of absent body iron stores.

Evaluation of Bone Marrow Iron Stores Although RE cell iron stores can be estimated from the iron stain of a bone marrow aspirate or biopsy, the measurement of serum ferritin has largely supplanted bone marrow aspirates for determination of storage iron (Table 98-3). The serum ferritin level is a better indicator of iron overload than the marrow iron stain. However, in addition to storage iron, the marrow iron stain provides information about the effective delivery of iron to developing erythroblasts. Normally, when the marrow smear is stained for iron, 20–40% of developing erythroblasts—called *sideroblasts*—will have visible ferritin granules in their cytoplasm. This represents iron in excess of that needed for hemoglobin synthesis. In states in which release of iron from storage sites is blocked, RE iron will be detectable, and there will be few or no sideroblasts. In the myelodysplastic syndromes, mitochondrial dysfunction can occur, and accumulation of iron in mitochondria appears in a necklace fashion around the nucleus of the erythroblast. Such cells are referred to as *ringed sideroblasts*.

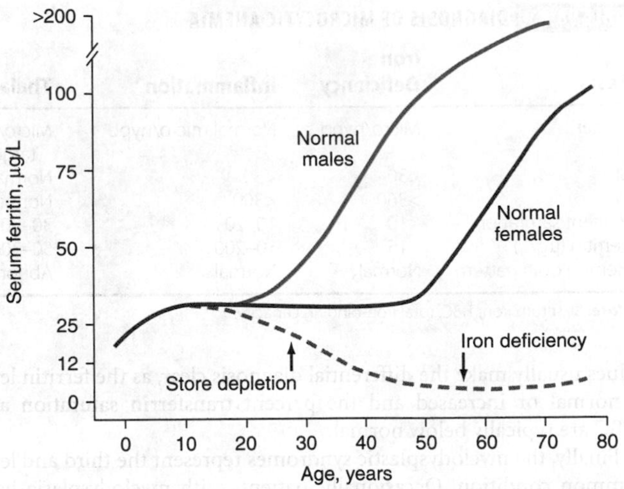

FIGURE 98-3 Serum ferritin levels as a function of sex and age. Iron store depletion and iron deficiency are accompanied by a fall in serum ferritin level below 20 μg/L. *(From Hillman et al, with permission.)*

Red Cell Protoporphyrin Levels Protoporphyrin is an intermediate in the pathway to heme synthesis. Under conditions in which heme synthesis is impaired, protoporphyrin accumulates within the red cell. This reflects an inadequate iron supply to erythroid precursors to support hemoglobin synthesis. Normal values are <30 μg/dL of red cells. In iron deficiency, values in excess of 100 μg/dL are seen. The most common causes of increased red cell protoporphyrin levels are absolute or relative iron deficiency and lead poisoning.

Serum Levels of Transferrin Receptor Protein Because erythroid cells have the highest numbers of transferrin receptors on their surface of any cell in the body, and because transferrin receptor protein (TRP) is released by cells into the circulation, serum levels of TRP reflect the total erythroid marrow mass. Another condition in which TRP levels are elevated is absolute iron deficiency. Normal values are 4–9 μg/L determined by immunoassay. This laboratory test is becoming increasingly available and, along with the serum ferritin, has been proposed to distinguish between iron deficiency and the anemia of chronic inflammation (see below).

DIFFERENTIAL DIAGNOSIS

Other than iron deficiency, only three conditions need to be considered in the differential diagnosis of a hypochromic microcytic anemia (Table 98-4). The first is an inherited defect in globin chain synthesis: the thalassemias. These are differentiated from iron deficiency most readily by serum iron values; normal or increased serum iron levels and transferrin saturation are characteristic of the thalassemias.

The second condition is the anemia of chronic inflammation with inadequate iron supply to the erythroid marrow. The distinction between true iron-deficiency anemia and the anemia associated with chronic inflammation is among the most common diagnostic problems encountered by clinicians (see below). Usually the anemia of chronic inflammation is normocytic and normochromic. The iron

TABLE 98-3 IRON STORE MEASUREMENTS

Iron Stores	Marrow Iron Stain, 0–4+	Serum Ferritin, μg/L
0	0	<15
1–300 mg	Trace to 1+	15–30
300–800 mg	2+	30–60
800–1000 mg	3+	60–150
1–2 g	4+	>150
Iron overload	—	>500–1000

TABLE 98-4 DIAGNOSIS OF MICROCYTIC ANEMIA

Tests	Iron Deficiency	Inflammation	Thalassemia	Sideroblastic Anemia
Smear	Micro/hypo	Normal micro/hypo	Micro/hypo with targeting	Variable
SI	<30	<50	Normal to high	Normal to high
TIBC	>360	<300	Normal	Normal
Percent saturation	<10	10–20	30–80	30–80
Ferritin (μg/L)	<15	30–200	50–300	50–300
Hemoglobin pattern	Normal	Normal	Abnormal	Normal

Note: SI, serum iron; TIBC, total iron-binding capacity.

values usually make the differential diagnosis clear, as the ferritin level is normal or increased and the percent transferrin saturation and TIBC are typically below normal.

Finally, the myelodysplastic syndromes represent the third and least common condition. Occasionally, patients with myelodysplasia have impaired hemoglobin synthesis with mitochondrial dysfunction, resulting in impaired iron incorporation into heme. The iron values again reveal normal stores and more than an adequate supply to the marrow, despite the microcytosis and hypochromia.

℞ IRON-DEFICIENCY ANEMIA

The severity and cause of iron-deficiency anemia will determine the appropriate approach to treatment. As an example, symptomatic elderly patients with severe iron-deficiency anemia and cardiovascular instability may require red cell transfusions. Younger individuals who have compensated for their anemia can be treated more conservatively with iron replacement. The foremost issue for the latter patient is the precise identification of the cause of the iron deficiency.

For the majority of cases of iron deficiency (pregnant women, growing children and adolescents, patients with infrequent episodes of bleeding, and those with inadequate dietary intake of iron), oral iron therapy will suffice. For patients with unusual blood loss or malabsorption, specific diagnostic tests and appropriate therapy take priority. Once the diagnosis of iron-deficiency anemia and its cause is made, there are three major therapeutic approaches.

RED CELL TRANSFUSION Transfusion therapy is reserved for individuals who have symptoms of anemia, cardiovascular instability, continued and excessive blood loss from whatever source, and require immediate intervention. The management of these patients is less related to the iron deficiency than it is to the consequences of the severe anemia. Not only do transfusions correct the anemia acutely, but the transfused red cells provide a source of iron for reutilization, assuming they are not lost through continued bleeding. Transfusion therapy will stabilize the patient while other options are reviewed.

ORAL IRON THERAPY In the asymptomatic patient with established iron-deficiency anemia, treatment with oral iron is usually adequate. Multiple preparations are available, ranging from simple iron salts to complex iron compounds designed for sustained release throughout the small intestine **(Table 98-5)**. While the various preparations contain different amounts of iron, they are generally all absorbed well and are effective in treatment. Some come with other compounds designed to enhance iron absorption, such as ascorbic acid. It is not clear whether the benefits of such compounds justify their costs. Typically, for iron replacement therapy, up to 300 mg of elemental iron per day is given, usually as three or four iron tablets (each containing 50–65 mg elemental iron) given over the course of the day. Ideally, oral iron preparations should be taken on an empty stomach, since foods may inhibit iron absorption. Some patients with gastric disease or prior gastric surgery require special treatment with iron solutions, since the retention capacity of the stomach may be reduced. The retention capacity is necessary for dissolving the shell of the iron tablet before the release of iron. A dose of 200–300 mg of elemental iron per day should result in the absorption of iron up to 50 mg/d. This supports a red cell production level of two to three times normal in an individual with a normally functioning marrow and appropriate erythropoietin stimulus. However, as the hemoglobin level rises, erythropoietin stimulation decreases, and the amount of iron absorbed is reduced. The goal of therapy in individuals with iron-deficiency anemia is not only to repair the anemia, but also to provide stores of at least 0.5–1.0 g of iron. Sustained treatment for a period of 6–12 months after correction of the anemia will be necessary to achieve this.

Of the complications of oral iron therapy, gastrointestinal distress is the most prominent and is seen in 15–20% of patients. Abdominal pain, nausea, vomiting, or constipation may lead to noncompliance. Although small doses of iron or iron preparations with delayed release may help somewhat, the gastrointestinal side effects are a major impediment to the effective treatment of a number of patients.

The response to iron therapy varies, depending on the erythropoietin (EPO) stimulus and the rate of absorption. Typically, the reticulocyte count should begin to increase within 4–7 days after initiation of therapy and peak at 1½ weeks. The absence of a response may be due to poor absorption, noncompliance (which is common), or a confounding diagnosis. A useful test in the clinic to determine the patient's ability to absorb iron is the *iron tolerance test*. Two iron tablets are given to the patient on an empty stomach, and the serum iron is measured serially over the subsequent 2 hours. Normal absorption will result in an increase in the serum iron of at least 100 μg/dL. If iron deficiency persists despite adequate treatment, it may be necessary to switch to parenteral iron therapy.

PARENTERAL IRON THERAPY Intravenous iron can be given to patients who are unable to tolerate oral iron; whose needs are relatively acute; or who need iron on an ongoing basis, usually due to persistent gastrointestinal blood loss. Parenteral iron use has been rising rapidly in the last several years with the recognition that recombinant erythropoietin therapy induces a large demand for iron—a demand that frequently cannot be met through the physiologic release of iron from RE sources. The safety of parenteral iron—particularly iron dextran—has been a concern. The serious adverse reaction rate to intravenous iron dextran is 0.7%. Fortunately, newer iron complexes are available in the United States, such as sodium ferric gluconate (Ferrlecit) and iron sucrose (Venofer), that have a much lower rate of adverse effects.

Parenteral iron is used in two ways: one is to administer the total dose of iron required to correct the hemoglobin deficit and provide the patient with at least 500 mg of iron stores; the second is to give repeated small doses of parenteral iron over a protracted period. The latter approach is common in dialysis centers, where it is not unusual for 100 mg of elemental iron to be given weekly for 10 weeks to augment the response to recombinant EPO therapy. The amount of iron needed by an individual patient is calculated by the following formula:

$$\text{Body weight (kg)} \times 2.3 \times (15 - \text{patient's hemoglobin, g/dL}) + 500 \text{ or } 1000 \text{ mg (for stores)}.$$

In administering intravenous iron dextran, anaphylaxis is a concern. Anaphylaxis is much rarer with the newer preparations. The factors that have correlated with an anaphylactic-like reaction include a history of multiple allergies or a prior allergic reaction to dextran (in the case of iron dextran). Generalized symptoms appearing several days after the infusion of a

TABLE 98-5 ORAL IRON PREPARATIONS

Generic Name	Tablet (Iron Content), mg	Elixir (Iron Content), mg in 5 mL
Ferrous sulfate	325 (65)	300 (60)
	195 (39)	90 (18)
Extended release	525 (105)	
Ferrous fumarate	325 (107)	
	195 (64)	100 (33)
Ferrous gluconate	325 (39)	300 (35)
Polysaccharide iron	150 (150)	100 (100)
	50 (50)	

large dose of iron can include arthralgias, skin rash, and low-grade fever. This may be dose-related, but it does not preclude the further use of parenteral iron in the patient. To date, patients with sensitivity to iron dextran have been safely treated with iron gluconate. If a large dose of iron dextran is to be given (>100 mg), the iron preparation should be diluted in 5% dextrose in water or 0.9% NaCl solution. The iron solution can then be infused over a 60- to 90-min period (for larger doses) or at a rate convenient for the attending nurse or physician. While a test dose (25 mg) of parenteral iron dextran is recommended, in reality a slow infusion of a larger dose of parenteral iron solution will afford the same kind of early warning as a separately injected test dose. Early in the infusion of iron, if chest pain, wheezing, a fall in blood pressure, or other systemic symptoms occur, the infusion of iron should be stopped immediately.

OTHER HYPOPROLIFERATIVE ANEMIAS

In addition to mild to moderate iron-deficiency anemia, the hypoproliferative anemias can be divided into four categories: (1) chronic inflammation, (2) renal disease, (3) endocrine and nutritional deficiencies (hypometabolic states), and (4) marrow damage (Chap. 102). With chronic inflammation, renal disease, or hypometabolism, endogenous EPO production is inadequate for the degree of anemia observed. For the anemia of chronic inflammation, the erythroid marrow also responds inadequately to stimulation, due in part to defects in *iron reutilization*. As a result of the lack of adequate EPO stimulation, an examination of the peripheral blood smear will disclose only an occasional polychromatophilic ("shift") reticulocyte. In cases of iron deficiency or marrow damage, appropriate elevations in endogenous EPO levels are typically found, and shift reticulocytes will be present on the blood smear.

ANEMIA OF ACUTE AND CHRONIC INFLAMMATION/INFECTION (THE ANEMIA OF CHRONIC DISEASE)

The anemia of chronic disease—which encompasses inflammation, infection, tissue injury, and conditions (such as cancer) associated with the release of proinflammatory cytokines—is one of the most common forms of anemia seen clinically and probably the most important in the differential diagnosis of iron deficiency, since many of the features of the anemia are brought about by inadequate iron delivery to the marrow, despite the presence of normal or increased iron stores. This is reflected by a low serum iron, increased red cell protoporphyrin, a hypoproliferative marrow, transferrin saturation in the range of 15–20%, and a normal or increased serum ferritin. The serum ferritin values are often the most distinguishing feature between true iron-deficiency anemia and the iron-deficient erythropoiesis associated with inflammation. Typically, serum ferritin values increase threefold over basal levels in the face of inflammation. All of these changes are due to the effects of inflammatory cytokines and hepcidin, the key iron regulatory hormone, acting at several levels of erythropoiesis (Fig. 98-4).

Interleukin 1 (IL-1) directly decreases EPO production in response to anemia. IL-1, acting through accessory cell release of interferon γ (IFN-γ), suppresses the response of the erythroid marrow to EPO—an effect that can be overcome by EPO administration in vitro and in vivo. In addition, tumor necrosis factor (TNF), acting through the release of IFN-γ by marrow stromal cells, also suppresses the response to EPO. Hepcidin, made by the liver, is increased in inflammation and acts to suppress iron absorption and iron release from storage sites. The overall result is a chronic hypoproliferative anemia with classic changes in iron metabolism. The anemia is further compounded by a mild to moderate shortening in red cell survival.

With chronic inflammation, the primary disease will determine the severity and characteristics of the anemia. For instance, many patients with cancer also have anemia that is typically normocytic and normochromic. In contrast, patients with long-standing active rheumatoid arthritis or chronic infections such as tuberculosis will have a microcytic, hypochromic anemia. In both cases, the bone marrow is hypoproliferative, but the differences in red cell indices reflect differences in the availability of iron for hemoglobin synthesis. Occasionally, conditions associated with chronic inflammation are also associated with chronic blood loss. Under these circumstances, a bone marrow aspirate stained for iron may be necessary to rule out absolute iron deficiency. However, the administration of iron in this case will correct the iron deficiency component of the anemia and leave the inflammatory component unaffected.

The anemia associated with acute infection or inflammation is typically mild but becomes more pronounced over time. Acute infection can produce a fall in hemoglobin levels of 2–3 g/dL within 1 or 2 days; this is largely related to the hemolysis of red cells near the end of their natural life span. The fever and cytokines released exert a selective pressure against cells with more limited capacity to maintain the red cell membrane. In most individuals the mild anemia is reasonably well tolerated, and symptoms, if present, are associated with the underlying disease. Occasionally, in patients with preexisting cardiac disease, moderate anemia (hemoglobin 10–11 g/dL) may be associated with angina, exercise intolerance, and shortness of breath. The erythropoietic profile that distinguishes the anemia of inflammation from the other causes of hypoproliferative anemias is shown in Table 98-6.

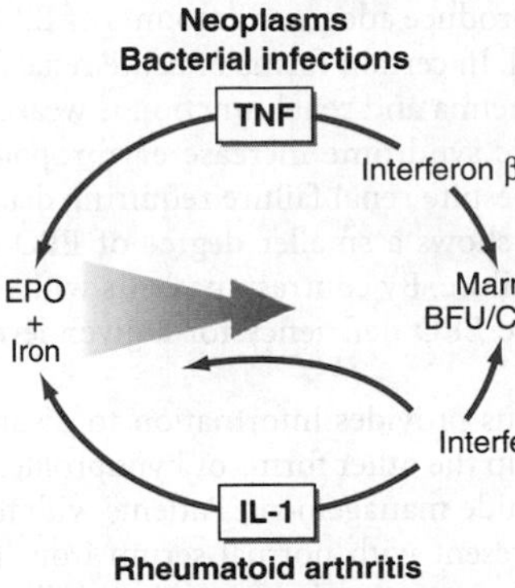

FIGURE 98-4 Suppression of erythropoiesis by inflammatory cytokines. Through the release of tumor necrosis factor (TNF) and interferon γ (IFN-γ), neoplasms and bacterial infections suppress erythropoietin (EPO) production and the proliferation of erythroid progenitors [erythroid burst-forming units and erythroid colony-forming units (BFU/CFU-E)]. The mediators in patients with vasculitis and rheumatoid arthritis include interleukin 1 (IL-1) and IFN-γ. The red arrows indicate sites of inflammatory cytokine inhibitory effects.

ANEMIA OF RENAL DISEASE

Chronic renal failure is usually associated with a moderate to severe hypoproliferative anemia; the level of the anemia correlates with the severity of the renal failure. Red cells are typically normocytic and normochromic, and reticulocytes are decreased. The anemia is pri-

TABLE 98-6 DIAGNOSIS OF HYPOPROLIFERATIVE ANEMIAS

Tests	Iron Deficiency	Inflammation	Renal Disease	Hypometabolic States
Anemia	Mild to severe	Mild	Mild to severe	Mild
MCV (fL)	60–90	80–90	90	90
Morphology	Normo-microcytic	Normocytic	Normocytic	Normocytic
SI	<30	<50	Normal	Normal
TIBC	>360	<300	Normal	Normal
Saturation (%)	<10	10–20	Normal	Normal
Serum ferritin (μg/L)	<15	30–200	115–150	Normal
Iron stores	0	2–4+	1–4+	Normal

Note: MCV, mean corpuscular volume; SI, serum iron; TIBC, total iron-binding capacity.

marily due to a failure to produce adequate amounts of EPO and a reduction in red cell survival. In certain forms of acute renal failure, the correlation between the anemia and renal function is weaker. Patients with the hemolytic-uremic syndrome increase erythropoiesis in response to the hemolysis, despite renal failure requiring dialysis. Polycystic kidney disease also shows a smaller degree of EPO deficiency for a given level of renal failure. By contrast, patients with diabetes or myeloma have more severe EPO deficiency for a given level of renal failure.

Assessment of iron status provides information to distinguish the anemia of renal disease from the other forms of hypoproliferative anemia (Table 98-6) and to guide management. Patients with the anemia of renal disease usually present with normal serum iron, TIBC, and ferritin levels. However, those maintained on chronic hemodialysis may develop iron deficiency from blood loss through the dialysis procedure. Iron must be replenished in these patients to ensure an adequate response to EPO therapy (see below).

ANEMIA IN HYPOMETABOLIC STATES

Patients who are starving, particularly for protein, and those with a variety of endocrine disorders that produce lower metabolic rates, may develop a mild to moderate hypoproliferative anemia. The release of EPO from the kidney is sensitive to the need for O_2, not just O_2 levels. Thus, EPO production is triggered at lower levels of blood O_2 content in disease states (such as hypothyroidism and starvation) where metabolic activity, and thus O_2 demand, is decreased.

Endocrine Deficiency States The difference in the levels of hemoglobin between men and women is related to the effects of androgen and estrogen on erythropoiesis. Testosterone and anabolic steroids augment erythropoiesis; castration and estrogen administration to males decrease erythropoiesis. Patients who are hypothyroid or have deficits in pituitary hormones also may develop a mild anemia. Pathogenesis may be complicated by other nutritional deficiencies since iron and folic acid absorption can be affected by these disorders. Usually, correction of the hormone deficiency reverses the anemia.

Anemia may be more severe in Addison's disease, depending on the level of thyroid and androgen hormone dysfunction; however, anemia may be masked by decreases in plasma volume. Once such patients are given cortisol and volume replacement, the hemoglobin level may fall rapidly. Mild anemia complicating hyperparathyroidism may be due to decreased EPO production as a consequence of the renal effects of hypercalcemia or to impaired proliferation of erythroid progenitors.

Protein Starvation Decreased dietary intake of protein may lead to mild to moderate hypoproliferative anemia; this form of anemia may be prevalent in the elderly. The anemia can be more severe in patients with a greater degree of starvation. In marasmus, where patients are both protein- and calorie-deficient, the release of EPO is impaired in proportion to the reduction in metabolic rate; however, the degree of anemia may be masked by volume depletion and becomes apparent after refeeding. Deficiencies in other nutrients (iron, folate) may also complicate the clinical picture but may not be apparent at diagnosis. Changes in the erythrocyte indices on refeeding should prompt evaluation of iron, folate, and B_{12} status.

Anemia in Liver Disease A mild hypoproliferative anemia may develop in patients with chronic liver disease from nearly any cause. The peripheral blood smear may show spur cells and stomatocytes from the accumulation of excess cholesterol in the membrane from a deficiency of lecithin cholesterol acyltransferase. Red cell survival is shortened, and the production of EPO is inadequate to compensate. In alcoholic liver disease, nutritional deficiencies are common and complicate the management. Folate deficiency from inadequate intake, as well as iron deficiency from blood loss and inadequate intake, can alter the red cell indices.

℞ HYPOPROLIFERATIVE ANEMIAS

Many patients with hypoproliferative anemias experience recovery of normal hemoglobin levels when the underlying disease is appropriately treated. For those in whom such reversals are not possible—such as patients with end-stage kidney disease, cancer, and chronic inflammatory diseases—symptomatic anemia requires treatment. The two major forms of treatment are transfusions and EPO.

TRANSFUSIONS Thresholds for transfusion should be altered based on the patient's symptoms. In general, patients without serious underlying cardiovascular or pulmonary disease can tolerate hemoglobin levels above 8 g/dL and do not require intervention until the hemoglobin falls below that level. Patients with more physiologic compromise may need to have their hemoglobin levels kept above 11 g/dL. A typical unit of packed red cells increases the hemoglobin level by 1 g/dL. Transfusions are associated with certain infectious risks (Chap. 107), and chronic transfusions can produce iron overload. Importantly, the liberal use of blood has been associated with increased morbidity and mortality, particularly in the intensive care setting. Therefore, in the absence of documented tissue hypoxia, a conservative approach to the use of red cell transfusions is preferable.

ERYTHROPOIETIN (EPO) EPO is particularly useful in anemias in which endogenous EPO levels are inappropriately low, such as the hypoproliferative anemias. Iron status must be evaluated and iron repleted to obtain optimal effects from EPO. In patients with chronic renal failure, the usual dose of EPO is 50–150 U/kg three times a week intravenously. Hemoglobin levels of 10–12 g/dL are usually reached within 4–6 weeks if iron levels are adequate; 90% of these patients respond. Once a target hemoglobin level is achieved, the EPO dose can be decreased. A fall in hemoglobin level occurring in the face of EPO therapy usually signifies the development of an infection or iron depletion. Aluminum toxicity and hyperparathyroidism can also compromise the EPO response. When an infection intervenes, it is best to interrupt the EPO therapy and rely on transfusion to correct the anemia until the infection is adequately treated. The dose needed to correct the anemia in patients with cancer is higher, up to 300 U/kg three times a week, and only about 60% of patients respond.

Longer-acting preparations of EPO can reduce the frequency of injections. Darbepoetin alfa, a molecularly modified EPO with additional carbohydrate, has a half-life in the circulation that is 3–4 times longer than epoetin alfa, permitting weekly or every other week dosing.

Acknowledgment

Dr. Robert S. Hillman was the author of this chapter in the 14th edition, and material from his chapter has been retained.

FURTHER READINGS

Bailie GR et al: Parenteral iron use in the management of anemia in end-stage renal disease patients. Am J Kidney Dis 35:1, 2000

Brugnara C: Iron deficiency and erythropoiesis: New diagnostic approaches. Clin Chem 49:1573, 2003

Fleming RE, Bacon BR: Orchestration of iron homeostasis. N Engl J Med 352:1741, 2005

Ganz T: Hepcidin, a key regulator of iron metabolism and mediator of inflammation. Blood 102:783, 2003

Hillman RS et al: *Hematology in Clinical Practice,* 4th ed. New York, McGraw-Hill, 2005

Stoltzfus RF: Iron deficiency: Global prevalence and consequences. Food Nutr Bull 24(Suppl 4):S99, 2003

Thomas C et al: The diagnostic plot: A concept for identifying different states of iron deficiency and monitoring the response to epoetin therapy. Med Oncol 23:23, 2006

99 Disorders of Hemoglobin

Edward J. Benz, Jr.

Hemoglobin is critical for normal oxygen delivery to tissues; it is also present in erythrocytes in such high concentrations that it can alter red cell shape, deformability, and viscosity. Hemoglobinopathies are disorders affecting the structure, function, or production of hemoglobin. These conditions are usually inherited and range in severity from asymptomatic laboratory abnormalities to death in utero. Different forms may present as hemolytic anemia, erythrocytosis, cyanosis, or vasoocclusive stigmata.

PROPERTIES OF THE HUMAN HEMOGLOBINS

HEMOGLOBIN STRUCTURE

Different hemoglobins are produced during embryonic, fetal, and adult life (Fig. 99-1). Each consists of a tetramer of globin polypeptide chains: a pair of α-like chains 141 amino acids long and a pair of β-like chains 146 amino acids long. The major adult hemoglobin, HbA, has the structure $\alpha_2\beta_2$. HbF ($\alpha_2\gamma_2$) predominates during most of gestation, and HbA_2 ($\alpha_2\delta_2$) is minor adult hemoglobin. Embryonic hemoglobins need not be considered here.

Each globin chain enfolds a single heme moiety, consisting of a protoporphyrin IX ring complexed with a single iron atom in the ferrous state (Fe^{2+}). Each heme moiety can bind a single oxygen molecule; a molecule of hemoglobin can transport up to four oxygen molecules.

The amino acid sequences of the various globins are highly homologous to one another. Each has a highly helical *secondary structure.* Their globular *tertiary structures* can cause the exterior surfaces to be rich in polar (hydrophilic) amino acids that enhance solubility and the interior to be lined with nonpolar groups, forming a hydrophobic pocket into which heme is inserted. The tetrameric *quaternary structure* of HbA contains two αβ dimers. Numerous tight interactions (i.e., $\alpha_1\beta_1$ contacts) hold the α and β chains together. The complete tetramer is held together by interfaces (i.e., $\alpha_1\beta_2$ contacts) between the α-like chain of one dimer and the non-α chain of the other dimer.

The hemoglobin tetramer is highly soluble but individual globin chains are insoluble. Unpaired globin precipitates, forming inclusions that damage the cell. Normal globin chain synthesis is balanced so that each newly synthesized α or non-α globin chain will have an available partner with which to pair.

Solubility and reversible oxygen binding are the key properties deranged in hemoglobinopathies. Both depend most on the hydrophilic surface amino acids, the hydrophobic amino acids lining the heme pocket, a key histidine in the F helix, and the amino acids forming the $\alpha_1\beta_1$ and $\alpha_1\beta_2$ contact points. Mutations in these strategic regions tend to be the ones that alter clinical behavior.

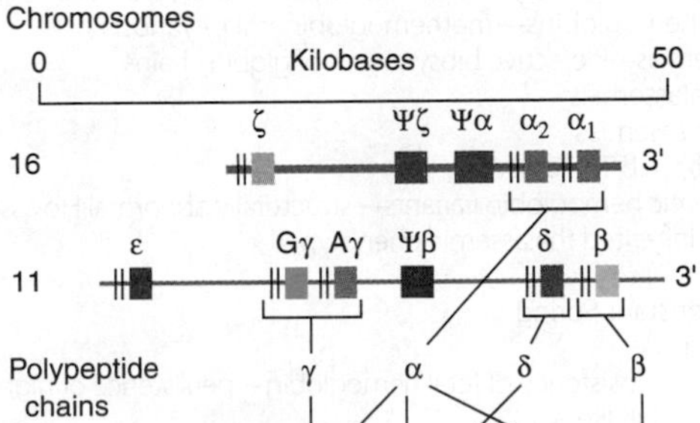

FIGURE 99-1 The globin genes. The α-like genes (α,ζ) are encoded on chromosome 16; the β-like genes (β,γ,δ,ε) are encoded on chromosome 11. The ζ and ε genes encode embryonic globins.

FUNCTION OF HEMOGLOBIN

To support oxygen transport, hemoglobin must bind O_2 efficiently at the partial pressure of oxygen (P_{O_2}) of the alveolus, retain it, and release it to tissues at the P_{O_2} of tissue capillary beds. Oxygen acquisition and delivery over a relatively narrow range of oxygen tensions depend on a property inherent in the tetrameric arrangement of heme and globin subunits within the hemoglobin molecule called *cooperativity* or *heme-heme interaction.*

At low oxygen tensions, the hemoglobin tetramer is fully deoxygenated (Fig. 99-2). Oxygen binding begins slowly as O_2 tension rises. However, as soon as some oxygen has been bound by the tetramer, an abrupt increase occurs in the slope of the curve. Thus, hemoglobin molecules that have bound some oxygen develop a higher oxygen affinity, greatly accelerating their ability to combine with more oxygen. This S-shaped oxygen equilibrium curve (Fig. 99-2), along which substantial amounts of oxygen loading *and unloading* can occur over a narrow range of oxygen tensions, is physiologically more useful than the high-affinity hyperbolic curve of individual monomers.

Oxygen affinity is modulated by several factors. The Bohr effect is the ability of hemoglobin to deliver more oxygen to tissues at low pH. It arises from the stabilizing action of protons on deoxyhemoglobin, which binds protons more readily than oxyhemoglobin because it is a weaker acid (Fig. 99-2). Thus, hemoglobin has a lower oxygen affinity at low pH. The major small molecule that alters oxygen affinity in humans is 2,3-bisphosphoglycerate (2,3-BPG, formerly 2,3-DPG), which lowers oxygen affinity when bound to hemoglobin. HbA has a reasonably high affinity for 2,3-BPG. HbF does not bind 2,3-BPG, so it tends to have a higher oxygen affinity in vivo. Hemoglobin also binds nitric oxide reversibly; this interaction may influence vascular tone, but its physiologic relevance remains unclear.

Proper oxygen transport depends on the tetrameric structure of the proteins, the proper arrangement of the charged amino acids, and interaction with protons or 2,3-BPG.

DEVELOPMENTAL BIOLOGY OF HUMAN HEMOGLOBINS

Red cells first appearing at about 6 weeks after conception contain the embryonic hemoglobins Hb Portland ($\zeta_2\gamma_2$), Hb Gower I ($\zeta_2\varepsilon_2$), and Hb Gower II ($\alpha_2\varepsilon_2$). At 10–11 weeks, fetal hemoglobin (HbF; $\alpha_2\gamma_2$) becomes predominant. The switch to nearly exclusive synthesis of adult hemoglobin (HbA; $\alpha_2\beta_2$) occurs at about 38 weeks (Fig. 99-1). Fetuses and newborns therefore require α-globin but not β-globin for normal gestation. Small amounts of HbF are produced during postnatal life. A few red cell clones called *F cells* are progeny of a small pool of immature committed erythroid precursors (BFU-e) that retain the ability to produce HbF. Profound erythroid stresses, such as severe hemolytic anemias, bone marrow transplant, or cancer chemotherapy, cause more of the F-potent BFU-e to be recruited. HbF levels thus tend to rise in some patients with sickle cell anemia or thalassemia. This phenomenon is also important because it probably explains the ability of hydroxyurea to increase levels of HbF in adults. Agents such as butyrate that inhibit histone deacetylase and modify chromatin structure can also activate fetal globin genes partially after birth.

GENETICS AND BIOSYNTHESIS OF HUMAN HEMOGLOBIN

The human hemoglobins are encoded in two tightly linked gene clusters; the α-like globin genes are clustered on chromosome 16, and the β-like genes on chromosome 11 (Fig. 99-1). The α-like cluster consists of two α-globin genes and a single copy of the ζ gene. The non-α gene cluster consists of a single ε gene, the Gγ and Aγ fetal globin genes, and the adult δ and β genes.

Important regulatory sequences flank each gene. Immediately upstream are typical promoter elements needed for the assembly of the transcription initiation complex. Sequences in the 5′ flanking region of the γ and the β genes appear to be crucial for the correct developmental regulation of these genes, while elements that function like classic enhancers and silencers are in the 3′ flanking regions. The locus control region (LCR) elements located far upstream appear to control the overall level of expression of each cluster. These elements achieve

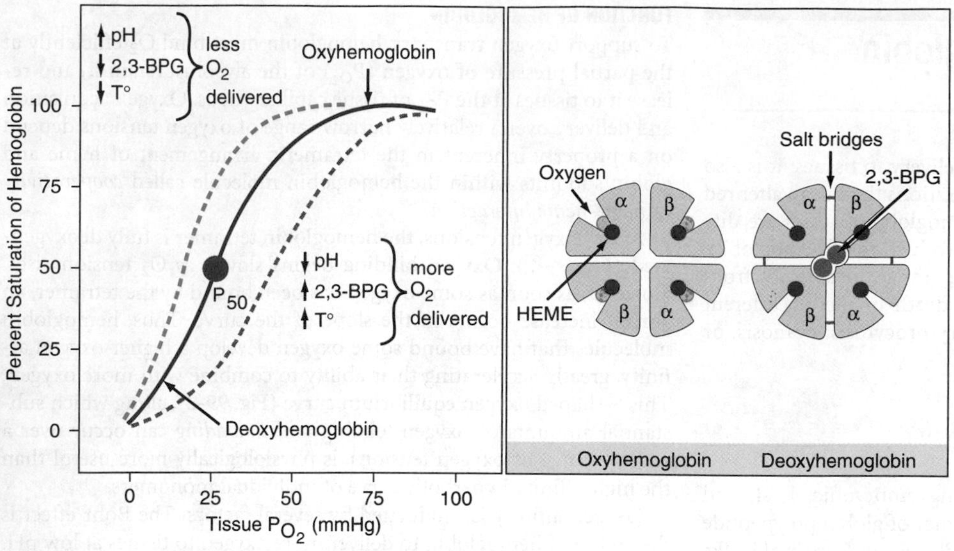

FIGURE 99-2 Hemoglobin-oxygen dissociation curve. The hemoglobin tetramer can bind up to four molecules of oxygen in the iron-containing sites of the heme molecules. As oxygen is bound, 2,3-BPG and CO_2 are expelled. Salt bridges are broken, and each of the globin molecules changes its conformation to facilitate oxygen binding. Oxygen release to the tissues is the reverse process, salt bridges being formed and 2,3-BPG and CO_2 bound. Deoxyhemoglobin does not bind oxygen efficiently until the cell returns to conditions of higher pH, the most important modulator of O_2 affinity (Bohr effect). When acid is produced in the tissues, the dissociation curve shifts to the right, facilitating oxygen release and CO_2 binding. Alkalosis has the opposite effect, reducing oxygen delivery.

their regulatory effects by interacting with *trans*-acting transcription factors. Some of these factors are ubiquitous (e.g., Sp1 and YY1), while others are more or less limited to erythroid cells or hematopoietic cells (e.g., GATA-1, NFE-2, and EKLF). The LCR controlling the α-globin gene cluster is modulated by a SWI/SNF-like protein called *ATRX*; this protein appears to influence chromatin remodeling and DNA methylation. The association of α thalassemia with mental retardation and myelodysplasia in some families appears to be related to mutations in the ATRX pathway. This pathway also modulates genes specifically expressed during erythropoiesis, such as those that encode the enzymes for heme biosynthesis. Normal red blood cell (RBC) differentiation requires the coordinated expression of the globin genes with the genes responsible for heme and iron metabolism. RBC precursors contain a protein, α-hemoglobin stabilizing protein (AHSP), that enhances the folding and solubility of α globin, which is otherwise easily denatured, leading to insoluble precipitates. These precipitates play an important role in the thalassemia syndromes and certain unstable hemoglobin disorders. Polymorphic variation in the amounts and/or functional capacity of AHSP might explain some of the clinical variability seen in patients inheriting identical thalassemia mutations. AHSP may be a therapeutic target, particularly in syndromes of intermediate severity.

CLASSIFICATION OF HEMOGLOBINOPATHIES

There are five major classes of hemoglobinopathies (Table 99-1). *Structural hemoglobinopathies* occur when mutations alter the amino acid sequence of a globin chain, altering the physiologic properties of the variant hemoglobins and producing the characteristic clinical abnormalities. The most clinically relevant variant hemoglobins polymerize abnormally, as in sickle cell anemia, or exhibit altered solubility or oxygen-binding affinity. *Thalassemia syndromes* arise from mutations that impair production or translation of globin mRNA, leading to deficient globin chain biosynthesis. Clinical abnormalities are attributable to the inadequate supply of hemoglobin and the imbalances in the production of individual globin chains, leading to premature destruction of erythroblasts and RBC. *Thalassemic hemoglobin variants* combine features of thalassemia (e.g., abnormal globin biosynthesis) and of structural hemoglobinopathies (e.g., an abnormal amino acid sequence). *Hereditary persistence of fetal hemoglobin* (HPFH) is characterized by synthesis of high levels of fetal hemoglobin in adult life. *Acquired hemoglobinopathies* include modifications of the hemoglobin molecule by toxins (e.g., acquired methemoglobinemia) and abnormal hemoglobin synthesis (e.g., high levels of HbF production in preleukemia and α thalassemia in myeloproliferative disorders).

EPIDEMIOLOGY

Hemoglobinopathies are especially common in areas in which malaria is endemic. This clustering of hemoglobinopathies is assumed to reflect a selective survival advantage for the abnormal RBC, which presumably provide a less hospitable environment during the obligate RBC stages of the parasitic life cycle. Very young children with α thalassemia are *more* susceptible to infection with the nonlethal *Plasmodium vivax*. Thalassemia might then favor a natural protection against infection with the more lethal *P. falciparum*.

Thalassemias are the most common genetic disorders in the world, affecting nearly 200 million people worldwide. About 15% of American blacks are silent carriers for α thalassemia; α-thalassemia trait (minor) occurs in 3% of American blacks and in 1–15% of persons of Mediterranean origin. β Thalassemia has a 10–15% incidence in individuals from the Mediterranean and Southeast Asia and 0.8% in American blacks. The number of severe cases of thalassemia in the United States is about 1000. Sickle cell disease is the most common structural hemoglobinopathy occurring in heterozygous form in ~8% of American blacks and in homozygous form in 1 in 400. Between 2 and 3% of American blacks carry a hemoglobin C allele.

INHERITANCE AND ONTOGENY

Hemoglobinopathies are autosomal co-dominant traits—compound heterozygotes who inherit a different abnormal mutant allele from

TABLE 99-1 CLASSIFICATION OF HEMOGLOBINOPATHIES

I. Structural hemoglobinopathies—hemoglobins with altered amino acid sequences that result in deranged function or altered physical or chemical properties
  - A. Abnormal hemoglobin polymerization—HbS, hemoglobin sickling
  - B. Altered O_2 affinity
    - 1. High affinity—polycythemia
    - 2. Low affinity—cyanosis, pseudoanemia
  - C. Hemoglobins that oxidize readily
    - 1. Unstable hemoglobins—hemolytic anemia, jaundice
    - 2. M hemoglobins—methemoglobinemia, cyanosis

II. Thalassemias—defective biosynthesis of globin chains
  - A. α Thalassemias
  - B. β Thalassemias
  - C. δβ, γδβ, αβ Thalassemias

III. Thalassemic hemoglobin variants—structurally abnormal Hb associated with co-inherited thalassemic phenotype
  - A. HbE
  - B. Hb Constant Spring
  - C. Hb Lepore

IV. Hereditary persistence of fetal hemoglobin—persistence of high levels of HbF into adult life

V. Acquired hemoglobinopathies
  - A. Methemoglobin due to toxic exposures
  - B. Sulfhemoglobin due to toxic exposures
  - C. Carboxyhemoglobin
  - D. HbH in erythroleukemia
  - E. Elevated HbF in states of erythroid stress and bone marrow dysplasia

each parent exhibit composite features of each. For example, patients inheriting sickle β thalassemia exhibit features of β thalassemia and sickle cell anemia. The α chain is present in HbA, HbA_2, and HbF; α-chain mutations thus cause abnormalities in all three. The α-globin hemoglobinopathies are symptomatic in utero and after birth because normal function of the α-globin gene is required throughout gestation and adult life. In contrast, infants with β-globin hemoglobinopathies tend to be asymptomatic until 3–9 months of age, when HbA has largely replaced HbF.

DETECTION AND CHARACTERIZATION OF HEMOGLOBINOPATHIES—GENERAL METHODS

Of the many methods available for hemoglobin analysis, electrophoretic techniques are used for routine clinical purposes. Electrophoresis at pH 8.6 on cellulose acetate membranes is especially simple, inexpensive, and reliable for initial screening. Agar gel electrophoresis at pH 6.1 in citrate buffer is often used as a complementary method because each method detects different variants. Comparison of results obtained in each system usually allows unambiguous diagnosis, but some important variants are electrophoretically silent. These mutant hemoglobins can usually be characterized by more specialized techniques such as isoelectric focusing and/or high-pressure liquid chromatography (HPLC).

Quantitation of the hemoglobin profile is often desirable. HbA_2 is frequently elevated in β-thalassemia trait and depressed in iron deficiency. HbF is elevated in HPFH, some β-thalassemia syndromes, and occasional periods of erythroid stress or marrow dysplasia. For characterization of sickle cell trait, sickle thalassemia syndromes, or HbSC disease, and for monitoring the progress of exchange transfusion therapy to lower the percentage of circulating HbS, quantitation of individual hemoglobins is also required. In most laboratories, quantitation is performed only if the test is specifically ordered.

Because some variants can comigrate with HbA or HbS (sickle hemoglobin), electrophoretic assessment should always be regarded as incomplete unless functional assays for hemoglobin sickling, solubility, or oxygen affinity are also performed, as dictated by the clinical presentation. The best sickling assays involve measurement of the degree to which the hemoglobin sample becomes insoluble, or gelated, as it is deoxygenated (i.e., sickle solubility test). Unstable hemoglobins are detected by their precipitation in isopropanol or after heating to 50°C. High-O_2 affinity and low-O_2 affinity variants are detected by quantitating the P_{50}, the partial pressure of oxygen at which the hemoglobin sample becomes 50% saturated with oxygen. Direct tests for the percent carboxyhemoglobin and methemoglobin, employing spectrophotometric techniques, can readily be obtained from most clinical laboratories on an urgent basis.

Complete characterization, including amino acid sequencing or gene cloning and sequencing, is available from several investigational laboratories around the world. Polymerase chain reaction (PCR), allele-specific oligonucleotide hybridization, and automated DNA sequencing allow identification of globin gene mutations in a few days.

Laboratory evaluation remains an adjunct, rather than the primary diagnostic aid. Diagnosis is best established by recognition of a characteristic history, physical findings, peripheral blood smear morphology, and abnormalities of the complete blood cell count (e.g., profound microcytosis with minimal anemia in thalassemia trait).

STRUCTURALLY ABNORMAL HEMOGLOBINS

SICKLE CELL SYNDROMES

The sickle cell syndromes are caused by a mutation in the β-globin gene that changes the sixth amino acid from glutamic acid to valine. HbS ($\alpha_2\beta_2^{6\ Glu \rightarrow Val}$) polymerizes reversibly when deoxygenated to form a gelatinous network of fibrous polymers that stiffen the RBC membrane, increase viscosity, and cause dehydration due to potassium leakage and calcium influx (Fig. 99-3). These changes also produce the sickle shape. Sickled cells lose the pliability needed to traverse small capillaries. They possess altered sticky membranes (especially reticulocytes) that are abnormally adherent to the endothelium of small venules. These abnormalities provoke unpredictable episodes of microvascular vasoocclusion and premature RBC destruction (hemolytic anemia). Hemolysis occurs because the spleen destroys the abnormal RBC. The rigid adherent cells also clog small capillaries and venules, causing tissue ischemia, acute pain, and gradual end-organ damage. This venoocclusive component usually dominates the clinical course. Prominent manifestations include episodes of ischemic pain (i.e., painful crises) and ischemic malfunction or frank infarction in the spleen, central nervous system, bones, liver, kidneys, and lungs (Fig. 99-3).

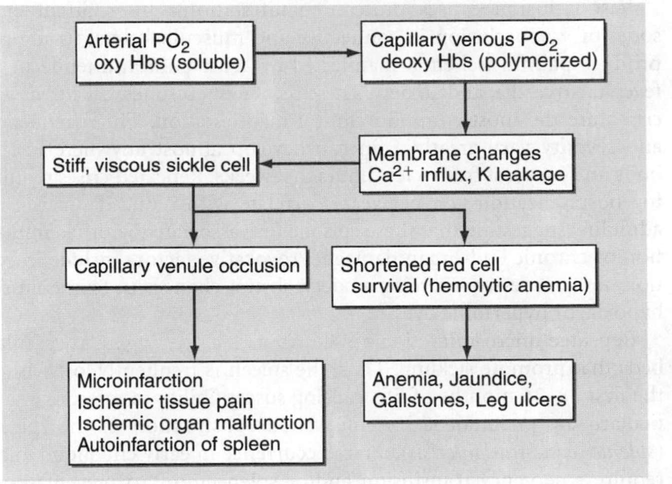

FIGURE 99-3 Pathophysiology of sickle cell crisis.

Several sickle syndromes occur as the result of inheritance of HbS from one parent and another hemoglobinopathy, such as β thalassemia or HbC ($\alpha_2\beta_2^{6\ Glu \rightarrow Lys}$), from the other parent. The prototype disease, sickle cell anemia, is the homozygous state for HbS (Table 99-2).

Clinical Manifestations of Sickle Cell Anemia Most patients with sickling syndromes suffer from hemolytic anemia, with hematocrits from 15–30%, and significant reticulocytosis. Anemia was once thought to exert protective effects against vasoocclusion by reducing blood viscosity. However, natural history and drug therapy trials suggest that an *increase* in the hematocrit and feedback inhibition of reticulocytosis might be beneficial, even at the expense of increased blood viscosity. The role of adhesive reticulocytes in vasoocclusion might account for these paradoxical effects.

Granulocytosis is common. The white count can fluctuate substantially and unpredictably during and between painful crises, infectious episodes, and other intercurrent illnesses.

TABLE 99-2 CLINICAL FEATURES OF SICKLE HEMOGLOBINOPATHIES

Condition	Clinical Abnormalities	Hemoglobin Level g/L (g/dL)	MCV, fL	Hemoglobin Electrophoresis
Sickle cell trait	None; rare painless hematuria	Normal	Normal	Hb S/A:40/60
Sickle cell anemia	Vasoocclusive crises with infarction of spleen, brain, marrow, kidney, lung; aseptic necrosis of bone; gallstones; priapism; ankle ulcers	70–100 (7–10)	80–100	Hb S/A:100/0 Hb F:2–25%
S/β° thalassemia	Vasoocclusive crises; aseptic necrosis of bone	70–100 (7–10)	60–80	Hb S/A:100/0 Hb F:1–10%
S/β⁺ thalassemia	Rare crises and aseptic necrosis	100–140 (10–14)	70–80	Hb S/A:60/40
Hemoglobin SC	Rare crises and aseptic necrosis; painless hematuria	100–140 (10–14)	80–100	Hb S/A:50/0 Hb C:50%

Vasoocclusion causes protean manifestations. Intermittent episodes of vasoocclusion in connective and musculoskeletal structures produce painful ischemia manifested by acute pain and tenderness, fever, tachycardia, and anxiety. These recurrent episodes, called *painful crises*, are the most common clinical manifestation. Their frequency and severity vary greatly. Pain can develop almost anywhere in the body and may last from a few hours to 2 weeks. Repeated crises requiring hospitalization (>3 per year) correlate with reduced survival in adult life, suggesting that these episodes are associated with accumulation of chronic end-organ damage. Provocative factors include infection, fever, excessive exercise, anxiety, abrupt changes in temperature, hypoxia, or hypertonic dyes.

Repeated micro-infarction can destroy tissues having microvascular beds that promote sickling. Thus, the spleen is frequently lost within the first 18–36 months of life, causing susceptibility to infection, particularly by pneumococci. Acute venous obstruction of the spleen (*splenic sequestration crisis*), a rare occurrence in early childhood, may require emergency transfusion and/or splenectomy to prevent trapping of the entire arterial output in the obstructed spleen. Occlusion of retinal vessels can produce hemorrhage, neovascularization, and eventual detachments. Renal papillary necrosis invariably produces isosthenuria. More widespread renal necrosis leads to renal failure in adults, a common late cause of death. Bone and joint ischemia can lead to aseptic necrosis, especially of the femoral or humeral heads; chronic arthropathy; and unusual susceptibility to osteomyelitis, which may be caused by organisms, such as *Salmonella*, rarely encountered in other settings. The *hand-foot syndrome* is caused by painful infarcts of the digits and dactylitis. Stroke is especially common in children; a small subset tend to suffer repeated episodes. Stroke is less common in adults and is often hemorrhagic. A particularly painful complication in males is priapism, due to infarction of the penile venous outflow tracts; permanent impotence is a frequent consequence. Chronic lower leg ulcers probably arise from ischemia and superinfection in the distal circulation.

Acute chest syndrome is a distinctive manifestation characterized by chest pain, tachypnea, fever, cough, and arterial oxygen desaturation. It can mimic pneumonia, pulmonary emboli, bone marrow infarction and embolism, myocardial ischemia, or in situ lung infarction. Acute chest syndrome is thought to reflect in situ sickling within the lung producing pain and temporary pulmonary dysfunction. Often it is difficult or impossible to distinguish among other possibilities. Pulmonary infarction and pneumonia are the most frequent underlying or concomitant conditions in patients with this syndrome. Repeated episodes of acute chest pain correlate with reduced survival. Acutely, reduction in arterial oxygen saturation is especially ominous because it promotes sickling on a massive scale. Chronic acute or subacute pulmonary crises lead to pulmonary hypertension and cor pulmonale, an increasingly common cause of death as patients survive longer.

Sickle cell syndromes are remarkable for their clinical heterogeneity. Some patients remain virtually asymptomatic into or even through adult life, while others suffer repeated crises requiring hospitalization from early childhood. Patients with sickle thalassemia and sickle-HbE tend to have similar, slightly milder, symptoms, perhaps because of the ameliorating effects of production of other hemoglobins within the RBC. Hemoglobin SC disease, one of the more common variants of sickle cell anemia, is frequently marked by lesser degrees of hemolytic anemia and a greater propensity for the development of retinopathy and aseptic necrosis of bones. In most respects, however, the clinical manifestations resemble sickle cell anemia. Some rare hemoglobin variants actually aggravate the sickling phenomenon. The clinical variability in different patients inheriting the same disease-causing mutation (sickle hemoglobin) has made sickle cell disease the focus of efforts to identify modifying genetic polymorphisms in other genes that might account for the heterogeneity. To date, these genome screening efforts have not yielded modifying genes, other than those known to affect the hemoglobin profile directly: e.g., persistence of fetal hemoglobin in adult life, α thalassemia, or co-inheritance of other hemoglobin structural variants. The complexity of the data obtained

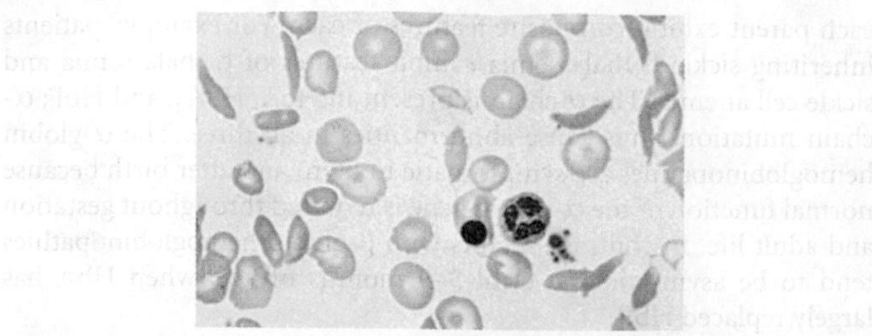

FIGURE 99-4 Sickle cell anemia. The elongated and crescent-shaped red blood cells seen on this smear represent circulating irreversibly sickled cells. Target cells and a nucleated red blood cell are also seen.

thus far undermines the expectation that genome-wide analysis will yield individualized profiles that predict a patient's clinical course.

Nevertheless, a number of interesting patterns have emerged from these modifying gene analyses. For example, genes affecting the inflammatory response or cytokine expression appear to be modifying candidates. Genes that affect transcriptional regulation of lymphocytes may be involved. Thus, it appears likely that key polymorphic changes in the patient's inflammatory response to the damages provoked by sickle red cells or in the response to chronic or recurrent infections may prove to be important for prognosticating the clinical severity of disease.

Clinical Manifestations of Sickle Cell Trait Sickle cell trait is usually asymptomatic. Anemia and painful crises are exceedingly rare. An uncommon but highly distinctive symptom is painless hematuria often occurring in adolescent males, probably due to papillary necrosis. Isosthenuria is a more common manifestation of the same process. Sloughing of papillae with urethral obstruction has been reported, as have isolated cases of massive sickling or sudden death due to exposure to high altitudes or extremes of exercise and dehydration.

Diagnosis Sickle cell syndromes are suspected on the basis of hemolytic anemia, RBC morphology (Fig. 99-4), and intermittent episodes of ischemic pain. Diagnosis is confirmed by hemoglobin electrophoresis and the sickling tests already discussed. Thorough characterization of the exact hemoglobin profile of the patient is important, because sickle thalassemia and hemoglobin SC disease have distinct prognoses or clinical features. Diagnosis is usually established in childhood, but occasional patients, often with compound heterozygous states, do not develop symptoms until the onset of puberty, pregnancy, or early adult life. Genotyping of family members and potential parental partners is critical for genetic counseling. Details of the childhood history establish prognosis and need for aggressive or experimental therapies. Factors associated with increased morbidity and reduced survival are more than three crises requiring hospitalization per year, chronic neutrophilia, a history of splenic sequestration or hand-foot syndrome, and second episodes of acute chest syndrome. Patients with a history of cerebrovascular accidents are at higher risk for repeated episodes and require especially close monitoring using Doppler carotid flow measurements. Patients with severe or repeated episodes of acute chest syndrome may need lifelong transfusion support, utilizing partial exchange transfusion, if possible.

Rx SICKLE CELL SYNDROMES

Patients with sickle cell syndromes require ongoing continuity of care. Familiarity with the pattern of symptoms provides the best safeguard against excessive use of the emergency room, hospitalization, and habituation to addictive narcotics. Additional preventive measures include regular slit-lamp examinations to monitor development of retinopathy; antibiotic prophylaxis appropriate for splenectomized patients during dental or other invasive procedures; and vigorous oral hydration during or in anticipation of periods of extreme exercise, exposure to heat or cold, emotional stress, or infection. Pneumococcal and *Haemophilus influenzae* vaccines are less effective in splenectomized individuals. Thus, patients with sickle cell anemia should be vaccinated early in life.

The management of acute painful crisis includes vigorous hydration, thorough evaluation for underlying causes (such as infection), and aggressive analgesia administered by a standing order and/or patient-controlled analgesia (PCA) pump. Morphine (0.1–0.15 mg/kg every 3–4 h) or meperidine (0.75–1.5 mg/kg every 2–4 h) should control severe pain. Meperidine should be used only for acute short-term pain control; as a chronic analgesic, it is unsuitable. Bone pain may respond as well to ketorolac (30–60 mg initial dose, then 15–30 mg every 6–8 h). Inhalation of nitrous oxide can provide short-term pain relief, but great care must be exercised to avoid hypoxia and respiratory depression. Nitrous oxide also elevates O_2 affinity, reducing O_2 delivery to tissues. Its use should be restricted to experts. Many crises can be managed at home with oral hydration and oral analgesia. Use of the emergency room should be reserved for especially severe symptoms or circumstances in which other processes, e.g., infection, are strongly suspected. Nasal oxygen should be employed as appropriate to protect arterial saturation. Most crises resolve in 1–7 days. Use of blood transfusion should be reserved for extreme cases: transfusions do not shorten the duration of the crisis.

No tests are definitive to diagnose acute painful crisis. Critical to good management is an approach that recognizes that most patients reporting crisis symptoms do indeed have crisis or another significant medical problem. Diligent diagnostic evaluation for underlying causes is imperative, even though these are found infrequently. In adults, the possibility of aseptic necrosis or sickle arthropathy must be considered, especially if pain and immobility become repeated or chronic at a single site. Nonsteroidal anti-inflammatory agents are often effective for sickle cell arthropathy.

Acute chest syndrome is a medical emergency that may require management in an intensive care unit. Hydration should be monitored carefully to avoid the development of pulmonary edema, and oxygen therapy should be especially vigorous for protection of arterial saturation. Diagnostic evaluation for pneumonia and pulmonary embolism should be especially thorough, since these may occur with atypical symptoms. Critical interventions are transfusion to maintain a hematocrit > 30, and emergency exchange transfusion if arterial saturation drops to <90%. As patients with sickle cell syndrome increasingly survive into their fifth and sixth decades, end-stage renal failure and pulmonary hypertension are becoming increasingly prominent causes of end-stage morbidity. A sickle cell cardiomyopathy and/or premature coronary artery disease may compromise cardiac function in later years. Sickle cell patients have received kidney transplants, but they often experience an increase in the frequency and severity of crises, possibly due to increased infection as a consequence of immunosuppression.

The most significant advance in the therapy of sickle cell anemia has been the introduction of hydroxyurea as a mainstay of therapy for patients with severe symptoms. Hydroxyurea (10–30 mg/kg per day) increases fetal hemoglobin and may also exert beneficial affects on RBC hydration, vascular wall adherence, and suppression of the granulocyte and reticulocyte counts; dosage is titrated to maintain a white cell count between 5000 and 8000 per μL. White cells and reticulocytes may play a major role in the pathogenesis of sickle cell crisis, and their suppression may be an important benefit of hydroxyurea therapy.

Hydroxyurea should be considered in patients experiencing repeated episodes of acute chest syndrome or with more than three crises per year requiring hospitalization. The utility of this agent for reducing the incidence of other complications (priapism, retinopathy) is under evaluation, as are the long-term side effects. Hydroxyurea offers broad benefits to most patients whose disease is severe enough to impair their functional status, and it may improve survival. HbF levels increase in most patients within a few months.

The antitumor drug, 5-azacytidine, was the first agent found to elevate HbF. It never achieved widespread use because of concerns about acute toxicity and carcinogenesis. However, low doses of the related agent, 5-deoxyazacytidine (decitabine) can elevate HbF with acceptable toxicity.

Bone marrow transplantation can provide definitive cures but is known to be effective and safe only in children. Prognostic features justifying bone marrow transplant are the presence of repeated crises early in life, a high neutrophil count, or the development of hand-foot syndrome. Children at risk for stroke can now be identified through the use of Doppler ultrasound techniques. Prophylactic exchange transfusion appears to substantially reduce the risk of stroke in this population. Children who do suffer a cerebrovascular accident should be maintained for at least 3–5 years on a program of vigorous exchange transfusion, as the risk of second strokes is extremely high.

Gene therapy for sickle cell anemia is being intensively pursued, but no safe measures are currently available. Agents blocking RBC dehydration or vascular adhesion, such as clotrimazole or magnesium, may have value as an adjunct to hydroxyurea therapy, pending the completion of ongoing trials. Combinations of clotrimazole and magnesium are being evaluated.

UNSTABLE HEMOGLOBINS

Amino acid substitutions that reduce solubility or increase susceptibility to oxidation produce unstable hemoglobins that precipitate, forming inclusion bodies injurious to the RBC membrane. Representative mutations are those that interfere with contact points between the α and β subunits [e.g., Hb Philly ($\beta^{35Tyr\rightarrow Phe}$)], alter the helical segments [e.g., Hb Genova ($\beta^{28Leu\rightarrow Pro}$)], or disrupt interactions of the hydrophobic pockets of the globin subunits with heme [e.g., Hb Koln ($\beta^{98Val\rightarrow Met}$)] (Table 99-3). The inclusions, called *Heinz bodies*, are clinically detectable by staining with supravital dyes such as crystal violet. Removal of these inclusions by the spleen generates pitted, rigid cells that have shortened life spans, producing hemolytic anemia of variable severity, sometimes requiring chronic transfusion support. Splenectomy may be needed to correct the anemia. Leg ulcers and premature gallbladder disease due to bilirubin load are frequent stigmata.

Unstable hemoglobins occur sporadically, often by spontaneous new mutations. Heterozygotes are often symptomatic because a significant Heinz body burden can develop even when the unstable variant accounts for a portion of the total hemoglobin. Symptomatic unstable hemoglobins tend to be β-globin variants, because sporadic mutations affecting only one of the four α globins would generate only 20–30% abnormal hemoglobin.

HEMOGLOBINS WITH ALTERED OXYGEN AFFINITY

High-affinity hemoglobins [e.g., Hb Yakima ($\beta^{99Asp\rightarrow His}$)] bind oxygen more readily but deliver less O_2 to tissues at normal capillary P_{O_2} levels (Fig. 99-2). Mild tissue hypoxia ensues, stimulating RBC production and erythrocytosis (Table 99-3). In extreme cases, the hematocrits can rise to 60–65%, increasing blood viscosity and producing typical symptoms (headache, somnolence, or dizziness). Phlebotomy may be required. Typical mutations alter interactions within the heme pocket or disrupt the Bohr effect or salt-bond site. Mutations that impair the interaction of HbA with 2,3-BPG can increase O_2 affinity because 2,3-BPG binding lowers O_2 affinity.

Low-affinity hemoglobins [e.g., Hb Kansas ($\beta^{102Asn\rightarrow Lys}$)] bind sufficient oxygen in the lungs, despite their lower oxygen affinity, to achieve nearly full saturation. At capillary oxygen tensions, they lose sufficient amounts of oxygen to maintain homeostasis at a low hematocrit (Fig. 99-2) (*pseudoanemia*). Capillary hemoglobin desaturation can also be sufficient to produce clinically apparent cyanosis. Despite these findings, patients usually require no specific treatment.

TABLE 99-3 REPRESENTATIVE ABNORMAL HEMOGLOBINS WITH ALTERED SYNTHESIS OR FUNCTION

Designation	Mutation	Population	Main Clinical Effects[a]
Sickle or S	$\beta^{6Glu\rightarrow Val}$	African	Anemia, ischemic infarcts
C	$\beta^{6Glu\rightarrow Lys}$	African	Mild anemia; interacts with HbS
E	$\beta^{26Glu\rightarrow Lys}$	Southeast Asian	Microcytic anemia, splenomegaly, thalassemic phenotype
Köln	$\beta^{98Val\rightarrow Met}$	Sporadic	Hemolytic anemia, Heinz bodies when splenectomized
Yakima	$\beta^{99Asp\rightarrow His}$	Sporadic	Polycythemia
Kansas	$\beta^{102Asn\rightarrow Lys}$	Sporadic	Mild anemia
M. Iwata	$\alpha^{87His\rightarrow Tyr}$	Sporadic	Methemoglobinemia

[a]See text for details.

METHEMOGLOBINEMIAS

Methemoglobin is generated by oxidation of the heme iron moieties to the ferric state, causing a characteristic bluish-brown muddy color resembling cyanosis. Methemoglobin has such high oxygen affinity that virtually no oxygen is delivered. Levels >50–60% are often fatal.

Congenital methemoglobinemia arises from globin mutations that stabilize iron in the ferric state [e.g., HbM Iwata ($\alpha^{87His \rightarrow Tyr}$), Table 99-3] or from mutations that impair the enzymes that reduce methemoglobin to hemoglobin (e.g., methemoglobin reductase, NADP diaphorase). Acquired methemoglobinemia is caused by toxins that oxidize heme iron, notably nitrate and nitrite-containing compounds.

DIAGNOSIS AND MANAGEMENT OF PATIENTS WITH UNSTABLE HEMOGLOBINS, HIGH-AFFINITY HEMOGLOBINS, AND METHEMOGLOBINEMIA

Unstable hemoglobin variants should be suspected in patients with nonimmune hemolytic anemia, jaundice, splenomegaly, or premature biliary tract disease. Severe hemolysis usually presents during infancy as neonatal jaundice or anemia. Milder cases may present in adult life with anemia or only as unexplained reticulocytosis, hepatosplenomegaly, premature biliary tract disease, or leg ulcers. Because spontaneous mutation is common, family history of anemia may be absent. The peripheral blood smear often shows anisocytosis, abundant cells with punctate inclusions, and irregular shapes (i.e., poikilocytosis).

The two best tests for diagnosing unstable hemoglobins are the Heinz body preparation and the isopropanol or heat stability test. Many unstable Hb variants are electrophoretically silent. A normal electrophoresis does not rule out the diagnosis.

Severely affected patients may require transfusion support for the first 3 years of life, because splenectomy before age 3 is associated with a significantly higher immune deficit. Splenectomy is usually effective thereafter, but occasional patients may require lifelong transfusion support. Even after splenectomy, patients can develop cholelithiasis and leg ulcers. Splenectomy can also be considered in patients exhibiting severe secondary complications of chronic hemolysis, even if anemia is absent. Precipitation of unstable hemoglobins is aggravated by oxidative stress, e.g., infection, antimalarial drugs.

High-O_2 affinity hemoglobin variants should be suspected in patients with erythrocytosis. The best test for confirmation is measurement of the P_{50}. A high-O_2 affinity Hb causes a significant left shift (i.e., lower numeric value of the P_{50}); confounding conditions, e.g., tobacco smoking or carbon monoxide exposure, can also lower the P_{50}.

High-affinity hemoglobins are often asymptomatic; rubor or plethora may be telltale signs. When the hematocrit reaches to 55–60%, symptoms of high blood viscosity and sluggish flow (headache, lethargy, dizziness, etc.) may be present. These persons may benefit from judicious phlebotomy. Erythrocytosis represents an appropriate attempt to compensate for the impaired oxygen delivery by the abnormal variant. Overzealous phlebotomy may stimulate increased erythropoiesis or aggravate symptoms by thwarting this compensatory mechanism. The guiding principle of phlebotomy should be to improve oxygen delivery by reducing blood viscosity and increasing blood flow rather than restoration of a normal hematocrit. Modest iron deficiency may aid in control.

Low-affinity hemoglobins should be considered in patients with cyanosis or a low hematocrit with no other reason apparent after thorough evaluation. The P_{50} test confirms the diagnosis. Counseling and reassurance are the interventions of choice.

Methemoglobin should be suspected in patients with hypoxic symptoms who appear cyanotic but have a Pa_{O_2} sufficiently high that hemoglobin should be fully saturated with oxygen. A history of nitrite or other oxidant ingestions may not always be available; some exposures may be unapparent to the patient, and others may result from suicide attempts. The characteristic muddy appearance of freshly drawn blood can be a critical clue. The best diagnostic test is methemoglobin assay, which is usually available on an emergency basis.

Methemoglobinemia often causes symptoms of cerebral ischemia at levels >15%; levels >60% are usually lethal. Intravenous injection of 1 mg/kg of methylene blue is effective emergency therapy. Milder cases and follow-up of severe cases can be treated orally with methylene blue (60 mg three to four times each day) or ascorbic acid (300–600 mg/d).

THALASSEMIA SYNDROMES

The thalassemia syndromes are inherited disorders of α- or β-globin biosynthesis. The reduced supply of globin diminishes production of hemoglobin tetramers, causing hypochromia and microcytosis. Unbalanced accumulation of α and β subunits occurs because the synthesis of the unaffected globins proceeds at a normal rate. Unbalanced chain accumulation dominates the clinical phenotype. Clinical severity varies widely, depending on the degree to which the synthesis of the affected globin is impaired, altered synthesis of other globin chains, and co-inheritance of other abnormal globin alleles.

CLINICAL MANIFESTATIONS OF β-THALASSEMIA SYNDROMES

Mutations causing thalassemia can affect any step in the pathway of globin gene expression: transcription, processing of the mRNA precursor, translation, and posttranslational metabolism of the β-globin polypeptide chain. The most common forms arise from mutations that derange splicing of the mRNA precursor or prematurely terminate translation of the mRNA.

Hypochromia and microcytosis characterize all forms of β thalassemia because of the reduced amounts of hemoglobin tetramers (Fig. 99-5). In heterozygotes (β-thalassemia trait), this is the only abnormality seen. Anemia is minimal. In more severe homozygous states, unbalanced α- and β-globin accumulation causes accumulation of highly insoluble unpaired α chains. They form toxic inclusion bodies that kill developing erythroblasts in the marrow. Few of the proerythroblasts beginning erythroid maturation survive. The few resulting RBCs bear a burden of inclusion bodies that are detected in the spleen, shortening the RBC life span and producing severe hemolytic anemia. The resulting profound anemia stimulates erythropoietin release and compensatory erythroid hyperplasia, but the marrow response is sabotaged by ineffective erythropoiesis. Anemia persists. Erythroid hyperplasia can become exuberant and produce masses of extramedullary erythropoietic tissue in the liver and spleen.

Massive bone marrow expansion deranges growth and development. Children develop characteristic "chipmunk" facies due to maxillary marrow hyperplasia and frontal bossing. Thinning and pathologic fracture of long bones and vertebrae may occur due to cortical invasion by erythroid elements and profound growth retardation. Hemolytic anemia causes hepatosplenomegaly, leg ulcers, gallstones, and high-output congestive heart failure. The conscription of caloric resources to support erythropoiesis leads to inanition, susceptibility to infection, endocrine dysfunction, and in the most severe cases, death during the first decade of life. Chronic transfusions with RBCs improves oxygen delivery, suppresses the excessive ineffective erythropoiesis, and prolongs life, but the inevitable side effects, notably iron overload, usually prove fatal by age 30.

Severity is highly variable. Known modulating factors are those that ameliorate the burden of unpaired α-globin inclusions. Alleles associated with milder synthetic defects and co-inheritance of α-thalassemia trait reduce clinical severity by reducing accumulation of excess α

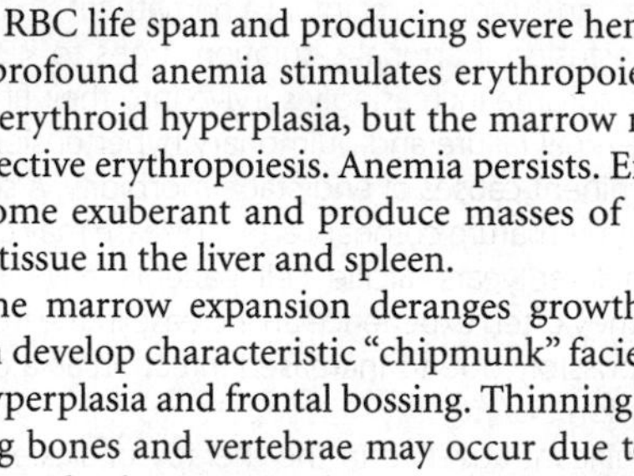

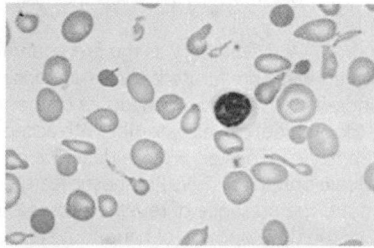

FIGURE 99-5 β-Thalassemia intermedia. Microcytic and hypochromic red blood cells are seen that resemble the red blood cells of severe iron deficiency anemia. Many elliptical and teardrop-shaped red blood cells are noted.

globin. HbF persists to various degrees in β thalassemias. γ-Globin gene chains can substitute for β chains, generating more hemoglobin and reducing the burden of α-globin inclusions. The terms *β-thalassemia major* and *β-thalassemia intermedia* are used to reflect the clinical heterogeneity. Patients with β-thalassemia major require intensive transfusion support to survive. Patients with β-thalassemia intermedia have a somewhat milder phenotype and can survive without transfusion. The terms *β-thalassemia minor* and *β-thalassemia trait* describe asymptomatic heterozygotes for β thalassemia.

TABLE 99-4 THE α THALASSEMIAS

Condition	Hemoglobin A, %	Hemoglobin H (β^4), %	Hemoglobin Level, g/L (g/dL)	MCV, fL
Normal	97	0	150 (15)	90
Silent thalassemia: –α/αα	98–100	0	150 (15)	90
Thalassemia trait: –α/–α homozygous α-thal-2[a] or ––/αα heterozygous α-thal-1[a]	85–95	Rare red blood cell inclusions	120–130 (12–13)	70–80
Hemoglobin H disease: ––/–α heterozygous α-thal-1/α-thal-2	70–95	5–30	60–100 (6–10)	60–70
Hydrops fetalis: ––/–– homozygous α-thal-1	0	5–10[b]	Fatal in utero or at birth	

[a]When both α alleles on one chromosome are deleted, the locus is called α-thal-1; when only a single α allele on one chromosome is deleted, the locus is called α-thal-2.
[b]90–95% of the hemoglobin is hemoglobin Barts (tetramers of γ chains).

α-THALASSEMIA SYNDROMES

The four classic α thalassemias, most common in Asians, are α-thalassemia-2 trait, in which one of the four α-globin loci is deleted; α-thalassemia-1 trait, with two deleted loci; HbH disease, with three loci deleted; and hydrops fetalis with Hb Bart's, with all four loci deleted (Table 99-4). Nondeletion forms of α thalassemia also exist.

α-Thalassemia-2 trait is an asymptomatic, silent carrier state. *α-Thalassemia-1 trait* resembles β-thalassemia minor. Offspring doubly heterozygous for α-thalassemia-2 and α-thalassemia-1 exhibit a more severe phenotype called *HbH disease.* Heterozygosity for a deletion that removes both genes from the same chromosome (*cis* deletion) is common in Asians and in those from the Mediterranean region, as is homozygosity for α-thalassemia-2 (*trans* deletion). Both produce asymptomatic hypochromia and microcytosis.

In *HbH disease,* HbA production is only 25–30% normal. Fetuses accumulate some unpaired β chains. In adults, unpaired β chains accumulate and are soluble enough to form β_4 tetramers called HbH. HbH forms few inclusions in erythroblasts and precipitates in circulating RBC. Patients with HbH disease have thalassemia intermedia characterized by moderately severe hemolytic anemia but milder ineffective erythropoiesis. Survival into mid-adult life without transfusions is common.

The homozygous state for the α-thalassemia-1 *cis* deletion (hydrops fetalis) causes total absence of α-globin synthesis. No physiologically useful hemoglobin is produced beyond the embryonic stage. Excess γ globin forms tetramers called *Hb Barts* (γ_4), which has a very high oxygen affinity. It delivers almost no O_2 to fetal tissues, causing tissue asphyxia, edema (hydrops fetalis), congestive heart failure, and death in utero. α-Thalassemia-2 trait is common (15–20%) among people of African descent. The *cis* α-thalassemia-1 deletion is almost never seen, however. Thus, α-thalassemia-2 and the *trans* form of α-thalassemia-1 are very common, but HbH disease and hydrops fetalis are almost never encountered.

It has been known for some time that some patients with myelodysplasia or erythroleukemia produce RBC clones containing HbH. This phenomenon is due to mutations in the ATRX pathway that affect the LCR of the α-globin gene cluster.

DIAGNOSIS AND MANAGEMENT OF THALASSEMIAS

The diagnosis of β-thalassemia major is readily made during childhood on the basis of severe anemia accompanied by the characteristic signs of massive ineffective erythropoiesis: hepatosplenomegaly, profound microcytosis, a characteristic blood smear (Fig. 99-5), and elevated levels of HbF, HbA_2, or both. Many patients require chronic hypertransfusion therapy designed to maintain a hematocrit of at least 27–30% so that erythropoiesis is suppressed. Splenectomy is required if the annual transfusion requirement (volume of RBCs per kilogram of body weight per year) increases by >50%. Folic acid supplements may be useful. Vaccination with Pneumovax in anticipation of eventual splenectomy is advised, as is close monitoring for infection, leg ulcers, and biliary tract disease. Many patients develop endocrine deficiencies as a result of iron overload. Early endocrine evaluation is required for glucose intolerance, thyroid dysfunction, and delayed onset of puberty or secondary sexual characteristics.

Patients with β-thalassemia intermedia exhibit similar stigmata but can survive without chronic hypertransfusion. Management is particularly challenging because a number of factors can aggravate the anemia, including infection, onset of puberty, and development of splenomegaly and hypersplenism. Some patients may eventually benefit from splenectomy. The expanded erythron can cause absorption of excessive dietary iron and hemosiderosis, even without transfusion.

β-Thalassemia minor (i.e., thalassemia trait) usually presents as profound microcytosis and hypochromia with target cells, but only minimal or mild anemia. The mean corpuscular volume is rarely >75 fL; the hematocrit is rarely <30–33%. Hemoglobin electrophoresis classically reveals an elevated HbA_2 (3.5–7.5%), but some forms are associated with normal HbA_2 and/or elevated HbF. Genetic counseling and patient education are essential. Patients with β-thalassemia trait should be warned that their blood picture resembles iron deficiency and can be misdiagnosed. They should eschew empirical use of iron; yet iron deficiency can develop during pregnancy or from chronic bleeding.

Persons with α-thalassemia trait may exhibit mild hypochromia and microcytosis usually without anemia. HbA_2 and HbF levels are normal. Affected individuals usually require only genetic counseling. HbH disease resembles β-thalassemia intermedia, with the added complication that the HbH molecule behaves like moderately unstable hemoglobin. Patients with HbH disease should undergo splenectomy if excessive anemia or a transfusion requirement develops. Oxidative drugs should be avoided. Iron overload leading to death can occur in more severely affected patients.

PREVENTION

Antenatal diagnosis of thalassemia syndromes is now widely available. DNA diagnosis is based on PCR amplification of fetal DNA, obtained by amniocentesis or chorionic villus biopsy followed by hybridization to allele-specific oligonucleotides probes. The probes can be designed to detect simultaneously the subset of mutations that account for 95–99% of the α- or β-thalassemias that occur in a particular group.

THALASSEMIC STRUCTURAL VARIANTS

Thalassemic structural variants are characterized by both defective synthesis and abnormal structure.

HEMOGLOBIN LEPORE

Hb Lepore $[\alpha_2(\delta\beta)_2]$ arises by an unequal crossover and recombination event that fuses the proximal end of the δ-gene with the distal end of the closely linked β-gene. The resulting chromosome contains only the fused δβ gene. The Lepore (δβ) globin is synthesized poorly because the fused gene is under the control of the weak δ-globin promoter. Hb Lepore alleles have a phenotype like β thalassemia, except for the added presence of 2–20% Hb Lepore. Compound heterozygotes for Hb Lepore and a classic β-thalassemia allele may also have severe thalassemia.

HEMOGLOBIN E

HbE (i.e., $\alpha_2\beta_2^{26Glu \rightarrow Lys}$) is extremely common in Cambodia, Thailand, and Vietnam. The gene has become far more prevalent in the United States as a result of immigration of Asian persons, especially in California, where HbE is the most common variant detected. HbE is mildly unstable but not enough to affect RBC life span significantly. The high frequency of the HbE gene may be a result of the thalassemia phenotype associated with its inheritance. Heterozygotes resemble individuals with mild β-thalassemia trait. Homozygotes have somewhat more marked abnormalities but are asymptomatic. Compound heterozygotes for HbE and a β-thalassemia gene can have β-thalassemia intermedia or β-thalassemia major, depending on the severity of the coinherited thalassemic gene.

The β^E allele contains a single base change in codon 26 that causes the amino acid substitution. However, this mutation activates a cryptic RNA splice site generating a structurally abnormal globin mRNA that cannot be translated from about 50% of the initial pre-mRNA molecules. The remaining 40–50% are normally spliced and generate functional mRNA that is translated into β^E-globin because the mature mRNA carries the base change that alters codon 26.

Genetic counseling of the persons at risk for HbE should focus on the interaction of HbE with β thalassemia rather than HbE homozygosity, a condition associated with asymptomatic microcytosis, hypochromia, and hemoglobin levels rarely <1 g/L (<10 g/dL).

HEREDITARY PERSISTENCE OF FETAL HEMOGLOBIN

HPFH is characterized by continued synthesis of high levels of HbF in adult life. No deleterious effects are apparent, even when all of the hemoglobin produced is HbF. These rare patients demonstrate convincingly that prevention or reversal of the fetal to adult hemoglobin switch would provide effective therapy for sickle cell anemia and β thalassemia.

ACQUIRED HEMOGLOBINOPATHIES

The two most important acquired hemoglobinopathies are carbon monoxide poisoning and methemoglobinemia (see above). Carbon monoxide has a higher affinity for hemoglobin than does oxygen; it can replace oxygen and diminish O_2 delivery. Chronic elevation of carboxyhemoglobin levels to 10 or 15%, as occurs in smokers, can lead to secondary polycythemia. Carboxyhemoglobin is cherry red in color and masks the development of cyanosis usually associated with poor O_2 delivery to tissues.

Abnormalities of hemoglobin biosynthesis have also been described in blood dyscrasias. In some patients with myelodysplasia, erythroleukemia, or myeloproliferative disorders, a mild form of HbH disease may also be seen. The abnormalities are not severe enough to alter the course of the underlying disease.

Rx TRANSFUSIONAL HEMOSIDEROSIS

Chronic blood transfusion can lead to blood-borne infection, alloimmunization, febrile reactions, and lethal iron overload (Chap. 107). A unit of packed RBCs contains 250–300 mg iron (1 mg/mL). The iron assimilated by a single transfusion of two units of packed RBCs is thus equal to a 1- to 2-year intake of iron. Iron accumulates in chronically transfused patients because no mechanisms exist for increasing iron excretion: an expanded erythron causes especially rapid development of iron overload because accelerated erythropoiesis promotes excessive absorption of dietary iron. Vitamin C should not be supplemented because it generates free radicals in iron excess states.

Patients who receive >100 units of packed RBCs usually develop hemosiderosis. The ferritin level rises, followed by early endocrine dysfunction (glucose intolerance and delayed puberty), cirrhosis, and cardiomyopathy. Liver biopsy shows both parenchymal and reticuloendothelial iron. The superconducting quantum-interference device (SQUID) is accurate at measuring hepatic iron but not widely available. Cardiac toxicity is often insidious. Early development of pericarditis is followed by dysrhythmia and pump failure. The onset of heart failure is ominous, often presaging death within a year (Chap. 351).

The decision to start long-term transfusion support should also prompt one to institute therapy with iron-chelating agents. Desferoxamine (Desferal) is for parenteral use. Its iron-binding kinetics require chronic slow infusion via a metering pump. The constant presence of the drug improves the efficiency of chelation and protects tissues from occasional releases of the most toxic fraction of iron—low-molecular-weight iron—which may not be sequestered by protective proteins.

Desferoxamine is relatively nontoxic. Occasional cataracts, deafness, and local skin reactions, including urticaria, occur. Skin reactions can usually be managed with antihistamines. Negative iron balance can be achieved, even in the face of a high transfusion requirement, but this alone does not prevent long-term morbidity and mortality in chronically transfused patients. Irreversible end-organ deterioration develops at relatively modest levels of iron overload, even if symptoms do not appear for many years thereafter. To enjoy a significant survival advantage, chelation must begin before 5–8 years of age in β-thalassemia major.

Deferasirox is a promising oral iron-chelating agent. Single daily doses of 20 or 30 mg deferasirox produced reductions in liver iron concentration comparable to desferoxamine in chronically transfused adult and pediatric patients. Deferasirox produces some elevations in liver enzymes and slight but persistent increases in serum creatinine, without apparent clinical consequence. Other toxicities are similar to those of desferoxamine. Its toxicity profile is acceptable, although long-term effects are still being evaluated.

EXPERIMENTAL THERAPIES

BONE MARROW TRANSPLANTATION, GENE THERAPY, AND MANIPULATION OF HbF

Bone marrow transplantation provides stem cells able to express normal hemoglobin; it has been used in a large number of patients with β thalassemia and a smaller number of patients with sickle cell anemia. Early in the course of disease, before end-organ damage occurs, transplantation is curative in 80–90% of patients. In highly experienced centers, the treatment-related mortality is <10%. Since survival into adult life is possible with conventional therapy, the decision to transplant is best made in consultation with specialized centers.

Gene therapy of thalassemia and sickle cell disease has proved to be an elusive goal. Uptake of gene vectors into the nondividing hematopoietic stem cells has been inefficient. Lentiviral-type vectors that can transduce nondividing cells may solve this problem.

Reestablishing high levels of fetal hemoglobin synthesis should ameliorate the symptoms of β thalassemia. Cytotoxic agents such as hydroxyurea and cytarabine promote high levels of HbF synthesis, probably by stimulating proliferation of the primitive HbF-producing progenitor cell population (i.e., F cell progenitors). Unfortunately, no regimen has yet been identified that ameliorates the clinical manifestations of β thalassemia. Butyrates stimulate HbF production, but only transiently. Pulsed or intermittent administration has been found to sustain HbF induction in the majority of patients with sickle cell disease. It is unclear whether butyrates will have similar activity in patients with β thalassemia.

APLASTIC AND HYPOPLASTIC CRISIS IN PATIENTS WITH HEMOGLOBINOPATHIES

Patients with hemolytic anemias sometimes exhibit an alarming decline in hematocrit during and immediately after acute illnesses. Bone marrow suppression occurs in almost everyone during acute inflammatory illnesses. In patients with short RBC life spans, suppression can affect RBC counts more dramatically. These hypoplastic crises are usually transient and self-correcting before intervention is required.

Aplastic crisis refers to a profound cessation of erythroid activity in patients with chronic hemolytic anemias. It is associated with a rapidly falling hematocrit. Episodes are usually self-limited. Aplastic crises are caused by infection with a particular strain of parvovirus, B19A. Children infected with this virus usually develop permanent immunity.

Aplastic crises do not often recur and are rarely seen in adults. Management requires close monitoring of the hematocrit and reticulocyte count. If anemia becomes symptomatic, transfusion support is indicated. Most crises resolve spontaneously within 1–2 weeks.

FURTHER READINGS

Ataga KI, Orringa EP: Hypercoagulability in sickle cell disease: A curious paradox. Am J Med 115:721, 2003

DeSimone J et al: Maintenance of elevated fetal hemoglobin levels by decitabine during dose interval treatment of sickle cell anemia. Blood 99:3905, 2002

Neufeld EJ: Oral chelators deferasirox and deferiprone for transfusional iron overload in thalassemia major: New data, new questions. Blood 107:3436, 2006

Quek L, Thein SL: Molecular therapies in beta-thalassaemia. Br J Haematol 136:353, 2007

Steinberg MH: Pathophysiologically based drug treatment of sickle cell disease. Trends Pharmacol Sci 27:204, 2006

Switzer JA et al: Pathophysiology and treatment of stroke in sickle-cell disease: Present and future. Lancet Neurol 5:501, 2006

Ware RE et al: Predictors of fetal hemoglobin response in children with sickle cell anemia receiving hydroxyurea therapy. Blood 99:10, 2002

100 Megaloblastic Anemias

A. Victor Hoffbrand

The megaloblastic anemias are a group of disorders characterized by the presence of distinctive morphologic appearances of the developing red cells in the bone marrow. The cause is usually deficiency of either cobalamin (vitamin B_{12}) or folate, but megaloblastic anemia may arise because of genetic or acquired abnormalities affecting the metabolism of these vitamins or because of defects in DNA synthesis not related to cobalamin or folate (Table 100-1). Cobalamin and folate absorption and metabolism are described next and then the biochemical basis, clinical and laboratory features, causes, and treatment of megaloblastic anemia. The marrow is usually cellular, and the anemia is based on ineffective erythropoiesis.

COBALAMIN

Cobalamin (vitamin B_{12}) exists in a number of different chemical forms. All have a cobalt atom at the center of a corrin ring. In nature, the vitamin is mainly in the 2-deoxyadenosyl (ado) form, which is located in mitochondria. It is the cofactor for the enzyme methylmalonyl CoA mutase. The other major natural cobalamin is methylcobalamin, the form in human plasma and in cell cytoplasm. It is the cofactor for methionine synthase. There are also minor amounts of hydroxocobalamin to which methyl- and adocobalamin are rapidly converted by exposure to light.

Dietary Sources and Requirements Cobalamin is synthesized solely by microorganisms. Ruminants obtain cobalamin from the foregut, but the only source for humans is food of animal origin, e.g., meat, fish, and dairy products. Vegetables, fruits, and other foods of non-animal origin are free from cobalamin unless they are contaminated by bacteria. A normal Western diet contains between 5 and 30 μg of cobalamin daily. Adult daily losses (mainly in the urine and feces) are between 1 and 3 μg (~0.1% of body stores) and, as the body does not have the ability to degrade cobalamin, daily requirements are also about 1–3 μg. Body stores are of the order of 2–3 mg, sufficient for 3–4 years if supplies are completely cut off.

TABLE 100-1 CAUSES OF MEGALOBLASTIC ANEMIA

Cobalamin deficiency or abnormalities of cobalamin metabolism (see Tables 100-3, 100-4)
Folate deficiency or abnormalities of folate metabolism (see Table 100-5)
Therapy with antifolate drugs (e.g., methotrexate)
Independent of either cobalamin or folate deficiency and refractory to cobalamin and folate therapy:
Some cases of acute myeloid leukemia, myelodysplasia
Therapy with drugs interfering with synthesis of DNA [e.g., cytosine arabinoside, hydroxyurea, 6-mercaptopurine, azidothymidine (AZT)]
Orotic aciduria (responds to uridine)
Thiamine-responsive

Absorption Two mechanisms exist for cobalamin absorption. One is passive, occurring equally through buccal, duodenal, and ileal mucosa; it is rapid but extremely inefficient, <1% of an oral dose being absorbed by this process. The normal physiologic mechanism is active; it occurs through the ileum and is efficient for small (a few micrograms) oral doses of cobalamin and is mediated by gastric intrinsic factor (IF). Dietary cobalamin is released from protein complexes by enzymes in the stomach, duodenum, and jejunum; it combines rapidly with a salivary glycoprotein that belongs to the family of cobalamin-binding proteins known as haptocorrins (HCs). In the intestine, the haptocorrin is digested by pancreatic trypsin and the cobalamin transferred to IF.

IF is produced in the gastric parietal cells of the fundus and body of the stomach, and its secretion parallels that of hydrochloric acid. The IF-cobalamin complex passes to the ileum, where IF attaches to a specific receptor (cubilin) on the microvillus membrane of the enterocytes. Cubilin is also present in yolk sac and renal proximal tubular epithclium. Cubulin appears to traffic by means of amnionless (AMN), an endocytic receptor protein that directs sublocalization and endocytosis of cubulin with its ligand IF-cobalamin complex. The cobalamin-IF complex enters the ileal cell where IF is destroyed. After a delay of about 6 h, the cobalamin appears in portal blood attached to transcobalamin (TC) II.

Between 0.5 and 5.0 μg of cobalamin enters the bile each day. This binds to IF, and a major portion of biliary cobalamin is normally reabsorbed together with cobalamin derived from sloughed intestinal cells. Because of the appreciable amount of cobalamin undergoing enterohepatic circulation, cobalamin deficiency develops more rapidly in individuals who malabsorb cobalamin than it does in vegans, in whom reabsorption of biliary cobalamin is intact.

Transport Two main cobalamin transport proteins exist in human plasma; they both bind cobalamin—one molecule for one molecule. One HC, known as TC I, is closely related to other cobalamin-binding HCs in milk, gastric juice, bile, saliva, and other fluids. These HCs differ from each other only in the carbohydrate moiety of the molecule. TC I is derived primarily from the specific granules in neutrophils. Normally, it is about two-thirds saturated with cobalamin, which it binds tightly. TC I does not enhance cobalamin entry into tissues. Glycoprotein receptors on liver cells are involved in the removal of TC I from plasma, and TC I may have a role in the transport of cobalamin analogues to the liver for excretion in bile.

The other major cobalamin transport protein in plasma is TC II. This is synthesized by liver and by other tissues, including macrophages, ileum, and endothelium. It normally carries only 20–60 ng of cobalamin per liter of plasma and readily gives up cobalamin to marrow, placenta, and other tissues, which it enters by receptor-mediated endocytosis.

FOLATE

Dietary Folate Folic (pteroylglutamic) acid is a yellow, crystalline, water-soluble substance. It is the parent compound of a large family of natural folate compounds, which differ from it in three respects:

TABLE 100-2 BIOCHEMICAL REACTIONS OF FOLATE COENZYMES

Reaction	Coenzyme Form of Folate Involved	Single Carbon Unit Transferred	Importance
Formate activation	THF	–CHO	Generation of 10-formyl-THF
Purine synthesis			
Formation of glycinamide ribonucleotide	5,10-MethyleneTHF	–CHO	Formation of purines needed for DNA, RNA synthesis, but reactions probably not rate limiting
Formylation of amino-imidazolecarboxamide-ribonucleotide (AICAR)	10-Formyl (CHO)THF		
Pyrimidine synthesis			
Methylation of deoxyuridine monophosphate (dUMP) to thymidine monophosphate (dTMP)	5,10-MethyleneTHF	$–CH_3$	Rate limiting in DNA synthesis Oxidizes THF to DHF Some breakdown of folate at the C-9–N-10 bond
Amino acid interconversion			
Serine–glycine interconversion	THF	$=CH_2$	Entry of single carbon units into active pool
Homocysteine to methionine	5-Methyl(M)THF	$–CH_3$	Demethylation of 5-MTHF to THF; also requires cobalamin, flavine adenine dinucleotide, ATP, and adenosylmethionine
Forminoglutamic acid to glutamic acid in histidine catabolism	THF	–HN–CH=	

DHF, dihydrofolate; THF, tetrahydrofolate.

(1) they are partly or completely reduced to di- or tetrahydrofolate (THF) derivatives; (2) they usually contain a single carbon unit (Table 100-2), and (3) 70–90% of natural folates are folate-polyglutamates.

Most foods contain some folate. The highest concentrations are found in liver, yeast, spinach, other greens, and nuts (>100 μg/100 g). The total folate content of an average Western diet is ~250 μg daily, but the amount varies widely according to the type of food eaten and the method of cooking. Folate is easily destroyed by heating, particularly in large volumes of water. Total-body folate in the adult is ~10 mg, the liver containing the largest store. Daily adult requirements are ~100 μg, so stores are only sufficient for 3–4 months in normal adults and severe folate deficiency may develop rapidly.

Absorption Folates are absorbed rapidly from the upper small intestine. The absorption of folate polyglutamates is less efficient than for monoglutamates; on average, ~50% of food folate is absorbed. Polyglutamate forms are hydrolysed to the monoglutamate derivatives, either in the lumen of the intestine or within the mucosa. All dietary folates are converted to 5-methylTHF (5-MTHF) within the small-intestinal mucosa before entering portal plasma. The monoglutamates are actively transported across the enterocyte by a carrier-mediated mechanism. Pteroylglutamic acid at doses >400 μg is absorbed largely unchanged and converted to natural folates in the liver. Lower doses are converted to 5-MTHF during absorption through the intestine.

About 60–90 μg of folate enters the bile each day and is excreted into the small intestine. Loss of this folate, together with the folate of sloughed intestinal cells, accelerates the speed with which folate deficiency develops in malabsorption conditions.

Transport Folate is transported in plasma; about one-third is loosely bound to albumin and two-thirds unbound. In all body fluids (plasma, cerebrospinal fluid, milk, bile) folate is largely, if not entirely, 5-MTHF in the monoglutamate form. Two types of folate-binding protein are involved in entry of MTHF into cells. A high-affinity folate receptor takes folate into cells by endocytosis, is internalized by clathrin-coated pits or in a vesicle (caveola), which is then acidified, releasing folate. Folate is then carried by the membrane folate transporter into the cytoplasm. The high-affinity receptor is attached to the outer surface of the cell membrane by glycosyl phosphatidylinositol linkages. It may be involved in transport of oxidized folates and folate breakdown products to the liver for excretion in bile. An independent low-affinity reduced-folate carrier also mediates uptake of physiologic folates into cells but also of methotrexate.

Biochemical Functions Folates (as the intracellular polyglutamate derivatives) act as coenzymes in the transfer of single-carbon units (Fig. 100-1 and Table 100-2). Two of these reactions are involved in purine and one in pyrimidine synthesis necessary for DNA and RNA replication. Folate is also a coenzyme for methionine synthesis, in which methylcobalamin is also involved and in which THF is regenerated. THF is the acceptor of single carbon units newly entering the active pool via conversion of serine to glycine. Methionine, the other product of the methionine synthase reaction, is the precursor for *S*-adenosylmethionine (SAM), the universal methyl donor involved in >100 methyltransferase reactions (Fig. 100-1).

During thymidylate synthesis, 5,10-methylene-THF is oxidized to DHF (dihydrofolate). The enzyme DHF reductase converts this to THF. The drugs methotrexate, pyrimethamine, and (mainly in bacteria) trimethoprim inhibit DHF reductase and so prevent formation of active THF coenzymes from DHF. A small fraction of the folate coenzyme is not recycled during thymidylate synthesis but is degraded.

BIOCHEMICAL BASIS OF MEGALOBLASTIC ANEMIA

The common feature of all megaloblastic anemias is a defect in DNA synthesis that affects rapidly dividing cells in the bone marrow. All conditions that give rise to megaloblastic changes share in common a disparity in the rate of synthesis or availability of the four immediate precursors of DNA: the deoxyribonucleoside triphosphates (dNTPs): dA(adenine)TP and dG(guanine)TP (purines), dT(thymine)TP and dC(cytosine)TP (pyrimidines). In deficiencies of either folate or cobalamin, there is failure to convert deoxyuridine monophosphate (dUMP) to deoxythymidine monophosphate (dTMP), the precursor of dTTP (Fig. 100-1). This is because folate is needed as the coenzyme 5,10-methylene-THF polyglutamate for conversion of dUMP to dTMP; the availability of 5,10-methylene-THF is reduced in either cobalamin or folate deficiency. An alternative theory for megaloblastic anemia in cobalamin or folate deficiency is misincorporation of uracil into DNA because of a build-up of deoxyuridine triphosphate (dUTP) at the DNA replication fork as a consequence of the block in conversion of dUMP to dTMP.

Cobalamin-Folate Relations Folate is required for many reactions in mammalian tissues. Only two reactions in the body are known to require cobalamin. Methylmalonyl CoA isomerization, which requires adocobalamin, and the methylation of homocysteine to methionine requires both methylcobalamin and both 5-MTHF (Fig. 100-1). This reaction is the first step in the pathway by which 5-MTHF, which enters bone marrow and other cells from plasma, is converted into all the intracellular folate coenzymes. The coenzymes are all polyglutamated (the larger size aiding retention in the cell), but the enzyme folate polyglutamate synthase can use only THF, not MTHF, as substrate. In cobalamin deficiency, MTHF accumulates in plasma, while intracellular folate concentrations fall due to failure of formation of THF, the substrate on which folate polyglutamates are built. This has been termed *THF starvation*, or the *methylfolate trap.*

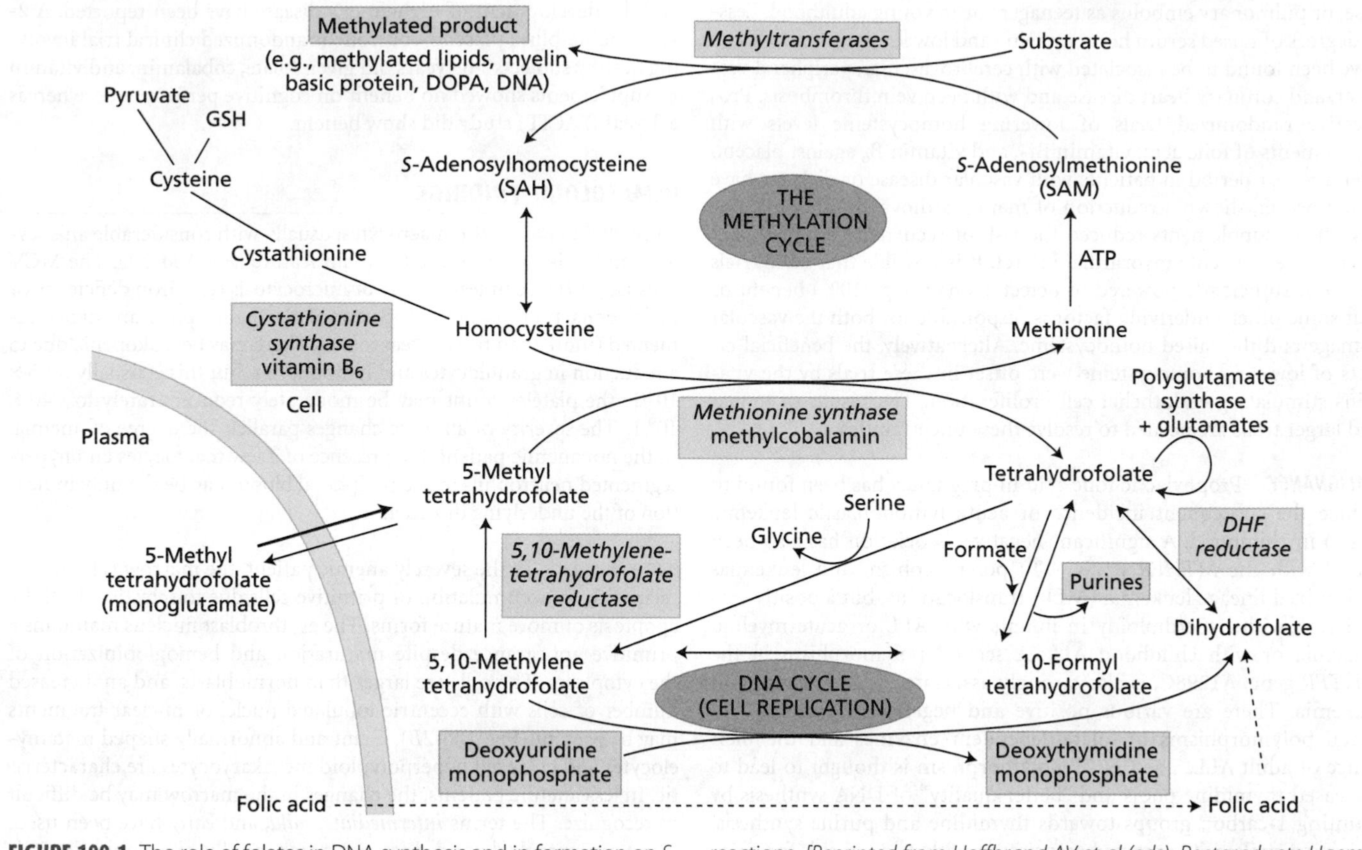

FIGURE 100-1 The role of folates in DNA synthesis and in formation on S-adenosylmethionine (SAM), which is involved in numerous methylation reactions. *[Reprinted from Hoffbrand AV et al (eds), Postgraduate Haematology, 5th ed, Blackwell Publishing, Oxford, UK 2005; with permission.]*

This theory explains the abnormalities of folate metabolism that occur in cobalamin deficiency [high serum folate, low cell folate, positive purine precursor aminomidazole carboxamide ribonucleotide (AICAR) excretion; Table 100-2] and also why the anemia of cobalamin deficiency will respond to folic acid in large doses.

CLINICAL FEATURES

Many symptomless patients are detected through the finding of a raised mean corpuscular volume (MCV) on a routine blood count. The main clinical features in more severe cases are those of anemia. Anorexia is usually marked and there may be weight loss, diarrhea, or constipation. Glossitis, angular cheilosis, a mild fever in the more severely anemic patients, jaundice (unconjugated), and reversible melanin skin hyperpigmentation may also occur with deficiency of either folate or cobalamin. Thrombocytopenia sometimes leads to bruising, and this may be aggravated by vitamin C deficiency or alcohol in malnourished patients. The anemia and low leukocyte count may predispose to infections, particularly of the respiratory or urinary tracts. Cobalamin deficiency has also been associated with impaired bactericidal function of phagocytes.

General Tissue Effects of Cobalamin and Folate Deficiencies • ***EPITHELIAL SURFACES*** After the marrow, the next most affected tissues are the epithelial cell surfaces of the mouth, stomach, and small intestine and the respiratory, urinary, and female genital tracts. The cells show macrocytosis, with increased numbers of multinucleate and dying cells. The deficiencies may cause cervical smear abnormalities.

COMPLICATIONS OF PREGNANCY The gonads are also affected, and infertility is common in both men and women with either deficiency. Maternal folate deficiency has been implicated as a cause of prematurity, and both folate and cobalamin deficiency have been implicated in recurrent fetal loss and neural tube defects, discussed below.

NEURAL TUBE DEFECTS Folic acid supplements at the time of conception and in the first 12 weeks of pregnancy reduce by ~70% the incidence of neural tube defects (NTDs) (anencephaly, meningomyelocele, encephalocele, and spina bifida) in the fetus. Most of this protective effect can be achieved by taking folic acid, 0.4 mg daily at the time of conception.

The incidence of cleft palate and harelip can also be reduced by prophylactic folic acid. There is no clear simple relationship between maternal folate status and these fetal abnormalities, although overall the lower the maternal folate, the greater the risk to the fetus. NTDs can also be caused by antifolate and antiepileptic drugs.

An underlying maternal folate metabolic abnormality has also been postulated. One abnormality has been identified: reduced activity of the enzyme 5,10-methylene-THF reductase (MTHFR) (Fig. 100-1) caused by a common 677C→T polymorphism in the *MTHFR* gene. In one study, the prevalence of this polymorphism was found to be higher in the parents of NTD fetuses and in the fetuses themselves: homozygosity for the TT mutation was found in 13% compared with 5% in control subjects. The polymorphism codes for a thermolabile form of MTHFR. The homozygous state results in a lower mean serum and red cell folate level compared with control subjects, as well as significantly higher serum homocysteine levels. Tests for mutations in other enzymes possibly associated with NTDs, e.g., methionine synthase or serine–glycine hydroxymethylase, have been negative.

Autoantibodies to folate receptors have, however, been detected in 9 of 12 women who were or had been pregnant with a fetus with a NTD, but in only 2 of 20 control women. Antiserum to folate receptors results in resorption or multiple developmental abnormalities in mouse embryos. It is possible, therefore, that the association of antibodies to maternal folate receptors and NTDs reflects a causal relation.

CARDIOVASCULAR DISEASE Children with severe homocystinuria (blood levels ≥100 μmol/L) due to deficiency of one of three enzymes, methionine synthase, MHTFR, or cystathionine synthase (Fig. 100-1), suffer from vascular disease, e.g., ischemic heart disease, cerebrovascular disease, or pulmonary embolus as teenagers or in young adulthood. Lesser degrees of raised serum homocysteine and low levels of serum folate have been found to be associated with cerebrovascular, peripheral vascular, and coronary heart disease and with deep vein thrombosis. Prospective randomized trials of lowering homocysteine levels with supplements of folic acid, vitamin B_{12}, and vitamin B_6 against placebo over a 5-year period in patients with vascular disease or diabetes have not, however, shown a reduction of major cardiovascular events, nor have these supplements reduced the risk of recurrent cardiovascular disease after an acute myocardial infarct. It is possible that these trials were not sufficiently powered to detect a small (e.g., 10%) benefit or that some other underlying factor is responsible for both the vascular damage and the raised homocysteine. Alternatively, the beneficial effects of lowering homocysteine were offset in these trials by the vitamins stimulating endothelial cell proliferation. The results of longer and larger trials are needed to resolve these uncertainties.

MALIGNANCY Prophylactic folic acid in pregnancy has been found to reduce the subsequent incidence of acute lymphoblastic leukemia (ALL) in childhood. A significant negative association has also been found with the *MTHFR* 677(C→T) polymorphism and leukemias with mixed lineage leukemia (MLL) translocations, but a positive association with hyperdiploidy in infants with ALL or acute myeloid leukemia or with childhood ALL. A second polymorphism in the *MHTFR* gene, A1298C, is also strongly associated with hyperdiploid leukemia. There are various positive and negative associations between polymorphisms in folate-dependent enzymes and the incidence of adult ALL. The C677T polymorphism is thought to lead to increased thymidine pools and "better quality" of DNA synthesis by shunting 1-carbon groups towards thymidine and purine synthesis. This may explain its reported association with a lower risk for colorectal cancer. Other tumors that have been associated with folate polymorphisms or status include follicular lymphoma, breast cancer, and gastric cancer.

NEUROLOGIC MANIFESTATIONS Cobalamin deficiency may cause a bilateral peripheral neuropathy or degeneration (demyelination) of the posterior and pyramidal tracts of the spinal cord and, less frequently, optic atrophy or cerebral symptoms.

The patient, more frequently male, presents with paresthesias, muscle weakness, or difficulty in walking and sometimes dementia, psychotic disturbances, or visual impairment. Long-term nutritional cobalamin deficiency in infancy leads to poor brain development and impaired intellectual development. Folate deficiency has been suggested to cause organic nervous disease but this is uncertain, although methotrexate injected into the cerebrospinal fluid may cause brain or spinal cord damage.

An important clinical problem is the nonanemic patient with neurologic or psychiatric abnormalities and a low or borderline serum cobalamin level. In such patients, it is necessary to try to establish whether or not there is significant cobalamin deficiency, e.g., by careful examination of the blood film, cobalamin absorption studies, tests for antibodies to IF or parietal cells, and serum methylmalonic acid (MMA) measurement if available. A trial of cobalamin therapy for at least 3 months will also usually be needed to determine whether the symptoms improve.

The biochemical basis for cobalamin neuropathy remains obscure. Its occurrence in the absence of methylmalonic aciduria in TC II deficiency suggests that the neuropathy is related to the defect in homocysteine-methionine conversion. Accumulation of *S*-adenosylhomocysteine in the brain, resulting in inhibition of transmethylation reactions, has been suggested.

Psychiatric disturbance is common in both folate and cobalamin deficiencies. This, like the neuropathy, has been attributed to a failure of the synthesis of SAM, which is needed in methylation of biogenic amines (e.g., dopamine) as well as of proteins, phospholipids, and neurotransmitters in the brain (Fig. 100-1). Associations between lower serum folate or cobalamin levels and higher homocysteine levels and the development of Alzheimer's disease have been reported. A 2-year double-blind placebo-controlled randomized clinical trial involving healthy subjects >65 years old given folate, cobalamin, and vitamin B_6 supplements showed no benefit on cognitive performance, whereas a 3-year (FACIT) study did show benefit.

HEMATOLOGIC FINDINGS

Peripheral Blood Oval macrocytes, usually with considerable anisocytosis and poikilocytosis, are the main feature (Fig. 100-2*A*). The MCV is usually >100 fL unless a cause of microcytosis (e.g., iron deficiency or thalassemia trait) is present. Some of the neutrophils are hypersegmented (more than five nuclear lobes). There may be leukopenia due to a reduction in granulocytes and lymphocytes, but this is usually $>1.5 \times 10^9$/L; the platelet count may be moderately reduced, rarely to $<40 \times 10^9$/L. The severity of all these changes parallels the degree of anemia. In the nonanemic patient, the presence of a few macrocytes and hypersegmented neutrophils in the peripheral blood may be the only indication of the underlying disorder.

Bone Marrow In the severely anemic patient, the marrow is hypercellular with an accumulation of primitive cells due to selective death by apoptosis of more mature forms. The erythroblast nucleus maintains a primitive appearance despite maturation and hemoglobinization of the cytoplasm. The cells are larger than normoblasts, and an increased number of cells with eccentric lobulated nuclei or nuclear fragments may be present (Fig. 100-2*B*). Giant and abnormally shaped metamyelocytes and enlarged hyperpolyploid megakaryocytes are characteristic. In less anemic patients, the changes in the marrow may be difficult to recognize. The terms *intermediate, mild*, and *early* have been used. The term *megaloblastoid* does not mean mildly megaloblastic. It is used to describe cells with both immature appearing nuclei and defective hemoglobinization and is usually seen in myelodysplasia.

Chromosomes Bone marrow cells, transformed lymphocytes, and other proliferating cells in the body show a variety of changes including random breaks, reduced contraction, spreading of the centromere, and exaggeration of secondary chromosomal constrictions and overprominent satellites. Similar abnormalities may be produced by antimetabolite drugs (e.g., cytosine arabinoside, hydroxyurea, and methotrexate) that either interfere with DNA replication or folate metabolism and that also cause megaloblastic appearances.

Ineffective Hemopoiesis There is an accumulation of unconjugated bilirubin in plasma due to the death of nucleated red cells in the marrow (ineffective erythropoiesis). Other evidence for this includes raised urine urobilinogen, reduced haptoglobins and positive urine hemosiderin, and a raised serum lactate dehydrogenase. A weakly positive direct antiglobulin test due to complement can lead to a false diagnosis of autoimmune hemolytic anemia.

CAUSES OF COBALAMIN DEFICIENCY

Cobalamin deficiency is usually due to malabsorption. The only other cause is inadequate dietary intake.

Inadequate Dietary Intake • ***ADULTS*** Dietary cobalamin deficiency arises in vegans who omit meat, fish, eggs, cheese, and other animal products from their diet. The largest group in the world consists of Hindus, and it is likely that many millions of Indians are at risk of deficiency of cobalamin on a nutritional basis. Subnormal serum cobalamin levels are found in up to 50% of randomly selected, young, adult Indian vegans, but the deficiency usually does not progress to megaloblastic anemia since the diet of most vegans is not totally lacking cobalamin and the enterohepatic circulation of cobalamin is intact. Dietary cobalamin deficiency may also arise rarely in nonvegetarian individuals who exist on grossly inadequate diets because of poverty or psychiatric disturbance.

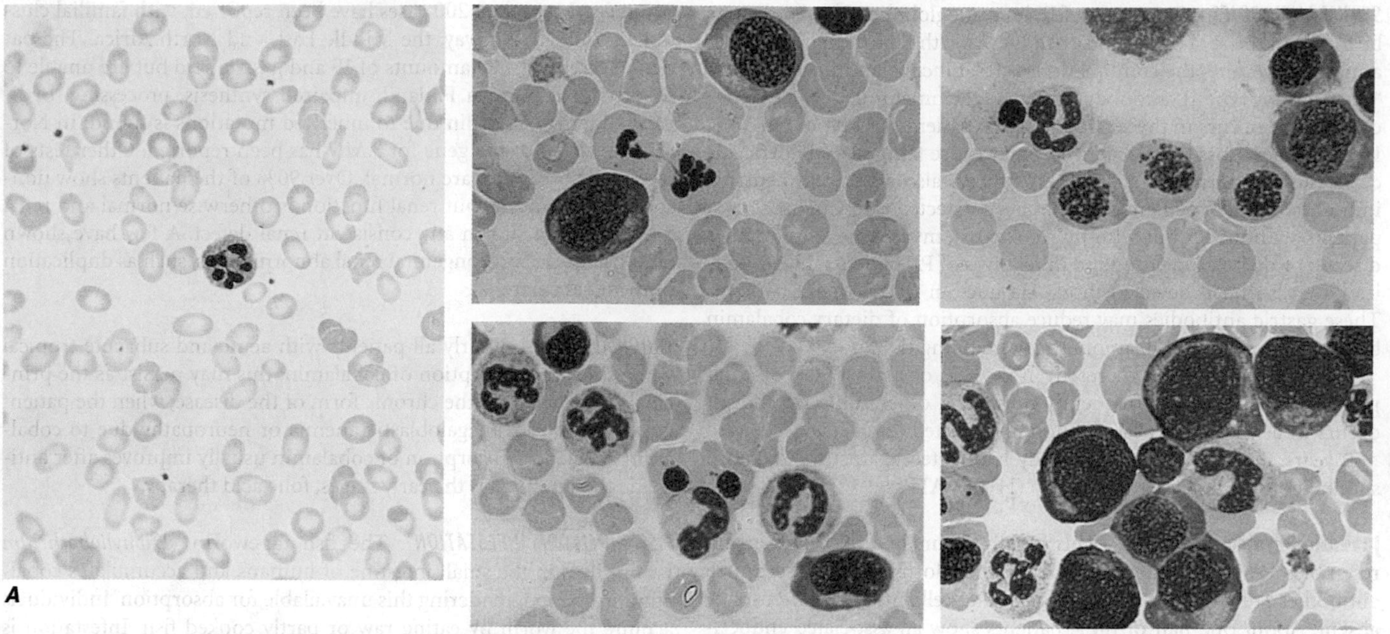

A

B

FIGURE 100-2 ***A.*** The peripheral blood in severe megaloblastic anemia. ***B.*** The bone marrow in severe megaloblastic anemia. *[Reprinted from Hoffbrand AV et al (eds) Postgraduate Haematology, 5th ed, Blackwell Publishing, Oxford, UK 2005; with permission.]*

INFANTS Cobalamin deficiency has been described in infants born to severely cobalamin-deficient mothers. These infants develop megaloblastic anemia at about 3–6 months of age, presumably because they are born with low stores of cobalamin and because they are fed breast milk of low cobalamin content. The babies have also shown growth retardation, impaired psychomotor development, and other neurologic sequelae.

Gastric Causes of Cobalamin Malabsorption See Tables 100-3 and 100-4.

PERNICIOUS ANEMIA Pernicious anemia (PA) may be defined as a severe lack of IF due to gastric atrophy. It is a common disease in north Europeans but occurs in all countries and ethnic groups. The overall incidence is about 120 per 100 000 population in the United Kingdom (UK). The ratio of incidence in men and women in Caucasians is ~1:1.6 and the peak age of onset is 60 years, with only 10% of patients being <40 years of age. However, in some ethnic groups, notably black individuals and Latin Americans, the age of onset of PA is generally lower. The disease occurs more commonly than by chance in close relatives and in persons with other organ-specific autoimmune diseases, e.g., thyroid diseases, vitiligo, hypoparathyroidism, and Addison's disease. It is also associated with hypogammaglobulinemia, with premature graying or blue eyes, and in persons of blood group A. An association with human leukocyte antigen (HLA) 3 has been reported in some but not all series and, in those with endocrine disease, with HLA-B8, -B12, and -BW15. The life expectancy is normal in women once regular treatment has begun. Men have a slightly subnormal life expectancy as a result of a higher incidence of carcinoma of the stomach than in control subjects. Gastric output of hydrochloric acid, pepsin, and IF are severely reduced. The serum gastrin level is raised, and serum pepsinogen I levels are low.

GASTRIC BIOPSY This usually shows atrophy of all layers of the body and fundus, with loss of glandular elements, an absence of parietal and chief cells and replacement by mucous cells, a mixed inflammatory cell infiltrate, and perhaps intestinal metaplasia. The infiltrate of plasma cells and lymphocytes contains an excess of CD4 cells. The antral mucosa is usually well preserved. *Helicobacter pylori* infection is infrequent in PA, but it has been suggested that *H. pylori* gastritis occurs at an early phase of atrophic gastritis and presents in younger patients as iron deficiency anemia but in older patients as PA. *H. pylori* is suggested to stimulate an autoimmune process directed against parietal cells, the *H. pylori* infection then being gradually replaced, in some individuals, by an autoimmune process.

TABLE 100-3 CAUSES OF COBALAMIN DEFICIENCY SUFFICIENTLY SEVERE TO CAUSE MEGALOBLASTIC ANEMIA

Nutritional	Vegans
Malabsorption	Pernicious anemia
Gastric causes	Congenital absence of intrinsic factor or functional abnormality
	Total or partial gastrectomy
Intestinal causes	Intestinal stagnant loop syndrome: jejunal diverticulosis, ileocolic fistula, anatomic blind loop, intestinal stricture, etc.
	Ileal resection and Crohn's disease
	Selective malabsorption with proteinuria
	Tropical sprue
	Transcobalamin II deficiency
	Fish tapeworm

TABLE 100-4 MALABSORPTION OF COBALAMIN MAY OCCUR IN THE FOLLOWING CONDITIONS BUT IS NOT USUALLY SUFFICIENTLY SEVERE AND PROLONGED TO CAUSE MEGALOBLASTIC ANEMIA

- Gastric causes
  - Simple atrophic gastritis (food cobalamin malabsorption)
  - Zollinger–Ellison syndrome
  - Gastric bypass surgery
  - Use of proton pump inhibitors
- Intestinal causes
  - Gluten-induced enteropathy
  - Severe pancreatitis
  - HIV infection
  - Radiotherapy
  - Graft-versus-host disease
- Deficiencies of cobalamin, folate, protein, ?riboflavin, ?nicotinic acid
- Therapy with colchicine, para-aminosalicylate, neomycin, slow-release potassium chloride, anticonvulsant drugs, metformin, phenformin, cytotoxic drugs
- Alcohol

SERUM ANTIBODIES Two types of IF immunoglobulin G antibody may be found in the sera of patients with PA. One, the "blocking," or type I, antibody, prevents the combination of IF and cobalamin, whereas the "binding," or type II, antibody prevents attachment of IF to ileal mucosa. Type I occurs in the sera of ~55% of patients and type II in 35%. IF antibodies cross the placenta and may cause temporary IF deficiency in the newborn infant. Patients with PA also show cell-mediated immunity to IF. Type I antibody has been detected rarely in the sera of patients without PA but with thyrotoxicosis, myxedema, Hashimoto's disease, or diabetes mellitus and in relatives of PA patients. IF antibodies have also been detected in gastric juice in ~80% of PA patients. These gastric antibodies may reduce absorption of dietary cobalamin by combining with small amounts of remaining IF.

Parietal cell antibody is present in the sera of almost 90% of adult patients with PA but is frequently present in other subjects. Thus, it occurs in as many as 16% of randomly selected female subjects aged >60 years. The parietal cell antibody is directed against the α and β subunits of the gastric proton pump (H^+,K^+-ATPase).

Juvenile Pernicious Anemia This usually occurs in older children and resembles PA of adults. Gastric atrophy, achlorhydria, and serum IF antibodies are all present, although parietal cell antibodies are usually absent. About one-half of these patients show an associated endocrinopathy such as autoimmune thyroiditis, Addison's disease, or hypoparathyroidism; in some, mucocutaneous candidiasis occurs.

Congenital Intrinsic Factor Deficiency or Functional Abnormality The affected child usually presents with megaloblastic anemia in the first to third year of life; a few have presented as late as the second decade. The child has no demonstrable IF but has a normal gastric mucosa and normal secretion of acid. The inheritance is autosomally recessive. Parietal cell and IF antibodies are absent. Variants have been described in which the child is born with IF that can be detected immunologically but is unstable or functionally inactive.

Gastrectomy Following total gastrectomy, cobalamin deficiency is inevitable, and prophylactic cobalamin therapy should be commenced immediately following the operation. After partial gastrectomy, 10–15% of patients also develop this deficiency. The exact incidence and time of onset are most influenced by the size of the resection and the preexisting size of cobalamin body stores.

Food Cobalamin Malabsorption Failure of release of cobalamin from binding proteins in food is believed to be responsible for this condition, more common in the elderly. It is associated with low serum cobalamin levels, with or without raised serum levels of MMA and homocysteine. Typically, these patients have normal cobalamin absorption, as measured with crystalline cobalamin, but show malabsorption when a modified test using food-bound cobalamin is used. The frequency of progression to severe cobalamin deficiency and reasons for this progression are not clear.

Intestinal Causes of Cobalamin Malabsorption • *INTESTINAL STAGNANT LOOP SYNDROME* Malabsorption of cobalamin occurs in a variety of intestinal lesions in which there is colonization of the upper small intestine by fecal organisms. This may occur in patients with jejunal diverticulosis, enteroanastomosis, or intestinal stricture or fistula or with an anatomic blood loop due to Crohn's disease, tuberculosis, or an operative procedure.

ILEAL RESECTION Removal of ≥1.2 m of terminal ileum causes malabsorption of cobalamin. In some patients following ileal resection, particularly if the ileocecal valve is incompetent, colonic bacteria may contribute further to the onset of cobalamin deficiency.

SELECTIVE MALABSORPTION OF COBALAMIN WITH PROTEINURIA (IMERSLUND SYNDROME: IMERSLUND-GRÄSBECK SYNDROME; CONGENITAL COBALAMIN MALABSORPTION; AUTOSOMAL RECESSIVE MEGALOBLASTIC ANEMIA, MGA1) This autosomally recessive disease is the most common cause of megaloblastic anemia due to cobalamin deficiency in infancy in Western countries. More than 200 cases have been reported, with familial clusters in Finland, Norway, the Middle East, and North Africa. The patients secrete normal amounts of IF and gastric acid but are unable to absorb cobalamin. In Finland, impaired synthesis, processing, or ligand binding of cubilin due to inherited mutations is found. In Norway, mutation of the gene for *AMN* has been reported. Other tests of intestinal absorption are normal. Over 90% of the patients show nonspecific proteinuria, but renal function is otherwise normal and renal biopsy has not shown any consistent renal defect. A few have shown aminoaciduria and congenital renal abnormalities, such as duplication of the renal pelvis.

TROPICAL SPRUE Nearly all patients with acute and subacute tropical sprue show malabsorption of cobalamin; this may persist as the principal abnormality in the chronic form of the disease, when the patient may present with megaloblastic anemia or neuropathy due to cobalamin deficiency. Absorption of cobalamin usually improves after antibiotic therapy and, in the early stages, folic acid therapy.

FISH TAPEWORM INFESTATION The fish tapeworm (*Diphyllobothrium latum*) lives in the small intestine of humans and accumulates cobalamin from food, rendering this unavailable for absorption. Individuals acquire the worm by eating raw or partly cooked fish. Infestation is common around the lakes of Scandinavia, Germany, Japan, North America, and Russia. Megaloblastic anemia or cobalamin neuropathy occurs only in those with a heavy infestation.

GLUTEN-INDUCED ENTEROPATHY Malabsorption of cobalamin occurs in ~30% of untreated patients (presumably those in whom the disease extends to the ileum). Cobalamin deficiency is not severe in these patients and is corrected with a gluten-free diet.

SEVERE CHRONIC PANCREATITIS In this condition, lack of trypsin is thought to cause dietary cobalamin attached to gastric non-IF (R) binder to be unavailable for absorption. It has also been proposed that in pancreatitis, the concentration of calcium ions in the ileum falls below the level needed to maintain normal cobalamin absorption.

HIV INFECTION Serum cobalamin levels tend to fall in patients with HIV infection and are subnormal in 10–35% of those with AIDS. Malabsorption of cobalamin not corrected by IF has been shown in some, but not all, patients with subnormal serum cobalamin levels. Cobalamin deficiency sufficiently severe to cause megaloblastic anemia or neuropathy is rare.

ZOLLINGER–ELLISON SYNDROME Malabsorption of cobalamin has been reported in the Zollinger–Ellison syndrome. It is thought that there is a failure to release cobalamin from R-binding protein due to inactivation of pancreatic trypsin by high acidity, as well as interference with IF binding of cobalamin.

RADIOTHERAPY Both total-body irradiation and local radiotherapy to the ileum (e.g., as a complication of radiotherapy for carcinoma of the cervix) may cause malabsorption of cobalamin.

GRAFT-VERSUS-HOST DISEASE This commonly affects the small intestine. Malabsorption of cobalamin due to abnormal gut flora, as well as damage to ileal mucosa, is frequent.

DRUGS The drugs that have been reported to cause malabsorption of cobalamin are listed in Table 100-4. Megaloblastic anemia due to these drugs is, however, rare.

Abnormalities of Cobalamin Metabolism • *CONGENITAL TRANSCOBALAMIN II DEFICIENCY OR ABNORMALITY* Infants with TC II deficiency usually present with megaloblastic anemia within a few weeks of birth. Serum cobalamin and folate levels are normal, but the anemia responds to massive (e.g., 1 mg three times weekly) injections of cobalamin. Some cases show neurologic complications. The protein may be present but functionally inert. Genetic abnormalities found include mutations of an intra-exonic cryptic splice site, extensive deletion, single nucleotide deletion, nonsense mutation, and an RNA editing defect. Malabsorption of cobalamin occurs in all cases and serum immunoglobulins are usually reduced. Failure to institute adequate cobalamin therapy or treatment with folic acid may lead to neurologic damage.

CONGENITAL METHYLMALONIC ACIDEMIA AND ACIDURIA The infants with this abnormality are ill from birth with vomiting, failure to thrive, severe metabolic acidosis, ketosis, and mental retardation. Anemia, if present, is normocytic and normoblastic. The condition may be due to a functional defect in either mitochondrial methylmalonyl CoA mutase or its cofactor adocobalamin. Mutations in the methylmalonyl CoA mutase are not responsive, or only poorly responsive, to treatment with cobalamin. A proportion of the infants with failure of adocobalamin synthesis respond to cobalamin in large doses. Some children have combined methylmalonic aciduria and homocystinuria due to defective formation of both cobalamin coenzymes. This usually presents in the first year of life with feeding difficulties, developmental delay, microcephaly, seizures, hypotonia, and megaloblastic anemia.

ACQUIRED ABNORMALITY OF COBALAMIN METABOLISM: NITROUS OXIDE INHALATION Nitrous oxide irreversibly oxidizes methylcobalamin to an inactive precursor; this inactivates methionine synthase. Megaloblastic anemia has occurred in patients undergoing prolonged N_2O anesthesia (e.g., in intensive care units). A neuropathy resembling cobalamin neuropathy has also been described in dentists and anesthetists who are repeatedly exposed to N_2O. Methylmalonic aciduria does not occur as adocobalamin is not inactivated by N_2O.

CAUSES OF FOLATE DEFICIENCY (Table 100-5)

Nutritional Dietary folate deficiency is common. Indeed, in most patients with folate deficiency a nutritional element is present. Certain individuals are particularly prone to have diets containing inadequate amounts of folate (Table 100-5). In the United States and other countries where fortification of the diet with folic acid has been adopted, the prevalence of folate deficiency has dropped dramatically and is now almost restricted to high-risk groups with increased folate needs. Nutritional folate deficiency occurs in kwashiorkor and scurvy and in infants with repeated infections or who are fed solely on goats' milk, which has a low folate content.

Malabsorption Malabsorption of dietary folate occurs in tropical sprue and in gluten-induced enteropathy. In the rare congenital syndrome of selective malabsorption of folate, there is an associated defect of folate transport into the cerebrospinal fluid, and these patients show megaloblastic anemia, which responds to physiologic doses of folic acid given parenterally but not orally. They also show mental retardation, convulsions, and other central nervous system abnormalities. Minor degrees of malabsorption may also occur following jejunal resection or partial gastrectomy, in Crohn's disease, and in systemic infections but, in these conditions, if severe deficiency occurs, it is usually largely due to poor nutrition. Malabsorption of folate has been described in patients receiving salazopyrine, cholestyramine, and triamterene.

Excess Utilization or Loss • ***PREGNANCY*** Folate requirements are increased by 200–300 μg to ~400 μg daily in a normal pregnancy, partly because of transfer of the vitamin to the fetus, but mainly because of increased folate catabolism due to cleavage of folate coenzymes in rapidly proliferating tissues. Megaloblastic anemia due to this deficiency is prevented by prophylactic folic acid therapy. It occurred in 0.5% of pregnancies in the UK and other Western countries before prophylaxis with folic acid, but the incidence is much higher in countries where the general nutritional status is poor.

TABLE 100-5 CAUSES OF FOLATE DEFICIENCY

Dietary[a]
Particularly in: old age, infancy, poverty, alcoholism, chronic invalids, and the psychiatrically disturbed; may be associated with scurvy or kwashiorkor
Malabsorption
Major causes of deficiency
Tropical sprue, gluten-induced enteropathy in children and adults, and in association with dermatitis herpetiformis, specific malabsorption of folate, intestinal megaloblastosis caused by severe cobalamin or folate deficiency
Minor causes of deficiency
Extensive jejunal resection, Crohn's disease, partial gastrectomy, congestive heart failure, Whipple's disease, scleroderma, amyloid, diabetic enteropathy, systemic bacterial infection, lymphoma, salazopyrine
Excess utilization or loss
Physiologic
Pregnancy and lactation, prematurity
Pathologic
Hematologic diseases: chronic hemolytic anemias, sickle cell anemia, thalassemia major, myelofibrosis
Malignant diseases: carcinoma, lymphoma, leukemia, myeloma
Inflammatory diseases: tuberculosis, Crohn's disease, psoriasis, exfoliative dermatitis, malaria
Metabolic disease: homocystinuria
Excess urinary loss: congestive heart failure, active liver disease
Hemodialysis, peritoneal dialysis
Antifolate drugs[b]
Anticonvulsant drugs (phenytoin, primidone, barbiturates), sulphasalazine
Nitrofurantoin, tetracycline, anti-tuberculosis (less well documented)
Mixed causes
Liver diseases, alcoholism, intensive care units

[a]In severely folate-deficient patients with causes other than those listed under Dietary, poor dietary intake is often present.
[b]Drugs inhibiting dihydrofolate reductase are discussed in the text.

PREMATURITY The newborn infant, whether full term or premature, has higher serum and red cell folate concentrations than the adult. However, the newborn infant's demand for folate has been estimated to be up to 10 times that of adults on a weight basis, and the neonatal folate level falls rapidly to the lowest values at about 6 weeks of age. The falls are steepest and are liable to reach subnormal levels in premature babies, a number of whom develop megaloblastic anemia responsive to folic acid at about 4–6 weeks of age. This occurs particularly in the smallest babies (<1500 g birth weight) and in those who have feeding difficulties or infections or who have undergone multiple exchange transfusions. In these babies, prophylactic folic acid should be given.

HEMATOLOGIC DISORDERS Folate deficiency frequently occurs in chronic hemolytic anemia, particularly in sickle cell disease, autoimmune hemolytic anemia, and congenital spherocytosis. In these and other conditions of increased cell turnover (e.g., myelofibrosis, malignancies) folate deficiency arises because it is not completely reutilized after performing coenzyme functions.

INFLAMMATORY CONDITIONS Chronic inflammatory diseases, such as tuberculosis, rheumatoid arthritis, Crohn's disease, psoriasis, exfoliative dermatitis, bacterial endocarditis, and chronic bacterial infections, cause deficiency by reducing the appetite and by increasing the demand for folate. Systemic infections may also cause malabsorption of folate. Severe deficiency is virtually confined to the patients with the most active disease and the poorest diet.

HOMOCYSTINURIA This is a rare metabolic defect in the conversion of homocysteine to cystathionine. Folate deficiency occurring in most of these patients may be due to excessive utilization because of compensatory increased conversion of homocysteine to methionine.

LONG-TERM DIALYSIS As folate is only loosely bound to plasma proteins, it is easily removed from plasma by dialysis. In patients with anorexia, vomiting, infections, and hemolysis, folate stores are particularly likely to become depleted. Routine folate prophylaxis is now given.

CONGESTIVE HEART FAILURE, LIVER DISEASE Excess urinary folate losses of >100 μg per day may occur in some of these patients. The explanation appears to be release of folate from damaged liver cells.

Antifolate Drugs A large number of epileptics, who are receiving long-term therapy with phenytoin or primidone, with or without barbiturates, develop low serum and red cell folate levels. The exact mechanism is unclear. Alcohol may also be a folate antagonist, as patients who are drinking spirits may develop megaloblastic anemia that will respond to normal quantities of dietary folate or to physiologic doses of folic acid only if alcohol is withdrawn. Macrocytosis of red cells is associated with chronic alcohol intake even when folate levels are normal. Inadequate folate intake is the major factor in the development of deficiency in spirit-drinking alcoholics. Beer is relatively folate-rich in some countries, depending on the technique used for brewing.

The drugs that inhibit DHF reductase include methotrexate, pyrimethamine, and trimethoprim. Methotrexate has the most powerful action against the human enzyme, whereas trimethoprim is most active against the bacterial enzyme and is only likely to cause megaloblastic anemia when used in conjunction with sulphamethoxazole in patients with preexisting folate or cobalamin deficiency. The activity of pyrimethamine is intermediate. The antidote to these drugs is folinic acid (5-formyl-THF).

Congenital Abnormalities of Folate Metabolism Some infants with congenital defects of folate enzymes (e.g., cyclohydrolase or methionine synthase) have had megaloblastic anemia.

DIAGNOSIS OF COBALAMIN AND FOLATE DEFICIENCIES

The diagnosis of cobalamin or folate deficiency has traditionally depended on the recognition of the relevant abnormalities in the peripheral blood and analysis of the blood levels of the vitamins.

Serum Cobalamin This is measured by an automated enzyme-linked immunoadsorbent (ELISA) assay. Normal serum levels range 118–148 pmol/L (160–200 ng/L) to ~738 pmol/L (1000 ng/L). In patients with megaloblastic anemia due to cobalamin deficiency, the level is usually <74 pmol/L (100 ng/L). In general, the more severe the deficiency, the lower the serum cobalamin level. In patients with spinal cord damage due to the deficiency, levels are very low even in the absence of anemia. Values of between 74 and 148 pmol/L (100 and 200 ng/L) are regarded as borderline. They may occur, for instance, in pregnancy, in patients with megaloblastic anemia due to folate deficiency. The serum cobalamin level is generally considered to be sufficiently robust, cost-effective, and most convenient to rule out cobalamin deficiency in the vast majority of patients suspected of having this problem.

Serum Methylmalonate and Homocysteine In patients with cobalamin deficiency sufficient to cause anemia or neuropathy, the serum MMA level is raised. Sensitive methods for measuring MMA and homocysteine in serum have been introduced and recommended for the early diagnosis of cobalamin deficiency, even in the absence of hematologic abnormalities or subnormal levels of serum cobalamin. Serum MMA levels fluctuate, however, in patients with renal failure. Mildly elevated serum MMA and/or homocysteine levels occur in up to 30% of apparently healthy volunteers, with serum cobalamin levels up to 258 pmol/L (350 ng/L) and normal serum folate levels; 15% of elderly subjects, even with cobalamin levels >258 pmol/L (>350 ng/L), have this pattern of raised metabolite levels. These findings bring into question the exact cut-off points for normal MMA and homocysteine levels. It is also unclear at present whether these mildly raised metabolite levels have clinical consequences.

Serum homocysteine is raised in both early cobalamin and folate deficiency but may be raised in other conditions, e.g., chronic renal disease, alcoholism, smoking, pyridoxine deficiency, hypothyroidism, therapy with steroids, cyclosporine, and other drugs. Levels are also higher in serum than in plasma, in men than in premenopausal women, in women taking hormone replacement therapy, or in oral contraceptive users and in elderly persons and patients with several inborn errors of metabolism affecting enzymes in trans-sulfuration pathways of homocysteine metabolism. Thus, homocysteine levels are not used for diagnosis of cobalamin or folate deficiency.

Cobalamin Absorption Studies of cobalamin absorption have been widely used, but difficulty in obtaining radioactive cobalamin and of ensuring IF preparations are free of viruses have led to reduced availability. For the urinary excretion (Schilling) test the patient is fasted overnight. Radioactive cyanocobalamin is given orally. Then, 2 h later an IM injection of cyanocobalamin or hydroxocobalamin (1 mg) is given ("flushing dose"). A 24-h urine specimen is collected for determination of radioactivity; low excretion shows malabsorption; the oral dose is then given again after 48 h with IF. The results distinguish between gastric and intestinal causes of cobalamin malabsorption.

Serum Folate This is also measured by an ELISA technique. In most laboratories, the normal range is from 11 nmol/L (2.0 μg/L) to ~82 nmol/L (15 μg/L). The serum folate level is low in all folate-deficient patients. It also reflects recent diet. Because of this, serum folate may be low before there is hematologic or biochemical evidence of deficiency. Serum folate rises in severe cobalamin deficiency because of the block in conversion of MTHF to THF inside cells; raised levels have also been reported in the intestinal stagnant loop syndrome, due to absorption of bacterially synthesized folate.

Red Cell Folate The red cell folate assay is a valuable test of body folate stores. It is less affected than the serum assay by recent diet and traces of hemolysis. In normal adults, concentrations range 880–3520 μmol/L (160–640 μg/L) of packed red cells. Subnormal levels occur in patients with megaloblastic anemia due to folate deficiency but also in nearly two-thirds of patients with severe cobalamin deficiency. False-normal results may occur if the folate-deficient patient has received a recent blood transfusion or if the patient has a raised reticulocyte count.

℞ MEGALOBLASTIC ANEMIA

It is usually possible to establish which of the two deficiencies, folate or cobalamin, is the cause of the anemia and to treat only with the appropriate vitamin. In patients who enter hospital severely ill, however, it may be necessary to treat with both vitamins in large doses once blood samples have been taken for cobalamin and folate assays and a bone marrow biopsy has been performed (if deemed necessary). Transfusion is usually unnecessary and inadvisable. If it is essential, packed red cells should be given slowly, one or two units only, with the usual treatment for heart failure if present. Potassium supplements have been recommended to obviate the danger of the hypokalemia that has been recorded in some patients during the initial hematologic response. Occasionally, an excessive rise in platelets occurs after 1–2 weeks of therapy. Antiplatelet therapy, e.g., aspirin should be considered if the platelet count rises to $>800 \times 10^9$/L.

TREATMENT OF COBALAMIN DEFICIENCY It is usually necessary to treat patients who have developed cobalamin deficiency with lifelong regular cobalamin injections. In the UK, the form used is hydroxocobalamin; in the United States, cyanocobalamin. In a few instances, the underlying cause of cobalamin deficiency can be permanently corrected, e.g., the fish tapeworm, tropical sprue, or an intestinal stagnant loop that is amenable to surgery. The indications for starting cobalamin therapy are a well-documented megaloblastic anemia or other hematologic abnormalities or neuropathy due to the deficiency. Patients with borderline serum cobalamin levels but no hematologic or other abnormality should be followed, e.g., at yearly intervals to make sure that the cobalamin deficiency does not progress. If malabsorption of cobalamin or rises in serum MMA levels have also been demonstrated, however, they should also be given regular maintenance cobalamin therapy. Cobalamin should be given routinely to all patients who have had a total gastrectomy or ileal resection.

Patients who have undergone gastric reduction for control of obesity or who are receiving long-term treatment with proton pump inhibitors should be screened and, if necessary, given cobalamin replacement.

Replenishment of body stores should be complete with six 1000-μg IM injections of hydroxocobalamin given at 3- to 7-day intervals. More frequent doses are usually used in patients with cobalamin neuropathy, but there is no evidence that these produce a better response. For maintenance therapy, 1000 μg hydroxocobalamin IM once every 3 months is satisfactory. Because of the poorer retention of cyanocobalamin, protocols generally use higher and more frequent doses, e.g., 1000 μg IM, monthly, for maintenance treatment.

Toxic reactions are extremely rare and are usually due to contamination in its preparation rather than to cobalamin itself. Because a small fraction of cobalamin can be absorbed passively through mucous membranes even when there is complete failure of physiological IF-dependent absorption, large daily oral doses (1000–2000 μg) of cyanocobalamin can be used in PA for replacement and maintenance of normal cobalamin status. Sublingual therapy has also been proposed for those in whom injections are difficult because of a bleeding tendency and may not tolerate oral therapy. If oral therapy is used, it is important to monitor compliance, particularly with elderly, forgetful patients.

TREATMENT OF FOLATE DEFICIENCY Oral doses of 5–15 mg folic acid daily are satisfactory, as sufficient folate is absorbed from these extremely large doses even in patients with severe malabsorption. The length of time therapy must be continued depends on the underlying disease. It is customary to continue therapy for about 4 months, when all folate-deficient red cells will have been eliminated and replaced by new folate-replete populations.

Before large doses of folic acid are given, cobalamin deficiency must be excluded and, if present, corrected, otherwise cobalamin neuropathy may develop, despite a response of the anemia of cobalamin deficiency to folate therapy. Studies in the United States, however, suggest that there is no increase in the proportion of individuals with low serum cobalamin levels and no anemia since food fortification with folic acid, but it is unknown if there has been a change in incidence of cobalamin neuropathy.

Long-term folic acid therapy is required when the underlying cause of the deficiency cannot be corrected and the deficiency is likely to recur, for instance, in chronic dialysis or hemolytic anemias. It may also be necessary in gluten-induced enteropathy if this does not respond to a gluten-free diet. Where mild but chronic folate deficiency occurs, it is preferable to encourage improvement in the diet after correcting the deficiency with a short course of folic acid. In any patient receiving long-term folic acid therapy, it is important to measure the serum cobalamin level at regular (e.g., once yearly) intervals to exclude the coincidental development of cobalamin deficiency.

Folinic Acid (5-Formyl-THF) This is a stable form of fully reduced folate. It is given orally or parenterally to overcome the toxic effects of methotrexate or other DHF reductase inhibitors.

PROPHYLACTIC FOLIC ACID In many countries, food is fortified with folic acid (in grain or flour) to prevent neural tube defects. It is also used in chronic dialysis patients and in parenteral feeds. Prophylactic folic acid has been used to reduce homocysteine levels to prevent cardiovascular disease, but further data are needed to assess the benefit for this and for cognitive function in the elderly.

Pregnancy Folic acid, 400 μg daily, should be given as a supplement before and throughout pregnancy. In women who have had a previous fetus with a neural tube defect, 5 mg daily is recommended when pregnancy is contemplated and throughout the subsequent pregnancy.

Infancy and Childhood The incidence of folate deficiency is so high in the smallest premature babies during the first 6 weeks of life that folic acid (e.g., 1 mg daily) should be given routinely to those weighing <1500 g at birth and to larger premature babies who require exchange transfusions or develop feeding difficulties, infections, or vomiting and diarrhea.

The World Health Organization currently recommends routine supplementation with iron and folic acid in children in countries where iron deficiency is common and child mortality, largely due to infectious diseases, is high. However, some studies suggest that where malaria rates are high, this approach may increase the incidence of severe illness and death. Even where malaria is rare, there appears to be no survival benefit.

MEGALOBLASTIC ANEMIA NOT DUE TO COBALAMIN OR FOLATE DEFICIENCY OR ALTERED METABOLISM

This may occur with many antimetabolic drugs (e.g.,. hydroxyurea, cytosine arabinoside, 6-mercaptopurine) that inhibit DNA replication. Antiviral nucleoside analogues used in treatment of HIV infection may also cause macrocytosis and megaloblastic marrow changes. In the rare disease orotic aciduria, two consecutive enzymes in purine synthesis are defective. The condition responds to therapy with uridine, which by-passes the block. In thiamine-responsive megaloblastic anemia, there is a genetic defect in the high-affinity thiamine transport (*SLC19A2*) gene. This causes defective RNA ribose synthesis through impaired activity of transketolase, a thiamine-dependent enzyme in the pentose cycle. This leads to reduced nucleic acid production. It may be associated with diabetes mellitus and deafness and the presence of many ringed sideroblasts in the marrow. The explanation is unclear for megaloblastic changes in the marrow in some patients with acute myeloid leukemia and myelodysplasia.

FURTHER READINGS

BAZZANO LA et al: Effect of folic acid supplementation on risk of cardiovascular diseases. JAMA 296:2720, 2006

BØNAA KH et al: Homocysteine lowering and cardiovascular events after acute myocardial infarction. N Engl J Med 354:1578, 2006

CHAN JCW et al: Pernicious anemia in Chinese: A study of 181 patients in a Hong Kong Hospital. Medicine 85:129, 2006

DURGA J et al: Effect of 3-year folic acid supplementation on cognitive function in older adults in the FACIT trial: A randomized double-blind, controlled trial. Lancet 369:208, 2007

HERSHKO C et al: Variable hematologic presentation of autoimmune gastritis: Age-related progression from iron deficiency to cobalamin depletion. Blood 107:1673, 2006

LONN E et al: Homocysteine lowering with folic acid and B vitamins in vascular disease. N Engl J Med 354:1567, 2006

MCMAHON JA et al: A controlled trial of homocysteine lowering and cognitive performance. N Engl J Med 354:2764, 2006

MILLS JL et al: Low vitamin B_{12} concentrations in patients without anemia: The effect of folic acid fortification of grain. Am J Clin Nutr 77:1474, 2003

ROTHENBERG SP et al: Autoantibodies against folate receptors in women with a pregnancy complicated by a neural tube defect. N Engl J Med 350:134, 2004

SAZAWAL S et al: Effects of routine prophylactic supplementation with iron and folic acid on admission to hospital and mortality in preschool child mortality in Southern Nepal: Community-based, cluster-randomized, placebo-controlled trial. Lancet 367:144, 2006

101 Hemolytic Anemias and Anemia Due to Acute Blood Loss

Lucio Luzzatto

DEFINITIONS

A finite life span is a distinct characteristic of red cells. Hence, a logical, time-honored classification of anemias comprises three groups: decreased production of red cells, increased destruction of red cells, and acute blood loss. Red cell destruction and acute loss, both associated with increased reticulocyte production, are covered in this chapter. Red cell production defects are discussed in Chaps. 98–100.

Physical loss of red cells from the bloodstream—which in most cases also means physical loss *from* the body—is fundamentally different from destruction of red cells *within* the body. Therefore the clinical aspects and the pathophysiology of anemia in these two groups of patients are quite different, and they will be considered separately.

HEMOLYTIC ANEMIAS

Anemias due to increased destruction of red cells, or hemolytic anemias (HAs), may be *inherited* or *acquired*. From the clinical point of view, they may be more *acute* or more *chronic*, and they may vary from mild to very severe. The site of hemolysis may be predominantly *intravascular* or *extravascular*. With respect to mechanisms, HAs may be due to *intracorpuscular* or *extracorpuscular* causes (Table 101-1); however, before reviewing the individual types of HAs, it is appropriate to consider what they have in common.

GENERAL CLINICAL AND LABORATORY FEATURES

The clinical presentation of a patient with anemia is greatly influenced by whether the onset is abrupt or gradual, and HA is no exception. A patient with autoimmune hemolytic anemia or with favism may be a medical emergency, whereas a patient with mild hereditary spherocytosis or with cold agglutinin disease may be diagnosed after years. This is due in large measure to the remarkable ability of the body to adapt to anemia when it is slowly progressing (Chap. 58).

What differentiates HA from other anemias is that the patient has signs and symptoms arising directly from hemolysis (Table 101-2). At the clinical level, the main sign is *jaundice;* in addition, the patient may report discoloration of the urine. In many cases of HA, the spleen is enlarged because it is a preferential site of hemolysis; in some cases the liver may be enlarged as well. In all severe congenital forms of HA, skeletal changes may be noted due to over-activity of the bone marrow (although they are never as severe as in thalassemia).

TABLE 101-1 CLASSIFICATION OF HEMOLYTIC ANEMIAS[a]

	Intracorpuscular Defects	Extracorpuscular Factors
Hereditary	Hemoglobinopathies Enzymopathies Membrane-cytoskeletal defects	Familial hemolytic uremic syndrome (HUS)
Acquired	Paroxysmal nocturnal hemoglobinuria (PNH)	Mechanical destruction (microangiopathic) Toxic agents Drugs Infectious Autoimmune

[a]There is a strong correlation between hereditary causes and intracorpuscular defects, because such defects are due to inherited mutations; the one exception is PNH, because the defect is due to an acquired somatic mutation. There is also a strong correlation between acquired causes and extracorpuscular factors; the one exception is familial HUS, because here an inherited abnormality allows excessive complement activation, with bouts of production of membrane attack complex capable of severely damaging normal cells.

TABLE 101-2 GENERAL FEATURES OF HEMOLYTIC DISORDERS

General examination	Jaundice, pallor
Other physical findings	Spleen may be enlarged; bossing of skull in severe congenital cases
Hemoglobin	From normal to severely reduced
MCV, MCH	Usually increased
Reticulocytes	Increased
Bilirubin	Increased (mostly unconjugated)
LDH	Increased (up to 10× normal with intravascular hemolysis)
Haptoglobin	Reduced to absent

Note: MCV, mean corpuscular volume; MCH, mean corpuscular hemoglobin; LDH, lactate dehydrogenase.

The laboratory features of HA are related to (1) hemolysis per se and (2) the erythropoietic response of the bone marrow. In the serum, hemolysis regularly produces an increased unconjugated bilirubin, increased lactate dehydrogenase (LDH), increased aspartate transaminase, and reduced haptoglobin. Urobilinogen will be increased in both urine and stool. If hemolysis is mainly intravascular, the telltale sign is hemoglobinuria, often associated with hemosiderinuria and an increase in serum hemoglobin; in contrast, the bilirubin level may be normal or only mildly elevated. The main sign of the erythropoietic response by the bone marrow is an increase in reticulocytes (a test all too often neglected in the initial workup of a patient with anemia). Usually the increase will be reflected in both the percentage of reticulocytes (the more commonly quoted figure) and the absolute reticulocyte count (the more definitive parameter). The increased number of reticulocytes is associated with an increased mean corpuscular volume (MCV) in the blood count. On the blood smear this is reflected in the presence of macrocytes; there is also polychromasia and sometimes nucleated red cells. In most cases a bone marrow aspirate is not necessary in the diagnostic workup; if it is done, it will show erythroid hyperplasia. In practice, once an HA is suspected, specific tests will usually be required for a definitive diagnosis of the specific type of HA.

GENERAL PATHOPHYSIOLOGY

The mature red cell is the product of a developmental pathway that brings the phenomenon of differentiation to an extreme. An orderly sequence of events produces synchronous changes whereby the gradual accumulation of a huge amount of hemoglobin in the cytoplasm (to a final level of 340 g/L, i.e., about 5 m*M*) goes hand in hand with the gradual loss of cellular organelles and of biosynthetic abilities. In the end the erythroid cell undergoes a process that has features of apoptosis, including nuclear pyknosis and actual loss of the nucleus. However, the final result is more altruistic than suicidal; the cytoplasmic body, instead of disintegrating, is now able to provide oxygen to all cells in the human organism for some remaining 120 days of the red cell "life" span.

As a result of this unique process of differentiation and maturation, intermediary metabolism is drastically curtailed in mature red cells (Fig. 101-1); for instance, cytochrome-mediated oxidative phosphorylation has been lost with the loss of mitochondria; therefore there is no backup to anaerobic glycolysis for the production of adenosine triphosphate (ATP). Also, the capacity of making protein has been lost with the loss of ribosomes. This places the cell's limited metabolic apparatus at risk because if any protein component deteriorates, it cannot be replaced as in most other cells; and in fact the activity of most enzymes gradually decreases as red cells age. Another consequence of the relative simplicity of red cells is that they have a very limited range of ways to manifest distress under hardship: in essence, any sort of metabolic failure will eventually lead either to structural damage to the membrane or to failure of the cation pump. In either case the life span of the red cell is reduced, which is the definition of a *hemolytic disorder*. If the rate of red cell destruction exceeds the capacity of the bone marrow to produce more red cells, the hemolytic disorder will manifest as *hemolytic anemia*.

Thus, the essential pathophysiologic process common to all HAs is an increased red cell turnover. The gold standard for proving that the

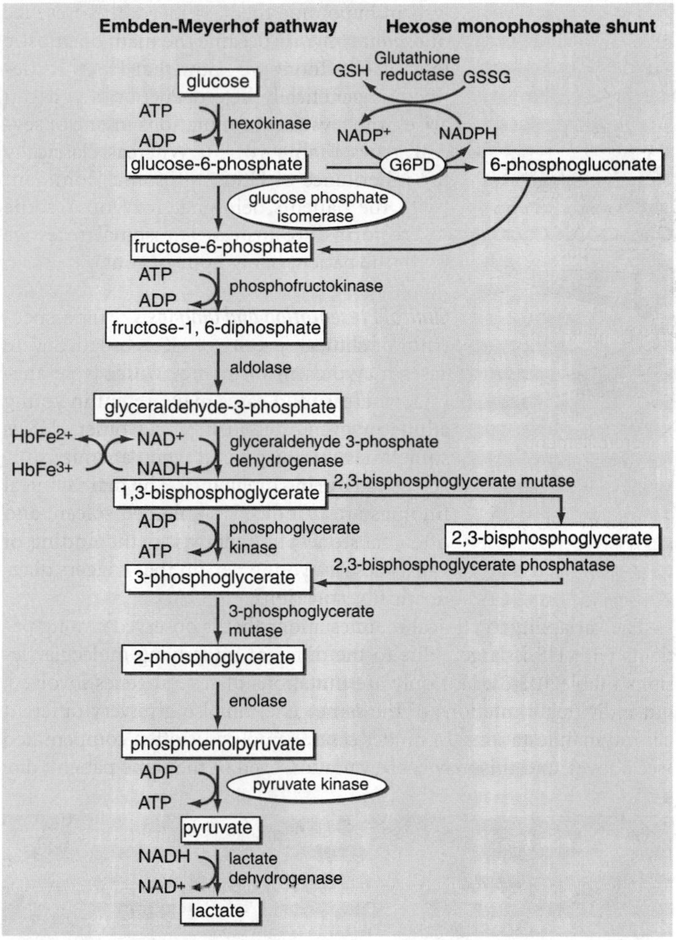

FIGURE 101-1 RBC metabolism. The Embden-Meyerhof pathway (glycolysis) generates ATP for energy and membrane maintenance. The generation of NADPH maintains hemoglobin in a reduced state. The hexose monophosphate shunt generates NADPH that is used to reduce glutathione, which protects the red cell against oxidant stress. Regulation of 2,3-bisphosphoglycerate levels is a critical determinant of oxygen affinity of hemoglobin. Enzyme deficiency states in order of prevalence: glucose-6-phosphate dehydrogenase (G6PD) >>> pyruvate kinase > glucose-6-phosphate isomerase > rare deficiencies of other enzymes in the pathway. The more common enzyme deficiencies are encircled.

life span of red cells is reduced (compared to the normal value of about 120 days) is a *red cell survival* study, which can be carried out by labeling the red cells with ^{51}Cr and measuring residual radioactivity over several days or weeks; however, this classic test is now available in very few centers and is rarely necessary. If the hemolytic event is transient, it does not usually cause any long-term consequences. However, if hemolysis is recurrent or persistent, the increased bilirubin production favors the formation of gallstones. If a considerable proportion of hemolysis takes place in the spleen, as is often the case, splenomegaly may become a prominent feature and hypersplenism may develop, with consequent neutropenia and/or thrombocytopenia.

The increased red cell turnover also has metabolic consequences. In normal subjects, the iron from effete red cells is very efficiently recycled by the body; however, with chronic intravascular hemolysis, the persistent hemoglobinuria will cause considerable iron loss, needing replacement. With chronic extravascular hemolysis, the opposite problem, iron overload, is more common, especially if the patient needs frequent blood transfusions. Chronic iron overload will cause secondary hemochromatosis; this will cause damage, particularly to the liver, eventually leading to cirrhosis, and to the heart muscle, eventually causing heart failure. The increased activity of the bone marrow also entails an increased requirement for erythropoietic factors, particularly folic acid.

Compensated Hemolysis versus HA Red cell destruction is a potent stimulus for erythropoiesis, which is mediated by erythropoietin (EPO) produced by the kidney. This mechanism is so effective that in many cases the increased output of red cells from the bone marrow can fully balance an increased destruction of red cells. In such cases we say that hemolysis is *compensated.* The pathophysiology of compensated hemolysis is similar to that just described, except there is no anemia. This notion is important from the diagnostic point of view, because a patient with a hemolytic condition, even an inherited one, may present without anemia. It is also important from the point of view of management because compensated hemolysis may become "decompensated"—i.e., anemia may suddenly appear—in certain circumstances—for instance, pregnancy, folate deficiency, renal failure interfering with adequate EPO production, or an acute infection depressing erythropoiesis. Another general feature of chronic HA is seen when any intercurrent condition depresses erythropoiesis. When this happens, in view of the increased rate of red cell turnover, the effect will be predictably much more marked than in a person who does not have hemolysis. The most dramatic example is infection by parvovirus B19, which may cause a rather precipitous fall in hemoglobin, an occurrence sometimes referred to as *aplastic crisis.*

INHERITED HEMOLYTIC ANEMIAS

There are three essential components in the red cell: (1) hemoglobin, (2) the membrane-cytoskeleton complex, and (3) the metabolic machinery necessary to keep (1) and (2) in working order. Here we will discuss diseases of the latter two components. Diseases caused by abnormalities of hemoglobin are discussed in Chap. 99.

Hemolytic Anemias Due to Abnormalities of the Membrane-Cytoskeleton Complex The detailed architecture of the red cell membrane is complex, but its basic design is relatively simple (Fig. 101-2). The lipid bilayer, which incorporates phospholipids and cholesterol, is spanned by a number of proteins that have their hydrophobic transmembrane domains embedded in the membrane. Most of these proteins have hydrophilic domains extending toward both the outside and the inside of the cell. Other proteins are tethered to the membrane through a glycosylphosphatidylinositol (GPI) anchor, and they have only an extracellular domain. These proteins are arranged roughly perpendicular to or lying across the membrane; they include ion channels, receptors for complement components, receptors for other ligands, and some of unknown function. The most abundant of these proteins are glycophorins and the so-called band 3, an anion transporter. The extracellular domains of many of these proteins are heavily glycosylated, and they carry antigenic determinants that correspond to blood groups. Underneath the membrane, and tangential to it, is a network of other proteins that make up the cytoskeleton. The main cytoskeletal protein is spectrin, the basic unit of which is a dimer of α-spectrin and β-spectrin. The membrane is physically linked to the cytoskeleton by a third set of proteins (including ankyrin and the so-called band 4.1 and band 4.2), which thus connect these two structures intimately.

The membrane-cytoskeleton complex is indeed so integrated that, not surprisingly, an abnormality of almost any of its components will be disturbing or disruptive, causing structural failure, which results ultimately in hemolysis. These abnormalities are almost invariably inherited mutations, and thus diseases of the membrane-cytoskeleton complex belong to the category of inherited hemolytic anemias. Before the red cells lyse, they often exhibit more or less specific morphologic changes that alter the normal biconcave disc shape. Thus, the majority of the diseases in this group have been known for over a century as *hereditary spherocytosis* (HS) and *hereditary elliptocytosis* (HE). Their molecular basis has been elucidated.

HEREDITARY SPHEROCYTOSIS This is a relatively common type of hemolytic anemia, with an estimated frequency of at least 1 in 5000.

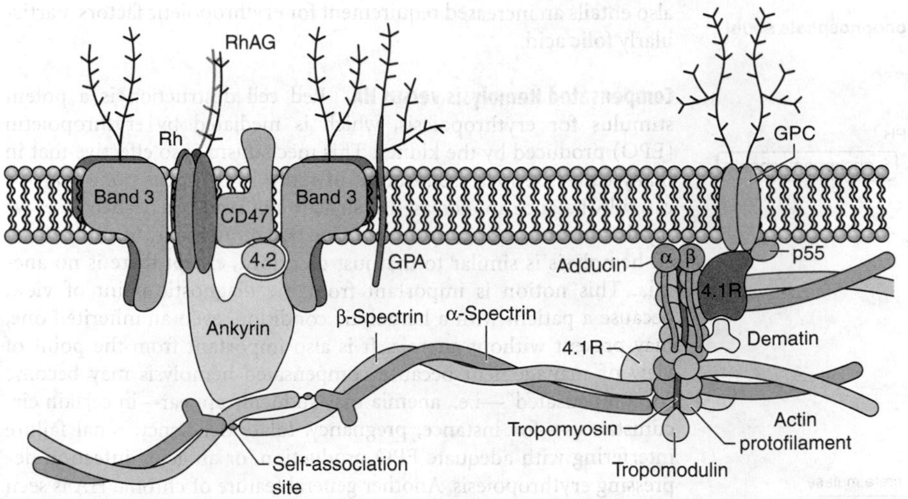

FIGURE 101-2 Diagram of red cell membrane/cytoskeleton. (For explanation see text.) *(From N Young et al: Clinical Hematology. Copyright Elsevier, 2006; with permission.)*

Its identification is credited to Minkowksy and Chauffard, who at the end of the 19th century reported families in whom HS was inherited as an autosomal dominant condition. From this seminal work, HS came to be defined as an inherited form of HA associated with the presence of spherocytes in the peripheral blood (**Fig. 101-3*A***). In addition, in vitro studies revealed that the red cells were abnormally susceptible to lysis in hypotonic media; indeed, the presence of *osmotic fragility* became the main diagnostic test for HS. Today we know that HS, thus defined, is genetically heterogeneous, i.e., it can arise from a variety of mutations in one of several genes (**Table 101-3**). Whereas classically the inheritance of HS is autosomal dominant (with the patients being heterozygous), some severe forms are instead autosomal recessive (with the patient being homozygous).

Clinical Presentation and Diagnosis The spectrum of clinical severity of HS is broad. Severe cases may present in infancy with severe anemia, whereas mild cases may present in young adults or even later in life. In women, HS is sometimes first diagnosed when anemia is investigated during pregnancy. The main clinical findings are jaundice, an enlarged spleen, and often gallstones; frequently it is the finding of gallstones in a young person that triggers diagnostic investigations.

The variability in clinical manifestations that is observed among patients with HS is largely due to the different underlying molecular lesions (Table 101-3). Not only are mutations of several genes involved, but individual mutations of the same gene can also give very different clinical manifestations. In milder cases, hemolysis is often compensated (see above), and this may cause variation even in the same patient, due

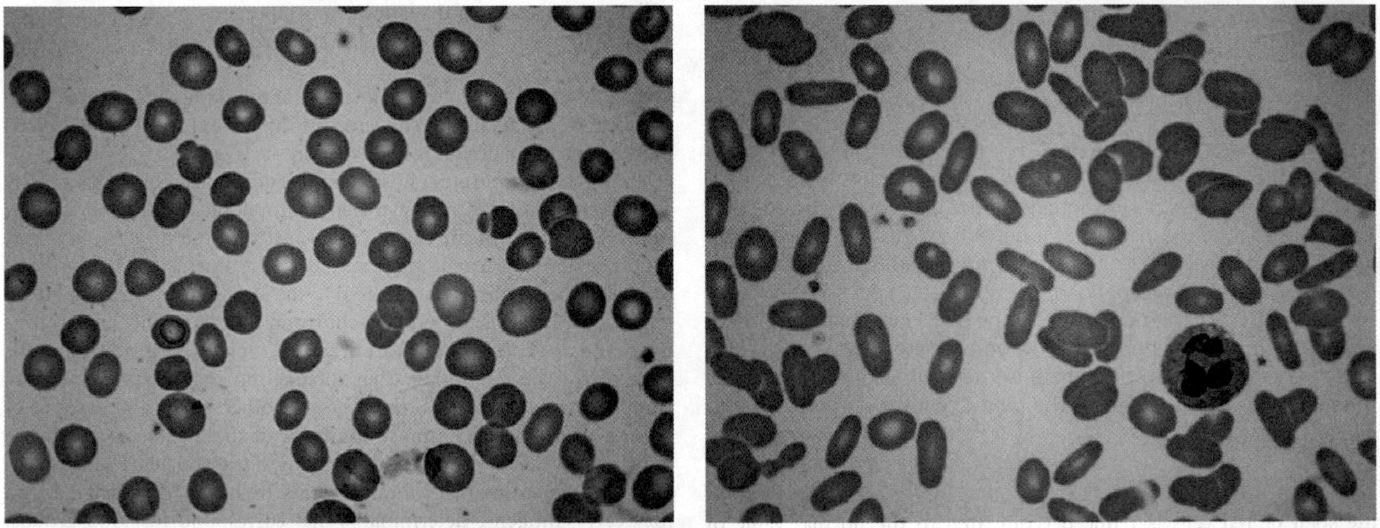

A ***B***

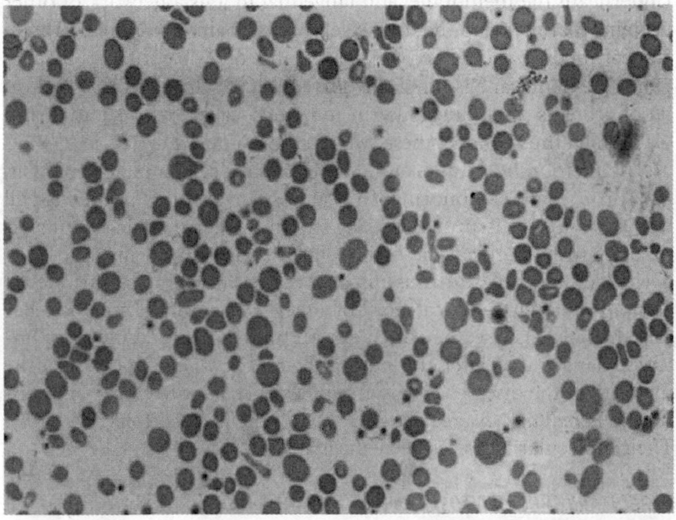

C

FIGURE 101-3 Peripheral blood smear from patients with membrane-cytoskeleton abnormalities. *A.* Hereditary spherocytosis. ***B.*** Hereditary elliptocytosis, heterozygote. ***C.*** Elliptocytosis, with both alleles of the α-spectrin gene mutated. *[From L Luzzatto, in J Gribben and D Pravan (eds): Molecular Hematology, 2d edition. Oxford, Blackwell, 2005; with permission.]*

TABLE 101-3 INHERITED DISEASES OF THE RED CELL MEMBRANE-CYTOSKELETON

Gene	Chromosomal Location	Protein Produced	Disease(s) with Certain Mutations (Inheritance)	Comments
SPTA1	1q22-q23	α-Spectrin	HS (recessive)	Rare.
			HE (dominant)	Mutations of this gene account for about 65% of HE. More severe forms may be due to coexistence of an otherwise silent mutant allele.
SPTB	14q23-q24.1	β-Spectrin	HS (dominant)	Rare.
			HE (dominant)	Mutations of this gene account for ~30% of HE, including some severe forms.
ANK1	8p11.2	Ankyrin	HS (dominant)	May account for majority of HS.
SLC4A1	17q21	Band 3 (anion channel)	HS (dominant)	Mutations of this gene may account for ~25% of HS.
			Southeast Asian ovalocytosis (dominant)	Polymorphic mutation (deletion of 9 amino acids); clinically asymptomatic; protective against *Plasmodium falciparum*.
EPB41	1p33-p34.2	Band 4.1	HE (dominant)	Mutations of this gene account for about 5% of HE, mostly with prominent morphology but no hemolysis in heterozygotes; severe hemolysis in homozygotes.
EPB42	15q15-q21	Band 4.2	HS (recessive)	Mutations of this gene account for about 3% of HS.
RHAG	6p21.1-p11	Rhesus antigen	Chronic nonspherocytic hemolytic anemia	Very rare; associated with total loss of all Rh antigens.

Note: HS, hereditary spherocytosis; HE, hereditary elliptocytosis.

to the fact that intercurrent conditions (e.g., infection) cause decompensation. The anemia is usually normocytic, with the characteristic morphology that gives the disease its name. A characteristic feature is an increase in mean corpuscular hemoglobin concentration (MCHC): this is almost the only condition in which high MCHC is seen.

When there is a family history, it is usually easy to suspect the diagnosis, but there may be no family history for at least two reasons: (1) The patient may have a de novo mutation, i.e., a mutation that has taken place in a germ cell of one of his parents or early after zygote formation; and (2) the patient may have a recessive form of HS (Table 101-3). In most cases the diagnosis is confirmed on the basis of red cell morphology and a test for osmotic fragility, a modified version of which is called the "pink test." In some cases a definitive diagnosis can be obtained only by molecular studies demonstrating a mutation in one of the genes underlying HS. This is carried out only in laboratories with special expertise in this area.

℞ HEREDITARY SPHEROCYTOSIS

There is currently no treatment aimed at the cause of HS; no way has yet been found to correct the basic defect in the membrane-cytoskeleton structure. However, it has been apparent for a long time that the spleen plays a special role in HS, through a dual mechanism. On one hand, as in many other HAs, the spleen itself is a major site of destruction; on the other hand, transit through the splenic circulation makes the defective red cells more spherocytic and therefore accelerates their demise, even though lysis may take place elsewhere. For these reasons, splenectomy has long been regarded as a prime, almost obligatory therapeutic measure in HS. However, it also increases the risk of certain infections, and therefore current guidelines (not evidence-based) are as follows.

1. Avoid splenectomy in mild cases.
2. Delay splenectomy until at least 4 years of age, after the risk of severe sepsis has peaked.
3. Antipneumococcal vaccination before splenectomy is imperative, whereas penicillin prophylaxis postsplenectomy is controversial.
4. HS patients often may require cholecystectomy. It used to be considered mandatory to combine this procedure with splenectomy, but this may not be always necessary.

HEREDITARY ELLIPTOCYTOSIS HE is at least as heterogeneous as HS, both from the genetic (Table 101-3) and from the clinical point of view. Again it is the shape of the red cells that gives the name to these conditions, but there is no direct correlation between elliptocytic morphology and clinical severity. In fact, some mild or even asymptomatic cases may have nearly 100% elliptocytes, whereas in severe cases, all sorts of bizarre poikilocytes may predominate (Fig. 101-3*B*, *C*). Clinical features and recommended management are similar to those for HS. Although the spleen may not have the specific role it has in HS, in severe cases splenectomy may be beneficial. The prevalence of HE causing clinical disease is similar to that of HS. However, an asymptomatic form, referred to as *Southeast Asian ovalocytosis*, has a frequency of up to 7% in certain populations, presumably as a result of malaria selection.

STOMATOCYTOSIS This rare condition with autosomal dominant inheritance draws its name (mouth-like cells) from the fact that the normally round-shaped central pallor of red cells is replaced by a linear-shaped central pallor. Hemolysis is usually relatively mild. Splenectomy is contraindicated as it has been followed in a majority of cases by severe thromboembolic complications.

Enzyme Abnormalities When there is an important defect in the membrane or in the cytoskeleton, hemolysis is a direct consequence of the fact that the very structure of the red cell is abnormal. Instead, when one of the enzymes is defective, the consequences will depend on the precise role of that enzyme in the metabolic machinery of the red cell, which, in its first approximation, has two important functions: (1) to provide energy in the form of ATP, and (2) to prevent oxidative damage to hemoglobin and to other proteins.

ABNORMALITIES OF THE GLYCOLYTIC PATHWAY (Fig. 101-1) Since red cells, in the course of their differentiation, have sacrificed not only their nucleus and their ribosomes but also their mitochondria, they rely exclusively on the anaerobic portion of the glycolytic pathway for producing energy in the form of ATP. Most of the ATP is required by the red cell for cation transport against a concentration gradient across the membrane. If this fails, due to a defect of any of the enzymes of the glycolytic pathway, the result will be hemolytic disease.

Pyruvate Kinase Deficiency Abnormalities of the glycolytic pathway are all inherited and all rare (Table 101-4). Among them, deficiency of pyruvate kinase (PK) is the least rare, with an estimated prevalence of 1:10,000. The clinical picture is that of an HA that often presents in the newborn with neonatal jaundice; the jaundice persists and is usually associated with a very high reticulocytosis. The anemia is of variable severity; sometimes it is so severe as to require regular blood transfusions; sometimes it is mild, bordering on a nearly compensated hemolytic disorder. As a result, the diagnosis may be delayed, and in some cases it is made in young adults—for instance, in a woman during her first pregnancy, when the anemia may get worse. In part the delay in diagnosis is due to the fact that the anemia is remarkably well-tolerated because the metabolic block at the last step in glycolysis causes an increase in bisphosphoglycerate (or DPG), a major effector of the hemoglobin-oxygen dissociation curve. Thus, the oxygen delivery to the tissues is increased.

TABLE 101-4 RED CELL ENZYME ABNORMALITIES CAUSING HEMOLYSIS

	Enzyme (Acronym)	Chromosomal Location	Prevalence of Enzyme Deficiency (Rank)	Clinical Manifestations Extra-Red Cell	Comments
Glycolytic pathway	*Hexokinase* (HK)	10q22	Very rare		Other isoenzymes known.
	Glucose 6-phosphate isomerase (G6PI)	19q31.1	Rare (4)	NM, CNS	
	Phosphofructokinase (PFK)	12q13	Very rare	Myopathy	
	Aldolase	16q22-24	Very rare		
	Triose phosphate isomerase (TPI)	12p13	Very rare	CNS (severe), NM	
	Glyceraldehyde 3-phosphate dehydrogenase (GAPD)	12p13.31–p13.1	Very rare	Myopathy	
	Diphosphoglycerate mutase (DPGM)	7q31-q34	Very rare		Erythrocytosis rather than hemolysis.
	Phosphoglycerate kinase (PGK)	Xq13	Very rare	CNS, NM	May benefit from splenectomy.
	Pyruvate kinase (PK)	1q21	Rare (2)		May benefit from splenectomy.
Redox	*Glucose 6-phosphate dehydrogenase* (G6PD)	Xq28	Common (1)	Very rarely granulocytes	In almost all cases only AHA from exogenous trigger.
	Glutathione synthase	20q11.2	Very rare	CNS	
	γ-Glutamylcysteine synthase	6p12	Very rare	CNS	
	Cytochrome b5 reductase	22q13.31–qter	Rare	CNS	Methemoglobinemia rather than hemolysis.
Nucleotide metabolism	*Adenylate kinase* (AK)	9q34.1	Very rare	CNS	
	Pyrimidine 5′-nucleotidase (P5N)	3q11–q12	Rare (3)		May benefit from splenectomy.

Note: CNS, central nervous system; AHA, acquired hemolytic anemia.

℞ PYRUVATE KINASE DEFICIENCY

Management of PK deficiency is mainly supportive. In view of the marked increase in red cell turnover, oral folic acid supplements should be given constantly. Blood transfusion should be used as necessary, and iron chelation may have to be added if the blood transfusion requirement is high enough to cause iron overload. In these patients, who have more severe disease, splenectomy may be beneficial. There is a single case report of curative treatment of PK deficiency by bone marrow transplantation from an HLA-identical PK normal sib: this seems a viable option for severe cases when a sib donor is available.

Other Glycolytic Enzyme Abnormalities All of these defects are rare to very rare (Table 101-4), and all cause HA of varying degrees of severity. It is not unusual for the presentation to be in the guise of severe neonatal jaundice, which may require exchange transfusion; if the anemia is less severe, it may present later in life or may even remain asymptomatic and be detected incidentally when a blood count is done for unrelated reasons. The spleen is often enlarged. When other systemic manifestations occur, they involve the central nervous system, sometimes entailing severe mental retardation (particularly in the case of triose phosphate isomerase deficiency) or the neuromuscular system, or both. The *diagnosis* of HA is usually not difficult, thanks to the triad of normo-macrocytic anemia, reticulocytosis, and hyperbilirubinemia. Enzymopathies should be considered in the differential diagnosis of any chronic Coombs-negative HA. In most cases of glycolytic enzymopathies, the morphologic abnormalities of red cells characteristically seen in membrane disorders are absent. A definitive diagnosis can be made only by demonstrating the deficiency of an individual enzyme by quantitative assays carried out in only a few specialized laboratories. If a particular molecular abnormality is already known in the family, then of course one could test directly for that defect at the DNA level, bypassing the need for enzyme assays.

ABNORMALITIES OF REDOX METABOLISM

G6PD Deficiency Glucose 6-phosphate dehydrogenase (G6PD) is a housekeeping enzyme critical in the redox metabolism of all aerobic cells (Fig. 101-4). In red cells, its role is even more critical because it is the only source of reduced nicotinamide adenine dinucleotide phosphate (NADPH), which, directly and via reduced glutathione (GSH), defends these cells against oxidative stress. G6PD deficiency is a prime example of an HA due to interaction between an intracorpuscular and an extracorpuscular cause, because in the majority of cases hemolysis is triggered by an exogenous agent. Although in G6PD-deficient subjects there is a decrease in G6PD activity in most tissues, this is less marked than in red cells, and it does not seem to produce symptoms.

GENETIC CONSIDERATIONS The *G6PD* gene is X-linked, and this has important implications. First, as males have only one *G6PD* gene (i.e., they are hemizygous for this gene), they must be either normal or G6PD-deficient. By contrast, females, having two *G6PD* genes, can be normal, deficient (homozygous), or intermediate (heterozygous). As a result of the phenomenon of X-chromosome inactivation, heterozygous females are genetic mosaics, with a highly variable ratio of G6PD-normal to G6PD-deficient cells and an equally variable degree of clinical expression; some heterozygotes can be just as affected as hemizygous males. The enzymatically active form of G6PD is either a dimer or a tetramer of a single protein subunit of 514 amino acids. G6PD-deficient subjects have been found invariably to have mutations in the coding region of the *G6PD* gene. Almost all of the 140 different mutations known are single missense point mutations, entailing single amino acid replacements in the G6PD protein. In most cases these mutations cause G6PD deficiency by decreasing the in vivo stability of the protein, and thus the physiologic decrease in G6PD

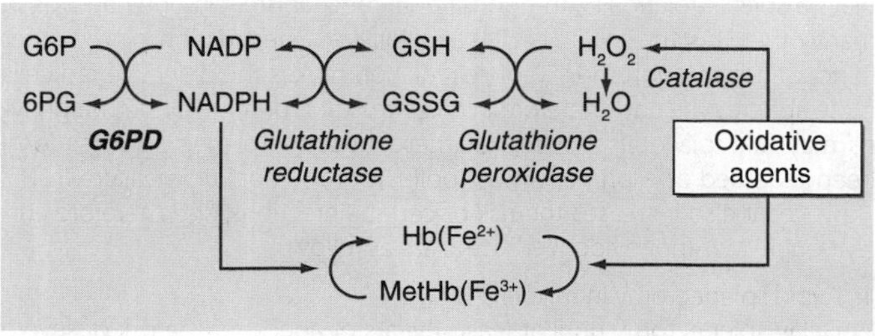

FIGURE 101-4 Diagram of redox metabolism in the red cell. G6P, glucose 6-phosphate; 6PG, 6-phosphogluconate; G6PD, glucose 6-phosphate dehydrogenase; GSH, reduced glutathione; GSSG, oxidized glutathione; Hb, hemoglobin; MetHb, methemoglobin; NADP, nicotinamide adenine dinucleotide phosphate; NADPH, reduced nicotinamide adenine dinucleotide phosphate.

activity that takes place with red cell ageing is greatly accelerated. In some cases an amino acid replacement can also affect the catalytic function of the enzyme.

Among the mutations, those underlying *chronic nonspherocytic hemolytic anemia* (CNSHA; see below) are a discrete subset. This much more severe clinical phenotype can be ascribed in some cases to adverse qualitative changes (for instance, a decreased affinity for the substrate, glucose 6-phosphate); or simply to the fact that the enzyme deficit is more extreme because it is more unstable. For instance, a cluster of mutations map at or near the dimer interface, and they prevent dimer formation.

TABLE 101-5 DRUGS THAT CARRY RISK OF CLINICAL HEMOLYSIS IN PERSONS WITH G6PD DEFICIENCY

	Definite Risk	Possible Risk	Doubtful Risk
Antimalarials	Primaquine Dapsone/chlorproguanil	Chloroquine	Quinine
Sulphonamides/sulphones	Sulphametoxazole Others Dapsone	Sulfasalazine Sulfadimidine	Sulfisoxazole Sulfadiazine
Antibacterial/antibiotics	Cotrimoxazole Nalidixic acid Nitrofurantoin Niridazole	Ciprofloxacin Norfloxacin	Chloramphenicol *p*-Aminosalicylic acid
Antipyretic/analgesics	Acetanilide Phenazopyridine (Pyridium)	Acetylsalicylic acid high dose (>3 g/d)	Acetylsalicylic acid <3 g/d Acetaminophen Phenacetin
Other	Naphthalene Methylene blue	Vitamin K analogues Ascorbic acid >1 g Rasburicase	Doxorubicin Probenecid

Epidemiology G6PD deficiency is widely distributed in tropical and subtropical parts of the world (Africa, Southern Europe, the Middle East, Southeast Asia, and Oceania) (Fig. 101-5) and wherever people from those areas have migrated; a conservative estimate is that at least 400 million people have a G6PD-deficiency gene. In several of these areas, the frequency of a G6PD-deficiency gene may be as high as 20% or more. It would be quite extraordinary for a trait that causes significant pathology to spread widely and reach high frequencies in many populations without conferring some biologic advantage. Indeed, G6PD is one of the best characterized examples of genetic polymorphisms in the human species. Clinical field studies and in vitro experiments strongly support the view that G6PD deficiency has been selected by *Plasmodium falciparum* malaria, by virtue of the fact that it confers a relative resistance against this highly lethal infection. Whether this protective effect is exerted mainly in hemizygous males or in females heterozygous for G6PD deficiency is still not clear. Different G6PD variants underlie G6PD deficiency in different parts of the world. Some of the more widespread variants are G6PD Mediterranean on the shores of the Mediterranean Sea, in the Middle East, and in India; G6PD A– in Africa and in Southern Europe; G6PD Vianchan and G6PD Mahidol in Southeast Asia; G6PD Canton in China; and G6PD Union worldwide. The heterogeneity of polymorphic G6PD variants is proof of their independent origin, and it supports the notion that they have been selected by a common environmental agent, in keeping with the concept of convergent evolution.

Clinical Manifestations The vast majority of people with G6PD deficiency remain clinically asymptomatic throughout their lifetime. However, all of them have an increased risk of developing neonatal jaundice (NNJ) and a risk of developing acute HA when challenged by a number of oxidative agents. NNJ related to G6PD deficiency is very rarely present at birth: the peak incidence of clinical onset is between day 2 and day 3, and in most cases the anemia is not severe. However, NNJ can be very severe in some G6PD-deficient babies, especially in association with prematurity, infection, and/or environmental factors (such as naphthalene-camphor balls used in babies' bedding and clothing). In these cases, if inadequately managed, NNJ associated with G6PD deficiency can produce kernicterus and permanent neurologic damage.

Acute HA can develop as a result of three types of triggers: (1) fava beans, (2) infections, and (3) drugs (Table 101-5). Typically, a hemolytic attack starts with malaise, weakness, and abdominal or lumbar pain. After an interval of several hours to 2–3 days, the patient develops jaundice and often dark urine, due to hemoglobinuria (Table 101-6). The onset can be extremely abrupt, especially with favism in children. The anemia is moderate to extremely severe, usually normocytic and normochromic, and due partly to intravascular hemolysis; hence, it is associated with hemoglobinemia, hemoglobinuria, and low or absent plasma haptoglobin. The blood film shows anisocytosis, polychromasia, and spherocytes (Fig. 101-6). The most typical feature is the presence of bizarre poikilocytes with red cells that appear to have unevenly distributed hemoglobin (hemighosts) and red cells that appear to have had parts of them bitten away (bite cells or blister cells). A classic test, now rarely carried out, is supravital staining with methyl violet, which, if done promptly, reveals the presence of Heinz bodies, consisting of precipitates of denatured hemoglobin and regarded as a signature of oxidative damage to red cells (except for the rare occurrence of an unstable hemoglobin). LDH is high and so is the unconjugated bilirubin, indicating that there is also extravascular hemolysis. The most serious threat from acute HA in adults is the development of acute renal failure (exceedingly rare in children). Once the threat of acute anemia is over, and in the absence of comorbidity, full recovery from acute HA associated with G6PD deficiency is the rule.

A very small minority of subjects with G6PD deficiency have CNSHA of variable severity. The patient is always a male, usually with a history of NNJ, who may present with anemia or unexplained jaundice, or because of gallstones later in life. The spleen may be enlarged. The severity of anemia ranges from borderline to transfusion-dependent. The anemia is

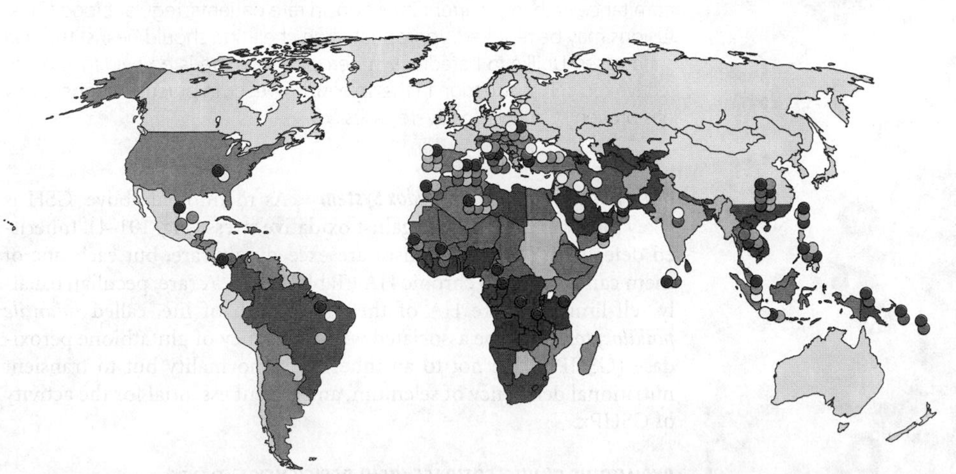

FIGURE 101-5 Epidemiology of G6PD deficiency throughout the world. The different shadings indicate increasingly high levels of prevalence, up to about 20%; the different colored symbols indicate individual genetic variants of G6PD, each one having a different mutation. *[From L Luzzatto et al in C Scriver et al (eds): The Metabolic & Molecular Bases of Inherited Disease, 8th edition. New York, McGraw-Hill, 2001.]*

TABLE 101-6 DISEASES/CLINICAL SITUATIONS WITH PREDOMINANTLY INTRAVASCULAR HEMOLYSIS

	Onset/Time Course	Main Mechanism	Appropriate Diagnostic Procedure	Comments
Mismatched blood transfusion	Abrupt	Nearly always ABO incompatibility	Repeat cross match	
Paroxysmal nocturnal hemoglobinuria (PNH)	Chronic with acute exacerbations	Complement (C)-mediated destruction of CD59(–) red cells	Flow cytometry to display a CD59(–) red cell population	Exacerbations due to C activation through any pathway
Paroxysmal cold hemoglobinuria (PCH)	Acute	Immune lysis of normal red cells	Test for Donath-Landsteiner antibody	Often triggered by viral infection
Septicemia	Very acute	Exotoxins produced by *Clostridium perfringens*	Blood cultures	Other organisms may be responsible
Microangiopathic	Acute or chronic	Red cell fragmentation	Red cell morphology on blood smear	Different causes ranging from endothelial damage to hemangioma to leaky prosthetic heart valve
March hemoglobinuria	Abrupt	Mechanical destruction	Targeted history taking	
Favism	Acute	Destruction of older fraction of G6PD-deficient red cells	G6PD assay	Triggered by ingestion of large dish of fava beans; but trigger can be infection or drug instead

usually normo-macrocytic, with reticulocytosis. Bilirubin and LDH are increased. Although hemolysis is, by definition, chronic in these patients, they are also vulnerable to acute oxidative damage, and therefore the same agents (see Table 101-5) that can cause acute HA in people with the ordinary type of G6PD deficiency will cause severe exacerbations in people with the severe form of G6PD deficiency. In some cases of CNSHA, the deficiency of G6PD is so severe in granulocytes that it becomes rate-limiting for their oxidative burst, with consequent increased susceptibility to bacterial infections.

Laboratory Diagnosis The suspicion of G6PD deficiency can be confirmed by semiquantitative methods often referred to as screening tests, which are suitable for population studies and can correctly classify male subjects, in the steady state, as G6PD-normal or G6PD-deficient. However, in clinical practice a diagnostic test is usually needed when the patient has had a hemolytic attack: this implies that the oldest, most G6PD-deficient red cells have been selectively destroyed, and young red cells, having higher G6PD activity, are being released into the circulation. Under these conditions, only a quantitative test can give a definitive result. In males this test will identify normal hemizygotes and G6PD-deficient hemizygotes; among females some heterozygotes will be missed, but those who are at most risk of hemolysis will be identified.

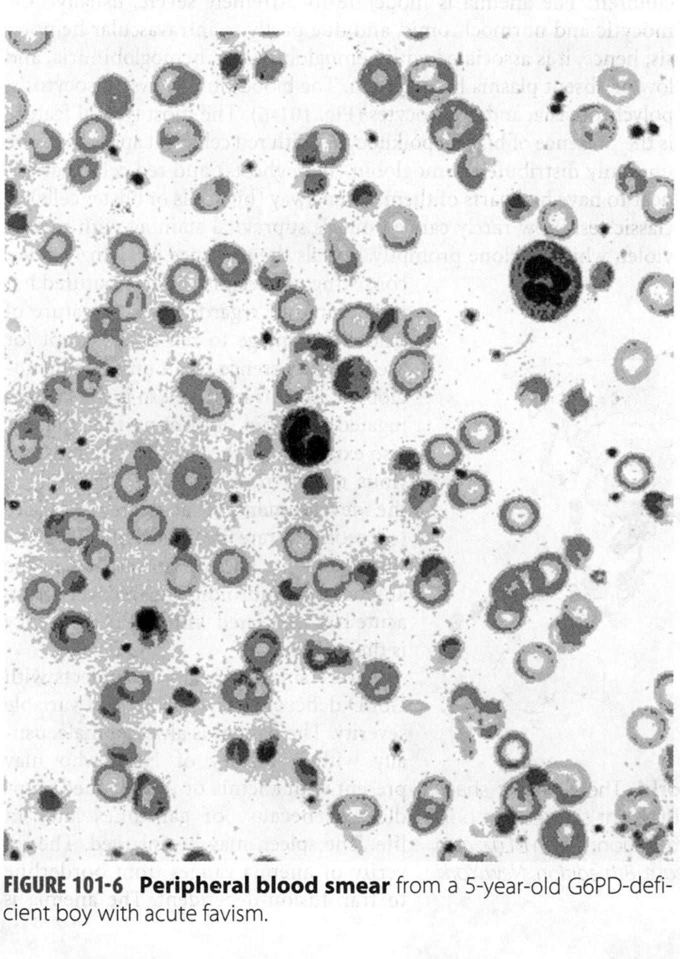

FIGURE 101-6 Peripheral blood smear from a 5-year-old G6PD-deficient boy with acute favism.

℞ G6PD DEFICIENCY

The acute HA of G6PD deficiency is largely preventable by avoiding exposure to triggering factors of previously screened subjects. Of course, the practicability and cost-effectiveness of screening depends on the prevalence of G6PD deficiency in each individual community. Favism is entirely preventable by not eating fava beans. Prevention of drug-induced hemolysis is possible in most cases by choosing alternative drugs. When acute HA develops and once its cause is recognized, no specific treatment is needed in most cases. However, if the anemia is severe, it may be a medical emergency, especially in children, requiring immediate action, including blood transfusion. If acute renal failure develops, hemodialysis may be necessary, but if there is no previous kidney disease, full recovery is the rule. The management of NNJ associated with G6PD deficiency is no different from that of NNJ due to other causes.

In cases with CNSHA, if the anemia is not severe, regular folic acid supplements and regular hematologic surveillance will suffice. It will be important to avoid exposure to potentially hemolytic drugs, and blood transfusion may be indicated when exacerbations occur, mostly in concomitance with intercurrent infection. In rare patients, regular blood transfusions may be required; appropriate iron chelation should be instituted in such cases. Unlike in hereditary spherocytosis, there is no evidence of selective red cell destruction in the spleen: however, in practice splenectomy has proven beneficial in severe cases.

Other Abnormalities of the Redox System As mentioned above, GSH is a key player in the defense against oxidative stress (Fig. 101-4). Inherited defects of GSH metabolism are exceedingly rare, but each one of them can give rise to chronic HA (Table 101-4). A rare, peculiar, usually self-limited severe HA of the first month of life, called *infantile poikilocytosis*, may be associated with deficiency of glutathione peroxidase (GSHPx) due not to an inherited abnormality but to transient nutritional deficiency of selenium, an element essential for the activity of GSHPx.

PYRIMIDINE 5′-NUCLEOTIDASE (P5N) DEFICIENCY P5N is a key enzyme in the catabolism of nucleotides arising from the degradation of nucleic acids that takes place in the final stages of red cell maturation. How exactly its deficiency causes HA is not well understood, but a highly distinctive feature of this condition is a morphologic abnormality of the red cells known as *basophilic stippling*. The condition is rare, but it probably ranks third in frequency among red cell enzyme defects (after G6PD deficiency and PK deficiency). The anemia is lifelong, of variable severity, and may benefit from splenectomy.

Familial Hemolytic Uremic Syndrome (HUS) This disorder is unique because, now that its basis has been elucidated, we can clearly see that hemolysis is due to an inherited defect, but this is external to red cells. HUS is defined as a microangiopathic hemolytic anemia with fragmented erythrocytes in the peripheral blood smear, thrombocytopenia (usually mild), and acute renal failure. An infection is usually the trigger of the syndrome, which tends to recur. When it does, the prognosis is serious. Although familial HUS is rare, studies of affected members from more than 100 families have revealed numerous mutations in any of three complement regulatory proteins: membrane cofactor protein, factor H, and factor I. It is thought that when complement is activated through the alternative pathway following damage to endothelial cells in the kidney, one of the results will be brisk hemolysis. Thus, the much more common Shiga toxin–related HUS can be regarded as a phenocopy of familial HUS.

ACQUIRED HEMOLYTIC ANEMIA

Mechanical Destruction of Red Cells Although red cells are characterized by the remarkable deformability that enables them to squeeze through capillaries narrower than themselves thousands of times in their lifetime, there are at least two situations in which they succumb to shear, if not to wear and tear; the result is intravascular hemolysis resulting in hemoglobinuria. One situation, *march hemoglobinuria*, is acute and self-inflicted. Why a marathon runner may sometimes develop this complication and at another time does not is unclear (perhaps the footwear needs attention). A similar syndrome may develop after prolonged barefoot ritual dancing or vigorous bongo drumming. The other situation, which has been called *microangiopathic hemolytic anemia*, (Table 101-6) is chronic and iatrogenic; it takes place in patients with prosthetic heart valves, especially when paraprosthetic regurgitation is present. If the hemolysis consequent to mechanical trauma to the red cells is mild, and provided the supply of iron is adequate, it may be largely compensated. If more than mild anemia develops, reintervention to correct regurgitation may be required.

Toxic Agents and Drugs A number of chemicals with oxidative potential, whether medicinal or not, can cause hemolysis even in people who are not G6PD-deficient (see above). Examples are hyperbaric oxygen (or 100% oxygen), nitrates, chlorates, methylene blue, dapsone, cisplatin, and numerous aromatic (cyclic) compounds. Other chemicals may be hemolytic through nonoxidative, largely unknown mechanisms; examples are arsine, stibine, copper, and lead. The HA caused by lead poisoning is characterized by basophilic stippling: it is in fact a phenocopy of that seen in P5N deficiency (see above), suggesting it is mediated at least in part by lead inhibiting this enzyme.

In these cases hemolysis appears to be mediated by a direct chemical action on red cells. But drugs can cause hemolysis through at least two other mechanisms. (1) A drug can behave as a hapten and induce antibody production. In rare subjects this happens, for instance, with penicillin. Upon a subsequent exposure, red cells are caught as innocent bystanders in the reaction between penicillin and antipenicillin antibodies. Hemolysis will subside as soon as penicillin administration is stopped. (2) A drug can trigger, perhaps through mimicry, the production of an antibody against a red cell antigen. The best-known example is methyldopa, an antihypertensive agent no longer in use, which in a small fraction of patients stimulated the production of the Rhesus antibody anti-e. In patients who have this antigen, the anti-e is a true autoantibody, which would then cause an autoimmune HA (see below). Usually HA would gradually subside once methyldopa was discontinued.

Nucleosides may also cause hemolysis by depletion of ATP. Ribavirin, a drug used in the treatment of hepatitis C, causes the destruction of red cells through this mechanism. Severe intravascular hemolysis can be caused by the venom of certain snakes (cobras and vipers), and HA can also follow spider bites.

Infection By far the most frequent infectious cause of hemolytic anemia in endemic areas is malaria (Chap. 203). In other parts of the world, the most frequent cause is probably Shiga toxin–producing *Escherichia coli* O157:H7, now recognized as the main etiologic agent of HUS, more common in children than in adults (Chap. 143). Life-threatening intravascular hemolysis due to a toxin with lecithinase activity occurs with *Clostridium perfringens* sepsis (Table 101-6), particularly with open wounds, following septic abortion, or as a disastrous accident due to a contaminated blood unit. Occasionally HA is seen, especially in children, with sepsis or endocarditis from a variety of organisms.

Autoimmune Hemolytic Anemia (AIHA) Except for countries where malaria is endemic, AIHA is the most common form of acquired hemolytic anemia. In fact, not quite appropriately, the two phrases are sometimes used synonymously.

PATHOPHYSIOLOGY AIHA is caused by an autoantibody directed against a red cell antigen, i.e., a molecule present on the surface of red cells. The autoantibody binds to the red cells. Once a red cell is coated by antibody, it will be destroyed by one or more mechanisms. In most cases the Fc portion of the antibody will be recognized by the Fc receptor of macrophages, and this will trigger erythrophagocytosis (Fig. 101-7). Thus, destruction of red cells will take place wherever macrophages are abundant—i.e., in the spleen, liver, and bone marrow. Because of the special anatomy of the spleen, this organ is particularly efficient in trapping antibody-coated red cells, and often this is the predominant site of red cell destruction. Although in severe cases even circulating monocytes can take part in this process, most of the phagocytosis-mediated red cell destruction takes place in the spleen and liver, and it is therefore called *extravascular hemolysis*. In some cases the nature of the antibody is such (usually an IgM antibody) that the antigen-antibody complex on the surface of red cells is able to activate complement (C). As a result, a large amount of membrane attack complex will form, and the red cells may be destroyed directly, known as *intravascular hemolysis*.

CLINICAL FEATURES The onset of AIHA is very often abrupt and can be dramatic. The hemoglobin level can drop, within days, to as low as 4 g/dL; the massive red cell removal will produce jaundice, and often the spleen will be enlarged. When this triad is present, the suspicion of AIHA must be high. When hemolysis is (in part) intravascular, the telltale sign will be hemoglobinuria, which the patient may report or for which the physician must test. The diagnostic test for AIHA is the antiglobulin test worked out in 1945 by R.R.A. Coombs and known since by his name. The beauty of this test is that it directly detects the pathogenetic mediator of the disease, i.e., the presence of antibody on the red cells themselves. When the test is positive, it clinches the diagnosis; when it is negative, the diagnosis is unlikely. However, the sensitivity of the Coombs test varies depending on the technology that is used, and in doubtful cases a repeat in a specialized lab is advisable; the term *Coombs-negative AIHA* is a last resort. In some cases the autoantibody has a defined identity: it may be specific for a Rhesus system antigen (often anti-e). In many cases it is regarded as "unspecific" because it reacts with virtually all types of red cells.

As in autoimmune diseases in general, the real cause of AIHA remains obscure. However, from the clinical point of view, an important feature is that AIHA can appear to be isolated, or it can develop as part of a more general autoimmune disease, particularly systemic lupus erythematosus (SLE), of which sometimes it may be the first manifestation. Therefore, when AIHA is diagnosed, a full screen for autoimmune disease is imperative. In some cases AIHA can be associated, on first presentation or subsequently, with autoimmune thrombocytopenia (Evans's syndrome).

Rx AUTOIMMUNE HEMOLYTIC ANEMIA

The first-line treatment of AIHA is glucocorticoids. A dose of prednisone of 1 mg/kg per day will cause a prompt remission in at least one-half of cases.

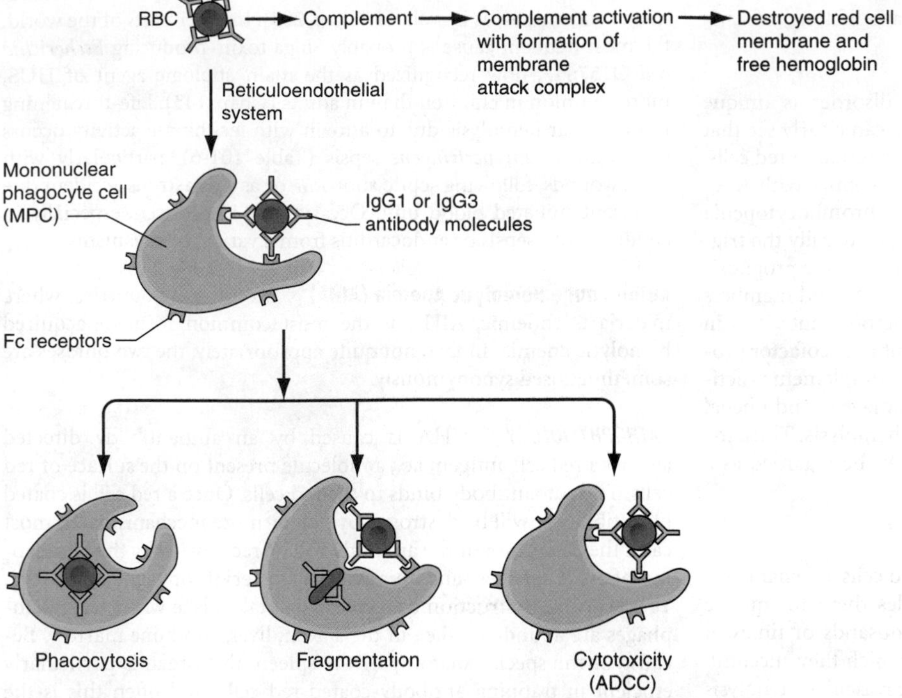

FIGURE 101-7 Mechanism of antibody-mediated immune destruction of red cells. *(From N Young et al: Clinical Hematology. Copyright Elsevier, 2006; with permission.)*

Whereas some patients are apparently cured, relapses are not uncommon. For patients who do not respond, and for those who have relapsed, second-line treatment measures include long-term immunosuppression with low-dose prednisone, azathioprine, or cyclosporine. In patients whose AIHA has become chronic, and sometimes even earlier, splenectomy is a viable option: although it does not cure the disease, it can produce significant benefit by removing a major site of hemolysis, thus improving the anemia and/or reducing the need for immunosuppressive agents. Most of the management of AIHA is not evidence-based. However, the anti-CD20 antibody rituximab has produced responses. Anecdotal reports suggest response to intravenous immunoglobulin. In severe refractory cases, either auto- or allohematopoietic stem cell transplantation has been used, sometimes successfully.

Severe acute AIHA can be a medical emergency. The immediate treatment almost invariably includes transfusion of red cells. This may pose a special problem because if the antibody involved is "unspecific," all the blood units cross-matched will be incompatible. In these cases it is often correct, paradoxically, to transfuse incompatible blood, the rationale being that the transfused red cells will be destroyed no less but no more than the patient's own red cells, and in the meantime the patient stays alive. Clearly this rather unique situation requires good liaison and understanding between the clinical unit treating the patient and the blood transfusion/serology lab.

PAROXYSMAL COLD HEMOGLOBINURIA (PCH) PCH is a rather rare form of AIHA occurring mostly in children, usually triggered by a viral infection, usually self-limited, and characterized by involvement of the so-called Donath-Landsteiner antibody. In vitro this antibody has unique serologic features: it has anti-P specificity and binds to red cells only at a low temperature (optimally at 4°C), but when the temperature is shifted to 37°C, lysis of red cells takes place in the presence of complement. Consequently, in vivo there is intravascular hemolysis, resulting in hemoglobinuria. Clinically, the differential diagnosis must include other causes of hemoglobinuria (Table 101-2), but the presence of the Donath-Landsteiner antibody will prove PCH. Active supportive treatment, including blood transfusion, is needed to control the anemia; subsequently, recovery is the rule.

COLD AGGLUTININ DISEASE (CAD) This designation is used for a form of chronic AIHA that usually affects the elderly and has special clinical and pathologic features. First, the term *cold* refers to the fact that the autoantibody involved reacts with red cells poorly or not at all at 37°C, whereas it reacts strongly at lower temperatures.[1] As a result, hemolysis is more prominent the more the body is exposed to cold. The antibody is usually an IgM, usually has an anti-I specificity (the I antigen is present on the red cells of almost everyone), and may have a very high titer (1:100,000 or more has been observed). Second, the antibody is produced by an expanded clone of B lymphocytes, and sometimes its concentration in the plasma is high enough to show up as a spike in plasma protein electrophoresis—i.e., as a monoclonal gammopathy. Third, since the antibody is IgM, CAD is related to Waldenström macroglobulinemia (WM; Chap. 106), although in most cases the other clinical features of this disease are not present. Thus, CAD must be regarded as a form of WM, i.e., as a low-grade mature B-cell lymphoma that manifests at an earlier stage because the unique biologic properties of the IgM that it produces give the clinical picture of chronic HA.

In mild forms of CAD, avoidance of exposure to cold may be all that is needed to enable the patient to live with a reasonably comfortable quality of life, but in more severe forms the management of CAD is not easy. Blood transfusion is not very effective because donor red cells are I-positive and will be removed rapidly. Immunosuppressive/cytotoxic treatment with prednisone, azathioprine, or cyclophosphamide can reduce the antibody titer, but clinical efficacy is limited, and in view of the chronic nature of the disease, the side effects may prove unacceptable. Plasma exchange is a rational approach, but it is laborious and must be carried out, in some patients, at very frequent intervals. The picture may be changing, as in a recent study rituximab gave a response rate of 60%. Given the long clinical course of CAD, it remains to be seen with what periodicity this agent will need to be administered.

Paroxysmal Nocturnal Hemoglobinuria (PNH) PNH is an acquired chronic HA characterized by persistent intravascular hemolysis subject to recurrent exacerbations (Table 101-6; Fig. 101-8). In addition to hemolysis, there is often pancytopenia and a risk of venous thrombosis. This triad makes PNH a truly unique clinical condition; however, when not all of these three features are manifest on presentation, the diagnosis is often delayed, although it can be always made by appropriate laboratory investigations (see below).

PNH has about the same frequency in men and women, and it is encountered in all populations throughout the world, but it is a rare disease: its prevalence is 1–5 per million (it may be somewhat less rare in Southeast Asia and in the Far East). There is no evidence of inherited susceptibility. PNH has never been reported as a congenital disease, but it can present in small children or in people in their seventies, although most patients are young adults.

CLINICAL FEATURES The patient may seek medical attention because one morning she or he has passed "blood instead of urine." This distressing event may be regarded as the classical presentation; however, more frequently this symptom is not noticed or is suppressed. Indeed, the patient often presents simply as a problem in the differential diagnosis of *anemia*, whether symptomatic or discovered incidentally. Sometimes the anemia is associated from the outset with neutropenia or thrombocytopenia, or both. Some patients may present with recurrent attacks of severe abdominal pain, defying a specific diagnosis and eventually found to be caused by thrombosis. When thrombosis af-

[1]In the past, this type of antibody was called a cold antibody, whereas the antibodies causing the more common form of AIHA were called warm antibodies.

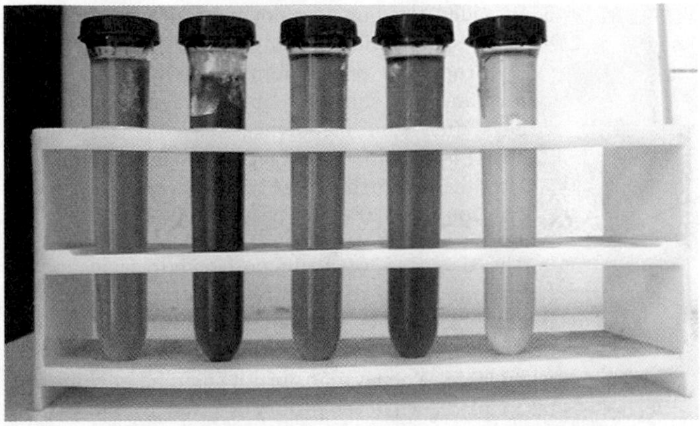

FIGURE 101-8 Consecutive urine samples from a patient with paroxysmal nocturnal hemoglobinuria (PNH). The variation in the severity of hemoglobinuria within hours is probably unique to this condition.

fects the hepatic veins, it may produce acute hepatomegaly and ascites, i.e., a full-fledged Budd-Chiari syndrome, which, in the absence of liver disease, ought to raise the suspicion of PNH.

The *natural history* of PNH can extend over decades. Without treatment, the median survival is ~8–10 years; in the past the commonest cause of death has been venous thrombosis followed by infection secondary to severe neutropenia and hemorrhage secondary to severe thrombocytopenia. PNH may evolve into aplastic anemia (AA), and PNH may manifest itself in patients who previously had AA. Rarely (estimated 1–2% of all cases), PNH may terminate in acute myeloid leukemia. On the other hand, full spontaneous recovery from PNH has been well documented, albeit rarely.

LABORATORY INVESTIGATIONS AND DIAGNOSIS The most consistent blood finding is anemia, which may range from mild to moderate to very severe. The anemia is usually normo-macrocytic, with unremarkable red cell morphology; if the MCV is high, it is usually largely accounted for by reticulocytosis, which may be quite marked (up to 20%, or up to 400,000/μL). The anemia may become microcytic if the patient is allowed to become iron-deficient as a result of chronic urinary blood loss through hemoglobinuria. Neutropenia and/or thrombocytopenia may or may not be present from the outset or may develop subsequently. Unconjugated bilirubin is mildly or moderately elevated, LDH is typically markedly elevated (values in the thousands are common), and haptoglobin is usually undetectable. All these findings make the diagnosis of HA compelling. Hemoglobinuria may be overt in a random urine sample; if it is not, it may be helpful to obtain serial urine samples, since hemoglobinuria can vary dramatically from day to day, and even from hour to hour (Fig. 101-8). The bone marrow is usually cellular with marked to massive erythroid hyperplasia, often with mild to moderate dyserythropoietic features (these do not justify confusing PNH with MDS). At some stage of the disease the marrow may become hypocellular or even frankly aplastic (see below).

The definitive diagnosis of PNH must be based on the demonstration that a substantial proportion of the patient's red cells have an increased susceptibility to complement (C), due to the deficiency on their surface of proteins (particularly CD59 and CD55) that normally protect the red cells from activated C. The sucrose hemolysis test is unreliable, and the acidified serum (Ham) test is carried out in few labs. The gold standard today is flow cytometry, which can be carried out on granulocytes as well as on red cells. A bimodal distribution of cells, with a discrete population that is CD59–, CD55–, is diagnostic of PNH. Usually this population is at least 5% of the total in the case of red cells and at least 20% of the total in the case of granulocytes.

PATHOPHYSIOLOGY Hemolysis in PNH is due to an intrinsic abnormality of the red cell, which makes it exquisitely sensitive to activated C, whether it is activated through the alternative pathway or through an antigen-antibody reaction. The former mechanism is mainly responsible for intravascular hemolysis in PNH. The latter mechanism explains why the hemolysis can be dramatically exacerbated in the course of a viral or bacterial infection. Hypersusceptibility to C is due to deficiency of several protective membrane proteins, of which CD59 is the most important because it hinders the insertion of C9 polymers into the membrane. The molecular basis for the deficiency of these proteins has been pinpointed not to a defect in any of the respective genes but rather to the shortage of a unique glycolipid molecule, GPI, which, through a peptide bond, anchors these proteins to the surface membrane of cells. The shortage of GPI is due in turn to a mutation in an X-linked gene, called *PIG-A*, required for an early step in GPI biosynthesis. In virtually each patient, the PIG-A mutation is different. This is not surprising, since these mutations are not inherited. Rather, each one takes place de novo in a hemopoietic stem cell (i.e., they are somatic mutations). As a result, the patient's marrow is a mosaic of mutant and nonmutant cells, and the peripheral blood always contains both PNH cells and normal (non-PNH) cells. Thrombosis is one of the most immediately life-threatening complications of PNH and yet one of the least understood in its pathogenesis. It could be that deficiency of CD59 on the PNH platelet causes inappropriate platelet activation; however, other mechanisms are possible.

BONE MARROW FAILURE—RELATIONSHIP BETWEEN PNH AND AA It is not unusual that patients with firmly established PNH have a previous history of well-documented AA. On the other hand, sometimes a patient with PNH becomes less hemolytic and more pancytopenic and ultimately has the clinical picture of AA. Since AA is probably an organ-specific autoimmune disease in which T cells cause damage to hematopoietic stem cells, the same may be true of PNH, with the specific proviso that the damage spares PNH stem cells. Skewing of the T cell repertoire in patients with PNH supports this notion. In addition, in mouse models, PNH stem cells do not expand when the rest of the bone marrow is normal, and by high-sensitivity flow cytometry technology, very rare PNH cells harboring PIG-A mutations can be demonstrated in normal people. In view of these facts, it seems that an element of bone marrow failure (BMF) in PNH is the rule rather than the exception. An extreme view is that PNH is a form of AA in which BMF is masked by the massive expansion of the PNH clone that populates the patient's bone marrow. The mechanism whereby PNH stem cells escape the damage suffered by non-PNH stem cells is not yet known.

℞ PAROXYSMAL NOCTURNAL HEMOGLOBINURIA

Unlike other acquired HAs, PNH may be lifelong and most patients receive supportive treatment only, including transfusion of filtered red cells[2] whenever necessary. Folic acid supplements (at least 3 mg/d) are mandatory; the serum iron should be checked periodically and iron supplements administered as appropriate. Long-term glucocorticoids are not indicated because there is no evidence that they have any effect on chronic hemolysis, and their side effects are considerable and potentially dangerous. The only form of treatment that can provide a cure for PNH is allogeneic bone marrow transplantation (BMT); when an HLA-identical sibling is available, BMT should be offered to any young patient with severe PNH.

A major advance in the management of PNH has been the development of a humanized monoclonal antibody, eculizumab, directed against the complement protein C5 (**Fig. 101-9**). By blocking the complement cascade downstream of C5, this antibody provides a medical intervention capable of controlling complement-dependent hemolysis in PNH. In an international multicenter placebo-controlled randomized trial on 87 patients who had been selected on grounds of having severe transfusion-dependent hemolysis, eculizumab completely abolished the need for blood transfusion in about one-half of the patients. Eculizumab administered intravenously at q2wk intervals also ameliorated the anemia in most patients and dramatically improved their quality of life.

---

[2]Now that filters with excellent removal of white cells are routinely used, the traditional washing of red cells, which aimed to avoid white cell reactions triggering hemolysis, is no longer necessary and considered wasteful.

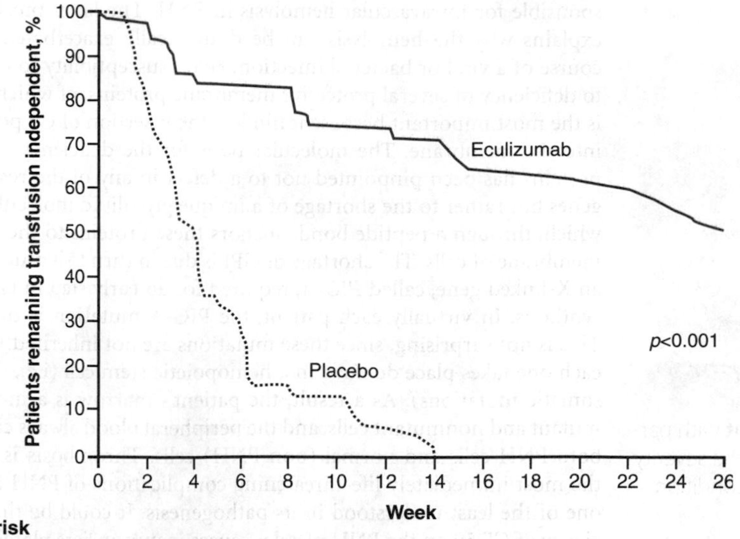

No. at risk

Placebo group	44	44	36	30	23	13	7	6	3	1	0	0	0	0	0	0
Eculizumab group	43	41	41	39	37	36	36	32	32	31	27	27	26	26	24	22

FIGURE 101-9 Therapeutic efficacy of an anti-C5 antibody on the anemia of paroxysmal nocturnal hemoglobinuria. *(From P Hillmen et al: N Engl J Med 355:1233, 2006; with permission.)*

For patients with PNH-AA syndrome, immunosuppressive treatment with antilymphocyte globulin (ALG or ATG) and cyclosporine A may be indicated. Although no formal trial has ever been conducted, this approach has helped particularly to relieve severe thrombocytopenia and/or neutropenia in patients in whom these were the main problem(s). By contrast, there is often little immediate effect on hemolysis. Thrombolytic therapy with tissue plasminogen activator may be indicated after severe thrombosis. Any patient who has had deep vein thrombosis at any site in the abdomen or in a limb should be on regular anticoagulant prophylaxis.

ANEMIA DUE TO ACUTE BLOOD LOSS

Blood loss causes anemia by two main mechanisms: first, by the direct loss of red cells; second, because if the loss of blood is protracted, it will gradually deplete the iron stores, eventually resulting in iron deficiency. Iron-deficiency anemia is discussed in Chap. 98.

Here we are concerned with *post-hemorrhagic anemia*, which follows *acute blood loss*. This can be *external* (as after trauma or due to postpartum hemorrhage) or *internal* (e.g., from bleeding in the gastrointestinal tract, rupture of the spleen, rupture of an ectopic pregnancy). In any of these cases—i.e., after the sudden loss of a large amount of blood—three clinical/pathophysiologic stages are noted.

1. At first, the dominant feature is hypovolemia, which poses a threat particularly to organs that normally have a high blood supply, such as the brain and the kidneys; therefore, loss of consciousness and acute renal failure are major threats. It is important to note that at this stage an ordinary blood count will not show anemia, as the hemoglobin concentration is not affected.
2. Next, as an emergency response, baroreceptors and stretch receptors will cause release of vasopressin and other peptides, and the body will shift fluid from the extravascular to the intravascular compartment, producing hemodilution. Thus, the hypovolemia gradually converts to anemia. The degree of anemia will reflect the amount of blood lost. If after 3 days the hemoglobin is, say, 7 g/dL, it means that about half of the entire blood volume had been lost.
3. Provided bleeding does not continue, the bone marrow response will gradually ameliorate the anemia if erythropoietin production, the erythroid progenitors, and iron supply are normal. Within about 2–3 days after acute hemorrhage, reticulocytes will increase in the blood and reach a maximum 7–10 days after the hemorrhage has been controlled. Reticulocyte counts of 20% may be achieved.

The diagnosis of acute post-hemorrhagic anemia (APHA) is usually straightforward, although sometimes internal bleeding episodes—after a traumatic injury or otherwise—may not be immediately obvious, even when large. Whenever an abrupt fall in hemoglobin has taken place, whatever history is given by the patient, APHA should be suspected. Supplementary history may have to be obtained by asking the appropriate questions, and appropriate investigations (e.g., a sonogram or an endoscopy) may have to be carried out. Internal bleeding may result in a rise in unconjugated bilirubin and a fall in serum haptoglobin.

℞ ANEMIA DUE TO BLOOD LOSS

With respect to treatment, a two-pronged approach is imperative. First, in many cases the blood lost needs to be replaced promptly. With many chronic anemias, finding and correcting the cause of the anemia is the first priority, and blood transfusion may not be even necessary, because the body is adapted to the anemia; with acute blood loss the reverse is true. Since the body is not adapted to the anemia, blood transfusion takes priority. Although fluorocarbon synthetic chemicals have shown promise, no "blood substitute" has yet become standard treatment. Second, while the emergency is being confronted, it is imperative to stop the hemorrhage and to eliminate its source.

ACKNOWLEDGMENT

H. Frank Bunn and Wendell Rosse contributed this chapter in the last edition and material from that chapter has been used here.

FURTHER READINGS

DACIE J: *The Haemolytic Anaemias*, 5 volumes. London, Churchill Livingstone, 1995

EBER S, LUX SE: Hereditary spherocytosis—defects in proteins that connect the membrane skeleton to the lipid bilayer. Semin Hematol 41:118, 2004

HEIER HE et al: Transfusion versus alternative treatment modalities in acute bleeding: A systematic review. Acta Anaesthesiol Scand 509:20, 2006

HILL A et al: Recent developments in the understanding and management of paroxysmal nocturnal hemoglobinuria. Br J Haematol 137:181, 2007

HILLMEN P, et al: The complement inhibitor eculizumab in paroxysmal nocturnal hemoglobinuria. N Engl J Med 355:1233, 2006

LUZZATTO L: Paroxysmal nocturnal hemoglobinuria, in *Clinical Hematology*, N Young, Gershon SL, High KA (eds). Philadelphia, Mosby, pp 326–339, 2006

ROSSE WF, HILLMEN P, SCHREIBER AD: Immune-mediated hemolytic anemia. *Hematology, Am Soc Hematol Educ Program* pp. 48–62, 2004

SHAPIRA Y et al: Erythropoietin can obviate the need for repeated heart valve replacement in high-risk patients with severe mechanical hemolytic anemia: Case reports and literature review. J Heart Valve Dis 10:431, 2001

102 Aplastic Anemia, Myelodysplasia, and Related Bone Marrow Failure Syndromes

Neal S. Young

The hypoproliferative anemias are normochromic, normocytic or macrocytic and are characterized by a low reticulocyte count. Deficient production of RBCs occurs with marrow damage and dysfunction, which may be secondary to infection, inflammation, and cancer. Hypoproliferative anemia is also a prominent feature of hematologic diseases that are described as bone marrow failure states; these include aplastic anemia, myelodysplasia (MDS), pure red cell aplasia (PRCA), and myelophthisis. Anemia in these disorders is often not a solitary or even the major hematologic finding. More frequent in bone marrow failure is pancytopenia: anemia, leukopenia, and thrombocytopenia. Low blood counts in the marrow failure diseases result from deficient hematopoiesis, as distinguished from blood count depression due to peripheral destruction of red cells (hemolytic anemias), platelets (idiopathic thrombocytopenic purpura or due to splenomegaly), and granulocytes (as in the immune leukopenias).

Hematopoietic failure syndromes are classified by dominant morphologic features of the bone marrow (Table 102-1). While practical distinction among these syndromes usually is clear, they can occur secondary to other diseases, and some processes are so closely related that the diagnosis may be complex. Patients may seem to suffer from two or three related diseases simultaneously, or one diagnosis may appear to evolve into another. Many of these syndromes share an immune-mediated mechanism of marrow destruction and some element of genomic instability resulting in a higher rate of malignant transformation.

APLASTIC ANEMIA

DEFINITION

Aplastic anemia is pancytopenia with bone marrow hypocellularity. Acquired aplastic anemia is distinguished from iatrogenic marrow aplasia, marrow hypocellularity after intensive cytotoxic chemotherapy for cancer. Aplastic anemia can also be constitutional: the genetic diseases Fanconi's anemia and dyskeratosis congenita, while frequently associated with typical physical anomalies and the development of pancytopenia early in life, can also present as marrow failure in normal-appearing adults. Acquired aplastic anemia is often stereotypical in its manifestations, with the abrupt onset of low blood counts in a previously well young adult; seronegative hepatitis or a course of an incriminated medical drug may precede the onset. The diagnosis in these instances is uncomplicated. Sometimes blood count depression is moderate or incomplete, resulting in anemia, leukopenia, and thrombocytopenia in some combination. Aplastic anemia is related to both paroxysmal nocturnal hemoglobinuria (PNH; Chap. 101) and to MDS, and in some cases a clear distinction among these disorders may not be possible.

TABLE 102-1 DIFFERENTIAL DIAGNOSIS OF PANCYTOPENIA

Pancytopenia with Hypocellular Bone Marrow	
Acquired aplastic anemia	
Constitutional aplastic anemia (Fanconi's anemia, dyskeratosis congenita)	
Some myelodysplasia	
Rare aleukemic leukemia (AML)	
Some acute lymphoid leukemia	
Some lymphomas of bone marrow	
Pancytopenia with Cellular Bone Marrow	
Primary bone marrow diseases	Secondary to systemic diseases
Myelodysplasia	Systemic lupus erythematosus
Paroxysmal nocturnal hemoglobinuria	Hypersplenism
Myelofibrosis	B_{12}, folate deficiency
Some aleukemic leukemia	Overwhelming infection
Myelophthisis	Alcohol
Bone marrow lymphoma	Brucellosis
Hairy cell leukemia	Sarcoidosis
	Tuberculosis
	Leishmaniasis
Hypocellular Bone Marrow ± Cytopenia	
Q fever	
Legionnaires' disease	
Anorexia nervosa, starvation	
Mycobacteria	

EPIDEMIOLOGY

The incidence of acquired aplastic anemia in Europe and Israel is two cases per million persons annually. In Thailand and China, rates of five to seven per million have been established. In general, men and women are affected with equal frequency, but the age distribution is biphasic, with the major peak in the teens and twenties and a second rise in the elderly.

ETIOLOGY

The origins of aplastic anemia have been inferred from several recurring clinical associations (Table 102-2); unfortunately, these relationships are not reliable in an individual patient and may not be etiologic. In addition, while most cases of aplastic anemia are idiopathic, little other than history separates these cases from those with a presumed etiology such as a drug exposure.

Radiation Marrow aplasia is a major acute sequela of radiation. Radiation damages DNA; tissues dependent on active mitosis are partic-

TABLE 102-2 CLASSIFICATION OF APLASTIC ANEMIA AND SINGLE CYTOPENIAS

Acquired	Inherited
Aplastic Anemia	
Secondary	Fanconi's anemia
Radiation	Dyskeratosis congenita
Drugs and chemicals	Shwachman-Diamond syndrome
Regular effects	Reticular dysgenesis
Idiosyncratic reactions	Amegakaryocytic thrombocytopenia
Viruses	Familial aplastic anemias
Epstein-Barr virus (infectious mononucleosis)	Preleukemia (monosomy 7, etc.)
	Nonhematologic syndrome (Down's, Dubowitz, Seckel)
Hepatitis (non-A, non-B, non-C hepatitis)	
Parvovirus B19 (transient aplastic crisis, PRCA)	
HIV-1 (AIDS)	
Immune diseases	
Eosinophilic fasciitis	
Hypoimmunoglobulinemia	
Thymoma/thymic carcinoma	
Graft-versus-host disease in immunodeficiency	
Paroxysmal nocturnal hemoglobinuria	
Pregnancy	
Idiopathic	
Cytopenias	
PRCA (see Table 102-4)	Congenital PRCA (Diamond-Blackfan anemia)
Neutropenia/Agranulocytosis	
Idiopathic	Kostmann's Syndrome
Drugs, toxins	Shwachman-Diamond syndrome
Pure white cell aplasia	Reticular dysgenesis
Thrombocytopenia	
Drugs, toxins	Amegakaryocytic thrombocytopenia
Idiopathic amegakaryocytic	Thrombocytopenia with absent radii

Note: PRCA, pure red cell aplasia.

ularly susceptible. Nuclear accidents can involve not only power plant workers but also employees of hospitals, laboratories, and industry (food sterilization, metal radiography, etc.), as well as innocents exposed to stolen, misplaced, or misused sources. While the radiation dose can be approximated from the rate and degree of decline in blood counts, dosimetry by reconstruction of the exposure can help to estimate the patient's prognosis and also to protect medical personnel from contact with radioactive tissue and excreta. MDS and leukemia, but probably not aplastic anemia, are late effects of radiation.

Chemicals Benzene is a notorious cause of bone marrow failure. Vast quantities of epidemiologic, clinical, and laboratory data link benzene to aplastic anemia, acute leukemia, and blood and marrow abnormalities. The occurrence of leukemia is roughly correlated with cumulative exposure, but susceptibility must also be important, as only a minority of even heavily exposed workers develop benzene myelotoxicity. The employment history is important, especially in industries where benzene is used for a secondary purpose, usually as a solvent. Benzene-related blood diseases have declined with regulation of industrial exposure. Although benzene is no longer generally available as a household solvent, exposure to its metabolites occurs in the normal diet and in the environment. The association between marrow failure and other chemicals is much less well substantiated.

Drugs (Table 102-3) Many chemotherapeutic drugs have marrow suppression as a major toxicity; effects are dose-dependent and will occur in all recipients. In contrast, idiosyncratic reactions to a large and diverse group of drugs may lead to aplastic anemia without a clear dose-response relationship. These associations rested largely on accumulated case reports until a large international study in Europe in the 1980s quantitated drug relationships, especially for nonsteroidal analgesics, sulfonamides, thyrostatic drugs, some psychotropics, penicillamine, allopurinol, and gold. Not all associations necessarily reflect causation: a drug may have been used to treat the first symptoms of bone marrow failure (antibiotics for fever or the preceding viral illness) or provoked the first symptom of a preexisting disease (petechiae by nonsteroidal anti-inflammatory agents administered to the thrombocytopenic patient). In the context of total drug use, idiosyncratic reactions, while individually devastating, are rare events. Chloramphenicol, the most infamous culprit, reportedly produced aplasia in only about 1/60,000 therapy courses, and even this number is almost certainly an overestimate (risks are almost invariably exaggerated when based on collections of cases; although the introduction of chloramphenicol was perceived to have created an epidemic of aplastic anemia, its diminished use was not followed by a changed frequency of marrow failure). Risk estimates are usually lower when determined in population-based studies; furthermore, the low absolute risk is also made more obvious: even a ten- or twentyfold increase in risk translates, in a rare disease, to but a handful of drug-induced aplastic anemia cases among hundreds of thousands of exposed persons.

TABLE 102-3 SOME DRUGS AND CHEMICALS ASSOCIATED WITH APLASTIC ANEMIA

Agents that regularly produce marrow depression as major toxicity in commonly employed doses or normal exposures:
Cytotoxic drugs used in cancer chemotherapy: *alkylating agents, antimetabolites, antimitotics*, some antibiotics
Agents that frequently but not inevitably produce marrow aplasia:
Benzene
Agents associated with aplastic anemia but with a relatively low probability:
Chloramphenicol
Insecticides
Antiprotozoals: *quinacrine* and chloroquine, mepacrine
Nonsteroidal anti-inflammatory drugs (including *phenylbutazone*, indomethacin, ibuprofen, sulindac, aspirin)
Anticonvulsants (*hydantoins, carbamazapine*, phenacemide, felbamate)
Heavy metals (*gold*, arsenic, bismuth, mercury)
Sulfonamides: some antibiotics, antithyroid drugs (methimazole, methylthiouracil, propylthiouracil), antidiabetes drugs (tolbutamide, chlorpropamide), carbonic anhydrase inhibitors (acetazolamide and methazolamide)
Antihistamines (*cimetidine*, chlorpheniramine)
D-Penicillamine
Estrogens (in pregnancy and in high doses in animals)
Agents whose association with aplastic anemia is more tenuous:
Other antibiotics (streptomycin, tetracycline, methicillin, mebendazole, trimethoprim/sulfamethoxazole, flucytosine)
Sedatives and tranquilizers (chlorpromazine, prochlorperazine, piperacetazine, chlordiazepoxide, meprobamate, methyprylon)
Allopurinol
Methyldopa
Quinidine
Lithium
Guanidine
Potassium perchlorate
Thiocyanate
Carbimazole

Note: Terms set in italic show the most consistent association with aplastic anemia.

Infections Hepatitis is the most common preceding infection, and posthepatitis marrow failure accounts for about 5% of etiologies in most series. Patients are usually young men who have recovered from a bout of liver inflammation 1 to 2 months earlier; the subsequent pancytopenia is very severe. The hepatitis is seronegative (non-A, non-B, non-C, non-G) and possibly due to a novel, as yet undiscovered, virus. Fulminant liver failure in childhood also follows seronegative hepatitis, and marrow failure occurs at a high rate in these patients. Aplastic anemia can rarely follow infectious mononucleosis, and Epstein-Barr virus has been found in the marrow of a few patients, some without a suggestive preceding history. Parvovirus B19, the cause of transient aplastic crisis in hemolytic anemias and of some PRCAs (see below), does not usually cause generalized bone marrow failure. Mild blood count depression is frequent in the course of many viral and bacterial infections but resolves with the infection.

Immunologic Diseases Aplasia is a major consequence and the inevitable cause of death in *transfusion-associated graft-versus-host disease* (GVDH), which can occur after infusion of unirradiated blood products to an immunodeficient recipient. Aplastic anemia is strongly associated with the rare collagen vascular syndrome called *eosinophilic fasciitis*, which is characterized by painful induration of subcutaneous tissues (Chap. 316). Pancytopenia with marrow hypoplasia can also occur in systemic lupus erythematosus.

Pregnancy Aplastic anemia very rarely may occur and recur during pregnancy and resolve with delivery or with spontaneous or induced abortion.

Paroxysmal Nocturnal Hemoglobinuria An acquired mutation in the *PIG-A* gene in a hematopoietic stem cell is required for the development of PNH, but *PIG-A* mutations probably occur commonly in normal individuals. If the PIG-A mutant stem cell proliferates, the result is a clone of progeny deficient in glycosylphosphatidylinositol-linked cell surface membrane proteins (Chap. 101). Such PNH cells are now accurately enumerated using fluorescence-activated flow cytometry of CD55 or CD59 expression on granulocytes rather than Ham or sucrose lysis tests on red cells. Small clones of deficient cells can be detected in about half of patients with aplastic anemia at the time of presentation [and PNH cells are also seen in MDS (see below)]; frank hemolysis and thrombotic episodes occur in patients with large PNH clones (>50%). Functional studies of bone marrow from PNH patients, even those with mainly hemolytic manifestations, show evidence of defective hematopoiesis. Patients with an initial clinical diagnosis of PNH, especially younger individuals, may later develop frank marrow aplasia and pancytopenia; patients with an initial diagnosis of aplastic anemia may suffer from hemolytic PNH years after recovery of blood counts. One popular but unproven explanation for the aplastic anemia/PNH syndrome is selection of the deficient clones because they are favored for proliferation in the peculiar environment of immune-mediated marrow destruction.

Constitutional Disorders Fanconi's anemia, an autosomal recessive disorder, manifests as congenital developmental anomalies, progressive pancytopenia, and an increased risk of malignancy. Chromosomes in Fanconi's anemia are peculiarly susceptible to DNA cross-linking agents, the basis for a diagnostic assay. Patients with Fanconi's anemia typically have short stature, café au lait spots, and anomalies involving the thumb, radius, and genitourinary tract. At least 12 different genetic defects (all but one with an identified gene) have been defined; the most common, type A Fanconi's anemia, is due to a mutation in *FANCA*. Most of the Fanconi's anemia gene products form a protein complex that activates FANCD2 by monoubiquitination to play a role in the cellular response to DNA damage and especially interstrand cross-linking, a response that includes BRCA1, ATM, and NBS1.

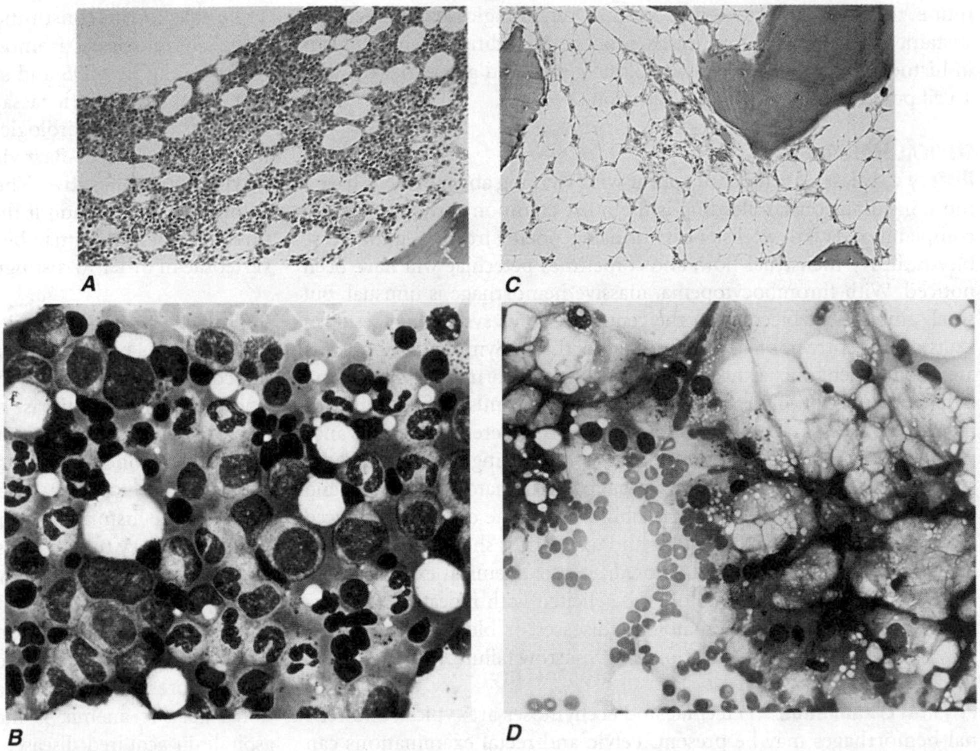

FIGURE 102-1 ***A.*** Normal bone marrow biopsy. ***B.*** Normal bone marrow aspirate smear. The marrow is normally 30–70% cellular, and there is a heterogeneous mix of myeloid, erythroid, and lymphoid cells. ***C.*** Aplastic anemia biopsy. ***D.*** Marrow smear in aplastic anemia. The marrow shows replacement of hematopoietic tissue by fat and only residual stromal and lymphoid cells.

Dyskeratosis congenita is characterized by mucous membrane leukoplasia, dystrophic nails, reticular hyperpigmentation, and the development of aplastic anemia during childhood. The X-linked variety is due to mutations in the *DKC1 (dyskerin)* gene; the more unusual autosomal dominant type is due to mutation in *hTERC*, which encodes an RNA template, and *hTERT*, which encodes the catalytic reverse transcriptase, telomerase; these gene products cooperate in a repair complex to maintain telomere length. In Shwachman-Diamond syndrome, marrow failure is seen with pancreatic insufficiency and malabsorption; most patients have compound heterozygous mutations in *SBDS*, which has been implicated in RNA processing.

PATHOPHYSIOLOGY

Bone marrow failure results from severe damage to the hematopoietic cell compartment. In aplastic anemia, replacement of the bone marrow by fat is apparent in the morphology of the biopsy specimen (Fig. 102-1) and MRI of the spine. Cells bearing the CD34 antigen, a marker of early hematopoietic cells, are greatly diminished, and in functional studies, committed and primitive progenitor cells are virtually absent; in vitro assays have suggested that the stem cell pool is reduced to ≤1% of normal in severe disease at the time of presentation.

An intrinsic stem cell defect exists for the constitutional aplastic anemias: cells from patients with Fanconi's anemia exhibit chromosome damage and death on exposure to certain chemical agents. Telomeres are short in a large proportion of patients with aplastic anemia, and mutations in genes of the telomere repair complex (*TERC* and *TERT*) can be identified in some adults with apparently acquired marrow failure and without physical anomalies or typical family history.

Aplastic anemia does not appear to result from defective stroma or growth factor production.

Drug Injury Extrinsic damage to the marrow follows massive physical or chemical insults such as high doses of radiation and toxic chemicals. For the more common idiosyncratic reaction to modest doses of medical drugs, altered drug metabolism has been invoked as a likely mechanism. The metabolic pathways of many drugs and chemicals, especially if they are polar and have limited water solubility, involve enzymatic degradation to highly reactive electrophilic compounds; these intermediates are toxic because of their propensity to bind to cellular macromolecules. For example, derivative hydroquinones and quinolones are responsible for benzene-induced tissue injury. Excessive generation of toxic intermediates or failure to detoxify the intermediates may be genetically determined and apparent only on specific drug challenge; the complexity and specificity of the pathways imply multiple susceptibility loci and would provide an explanation for the rarity of idiosyncratic drug reactions.

Immune-Mediated Injury The recovery of marrow function in some patients prepared for bone marrow transplantation with antilymphocyte globulin (ALG) first suggested that aplastic anemia might be immune-mediated. Consistent with this hypothesis was the frequent failure of simple bone marrow transplantation from a syngeneic twin, without conditioning cytotoxic chemotherapy, which also argued both *against* simple stem cell absence as the cause and *for* the presence of a host factor producing marrow failure. Laboratory data support an important role for the immune system in aplastic anemia. Blood and bone marrow cells of patients can suppress normal hematopoietic progenitor cell growth, and removal of T cells from aplastic anemia bone marrow improves colony formation in vitro. Increased numbers of activated cytotoxic T cells are observed in aplastic anemia patients and usually decline with successful immunosuppressive therapy; cytokine measurements show a T_H1 immune response (interferon γ and tumor necrosis factor). Interferon and tumor necrosis factor induce Fas expression on CD34 cells, leading to apoptotic cell death; localization of activated T cells to bone marrow and local production of their soluble factors are probably important in stem cell destruction.

Early immune system events in aplastic anemia are not well understood. Analysis of T cell receptor expression suggests an oligoclonal, antigen-driven cytotoxic T cell response. Many different exogenous antigens appear capable of initiating a pathologic immune response, but at least some of the T cells may recognize true self-antigens. The rarity of aplastic anemia despite common exposures (medicines, hepatitis virus) suggests that genetically determined features of the immune response can convert a normal physiologic response into a sustained abnormal autoimmune process, including polymorphisms in histocompatibility antigens, cytokine genes, and genes that regulate T cell polarization and effector function.

CLINICAL FEATURES

History Aplastic anemia can appear with seeming abruptness or have a more insidious onset. Bleeding is the most common early symptom; a complaint of days to weeks of easy bruising, oozing from the gums, nose bleeds, heavy menstrual flow, and sometimes petechiae will have been noticed. With thrombocytopenia, massive hemorrhage is unusual, but small amounts of bleeding in the central nervous system can result in catastrophic intracranial or retinal hemorrhage. Symptoms of anemia are also frequent, including lassitude, weakness, shortness of breath, and a pounding sensation in the ears. Infection is an unusual first symptom in aplastic anemia (unlike in agranulocytosis, where pharyngitis, anorectal infection, or frank sepsis occur early). A striking feature of aplastic anemia is the restriction of symptoms to the hematologic system, and patients often feel and look remarkably well despite drastically reduced blood counts. Systemic complaints and weight loss should point to other etiologies of pancytopenia. Prior drug use, chemical exposure, and preceding viral illnesses must often be elicited with repeated questioning. A family history of hematologic diseases or blood abnormalities may indicate a constitutional etiology of marrow failure.

Physical Examination Petechiae and ecchymoses are typical, and retinal hemorrhages may be present. Pelvic and rectal examinations can often be deferred but, when performed, should be undertaken with great gentleness to avoid trauma; these will often show bleeding from the cervical os and blood in the stool. Pallor of the skin and mucous membranes is common except in the most acute cases or those already transfused. Infection on presentation is unusual but may occur if the patient has been symptomatic for a few weeks. Lymphadenopathy and splenomegaly are highly atypical of aplastic anemia. Café au lait spots and short stature suggest Fanconi's anemia; peculiar nails and leukoplakia suggest dyskeratosis congenita.

LABORATORY STUDIES

Blood The smear shows large erythrocytes and a paucity of platelets and granulocytes. Mean corpuscular volume (MCV) is commonly increased. Reticulocytes are absent or few, and lymphocyte numbers may be normal or reduced. The presence of immature myeloid forms suggests leukemia or MDS; nucleated red blood cells suggest marrow fibrosis or tumor invasion; abnormal platelets suggest either peripheral destruction or MDS.

Bone Marrow The bone marrow is usually readily aspirated but dilute on smear, and the fatty biopsy specimen may be grossly pale on withdrawal; a "dry tap" instead suggests fibrosis or myelophthisis. In severe aplasia the smear of the aspirated specimen shows only red cells, residual lymphocytes, and stromal cells; the biopsy (which should be >1 cm in length) is superior for determination of cellularity and shows mainly fat under the microscope, with hematopoietic cells occupying <25% of the marrow space; in the most serious cases the biopsy is virtually 100% fat. The correlation between marrow cellularity and disease severity is imperfect, in part because marrow cellularity declines physiologically with aging. Additionally, some patients with moderate disease by blood counts will have empty iliac crest biopsies, while "hot spots" of hematopoiesis may be seen in severe cases. If an iliac crest specimen is inadequate, cells may also be obtained by aspiration from the sternum. Residual hematopoietic cells should have normal morphology, except for mildly megaloblastic erythropoiesis; megakaryocytes are invariably greatly reduced and usually absent. Areas adjacent to the spicule should be searched for myeloblasts. Granulomas (in cellular specimens) may indicate an infectious etiology of the marrow failure.

Ancillary Studies Chromosome breakage studies of peripheral blood using diepoxybutane or mitomycin C should be performed on children and younger adults to exclude Fanconi's anemia. Genetic analysis applicable to the constitutional marrow failure states is available in some laboratories. Chromosome studies of bone marrow cells are often revealing in MDS and should be negative in typical aplastic anemia. Flow cytometric assays have replaced the Ham test for the diagnosis of PNH. Serologic studies may show evidence of viral infection, such as Epstein-Barr virus and HIV. Posthepatitis aplastic anemia is typically seronegative. The spleen size should be determined by CT scanning or ultrasound if the physical examination of the abdomen is unsatisfactory. MRI may be helpful to assess the fat content of a few vertebrae in order to distinguish aplasia from MDS.

DIAGNOSIS

The diagnosis of aplastic anemia is usually straightforward, based on the combination of pancytopenia with a fatty, empty bone marrow. Aplastic anemia is a disease of the young and should be a leading diagnosis in the pancytopenic adolescent or young adult. When pancytopenia is secondary, the primary diagnosis is usually obvious from either history or physical examination: the massive spleen of alcoholic cirrhosis, the history of metastatic cancer or systemic lupus erythematosus, or miliary tuberculosis on chest radiograph (Table 102-1).

Diagnostic problems can occur with atypical presentations and among related hematologic diseases. While pancytopenia is most common, some patients with bone marrow hypocellularity have depression of only one or two of three blood lines, sometimes showing later progression to more recognizable aplastic anemia. The bone marrow in constitutional aplastic anemia is indistinguishable morphologically from the aspirate in acquired disease. The diagnosis can be suggested by family history, abnormal blood counts since childhood, or the presence of associated physical anomalies. Aplastic anemia may be difficult to distinguish from the hypocellular variety of MDS: MDS is favored by finding morphologic abnormalities, particularly of megakaryocytes and myeloid precursor cells, and typical cytogenetic abnormalities (see below).

PROGNOSIS

The natural history of severe aplastic anemia is rapid deterioration and death. Provision first of red blood cell and later of platelet transfusions and effective antibiotics are of some benefit, but few patients show spontaneous recovery. The major prognostic determinant is the blood count; severe disease is defined by the presence of two of three parameters: absolute neutrophil count <500/μL, platelet count <20,000/μL, and corrected reticulocyte count <1% (or absolute reticulocyte count <60,000/μL). Survival of patients who fulfill these criteria is about 20% at 1 year after diagnosis with only supportive care; patients with very severe disease, defined by an absolute neutrophil count <200/μL, fare even more poorly. Treatment has markedly improved survival in this disease.

Rx APLASTIC ANEMIA

Severe acquired aplastic anemia can be cured by replacement of the absent hematopoietic cells (and the immune system) by stem cell transplant, or it can be ameliorated by suppression of the immune system to allow recovery of the patient's residual bone marrow function. Hematopoietic growth factors have limited usefulness and glucocorticoids are of no value. Suspect exposures to drugs or chemicals should be discontinued; however, spontaneous recovery of severe blood count depression is rare, and a waiting period before beginning treatment may not be advisable unless the blood counts are only modestly depressed.

HEMATOPOIETIC STEM CELL TRANSPLANTATION This is the best therapy for the young patient with a fully histocompatible sibling donor (Chap. 108). Human leukocyte antigen (HLA) typing should be ordered as soon as the diagnosis of aplastic anemia is established in a child or younger adult. In transplant candidates, transfusion of blood from family members should be avoided so as to prevent sensitization to histocompatibility antigens; while transfusions in general should be minimized, limited numbers of blood products probably do not seriously affect outcome.

For allogeneic transplant from fully matched siblings, long-term survival rates for children are 80–90%. Transplant morbidity and mortality are increased among adults, due mainly to the higher risk of chronic GVHD and serious infections. Graft rejection was historically a major determinant of outcome in transplant for aplastic anemia, perhaps related to the underlying pathophysiology as well as to alloimmunization from transfusions (the latter now much improved by leukocyte depletion before blood product administration).

Most patients do not have a suitable sibling donor. Occasionally, a full phenotypic match can be found within the family and serve as well. Far more available are other alternative donors, either unrelated but histocompatible volunteers or closely but not perfectly matched family members. Survival using alternative donors is about half that of conventional sibling transplants but improving with higher-resolution HLA matching and more effective conditioning regimens and GVHD prophylaxis. Patients will be at risk for late complications, especially a higher rate of cancer, if radiation is used as a component of conditioning.

IMMUNOSUPPRESSION Used alone, ALG or antithymocyte globulin (ATG) induces hematologic recovery (independence from transfusion and a leukocyte count adequate to prevent infection) in about 50% of patients. The addition of cyclosporine to either ALG or ATG has further increased response rates to about 70% and especially improved outcomes for children and for severely neutropenic patients. Such combined treatment is now standard for patients with severe disease. An early robust hematologic response strongly correlates with long-term survival. Improvement in granulocyte number is generally apparent within 2 months of treatment. Most recovered patients continue to have some degree of blood count depression, the MCV remains elevated, and the bone marrow cellularity returns toward normal only very slowly, if at all. Relapse (recurrent pancytopenia) is frequent, often occurring as cyclosporine is discontinued; most, but not all, patients respond to reinstitution of immunosuppression, but some responders become dependent on continued cyclosporine administration. Development of MDS, with typical marrow morphologic or cytogenetic abnormalities, occurs in about 15% of treated patients, usually but not invariably associated with a return of pancytopenia, and some patients develop leukemia. A laboratory diagnosis of PNH can generally be made at the time of presentation of aplastic anemia by flow cytometry; recovered patients may have frank hemolysis if the PNH clone expands. Bone marrow examinations should be performed if there is an unfavorable change in blood counts.

Horse ATG is given at 40 mg/kg per day for 4 days; rabbit ALG is administered at 3.5 mg/kg per day for 5 days. For ATG, anaphylaxis is a rare but occasionally fatal complication; allergy can be tested by a skin-prick test with an undiluted solution and immediate observation; desensitization is feasible. ATG binds to peripheral blood cells; therefore, platelet and granulocyte numbers may fall further during active treatment. Serum sickness, a flu-like illness with a characteristic cutaneous eruption and arthralgia, often develops about 10 days after initiating treatment. Methylprednisolone, 1 mg/kg per day for 2 weeks, can ameliorate the immune consequences of heterologous protein infusion. Excessive or extended glucocorticoid therapy is associated with avascular joint necrosis. Cyclosporine is administered orally at an initial dose of 12 mg/kg per day in adults (15 mg/kg per day in children), with subsequent adjustment according to blood levels obtained every 2 weeks. Trough levels should be between 150 and 200 ng/mL. The most important side effects of chronic cyclosporine treatment are nephrotoxicity, hypertension, seizures, and opportunistic infections, especially *Pneumocystis carinii* (prophylactic treatment with monthly inhaled pentamidine is recommended).

Most patients with aplastic anemia lack a suitable marrow donor, and immunosuppression is the treatment of choice. Overall survival is equivalent with transplantation and immunosuppression. However, successful transplant cures marrow failure, while patients who recover adequate blood counts after immunosuppression remain at risk of relapse and malignant evolution. Because of excellent results in children and younger adults, allogeneic transplant should be performed if a suitable sibling donor is available. Increasing age and the severity of neutropenia are the most important factors weighing in the decision between transplant and immunosuppression in adults who have a matched family donor: older patients do better with ATG and cyclosporine, whereas transplant is preferred if granulocytopenia is profound. Some patients may prefer immunosuppression; transplant is used for failure to recover blood counts or occurrence of late complications.

Outcomes following both transplant and immunosuppression have improved with time. High doses of cyclophosphamide, without stem cell rescue, have been reported to produce durable hematologic recovery, without relapse or evolution to MDS, but this treatment can produce sustained severe fatal neutropenia and response is often delayed. New immunosuppressive drugs in clinical trial may further improve outcome.

OTHER THERAPIES The effectiveness of androgens has not been verified in controlled trials, but occasional patients will respond or even demonstrate blood count dependence on continued therapy. For patients with moderate disease or those with severe pancytopenia in whom immunosuppression has failed, a 3–4-month trial is appropriate. Hematopoietic growth factors, granulocyte colony-stimulating factor (G-CSF), granulocyte-macrophage CSF (GM-CSF), and interleukin 3 (IL-3) are not recommended as initial therapy for severe aplastic anemia, and even their role as adjuncts to immunosuppression is not well defined. Some patients may respond to combinations of growth factors after immunosuppression has failed.

SUPPORTIVE CARE Meticulous medical attention is required so that the patient may survive to benefit from definitive therapy or, having failed treatment, to maintain a reasonable existence in the face of pancytopenia. First and most important, infection in the presence of severe neutropenia must be aggressively treated by prompt institution of parenteral, broad-spectrum antibiotics, usually ceftazidime or a combination of an aminoglycoside, cephalosporin, and semisynthetic penicillin. Therapy is empirical and must not await results of culture, although specific foci of infection such as oropharyngeal or anorectal abscesses, pneumonia, sinusitis, and typhlitis (necrotizing colitis) should be sought on physical examination and with radiographic studies. When indwelling plastic catheters become contaminated, vancomycin should be added. Persistent or recrudescent fever implies fungal disease: *Candida* and *Aspergillus* are common, especially after several courses of antibacterial antibiotics, and a progressive course may be averted by timely initiation of antifungal therapy. Granulocyte transfusions using G-CSF–mobilized peripheral blood have appeared to be effective in the treatment of overwhelming or refractory infections in a few patients. Hand washing, the single best method of preventing the spread of infection, remains a neglected practice. Nonabsorbed antibiotics for gut decontamination are poorly tolerated and not of proven value. Total reverse isolation does not reduce mortality from infections.

Both platelet and erythrocyte numbers can be maintained by transfusion. Alloimmunization historically limited the usefulness of platelet transfusions and is now minimized by several strategies, including use of single donors to reduce exposure and physical or chemical methods to diminish leukocytes in the product; HLA-matched platelets are often effective in patients refractory to random donor products. Inhibitors of fibrinolysis such as aminocaproic acid have not been shown to relieve mucosal oozing; the use of low-dose glucocorticoids to induce "vascular stability" is unproven and not recommended. Whether platelet transfusions are better used prophylactically or only as needed remains unclear. Any rational regimen of prophylaxis requires transfusions once or twice weekly in order to maintain the platelet count >10,000/μL (oozing from the gut, and presumably also from other vascular beds, increases precipitously at counts <5000/μL). Menstruation should be suppressed either by oral estrogens or nasal follicle-stimulating hormone/luteinizing hormone (FSH/LH) antagonists. Aspirin and other nonsteroidal anti-inflammatory agents inhibit platelet function and must be avoided.

Red blood cells should be transfused to maintain a normal level of activity, usually at a hemoglobin value of 70 g/L (90 g/L if there is underlying cardiac or pulmonary disease); a regimen of 2 units every 2 weeks will replace normal losses in a patient without a functioning bone marrow. In chronic anemia, the iron chelators deferoxamine and deferasirox should be added at around the fiftieth transfusion in order to avoid secondary hemochromatosis.

PURE RED CELL APLASIA

Other, more restricted forms of marrow failure occur, in which only a single circulating cell type is affected and the aregenerative marrow shows corresponding absence or decreased numbers of specific precursor cells: aregenerative anemia as in PRCA (see below), thrombocytopenia with amegakaryocytosis (Chap. 109), and neutropenia without marrow myeloid cells in agranulocytosis (Chap. 61). In general, and in contrast to aplastic anemia and MDS, the unaffected lineages appear quantitatively and qualitatively normal. Agranulocytosis, the most frequent of these syndromes, is usually a complication of medical drug use (with agents similar to those related to aplastic anemia), either by a mechanism of direct chemical toxicity or by immune destruction. Agranulocytosis has an incidence similar to aplastic anemia but is especially frequent among the elderly and in women. The syndrome should resolve with discontinuation of exposure, but significant mortality is attached to neutropenia in the older and often previously unwell patient. Both pure white cell aplasia (agranulocytosis without incriminating drug exposure) and amegakaryocytic thrombocytopenia are exceedingly rare and, like PRCA, appear to be due to destructive antibodies or lymphocytes and can respond to immunosuppressive therapies. In all the single lineage failure syndromes, progression to pancytopenia or leukemia is unusual.

DEFINITION AND DIFFERENTIAL DIAGNOSIS

PRCA is characterized by anemia, reticulocytopenia, and absent or rare erythroid precursor cells in the bone marrow. The classification of PRCA is shown in Table 102-4. In adults, PRCA is acquired. An identical syndrome can occur constitutionally: Diamond-Blackfan anemia, or congenital PRCA, is diagnosed at birth or in early childhood and often responds to glucocorticoid treatment; a minority of patients have etiologic mutations in a ribosomal RNA processing gene called *RPS19*. Temporary red cell failure occurs in transient aplastic crisis of hemolytic anemias due to acute parvovirus infection (Chap. 177) and in transient erythroblastopenia of childhood, which affects normal children.

CLINICAL ASSOCIATIONS AND ETIOLOGY

PRCA has important associations with immune system diseases. A small minority of cases occur with a thymoma. More frequently, red cell aplasia can be the major manifestation of large granular lymphocytosis or may occur in chronic lymphocytic leukemia. Some patients may be hypogammaglobulinemic. As with agranulocytosis, PRCA can be due to an idiosyncratic reaction to a drug. Subcutaneous administration of erythropoietin can lead to PRCA mediated by neutralizing antibodies.

Like aplastic anemia, PRCA results from diverse mechanisms. Antibodies to red blood cell precursors are frequently present in the blood, but T cell inhibition is probably the more common immune mechanism. Cytotoxic lymphocyte activity restricted by histocompatibility locus or specific for human T cell leukemia/lymphoma virus I–infected cells, as well as natural killer cell activity inhibitory of erythropoiesis, have been demonstrated in particularly well-studied individual cases.

TABLE 102-4 CLASSIFICATION OF PURE RED CELL APLASIA

Self-limited
- Transient erythroblastopenia of childhood
- Transient aplastic crisis of hemolysis (acute B19 parvovirus infection)

Fetal red blood cell aplasia
- Nonimmune hydrops fetalis (in utero B19 parvovirus infection)

Hereditary pure red cell aplasia
- Congenital pure red cell aplasia (Diamond-Blackfan syndrome)

Acquired pure red cell aplasia
- Thymoma and malignancy
  - Thymoma
  - Lymphoid malignancies (and more rarely other hematologic diseases)
  - Paraneoplastic to solid tumors
- Connective tissue disorders with immunologic abnormalities
  - Systemic lupus erythematosus, juvenile rheumatoid arthritis, rheumatoid arthritis
  - Multiple endocrine gland insufficiency
- Virus
  - Persistent B19 parvovirus, hepatitis, adult T cell leukemia virus, Epstein-Barr virus
- Pregnancy
- Drugs
  - Especially phenytoin, azathioprine, chloramphenicol, procainamide, isoniazid
  - Erythropoietin

Idiopathic

Persistent Parvovirus B19 Infection Chronic parvovirus infection is an important, treatable cause of PRCA. This common virus causes a benign exanthem of childhood (fifth disease) and a polyarthralgia/arthritis syndrome in adults. In patients with underlying hemolysis (or any condition that increases demand for red blood cell production), parvovirus infection can cause a transient aplastic crisis and an abrupt but temporary worsening of the anemia due to failed erythropoiesis. In normal individuals, acute infection is resolved by production of neutralizing antibodies to the virus, but in the setting of congenital, acquired, or iatrogenic immunodeficiency, persistent viral infection may occur. The bone marrow shows red cell aplasia and the presence of giant pronormoblasts (Fig. 102-2), which is the cytopathic sign of B19 parvovirus infection. Viral tropism for human erythroid progenitor cells is due to its use of erythrocyte P antigen as a cellular receptor for entry. Direct cytotoxicity of virus causes anemia if demands on erythrocyte production are high; in normal individuals, the temporary cessation of red cell production is not clinically apparent, and skin and joint symptoms are mediated by immune complex deposition.

℞ PURE RED CELL APLASIA

History, physical examination, and routine laboratory studies may disclose an underlying disease or a suspect drug exposure. Thymoma should be sought by radiographic procedures. Tumor excision is indicated, but anemia does not necessarily improve with surgery. The diagnosis of parvovirus infection requires detection of viral DNA sequences in the blood (IgG and IgM antibodies are commonly absent). The presence of erythroid colonies has been considered predictive of response to immunosuppressive therapy in idiopathic PRCA.

Red cell aplasia is compatible with long survival with supportive care alone: a combination of erythrocyte transfusions and iron chelation. For persistent B19 parvovirus infection, almost all patients respond to intravenous immunoglobulin therapy (for example, 0.4 g/kg daily for 5 days), although relapse and retreatment may be expected, especially in patients with AIDS. The majority of patients with idiopathic PRCA respond favorably to immunosuppression. Most first receive a course of glucocorticoids. Also effective are cyclosporine, ATG, azathioprine, cyclophosphamide, and the monoclonal antibody daclizumab, an antibody to the IL-2 receptor. PRCA developing on erythropoietin therapy should be treated with immunosuppression and withdrawal of erythropoietin.

MYELODYSPLASIA

DEFINITION

The myelodysplasias (MDSs) are a heterogeneous group of hematologic disorders broadly characterized by cytopenias associated with a dysmorphic (or abnormal appearing) and usually cellular bone marrow, and by consequent ineffective blood cell production. A clinically useful nosology of these entities was first developed by the French-American-British Cooperative Group in 1983. Five entities were defined: refractory anemia (RA), refractory anemia with ringed sideroblasts (RARS), refractory anemia with excess blasts (RAEB), refractory anemia with excess blasts in transformation (RAEB-t), and chronic myelomonocytic leukemia (CMML). The World Health Organization classification (2002) recognizes that the distinction between RAEB-t and acute myeloid leukemia is arbitrary and groups them together as acute leukemia, notes that CMML behaves as a myeloproliferative disease, and separates refractory anemias with dysmorphic change restricted to erythroid lineage from those with multilineage changes (Table 102-5).

EPIDEMIOLOGY

Idiopathic MDS is a disease of the elderly; the mean age at onset is 68 years. There is a slight male preponderance. MDS is a relatively common form of bone marrow failure, with reported incidence rates of 35 to >100 per million persons in the general population and 120 to >500 per million in the elderly. MDS is rare in children, but monocytic leukemia can be seen. Therapy-related MDS is not age-related and may

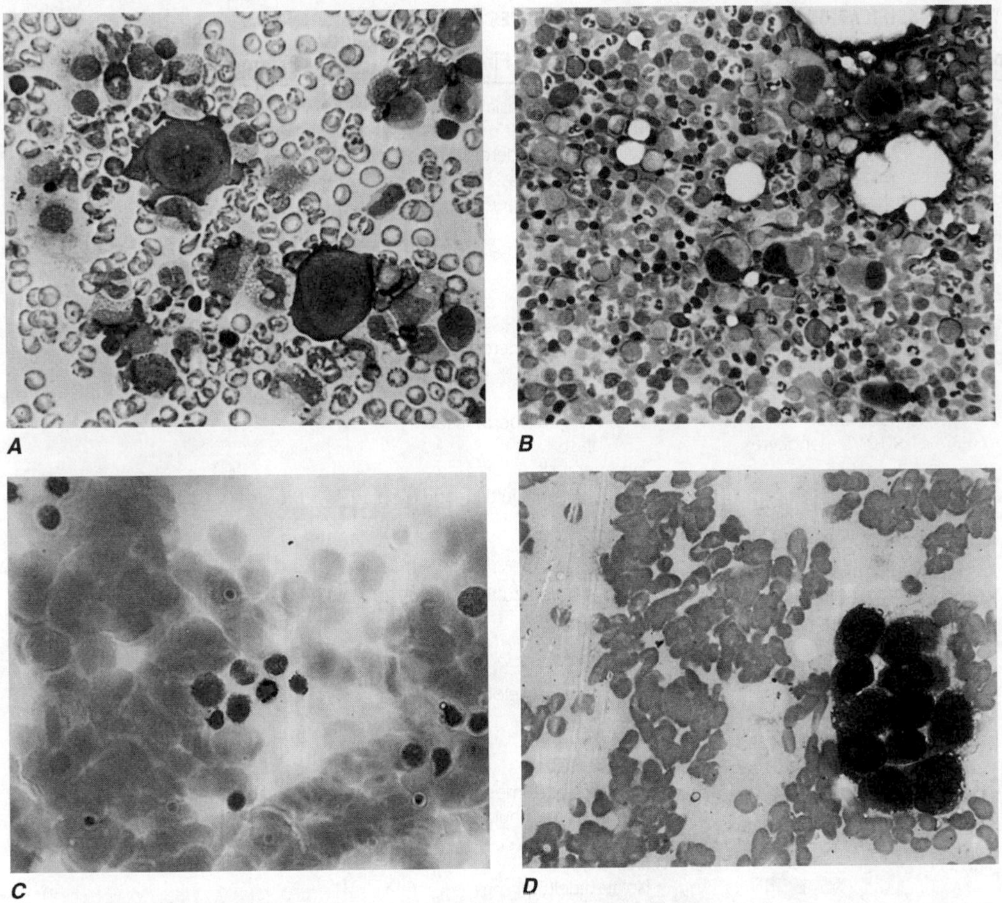

FIGURE 102-2 Pathognomonic cells in marrow failure syndromes. ***A.*** Giant pronormoblast, the cytopathic effect of B19 parvovirus infection of the erythroid progenitor cell. ***B.*** Uninuclear megakaryocyte and microblastic erythroid precursors typical of the 5q− myelodysplasia syndrome. ***C.*** Ringed sideroblast showing perinuclear iron granules. ***D.*** Tumor cells present on a touch preparation made from the marrow biopsy of a patient with metastatic carcinoma.

occur in as many as 15% of patients within a decade following intensive combined modality treatment for cancer. Rates of MDS have increased over time, due to the recognition of the syndrome by physicians and the aging of the population.

ETIOLOGY AND PATHOPHYSIOLOGY

MDS is caused by environmental exposures such as radiation and benzene; other risk factors have been reported inconsistently. Secondary MDS occurs as a late toxicity of cancer treatment, usually with a combination of radiation and the radiomimetic alkylating agents such as busulfan, nitrosourea, or procarbazine (with a latent period of 5–7 years) or the DNA topoisomerase inhibitors (2 years). Both acquired aplastic anemia following immunosuppressive treatment and Fanconi's anemia can evolve into MDS.

MDS is a clonal hematopoietic stem cell disorder leading to impaired cell proliferation and differentiation. Cytogenetic abnormalities are found in about half of patients, and some of the same specific lesions are also seen in frank leukemia; aneuploidy is more frequent than translocations. Both presenting and evolving hematologic manifestations result from the accumulation of multiple genetic lesions: loss of tumor suppressor genes, activating oncogene mutations, or other harmful alterations. Cytogenetic abnormalities are not random (loss of all or part of 5, 7, and 20, trisomy of 8) and may be related to etiology (11q23 following topoisomerase II inhibitors); chronic myelomonocytic leukemia is often associated with t(5;12) that creates a chimeric *tel-PDGFβ* gene. The type and number of cytogenetic abnormalities strongly correlate with the probability of leukemic transformation and survival. Mutations of N-*ras* (an oncogene), *p53* and *IRF-1* (tumor suppressor genes), *Bcl-2* (an antiapoptotic gene), and others have been reported in some patients but likely occur late in the sequence leading to leukemic transformation. Apoptosis of marrow cells is increased in MDS, presumably due to these acquired genetic alterations or possibly to an overlaid immune response. An immune pathophysiology has been suggested for trisomy 8 MDS, which often responds clinically to immunosuppressive therapy. Such patients have T cell activity directed to the cytogenetically aberrant clone. Sideroblastic anemia may be related to mutations in mitochondrial genes; ineffective erythropoiesis and disordered iron metabolism are the functional consequences of the genetic alterations.

CLINICAL FEATURES

Anemia dominates the early course. Most symptomatic patients complain of the gradual onset of fatigue and weakness, dyspnea, and pallor, but at least half the patients are asymptomatic and their MDS is discovered only incidentally on routine blood counts. Previous chemotherapy or radiation exposure is an important historic fact. Fever and weight loss should point to a myeloproliferative rather than myelodysplastic process. Children with Down syndrome are susceptible to MDS, and a family history may indicate a hereditary form of sideroblastic anemia or Fanconi's anemia.

The physical examination is remarkable for signs of anemia; about 20% of patients have splenomegaly. Some unusual skin lesions, including Sweet's syndrome (febrile neutrophilic dermatosis), occur with MDS. Autoimmune syndromes are not infrequent.

LABORATORY STUDIES

Blood Anemia is present in the majority of cases, either alone or as part of bi- or pancytopenia; isolated neutropenia or thrombocytopenia is more unusual. Macrocytosis is common, and the smear may be dimorphic with a distinctive population of large red blood cells. Platelets are also large and lack granules. In functional studies, they may show marked abnormalities, and patients may have bleeding symptoms despite seemingly adequate numbers. Neutrophils are hypogranulated; have hyposegmented, ringed, or abnormally segmented nuclei; contain Dohle bodies; and may be functionally deficient. Circulating myeloblasts usually correlate with marrow blast numbers, and their quantitation is important for classification and prognosis. The total white blood cell count is usually normal or low, except in chronic myelomonocytic leukemia. As in aplastic anemia, MDS can be associated with a clonal population of PNH cells.

Bone Marrow The bone marrow is usually normal or hypercellular, but in 20% of cases it is sufficiently hypocellular to be confused with aplasia. No single characteristic feature of marrow morphology distinguishes MDS, but the following are commonly observed: dyserythropoietic changes (especially nuclear abnormalities) and ringed sideroblasts in the erythroid lineage; hypogranulation and hyposegmentation in granulocytic precursors, with an increase in myeloblasts; and megakaryocytes showing reduced numbers or disorganized nuclei. Megaloblastic nuclei associated with defective hemoglobinization

TABLE 102-5 WORLD HEALTH ORGANIZATION CLASSIFICATION OF MYELODYSPLASTIC SYNDROMES

Disease	Frequency	Blood Findings	Bone Marrow Findings	Prognosis
Refractory anemia (RA)	5–10%	Anemia No or rare blasts	Erythroid dysplasia only <5% blasts <15% ringed sideroblasts	Protracted course Leukemic transformation in ~6%
Refractory anemia with ringed sideroblasts (RARS)	10–12%	Anemia No blasts	Erythroid dysplasia only ≥15% ringed sideroblasts <5% blasts	Protracted course Leukemia in ~1–2%
Refractory cytopenia with multilineage dysplasia (RCMD)	24%	Cytopenias (2 or 3 lineages) No or rare blasts No Auer rods $<1 \times 10^9$/L monocytes	Dysplasia in ≥10% of cells in ≥2 lineages <5% blasts No Auer rods <15% ringed sideroblasts	Variable clinical course Leukemia in ~11%
RCMD with ringed sideroblasts (RCMD-RS)	15%	Cytopenias (2 or 3 lineages) No or rare blasts No Auer rods $<1 \times 10^9$/L monocytes	Dysplasia in ≥10% of cells in ≥2 lineages ≥15% ringed sideroblasts <5% blasts No Auer rods	
Refractory anemia with excess blasts-1 (RAEB-1)	40% (RAEB-1 +2)	Cytopenias <5% blasts No Auer rods $<1 \times 10^9$/L monocytes	Unilineage or multilineage dysplasia 5–9% blasts No Auer rods	Progressive BM failure Leukemia in ~25%
Refractory anemia with excess blasts-2 (RAEB-2)		Cytopenias 5–19% blasts ±Auer rods $<1 \times 10^9$/L monocytes	Unilineage or multilineage dysplasia 10–19% blasts ±Auer rods	Progressive BM failure Leukemia in ~33%
Myelodysplastic syndrome, unclassified (MDS-U)	Unknown	Cytopenias No or rare blasts No Auer rods	Dysplasia in myeloid or platelet lineage <5% blasts No Auer rods	Unknown
MDS with isolated del(5q)	Unknown	Anemia <5% blasts Platelets nl or increased	Nl or increased megakaryocytes with hypolobated nuclei <5% blasts No Auer rods Isolated del(5q)	Long survival

Note: BM, bone marrow.
Source: Extracted from Jaffe ES et al (eds): *Pathology and Genetics of Tumors of Haematopoietic and Lymphoid Tissues*. Lyon, IARC Press, 2001.

in the erythroid lineage are common. Prognosis strongly correlates with the proportion of marrow blasts. Cytogenetic analysis and fluorescent in situ hybridization can identify chromosomal abnormalities.

DIFFERENTIAL DIAGNOSIS

Deficiencies of vitamin B_{12} or folate should be excluded by appropriate blood tests; vitamin B_6 deficiency can be assessed by a therapeutic trial of pyridoxine if the bone marrow shows ringed sideroblasts. Marrow dysplasia can be observed in acute viral infections, drug reactions, or chemical toxicity but should be transient. More difficult are the distinctions between hypocellular MDS and aplasia or between refractory anemia with excess blasts and early acute leukemia. The World Health Organization considers the presence of 20% blasts in the marrow as the criterion that separates acute myeloid leukemia from MDS.

PROGNOSIS

The median survival varies greatly from years for patients with 5q– or sideroblastic anemia to a few months in refractory anemia with excess blasts or severe pancytopenia associated with monosomy 7; an International Prognostic Scoring System (Table 102-6) assists in making predictions. Most patients die as a result of complications of pancytopenia and not due to leukemic transformation; perhaps one-third will succumb to other diseases unrelated to their MDS. Precipitous worsening of pancytopenia, acquisition of new chromosomal abnormalities on serial cytogenetic determination, and increase in the number of blasts are all poor prognostic indicators. The outlook in therapy-related MDS, regardless of type, is very poor, and most patients will progress within a few months to refractory acute myeloid leukemia.

Rx MYELODYSPLASIA

The therapy of MDS has been unsatisfactory. Only stem cell transplantation offers cure: survival rates of 50% at 3 years have been reported, but older patients are particularly prone to develop treatment-related mortality and morbidity. Results of transplant using matched unrelated donors are comparable, although most series contain younger and more highly selected cases.

MDS has been regarded as particularly refractory to cytotoxic chemotherapy regimens but is probably no more resistant to effective treatment than acute myeloid leukemia in the elderly, in whom drug toxicity is often fatal and remissions, if achieved, are brief.

TABLE 102-6 INTERNATIONAL PROGNOSTIC SCORING SYSTEM

	Score Value				
Prognostic Variable	**0**	**0.5**	**1.0**	**1.5**	**2.0**
Bone marrow blasts (%)	<5%	5–10%		11–20%	21–30%
Karyotype[a]	Good	Intermediate	Poor		
Cytopenia[b] (lineages affected)	0 or 1	2 or 3			
Risk Group Scores	**Score**				
Low	0				
Intermediate-1	0.5–1.0				
Intermediate-2	1.5–2.0				
High	≥2.5				

[a]Good, normal, -Y, del(5q), del (20q); poor, complex (≥3 abnormalities) or chromosome 7 abnormalities; intermediate, all other abnormalities.
[b]Cytopenias defined as Hb <100 g/L, platelet count < 100,000/μL, absolute neutrophil count <1500/μL.

Low doses of cytotoxic drugs have been administered for their "differentiating" potential, and from this experience has emerged drug therapies based on pyrimidine analogues. Azacitidine is directly cytotoxic but also inhibits DNA methylation, thereby altering gene expression. Azacitidine improves blood counts and modestly improves survival in about 16% of MDS patients, compared to best supportive care. Azacitidine is administered subcutaneously at a dose of 75 mg/m^2, daily for 7 days, at 4-week intervals, for at least four cycles, although further cycles may be required to observe a response. Decitabine is closely related to azacitidine and more potent. Similar to azacitidine, about 20% of patients show responses in blood counts, with a duration of response of almost a year. Activity may be higher in more advanced MDS subtypes. Decitabine dose is 15 mg/m^2 by continuous intravenous infusion, every eight hours for three days, repeating the cycle every 6 weeks for at least four cycles. The major toxicity of both azacitidine and decitabine is myelosuppression, leading to worsened blood counts. Other symptoms associated with cancer chemotherapy frequently occur. Ironically, it has been difficult to establish that either agent acts in patients by a mechanism of DNA demethylation.

Thalidomide, a drug with many activities including antiangiogenesis and immunomodulation, has modest biologic activity in MDS. Lenalidomide, a thalidomide derivative with a more favorable toxicity profile, is particularly effective in reversing anemia in MDS patients with 5q– syndrome; not only do a high proportion of these patients become transfusion-independent with normal or near-normal hemoglobin levels, but their cytogenetics also become normal. Lenalidomide is administered orally, 10 mg daily. Most patients will improve within 3 months of initiating therapy. Toxicities include myelosuppression (worsening thrombocytopenia and neutropenia, necessitating blood count monitoring) and an increased risk of deep vein thrombosis and pulmonary embolism.

Other treatments for MDS include amifostine, an organic thiophosphonate that blocks apoptosis; it can improve blood counts but has significant toxicities. ATG and cyclosporine, as employed in aplastic anemia, also may produce sustained independence from transfusion, especially in younger MDS patients with more favorable International Prognostic Scoring System (IPSS) scores.

Hematopoietic growth factors can improve blood counts but, as in most other marrow failure states, have been most beneficial to patients with the least severe pancytopenia. G-CSF treatment alone failed to improve survival in a controlled trial. Erythropoietin alone or in combination with G-CSF can improve hemoglobin levels, but mainly in those with low serum erythropoietin levels who have no or only a modest need for transfusions.

The same principles of supportive care described for aplastic anemia apply to MDS. Despite improvements in drug therapy, many patients will be anemic for years. RBC transfusion support should be accompanied by iron chelation in order to prevent secondary hemochromatosis.

MYELOPHTHISIC ANEMIAS

Fibrosis of the bone marrow (see Fig. 103-2), usually accompanied by a characteristic blood smear picture called *leukoerythroblastosis*, can occur as a primary hematologic disease, called *myelofibrosis* or *myeloid metaplasia* (Chap. 103), and as a secondary process, called *myelophthisis*. Myelophthisis, or secondary myelofibrosis, is reactive. Fibrosis can be a response to invading tumor cells, usually an epithelial cancer of breast, lung, a prostate origin or neuroblastoma. Marrow fibrosis may occur with infection of mycobacteria (both *Mycobacterium tuberculosis* and *M. avium*), fungi, or HIV, and in sarcoidosis. Intracellular lipid deposition in Gaucher disease and obliteration of the marrow space related to absence of osteoclast remodeling in congenital osteopetrosis also can produce fibrosis. Secondary myelofibrosis is a late consequence of radiation therapy or treatment with radiomimetic drugs. Usually the infectious or malignant underlying processes are obvious. Marrow fibrosis can also be a feature of a variety of hematologic syndromes, especially chronic myeloid leukemia, multiple myeloma, lymphomas, myeloma, and hairy cell leukemia.

The pathophysiology has three distinct features: proliferation of fibroblasts in the marrow space (myelofibrosis); the extension of hematopoiesis into the long bones and into extramedullary sites, usually the spleen, liver, and lymph nodes (myeloid metaplasia); and ineffective erythropoiesis. The etiology of the fibrosis is unknown but most likely involves dysregulated production of growth factors: platelet-derived growth factor and transforming growth factor β have been implicated. Abnormal regulation of other hematopoietins would lead to localization of blood-producing cells in nonhematopoietic tissues and uncoupling of the usually balanced processes of stem cell proliferation and differentiation. Myelofibrosis is remarkable for pancytopenia despite very large numbers of circulating hematopoietic progenitor cells.

Anemia is dominant in secondary myelofibrosis, usually normocytic and normochromic. The diagnosis is suggested by the characteristic leukoerythroblastic smear (see Fig. 103-1). Erythrocyte morphology is highly abnormal, with circulating nucleated red blood cells, teardrops, and shape distortions. White blood cell numbers are often elevated, sometimes mimicking a leukemoid reaction, with circulating myelocytes, promyelocytes, and myeloblasts. Platelets may be abundant and are often of giant size. Inability to aspirate the bone marrow, the characteristic "dry tap," can allow a presumptive diagnosis in the appropriate setting before the biopsy is decalcified.

The course of secondary myelofibrosis is determined by its etiology, usually a metastatic tumor or an advanced hematologic malignancy. Treatable causes must be excluded, especially tuberculosis and fungus. Transfusion support can relieve symptoms.

FURTHER READINGS

BAGBY GC, ALTER BP: Fanconi anemia. Semin Hematol 43:147, 2006

ESTEY E et al: Acute myeloid leukemia and myelodysplastic syndromes in older patients. J Clin Oncol 25:1908, 2007

FISCH P et al: Pure red cell aplasia. Br J Haematol 111:1010, 2000

LIPTON JM: Diamond Blackfan anemia: New paradigms for a "not so pure" inherited red cell aplasia. Semin Hematol 43:167, 2006

LIST A et al: Efficacy of lenalidomide in myelodysplastic syndromes. N Engl J Med 352:549, 2005

YOUNG NS, BROWN KE: Parvovirus B19. N Engl J Med 350:586, 2004

——— et al: Current concepts in the pathophysiology and treatment of aplastic anemia. Blood 108:2509, 2006

103 Polycythemia Vera and Other Myeloproliferative Diseases

Jerry L. Spivak

The World Health Organization (WHO) classification of the chronic myeloproliferative diseases includes seven disorders, some of which are rare or poorly characterized (Table 103-1) but all of which share an origin in a multipotent hematopoietic progenitor cell, overproduction of one or more of the formed elements of the blood without significant dysplasia, a predilection to extramedullary hematopoiesis, myelofibrosis, and transformation at varying rates to acute leukemia. Within this broad classification, however, significant phenotypic heterogeneity exists. Some diseases, such as chronic myelogenous leukemia (CML), chronic neutrophilic leukemia (CNL) and chronic eosinophilic leukemia (CEL) express primarily a myeloid phenotype, while in others, such as polycythemia vera (PV), idiopathic myelofibrosis (IMF), and essential thrombocytosis (ET), erythroid or megakaryocytic hyperplasia predominates. The latter three disorders, in contrast to the former three, also appear capable of transforming into each other.

This phenotypic heterogeneity has a genetic basis; CML is the consequence of the balanced translocation between chromosomes 9 and

TABLE 103-1 WHO CLASSIFICATION OF CHRONIC MYELOPROLIFERATIVE DISORDERS

Chronic myelogenous leukemia, [Ph chromosome t(9;22)(q34;11), BCR/ABL-positive]
Chronic neutrophilic leukemia
Chronic eosinophilic leukemia (and the hypereosinophilic syndrome)
Polycythemia vera
Chronic idiopathic myelofibrosis (with extramedullary hematopoiesis)
Essential thrombocythemia
Chronic myeloproliferative disease, unclassifiable

22 [t(9;22)(q34;11)]; CNL has been associated with a t(15:19) translocation, and CEL with a deletion or balanced translocations involving the PDGFRα gene. By contrast, to a greater or lesser extent, PV, IMF, and ET are characterized by expression of a JAK2 mutation, V617F, which causes constitutive activation of this tyrosine kinase that is essential for the function of the erythropoietin and thrombopoietin receptors but not the granulocyte colony–stimulating factor receptor. This essential distinction is also reflected in the natural history of CML, CNL, and CEL, which is usually measured in years, and their high rate of transformation into acute leukemia. By contrast, the natural history of PV, IMF, and ET is usually measured in decades, and transformation to acute leukemia is uncommon in the absence of exposure to mutagenic agents. This chapter, therefore, will focus only on PV, IMF, and ET, because their clinical overlap is substantial and their clinical courses are distinctly different. **Other chronic myeloproliferative disorders will be discussed in Chapter 104.**

POLYCYTHEMIA VERA

Polycythemia vera (PV) is a clonal disorder involving a multipotent hematopoietic progenitor cell in which phenotypically normal red cells, granulocytes, and platelets accumulate in the absence of a recognizable physiologic stimulus. The most common of the chronic myeloproliferative disorders, PV occurs in 2 per 100,000 persons, sparing no adult age group and increasing with age to rates as high as 18/100,000. Familial transmission occurs but is infrequent. A slight overall male predominance has been observed, but women predominate within the reproductive age range.

ETIOLOGY

The etiology of PV is unknown. Although nonrandom chromosome abnormalities such as 20q, trisomy 8, and especially 9p, have been documented in up to 30% of untreated PV patients, unlike CML no consistent cytogenetic abnormality has been associated with the disorder. However, a mutation in the autoinhibitory, pseudokinase domain of the tyrosine kinase JAK2—which replaces valine with phenylalanine (V617F), causing constitutive activation of the kinase—appears to have a central role in the pathogenesis of PV.

JAK2 is a member of an evolutionarily well-conserved, nonreceptor tyrosine kinase family and serves as the cognate tyrosine kinase for the erythropoietin and thrombopoietin receptors. It also functions as an obligate chaperone for these receptors in the Golgi apparatus and is responsible for their cell-surface expression. The conformational change induced in the erythropoietin and thrombopoietin receptors following binding to erythropoietin or thrombopoietin leads to JAK2 autophosphorylation, receptor phosphorylation, and phosphorylation of proteins involved in cell proliferation, differentiation, and resistance to apoptosis. Transgenic animals lacking JAK2 die as embryos from severe anemia. Constitutive activation of JAK2 can explain the erythropoietin-independent erythroid colony formation, and the hypersensitivity of PV erythroid progenitor cells to erythropoietin and other hematopoietic growth factors, their resistance to apoptosis in vitro in the absence of erythropoietin, their rapid terminal differentiation, and their increase in Bcl-X_L expression, all of which are characteristic in PV.

Importantly, the JAK2 gene is located on the short arm of chromosome 9, and loss of heterozygosity on chromosome 9p, due to uniparental disomy is the most common cytogenetic abnormality in PV. The segment of 9p involved contains the JAK2 locus; loss of heterozygosity in this region leads to homozygosity for the mutant JAK2 V617F. Over 90% of PV patients express this mutation, as do approximately 45% of IMF and ET patients. Homozygosity for the mutation occurs in approximately 30% of PV patients and 60% of IMF patients; homozygosity is rare in ET. Over time, a portion of PV JAK2 V617F heterozygotes become homozygotes, but usually not after 10 years of the disease. PV patients who do not express JAK2 V617F are not clinically different than those who do, nor do JAK2 V617F heterozygotes differ clinically from homozygotes. In general, patients who express JAK2 V617F are older than those who do not, but they do not have a longer duration of disease.

JAK2 V617F is the basis for many of the phenotypic and biochemical characteristics of PV, such as elevation of the leukocyte alkaline phosphatase (LAP) score and increased expression of the mRNA of PVR-1, a glycosylphosphatidylinositol (GPI)-linked membrane protein; however, it cannot solely account for the entire PV phenotype. First, PV patients with the same phenotype and documented clonal disease lack this mutation. Second, IMF patients have the same mutation but a different clinical phenotype. Third, familial PV can occur without the mutation, even when other members of the same family express it. Fourth, not all the cells of the malignant clone express JAK2 V617F. Fifth, JAK2 V617F has been observed in patients with long-standing idiopathic erythrocytosis. However, while JAK2 V617F alone may not be sufficient to cause PV, it is essential for the transformation of ET to PV, though not for its transformation to IMF.

CLINICAL FEATURES

Although splenomegaly may be the initial presenting sign in PV, most often the disorder is first recognized by the incidental discovery of a high hemoglobin or hematocrit. With the exception of aquagenic pruritus, no symptoms distinguish PV from other causes of erythrocytosis.

Uncontrolled erythrocytosis causes hyperviscosity, leading to neurologic symptoms such as vertigo, tinnitus, headache, visual disturbances, and transient ischemic attacks (TIAs). Systolic hypertension is also a feature of the red cell mass elevation. In some patients, venous or arterial thrombosis may be the presenting manifestation of PV. Any vessel can be affected, but cerebral, cardiac, or mesenteric vessels are most commonly involved. Intraabdominal venous thrombosis is particularly common in young women and may be catastrophic if a sudden and complete obstruction of the hepatic vein occurs. Indeed, PV should be suspected in any patient who develops hepatic vein thrombosis. Digital ischemia, easy bruising, epistaxis, acid-peptic disease, or gastrointestinal hemorrhage may occur due to vascular stasis or thrombocytosis. Erythema, burning, and pain in the extremities, a symptom complex known as erythromelalgia, is another complication of the thrombocytosis of PV. Given the large turnover of hematopoietic cells, hyperuricemia with secondary gout, uric acid stones, and symptoms due to hypermetabolism can also complicate the disorder.

The plasma erythropoietin level is a useful diagnostic test in patients with isolated erythrocytosis, because an elevated level excludes PV as the cause for the erythrocytosis.

DIAGNOSIS

When PV presents with erythrocytosis in combination with leukocytosis, thrombocytosis, or both, the diagnosis is apparent. However, when patients present with an elevated hemoglobin or hematocrit alone, or with thrombocytosis alone, the diagnostic evaluation is more complex because of the many diagnostic possibilities **(Table 103-2)**. Furthermore, unless the hemoglobin level is ≥20 gm% (hematocrit ≥60%), it is not possible to distinguish PV from disorders causing plasma volume contraction. Uniquely in PV, an expanded plasma volume can mask an elevated red cell mass; thus, red cell mass and plasma volume determinations are mandatory to establish the presence of an absolute erythrocytosis and to distinguish this from relative erythrocytosis due to a reduction in plasma volume alone (also known as *stress* or *spurious erythrocytosis* or *Gaisböck's syndrome*). This is true even in with the discovery of the JAK2 V617F mutation, because not very patient with PV expresses this mutation, while

TABLE 103-2 CAUSES OF ERYTHROCYTOSIS

Relative erythrocytosis: Hemoconcentration secondary to dehydration, androgens, or tobacco abuse
Absolute erythrocytosis
Hypoxia
Carbon monoxide intoxication
High affinity hemoglobin
High altitude
Pulmonary disease
Right-to-left shunts
Sleep-apnea syndrome
Neurologic disease
Renal disease
Renal artery stenosis
Focal sclerosing or membranous glomerulonephritis
Renal transplantation
Tumors
Hypernephroma
Hepatoma
Cerebellar hemangioblastoma
Uterine fibromyoma
Adrenal tumors
Meningioma
Pheochromocytoma
Drugs
Androgens
Recombinant erythropoietin
Familial (with normal hemoglobin function, Chuvash, erythropoietin receptor mutations)
Polycythemia vera

patients without PV do. Figure 58-18 illustrates a diagnostic algorithm for the evaluation of suspected erythrocytosis.

Once absolute erythrocytosis has been established, its cause must be determined. An elevated plasma erythropoietin level suggests either a hypoxic cause for erythrocytosis or autonomous erythropoietin production, in which case assessment of pulmonary function and an abdominal CT scan to evaluate renal and hepatic anatomy are appropriate. A normal erythropoietin level does not exclude a hypoxic cause for erythrocytosis. In PV, in contrast to hypoxic erythrocytosis, the arterial oxygen saturation is normal. However, a normal oxygen saturation does not exclude a high-affinity hemoglobin as a cause for erythrocytosis; documentation of previous hemoglobin levels and a family study are important.

Other laboratory studies that may aid in diagnosis include the red cell count, mean corpuscular volume, and red cell distribution width (RDW). Only three situations cause microcytic erythrocytosis: β-thalassemia trait, hypoxic erythrocytosis, and PV. With β-thalassemia trait the RDW is normal, whereas with hypoxic erythrocytosis and PV, the RDW is usually elevated due to iron deficiency. In many patients, the LAP level is also increased, as is the uric acid level. Elevated serum vitamin B_{12} or B_{12}-binding capacity may be present. In patients with associated acid-peptic disease, occult gastrointestinal bleeding may lead to presentation with hypochromic, microcytic anemia.

A bone marrow aspirate and biopsy provide no specific diagnostic information since these may be normal or indistinguishable from ET or IMF, and unless there is a need to establish the presence of myelofibrosis or exclude some other disorder, these procedures need not be done. Although the presence of a cytogenetic abnormality such as trisomy 8 or 9 or 20q– in the setting of an expanded red cell mass supports a clonal etiology, no specific cytogenetic abnormality is associated with PV, and the absence of a cytogenetic marker does not exclude the diagnosis.

COMPLICATIONS

The major clinical complications of PV relate directly to the increase in blood viscosity associated with red cell mass elevation and indirectly to the increased turnover of red cells, leukocytes, and platelets with the attendant increase in uric acid and cytokine production. The latter appears to be responsible for the increase in peptic ulcer disease and for the pruritus associated with this disorder, although formal proof for this has not been obtained. A sudden massive increase in spleen size can be associated with splenic infarction or progressive cachexia. Myelofibrosis appears to be part of the natural history of the disease but is a reactive, reversible process that does not itself impede hematopoiesis and by itself has no prognostic significance. In some patients, however, the myelofibrosis is accompanied by significant extramedullary hematopoiesis, hepatosplenomegaly, and transfusion-dependent anemia. The organomegaly can cause significant mechanical discomfort, portal hypertension, and cachexia. Although the incidence of acute nonlymphocytic leukemia is increased in PV, the incidence of acute leukemia in patients not exposed to chemotherapy or radiation is low, and the development of leukemia is related to older age but not disease duration, suggesting that the treatment exposure may be a more important risk factor than the disease itself.

Erythromelalgia is a curious syndrome of unknown etiology associated with thrombocytosis, primarily involving the lower extremities and manifested usually by erythema, warmth, and pain of the affected appendage and occasionally digital infarction. It occurs with a variable frequency in myeloproliferative disorder patients and is usually responsive to salicylates. Some of the central nervous system symptoms observed in patients with PV, such as ocular migraine, may represent a variant of erythromelalgia.

If left uncontrolled, erythrocytosis can lead to thrombosis involving vital organs such as the liver, heart, brain, or lungs. Patients with massive splenomegaly are particularly prone to thrombotic events because the associated increase in plasma volume masks the true extent of the red cell mass elevation as measured by the hematocrit or hemoglobin level. A "normal" hematocrit or hemoglobin level in a PV patient with massive splenomegaly should be considered indicative of an elevated red cell mass until proven otherwise.

℞ POLYCYTHEMIA VERA

PV is generally an indolent disorder whose clinical course is measured in decades, and its medical management should reflect its tempo. Thrombosis due to erythrocytosis is the most significant complication, and maintenance of the hemoglobin level at ≤140 g/L (14 g/dL; hematocrit <45%) in men and ≤120 g/L (12 g/dL; hematocrit <42%) in women is mandatory to avoid thrombotic complications. Phlebotomy serves initially to reduce hyperviscosity by bringing the red cell mass into the normal range. Periodic phlebotomies thereafter serve to maintain the red cell mass within the normal range and to induce a state of iron deficiency, which prevents an accelerated reexpansion of the red cell mass. In most PV patients, once an iron-deficient state is achieved, phlebotomy is usually only required at 3-month intervals. Neither phlebotomy nor iron deficiency increases the platelet count relative to the effect of the disease itself, and thrombocytosis is not correlated with thrombosis in PV, in contrast to the strong correlation between erythrocytosis and thrombosis in this disease. The use of salicylates as a tonic against thrombosis in PV patients is potentially harmful if the red cell mass is not controlled by phlebotomy. Anticoagulants are only indicated when a thrombosis has occurred and can be difficult to monitor owing to the artifactual imbalance between the test tube anticoagulant and plasma that occurs when blood from these patients is assayed for prothrombin or partial thromboplastin activity. Asymptomatic hyperuricemia (<10 mg%) requires no therapy, but allopurinol should be administered to avoid further elevation of the uric acid when chemotherapy is employed to reduce splenomegaly or leukocytosis or to treat pruritus. Generalized pruritus intractable to antihistamines or antidepressants such as doxepin can be a major problem in PV; hydroxyurea, interferon α (IFN-α), and psoralens with ultraviolet light in the A range (PUVA) therapy are other methods of palliation. Asymptomatic thrombocytosis requires no therapy unless the platelet count is sufficiently high to cause an acquired form of von Willebrand's disease due to proteolysis of high-molecular-weight vWF multimers. Symptomatic splenomegaly can be treated with IFN-α. Although the drug can be associated with significant side effects when used chronically, IFN-α reduces JAK2 V617F expression in PV patients, and its role in this disorder may be expanding. Anagrelide, a phosphodiesterase inhibitor, can reduce the platelet count and, if tolerated, is preferable to hydroxyurea because it lacks marrow toxicity. A reduction in platelet number may be necessary in the treatment of erythromelalgia or ocular migraine if salicylates are not effective or the platelet count is sufficiently high to cause an hemorrhagic diathesis. Alkylating agents and radioactive sodium phosphate (^{32}P) are leukemogenic in PV, and their use should be avoided. If a cytotoxic agent must be used, hydroxyurea is preferred, but this drug does not prevent either thrombosis or myelofibrosis in this disorder. Chemotherapy should be used for as short a time as possible. In some patients, massive splenomegaly unresponsive to reduction by hydroxyurea or IFN-α therapy and associated with intractable weight loss will require splenectomy. In some patients with end-stage disease, pulmonary hypertension may develop due to fibrosis and extramedullary hematopoiesis. Allogeneic bone marrow transplantation may be curative in young patients.

Most patients with PV can live long lives without functional impairment when their red cell mass is effectively managed with phlebotomy. Chemotherapy is never indicated to control the red cell mass unless venous access is inadequate.

CHRONIC IDIOPATHIC MYELOFIBROSIS

Chronic IMF (other designations include *agnogenic myeloid metaplasia* or *myelofibrosis with myeloid metaplasia*) is a clonal disorder of a multipotent hematopoietic progenitor cell of unknown etiology characterized by marrow fibrosis, extramedullary hematopoiesis, and splenomegaly. Chronic IMF is the least common chronic myeloproliferative disorder, and establishing this diagnosis in the absence of a specific clonal marker is difficult because myelofibrosis and splenomegaly are also features of both PV and CML. Furthermore, myelofibrosis and splenomegaly also occur in a variety of benign and malignant disorders (Table 103-3), many of which are amenable to specific therapies not effective in chronic IMF. In contrast to the other chronic myeloproliferative disorders and so-called acute or malignant myelofibrosis, which can occur at any age, chronic IMF primarily afflicts individuals in their sixth decade or later.

ETIOLOGY

The etiology of chronic IMF is unknown. Nonrandom chromosome abnormalities such as 9p, 20q–, 13q–, trisomy 8 or 9, or partial trisomy 1q are common, but no cytogenetic abnormality specific to the disease has been identified. The degree of myelofibrosis and the extent of extramedullary hematopoiesis are also not related. Fibrosis in this disorder is associated with overproduction of transforming growth factor β and tissue inhibitors of metalloproteinases, while osteosclerosis is associated with overproduction of osteoprotegerin, an osteoclast inhibitor. Marrow angiogenesis occurs due to increased production of vascular endothelial growth factor (VEGF). Importantly, fibroblasts in chronic IMF are polyclonal and not part of the neoplastic clone.

CLINICAL FEATURES

No signs or symptoms are specific for chronic IMF. Many patients are asymptomatic at presentation, and the disease is usually detected by the discovery of splenic enlargement and/or abnormal blood counts during a routine examination. However, in contrast to its companion myeloproliferative disorders, night sweats, fatigue, and weight loss may be presenting complaints. A blood smear shows the characteristic features of extramedullary hematopoiesis: teardrop-shaped red cells, nucleated red cells, myelocytes, and promyelocytes; myeloblasts may also be present (Fig. 103-1). Anemia, usually mild initially, is the rule, while the leukocyte and platelet counts are either normal or increased, but either can be depressed. Mild hepatomegaly may accompany the splenomegaly but is unusual in the absence of splenic enlargement; isolated lymphadenopathy should suggest another diagnosis. Both serum lactate dehydrogenase and alkaline phosphatase levels can be elevated. The LAP score can be low, normal, or high. Marrow is usually inaspirable due to the myelofibrosis (Fig. 103-2), and bone x-rays may reveal osteosclerosis. Exuberant extramedullary hematopoiesis can cause ascites, portal, pulmonary or intracranial hypertension, intestinal or ureteral obstruction, pericardial tamponade, spinal cord compression, or skin nodules. Splenic enlargement can be sufficiently rapid to cause splenic infarction with fever and pleuritic chest pain. Hyperuricemia and secondary gout may ensue.

TABLE 103-3 DISORDERS CAUSING MYELOFIBROSIS

Malignant	Nonmalignant
Acute leukemia (lymphocytic, myelogenous, megakaryocytic)	HIV infection
Chronic myelogenous leukemia	Hyperparathyroidism
Hairy cell leukemia	Renal osteodystrophy
Hodgkin disease	Systemic lupus erythematosus
Idiopathic myelofibrosis	Tuberculosis
Lymphoma	Vitamin D deficiency
Multiple myeloma	Thorium dioxide exposure
Myelodysplasia	Gray platelet syndrome
Metastatic carcinoma	
Polycythemia vera	
Systemic mastocytosis	

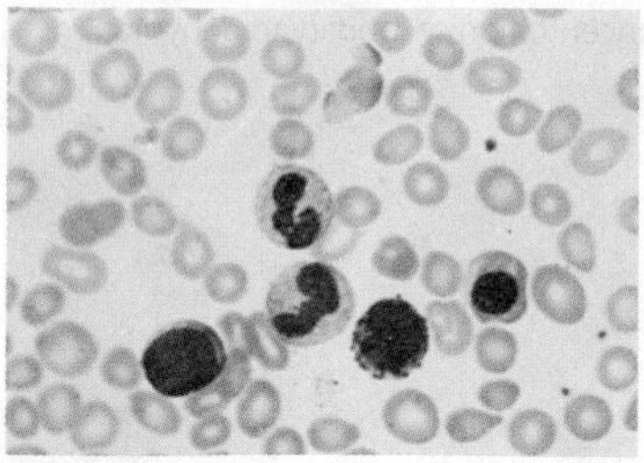

FIGURE 103-1 Teardrop-shaped red blood cells indicative of membrane damage from passage through the spleen, a nucleated red blood cell, and immature myeloid cells indicative of extramedullary hematopoiesis are noted. This peripheral blood smear is related to any cause of extramedullary hematopoiesis.

DIAGNOSIS

While the clinical picture described above is characteristic of chronic IMF, all of the clinical features described can also be observed in PV or CML. Massive splenomegaly commonly masks erythrocytosis in PV, and reports of intraabdominal thromboses in chronic IMF most likely represent instances of unrecognized PV. In some patients with chronic IMF, erythrocytosis has developed during the course of the disease. Furthermore, since many other disorders have features that overlap with chronic IMF but respond to distinctly different therapies, the diagnosis of chronic IMF is one of exclusion, which requires that the disorders listed in Table 103-3 be ruled out. A diagnostic algorithm has been proposed but does not distinguish one disease causing myeloid metaplasia from another.

The presence of teardrop-shaped red cells, nucleated red cells, myelocytes, and promyelocytes establishes the presence of extramedullary hematopoiesis, while the presence of leukocytosis, thrombocytosis with large and bizarre platelets, and circulating myelocytes suggests the presence of a myeloproliferative disorder as opposed to a secondary form of myelofibrosis (Table 103-3). Marrow is usually not aspirable due to increased marrow reticulin, but marrow biopsy will reveal a hypercellular marrow with trilineage hyperplasia and, in particular, increased numbers of megakaryocytes in clusters and with large, dysplastic nuclei However, there are no characteristic morphologic abnormalities that distinguish IMF from the other chronic myeloproliferative disorders. Splenomegaly due to extramedullary hematopoiesis may be sufficiently massive to cause portal hypertension and variceal formation. In some patients, exuberant extramedullary hematopoiesis can dominate the

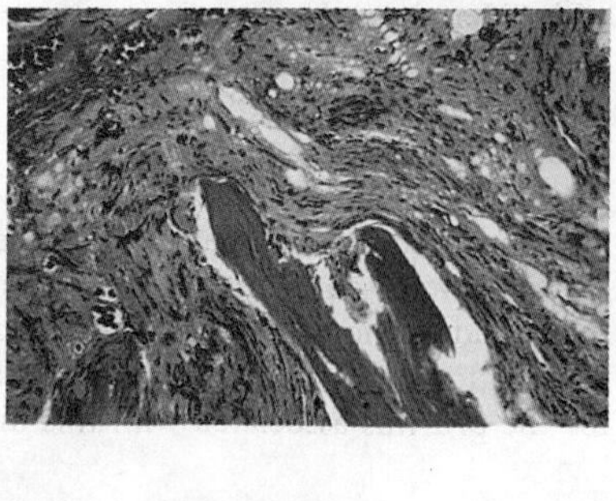

FIGURE 103-2 This marrow section shows the marrow cavity replaced by fibrous tissue composed of reticulin fibers and collagen. When this fibrosis is due to a primary hematologic process, it is called *myelofibrosis*. When the fibrosis is secondary to a tumor or a granulomatous process, it is called *myelophthisis*.

clinical picture. An intriguing feature of chronic IMF is the occurrence of autoimmune abnormalities such as immune complexes, antinuclear antibodies, rheumatoid factor, or a positive Coombs' test. Whether these represent a host reaction to the disorder or are involved in its pathogenesis is unknown. Cytogenetic analysis of blood is useful both to exclude CML and for prognostic purposes, because complex karyotype abnormalities portend a poor prognosis in chronic IMF. For unknown reasons, the number of circulating CD34+ cells is markedly increased in chronic IMF (>15,000/μL) compared to the other chronic myeloproliferative disorders, unless they too develop myeloid metaplasia.

Importantly, approximately 45% of chronic IMF patients, like patients with its companion myeloproliferative disorders PV and ET, express the JAK2 V617F mutation, often as homozygotes. Such patients had a poorer survival in one retrospective study but not in another, where they were found to be older and to have higher hematocrits than those patients who were JAK2 V617F-negative.

COMPLICATIONS

Survival in chronic IMF varies according to specific clinical features (Table 103-4) but is shorter than in patients with PV or ET. The natural history of chronic IMF is one of increasing marrow failure with transfusion-dependent anemia and increasing organomegaly due to extramedullary hematopoiesis. As with CML, chronic IMF can evolve from a chronic phase to an accelerated phase with constitutional symptoms and increasing marrow failure. About 10% of patients develop an aggressive form of acute leukemia for which therapy is usually ineffective. Important prognostic factors for disease acceleration include anemia, leukocytosis, thrombocytopenia, the presence of circulating myeloblasts, older age, the presence of complex cytogenetic abnormalities, and constitutional symptoms such as unexplained fever, night sweats, or weight loss.

TABLE 103-4 RISK STRATIFICATION FOR IDIOPATHIC MYELOFIBROSIS

A. Prognostic factors[a]		
Hemoglobin <10 gm%		
White cell count < 4000/μL or > 30,000/μL		
Number of prognostic factors	**Risk group**	**Median survival (months)**
0	Low	93
1–2	High	17
B. Prognostic factors[b]		
Hemoglobin < 10 gm%		
Constitutional symptoms		
Blast cells > 1%		
Number of prognostic factors	**Risk group**	**Median survival (months)**
0–1	Low	99
2–3	High	21
C. Prognostic factors[c]	**Median survival (months)**	
Age <65 years		
Hemoglobin ≤10 gm%		
Karyotype: Normal	54	
Abnormal	22	
Age <65 years		
Hemoglobin >10 gm%		
Karyotype: Normal	180	
Abnormal	72	
Age >65 years		
Hemoglobin ≤10 gm%		
Karyotype: Normal	44	
Abnormal	16	
Age >65 years		
Hemoglobin >10 gm%		
Karyotype: Normal	70	
Abnormal	78	

[a]From B Dupriez et al. Blood 88:1013, 1996.
[b]From F Cervantes et al. Br J Haematol 102:684, 1998.
[c]From JT Reilly et al. Br J Haematol 98:96, 1997.

℞ CHRONIC IDIOPATHIC MYELOFIBROSIS

No specific therapy exists for chronic IMF. Anemia may be due to gastrointestinal blood loss and exacerbated by folic acid deficiency, and in rare instances, pyridoxine therapy has been effective. However, anemia is more often due to ineffective erythropoiesis uncompensated by extramedullary hematopoiesis in the spleen and liver. Neither recombinant erythropoietin nor androgens, such as Danazol, have proved consistently effective as therapy for anemia. Erythropoietin may worsen splenomegaly and will be ineffective if the serum erythropoietin level is >125 mU/L. A red cell splenic sequestration study can establish the presence of hypersplenism, for which splenectomy is indicated. Splenectomy may also be necessary if splenomegaly impairs alimentation and should be performed before cachexia sets in. In this situation, splenectomy should not be avoided because of concern over rebound thrombocytosis, loss of hematopoietic capacity, or compensatory hepatomegaly. However, for unexplained reasons, splenectomy increases the risk of blastic transformation. Splenic irradiation is, at best, temporarily palliative and associated with a significant risk of neutropenia and infection. Allopurinol can control significant hyperuricemia, and hydroxyurea has proved useful for controlling organomegaly in some patients. The role of IFN-α is still undefined and its side effects are more pronounced in the older individuals who are usually afflicted with this disorder. Glucocorticoids have been used to control constitutional symptoms and autoimmune complications and may ameliorate anemia alone or in combination with low dose thalidomide (50–100 mg/d). Allogeneic bone marrow transplantation is the only curative treatment and should be considered in younger patients; reduced-intensity conditioning regimens may permit hematopoietic cell transplantation to be extended to older individuals.

ESSENTIAL THROMBOCYTOSIS

Essential thrombocytosis (other designations include *essential thrombocythemia, idiopathic thrombocytosis, primary thrombocytosis, hemorrhagic thrombocythemia*) is a clonal disorder of unknown etiology involving a multipotent hematopoietic progenitor cell manifested clinically by overproduction of platelets without a definable cause. ET is an uncommon disorder, with an incidence of 1–2/100,000 and a distinct female predominance, in contrast to the other chronic myeloproliferative disorders. No clonal marker is available to consistently distinguish ET from the more common nonclonal, reactive forms of thrombocytosis (Table 103-5), making its diagnosis difficult. Once considered a disease of the elderly and responsible for significant morbidity due to hemorrhage or thrombosis, with the widespread use of electronic cell counters, it is now clear that ET can occur at any age in adults and often without symptoms or disturbances of hemostasis. There is an unexplained female predominance in contrast to the other chronic myeloproliferative disorders or the reactive forms of thrombocytosis where no sex difference exists. Because no specific clonal marker is available, clinical criteria have been proposed to distinguish ET from the other chronic myeloproliferative disorders, which may also present with thrombocytosis but have differing prognoses and therapy (Table 103-5). These criteria do not establish clonality; therefore, they

TABLE 103-5 CAUSES OF THROMBOCYTOSIS

- Tissue inflammation: collagen vascular disease, inflammatory bowel disease
- Malignancy
- Infection
- Myeloproliferative disorders: polycythemia vera, idiopathic myelofibrosis, essential thrombocytosis, chronic myelogenous leukemia
- Myelodysplastic disorders: 5q-syndrome, idiopathic refractory sideroblastic anemia
- Postsplenectomy or hyposplenism
- Hemorrhage
- Iron deficiency anemia
- Surgery
- Rebound: Correction of vitamin B_{12} or folate deficiency, post-ethanol abuse
- Hemolysis
- Familial: Thrombopoietin overproduction, constitutive Mpl activation

are truly useful only in identifying disorders such as CML, PV, or myelodysplasia, which can masquerade as ET, as opposed to actually establishing the presence of ET. Furthermore, as with "idiopathic" erythrocytosis, nonclonal benign forms of thrombocytosis exist (such as hereditary overproduction of thrombopoietin) that are not widely recognized because we currently lack adequate diagnostic tools.

ETIOLOGY

Megakaryocytopoiesis and platelet production depend upon thrombopoietin and its receptor, Mpl. As in the case of early erythroid and myeloid progenitor cells, early megakaryocytic progenitors require the presence of interleukin 3 (IL-3) and stem cell factor for optimal proliferation in addition to thrombopoietin. Their subsequent development is also enhanced by the chemokine stromal cell–derived factor 1 (SDF-1). However, megakaryocyte maturation and differentiation require thrombopoietin.

Megakaryocytes are unique among hematopoietic progenitor cells because reduplication of their genome is endomitotic rather than mitotic. In the absence of thrombopoietin, endomitotic megakaryocytic reduplication and, by extension, the cytoplasmic development necessary for platelet production are impaired. Like erythropoietin, thrombopoietin is produced in both the liver and the kidneys, and an inverse correlation exists between the platelet count and plasma thrombopoietic activity. Like erythropoietin, plasma levels of thrombopoietin are controlled largely by the size of its progenitor cell pool. In contrast to erythropoietin, but like its myeloid counterparts, granulocyte- and granulocyte-macrophage colony-stimulating factors, thrombopoietin not only enhances the proliferation of its target cells but also enhances the reactivity of their end-stage product, the platelet. In addition to its role in thrombopoiesis, thrombopoietin also enhances the survival of multipotent hematopoietic stem cells.

The clonal nature of ET was established by analysis of glucose-6-phosphate dehydrogenase isoenzyme expression in patients hemizygous for this gene, by analysis of X-linked DNA polymorphisms in informative women patients, and by the expression in patients of nonrandom, though variable, cytogenetic abnormalities. Although thrombocytosis is its principal manifestation, like the other chronic myeloproliferative disorders, a multipotent hematopoietic progenitor cell is involved in ET. Furthermore, a number of families have been described in which ET was inherited, in one instance as an autosomal dominant trait. In addition to ET, IMF and PV have also been observed in some kindreds.

CLINICAL FEATURES

Clinically, ET is most often identified incidentally when a platelet count is obtained during the course of a routine medical evaluation. Occasionally, review of previous blood counts will reveal that an elevated platelet count was present but overlooked for many years. No symptoms or signs are specific for ET, but these patients can have hemorrhagic and thrombotic tendencies expressed as easy bruising for the former and microvascular occlusions for the latter, such as erythromelalgia, ocular migraine, or TIAs. Physical examination is generally unremarkable except occasionally for mild splenomegaly. Massive splenomegaly is more indicative of another myeloproliferative disorder, in particular PV, IMF, or CML.

Anemia is unusual, but a mild neutrophilic leukocytosis is not. The blood smear is most remarkable for the number of platelets present, some of which may be very large. The LAP score is either normal or elevated. The large mass of circulating platelets may prevent the accurate measurement of serum potassium due to release of platelet potassium upon blood clotting. This type of hyperkalemia is a laboratory artifact and not associated with electrocardiographic abnormalities. Similarly, arterial oxygen measurements can be inaccurate unless thrombocythemic blood is collected on ice. The prothrombin and partial thromboplastin times are normal, while abnormalities of platelet function such as a prolonged bleeding time and impaired platelet aggregation can be present. However, in spite of much study, no platelet function abnormalities are characteristic of ET, and no platelet function test predicts the risk of clinically significant bleeding or thrombosis.

The elevated platelet count may hinder marrow aspiration, but marrow biopsy usually reveals megakaryocyte hyperplasia and hypertrophy, as well as an overall increase in marrow cellularity. If marrow reticulin is increased, another diagnosis should be considered. The absence of stainable iron demands an explanation because iron deficiency alone can cause thrombocytosis, and absent marrow iron in the presence of marrow hypercellularity is a feature of PV.

Nonrandom cytogenetic abnormalities occur in ET but are uncommon, and no specific or consistent abnormality is notable, even those involving chromosomes 3 and 1, where the genes for thrombopoietin and its receptor Mpl, respectively, are located.

DIAGNOSIS

Thrombocytosis is encountered in a broad variety of clinical disorders (Table 103-5) in many of which production of cytokines is increased. The absolute level of the platelet count is not a useful diagnostic aid for distinguishing between benign and clonal causes of thrombocytosis. About 50% of ET patients express the JAK2 V617F mutation. When JAK2 V617F is absent, cytogenetic evaluation is mandatory to determine if the thrombocytosis is due to CML or a myelodysplastic disorder such as the 5q– syndrome. Because the bcr-abl translocation can be present in the absence of the Ph chromosome, and because bcr-abl RT-PCR is associated with false-positive results, fluorescence in situ hybridization (FISH) analysis for bcr-abl is the preferred assay in patients with thrombocytosis in whom a cytogenetic study for the Ph chromosome is negative. Anemia and ringed sideroblasts are not features of ET, but they are features of idiopathic refractory sideroblastic anemia, and in some of these patients the thrombocytosis occurs in association with JAK2 V617F expression. Massive splenomegaly should suggest the presence of another myeloproliferative disorder, and in this setting a red cell mass determination should be performed because splenomegaly can mask the presence of erythrocytosis. Importantly, what appears to be ET can evolve into PV or IMF after a period of many years, revealing the true nature of the underlying myeloproliferative disorder.

COMPLICATIONS

Perhaps no other condition in clinical medicine has caused otherwise astute physicians to intervene inappropriately more often than thrombocytosis, particularly if the platelet count is $>1 \times 10^6/\mu L$. It is commonly believed that a high platelet count causes intravascular stasis and thrombosis; however, no controlled clinical study has ever established this association, and in patients younger than age 60, the incidence of thrombosis was not greater in patients with thrombocytosis than in age-matched controls.

To the contrary, very high platelet counts are associated primarily with hemorrhage due to acquired von Willebrand disease. This is not meant to imply that an elevated platelet count cannot cause symptoms in a patient with ET, but rather that the focus should be on the patient, not the platelet count. For example, some of the most dramatic neurologic problems in ET are migraine-related and respond only to lowering of the platelet count, while other symptoms such as erythromelalgia respond simply to platelet cyclooxygenase 1 inhibitors such as aspirin or ibuprofen, without a reduction in platelet number. Still others may represent an interaction between an atherosclerotic vascular system and a high platelet count, and others may have no relationship to the platelet count whatsoever. Recognition that PV can present with thrombocytosis as well as the discovery of previously unrecognized causes of hypercoagulability (Chap. 111) make the older literature on the complications of thrombocytosis unreliable.

Rx ESSENTIAL THROMBOCYTOSIS

Survival of patients with ET is not different than for the general population. An elevated platelet count in an asymptomatic patient without cardiovascular risk factors requires no therapy. Indeed, before any therapy is initiated in a patient with thrombocytosis, the cause of symptoms must be clearly identified as due to the elevated platelet count. When the platelet count rises above $1 \times 10^6/\mu L$, a substantial quantity of high-molecular-weight von

Willebrand multimers are removed from the circulation and destroyed by the platelets, resulting in an acquired form of von Willebrand disease. This can be identified by a reduction in ristocetin cofactor activity. In this situation, aspirin could promote hemorrhage. Bleeding in this situation usually responds to ε-aminocaproic acid, which can be given prophylactically before and after elective surgery. Plateletpheresis is at best a temporary and inefficient remedy that is rarely required. Importantly, ET patients treated with ^{32}P or alkylating agents are at risk of developing acute leukemia without any proof of benefit; combining either therapy with hydroxyurea increases this risk. If platelet reduction is deemed necessary on the basis of symptoms refractory to salicylates alone, IFN-α, the quinazoline derivative, anagrelide, or hydroxyurea can be used to reduce the platelet count, but none of these is uniformly effective nor without significant side effects. Hydroxyurea and aspirin are more effective than anagrelide and aspirin for prevention of TIAs but not more effective for the prevention of other types of arterial thrombosis and actually less effective for venous thrombosis. Normalizing the platelet count does not prevent either arterial or venous thrombosis. Risk of gastrointestinal bleeding is also higher when aspirin is combined with anagrelide.

As more clinical experience is acquired, ET is more benign than previously thought. Evolution to acute leukemia is more likely to be a consequence of therapy than of the disease itself. In managing patients with thrombocytosis, the physician's first obligation is to do no harm.

FURTHER READINGS

Buss DH et al: The incidence of thrombotic and hemorrhagic disorders in association with extreme thrombocytosis: An analysis of 129 cases. Am J Hematol 20:365, 1985

Elliot MA et al: Thrombosis and hemorrhage in polycythemia vera and essential thrombocythaemia. Br J Haematol 128:275, 2005

Levine RL, Gilliland DG: JAK-2 mutations and their relevance to myeloproliferative disease. Curr Opin Hematol 14:43, 2007

Reilly JT: Idiopathic myelofibrosis: Pathogenesis to treatment. Hematol Oncol 24:56, 2006

Spivak JL: Polycythemia vera: Myths, mechanisms, and management. Blood 100:4272, 2002

Vainchenker W et al: A unique activating mutation in JAK2 (V617F) is at the origin of polycythemia vera and allows a new classification of myeloproliferative diseases. Hematology (Am Soc Hematol Educ Program):195, 2005

104 Acute and Chronic Myeloid Leukemia

Meir Wetzler, John C. Byrd, Clara D. Bloomfield

The myeloid leukemias are a heterogeneous group of diseases characterized by infiltration of the blood, bone marrow, and other tissues by neoplastic cells of the hematopoietic system. In 2006 the estimated number of new myeloid leukemia cases in the United States was 16,430. These leukemias comprise a spectrum of malignancies that, untreated, range from rapidly fatal to slowly growing. Based on their untreated course, the myeloid leukemias have traditionally been designated acute or chronic.

ACUTE MYELOID LEUKEMIA

INCIDENCE

The incidence of acute myeloid leukemia (AML) is ~3.7 per 100,000 people per year, and the age-adjusted incidence is higher in men than in women (4.6 versus 3.0). AML incidence increases with age; it is 1.9 in individuals <65 years and 18.6 in those >65. A significant increase in AML incidence has occurred over the past 10 years.

ETIOLOGY

Heredity, radiation, chemical and other occupational exposures, and drugs have been implicated in the development of AML. No direct evidence suggests a viral etiology.

Heredity Certain syndromes with somatic cell chromosome aneuploidy, such as trisomy 21 noted in Down syndrome, are associated with an increased incidence of AML. Inherited diseases with defective DNA repair, e.g., Fanconi anemia, Bloom syndrome, and ataxia telangiectasia, are also associated with AML. Congenital neutropenia (Kostmann syndrome) is a disease with mutations in the granulocyte colony-stimulating factor (G-CSF) receptor and, often, neutrophil elastase that may evolve into AML. Myeloproliferative syndromes may also evolve into AML (Chap. 103). Germ-line mutations of CCAAT/enhancer-binding protein α (C/EBP α), runt-related transcription factor 1 (RUNX1), and tumor protein p53 (TP53) have also been associated with a higher predisposition to AML in some series.

Radiation Survivors of the atomic bomb explosions in Japan had an increased incidence of myeloid leukemias that peaked 5–7 years after exposure. Therapeutic radiation alone seems to add little risk of AML but can increase the risk in people also exposed to alkylating agents.

Chemical and Other Exposures Exposure to benzene, a solvent used in the chemical, plastic, rubber, and pharmaceutical industries, is associated with an increased incidence of AML. Smoking and exposure to petroleum products, paint, embalming fluids, ethylene oxide, herbicides, and pesticides, have also been associated with an increased risk of AML.

Drugs Anticancer drugs are the leading cause of therapy-associated AML. Alkylating agent–associated leukemias occur on average 4–6 years after exposure, and affected individuals have aberrations in chromosomes 5 and 7. Topoisomerase II inhibitor–associated leukemias occur 1–3 years after exposure, and affected individuals often have aberrations involving chromosome 11q23. Chloramphenicol, phenylbutazone, and, less commonly, chloroquine and methoxypsoralen can result in bone marrow failure that may evolve into AML.

CLASSIFICATION

The World Health Organization (WHO) classification (Table 104-1) includes different biologically distinct groups based on immunophenotype, clinical features, and cytogenetic and molecular abnormalities in addition to morphology. In contrast to the previously used French-American-British (FAB) schema, the WHO classification places limited reliance on cytochemistry. Since much of the recent literature and some ongoing studies use the FAB classification, a description of this system is also provided in Table 104-1. A major difference between the WHO and FAB systems is the blast cutoff for a diagnosis of AML as opposed to myelodysplastic syndrome (MDS); it is 20% in the WHO classification and 30% in the FAB. AML with 20–30% blasts as defined by the WHO classification can benefit from approved therapies for MDS (such as decitabine or 5-azacytidine) that were approved in the past by the Food and Drug Administration (FDA) for marketing based on trials using the FAB criteria.

Importantly, the WHO schema is the first leukemia classification system to consider genetic along with morphologic features to define different subsets of AML.

Immunophenotype and Relevance to the WHO Classification The immunophenotype of human leukemia cells can be studied by multiparameter flow cytometry after the cells are labeled with monoclonal antibodies to cell-surface antigens. This can be important for separating AML from acute lymphoblastic leukemia (ALL) and identifying some types of AML. For example, AML that is minimally differentiat-

TABLE 104-1 ACUTE MYELOID LEUKEMIA (AML) CLASSIFICATION SYSTEMS

World Health Organization Classification[a]
I. AML with recurrent genetic abnormalities
AML with t(8;21)(q22;q22);*RUNX1/RUNX1T1*[b]
AML with abnormal bone marrow eosinophils [inv(16)(p13q22) or t(16;16)(p13;q22);*CBFB/MYH11*][b]
Acute promyelocytic leukemia [AML with t(15;17)(q22;q12) (*PML/RARA*) and variants][b]
AML with 11q23 (*MLL*) abnormalities
II. AML with multilineage dysplasia
Following a myelodysplastic syndrome or myelodysplastic syndrome/myeloproliferative disorder
Without antecedent myelodysplastic syndrome
III. AML and myelodysplastic syndromes, therapy-related
Alkylating agent–related
Topoisomerase type II inhibitor–related
Other types
IV. AML not otherwise categorized
AML minimally differentiated
AML without maturation
AML with maturation
Acute myelomonocytic leukemia
Acute monoblastic and monocytic leukemia
Acute erythroid leukemia
Acute megakaryoblastic leukemia
Acute basophilic leukemia
Acute panmyelosis with myelofibrosis
Myeloid sarcoma

French-American-British (FAB) Classification[c]	Incidence
M0: Minimally differentiated leukemia	5%
M1: Myeloblastic leukemia without maturation	20%
M2: Myeloblastic leukemia with maturation	30%
M3: Hypergranular promyelocytic leukemia	10%
M4: Myelomonocytic leukemia	20%
M4Eo: Variant: Increase in abnormal marrow eosinophils	
M5: Monocytic leukemia	10%
M6: Erythroleukemia (DiGuglielmo's disease)	4%
M7: Megakaryoblastic leukemia	1%

[a]ES Jaffe et al: *World Health Organization Classification of Tumours.* Lyon, IARC Press, 2001.
[b]Diagnosis is AML regardless of blast count.
[c]JM Bennett et al: Ann Intern Med 103:620, 1985.

ed (immature morphology and no lineage-specific cytochemical reactions) is diagnosed by flow-cytometric demonstration of the myeloid-specific antigens cluster designation (CD) 13 or 33. Similarly, acute megakaryoblastic leukemia can often be diagnosed only by expression of the platelet-specific antigens CD41 and/or CD61. While flow cytometry is useful, widely used, and, in some cases, essential for the diagnosis of AML, it is only supportive in establishing the different subtypes of AML through the WHO classification.

Clinical Features and Relevance to the WHO Classification The WHO classification considers clinical features in subdividing AML. For example, it identifies therapy-related AML as a separate entity and subclassifies this group based on the specific types of prior chemotherapy received. It also divides AML with multilineage dysplasia based upon the presence or absence of an antecedent MDS. These clinical features contribute to the prognosis of the specific type of AML.

Genetic Findings and Relevance to the WHO Classification The WHO classification is the first AML classification to incorporate genetic (chromosomal and molecular) information. Indeed, AML is first subclassified based on the presence or absence of specific recurrent genetic abnormalities. For example, AML FAB M3 is now designated *acute promyelocytic leukemia* (APL), based on the presence of either the t(15;17)(q22;q12) cytogenetic rearrangement or the *PML/RARα* product of the translocation. Thus, the WHO classification separates APL from all other types of AML as a first step and forces the clinician to correctly identify the entity and tailor treatment(s) accordingly.

CHROMOSOMAL ANALYSES Chromosomal analysis of the leukemic cell provides the most important pretreatment prognostic information in AML. Two cytogenetic abnormalities have been invariably associated with specific morphologic features: t(l5;17)(q22;q12) with APL and inv(16)(p13q22) with AML with abnormal bone marrow eosinophils. Many other chromosomal abnormalities have been associated primarily with one morphologic/immunophenotypic group, including t(8;21)(q22;q22) with slender Auer rods, expression of CD19, and abundance of normal eosinophils, and t(9;11)(p22;q23), as well as other translocations involving 11q23, with monocytic features. Many of the recurring chromosomal abnormalities in AML have been associated with specific clinical characteristics. More commonly associated with younger age are t(8;21) and t(l5;17); with older age, del(5q) and del(7q). Myeloid sarcomas (see below) are associated with t(8;21) and disseminated intravascular coagulation (DIC) with t(15;17).

Molecular Classification Molecular study of many recurring cytogenetic abnormalities has revealed genes that may be involved in leukemogenesis; this information is increasingly being incorporated into the WHO classification. For instance, the t(15;17) encodes a chimeric protein, promyelocytic leukemia (Pml)/retinoic acid receptor α (Rarα), which is formed by the fusion of the retinoic acid receptor α (*RARα*) gene from chromosome 17 and the promyelocytic leukemia (*PML*) gene from chromosome 15. The *RARα* gene encodes a member of the nuclear hormone receptor family of transcription factors. After binding retinoic acid, *RARα* can promote expression of a variety of genes. The 15;17 translocation juxtaposes *PML* with *RARα* in a head-to-tail configuration that is under the transcriptional control of *PML*. Three different breakpoints in the *PML* gene lead to various fusion proteins. The Pml-Rarα fusion protein tends to suppress gene transcription and blocks differentiation of the cells. Pharmacologic doses of the Rarα ligand, all-*trans*-retinoic acid (tretinoin), relieve the block and promote differentiation (see below). Similar examples exist with a variety of other balanced translocations and inversions, including the t(8;21), t(9;11), t(6;9), and inv(16).

Molecular aberrations are also being identified that are useful for classifying risk of relapse in patients without cytogenetic abnormalities. A partial tandem duplication (PTD) of the *MLL* gene is found in 5–10% of patients with normal cytogenetics and results in short remission duration. FMS-like tyrosine kinase 3 (Flt3) is a tyrosine kinase receptor important in the development of myeloid and lymphoid lineages. Activating mutations of the gene *FLT3* are present in ~30% of adult AML patients due to internal tandem duplications (ITDs) in the juxtamembrane domain or mutations of the activating loop of the kinase. These occur more commonly in patients with normal karyotype. Continuous activation of Flt3 and downstream target kinases, including signal transducer and activator of transcription protein 5, Ras/mitogen-activated protein kinase, and phosphatidylinositol 3-kinase/Akt, provides increased proliferation and antiapoptotic signals to the myeloid progenitor cell. Presence of *FLT3* ITD in patients with normal cytogenetics predicts for short remission duration and inferior survival. Other molecular prognostic factors in patients with normal karyotype AML include mutations of the nucleophosmin gene (*NPM1*) and *C/EBPα* that are associated with improved treatment outcome. In contrast, overexpression of genes such as brain and acute leukemia, cytoplasmic (*BAALC*) predicts for poor outcome. Gene expression profiles to predict outcome in normal karyotype AML patients are under active investigation.

CLINICAL PRESENTATION

Symptoms Patients with AML most often present with nonspecific symptoms that begin gradually or abruptly and are the consequence of anemia, leukocytosis, leukopenia or leukocyte dysfunction, or thrombocytopenia. Nearly half have had symptoms for ≤3 months before the leukemia was diagnosed.

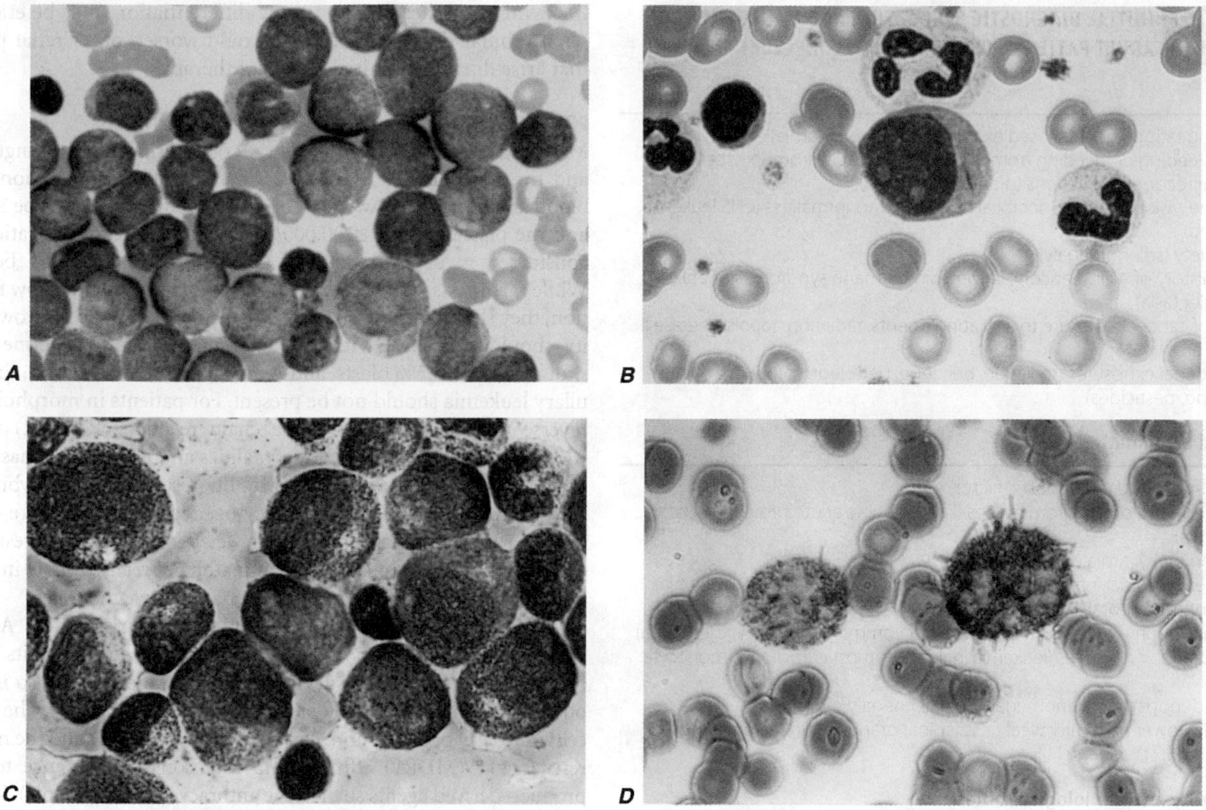

FIGURE 104-1 Morphology of AML cells. ***A.*** Uniform population of primitive myeloblasts with immature chromatin, nucleoli in some cells, and primary cytoplasmic granules. ***B.*** Leukemic myeloblast containing an Auer rod. ***C.*** Promyelocytic leukemia cells with prominent cytoplasmic primary granules. ***D.*** Peroxidase stain shows dark blue color characteristic of peroxidase in granules in AML.

Half mention fatigue as the first symptom, but most complain of fatigue or weakness at the time of diagnosis. Anorexia and weight loss are common. Fever with or without an identifiable infection is the initial symptom in ~10% of patients. Signs of abnormal hemostasis (bleeding, easy bruising) are noted first in 5% of patients. On occasion, bone pain, lymphadenopathy, nonspecific cough, headache, or diaphoresis is the presenting symptom.

Rarely patients may present with symptoms from a mass lesion located in the soft tissues, breast, uterus, ovary, cranial or spinal dura, gastrointestinal tract, lung, mediastinum, prostate, bone, or other organs. The mass lesion represents a tumor of leukemic cells and is called a *granulocytic sarcoma*, or *chloroma*. Typical AML may occur simultaneously, later, or not at all in these patients. This rare presentation is more common in patients with t(8;21).

Physical Findings Fever, splenomegaly, hepatomegaly, lymphadenopathy, sternal tenderness, and evidence of infection and hemorrhage are often found at diagnosis. Significant gastrointestinal bleeding, intrapulmonary hemorrhage, or intracranial hemorrhage occur most often in APL. Bleeding associated with coagulopathy may also occur in monocytic AML and with extreme degrees of leukocytosis or thrombocytopenia in other morphologic subtypes. Retinal hemorrhages are detected in 15% of patients. Infiltration of the gingivae, skin, soft tissues, or the meninges with leukemic blasts at diagnosis is characteristic of the monocytic subtypes and those with 11q23 chromosomal abnormalities.

Hematologic Findings Anemia is usually present at diagnosis and can be severe. The degree varies considerably, irrespective of other hematologic findings, splenomegaly, or duration of symptoms. The anemia is usually normocytic normochromic. Decreased erythropoiesis often results in a reduced reticulocyte count, and red blood cell (RBC) survival is decreased by accelerated destruction. Active blood loss also contributes to the anemia.

The median presenting leukocyte count is about 15,000/μL. Between 25 and 40% of patients have counts <5000/μL, and 20% have counts >100,000/μL. Fewer than 5% have no detectable leukemic cells in the blood. The morphology of the malignant cell varies in difference subsets. In AML the cytoplasm often contains primary (nonspecific) granules, and the nucleus shows fine, lacy chromatin with one or more nucleoli characteristic of immature cells. Abnormal rod-shaped granules called Auer rods are not uniformly present, but when they are, myeloid lineage is virtually certain (Fig 104-1). Poor neutrophil function may be noted by impaired phagocytosis and migration and morphologically by abnormal lobulation and deficient granulation.

Platelet counts <100,000/μL are found at diagnosis in ~75% of patients, and about 25% have counts <25,000/μL. Both morphologic and functional platelet abnormalities can be observed, including large and bizarre shapes with abnormal granulation and inability of platelets to aggregate or adhere normally to one another.

Pretreatment Evaluation Once the diagnosis of AML is suspected, a rapid evaluation and initiation of appropriate therapy should follow (Table 104-2). In addition to clarifying the subtype of leukemia, initial studies should evaluate the overall functional integrity of the major organ systems, including the cardiovascular, pulmonary, hepatic, and renal systems. Factors that have prognostic significance, either for achieving complete remission (CR) or for predicting the duration of CR, should also be assessed before initiating treatment. Leukemic cells should be obtained from all patients and cryopreserved for future use as new tests and therapeutics become available. All patients should be evaluated for infection.

Most patients are anemic and thrombocytopenic at presentation. Replacement of the appropriate blood components, if necessary, should begin promptly. Because qualitative platelet dysfunction or the presence of an infection may increase the likelihood of bleeding, evidence of hemorrhage justifies the immediate use of platelet transfusion, even if the platelet count is only moderately decreased.

TABLE 104-2 INITIAL DIAGNOSTIC EVALUATION AND MANAGEMENT OF ADULT PATIENTS WITH ACUTE MYELOID LEUKEMIA

History
Increasing fatigue or decreased exercise tolerance (anemia)
Excess bleeding or bleeding from unusual sites (DIC, thrombocytopenia)
Fevers or recurrent infections (granulocytopenia)
Headache, vision changes, nonfocal neurologic abnormalities (CNS leukemia or bleed)
Early satiety (splenomegaly)
Family history of AML (Fanconi, Bloom, or Kostmann syndromes or ataxia telangiectasia)
History of cancer (exposure to alkylating agents, radiation, topoisomerase II inhibitors)
Occupational exposures (radiation, benzene, petroleum products, paint, smoking, pesticides)
Physical Examination
Performance status (prognostic factor)
Ecchymosis and oozing from IV sites (DIC, possible acute promyelocytic leukemia)
Fever and tachycardia (signs of infection)
Papilledema, retinal infiltrates, cranial nerve abnormalities (CNS leukemia)
Poor dentition, dental abscesses
Gum hypertrophy (leukemic infiltration, most common in monocytic leukemia)
Skin infiltration or nodules (leukemia infiltration, most common in monocytic leukemia)
Lymphadenopathy, splenomegaly, hepatomegaly
Back pain, lower extremity weakness [spinal granulocytic sarcoma, most likely in t(8;21) patients]
Laboratory and Radiologic Studies
CBC with manual differential cell count
Chemistry tests (electrolytes, creatinine, BUN, calcium, phosphorus, uric acid, hepatic enzymes, bilirubin, LDH, amylase, lipase)
Clotting studies (prothrombin time, partial thromboplastin time, fibrinogen, D-dimer)
Viral serologies (CMV, HSV-1, varicella zoster)
RBC type and screen
HLA typing of patient, siblings, and parents for potential allogeneic SCT
Bone marrow aspirate and biopsy (morphology, cytogenetics, flow cytometry, molecular studies)
Cryopreservation of viable leukemia cells
Echocardiogram or heart scan
PA and lateral chest radiograph
Placement of central venous access device
Interventions for Specific Patients
Dental evaluation (for those with poor dentition)
Lumbar puncture (for those with symptoms of CNS involvement)
Screening spine MRI (for patients with back pain, lower extremity weakness, paresthesias)
Social work referral for patient and family psychosocial support
Counseling for All Patients
Provide patient with information regarding his/her disease, financial counseling, and support group contacts

Abbreviations: BUN, blood urea nitrogen; CBC, complete blood count; CMV, cytomegalovirus; CNS, central nervous system; DIC, disseminated intravascular coagulation; HLA, human leukocyte antigen; HSV, herpes simplex virus; LDH, lactate dehydrogenase; MRI, magnetic resonance imaging; PA, posteroanterior; RBC, red blood (cell) count; SCT, stem cell transplant.

About 50% of patients have a mild to moderate elevation of serum uric acid at presentation. Only 10% have marked elevations, but renal precipitation of uric acid and the nephropathy that may result is a serious but uncommon complication. The initiation of chemotherapy may aggravate hyperuricemia, and patients are usually started immediately on allopurinol and hydration at diagnosis. Rasburicase (recombinant uric oxidase) is also useful for treating uric acid nephropathy and often can normalize the serum uric acid level within hours with a single dose of treatment. The presence of high concentrations of lysozyme, a marker for monocytic differentiation, may be etiologic in renal tubular dysfunction, which could worsen other renal problems that arise during the initial phases of therapy.

PROGNOSTIC FACTORS

Many factors influence the likelihood of entering CR, the length of CR, and the curability of AML. CR is defined after examination of both blood and bone marrow. The blood neutrophil count must be ≥1000/μL and the platelet count ≥100,000/μL. Hemoglobin concentration is not considered in determining CR. Circulating blasts should be absent. While rare blasts may be detected in the blood during marrow regeneration, they should disappear on successive studies. Bone marrow cellularity should be >20% with trilineage maturation. The bone marrow should contain <5% blasts, and Auer rods should be absent. Extramedullary leukemia should not be present. For patients in morphologic CR, reverse transcriptase polymerase chain reaction (RT-PCR) to detect AML-associated molecular abnormalities and either metaphase cytogenetics or interphase cytogenetics by fluorescence in situ hybridization (FISH) to detect AML-associated cytogenetic aberrations are currently used to detect residual disease. Such detection of minimal residual disease may become a reliable discriminator between patients in CR who do or do not require additional and/or alternative therapies.

Age at diagnosis is among the most important risk factors. Advancing age is associated with a poorer prognosis, in part because of its influence on the patient's ability to survive induction therapy. Age also influences outcome because AML in older patients differs biologically. The leukemic cells in elderly patients more commonly express CD34 and the multidrug resistance 1 (MDR1) efflux pump that conveys resistance to natural product–derived agents such as the anthracyclines (see below). With each successive decade of age, a greater proportion of patients have more resistant disease. Chronic and intercurrent diseases impair tolerance to rigorous therapy; acute medical problems at diagnosis reduce the likelihood of survival. Performance status, independent of age, also influences ability to survive induction therapy and thus respond to treatment.

Chromosome findings at diagnosis are important independent prognostic factors. Patients with t(15;17) have a very good prognosis (approximately 85% cured), and those with t(8;21) and inv(16) a good prognosis (approximately 50% cured), while those with no cytogenetic abnormality have a moderately favorable outcome (approximately 40% cured). Patients with a complex karyotype, t(6;9), inv(3), or 7 have a very poor prognosis. This emphasizes the importance of cytogenetic as well as the previously discussed molecular assessment of the leukemia cells at diagnosis and relevance of storing samples for potential later use.

A prolonged symptomatic interval with cytopenias preceding diagnosis or a history of an antecedent hematologic disorder is another pretreatment clinical feature associated with a lower CR rate and shorter survival time. The CR rate is lower in patients who have had anemia, leukopenia, and/or thrombocytopenia for >3 months before the diagnosis of AML when compared to those without such a history. Responsiveness to chemotherapy declines as the duration of the antecedent disorder(s) increases. Secondary AML developing after treatment with cytotoxic agents for other malignancies is usually difficult to treat successfully.

A high presenting leukocyte count is an independent prognostic factor for attaining a CR. Among patients with hyperleukocytosis (>100,000/μL), early central nervous system bleeding and pulmonary leukostasis contribute to poor outcome with initial therapy.

In addition to pretreatment variables such as age, cytogenetics, and leukocyte count, several treatment factors correlate with prognosis in AML, including, most importantly, achievement of CR. In addition, patients who achieve CR after one induction cycle have longer CR durations than those requiring multiple cycles.

℞ ACUTE MYELOID LEUKEMIA

Treatment of the newly diagnosed patient with AML is usually divided into two phases, induction and postremission management **(Fig. 104-2)**. The initial goal is to quickly induce CR. Once CR is obtained, further therapy must

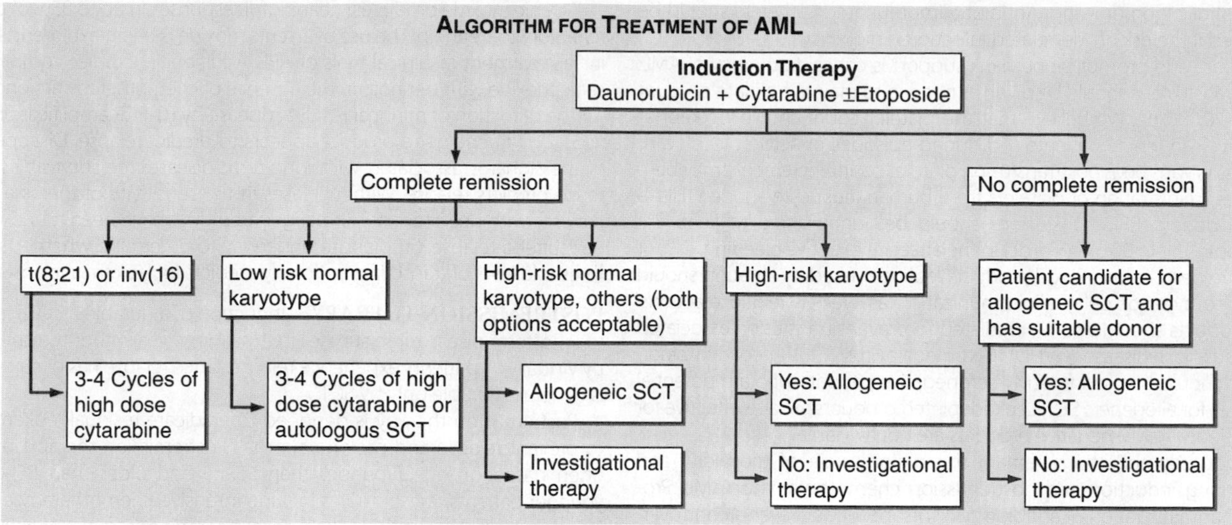

FIGURE 104-2 Flow chart for the therapy of newly diagnosed acute myeloid leukemia. For all forms of AML except acute promyelocytic leukemia (APL), standard therapy includes a 7-day continuous infusion of cytarabine (100–200 mg/m^2 per day) and a 3-day course of daunorubicin (45–60 mg/m^2 per day) or idarubicin (12–13 mg/m^2 per day) with or without 3 days of etoposide. Patients who achieve complete remission undergo postremission consolidation therapy, including sequential courses of high-dose cytarabine, autologous stem cell transplant (SCT), high-dose combination chemotherapy with allogeneic SCT, or novel therapies, based on their predicted risk of relapse (i.e., risk-stratified therapy). Patients with APL usually receive tretinoin together with anthracycline chemotherapy for remission induction and then consolidation chemotherapy (daunorubicin) followed by maintenance tretinoin, with or without chemotherapy. The role of cytarabine in APL induction and consolidation is controversial.

be used to prolong survival and achieve cure. The initial induction treatment and subsequent postremission therapy are often chosen based on the patient's age. The influence of intensifying therapy with traditional chemotherapy agents such as cytarabine and anthracyclines in younger patients (<60 years) appears to increase the cure rate of AML. In older patients the benefit of intensive therapy is controversial; novel therapies are being pursued.

INDUCTION CHEMOTHERAPY The most commonly used CR induction regimens (for patients other than those with APL) consist of combination chemotherapy with cytarabine and an anthracycline. Cytarabine is a cell cycle S-phase–specific antimetabolite that becomes phosphorylated intracellularly to an active triphosphate form that interferes with DNA synthesis. Anthracyclines are DNA intercalaters. Their primary mode of action is thought to be inhibition of topoisomerase II, leading to DNA breaks. Cytarabine is usually administered as a continuous intravenous infusion for 7 days. Anthracycline therapy generally consists of daunorubicin intravenously on days 1, 2, and 3 (the 7 and 3 regimen). Treatment with idarubicin for 3 days in conjunction with cytarabine by 7-day continuous infusion is at least as effective and may be superior to daunorubicin in younger patients. The addition of etoposide may improve the CR duration.

After induction chemotherapy, the bone marrow is examined to determine if the leukemia has been eliminated. If ≥5% blasts exist with ≥20% cellularity, the patient is usually re-treated with cytarabine and an anthracycline in doses similar to those given initially, but for 5 and 2 days, respectively. Our recommendation, however, is to change therapy in this setting. Patients who fail to attain CR after two induction courses should immediately proceed to an allogeneic stem cell transplant (SCT) if an appropriate donor exists. This approach is only applied to patients under the age of 70 with acceptable end-organ function.

With the 7 and 3 cytarabine/daunorubicin regimen outlined above, 65–75% of adults with de novo AML under the age of 60 years achieve CR. Two-thirds achieve CR after a single course of therapy, and one-third require two courses. About 50% of patients who do not achieve CR have a drug-resistant leukemia, and 50% do not achieve CR because of fatal complications of bone marrow aplasia or impaired recovery of normal stem cells. Higher induction treatment–related mortality and frequency of resistant disease have been observed with increasing age and in patients with prior hematologic disorders (MDS or myeloproliferative syndromes) or chemotherapy treatment for another malignancy.

High-dose cytarabine-based regimens have very high CR rates after a single cycle of therapy. When given in high doses, more cytarabine may enter the cells, saturate the cytarabine-inactivating enzymes, and increase the intracellular levels of 1-β-D-arabinofuranylcytosine-triphosphate, the active metabolite incorporated into DNA. Thus, higher doses of cytarabine may increase the inhibition of DNA synthesis and thereby overcome resistance to standard-dose cytarabine. In two randomized studies, high-dose cytarabine with an anthracycline produced CR rates similar to those achieved with standard 7 and 3 regimens. However, the CR duration was longer after high-dose cytarabine than after standard-dose cytarabine.

The hematologic toxicity of high-dose cytarabine-based induction regimens has typically been greater than that associated with 7 and 3 regimens. Toxicity with high-dose cytarabine includes myelosuppression, pulmonary toxicity, and significant and occasionally irreversible cerebellar toxicity. All patients treated with high-dose cytarabine must be closely monitored for cerebellar toxicity. Full cerebellar testing should be performed before each dose, and further high-dose cytarabine should be withheld if evidence of cerebellar toxicity develops. This toxicity occurs more commonly in patients with renal impairment and in those over age 60. The increased toxicity observed with high-dose cytarabine has limited the use of this therapy in elderly AML patients.

SUPPORTIVE CARE Measures geared to supporting patients through several weeks of granulocytopenia and thrombocytopenia are critical to the success of AML therapy. Patients with AML should be treated in centers expert in providing supportive measures.

Recombinant hematopoietic growth factors have been incorporated into clinical trials in AML. These trials have been designed to lower the infection rate after chemotherapy. Both G-CSF and granulocyte-macrophage colony-stimulating factor (GM-CSF) have reduced the median time to neutrophil recovery by an average of 5–7 days. This accelerated rate of neutrophil recovery, however, has not generally translated into significant reductions in infection rates or shortened hospitalizations. In most randomized studies, both G-CSF and GM-CSF have failed to improve the CR rate, disease-free survival, or overall survival. Although receptors for both G-CSF and GM-CSF are present on AML blasts, therapeutic efficacy is neither enhanced nor inhibited by these agents. The use of growth factors as supportive care for AML patients is controversial. We favor their use in elderly patients with complicated courses, those receiving intensive postremission regimens, patients with uncontrolled infections, or those participating in clinical trials.

Multilumen right atrial catheters should be inserted as soon as patients with newly diagnosed AML have been stabilized. They should be used thereafter for administration of intravenous medications and transfusions, as well as for blood drawing. Antibiotic-impregnated catheters should be considered if the risk of line-related infection is high.

Adequate and prompt blood bank support is critical to therapy of AML. Platelet transfusions should be given as needed to maintain a platelet count >10,000–20,000/μL. We believe that the platelet count should be kept at higher levels in febrile patients and during episodes of active bleeding or DIC. Patients with poor posttransfusion platelet count increments may benefit from administration of platelets from human leukocyte antigen (HLA)-matched donors. RBC transfusions should be administered to keep the hemoglobin level >80 g/L (8 g/dL) in the absence of active bleeding, DIC, or congestive heart failure. Blood products leukodepleted by filtration should be used to avert or delay alloimmunization as well as febrile reactions. Blood products should also be irradiated to prevent transfusion associated graft-versus-host disease (GVHD). Cytomegalovirus (CMV)-negative blood products should be used for CMV-seronegative patients who are potential candidates for allogeneic SCT. Leukodepleted products are also effective for these patients if CMV-negative products are not available.

Infectious complications remain the major cause of morbidity and death during induction and postremission chemotherapy for AML. Prophylactic administration of antibiotics in the absence of fever is controversial. Oral nystatin or clotrimazole is recommended to prevent localized candidiasis. For patients who are herpes simplex virus antibody titer–positive, acyclovir prophylaxis is effective in preventing reactivation of latent oral herpes infections.

Fever develops in most patients with AML, but infections are documented in only half of febrile patients. Early initiation of empirical broad-spectrum antibacterial and antifungal antibiotics has significantly reduced the number of patients dying of infectious complications (Chap. 82). An antibiotic regimen adequate to treat gram-negative organisms should be instituted at the onset of fever in a granulocytopenic patient after clinical evaluation, including a detailed physical examination with inspection of the indwelling catheter exit site and a perirectal examination, as well as procurement of cultures and radiographs aimed at documenting the source of fever. Specific antibiotic regimens should be based on antibiotic sensitivity data obtained from the institution at which the patient is being treated. Acceptable regimens include imipenem-cilastin; an antipseudomonal semisynthetic penicillin (e.g., piperacillin) combined with an aminoglycoside; a third-generation cephalosporin with antipseudomonal activity (i.e., ceftazidime or cefepime); or double β-lactam combinations (ceftazidime and piperacillin). Aminoglycosides should be avoided if possible in patients with renal insufficiency. For patients with known immediate-type hypersensitivity reactions to penicillin, aztreonam may be substituted for β-lactams. Aztreonam should be combined with an aminoglycoside or a quinolone antibiotic rather than used alone.

Empirical vancomycin is not given initially in the absence of suspected gram-positive infection or mucositis but should be initiated in neutropenic patients who remain febrile for 3 days; empirical systemic antifungal therapy is added at 7 days if fever persists. Voriconazole has been shown to be equivalent in efficacy and less toxic than amphotericin-B. Caspofungin or liposomal amphotericin are also considered for fungal infections not responsive to first-line therapy or when such therapy is not tolerated. Antibacterial and antifungal antibiotics should be continued until patients are no longer neutropenic, regardless of whether a specific source has been found for the fever.

TREATMENT OF PROMYELOCYTIC LEUKEMIA Tretinoin is an oral drug that induces the differentiation of leukemic cells bearing the t(15;17). APL is responsive to cytarabine and daunorubicin, but about 10% of patients treated with these drugs die from DIC induced by the release of granule components by dying tumor cells. Tretinoin does not produce DIC but produces another complication called the *retinoic acid syndrome*. Occurring within the first 3 weeks of treatment, it is characterized by fever, dyspnea, chest pain, pulmonary infiltrates, pleural and pericardial effusions, and hypoxia. The syndrome is related to adhesion of differentiated neoplastic cells to the pulmonary vasculature endothelium. Glucocorticoids, chemotherapy, and/or supportive measures can be effective for management of the retinoic acid syndrome. The mortality of this syndrome is about 10%.

Tretinoin (45 mg/m^2 per day orally until remission is documented) plus concurrent anthracycline chemotherapy appears to be among the safest and most effective treatments for APL. Unlike patients with other types of AML, patients with this subtype benefit from maintenance therapy with either tretinoin or chemotherapy.

Arsenic trioxide produces meaningful responses in up to 85% of patients refractory to tretinoin. The use of arsenic trioxide is being explored as part of initial treatment in clinical trials of APL. Additionally, studies combining arsenic trioxide with tretinoin in the absence of chemotherapy are ongoing.

The detection of minimal residual disease by RT-PCR amplification of the t(15;17) chimeric gene product appears to predict relapse. Disappearance of the signal is associated with long-term disease-free survival; its persistence predicts relapse. With increases in the sensitivity of the assay, some patients with persistent abnormal gene product have been found who do not suffer a relapse. Studies are underway to determine whether a critical threshold level of transcripts uniformly predicts for leukemia relapse.

POSTREMISSION THERAPY Induction of a durable first CR is critical to long-term disease-free survival in AML. However, without further therapy virtually all patients experience relapse. Once relapse has occurred, AML is generally curable only by SCT.

Postremission therapy is designed to eradicate residual leukemic cells to prevent relapse and prolong survival. Postremission therapy in AML is often based on age (younger than 55–65 and older than 55–65). For younger patients, most studies include intensive chemotherapy and allogeneic or autologous SCT. High-dose cytarabine is more effective than standard-dose cytarabine. The Cancer and Leukemia Group B (CALGB), for example, compared the duration of CR in patients randomly assigned post-remission to four cycles of high (3 g/m^2, every 12 h on days 1, 3, and 5), intermediate (400 mg/m^2 for 5 days by continuous infusion), or standard (100 mg/m^2 per day for 5 days by continuous infusion) doses of cytarabine. A dose-response effect for cytarabine in patients with AML who were ≤60 years was demonstrated. High-dose cytarabine significantly prolonged CR and increased the fraction cured in patients with favorable [t(8;21) and inv(16)] and normal cytogenetics, but it had no significant effect on patients with other abnormal karyotypes. For older patients, exploration of attenuated intensive therapy that includes either chemotherapy or reduced intensity allogeneic SCT has been pursued. Postremission therapy is a setting for introduction of new agents **(Table 104-3)**.

Allogeneic SCT is used in patients <70 years old with an HLA-compatible donor who have high-risk cytogenetics. In the subset with normal cytogenetics and high-risk molecular features such as *FLT3* ITD, allogeneic SCT is best applied in the context of clinical trials, as the impact of aggressive therapy on outcome is unknown. Relapse following allogeneic SCT occurs in only a small fraction of patients, but toxicity is relatively high from treatment; complications include venoocclusive disease, GVHD, and infections. Autologous transplantation can be administered in young and older patients and uses the same preparative regimens. Patients subsequently receive their own stem cells collected while in remission. The toxicity is lower with autologous SCT (5% mortality rate), but the relapse rate is higher than with allogeneic SCT, and randomized studies have not demonstrated outcome superior to postremission conventional-dose chemotherapy. The increased relapse rate is due to the absence of the graft-versus-leuke-

TABLE 104-3 SELECTED NEW AGENTS UNDER STUDY FOR TREATMENT OF ADULTS WITH AML

Class of Drugs	Example Agent(s)
MDR1 modulators	Cyclosporine, LY335979
Demethylating agents	Decitabine, 5-azacytidine, zebularine
Histone deacetylase inhibitors	Suberoylanilide hydroxamic acid (SAHA), MS275, LBH589, valproic acid
Heavy metals	Arsenic trioxide, antimony
Farnesyl transferase inhibitors	R115777, SCH66336
FLT3 inhibitors	SU11248, PKC412, MLN518, CHIR-258
HSP-90 antagonists	17-allylaminogeldanamycin (17-AAG) or derivatives
BCR-ABL PDGFR/KIT inhibitors	Imatinib (ST1571, Gleevec), dasatinib, nilotinib
Telomerase inhibitor	GRN163L
Cell cycle inhibitors	Flavopiridol, CYC202 (R-Roscovitine), SNS-032
Nucleoside analogues	Clofarabine, troxacitabine
Humanized antibodies	Anti-CD33 (SGN33), anti-DR4, anti-DR5, anti-KiR
Toxin-conjugated antibodies	Gemtuzumab ozogamicin (Mylotarg)
Radiolabeled antibodies	Yttrium-90-labeled human M195

mia (GVL) effect seen with allogeneic SCT and possible contamination of the autologous stem cells with tumor cells. Purging tumor from the autologous stem cells has not lowered the relapse rate with autologous SCT.

Randomized trials comparing intensive chemotherapy and autologous and allogeneic SCT have shown improved duration of remission with allogeneic SCT compared to autologous SCT or chemotherapy alone. However, overall survival is generally not different; the improved disease control with allogeneic SCT is erased by the increase in fatal toxicity. While stem cells were previously harvested from the bone marrow, virtually all efforts currently collect these from the blood following mobilization regimens, including growth factors with or without chemotherapy. Prognostic factors may help select patients in first CR for whom transplant is most effective.

Our approach includes considering allogeneic SCT in first CR for patients with high-risk karyotypes. Patients with normal karyotypes who have other poor risk factors (e.g., an antecedent hematologic disorder, failure to attain remission with a single induction course, PTD of the *MLL* gene, ITD of the *FLT3* gene, overexpression of *BAALC*) are also potential candidates. If a suitable HLA donor does not exist, novel therapeutic approaches are considered. Other novel transplant strategies, including reduced-intensity SCT, are being explored for consolidation of high-risk AML patients. Patients with t(8;21) and inv(16) are treated with repetitive doses of high-dose cytarabine, which offers a high frequency of cure without the morbidity of transplant. In AML patients with t(8;21) and inv(16), those with *KIT* mutations may be considered for novel investigational studies.

Autologous SCT is generally applied to AML patients only in the context of a clinical trial or when the risk of repetitive intensive chemotherapy represents a higher risk than the autologous SCT (e.g., in patients with severe platelet alloimmunization).

RELAPSE Once relapse occurs, patients are rarely cured with further standard-dose chemotherapy. Patients eligible for allogeneic SCT should receive transplants expeditiously at the first sign of relapse. Long-term disease-free survival is approximately the same (30–50%) with allogeneic SCT in first relapse or in second remission. Autologous SCT rescues about 20% of relapsed patients with AML who have chemosensitive disease. The most important factors predicting response at relapse are the length of the previous CR, whether initial CR was achieved with one or two courses of chemotherapy, and the type of postremission therapy.

Because of the poor outcome of patients in early first relapse (<12 months), it is justified (for patients without HLA-compatible donors) to explore innovative approaches, such as new drugs or immunotherapies (Table 104-3). Patients with longer first CR (>12 months) generally relapse with drug-sensitive disease and have a higher chance of attaining a CR. However, cure is uncommon, and treatment with novel approaches should be considered if SCT is not possible. One promising therapy is decitabine, a nucleoside analog that inhibits DNA methyltransferase and subsequently reverses aberrant methylation in AML cells. Interestingly, inhibiting DNA methyltransferase occurs at a much lower dose than previously used to produce a cytotoxic effect in AML. Low-dose decitabine yields CR in a small subset of patients with relapsed AML, including those with unfavorable karyotypes. New agents are needed.

For elderly patients (age >60) for whom clinical trials are not available, gemtuzumab ozogamicin (Mylotarg) is another alternative. This therapy is an antibody-targeted chemotherapy consisting of the humanized anti-CD33 antibody linked to calicheamicin, a potent antitumor antibiotic. The CR rate is ~30%. Its effectiveness in early relapsing (<6 months) or refractory AML patients is limited, possibly due to calicheamicin being a potent MDR1 substrate. Toxicity, including myelosuppression, infusion toxicity, and venoocclusive disease, can be observed with gemtuzumab ozogamicin. Pretreatment with glucocorticoids can diminish many of the infusion reactions associated with gemtuzumab ozogamicin. Studies are examining this treatment in combination with chemotherapy for both young and older patients with previously untreated AML.

CHRONIC MYELOGENOUS LEUKEMIA

INCIDENCE

The incidence of chronic myelogenous leukemia (CML) is 1.5 per 100,000 people per year, and the age-adjusted incidence is higher in men than in women (2.0 versus 1.2). The incidence of CML increases slowly with age until the middle forties, when it starts to rise rapidly. CML incidence for males decreased slightly (4.4%) between 1997 and 2003 as compared to 1977–1997.

DEFINITION

The diagnosis of CML is established by identifying a clonal expansion of a hematopoietic stem cell possessing a reciprocal translocation between chromosomes 9 and 22. This translocation results in the head-to-tail fusion of the breakpoint cluster region (*BCR*) gene on chromosome 22q11 with the *ABL* (named after the abelson murine leukemia virus) gene located on chromosome 9q34. Untreated, the disease is characterized by the inevitable transition from a chronic phase to an accelerated phase and on to blast crisis in a median time of 4 years.

ETIOLOGY

No clear correlation with exposure to cytotoxic drugs has been found, and no evidence suggests a viral etiology. In the pre-imatinib era, cigarette smoking accelerated the progression to blast crisis and therefore adversely affected survival in CML. Atomic bomb survivors had an increased incidence; the development of a CML cell mass of 10,000/μL took 6.3 years. No increase in CML incidence was found in the survivors of the Chernobyl accident, suggesting that only large doses of radiation can induce CML.

PATHOPHYSIOLOGY

The product of the fusion gene resulting from the t(9;22) plays a central role in the development of CML. This chimeric gene is transcribed into a hybrid *BCR/ABL* mRNA in which exon 1 of *ABL* is replaced by variable numbers of 5′ *BCR* exons. Bcr/Abl fusion proteins, $p210^{BCR/ABL}$, are produced that contain NH_2-terminal domains of Bcr and the COOH-terminal domains of Abl. A rare breakpoint, occurring within the 3′ region of the *BCR* gene, yields a fusion protein of 230 kDa, $p230^{BCR/ABL}$. Bcr/Abl fusion proteins can transform hematopoietic progenitor cells in vitro. Furthermore, reconstituting lethally irradiated mice with bone marrow cells infected with retrovirus carrying the gene encoding the $p210^{BCR/ABL}$ leads to the development of a myeloproliferative syndrome resembling CML in 50% of the mice. Specific antisense oligomers to the *BCR/ABL* junction inhibit the growth of t(9;22)-positive leukemic cells without affecting normal colony formation.

The mechanism(s) by which $p210^{BCR/ABL}$ promotes the transition from the benign state to the fully malignant one is still unclear. Messenger RNA for *BCR/ABL* can occasionally be detected in normal individuals. However, attachment of the *BCR* sequences to *ABL* results in three critical functional changes: (1) the Abl protein becomes constitutively active as a tyrosine kinase (TK) enzyme, activating downstream kinases that prevent apoptosis; (2) the DNA-protein-binding activity of Abl is attenuated; and (3) the binding of Abl to cytoskeletal actin microfilaments is enhanced.

Disease Progression The events associated with transition to the acute phase, a common occurrence in the pre-imatinib era, were extensively studied. Chromosomal instability of the malignant clone, resulting, for example, in the acquisition of an additional t(9;22), trisomy 8, or 17p- (p53 loss), is a basic feature of CML. Acquisition of these additional genetic and/or molecular abnormalities is critical to the phenotypic transformation. Large deletions adjacent to the translocation breakpoint on the derivative 9 chromosome, detected by microsatellite polymerase chain reaction (PCR) or FISH, are associated with shorter survival times. Heterogeneous structural alterations of the p53 gene, as well as structural alterations and lack of protein production of the retinoblastoma gene and the catalytic component of telomerase, have been associated with disease progression in a subset of patients. Rare patients show alterations in the rat sarcoma viral oncogene homolog (*RAS*). Sporadic reports also document the presence of an altered *MYC* (named after the myelocytomatosis virus) gene. Progressive de novo DNA methylation at the *BCR/ABL* locus and hypomethylation of the *LINE-1* retrotransposon promoter herald blastic transformation. Further, interleukin 1β may be involved in the progression of CML to the blastic phase. In addition, functional inactivation of the tumor suppressor protein phosphatase A2 may be required for blastic transformation. Finally, CML that develops resistance to imatinib is at an increased risk of progressing to accelerated/blast crisis. Multiple pathways to disease transformation exist, but the exact timing and relevance of each remain unclear.

CLINICAL PRESENTATION

Symptoms The clinical onset of the chronic phase is generally insidious. Accordingly, some patients are diagnosed while still asymptomatic, during health-screening tests; other patients present with fatigue, malaise, and weight loss or have symptoms resulting from splenic enlargement, such as early satiety and left upper quadrant pain or mass. Less common are features related to granulocyte or platelet dysfunction, such as infections, thrombosis, or bleeding. Occasionally, patients present with leukostatic manifestations due to severe leukocytosis or thrombosis such as vasoocclusive disease, cerebrovascular accidents, myocardial infarction, venous thrombosis, priapism, visual disturbances, and pulmonary insufficiency. Patients with $p230^{BCR/ABL}$-positive CML have a more indolent course.

Progression of CML is associated with worsening symptoms. Unexplained fever, significant weight loss, increasing dose requirement of the drugs controlling the disease, bone and joint pain, bleeding, thrombosis, and infections suggest transformation into accelerated or blastic phases. Fewer than 10–15% of newly diagnosed patients present with accelerated disease or with de novo blastic phase CML.

Physical Findings Minimal to moderate splenomegaly is the most common physical finding; mild hepatomegaly is found occasionally. Persistent splenomegaly despite continued therapy is a sign of disease acceleration. Lymphadenopathy and myeloid sarcomas are unusual except late in the course of the disease; when they are present, the prognosis is poor.

Hematologic Findings Elevated white blood cell counts (WBCs), with increases in both immature and mature granulocytes, are present at diagnosis. Usually <5% circulating blasts and <10% blasts and promyelocytes are noted with the majority of cells being myelocytes, metamyelocytes and band forms. Cycling of the counts may be observed in patients followed without treatment. Platelet counts are almost always elevated at diagnosis, and a mild degree of normocytic normochromic anemia is present. Leukocyte alkaline phosphatase is low in CML cells. Serum levels of vitamin B_{12} and vitamin B_{12}–binding proteins are elevated. Phagocytic functions are usually normal at diagnosis and remain normal during the chronic phase. Histamine production secondary to basophilia is increased in later stages, causing pruritus, diarrhea, and flushing.

At diagnosis, bone marrow cellularity is increased, with an increased myeloid to erythroid ratio. The marrow blast percentage is generally normal or slightly elevated. Marrow or blood basophilia, eosinophilia, and monocytosis may be present. While collagen fibrosis in the marrow is unusual at presentation, significant degrees of reticulin stain–measured fibrosis are noted in about half of the patients.

Disease acceleration is defined by the development of increasing degrees of anemia unaccounted for by bleeding or therapy; cytogenetic clonal evolution; or blood or marrow blasts between 10 and 20%, blood or marrow basophils ≥20%, or platelet count <100,000/μL. *Blast crisis* is defined as acute leukemia, with blood or marrow blasts ≥20%. Hyposegmented neutrophils may appear (Pelger-Huet anomaly). Blast cells can be classified as myeloid, lymphoid, erythroid, or undifferentiated, based on morphologic, cytochemical, and immunologic features. Occurrence of de novo blast crisis or following imatinib therapy is rare.

Chromosomal Findings The cytogenetic hallmark of CML, found in 90–95% of patients, is the t(9;22)(q34;q11.2). Originally, this was recognized by the presence of a shortened chromosome 22 (22q-), designated as the *Philadelphia chromosome*, that arises from the reciprocal t(9;22). Some patients may have complex translocations (designated as *variant translocations*) involving three, four, or five chromosomes (usually including chromosomes 9 and 22). However, the molecular consequences of these changes are similar to those resulting from the typical t(9;22). All patients should have evidence of the translocation molecularly or by cytogenetics or FISH to make a diagnosis of CML.

PROGNOSTIC FACTORS

The clinical outcome of patients with CML is variable. Before imatinib mesylate, death was expected in 10% of patients within 2 years and in about 20% yearly thereafter, and the median survival time was ~4 years. Therefore, several prognostic models that identify different risk groups in CML were developed. The most commonly used staging systems have been derived from multivariate analyses of prognostic factors. The *Sokal index* identified percentage of circulating blasts, spleen size, platelet count, age, and cytogenetic clonal evolution as the most important prognostic indicators. This system was developed based on chemotherapy-treated patients. The *Hasford system* was developed on interferon (IFN) α–treated patients. It identified percentage of circulating blasts, spleen size, platelet count, age, and percentage of eosinophils and basophils as the most important prognostic indicators. This system differs from the Sokal index by ignoring clonal evolution and incorporating percentage of eosinophils and basophils. When applied to a data set of 272 patients treated with IFN-α, the Hasford system was better than the Sokal score for predicting survival time; it identified more low-risk patients but left only a small number of cases in the high-risk group. Preliminary results suggest that both the Sokal and the Hasford systems are applicable to imatinib-treated patients.

℞ CHRONIC MYELOGENOUS LEUKEMIA

The therapy of CML is changing rapidly because we have a proven curative treatment (allogeneic transplantation) that has significant toxicity and a new targeted treatment (imatinib) with excellent outcome based on 5-year follow-up data. Therefore, physician experience and patient preference must be factored into the treatment selection process. Discussion of both treatment options with a patient is indicated. The decision should focus on the outcomes, risks, and toxicities of the various approaches.

At present, the goal of therapy in CML is to achieve prolonged, durable, nonneoplastic, nonclonal hematopoiesis, which entails the eradication of any residual cells containing the *BCR/ABL* transcript. Hence the goal is complete molecular remission and cure. A proposed imatinib treatment algorithm for the newly diagnosed CML patient is presented in **Table 104-4**.

TABLE 104-4 IMATINIB TREATMENT MILESTONES FOR NEWLY DIAGNOSED CML PATIENTS

		Proposed Course of Action[a]	
		Transplantation from an HLA-compatible (related or unrelated) donor, dasatinib, new drugs	Continue same[b] or increase dose[c]
Time, months	**Milestones**		
3	No complete hematologic remission	Complete hematologic remission[b,d]	
6	No cytogenetic remission	Any cytogenetic remission[c]	
12	Minor[e] or no cytogenetic remission	Complete[b,f] or partial[c,g] cytogenetic remission	
18	Partial, minor, or no cytogenetic remission	Complete cytogenetic remission[b]	
Anytime	Loss of previously achieved hematologic, cytogenetic, or molecular remission		

[a]Nutritional Comprehensive Cancer Network, Chronic myelogenous leukemia.
[b]Denotes that at the indicated milestones, patients should stay on the same dose.
[c]Denotes that at the indicated milestones, for patients on 400 mg/d, one can either continue the same or increase the dose to a maximum of 600–800 mg, as tolerated.
[d]Complete hematologic remission, WBC <10,000/μL, normal blood morphology, hemoglobin and platelet counts, and disappearance of splenomegaly.
[e]Minor cytogenetic remission, 36–85% bone marrow metaphases with t(9;22).
[f]Complete cytogenetic remission, no bone marrow metaphases with t(9;22).
[g]Partial cytogenetic remission, 1–35% bone marrow metaphases with t(9;22).
Abbreviations: HLA, human leukocyte antigen; WBC, white blood cell count.

ALLOGENEIC SCT Allogeneic SCT is complicated by early mortality owing to the transplant procedure. Outcome of SCT depends on multiple factors including: (1) the patient (e.g., age and phase of disease); (2) the type of donor [e.g., syngeneic (monozygotic twins) or HLA-compatible allogeneic, related or unrelated]; (3) the preparative regimen (myeloblative or reduced intensity); (4) GVHD; and (5) posttransplantation treatment.

The Patient Patients should have acceptable end-organ function, be <70 years, and have a healthy, histocompatible donor. Furthermore, survival after SCT in the accelerated and blastic phases of the disease is significantly diminished and is associated with high rates of relapse. Bone marrow transplantation (BMT) early in the chronic phase (1–2 years from diagnosis) is superior to later BMT. In the imatinib era, allogeneic transplantation should be used when possible for patients with accelerated/blastic phases of the disease or those whose disease fails to respond or progresses on imatinib.

The Donor Transplantation from a family donor, who is either fully matched or mismatched at only one HLA locus, should be considered for any patient with CML who is a candidate for an HLA-related sibling transplant. Syngeneic BMT in patients with chronic-phase CML results in 7-year disease-free survival in 55% of patients, with a 30% relapse rate. BMT with an HLA-identical sibling in the chronic phase achieves 5-year disease-free survival in 40–70% of patients, with a 25% relapse rate. BMT from an HLA-matched unrelated donor in chronic phase <1 year from diagnosis and <30 years of age results in 5-year disease-free survival similar to matched-sibling donor transplantation. For all other groups, patients receiving BMT from unrelated donors have higher rates of graft failure and acute and chronic GVHD and prolonged convalescence after treatment, compared to those who receive allogeneic transplants from related donors.

Sex mismatch has an adverse effect on transplantation, with worse outcome associated with a female donor and male recipient. This has been attributed to GVHD against the male histocompatibility Y antigen.

Peripheral blood is now being studied as a source of hematopoietic progenitor cells; it may offer rapid engraftment and less risk for the donor. With unrelated donors, some studies demonstrated no difference in GVHD and improved disease-free survival when comparing peripheral blood to bone marrow stem cells. Using matched sibling donors in chronic-phase CML, marrow stem cells led to a higher cumulative incidence of relapse at 3 years, while peripheral blood stem cell recipients had a higher cumulative incidence of chronic GVHD. At the current time, some centers collect bone marrow and some peripheral blood from sibling donors for newly diagnosed chronic-phase CML patients. Patients with more advanced stages are offered peripheral blood SCT. Umbilical-cord blood may permit mismatched SCT with notably less GVHD; GVL effects do not appear to be impaired. A problem with cord blood is obtaining a sufficient number of progenitor cells to reconstitute hematopoiesis in an adult.

Preparative Regimens Myeloablative regimens have been studied by several groups. Cyclophosphamide plus total-body irradiation is comparable to busulphan plus cyclophosphamide in the 3-year probabilities of survival, relapse, event-free survival, speed of engraftment, and incidence of venoocclusive disease of the liver. Significantly more patients in the total-body irradiation arm experienced major elevations of creatinine, acute GVHD, longer periods of fever, positive blood cultures, hospital admissions, and longer inpatient hospital stays. However, increased chronic GVHD, obstructive bronchiolitis, and alopecia were noted with busulphan. Measurement of busulphan levels revealed no significant association between busulphan levels and regimen-related toxicity, but low levels were associated with an increased risk of relapse. Intravenous busulphan allows better control of serum levels.

Reduced-intensity transplants in which the preparative regimen is aimed at eliminating host lymphocytes rather than bone marrow have been reported by numerous groups. No randomized trials comparing the two approaches have been published. Retrospective comparisons reveal that reduced-intensity conditioning regimens produce equivalent or acceptable results (in toxicity as well as outcome). Reduced toxicity with preserved antitumor efficacy is the goal, and therefore reduced-intensity transplantation is our recommendation.

Development and Type of GVHD Development of grade I GVHD (Chap. 108) decreases the risk of relapse compared to no GVHD. An even lower relapse rate was observed in patients with grade II GVHD but was accompanied by a substantially higher transplant-related mortality rate. The decreased relapse rate may be caused by a GVL effect. Depletion of T lymphocytes from donor marrow can prevent GVHD but results in an increased risk of relapse, which exceeds the relapse rate after syngeneic SCT. Thus, T lymphocytes from the donor marrow mediate a significant antileukemic or GVL effect, and even syngeneic marrow may exhibit limited GVL activity in CML.

Posttransplantation Treatment *BCR/ABL* transcript levels have served as early predictors for hematologic relapse following transplantation. These should facilitate risk-adapted approaches with immunosuppression or TK inhibitor(s), or a combination of the two. Donor leukocyte infusions (without any preparative chemotherapy or GVHD prophylaxis) can induce hematologic and cytogenetic remissions in patients with CML who have relapsed after allogeneic SCT.

Imatinib can control CML that has recurred after allogeneic SCT but is sometimes associated with myelosuppression and recurrence of severe GVHD. Imatinib after allogeneic SCT is being studied for prevention of relapse in patients with advanced disease at the time of transplantation (i.e., patients at high risk for relapse), patients undergoing reduced-intensity transplants, or patients with slow reduction of *BCR/ABL* message following transplantation. Imatinib has also been combined with donor lymphocytes to induce rapid molecular remissions in CML patients with disease relapse after allogeneic SCT. Of interest are studies with newer TK inhibitors following transplantation for imatinib-resistant CML.

IMATINIB MESYLATE Imatinib mesylate (Gleevec) functions through competitive inhibition at the ATP binding site of the Abl kinase in the inactive conformation, which leads to inhibition of tyrosine phosphorylation of proteins involved in Bcr/Abl signal transduction. It shows specificity for Bcr/Abl, the receptor for platelet-derived growth factor, and Kit tyrosine kinases. Imatinib induces apoptosis in cells expressing Bcr/Abl.

In newly diagnosed CML, imatinib (400 mg/d) is more effective than IFN-α and cytarabine. The complete hematologic remission rate, at 18 months, of patients treated with imatinib was 97% compared to 69% in patients treated with IFN-α and cytarabine. Similarly, the complete cytogenetic remission rate was 76% with imatinib compared to 14% with IFN-α and cytarabine.

All imatinib-treated patients who achieved major molecular remission (26%), defined as ≥3 log reduction in *BCR/ABL* transcript level at 18 months compared to pretreatment level, were progression-free at 5 years. The progression-free survival (PFS) at 5 years for patients achieving complete cytogenetic remission but less pronounced molecular remission is 98%. The 5-year PFS for patients not achieving complete cytogenetic remission at 18 months was 87%. These results have led to a consensus that molecular responses can be used as a treatment goal in CML. Specific milestones have been developed for chronic-phase CML patients (Table 104-4). For example, chronic-phase CML patients who do not achieve any cytogenetic remission following six months of imatinib are unlikely to achieve major molecular remission and should be offered other treatment approaches.

Progression to accelerated/blastic phases of the disease was noted in 3% of patients treated with imatinib as compared to 8.5% of patients treated with IFN-α and cytarabine during the first year. Over time, the annual incidence of disease progression on imatinib decreased gradually to <1% during the fourth and fifth years, and no patient who achieved complete cytogenetic remission during the first year of imatinib treatment progressed to the accelerated/blastic phases of the disease.

Imatinib is administered orally. The main side effects are fluid retention, nausea, muscle cramps, diarrhea, and skin rashes. The management of these side effects is usually supportive. Myelosuppression is the most common hematologic side effect. Myelosuppression, while rare, may require holding drug and/or growth factor support. Doses <300 mg/d seem ineffective and may lead to development of resistance.

Four mechanisms of resistance to imatinib have been described to date. These are (1) gene amplification, (2) mutations at the kinase site, (3) enhanced expression of multidrug exporter proteins, and (4) alternative signaling pathways functionally compensating for the imatinib-sensitive mechanisms. All four mechanisms are being targeted in clinical trials.

BCR/ABL gene amplification and decreased intracellular imatinib concentrations are addressed by intensifying the therapy with higher (up to 800 mg/d) imatinib doses. Response in some patients has led to early intensification of imatinib dosage in newly diagnosed CML patients, resulting in improved major molecular remissions when retrospectively compared to controls treated with 400 mg/d. Randomized studies comparing 400 mg/d doses to 800 mg/d in newly diagnosed CML patients are ongoing.

Mutations at the kinase domain are being targeted by novel TK inhibitors that have a different conformation than imatinib, demonstrating activity against most imatinib-resistant mutations. Nilotinib (Tasigma), like imatinib, binds to the kinase domain in the inactive conformation. Dasatinib (Sprycel) binds to the kinase domain in the open conformation and also inhibits the SRC (sarcoma) family of kinases, addressing the last mechanism of resistance. CML with the T315I mutation is resistant to imatinib, nilotinib, and dasatinib.

Dasatinib is approved by the FDA for the treatment of all stages of CML with resistance or intolerance to prior therapy, including imatinib. Nilotinib will likely follow suit. Both are oral agents given twice daily, with toxicity profiles similar to imatinib with small but significant differences. Dasatinib was shown to cause pleural effusion in 22% of patients with 7% developing grade 3-4 toxicity. Nilotinib was associated with sudden death in six of approximately 550 CML patients. A suspected relationship to nilotinib was reported in two of these cases.

These new agents have changed the treatment algorithm of CML. For example, patients who do not achieve any cytogenetic remission at six months on imatinib will now be offered either dasatinib or SCT. IFN-α, though FDA-approved for CML, will only be offered if all other options have failed.

The encouraging results with imatinib have led clinicians to offer it as first-line therapy for newly diagnosed CML patients, including those who otherwise would have benefited from transplant (e.g., young patients with a matched sibling donor). Prior exposure to imatinib does not affect transplant outcome. However, delaying BMT for high-risk patients (Sokal/Hasford criteria) may result in disease progression. SCT after disease progression is associated with poorer outcome. Therefore, we recommend close monitoring of imatinib response, especially in these patients (Table 104-4).

INTERFERON Before imatinib, when allogeneic SCT was not feasible, IFN-α therapy was the treatment of choice. Only longer follow-up of patients treated with imatinib will prove whether IFN-α will still have a role in the treatment of CML. Its mode(s) of action in CML is still unknown.

CHEMOTHERAPY Initial management of patients with chemotherapy is currently reserved for rapid lowering of WBCs, reduction of symptoms, and reversal of symptomatic splenomegaly. Hydroxyurea, a ribonucleotide reductase inhibitor, induces rapid disease control. The initial dose is 1–4 g/d; the dose should be halved with each 50% reduction of the leukocyte count. Unfortunately, cytogenetic remissions with hydroxyurea are uncommon. Busulphan, an alkylating agent that acts on early progenitor cells, has a more prolonged effect. However, we do not recommend its use because of its serious side effects, which include unexpected, and occasionally fatal, myelosuppression in 5–10% of patients; pulmonary, endocardial, and marrow fibrosis; and an Addison-like wasting syndrome.

AUTOLOGOUS SCT Autologous SCT could potentially cure CML if a means to select the residual normal progenitors, which coexist with their malignant counterparts, could be developed. As a source of autologous hematopoietic stem cells for transplantation, blood offers certain advantages over marrow (e.g., faster engraftment for the patient and no general anesthesia for the donor). Normal hematopoietic stem cells appear with increased frequency in the blood of patients with CML during the recovery phase after chemotherapy and G-CSF. A role for imatinib before stem cell collection to achieve minimal residual disease and following transplantation to maintain this status is currently being investigated. Specifically, several groups store peripheral blood stem cells from patients in major or complete molecular remissions. However, only a few cases have been transplanted following imatinib therapy. Therefore, such approaches should be performed only in clinical trials.

LEUKAPHERESIS AND SPLENECTOMY Intensive leukapheresis may control the blood counts in chronic-phase CML; however, it is expensive and cumbersome. It is useful in emergencies where leukostasis-related complications such as pulmonary failure or cerebrovascular accidents are likely. It may also have a role in the treatment of pregnant women in whom it is important to avoid potentially teratogenic drugs.

Splenectomy was used in CML in the past because of the suggestion that evolution to the acute phase might occur in the spleen. However, this does not appear to be the case, and splenectomy is now reserved for symptomatic relief of painful splenomegaly unresponsive to imatinib or chemotherapy, or for significant anemia or thrombocytopenia associated with hypersplenism. Splenic radiation is used rarely to reduce the size of the spleen.

MINIMAL RESIDUAL DISEASE The kinetics of *BCR/ABL* transcript elimination are currently replacing qualitative detection of the *BCR/ABL* message, in spite of a lack of standard acceptable methodology. A consensus panel has proposed ways to harmonize the different methods and to use a conversion factor so that individual laboratories will be able to express *BCR/ABL* transcript levels on an agreed upon scale.

Slow reduction of *BCR/ABL* transcripts following SCT correlates with the possibility of hematologic relapse. However, the definition of "slow reduction" depends on the preparative regimen (reduced-intensity versus fully myeloablative) and the selection of time-points to measure the transcript levels. While persistent RT-PCR positivity at 6 months was regarded as an indication for additional therapy in the past, current studies utilize periods between engraftment and day 100 for evaluating the clearance rate of *BCR/ABL* transcripts and recommending additional therapies. Large trials with longer follow-up are needed to establish consensus guidelines.

The randomized trial of imatinib versus IFN-α and cytarabine was the first to establish the concept of $\log_{10}$ reduction of *BCR/ABL* transcript from a standardized baseline for untreated patients. This measurement unit was developed instead of either the transcript numbers expressed per μg of leukocyte RNA or the ratio of *BCR/ABL* to a housekeeping gene on a log scale. In this randomized trial, patients who achieved ≥3 log reduction of BCR/ABL message had an extremely low probability of relapse, with a median follow-up of 60 months. It is unclear whether achieving complete molecular remission should still be the goal of treatment in this disease.

These studies also established the value and convenience of using peripheral blood instead of bone marrow testing as a means to assess disease status in patients who achieve complete cytogenetic responses. However, one still needs to consider following CML patients in complete cytogenetic remission and at least major molecular remission with annual cytogenetic bone marrow testing, as these patients are at risk of developing cytogenetic aberrations in t(9;22)-negative cells and secondary MDS/AML. These aberrations in the t(9;22)-negative cells are frequently transient, and their clinical significance is unclear. Such aberrations may occur in 7–10% of imatinib-treated patients. Development of MDS/AML is rare.

TREATMENT OF BLAST CRISIS Treatments for primary blast crisis, including imatinib, are generally ineffective. Only 52% of patients treated with imatinib achieved hematologic remission (21% complete hematologic remission), and the median overall survival was 6.6 months. Patients who achieve complete hematologic remission or whose disease returns to a second chronic phase should be considered for allogeneic SCT. Other approaches include induction chemotherapy tailored to the phenotype of the blast cell followed by imatinib, with or without additional chemotherapy and SCT. Blast crisis following initial therapy with imatinib carries a dismal prognosis even if treated with dasatinib or nilotinib.

FURTHER READINGS

AML

FROHLING S et al: Genetics of myeloid malignancies: Pathogenetic and clinical implications. J Clin Oncol 23:6285, 2005

NATIONAL COMPREHENSIVE CANCER NETWORK: Acute myeloid leukemia. Clinical Practice Guidelines in Oncology, Version 1. 2006. *http://www.nccn.org/professionals/physician_gls/PDF/aml.pdf*

SANZ MA et al: Tricks of the trade for the appropriate management of newly diagnosed acute promyelocytic leukemia. Blood 105:3019, 2005

TALLMAN MS et al: Drug therapy for acute myeloid leukemia. Blood 106:1154, 2005

CML

CORTES J, KANTARJIAN H: New targeted approaches in chronic myeloid leukemia. J Clin Oncol 23:6316, 2005

HUGHES TP et al: Monitoring CML patients responding to treatment with tyrosine kinase inhibitors. Review and recommendations for 'harmonizing' current methodology for detecting BCR-ABL transcripts and kinase domain mutations and for expressing results. Blood 108:28, 2006

NATIONAL COMPREHENSIVE CANCER NETWORK: Chronic myelogenous leukemia. Clinical Practice Guidelines in Oncology, Version 1. 2007. *http://www.nccn.org/professionals/physician_gls/PDF/cml.pdf*

105 Malignancies of Lymphoid Cells

Dan L. Longo

Malignancies of lymphoid cells range from the most indolent to the most aggressive human malignancies. These cancers arise from cells of the immune system at different stages of differentiation, resulting in a wide range of morphologic, immunologic, and clinical findings. Insights on the normal immune system have allowed a better understanding of these sometimes confusing disorders.

Some malignancies of lymphoid cells almost always present as leukemia (i.e., primary involvement of bone marrow and blood), while others almost always present as lymphomas (i.e., solid tumors of the immune system). However, other malignancies of lymphoid cells can present as either leukemia or lymphoma. In addition, the clinical pattern can change over the course of the illness. This change is more often seen in a patient who seems to have a lymphoma and then develops the manifestations of leukemia over the course of the illness.

BIOLOGY OF LYMPHOID MALIGNANCIES: CONCEPTS OF THE WHO CLASSIFICATION OF LYMPHOID MALIGNANCIES

The classification of lymphoid cancers evolved steadily throughout the twentieth century. The distinction between leukemia and lymphoma was made early, and separate classification systems were developed for each. Leukemias were first divided into acute and chronic subtypes based on average survival. Chronic leukemias were easily subdivided into those of lymphoid or myeloid origin based on morphologic characteristics. However, a spectrum of diseases that were formerly all called *chronic lymphoid leukemia* has become apparent (Table 105-1). The acute leukemias were usually malignancies of blast cells with few identifying characteristics. When cytochemical stains became available, it was possible to divide these objectively into myeloid malignancies and acute leukemias of lymphoid cells. Acute leukemias of lymphoid cells have been subdivided based on morphologic characteristics by the French-American-British (FAB) group (Table 105-2). Using this system, lymphoid malignancies of small uniform blasts (e.g., typical childhood acute lymphoblastic leukemia) were called L1, lymphoid malignancies with larger and more variable size cells were called L2, and lymphoid malignancies of uniform cells with basophilic and sometimes vacuolated cytoplasm were called L3 (e.g., typical Burkitt's lymphoma cells). Acute leukemias of lymphoid cells have also been subdivided based on immunologic (i.e., T cell vs. B cell) and cytogenetic abnormalities (Table 105-2). Major cytogenetic subgroups include the t(9;22) (e.g., Philadelphia chromosome–positive acute lymphoblastic leukemia) and the t(8;14) found in the L3 or Burkitt's leukemia.

Non-Hodgkin's lymphomas were separated from Hodgkin's disease by recognition of the Sternberg-Reed cells early in the twentieth century. The histologic classification for non-Hodgkin's lymphomas has been one of the most contentious issues in oncology. Imperfect morphologic systems were supplanted by imperfect immunologic systems, and poor reproducibility of diagnosis has hampered progress. In 1999, the World Health Organization (WHO) classification of lymphoid malignancies was devised through a process of consensus development among international leaders in hematopathology and clinical oncology. The WHO classification takes into account morphologic, clinical, immunologic, and genetic information and attempts to divide non-Hodgkin's lymphomas and other lymphoid malignancies into clinical/pathologic entities that have clinical and therapeutic relevance. This system is presented in Table 105-3. This system is clinically relevant and has a higher degree of diagnostic accuracy than those used previously. The possibilities for subdividing lymphoid malignancies are extensive. However, Table 105-3 presents in bold those malignancies that occur in at least 1% of patients. Specific lymphoma subtypes will be dealt with in more detail below. Lymphomas associated with HIV infection are discussed in Chap. 182.

TABLE 105-1 LYMPHOID DISORDERS THAT CAN PRESENT AS "CHRONIC LEUKEMIA" AND BE CONFUSED WITH TYPICAL B CELL CHRONIC LYMPHOID LEUKEMIA

Follicular lymphoma	Prolymphocytic leukemia (B cell or T cell)
Splenic marginal zone lymphoma	Lymphoplasmacytic lymphoma
Nodal marginal zone lymphoma	Sézary syndrome
Mantle cell lymphoma	Smoldering adult T cell leukemia/lymphoma
Hairy cell leukemia	

TABLE 105-2 CLASSIFICATION OF ACUTE LYMPHOID LEUKEMIA (ALL)

Immunologic Subtype	% of Cases	FAB Subtype	Cytogenetic Abnormalities
Pre-B ALL	75	L1, L2	t(9;22), t(4;11), t(1;19)
T cell ALL	20	L1, L2	14q11 or 7q34
B cell ALL	5	L3	t(8;14), t(8;22), t(2;8)

Note: FAB, French-American-British classification.

GENERAL ASPECTS OF LYMPHOID MALIGNANCIES

ETIOLOGY AND EPIDEMIOLOGY

The relative frequency of the various lymphoid malignancies is shown in Fig. 105-1. Chronic lymphoid leukemia (CLL) is the most prevalent form of leukemia in western countries. It occurs most frequently in older adults and is exceedingly rare in children. In 2007, 15,340 new cases were diagnosed in the United States, but because of the prolonged survival associated with this disorder, the total prevalence is many times higher. CLL is more common in men than in women and more common in whites than in blacks. This is an uncommon malignancy in Asia. The etiologic factors for typical CLL are unknown.

In contrast to CLL, acute lymphoid leukemias (ALLs) are predominantly cancers of children and young adults. The L3 or Burkitt's leukemia occurring in children in developing countries seems to be associated with infection by the Epstein-Barr virus (EBV) in infancy. However, the explanation for the etiology of more common subtypes of ALL is much less certain. Childhood ALL occurs more often in higher socioeconomic subgroups. Children with trisomy 21 (Down's syndrome) have an increased risk for childhood acute lymphoblastic leukemia as well as acute myeloid leukemia. Exposure to high-energy radiation in early childhood increases the risk of developing T cell acute lymphoblastic leukemia.

The etiology of ALL in adults is also uncertain. ALL is unusual in middle-aged adults but increases in incidence in the elderly. However, acute myeloid leukemia is still much more common in older patients. Environmental exposures including certain industrial exposures, exposure to agricultural chemicals, and smoking might increase the risk of developing ALL as an adult. ALL was diagnosed in 5200 persons and AML in 13,410 persons in the United States in 2007.

The preponderance of evidence suggests that Hodgkin's disease is of B cell origin. The incidence of Hodgkin's disease appears fairly stable, with 8190 new cases diagnosed in 2007 in the United States. Hodgkin's disease is more common in whites than in blacks and more common in males than in females. A bimodal distribution of age at diagnosis has been observed, with one peak incidence occurring in patients in their twenties and the other in those in their eighties. Some of the late age peak may be attributed to confusion among entities with similar appearance such as anaplastic large cell lymphoma and T cell–rich B cell lymphoma. Patients in the younger age groups diagnosed in the United States largely have the nodular sclerosing subtype of Hodgkin's disease. Elderly patients, patients infected with HIV, and patients in third world countries more commonly have mixed-cellularity Hodgkin's disease or lymphocyte-depleted Hodgkin's disease. Infection by HIV is a risk factor for developing Hodgkin's disease. In addition, an association between infection by EBV and Hodgkin's disease has been suggested. A monoclonal or oligoclonal proliferation of EBV-

TABLE 105-3 WHO CLASSIFICATION OF LYMPHOID MALIGNANCIES

B Cell	T Cell	Hodgkin's Disease
Precursor B cell neoplasm	Precursor T cell neoplasm	Nodular lymphocyte-predominant Hodgkin's disease
Precursor B lymphoblastic leukemia/lymphoma (precursor B cell acute lymphoblastic leukemia)	**Precursor T lymphoblastic lymphoma/leukemia (precursor T cell acute lymphoblastic leukemia)**	
Mature (peripheral) B cell neoplasms	Mature (peripheral) T cell neoplasms	Classical Hodgkin's disease
B cell chronic lymphocytic leukemia/small lymphocytic lymphoma	T cell prolymphocytic leukemia	Nodular sclerosis Hodgkin's disease
B cell prolymphocytic leukemia	T cell granular lymphocytic leukemia	Lymphocyte-rich classic Hodgkin's disease
Lymphoplasmacytic lymphoma	Aggressive NK cell leukemia	Mixed-cellularity Hodgkin's disease
Splenic marginal zone B cell lymphoma (± villous lymphocytes)	Adult T cell lymphoma/leukemia (HTLV-I+)	Lymphocyte-depletion Hodgkin's disease
Hairy cell leukemia	Extranodal NK/T cell lymphoma, nasal type	
Plasma cell myeloma/plasmacytoma	Enteropathy-type T cell lymphoma	
Extranodal marginal zone B cell lymphoma of MALT type	Hepatosplenic γδ T cell lymphoma	
Mantle cell lymphoma	Subcutaneous panniculitis-like T cell lymphoma	
Follicular lymphoma	**Mycosis fungoides/Sézary syndrome**	
Nodal marginal zone B cell lymphoma (± monocytoid B cells)	Anaplastic large cell lymphoma, primary cutaneous type	
Diffuse large B cell lymphoma	**Peripheral T cell lymphoma, not otherwise specified (NOS)**	
Burkitt's lymphoma/Burkitt cell leukemia	**Angioimmunoblastic T cell lymphoma**	
	Anaplastic large cell lymphoma, primary systemic type	

Note: HTLV, human T cell lymphotropic virus; MALT, mucosa-associated lymphoid tissue; NK, natural killer; WHO, World Health Organization.
Malignancies in bold occur in at least 1% of patients.
Source: Adapted from Harris et al.

infected cells in 20–40% of the patients with Hodgkin's disease has led to proposals for this virus having an etiologic role in Hodgkin's disease. However, the matter is not settled definitively.

For unknown reasons, non-Hodgkin's lymphomas increased in frequency in the United States at the rate of 4% per year between 1950 and the late 1990s. The rate of increase in the past few years seems to be decreasing. About 63,190 new cases of non-Hodgkin's lymphoma were diagnosed in the United States in 2007. Non-Hodgkin's lymphomas are more frequent in the elderly and more frequent in men. Patients with both primary and secondary immunodeficiency states are predisposed to developing non-Hodgkin's lymphomas. These include patients with HIV infection; patients who have undergone organ transplantation; and patients with inherited immune deficiencies, the sicca syndrome, and rheumatoid arthritis.

The incidence of non-Hodgkin's lymphomas and the patterns of expression of the various subtypes differ geographically. T cell lymphomas are more common in Asia than in western countries, while certain subtypes of B cell lymphomas such as follicular lymphoma are more common in western countries. A specific subtype of non-Hodgkin's lymphoma known as the angiocentric nasal T/natural killer (NK) cell lymphoma has a striking geographic occurrence, being most frequent in Southern Asia and parts of Latin America. Another subtype of non-Hodgkin's lymphoma associated with infection by human T cell lymphotropic virus (HTLV) I is seen particularly in southern Japan and the Caribbean (Chap. 181).

A number of environmental factors have been implicated in the occurrence of non-Hodgkin's lymphoma, including infectious agents, chemical exposures, and medical treatments. Several studies have demonstrated an association between exposure to agricultural chemicals and an increased incidence in non-Hodgkin's lymphoma. Patients treated for Hodgkin's disease can develop non-Hodgkin's lymphoma; it is unclear whether this is a consequence of the Hodgkin's disease or its treatment. However, a number of non-Hodgkin's lymphomas are associated with infectious agents (Table 105-4). HTLV-I infects T cells and leads directly to the development of adult T cell lymphoma (ATL) in a small percentage of infected patients. The cumulative lifetime risk of developing lymphoma in an infected patient is 2.5%. The virus is transmitted by infected lymphocytes ingested by nursing babies of infected mothers, blood-borne transmission, or sexually. The median age of patients with ATL is ~56 years, emphasizing the long latency. HTLV-I is also the cause of tropical spastic paraparesis—a neurologic disorder that occurs somewhat more frequently than lymphoma and with shorter latency and usually from transfusion-transmitted virus (Chap. 181).

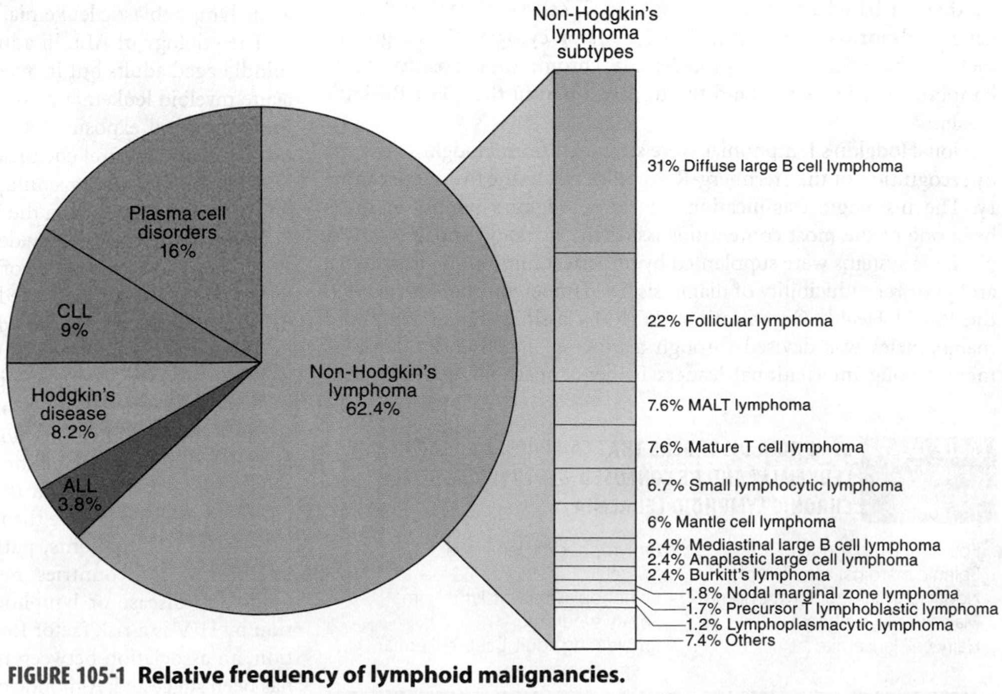

FIGURE 105-1 Relative frequency of lymphoid malignancies.

TABLE 105-4 INFECTIOUS AGENTS ASSOCIATED WITH THE DEVELOPMENT OF LYMPHOID MALIGNANCIES

Infectious Agent	Lymphoid Malignancy
Epstein-Barr virus	Burkitt's lymphoma
	Post–organ transplant lymphoma
	Primary CNS diffuse large B cell lymphoma
	Hodgkin's disease
	Extranodal NK/T cell lymphoma, nasal type
HTLV-I	Adult T cell leukemia/lymphoma
HIV	Diffuse large B cell lymphoma
	Burkitt's lymphoma
Hepatitis C virus	Lymphoplasmacytic lymphoma
Helicobacter pylori	Gastric MALT lymphoma
Human herpesvirus 8	Primary effusion lymphoma
	Multicentric Castleman's disease

Note: CNS, central nervous system; HTLV, human T cell lymphotropic virus; MALT, mucosa-associated lymphoid tissue; NK, natural killer.

TABLE 105-5 DISEASES OR EXPOSURES ASSOCIATED WITH INCREASED RISK OF DEVELOPMENT OF MALIGNANT LYMPHOMA

Inherited immunodeficiency disease	Autoimmune disease
Klinefelter's syndrome	Sjögren's syndrome
Chédiak-Higashi syndrome	Celiac sprue
Ataxia telangiectasia syndrome	Rheumatoid arthritis and systemic lupus erythematosus
Wiscott-Aldrich syndrome	Chemical or drug exposures
Common variable immunodeficiency disease	Phenytoin
Acquired immunodeficiency diseases	Dioxin, phenoxyherbicides
Iatrogenic immunosuppression	Radiation
HIV-1 infection	Prior chemotherapy and radiation therapy
Acquired hypogammaglobulinemia	

EBV is associated with the development of Burkitt's lymphoma in Central Africa and the occurrence of aggressive non-Hodgkin's lymphomas in immunosuppressed patients in western countries. The majority of primary central nervous system (CNS) lymphomas are associated with EBV. EBV infection is strongly associated with the occurrence of extranodal nasal T/NK cell lymphomas in Asia and South America. Infection with HIV predisposes to the development of aggressive, B cell non-Hodgkin's lymphoma. This may be through overexpression of interleukin 6 by infected macrophages. Infection of the stomach by the bacterium *Helicobacter pylori* induces the development of gastric MALT (mucosa-associated lymphoid tissue) lymphomas. This association is supported by evidence that patients treated with antibiotics to eradicate *H. pylori* have regression of their MALT lymphoma. The bacterium does not transform lymphocytes to produce the lymphoma; instead, a vigorous immune response is made to the bacterium, and the chronic antigenic stimulation leads to the neoplasia. MALT lymphomas of the skin may be related to *Borrelia* sp. infections, those of the eyes to *Chlamydophila psittaci*, and those of the small intestine to *Campylobacter jejuni*.

Chronic hepatitis C virus infection has been associated with the development of lymphoplasmacytic lymphoma. Human herpesvirus 8 is associated with primary effusion lymphoma in HIV-infected persons and multicentric Castleman's disease, a diffuse lymphadenopathy associated with systemic symptoms of fever, malaise, and weight loss.

In addition to infectious agents, a number of other diseases or exposures may predispose to developing lymphoma (Table 105-5).

IMMUNOLOGY

All lymphoid cells are derived from a common hematopoietic progenitor that gives rise to lymphoid, myeloid, erythroid, monocyte, and megakaryocyte lineages. Through the ordered and sequential activation of a series of transcription factors, the cell first becomes committed to the lymphoid lineage and then gives rise to B and T cells. About 75% of all lymphoid leukemias and 90% of all lymphomas are of B cell origin. A cell becomes committed to B cell development when it begins to rearrange its immunoglobulin genes. The sequence of cellular changes, including changes in cell-surface phenotype, that characterizes normal B cell development is shown in Fig. 105-2. A cell becomes committed to T cell differentiation upon migration to the thymus and rearrangement of T cell antigen receptor genes. The sequence of the events that characterize T cell development is depicted in Fig. 105-3.

Although lymphoid malignancies often retain the cell-surface phenotype of lymphoid cells at particular stages of differentiation, this information is of little consequence. The so-called stage of differentiation of a malignant lymphoma does not predict its natural history. For example, the clinically most aggressive lymphoid leukemia is Burkitt's

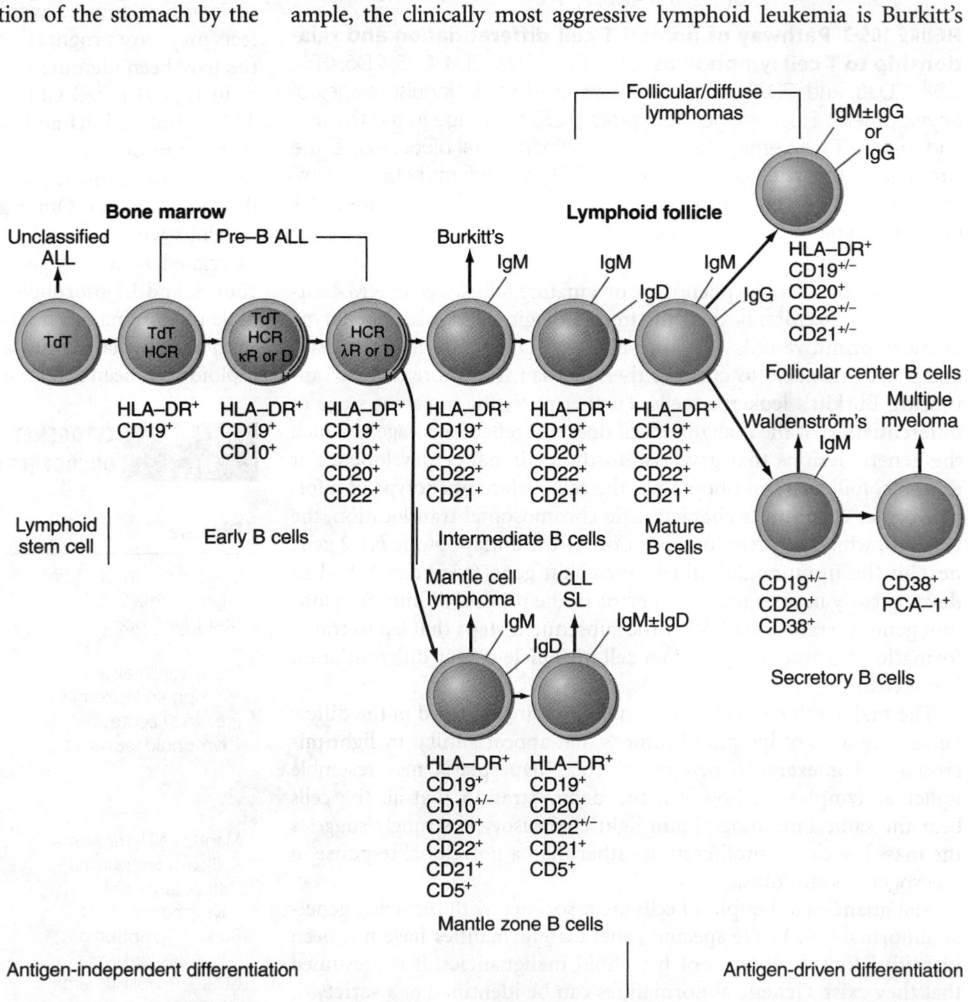

FIGURE 105-2 Pathway of normal B cell differentiation and relationship to B cell lymphomas. HLA-DR, CD10, CD19, CD20, CD21, CD22, CD5, and CD38 are cell markers used to distinguish stages of development. Terminal transferase (TdT) is a cellular enzyme. Immunoglobulin heavy chain gene rearrangement (HCR) and light chain gene rearrangement or deletion (κR or D, λR or D) occur early in B cell development. The approximate normal stage of differentiation associated with particular lymphomas is shown. ALL, acute lymphoid leukemia; CLL, chronic lymphoid leukemia; SL, small lymphocytic lymphoma.

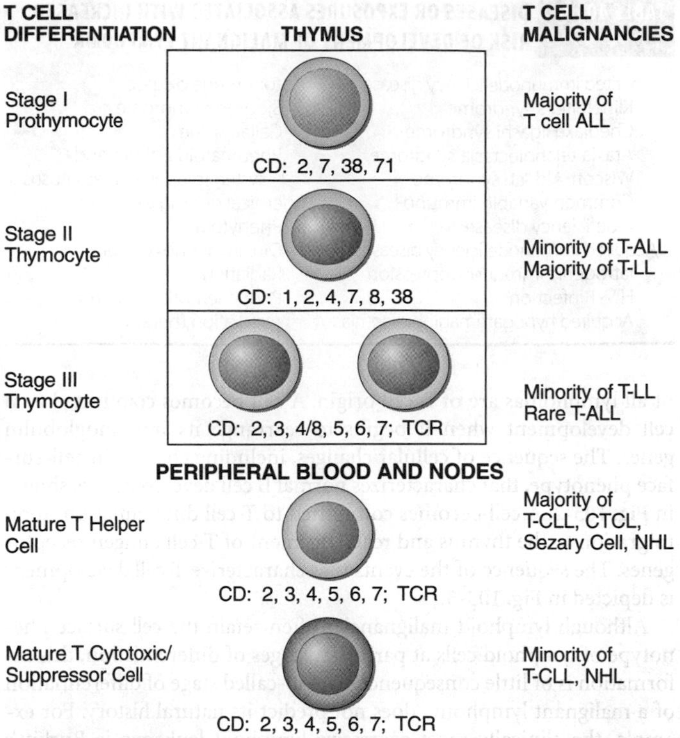

FIGURE 105-3 Pathway of normal T cell differentiation and relationship to T cell lymphomas. CD1, CD2, CD3, CD4, CD5, CD6, CD7, CD8, CD38, and CD71 are cell markers used to distinguish stages of development. T cell antigen receptors (TCR) rearrange in the thymus, and mature T cells emigrate to nodes and peripheral blood. ALL, acute lymphoid leukemia; T-ALL, T cell ALL; T-LL, T cell lymphoblastic lymphoma; T-CLL, T cell chronic lymphoid leukemia; CTCL, cutaneous T cell lymphoma; NHL, non-Hodgkin's lymphoma.

leukemia, which has the phenotype of a mature follicle center IgM-bearing B cell. Leukemias bearing the immunologic cell-surface phenotype of more primitive cells (e.g., pre-B ALL, CD10+) are less aggressive and more amenable to curative therapy than the "more mature" appearing Burkitt's leukemia cells. Furthermore, the apparent stage of differentiation of the malignant cell does not reflect the stage at which the genetic lesions that gave rise to the malignancy developed. For example, follicular lymphoma has the cell-surface phenotype of a follicle center cell, but its characteristic chromosomal translocation, the t(14;18), which involves juxtaposition of the antiapoptotic *bcl-2* gene next to the immunoglobulin heavy chain gene (see below), had to develop early in ontogeny as an error in the process of immunoglobulin gene rearrangement. Why the subsequent steps that led to transformation became manifest in a cell of follicle center differentiation is not clear.

The major value of cell-surface phenotyping is to aid in the differential diagnosis of lymphoid tumors that appear similar by light microscopy. For example, benign follicular hyperplasia may resemble follicular lymphoma; however, the demonstration that all the cells bear the same immunoglobulin light chain isotype strongly suggests the mass is a clonal proliferation rather than a polyclonal response to an exogenous stimulus.

Malignancies of lymphoid cells are associated with recurring genetic abnormalities. While specific genetic abnormalities have not been identified for all subtypes of lymphoid malignancies, it is presumed that they exist. Genetic abnormalities can be identified at a variety of levels including gross chromosomal changes (i.e., translocations, additions, or deletions); rearrangement of specific genes that may or may not be apparent from cytogenetic studies; and overexpression, underexpression, or mutation of specific oncogenes. Altered expression or mutation of specific proteins is particularly important. Many lymphomas contain balanced chromosomal translocations involving the antigen receptor genes; immunoglobulin genes on chromosomes 2, 14, and 22 in B cells; and T cell antigen receptor genes on chromosomes 7 and 14 in T cells. The rearrangement of chromosome segments to generate mature antigen receptors must create a site of vulnerability to aberrant recombination. B cells are even more susceptible to acquiring mutations during their maturation in germinal centers; the generation of antibody of higher affinity requires the introduction of mutations into the variable region genes in the germinal centers. Other nonimmunoglobulin genes, e.g., *bcl-6*, may acquire mutations as well.

In the case of diffuse large B cell lymphoma, the translocation t(14; 18) occurs in ~30% of patients and leads to overexpression of the *bcl-2* gene found on chromosome 18. Some other patients without the translocation also overexpress the BCL-2 protein. This protein is involved in suppressing apoptosis—i.e., the mechanism of cell death most often induced by cytotoxic chemotherapeutic agents. A higher relapse rate has been observed in patients whose tumors overexpress the BCL-2 protein, but not in those patients whose lymphoma cells show only the translocation. Thus, particular genetic mechanisms have clinical ramifications.

Table 105-6 presents the best documented translocations and associated oncogenes for various subtypes of lymphoid malignancies. In some cases, such as the association of the t(14;18) in follicular lymphoma, the t(2;5) in anaplastic large T/null cell lymphoma, the t(8;14) in Burkitt's lymphoma, and the t(11;14) in mantle cell lymphoma, the great majority of tumors in patients with these diagnoses display these abnormalities. In other types of lymphoma where a minority of the patients have tumors expressing specific genetic abnormalities, the defects may have prognostic significance. No specific genetic abnormalities have been identified in Hodgkin's disease other than aneuploidy.

In typical B cell CLL, trisomy 12 conveys a poorer prognosis. In ALL in both adults and children, genetic abnormalities have important prognostic significance. Patients whose tumor cells display the t(9;22) have a much poorer outlook than patients who do not have this translocation. Other genetic abnormalities that occur frequently in adults with ALL include the t(4;11) and the t(8;14). The t(4;11) is associated with younger age, female predominance, high white cell counts, and L1 morphology. The t(8;14) is associated with older age, male predominance, frequent CNS involvement, and L3 morphology. Both are associated with a poor prognosis. In childhood ALL, hyperdiploidy has been shown to have a favorable prognosis.

TABLE 105-6 CYTOGENETIC TRANSLOCATION AND ASSOCIATED ONCOGENES OFTEN SEEN IN LYMPHOID MALIGNANCIES

Disease	Cytogenetic Abnormality	Oncogene
CLL/small lymphocytic lymphoma	t(14;15)(q32;q13)	—
MALT lymphoma	t(11;18)(q21;q21)	API2/MALT, BCL-10
Precursor B cell acute lymphoid leukemia	t(9;22)(q34;q11) or variant t(4;11)(q21;q23)	BCR/ABL AF4, ALLI
Precursor acute lymphoid leukemia	t(9;22) t(1;19) t(17;19) t(5;14)	BCR, ABL E2A, PBX HLF, E2A HOX11L2, CTIP2
Mantle cell lymphoma	t(11;14)(q13;q32)	BCL-1, IgH
Follicular lymphoma	t(14;18)(q32;q21)	BCL-2, IgH
Diffuse large cell lymphoma	t(3;-)(q27;-)[a] t(17;-)(p13;-)	BCL-6 p53
Burkitt's lymphoma, Burkitt's leukemia	t(8;-)(q24;-)[a]	C-MYC
CD30+ Anaplastic large cell lymphoma	t(2;5)(p23;q35)	ALK
Lymphoplasmacytoid lymphoma	t(9;14)(p13;q32)	PAX5, IgH

[a]Numerous sites of translocation may be involved with these genes.

Note: CLL, chronic lymphoid leukemia; MALT, mucosa-associated lymphoid tissue; IgH, immunoglobulin heavy chain.

Gene profiling using array technology allows the simultaneous assessment of the expression of thousands of genes. This technology provides the possibility to identify new genes with pathologic importance in lymphomas, the identification of patterns of gene expression with diagnostic and/or prognostic significance, and the identification of new therapeutic targets. Recognition of patterns of gene expression is complicated and requires sophisticated mathematical techniques. Early successes using this technology in lymphoma include the identification of previously unrecognized subtypes of diffuse large B cell lymphoma whose gene expression patterns resemble either those of follicular center B cells or activated peripheral blood B cells. Patients whose lymphomas have a germinal center B cell pattern of gene expression have a considerably better prognosis than those whose lymphomas have a pattern resembling activated peripheral blood B cells. This improved prognosis is independent of other known prognostic factors. Similar information is being generated in follicular lymphoma and mantle cell lymphoma. The challenge remains to provide information from such techniques in a clinically useful time frame.

APPROACH TO THE PATIENT: Lymphoid Cell Malignancies

Regardless of the type of lymphoid malignancy, the initial evaluation of the patient should include performance of a careful history and physical examination. These will help confirm the diagnosis, identify those manifestations of the disease that might require prompt attention, and aid in the selection of further studies to optimally characterize the patient's status to allow the best choice of therapy. It is difficult to overemphasize the importance of a carefully done history and physical examination. They might provide observations that lead to reconsidering the diagnosis, provide hints at etiology, clarify the stage, and allow the physician to establish rapport with the patient that will make it possible to develop and carry out a therapeutic plan.

For patients with ALL, evaluation is usually completed after a complete blood count, chemistry studies reflecting major organ function, a bone marrow biopsy with genetic and immunologic studies, and a lumbar puncture. The latter is necessary to rule out occult CNS involvement. At this point, most patients would be ready to begin therapy. In ALL, prognosis is dependent upon the genetic characteristics of the tumor, the patient's age, the white cell count, and the patient's overall clinical status and major organ function.

In CLL, the patient evaluation should include a complete blood count, chemistry tests to measure major organ function, serum protein electrophoresis, and a bone marrow biopsy. However, some physicians believe that the diagnosis would not always require a bone marrow biopsy. Patients often have imaging studies of the chest and abdomen looking for pathologic lymphadenopathy. Patients with typical B cell CLL can be subdivided into three major prognostic groups. Those patients with only blood and bone marrow involvement by leukemia but no lymphadenopathy, organomegaly, or signs of bone marrow failure have the best prognosis. Those with lymphadenopathy and organomegaly have an intermediate prognosis, and patients with bone marrow failure, defined as hemoglobin <100 g/L (10 g/dL) or platelet count <100,000/μL, have the worst prognosis. The pathogenesis of the anemia or thrombocytopenia is important to discern. The prognosis is adversely affected when either or both of these abnormalities are due to progressive marrow infiltration and loss of productive marrow. However, either or both may be due to autoimmune phenomena or to hypersplenism that can develop during the course of the disease. These destructive mechanisms are usually completely reversible (glucocorticoids for autoimmune disease; splenectomy for hypersplenism) and do not influence disease prognosis.

Two popular staging systems have been developed to reflect these prognostic groupings (Table 105-7). Patients with typical B cell CLL can have their course complicated by immunologic abnormalities including autoimmune hemolytic anemia, autoimmune thrombocytopenia, and hypogammaglobulinemia. Patients with hypogammaglobulinemia benefit from regular (monthly) γ globulin administration. Because of expense, γ globulin is often withheld until the patient experiences a significant infection. These abnormalities do not have a clear prognostic significance and should not be used to assign a higher stage.

Two other features may be used to assess prognosis in B cell CLL, but neither has yet been incorporated into a staging classification. At least two subsets of CLL have been identified based on the cytoplasmic expression of ZAP-70; expression of this protein, which is usually expressed in T cells, identifies a subgroup with poorer prognosis. A less powerful subsetting tool is CD38 expression. CD38+ tumors tend to have a poorer prognosis than CD38– tumors.

The initial evaluation of a patient with Hodgkin's disease or non-Hodgkin's lymphoma is similar. In both situations, the determination of an accurate anatomic stage is an important part of the evaluation. The staging system is the Ann Arbor staging system originally developed for Hodgkin's disease (Table 105-8).

TABLE 105-7 STAGING OF TYPICAL B CELL LYMPHOID LEUKEMIA

Stage	Clinical Features	Median Survival, Years
RAI System		
0: Low risk	Lymphocytosis only in blood and marrow	>10
I: Intermediate risk	Lymphocytosis + lymphadenopathy + splenomegaly ± hepatomegaly	7
II		
III: High risk	Lymphocytosis + anemia	1.5
IV	Lymphocytosis + thrombocytopenia	
Binet System		
A	Fewer than three areas of clinical lymphadenopathy; no anemia or thrombocytopenia	>10
B	Three or more involved node areas; no anemia or thrombocytopenia	7
C	Hemoglobin ≤10 g/dL and/or platelets <100,000/μL	2

TABLE 105-8 THE ANN ARBOR STAGING SYSTEM FOR HODGKIN'S DISEASE

Stage	Definition
I	Involvement of a single lymph node region or lymphoid structure (e.g., spleen, thymus, Waldeyer's ring)
II	Involvement of two or more lymph node regions on the same side of the diaphragm (the mediastinum is a single site; hilar lymph nodes should be considered "lateralized" and, when involved on both sides, constitute stage II disease)
III	Involvement of lymph node regions or lymphoid structures on both sides of the diaphragm
III_1	Subdiaphragmatic involvement limited to spleen, splenic hilar nodes, celiac nodes, or portal nodes
III_2	Subdiaphragmatic involvement includes paraaortic, iliac, or mesenteric nodes plus structures in III_1
IV	Involvement of extranodal site(s) beyond that designated as "E" More than one extranodal deposit at any location Any involvement of liver or bone marrow
A	No symptoms
B	Unexplained weight loss of >10% of the body weight during the 6 months before staging investigation Unexplained, persistent, or recurrent fever with temperatures >38°C during the previous month Recurrent drenching night sweats during the previous month
E	Localized, solitary involvement of extralymphatic tissue, excluding liver and bone marrow

TABLE 105-9 INTERNATIONAL PROGNOSTIC INDEX FOR NHL

Five clinical risk factors:	
Age ≥ 60 years	
Serum lactate dehydrogenase levels elevated	
Performance status ≥2 (ECOG) or ≤ 70 (Karnofsky)	
Ann Arbor stage III or IV	
>1 site of extranodal involvement	
Patients are assigned a number for each risk factor they have	
Patients are grouped differently based upon the type of lymphoma	
For diffuse large B cell lymphoma:	
0, 1 factor = low risk:	35% of cases; 5-year survival, 73%
2 factors = low-intermediate risk:	27% of cases; 5-year survival, 51%
3 factors = high-intermediate risk:	22% of cases; 5-year survival, 43%
4, 5 factors = high risk:	16% of cases; 5-year survival, 26%
For diffuse large B cell lymphoma treated with R-CHOP:	
0 factor = very good:	10% of cases; 5-year survival, 94%
1, 2 factors = good:	45% of cases; 5-year survival, 79%
3, 4, 5 factors = poor:	45% of cases; 5-year survival, 55%

Evaluation of patients with Hodgkin's disease will typically include a complete blood count; erythrocyte sedimentation rate; chemistry studies reflecting major organ function; CT scans of the chest, abdomen, and pelvis; and a bone marrow biopsy. Neither a positron emission tomography (PET) scan nor a gallium scan is absolutely necessary for primary staging, but one performed at the completion of therapy allows evaluation of persisting radiographic abnormalities, particularly the mediastinum. Knowing that the PET scan or gallium scan is abnormal before treatment can help in this assessment. In most cases, these studies will allow assignment of anatomic stage and the development of a therapeutic plan.

In patients with non-Hodgkin's lymphoma, the same evaluation described for patients with Hodgkin's disease is usually carried out. In addition, serum levels of lactate dehydrogenase (LDH) and β_2-microglobulin and serum protein electrophoresis are often included in the evaluation. Anatomic stage is assigned in the same manner as used for Hodgkin's disease. However, the prognosis of patients with non-Hodgkin's lymphoma is best assigned using the International Prognostic Index (IPI) (Table 105-9). This is a powerful predictor of outcome in all subtypes of non-Hodgkin's lymphoma. Patients are assigned an IPI score based on the presence or absence of five adverse prognostic factors and may have none or all five of these adverse prognostic factors. Figure 105-4 shows the prognostic significance of this score in 1300 patients with all types of non-Hodgkin's lymphoma. With the addition of rituximab to CHOP, treatment outcomes have improved and the original IPI has lost some of its discrimination power. A revised IPI has been proposed that better predicts outcome of rituximab plus chemotherapy-based programs (Table 105-9). CT scans are routinely used in the evaluation of patients with all subtypes of non-Hodgkin's lymphoma, but PET and gallium scans are much more useful in aggressive

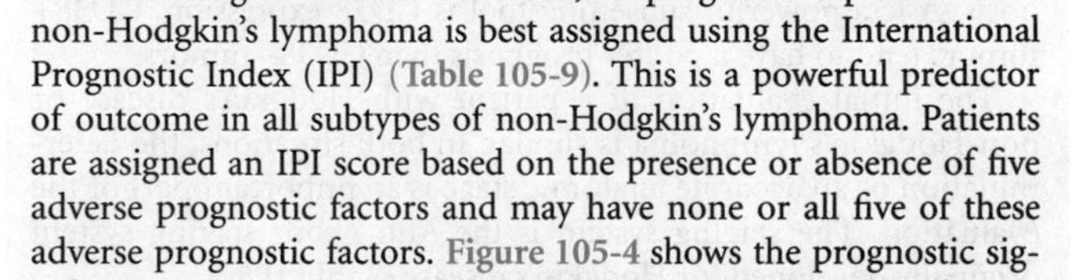

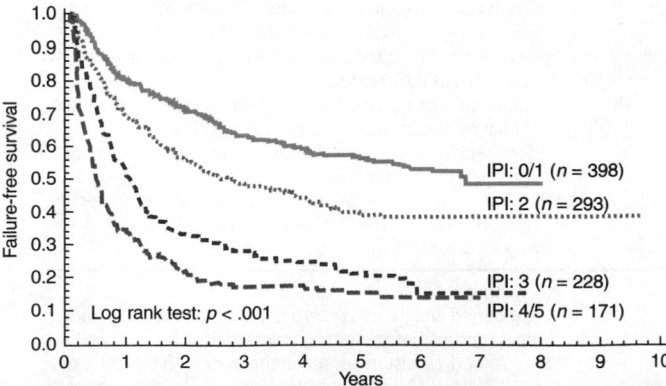

FIGURE 105-4 Relationship of International Prognostic Index (IPI) to survival. Kaplan-Meier survival curves for 1300 patients with various kinds of lymphoma stratified according to the IPI.

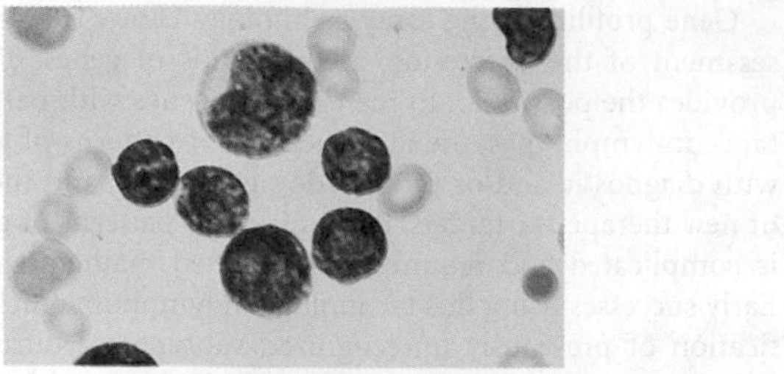

FIGURE 105-5 Acute lymphoblastic leukemia. The cells are heterogeneous in size, have round or convoluted nuclei, high nuclear/cytoplasmic ratio, and absence of cytoplasmic granules.

subtypes such as diffuse large B cell lymphoma than in more indolent subtypes such a follicular lymphoma or small lymphocytic lymphoma. While the IPI does divide patients with follicular lymphoma into subsets with distinct prognoses, the distribution of such patients is skewed toward lower-risk categories. A follicular lymphoma–specific IPI (FLIPI) has been proposed that replaces performance status with hemoglobin level [<120 g/L (<12 g/dL)] and number of extranodal sites with number of nodal sites (more than four). Low risk (zero or one factor) was assigned to 36% of patients, intermediate risk (two factors) to 37%, and poor risk (more than two factors) to 27% of patients.

CLINICAL FEATURES, TREATMENT, AND PROGNOSIS OF SPECIFIC LYMPHOID MALIGNANCIES

PRECURSOR CELL B CELL NEOPLASMS

Precursor B Cell Lymphoblastic Leukemia/Lymphoma The most common cancer in childhood is B cell ALL. Although this disorder can also present as a lymphoma in either adults or children, presentation as lymphoma is rare.

The malignant cells in patients with precursor B cell lymphoblastic leukemia are most commonly of pre-B cell origin. Patients typically present with signs of bone marrow failure such as pallor, fatigue, bleeding, fever, and infection related to peripheral blood cytopenias. Peripheral blood counts regularly show anemia and thrombocytopenia but might show leukopenia, a normal leukocyte count, or leukocytosis based largely on the number of circulating malignant cells (Fig. 105-5). Extramedullary sites of disease are frequently involved in patients who present with leukemia, including lymphadenopathy, hepato- or splenomegaly, CNS disease, testicular enlargement, and/or cutaneous infiltration.

The diagnosis is usually made by bone marrow biopsy, which shows infiltration by malignant lymphoblasts. Demonstration of a pre-B cell immunophenotype (Fig. 105-2) and, often, characteristic cytogenetic abnormalities (Table 105-6) confirm the diagnosis. An adverse prognosis in patients with precursor B cell ALL is predicted by a very high white cell count, the presence of symptomatic CNS disease, and unfavorable cytogenetic abnormalities. For example, t(9;22), frequently found in adults with B cell ALL, has been associated with a very poor outlook. The bcr/abl kinase inhibitors have improved the prognosis.

℞ PRECURSOR B CELL LYMPHOBLASTIC LEUKEMIA

The treatment of patients with precursor B cell ALL involves remission induction with combination chemotherapy, a consolidation phase that includes administration of high-dose systemic therapy and treatment to eliminate disease in the CNS, and a period of continuing therapy to prevent relapse and effect cure. The overall cure rate in children is 90%, while ~50% of adults are long-term disease-free survivors. This reflects the high proportion of adverse cytogenetic abnormalities seen in adults with precursor B cell ALL.

Precursor B cell lymphoblastic lymphoma is a rare presentation of precursor B cell lymphoblastic malignancy. These patients often have a rapid transformation to leukemia and should be treated as though they had presented with leukemia. The few patients who present with the disease confined to lymph nodes have a high cure rate.

TABLE 105-10 CLINICAL CHARACTERISTICS OF PATIENTS WITH COMMON TYPES OF NON-HODGKIN'S LYMPHOMAS (NHL)

Disease	Median Age, years	Frequency in Children	% Male	Stage I/II vs III/IV, %	B Symptoms, %	Bone Marrow Involvement, %	Gastrointestinal Tract Involvement, %	% Surviving 5 years
B cell chronic lymphocytic leukemia/small lymphocytic lymphoma	65	Rare	53	9 vs 91	33	72	3	51
Mantle cell lymphoma	63	Rare	74	20 vs 80	28	64	9	27
Extranodal marginal zone B cell lymphoma of MALT type	60	Rare	48	67 vs 33	19	14	50	74
Follicular lymphoma	59	Rare	42	33 vs 67	28	42	4	72
Diffuse large B cell lymphoma	64	~25% of childhood NHL	55	54 vs 46	33	16	18	46
Burkitt's lymphoma	31	~30% of childhood NHL	89	62 vs 38	22	33	11	45
Precursor T cell lymphoblastic lymphoma	28	~40% of childhood NHL	64	11 vs 89	21	50	4	26
Anaplastic large T/null cell lymphoma	34	Common	69	51 vs 49	53	13	9	77
Peripheral T cell non-Hodgkin's lymphoma	61	~5% of childhood NHL	55	20 vs 80	50	36	15	25

Note: MALT, mucosa-associated lymphoid tissue.

MATURE (PERIPHERAL) B CELL NEOPLASMS

B Cell Chronic Lymphoid Leukemia/Small Lymphocytic Lymphoma B cell CLL/small lymphocytic lymphoma represents the most common lymphoid leukemia, and when presenting as a lymphoma, it accounts for ~7% of non-Hodgkin's lymphomas. Presentation can be as either leukemia or lymphoma. The major clinical characteristics of B cell CLL/small lymphocytic lymphoma are presented in Table 105-10.

The diagnosis of typical B cell CLL is made when an increased number of circulating lymphocytes (i.e., $>4 \times 10^9$/L and usually $>10 \times 10^9$/L) is found (Fig. 105-6) that are monoclonal B cells expressing the CD5 antigen. Finding bone marrow infiltration by the same cells confirms the diagnosis. The peripheral blood smear in such patients typically shows many "smudge" or "basket" cells, nuclear remnants of cells damaged by the physical shear stress of making the blood smear. If cytogenetic studies are performed, trisomy 12 is found in 25–30% of patients. Abnormalities in chromosome 13 are also seen.

If the primary presentation is lymphadenopathy and a lymph node biopsy is performed, pathologists usually have little difficulty in making the diagnosis of small lymphocytic lymphoma based on morphologic findings and immunophenotype. However, even in these patients, 70–75% will be found to have bone marrow involvement and circulating monoclonal B lymphocytes are often present.

The differential diagnosis of typical B cell CLL is extensive (Table 105-1). Immunophenotyping will eliminate the T cell disorders and can often help sort out other B cell malignancies. For example, only mantle cell lymphoma and typical B cell CLL are usually CD5 positive. Typical B cell small lymphocytic lymphoma can be confused with other B cell disorders including lymphoplasmacytic lymphoma (i.e., the tissue manifestation of Waldenström's macroglobulinemia), nodal marginal zone B cell lymphoma, and mantle cell lymphoma. In addition, some small lymphocytic lymphomas have areas of large cells that can lead to confusion with diffuse large B cell lymphoma. An expert hematopathologist is vital for making this distinction.

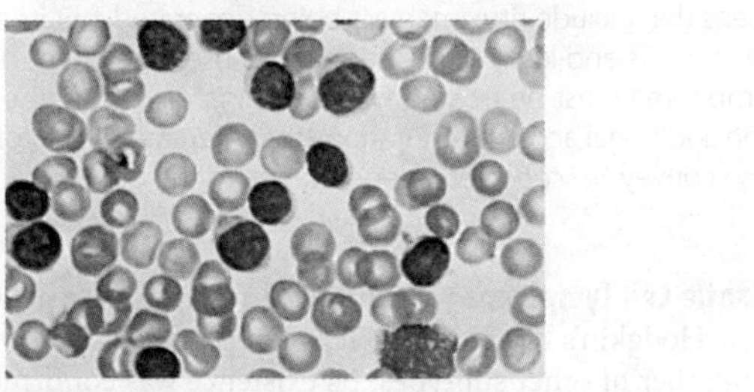

FIGURE 105-6 Chronic lymphocytic leukemia. The peripheral white blood cell count is high due to increased numbers of small, well-differentiated, normal-appearing lymphocytes. The leukemia lymphocytes are fragile, and substantial numbers of broken, smudged cells are usually also present on the blood smear.

Typical B cell CLL is often found incidentally when a complete blood count is done for another reason. However, complaints that might lead to the diagnosis include fatigue, frequent infections, and new lymphadenopathy. The diagnosis of typical B cell CLL should be considered in a patient presenting with an autoimmune hemolytic anemia or autoimmune thrombocytopenia. B cell CLL has also been associated with red cell aplasia. When this disorder presents as lymphoma, the most common abnormality is asymptomatic lymphadenopathy, with or without splenomegaly. The staging systems predict prognosis in patients with typical B cell CLL (Table 105-7). The evaluation of a new patient with typical B cell CLL/small lymphocytic lymphoma will include many of the studies (Table 105-11) that are used in patients with other non-Hodgkin's lymphomas. In addition, particular attention needs to be given to detecting immune abnormalities such as autoimmune hemolytic anemia, autoimmune thrombocytopenia, hypogammaglobulinemia, and red cell aplasia. Molecular analysis of immunoglobulin gene sequences in CLL has demonstrated that about half the patients have tumors expressing mutated immunoglobulin genes and half have tumors expressing unmutated or germ-line immunoglobulin sequences. Patients with unmutated immunoglobulins tend to have a more aggressive clinical course and are less responsive to therapy. Unfortunately, immunoglobulin gene sequencing is not routinely available. CD38 expression is said to be low in the better-

TABLE 105-11 STAGING EVALUATION FOR NON-HODGKIN'S LYMPHOMA

Physical examination
Documentation of B symptoms
Laboratory evaluation
- Complete blood counts
- Liver function tests
- Uric acid
- Calcium
- Serum protein electrophoresis
- Serum β_2-microglobulin

Chest radiograph
CT scan of abdomen, pelvis, and usually chest
Bone marrow biopsy
Lumbar puncture in lymphoblastic, Burkitt's, and diffuse large B cell lymphoma with positive marrow biopsy
Gallium scan (SPECT) or PET scan in large cell lymphoma

Note: SPECT, single photon emission CT; PET, positron emission tomography.

prognosis patients expressing mutated immunoglobulin and high in poorer-prognosis patients expressing unmutated immunoglobulin, but this test has not been confirmed as a reliable means of distinguishing the two groups. ZAP-70 expression correlates with the presence of unmutated immunoglobulin genes, but the assay is not yet standardized and widely available.

Rx B CELL CHRONIC LYMPHOID LEUKEMIA/SMALL LYMPHOCYTIC LYMPHOMA

Patients whose presentation is typical B cell CLL with no manifestations of the disease other than bone marrow involvement and lymphocytosis (i.e., Rai stage O and Binet stage A; Table 105-7) can be followed without specific therapy for their malignancy. These patients have a median survival >10 years, and some will never require therapy for this disorder. If the patient has an adequate number of circulating normal blood cells and is asymptomatic, many physicians would not initiate therapy for patients in the intermediate stage of the disease manifested by lymphadenopathy and/or hepatosplenomegaly. However, the median survival for these patients is ~7 years, and most will require treatment in the first few years of follow-up. Patients who present with bone marrow failure (i.e., Rai stage III or IV or Binet stage C) will require initial therapy in almost all cases. These patients have a serious disorder with a median survival of only 1.5 years. It must be remembered that immune manifestations of typical B cell CLL should be managed independently of specific antileukemia therapy. For example, glucocorticoid therapy for autoimmune cytopenias and γ globulin replacement for patients with hypogammaglobulinemia should be used whether or not antileukemia therapy is given.

Patients who present primarily with lymphoma and have a low IPI score have a 5-year survival of ~75%, but those with a high IPI score have a 5-year survival of <40% and are more likely to require early therapy.

The most common treatments for patients with typical B cell CLL/small lymphocytic lymphoma have been chlorambucil or fludarabine, alone or in combination. Chlorambucil can be administered orally with few immediate side effects, while fludarabine is administered IV and is associated with significant immune suppression. However, fludarabine is by far the more active agent and is the only drug associated with a significant incidence of complete remission. The combination of rituximab (375–500 mg/m^2 day 1), fludarabine (25 mg/m^2 days 2–4 on cycle 1 and 1–3 in subsequent cycles), and cyclophosphamide (250 mg/m^2 with fludarabine) achieves complete responses in 69% of patients, and those responses are associated with molecular remissions in half of the cases. Half the patients experience grade III or IV neutropenia. For young patients presenting with leukemia requiring therapy, regimens containing fludarabine are the treatment of choice. Because fludarabine is an effective second-line agent in patients with tumors unresponsive to chlorambucil, the latter agent is often chosen in elderly patients who require therapy. Many patients who present with lymphoma will receive a combination chemotherapy regimen used in other lymphomas such as CVP (cyclophosphamide, vincristine, and prednisone) or CHOP (cyclophosphamide, doxorubicin, vincristine, and prednisone), although fludarabine-containing regimens may be preferable. Alemtuzimab (anti-CD52) is an antibody with activity in the disease, but it kills both B and T cells and is associated with more immune compromise than rituximab. Young patients with this disease can be candidates for bone marrow transplantation. Allogeneic bone marrow transplantation can be curative but is associated with a significant treatment-related mortality. Mini-transplants using immunosuppressive rather than myeloablative doses of preparative drugs are being studied (Chap. 108). The use of autologous transplantation in patients with this disorder has been discouraging.

Extranodal Marginal Zone B Cell Lymphoma of MALT Type Extranodal marginal zone B cell lymphoma of MALT type (MALT lymphoma) makes up ~8% of non-Hodgkin's lymphomas. This small cell lymphoma presents in extranodal sites. It was previously considered a small lymphocytic lymphoma or sometimes a pseudolymphoma. The recognition that the gastric presentation of this lymphoma was associated with *H. pylori* infection was an important step in recognizing it as a separate entity. The clinical characteristics of MALT lymphoma are presented in Table 105-10.

The diagnosis of MALT lymphoma can be made accurately by an expert hematopathologist based on a characteristic pattern of infiltration of small lymphocytes that are monoclonal B cells and CD5 negative. In some cases, transformation to diffuse large B cell lymphoma occurs, and both diagnoses may be made in the same biopsy. The differential diagnosis includes benign lymphocytic infiltration of extranodal organs and other small cell B cell lymphomas.

MALT lymphoma may occur in the stomach, orbit, intestine, lung, thyroid, salivary gland, skin, soft tissues, bladder, kidney, and CNS. It may present as a new mass, be found on routine imaging studies, or be associated with local symptoms such as upper abdominal discomfort in gastric lymphoma. Most MALT lymphomas are gastric in origin. At least two genetic forms of gastric MALT exist: one (accounting for ~50% of cases) characterized by t(11;18)(q21;q21) that juxtaposes the amino terminal of the *API2* gene with the carboxy terminal of the *MALT1* gene creating an API2/MALT1 fusion product, and the other characterized by multiple sites of genetic instability including trisomies of chromosomes 3, 7, 12, and 18. About 95% of gastric MALT lymphomas are associated with *H. pylori* infection, and those that are do not usually express t(11;18). The t(11;18) usually results in activation of NF-κB, which acts a survival factor for the cells. Lymphomas with t(11;18) translocations are genetically stable and do not evolve to diffuse large B cell lymphoma. By contrast, t(11;18)-negative MALT lymphomas often acquire *BCL6* mutations and progress to aggressive histology lymphoma. MALT lymphomas are localized to the organ of origin in ~40% of cases and to the organ and regional lymph nodes in ~30% of patients. However, distant metastasis can occur—particularly with transformation to diffuse large B cell lymphoma. Many patients who develop this lymphoma will have an autoimmune or inflammatory process such as Sjögren's syndrome (salivary gland MALT), Hashimoto's thyroiditis (thyroid MALT), *Helicobacter* gastritis (gastric MALT), *C. psittaci* conjunctivitis (ocular MALT), or *Borelia* skin infections (cutaneous MALT).

Evaluation of patients with MALT lymphoma follows the pattern (Table 105-11) for staging a patient with non-Hodgkin's lymphoma. In particular, patients with gastric lymphoma need to have studies performed to document the presence or absence of *H. pylori* infection. Endoscopic studies including ultrasound can help define the extent of gastric involvement. Most patients with MALT lymphoma have a good prognosis, with a 5-year survival of ~75%. In patients with a low IPI score, the 5-year survival is ~90%, while it drops to ~40% in patients with a high IPI score.

Rx MUCOSA-ASSOCIATED LYMPHOID TISSUE LYMPHOMA

MALT lymphoma is often localized. Local therapy such as radiation or surgery can effect cure, and this is one of the few times where surgery might be a reasonable primary therapy for a patient with non-Hodgkin's lymphoma. Patients with gastric MALT lymphomas who are infected with *H. pylori* can achieve remission in the majority of cases with eradication of the infection. These remissions can be durable, but molecular evidence of persisting neoplasia is frequent and the long-term outcome is uncertain. Patients who present with more extensive disease are most often treated with single-agent chemotherapy such as chlorambucil. Data on combination regimens that include rituximab are being generated, but its efficacy in other B cell tumors and low toxicity support its use. Coexistent diffuse large B cell lymphoma must be treated with combination chemotherapy (see below). The additional acquired mutations that mediate the histologic progression also convey *Helicobacter* independence to the growth.

Mantle Cell Lymphoma Mantle cell lymphoma makes up ~6% of all non-Hodgkin's lymphomas. This lymphoma was previously placed in a number of other subtypes. Its existence was confirmed by the recognition that these lymphomas have a characteristic chromosomal translocation, t(11;14), between the immunoglobulin heavy chain gene on chromosome 14 and the *bcl-1* gene on chromosome 11, and regularly overexpress the BCL-1 protein, also known as cyclin D1. Table 105-10 shows the clinical characteristics of mantle cell lymphoma.

The diagnosis of mantle cell lymphoma can be made accurately by an expert hematopathologist. As with all subtypes of lymphoma, an adequate biopsy is important. The differential diagnosis of mantle cell lymphoma includes other small cell B cell lymphomas. In particular, mantle cell lymphoma and small lymphocytic lymphoma share a characteristic expression of CD5. Mantle cell lymphoma usually has a slightly indented nucleus.

The most common presentation of mantle cell lymphoma is with palpable lymphadenopathy, frequently accompanied by systemic symptoms. Approximately 70% of patients will be stage IV at the time of diagnosis, with frequent bone marrow and peripheral blood involvement. Of the extranodal organs that can be involved, gastrointestinal involvement is particularly important to recognize. Patients who present with lymphomatosis polyposis in the large intestine usually have mantle cell lymphoma. Table 105-11 outlines the evaluation of patients with mantle cell lymphoma. Patients who present with gastrointestinal tract involvement often have Waldeyer's ring involvement, and vice versa. The 5-year survival for all patients with mantle cell lymphoma is ~25%, with only occasional patients who present with a high IPI score surviving 5 years and ~50% of patients with a low IPI score surviving 5 years.

℞ MANTLE CELL LYMPHOMA

Current therapies for mantle cell lymphoma are unsatisfactory. Patients with localized disease might be treated with combination chemotherapy followed by radiotherapy; however, these patients are exceedingly rare. For the usual presentation with disseminated disease, treatments have been unsatisfactory, with the minority of patients achieving complete remission. Aggressive combination chemotherapy regimens followed by autologous or allogeneic bone marrow transplantation are frequently offered to younger patients. For the occasional elderly, asymptomatic patient, observation followed by single-agent chemotherapy might be the most practical approach. An intensive combination chemotherapy regimen originally used in the treatment of acute leukemia, HyperC-VAD (cyclophosphamide, vincristine, doxorubicin, dexamethasone, cytarabine, and methotrexate), in combination with rituximab seems to be associated with better response rates—particularly in younger patients. CHOP plus rituximab has shown better response rates than CHOP alone, but long-term follow-up is lacking. Bortezomib induces transient partial responses in a minority of patients.

Follicular Lymphoma Follicular lymphomas make up 22% of non-Hodgkin's lymphomas worldwide and at least 30% of non-Hodgkin's lymphomas diagnosed in the United States. This type of lymphoma can be diagnosed accurately on morphologic findings alone and has been the diagnosis in the majority of patients in therapeutic trials for "low-grade" lymphoma in the past. The clinical characteristics of follicular lymphoma are presented in Table 105-10.

Evaluation of an adequate biopsy by an expert hematopathologist is sufficient to make a diagnosis of follicular lymphoma. The tumor is composed of small cleaved and large cells in varying proportions organized in a follicular pattern of growth (Fig. 105-7). Confirmation of B cell immunophenotype and the existence of the t(14;18) and abnormal expression of BCL-2 protein are confirmatory. The major differential diagnosis is between lymphoma and reactive follicular hyperplasia. The coexistence of diffuse large B cell lymphoma must be considered. Patients with follicular lymphoma are often subclassified into those with predominantly small cells, those with a mixture of small and large cells, and those with predominantly large cells. While this distinction cannot be made simply or very accurately, these subdivisions do have prognostic significance. Patients with follicular lymphoma with predominantly large cells have a higher proliferative fraction, progress more rapidly, and have a shorter overall survival with simple chemotherapy regimens.

The most common presentation for follicular lymphoma is with new, painless lymphadenopathy. Multiple sites of lymphoid involvement are typical, and unusual sites such as epitrochlear nodes are sometimes seen. However, essentially any organ can be involved, and extranodal presentations do occur. Most patients do not have fevers,

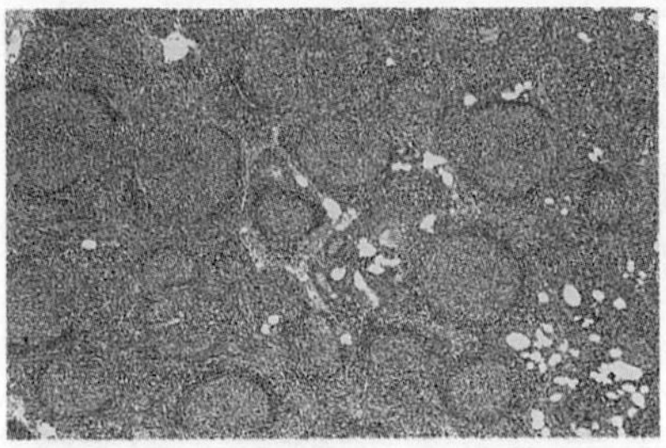

FIGURE 105-7 Follicular lymphoma. The normal nodal architecture is effaced by nodular expansions of tumor cells. Nodules vary in size and contain predominantly small lymphocytes with cleaved nuclei along with variable numbers of larger cells with vesicular chromatin and prominent nucleoli.

sweats, or weight loss, and an IPI score of 0 or 1 is found in ~50% of patients. Fewer than 10% of patients have a high (i.e., 4 or 5) IPI score. The staging evaluation for patients with follicular lymphoma should include the studies included in Table 105-11.

℞ FOLLICULAR LYMPHOMA

Follicular lymphoma is one of the malignancies most responsive to chemotherapy and radiotherapy. In addition, tumors in as many as 25% of the patients undergo spontaneous regression—usually transient—without therapy. In an asymptomatic patient, no initial treatment and watchful waiting can be an appropriate management strategy and is particularly likely to be adopted for older patients with advanced stage disease. For patients who do require treatment, single-agent chlorambucil or cyclophosphamide or combination chemotherapy with CVP or CHOP are most frequently used. With adequate treatment, 50–75% of patients will achieve a complete remission. While most patients relapse (median response duration is ~2 years), at least 20% of complete responders will remain in remission for >10 years. For the rare patient (15%) with localized follicular lymphoma, involved field radiotherapy produces long-term disease-free survival in the majority.

A number of therapies have been shown to be active in the treatment of patients with follicular lymphoma. These include cytotoxic agents such as fludarabine, and biologic agents such as interferon α, monoclonal antibodies with or without radionuclides, and lymphoma vaccines. In patients treated with a doxorubicin-containing combination chemotherapy regimen, interferon α given to patients in complete remission seems to prolong survival. The monoclonal antibody rituximab can cause objective responses in 35–50% of patients with relapsed follicular lymphoma, and radiolabeled antibodies appear to have response rates well in excess of 50%. The addition of rituximab to CHOP and other effective combination chemotherapy programs is beginning to show prolonged overall survival and a decreased risk of histologic progression. Trials with tumor vaccines have been encouraging. Both autologous and allogeneic hematopoietic stem cell transplantation yield high complete response rates in patients with relapsed follicular lymphoma, and long-term remissions can occur.

Patients with follicular lymphoma with a predominance of large cells have a shorter survival when treated with single-agent chemotherapy but seem to benefit from receiving an anthracycline-containing combination chemotherapy regimen plus rituximab. When their disease is treated aggressively, the overall survival for such patients is no lower than for patients with other follicular lymphomas, and the failure-free survival is superior.

Patients with follicular lymphoma have a high rate of histologic transformation to diffuse large B cell lymphoma (5–7% per year). This is recognized ~40% of the time during the course of the illness by repeat biopsy and is present in almost all patients at autopsy. This transformation is usually heralded by rapid growth of lymph nodes—often localized—and the development of systemic symptoms such as fevers, sweats, and weight loss. Although these patients have a poor prognosis, aggressive combination chemotherapy regimens can sometimes cause a complete remission in the diffuse large B cell lymphoma, at times leaving the patient with persisting follicular lymphoma.

Diffuse Large B Cell Lymphoma Diffuse large B cell lymphoma is the most common type of non-Hodgkin's lymphoma, representing ap-

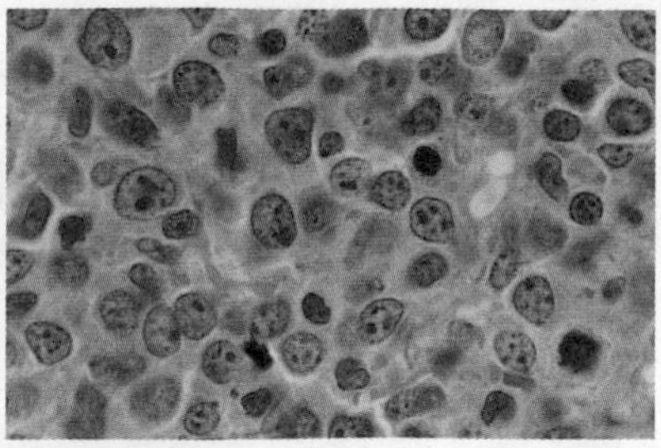

FIGURE 105-8 Diffuse large B cell lymphoma. The neoplastic cells are heterogeneous but predominantly large cells with vesicular chromatin and prominent nucleoli.

proximately one-third of all cases. This lymphoma makes up the majority of cases in previous clinical trials of "aggressive" or "intermediate-grade" lymphoma. Table 105-10 shows the clinical characteristics of diffuse large B cell lymphoma.

The diagnosis of diffuse large B cell lymphoma can be made accurately by an expert hematopathologist (Fig. 105-8). Cytogenetic and molecular genetic studies are not necessary for diagnosis, but some evidence has accumulated that patients whose tumors overexpress the BCL-2 protein might be more likely to relapse than others. Patients with prominent mediastinal involvement are sometimes diagnosed as a separate subgroup having primary mediastinal diffuse large B cell lymphoma. This latter group of patients has a younger median age (i.e., 37 years) and a female predominance (66%). Subtypes of diffuse large B cell lymphoma, including those with an immunoblastic subtype and tumors with extensive fibrosis, are recognized by pathologists but do not appear to have important independent prognostic significance.

Diffuse large B cell lymphoma can present as either primary lymph node disease or at extranodal sites. More than 50% of patients will have some site of extranodal involvement at diagnosis, with the most common sites being the gastrointestinal tract and bone marrow, each being involved in 15–20% of patients. Essentially any organ can be involved, making a diagnostic biopsy imperative. For example, diffuse large B cell lymphoma of the pancreas has a much better prognosis than pancreatic carcinoma but would be missed without biopsy. Primary diffuse large B cell lymphoma of the brain is being diagnosed with increasing frequency. Other unusual subtypes of diffuse large B cell lymphoma such as pleural effusion lymphoma and intravascular lymphoma have been difficult to diagnose and associated with a very poor prognosis.

Table 105-11 shows the initial evaluation of patients with diffuse large B cell lymphoma. After a careful staging evaluation, ~50% of patients will be found to have stage I or II disease and ~50% will have widely disseminated lymphoma. Bone marrow biopsy shows involvement by lymphoma in ~15% of cases, with marrow involvement by small cells more frequent than by large cells.

℞ DIFFUSE LARGE B CELL LYMPHOMA

The initial treatment of all patients with diffuse large B cell lymphoma should be with a combination chemotherapy regimen. The most popular regimen in the United States is CHOP plus rituximab, although a variety of other anthracycline-containing combination chemotherapy regimens appear to be equally efficacious. Patients with stage I or nonbulky stage II can be effectively treated with three to four cycles of combination chemotherapy followed by involved field radiotherapy. The need for radiation therapy is unclear. Cure rates of 70–80% in stage II disease and 85–90% in stage I disease can be expected.

For patients with bulky stage II, stage III, or stage IV disease, six to eight cycles of CHOP plus rituximab are usually administered. A large randomized trial showed the superiority of CHOP combined with rituximab over CHOP alone in elderly patients. A frequent approach would be to administer four cycles of therapy and then reevaluate. If the patient has achieved a complete remission after four cycles, two more cycles of treatment might be given and then therapy discontinued. Using this approach, 70–80% of patients can be expected to achieve a complete remission, and 50–70% of complete responders will be cured. The chances for a favorable response to treatment are predicted by the IPI. In fact, the IPI was developed based on the outcome of patients with diffuse large B cell lymphoma treated with CHOP-like regimens. For the 35% of patients with a low IPI score of 0–1, the 5-year survival is >70%, while for the 20% of patients with a high IPI score of 4–5, the 5-year survival is ~20%. The addition of rituximab to CHOP has improved each of those numbers by ~15%. A number of other factors, including molecular features of the tumor, levels of circulating cytokines and soluble receptors, and other surrogate markers, have been shown to influence prognosis. However, they have not been validated as rigorously as the IPI and have not been uniformly applied clinically.

Because a number of patients with diffuse large B cell lymphoma are either initially refractory to therapy or relapse after apparently effective chemotherapy, 30–40% of patients will be candidates for salvage treatment at some point. Alternative combination chemotherapy regimens can induce complete remission in as many as 50% of these patients, but long-term disease-free survival is seen in ≤10%. Autologous bone marrow transplantation is superior to salvage chemotherapy at usual doses and leads to long-term disease-free survival in ~40% of patients whose lymphomas remain chemotherapy-sensitive after relapse.

Burkitt's Lymphoma/Leukemia Burkitt's lymphoma/leukemia is a rare disease in adults in the United States, making up <1% of non-Hodgkin's lymphomas, but it makes up ~30% of childhood non-Hodgkin's lymphoma. Burkitt's leukemia, or L3 ALL, makes up a small proportion of childhood and adult acute leukemias. Table 105-10 shows the clinical features of Burkitt's lymphoma.

Burkitt's lymphoma can be diagnosed morphologically by an expert hematopathologist with a high degree of accuracy. The cells are homogeneous in size and shape (Fig. 105-9). Demonstration of a very high proliferative fraction and the presence of the t(8;14) or one of its variants, t(2;8) (*c-myc* and the λ light chain gene) or t(8;22) (*c-myc* and the κ light chain gene), can be confirmatory. Burkitt's cell leukemia is recognized by the typical monotonous mass of medium-sized cells with round nuclei, multiple nucleoli, and basophilic cytoplasm with cytoplasmic vacuoles. Demonstration of surface expression of immunoglobulin and one of the above-noted cytogenetic abnormalities is confirmatory.

Three distinct clinical forms of Burkitt's lymphoma are recognized; endemic, sporadic, and immunodeficiency-associated. Endemic and sporadic Burkitt's lymphomas occur frequently in children in Africa, and the sporadic form in western countries. Immunodeficiency-associated Burkitt's lymphoma is seen in patients with HIV infection.

Pathologists sometimes have difficulty distinguishing between Burkitt's lymphoma and diffuse large B cell lymphoma. In the past, a separate subgroup of non-Hodgkin's lymphoma intermediate between the two was recognized. When tested, this subgroup could not be diagnosed accurately. Distinction between the two major types of B cell aggressive non-Hodgkin's lymphoma can sometimes be made based on the extremely high proliferative fraction seen in patients with Burkitt's lymphoma (i.e., essentially 100% of tumor cells are in cycle) caused by *c-myc* deregulation.

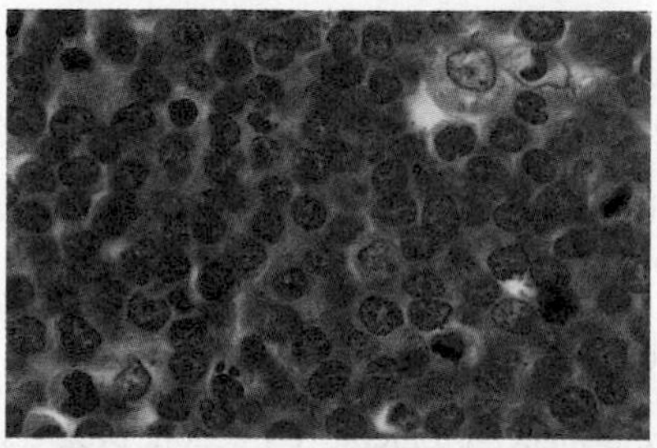

FIGURE 105-9 Burkitt's lymphoma. The neoplastic cells are homogenous, medium-sized B cells with frequent mitotic figures, a morphologic correlate of high growth fraction. Reactive macrophages are scattered through the tumor and their pale cytoplasm in a background of blue-staining tumor cells give the tumor a so-called starry sky appearance.

Most patients in the United States with Burkitt's lymphoma present with peripheral lymphadenopathy or an intraabdominal mass. The disease is rapidly progressive and has a propensity to metastasize to the CNS. Initial evaluation should always include an examination of cerebral spinal fluid to rule out metastasis in addition to the other staging evaluations noted in Table 105-11. Once the diagnosis of Burkitt's lymphoma is suspected, a diagnosis must be made promptly and staging evaluation must be accomplished expeditiously. This is the most rapidly progressive human tumor, and any delay in initiating therapy can adversely affect the patient's prognosis.

℞ BURKITT'S LYMPHOMA

Treatment of Burkitt's lymphoma in both children and adults should begin within 48 h of diagnosis and involves the use of intensive combination chemotherapy regimens incorporating high doses of cyclophosphamide. Prophylactic therapy to the CNS is mandatory. Burkitt's lymphoma was one of the first cancers shown to be curable by chemotherapy. Today, cure can be expected in 70–80% of both children and young adults when effective therapy is administered precisely. Salvage therapy has been generally ineffective in patients failing the initial treatment, emphasizing the importance of the initial treatment approach.

Other B Cell Lymphoid Malignancies *B cell prolymphocytic leukemia* involves blood and marrow infiltration by large lymphocytes with prominent nucleoli. Patients typically have a high white cell count, splenomegaly, and minimal lymphadenopathy. The chances for a complete response to therapy are poor.

Hairy cell leukemia is a rare disease that presents predominantly in older males. Typical presentation involves pancytopenia, although occasional patients will have a leukemic presentation. Splenomegaly is usual. The malignant cells appear to have "hairy" projections on light and electron microscopy and show a characteristic staining pattern with tartrate-resistant acid phosphatase. Bone marrow is typically not able to be aspirated, and biopsy shows a pattern of fibrosis with diffuse infiltration by the malignant cells. Patients with this disorder are prone to unusual infections, including infection by *Mycobacterium avium intracellulare*, and to vasculitic syndromes. Hairy cell leukemia is responsive to chemotherapy with interferon α, pentostatin, or cladribine, with the latter being the usually preferred treatment. Clinical complete remissions with cladribine occur in the majority of patients, and long-term disease-free survival is frequent.

Splenic marginal zone lymphoma involves infiltration of the splenic white pulp by small, monoclonal B cells. This is a rare disorder that can present as leukemia as well as lymphoma. Definitive diagnosis is often made at splenectomy, which is also an effective therapy. This is an extremely indolent disorder, but when chemotherapy is required, the most usual treatment has been chlorambucil.

Lymphoplasmacytic lymphoma is the tissue manifestation of Waldenström's macroglobulinemia (Chap. 106). This type of lymphoma has been associated with chronic hepatitis C virus infection, and an etiologic association has been proposed. Patients typically present with lymphadenopathy, splenomegaly, bone marrow involvement, and occasionally peripheral blood involvement. The tumor cells do not express CD5. Patients often have a monoclonal IgM protein, high levels of which can dominate the clinical picture with the symptoms of hyperviscosity. Treatment of lymphoplasmacytic lymphoma can be aimed primarily at reducing the abnormal protein, if present, but will usually also involve chemotherapy. Chlorambucil, fludarabine, and cladribine have been utilized. The median 5-year survival for patients with this disorder is ~60%.

Nodal marginal zone lymphoma, also known as *monocytoid B cell lymphoma*, represents ~1% of non-Hodgkin's lymphomas. This lymphoma has a slight female predominance and presents with disseminated disease (i.e., stage III or IV) in 75% of patients. Approximately one-third of patients have bone marrow involvement, and a leukemic presentation occasionally occurs. The staging evaluation and therapy should use the same approach as used for patients with follicular lymphoma. Approximately 60% of the patients with nodal marginal zone lymphoma will survive 5 years after diagnosis.

PRECURSOR CELL T CELL MALIGNANCIES

Precursor T Cell Lymphoblastic Leukemia/Lymphoma Precursor T cell malignancies can present either as ALL or as an aggressive lymphoma. These malignancies are more common in children and young adults, with males more frequently affected than females.

Precursor T cell ALL can present with bone marrow failure, although the severity of anemia, neutropenia, and thrombocytopenia is often less than in precursor B cell ALL. These patients sometimes have very high white cell counts, a mediastinal mass, lymphadenopathy, and hepatosplenomegaly. Precursor T cell lymphoblastic lymphoma is most often found in young men presenting with a large mediastinal mass and pleural effusions. Both presentations have a propensity to metastasize to the CNS, and CNS involvement is often present at diagnosis.

℞ PRECURSOR T CELL LYMPHOBLASTIC LEUKEMIA/LYMPHOMA

Children with precursor T cell ALL seem to benefit from very intensive remission induction and consolidation regimens. The majority of patients treated in this manner can be cured. Older children and young adults with precursor T cell lymphoblastic lymphoma are also often treated with "leukemia-like" regimens. Patients who present with localized disease have an excellent prognosis. However, advanced age is an adverse prognostic factor. Adults with precursor T cell lymphoblastic lymphoma who present with high LDH levels or bone marrow or CNS involvement are often offered bone marrow transplantation as part of their primary therapy.

MATURE (PERIPHERAL) T CELL DISORDERS

Mycosis Fungoides Mycosis fungoides is also known as *cutaneous T cell lymphoma*. This lymphoma is more often seen by dermatologists than internists. The median age of onset is in the mid-fifties, and the disease is more common in males and in blacks.

Mycosis fungoides is an indolent lymphoma with patients often having several years of eczematous or dermatitic skin lesions before the diagnosis is finally established. The skin lesions progress from patch stage to plaque stage to cutaneous tumors. Early in the disease, biopsies are often difficult to interpret, and the diagnosis may only become apparent by observing the patient over time. In advanced stages, the lymphoma can spread to lymph nodes and visceral organs. Patients with this lymphoma may develop generalized erythroderma and circulating tumor cells, called *Sézary's syndrome*.

Rare patients with localized early stage mycosis fungoides can be cured with radiotherapy, often total-skin electron beam irradiation. More advanced disease has been treated with topical glucocorticoids, topical nitrogen mustard, phototherapy, psoralen with ultraviolet A (PUVA), electron beam radiation, interferon, antibodies, fusion toxins, and systemic cytotoxic therapy. Unfortunately, these treatments are palliative.

Adult T Cell Lymphoma/Leukemia Adult T cell lymphoma/leukemia is one manifestation of infection by the HTLV-I retrovirus. Patients can be infected through transplacental transmission, mother's milk, blood transfusion, and by sexual transmission of the virus. Patients who acquire the virus from their mother through breast milk are most likely to develop lymphoma, but the risk is still only 2.5% and the latency averages 55 years. Nationwide testing for HTLV-I antibodies and the aggressive implementation of public health measures could theoretically lead to the disappearance of adult T cell lymphoma/leukemia. Tropical spastic paraparesis, another manifestation of HTLV-I infection (Chap. 181), occurs after a shorter latency (1–3 years) and is most common in individuals who acquire the virus during adulthood from transfusion or sex.

The diagnosis of adult T cell lymphoma/leukemia is made when an expert hematopathologist recognizes the typical morphologic picture, a T cell immunophenotype (i.e., CD4 positive), and the presence in se-

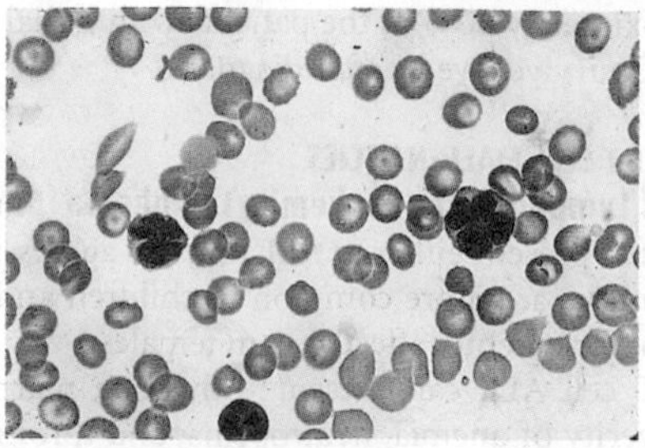

FIGURE 105-10 Adult T cell leukemia/lymphoma. Peripheral blood smear showing leukemia cells with typical "flower-shaped" nucleus.

rum of antibodies to HTLV-I. Examination of the peripheral blood will usually reveal characteristic, pleomorphic abnormal CD4-positive cells with indented nuclei, which have been called "flower" cells (Fig. 105-10).

A subset of patients have a smoldering clinical course and long survival, but most patients present with an aggressive disease manifested by lymphadenopathy, hepatosplenomegaly, skin infiltration, pulmonary infiltrates, hypercalcemia, lytic bone lesions, and elevated LDH levels. The skin lesions can be papules, plaques, tumors, and ulcerations. Lung lesions can be either tumor or opportunistic infection in light of the underlying immunodeficiency in the disease. Bone marrow involvement is not usually extensive, and anemia and thrombocytopenia are not usually prominent. Although treatment by combination chemotherapy regimens can result in objective responses, true complete remissions are unusual, and the median survival of patients is ~7 months.

Anaplastic Large T/Null Cell Lymphoma Anaplastic large T/null cell lymphoma was previously usually diagnosed as undifferentiated carcinoma or malignant histiocytosis. Discovery of the CD30 (Ki-1) antigen and the recognition that some patients with previously unclassified malignancies displayed this antigen led to the identification of a new type of lymphoma. Subsequently, discovery of the t(2;5) and the resultant frequent overexpression of the anaplastic lymphoma kinase (ALK) protein confirmed the existence of this entity. This lymphoma accounts for ~2% of all non-Hodgkin's lymphomas. Table 105-10 shows the clinical characteristics of patients with anaplastic large T/null cell lymphoma.

The diagnosis of anaplastic large T/null cell lymphoma is made when an expert hematopathologist recognizes the typical morphologic picture and a T cell or null cell immunophenotype with CD30 positivity. Documentation of the t(2;5) and/or overexpression of ALK protein confirm the diagnosis. Some diffuse large B cell lymphomas can also have an anaplastic appearance but have the same clinical course or response to therapy as other diffuse large B cell lymphomas.

Patients with anaplastic large T/cell null cell lymphoma are typically young (median age, 33 years) and male (~70%). Some 50% of patients present in stage I/II, and the remainder with more extensive disease. Systemic symptoms and elevated LDH levels are seen in about one-half of patients. Bone marrow and the gastrointestinal tract are rarely involved, but skin involvement is frequent. Some patients with disease confined to the skin have a different and more indolent disorder that has been termed *cutaneous anaplastic large T/null cell lymphoma* and might be related to lymphomatoid papulosis.

℞ ANAPLASTIC LARGE T/NULL CELL LYMPHOMA

Treatment regimens appropriate for other aggressive lymphomas, such as diffuse large B cell lymphoma, should be utilized in patients with anaplastic large T/null cell lymphoma, with the exception that the B cell–specific antibody, rituximab, is omitted. Surprisingly, given the anaplastic appearance, this disorder has the best survival rate of any aggressive lymphoma. The 5-year survival is >75%. While traditional prognostic factors such as the IPI predict treatment outcome, overexpression of the ALK protein is an important prognostic factor, with patients overexpressing this protein having a superior treatment outcome.

Peripheral T Cell Lymphoma The peripheral T cell lymphomas make up a heterogeneous morphologic group of aggressive neoplasms that share a mature T cell immunophenotype. They represent ~7% of all cases of non-Hodgkin's lymphoma. A number of distinct clinical syndromes are included in this group of disorders. Table 105-10 shows the clinical characteristics of patients with peripheral T cell lymphoma.

The diagnosis of peripheral T cell lymphoma, or any of its specific subtypes, requires an expert hematopathologist, an adequate biopsy, and immunophenotyping. Most peripheral T cell lymphomas are CD4+, but a few will be CD8+, both CD4+ and CD8+, or have an NK cell immunophenotype. No characteristic genetic abnormalities have yet been identified, but translocations involving the T cell antigen receptor genes on chromosomes 7 or 14 may be detected. The differential diagnosis of patients suspected of having peripheral T cell lymphoma includes reactive T cell infiltrative processes. In some cases, demonstration of a monoclonal T cell population using T cell receptor gene rearrangement studies will be required to make a diagnosis.

The initial evaluation of a patient with a peripheral T cell lymphoma should include the studies in Table 105-11 for staging patients with non-Hodgkin's lymphoma. Unfortunately, patients with peripheral T cell lymphoma usually present with adverse prognostic factors, with >80% of patients having an IPI score ≥2 and >30% having an IPI score ≥4. As this would predict, peripheral T cell lymphomas are associated with a poor outcome, and only 25% of the patients survive 5 years after diagnosis. Treatment regimens are the same as those used for diffuse large B cell lymphoma (omitting rituximab), but patients with peripheral T cell lymphoma have a poorer response to treatment. Because of this poor treatment outcome, hematopoietic stem cell transplantation is often considered early in the care of young patients.

A number of specific clinical syndromes are seen in the peripheral T cell lymphomas. *Angioimmunoblastic T cell lymphoma* is one of the more common subtypes, making up ~20% of T cell lymphomas. These patients typically present with generalized lymphadenopathy, fever, weight loss, skin rash, and polyclonal hypergammaglobulinemia. In some cases, it is difficult to separate patients with a reactive disorder from those with true lymphoma.

Extranodal T/NK cell lymphoma of nasal type has also been called *angiocentric lymphoma* and was previously termed *lethal midline granuloma*. This disorder is more frequent in Asia and South America than in the United States and Europe. EBV is thought to play an etiologic role. Although most frequent in the upper airway, it can involve other organs. The course is aggressive, and patients frequently have the hemophagocytic syndrome. When marrow and blood involvement occur, distinction between this disease and leukemia might be difficult. Some patients will respond to aggressive combination chemotherapy regimens, but the overall outlook is poor.

Enteropathy-type intestinal T cell lymphoma is a rare disorder that occurs in patients with untreated gluten-sensitive enteropathy. Patients are frequently wasted and sometimes present with intestinal perforation. The prognosis is poor. *Hepatosplenic γδ T cell lymphoma* is a systemic illness that presents with sinusoidal infiltration of the liver, spleen, and bone marrow by malignant T cells. Tumor masses generally do not occur. The disease is associated with systemic symptoms and is often difficult to diagnosis. Treatment outcome is poor. *Subcutaneous panniculitis-like T cell lymphoma* is a rare disorder that is often confused with panniculitis. Patients present with multiple subcutaneous nodules, which progress and can ulcerate. Hemophagocytic syndrome is common. Response to therapy is poor. The development of the hemophagocytic syndrome (profound anemia, ingestion of erythrocytes by monocytes and macrophages) in the course of any peripheral T cell lymphoma is generally associated with a fatal outcome.

HODGKIN'S DISEASE

Classical Hodgkin's Disease Hodgkin's disease occurs in 8000 patients in the United States each year, and the disease does not appear to be increasing in frequency. Most patients present with palpable lymphadenopathy that is nontender; in most patients, these lymph nodes are in the neck, supraclavicular area, and axilla. More than half the patients will

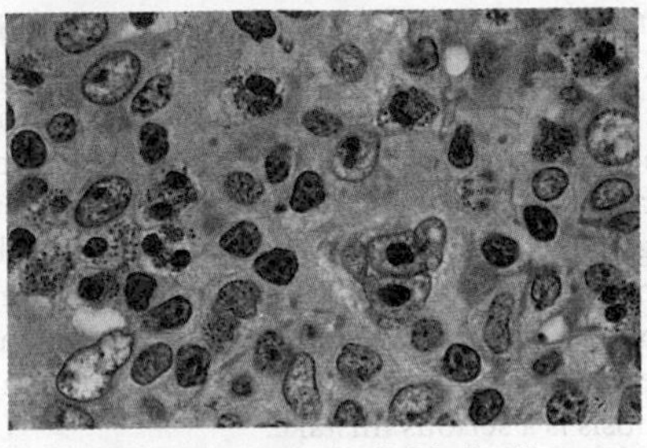

FIGURE 105-11 Mixed cellularity Hodgkin's disease. A Reed-Sternberg cell is present near the center of the field; a large cell with a bilobed nucleus and prominent nucleoli giving an "owl's eyes" appearance. The majority of the cells are normal lymphocytes, neutrophils, and eosinophils that form a pleiomorphic cellular infiltrate.

have mediastinal adenopathy at diagnosis, and this is sometimes the initial manifestation. Subdiaphragmatic presentation of Hodgkin's disease is unusual and more common in older males. One-third of patients present with fevers, night sweats, and/or weight loss—B symptoms in the Ann Arbor staging classification (Table 105-8). Occasionally, Hodgkin's disease can present as a fever of unknown origin. This is more common in older patients who are found to have mixed-cellularity Hodgkin's disease in an abdominal site. Rarely, the fevers persist for days to weeks, followed by afebrile intervals and then recurrence of the fever. This pattern is known as *Pel-Ebstein fever*. Hodgkin's disease can occasionally present with unusual manifestations. These include severe and unexplained itching, cutaneous disorders such as erythema nodosum and ichthyosiform atrophy, paraneoplastic cerebellar degeneration and other distant effects on the CNS, nephrotic syndrome, immune hemolytic anemia and thrombocytopenia, hypercalcemia, and pain in lymph nodes on alcohol ingestion.

The diagnosis of Hodgkin's disease is established by review of an adequate biopsy specimen by an expert hematopathologist. In the United States, most patients have nodular sclerosing Hodgkin's disease, with a minority of patients having mixed-cellularity Hodgkin's disease. Lymphocyte-predominant and lymphocyte-depleted Hodgkin's disease are rare. Mixed-cellularity Hodgkin's disease or lymphocyte-depletion Hodgkin's disease are seen more frequently in patients infected by HIV (Fig. 105-11). The differential diagnosis of a lymph node biopsy suspicious for Hodgkin's disease includes inflammatory processes, mononucleosis, non-Hodgkin's lymphoma, phenytoin-induced adenopathy, and nonlymphomatous malignancies.

The staging evaluation for a patient with Hodgkin's disease would typically include a careful history and physical examination; complete blood count; erythrocyte sedimentation rate; serum chemistry studies including LDH; chest radiograph; CT scan of the chest, abdomen, and pelvis; and bone marrow biopsy. Many patients would also have a PET scan or a gallium scan. Although rarely utilized, a bipedal lymphangiogram can be helpful. PET and gallium scans are most useful to document remission. Staging laparotomies were once popular for most patients with Hodgkin's disease but are now done rarely because of an increased reliance on systemic rather than local therapy.

℞ CLASSICAL HODGKIN'S DISEASE

Patients with localized Hodgkin's disease are cured >90% of the time. In patients with good prognostic factors, extended-field radiotherapy has a high cure rate. Increasingly, patients with all stages of Hodgkin's disease are treated initially with chemotherapy. Patients with localized or good-prognosis disease receive a brief course of chemotherapy followed by radiotherapy to sites of node involvement. Patients with more extensive disease or those with B symptoms receive a complete course of chemotherapy. The most popular chemotherapy regimens used in Hodgkin's disease include doxorubicin, bleomycin, vinblastine, and dacarbazine (ABVD) and mechlorethamine, vincristine, procarbazine, and prednisone (MOPP), or combinations of the drugs in these two regimens. Today, most patients in the United States receive ABVD, but a weekly chemotherapy regimen administered for 12 weeks called *Stanford V* is becoming increasingly popular, but includes radiation therapy, which has been associated with life-threatening late toxicities such as premature coronary artery disease and second solid tumors. In Europe a high-dose regimen called *BEACOPP* incorporating alkylating agents has become popular and might have a better response rate in very high risk patients. Long-term disease-free survival in patients with advanced disease can be achieved in >75% of patients who lack systemic symptoms and in 60–70% of patients with systemic symptoms.

Patients who relapse after primary therapy of Hodgkin's disease can frequently still be cured. Patients who relapse after initial treatment only with radiotherapy have an excellent outcome when treated with chemotherapy. Patients who relapse after an effective chemotherapy regimen are usually not curable with subsequent chemotherapy administered at standard doses. However, patients with a long initial remission can be an exception to this rule. Autologous bone marrow transplantation can cure half of patients who fail effective chemotherapy regimens.

Because of the very high cure rate in patients with Hodgkin's disease, long-term complications have become a major focus for clinical research. In fact, in some series of patients with early-stage disease, more patients died from late complications of therapy than from Hodgkin's disease itself. This is particularly true in patients with localized disease. The most serious late side effects include second malignancies and cardiac injury. Patients are at risk for the development of acute leukemia in the first 10 years after treatment with combination chemotherapy regimens that contain alkylating agents plus radiation therapy. The risk for development of acute leukemia appears to be greater after MOPP-like regimens than with ABVD. The risk of development of acute leukemia after treatment for Hodgkin's disease is also related to the number of exposures to potentially leukemogenic agents (i.e., multiple treatments after relapse) and the age of the patient being treated, with those >60 years at particularly high risk. The development of carcinomas as a complication of treatment for Hodgkin's disease has become a major problem. These tumors usually occur ≥10 years after treatment and are associated with use of radiotherapy. For this reason, young women treated with thoracic radiotherapy for Hodgkin's disease should institute screening mammograms 5–10 years after treatment, and all patients who receive thoracic radiotherapy for Hodgkin's disease should be discouraged from smoking. Thoracic radiation also accelerates coronary artery disease, and patients should be encouraged to minimize risk factors for coronary artery disease such as smoking and elevated cholesterol levels.

A number of other late side effects from the treatment of Hodgkin's disease are well known. Patients who receive thoracic radiotherapy are at very high risk for the eventual development of hypothyroidism and should be observed for this complication; intermittent measurement of thyrotropin should be made to identify the condition before it becomes symptomatic. Lhermitte's syndrome occurs in ~15% of patients who receive thoracic radiotherapy. This syndrome is manifested by an "electric shock" sensation into the lower extremities on flexion of the neck. Infertility is a concern for all patients undergoing treatment for Hodgkin's disease. In both women and men, the risk of permanent infertility is age-related, with younger patients more likely to recover fertility. In addition, treatment with ABVD rather than MOPP increases the chances to retain fertility.

Nodular Lymphocyte-Predominant Hodgkin's Disease Nodular lymphocyte-predominant Hodgkin's disease is now recognized as an entity distinct from classical Hodgkin's disease. Previous classification systems recognized that biopsies from a subset of patients diagnosed as having Hodgkin's disease contained a predominance of small lymphocytes and rare Reed-Sternberg cells. A subset of these patients have tumors with nodular growth pattern and a clinical course that varied from that of patients with classical Hodgkin's disease. This is an unusual clinical entity and represents <5% of cases of Hodgkin's disease.

Nodular lymphocyte-predominant Hodgkin's disease has a number of characteristics that suggest its relationship to non-Hodgkin's lymphoma. These include a clonal proliferation of B cells and a distinctive immunophenotype; tumor cells express J chain and display CD45 and epithelial membrane antigen (ema) and do not express two markers normally found on Sternberg-Reed cells, CD30 and CD15. This lymphoma tends to have a chronic, relapsing course and sometimes transforms to diffuse large B cell lymphoma.

The treatment of patients with nodular lymphocyte-predominant Hodgkin's disease is controversial. Some clinicians favor no treatment and merely close follow-up. In the United States, most physicians will treat localized disease with radiotherapy and disseminated disease with regimens utilized for patients with classical Hodgkin's disease. Regardless of the therapy utilized, most series report a long-term survival of >80%.

LYMPHOMA-LIKE DISORDERS

The most common condition that pathologists and clinicians might confuse with lymphoma is reactive, atypical lymphoid hyperplasia. Patients might have localized or disseminated lymphadenopathy and might have the systemic symptoms characteristic of lymphoma. Underlying causes include a drug reaction to phenytoin or carbamazepine. Immune disorders such as rheumatoid arthritis and lupus erythematosus, viral infections such as cytomegalovirus and EBV, and bacterial infections such as cat-scratch disease may cause adenopathy (Chap. 60). In the absence of a definitive diagnosis after initial biopsy, continued follow-up, further testing, and repeated biopsies, if necessary, are the appropriate approach rather than instituting therapy.

Specific conditions that can be confused with lymphoma include *Castleman's disease*, which can present with localized or disseminated lymphadenopathy; some patients have systemic symptoms. The disseminated form is often accompanied by anemia and polyclonal hypergammaglobulinemia, and the condition has been associated with overproduction of interleukin 6, possibly produced by human herpesvirus 8. Patients with localized disease can be treated effectively with local therapy, while the initial treatment for patients with disseminated disease is usually with systemic glucocorticoids.

Sinus histiocytosis with massive lymphadenopathy (*Rosai-Dorfman's disease*) usually presents with bulky lymphadenopathy in children or young adults. The disease is usually nonprogressive and self-limited, but patients can manifest autoimmune hemolytic anemia.

Lymphomatoid papulosis is a cutaneous lymphoproliferative disorder that is often confused with anaplastic large cell lymphoma involving the skin. The cells of lymphomatoid papulosis are similar to those seen in lymphoma and stain for CD30, and T cell receptor gene rearrangements are sometimes seen. However, the condition is characterized by waxing and waning skin lesions that usually heal, leaving small scars. In the absence of effective communication between the clinician and the pathologist regarding the clinical course in the patient, this disease will be misdiagnosed. Since the clinical picture is usually benign, misdiagnosis is a serious mistake.

ACKNOWLEDGMENT

James Armitage was a coauthor of this chapter in prior editions, and substantial material from those editions has been included here.

FURTHER READINGS

ANSEL SM, ARMITAGE JO: Management of Hodgkin lymphoma. Mayo Clin Proc 81:419, 2006

ARMITAGE JO et al: Lymphoma 2006: Classification and treatment. Oncology 20:231, 2006

BREPOELS L et al: PET and PET/CT for response evaluation in lymphoma: Current practice and developments. Leuk Lymphoma 48:270, 2007

HARRIS NL et al: World Health Organization classification of neoplastic diseases of the hematopoietic and lymphoid tissues: Report of the Clinical Advisory Committee Meeting, Airlie House, Virginia, November, 1997. J Clin Oncol 17:3835, 1999

SEHN LH et al: The revised International Prognostic Index (R-IPI) is a better predictor of outcome than the standard IPI for patients with diffuse large B-cell lymphoma treated with R-CHOP. Blood 109:1857, 2007

URBA WJ, LONGO DL: Hodgkin's disease. N Engl J Med 326:678, 1992

106 Plasma Cell Disorders

Nikhil C. Munshi, Dan L. Longo, Kenneth C. Anderson

The *plasma cell disorders* are monoclonal neoplasms related to each other by virtue of their development from common progenitors in the B lymphocyte lineage. Multiple myeloma, Waldenström's macroglobulinemia, primary amyloidosis (Chap. 324), and the heavy chain diseases comprise this group and may be designated by a variety of synonyms such as *monoclonal gammopathies*, *paraproteinemias*, *plasma cell dyscrasias*, and *dysproteinemias*. Mature B lymphocytes destined to produce IgG bear surface immunoglobulin molecules of both M and G heavy chain isotypes with both isotypes having identical idiotypes (variable regions). Under normal circumstances, maturation to antibody-secreting plasma cells is stimulated by exposure to the antigen for which the surface immunoglobulin is specific; however, in the plasma cell disorders the control over this process is lost. The clinical manifestations of all the plasma cell disorders relate to the expansion of the neoplastic cells, to the secretion of cell products (immunoglobulin molecules or subunits, lymphokines), and to some extent to the host's response to the tumor. **Normal development of B lymphocytes is discussed in Chap. 308.**

There are three categories of structural variation among immunoglobulin molecules that form antigenic determinants, and these are used to classify immunoglobulins (Chap. 308). *Isotypes* are those determinants that distinguish among the main classes of antibodies of a given species and are the same in all normal individuals of that species. Therefore, isotypic determinants are, by definition, recognized by antibodies from a distinct species (heterologous sera) but not by antibodies from the same species (homologous sera). There are five heavy chain isotypes (M, G, A, D, E) and two light chain isotypes (κ, λ). *Allotypes* are distinct determinants that reflect regular small differences between individuals of the same species in the amino acid sequences of otherwise similar immunoglobulins. These differences are determined by allelic genes; by definition, they are detected by antibodies made in the same species. *Idiotypes* are the third category of antigenic determinants. They are unique to the molecules produced by a given clone of antibody-producing cells. Idiotypes are formed by the unique structure of the antigen-binding portion of the molecule.

Antibody molecules (Fig. 308-9) are composed of two heavy chains (mol wt ~ 50,000) and two light chains (mol wt ~ 25,000). Each chain has a constant portion (limited amino acid sequence variability) and a variable region (extensive sequence variability). The light and heavy chains are linked by disulfide bonds and are aligned so that their variable regions are adjacent to one another. This variable region forms the antigen recognition site of the antibody molecule; its unique structural features form a particular set of determinants, or idiotypes, that are reliable markers for a particular clone of cells because each antibody is formed and secreted by a single clone. Each chain is specified by distinct genes, synthesized separately, and assembled into an intact antibody molecule after translation. Because of the mechanics of the gene rearrangements necessary to specify the immunoglobulin variable regions (VDJ joining for the heavy chain, VJ joining for the light chain), a particular clone rearranges only one of the two chromosomes to produce an immunoglobulin molecule of only one light chain isotype and only one allotype (allelic exclusion). After exposure to antigen, the variable region may become associated with a new heavy chain isotype (class switch). Each clone of cells performs these sequential gene arrangements in a unique way. This results in each clone producing a unique immunoglobulin molecule. In most cells, light chains are synthesized in slight excess, are secreted as free light chains by plasma cells, and are cleared by the kidney, but <10 mg of such light chains is excreted per day.

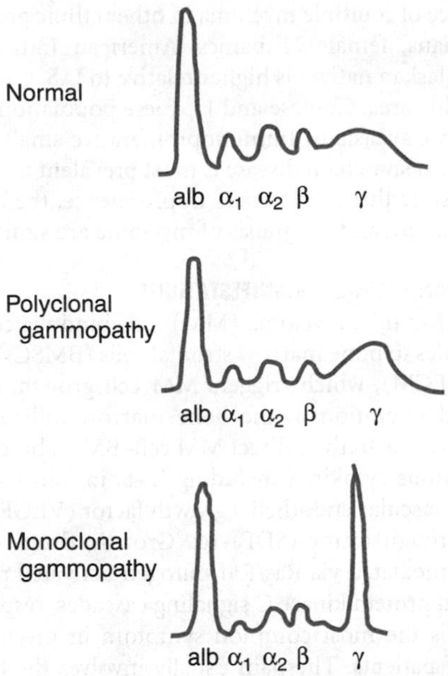

FIGURE 106-1 Representative patterns of serum electrophoresis. The upper panel illustrates the normal pattern of serum protein on electrophoresis. Since there are many different immunoglobulins in the serum, their differing mobilities in an electric field produce a broad peak. In conditions associated with increases in polyclonal immunoglobulin, the broad peak is more prominent (middle panel). In monoclonal gammopathies, the predominance of a product of a single cell produces a "church spire" sharp peak, usually in the γ globulin region (bottom panel).

Electrophoretic analysis of components of the serum proteins permits determination of the amount of immunoglobulin in the serum (Fig. 106-1). The immunoglobulins move heterogeneously in an electric field and form a broad peak in the gamma region. The γ globulin region of the electrophoretic pattern is usually increased in the sera of patients with plasma cell tumors. There is a sharp spike in this region called an *M component* (M for monoclonal). Less commonly, the M component may appear in the β_2 or α_2 globulin region. The antibody must be present at a concentration of at least 5 g/L (0.5 g/dL) to be detectable by this method. This corresponds to ~10^9 cells producing the antibody. Confirmation that such an M component is truly monoclonal relies on the use of immunoelectrophoresis that shows a single light and heavy chain type. Hence immunoelectrophoresis and electrophoresis provide qualitative and quantitative assessment of the M component, respectively. Once the presence of an M component has been confirmed, electrophoresis provides the more practical information for managing patients with monoclonal gammopathies. In a given patient, the amount of M component in the serum is a reliable measure of the tumor burden. This makes the M component an excellent tumor marker, yet it is not specific enough to be used to screen asymptomatic patients. In addition to the plasma cell disorders, M components may be detected in other lymphoid neoplasms such as chronic lymphocytic leukemia and lymphomas of B or T cell origin; nonlymphoid neoplasms such as chronic myeloid leukemia, breast cancer, and colon cancer; a variety of nonneoplastic conditions such as cirrhosis, sarcoidosis, parasitic diseases, Gaucher disease, and pyoderma gangrenosum; and a number of autoimmune conditions, including rheumatoid arthritis, myasthenia gravis, and cold agglutinin disease. At least two very rare skin diseases—lichen myxedematosus, or papular mucinosis, and necrobiotic xanthogranuloma—are associated with a monoclonal gammopathy. In papular mucinosis, highly cationic IgG is deposited in the dermis of patients. This organ specificity may reflect the specificity of the antibody for some antigenic component of the dermis. Necrobiotic xanthogranuloma is a histiocytic infiltration of the skin, usually of the face, that produces red or yellow nodules that can enlarge to plaques. Some 10% progress to myeloma.

The nature of the M component is variable in plasma cell disorders. It may be an intact antibody molecule of any heavy chain subclass, or it may be an altered antibody or fragment. Isolated light or heavy chains may be produced. In some plasma cell tumors such as extramedullary or solitary bone plasmacytomas, <1/3 of patients will have an M component. In ~20% of myelomas, only light chains are produced and in most cases are secreted in the urine as Bence Jones proteins. The frequency of myelomas of a particular heavy chain class is roughly proportional to the serum concentration, and therefore IgG myelomas are more common than IgA and IgD myelomas.

MULTIPLE MYELOMA

DEFINITION

Multiple myeloma represents a malignant proliferation of plasma cells derived from a single clone. The terms *multiple myeloma* and *myeloma* may be used interchangeably. The tumor, its products, and the host response to it result in a number of organ dysfunctions and symptoms of bone pain or fracture, renal failure, susceptibility to infection, anemia, hypercalcemia, and occasionally clotting abnormalities, neurologic symptoms, and manifestations of hyperviscosity.

ETIOLOGY

The cause of myeloma is not known. Myeloma occurred with increased frequency in those exposed to the radiation of nuclear warheads in World War II after a 20-year latency. A variety of chromosomal alterations have been found in patients with myeloma; 13q14 deletions, 17p13 deletions, and 11q abnormalities predominate. The most common translocations are t(11;14)(q13;q32) and t(4;14)(p16;q32), and evidence is strong that errors in switch recombination—the genetic mechanism to change antibody heavy chain isotype—participate in the transformation pathway. Overexpression of *myc* or *ras* genes has been noted in some cases. Mutations in p53 and Rb-1 have also been described, but no common molecular pathogenesis has yet emerged.

Myeloma has been seen more commonly than expected among farmers, wood workers, leather workers, and those exposed to petroleum products. The neoplastic event in myeloma may involve cells earlier in B cell differentiation than the plasma cell. Circulating B cells bearing surface immunoglobulin that share the idiotype of the M component are present in myeloma patients. Interleukin (IL) 6 may play a role in driving myeloma cell proliferation; a large fraction of myeloma cells exposed to IL-6 in vitro respond by proliferating. The IL-6 dependency of myeloma is controversial. It remains difficult to distinguish benign from malignant plasma cells on the basis of morphologic criteria in all but a few cases (Fig. 106-2).

INCIDENCE AND PREVALENCE

About 19,900 cases of myeloma were diagnosed in 2007, and 10,790 people died from the disease in the United States. Myeloma increases in incidence with age. The median age at diagnosis is 68 years; it is uncommon under age 40. The yearly incidence is around 4 per 100,000 and remarkably similar throughout the world.

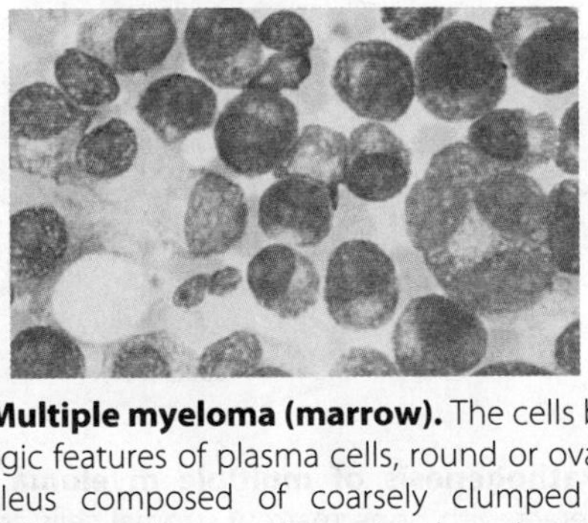

FIGURE 106-2 Multiple myeloma (marrow). The cells bear characteristic morphologic features of plasma cells, round or oval cells with an eccentric nucleus composed of coarsely clumped chromatin, a densely basophilic cytoplasm, and a perinuclear clear zone (hof) containing the Golgi apparatus. Binucleate and multinucleate malignant plasma cells can be seen.

TABLE 106-1 CLINICAL FEATURES OF MULTIPLE MYELOMA

Clinical Finding	Underlying Cause and Pathogenetic Mechanism
Hypercalcemia, osteoporosis, pathologic fractures, lytic bone lesions, bone pain	Tumor expansion, production of osteoclast activating factor by tumor cells, osteoblast inhibitory factors
Renal failure	Hypercalcemia, light chain deposition, amyloidosis, urate nephropathy, drug toxicity (nonsteroidal anti-inflammatory agents, bisphosphonates), contrast dye
Easy fatigue—anemia	Bone marrow infiltration, production of inhibitory factors, hemolysis, decreased red cell production, decreased erythropoietin levels
Recurrent infections	Hypogammaglobulinemia, low CD4 count, decreased neutrophil migration
Neurologic symptoms	Hyperviscosity, cryoglobulinemia, amyloid deposits, hypercalcemia, nerve compression, anti-neuronal antibody, POEMS syndrome, therapy-related toxicity
Nausea and vomiting	Renal failure, hypercalcemia
Bleeding/clotting disorder	Interference with clotting factors, antibody to clotting factors, amyloid damage of endothelium, platelet dysfunction, antibody coating of platelet, therapy-related hypercoagulable defects

Note: POEMS, polyneuropathy, organomegaly, endocrinopathy, multiple myeloma, and skin changes.

Males are more commonly affected than females, and blacks have nearly twice the incidence of whites. Myeloma accounts for ~1% of all malignancies in whites and 2% in blacks; 13% of all hematologic cancers in whites and 33% in blacks.

The incidence of myeloma is highest in African-American and Pacific islanders; intermediate in Europeans and North American Caucasians; and lowest in developing countries including Asia. The higher incidence in more developed countries may result from the combination of a longer life expectancy and more frequent medical surveillance. Incidence of multiple myeloma in other ethnic groups including native Hawaiians, female Hispanics, American Indians from New Mexico, and Alaskan natives is higher relative to U.S. Caucasians in the same geographic area. Chinese and Japanese populations have a lower incidence than Caucasians. Immunoproliferative small intestinal disease with alpha heavy chain disease is most prevalent in the Mediterranean area. Despite these differences in prevalence, the characteristics, response to therapy, and prognosis of myeloma are similar worldwide.

PATHOGENESIS AND CLINICAL MANIFESTATIONS

(Table 106-1) Multiple myeloma (MM) cells bind via cell-surface adhesion molecules to bone marrow stromal cells (BMSCs) and extracellular matrix (ECM), which triggers MM cell growth, survival, drug resistance, and migration in the bone marrow milieu (Fig. 106-3). These effects are due both to direct MM cell–BMSC binding and to induction of various cytokines including IL-6, insulin-like growth factor-1 (IGF-1), vascular endothelial growth factor (VEGF), and stromal cell–derived growth factor (SDF)-1α. Growth, drug resistance, and migration are mediated via Ras/Raf/mitogen-activated protein kinase, PI3-K/Akt, and protein kinase C signaling cascades, respectively.

Bone pain is the most common symptom in myeloma, affecting nearly 70% of patients. The pain usually involves the back and ribs, and unlike the pain of metastatic carcinoma, which often is worse at night, the pain of myeloma is precipitated by movement. Persistent localized pain in a patient with myeloma usually signifies a pathologic fracture. The bone lesions of myeloma are caused by the proliferation of tumor cells, activation of osteoclasts that destroy bone, and suppression of osteoblasts that form new bone. The osteoclasts respond to osteoclast activating factors (OAF) made by the myeloma cells [OAF activity can be mediated by several cytokines, including IL-1, lymphotoxin, VEGF, receptor activator of NF-κB (RANK) ligand, macrophage inhibitory factor (MIP)-1α, and tumor necrosis factor (TNF)]. However, production of these factors decreases following administration of glucocorticoids or interferon (IFN) α. The bone lesions are lytic in nature and are rarely associated with osteoblastic new bone formation. Therefore, radioisotopic bone scanning is less useful in diagnosis than is plain radiography. The bony lysis results in substantial mobilization

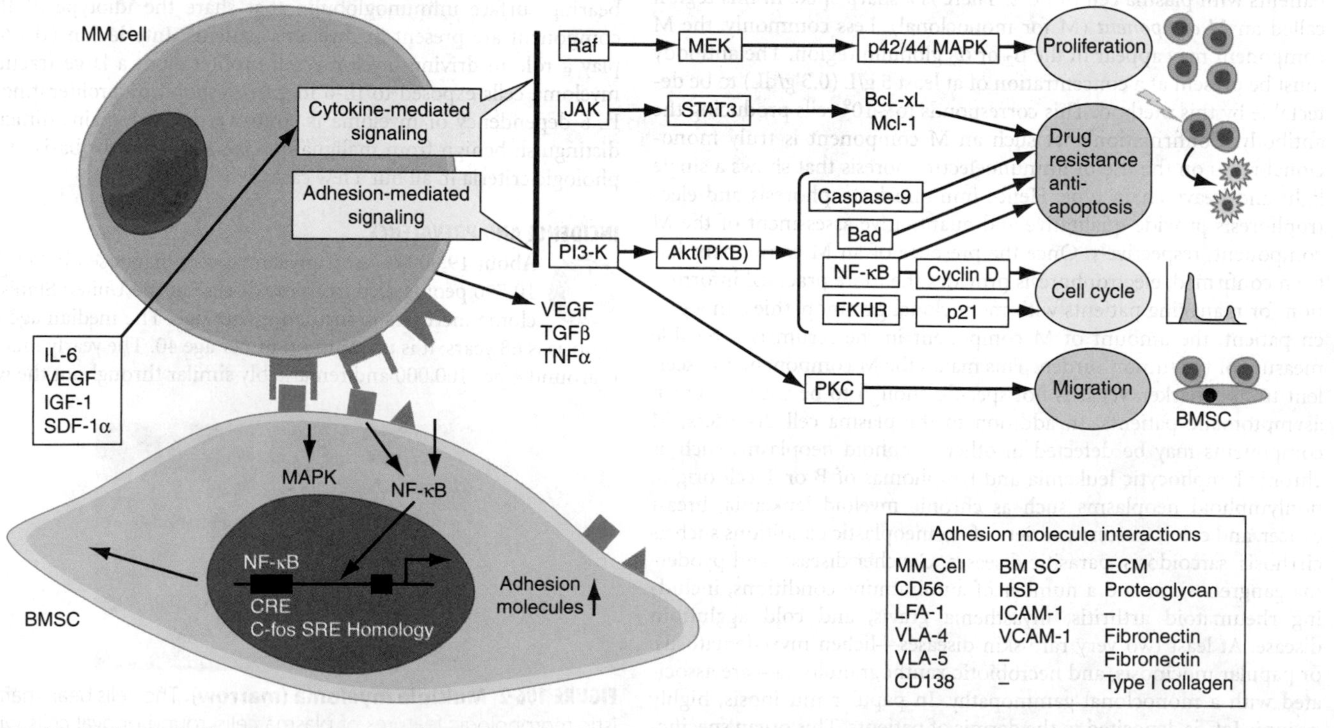

FIGURE 106-3 Pathogenesis of multiple myeloma. Multiple myeloma cells interact with bone marrow stromal cells and extracellular matrix proteins via adhesion molecules, triggering adhesion-mediated signaling as well as cytokine production. This triggers cytokine-mediated signaling that provides growth, survival, and anti-apoptotic effects as well as development of drug resistance. HSP, heparin sulfate proteoglycan.

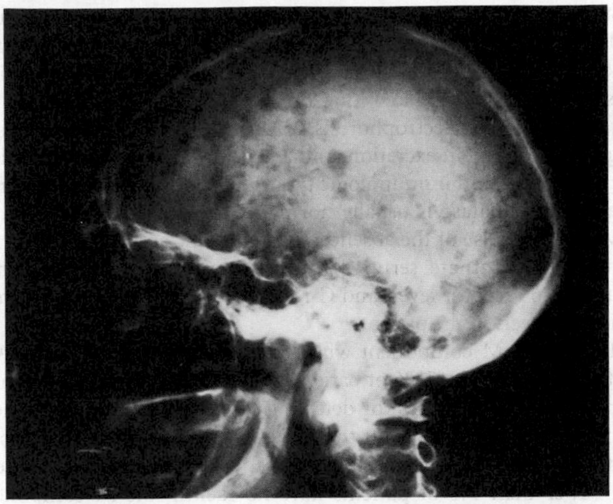

FIGURE 106-4 Bony lesions in multiple myeloma. The skull demonstrates the typical "punched out" lesions characteristic of multiple myeloma. The lesion represents a purely osteolytic lesion with little or no osteoblastic activity. *(Courtesy of Dr. Geraldine Schechter; with permission.)*

of calcium from bone, and serious acute and chronic complications of hypercalcemia may dominate the clinical picture (see below). Localized bone lesions may expand to the point that mass lesions may be palpated, especially on the skull (Fig. 106-4), clavicles, and sternum, and the collapse of vertebrae may lead to spinal cord compression.

The next most common clinical problem in patients with myeloma is susceptibility to bacterial infections. The most common infections are pneumonias and pyelonephritis, and the most frequent pathogens are *Streptococcus pneumoniae*, *Staphylococcus aureus*, and *Klebsiella pneumoniae* in the lungs and *Escherichia coli* and other gram-negative organisms in the urinary tract. In ~25% of patients, recurrent infections are the presenting features, and >75% of patients will have a serious infection at some time in their course. The susceptibility to infection has several contributing causes. First, patients with myeloma have diffuse hypogammaglobulinemia if the M component is excluded. The hypogammaglobulinemia is related to both decreased production and increased destruction of normal antibodies. Moreover, some patients generate a population of circulating regulatory cells in response to their myeloma that can suppress normal antibody synthesis. In the case of IgG myeloma, normal IgG antibodies are broken down more rapidly than normal because the catabolic rate for IgG antibodies varies directly with the serum concentration. The large M component results in fractional catabolic rates of 8–16% instead of the normal 2%. These patients have very poor antibody responses, especially to polysaccharide antigens such as those on bacterial cell walls. Most measures of T cell function in myeloma are normal, but a subset of CD4+ cells may be decreased. Granulocyte lysozyme content is low, and granulocyte migration is not as rapid as normal in patients with myeloma, probably the result of a tumor product. There are also a variety of abnormalities in complement functions in myeloma patients. All these factors contribute to the immune deficiency of these patients. Some commonly used therapeutic agents, e.g., dexamethasone, suppress immune responses and increase susceptibility to infection.

Renal failure occurs in nearly 25% of myeloma patients, and some renal pathology is noted in over half. Many factors contribute to this. Hypercalcemia is the most common cause of renal failure. Glomerular deposits of amyloid, hyperuricemia, recurrent infections, frequent use of nonsteroidal anti-inflammatory agents for pain control, use of iodinated contrast dye for imaging, bisphosphonate use, and occasional infiltration of the kidney by myeloma cells all may contribute to renal dysfunction. However, tubular damage associated with the excretion of light chains is almost always present. Normally, light chains are filtered, reabsorbed in the tubules, and catabolized. With the increase in the amount of light chains presented to the tubule, the tubular cells become overloaded with these proteins, and tubular damage results either directly from light chain toxic effects or indirectly from the release of intracellular lysosomal enzymes. The earliest manifestation of this tubular damage is the adult Fanconi syndrome (a type 2 proximal renal tubular acidosis), with loss of glucose and amino acids, as well as defects in the ability of the kidney to acidify and concentrate the urine. The proteinuria is not accompanied by hypertension, and the protein is nearly all light chains. Generally, very little albumin is in the urine because glomerular function is usually normal. When the glomeruli are involved, nonselective proteinuria is also observed. Patients with myeloma also have a decreased anion gap [i.e., $Na^+ - (Cl^- + HCO_3^-)$] because the M component is cationic, resulting in retention of chloride. This is often accompanied by hyponatremia that is felt to be artificial (pseudohyponatremia) because each volume of serum has less water as a result of the increased protein. Renal dysfunction due to light chain deposition disease, light chain cast nephropathy, and amyloidosis is partially reversible with effective therapy. Myeloma patients are susceptible to developing acute renal failure if they become dehydrated.

Anemia occurs in ~80% of myeloma patients. It is usually normocytic and normochromic and related both to the replacement of normal marrow by expanding tumor cells and to the inhibition of hematopoiesis by factors made by the tumor. In addition, mild hemolysis may contribute to the anemia. A larger than expected fraction of patients may have megaloblastic anemia due to either folate or vitamin B_{12} deficiency. Granulocytopenia and thrombocytopenia are very rare. Clotting abnormalities may be seen due to the failure of antibody-coated platelets to function properly or to the interaction of the M component with clotting factors I, II, V, VII, or VIII. Deep venous thrombosis is also observed with use of thalidomide or lenalidomide in combination with dexamethasone. Raynaud's phenomenon and impaired circulation may result if the M component forms cryoglobulins, and hyperviscosity syndromes may develop depending on the physical properties of the M component (most common with IgM, IgG3, and IgA paraproteins). Hyperviscosity is defined on the basis of the relative viscosity of serum as compared with water. Normal relative serum viscosity is 1.8 (i.e., serum is normally almost twice as viscous as water). Symptoms of hyperviscosity occur at a level of 5–6, a level usually reached at paraprotein concentrations of ~40 g/L (4 g/dL) for IgM, 50 g/L (5 g/dL) for IgG3, and 70 g/L (7 g/dL) for IgA.

Although neurologic symptoms occur in a minority of patients, they may have many causes. Hypercalcemia may produce lethargy, weakness, depression, and confusion. Hyperviscosity may lead to headache, fatigue, visual disturbances, and retinopathy. Bony damage and collapse may lead to cord compression, radicular pain, and loss of bowel and bladder control. Infiltration of peripheral nerves by amyloid can be a cause of carpal tunnel syndrome and other sensorimotor mono- and polyneuropathies. Sensory neuropathy is also a side effect of thalidomide and bortezomib therapy.

Many of the clinical features of myeloma, e.g., cord compression, pathologic fractures, hyperviscosity, sepsis, and hypercalcemia, can present as medical emergencies. Despite the widespread distribution of plasma cells in the body, tumor expansion is dominantly within bone and bone marrow and, for reasons unknown, rarely causes enlargement of spleen, lymph nodes, or gut-associated lymphatic tissue.

DIAGNOSIS AND STAGING

The classic triad of myeloma is marrow plasmacytosis (>10%), lytic bone lesions, and a serum and/or urine M component. Bone marrow plasma cells are CD138+ and monoclonal. The most important differential diagnosis in patients with myeloma involves their separation from individuals with monoclonal gammopathies of uncertain significance (MGUS). MGUS are vastly more common than myeloma, occurring in 1% of the population over age 50 and in up to 10% individuals over age 75. The diagnostic criteria for MGUS, smoldering myeloma, and myeloma are described in Table 106-2. When bone marrow cells are exposed to radioactive thymidine in order to quantitate dividing cells, patients with MGUS always have a labeling index < 1%; patients with myeloma always have a labeling index > 1%. With long-term follow-up, ~1% per year of patients with MGUS go on to

TABLE 106-2 DIAGNOSTIC CRITERIA FOR MULTIPLE MYELOMA, MYELOMA VARIANTS, AND MONOCLONAL GAMMOPATHY OF UNKNOWN SIGNIFICANCE

Monoclonal gammopathy of undetermined significance (MGUS)
M protein in serum < 30 g/L
Bone marrow clonal plasma cells < 10%
No evidence of other B cell proliferative disorders
No myeloma-related organ or tissue impairment (no end organ damage, including bone lesions)[a]
Asymptomatic myeloma (smouldering myeloma)
M protein in serum ≥ 30 g/L *and/or*
Bone marrow clonal plasma cells ≥ 10%
No myeloma-related organ or tissue impairment (no end organ damage, including bone lesions)[a] or symptoms
Symptomatic multiple myeloma
M protein in serum and/or urine
Bone marrow (clonal) plasma cells[b] or plasmacytoma
Myeloma-related organ or tissue impairment (end organ damage, including bone lesions)
Nonsecretory myeloma
No M protein in serum and/or urine with immunofixation
Bone marrow clonal plasmacytosis ≥ 10% or plasmacytoma
Myeloma-related organ or tissue impairment (end organ damage, including bone lesions)[a]
Solitary plasmacytoma of bone
No M protein in serum and/or urine[c]
Single area of bone destruction due to clonal plasma cells
Bone marrow not consistent with multiple myeloma
Normal skeletal survey (and MRI of spine and pelvis if done)
No related organ or tissue impairment (no end organ damage other than solitary bone lesion)[a]

[a]Myeloma-related organ or tissue impairment (end organ damage) (ROTI): Calcium levels increased: serum calcium > 0.25 mmol/L above the upper limit of normal or > 2.75 mmol/L; renal insufficiency: creatinine > 173 mmol/L; anemia: hemoglobin 2 g/dL below the lower limit of normal or hemoglobin < 10 g/dL; bone lesions: lytic lesions or osteoporosis with compression fractures (MRI or CT may clarify); other: symptomatic hyperviscosity, amyloidosis, recurrent bacterial infections (>2 episodes in 12 months).

[b]If flow cytometry is performed, most plasma cells (>90%) will show a "neoplastic" phenotype.

[c]A small M component may sometimes be present.

develop myeloma. Non-IgG subtype, abnormal kappa/lambda free light chain ratio, and serum M protein > 15 g/L (1.5 g/dL) are associated with higher incidence of progression of MGUS to myeloma. Typically, patients with MGUS require no therapy. Their survival is ~2 years shorter than age-matched controls without MGUS. There are two important variants of myeloma, solitary bone plasmacytoma and extramedullary plasmacytoma. These lesions are associated with an M component in <30% of the cases, they may affect younger individuals, and both are associated with median survivals of ≥10 years. Solitary bone plasmacytoma is a single lytic bone lesion without marrow plasmacytosis. Extramedullary plasmacytomas usually involve the submucosal lymphoid tissue of the nasopharynx or paranasal sinuses without marrow plasmacytosis. Both tumors are highly responsive to local radiation therapy. If an M component is present, it should disappear after treatment. Solitary bone plasmacytomas may recur in other bony sites or evolve into myeloma. Extramedullary plasmacytomas rarely recur or progress.

The clinical evaluation of patients with myeloma includes a careful physical examination searching for tender bones and masses. Only a small minority of patients has an enlargement of the spleen and lymph nodes, the physiologic sites of antibody production. Chest and bone radiographs may reveal lytic lesions or diffuse osteopenia. MRI offers a sensitive means to document extent of bone marrow infiltration and cord or root compression in patients with pain syndromes. A complete blood count with differential may reveal anemia. Erythrocyte sedimentation rate is elevated. Rare patients (~2%) may have plasma cell leukemia with >2000 plasma cells/μL. This may be seen in disproportionate frequency in IgD (12%) and IgE (25%) myelomas. Serum calcium, urea nitrogen, creatinine, and uric acid levels may be elevated. Protein electrophoresis and measurement of serum immunoglobulins and free light chains are useful for detecting and characterizing M spikes, supplemented by immunoelectrophoresis, which is especially sensitive for identifying low concentrations of M components not detectable by protein electrophoresis. A 24-h urine specimen is necessary to quantitate protein excretion, and a concentrated aliquot is used for electrophoresis and immunologic typing of any M component. Serum alkaline phosphatase is usually normal even with extensive bone involvement because of the absence of osteoblastic activity. It is also important to quantitate serum β_2-microglobulin (see below). Serum soluble IL-6 receptor levels and C-reactive protein may reflect physiologic IL-6 levels in the patient.

The serum M component will be IgG in 53% of patients, IgA in 25%, and IgD in 1%; 20% of patients will have only light chains in serum and urine. Dipsticks for detecting proteinuria are not reliable at identifying light chains, and the heat test for detecting Bence Jones protein is falsely negative in ~50% of patients with light chain myeloma. Fewer than 1% of patients have no identifiable M component; these patients usually have light chain myeloma in which renal catabolism has made the light chains undetectable in the urine. IgD myeloma may also present as light chain myeloma. About two-thirds of patients with serum M components also have urinary light chains. The light chain isotype may have an impact on survival. Patients secreting lambda light chains have a significantly shorter overall survival than those secreting kappa light chains. It is not clear whether this is due to some genetically important determinant of cell proliferation or because lambda light chains are more likely to cause renal damage and form amyloid than are kappa light chains. The heavy chain isotype may have an impact on patient management as well. About half of patients with IgM paraproteins develop hyperviscosity compared with only 2–4% of patients with IgA and IgG M components. Among IgG myelomas, it is the IgG3 subclass that has the highest tendency to form both concentration- and temperature-dependent aggregates, leading to hyperviscosity and cold agglutination at lower serum concentrations.

The various staging systems for patients with myeloma (Table 106-3) are functional systems for predicting survival and are based on a variety of clinical and laboratory tests, unlike the anatomic staging systems for solid tumors. The Durie-Salmon staging system is based on the hemoglobin, calcium, M component, and degree of skeletal involvement; the total-body tumor burden is estimated to be low (stage I), intermediate (stage II), or high (stage III), and the stages are further subdivided on the basis of renal function [A if serum creatinine <177 mol/L (<2 mg/dL), B if >177 (>2)]. Patients in stage IA have a median survival of >5 years and those in stage IIIB about 15 months. This staging system has been found not to predict prognosis after treatment with high-dose therapy or the novel targeted therapies that have emerged.

Serum β_2-microglobulin is a protein of 11,000 mol wt with homologies with the constant region of immunoglobulins that is the light chain of the class I major histocompatibility antigens (HLA-A, -B, -C) on the surface of every cell. Serum β_2-microglobulin is the single most powerful predictor of survival and can substitute for staging. Patients with β_2-microglobulin levels <0.004 g/L have a median survival of 43 months and those with levels >0.004 g/L only 12 months. Serum β_2-microglobulin and albumin levels are the basis for a three-stage International Staging System (ISS). It is also felt that once the diagnosis of myeloma is firm, histologic features of atypia may also exert an influence on prognosis. IL-6 may be an autocrine and/or paracrine growth factor for myeloma cells; elevated levels are associated with more aggressive disease. High labeling index and high levels of lactate dehydrogenase are also associated with poor prognosis.

Other factors that may influence prognosis are the number of cytogenetic abnormalities including hyperploidy, chromosome 13q and 17p deletion, t(4;14) and t(11;14); % plasma cells in the marrow; circulating plasma cells; performance status; as well as serum levels of soluble IL-6 receptor, C-reactive protein, hepatocyte growth factor, C-terminal cross-linked telopeptide of collagen I, transforming growth factor (TGF) β, and syndecan-1. Microarray profiling and comparative genomic hybridization have formed the basis for RNA- and DNA-

TABLE 106-3 MYELOMA STAGING SYSTEMS

Durie-Salmon Staging System

Stage	Criteria	Estimated Tumor Burden, $\times 10^{12}$ cells/m^2
I	All of the following: 1. Hemoglobin >100 g/L (>10 g/dL) 2. Serum calcium <3 mmol/L (<12 mg/dL) 3. Normal bone x-ray or solitary lesion 4. Low M-component production a. IgG level <50 g/L (<5 g/dL) b. IgA level <30 g/L (<3 g/dL) c. Urine light chain <4 g/24 h	<0.6 (low)
II	Fitting neither I nor III	0.6–1.20 (intermediate)
III	One or more of the following: 1. Hemoglobin <85 g/L (<8.5 g/dL) 2. Serum calcium >3 mmol/L (>12 mg/dL) 3. Advanced lytic bone lesions 4. High M-component production a. IgG level >70 g/L (>7 g/dL) b. IgA level >50 g/L (>5 g/dL) c. Urine light chains >12 g/24 h	>1.20 (high)

Level	Stage	Median Survival, Months
Subclassification based on serum creatinine levels		
A < 177 μmol/L (<2 mg/dL)	IA	61
B > 177 μmol/L (>2 mg/dL)	IIA, B	55
	IIIA	30
	IIIB	15
International Staging System		
β_2M < 3.5, alb ≥ 3.5	I (28%)	62
β_2M < 3.5, alb < 3.5 *or* β_2M = 3.5–5.5	II (39%)	44
β_2M > 5.5	III (33%)	29

Note: β_2M, serum β_2-microglobulin in mg/L; alb, serum albumin in g/dL; (#), % patients presenting at each stage.

based prognostic staging systems, respectively. The ISS system is the most widely used method of assessing prognosis (Table 106-3).

℞ MULTIPLE MYELOMA

About 10% of patients with myeloma will have an indolent course demonstrating only very slow progression of disease over many years. Such patients only require antitumor therapy when the disease becomes symptomatic with development of anemia, hypercalcemia, progressive lytic bone lesions (including vertebral compression fractures), progressive rise in serum myeloma protein levels and/or Bence Jones proteinuria, or recurrent infections. Patients with solitary bone plasmacytomas and extramedullary plasmacytomas may be expected to enjoy prolonged disease-free survival after local radiation therapy to a dose of around 40 Gy. There is a low incidence of occult marrow involvement in patients with solitary bone plasmacytoma. Such patients are usually detected because their serum M component falls slowly or disappears initially only to return after a few months. These patients respond well to systemic chemotherapy.

Patients with symptomatic and/or progressive myeloma require therapeutic intervention. In general such therapy is of two sorts: systemic therapy to control the progression of myeloma, and symptomatic supportive care to prevent serious morbidity from the complications of the disease. Therapy can significantly prolong survival and improve the quality of life for myeloma patients.

The initial standard treatment for newly diagnosed myeloma is dependent on whether or not the patient is a candidate for high-dose chemotherapy with autologous stem cell transplant.

In patients who are transplant candidates, alkylating agents such as melphalan should be avoided since they damage stem cells, leading to decreased ability to collect stem cells for autologous transplant. High-dose pulsed glucocorticoids have been used either alone (dexamethasone 40 mg for 4 days every 2 weeks) or in combination VAD chemotherapy (vincristine, 0.4 mg/d in a 4-day continuous infusion; doxorubicin, 9 mg/m^2 per day in a 4-day continuous infusion; dexamethasone, 40 mg/d for 4 days per week for 3 weeks) for initial cytoreduction. However, two studies have combined thalidomide with dexamethasone as initial therapy for newly diagnosed multiple myeloma in transplant candidates and reported rapid responses in two-thirds of patients, while allowing for successful harvesting of peripheral blood stem cells for transplantation. A randomized phase III trial showed statistically significantly higher response rates for thalidomide (200 mg PO qhs) plus dexamethasone (40 mg for 4 days every 2 weeks) compared to dexamethasone alone, setting the stage for use of this combination as standard therapy in newly diagnosed patients. Initial therapy is continued until maximal cytoreduction. Importantly, novel agents bortezomib, a proteasome inhibitor, and lenalidomide, an immunomodulatory derivative of thalidomide, have similarly been combined with dexamethasone and obtained high response rates without compromising collection of stem cells for transplantation.

In patients who are not transplant candidates, therapy has consisted of intermittent pulses of an alkylating agent, L-phenylalanine mustard (L-PAM, melphalan) and prednisone administered for 4–7 days every 4–6 weeks. The usual doses of melphalan/prednisone (MP) are melphalan, 8 mg/m^2 per day, and prednisone, 25–60 mg/m^2 per day for 4 days. Doses may need adjustment due to unpredictable absorption and based on marrow tolerance. Patients responding to therapy generally have a prompt and gratifying reduction in bone pain, hypercalcemia, and anemia, and often have fewer infections. The serum M component lags substantially behind the symptomatic improvement, often taking 4–6 weeks to fall. This fall depends on the rate of tumor kill and the fractional catabolic rate of immunoglobulin, which in turn depends on the serum concentration (for IgG). Light chain excretion, with a functional half-life of ~6 h, may fall within the first week of treatment. However, since urine light chain levels may relate to renal tubular function, they are not a reliable measure of tumor cell kill. Calculations of tumor cell kill are made by extrapolation of the serum M component level and rely heavily on the assumption that every tumor cell produces immunoglobulin at a constant rate. About 60% of patients will achieve at least a 75% reduction in serum M component level and tumor cell mass in response to melphalan and prednisone. Although this is a tumor reduction of <1 log, clinical responses may last many months. The important feature of the level of the M protein is not how far or how fast it falls, but the rate of its increase after therapy. Efforts to improve the fraction of patients responding and the degree of response have involved adding other active agents to the treatment program. In patients >65 years, combining thalidomide with MP (MPT) obtains higher response rates and overall survival than MP alone, and MPT is the standard therapy for patients who are not transplant candidates.

Randomized studies comparing standard-dose therapy to high-dose melphalan therapy (HDT) with hematopoietic stem cell support have shown that HDT can achieve high overall response rates and prolonged progression-free and overall survival; however, few, if any, patients are cured. Although complete responses are rare (<5%) with standard-dose chemotherapy, HDT achieves 25–40% complete responses. In randomized studies, HDT produced better median event-free survival in four of five studies, higher complete response rate in four of five trials, and better overall survival in three of five studies. Two successive HDTs (tandem transplants) are more effective than single HDT in the subset of patients who do not achieve a complete or very good partial response to the first transplant. Allogeneic transplants may also produce high response rates, but treatment-related mortality may be as high as 40%. Non-myeloablative allogeneic transplantation is now under evaluation to reduce toxicity, while permitting an immune graft-vs.-myeloma effect.

There is no standard maintenance therapy to prolong time to progression. IFN-α has allowed modest benefit but has significant side effects. Oral prednisone maintenance therapy was effective in a single trial. Ongoing studies are evaluating maintenance thalidomide and lenalidomide to prolong progression-free survival post-transplant.

Relapsed myeloma can be treated with novel agents including lenalidomide and/or bortezomib. These agents target not only the tumor cell but also the tumor cell–bone marrow interaction and the bone marrow milieu. These agents in combination with dexamethasone can achieve up to 60% partial responses and 10–15% complete responses in patients with relapsed disease. The combination of bortezomib and liposomal doxorubicin is active in relapsed myeloma. Thalidomide, if not used as initial therapy, can achieve responses in refractory cases. High-dose melphalan and stem cell transplant, if not used earlier, also have activity in patients with refractory disease.

The median overall survival of patients with myeloma is 5–6 years, with subsets of patients surviving over 10 years. The major causes of death are progressive myeloma, renal failure, sepsis, or therapy-related acute leukemia or myelodysplasia. Nearly a quarter of patients die of myocardial infarction, chronic lung disease, diabetes, or stroke, all intercurrent illnesses related more to the age of the patient group than to the tumor.

Supportive care directed at the anticipated complications of the disease may be as important as primary antitumor therapy. The hypercalcemia generally responds well to bisphosphonates, glucocorticoid therapy, hydration, and natriuresis. Calcitonin may add to the inhibitory effects of glucocorticoids on bone resorption. Bisphosphonates (e.g., pamidronate 90 mg or zoledronate 4 mg once a month) reduce osteoclastic bone resorption and preserve performance status and quality of life, decrease bone-related complications, and may also have antitumor effects. Treatments aimed at strengthening the skeleton, such as fluorides, calcium, and vitamin D, with or without androgens, have been suggested but are not of proven efficacy. Iatrogenic worsening of renal function may be prevented by maintaining a high fluid intake to prevent dehydration and to help excrete light chains and calcium. In the event of acute renal failure, plasmapheresis is ~10 times more effective at clearing light chains than peritoneal dialysis; however, its role in reversing renal failure remains controversial. Importantly, reducing the protein load by effective antitumor therapy with agents such as bortezomib may result in functional improvement. Urinary tract infections should be watched for and treated early. Plasmapheresis may be the treatment of choice for hyperviscosity syndromes. Although the pneumococcus is a dreaded pathogen in myeloma patients, pneumococcal polysaccharide vaccines may not elicit an antibody response. Prophylactic administration of IV γ globulin preparations is used in the setting of recurrent serious infections. Chronic oral antibiotic prophylaxis is probably not warranted. Patients developing neurologic symptoms in the lower extremities, severe localized back pain, or problems with bowel and bladder control may need emergency MRI and radiation therapy for palliation. Most bone lesions respond to analgesics and chemotherapy, but certain painful lesions may respond most promptly to localized radiation. The anemia associated with myeloma may respond to erythropoietin along with hematinics (iron, folate, cobalamin). The pathogenesis of the anemia should be established and specific therapy instituted, where possible.

WALDENSTRÖM'S MACROGLOBULINEMIA

In 1948, Waldenström described a malignancy of lymphoplasmacytoid cells that secreted IgM. In contrast to myeloma, the disease was associated with lymphadenopathy and hepatosplenomegaly, but the major clinical manifestation was the hyperviscosity syndrome. The disease resembles the related diseases chronic lymphocytic leukemia, myeloma, and lymphocytic lymphoma. It originates from a post–germinal center B cell that has undergone somatic mutations and antigenic selection in the lymphoid follicle and has the characteristics of an IgM-bearing memory B cell. Waldenström's macroglobulinemia and IgM myeloma follow a similar clinical course, but therapeutic options are different. The diagnosis of IgM myeloma is usually reserved for patients with lytic bone lesions and predominant infiltration with CD138+ plasma cells in the bone marrow. Such patients are at greater risk of pathologic fractures than patients with Waldenström's macroglobulinemia.

The cause of macroglobulinemia is unknown. The disease is similar to myeloma in being slightly more common in men and occurring with increased incidence with age (median 64 years). There have been reports that the IgM in some patients with macroglobulinemia may have specificity for myelin-associated glycoprotein (MAG), a protein that has been associated with demyelinating disease of the peripheral nervous system and may be lost earlier and to a greater extent than the better known myelin basic protein in patients with multiple sclerosis. Sometimes patients with macroglobulinemia develop a peripheral neuropathy before the appearance of the neoplasm. There is speculation that the whole process begins with a viral infection that may elicit an antibody response that cross-reacts with a normal tissue component.

Like myeloma, the disease involves the bone marrow, but unlike myeloma, it does not cause bone lesions or hypercalcemia. Like myeloma, a serum M component is present in the serum in excess of 30 g/L (3 g/dL), but unlike myeloma, the size of the IgM paraprotein results in little renal excretion, and only ~20% of patients excrete light chains. Therefore, renal disease is not common. The light chain isotype is kappa in 80% of the cases. Patients present with weakness, fatigue, and recurrent infections, similar to myeloma patients, but epistaxis, visual disturbances, and neurologic symptoms such as peripheral neuropathy, dizziness, headache, and transient paresis are much more common in macroglobulinemia. Physical examination reveals adenopathy and hepatosplenomegaly, and ophthalmoscopic examination may reveal vascular segmentation and dilatation of the retinal veins characteristic of hyperviscosity states. Patients may have a normocytic, normochromic anemia, but rouleaux formation and a positive Coombs' test are much more common than in myeloma. Malignant lymphocytes are usually present in the peripheral blood. About 10% of macroglobulins are cryoglobulins. These are pure M components and are not the mixed cryoglobulins seen in rheumatoid arthritis and other autoimmune diseases. Mixed cryoglobulins are composed of IgM or IgA complexed with IgG, for which they are specific. In both cases, Raynaud's phenomenon and serious vascular symptoms precipitated by the cold may occur, but mixed cryoglobulins are not commonly associated with malignancy. Patients suspected of having a cryoglobulin based on history and physical examination should have their blood drawn into a warm syringe and delivered to the laboratory in a container of warm water to avoid errors in quantitating the cryoglobulin.

℞ WALDENSTRÖM'S MACROGLOBULINEMIA

Control of serious hyperviscosity symptoms such as an altered state of consciousness or paresis can be achieved acutely by plasmapheresis because 80% of the IgM paraprotein is intravascular. The median survival is ~50 months, similar to that of multiple myeloma. However, many individuals with Waldenström's macroglobulinemia have indolent disease that does not require therapy. Pretreatment parameters including older age, male sex, general symptoms, and cytopenias define a high-risk population. Fludarabine (25 mg/m^2 per day for 5 days every 4 weeks) or cladribine (0.1 mg/kg per day for 7 days every 4 weeks) are highly effective single agents. About 80% of patients respond to chemotherapy, and their median survival is >3 years. Rituximab (anti-CD20) can produce responses alone or combined with chemotherapy. As in multiple myeloma, bortezomib and lenalidomide also have activity.

POEMS SYNDROME

The features of this syndrome are *p*olyneuropathy, *o*rganomegaly, *e*ndocrinopathy, *m*ultiple myeloma, and *s*kin changes (POEMS). Patients usually have a severe, progressive sensorimotor polyneuropathy associated with sclerotic bone lesions from myeloma. Polyneuropathy occurs in ~1.4% of myelomas, but the POEMS syndrome is only a rare subset of that group. Unlike typical myeloma, hepatomegaly and lymphadenopathy occur in about two-thirds of patients, and splenomegaly is seen in one-third. The lymphadenopathy frequently resembles Castleman's disease histologically, a condition that has been linked to IL-6 overproduction. The endocrine manifestations include amenorrhea in women and impotence and gynecomastia in men. Hyperprolactinemia due to loss of normal inhibitory control by the hypothalamus may be associated with other central nervous system manifestations such as papilledema and elevated cerebrospinal fluid pressure and protein. Type 2 diabetes mellitus occurs in about one-third of patients. Hypothyroidism and adrenal insufficiency are occasionally noted. Skin changes are diverse: hyperpigmentation, hypertrichosis, skin thickening, and digital clubbing. Other manifestations include peripheral edema, ascites, pleural effusions, fever, and thrombocytosis.

The pathogenesis of the disease is unclear, but high circulating levels of the proinflammatory cytokines IL-1, IL-6, VEGF, and TNF have been documented and levels of the inhibitory cytokine TGF-β are lower than expected. Treatment of the myeloma may result in an improvement in the other disease manifestations.

Patients are often treated similarly to those with myeloma. Plasmapheresis does not appear to be of benefit in POEMS syndrome. Patients presenting with isolated sclerotic lesions may have resolution of neuropathic symptoms after local therapy for plasmacytoma with radiotherapy. Similar to multiple myeloma, novel agents as well as high-dose therapy with autologous stem cell transplant have been pursued in selected patients and have been associated with prolonged progression-free survival.

HEAVY CHAIN DISEASES

The heavy chain diseases are rare lymphoplasmacytic malignancies. Their clinical manifestations vary with the heavy chain isotype. Patients secrete a defective heavy chain that usually has an intact Fc fragment and a deletion in the Fd region. Gamma, alpha, and mu heavy chain diseases have been described, but no reports of delta or epsilon heavy chain diseases have appeared. Molecular biologic analysis of these tumors has revealed structural genetic defects that may account for the aberrant chain secreted.

GAMMA HEAVY CHAIN DISEASE (FRANKLIN'S DISEASE)

This disease affects individuals of widely different age groups and countries of origin. It is characterized by lymphadenopathy, fever, anemia, malaise, hepatosplenomegaly, and weakness. Its most distinctive symptom is palatal edema, resulting from involvement of nodes in Waldeyer's ring, and this may progress to produce respiratory compromise. The diagnosis depends on the demonstration of an anomalous serum M component [often <20 g/L (<2 g/dL)] that reacts with anti-IgG but not anti-light chain reagents. *The M component is typically present in both serum and urine.* Most of the paraproteins have been of the $gamma_1$ subclass, but other subclasses have been seen. The patients may have thrombocytopenia, eosinophilia, and nondiagnostic bone marrow. Patients usually have a rapid downhill course and die of infection; however, some patients have survived 5 years with chemotherapy.

ALPHA HEAVY CHAIN DISEASE (SELIGMANN'S DISEASE)

This is the most common of the heavy chain diseases. It is closely related to a malignancy known as *Mediterranean lymphoma*, a disease that affects young persons in parts of the world where intestinal parasites are common, such as the Mediterranean, Asia, and South America. The disease is characterized by an infiltration of the lamina propria of the small intestine with lymphoplasmacytoid cells that secrete truncated alpha chains. Demonstrating alpha heavy chains is difficult because the alpha chains tend to polymerize and appear as a smear instead of a sharp peak on electrophoretic profiles. Despite the polymerization, hyperviscosity is not a common problem in alpha heavy chain disease. Without J chain–facilitated dimerization, viscosity does not increase dramatically. Light chains are absent from serum and urine. The patients present with chronic diarrhea, weight loss, and malabsorption and have extensive mesenteric and paraaortic adenopathy. Respiratory tract involvement occurs rarely. Patients may vary widely in their clinical course. Some may develop diffuse aggressive histologies of malignant lymphoma. Chemotherapy may produce long-term remissions. Rare patients appear to have responded to antibiotic therapy, raising the question of the etiologic role of antigenic stimulation, perhaps by some chronic intestinal infection. Chemotherapy plus antibiotics may be more effective than chemotherapy alone. Immunoproliferative small intestinal disease (IPSID) is recognized as an infectious pathogen–associated human lymphoma that has association with *Campylobacter jejuni*. It involves mainly the proximal small intestine resulting in malabsorption, diarrhea, and abdominal pain. IPSID is associated with excessive plasma cell differentiation and produces truncated alpha heavy chain proteins lacking the light chains as well as the first constant domain. Early-stage IPSID responds to antibiotics (30–70% complete remission). Most untreated IPSID patients progress to lymphoplasmacytic and immunoblastic lymphoma.

MU HEAVY CHAIN DISEASE

The secretion of isolated mu heavy chains into the serum appears to occur in a very rare subset of patients with chronic lymphocytic leukemia. The only features that may distinguish patients with mu heavy chain disease are the presence of vacuoles in the malignant lymphocytes and the excretion of kappa light chains in the urine. The diagnosis requires ultracentrifugation or gel filtration to confirm the nonreactivity of the paraprotein with the light chain reagents, because some intact macroglobulins fail to interact with these serums. The tumor cells seem to have a defect in the assembly of light and heavy chains, because they appear to contain both in their cytoplasm. There is no evidence that such patients should be treated differently from other patients with chronic lymphocytic leukemia (Chap. 105).

FURTHER READINGS

GHOBRIAL IM et al: Waldenström macroglobulinaemia. Lancet Oncol 4:679, 2003

HAROUSSEAU JL, MOREAU P: Evolving role of stem cell transplantation in multiple myeloma. Clin Lymphoma Myeloma 6:89, 2005

HIDESHIMA T et al: Understanding multiple myeloma pathogenesis in the bone marrow to identify new therapeutic targets. Nature Rev Cancer 7:585, 2007

THE INTERNATIONAL MYELOMA WORKING GROUP: Criteria for the classification of monoclonal gammopathies, multiple myeloma and related disorders: A report of the International Myeloma Working Group. Br J Haematol 121:749, 2003

KUEHL WM, BERGSAGEL PL: Multiple myeloma: Evolving genetic events and host interactions. Nature Rev Cancer 2:175, 2002

KYLE RA, RAJKUMAR SV: Multiple myeloma. N Engl J Med 351:1860, 2004

——— et al: Prevalence of monoclonal gammopathy of undetermined significance. N Engl J Med 354:1362, 2006

——— et al: American Society of Clinical Oncology 2007 clinical practice guideline update on the role of bisphosphonates in multiple myeloma. J Clin Oncol 25:2464, 2007

MITSIADES CS et al: Focus on multiple myeloma. Cancer Cell 6:439, 2005

MUNSHI NC, ANDERSON KC: Plasma cell neoplasm, in *Principles and Practice of Oncology*, 7th ed, V DeVita, S Rosenberg, S Hellman (eds). Philadelphia, Lippincott–Raven Publishers, 2005

TREON SP et al: Update on treatment recommendations from the Third International Workshop on Waldenström's macroglobulinemia. Blood 107:3442, 2006

WAHNER-ROEDLER DL et al: Gamma-heavy chain disease: Review of 23 cases. Medicine 82:236, 2003

107 Transfusion Biology and Therapy

Jeffery S. Dzieczkowski, Kenneth C. Anderson

BLOOD GROUP ANTIGENS AND ANTIBODIES

The study of red blood cell (RBC) antigens and antibodies forms the foundation of transfusion medicine. Serologic studies initially characterized these antigens, but now the molecular composition and structure of many are known. Antigens, either carbohydrate or protein, are assigned to a blood group system based on the structure and similarity of the determinant epitopes. Other cellular blood elements and plasma proteins are also antigenic and can result in *alloimmunization*, the production of antibodies directed against the blood group antigens of another individual. These antibodies are called *alloantibodies*.

Antibodies directed against RBC antigens may result from "natural" exposure, particularly to carbohydrates that mimic some blood group antigens. Those antibodies that occur via natural stimuli are usually produced by a T cell–independent response (thus, generating no memory) and are IgM isotype. *Autoantibodies* (antibodies against autologous blood group antigens) arise spontaneously or as the result of infectious sequelae (e.g., from *Mycoplasma pneumoniae*) and are also often IgM. These antibodies are often clinically insignificant due to their low affinity for antigen at body temperature. However, IgM antibodies can activate the complement cascade and result in hemolysis. Antibodies that result from allogeneic exposure, such as transfusion or pregnancy, are usually IgG. IgG antibodies commonly bind to antigen at warmer temperatures and may hemolyze RBCs. Unlike IgM antibodies, IgG antibodies can cross the placenta and bind fetal erythrocytes bearing the corresponding antigen, resulting in hemolytic disease of the newborn, or *hydrops fetalis.*

Alloimmunization to leukocytes, platelets, and plasma proteins may also result in transfusion complications such as fevers and urticaria but generally does not cause hemolysis. Assay for these other alloantibodies is not routinely performed; however, they may be detected using special assays.

ABO ANTIGENS AND ANTIBODIES

The first blood group antigen system, recognized in 1900, was ABO, the most important in transfusion medicine. The major blood groups of this system are A, B, AB, and O. O type RBCs lack A or B antigens. These antigens are carbohydrates attached to a precursor backbone, may be found on the cellular membrane either as glycosphingolipids or glycoproteins, and are secreted into plasma and body fluids as glycoproteins. H substance is the immediate precursor on which the A and B antigens are added. This H substance is formed by the addition of fucose to the glycolipid or glycoprotein backbone. The subsequent addition of *N*-acetylgalactosamine creates the A antigen, while the addition of galactose produces the B antigen.

The genes that determine the A and B phenotypes are found on chromosome 9p and are expressed in a Mendelian codominant manner. The gene products are glycosyl transferases, which confer the enzymatic capability of attaching the specific antigenic carbohydrate. Individuals who lack the "A" and "B" transferases are phenotypically type "O," while those who inherit both transferases are type "AB." Rare individuals lack the H gene, which codes for fucose transferase, and cannot form H substance. These individuals are homozygous for the silent h allele (hh) and have Bombay phenotype (O_h).

The ABO blood group system is important because essentially all individuals produce antibodies to the ABH carbohydrate antigen that they lack. The naturally occurring anti-A and anti-B antibodies are termed *isoagglutinins*. Thus, type A individuals produce anti-B, while type B individuals make anti-A. Neither isoagglutinin is found in type AB individuals, while type O individuals produce both anti-A and anti-B. Thus, persons with type AB are "universal recipients" because they do not have antibodies against any ABO phenotype, while persons with type O blood can donate to essentially all recipients because their cells are not recognized by any ABO isoagglutinins. The rare individuals with Bombay phenotype produce antibodies to H substance (which is present on all red cells except those of hh phenotype) as well as to both A and B antigens and are therefore compatible only with other hh donors.

In most people, A and B antigens are secreted by the cells and are present in the circulation. Nonsecretors are susceptible to a variety of infections (e.g., *Candida albicans, Neisseria meningitidis, Streptococcus pneumoniae, Haemophilus influenzae*) as many organisms may bind to polysaccharides on cells. Soluble blood group antigens may block this binding.

Rh SYSTEM

The Rh system is the second most important blood group system in pretransfusion testing. The Rh antigens are found on a 30- to 32-kDa RBC membrane protein that has no defined function. Although >40 different antigens in the Rh system have been described, five determinants account for the vast majority of phenotypes. The presence of the D antigen confers Rh "positivity," while persons who lack the D antigen are Rh negative. Two allelic antigen pairs, E/e and C/c, are also found on the Rh protein. The three Rh genes, E/e, D, and C/c, are arranged in tandem on chromosome 1 and inherited as a haplotype, i.e., cDE or Cde. Two haplotypes can result in the phenotypic expression of two to five Rh antigens.

The D antigen is a potent alloantigen. About 15% of individuals lack this antigen. Exposure of these Rh-negative people to even small amounts of Rh-positive cells, by either transfusion or pregnancy, can result in the production of anti-D alloantibody.

TABLE 107-1 RBC BLOOD GROUP SYSTEMS AND ALLOANTIGENS

Blood Group System	Antigen	Alloantibody	Clinical Significance
Rh (D, C/c, E/e)	RBC protein	IgG	HTR, HDN
Lewis (Le^a, Le^b)	Oligosaccharide	IgM/IgG	Rare HTR
Kell (K/k)	RBC protein	IgG	HTR, HDN
Duffy (Fy^a/Fy^b)	RBC protein	IgG	HTR, HDN
Kidd (Jk^a/Jk^b)	RBC protein	IgG	HTR (often delayed), HDN (mild)
I/i	Carbohydrate	IgM	None
MNSsU	RBC protein	IgM/IgG	Anti-M rare HDN, anti-S, -s, and -U HDN, HTR

Note: RBC, red blood cell; HDN, hemolytic disease of the newborn; HTR, hemolytic transfusion reaction.

OTHER BLOOD GROUP SYSTEMS AND ALLOANTIBODIES

More than 100 blood group systems are recognized, composed of more than 500 antigens. The presence or absence of certain antigens has been associated with various diseases and anomalies; antigens also act as receptors for infectious agents. Alloantibodies of importance in routine clinical practice are listed in Table 107-1.

Antibodies to *Lewis system* carbohydrate antigens are the most common cause of incompatibility during pretransfusion screening. The Lewis gene product is a fucosyl transferase and maps to chromosome 19. The antigen is not an integral membrane structure but is adsorbed to the RBC membrane from the plasma. Antibodies to Lewis antigens are usually IgM and cannot cross the placenta. Lewis antigens may be adsorbed onto tumor cells and may be targets of therapy.

I system antigens are also oligosaccharides related to H, A, B, and Le. I and i are not allelic pairs but are carbohydrate antigens that differ only in the extent of branching. The i antigen is an unbranched chain that is converted by the I gene product, a glycosyltransferase, into a branched chain. The branching process affects all the ABH antigens, which become progressively more branched in the first 2 years of life. Some patients with cold agglutinin disease or lymphomas can produce anti-I autoantibodies that cause RBC destruction. Occasional patients with mononucleosis or *Mycoplasma* pneumonia may develop cold agglutinins of either anti-I or anti-i specificity. Most adults lack i expression; thus, finding a donor for patients with anti-i is not difficult. Even though most adults express I antigen, binding is generally low at body temperature. Thus, administration of warm blood prevents isoagglutination.

The *P system* is another group of carbohydrate antigens controlled by specific glycosyltransferases. Its clinical significance is in rare cases of syphilis and viral infection that lead to paroxysmal cold hemoglobinuria. In these cases, an unusual autoantibody to P is produced that binds to RBCs in the cold and fixes complement upon warming. Antibodies with these biphasic properties are called *Donath-Landsteiner antibodies*. The P antigen is the cellular receptor of parvovirus B19 and also may be a receptor for *Escherichia coli* binding to urothelial cells.

The *MNSsU system* is regulated by genes on chromosome 4. M and N are determinants on glycophorin A, an RBC membrane protein, and S and s are determinants on glycophorin B. Anti-S and anti-s IgG antibodies may develop after pregnancy or transfusion and lead to hemolysis. Anti-U antibodies are rare but problematic; virtually every donor is incompatible because nearly all persons express U.

The *Kell* protein is very large (720 amino acids), and its secondary structure contains many different antigenic epitopes. The immunogenicity of Kell is third behind the ABO and Rh systems. The absence of the Kell precursor protein (controlled by a gene on X) is associated with acanthocytosis, shortened RBC survival, and a progressive form of muscular dystrophy that includes cardiac defects. This rare condition is called the *McLeod phenotype*. The K_x gene is linked to the 91-kDa component of the NADPH-oxidase on the X chromosome, deletion or mutation of which accounts for about 60% of cases of chronic granulomatous disease.

The *Duffy* antigens are codominant alleles, Fy^a and Fy^b, that also serve as receptors for *Plasmodium vivax*. More than 70% of persons in malaria-endemic areas lack these antigens, probably from selective influences of the infection on the population.

The *Kidd* antigens, Jk^a and Jk^b, may elicit antibodies transiently. A delayed hemolytic transfusion reaction that occurs with blood tested as compatible is often related to delayed appearance of anti-Jk^a.

PRETRANSFUSION TESTING

Pretransfusion testing of a potential recipient consists of the "type and screen." The "forward type" determines the ABO and Rh phenotype of the recipient's RBC by using antisera directed against the A, B, and D antigens. The "reverse type" detects isoagglutinins in the patient's serum and should correlate with the ABO phenotype, or forward type.

The alloantibody screen identifies antibodies directed against other RBC antigens. The alloantibody screen is performed by mixing patient serum with type O RBCs that contain the major antigens of most blood group systems and whose extended phenotype is known. The specificity of the alloantibody is identified by correlating the presence or absence of antigen with the results of the agglutination.

Cross-matching is ordered when there is a high probability that the patient will require a packed RBC (PRBC) transfusion. Blood selected for cross-matching must be ABO compatible and lack antigens for which the patient has alloantibodies. Nonreactive cross-matching confirms the absence of any major incompatibility and reserves that unit for the patient.

In the case of Rh-negative patients, every attempt must be made to provide Rh-negative blood components to prevent alloimmunization to the D antigen. In an emergency, Rh-positive blood can be safely transfused to an Rh-negative patient who lacks anti-D; however, the recipient is likely to become alloimmunized and produce anti-D. Rh-negative women of childbearing age who are transfused with products containing Rh-positive RBCs should receive passive immunization with anti-D (RhoGam or WinRho) to reduce or prevent sensitization.

BLOOD COMPONENTS

Blood products intended for transfusion are routinely collected as whole blood (450 mL) in various anticoagulants. Most donated blood is processed into components: PRBCs, platelets, and fresh-frozen plasma (FFP) or cryoprecipitate (Table 107-2). Whole blood is first separated into PRBCs and platelet-rich plasma by slow centrifugation. The platelet-rich plasma is then centrifuged at high speed to yield one unit of random donor (RD) platelets and one unit of FFP. Cryoprecipitate is produced by thawing FFP to precipitate the plasma proteins, then separated by centrifugation.

Apheresis technology is used for the collection of multiple units of platelets from a single donor. These single-donor apheresis platelets (SDAP) contain the equivalent of at least six units of RD platelets and have fewer contaminating leukocytes than pooled RD platelets.

Plasma may also be collected by apheresis. Plasma derivatives such as albumin, intravenous immunoglobulin, antithrombin, and coagulation factor concentrates are prepared from pooled plasma from many donors and are treated to eliminate infectious agents.

WHOLE BLOOD

Whole blood provides both oxygen-carrying capacity and volume expansion. It is the ideal component for patients who have sustained acute hemorrhage of ≥25% total blood volume loss. Whole blood is stored at 4°C to maintain erythrocyte viability, but platelet dysfunction and degradation of some coagulation factors occurs. In addition, 2,3-bisphosphoglycerate levels fall over time, leading to an increase in the oxygen affinity of the hemoglobin and a decreased capacity to deliver oxygen to the tissues, a problem with all red cell storage. Whole blood is not readily available since it is routinely processed into components.

PACKED RED BLOOD CELLS

This product increases oxygen-carrying capacity in the anemic patient. Adequate oxygenation can be maintained with a hemoglobin content of 70 g/L in the normovolemic patient without cardiac disease; however, comorbid factors often necessitate transfusion at a higher threshold. The decision to transfuse should be guided by the clinical situation and not by an arbitrary laboratory value. In the critical care setting, liberal use of transfusions to maintain near-normal levels of hemoglobin may have unexpected negative effects on survival. In most patients requiring transfusion, levels of hemoglobin of 100 g/L are sufficient to keep oxygen supply from being critically low.

PRBCs may be modified to prevent certain adverse reactions. Leukocyte reduction of cellular blood products is increasingly common, and universal prestorage leukocyte reduction has been recommended. Prestorage filtration appears superior to bedside filtration as smaller amounts of cytokines are generated in the stored product. These PRBC units contain $<5 \times 10^6$ donor white blood cells (WBCs), and their use lowers the incidence of posttransfusion fever, cytomegalovirus (CMV) infections, and alloimmunization. Other theoretical benefits include less immunosuppression in the recipient and lower risk of infections. Plasma, which may cause allergic reactions, can be removed from cellular blood components by washing.

PLATELETS

Thrombocytopenia is a risk factor for hemorrhage, and platelet transfusion reduces the incidence of bleeding. The threshold for prophylactic platelet transfusion is 10,000/μL. In patients without fever or infections, a threshold of 5000/μL may be sufficient to prevent spontaneous hemorrhage. For invasive procedures, 50,000/μL platelets is the usual target level.

Platelets are given either as pools prepared from five to eight RDs or as SDAPs from a single donor. In an unsensitized patient without increased platelet consumption [splenomegaly, fever, disseminated intravascular coagulation (DIC)], six to eight units of RD platelets (about 1 unit per 10 kg body weight) are transfused, and each unit is anticipated to increase the platelet count 5000–10,000/μL. Patients who have received multiple transfusions may be alloimmunized to many HLA- and platelet-specific antigens and have little or no increase in their posttransfusion platelet counts. Patients who may require multiple transfusions are best served by receiving SDAP and leukocyte-reduced components to lower the risk of alloimmunization.

Refractoriness to platelet transfusion may be evaluated using the corrected count increment (CCI):

$$\text{CCI} = \frac{\text{posttransfusion count} - \text{pretransfusion count}}{\text{number of platelets transfused} \times 10^{11}} \times \text{BSA}$$

TABLE 107-2 CHARACTERISTICS OF SELECTED BLOOD COMPONENTS

Component	Volume, mL	Content	Clinical Response
PRBC	180–200	RBCs with variable leukocyte content and small amount of plasma	Increase hemoglobin 10 g/L and hematocrit 3%
Platelets	50–70	5.5×10^{10}/RD unit	Increase platelet count 5000–10,000/μL
	200–400	$\geq 3.0 \times 10^{11}$/SDAP product	CCI $\geq 10 \times 10^9$/L within 1 h and $\geq 7.5 \times 10^9$/L within 24 h posttransfusion
FFP	200–250	Plasma proteins—coagulation factors, proteins C and S, antithrombin	Increases coagulation factors about 2%
Cryoprecipitate	10–15	Cold-insoluble plasma proteins, fibrinogen, factor VIII, vWF	Topical fibrin glue, also 80 IU factor VIII

Note: PRBC, packed red blood cells; RBC, red blood cell; RD, random donor; SDAP, single-donor apheresis platelets; CCI, corrected count increment; FFP, fresh-frozen plasma; vWF, von Willebrand factor.

where BSA is body surface area measured in square meters. The platelet count performed 1 h after the transfusion is acceptable if the CCI is 10 $\times 10^9$/mL, and after 18–24 h an increment of 7.5×10^9/mL is expected. Patients who have suboptimal responses are likely to have received multiple transfusions and have antibodies directed against class I HLA antigens. Refractoriness can be investigated by detecting anti-HLA antibodies in the recipient's serum. Patients who are sensitized will often react with 100% of the lymphocytes used for the HLA-antibody screen, and HLA-matched SDAPs should be considered for those patients who require transfusion. Although ABO-identical HLA-matched SDAPs provide the best chance for increasing the platelet count, locating these products is difficult. Platelet cross-matching is available in some centers. Additional clinical causes for a low platelet CCI include fever, bleeding, splenomegaly, DIC, or medications in the recipient.

FRESH-FROZEN PLASMA

FFP contains stable coagulation factors and plasma proteins: fibrinogen, antithrombin, albumin, as well as proteins C and S. Indications for FFP include correction of coagulopathies, including the rapid reversal of warfarin; supplying deficient plasma proteins; and treatment of thrombotic thrombocytopenic purpura. FFP should not be routinely used to expand blood volume. FFP is an acellular component and does not transmit intracellular infections, e.g., CMV. Patients who are IgA-deficient and require plasma support should receive FFP from IgA-deficient donors to prevent anaphylaxis (see below).

CRYOPRECIPITATE

Cryoprecipitate is a source of fibrinogen, factor VIII, and von Willebrand factor (vWF). It is ideal for supplying fibrinogen to the volume-sensitive patient. When factor VIII concentrates are not available, cryoprecipitate may be used since each unit contains approximately 80 units of factor VIII. Cryoprecipitate may also supply vWF to patients with dysfunctional (type II) or absent (type III) von Willebrand disease.

PLASMA DERIVATIVES

Plasma from thousands of donors may be pooled to derive specific protein concentrates, including albumin, intravenous immunoglobulin, antithrombin, and coagulation factors. In addition, donors who have high-titer antibodies to specific agents or antigens provide hyperimmune globulins, such as anti-D (RhoGam, WinRho), and antisera to hepatitis B virus (HBV), varicella-zoster virus, CMV, and other infectious agents.

ADVERSE REACTIONS TO BLOOD TRANSFUSION

Adverse reactions to transfused blood components occur despite multiple tests, inspections, and checks. Fortunately, the most common reactions are not life-threatening, although serious reactions can present with mild symptoms and signs. Some reactions can be reduced or prevented by modified (filtered, washed, or irradiated) blood components. When an adverse reaction is suspected, the transfusion should be stopped and reported to the blood bank for investigation.

Transfusion reactions may result from immune and nonimmune mechanisms. Immune-mediated reactions are often due to preformed donor or recipient antibody; however, cellular elements may also cause adverse effects. Nonimmune causes of reactions are due to the chemical and physical properties of the stored blood component and its additives.

Transfusion-transmitted viral infections are increasingly rare due to improved screening and testing. As the risk of viral infection is reduced, the relative risk of other reactions increases, such as hemolytic transfusion reactions and sepsis from bacterially contaminated components. More effort is being directed at improving pretransfusion quality assurance to further increase the safety of transfusion therapy. Infections, like any adverse transfusion reaction, must be brought to the attention of the blood bank for appropriate studies (Table 107-3).

TABLE 107-3 RISKS OF TRANSFUSION COMPLICATIONS

	Frequency, Episodes:Unit
Reactions	
Febrile (FNHTR)	1–4:100
Allergic	1–4:100
Delayed hemolytic	1:1000
TRALI	1:5000
Acute hemolytic	1:12,000
Fatal hemolytic	1:100,000
Anaphylactic	1:150,000
Infections[a]	
Hepatitis B	1:63,000
Hepatitis C	1:1,600,000
HIV-1	1:1,960,000
HIV-2	None reported
HTLV-I and -II	1:641,000
Malaria	1:4,000,000
Other complications	
RBC allosensitization	1:100
HLA allosensitization	1:10
Graft-versus-host disease	Rare

[a]Infectious agents rarely associated with transfusion, theoretically possible or of unknown risk include: Hepatitis A virus, parvovirus B-19, *Babesia microti* (babesiosis), *Borrelia burgdorferi* (Lyme disease), *Trypanosoma cruzi* (Chagas disease), and *Treponema pallidum*, human herpesvirus-8 and hepatitis G virus.

Note: FNHTR, febrile nonhemolytic transfusion reaction; TRALI, transfusion-related acute lung injury; HTLV, human T lymphotropic virus; RBC, red blood cell.

IMMUNE-MEDIATED REACTIONS

Acute Hemolytic Transfusion Reactions Immune-mediated hemolysis occurs when the recipient has preformed antibodies that lyse donor erythrocytes. The ABO isoagglutinins are responsible for the majority of these reactions, although alloantibodies directed against other RBC antigens, i.e., Rh, Kell, and Duffy, may result in hemolysis.

Acute hemolytic reactions may present with hypotension, tachypnea, tachycardia, fever, chills, hemoglobinemia, hemoglobinuria, chest and/or flank pain, and discomfort at the infusion site. Monitoring the patient's vital signs before and during the transfusion is important to identify reactions promptly. When acute hemolysis is suspected, the transfusion must be stopped immediately, intravenous access maintained, and the reaction reported to the blood bank. A correctly labeled posttransfusion blood sample and any untransfused blood should be sent to the blood bank for analysis. The laboratory evaluation for hemolysis includes the measurement of serum haptoglobin, lactate dehydrogenase (LDH), and indirect bilirubin levels.

The immune complexes that result in RBC lysis can cause renal dysfunction and failure. Diuresis should be induced with intravenous fluids and furosemide or mannitol. Tissue factor released from the lysed erythrocytes may initiate DIC. Coagulation studies including prothrombin time (PT), activated partial thromboplastin time (aPTT), fibrinogen, and platelet count should be monitored in patients with hemolytic reactions.

Errors at the patient's bedside, such as mislabeling the sample or transfusing the wrong patient, are responsible for the majority of these reactions. The blood bank investigation of these reactions includes examination of the pre- and posttransfusion samples for hemolysis and repeat typing of the patient samples; direct antiglobulin test (DAT), sometimes called the *direct Coombs test*, of the posttransfusion sample; repeating the cross-matching of the blood component; and checking all clerical records for errors. DAT detects the presence of antibody or complement bound to RBCs in vivo.

Delayed Hemolytic and Serologic Transfusion Reactions Delayed hemolytic transfusion reactions (DHTRs) are not completely preventable. These reactions occur in patients previously sensitized to RBC alloantigens who have a negative alloantibody screen due to low antibody levels. When the patient is transfused with antigen-positive blood, an anamnestic response results in the early production of alloantibody that binds donor RBCs. The alloantibody is detectable 1–2 weeks following the transfusion, and the posttransfusion DAT may become positive due to circulating donor RBCs coated with antibody or complement. The transfused, alloantibody-coated erythrocytes are cleared by the reticuloendothelial system. These reactions are detected most commonly in the blood bank when a subsequent patient sample reveals a positive alloantibody screen or a new alloantibody in a recently transfused recipient.

No specific therapy is usually required, although additional RBC transfusions may be necessary. Delayed serologic transfusion reactions are similar to DHTR, as the DAT is positive and alloantibody is detected; however, RBC clearance is not increased.

Febrile Nonhemolytic Transfusion Reaction The most frequent reaction associated with the transfusion of cellular blood components is a febrile nonhemolytic transfusion reaction (FNHTR). These reactions are characterized by chills and rigors and a ≥1°C rise in temperature. FNHTR is diagnosed when other causes of fever in the transfused patient are ruled out. Antibodies directed against donor leukocyte and HLA antigens may mediate these reactions; thus, multiply transfused patients and multiparous women are felt to be at increased risk. Although antibodies may be demonstrated in the recipient's serum, investigation is not routinely done because of the mild nature of most FNHTR. The use of leukocyte-reduced blood products may prevent or delay sensitization to leukocyte antigens and thereby reduce the incidence of these febrile episodes. Cytokines released from cells within stored blood components may mediate FNHTR; thus, leukoreduction before storage may prevent these reactions. The incidence and severity of these reactions can be decreased in patients with recurrent reactions by premedicating with acetaminophen or other antipyretic agents.

Allergic Reactions Urticarial reactions are related to plasma proteins found in transfused components. Mild reactions may be treated symptomatically by temporarily stopping the transfusion and administering antihistamines (diphenhydramine, 50 mg orally or intramuscularly). The transfusion may be completed after the signs and/or symptoms resolve. Patients with a history of allergic transfusion reaction should be premedicated with an antihistamine. Cellular components can be washed to remove residual plasma for the extremely sensitized patient.

Anaphylactic Reaction This severe reaction presents after transfusion of only a few milliliters of the blood component. Symptoms and signs include difficulty breathing, coughing, nausea and vomiting, hypotension, bronchospasm, loss of consciousness, respiratory arrest, and shock. Treatment includes stopping the transfusion, maintaining vascular access, and administering epinephrine (0.5–1.0 mL of 1:1000 dilution subcutaneously). Glucocorticoids may be required in severe cases.

Patients who are IgA-deficient, <1% of the population, may be sensitized to this Ig class and are at risk for anaphylactic reactions associated with plasma transfusion. Individuals with severe IgA deficiency should therefore receive only IgA-deficient plasma and washed cellular blood components. Patients who have anaphylactic or repeated allergic reactions to blood components should be tested for IgA deficiency.

Graft-versus-Host Disease Graft-versus-host disease (GVHD) is a frequent complication of allogeneic stem cell transplantation, in which lymphocytes from the donor attack and cannot be eliminated by an immunodeficient host. Transfusion-related GVHD is mediated by donor T lymphocytes that recognize host HLA antigens as foreign and mount an immune response, which is manifested clinically by the development of fever, a characteristic cutaneous eruption, diarrhea, and liver function abnormalities. GVHD can also occur when blood components that contain viable T lymphocytes are transfused to immunodeficient recipients or to immunocompetent recipients who share HLA antigens with the donor (e.g., a family donor). In addition to the aforementioned clinical features of GVHD, transfusion-associated GVHD (TA-GVHD) is characterized by marrow aplasia and pancytopenia. TA-GVHD is highly resistant to treatment with immunosuppressive therapies, including glucocorticoids, cyclosporine, antithymocyte globulin, and ablative therapy followed by allogeneic bone marrow transplantation. Clinical manifestations appear at 8–10 days, and death occurs at 3–4 weeks posttransfusion.

TA-GVHD can be prevented by irradiation of cellular components (minimum of 2500 cGy) before transfusion to patients at risk. Patients at risk for TA-GVHD include fetuses receiving intrauterine transfusions, selected immunocompetent (e.g., lymphoma patients) or immunocompromised recipients, recipients of donor units known to be from a blood relative, and recipients who have undergone marrow transplantation. Directed donations by family members should be discouraged (they are not less likely to transmit infection); lacking other options, the blood products from family members should always be irradiated.

Transfusion-Related Acute Lung Injury This uncommon reaction results from the transfusion of donor plasma that contains high-titer anti-HLA antibodies that bind recipient leukocytes. The leukocytes aggregate in the pulmonary vasculature and release mediators that increase capillary permeability. The recipient develops symptoms of respiratory compromise and signs of noncardiogenic pulmonary edema, including bilateral interstitial infiltrates on chest x-ray. Treatment is supportive, and patients usually recover without sequelae. Testing the donor's plasma for anti-HLA antibodies can support this diagnosis. The implicated donors are frequently multiparous women, and transfusion of their plasma component should be avoided.

Posttransfusion Purpura This reaction presents as thrombocytopenia 7–10 days after platelet transfusion and occurs predominantly in women. Platelet-specific antibodies are found in the recipient's serum, and the most frequently recognized antigen is HPA-1a found on the platelet glycoprotein IIIa receptor. The delayed thrombocytopenia is due to the production of antibodies that react to both donor and recipient platelets. Additional platelet transfusions can worsen the thrombocytopenia and should be avoided. Treatment with intravenous immunoglobulin may neutralize the effector antibodies, or plasmapheresis can be used to remove the antibodies.

Alloimmunization A recipient may become alloimmunized to a number of antigens on cellular blood elements and plasma proteins. Alloantibodies to RBC antigens are detected during pretransfusion testing, and their presence may delay finding antigen-negative crossmatch-compatible products for transfusion. Women of childbearing age who are sensitized to certain RBC antigens (i.e., D, c, E, Kell, or Duffy) are at risk for bearing a fetus with hemolytic disease of the newborn. Matching for D antigen is the only pretransfusion selection test to prevent RBC alloimmunization.

Alloimmunization to antigens on leukocytes and platelets can result in refractoriness to platelet transfusions. Once alloimmunization has developed, HLA-compatible platelets from donors who share similar antigens with the recipient may be difficult to find. Hence, prudent transfusion practice is directed at preventing sensitization through the use of leukocyte-reduced cellular components, as well as limiting antigenic exposure by the judicious use of transfusions and use of SDAPs.

NONIMMUNOLOGIC REACTIONS

Fluid Overload Blood components are excellent volume expanders, and transfusion may quickly lead to volume overload. Monitoring the rate and volume of the transfusion and using a diuretic can minimize this problem.

Hypothermia Refrigerated (4°C) or frozen (–18°C or below) blood components can result in hypothermia when rapidly infused. Cardiac dysrhythmias can result from exposing the sinoatrial node to cold fluid. Use of an in-line warmer will prevent this complication.

Electrolyte Toxicity RBC leakage during storage increases the concentration of potassium in the unit. Neonates and patients in renal failure are at risk for hyperkalemia. Preventive measures, such as using fresh or washed RBCs, are warranted for neonatal transfusions because this complication can be fatal.

Citrate, commonly used to anticoagulate blood components, chelates calcium and thereby inhibits the coagulation cascade. Hypocalcemia, manifested by circumoral numbness and/or tingling sensation of the fingers and toes, may result from multiple rapid transfusions. Because citrate is quickly metabolized to bicarbonate, calcium infusion is seldom required in this setting. If calcium or any other intravenous infusion is necessary, it must be given through a separate line.

Iron Overload Each unit of RBCs contains 200–250 mg of iron. Symptoms and signs of iron overload affecting endocrine, hepatic, and cardiac function are common after 100 units of RBCs have been transfused (total-body iron load of 20 g). Preventing this complication by using alternative therapies (e.g., erythropoietin) and judicious transfusion is preferable and cost effective. Deferoxamine and other chelating agents are available, but the response is often suboptimal.

Hypotensive Reactions Transient hypotension may be noted among transfused patients who take angiotensin-converting enzyme (ACE) inhibitors. Since blood products contain bradykinin that is normally degraded by ACE, patients on ACE inhibitors may have increased bradykinin levels that cause hypotension. The blood pressure typically returns to normal without intervention.

Immunomodulation Transfusion of allogeneic blood is immunosuppressive. Multiply transfused renal transplant recipients are less likely to reject the graft, and transfusion may result in poorer outcomes in cancer patients and increase the risk of infections. Transfusion-related immunomodulation is thought to be mediated by transfused leukocytes. Leukocyte-depleted cellular products may cause less immunosuppression, though controlled data have not been obtained and are unlikely to be obtained as the blood supply becomes universally leukocyte-depleted.

INFECTIOUS COMPLICATIONS

Nucleic acid amplification testing (NAT) began in 1999 to screen donated blood for the presence of HIV and hepatitis C virus (HCV) RNA. Since 2003 NAT has been used to detect West Nile virus (WNV) RNA in donated blood.

Viral Infections • ***HEPATITIS C VIRUS*** Blood donations are tested for antibodies to HCV and HCV RNA. Fewer than 200 HCV RNA-positive, antibody-negative donors have been found. The risk of acquiring HCV through transfusion is now calculated to be approximately 1 in 2,000,000 units. Infection with HCV may be asymptomatic or lead to chronic active hepatitis, cirrhosis, and liver failure.

HUMAN IMMUNODEFICIENCY VIRUS TYPE 1 Donated blood is tested for antibodies to HIV-1, HIV-1 p24 antigen, and HIV RNA using NAT. Approximately a dozen seronegative donors have been shown to harbor HIV RNA. The risk of HIV-1 infection per transfusion episode is 1 in 2 million. Antibodies to HIV-2 are also measured in donated blood. No cases of HIV-2 infection have been reported in the United States since 1992.

HEPATITIS B VIRUS Donated blood is screened for HBV using assays for hepatitis B surface antigen (HbsAg). NAT testing is not practical because of slow viral replication and lower levels of viremia. The risk of transfusion-associated HBV infection is 1 in 63,000 units, twenty-fold greater than for HCV. Vaccination of individuals who require long-term transfusion therapy can prevent this complication.

OTHER HEPATITIS VIRUSES Hepatitis A virus is rarely transmitted by transfusion; infection is typically asymptomatic and does not lead to chronic disease. Other transfusion-transmitted viruses—TTV, SEN-V, and GBV-C—do not cause chronic hepatitis or other disease states. Routine testing does not appear to be warranted.

WEST NILE VIRUS Transfusion-transmitted WNV infections were documented in 2002. This RNA virus can be detected using NAT; routine screening began in 2003, and more than 1000 blood donors have tested positive. WNV infections range in severity from asymptomatic to fatal, with the older population at greater risk.

CYTOMEGALOVIRUS This ubiquitous virus infects ≥50% of the general population and is transmitted by the infected "passenger" WBCs found in transfused PRBCs or platelet components. Cellular components that are leukocyte-reduced have a decreased risk of transmitting CMV, regardless of the serologic status of the donor. Groups at risk for CMV infections include immunosuppressed patients, CMV-seronegative transplant recipients, and neonates; these patients should receive leukocyte-depleted components or CMV seronegative products.

HUMAN T LYMPHOTROPIC VIRUS (HTLV) TYPE I Assays to detect HTLV-I and -II are used to screen all donated blood. HTLV-I is associated with adult T cell leukemia/lymphoma and tropical spastic paraparesis in a small percentage of infected persons (Chap. 181). The risk of HTLV-I infection via transfusion is 1 in 641,000 transfusion episodes. HTLV-II is not clearly associated with any disease.

PARVOVIRUS B-19 Blood components and pooled plasma products can transmit this virus, the etiologic agent of erythema infectiosum, or fifth disease, in children. Parvovirus B-19 shows tropism for erythroid precursors and inhibits both erythrocyte production and maturation. Pure red cell aplasia, presenting either as acute aplastic crisis or chronic anemia with shortened RBC survival, may occur in individuals with an underlying hematologic disease, such as sickle cell disease or thalassemia (Chap. 102). The fetus of a seronegative woman is at risk for developing hydrops from this virus.

Bacterial Contamination The relative risk of transfusion-transmitted bacterial infection has increased as the absolute risk of viral infections has dramatically decreased.

Most bacteria do not grow well at cold temperatures; thus, PRBCs and FFP are not common sources of bacterial contamination. However, some gram-negative bacteria can grow at 1° to 6°C. *Yersinia, Pseudomonas, Serratia, Acinetobacter* and *Escherichia* species have all been implicated in infections related to PRBC transfusion. Platelet concentrates, which are stored at room temperature, are more likely to contain skin contaminants such as gram-positive organisms, including coagulase-negative staphylococci. It is estimated that 1 in 1000–2000 platelet components is contaminated with bacteria. The risk of death due to transfusion-associated sepsis has been calculated at 1 in 17,000 for single-unit platelets derived from whole blood donation and 1 in 61,000 for apheresis product. Since 2004, blood banks have instituted methods to detect contaminated platelet components.

Recipients of transfusion contaminated with bacteria may develop fever and chills, which can progress to septic shock and DIC. These reactions may occur abruptly, within minutes of initiating the transfusion, or after several hours. The onset of symptoms and signs is often sudden and fulminant, which distinguishes bacterial contamination from an FNHTR. The reactions, particularly those related to gram-negative contaminants, are the result of infused endotoxins formed within the contaminated stored component.

When these reactions are suspected, the transfusion must be stopped immediately. Therapy is directed at reversing any signs of shock, and broad-spectrum antibiotics should be given. The blood bank should be notified to identify any clerical or serologic error. The blood component bag should be sent for culture and Gram stain.

Other Infectious Agents Various parasites, including those causing malaria, babesiosis, and Chagas disease, can be transmitted by blood transfusion. Geographic migration and travel of donors shift the incidence of these rare infections. Other agents implicated in transfusion transmission include Lyme disease and variant Creutzfeldt-Jakob disease. These infections should be considered in the transfused patient in the appropriate clinical setting.

ALTERNATIVES TO TRANSFUSION

Alternatives to allogeneic blood transfusions that avoid homologous donor exposures with attendant immunologic and infectious risks remain attractive. Autologous blood is the best option when transfusion is anticipated. However, the cost:benefit ratio of autologous transfusion remains high. No transfusion is a zero-risk event; clerical errors and bacterial contamination remain potential complications even with autologous transfusions. Additional methods of autologous transfusion in the surgical patient include preoperative hemodilution, recovery of shed blood from sterile surgical sites, and postoperative drainage collection. Directed or designated donation from friends and family of the potential recipient has not been safer than volunteer donor component transfusions. Such directed donations may in fact place the recipient at higher risk for complications such as GVHD and alloimmunization.

Granulocyte and granulocyte-macrophage colony-stimulating factor are clinically useful to hasten leukocyte recovery in patients with leukopenia related to high-dose chemotherapy. Erythropoietin stimulates erythrocyte production in patients with anemia of chronic renal failure and other conditions, thus avoiding or reducing the need for transfusion. This hormone can also stimulate erythropoiesis in the autologous donor to enable additional donation.

FURTHER READINGS

Blajchman MA: The clinical benefits of the leukoreduction of blood products. J Trauma 60:S83, 2006

Brecher ME, Hay SN: Bacterial contamination of blood components. Clin Micro Rev 18:195, 2005

———et al: *The Technical Manual*, 15th ed. Arlington, VA, American Association of Blood Banks, 2005

Busch MP et al: A new strategy for estimating risks of transfusion transmitted viral infections based on rates of detection of recently infected donors. Transfusion 45:254, 2005

Raghavana M, Marik PE: Anemia, allogeneic blood transfusion, and immunomodulation in the critically ill. Chest 127:295, 2005

Sheppard CA et al: Transfusion-related acute lung injury. Hematol Oncol Clin North Am 21:163, 2007

108 Hematopoietic Cell Transplantation

Frederick R. Appelbaum

Bone marrow transplantation was the original term used to describe the collection and transplantation of hematopoietic stem cells, but with the demonstration that the peripheral blood and umbilical cord blood are also useful sources of stem cells, *hematopoietic cell transplantation* has become the preferred generic term for this process. The procedure is usually carried out for one of two purposes: (1) to replace an abnormal but nonmalignant lymphohematopoietic system with one from a normal donor, or (2) to treat malignancy by allowing the administration of higher doses of myelosuppressive therapy than would otherwise be possible. The use of hematopoietic cell transplantation has been increasing, both because of its efficacy in selected diseases and because of increasing availability of donors. The International Bone Marrow Transplant Registry (*http://www.ibmtr.org*) estimates that about 50,000 transplants are performed each year.

THE HEMATOPOIETIC STEM CELL

Several features of the hematopoietic stem cell make transplantation clinically feasible, including its remarkable regenerative capacity, its ability to home to the marrow space following intravenous injection, and the ability of the stem cell to be cryopreserved. Transplantation of a single stem cell can replace the entire lymphohematopoietic system of an adult mouse. In humans, transplantation of a few percent of a donor's bone marrow volume regularly results in complete and sustained replacement of the recipient's entire lymphohematopoietic system, including all red cells, granulocytes, B and T lymphocytes, and platelets, as well as cells comprising the fixed macrophage population, including Kupffer cells of the liver, pulmonary alveolar macrophages, osteoclasts, Langerhans cells of the skin, and brain microglial cells. The ability of the hematopoietic stem cell to home to the marrow following intravenous injection is mediated, at least in part, by the interaction of cell-surface molecules, termed *selectins*, on bone marrow endothelial cells with ligands, termed *integrins*, on early hematopoietic cells. Human hematopoietic stem cells can survive freezing and thawing with little, if any, damage, making it possible to remove and store a portion of the patient's own bone marrow for later reinfusion following treatment of the patient with high-dose myelotoxic therapy.

CATEGORIES OF HEMATOPOIETIC CELL TRANSPLANTATION

Hematopoietic cell transplantation can be described according to the relationship between the patient and the donor and by the anatomic source of stem cells. In ~1% of cases, patients have identical twins who can serve as donors. With the use of syngeneic donors, there is no risk of graft-versus-host disease (GVHD) that often complicates allogeneic transplantation, and unlike the use of autologous marrow, there is no risk that the stem cells are contaminated with tumor cells.

Allogeneic transplantation involves a donor and recipient who are not immunologically identical. Following allogeneic transplantation, immune cells transplanted with the stem cells or developing from them can react against the patient, causing GVHD. Alternatively, if the immunosuppressive preparative regimen used to treat the patient before transplant is inadequate, immunocompetent cells of the patient can cause graft rejection. The risks of these complications are greatly influenced by the degree of matching between donor and recipient for antigens encoded by genes of the major histocompatibility complex.

The human leukocyte antigen (HLA) molecules are responsible for binding antigenic proteins and presenting them to T cells. The antigens presented by HLA molecules may derive from exogenous sources (e.g., during active infections) or may be endogenous proteins. If individuals are not HLA-matched, T cells from one individual will react strongly to the mismatched HLA, or "major antigens," of the second. Even if the individuals are HLA-matched, the T cells of the donor may react to differing endogenous, or "minor antigens," presented by the HLA of the recipient. Reactions to minor antigens tend to be less vigorous. The genes of major relevance to transplantation include HLA-A, -B, -C, and -D; they are closely linked and therefore tend to be inherited as haplotypes, with only rare crossovers between them. Thus, the odds that any one full sibling will match a patient are one in four, and the probability that the patient has an HLA-identical sibling is $1 - (0.75)^n$, where n equals the number of siblings.

With current techniques, the risk of graft rejection is 1–3%, and the risk of severe, life-threatening acute GVHD is ~15% following transplantation between HLA-identical siblings. The incidence of graft rejection and GVHD increases progressively with the use of family member donors mismatched for one, two, or three antigens. While survival following a one-antigen mismatched transplant is not markedly altered, survival following two- or three-antigen mismatched transplants is significantly reduced, and such transplants should be performed only as part of clinical trials.

Since the formation of the National Marrow Donor Program, it has become possible to identify HLA-matched unrelated donors for many patients. The genes encoding HLA antigens are highly polymorphic, and thus the odds of any two unrelated individuals being HLA-identical are extremely low, somewhat less than 1 in 10,000. However, by identifying and typing >7 million volunteer donors, HLA-matched donors can now be found for ~50% of patients for whom a search is initiated. It takes, on average, 3–4 months to complete a search and schedule and initiate an unrelated donor transplant. Results so far suggest that GVHD is somewhat increased and survival somewhat poorer with such donors than with HLA-matched siblings.

Autologous transplantation involves the removal and storage of the patient's own stem cells with subsequent reinfusion after the patient receives high-dose myeloablative therapy. Unlike allogeneic transplantation, there is no risk of GVHD or graft rejection with autologous transplantation. On the other hand, autologous transplantation lacks a graft-versus-tumor (GVT) effect, and the autologous stem cell product can be contaminated with tumor cells that could lead to relapse. A variety of techniques have been developed to "purge" autologous products of tumor cells. Some use antibodies directed at tumor-associated antigens plus complement, antibodies linked to toxins, or antibodies conjugated to immunomagnetic beads. In vitro incubation with certain chemotherapeutic agents such as 4-hydroperoxycyclophosphamide and long-term culture of bone marrow have also been shown to diminish tumor cell numbers in stem cell products. Another technique is positive selection of stem cells using antibodies to CD34, with subsequent column adherence or flow techniques to select normal stem cells while leaving tumor cells behind. All these approaches can reduce the number of tumor cells from 1000- to 10,000-fold and are clinically feasible; however, no prospective randomized trials have yet shown that any of these approaches results in a decrease in relapse rates or improvements in disease-free or overall survival.

Bone marrow aspirated from the posterior and anterior iliac crests has traditionally been the source of hematopoietic stem cells for transplantation. Typically, anywhere from 1.5 to 5×10^8 nucleated marrow cells per kilogram are collected for allogeneic transplantation. Several studies have found improved survival in the settings of both matched sibling and unrelated transplantation by transplanting higher numbers of bone marrow cells.

Hematopoietic stem cells circulate in the peripheral blood but in very low concentrations. Following the administration of certain hematopoietic growth factors, including granulocyte colony-stimulating factor (G-CSF) or granulocyte-macrophage colony-stimulating factor (GM-CSF), and during recovery from intensive chemotherapy, the concentration of hematopoietic progenitor cells in blood, as measured either by colony-forming units or expression of the CD34 antigen, increases markedly. This has made it possible to harvest adequate numbers of stem cells from the peripheral blood for transplantation. Donors are typically treated with 4 or 5 days of hematopoietic growth factor, following which stem cells are collected in one or two 4-h pheresis sessions. In the autologous setting, transplantation of $>2.5 \times 10^6$ CD34 cells per kilogram, a number easily collected in most circumstances, leads to rapid and sustained engraftment in virtually all cases. Compared to the use of autologous marrow, use of peripheral blood stem cells results in more rapid hematopoietic recovery, with granulocytes recovering to 500/μL by day 12 and platelets recovering to 20,000/μL by day 14. While this more rapid recovery diminishes the morbidity of transplantation, no studies show improved survival.

Hesitation in studying the use of peripheral blood stem cells for allogeneic transplantation was because peripheral blood stem cell products contain as much as one log more T cells than are contained in the typical marrow harvest; in animal models, the incidence of GVHD is related to the number of T cells transplanted. Nonetheless, clinical trials have shown that the use of growth factor–mobilized peripheral blood stem cells from HLA-matched family members leads to faster engraftment without an increase in acute GVHD. Chronic GVHD may be increased with peripheral blood stem cells, but in trials conducted so far, this has been more than balanced by reductions in relapse rates and nonrelapse mortality, with the use of peripheral blood stem cells resulting in improved overall survival.

Umbilical cord blood contains a high concentration of hematopoietic progenitor cells, allowing for its use as a source of stem cells for transplantation. Cord blood transplantation from family members has been explored in the setting where the immediate need for transplantation precludes waiting the 9 or so months generally required for the baby to mature to the point of donating marrow. Use of cord blood results in slower engraftment and peripheral count recovery than seen with marrow but a low incidence of GVHD, perhaps reflecting the low number of T cells in cord blood. Several banks have been developed to harvest and store cord blood for possible transplantation to unrelated patients from material that would otherwise be discarded. A summary of the first 562 unrelated cord blood transplants, facilitated by the New York Blood Center, reported engraftment in ~85% of patients but at a slower pace than seen with marrow. Severe GVHD was seen in 23% of patients. The risk of graft failure was related to the dose of cord blood cells per kilogram infused. The low cell content of most cord blood collections has limited the use of this approach for adult patients.

THE TRANSPLANT PREPARATIVE REGIMEN

The treatment regimen administered to patients immediately preceding transplantation is designed to eradicate the patient's underlying disease and, in the setting of allogeneic transplantation, immunosuppress the patient adequately to prevent rejection of the transplanted marrow. The appropriate regimen therefore depends on the disease setting and source of marrow. For example, when transplantation is performed to treat severe combined immunodeficiency and the donor is a histocompatible sibling, no treatment is required because no host cells require eradication and the patient is already too immunoincompetent to reject the transplanted marrow. For aplastic anemia, there is no large population of cells to eradicate, and high-dose cyclophosphamide plus antithymocyte globulin are sufficient to immunosuppress the patient adequately to accept the marrow graft. In the setting of thalassemia and sickle cell anemia, high-dose busulfan is frequently added to cyclophosphamide in order to eradicate hyperplastic host hematopoiesis. A variety of different regimens have been developed to treat malignant diseases. Most of these regimens include agents that have high activity against the tumor in question at conventional doses and have myelosuppression as their predominant dose-limiting toxicity. Therefore, these regimens commonly include busulfan, cyclophosphamide, melphalan, thiotepa, carmustine, etoposide, and total-body irradiation in various combinations.

Although high-dose treatment regimens have typically been used in transplantation, the understanding that much of the antitumor effect of transplantation derives from an immunologically mediated GVT response has led investigators to ask if less-intensive "nonmyeloablative" regimens might be effective and more tolerable. Evidence for a GVT effect comes from studies showing that posttransplant relapse rates are lowest in patients who develop acute and chronic GVHD, higher in those without GVHD, and higher still in recipients of T cell–depleted allogeneic or syngeneic marrow. The demonstration that complete remissions can be obtained in many patients who have relapsed posttransplant by simply administering viable lymphocytes from the original donor further strengthens the argument for a potent GVT effect. Accordingly, a variety of less-intensive nonmyeloablative regimens have been studied, ranging in intensity from the very minimum required to achieve engraftment (e.g., fludarabine plus 200 cGy total-body irradiation) to regimens of more immediate intensity (e.g., fludarabine plus melphalan). Studies to date document that engraftment can be readily achieved with less toxicity than seen with conventional transplantation. Furthermore, the severity of GVHD appears to be decreased because less tissue damage is done by the lower doses of drugs in the preparative regimen. Complete sustained responses have been documented in many patients, particularly those with more indolent hematologic malignancies. The role of nonmyeloablative transplants in any disease, however, has not been fully defined.

THE TRANSPLANT PROCEDURE

Marrow is usually collected from the donor's posterior and sometimes anterior iliac crests with the donor under general or spinal anesthesia. Typically, 10–15 mL/kg of marrow is aspirated, placed in heparinized media, and filtered through 0.3- and 0.2-mm screens to remove fat and bony spicules. The collected marrow may undergo further processing depending on the clinical situation, such as the removal of red cells to prevent hemolysis in ABO-incompatible transplants, the removal of donor T cells to prevent GVHD, or attempts to remove possible contaminating tumor cells in autologous transplantation. Marrow donation is safe, with only very rare complications reported.

Peripheral blood stem cells are collected by leukophoresis after the donor has been treated with hematopoietic growth factors or, in the setting of autologous transplantation, sometimes after treatment with a combination of chemotherapy and growth factors. Stem cells for transplantation are generally infused through a large-bore central venous catheter. Such infusions are usually well tolerated, although occasionally patients develop fever, cough, or shortness of breath. These symptoms usually resolve with slowing of the infusion. When the stem cell product has been cryopreserved using dimethyl sulfoxide, patients more often experience short-lived nausea or vomiting due to the odor and taste of the cryoprotectant.

ENGRAFTMENT

Peripheral blood counts usually reach their nadir several days to a week posttransplant as a consequence of the preparative regimen, then cells produced by the transplanted stem cells begin to appear in the peripheral blood. The rate of recovery depends on the source of stem cells, the use of posttransplant growth factors, and the form of GVHD prophylaxis employed. If marrow is the source of stem cells, recovery to 100 granulocytes/μL occurs by day 16 and to 500/μL by day 22. Use of G-CSF–mobilized peripheral blood stem cells speeds the rate of recovery by ~1 week when compared to marrow. Use of a myeloid growth factor (G-CSF or GM-CSF) posttransplant can further accelerate recovery by 3–5 days, while use of methotrexate to prevent GVHD delays engraftment by a similar period. Following allogeneic transplantation, engraftment can be documented using fluorescence in situ hybridization of sex chromosomes if donor and recipient are sex-mismatched, HLA-typing if HLA-mismatched, or restriction fragment length polymorphism analysis if sex- and HLA-matched.

COMPLICATIONS FOLLOWING HEMATOPOIETIC CELL TRANSPLANT

Early Direct Chemoradiotoxicities The transplant preparative regimens commonly used cause a spectrum of acute toxicities that vary according to the specific regimen but frequently result in nausea, vomiting, and mild skin erythema (Fig. 108-1). Regimens that include high-dose cyclophosphamide can result in hemorrhagic cystitis, which can usually be prevented by bladder irrigation or with the sulfhydryl compound mercaptoethanesulfonate (MESNA); rarely, acute hemorrhagic carditis is seen. Most preparative regimens will result in oral mucositis, which typically develops 5–7 days posttransplant and often requires

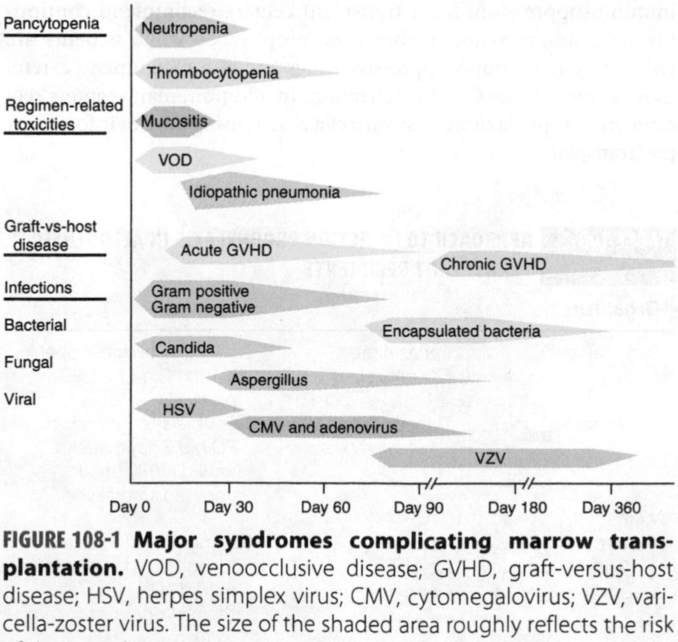

FIGURE 108-1 Major syndromes complicating marrow transplantation. VOD, venoocclusive disease; GVHD, graft-versus-host disease; HSV, herpes simplex virus; CMV, cytomegalovirus; VZV, varicella-zoster virus. The size of the shaded area roughly reflects the risk of the complication.

narcotic analgesia. Use of a patient-controlled analgesic pump provides the greatest patient satisfaction and results in a lower cumulative dose of narcotic. Patients begin losing their hair 5–6 days posttransplant and by 1 week are usually profoundly pancytopenic.

Approximately 10% of patients will develop venoocclusive disease of the liver, a syndrome resulting from direct cytotoxic injury to hepatic-venular and sinusoidal endothelium, with subsequent deposition of fibrin and the development of a local hypercoagulable state. This chain of events results in the clinical symptoms of tender hepatomegaly, ascites, jaundice, and fluid retention. These symptoms can develop any time during the first month posttransplant, with the peak incidence at day 16. Predisposing factors include prior exposure to intensive chemotherapy, pretransplant hepatitis of any cause, and use of more intense conditioning regimens. The mortality of venoocclusive disease is ~30%, with progressive hepatic failure culminating in a terminal hepatorenal syndrome. Both thrombolytic and antithrombotic agents, such as tissue plasminogen activator, heparin, and prostaglandin E, have been studied as therapy, but none has proven of consistent major benefit in controlled trials, and all have significant toxicity. Early studies with defibrotide, a polydeoxyribonucleotide, seem encouraging.

Although most pneumonias developing posttransplant are caused by infectious agents, in ~5% of patients a diffuse interstitial pneumonia will develop that is thought to be the result of direct toxicity of the preparative regimen. Bronchoalveolar lavage typically shows alveolar hemorrhage, and biopsies are typically characterized by diffuse alveolar damage, although some cases may have a more clearly interstitial pattern. High-dose glucocorticoids are often used as treatment, although randomized trials testing their utility have not been reported.

Late Direct Chemoradiotoxicities Late complications of the preparative regimen include decreased growth velocity in children and delayed development of secondary sex characteristics. These complications can be partly ameliorated with the use of appropriate growth and sex hormone replacement. Most men become azoospermic, and most postpubertal women will develop ovarian failure, which should be treated. Thyroid dysfunction, usually well compensated, is sometimes seen. Cataracts develop in 10–20% of patients and are most common in patients treated with total-body irradiation and those who receive glucocorticoid therapy posttransplant for treatment of GVHD. Aseptic necrosis of the femoral head is seen in 10% of patients and is particularly frequent in those receiving chronic glucocorticoid therapy.

Graft-Versus-Host Disease GVHD is the result of allogeneic T cells that were either transferred with the donor's stem cell inoculum or develop from it, reacting with antigenic targets on host cells. GVHD developing within the first 3 months posttransplant is termed *acute GVHD*, while GVHD developing or persisting beyond 3 months posttransplant is termed *chronic GVHD*. Acute GVHD most often first becomes apparent 2–4 weeks posttransplant and is characterized by an erythematous maculopapular rash; persistent anorexia or diarrhea, or both; and by liver disease with increased serum levels of bilirubin, alanine and aspartate aminotransferase, and alkaline phosphatase. Since many conditions can mimic acute GVHD, diagnosis usually requires skin, liver, or endoscopic biopsy for confirmation. In all these organs, endothelial damage and lymphocytic infiltrates are seen. In skin, the epidermis and hair follicles are damaged; in liver, the small bile ducts show segmental disruption; and in intestines, destruction of the crypts and mucosal ulceration may be noted. A commonly used rating system for acute GVHD is shown in Table 108-1. Grade I acute GVHD is of little clinical significance, does not affect the likelihood of survival, and does not require treatment. In contrast, grades II to IV GVHD are associated with significant symptoms and a poorer probability of survival, and they require aggressive therapy. The incidence of acute GVHD is higher in recipients of stem cells from mismatched or unrelated donors, in older patients, and in patients unable to receive full doses of drugs used to prevent the disease.

One general approach to the prevention of GVHD is the administration of immunosuppressive drugs early after transplant. Combina-

TABLE 108-1 CLINICAL STAGING AND GRADING OF ACUTE GRAFT-VERSUS-HOST DISEASE

Clinical Stage	Skin	Liver—Bilirubin, μmol/L (mg/dL)	Gut
1	Rash <25% body surface	34–51 (2–3)	Diarrhea 500–1000 mL/d
2	Rash 25–50% body surface	51–103 (3–6)	Diarrhea 1000–1500 mL/d
3	Generalized erythroderma	103–257 (6–15)	Diarrhea >1500 mL/d
4	Desquamation and bullae	>257 (> 15)	Ileus

Overall Clinical Grade	Skin Stage	Liver Stage	Gut Stage
I	1–2	0	0
II	1–3	1	1
III	1–3	2–3	2–3
IV	2–4	2–4	2–4

tions of methotrexate and either cyclosporine or tacrolimus are among the most effective and widely used regimens. Prednisone, anti–T cell antibodies, mycophenolate mofetil, and other immunosuppressive agents have also been or are being studied in various combinations. A second general approach to GVHD prevention is removal of T cells from the stem cell inoculum. While effective in preventing GVHD, T cell depletion is associated with an increased incidence of graft failure and of tumor recurrence posttransplant; as yet, little evidence suggests that T-cell depletion improves cure rates in any specific setting.

Despite prophylaxis, significant acute GVHD will develop in ~30% of recipients of stem cells from matched siblings and in as many as 60% of those receiving stem cells from unrelated donors. The disease is usually treated with glucocorticoids, antithymocyte globulin, or monoclonal antibodies targeted against T cells or T cell subsets.

Between 20 and 50% of patients surviving >6 months after allogeneic transplantation will develop chronic GVHD. The disease is more common in older patients, in recipients of mismatched or unrelated stem cells, and in those with a preceding episode of acute GVHD. The disease resembles an autoimmune disorder with malar rash, sicca syndrome, arthritis, obliterative bronchiolitis, and bile duct degeneration and cholestasis. Single-agent prednisone or cyclosporine is standard treatment at present, although trials of other agents are under way. In most patients, chronic GVHD resolves, but it may require 1–3 years of immunosuppressive treatment before these agents can be withdrawn without the disease recurring. Because patients with chronic GVHD are susceptible to significant infection, they should receive prophylactic trimethoprim-sulfamethoxazole, and all suspected infections should be investigated and treated aggressively.

Graft Failure While complete and sustained engraftment is usually seen posttransplant, occasionally marrow function either does not return or, after a brief period of engraftment, is lost. Graft failure after autologous transplantation can be the result of inadequate numbers of stem cells being transplanted, damage during ex vivo treatment or storage, or exposure of the patient to myelotoxic agents posttransplant. Infections with cytomegalovirus (CMV) or human herpes virus type 6 have also been associated with loss of marrow function. Graft failure after allogeneic transplantation can also be due to immunologic rejection of the graft by immunocompetent host cells. Immunologically based graft rejection is more common following use of less-immunosuppressive preparative regimens, in recipients of T cell–depleted stem cell products, and in patients receiving grafts from HLA-mismatched donors.

Treatment of graft failure usually involves removing all potentially myelotoxic agents from the patient's regimen and attempting a short trial of a myeloid growth factor. Persistence of lymphocytes of host origin in allogeneic transplant recipients with graft failure indicates immunologic rejection. Reinfusion of donor stem cells in such patients is usually unsuccessful unless preceded by a second immunosuppressive preparative regimen. Standard preparative regimens are generally tolerated poorly if administered within 100 days of a first transplant because of cumulative toxicities. However, use of regimens combining, for example, anti-CD3 antibodies with high-dose glucocorticoids, fludarabine plus low-dose total-body irradiation, or cyclophosphamide plus antithymocyte globulin have been effective in some cases.

Infection Posttransplant patients, particularly recipients of allogeneic transplantation, require unique approaches to the problem of infection. Early after transplantation, patients are profoundly neutropenic, and because the risk of bacterial infection is so great, most centers initiate antibiotic treatment once the granulocyte count falls to <500/μL. Fluconazole prophylaxis at a dose of 200–400 mg/kg per day reduces the risk of candidal infections. Patients seropositive for herpes simplex should receive acyclovir prophylaxis. One approach to infection prophylaxis is shown in Table 108-2. Despite these prophylactic measures, most patients will develop fever and signs of infection posttransplant. The management of patients who become febrile despite bacterial and fungal prophylaxis is a difficult challenge and is guided by individual aspects of the patient and by the institution's experience. **The general problem of infection in the immunocompromised host is discussed in Chap. 126.**

Once patients engraft, the incidence of bacterial infection diminishes; however, patients, particularly allogeneic transplant recipients, remain at significant risk of infection. During the period from engraftment until about 3 months posttransplant, the most common causes of infection are gram-positive bacteria, fungi (particularly *Aspergillus*) and viruses including CMV. CMV infection, which in the past was frequently seen and often fatal, can be prevented in seronegative patients by the use of seronegative blood products. The use of ganciclovir, either as prophylaxis beginning at the time of engraftment or initiated when CMV first reactivates as evidenced by development of antigenemia, can significantly reduce the risk of CMV disease in seropositive patients. Elimination of white blood cells from transfused blood products is another method to prevent CMV transmission. Foscarnet is effective for some patients who develop CMV antigenemia or infection despite the use of ganciclovir or who cannot tolerate the drug.

Pneumocystis jiroveci pneumonia, once seen in 5–10% of patients, can be prevented by treating patients with oral trimethoprim-sulfamethoxazole for 1 week pretransplant and resuming the treatment once patients have engrafted.

The risk of infection diminishes considerably beyond 3 months after transplant unless chronic GVHD develops, requiring continuous immunosuppression. Most transplant centers recommend continuing trimethoprim-sulfamethoxazole prophylaxis while patients are receiving any immunosuppressive drugs and also recommend careful monitoring for late CMV reactivation. In addition, many centers recommend prophylaxis against varicella zoster, using acyclovir for 1 year posttransplant.

TABLE 108-2 APPROACH TO INFECTION PROPHYLAXIS IN ALLOGENEIC TRANSPLANT RECIPIENTS

Organism		Approach
Bacterial	Ceftazidime	2 g IV q8h while neutropenic
Fungal	Fluconazole	400 mg PO qd to day 75 posttransplant
Pneumocystis carinii	Trimethoprim-sulfamethoxazole	1 double-strength tablet PO bid 2 days/week until day 180 or off immunosuppression
Viral		
Herpes simplex	Acyclovir	800 mg PO bid to day 30
Varicella zoster	Acyclovir	800 mg PO bid to day 365
Cytomegalovirus	Ganciclovir	5 mg/kg IV bid for 7 days, then 5 (mg/kg)/d 5 days/week to day 100

TREATMENT OF SPECIFIC DISEASES USING HEMATOPOIETIC CELL TRANSPLANTATION

℞ NONMALIGNANT DISEASES

IMMUNODEFICIENCY DISORDERS By replacing abnormal stem cells with cells from a normal donor, hematopoietic cell transplantation can cure patients of a variety of immunodeficiency disorders including severe combined immunodeficiency, Wiskott-Aldrich syndrome, and Chédiak-Higashi syndrome. The widest experience has been with severe combined immunodeficiency disease, where cure rates of 90% can be expected with HLA-identical donors and success rates of 50–70% have been reported using haplotype-mismatched parents as donors (**Table 108-3**).

APLASTIC ANEMIA Transplantation from matched siblings after a preparative regimen of high-dose cyclophosphamide and antithymocyte globulin can cure up to 90% of patients <40 years with severe aplastic anemia. Results in older patients and in recipients of mismatched family member or unrelated marrow are less favorable; therefore, a trial of immunosuppressive therapy is generally recommended for such patients before considering transplantation. Transplantation is effective in all forms of aplastic anemia including, for example, the syndromes associated with paroxysmal nocturnal hemoglobinuria and Fanconi's anemia. Patients with Fanconi's anemia are abnormally sensitive to the toxic effects of alkylating agents and so less intensive preparative regimens must be used in their treatment (Chap. 102).

HEMOGLOBINOPATHIES Marrow transplantation from an HLA-identical sibling following a preparative regimen of busulfan and cyclophosphamide can cure 70–90% of patients with thalassemia major. The best outcomes can be expected if patients are transplanted before they develop hepatomegaly or portal fibrosis and if they have been given adequate iron chelation therapy. Among such patients, the probabilities of 5-year survival and disease-free survival are 95 and 90%, respectively. Although prolonged survival can be achieved with aggressive chelation therapy, transplantation is the only curative treatment for thalassemia. Transplantation is being studied as a curative approach to patients with sickle cell anemia. Two-year survival and disease-free survival rates of 90 and 80%, respectively, have been reported following matched sibling transplantation. Decisions about patient selection and the timing of transplantation remain difficult, but transplantation represents a reasonable option for younger patients who suffer repeated crises or other significant complications and who have not responded to other interventions (Chap. 99).

TABLE 108-3 ESTIMATED 5-YEAR SURVIVAL RATES FOLLOWING TRANSPLANTATION[a]

Disease	Allogeneic, %	Autologous, %
Severe combined immunodeficiency	90	N/A
Aplastic anemia	90	N/A
Thalassemia	90	N/A
Acute myeloid leukemia		
First remission	55–60	50
Second remission	40	30
Acute lymphocytic leukemia		
First remission	50	40
Second remission	40	30
Chronic myeloid leukemia		
Chronic phase	70	ID
Accelerated phase	40	ID
Blast crisis	15	ID
Chronic lymphocytic leukemia	50	ID
Myelodysplasia	45	ID
Multiple myeloma	30	35
Non-Hodgkin's lymphoma		
First relapse/second remission	40	40
Hodgkin's disease		
First relapse/second remission	40	50
Breast cancer		
High-risk stage II	N/A	70
Stage IV	N/A	15

[a]These estimates are generally based on data reported by the International Bone Marrow Transplant Registry. The analysis has not been reviewed by their Advisory Committee.

Note: N/A, not applicable; ID, insufficient data.

OTHER NONMALIGNANT DISEASES Theoretically, hematopoietic cell transplantation should be able to cure any disease that results from an inborn error of the lymphohematopoietic system. Transplantation has been used successfully to treat congenital disorders of white blood cells such as Kostmann's syndrome, chronic granulomatous disease, and leukocyte adhesion deficiency. Congenital anemias such as Blackfan-Diamond anemia can also be cured with transplantation. Infantile malignant osteopetrosis is due to an inability of the osteoclast to resorb bone, and since osteoclasts derive from the marrow, transplantation can cure this rare inherited disorder.

Hematopoietic cell transplantation has been used as treatment for a number of storage diseases caused by enzymatic deficiencies, such as Gaucher's disease, Hurler's syndrome, Hunter's syndrome, and infantile metachromatic leukodystrophy. Transplantation for these diseases has not been uniformly successful, but treatment early in the course of these diseases, before irreversible damage to extramedullary organs has occurred, increases the chance for success.

Transplantation is being explored as a treatment for severe acquired autoimmune disorders. These trials are based on studies demonstrating that transplantation can reverse autoimmune disorders in animal models and on the observation that occasional patients with coexisting autoimmune disorders and hematologic malignancies have been cured of both with transplantation.

℞ MALIGNANT DISEASES

ACUTE LEUKEMIA Allogeneic hematopoietic cell transplantation cures 15–20% of patients who do not achieve complete response from induction chemotherapy for acute myeloid leukemia (AML) and is the only form of therapy that can cure such patients. Cure rates of 30–35% are seen when patients are transplanted in second remission or in first relapse. The best results with allogeneic transplantation are achieved when applied during first remission, with disease-free survival rates averaging 55–60%. Chemotherapy alone can cure a portion of AML patients, and so the relative merits of transplanting all patients during first remission versus only transplanting very-high-risk patients and those who relapse continue to be discussed. Autologous transplantation is also able to cure a portion of patients with AML. The rates of disease recurrence with autologous transplantation are higher than those seen after allogeneic transplantation, and cure rates are somewhat less.

Similar to patients with AML, adults with acute lymphocytic leukemia who do not achieve a complete response to induction chemotherapy can be cured in 15–20% of cases with immediate transplantation. Cure rates improve to 30–50% in second remission, and therefore transplantation can be recommended for adults who have persistent disease after induction chemotherapy or who have subsequently relapsed. Transplantation in first remission results in cure rates around 55%. While transplantation appears to offer a clear advantage over chemotherapy for patients with high-risk disease, such as those with Philadelphia chromosome–positive disease, debate continues about whether adults with standard-risk disease should be transplanted in first remission or whether transplantation should be reserved until relapse. Autologous transplantation is associated with a higher relapse rate but a somewhat lower risk of nonrelapse mortality when compared to allogeneic transplantation. On balance, most experts recommend use of allogeneic stem cells if an appropriate donor is available.

CHRONIC LEUKEMIA Allogeneic hematopoietic cell transplantation is the only therapy shown to cure a substantial portion of patients with chronic myeloid leukemia (CML). Five-year disease-free survival rates are 15–20% for patients transplanted for blast crisis, 25–50% for accelerated-phase patients, and 60–70% for chronic phase patients, with cure rates as high as 80% at selected centers. Use of unrelated donors results in more GVHD and slightly worse survival than seen with matched siblings, although 3-year disease-free survival rates of 70% have been reported at some large centers. The timing of transplantation in CML has become more complicated with the introduction of imatinib mesylate, a remarkably effective, relatively nontoxic oral agent. Even though imatinib is not generally regarded as curative, given its favorable toxicity profile, most physicians favor its use as initial therapy for CML, with transplantation being reserved for those who fail to achieve a complete cytogenetic response with imatinib, relapse after an initial response, or are intolerant of the drug (Chap. 104).

Allogeneic transplantation has been used to only a limited extent for chronic lymphocytic leukemia, in large part because of the chronic nature of the disease and because of the age profile of patients. With allogeneic transplantation, complete remissions have been achieved in the majority of patients so far reported, with disease-free survival rates of ~50% at 3 years. However, treatment-related mortality has been substantial, and further follow-up is needed. Encouraging results have been seen using reduced intensity preparative regimens before allogeneic transplantation.

MYELODYSPLASIA Between 40 and 50% of patients with myelodysplasia appear to be cured with allogeneic transplantation. Results are better among younger patients and those with less-advanced disease. However, some patients with myelodysplasia can live for extended periods without intervention, and so transplantation is generally recommended only for patients with disease categorized as intermediate risk I or greater according to the International Prognostic Scoring System (Chap. 102).

LYMPHOMA Patients with disseminated intermediate- or high-grade non-Hodgkin's lymphoma who have not been cured by first-line chemotherapy and are transplanted in first relapse or second remission can still be cured in 40–50% of cases. This represents a clear advantage over results obtained with conventional-dose salvage chemotherapy. It is unsettled whether patients with high-risk disease benefit from transplantation in first remission. Most experts favor the use of autologous rather than allogeneic transplantation for patients with intermediate or high grade non-Hodgkin's lymphoma, because fewer complications occur with this approach and survival appears equivalent. For patients with recurrent disseminated indolent non-Hodgkin's lymphoma, autologous transplantation results in high response rates and improved progression-free survival compared to salvage chemotherapy. However, late relapses are seen after transplantation. The role of autologous transplantation in the initial treatment of patients is under study. Nonmyeloablative preparative regimens followed by allogeneic transplantation result in high response rates in patients with indolent lymphomas, but the exact role of this approach remains to be defined.

The role of transplantation in Hodgkin's disease is similar to that in intermediate- and high-grade non-Hodgkin's lymphoma. With transplantation, 5-year disease-free survival is 20–30% in patients who never achieve a first remission with standard chemotherapy and up to 70% for those transplanted in second remission. Transplantation has no defined role in first remission in Hodgkin's disease.

MYELOMA Patients with myeloma who have progressed on first-line therapy can sometimes benefit from allogeneic or autologous transplantation. Autologous transplantation has been studied as part of the initial therapy of patients, and both disease-free survival as well as overall survival were improved with this approach in randomized trials. The use of autologous transplantation followed by nonmyeloablative allogeneic transplantation has shown encouraging results.

SOLID TUMORS Among women with metastatic breast cancer, 15–20% disease-free survival rates at 3 years have been reported, with better results seen in younger patients who have responded completely to standard-dose therapy before undergoing transplantation. Randomized trials have not shown superior survival for patients treated for metastatic disease with high-dose chemotherapy plus stem cell support. Randomized trials evaluating transplantation as treatment for primary breast cancer have yielded mixed results. No role for autologous transplantation has been established in the treatment of breast cancer.

Patients with testicular cancer who have failed first-line chemotherapy have been treated with autologous transplantation; ~10–20% of such patients apparently have been cured with this approach.

The use of high-dose chemotherapy with autologous stem cell support is being studied for several other solid tumors, including ovarian cancer, small cell lung cancer, neuroblastoma, and pediatric sarcomas. As in most other settings, the best results have been obtained in patients with limited amounts of disease and where the remaining tumor remains sensitive to conventional-dose chemotherapy. Few randomized trials of transplantation in these diseases have been completed.

Partial and complete responses have been reported following nonmyeloablative allogeneic transplantation for some solid tumors, most notably renal cell cancers. The GVT effect, well documented in the treatment of hematologic malignancies, may apply to selected solid tumors under certain circumstances.

POSTTRANSPLANT RELAPSE Patients who relapse following autologous transplantation sometimes respond to further chemotherapy, particularly if the remission following transplantation was long. More options are available for patients who relapse following allogeneic transplantation. Of particular interest are the response rates seen with infusion of unirradiated donor lymphocytes. Complete responses in as many as 75% of patients with chronic myeloid leukemia, 40% in myelodysplasia, 25% in AML, and 15% in myeloma have been reported. Major complications of donor lymphocyte infusions include transient myelosuppression and the development of GVHD. These complications depend on the number of donor lymphocytes given and the schedule of infusions, with less GVHD seen with lower dose, fractionated schedules.

FURTHER READINGS

APPELBAUM FR: Haematopoietic cell transplantation as immunotherapy. Nature 411:385, 2001

BARON F, STORB R: Hematopoietic stem cell transplantation after reduced-intensity conditioning for older adults with acute myeloid leukemia. Curr Opin Hematol 14:145, 2007

BENSINGER WI et al: Transplantation of bone marrow as compared with peripheral-blood cells from HLA-identical relatives in patients with hematologic cancers. N Engl J Med 344:175, 2001

COPELAN EA: Hematopoietic stem-cell transplantation. N Engl J Med 354:1813, 2006

PETERSDORF EW et al: Major-histocompatibility-complex class I alleles and antigens in hematopoietic-cell transplantation. N Engl J Med 345:1794, 2001

SECTION 3 DISORDERS OF HEMOSTASIS

109 Disorders of Platelets and Vessel Wall

Barbara A. Konkle

Hemostasis is a dynamic process in which the platelet and the blood vessel wall play key roles. Platelets become activated upon adhesion to von Willebrand factor (vWF) and collagen in the exposed subendothelium after injury. Platelet activation is also mediated through shear forces imposed by blood flow itself, particularly in areas where the vessel wall is diseased, and is also affected by the inflammatory state of the endothelium. The activated platelet surface provides the major physiologic site for coagulation factor activation, which results in further platelet activation and fibrin formation. Genetic and acquired influences on the platelet and vessel wall, as well as on the coagulation and fibrinolytic systems, determine whether normal hemostasis, or bleeding or clotting symptoms, will result.

THE PLATELET

Platelets are released from the megakaryocyte, likely under the influence of flow in the capillary sinuses. The normal blood platelet count is 150,000–450,000/μL. The major regulator of platelet production is the hormone thrombopoietin (TPO), which is synthesized in the liver. Synthesis is increased with inflammation and specifically by interleukin 6. TPO binds to its receptor on platelets and megakaryocytes, by which it is removed from the circulation. Thus, a reduction in platelet and megakaryocyte mass increases the level of TPO, which then stimulates platelet production. Platelets circulate with an average life span of 7–10 days. Approximately one-third of the platelets reside in the spleen, and this number increases in proportion to splenic size, although the platelet count rarely decreases to <40,000/μL as the spleen enlarges. Platelets are physiologically very active but are anucleate, and thus they have limited capacity to synthesize new proteins.

Normal vascular endothelium contributes to preventing thrombosis by inhibiting platelet function (Chap. 59). When vascular endothelium is injured, these inhibitory effects are overcome, and platelets adhere to the exposed intimal surface primarily through vWF, a large multimeric protein present in both plasma and in the extracellular matrix of the subendothelial vessel wall. Platelet adhesion results in the generation of intracellular signals that lead to activation of the platelet glycoprotein (Gp) IIb/IIIa ($\alpha_{IIb}\beta_3$) receptor and resultant platelet aggregation.

Activated platelets undergo release of their granule contents, including nucleotides, adhesive proteins, growth factors, and procoagulants that serve to promote platelet aggregation and blood clot formation, and influence the environment of the forming clot. During platelet aggregation, additional platelets are recruited to the site of injury, leading to the formation of an occlusive platelet thrombus. The platelet plug is stabilized by the fibrin mesh that develops simultaneously as the product of the coagulation cascade.

THE VESSEL WALL

Endothelial cells line the surface of the entire circulatory tree, totaling 1–6 × 10^{13} cells, enough to cover a surface area equivalent to about six tennis courts. The endothelium is physiologically active, controlling vascular permeability, flow of biologically active molecules and nutrients, blood cell interactions with the vessel wall, the inflammatory response, and angiogenesis.

The endothelium normally presents an antithrombotic surface (Chap. 59) but rapidly becomes prothrombotic when stimulated, which promotes coagulation, inhibits fibrinolysis, and activates platelets. In many cases, endothelium-derived vasodilators are also platelet inhibitors (e.g., nitric oxide) and, conversely, endothelium-derived vasoconstrictors (e.g., endothelin) can also be platelet activators. The net effect of vasodilation and inhibition of platelet function is to promote blood fluidity, whereas the net effect of vasoconstriction and platelet activation is to promote hemostasis. Thus, blood fluidity and hemostasis are regulated by the balance of antithrombotic/prothrombotic and vasodilatory/vasoconstrictor properties of endothelial cells.

DISORDERS OF PLATELETS

THROMBOCYTOPENIA

Thrombocytopenia results from one or more of three processes: (1) decreased bone marrow production; (2) sequestration, usually in an enlarged spleen; and/or (3) increased platelet destruction. Disorders of production may be either inherited or acquired. In evaluating a patient with thrombocytopenia, a key step is to review the peripheral blood smear and to first rule out "pseudothrombocytopenia," particularly in a patient without an apparent cause for the thrombocytopenia. Pseudothrombocytopenia (Fig. 109-1*B*) is an in vitro artifact resulting from platelet agglutination via antibodies (usually IgG, but also IgM and IgA) when the calcium content is decreased by blood collection in ethylenediamine tetraacetic (EDTA), the anticoagulant present in tubes (purple top, often) used to collect blood for complete blood counts (CBCs). If a low platelet count is obtained in EDTA-anticoagulated blood, a blood smear can be evaluated and a platelet count determined in blood collected into sodium citrate (blue-top tube) or heparin (green-top tube), or ideally a smear of freshly obtained unanticoagulated blood, such as from a finger stick, can be examined.

APPROACH TO THE PATIENT: Thrombocytopenia

The history and physical examination, results of the CBC, and review of the peripheral blood smear are all critical components in the initial evaluation of the thrombocytopenic patients (Fig. 109-2). The overall health of the patient and whether he/she is receiving drug treatment will influence the differential diagnosis. A healthy young adult with thrombocytopenia will have a much more limited differential diagnosis than an ill hospitalized patient who is receiving multiple medications. Except in unusual inherited disorders, decreased platelet production usually results from bone marrow disorders that also affect red blood cell (RBC) and/or white blood cell (WBC) production. Because myelodysplasia can present with isolated thrombocytopenia, the bone marrow should be examined in patients presenting with isolated thrombocytopenia who are older than 60 years. While inherited thrombocytopenia is rare, any prior platelet counts should be retrieved and a family history regarding thrombocytopenia obtained. A careful history of drug ingestion should be obtained, including nonprescription and herbal remedies, as drugs are the most common cause of thrombocytopenia.

The physical examination can document an enlarged spleen, evidence of chronic liver disease, and other underlying disorders. Mild to moderate splenomegaly may be difficult to appreciate in many individuals due to body habitus and/or obesity but can be easily assess by abdominal ultrasound. A platelet count of approximately 5000–10,000 is required to maintain vascular integrity in the microcirculation. When the platelet count is markedly decreased, petechiae first appear in areas of increased venous pressure, the ankles and feet in an ambulatory patient. Petechiae are pinpoint, nonblanching hemorrhages and are usually a sign of a decreased platelet number and not platelet dysfunction. Wet purpura, blood blisters that form on the oral mucosa, are thought to denote an increased risk of life-threatening hemorrhage in the thrombocytopenic patient. Excessive bruising is seen in disorders of both platelet number and function.

Infection-Induced Thrombocytopenia Many viral and bacterial infections result in thrombocytopenia and are the most common noniatrogenic cause of thrombocytopenia. This may or may not be associated with laboratory evidence of disseminated intravascular coagulation (DIC), which is most commonly seen in patients with systemic infections with gram negative bacteria. Infections can affect both platelet production and platelet survival. In addition, immune mechanisms can be at work, as in infectious mononucleosis and early HIV infection. Late in HIV infection, pancytopenia and decreased and dysplastic platelet production is more common. Immune-mediated thrombocytopenia (ITP2) in children usually follows a viral infection and almost always resolves spontaneously. This association of infection with ITP is less clear in adults.

Bone marrow examination is often requested for evaluation of occult infections. A study evaluating the role of bone marrow examination in fever of unknown origin in HIV-infected patients found that for 86% of patients, the same diagnosis was established by less-invasive techniques, notably blood culture. In some instances, however, the diagnosis can be made earlier; thus, a bone marrow examination and culture is recommended when the diagnosis is needed urgently or when other, less-invasive methods have been unsuccessful.

Drug-Induced Thrombocytopenia Many drugs have been associated with thrombocytopenia. A predictable decrease in platelet count occurs after treatment with many chemotherapeutic drugs due to bone marrow suppression (Chap. 81). Other commonly used drugs that cause isolated thrombocytopenia are listed in Table 109-1, but all drugs should be suspect in a patient with thrombocytopenia without an apparent cause and should be stopped, or substituted, if possible. A helpful website, Platelets on the Internet (*http://moon.ouhsc.edu/jgeorge*), lists drugs reported to have caused thrombocytopenia and the level of evidence supporting the association. Although not well studied, herbal and over-the-counter

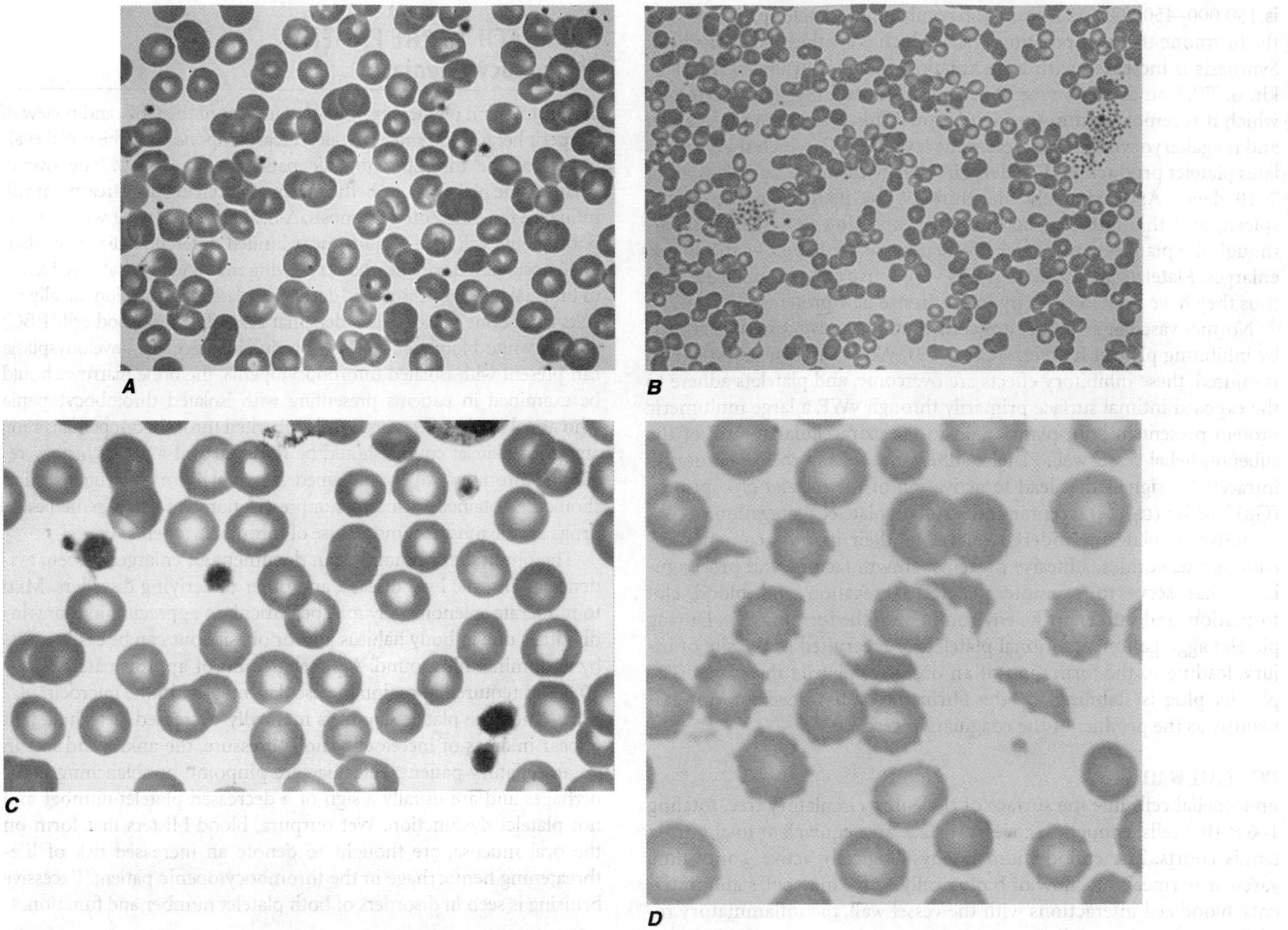

FIGURE 109-1 Photomicrographs of peripheral blood smears. ***A.*** Normal peripheral blood. ***B.*** Platelet clumping in pseudothrombocytopenia. ***C.*** Abnormal large platelet in autosomal dominant macrothrombocytopenia. ***D.*** Schistocytes and decreased platelets in microangiopathic hemolytic anemia.

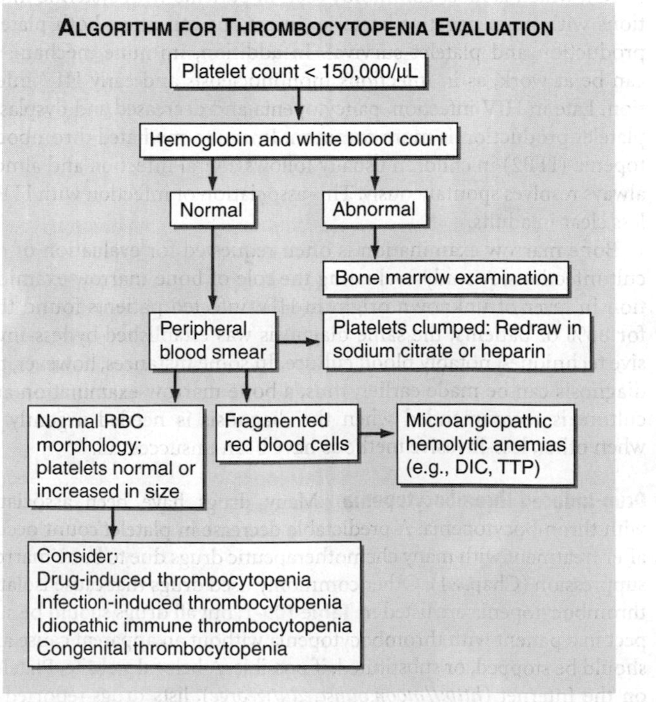

FIGURE 109-2 Algorithm for evaluating the thrombocytopenic patient.

preparations may also result in thrombocytopenia and should be discontinued in patients who are thrombocytopenic.

Classic drug-dependent antibodies are antibodies that react with specific platelet surface antigens and result in thrombocytopenia only when the drug is present. Many drugs are capable of inducing these antibodies, but for some reason they are more common with quinine and sulfonamides. Drug-dependent antibody binding can be demonstrated by laboratory assays, showing antibody binding in the presence of, but not without, the

TABLE 109-1 DRUGS DEFINITIVELY REPORTED TO CAUSE ISOLATED THROMBOCYTOPENIA[a]

Abciximab	Digoxin
Acetaminophen	Eptifibatide
Acyclovir	Hydrochlorothiazide
Aminosalicylic acid	Ibuprofen
Amiodarone	Levamisole
Amphotericin B	Octreotide
Ampicillin	Phenytoin
Carbamazepine	Quinine
Chlorpropamide	Rifampin
Danazol	Tamoxifen
Diatrizoate meglumine (Hypaque Meglumine)	Tirofiban
	Trimethoprim/sulfamethoxazole
Diclofenac	Vancomycin

[a]Drugs that preceded thrombocytopenia and full recovery occurred after drug discontinuation, but recurred with re-introduction of the drug, and other causes, including other drugs were excluded.

Source: Data from George and colleagues, *http://moon.ouhsc.edu/jgeorge.*

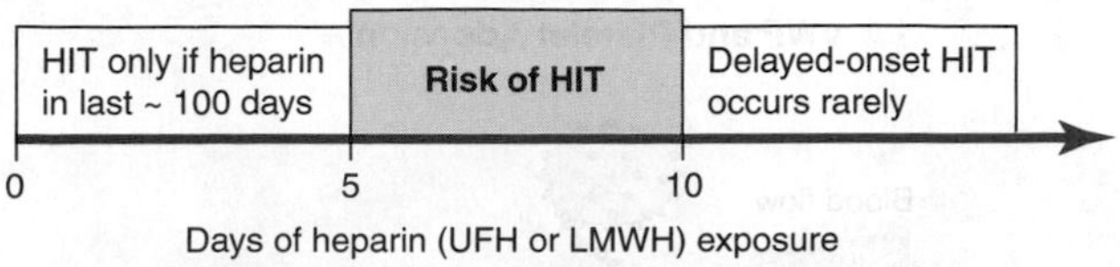

FIGURE 109-3 Time course of heparin-induced thrombocytopenia (HIT) development after heparin exposure. The timing of development after heparin exposure is a critical factor in determining the likelihood of HIT in a patient. HIT occurs early in heparin exposure only in the presence of preexisting heparin/platelet factor 4 (PF4) antibodies, which disappear from circulation by ~100 days following a prior exposure. Rarely, HIT may occur later after heparin exposure (termed *delayed-onset HIT*). In this setting, heparin/PF4 antibody testing is markedly positive. HIT can occur after exposure to either unfractionated heparin (UFH) or low-molecular-weight heparin (LMWH).

drug present in the assay. The thrombocytopenia typically occurs after a period of initial exposure (median length 21 days), or upon reexposure, and usually resolves in 7–10 days after drug withdrawal. The thrombocytopenia caused by the platelet GpIIbIIIa inhibitory drugs, such as abciximab, differs in that it may occur within 24 hours of initial exposure. This appears to be due to the presence of naturally occurring antibodies that cross-react with the drug bound to the platelet.

Heparin-Induced Thrombocytopenia Drug-induced thrombocytopenia due to heparin differs from that seen with other drugs in two major ways. (1) The thrombocytopenia is not usually severe, with nadir counts rarely <20,000/μL. (2) Heparin-induced thrombocytopenia (HIT) is not associated with bleeding and, in fact, markedly increases the risk of thrombosis. HIT results from antibody formation to a complex of the platelet-specific protein platelet factor 4 (PF4) and heparin. The antiheparin/PF4 antibody can activate platelets through the FcγRIIa receptor and also likely activates endothelial cells. Many patients exposed to heparin develop antibodies to heparin/PF4, but do not appear to have adverse consequences. A fraction of those who develop antibodies will develop thrombocytopenia, and a portion of those (up to 50%) will develop HIT and thrombosis (HITT).

HIT can occur after exposure to low-molecular-weight heparin (LMWH), as well as unfractionated heparin (UFH), although it is about 10 times more common with the latter. Most patients develop HIT after exposure to heparin for 5–10 days (Fig. 109-3). It occurs before 5 days only in those who were exposed to heparin in the prior few weeks or months (< ~100 days) and have circulating antiheparin/PF4 antibodies. Rarely, thrombocytopenia and thrombosis begin several days after all heparin has been stopped (termed *delayed onset HIT*). The 4 "T"s have been recommended to be used in a diagnostic algorithm for HIT: *t*hrombocytopenia, *t*iming of platelet count drop, *t*hrombosis and other sequelae such as localized skin reactions, and o*t*her cause of thrombocytopenia not evident.

LABORATORY TESTING FOR HIT HIT (antiheparin/PF4) antibodies can be detected using two types of assays. The most widely available is an enzyme-linked immunoassay (ELISA) with PF4/polyanion complex as the antigen. Since many patients develop antibodies but do not develop clinical HIT, the test has a low specificity for the diagnosis of HIT. This is especially true in patients who have undergone cardiopulmonary bypass surgery, where approximately 50% of patients develop these antibodies postoperatively. The other assay is a platelet activation assay that measures the ability of the patients' serum to activate platelets in the presence of heparin in a concentration-dependent manner. This test has lower sensitivity but higher specificity than the ELISA. However, HIT remains a clinical diagnosis. The main value in testing is in excluding the diagnosis with negative tests, particularly ELISA.

Rx HEPARIN-INDUCED THROMBOCYTOPENIA

Early recognition is key in treatment of HIT, with prompt discontinuation of heparin and use of alternative anticoagulants. Thrombosis is a common complication of HIT, even after heparin discontinuation, and can occur in both the venous and arterial systems. In patients diagnosed with HIT, imaging studies to evaluate the presence of thrombosis (at least lower-extremity duplex dopplers) are recommended. Patients requiring anticoagulation should be switched from heparin to an alternative anticoagulant. The direct thrombin inhibitors (DTIs) argatroban and lepirudin are effective in HITT. The DTI bivalirudin and the antithrombin-binding pentasaccharide fondaparinux appear to be effective but are not yet approved by the U.S. Food and Drug Administration (FDA) for this indication. Danaparoid, a mixture of glycosoaminoglycans with anti-Xa activity, has been used extensively for the treatment of HITT; it is no longer available in the United States but is in other countries. HIT antibodies cross-react with LMWH, and these preparations should not be used in the treatment of HIT.

Because of the high rate of thrombosis in patients with HIT, anticoagulation should be strongly considered, even in the absence of thrombosis. In patients with thrombosis, patients can be transitioned to warfarin, with treatment usually for 3–6 months. In patients without thrombosis, the duration of anticoagulation needed is undefined. An increased risk of thrombosis is present for at least 1 month after diagnosis; however, most thromboses occur early, and whether thrombosis occurs later if the patient is initially anticoagulated is unknown. Options include continuing anticoagulation until a few days after platelet recovery or for one month. Introduction of warfarin alone in the setting of HIT or HITT may precipitate thrombosis, particularly venous gangrene, presumably due to clotting activation and severely reduced levels of proteins C and S. Warfarin should only be started after alternative anticoagulation has been given for several days and the prothrombotic state has lessened.

Immune Thrombocytopenic Purpura (ITP) Immune thrombocytopenic purpura (ITP; also termed *idiopathic thrombocytopenic purpura*) is an acquired disorder leading to immune-mediated destruction of platelets and possibly inhibition of platelet release from the megakaryocyte. In children it is usually an acute disease, most commonly following an infection, and with a self-limited course. In adults it usually runs a more chronic course. The exact nature of the immune dysfunction is generally not known. ITP is termed *secondary* if it is associated with an underlying disorder; autoimmune disorders, particularly systemic lupus erythematosis (SLE), and infections, such as HIV and hepatitis C, are common causes. The association of ITP with *Helicobacter pylori* infection is unclear.

ITP is characterized by mucocutaneous bleeding and a low, often very low, platelet count, with otherwise normal peripheral blood cells and smear. Patients usually present either with ecchymoses and petechiae, or with thrombocytopenia incidentally found on a routine CBC. Mucocutaneous bleeding, such as oral mucosa, gastrointestinal, or heavy menstrual bleeding, may be present. Rarely, life-threatening bleeding, including in the central nervous system, can occur. Wet purpura (blood blisters in the mouth) and retinal hemorrhages may herald life-threatening bleeding.

LABORATORY TESTING IN ITP Laboratory testing for antibodies (serologic testing) is usually not helpful due to the low sensitivity and specificity of the tests. Bone marrow examination can be reserved for older adults (usually >60 years) or those who have other signs or laboratory abnormalities not explained by ITP, or in patients who do not respond to initial therapy. The peripheral blood smear may show large platelets, with otherwise normal morphology. Depending on the bleeding history, iron deficiency anemia may be present.

Laboratory testing is performed to evaluate for secondary causes of ITP and should include testing for HIV infection and hepatitis C (and other infections if indicated); serologic testing for SLE; serum protein electrophoresis and immunoglobulin levels to potentially detect hypogammaglobulinemia, IgA deficiency, or monoclonal gammopathies; and, if anemia is present, direct antiglobulin testing (Coombs test) to rule out combined autoimmune hemolytic anemia with ITP (Evans's syndrome).

Rx IMMUNE THROMBOCYTOPENIC PURPURA

The treatment of ITP utilizes drugs that decrease reticuloendothelial uptake of the antibody-bound platelet and/or decrease antibody production.

However, the diagnosis of ITP does not necessarily mean that treatment must be instituted. Patients with platelet counts >30,000/μL appear not to have increased mortality related to the thrombocytopenia.

Initial treatment in patients without significant bleeding symptoms, severe thrombocytopenia (<5000/μL), or signs of impending bleeding (such as retinal hemorrhage or large oral mucosal hemorrhages) can be instituted as an outpatient using single agents. Traditionally this has been prednisone at 1 mg/kg, although Rh_0(D) immune globulin therapy (WinRho SDF) at 50–75 μg/kg is also being used in this setting. Rh_0(D) immune globulin must be used only in Rh+ patients as the mechanism of action is production of limited hemolysis, with antibody-coated cells "saturating" the Fc receptors, inhibiting Fc receptor function. Hemoglobin levels usually decrease (mean 1.7 g/dL), although severe intravascular hemolysis is a rare complication. Doses are reduced if given to anemic patients. Intravenous gamma globulin (IVIgG), which is pooled, primarily IgG antibodies, also blocks the Fc receptor system, but appears to work primarily through different mechanism(s). IVIgG has more efficacy than anti-Rh_0(D) in post-splenectomized patients. IVIgG is dosed at 2 g/kg total, given in divided doses over 2–5 days. Side effects are usually related to the volume of infusion and infrequently include aseptic meningitis and renal failure. All immunoglobulin preparations are derived from human plasma and undergo treatment for viral inactivation.

For patients with severe ITP and/or symptoms of bleeding, hospital admission and combined modality therapy are given using high-dose glucocorticoids with IVIgG or anti-Rh_0D therapy, and, as needed, additional immunosuppressive agents. Rituximab, an anti-CD20 (B cell) antibody, has shown efficacy in the treatment of refractory ITP.

Splenectomy has been used for treatment of patients who relapse after glucocorticoids are tapered. Splenectomy remains an important treatment option; however, more patients than previously thought will go into a remission over time. Observation, if the platelet count is high enough, or intermittent treatment with anti-Rh_0(D) or IVIgG may be a reasonable approach to see if the ITP will resolve. Vaccination against encapsulated organisms (especially pneumococcus, but also menningococcus and *Haemophilus influenzae*, depending on patient age and potential exposure) is recommended before splenectomy. Accessory spleen(s) are a very rare cause of relapse.

New drugs for ITP include TPO receptor agonists. This approach to treatment of ITP stems from the finding that many patients with ITP do not have increased TPO levels, as was previously hypothesized, nor do they all have increased platelet destruction. Two agents, one administered subcutaneously and another orally, have shown response in many patients with refractory ITP. Roles for these agents in ITP treatment are not fully defined.

Inherited Thrombocytopenia Thrombocytopenia is rarely inherited, either as an isolated finding or as part of a syndrome, and may be inherited in an autosomal dominant, autosomal recessive, or X-linked pattern. Many forms of autosomal dominant thrombocytopenia are now known to be associated with mutations in the nonmuscle myosin heavy chain *MYH9* gene. Interestingly, these include the May-Hegglin anomaly and Sebastian, Epstein's, and Fechtner syndromes, all of which have distinct distinguishing features. A common feature of these disorders is large platelets (Fig. 109-1*C*). Autosomal recessive disorders include congenital amegakaryocytic thrombocytopenia, thrombocytopenia with absent radii, and Bernard Soulier syndrome. The latter is primarily a functional platelet disorder due to absence of GPIb-IX-V, the vWF adhesion receptor. X-linked disorders include Wiskott-Aldrich syndrome and a dyshematopoietic syndrome resulting from a mutation in GATA-1, an important transcriptional regulator of hematopoiesis.

THROMBOTIC THROMBOCYTOPENIC PURPURA AND HEMOLYTIC UREMIC SYNDROME

Thrombotic thrombocytopenic microangiopathies are a group of disorders characterized by thrombocytopenia, a microangiopathic hemolytic anemia evident by fragmented RBCs (Fig. 109-1*D*) and laboratory evidence of hemolysis, and microvascular thrombosis. This includes thrombotic thrombocytopenic purpura (TTP) and hemolytic uremic syndrome (HUS), as well as syndromes complicating bone marrow transplantation, certain medications and infections, pregnancy, and vasculitis. In DIC, while thrombocytopenia and microangiopathy are seen, a coagulopathy predominates, with consumption of clotting factors and fibrinogen resulting in an elevated prothrombin time (PT) and often activated partial thromboplastin time (aPTT). The PT and aPTT are characteristically normal in TTP or HUS.

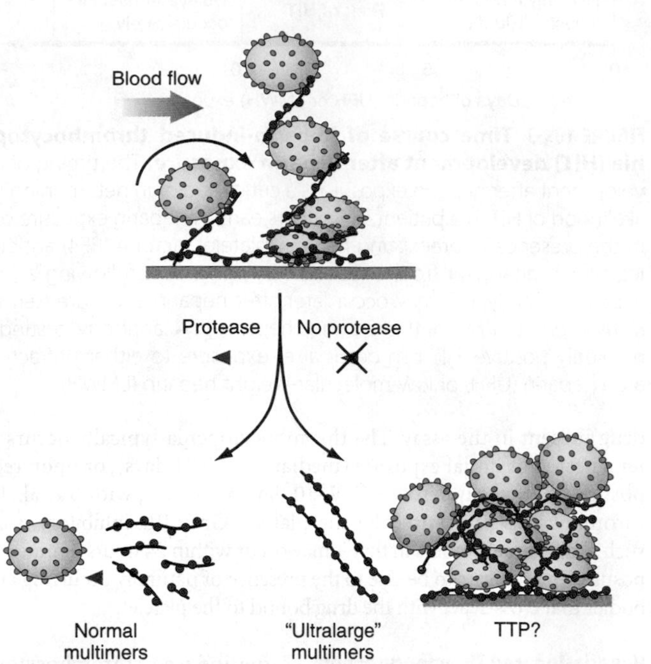

FIGURE 109-4 Pathogenesis of thrombotic thrombocytopenic purpura (TTP). Normally the ultra-high molecular-weight multimers of von Willebrand factor (vWF) produced by the endothelial cells are processed into smaller multimers by a plasma metalloproteinase called *ADAMTS13*. In TTP the activity of the protease is inhibited, and the ultra-high molecular-weight multimers of vWF initiate platelet aggregation and thrombosis. *(From Vesely et al., Copyright American Society of Hematology.)*

Thrombotic Thrombocytopenic Purpura TTP and HUS were previously considered overlap syndromes. However, in the past few years the pathophysiology of inherited and idiopathic TTP has become better understood and clearly differs from HUS. TTP was first described in 1924 by Eli Moschcowitz and characterized by a pentad of findings that include microangiopathic hemolytic anemia, thrombocytopenia, renal failure, neurologic findings, and fever. The full-blown syndrome is less commonly seen now, probably due to earlier diagnosis. The introduction of treatment with plasma exchange markedly improved the prognosis in patients, with a decrease in mortality from 85–100% to 10–30%.

The pathogenesis of inherited (Upshaw-Schulman syndrome) and idiopathic TTP is related to a deficiency of, or antibodies to, a metalloprotease that cleaves vWF and ADAMTS13, respectively. vWF is normally secreted as ultra-large multimers, which are then cleaved by ADAMTS13. The persistence of ultra-large vWF molecules are thought to contribute to pathogenic platelet adhesion and aggregation (Fig. 109-4). This defect alone, however, is not sufficient to result in TTP as individuals with a congenital absence of ADAMTS13 develop TTP only episodically. Additional provocative factors have not been defined. The level of ADAMTS13 activity, as well as antibodies, can now be detected by laboratory assays. However, assays with sufficient sensitivity and specificity to direct clinical management have yet to be defined.

Idiopathic TTP appears to be more common in women than in men. No geographic or racial distribution has been defined. TTP is more common in patients with HIV infection and in pregnant women. Medication-related TTP may be secondary to antibody formation (ticlopidine and possibly clopidogrel) or direct endothelial toxicity (cyclosporine, mitomycin C, tacrolimus, quinine), although this is not always so clear, and fear of withholding treatment, as well as lack of other treatment alternatives, results in broad application of plasma exchange. However, withdrawal, or reduction in dose, of endothelial toxic agents may decrease the microangiopathy.

℞ THROMBOTIC THROMBOCYTOPENIC PURPURA

TTP is a devastating disease if not diagnosed and treated promptly. In patients presenting with new thrombocytopenia, with or without evidence of renal insufficiency and other elements of classic TTP, laboratory data should be obtained to rule out DIC and to evaluate for evidence of microangiopathic hemolytic anemia. Findings to support the TTP diagnosis include an increased lactate dehydrogenase and indirect bilirubin, decreased haptoglobin, and increased reticulocyte count, with a negative direct antiglobulin test. The peripheral smear should be examined for evidence of schistocytes (Fig. 109-1*D*). Polychromasia is usually also present due to the increased number of young red blood cells, and nucleated RBCs are often present, which is thought to be due to infarction in the microcirculatory system of the bone marrow.

Plasma exchange remains the mainstay of treatment of ITP. ADAMTS13 antibody–mediated TTP (idiopathic TTP) appears to respond best to plasma exchange. Plasma exchange is continued until the platelet count is normal and signs of hemolysis are resolved for at least 2 days. While never evaluated in clinical trial, the use of glucocorticoids seems a reasonable approach, but they should only be used as an adjunct to plasma exchange. Additionally, other immunomodulatory therapies have been reported to be successful in refractory or relapsing TTP, including rituximab, vincristine, cyclophosphamide, and splenectomy. The role of rituximab in the treatment of this disorder needs to be defined. A significant relapse rate is noted: 25–45% within 30 days of initial "remission" and 12–40% with late relapses. Relapses may be more frequent in patients with severe ADAMTS13 deficiency at presentation.

Hemolytic Uremic Syndrome HUS is a syndrome characterized by acute renal failure, microangiopathic hemolytic anemia, and thrombocytopenia. It is seen predominantly in children and in most cases is preceded by an episode of diarrhea, often hemorrhagic in nature. *Escherichia coli* O157:H7 is the most frequent, although not only, etiologic serotype. HUS not associated with diarrhea (termed *DHUS*) is more heterogeneous in presentation and course. Some children who develop DHUS have been found to have mutations in genes encoding Factor H, a soluble complement regulator, and membrane cofactor protein that is mainly expressed in the kidney.

℞ HEMOLYTIC UREMIC SYNDROME

Treatment of HUS is primarily supportive. In D+HUS, many (~40%) children require at least some period of support with dialysis; however, the overall mortality is <5%. In D–HUS the mortality is higher, approximately 26%. Plasma infusion or plasma exchange has not been shown to alter the overall course. ADAMTS13 levels are generally reported to be normal in HUS, although occasionally they have been reported to be decreased. As ADAMTS13 assays improve, they may help in defining a subset that better fits a TTP diagnosis and may respond to plasma exchange.

THROMBOCYTOSIS

Thrombocytosis is almost always due to (1) iron deficiency; (2) inflammation, cancer, or infection (reactive thrombocytosis); or (3) an underlying myeloproliferative process [essential thrombocythemia or polycythemia vera (Chap. 103)] or, rarely, the 5q-myelodysplastic process (Chap. 102). Patients presenting with an elevated platelet count should be evaluated for underlying inflammation or malignancy, and iron deficiency should be ruled out. Thrombocytosis in response to acute or chronic inflammation has not been associated with an increased thrombotic risk. In fact, patients with markedly elevated platelet counts (>1.5 million), usually seen in the setting of a myeloproliferative disorder, have an increased risk of bleeding. This appears to be due, at least in part, to acquired von Willebrand disease (vWD) due to platelet-vWF adhesion and removal.

QUALITATIVE DISORDERS OF PLATELET FUNCTION

Inherited Disorders of Platelet Function Inherited platelet function disorders are thought to be relatively rare, although the prevalence of mild disorders of platelet function is unclear, in part because our testing for such disorders is suboptimal. Rare qualitative disorders include the autosomal recessive disorders Glanzmann's thrombasthenia (absence of the platelet GpIIbIIIa receptor) and Bernard Soulier syndrome (absence of the platelet GpIb-IX-V receptor). Both are inherited in an autosomal recessive fashion and present with bleeding symptoms in childhood.

Platelet storage pool disorder (SPD) is the classic autosomal dominant qualitative platelet disorder. This results from abnormalities of platelet granule formation. It is also seen as a part of inherited disorders of granule formation, such as Hermansky-Pudlak syndrome. Bleeding symptoms in SPD are variable but often mild. The most common inherited disorders of platelet function are disorders that prevent normal secretion of granule content. Few of the abnormalities have been dissected at the molecular level, but these are likely due to multiple abnormalities. They are usually described as *secretion defects*. Bleeding symptoms are usually mild in nature.

℞ INHERITED DISORDERS OF PLATELET DYSFUNCTION

Bleeding symptoms or prevention of bleeding in patients with severe dysfunction frequently requires platelet transfusion. Care is taken to limit the risk of alloimmunization by limiting exposure and using prestorage leukodepleted platelets for transfusion. Platelet disorders associated with milder bleeding symptoms frequently respond to desmopressin [1-deamino-8-D-arginine vasopressin (DDAVP)]. DDAVP increases plasma vWF and FVIII levels; whether it also has a direct effect on platelet function is unknown. Particularly for mucosal bleeding symptoms, antifibrinolytic therapy (epsilon-aminocaproic acid or tranexamic acid) is used alone or in conjunction with DDAVP or platelet therapy.

Acquired Disorders of Platelet Function Acquired platelet dysfunction is common, usually due to medications, either intentionally, as with antiplatelet therapy, or unintentionally, as with high dose penicillins. Acquired platelet dysfunction occurs in uremia. This is likely multifactorial, but the resultant effect is defective adhesion and activation. The platelet defect is improved most by dialysis, but may also be improved by increasing the hematocrit to 27–32%, giving DDAVP (0.3 μg/kg), or use of conjugated estrogens. Platelet dysfunction also occurs with cardiopulmonary bypass due to the effect of the artificial circuit on platelets, and bleeding symptoms respond to platelet transfusion. Platelet dysfunction seen with underlying hematologic disorders can result from nonspecific interference by circulating paraproteins or intrinsic platelet defects in myeloproliferative and myelodysplastic syndromes.

VON WILLEBRAND DISEASE

vWD is the most common inherited bleeding disorder. Estimates from laboratory data suggest a prevalence of approximately 1%, but data based on symptomatic individuals suggest that it is closer to 0.1% of the population. vWF serves two roles: (1) as the major adhesion molecule that tethers the platelet to the exposed subendothelium; and (2) as the binding protein for FVIII, resulting in significant prolongation of the FVIII half-life in circulation. The platelet-adhesive function of vWF is critically dependent on the presence of large vWF multimers, while FVIII binding is not. Most of the symptoms of vWD are "platelet-like" except in more severe vWD when the FVIII is low enough to produce symptoms similar to those found in Factor VIII deficiency (hemophilia A).

vWD has been classified into three major types, with four subtypes of type 2 (Table 109-2). By far the most common type of vWD is type 1 disease, with a parallel decrease in vWF protein, vWF function, and

TABLE 109-2 LABORATORY DIAGNOSIS OF VON WILLEBRAND DISEASE

Type	aPTT	vWF Antigen	vWF Activity	FVIII Activity	Multimer
1	Nl or ↑	↓	↓	↓	Normal distribution, decreased in quantity
2A	Nl or ↑	↓	↓↓	↓	Loss of high and intermediate MW multimers
2B[a]	Nl or ↑	↓	↓↓	↓	Loss of high MW multimers
2M	Nl or ↑	↓	↓↓	↓	Normal distribution, decreased in quantity
2N	↑↑	Nl or ↓[b]	Nl or ↓[b]	↓↓	Normal distribution
3	↑↑	↓↓	↓↓	↓↓	Absent

[a]Usually also decreased platelet count.
[b]For type 2N, in the homozygous state, FVIII is very low; in the heterozygous state, only seen in conjunction with type 1 vWD.
Abbreviations: aPTT, activated partial thromboplastin time; vWF, von Willebrand factor; F, Factor; Nl, normal; MW, molecular weight.

FVIII levels, accounting for at least 80% of cases. Patients have predominantly mucosal bleeding symptoms, although postoperative bleeding can also be seen. Bleeding symptoms are very uncommon in infancy and usually manifest later in childhood with excessive bruising and epistaxis. Since these symptoms occur commonly in childhood, the clinician should particularly note bruising at sites unlikely to be traumatized and/or prolonged epistaxis requiring medical attention. Menorrhagia is a common manifestation of vWD. Menstrual bleeding resulting in anemia should warrant an evaluation for vWD and, if negative, functional platelet disorders. Frequently, mild type 1 vWD first manifests with dental extractions, particularly wisdom tooth extraction, or tonsillectomy.

Not all patients with low vWF levels have bleeding symptoms. Whether patients bleed or not will depend on the overall hemostatic balance they have inherited, along with environmental influences and the type of hemostatic challenges they experience. Although the inheritance of vWD is autosomal, many factors influence both vWF levels and bleeding symptoms. These have not all been defined but include blood type, thyroid hormone status, race, stress, exercise, and hormonal (both endogenous and exogenous) influences. Patients with type O blood have vWF protein levels about one-half those of patients with AB blood type; in fact, the normal range for patients with type O blood overlaps that usually considered diagnostic for vWD. A mildly decreased vWF level should perhaps be viewed more as a risk factor for bleeding than as an actual disease.

Patients with type 2 vWD have functional defects; thus, the vWF antigen measurement is significantly higher than the test of function. For types 2A, 2B, and 2M, vWF activity is decreased, measured as ristocetin cofactor or collagen binding activity. In type 2A vWD, the impaired function is due either to increased susceptibility to cleavage by ADAMTS13, resulting in loss of intermediate- and high-molecular weight (M.W.) multimers, or to decreased secretion of these multimers by the cell. Type 2B vWD results from gain of function mutations that result in increased spontaneous binding of vWF to platelets in circulation, with subsequent clearance of this complex by the reticuloendothelial system. The resulting vWF in the patients' plasma lacks the highest M.W. multimers, and the platelet count is usually modestly reduced. Type 2M results from a group of mutations that cause dysfunction of the molecule but do not affect multimer structure.

Type 2N vWD reflects mutations in vWF that preclude binding of FVIII. As FVIII is stabilized by binding to vWF, the FVIII in patients with type 2N vWD has a very short half-life, and the FVIII level is markedly decreased. This is sometimes termed *autosomal hemophilia*. Type 3 vWD, or severe vWD, describes patients with virtually no vWF antigen (usually <10%). Patients experience mucosal and joint postoperative symptoms as well as other bleeding symptoms. Some patients with type 3 vWD, particularly those with large vWF gene deletions, are at risk of developing antibodies to infused vWF.

Acquired vWD is a rare disorder, most commonly seen in patients with underlying lymphoproliferative disorders, including monoclonal gammopathies of undetermined significance (MGUS), multiple myeloma, and Waldenstrom's macroglobulinemia. It is seen most commonly in the setting of MGUS and should be suspected in patients, particularly elderly patients, with a new onset of severe mucosal bleeding symptoms.

Heyde's syndrome (aortic stenosis with gastrointestinal bleeding) is attributed to the presence of angiodysplasia of the gastrointestinal tract in patients with aortic stenosis. However, the shear stress on blood passing through the stenotic aortic valve appears to produce a change in vWF, making it susceptible to serum proteases. Consequently, large multimer forms are lost, leading to an acquired type 2 vWD, but return when the stenotic valve is replaced.

℞ VON WILLEBRAND DISEASE

The mainstay of treatment for type 1 vWD is 1-deamino-8-D-arginine vasopressin (DDAVP, or desmopressin), which results in release of vWF and FVIII from endothelial stores. DDAVP can be given intravenously or by an intranasal spray (1.5 mg/mL). The peak activity when given intravenously is approximately 30 min, while it is 2 h when given intranasally. The usual dose is 0.3 μg/kg intravenously or 2 squirts (1 in each nostril) for patients >50 kg (1 squirt for those <50 kg). It is recommended that patients with vWD be tested with DDAVP to assess their response before using it. In patients who respond well (increase in values of two- to fourfold), it can be used for procedures with minor-to-moderate risk of bleeding. Depending on the procedure, additional doses may be needed; it is usually given every 12–24 h. Less frequent dosing may result in less tachyphylaxis, which occurs when synthesis cannot compensate for the released stores. The major side effect of DDAVP is hyponatremia due to decreased free water clearance. This occurs most commonly in the very young and the very old, but fluid restriction should be advised for all patients for the 24 hours following each dose.

Some patients with types 2A and 2M vWD respond to DDAVP such that it can be used for minor procedures. For the other subtypes, for type 3 disease, and for major procedures requiring longer periods of normal hemostasis, vWF replacement can be given. Virally inactivated vWF-containing factor concentrates are thought to be safer than cryoprecipitate as the replacement product. Humate-P is the only FDA-approved product for this indication in the United States. Other concentrates have been studied in vWD, and a vWF concentrate is available in some countries in Europe.

Antifibrinolytic therapy, using either epsilon-aminocaproic acid or tranexamic acid, is an important therapy, either alone or in an adjunctive capacity, particularly for the prevention or treatment of mucosal bleeding. These agents are particularly useful in prophylaxis for dental procedures, with DDAVP for dental extractions and tonsillectomy, menorrhagia, and prostate procedures. It is contraindicated in the setting of upper urinary tract bleeding, due to the risk of ureteral obstruction.

DISORDERS OF THE VESSEL WALL

The vessel wall is an integral part of hemostasis, and separation of a fluid phase is artificial, particularly in disorders such as TTP or HIT that clearly involve the endothelium as well. Inflammation localized to the vessel wall, such as vasculitis, or inherited connective tissue disorders are abnormalities inherent to the vessel wall.

METABOLIC AND INFLAMMATORY DISORDERS

Acute febrile illnesses may result in vascular damage. This can result from immune complexes containing viral antigens or the viruses themselves. Certain pathogens, such as the rickettsiae causing Rocky Mountain spotted fever, replicate in endothelial cells and damage them. Vascular purpura may occur in patients with polyclonal gammopathies but more commonly in those with monoclonal gammopathies, including Waldenstrom's macroglobulinemia, multiple myeloma, and cryoglobulinemia. Patients with mixed cryoglobulinemia develop a more extensive maculopapular rash due to immune complex-mediated damage to the vessel wall.

Patients with scurvy (vitamin C deficiency) develop painful episodes of perifollicular skin bleeding as well as more systemic bleeding symptoms. Vitamin C is needed to synthesize hydroxyproline, an essential constituent of collagen. Patients with Cushing's syndrome or on chronic glucocorticoid therapy develop skin bleeding and easy bruising due to atrophy of supporting connective tissue. A similar phenomena is seen with aging, where, following minor trauma, blood spreads superficially under the epidermis. This has been termed *senile purpura,* and it is most common on skin that has been previously damaged by sun exposure.

Henoch-Schönlein, or anaphylactoid, purpura is a distinct, self-limited type of vasculitis that occurs in children and young adults. Patients have an acute inflammatory reaction with IgA and complement components in capillaries, mesangial tissues, and small arterioles, leading to increased vascular permeability and localized hemorrhage. The syndrome is often preceded by an upper respiratory infection, commonly with streptococcal pharyngitis, or is triggered by drug or food allergies. Patients develop a purpuric rash on the extensor surfaces of the arms and legs, usually accompanied by polyarthralgias or arthritis, abdominal pain, and hematuria from focal glomerulonephritis. All coagulation tests are normal, but renal impairment may occur. Glucocorticoids can provide symptomatic relief but do not alter the course of the illness.

INHERITED DISORDERS OF THE VESSEL WALL

Patients with inherited disorders of the connective tissue matrix, such as Marfan's syndrome, Ehlers-Danlos syndrome, and pseudoxanthoma elasticum, frequently report easy bruising. Inherited vascular abnormalities can result in increased bleeding. This is notably seen in hereditary hemorrhagic telangiectasia (HHT, or Osler-Weber-Rendu disease), a disorder where abnormal telangiectatic capillaries result in frequent bleeding episodes, primarily from the nose and gastrointestinal tract. Arteriovenous malformation (AVM) in the lung, brain, and liver may also occur in HHT. The telangiectasia can often be visualized on the oral and nasal mucosa. Two genes involved in the pathogenesis are *eng* (endoglin) on chromosome 9q33-34 (so-called HHT type 1), associated with pulmonary AVM in 40% of cases; and *alk1* (activin-receptor-like kinase 1) on chromosome 12q13, associated with a much lower risk of pulmonary AVM.

ACKNOWLEDGMENT

Robert Handin, MD, contributed this chapter in HPIM, 16e, and some materials from his chapter are included here.

FURTHER READINGS

AREPALLY GM, ORTEL TL: Clinical practice. Heparin-induced thrombocytopenia. N Engl J Med 355:809, 2006

ARMSTRONG E, KONKLE BA: Von Willebrand Disease, in *Clinical Hematology*, 1st ed, NS Young et al (eds). Philadelphia, Mosby Elsevier, 2006, pp 830–841

CINES DB, MCMILLAN R: Management of adult idiopathic thrombocytopenic purpura. Annu Rev Med 56:425, 2005

GEORGE JN: Clinical practice. Thrombotic thrombocytopenic purpura. N Engl J Med 354:1927, 2006

RAO AK et al: Inherited defects in platelet signaling mechanisms. Semin Thromb Hemostas 30:525, 2004

SADLER JE: New concepts in von Willebrand disease. Annu Rev Med 56:173, 2005

WARKENTIN TE: Heparin-induced thrombocytopenia. Disease-A-Month 51:141, 2005

110 Coagulation Disorders

Valder Arruda, Katherine A. High

Deficiencies of coagulation factors have been recognized for centuries. Patients with genetic deficiencies of plasma coagulation factors exhibit lifelong recurrent bleeding episodes into joints, muscles, and closed spaces, either spontaneously or following an injury. The most common inherited factor deficiencies are the hemophilias, X-linked diseases caused by deficiency of Factor (F) VIII (hemophilia A) or Factor IX (FIX, hemophilia B). Rare congenital bleeding disorders due to deficiencies of other factors, including FII (prothrombin), FV, FVII, FX, FXI, FXIII, and fibrinogen are usually inherited in an autosomal recessive manner (Table 110-1). Advances in characterization of the molecular bases of clotting factor deficiencies have contributed to a better understanding of the disease phenotypes and may allow more targeted therapeutic approaches through the development of small molecules, recombinant proteins, or cell and gene-based therapies.

Commonly used tests of hemostasis provide the initial screening for clotting factor activity (Fig. 110-1), and disease phenotype often correlates with the level of clotting activity. An isolated abnormal prothrombin time (PT) suggests FVII deficiency, whereas a prolonged activated partial thromboplastin time (aPTT) indicates most commonly hemophilia or FXI deficiency (Fig. 110-1). The prolongation of both PT and aPTT suggests deficiency of FV, FX, FII, or fibrinogen abnormalities. The addition of the missing factor to the subject's plasma at a range of doses will correct the abnormal clotting times; the result is expressed as percent of the activity observed in normal subjects.

Acquired deficiencies of plasma coagulation are more frequent than congenital disorders; the most common disorders include hemorrhagic diathesis of liver disease, disseminated intravascular coagulation (DIC), and vitamin K deficiency. In these disorders, blood coagulation is hampered by the deficiency of more than one clotting factor, and the bleeding episodes result from perturbation of both primary (e.g., platelet and vessel wall interactions) and secondary (coagulation) hemostasis.

TABLE 110-1 GENETIC AND LABORATORY CHARACTERISTICS OF INHERITED COAGULATION DISORDERS

Clotting Factor Deficiency	Inheritance	Prevalence in General Population	Laboratory Abnormality[a]			Minimum Hemostatic Levels	Treatment	Plasma Half-Life
			aPTT	PT	TT			
Fibrinogen	AR	1 in 1,000,000	+	+	+	100 mg/dL	Cryoprecipitate	2–4 d
Prothrombin	AR	1 in 2,000,000	+	+	–	20–30%	FFP/PCCs	3–4 d
Factor V	AR	1 in 1,000,000	+/–	+/–	–	15–20%	FFP	36 h
Factor VII	AR	1 in 500,000	–	+	–	15–20%	FFP/PCCs	4–6 h
Factor VIII	X-linked	1 in 5,000	+	–	–	30%	FVIII concentrates	8–12 h
Factor IX	X-linked	1 in 30,000	+	–	–	30%	FIX concentrates	18–24 h
Factor X	AR	1 in 1,000,000	+/–	+/–	–	15–20%	FFP/PCCs	40–60 h
Factor XI	AR	1 in 1,000,000	+	–	–	15–20%	FFP	40–70 h
Factor XII	AR	ND	+	–	–	[b]	[b]	60 h
HK	AR	ND	+	–	–	[b]	[b]	150 h
Prekallikrein	AR	ND	+	–	–	[b]	[b]	35 h
Factor XIII	AR	1 in 2,000,000	–	–	+/–	2–5%	Cryoprecipitate	11–14 d

[a]Values within normal range (–) or prolonged (+).

[b]No risk for bleeding, treatment is not indicated.

Abbreviations: HK, high-molecular weight kininogen; AR, autosomal recessive; aPTT, activated partial thromboplastin time; PT, prothrombin time; TT, thrombin time; ND, not determined; FFP, fresh frozen plasma; PCCs, prothrombin complex concentrates.

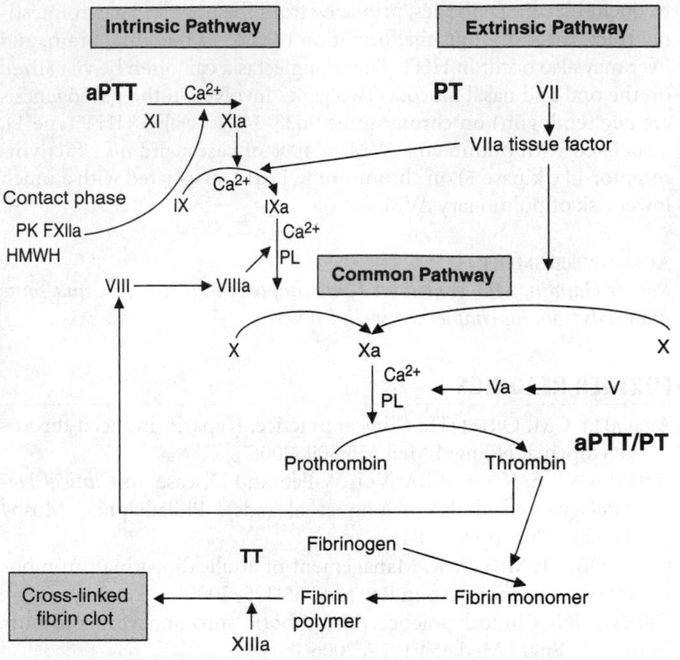

FIGURE 110-1 Coagulation cascade and laboratory assessment of clotting factor deficiency by activated partial prothrombin time (aPTT), prothrombin time (PT), and thrombin time (TT).

The development of antibodies to coagulation plasma proteins, clinically termed *inhibitors*, is a relatively rare problem that most often affects hemophilia A or B and FXI-deficient patients who receive repeated doses of the missing protein to control bleeding episodes. Inhibitors also occur among subjects without genetic deficiency of clotting factors—for example, in the postpartum setting, as a manifestation of underlying autoimmune or neoplastic disease, or idiopathically. Rare cases of inhibitors to thrombin or FV have been reported in patients receiving topical bovine thrombin preparation as a local hemostatic agent in complex surgeries. The diagnosis of inhibitors is based on the same tests as those used to diagnose inherited plasma coagulation factor deficiencies. However, the addition of the missing protein to the plasma of a subject with an inhibitor does not correct the abnormal aPTT and/or PT tests. This is the major laboratory difference between deficiencies and inhibitors. Additional tests are required to measure the specificity of the inhibitor and its titer.

The treatment of these bleeding disorders often requires replacement of the deficient protein using recombinant or purified plasma-derived products or fresh frozen plasma. Therefore, it is imperative to arrive at a proper diagnosis to optimize patient care without unnecessary exposure to the risks of bloodborne disease.

HEMOPHILIA

PATHOGENESIS AND CLINICAL MANIFESTATIONS

Hemophilia is an X-linked recessive hemorrhagic disease due to mutations in the *F8* gene (hemophilia A or classic hemophilia) or *F9* gene (hemophilia B). The disease affects 1 in 10,000 males worldwide, in all ethnic groups; hemophilia A represents 80% of all cases. Male subjects are clinically affected; women, who carry a single mutated gene, are generally asymptomatic. Family history of the disease is absent in approximately 30% of cases. In these cases, 80% of the mothers are carriers of the de novo mutated allele. More than 500 different mutations have been identified in the *F8* or *F9* genes. One of the most common hemophilia A mutations results from an inversion of the intron 22 sequence, which is present in 40% of cases of severe hemophilia A. Advances in molecular diagnosis now permit precise identification of mutations, allowing accurate diagnosis of women carriers of the hemophilia gene in affected families.

Clinically, hemophilia A and hemophilia B are indistinguishable. The disease phenotype correlates with the residual activity of FVIII or FIX and can be classified as severe (< 1%), moderate (1–5%), or mild (6–30%). In the severe and moderate forms, the disease is characterized by bleeding episodes into the joints (hemarthroses), soft tissues, and muscles after minor trauma or even spontaneously. Patients with mild disease experience infrequent bleeding that is usually secondary to trauma. Among those with residual FVIII or FIX activity >25% of normal, the disease is discovered only by bleeding after major trauma or during routine presurgery laboratory tests. Typically, the global tests of coagulation show only an isolated prolongation of the aPTT assay. Patients with hemophilia have normal bleeding times and platelet counts. The diagnosis is made after specific determination of FVIII or FIX clotting activity.

Early in life, bleeding may present after circumcision or rarely as intracranial hemorrhages. The disease is more evident when children begin to walk or crawl. In the severe form, the most common bleeding manifestations are the recurrent hemarthroses, which can affect every joint but mainly affect knees, elbows, ankles, shoulders, and hips. Acute hemarthroses are painful, and clinical signs are local swelling and erythema. To avoid pain, the patient may adopt a fixed position, which leads eventually to muscle contractures. Very young children unable to communicate verbally show irritability and a lack of movement of the affected joint. Chronic hemarthroses are debilitating, with synovial thickening and synovitis in response to the intraarticular blood. After a joint has been damaged, recurrent bleeding episodes result in the clinically recognized "target joint," which then establishes a vicious cycle of bleeding, resulting in progressive joint deformity that in critical cases requires surgery as the only therapeutic option. Hematomas into the muscle of distal parts of the limbs may lead to external compression of arteries, veins, or nerves, which can evolve to a compartment syndrome.

Bleeding into the oropharyngeal spaces, central nervous system, or the retroperitoneum is life-threatening and requires immediate therapy. Retroperitoneal hemorrhages can accumulate large quantities of blood along with formation of masses with calcification and inflammatory tissue reaction (pseudotumor syndrome), and they can also result in damage to the femoral nerve. Pseudotumors can also form in bones, especially long bones of the lower limbs. Hematuria is frequent among hemophilia patients, even in the absence of genitourinary pathology. It is often self-limited and may not require specific therapy.

Rx HEMOPHILIA

Without treatment, patients with severe hemophilia have a limited life expectancy. Advances in the blood fractionation industry during World War II resulted in the realization that plasma could be used to treat hemophilia, but the volumes required to achieve even modest elevation of circulating factor levels limits the utility of plasma infusion as an approach to disease management. The discovery in the 1960s that cryoprecipitate fraction of plasma was enriched for FVIII, in addition to the eventual purification of FVIII and FIX from plasma, led to the introduction of home infusion therapy with factor concentrates in the 1970s. The availability of factor concentrates resulted in a dramatic improvement in life expectancy and in quality of life for people with severe hemophilia. However, the contamination of the blood supply with hepatitis viruses and, subsequently, HIV resulted in widespread transmission of these bloodborne infections within the hemophilia population; complications of HIV and of hepatitis C are now the leading causes of death among US adults with severe hemophilia. The introduction of viral inactivation steps in the preparation of plasma-derived products in the mid-1980s greatly reduced the risk of HIV and hepatitis, and the risks were further reduced by the successful production of recombinant FVIII and FIX proteins, both licensed in the 1990s. It is uncommon for hemophilic patients born after 1985 to have contracted either hepatitis or HIV, and for these individuals, life expectancy is in the range of 65 years of age.

Factor replacement therapy for hemophilia can be provided either in response to a bleeding episode or as a prophylactic treatment. Primary prophylaxis is defined as a strategy for maintaining the missing clotting factor at levels ~1% or higher on a regular basis in order to prevent bleeds, especially the onset of hemarthroses. Hemophilic boys receiving regular infusions of FVIII (3 days/week) or FIX (2 days/week) can reach puberty without detectable joint abnormalities. Although highly recommended, this regimen is performed for <30% of patients because of the high cost, difficulties in accessing peripheral veins in young patients, and the potential infectious and thrombotic risks of long-term central vein catheters.

General considerations regarding the treatment of bleeds in hemophilia include (1) the need to begin the treatment as soon as possible because symptoms often precede objective evidence of bleeding; because of the superior efficacy of early therapeutic intervention, classic symptoms of bleeding into the joint in a reliable patient, headaches, or automobile or other accidents, require prompt replacement and further laboratory investigation; and (2) the need to avoid drugs that hamper platelet function such as aspirin or aspirin-containing drugs; to control pain, drugs such as ibuprofen or propoxyphene are preferred.

Factor VIII and Factor IX are dosed in units. One unit is by definition the amount of FVIII (100 ng/mL) or FIX (5 μg/mL) in 1 mL of normal plasma. One unit of FVIII per kilogram of body weight increases the plasma FVIII level by 2%. One can calculate the dose needed to increase FVIII levels to 100% in a 70-kg severe hemophilia patient (<1%) using the simple formula below. Thus, 3500 units of FVIII will raise the circulating level to 100%.

$$\text{FVIII dose (IU)} = \text{Target FVIII levels} - \text{FVIII baseline levels} \times \text{body weight (kg)} \times 0.5 \text{ unit/kg}$$

The doses for FIX replacement are different from those for FVIII, because FIX recovery postinfusion is usually only 50% of the predicted value. Therefore, the formula for FIX replacement is

$$\text{FIX dose (IU)} = \text{Target FIX levels} - \text{FIX baseline levels} \times \text{body weight (kg)} \times 1.0 \text{ unit/kg}$$

The FVIII half-life of 8–12 h requires injections twice a day to maintain therapeutic levels, whereas the FIX half-life is longer, ~24 h, so that once-a-day injection is sufficient. In specific situations such as postsurgery, continuous infusion of factor may be desirable because of its safety in achieving sustained factor levels at a lower total cost.

Cryoprecipitate is enriched with FVIII protein (each bag contains ~80 IU of FVIII) and was commonly used for the treatment of hemophilia A decades ago; it is still in use in some developing countries, but because of the risk of bloodborne diseases, this product should be avoided in hemophilia patients when factor concentrates are available.

Mild bleeds such as uncomplicated hemarthroses or superficial hematomas require initial therapy with factor levels of 30–50%. Additional doses to maintain levels of 15–25% for 2 or 3 days are indicated for severe hemarthroses, especially when these episodes affect the "target joint." Large hematomas, or bleeds into deep muscles, require factor levels of 50% or even higher if the clinical symptoms do not improve, and factor replacement may be required for a period of 1 week or longer. The control of serious bleeds, including those that affect the oropharyngeal spaces, central nervous system, and the retroperitoneum, require sustained protein levels of 50–100% for 7–10 days. Prophylactic replacement for surgery is aimed at achieving normal factor levels (100%) for a period of 7–10 days; replacement can then be tapered depending on the extent of the surgical wounds. Oral surgery is associated with extensive tissue damage, which usually requires factor replacement for 1–3 days coupled with oral antifibrinolytic drugs.

NON-TRANSFUSION THERAPY IN HEMOPHILIA **DDAVP (1-deamino-8-D-arginine vasopressin)** DDAVP is a synthetic vasopressin analogue that causes a transient rise in FVIII and von Willebrand factor (vWF), but not FIX, through a mechanism involving release from endothelial cells. Patients with moderate or mild hemophilia A should be tested to determine if they respond to DDAVP before a therapeutic application. DDAVP at doses of 0.3 μg/kg body weight infused over a 20-min period is expected to raise FVIII levels by two- to threefold over baseline, peaking between 30–60 min postinfusion. DDAVP does not improve FVIII levels in severe hemophilia A patients, as there are no stores to release. Repeated dosing of DDAVP results in tachyphylaxis because the mechanism is an increase in release rather than de novo synthesis of FVIII and vWF. More than three consecutive doses become ineffective and if further therapy is indicated, FVIII replacement is required to achieve hemostasis.

Antifibrinolytic Drugs Bleeding in the gums, in the gastrointestinal tract, and during oral surgery requires the use of oral antifibrinolytic drugs such as ε-aminocaproic acid (EACA) or tranexamic acid to control local hemostasis. The duration of the treatment depending on the clinical indication is 1 week or longer. Tranexamic acid is given at doses of 25 mg/kg three to four times a day. EACA treatment requires a loading dose of 200 mg/kg (maximum of 10 g) followed by 100 mg/kg (maximum 30 g/d) every 6 h. These drugs are not indicated to control hematuria because of the risk of formation of an occlusive clot in the lumen of genitourinary tract structures.

COMPLICATIONS **Inhibitor Formation** The formation of alloantibodies to FVIII or FIX is currently the major complication of hemophilia treatment. The prevalence of inhibitors to FVIII is estimated at 5–10% of all cases and approximately 20% of severe hemophilia A patients. Inhibitors to FIX are detected in only 3–5% of all hemophilia B patients. The high-risk group for inhibitor formation includes severe deficiency (>80% of all cases of inhibitors), familial history of inhibitors, African descent, mutations in the FVIII or FIX gene resulting in deletion of large coding regions, or gross gene rearrangements. Inhibitors usually appear early in life, at a median of two years of age, and after 10 cumulative days of exposure.

The clinical diagnosis of inhibitor is suspected when patients do not respond to factor replacement at therapeutic doses. Inhibitors increase both morbidity and mortality in hemophilia. Because early detection of an inhibitor is critical to a successful correction of the bleeding or to eradication of the antibody, most hemophilia centers perform annual screening for inhibitors. The laboratory test required to confirm the presence of an inhibitor is an aPTT mixed with normal plasma. In most hemophilia patients, a 1:1 mix with normal plasma completely corrects the aPTT. In inhibitor patients, the aPTT on a 1:1 mix is abnormally prolonged, because the inhibitor neutralizes the FVIII clotting activity of the normal plasma. The Bethesda assay uses a similar principle and defines the specificity of the inhibitor and its titer. The results are expressed in Bethesda units (BU), in which 1 BU is the amount of antibody that neutralizes 50% of the FVIII or FIX present in normal plasma after 2 h of incubation at 37°C. Clinically, inhibitor patients are classified as low responders or high responders, which provides guidelines for optimal therapy. Therapy for inhibitor patients has two goals: the control of acute bleeding episodes and the eradication of the inhibitor. For the control of bleeding episodes, low responders, those with titers <5 BU, respond well to high doses of human or porcine FVIII (50–100 U/kg) with minimal or no increase in the inhibitor titers. However, high-responder patients—those with initial inhibitor titer >10 BU or an anamnestic response in the antibody titer to >10 BU even if low titer initially—do not respond to FVIII or FIX concentrates. The control of bleeding episodes in high-responder patients can be achieved by using concentrates enriched for prothrombin, FVII, FIX, FX [prothrombin complex concentrates (PCCs) or activated PCCs], and more recently by recombinant activated Factor VII (FVIIa) (Fig. 110-1). The rates of therapeutic success have been higher for FVIIa than for PCC or aPCC. For eradication of the inhibitory antibody, immunosuppression is not effective. The most effective strategy is immune tolerance induction (ITI) based on daily infusion of the missing protein until the inhibitor disappears, typically requiring periods longer than one year, with success rates in the range of 60%. Promising results have been obtained by adding anti-CD20 monoclonal antibody (rituximab) as a coadjuvant for the eradication of high levels of antibody in patients undergoing ITI.

Infectious Diseases Hepatitis C virus (HCV) infection is the major cause of morbidity and the second leading cause of death in hemophilia patients exposed to older clotting factor concentrates. The vast majority of young patients treated with plasma-derived products from 1970 to 1985 became infected with HCV. It has been estimated that >80% of patients older than 20 years of age are HCV antibody positive as of 2006. The comorbidity of the underlying liver disease in hemophilia patients is clear when these individuals require invasive procedures; correction of both genetic and acquired (secondary to liver disease) deficiencies may be needed. Infection with HIV also swept the population of patients treated with plasma-derived concentrates two decades ago. Co-infection of HCV and HIV, present in almost 50% of hemophilia patients, is an aggravating factor for the evolution of liver disease. The response to HCV antiviral therapy in hemophilia is restricted to <30% of patients and is even poorer among those with both HCV and HIV infection. End-stage liver disease requiring organ transplantation may be curative for both the liver disease and for hemophilia.

FACTOR XI DEFICIENCY

Factor XI is a zymogen of an active serine protease (FXIa) in the intrinsic pathway of blood coagulation that activates FIX (Fig. 110-1). There are two pathways for the formation of FXIa. In an aPTT-based assay, the protease is the result of activation by FXIIa in conjunction with high-molecular-weight kininogen and kallikrein. Thrombin appears to be the physiologic activator of FXI. The generation of thrombin by the tissue-factor/Factor VIIa pathway activates FXI on the platelet surface, which contributes to additional thrombin generation after the clot has formed and thus augments resistance to fibrinolysis through a thrombin-activated fibrinolytic inhibitor (TAFI).

Factor XI deficiency is a rare bleeding disorder that occurs in the general population at a frequency of one in a million. However, the disease is highly prevalent among Ashkenazi and Iraqi Jewish populations, reaching a frequency of 6% as heterozygotes and 0.1–0.3% as homozygotes. More than 65 mutations in the *FXI* gene have been reported, whereas two to three mutations are found among affected Jewish populations.

Normal FXI clotting activity levels range from 70 to 150 U/dL. In heterozygous patients with moderate deficiency, FXI ranges from 20 to 70 U/dL, whereas in homozygous or double heterozygote patients, FXI levels are <1–20 U/dL. Patients with FXI levels <10% of normal have a high risk of bleeding, but the disease phenotype does not always correlate with residual FXI clotting activity. A family history is indicative of the risk of bleeding in the propositus. Clinically, the presence of mucocutaneous hemorrhages such as bruises, gum bleeding, epistaxis, hematuria, and menorrhagia are common, especially following trauma. This hemorrhagic phenotype suggests that tissues rich in fibrinolytic activity are more susceptible to FXI deficiency. Postoperative bleeding is common but not always present, even among patients with very low FXI levels.

℞ FACTOR XI DEFICIENCY

The treatment of FXI deficiency is based on the infusion of FFP at doses of 15–20 mL/kg to maintain trough levels ranging from 10 to 20%. Because FXI has a half-life of 40–70 h, the replacement therapy can be given on alternate days. The use of antifibrinolytic drugs is beneficial to control bleeds, with the exception of hematuria or bleeds in the bladder. The development of a FXI inhibitor was observed in 10% of severely FXI-deficient patients who received replacement therapy.

OTHER RARE BLEEDING DISORDERS

Collectively, the inherited disorders resulting from deficiencies of clotting factors other than FVIII, FIX, and FXI (Table 110-1) represent a group of rare bleeding diseases. The bleeding symptoms in these patients vary from asymptomatic (dysfibrinogenemia or FVII deficiency) to life-threatening (FX or FXIII deficiency). There is no pathognomonic clinical manifestation that suggests one specific disease, but overall, in contrast to hemophilia, hemarthrosis is a rare event, and bleeding in the mucosal tract or after umbilical cord clamping is common. Individuals heterozygous for plasma coagulation deficiencies are often asymptomatic. The laboratory assessment for the specific deficient factor following screening with general coagulation tests (Table 110-1) will establish the diagnosis.

Replacement therapy using fresh frozen plasma (FFP) or PCCs (containing prothrombin, FVII, FIX and FX) provides adequate hemostasis in response to bleeds or as prophylactic treatment. The use of PCCs should be carefully monitored and avoided in patients with underlying liver disease or those at high risk for thrombosis because of the risk of DIC.

FAMILIAL MULTIPLE COAGULATION DEFICIENCIES

Several bleeding disorders are characterized by the inherited deficiency of more than one plasma coagulation factor. To date, the genetic defects in two of these diseases have been characterized, and they provide new insights into the regulation of hemostasis by genes encoding proteins outside blood coagulation.

Combined Deficiency of FV and FVIII Patients with combined FV and FVIII deficiency exhibit ~5% of residual clotting activity of each factor. Interestingly, the disease phenotype is a mild bleeding tendency, often following trauma. An underlying mutation has been identified in the endoplasmic reticulum/Golgi intermediate compartment (ERGIC-53) gene, a mannose-binding protein localized in the Golgi apparatus that functions as a chaperone for both FV and FVIII. In other families, mutations in the multiple coagulation factor deficiency 2 (MCFD2) gene have been defined; this gene encodes a protein that forms a Ca^{2+}-dependent complex with ERGIC-53 and provides cofactor activity in the intracellular mobilization of both FV and FVIII.

Multiple Deficiencies of Vitamin K–Dependent Coagulation Factors Two enzymes involved in vitamin K metabolism have been associated with combined deficiency of all vitamin K–dependent proteins, including the procoagulant proteins prothrombin, VII, IX, and X and the anticoagulants protein C and protein S. Vitamin K is a fat-soluble vitamin that is a cofactor for carboxylation of the gamma carbon of the glutamic acid residues in the vitamin K dependent–factors, a critical step for calcium and phospholipid binding of these proteins (Fig. 110-2). The enzymes γ-glutamylcarboxylase and epoxide reductase are critical for the metabolism and regeneration of vitamin K. Mutations in the genes encoding the gamma-carboxylase (GGCX) or vitamin K epoxide reductase complex 1 (VKORC1) result in defective enzymes and thus in vitamin K–dependent factors with reduced activity, varying from 1 to 30% of normal. The disease phenotype is characterized by mild to severe bleeding episodes present from birth. Some patients respond to high doses of vitamin K. For severe bleeding, replacement therapy with FFP or PCCs may be necessary for achieving full hemostatic control.

DISSEMINATED INTRAVASCULAR COAGULATION

DIC is a clinicopathologic syndrome characterized by widespread intravascular fibrin formation in response to excessive blood protease activity that overcomes the natural anticoagulant mechanisms. DIC is associated with several underlying pathologies (Table 110-2). The most common causes are bacterial sepsis, malignant disorders such as solid tumors or acute promyelocytic leukemia (APL), and obstetric causes. DIC is diagnosed in almost half of pregnant women with abruptio placentae or with amniotic fluid embolism. Trauma, particularly to the brain, can also result in DIC. The exposure of blood to phospholipids from damaged tissue, hemolysis, and endothelial damage are all contributing factors to the development of DIC in this setting. Purpura fulminans is a severe form of DIC resulting from thrombosis of extensive areas of the skin; it affects predominantly young children following viral or bacterial infection, particularly those

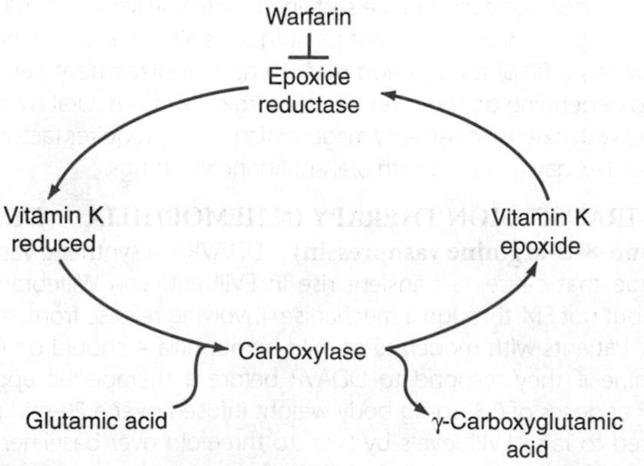

FIGURE 110-2 The vitamin K cycle. Vitamin K is a cofactor for the formation of γ-carboxyglutamic acid residues on coagulation proteins. Vitamin K–dependent γ-glutamylcarboxylase, the enzyme that catalyzes the vitamin K epoxide reductase, regenerates reduced vitamin K. Warfarin blocks the action of the reductase and competitively inhibits the effects of vitamin K.

TABLE 110-2 COMMON CLINICAL CAUSES OF DISSEMINATED INTRAVASCULAR COAGULATION

Sepsis	**Immunologic disorders**
Bacterial	Acute hemolytic transfusion reaction
Staphylococci, streptococci, pneumococci, meningococci, gram-negative bacilli	Organ or tissue transplant rejection
Viral	Graft-versus-host disease
Mycotic	
Parasitic	
Rickettsial	
Trauma and tissue injury	**Drugs**
Brain injury (gunshot)	Fibrinolytic agents
Extensive burns	Aprotinin
Fat embolism	Warfarin (especially in neonates with protein C deficiency)
Rhabdomyolysis	Prothrombin complex concentrates
	Recreational drugs (amphetamines)
Vascular disorders	**Envenomation**
Giant hemangiomas (Kasabach-Merrit syndrome)	Snake
Large vessel aneurysms (e.g., aorta)	Insects
Obstetric complications	**Liver disease**
Abruptio placentae	Fulminant hepatic failure
Amniotic fluid embolism	Cirrhosis
Dead fetus syndrome	Fatty liver of pregnancy
Septic abortion	
Cancer	**Miscellaneous**
Adenocarcinoma (prostate, pancreas, etc)	Shock
Hematologic malignancies (acute promyelocytic leukemia)	Respiratory distress syndrome
	Massive transfusion

with inherited or acquired hypercoagulability due to deficiencies of the components of the protein C pathway. Neonates homozygous for protein C deficiency also present high risk for purpura fulminans, with or without thrombosis of large vessels.

The central mechanism of DIC is the uncontrolled generation of thrombin by exposure of the blood to pathologic levels of tissue factor (Fig. 110-3). Simultaneous suppression of physiologic anticoagulant mechanisms and abnormal fibrinolysis further accelerate the process. Together these abnormalities contribute to systemic fibrin deposition in small and mid-sized vessels. The duration and intensity of the fibrin deposition can compromise the blood supply of many organs, especially the lung, kidney, liver, and brain, with consequent organ failure. The sustained activation of coagulation results in consumption of clotting factors and platelets, which in turn leads to systemic bleeding. This is further aggravated by secondary hyperfibrinolysis. Studies in animals demonstrate that the fibrinolytic system is indeed suppressed at the time of maximal activation of coagulation. Interestingly, in patients with APL, a severe hyperfibrinolytic state often occurs in addition to the coagulation activation. The release of several proinflammatory cytokines such as interleukin 6 and tumor necrosis factor α play central roles in mediating the coagulation defects in DIC and symptoms associated with systemic inflammatory response syndrome.

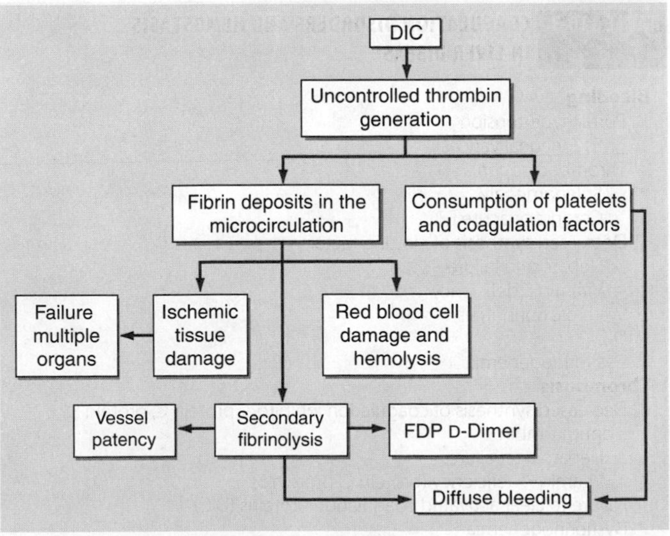

FIGURE 110-3 The pathophysiology of disseminated intravascular coagulation (DIC). Interactions between coagulation and fibrinolytic pathways result in bleeding and thrombosis in the microcirculation in patients with DIC.

Clinical manifestations of DIC are related to the magnitude of the imbalance of hemostasis, to the underlying disease, or to both. The most common findings are bleeding ranging from oozing from venipuncture sites, petechiae, and ecchymoses to severe hemorrhage from the gastrointestinal tract or lung or into the central nervous system. In chronic DIC the bleeding symptoms are discreet and restricted to skin or mucosal surfaces. The hypercoagulability of DIC manifests as the occlusion of vessels in the microcirculation and resulting organ failure. Thrombosis of large vessels and cerebral embolism can also occur. Hemodynamic complications and shock are common among patients with acute DIC. The mortality ranges from 30 to >80% depending on the underlying disease, the severity of the DIC, and the age of the patient.

The diagnosis of clinically significant DIC is based on the presence of clinical and/or laboratory abnormalities of coagulation or thrombocytopenia. The laboratory diagnosis of DIC should prompt a search for the underlying disease if it is not already apparent. No single test establishes the diagnosis of DIC. The laboratory investigation should include coagulation tests [aPTT, PT, thrombin time (TT)] and markers of fibrin degradation products (FDP), in addition to platelet and red cell count and analysis of the blood smear. These tests should be repeated over a period of 6–8 h because an initially mild abnormality can changed dramatically in patients with severe DIC.

Common findings include the prolongation of PT and/or aPTT; platelet counts ≤ 100,000/mm^3, or a rapid decline in platelet numbers; the presence of schistocytes (fragmented red cells) in the blood smear; and elevated levels of FDP. The most sensitive test for DIC is the FDP level. DIC is an unlikely diagnosis in the presence of normal levels of FDP. The D-dimer test is more specific for detection of fibrin (but not fibrinogen) degradation products and indicates that the cross-linked fibrin has been digested by plasmin. Because fibrinogen has a prolonged half-life, plasma levels diminish acutely only in severe cases of DIC. High-grade DIC is also associated with levels of antithrombin III or plasminogen activity <60% of normal.

Chronic DIC Low-grade, compensated DIC can occur in certain clinical situations, including giant hemangioma, metastatic carcinoma, or the dead fetus syndrome. Plasma levels of FDP or D-dimers are elevated. aPTT, PT, and fibrinogen values are within the normal range or high. Mild thrombocytopenia or normal platelet counts are also common findings. Red cell fragmentation is often detected but at a lower degree than in acute DIC.

Differential Diagnosis The differential diagnosis between DIC and severe liver disease is challenging and requires serial measurements of the laboratory parameters of DIC. Patients with severe liver disease are at risk for bleeding and manifest laboratory features including thrombocytopenia (due to platelet sequestration, portal hypertension, or hypersplenism), decreased synthesis of coagulation factors and natural anticoagulants, and elevated levels of FDP due to reduced hepatic clearance. However, in contrast to DIC, these laboratory parameters in liver disease do not change rapidly. Other important differential findings include the presence of portal hypertension or other clinical or laboratory evidence of underlying liver disease.

Microangiopathic disorders such as thrombotic thrombocytopenic purpura present an acute clinical onset of illness accompanied by thrombocytopenia, red cell fragmentation, and multiorgan failure. There is, however, no consumption of clotting factors or hyperfibrinolysis.

Rx DISSEMINATED INTRAVASCULAR COAGULATION

The morbidity and mortality associated with DIC are primarily related to the underlying disease rather than the complications of the DIC. The control or elimination of the underlying cause should therefore be the primary concern. Patients with severe DIC require control of hemodynamic parameters, respiratory support, and sometimes invasive surgical procedures. Attempts to treat DIC without accompanying treatment of the causative disease are likely to fail.

MANAGEMENT OF HEMORRHAGIC SYMPTOMS The control of bleeding in DIC patients with marked thrombocytopenia (platelet counts <10,000–20,000/mm³) and low levels of coagulation factors will require replacement therapy. The PT (>1.5 × normal) provides a good indicator of the severity of the clotting factor consumption. Replacement with FFP is indicated (1 unit of FFP increases most coagulation factors by 3% in an adult without DIC). Low levels of fibrinogen (<100 mg/dL) or brisk hyperfibrinolysis will require infusion of cryoprecipitate (plasma fraction enriched for fibrinogen, FVIII, and vWF). The replacement of 10 U of cryoprecipitate for every 2–3 U of FFP is sufficient to correct the hemostasis. The transfusion scheme must be adjusted according to the patient's clinical and laboratory evolution. Platelet concentrates at a dose of 1–2 U/10 kg body weight are sufficient for most DIC patients with severe thrombocytopenia.

Clotting factor concentrates are not recommended for control of bleeding in DIC because of the limited efficacy afforded by replacement of single factors (factor VIII or IX concentrates) and the high risk of products containing traces of activated blood proteases (PCCs), which further aggravates the disease.

REPLACEMENT OF COAGULATION OR FIBRINOLYSIS INHIBITORS Drugs to control coagulation such as heparin, antithrombin III (ATIII) concentrates, or antifibrinolytic drugs have all been tried in the treatment of DIC. Low doses of continuous infusion heparin (5–10 U/kg per h) may be effective in patients with low-grade DIC associated with solid tumor or APL or in a setting with recognized thrombosis. Heparin is also indicated for the treatment of purpura fulminans, during the surgical resection of giant hemangiomas, and during removal of a dead fetus. In acute DIC, the use of heparin is likely to aggravate bleeding. To date, the use of heparin in severe DIC patients is of no proven survival benefit.

The use of antifibrinolytic drugs, EACA, or tranexamic acid to prevent fibrin degradation by plasmin may reduce bleeding episodes in patients with DIC and confirmed hyperfibrinolysis. However, these drugs can increase the risk of thrombosis, and concomitant use of heparin is indicated. Patients with APL or those with chronic DIC associated with giant hemangiomas are among the few patients who may benefit from this therapy.

The use of protein C concentrates to treat purpura fulminans associated with acquired protein C deficiency or meningococcemia has been proved effective. The results from the replacement of ATIII in early phase studies are promising but require further study.

VITAMIN K DEFICIENCY

Vitamin K–dependent proteins are a heterogenous group, including clotting factor proteins and also proteins found in bone, lung, kidney, and placenta. Vitamin K mediates posttranslational modification of glutamate residues to γ-carboxylglutamate, a critical step for the activity of vitamin K–dependent proteins for calcium binding and proper assembly to phospholipid membranes (Fig. 110-2). Inherited deficiency of the functional activity of the enzymes involved in vitamin K metabolism, notably the GGCX or VKOR-1 (see above), results in bleeding disorders. The amount of vitamin K in the diet is often limiting for the carboxylation reaction, and thus recycling of the vitamin K is essential to maintain normal levels of vitamin K–dependent proteins. In adults, low dietary intake alone is seldom reason for severe vitamin K deficiency but may become common in association with the use of broad-spectrum antibiotics. Disease or surgical interventions that affect the ability of the intestinal tract to absorb vitamin K, either through anatomic alterations or by changing the fat content of bile salts and pancreatic juices in the proximal small bowel, can result in significant reduction of vitamin K levels. Chronic liver diseases such as primary biliary cirrhosis also deplete vitamin K stores. Neonatal vitamin K deficiency and the resulting hemorrhagic disease of the newborn have been almost entirely eliminated by routine administration of vitamin K to all neonates. Prolongation of PT values is the most common and earliest finding in vitamin K–deficient patients due to reduction in prothrombin, FVII, FIX, and FX levels. FVII has the shortest half-life among these factors, which can prolong the PT before changes in the aPTT. Parenteral administration of vitamin K at a total dose of 10 mg is sufficient to restore normal levels of clotting factor within 8–10 h. In the presence of ongoing bleeding or a need for immediate correction before an invasive procedure, replacement with FFP or PCC is required. PCC should be avoided in patients with severe underlying liver disorders due to high risk of thrombosis. The reversal of excessive anticoagulant therapy with warfarin or warfarin-like drugs can be achieved by minimal doses of vitamin K (1 mg orally or by intravenous injection) for asymptomatic patients. This strategy can diminish the risk of bleeding while maintaining therapeutic anticoagulation for an underlying prothrombotic state.

COAGULATION DISORDERS ASSOCIATED WITH LIVER FAILURE

The liver is central to hemostasis because it is the site of synthesis and clearance of most procoagulant and natural anticoagulant proteins and of essential components of the fibrinolytic system. Liver failure is associated with a high risk of bleeding due to deficient synthesis of procoagulant factors and enhanced fibrinolysis. Thrombocytopenia is common in patients with liver disease and may be due to congestive splenomegaly (hypersplenism), or immune-mediated shortened platelet life span (primary biliary cirrhosis). In addition, several anatomic abnormalities secondary to underlying liver disease further promote the occurrence of hemorrhage (Table 110-3). Dysfibrinogenemia is a relatively common finding in patients with liver disease due to impaired fibrin polymerization. The development of DIC concomitant to chronic liver disease is not uncommon and may enhance the risk for bleeding. Laboratory evaluation is mandatory for an optimal therapeutic strategy, either to control ongoing bleeding or to prepare the patients with liver disease for invasive procedures. Typically these patients present with prolonged PT, aPTT, and TT, depending on the degree of liver damage, thrombocytopenia, and normal or slight increase of FDP. Fibrinogen levels are diminished only in fulminant hepatitis, decompensated cirrhosis, or advanced

TABLE 110-3 COAGULATION DISORDERS AND HEMOSTASIS IN LIVER DISEASE

Bleeding
- Portal hypertension
  - Esophageal varices
- Thrombocytopenia
  - Splenomegaly
  - Chronic or acute DIC
- Decreased synthesis of clotting factors
  - Hepatocyte failure
  - Vitamin K deficiency
- Systemic fibrinolysis
- DIC
- Dysfibrinogenemia

Thrombosis
- Decreased synthesis of coagulation inhibitors: protein C, protein S, antithrombin
  - Hepatocyte failure
  - Vitamin K deficiency (protein C, protein S)
- Failure to clear activated coagulation proteins (DIC)
- Dysfibrinogenemia
- Iatrogenic: Transfusion of prothrombin complex concentrates
  - Antifibrinolytic agents: ε-aminocaproic acid (EACA), tranexamic acid

Note: DIC, disseminated intravascular coagulation.

liver disease, or in the presence of DIC. The presence of prolonged TT, normal fibrinogen, and FDP levels suggests dysfibrinogenemia. FVIII levels are often normal or elevated in patients with liver failure, and decreased levels suggest superimposing DIC. Because FV is only synthesized in the hepatocyte and is not a vitamin K–dependent protein, reduced levels of FV may be an indicator of hepatocyte failure. Normal levels of FV and low levels of FVII suggest vitamin K deficiency. Vitamin K levels may be reduced in patients with liver failure due to compromised storage in hepatocellular disease, changes in bile acids, or cholestasis that can diminish the absorption of vitamin K. Replacement of vitamin K may be desirable (10 mg given by slow intravenous injection) to improve hemostasis.

Treatment with FFP is the most effective way to correct hemostasis in patients with liver failure. Infusion of FFP (5–10 mL/kg; each bag contains ~200 mL) is sufficient to ensure 10–20% of normal levels of clotting factors but not correction of PT or aPTT. Even high doses of FFP (20 mL/kg) do not correct the clotting times in all patients. Monitoring for clinical symptoms and clotting times will determine if repeated doses are required 8–12 h after the first infusion. Platelet concentrates are indicated when platelet counts are <10,000–20,000/mm^3 to control an ongoing bleed or immediately before an invasive procedure if counts are <50,000/mm^3. Cryoprecipitate is indicated only when fibrinogen levels are <100 mg/mL; dosing is six bags for a 70-kg patient daily. As noted above, PCC infusion in patients with liver failure should be avoided due to the high risk of thrombotic complications. The safety of antifibrinolytic drugs to control bleeding in patients with liver failure is not yet well-defined and should be avoided.

ACQUIRED INHIBITORS OF COAGULATION FACTORS

An *acquired inhibitor* is an immune-mediated disease characterized by the presence of an autoantibody against a specific clotting factor. FVIII is the most common target of antibody formation, but inhibitors to prothrombin, FV, FIX, FX, and FXI are also reported. The disease occurs predominantly in older adults (median age of 60 years) but occasionally in pregnant or postpartum women with no previous history of bleeding. In 50% of patients with inhibitors, no underlying disease is identified at the time of diagnosis. In the remaining half, the causes are autoimmune diseases, malignancies (lymphomas, prostate cancer), dermatologic diseases, and pregnancy. Previous history of open surgery in which topical thrombin is used, especially preparations containing bovine FV, is sometimes associated. Bleeding episodes occur commonly into soft tissues and in the gastrointestinal or urinary tracts and skin. In contrast to hemophilia, hemarthrosis is rare. Retroperitoneal hemorrhages and other life-threatening bleeding may appear suddenly. The overall mortality in untreated patients ranges from 8 to 22%, and most deaths occur within the first few weeks after presentation. The diagnosis is based on the prolonged aPTT with normal PT and TT. The aPTT remains prolonged after mixture of the test plasma with equal amounts of pooled normal plasma for 2 h at 37°C. The Bethesda assay using FVIII-deficient plasma as performed for inhibitor detection in hemophilia will confirm the diagnosis. Major bleeding is treated with high doses of human or porcine FVIII, PCC/PCCa, or recombinant FVIIa. High-dose intravenous gamma globulin and anti-CD20 monoclonal antibody (rituximab) have been reported to be effective in patients with autoantibodies to FVIII. In contrast to hemophilia, inhibitors in nonhemophilia patients are sometimes responsive to prednisone alone or in association with cytotoxic therapy (e.g., cyclophosphamide).

The presence of lupus anticoagulant can be associated with venous or arterial thrombotic disease. However, bleeding has also been reported in lupus anticoagulant; it is due to the presence of antibodies to prothrombin, which results in hypoprothrombinemia. Both disorders show a prolonged PTT that does not correct on mixing. To distinguish acquired inhibitors from lupus anticoagulants, the dilute Russell's viper venom test and the hexagonal-phase phospholipids test will be negative in patients with an acquired inhibitor and positive in patients with lupus anticoagulants. Moreover, lupus anticoagulant interferes with the clotting activity of many factors (FVIII, FIX, FXII, FXI), whereas acquired inhibitors are specific to a single factor.

FURTHER READINGS

CALDWELL SH et al: Coagulation disorders and hemostasis in liver disease: Pathophysiology and critical assessment of current management. Hepatology 44:1039, 2006

HOYER LW: Hemophilia A. N Engl J Med 330:39, 1994

KEY NS, NEGRIER C: Coagulation factor concentrates: Past, present, and future. Lancet 370:439, 2007

LEVI M, OPAL SM: Coagulation abnormalities in critically ill patients. Critical Care 10:222, 2006

MANNUCCI PM, et al: Recessively inherited coagulation disorders. Blood 104:1243, 2004

STAFFORD DW: The vitamin K cycle. J Thromb Haemost 3:1873, 2005

111 Venous Thrombosis

F.R. Rosendaal, H.R. Büller

Venous thrombosis is the result of occlusive clot formation in the veins. It occurs mainly in the deep veins of the leg (deep vein thrombosis, DVT), from which parts of the clot frequently embolize to the lungs (pulmonary embolism, PE). Fewer than 5% of all venous thromboses occur at other sites (see "Thrombosis at Rare Sites," and "Superficial Thrombophlebitis," below). Venous thrombosis is common and often occurs spontaneously, but it also frequently accompanies medical and surgical conditions, both in the community and the hospital.

The symptoms of venous thrombosis are nonspecific, and therefore the clinical diagnosis is difficult and requires objective testing by imaging. Major complications of thrombosis include a disabling post-thrombotic syndrome and death due to fatal PE. Treatment with anticoagulants should be prompt and adequate.

Many risk factors for thrombosis are known, all of them related either to immobilization or to hypercoagulability. While it has no utility to assess the risk factor status after thrombosis has occurred, several acquired risk factors are so strong that they warrant prophylactic anticoagulation, in both those with and without a history of thrombosis. Detailed guidelines for primary prevention are available.

Venous thrombosis tends to recur. The risk factors for a first venous thrombosis are not the same as for recurrent venous thrombosis and to a large extent are unknown. Individuals from families with inherited thrombophilia tend to develop thrombosis at a young age and to have frequent recurrences.

EPIDEMIOLOGY

The incidence of a first venous thrombosis is 1–3 per 1000 persons per year. Around two-thirds manifest as DVT of the leg, and one-third as PE. Up to half of patients with PE have no signs of DVT. From 1–10% of venous thromboses prove fatal, with deaths predominantly, but not exclusively, among the elderly or in patients with severe underlying disease, notably cancer. The incidence of venous thrombosis is exponentially related to age, where a rule of 10 applies: in children the incidence is 1 per 100,000 per year; in young adults, 1 in 10,000 per year; in the middle-aged, 1 per 1000 per year; in the elderly the incidence is 1% per year, up to nearly 10% per year in the very oldest. The recurrence rate of venous thrombosis is 3–10% per year.

TABLE 111-1 RISK FACTORS FOR VENOUS THROMBOSIS

Acquired	Inherited	Mixed/Unknown
Orthopedic surgery	Antithrombin deficiency	High levels of factor VIII
Neurosurgery	Protein C deficiency	High levels of factor IX
Major abdominal surgery	Protein S deficiency	High levels of factor XI
Major trauma	Factor V Leiden (FVL)	High levels of fibrinogen
Central venous catheters	Prothrombin 20210A	High levels of TAFI
Malignancy	Non-O blood group	Low levels of TFPI
Antiphospholipid syndrome	Dysfibrinogenemia	APC resistance in the absence of FVL
Puerperium	Factor XIII 34val	
Prolonged bed rest		Hyperhomocysteinemia
Pregnancy		High levels of PCI (PAI-3)
Obesity		
Plaster cast		
Oral contraceptives		
Hormonal replacement therapy		
Myeloproliferative disorders		
Polycythemia vera		
Long-haul travel		
Age		

Note: TAFI, thrombin activatable fibrinolysis inhibitor; TFPI, tissue factor pathway inhibitor; PCI, protein C inhibitor; PAI-3, plasminogen activator inhibitor-3; APC, activated protein C.

ETIOLOGY

The causes of thrombosis can be divided into those associated with immobilization, which are usually acquired, and those associated with hypercoagulability, which can be either genetic or acquired (**Table 111-1**). Venous thrombosis is a multicausal disease that occurs when several risk factors are present simultaneously in a particular combination. Often, long-term risk factors, e.g., genetic defects, are joined by short-term acquired factors (**Fig. 111-1**). While many factors simply add to the risk, contributing to an individual's "thrombosis potential," some factors may interact synergistically, when the combination adds more to the risk than the sum of the separate contributions of the risk factors (e.g., factor V Leiden and oral contraceptive use).

Several acquired risk factors are very strong, causing thrombosis in several percent of those afflicted, which implies a relative risk of ≥50. These are orthopedic, neurosurgical, and major abdominal interventions; major trauma with multiple fractures; central venous catheters; and metastasized cancer, particularly adenocarcinomas. Moderate risk factors are antiphospholipid antibody syndrome, puerperium, prolonged bedrest, and nonmetastasized cancers; pregnancy, oral contraceptive use, hormone replacement therapy, obesity, and long-distance travel are mild risk factors, with a two- to fivefold increased risk.

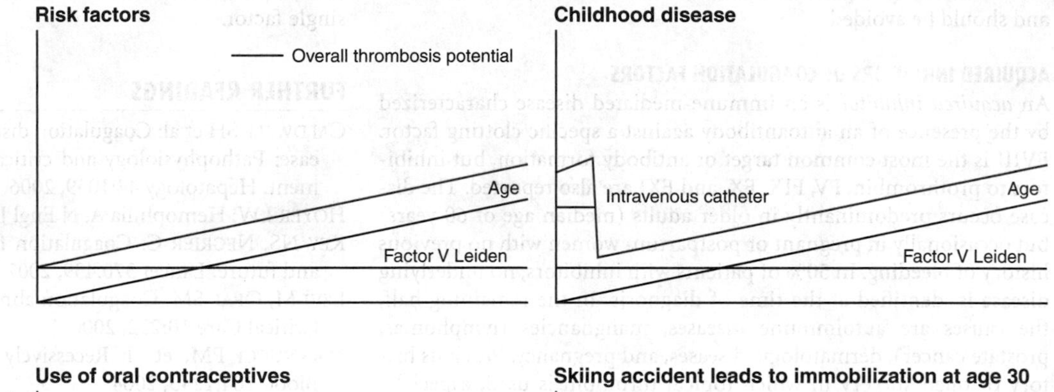

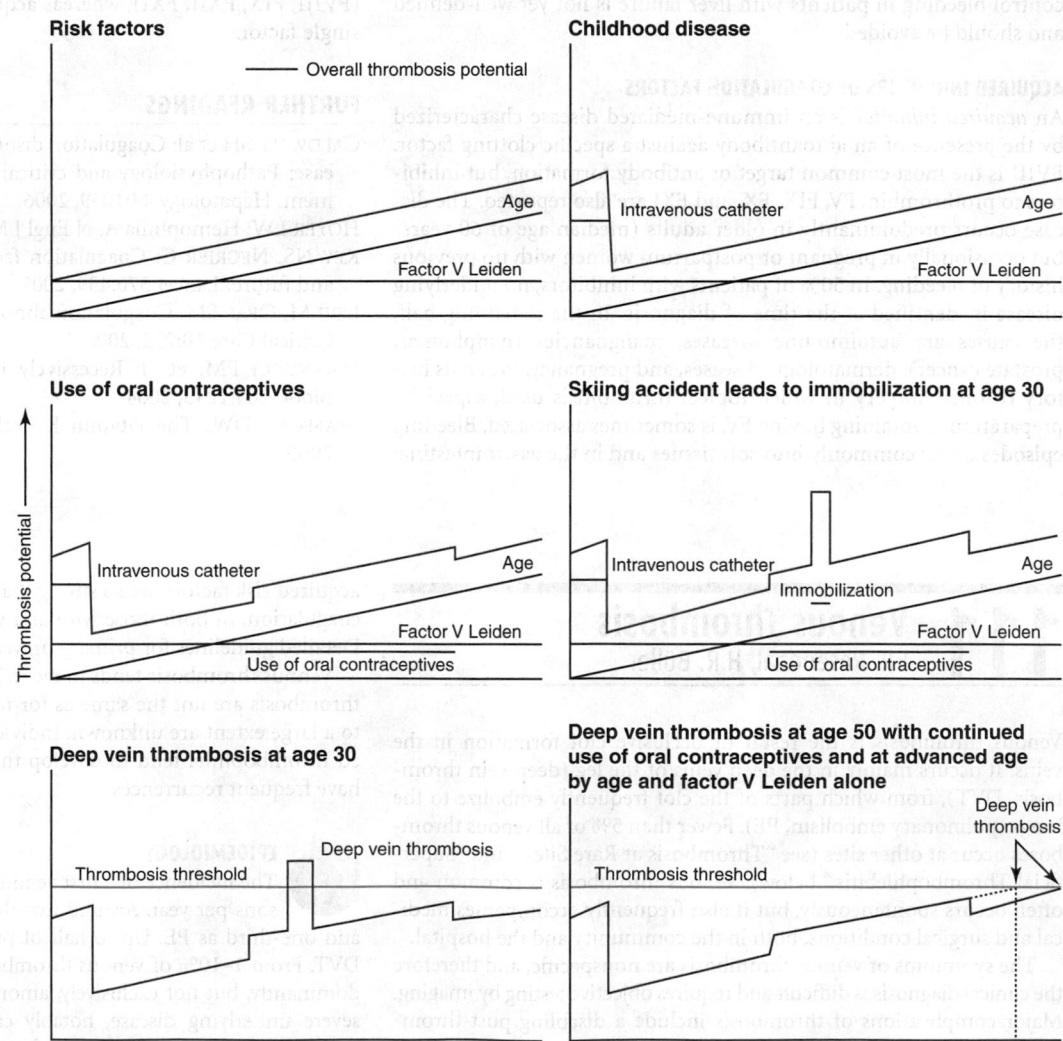

FIGURE 111-1 Models of thrombosis risk. In each panel, the figure shows the thrombosis (black) potential of each risk factor present during an individual's life and the resultant thrombosis potential (red). *(From FR Rosendaal: Venous thrombosis: A multicausal disease. Lancet 353:1167, 1999; with permission.)*

Homozygous protein C or protein S deficiency leads to potentially fatal purpura fulminans directly after birth, while homozygous antithrombin deficiency is not compatible with life. These are exceedingly rare, except in communities with a high frequency of consanguinity. Heterozygous antithrombin deficiency and homozygous factor V Leiden are the strongest genetic risk factors, increasing the risk of thrombosis 20- to 50-fold. Heterozygous protein C and protein S deficiencies are moderate contributors to risk, with a relative risk of 10. Other genetic factors that are associated with venous thrombosis are either mild and increase the risk two- to fivefold (as is the case for factor V Leiden, prothrombin 20210A, and non-O blood groups) or have negligible effects on risk that are only of academic interest (MTHFR 677T, factor V HR2, FXIII val34leu, PAI-1 4G/5G).

Mildly increased risks are also present for abnormalities in the coagulation system of which the origin is unclear, such as elevated levels of procoagulant factors (fibrinogen, II, von Willebrand factor, VIII, IX, X, and XI) and antifibrinolytic factors (TAFI), and low levels of anticoagulant factors (TFPI) (Table 111-1).

PROGNOSIS

Patients who have had a venous thrombosis have a high risk (3–10% per year) of another. Up to half of the recurrences after a first thrombosis in one leg occur in the other, indicating that systemic changes rather than residual local damage are associated with rethrombosis. Nevertheless, few of the established risk factors associated with a hypercoagulable state (such as factor V Leiden, prothrombin 20210A, and elevated levels of clotting factors VIII, IX, and XI) are associated with recurrence risk. Even the strongest prothrombotic abnormalities—antithrombin, protein C, and protein S deficiencies—increase the risk of recurrent thrombosis by 50% at most. The only two clear risk factors for recurrence are male sex (increasing risk three- to fourfold) and the absence of a clear precipitating factor at the first event (doubling recurrence risk); in other words, a first thrombosis following surgery or plaster cast is unlikely to recur.

Acquired risk factors, such as surgery, immobilization, and cancer, increase the risk of recurrent thrombosis—as they increase the risk of a first event.

PREVENTION

The presence of prothrombotic defects or a history of thrombosis does not usually lead to different preventative strategies, with the exception of the postpartum period, where anticoagulation seems indicated, particularly for antithrombin deficiency. Similarly, the decision for long-term or lifelong anticoagulation, i.e., beyond the period of increased risk, depends on the clinical presentation rather than on the presence of prothrombotic abnormalities. Before prescribing long-term anticoagulation, clinicians should be aware of the cumulative annual risk of major hemorrhage of 1–2%.

Patients with a history of thrombosis should not use estrogen-containing drugs, i.e., hormone replacement therapy is contraindicated and for contraception, mechanical methods are preferred.

Thrombophilia Testing Testing for prothrombotic abnormalities outside the setting of abundant familial thrombophilia serves no purpose. A positive test does not help in the diagnosis of thrombosis, nor does it predict the risk of recurrent thrombosis, nor, therefore, does it affect long-term preventive strategies.

HEREDITARY THROMBOPHILIA

Individuals from families with a hereditary tendency for venous thrombosis generally have a more severe thrombotic tendency than individuals not from such families. Even when the genetic defect is the same in the two groups, those with hereditary thrombophilia from affected families have their first thrombosis at a young age (20–35 years), few fail to develop thrombosis in their lifetime, and many have recurrent disease. Early studies on thrombotic risk associated with prothrombotic defects were based on such families and overestimated risks for all patients with thrombophilic defects. Generally, individuals from such families need not be treated differently than others, except (1) oral contraceptives containing estrogens should be discouraged in all, and (2) postpartum anticoagulant prophylaxis should be considered in those with prothrombotic defects. Long-term treatment can be considered after a first episode of thrombosis, but only in high-risk families, particularly those with antithrombin deficiency.

THROMBOSIS AT RARE SITES

One in 25 venous thromboses occurs in the arm, while other, even more rare locations are the brain (cerebral vein thrombosis), the digestive system (mesenteric vein thrombosis), and the liver (portal vein thrombosis, and hepatic vein thrombosis, also known as *Budd-Chiari syndrome*). Thrombosis of the arm is almost invariably associated with central venous catheters. Deteriorating liver function and portal hypertension may point to thrombosis in the hepatic or portal veins, neurologic defects to cerebral vein thrombosis, and severe abdominal complaints to mesenteric vein thrombosis. In rare cases, DVT may be associated with embolic stroke, when a patent foramen ovale is present (paradoxical stroke). Although local abnormalities often play a role, a procoagulant state due to cancer or hereditary abnormalities increases the incidence of thrombosis in rare locations. In all these cases diagnosis is based on imaging, and treatment should consist of anticoagulation similar to that of more common forms of thrombosis, as well as treatment of local causes and consequences.

SUPERFICIAL THROMBOPHLEBITIS

A painful red string is a clear sign of superficial thrombophlebitis. This is the only type of venous thrombosis that can reliably be diagnosed without imaging techniques. Although research is limited, the causes of superficial thrombophlebitis appear similar to those of other forms of venous thrombosis, and extension to the deep vein occurs. Treatment options are a matter of debate and vary from anticoagulants to an expectant approach.

GLOBAL DATA

Venous thrombosis occurs in all ethnic groups, with possibly a somewhat higher incidence in Africans than in whites and Asians. Whereas acquired risk factors are largely identical in these large ethnic groups, the two most common genetic risk factors (factor V Leiden and prothrombin 20210A) are found only in whites. These are unique gain-of-function mutations with a very low mutation rate (i.e., they occurred only once). Loss-of-function mutations leading to deficiencies of antithrombin, protein C, and protein S do not differ much by ethnic group. Due to founder effects, prevalences of factor V Leiden and prothrombin 20210A may vary widely in ethnic subpopulations, i.e., in various European populations the prevalence of factor V Leiden varies between 1% (Italy) and 15% (southern Sweden). Acquired risk factors may vary by local circumstances, e.g., hyperhomocysteinemia due to differences in diet, reproductive factors due to number of pregnancies, and use of oral contraceptives. The literature on Africans and Asians is sparse.

DIAGNOSIS

The true prevalence of thrombosis in patients presenting with either clinically suspected DVT of the leg or PE is ~15–25%. Therefore, the diagnostic workup for both these diseases has two objectives: (1) to exclude the disease quickly and safely in as many patients as possible, preferably with noninvasive and easy-to-use and cost-effective methods; and (2) to confirm the presence of thrombosis in the remaining patients with an accurate imaging technique. The purpose of the first step is to withhold both unnecessary further diagnostic testing and anticoagulant treatment. Although the diagnostic workup of DVT and PE have much in common, they will be discussed separately.

Deep Vein Thrombosis The signs and symptoms of DVT, such as swelling, pain, redness, superficial venous dilatation, and Homan's sign (pain in the calf or behind the knee on dorsiflexion of the ankle), are nonspecific and consequently insufficient for ruling the disease in or out. The classic "gold standard" is contrast venography. Although very accurate, this method requires radiologic facilities and expertise and is invasive and sometimes uncomfortable for the patient. Ultrasonography, with noncompressibility of the vein as the sole criterion, has largely replaced contrast venography. The investigation is limited to the femoral vein in the groin and the popliteal vein in the popliteal fossa. This method has a very high sensitivity and specificity (95–100%) in symptomatic patients for proximal DVT. For isolated DVT in the calf veins the method is less accurate. This latter characteristic of compression ultrasonography explains the necessity of repeating the test after ~1 week in those patients with an initial normal test result in order to detect extending calf thrombi. However, the first objective of the diagnostic workup was to rule out DVT quickly and safely. For this purpose the combination of the assessment of clinical probability and the measurement of the D-dimer blood concentration has been shown to be very useful. The clinical probability can be best assessed by the

TABLE 111-2 CLINICAL DECISION RULE FOR DIAGNOSING THROMBOSIS

Decision rule for clinically suspected deep vein thrombosis (DVT)	Points
Active cancer (patient receiving treatment for cancer within the previous 6 months or currently receiving palliative treatment)	1
Paralysis, paresis, or recent plaster immobilization of the lower extremities	1
Recently bedridden for ≥3 days or major surgery within the previous 12 weeks requiring general or regional anesthesia	1
Localized tenderness along the distribution of the deep venous system	1
Entire leg swollen	1
Calf swelling at least 3 cm larger than that on the asymptomatic side (measured 10 cm below tibial tuberosity)	1
Pitting edema confined to the symptomatic leg	1
Collateral superficial veins (nonvaricose)	1
Previously documented deep vein thrombosis	1
Alternative diagnosis at least as likely as deep vein thrombosis	−2
Score <2: DVT unlikely	
≥2: DVT likely	
Decision rule for clinically suspected pulmonary embolism (PE)	Points
Clinical signs and symptoms of deep vein thrombosis (minimum of leg swelling and pain with palpation of the deep veins)	3
Alternative diagnosis less likely than pulmonary embolism	3
Heart rate > 100/min	1.5
Immobilization (>3 days) or surgery in the previous 4 weeks	1.5
Previous pulmonary embolism or deep vein thrombosis	1.5
Hemoptysis	1
Malignancy (receiving treatment, treated in the last 6 months or palliative)	1
Score ≤4: PE unlikely	
>4: PE likely	

rule shown in Table 111-2, which results in a classification of either DVT likely or DVT unlikely. D-Dimer is a degradation product of cross-linked fibrin and therefore concentrations of D-dimer below a certain cut-off level are considered to indicate the absence of thrombosis. Elevations of D-dimer in patients > 70 years who do not have thrombosis make the test less useful in this population.

Withholding further diagnostic testing and anticoagulant treatment in those patients with an unlikely clinical probability and a normal D-dimer level, which constitutes 30–50% of all referred patients, is safe. The remaining patients need to undergo (repeated) compression ultrasonography. An alternative approach is to perform a whole-leg imaging test on the day of referral. The advantage of this approach is that it eliminates the need for a repeat test (and may even obviate the probability assessment and D-dimer testing). The major disadvantage is the detection and likely treatment of a substantial number of isolated calf DVTs that may otherwise have lysed spontaneously.

Pulmonary Embolism The signs and symptoms of PE, such as dyspnea, pleuritic chest pain, cough, and hemoptysis, are nonspecific and, as for DVT, insufficiently accurate to confirm or refute the diagnosis of PE. The classic gold standard is pulmonary angiography, which is an invasive method requiring expertise. Hence, very similar to the developments in the diagnosis of DVT, two (complementary) strategies have evolved. The first is the combination of the assessment of clinical probability and the measurement of the D-dimer blood level; the second is the introduction of spiral CT of the chest. The clinical probability can be categorized accurately using the rule developed for suspected PE (Table 111-2). In those with an unlikely probability, a D-dimer test should be performed and, if normal, the disease can be safely ruled out and no anticoagulant therapy is indicated. Depending on the referral pattern of patients, this combination rules out PE in 30–60% of all referred patients. Those with either a likely clinical probability at presentation or an abnormal D-dimer (and unlikely probability) need to undergo an imaging test.

At present the most attractive method is the multi-slice spiral CT of the chest. This technique accurately detects pulmonary embolism and, if normal, has been shown to also safely rule out the presence of emboli. Another advantage is the possibility of detecting an alternative disease in the thorax in those in whom PE is excluded, which may provide an explanation for the presenting symptoms. Alternative diagnostic methods in the workup of suspected PE are perfusion-ventilation scintigraphy, ultrasonography of the legs, and pulmonary angiography. Although a normal perfusion scan adequately rules out PE and a high probability perfusion-ventilation scan adequately rules in PE, the major disadvantages are the high proportion of nondiagnostic test results (~50%) and therefore the need for additional (costly) testing, usually with pulmonary angiography.

The role of compression ultrasonography of the legs before angiography or spiral CT is limited, as only a small fraction of patients have abnormal results and it further complicates the workup.

℞ DEEP VEIN THROMBOSIS AND PULMONARY EMBOLISM

The objectives of anticoagulant treatment for DVT and PE are to minimize local extension of the disease in the acute phase and to reduce the risk of recurrence of the disease in the months to years after the initial episode. In addition, in DVT, treatment lowers the risk of the development of the post-thrombotic syndrome (swelling, stasis dermatitis, ulceration, venous claudication); in PE, treatment reduces the risk of pulmonary hypertension.

A spectrum of treatment options is available. At one end an expectant approach is indicated with no treatment in the setting of minimal disease without a tendency to extend or recur (as is the case, for example, with small calf thrombi). At the other end is the DVT or PE that is massive, either with serious compromise of lung perfusion or with impending gangrene of the leg. In these circumstances, aggressive treatment with either thrombolysis or even surgical intervention may be required. However, the vast majority of patients with DVT or PE require treatment in the middle part of the spectrum, which consists of the use of anticoagulants, usually low-molecular-weight heparin (LMWH) and a vitamin K antagonist (VKA) such as warfarin. Although the treatments of DVT and PE have much in common, they will be discussed separately.

DEEP VEIN THROMBOSIS The standard treatment for DVT consists of an initial course of LMWH, given once or twice daily via SC injection at a dose of 100 U/kg, followed by a VKA. Unfractionated heparin given IV is an alternative for LMWH but is less and less used these days. LMWH does not require laboratory monitoring and is given in a fixed dose, usually adapted for body weight (categories). An alternative for the initial LMWH therapy is the short-acting synthetic pentasaccharide fondaparinux, which can be given as a once-a-day SC injection of 2.5 mg, without laboratory monitoring. Therapy with LMWH or fondaparinux should be started as soon as the diagnosis is confirmed or during the diagnostic workup if the clinical suspicion is high. VKA (warfarin) can be safely started at the same day and the dose is titrated according to the international normalized ratio (INR) with a target of 2.5 (range 2–3). LMWH therapy should be continued for at least 5 days and can be discontinued if the INR is >2 on two consecutive measurements at least 24 h apart. The recommendations for the duration of VKA treatment for a first episode of DVT are summarized in **Table 111-3**. For a first DVT secondary to a transient (reversible) risk factor, such as following surgery, after immobilization, or associated with oral contraceptive use, a treatment duration of 3 months with a VKA is recommended. For patients with a first episode of idiopathic DVT, the recommendation is to treat for 6–12 months. At present, evidence is insufficient to treat patients with a first episode of DVT and a documented thrombophilic abnormality differently from those with idiopathic thrombosis. Hence, the recommendation is also 6–12 months of VKA. A duration of 12 months is recommended for patients with a first episode of DVT with documented antiphospholipid antibodies or two or more thrombophilic abnormalities. The decision to continue VKA treatment after 6–12 months requires the balancing of the risks of recurrence and bleeding and should take the patient's preference into account. No strong recommendations exist about the treatment duration for a second episode of DVT, but minimally 12

TABLE 111-3 LONG-TERM TREATMENT WITH VITAMIN K ANTAGONISTS FOR DEEP VEIN THROMBOSIS (DVT) AND PULMONARY EMBOLISM (PE)

Patient Categories	Duration, months	Comments
First episode of DVT or PE secondary to a transient (reversible) risk factor	3	Recommendation applies to both proximal and calf vein thrombosis
First episode of idiopathic DVT or PE	6–12	Continuation of anticoagulant therapy after 6–12 months may be considered
First episode of DVT or PE with a documented thrombophilic abnormality	6–12	Continuation of anticoagulant therapy after 6–12 months may be considered
First episode of DVT or PE with documented antiphospholipid or two or more thrombophilic abnormalities	12	Continuation of anticoagulant therapy after 12 months may be considered

months are usually given and often treatment is continued longer. Again, this decision requires the balancing of risk and benefit.

The preferred intensity of VKA treatment for DVT is an INR between 2 and 3. Higher intensities are not more effective, whereas lower intensities are less effective with a similar bleeding risk. Although VKAs are generally used for long-term treatment, LMWH is preferred in patients with DVT and concomitant cancer. This treatment is associated with a lower risk of recurrent thrombosis than VKA and a similar risk of bleeding.

The role of thrombolytic therapy as well as surgical removal of the thrombus in the initial treatment of DVT is controversial; the current recommendations are to refrain from their use with the single exception of patients with massive, recent ileofemoral DVT at risk of limb gangrene.

Patients with DVT are at risk of developing the postthrombotic syndrome in the first years after the initial episode. This syndrome can range from mild, with some swelling and pain at the end of the day, to severe, with massive swelling and skin ulceration. Graduated elastic compression stockings to the knee with an ankle pressure of 30–40 mmHg fitted in the first weeks after the initial thrombosis and worn for 2 years reduce the risk of the postthrombotic syndrome by ~50%.

As a result of the introduction of LMWH for the initial treatment of DVT, most patients with DVT can be treated at home either entirely or after a short hospital stay. The LMWH can be self-injected or given by family members or visiting nurses.

PULMONARY EMBOLISM The initial treatment with LMWH followed by a VKA for patients with PE is identical to that for patients with DVT. The intensity and duration of VKA treatment is also no different (Table 111-3). An alternative for LMWH is unfractionated heparin, which is still often used. The main disadvantage of unfractionated heparin is the need for continuous IV infusion and the requirement of frequent laboratory monitoring and dose adjustments. In contrast, LMWH can be given in fixed doses adjusted only for body weight. Another alternative for the initial LMWH therapy is fondaparinux, which can be given as a 2.5-mg once-a-day SC injection, without laboratory monitoring.

The treatment with LWMH or fondaparinux followed by VKA is indicated for PE patients who are hemodynamically stable—the great majority of patients. However, for those patients with PE who are hemodynamically unstable (usually defined as a systolic blood pressure <90–100 mmHg), a course of thrombolytic therapy should be considered. When no contraindications for thrombolysis (such as recent surgery or a bleeding diathesis) exist, this therapy reduces the short-term risk of recurrent PE or death by ~50% as compared to heparin. Although streptokinase and urokinase have been used in patients with PE, the most widely applied regimen is recombinant tissue plasminogen activator r(tPA) (bolus of 10 mg IV, followed by 90 mg in 2 h).

A controversial area is the best therapy for PE patients who are hemodynamically stable, but who have echocardiographic evidence of right ventricular dysfunction (usually defined as paradoxical interventricular septal motion and right ventricular dilatation and impaired systolic function). Although these patients have a higher mortality risk compared to patients without right ventricular dysfunction, it is unclear whether more aggressive therapy (with thrombolytic therapy or catheter removal of thrombus) is beneficial in terms of mortality, recurrent PE, and major hemorrhage.

Another area of controversy is vena caval interruption, usually with caval filters. The current recommendation is that a filter, preferably removable, should be considered only for patients with a contraindication for anticoagulant therapy, as well as in those with recurrent PE despite adequate treatment.

FURTHER READINGS

PRANDONI P: Links between arterial and venous disease. J Intern Med 262:341, 2007

ROSENDAAL FR: Venous thrombosis, a multicausal disease. Lancet 353:1167, 1999

The Seventh ACCP Conference on Antithrombotic and Thrombolytic Therapy. Chest 126(3 Suppl):167S, 2004

112 Antiplatelet, Anticoagulant, and Fibrinolytic Drugs

Jeffrey I. Weitz

Arterial and venous thromboses are major causes of morbidity and mortality. Arterial thrombosis is the most common cause of acute myocardial infarction, ischemic stroke, and limb gangrene, whereas deep vein thrombosis leads to pulmonary embolism (PE), which can be fatal, and to the postphlebitic syndrome. Most arterial thrombi are superimposed on disrupted atherosclerotic plaque because plaque rupture exposes thrombogenic material in the plaque core to the blood. This material then triggers platelet aggregation and fibrin formation, which results in the generation of a platelet-rich thrombus that can temporarily or permanently occlude blood flow. In contrast to arterial thrombi, venous thrombi rarely form at sites of obvious vascular disruption. Although they can develop after surgical trauma to veins or secondary to indwelling venous catheters, venous thrombi usually originate in the valve cusps of the deep veins of the calf or in the muscular sinuses, where they are triggered by stasis. Sluggish blood flow in these veins reduces the oxygen supply to the avascular valve cusps. Endothelial cells lining these valve cusps become activated and express adhesion molecules on their surface. Tissue factor–bearing leukocytes and microparticles adhere to these activated cells and induce coagulation. Local thrombus formation is exacerbated by reduced clearance of activated clotting factors as a result of impaired blood flow. If the thrombi extend into more proximal veins of the leg, thrombus fragments can dislodge, travel to the lungs, and produce a PE.

Arterial and venous thrombi are composed of platelets and fibrin, but the proportions differ. Arterial thrombi are rich in platelets because of the high shear in the injured arteries. In contrast, venous thrombi, which form under low shear conditions, contain relatively few platelets and are predominantly composed of fibrin and trapped red cells. Because of the predominance of platelets, arterial thrombi appear white, whereas venous thrombi are red in color, reflecting the trapped red cells.

Antithrombotic drugs are used for prevention and treatment of thrombosis. Targeting the components of thrombi, these agents include (1) antiplatelet drugs, (2) anticoagulants, and (3) fibrinolytic agents (Fig. 112-1). With the predominance of platelets in arterial thrombi, strategies to inhibit or treat arterial thrombosis focus mainly

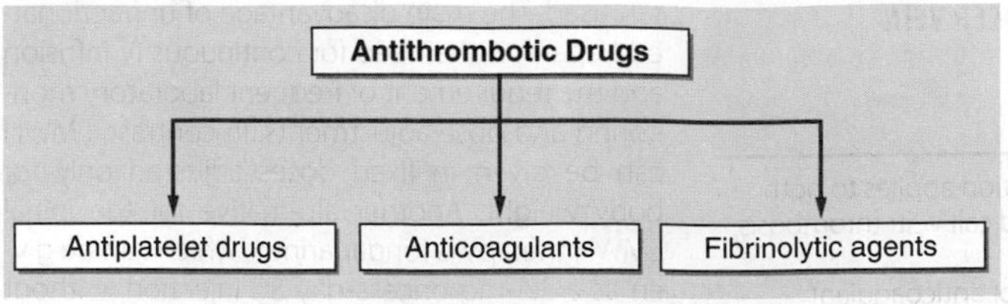

FIGURE 112-1 Classification of antithrombotic drugs.

on antiplatelet agents, although, in the acute setting, they often include anticoagulants and fibrinolytic agents. Anticoagulants are the mainstay of prevention and treatment of venous thromboembolism because fibrin is the predominant component of venous thrombi. Antiplatelet drugs are less effective than anticoagulants in this setting because of the limited platelet content of venous thrombi. Fibrinolytic therapy is used in selected patients with venous thromboembolism. For example, patients with massive or submassive PE can benefit from systemic or catheter-directed fibrinolytic therapy. The latter can also be used as an adjunct to anticoagulants for treatment of patients with extensive iliofemoral vein thrombosis.

ANTIPLATELET DRUGS

ROLE OF PLATELETS IN ARTERIAL THROMBOSIS

In healthy vasculature, circulating platelets are maintained in an inactive state by nitric oxide (NO) and prostacyclin released by endothelial cells lining the blood vessels. In addition, endothelial cells also express adenosine diphosphatase (ADPase) on their surface, which degrades ADP released from activated platelets. When the vessel wall is damaged, release of these substances is impaired and subendothelial matrix is exposed. Platelets adhere to exposed collagen, von Willebrand factor (vWF), and fibronectin via $\alpha_2\beta_1$, glycoprotein (GP) Ib-IX, and $\alpha_5\beta_1$ receptors, respectively, which are constitutively expressed on the platelet surface. Adherent platelets undergo a change in shape, secrete ADP from their dense granules, and synthesize and release thromboxane A_2. Released ADP and thromboxane A_2, which are platelet agonists, activate ambient platelets and recruit them to the site of vascular injury (Fig. 112-2).

Disruption of the vessel wall also exposes tissue factor–expressing cells to the blood. Tissue factor initiates coagulation. Activated platelets potentiate coagulation by binding clotting factors and supporting the assembly of activation complexes that enhance thrombin generation. In addition to converting fibrinogen to fibrin, thrombin also serves as a potent platelet agonist and recruits more platelets to the site of vascular injury.

When platelets are activated, GPIIb/IIIa, the most abundant receptor on the platelet surface, undergoes a conformational change that enables it to bind fibrinogen. Divalent fibrinogen molecules bridge adjacent platelets together to form platelet aggregates. Fibrin strands, generated through the action of thrombin, then weave these aggregates together to form a platelet/fibrin mesh.

Antiplatelet drugs target various steps in this process. The commonly used drugs include aspirin, thienopyridines (clopidogrel and ticlopidine), dipyridimole, and GPIIb/IIIa antagonists.

ASPIRIN

The most widely used antiplatelet agent worldwide is aspirin. As a cheap and effective antiplatelet drug, aspirin serves as the foundation of most antiplatelet strategies.

MECHANISM OF ACTION Aspirin produces its antithrombotic effect by irreversibly acetylating and inhibiting platelet cyclooxygenase (COX)-1 (Fig. 112-3), a critical enzyme in the biosynthesis of thromboxane A_2. At high doses (~1 g/d), aspirin also inhibits COX-2, an inducible COX isoform found in endothelial cells and inflammatory cells. In endothelial cells, COX-2 initiates the synthesis of prostacyclin, a potent vasodilator and inhibitor of platelet aggregation.

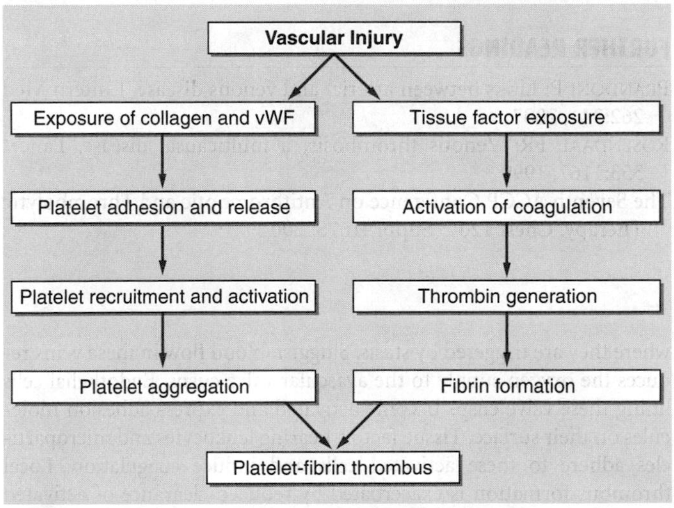

FIGURE 112-2 Coordinated role of platelets and the coagulation system in thrombogenesis. Vascular injury simultaneously triggers platelet activation and aggregation and activation of the coagulation system. Platelet activation is initiated by exposure of subendothelial collagen and von Willebrand factor (vWF) onto which platelets adhere. Adherent platelets become activated and release ADP and thromboxane A_2, platelet agonists that activate ambient platelets and recruit them to the site of injury. When platelets are activated, glycoprotein IIb/IIIa on their surface undergoes a conformational change that enables it to ligate fibrinogen and mediate platelet aggregation. Coagulation is triggered by tissue factor exposed at the site of injury. Tissue factor triggers thrombin generation. As a potent platelet agonist, thrombin amplifies platelet recruitment to the site of injury. Thrombin also converts fibrinogen to fibrin, and the fibrin strands then weave the platelet aggregates together to form a platelet/fibrin thrombus.

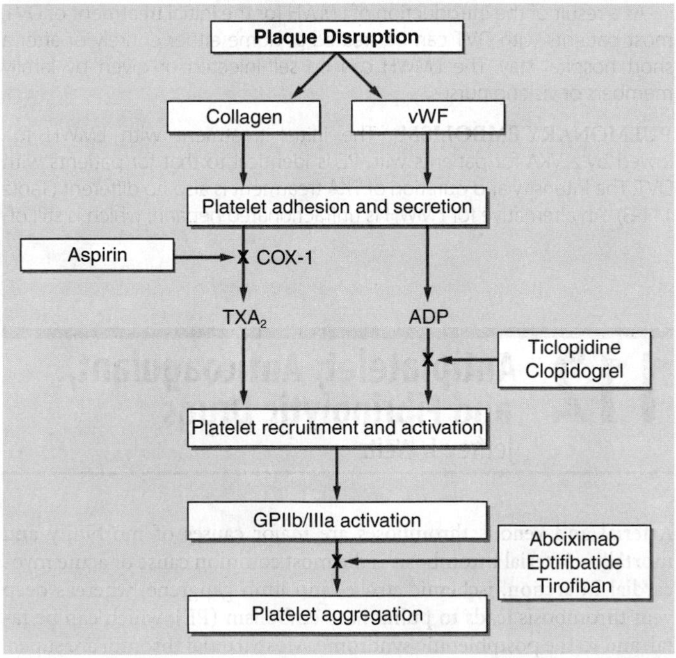

FIGURE 112-3 Site of action of antiplatelet drugs. Aspirin inhibits thromboxane A_2 (TXA_2) synthesis by irreversibly acetylating cyclooxygenase-1 (COX-1). Reduced TXA_2 release attenuates platelet activation and recruitment to the site of vascular injury. Ticlopidine and clopidogrel irreversibly block $P2Y_{12}$, a key ADP receptor on the platelet surface. Therefore, these agents also attenuate platelet recruitment. Abciximab, eptifibatide, and tirofiban inhibit the final common pathway of platelet aggregation by blocking fibrinogen binding to activated glycoprotein (GP) IIb/IIIa.

COX-2 inhibitors were developed to block the production of inflammatory prostaglandins without affecting platelet function. The various COX-2 inhibitors differ in their selectivity for COX-2 relative to COX-1. By blocking prostacyclin synthesis without concomitant inhibition of thromboxane A_2 production, highly selective inhibitors of COX-2 increase the risk of cardiovascular events. Thus, long-term rofecoxib therapy increases the risk of myocardial infarction (MI) three- to fivefold, a finding that led to the withdrawal of this drug from the market.

INDICATIONS Aspirin is widely used for secondary prevention of cardiovascular events in patients with coronary artery, cerebrovascular, or peripheral vascular disease. Compared with placebo, aspirin produces a 25% reduction in the risk of cardiovascular death, MI, or stroke. Aspirin is also used for primary prevention in patients whose estimated annual risk of MI is >1%, a point where its benefits are likely to outweigh harms. This includes patients over the age of 40 with two or more major risk factors for cardiovascular disease or those over the age of 50 with one or more such risk factor. Aspirin is equally effective in men and women. In men, aspirin mainly reduces the risk of MI, while in women aspirin lowers the risk of stroke.

DOSAGES Aspirin is usually administered at doses of 75–325 mg once daily. Higher dose aspirin is not more effective than lower aspirin doses, and some analyses suggest reduced efficacy with higher doses. Because the side effects of aspirin are dose-related, daily aspirin doses of 75–100 mg are recommended for most indications. When rapid platelet inhibition is required, an initial aspirin dose of at least 160 mg should be given.

SIDE EFFECTS Most common side effects are gastrointestinal and range from dyspepsia to erosive gastritis or peptic ulcers with bleeding and perforation. These side effects are dose-related. Use of enteric-coated or buffered aspirin in place of plain aspirin does not eliminate the risk of gastrointestinal side effects. The overall risk of major bleeding with aspirin is 1–3% per year. The risk of bleeding is increased when aspirin is given in conjunction with anticoagulants, such as warfarin. When dual therapy is used, low-dose aspirin should be given (75–100 mg daily). Eradication of *Helicobacter pylori* infection and administration of proton pump inhibitors may reduce the risk of aspirin-induced gastrointestinal bleeding in patients with peptic ulcer disease.

Aspirin should not be administered to patients with a history of aspirin allergy characterized by bronchospasm. This problem occurs in ~0.3% of the general population but is more common in those with chronic urticaria or asthma, particularly in individuals with nasal polyps or chronic rhinitis. Hepatic and renal toxicity are observed with aspirin overdose.

ASPIRIN RESISTANCE Clinical aspirin resistance is defined as the failure of aspirin to protect patients from ischemic vascular events. This is not a helpful definition because it is made after the event occurs. Furthermore, it is not realistic to expect aspirin, which only blocks thromboxane A_2–induced platelet activation, to prevent all vascular events.

Aspirin resistance has also been described biochemically as failure of the drug to produce its expected inhibitory effects on tests of platelet function, such as thromboxane A_2 synthesis or arachidonic acid–induced platelet aggregation. However, the tests of platelet function used for diagnosis of biochemical aspirin resistance have not been well standardized. Furthermore, these tests are not proven to identify patients at risk of recurrent vascular events. In addition, resistance is not reversed by either giving higher doses of aspirin or adding other antiplatelet drugs. Thus, testing for aspirin resistance remains a research tool.

THIENOPYRIDINES

The thienopyridines include ticlopidine and clopidogrel, drugs that target $P2Y_{12}$, a key ADP receptor on platelets.

MECHANISM OF ACTION The thienopyridines are structurally related drugs that selectively inhibit ADP-induced platelet aggregation by irreversibly blocking $P2Y_{12}$ (Fig. 112-3). Ticlopidine and clopidogrel are both prodrugs that must be metabolized by the hepatic cytochrome P450 (CYP) enzyme system to acquire activity. Consequently, when given in usual doses, their onset of action is delayed for several days.

INDICATIONS Like aspirin, ticlopidine is more effective than placebo at reducing the risk of cardiovascular death, MI, and stroke in patients with atherosclerotic disease. Because of its delayed onset of action, ticlopidine is not recommended in patients with acute MI. Ticlopidine was used routinely as an adjunct to aspirin after coronary artery stenting and as an aspirin substitute in those intolerant to aspirin. Because clopidogrel is more potent than ticlopidine and has a better safety profile, clopidogrel has replaced ticlopidine.

When compared with aspirin in patients with recent ischemic stroke, MI, or peripheral arterial disease, clopidogrel reduced the risk of cardiovascular death, MI, and stroke by 8.7%. Therefore, clopidogrel is more effective than aspirin but is also more expensive. In some patients, clopidogrel and aspirin are combined to capitalize on their capacity to block complementary pathways of platelet activation. For example, the combination of aspirin plus clopidogrel is recommended for at least 4 weeks after implantation of a bare metal stent in a coronary artery and longer in those with a drug-eluting stent. Concerns about late in-stent thrombosis with drug-eluting stents have led some experts to recommend long-term use of clopidogrel plus aspirin for this indication.

The combination of clopidogrel and aspirin is also effective in patients with unstable angina. Thus, in 12,562 such patients, the risk of cardiovascular death, MI, or stroke was 9.3% in those randomized to the combination of clopidogrel and aspirin and 11.4% in those given aspirin alone. This 20% relative risk reduction with combination therapy was highly statistically significant. However, combining clopidogrel with aspirin increases the risk of major bleeding to about 2% per year. This bleeding risk persists even if the daily dose of aspirin is ≤100 mg. Therefore, the combination of clopidogrel and aspirin should only be used when there is a clear benefit. For example, this combination has not proven to be superior to clopidogrel alone in patients with acute ischemic stroke or to aspirin alone for primary prevention in those at risk for cardiovascular events.

DOSING Ticlopidine is given twice daily at a dose of 250 mg. The more potent clopidogrel is given once daily at a dose of 75 mg. Loading doses of clopidogrel are given when rapid ADP receptor blockade is desired. For example, patients undergoing coronary stenting are often given a loading dose of 300 mg, which effects inhibition of ADP-induced platelet aggregation in about 6 h. Loading doses of 600 or 900 mg produce an even more rapid effect.

SIDE EFFECTS The most common side effects of ticlopidine are gastrointestinal. More serious are the hematologic side effects, which include neutropenia, thrombocytopenia, and thrombotic thrombocytopenic purpura. These side effects usually occur within the first few months of starting treatment. Therefore, blood counts must be carefully monitored when initiating therapy with ticlopidine. Gastrointestinal and hematologic side effects are rare with clopidogrel.

THIENOPYRIDINE RESISTANCE There is between-subject variability in the capacity of the thienopyridines to inhibit ADP-induced platelet aggregation. This variability reflects, at least in part, genetic polymorphisms in the CYP isoenzymes involved in the metabolic activation of the drugs. For example, subjects with the *CYP2C19*2* allele exhibit decreased responsiveness to clopidogrel, as do those with reduced CYP3A4 activity. These findings raise the possibility that pharmacogenomic profiling may help identify clopidogrel-resistant patients. Point-of-care devices that assess the extent of platelet inhibition may also help to identify these patients. It is currently unknown, however, whether patients with biochemical evidence of clopidogrel resistance have a poorer outcome and whether administration of higher doses of clopidogrel to these patients overcomes this problem.

DIPYRIDAMOLE

Dipyridamole is a relatively weak antiplatelet agent on its own, but an extended-release formulation of dipyridamole combined with low-dose aspirin, a preparation known as *Aggrenox*, is used for prevention of stroke in patients with transient ischemic attacks.

MECHANISM OF ACTION By inhibiting phosphodiesterase, dipyridamole blocks the breakdown of cAMP. Increased levels of cAMP reduce intracellular calcium and inhibit platelet activation. Dipyridamole also blocks the uptake of adenosine by platelets and other cells. This produces a further increase in local cAMP levels because the platelet adenosine A_2 receptor is coupled to adenylate cyclase (Fig. 112-4).

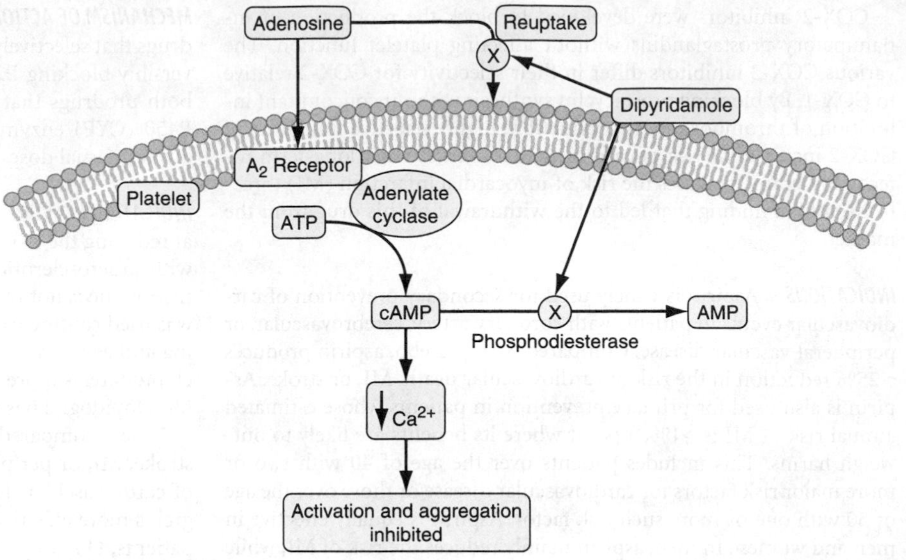

FIGURE 112-4 Mechanism of action of dipyridamole. Dipyridamole increases levels of cyclic AMP in platelets by (1) blocking the reuptake of adenosine, and (2) inhibiting phosphodiesterase-mediated cyclic AMP degradation. By promoting calcium uptake, cyclic AMP reduces intracellular levels of calcium. This, in turn, inhibits platelet activation and aggregation.

DOSING Aggrenox is given twice daily. Each capsule contains 200 mg of extended-release dipyridamole and 25 mg of aspirin.

SIDE EFFECTS Because dipyridamole has vasodilatory effects, it must be used with caution in patients with coronary artery disease. Gastrointestinal complaints, headache, facial flushing, dizziness, and hypotension can also occur. These symptoms often subside with continued use of the drug.

INDICATIONS Dipyridamole plus aspirin was compared with aspirin or dipyridamole alone, or with placebo, in patients with an ischemic stroke or transient ischemic attack. The combination reduced the risk of stroke by 22.1% compared with aspirin and by 24.4% compared with dipyridamole. A second trial compared dipyridamole plus aspirin with aspirin alone for secondary prevention in patients with ischemic stroke. Vascular death, stroke, or MI occurred in 13% of patients given combination therapy and in 16% of those treated with aspirin alone. Based on these data, Aggrenox is often used for stroke prevention. However, because of its vasodilatory effects and the paucity of data supporting the use of dipyridamole in patients with symptomatic coronary artery disease, Aggrenox should not be used for stroke prevention in such patients.

GPIIB/IIIA RECEPTOR ANTAGONISTS

As a class, parenteral GPIIb/IIIa receptor antagonists have an established niche in patients with acute coronary syndromes. The three agents in this class are abciximab, eptifibatide, and tirofiban.

MECHANISM OF ACTION A member of the integrin family of adhesion receptors, GPIIb/IIIa is found on the surface of platelets and megakaryocytes. With about 80,000 copies per platelet, GPIIb/IIIa is the most abundant receptor. Consisting of a non-covalently linked heterodimer, GPIIb/IIIa is inactive on resting platelets. When platelets are activated, inside-outside signal transduction pathways trigger a conformational activation of the receptor. Once activated, GPIIb/IIIa binds adhesive molecules, such as fibrinogen and, under high shear conditions, vWF. Binding is mediated by the Arg-Gly-Asp (RGD) sequence found on the α chains of fibrinogen and on vWF, and by the Lys-Gly-Asp (KGD) sequence located within a unique dodecapeptide domain on the γ chains of fibrinogen. Once bound, fibrinogen and/or vWF bridge adjacent platelets together to induce platelet aggregation.

Although abciximab, eptifibatide, and tirofiban all target the GPIIb/IIIa receptor, they are structurally and pharmacologically distinct (Table 112-1). Abciximab is a Fab fragment of a humanized murine monoclonal antibody directed against the activated form of GPIIb/IIIa. Abciximab binds to the activated receptor with high affinity and blocks the binding of adhesive molecules. In contrast to abciximab, eptifibatide and tirofiban are synthetic small molecules. Eptifibatide is a cyclic heptapeptide that binds GPIIb/IIIa because it incorporates the KGD motif, whereas tirofiban is a nonpeptidic tyrosine derivative that acts as a RGD mimetic. Abciximab has a long half-life and can be detected on the surface of platelets for up to 2 weeks. Eptifibatide and tirofiban have shorter half-lives.

In addition to targeting the GPIIb/IIIa receptor, abciximab also inhibits the closely related $\alpha_v\beta_3$ receptor, which binds vitronectin, and $\alpha_M\beta_2$, a leukocyte integrin. In contrast, eptifibatide and tirofiban are specific for GPIIb/IIIa. Inhibition of $\alpha_v\beta_3$ and $\alpha_M\beta_2$ may endow abciximab with anti-inflammatory and/or antiproliferative properties that extend beyond platelet inhibition.

DOSING All of the GPIIb/IIIa antagonists are given as an IV bolus followed by an infusion. Because they are cleared by the kidneys, the doses of eptifibatide and tirofiban must be reduced in patients with renal insufficiency.

SIDE EFFECTS In addition to bleeding, thrombocytopenia is the most serious complication. Thrombocytopenia is immune-mediated and is

TABLE 112-1 FEATURES OF GPIIb/IIIa ANTAGONISTS

Feature	Abciximab	Eptifibatide	Tirofiban
Description	Fab fragment of humanized mouse monoclonal antibody	Cyclical KGD-containing heptapeptide	Nonpeptidic RGD mimetic
Specific for GPIIb/IIIa	No	Yes	Yes
Plasma half-life	Short (min)	Long (2.5 h)	Long (2.0 h)
Platelet-bound half-life	Long (days)	Short (s)	Short (s)
Renal clearance	No	Yes	Yes

Note: KGD, Lys-Gly-Asp; RGD, Arg-Gly-Asp.

caused by antibodies directed against neoantigens on GPIIb/IIIa that are exposed upon antagonist binding. With abciximab, thrombocytopenia occurs in up to 5% of patients. Thrombocytopenia is severe in ~1% of these individuals. Thrombocytopenia is less common with the other two agents, occurring in ~1% of patients.

INDICATIONS Abciximab and eptifibatide are used in patients undergoing percutaneous coronary interventions, particularly those with acute MI. Tirofiban is used in high-risk patients with unstable angina. Eptifibatide also can be used for this indication.

NEW ANTIPLATELET AGENTS

Thienopyridines that produce more predictable suppression of ADP-induced platelet aggregation are under investigation. Direct-acting reversible $P2Y_{12}$ antagonists have also been developed. These agents can be given orally or parenterally and have a rapid onset of action because they are not prodrugs. Finally, orally active inhibitors of the type 1 protease activated receptor (PAR-1), the major thrombin receptor on platelets, are also entering clinical trials.

ANTICOAGULANTS

There are both parenteral and oral anticoagulants. Currently available parenteral anticoagulants include heparin, low-molecular-weight heparin (LMWH), and fondaparinux, a synthetic pentasaccharide. The only available oral anticoagulants are the vitamin K antagonists, of which warfarin is the agent most often used in North America.

PARENTERAL ANTICOAGULANTS

Heparin Heparin is a sulfated polysaccharide and is isolated from mammalian tissues rich in mast cells. Most commercial heparin is derived from porcine intestinal mucosa and is a polymer of alternating D-glucuronic acid and *N*-acetyl-D-glucosamine residues.

MECHANISM OF ACTION Heparin acts as an anticoagulant by activating antithrombin (previously known as antithrombin III) and accelerating the rate at which antithrombin inhibits clotting enzymes, particularly thrombin and factor Xa. Antithrombin, the obligatory plasma cofactor for heparin, is a member of the serine protease inhibitor (serpin) superfamily. Synthesized in the liver and circulating in plasma at a concentration of 2.6 ± 0.4 μ*M*, antithrombin acts as a suicide substrate for its target enzymes.

To activate antithrombin, heparin binds to the serpin via a unique pentasaccharide sequence that is found on one-third of the chains of commercial heparin (Fig. 112-5). The remainder of the heparin chains that lack this pentasaccharide sequence have little or no anticoagulant activity. Once bound to antithrombin, heparin induces a conformational change in the reactive center loop of antithrombin that renders it more readily accessible to its target proteases. This conformational change enhances the rate at which antithrombin inhibits factor Xa by at least two orders of magnitude but has little effect on the rate of thrombin inhibition by antithrombin. To catalyze thrombin inhibition, heparin serves as a template that binds antithrombin and thrombin simultaneously. Formation of this ternary complex brings the enzyme in close apposition to the inhibitor, thereby promoting the formation of a stable covalent thrombin-antithrombin complex.

Only pentasaccharide-containing heparin chains composed of at least 18 saccharide units (which correspond to a molecular weight of 5400) are of sufficient length to bridge thrombin and antithrombin together. With a mean molecular weight of 15,000, and a range of 5000–30,000, almost all of the chains of unfractionated heparin are long enough to effect this bridging function. Consequently, by definition, heparin has equal capacity to promote the inhibition of thrombin and factor Xa by antithrombin and is assigned an anti-factor Xa to anti-factor IIa (thrombin) ratio of 1:1.

Heparin causes the release of tissue factor pathway inhibitor (TFPI) from the endothelium. A factor Xa–dependent inhibitor of tissue factor–bound factor VIIa, TFPI may contribute to the antithrombotic activity of heparin. Longer heparin chains induce the release of more TFPI than shorter chains.

PHARMACOLOGY Heparin must be given parenterally. It is usually administered SC or by continuous IV infusion. When used for therapeutic purposes, the IV route is most often employed. If heparin is given SC for treatment of thrombosis, the dose of heparin must be high enough to overcome the limited bioavailability associated with this method of delivery.

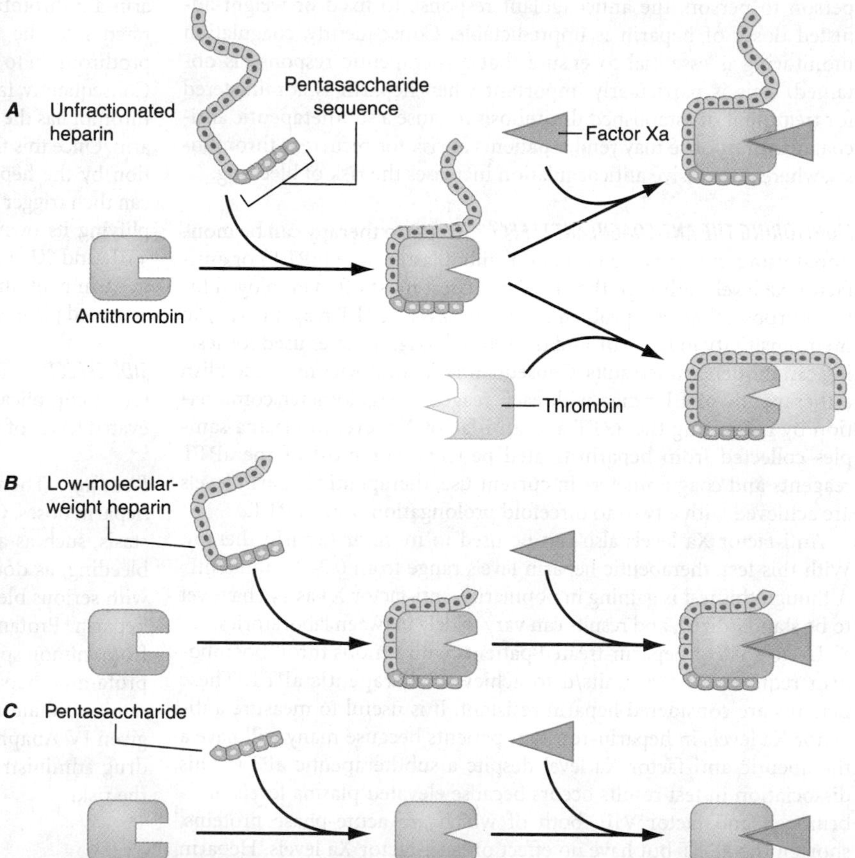

FIGURE 112-5 Mechanism of action of heparin, low-molecular-weight heparin (LMWH), and fondaparinux, a synthetic pentasaccharide. *A.* Heparin binds to antithrombin via its pentasaccharide sequence. This induces a conformational change in the reactive center loop of antithrombin that accelerates its interaction with factor Xa. To potentiate thrombin inhibition, heparin must simultaneously bind to antithrombin and thrombin. Only heparin chains composed of at least 18 saccharide units, which corresponds to a molecular weight of 5400, are of sufficient length to perform this bridging function. With a mean molecular weight of 15,000, all of the heparin chains are long enough to do this. ***B.*** LMWH has greater capacity to potentiate factor Xa inhibition by antithrombin than thrombin because, with a mean molecular weight of 4500–5000, at least half of the LMWH chains are too short to bridge antithrombin to thrombin. ***C.*** The pentasaccharide only accelerates factor Xa inhibition by antithrombin because the pentasaccharide is too short to bridge antithrombin to thrombin.

In the circulation, heparin binds to the endothelium and to plasma proteins other than antithrombin. Heparin binding to endothelial cells explains its dose-dependent clearance. At low doses, the half-life of heparin is short because it binds rapidly to the endothelium. With higher doses of heparin, the half-life is longer because heparin is cleared more slowly once the endothelium is saturated. Clearance is mainly extrarenal; heparin binds to macrophages, which internalize and depolymerize the long heparin chains and secrete shorter chains back into the circulation. Because of its dose-dependent clearance mechanism, the plasma half-life of heparin ranges from 30–60 min with bolus IV doses of 25 and 100 U/kg, respectively.

Once heparin enters the circulation, it binds to plasma proteins other than antithrombin, a phenomenon that reduces its anticoagulant activity. Some of the heparin-binding proteins found in plasma are acute-phase reactants whose levels are elevated in ill patients. Others, such as high-molecular-weight multimers of vWF, are released from activated platelets or endothelial cells. Activated platelets also release platelet factor 4 (PF4), a highly cationic protein that binds heparin with high affinity. The large amounts of PF4 found in the vicinity of platelet-rich arterial thrombi can neutralize the anticoagulant activity of heparin. This phenomenon may attenuate heparin's capacity to suppress thrombus growth.

Because the levels of heparin-binding proteins in plasma vary from person to person, the anticoagulant response to fixed or weight-adjusted doses of heparin is unpredictable. Consequently, coagulation monitoring is essential to ensure that a therapeutic response is obtained. This is particularly important when heparin is administered for treatment of established thrombosis because a subtherapeutic anticoagulant response may render patients at risk for recurrent thrombosis, whereas excessive anticoagulation increases the risk of bleeding.

MONITORING THE ANTICOAGULANT EFFECT Heparin therapy can be monitored using the activated partial thromboplastin time (aPTT) or anti-factor Xa level. Although the aPTT is the test most often employed for this purpose, there are problems with this assay. aPTT reagents vary in their sensitivity to heparin, and the type of coagulometer used for testing can influence the results. Consequently, laboratories must establish a therapeutic aPTT range with each reagent-coagulometer combination by measuring the aPTT and anti-factor Xa level in plasma samples collected from heparin-treated patients. For most of the aPTT reagents and coagulometers in current use, therapeutic heparin levels are achieved with a two- to threefold prolongation of the aPTT.

Anti-factor Xa levels also can be used to monitor heparin therapy. With this test, therapeutic heparin levels range from 0.3–0.7 units/mL. Although this test is gaining in popularity, anti-factor Xa assays have yet to be standardized, and results can vary widely between laboratories.

Up to 25% of heparin-treated patients with venous thromboembolism require >35,000 units/d to achieve a therapeutic aPTT. These patients are considered heparin resistant. It is useful to measure anti-factor Xa levels in heparin-resistant patients because many will have a therapeutic anti-factor Xa level despite a subtherapeutic aPTT. This dissociation in test results occurs because elevated plasma levels of fibrinogen and factor VIII, both of which are acute-phase proteins, shorten the aPTT but have no effect on anti-factor Xa levels. Heparin therapy in patients who exhibit this phenomenon is best monitored using anti-factor Xa levels instead of the aPTT. Patients with congenital or acquired antithrombin deficiency and those with elevated levels of heparin-binding proteins may also need high doses of heparin to achieve a therapeutic aPTT or anti-factor Xa level. If there is good correlation between the aPTT and the anti-factor Xa levels, either test can be used to monitor heparin therapy.

DOSING For prophylaxis, heparin is usually given in fixed doses of 5000 units SC two or three times daily. With these low doses, coagulation monitoring is unnecessary. In contrast, monitoring is essential when the drug is given in therapeutic doses. Fixed-dose or weight-based heparin nomograms are used to standardize heparin dosing and to shorten the time required to achieve a therapeutic anticoagulant response. At least two heparin nomograms have been validated in patients with venous thromboembolism and reduce the time required to achieve a therapeutic aPTT. Weight-adjusted heparin nomograms have also been evaluated in patients with acute coronary syndromes. After an IV heparin bolus of 5000 units or 70 units/kg, a heparin infusion rate of 12–15 units/kg per hour is usually administered. In contrast, weight-adjusted heparin nomograms for patients with venous thromboembolism use an initial bolus of 5000 units or 80 units/kg, followed by an infusion of 18 units/kg per hour. Thus, patients with venous thromboembolism appear to require higher doses of heparin to achieve a therapeutic aPTT than do patients with acute coronary syndromes. This may reflect differences in the thrombus burden. Heparin binds to fibrin, and the fibrin content of extensive deep vein thrombi is greater than that of small coronary thrombi.

LIMITATIONS Heparin has pharmacokinetic and biophysical limitations (Table 112-2). The pharmacokinetic limitations reflect heparin's propensity to bind in a pentasaccharide-independent fashion to cells and plasma proteins. Heparin binding to endothelial cells explains its dose-dependent clearance, whereas binding to plasma proteins results in a variable anticoagulant response and can lead to heparin resistance.

The biophysical limitations of heparin reflect the inability of the heparin-antithrombin complex to (1) inhibit factor Xa when it is incorporated into the prothrombinase complex, the complex that converts prothrombin to thrombin; and (2) to inhibit thrombin bound to fibrin. Consequently, factor Xa bound to activated platelets within platelet-rich thrombi has the potential to generate thrombin, even in the face of heparin. Once this thrombin binds to fibrin, it too is protected from inhibition by the heparin-antithrombin complex. Clot-associated thrombin can then trigger thrombus growth by locally activating platelets and amplifying its own generation through feedback activation of factors V, VIII, and XI. Further compounding the problem is the potential for heparin neutralization by the high concentrations of PF4 released from activated platelets within the platelet-rich thrombus.

SIDE EFFECTS The most common side effect of heparin is bleeding. Other complications include thrombocytopenia, osteoporosis, and elevated levels of transaminases.

Bleeding The risk of heparin-induced bleeding increases with higher heparin doses. Concomitant administration of drugs that affect hemostasis, such as antiplatelet or fibrinolytic agents, increases the risk of bleeding, as does recent surgery or trauma. Heparin-treated patients with serious bleeding can be given protamine sulfate to neutralize the heparin. Protamine sulfate, a mixture of basic polypeptides isolated from salmon sperm, binds heparin with high affinity, and the resultant protamine-heparin complexes are then cleared. Typically, 1 mg of protamine sulfate neutralizes 100 units of heparin. Protamine sulfate is given IV. Anaphylactoid reactions to protamine sulfate can occur, and drug administration by slow IV infusion is recommended to reduce the risk.

TABLE 112-2 PHARMACOKINETIC AND BIOPHYSICAL LIMITATIONS OF HEPARIN

Limitations	Mechanism
Poor bioavailability at low doses	Binds to proteins in subcutaneous depot site
Dose-dependent clearance	Binds to macrophages
Variable anticoagulant response	Binds to plasma proteins whose levels vary from patient to patient
Reduced activity in the vicinity of platelet-rich thrombi	Neutralized by platelet factor 4 released from activated platelets
Limited activity against factor Xa incorporated in the prothrombinase complex and thrombin bound to fibrin	Reduced capacity of heparin-antithrombin complex to inhibit factor Xa bound to activated platelets and thrombin bound to fibrin

Thrombocytopenia Heparin can cause thrombocytopenia. Heparin-induced thrombocytopenia (HIT) is an antibody-mediated process that is triggered by antibodies directed against neoantigens on PF4 that are exposed when heparin binds to this protein. These antibodies, which are usually of the IgG isotype, bind simultaneously to the heparin-PF4 complex and to platelet Fc receptors. Such binding activates the platelets and generates platelet microparticles. Circulating microparticles are prothrombotic because they express anionic phospholipids on their surface and can bind clotting factors and promote thrombin generation.

The clinical features of HIT are illustrated in Table 112-3. Typically, HIT occurs 5–14 days after initiation of heparin therapy, but it can manifest earlier if the patient has received heparin within the past 3 months. It is rare for the platelet count to fall below 100,000/μL in patients with HIT, and even a 50% decrease in the platelet count from the pretreatment value should raise the suspicion of HIT in those receiving heparin. HIT is more common in surgical patients than in medical patients and, like many autoimmune disorders, occurs more frequently in females than in males.

HIT can be associated with thrombosis, either arterial or venous. Venous thrombosis, which manifests as DVT and/or PE, is more common than arterial thrombosis. Arterial thrombosis can manifest as ischemic stroke or acute MI. Rarely, platelet-rich thrombi in the distal aorta or iliac arteries can cause critical limb ischemia.

The diagnosis of HIT is established using enzyme-linked assays to detect antibodies against heparin-PF4 complexes or with platelet activation assays. Enzyme-linked assays are sensitive but can be positive in the absence of any clinical evidence of HIT. The most specific diagnostic test is the serotonin release assay. This test is performed by quantifying serotonin release when washed platelets loaded with labeled serotonin are exposed to patient serum in the absence or presence of varying concentrations of heparin. If the patient serum contains the HIT antibody, heparin addition induces platelet activation and serotonin release.

Management of HIT is outlined in Table 112-4. Heparin should be stopped in patients with suspected or documented HIT, and an alternative anticoagulant should be administered to prevent or treat thrombosis. The agents most often used for this indication are parenteral direct thrombin inhibitors, such as lepirudin, argatroban, or bivalirudin, or factor Xa inhibitors, such as fondaparinux or danaparoid.

Patients with HIT, particularly those with associated thrombosis, often have evidence of increased thrombin generation that can lead to consumption of protein C. If these patients are given warfarin without a concomitant parenteral anticoagulant to inhibit thrombin or thrombin generation, the further decrease in protein C levels induced by the vitamin K antagonist can trigger skin necrosis. To avoid this problem, patients with HIT should be treated with a direct thrombin inhibitor or fondaparinux until the platelet count returns to normal levels. At this point, low-dose warfarin therapy can be introduced, and the thrombin inhibitor can be discontinued when the anticoagulant response to warfarin has been therapeutic for at least 2 days.

Osteoporosis Treatment with therapeutic doses of heparin for >1 month can cause a reduction in bone density. This complication has been reported in up to 30% of patients given long-term heparin therapy, and symptomatic vertebral fractures occur in 2–3% of these individuals.

TABLE 112-3 FEATURES OF HEPARIN-INDUCED THROMBOCYTOPENIA

Features	Details
Thrombocytopenia	Platelet count of ≤100,000/μL or a decrease in platelet count of ≥50%
Timing	Platelet count falls 5–10 days after starting heparin
Type of heparin	More common with unfractionated heparin than with low-molecular-weight heparin
Type of patient	More common in surgical patients than medical patients; more common in women than in men.
Thrombosis	Venous thrombosis more common than arterial thrombosis

TABLE 112-4 MANAGEMENT OF HEPARIN-INDUCED THROMBOCYTOPENIA

Stop all heparin
Give an alternative anticoagulant, such as lepirudin, argatroban, bivalirudin, danaparoid, or fondaparinux
Do not give platelet transfusions
Do not give warfarin until the platelet count returns to its baseline level; if warfarin is administered, give vitamin K to restore the INR to normal
Evaluate for thrombosis, particularly deep vein thrombosis

Heparin causes bone loss both by decreasing bone formation and by enhancing bone resorption. Thus, heparin affects the activity of both osteoblasts and osteoclasts.

Elevated Levels of Transaminases Therapeutic doses of heparin frequently cause modest elevation in the serum levels of hepatic transaminases, without a concomitant increase in the level of bilirubin. The levels of transaminases rapidly return to normal when the drug is stopped. The mechanism of this phenomenon is unknown.

Low-Molecular-Weight Heparin Consisting of smaller fragments of heparin, LMWH is prepared from unfractionated heparin by controlled enzymatic or chemical depolymerization. The mean molecular weight of LMWH is 5000, one-third the mean molecular weight of unfractionated heparin. LMWH has advantages over heparin (Table 112-5) and has replaced heparin for most indications.

MECHANISM OF ACTION Like heparin, LMWH exerts its anticoagulant activity by activating antithrombin. With a mean molecular weight of 5000, which corresponds to about 17 saccharide units, at least half of the pentasaccharide-containing chains of LMWH are too short to bridge thrombin to antithrombin (Fig. 112-5). However, these chains retain the capacity to accelerate factor Xa inhibition by antithrombin because this activity is largely the result of the conformational changes in antithrombin evoked by pentasaccharide binding. Consequently, LMWH catalyzes factor Xa inhibition by antithrombin more than thrombin inhibition. Depending on their unique molecular weight distributions, LMWH preparations have anti-factor Xa to anti-factor IIa ratios ranging from 2:1–4:1.

PHARMACOLOGY Although usually given SC, LMWH also can be administered IV if a rapid anticoagulant response is needed. LMWH has pharmacokinetic advantages over heparin. These advantages reflect the fact that shorter heparin chains bind less avidly to endothelial cells, macrophages, and heparin-binding plasma proteins. Reduced binding to endothelial cells and macrophages eliminates the rapid, dose-dependent, and saturable mechanism of clearance that is a characteristic of unfractionated heparin. Instead, the clearance of LMWH is dose-independent and its plasma half-life is longer. Based on measurement of anti-factor Xa levels, LMWH has a plasma half-life of ~4 h. LMWH is cleared almost exclusively by the kidneys, and the drug can accumulate in patients with renal insufficiency.

LMWH exhibits about 90% bioavailability after SC injection. Because LMWH binds less avidly to heparin-binding proteins in plasma

TABLE 112-5 ADVANTAGES OF LMWH[a] OVER HEPARIN

Advantage	Consequence
Better bioavailability and longer half-life after SC injection	Can be given SC once or twice daily for both prophylaxis and treatment
Dose-independent clearance	Simplified dosing
Predictable anticoagulant response	Coagulation monitoring is unnecessary in most patients
Lower risk of heparin-induced thrombocytopenia	Safer than heparin for short- or long-term administration
Lower risk of osteoporosis	Safer than heparin for extended administration

[a]LMWH, low-molecular-weight heparin.

than heparin, LMWH produces a more predictable dose response, and resistance to LMWH is rare. With a longer half-life and more predictable anticoagulant response, LMWH can be given SC once or twice daily without coagulation monitoring, even when the drug is given in treatment doses. These properties render LMWH more convenient than unfractionated heparin. Capitalizing on this feature, studies in patients with venous thromboembolism have shown that home treatment with LMWH is as effective and safe as in-hospital treatment with continuous IV infusions of heparin. Outpatient treatment with LMWH streamlines care, reduces health care costs, and increases patient satisfaction.

MONITORING In the majority of patients, LMWH does not require coagulation monitoring. If monitoring is necessary, anti-factor Xa levels must be measured because most LMWH preparations have little effect on the aPTT. Therapeutic anti-factor Xa levels with LMWH range from 0.5–1.2 units/mL when measured 3–4 h after drug administration. When LMWH is given in prophylactic doses, peak anti-factor Xa levels of 0.2–0.5 units/mL are desirable.

Indications for LMWH monitoring include renal insufficiency and obesity. LMWH monitoring in patients with a creatinine clearance of ≤50 mL/min is advisable to ensure that there is no drug accumulation. Although weight-adjusted LMWH dosing appears to produce therapeutic anti-factor Xa levels in patients who are overweight, this approach has not been extensively evaluated in those with morbid obesity. It may also be advisable to monitor the anticoagulant activity of LMWH during pregnancy because dose requirements can change, particularly in the third trimester. Monitoring should also be considered in high-risk settings, such as in patients with mechanical heart valves who are given LMWH for prevention of valve thrombosis, and when LMWH is used in treatment doses in infants or children.

DOSING The doses of LMWH recommended for prophylaxis or treatment vary depending on the LMWH preparation. For prophylaxis, once-daily SC doses of 4000–5000 units are often used, whereas doses of 2500–3000 units are given when the drug is administered twice daily. For treatment of venous thromboembolism, a dose of 150–200 units/kg is given if the drug is administered once daily. If a twice-daily regimen is employed, a dose of 100 units/kg is given. In patients with unstable angina, LMWH is given SC on a twice-daily basis at a dose of 100–120 units/kg.

SIDE EFFECTS The major complication of LMWH is bleeding. Meta-analyses suggest that the risk of major bleeding is lower with LMWH than with unfractionated heparin. HIT and osteoporosis are less common with LMWH than with unfractionated heparin.

Bleeding Like the situation with heparin, bleeding with LMWH is more common in patients receiving concomitant therapy with antiplatelet or fibrinolytic drugs. Recent surgery, trauma, or underlying hemostatic defects also increase the risk of bleeding with LMWH.

Although protamine sulfate can be used as an antidote for LMWH, protamine sulfate incompletely neutralizes the anticoagulant activity of LMWH because it only binds the longer chains of LMWH. Because longer chains are responsible for catalysis of thrombin inhibition by antithrombin, protamine sulfate completely reverses the anti-factor IIa activity of LMWH. In contrast, protamine sulfate only partially reverses the anti-factor Xa activity of LMWH because the shorter pentasaccharide-containing chains of LMWH do not bind to protamine sulfate. Consequently, patients at high risk for bleeding may be more safely treated with continuous IV unfractionated heparin than with SC LMWH.

Thrombocytopenia The risk of HIT is about fivefold lower with LMWH than with heparin. LMWH binds less avidly to platelets and causes less PF4 release. Furthermore, with lower affinity for PF4 than heparin, LMWH is less likely to induce the conformational changes in PF4 that trigger the formation of HIT antibodies.

LMWH should not be used to treat HIT patients because most HIT antibodies exhibit cross-reactivity with LMWH. This in vitro cross-reactivity is not simply a laboratory phenomenon because there are case reports of thrombosis when HIT patients are treated with LMWH.

Osteoporosis The risk of osteoporosis is lower with long-term LMWH than with heparin. For extended treatment, therefore, LMWH is a better choice than heparin because of the lower risk of osteoporosis and HIT.

Fondaparinux A synthetic analogue of the antithrombin-binding pentasaccharide sequence, fondaparinux differs from LMWH in several ways (Table 112-6). Fondaparinux is licensed for thromboprophylaxis in general surgical and high-risk orthopedic patients and as an alternative to heparin or LMWH for initial treatment of patients with established venous thromboembolism. It is likely that fondaparinux will also be approved for treatment of patients with acute coronary syndromes.

MECHANISM OF ACTION As a synthetic analogue of the antithrombin-binding pentasaccharide sequence found in heparin and LMWH, fondaparinux has a molecular weight of 1728. Fondaparinux binds only to antithrombin (Fig. 112-5) and is too short to bridge thrombin to antithrombin. Consequently, fondaparinux catalyzes factor Xa inhibition by antithrombin and does not enhance the rate of thrombin inhibition.

PHARMACOLOGY Fondaparinux exhibits complete bioavailability after SC injection. With no binding to endothelial cells or plasma proteins, the clearance of fondaparinux is dose independent and its plasma half-life is 17 h. The drug is given SC once daily. Because fondaparinux is cleared unchanged via the kidneys, it is contraindicated in patients with a creatinine clearance < 30 mL/min and should be used with caution in those with a creatinine clearance < 50 mL/min.

Fondaparinux produces a predictable anticoagulant response after administration in fixed doses because it does not bind to plasma proteins. The drug is given at a dose of 2.5 mg once daily for prevention of venous thromboembolism. For initial treatment of established venous thromboembolism, fondaparinux is given at a dose of 7.5 mg once daily. The dose can be reduced to 5 mg once daily for those weighing <50 kg and increased to 10 mg for those >100 kg. When given in these doses, fondaparinux is as effective as heparin or LMWH for initial treatment of patients with DVT or PE and produces similar rates of bleeding.

Fondaparinux is used at a dose of 2.5 mg once daily in patients with acute coronary syndromes. When this prophylactic dose of fondaparinux was compared with treatment doses of enoxaparin in patients with non-ST-segment elevation acute coronary syndromes, there was no difference in the rate of cardiovascular death, MI, or stroke at 9 days. However, the rate of major bleeding was 50% lower with fondaparinux than with enoxaparin, a difference that likely reflects the fact that the dose of fondaparinux was lower than that of enoxaparin. In acute coronary syndrome patients who require percutaneous coronary

TABLE 112-6 COMPARISON OF LMWH[a] AND FONDAPARINUX

Features	LMWH	Fondaparinux
Number of saccharide units	15–17	5
Catalysis of factor Xa inhibition	Yes	Yes
Catalysis of thrombin inhibition	Yes	No
Bioavailability after subcutaneous administration (%)	90	100
Plasma half-life (h)	4	17
Renal excretion	Yes	Yes
Induces release of tissue factor pathway inhibitor	Yes	No
Neutralized by protamine sulfate	Partially	No

[a]LMWH, low-molecular-weight heparin.

interventions, there is a risk of catheter thrombosis with fondaparinux, unless adjunctive heparin is given.

SIDE EFFECTS Fondaparinux does not cause HIT because it does not bind to PF4. In contrast to LMWH, there is no cross-reactivity of fondaparinux with HIT antibodies. Consequently, fondaparinux appears to be effective for treatment of HIT patients, although large clinical trials supporting its use are lacking.

The major side effect of fondaparinux is bleeding. There is no antidote for fondaparinux. Protamine sulfate has no effect on the anticoagulant activity of fondaparinux because it fails to bind to the drug. Recombinant activated factor VII reverses the anticoagulant effects of fondaparinux in volunteers, but it is unknown whether this agent will control fondaparinux-induced bleeding.

Parenteral Direct Thrombin Inhibitors Heparin and LMWH are indirect inhibitors of thrombin because their activity is mediated by antithrombin. In contrast, direct thrombin inhibitors do not require a plasma cofactor; instead, these agents bind directly to thrombin and block its interaction with its substrates. Approved parenteral direct thrombin inhibitors include lepirudin, argatroban, and bivalirudin (Table 112-7). Lepirudin and argatroban are licensed for treatment of patients with HIT, whereas bivalirudin is approved as an alternative to heparin in patients undergoing percutaneous coronary interventions, including those with HIT.

LEPIRUDIN A recombinant form of hirudin, lepirudin is a bivalent direct thrombin inhibitor that interacts with both the active site and exosite 1, the substrate binding site, on thrombin. For rapid anticoagulation, lepirudin is given by continuous IV infusion, but the drug can be given SC for thromboprophylaxis. Lepirudin has a plasma half-life of 60 min after IV infusion and is cleared by the kidneys. Consequently, lepirudin accumulates in patients with renal insufficiency. A high proportion of lepirudin-treated patients develop antibodies against the drug. Although these antibodies rarely cause problems, in a small subset of patients they can delay lepirudin clearance and enhance its anticoagulant activity. Serious bleeding has been reported in some of these patients.

Lepirudin is usually monitored using the aPTT, and the dose is adjusted to maintain an aPTT that is 1.5–2.5 times the control. The aPTT is not an ideal test for monitoring lepirudin therapy because the clotting time plateaus with higher drug concentrations. Although the ecarin clotting time provides a better index of lepirudin dose than the aPTT, the ecarin clotting time has yet to be standardized.

ARGATROBAN A univalent inhibitor that targets the active site of thrombin, argatroban is metabolized in the liver. Consequently, this drug must be used with caution in patients with hepatic insufficiency. Argatroban is not cleared via the kidneys, so this drug is safer than lepirudin for HIT patients with renal insufficiency.

Argatroban is administered by continuous IV infusion and has a plasma half-life of ~45 min. The aPTT is used to monitor its anticoagulant effect, and the dose is adjusted to achieve an aPTT 1.5–3 times the baseline value, but not to exceed 100 sec. Argatroban also prolongs the international normalized ratio (INR), a feature that can complicate the transitioning of patients to warfarin. This problem can be circumvented by using the levels of factor X to monitor warfarin in place of the INR. Alternatively, argatroban can be stopped for 2–3 h prior to INR determination.

BIVALIRUDIN A synthetic 20-amino-acid analogue of hirudin, bivalirudin is a divalent thrombin inhibitor. Thus, the N-terminal portion of bivalirudin interacts with the active site of thrombin, whereas its C-terminal tail binds to exosite 1, the substrate-binding domain on thrombin. Bivalirudin has a plasma half-life of 25 min, the shortest half-life of all the parenteral direct thrombin inhibitors. Bivalirudin is degraded by peptidases and is partially excreted via the kidneys. When given in high doses in the cardiac catheterization laboratory, the anticoagulant activity of bivalirudin is monitored using the activated clotting time. With lower doses, its activity can be assessed using the aPTT.

TABLE 112-7 COMPARISON OF THE PROPERTIES OF HIRUDIN, BIVALIRUDIN, AND ARGATROBAN

	Hirudin	Bivalirudin	Argatroban
Molecular mass	7000	1980	527
Site(s) of interaction with thrombin	Active site and exosite 1	Active site and exosite 1	Active site
Renal clearance	Yes	No	No
Hepatic metabolism	No	No	Yes
Plasma half-life (min)	60	25	45

Studies comparing bivalirudin with heparin suggest that bivalirudin produces less bleeding. This feature plus its short half-life make bivalirudin an attractive alternative to heparin in patients undergoing percutaneous coronary interventions. Bivalirudin also has been used successfully in HIT patients who require percutaneous coronary interventions.

ORAL ANTICOAGULANTS

Current oral anticoagulant practice dates back almost 60 years to when the vitamin K antagonists were discovered as a result of investigations into the cause of hemorrhagic disease in cattle. Characterized by a decrease in prothrombin levels, this disorder is caused by ingestion of hay containing spoiled sweet clover. Hydroxycoumarin, which was isolated from bacterial contaminants in the hay, interferes with vitamin K metabolism, thereby causing a syndrome similar to vitamin K deficiency.

Warfarin A water-soluble vitamin K antagonist initially developed as a rodenticide, warfarin is the coumarin derivative most often prescribed in North America. Like other vitamin K antagonists, warfarin interferes with the synthesis of the vitamin K–dependent clotting proteins, which include prothrombin (factor II) and factors VII, IX, and X. The synthesis of the vitamin K–dependent anticoagulant proteins, proteins C and S, is also reduced by vitamin K antagonists.

MECHANISM OF ACTION All of the vitamin K–dependent clotting factors possess glutamic acid residues at their N termini. A posttranslational modification adds a carboxyl group to the γ-carbon of these residues to generate γ-carboxyglutamic acid. This modification is essential for expression of the activity of these clotting factors because it permits their calcium-dependent binding to negatively charged phospholipid surfaces. The γ-carboxylation process is catalyzed by a vitamin K–dependent carboxylase. Thus, vitamin K from the diet is reduced to vitamin K hydroquinone by vitamin K reductase (Fig. 112-6). Vitamin K hydroquinone serves as a cofactor for the carboxylase enzyme, which in the presence of carbon dioxide replaces the hydrogen on the γ-carbon of glutamic acid residues with a carboxyl group. During this process, vitamin K hydroquinone is oxidized to vitamin K epoxide, which is then reduced to vitamin K by vitamin K epoxide reductase.

Warfarin inhibits vitamin K epoxide reductase (VKOR), thereby blocking the γ-carboxylation process. This results in the synthesis of vitamin K–dependent clotting proteins that are only partially γ-carboxylated. Warfarin acts as an anticoagulant because these partially γ-carboxylated proteins have reduced or absent biologic activity. The onset of action of warfarin is delayed until the newly synthesized clotting factors with reduced activity gradually replace their fully active counterparts.

The antithrombotic effect of warfarin depends on a reduction in the functional levels of factor X and prothrombin, clotting factors that have half-lives of 24 and 72 h, respectively. Because of the delay in achieving an antithrombotic effect, initial treatment with warfarin is supported by concomitant administration of a rapidly acting parenteral anticoagulant, such as heparin, LMWH, or fondaparinux, in patients with established thrombosis or at high risk for thrombosis.

PHARMACOLOGY Warfarin is a racemic mixture of R and S isomers. Warfarin is rapidly and almost completely absorbed from the gas-

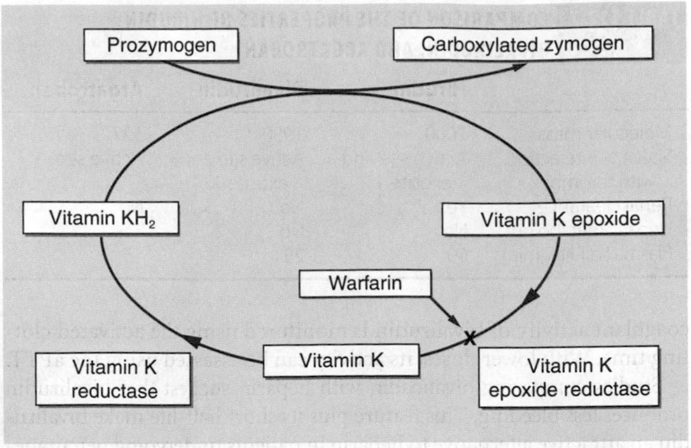

FIGURE 112-6 Mechanism of action of warfarin. By blocking vitamin K epoxide reductase, warfarin inhibits vitamin K–dependent γ-carboxylation of factors II, VII, IX, and X. Dietary vitamin K is reduced to vitamin K hydroquinone (vitamin KH_2) by vitamin K reductase. Vitamin KH_2 serves as a cofactor for a vitamin K–dependent carboxylase that catalyzes the γ-carboxylation process, thereby converting prozymogens to zymogens capable of binding calcium and interacting with anionic phospholipid surfaces. During this process, vitamin KH_2 is oxidized to vitamin K epoxide, which is then reduced to vitamin K by vitamin K epoxide reductase.

trointestinal tract. Levels of warfarin in the blood peak about 90 min after drug administration. Racemic warfarin has a plasma half-life of 36–42 h, and >97% of circulating warfarin is bound to albumin. It is only the small fraction of unbound warfarin that is biologically active.

Warfarin accumulates in the liver where the two isomers are metabolized via distinct pathways. Oxidative metabolism of the more active S-isomer is effected by CYP2C9. Two relatively common variants, *CYP2C9*2* and *CYP2C9*3*, have reduced activity. Patients with these variants require lower maintenance dose of warfarin. Polymorphisms in VKORC1 can also influence the anticoagulant response to warfarin. These findings have prompted the recommendation that patients starting on warfarin should be tested for these polymorphisms and that this information should be incorporated into their warfarin dosing algorithms.

In addition to genetic factors, the anticoagulant effect of warfarin is influenced by diet, drugs, and various disease states. Fluctuations in dietary vitamin K intake affect the activity of warfarin. A wide variety of drugs can alter absorption, clearance, or metabolism of warfarin. Because of the variability in the anticoagulant response to warfarin, coagulation monitoring is essential to ensure that a therapeutic response is obtained.

MONITORING Warfarin therapy is most often monitored using the prothrombin time, a test that is sensitive to reductions in the levels of prothrombin, factor VII, and factor X. The test is performed by adding thromboplastin, a reagent that contains tissue factor, phospholipid, and calcium, to citrated plasma and determining the time to clot formation. Thromboplastins vary in their sensitivity to reductions in the levels of the vitamin K–dependent clotting factors. Thus, less sensitive thromboplastins will trigger the administration of higher doses of warfarin to achieve a target prothrombin time. This is problematic because higher doses of warfarin increase the risk of bleeding.

The INR was developed to circumvent many of the problems associated with the prothrombin time. To calculate the INR, the patient's prothrombin time is divided by the mean normal prothrombin time, and this ratio is then multiplied by the international sensitivity index (ISI), an index of the sensitivity of the thromboplastin used for prothrombin time determination to reductions in the levels of the vitamin K–dependent clotting factors. Highly sensitive thromboplastins have an ISI of 1.0. Most current thromboplastins have ISI values that range from 1.0–1.4.

Although the INR has helped to standardize anticoagulant practice, problems persist. The precision of INR determination varies depending on reagent-coagulometer combinations. This leads to variability in the INR results. Also complicating INR determination is unreliable reporting of the ISI by thromboplastin manufacturers. Furthermore, every laboratory must establish the mean normal prothrombin time with each new batch of thromboplastin reagent. To accomplish this, the prothrombin time must be measured in fresh plasma samples from at least 20 healthy volunteers using the same coagulometer that is used for patient samples.

For most indications, warfarin is administered in doses that produce a target INR of 2.0–3.0. An exception is patients with mechanical heart valves, where a target INR of 2.5–3.5 is recommended. Studies in atrial fibrillation demonstrate an increased risk of cardioembolic stroke when the INR falls to <1.7 and an increase in bleeding with INR values >4.5. These findings highlight the fact that vitamin K antagonists have a narrow therapeutic window. In support of this concept, a study in patients receiving long-term warfarin therapy for unprovoked venous thromboembolism demonstrated a higher rate of recurrent venous thromboembolism with a target INR of 1.5–1.9 compared with a target INR of 2.0–3.0.

DOSING Warfarin is usually started at a dose of 5–10 mg. The dose is then titrated to achieve the desired target INR. Because of its delayed onset of action, patients with established thrombosis or those at high risk for thrombosis are given concomitant treatment with a rapidly acting parenteral anticoagulant, such as heparin, LMWH, or fondaparinux. Initial prolongation of the INR reflects reduction in the functional levels of factor VII. Consequently, concomitant treatment with the parenteral anticoagulant should be continued until the INR has been therapeutic for at least two consecutive days. A minimum 5-day course of parenteral anticoagulation is recommended to ensure that the levels of prothrombin have been reduced into the therapeutic range with warfarin.

Because warfarin has a narrow therapeutic window, frequent coagulation monitoring is essential to ensure that a therapeutic anticoagulant response is obtained. Even patients with stable warfarin dose requirements should have their INR determined every 2–3 weeks. More frequent monitoring is necessary when new medications are introduced because so many drugs enhance or reduce the anticoagulant effects of warfarin.

SIDE EFFECTS Like all anticoagulants, the major side effect of warfarin is bleeding. A rare complication is skin necrosis. Warfarin crosses the placenta and can cause fetal abnormalities. Consequently, warfarin should not be used during pregnancy.

Bleeding At least half of the bleeding complications with warfarin occur when the INR exceeds the therapeutic range. Bleeding complications may be mild, such as epistaxis or hematuria, or more severe, such as retroperitoneal or gastrointestinal bleeding. Life-threatening intracranial bleeding can also occur.

To minimize the risk of bleeding, the INR should be maintained in the therapeutic range. In asymptomatic patients whose INR is between 3.5 and 4.5, warfarin should be withheld until the INR returns to the therapeutic range. If the INR is >4.5, a therapeutic INR can be achieved more rapidly by administration of low doses of sublingual vitamin K. A vitamin K dose of 1 mg is usually adequate for patients with an INR between 4.9 and 9, whereas 2–3 mg can be used for those with an INR > 9. Higher doses of vitamin K can be administered if more rapid reversal of the INR is required or if the INR is excessively high.

Patients with serious bleeding need more aggressive treatment. These patients should be given 10 mg of vitamin K by slow IV infusion. Additional vitamin K should be given until the INR is in the normal range. Treatment with vitamin K should be supplemented with fresh-frozen plasma as a source of the vitamin K–dependent clotting proteins. For life-threatening bleeds, or if patients cannot tolerate the volume load, recombinant factor VIIa or prothrombin complex concentrates can be used.

Warfarin-treated patients who experience bleeding when their INR is in the therapeutic range require investigation into the cause of the bleeding. Those with gastrointestinal bleeding often have underlying peptic ulcer disease or a tumor. Similarly, investigation of hematuria or uterine bleeding in patients with a therapeutic INR may unmask a tumor of the genitourinary tract.

Skin Necrosis A rare complication of warfarin, skin necrosis usually is seen 2–5 days after initiation of therapy. Well-demarcated erythematous lesions form on the thighs, buttocks, breasts, or toes. Typically, the center of the lesion becomes progressively necrotic. Examination of skin biopsies taken from the border of these lesions reveals thrombi in the microvasculature.

Warfarin-induced skin necrosis is seen in patients with congenital or acquired deficiencies of protein C or protein S. Initiation of warfarin therapy in these patients produces a precipitous fall in plasma levels of proteins C or S, thereby eliminating this important anticoagulant pathway before warfarin exerts an antithrombotic effect through lowering of the functional levels of factor X and prothrombin. The resultant procoagulant state triggers thrombosis. Why the thrombosis is localized to the microvasculature of fatty tissues is unclear.

Treatment involves discontinuation of warfarin and reversal with vitamin K, if needed. An alternative anticoagulant, such as heparin or LMWH, should be given in patients with thrombosis. Protein C concentrates or recombinant activated protein C can be given to protein C–deficient patients to accelerate healing of the skin lesions; fresh-frozen plasma may be of value for those with protein S deficiency. Occasionally, skin grafting is necessary when there is extensive skin loss.

Because of the potential for skin necrosis, patients with known protein C or protein S deficiency require overlapping treatment with a parenteral anticoagulant when initiating warfarin therapy. Warfarin should be started in low doses in these patients, and the parenteral anticoagulant should be continued until the INR is therapeutic for at least two to three consecutive days.

Pregnancy Warfarin crosses the placenta and can cause fetal abnormalities or bleeding. The fetal abnormalities include a characteristic embryopathy, which consists of nasal hypoplasia and stippled epiphyses. The risk of embryopathy is highest if warfarin is given in the first trimester of pregnancy. Central nervous system abnormalities can also occur with exposure to coumarins at any time during pregnancy. Finally, maternal administration of warfarin produces an anticoagulant effect in the fetus that can cause bleeding. This is of particular concern at delivery when trauma to the head during passage through the birth canal can lead to intracranial bleeding. Because of these potential problems, warfarin is contraindicated in pregnancy, particularly in the first and third trimesters. Instead, heparin, LMWH, or fondaparinux can be given during pregnancy for prevention or treatment of thrombosis.

Warfarin does not pass into the breast milk. Consequently, warfarin can safely be given to nursing mothers.

Special Problems Patients with a lupus anticoagulant or those who need urgent or elective surgery present special challenges. Although observational studies suggested that patients with thrombosis complicating the antiphospholipid antibody syndrome required higher intensity warfarin regimens to prevent recurrent thromboembolic events, two randomized trials showed that targeting an INR of 2.0–3.0 is as effective as higher intensity treatment and produces less bleeding. Monitoring warfarin therapy can be problematic in patients with antiphospholipid antibody syndrome if the lupus anticoagulant prolongs the baseline INR.

If patients receiving long-term warfarin treatment require an elective invasive procedure, warfarin can be stopped 5 days before the procedure to allow the INR to return to normal levels. Those at high risk for recurrent thrombosis can be bridged with once- or twice-daily SC injections of LMWH when the INR falls to <2.0. The last dose of LMWH should be given 12–24 h before the procedure, depending on whether LMWH is administered twice or once daily. After the procedure, treatment with warfarin can be restarted.

New Oral Anticoagulants New oral anticoagulants that target thrombin or factor Xa are under development. These drugs have a rapid onset of action and have half-lives that permit once- or twice-daily administration. Designed to produce a predictable level of anticoagulation, these new oral agents can be given in fixed doses without coagulation monitoring. Therefore, these drugs will be more convenient to administer than warfarin. The results of ongoing phase II and III clinical trials will determine the role of these new oral anticoagulants in the prevention and treatment of thrombosis.

FIBRINOLYTIC DRUGS

ROLE OF FIBRINOLYTIC THERAPY

Fibrinolytic drugs can be used to degrade thrombi and are administered systemically or can be delivered via catheters directly into the substance of the thrombus. Systemic delivery is used for treatment of acute MI, acute ischemic stroke, and most cases of massive PE. The goal of therapy is to produce rapid thrombus dissolution, thereby restoring antegrade blood flow. In the coronary circulation, restoration of blood flow reduces morbidity and mortality by limiting myocardial damage, whereas in the cerebral circulation, rapid thrombus dissolution decreases the neuronal death and brain infarction that produce irreversible brain injury. For patients with massive PE, the goal of thrombolytic therapy is to restore pulmonary artery perfusion.

Peripheral arterial thrombi and thrombi in the proximal deep veins of the leg are most often treated using catheter-directed thrombolytic therapy. Catheters with multiple side holes can be utilized to enhance drug delivery. In some cases, intravascular devices that fragment and extract the thrombus are used to hasten treatment. These devices can be used alone or in conjunction with fibrinolytic drugs.

MECHANISM OF ACTION

Currently approved fibrinolytic agents include streptokinase; acylated plasminogen streptokinase activator complex (anistreplase); urokinase; recombinant tissue-type plasminogen activator (rt-PA), which is also known as alteplase or activase; and two recombinant derivatives of rt-PA, tenecteplase and reteplase. All of these agents act by converting the proenzyme, plasminogen, to plasmin, the active enzyme (Fig. 112-7). Plasmin then degrades the fibrin matrix of thrombi and produces soluble fibrin degradation products.

Endogenous fibrinolysis is regulated at two levels. Plasminogen activator inhibitors, particularly the type 1 form (PAI-1), prevent excessive plasminogen activation by regulating the activity of t-PA and urokinase-type plasminogen activator (u-PA). Once plasmin is generated, it is regulated by plasmin inhibitors, the most important of which is α_2-antiplasmin. The plasma concentration of plasminogen is twofold higher than that of α_2-antiplasmin. Consequently, with pharmacologic doses of plasmino-

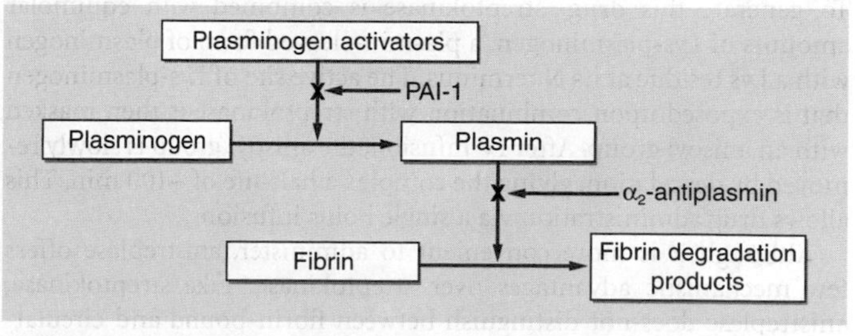

FIGURE 112-7 The fibrinolytic system and its regulation. Plasminogen activators convert plasminogen to plasmin. Plasmin then degrades fibrin into soluble fibrin degradation products. The system is regulated at two levels. Type 1 plasminogen activator inhibitor (PAI-1) regulates the plasminogen activators, whereas α_2-antiplasmin serves as the major inhibitor of plasmin.

gen activators, the concentration of plasmin that is generated can exceed that of α_2-antiplasmin. In addition to degrading fibrin, unregulated plasmin can also degrade fibrinogen and other clotting factors. This process, which is known as the *systemic lytic state*, reduces the hemostatic potential of the blood and increases the risk of bleeding.

The endogenous fibrinolytic system is geared to localize plasmin generation to the fibrin surface. Both plasminogen and t-PA bind to fibrin to form a ternary complex that promotes efficient plasminogen activation. In contrast to free plasmin, plasmin generated on the fibrin surface is relatively protected from inactivation by α_2-antiplasmin, a feature that promotes fibrin dissolution. Furthermore, C-terminal lysine residues exposed as plasmin degrades fibrin serve as binding sites for additional plasminogen and t-PA molecules. This creates a positive feedback that enhances plasmin generation. When used pharmacologically, the various plasminogen activators capitalize on these mechanisms to a lesser or greater extent.

Plasminogen activators that preferentially activate fibrin-bound plasminogen are considered fibrin-specific. In contrast, nonspecific plasminogen activators do not discriminate between fibrin-bound and circulating plasminogen. Activation of circulating plasminogen results in the generation of unopposed plasmin that can trigger the systemic lytic state. Alteplase and its derivatives are fibrin-specific plasminogen activators, whereas streptokinase, anistreplase, and urokinase are nonspecific agents.

STREPTOKINASE

Unlike other plasminogen activators, streptokinase is not an enzyme and does not directly convert plasminogen to plasmin. Instead, streptokinase forms a 1:1 stoichiometric complex with plasminogen. Formation of this complex induces a conformational change in plasminogen that exposes its active site (Fig. 112-8). This conformationally altered plasminogen then converts additional plasminogen molecules to plasmin.

Streptokinase has no affinity for fibrin, and the streptokinase-plasminogen complex activates both free and fibrin-bound plasminogen. Activation of circulating plasminogen generates sufficient amounts of plasmin to overwhelm α_2-antiplasmin. Unopposed plasmin not only degrades fibrin in the occlusive thrombus but also induces a systemic lytic state.

When given systemically to patients with acute MI, streptokinase reduces mortality. For this indication, the drug is usually given as an IV infusion of 1.5 million units over 30–60 min. Patients who receive streptokinase can develop antibodies against the drug, as can patients with prior streptococcal injection. These antibodies can reduce the effectiveness of streptokinase.

Allergic reactions occur in ~5% of patients treated with streptokinase. These may manifest as a rash, fever, chills, and rigors. Although anaphylactic reactions can occur, these are rare. Transient hypotension is common with streptokinase and has been attributed to plasmin-mediated release of bradykinin from kallikrein. The hypotension usually responds to leg elevation and administration of IV fluids and low-doses of vasopressors, such as dopamine or norepinephrine.

ANISTREPLASE

To generate this drug, streptokinase is combined with equimolar amounts of Lys-plasminogen, a plasmin-cleaved form of plasminogen with a Lys residue at its N terminus. The active site of Lys-plasminogen that is exposed upon combination with streptokinase is then masked with an anisoyl group. After IV infusion, the anisoyl group is slowly removed by deacylation, giving the complex a half-life of ~100 min. This allows drug administration via a single bolus infusion.

Although it is more convenient to administer, anistreplase offers few mechanistic advantages over streptokinase. Like streptokinase, anistreplase does not distinguish between fibrin-bound and circulating plasminogen. Consequently, it too produces a systemic lytic state. Likewise, allergic reactions and hypotension are just as frequent with anistreplase as they are with streptokinase.

When anistreplase was compared with alteplase in patients with acute MI, reperfusion was obtained more rapidly with alteplase than with anistreplase. Improved reperfusion was associated with a trend toward better clinical outcomes and reduced mortality with alteplase. These results and the high cost of anistreplase have dampened the enthusiasm for its use.

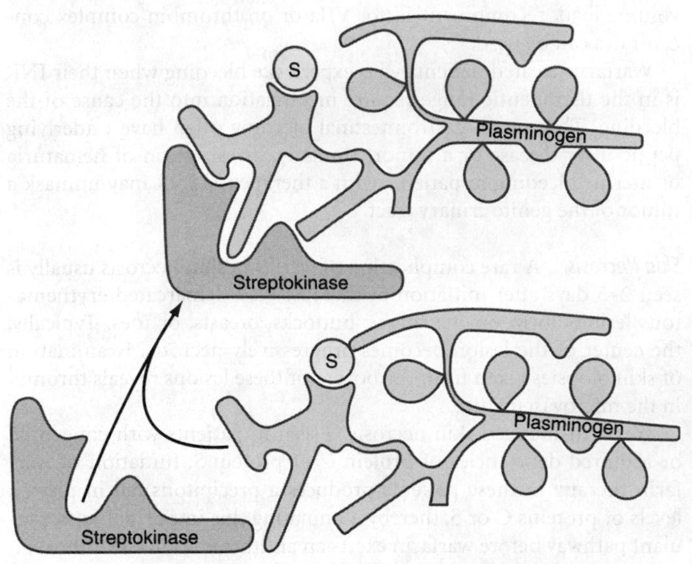

FIGURE 112-8 Mechanism of action of streptokinase. Streptokinase binds to plasminogen and induces a conformational change in plasminogen that exposes its active site. The streptokinase/plasmin(ogen) complex then serves as the activator of additional plasminogen molecules.

UROKINASE

Urokinase is a two-chain serine protease derived from cultured fetal kidney cells with a molecular weight of 34,000. Urokinase converts plasminogen to plasmin directly by cleaving the Arg560-Val561 bond. Unlike streptokinase, urokinase is not immunogenic and allergic reactions are rare. Urokinase produces a systemic lytic state because it does not discriminate between fibrin-bound and circulating plasminogen.

Despite many years of use, urokinase has never been systemically evaluated for coronary thrombolysis. Instead, urokinase is often employed for catheter-directed lysis of thrombi in the deep veins or the peripheral arteries. Because of production problems, the availability of urokinase is limited.

ALTEPLASE

A recombinant form of single-chain t-PA, alteplase has a molecular weight of 68,000. Alteplase is rapidly converted into its two-chain form by plasmin. Although single- and two-chain forms of t-PA have equivalent activity in the presence of fibrin, in its absence, single-chain t-PA has tenfold lower activity.

Alteplase consists of five discrete domains (Fig. 112-9); the N-terminal A chain of two-chain alteplase contains four of these domains. Residues 4 through 50 make up the finger domain, a region that resembles the finger domain of fibronectin; residues 50 through 87 are homologous with epidermal growth factor, whereas residues 92 through 173 and 180 through 261, which have homology to the kringle domains of plasminogen, are designated as the first and second kringle, respectively. The fifth alteplase domain is the protease domain; it is located on the C-terminal B chain of two-chain alteplase.

The interaction of alteplase with fibrin is mediated by the finger domain and, to a lesser extent, by the second kringle domain. The affinity of alteplase for fibrin is considerably higher than that for fibrinogen. Consequently, the catalytic efficiency of plasminogen activation by alteplase is two to three orders of magnitude higher in the presence of fibrin than in the presence of fibrinogen. This phenomenon helps to localize plasmin generation to the fibrin surface.

Although alteplase preferentially activates plasminogen in the presence of fibrin, alteplase is not as fibrin-selective as was first predicted. Its fibrin specificity is limited because like fibrin, (DD)E, the major soluble degradation product of cross-linked fibrin, binds alteplase and plasminogen with high affinity. Consequently, (DD)E is as potent as fibrin as a stimula-

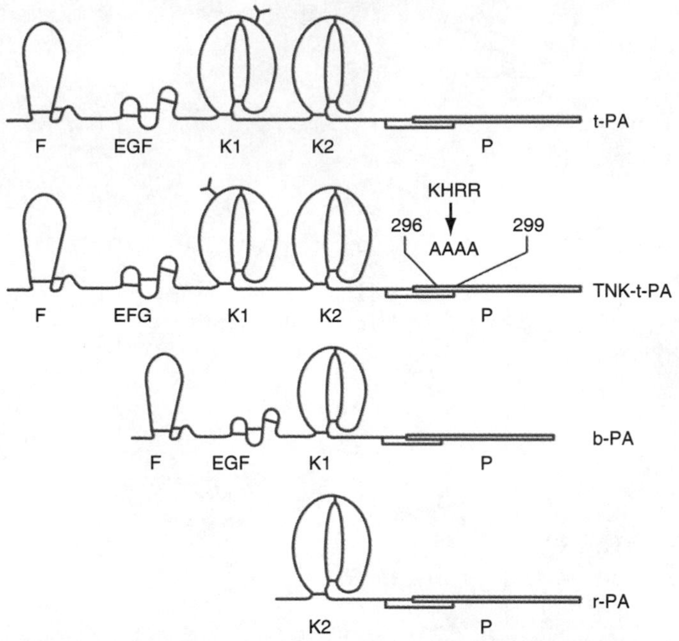

FIGURE 112-9 Domain structures of alteplase (t-PA), tenecteplase (TNK-t-PA), desmoteplase (b-PA), and reteplase (r-PA). The finger (F), epidermal growth factor (EGF), first and second kringles (K1 and K2, respectively), and protease (P) domains are illustrated. The glycosylation site (Y) on K1 has been repositioned in tenecteplase to endow it with a longer half-life. In addition, a tetra-alanine substitution in the protease domain renders tenecteplase resistant to PAI-1 inhibition. Desmoteplase differs from alteplase and tenecteplase in that it lacks a K2 domain. Reteplase is a truncated variant that lacks the F, EGF, and K1 domains.

tor of plasminogen activation by alteplase. Whereas plasmin generated on the fibrin surface results in thrombolysis, plasmin generated on the surface of circulating (DD)E degrades fibrinogen. Fibrinogenolysis results in the accumulation of fragment X, a high-molecular-weight clottable fibrinogen degradation product. Incorporation of fragment X into hemostatic plugs formed at sites of vascular injury renders them susceptible to lysis. This phenomenon may contribute to alteplase-induced bleeding.

A trial comparing alteplase with streptokinase for treatment of patients with acute MI demonstrated significantly lower mortality with alteplase than with streptokinase, although the absolute difference was small. The greatest benefit was seen in patients <75 years with anterior MI who presented <6 h after symptom onset.

For treatment of acute MI or acute ischemic stroke, alteplase is given as an IV infusion over 60–90 min. The total dose of alteplase usually ranges from 90–100 mg. Allergic reactions and hypotension are rare, and alteplase is not immunogenic.

TENECTEPLASE

Tenecteplase is a genetically engineered variant of t-PA and was designed to have a longer half-life than t-PA and to be resistant to inactivation by PAI-1. To prolong its half-life, a new glycosylation site was added to the first kringle domain (Fig. 112-9). Because addition of this extra carbohydrate side chain reduced fibrin affinity, the existing glycosylation site on the first kringle domain was removed. To render the molecule resistant to inhibition by PAI-1, a tetra-alanine substitution was introduced at residues 296–299 in the protease domain, the region responsible for the interaction of t-PA with PAI-1.

Tenecteplase is more fibrin-specific than t-PA. Although both agents bind to fibrin with similar affinity, the affinity of tenecteplase for (DD)E is significantly lower than that of t-PA. Consequently, (DD)E does not stimulate systemic plasminogen activation by tenecteplase to the same extent as t-PA. As a result, tenecteplase produces less fibrinogenolysis than t-PA.

For coronary thrombolysis, tenecteplase is given as a single IV bolus. In a large phase III trial that enrolled >16,000 patients, the 30-day mortality rate with single-bolus tenecteplase was similar to that with accelerated dose t-PA. Although rates of intracranial hemorrhage were also similar with both treatments, patients given tenecteplase had fewer noncerebral bleeds and a reduced need for blood transfusions than those treated with t-PA. The improved safety profile of tenecteplase likely reflects its enhanced fibrin specificity.

RETEPLASE

Reteplase is a recombinant t-PA derivative and is a single-chain variant that lacks the finger, epidermal growth factor, and first kringle domains (Fig. 112-9). This truncated derivative has a molecular weight of 39,000. Reteplase binds fibrin more weakly than t-PA because it lacks the finger domain. Because it is produced in *Escherichia coli*, reteplase is not glycosylated. This endows it with a plasma half-life longer than that of t-PA. Consequently, reteplase is given as two IV boluses, which are separated by 30 min. Clinical trials have demonstrated that reteplase is at least as effective as streptokinase for treatment of acute MI, but the agent is not superior to t-PA.

NEW FIBRINOLYTIC AGENTS

Several new drugs are under investigation. These include desmoteplase (Fig. 112-9), a recombinant form of the full-length plasminogen activator isolated from the saliva of the vampire bat, and alfimeprase, a truncated form of fibrolase, an enzyme isolated from the venom of the southern copperhead snake. Desmoteplase, which is more fibrin-specific than t-PA, is being investigated for the treatment of acute ischemic stroke. With a potential for enhanced safety, desmoteplase may extend the window for treatment beyond 3 h. An ongoing phase III clinical trial is exploring this possibility. Alfimeprase is a metalloproteinase that degrades fibrin in a plasmin-independent fashion. Because of its unique mechanism of action, it was hoped that alfimeprase would provide more rapid degradation of thrombi. However, a phase III trial investigating the use of this agent in patients with peripheral arterial occlusion has been halted, at least temporarily. Therefore, the future of this drug is uncertain.

CONCLUSIONS AND FUTURE DIRECTIONS

Arterial and venous thromboses reflect a complex interplay among the vessel wall, platelets, the coagulation system, and the fibrinolytic pathways. Activation of coagulation also triggers inflammatory pathways that may contribute to thrombogenesis. A better understanding of the biochemistry of blood coagulation and advances in structure-based drug design have identified new targets and resulted in the development of novel antithrombotic drugs. Well-designed clinical trials have provided detailed information on which drugs to use and when to use them. Despite these advances, however, thromboembolic disorders remain a major cause of morbidity and mortality. Therefore, the search for better targets and more potent antiplatelet, anticoagulant, and fibrinolytic drugs continues.

FURTHER READINGS

KAMALI F: Genetic influences on the response to warfarin. Curr Opin Hematol 13:357, 2006

KEELING D et al: The management of heparin-induced thrombocytopenia. Br J Haematol 133:259, 2006

LIM W et al: Management of antiphospholipid antibody syndrome: A systematic review. JAMA 295:1050, 2006

MEADOWS TA, BHATT DL: Clinical aspects of platelet inhibitors and thrombus formation. Circ Res 100:1261, 2007

PALARETI G et al: D-Dimer testing to determine the duration of anticoagulation therapy. N Engl J Med 355:1780, 2006

SEGAL JB et al: Management of venous thromboembolism: A systematic review for a practice guideline. Ann Intern Med 146:211, 2007

SIMIONI P, TORMENE D: Inherited thrombophilia and venous thromboembolism. Semin Thromb Hemost 32:700, 2006

YUSUF S, MEHTA SR: Comparison of fondaparinux and enoxaparin in acute coronary syndromes. N Engl J Med 354:1464, 2006

SECTION 1 BASIC CONSIDERATIONS IN INFECTIOUS DISEASES

113 Introduction to Infectious Diseases: Host–Pathogen Interactions

Lawrence C. Madoff, Dennis L. Kasper

Despite decades of dramatic progress in their treatment and prevention, infectious diseases remain a major cause of death and debility and are responsible for worsening the living conditions of many millions of people around the world. Infections frequently challenge the physician's diagnostic skill and must be considered in the differential diagnoses of syndromes affecting every organ system.

CHANGING EPIDEMIOLOGY OF INFECTIOUS DISEASES

With the advent of antimicrobial agents, some medical leaders believed that infectious diseases would soon be eliminated and become of historic interest only. Indeed, the hundreds of chemotherapeutic agents developed since World War II, most of which are potent and safe, include drugs effective not only against bacteria but also against viruses, fungi, and parasites. Nevertheless, we now realize that as we developed antimicrobial agents, microbes developed the ability to elude our best weapons and to counterattack with new survival strategies. Antibiotic resistance occurs at an alarming rate among all classes of mammalian pathogens. Pneumococci resistant to penicillin and enterococci resistant to vancomycin have become commonplace. Even *Staphylococcus aureus* strains resistant to vancomycin have appeared. Such pathogens present real clinical problems in managing infections that were easily treatable just a few years ago. Diseases once thought to have been nearly eradicated from the developed world—tuberculosis, cholera, and rheumatic fever, for example—have rebounded with renewed ferocity. Newly discovered and emerging infectious agents appear to have been brought into contact with humans by changes in the environment and by movements of human and animal populations. An example of the propensity for pathogens to escape from their usual niche is the alarming 1999 outbreak in New York of encephalitis due to West Nile virus, which had never previously been isolated in the Americas. In 2003, severe acute respiratory syndrome (SARS) was first recognized. This emerging clinical entity is caused by a novel coronavirus that may have jumped from an animal niche to become a significant human pathogen. By 2006, H5N1 avian influenza, having spread rapidly through poultry farms in Asia and having caused deaths in exposed humans, had reached Europe and Africa, heightening fears of a new influenza pandemic.

Many infectious agents have been discovered only in recent decades (Fig. 113-1). Ebola virus, human metapneumovirus, *Anaplasma phagocytophila* (the agent of human granulocytotropic ehrlichiosis), and retroviruses such as HIV humble us despite our deepening understanding of pathogenesis at the most basic molecular level. Even in developed countries, infectious diseases have made a resurgence. Between 1980 and 1996, mortality from infectious diseases in the United States increased by 64% to levels not seen since the 1940s.

The role of infectious agents in the etiology of diseases once believed to be noninfectious is increasingly recognized. For example, it is now widely accepted that *Helicobacter pylori* is the causative agent of peptic ulcer disease and perhaps of gastric malignancy. Human papillomavirus is likely to be the most important cause of invasive cervical cancer. Human herpesvirus type 8 is believed to be the cause of most cases of Kaposi's sarcoma. Epstein-Barr virus is a cause of certain lymphomas and may play a role in the genesis of Hodgkin's disease. The possibility certainly exists that other diseases of unknown cause, such as rheumatoid arthritis, sarcoidosis, or inflammatory bowel disease, have infectious etiologies. There is even evidence that atherosclerosis may have an infectious component. In contrast, there are data to suggest that decreased exposures to pathogens in childhood may be contributing to an increase in the observed rates of allergic diseases.

Medical advances against infectious diseases have been hindered by changes in patient populations. Immunocompromised hosts now constitute a significant proportion of the seriously infected population. Physicians immunosuppress their patients to prevent the rejection of transplants and to treat neoplastic and inflammatory diseases. Some infections, most notably that caused by HIV, immunocompromise the host in and of themselves. Lesser degrees of immunosuppression are associated with other infections, such as influenza and syphilis. Infectious agents that coexist peacefully with immunocompetent hosts wreak havoc in those who lack a complete immune system. AIDS has brought to prominence once-obscure organisms such as *Pneumocystis*, *Cryptosporidium parvum*, and *Mycobacterium avium*.

HOST FACTORS IN INFECTION

For any infectious process to occur, the pathogen and the host must first encounter each other. Factors such as geography, environment, and behavior thus influence the likelihood of infection. Although the initial encounter between a susceptible host and a virulent organism frequently results in disease, some organisms can be harbored in the host for years before disease becomes clinically evident. For a complete view, individual patients must be considered in the context of the population to which they belong. Infectious diseases do not often occur in isolation; rather, they spread through a group exposed from a point source (e.g., a contaminated water supply) or from one individual to another (e.g., via respiratory droplets). Thus, the clinician must be alert to infections prevalent in the community as a whole. A detailed history, including information on travel, behavioral factors, exposures to animals or potentially contaminated environments, and living and occupational conditions, must be elicited. For example, the likelihood of infection by *Plasmodium falciparum* can be significantly affected by altitude, climate, terrain, season, and even time of day. Antibiotic-resistant strains of *P. falciparum* are localized to specific geographic regions, and a seemingly minor alteration in a travel itinerary can dramatically influence the likelihood of acquiring chloroquine-resistant malaria. If such important details in the history are overlooked, inappropriate treatment may result in the death of the patient. Likewise, the chance of acquiring a sexually transmitted disease can be greatly affected by a relatively minor variation in sexual practices, such as the method used for contraception. Knowledge of the relationship between specific risk factors and disease allows the physician to influence a patient's health even before the development of infection by modification of these risk factors and—when a vaccine is available—by immunization.

Many specific host factors influence the likelihood of acquiring an infectious disease. Age, immunization history, prior illnesses, level of nutrition, pregnancy, coexisting illness, and perhaps emotional state all have some impact on the risk of infection after exposure to a potential pathogen. The importance of individual host defense mechanisms, either specific or nonspecific, becomes apparent in their absence, and

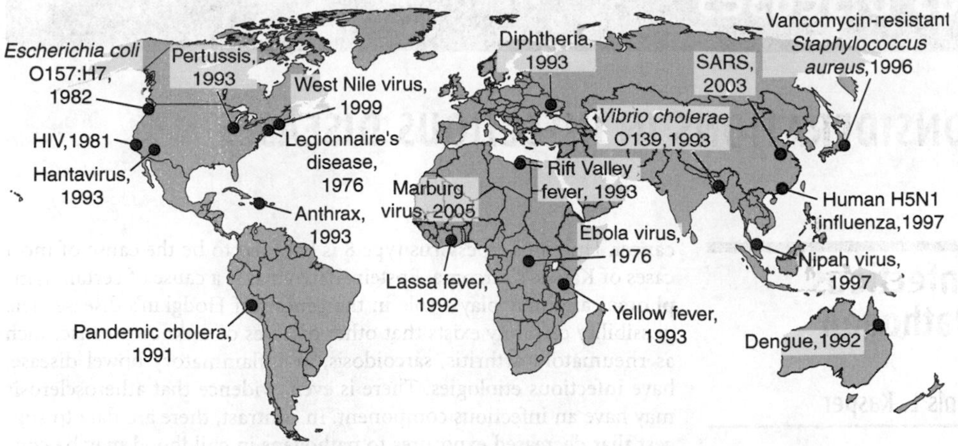

FIGURE 113-1 Map of the world showing examples of geographic locales where infectious diseases were noted to have emerged or resurged. *(Adapted from Addressing Emerging Infectious Disease Threats: A Prevention Strategy for the United States, Department of Health and Human Services, Centers for Disease Control and Prevention, 1994.)*

our understanding of these immune mechanisms is enhanced by studies of clinical syndromes developing in immunodeficient patients (Table 113-1). For example, the higher attack rate of meningococcal disease among people with deficiencies in specific complement proteins of the so-called membrane attack complex (see "Adaptive Immunity," below) than in the general population underscores the importance of an intact complement system in the prevention of meningococcal infection.

Medical care itself increases the patient's risk of acquiring an infection in several ways: (1) through contact with pathogens during hospitalization, (2) through breaching of the skin (with intravenous devices or surgical incisions) or mucosal surfaces (with endotracheal tubes or bladder catheters), (3) through introduction of foreign bodies, (4) through alteration of the natural flora with antibiotics, and (5) through treatment with immunosuppressive drugs.

Infection involves complicated interactions of microbe and host and inevitably affects both. In most cases, a pathogenic process consisting of several steps is required for the development of infections. Since the competent host has a complex series of barricades in place to prevent infection, the successful pathogen must use specific strategies at each of these steps. The specific strategies used by bacteria, viruses, and parasites (Chap. 114) have some remarkable conceptual similarities, but the strategic details are unique not only for each class of microorganism but also for individual species within a class.

THE IMMUNE RESPONSE

INNATE IMMUNITY

As they have co-evolved with microbes, higher organisms have developed mechanisms for recognizing and responding to microorganisms. Many of these mechanisms, referred to together as *innate immunity*, are evolutionarily ancient, having been conserved from insects to humans. In general, innate immune mechanisms exploit molecular patterns found specifically in pathogenic microorganisms. These "pathogen signatures" are recognized by host molecules that either directly interfere with the pathogen or initiate a response that does so. Innate immunity serves to protect the host without prior exposure to an infectious agent—i.e., before specific or adaptive immunity has had a chance to develop. Innate immunity also functions as a warning system that activates components of adaptive immunity early in the course of infection.

Toll-like receptors (TLRs) are instructive in illustrating how organisms are detected and send signals to the immune system. There are at least 11 TLRs, each specific to different biologic classes of molecules. For example, even minuscule amounts of lipopolysaccharide (LPS), a molecule found uniquely in gram-negative bacteria, are detected by LPS-binding protein, CD14, and TLR4 (see Fig. 114-3). The interaction of LPS with these components of the innate immune system prompts macrophages, via the transcriptional activator nuclear factor κB (NF-κB), to produce cytokines that lead to inflammation and enzymes that enhance the clearance of microbes. These initial responses serve not only to limit infection but also to initiate specific or adaptive immune responses.

ADAPTIVE IMMUNITY

Once in contact with the host immune system, the microorganism faces the host's tightly integrated cellular and humoral immune responses. Cellular immunity (Chap. 308), comprising T lymphocytes, macrophages, and natural killer cells, primarily recognizes and combats pathogens that proliferate intracellularly. Cellular immune mechanisms are important in immunity to all classes of infectious agents, including most viruses and many bacteria (e.g., *Mycoplasma*, *Chlamydophila*, *Listeria*, *Salmonella*, and *Mycobacterium*), parasites (e.g., *Trypanosoma*, *Toxoplasma*, and *Leishmania*), and fungi (e.g., *Histoplasma*, *Cryptococcus*, and *Coccidioides*). Usually, T lymphocytes are activated by macrophages and B lymphocytes, which present foreign antigens along with the host's own major histocompatibility complex antigen to the T cell receptor. Activated T cells may then act in several ways to fight infection. *Cytotoxic* T cells may directly attack and lyse host cells that express foreign antigens. *Helper* T cells stimulate the proliferation of B cells and the production of immunoglobulins. Antigen-presenting cells and T cells communicate with each other via a variety of signals, acting coordinately to instruct the immune system to respond in a specific fashion. T cells elaborate cytokines (e.g., interferon) that directly inhibit the growth of pathogens or stimulate killing by host macrophages and cytotoxic cells. Cytokines also augment the host's immunity by stimulating the inflammatory response (fever, the production of acute-phase serum components, and the proliferation of leukocytes). Cytokine stimulation does not always result in a favorable response in the host; septic shock (Chap. 265) and toxic shock syndrome (Chaps. 129 and 130) are among the conditions that are mediated by these inflammatory substances.

The immune system has also developed cells that specialize in controlling or downregulating immune responses. For example, T_{reg} cells, a subgroup of CD4+ T cells, prevent autoimmune responses by other T cells and are thought to be important in downregulating immune responses to foreign antigens. There appear to be both naturally occurring and acquired T_{reg} cells.

The reticuloendothelial system comprises monocyte-derived phagocytic cells that are located in the liver (Kupffer cells), lung (alveolar macrophages), spleen (macrophages and dendritic cells), kidney (mesangial cells), brain (microglia), and lymph nodes (macrophages and dendritic cells) and that clear circulating microorganisms. Although these tissue macrophages and polymorphonuclear leukocytes (PMNs) are capable of killing microorganisms without help, they function much more efficiently when pathogens are first *opsonized* (Greek, "to prepare for eating") by components of the complement system such as C3b and/or by antibodies.

Extracellular pathogens, including most encapsulated bacteria (those surrounded by a complex polysaccharide coat), are attacked by the humoral immune system, which includes antibodies, the complement cascade, and phagocytic cells. *Antibodies* are complex glycoproteins (also called *immunoglobulins*) that are produced by mature B lymphocytes, circulate in body fluids, and are secreted on mucosal surfaces. Antibodies specifically recognize and bind to foreign antigens. One of the most impressive features of the immune system is the ability to

TABLE 113-1 INFECTIONS ASSOCIATED WITH SELECTED DEFECTS IN IMMUNITY

Host Defect	Disease or Therapy Associated with Defect	Common Etiologic Agent of Infection
Nonspecific Immunity		
Impaired cough	Rib fracture, neuromuscular dysfunction	Bacteria causing pneumonia, aerobic and anaerobic oral flora
Loss of gastric acidity	Achlorhydria, histamine blockade	*Salmonella* spp., enteric pathogens
Loss of cutaneous integrity	Penetrating trauma, athlete's foot	*Staphylococcus* spp., *Streptococcus* spp.
	Burn	*Pseudomonas aeruginosa*
	Intravenous catheter	*Staphylococcus* spp., *Streptococcus* spp., gram-negative rods, coagulase-negative staphylococci
Implantable device	Heart valve	*Streptococcus* spp., coagulase-negative staphylococci, *Staphylococcus aureus*
	Artificial joint	*Staphylococcus* spp., *Streptococcus* spp., gram-negative rods
Loss of normal bacterial flora	Antibiotic use	*Clostridium difficile*, *Candida* spp.
Impaired clearance		
Poor drainage	Urinary tract infection	*Escherichia coli*
Abnormal secretions	Cystic fibrosis	Chronic pulmonary infection with *P. aeruginosa*
Inflammatory Response		
Neutropenia	Hematologic malignancy, cytotoxic chemotherapy, aplastic anemia, HIV infection	Gram-negative enteric bacilli, *Pseudomonas* spp., *Staphylococcus* spp., *Candida* spp.
Chemotaxis	Chédiak-Higashi syndrome, Job's syndrome, protein-calorie malnutrition	*S. aureus*, *Streptococcus pyogenes*, *Haemophilus influenzae*, gram-negative bacilli
	Leukocyte adhesion defects 1 and 2	Bacteria causing skin and systemic infections, gingivitis
Phagocytosis (cellular)	Systemic lupus erythematosus (SLE), chronic myelogenous leukemia, megaloblastic anemia	*Streptococcus pneumoniae*, *H. influenzae*
Splenectomy		*H. influenzae*, *S. pneumoniae*, other streptococci, *Capnocytophaga* spp., *Babesia microti*, *Salmonella* spp.
Microbicidal defect	Chronic granulomatous disease	Catalase-positive bacteria and fungi: staphylococci, *E. coli*, *Klebsiella* spp., *P. aeruginosa*, *Aspergillus* spp., *Nocardia* spp.
	Chédiak-Higashi syndrome	*S. aureus*, *S. pyogenes*
	Interferon γ receptor defect, interleukin 12 deficiency, interleukin 12 receptor defect	*Mycobacterium* spp., *Salmonella* spp.
Innate Immunity		
Complement system		
C3	Congenital liver disease, SLE, nephrotic syndrome	*S. aureus*, *S. pneumoniae*, *Pseudomonas* spp., *Proteus* spp.
C5	Congenital	*Neisseria* spp., gram-negative rods
C6, C7, C8	Congenital, SLE	*Neisseria meningitidis*, *N. gonorrhoeae*
Alternative pathway	Sickle cell disease	*S. pneumoniae*, *Salmonella* spp.
Toll-like receptor 4	Congenital	Gram-negative bacilli
Interleukin 1 receptor–associated kinase (IRAK) 4	Congenital	*S. pneumoniae*, *S. aureus*, other bacteria
Mannan-binding lectin	Congenital	*N. meningitidis*, other bacteria
Adaptive Immunity		
T lymphocyte deficiency/dysfunction	Thymic aplasia, thymic hypoplasia, Hodgkin's disease, sarcoidosis, lepromatous leprosy	*Listeria monocytogenes*, *Mycobacterium* spp., *Candida* spp., *Aspergillus* spp., *Cryptococcus neoformans*, herpes simplex virus, varicella-zoster virus
	AIDS	*Pneumocystis*, cytomegalovirus, herpes simplex virus, *Mycobacterium avium-intracellulare*, *C. neoformans*, *Candida* spp.
	Mucocutaneous candidiasis	*Candida* spp.
	Purine nucleoside phosphorylase deficiency	Fungi, viruses
B cell deficiency/dysfunction	Bruton's X-linked agammaglobulinemia	*S. pneumoniae*, other streptococci
	Agammaglobulinemia, chronic lymphocytic leukemia, multiple myeloma, dysglobulinemia	*H. influenzae*, *N. meningitidis*, *S. aureus*, *Klebsiella pneumoniae*, *E. coli*, *Giardia lamblia*, *Pneumocystis*, enteroviruses
	Selective IgM deficiency	*S. pneumoniae*, *H. influenzae*, *E. coli*
	Selective IgA deficiency	*G. lamblia*, hepatitis virus, *S. pneumoniae*, *H. influenzae*
Mixed T and B cell deficiency/dysfunction	Common variable hypogammaglobulinemia	*Pneumocystis*, cytomegalovirus, *S. pneumoniae*, *H. influenzae*, various other bacteria
	Ataxia-telangiectasia	*S. pneumoniae*, *H. influenzae*, *S. aureus*, rubella virus, *G. lamblia*
	Severe combined immunodeficiency	*S. aureus*, *S. pneumoniae*, *H. influenzae*, *Candida albicans*, *Pneumocystis*, varicella-zoster virus, rubella virus, cytomegalovirus
	Wiskott-Aldrich syndrome	Agents of infections associated with T and B cell abnormalities
	X-linked hyper-IgM syndrome	*Pneumocystis*, cytomegalovirus, *Cryptosporidium parvum*

generate an incredible diversity of antibodies capable of recognizing virtually every foreign antigen yet not reacting with self. In addition to being exquisitely specific for antigens, antibodies come in different structural and functional classes: IgG predominates in the circulation and persists for many years after exposure; IgM is the earliest specific antibody to appear in response to infection; secretory IgA is important in immunity at mucosal surfaces, while monomeric IgA appears in the serum; and IgE is important in allergic and parasitic diseases. Antibodies may directly impede the function of an invading organism, neutralize secreted toxins and enzymes, or facilitate the removal of the antigen (invading organism) by phagocytic cells. Immunoglobulins participate in cell-mediated immunity by promoting the antibody-dependent cellular cytotoxicity functions of certain T lymphocytes. Antibodies also promote the deposition of complement components on the surface of the invader.

The *complement* system (Chap. 308) consists of a group of serum proteins functioning as a cooperative, self-regulating cascade of enzymes that adhere to—and in some cases disrupt—the surface of invading organisms. Some of these surface-adherent proteins (e.g., C3b) can then act as opsonins for destruction of microbes by phagocytes. The later, "terminal" components (C7, C8, and C9) can directly kill some bacterial invaders (notably, many of the neisseriae) by forming a membrane attack complex and disrupting the integrity of the bacterial membrane, thus causing bacteriolysis. Other complement components, such as C5a, act as chemoattractants for PMNs (see below). Complement activation and deposition occur by either or both of two pathways: the *classic* pathway is activated primarily by immune complexes (i.e., antibody bound to antigen), and the *alternative* pathway is activated by microbial components, frequently in the absence of antibody. PMNs have receptors for both antibody and C3b, and antibody and complement function together to aid in the clearance of infectious agents.

PMNs, short-lived white blood cells that engulf and kill invading microbes, are first attracted to inflammatory sites by chemoattractants such as C5a, which is a product of complement activation at the site of infection. PMNs localize to the site of infection by adhering to cellular adhesion molecules expressed by endothelial cells. Endothelial cells express these receptors, called *selectins* (CD-62, ELAM-1), in response to inflammatory cytokines such as tumor necrosis factor α and interleukin 1. The binding of these selectin molecules to specific receptors on PMNs results in the adherence of the PMNs to the endothelium. Cytokine-mediated upregulation and expression of intercellular adhesion molecule 1 (ICAM 1) on endothelial cells then take place, and this latter receptor binds to β_2 integrins on PMNs, thereby facilitating diapedesis into the extravascular compartment. Once the PMNs are in the extravascular compartment, various molecules (e.g., arachidonic acids) further enhance the inflammatory process.

APPROACH TO THE PATIENT: Infectious Diseases

The clinical manifestations of infectious diseases at presentation are myriad, varying from fulminant life-threatening processes to brief and self-limited conditions to indolent chronic maladies. A careful history is essential and must include details on underlying chronic diseases, medications, occupation, and travel. Risk factors for exposure to certain types of pathogens may give important clues to diagnosis. A sexual history may reveal risks for exposure to HIV and other sexually transmitted pathogens. A history of contact with animals may suggest numerous diagnoses, including rabies, Q fever, bartonellosis, *Escherichia coli* O157 infection, or cryptococcosis. Blood transfusions have been linked to diseases ranging from viral hepatitis to malaria to prion disease. A history of exposure to insect vectors (coupled with information about the season and geographic site of exposure) may lead to consideration of such diseases as Rocky Mountain spotted fever, other rickettsial diseases, tularemia, Lyme disease, babesiosis, malaria, trypanosomiasis, and numerous arboviral infections. Ingestion of contaminated liquids or foods may lead to enteric infection with *Salmonella*, *Listeria*, *Campylobacter*, amebas, cryptosporidia, or helminths. Since infectious diseases may involve many organ systems, a careful review of systems may elicit important clues as to the disease process.

The physical examination must be thorough, and attention must be paid to seemingly minor details, such as a soft heart murmur that might indicate bacterial endocarditis or a retinal lesion that suggests disseminated candidiasis or cytomegalovirus (CMV) infection. Rashes are extremely important clues to infectious diagnoses and may be the only sign pointing to a specific etiology (Chap. 18; **Chap. e5**). Certain rashes are so specific as to be pathognomonic—e.g., the childhood exanthems (measles, rubella, varicella), the target lesion of erythema migrans (Lyme disease), ecthyma gangrenosum (*Pseudomonas aeruginosa*), and eschars (rickettsial diseases). Other rashes, although less specific, may be exceedingly important diagnostic indicators. The prompt recognition of the early scarlatiniform and later petechial rashes of meningococcal infection or of the subtle embolic lesions of disseminated fungal infections in immunosuppressed patients can hasten life-saving therapy. Fever (Chaps. 17, 18, and 19) is a common manifestation of infection and may be its sole apparent indication. Sometimes the pattern of fever or its temporally associated findings may help refine the differential diagnosis. For example, fever occurring every 48–72 h is suggestive of malaria (Chap. 203). The elevation in body temperature in fever (through resetting of the hypothalamic setpoint mediated by cytokines) must be distinguished from elevations in body temperature from other causes such as drug toxicity (Chap. 19) or heat stroke (Chap. 17).

LABORATORY INVESTIGATIONS

Laboratory studies must be carefully considered and directed toward establishing an etiologic diagnosis in the shortest possible time, at the lowest possible cost, and with the least possible discomfort to the patient. Since mucosal surfaces and the skin are colonized with many harmless or beneficial microorganisms, cultures must be performed in a manner that minimizes the likelihood of contamination with this normal flora while maximizing the yield of pathogens. A sputum sample is far more likely to be valuable when elicited with careful coaching by the clinician than when collected in a container simply left at the bedside with cursory instructions. Gram's stains of specimens should be interpreted carefully and the quality of the specimen assessed. The findings on Gram's staining should correspond to the results of culture; a discrepancy may suggest diagnostic possibilities such as infection due to fastidious or anaerobic bacteria.

The microbiology laboratory must be an ally in the diagnostic endeavor. Astute laboratory personnel will suggest optimal culture and transport conditions or alternative tests to facilitate diagnosis. If informed about specific potential pathogens, an alert laboratory staff will allow sufficient time for these organisms to become evident in culture, even when the organisms are present in small numbers or are slow-growing. The parasitology technician who is attuned to the specific diagnostic considerations relevant to a particular case may be able to detect the rare, otherwise-elusive egg or cyst in a stool specimen. In cases where a diagnosis appears difficult, serum should be stored during the early acute phase of the illness so that a diagnostic rise in titer of antibody to a specific pathogen can be detected later. Bacterial and fungal antigens can sometimes be detected in body fluids, even when cultures are negative or are rendered sterile by antibiotic therapy. Techniques such as the polymerase chain reaction allow the amplification of specific DNA sequences so that minute quantities of foreign nucleic acids can be recognized in host specimens.

℞ INFECTIOUS DISEASES

Optimal therapy for infectious diseases requires a broad knowledge of medicine and careful clinical judgment. Life-threatening infections such as bacterial meningitis or sepsis, viral encephalitis, or falciparum malaria must be treated immediately, often before a specific causative organism is identified. Antimicrobial agents must be chosen empirically and must be active against the range of potential infectious agents consistent with the clinical scenario. In contrast, good clinical judgment sometimes dictates withholding of antimicrobial drugs in a self-limited process or until a specific diagnosis is made. The dictum *primum non nocere* should be adhered to, and it should be remembered that all antimicrobial agents carry a risk (and a cost) to the patient. Direct toxicity may be encountered—e.g., ototoxicity due to aminoglycosides, lipodystrophy due to antiretroviral agents, and hepatotoxicity due to antituberculous agents such as isoniazid and rifampin. Allergic reactions are common and can be serious. Since superinfection sometimes follows the eradication of the normal flora and colonization by a resistant organism, one invariant principle is that infectious disease therapy should be directed toward as narrow a spectrum of infectious agents as possible. Treatment specific for the pathogen should result in as little perturbation as possible of the host's microflora. Indeed, future therapeutic agents may act not by killing a microbe, but by interfering with one or more of its virulence factors.

With few exceptions, abscesses require surgical or percutaneous drainage for cure. Foreign bodies, including medical devices, must generally be removed in order to eliminate an infection of the device or of the adjacent tissue. Other infections, such as necrotizing fasciitis, peritonitis due to a perforated organ, gas gangrene, and chronic osteomyelitis, require surgery as the primary means of cure; in these conditions, antibiotics play only an adjunctive role.

The role of immunomodulators in the management of infectious diseases has received increasing attention. Glucocorticoids have been shown to be of benefit in the adjunctive treatment of bacterial meningitis and in therapy for *Pneumocystis* pneumonia in patients with AIDS. The use of these agents in other infectious processes remains less clear and in some cases (in cerebral malaria, for example) is detrimental. Activated protein C (drotrecogin alfa, activated) is the first immunomodulatory agent widely available for the treatment of severe sepsis. Its usefulness demonstrates the interrelatedness of the clotting cascade and systemic immunity. Other agents that modulate the immune response include prostaglandin inhibitors, specific lymphokines, and tumor necrosis factor inhibitors. Specific antibody therapy plays a role in the treatment and prevention of many diseases. Specific immunoglobulins have long been known to prevent the development of symptomatic rabies and tetanus. More recently, CMV immune globulin has been recognized as important not only in preventing the transmission of the virus during organ transplantation but also in treating CMV pneumonia in bone marrow transplant recipients. There is a strong need for well-designed clinical trials to evaluate each new interventional modality.

PERSPECTIVE

The genetic simplicity of many infectious agents allows them to undergo rapid evolution and to develop selective advantages that result in constant variation in the clinical manifestations of infection. Moreover, changes in the environment and the host can predispose new populations to a particular infection. The dramatic march of West Nile virus from a single focus in New York City in 1999 to locations throughout the North American continent by the summer of 2002 caused widespread alarm, illustrating the fear that new plagues induce in the human psyche. The intentional release of deadly spores of *Bacillus anthracis* via the U.S. Postal Service awakened many from a sense of complacency regarding biologic weapons.

"The terror of the unknown is seldom better displayed than by the response of a population to the appearance of an epidemic, particularly when the epidemic strikes without apparent cause." Edward H. Kass made this statement in 1977 in reference to the newly discovered Legionnaire's disease, but it could apply equally to SARS, H5N1 (avian) influenza, or any other new and mysterious disease. The potential for infectious agents to emerge in novel and unexpected ways requires that physicians and public health officials be knowledgeable, vigilant, and open-minded in their approach to unexplained illness. The emergence of antimicrobial-resistant pathogens (e.g., enterococci that are resistant to all known antimicrobial agents and cause infections that are essentially untreatable) has led some to conclude that we are entering the "postantibiotic era." Others have held to the perception that infectious diseases no longer represent as serious a concern to world health as they once did. The progress that science, medicine, and society as a whole have made in combating these maladies is impressive, and it is ironic that, as we stand on the threshold of an understanding of the most basic biology of the microbe, infectious diseases are posing renewed problems. We are threatened by the appearance of new diseases such as SARS, hepatitis C, and Ebola virus infection and by the reemergence of old foes such as tuberculosis, cholera, plague, and *Streptococcus pyogenes* infection. True students of infectious diseases were perhaps less surprised than anyone else by these developments. Those who know pathogens are aware of their incredible adaptability and diversity. As ingenious and successful as therapeutic approaches may be, our ability to develop methods to counter infectious agents so far has not matched the myriad strategies employed by the sea of microbes that surrounds us. Their sheer numbers and the rate at which they can evolve are daunting. Moreover, environmental changes, rapid global travel, population movements, and medicine itself—through its use of antibiotics and immunosuppressive agents—all increase the impact of infectious diseases. Although new vaccines, new antibiotics, improved global communication, and new modalities for treating and preventing infection will be developed, pathogenic microbes will continue to develop new strategies of their own, presenting us with an unending and dynamic challenge.

FURTHER READINGS

ARMSTRONG G et al: Trends in infectious disease mortality in the United States during the 20th century. JAMA 281:61, 1999

BARTLETT JG: Update in infectious diseases. Ann Intern Med 144:49, 2006

BLASER MJ: Introduction to bacteria and bacterial diseases, in *Principles and Practice of Infectious Diseases*, 6th ed, GL Mandell et al (eds). Philadelphia, Elsevier, 2005, p 2319

HENDERSON DA: Countering the posteradication threat of smallpox and polio. Clin Infect Dis 34:79, 2002

HOFFMAN J et al: Phylogenetic perspectives in innate immunity. Science 284:1313, 1999

HUNG DT et al: Small-molecule inhibitor of *Vibrio cholerae* virulence and intestinal colonization. Science 310:670, 2005

PROMED-MAIL: The Program for Monitoring Emerging Diseases. *www.promedmail.org*

PUCK JM: Primary immunodeficiency diseases. JAMA 278:1835, 1997

TYLER KL, NATHANSON N: Pathogenesis of viral infections, in *Fields Virology*, DM Knipe, PM Howley (eds). Philadelphia, Lippincott Williams & Wilkins, 2001, pp 199–244

WEISS ST: Eat dirt—the hygiene hypothesis and allergic diseases. N Engl J Med 347:930, 2002

114 Molecular Mechanisms of Microbial Pathogenesis

Gerald B. Pier

Over the past three decades, molecular studies of the pathogenesis of microorganisms have yielded an explosion of information about the various microbial and host molecules that contribute to the processes of infection and disease. These processes can be classified into several stages: microbial encounter with and entry into the host; microbial growth after entry; avoidance of innate host defenses; tissue invasion and tropism; tissue damage; and transmission to new hosts. *Virulence* is the measure of an organism's capacity to cause disease and is a function of the pathogenic factors elaborated by microbes. These factors promote *colonization* (the simple presence of potentially pathogenic microbes in or on a host), *infection* (attachment and growth of pathogens and avoidance of host defenses), and *disease* (often, but not always, the result of activities of secreted toxins or toxic metabolites). In addition, the host's inflammatory response to infection greatly contributes to disease and its attendant clinical signs and symptoms.

MICROBIAL ENTRY AND ADHERENCE

ENTRY SITES

A microbial pathogen can potentially enter any part of a host organism. In general, the type of disease produced by a particular microbe is often a direct consequence of its route of entry into the body. The most common sites of entry are mucosal surfaces (the respiratory, alimentary, and urogenital tracts) and the skin. Ingestion, inhalation, and sexual contact are typical routes of microbial entry. Other portals of entry include sites of skin injury (cuts, bites, burns, trauma) along with injection via natural (i.e., vector-borne) or artificial (i.e., needlestick) routes. A few pathogens, such as *Schistosoma* spp., can penetrate unbroken skin. The conjunctiva can serve as an entry point for pathogens of the eye.

Microbial entry usually relies on the presence of specific microbial factors needed for persistence and growth in a tissue. Fecal-oral spread via the alimentary tract requires a biology consistent with survival in the varied environments of the gastrointestinal tract (including the low pH of the stomach and the high bile content of the intestine) as well as in contaminated food or water outside the host. Organisms that gain entry via the respiratory tract survive well in small moist droplets produced during sneezing and coughing. Pathogens that enter by venereal routes often survive best on the warm moist environment of the urogenital mucosa and have restricted host ranges (e.g., *Neisseria gonorrhoeae*, *Treponema pallidum*, and HIV).

The biology of microbes entering through the skin is highly varied. Some organisms can survive in a broad range of environments, such as the salivary glands or alimentary tracts of arthropod vectors, the mouths of larger animals, soil, and water. A complex biology allows protozoan parasites such as *Plasmodium*, *Leishmania*, and *Trypanosoma* spp. to undergo morphogenic changes that permit transmission to mammalian hosts during insect feeding for blood meals. Plasmodia are injected as infective sporozoites from the salivary glands during mosquito feeding. *Leishmania* parasites are regurgitated as promastigotes from the alimentary tract of sandflies and are injected by bite into a susceptible host. Trypanosomes are ingested from infected hosts by reduviid bugs, multiply in the insects' gastrointestinal tract, and are released in feces onto the host's skin during subsequent feedings. Most microbes that land directly on intact skin are destined to die, as survival on the skin or in hair follicles requires resistance to fatty acids, low pH, and other antimicrobial factors on skin. Once it is damaged (and particularly if it becomes necrotic), the skin can be a major portal of entry and growth for pathogens and elaboration of their toxic products. Burn wound infections and tetanus are clear examples. After animal bites, pathogens resident in the animal's saliva gain access to the victim's tissues through the damaged skin. Rabies is the paradigm for this pathogenic process; rabies virus grows in striated muscle cells at the site of inoculation.

MICROBIAL ADHERENCE

Once in or on a host, most microbes must anchor themselves to a tissue or tissue factor; the possible exceptions are organisms that directly enter the bloodstream and multiply there. Specific ligands or adhesins for host receptors constitute a major area of study in the field of microbial pathogenesis. Adhesins comprise a wide range of surface structures, not only anchoring the microbe to a tissue and promoting cellular entry where appropriate but also eliciting host responses critical to the pathogenic process (Table 114-1). Most microbes produce multiple adhesins specific for multiple host receptors. These adhesins are often redundant, are serologically variable, and act additively or synergistically with other microbial factors to promote microbial sticking to host tissues. In addition, some microbes adsorb host proteins onto their surface and utilize the natural host protein receptor for microbial binding and entry into target cells.

Viral Adhesins (See also Chap. 161) All viral pathogens must bind to host cells, enter them, and replicate within them. Viral coat proteins serve as the ligands for cellular entry, and more than one ligand-receptor interaction may be needed; for example, HIV uses its envelope glycoprotein (gp) 120 to enter host cells by binding to both CD4 and one of two receptors for chemokines (designated CCR5 and CXCR4). Similarly, the measles virus H glycoprotein binds to both CD46 and the membrane-organizing protein moesin on host cells. The gB and gC proteins on herpes simplex virus bind to heparan sulfate; this adherence is not essential for entry but rather serves to concentrate virions close to the cell surface. This step is followed by attachment to mammalian cells mediated by the viral gD protein. Herpes simplex virus can use a number of eukaryotic cell surface receptors for entry, including the herpesvirus entry mediator (related to the tumor necrosis factor receptor); members of the immunoglobulin superfamily; two proteins called nectin-1 and nectin-2; and modified heparan sulfate.

Bacterial Adhesins Among the microbial adhesins studied in greatest detail are bacterial pili and flagella (Fig. 114-1). *Pili* or *fimbriae* are commonly used by gram-negative and gram-positive bacteria for attachment to host cells and tissues. In electron micrographs, these hair-like projections (up to several hundred per cell) may be confined to one end of the organism (polar pili) or distributed more evenly over the surface. An individual cell may have pili with a variety of functions. Most pili are made up of a major pilin protein subunit (molecular weight, 17,000–30,000) that polymerizes to form the pilus. Many strains of *Escherichia coli* isolated from urinary tract infections express mannose-binding type 1 pili, whose binding to the integral membrane glycoproteins called *uroplakins* that coat the cells in the bladder epithelium is inhibited by D-mannose. Other strains produce the Pap (pyelonephritis-associated) or P pilus adhesin that mediates binding to

TABLE 114-1 EXAMPLES OF MICROBIAL LIGAND-RECEPTOR INTERACTIONS

Microorganism	Type of Microbial Ligand	Host Receptor
Viral Pathogens		
Influenza virus	Hemagglutinin	Sialic acid
Measles virus		
Vaccine strain	Hemagglutinin	CD46/moesin
Wild-type strains	Hemagglutinin	Signaling lymphocytic activation molecule (SLAM)
Human herpesvirus type 6	?	CD46
Herpes simplex virus	Glycoprotein C	Heparan sulfate
HIV	Surface glycoprotein	CD4 and chemokine receptors (CCR5 and CXCR4)
Epstein-Barr virus	Envelope protein	CD21 (=CR2)
Adenovirus	Fiber protein	Coxsackie-adenovirus receptor (CAR)
Coxsackievirus	Viral coat proteins	CAR and major histocompatibility class I antigens
Bacterial Pathogens		
Neisseria spp.	Pili	Membrane cofactor protein (CD46)
Pseudomonas aeruginosa	Pili and flagella	Asialo-GM1
	Lipopolysaccharide	Cystic fibrosis transmembrane conductance regulator (CFTR)
Escherichia coli	Pili	Ceramides/mannose and digalactosyl residues
Streptococcus pyogenes	Hyaluronic acid capsule	CD44
Yersinia spp.	Invasin/accessory invasin locus	β_1 Integrins
Bordetella pertussis	Filamentous hemagglutinin	CR3
Legionella pneumophila	Adsorbed C3bi	CR3
Mycobacterium tuberculosis	Adsorbed C3bi	CR3; DC-SIGN[a]
Fungal Pathogens		
Blastomyces dermatitidis	WI-1	Possibly matrix proteins and integrins
Candida albicans	Int1p	Extracellular matrix proteins
Protozoal Pathogens		
Plasmodium vivax	Merozoite form	Duffy Fy antigen
Plasmodium falciparum	Erythrocyte-binding protein 175 (EBA-175)	Glycophorin A
Entamoeba histolytica	Surface lectin	*N*-Acetylglucosamine

[a] A novel dendritic cell–specific C-type lectin.

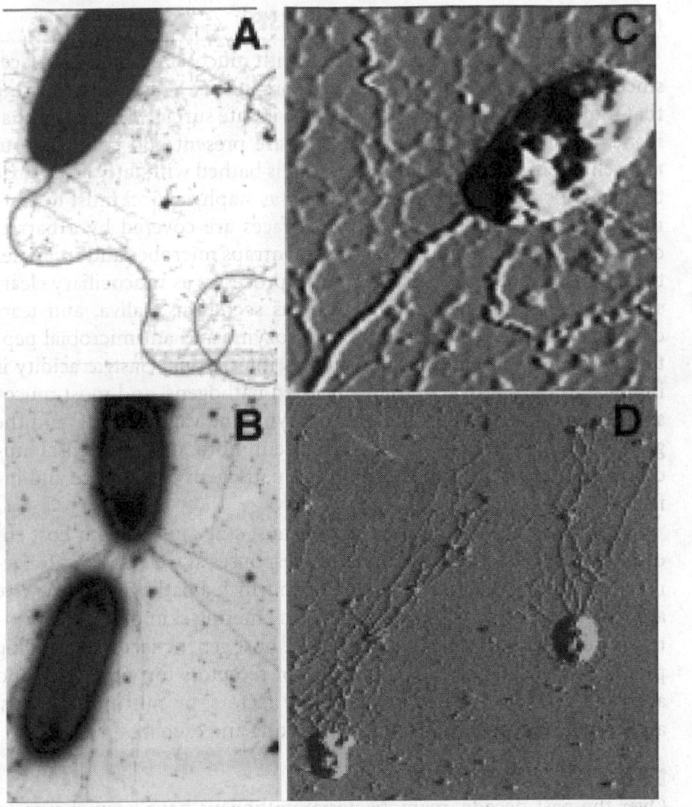

FIGURE 114-1 Bacterial surface structures. *A* and *B*. Traditional electron micrographic images of fixed cells of *Pseudomonas aeruginosa*. Flagella ***(A)*** and pili ***(B)*** projecting out from the bacterial poles can be seen. ***C*** and ***D***. Atomic force microscopic image of live *P. aeruginosa* freshly planted onto a smooth mica surface. This technology reveals the fine, three-dimensional detail of the bacterial surface structures. *(Images courtesy of Dr. Martin Lee and Dr. Milan Bajmoczi, Harvard Medical School; with permission.)*

digalactose (gal-gal) residues on globosides of the human P blood groups. Both of these types of pili have proteins located at the tips of the main pilus unit that are critical to the binding specificity of the whole pilus unit. It is interesting that, although immunization with the mannose-binding tip protein (FimH) of type 1 pili prevents experimental *E. coli* bladder infections in mice and monkeys, a trial of this vaccine in humans was not successful. *E. coli* cells causing diarrheal disease express pilus-like receptors for enterocytes on the small bowel, along with other receptors termed *colonization factors*.

The type IV pilus, a common type of pilus found in *Neisseria* spp., *Moraxella* spp., *Vibrio cholerae, Legionella pneumophila, Salmonella enterica* serovar *typhi*, enteropathogenic *E. coli*, and *Pseudomonas aeruginosa*, mediates adherence of these organisms to target surfaces. These pili tend to have a relatively conserved amino-terminal region and a more variable carboxyl-terminal region. For some species (e.g., *N. gonorrhoeae, Neisseria meningitidis*, and enteropathogenic *E. coli*), the pili are critical for attachment to mucosal epithelial cells. For others, such as *P. aeruginosa*, the pili only partially mediate the cells' adherence to host tissues. Whereas interference with this stage of colonization would appear to be an effective antibacterial strategy, attempts to develop pilus-based vaccines for human diseases have not been highly successful to date.

Flagella are long appendages attached at either one or both ends of the bacterial cell (polar flagella) or distributed over the entire cell surface (peritrichous flagella). Flagella, like pili, are composed of a polymerized or aggregated basic protein. In flagella, the protein subunits form a tight helical structure and vary serologically with the species. Spirochetes such as *T. pallidum* and *Borrelia burgdorferi* have axial filaments similar to flagella running down the long axis of the center of the cell, and they "swim" by rotation around these filaments. Some bacteria can glide over a surface in the absence of obvious motility structures.

Other bacterial structures involved in adherence to host tissues include specific staphylococcal and streptococcal proteins that bind to human extracellular matrix proteins such as fibrin, fibronectin, fibrinogen, laminin, and collagen. Fibronectin appears to be a commonly used receptor for various pathogens; a particular amino acid sequence in fibronectin (Arg-Gly-Asp, or RGD) is critical for bacterial binding. Binding of the highly conserved *Staphylococcus aureus* surface protein clumping factor A (ClfA) to fibrinogen has been implicated in many aspects of pathogenesis. The conserved outer-core portion of the lipopolysaccharide (LPS) of *P. aeruginosa* mediates binding to the cystic fibrosis transmembrane conductance regulator (CFTR) on airway epithelial cells—an event that appears to be critical for normal host resistance to infection. A number of bacterial pathogens, including coagulase-negative staphylococci, *S. aureus*, and uropathogenic *E. coli* as well as *Yersinia pestis, Y. pseudotuberculosis*, and *Y. enterocolitica*, express a surface polysaccharide composed of poly-*N*-acetylglucosamine. One function of this polysaccharide is to promote binding to materials used in catheters and other types of implanted devices; poly-*N*-acetylglucosamine may be a critical factor in the establishment of device-related infections by pathogens such as staphylococci and *E. coli*. High-powered imaging techniques (e.g., atomic force microscopy) have revealed that bacterial cells have a nonhomogeneous surface that is probably attributable to different concentrations of cell surface molecules, including microbial adhesins, at specific places on the cell surface (Fig114-1*D*).

Fungal Adhesins Several fungal adhesins have been described that mediate colonization of epithelial surfaces, particularly adherence to structures like fibronectin, laminin, and collagen. The product of the *Candida albicans INT1* gene, Int1p, bears similarity to mammalian integrins that bind to extracellular matrix proteins. Transformation of normally nonadherent *Saccharomyces cerevisiae* with this gene allows these yeast cells to adhere to human epithelial cells. The agglutinin-like sequence (ALS) adhesins are large cell-surface glycoproteins mediating adherence of pathogenic *Candida* to host tissues. These adhesins are expressed under certain environmental conditions (often associated with stress) and are crucial for pathogenesis of fungal infections.

For several fungal pathogens that initiate infections after inhalation, the inoculum is ingested by alveolar macrophages, in which the fungal cells transform to pathogenic phenotypes.

Eukaryotic Pathogen Adhesins Eukaryotic parasites use complicated surface glycoproteins as adhesins, some of which are lectins (proteins that bind to specific carbohydrates on host cells). For example, *Plasmodium vivax* binds (via Duffy-binding protein) to the Duffy blood group carbohydrate antigen Fy on erythrocytes. *Entamoeba histolytica* expresses two proteins that bind to the disaccharide galactose/*N*-acetylgalactosamine. Reports indicate that children with mucosal IgA antibody to one of these lectins are resistant to reinfection with virulent *E. histolytica*. A major surface glycoprotein (gp63) of *Leishmania* promastigotes is needed for these parasites to enter human macrophages—the principal target cell of infection. This glycoprotein promotes complement binding but inhibits complement lytic activity, allowing the parasite to use complement receptors for entry into macrophages; gp63 also binds to fibronectin receptors on macrophages. In addition, the pathogen can express a carbohydrate that mediates binding to host cells. Evidence suggests that, as part of hepatic granuloma formation, *Schistosoma mansoni* expresses a carbohydrate epitope related to the Lewis X blood group antigen that promotes adherence of helminthic eggs to vascular endothelial cells under inflammatory conditions.

HOST RECEPTORS

Host receptors are found both on target cells (e.g., epithelial cells lining mucosal surfaces) and within the mucous layer covering these cells. Microbial pathogens bind to a wide range of host receptors to establish infection (Table 114-1). Selective loss of host receptors for a pathogen may confer natural resistance to an otherwise susceptible population. For example, 70% of individuals in West Africa lack Fy antigens and are resistant to *P. vivax* infection. *S. enterica* serovar *typhi*, the etiologic agent of typhoid fever, uses CFTR to enter the gastrointestinal submucosa after being ingested. As homozygous mutations in *CFTR* are the cause of the life-shortening disease cystic fibrosis, heterozygote carriers (e.g., 4–5% of individuals of European ancestry) may have had a selective advantage due to decreased susceptibility to typhoid fever.

Numerous virus–target cell interactions have been described, and it is now clear that different viruses can use similar host-cell receptors for entry. The list of certain and likely host receptors for viral pathogens is long. Among the host membrane components that can serve as receptors for viruses are sialic acids, gangliosides, glycosaminoglycans, integrins and other members of the immunoglobulin superfamily, histocompatibility antigens, and regulators and receptors for complement components. A notable example of the effect of host receptors on the pathogenesis of infection comes from comparative binding studies of avian influenza A virus subtype H5N1 and influenza A virus strains expressing hemagglutinin subtype H1. The H1-subtype strains, which tend to be highly pathogenic and transmissible from human to human, bind to a receptor composed of two sugar molecules: sialic acid linked α-2-6 to galactose. This receptor is highly expressed in the airway epithelium. When virus is shed from this surface, its transmission via coughing and aerosol droplets is readily facilitated. In contrast, H5N1 avian influenza virus binds to sialic acid linked α-2-3 to galactose, and this receptor is highly expressed in pneumocytes in the alveoli. Alveolar infection is thought to underlie not only the high mortality rate associated with avian influenza but also the low human-to-human transmissibility rate of this strain, which is not readily transported to the airways (from which it could be expelled by coughing).

MICROBIAL GROWTH AFTER ENTRY

Once established on a mucosal or skin site, pathogenic microbes must replicate before causing full-blown infection and disease. Within cells, viral particles release their nucleic acids, which may be directly translated into viral proteins (positive-strand RNA viruses), transcribed from a negative strand of RNA into a complementary mRNA (negative-strand RNA viruses), or transcribed into a complementary strand of DNA (retroviruses); for DNA viruses, mRNA may be transcribed directly from viral DNA, either in the cell nucleus or in the cytoplasm. To grow, bacteria must acquire specific nutrients or synthesize them from precursors in host tissues. Many infectious processes are usually confined to specific epithelial surfaces—e.g., H1-subtype influenza to the respiratory mucosa, gonorrhea to the urogenital epithelium, and shigellosis to the gastrointestinal epithelium. While there are multiple reasons for this specificity, one important consideration is the ability of these pathogens to obtain from these specific environments the nutrients needed for growth and survival.

Temperature restrictions also play a role in limiting certain pathogens to specific tissues. Rhinoviruses, a cause of the common cold, grow best at 33°C and replicate in cooler nasal tissues but not as well in the lung. Leprosy lesions due to *Mycobacterium leprae* are found in and on relatively cool body sites. Fungal pathogens that infect the skin, hair follicles, and nails (dermatophyte infections) remain confined to the cooler, exterior, keratinous layer of the epithelium.

Many bacterial, fungal, and protozoal species grow in multicellular masses referred to as *biofilms*. These masses are biochemically and morphologically quite distinct from the free-living individual cells referred to as *planktonic cells*. Growth in biofilms leads to altered microbial metabolism, production of extracellular virulence factors, and decreased susceptibility to biocides, antimicrobial agents, and host defense molecules and cells. *P. aeruginosa* growing on the bronchial mucosa during chronic infection, staphylococci and other pathogens growing on implanted medical devices, and dental pathogens growing on tooth surfaces to form plaques represent several examples of microbial biofilm growth associated with human disease. Many other pathogens can form biofilms during in vitro growth, and it is increasingly accepted that this mode of growth contributes to microbial virulence and induction of disease.

AVOIDANCE OF INNATE HOST DEFENSES

As microbes have probably interacted with mucosal/epithelial surfaces since the emergence of multicellular organisms, it is not surprising that multicellular hosts have a variety of innate surface defense mechanisms that can sense when pathogens are present and contribute to their elimination. The skin is acidic and is bathed with fatty acids toxic to many microbes. Skin pathogens such as staphylococci must tolerate these adverse conditions. Mucosal surfaces are covered by a barrier composed of a thick mucous layer that entraps microbes and facilitates their transport out of the body by such processes as mucociliary clearance, coughing, and urination. Mucous secretions, saliva, and tears contain antibacterial factors such as lysozyme and antimicrobial peptides as well as antiviral factors such as interferons. Gastric acidity is inimical to the survival of many ingested pathogens, and most mucosal surfaces—particularly the nasopharynx, the vaginal tract, and the gastrointestinal tract—contain a resident flora of commensal microbes that interfere with the ability of pathogens to colonize and infect a host.

Pathogens that survive these factors must still contend with host endocytic, phagocytic, and inflammatory responses as well as with host genetic factors that determine the degree to which a pathogen can survive and grow. The growth of viral pathogens entering skin or mucosal epithelial cells can be limited by a variety of host genetic factors, including production of interferons, modulation of receptors for viral entry, and age- and hormone-related susceptibility factors; by nutritional status; and even by personal habits such as smoking and exercise.

ENCOUNTERS WITH EPITHELIAL CELLS

Over the past decade, many bacterial pathogens have been shown to enter epithelial cells (Fig. 114-2); the bacteria often use specialized surface structures that bind to receptors, with consequent internalization. However, the exact role and the importance of this process in infection and disease are not well defined for most of these pathogens. Bacterial entry into host epithelial cells is seen as a means for dissemination to adjacent or deeper tissues or as a route to sanctuary to avoid ingestion and killing by professional phagocytes. Epithelial cell entry appears, for instance, to be a critical aspect of dysentery induction by *Shigella*.

Curiously, the less virulent strains of many bacterial pathogens are more adept at entering epithelial cells than are more virulent strains; examples include pathogens that lack the surface polysaccharide capsule needed to cause serious disease. Thus, for *Haemophilus influenzae*, *Streptococcus pneumoniae*, *Streptococcus agalactiae* (group B *Streptococcus*), and *Streptococcus pyogenes*, isogenic mutants or variants lacking capsules enter epithelial cells better than the wild-type, encapsulated parental forms that cause disseminated disease. These observations have led to the proposal that epithelial cell entry may be primarily a manifestation of host defense, resulting in bacterial clearance by both shedding of epithelial cells containing internalized bacteria and initiation of a protective and nonpathogenic inflammatory response. However, a possible consequence of this process could be the opening of a hole in the epithelium, potentially allowing uningested organisms to enter the submucosa. This scenario has been documented in murine *S. enterica* serovar *typhimurium* infections and in experimental bladder infections with uropathogenic *E. coli*. In the latter system, bacterial pilus–mediated attachment to uroplakins induces exfoliation of the cells with attached bacteria. Subsequently, infection is produced by residual bacterial cells that invade the superficial bladder epithelium, where they can grow intracellularly into biofilm-like masses encased in an extracellular polysaccharide-rich matrix and surrounded by uroplakin. This mode of growth produces structures that have been referred to as *bacterial pods*. At low bacterial inocula, epithelial cell ingestion and subclinical inflammation are probably efficient means to eliminate pathogens; in contrast, at higher inocula, a proportion of surviving bacterial cells enter host tissue through the damaged mucosal surface and multiply, producing disease. Alternatively, failure of the appropriate epithelial cell response to a pathogen may allow the organism to survive on a mucosal surface where, if it avoids other host defenses, it can grow and cause a local infection. Along these lines, as

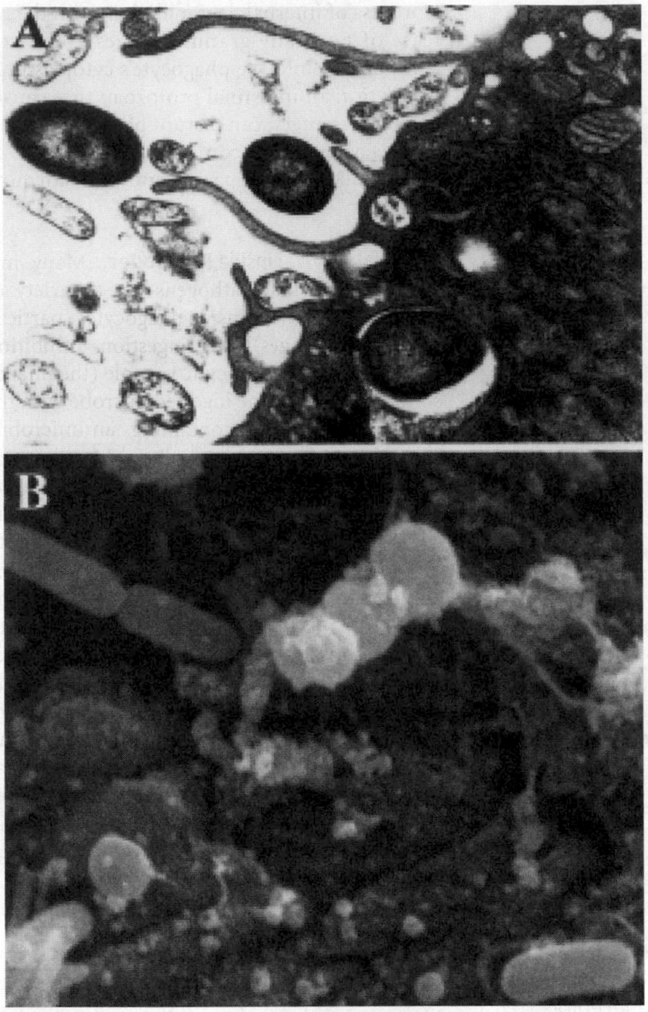

FIGURE 114-2 Entry of bacteria into epithelial cells. ***A.*** Internalization of *P. aeruginosa* by cultured human airway epithelial cells expressing wild-type cystic fibrosis transmembrane conductance regulator (CFTR), the cell receptor for bacterial ingestion. ***B.*** Entry of *P. aeruginosa* into murine tracheal epithelial cells after infection by the intranasal route.

noted above, *P. aeruginosa* is taken into epithelial cells by CFTR, a protein missing or nonfunctional in most severe cases of cystic fibrosis. The major clinical consequence is chronic airway-surface infection with *P. aeruginosa* in 80–90% of patients with cystic fibrosis. The failure of airway epithelial cells to ingest and promote the removal of *P. aeruginosa* via a properly regulated inflammatory response has been proposed as a key component of the hypersusceptibility of these patients to chronic airway infection with this organism.

ENCOUNTERS WITH PHAGOCYTES

Phagocytosis and Inflammation Phagocytosis of microbes is a major innate host defense that limits the growth and spread of pathogens. Phagocytes appear rapidly at sites of infection in conjunction with the initiation of inflammation. Ingestion of microbes by both tissue-fixed macrophages and migrating phagocytes probably accounts for the limited ability of most microbial agents to cause disease. A family of related molecules called *collectins*, *soluble defense collagens*, or *pattern-recognition molecules* are found in blood (mannose-binding lectins), in lung (surfactant proteins A and D), and most likely in other tissues as well and bind to carbohydrates on microbial surfaces to promote phagocyte clearance. Bacterial pathogens seem to be ingested principally by polymorphonuclear neutrophils (PMNs), while eosinophils are frequently found at sites of infection with protozoan or multicellular parasites. Successful pathogens, by definition, must avoid being cleared by professional phagocytes. One of several antiphagocytic strategies employed by bacteria and by the fungal pathogen *Cryptococcus neoformans* is to elaborate large-molecular-weight surface polysaccharide antigens, often in the form of a capsule that coats the cell surface. Most pathogenic bacteria produce such antiphagocytic capsules. On occasion, proteins or polypeptides form capsule-like coatings on organisms such as *Bacillus anthracis*.

As activation of local phagocytes in tissues is a key step in initiating inflammation and migration of additional phagocytes into infected sites, much attention has been paid to microbial factors that initiate inflammation. Encounters with phagocytes are governed largely by the structure of the microbial constituents that elicit inflammation, and detailed knowledge of these structures for bacterial pathogens has contributed greatly to our understanding of molecular mechanisms of microbial pathogenesis (Fig. 114-3). One of the best-studied systems involves the interaction of LPS from gram-negative bacteria and the glycosylphosphatidylinositol (GPI)-anchored membrane protein CD14 found on the surface of professional phagocytes, including migrating and tissue-fixed macrophages and PMNs. A soluble form of CD14 is also found in plasma and on mucosal surfaces. A plasma protein, LPS-binding protein (LBP), transfers LPS to membrane-bound CD14 on myeloid cells and promotes binding of LPS to soluble CD14. Soluble CD14/LPS/LBP complexes bind to many cell types and may be internalized to initiate cellular responses to microbial pathogens. It has been shown that peptidoglycan and lipoteichoic acid from gram-positive bacteria and cell-surface products of mycobacteria and spirochetes can interact with CD14 (Fig. 114-3). Additional molecules, such as MD-2, also participate in the recognition of bacterial activators of inflammation.

GPI-anchored receptors do not have intracellular signaling domains. Instead, the mammalian Toll-like receptors (TLRs) transduce signals for cellular activation due to LPS binding. It has recently been shown that binding of microbial factors to TLRs to activate signal transduction occurs not on the cell surface, but rather in the phagosome of cells that have internalized the microbe. This interaction is probably due to the release of the microbial surface factor from the cell in the environment of the phagosome, where the liberated factor can bind to its cognate TLRs. TLRs initiate cellular activation through a series of signal-transducing molecules (Fig. 114-3) that lead to nuclear translocation of the transcription factor nuclear factor κB (NF-κB), a master-switch for production of important inflammatory cytokines such as tumor necrosis factor α (TNF-α) and interleukin (IL) 1.

Inflammation can be initiated not only with LPS and peptidoglycan but also with viral particles and other microbial products such as polysaccharides, enzymes, and toxins. Bacterial flagella activate inflammation by binding of a conserved sequence to TLR5. Some pathogens, including *Campylobacter jejuni*, *Helicobacter pylori*, and *Bartonella bacilliformis*, make flagella that lack this sequence and thus do not bind to TLR5. The result is a lack of efficient host response to infection. Bacteria also produce a high proportion of DNA molecules with unmethylated CpG residues that activate inflammation through TLR9. TLR3 recognizes double-strand RNA, a pattern-recognition molecule produced by many viruses during their replicative cycle. TLR1 and TLR6 associate with TLR2 to promote recognition of acylated microbial proteins and peptides.

The myeloid differentiation factor 88 (MyD88) molecule is a generalized adaptor protein that binds to the cytoplasmic domains of all known TLRs and also to receptors that are part of the IL-1 receptor (IL-1Rc) family. Numerous studies have shown that MyD88-mediated transduction of signals from TLRs and IL-1Rc is critical for innate resistance to infection. Mice lacking MyD88 are more susceptible than normal mice to infection with group B *Streptococcus*, *Listeria monocytogenes*, and *Mycobacterium tuberculosis*. However, it is now appreciated that some of the TLRs (e.g., TLR3 and TLR4) can activate signal transduction via an MyD88-independent pathway.

Additional Interactions of Microbial Pathogens and Phagocytes Other ways that microbial pathogens avoid destruction by phagocytes include production of factors that are toxic to phagocytes or that interfere with the chemotactic and ingestion function of phagocytes.

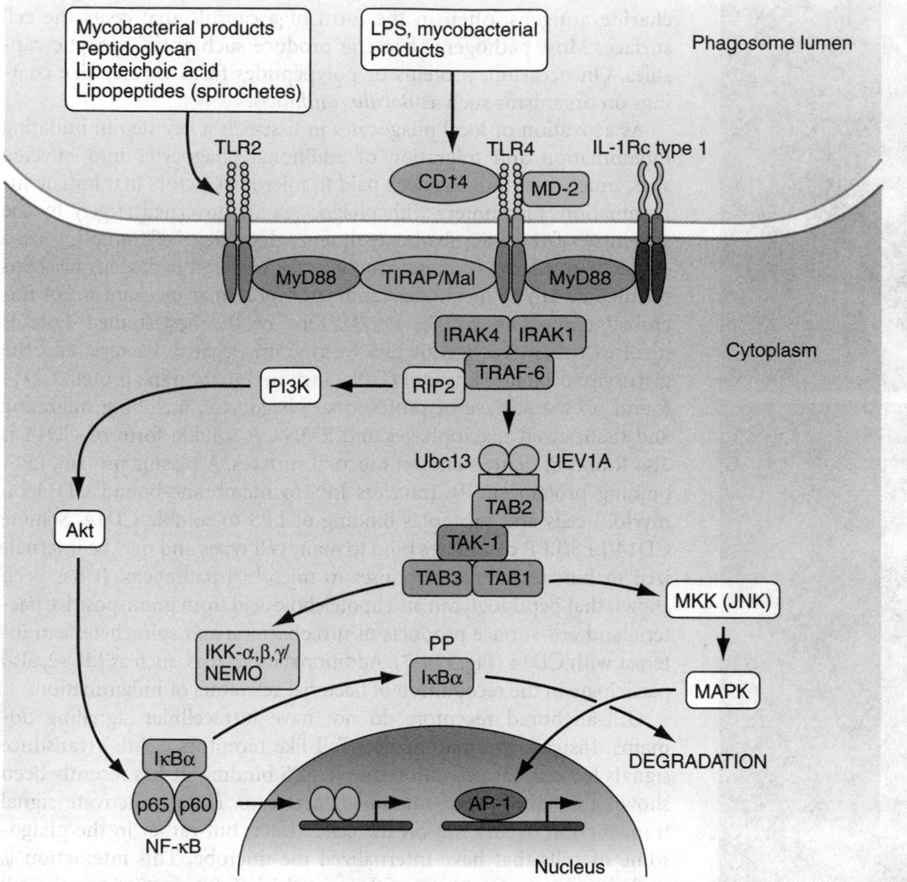

FIGURE 114-3 Cellular signaling pathways for production of inflammatory cytokines in response to microbial products. Various microbial cell-surface constituents interact with CD14, which in turn interacts in a currently unknown fashion with Toll-like receptors (TLRs). Some microbial factors do not need CD14 to interact with TLRs. Associating with TLR4 (and to some extent with TLR2) is MD-2, a cofactor that facilitates the response to lipopolysaccharide (LPS). Both CD14 and TLRs contain extracellular leucine-rich domains that become localized to the lumen of the phagosome upon uptake of bacterial cells; there, the TLRs can bind to microbial products. The TLRs are oligomerized, usually forming homodimers, and then bind to the general adaptor protein MyD88 via the C-terminal Toll/IL-1R (TIR) domains, which also bind to TIRAP (TIR domain-containing adaptor protein), a molecule that participates in the transduction of signals from TLR4. The MyD88/TIRAP complex activates signal-transducing molecules such as IRAK1 and IRAK4 (IL-1Rc-associated kinases 1 and 4); TRAF-6 (tumor necrosis factor receptor–associated factor 6); TAK-1 (transforming growth factor β–activating kinase 1); and TAB1, TAB2, and TAB3 (TAK1-binding proteins 1, 2, and 3). This signaling complex associates with the ubiquitin-conjugating enzyme Ubc13 and the Ubc-like protein UEV1A to catalyze the formation of a polyubiquitin chain on TRAF6. Polyubiquitination of TRAF6 activates TAK1, which, along with TAB2 (a protein that binds to lysine residue 63 in polyubiquitin chains via a conserved zinc-finger domain), phosphorylates the inducible kinase complex IKK-α, -β, and -γ. IKK-γ is also called NEMO [nuclear factor κB (NF-κB) essential modulator]. This large complex then phosphorylates the inhibitory component of NF-κB, IκBα, resulting in release of IκBα from NF-κB. Phosphorylated (PP) IκB is then degraded, and the two components of NF-κB, p50 and p65, translocate to the nucleus, where they bind to regulatory transcriptional sites on target genes, many of which encode inflammatory proteins. In addition to inducing NF-κB nuclear translocation, TAK1 also activates MAP kinase transducers such as the c-Jun N-terminal kinase (JNK) pathway, which can lead to nuclear translocation of the transcription factor AP1. Via the RIP2 protein, TRAF6 bound to IRAK can activate phosphatidylinositol-3 kinase (PI3K) and the regulatory protein Akt to dissociate NF-κB from IκBα, an event followed by translocation of the active NF-κB to the nucleus. *(Figure modified from an original produced by Dr. Terry Means and Dr. Douglas Golenbock.)*

Hemolysins, leukocidins, and the like are microbial proteins that can kill phagocytes that are attempting to ingest organisms elaborating these substances. For example, staphylococcal hemolysins inhibit macrophage chemotaxis and kill these phagocytes. Streptolysin O made by *S. pyogenes* binds to cholesterol in phagocyte membranes and initiates a process of internal degranulation, with the release of normally granule-sequestered toxic components into the phagocyte's cytoplasm. *E. histolytica*, an intestinal protozoan that causes amebic dysentery, can disrupt phagocyte membranes after direct contact via the release of protozoal phospholipase A and pore-forming peptides.

Microbial Survival inside Phagocytes Many important microbial pathogens use a variety of strategies to survive inside phagocytes (particularly macrophages) after ingestion. Inhibition of fusion of the phagocytic vacuole (the phagosome) containing the ingested microbe with the lysosomal granules containing antimicrobial substances (the lysosome) allows *M. tuberculosis*, *S. enterica* serovar *typhi*, and *Toxoplasma gondii* to survive inside macrophages. Some organisms, such as *L. monocytogenes*, escape into the phagocyte's cytoplasm to grow and eventually spread to other cells. Resistance to killing within the macrophage and subsequent growth are critical to successful infection by herpes-type viruses, measles virus, poxviruses, *Salmonella*, *Yersinia*, *Legionella*, *Mycobacterium*, *Trypanosoma*, *Nocardia*, *Histoplasma*, *Toxoplasma*, and *Rickettsia*. *Salmonella* spp. use a master regulatory system, in which the *PhoP/PhoQ* genes control other genes, to enter and survive within cells; intracellular survival entails structural changes in the cell envelope LPS.

TISSUE INVASION AND TISSUE TROPISM

TISSUE INVASION

Most viral pathogens cause disease by growth at skin or mucosal entry sites, but some pathogens spread from the initial site to deeper tissues. Virus can spread via the nerves (rabies virus) or plasma (picornaviruses) or within migratory blood cells (poliovirus, Epstein-Barr virus, and many others). Specific viral genes determine where and how individual viral strains can spread.

Bacteria may invade deeper layers of mucosal tissue via intracellular uptake by epithelial cells, traversal of epithelial cell junctions, or penetration through denuded epithelial surfaces. Among virulent *Shigella* strains and invasive *E. coli*, outer-membrane proteins are critical to epithelial cell invasion and bacterial multiplication. *Neisseria* and *Haemophilus* spp. penetrate mucosal cells by poorly understood mechanisms before dissemination into the bloodstream. Staphylococci and streptococci elaborate a variety of extracellular enzymes, such as hyaluronidase, lipases, nucleases, and hemolysins, that are probably important in breaking down cellular and matrix structures and allowing the bacteria access to deeper tissues and blood. Organisms that colonize the gastrointestinal tract can often translocate through the mucosa into the blood and, under circumstances in which host defenses are inadequate, cause bacteremia. *Y. enterocolitica* can invade the mucosa through the activity of the invasin protein. Some bacteria (e.g., *Brucella*) can be carried from a mucosal site to a distant site by phagocytic cells (e.g., PMNs) that ingest but fail to kill the bacteria.

Fungal pathogens almost always take advantage of host immunocompromise to spread hematogenously to deeper tissues. The AIDS epidemic has resoundingly illustrated this principle: the immunodeficiency of many HIV-infected patients permits the development of life-threatening fungal infections of the lung, blood, and brain. Other than the capsule of *C. neoformans*, specific fungal antigens involved in tissue invasion are not well characterized. Both fungal and protozoal pathogens undergo morphologic changes to spread within a host. Yeast-cell forms of *C. albicans* transform into hyphal forms when invading deeper tissues. Malarial parasites grow in liver cells as merozoites and are released into the blood to invade erythrocytes and become trophozoites. *E. histolytica* is found as both a cyst and a trophozoite in the intestinal lumen, through which this pathogen enters the host, but only the trophozoite form can spread systemically to cause amebic liver abscesses. Other protozoal pathogens, such as *T. gondii*, *Giardia lamblia*, and *Cryptosporidium*, also undergo extensive morphologic changes after initial infection to spread to other tissues.

TISSUE TROPISM

The propensity of certain microbes to cause disease by infecting specific tissues has been known since the early days of bacteriology, yet the molecular basis for this propensity is understood somewhat better for viral pathogens than for other agents of infectious disease. Specific receptor-ligand interactions clearly underlie the ability of certain viruses to enter cells within tissues and disrupt normal tissue function, but the mere presence of a receptor for a virus on a target tissue is not sufficient for tissue tropism. Factors in the cell, route of viral entry, viral capacity to penetrate into cells, viral genetic elements that regulate gene expression, and pathways of viral spread in a tissue all affect tissue tropism. Some viral genes are best transcribed in specific target cells, such as hepatitis B genes in liver cells and Epstein-Barr virus genes in B lymphocytes. The route of inoculation of poliovirus determines its neurotropism, although the molecular basis for this circumstance is not understood.

The lesser understanding of the tissue tropism of bacterial and parasitic infections is exemplified by *Neisseria* spp. There is no well-accepted explanation of why *N. gonorrhoeae* colonizes and infects the human genital tract while the closely related species *N. meningitidis* principally colonizes the human oropharynx. *N. meningitidis* expresses a capsular polysaccharide, while *N. gonorrhoeae* does not; however, there is no indication that this property plays a role in the different tissue tropisms displayed by these two bacterial species. *N. gonorrhoeae* can use cytidine monophosphate *N*-acetylneuraminic acid from host tissues to add *N*-acetylneuraminic acid (sialic acid) to its lipooligosaccharide (LOS) O side chain, and this alteration appears to make the organism resistant to host defenses. Lactate, present at high levels on genital mucosal surfaces, stimulates sialylation of gonococcal LOS. Bacteria with sialic acid sugars in their capsules, such as *N. meningitidis*, *E. coli* K1, and group B streptococci, have a propensity to cause meningitis, but this generalization has many exceptions. For example, all recognized serotypes of group B streptococci contain sialic acid in their capsules, but only one serotype (III) is responsible for most cases of group B streptococcal meningitis. Moreover, both *H. influenzae* and *S. pneumoniae* can readily cause meningitis, but these organisms do not have sialic acid in their capsules.

TISSUE DAMAGE AND DISEASE

Disease is a complex phenomenon resulting from tissue invasion and destruction, toxin elaboration, and host response. Viruses cause much of their damage by exerting a cytopathic effect on host cells and inhibiting host defenses. The growth of bacterial, fungal, and protozoal parasites in tissue, which may or may not be accompanied by toxin elaboration, can also compromise tissue function and lead to disease. For some bacterial and possibly some fungal pathogens, toxin production is one of the best-characterized molecular mechanisms of pathogenesis, while host factors such as IL-1, TNF-α, kinins, inflammatory proteins, products of complement activation, and mediators derived from arachidonic acid metabolites (leukotrienes) and cellular degranulation (histamines) readily contribute to the severity of disease.

VIRAL DISEASE

See Chap. 170.

BACTERIAL TOXINS

Among the first infectious diseases to be understood were those due to toxin-elaborating bacteria. Diphtheria, botulism, and tetanus toxins are responsible for the diseases associated with local infections due to *Corynebacterium diphtheriae*, *Clostridium botulinum*, and *Clostridium tetani*, respectively. Enterotoxins produced by *E. coli*, *Salmonella*, *Shigella*, *Staphylococcus*, and *V. cholerae* contribute to diarrheal disease caused by these organisms. Staphylococci, streptococci, *P. aeruginosa*, and *Bordetella* elaborate various toxins that cause or contribute to disease, including toxic shock syndrome toxin 1 (TSST-1); erythrogenic toxin; exotoxins A, S, T, and U; and pertussis toxin. A number of these toxins (e.g., cholera toxin, diphtheria toxin, pertussis toxin, *E. coli* heat-labile toxin, and *P. aeruginosa* exotoxins A, S, and T) have adenosine diphosphate (ADP)-ribosyltransferase activity—i.e., the toxins enzymatically catalyze the transfer of the ADP-ribosyl portion of nicotinamide adenine diphosphate to target proteins and inactivate them. The staphylococcal enterotoxins, TSST-1, and the streptococcal pyogenic exotoxins behave as superantigens, stimulating certain T cells to proliferate without processing of the protein toxin by antigen-presenting cells. Part of this process involves stimulation of the antigen-presenting cells to produce IL-1 and TNF-α, which have been implicated in many of the clinical features of diseases like toxic shock syndrome and scarlet fever. A number of gram-negative pathogens (*Salmonella*, *Yersinia*, and *P. aeruginosa*) can inject toxins directly into host target cells by means of a complex set of proteins referred to as the type III secretion system. Loss or inactivation of this virulence system usually greatly reduces the capacity of a bacterial pathogen to cause disease.

ENDOTOXIN

The lipid A portion of gram-negative LPS has potent biologic activities that cause many of the clinical manifestations of gram-negative bacterial sepsis, including fever, muscle proteolysis, uncontrolled intravascular coagulation, and shock. The effects of lipid A appear to be mediated by the production of potent cytokines due to LPS binding to CD14 and signal transduction via TLRs, particularly TLR4. Cytokines exhibit potent hypothermic activity through effects on the hypothalamus; they also increase vascular permeability, alter the activity of endothelial cells, and induce endothelial-cell procoagulant activity. Numerous therapeutic strategies aimed at neutralizing the effects of endotoxin are under investigation, but so far the results have been disappointing. One drug, activated protein C (drotrecogin alfa, activated), was found to reduce mortality by ~20% during severe sepsis—a condition that can be induced by endotoxin during gram-negative bacterial sepsis.

INVASION

Many diseases are caused primarily by pathogens growing in tissue sites that are normally sterile. Pneumococcal pneumonia is mostly attributable to the growth of *S. pneumoniae* in the lung and the attendant host inflammatory response, although specific factors that enhance this process (e.g., pneumolysin) may be responsible for some of the pathogenic potential of the pneumococcus. Disease that follows bacteremia and invasion of the meninges by meningitis-producing bacteria such as *N. meningitidis*, *H. influenzae*, *E. coli* K1, and group B streptococci appears to be due solely to the ability of these organisms to gain access to these tissues, multiply in them, and provoke cytokine production leading to tissue-damaging host inflammation.

Specific molecular mechanisms accounting for tissue invasion by fungal and protozoal pathogens are less well described. Except for studies pointing to factors like capsule and melanin production by *C. neoformans* and (possibly) levels of cell wall glucans in some pathogenic fungi, the molecular basis for fungal invasiveness is not well defined. Melanism has been shown to protect the fungal cell against death caused by phagocyte factors such as nitric oxide, superoxide, and hypochlorite. Morphogenic variation and production of proteases (e.g., the *Candida* aspartyl proteinase) have been implicated in fungal invasion of host tissues.

If pathogens are effectively to invade host tissues (particularly the blood), they must avoid the major host defenses represented by complement and phagocytic cells. Bacteria most often avoid these defenses through their cell surface polysaccharides—either capsular polysaccharides or long O-side-chain antigens characteristic of the smooth LPS of gram-negative bacteria. These molecules can prevent the activation and/or deposition of complement opsonins or limit the access of phagocytic cells with receptors for complement opsonins to these molecules when they are deposited on the bacterial surface below the capsular layer. Another potential mechanism of microbial virulence is the ability of some organisms to present the capsule as an apparent self antigen through molecular mimicry. For example, the polysialic acid capsule of group B *N. meningitidis* is chemically identical to an oligosaccharide found on human brain cells.

Immunochemical studies of capsular polysaccharides have led to an appreciation of the tremendous chemical diversity that can result from the linking of a few monosaccharides. For example, three hexoses can link up in more than 300 different and potentially serologically distinct ways, while three amino acids have only six possible peptide combinations. Capsular polysaccharides, which have been used as effective vaccines against meningococcal meningitis as well as against pneumococcal and *H. influenzae* infections, may prove to be of value as vaccines against any organisms that express a nontoxic, immunogenic capsular polysaccharide. In addition, most encapsulated pathogens become virtually avirulent when capsule production is interrupted by genetic manipulation; this observation emphasizes the importance of this structure in pathogenesis.

HOST RESPONSE

The inflammatory response of the host is critical for interruption and resolution of the infectious process but also is often responsible for the signs and symptoms of disease. Infection promotes a complex series of host responses involving the complement, kinin, and coagulation pathways. The production of cytokines such as IL-1, TNF-α, and other factors regulated in part by the NF-κ*B* transcription factor leads to fever, muscle proteolysis, and other effects, as noted above. An inability to kill or contain the microbe usually results in further damage due to the progression of inflammation and infection. In many chronic infections, degranulation of host inflammatory cells can lead to release of host proteases, elastases, histamines, and other toxic substances that can degrade host tissues. Chronic inflammation in any tissue can lead to the destruction of that tissue and to clinical disease associated with loss of organ function; an example is sterility from pelvic inflammatory disease caused by chronic infection with *N. gonorrhoeae*.

The nature of the host response elicited by the pathogen often determines the pathology of a particular infection. Local inflammation produces local tissue damage, while systemic inflammation, such as that seen during sepsis, can result in the signs and symptoms of septic shock. The severity of septic shock is associated with the degree of production of host effectors. Disease due to intracellular parasitism results from the formation of granulomas, wherein the host attempts to wall off the parasite inside a fibrotic lesion surrounded by fused epithelial cells that make up so-called multinucleated giant cells. A number of pathogens, particularly anaerobic bacteria, staphylococci, and streptococci, provoke the formation of an abscess, probably because of the presence of zwitterionic surface polysaccharides such as the capsular polysaccharide of *Bacteroides fragilis*. The outcome of an infection depends on the balance between an effective host response that eliminates a pathogen and an excessive inflammatory response that is associated with an inability to eliminate a pathogen and with the resultant tissue damage that leads to disease.

TRANSMISSION TO NEW HOSTS

As part of the pathogenic process, most microbes are shed from the host, often in a form infectious for susceptible individuals. However, the rate of transmissibility may not necessarily be high, even if the disease is severe in the infected individual, as transmissibility and virulence are not linked traits. Most pathogens exit via the same route by which they entered: respiratory pathogens by aerosols from sneezing or coughing or through salivary spread, gastrointestinal pathogens by fecal-oral spread, sexually transmitted diseases by venereal spread, and vector-borne organisms by either direct contact with the vector through a blood meal or indirect contact with organisms shed into environmental sources such as water. Microbial factors that specifically promote transmission are not well characterized. Respiratory shedding is facilitated by overproduction of mucous secretions, with consequently enhanced sneezing and coughing. Diarrheal toxins such as cholera toxin, *E. coli* heat-labile toxins, and *Shigella* toxins probably facilitate fecal-oral spread of microbial cells in the high volumes of diarrheal fluid produced during infection. The ability to produce phenotypic variants that resist hostile environmental factors (e.g., the highly resistant cysts of *E. histolytica* shed in feces) represents another mechanism of pathogenesis relevant to transmission. Blood parasites such as *Plasmodium* spp. change phenotype after ingestion by a mosquito—a prerequisite for the continued transmission of this pathogen. Venereally transmitted pathogens may undergo phenotypic variation due to the production of specific factors to facilitate transmission, but shedding of these pathogens into the environment does not result in the formation of infectious foci.

In summary, the molecular mechanisms used by pathogens to colonize, invade, infect, and disrupt the host are numerous and diverse. Each phase of the infectious process involves a variety of microbial and host factors interacting in a manner that can result in disease. Recognition of the coordinated genetic regulation of virulence factor elaboration when organisms move from their natural environment into the mammalian host emphasizes the complex nature of the host-parasite interaction. Fortunately, the need for diverse factors in successful infection and disease implies that a variety of therapeutic strategies may be developed to interrupt this process and thereby prevent and treat microbial infections.

FURTHER READINGS

CAMILLI A, BASSLER BL: Bacterial small-molecule signaling pathways. Science 311:1113, 2006

FINLAY BB, MCFADDEN G: Anti-immunology: Evasion of the host immune system by bacterial and viral pathogens. Cell 124:767, 2006

HAN J, ULEVITCH RJ: Limiting inflammatory responses during activation of innate immunity. Nat Immunol 6:1198, 2005

KAWAI T, AKIRA S: Innate immune recognition of viral infection. Nat Immunol 7:131, 2006

KNIREL YA et al: Structural features and structural variability of the lipopolysaccharide of *Yersinia pestis*, the cause of plague. J Endotoxin Res 12:3, 2006

MENDES-GIANNINI MJ et al: Interaction of pathogenic fungi with host cells: Molecular and cellular approaches. FEMS Immunol Med Microbiol 45:383, 2005

PIZARRO-CERDA J, COSSART P: Bacterial adhesion and entry into host cells. Cell 124:715, 2006

SPEAR PG et al: Different receptors binding to distinct interfaces on herpes simplex virus gD can trigger events leading to cell fusion and viral entry. Virology 344:17, 2006

TAKAHASHI K et al: The mannose-binding lectin: A prototypic pattern recognition molecule. Curr Opin Immunol 18:16, 2006

115 Approach to the Acutely Ill Infected Febrile Patient

Tamar F. Barlam, Dennis L. Kasper

The physician treating the acutely ill febrile patient must be able to recognize infections that require emergent attention. If such infections are not adequately evaluated and treated at initial presentation, the opportunity to alter an adverse outcome may be lost. In this chapter, the clinical presentations of and approach to patients with relatively common infectious disease emergencies are discussed. These infectious processes and their treatments are discussed in detail in other chapters. Noninfectious causes of fever are not covered in this chapter; information on the approach to fever of unknown origin, including that eventually shown to be of noninfectious etiology, is presented in Chap. 19.

APPROACH TO THE PATIENT: Acute Febrile Illness

A physician must have a consistent approach to acutely ill patients. Even before the history is elicited and a physical examination performed, an immediate assessment of the patient's general appearance yields valuable information. The perceptive physician's subjective sense that a patient is septic or toxic often proves accurate. Visible agitation or anxiety in a febrile patient can be a harbinger of critical illness.

HISTORY Presenting symptoms are frequently nonspecific. Detailed questions should be asked about the onset and duration of symptoms and about changes in severity or rate of progression over time. Host factors and comorbid conditions may enhance the risk of infection with certain organisms or of a more fulminant course than is usually seen. Lack of splenic function, alcoholism with significant liver disease, intravenous drug use, HIV infection, diabetes, malignancy, and chemotherapy all predispose to specific infections and frequently to increased severity. The patient should be questioned about factors that might help identify a nidus for invasive infection, such as recent upper respiratory tract infections, influenza, or varicella; prior trauma; disruption of cutaneous barriers due to lacerations, burns, surgery, or decubiti; and the presence of foreign bodies, such as nasal packing after rhinoplasty, barrier contraceptives, tampons, arteriovenous fistulas, or prosthetic joints. Travel, contact with pets or other animals, or activities that might result in tick exposure can lead to diagnoses that would not otherwise be considered. Recent dietary intake, medication use, social or occupational contact with ill individuals, vaccination history, recent sexual contacts, and menstrual history may be relevant. A review of systems should focus on any neurologic signs or sensorium alterations, rashes or skin lesions, and focal pain or tenderness and should also include a general review of respiratory, gastrointestinal, or genitourinary symptoms.

PHYSICAL EXAMINATION A complete physical examination should be performed, with special attention to several areas that are sometimes given short shrift in routine examinations. Assessment of the patient's general appearance and vital signs, skin and soft tissue examination, and the neurologic evaluation are of particular importance.

The patient may appear either anxious and agitated or lethargic and apathetic. Fever is usually present, although elderly patients and compromised hosts [e.g., patients who are uremic or cirrhotic and those who are taking glucocorticoids or nonsteroidal anti-inflammatory drugs (NSAIDs)] may be afebrile despite serious underlying infection. Measurement of blood pressure, heart rate, and respiratory rate helps determine the degree of hemodynamic and metabolic compromise. The patient's airway must be evaluated to rule out the risk of obstruction from an invasive oropharyngeal infection.

The etiologic diagnosis may become evident in the context of a thorough skin examination (Chap. 18). Petechial rashes are typically seen with meningococcemia or Rocky Mountain spotted fever (RMSF); erythroderma is associated with toxic shock syndrome (TSS) and drug fever. The soft tissue and muscle examination is critical. Areas of erythema or duskiness, edema, and tenderness may indicate underlying necrotizing fasciitis, myositis, or myonecrosis. The neurologic examination must include a careful assessment of mental status for signs of early encephalopathy. Evidence of nuchal rigidity or focal neurologic findings should be sought.

DIAGNOSTIC WORKUP After a quick clinical assessment, diagnostic material should be obtained rapidly and antibiotic and supportive treatment begun. Blood (for cultures; baseline complete blood count with differential; measurement of serum electrolytes, blood urea nitrogen, serum creatinine, and serum glucose; and liver function tests) can be obtained at the time an intravenous line is placed and before antibiotics are administered. Three sets of blood cultures should be performed for patients with possible acute endocarditis. Asplenic patients should have a blood smear examined to confirm the presence of Howell-Jolly bodies (indicating the absence of splenic function) and a buffy coat examined for bacteria; these patients can have $>10^6$ organisms per milliliter of blood (compared with 10^4/mL in patients with an intact spleen). Blood smears from patients at risk for severe parasitic disease, such as malaria or babesiosis, must be examined for the diagnosis and quantitation of parasitemia. Blood smears may also be diagnostic in ehrlichiosis.

Patients with possible meningitis should have cerebrospinal fluid (CSF) obtained before the initiation of antibiotic therapy. Focal findings, depressed mental status, or papilledema should be evaluated by brain imaging prior to lumbar puncture, which, in this setting, could initiate herniation. *Antibiotics should be administered before imaging but after blood for cultures has been drawn.* If CSF cultures are negative, blood cultures will provide the diagnosis in 50–70% of cases.

Focal abscesses necessitate immediate CT or MRI as part of an evaluation for surgical intervention. Other diagnostic procedures, such as cultures of wounds or scraping of skin lesions, should not delay the initiation of treatment for more than minutes. Once emergent evaluation, diagnostic procedures, and (if appropriate) surgical consultation (see below) have been completed, other laboratory tests can be conducted. Appropriate radiography, computed axial tomography, MRI, urinalysis, erythrocyte sedimentation rate (ESR) determination, and transthoracic or transesophageal echocardiography may all prove important.

Rx THE ACUTELY ILL PATIENT

In the acutely ill patient, empirical antibiotic therapy is critical and should be administered without undue delay. Increased prevalence of antibiotic resistance in community-acquired bacteria must be considered when antibiotics are selected. **Table 115-1** lists first-line treatments for infections considered in this chapter. In addition to the rapid initiation of antibiotic therapy, several of these infections require urgent surgical attention. Neurosurgical evaluation for subdural empyema or spinal epidural abscess, otolaryngologic surgery for possible mucormycosis, and cardiothoracic surgery for critically ill patients with acute endocarditis are as important as antibiotic therapy. For infections such as necrotizing fasciitis and clostridial myonecrosis, rapid surgical intervention supersedes other diagnostic or therapeutic maneuvers.

Adjunctive treatments may reduce morbidity and mortality and include dexamethasone for bacterial meningitis; intravenous immunoglobulin (IVIg) for TSS and necrotizing fasciitis caused by group A *Streptococcus*; low-dose hydrocortisone and fludrocortisone for septic shock; and drotrecogin alfa (activated), also known as recombinant human activated protein C, for meningococcemia and severe sepsis. Adjunctive therapies should usually be initiated within the first hours of treatment; however, dexamethasone for bacterial meningitis must be given before or at the time of the first dose of antibiotic.

TABLE 115-1 EMPIRICAL TREATMENT FOR COMMON INFECTIOUS DISEASE EMERGENCIES

Clinical Syndrome	Possible Etiologies	Treatment	Comments	See Chap.
Sepsis without a Clear Focus				
Septic shock	*Pseudomonas* spp., gram-negative enteric bacilli, *Staphylococcus* spp., *Streptococcus* spp.	Vancomycin (1 g q12h) ***plus*** Gentamicin (5 mg/kg per day) ***plus either*** Piperacillin/tazobactam (3.375 g q4h) ***or*** Cefepime (2 g q12h)	Adjust treatment when culture data become available. Drotrecogin alfa (activated)[a] or low-dose hydrocortisone and fludrocortisone[b] may improve outcome in patients with septic shock.	129, 130, 143, 145, 265
Overwhelming postsplenectomy sepsis	*Streptococcus pneumoniae, Haemophilus influenzae, Neisseria meningitidis*	Ceftriaxone (2 g q12h) ***plus*** Vancomycin (1 g q12h)	If a β-lactam–sensitive strain is identified, vancomycin can be discontinued.	265
Babesiosis	*Babesia microti* (U.S.), *B. divergens* (Europe)	***Either:*** Clindamycin (600 mg tid) ***plus*** Quinine (650 mg tid) ***or*** Atovaquone (750 mg q12h) ***plus*** Azithromycin (500-mg loading dose, then 250 mg/d)	Atovaquone and azithromycin are as effective as clindamycin and quinine and are associated with fewer side effects. Treatment with doxycycline (100 mg bid[c]) for potential coinfection with *Borrelia burgdorferi* or *Ehrlichia* spp. may be prudent.	201, 204
Sepsis with Skin Findings				
Meningococcemia	*N. meningitidis*	Penicillin (4 mU q4h) ***or*** Ceftriaxone (2 g q12h)	Consider protein C replacement in fulminant meningococcemia.	136, 167
Rocky Mountain spotted fever (RMSF)	*Rickettsia rickettsii*	Doxycycline (100 mg bid)	If both meningococcemia and RMSF are being considered, use chloramphenicol alone (50–75 mg/kg per day in four divided doses) ***or*** ceftriaxone (2 g q12h) ***plus*** doxycycline (100 mg bid[c]). If RMSF is diagnosed, doxycycline is the proven superior agent.	
Purpura fulminans	*S. pneumoniae, H. influenzae, N. meningitidis*	Ceftriaxone (2 g q12h) ***plus*** Vancomycin (1 g q12h)	If a β-lactam–sensitive strain is identified, vancomycin can be discontinued.	136, 265
Erythroderma: toxic shock syndrome	Group A *Streptococcus*, *Staphylococcus aureus*	Vancomycin (1 g q12h) ***plus*** Clindamycin (600 mg q8h)	If a penicillin- or oxacillin-sensitive strain is isolated, those agents are superior to vancomycin (penicillin, 2 mU q4h; or oxacillin, 2 g q4h). The site of toxigenic bacteria should be debrided; IV immunoglobulin can be used in severe cases.[d]	129, 130
Sepsis with Soft Tissue Findings				
Necrotizing fasciitis	Group A *Streptococcus*, mixed aerobic/anaerobic flora	Penicillin (2 mU q4h) ***plus*** Clindamycin (600 mg q8h) ***plus*** Gentamicin (5 mg/kg per day)	Urgent surgical evaluation is critical. If community-acquired methicillin-resistant *S. aureus* is a concern, vancomycin (1 g q12h) can be substituted for penicillin while culture data are pending.	119, 130
Clostridial myonecrosis	*Clostridium perfringens*	Penicillin (2 mU q4h) ***plus*** Clindamycin (600 mg q8h)	Urgent surgical evaluation is critical.	135
Neurologic Infections				
Bacterial meningitis	*S. pneumoniae, N. meningitidis*	Ceftriaxone (2 g q12h) ***plus*** Vancomycin (1 g q12h)	If a β-lactam–sensitive strain is identified, vancomycin can be discontinued. If the patient is >50 years old or has comorbid disease, add ampicillin (2 g q4h) for *Listeria* coverage. Dexamethasone (10 mg q6h × 4 days) improves outcome in adult patients with meningitis (especially pneumococcal) and cloudy CSF, positive CSF Gram's stain, or a CSF leukocyte count >1000/μL.	376
Brain abscess, suppurative intracranial infections	*Streptococcus* spp., *Staphylococcus* spp., anaerobes, gram-negative bacilli	Vancomycin (1 g q12h) ***plus*** Metronidazole (500 mg q8h) ***plus*** Ceftriaxone (2 g q12h)	Urgent surgical evaluation is critical. If a penicillin- or oxacillin-sensitive strain is isolated, those agents are superior to vancomycin (penicillin, 4 mU q4h; or oxacillin, 2 g q4h).	376
Cerebral malaria	*Plasmodium falciparum*	Quinine (650 mg tid) ***plus*** Tetracycline (250 mg tid)	Do not use glucocorticoids.	201, 203

(continued)

TABLE 115-1 EMPIRICAL TREATMENT FOR COMMON INFECTIOUS DISEASE EMERGENCIES (CONTINUED)

Clinical Syndrome	Possible Etiologies	Treatment	Comments	See Chap.
Spinal epidural abscess	*Staphylococcus* spp., gram-negative bacilli	Vancomycin (1 g q12h) ***plus*** Ceftriaxone (2 g q24h)	Surgical evaluation is essential. If a penicillin- or oxacillin-sensitive strain is isolated, those agents are superior to vancomycin (penicillin, 4 mU q4h; or oxacillin, 2 g q4h).	372
Focal Infections				
Acute bacterial endocarditis	*S. aureus*, β-hemolytic streptococci, HACEK group,[e] *Neisseria* spp., *S. pneumoniae*	Ceftriaxone (2 g q12h) ***plus*** Vancomycin (1 g q12h)	Adjust treatment when culture data become available. Surgical evaluation is essential.	118

[a]Drotrecogin alfa (activated) is administered at a dose of 24 μg/kg per hour for 96 h. It has been approved for use in patients with severe sepsis and a high risk of death as defined by an Acute Physiology and Chronic Health Evaluation II (APACHE II) score of ≥25 and/or multiorgan failure.

[b]Hydrocortisone (50-mg IV bolus q6h) with fludrocortisone (50-μg tablet daily for 7 days) may improve outcomes of severe sepsis, particularly in the setting of relative adrenal insufficiency.

[c]Tetracyclines can be antagonistic in action to β-lactam agents. Adjust treatment as soon as the diagnosis is confirmed.

[d]The optimal dose of IV immunoglobulin has not been determined, but the median dose in observational studies is 2 g/kg (total dose administered over 1–5 days).

[e]*Haemophilus aphrophilus, H. paraphrophilus, H. parainfluenzae, Actinobacillus actinomycetemcomitans, Cardiobacterium hominis, Eikenella corrodens,* and *Kingella kingae*.

SPECIFIC PRESENTATIONS

The infections considered below according to common clinical presentation can have rapidly catastrophic outcomes, and their immediate recognition and treatment can be life-saving. Recommended empirical therapeutic regimens are presented in Table 115-1.

SEPSIS WITHOUT AN OBVIOUS FOCUS OF PRIMARY INFECTION

These patients initially have a brief prodrome of nonspecific symptoms and signs that progresses quickly to hemodynamic instability with hypotension, tachycardia, tachypnea, respiratory distress, and altered mental status. Disseminated intravascular coagulation (DIC) with clinical evidence of a hemorrhagic diathesis is a poor prognostic sign.

Septic Shock (See also Chap. 265) Patients with bacteremia leading to septic shock may have a primary site of infection (e.g., pneumonia, pyelonephritis, or cholangitis) that is not evident initially. Elderly patients with comorbid conditions, hosts compromised by malignancy and neutropenia, and patients who have recently undergone a surgical procedure or hospitalization are at increased risk for an adverse outcome. Gram-negative bacteremia with organisms such as *Pseudomonas aeruginosa* or *Escherichia coli* and gram-positive infection with organisms such as *Staphylococcus aureus* or group A streptococci can present as intractable hypotension and multiorgan failure. Treatment can usually be initiated empirically on the basis of the presentation (Table 265-3). Adjunctive therapy with either drotrecogin alfa (activated) or glucocorticoids should be considered for patients with severe sepsis.

Overwhelming Infection in Asplenic Patients (See also Chap. 265) Patients without splenic function are at risk for overwhelming bacterial sepsis. Asplenic adult patients succumb to sepsis at 58 times the rate of the general population; 50–70% of cases occur within the first 2 years after splenectomy, with a mortality rate of up to 80%, but the increased risk persists throughout life. In asplenia, encapsulated bacteria cause the majority of infections. Adults, who are more likely to have antibody to these organisms, are at lower risk than children. *Streptococcus pneumoniae* is the most common isolate, causing 50–70% of cases, but the risk of infection with *Haemophilus influenzae* or *Neisseria meningitidis* is also high. Severe clinical manifestations of infections due to *E. coli, S. aureus*, group B streptococci, *P. aeruginosa, Capnocytophaga, Babesia*, and *Plasmodium* have been described.

Babesiosis (See also Chap. 204) A history of recent travel to endemic areas raises the possibility of infection with *Babesia*. Between 1 and 4 weeks after a tick bite, the patient experiences chills, fatigue, anorexia, myalgia, arthralgia, shortness of breath, nausea, and headache; ecchymosis and/or petechiae are occasionally seen. The tick that most commonly transmits *Babesia, Ixodes scapularis*, also transmits *Borrelia burgdorferi* (the agent of Lyme disease) and *Ehrlichia*; co-infection can occur, resulting in more severe disease. Infection with the European species *Babesia divergens* is more frequently fulminant than that due to the U.S. species *Babesia microti. B. divergens* causes a febrile syndrome with hemolysis, jaundice, hemoglobinemia, and renal failure and is associated with a mortality rate of >50%. Severe babesiosis is especially common in asplenic hosts but does occur in hosts with normal splenic function, particularly at >60 years of age. Complications include renal failure, acute respiratory failure, and DIC.

Other Sepsis Syndromes Tularemia (Chap. 151) is seen throughout the United States but occurs primarily in Arkansas, Oklahoma, and Missouri. This disease is associated with wild rabbit, tick, and tabanid fly contact. The uncommon typhoidal form can be associated with gram-negative septic shock and a mortality rate of >30%. In the United States, plague (Chap. 152) occurs primarily in New Mexico, Arizona, and Colorado after contact with ground squirrels, prairie dogs, or chipmunks. Plague can occur with greater frequency outside the United States, especially in developing countries in Africa and Asia. The septic form is particularly rare and is associated with shock, multiorgan failure, and a 30% mortality rate. These rare infections should be considered in the appropriate epidemiologic setting. The Centers for Disease Control and Prevention lists tularemia and plague, along with anthrax, as important agents that might be used for bioterrorism (Chap. 214).

SEPSIS WITH SKIN MANIFESTATIONS

(See also Chap. 18) Maculopapular rashes may reflect early meningococcal or rickettsial disease but are usually associated with nonemergent infections. Exanthems are usually viral. Primary HIV infection commonly presents with a rash that is typically maculopapular and involves the upper part of the body but can spread to the palms and soles. The patient is usually febrile and can have lymphadenopathy, severe headache, dysphagia, diarrhea, myalgias, and arthralgias. Recognition of this syndrome provides an opportunity to prevent transmission and to institute treatment and monitoring early on.

Petechial rashes caused by viruses are seldom associated with hypotension or a toxic appearance, although severe measles can be an exception. In other settings, petechial rashes require more urgent attention.

Meningococcemia (See also Chap. 136) Almost three-quarters of patients with bacteremic *N. meningitidis* infection have a rash. Meningococcemia most often affects young children (i.e., those 6 months to 5 years old). In sub-Saharan Africa, the high prevalence of serogroup A meningococcal disease has been a threat to public health for more than a century. In addition, epidemic outbreaks occur every 8–12 years. In the United States, sporadic cases and outbreaks occur in day-care centers, schools (grade school through college), and army barracks. Household members of index cases are at 400–800 times greater risk of disease than the general population. Patients may exhibit fever, headache, nausea, vomiting, myalgias, changes in mental status, and meningismus. However, the rapidly progressive form of disease is not usually associated with meningitis. The rash is initially pink, blanching, and maculopapular, appearing on the trunk and extremities, but then becomes hemorrhagic, forming petechiae. Petechiae are first seen at the ankles, wrists, axillae, mucosal surfaces, and palpebral and bulbar conjunctiva, with subsequent spread to the lower extremities and trunk. A cluster of petechiae may be seen at pressure points—e.g., where a blood pressure cuff has been inflated. In rapidly progressive meningococcemia (10–20% of cases), the petechial rash quickly becomes purpuric (see Fig. 52-5), and patients develop DIC, multiorgan failure, and shock. Of these patients, 50–60% die, and survivors often require extensive debridement or amputation of gangrenous extremities. Hypotension with petechiae for <12 h is associated with significant mortality. The mortality rate can exceed 90% among patients without meningitis who have rash, hypotension, and a normal or low white blood cell (WBC) count and ESR. Cyanosis, coma, oliguria, metabolic acidosis, and elevated partial thromboplastin time are also associated with a fatal outcome. Correction of protein C deficiency may improve outcome. Antibiotics given in the office by the primary care provider before hospital evaluation and admission may improve prognosis; this observation suggests that early initiation of treatment may be life-saving.

Rocky Mountain Spotted Fever (See also Chap. 167) RMSF is a tick-borne disease caused by *Rickettsia rickettsii* that occurs throughout North and South America. A history of known tick bite is common; however, if such a history is lacking, a history of travel or outdoor activity (e.g., camping in tick-infested areas) can be ascertained. For the first 3 days, headache, fever, malaise, myalgias, nausea, vomiting, and anorexia are present. By day 3, half of patients have skin findings. Blanching macules develop initially on the wrists and ankles and then spread over the legs and trunk. The lesions become hemorrhagic and are frequently petechial. The rash spreads to palms and soles later in the course. The centripetal spread is a classic feature of RMSF. However, 10–15% of patients with RMSF never develop a rash. The patient can be hypotensive and develop noncardiogenic pulmonary edema, confusion, lethargy, and encephalitis progressing to coma. The CSF contains 10–100 cells/μL, usually with a predominance of mononuclear cells. The CSF glucose level is often normal; the protein concentration may be slightly elevated. Renal and hepatic injury and bleeding secondary to vascular damage are noted. Untreated infection has a mortality rate of 30%.

Although RMSF is the most severe rickettsial disease, other rickettsial diseases cause significant morbidity and mortality worldwide. *Mediterranean spotted fever* caused by *Rickettsia conorii* is found in Africa, southwestern and south-central Asia, and southern Europe. Patients have fever, flu-like symptoms, and an inoculation eschar at the site of the tick bite. A maculopapular rash develops within 1–7 days, involving the palms and soles but sparing the face. Elderly patients or those with diabetes, alcoholism, uremia, or congestive heart failure are at risk for severe disease characterized by neurologic involvement, respiratory distress, and gangrene of the digits. Mortality rates associated with this severe form of disease approach 50%. *Epidemic typhus*, caused by *Rickettsia prowazekii*, is transmitted in louse-infested environments and emerges in conditions of extreme poverty, war, and natural disaster. Patients experience a sudden onset of high fevers, severe headache, cough, myalgias, and abdominal pain. A maculopapular rash develops (primarily on the trunk) in more than half of patients and can progress to petechiae and purpura. Serious signs include delirium, coma, seizures, noncardiogenic pulmonary edema, skin necrosis, and peripheral gangrene. Mortality rates approached 60% in the preantibiotic era and continue to exceed 10–15% in contemporary outbreaks. *Scrub typhus*, caused by *Orientia tsutsugamushi*—a separate genus in the family Rickettsiaceae—is transmitted by larval mites or chiggers and is one of the most common infections in southeastern Asia and the western Pacific. The organism is found in areas of heavy scrub vegetation (e.g., along riverbanks). Patients present with fever and lymphadenopathy, may have an inoculation eschar, and may develop a maculopapular rash. Severe cases progress to pneumonia, meningoencephalitis, DIC, and renal failure. Mortality rates range from 1% to 35%.

If recognized in a timely fashion, rickettsial disease is very responsive to treatment. Doxycycline (100 mg twice daily for 3–14 days) is the treatment of choice for both adults and children. The newer macrolides and chloramphenicol may be suitable alternatives.

Purpura Fulminans (See also Chaps. 136 and 265) Purpura fulminans is the cutaneous manifestation of DIC and presents as large ecchymotic areas and hemorrhagic bullae. Progression of petechiae to purpura, ecchymoses, and gangrene is associated with congestive heart failure, septic shock, acute renal failure, acidosis, hypoxia, hypotension, and death. Purpura fulminans has been associated primarily with *N. meningitidis* but, in splenectomized patients, may be associated with *S. pneumoniae* and *H. influenzae*. Several small studies have suggested that correction of the protein C deficiency evident in meningococcal purpura fulminans with drotrecogin alfa (activated) may dramatically improve outcome.

Ecthyma Gangrenosum Septic shock caused by *P. aeruginosa* or *Aeromonas hydrophila* can be associated with ecthyma gangrenosum (see Fig. 145-1): hemorrhagic vesicles surrounded by a rim of erythema with central necrosis and ulceration. These gram-negative bacteremias are most common among patients with neutropenia, extensive burns, and hypogammaglobulinemia.

Other Emergent Infections Associated with Rash *Vibrio vulnificus* and other noncholera *Vibrio* bacteremic infections (Chap. 149) can cause focal skin lesions and overwhelming sepsis in hosts with liver disease. After ingestion of contaminated shellfish, there is a sudden onset of malaise, chills, fever, and hypotension. The patient develops bullous or hemorrhagic skin lesions, usually on the lower extremities, and 75% of patients have leg pain. The mortality rate can be as high as 50–60%. *Capnocytophaga canimorsus* can cause septic shock in asplenic patients. Infection with this fastidious gram-negative rod typically presents after a dog bite as fever, chills, myalgia, vomiting, diarrhea, dyspnea, confusion, and headache. Findings can include an exanthem or erythema multiforme (see Fig. 52-9), cyanotic mottling or peripheral cyanosis, petechiae, and ecchymosis. About 30% of patients with this fulminant form die of overwhelming sepsis and DIC, and survivors may require amputation because of gangrene.

Erythroderma TSS (Chaps. 129 and 130) is usually associated with erythroderma. The patient presents with fever, malaise, myalgias, nausea, vomiting, diarrhea, and confusion. There is a sunburn-type rash that may be subtle and patchy but is usually diffuse and is found on the face, trunk, and extremities. Erythroderma, which desquamates after 1–2 weeks, is more common in *Staphylococcus*-associated than in *Streptococcus*-associated TSS. Hypotension develops rapidly—often within hours—after the onset of symptoms. Multiorgan failure is seen. Early renal failure may precede hypotension and distinguishes this syndrome from other septic shock syndromes. Commonly there is no indication of a primary focal infection, although possible cutaneous or mucosal portals of entry for the organism can be ascertained when a careful history is taken. Colonization rather than overt infection of the vagina or a postoperative wound, for example, is typical with staphylococcal TSS, and the mucosal areas appear hyperemic but not infected. The diagnosis of TSS is defined by the clinical criteria of fever, rash, hypotension, and multiorgan involvement. The mortality rate is 5% for menstruation-associated TSS, 10–15% for nonmenstrual TSS, and 30–70% for streptococcal TSS.

Viral Hemorrhagic Fevers Viral hemorrhagic fevers (Chaps. 189 and 190) are zoonotic illnesses caused by viruses that reside in either animal reservoirs or arthropod vectors. These diseases occur worldwide and are restricted to areas where the host species live.

They are caused by four major groups of viruses: Arenaviridae (e.g., Lassa fever in Africa), Bunyaviridae (e.g., Rift Valley fever in Africa or hantavirus hemorrhagic fever with renal syndrome in Asia), Filoviridae (e.g., Ebola and Marburg virus infections in Africa), and Flaviviridae (e.g., yellow fever in Africa and South America and dengue in Asia, Africa, and the Americas). Lassa fever as well as Ebola and Marburg virus infections are also transmitted from person to person. The vectors for most viral fevers are found in rural areas; dengue and yellow fever are important exceptions. After a prodrome of fever, myalgias, and malaise, patients develop evidence of vascular damage, petechiae, and local hemorrhage. Shock, multifocal hemorrhaging, and neurologic signs (e.g., seizures or coma) predict a poor prognosis. Although supportive care to maintain blood pressure and intravascular volume is key, ribavirin may be useful against Arenaviridae and Bunyaviridae. Dengue (Chap. 189) is the most common arboviral disease worldwide. More than a quarter of a million cases of dengue hemorrhagic fever occur each year, with 25,000 deaths. Patients have a triad of symptoms: hemorrhagic manifestations, evidence of plasma leakage, and platelet counts <100,000/μL. Mortality rates are 10–20%. If dengue shock syndrome develops, mortality can reach 40%. Immediate supportive care and volume-replacement therapy are life-saving.

SEPSIS WITH A SOFT TISSUE/MUSCLE PRIMARY FOCUS

See also Chap. 119.

Necrotizing Fasciitis This infection may arise at a site of minimal trauma or postoperative incision and may also be associated with recent varicella, childbirth, or muscle strain. The most common causes of necrotizing fasciitis are group A streptococci alone (Chap. 130) and a mixed facultative and anaerobic flora (Chap. 119). Diabetes mellitus, peripheral vascular disease, and intravenous drug use are associated risk factors. Use of NSAIDs has been reported to allow progression of skin or soft tissue infections; however, prospective studies have not shown that NSAIDs increase the risk of disease or exacerbate established infection. The patient may have bacteremia and hypotension without other organ-system failure. Physical findings are minimal compared with the severity of pain and the degree of fever. The examination is often unremarkable except for soft tissue edema and erythema. The infected area is red, hot, shiny, swollen, and exquisitely tender. In untreated infection, the overlying skin develops blue-gray patches after 36 h, and cutaneous bullae and necrosis develop after 3–5 days. Necrotizing fasciitis due to a mixed flora, but not that due to group A streptococci, can be associated with gas production. Without treatment, pain decreases because of thrombosis of the small blood vessels and destruction of the peripheral nerves—an ominous sign. The mortality rate is 25–30% overall, >70% in association with TSS, and nearly 100% without surgical intervention. Life-threatening necrotizing fasciitis may also be due to *Clostridium perfringens* (Chap. 135); in this condition, the patient is extremely toxic and the mortality rate is high. Within 48 h, rapid tissue invasion and systemic toxicity associated with hemolysis and death ensue. The distinction between this entity and clostridial myonecrosis is made by muscle biopsy. Necrotizing fasciitis caused by community-acquired methicillin-resistant *S. aureus* (MRSA) was recently described. The MRSA-infected patients required extensive surgical debridement, but there were no deaths.

Clostridial Myonecrosis (See also Chap. 135) Myonecrosis is often associated with trauma or surgery but can be spontaneous. The incubation period is usually 12–24 h long, and massive necrotizing gangrene develops within hours of onset. Systemic toxicity, shock, and death can occur within 12 h. The patient's pain and toxic appearance are out of proportion to physical findings. On examination, the patient is febrile, apathetic, tachycardic, and tachypneic and may express a feeling of impending doom. Hypotension and renal failure develop later, and hyperalertness is evident preterminally. The skin over the affected area is bronze-brown, mottled, and edematous. Bullous lesions with serosanguineous drainage and a mousy or sweet odor can be present. Crepitus can occur secondary to gas production in muscle tissue. The mortality rate is >65% with spontaneous myonecrosis, which is often associated with *Clostridium septicum* and underlying malignancy. The mortality rates associated with trunk and limb infection are 63% and 12%, respectively, and any delay in surgical treatment increases the risk of death.

NEUROLOGIC INFECTIONS WITH OR WITHOUT SEPTIC SHOCK

Bacterial Meningitis (See also Chap. 376) Bacterial meningitis is one of the most common infectious disease emergencies involving the central nervous system. Although hosts with cell-mediated immune deficiency (including transplant recipients, diabetic patients, elderly patients, and cancer patients receiving certain chemotherapeutic agents) are at particular risk for *Listeria monocytogenes* meningitis, most cases in adults are due to *S. pneumoniae* (30–50%) and *N. meningitidis* (10–35%). The classic presentation of headache, meningismus, and fever is seen in only one-half to two-thirds of patients. The elderly can present without fever or meningeal signs despite lethargy and confusion. Cerebral dysfunction is evidenced by confusion, delirium, and lethargy that can progress to coma. A fulminant presentation with sepsis and brain edema occurs in some cases; papilledema at presentation is unusual and suggests another diagnosis (e.g., an intracranial lesion). Focal signs, including cranial nerve palsies (IV, VI, VII), can be seen in 10–20% of cases; 50–70% of patients have bacteremia. A poor outcome is associated with coma, hypotension, meningitis due to *S. pneumoniae*, respiratory distress, a CSF glucose level of <0.6 mmol/L (<10 mg/dL), a CSF protein level of >2.5 g/L, a peripheral WBC count of <5000/μL, and a serum sodium level of <135 mmol/L.

Suppurative Intracranial Infections (See also Chap. 376) In suppurative intracranial infections, rare intracranial lesions present along with sepsis and hemodynamic instability. Rapid recognition of the toxic patient with central neurologic signs is crucial to improvement of the dismal prognosis of these entities. *Subdural empyema* arises from the paranasal sinus in 60–70% of cases. Microaerophilic streptococci and staphylococci are the predominant etiologic organisms. The patient is toxic, with fever, headache, and nuchal rigidity. Of all patients, 75% have focal signs and 6–20% die. Despite improved survival rates, 15–44% of patients are left with permanent neurologic deficits. *Septic cavernous sinus thrombosis* follows a facial or sphenoid sinus infection; 70% of cases are due to staphylococci, and the remainder are due primarily to aerobic or anaerobic streptococci. A unilateral or retroorbital headache progresses to a toxic appearance and fever within days. Three-quarters of patients have unilateral periorbital edema that becomes bilateral and then progresses to ptosis, proptosis, ophthalmoplegia, and papilledema. The mortality rate is as high as 30%. *Septic thrombosis of the superior sagittal sinus* spreads from the ethmoid or maxillary sinuses and is caused by *S. pneumoniae*, other streptococci, and staphylococci. The fulminant course is characterized by headache, nausea, vomiting, rapid progression to confusion and coma, nuchal rigidity, and brainstem signs. If the sinus is totally thrombosed, the mortality rate exceeds 80%.

Brain Abscess (See also Chap. 376) Brain abscess often occurs without systemic signs. Almost half of patients are afebrile, and presentations are more consistent with a space-occupying lesion in the brain; 70% of patients have headache, 50% have focal neurologic signs, and 25% have papilledema. Abscesses can present as single or multiple lesions resulting from contiguous foci or hematogenous infection, such as endocarditis. The infection progresses over several days from cerebritis to an abscess with a mature capsule. More than half of infections are polymicrobial, with an etiology consisting of aerobic bacteria (primarily streptococcal species) and anaerobes. Abscesses arising hematogenously are especially apt to rupture into the ventricular space, causing a sudden and severe deterioration in clinical status and high mortality. Otherwise, mortality is low but morbidity is high (30–55%). Patients presenting with stroke and a parameningeal infectious focus, such as sinusitis or otitis, may have a brain abscess, and physicians must maintain a high level of suspicion. Prognosis worsens in patients with a fulminant course, delayed diagnosis, abscess rupture into the ventricles, multiple abscesses, or abnormal neurologic status at presentation.

Cerebral Malaria (See also Chap. 203) This entity should be urgently considered if patients who have recently traveled to areas endemic for malaria present with a febrile illness and lethargy or other neurologic signs. Fulminant malaria is caused by *Plasmodium falciparum* and is associated with temperatures of >40°C (>104°F), hypotension, jaundice, adult respiratory distress syndrome, and bleeding. By definition, any patient with a change in mental status or repeated seizure in the setting of fulminant malaria has cerebral malaria. In adults, this nonspecific febrile illness progresses to coma over several days; occasionally, coma occurs within hours and death within 24 h. Nuchal rigidity and photophobia are rare. On physical examination, symmetric encephalopathy is typical, and upper motor neuron dysfunction with decorticate and decerebrate posturing can be seen in advanced disease. Unrecognized infection results in a 20–30% mortality rate.

Spinal Epidural Abscesses (See also Chap. 372) Patients with spinal epidural abscesses often present with back pain and develop neurologic deficits late in their course. At-risk patients include those with diabetes mellitus; intravenous drug use; chronic alcohol abuse; recent spinal trauma, surgery, or epidural anesthesia; and other comorbid conditions, such as HIV infection. The thoracic or lumbar spine is the most common location; cervical spine infections are associated with worse outcomes. Staphylococci are the most common etiologic agents. This diagnosis must immediately be considered in patients with a history of antecedent back pain and new neurologic symptoms. Almost 60% of patients have fever, and almost 90% have back pain. Paresthesia, bowel and bladder dysfunction, radicular pain, and weakness are frequent neurologic complaints, and examination of the patient may reveal abnormal reflexes and motor and sensory deficits. The ESR and leukocyte counts are usually elevated. Rapid recognition and treatment, which may include surgical drainage, can prevent or minimize permanent neurologic sequelae.

OTHER FOCAL SYNDROMES WITH A FULMINANT COURSE

Infection at virtually any primary focus (e.g., osteomyelitis, pneumonia, pyelonephritis, or cholangitis) can result in bacteremia and sepsis. TSS has been associated with focal infections such as septic arthritis, peritonitis, sinusitis, and wound infection. Rapid clinical deterioration and death can be associated with destruction of the primary site of infection, as is seen in endocarditis and in necrotizing infections of the oropharynx (in which edema suddenly compromises the airway).

Rhinocerebral Mucormycosis (See also Chap. 198) Patients with diabetes or malignancy are at risk for invasive rhinocerebral mucormycosis. Patients present with low-grade fever, dull sinus pain, diplopia, decreased mental status, decreased ocular motion, chemosis, proptosis, dusky or necrotic nasal turbinates, and necrotic hard-palate lesions that respect the midline. Without rapid recognition and intervention, the process continues on an inexorable invasive course, with high mortality.

Acute Bacterial Endocarditis (See also Chap. 118) This entity presents with a much more aggressive course than subacute endocarditis. Bacteria such as *S. aureus, S. pneumoniae, L. monocytogenes, Haemophilus* spp., and streptococci of groups A, B, and G attack native valves. Mortality rates range from 10% to 40%. The host may have comorbid conditions such as underlying malignancy, diabetes mellitus, intravenous drug use, or alcoholism. The patient presents with fever, fatigue, and malaise <2 weeks after onset of infection. On physical examination, a changing murmur and congestive heart failure may be noted. Hemorrhagic macules on palms or soles (*Janeway lesions*) sometimes develop. Petechiae, Roth's spots, splinter hemorrhages, and splenomegaly are unusual. Rapid valvular destruction, particularly of the aortic valve, results in pulmonary edema and hypotension. Myocardial abscesses can form, eroding through the septum or into the conduction system and causing life-threatening arrhythmias or high-degree conduction block. Large friable vegetations can result in major arterial emboli, metastatic infection, or tissue infarction. Emboli can lead to stroke, changes in mental status, visual disturbances, aphasia, ataxia, headache, meningismus, brain abscess, cerebritis, spinal cord infarct with paraplegia, arthralgia, osteomyelitis, splenic abscess, septic arthritis, and hematuria. Older patients with *S. aureus* endocarditis are especially likely to present with nonspecific symptoms—a circumstance that delays diagnosis and worsens prognosis. Rapid intervention is crucial for a successful outcome.

Inhalational Anthrax (See also Chap. 214) Inhalational anthrax, the most severe form of disease caused by *Bacillus anthracis*, had not been reported in the United States for more than 25 years until the recent use of this organism as an agent of bioterrorism (Chap. 214). Patients presented with malaise, fever, cough, nausea, drenching sweats, shortness of breath, and headache. Rhinorrhea was unusual. All patients had abnormal chest roentgenograms at presentation. Pulmonary infiltrates, mediastinal widening, and pleural effusions were the most common findings. Hemorrhagic meningitis was seen in 38% of these patients. Survival was more likely when antibiotics were given during the prodromal period and if multidrug regimens were used. In the absence of urgent intervention with antimicrobial agents and supportive care, inhalational anthrax progresses rapidly to hypotension, cyanosis, and death.

Avian Influenza (H5N1) Infection (See also Chap. 180) Human cases of avian influenza were first reported in Hong Kong. Recent cases have occurred primarily in Southeast Asia, particularly Vietnam. However, evidence of a rapidly expanding geographic distribution of the virus throughout the world is of grave concern. Avian influenza should be considered in patients with severe respiratory tract illness, particularly if they have been exposed to poultry. To date, human-to-human transmission is rare. Patients present with high fever, an influenza-like illness, and lower respiratory tract symptoms. Watery diarrhea may develop and may precede respiratory symptoms. Dyspnea develops a median of 5 days after the onset of symptoms and can progress to respiratory distress syndrome, multiorgan failure, and death within 9–10 days after the onset of illness. Early antiviral treatment with neuraminidase inhibitors should be initiated along with aggressive supportive measures.

Hantavirus Pulmonary Syndrome (See also Chap. 189) Hantavirus pulmonary syndrome (HPS) has been documented in the United States (primarily the southwestern states), Canada, and South America. Most cases occur in rural areas and are associated with exposure to rodents. Patients present with a nonspecific viral prodrome of fever, malaise, myalgias, nausea, vomiting, and dizziness that may progress to pulmonary edema and respiratory failure. HPS causes myocardial depression and increased pulmonary vascular permeability; therefore, careful fluid resuscitation and use of pressor agents are crucial. Aggressive cardiopulmonary support during the first few hours of illness can be life-saving.

CONCLUSION

Acutely ill febrile patients with the syndromes discussed in this chapter require close observation, aggressive supportive measures, and—in most cases—admission to intensive care units. The most important task of the physician is to distinguish these patients from other infected febrile patients who will not progress to fulminant disease. The alert physician must recognize the acute infectious disease emergency and then proceed with appropriate urgency.

FURTHER READINGS

BEIGEL JH et al: Avian influenza A (H5N1) infection in humans. N Engl J Med 353:1374, 2005

DAROUICHE RO: Spinal epidural abscess. N Engl J Med 355:2012, 2006

Hasham S et al: Necrotising fasciitis. BMJ 330:830, 2005

Idro R et al: Pathogenesis, clinical features, and neurological outcome of cerebral malaria. Lancet Neurol 4:827, 2005

Kyaw MH et al: Evaluation of severe infection and survival after splenectomy. Am J Med 119:276.e1, 2006

Nguyen HB et al: Severe sepsis and septic shock: Review of the literature and emergency department management guidelines. Ann Emerg Med 48:28, 2006

Osborn MK, Steinberg JP: Subdural empyema and other suppurative complications of paranasal sinusitis. Lancet Infect Dis 7:62, 2007

Stephens DS et al: Epidemic meningitis, meningococcaemia, and *Neisseria meningitidis*. Lancet 369:2196, 2007

van de Beek D et al: Community-acquired bacterial meningitis in adults. N Engl J Med 354:44, 2006

Wills BA et al: Comparison of three fluid solutions for resuscitation in dengue shock syndrome. N Engl J Med 353:877, 2005

116 Immunization Principles and Vaccine Use

Gerald T. Keusch, Kenneth J. Bart, Mark Miller

Vaccines play a special role in the health and security of nations. The World Health Organization (WHO) cites immunization and the provision of clean water as the two public health interventions that have had the greatest impact on the world's health, and the World Bank notes that vaccines are among the most cost-effective health interventions available. Over the past century, the integration of immunization into routine health care services in many countries has provided caregivers with some degree of control over disease-related morbidity and mortality, especially among infants and children.

Despite these extraordinary successes, vaccines and their constituents (e.g., the mercury compound thimerosal, formerly used as a preservative) have come under attack in some countries as causes of neurodevelopmental disorders, such as autism and attention-deficit hyperactivity disorder; diabetes; and a variety of allergic and autoimmune diseases. Although millions of lives are saved by vaccines each year and countless cases of postinfection disability are averted, some segments of the public are increasingly unwilling to accept any risk whatsoever of vaccine-associated complications (severe or otherwise), and resistance to vaccination is growing.

No medical procedure is absolutely risk-free, and the risk to the individual must always be balanced with benefits to the individual and to the population at large. This dichotomy poses two essential challenges for the medical and public health communities with respect to vaccines: (1) to create more effective and ever-safer vaccines, and (2) to educate patients and the general public more fully about the benefits as well as the risks of vaccine use. Because immunity to infectious diseases is acquired only by infection itself or by immunization, sustained vaccination programs for each birth cohort will continue to be necessary to control vaccine-preventable infectious diseases until and unless their etiologic agents can be eradicated from every region of the world.

An unwavering scientific and public health commitment to immunization is essential in countering public distrust and political pressure to legislate well-intentioned but ill-informed vaccine safety laws in response to the concerns of organized antivaccine advocacy groups. Ironically, it is the public health success of vaccines that has created a significant part of the problem: because the major fatal and disabling diseases of childhood are only rarely seen today in the United States, parents and young practitioners most likely will never have seen tetanus, diphtheria, *Haemophilus influenzae* disease, polio, or measles. Under these circumstances, the risks of immunization can easily (if erroneously) be perceived to outweigh the benefits, and this perception can be fueled by inaccurate information, poor science, and zealous advocacy. Caregivers must be prepared to educate parents about the importance of childhood immunization and to address their concerns effectively.

The medical community must also appreciate public concern about the sheer number of vaccines now licensed and the attendant fear that the more vaccines are administered, the more likely it is that complications and adverse immunologic consequences will occur. More than 50 biologic products are presently licensed in the United States, and dozens of antigens (many of them components of vaccine-combination products) are recommended for routine immunization of infants, children, adolescents, and adults (Figs. 116-1 and 116-2). Moreover, new vaccines are continually becoming available—e.g., human papillomavirus (HPV) vaccine for use in adolescent girls to prevent cervical cancer (Chap. 178) and a herpes zoster vaccine to prevent zoster (Chap. 173). Still other vaccines are used in special situations, including responses to outbreaks (e.g., polio), prophylaxis in travelers (e.g., yellow fever), and fulfillment of regional requirements (e.g., Japanese B encephalitis).

Of course, for many serious infectious agents, such as eukaryotic pathogens (protozoa and helminths) and HIV, effective and safe vaccines remain only a hope for the future. Current concern about the potential for a human pandemic of H5N1 avian influenza, against which a vaccine product is lacking, underscores the lag time between emerging public health needs and vaccine development programs.

The U.S. government's document *Healthy People 2010 Objectives for the Nation* includes a set of immunization indicators. The goals are for 80% of children to receive diphtheria–tetanus–acellular pertussis (DTaP), poliovirus, measles-mumps-rubella (MMR), *H. influenzae* type b (Hib), and hepatitis B vaccines and for 90% of adults to receive influenza and pneumococcal vaccines by 2010. Unfortunately, even these modest goals may not be attained in the United States.

IMPACT OF IMMUNIZATION

The epidemiologically appropriate use of vaccine resulted in the global eradication of smallpox, permitting the cessation of routine smallpox vaccination. Unfortunately, recent concerns about the potential use of smallpox virus for bioterrorism have led to renewed consideration of the need for routine smallpox immunization and for a new, effective, and much safer smallpox vaccine. Immunization has eliminated naturally transmitted poliomyelitis from the Western Hemisphere, Europe, and the western Pacific. However, polio has recrudesced in some countries in Africa, the Middle East, and parts of Asia because of interruption (for a variety of reasons) of immunization programs. Measles, which affected nearly 100% of children in the prevaccination era, has been effectively eliminated from most of the Western Hemisphere by widespread immunization; a global campaign to reduce measles mortality rates elsewhere is under way. The virtual elimination of rubella and congenital rubella syndrome, neonatal tetanus, and diphtheria in the United States is entirely due to vaccination. The introduction of Hib conjugate vaccines for immunization of infants has all but eliminated invasive Hib infections (including meningitis and pneumonia) among children <5 years of age. This vaccine both elicits durable immunity by the time maternal-derived antibodies dissipate and reduces nasopharyngeal carriage of Hib, thus diminishing the risk of transmission. The introduction of polyvalent pneumococcal polysaccharide conjugate vaccine is beginning to have a significant impact on serious invasive pneumococcal diseases, including otitis media. Vaccine has reduced the incidence of varicella by 70–87% in high-coverage areas. In short, vaccines work.

DEFINITIONS

The terms *vaccination* and *immunization* are often used interchangeably, although technically the former denotes the administration of a vaccine, whereas the latter refers to the induction or provision of immunity by any means, active or passive. Thus vaccination does not guarantee immunization, and immunization may not involve vaccine.

Recommended Immunization Schedule for Persons Aged 0–6 Years
UNITED STATES • 2007

Vaccine ▼ / Age ▶	Birth	1 month	2 months	4 months	6 months	12 months	15 months	18 months	19–23 months	2–3 years	4–6 years
Hepatitis B[1]	HepB	HepB		see footnote 1	HepB				HepB Series		
Rotavirus[2]			Rota	Rota	Rota						
Diphtheria, Tetanus, Pertussis[3]			DTaP	DTaP	DTaP		DTaP				DTaP
Haemophilus influenzae type b[4]			Hib	Hib	*Hib*[4]	Hib		Hib			
Pneumococcal[5]			PCV	PCV	PCV	PCV				PCV PPV	
Inactivated Poliovirus			IPV	IPV	IPV						IPV
Influenza[6]					Influenza (Yearly)						
Measles, Mumps, Rubella[7]						MMR					MMR
Varicella[8]						Varicella					Varicella
Hepatitis A[9]						HepA (2 doses)				HepA Series	
Meningococcal[10]										MPSV4	

A

Range of recommended ages — Catch-up immunization — Certain high-risk groups

FIGURE 116-1 These schedules indicate the recommended ages for routine administration of currently licensed childhood vaccines, as of December 1, 2006, for children aged 0–6 and 7–18 years. Additional information is available at http://www.cdc.gov/nip/recs/child-schedule.htm. Any dose not administered at the recommended age should be administered at any subsequent visit, when indicated and feasible. Additional vaccines may be licensed and recommended during the year. Licensed combination vaccines may be used whenever any components of the combination are indicated and other components of the vaccine are not contraindicated and if approved by the Food and Drug Administration for that dose of the series. Providers should consult the respective Advisory Committee on Immunization Practices statement for detailed recommendations. Clinically significant adverse events that follow immunization should be reported to the Vaccine Adverse Event Reporting System (VAERS). Guidance about how to obtain and complete a VAERS form is available at http://www.vaers.hhs.gov or by telephone, 800-822-7967.

A. Recommended immunization schedule for persons aged 0–6 years—United States, 2006–2007. **1. Hepatitis B vaccine (HepB).** *(Minimum age: birth)* **At birth:** Administer monovalent HepB to all newborns before hospital discharge. If mother is hepatitis surface antigen (HBsAg)-positive, administer HepB and 0.5 mL of hepatitis B immune globulin (HBIG) within 12 hours of birth. If mother's HBsAg status is unknown, administer HepB within 12 hours of birth. Determine the HBsAg status as soon as possible and if HBsAg-positive, administer HBIG (no later than age 1 week). If mother is HBsAg-negative, the birth dose can only be delayed with physician's order and mother's negative HBsAg laboratory report documented in the infant's medical record. **After the birth dose:** The HepB series should be completed with either monovalent HepB or a combination vaccine containing HepB. The second dose should be administered at age 1–2 months. The final dose should be administered at age ≥24 weeks. Infants born to HBsAg-positive mothers should be tested for HBsAg and antibody to HBsAg after completion of ≥3 doses of a licensed HepB series, at age 9–18 months (generally at the next well-child visit). **4-month dose:** It is permissible to administer 4 doses of HepB when combination vaccines are administered after the birth dose. If monovalent HepB is used for doses after the birth dose, a dose at age 4 months is not needed. **2. Rotavirus vaccine (Rota).** *(Minimum age: 6 weeks)* Administer the first dose at age 6–12 weeks. Do not start the series later than age 12 weeks. Administer the final dose in the series by age 32 weeks. Do not administer a dose later than age 32 weeks. Data on safety and efficacy outside of these age ranges are insufficient. **3. Diphtheria and tetanus toxoids and acellular pertussis vaccine (DTaP).** *(Minimum age: 6 weeks)* The fourth dose of DTaP may be administered as early as age 12 months, provided 6 months have elapsed since the third dose. Administer the final dose in the series at age 4–6 years. **4. *Haemophilus influenzae* type b conjugate vaccine (Hib).** *(Minimum age: 6 weeks)* If PRP-OMP (PedvaxHIB or ComVax [Merck]) is administered at ages 2 and 4 months, a dose at age 6 months is not required. TriHiBit (DTaP/Hib) combination products should not be used for primary immunization but can be used as boosters following any Hib vaccine in children aged ≥12 months. **5. Pneumococcal vaccine.** *(Minimum age: 6 weeks for pneumococcal conjugate vaccine [PCV]; 2 years for pneumococcal polysaccharide vaccine [PPV]).* Administer PCV at ages 24–59 months in certain high-risk groups. Administer PPV to children aged ≥2 years in certain high-risk groups. See MMWR 2000;49(No. RR-9):1–35. **6. Influenza vaccine.** *(Minimum age: 6 months for trivalent inactivated influenza vaccine [TIV]; 5 years for live, attenuated influenza vaccine [LAIV]).* All children aged 6–59 months and close contacts of all children aged 0–59 months are recommended to receive influenza vaccine. Influenza vaccine is recommended annually for children aged ≥59 months with certain risk factors, health-care workers, and other persons (including household members) in close contact with persons in groups at high risk. See MMWR 2006;55(No. RR-10):1–41. For healthy persons aged 5–49 years, LAIV may be used as an alternative to TIV. Children receiving TIV should receive 0.25 mL if aged 6–35 months or 0.5 mL if aged ≥3 years. Children aged <9 years who are receiving influenza vaccine for the first time should receive 2 doses (separated by ≥4 weeks for TIV and ≥6 weeks for LAIV). **7. Measles, mumps, and rubella vaccine (MMR).** *(Minimum age: 12 months)* Administer the second dose of MMR at age 4–6 years. MMR may be administered before age 4–6 years, provided ≥4 weeks have elapsed since the first dose and both doses are administered at age ≥12 months. **8. Varicella vaccine.** *(Minimum age: 12 months)* Administer the second dose of varicella vaccine at age 4–6 years. Varicella vaccine may be administered before age 4–6 years, provided that ≥3 months have elapsed since the first dose and both doses are administered at age ≥12 months. If second dose was administered ≥28 days following the first dose, the second dose does not need to be repeated.

(continued)

Recommended Immunization Schedule for Persons Aged 7–18 Years
UNITED STATES • 2007

Vaccine ▼ / Age ▶	7–10 years	11–12 YEARS	13–14 years	15 years	16–18 years
Tetanus, Diphtheria, Pertussis [1]	see footnote 1	Tdap		Tdap	
Human Papillomavirus [2]	see footnote 2	HPV (3 doses)		HPV Series	
Meningococcal [3]	MPSV4	MCV4		MCV4 [3] MCV4	
Pneumococcal [4]		PPV			
Influenza [5]		Influenza (Yearly)			
Hepatitis A [6]		HepA Series			
Hepatitis B [7]		HepB Series			
Inactivated Poliovirus [8]		IPV Series			
Measles, Mumps, Rubella [9]		MMR Series			
Varicella [10]		Varicella Series			

B

Range of recommended ages — Catch-up immunization — Certain high-risk groups

FIGURE 116-1 ***(Continued)***

9. Hepatitis A vaccine (HepA). *(Minimum age: 12 months)* HepA is recommended for all children aged 1 year (i.e., aged 12–23 months). The 2 doses in the series should be administered at least 6 months apart. Children not fully vaccinated by age 2 years can be vaccinated at subsequent visits. HepA is recommended for certain other groups of children, including in areas where vaccination programs target older children. See MMWR 2006;55(No. RR-7):1–23. **10. Meningococcal polysaccharide vaccine (MPSV4).** *(Minimum age: 2 years)* Administer MPSV4 to children aged 2–10 years with terminal complement deficiencies or anatomic or functional asplenia and certain other high-risk groups. See MMWR 2005;54(No. RR-7):1–21.

B. Recommended immunization schedule for persons aged 7–18 years—United States, 2006–2007. **1. Tetanus and diphtheria toxoids and acellular pertussis vaccine (Tdap).** *(Minimum age: 10 years for BOOSTRIX and 11 years for ADACEL)* Administer at age 11–12 years for those who have completed the recommended childhood DTP/DTaP vaccination series and have not received a tetanus and diphtheria toxoids vaccine (Td) booster dose. Adolescents aged 13–18 years who missed the 11–12 year Td/Tdap booster dose should also receive a single dose of Tdap if they have completed the recommended childhood DTP/DTaP vaccination series. **2. Human papillomavirus vaccine (HPV).** *(Minimum age: 9 years)* Administer the first dose of the HPV vaccine series to females at age 11–12 years. Administer the second dose 2 months after the first dose and the third dose 6 months after the first dose. Administer the HPV vaccine series to females at age 13–18 years if not previously vaccinated. **3. Meningococcal vaccine.** *(Minimum age: 11 years for meningococcal conjugate vaccine [MCV4]; 2 years for meningococcal polysaccharide vaccine [MPSV4]).* Administer MCV4 at age 11–12 years and to previously unvaccinated adolescents at high school entry (at approximately age 15 years). Administer MCV4 to previously unvaccinated college freshmen living in dormitories; MPSV4 is an acceptable alternative. Vaccination against invasive meningococcal disease is recommended for children and adolescents aged ≥2 years with terminal complement deficiencies or anatomic or functional asplenia and certain other high-risk groups. See MMWR 2005;54(No. RR-7):1–21. Use MPSV4 for children aged 2–10 years and MCV4 or MPSV4 for older children. **4. Pneumococcal polysaccharide vaccine (PPV).** *(Minimum age: 2 years)* Administer for certain high-risk groups. See MMWR 1997;46(No. RR-8):1–24, and MMWR 2000;49(No. RR-9):1–35. **5. Influenza vaccine.** *(Minimum age: 6 months for trivalent inactivated influenza vaccine [TIV]; 5 years for live, attenuated influenza vaccine [LAIV]).* Influenza vaccine is recommended annually for persons with certain risk factors, health-care workers, and other persons (including household members) in close contact with persons in groups at high risk. See MMWR 2006;55 (No. RR-10):1–41. For healthy persons aged 5–49 years, LAIV may be used as an alternative to TIV. Children aged <9 years who are receiving influenza vaccine for the first time should receive 2 doses (separated by ≥4 weeks for TIV and ≥6 weeks for LAIV). **6. Hepatitis A vaccine (HepA).** *(Minimum age: 12 months)* The 2 doses in the series should be administered at least 6 months apart. HepA is recommended for certain other groups of children, including in areas where vaccination programs target older children. See MMWR 2006;55 (No. RR-7):1–23. **7. Hepatitis B vaccine (HepB).** *(Minimum age: birth)* Administer the 3-dose series to those who were not previously vaccinated. A 2-dose series of Recombivax HB is licensed for children aged 11–15 years. **8. Inactivated poliovirus vaccine (IPV).** *(Minimum age: 6 weeks)* For children who received an all-IPV or all-oral poliovirus (OPV) series, a fourth dose is not necessary if the third dose was administered at age ≥4 years. If both OPV and IPV were administered as part of a series, a total of 4 doses should be administered, regardless of the child's current age. **9. Measles, mumps, and rubella vaccine (MMR).** *(Minimum age: 12 months)* If not previously vaccinated, administer 2 doses of MMR during any visit, with ≥4 weeks between the doses. **10. Varicella vaccine.** *(Minimum age: 12 months)* Administer 2 doses of varicella vaccine to persons without evidence of immunity. Administer 2 doses of varicella vaccine to persons aged <13 years at least 3 months apart. Do not repeat the second dose, if administered ≥28 days after the first dose. Administer 2 doses of varicella vaccine to persons aged ≥13 years at least 4 weeks apart.

Recommended Adult Immunization Schedule
United States, October 2006–September 2007

Recommended adult immunization schedule, by vaccine and age group

Vaccine ▼ / Age group (yrs) ►	19–49 years	50–64 years	≥65 years
Tetanus, diphtheria, pertussis (Td/Tdap)[1]*	1-dose Td booster every 10 yrs; Substitute 1 dose of Tdap for Td	1-dose Td booster every 10 yrs; Substitute 1 dose of Tdap for Td	1-dose Td booster every 10 yrs
Human papillomavirus (HPV)[2]*	3 doses (females)		
Measles, mumps, rubella (MMR)[3]*	1 or 2 doses	1 dose	1 dose
Varicella[4]*	2 doses (0, 4–8 wks)	2 doses (0, 4–8 wks)	
Influenza[5]*	1 dose annually	1 dose annually	1 dose annually
Pneumococcal (polysaccharide)[6,7]	1–2 doses	1–2 doses	1 dose
Hepatitis A[8]*	2 doses (0, 6–12 mos, or 0, 6–18 mos)	2 doses (0, 6–12 mos, or 0, 6–18 mos)	2 doses (0, 6–12 mos, or 0, 6–18 mos)
Hepatitis B[9]*	3 doses (0, 1–2, 4–6 mos)	3 doses (0, 1–2, 4–6 mos)	3 doses (0, 1–2, 4–6 mos)
Meningococcal[10]	1 or more doses	1 or more doses	1 or more doses

Light bar: For all persons in this category who meet the age requirements and who lack evidence of immunity (e.g., lack documentation of vaccination or have no evidence of prior infection)

Dark bar: Recommended if some other risk factor is present (e.g., on the basis of medical, occupational, lifestyle, or other indications)

FIGURE 116-2 Recommended adult immunization schedule, by vaccine and age group—United States, 2006–2007. This schedule indicates the recommended age groups for routine administration of currently licensed vaccines for persons aged ≥19 years, as of October 1, 2006. Licensed combination vaccines may be used whenever any components of the combination are indicated and when the vaccine's other components are not contraindicated. For detailed recommendations on all vaccines, including those used primarily for travelers or that are issued during the year, consult the manufacturers' package inserts and the complete statements from the Advisory Committee on Immunization Practices (*http://www.cdc.gov/nip/publications/acip-list.htm*). Report all clinically significant postvaccination reactions to the Vaccine Adverse Event Reporting System (VAERS). Reporting forms and instructions on filing a VAERs report are available at *http://vaers.hhs.gov* or by telephone, 800-822-7967. Information on how to file a Vaccine Injury Compensation Program claim is available at *http://www.hrsa.gov/vaccinecompensation* or by telephone, 800-338-2382. To file a claim for vaccine injury, contact the U.S. Court of Federal Claims, 717 Madison Place, N.W., Washington, DC, 20005; telephone, 202-357-6400. Additional information about the vaccines in this schedule and contraindications for vaccination is also available at *http://www.cdc.gov/nip* or from the CDC-INFO Contact Center at 800-CDC-INFO (800-232-4636) in English and Spanish, 24 hours a day, 7 days a week.

1. Tetanus, diphtheria, and acellular pertussis (Td/Tdap) vaccination. Adults with uncertain histories of a complete primary vaccination series with diphtheria and tetanus toxoid–containing vaccines should begin or complete a primary vaccination series. A primary series for adults is 3 doses; administer the first 2 doses at least 4 weeks apart and the third dose 6–12 months after the second. Administer a booster dose to adults who have completed a primary series and if the last vaccination was received ≥10 years previously. Tdap or tetanus and diphtheria (Td) vaccine may be used; Tdap should replace a single dose of Td for adults aged <65 years who have not previously received a dose of Tdap (either in the primary series, as a booster, or for wound management). Only one of two Tdap products (Adacel [sanofi pasteur]) is licensed for use in adults. If the person is pregnant and received the last Td vaccination ≥10 years previously, administer Td during the second or third trimester; if the person received the last Td vaccination in <10 years, administer Tdap during the immediate postpartum period. A one-time administration of 1 dose of Tdap with an interval as short as 2 years from a previous Td vaccination is recommended for postpartum women, close contacts of infants aged <12 months, and all healthcare workers with direct patient contact. In certain situations, Td can be deferred during pregnancy and Tdap substituted in the immediate postpartum period, or Tdap can be given instead of Td to a pregnant woman after an informed discussion with the woman (see *www.cdc.gov/nip/publications/acip-list.htm*). Consult the ACIP statement for recommendations for administering Td as prophylaxis in wound management (*www.cdc.gov/mmwr/preview/mmwrhtml/00041645.htm*). **2. Human papillomavirus (HPV) vaccination.** HPV vaccination is recommended for all women aged ≤ 26 years who have not completed the vaccine series. Ideally, vaccine should be administered before potential exposure to HPV through sexual activity; however, women who are sexually active should still be vaccinated. Sexually active women who have not been infected with any of the HPV vaccine types receive the full benefit of the vaccination. Vaccination is less beneficial for women who have already been infected with one or more of the four HPV vaccine types. A complete series consists of 3 doses. The second dose should be administered 2 months after the first dose; the third dose should be administered 6 months after the first dose. Vaccination is not recommended during pregnancy. If a woman is found to be pregnant after initiating the vaccination series, the remainder of the 3-dose regimen should be delayed until after completion of the pregnancy. **3. Measles, mumps, rubella (MMR) vaccination.** *Measles component:* adults born before 1957 can be considered immune to measles. Adults born during or after 1957 should receive ≥1 dose of MMR unless they have a medical contraindication, documentation of ≥1 dose, history of measles based on healthcare provider diagnosis, or laboratory evidence of immunity. A second dose of MMR is recommended for adults who (1) have been recently exposed to measles or in an outbreak setting; (2) have been previously vaccinated with killed measles vaccine; (3) have been vaccinated with an unknown type of measles vaccine during 1963–1967; (4) are students in postsecondary educational institutions; (5) work in a healthcare facility; or (6) plan to travel internationally. Withhold MMR or other measles-containing vaccines from HIV-infected persons with severe immunosuppression. *Mumps component:* adults born before 1957 can generally be considered immune to mumps. Adults born during or after 1957 should receive 1 dose of MMR unless they have a medical contraindication, history of mumps based on healthcare provider diagnosis, or laboratory evidence of immunity.

(continued)

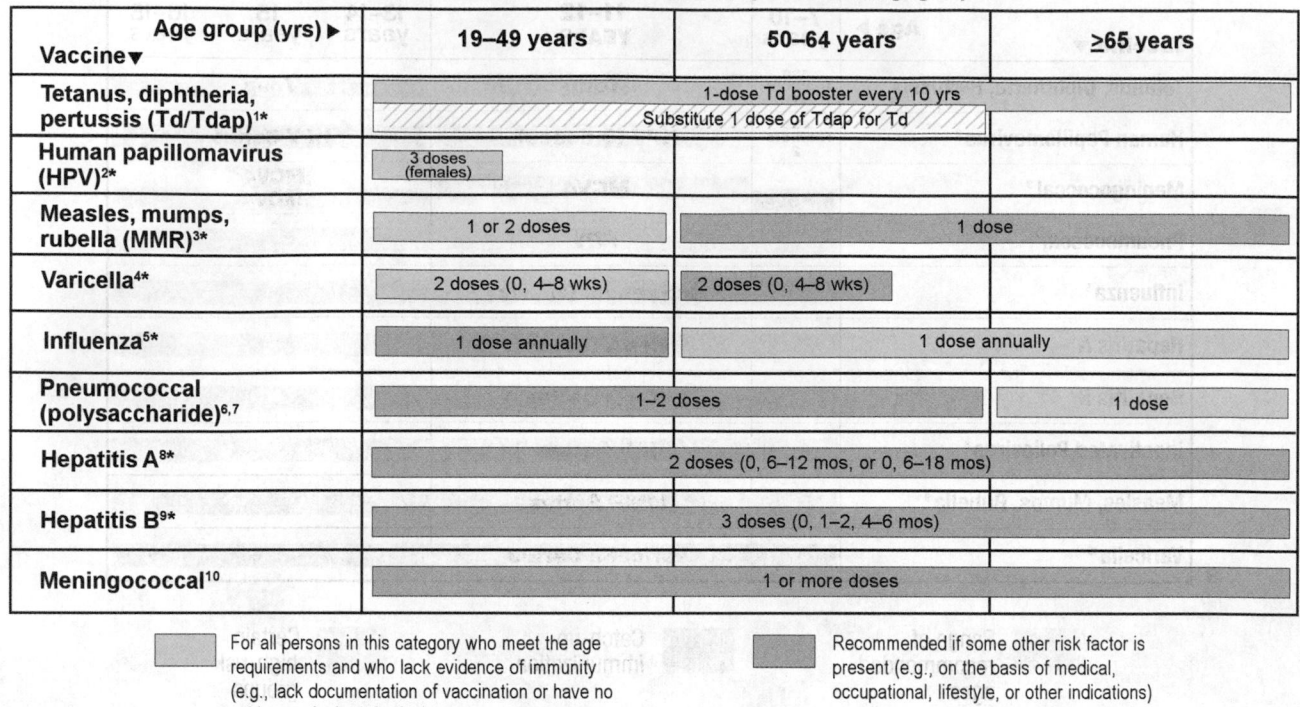

FIGURE 116-2 (*Continued*)

A second dose of MMR is recommended for adults who (1) are in an age group that is affected during a mumps outbreak; (2) are students in postsecondary educational institutions; (3) work in a healthcare facility; or (4) plan to travel internationally. For unvaccinated healthcare workers born before 1957 who do not have other evidence of mumps immunity, consider giving 1 dose on a routine basis and strongly consider giving a second dose during an outbreak. *Rubella component:* administer 1 dose of MMR vaccine to women whose rubella vaccination history is unreliable or who lack laboratory evidence of immunity. For women of childbearing age, regardless of birth year, routinely determine rubella immunity and counsel women regarding congenital rubella syndrome. Do not vaccinate women who are pregnant or who might become pregnant within 4 weeks of receiving vaccine. Women who do not have evidence of immunity should receive MMR vaccine upon completion or termination of pregnancy and before discharge from the healthcare facility. **4. Varicella vaccination.** All adults without evidence of immunity to varicella should receive 2 doses of varicella vaccine. Special consideration should be given to those who (1) have close contact with persons at high risk for severe disease (e.g., healthcare workers and family contacts of immunocompromised persons) or (2) are at high risk for exposure or transmission (e.g., teachers of young children; child care employees; residents and staff members of institutional settings, including correctional institutions; college students; military personnel; adolescents and adults living in households with children; nonpregnant women of childbearing age; and international travelers). Evidence of immunity to varicella in adults includes any of the following: (1) documentation of 2 doses of varicella vaccine at least 4 weeks apart; (2) U.S.-born before 1980 (although for healthcare workers and pregnant women, birth before 1980 should not be considered evidence of immunity); (3) history of varicella based on diagnosis or verification of varicella by a healthcare provider (for a patient reporting a history of or presenting with an atypical case, a mild case, or both, healthcare providers should seek either an epidemiologic link with a typical varicella case or evidence of laboratory confirmation, if it was performed at the time of acute disease); (4) history of herpes zoster based on healthcare provider diagnosis; or (5) laboratory evidence of immunity or laboratory confirmation of disease. Do not vaccinate women who are pregnant or might become pregnant within 4 weeks of receiving the vaccine. Assess pregnant women for evidence of varicella immunity. Women who do not have evidence of immunity should receive dose 1 of varicella vaccine upon completion or termination of pregnancy and before discharge from the healthcare facility. Dose 2 should be administered 4–8 weeks after dose 1. **5. Influenza vaccination.** *Medical indications:* chronic disorders of the cardiovascular or pulmonary systems, including asthma; chronic metabolic diseases, including diabetes mellitus, renal dysfunction, hemoglobinopathies, or immunosuppression (including immunosuppression caused by medications or HIV); any condition that compromises respiratory function or the handling of respiratory secretions or that can increase the risk of aspiration (e.g., cognitive dysfunction, spinal cord injury, or seizure disorder or other neuromuscular disorder); and pregnancy during the influenza season. No data exist on the risk for severe or complicated influenza disease among persons with asplenia; however, influenza is a risk factor for secondary bacterial infections that can cause severe disease among persons with asplenia. *Occupational indications:* healthcare workers and employees of long-term-care and assisted living facilities. *Other indications:* residents of nursing homes and other long-term–care and assisted living facilities; persons likely to transmit influenza to persons at high risk (e.g., in-home household contacts and caregivers of children aged 0–59 months, or persons of all ages with high-risk conditions); and anyone who would like to be vaccinated. Healthy, nonpregnant persons aged 5–49 years without high-risk medical conditions who are not contacts of severely immunocompromised persons in special care units can receive either intranasally administered influenza vaccine (FluMist) or inactivated vaccine. Other persons should receive the inactivated vaccine. **6. Pneumococcal polysaccharide vaccination.** *Medical indications:* chronic disorders of the pulmonary system (excluding asthma); cardiovascular diseases; diabetes mellitus; chronic liver diseases, including liver disease as a result of alcohol abuse (e.g., cirrhosis); chronic renal failure or nephrotic syndrome; functional or anatomic asplenia (e.g., sickle cell disease or splenectomy [if elective splenectomy is planned, vaccinate at least 2 weeks before surgery]); immunosuppressive conditions (e.g., congenital immunodeficiency, HIV infection [vaccinate as close to diagnosis as possible when CD4 cell counts are highest], leukemia, lymphoma, multiple myeloma, Hodgkin disease, generalized malignancy, or organ or bone marrow transplantation); chemotherapy with alkylating agents, antimetabolites, or high-dose, long-term corticosteroids; and cochlear implants. *Other indications:* Alaska Natives and certain American Indian populations and residents of nursing homes or other long-term–care facilities. **7. Revaccination with pneumococcal polysaccharide vaccine.** One-time revaccination after 5 years for persons with chronic renal failure or nephrotic syndrome; functional or anatomic asplenia (e.g., sickle cell disease or splenectomy); immunosuppressive conditions (e.g., congenital immunodeficiency, HIV infection, leukemia, lymphoma, multiple myeloma, Hodgkin disease, generalized malignancy, or organ or bone marrow transplantation); or chemotherapy with alkylating agents, antimetabolites, or high-dose, long-term corticosteroids. For persons aged ≥65 years, one-time revaccination if they were vaccinated ≥5 years previously and were aged <65 years at the time of primary vaccination. **8. Hepatitis A vaccination.** *Medical indications:* persons with chronic liver disease and persons who receive clotting factor concentrates. *Behavioral indications:* men who have sex with men and persons who use illegal drugs. *Occupational indications:* persons working with hepatitis A virus (HAV)–infected primates or with HAV in a research laboratory setting. *Other indications:* persons traveling to or working in countries that have high or intermediate endemicity of hepatitis A (a list of countries is available at *www.cdc.gov/travel/diseases.htm*) and any person who would like to obtain immunity. Current vaccines should be administered in a 2-dose schedule at either 0 and 6–12 months, or 0 and 6–18 months. If the combined hepatitis A and hepatitis B vaccine is used, administer 3 doses at 0, 1, and 6 months. **9. Hepatitis B vaccination.** *Medical indications:* persons with end-stage renal disease, including patients receiving hemodialysis; persons seeking evaluation or treatment for a sexually transmitted disease (STD); persons with HIV infection; persons with chronic liver disease; and persons who receive clotting factor concentrates. *Occupational indications:* healthcare workers and public-safety workers who are exposed to blood or other potentially infectious body fluids. *Behavioral indications:* sexually active persons who are not in a long-term, mutually monogamous relationship (i.e., persons with >1 sex partner during the previous 6 months); current or recent injection-drug users; and men who have sex with men. *Other indications:* household contacts and sex partners of persons with chronic hepatitis B virus (HBV) infection; clients and staff members of institutions for persons with developmental disabilities; all clients of STD clinics; international travelers to countries with high or intermediate prevalence of chronic HBV infection (a list of countries is available at *www.cdc.gov/travel/diseases.htm*); and any adult seeking protection from HBV infection. Settings where hepatitis B vaccination is recommended for all adults: STD treatment facilities; HIV testing and treatment facilities; facilities providing drug-abuse treatment and prevention services; healthcare settings providing services for injection-drug users or men who have sex with men; correctional facilities; end-stage renal disease programs and facilities for chronic hemodialysis patients; and institutions and nonresidential daycare facilities for persons with developmental disabilities. *Special formulation indications:* for adult patients receiving hemodialysis and other immunocompromised adults, 1 dose of 40 μg/mL (Recombivax HB) or 2 doses of 20 μg/mL (Engerix-B). **10. Meningococcal vaccination.** *Medical indications:* adults with anatomic or functional asplenia, or terminal complement component deficiencies. *Other indications:* first-year college students living in dormitories; microbiologists who are routinely exposed to isolates of *Neisseria meningitidis*; military recruits; and persons who travel to or live in countries in which meningococcal disease is hyperendemic or epidemic (e.g., the "meningitis belt" of sub-Saharan Africa during the dry season [December–June]), particularly if their contact with local populations will be prolonged. Vaccination is required by the government of Saudi Arabia for all travelers to Mecca during the annual Hajj. Meningococcal conjugate vaccine is preferred for adults with any of the preceding indications who are aged ≤ 55 years, although meningococcal polysaccharide vaccine (MPSV4) is an acceptable alternative. Revaccination after 5 years might be indicated for adults previously vaccinated with MPSV4 who remain at high risk for infection (e.g., persons residing in areas in which disease is epidemic).

The immune system, composed of a variety of cell types and soluble factors, is geared toward the recognition of and response to "foreign" substances termed *antigens*. Vaccines convey antigens from living or killed microorganisms (or protein or carbohydrate molecules derived from these antigens) to elicit immune responses that are generally protective but can occasionally backfire and cause harm to the recipient. Specific immune responses, which interrupt the infectious process, generally take the form of immunoglobulin proteins called *antibodies* and/or activated immune cells that recognize particular antigens from an infectious agent. Immunity is medically induced by active or passive immunization. *Active immunization*—i.e., the administration of a vaccine—induces immunity that is usually long-lasting and is sometimes life-long. In contrast, *passive immunization*—i.e., the administration of exogenously produced immune substances or of protective products made in animals—elicits temporary immunity that dissipates with the turnover of the administered protective substances. Used together, the two methods can produce a complementary effect; this is the case, for example, with the coadministration of hepatitis B vaccine and hepatitis B immune globulin. Caution is required, however: the combination of active and passive immunization can also interfere with the development of immunity—e.g., when measles vaccine is administered within 6 weeks of measles immunoglobulin.

When multiple species or serotypes of an organism exist and share common, cross-reactive antigens, vaccination may induce broad immunity to all or most of the related forms or may result in serotype-specific immunity against the immunizing strain alone. One of the virtues of whole-organism vaccines is their potential to contain all the protective antigens of the organism. This advantage is balanced by the possibility of adverse responses to reactive but nonprotective antigens present in the mix. Because the immune response is genetically controlled, all individuals cannot be expected to respond identically to the same vaccine. Additional vaccine constituents affect immunogenicity, efficacy, and safety and may render one formulation superior to another formulation of the same antigens (see "Adjuvants," below).

Approaches to Active Immunization The two standard approaches to active immunization are (1) the use of live, generally attenuated infectious agents (e.g., measles virus); and (2) the use of inactivated agents (e.g., influenza virus), their constituents (e.g., *Bordetella pertussis*), or their products, which are now commonly obtainable through genetic engineering (e.g., hepatitis B vaccine). For many diseases (e.g., poliomyelitis), both live and inactivated vaccines have been employed, each offering advantages and disadvantages.

Live attenuated vaccines consisting of selected or genetically altered organisms that are avirulent or dramatically attenuated, yet remain immunogenic, typically generate long-lasting immunity. These vaccines are designed to cause a subclinical or mild illness and an immune response that mimics natural infection. They offer the advantage of microbial replication in vivo, which simulates natural infection; they may confer life-long protection with one dose; they can present all potential antigens, including those made only in vivo, thus overcoming immunogenetic restrictions in some hosts; and they can reach the local sites most relevant to the induction of protective immunity.

Nonliving vaccines typically require multiple doses and periodic boosters for the maintenance of immunity. The exceptions to this rule are the pure polysaccharide vaccines, whose effects cannot be boosted by additional exposures because polysaccharides do not elicit immunologic memory. Nonliving vaccines administered parenterally fail to induce mucosal immunity because they lack a delivery system that can effectively transport them to local mucosal antigen-processing cells. Nonetheless, nonliving parenteral vaccines can be extremely efficacious. For example, hepatitis A vaccine appears to be effective in nearly 100% of recipients. Currently available nonliving vaccines consist of inactivated whole organisms (e.g., plague vaccine), detoxified protein exotoxins (e.g., tetanus toxoid), recombinant protein antigens (e.g., hepatitis B vaccine), or carbohydrate antigens—either soluble purified capsular material (e.g., serotype-specific *Streptococcus pneumoniae* polysaccharides) or polysaccharide conjugated to a protein carrier to induce a memory response (e.g., Hib polysaccharide conjugated to a suitable protein moiety).

Despite their many advantages, live vaccines are not always preferable. For example, after several decades of extensive use, live oral polio vaccine (OPV) is no longer recommended in the United States because of the rare but real risk of vaccine-associated polio due to reversion to virulence. However, the WHO continues to recommend OPV for use in the developing world because of lower costs and logistical advantages.

Approaches to Passive Immunization Passive immunization is generally used to provide temporary immunity in a person exposed to an infectious disease who has not been actively immunized; this situation can arise when active immunization is unavailable (e.g., for respiratory syncytial virus) or when active immunization simply has not been implemented before exposure (e.g., for rabies). Passive immunization is used in the treatment of certain illnesses associated with toxins (e.g., diphtheria) as well as for some snake and spider bites and as a specific or nonspecific immunosuppressant [Rho(D) immune globulin and antilymphocyte globulin, respectively]. Three types of preparations can be used in passive immunization: (1) standard human immune serum globulin for IM or IV administration; (2) special immune serum globulins with a known content of antibody to specific agents (e.g., hepatitis B virus or varicella-zoster immune globulin); and (3) specific animal antisera and antitoxins.

Postexposure Immunization For certain infections, active or passive immunization soon after exposure can prevent or attenuate disease expression. Recommended postexposure immunization regimens are shown in Table 116-1. For example, giving either measles immune globulin within 6 days of exposure or measles vaccine within the first few days after exposure may prevent symptomatic infection. Nonimmune pregnant women exposed to rubella can minimize clinical illness by postexposure passive immunization; however, this measure may fail to prevent viremia and infection of the fetus and thus may be followed by the congenital rubella syndrome. Proper immunization for tetanus plays an important role in dirty-wound management. The need for active immunization—with or without passive immunization—depends on the wound's condition and the patient's immunization history. Tetanus is rare among persons with documented receipt of a primary series of tetanus toxoid doses. Tetanus immune globulin is helpful in patients with clinical tetanus, but survivors must be actively immunized since the disease does not stimulate protective levels of antitoxin antibody. Administration of rabies immune globulin plus rabies vaccine in the immediate postexposure period is highly effective in preventing disease. Similarly, for persons who have not been actively immunized, administration of hepatitis A immune globulin within 2 weeks of exposure to hepatitis A virus is likely to prevent clinical illness. Evidence also supports the efficacy of human hepatitis B immune globulin in preventing disease after exposure. While no high-titer preparation is available for postexposure protection against non-A, non-B hepatitis, standard human immune serum globulin is efficacious. VariZIG, a highly purified preparation of human antibody to varicella-zoster virus (VZV), is licensed in Canada for the prevention of varicella in nonimmune pregnant women who are exposed to infected individuals. At the time of this writing, this product is available in the United States from the Centers for Disease Control and Prevention (CDC) under an investigational new drug (IND) protocol or under an expanded-access program through the U.S. Food and Drug Administration.

THE IMMUNE RESPONSE

While many constituents of infectious microorganisms and their products (e.g., exotoxins) are or can be rendered immunogenic, only some stimulate protective immune responses that can prevent infection and/or clinical illness or (as in the case of rotavirus) can attenuate illness, providing protection against severe disease but not against infection or mild illness. The immune system is complex, and many factors—including antigen composition and presentation as well as host

TABLE 116-1 RECOMMENDED POSTEXPOSURE IMMUNIZATION WITH IMMUNOGLOBULIN PREPARATIONS IN THE UNITED STATES

Disease	Indicated	Comments
Measles	Yes	Standard human immune globulin is recommended for exposed infants and adults with normal immunocompetence (but with a contraindication to measles vaccine) and for immunocompromised patients exposed to measles (regardless of immunization status). Patients should be actively immunized 3–6 months after immunoglobulin administration. Recommended dose: 0.25–0.50 mL/kg (40–80 mg of IgG/kg) IM; 80 mg of IgG/kg for immunocompromised contact; maximum, 15 mL.
Rubella	No	Efficacy is unreliable; therefore, standard human immune globulin is recommended for administration only to antibody-negative pregnant women in the first trimester who have a documented rubella exposure and will not consider terminating the pregnancy. Recommended dose is 0.55 mL/kg (90 mg of IgG/kg) IM.
Tetanus	Yes	Human tetanus immune globulin (TIG) has replaced equine tetanus antitoxin because of the risk of serum sickness with equine serum. Recommended dose for postexposure prophylaxis is 250–500 units of TIG (10–20 mg of IgG/kg) IM. Recommended dose for treatment of tetanus is 3000–6000 units of TIG IM.
Rabies	Yes	Human rabies immune globulin (RIG) is preferred over equine rabies antiserum because of the risk of serum sickness with equine serum. RIG or antiserum is recommended for nonimmunized individuals with animal bites in whom rabies cannot be ruled out and with other exposures to known rabid animals. Recommended dose of RIG is 20 IU/kg (22 mg of IgG/kg). Recommended dose of antiserum is 40 IU/kg. Rabies vaccine is given as well at 0, 3, 7, 14, and 28 days.
Hepatitis A	Yes	Standard immune serum globulin is given in a single dose of 0.02–0.04 mL/kg or (for continuous exposure) in a dose up to 0.06 mL/kg every 5 months. Postexposure treatment with hepatitis A immune globulin has not been studied.
Varicella	Yes	VariZIG, a new Canadian purified human immune globulin containing high-titer IgG antibody to varicella-zoster virus, is intended for patients without evidence of immunity to varicella who are exposed to infection and who are at high risk for severe disease and complications. It is not currently licensed in the United States but instead has investigational new drug status. VariZIG may be obtained under expanded-access provisions for patients who meet the enrollment criteria and choose to participate. Maximal benefit requires administration within 96 h of exposure. The recommended dose is 125 units/10 kg of body weight, up to a maximum of 625 units.

characteristics—are critical for stimulation of the desired immune responses (Chap. 308).

The Primary Response The primary response to a vaccine antigen includes an apparent latent period of several days before immune responses can be detected. Although the immune system is rapidly activated, it takes 7–10 days for activated B lymphocytes to produce enough antibody to be detected in the circulation. The primarily IgM antibodies seen initially are rapidly produced but have only a low affinity for the antigen. After the first week, high-affinity IgG antibodies begin to be produced in quantity; this switch from IgM to IgG production requires the participation of CD4+ T-helper lymphocytes—the "middle men" of the immune response. Because precursors for T cells mature within the thymus gland, antigens that stimulate T cells are referred to as *T* or *thymus-dependent* antigens. Circulating antigen-specific T lymphocytes that implement cell-mediated immune responses are identified in the peripheral bloodstream only after several days but begin to increase in number immediately after antigenic stimulation.

Activation of these responses typically requires co-recognition of the antigen by specific molecular species of HLA, the major histocompatibility complex, which is present on the surface of lymphocytes and macrophages. Some individuals cannot respond to one or more antigens, even when repeatedly exposed, because they do not have the genes for the particular HLA type involved in antigen recognition, processing, and presentation for an immune response. This situation is known as *primary vaccine failure.*

The Secondary Response Stronger and faster humoral or cell-mediated responses are elicited by a second exposure to the same antigen and are detectable within days of the "booster" dose. The secondary response depends on immunologic memory induced by the primary exposure and is characterized by a marked proliferation of IgG antibody–producing B lymphocytes and/or effector T cells. Pure polysaccharide antigens, such as the first-generation pneumococcal vaccine, evoke immune responses that are independent of T cells and are not enhanced by repeated administration. However, conjugation of the same polysaccharide to a suitable protein converts the carbohydrate antigen into one that is T cell–dependent and able to induce immunologic memory and secondary responses to reexposure. Although levels of vaccine-induced antibodies may decline over time, revaccination or infection generally elicits a rapid (anamnestic) protective secondary response consisting of IgG antibodies, with little or no detectable IgM. Thus, a lack of measurable antibody in an immunized individual does not necessarily indicate secondary vaccine failure. Similarly, the mere presence of detectable antibodies after immunization does not ensure clinical protection: the level of circulating antibody may need to exceed a threshold value in order to mediate protection (e.g., 0.01 IU/mL for tetanus antitoxin).

Mucosal Immunity Some pathogens are confined to and replicate only at mucosal surfaces (e.g., *Vibrio cholerae*), whereas others first encounter the host at a mucosal surface before they invade systemically (e.g., influenza virus). A distinctive immunoglobulin, *secretory IgA*, is produced at mucosal surfaces and is adapted to resist degradation and to function at these sites. Vaccines may be specifically designed to induce secretory IgA and thereby to block the essential initial steps in disease pathogenesis that occur on mucosal surfaces. Given its complexity, mucosal immunology has become a separate branch of the field of immunology.

Measurement of the Immune Response Immune responses to vaccines are often gauged by the concentration of specific antibody in serum. Although seroconversion (i.e., transition from antibody-negative to antibody-positive status) serves as a dependable indicator of an immune response, it does not necessarily correlate with protection unless serum antibody is the critical mechanism in vivo and the levels achieved are sufficient (e.g., against measles). In some instances, serum antibody correlates with clinical protection but does not directly mediate it (e.g., vibriocidal serum antibodies in cholera).

Herd Immunity Successful vaccination protects immunized individuals from infection, thereby decreasing the percentage of susceptible persons within a population and reducing the possibility of infection transmission to others. At a definable prevalence of immunity, an infectious organism can no longer circulate freely among the remaining susceptibles. This indirect protection of unvaccinated (nonimmune) persons is called the *herd immunity effect*; through this effect, vaccination programs may confer societal benefits that exceed individual costs. The level of vaccine coverage needed to elicit herd immunity depends on the patterns of interaction among individuals within the population and the biology of the specific infectious agent. For example, measles virus and VZV have high transmission rates and require a higher level of vaccine coverage for herd immunity than do organisms with lower transmission rates, such as *S. pneumoniae.* Wherever herd immunity for poliomyelitis and measles has been induced with vaccines, transmission of infection has ceased; however, herd immunity may wane if immunization programs are interrupted (as was the case for diphtheria in the former Soviet Union) or if a sufficient percentage of individuals refuse to be immunized because of a fear of vaccine-related adverse events (as occurred for pertussis in the United Kingdom and Japan). In either setting, the loss of herd immunity has led to renewed circulation of the organism and subsequent large outbreaks with serious consequences.

PRINCIPLES OF VACCINE USE

Route of Administration Microbes differ in their routes of infection, patterns of transmission, and predispositions for certain age groups. The route of vaccine administration (oral, intranasal, intradermal, transdermal, subcutaneous, or intramuscular) takes these factors into account in order to maximize protection and minimize adverse events. Vaccine development is more a pragmatic undertaking than an exact science, guided only in part by immunologic principles and shaped largely by the results of clinical trials. While vaccines can theoretically be given by any route, each vaccine has unique characteristics adapted to a particular route and, in practice, must be given by the licensed route, for which optimal immunogenicity and safety have been documented. For example, vaccines containing adjuvants are designed for injection into the muscle mass. Mucosal administration of vaccines designed for parenteral administration may not induce good systemic responses because such vaccines do not induce mucosal secretory IgA. Administration of hepatitis B vaccine into the gluteal rather than the deltoid muscle may fail to induce an adequate immune response, while SC rather than IM administration of DTaP vaccine increases the risk of adverse reactions. Injectable biologicals should be administered at sites where the likelihood of local, neural, vascular, or tissue injury is minimized.

Age Because age influences the response to vaccines, schedules for immunization are based on age-dependent responses determined empirically in clinical trials. The presence of high levels of maternal antibody and/or the immaturity of the immune system in the early months of life impairs the initial immune response to some vaccines (e.g., measles and pneumococcal polysaccharide vaccines) but not to others (e.g., hepatitis B vaccine). In the elderly, vaccine responses may be diminished because of the natural waning of the immune system, and larger amounts of an antigen may be required to produce the desired response (e.g., in vaccination against influenza). In contrast, in some age groups, the use of substandard amounts of antigen is sufficient for immunity induction and reduces the risk of adverse effects (e.g., a reduced dose of diphtheria toxoid for persons ≥7 years of age). Age-related adverse events are discussed in a later section.

Target Populations and Timing of Administration Disease attack rates differ across the human life span, and the timing of immunization must consider these variations along with the age-specific response to vaccines, the durability of the immune response, and the logistics for optimal identification and vaccination of the groups at risk. Aside from immunologic parameters, many factors are involved, including demographic features; thus, vaccination programs are really as much community as individual endeavors. Schedules for immunization are ultimately derived from careful consideration of the many relevant variables and may ultimately depend on the best opportunities to reach the target groups (e.g., infancy, school entry, puberty, college enrollment, military induction, entry into the workplace). Health care workers administering vaccines or caring for patients with vaccine-preventable diseases have a special responsibility to be adequately immunized themselves and to take all necessary precautions to minimize the risk of spreading infection (e.g., hand washing between immunizations or other interactions with patients). Catch-up immunization schedules for infants and children through the age of 18 years have been approved by the CDC (Fig. 116-3).

For common and highly communicable childhood diseases such as measles, the target population is the universe of susceptible individuals, and the time to immunize is as early in life as is feasible and effective. In the industrialized world, immunization with live-virus vaccine at 12–15 months of age has become the norm because the vaccine protects >95% of children immunized at this age and there is little measles morbidity or mortality among infants <1 year of age. In contrast, under crowded conditions in the developing world, measles remains a significant cause of death among young infants. For optimal benefit in this situation, it is necessary to immunize early enough to narrow the window of vulnerability between the rapid decline of maternal antibody 4–6 months after birth and the development of vaccine-induced active immunity; this choice must be made despite the less efficient immune response in children <1 year old.

Invasive infections due to Hib (meningitis, pneumonia, and epiglottitis) occur primarily in young children, with rates rising sharply after the disappearance of maternally derived antibody. First-generation Hib polysaccharide vaccines often failed when administered during infancy because very young children cannot respond to pure polysaccharides. This problem has been overcome by conjugating the capsular polysaccharide with a protein to create a T cell–dependent antigen, to which infants effectively respond.

In contrast, rubella is primarily a threat to the fetus rather than to infants and young children. The ideal strategy would be to immunize all women of reproductive age before they became pregnant. Because it is difficult to ensure this type of coverage, rubella is included in a combination vaccine with measles and mumps (MMR) that is administered during infancy and boosted at the age of 4–6 years. It is recommended that pregnant women be screened for rubella antibodies and that seronegative women be given rubella vaccine after delivery. Similar considerations apply to the use of the vaccine against HPV that was recently approved in the United States and is intended primarily to prevent cervical cancer in women. Accordingly, it is recommended that the vaccine be given at the age of 11–12 years (or as early as 9 years), so that all are immunized before becoming sexually active.

Some vaccines, such as the influenza and polyvalent pneumococcal polysaccharide products, were originally formulated to prevent pneumonia hospitalizations and deaths among the elderly. These products have been consistently underused, in large part because physicians and otherwise-healthy older individuals ignore the recommendations but also because vaccines continue to be thought of as interventions for infants and children. There is considerable debate about alternative strategies to reduce the burden of these diseases in the elderly by indirectly protecting them through childhood vaccination, which would reduce transmission. The development of new vaccines and the exploitation of new routes of administration may facilitate this approach; examples include the development of pneumococcal conjugate vaccines and the administration of influenza vaccine by the intranasal route, respectively. The pneumococcal conjugate vaccine has made it possible to immunize young infants at risk of pneumococcal pneumonia, meningitis, and otitis media, but whether immunity will persist or will need boosting in adulthood remains to be determined. What is clear is that the number of recommended vaccines and the strategies for their deployment are undergoing constant revision.

Adjuvants The immune response to some antigens is enhanced by the addition of adjuvants—nonspecific boosters of immune responses. Adjuvants include aluminum salts or, in the case of polysaccharides such as the polyribose phosphate oligosaccharide of Hib, a carrier protein to which the polysaccharide is conjugated. Adjuvants are essential to the efficacy of a number of inactivated vaccines, including diphtheria and tetanus toxoids, acellular pertussis vaccine, and hepatitis B vaccine; they also appear to be required for enhancement of the response to killed H5N1 avian influenza vaccines. The mechanism by which adjuvants enhance immunogenicity is not well defined but appears to relate to the ability of the adjuvant to activate antigen-presenting cells, frequently through stimulation of Toll-like receptors. Other reported mechanisms for adjuvant effects include rendering of soluble antigens into a particulate form, the mobilization of phagocytes to the site of antigen deposition, and the slowing down of antigen release in order to prolong stimulation of the immune response. Identification of new adjuvants that are safe, more effective, and inexpensive is a high priority for vaccine researchers and manufacturers.

Catch-up Immunization Schedule UNITED STATES • 2007
for Persons Aged 4 Months–18 Years Who Start Late or Who Are More Than One Month Behind

The table below provides catch-up schedules and minimum intervals between doses for children whose vaccinations have been delayed. A vaccine series does not need to be restarted, regardless of the time that has elapsed between doses. Use the section appropriate for the child's age.

Vaccine	Minimum Age for Dose 1	Minimum Interval Between Doses: Dose 1 to Dose 2	Dose 2 to Dose 3	Dose 3 to Dose 4	Dose 4 to Dose 5
CATCH-UP SCHEDULE FOR PERSONS AGED 4 MONTHS–6 YEARS					
Hepatitis B[1]	Birth	4 weeks	8 weeks (and 16 weeks after first dose)		
Rotavirus[2]	6 wks	4 weeks	4 weeks		
Diphtheria, Tetanus, Pertussis[3]	6 wks	4 weeks	4 weeks	6 months	6 months[3]
Haemophilus influenzae type b[4]	6 wks	4 weeks if first dose administered at age < 12 months 8 weeks (as final dose) if first dose administered at age 12-14 months No further doses needed if first dose administered at age ≥ 15 months	4 weeks[4] if current age < 12 months 8 weeks (as final dose)[4] if current age ≥ 12 months and second dose administered at age < 15 months No further doses needed if previous dose administered at age ≥ 15 months	8 weeks (as final dose) This dose only necessary for children aged 12 months–5 years who received 3 doses before age 12 months	
Pneumococcal[5]	6 wks	4 weeks if first dose administered at age < 12 months and current age < 24 months 8 weeks (as final dose) if first dose administered at age ≥ 12 months or current age 24–59 months No further doses needed for healthy children if first dose administered at age ≥ 24 months	4 weeks if current age < 12 months 8 weeks (as final dose) if current age ≥ 12 months No further doses needed for healthy children if previous dose administered at age ≥ 24 months	8 weeks (as final dose) This dose only necessary for children aged 12 months–5 years who received 3 doses before age 12 months	
Inactivated Poliovirus[6]	6 wks	4 weeks	4 weeks	4 weeks[6]	
Measles, Mumps, Rubella[7]	12 mos	4 weeks			
Varicella[8]	12 mos	3 months			
Hepatitis A[9]	12 mos	6 months			
CATCH-UP SCHEDULE FOR PERSONS AGED 7–18 YEARS					
Tetanus, Diphtheria/ Tetanus, Diphtheria, Pertussis[10]	7 yrs[10]	4 weeks	8 weeks if first dose administered at age < 12 months 6 months if first dose administered at age ≥ 12 months	6 months if first dose administered at age < 12 months	
Human Papillomavirus[11]	9 yrs	4 weeks	12 weeks		
Hepatitis A[9]	12 mos	6 months			
Hepatitis B[1]	Birth	4 weeks	8 weeks (and 16 weeks after first dose)		
Inactivated Poliovirus[6]	6 wks	4 weeks	4 weeks	4 weeks[6]	
Measles, Mumps, Rubella[7]	12 mos	4 weeks			
Varicella[8]	12 mos	4 weeks if first dose administered at age ≥ 13 years 3 months if first dose administered at age < 13 years			

FIGURE 116-3 Catch-up immunization schedule for persons aged 4 months–18 years who start late or who are more than 1 month behind. 1. Hepatitis B vaccine (HepB). *(Minimum age: birth)* Administer the 3-dose series to those who were not previously vaccinated. A 2-dose series of Recombivax HB is licensed for children aged 11–15 years. **2. Rotavirus vaccine (Rota).** *(Minimum age: 6 weeks)* Do not start the series later than age 12 weeks. Administer the final dose in the series by age 32 weeks. Do not administer a dose later than age 32 weeks. Data on safety and efficacy outside of these age ranges are insufficient. **3. Diphtheria and tetanus toxoids and acellular pertussis vaccine (DTaP).** *(Minimum age: 6 weeks)* The fifth dose is not necessary if the fourth dose was administered at age ≥4 years. DTaP is not indicated for persons aged ≥7 years. **4. *Haemophilus influenzae* type b conjugate vaccine (Hib).** *(Minimum age: 6 weeks)* Vaccine is not generally recommended for children aged ≥5 years. If current age <12 months and the first 2 doses were PRP-OMP (PedvaxHIB or ComVax [Merck]), the third (and final) dose should be administered at age 12–15 months and at least 8 weeks after the second dose. If first dose was administered at age 7–11 months, administer 2 doses separated by 4 weeks plus a booster at age 12–15 months. **5. Pneumococcal conjugate vaccine (PCV).** *(Minimum age: 6 weeks)* Vaccine is not generally recommended for children aged ≥5 years. **6. Inactivated poliovirus vaccine (IPV).** *(Minimum age: 6 weeks)* For children who received an all-IPV or all-oral poliovirus (OPV) series, a fourth dose is not necessary if third dose was administered at age ≥4 years. If both OPV and IPV were administered as part of a series, a total of 4 doses should be administered, regardless of the child's current age. **7. Measles, mumps, and rubella vaccine (MMR).** *(Minimum age: 12 months)* The second dose of MMR is recommended routinely at age 4–6 years but may be administered earlier if desired. If not previously vaccinated, administer 2 doses of MMR during any visit with ≥4 weeks between the doses. **8. Varicella vaccine.** *(Minimum age: 12 months)* The second dose of varicella vaccine is recommended routinely at age 4–6 years but may be administered earlier if desired. Do not repeat the second dose in persons aged <13 years if administered ≥28 days after the first dose. **9. Hepatitis A vaccine (HepA).** *(Minimum age: 12 months)* HepA is recommended for certain groups of children, including in areas where vaccination programs target older children. See MMWR 2006;55(No. RR-7):1–23. **10. Tetanus and diphtheria toxoids vaccine (Td) and tetanus and diphtheria toxoids and acellular pertussis vaccine (Tdap).** *(Minimum ages: 7 years for Td, 10 years for BOOSTRIX, and 11 years for ADACEL)* Tdap should be substituted for a single dose of Td in the primary catch-up series or as a booster if age appropriate; use Td for other doses. A 5-year interval from the last Td dose is encouraged when Tdap is used as a booster dose. A booster (fourth) dose is needed if any of the previous doses were administered at age <12 months. Refer to ACIP recommendations for further information. See MMWR 2006;55(No. RR-3). **11. Human papillomavirus vaccine (HPV).** *(Minimum age: 9 years)* Administer the HPV vaccine series to females at age 13–18 years if not previously vaccinated.

RECOMMENDATIONS FOR USE

Two or more vaccines should not be mixed in the same syringe in an effort to diminish the number of needle sticks unless such a practice is specifically endorsed by licensure. Disposable needles and syringes must be safely discarded to prevent inadvertent needle stick injury. While the importance of using a new syringe and needle for each vaccine recipient is obvious, reuse of contaminated equipment is a common reality in resource-poor settings. One-time-use, "auto-destruct" needles and syringes have been designed to prevent this practice, but their use adds to the cost of vaccine delivery.

Wherever effective primary health care systems ensure access to medical services for the majority and the population is educated about the need for and efficacy of vaccines, coverage rates for basic immunizations are usually high, regardless of the route of vaccine administration or the number of doses necessary. However, without systematic attention to the completion of multiple-dose vaccine schedules, coverage rates for second, third, and booster doses may drop off, and the efficacy of immunization may be significantly diminished.

RISK ASSESSMENT

Vaccines are considered safe when the risk of use is judged to be acceptable in relation to the benefits. For vaccines given to healthy individuals for diseases that are no longer common, acceptable risks are set at very low levels—indeed, far lower than for most medical products. However, "safety" does not and cannot ever mean "zero risk." The determination of safety is thus based on a scientific assessment of the data and a considered judgment of all the issues involved, including benefits and risks. Communities and individuals may differ, both among themselves and from health care professionals, in how they perceive the risks, benefits, and acceptability of vaccines and in how they judge the amount of uncertainty that is tolerable. Some parent advocacy groups, such as those that oppose mandatory vaccination, feel that no amount of risk is acceptable, especially for childhood vaccines.

SOURCES OF IMMUNIZATION RECOMMENDATIONS

Harmonized recommendations for vaccine use in the United States are developed by several professional groups. Schedules for immunization of children and adolescents and of adults are shown in Figs. 116-1 and 116-2, respectively. Vaccines recommended for special use are shown in Table 116-2.

As noted above, the number of licensed vaccines and the strategies for their best use change constantly as new products, new indications, and new information become available. The Advisory Committee on Immunization Practices (ACIP) regularly amends immunization recommendations to reflect the evolution of vaccines and vaccination policy in the United States. Changes for 2006 include the following points:

- to implement standing orders to administer hepatitis B vaccine—soon after birth and before hospital discharge—to all infants except those with documented hepatitis B–negative mothers;
- to target adults at high risk for hepatitis B vaccination;
- to use a new tetanus toxoid/reduced-dose diphtheria toxoid plus acellular pertussis combination vaccine (Tdap) formulated for adolescents and adults in place of Td;
- to provide meningococcal conjugate vaccine (MCV4) to all children at 11–12 years of age, to unvaccinated adolescents at age 15, and to all college freshmen living in dormitories;
- to administer hepatitis A vaccine to all children at 1 year of age;
- to administer three doses of the newly licensed rotavirus vaccine at 2, 4, and 6 months of age, with the first dose given by 12 weeks of age and the last by 32 weeks of age;
- to immunize children 6 months to 5 years of age with influenza vaccine and to expand routine use of the vaccine for their household contacts and out-of-home caregivers;
- to administer Tdap to protect health care personnel from pertussis and to reduce their potential to transmit nosocomial infections, assigning the highest priority to those who have direct contact with infants <1 year old; and
- to administer HPV vaccine routinely to girls at 11–12 years of age.

VACCINES FOR ROUTINE USE

Infants and Children It is current practice for all children in the United States to receive DTaP, poliovirus, MMR, Hib, hepatitis B, and varicella vaccines and to receive pneumococcal conjugate, hepatitis A, and rotavirus vaccines in the absence of specific contraindications (Fig. 116-1; *www.cdc.gov/vaccines/vpd-vac/vaccines-list.htm*). Annual influenza seasonal vaccine is recommended for all children 6 months to 5 years old and to other children who have certain risk factors or who reside with persons with certain chronic disorders. In several European countries, meningococcal C conjugate vaccine is routinely recommended for children.

Teenagers It is now recommended that all adolescents routinely receive quadrivalent meningococcal conjugate vaccine for serogroups A, C, Y, and W135 and the new-formulation Tdap vaccine. Girls should be given HPV vaccine, ideally at the age of 11–12 years but certainly before becoming sexually active (Fig. 116-1; *www.cdc.gov/vaccines/recs/schedules/teen-schedule.htm*).

Adults, Including College Students (Fig. 116-2) Immunization recommendations for adults (≥18 years old) fall into four categories: (1) routine vaccines for all adults; (2) vaccines for high-risk exposure groups (health care and other institutional workers, prisoners, students, military personnel, travelers to endemic areas, injection drug users, and men who have sex with men); (3) vaccines for persons at high risk for severe outcomes of infection (pregnant women; the elderly; persons with chronic medical conditions, including diabetes, alcoholism, immunodeficiency, and renal, hepatic, respiratory, or cardiac disease); and (4) vaccines for household contacts of persons in group 3.

Because a substantial proportion of adults in the United States no longer have protective levels of antibodies to tetanus or diphtheria, all adults should receive routine booster doses of Td every 10 years. For those under age 65 years, one-time substitution of Tdap suitable for adults (Adacel, Sanofi-Pasteur) in place of the usual Td booster is recommended. Pregnant women who received their last Td booster >10 years previously may receive Td during the second or third trimester; those boosted <10 years previously (and as recently as 2 years before) should receive Tdap after delivery. Adults who have contact with infants <12 months of age should receive a single dose of Tdap—ideally at least 2 weeks before contact begins—if the most recent Td booster was ≥2 years earlier. If not previously immunized, adults require a primary immunizing course of Td. Young adults without laboratory evidence or a reliable history of past vaccination or disease should be immunized against measles, mumps, rubella, and varicella. A second dose of MMR vaccine is recommended for groups with a higher risk of exposure and for health care workers with certain other indications. Unless they have documented proof of immunity, rubella vaccine should be given to all nonpregnant women of childbearing age. Rubella-susceptible pregnant women should be vaccinated as early as possible in the postpartum period. Live-virus vaccines, such as MMR and varicella vaccines, are contraindicated in pregnant women and immunosuppressed individuals. Routine immunization against polio (with inactivated vaccine) is not recommended for adults unless they are at particular risk of exposure because of travel to the remaining endemic areas. College students, particularly freshmen living in dormitory settings, are at increased risk of meningococcal meningitis, as are military recruits; individuals in both of these groups should be offered the meningococcal polysaccharide or conjugate vaccine for serogroups A, C, Y, and W-135.

Current recommendations also include influenza vaccine for routine annual administration to individuals with chronic illness at any age, to persons living in the same household as chronically ill individuals, and to all adults >50 years of age. Polyvalent pneumococcal polysaccharide vaccine is similarly recommended for adults ≥65 years of age and for all chronically ill persons. Hepatitis B vaccine should be given to adults at high risk from clinical, occupational, behavioral, or

TABLE 116-2 SPECIAL VACCINES FOR INFANTS, CHILDREN, AND ADULTS

Vaccine	Vaccine Type	Route of Administration	Indications	Efficacy	Adverse Events
Anthrax	Inactivated avirulent bacteria	SC (6 doses primary plus annual booster)	For high risk of exposure (e.g., persons in contact with or involved in manufacture of animal hides, furs, bone meal, wool, goat hair) and military risk of biowarfare exposure	90% antibody response; efficacy uncertain	No serious adverse effects known
Tuberculosis (BCG)	Live bacteria (attenuated *Mycobacterium bovis*)	ID	Not generally recommended in U.S. because of low risk of TB and interference with PPD test Consider for PPD-negative children in prolonged contact with ineffectively treated adult TB patients or those with drug-resistant TB and for health care workers in high-risk settings. Not for immunosuppressed individuals	Variable for adult pulmonary TB; best used to prevent childhood TB, meningitis, and miliary disease	Regional adenitis, disseminated BCG infection in immunocompromised hosts
Cholera	Killed whole bacteria	Oral	Travelers to endemic areas; however, not recommended for use by U.S. citizens because of extremely low risk. Not available in the U.S.	60–85%, short duration	Frequent fever and local reactions, pain, swelling
Plague	Inactivated bacteria	IM	Laboratory workers; foresters in endemic areas; ?travelers	90% antibody response; efficacy uncertain	10% local reactions; rare sterile abscess and hypersensitivity
Rabies	Inactivated virus grown in cell culture (human diploid cell or purified chick embryo cell) or grown in cell culture and adsorbed to aluminum phosphate	IM or ID	Preexposure immunization for travelers to high-risk countries, laboratory workers, and veterinarians or postexposure immunization following a bite from a proven or suspected rabies-infected animal	Virtually 100% for pre- or postexposure immunization	25% local reactions; 6% of patients receiving booster doses may develop immune complex reactions with arthropathy, arthritis, angioedema
Yellow fever	Live attenuated virus	SC	Travelers to endemic areas; laboratory workers	High	Rare associated neurologic complications (encephalitis, encephalopathy) or viscerotropic disease (fever; hypotension; respiratory, renal, or hepatic failure; lymphocytopenia; thrombocytopenia; and high risk of death)
Japanese B encephalitis	Inactivated virus	SC	Travelers to endemic areas	80–90%	Anaphylaxis/severe delayed allergic reactions common; recipients should be observed for 10 days
Typhoid	Purified Vi polysaccharide (not for children <2 years of age)	IM	Travelers (≥2 years old) to high-risk areas (southern Asia and other developing areas) except febrile patients	50–80%	Local reactions, mild
	Oral live attenuated Ty21a strain	Oral	Travelers (≥6 years old) to high-risk areas as above, except within 24 h of antibiotic ingestion or in febrile patients	50–80%	Nil

Note: SC, subcutaneous; BCG, bacille Calmette-Guérin; ID, intradermal; PPD, purified protein derivative; TB, tuberculosis.

Source: Recommendations of the Advisory Committee on Immunization Practices of the Centers for Disease Control and Prevention, American Academy of Pediatrics, American College of Physicians.

travel exposures, including patients undergoing hemodialysis, routine recipients of clotting factors, health care workers exposed to potentially infected blood or blood products, individuals living and working in institutions for the mentally handicapped, travelers to highly endemic countries, persons at excess risk for sexually transmitted diseases, injection drug users, and household contacts of known carriers of hepatitis B surface antigen. Hepatitis A vaccine is recommended for these same groups and for persons with clotting disorders or chronic liver disease. There are a number of other special-use vaccines whose administration is related to travel and occupational exposures (e.g., Japanese B encephalitis, typhoid fever, yellow fever, and rabies); specific recommendations for the use of these vaccines in the United States can be found at *www.cdc.gov/nip/recs/adult-schedule.htm*.

Simultaneous Administration of Multiple Vaccines There are no contraindications to the simultaneous administration of multiple individual vaccines, although the use of licensed combination vaccines can significantly reduce the required number of injections during the first 2 years of life. Combination DTaP/Hib vaccine should not be used for primary immunization of infants because it results in a blunted, suboptimal response to Hib; the combination may be used for booster immunizations.

Simultaneous administration of the most widely used live and inactivated vaccines has not resulted in impaired antibody responses or in elevated rates of adverse reactions. In fact, this approach increases the likelihood that a child will ultimately be fully immunized. The simultaneous administration of vaccines is useful in any age group when the potential exists for exposure to multiple infectious diseases during travel to endemic countries. Live-virus vaccines may be given together on the same day; if this approach is not feasible, an interval of at least 30 days should be allowed to avoid interference in the response to one or another of the administered vaccine strains.

Because high doses of immune globulin can inhibit the efficacy of measles and rubella vaccines, an interval of at least 3 months is recommended between the administration of immune globulin and that of MMR vaccine or its components. However, postpartum vaccination of rubella-susceptible women should not be delayed because of the administration of anti-Rho(D) immune globulin or any other blood product during the last trimester or at delivery. Should the administration of an immune globulin preparation become necessary after vaccination, it should be postponed, if at all possible, for at least 14 days to allow time for vaccine-virus replication and development of immunity. In general, there is little interaction of immune globulin with inactivated vaccines, and postexposure passive prophylaxis can be given together with hepatitis B vaccine or tetanus toxoid, resulting in both immediate and long-lasting protection.

Adverse Events Vaccines are generally very safe. Serious adverse events proven to be due to currently licensed vaccines are rare. Concerns about vaccine safety have at times become inflated in conjunction with complacency about the consequences of infections no longer routinely transmitted in the United States. As a result, some parents have refused to have their infants and children immunized.

An *adverse reaction* or *vaccine side effect* is an untoward vaccine effect that is extraneous to the vaccine's primary purpose (to produce immunity). An adverse event can be either a true vaccine reaction or an event whose occurrence is temporally related to a vaccine dose but is entirely unrelated to the vaccine itself. As vaccines are routinely administered through childhood, coincidental events are inevitable. Because our understanding of the underlying biologic mechanisms that cause adverse events remains limited, a few highly publicized claims—unsubstantiated by validated data or analysis—can easily heighten the suspicion that some or all vaccines routinely cause unacceptable adverse events. Antivaccine advocacy groups actively encourage the avoidance of immunization because they believe that vaccines cause certain disorders (e.g., autism). This situation presents a challenge to physicians and public health officials who must educate parents and practitioners about vaccine benefits and risks.

It is true that modern vaccines, while remarkably safe and effective, are associated with adverse events in some recipients and that these events range from frequent and mild to rare and serious or even life-threatening. The decision to recommend a vaccine involves an assessment of the risks of disease and its complications for those who remain unimmunized and the benefit-to-risk ratio of vaccination itself. Because these factors may change over time, the balance between societal benefits and individual risks must be continually evaluated. Valid and invalid contraindications to childhood immunization and appropriate precautions in the use of specific vaccines are reported by the CDC (Table 116-3); updated information can be found at *www.cdc.gov/vaccines/recs/vac-admin/downloads/contraindications_guide.pdf*. A putative link between measles immunization and autism has been the subject of intense international controversy. The Institute of Medicine of the U.S. National Academies of Science has issued four recent reports whose findings (1) fail to support hypotheses that vaccines are associated with multiple sclerosis, neurodevelopmental disorders (e.g., autism), or immune dysfunction; (2) provide no evidence for a temporal association of these conditions with vaccination; and (3) elucidate no biologically plausible basis for the purported relationships.

An illuminating example is the case of Rotashield, a rhesus reassortant rotavirus vaccine, which was introduced for routine use in the United States in the late 1990s. Within 9 months of its introduction, cases of intussusception were reported by the CDC to be temporally associated with the administration of the initial vaccine dose. This report led first to the cessation of the vaccine's use and subsequently to its withdrawal from the market and the discontinuation of its production. The withdrawal of the vaccine in the United States made its use impossible in developing countries, where the risk of any increase in intussusception would have been dramatically outweighed by the benefit of decreased rotavirus mortality rates. It is now apparent that the susceptibility to intussception is age related, with virtually no events in children <90 days of age. Almost a decade later, a new rotavirus vaccine has been licensed in the United States and recommended for routine use beginning at ≤2 months of age. In the interim, some 4–5 million infants have died of rotavirus diarrhea in the developing world; most of these deaths could have been prevented by the original rhesus rotavirus vaccine.

Vaccine components, including protective antigens, animal proteins introduced during vaccine production, and antibiotics or other preservatives or stabilizers, can certainly cause allergic reactions in some recipients. These reactions may be local or systemic, including urticaria and serious anaphylaxis. The most common extraneous allergen is egg protein derived from the growth of measles, mumps, influenza, and yellow fever viruses in embryonated eggs. Gelatin, used as a heat stabilizer, has been implicated in rare but severe allergic reactions. Local or systemic reactions (probably due to antigen-antibody complexes) can result from the too frequent administration of vaccines such as Td or rabies vaccine. Because live-virus vaccines can interfere with tuberculin test responses, necessary tuberculin testing should be done either on the day of immunization or at least 6 weeks later.

USE OF VACCINES IN SPECIAL CIRCUMSTANCES

Breast Feeding Neither killed nor live vaccines affect the safety of breast feeding for either mother or infant. Breast-fed infants can be immunized on a normal schedule. Even premature infants can be immunized at their appropriate chronologic age. Seroconversion in response to hepatitis vaccine at birth may be impaired in some premature infants with birth weights of <2000 g. By a chronologic age of 1 month, however, premature infants—regardless of initial birth weight or gestational age—are as likely to respond adequately to vaccines as older and larger infants.

Occupational Exposure Immunization recommendations for most occupational groups remain to be developed. Specific practices for the immunization of U.S. health care workers against hepatitis B are mandated by the Occupational Safety and Health Administration. Persons employed in caring for patients with chronic diseases can transmit influenza and should be vaccinated annually, independent of age. Rubella is transmitted to and from health care workers in medical facilities, particularly in pediatric practice. Health care workers who might transmit rubella to pregnant patients should be documented to be immune to rubella; susceptible individuals should be promptly immunized. Persons providing health care are also at greater risk from measles and varicella than the general public, and those who are likely to come into contact with measles- and varicella-infected patients should be documented to be immune or be immunized.

HIV Infection and Other Medical Conditions Limited studies in HIV-infected individuals have found no increase in the risk of adverse events from the use of live or inactivated vaccines. It is not surprising that immune responses may not be as vigorous in immunocompromised individuals as in those with a normal immune system; therefore, persons known to be infected with HIV should be immunized with recommended vaccines in the same manner as individuals with a normal immune system and as early in the course of their disease as possible, before immune function becomes significantly impaired. If MMR immunization is indicated, HIV-infected patients may receive the standard attenuated vaccine; if polio vaccination is required, these patients and their household contacts should receive inactivated polio vaccine.

Albeit prudent, it is not necessary to test for HIV before making decisions about the immunization of asymptomatic individuals from known HIV risk groups. Live attenuated vaccines are contraindicated in other immunocompromised patients, including those with congenital immunodeficiency syndromes, those who have undergone splenectomy, and those who are receiving immunosuppressive therapy. Passive immunization with immunoglobulin preparations or antitoxins can be considered in individual cases, either as postexposure prophylaxis or as part of the treatment of established infection.

Travel (See also Chap. 117) The International Sanitary Regulations allow countries to impose requirements for yellow fever and killed

TABLE 116-3 VALID AND INVALID CONTRAINDICATIONS TO VACCINATION

Vaccine	Valid Contraindication[a]	Invalid Contraindication
All vaccines in general	Serious allergic reactions (e.g., anaphylaxis) to a previous vaccine dose or a vaccine component *Precaution:* Moderate or severe concurrent illness with or without fever	Mild acute illness with or without fever Mild to moderate local reactions; low-grade or moderate fever after a previous dose Lack of previous physical examination in a well-appearing person Current antimicrobial therapy (except certain live bacterial vaccines) Convalescent phase of illness Premature birth (except hepatitis B in some circumstances) Recent exposure to infectious diseases History of penicillin allergy, other nonvaccine allergies; relatives with allergies; receiving desensitization treatment
DTaP[b]	Severe allergic reaction to a previous dose or a vaccine component Encephalopathy (e.g., coma, decreased level of consciousness, prolonged seizures) within 7 days of a previous dose of DTP or DTaP Progressive neurologic disorder, including infantile spasms, uncontrolled epilepsy, progressive encephalopathy: defer DTaP until neurologic status is clarified and stabilized *Precaution:* Fever of ≥40.5°C at ≤48 h after a previous dose of DTP or DTaP Collapse or shock-like state (i.e., hypotonic hyporesponsive episode ≤48 h after a previous dose of DTP or DTaP) Seizure ≤3 days after a previous dose of DTP or DTaP Persistent, inconsolable crying lasting ≥3 h/≤48 h after a previous dose of DTP or DTaP Moderate or severe acute illness with or without fever	Temperature of <40.5°C; fussiness; mild drowsiness after a prior dose of DTP or DTaP Family history of seizures, sudden infant death syndrome, or adverse event after DTP or DTaP Stable neurologic conditions (e.g., cerebral palsy, well-controlled convulsions, developmental delay)
DT, Td	Severe allergic reaction after a previous dose or to a vaccine component *Precaution:* Guillain-Barré syndrome ≤6 weeks after a previous dose of tetanus toxoid–containing vaccine Moderate or severe acute illness with or without fever	
IPV	Severe allergic reaction to a previous dose or a vaccine component *Precautions:* Pregnancy; moderate or severe acute illness with or without fever	
MMR	Severe allergic reaction to a previous dose or a vaccine component Pregnancy Known severe immunodeficiency (e.g., hematologic and solid tumors, congenital immunodeficiency, long-term immunosuppressive therapy, or severely symptomatic HIV infection) *Precautions:* Recent (≤11 months) receipt of antibody-containing blood products (specific interval depends on product); history of thrombocytopenia and thrombocytopenic purpura; moderate or severe acute illness with or without fever	Positive tuberculin skin test; simultaneous TB skin testing Breast-feeding Pregnancy of recipient's mother or other close or household contact; recipient is childbearing-age female or immunodeficient family member or household contact; asymptomatic or mildly symptomatic HIV infection; allergy to eggs
Hib	Severe allergic reaction to a previous dose or a vaccine component Age <6 weeks *Precaution:* Moderate or severe acute illness with or without fever	
Hepatitis B	Severe allergic reaction to a previous dose or a vaccine component *Precautions:* Infant weighing <2000 g; moderate or severe acute illness with or without fever	Pregnancy; autoimmune disease (e.g., systemic lupus erythematosus or rheumatoid arthritis)
Hepatitis A	Severe allergic reaction to a previous dose or a vaccine component *Precaution:* Pregnancy; moderate or severe acute illness with or without fever	
Varicella	Severe allergic reaction to a previous dose or a vaccine component Substantial suppression of cellular immunity Pregnancy *Precaution:* Recent (≤11 months) receipt of antibody-containing blood products (specific interval depends on product)	Pregnancy of recipient's mother or another close or household contact Immunodeficient family member or household contact; asymptomatic or mildly symptomatic HIV infection
Pneumococcal conjugate vaccines	Severe allergic reaction to a previous dose or a vaccine component *Precaution:* Moderate or severe acute illness with or without fever	
Influenza	Severe allergic reaction to a previous dose or a vaccine component, including egg protein *Precaution:* Moderate or severe acute illness with or without fever	Nonsevere (e.g., contact) allergy to latex or thimerosal; concurrent administration of warfarin or aminophylline
Pneumococcal polysaccharide vaccines	Severe allergic reaction to a previous dose or a vaccine component *Precaution:* Moderate or severe acute illness with or without fever	

[a]Events or conditions listed as precautions should be reviewed carefully. Benefits and risks of administering a specific vaccine to a person under these circumstances should be considered. If the risk from the vaccine is believed to outweigh the benefit, the vaccine should not be administered. If the benefit of vaccination is believed to outweigh the risk, the vaccine should be administered.

[b]Whether and when to administer DTaP to children with proven or suspected underlying neurologic disorders should be decided on a case-by-case basis.

Note: DTP, diphtheria and tetanus toxoids and whole-cell pertussis vaccine; DTaP, diphtheria and tetanus toxoids and acellular pertussis vaccine; DT, diphtheria and tetanus toxoids; Td, tetanus and reduced-dose diphtheria toxoids, adsorbed; IPV, inactivated polio vaccine; MMR, measles, mumps, and rubella vaccine; Hib, *Haemophilus influenzae* type b vaccine.

Source: General Recommendations on Immunization. MMWR 51(RR02): 1, 2002.

cholera vaccines as a condition for admission, even though the latter vaccine is not an effective public health tool. Travelers should know whether these vaccines are required for entry into the countries on their itinerary to avoid being turned back or immunized on the spot, with the inherent danger of unsafe injections in poor developing countries. Infants, children, and adults should have all routine immunizations updated before traveling, especially to developing countries, with particular attention to polio, measles, and DTaP or Tdap, depending on age. Immunity to hepatitis A and hepatitis B is advisable for travelers. Special-use vaccines (Table 116-2), including rabies, typhoid, Japanese B encephalitis, and plague vaccines, should be considered for those individuals who expect to go beyond the usual tourist routes or to spend extended periods in rural areas in disease-endemic regions. Most U.S. cities have travel clinics that maintain up-to-date epidemiologic information and can provide the appropriate vaccines. The CDC maintains a useful website for travelers (*www.cdc.gov/travel*).

CURRENT CONTROVERSIES

Even though vaccines are very safe and serious adverse events proven to be due to licensed vaccines are rare, the recent rise in the reporting of autism spectrum disorders has led some parents of affected children to claim that thimerosal—used as a preservative—is the cause of the problem. No study has yet implicated thimerosal or the vaccines in which it has been used as a likely cause of these disorders; however, fully 50% of cases before the Vaccine Injury Compensation Program concern autism allegedly due to mercury. In 1999, thimerosal was removed from single-dose formulations of recommended childhood vaccines in the United States; the exception is influenza vaccine, for which thimerosal-free preparations have been in short supply. There is no evidence that the frequency of autism diagnoses has changed since the discontinuation of thimerosal use, but further observation is necessary. It is important to resolve these controversies, particularly because it may be difficult to ensure product sterility in developing countries—where multidose vials of vaccine are most cost-effective—without the use of preservative.

Disparities in vaccine coverage among the majority and minority communities in the United States persist. Reasons for underimmunization include limited access to health care, lack of insurance, assignment of a low priority to preventive measures, and insufficient knowledge about vaccines and the importance of being vaccinated. The persistence of wild poliovirus in immunocompromised individuals and the reversion of live poliovirus vaccine to virulence in several communities have catalyzed debate about whether it really is possible to eradicate poliovirus from the world (thus allowing the cessation of immunization) or whether the best that can be hoped for is the worldwide elimination of clinical disease, with continued routine immunization to keep the risk low.

The addition of new, individually injectable vaccines to the childhood immunization schedule has heightened parental concerns about multiple injections at a single clinic visit. The continued development and testing of vaccine combinations aim to mitigate these concerns. Even when multiple injections are required, providers must make every effort to administer all indicated vaccines at each visit.

DELIVERY OF VACCINES

Over the past 25 years, considerable progress has been made to ensure that every child in the United States is fully immunized by the time of school entry. All 50 states now require immunization for school entry, and most have laws addressing attendance at preschools and day-care centers. Despite the dramatic impact of immunization and of other improvements in health care on the incidence of vaccine-preventable illness in the United States, many children still are not fully immunized, both in poor communities with inadequate health services and in affluent communities where parental concern about potential adverse events may exceed concern about now-uncommon diseases. The failure to vaccinate preschool children was largely responsible for the resurgence of measles in the United States in 1989–1991, with >55,000 cases and >130 measles-related deaths. Outbreaks of pertussis, mumps, and congenital rubella syndrome have occurred wherever immunization rates among preschool children are low. While indigenous transmission of polio, measles, and rubella has been eliminated in the United States, the risk of imported infection and spread to vaccine-naïve susceptible persons persists.

ACCESS TO IMMUNIZATION

Four major barriers to infant and childhood immunization have been identified within the health care system: (1) low public awareness and lack of public demand for immunization, (2) inadequate access to immunization services, (3) missed opportunities to administer vaccines, and (4) inadequate resources for public health and preventive programs. National outreach and educational campaigns promote parental awareness of the value of vaccination and encourage health care providers to use every opportunity to vaccinate the children in their care.

HANDLING OF VACCINES

Vaccines must be handled and stored with care. Attention to the entire "cold chain"—from storage, shelf life, reconstitution, and shelf life after reconstitution and opening—is essential to ensuring that clients receive potent vaccines. Vaccines should be kept at 2°–8°C and, with the exception of varicella vaccine and live attenuated influenza vaccine, should not be frozen. The latter two vaccines should be kept frozen at –15°C. Measles vaccine must be protected from light, which inactivates the virus.

STANDARDS FOR IMMUNIZATION PRACTICE

National standards of immunization for childhood, adolescent, and adult practice have been established to define common policies and practices for public health clinics and physicians' private offices (Table 116-4). These standards represent the most desirable immunization practices and highlight the need to distinguish between valid contraindications and conditions that are often considered to be but are not in fact contraindications (*www.cdc.gov/vaccines/recs/vac-admin/downloads/contraindications_guide.pdf*).

Among the valid contraindications applicable to all vaccines are a history of anaphylaxis or other serious allergic reactions to a vaccine or vaccine component and the presence of a moderate or severe illness, with or without fever. Infants who develop encephalopathy within 72 h of a dose of DTP or DTaP should not receive further doses; those who experience a "precaution" event should not normally receive further doses. Because of theoretical risks to the fetus, pregnant women should not receive MMR or varicella vaccine. Diarrhea, minor respiratory illness (with or without fever), mild to moderate local reactions to a previous dose of vaccine, the concurrent or recent use of antimicrobial agents, mild to moderate malnutrition, and the convalescent phase of an acute illness are not valid contraindications to routine immunization. Failure to vaccinate children because of these conditions is increasingly viewed as a missed opportunity for immunization.

CONTROL OF VACCINE-PREVENTABLE DISEASE

A continuing task of public health practice is to maintain individual and herd immunity, and the job is not over once a population is fully vaccinated. Rather, it is imperative to immunize each subsequent generation as long as the threat of the reintroduction of the disease from anywhere in the world persists. Ongoing surveillance and prompt reporting of disease to local or state health departments are essential to this goal, ensuring a continuing awareness of the possibility of vaccine-preventable illness. Nearly all vaccine-preventable diseases are notifiable, and individual case data are routinely forwarded to the CDC. These data are used to detect outbreaks or other unusual events that require investigation and to evaluate prevention and control policies, practices, and strategies.

INTERNATIONAL CONSIDERATIONS

Since the establishment of the Expanded Programme on Immunization (EPI) by the WHO in 1981 and the involvement of UNICEF in the program's implementation, levels of coverage for the

TABLE 116-4 STANDARDS FOR IMMUNIZATION PRACTICE

Child and Adolescent Immunization Practice

1. Immunization services are readily available.
2. Vaccinations are coordinated with other health care services and provided in a "medical home" when possible.
3. Barriers to vaccination are identified and minimized.
4. Patient's costs are minimized.
5. Health care professionals review the vaccination and health status of patients at every encounter to determine which vaccines are indicated.
6. Health care professionals assess for and follow only medically accepted contraindications.
7. Parents/guardians and patients are educated about the benefits and risks of vaccination in a culturally appropriate manner and in easy-to-understand language.
8. Health care professionals follow appropriate procedures for vaccine storage and handling.
9. Up-to-date written vaccination protocols are accessible at all locations where vaccines are administered.
10. Persons who administer vaccines and staff who manage or support vaccine administration are knowledgeable and receive ongoing education.
11. Health care professionals simultaneously administer as many indicated vaccine doses as possible.
12. Vaccination records for patients are accurate, complete, and easily accessible.
13. Health care professionals report adverse events following vaccination promptly and accurately to the VAERS and are aware of the VICP.
14. All personnel who have contact with patients are appropriately vaccinated.
15. Systems are used to remind parents/guardians, patients, and health care professionals when vaccinations are due and to recall patients whose vaccinations are overdue.
16. Office- or clinic-based patient record reviews and vaccination coverage assessments are performed annually.
17. Health care professionals practice community-based approaches.

Adult Immunization Practice

1. Adult immunization services are readily available.
2. Barriers to receiving vaccines are identified and minimized.
3. Patient's out-of-pocket costs are minimized.
4. Health care professionals routinely review the vaccination status of patients.
5. Health care professionals assess for valid contraindications.
6. Patients are educated about risks and benefits of vaccination in easy-to-understand language.
7. Written vaccination protocols are available at all locations where vaccinations are administered.
8. Persons who administer vaccines are properly trained.
9. Health care professionals recommend simultaneous administration of all indicated vaccine doses.
10. Vaccination records for patients are accurate and easily accessible.
11. All personnel who have contact with patients are appropriately vaccinated.
12. Systems are developed and used to remind patients and health care professionals when vaccinations are due and to recall patients whose vaccinations are overdue.
13. Standing orders for vaccinations are employed.
14. Regular assessments of vaccination coverage levels are conducted in the provider's practice.
15. Patient-oriented and community-based approaches are used to reach target populations.

Note: VAERS, Vaccine Adverse Events Reporting System; VICP, Vaccine Injury Compensation Program.
Source: Centers for Disease Control and Prevention, in *Epidemiology and Prevention of Vaccine-Preventable Diseases*, 2006, Appendix H. These standards can be found at *www.cdc.gov/nip/publications*.

recommended basic children's vaccines (bacille Calmette-Guérin, poliomyelitis, DTP/DTaP, and measles) have risen from 5% to ~80% worldwide, although coverage does not necessarily translate into protective immunity. Each year, at least 2.7 million deaths from measles, neonatal tetanus, and pertussis and 200,000 cases of paralysis due to polio are prevented by immunization. Despite the successes of this program, many vaccine-preventable diseases remain prevalent in the developing world. Measles, for example, continues to kill an estimated 500,000 children each year, and diphtheria, whooping cough, polio, and neonatal tetanus still occur at unacceptably high rates. An estimated 20–35% of all deaths of children are due to vaccine-preventable diseases.

In addition to the antigens included in the EPI for routine use in the developing world, others (hepatitis B, Hib, Japanese B encephalitis, yellow fever, meningococcal, mumps, and rubella) are used regionally, depending on disease epidemiology and resources. The rationale for inclusion of hepatitis B vaccine in Africa and Asia is to prevent the subsequent development of hepatocellular carcinoma, which is strongly linked with the persistence of hepatitis B virus from early childhood. The delivery of vaccines in mass campaigns on national immunization days, superseding even civil wars and insurgencies, has resulted in the cessation of transmission of poliomyelitis in the Western Hemisphere, the western Pacific, and Europe and in the virtual elimination of clinical measles from the Western Hemisphere. Periodic vaccination campaigns complement routine infant and childhood vaccination services under the rubric "catch up, follow up, and keep up." Despite these successes, concerns remain about the adequacy of long-term strategies to ensure continuity, the impact of vaccine campaigns on the provision of routine services, and unsafe injection practices.

Because infectious diseases know no geographic or political boundaries, uncontrolled disease anywhere in the world poses a threat to the United States, even without bioterrorism. Vaccines offer the opportunity to effectively control and even eliminate some diseases through individual and herd protection. Vaccines also represent the best societal hope for stopping the pandemic of HIV infection throughout the world and for efficiently controlling malaria and tuberculosis. Issues of cost, liability, risk, and profitability limit the interest of the pharmaceutical industry in the development of vaccines for infectious diseases of the poor.

SOURCES OF INFORMATION ON IMMUNIZATION

- Official vaccine package circulars and Vaccine Administration Statements from the CDC
- Report of the Committee on Infectious Diseases of the American Academy of Pediatrics ("Red Book")
- Recommendations of the Advisory Committee on Immunization Practices, CDC
- Guide for Adult Immunization, American College of Physicians
- Health Information for International Travel (published yearly) and Advisory Memoranda on Travel (published periodically), CDC
- Control of Communicable Diseases in Man, American Public Health Association
- Technical Bulletin of the College of Obstetrics and Gynecology
- National Network for Immunization Information, Infectious Diseases Society of America/Pediatric Infectious Diseases Society/American Academy of Pediatrics/American Nurses Association

FURTHER READINGS

BONHOEFFER J, HEININGER U: Immunization: Perception and evidence. Curr Opin Infect Dis 20:237, 2007

BROWN NJ et al: Vaccination, seizures and "vaccine damage." Curr Opin Neurol 20:181, 2007

BRUCE AYLWARD R et al: Risk management in a polio-free world. Risk Anal 26:1441, 2006

GOLDIE S: A public health approach to cervical cancer control: Considerations of screening and vaccination strategies. Int J Gynaecol Obstet 94(Suppl 1):S95, 2006

JACOBSON RM et al: Why is evidence-based medicine so harsh on vaccines? An exploration of the method and its natural biases. Vaccine 25:3165, 2007

KAUFMANN SH: The contribution of immunology to the rational design of novel antibacterial vaccines. Nat Rev Microbiol 5:491, 2007

KIMMEL SR et al: Addressing immunization barriers, benefits, and risks. J Fam Pract 56:S61, 2007

REELER AV: Anthropological perspectives on injections: A reivew. Bull World Health Organ 78:135, 2000

THOMPSON KM, TEBBENS RJ: Eradication versus control for poliomyelitis: An economic anlysis. Lancet 369:1363, 2007

VAN DER ZEIJST BA et al: On the design of national vaccination programmes. Vaccine 25:3143, 2007

117 Health Advice for International Travel

Jay S. Keystone, Phyllis E. Kozarsky

According to the World Tourism Organization, the number of international tourist arrivals in 2004 reached an all-time record of 763 million. This number represents an increase over the 2003 figure of almost 11%—the highest and the only double-digit percentage increase since 1980, when these statistics were first collected. Not only are more people traveling; travelers are seeking more exotic and remote destinations. Studies show that 50–75% of short-term travelers to the tropics or subtropics report some health impairment. Most of these health problems are minor: only 5% require medical attention, and <1% require hospitalization. Although infectious agents contribute substantially to morbidity among travelers, these pathogens account for only ~1% of deaths in this population. Cardiovascular disease and injuries are the most frequent causes of death among travelers from the United States, accounting for 49% and 22% of deaths, respectively. Age-specific rates of death due to cardiovascular disease are similar among travelers and nontravelers. In contrast, rates of death due to injury (the majority from motor vehicle, drowning, or aircraft accidents) are several times higher among travelers. Figure 117-1 summarizes the monthly incidence of health problems during travel in developing countries.

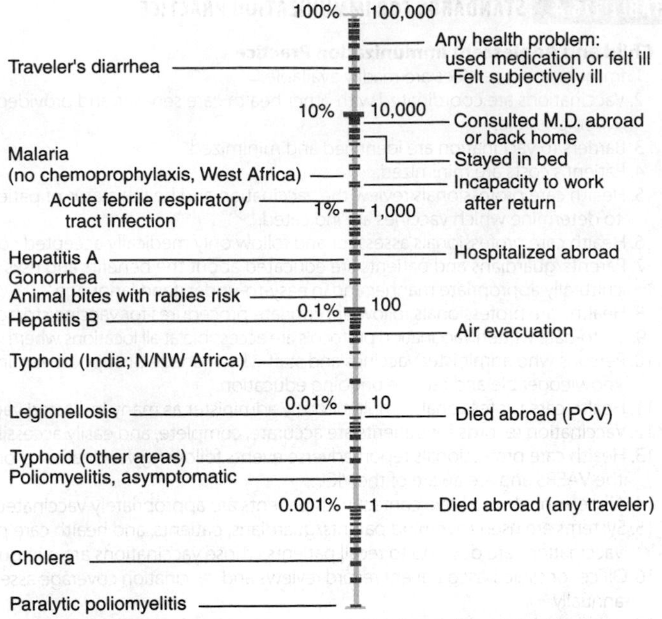

FIGURE 117-1 Incidence rate, per month, of health problems during a stay in developing countries. PCV, Peace Corps volunteer. *(From Steffen R, Lobel HO: Epidemiologic basis for the practice of travel medicine. J Wilderness Med 5:56, 1994. Reprinted with permission from Chapman and Hall, New York.)*

GENERAL ADVICE

Health maintenance recommendations are based not only on the traveler's destination but also on assessment of risk, which is determined by health status, specific itinerary, and lifestyle during travel. Detailed information regarding country-specific risks and recommendations may be obtained from the Centers for Disease Control and Prevention (CDC) publication *Health Information for International Travel* (available at *www.cdc.gov/travel/yb/*).

Fitness for travel is an issue of growing concern in view of the increased numbers of elderly and chronically ill individuals journeying to exotic destinations (see "Travel and Special Hosts," below). Since most commercial aircraft are pressurized to 2500 m (8000 ft) above sea level (corresponding to a Pa_{O_2} of ~55 mmHg), individuals with serious cardiopulmonary problems or anemia should be evaluated before travel. In addition, those who have recently had surgery, a myocardial infarction, a cerebrovascular accident, or a deep-vein thrombosis may be at high risk for adverse events during flight. A summary of current recommendations regarding fitness to fly has been published by the Aerospace Medical Association Air Transport Medicine Committee (*www.asma.org/publications/*). A pretravel health assessment may be advisable for individuals considering particularly adventurous recreational activities, such as mountain climbing and scuba diving.

IMMUNIZATIONS FOR TRAVEL

Immunizations for travel fall into three broad categories: *routine* (childhood/adult boosters that are necessary regardless of travel), *required* (immunizations that are mandated by international regulations for entry into certain areas or for border crossings), and *recommended* (immunizations that are desirable because of travel-related risks). Vaccines commonly given to travelers are listed in Table 117-1.

Routine Immunizations • ***DIPHTHERIA, TETANUS, AND POLIO*** Diphtheria (Chap. 131) continues to be a problem worldwide. Large outbreaks have occurred over the past decade in the independent states formerly encompassed by the Soviet Union. Serologic surveys show that tetanus (Chap. 133) antitoxin is lacking in many North Americans, especially in women over the age of 50. The risk of polio (Chap. 184) to the international traveler is extremely low, and wild-type poliovirus has been eradicated from the western hemisphere and Europe. However, studies in the United States suggest that 12% of adult travelers are unprotected against at least one poliovirus serogroup. Foreign travel offers an ideal opportunity to have these immunizations updated. With the recent increase in pertussis in adults, the diphtheria-tetanus-acellular pertussis (Tdap) combination may replace the Td vaccine as a 10-year booster once an adult polio immunization has been administered.

MEASLES Measles (rubeola) continues to be a major cause of morbidity and mortality in the developing world (Chap. 185). Several outbreaks of measles in the United States have been linked to imported cases. The group at highest risk consists of persons born after 1956 and vaccinated before 1980, in many of whom primary vaccination failed.

INFLUENZA Influenza—possibly the most common vaccine-preventable infection in travelers—occurs year-round in the tropics and during the summer months in the southern hemisphere (coinciding with the winter months in the northern hemisphere). One prospective study showed that influenza developed in 1% of travelers to Southeast Asia per month of stay. Vaccination should be considered for all travelers to these regions, particularly those who are elderly or chronically ill. Travel-related influenza continues to occur during summer months in Alaska and the Northwest Territories of Canada among cruise-ship passengers and staff (Chap. 180).

PNEUMOCOCCAL INFECTION Regardless of travel, pneumococcal vaccine should be administered routinely to the elderly and to persons at high risk of serious infection, including those with chronic heart, lung, or renal disease and those who have been splenectomized or have sickle cell disease (Chap. 128).

Required Immunizations • ***YELLOW FEVER*** Documentation of vaccination against yellow fever (Chap. 189) may be required as a condition of entry into or passage through countries of sub-Saharan Africa and equatorial South America, where the disease is endemic or epidemic, or for entry into countries at risk of having the infection introduced. This vaccine is given only by state-authorized yellow fever centers, and its administration must be documented on an official International Certificate of Vaccination. A registry of U.S. clinics that provide the vac-

TABLE 117-1 VACCINES COMMONLY USED FOR TRAVEL

Vaccine	Primary Series	Booster Interval
Cholera, live oral (CVD 103 - HgR)	1 dose	6 months
Hepatitis A (Havrix), 1440 enzyme immunoassay U/mL	2 doses, 6–12 months apart, IM	None required
Hepatitis A (VAQTA, AVAXIM, EPAXAL)	2 doses, 6–12 months apart, IM	None required
Hepatitis A/B combined (Twinrix)	3 doses at 0, 1, and 6–12 months *or* 0, 7, and 21 days plus booster at 1 year, IM	None required *except* 12 months (once only, for accelerated schedule)
Hepatitis B (Engerix B): accelerated schedule	3 doses at 0, 1, and 2 months *or* 0, 7, and 21 days plus booster at 1 year, IM	12 months, once only
Hepatitis B (Engerix B or Recombivax): standard schedule	3 doses at 0, 1, and 6 months, IM	None required
Immune globulin (hepatitis A prevention)	1 dose IM	Intervals of 3–5 months, depending on initial dose
Japanese encephalitis (JEV, Biken)	3 doses, 1 week apart, SC	12–18 months (first booster), then 4 years
Meningococcus, quadrivalent [Menimmune (polysaccharide), Menactra (conjugate)]	1 dose SC	>3 years (optimum booster schedule not yet determined)
Rabies (HDCV), rabies vaccine absorbed (RVA), or purified chick embryo cell vaccine (PCEC)	3 doses at 0, 7, and 21 or 28 days, IM	None required except with exposure
Typhoid Ty21a, oral live attenuated (Vivotif)	1 capsule every other day × 4 doses	5 years
Typhoid Vi capsular polysaccharide, injectable (Typhim Vi)	1 dose IM	2 years
Yellow fever	1 dose SC	10 years

cine is available from the CDC (*www.cdc.gov/travel/*). Recent data suggest that fewer than 50% of travelers entering areas endemic for yellow fever are immunized. Severe adverse events associated with this vaccine have recently increased in incidence. First-time vaccine recipients may present with a syndrome characterized as either neurotropic (1 case per 150,000–250,000 doses) or viscerotropic (1 case per 200,000–300,000 doses; among persons >60 years of age, 1 case per 40,000–50,000). Advanced age and thymic disease seem to increase the risk for these adverse events (*www.cdc.gov/nip/publications/VIS/vis-yf.pdf*).

MENINGOCOCCAL MENINGITIS Protection against meningitis (using one of the quadrivalent vaccines) is required for entry into Saudi Arabia during the Hajj (Chap. 136).

Recommended Immunizations • ***HEPATITIS A AND B*** Hepatitis A (Chap. 298) is one of the most frequent vaccine-preventable infections of travelers. The risk is six times greater for travelers who stray from the usual tourist routes. The mortality rate for hepatitis A increases with age, reaching almost 3% among individuals over age 50. Of the four hepatitis A vaccines currently available in North America (two in the United States), all are interchangeable and have an efficacy rate of >95%.

Long-stay overseas workers appear to be at considerable risk for hepatitis B infection (Chap. 298). The recommendation that all travelers be immunized against hepatitis B before departure is supported by two recent studies showing that 17% of the assessed travelers who received health care abroad had some type of injection; according to the World Health Organization, nonsterile equipment is used for up to 75% of all injections given in the developing world. A combined hepatitis A and B vaccine is now available in the United States and has been approved for administration on a 3-week accelerated schedule. It seems prudent to consider immunization of all travelers against hepatitis A and B.

TYPHOID FEVER The attack rate for typhoid fever (Chap. 146) is 1 case per 30,000 per month of travel to the developing world. However, the attack rates in India, Senegal, and North Africa are tenfold higher and are especially high among travelers to relatively remote destinations and among VFRs (immigrants returning to their homelands to visit friends or relatives). Between 1994 and 1999 in the United States, 77% of imported cases involved the latter group. Both of the available vaccines—one oral (live) and the other injectable (polysaccharide)—have efficacy rates of ~70%. In some countries, a combined hepatitis A/typhoid vaccine is available.

MENINGOCOCCAL MENINGITIS Although the risk of meningococcal disease among travelers has not been quantified, it is likely to be higher among travelers who live with poor indigenous populations in overcrowded conditions (Chap. 136). Either the older polysaccharide vaccine or the newer quadrivalent conjugate vaccine is recommended for persons traveling to sub-Saharan Africa during the dry season or to areas of the world where there are epidemics. The vaccine, which protects against serogroups A, C, Y, and W-135, has an efficacy rate of >90%.

JAPANESE ENCEPHALITIS The risk of Japanese encephalitis (Chap. 189), an infection transmitted by mosquitoes in rural Asia and Southeast Asia, is ~1 case per 5000 travelers per month of stay in an endemic area. Most symptomatic infections among U.S. residents have involved military personnel or their families. The vaccine efficacy rate is >90%; serious allergic reactions occur only rarely. The vaccine is recommended for persons staying >1 month in rural endemic areas or for shorter periods if their activities (e.g., camping, bicycling, hiking) in these areas will increase exposure risk. A Vero cell vaccine may be licensed in the United States within the next 2 years.

CHOLERA The risk of cholera (Chap. 149) is extremely low, with ~1 case per 500,000 journeys to endemic areas. Cholera vaccine, no longer available in the United States, was rarely recommended but was considered for aid and health care workers in refugee camps or in disaster-stricken/war-torn areas. A more effective oral cholera vaccine is available in other countries.

RABIES Domestic animals, primarily dogs, are the major transmitters of rabies in developing countries (Chap. 188). Several studies have shown that the risk of rabies posed by a dog bite in an endemic area translates into 1–3.6 cases per 1000 travelers per month of stay. Countries where canine rabies is highly endemic include Mexico, the Philippines, Sri Lanka, India, Thailand, and Vietnam. The three vaccines available in the United States provide >90% protection. Rabies vaccine is recommended for long-stay travelers, particularly children, and persons who may be occupationally exposed to rabies in endemic areas. Even after receipt of a preexposure rabies vaccine series, two postexposure doses are required. Travelers who have had the preexposure series will not require rabies immune globulin (which is often unavailable in developing countries) if they are exposed to the disease.

PREVENTION OF MALARIA AND OTHER INSECT-BORNE DISEASES

It is estimated that more than 30,000 American and European travelers develop malaria each year (Chap. 203). The risk to travelers is highest in Oceania and sub-Saharan Africa (estimated at 1:5 and 1:50 per month of stay, respectively, among persons not using chemoprophylaxis); intermediate in malarious areas on the Indian subcontinent and in Southeast Asia (1:250–1:1000 per month); and low in South and Central America (1:2500–1:10,000 per month). Of the more than 1000 cases of malaria reported annually in the United States, 90% of those due to *Plasmodium falciparum* occur in travelers returning or immigrating from Africa and

Oceania. VFRs are at the highest risk of acquiring malaria. With the worldwide increase in chloroquine- and multidrug-resistant falciparum malaria, decisions about chemoprophylaxis have become more difficult. In addition, the spread of malaria due to primaquine- and chloroquine-resistant strains of *Plasmodium vivax* has added to the complexity of treatment. The case-fatality rate of falciparum malaria in the United States is 4%; however, in only one-third of patients who die is the diagnosis of malaria considered before death.

Several studies indicate that fewer than 50% of travelers adhere to basic recommendations for malaria prevention. Keys to the prevention of malaria include both personal protection measures against mosquito bites (especially between dusk and dawn) and malaria chemoprophylaxis. The former measures include the use of DEET-containing insect repellents, permethrin-impregnated bed-nets and clothing, screened sleeping accommodations, and protective clothing. A new insect repellent containing picaridin as an active ingredient appears to be quite efficacious and is available in the United States only in low-concentration formulations that require frequent reapplications. Thus, in regions where infections such as malaria are transmitted, DEET products (25–50%) are recommended, even for children and infants >2 months of age. Personal protection measures also help prevent other insect-transmitted illnesses, such as dengue fever (Chap. 189). Over the past decade, the incidence of dengue has increased, particularly in the Caribbean region, Latin America, and Southeast Asia. Dengue virus is transmitted by an urban-dwelling mosquito that bites primarily at dawn and dusk.

Table 117-2 lists the currently recommended drugs of choice for prophylaxis of malaria, by destination.

PREVENTION OF GASTROINTESTINAL ILLNESS

Diarrhea, the leading cause of illness in travelers (Chap. 122), is usually a short-lived, self-limited condition; however, 40% of affected individuals need to alter their scheduled activities, and another 20% are confined to bed. The most important determinant of risk is the destination. Incidence rates per 2-week stay have been reported to be as low as 8% in industrialized countries and as high as 55% in parts of Africa, Central and South America, and Southeast Asia. Infants and young adults are at particularly high risk. A recent review suggested that there is little correlation between dietary indiscretions and the occurrence of travelers' diarrhea. Earlier studies of U.S. students in Mexico showed that eating meals in restaurants and cafeterias or consuming food from street vendors was associated with increased risk.

Etiology (See also Table 122-3) The most frequently identified pathogens causing travelers' diarrhea are toxigenic *Escherichia coli* and enteroaggregative *E. coli* (Chap. 143), although in some parts of the world (notably northern Africa and Southeast Asia) *Campylobacter* infections (Chap. 148) appear to predominate. Other common causative organisms include *Salmonella* (Chap. 146), *Shigella* (Chap. 147), rotavirus (Chap. 183), and norovirus (Chap. 183). The latter virus has caused numerous outbreaks on cruise ships. Except for giardiasis (Chap. 208), parasitic infections are uncommon causes of travelers' diarrhea. A growing problem for travelers is the development of antibiotic resistance among many bacterial pathogens. Examples include strains of *Campylobacter* resistant to quinolones and strains of *E. coli*, *Shigella*, and *Salmonella* resistant to trimethoprim-sulfamethoxazole.

TABLE 117-2 MALARIA CHEMOSUPPRESSIVE REGIMENS ACCORDING TO GEOGRAPHIC AREA[a]

Geographic Area	Drug of Choice	Alternatives
Central America (north of Panama), Haiti, Dominican Republic, Iraq, Egypt, Turkey, northern Argentina, and Paraguay	Chloroquine	Mefloquine Doxycycline Atovaquone/proguanil
South America including Panama (except northern Argentina and Paraguay); Asia (including Southeast Asia); Africa; and Oceania	Mefloquine Doxycycline Atovaquone-proguanil (Malarone)	Primaquine
Thai-Myanmar and Thai-Cambodian borders	Doxycycline Atovaquone-proguanil (Malarone)	

[a]See CDC's *Health Information for International Travel 2005–2006.*
Note: See also Chap. 203.

Precautions Although the mainstay of prevention of travelers' diarrhea involves food and water precautions, the literature has repeatedly documented dietary indiscretions by 98% of travelers within the first 72 h after arrival at their destination. The maxim "Boil it, cook it, peel it, or forget it!" is easy to remember but apparently difficult to follow. General food and water precautions include eating foods piping hot; avoiding foods that are raw, poorly cooked, or sold by street vendors; and drinking only boiled or commercially bottled beverages, particularly those that are carbonated. Heating kills diarrhea-causing organisms, whereas freezing does not; therefore, ice cubes made from unpurified water should be avoided.

Self-Treatment (See also Table 122-5) As travelers' diarrhea often occurs despite rigorous food and water precautions, travelers should carry medications for self-treatment. An antibiotic is useful in reducing the frequency of bowel movements and duration of illness in moderate to severe diarrhea. The standard regimen is a 3-day course of a quinolone taken twice daily (or, in the case of some newer formulations, once daily). However, studies have shown that a single double dose of a quinolone may be equally effective. For diarrhea acquired in areas such as Thailand, where >90% of *Campylobacter* infections are quinolone resistant, azithromycin may be a better alternative. Rifaximin, a poorly absorbed rifampin derivative, is highly effective against noninvasive bacterial pathogens such as toxigenic and enteroaggregative *E. coli.*

The current approach to self-treatment of travelers' diarrhea is for the traveler to carry three once-daily doses of an antibiotic and to use as many doses as necessary to resolve the illness. If neither high fever nor blood in the stool accompanies the diarrhea, loperamide may be taken in combination with the antibiotic.

Prophylaxis Prophylaxis of travelers' diarrhea with bismuth subsalicylate is widely used but only ~60% effective. For certain individuals (e.g., athletes, persons with a repeated history of travelers' diarrhea, and persons with chronic diseases), a single daily dose of a quinolone or azithromycin or a once-daily rifaximin regimen during travel of <1 month's duration is 75–90% efficacious in preventing travelers' diarrhea.

Illness after Return Although extremely common, acute travelers' diarrhea is usually self-limited or amenable to antibiotic therapy. Persistent bowel problems after the traveler returns home have a less well-defined etiology and may require medical attention from a specialist. Infectious agents (e.g., *Giardia lamblia*, *Cyclospora cayetanensis*, *Entamoeba histolytica*) appear to be responsible for only a small proportion of cases with persistent bowel symptoms. By far the most frequent causes of persistent diarrhea after travel are postinfectious sequelae such as lactose intolerance or irritable bowel syndrome. A recent meta-analysis showed that postinfectious irritable bowel syndrome may occur in as many as 4–13% of cases. When no infectious etiology can be identified, a trial of metronidazole therapy for presumed giardiasis, a strict lactose-free diet for 1 week, or a several-week trial of high-dose hydrophilic mucilloid (plus lactulose for persons with constipation) relieves the symptoms of many patients.

PREVENTION OF OTHER TRAVEL-RELATED PROBLEMS

Travelers are at high risk for *sexually transmitted diseases* (Chap. 124). Surveys have shown that large numbers engage in casual sex, and there is a reluctance to use condoms consistently. An increasing number of travelers are being diagnosed with *schistosomiasis* (Chap. 212). Travelers should be cautioned to avoid bathing, swimming, or wading in freshwater lakes, streams, or rivers in parts of tropical South America, the Caribbean, Africa, and Southeast Asia. Prevention of *travel-associated injury* depends mostly on common-sense precautions. Riding on motorcycles (especially without helmets) and in overcrowded public vehicles is not recommended; individuals should not travel in developing countries by road after dark, particularly in rural areas. In addition to its association with motor vehicle accidents, excessive alcohol use has been a significant factor in drownings, assaults, and injuries. Travelers are cautioned to avoid walking barefoot because of the risk of hookworm and *Strongyloides* infections (Chap. 210) and snakebites (Chap. 391).

THE TRAVELER'S MEDICAL KIT

A traveler's medical kit is strongly advisable. The contents may vary widely, depending on the itinerary, duration of stay, style of travel, and local medical facilities. While many medications are available abroad (often over the counter), directions for their use may be nonexistent or in a foreign language, or a product may be outdated or counterfeit. For example, a recent multicountry study in Southeast Asia showed that a mean of 53% (range, 21–92%) of antimalarial products were counterfeit or contained inadequate amounts of active drug. In the medical kit, the short-term traveler should consider carrying an analgesic; an antidiarrheal agent and an antibiotic for self-treatment of travelers' diarrhea; antihistamines; a laxative; oral rehydration salts; a sunscreen with a skin-protection factor of at least 30; a DEET-containing insect repellent for the skin; an insecticide for clothing (permethrin); and, if necessary, an antimalarial drug. To these medications, the long-stay traveler might add a broad-spectrum general-purpose antibiotic (levofloxacin or azithromycin), an antibacterial eye and skin ointment, and a topical antifungal cream. Regardless of the duration of travel, a first-aid kit containing such items as scissors, tweezers, and bandages should be considered. A practical approach to self-treatment of infections in the long-stay traveler who carries a once-daily dose of antibiotics is to use 3 tablets "below the waist" (bowel and bladder infections) and 6 tablets "above the waist" (skin and respiratory infections).

TRAVEL AND SPECIAL HOSTS

PREGNANCY AND TRAVEL

(See also Chap. 7) A woman's medical history and itinerary, the quality of medical care at her destinations, and her degree of flexibility determine whether travel is wise during pregnancy. According to the American College of Obstetrics and Gynecology, the safest part of pregnancy in which to travel is between 18 and 24 weeks, when there is the least danger of spontaneous abortion or premature labor. Some obstetricians prefer that women stay within a few hundred miles of home after the 28th week of pregnancy in case problems arise. In general, however, healthy women may be advised that it is acceptable to travel.

Relative contraindications to international travel during pregnancy include a history of miscarriage, premature labor, incompetent cervix, or toxemia. General medical problems such as diabetes, heart failure, severe anemia, or a history of thromboembolic disease should also prompt the pregnant woman to postpone her travels. Finally, regions in which the pregnant woman and her fetus may be at excessive risk (e.g., those at high altitudes and those where live-virus vaccines are required or where multidrug-resistant malaria is endemic) are not ideal destinations during any trimester.

Malaria Malaria during pregnancy carries a significant risk of morbidity and death. Levels of parasitemia are highest and failure to clear the parasites after treatment is most frequent among primigravidae. Severe disease, with complications such as cerebral malaria, massive hemolysis, and renal failure, is especially likely in pregnancy. Fetal sequelae include spontaneous abortion, stillbirth, preterm delivery, and congenital infection.

Travelers' Diarrhea Pregnant travelers must be extremely cautious regarding their food and beverage intake. Dehydration due to travelers' diarrhea can lead to inadequate placental blood flow. Infections such as toxoplasmosis, hepatitis E, and listeriosis can also have serious sequelae in pregnancy.

The mainstay of therapy for travelers' diarrhea is rehydration. Loperamide may be used if necessary. For self-treatment, azithromycin may be the best option. Although quinolones are increasingly being used safely during pregnancy and rifaximin is poorly absorbed from the gastrointestinal tract, they are not approved for this indication.

Because of the major problems encountered when infants are given local foods and beverages, women are strongly encouraged to breast-feed when traveling with a neonate. A nursing mother with travelers' diarrhea should not stop breast-feeding but should increase her fluid intake.

Air Travel and High-Altitude Destinations Commercial air travel is not a risk to the healthy pregnant woman or to the fetus. The higher radiation levels reported at altitudes of >10,500 m (>35,000 ft) should pose no problem to the healthy pregnant traveler. Since each airline has a policy regarding pregnancy and flying, it is best to check with the specific carrier when booking reservations. Domestic air travel is usually permitted until the 36th week, whereas international air travel is generally curtailed after the 32nd week.

There are no known risks for pregnant women who travel to high-altitude destinations and stay for short periods. However, there are likewise no data on the safety of pregnant women at altitudes of >4500 m (15,000 ft).

THE HIV-INFECTED TRAVELER

(See also Chap. 182) The HIV-infected traveler is at special risk of serious infections due to a number of pathogens that may be more prevalent at travel destinations than at home. However, the degree of risk depends primarily on the state of the immune system at the time of travel. For persons whose CD4+ T cell counts are normal or >500/μL, no data suggest a greater risk during travel than for persons without HIV infection. Individuals with AIDS (CD4+ T cell counts of <200/μL) and others who are symptomatic need special counseling and should visit a travel medicine practitioner before departure, especially when traveling to the developing world.

Several countries now routinely deny entry to HIV-positive individuals, even though these restrictions do not appear to decrease rates of transmission of the virus. In general, HIV testing is required of those individuals who wish to stay abroad >3 months or who intend to work or study abroad. Some countries will accept an HIV serologic test done within 6 months of departure, whereas others will not accept a blood test done at any time in the traveler's home country. Border officials often have the authority to make inquiries of individuals entering a country and to check the medications they are carrying. If a drug such as zidovudine is identified, the person may be barred from entering the country. Information on testing requirements for specific countries is available from consular offices but is subject to frequent change.

Immunizations All of the HIV-infected traveler's routine immunizations should be up to date (Chap. 116). The response to immunization may be impaired at CD4+ T cell counts of <200/μL (and in some cases at even higher counts). Thus HIV-infected persons should be vaccinated as early as possible to ensure adequate immune responses to all vaccines. In patients receiving highly active antiretroviral therapy, at least 3 months must elapse before regenerated CD4+ T cells can be considered fully functional; therefore, in these patients, vaccinations should be delayed. However, when the risk of illness is high or the sequelae of illness are serious, immunization is recommended. In certain circumstances, it may be prudent to check the adequacy of the serum antibody response before departure.

Because of the increased risk of infections due to *Streptococcus pneumoniae* and other bacterial pathogens that cause pneumonia following influenza, pneumococcal polysaccharide and influenza vaccines should be administered. The estimated rates of response to influenza vaccine are >80% among persons with asymptomatic HIV infection and <50% among those with AIDS.

In general, live attenuated vaccines are contraindicated for persons with immune dysfunction. Because measles (rubeola) can be a severe and lethal infection in HIV-positive patients, these patients should receive the measles vaccine (or the combination measles-mumps-rubella vaccine) unless the CD4+ T cell count is <200/μL. Between 18% and 58% of symptomatic HIV-infected vaccinees develop adequate antibody titers, and 50–100% of asymptomatic HIV-infected persons seroconvert.

It is recommended that the live yellow fever vaccine not be given to HIV-infected travelers. Although the potential adverse effects of a live vaccine in an HIV-infected individual are always a consideration, there appear to have been no reported cases of illness in those who have inadvertently received this vaccine. Nonetheless, if the CD4+ T cell count is <200/μL, an alternative itinerary that poses no risk of exposure to yellow fever is recommended. If the traveler is passing through or traveling to an area where the vaccine is required but the disease risk is low, a physician's waiver should be issued.

A transient increase in viremia (lasting days to weeks) has been demonstrated in HIV-infected individuals following immunization against influenza, pneumococcal infection, and tetanus (Chap. 182). However, at this point, there is no evidence that this transient increase is detrimental.

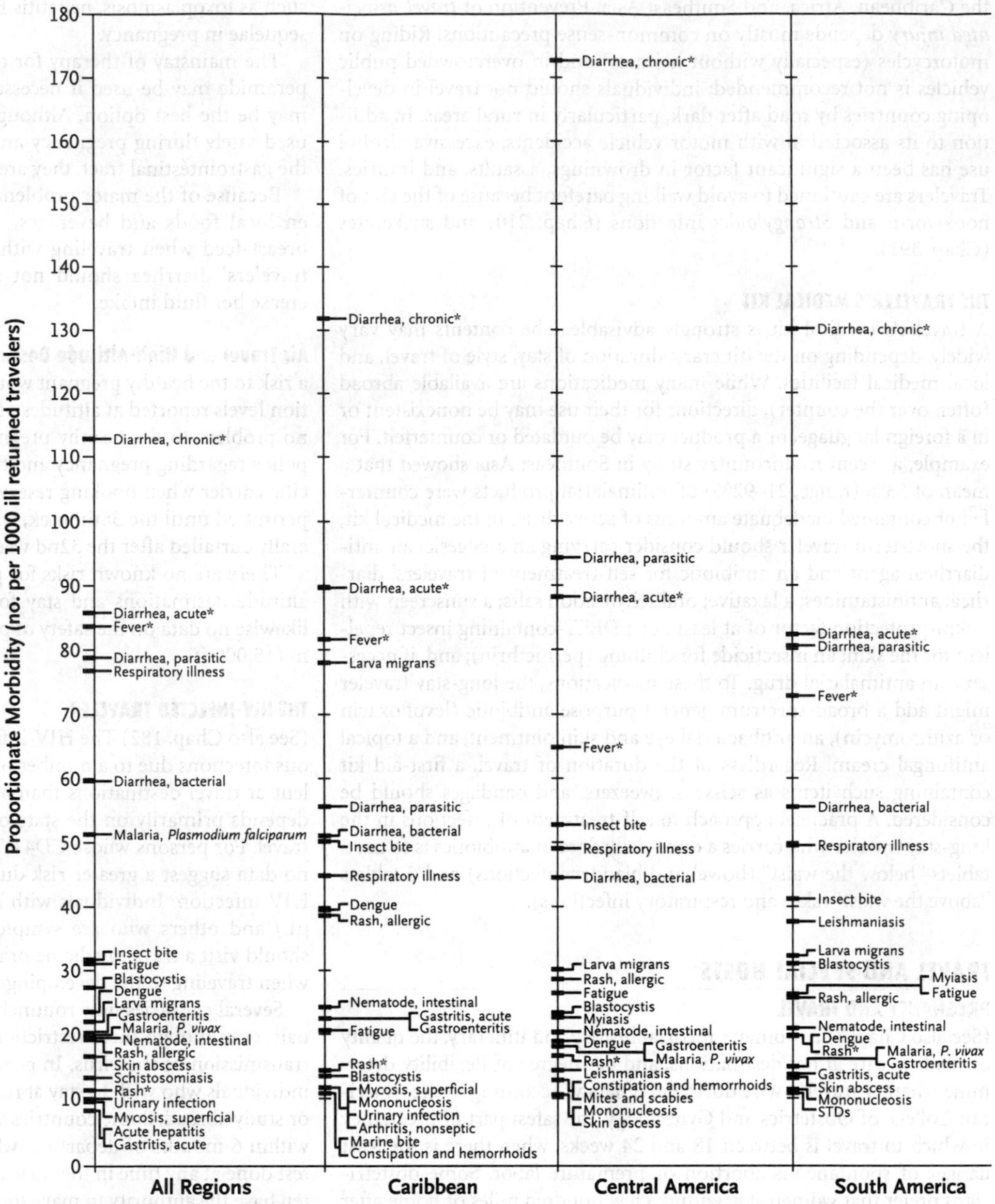

FIGURE 117-2 Proportionate morbidity among ill travelers returning from the developing world, according to region of travel. The proportions (not incidence rates) are shown for each of the top 22 specific diagnoses among all ill returned travelers within each region.

Gastrointestinal Illness Decreased levels of gastric acid, abnormal gastrointestinal mucosal immunity, other complications of HIV infection, and medications taken by HIV-infected patients make travelers' diarrhea especially problematic in these individuals. Travelers' diarrhea is likely to occur more frequently, be more severe, be accompanied by bacteremia, and be more difficult to treat. Although uncommon, *Cryptosporidium, Isospora belli, and Microsporidium* infections are associated with increased morbidity and mortality in AIDS patients.

The HIV-infected traveler must be careful to consume only appropriately prepared foods and beverages and may benefit from antibiotic prophylaxis for travelers' diarrhea. Sulfonamides (as used to prevent pneumocystosis) are ineffective because of widespread resistance.

Other Travel-Related Infections Data are lacking on the severity of many vector-borne diseases in HIV-infected individuals. Malaria is especially severe in asplenic persons and in those with AIDS. The HIV load doubles during malaria, with subsidence in ~8–9 weeks; the significance of this increase in viral load is unknown.

Visceral leishmaniasis (Chap. 205) has been reported in numerous HIV-infected travelers. Diagnosis may be difficult, given that splenomegaly and hyperglobulinemia are often lacking and serologic results are frequently negative. Sandfly bites may be prevented by evening use of insect repellents.

Certain respiratory illnesses, such as histoplasmosis and coccidioidomycosis, cause greater morbidity and mortality among patients with AIDS. Although tuberculosis is common among HIV-infected persons (especially in developing countries), its acquisition by the short-term HIV-infected traveler has not been reported as a major problem.

Medications Adverse events due to medications and drug interactions are common and raise complex issues for HIV-infected persons. Rates of cutaneous reaction (e.g., increased cutaneous sensitivity to sulfonamides) are unusually high among patients with AIDS. Since zidovudine is metabolized by hepatic glucuronidation, inhibitors of this process may elevate serum levels of the drug. Concomitant administration of the antimalarial drug mefloquine and the antiretroviral agent ritonavir may result in decreased plasma levels of ritonavir. In contrast, no significant influence of concomitant mefloquine administration on plasma levels of indinavir or nelfinavir was detected in two HIV-infected travelers. There is a strong theoretical concern that the

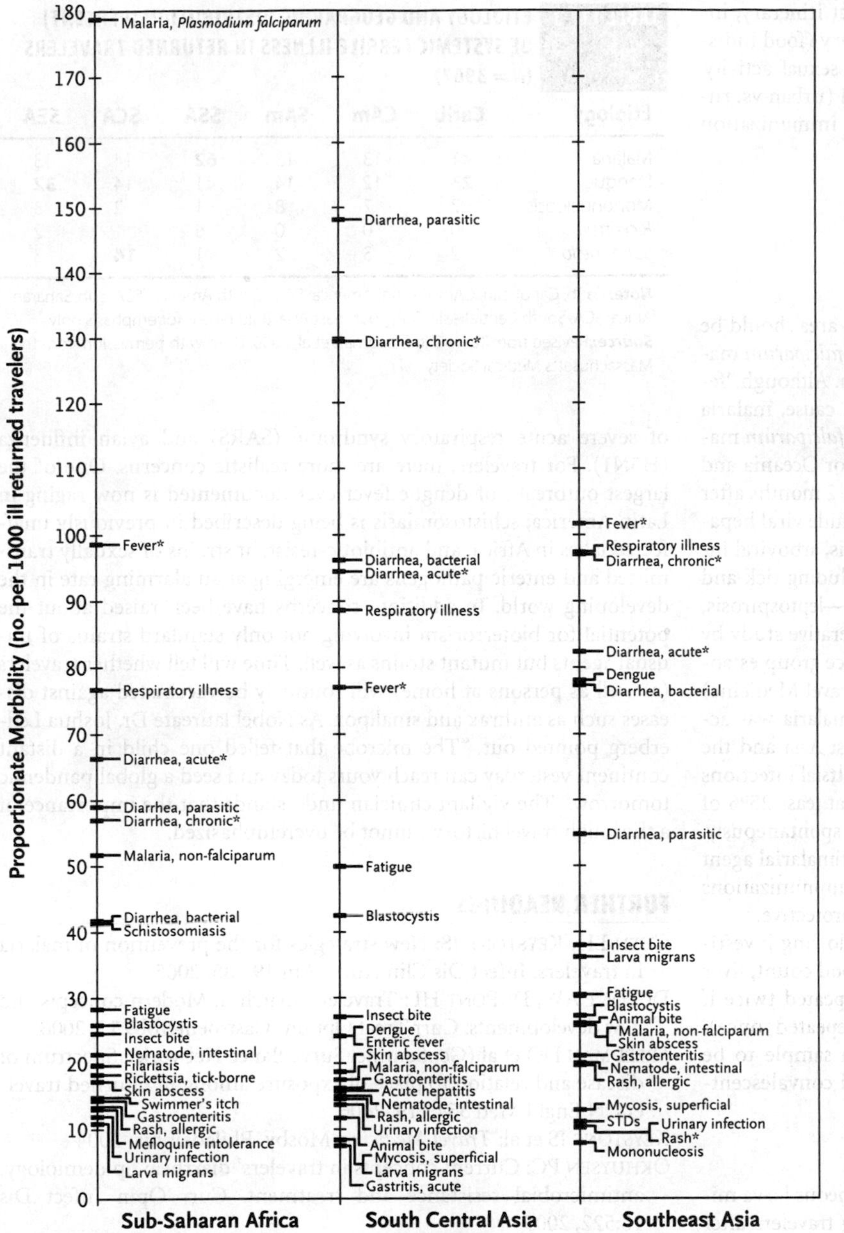

FIGURE 117-2 ***(Continued)*** STDs, sexually transmitted diseases. Asterisks indicate syndromic diagnoses for which specific etiologies could not be assigned. *(Reprinted with permission from Freedman et al. © 2006 Massachusetts Medical Society.)*

antimalarial drugs lumefantrine (combined with artemisinin in Coartem and Riamet) and halofantrine may interact with HIV protease inhibitors and nonnucleoside reverse transcriptase inhibitors since the latter are known to be potent inhibitors of cytochrome P450.

CHRONIC ILLNESS, DISABILITY, AND TRAVEL

Chronic health problems need not prevent travel, but special measures can make the journey safer and more comfortable.

Heart Disease Cardiovascular events are the main cause of deaths among travelers and of in-flight emergencies on commercial aircraft. Extra supplies of all medications should be kept in carry-on luggage, along with a copy of a recent electrocardiogram and the name and telephone number of the traveler's physician at home. Pacemakers are not affected by airport security devices, although electronic telephone checks of pacemaker function cannot be transmitted by international satellites. Travelers with electronic defibrillators should carry a note to that effect and ask for hand screening. A traveler may benefit from supplemental oxygen; since oxygen delivery systems are not standard, supplementary oxygen should be ordered by the traveler's physician well before flight time. Travelers may benefit from aisle seating and should walk, perform stretching and flexing exercises, consider wearing support hose, and remain hydrated during the flight to prevent venous thrombosis and pulmonary embolism.

Chronic Lung Disease Chronic obstructive pulmonary disease is one of the most common diagnoses in patients who require emergency-department evaluation for symptoms occurring during airline flights. The best predictor of the development of in-flight problems is the sea-level Pa_{O_2}. A Pa_{O_2} of at least 72 mmHg corresponds to an in-flight arterial Pa_{O_2} of ~55 mmHg when the cabin is pressurized to 2500 m (8000 ft). If the traveler's baseline Pa_{O_2} is <72 mmHg, the provision of supplemental oxygen should be considered. Contraindications to flight include active bronchospasm, lower respiratory infection, lower-limb deep-vein phlebitis, pulmonary hypertension, and recent thoracic surgery (within the preceding 3 weeks) or pneumothorax. Decreased outdoor activity at the destination should be considered if air pollution is excessive.

Diabetes Mellitus Alterations in glucose control and changes in insulin requirements are common problems among patients with diabetes who travel. Changes in time zone, in the amount and timing of food intake, and in physical activity demand vigilant assessment of metabolic control. The traveler with diabetes should pack medication (including a bottle of regular insulin for emergencies), insulin syringes and needles, equipment and supplies for glucose monitoring, and snacks in carry-on luggage. Insulin is stable for ~3 months at room temperature but should be kept as cool as possible. The name and telephone number of the home physician and a card and bracelet listing the patient's medical problems and the type and dose of insulin used should accompany the traveler. In traveling eastward (e.g., from the United States to Europe), the morning insulin dose on arrival may need to be decreased. The blood glucose can then be checked during the day to determine whether additional insulin is required. For flights westward, with lengthening of the day, an additional dose of regular insulin may be required.

Other Special Groups Other groups for whom special travel measures are encouraged include patients undergoing dialysis, those with transplants, and those with other disabilities. Up to 13% of travelers have some disability, but few advocacy groups and tour companies dedicate themselves to this growing population. Medication interactions are a source of serious concern for these travelers, and appropriate medical information should be carried, along with the home physician's name and telephone number. Some travelers taking glucocorticoids carry stress doses in case they become ill. Immunization of these immunocompromised travelers may result in less than adequate protection. Thus the traveler and the physician must carefully consider which destinations are appropriate.

PROBLEMS AFTER RETURN

The most common medical problems encountered by travelers after their return home are diarrhea, fever, respiratory illnesses, and skin diseases (Fig. 117-2). Frequently ignored problems are fatigue and emotional stress, especially in long-stay travelers. The approach to diagnosis requires some knowledge of geographic medicine, in particular the epidemiology and clinical presentation of infectious disorders. A geographic history should focus on the traveler's exact itinerary, including dates of arrival and departure; exposure history (food indiscretions, drinking-water sources, freshwater contact, sexual activity, animal contact, insect bites); location and style of travel (urban vs. rural, first-class hotel accommodation vs. camping); immunization history; and use of antimalarial chemosuppression.

DIARRHEA

See "Prevention of Gastrointestinal Illness," above.

FEVER

Fever in a traveler who has returned from a malarious area should be considered a medical emergency because death from *P. falciparum* malaria can follow an illness of only several days' duration. Although "fever from the tropics" does not always have a tropical cause, malaria should be the first diagnosis considered. The risk of *P. falciparum* malaria is highest among travelers returning from Africa or Oceania and among those who become symptomatic within the first 2 months after return. Other important causes of fever after travel include viral hepatitis (hepatitis A and E), typhoid fever, bacterial enteritis, arboviral infections (e.g., dengue fever), rickettsial infections (including tick and scrub typhus and Q fever), and—in rare instances—leptospirosis, acute HIV infection, and amebic liver abscess. A cooperative study by GeoSentinel (an emerging infectious disease surveillance group established by the CDC and the International Society of Travel Medicine) showed that, among 3907 febrile returned travelers, malaria was acquired most often from Africa, dengue from Southeast Asia and the Caribbean, typhoid fever from southern Asia, and rickettsial infections (tick typhus) from southern Africa (**Table 117-3**). In at least 25% of cases, no etiology can be found, and the illness resolves spontaneously. Clinicians should keep in mind that no present-day antimalarial agent guarantees protection from malaria and that some immunizations (notably, that against typhoid fever) are only partially protective.

When no specific diagnosis is forthcoming, the following investigations, where applicable, are suggested: complete blood count, liver function tests, thick/thin blood films for malaria (repeated twice if necessary), urinalysis, urine and blood cultures (repeated once), chest x-ray, and collection of an acute-phase serum sample to be held for subsequent examination along with a paired convalescent-phase serum sample.

SKIN DISEASES

Pyodermas, sunburn, insect bites, skin ulcers, and cutaneous larva migrans are the most common skin conditions affecting travelers after their return home. In those with persistent skin ulcers, a diagnosis of cutaneous leishmaniasis, mycobacterial infection, or fungal infection should be considered. Careful, complete inspection of the skin is important in detecting the rickettsial eschar in a febrile patient or the central breathing hole in a "boil" due to myiasis.

EMERGING INFECTIOUS DISEASES

In recent years, travel and commerce have fostered the worldwide spread of HIV infection, led to the reemergence of cholera as a global health threat, and created considerable fear about the possible spread of severe acute respiratory syndrome (SARS) and avian influenza (H5N1). For travelers, there are more realistic concerns. One of the largest outbreaks of dengue fever ever documented is now raging in Latin America; schistosomiasis is being described in previously unaffected lakes in Africa; and antibiotic-resistant strains of sexually transmitted and enteric pathogens are emerging at an alarming rate in the developing world. In addition, concerns have been raised about the potential for bioterrorism involving not only standard strains of unusual agents but mutant strains as well. Time will tell whether travelers (as well as persons at home) will routinely be vaccinated against diseases such as anthrax and smallpox. As Nobel laureate Dr. Joshua Lederberg pointed out, "The microbe that felled one child in a distant continent yesterday can reach yours today and seed a global pandemic tomorrow." The vigilant clinician understands that the importance of a thorough travel history cannot be overemphasized.

TABLE 117-3 ETIOLOGY AND GEOGRAPHIC DISTRIBUTION (PERCENT) OF SYSTEMIC FEBRILE ILLNESS IN RETURNED TRAVELERS (*N* = 3907)

Etiology	Carib	CAm	SAm	SSA	SCA	SEA
Malaria	<1	13	13	**62**	14	13
Dengue	**23**	12	14	<1	14	**32**
Mononucleosis	7	7	8	1	2	3
Rickettsia	0	0	0	**6**	1	2
Salmonella	2	3	2	<1	**14**	3

Note: Carib, Caribbean; CAm, Central America; SAm, South America; SSA, Sub-Saharan Africa; SCA, South Central Asia; SEA, Southeast Asia. Bold type is for emphasis only.
Source: Revised from Table 2 in Freedman et al, 2006. Used with permission from the Massachusetts Medical Society.

FURTHER READINGS

CHEN LH, KEYSTONE JS: New strategies for the prevention of malaria in travelers. Infect Dis Clin North Am 19:185, 2005

DUPONT AW, DUPONT HL: Travelers' diarrhea: Modern concepts and new developments. Curr Treat Options Gastroenterol 9:13, 2006

FREEDMAN DO et al (GeoSentinel Surveillance Network): Spectrum of disease and relation to place of exposure among ill returned travelers. N Engl J Med 354:119, 2006

KEYSTONE JS et al: *Travel Medicine*. Mosby, Philadelphia, 2004

OKHUYSEN PC: Current concepts in travelers' diarrhea: Epidemiology, antimicrobial resistance and treatment. Curr Opin Infect Dis 18:522, 2005

RYAN ET et al: Illness after international travel. N Engl J Med 347:505, 2002

SHLIM DR: Update in traveler's diarrhea. Infect Dis Clin North Am 19:137, 2005

SOHAIL MR, FISCHER PR: Health risks to air travelers. Infect Dis Clin North Am 19:67, 2005

WILSON ME, CHEN LH: Dermatologic infectious diseases in international travelers. Curr Infect Dis Rep 6:54, 2004

WEBSITES OF INTEREST: Chronic renal failure: *www.kidney.org*. Diabetes: *www.diabetesmonitor.com/other-14.htm*. Dialysis: *www.dialysisfinder.com*. Disability: *www.access-able.com*. HIV: *www.aegis.com*

118 Infective Endocarditis

Adolf W. Karchmer

The prototypic lesion of infective endocarditis, the *vegetation* (Fig. 118-1), is a mass of platelets, fibrin, microcolonies of microorganisms, and scant inflammatory cells. Infection most commonly involves heart valves (either native or prosthetic) but may also occur on the low-pressure side of the ventricular septum at the site of a defect, on the mural endocardium where it is damaged by aberrant jets of blood or foreign bodies, or on intracardiac devices themselves. The analogous process involving arteriovenous shunts, arterioarterial shunts (patent ductus arteriosus), or a coarctation of the aorta is called *infective endarteritis.*

Endocarditis may be classified according to the temporal evolution of disease, the site of infection, the cause of infection, or a predisposing risk factor such as injection drug use. While each classification criterion provides therapeutic and prognostic insight, none is sufficient alone. *Acute endocarditis* is a hectically febrile illness that rapidly damages cardiac structures, hematogenously seeds extracardiac sites, and, if untreated, progresses to death within weeks. *Subacute endocarditis* follows an indolent course; causes structural cardiac damage only slowly, if at all; rarely metastasizes; and is gradually progressive unless complicated by a major embolic event or ruptured mycotic aneurysm.

In developed countries, the incidence of endocarditis ranges from 2.6 to 7.0 cases per 100,000 population per year and remained relatively stable from 1950 to 2000. While rates of congenital heart diseases remain constant, other predisposing conditions in developed countries have shifted from chronic rheumatic heart disease to illicit IV drug use, degenerative valve disease, intracardiac devices, and health care–associated infection. The incidence of endocarditis is notably increased among the elderly. In reported series, 10–30% of endocarditis cases involve prosthetic valves. The risk of prosthesis infection is greatest during the first 6 months after valve replacement; gradually declines to a low, stable rate thereafter; and is similar for mechanical and bioprosthetic devices.

ETIOLOGY

Although many species of bacteria and fungi cause sporadic episodes of endocarditis, only a few bacterial species cause the majority of cases (Table 118-1). The pathogens vary somewhat with the clinical types of endocarditis, in part because of different portals of entry. The oral cavity, skin, and upper respiratory tract are the respective primary portals for the viridans streptococci, staphylococci, and HACEK organisms (*Haemophilus*, *Actinobacillus*, *Cardiobacterium*, *Eikenella*, and *Kingella*) causing community-acquired native valve endocarditis. *Streptococcus bovis* originates from the gastrointestinal tract, where it is associated with polyps and colonic tumors, and enterococci enter the bloodstream from the genitourinary tract. Health care–associated native valve endocarditis is the consequence of bacteremia arising from intravascular catheter infections, nosocomial wound and urinary tract infections, and chronic invasive procedures such as hemodialysis. Endocarditis complicates 6–25% of episodes of catheter-associated *Staphylococcus aureus* bacteremia; the higher rates are detected by careful transesophageal echocardiography (TEE) screening (see "Echocardiography," below).

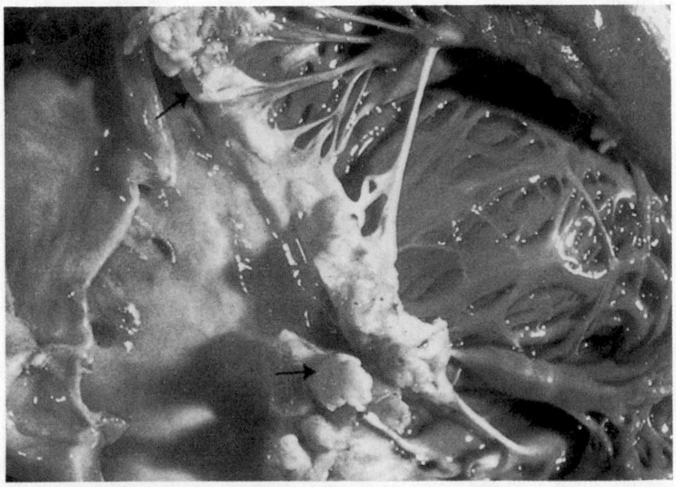

FIGURE 118-1 Vegetations (*arrows*) due to viridans streptococcal endocarditis involving the mitral valve.

Prosthetic valve endocarditis arising within 2 months of valve surgery is generally the result of intraoperative contamination of the prosthesis or a bacteremic postoperative complication. The nosocomial nature of these infections is reflected in their primary microbial causes: coagulase-negative staphylococci (CoNS), *S. aureus*, facultative gram-negative bacilli, diphtheroids, and fungi. The portals of entry and organisms causing cases beginning >12 months after surgery are similar to those in community-acquired native valve endocarditis. Epidemiologic evidence suggests that prosthetic valve endocarditis due to CoNS that presents 2–12 months after surgery often represents delayed-onset nosocomial infection. At least 85% of CoNS strains that cause prosthetic valve endocarditis within 12 months of surgery are methicillin-resistant; the rate of methicillin resistance decreases to 25% among CoNS strains causing prosthetic valve endocarditis that presents >1 year after valve surgery.

Transvenous pacemaker lead– and/or implanted defibrillator–associated endocarditis is usually nosocomial. The majority of episodes occur within weeks of implantation or generator change and are caused by *S. aureus* or CoNS.

Endocarditis occurring among injection drug users, especially when infection involves the tricuspid valve, is commonly caused by *S. aureus* strains, many of which are methicillin-resistant. Left-sided valve infections in addicts have a more varied etiology and involve abnormal valves, often ones damaged by prior episodes of endocarditis. A number of these cases are caused by *Pseudomonas aeruginosa* and *Candida* species, and sporadic cases are due to unusual organisms such as *Bacillus*, *Lactobacillus*, and *Corynebacterium* species. Polymicrobial endocarditis is more common among injection drug users than among patients who do not inject drugs. The presence of HIV in the former population does not significantly influence the causes of endocarditis.

From 5 to 15% of patients with endocarditis have negative blood cultures; in one-third to one-half of these cases, cultures are negative because of prior antibiotic exposure. The remainder of these patients are infected by fastidious organisms, such as nutritionally variant organisms (now designated *Granulicatella* and *Abiotrophia* species), HACEK organisms, and *Bartonella* species. Some fastidious organisms that cause endocarditis do so in characteristic epidemiologic settings (e.g., *Coxiella burnetii* in Europe, *Brucella* species in the Middle East). *Tropheryma whipplei* causes an indolent, culture-negative, afebrile form of endocarditis.

PATHOGENESIS

Unless it is injured, the endothelium is resistant to infection by most bacteria and to thrombus formation. Endothelial injury (e.g., at the site of impact of high-velocity blood jets or on the low-pressure side of a cardiac structural lesion) causes aberrant flow and allows either direct infection by virulent organisms or the development of an uninfected

TABLE 118-1 ORGANISMS CAUSING MAJOR CLINICAL FORMS OF ENDOCARDITIS

	Percent of Cases							
	Native Valve Endocarditis		Prosthetic Valve Endocarditis at Indicated Time of Onset (Months) after Valve Surgery			Endocarditis in Injection Drug Users		
Organism	Community-Acquired (*n* = 683)	Health Care–Associated (*n* = 128)	< 2 (*n* = 144)	2–12 (*n* = 31)	> 12 (*n* = 194)	Right-Sided (*n* = 346)	Left-Sided (*n* = 204)	Total (*n* = 675)[a]
Streptococci[b]	32	8	1	9	31	5	15	12
Pneumococci	1	—	—	—	—	—	—	—
Enterococci	8	16	8	12	11	2	24	9
Staphylococcus aureus	35	44[c]	22	12	18	77	23	57
Coagulase-negative staphylococci	4	15	33	32	11	—	—	—
Fastidious gram-negative coccobacilli (HACEK group)[d]	3	—	—	—	6	—	—	—
Gram-negative bacilli	3	5	13	3	6	5	13	7
Candida spp.	1	6	8	12	1	—	12	4
Polymicrobial/miscellaneous	6	1	3	6	5	8	10	7
Diphtheroids	—	—	6	—	3	—	—	0.1
Culture-negative	5	5	5	6	8	3	3	3

[a]The total number of cases is larger than the sum of right- and-left-sided cases because the location of infection was not specified in some cases.
[b]Includes viridans streptococci; *Streptococcus bovis*; other non–group A, groupable streptococci; and *Abiotrophia* spp. (nutritionally variant, pyridoxal-requiring streptococci).
[c]Methicillin resistance is common among these *S. aureus* strains.
[d]Includes *Haemophilus* spp., *Actinobacillus actinomycetemcomitans*, *Cardiobacterium hominis*, *Eikenella* spp., and *Kingella* spp.
Note: Data are compiled from multiple studies.

platelet-fibrin thrombus—a condition called *nonbacterial thrombotic endocarditis* (NBTE). The thrombus subsequently serves as a site of bacterial attachment during transient bacteremia. The cardiac conditions most commonly resulting in NBTE are mitral regurgitation, aortic stenosis, aortic regurgitation, ventricular septal defects, and complex congenital heart disease. These conditions result from rheumatic heart disease (particularly in the developing world, where rheumatic fever remains prevalent), mitral valve prolapse, degenerative heart disease, and congenital malformations. NBTE also arises as a result of a hypercoagulable state; this phenomenon gives rise to the clinical entity of *marantic endocarditis* (uninfected vegetations seen in patients with malignancy and chronic diseases) and to bland vegetations complicating systemic lupus erythematosus and the antiphospholipid antibody syndrome.

Organisms that cause endocarditis generally enter the bloodstream from mucosal surfaces, the skin, or sites of focal infection. Except for more virulent bacteria (e.g., *S. aureus*) that can adhere directly to intact endothelium or exposed subendothelial tissue, microorganisms in the blood adhere to sites at NBTE. If resistant to the bactericidal activity of serum and the microbicidal peptides released locally by platelets, the organisms proliferate and induce a procoagulant state at the site by eliciting tissue factor from adherent monocytes or, in the case of *S. aureus*, from monocytes and from intact endothelium. Fibrin deposition combines with platelet aggregation, stimulated by tissue factor and independently by proliferating microorganisms, to generate an infected vegetation. The organisms that commonly cause endocarditis have surface adhesin molecules, collectively called microbial surface components recognizing adhesin matrix molecules (MSCRAMMs), that mediate adherence to NBTE sites or injured endothelium. Fibronectin-binding proteins present on many gram-positive bacteria, clumping factor (a fibrinogen- and fibrin-binding surface protein) on *S. aureus*, and glucans or FimA (a member of the family of oral mucosal adhesins) on streptococci facilitate adherence. Fibronectin-binding proteins are required for *S. aureus* invasion of intact endothelium; thus these surface proteins may facilitate infection of previously normal valves. In the absence of host defenses, organisms enmeshed in the growing platelet-fibrin vegetation proliferate to form dense microcolonies. Organisms deep in vegetations are metabolically inactive (nongrowing) and relatively resistant to killing by antimicrobial agents. Proliferating surface organisms are shed into the bloodstream continuously.

The pathophysiologic consequences and clinical manifestations of endocarditis—other than constitutional symptoms, which probably result from cytokine production—arise from damage to intracardiac structures; embolization of vegetation fragments, leading to infection or infarction of remote tissues; hematogenous infection of sites during bacteremia; and tissue injury due to the deposition of circulating immune complexes or immune responses to deposited bacterial antigens.

CLINICAL MANIFESTATIONS

The clinical syndrome of infective endocarditis is highly variable and spans a continuum between acute and subacute presentations. Native valve endocarditis (whether acquired in the community or in association with health care), prosthetic valve endocarditis, and endocarditis due to injection drug use share clinical and laboratory manifestations (Table 118-2). The causative microorganism is primarily responsible for the temporal course of endocarditis. β-Hemolytic streptococci, *S. aureus*, and pneumococci typically result in an acute course, although

TABLE 118-2 CLINICAL AND LABORATORY FEATURES OF INFECTIVE ENDOCARDITIS

Feature	Frequency, %
Fever	80–90
Chills and sweats	40–75
Anorexia, weight loss, malaise	25–50
Myalgias, arthralgias	15–30
Back pain	7–15
Heart murmur	80–85
New/worsened regurgitant murmur	10–40
Arterial emboli	20–50
Splenomegaly	15–50
Clubbing	10–20
Neurologic manifestations	20–40
Peripheral manifestations (Osler's nodes, subungual hemorrhages, Janeway lesions, Roth's spots)	2–15
Petechiae	10–40
Laboratory manifestations	
Anemia	70–90
Leukocytosis	20–30
Microscopic hematuria	30–50
Elevated erythrocyte sedimentation rate	>90
Elevated C-reactive protein level	>90
Rheumatoid factor	50
Circulating immune complexes	65–100
Decreased serum complement	5–40

S. aureus occasionally causes subacute disease. Endocarditis caused by *Staphylococcus lugdunensis* (a coagulase-negative species) or by enterococci may present acutely. Subacute endocarditis is typically caused by viridans streptococci, enterococci, CoNS, and the HACEK group. Endocarditis caused by *Bartonella* species and the agent of Q fever, *C. burnetii*, is exceptionally indolent.

The clinical features of endocarditis are nonspecific. However, these symptoms in a febrile patient with valvular abnormalities or a behavior pattern that predisposes to endocarditis (e.g., injection drug use) suggest the diagnosis, as do bacteremia with organisms that frequently cause endocarditis, otherwise-unexplained arterial emboli, and progressive cardiac valvular incompetence. In patients with subacute presentations, fever is typically low-grade and rarely exceeds 39.4°C (103°F); in contrast, temperatures of 39.4°–40°C (103°–104°F) are often noted in acute endocarditis. Fever may be blunted or absent in patients who are elderly or severely debilitated or who have marked cardiac or renal failure.

Cardiac Manifestations Although heart murmurs are usually indicative of the predisposing cardiac pathology rather than of endocarditis, valvular damage and ruptured chordae may result in new regurgitant murmurs. In acute endocarditis involving a normal valve, murmurs are heard on presentation in only 30–45% of patients but ultimately are detected in 85%. Congestive heart failure develops in 30–40% of patients; it is usually a consequence of valvular dysfunction but occasionally is due to endocarditis-associated myocarditis or an intracardiac fistula. Heart failure due to aortic valve dysfunction progresses more rapidly than does that due to mitral valve dysfunction. Extension of infection beyond valve leaflets into adjacent annular or myocardial tissue results in perivalvular abscesses, which in turn may cause fistulae (from the root of the aorta into cardiac chambers or between cardiac chambers) with new murmurs. Abscesses may burrow from the aortic valve annulus through the epicardium, causing pericarditis. Extension of infection into paravalvular tissue adjacent to either the right or the noncoronary cusp of the aortic valve may interrupt the conduction system in the upper interventricular septum, leading to varying degrees of heart block. Although perivalvular abscesses arising from the mitral valve may potentially interrupt conduction pathways near the atrioventricular node or in the proximal bundle of His, such interruption occurs infrequently. Emboli to a coronary artery may result in myocardial infarction; nevertheless, embolic transmural infarcts are rare.

Noncardiac Manifestations The classic nonsuppurative peripheral manifestations of subacute endocarditis are related to the duration of infection and, with early diagnosis and treatment, have become infrequent. In contrast, septic embolization mimicking some of these lesions (subungual hemorrhage, Osler's nodes) is common in patients with acute *S. aureus* endocarditis (Fig. 118-2). Musculoskeletal symptoms, including nonspecific inflammatory arthritis and back pain, usually remit promptly with treatment but must be distinguished from focal metastatic infection. Hematogenously seeded focal infection may involve any organ but most often is clinically evident in the skin, spleen, kidneys, skeletal system, and meninges. Arterial emboli are clinically apparent in up to 50% of patients. Vegetations >10 mm in diameter (as measured by echocardiography) and those located on the mitral valve are more likely to embolize than are smaller or nonmitral vegetations. Embolic events—often with infarction—involving the extremities, spleen, kidneys, bowel, or brain are often noted at presentation. With effective antibiotic treatment, the frequency of embolic events decreases from 13 per 1000 patient-days during the initial week to 1.2 per 1000 patient-days after the third week. Emboli occurring late during or after effective therapy do not in themselves constitute evidence of failed antimicrobial treatment. Neurologic symptoms, most often resulting from embolic strokes, occur in up to 40% of patients. Other neurologic complications include aseptic or purulent meningitis, intracranial hemorrhage due to hemorrhagic infarcts or ruptured mycotic aneurysms, seizures, and encephalopathy. (*Mycotic aneurysms* are focal dilations of arteries occurring at points in the artery wall that have been weakened by infection in the vasa vasorum or where septic emboli have lodged.) Microabscesses in brain and meninges occur commonly in *S. aureus* endocarditis; surgically drainable intracerebral abscesses are infrequent.

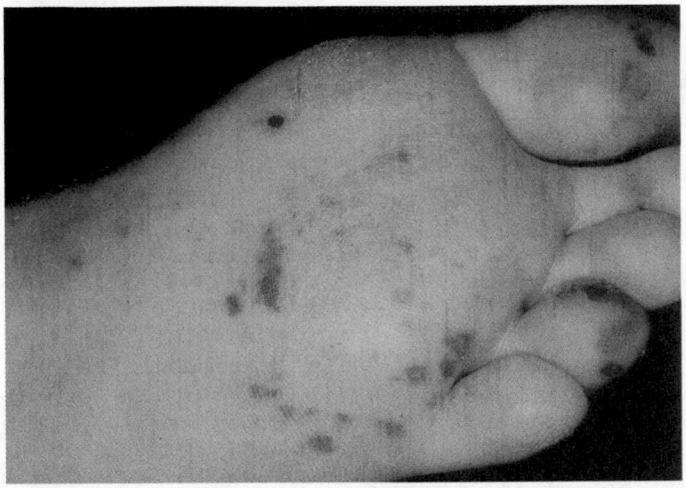

FIGURE 118-2 Septic emboli with hemorrhage and infarction due to acute *Staphylococcus aureus* endocarditis. *(Used with permission of L. Baden.)*

Immune complex deposition on the glomerular basement membrane causes diffuse hypocomplementemic glomerulonephritis and renal dysfunction, which typically improve with effective antimicrobial therapy. Embolic renal infarcts cause flank pain and hematuria but rarely cause renal dysfunction.

Manifestations of Specific Predisposing Conditions In almost 50% of patients who have endocarditis associated with injection drug use, infection is limited to the tricuspid valve. These patients present with fever, faint or no murmur, and (in 75% of cases) prominent pulmonary findings related to septic emboli, including cough, pleuritic chest pain, nodular pulmonary infiltrates, and occasionally pyopneumothorax. Infection involving valves on the left side of the heart presents with the typical clinical features of endocarditis.

Health care–associated endocarditis (defined as that which is nosocomial, arises after recent hospitalization, or is a direct consequence of long-term indwelling devices) has typical manifestations if it is not associated with a retained intracardiac device. Endocarditis associated with flow-directed pulmonary artery catheters is often cryptic, with symptoms masked by comorbid critical illness, and is commonly diagnosed at autopsy. Transvenous pacemaker lead– and/or implanted defibrillator–associated endocarditis may be associated with obvious or cryptic generator pocket infection and results in fever, minimal murmur, and pulmonary symptoms due to septic emboli.

Late-onset prosthetic valve endocarditis presents with typical clinical features. Cases arising within 60 days of valve surgery (early onset) lack peripheral vascular manifestations, and typical symptoms may be obscured by comorbidity associated with recent surgery. In both early-onset and more delayed presentations, paravalvular infection is common and often results in partial valve dehiscence, regurgitant murmurs, congestive heart failure, or disruption of the conduction system.

DIAGNOSIS

The Duke Criteria The diagnosis of infective endocarditis is established with certainty only when vegetations obtained at cardiac surgery, at autopsy, or from an artery (an embolus) are examined histologically and microbiologically. Nevertheless, a highly sensitive and specific diagnostic schema—known as the *Duke criteria*—has been developed on the basis of clinical, laboratory, and echocardiographic findings (Table 118-3). Documentation of two major criteria, of one major and three minor criteria, or of five minor criteria allows a clinical diagnosis of definite endocarditis. The diagnosis of endocarditis is rejected if an alternative

TABLE 118-3 THE DUKE CRITERIA FOR THE CLINICAL DIAGNOSIS OF INFECTIVE ENDOCARDITIS

Major Criteria

1. Positive blood culture
   - Typical microorganism for infective endocarditis from two separate blood cultures
     - Viridans streptococci, *Streptococcus bovis*, HACEK group, *Staphylococcus aureus*, *or*
     - Community-acquired enterococci in the absence of a primary focus, *or*
   - Persistently positive blood culture, defined as recovery of a microorganism consistent with infective endocarditis from:
     - Blood cultures drawn >12 h apart; *or*
     - All of three or a majority of four or more separate blood cultures, with first and last drawn at least 1 h apart
   - Single positive blood culture for *Coxiella burnetii* or phase I IgG antibody titer of >1:800
2. Evidence of endocardial involvement
   - Positive echocardiogram[a]
     - Oscillating intracardiac mass on valve or supporting structures or in the path of regurgitant jets or in implanted material, in the absence of an alternative anatomic explanation, *or*
     - Abscess, *or*
     - New partial dehiscence of prosthetic valve, *or*
   - New valvular regurgitation (increase or change in preexisting murmur not sufficient)

Minor Criteria

1. Predisposition: predisposing heart condition or injection drug use
2. Fever ≥38.0°C (≥100.4°F)
3. Vascular phenomena: major arterial emboli, septic pulmonary infarcts, mycotic aneurysm, intracranial hemorrhage, conjunctival hemorrhages, Janeway lesions
4. Immunologic phenomena: glomerulonephritis, Osler's nodes, Roth's spots, rheumatoid factor
5. Microbiologic evidence: positive blood culture but not meeting major criterion as noted previously[b] or serologic evidence of active infection with organism consistent with infective endocarditis

[a]Transesophageal echocardiography is recommended for assessing possible prosthetic valve endocarditis or complicated endocarditis.
[b]Excluding single positive cultures for coagulase-negative staphylococci and diphtheroids, which are common culture contaminants, and organisms that do not cause endocarditis frequently, such as gram-negative bacilli.
Note: HACEK, *Haemophilus* spp., *Actinobacillus actinomycetemcomitans*, *Cardiobacterium hominis*, *Eikenella corrodens*, *Kingella* species.
Source: Adapted from Li et al., with permission from the University of Chicago Press.

diagnosis is established, if symptoms resolve and do not recur with ≤4 days of antibiotic therapy, or if surgery or autopsy after ≤4 days of antimicrobial therapy yields no histologic evidence of endocarditis. Illnesses not classified as definite endocarditis or rejected are considered cases of possible infective endocarditis when either one major and one minor criterion or three minor criteria are identified. Requiring the identification of clinical features of endocarditis for classification as possible infective endocarditis increases the specificity of the schema without significantly reducing its sensitivity.

The roles of bacteremia and echocardiographic findings in the diagnosis of endocarditis are appropriately emphasized in the Duke criteria. The requirement for multiple positive blood cultures over time is consistent with the continuous low-density bacteremia characteristic of endocarditis (≤100 organisms/mL). Among patients with untreated endocarditis who ultimately have a positive blood culture, 95% of all blood cultures are positive; in 98% of these cases, one of the initial two sets of cultures yields the microorganism. The diagnostic criteria attach significance to the species of organism isolated from blood cultures. To fulfill a major criterion, the isolation of an organism that causes both endocarditis and bacteremia in the absence of endocarditis (e.g., *S. aureus*, enterococci) must take place repeatedly (i.e., persistent bacteremia) and in the absence of a primary focus of infection. Organisms that rarely cause endocarditis but commonly contaminate blood cultures (e.g., diphtheroids, CoNS) must be isolated repeatedly if their isolation is to serve as a major criterion.

Blood Cultures Isolation of the causative microorganism from blood cultures is critical not only for diagnosis but also for determination of antimicrobial susceptibility and planning of treatment. In the absence of prior antibiotic therapy, three blood culture sets (with two bottles per set), separated from each other by at least 1 h, should be obtained from different venipuncture sites over 24 h. If the cultures remain negative after 48–72 h, two or three additional blood culture sets should be obtained, and the laboratory should be consulted for advice regarding optimal culture techniques. Empirical antimicrobial therapy should not be administered initially to hemodynamically stable patients with subacute endocarditis, especially those who have received antibiotics within the preceding 2 weeks; thus, if necessary, additional blood culture sets can be obtained without the confounding effect of empirical treatment. Patients with acute endocarditis or with deteriorating hemodynamics who may require urgent surgery should be treated empirically immediately after three sets of blood cultures are obtained over several hours.

Non-Blood-Culture Tests Serologic tests can be used to implicate causally some organisms that are difficult to recover by blood culture: *Brucella*, *Bartonella*, *Legionella*, and *C. burnetii*. Pathogens can also be identified in surgically recovered vegetations or emboli by culture, by microscopic examination with special stains (i.e., the periodic acid–Schiff stain for *T. whipplei*), and by use of polymerase chain reaction (PCR) to recover unique microbial DNA or 16S rRNA that, when sequenced, allows identification of organisms.

Echocardiography Imaging with echocardiography allows anatomic confirmation of infective endocarditis, sizing of vegetations, detection of intracardiac complications, and assessment of cardiac function (Fig. 118-3). Transthoracic echocardiography (TTE) is noninvasive and exceptionally specific; however, it cannot image vegetations <2 mm in diameter, and in 20% of patients it is technically inadequate because of emphysema or body habitus. Thus, TTE detects vegetations in only 65% of patients with definite clinical endocarditis; i.e., it has a sensitivity of 65%. Moreover, TTE is not adequate for evaluating prosthetic valves or detecting intracardiac complications. TEE is safe and significantly more sensitive than TTE. It detects vegetations in >90% of patients with definite endocarditis; nevertheless, false-negative studies are noted in 6–18% of endocarditis patients. TEE is the optimal method for the diagnosis of prosthetic endocarditis or the detection of myocardial abscess, valve perforation, or intracardiac fistulae.

Experts favor echocardiographic evaluation of all patients with a clinical diagnosis of endocarditis; however, the test should not be used to screen patients with a low probability of endocarditis (e.g., patients with unexplained fever). An American Heart Association approach to the use of echocardiography for evaluation of patients with suspected endocarditis is illustrated in Fig. 118-4. A negative TEE when endocarditis is likely does not exclude the diagnosis but rather warrants repetition of the study in 7–10 days.

Other Studies Many laboratory studies that are not diagnostic—i.e., complete blood count, creatinine determination, liver function tests, chest radiography, and electrocardiography—are nevertheless important in the management of patients with endocarditis. The erythrocyte sedimentation rate, C-reactive protein level, and circulating immune complex titer are commonly increased in endocarditis (Table 118-2). Cardiac catheterization is useful primarily to assess coronary artery patency in older individuals who are to undergo surgery for endocarditis.

Rx INFECTIVE ENDOCARDITIS

ANTIMICROBIAL THERAPY It is difficult to eradicate bacteria from the avascular vegetation in infective endocarditis because this site is relatively deficient in host defenses and because the largely nongrowing, metabolically inactive bacteria are less easily killed by antibiotics. To cure endocarditis, all bacteria in the vegetation must be killed; therefore, therapy must be bactericidal and prolonged. Antibiotics are generally given

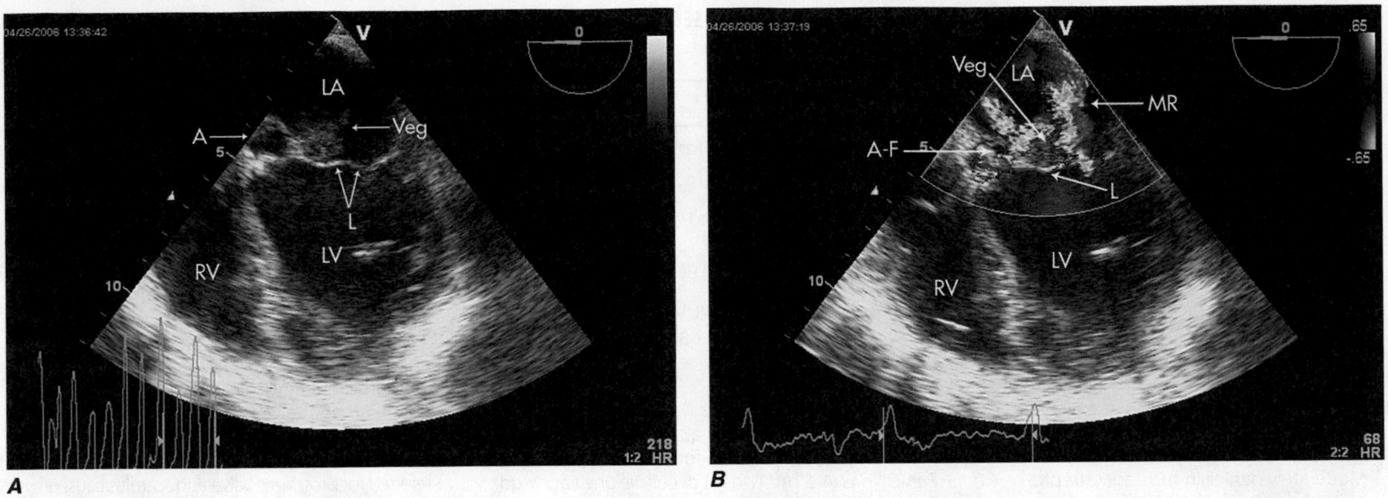

FIGURE 118-3 Imaging of a mitral valve infected with *Staphylococcus aureus* by low-esophageal four-chamber-view transesophageal echocardiography (TEE). ***A.*** Two-dimensional echocardiogram showing a large vegetation with an adjacent echolucent abscess cavity. ***B.*** Color-flow Doppler image showing severe mitral regurgitation through both the abscess-fistula and the central valve orifice. A, abscess; A-F, abscess-fistula; L, valve leaflets; LA, left atrium; LV, left ventricle; MR, mitral central valve regurgitation; RV, right ventricle; veg, vegetation. *(With permission of Andrew Burger, M.D.)*

parenterally and must reach high serum concentrations that will, through passive diffusion, lead to effective concentrations in the depths of the vegetation. The choice of effective therapy requires precise knowledge of the susceptibility of the causative microorganisms. The decision to initiate treatment before a cause is defined must balance the need to establish a microbiologic diagnosis against the potential progression of disease or the need for urgent surgery (see "Blood Cultures," above). The individual vulnerabilities of the patient should be weighed in the selection of therapy—e.g., simultaneous infection at other sites (such as meningitis), allergies, end-organ dysfunction, interactions with concomitant medications, and risks of adverse events.

Although given for several weeks longer, the regimens recommended for the treatment of endocarditis involving prosthetic valves (except for staphylococcal infections) are similar to those used to treat native valve infection **(Table 118-4)**. Recommended doses and durations of therapy should be adhered to unless alterations are required by adverse events.

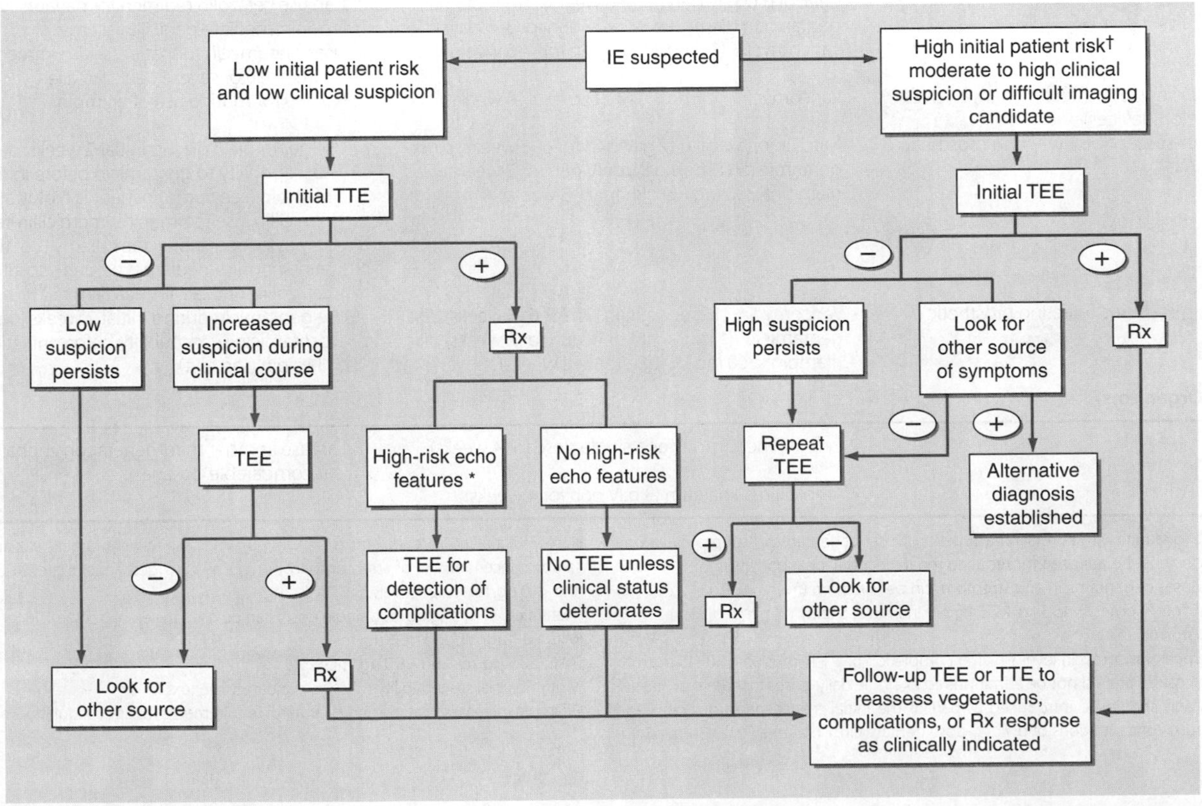

FIGURE 118-4 The diagnostic use of transesophageal and transtracheal echocardiography (TEE and TTE, respectively). †High initial patient risk for endocarditis as listed in Table 118-8 or evidence of intracardiac complications (new regurgitant murmur, new electrocardiographic conduction changes, or congestive heart failure). *High-risk echocardiographic features include large vegetations, valve insufficiency, paravalvular infection, or ventricular dysfunction. Rx indicates initiation of antibiotic therapy. *[Reproduced with permission from Diagnosis and Management of Infective Endocarditis and Its Complications (Circulation 1998; 98:2936-2948. © 1998 American Heart Association.)]*

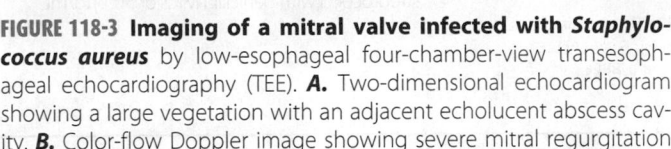

TABLE 118-4 ANTIBIOTIC TREATMENT FOR INFECTIVE ENDOCARDITIS CAUSED BY COMMON ORGANISMS[a]

Organism	Drug (Dose, Duration)	Comments
Streptococci		
Penicillin-susceptible[b] streptococci, *S. bovis*	• Penicillin G (2–3 mU IV q4h for 4 weeks)	—
	• Ceftriaxone (2 g/d IV as a single dose for 4 weeks)	Can use ceftriaxone in patients with nonimmediate penicillin allergy
	• Vancomycin[c] (15 mg/kg IV q12h for 4 weeks)	Use vancomycin in patients with severe or immediate β-lactam allergy
	• Penicillin G (2–3 mU IV q4h) *or* ceftriaxone (2 g IV qd) for 2 weeks *plus* gentamicin[d] (3 mg/kg qd IV or IM, as a single dose[e] or divided into equal doses q8h for 2 weeks)	Avoid 2-week regimen when risk of aminoglycoside toxicity is increased and in prosthetic valve or complicated endocarditis
Relatively penicillin-resistant[f] streptococci	• Penicillin G (4 mU IV q4h) *or* ceftriaxone (2 g IV qd) for 4 weeks *plus* gentamicin[d] (3 mg/kg qd IV or IM, as a single dose[e] or divided into equal doses q8h for 2 weeks)	Penicillin alone at this dose for 6 weeks or with gentamicin during initial 2 weeks preferred for prosthetic valve endocarditis caused by streptococci with penicillin MIC ≤0.1 μg/mL
	Vancomycin[c] as noted above for 4 weeks	—
Moderately penicillin-resistant[g] streptococci, nutritionally variant organisms, or *Gemella morbillorum*	• Penicillin G (4–5 mU IV q4h) *or* ceftriaxone (2 g IV qd) for 6 weeks *plus* gentamicin[d] (3 mg/kg qd IV or IM as a single dose[e] or divided into equal doses q8h for 6 weeks)	Preferred for prosthetic valve endocarditis caused by streptococci with penicillin MICs of >0.1 μg/mL
	• Vancomycin[c] as noted above for 4 weeks	—
Enterococci[h]		
	• Penicillin G (4–5 mU IV q4h) *plus* gentamicin[d] (1 mg/kg IV q8h), both for 4–6 weeks	Can use streptomycin (7.5 mg/kg q12h) in lieu of gentamicin if there is not high-level resistance to streptomycin
	• Ampicillin (2 g IV q4h) *plus* gentamicin[d] (1 mg/kg IV q8h), both for 4–6 weeks	—
	• Vancomycin[c] (15 mg/kg IVq12h) *plus* gentamicin[d] (1 mg/kg IV q8h), both for 4–6 weeks	Use vancomycin plus gentamicin for penicillin-allergic patients, or desensitize to penicillin
Staphylococci		
Methicillin-susceptible, infecting native valves (no foreign devices)	• Nafcillin or oxacillin (2 g IV q4h for 4–6 weeks) *plus* (optional) gentamicin[d] (1 mg/kg IM or IV q8h for 3–5 days)	Can use penicillin (4 mU q4h) if isolate is penicillin-susceptible (does not produce β-lactamase)
	• Cefazolin (2 g IV q8h for 4–6 weeks) *plus* (optional) gentamicin[d] (1 mg/kg IM or IV q8h for 3–5 days)	Can use cefazolin regimen for patients with nonimmediate penicillin allergy
	• Vancomycin[c] (15 mg/kg IV q12h for 4–6 weeks)	Use vancomycin for patients with immediate (urticarial) or severe penicillin allergy
Methicillin-resistant, infecting native valves (no foreign devices)	• Vancomycin[c] (15 mg/kg IV q12h for 4–6 weeks)	No role for routine use of rifampin
Methicillin-susceptible, infecting prosthetic valves	• Nafcillin or oxacillin (2 g IV q4h for 6–8 weeks) *plus* gentamicin[d] (1 mg/kg IM or IV q8h for 2 weeks) *plus* rifampin[i] (300 mg PO q8h for 6–8 weeks)	Use gentamicin during initial 2 weeks; determine susceptibility to gentamicin before initiating rifampin (see text); if patient is highly allergic to penicillin, use regimen for methicillin-resistant staphylococci; if β-lactam allergy is of the minor, nonimmediate type, can substitute cefazolin for oxacillin/nafcillin
Methicillin-resistant, infecting prosthetic valves	• Vancomycin[c] (15 mg/kg IV q12h for 6–8 weeks) *plus* gentamicin[d] (1 mg/kg IM or IV q8h for 2 weeks) *plus* rifampin[i] (300 mg PO q8h for 6–8 weeks)	Use gentamicin during initial 2 weeks; determine gentamicin susceptibility before initiating rifampin (see text)
HACEK Organisms		
	• Ceftriaxone (2 g/d IV as a single dose for 4 weeks)	Can use another third-generation cephalosporin at comparable dosage
	• Ampicillin/sulbactam (3 g IV q6h for 4 weeks)	—

[a]Doses are for adults with normal renal function. Doses of gentamicin, streptomycin, and vancomycin must be adjusted for reduced renal function. Ideal body weight is used to calculate doses of gentamicin and streptomycin per kilogram (men = 50 kg + 2.3 kg per inch over 5 feet; women = 45.5 kg + 2.3 kg per inch over 5 feet).
[b]MIC, ≤0.1 μg/mL.
[c]Desirable peak vancomycin level 1 h after completion of a 1-h infusion is 30–45 μg/mL.
[d]Aminoglycosides should not be administered as single daily doses for enterococcal endocarditis and should be introduced as part of the initial treatment. Target peak and trough serum concentrations of divided-dose gentamicin 1 h after a 20- to 30-min infusion or IM injection are ~3.5 μg/mL and ≤1 μg/mL, respectively; target peak and trough serum concentrations of streptomycin (timing as with gentamicin) are 20–35 μg/mL and <10 μg/mL, respectively.
[e]Netilmicin (4 mg/kg qd, as a single dose) can be used in lieu of gentamicin.
[f]MIC, >0.1 μg/mL and <0.5 μg/mL.
[g]MIC, ≥0.5 μg/mL and <8.0 μg/mL.
[h]Antimicrobial susceptibility must be evaluated; see text.
[i]Rifampin increases warfarin and dicumarol requirements for anticoagulation.

Organism-Specific Therapies ***Streptococci*** To select the optimal therapy for streptococcal endocarditis, the minimum inhibitory concentration (MIC) of penicillin for the causative isolate must be determined (Table 118-4). The 2-week penicillin/gentamicin or ceftriaxone/gentamicin regimens should not be used to treat complicated native valve infection or prosthetic valve endocarditis. The regimen recommended for relatively penicillin-resistant streptococci is advocated for treatment of endocarditis caused by organisms of group B, C, or G. Endocarditis caused by nutritionally variant organisms (*Granulicatella* or *Abiotrophia* species) and *Gemella morbillorum* is treated with the regimen for moderately penicillin-resistant streptococci, as is prosthetic valve endocarditis caused by these organisms or by streptococci with a penicillin MIC of >0.1 μg/mL (Table 118-4).

Enterococci Enterococci are resistant to oxacillin, nafcillin, and the cephalosporins and are only inhibited—not killed—by penicillin, ampicillin, teicoplanin (not available in the United States), and vancomycin. To kill enterococci requires the synergistic interaction of a cell wall–active antibiotic (penicillin, ampicillin, vancomycin, or teicoplanin) that is effective at achievable serum concentrations and an aminoglycoside (gentamicin or streptomycin) to which the isolate does not exhibit high-level resistance. An isolate's resistance to cell wall–active agents or its ability to replicate in the presence of gentamicin at ≥500 μg/mL or streptomycin at 1000–2000 μg/mL—a phenomenon called *high-level aminoglycoside resistance*—indicates that the ineffective antimicrobial agent cannot participate in the interaction to produce killing. High-level resistance to gentamicin predicts that tobramycin, netilmicin, amikacin, and kanamycin also will be ineffective. In fact, even when enterococci are not highly resistant to gentamicin, it is difficult to predict the ability of these other aminoglycosides to participate in synergistic killing; consequently, they should not in general be used to treat enterococcal endocarditis.

Enterococci causing endocarditis must be tested for high-level resistance to streptomycin and gentamicin, β-lactamase production, and susceptibility to penicillin and ampicillin (MIC ≤16 μg/mL) and to vancomycin (MIC ≤8 μg/mL). If the isolate produces β-lactamase, ampicillin/sulbactam or vancomycin can be used as the cell wall–active component; if the penicillin/ampicillin MIC is >16 μg/mL, vancomycin can be considered; and if the vancomycin MIC is >8 μg/mL, penicillin or ampicillin may be considered. In the absence of high-level resistance, gentamicin or streptomycin should be used as the aminoglycoside (Table 118-4). If there is high-level resistance to both these drugs, no aminoglycoside should be given; instead, an 8- to 12-week course of a single cell wall–active agent is suggested—or, for *E. faecalis*, high doses of ampicillin plus either ceftriaxone or cefotaxime. If this alternative therapy fails or the isolate is resistant to all of the commonly used agents, surgical treatment is advised. The role of newer agents potentially active against multidrug-resistant enterococci [quinupristin/dalfopristin (*E. faecium* only), linezolid, and daptomycin] in the treatment of endocarditis has not been established. Although the dose of gentamicin used to achieve bactericidal synergy in treating enterococcal endocarditis is smaller than that used in standard therapy, nephrotoxicity is not uncommon during treatment for 4–6 weeks. Regimens wherein the aminoglycoside component of treatment has been truncated at 2–3 weeks because of toxicity have been curative. Thus, discontinuation of the aminoglycoside is recommended when toxicity develops in patients with enterococcal endocarditis who have responded satisfactorily to therapy.

Staphylococci The regimens used to treat staphylococcal endocarditis (Table 118-4) are based not on coagulase production but rather on the presence or absence of a prosthetic valve or foreign device, the native valve(s) involved, and the resistance of the isolate to penicillin and methicillin. Penicillinase is produced by 95% of staphylococci; thus, all isolates should be considered penicillin-resistant until shown not to produce this enzyme. Similarly, methicillin resistance has become so prevalent among staphylococci, including *S. aureus*, that therapy should be initiated with a regimen for methicillin-resistant organisms and subsequently revised if the strain proves to be susceptible to methicillin. The addition of gentamicin (if the isolate is susceptible) to a β-lactam antibiotic to enhance therapy for native mitral or aortic valve endocarditis is optional. Its addition hastens eradication of bacteremia but does not improve survival rates. If added, gentamicin should be limited to the initial 3–5 days of therapy to minimize nephrotoxicity. Gentamicin generally is not added to the vancomycin regimen in this setting. The efficacy of linezolid or daptomycin as an alternative to vancomycin for left-sided, methicillin-resistant *S. aureus* (MRSA) endocarditis has not been established.

Methicillin-susceptible *S. aureus* endocarditis that is uncomplicated and limited to the tricuspid or pulmonic valve—a condition occurring almost exclusively in injection drug users—can often be treated with a 2-week course that combines oxacillin or nafcillin (but not vancomycin) with gentamicin. Prolonged fevers (≥5 days) during therapy suggest that these patients should receive standard therapy. Right-sided endocarditis caused by MRSA is treated for 4 weeks with standard doses of vancomycin or daptomycin (6 mg/kg as a single daily dose).

Staphylococcal prosthetic valve endocarditis is treated for 6–8 weeks with a multidrug regimen. Rifampin is an essential component because it kills staphylococci that are adherent to foreign material. Two other agents (selected on the basis of susceptibility testing) are combined with rifampin to prevent in vivo emergence of resistance. Because many staphylococci (particularly MRSA and *S. epidermidis*) are resistant to gentamicin, the utility of gentamicin or an alternative agent should be established before rifampin treatment is begun. If the isolate is resistant to gentamicin, another aminoglycoside or a fluoroquinolone (chosen in light of susceptibility results) or another active agent should be substituted for gentamicin.

Other Organisms In the absence of meningitis, endocarditis caused by *Streptococcus pneumoniae* with a penicillin MIC of ≤1.0 can be treated with IV penicillin (4 million units every 4 h), ceftriaxone (2 g/d as a single dose), or cefotaxime (at a comparable dosage). Infection caused by pneumococcal strains with a penicillin MIC of ≥2.0 should be treated with vancomycin. Until the strain's susceptibility to penicillin is established, therapy should consist of vancomycin plus ceftriaxone, especially if concurrent meningitis is suspected. *P. aeruginosa* endocarditis is treated with an antipseudomonal penicillin (ticarcillin or piperacillin) and high doses of tobramycin (8 mg/kg per day in three divided doses). Endocarditis caused by Enterobacteriaceae is treated with a potent β-lactam antibiotic plus an aminoglycoside. Corynebacterial endocarditis is treated with penicillin plus an aminoglycoside (if the organism is susceptible to the aminoglycoside) or with vancomycin, which is highly bactericidal for most strains. Therapy for *Candida* endocarditis consists of amphotericin B plus flucytosine and early surgery; long-term (if not indefinite) suppression with an oral azole is advised. Caspofungin treatment of *Candida* endocarditis has been effective in sporadic cases; nevertheless, the role of echinocandins in this setting has not been established.

Empirical Therapy In designing and executing therapy without culture data (i.e., before culture results are known or when cultures are negative), clinical and epidemiologic clues to etiology must be weighed, and both the pathogens associated with the specific endocarditis syndrome and the hazards of suboptimal therapy must be considered. Thus, empirical therapy for acute endocarditis in an injection drug user should cover MRSA and gram-negative bacilli. The initiation of treatment with vancomycin plus gentamicin immediately after blood is obtained for cultures covers these as well as many other potential causes. In the treatment of culture-negative episodes, marantic endocarditis must be excluded and fastidious organisms sought serologically. In the absence of confounding prior antibiotic therapy, it is unlikely that *S. aureus*, CoNS, or enterococcal infection will present with negative blood cultures. Thus, in this situation, these organisms are not the determinants of therapy for subacute endocarditis. Pending the availability of diagnostic data, blood culture–negative subacute native valve endocarditis is treated with ceftriaxone plus gentamicin; these two antimicrobial agents plus vancomycin should be used if prosthetic valves are involved.

Outpatient Antimicrobial Therapy Fully compliant patients who have sterile blood cultures, are afebrile during therapy, and have no clinical or echocardiographic findings that suggest an impending complication may complete therapy as outpatients. Careful follow-up and a stable home setting are necessary, as are predictable IV access and use of antimicrobial agents that are stable in solution.

Monitoring Antimicrobial Therapy The serum bactericidal titer—the highest dilution of the patient's serum during therapy that kills 99.9% of the standard inoculum of the infecting organism—is no longer recommended for assessment of standard regimens. However, in the treatment of endocarditis caused by unusual organisms, this measurement, although not standardized and difficult to interpret, may provide a patient-specific assessment of in vivo antibiotic effect. Serum concentrations of aminoglycosides and vancomycin should be monitored.

Antibiotic toxicities, including allergic reactions, occur in 25–40% of patients and commonly arise during the third week of therapy. Blood tests to detect renal, hepatic, and hematologic toxicity should be performed periodically.

In most patients, effective antibiotic therapy results in subjective improvement and resolution of fever within 5–7 days. Blood cultures should be repeated daily until sterile, rechecked if there is recrudescent fever, and performed again 4–6 weeks after therapy to document cure. Blood cultures become sterile within 2 days after the start of appropriate therapy when infection is caused by viridans streptococci, enterococci, or HACEK organisms. In *S. aureus* endocarditis, β-lactam therapy results in sterile cultures in 3–5 days, whereas positive cultures may persist for 7–9 days with vancomycin treatment. When fever persists for 7 days despite appropriate antibiotic therapy, patients should be evaluated for paravalvular abscess and for extracardiac abscesses (spleen, kidney) or complications (embolic events). Recrudescent fever raises the question of these complications but also of drug reactions or complications of hospitalization. Serologic abnormalities (e.g., in C-reactive protein level, erythrocyte sedimentation rate, rheumatoid factor) resolve slowly and do not reflect response to treatment. Vegetations become smaller with effective therapy, but at 3 months after cure half are unchanged and 25% are slightly larger.

SURGICAL TREATMENT Intracardiac and central nervous system complications of endocarditis are important causes of morbidity and death associated with this infection. In some cases, effective treatment for these complications requires surgery. Most of the clinical indications for surgical treatment of endocarditis are not absolute **(Table 118-5)**. The risks and benefits as well as the timing of surgical treatment must therefore be individualized **(Table 118-6)**.

Intracardiac Surgical Indications Most surgical interventions are warranted by intracardiac findings, detected most reliably by TEE. Because of the highly invasive nature of prosthetic valve endocarditis, as many as 40% of affected patients merit surgical treatment. In many patients, coincident rather than single intracardiac events necessitate surgery.

Congestive Heart Failure Moderate to severe refractory congestive heart failure caused by new or worsening valve dysfunction is the major indication for cardiac surgical treatment of endocarditis. Of patients with moderate to severe heart failure due to valve dysfunction who are treated medically, 60–90% die within 6 months. In this setting, surgical treatment improves outcome, with mortality rates of 20% in native valve endocarditis and 35–55% in prosthetic valve infection. Surgery can relieve functional stenosis due to large vegetations or restore competence to damaged regurgitant valves.

Perivalvular Infection This complication, which occurs in 10–15% of native valve and 45–60% of prosthetic valve infections, is suggested by persistent unexplained fever during appropriate therapy, new electrocardiographic conduction disturbances, and pericarditis. Extension can occur from any valve but is most common with aortic valve infection. TEE with color Doppler is the test of choice to detect perivalvular abscesses (sensitivity, ≥85%). Although occasional perivalvular infections are cured medically, surgery is warranted when fever persists, fistulae develop, prostheses are dehisced and unstable, and invasive infection relapses after appropriate treatment. Cardiac rhythm must be monitored since high-grade heart block may require insertion of a pacemaker.

Uncontrolled Infection Continued positive blood cultures or otherwise-unexplained persistent fevers (in patients with either blood culture–positive or –negative endocarditis) despite optimal antibiotic therapy may reflect uncontrolled infection and may warrant surgery. Surgical treatment is also advised for endocarditis caused by organisms against which clinical experience indicates that effective antimicrobial therapy is lacking. This category includes infections caused by yeasts, fungi, *P. aeruginosa*, other highly resistant gram-negative bacilli, *Brucella* species, and probably *C. burnetii*.

TABLE 118-5 INDICATIONS FOR CARDIAC SURGICAL INTERVENTION IN PATIENTS WITH ENDOCARDITIS

Surgery required for optimal outcome
- Moderate to severe congestive heart failure due to valve dysfunction
- Partially dehisced unstable prosthetic valve
- Persistent bacteremia despite optimal antimicrobial therapy
- Lack of effective microbicidal therapy (e.g., fungal or *Brucella* endocarditis)
- *S. aureus* prosthetic valve endocarditis with an intracardiac complication
- Relapse of prosthetic valve endocarditis after optimal antimicrobial therapy

Surgery to be strongly considered for improved outcome[a]
- Perivalvular extension of infection
- Poorly responsive *S. aureus* endocarditis involving the aortic or mitral valve
- Large (>10-mm diameter) hypermobile vegetations with increased risk of embolism
- Persistent unexplained fever (≥10 days) in culture-negative native valve endocarditis
- Poorly responsive or relapsed endocarditis due to highly antibiotic-resistant enterococci or gram-negative bacilli

[a]Surgery must be carefully considered; findings are often combined with other indications to prompt surgery.

TABLE 118-6 TIMING OF CARDIAC SURGICAL INTERVENTION IN PATIENTS WITH ENDOCARDITIS

	Indication for Surgical Intervention	
Timing	**Strong Supporting Evidence**	**Conflicting Evidence, but Majority of Opinions Favor Surgery**
Emergent (same day)	Acute aortic regurgitation plus preclosure of mitral valve Sinus of Valsalva abscess ruptured into right heart Rupture into pericardial sac	
Urgent (within 1–2 days)	Valve obstruction by vegetation Unstable (dehisced) prosthesis Acute aortic or mitral regurgitation with heart failure (New York Heart Association class III or IV) Septal perforation Perivalvular extension of infection with/without new electrocardiographic conduction system changes Lack of effective antibiotic therapy	Major embolus plus persisting large vegetation (>10 mm in diameter)
Elective (earlier usually preferred)	Progressive paravalvular prosthetic regurgitation Valve dysfunction plus persisting infection after ≥7–10 days of antimicrobial therapy Fungal (mold) endocarditis	Staphylococcal PVE Early PVE (≤2 months after valve surgery) Fungal endocarditis (*Candida* spp.) Antibiotic-resistant organisms

Abbreviation: PVE, prosthetic valve endocarditis.
Source: Adapted from L Olaison, G Pettersson: Infect Dis Clin North Am 16:453, 2002.

S. aureus *Endocarditis* Mortality rates for *S. aureus* prosthetic valve endocarditis exceed 70% with medical treatment but are reduced to 25% with surgical treatment. In patients with intracardiac complications associated with *S. aureus* prosthetic valve infection, surgical treatment reduces the mortality rate twentyfold. Surgical treatment should be considered for patients with *S. aureus* native aortic or mitral valve infection who have TTE-demonstrable vegetations and remain septic during the initial week of therapy. Isolated tricuspid valve endocarditis, even with persistent fever, rarely requires surgery.

Prevention of Systemic Emboli Death and persisting morbidity due to emboli are largely limited to patients suffering occlusion of cerebral or coronary arteries. Echocardiographic determination of vegetation size and anatomy, although predictive of patients at high risk of systemic emboli, does not identify those patients in whom the benefits of surgery to prevent emboli clearly exceed the risks of the surgical procedure and an implanted prosthetic valve. Net benefits favoring surgery are most likely when the risk of embolism is high and other surgical benefits can be achieved simultaneously—e.g., repair of a moderately dysfunctional valve or debridement of a paravalvular abscess. Reduced overall risks of surgical intervention (e.g., use of vegetation resection and valve repair to avoid insertion of a prosthesis) make the benefit-to-risk ratio more favorable and this intervention more attractive.

Timing of Cardiac Surgery In general, when indications for surgical treatment of infective endocarditis are identified, surgery should not be delayed simply to permit additional antibiotic therapy, since this course of action increases the risk of death (Table 118-6). Delay is justified only when infection is controlled and congestive heart failure is fully compensated with medical therapy. After 14 days of recommended antibiotic therapy, excised valves are culture-negative in 99% and 50% of patients with streptococcal and *S. aureus* endocarditis, respectively. Recrudescent endocarditis involving a new implanted prosthetic valve follows surgery in 2% of patients with culture-positive native valve endocarditis and in 6–15% of patients with active prosthetic valve endocarditis. These risks are more acceptable than the high mortality rates that result when surgery is inappropriately delayed or not performed.

Among patients who have experienced a neurologic complication of endocarditis, further neurologic deterioration can occur as a consequence of cardiac surgery. The risk of significant neurologic exacerbation is related to the interval between the complication and the surgery. Whenever feasible, cardiac surgery should be delayed for 2–3 weeks after a nonhemorrhagic embolic stroke and for 4 weeks after a hemorrhagic embolic stroke. A ruptured mycotic aneurysm should be clipped and cerebral edema allowed to resolve before cardiac surgery.

Antibiotic Therapy after Cardiac Surgery Bacteria visible in Gram-stained preparations of excised valves do not necessarily indicate a failure of antibiotic therapy. Organisms have been detected on Gram's stain—or their DNA has been detected by PCR—in excised valves from 45% of patients who have successfully completed the recommended therapy for endocarditis. In only 7% of these patients are the organisms, most of which are unusual and antibiotic resistant, cultured from the valve. Despite the detection of organisms or their DNA, relapse of endocarditis after surgery is uncommon. Thus, for uncomplicated native valve infection caused by susceptible organisms in conjunction with negative valve cultures, the duration of preoperative plus postoperative treatment should equal the total duration of recommended therapy, with ~2 weeks of treatment administered after surgery. For endocarditis complicated by paravalvular abscess, partially treated prosthetic valve infection, or cases with culture-positive valves, a full course of therapy should be given postoperatively.

Extracardiac Complications Splenic abscess develops in 3–5% of patients with endocarditis. Effective therapy requires either image-guided percutaneous drainage or splenectomy. Mycotic aneurysms occur in 2–15% of endocarditis patients; half of these cases involve the cerebral arteries and present as headaches, focal neurologic symptoms, or hemorrhage. Cerebral aneurysms should be monitored by angiography. Some will resolve with effective antimicrobial therapy, but those that persist, enlarge, or leak should be treated surgically if possible. Extracerebral aneurysms present as local pain, a mass, local ischemia, or bleeding; these aneurysms are treated by resection.

OUTCOME

Older age, severe comorbid conditions, delayed diagnosis, involvement of prosthetic valves or the aortic valve, an invasive (*S. aureus*) or antibiotic-resistant (*P. aeruginosa*, yeast) pathogen, intracardiac complications, and major neurologic complications adversely impact outcome. Death and poor outcome often are related not to failure of antibiotic therapy but rather to the interactions of comorbidities and endocarditis-related end-organ complications. Overall survival rates for patients with native valve endocarditis caused by viridans streptococci, HACEK organisms, or enterococci (susceptible to synergistic therapy) are 85–90%. For *S. aureus* native valve endocarditis in patients who do not inject drugs, survival rates are 55–70%, whereas 85–90% of injection drug users survive this infection. Prosthetic valve endocarditis beginning within 2 months of valve replacement results in mortality rates of 40–50%, whereas rates are only 10–20% in later-onset cases.

PREVENTION

Antibiotic prophylaxis has been recommended by the American Heart Association in conjunction with selected procedures considered to entail a risk for bacteremia and endocarditis. The benefits of prophylaxis, however, are not established and in fact may be modest: only 50% of patients presenting with native valve endocarditis know that they have a predisposing valve lesion, most endocarditis cases do not follow a procedure, and 35% of cases are caused by organisms not targeted by prophylaxis. Dental treatments, the procedures most widely accepted as predisposing to endocarditis, are no more frequent during the 3 months preceding endocarditis than in uninfected matched controls. Furthermore, the frequency and magnitude of bacteremia associated with dental procedures and routine daily activities (e.g., tooth brushing and flossing) are similar. Because patients undergo dental procedures infrequently, exposure of endocarditis-vulnerable cardiac structures to bacteremia-causing oral cavity organisms is notably greater from routine daily activities than from dental care. It is estimated that annual exposure of heart valves to bacteremia-causing organisms may be 5.6 million times greater from routine daily activity than from a tooth extraction. The relation of gastrointestinal and genitourinary procedures to subsequent endocarditis is more tenuous than that of dental procedures.

Antibiotic prophylaxis, if 100% effective, likely prevents only a small number of cases of endocarditis; nevertheless, it is possible that rare cases are prevented. Weighing the potential benefits, potential adverse events, and costs associated with antibiotic prophylaxis, the expert committee of the American Heart Association has dramatically restricted the recommendations for antibiotic prophylaxis. Prophylactic antibiotics (Table 118-7) are advised only for those patients at highest risk for severe morbidity or death from endocarditis (Table 118-8). Prophylaxis is recommended only for dental procedures wherein there is manipulation of gingival tissue or the periapical region of the teeth or perforation of the oral mucosa (including surgery on the respiratory tract). Although prophylaxis is not advised for patients undergoing gastrointestinal or genitourinary tract procedures, it is recommended that effective treatment be given to these high-risk patients before or when they undergo procedures on an infected genitourinary tract or on infected skin and related soft tissue. Maintaining good dental hygiene is also advised. (For further details, see *http://www.americanheart.org/presenter.jhtml?identifier=3047083.*)

TABLE 118-7 ANTIBIOTIC REGIMENS FOR PROPHYLAXIS OF ENDOCARDITIS IN ADULTS WITH HIGH-RISK CARDIAC LESIONS[a,b]

A. Standard oral regimen
1. Amoxicillin 2.0 g PO 1 h before procedure
B. Inability to take oral medication
1. Ampicillin 2.0 g IV or IM within 1 h before procedure
C. Penicillin allergy
1. Clarithromycin or azithromycin 500 mg PO 1 h before procedure
2. Cephalexin[c] 2.0 g PO 1 h before procedure
3. Clindamycin 600 mg PO 1 h before procedure
D. Penicillin allergy, inability to take oral medication
1. Cefazolin[c] or ceftriaxone[c] 1.0 g IV or IM 30 min before procedure
2. Clindamycin 600 mg IV or IM 1 h before procedure

[a]Dosing for children: for amoxicillin, ampicillin, cephalexin, or cefadroxil, use 50 mg/kg PO; cefazolin, 25 mg/kg IV; clindamycin, 20 mg/kg PO, 25 mg/kg IV; clarithromycin, 15 mg/kg PO; and vancomycin, 20 mg/kg IV.
[b]For high-risk lesions, see Table 118-8. Prophylaxis is not advised for other lesions.
[c]Do not use cephalosporins in patients with immediate hypersensitivity (urticaria, angioedema, anaphylaxis) to penicillin.
Source: W Wilson et al: Circulation, published online 4/19/07.

TABLE 118-8 HIGH-RISK CARDIAC LESIONS FOR WHICH ENDOCARDITIS PROPHYLAXIS IS ADVISED BEFORE DENTAL PROCEDURES

Prosthetic heart valves
Prior endocarditis
Unrepaired cyanotic congenital heart disease, including palliative shunts or conduits
Completely repaired congenital heart defects during the 6 months after repair
Incompletely repaired congenital heart disease with residual defects adjacent to prosthetic material
Valvulopathy developing after cardiac transplantation

Source: W Wilson et al: Circulation, published online 4/19/07.

BADDOUR LM et al: Diagnosis, antimicrobial therapy, and management of complications. A statement for healthcare professionals from the Committee on Rheumatic Fever, Endocarditis, and Kawasaki Disease, Council on Cardiovascular Disease in the Young, and the Councils on Clinical Cardiology, Stroke, and Cardiovascular Surgery and Anesthesia, American Heart Association. Circulation 111:e394, 2005

DURACK DT (ed): Infective endocarditis. Infect Dis Clin North Am 16:255, 2002

FOWLER VG JR et al: Endocarditis and intravascular infections, in *Principles and Practice of Infectious Diseases*, 6th ed, GL Mandell et al (eds). Philadelphia, Elsevier Churchill Livingstone, 2005, pp 975–1021

HORSTKOTTE D et al: Guidelines on prevention, diagnosis and treatment of infective endocarditis. Executive summary, The Task Force on Infective Endocarditis of the European Society of Cardiology. Eur Heart J 25:267, 2004

KARCHMER AW: Infective endocarditis, in *Heart Disease*, 8th ed, E Braunwald et al (eds). Philadelphia, Elsevier Saunders, 2007, in press

———, LONGWORTH DL: Infections of intracardiac devices. Cardiol Clin 21:253, 2003

LI JS et al: Proposed modifications to the Duke criteria for the diagnosis of infective endocarditis. Clin Infect Dis 30:633, 2000

MOREILLON P, QUE YA: Infective endocarditis. Lancet 363:139, 2004

MORRIS AJ et al: Bacteriological outcome after valve surgery for active infective endocarditis: Implications for duration of treatment after surgery (abstract). Clin Infect Dis 41:187, 2005

VIKRAM HR et al: Impact of valve surgery on 6-month mortality in adults with complicated, left-sided native valve endocarditis: A propensity analysis. JAMA 290:3207, 2003

WILSON W et al: Prevention of infective endocarditis. Guidelines from the American Heart Association. A guideline from the American Heart Association Rheumatic Fever, Endocarditis, and Kawasaki Disease Committee, Council on Cardiovascular Disease in the Young, and the Council on Clinical Cardiology, Council on Cardiovascular Surgery and Anesthesia, and the Quality of Care and Outcomes Research Interdisciplinary Working Group. Circulation, April 19, 2007 (epub ahead of print) (*http://www.americanheart.org/presenter.jhtml?identifier=3047083*)

119 Infections of the Skin, Muscle, and Soft Tissues

Dennis L. Stevens

ANATOMIC RELATIONSHIPS: CLUES TO THE DIAGNOSIS OF SOFT TISSUE INFECTIONS

Protection against infection of the epidermis depends on the mechanical barrier afforded by the stratum corneum, since the epidermis itself is devoid of blood vessels (Fig. 119-1). Disruption of this layer by burns or bites, abrasions, foreign bodies, primary dermatologic disorders (e.g., herpes simplex, varicella, ecthyma gangrenosum), surgery, or vascular or pressure ulcer allows penetration of bacteria to the deeper structures. Similarly, the hair follicle can serve as a portal either for components of the normal flora (e.g., *Staphylococcus*) or for extrinsic bacteria (e.g., *Pseudomonas* in hot-tub folliculitis). Intracellular infection of the squamous epithelium with vesicle formation may arise from cutaneous inoculation, as in infection with herpes simplex virus (HSV)

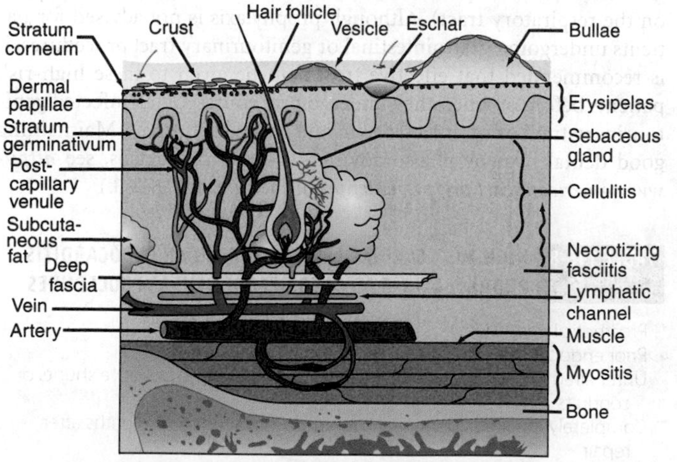

FIGURE 119-1 Structural components of the skin and soft tissue, superficial infections, and infections of the deeper structures. The rich capillary network beneath the dermal papillae plays a key role in the localization of infection and in the development of the acute inflammatory reaction.

type 1; from the dermal capillary plexus, as in varicella and infections due to other viruses associated with viremia; or from cutaneous nerve roots, as in herpes zoster. Bacteria infecting the epidermis, such as *Streptococcus pyogenes*, may be translocated laterally to deeper structures via lymphatics, an event that results in the rapid superficial spread of erysipelas. Later, engorgement or obstruction of lymphatics causes flaccid edema of the epidermis, another characteristic of erysipelas.

The rich plexus of capillaries beneath the dermal papillae provides nutrition to the stratum germinativum, and physiologic responses of this plexus produce important clinical signs and symptoms. For example, infective vasculitis of the plexus results in petechiae, Osler's nodes, Janeway lesions, and palpable purpura, which, if present, are important clues to the existence of endocarditis (Chap. 118). In addition, metastatic infection within this plexus can result in cutaneous manifestations of disseminated fungal infection (Chap. 196), gonococcal infection (Chap. 137), *Salmonella* infection (Chap. 146), *Pseudomonas* infection (i.e., ecthyma gangrenosum; Chap. 145), meningococcemia (Chap. 136), and staphylococcal infection (Chap. 129). The plexus also provides bacteria with access to the circulation, thereby facilitating local spread or bacteremia. The postcapillary venules of this plexus are a major site of polymorphonuclear leukocyte sequestration, diapedesis, and chemotaxis to the site of cutaneous infection.

Exaggeration of these physiologic mechanisms by excessive levels of cytokines or bacterial toxins causes leukostasis, venous occlusion, and pitting edema. Edema with purple bullae, ecchymosis, and cutaneous anesthesia suggests loss of vascular integrity and necessitates exploration of the deeper structures for evidence of necrotizing fasciitis or myonecrosis. An early diagnosis requires a high level of suspicion in instances of unexplained fever and of pain and tenderness in the soft tissue, even in the absence of acute cutaneous inflammation.

Table 119-1 indicates the chapters in which the infections described below are discussed in greater detail. Many of these infections are illustrated in the chapters cited or in **Chap. e5** (Atlas of Rashes Associated with Fever).

INFECTIONS ASSOCIATED WITH VESICLES

(Table 119-1) Vesicle formation due to infection is caused by viral proliferation within the epidermis. In varicella and variola, viremia precedes the onset of a diffuse centripetal rash that progresses from macules to vesicles, then to pustules, and finally to scabs over the course of 1–2 weeks. Vesicles of varicella have a "dewdrop" appearance and develop in crops randomly about the trunk, extremities, and face over 3–4 days. Herpes zoster occurs in a single dermatome; the ap-

TABLE 119-1 SKIN AND SOFT TISSUE INFECTIONS

Lesion, Clinical Syndrome	Infectious Agent	Chapter(s)
Vesicles		
Smallpox	Variola virus	214
Chickenpox	Varicella-zoster virus	173
Shingles (herpes zoster)	Varicella-zoster virus	173
Cold sores, herpetic whitlow, herpes gladiatorum	Herpes simplex virus	172
Hand-foot-and-mouth disease	Coxsackievirus A16	184
Orf	Parapoxvirus	176
Molluscum contagiosum	Pox-like virus	176
Rickettsialpox	*Rickettsia akari*	167
Blistering distal dactylitis	*Staphylococcus aureus* or *Streptococcus pyogenes*	129, 130
Bullae		
Staphylococcal scalded-skin syndrome	*S. aureus*	129
Necrotizing fasciitis	*S. pyogenes, Clostridium* spp., mixed aerobes and anaerobes	157
Gas gangrene	*Clostridium* spp.	135
Halophilic vibrio	*Vibrio vulnificus*	149
Crusted lesions		
Bullous impetigo/ecthyma	*S. aureus*	129
Impetigo contagiosa	*S. pyogenes*	130
Ringworm	Superficial dermatophyte fungi	199
Sporotrichosis	*Sporothrix schenckii*	199
Histoplasmosis	*Histoplasma capsulatum*	192
Coccidioidomycosis	*Coccidioides immitis*	193
Blastomycosis	*Blastomyces dermatitidis*	194
Cutaneous leishmaniasis	*Leishmania* spp.	205
Cutaneous tuberculosis	*Mycobacterium tuberculosis*	158
Nocardiosis	*Nocardia asteroides*	155
Folliculitis		
Furunculosis	*S. aureus*	129
Hot-tub folliculitis	*Pseudomonas aeruginosa*	145
Swimmer's itch	*Schistosoma* spp.	212
Acne vulgaris	*Propionibacterium acnes*	53
Papular and nodular lesions		
Fish-tank or swimming-pool granuloma	*Mycobacterium marinum*	160
Creeping eruption (cutaneous larva migrans)	*Ancylostoma braziliense*	209
Dracunculiasis	*Dracunculus medinensis*	211
Cercarial dermatitis	*Schistosoma mansoni*	212
Verruca vulgaris	Human papillomaviruses 1, 2, 4	178
Condylomata acuminata (anogenital warts)	Human papillomaviruses 6, 11, 16, 18	178
Onchocerciasis nodule	*Onchocerca volvulus*	211
Cutaneous myiasis	*Dermatobia hominis*	e35
Verruca peruana	*Bartonella bacilliformis*	153
Cat-scratch disease	*Bartonella henselae*	153
Lepromatous leprosy	*Mycobacterium leprae*	159
Secondary syphilis (papulosquamous, nodular, and condylomata lata lesions)	*Treponema pallidum*	162
Tertiary syphilis (nodular gummatous lesions)	*T. pallidum*	162
Ulcers with or without eschars		
Anthrax	*Bacillus anthracis*	214
Ulceroglandular tularemia	*Francisella tularensis*	151, 214
Bubonic plague	*Yersinia pestis*	152, 214
Buruli ulcer	*Mycobacterium ulcerans*	160
Leprosy	*M. leprae*	159
Cutaneous tuberculosis	*M. tuberculosis*	158
Chancroid	*Haemophilus ducreyi*	139
Primary syphilis	*T. pallidum*	162
Erysipelas	*S. pyogenes*	130
Cellulitis	*Staphylococcus* spp., *Streptococcus* spp., various other bacteria	Various
Necrotizing fasciitis		
Streptococcal gangrene	*S. pyogenes*	130
Fournier's gangrene	Mixed aerobic and anaerobic bacteria	157
Staphylococcal necrotizing fasciitis	Methicillin-resistant *S. aureus*	129
Myositis and myonecrosis		
Pyomyositis	*S. aureus*	129
Streptococcal necrotizing myositis	*S. pyogenes*	130
Gas gangrene	*Clostridium* spp.	135
Nonclostridial (crepitant) myositis	Mixed aerobic and anaerobic bacteria	157
Synergistic nonclostridial anaerobic myonecrosis	Mixed aerobic and anaerobic bacteria	157

pearance of vesicles is preceded by pain for several days. Zoster may occur in persons of any age but is most common among immunosuppressed individuals and elderly patients, whereas most cases of varicella occur in young children. Vesicles due to HSV are found on or around the lips (HSV-1) or genitals (HSV-2) but may appear on the head and neck of young wrestlers (herpes gladiatorum) or on the digits of health care workers (herpetic whitlow). Recurrent herpes labialis (HSV-1) and herpes genitalis commonly follow primary infection. Coxsackievirus A16 characteristically causes vesicles on the hands, feet, and mouth of children. Orf is caused by a DNA virus related to smallpox virus and infects the fingers of individuals who work around goats and sheep. Molluscum contagiosum virus induces flaccid vesicles on the skin of healthy and immunocompromised individuals. Although variola (smallpox) in nature was eradicated as of 1977, recent terrorist events have renewed interest in this devastating infection (Chap. 214). Viremia beginning after an incubation period of 12 days is followed by a diffuse maculopapular rash, with rapid evolution to vesicles, pustules, and then scabs. Secondary cases can occur among close contacts.

Rickettsialpox begins after mite-bite inoculation of *Rickettsia akari* into the skin. A papule with a central vesicle evolves to form a 1- to 2.5-cm painless crusted black eschar with an erythematous halo and proximal adenopathy. While more common in the northeastern United States and the Ukraine in 1940–1950, rickettsialpox has recently been described in Ohio, Arizona, and Utah. Blistering dactylitis is a painful, vesicular, localized *Staphylococcus aureus* or group A streptococcal infection of the pulps of the distal digits of the hands.

INFECTIONS ASSOCIATED WITH BULLAE

(Table 119-1) Staphylococcal scalded-skin syndrome (SSSS) in neonates is caused by a toxin (exfoliatin) from phage group II *S. aureus.* SSSS must be distinguished from toxic epidermal necrolysis (TEN), which occurs primarily in adults, is drug-induced, and is associated with a higher mortality rate. Punch biopsy with frozen section is useful in making this distinction since the cleavage plane is the stratum corneum in SSSS and the stratum germinativum in TEN (Fig. 119-1). Intravenous γ-globulin is a promising treatment for TEN. Necrotizing fasciitis and gas gangrene also induce bulla formation (see "Necrotizing Fasciitis," below). Halophilic vibrio infection can be as aggressive and fulminant as necrotizing fasciitis; a helpful clue in its diagnosis is a history of exposure to waters of the Gulf of Mexico or the Atlantic seaboard or (in a patient with cirrhosis) the ingestion of raw seafood. The etiologic organism (*Vibrio vulnificus*) is highly susceptible to tetracycline.

INFECTIONS ASSOCIATED WITH CRUSTED LESIONS

(Table 119-1) Impetigo contagiosa is caused by *S. pyogenes*, and bullous impetigo is due to *S. aureus*. Both skin lesions may have an early bullous stage but then appear as thick crusts with a golden-brown color. Epidemics of impetigo caused by methicillin-resistant *S. aureus* (MRSA) have been reported. Streptococcal lesions are most common among children 2–5 years of age, and epidemics may occur in settings of poor hygiene, particularly among children of lower socioeconomic status in tropical climates. It is important to recognize impetigo contagiosa because of its relationship to poststreptococcal glomerulonephritis. Rheumatic fever is not a complication of skin infection caused by *S. pyogenes*. Superficial dermatophyte infection (ringworm) can occur on any skin surface, and skin scrapings with KOH staining are diagnostic. Primary infections with dimorphic fungi such as *Blastomyces dermatitidis* and *Sporothrix schenckii* can initially present as crusted skin lesions resembling ringworm. Disseminated infection with *Coccidioides immitis* can also involve the skin, and biopsy and culture should be performed on crusted lesions in patients from endemic areas. Crusted nodular lesions caused by *Mycobacterium chelonei* have been described in HIV-seropositive patients. Treatment with clarithromycin looks promising.

FOLLICULITIS

(Table 119-1) Hair follicles serve as portals for a number of bacteria, although *S. aureus* is the most common cause of localized folliculitis. Sebaceous glands empty into hair follicles and ducts and, if blocked, form sebaceous cysts, which may resemble staphylococcal abscesses or may become secondarily infected. Infection of sweat glands (hidradenitis suppurativa) can also mimic infection of hair follicles, particularly in the axillae. Chronic folliculitis is uncommon except in acne vulgaris, where constituents of the normal flora (e.g., *Propionibacterium acnes*) may play a role.

Diffuse folliculitis occurs in two settings. Hot-tub folliculitis is caused by *Pseudomonas aeruginosa* in waters that are insufficiently chlorinated and maintained at temperatures of 37–40°C. Infection is usually self-limited, although bacteremia and shock have been reported. Swimmer's itch occurs when a skin surface is exposed to water infested with freshwater avian schistosomes. Warm water temperatures and alkaline pH are suitable for mollusks that serve as intermediate hosts between birds and humans. Free-swimming schistosomal cercariae readily penetrate human hair follicles or pores but quickly die and elicit a brisk allergic reaction, causing intense itching and erythema.

PAPULAR AND NODULAR LESIONS

(Table 119-1) Raised lesions of the skin occur in many different forms. *Mycobacterium marinum* infections of the skin may present as cellulitis or as raised erythematous nodules. Erythematous papules are early manifestations of cat-scratch disease (with lesions developing at the primary site of inoculation of *Bartonella henselae*) and bacillary angiomatosis (also caused by *B. henselae*). Raised serpiginous or linear eruptions are characteristic of cutaneous larva migrans, which is caused by burrowing larvae of dog or cat hookworms (*Ancylostoma braziliense*) and which humans acquire through contact with soil that has been contaminated with dog or cat feces. Similar burrowing raised lesions are present in dracunculiasis caused by migration of the adult female nematode *Dracunculus medinensis*. Nodules caused by *Onchocerca volvulus* measure 1–10 cm in diameter and occur mostly in persons bitten by *Simulium* flies in Africa. The nodules contain the adult worm encased in fibrous tissue. Migration of microfilariae into the eyes may result in blindness. Verruca peruana is caused by *Bartonella bacilliformis*, which is transmitted to humans by the sandfly *Phlebotomus*. This condition can take the form of single gigantic lesions (several centimeters in diameter) or multiple small lesions (several millimeters in diameter). Numerous subcutaneous nodules may also be present in cysticercosis caused by larvae of *Taenia solium*. Multiple erythematous papules develop in schistosomiasis; each represents a cercarial invasion site. Skin nodules as well as thickened subcutaneous tissue are prominent features of lepromatous leprosy. Large nodules or gummas are features of tertiary syphilis, whereas flat papulosquamous lesions are characteristic of secondary syphilis. Human papillomavirus may cause singular warts (verruca vulgaris) or multiple warts in the anogenital area (condylomata acuminata). The latter are major problems in HIV-infected individuals.

ULCERS WITH OR WITHOUT ESCHARS

(Table 119-1) Cutaneous anthrax begins as a pruritic papule, which develops within days into an ulcer with surrounding vesicles and edema and then into an enlarging ulcer with a black eschar. Cutaneous anthrax may cause chronic nonhealing ulcers with an overlying dirty-gray membrane, although lesions may also mimic psoriasis, eczema, or impetigo. Ulceroglandular tularemia may have associated ulcerated skin lesions with painful regional adenopathy. Although buboes are the major cutaneous manifestation of plague, ulcers with eschars, papules, or pustules are also present in 25% of cases.

Mycobacterium ulcerans typically causes chronic skin ulcers on the extremities of individuals living in the tropics. *Mycobacterium leprae* may be associated with cutaneous ulcerations in patients with lepromatous leprosy related to Lucio's phenomenon, in which immune-mediated destruction of tissue bearing high concentrations of *M. leprae* bacilli occurs, usually several months after initiation of effective therapy. *Mycobacterium tuberculosis* may also cause ulcerations, papules, or erythematous macular lesions of the skin in both normal and immunocompromised patients.

Decubitus ulcers are due to tissue hypoxia secondary to pressure-induced vascular insufficiency and may become secondarily infected with components of the skin and gastrointestinal flora, including anaerobes. Ulcerative lesions on the anterior shins may be due to pyoderma gangrenosum, which must be distinguished from similar lesions of infectious etiology by histologic evaluation of biopsy sites. Ulcerated lesions on the genitals may be either painful (chancroid) or painless (primary syphilis).

ERYSIPELAS

(Table 119-1) Erysipelas is due to *S. pyogenes* and is characterized by an abrupt onset of fiery-red swelling of the face or extremities. The distinctive features of erysipelas are well-defined indurated margins, particularly along the nasolabial fold; rapid progression; and intense pain. Flaccid bullae may develop during the second or third day of illness, but extension to deeper soft tissues is rare. Treatment with penicillin is effective; swelling may progress despite appropriate treatment, although fever, pain, and the intense red color diminish. Desquamation of the involved skin occurs 5–10 days into the illness. Infants and elderly adults are most commonly afflicted, and the severity of systemic toxicity varies.

CELLULITIS

(Table 119-1) Cellulitis is an acute inflammatory condition of the skin that is characterized by localized pain, erythema, swelling, and heat. Cellulitis may be caused by indigenous flora colonizing the skin and appendages (e.g., *S. aureus* and *S. pyogenes*) or by a wide variety of exogenous bacteria. Because the exogenous bacteria involved in cellulitis occupy unique niches in nature, a thorough history (including epidemiologic data) provides important clues to etiology. When there is drainage, an open wound, or an obvious portal of entry, Gram's stain and culture provide a definitive diagnosis. In the absence of these findings, the bacterial etiology of cellulitis is difficult to establish, and in some cases staphylococcal and streptococcal cellulitis may have similar features. Even with needle aspiration of the leading edge or a punch biopsy of the cellulitis tissue itself, cultures are positive in only 20% of cases. This observation suggests that relatively low numbers of bacteria may cause cellulitis and that the expanding area of erythema within the skin may be a direct effect of extracellular toxins or of the soluble mediators of inflammation elicited by the host.

Bacteria may gain access to the epidermis through cracks in the skin, abrasions, cuts, burns, insect bites, surgical incisions, and intravenous catheters. Cellulitis caused by *S. aureus* spreads from a central localized infection, such as an abscess, folliculitis, or an infected foreign body (e.g., a splinter, a prosthetic device, or an intravenous catheter). MRSA is rapidly replacing methicillin-sensitive *S. aureus* (MSSA) as a cause of cellulitis in both inpatient and outpatient settings. In contrast, cellulitis due to *S. pyogenes* is a more rapidly spreading, diffuse process frequently associated with lymphangitis and fever. Recurrent streptococcal cellulitis of the lower extremities may be caused by organisms of group A, C, or G in association with chronic venous stasis or with saphenous venectomy for coronary artery bypass surgery. Streptococci also cause recurrent cellulitis among patients with chronic lymphedema resulting from elephantiasis, lymph node dissection, or Milroy's disease. Recurrent staphylococcal cutaneous infections are more common among individuals who have eosinophilia and elevated serum levels of IgE (Job's syndrome) and among nasal carriers of staphylococci. Cellulitis caused by *Streptococcus agalactiae* (group B *Streptococcus*) occurs primarily in elderly patients and those with diabetes mellitus or peripheral vascular disease. *Haemophilus influenzae* typically causes periorbital cellulitis in children in association with sinusitis, otitis media, or epiglottitis. It is unclear whether this form of cellulitis will (like meningitis) become less common as a result of the impressive efficacy of the *H. influenzae* type b vaccine.

Many other bacteria also cause cellulitis. Fortunately, these organisms occur in such characteristic settings that a good history provides useful clues to the diagnosis. Cellulitis associated with cat bites and, to a lesser degree, with dog bites is commonly caused by *Pasteurella multocida*, although in the latter case *Staphylococcus intermedius* and *Capnocytophaga canimorsus* (formerly DF-2) must also be considered. Sites of cellulitis and abscesses associated with dog bites and human bites also contain a variety of anaerobic organisms, including *Fusobacterium*, *Bacteroides*, aerobic and anaerobic streptococci, and *Eikenella corrodens*. *Pasteurella* is notoriously resistant to dicloxacillin and nafcillin but is sensitive to all other β-lactam antimicrobial agents as well as to quinolones, tetracycline, and erythromycin. Ampicillin/clavulanate, ampicillin/sulbactam, and cefoxitin are good choices for the treatment of animal or human bite infections. *Aeromonas hydrophila* causes aggressive cellulitis in tissues surrounding lacerations sustained in freshwater (lakes, rivers, and streams). This organism remains sensitive to aminoglycosides, fluoroquinolones, chloramphenicol, trimethoprim-sulfamethoxazole, and third-generation cephalosporins; it is resistant to ampicillin, however.

P. aeruginosa causes three types of soft tissue infection: ecthyma gangrenosum in neutropenic patients, hot-tub folliculitis, and cellulitis following penetrating injury. Most commonly, *P. aeruginosa* is introduced into the deep tissues when a person steps on a nail. Treatment includes surgical inspection and drainage, particularly if the injury also involves bone or joint capsule. Choices for empirical treatment while antimicrobial susceptibility data are awaited include an aminoglycoside, a third-generation cephalosporin (ceftazidime, cefoperazone, or cefotaxime), a semisynthetic penicillin (ticarcillin, mezlocillin, or piperacillin), or a fluoroquinolone (although drugs of the last class are not indicated for the treatment of children <13 years old).

Gram-negative bacillary cellulitis, including that due to *P. aeruginosa*, is most common among hospitalized, immunocompromised hosts. Cultures and sensitivity tests are critically important in this setting because of multidrug resistance (Chap. 145).

The gram-positive aerobic rod *Erysipelothrix rhusiopathiae* is most often associated with fish and domestic swine and causes cellulitis primarily in bone renderers and fishmongers. *E. rhusiopathiae* remains susceptible to most β-lactam antibiotics (including penicillin), erythromycin, clindamycin, tetracycline, and cephalosporins but is resistant to sulfonamides, chloramphenicol, and vancomycin. Its resistance to vancomycin, which is unusual among gram-positive bacteria, is of potential clinical significance since this agent is sometimes used in empirical therapy for skin infection. Fish food containing the water flea *Daphnia* is sometimes contaminated with *M. marinum*, which can cause cellulitis or granulomas on skin surfaces exposed to the water in aquariums or injured in swimming pools. Rifampin plus ethambutol has been an effective therapeutic combination in some cases, although no comprehensive studies have been undertaken. In addition, some strains of *M. marinum* are susceptible to tetracycline or to trimethoprim-sulfamethoxazole.

NECROTIZING FASCIITIS

(Table 119-1) Necrotizing fasciitis, formerly called streptococcal gangrene, may be associated with group A *Streptococcus* or mixed aerobic-anaerobic bacteria or may occur as part of gas gangrene caused by *Clostridium perfringens*. Strains of MRSA that produce the Panton-Valentine leukocidin have been reported to cause necrotizing fasciitis. Early diagnosis may be difficult when pain or unexplained fever is the only presenting manifestation. Swelling then develops and is followed by brawny edema and tenderness. With progression, dark-red induration of the epidermis appears, along with bullae filled with blue or purple fluid. Later the skin becomes friable and takes on a bluish, maroon, or black color. By this stage, thrombosis of blood vessels in the dermal papillae (Fig. 119-1) is extensive. Extension of infection to the level of the deep fascia causes this tissue to take on a brownish-gray appearance. Rapid spread occurs along fascial planes, through venous channels and lymphatics. Patients in the later stages are toxic and frequently manifest shock and multiorgan failure.

Necrotizing fasciitis caused by mixed aerobic-anaerobic bacteria begins with a breach in the integrity of a mucous membrane barrier, such as the mucosa of the gastrointestinal or genitourinary tract. The portal can be a malignancy, diverticulum, hemorrhoid, anal fissure, or urethral tear. Other predisposing factors include peripheral vascular disease, diabetes mellitus, surgery, and penetrating injury to the abdomen. Leakage into the perineal area results in a syndrome called *Fournier's gangrene*, characterized by massive swelling of the scrotum and penis with extension into the perineum or the abdominal wall and legs.

Necrotizing fasciitis caused by *S. pyogenes* has increased in frequency and severity since 1985. It often begins deep at the site of a nonpenetrating minor trauma, such as a bruise or a muscle strain. Seeding of the site via transient bacteremia is likely, although most patients deny antecedent streptococcal infection. Alternatively, *S. pyogenes* may reach the deep fascia from a site of cutaneous infection or penetrating trauma. Toxicity is severe, and renal impairment may precede the development of shock. In 20–40% of cases, myositis occurs concomitantly, and, as in gas gangrene (see below), serum creatine phosphokinase levels may be markedly elevated. Necrotizing fasciitis due to mixed aerobic-anaerobic bacteria may be associated with gas in deep tissue, but gas usually is not present when the cause is *S. pyogenes* or MRSA. Prompt surgical exploration down to the deep fascia and muscle is essential. Necrotic tissue must be surgically removed, and Gram's staining and culture of excised tissue are useful in establishing whether group A streptococci, mixed aerobic-anaerobic bacteria, MRSA, or *Clostridium* species are present (see "Treatment," below).

MYOSITIS/MYONECROSIS

(Table 119-1) Muscle involvement can occur with viral infection (e.g., influenza, dengue, or coxsackievirus B infection) or parasitic invasion (e.g., trichinellosis, cysticercosis, or toxoplasmosis). Although myalgia can occur in most of these infections, severe muscle pain is the hallmark of pleurodynia (coxsackievirus B), trichinellosis, and bacterial infection. Acute rhabdomyolysis predictably occurs with clostridial and streptococcal myositis but may also be associated with influenza virus, echovirus, coxsackievirus, Epstein-Barr virus, and *Legionella* infections.

Pyomyositis is usually due to *S. aureus*, is common in tropical areas, and generally has no known portal of entry. Infection remains localized, and shock does not develop unless organisms produce toxic shock syndrome toxin 1 or certain enterotoxins and the patient lacks antibodies to the toxin produced by the infecting organisms. In contrast, *S. pyogenes* may induce primary myositis (referred to as *strepto-*

coccal necrotizing myositis) in association with severe systemic toxicity. Myonecrosis occurs concomitantly with necrotizing fasciitis in ~50% of cases. Both are part of the streptococcal toxic shock syndrome.

Gas gangrene usually follows severe penetrating injuries that result in interruption of the blood supply and introduction of soil into wounds. Such cases of traumatic gangrene are usually caused by the clostridial species *C. perfringens*, *C. septicum*, and *C. histolyticum*. Rarely, latent or recurrent gangrene can occur years after penetrating trauma; dormant spores that reside at the site of previous injury are most likely responsible. Spontaneous nontraumatic gangrene among patients with neutropenia, gastrointestinal malignancy, diverticulosis, or recent radiation therapy to the abdomen is caused by several clostridial species, of which *C. septicum* is the most commonly involved. The tolerance of this anaerobe to oxygen probably explains why it can initiate infection spontaneously in normal tissue anywhere in the body.

Synergistic nonclostridial anaerobic myonecrosis, also known as necrotizing cutaneous myositis and synergistic necrotizing cellulitis, is a variant of necrotizing fasciitis caused by mixed aerobic and anaerobic bacteria with the exclusion of clostridial organisms (see "Necrotizing Fasciitis," above).

DIAGNOSIS

This chapter has emphasized the physical appearance and location of lesions within the soft tissues as important diagnostic clues. The temporal progression of the lesions as well as the patient's travel history, animal exposure or bite history, age, underlying disease status, and lifestyle are

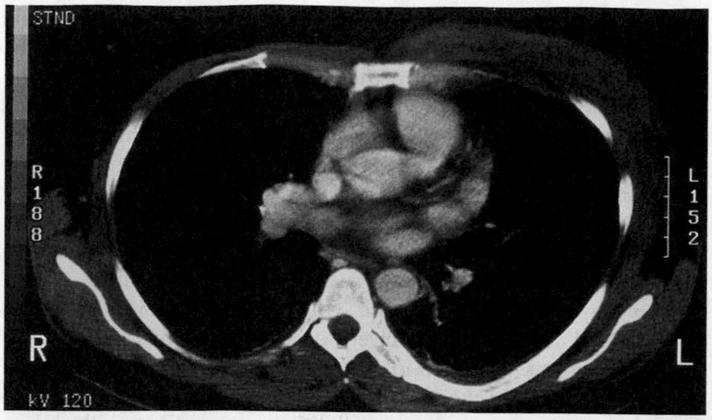

FIGURE 119-2 Computed tomography showing edema and inflammation of the left chest wall in a patient with necrotizing fasciitis and myonecrosis caused by group A *Streptococcus*.

also crucial considerations in the formulation of a narrowed differential diagnosis. However, even the astute clinician may find it challenging to diagnose all infections of the soft tissues by history and inspection alone. Soft tissue radiography, computed tomography (Fig. 119-2), and magnetic resonance imaging may be useful in determining the depth of infection and should be performed in patients with rapidly progressing lesions or evidence of systemic inflammatory response syndrome. These

TABLE 119-2 TREATMENT OF COMMON INFECTIONS OF THE SKIN

Diagnosis/Condition	Primary Treatment	Alternative Treatment	See Also Chap(s).
Animal bite (prophylaxis or early infection)[a]	Amoxicillin/clavulanate, 875/125 mg PO bid	Doxycycline, 100 mg PO bid	**e15**
Animal bite[a] (established infection)	Ampicillin/sulbactam, 1.5–3.0 g IV q6h	Clindamycin, 600–900 mg IV q8h *plus* Ciprofloxacin, 400 mg IV q12h *or* Cefoxitin, 2 g IV q6h	**e15**
Bacillary angiomatosis	Erythromycin, 500 mg PO qid	Doxycycline, 100 mg PO bid	153
Herpes simplex (primary genital)	Acyclovir, 400 mg PO tid for 10 days	Famciclovir, 250 mg PO tid for 5–10 days *or* Valacyclovir, 1000 mg PO bid for 10 days	172
Herpes zoster (immunocompetent host >50 years of age)	Acyclovir, 800 mg PO 5 times daily for 7–10 days	Famciclovir, 500 mg PO tid for 7–10 days *or* Valacyclovir, 1000 mg PO tid for 7 days	173
Cellulitis (staphylococcal or streptococcal[b,c])	Nafcillin or oxacillin, 2 g IV q4–6h	Cefazolin, 1–2 g q8h *or* Ampicillin/sulbactam, 1.5–3.0 g IV q6h *or* Erythromycin, 0.5–1.0 g IV q6h *or* Clindamycin, 600–900 mg IV q8h	129, 130
MRSA skin infection[d]	Vancomycin, 1 g IV q12h	Linezolid, 600 mg IV q12h	129
Necrotizing fasciitis (group A streptococcal[b])	Clindamycin, 600–900 mg IV q6–8h *plus* Penicillin G, 4 million units IV q4h	Clindamycin, 600–900 mg IV q6–8h *plus* Cephalosporin (first- or second-generation)	130
Necrotizing fasciitis (mixed aerobes and anaerobes)	Ampicillin, 2 g IV q4h *plus* Clindamycin, 600–900 mg IV q6–8h *plus* Ciprofloxacin, 400 mg IV q6–8h	Vancomycin, 1 g IV q6h *plus* Metronidazole, 500 mg IV q6h *plus* Ciprofloxacin, 400 mg IV q6–8h	157
Gas gangrene	Clindamycin, 600–900 mg IV q6–8h *plus* Penicillin G, 4 million units IV q4–6h	Clindamycin, 600–900 mg IV q6–8h *plus* Cefoxitin, 2 g IV q6h	135

[a]*Pasteurella multocida*, a species commonly associated with both dog and cat bites, is resistant to cephalexin, dicloxacillin, clindamycin, and erythromycin. *Eikenella corrodens*, a bacterium commonly associated with human bites, is resistant to clindamycin, penicillinase-resistant penicillins, and metronidazole but is sensitive to trimethoprim-sulfamethoxazole and fluoroquinolones.

[b]The frequency of erythromycin resistance in group A *Streptococcus* is currently ~5% in the United States but has reached 70–100% in some other countries. Most, but not all, erythromycin-resistant group A streptococci are susceptible to clindamycin. Approximately 90–95% of *Staphylococcus aureus* strains are sensitive to clindamycin.

[c]Severe hospital-acquired *S. aureus* infections or community-acquired *S. aureus* infections that are not responding to the β-lactam antibiotics recommended in this table may be caused by methicillin-resistant strains, requiring a switch to vancomycin or linezolid.

[d]Some strains of methicillin-resistant *S. aureus* (MRSA) remain sensitive to tetracycline and trimethoprim-sulfamethoxazole. Daptomycin (4 mg/kg IV q24h) or tigecycline (100-mg loading dose followed by 50 mg IV q12h) are alternative treatments for MRSA.

tests are particularly valuable for defining a localized abscess or detecting gas in tissue. Unfortunately, they may reveal only soft tissue swelling and thus are not specific for fulminant infections such as necrotizing fasciitis or myonecrosis caused by group A *Streptococcus* (Fig. 119-2), where gas is not found in lesions.

Aspiration of the leading edge or punch biopsy with frozen section may be helpful if the results are positive, but false-negative results occur in ~80% of cases. There is some evidence that aspiration alone may be superior to injection and aspiration with normal saline. Frozen sections are especially useful in distinguishing SSSS from TEN and are quite valuable in cases of necrotizing fasciitis. Open surgical inspection with debridement as indicated is clearly the best way to determine the extent and severity of infection and to obtain material for Gram's staining and culture. Such an aggressive approach is important and may be lifesaving if undertaken early in the course of fulminant infections where there is evidence of systemic toxicity.

Rx INFECTIONS OF THE SKIN, MUSCLE, AND SOFT TISSUES

A full description of the treatment of all the clinical entities described herein is beyond the scope of this chapter. As a guide to the clinician in selecting appropriate treatment, the antimicrobial agents useful in the most common and the most fulminant cutaneous infections are listed in **Table 119-2**.

Early and aggressive surgical exploration is essential in patients with suspected necrotizing fasciitis, myositis, or gangrene in order to (1) visualize the deep structures, (2) remove necrotic tissue, (3) reduce compartment pressure, and (4) obtain suitable material for Gram's staining and for aerobic and anaerobic cultures. Appropriate empirical antibiotic treatment for mixed aerobic-anaerobic infections could consist of ampicillin/sulbactam, cefoxitin, or the following combination: (1) clindamycin (600–900 mg intravenously every 8 h) or metronidazole (750 mg every 6 h) plus (2) ampicillin or ampicillin/sulbactam (2–3 g intravenously every 6 h) plus (3) gentamicin (1.0–1.5 mg/kg every 8 h). Group A streptococcal and clostridial infection of the fascia and/or muscle carries a mortality rate of 20–50% with penicillin treatment. In experimental models of streptococcal and clostridial necrotizing fasciitis/myositis, clindamycin has exhibited markedly superior efficacy, but no comparative trials have been performed in humans. Hyperbaric oxygen treatment may also be useful in gas gangrene due to clostridial species. Antibiotic treatment should be continued until all signs of systemic toxicity have resolved, all devitalized tissue has been removed, and granulation tissue has developed (Chaps. 130, 135, and 157).

In summary, infections of the skin and soft tissues are diverse in presentation and severity and offer a great challenge to the clinician. This chapter provides an approach to diagnosis and understanding of the pathophysiologic mechanisms involved in these infections. More in-depth information is found in chapters on specific infections.

FURTHER READINGS

BISNO AI, STEVENS DL: Streptococcal infections in skin and soft tissues. N Engl J Med 334:240, 1996

BREMAN JG, HENDERSON DA: Diagnosis and management of smallpox. N Engl J Med 346:1300, 2002

CARPENTER CF, CHAMBERS HF: Daptomycin: Another novel agent for treating infections due to drug-resistant gram-positive pathogens. Clin Infect Dis 38:994, 2004

ELLIS-GROSSE EJ et al: The efficacy and safety of tigecycline in the treatment of skin and skin-structure infections: Results of 2 double-blind phase 3 comparison studies with vancomycin-aztreonam. Clin Infect Dis 41(Suppl 5):S341, 2005

FRIDKIN SK et al: Methicillin-resistant *Staphylococcus aureus* disease in three communities. N Engl J Med 352:1436, 2005

MILLER LG et al: Necrotizing fasciitis caused by community-associated methicillin-resistant *Staphylococcus aureus* in Los Angeles. N Engl J Med 352:1445, 2005

NORRBY-TEGLUND A, STEVENS DL: Novel therapies in streptococcal toxic shock syndrome: Attenuation of virulence factor expression and modulation of host response. Curr Opin Infect Dis 11:285, 1998

STEVENS DL: Streptococcal toxic shock syndrome associated with necrotizing fasciitis. Annu Rev Med 51:271, 2000

———: Necrotizing soft tissue infections. Curr Treat Opt Infect Dis 2:359, 2000

TALAN DA et al: Bacteriologic analysis of infected dog and cat bites. Emergency Medicine Animal Bite Infection Study Group. N Engl J Med 340:85, 1999

120 Osteomyelitis

Jeffrey Parsonnet

Osteomyelitis, an infection of bone, is caused most commonly by pyogenic bacteria and mycobacteria. As a useful framework for evaluating a patient and planning treatment, cases are classified on the basis of the causative agent; the route by which organisms gain access to bone; the duration of infection; the anatomic location of infection; and the local and systemic host factors that have a bearing on pathogenesis and outcome.

PATHOGENESIS AND PATHOLOGY

Microorganisms enter bone by hematogenous dissemination, by spread from a contiguous focus of infection, or by a penetrating wound. Trauma, ischemia, and foreign bodies enhance the susceptibility of bone to microbial invasion by exposing sites to which bacteria can bind and by impeding host defenses. Phagocytes attempt to contain the infection and, in the process, release enzymes that lyse bone. Bacteria escape host defenses by adhering tightly to damaged bone, by entering and persisting within osteoblasts, and by coating themselves and underlying surfaces with a protective polysaccharide-rich biofilm. Pus spreads into vascular channels, raising intraosseous pressure and impairing the flow of blood; as the untreated infection becomes chronic, ischemic necrosis of bone results in the separation of large devascularized fragments (*sequestra*). When pus breaks through the cortex, subperiosteal or soft tissue abscesses form, and the elevated periosteum deposits new bone (an *involucrum*) around the sequestrum.

Microorganisms, infiltrates of neutrophils, and congested or thrombosed blood vessels are the principal histologic findings of acute osteomyelitis. The distinguishing feature of chronic osteomyelitis is necrotic bone, which is characterized by the absence of living osteocytes. Mononuclear cells predominate in chronic infections, and granulation and fibrous tissues replace bone that has been resorbed by osteoclasts. In the chronic stage, organisms may be too few to be seen on staining.

HEMATOGENOUS OSTEOMYELITIS

Hematogenous infection accounts for ~20% of cases of osteomyelitis and primarily affects children, in whom the long bones are infected, and older adults and IV drug users, in whom the spine is the most common site of infection.

ACUTE HEMATOGENOUS OSTEOMYELITIS

Infection usually involves a single bone, most commonly the tibia, femur, or humerus in children and vertebral bodies in injection drug users and older adults. Bacteria settle in the well-perfused metaphysis of growing bones, a network of venous sinusoids slows the flow of blood, and fenestrations in capillaries allow organisms to escape into the extravascular space. Because vascular anatomy changes with age, hematogenous infection of long bones is uncommon during adulthood and, when it occurs, usually involves the diaphysis.

On presentation, the child with osteomyelitis usually appears acutely ill, with fever, chills, localized pain and tenderness, and—in many cases—restriction of movement or difficulty bearing weight. Overlying erythema and swelling indicate extension of pus through the cortex. During infancy and after puberty, infection may spread through the epiphysis into the joint space. In children of other ages, extension of infection through the cortex results in involvement of joints if the metaphysis is intracapsular. Thus, septic arthritis of the elbow, shoulder, and hip may complicate osteomyelitis of the proximal radius, humerus, and femur, respectively. In children, the source of bacteremia is usually inapparent. A history is often obtained of recent blunt trauma to the area involved; presumably, this event results in a small intraosseous hematoma or vascular obstruction that predisposes to infection. Adults with hematogenous osteomyelitis may present either in the context of an infection elsewhere (e.g., the respiratory or urinary tract, a heart valve, or an intravascular catheter site) or without an obvious source of bacteremia.

Plain radiographs obtained early in the course of infection may show soft tissue swelling, but the first change in bone—a periosteal reaction—is not evident until at least 10 days after the onset of infection. Lytic changes can be detected only after 2–6 weeks, when 50–75% of bone density has been lost. Rarely, a well-circumscribed lytic lesion, or *Brodie's abscess*, is seen in a child who has been in pain for several months but has had no fever.

VERTEBRAL OSTEOMYELITIS

The vertebrae are the most common sites of hematogenous osteomyelitis in adults. Organisms reach the well-perfused vertebral body via spinal arteries and quickly spread from the end plate into the disk space and then to the adjacent vertebral body. Sources of bacteremia include the urinary tract (especially among men over age 50), dental abscesses, soft tissue infections, and contaminated IV lines, but the source of bacteremia is not evident in more than half of patients. Diabetes mellitus requiring insulin injection, a recent invasive medical procedure, hemodialysis, and injection drug use carry an increased risk of spinal infection. Many patients have a history of degenerative joint disease involving the spine, and some report an episode of trauma preceding the onset of infection. Penetrating injuries and surgical procedures involving the spine may cause nonhematogenous vertebral osteomyelitis or infection localized to a disk.

Most patients with vertebral osteomyelitis report neck or back pain; patients may describe atypical pain in the chest, the abdomen, or an extremity that is due to irritation of nerve roots. Symptoms are localized to the lumbar spine more often than to the thoracic spine (>50% vs. 35% of cases) or the cervical spine in pyogenic infections, but the thoracic spine is involved most commonly in tuberculous spondylitis (Pott's disease). More than 50% of patients experience a subacute illness in which a vague, dull pain gradually intensifies over 2–3 months. Fever is usually low-grade or absent, but some patients recall having had an episode of fever and chills prior to or at the onset of pain. An acute presentation with high fever and toxicity is less common and suggests ongoing bacteremia. Percussion over the involved vertebra elicits tenderness, and physical examination may reveal spasm of the paraspinal muscles and limitation of motion.

Laboratory findings at the time of presentation include a normal or modestly elevated white blood cell count, anemia, and, almost invariably, an increased erythrocyte sedimentation rate (ESR) and C-reactive protein (CRP) level. Blood cultures are positive only 20–50% of the time.

By the time the patient seeks medical attention, plain radiographs often show irregular erosions in the end plates of adjacent vertebral bodies and narrowing of the intervening disk space. This radiographic pattern is virtually diagnostic of bacterial infection because tumors and other diseases of the spine rarely cross the disk space. CT or MRI may demonstrate epidural, paraspinal, retropharyngeal, mediastinal, retroperitoneal, or psoas abscesses that originate in the spine.

A spinal epidural abscess may evolve suddenly or over several weeks; the classic clinical presentation is spinal pain progressing to radicular pain and/or weakness. Irreversible paralysis may result from failure to recognize epidural abscess before the development of neurologic deficits. MRI is the best procedure for detection of epidural abscess and should be performed in all cases of vertebral osteomyelitis accompanied by subjective weakness or objective neurologic abnormalities.

MICROBIOLOGY

More than 95% of cases of hematogenous osteomyelitis are caused by a single organism, with *Staphylococcus aureus* accounting for 50% of cases. Other common pathogens in children are group A streptococci and, during the neonatal period, group B streptococci and *Escherichia coli*. In adults, vertebral osteomyelitis is caused by *E. coli* and other enteric bacilli in ~25% of cases. *S. aureus*, *Pseudomonas aeruginosa*, *Serratia*, and *Candida albicans* infections are associated with injection drug use and may involve the sacroiliac, sternoclavicular, or pubic joints as well as the spine. *Salmonella* spp. and *S. aureus* are the major causes of long-bone osteomyelitis complicating sickle cell anemia and other hemoglobinopathies. Tuberculosis and brucellosis affect the spine more often than other bones. Other common sites of tuberculous osteomyelitis include the small bones of the hands and feet, the metaphyses of long bones, the ribs, and the sternum.

Unusual causes of hematogenous osteomyelitis include disseminated histoplasmosis, coccidioidomycosis, and blastomycosis in endemic areas. Immunocompromised persons may rarely develop osteomyelitis due to atypical mycobacteria, *Bartonella henselae*, or opportunistic fungi. Hematogenous osteomyelitis with *Mycobacterium bovis* has been reported following intravesicular instillation of bacille Calmette-Guérin (BCG) for cancer of the bladder. The etiology of chronic relapsing multifocal osteomyelitis, an inflammatory condition of children that is characterized by recurrent episodes of painful lytic lesions in multiple bones, has not been identified.

OSTEOMYELITIS SECONDARY TO A CONTIGUOUS FOCUS OF INFECTION

CLINICAL FEATURES

This broad category of osteomyelitis accounts for ~80% of all cases and occurs most commonly in adults. It includes infections introduced by penetrating injuries, such as bites, puncture wounds, and open fractures; by surgical procedures; and by direct extension of infection from adjacent soft tissues. Generalized vascular insufficiency and the presence of a foreign body are important predisposing factors and also make infection more difficult to cure.

Frequently, the diagnosis of this type of osteomyelitis is not made until the infection has already become chronic. The pain, fever, and inflammatory signs due to bony infection may be attributed to the original injury, to underlying bone or joint disease (such as degenerative arthritis), or to overlying soft tissue infection. Osteomyelitis may become apparent only weeks or months later, when a sinus tract develops, a surgical wound breaks down, or a fracture fails to heal. It may be impossible to distinguish radiographic abnormalities due to osteomyelitis from those due to the precipitating condition.

A special type of contiguous-focus osteomyelitis occurs in the setting of peripheral vascular disease and nearly always involves the small bones of the feet of adults with diabetes. This type of infection is a major cause of morbidity for patients with diabetes and results in many thousands of amputations per year. Diabetic neuropathy exposes the foot to frequent trauma and pressure sores, and the patient may be unaware of infection as it spreads into bone. Poor tissue perfusion impairs normal inflammatory responses and wound healing and creates a milieu that is conducive to anaerobic infections. It is often during the evaluation of a nonhealing ulcer, a swollen toe, or acute cellulitis that a radiograph provides the first evidence of osteomyelitis. If bone is palpable during examination of the base of an ulcer with a blunt surgical probe, osteomyelitis is likely.

MICROBIOLOGY

S. aureus is a pathogen in more than half of cases of contiguous-focus osteomyelitis. However, in contrast to hematogenous osteomyelitis,

TABLE 120-1 DIAGNOSTIC IMAGING STUDIES FOR OSTEOMYELITIS

Type of Study	Comments
Plain radiographs	Insensitive, especially in early osteomyelitis. May show periosteal elevation after 10 days, lytic changes after 2–6 weeks. Useful to look for anatomic abnormalities (e.g., fractures, bony variants, or deformities), foreign bodies, and soft tissue gas.
Three-phase bone scan (^{99m}Tc-MDP)	Characteristic finding in osteomyelitis: increased uptake in all three phases of scan. Highly sensitive (~95%) in acute infection; somewhat less sensitive if blood flow to bone is poor. Specificity moderate if plain films are normal, but poor in presence of neuropathic arthropathy, fractures, tumor, infarction.
Other radionuclide scans	Examples: ^{67}Ga-citrate, ^{111}In-labeled WBCs. ^{111}In-WBCs more specific than gallium but not always available. Often used in conjunction with bone scan because its greater specificity for inflammation than ^{99m}Tc-MDP helps to distinguish infectious from noninfectious processes. Lack of consensus over role; often supplanted by MRI when the latter is available.
Ultrasound	May detect subperiosteal fluid collection or soft tissue abscess adjacent to bone, but largely supplanted by CT and MRI.
CT	Limited role in acute osteomyelitis. In chronic osteomyelitis, excellent for detection of sequestra, cortical destruction, soft tissue abscesses, and sinus tracts. Use limited in the presence of a metallic foreign body.
MRI	As sensitive as ^{99m}Tc-MDP bone scan for acute osteomyelitis (~95%); detects changes in water content of marrow before disruption of cortical bone. High specificity (~87%), with better anatomic detail than nuclear studies. Procedure of choice for vertebral osteomyelitis because of high sensitivity for epidural abscess. Use may be limited by a metallic foreign body.

Abbreviations: MDP, monodiphosphonate; WBCs, white blood cells.

these infections are often polymicrobial and are more likely to involve gram-negative and anaerobic bacteria. Hence a mixture of staphylococci, streptococci, enteric organisms, and anaerobic bacteria may be isolated from a diabetic foot infection or pelvic osteomyelitis underlying a decubitus ulcer. Aerobic and anaerobic bacteria cause osteomyelitis following surgery or soft tissue infection of the oropharynx, paranasal sinuses, gastrointestinal tract, or female genital tract. A human bite may result in mixed infection of the hand, with anaerobes included among the etiologic agents. *S. aureus* is the principal cause of postoperative infections; coagulase-negative staphylococci are common pathogens after implantation of orthopedic appliances; and these organisms as well as gram-negative enteric bacilli, atypical mycobacteria, and *Mycoplasma* may cause sternal osteomyelitis after cardiac surgery. Infection with *P. aeruginosa* is frequently associated with puncture wounds of the foot, especially when a nail passes through a sneaker, and *Pasteurella multocida* infection commonly follows cat bites.

CHRONIC OSTEOMYELITIS

With prompt treatment, <5% of cases of acute hematogenous osteomyelitis progress to chronic osteomyelitis. Chronic infection is more likely to develop in contiguous-focus than in hematogenous osteomyelitis. The presence of a foreign body makes establishment of chronic infection especially likely.

A protracted clinical course, long periods of quiescence, and recurrent exacerbations are characteristic of chronic osteomyelitis. Sinus tracts between bone and skin may drain purulent material and occasionally pieces of necrotic bone. An increase in drainage, pain, or swelling signals an exacerbation, which is usually accompanied by increases in CRP level and ESR. Fever is unusual except when obstruction of a sinus tract leads to soft tissue infection. Rare late complications include pathologic fractures, squamous cell carcinoma of the sinus tract, and amyloidosis.

DIAGNOSIS

Early diagnosis of acute osteomyelitis is critical because prompt antibiotic therapy may prevent necrosis of bone. The ESR and the CRP level are elevated in most cases of active osteomyelitis, including those in which constitutional symptoms and leukocytosis are lacking. These findings are not specific to osteomyelitis, however, and the ESR is occasionally normal in early infections. Baseline values are often useful in monitoring the efficacy of treatment.

A variety of radiologic tests are available for evaluation of osteomyelitis (Table 120-1). Evaluation usually begins with plain radiographs because of their ready availability, although they typically show no abnormalities during early infection. Three-phase bone scans (^{99}Tc-monodiphosphonate) offer high sensitivity but are often of low specificity, especially in the presence of underlying bone abnormalities. There is a lack of consensus over the optimal use of other radionuclide studies, and there is considerable variation between institutions in their use. Use of MRI (Fig. 120-1) is expanding because of its high sensitivity and specificity as well as its ability to demonstrate associated soft tissue abnormalities, but this modality is not available at all institutions.

The role of diagnostic imaging in chronic osteomyelitis is to detect active infection and delineate the extent of debridement necessary to remove necrotic bone and abnormal soft tissues. CT is more sensitive than plain films for the detection of sequestra, sinus tracts, and soft tissue abscesses. Both CT and ultrasound are useful for guiding percutaneous aspiration of subperiosteal and soft tissue fluid collections. Sequential technetium and gallium or indium scans may help determine whether infection is active and may distinguish infection from noninflammatory bone changes. MRI provides superior information about the anatomic extent of infection but does not always distinguish osteomyelitis from healing fractures and tumors. MRI is particularly useful in distinguishing cellulitis from osteomyelitis in the diabetic foot; however, no imaging modality consistently distinguishes infection from neuropathic osteopathy.

Appropriate samples for microbiologic studies should be obtained in all cases of suspected osteomyelitis before the initiation of antimicrobial therapy. Blood cultures are indicated in acute cases and are

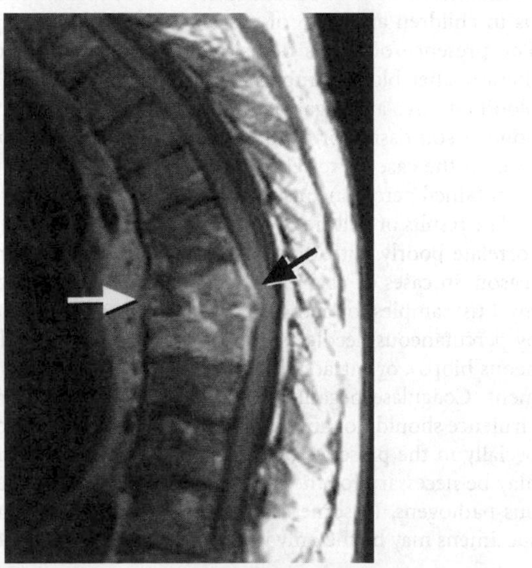

FIGURE 120-1 Osteomyelitis of the thoracic spine demonstrated on a sagittal, fat-suppressed T1-weighted magnetic resonance image after the administration of IV gadolinium. At T8–T9, there is involvement of the adjacent vertebral bodies and intervening disk. Abnormally enhancing inflammatory tissue extends from the disk space anteriorly (*white arrow*) as well as posteriorly into the epidural space, compressing the thecal sac (*black arrow*).

TABLE 120-2 SELECTION OF ANTIBIOTICS FOR TREATMENT OF ACUTE OSTEOMYELITIS

	Suggested Regimen[a]	
Organism	**Primary**	**Alternatives[b]**
Staphylococcus aureus		
Penicillin-resistant, methicillin-sensitive (MSSA)	Nafcillin or oxacillin, 2 g IV q4h	Cefazolin, 1 g IV q8h; ceftriaxone, 1 g IV q24h; clindamycin, 900 mg IV q8h[c]
Penicillin-sensitive	Penicillin, 3–4 million U IV q4h	Cefazolin, ceftriaxone, clindamycin (as above)
Methicillin-resistant (MRSA)	Vancomycin, 15 mg/kg IV q12h; rifampin, 300 mg PO q12h (see text)	Clindamycin[c] (as above); linezolid, 600 mg IV or PO q12h[d]; daptomycin, 4–6 mg/kg IV q24h[d]
Streptococci (including *S. milleri*, β-hemolytic streptococci)	Penicillin (as above)	Cefazolin, ceftriaxone, clindamycin (as above)
Gram-negative aerobic bacilli		
Escherichia coli, other "sensitive" species	Ampicillin, 2 g IV q4h; cefazolin, 1 g IV q8h	Ceftriaxone, 1 g IV q24h; parenteral or oral fluoroquinolone (e.g., ciprofloxacin, 400 mg IV or 750 mg PO q12h)[e]
Pseudomonas aeruginosa	Extended-spectrum β-lactam agent (e.g., piperacillin, 3–4 g IV q4–6h; or ceftazidime, 2 g IV q12h) *plus* tobramycin, 5–7 mg/kg q24h[f]	May substitute parenteral or oral fluoroquinolone for β-lactam agents (if patient is allergic) or for tobramycin (in relation to nephrotoxicity)
Enterobacter spp., other "resistant" species	Extended-spectrum β-lactam agent IV or fluoroquinolone IV or PO[e] (as above)	
Mixed infections possibly involving anaerobic bacteria	Ampicillin/sulbactam, 1.5–3 g IV q6h; piperacillin/tazobactam, 3.375 g IV q6h	Carbapenem antibiotic or a combination of a fluoroquinolone plus clindamycin (as above) or metronidazole, 500 mg PO tid

[a]Duration of treatment is discussed in the text.
[b]Cephalosporins may be used for the treatment of patients allergic to penicillin whose reaction did not consist of anaphylaxis or urticaria (immediate-type hypersensitivity).
[c]Because of the possibility of inducible resistance, clindamycin must be used with caution for the treatment of strains resistant to erythromycin. Consult clinical microbiology laboratory.
[d]Experience is limited; there are anecdotal reports of efficacy.
[e]Oral fluoroquinolones must not be coadministered with divalent cations (calcium, magnesium, iron, aluminum), which block the drugs' absorption.
[f]Tobramycin levels and renal function must be monitored closely to minimize the risks of nephro- and ototoxicity.

positive in more than one-third of cases of hematogenous osteomyelitis in children and 25% of cases of vertebral osteomyelitis in adults. The presence of sepsis occasionally requires initiation of empirical therapy after blood samples alone have been obtained for culture. If blood cultures are negative, samples from needle aspiration of pus in bone or soft tissues or from a bone biopsy should be obtained for culture; in the case of vertebral osteomyelitis, these samples can usually be obtained percutaneously with the guidance of fluoroscopy or CT.

The results of culture of swabs of a sinus tract or the base of an ulcer correlate poorly with those of samples of the infected bone. For this reason, in cases of chronic osteomyelitis and contiguous-focus osteomyelitis, samples for aerobic and anaerobic culture should be obtained by percutaneous needle aspiration through uninfected tissue, percutaneous biopsy, or intraoperative biopsy at the time of surgical debridement. Coagulase-negative staphylococci and other organisms of low virulence should not automatically be disregarded as contaminants, especially in the presence of prosthetic materials. Special culture media may be necessary for the isolation of mycobacteria, fungi, and fastidious pathogens. In some cases, histopathologic examination of biopsy specimens may be the only way to confirm a diagnosis of osteomyelitis.

Rx TREATMENT

ANTIBIOTIC THERAPY (Table 120-2) Antibiotics should be administered only after appropriate specimens have been obtained for culture. Use of bactericidal agents has been recommended, although controlled data for this recommendation are lacking. Antibiotics should be given at a high dose; thus, for most agents, parenteral administration is required. Empirical therapy is guided by findings on Gram's staining of a specimen from the bone or abscess or is chosen to cover the most likely pathogens; such therapy should usually include high doses of an agent active against *S. aureus* (such as oxacillin, nafcillin, cefazolin, or vancomycin) or—if gram-negative organisms are likely to be involved—a third-generation cephalosporin, an aminoglycoside, or a fluoroquinolone. Empirical therapy should also include an agent active against anaerobes in the setting of a decubitus ulcer or diabetic foot infection.

Specific therapy is ultimately based on in vitro susceptibility testing of the organism(s) isolated from bone or blood. Outpatient parenteral antimicrobial therapy (OPAT) is appropriate for motivated and medically stable patients and represents a significant advance in management. Antibiotics that require infrequent dosing, such as ceftriaxone, ertapenem, daptomycin, and vancomycin, may facilitate home therapy, but these choices often have an overly broad spectrum of activity. Fortunately, many antibiotics can be given automatically by means of a portable infusion pump, which decreases the disruption otherwise caused by frequent administration of a drug. Use of a peripherally inserted central catheter (PICC line) also greatly facilitates outpatient drug administration. OPAT requires close coordination of nursing, pharmacy, and physician care, with clear delineations of responsibility for monitoring of safety and efficacy.

After administration of parenteral therapy for 5–10 days and after resolution of signs of active infection, oral antibiotics have been used with great success in children with hematogenous osteomyelitis. The doses of oral penicillins or cephalosporins required for the treatment of pediatric osteomyelitis are high, and adults may not tolerate such doses as well as children. With the exception of the fluoroquinolones, rifampin, and linezolid, few data support the use of oral antibiotics for adults with osteomyelitis. For treatment of infection due to Enterobacteriaceae, oral administration of a fluoroquinolone has been as successful as IV administration of β-lactam antibiotics. Caution should be exercised in the use of fluoroquinolones as the sole agents for treatment of infection due to *S. aureus* or *P. aeruginosa* because resistance may develop during therapy. Addition of oral rifampin (300 mg bid) to a fluoroquinolone has yielded encouraging results in infections due to *S. aureus*, but potential drug toxicity and drug interactions make this option desirable only for selected patients, such as those for whom parenteral therapy poses unacceptable logistical or financial hardship. Oral administration of metronidazole (500 mg every 8 h) results in high drug levels in serum and can take the place of IV regimens for the treatment of *Bacteroides* infections. The bacteriostatic drug linezolid (600 mg by mouth every 12 h) has been used successfully in uncontrolled studies involving moderate numbers of patients with infection caused by methicillin-resistant *S. aureus* (MRSA) and vancomycin-resistant enterococci, but data are currently insufficient to recommend the routine use of this agent. Data do not support the routine use of the serum minimal bactericidal concentration in guiding therapy.

Osteomyelitis caused by MRSA is a growing problem that poses unique challenges in terms of treatment. Vancomycin has historically been the drug of choice for MRSA osteomyelitis, but only because of a lack of acceptable alternatives. The drug is less effective than β-lactam agents in treating infections cause by methicillin-susceptible *S. aureus* (MSSA), and this low efficacy extends to infections caused by MRSA. Vancomycin should not be used for treatment of osteomyelitis caused by MSSA, and oral rifampin should be coadministered with vancomycin when the latter drug is used for MRSA infection unless there are compelling contraindications. Linezolid has performed reasonably well in uncontrolled studies of staphylococcal osteomyelitis. However, side effects and hematologic toxicity are common with this agent; thus, in the absence of controlled studies, its routine use is discouraged. Daptomycin, a bactericidal drug with favorable pharmacokinetics, has also been used successfully. Unfortunately, because resistance can develop during therapy (with resultant treatment failure), the routine use of this drug is not recommended. Trimethoprim-sulfamethoxazole, clindamycin, and tetracycline derivatives (doxycycline and minocycline) are often used—seemingly to good advantage—as "continuation therapy" for MRSA osteomyelitis after a course of a parenteral agent, but no controlled data are available to support this approach.

ACUTE HEMATOGENOUS OSTEOMYELITIS Early treatment of acute hematogenous osteomyelitis of childhood with 4–6 weeks of an appropriate antibiotic is usually successful; treatment for <3 weeks has resulted in a tenfold greater rate of failure. Surgical intervention in childhood cases is indicated for intraosseous or subperiosteal abscesses, concomitant septic arthritis, and lack of improvement of the acute signs of infection in 24–48 h. Acute hematogenous osteomyelitis of bones other than the spine in adults often requires surgical debridement.

VERTEBRAL OSTEOMYELITIS A 6- to 8-week course of treatment with an appropriate antibiotic is usually sufficient to cure vertebral osteomyelitis. Failure of the ESR to drop by two-thirds or more of its pretreatment level or of the CRP level to normalize is an indication for reevaluation and (possibly) longer treatment. Surgery is seldom necessary, even in cases of many months' duration, except in instances of spinal instability, new or progressive neurologic deficits, or large soft-tissue abscesses that cannot be drained percutaneously. All but small and asymptomatic epidural abscesses should be surgically drained. Patients should maintain bed rest until back pain has declined to the point at which ambulation is possible. Body casts are no longer used except for comfort.

CONTIGUOUS-FOCUS OSTEOMYELITIS Even when diagnosed early, contiguous-focus osteomyelitis usually requires surgery in addition to 4–6 weeks of appropriate antibiotic therapy because of underlying soft tissue infection or damage to bone from an injury or surgery. A 2-week course of antibiotics after thorough debridement and soft tissue coverage has yielded adequate results in the treatment of superficial osteomyelitis involving only the outer cortex of bone.

CHRONIC OSTEOMYELITIS The risks and benefits of aggressive therapy for chronic osteomyelitis should be weighed before any attempt is made to eradicate the infection. Some patients with extensive disease prefer to live with their infections rather than undergo multiple surgical procedures, take prolonged courses of antimicrobial therapy, and face the risk of loss of an extremity. Such persons often benefit from intermittent courses of oral antibiotics to suppress acute exacerbations.

Once the decision has been made to treat chronic osteomyelitis aggressively, the patient's nutritional and metabolic status should be optimized to expedite healing of soft tissues and bone. Antibiotic administration should be started several days before surgery to reduce inflammation if the etiology of the infection is known; if not, antibiotic therapy should be withheld until debridement. A 4- to 6-week course of appropriate antibiotic therapy is given postoperatively on the basis of the susceptibility pattern of organisms isolated from bone. A subsequent prolonged course of oral antibiotic therapy is often prescribed, especially in the setting of a foreign body, but controlled data for this approach are lacking. There are insufficient data to recommend either the routine use of hyperbaric oxygen or the use of antibiotic-impregnated methacrylate beads or other depots to deliver high levels of antibiotics to the bone. The success of therapy for chronic osteomyelitis still rests largely on the complete surgical removal of necrotic bone and abnormal soft tissues. In the past, the inability to repair large defects in bone and soft tissue limited the extent of debridement. Muscle flaps and skin grafts are now used routinely to cover large soft-tissue defects and to fill dead space, and bone grafts and vascularized bone transfer may restore a seriously compromised bone to a functional state.

In infections of recent fractures requiring internal fixators, such devices are often left in place and the infection is controlled by limited debridement and "suppressive" antibiotic therapy. Definitive surgical/antimicrobial therapy is delayed until bony union of the fracture has been achieved. If there is persistent nonunion of the fracture or loosening of the fixator, the appliance must be removed, the bone debrided, and an external fixator or a new internal fixator applied.

Osteomyelitis of the small bones of the feet in persons with vascular disease usually requires surgical treatment. The effectiveness of the surgery is limited by the blood supply to the site and the body's ability to heal the wound. Revascularization of the extremity is indicated if the vascular disease involves large arteries. In cases of decreased perfusion due to small-vessel disease, foot-sparing surgery may fail, and the best option is often suppressive therapy or amputation. The duration of antibiotic therapy depends on the surgical procedure performed. When the infected bone is removed entirely but residual infection of soft tissues remains, antibiotic therapy should be given for 2 weeks; if amputation eliminates infected bone and soft tissue, standard surgical prophylaxis is given; otherwise, postoperative antibiotics must be given for 4–6 weeks.

ACKNOWLEDGMENT

The substantial contributions of Dr. James H. Maguire to this chapter in previous editions are gratefully acknowledged.

FURTHER READINGS

Darouiche RO: Spinal epidural abscess. N Engl J Med 355:2012, 2006

Kaim AH et al: Imaging of chronic posttraumatic osteomyelitis. Eur Radiol 12:1193, 2002

Khatri G et al: Effect of bone biopsy in guiding antimicrobial therapy for osteomyelitis complicating open wounds. Am J Med Sci 321:367, 2001

Lew DP, Waldvogel FA: Osteomyelitis. N Engl J Med 336:999, 1997

Lipsky BA: Osteomyelitis of the foot in diabetic patients. Clin Infect Dis 25:1318, 1997

McHenry MC et al: Vertebral osteomyelitis: Long-term outcome for 253 patients from 7 Cleveland-area hospitals. Clin Infect Dis 34:1342, 2002

Rissing JP: Antimicrobial therapy for chronic osteomyelitis in adults: Role of the quinolones. Clin Infect Dis 25:1327, 1997

Tice AD et al: Outcomes of osteomyelitis among patients treated with outpatient parenteral antimicrobial therapy. Am J Med 114:723, 2003

Tsukayama DT: Pathophysiology of posttraumatic osteomyelitis. Clin Orthop 360:22, 1999

Zarrouk V et al: Imaging does not predict the clinical outcome of bacterial osteomyelitis. Rheumatology 46:292, 2007

121 Intraabdominal Infections and Abscesses

Miriam J. Baron, Dennis L. Kasper

Intraperitoneal infections generally arise because a normal anatomic barrier is disrupted. This disruption may occur when the appendix, a diverticulum, or an ulcer ruptures; when the bowel wall is weakened by ischemia, tumor, or inflammation (e.g., in inflammatory bowel disease); or with adjacent inflammatory processes, such as pancreatitis or pelvic inflammatory disease, in which enzymes (in the former case) or organisms (in the latter) may leak into the peritoneal cavity. Whatever the inciting event, once inflammation develops and organisms usually contained within the bowel or another organ enter the normally sterile peritoneal space, a predictable series of events takes place. Intraabdominal infections occur in two stages: peritonitis and—if the patient survives this stage and goes untreated—abscess formation. The types of microorganisms predominating in each stage of infection are responsible for the pathogenesis of disease.

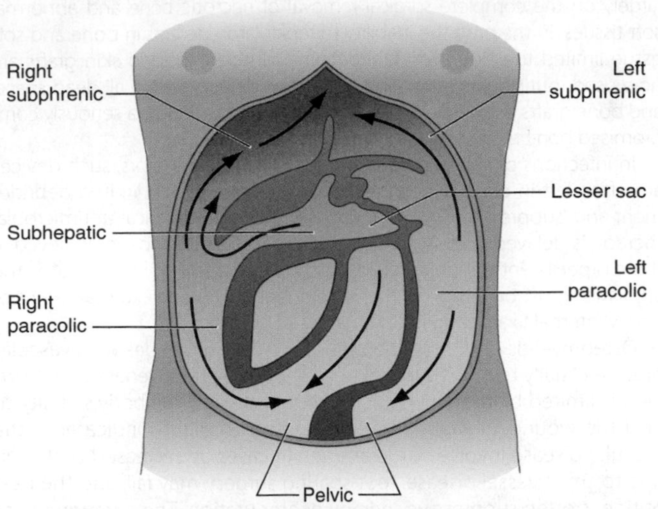

FIGURE 121-1 Diagram of the intraperitoneal spaces, showing the circulation of fluid and potential areas for abscess formation. Some compartments collect fluid or pus more often than others. These compartments include the pelvis (the lowest portion), the subphrenic spaces on the right and left sides, and Morrison's pouch, which is a posterosuperior extension of the subhepatic spaces and is the lowest part of the paravertebral groove when a patient is recumbent. The falciform ligament separating the right and left subphrenic spaces appears to act as a barrier to the spread of infection; consequently, it is unusual to find bilateral subphrenic collections. *[Reprinted with permission from B Lorber (ed): Atlas of Infectious Diseases, vol VII: Intra-abdominal Infections, Hepatitis, and Gastroenteritis. Philadelphia, Current Medicine, 1996, p 1.13.]*

PERITONITIS

Peritonitis is a life-threatening event that is often accompanied by bacteremia and sepsis syndrome (Chap. 265). The peritoneal cavity is large but is divided into compartments. The upper and lower peritoneal cavities are divided by the transverse mesocolon; the greater omentum extends from the transverse mesocolon and from the lower pole of the stomach to line the lower peritoneal cavity. The pancreas, duodenum, and ascending and descending colon are located in the anterior retroperitoneal space; the kidneys, ureters, and adrenals are found in the posterior retroperitoneal space. The other organs, including liver, stomach, gallbladder, spleen, jejunum, ileum, transverse and sigmoid colon, cecum, and appendix, are within the peritoneal cavity. The cavity is lined with a serous membrane that can serve as a conduit for fluids—a property exploited in peritoneal dialysis (Fig. 121-1). A small amount of serous fluid is normally present in the peritoneal space, with a protein content (consisting mainly of albumin) of <30 g/L and <300 white blood cells (WBCs, generally mononuclear cells) per microliter. In bacterial infections, leukocyte recruitment into the infected peritoneal cavity consists of an early influx of polymorphonuclear leukocytes (PMNs) and a prolonged subsequent phase of mononuclear cell migration. The phenotype of the infiltrating leukocytes during the course of inflammation is regulated primarily by resident-cell chemokine synthesis.

PRIMARY (SPONTANEOUS) BACTERIAL PERITONITIS

Peritonitis is either primary (without an apparent source of contamination) or secondary. The types of organisms found and the clinical presentations of these two processes are different. In adults, primary bacterial peritonitis (PBP) occurs most commonly in conjunction with cirrhosis of the liver (frequently the result of alcoholism). However, the disease has been reported in adults with metastatic malignant disease, postnecrotic cirrhosis, chronic active hepatitis, acute viral hepatitis, congestive heart failure, systemic lupus erythematosus, and lymphedema as well as in patients with no underlying disease. Although PBP virtually always develops in patients with preexisting ascites, it is, in general, an uncommon event, occurring in ≤10% of cirrhotic patients. The cause of PBP has not been established definitively but is believed to involve hematogenous spread of organisms in a patient in whom a diseased liver and altered portal circulation result in a defect in the usual filtration function. Organisms multiply in ascites, a good medium for growth. The proteins of the complement cascade have been found in peritoneal fluid, with lower levels in cirrhotic patients than in patients with ascites of other etiologies. The opsonic and phagocytic properties of PMNs are diminished in patients with advanced liver disease.

The presentation of PBP differs from that of secondary peritonitis. The most common manifestation is fever, which is reported in up to 80% of patients. Ascites is found but virtually always predates infection. Abdominal pain, an acute onset of symptoms, and peritoneal irritation during physical examination can be helpful diagnostically, but the absence of any of these findings does not exclude this often-subtle diagnosis. Nonlocalizing symptoms (such as malaise, fatigue, or encephalopathy) without another clear etiology should also prompt consideration of PBP in a susceptible patient. It is vital to sample the peritoneal fluid of any cirrhotic patient with ascites and fever. The finding of >250 PMNs/μL is diagnostic for PBP, according to Conn (*http://jac.oxfordjournals.org/cgi/content/full/47/3/369*). This criterion does not apply to secondary peritonitis (see below). The microbiology of PBP is also distinctive. While enteric gram-negative bacilli such as *Escherichia coli* are most commonly encountered, gram-positive organisms such as streptococci, enterococci, or even pneumococci are sometimes found. In PBP, a single organism is typically isolated; anaerobes are found less frequently in PBP than in secondary peritonitis, in which a mixed flora including anaerobes is the rule. In fact, if PBP is suspected and multiple organisms including anaerobes are recovered from the peritoneal fluid, the diagnosis must be reconsidered and a source of secondary peritonitis sought.

The diagnosis of PBP is not easy. It depends on the exclusion of a primary intraabdominal source of infection. Contrast-enhanced CT is useful in identifying an intraabdominal source for infection. It may be difficult to recover organisms from cultures of peritoneal fluid, presumably because the burden of organisms is low. However, the yield can be improved if 10 mL of peritoneal fluid is placed directly into a blood culture bottle. Since bacteremia frequently accompanies PBP, blood should be cultured simultaneously. No specific radiographic studies are helpful in the diagnosis of PBP. A plain film of the abdomen would be expected to show ascites. Chest and abdominal radiography should be performed in patients with abdominal pain to exclude free air, which signals a perforation (Fig. 121-2).

Rx PRIMARY BACTERIAL PERITONITIS

Treatment for PBP is directed at the isolate from blood or peritoneal fluid. Gram's staining of peritoneal fluid often gives negative results in PBP. Therefore, until culture results become available, therapy should cover gram-negative aerobic bacilli and gram-positive cocci. Third-generation cephalosporins such as cefotaxime (2 g q8h, administered IV) provide reasonable initial coverage in moderately ill patients. Broad-spectrum antibiotics, such as penicillin/β-lactamase inhibitor combinations (e.g., piperacillin/tazobactam, 3.375 g q6h IV for adults with normal renal function) or ceftriaxone (2 g q24h IV), are also options. Empirical coverage for anaerobes is not necessary. After the infecting organism is identified, therapy should be narrowed to target the specific pathogen. Patients with PBP usually respond within 72 h to appropriate antibiotic therapy. Antimicrobial therapy can be administered for as little as 5 days if rapid improvement occurs and blood cultures are negative, but a course of up to 2 weeks may be required for patients with bacteremia and for those whose improvement is slow. Persistence of WBCs in the ascitic fluid after therapy should prompt a search for additional diagnoses.

Prevention PBP has a high rate of recurrence. Up to 70% of patients experience a recurrence within 1 year. Antibiotic prophylaxis reduces

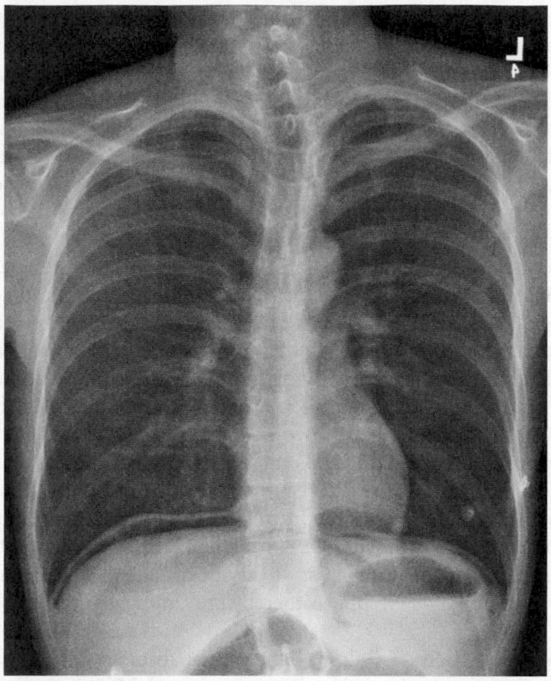

FIGURE 121-2 Pneumoperitoneum. Free air under the diaphragm on an upright chest film suggests the presence of a bowel perforation and associated peritonitis. *(Image courtesy of Dr. John Braver; with permission.)*

this rate to <20%. Prophylactic regimens for adults with normal renal function include fluoroquinolones (ciprofloxacin, 750 mg weekly; norfloxacin, 400 mg/d) or trimethoprim-sulfamethoxazole (one double-strength tablet daily). However, long-term administration of broad-spectrum antibiotics in this setting has been shown to increase the risk of severe staphylococcal infections.

SECONDARY PERITONITIS

Secondary peritonitis develops when bacteria contaminate the peritoneum as a result of spillage from an intraabdominal viscus. The organisms found almost always constitute a mixed flora in which facultative gram-negative bacilli and anaerobes predominate, especially when the contaminating source is colonic. Early in the course of infection, when the host response is directed toward containment of the infection, exudate containing fibrin and PMNs is found. Early death in this setting is attributable to gram-negative bacillary sepsis and to potent endotoxins circulating in the bloodstream (Chap. 265). Gram-negative bacilli, particularly *E. coli*, are common bloodstream isolates, but *Bacteroides fragilis* bacteremia also occurs. The severity of abdominal pain and the clinical course depend on the inciting process. The organisms isolated from the peritoneum also vary with the source of the initial process and the normal flora at that site. Secondary peritonitis can result primarily from chemical irritation and/or bacterial contamination. For example, as long as the patient is not achlorhydric, a ruptured gastric ulcer will release low-pH gastric contents that will serve as a chemical irritant. The normal flora of the stomach comprises the same organisms found in the oropharynx (Chap. 157) but in lower numbers. Thus, the bacterial burden in a ruptured ulcer is negligible compared with that in a ruptured appendix. The normal flora of the colon below the ligament of Treitz contains ~10^{11} anaerobic organisms/g of feces but only 10^8 aerobes/g; therefore, anaerobic species account for 99.9% of the bacteria. Leakage of colonic contents (pH 7–8) does not cause significant chemical peritonitis, but infection is intense because of the heavy bacterial load.

Depending on the inciting event, local symptoms may occur in secondary peritonitis—for example, epigastric pain from a ruptured gastric ulcer. In appendicitis (Chap. 294), the initial presenting symptoms are often vague, with periumbilical discomfort and nausea followed in a number of hours by pain more localized to the right lower quadrant. Unusual locations of the appendix (including a retrocecal position) can complicate this presentation further. Once infection has spread to the peritoneal cavity, pain increases, particularly with infection involving the parietal peritoneum, which is innervated extensively. Patients usually lie motionless, often with knees drawn up to avoid stretching the nerve fibers of the peritoneal cavity. Coughing and sneezing, which increase pressure within the peritoneal cavity, are associated with sharp pain. There may or may not be pain localized to the infected or diseased organ from which secondary peritonitis has arisen. Patients with secondary peritonitis generally have abnormal findings on abdominal examination, with marked voluntary and involuntary guarding of the anterior abdominal musculature. Later findings include tenderness, especially rebound tenderness. In addition, there may be localized findings in the area of the inciting event. In general, patients are febrile, with marked leukocytosis and a left shift of the WBCs to band forms.

While recovery of organisms from peritoneal fluid is easier in secondary than in primary peritonitis, a tap of the abdomen is rarely the procedure of choice in secondary peritonitis. An exception is in cases involving trauma, where the possibility of a hemoperitoneum may need to be excluded early. Emergent studies (such as abdominal CT) to find the source of peritoneal contamination should be undertaken if the patient is hemodynamically stable; unstable patients may require surgical intervention without prior imaging.

℞ SECONDARY PERITONITIS

Treatment for secondary peritonitis includes early administration of antibiotics aimed particularly at aerobic gram-negative bacilli and anaerobes (see below). Mild to moderate disease can be treated with many drugs covering these organisms, including broad-spectrum penicillin/β-lactamase inhibitor combinations (e.g., ticarcillin/clavulanate, 3.1 g q4–6h IV) or cefoxitin (2 g q4–6h IV). Patients in intensive care units should receive imipenem (500 mg q6h IV), meropenem (1 g q8h IV), or combinations of drugs, such as ampicillin plus metronidazole plus ciprofloxacin. The role of enterococci and *Candida* spp. in mixed infections is controversial. Secondary peritonitis usually requires both surgical intervention to address the inciting process and antibiotics to treat early bacteremia, to decrease the incidence of abscess formation and wound infection, and to prevent distant spread of infection. While surgery is rarely indicated in PBP in adults, it may be life-saving in secondary peritonitis.

Peritonitis may develop as a complication of abdominal surgeries. These infections may be accompanied by localizing pain and/or nonlocalizing symptoms such as fever, malaise, anorexia, and toxicity. As a nosocomial infection, postoperative peritonitis may be associated with organisms such as staphylococci, components of the gram-negative hospital microflora, and the microbes that cause PBP and secondary peritonitis, as described above.

PERITONITIS IN PATIENTS UNDERGOING CAPD

A third type of peritonitis arises in patients who are undergoing continuous ambulatory peritoneal dialysis (CAPD). Unlike PBP and secondary peritonitis, which are caused by endogenous bacteria, CAPD-associated peritonitis usually involves skin organisms. The pathogenesis of infection is similar to that of intravascular device–related infection, in which skin organisms migrate along the catheter, which both serves as an entry point and exerts the effects of a foreign body. Exit-site or tunnel infection may or may not accompany CAPD-associated peritonitis. Like PBP, CAPD-associated peritonitis is usually caused by a single organism. Peritonitis is, in fact, the most common reason for discontinuation of CAPD. Improvements in equipment design, especially the Y-set connector, have resulted in a decrease from one case of peritonitis per 9 months of CAPD to one case per 15 months.

The clinical presentation of CAPD peritonitis resembles that of secondary peritonitis in that diffuse pain and peritoneal signs are common. The dialysate is usually cloudy and contains >100 WBCs/μL, >50% of which are neutrophils. The most common organisms are *Staphylococcus* spp., which accounted for ~45% of cases in one recent series. Historically, coagulase-negative staphylococcal species were identified most commonly in these infections, but more recently these isolates have been decreasing in frequency. *Staphylococcus aureus* is more often involved among patients who are nasal carriers of the organism than among those who are not, and this organism is the most common pathogen in overt exit-site infections. Gram-negative bacilli and fungi such as *Candida* spp. are also found. Vancomycin-resistant enterococci and vancomycin-intermediate *S. aureus* have been reported to produce peritonitis in CAPD patients. The finding of more than one organism in dialysate culture should prompt evaluation for secondary peritonitis. As with PBP, culture of dialysate fluid in blood culture bottles improves the yield. To facilitate diagnosis, several hundred milliliters of removed dialysis fluid should be concentrated by centrifugation before culture.

℞ CAPD PERITONITIS

Empirical therapy for CAPD peritonitis should be directed at *S. aureus*, coagulase-negative *Staphylococcus*, and gram-negative bacilli until the results of cultures are available. Guidelines issued in 2005 suggest that agents should be chosen on the basis of local experience with resistant organisms. In some centers, a first-generation cephalosporin such as cefazolin (for gram-positive bacteria) and a fluoroquinolone or a third-generation cephalosporin such as ceftazidime (for gram-negative bacteria) may be reasonable; in areas with high rates of infection with methicillin-resistant *S. aureus*, vancomycin should be used instead of cefazolin, and gram-negative coverage may need to be broadened. Broad coverage including vancomycin should be particularly considered for toxic patients and for those with exit-site infections. Loading doses are administered intraperitoneally; doses depend on the dialysis method and the patient's renal function. Antibiotics are given either continuously (i.e., with each exchange) or intermittently (i.e., once daily, with the dose allowed to remain in the peritoneal cavity for at least 6 h). If the patient is severely ill, IV antibiotics should be added at doses appropriate for the patient's degree of renal failure. The clinical response to an empirical treatment regimen should be rapid; if the patient has not responded after 48 h of treatment, catheter removal should be considered.

TUBERCULOUS PERITONITIS

See Chap. 158.

INTRAABDOMINAL ABSCESSES

INTRAPERITONEAL ABSCESSES

Abscess formation is common in untreated peritonitis if overt gram-negative sepsis either does not develop or develops but is not fatal. In experimental models of abscess formation, mixed aerobic and anaerobic organisms have been implanted intraperitoneally. Without therapy directed at anaerobes, animals develop intraabdominal abscesses. As in humans, these experimental abscesses may stud the peritoneal cavity, lie within the omentum or mesentery, or even develop on the surface of or within viscera such as the liver.

Pathogenesis and Immunity There is often disagreement about whether an abscess represents a disease state or a host response. In a sense, it represents both: while an abscess is an infection in which viable infecting organisms and PMNs are contained in a fibrous capsule, it is also a process by which the host confines microbes to a limited space, thereby preventing further spread of infection. In any event, abscesses do cause significant symptoms, and patients with abscesses can be quite ill. Experimental work has helped to define both the host cells and the bacterial virulence factors responsible—most notably, in the case of *B. fragilis*. This organism, although accounting for only 0.5% of the normal colonic flora, is the anaerobe most frequently isolated from intraabdominal infections, is especially prominent in abscesses, and is the most common anaerobic bloodstream isolate. On clinical grounds, therefore, *B. fragilis* appears to be uniquely virulent. Moreover, *B. fragilis* acts alone to cause abscesses in animal models of intraabdominal infection, whereas most other *Bacteroides* species must act synergistically with a facultative organism to induce abscess formation.

Of the several virulence factors identified in *B. fragilis*, one is critical: the capsular polysaccharide complex (CPC) found on the bacterial surface. The CPC comprises at least eight distinct surface polysaccharides. Structural analysis of these polysaccharides has shown an unusual motif of oppositely charged sugars. Polysaccharides having these *zwitterionic* characteristics, such as polysaccharide A (PSA), evoke a host response in the peritoneal cavity that localizes bacteria into abscesses. *B. fragilis* and PSA have been found to adhere to primary mesothelial cells in vitro; this adherence, in turn, stimulates the production of tumor necrosis factor α (TNF-α) and intercellular adhesion molecule 1 (ICAM-1) by peritoneal macrophages. Although abscesses characteristically contain PMNs, the process of abscess induction depends on the stimulation of T lymphocytes by these unique zwitterionic polysaccharides. The stimulated CD4+ T lymphocytes secrete leukoattractant cytokines and chemokines. The alternative pathway of complement and fibrinogen also participate in abscess formation.

While antibodies to the CPC enhance bloodstream clearance of *B. fragilis*, CD4+ T cells are critical in immunity to abscesses. When administered subcutaneously, *B. fragilis* PSA has immunomodulatory characteristics and stimulates CD4+ T regulatory cells via an interleukin (IL) 2–dependent mechanism to produce IL-10. IL-10 downregulates the inflammatory response, thereby preventing abscess formation.

Clinical Presentation Of all intraabdominal abscesses, 74% are intraperitoneal or retroperitoneal and are not visceral. Most intraperitoneal abscesses result from fecal spillage from a colonic source, such as an inflamed appendix. Abscesses can also arise from other processes. They usually form within weeks of the development of peritonitis and may be found in a variety of locations—from omentum to mesentery, pelvis to psoas muscles, and subphrenic space to a visceral organ such as the liver, where they may develop either on the surface of the organ or within it. Periappendiceal and diverticular abscesses occur commonly. Diverticular abscesses are least likely to rupture. Infections of the female genital tract and pancreatitis are also among the more common causative events. When abscesses occur in the female genital tract—either as a primary infection (e.g., tuboovarian abscess) or as an infection extending into the pelvic cavity or peritoneum—*B. fragilis* figures prominently among the organisms isolated. *B. fragilis* is not found in large numbers in the normal vaginal flora. For example, it is encountered less commonly in pelvic inflammatory disease and endometritis without an associated abscess. In pancreatitis with leakage of damaging pancreatic enzymes, inflammation is prominent. Therefore, clinical findings such as fever, leukocytosis, and even abdominal pain do not distinguish pancreatitis itself from complications such as pancreatic pseudocyst, pancreatic abscess (Chap. 307), or intraabdominal collections of pus. Especially in cases of necrotizing pancreatitis, in which the incidence of local pancreatic infection may be as high as 30%, needle aspiration under CT guidance is performed to sample fluid for culture. Many centers prescribe preemptive antibiotics for patients with necrotizing pancreatitis. Imipenem is frequently used for this purpose since it reaches high tissue levels in the pancreas (although it is not unique in this regard). If needle aspiration yields infected fluid, most experts agree that surgery is superior to percutaneous drainage.

Diagnosis Scanning procedures have considerably facilitated the diagnosis of intraabdominal abscesses. Abdominal CT probably has the highest yield, although ultrasonography is particularly useful for the right upper quadrant, kidneys, and pelvis. Both indium-labeled WBCs and gallium tend to localize in abscesses and may be useful in finding a collection. Since gallium is taken up in the bowel, indium-labeled WBCs may have a slightly greater yield for abscesses near the bowel. Neither indium-labeled WBC nor gallium scans serve as a basis for a definitive diagnosis, however; both need to be followed by other, more specific studies, such as CT, if an area of possible abnormality is identified. Abscesses contiguous with or contained within diverticula are particularly difficult to diagnose with scanning procedures. Occasionally, a barium enema may detect a diverticular abscess not diagnosed by other procedures, although barium should not be injected if a perforation is sus-

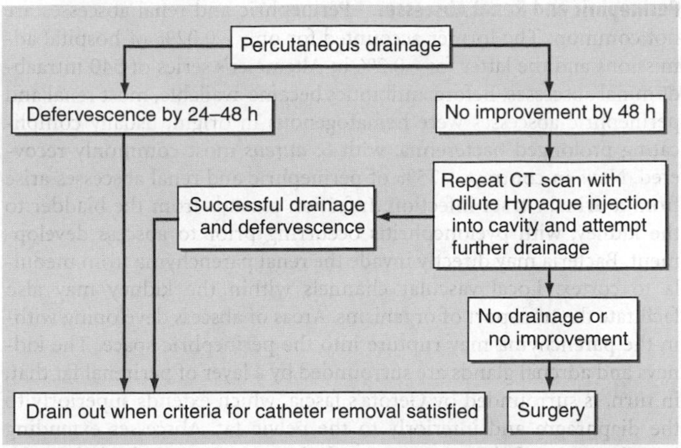

FIGURE 121-3 Algorithm for the management of patients with intraabdominal abscesses using percutaneous drainage. Antimicrobial therapy should be administered concomitantly. *[Reprinted with permission from B Lorber (ed): Atlas of Infectious Diseases, vol VII: Intra-abdominal Infections, Hepatitis, and Gastroenteritis. Philadelphia, Current Medicine, 1996, p 1.30, as adapted from OD Rotstein, RL Simmons, in SL Gorbach et al (eds): Infectious Diseases. Philadelphia, Saunders, 1992, p 668.]*

pected. If one study is negative, a second study sometimes reveals a collection. Although exploratory laparotomy has been less commonly used since the advent of CT, this procedure still must be undertaken on occasion if an abscess is strongly suspected on clinical grounds.

℞ INTRAPERITONEAL ABSCESSES

An algorithm for the management of patients with intraabdominal (including intraperitoneal) abscesses is presented in **Fig. 121-3**. The treatment of intraabdominal infections involves the determination of the initial focus of infection, the administration of broad-spectrum antibiotics targeting the organisms involved, and the performance of a drainage procedure if one or more definitive abscesses have formed. Antimicrobial therapy, in general, is adjunctive to drainage and/or surgical correction of an underlying lesion or process in intraabdominal abscesses. Unlike the intraabdominal abscesses resulting from most causes, for which drainage of some kind is generally required, abscesses associated with diverticulitis usually wall off locally after rupture of a diverticulum, so that surgical intervention is not routinely required.

A number of agents exhibit excellent activity against aerobic gram-negative bacilli. Since mortality in intraabdominal sepsis is linked to gram-negative bacteremia, empirical therapy for intraabdominal infection always needs to include adequate coverage of gram-negative aerobic, facultative, and anaerobic organisms. Even if anaerobes are not cultured from clinical specimens, they still must be covered by the therapeutic regimen. Empirical antibiotic therapy should be the same as that discussed above for secondary peritonitis.

VISCERAL ABSCESSES

Liver Abscesses The liver is the organ most subject to the development of abscesses. In one study of 540 intraabdominal abscesses, 26% were visceral. Liver abscesses made up 13% of the total number, or 48% of all visceral abscesses. Liver abscesses may be solitary or multiple; they may arise from hematogenous spread of bacteria or from local spread from contiguous sites of infection within the peritoneal cavity. In the past, appendicitis with rupture and subsequent spread of infection was the most common source for a liver abscess. Currently, associated disease of the biliary tract is most common. Pylephlebitis (suppurative thrombosis of the portal vein), usually arising from infection in the pelvis but sometimes from infection elsewhere in the peritoneal cavity, is another common source for bacterial seeding of the liver.

Fever is the most common presenting sign of liver abscess. Some patients, particularly those with associated disease of the biliary tract, have symptoms and signs localized to the right upper quadrant, including pain, guarding, punch tenderness, and even rebound tenderness. Nonspecific symptoms, such as chills, anorexia, weight loss, nausea, and vomiting, may also develop. Only 50% of patients with liver abscesses, however, have hepatomegaly, right-upper-quadrant tenderness, or jaundice; thus, half of patients have no symptoms or signs to direct attention to the liver. Fever of unknown origin (FUO) may be the only manifestation of liver abscess, especially in the elderly. Diagnostic studies of the abdomen, especially the right upper quadrant, should be a part of any FUO workup. The single most reliable laboratory finding is an elevated serum concentration of alkaline phosphatase, which is documented in 70% of patients with liver abscesses. Other tests of liver function may yield normal results, but 50% of patients have elevated serum levels of bilirubin, and 48% have elevated concentrations of aspartate aminotransferase. Other laboratory findings include leukocytosis in 77% of patients, anemia (usually normochromic, normocytic) in 50%, and hypoalbuminemia in 33%. Concomitant bacteremia is found in one-third of patients. A liver abscess is sometimes suggested by chest radiography, especially if a new elevation of the right hemidiaphragm is seen; other suggestive findings include a right basilar infiltrate and a right pleural effusion.

Imaging studies are the most reliable methods for diagnosing liver abscesses. These studies include ultrasonography, CT (Fig. 121-4), indium-labeled WBC or gallium scan, and MRI. More than one such study may be required. Organisms recovered from liver abscesses vary with the source. In liver infection arising from the biliary tree, enteric gram-negative aerobic bacilli and enterococci are common isolates. Unless previous surgery has been performed, anaerobes are not generally involved in liver abscesses arising from biliary infections. In contrast, in liver abscesses arising from pelvic and other intraperitoneal sources, a mixed flora including both aerobic and anaerobic species is common; *B. fragilis* is the species most frequently isolated. With hematogenous spread of infection, usually only a single organism is encountered; this species may be *S. aureus* or a streptococcal species such as *S. milleri*. Results of cultures obtained from drain sites are not reliable for defining the etiology of infections. Liver abscesses may also be caused by *Candida* spp.; such abscesses usually follow fungemia in patients receiving chemotherapy for cancer and often present when PMNs return after a period of neutropenia. Amebic liver abscesses are not an uncommon problem (Chap. 202). Amebic serologic testing gives positive results in >95% of cases; thus, a negative result helps to exclude this diagnosis.

℞ LIVER ABSCESSES (FIG. 121-3)

While drainage—either percutaneous (with a pigtail catheter kept in place) or surgical—is the mainstay of therapy for intraabdominal abscesses (in-

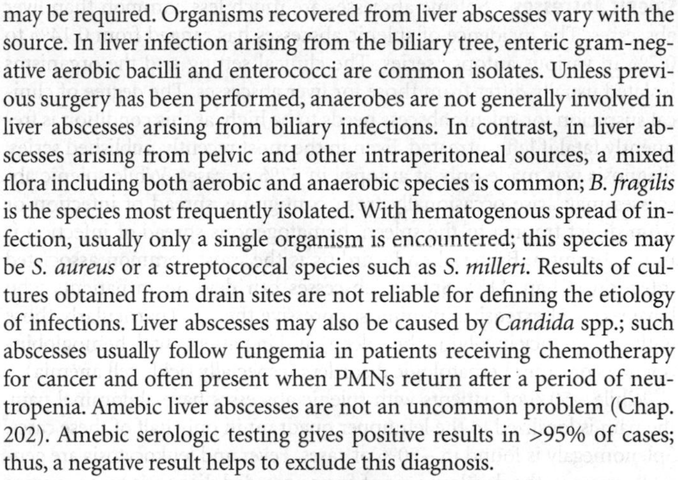

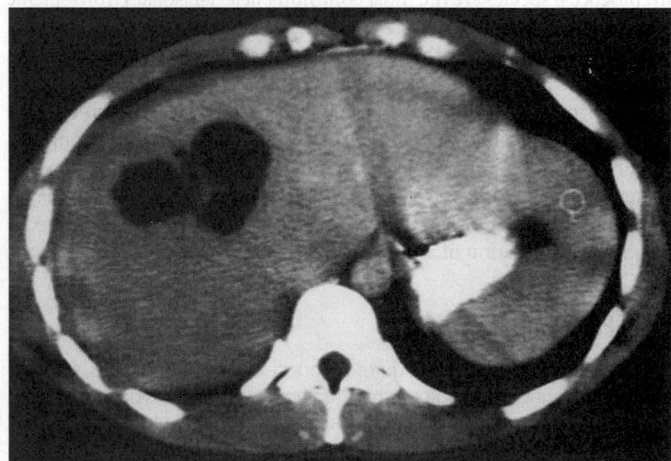

FIGURE 121-4 Multilocular liver abscess on CT scan. Multiple or multilocular abscesses are more common than solitary abscesses. *[Reprinted with permission from B Lorber (ed): Atlas of Infectious Diseases, Vol VII: Intra-abdominal Infections, Hepatitis, and Gastroenteritis. Philadelphia, Current Medicine, 1996, Fig. 1.22.]*

cluding liver abscesses), there is growing interest in medical management alone for pyogenic liver abscesses. The drugs used for empirical therapy include the same ones used in intraabdominal sepsis and secondary bacterial peritonitis. Usually, a diagnostic aspirate of abscess contents should be obtained before the initiation of empirical therapy, with antibiotic choices adjusted when the results of Gram's staining and culture become available. Cases treated without definitive drainage generally require longer courses of antibiotic therapy. When percutaneous drainage was compared with open surgical drainage, the average length of hospital stay for the former was almost twice that for the latter, although both the time required for fever to resolve and the mortality rate were the same for the two procedures. Mortality was appreciable despite treatment, averaging 15%. Several factors predict the failure of percutaneous drainage and therefore may favor primary surgical intervention. These factors include the presence of multiple, sizable abscesses; viscous abscess contents that tend to plug the catheter; associated disease (e.g., disease of the biliary tract) requiring surgery; or the lack of a clinical response to percutaneous drainage in 4–7 days.

Treatment of candidal liver abscesses often entails initial administration of amphotericin B or liposomal amphotericin, with subsequent fluconazole therapy (Chap. 196). In some cases, therapy with fluconazole alone (6 mg/kg daily) may be used—e.g., in clinically stable patients whose infecting isolate is susceptible to this drug.

Splenic Abscesses Splenic abscesses are much less common than liver abscesses. The incidence of splenic abscesses has ranged from 0.14% to 0.7% in various autopsy series. The clinical setting and the organisms isolated usually differ from those for liver abscesses. The degree of clinical suspicion for splenic abscess needs to be high, as this condition is frequently fatal if left untreated. Even in the most recently published series, diagnosis was made only at autopsy in 37% of cases. While splenic abscesses may arise occasionally from contiguous spread of infection or from direct trauma to the spleen, hematogenous spread of infection is more common. Bacterial endocarditis is the most common associated infection (Chap. 118). Splenic abscesses can develop in patients who have received extensive immunosuppressive therapy (particularly those with malignancy involving the spleen) and in patients with hemoglobinopathies or other hematologic disorders (especially sickle cell anemia).

While ~50% of patients with splenic abscesses have abdominal pain, the pain is localized to the left upper quadrant in only half of these cases. Splenomegaly is found in ~50% of cases. Fever and leukocytosis are generally present; the development of fever preceded diagnosis by an average of 20 days in one series. Left-sided chest findings may include abnormalities to auscultation, and chest radiographic findings may include an infiltrate or a left-sided pleural effusion. CT scan of the abdomen has been the most sensitive diagnostic tool. Ultrasonography can yield the diagnosis but is less sensitive. Liver-spleen scan or gallium scan may also be useful. Streptococcal species are the most common bacterial isolates from splenic abscesses, followed by *S. aureus*—presumably reflecting the associated endocarditis. An increase in the prevalence of gram-negative aerobic isolates from splenic abscesses has been reported; these organisms often derive from a urinary tract focus, with associated bacteremia, or from another intraabdominal source. *Salmonella* species are seen fairly commonly, especially in patients with sickle cell hemoglobinopathy. Anaerobic species accounted for only 5% of isolates in the largest collected series, but the reporting of a number of "sterile abscesses" may indicate that optimal techniques for the isolation of anaerobes were not employed.

℞ SPLENIC ABSCESSES

Because of the high mortality figures reported for splenic abscesses, splenectomy with adjunctive antibiotics has traditionally been considered standard treatment and remains the best approach for complex, multilocular abscesses or multiple abscesses. However, percutaneous drainage has worked well for single, small (<3-cm) abscesses in some studies and may also be useful for patients with high surgical risk. Patients undergoing splenectomy should be vaccinated against encapsulated organisms (*Streptococcus pneumoniae, Haemophilus influenzae, Neisseria meningitidis*). The most important factor in successful treatment of splenic abscesses is early diagnosis.

Perinephric and Renal Abscesses Perinephric and renal abscesses are not common: The former accounted for only ~0.02% of hospital admissions and the latter for ~0.2% in Altemeier's series of 540 intraabdominal abscesses. Before antibiotics became available, most renal and perinephric abscesses were hematogenous in origin, usually complicating prolonged bacteremia, with *S. aureus* most commonly recovered. Now, in contrast, >75% of perinephric and renal abscesses arise from a urinary tract infection. Infection ascends from the bladder to the kidney, with pyelonephritis occurring prior to abscess development. Bacteria may directly invade the renal parenchyma from medulla to cortex. Local vascular channels within the kidney may also facilitate the transport of organisms. Areas of abscess developing within the parenchyma may rupture into the perinephric space. The kidneys and adrenal glands are surrounded by a layer of perirenal fat that, in turn, is surrounded by Gerota's fascia, which extends superiorly to the diaphragm and inferiorly to the pelvic fat. Abscesses extending into the perinephric space may track through Gerota's fascia into the psoas or transversalis muscles, into the anterior peritoneal cavity, superiorly to the subdiaphragmatic space, or inferiorly to the pelvis. Of the risk factors that have been associated with the development of perinephric abscesses, the most important is concomitant nephrolithiasis obstructing urinary flow. Of patients with perinephric abscess, 20–60% have renal stones. Other structural abnormalities of the urinary tract, prior urologic surgery, trauma, and diabetes mellitus have also been identified as risk factors.

The organisms most frequently encountered in perinephric and renal abscesses are *E. coli*, *Proteus* spp., and *Klebsiella* spp. *E. coli*, the aerobic species most commonly found in the colonic flora, seems to have unique virulence properties in the urinary tract, including factors promoting adherence to uroepithelial cells. The urease of *Proteus* spp. splits urea, thereby creating a more alkaline and more hospitable environment for bacterial proliferation. *Proteus* spp. are frequently found in association with large struvite stones caused by the precipitation of magnesium ammonium sulfate in an alkaline environment. These stones serve as a nidus for recurrent urinary tract infection. While a single bacterial species is usually recovered from a perinephric or renal abscess, multiple species may also be found. If a urine culture is not contaminated with periurethral flora and is found to contain more than one organism, a perinephric abscess or renal abscess should be considered in the differential diagnosis. Urine cultures may also be polymicrobial in cases of bladder diverticulum.

Candida spp. can cause renal abscesses. This fungus may spread to the kidney hematogenously or by ascension from the bladder. The hallmark of the latter route of infection is ureteral obstruction with large fungal balls.

The presentation of perinephric and renal abscesses is quite nonspecific. Flank pain and abdominal pain are common. At least 50% of patients are febrile. Pain may be referred to the groin or leg, particularly with extension of infection. The diagnosis of perinephric abscess, like that of splenic abscess, is frequently delayed, and the mortality rate in some series is appreciable, although lower than in the past. Perinephric or renal abscess should be most seriously considered when a patient presents with symptoms and signs of pyelonephritis and remains febrile after 4 or 5 days of treatment. Moreover, when a urine culture yields a polymicrobial flora, when a patient is known to have renal stones, or when fever and pyuria coexist with a sterile urine culture, these diagnoses should be entertained.

Renal ultrasonography and abdominal CT are the most useful diagnostic modalities. If a renal or perinephric abscess is diagnosed, nephrolithiasis should be excluded, especially when a high urinary pH suggests the presence of a urea-splitting organism.

℞ PERINEPHRIC AND RENAL ABSCESSES

Treatment for perinephric and renal abscesses, like that for other intraabdominal abscesses, includes drainage of pus and antibiotic therapy directed at the organism(s) recovered. For perinephric abscesses, percutaneous drainage is usually successful.

Psoas Abscesses The psoas muscle is another location in which abscesses are encountered. Psoas abscesses may arise from a hematogenous source, by contiguous spread from an intraabdominal or pelvic process, or by contiguous spread from nearby bony structures (e.g., vertebral bodies). Associated osteomyelitis due to spread from bone to muscle or from muscle to bone is common in psoas abscesses. When Pott's disease was common, *Mycobacterium tuberculosis* was a frequent cause of psoas abscess. Currently, either *S. aureus* or a mixture of enteric organisms including aerobic and anaerobic gram-negative bacilli is usually isolated from psoas abscesses in the United States. *S. aureus* is most likely to be isolated when a psoas abscess arises from hematogenous spread or a contiguous focus of osteomyelitis; a mixed enteric flora is the most likely etiology when the abscess has an intraabdominal or pelvic source. Patients with psoas abscesses frequently present with fever, lower abdominal or back pain, or pain referred to the hip or knee. CT is the most useful diagnostic technique.

Rx PSOAS ABSCESSES

Treatment includes surgical drainage and the administration of an antibiotic regimen directed at the inciting organism(s).

Pancreatic Abscesses See Chap. 307.

ACKNOWLEDGMENT

The substantial contributions of Dori F. Zaleznik, MD, to this chapter in previous editions are gratefully acknowledged.

FURTHER READINGS

CAMPILLO B et al: Epidemiology of severe hospital-acquired infections in patients with liver cirrhosis: Effect of long-term administration of norfloxacin. Clin Infect Dis 26:1066, 1998

GIBSON FC III et al: Cellular mechanism of intraabdominal abscess formation by *Bacteroides fragilis*. J Immunol 160:5000, 1998

JOHANSSEN EC, MADOFF LC: Infections of the liver and biliary system, in *Principles and Practice of Infectious Diseases*, 6th ed, GL Mandell et al (eds). Philadelphia, Elsevier Churchill Livingstone, 2005, pp 951–959

LEVISON ME, BUSH LM: Peritonitis and intraperitoneal abscesses, in *Principles and Practice of Infectious Diseases*, 6th ed, GL Mandell et al (eds). Philadelphia, Elsevier Churchill Livingstone, 2005, pp 927-945

PAPPAS PG et al: Guidelines for treatment of candidiasis. Clin Infect Dis 38:161, 2004

PIRAINO B et al: Peritoneal dialysis–related infections recommendations: 2005 update. Perit Dial Int 25:107, 2005

RAHIMIAN J et al: Pyogenic liver abscess: Recent trends in etiology and mortality. Clin Infect Dis 39:1654, 2004

SOLOMKIN JS et al: Guidelines for the selection of anti-infective agents for complicated intra-abdominal infections. Clin Infect Dis 37:997, 2003

TZIANABOS AO, KASPER DL: Anaerobic infections: General concepts, in *Principles and Practice of Infectious Diseases*, 6th ed, GL Mandell et al (eds). Philadelphia, Elsevier Churchill Livingstone, 2005, pp 2810–2816

TZIANABOS AO et al: T cells activated by zwitterionic molecules prevent abscesses induced by pathogenic bacteria. J Biol Chem 275:6733, 2000

VAN RULER O et al: Comparison of on-demand vs planned relaparotomy strategy in patients with severe peritonitis: A randomized trial. JAMA 298:865, 2007

122 Acute Infectious Diarrheal Diseases and Bacterial Food Poisoning

Joan R. Butterton, Stephen B. Calderwood

Ranging from mild annoyances during vacations to devastating dehydrating illnesses that can kill within hours, acute gastrointestinal illnesses rank second only to acute upper respiratory illnesses as the most common diseases worldwide. In children <5 years old, attack rates range from 2–3 illnesses per child per year in developed countries to as high as 10–18 illnesses per child per year in developing countries. In Asia, Africa, and Latin America, acute diarrheal illnesses are not only a leading cause of morbidity in children—with an estimated 1 billion cases per year—but also a major cause of death. These illnesses are responsible for 4–6 million deaths per year, or a sobering total of 12,600 deaths per day. In some areas, >50% of childhood deaths are directly attributable to acute diarrheal illnesses. In addition, by contributing to malnutrition and thereby reducing resistance to other infectious agents, gastrointestinal illnesses may be indirect factors in a far greater burden of disease.

The wide range of clinical manifestations of acute gastrointestinal illnesses is matched by the wide variety of infectious agents involved, including viruses, bacteria, and parasitic pathogens (Table 122-1). This chapter discusses factors that enable gastrointestinal pathogens to cause disease, reviews host defense mechanisms, and delineates an approach to the evaluation and treatment of patients presenting with acute diarrhea. Individual organisms causing acute gastrointestinal illnesses are discussed in detail in subsequent chapters.

PATHOGENIC MECHANISMS

Enteric pathogens have developed a variety of tactics to overcome host defenses. Understanding the virulence factors employed by these organisms is important in the diagnosis and treatment of clinical disease.

Inoculum Size The number of microorganisms that must be ingested to cause disease varies considerably from species to species. For *Shigella*, enterohemorrhagic *Escherichia coli*, *Giardia lamblia*, or *Entamoeba*, as few as 10–100 bacteria or cysts can produce infection, while 10^5–10^8 *Vibrio cholerae* organisms must be ingested orally to cause disease. The infective dose of *Salmonella* varies widely, depending on the species, host, and food vehicle. The ability of organisms to overcome host defenses has important implications for transmission; *Shigella*, enterohemorrhagic *E. coli*, *Entamoeba*, and *Giardia* can spread by person-to-person contact, whereas under some circumstances *Salmonella* may have to grow in food for several hours before reaching an effective infectious dose.

Adherence Many organisms must adhere to the gastrointestinal mucosa as an initial step in the pathogenic process; thus, organisms that can compete with the normal bowel flora and colonize the mucosa have an important advantage in causing disease. Specific cell-surface proteins involved in attachment of bacteria to intestinal cells are important virulence determinants. *V. cholerae*, for example, adheres to the brush border of small-intestinal enterocytes via specific surface adhesins, including the toxin-coregulated pilus and other accessory colonization factors. Enterotoxigenic *E. coli*, which causes watery diarrhea, produces an adherence protein called *colonization factor antigen* that is necessary for colonization of the upper small intestine by the organism prior to the production of enterotoxin. Enteropathogenic *E. coli*, an agent of diarrhea in young children, and enterohemorrhagic *E. coli*, which causes hemorrhagic colitis and the hemolytic-uremic syndrome, produce virulence determinants that allow these organisms to attach to and efface the brush border of the intestinal epithelium.

Toxin Production The production of one or more exotoxins is important in the pathogenesis of numerous enteric organisms. Such toxins include *enterotoxins*, which cause watery diarrhea by acting directly on secretory mechanisms in the intestinal mucosa; *cytotoxins*, which cause destruction of mucosal cells and associated inflammatory diarrhea; and *neurotoxins*, which act directly on the central or peripheral nervous system.

TABLE 122-1 GASTROINTESTINAL PATHOGENS CAUSING ACUTE DIARRHEA

Mechanism	Location	Illness	Stool Findings	Examples of Pathogens Involved
Noninflammatory (enterotoxin)	Proximal small bowel	Watery diarrhea	No fecal leukocytes; mild or no increase in fecal lactoferrin	*Vibrio cholerae*, enterotoxigenic *Escherichia coli* (LT and/or ST), enteroaggregative *E. coli, Clostridium perfringens, Bacillus cereus, Staphylococcus aureus, Aeromonas hydrophila, Plesiomonas shigelloides*, rotavirus, norovirus, enteric adenoviruses, *Giardia lamblia, Cryptosporidium* spp., *Cyclospora* spp., microsporidia
Inflammatory (invasion or cytotoxin)	Colon or distal small bowel	Dysentery or inflammatory diarrhea	Fecal polymorphonuclear leukocytes; substantial increase in fecal lactoferrin	*Shigella* spp., *Salmonella* spp., *Campylobacter jejuni*, enterohemorrhagic *E. coli*, enteroinvasive *E. coli, Yersinia enterocolitica, Vibrio parahaemolyticus, Clostridium difficile, ?A. hydrophila, ?P. shigelloides, Entamoeba histolytica*
Penetrating	Distal small bowel	Enteric fever	Fecal mononuclear leukocytes	*Salmonella typhi, Y. enterocolitica, ?Campylobacter fetus*

Abbreviations: LT, heat-labile enterotoxin; ST, heat-stable enterotoxin.

Source: After Guerrant and Steiner.

The prototypical enterotoxin is cholera toxin, a heterodimeric protein composed of one A and five B subunits. The A subunit contains the enzymatic activity of the toxin, while the B subunit pentamer binds holotoxin to the enterocyte surface receptor, the ganglioside G_{M1}. After the binding of holotoxin, a fragment of the A subunit is translocated across the eukaryotic cell membrane into the cytoplasm, where it catalyzes the ADP-ribosylation of a GTP-binding protein and causes persistent activation of adenylate cyclase. The end result is an increase of cyclic AMP in the intestinal mucosa, which increases Cl^- secretion and decreases Na^+ absorption, leading to loss of fluid and the production of diarrhea.

Enterotoxigenic strains of *E. coli* may produce a protein called *heat-labile enterotoxin* (LT) that is similar to cholera toxin and causes secretory diarrhea by the same mechanism. Alternatively, enterotoxigenic strains of *E. coli* may produce *heat-stable enterotoxin* (ST), one form of which causes diarrhea by activation of guanylate cyclase and elevation of intracellular cyclic GMP. Some enterotoxigenic strains of *E. coli* produce both LT and ST.

Bacterial cytotoxins, in contrast, destroy intestinal mucosal cells and produce the syndrome of dysentery, with bloody stools containing inflammatory cells. Enteric pathogens that produce such cytotoxins include *Shigella dysenteriae* type 1, *Vibrio parahaemolyticus*, and *Clostridium difficile. S. dysenteriae* type 1 and Shiga toxin–producing strains of *E. coli* produce potent cytotoxins and have been associated with outbreaks of hemorrhagic colitis and hemolytic-uremic syndrome.

Neurotoxins are usually produced by bacteria outside the host and therefore cause symptoms soon after ingestion. Included are the staphylococcal and *Bacillus cereus* toxins, which act on the central nervous system to produce vomiting.

Invasion Dysentery may result not only from the production of cytotoxins but also from bacterial invasion and destruction of intestinal mucosal cells. Infections due to *Shigella* and enteroinvasive *E. coli* are characterized by the organisms' invasion of mucosal epithelial cells, intraepithelial multiplication, and subsequent spread to adjacent cells. *Salmonella* causes inflammatory diarrhea by invasion of the bowel mucosa but generally is not associated with the destruction of enterocytes or the full clinical syndrome of dysentery. *Salmonella typhi* and *Yersinia enterocolitica* can penetrate intact intestinal mucosa, multiply intracellularly in Peyer's patches and intestinal lymph nodes, and then disseminate through the bloodstream to cause enteric fever, a syndrome characterized by fever, headache, relative bradycardia, abdominal pain, splenomegaly, and leukopenia.

HOST DEFENSES

Given the enormous number of microorganisms ingested with every meal, the normal host must combat a constant influx of potential enteric pathogens. Studies of infections in patients with alterations in defense mechanisms have led to a greater understanding of the variety of ways in which the normal host can protect itself against disease.

Normal Flora The large numbers of bacteria that normally inhabit the intestine act as an important host defense by preventing colonization by potential enteric pathogens. Persons with fewer intestinal bacteria, such as infants who have not yet developed normal enteric colonization or patients receiving antibiotics, are at significantly greater risk of developing infections with enteric pathogens. The composition of the intestinal flora is as important as the number of organisms present. More than 99% of the normal colonic flora is made up of anaerobic bacteria, and the acidic pH and volatile fatty acids produced by these organisms appear to be critical elements in resistance to colonization.

Gastric Acid The acidic pH of the stomach is an important barrier to enteric pathogens, and an increased frequency of infections due to *Salmonella, G. lamblia*, and a variety of helminths has been reported among patients who have undergone gastric surgery or are achlorhydric for some other reason. Neutralization of gastric acid with antacids or H_2 blockers—a common practice in the management of hospitalized patients—similarly increases the risk of enteric colonization. In addition, some microorganisms can survive the extreme acidity of the gastric environment; rotavirus, for example, is highly stable to acidity.

Intestinal Motility Normal peristalsis is the major mechanism for clearance of bacteria from the proximal small intestine. When intestinal motility is impaired (e.g., by treatment with opiates or other antimotility drugs, anatomic abnormalities, or hypomotility states), the frequency of bacterial overgrowth and infection of the small bowel with enteric pathogens is increased. Some patients whose treatment for *Shigella* infection consists of diphenoxylate hydrochloride with atropine (Lomotil) experience prolonged fever and shedding of organisms, while patients treated with opiates for mild *Salmonella* gastroenteritis have a higher frequency of bacteremia than those not treated with opiates.

Immunity Both cellular immune responses and antibody production play important roles in protection from enteric infections. The wide spectrum of viral, bacterial, parasitic, and fungal gastrointestinal infections in patients with AIDS highlights the significance of cell-mediated immunity in protection from these pathogens. Humoral immunity is also important and consists of systemic IgG and IgM as well as secretory IgA. The mucosal immune system may be the first line of defense against many gastrointestinal pathogens. The binding of bacterial antigens to the luminal surface of M cells in the distal small bowel and the subsequent presentation of antigens to subepithelial lymphoid tissue lead to the proliferation of sensitized lymphocytes. These lymphocytes circulate and populate all of the mucosal tissues of the body as IgA-secreting plasma cells.

Genetic Determinants The mechanisms underlying genetic variation in host susceptibility remain poorly understood. People with blood group O show increased susceptibility to cholera, shigellosis, and norovirus infection. A polymorphism in the interleukin 8 gene is associated with increased risk of diarrhea from enteroaggregative *E. coli*.

APPROACH TO THE PATIENT: Infectious Diarrhea or Bacterial Food Poisoning

The approach to the patient with possible infectious diarrhea or bacterial food poisoning is shown in Fig. 122-1.

HISTORY The answers to questions with high discriminating value can quickly narrow the range of potential causes of diarrhea and help determine whether treatment is needed. Important elements of the narrative history are detailed in Fig. 122-1.

PHYSICAL EXAMINATION The examination of patients for signs of dehydration provides essential information about the severity of the diarrheal illness and the need for rapid therapy. Mild dehydration is indicated by thirst, dry mouth, decreased axillary sweat, decreased urine output, and slight weight loss. Signs of moderate dehydration include an orthostatic fall in blood pressure, skin tenting, and sunken eyes (or, in infants, a sunken fontanelle). Signs of severe dehydration range from hypotension and tachycardia to confusion and frank shock.

DIAGNOSTIC APPROACH After the severity of illness is assessed, the clinician must distinguish between *inflammatory* and *noninflammatory* disease. Using the history and epidemiologic features of the case as guides, the clinician can then rapidly evaluate the need for further efforts to define a specific etiology and for therapeutic intervention. Examination of a stool sample may supplement the narrative history. Grossly bloody or mucoid stool suggests an inflammatory process. A test for fecal leukocytes (preparation of a thin smear of stool on a glass slide, addition of a drop of methylene blue, and examination of the wet mount) can suggest inflammatory disease in patients with diarrhea, although the predictive value of this test is still debated. A test for fecal lactoferrin, which is a marker of fecal leukocytes, is more sensitive and is available in latex agglutination and enzyme-linked immunosorbent assay formats. Causes of acute infectious diarrhea, categorized as inflammatory and noninflammatory, are listed in Table 122-1.

POST-DIARRHEA COMPLICATIONS Chronic complications may follow the resolution of an acute diarrheal episode. The clinician should inquire about prior diarrheal illness if the conditions listed in Table 122-2 are observed.

EPIDEMIOLOGY

Travel History Of the several million people who travel from temperate industrialized countries to tropical regions of Asia, Africa, and Central and South America each year, 20–50% experience a sudden onset of abdominal cramps, anorexia, and watery diarrhea; thus *traveler's diarrhea* is the most common travel-related illness (Chap. 117). The time of onset is usually 3 days to 2 weeks after the traveler's arrival in a tropical area; most cases begin within the first 3–5 days. The illness is generally self-limited, lasting 1–5 days. The high rate of diarrhea among travelers to underdeveloped areas is related to the ingestion of contaminated food or water.

The organisms that cause traveler's diarrhea vary considerably with location (Table 122-3). In all areas, enterotoxigenic and enteroaggregative *E. coli* are the most common isolates from persons with the classic secretory traveler's diarrhea syndrome.

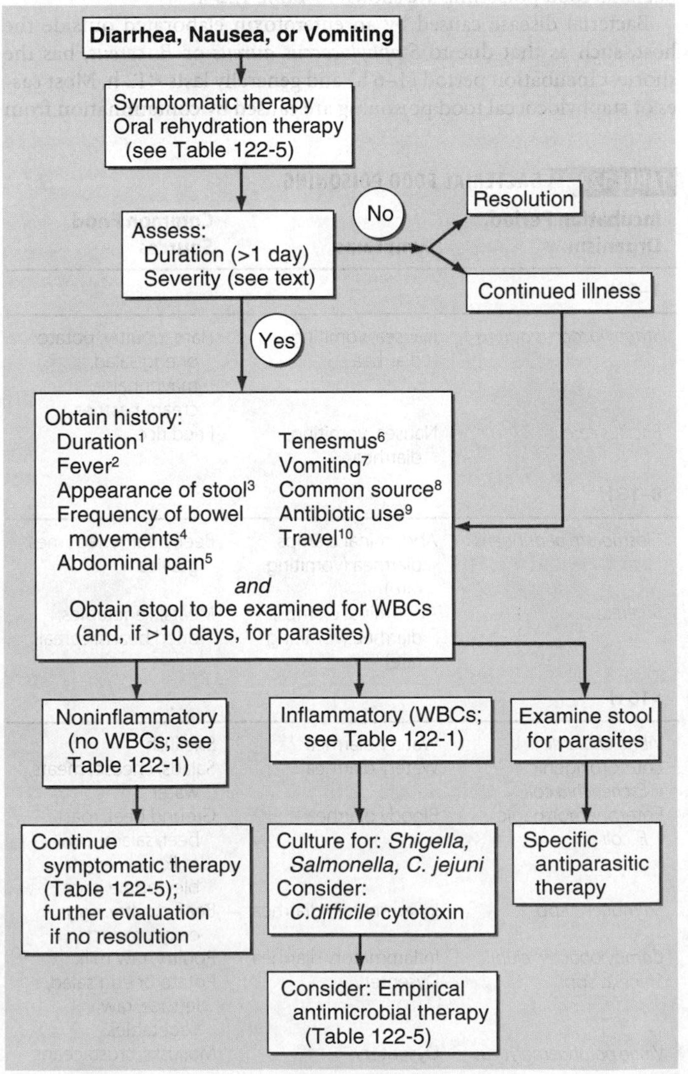

FIGURE 122-1 Clinical algorithm for the approach to patients with community-acquired infectious diarrhea or bacterial food poisoning. Key to superscripts: **1.** Diarrhea lasting >2 weeks is generally defined as chronic; in such cases, many of the causes of acute diarrhea are much less likely, and a new spectrum of causes needs to be considered. **2.** Fever often implies invasive disease, although fever and diarrhea may also result from infection outside the gastrointestinal tract, as in malaria. **3.** Stools that contain blood or mucus indicate ulceration of the large bowel. Bloody stools without fecal leukocytes should alert the laboratory to the possibility of infection with Shiga toxin–producing enterohemorrhagic *Escherichia coli*. Bulky white stools suggest a small-intestinal process that is causing malabsorption. Profuse "rice-water" stools suggest cholera or a similar toxigenic process. **4.** Frequent stools over a given period can provide the first warning of impending dehydration. **5.** Abdominal pain may be most severe in inflammatory processes like those due to *Shigella*, *Campylobacter*, and necrotizing toxins. Painful abdominal muscle cramps, caused by electrolyte loss, can develop in severe cases of cholera. Bloating is common in giardiasis. An appendicitis-like syndrome should prompt a culture for *Yersinia enterocolitica* with cold enrichment. **6.** Tenesmus (painful rectal spasms with a strong urge to defecate but little passage of stool) may be a feature of cases with proctitis, as in shigellosis or amebiasis. **7.** Vomiting implies an acute infection (e.g., a toxin-mediated illness or food poisoning) but can also be prominent in a variety of systemic illnesses (e.g., malaria) and in intestinal obstruction. **8.** Asking patients whether anyone else they know is sick is a more efficient means of identifying a common source than is constructing a list of recently eaten foods. If a common source seems likely, specific foods can be investigated. See text for a discussion of bacterial food poisoning. **9.** Current antibiotic therapy or a recent history of treatment suggests *Clostridium difficile* diarrhea (Chap. 123). Stop antibiotic treatment if possible and consider tests for *C. difficile* toxins. Antibiotic use may increase the risk of other infections, such as salmonellosis. **10.** See text (and Chap. 117) for a discussion of traveler's diarrhea. (*After Guerrant and Steiner; RL Guerrant, DA Bobak: N Engl J Med 325:327, 1991; with permission.*)

TABLE 122-2 POST-DIARRHEA COMPLICATIONS OF ACUTE INFECTIOUS DIARRHEAL ILLNESS

Complication	Comments
Chronic diarrhea • Lactase deficiency • Small-bowel bacterial overgrowth • Malabsorption syndromes (tropical and celiac sprue)	Occurs in ~1% of travelers with acute diarrhea • Protozoa account for ~1/3 of cases
Initial presentation or exacerbation of inflammatory bowel disease	May be precipitated by traveler's diarrhea
Irritable bowel syndrome	Occurs in ~10% of travelers with traveler's diarrhea
Reiter's syndrome (reactive arthritis)	Particularly likely after infection with invasive organisms (*Shigella, Salmonella, Campylobacter*)
Hemolytic-uremic syndrome (hemolytic anemia, thrombocytopenia, and renal failure)	Follows infection with Shiga toxin–producing bacteria (*Shigella dysenteriae* type 1 and enterohemorrhagic *Escherichia coli*)

Location Day-care centers have particularly high attack rates of enteric infections. Rotavirus is most common among children <2 years old, with attack rates of 75–100% among those exposed. *G. lamblia* is more common among older children, with somewhat lower attack rates. Other common organisms, often spread by fecal-oral contact, are *Shigella*, *Campylobacter jejuni*, and *Cryptosporidium*. A characteristic feature of infection among children attending day-care centers is the high rate of secondary cases among family members.

Similarly, hospitals are sites in which enteric infections are concentrated. In medical intensive-care units and pediatric wards, diarrhea is one of the most common manifestations of nosocomial infections. *C. difficile* is the predominant cause of nosocomial diarrhea among adults in the United States. Viral pathogens, especially rotavirus, can spread rapidly in pediatric wards. Enteropathogenic *E. coli* has been associated with outbreaks of diarrhea in nurseries for newborns. One-third of elderly patients in chronic-care institutions develop a significant diarrheal illness each year; more than half of these cases are caused by cytotoxin-producing *C. difficile*. Antimicrobial therapy can predispose to pseudomembranous colitis by altering the normal colonic flora and allowing the multiplication of *C. difficile* (Chap. 123).

Age Most of the morbidity and mortality from enteric pathogens involves children <5 years of age. Breast-fed infants are protected from contaminated food and water and derive some protection from maternal antibodies, but their risk of infection rises dramatically when they begin to eat solid foods. Infants and younger children are more likely than adults to develop rotavirus disease, while older children and adults are more commonly infected with norovirus. Other organisms with higher attack rates among children than among adults include enterotoxigenic, enteropathogenic, and enterohemorrhagic *E. coli*; *C. jejuni*; and *G. lamblia*. In children, the incidence of *Salmonella* infections is highest among those <1 year of age, while the attack rate for *Shigella* infections is greatest among those 6 months to 4 years of age.

Bacterial Food Poisoning If the history and the stool examination indicate a noninflammatory etiology of diarrhea and there is evidence of a common-source outbreak, questions concerning the ingestion of specific foods and the time of onset of the diarrhea after a meal can provide clues to the bacterial cause of the illness. Potential causes of bacterial food poisoning are shown in Table 122-4.

Bacterial disease caused by an enterotoxin elaborated outside the host, such as that due to *Staphylococcus aureus* or *B. cereus*, has the shortest incubation period (1–6 h) and generally lasts <12 h. Most cases of staphylococcal food poisoning are caused by contamination from

TABLE 122-3 EPIDEMIOLOGY OF TRAVELER'S DIARRHEA

Etiologic Agent	Approximate Percentage of Cases	Comments
Enterotoxigenic *Escherichia coli*	15–50	Single most important agent, particularly in summertime in semitropical areas; percentage of cases ranges from 15% in Asia to 50% in Latin America
Enteroaggregative *E. coli*	20–35	Emerging enteric pathogen of worldwide distribution
Shigella and enteroinvasive *E. coli*	10–25	Major causes of fever and dysentery
Salmonella	5–10	Causes fever and dysentery
Campylobacter jejuni	3–15	More common in winter in semitropical areas; more common in Asia
Aeromonas	5	Important in Thailand
Plesiomonas	5	Related to tropical travel and seafood consumption
Vibrio cholerae	0–10	Most common in India and Asia; also common in Central and South America
Rotavirus and norovirus	10–40	Latin America, Asia, and Africa; norovirus associated with seafood ingestion on cruise ships
Entamoeba histolytica	5	Particularly important in Mexico and Thailand
Giardia lamblia	<2	Zoonotic reservoirs in northern United States; affects hikers and campers who drink from freshwater streams; contaminates water supplies in Russia
Cryptosporidium	2	Affects travelers to Russia, Mexico, and Africa; causes large-scale urban outbreaks in United States
Cyclospora	<1	Affects travelers to Nepal, Haiti, and Peru; contaminates water or food
Unknown	20	Illness improves with antibacterial therapy, implicating bacterial diarrhea

Source: After Dupont.

TABLE 122-4 BACTERIAL FOOD POISONING

Incubation Period, Organism	Symptoms	Common Food Sources
1–6 H		
Staphylococcus aureus	Nausea, vomiting, diarrhea	Ham, poultry, potato or egg salad, mayonnaise, cream pastries
Bacillus cereus	Nausea, vomiting, diarrhea	Fried rice
8–16 H		
Clostridium perfringens	Abdominal cramps, diarrhea (vomiting rare)	Beef, poultry, legumes, gravies
B. cereus	Abdominal cramps, diarrhea (vomiting rare)	Meats, vegetables, dried beans, cereals
>16 H		
Vibrio cholerae	Watery diarrhea	Shellfish
Enterotoxigenic *Escherichia coli*	Watery diarrhea	Salads, cheese, meats, water
Enterohemorrhagic *E. coli*	Bloody diarrhea	Ground beef, roast beef, salami, raw milk, raw vegetables, apple juice
Salmonella spp.	Inflammatory diarrhea	Beef, poultry, eggs, dairy products
Campylobacter jejuni	Inflammatory diarrhea	Poultry, raw milk
Shigella spp.	Dysentery	Potato or egg salad, lettuce, raw vegetables
Vibrio parahaemolyticus	Dysentery	Mollusks, crustaceans

infected human carriers. Staphylococci can multiply at a wide range of temperatures; thus, if food is left to cool slowly and remains at room temperature after cooking, the organisms will have the opportunity to form enterotoxin. Outbreaks following picnics where potato salad, mayonnaise, and cream pastries have been served offer classic examples of staphylococcal food poisoning. Diarrhea, nausea, vomiting, and abdominal cramping are common, while fever is less so.

B. cereus can produce either a syndrome with a short incubation period—the *emetic* form, mediated by a staphylococcal type of enterotoxin—or one with a longer incubation period (8–16 h)—the *diarrheal* form, caused by an enterotoxin resembling *E. coli* LT, in which diarrhea and abdominal cramps are characteristic but vomiting is uncommon. The emetic form of *B. cereus* food poisoning is associated with contaminated fried rice; the organism is common in uncooked rice, and its heat-resistant spores survive boiling. If cooked rice is not refrigerated, the spores can germinate and produce toxin. Frying before serving may not destroy the preformed, heat-stable toxin.

Food poisoning due to *Clostridium perfringens* also has a slightly longer incubation period (8–14 h) and results from the survival of heat-resistant spores in inadequately cooked meat, poultry, or legumes. After ingestion, toxin is produced in the intestinal tract, causing moderately severe abdominal cramps and diarrhea; vomiting is rare, as is fever. The illness is self-limited, rarely lasting >24 h.

Not all food poisoning has a bacterial cause. Nonbacterial agents of short-incubation food poisoning include capsaicin, which is found in hot peppers, and a variety of toxins found in fish and shellfish (Chap. 391).

LABORATORY EVALUATION

Many cases of noninflammatory diarrhea are self-limited or can be treated empirically, and in these instances the clinician may not need to determine a specific etiology. Potentially pathogenic *E. coli* cannot be distinguished from normal fecal flora by routine culture, and tests to detect enterotoxins are not available in most clinical laboratories. In situations in which cholera is a concern, stool should be cultured on thiosulfate–citrate–bile salts–sucrose (TCBS) agar. A latex agglutination test has made the rapid detection of rotavirus in stool practical for many laboratories, while reverse-transcriptase polymerase chain reaction and specific antigen enzyme immunoassays have been developed for the identification of norovirus. At least three stool specimens should be examined for *Giardia* cysts or stained for *Cryptosporidium* if the level of clinical suspicion regarding the involvement of these organisms is high.

All patients with fever and evidence of inflammatory disease acquired outside the hospital should have stool cultured for *Salmonella*, *Shigella*, and *Campylobacter*. *Salmonella* and *Shigella* can be selected on MacConkey's agar as non-lactose-fermenting (colorless) colonies or can be grown on *Salmonella-Shigella* agar or in selenite enrichment broth, both of which inhibit most organisms except these pathogens. Evaluation of nosocomial diarrhea should initially focus on *C. difficile*; stool culture for other pathogens in this setting has an extremely low yield and is not cost-effective. Toxins A and B produced by pathogenic strains of *C. difficile* can be detected by rapid enzyme immunoassays and latex agglutination tests (Chap. 123). Isolation of *C. jejuni* requires inoculation of fresh stool onto selective growth medium and incubation at 42°C in a microaerophilic atmosphere. In many laboratories in the United States, *E. coli* O157:H7 is among the most common pathogens isolated from visibly bloody stools. Strains of this enterohemorrhagic serotype can be identified in specialized laboratories by serotyping but also can be identified presumptively in hospital laboratories as lactose-fermenting, indole-positive colonies of sorbitol nonfermenters (white colonies) on sorbitol MacConkey plates. Fresh stools should be examined for amebic cysts and trophozoites.

Rx INFECTIOUS DIARRHEA OR BACTERIAL FOOD POISONING

In many cases, a specific diagnosis is not necessary or not available to guide treatment. The clinician can proceed with the information obtained from the history, stool examination, and evaluation of dehydration severity. Empirical regimens for the treatment of traveler's diarrhea are listed in **Table 122-5**.

The mainstay of treatment is adequate rehydration. The treatment of cholera and other dehydrating diarrheal diseases was revolutionized by

TABLE 122-5 TREATMENT OF TRAVELER'S DIARRHEA ON THE BASIS OF CLINICAL FEATURES

Clinical Syndrome	Suggested Therapy
Watery diarrhea (no blood in stool, no fever), 1 or 2 unformed stools per day without distressing enteric symptoms	Oral fluids (Pedialyte, Lytren, or flavored mineral water) and saltine crackers
Watery diarrhea (no blood in stool, no fever), 1 or 2 unformed stools per day with distressing enteric symptoms	Bismuth subsalicylate (for adults): 30 mL or 2 tablets (262 mg/tablet) every 30 min for 8 doses; or loperamide[a]: 4 mg initially followed by 2 mg after passage of each unformed stool, not to exceed 8 tablets (16 mg) per day (prescription dose) or 4 caplets (8 mg) per day (over-the-counter dose); drugs can be taken for 2 days
Watery diarrhea (no blood in stool, no distressing abdominal pain, no fever), >2 unformed stools per day	Antibacterial drug[b] plus (for adults) loperamide[a] (see dose above)
Dysentery (passage of bloody stools) or fever (>37.8°C)	Antibacterial drug[b]
Vomiting, minimal diarrhea	Bismuth subsalicylate (for adults; see dose above)
Diarrhea in infants (<2 y old)	Fluids and electrolytes (Pedialyte, Lytren); continue feeding, especially with breast milk; seek medical attention for moderate dehydration, fever lasting >24 h, bloody stools, or diarrhea lasting more than several days
Diarrhea in pregnant women	Fluids and electrolytes; can consider attapulgite, 3 g initially, with dose repeated after passage of each unformed stool or every 2 h (whichever is earlier), for a total dosage of 9 g/d; seek medical attention for persistent or severe symptoms
Diarrhea despite trimethoprim-sulfamethoxazole prophylaxis	Fluoroquinolone—with loperamide[a] (see dose above) if no fever and no blood in stool, alone in cases of fever/dysentery
Diarrhea despite fluoroquinolone prophylaxis	Bismuth subsalicylate (see dose above) for mild to moderate disease; consult physician for moderate to severe disease or if disease persists

[a]Loperamide should not be used by patients with fever or dysentery; its use may prolong diarrhea in patients with infection due to *Shigella* or other invasive organisms.

[b]The recommended antibacterial drugs are as follows:

Travel to high-risk country other than Thailand:

Adults: (1) A fluoroquinolone such as ciprofloxacin, 750 mg as a single dose or 500 mg bid for 3 days; levofloxacin, 500 mg as a single dose or 500 mg qd for 3 days; or norfloxacin, 800 mg as a single dose or 400 mg bid for 3 days. (2) Azithromycin, 1000 mg as a single dose or 500 mg qd for 3 days. (3) Rifaximin, 200 mg tid or 400 mg bid for 3 days (not recommended for use in dysentery).

Children: Azithromycin, 10 mg/kg on day 1, 5 mg/kg on days 2 and 3 if diarrhea persists. Alternative agent: furazolidone, 7.5 mg/kg per day in four divided doses for 5 days.

Travel to Thailand (with risk of fluoroquinolone-resistant *Campylobacter*):

Adults: Azithromycin (at above dose for adults). Alternative agent: a fluoroquinolone (at above doses for adults).

Children: Same as for children traveling to other areas (see above).

All patients should take oral fluids (Pedialyte, Lytren, or flavored mineral water) plus saltine crackers. If diarrhea becomes moderate or severe, if fever persists, or if bloody stools or dehydration develops, the patient should seek medical attention.

Source: After Dupont.

the promotion of oral rehydration solutions, the efficacy of which depends on the fact that glucose-facilitated absorption of sodium and water in the small intestine remains intact in the presence of cholera toxin. The use of oral rehydration solutions has reduced mortality due to cholera from >50% (in untreated cases) to <1%. The World Health Organization recommends a solution containing 3.5 g sodium chloride, 2.5 g sodium bicarbonate, 1.5 g potassium chloride, and 20 g glucose (or 40 g sucrose) per liter of water. Oral rehydration solutions containing rice or cereal as the carbohydrate source may be even more effective than glucose-based solutions, and the addition of L-histidine may reduce the frequency and volume of stool output. Patients who are severely dehydrated or in whom vomiting precludes the use of oral therapy should receive IV solutions such as Ringer's lactate.

Although most secretory forms of traveler's diarrhea—usually due to enterotoxigenic and enteroaggregative *E. coli*—can be treated effectively with rehydration, bismuth subsalicylate, or antiperistaltic agents, antimicrobial agents can shorten the duration of illness from 3–4 days to 24–36 h. Changes in diet have not been shown to have an impact on the duration of illness, while the efficacy of probiotics continues to be debated.

Antibiotic treatment for children who present with bloody diarrhea raises special concerns. Laboratory studies of enterohemorrhagic *E. coli* strains have demonstrated that a number of antibiotics induce replication of Shiga toxin–producing lambdoid bacteriophages, significantly increasing toxin production by these strains. Clinical studies have supported these laboratory results, and antibiotics are not recommended for the treatment of enterohemorrhagic *E. coli* infections in children.

PROPHYLAXIS

Improvements in hygiene to limit fecal-oral spread of enteric pathogens will be necessary if the prevalence of diarrheal diseases is to be significantly reduced in developing countries. Travelers can reduce their risk of diarrhea by eating only hot, freshly cooked food; by avoiding raw vegetables, salads, and unpeeled fruit; and by drinking only boiled or treated water and avoiding ice. Historically, few travelers to tourist destinations adhere to these dietary restrictions. However, an intensive hygienic effort in Jamaica involving government, hotel, and tourism agencies led to a decrease in the incidence of traveler's diarrhea by 72% from 1996 to 2002.

Bismuth subsalicylate is an inexpensive agent for the prophylaxis of traveler's diarrhea; it is taken at a dosage of 2 tablets (525 mg) four times a day. Treatment appears to be effective and safe for up to 3 weeks. Prophylactic antimicrobial agents, although effective, are not generally recommended for the prevention of traveler's diarrhea, except when travelers are immunosuppressed or have other underlying illnesses that place them at high risk for morbidity from gastrointestinal infection. The risk of side effects and the possibility of developing an infection with a drug-resistant organism or with more harmful, invasive bacteria make it more reasonable to institute an empirical short course of treatment if symptoms develop. The recent availability of effective nonabsorbed antibiotics such as rifaximin may lead to new prophylactic options.

The possibility of exerting a major impact on the worldwide morbidity and mortality associated with diarrheal diseases has led to intense efforts to develop effective vaccines against the common bacterial and viral enteric pathogens. Recent research has yielded promising advances in the development of vaccines against rotavirus, *Shigella*, *V. cholerae*, *S. typhi*, and enterotoxigenic *E. coli*.

FURTHER READINGS

AL-ABRI SS et al: Traveller's diarrhoea. Lancet Infect Dis 5:349, 2005

BARTLETT JG: Clinical practice. Antibiotic-associated diarrhea. N Engl J Med 346:334, 2002

DUPONT HL: Travelers' diarrhea, in *Infections of the Gastrointestinal Tract*, 2d ed, MJ Blaser et al (eds). Philadelphia, Lippincott Williams & Wilkins, 2002, Chap 19

GUERRANT RL, STEINER TS: Principles and syndromes of enteric infection, in *Mandell, Douglas and Bennett's Principles and Practice of Infectious Diseases*, 5th ed, GL Mandell et al (eds). Philadelphia, Churchill Livingstone, 2000, Chap 81

KOO HL, DUPONT HL: Current and future developments in travelers' diarrhea therapy. Expert Rev Anti Infect Ther 4:417, 2006

MUSHER DM, MUSHER BL: Contagious acute gastrointestinal infections. N Engl J Med 351:2417, 2004

OKHUYSEN PC: Current concepts in travelers' diarrhea: Epidemiology, antimicrobial resistance and treatment. Curr Opin Infect Dis 18:522, 2005

SAZAWAL S et al: Efficacy of probiotics in prevention of acute diarrhoea: A meta-analysis of masked, randomised, placebo-controlled trials. Lancet Infect Dis 6:374, 2006

TAUXE RV et al: Foodborne disease, in *Mandell, Douglas and Bennett's Principles and Practice of Infectious Diseases*, 5th ed, GL Mandell et al (eds). Philadelphia, Churchill Livingstone, 2000, Chap 87

WONG CS et al: The risk of the hemolytic-uremic syndrome after antibiotic treatment of *Escherichia coli* O157:H7 infections. N Engl J Med 342:1930, 2000

123 *Clostridium difficile*-Associated Disease, Including Pseudomembranous Colitis

Dale N. Gerding, Stuart Johnson

DEFINITION

Clostridium difficile–associated disease (CDAD) is a unique colon infection that is acquired almost exclusively in association with antimicrobial use and the consequent disruption of the normal colonic flora. The most commonly diagnosed diarrheal illness acquired in the hospital, CDAD results from the ingestion of spores of *C. difficile* that vegetate, multiply, and secrete toxins, causing diarrhea and pseudomembranous colitis (PMC).

ETIOLOGY AND EPIDEMIOLOGY

C. difficile is an obligately anaerobic, gram-positive, spore-forming bacillus whose spores are found widely in nature, particularly in the environment of hospitals and chronic-care facilities. CDAD occurs most frequently in hospitals and nursing homes where the level of antimicrobial use is high and the environment is contaminated by *C. difficile* spores.

Clindamycin, ampicillin, and cephalosporins were the first antibiotics associated with CDAD. The second- and third-generation cephalosporins, particularly cefotaxime, ceftriaxone, cefuroxime, and ceftazidime, are agents frequently responsible for this condition, and the fluoroquinolones (ciprofloxacin, levofloxacin, gatifloxacin, and moxifloxacin) are the most recent drug class to be implicated in hospital outbreaks. Penicillin/β-lactamase-inhibitor combinations such as ticarcillin/clavulanate and piperacillin/tazobactam pose significantly less risk. However, all antibiotics, including vancomycin and metronidazole (the agents most commonly used to treat CDAD), have been found to carry a risk of subsequent CDAD. Rare cases are reported in patients without prior antibiotic exposure.

C. difficile is acquired exogenously, most frequently in the hospital, and is carried in the stool of symptomatic and asymptomatic patients. The rate of fecal colonization is often ≥20% among adult patients hospitalized for >1 week; in contrast, the rate is 1–3% among community residents. The risk of *C. difficile* acquisition increases in proportion to length of hospital stay. Asymptomatic fecal carriage of *C. difficile* in healthy neonates is very common, with rates often exceeding 50% during the first 6 months of life, but associated disease in this population is rare. Spores of *C. difficile* are found on environmental surfaces (where the organism can persist for months) and on the hands of hospital personnel who fail to practice good hand hygiene. Hospital epidemics of CDAD have been attributed to a single *C. difficile* strain and to multiple strains present simultaneously. Other identified risk factors for CDAD include older age, greater severity of underlying illness, gastrointestinal surgery, use of electronic rectal thermometers, enteral tube feeding, and antacid treatment. Use of proton pump inhibitors may be a risk factor.

PATHOLOGY AND PATHOGENESIS

Spores of toxigenic *C. difficile* are ingested, survive gastric acidity, germinate in the small bowel, and colonize the lower intestinal tract, where they elaborate two large toxins: toxin A, an enterotoxin, and toxin B, a cytotoxin. These toxins initiate processes resulting in the disruption of epithelial-cell barrier function, diarrhea, and pseudomembrane formation. Toxin A is a potent neutrophil chemoattractant, and both toxins glucosylate the GTP-binding proteins of the Rho subfamily that regulate the actin cell cytoskeleton. Disruption of the cytoskeleton results in loss of cell shape, adherence, and tight junctions, with consequent fluid leakage. A third toxin, binary toxin CDT, was previously found in only ~6% of strains but is present in all isolates of the newly recognized epidemic strain (see "Global Considerations," below); this toxin is related to *C. perfringens* iota toxin. Its role in the pathogenesis of CDAD has not yet been defined.

The pseudomembranes of PMC are confined to the colonic mucosa and initially appear as 1- to 2-mm whitish-yellow plaques. The intervening mucosa appears unremarkable, but, as the disease progresses, the pseudomembranes coalesce to form larger plaques and become confluent over the entire colon wall (Fig. 123-1). The whole colon is usually involved, but 10% of patients have rectal sparing. Viewed microscopically, the pseudomembranes have a mucosal attachment point and contain necrotic leukocytes, fibrin, mucus, and cellular debris. The epithelium is eroded and necrotic in focal areas, with neutrophil infiltration of the mucosa.

Patients colonized with *C. difficile* were initially thought to be at high risk for CDAD. However, four prospective studies have shown that colonized patients actually have a decreased risk of subsequent CDAD. At least three events are proposed as essential for the development of CDAD (Fig. 123-2). Exposure to antimicrobial agents is the first event and establishes susceptibility to *C. difficile* infection. The second event is exposure to toxigenic *C. difficile*. Given that the majority of patients do not develop CDAD after the first two events, a third event is clearly essential for its occurrence. Candidate third events include exposure to a *C. difficile* strain of particular virulence, exposure to antimicrobial agents especially likely to cause CDAD, and an inadequate host immune response. The host anamnestic serum IgG antibody response to toxin A of *C. difficile* is the most likely third event that determines which patients develop diarrhea and which patients remain asymptomatic. The majority of humans first develop antibody to *C. difficile* toxins when colonized asymptomatically during the first year of life. Infants are thought not to develop symptomatic CDAD because they lack suitable mucosal toxin receptors that develop later in life. In adulthood, serum levels of IgG antibody to toxin A increase more in response to infection in individuals who become asymptomatic carriers than in those who develop CDAD. For persons who develop CDAD, increasing levels of antitoxin A during treatment correlate with a lower risk of recurrence of CDAD.

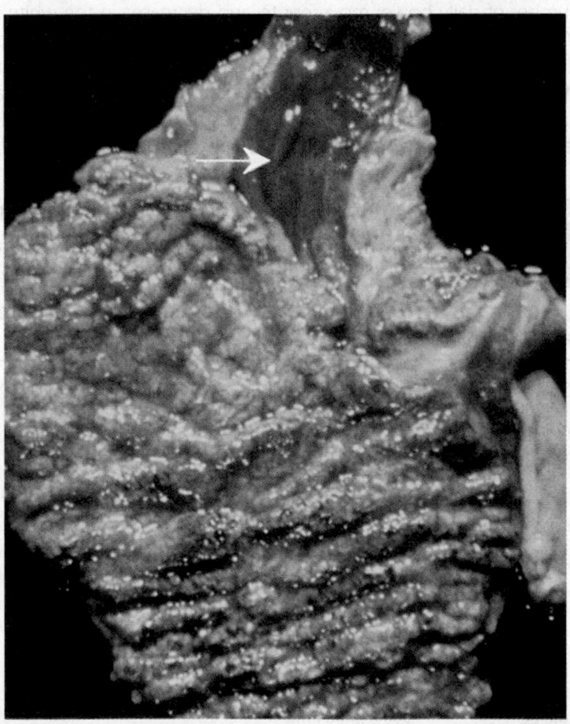

FIGURE 123-1 Autopsy specimen showing confluent pseudomembranes covering the cecum of a patient with pseudomembranous colitis. Note the sparing of the terminal ileum (*arrow*).

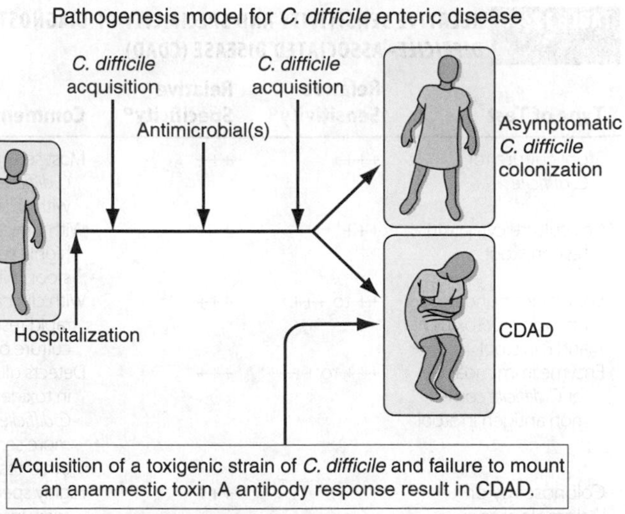

FIGURE 123-2 Pathogenesis model for hospital-acquired *Clostridium difficile*–associated diarrhea (CDAD). At least three events are integral to *C. difficile* pathogenesis. Exposure to antibiotics establishes susceptibility to infection. Once susceptible, the patient may acquire nontoxigenic (nonpathogenic) or toxigenic strains of *C. difficile* as a second event. Acquisition of toxigenic *C. difficile* may be followed by asymptomatic colonization or CDAD, depending on one or more additional events, including an inadequate host anamnestic IgG response to *C. difficile* toxin A.

GLOBAL CONSIDERATIONS

Rates and severity of CDAD in the United States, Canada, and Europe have increased markedly since the year 2000. Rates in U.S. hospitals tripled between 2000 and 2005. Hospitals in Montreal, Quebec, have reported rates four times higher than the 1997 baseline, with directly attributable mortality of 6.9% (increased from 1.5% previously). An epidemic strain, variously known as toxinotype III, REA type BI, PCR ribotype 027, and pulsed-field type NAP1, is thought to account for much of the increase in incidence and has been found in the United States, Canada, and Europe. The epidemic organism is characterized by (1) an ability to produce 16–23 times as much toxin A and toxin B as control strains in vitro; (2) the presence of a third toxin (binary toxin CDT); and (3) high-level resistance to all fluoroquinolones.

CLINICAL MANIFESTATIONS

Diarrhea is the most common manifestation caused by *C. difficile*. Stools are almost never grossly bloody and range from soft and unformed to watery or mucoid in consistency, with a characteristic odor. Patients may have as many as 20 bowel movements per day. Clinical and labora-

TABLE 123-1 RELATIVE SENSITIVITY AND SPECIFICITY OF DIAGNOSTIC TESTS FOR *CLOSTRIDIUM DIFFICILE*–ASSOCIATED DISEASE (CDAD)

Type of Test	Relative Sensitivity[a]	Relative Specificity[a]	Comment
Stool culture for *C. difficile*	++++	+++	Most sensitive test; specificity is ++++ if the *C. difficile* isolate tests positive for toxin; with clinical data, is diagnostic of CDAD
Cell culture cytotoxin test on stool	+++	++++	With clinical data, is diagnostic of CDAD; highly specific but not as sensitive as stool culture
Enzyme immunoassay for toxin A or toxins A and B in stool	++ to +++	+++	With clinical data, is diagnostic of CDAD; rapid results, but not as sensitive as stool culture or cell culture cytotoxin test
Enzyme immunoassay for *C. difficile* common antigen in stool	+++ to ++++	+++	Detects glutamate dehydrogenase found in toxigenic and nontoxigenic strains of *C. difficile* and other stool organisms; more sensitive and less specific than other tests; rapid results
Colonoscopy or sigmoidoscopy	+	++++	Highly specific if pseudomembranes are seen; insensitive compared with other tests

[a]According to both clinical and test-based criteria.
Note: ++++, >90%; +++, 71–90%; ++, 51–70%; +, ~50%.

tory findings include fever in 28% of cases, abdominal pain in 22%, and leukocytosis in 50%. When adynamic ileus (which is seen on x-ray in ~20% of cases) results in cessation of stool passage, the diagnosis of CDAD is frequently overlooked. A clue to the presence of unsuspected CDAD in these patients is unexplained leukocytosis, with ≥15,000 cells/μL. Such patients are at high risk for complications of *C. difficile* infection, particularly toxic megacolon and sepsis.

C. difficile diarrhea recurs after treatment in ~15–30% of cases, and this figure may be increasing. Recurrences may represent either relapses due to the same strain or reinfections with a new strain. Recurrence of clinical CDAD is likely to be a result of continued disruption of the normal fecal flora by the antibiotic used to treat CDAD.

DIAGNOSIS

The diagnosis of CDAD is based on a combination of clinical criteria: (1) diarrhea (≥3 unformed stools per 24 h for ≥2 days), with no other recognized cause; plus (2) toxin A or B detected in the stool, toxin-producing *C. difficile* detected by stool culture, or pseudomembranes seen in the colon. PMC is a more advanced form of CDAD and is visualized at endoscopy in only ~50% of patients with diarrhea who have a positive stool culture and toxin assay for *C. difficile* (Table 123-1). Endoscopy is a rapid diagnostic tool in seriously ill patients with suspected PMC and an acute abdomen, but a negative result in this examination does not rule out CDAD.

Despite the array of tests available for *C. difficile* and its toxins (Table 123-1), no single test has high sensitivity, high specificity, and rapid turnaround. The turnaround time for reporting of a positive result in the cell cytotoxicity test can be shortened to <24 h if cell cultures are examined at intervals as short as 4 h. However, this approach is labor intensive, and observation for 48 h is required for a conclusive test result. Most laboratory tests for toxins lack sensitivity. However, testing of multiple additional stool specimens is not recommended. Empirical treatment is appropriate if CDAD is strongly suspected on clinical grounds. Testing of asymptomatic patients is not recommended except for epidemiologic study purposes. In particular, so-called tests of cure following treatment are not recommended because many patients continue to harbor the organism and toxin after diarrhea has ceased and test results do not always predict recurrence of CDAD. Thus these results should not be used to restrict placement of patients in long-term-care or nursing home facilities.

Rx *CLOSTRIDIUM DIFFICILE*–ASSOCIATED DISEASE

PRIMARY CDAD When possible, discontinuation of any ongoing antimicrobial administration is recommended as the first step in treatment of CDAD. Earlier studies indicated that 15–23% of patients respond to this simple measure. However, with the advent of the current epidemic strain and the associated rapid clinical deterioration of some patients, prompt initiation of specific CDAD treatment has become the standard. General treatment guidelines include hydration and the avoidance of antiperistaltic agents and opiates, which may mask symptoms and possibly worsen disease. Nevertheless, antiperistaltic agents have been used safely with vancomycin or metronidazole for mild to moderate CDAD.

Although limited prospective randomized clinical trials showed no statistical differences among treatment agents for cessation of diarrhea (the primary outcome endpoint; **Table 123-2**), later observational studies suggest that response rates to metronidazole may have decreased. The clinical response rate for bacitracin is 10–20% lower than that for vancomycin; therefore, bacitracin use for first-line therapy is discouraged. All drugs, particularly vancomycin, should be given orally if possible. When IV metronidazole is administered, fecal bactericidal drug concentrations are achieved during acute diarrhea, and CDAD treatment has been successful; however, in the presence of adynamic ileus, IV metronidazole treatment of PMC has failed. In previous randomized trials, diarrhea response rates to oral therapy with vancomycin or metronidazole were ≥94%, but two recent observational studies found that metronidazole response rates had declined to 74% and 78%. Although the mean time to resolution of diarrhea is 2–4 days, the response to metronidazole may be much slower. Treatment should not be deemed a failure until a drug has been given for at least 6 days. On the basis of data for shorter courses of vancomycin (Table 123-2), it is recommended that metronidazole and vancomycin be given for at least 10 days, although no controlled comparisons are available. Although metronidazole is not approved for this indication by the U.S. Food and Drug Administration (FDA), most patients with mild to moderate illness respond to 500 mg given by mouth three times a day for 10 days; extension of the treatment period may be needed for slow responders. Because of the recent increase in metronidazole failures, patients treated with this drug should be monitored carefully for progressive defervescence (if fever is present), alleviation of abdominal pain and tenderness, decreases in the number of daily bowel movements, and decreases in the white blood cell (WBC) count. Clinical deterioration, with worsening signs and symptoms, or an unexplained increase in the WBC count during treatment are indications for a switch to vancomycin (usual dose, 125 mg orally four times a day). Although the use of vancomycin is discouraged for treatment of mildly to moderately ill patients, it is appropriate to use this agent for the initial treat-

TABLE 123-2 EXPECTED TREATMENT OUTCOMES BASED ON RANDOMIZED COMPARATIVE TRIALS OF ORAL THERAPY FOR *CLOSTRIDIUM DIFFICILE*–ASSOCIATED DISEASE

Treatment	Dose and Duration	Resolution of Diarrhea, %	Recurrence, %
Placebo or discontinuation of offending antibiotics	None	21	Unknown
Metronidazole	250 mg qid × 10 d	95	5
	250 mg qid × 10 d[a]	82	30
	500 mg tid × 10 d	94	17
Vancomycin	500 mg tid × 10 d	94	17
	500 mg qid × 10 d	100	15
	125 mg qid × 10 d[a]	91	19
	125 mg qid × 7 d	86	33
	125 mg qid × 5 d	75	Unknown
Teicoplanin	400 mg bid × 10 d	96	7
	100 mg bid × 10 d	96	8
Nitazoxanide	500 mg bid × 10 d[a]	89	22
Fusidic acid	500 mg tid × 10 d	93	28
Bacitracin	25,000 U qid × 10 d	80	42

[a]Data from randomized trials reported in 2006.

ment of patients who appear seriously ill, particularly if they have a high WBC count (>15,000/μL); controlled clinical outcome data on vancomycin use against the epidemic strain are not available. A randomized prospective trial of the antiparasitic drug nitazoxanide showed that (although not approved by the FDA for this indication) it was at least as effective as metronidazole for the treatment of CDAD, providing a potential alternative to vancomycin and metronidazole.

RECURRENT CDAD Overall, ~15–30% of patients experience recurrences of CDAD, either as relapses caused by the original organism or as reinfections following treatment (Table 123-2). Recurrence rates are higher among patients ≥65 years old and among patients who remain in the hospital after the initial episode of CDAD. Patients who have a first recurrence of CDAD have a high rate of second recurrence (33–65%). In the first recurrence, re-treatment with metronidazole is comparable to treatment with vancomycin. Recurrent disease, once thought to be relatively mild, has been documented to pose a significant (11%) risk of serious complications (shock, megacolon, perforation, colectomy, or death within 30 days). There is no standard treatment for multiple recurrences, but long or repeated metronidazole courses should be avoided because of potential neurotoxicity. Approaches include the administration of vancomycin followed by the yeast *Saccharomyces boulardii*; the administration of vancomycin followed by synthetic fecal bacterial enema; and the intentional colonization of the patient with a nontoxigenic strain of *C. difficile*. None of these biotherapeutic approaches has been approved by the FDA for use in the United States. Other strategies include (1) the use of vancomycin in tapering doses or with pulse dosing every other day for 4–6 weeks and (2) sequential treatment with vancomycin (125 mg four times daily) followed by rifaximin (400 mg twice daily) for 14 days. IV immunoglobulin, which has also been used with some success, presumably provides antibodies to *C. difficile* toxins.

FULMINANT CDAD Fulminant (rapidly progressive and severe) CDAD presents the most difficult treatment challenge. Patients with fulminant disease often do not have diarrhea, and their illness mimics an acute surgical abdomen. Sepsis (hypotension, fever, tachycardia, leukocytosis) may result from severe CDAD. An acute abdomen (with or without toxic megacolon) may include signs of obstruction, ileus, colon-wall thickening, and ascites on abdominal CT, often with peripheral-blood leukocytosis (≥20,000 cells/μL). Whether or not the patient has diarrhea, the differential diagnosis of an acute abdomen, sepsis, or toxic megacolon should include CDAD if the patient has received antibiotics in the past 2 months. Cautious sigmoidoscopy or colonoscopy to visualize PMC and an abdominal CT examination are the best diagnostic tests in patients without diarrhea.

Medical management of fulminant CDAD is suboptimal because of the difficulty of delivering metronidazole or vancomycin to the colon by the oral route in the presence of ileus. Vancomycin (given via nasogastric tube and by retention enema) plus IV metronidazole have been used in uncontrolled studies with some success, but surgical colectomy may be life-saving if there is no response to medical management. The incidence of fulminant CDAD requiring colectomy appears to be increasing in the evolving epidemic.

PROGNOSIS

The mortality rate attributed to CDAD, previously found to be 0.6–3.5%, has reached 6.9% in recent outbreaks and is progressively higher with increasing age. Most patients recover, but recurrences are common.

PREVENTION AND CONTROL

Strategies for the prevention of CDAD are of two types: those aimed at preventing transmission of the organism to the patient and those aimed at reducing the risk of CDAD if the organism is transmitted. Transmission of *C. difficile* in clinical practice has been prevented by gloving of personnel, elimination of the use of contaminated electronic thermometers, and use of hypochlorite (bleach) solution for environmental decontamination of patients' rooms. Hand hygiene is critical; hand washing is recommended in CDAD outbreaks because alcohol hand gels are not sporicidal. CDAD outbreaks have been best controlled by restricting the use of specific antibiotics, such as clindamycin and second- and third-generation cephalosporins. Outbreaks of CDAD due to clindamycin-resistant strains have resolved promptly when clindamycin use was restricted.

FURTHER READINGS

Hubert B et al: A portrait of the geographic dissemination of the *Clostridium difficile* North American pulsed-field type 1 strain and the epidemiology of *C. difficile*–associated disease in Quebec. Clin Infect Dis 44:238, 2007

Johnson S et al: Interruption of recurrent *Clostridium difficile*–associated diarrhea episodes by serial therapy with vancomycin and rifaximin. Clin Infect Dis 44:846, 2007

Kyne L et al: Association between antibody response to toxin A and protection against recurrent *Clostridium difficile* diarrhea. Lancet 357:189, 2001

——— et al: Asymptomatic carriage of *Clostridium difficile* and serum levels of IgG antibody against toxin A. N Engl J Med 342:390, 2000

Loo VG et al: A predominantly clonal multi-institutional outbreak of *Clostridium difficile*–associated diarrhea with high morbidity and mortality. N Engl J Med 353:2442, 2005

McDonald LC et al: *Clostridium difficile* infection in patients discharged from US short-stay hospitals, 1996-2003. Emerg Infect Dis 12:409, 2006

——— et al: An epidemic, toxin gene–variant strain of *Clostridium difficile*. N Engl J Med 353:2433, 2005

McFarland LV: Alternative treatments for *Clostridium difficile* disease: What really works? J Med Microbiol 54:101, 2005

Pepin J et al: The management and outcomes of a first recurrence of *Clostridium difficile* associated disease in Quebec. Clin Infect Dis 42:758, 2006

Zar FA et al: A comparison of vancomycin and metronidazole for the treatment of *Clostridium difficile*–associated diarrhea, stratified by disease severity. Clin Infect Dis 45:302, 2007

124 Sexually Transmitted Infections: Overview and Clinical Approach

King K. Holmes

CLASSIFICATION AND EPIDEMIOLOGY

Worldwide, most adults acquire at least one sexually transmitted infection (STI), and many remain at risk for complications. Each year, for example, an estimated 6.2 million persons in the United States acquire a new genital human papillomavirus (HPV) infection, and many of these individuals are at risk for genital neoplasias. Certain STIs, such as syphilis, gonorrhea, HIV infection, hepatitis B, and chancroid, are most concentrated within "core populations" characterized by high rates of partner change, multiple concurrent partners, or "dense," highly connected sexual networks—e.g., involving prostitutes and their clients, some homosexual men, and persons involved in the use of illicit drugs, particularly crack cocaine and methamphetamine. Other STIs are distributed more evenly throughout societies. For example, chlamydial infections, genital infections with HPV, and genital herpes can spread widely, even in relatively low-risk populations.

In general, the product of three factors determines the initial rate of spread of any STI within a population: rate of sexual exposure of susceptible to infectious people, efficiency of transmission per exposure, and duration of infectivity of those infected. Accordingly, efforts to prevent and control STIs aim to decrease the rate of sexual exposure of susceptibles to infected persons (e.g., through individual counseling and efforts to change the norms of sexual behavior), to decrease the duration of infectivity (through early diagnosis and curative or suppressive treatment), and to decrease the efficiency of transmission (e.g., through promotion of condom use and safer sexual practices and recently through male circumcision).

TABLE 124-1 SEXUALLY TRANSMITTED AND SEXUALLY TRANSMISSIBLE MICROORGANISMS

Bacteria	Viruses	Other[a]
Transmitted in Adults Predominantly by Sexual Intercourse		
Neisseria gonorrhoeae	HIV (types 1 and 2)	*Trichomonas vaginalis*
Chlamydia trachomatis	Human T-cell lymphotropic virus type I	*Phthirus pubis*
Treponema pallidum	Herpes simplex virus type 2	
Haemophilus ducreyi	Human papillomavirus (multiple genotypes)	
Calymmatobacterium granulomatis	Hepatitis B virus[b]	
	Molluscum contagiosum virus	
Ureaplasma urealyticum		
Sexual Transmission Repeatedly Described but Not Well Defined or Not the Predominant Mode		
Mycoplasma hominis	Cytomegalovirus	*Candida albicans*
Mycoplasma genitalium	Human T-cell lymphotropic virus type II	*Sarcoptes scabiei*
Gardnerella vaginalis and other vaginal bacteria	(?) Hepatitis C, D viruses	
	Herpes simplex virus type 1	
Group B *Streptococcus*	(?) Epstein-Barr virus	
Mobiluncus spp.	Human herpesvirus type 8	
Helicobacter cinaedi		
Helicobacter fennelliae		
Transmitted by Sexual Contact Involving Oral-Fecal Exposure; of Declining Importance in Homosexual Men		
Shigella spp.	Hepatitis A virus	*Giardia lamblia*
Campylobacter spp.		*Entamoeba histolytica*

[a]Includes protozoa, ectoparasites, and fungi.
[b]Among U.S. patients for whom a risk factor can be ascertained, most hepatitis B virus infections are transmitted sexually or by injection drug use.

In all societies, STIs rank among the most common of all infectious diseases, with >30 infections now classified as predominantly sexually transmitted or as frequently sexually transmissible (Table 124-1). In developing countries, with three-quarters of the world's population and 90% of the world's STIs, such factors as population growth (especially in adolescent and young-adult age groups), rural-to-urban migration, wars, and poverty create exceptional vulnerability to disease resulting from risky sexual behaviors. During the 1990s, in China, Russia, the other states of the former Soviet Union, and South Africa, internal social structures changed rapidly as borders opened to the West, unleashing enormous new epidemics of HIV infection and other STIs. HIV has become the leading cause of death in some developing countries, and HPV and hepatitis B virus (HBV) remain important causes of cervical and hepatocellular carcinoma, respectively—two of the most common malignancies in the developing world. Sexually transmitted herpes simplex virus (HSV) infections now cause most genital ulcer disease throughout the world and an increasing proportion of cases of genital herpes in developing countries with generalized HIV epidemics, where the positive feedback loop between HSV and HIV transmission is a growing, intractable problem. Randomized trials of the efficacy of therapy against HSV-2 in preventing the acquisition or transmission of HIV infection will be completed in 2007–2008, and the outcome will help shape future efforts to prevent HIV infection. Globally, five curable STIs—gonorrhea, chlamydial infection, syphilis, chancroid, and trichomoniasis—caused ~350 million new infections annually in the mid-1990s. Up to 50% of women of reproductive age in developing countries have bacterial vaginosis (arguably acquired sexually). All six of these curable infections have been associated with increased risk of HIV transmission or acquisition.

In the United States, the prevalence of antibody to HSV-2 has begun to fall only recently (since the late 1990s), especially among adolescents and young adults; the decline is presumably due to delayed sexual debut, increased condom use, and lower rates of multiple (≥4) sex partners, as is well documented in the U.S. Youth Risk Behavior Surveillance System (YRBSS). Genital HPV remains the most common sexually transmitted pathogen in this country, infecting 60% of a cohort of initially HPV-negative, sexually active Washington state college women within 5 years in a study conducted from 1990 to 2000.

In industrialized countries, fear of HIV infection since the mid-1980s, coupled with widespread behavioral interventions and better-organized systems of care for the curable STIs, has helped curb the transmission of the latter diseases. Nonetheless, foci of hyperendemic transmission persist in the southeastern United States and in most large U.S. cities. Rates of gonorrhea and syphilis remain higher in the United States than in any other Western industrialized country. The remarkable resurgence of gonorrhea and syphilis among homosexual and bisexual men in many parts of the United States and Europe since the 1990s reflects increased risk-taking following the advent of potent antiretroviral therapy and has been accompanied by increasing HIV transmission in this group.

In the United States, the Centers for Disease Control and Prevention (CDC) has compiled reported rates of STIs since 1941. The incidence of reported gonorrhea peaked at 468 cases per 100,000 population in the mid-1970s, fell to a low of 112 cases per 100,000 in 2004, and rose slightly in 2005. Because of increased testing and more sensitive tests, the incidence of reported *Chlamydia trachomatis* infection has been increasing steadily since reporting began in 1984, reaching 333 cases per 100,000 in 2005. The incidence of primary and secondary syphilis per 100,000 peaked at 71 cases in 1946, fell rapidly to 3.9 cases in 1956, ranged from ~10 to 15 cases through 1987 (with markedly increased rates among homosexual men and African Americans), and then fell to a nadir of 2.1 cases in 2000–2001 (with rates falling most rapidly among heterosexual African Americans). Unfortunately, since 1996, with the introduction of highly active antiretroviral therapy and the increased use of "serosorting" (i.e., the avoidance by some homosexual men of unprotected sex with HIV-serodiscordant partners but not with HIV-seroconcordant partners, a strategy that provides no protection against STIs other than HIV infection), gonorrhea, syphilis, and chlamydial infection have had a remarkable resurgence among homosexual men in North America and Europe, and an outbreak of a rare type of chlamydial infection (lymphogranuloma venereum; LGV) that had virtually disappeared during the AIDS era has occurred.

MANAGEMENT OF COMMON SEXUALLY TRANSMITTED DISEASE (STD) SYNDROMES

Although other chapters discuss management of specific STIs, delineating treatment based on diagnosis of a specific infection, most patients are actually managed (at least initially) on the basis of presenting symptoms and signs and associated risk factors, even in industrialized countries. Table 124-2 lists some of the most common clinical STD syndromes and their microbial etiologies. Strategies for their management are outlined below. **Chapters 181 and 182 address the management of infections with human retroviruses.**

STD care and management begin with risk assessment and proceed to clinical assessment, diagnostic testing or screening, treatment, and prevention. Indeed, the routine care of any patient begins with risk assessment (e.g., for risk of heart disease, cancer). STD/HIV risk assessment is important in primary care, urgent care, and emergency care settings as well as in specialty clinics providing adolescent, prenatal, and family planning services. STD/HIV risk assessment guides interpretation of symptoms that could reflect an STD; decisions on screening or prophylactic/preventive treatment; risk reduction counseling and intervention (e.g., hepatitis B vaccination); and notification of partners of patients with known infections. Consideration of routine demographic data (e.g., gender, age, marital status, area of residence) is

TABLE 124-2 MAJOR STD SYNDROMES AND SEXUALLY TRANSMITTED MICROBIAL ETIOLOGIES

Syndrome	ST Microbial Etiologies
AIDS	HIV types 1 and 2
Urethritis: males	*Neisseria gonorrhoeae, Chlamydia trachomatis, Mycoplasma genitalium, Ureaplasma urealyticum* (?subspecies *urealyticum*), *Trichomonas vaginalis*, HSV
Epididymitis	*C. trachomatis, N. gonorrhoeae*
Lower genital tract infections: females	
Cystitis/urethritis	*C. trachomatis, N. gonorrhoeae*, HSV
Mucopurulent cervicitis	*C. trachomatis, N. gonorrhoeae, M. genitalium*
Vulvitis	*Candida albicans*, HSV
Vulvovaginitis	*C. albicans, T. vaginalis*
Bacterial vaginosis (BV)	BV-associated bacteria (see text)
Acute pelvic inflammatory disease	*N. gonorrhoeae, C. trachomatis*, BV-associated bacteria, *M. genitalium*, group B streptococci
Infertility	*N. gonorrhoeae, C. trachomatis*, BV-associated bacteria
Ulcerative lesions of the genitalia	HSV-1, HSV-2, *Treponema pallidum, Haemophilus ducreyi, C. trachomatis* (LGV strains), *Calymmatobacterium granulomatis*
Complications of pregnancy/puerperium	Several agents implicated
Intestinal infections	
Proctitis	*C. trachomatis, N. gonorrhoeae*, HSV, *T. pallidum*
Proctocolitis or enterocolitis	*Campylobacter* spp., *Shigella* spp., *Entamoeba histolytica*, other enteric pathogens
Enteritis	*Giardia lamblia*
Acute arthritis with urogenital infection or viremia	*N. gonorrhoeae* (e.g., DGI), *C. trachomatis* (e.g., Reiter's syndrome), HBV
Genital and anal warts	HPV (30 genital types)
Mononucleosis syndrome	CMV, HIV, EBV
Hepatitis	Hepatitis viruses, *T. pallidum*, CMV, EBV
Neoplasias	
Squamous cell dysplasias and cancers of the cervix, anus, vulva, vagina, or penis	HPV (especially types 16, 18, 31, 45)
Kaposi's sarcoma, body-cavity lymphomas	HHV-8
T cell leukemia	HTLV-I
Hepatocellular carcinoma	HBV
Tropical spastic paraparesis	HTLV-I
Scabies	*Sarcoptes scabiei*
Pubic lice	*Phthirus pubis*

Note: HSV, herpes simplex virus; LGV, lymphogranuloma venereum; DGI, disseminated gonococcal infection; HPV, human papillomavirus; CMV, cytomegalovirus; EBV, Epstein-Barr virus; HBV, hepatitis B virus; HTLV, human T-cell lymphotropic virus; HHV-8, human herpesvirus type 8.

TABLE 124-3 TEN-QUESTION STD/HIV RISK ASSESSMENT

Framing Statement:
In order to provide the best care for you today and to understand your risk for certain infections, it is necessary for us to talk about your sexual behavior.

Screening Questions:
(1) Do you have any reason to think you might have a sexually transmitted disease? If so, what reason?
(2) For all adolescents <18 years old: Have you begun having any kind of sex yet?

STD History:
(3) Have you ever had any sexually transmitted diseases or any genital infections? If so, which ones?

Sexual Preference:
(4) Have you had sex with men, women, or both?

Injection Drug Use:
(5) Have you ever injected yourself ("shot up") with drugs? (If yes, have you ever shared needles or injection equipment?)
(6) Have you ever had sex with a gay or bisexual man or with anyone who had ever injected drugs?

Characteristics of Partner(s):
(7) Has your sex partner(s) had any sexually transmitted infections? If so, which ones?

STD Symptoms Checklist:
(8) Have you recently developed any of these symptoms?

For Men	For Women
(a) Discharge of pus (drip) from the penis	(a) Abnormal vaginal discharge (increased amount, abnormal odor, abnormal yellow color)
(b) Genital sores (ulcers) or rash	(b) Genital sores (ulcers), rash, or itching

Sexual Practices, Past 2 Months (for patients answering yes to any of the above questions, to guide examination and testing):
(9) Now I'd like to ask what parts of your body may have been sexually exposed to an STD (e.g., your penis, mouth, vagina, anus)?

Query about Interest in STD Screening Tests (for patients answering no to all of the above questions):
(10) Would you like to be tested for HIV or any other STDs today? (If yes, clinician can explore which STD and why.)

Source: Adapted from JR Curtis, KK Holmes, in KK Holmes et al (eds): *Sexually Transmitted Diseases*, 3d ed. New York, McGraw-Hill, 1999.

a simple first step in STD/HIV risk assessment. For example, national guidelines now recommend routine screening of sexually active females ≤25 years of age for *C. trachomatis* infection. Table 124-3 provides a set of 10 STD/HIV risk-assessment questions that clinicians can pose verbally or that health care systems can adapt (with yes/no responses) into a routine self-administered questionnaire for use in clinics. The initial framing statement gives permission to discuss taboo topics.

Risk assessment is followed by clinical assessment (elicitation of information on specific current symptoms and signs of STDs). Confirmatory diagnostic tests (for persons with symptoms or signs) or screening tests (for those without symptoms or signs) may involve microscopic examination, culture, antigen detection tests, genetic probe or amplification tests, or serology. Initial syndrome-based treatment should cover the most likely causes. For certain syndromes, results of rapid tests can narrow the spectrum of this initial therapy (e.g., wet mount of vaginal fluid for women with vaginal discharge, Gram's stain of urethral discharge for men with urethral discharge, rapid plasma reagin test for genital ulcer). After the institution of treatment, STD management proceeds to the "4 C's" of prevention and control: *c*ontact tracing (see "Prevention and Control of STIs," below), ensuring *c*ompliance with therapy, and *c*ounseling on risk reduction, including *c*ondom promotion and provision.

URETHRITIS IN MEN

Urethritis in men produces urethral discharge, dysuria, or both, usually without frequency of urination. Causes include *Neisseria gonorrhoeae, C. trachomatis, Mycoplasma genitalium, Ureaplasma urealyticum, Trichomonas vaginalis*, HSV, and perhaps adenovirus.

Until recently, *C. trachomatis* caused ~30–40% of cases of nongonococcal urethritis (NGU); however, the proportion of cases due to this organism may have declined in some populations served by effective chlamydial-control programs, and older men with urethritis appear less likely to have chlamydial infection. HSV and *T. vaginalis* each cause a small proportion of NGU cases in the United States. Recently, multiple studies have consistently implicated *M. genitalium* as a probable cause of many *Chlamydia*-negative cases. Fewer studies than in the past have implicated *Ureaplasma*; the ureaplasmas have been differentiated into *U. urealyticum* and *U. parvum*, and a few studies suggest that *U. urealyticum*—but not *U. parvum*—is associated with NGU. Coliform bacteria can cause urethritis in men who practice insertive anal intercourse. The initial diagnosis of urethritis in men currently includes specific tests only for *N. gonorrhoeae* and *C. trachomatis*. The following summarizes the approach to the patient with suspected urethritis:

1. *Establish the presence of urethritis.* If proximal-to-distal "milking" of the urethra does not express a purulent or mucopurulent discharge, even after the patient has not voided for several hours (or preferably overnight), a Gram's-stained smear of overt discharge or of an anterior urethral specimen obtained by passage of a small

urethrogenital swab 2–3 cm into the urethra usually reveals ≥5 neutrophils per 1000× field in areas containing cells; in gonococcal infection, such a smear usually reveals gram-negative intracellular diplococci as well. Alternatively, the centrifuged sediment of the first 20–30 mL of voided urine—ideally collected as the first morning specimen—can be examined for inflammatory cells, either by microscopy showing ≥10 leukocytes per high-power field or by the leukocyte esterase test. Patients with symptoms who lack objective evidence of urethritis may have functional rather than organic problems and generally do not benefit from repeated courses of antibiotics.

2. *Evaluate for complications or alternative diagnoses.* A brief history and examination will exclude epididymitis and systemic complications, such as disseminated gonococcal infection (DGI) and Reiter's syndrome. Although digital examination of the prostate gland seldom contributes to the evaluation of sexually active young men with urethritis, men with dysuria who lack evidence of urethritis as well as sexually inactive men with urethritis should undergo prostate palpation, urinalysis, and urine culture to exclude bacterial prostatitis and cystitis.
3. *Evaluate for gonococcal and chlamydial infection.* An absence of typical gram-negative diplococci on Gram's-stained smear of urethral exudate containing inflammatory cells warrants a preliminary diagnosis of NGU and should lead to testing of the urethral specimen for *C. trachomatis*. However, an increasing proportion of men with symptoms and/or signs of urethritis are simultaneously assessed for infection with *N. gonorrhoeae* and *C. trachomatis* by "multiplex" nucleic acid amplification tests (NAATs) of early-morning first-voided urine. Culture or NAAT for *N. gonorrhoeae* may be positive when Gram's staining is negative; certain strains of *N. gonorrhoeae* can result in negative urethral Gram's stains in up to 30% of cases of urethritis. Results of tests for gonococcal and chlamydial infection predict the patient's prognosis (with greater risk for recurrent NGU if neither chlamydiae nor gonococci are found than if either is detected) and can guide both the counseling given to the patient and the management of the patient's sexual partner(s).
4. *Treat urethritis promptly, while test results are pending.*

Table 124-4 summarizes the steps in management of sexually active men with urethral discharge and/or dysuria.

TABLE 124-4 MANAGEMENT OF URETHRAL DISCHARGE IN MEN

Usual causes	**Usual initial evaluation**
Chlamydia trachomatis	Demonstration of urethral discharge or pyuria
Neisseria gonorrhoeae	Exclusion of local or systemic complications
Mycoplasma genitalium	Urethral Gram's stain to confirm urethritis, detect gram-negative diplococci
Ureaplasma urealyticum	
Trichomonas vaginalis	Test for *N. gonorrhoeae*, *C. trachomatis*
Herpes simplex virus	

Initial Treatment for Patient and Partners

Treat gonorrhea (unless excluded):	plus	**Treat chlamydial infection:**
Ceftriaxone, 125 mg IM; *or*		Azithromycin, 1 g PO; *or*
Cefpodoxime, 400 mg PO;		Doxycycline, 100 mg bid for 7 days
or		
Cefixime, 400 mg PO[a]		

Management of Recurrence

Confirm objective evidence of urethritis. If patient was reexposed to untreated or new partner, repeat treatment of patient and partner.
If patient was not reexposed, consider infection with *T. vaginalis*[b] or doxycycline-resistant *M. genitalium* or *Ureaplasma*, and consider treatment with metronidazole, azithromycin, or both.

[a]Updates on the availability of cefixime can be obtained from the Centers for Disease Control and Prevention or state health departments.
[b]In men, the diagnosis of *T. vaginalis* infection requires culture (or nucleic acid amplification test, where available) of early-morning first-voided urine sediment or of a urethral swab specimen obtained before voiding.

℞ URETHRITIS IN MEN

In practice, if Gram's stain does not reveal gonococci, urethritis is treated with a regimen effective for NGU, such as azithromycin (1.0 g PO in a single dose) or doxycycline (100 mg PO bid for 7 days). Both are effective, although azithromycin may give better results in *M. genitalium* infection. If gonococci are demonstrated by Gram's stain or if no diagnostic tests are performed to exclude gonorrhea definitively, treatment should include a single-dose regimen for gonorrhea (Chap. 137) plus azithromycin or doxycycline treatment for *C. trachomatis*, which frequently occurs as a urethral co-infection in men with gonococcal urethritis. Sexual partners should be tested for gonorrhea and chlamydial infection and should receive the same regimen given to the male index case. Patients with confirmed persistence or recurrence of urethritis after treatment should be re-treated with the initial regimen if they did not comply with the original treatment or were reexposed to an untreated partner. Otherwise, an intraurethral swab specimen and a first-voided urine sample should be tested for *T. vaginalis* (currently best done by culture, although NAATs appear to be more sensitive and are likely to become commercially available in the future). If compliance with initial treatment is confirmed and reexposure excluded, the recommended treatment is with metronidazole or tinidazole (2 g PO in a single dose) plus azithromycin (1 g PO in a single dose); the azithromycin component is especially important if this drug has not been given during initial therapy.

EPIDIDYMITIS

Acute epididymitis, almost always unilateral, produces pain, swelling, and tenderness of the epididymis, with or without symptoms or signs of urethritis. This condition must be differentiated from testicular torsion, tumor, and trauma. Torsion, a surgical emergency, usually occurs in the second or third decade of life and produces a sudden onset of pain, elevation of the testicle within the scrotal sac, rotation of the epididymis from a posterior to an anterior position, and absence of blood flow on Doppler examination or ^{99m}Tc scan. Persistence of symptoms after a course of therapy for epididymitis suggests the possibility of testicular tumor or of a chronic granulomatous disease, such as tuberculosis. In sexually active men under age 35, acute epididymitis is caused most frequently by *C. trachomatis* and less commonly by *N. gonorrhoeae* and is usually associated with overt or subclinical urethritis. Acute epididymitis occurring in older men or following urinary tract instrumentation is usually caused by urinary pathogens. Similarly, epididymitis in men who have practiced insertive rectal intercourse is often caused by Enterobacteriaceae. These men usually have no urethritis but do have bacteriuria.

℞ EPIDIDYMITIS

Ceftriaxone (250 mg as a single dose IM) followed by doxycycline (100 mg PO twice daily for 10 days) constitutes effective treatment for epididymitis caused by *N. gonorrhoeae* or *C. trachomatis*. Fluoroquinolones are no longer recommended for treatment of gonorrhea in the United States because of the emergence of resistant strains of *N. gonorrhoeae*, especially (but not only) among homosexual men (**Fig. 124-1**). Levofloxacin (500 mg PO once daily for 10 days) is also effective for syndrome-based initial treatment of epididymitis when infection with Enterobacteriaceae is suspected; however, this regimen should probably be combined with effective therapy for possible gonococcal or chlamydial infection unless bacteriuria with Enterobacteriaceae is confirmed.

URETHRITIS AND THE URETHRAL SYNDROME IN WOMEN

C. trachomatis, *N. gonorrhoeae*, and occasionally HSV cause symptomatic urethritis—known as the urethral syndrome in women—that is characterized by "internal" dysuria (usually without urinary urgency or frequency), pyuria, and an absence of *Escherichia coli* and other uropathogens in urine at counts of ≥10^2/mL. In contrast, the dysuria associated with vulvar herpes or vulvovaginal candidiasis (and perhaps with trichomoniasis) is often described as "external," being caused by painful contact of urine with the inflamed or ulcerated labia

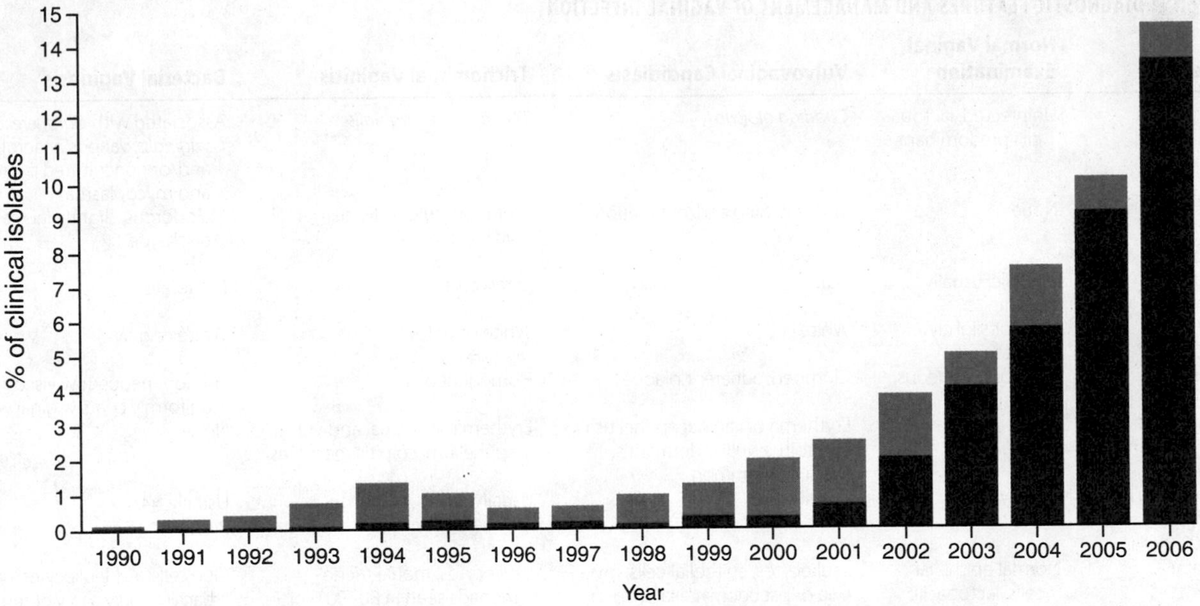

FIGURE 124-1 Percentage of *N. gonorrhoeae* isolates with intermediate resistance or resistance to ciprofloxacin, by year: Gonococcal Isolate Surveillance Project, United States, 1990–2006. Data for 2006 are preliminary (January–June only). ■, Intermediate resistance [ciprofloxacin minimum inhibitory concentrations (MICs) of 0.125–0.500 μg/mL]. ■, Resistance (ciprofloxacin MICs of ≥1.0 μg/mL). *(From Centers for Disease Control and Prevention: MMWR 56:332, 2007.)*

or introitus. Acute onset, association with urinary urgency or frequency, hematuria, or suprapubic bladder tenderness suggests bacterial cystitis. Among women with symptoms of acute bacterial cystitis, costovertebral pain and tenderness or fever suggests acute pyelonephritis. The management of bacterial urinary tract infection (UTI) is discussed in Chap. 282.

Signs of vulvovaginitis, coupled with symptoms of external dysuria, suggest vulvar infection (e.g., with HSV or *Candida albicans*). Among dysuric women without signs of vulvovaginitis, bacterial UTI must be differentiated from the urethral syndrome by assessment of risk, evaluation of the pattern of symptoms and signs, and specific microbiologic testing. An STI etiology of the urethral syndrome is suggested by young age, more than one current sexual partner, a new partner within the past month, a partner with urethritis, or coexisting mucopurulent cervicitis (see below). The finding of a single urinary pathogen, such as *E. coli* or *Staphylococcus saprophyticus*, at a concentration of $\geq 10^2$/mL in a properly collected specimen of midstream urine from a dysuric woman with pyuria indicates probable bacterial UTI, whereas pyuria with $<10^2$ conventional uropathogens per milliliter of urine ("sterile" pyuria) suggests acute urethral syndrome due to *C. trachomatis* or *N. gonorrhoeae*. Gonorrhea and chlamydial infection should be sought by specific tests (e.g., NAATs on the first 10 mL of voided urine). Among dysuric women with sterile pyuria caused by infection with *N. gonorrhoeae* or *C. trachomatis*, appropriate treatment alleviates dysuria.

VULVOVAGINAL INFECTIONS

Abnormal Vaginal Discharge If directly questioned about vaginal discharge during routine health checkups, many women acknowledge having nonspecific symptoms of vaginal discharge that do not correlate with objective signs of inflammation or with actual infection. However, unsolicited reporting of abnormal vaginal discharge does suggest bacterial vaginosis or trichomoniasis. Specifically, an abnormally increased amount or an abnormal odor of the discharge is associated with one or both of these conditions. Cervical infection with *N. gonorrhoeae* or *C. trachomatis* does not appear to cause an increased amount or abnormal odor of discharge, but cervicitis, like trichomoniasis, can include the production of an increased number of neutrophils in vaginal fluid, resulting in a yellow color. Vulvar conditions such as genital herpes or vulvovaginal candidiasis can cause vulvar pruritus, burning, irritation, or lesions as well as external dysuria (as urine passes over the inflamed vulva) or vulvar dyspareunia.

Certain vulvovaginal infections may have serious sequelae. Trichomoniasis, bacterial vaginosis, and vulvovaginal candidiasis have all been associated with increased risk of acquisition of HIV infection. Vaginal trichomoniasis and bacterial vaginosis early in pregnancy independently predict premature onset of labor. Bacterial vaginosis can also lead to anaerobic bacterial infection of the endometrium and salpinges. Vaginitis may be an early and prominent feature of toxic shock syndrome, and recurrent or chronic vulvovaginal candidiasis develops with increased frequency among women with systemic illnesses, such as diabetes mellitus or HIV-related immunosuppression (although only a very small proportion of women with recurrent vulvovaginal candidiasis in industrialized countries actually have a serious predisposing illness).

Thus vulvovaginal symptoms or signs warrant careful evaluation, including pelvic examination, simple rapid diagnostic tests, and appropriate therapy specific for the anatomic site and type of infection. Unfortunately, a survey in the United States indicated that clinicians seldom perform the tests required to establish the cause of such symptoms. Further, comparison of telephone and office management of vulvovaginal symptoms has documented the inaccuracy of the former, and comparison of evaluations by nurse-midwives with those by physician-practitioners showed that the practitioners' clinical evaluations correlated poorly both with the nurses' evaluations and with diagnostic tests. The diagnosis and treatment of the three most common types of vaginal infection are summarized in Table 124-5.

Inspection of the vulva and perineum may reveal tender genital ulcerations (typically due to HSV infection, occasionally due to chancroid) or fissures (typically due to vulvovaginal candidiasis) or discharge visible at the introitus before insertion of a speculum (suggestive of bacterial vaginosis or trichomoniasis). Speculum examination permits the clinician to discern whether the discharge in fact looks abnormal and whether any abnormal discharge in the vagina emanates from the cervical os (mucoid and, if abnormal, yellow) or from the vagina (not mucoid, since the vaginal epithelium does not produce mucus). Symptoms or signs of abnormal vaginal discharge should prompt testing of vaginal fluid for pH, for a fishy odor when mixed with 10% KOH, and for certain microscopic features when mixed with saline (motile trichomonads and/or "clue cells") and with

TABLE 124-5 DIAGNOSTIC FEATURES AND MANAGEMENT OF VAGINAL INFECTION

Feature	Normal Vaginal Examination	Vulvovaginal Candidiasis	Trichomonal Vaginitis	Bacterial Vaginosis
Etiology	Uninfected; lactobacilli predominant	*Candida albicans*	*Trichomonas vaginalis*	Associated with *Gardnerella vaginalis*, various anaerobic and/or noncultured bacteria, and mycoplasmas
Typical symptoms	None	Vulvar itching and/or irritation	Profuse purulent discharge; vulvar itching	Malodorous, slightly increased discharge
Discharge				
Amount	Variable; usually scant	Scant	Often profuse	Moderate
Color[a]	Clear or slightly white	White	White or yellow	White or gray
Consistency	Nonhomogeneous, floccular	Clumped; adherent plaques	Homogeneous	Homogeneous, low viscosity; uniformly coats vaginal walls
Inflammation of vulvar or vaginal epithelium	None	Erythema of vaginal epithelium, introitus; vulvar dermatitis, fissures common	Erythema of vaginal and vulvar epithelium; colpitis macularis	None
pH of vaginal fluid[b]	Usually ≤4.5	Usually ≤4.5	Usually ≥5.0	Usually >4.5
Amine ("fishy") odor with 10% KOH	None	None	May be present	Present
Microscopy[c]	Normal epithelial cells; lactobacilli predominant	Leukocytes, epithelial cells; mycelia or pseudomycelia in up to 80% of *C. albicans* culture-positive persons with typical symptoms	Leukocytes; motile trichomonads seen in 80–90% of symptomatic patients, less often in the absence of symptoms	Clue cells; few leukocytes; no lactobacilli or only a few outnumbered by profuse mixed flora, nearly always including *G. vaginalis* plus anaerobic species on Gram's stain (Nugent's score ≥7)
Other laboratory findings		Isolation of *Candida* spp.	Isolation of *T. vaginalis* or positive NAAT[d]	
Usual treatment	None	Azole cream, tablet, or suppository—e.g., miconazole 100-mg vaginal suppository or clotrimazole 100-mg vaginal tablet, once daily for 7 days Fluconazole, 150 mg orally (single dose)	Metronidazole or tinidazole, 2 g orally (single dose) Metronidazole, 500 mg PO bid for 7 days	Metronidazole, 500 mg PO bid for 7 days Clindamycin, 2% cream, one full applicator vaginally each night for 7 days
Usual management of sexual partner	None	None; topical treatment if candidal dermatitis of penis is detected	Examination for STD; treatment with metronidazole, 2 g PO (single dose)	Examination for STD; no treatment if normal

[a]Color of discharge is best determined by examination against the white background of a swab.
[b]pH determination is not useful if blood is present.
[c]To detect fungal elements, vaginal fluid is digested with 10% KOH prior to microscopic examination; to examine for other features, fluid is mixed (1:1) with physiologic saline. Gram's stain is also excellent for detecting yeasts (less predictive of vulvovaginitis) and pseudomycelia or mycelin (strongly predictive of vulvovaginitis) and for distinguishing normal flora from the mixed flora seen in bacterial vaginosis, but it is less sensitive than the saline preparation for detection of *T. vaginalis*.
[d]NAAT, nucleic acid amplification test (where available).

10% KOH (pseudohyphae or hyphae indicative of vulvovaginal candidiasis). Additional objective laboratory tests useful for establishing the cause of abnormal vaginal discharge include Gram's staining to detect alterations in the vaginal flora; card tests for bacterial vaginosis, as described below; and a DNA probe test (the Affirm test) to detect *T. vaginalis* and *C. albicans* as well as the increased concentrations of *Gardnerella vaginalis* associated with bacterial vaginosis.

℞ VAGINAL DISCHARGE

Patterns of treatment for vaginal discharge vary widely. In developing countries, where clinics or pharmacies often dispense treatment based on symptoms alone without examination or testing, oral treatment with metronidazole—either as a 2-g single dose or as a 7-day regimen—provides reasonable coverage against both trichomoniasis and bacterial vaginosis, the usual causes of symptoms of vaginal discharge; metronidazole treatment of sex partners prevents reinfection of women with trichomoniasis, even though it does not help prevent the recurrence of bacterial vaginosis. Guidelines promulgated during the 1990s by the World Health Organization suggested treatment for cervical infection and for vulvovaginal candidiasis in women with symptoms of abnormal vaginal discharge; in retrospect, these recommendations were faulty, since these conditions seldom produce such symptoms.

In industrialized countries, clinicians treating symptoms and signs of abnormal vaginal discharge should at least differentiate between bacterial vaginosis and trichomoniasis, because optimal management of patients and partners differs for these two conditions (as discussed briefly below).

Vaginal Trichomoniasis (See also Chap. 208) Symptomatic trichomoniasis characteristically produces a profuse, yellow, purulent, homogeneous vaginal discharge and vulvar irritation, often with visible inflammation of the vaginal and vulvar epithelium and petechial lesions on the cervix (the so-called strawberry cervix, usually evident only by colposcopy). The pH of vaginal fluid usually rises to ≥5.0. In women with typical symptoms and signs of trichomoniasis, microscopic examination of vaginal discharge mixed with saline reveals motile trichomonads in most culture-positive cases. However, in the absence of symptoms or signs, culture is often required for detection of the organism. NAAT for *T. vaginalis* is as sensitive as or more sensitive than culture, and NAAT of urine has disclosed surprisingly high prevalences of this pathogen among men at several STD clinics in the United States. Treatment of asymptomatic as well as symptomatic cases reduces rates of transmission and prevents later development of symptoms.

℞ VAGINAL TRICHOMONIASIS

Only nitroimidazoles (e.g., metronidazole and tinidazole) consistently cure trichomoniasis. A single 2-g oral dose of metronidazole is effective and much less expensive than the alternatives. Tinidazole has a longer half-life than metronidazole and is useful in treating trichomoniasis that fails to respond to metronidazole. Treatment of male sexual partners—often facilitated by dispensing metronidazole to the female patient to give to her partner(s), with a warning about avoiding the concurrent use of alcohol—significantly reduces both the risk of reinfection and the reservoir of infection; treating the partner is the standard of care. Treatment with 0.75% metronidazole gel intravaginally, although moderately effective for bacterial vaginosis, is not reliable for vaginal trichomoniasis. Systemic use of metronidazole is not recommended during the first trimester of pregnancy but is considered safe thereafter. In a large randomized trial, metronidazole treatment of trichomoniasis during pregnancy did not reduce—and in fact actually increased—the frequency of perinatal morbidity.

Bacterial Vaginosis This syndrome (formerly termed *nonspecific vaginitis, Haemophilus vaginitis, anaerobic vaginitis*, or *Gardnerella-associated vaginal discharge*) is characterized by symptoms of vaginal malodor and a slightly to moderately increased white discharge, which appears homogeneous, is low in viscosity, and evenly coats the vaginal mucosa. An interesting observation is that new genital HPV infection in young women is associated with increased subsequent risk of developing bacterial vaginosis. Other risk factors include multiple sexual partners and recent intercourse with a new partner, but metronidazole treatment of male partners has not reduced the rate of recurrence among affected women.

Among women with bacterial vaginosis, culture of vaginal fluid has shown markedly increased prevalences and concentrations of *G. vaginalis, Mycoplasma hominis*, and several anaerobic bacteria [e.g., *Mobiluncus* spp., *Prevotella* spp. (formerly *Bacteroides* spp.), and some *Peptostreptococcus* spp.] as well as an absence of hydrogen peroxide–producing *Lactobacillus* spp., which constitute most of the normal vaginal flora and perhaps help protect against certain cervical and vaginal infections. The use of broad-range polymerase chain reaction (PCR) amplification of 16S rDNA in vaginal fluid, with subsequent identification of specific bacterial species by various methods, has documented an even greater and unexpected bacterial diversity, including several unique species not previously cultivated [e.g., three species in the order Clostridiales that appear to be specific for bacterial vaginosis (Fig. 124-2)]. Also detected are DNA sequences related to *Atopobium vaginae*, an organism that is strongly associated with bacterial vaginosis, is resistant to metronidazole, and is associated with recurrent bacterial vaginosis after metronidazole treatment. Other species newly implicated in bacterial vaginosis include *Lactobacillus iners, Megasphaera, Leptotrichia, Eggerthella*, and *Dialister*.

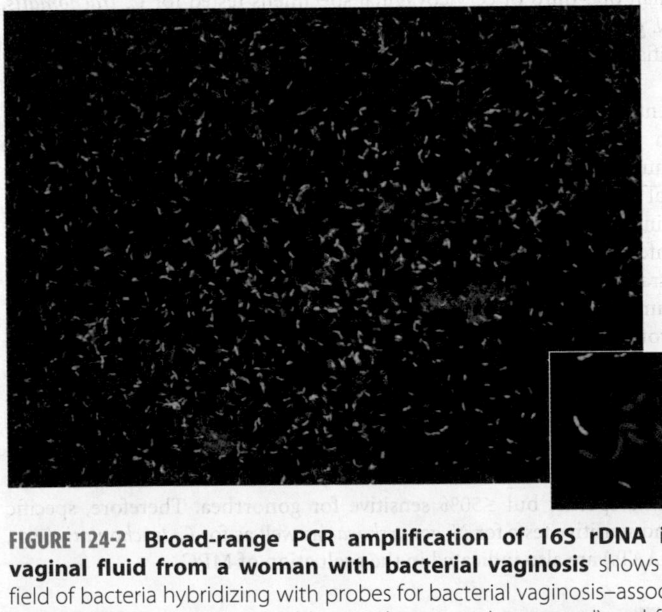

FIGURE 124-2 Broad-range PCR amplification of 16S rDNA in vaginal fluid from a woman with bacterial vaginosis shows a field of bacteria hybridizing with probes for bacterial vaginosis–associated bacterium 1 (BVAB1, visible as a thin, curved green rod) and for *Mobiluncus* (red). The inset shows that *Mobiluncus* (red) is larger than BVAB1 (green) but that the two have a similar morphology (curved rod). (*Reprinted with permission from DN Fredricks et al.*)

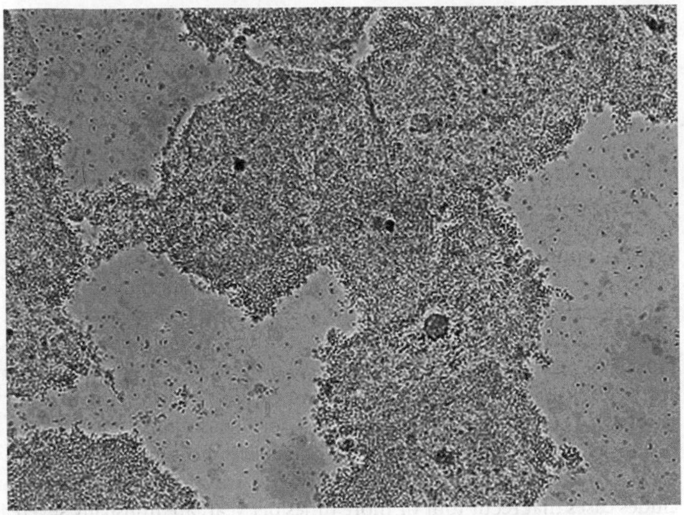

FIGURE 124-3 Wet mount of vaginal fluid showing typical clue cells from a woman with bacterial vaginosis. Note the obscured epithelial cell margins and the granular appearance attributable to many adherent bacteria (× 400). [*Photograph provided by Lorna K. Rabe, reprinted with permission from S Hillier et al, in KK Holmes et al (eds). Sexually Transmitted Diseases, 4th ed. New York, McGraw-Hill, 2008.*]

Bacterial vaginosis is conventionally diagnosed clinically with the Amsel criteria, which include any three of the following four clinical abnormalities: (1) objective signs of increased white homogeneous vaginal discharge; (2) a vaginal discharge pH of >4.5; (3) liberation of a distinct fishy odor (attributable to volatile amines such as trimethylamine) immediately after vaginal secretions are mixed with a 10% solution of KOH; and (4) microscopic demonstration of "clue cells" (vaginal epithelial cells coated with coccobacillary organisms, which have a granular appearance and indistinct borders; Fig. 124-3) on a wet mount prepared by mixing vaginal secretions with normal saline in a ratio of ~1:1.

℞ BACTERIAL VAGINOSIS

The standard dosage of metronidazole for the treatment of bacterial vaginosis is 500 mg PO twice daily for 7 days. The single 2-g oral dose of metronidazole recommended for trichomoniasis produces somewhat lower short-term cure rates. Intravaginal treatment with 2% clindamycin cream [one full applicator (5 g containing 100 mg of clindamycin phosphate) each night for 7 nights] or with 0.75% metronidazole gel [one full applicator (5 g containing 37.5 mg of metronidazole) twice daily for 5 days] is also approved for use in the United States and does not elicit systemic adverse reactions. Oral clindamycin (300 mg bid for 7 days) and clindamycin ovules (100 g intravaginally once at bedtime for 3 days) have also been approved. Unfortunately, long-term recurrence (i.e., several months later) is distressingly common after either oral or intravaginal treatment. A randomized trial comparing this intravaginal gel containing 37.5 mg of metronidazole with a suppository containing 500 mg of metronidazole plus nystatin (the latter not marketed in the United States) showed significantly higher rates of recurrent bacterial vaginosis with the 37.5-mg regimen; this result suggests that higher metronidazole dosages may be important in topical intravaginal therapy. Treatment of male partners with metronidazole does not prevent recurrence of bacterial vaginosis.

A randomized trial of orally ingested lactobacilli found reduced rates of recurrent bacterial vaginosis; however, this result has not yet been either confirmed or refuted. A randomized multicenter trial in the United States found no benefit of repeated intravaginal inoculation of a vaginal peroxide-producing *Lactobacillus* species following treatment of bacterial vaginosis with metronidazole. A meta-analysis of 18 studies concluded that bacterial vaginosis during pregnancy substantially increased the risk of preterm delivery and of spontaneous abortion. However, most studies of topical intravaginal treatment of bacterial vaginosis with clindamycin during pregnancy have not reduced adverse pregnancy outcomes. Numerous trials of oral metronidazole treatment during pregnancy have given inconsistent results, and a 2007 Cochrane review concluded that antenatal treatment of women with bacterial vaginosis—even those with previous preterm delivery—did not reduce the risk of preterm delivery.

Vulvovaginal Pruritus, Burning, or Irritation Vulvovaginal candidiasis produces vulvar pruritus, burning, or irritation, generally without symptoms of increased vaginal discharge or malodor. Genital herpes can produce similar symptoms, with lesions sometimes difficult to distinguish from the fissures and inflammation caused by candidiasis. Signs of vulvovaginal candidiasis include vulvar erythema, edema, fissures, and tenderness. With candidiasis, a white scanty vaginal discharge sometimes takes the form of white thrush-like plaques or cottage cheese–like curds adhering loosely to the vaginal mucosa. *C. albicans* accounts for nearly all cases of symptomatic vulvovaginal candidiasis, which probably arise from endogenous strains of *C. albicans* that have colonized the vagina or the intestinal tract. Complicated vulvovaginal candidiasis includes cases that recur four or more times per year; are unusually severe; are caused by non-*albicans Candida* spp.; or occur in women with uncontrolled diabetes, debilitation, immunosuppression, or pregnancy.

The diagnosis of vulvovaginal candidiasis usually involves the demonstration of pseudohyphae or hyphae by microscopic examination of vaginal fluid mixed with saline or 10% KOH or subjected to Gram's staining. Microscopic examination is less sensitive than culture but correlates better with symptoms.

℞ VULVOVAGINAL PRURITUS, BURNING, OR IRRITATION

Symptoms and signs of vulvovaginal candidiasis warrant treatment, usually intravaginal administration of any of several imidazole antibiotics (e.g., miconazole or clotrimazole) for 3–7 days (Table 124-5). Over-the-counter marketing of such preparations has reduced the cost of care and made treatment more convenient for many women with recurrent yeast vulvovaginitis. However, most women who purchase these preparations do not have vulvovaginal candidiasis, while many do have other vaginal infections that require different treatment. Therefore, only women with classic symptoms of vulvar pruritus and a history of previous episodes of yeast vulvovaginitis documented by an experienced clinician should self-treat. Short-course topical intravaginal azole drugs are effective for the treatment of uncomplicated vulvovaginal candidiasis (e.g., clotrimazole, two 100-mg vaginal tablets daily for 3 days; or miconazole, a 1200-mg vaginal suppository as a single dose). Single-dose oral treatment with fluconazole (150 mg) is also effective and is preferred by many patients. Management of complicated cases (see above) and those that do not respond to the usual intravaginal or single-dose oral therapy often involves prolonged or periodic oral therapy; this situation is discussed extensively in the 2006 STD treatment guidelines published by the CDC. Treatment of sexual partners is not routinely indicated.

Other Causes of Vaginal Discharge or Vaginitis In the ulcerative vaginitis associated with staphylococcal toxic shock syndrome, *Staphylococcus aureus* should be promptly identified in vaginal fluid by Gram's stain and by culture. In desquamative inflammatory vaginitis, smears of vaginal fluid reveal neutrophils, massive vaginal epithelial-cell exfoliation with increased numbers of parabasal cells, and gram-positive cocci; this syndrome may respond to treatment with 2% clindamycin cream. Additional causes of vaginitis and vulvovaginal symptoms include retained foreign bodies (e.g., tampons), cervical caps, vaginal spermicides, vaginal antiseptic preparations or douches, vaginal epithelial atrophy (in postmenopausal women or during prolonged breast-feeding in the postpartum period), allergic reactions to latex condoms, vaginal aphthae associated with HIV infection or Behçet's syndrome, and vestibulitis (a poorly understood syndrome).

MUCOPURULENT CERVICITIS

Mucopurulent cervicitis (MPC) refers to inflammation of the columnar epithelium and subepithelium of the endocervix and of any contiguous columnar epithelium that lies exposed in an ectopic position on the exocervix. MPC in women represents the "silent partner" of urethritis in men, being equally common and often caused by the same agents (*N. gonorrhoeae*, *C. trachomatis*, or—as shown by case-control studies—*M. genitalium*); however, MPC is more difficult than urethritis to recognize. As the most common manifestation of these serious bacterial infections in women, MPC can be a harbinger or sign of upper genital tract infection, also known as *pelvic inflammatory disease* (PID; see below). In pregnant women, MPC can lead to obstetric complications. In a prospective study in Seattle of 167 consecutive patients with MPC [defined on the basis of yellow endocervical mucopus or ≥30 polymorphonuclear leukocytes (PMNs)/1000× microscopic field] who were seen at STD clinics during the 1980s, slightly more than one-third of cervicovaginal specimens tested for *C. trachomatis*, *N. gonorrhoeae*, *M. genitalium*, HSV, and *T. vaginalis* revealed no identifiable etiology (Fig. 124-4).

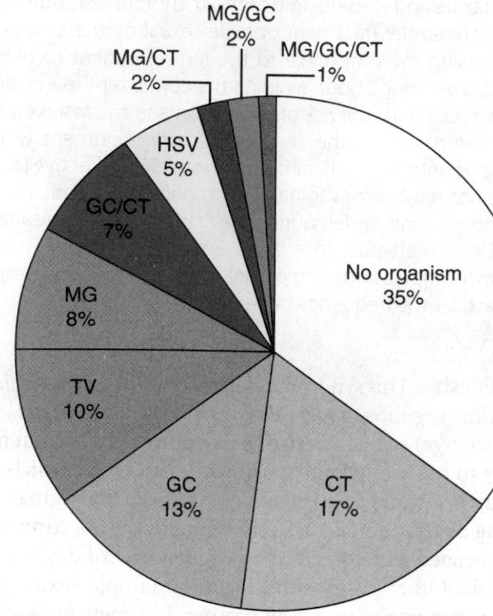

FIGURE 124-4 Organisms detected among female STD clinic patients with mucopurulent cervicitis (n = 167). GC, gonococcus; CT, *Chlamydia trachomatis*; MG, *Mycoplasma genitalium*; TV, *Trichomonas vaginalis*; HSV, herpes simplex virus. (*Courtesy of Dr. Lisa Manhart; with permission.*)

The diagnosis of MPC rests on the detection of yellow mucopurulent discharge from the cervical os or of increased numbers of PMNs in Gram's-stained or Papanicolaou-stained smears of endocervical mucus. MPC due to *C. trachomatis* can also produce edematous cervical ectopy (see below) and endocervical bleeding upon gentle swabbing. Unlike the endocervicitis produced by gonococcal or chlamydial infection, cervicitis caused by HSV produces ulcerative lesions on the stratified squamous epithelium of the exocervix as well as on the columnar epithelium. Yellow cervical mucus on a white swab removed from the endocervix indicates the presence of PMNs. The mucus should be rolled thinly on a slide for Gram's staining. The presence of ≥20 PMNs/1000× microscopic field within strands of cervical mucus not contaminated by vaginal squamous epithelial cells or vaginal bacteria indicates endocervicitis (Fig. 124-5). Detection of intracellular gram-negative diplococci in carefully collected endocervical mucus is quite specific but ≤50% sensitive for gonorrhea. Therefore, specific and sensitive tests for *N. gonorrhoeae* as well as for *C. trachomatis* (e.g., NAATs) are also indicated in the evaluation of MPC.

℞ MUCOPURULENT CERVICITIS

Although the above criteria for MPC are neither highly specific nor highly predictive of gonococcal or chlamydial infection in some settings, the

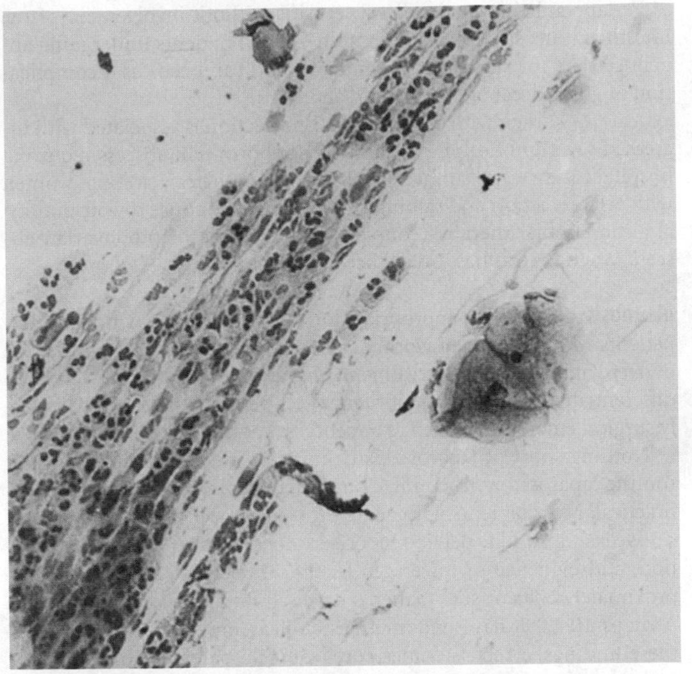

FIGURE 124-5 Gram's stain of cervical mucus, showing a strand of cervical mucus containing many polymorphonuclear leukocytes. This picture is typical of mucopurulent cervicitis. Note that leukocytes are not seen in areas of the slide containing vaginal epithelial cells, adjacent to the mucus strands.

2006 CDC guidelines call for consideration of empirical treatment for MPC, pending test results, in certain patients. Treatment with antibiotics active against *C. trachomatis* should be provided for women at increased risk for this common STI (risk factors: age <25 years, new or multiple sex partners, and unprotected sex), especially if follow-up connot be ensured and if a relatively insensitive diagnostic test (not a NAAT) is used. Concurrent therapy for gonorrhea is indicated if the prevalence of this infection is high (>5%) in the relevant patient population (e.g., young adults, a clinic with documented high prevalence). In this situation, therapy should include a single-dose regimen effective for gonorrhea plus treatment for chlamydial infection, as outlined in Table 124-4 for the treatment of urethritis. In settings where gonorrhea is much less common than chlamydial infection, initial therapy for chlamydial infection alone suffices, pending test results for gonorrhea. The etiology and potential benefit of treatment for endocervicitis not associated with gonorrhea or chlamydial infection have not been established. Although the antimicrobial susceptibility of *M. genitalium* is not yet well defined, the organism frequently persists after doxycycline therapy, and it currently seems reasonable to use azithromycin to treat possible *M. genitalium* infection in such cases. The sexual partner(s) of a woman with MPC should be examined and given a regimen similar to that chosen for the woman unless results of tests for gonorrhea or chlamydial infection in either partner warrant different therapy or no therapy.

CERVICAL ECTOPY

Cervical ectopy, often mislabeled "cervical erosion," is easily confused with infectious endocervicitis. Ectopy represents the presence of the one-cell-thick columnar epithelium extending from the endocervix out onto the visible ectocervix. In ectopy, the cervical os may contain clear or slightly cloudy mucus but usually not yellow mucopus. Colposcopy shows intact epithelium. Normally found during adolescence and early adulthood, ectopy gradually recedes through the second and third decades of life, as squamous metaplasia replaces the ectopic columnar epithelium. Oral contraceptive use favors the persistence or reappearance of ectopy, while smoking apparently accelerates squamous metaplasia. Cauterization of ectopy is not warranted. Ectopy may render the cervix more susceptible to infection with *N. gonorrhoeae*, *C. trachomatis*, or HIV.

PELVIC INFLAMMATORY DISEASE

The term *pelvic inflammatory disease* usually refers to infection that ascends from the cervix or vagina to involve the endometrium and/or fallopian tubes. Infection can extend beyond the reproductive tract to cause pelvic peritonitis, generalized peritonitis, perihepatitis, perisplenitis, or pelvic abscess. Rarely in young women, infection not related to STI extends secondarily to the pelvic organs (1) from adjacent foci of inflammation (e.g., appendicitis, regional ileitis, or diverticulitis), (2) as a result of hematogenous dissemination (e.g., of tuberculosis), or (3) as a complication of certain tropical diseases (e.g., schistosomiasis). Intrauterine infection can be primary (spontaneously occurring and usually sexually transmitted) or secondary to invasive intrauterine surgical procedures [e.g., dilatation and curettage, termination of pregnancy, insertion of an intrauterine device (IUD), or hysterosalpingography] or to parturition.

Etiology The agents most often implicated in acute PID include the primary causes of endocervicitis (e.g., *N. gonorrhoeae* and *C. trachomatis*) and organisms that can be regarded as components of an altered vaginal flora. In general, PID is most often caused by *N. gonorrhoeae* where there is a high incidence of gonorrhea—e.g., in developing countries and in indigent inner-city populations in the United States. In recent case-control studies, *M. genitalium* has also been significantly associated with histopathologic diagnoses of endometritis and with salpingitis.

Anaerobic and facultative organisms (especially *Prevotella* species, peptostreptococci, *E. coli*, *Haemophilus influenzae*, and group B streptococci) as well as genital mycoplasmas have been isolated from the peritoneal fluid or fallopian tubes in a varying proportion (typically one-fourth to one-third) of women with PID studied in the United States. The difficulty of determining the exact microbial etiology of an individual case of PID—short of using invasive procedures for specimen collection—has implications for the approach to empirical antimicrobial treatment of this infection.

Epidemiology In the United States, the estimated annual number of initial visits to physicians' offices for PID by women 15–44 years of age fell from an average of 400,000 during the 1980s to 250,000 in 1999 and then to 176,000 in 2005. Hospitalizations for acute PID in the United States also declined steadily throughout the 1980s and early 1990s but have remained fairly constant at 70,000–100,000 per year since 1995. Important risk factors for acute PID include the presence of endocervical infection or bacterial vaginosis, a history of salpingitis or of recent vaginal douching, and the use of an IUD (especially among nulliparous women, during the first few months after IUD insertion, and among women with multiple sex partners). Certain other iatrogenic factors, such as dilatation and curettage or cesarean section, can increase the risk of PID, especially among women with endocervical gonococcal or chlamydial infection or bacterial vaginosis. Symptoms of *N. gonorrhoeae*–associated and *C. trachomatis*–associated PID often begin during or soon after the menstrual period; this timing suggests that menstruation is a risk factor for ascending infection from the cervix and vagina. Experimental inoculation of the fallopian tubes of lower primates has shown that repeated exposure to *C. trachomatis* leads to the greatest degree of tissue inflammation and damage; thus, immunopathology probably contributes to the pathogenesis of chlamydial salpingitis. Women using oral contraceptives appear to be at decreased risk of symptomatic PID, and tubal sterilization reduces the risk of salpingitis by preventing intraluminal spread of infection into the tubes.

Clinical Manifestations • ***ENDOMETRITIS: A CLINICAL PATHOLOGIC SYNDROME*** A study of women with clinically suspected PID who were undergoing both endometrial biopsy and laparoscopy showed that those with endometritis alone differed from those who also had salpingitis in significantly less often having lower quadrant, adnexal, or cervical motion or abdominal rebound tenderness; fever; or elevated C-reactive protein levels. In addition, women with endometritis alone differed from those with neither endometritis nor salpingitis in more often having gonorrhea, chlamydial infection, and risk factors such as douching or IUD use. Thus, women with endometritis alone were intermediate between those with neither endometritis nor salpingitis and those with salpingitis with respect to risk factors, clinical manifestations, cervical infection prevalence, and elevated C-reactive protein level. Women with endometritis alone are at lower risk of subsequent tubal occlusion and resulting infertility than are those with salpingitis.

SALPINGITIS Symptoms of nontuberculous salpingitis classically evolve from a yellow or malodorous vaginal discharge caused by MPC and/or bacterial vaginosis to midline abdominal pain and abnormal vaginal bleeding caused by endometritis and then to bilateral lower abdominal and pelvic pain caused by salpingitis, with nausea, vomiting, and increased abdominal tenderness if peritonitis develops.

The abdominal pain in nontuberculous salpingitis is usually described as dull or aching. In some cases, pain is lacking or atypical, but active inflammatory changes are found in the course of an unrelated evaluation or procedure, such as a laparoscopic evaluation for infertility. Abnormal uterine bleeding precedes or coincides with the onset of pain in ~40% of women with PID, symptoms of urethritis (dysuria) occur in 20%, and symptoms of proctitis (anorectal pain, tenesmus, and rectal discharge or bleeding) are occasionally seen in women with gonococcal or chlamydial infection.

Speculum examination shows evidence of MPC (yellow endocervical discharge, easily induced endocervical bleeding) in the majority of women with gonococcal or chlamydial PID. Cervical motion tenderness is produced by stretching of the adnexal attachments on the side toward which the cervix is pushed. Bimanual examination reveals uterine fundal tenderness due to endometritis and abnormal adnexal tenderness due to salpingitis that is usually, but not necessarily, bilateral. Adnexal swelling is palpable in about one-half of women with acute salpingitis, but evaluation of the adnexae in a patient with marked tenderness is not reliable. The initial temperature is >38°C in only about one-third of patients with acute salpingitis. Laboratory findings include elevation of the erythrocyte sedimentation rate (ESR) in 75% of patients with acute salpingitis and elevation of the peripheral white blood cell count in up to 60%.

Unlike nontuberculous salpingitis, genital tuberculosis often occurs in older women, many of whom are postmenopausal. Presenting symptoms include abnormal vaginal bleeding, pain (including dysmenorrhea), and infertility. About one-quarter of these women have had adnexal masses. Endometrial biopsy shows tuberculous granulomas and provides optimal specimens for culture.

PERIHEPATITIS AND PERIAPPENDICITIS Pleuritic upper abdominal pain and tenderness (usually localized to the right upper quadrant) develop in 3–10% of women with acute PID. Symptoms of perihepatitis arise during or after the onset of symptoms of PID and may overshadow lower abdominal symptoms, thereby leading to a mistaken diagnosis of cholecystitis. In perhaps 5% of cases of acute salpingitis, early laparoscopy reveals perihepatic inflammation ranging from edema and erythema of the liver capsule to exudate with fibrinous adhesions between the visceral and parietal peritoneum. When treatment is delayed and laparoscopy is performed late, dense "violin-string" adhesions can be seen over the liver; chronic exertional or positional right upper quadrant pain ensues when traction is placed on the adhesions. Although perihepatitis, also known as the *Fitz-Hugh–Curtis syndrome*, was for many years specifically attributed to gonococcal salpingitis, most cases are now attributed to chlamydial salpingitis. In patients with chlamydial salpingitis, serum titers of microimmunofluorescent antibody to *C. trachomatis* are typically much higher when perihepatitis is present than when it is absent.

Physical findings include right upper quadrant tenderness and usually include adnexal tenderness and cervicitis, even in patients whose symptoms do not suggest salpingitis. Results of liver function tests and right upper quadrant ultrasonography are nearly always normal. The presence of MPC and pelvic tenderness in a young woman with subacute pleuritic right upper quadrant pain and normal ultrasonography of the gallbladder points to a diagnosis of perihepatitis.

Periappendicitis (appendiceal serositis without involvement of the intestinal mucosa) has been found in ~5% of patients undergoing appendectomy for suspected appendicitis and can occur as a complication of gonococcal or chlamydial salpingitis.

Among women with salpingitis, HIV infection is associated with increased severity of salpingitis and with tuboovarian abscess requiring hospitalization and surgical drainage. Nonetheless, among women with HIV infection and salpingitis, the clinical reponse to conventional antimicrobial therapy (coupled with drainage of tuboovarian abscess, when found) has usually been satisfactory.

Diagnosis Treatment appropriate for PID must not be withheld from patients who have an equivocal diagnosis; it is better to err on the side of overdiagnosis and overtreatment. On the other hand, it is essential to differentiate between salpingitis and other pelvic pathology, particularly surgical emergencies such as appendicitis and ectopic pregnancy.

Nothing short of laparoscopy definitively identifies salpingitis, but routine laparoscopy to confirm suspected salpingitis is generally impractical. Most patients with acute PID have lower abdominal pain of <3 weeks' duration, pelvic tenderness on bimanual pelvic examination, and evidence of lower genital tract infection (e.g., MPC). Approximately 60% of such patients have salpingitis at laparoscopy, and perhaps 10–20% have endometritis alone. Among the patients with these findings, a rectal temperature >38°C, a palpable adnexal mass, and elevation of the ESR to >15 mm/h also raise the probability of salpingitis, which has been found at laparoscopy in 68% of patients with one of these additional findings, 90% of patients with two, and 96% of patients with three. However, only 17% of all patients with laparoscopy-confirmed salpingitis have had all three additional findings.

In a woman with pelvic pain and tenderness, increased numbers of PMNs (30 per 1000× microscopic field in strands of cervical mucus) or leukocytes outnumbering epithelial cells in vaginal fluid (in the absence of trichomonal vaginitis, which also produces PMNs in vaginal discharge) increase the predictive value of a clinical diagnosis of acute PID, as do onset with menses, history of recent abnormal menstrual bleeding, presence of an IUD, history of salpingitis, and sexual exposure to a male with urethritis. Appendicitis or another disorder of the gut is favored by the early onset of anorexia, nausea, or vomiting; the onset of pain later than day 14 of the menstrual cycle; or unilateral pain limited to the right or left lower quadrant. Whenever the diagnosis of PID is being considered, serum assays for human β-chorionic gonadotropin should be performed; these tests are usually positive with ectopic pregnancy. Ultrasonography and MRI can be useful for the identification of tuboovarian or pelvic abscess. MRI of the tubes can also show increased tubal diameter, intratubal fluid, or tubal wall thickening in cases of salpingitis.

The primary and uncontested value of laparoscopy in women with lower abdominal pain is for the exclusion of other surgical problems. Some of the most common or serious problems that may be confused with salpingitis (e.g., acute appendicitis, ectopic pregnancy, corpus luteum bleeding, ovarian tumor) are unilateral. Unilateral pain or pelvic mass, although not incompatible with PID, is a strong indication for laparoscopy unless the clinical picture warrants laparotomy instead. Atypical clinical findings, such as the absence of lower genital tract infection, a missed menstrual period, a positive pregnancy test, or failure to respond to appropriate therapy, are other common indications for laparoscopy. Endometrial biopsy is relatively sensitive and specific for the diagnosis of endometritis, which correlates well with the presence of salpingitis.

Endocervical swab specimens should be examined by Gram's staining for PMNs and gram-negative diplococci and by NAATs for *N. gonorrhoeae* and *C. trachomatis*. The clinical diagnosis of PID made by expert gynecologists is confirmed by laparoscopy or endometrial biopsy in ~90% of women who also have cultures positive for *N. gonorrhoeae* or *C. trachomatis*. Even among women with no symptoms suggestive of acute PID who were attending an STD clinic or a gynecology clinic in Pittsburgh, endometritis was significantly associated with endocervical gonorrhea or chlamydial infection or with bacterial vaginosis, being detected in 26%, 27%, and 15% of women with these conditions, respectively.

℞ PELVIC INFLAMMATORY DISEASE

The 2006 CDC guidelines recommend initiation of empirical treatment for PID in sexually active young women and other women at risk for PID if they are experiencing pelvic or lower abdominal pain, if no other cause for the pain can be identified, and if pelvic examination reveals one or more of the following criteria for PID: cervical motion tenderness, uterine tenderness, or adnexal tenderness.

Women with suspected PID can be treated as either outpatients or inpatients. In the multicenter Pelvic Inflammatory Disease Evaluation and Clinical Health (PEACH) trial, 831 women with mild to moderately severe symptoms and signs of PID were randomized to receive either inpatient treatment with IV cefoxitin and doxycycline or outpatient treatment with a single IM dose of cefoxitin plus oral doxycycline. Short-term clinical and microbiologic outcomes and long-term outcomes were equivalent in the two groups. Nonetheless, hospitalization should be considered when (1) the diagnosis is uncertain and surgical emergencies such as appendicitis and ectopic pregnancy cannot be excluded, (2) the patient is pregnant, (3) pelvic abscess is suspected, (4) severe illness or nausea and vomiting preclude outpatient management, (5) the patient has HIV infection, (6) the patient is assessed as unable to follow or tolerate an outpatient regimen, or (7) the patient has failed to respond to outpatient therapy. Some experts also prefer to hospitalize adolescents with PID for initial therapy, although younger women do as well as older women on outpatient therapy.

Recommended combination regimens for ambulatory or parenteral management of PID are presented in **Table 124-6**. Women managed as outpatients should receive a combined regimen with broad activity, such as ceftriaxone to cover possible gonococcal infection followed by doxycycline to cover possible chlamydial infection. Metronidazole can be added, if tolerated, to enhance activity against anaerobes. Neither doxycycline nor the fluoroquinolones provide reliable coverage for gonococcal infection today. Although the 2006 CDC guidelines for ambulatory treatment of PID included the option of using an oral fluoroquinolone, with or without metronidazole, for 14 days, these guidelines are already outdated because of emerging gonococcal resistance to the fluoroquinolones. Although few methodologically sound clinical trials (especially with prolonged follow-up) have been conducted, one meta-analysis suggested a benefit of providing good coverage against anaerobes.

For hospitalized patients, the following two parenteral regimens have given nearly identical results in a multicenter randomized trial:

1. Doxycycline (100 mg twice daily, given IV or PO) plus cefotetan (2.0 g IV every 12 h) or cefoxitin (2.0 g IV every 6 h). Administration of these drugs should be continued by the IV route for at least 48 h after the patient's condition improves and then followed with oral doxycycline (100 mg twice daily) to complete 14 days of therapy.
2. Clindamycin (900 mg IV every 8 h) plus gentamicin (2.0 mg/kg IV or IM, followed by 1.5 mg/kg every 8 h) in patients with normal renal function. Once-daily dosing of gentamicin (with combination of the total daily dose into a single daily dose) has not been evaluated in PID but has been efficacious in other serious infections and could be substituted.

Treatment with these drugs should be continued for at least 48 h after the patient's condition improves and then followed with oral doxycycline (100 mg twice daily) or clindamycin (450 mg four times daily) to complete 14 days of therapy. In cases with tuboovarian abscess, clindamycin rather than doxycycline for continued therapy provides better coverage for anaerobic infection.

FOLLOW-UP Hospitalized patients should show substantial clinical improvement within 3–5 days. Women treated as outpatients should be clinically reevaluated within 72 h. A follow-up telephone survey of women seen in an emergency room and given a prescription for 10 days of oral doxycycline for PID found that 28% never filled the prescription and 41% stopped taking the medication early (after an average of 4.1 days), often because of persistent symptoms, lack of symptoms, or side effects. Women not responding favorably to ambulatory therapy should be hospitalized for parenteral therapy and further diagnostic evaluations, including a consideration of laparoscopy. Male sex partners should be evaluated and treated empirically for gonorrhea and chlamydial infection. After completion of treatment, tests for persistent or recurrent infection with *N. gonorrhoeae* or *C. trachomatis* should be performed if symptoms persist or recur or if the patient has not complied with therapy or has been reexposed to an untreated sex partner.

TABLE 124-6 COMBINATION ANTIMICROBIAL REGIMENS RECOMMENDED FOR OUTPATIENT TREATMENT OR FOR PARENTERAL TREATMENT OF PID

Outpatient Regimens	Parenteral Regimens
	Initiate parenteral therapy with either of the following regimens; continue parenteral therapy until 48 h after clinical improvement; then change to outpatient therapy, as described in the text.
Regimen A Ofloxacin 400 mg PO bid for 14 days *or* Levofloxacin 500 mg PO once daily for 14 days *plus*[a] Metronidazole 500 mg PO bid for 14 days	**Regimen A** Cefotetan 2 g IV q12h *or* Cefoxitin 2 g IV q6h *plus* Doxycycline 100 mg IV or PO q12h
Regimen B Ceftriaxone 250 mg IM once *plus* Doxycycline 100 mg PO bid for 14 days *plus*[a] Metronidazole 500 mg PO bid for 14 days	**Regimen B** Clindamycin 900 mg IV q8h *plus* Gentamicin, loading dose of 2 mg/kg IV or IM, then maintenance dose of 1.5 mg/kg q8h

[a]The addition of metronidazole is recommended by some experts.

Source: Adapted from Centers for Disease Control and Prevention: MMWR Recomm Rep 55(RR-11):1, 2006.

SURGERY Surgery is necessary for the treatment of salpingitis only in the face of life-threatening infection (such as rupture or threatened rupture of a tuboovarian abscess) or for drainage of an abscess. Conservative surgical procedures are usually sufficient. Pelvic abscesses can often be drained by posterior colpotomy, and peritoneal lavage can be used for generalized peritonitis.

Prognosis Late sequelae include infertility due to bilateral tubal occlusion, ectopic pregnancy due to tubal scarring without occlusion, chronic pelvic pain, and recurrent salpingitis. The overall postsalpingitis risk of infertility due to tubal occlusion in a large study in Sweden was 11% after one episode of salpingitis, 23% after two episodes, and 54% after three or more episodes. A University of Washington study found a sevenfold increase in the risk of ectopic pregnancy and an eightfold increase in the rate of hysterectomy after PID.

Prevention A randomized controlled trial designed to determine whether selective screening for chlamydial infection reduced the risk of subsequent PID showed that women randomized to undergo screening had a 56% lower rate of PID over the following year than did women receiving the usual care without screening. This report helped prompt U.S. national guidelines for risk-based chlamydial screening of young women to reduce the incidence of PID and the prevalence of post-PID sequelae, while also reducing sexual transmission of *C. trachomatis*.

ULCERATIVE GENITAL OR PERIANAL LESIONS

Genital ulceration reflects a set of important STIs, most of which sharply increase the risk of sexual acquisition and shedding of HIV. In a 1996 study of genital ulcers in 10 of the U.S. cities with the highest rates of primary syphilis, PCR testing of ulcer specimens demonstrated HSV in 62% of patients, *Treponema pallidum* in 13%, and *Haemophilus ducreyi* in 12–20%. Today, genital herpes probably represents an even higher proportion of genital ulcers in the United States and other industrialized countries.

In Asia and Africa, chancroid (Fig. 124-6) was once considered the most common type of genital ulcer, followed in frequency by primary syphilis and then genital herpes. With increased efforts to control chancroid and syphilis, together with more frequent re-

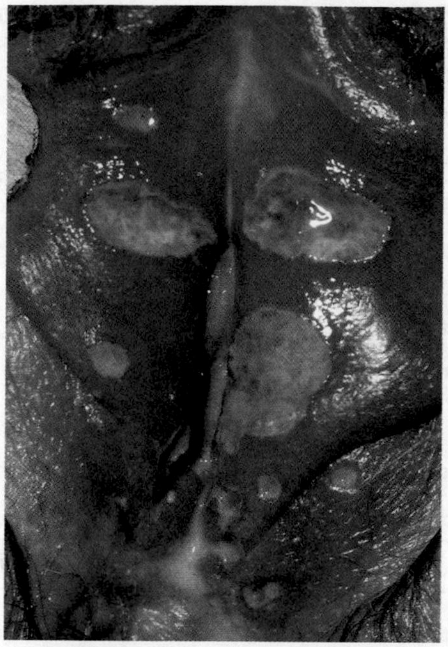

FIGURE 124-6 Chancroid: multiple, painful, punched-out ulcers with undermined borders on the labia occurring after autoinoculation.

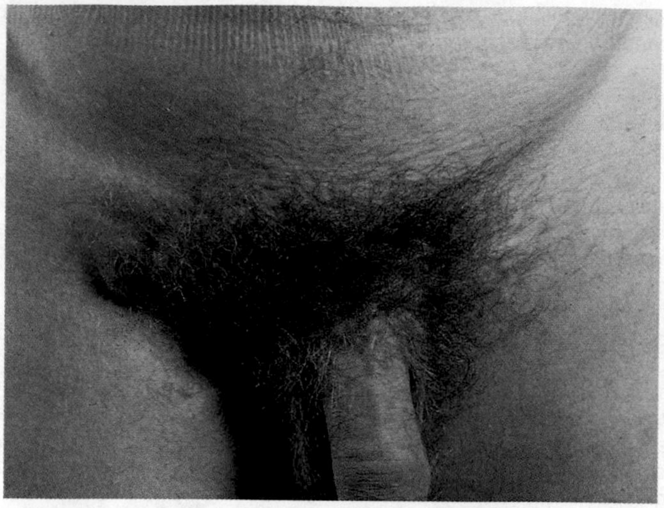

FIGURE 124-7 Lymphogranuloma venereum: striking tender lymphadenopathy occurring at the femoral and inguinal lymph nodes, separated by a groove made by Poupart's ligament. This "sign-of-the-groove" is not considered specific for LGV; for example, lymphomas may present with this sign.

currences or persistence of genital herpes attributable to HIV infection, PCR testing of genital ulcers now clearly implicates genital herpes as the most common cause of genital ulceration in most developing countries. LGV (Fig. 124-7) and donovanosis (granuloma inguinale) continue to cause genital ulceration in developing countries. LGV virtually disappeared in industrialized countries during the first 20 years of the HIV pandemic, but outbreaks are again occurring in Europe (including the United Kingdom), in North America, and in Australia. In these outbreaks, LGV is usually causing anal and rectal disease in homosexual men, very often in association with HIV and/or hepatitis C virus infections. Other causes of genital ulcer include (1) candidiasis and traumatized genital warts—both readily recognized; (2) lesions due to genital involvement by more widespread dermatoses; and (3) cutaneous manifestations of systemic diseases, such as genital mucosal ulceration in Stevens-Johnson syndrome or Behçet's disease.

Diagnosis Although most genital ulcerations cannot be diagnosed confidently on clinical grounds alone, clinical findings plus epidemiologic considerations (Table 124-7) can usually guide initial management (Table 124-8) pending results of further tests. Clinicians should order a rapid serologic test for syphilis in all cases of genital ulcer and a dark-field or direct immunofluorescence test (or PCR test, where available) for *T. pallidum* in all lesions except those highly characteristic of infection with HSV (i.e., those with herpetic vesicles). All patients presenting with genital ulceration should be counseled and tested for HIV infection.

Typical vesicles or pustules or a cluster of painful ulcers preceded by vesiculopustular lesions suggests genital herpes. These typical clinical manifestations make detection of the virus optional; however, many patients want confirmation of the diagnosis, and differentiation of HSV-1 from HSV-2 has prognostic implications, since the latter causes more frequent genital recurrences.

Painless, nontender, indurated ulcers with firm, nontender inguinal adenopathy suggest primary syphilis. If dark-field examination and a rapid serologic test for syphilis are initially negative and the patient will comply with follow-up and sexual abstinence, the performance of two more dark-field examinations on successive days before treatment is begun will improve the sensitivity of the diagnosis of syphilis, and repeated serologic testing for syphilis 1 or 2 weeks after treatment of seronegative primary syphilis usually demonstrates seroconversion.

"Atypical" or clinically trivial ulcers may be more common manifestations of genital herpes than classic vesiculopustular lesions. Specific tests for HSV in such lesions are therefore indicated (Chap. 172).

TABLE 124-7 CLINICAL FEATURES OF GENITAL ULCERS

Feature	Syphilis	Herpes	Chancroid	Lymphogranuloma Venereum	Donovanosis
Incubation period	9–90 days	2–7 days	1–14 days	3 days–6 weeks	1–4 weeks (up to 6 months)
Early primary lesions	Papule	Vesicle	Pustule	Papule, pustule, or vesicle	Papule
No. of lesions	Usually one	Multiple	Usually multiple, may coalesce	Usually one; often not detected, despite lymphadenopathy	Variable
Diameter	5–15 mm	1–2 mm	Variable	2–10 mm	Variable
Edges	Sharply demarcated, elevated, round, or oval	Erythematous	Undermined, ragged, irregular	Elevated, round, or oval	Elevated, irregular
Depth	Superficial or deep	Superficial	Excavated	Superficial or deep	Elevated
Base	Smooth, nonpurulent, relatively nonvascular	Serous, erythematous, nonvascular	Purulent, bleeds easily	Variable, nonvascular	Red and velvety, bleeds readily
Induration	Firm	None	Soft	Occasionally firm	Firm
Pain	Uncommon	Frequently tender	Usually very tender	Variable	Uncommon
Lymphadenopathy	Firm, nontender, bilateral	Firm, tender, often bilateral with initial episode	Tender, may suppurate, loculated, usually unilateral	Tender, may suppurate, loculated, usually unilateral	None; pseudobuboes

Source: From RM Ballard, in KK Holmes et al (eds): *Sexually Transmitted Diseases*, 4th ed. New York, McGraw-Hill, 2008.

TABLE 124-8 INITIAL MANAGEMENT OF GENITAL OR PERIANAL ULCER

Usual causes
- Herpes simplex virus (HSV)
- *Treponema pallidum* (primary syphilis)
- *Haemophilus ducreyi* (chancroid)

Usual initial laboratory evaluation
- Dark-field exam, direct FA, or PCR for *T. pallidum*; RPR or VDRL test for syphilis (if negative but primary syphilis suspected, repeat in 1 week); culture, direct FA, ELISA, or PCR for HSV; consider HSV-2-specific serology. In chancroid-endemic area: PCR or culture for *H. ducreyi*

Initial Treatment

Herpes confirmed or suspected (history or sign of vesicles):
- Treat for genital herpes with acyclovir, valacyclovir, or famciclovir

Syphilis confirmed (dark-field, FA, or PCR showing *T. pallidum*, or RPR reactive):
- Benzathine penicillin 2.4 million units IM once to patient, recent (e.g., within 3 months) seronegative partner(s), and all seropositive partners

Chancroid confirmed or suspected (diagnostic test positive, or HSV and syphilis excluded, and lesion persists):
- Ciprofloxacin 500 mg PO as single dose *or*
- Ceftriaxone 250 mg IM as single dose *or*
- Azithromycin 1 g PO as single dose

Note: FA, fluorescent antibody; PCR, polymerase chain reaction; RPR, rapid plasma reagin; ELISA, enzyme-linked immunosorbent assay; HSV, herpes simplex virus; VDRL, Venereal Disease Research Laboratory.

Type-specific serologic tests for serum antibody to HSV-2, now commercially available, may give negative results, especially when patients present early with the initial episode of genital erpes or when HSV-1 is the cause of genital herpes (as is often the case today). Furthermore, a positive test for antibody to HSV-2 does not prove that the current lesions are herpetic, since nearly one-fourth of the general population of the United States (and no doubt a higher proportion of those at risk for other STIs) becomes seropositive for HSV-2 during early adulthood. Although even type-specific tests for HSV-2 that are commercially available in the United States are not 100% specific, a positive HSV-2 serology does enable the clinician to tell the patient that he or she has probably had genital herpes, should learn to recognize symptoms, should avoid sex during recurrences, and should consider use of condoms or suppressive antiviral therapy, both of which can reduce transmission to a sexual partner.

Demonstration of *H. ducreyi* by culture (or by PCR test, when available) is most useful when ulcers are painful and purulent, especially if inguinal lymphadenopathy with fluctuance or overlying erythema is noted; if chancroid is prevalent in the community; or if the patient has recently had a sexual exposure elsewhere in a chancroid-endemic area (e.g., a developing country). Enlarged, fluctuant lymph nodes should be aspirated for culture or PCR tests to detect *H. ducreyi* as well as for Gram's staining and culture to rule out the presence of other pyogenic bacteria.

When genital ulcers persist beyond the natural history of initial episodes of herpes (2–3 weeks) or of chancroid or syphilis (up to 6 weeks) and do not resolve with syndrome-based antimicrobial therapy, then—in addition to the usual tests for herpes, syphilis, and chancroid—biopsy is indicated to exclude donovanosis, carcinoma, and other nonvenereal dermatoses. HIV serology should also be undertaken, since chronic, persistent genital herpes is common in AIDS.

℞ ULCERATIVE GENITAL OR PERIANAL LESIONS

Immediate syndrome-based treatment for acute genital ulcerations (after collection of all necessary hdiagnostic specimens at the first visit) is often appropriate before all test results become available, because patients with typical initial or recurrent episodes of genital or anorectal herpes can benefit from prompt oral antiviral therapy (Chap. 172); because early treatment of sexually transmitted causes of genital ulcers decreases further transmission; and because some patients do not return for test results and treatment. The patient with nonvesicular ulcerative lesions who may not return for follow-up or may not discontinue sexual activity should receive initial treatment for syphilis, together with empirical therapy for chancroid if there has been an exposure in an area where chancroid occurs or if regional lymph node suppuration is evident. In resource-poor settings lacking ready access to diagnostic tests, this approach to syndromic treatment for syphilis and chancroid has helped bring these two diseases under control. Finally, empirical antimicrobial therapy may be indicated if ulcers persist and the diagnosis remains unclear after a week of observation despite attempts to diagnose herpes, syphilis, and chancroid.

PROCTITIS, PROCTOCOLITIS, ENTEROCOLITIS, AND ENTERITIS

Sexually acquired *proctitis*, with inflammation limited to the rectal mucosa (the distal 10–12 cm), results from direct rectal inoculation of typical STD pathogens. In contrast, inflammation extending from the rectum to the colon (*proctocolitis*), involving both the small and the large bowel (*enterocolitis*), or involving the small bowel alone (*enteritis*) can result from ingestion of typical intestinal pathogens through oral-anal exposure during sexual contact. Anorectal pain and mucopurulent, bloody rectal discharge suggest proctitis or proctocolitis. Proctitis commonly produces tenesmus (causing frequent attempts to defecate, but not true diarrhea) and constipation, whereas proctocolitis and enterocolitis more often cause true diarrhea. In all three conditions, anoscopy usually shows mucosal exudate and easily induced mucosal bleeding (i.e., a positive "wipe test"), sometimes with petechiae or mucosal ulcers. Exudate should be sampled for Gram's staining and other microbiologic studies. Sigmoidoscopy or colonoscopy shows inflammation limited to the rectum in proctitis or disease extending at least up into the sigmoid colon in proctocolitis.

The AIDS era brought an extraordinary shift in the clinical and etiologic spectrum of intestinal infections among homosexual men. The number of cases of the acute intestinal STIs described above fell as high-risk sexual behaviors became less common in this group. At the same time, the number of AIDS-related opportunistic intestinal infections increased rapidly, many associated with chronic or recurrent symptoms. The incidence of these infections has since fallen with increasingly effective antiretroviral therapy. Two species initially isolated in association with intestinal symptoms in homosexual men are now known as *Helicobacter cinaedi* and *Helicobacter fennelliae*, and both have subsequently been isolated from the blood of HIV-infected men with a syndrome of multifocal dermatitis and arthritis.

Acquisition of HSV, *N. gonorrhoeae*, or *C. trachomatis* (now again including LGV strains of *C. trachomatis*) during receptive anorectal intercourse causes most cases of infectious proctitis in women and homosexual men. Primary and secondary syphilis can also produce anal or anorectal lesions, with or without symptoms. Gonococcal or chlamydial proctitis typically involves the most distal rectal mucosa and the anal crypts and is clinically mild, without systemic manifestations. In contrast, primary proctitis due to HSV and proctocolitis due to the strains of *C. trachomatis* that cause LGV usually produce severe anorectal pain and often cause fever. Perianal ulcers and inguinal lymphadenopathy, most commonly due to HSV, can also occur in LGV or syphilis. Sacral nerve root radiculopathies, usually presenting as urinary retention, laxity of the anal sphincter, or constipation, may complicate primary herpetic proctitis. In LGV, rectal biopsy typically shows crypt abscesses, granulomas, and giant cells—findings resembling those in Crohn's disease; such findings should always prompt rectal culture and serology for LGV, which is a curable infection. Syphilis can also produce rectal granulomas, usually in association with infiltration by plasma cells or other mononuclear cells. Syphilis, LGV, and HSV infection involving the rectum can produce perirectal adenopathy that is sometimes mistaken for malignancy; syphilis, LGV, HSV infection, and chancroid involving the anus can produce inguinal adenopathy, because anal lymphatics drain to inguinal lymph nodes.

Diarrhea and abdominal bloating or cramping pain without anorectal symptoms and with normal findings on anoscopy and sigmoidoscopy occur with inflammation of the small intestine (enteritis) or with proximal colitis. In homosexual men without HIV infection, enteritis is often attributable to *Giardia lamblia*. Sexually acquired proctocolitis is most often due to *Campylobacter* or *Shigella* spp.

℞ PROCTITIS, PROCTOCOLITIS, ENTEROCOLITIS, AND ENTERITIS

Acute proctitis in persons who have practiced receptive anorectal intercourse is usually sexually acquired. Such patients should undergo anoscopy to detect rectal ulcers or vesicles and petechiae after swabbing of the rectal mucosa; to examine rectal exudates for PMNs and gram-negative diplococci; and to obtain rectal swab specimens for testing for rectal gonorrhea, chlamydial infection, herpes, and syphilis. Pending test results, patients with proctitis should receive empirical syndromic treatment—e.g., with ceftriaxone (a single IM dose of 125 mg for gonorrhea) plus doxycycline (100 mg PO twice daily for 7 days for possible chlamydial infection) plus treatment for herpes or syphilis if indicated.

PREVENTION AND CONTROL OF STIS

Prevention and control of STIs require the following:

1. Reduction of the average rate of sexual exposure to STIs through alteration of sexual risk behaviors and behavioral norms among both susceptible and infected persons in all population groups. The necessary changes include reduction in the total number of sexual partners and the number of concurrent sexual partners.
2. Reduction of the efficiency of transmission through the promotion of safer sexual practices, the use of condoms during casual or commercial sex, vaccination against HBV and HPV infection, male circumcision, and a growing number of other approaches (e.g., early detection and treatment of other STIs to reduce the efficiency of sexual transmission of HIV). We now know from longitudinal studies over the past decade that consistent condom use is associated with significant protection of both males and females against all STIs that have been examined, including HIV, HPV, and HSV infections as well as gonorrhea and chlamydial infection. The only exceptions are probably sexually transmitted *Phthirus pubis* and *Sarcoptes scabiei* infestations.
3. Shortening of the duration of infectivity of STIs through early detection and curative or suppressive treatment of patients and their sexual partners.

Financial and time constraints imposed by managed-care practice patterns, along with the reluctance of some clinicians to ask questions about stigmatized sexual behaviors, often curtail screening and prevention services. As outlined in Fig. 124-8, the success of clinicians' efforts to detect and treat STIs depends in part on societal efforts to teach young people how to recognize symptoms of STIs; to motivate those with symptoms to seek care promptly; and to make high-quality, appropriate care accessible, affordable, and acceptable, especially to the young indigent patients most likely to acquire an STI.

Since many infected individuals develop no symptoms or fail to recognize and report symptoms, clinicians should routinely perform an STI risk assessment for teenagers and young adults as a guide to selective screening. U.S. Preventive Services Task Force Guidelines recommend screening sexually active female patients ≤25 years of age for *C. trachomatis* whenever they present for health care (at least once a year); older women should be tested if they have more than one sexual partner, have begun a new sexual relationship since the previous test, or have another STI diagnosed. In the United States, widespread selective screening of young women for cervical *C. trachomatis* infection in some regions has been associated with a 50–60% drop in prevalence, and such screening also protects the individual woman from PID. Sensitive urine-based genetic amplification tests permit expansion of screening to men, teenage boys, and girls in settings where examination is not planned or is impractical (e.g., during pre-participation sports examinations or during initial medical evaluation of adolescent girls).

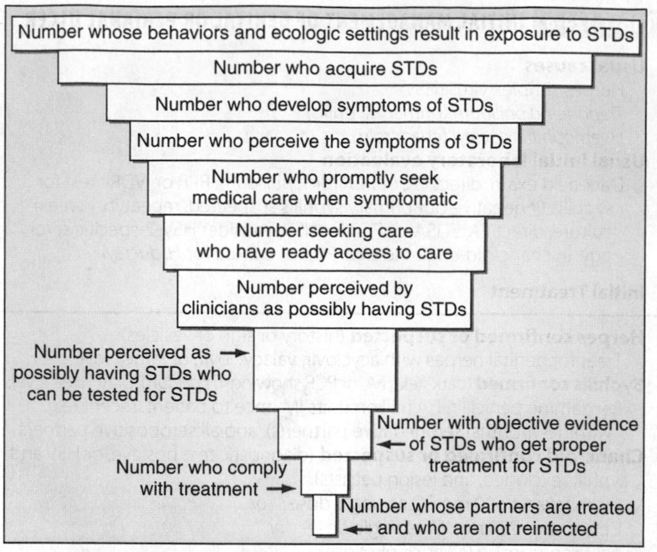

FIGURE 124-8 Critical control points for preventive and clinical interventions against sexually transmitted diseases (STDs). *[Adapted from HT Waller and MA Piot: Bull World Health Organ 41:75, 1969 and 43:1, 1970; and from "Resource allocation model for public health planning—a case study of tuberculosis control," Bull World Health Organ 84(Suppl), 1973.]*

Although gonorrhea is now substantially less common than chlamydial infection in industrialized countries, screening tests for *N. gonorrhoeae* are still appropriate for women and teenage girls attending STD clinics and for sexually active teens and young women from areas of high gonorrhea prevalence. Multiplex NAATs that combine screening for *N. gonorrhoeae* and *C. trachomatis* in a single low-cost assay now facilitate the prevention and control of both infections in populations at high risk.

All patients with newly detected STIs or at high risk for STIs according to routine risk assessment as well as all pregnant women should be encouraged to undergo serologic testing for syphilis and HIV infection, with appropriate HIV counseling before and after testing. Randomized trials have shown that risk-reduction counseling of patients with STIs significantly lowers subsequent risk of acquiring an STI; such counseling should now be considered a standard component of STI management. Preimmunization serologic testing for antibody to HBV is indicated for unvaccinated persons who are known to be at high risk, such as homosexually active men and injection drug users. In most young persons, however, it is more cost-effective to vaccinate against HBV without serologic screening. In 2006, the Advisory Committee on Immunization Practices (ACIP) of the CDC recommended the following: (1) Universal hepatitis B vaccination should be implemented for all unvaccinated adults in settings in which a high proportion of adults have risk factors for HBV infection (e.g., STD clinics, HIV testing and treatment facilities, drug-abuse treatment and prevention settings, health care settings targeting services to injection drug users or men who have sex with men, and correctional facilities). (2) In other primary care and specialty medical settings in which adults at risk for HBV infection receive care, health care providers should inform all patients about the health benefits of vaccination, the risk factors for HBV infection, and the persons for whom vaccination is recommended and should vaccinate adults who report risk factors for HBV infection as well as any adult who requests protection from HBV infection. To promote vaccination in all settings, health care providers should implement standing orders to identify adults recommended for hepatitis B vaccination, should administer HBV vaccination as part of routine clinical services, should not require acknowledgment of an HBV infection risk factor for adult vaccination, and should use available reimbursement mechanisms to remove financial barriers to hepatitis B vaccination.

In 2007, the ACIP recommended routine immunization of 9- to 26-year-old girls and women with the quadrivalent HPV vaccine (against

HPV types 6, 11, 16, and 18) approved by the U.S. Food and Drug Administration; the optimal age for recommended vaccination is 11–12 years because of the very high risk of HPV infection after sexual debut.

Partner notification is the process of identifying and informing partners of infected patients about possible exposure to an STI and of examining, testing, and treating partners as appropriate. In a series of 22 reports concerning partner notification during the 1990s, index patients with gonorrhea or chlamydial infection named a mean of 0.75–1.6 partners, of whom one-fourth to one-third were infected; those with syphilis named 1.8–6.3 partners, with one-third to one-half infected; and those with HIV infection named 0.76–5.31 partners, with up to one-fourth infected. Persons who transmit infection or who have recently been infected and are still in the incubation period usually have no symptoms or only mild symptoms and seek medical attention only when notified of their exposure. Therefore, the clinician must encourage patients to participate in partner notification, must ensure that exposed persons are notified, and must guarantee confidentiality to all involved. In the United States, local health departments often offer assistance in partner notification, treatment, and/or counseling. It seems both feasible and most useful to notify those partners exposed within the patient's likely period of infectiousness, which is often considered the preceding 1 month for gonorrhea, 1–2 months for chlamydial infection, and up to 3 months for early syphilis.

Persons with a new-onset STI always have a *source* contact who gave them the infection; in addition, they may have a *secondary* (*spread* or *exposed*) contact with whom they had sex after becoming infected. The identification and treatment of these two types of contacts have different objectives. Treatment of the source contact (often a casual contact) benefits the community by preventing further transmission; treatment of the recently exposed secondary contact (typically a spouse or another steady sexual partner) prevents both the development of serious complications (such as PID) in the partner and reinfection of the index patient. A survey of a random sample of U.S. physicians found that most instructed patients to abstain from sex during treatment, to use condoms, and to inform their sex partners after being diagnosed with gonorrhea, chlamydial infection, or syphilis; physicians sometimes gave the patients drugs for their partners. However, follow-up of the partners by physicians was infrequent. A randomized trial compared patients' delivery of therapy to partners exposed to gonorrhea or chlamydial infection with conventional notification and advice to partners to seek evaluation for STD; patients' delivery of partners' therapy (PDPT), also known as *expedited partner therapy* (EPT), significantly reduced combined rates of reinfection of the index patient with *N. gonorrhoeae* or *Chlamydia.* State-by-state variations in regulations governing this approach have not been well defined, but the 2006 CDC STD treatment guidelines and the EPT final report of 2006 (*http://www.cdc.gov/std/treatment/EPTFinalReport2006.pdf*) describe its potential use. Currently, EPT is commonly used by many practicing physicians; it is not feasible in some settings and lacks clear legal sanctioning in some states.

In summary, clinicians and public health agencies share responsibility for the prevention and control of STIs. In the managed-care era, the role of primary care clinicians has become increasingly important in prevention as well as in diagnosis and treatment.

FURTHER READINGS

Centers for Disease Control and Prevention: Sexually transmitted diseases treatment guidelines, 2006. MMWR Recomm Rep 55(RR-11):1, 2006 (Erratum in MMWR Recomm Rep 55(36):997, 2006)

Fredricks DN et al: Molecular identification of bacteria associated with bacterial vaginosis. N Engl J Med 353:1899, 2005

FUTURE II Group: Quadrivalent vaccine against human papillomavirus to prevent high-grade cervical lesions. N Engl J Med 356:1915, 2007

Golden MR et al: Effect of expedited treatment of sex partners on recurrent or persistent gonorrhea or chlamydial infection. N Engl J Med 352:676, 2005

Holmes KK et al (eds): *Sexually Transmitted Diseases*, 4th ed. New York, McGraw-Hill, 2008

Manhart LE, Holmes KK: Randomized controlled trials of individual-level, population-level, and multilevel interventions for preventing sexually transmitted infections: What has worked? J Infect Dis 191(Suppl 1):S7, 2005

Markowitz LE et al: Quadrivalent human papillomavirus vaccine: Recommendations of the Advisory Committee on Immunization Practices (ACIP). MMWR Recomm Rep 56(RR-2):1, 2007

Mast EE et al: A comprehensive immunization strategy to eliminate transmission of hepatitis B virus infection in the United States: Recommendations of the Advisory Committee on Immunization Practices (ACIP) Part II: Immunization of adults. MMWR Recomm Rep 55(RR-16):1, 2006

Workowski KA: Sexually transmitted disease treatment guidelines. Clin Infect Dis 44(Suppl 3):S1, 2007

World Health Organization: Sexually transmitted diseases diagnostics initiative. Geneva, WHO, 2001 (*http://www.who.int/std_diagnostics/news/SDI_founding_members.htm*)

SECTION 3 CLINICAL SYNDROMES: HEALTH CARE–ASSOCIATED INFECTIONS

125 Health Care–Associated Infections

Robert A. Weinstein

The costs of hospital-acquired (nosocomial) and other health care–associated infections are great. It is estimated that these infections affect >2 million patients, cost $4.5 billion, and contribute to 88,000 deaths in U.S. hospitals annually. Efforts to lower infection risks have been challenged by the growing numbers of immunocompromised patients, antibiotic-resistant bacteria, fungal and viral superinfections, and invasive devices and procedures. Nevertheless, evidence-based guidelines for prevention and control are available (Table 125-1); according to some estimates, consistent application of these guidelines may reduce the risk of health care–associated infection by more than one-third, and the growing viewpoint of consumer advocates is that almost all such infections are preventable. This chapter reviews health care–acquired and device-related infections and the basic surveillance, prevention, control, and treatment activities that have been developed to deal with these problems.

ORGANIZATION, RESPONSIBILITIES, AND INCREASING SCRUTINY OF INFECTION-CONTROL PROGRAMS

The standards of the Joint Commission on Accreditation of Healthcare Organizations require all accredited hospitals to have an active program for surveillance, prevention, and control of nosocomial infections. Education of physicians in infection control and health care epidemiology is required in infectious disease fellowship programs and is available by online courses. Diagnosis-related reimbursement has led hospital administrators to place increased emphasis on infection control. Federal concerns over "patient safety" have led to legislation that would limit re-

TABLE 125-1 SOURCES OF INFECTION-CONTROL GUIDANCE AND OVERSIGHT

Organization	Role	Major Constituents	Web Site
JCAHO	Regulatory	Hospitals, long-term-care facilities, laboratories	http://www.jcaho.org
CAP	Regulatory	Laboratories	http://www.cap.org
OSHA	Regulatory	Workers	http://www.osha.gov
CMS (formerly HCFA)	Regulatory	Medicare/Medicaid providers	http://www.cms.hhs.gov
CDC			
DHQP	Advisory	Health care facilities and personnel	http://www.cdc.gov/ncidod/hip/default.htm
HICPAC	Advisory	Health care facilities and personnel	http://www.cdc.gov/ncidod/hip/HICPAC/hicpac.htm
NIOSH	Advisory	Workers	http://www.cdc.gov/niosh/homepage.htm
AHRQ	Advisory	Broad (e.g., health care personnel)	http://www.ahrq.org
NQF	Advisory	Broad (e.g., health care personnel)	http://www.qualityforum.org
IOM	Advisory	Broad (e.g., health care personnel)	http://www.iom.edu
IDSA	Professional society	Infectious disease physicians/researchers	http://www.idsociety.org
SHEA	Professional society	Hospital epidemiologists	http://www.shea-online.org
APIC	Professional society	Infection-control practitioners	http://www.apic.org
MedQIC	Quality improvement	Broad (e.g., health care personnel)	http://www.medqic.org
IHI	Quality improvement	Broad (e.g., health care personnel)	http://www.ihi.org

Abbreviations: JCAHO, Joint Commission on Accreditation of Healthcare Organizations; CAP, College of American Pathologists; OSHA, Occupational Safety & Health Administration; CMS, Centers for Medicare & Medicaid Services; HCFA, Health Care Financing Administration; CDC, Centers for Disease Control and Prevention; DHQP, Division of Healthcare Quality Promotion; HICPAC, Healthcare Infection Control Practices Advisory Committee; NIOSH, National Institute for Occupational Safety and Health; AHRQ, Agency for Healthcare Research and Quality; NQF, National Quality Forum; IOM, Institute of Medicine; IDSA, Infectious Diseases Society of America; SHEA, Society for Healthcare Epidemiology of America, Inc.; APIC, Association for Professionals in Infection Control and Epidemiology, Inc.; MedQIC, Medicare Quality Improvement Community; IHI, Institute for Healthcare Improvement.

imbursement for hospital costs resulting from at least two (yet-to-be-determined) nosocomial infections. The patient safety movement has prompted major national efforts to improve, measure, and publicly report on processes of patient care (e.g., timely administration and appropriateness of perioperative antibiotic prophylaxis) and patient outcomes (e.g., surgical wound infection rates).

SURVEILLANCE

Traditionally, infection-control practitioners have surveyed inpatients for infections acquired in hospitals (defined as those neither present nor incubating at the time of admission). Surveillance involves review of microbiology laboratory results, "shoe-leather" epidemiology on nursing wards, and application of standardized definitions of infection. Some infection-control programs use computerized hospital databases for algorithm-driven electronic surveillance (e.g., of vascular catheter and surgical wound infections). Commercial health care information systems that facilitate these functions are considered "value-added" products.

Most hospitals aim surveillance at infections associated with a high level of morbidity or expense. Quality-improvement activities in infection control have led to increased surveillance of personnel compliance with infection-control policies (e.g., adherence to influenza vaccination recommendations). The growing number of states that require public reporting of processes for prevention of health care–associated infection and/or patient outcomes has added new complexity to what hospitals measure and how they measure it.

Results of surveillance are expressed as rates. In general, 5–10% of patients develop nosocomial infections—a rate that, as patient advocates emphasize, has remained unchanged for 20–30 years. However, such broad statistics have little value unless qualified by duration of risk, by site of infection, by patient population, and by exposure to risk factors. Meaningful denominators for infection rates include the number of patients exposed to a specific risk (e.g., patients using mechanical ventilators) or the number of intervention days (e.g., 1000 patient-days on a ventilator).

Temporal trends in rates should be reviewed, and rates should be compared with regional and national benchmarks. However, even comparison rates generated by the National Healthcare Safety Network (NHSN) have not been validated independently and represent a nonrandom sample of hospitals. [NHSN is the successor to the National Nosocomial Infections Surveillance System, a program of the Centers for Disease Control and Prevention (CDC) that collected data from more than 350 hospitals that use standardized definitions of nosocomial infections.] Interhospital comparisons may be misleading because of the wide range in risk factors and severity of underlying illnesses. Although systems for making adjustments for these factors either are rudimentary or have not been well validated, process measures (e.g., adherence to hand hygiene) do not usually require risk adjustment, and outcome measures (e.g., cardiac surgery wound infection rates) can identify hospitals with higher infection rates (e.g., in the top quartile) for further evaluation. Moreover, temporal analysis of an individual hospital's process and infection outcome rates helps to determine whether control measures are succeeding and where increased efforts should be focused.

EPIDEMIOLOGIC BASIS AND GENERAL MEASURES FOR PREVENTION AND CONTROL

Nosocomial infections follow basic epidemiologic patterns that can help to direct prevention and control measures. Nosocomial pathogens have reservoirs, are transmitted by predictable routes, and require susceptible hosts. Reservoirs and sources exist in the inanimate environment (e.g., tap water contaminated with *Legionella*) and in the animate environment (e.g., infected or colonized health care workers, patients, and hospital visitors). The mode of transmission usually is either cross-infection (e.g., indirect spread of pathogens from one patient to another on the inadequately cleaned hands of hospital personnel) or autoinoculation (e.g., aspiration of oropharyngeal flora into the lung along an endotracheal tube). Occasionally, pathogens (e.g., group A streptococci and many respiratory viruses) are spread from person to person via infectious droplets released by coughing or sneezing. Much less common—but often devastating in terms of epidemic risk—is true airborne spread of droplet nuclei (as in nosocomial chickenpox) or common-source spread by contaminated materials (e.g., contaminated intravenous fluids). Factors that increase host susceptibility include underlying conditions and the many medical-surgical interventions and procedures that bypass or compromise normal host defenses.

Through their programs, hospitals' infection-control committees must determine general and specific control measures. Given the prominence of cross-infection, hand hygiene is the single most important preventive measure in hospitals. Health care workers' rates of adherence to hand-hygiene recommendations are abysmally low (<50%). Reasons cited include inconvenience, time pressures, and skin damage from frequent washing. Sinkless alcohol rubs are quick and highly effective and actually improve hand condition since they contain emollients and allow the retention of natural protective oils that would be removed with repeated rinsing. Use of alcohol hand rubs between patient contacts is now recommended for all health care workers except when the hands are visibly soiled, in which case washing with soap and water is still required.

NOSOCOMIAL AND DEVICE-RELATED INFECTIONS

The fact that 25–50% or more of nosocomial infections are due to the combined effect of the patient's own flora and invasive devices highlights the importance of improvements in the use and design of such devices. Intensive education and "bundling" of evidence-based interventions (Table 125-2) can reduce infection rates through improved asepsis in handling and earlier removal of invasive devices, but the maintenance of such gains requires ongoing efforts. It is especially noteworthy that turnover or shortages of trained personnel jeopardize safe and effective patient care and have been associated with increased infection rates.

Urinary Tract Infections Urinary tract infections (UTIs) account for as many as 40–45% of nosocomial infections; up to 3% of bacteriuric patients develop bacteremia. Although UTIs contribute only 10–15% to prolongation of hospital stay and to extra costs, these infections are important reservoirs and sources for spread of antibiotic-resistant bacteria in hospitals. Almost all nosocomial UTIs are associated with preceding instrumentation or indwelling bladder catheters, which create a 3–10% risk of infection each day. UTIs generally are caused by pathogens that spread up the periurethral space from the patient's perineum or gastrointestinal tract—the most common pathogenesis in women—or via intraluminal contamination of urinary catheters, usually due to cross-infection by caregivers who are irrigating catheters or emptying drainage bags. Pathogens come occasionally from inadequately disinfected urologic equipment and rarely from contaminated supplies.

TABLE 125-2 EXAMPLES OF "BUNDLED INTERVENTIONS" TO PREVENT COMMON HEALTH CARE–ASSOCIATED INFECTIONS AND OTHER ADVERSE EVENTS

Prevention of Central Venous Catheter Infections
Educate personnel about catheter insertion and care.
Use chlorhexidine to prepare the insertion site.
Use maximum barrier precautions during catheter insertion.
Ask daily: Is the catheter needed?
Prevention of Ventilator-Associated Pneumonia and Complications
Elevate head of bed to 30–45 degrees.
Give "sedation vacation" and assess readiness to extubate daily.
Use peptic ulcer disease prophylaxis.
Use deep-vein thrombosis prophylaxis (unless contraindicated).
Prevention of Surgical-Site Infections
Administer prophylactic antibiotics within 1 h before surgery; discontinue within 24 h.
Limit any hair removal to the time of surgery; use clippers or do not remove hair at all.
Maintain normal perioperative glucose levels (cardiac surgery patients).[a]
Maintain perioperative normothermia (colorectal surgery patients).[a]
Prevention of Urinary Tract Infections
Place bladder catheters only when absolutely needed (e.g., to relieve obstruction), not solely for the provider's convenience.
Use aseptic technique for catheter insertion and urinary tract instrumentation.
Minimize manipulation or opening of drainage systems.
Remove bladder catheters as soon as is feasible.

[a]These components of care are supported by clinical trials and experimental evidence in the specified populations; they may prove valuable for other surgical patients as well.

Source: Adapted from information presented at the following websites: *www.cdc.gov/ncidod/dhqp/gl_intravascular.html; www.cdc.gov/ncidod/dhqp/gl_hcpneumonia.html; www.cdc.gov/ncidod/dhqp/gl_surgicalsite.html; www.cdc.gov/ncidod/dhqp/gl_catheter_assoc.html; www.ihi.org; www.medqic.org/scip.*

Hospitals should closely monitor essential performance measures for preventing nosocomial UTIs (Table 125-2). Sealed catheter–drainage tube junctions can help to prevent breaks in the system. Approaches to the prevention of UTIs also have included use of topical meatal antimicrobials, drainage bag disinfectants, and anti-infective catheters. None of the latter three measures is considered routine. In fact, a recent meta-analysis suggests that silver alloy–coated anti-infective catheters do not reduce the incidence of bacteriuria from that occurring with silicone catheters.

Administration of systemic antimicrobial agents for other purposes decreases the risk of UTI during the first 4 days of catheterization, after which resistant bacteria or yeasts emerge as pathogens. Selective decontamination of the gut is also associated with a reduced risk. Again, however, neither approach is routine.

Irrigation of catheters, with or without antimicrobial agents, may actually increase the risk of infection. A condom catheter for men without bladder obstruction may be more acceptable than an indwelling catheter, but the infection risks with the two types are similar unless the condom catheter is carefully maintained. The role of suprapubic catheters in preventing infection is not well defined.

Treatment of UTIs is based on the results of quantitative urine cultures (Chap. 282). The most common pathogens are *Escherichia coli*, nosocomial gram-negative bacilli, enterococci, and *Candida*. Several caveats apply in the treatment of institutionally acquired infection. First, in patients with chronic indwelling bladder catheters, especially those in long-term-care facilities, "catheter flora"—microorganisms living on encrustations within the catheter lumen—may differ from actual urinary tract pathogens. Therefore, for suspected infection in the setting of chronic catheterization (especially in women), it is useful to replace the bladder catheter and to obtain a freshly voided urine specimen. Second, as in all nosocomial infections, at the time treatment is initiated on the basis of a positive culture, it is useful to repeat the culture to verify the persistence of infection. Third, the frequency with which UTIs occur may lead to the erroneous assumption that this site alone is the source of infection in a febrile hospitalized patient. Fourth, recovery of *Staphylococcus aureus* from urine cultures may result from hematogenous seeding and may indicate an occult systemic infection. Finally, although *Candida* is now the most common pathogen in nosocomial UTIs in patients on intensive care units (ICUs), treatment of candiduria is often unsuccessful and is recommended only when there is upper-pole invasion, obstruction, neutropenia, or immunosuppression.

Pneumonia Pneumonia accounts for 15–20% of nosocomial infections but has been responsible for 24% of extra hospital days and 39% of extra costs—i.e., 6 days and the associated costs per episode. Almost all cases of bacterial nosocomial pneumonia are caused by aspiration of endogenous or hospital-acquired oropharyngeal (and occasionally gastric) flora. Nosocomial pneumonias are associated with more deaths than are infections at any other body site. However, attributable mortality for ventilator-associated pneumonia—the most common and lethal form of nosocomial pneumonia—is in the 6–14% range; this figure suggests that the risk of dying from nosocomial pneumonia is affected greatly by other factors, including comorbidities, inadequate antibiotic treatment, and the involvement of specific pathogens (particularly *Pseudomonas aeruginosa* and *Acinetobacter*). Surveillance and accurate diagnosis of pneumonia are often problematic in hospitals because many patients, especially those in the ICU, have abnormal chest roentgenographs, fever, and leukocytosis potentially attributable to multiple causes. Viral pneumonias, which are particularly important in pediatric and immunocompromised patients, are discussed in the virology section and in Chap. 251.

Risk factors for nosocomial pneumonia, particularly ventilator-associated pneumonia, include those events that increase colonization by potential pathogens (e.g., prior antimicrobial therapy, contaminated ventilator circuits or equipment, or decreased gastric acidity); those that facilitate aspiration of oropharyngeal contents into the lower respiratory tract (e.g., intubation, decreased levels of consciousness, or presence of a nasogastric tube); and those that reduce host defense mechanisms in the lung and permit overgrowth of aspirated pathogens (e.g., chronic obstructive pulmonary disease, old age, or upper abdominal surgery).

Control measures for pneumonia (Table 125-2) are aimed at the remediation of risk factors in general patient care (e.g., minimizing aspiration-prone supine positioning) and at meticulous aseptic care of respirator equipment (e.g., disinfecting or sterilizing all inline reusable components such as nebulizers, replacing tubing circuits at intervals of >48 h—rather than more frequently—to lessen the number of breaks in the system, and teaching aseptic technique for suctioning). The benefits of selective decontamination of the oropharynx and gut with nonabsorbable antimicrobial agents and/or use of short-course postintubation systemic antibiotics have been controversial. Among the logical preventive measures that require further investigation are the use of endotracheal tubes that provide channels for subglottic drainage of secretions and the use of noninvasive mechanical ventilation whenever feasible. It is noteworthy that reducing the rate of ventilator-associated pneumonia most often has not reduced overall ICU mortality; this fact suggests that this infection is a marker for patients with an otherwise-heightened risk of death.

The most likely pathogens for nosocomial pneumonia and treatment options are discussed in Chap. 251. Several considerations regarding diagnosis and treatment are worth emphasizing. Clinical criteria for diagnosis (e.g., fever, leukocytosis, development of purulent secretions, new or changing radiographic infiltrates, changes in oxygen requirement or ventilator settings) have high sensitivity but relatively low specificity. These criteria are most useful for selecting patients for bronchoscopic or nonbronchoscopic procedures that yield lower respiratory tract samples protected from upper-tract contamination; quantitative cultures of such specimens have diagnostic sensitivities in the range of 80%. Early-onset nosocomial pneumonia, which manifests within the first 4 days of hospitalization, is most often caused by community-acquired pathogens, such as *Streptococcus pneumoniae* and *Haemophilus* species. Late-onset pneumonias most commonly are due to *S. aureus*, *P. aeruginosa*, *Enterobacter* species, *Klebsiella pneumoniae*, or *Acinetobacter*—a pathogen of increasing concern in many ICUs. When invasive techniques are used to diagnose ventilator-associated pneumonia, the proportion of isolates accounted for by gram-negative bacilli decreases from 50–70% to 35–45%. Infection is polymicrobial in as many as 20–40% of cases. The role of anaerobic bacteria in ventilator-associated pneumonia is not well defined. A recent study suggested that 8 days is an appropriate duration of therapy for nosocomial pneumonia, with a longer duration (15 days in this study) when the pathogen is *Acinetobacter* or *P. aeruginosa*. Finally, in febrile patients (particularly those who have endotracheal and/or nasogastric tubes), more occult sources of respiratory tract infection, especially bacterial sinusitis and otitis media, should be considered.

Surgical Wound Infections Wound infections account for up to 20–30% of nosocomial infections but contribute up to 57% of extra hospital days and 42% of extra costs. The average wound infection has an incubation period of 5–7 days (longer than many postoperative stays), and many procedures are now performed on an outpatient basis. Thus the incidence of wound infections has become difficult to assess. These infections usually are caused by the patient's endogenous or hospital-acquired skin and mucosal flora and occasionally are due to airborne spread of skin squames that may be shed into the wound from members of the operating-room team. True airborne spread of infection through droplet nuclei is rare in operating rooms unless there is a "disseminator" (e.g., of group A streptococci or staphylococci) among the staff. In general, the most common risks for postoperative wound infection are related to the surgeon's technical skill, the patient's underlying diseases (e.g., diabetes mellitus, obesity) or advanced age, and inappropriate timing of antibiotic prophylaxis. Additional risk factors include the presence of drains, prolonged preoperative hospital stays, shaving of the operative site by razor the day before surgery, a long duration of surgery, and infection at remote sites (e.g., untreated UTI).

The substantial literature related to risk factors for surgical-site infections and the recognized morbidity and cost of these infections have led to national prevention efforts—the Surgical Infection Prevention (SIP) Project, the Institute for Healthcare Improvement (IHI) 100,000 Lives Campaign, and the Surgical Care Improvement Project (SCIP)—and to recommendations for "bundling" of evidence-based preventive measures (Table 125-2). Additional measures include attention to technical surgical issues and operating-room asepsis (e.g., avoiding open or prophylactic drains) and preoperative therapy for active infection. Reporting of surveillance results to surgeons has been associated with reductions in infection rates. The use of preoperative intranasal mupirocin to eliminate that reservoir for *S. aureus*, preoperative antiseptic bathing, and supplemental intra- and postoperative oxygen remain controversial because of conflicting study results.

The increasingly extensive review of infection rates by regulatory agencies and third-party payers emphasizes the importance of stratifying rates by patient-related risk factors and of developing meaningful systems for wound surveillance after the patient's discharge from the hospital or clinic (when >50% of infections first become apparent) or for use of surrogate markers of wound infection (e.g., prolonged postoperative antibiotic courses).

The epidemic of mad cow disease, centered in the United Kingdom, and associated human cases of variant Creutzfeldt-Jakob disease (Chap. 378) caused by disinfection-resistant prion agents have led to revised recommendations for decontaminating surgical instruments, especially those used for operations on the central nervous system or in patients with dementing illness of unknown etiology.

The process of diagnosing and treating wound infections begins with a careful assessment of the surgical site in the febrile postoperative patient. Clinical findings range from obvious cellulitis or abscess formation to subtler clues such as a sternal "click" following open heart surgery. Diagnosis of deeper organ-space infections or subphrenic abscesses requires a high index of suspicion and the use of CT or MRI. Diagnosis of infections of prosthetic devices, such as orthopedic implants, may be particularly difficult and often requires the use of interventional radiographic techniques to obtain periprosthetic specimens for culture. The most common pathogens in postoperative wound infections are *S. aureus*, coagulase-negative staphylococci, and enteric and anaerobic bacteria. In rapidly progressing postoperative infections, which manifest within 24–48 h of a surgical procedure, the level of suspicion regarding group A streptococcal or clostridial infection (Chaps. 130 and 135) should be high. Treatment of postoperative wound infections requires drainage or surgical excision of infected or necrotic material and antibiotic therapy aimed at the most likely or laboratory-confirmed pathogens.

Infections Related to Vascular Access and Monitoring Intravascular devices are common causes of local site infection and cause up to 50% of nosocomial bacteremias; central vascular catheters (CVCs) account for 80–90% of these infections. National estimates indicate that as many as 200,000 bloodstream infections associated with CVCs occur each year in the United States, with an attributable mortality of 12–25% and an estimated cost of $25,000 per episode; one-third to one-half of these episodes occur in ICUs. With increasing care of seriously ill patients in the community, vascular catheter–associated bloodstream infections acquired in outpatient settings may become as frequent as those acquired in hospitals. This possibility emphasizes the need to broaden surveillance activities.

Catheter-related bloodstream infections derive largely from the cutaneous microflora of the insertion site, with pathogens migrating extraluminally to the catheter tip, usually during the first week after insertion. In addition, contamination of hubs of CVCs or of the ports of "needleless" systems may lead to intraluminal infection over longer periods, particularly with surgically implanted or cuffed catheters. Intrinsic contamination of infusate, although rare, is the most common cause of epidemic device-related bloodstream infection; extrinsic contamination may cause up to half of endemic bacteremias related to arterial infusions used for hemodynamic monitoring. The most common pathogens isolated from vascular device–associated bacteremias include coagulase-negative staphylococci, *S. aureus* (with up to 50% or more of isolates in the United States resistant to methicillin), enterococci, nosocomial gram-negative bacilli, and *Candida*. Many pathogens, especially staphylococci, produce extracellular polysaccharide biofilms that facilitate attachment to catheters and provide sanctuary from antimicrobial agents. "Quorum-sensing" proteins help bacterial cells communicate during biofilm development.

Infections related to vascular catheters and monitoring devices may be the most preventable of nosocomial infections. Evidence-based bundles of control measures (Table 125-2) have been strikingly effective, eliminating all infections in one ICU study. Hospitals should periodically monitor adherence to these performance indicators. Use of antimicrobial- or antiseptic-impregnated CVCs does not appear necessary if the prevention bundle is fully implemented. Additional control measures for infections associated with vascular access include using a chlorhexidine-impregnated patch at the skin-catheter junction; avoiding the femoral site for catheterization because of higher risk of infection (most likely related to the density of the skin flora); moving peripheral catheters to a new site at specified intervals (e.g., every 72–96 h), which may be facilitated by use of an IV therapy team; and applying disposable transducers for pressure monitoring and aseptic technique for accessing transducers or other vascular ports. Improvements in composition of semitransparent access-site dressings and potential nursing benefits (ease of bathing and site inspection, protection of site from secretions) favor the use of such coverings. Unresolved issues include the best frequency for rotation of CVC sites (given that guidewire-assisted catheter changes at the same site do not lessen and may even increase infection risk); the appropriate role of mupirocin ointment, a topical antibiotic with excellent antistaphylococcal activity, in site care; the relative degrees of risk posed by peripherally inserted central catheters (PICC lines); and the risk-benefit of prophylactic use of heparin (to avoid catheter thrombi, which may be associated with increased risk of infection) or of vancomycin or alcohol (as catheter flushes or "locks"—i.e., concentrated anti-infective solutions instilled into the catheter lumen) for high-risk patients.

Vascular device–related infection is suspected on the basis of the appearance of the catheter site or the presence of fever or bacteremia without another source in patients with vascular catheters. The diagnosis is confirmed by the recovery of the same species of microorganism from peripheral-blood cultures (preferably two cultures drawn from peripheral veins by separate venipunctures) and from semiquantitative or quantitative cultures of the vascular catheter tip. Less commonly used diagnostic measures include differential time to positivity (>2 h) for blood drawn through the vascular access device compared with a sample from a peripheral vein or differences in quantitative cultures (a 5- to 10-fold or greater "step-up") for blood samples drawn simultaneously from a peripheral vein and from a CVC. When infusion-related sepsis is considered (e.g., because of the abrupt onset of fever or shock temporally related to infusion therapy), a sample of the infusate or blood product should be retained for culture.

Therapy for vascular access–related infection is directed at the pathogen recovered from the blood and/or infected site. Important considerations in treatment are the need for an echocardiogram (to evaluate the patient for bacterial endocarditis), the duration of therapy, and the need to remove potentially infected catheters. In one report, approximately one-fourth of patients with intravascular catheter–associated *S. aureus* bacteremia who were studied by transesophageal echocardiography had evidence of endocarditis; this test may be useful in determining the appropriate duration of treatment.

Detailed consensus guidelines for the management of intravascular catheter–related infections have been published and recommend catheter removal in most cases of bacteremia or fungemia due to nontunneled CVCs. When attempting to salvage a potentially infected catheter, some clinicians use the "antibiotic lock" technique, which may facilitate penetration of infected biofilms, in addition to systemic antimicrobial therapy. In one study of hemodialysis catheters, only about one-third of salvage attempts were successful, although delayed removal did not appear to increase the risk of complications.

Often, a potentially infected CVC may be exchanged over a guidewire. If cultures of the removed catheter tip are positive, the replacement catheter will be moved to a new site; if the tip cultures are negative, the replacement catheter may remain in the original site but may be at increased risk of subsequent infection due to this manipulation.

The authors of the consensus guidelines advise that the decision to remove a tunneled catheter or implanted device suspected of being the source of bacteremia or fungemia should be based on the severity of the patient's illness, the strength of the evidence that the device is infected, an assessment of the specific pathogens, and the presence of local or systemic complications. For patients with track-site infection, successful therapy without catheter removal is unusual. For patients with suppurative venous thrombophlebitis, excision of the affected vein is usually required.

ISOLATION TECHNIQUES

Written policies for the isolation of infectious patients are a standard component of infection-control programs. In 1996, the CDC revised its isolation guidelines to make them simpler; to recognize the importance of all body fluids, secretions, and excretions in the transmission of nosocomial pathogens; and to focus precautions on the major routes of infection transmission. These policies are currently being updated by the CDC to include integrated guidelines for control of multidrug-resistant organisms.

Standard precautions are designed for the care of all patients in hospitals and aim to reduce the risk of transmission of microorganisms from both recognized and unrecognized sources. These precautions include gloving as well as hand cleansing for potential contact with (1) blood; (2) all other body fluids, secretions, and excretions, whether or not they contain visible blood; (3) nonintact skin; and (4) mucous membranes. Depending on exposure risks, standard precautions also include use of masks, eye protection, and gowns.

Precautions for the care of patients with potentially contagious clinical syndromes (e.g., acute diarrhea) or with suspected or diagnosed colonization or infection with transmissible pathogens are based on probable routes of transmission: *airborne*, *droplet*, and *contact*. Sets of precautions may be combined for diseases that have more than one route of transmission (e.g., varicella).

Because some prevalent antibiotic-resistant pathogens, particularly vancomycin-resistant enterococci (VRE), may be present on *intact* skin of patients in hospitals, some experts recommend gloving for all contact with patients who are acutely ill and/or from high-risk units, such as ICUs. Wearing gloves does not replace the need for hand hygiene because hands occasionally become contaminated during wearing or removal of gloves. Some studies have suggested that use of gowns and gloves compared with routine care of patients (i.e., using neither of these barriers) decreases the risk of nosocomial infection; however, the benefit of gowning by personnel beyond that conferred by gloving and hand hygiene is controversial. Nevertheless, requiring increased precaution levels can improve the compliance of health care workers with isolation recommendations by 30%.

EPIDEMIC AND EMERGING PROBLEMS

Outbreaks and emerging pathogens are always big news but probably account for <5% of nosocomial infections. Concern about emerging pathogens often prompts authorities to require hospitals to develop contingency and response plans. The investigation and control of nosocomial epidemics require that infection-control personnel develop a case definition, confirm that an outbreak really exists (since many apparent epidemics are actually pseudo-outbreaks due to surveillance or laboratory artifacts), review aseptic practices and disinfectant use, determine the extent of the outbreak, perform an epidemiologic investigation to determine modes of transmission, work closely with microbiology personnel to culture for common sources or personnel carriers as appropriate and to type epidemiologically important isolates, and heighten surveillance to judge the effect of control measures. Control measures generally include reinforcing routine aseptic practices and hand hygiene during a search for compliance problems that may have fostered the outbreak, ensuring appropriate isolation of cases (and instituting cohort isolation and nursing if needed), and implementing further controls on the basis of the investigation's findings. Examples of some emerging and potential epidemic problems follow.

Viral Respiratory Infections: SARS and Influenza Infections caused by the severe acute respiratory syndrome (SARS)–associated coronavirus challenged health care systems globally in 2003 (Chap. 179). Basic infection-control measures helped to keep the worldwide case and death counts at ~8000 and ~800, respectively, although SARS was unforgiving of lapses in protocol adherence or laboratory biosafety. The epidemiology of SARS—spread largely in households once patients were ill or in hospitals—contrasts markedly with that of influenza (Chap. 180), which is often contagious a day before symptom onset, can spread rapidly in the community among nonimmune persons, and kills as many as 30,000 persons each year in the United States. Control of influenza has depended on (1) the use of effective vaccines, with increasingly broad recommendations for vaccination and emphasis on vaccination of health care workers; (2) the use of antiviral medications for early treatment and for prophylaxis as part of outbreak control, especially in high-risk settings like nursing homes or hospitals; and (3) infection control (surveillance and droplet precautions) for symptomatic patients.

Concerns about avian (H5N1) and pandemic influenza have led to recommendations for "respiratory hygiene and cough etiquette" and "source containment" (e.g., use of face masks and spatial separation) for outpatients with potentially infectious respiratory illnesses; to the concept of "social distancing" (e.g., closing community venues such as shopping malls) in the event of a pandemic; and to debate about the level of avian influenza respiratory protection required for health care workers—i.e., whether to use the higher-efficiency N95 respirators recommended for airborne isolation rather than the surgical masks used for droplet precautions.

Nosocomial Diarrhea A new, more virulent strain of *Clostridium difficile* has emerged in North America, and overall rates of *C. difficile*–associated diarrhea (Chap. 123) have increased in U.S. hospitals during the past few years. The potential role of exposure to newer fluoroquinolone antibiotics in driving these changes is being investigated. *C. difficile* control measures include judicious use of all antibiotics; heightened suspicion for "atypical" presentations (e.g., toxic megacolon or leukemoid reaction without diarrhea); and early diagnosis, treatment, and contact precautions.

Outbreaks of norovirus infection (Chap. 183) in U.S. and European health care facilities appear to be increasing in frequency, with the virus often introduced by ill visitors or health care workers. This pathogen should be suspected when nausea and vomiting are prominent aspects of bacterial culture–negative diarrheal syndromes. Contact precautions may need to be augmented by aggressive environmental cleaning (given the persistence of norovirus on inanimate objects) and active exclusion of ill staff and visitors.

Chickenpox Infection-control practitioners institute a varicella exposure investigation and control plan whenever health care workers either (1) are exposed to chickenpox (Chap. 173) in the community or through patients with initially unrecognized infections or (2) work during the 24 h before developing chickenpox. The names of exposed workers and patients are obtained; medical histories are reviewed, and (if necessary) serologic tests for immunity are conducted; physicians are notified of susceptible exposed patients; postexposure prophylaxis with varicella-zoster immune globulin (VZIG) is considered for immunocompromised or pregnant contacts (see Table 173-1); varicella vaccine is recommended or preemptive use of acyclovir is considered as an alternative strategy in other susceptible persons; and susceptible exposed employees are furloughed during the at-risk period for disease (8–21 days or—if VZIG has been administered—28 days). Routine varicella vaccination of children and susceptible employees can markedly decrease risk and frequency of exposures.

Tuberculosis Important measures for the control of tuberculosis (Chap. 158) include prompt recognition, isolation, and treatment of cases; recognition of atypical presentations (e.g., lower-lobe infiltrates without cavitation); use of negative-pressure, 100% exhaust, private isolation rooms with closed doors and 6–12 or more air changes per hour; use of N95 "respirators" (approved by the National Institute for Occupational Safety and Health) by caregivers entering isolation rooms; possible use of high-efficiency particulate air filter units and/or ultraviolet lights for disinfecting air when other engineering controls are not feasible or reliable; and follow-up skin-testing of susceptible personnel who have been exposed to infectious patients before isolation. The use of new serologic tests, rather than skin tests, in the diagnosis of latent tuberculosis for infection control purposes is being studied.

Group A Streptococcal Infections The potential for an outbreak of group A streptococcal infection (Chap. 130) should be considered when even a single nosocomial case occurs. Most outbreaks involve surgical wounds and are due to the presence of an asymptomatic carrier in the operating room. Investigation can be confounded by carriage at extrapharyngeal sites such as the rectum and vagina. Health care workers in whom carriage has been linked to nosocomial transmission of group A streptococci are removed from the patient-care setting and are not permitted to return until carriage has been eliminated by antimicrobial therapy.

Fungal Infections Fungal spores are common in the environment, particularly on dusty surfaces. When dusty areas are disturbed during hospital repairs or renovation, the spores become airborne. Inhalation of spores by immunosuppressed (especially neutropenic) patients creates a risk of pulmonary and/or paranasal sinus infection and disseminated aspergillosis (Chap. 197). Routine surveillance among neutropenic patients for infections with filamentous fungi, such as *Aspergillus* and *Fusarium*, helps hospitals to determine whether they are facing unduly extensive environmental risks. As a matter of routine, hospitals should inspect and clean air-handling equipment, review all planned renovations with infection-control personnel and subsequently construct appropriate barriers, remove immunosuppressed patients from renovation sites, and consider the use of high-efficiency particulate air intake filters for rooms housing immunosuppressed patients.

Legionellosis Nosocomial *Legionella* pneumonia (Chap. 141) is most often due to contamination of potable water and predominantly affects immunosuppressed patients, particularly those receiving glucocorticoid medication. The risk varies greatly within and among geographic regions, depending on the extent of hospital hot-water contamination and on specific hospital practices (e.g., inappropriate use of nonsterile water in respiratory therapy equipment). Laboratory-based surveillance for nosocomial *Legionella* should be performed, and a diagnosis of legionellosis should probably be considered more often than it is. If cases are detected, environmental samples (e.g., tap water) should be cultured. If cultures yield *Legionella* and if typing of clinical and environmental isolates reveals a correlation, eradication measures should be pursued. An alternative approach is to periodically culture tap water in wards housing high-risk patients. If *Legionella* is found, a concerted effort should be made to culture samples from all patients with nosocomial pneumonia for *Legionella*.

Antibiotic-Resistant Bacteria Control of antibiotic resistance, particularly in outbreaks (Table 125-3), depends on close laboratory surveillance, with early detection of problems; on aggressive reinforcement of routine asepsis (e.g., hand hygiene); on implementation of barrier precautions for all colonized and/or infected patients; on use of patient-surveillance cultures to more fully ascertain the extent of patient

TABLE 125-3 CONTROLLING ANTIBIOTIC RESISTANCE: APPROACHES TO CONSIDER

Conduct surveillance for antibiotic resistance.
Perform molecular typing (e.g., pulsed-field gel electrophoresis) when rates increase.
For clonal expansion (e.g., single-strain outbreaks): Stress hand hygiene (alcohol hand rub and universal gloving); monitor adherence and give feedback.
For polyclonal expansion (e.g., multistrain outbreaks): Stress antibiotic prudence (consider antibiotic rotation for ICUs); monitor adherence and give feedback.
For continued problems: Obtain patient-surveillance cultures and isolate or provide cohort nursing for colonized/infected patients.
Control device-related infections.
Enlist administrative support proactively.

Source: *Adapted from: RA Weinstein, Emerg Infect Dis 7:188, 2001; see also www.cdc.gov/ncidod/dhqp/pdf/ar/mdroGuideline2006.pdf.*

colonization; and on timely initiation of an epidemiologic investigation when rates increase. Colonized personnel who are implicated in nosocomial transmission and patients who pose a threat may be decontaminated. In a few ICUs, selective decontamination of patients has been used successfully as a temporary emergency control measure for outbreaks of infection due to gram-negative bacilli. Other promising ICU control measures include daily bathing of patients with chlorhexidine and enforcement of environmental cleaning; in recent trials, each of these measures reduced cross-transmission of VRE. The value of "search-and-destroy" methods—i.e., the use of active surveillance cultures to detect and isolate the "resistance iceberg" of patients colonized with methicillin-resistant *S. aureus* (MRSA) or VRE—in non-outbreak settings has been controversial but is credited with elimination of nosocomial MRSA in the Netherlands and Denmark.

Currently, several antibiotic resistance problems are of particular health care concern. First, the emergence of community-acquired MRSA has been dramatic in many countries, with as many as 50% of community-acquired "staph infections" in some U.S. cities now caused by strains resistant to β-lactam antibiotics (Chap. 129). The potential incursion of these strains into hospitals and the resulting impact on control of nosocomial MRSA infections are of enormous concern. Second, in the ongoing global reemergence of nosocomial multidrug-resistant gram-negative bacilli, new problems include plasmid-mediated resistance to fluoroquinolones, metallo-β-lactamase-mediated resistance to carbapenems, and panresistant strains of *Acinetobacter*. Many of these multidrug-resistant strains are susceptible only to colistin, which has led to a "rediscovery" and renewed use of this drug. Finally, clinical infections with MRSA strains exhibiting high-level vancomycin resistance due to VRE-derived plasmids have been reported in several patients in the United States, often in the setting of prolonged or repeated treatment with vancomycin and/or VRE colonization. The detection of any of these current problems should trigger an epidemiologic investigation and aggressive infection-control measures.

Because the excessive use of broad-spectrum antibiotics underlies many resistance problems, aggressive antibiotic-control policies must be considered a cornerstone of resistance-control efforts. Recommendations for "antibiotic stewardship" are being promulgated by the Infectious Diseases Society of America. Although the efficacy of antibiotic-control measures in reducing rates of antimicrobial resistance has not been proven in prospective controlled trials, it seems worthwhile to restrict the use of particular agents to narrowly defined indications in order to limit selective pressure on the nosocomial flora.

Bioterrorism and Other "Surge-Event" Preparedness The horrific attack on the World Trade Center in New York City on September 11, 2001; the subsequent mailings of anthrax spores in the United States; and recently exposed terrorist plans and activities in the United Kingdom and elsewhere have made bioterrorism a prominent source of concern to hospital infection-control programs. The essentials for hospital preparedness (Table 125-4) entail education, internal and external communication, and risk assessment. Up-to-date information on a variety of bioterrorism-associated issues is available from the CDC (see *www.bt.cdc.gov*).

TABLE 125-4 HIGHLIGHTS OF HOSPITAL PREPAREDNESS FOR BIOTERRORISM AND OTHER "SURGE EVENTS"

Emergency Department: Educate (bioterrorism diagnoses, case definitions, and appropriate syndrome-based isolation precautions)
Laboratory: Identify protocols and laboratory safety procedures for agents of bioterrorism
Pharmacy: Develop medication and vaccine par stock, allocation, and delivery plans
Nursing: Assess bed and isolation surge capacity; help develop contingency plans to free bed space (e.g., early discharges)
Hospital Police: Plan for responsibilities as first responders and providers of risk assessment
Engineering/Buildings and Grounds: Evaluate air-handling systems and ensure familiarity with shutoffs and controls; educate about environmental decontamination
Outpatient Areas: Develop plans for delivery of prophylactic medications and/or vaccines
Public Health: Open lines of communication, education, and surveillance
The Community: Plan for infection-control practitioners to serve as liaisons for emergency departments, laboratories, and community providers
Administration: Perform resource assessment (e.g., medical supplies, transportation capabilities, potable water, sanitation facilities, provider backup, bed-space backup); oversee development of an incident command system
"Morale Officer": Keep staff functioning

EMPLOYEE HEALTH SERVICE ISSUES

An institution's employee health service is a critical component of its infection-control efforts. New employees should be processed through the service, where a contagious-disease history can be taken; evidence of immunity to a variety of diseases, such as hepatitis B, chickenpox, measles, mumps, and rubella, can be sought; immunizations for hepatitis B, measles, mumps, rubella, and varicella can be given as needed and a reminder about the need for yearly influenza immunization can be imparted; baseline and "booster" PPD (purified protein derivative of tuberculin) skin-testing or serologic testing for tuberculosis can be performed; and education about personal responsibility for infection control can be initiated. Evaluations of employees should be codified to meet the requirements of accrediting and regulatory agencies.

The employee health service must have protocols for dealing with workers who have been exposed to contagious diseases, such as those percutaneously or mucosally exposed to the blood of patients infected with HIV or hepatitis B or C virus. For example, postexposure HIV prophylaxis with a combination of two or three antiretroviral agents is recommended; free consultation is available from the CDC PEPLine (888-HIV-4911). Protocols are also needed for dealing with caregivers who have common contagious diseases (such as chickenpox, group A streptococcal infections, respiratory infections, and infectious diarrhea) and for those who have less common but high-visibility public health problems (such as chronic hepatitis B or C or HIV infection) for which exposure-control guidelines have been published by the CDC and by the Society for Healthcare Epidemiology of America.

FURTHER READINGS

BRATZLER DW, HUNT DR: The Surgical Infection Prevention and Surgical Care Improvement Projects: National initiatives to improve outcomes for patients having surgery. Clin Infect Dis 43:322, 2006

CENTERS FOR DISEASE CONTROL AND PREVENTION: Environmental infection control guidelines. Recommendations of the Healthcare Infection Control Practices Advisory Committee. MMWR 52(RR10):1, 2003

———: Guideline for hand hygiene in health-care settings: Recommendations of the Healthcare Infection Control Practices Advisory Committee and the HICPAC/SHEA/APIC/IDSA Hand Hygiene Task Force. MMWR 51(RR-16):1, 2002

———: Guidelines for preventing opportunistic infections among hematopoietic stem cell transplant recipients: Recommendations of CDC, the Infectious Diseases Society of America, and the American Society of Blood and Marrow Transplantation. MMWR 49(RR-10):1, 2000

HOTA B, WEINSTEIN RA: Basics work: Preventing infections in ICUs in developing countries. Crit Care Med 33:2133, 2005

MCKIBBEN L et al: Guidance on public reporting of healthcare-associated recommendations of the Healthcare Infection Control Practices Advisory Committee. Infect Control Hosp Epidemiol 26:580, 2005

MERMEL LA et al: Guidelines for the management of intravascular catheter–related infections. Clin Infect Dis 32:1249, 2001

STRAUSBAUGH LJ et al: Preventing transmission of multidrug-resistant bacteria in health care settings: A tale of two guidelines. Clin Infect Dis 42:828, 2006

WEINSTEIN RA et al: Infection control report cards—securing patient safety. N Engl J Med 353:225, 2005

———, BONTEN MJ: Controlling antibiotic resistant bacteria: What's an intensivist to do? Crit Care Med 33:2446, 2005

126 Infections in Transplant Recipients

Robert Finberg, Joyce Fingeroth

The evaluation of infections in transplant recipients involves consideration of both the donor and the recipient of the transplanted organ. Infections following transplantation are complicated by the use of drugs that are necessary to enhance the likelihood of survival of the transplanted organ but that also cause the host to be immunocompromised. Thus, what might have been a latent or asymptomatic infection in an immunocompetent donor or in the recipient prior to therapy can become a life-threatening problem when the recipient becomes immunosuppressed.

PRETRANSPLANTATION EVALUATION

A variety of organisms have been transmitted by organ transplantation (Table 126-1). Careful attention to the sterility of the medium used to process the organ combined with meticulous microbiologic evaluation reduces rates of transmission of bacteria that may be present or grow in the organ culture medium. From 2% to >20% of donor kidneys are estimated to be contaminated with bacteria—in most cases, with the organisms that colonize the skin or grow in the tissue culture medium used to bathe the donor kidney while it awaits implantation. The reported rate of bacterial contamination of transplanted stem cells (bone marrow, peripheral blood, cord blood) is as high as 17% but is most commonly ~1%. The use of enrichment columns and monoclonal-antibody depletion procedures results in a higher incidence of contamination. In one series of patients receiving contaminated products, 14% had fever or bacteremia, but none died. Results of cultures performed at the time of cryopreservation and at the time of thawing were helpful in guiding therapy for the recipient.

In many transplantation centers, transmission of infections that may be latent or clinically inapparent in the donor organ has resulted in the development of specific donor-screening protocols. In addition to ordering serologic studies focused on viruses such as herpes-group viruses [herpes simplex virus types 1 and 2 (HSV-1, HSV-2), varicella-zoster virus (VZV), cytomegalovirus (CMV), human herpesvirus (HHV) type 6, Epstein-Barr virus (EBV), and Kaposi's sarcoma–associated herpesvirus (KSHV)] as well as hepatitis B and C viruses, human immunodeficiency virus (HIV), human T cell lymphotropic virus type I, and West Nile virus, donors should be screened for parasites such as *Toxoplasma gondii and Trypanosoma cruzi* (the latter particularly in Latin America). Clinicians caring for prospective organ donors should also consider assessing stool for parasites, should examine chest radiographs for evidence of granulomatous disease, and should perform purified protein derivative (PPD) skin testing or obtain blood for immune cell–based assays that detect active or latent *Mycobacterium tuberculosis* infection. An investigation of the donor's dietary habits (e.g., consumption of raw meat or fish or of unpasteurized dairy products), occupations or avocations (e.g., gardening or spelunking), and travel history (e.g., travel to areas with endemic fungi) is also mandatory. It is expected that the recipient will have been likewise assessed. Because of immune dysfunction resulting from chemotherapy or underlying chronic

TABLE 126-1 ORGANISMS TRANSMITTED BY ORGAN TRANSPLANTATION AND THEIR PRIMARY SITES OF REACTIVATION DISEASE[a]

	Blood	Lungs	Heart	Brain	Liver/Spleen	Skin
Viruses						
Cytomegalovirus[b]	+	+	±	±	+	±
Epstein-Barr virus[c]	+	+	±	±	+	±
Herpes simplex virus		+		±	+	+
Human herpesvirus type 6	+	+		+		+
Kaposi's sarcoma–associated herpesvirus	+	±			±	+
Hepatitis B and C viruses					+	
Rabies virus[d]				+		
West Nile virus	+			+		
Fungi						
Candida albicans	+	+			+	+
Histoplasma capsulatum	+	+			+	+
Cryptococcus neoformans	+	+		+	±	+
Parasites						
Toxoplasma gondii[e]		+	+	+		
Strongyloides stercoralis[f,g]		+				
Trypanosoma cruzi[g]			+			
Plasmodium falciparum[g]	+					
Prion Diseases						
Creutzfeldt-Jakob disease (CJD)[h]				+		
Variant CJD/bovine spongiform encephalopathy[i]				+		

[a]+, well documented; ±, probably occurs.

[b]Cytomegalovirus reactivation is prone to occur in the transplanted organ. The same may be true for Kaposi's sarcoma–associated herpesvirus.

[c]Epstein-Barr virus reactivation usually presents as an extranodal proliferation of transformed B cells and can be present either as a diffuse disease or as a mass lesion in a single organ.

[d]Rabies virus has been transmitted through corneal transplants.

[e]*T. gondii* usually causes disease in the brain. In hematopoietic stem cell transplant recipients, acute pulmonary disease may also occur. Heart transplant recipients develop disease in the allograft.

[f]*Strongyloides* "hyperinfection" may present with pulmonary disease—often associated with gram-negative bacterial pneumonia.

[g]While transmission with organs has been described, it is unusual.

[h]CJD (sporadic and familial) has been transmitted with corneal transplants. Whether it can be transmitted with blood is not known.

[i]Variant CJD can be transmitted with transfused non-leukodepleted blood, posing a theoretical risk to transplant recipients.

TABLE 126-2 COMMON SOURCES OF INFECTIONS AFTER HEMATOPOIETIC STEM CELL TRANSPLANTATION

	Period after Transplantation		
Infection Site	**Early (<1 Month)**	**Middle (1–4 Months)**	**Late (>6 Months)**
Disseminated	Aerobic gram-negative, gram-positive bacteria	*Nocardia* *Candida, Aspergillus*	Encapsulated bacteria (*Streptococcus pneumoniae, Haemophilus influenzae, Neisseria meningitidis*)
Skin and mucous membranes	HSV	HHV-6	VZV
Lungs	Aerobic gram-negative, gram-positive bacteria *Candida, Aspergillus* HSV	CMV, seasonal respiratory viruses *Pneumocystis* *Toxoplasma*	*Pneumocystis*
Gastrointestinal tract		CMV	
Kidney		BK virus, adenovirus	BK virus
Brain	HHV-6	HHV-6 *Toxoplasma*	*Toxoplasma* JC virus
Bone marrow	HHV-6		

Note: CMV, cytomegalovirus; HHV-6, human herpesvirus type 6; HSV, herpes simplex virus; VZV, varicella-zoster virus.

disease, however, direct testing of the recipient may prove less reliable. This chapter considers aspects of infection unique to various transplantation settings.

INFECTIONS IN HEMATOPOIETIC STEM CELL TRANSPLANT (HSCT) RECIPIENTS

Transplantation of hematopoietic stem cells from bone marrow or from peripheral or cord blood for cancer, immunodeficiency, or autoimmune disease results in a transient state of complete immunologic incompetence. Immediately after transplantation, both phagocytes and adaptive immune cells (T and B cells) are absent, and the host is extremely susceptible to infection. The reconstitution that follows transplantation has been likened to maturation of the immune system in neonates. The analogy does not entirely predict infections seen in HSCT recipients, however, because the new cells mature in an old host who has several latent infections already. Nevertheless, most infections occur in a predictable time frame after transplantation (Table 126-2).

BACTERIAL INFECTIONS

In the first month after hematopoietic stem cell transplantation, infectious complications are similar to those in granulocytopenic patients receiving chemotherapy for acute leukemia (Chap. 82). Because of the anticipated 1- to 3-week duration of neutropenia and the high rate of bacterial infection in this population, many centers give prophylactic antibiotics to patients upon initiation of myeloablative therapy. Quinolones decrease the incidence of gram-negative bacteremia among these patients. Bacterial infections are common in the first few days after hematopoietic stem cell transplantation. The organisms involved are predominantly those found on the skin or in IV catheters (*Staphylococcus aureus*, coagulase-negative staphylococci) and aerobic bacteria that colonize the bowel (*Escherichia coli, Klebsiella, Pseudomonas*). Beyond the first few days of neutropenia, infections with filamentous bacteria such as *Nocardia* become more common. Episodes of bacteremia due to encapsulated organisms mark the late posttransplantation period (>6 months after hematopoietic stem cell reconstitution). Chemotherapy and use of broad-spectrum antibiotics place HSCT patients at risk for diarrhea and colitis caused by *Clostridium difficile* overgrowth and toxin production.

FUNGAL INFECTIONS

Beyond the first week after transplantation, fungal infections become increasingly common, particularly among patients who have received broad-spectrum antibiotics. As in most granulocytopenic patients, *Candida* infections are most commonly seen in this setting. With increased use of prophylactic fluconazole, infections with resistant fungi—in particular, *Aspergillus* and other molds (*Fusarium, Scedosporium, Penicillium*)—have become more common, prompting some centers to replace fluconazole with agents such as caspofungin, voriconazole, and posaconazole. The role of antifungal prophylaxis with these different agents, in contrast to empirical treatment for suspected or documented infection, remains controversial (Chap. 82). In patients with graft-versus-host disease (GVHD) who require prolonged or indefinite courses of glucocorticoids and other immunosuppressive agents [e.g., cyclosporine, FK506 (tacrolimus), mycophenolate, rapamycin (sirolimus), antithymocyte globulin, or anti-CD52 antibody (alemtuzumab, an anti-lymphocyte and antimonocyte monoclonal antibody)], there is a high risk of fungal infection (usually with *Candida* or *Aspergillus*), even after engraftment and resolution of neutropenia. These patients are also at high risk for reactivation of latent fungal infection (histoplasmosis, coccidioidomycosis, blastomycosis) in areas where endemic fungi reside and if they have been involved in activities such as gardening or caving. Prolonged use of central venous catheters for parenteral nutrition (lipids) increases the risk of fungemia with *Malassezia*. Some centers administer prophylactic antifungal agents to these patients. Because of the high and prolonged risk of *Pneumocystis jiroveci* pneumonia (especially among patients being treated for hematologic malignancies), most patients receive maintenance prophylaxis with trimethoprim-sulfamethoxazole (TMP-SMX) starting 1 month after engraftment and continuing for at least 1 year.

PARASITIC INFECTIONS

The regimen just described for the fungal pathogen *Pneumocystis* may also protect patients seropositive for the parasite *T. gondii*, which may cause pneumonia or, more commonly, central nervous system (CNS) lesions. The advantages of maintaining HSCT recipients on daily TMP-SMX for 1 year after transplantation include some protection against *Listeria monocytogenes* and nocardial disease as well as late infections with *Streptococcus pneumoniae* and *Haemophilus influenzae*, which are a consequence of the inability of the immature immune system to respond to polysaccharide antigens.

VIRAL INFECTIONS

HSCT recipients are susceptible to infection with a variety of viruses, including primary and reactivation syndromes caused by most HHVs (Table 126-3) and acute infections caused by viruses that circulate in the community.

Herpes Simplex Virus Within the first 2 weeks after transplantation, most patients who are seropositive for HSV-1 excrete the virus from the oropharynx. The ability to isolate HSV declines with time. Administration of prophylactic acyclovir (or valacyclovir) to seropositive HSCT recipients has been shown to reduce mucositis and prevent HSV pneumonia (a rare condition reported almost exclusively in allogeneic HSCT recipients). Both esophagitis (usually due to HSV-1) and anogenital disease (commonly induced by HSV-2) may be prevented with acyclovir prophylaxis. For further discussion, see Chap. 172.

Varicella-Zoster Virus Reactivation of herpes zoster may occur within the first month but more commonly occurs several months after transplantation. Reactivation rates are ~40% for allogeneic recipients and 25% for autologous recipients. Localized zoster can spread rapidly in an immunosuppressed patient. Fortunately, disseminated disease can usually be controlled with high doses of acyclovir. Because of frequent dissemination among patients with skin lesions, acyclovir is given prophylactically in some centers to prevent severe disease. Low doses of acyclovir (400 mg orally, three times daily) appear to be effec-

TABLE 126-3 COMMON HERPESVIRUS SYNDROMES IN TRANSPLANT RECIPIENTS

Virus	Reactivation Disease
Herpes simplex virus type 1	Oral lesions Esophageal lesions Pneumonia (only in hematopoietic stem cell transplant recipients) Hepatitis
Herpes simplex virus type 2	Anogenital lesions Hepatitis
Varicella-zoster virus	Zoster (potentially disseminated)
Cytomegalovirus	Associated graft rejection Fever Bone marrow failure Pneumonitis Gastrointestinal disease Other
Epstein-Barr virus	B cell lymphoproliferative disease/lymphoma Oral hairy leukoplakia (rare)
Human herpesvirus type 6	Fever Delayed monocyte/platelet engraftment Encephalitis (controversial)
Human herpesvirus type 7	Undefined
Kaposi's sarcoma–associated virus	Kaposi's sarcoma Primary effusion lymphoma (rare) Multicentric Castleman's disease (rare) Marrow aplasia

tive in preventing reactivation of VZV. However, acyclovir can also suppress the development of VZV-specific immunity. Thus, its administration for only 6 months after transplantation does not prevent zoster from occurring when treatment is stopped. Some data suggest that administration of low doses of acyclovir for an entire year after transplantation is effective and may eliminate most cases of posttransplantation zoster. **For further discussion, see Chap. 173.**

Cytomegalovirus The onset of CMV disease (interstitial pneumonia, bone marrow suppression, graft failure, hepatitis/colitis) usually begins 30–90 days after transplantation, when the granulocyte count is adequate but immunologic reconstitution has not occurred. CMV disease rarely develops earlier than 14 days after transplantation and may become evident as late as 4 months after the procedure. It is of greatest concern in the second month after transplantation, particularly in allogeneic HSCT recipients. In cases in which the donor marrow is depleted of T cells (to prevent GVHD or eliminate a T cell tumor), the disease may be manifested earlier. The use of alemtuzumab to prevent GVHD in nonmyeloablative transplantation has been associated with an increase in CMV disease. Patients who receive ganciclovir for prophylaxis, preemptive treatment, or treatment (see below) may develop recurrent CMV infection even later than 4 months after transplantation, as treatment appears to delay the development of the normal immune response to CMV infection. Although CMV disease may present as isolated fever, granulocytopenia, thrombocytopenia, or gastrointestinal disease, the foremost cause of death from CMV infection in the setting of hematopoietic stem cell transplantation is pneumonia.

With the standard use of CMV-negative or filtered blood products, primary CMV infection should be a risk in allogeneic transplantation only when the donor is CMV-seropositive and the recipient is CMV-seronegative. Reactivation disease or superinfection with another strain from the donor is also common in CMV-positive recipients, and most seropositive patients who undergo hematopoietic stem cell transplantation excrete CMV, with or without clinical findings. Serious CMV disease is much more common among allogeneic than autologous recipients and is often associated with GVHD. In addition to pneumonia and marrow suppression (and, less often, graft failure), manifestations of CMV disease in HSCT recipients include fever with or without arthralgias, myalgias, hepatitis, and esophagitis. CMV ulcerations occur in both the lower and the upper gastrointestinal tract, and it may be difficult to distinguish diarrhea due to GVHD from that due to CMV infection. The finding of CMV in the liver of a patient with GVHD does not necessarily mean that CMV is responsible for hepatic enzyme abnormalities. It is interesting that the ocular and neurologic manifestations of CMV infections are uncommon in these patients.

Management of CMV disease in HSCT recipients includes strategies directed at prophylaxis and preemptive therapy (suppression of silent replication) and at treatment of disease. Prophylaxis results in a lower incidence of disease at the cost of treating many patients who otherwise would not require therapy. Because of the high fatality rate associated with CMV pneumonia in these patients and the difficulty of early diagnosis of CMV infection, prophylactic IV ganciclovir (or oral valganciclovir) has been used in some centers and has been shown to abort CMV disease during the period of maximal vulnerability (from engraftment to day 120 after transplantation). Ganciclovir also prevents HSV reactivation and reduces the risk of VZV reactivation; thus acyclovir prophylaxis should be discontinued when ganciclovir is administered. The foremost problem with the administration of ganciclovir relates to adverse effects, which include dose-related bone marrow suppression (thrombocytopenia, leukopenia, anemia, and pancytopenia). Because the frequency of CMV pneumonia is lower among autologous HSCT recipients (2–7%) than among allogeneic HSCT recipients (10–40%), prophylaxis in the former group will not become the rule until a less toxic oral antiviral agent becomes available. Promising new drugs that are now being assessed in clinical trials include maribavir, a benzimidazole riboside that inhibits a viral protein kinase activity (UL97).

Like prophylaxis, preemptive treatment, which targets patients with polymerase chain reaction (PCR) evidence of CMV entails the unnecessary treatment of many individuals (on the basis of a laboratory test that is not highly predictive of disease) with drugs that have adverse effects. Currently, because of the neutropenia associated with ganciclovir in HSCT recipients, a preemptive approach—that is, treatment of those patients in whose blood CMV is detected by an antigen or nucleic acid amplification test—is used at most centers. This approach is almost as effective as prophylaxis and causes less toxicity. Quantitative viral load assays, which are not dependent on circulating polymorphonuclear leukocytes, have supplanted antigen-based assays and are used by most centers. A positive test (or increasing viral load) prompts the initiation of preemptive therapy. When prophylaxis or preemptive therapy is stopped, late disease may occur, although by then the patient is often equipped with improved graft function and is better able to combat disease.

Treatment of CMV pneumonia in HSCT recipients (unlike that in other clinical settings) involves both IV immune globulin (IVIg) and ganciclovir. In patients who cannot tolerate ganciclovir, foscarnet is a useful alternative, although it may produce nephrotoxicity and electrolyte imbalance. When neither ganciclovir nor foscarnet is clinically tolerated, cidofovir can be used; however, its efficacy is less well established, and its side effects include nephrotoxicity. Case reports have suggested that the immunosuppressive agent leflunomide may be active in this setting, but controlled studies are lacking. Maribavir is under investigation for treatment as well as prophylaxis. Transfusion of CMV-specific T cells from the donor decreased viral load in a small series of patients; this result suggests that immunotherapy may play a role in the treatment of this disease in the future. **For further discussion, see Chap. 175.**

Human Herpesviruses 6 and 7 HHV-6, the cause of roseola in children, is a ubiquitous herpesvirus that reactivates (as determined by quantitative plasma PCR) in ~50% of HSCT recipients 2–4 weeks after transplantation. Reactivation is more common among patients requiring glucocorticoids for GVHD and among those receiving second transplants. Reactivation of HHV-6 (primarily type B) appears to be associated with delayed monocyte and platelet engraftment. Although encephalitis developing after transplantation has been associated with HHV-6 in cerebrospinal fluid (CSF), the causality of the association is not well defined. In several cases, plasma viremia was detected long before the onset of encephalitis; nevertheless, patients with encephalitis did tend to have very high viral loads in plasma at the time of CNS illness. HHV-6 DNA is sometimes found in lung samples after transplantation. However, its role in pneumonitis is also unclear. While HHV-6 has been shown to be susceptible to foscarnet (and possibly to ganciclovir) in vitro, the efficacy of antiviral treatment has not been well studied. Little is known about the related herpesvirus HHV-7 or its role in posttransplantation infection. For further discussion, see Chap. 175.

Epstein-Barr Virus Primary EBV infection can be fatal to HSCT recipients; EBV reactivation can cause EBV–B cell lymphoproliferative disease (EBV-LPD), which may also be fatal to patients taking immunosuppressive drugs. Latent EBV infection of B cells leads to several interesting phenomena in HSCT recipients. The marrow ablation that occurs as part of the HSCT procedure may sometimes eliminate latent EBV from the host. Infection can then be reacquired immediately after transplantation by transfer of infected donor B cells. Rarely, transplantation from a seronegative donor may result in cure. The recipient is then at risk for a second primary infection.

EBV-LPD can develop in the recipient's B cells (if any survive marrow ablation) but is more likely to be a consequence of outgrowth of infected donor cells. Both lytic and latent EBV replication are more likely during immunosuppression (e.g., they are associated with GVHD and the use of antibodies to T cells). Although less likely in autologous transplantation, reactivation can occur in T cell–depleted autologous recipients (e.g., patients being given antibodies to T cells for the treatment of a T cell lymphoma with marrow depletion). EBV-LPD, which can become apparent as early as 1–3 months after engraftment, can cause high fevers and cervical adenopathy resembling the symptoms of infectious mononucleosis but more commonly presents as an extranodal mass. The incidence of EBV-LPD among allogeneic HSCT recipients is 0.6–1%, which contrasts with figures of ~5% for renal transplant recipients and up to 20% for cardiac transplant patients. In all cases, EBV-LPD is more likely to occur with high-dose, prolonged immunosuppression, especially that caused by the use of antibodies to T cells, glucocorticoids, and calcineurin inhibitors (e.g., cyclosporine, FK506).

PCR can be used to monitor EBV production after hematopoietic stem cell transplantation. High or increasing viral loads predict an enhanced likelihood of developing EBV-LPD and should prompt rapid reduction of immunosuppression and search for a focus of disease. If reduction of immunosuppression does not have the desired effect, administration of a monoclonal antibody to CD20 (rituximab or others) for the treatment of B cell lymphomas that express this surface protein has elicited dramatic responses and currently constitutes first-line therapy for CD20-positive EBV-LPD. However, long-term suppression of new antibody responses accompanies therapy, and recurrences are not infrequent. Additional B cell–directed antibodies, including anti-CD22, are under study. The role of antivirals is uncertain because no available agents have been documented to have activity against the different forms of latent EBV infection. Preventing lytic replication in these patients would theoretically produce a statistical decrease in the frequency of latent disease by decreasing the number of virions available to cause additional infection. In case reports and small animal studies, ganciclovir and/or high-dose zidovudine together with other agents has been used to eradicate EBV-LPD and CNS lymphomas, another EBV-associated complication of transplantation. Both interferon and retinoic acid have been employed in the treatment of EBV-LPD, as has IVIg, but no large prospective studies have assessed the efficacy of any of these agents. Several additional drugs are undergoing preclinical evaluation. Standard chemotherapeutic regimens have been used as a last resort, even though patients' tolerance and long-term results have been disappointing. EBV-specific T cells generated from the donor have been used experimentally to prevent and to treat EBV-LPD in allogeneic recipients, and efforts are under way to increase the activity and specificity of ex vivo–generated T cells. For further discussion, see Chap. 174.

Human Herpesvirus 8 The EBV-related gammaherpesvirus KSHV, which is causally associated with Kaposi's sarcoma, with primary effusion lymphoma, and with multicentric Castleman's disease, has rarely resulted in disease in HSCT recipients, although some cases of virus-associated marrow aplasia have been reported in the peritransplantation period. The relatively low seroprevalence of KSHV in the population and the limited duration of profound T cell suppression after hematopoietic stem cell transplantation provide a probable explanation for the currently low incidence of KSHV disease. For further discussion, see Chap. 175.

Other (Nonherpes) Viruses The diagnosis of pneumonia in HSCT recipients poses some special problems. Because patients have undergone treatment with multiple chemotherapeutic agents and sometimes irradiation, their differential diagnosis should include—in addition to bacterial and fungal pneumonia—CMV pneumonitis, pneumonia of other viral etiologies, parasitic pneumonia, diffuse alveolar hemorrhage, and chemical- or radiation-associated pneumonitis. Since fungi and viruses [e.g., influenza A and B viruses, respiratory syncytial virus (RSV), parainfluenza virus (types 1, 2, and 3), metapneumoviruses, and adenoviruses] are also causes of pneumonia in this setting, it is important to diagnose CMV specifically (see "Cytomegalovirus," above). *M. tuberculosis* has been an uncommon cause of pneumonia among HSCT recipients in Western countries (accounting for <0.1–0.2% of cases) but is common in Hong Kong (5.5%) and in countries where the prevalence of tuberculosis is high. The recipient's exposure history is clearly critical in an assessment of posttransplantation infections.

Both RSV and parainfluenza viruses, particularly type 3, can cause severe or even fatal pneumonia in HSCT recipients. Infections with both of these agents sometimes occur as disastrous nosocomial epidemics. Preemptive treatment of upper airway infection and therapy for established lower tract invasion with aerosolized ribavirin and/or the anti-RSV monoclonal antibody palivizumab have been reported to lessen the severity of RSV disease in some studies. (Respigam, a polyclonal anti-RSV preparation, is no longer available.) However, no large prospective studies establishing the efficacy of these agents in HSCT recipients have been performed. Aerosolized ribavirin is difficult to administer. Antibody in particular may prove more active in immunocompromised hosts, but relevant evaluation is lacking.

Influenza also occurs in HSCT recipients and generally mirrors the presence of infection in the community. Progression to pneumonia is more common when infection occurs early after transplantation and when the recipient is lymphopenic. Several drugs are available for the treatment of influenza. Amantadine and rimantadine have limited effects, primarily reducing symptoms and shortening the duration of illness caused by sensitive strains of influenza A virus. The neuraminidase inhibitors oseltamivir (oral) and zanamivir (aerosolized) are active against both influenza A virus and influenza B virus and are a reasonable treatment option. Parenteral forms of neuraminidase inhibitors are undergoing clinical trials. An important preventive measure is immunization of household members, hospital staff members, and other frequent contacts.

Human metapneumovirus, a paramyxovirus, can sometimes cause severe pneumonia and respiratory failure in HSCT recipients; however, mild or even asymptomatic infection may be more common. At present, the overall contribution of human metapneumovirus to the burden of lower respiratory tract disease in HSCT recipients is unknown.

Adenovirus can be isolated from HSCT recipients at rates varying from 5 to 18%. Although hemorrhagic cystitis, pneumonia, gastroenteritis, and fatal disseminated infection have been reported, adenovirus infection, which (like CMV infection) usually occurs in the first or second month after transplantation, is often asymptomatic. A role for cidofovir therapy has been suggested, but the efficacy of this agent is unproven.

Infections with parvovirus B19 (presenting as anemia or occasionally as pancytopenia) and enteroviruses (sometimes fatal) can occur. Parvovirus infection may possibly respond to IVIg (Chap. 177). Intranasal pleconaril, a capsid-binding agent, is being studied for the treatment of enterovirus infection.

Rhinoviruses and coronaviruses are frequent co-pathogens in HSCT recipients; however, whether they independently contribute to significant pulmonary infection is not known. Rotaviruses are a common cause of gastroenteritis in these patients. The polyomavirus BK virus is found at high titers in the urine of patients who are profoundly immunosuppressed. BK viruria may be associated with hemorrhagic cystitis in these patients. Compared with the incidence among patients with impaired T cell function due to HIV infection, progressive multifocal leukoencephalopathy caused by the related JC virus is rare among HSCT recipients (Chap. 376). When transmitted by mosquitoes or by blood transfusion, West Nile virus can cause encephalitis and death after hematopoietic stem cell transplantation.

INFECTIONS IN SOLID ORGAN TRANSPLANT (SOT) RECIPIENTS

Morbidity and mortality among SOT recipients are reduced by the use of effective antibiotics. The organisms that cause acute infections in recipients of SOT are different from those that infect HSCT recipients because SOT recipients do not go through a period of neutropenia. As the transplantation procedure involves major surgery, however, SOT recipients are subject to infections at anastomotic sites and to wound infections. Compared with HSCT recipients, SOT patients are immunosuppressed for longer periods (often permanently). Thus they are susceptible to many of the same organisms as patients with chronically impaired T cell immunity (Chap. 82, especially Table 82-1).

During the early period (<1 month after transplantation), infections are most commonly caused by extracellular bacteria (staphylococci, streptococci, enterococci, *E. coli*, other gram-negative organisms), which often originate in surgical wound or anastomotic sites. The type of transplant largely determines the spectrum of infection.

In subsequent weeks, the consequences of the administration of agents that suppress cell-mediated immunity become apparent, and acquisition or reactivation of viruses and parasites (from the recipient or from the transplanted organ) can occur. CMV infection is often a problem, particularly in the first 6 months after transplantation and may present as severe systemic disease or as infection of the transplanted organ. HHV-6 reactivation (assessed by plasma PCR) occurs within the first 2–4 weeks after transplantation and may be associated with fever, leukopenia, and possibly encephalitis. Data suggest that replication of HHV-6 and HHV-7 may exacerbate CMV-induced disease. CMV is associated not only with generalized immunosuppression but also with organ-specific, rejection-related syndromes: glomerulopathy in kidney transplant recipients, bronchiolitis obliterans in lung transplant recipients, vasculopathy in heart transplant recipients, and the vanishing bile duct syndrome in liver transplant recipients. A complex interplay between increased CMV replication and enhanced graft rejection is well established: increasing immunosuppression leads to increased CMV replication, which is associated with graft rejection. For this reason, considerable attention has been focused on the diagnosis, prophylaxis, and treatment of CMV infection in SOT recipients. Early transmission of West Nile virus to transplant recipients from an organ donor has been reported; however, the risk of West Nile acquisition has been reduced by implementation of screening procedures.

Beyond 6 months after transplantation, infections characteristic of patients with defects in cell-mediated immunity—e.g., infections with *Listeria*, *Nocardia*, *Rhodococcus*, various fungi, and other intracellular pathogens—may be a problem. International patients and global travelers may experience reactivation of dormant infections with trypanosomes, *Leishmania*, *Plasmodium*, *Strongyloides*, and other parasites. Elimination of these late infections will not be possible until the patient develops specific tolerance to the transplanted organ in the absence of drugs that lead to generalized immunosuppression. Meanwhile, vigilance, prophylaxis/preemptive therapy (when indicated), and rapid diagnosis and treatment of infections can be lifesaving in SOT recipients, who, unlike most HSCT recipients, continue to be immunosuppressed.

SOT recipients are susceptible to EBV-LPD from as early as 2 months to many years after transplantation. The prevalence of this complication is increased by potent and prolonged use of T cell–suppressive drugs. Decreasing the degree of immunosuppression may in some cases reverse the condition. Among SOT patients, those with heart and lung transplants—who receive the most intensive immunosuppressive regimens—are most likely to develop EBV-LPD, particularly in the lungs. Although the disease usually originates in recipient B cells, several cases of donor origin, particularly in the transplanted organ, have been noted. High organ-specific content of B lymphoid tissues (e.g., bronchial-associated lymphoid tissue in the lung), anatomic factors (e.g., lack of access of host T cells to the transplanted organ because of disturbed lymphatics), and differences in major histocompatibility loci between the host T cells and the organ (e.g., lack of cell migration or lack of effective T cell/macrophage cooperation) may result in defective elimination of EBV-infected B cells. SOT recipients are also highly susceptible to the development of Kaposi's sarcoma and less frequently to the B cell proliferative disorders associated with KSHV, such as primary effusion lymphoma and multicentric Castleman's disease. Kaposi's sarcoma is much more common (in fact, 550–1000 times more common than in the general population), can develop very rapidly after transplantation, and can also occur in the allograft. However, because the seroprevalence of KSHV is very low in Western countries, Kaposi's sarcoma is not often observed.

KIDNEY TRANSPLANTATION

(See **Table 126-4**)

Early Infections Bacteria often cause infections that develop in the period immediately after kidney transplantation. There is a role for perioperative antibiotic prophylaxis, and many centers give cephalosporins to decrease the risk of postoperative complications. Urinary tract infections developing soon after transplantation are usually related to anatomic alterations resulting from surgery. Such early infections may require prolonged treatment (e.g., 6 weeks of antibiotic administration for pyelonephritis). Urinary tract infections that occur >6 months after transplantation may be treated for shorter periods because they do not seem to be associated with the high rate of pyelonephritis or relapse seen with infections that occur in the first 3 months.

Prophylaxis with TMP-SMX [1 double-strength tablet (800 mg of sulfamethoxazole, 160 mg of trimethoprim) per day] for the first 4–6 months after transplantation decreases the incidence of early and middle-period infections (see below, Table 126-4, and **Table 126-5**).

Middle-Period Infections Because of continuing immunosuppression, kidney transplant recipients are predisposed to lung infections characteristic of those in patients with T cell deficiency (i.e., infections

TABLE 126-4 COMMON INFECTIONS AFTER KIDNEY TRANSPLANTATION

	Period after Transplantation		
Infection Site	**Early (<1 Month)**	**Middle (1–4 Months)**	**Late (>6 Months)**
Urinary tract	Bacteria (*Escherichia coli*, *Klebsiella*, Enterobacteriaceae, *Pseudomonas*, *Enterococcus*) associated with bacteremia and pyelonephritis; *Candida*	CMV (fever, bone marrow suppression, hepatitis); BK virus (nephropathy, graft failure, vasculopathy)	Bacteria (late urinary tract infections usually not associated with bacteremia); BK virus (nephropathy, graft failure, generalized vasculopathy)
Lungs	Bacteria (*Legionella* in endemic settings)	CMV disease; *Pneumocystis*; *Legionella*	*Nocardia*; invasive fungi
Central nervous system		*Listeria* (meningitis); *Toxoplasma gondii*	CMV disease; *Listeria* (meningitis); *Cryptococcus* (meningitis); *Nocardia*

Note: CMV, cytomegalovirus.

TABLE 126-5 PROPHYLAXIS OF INFECTIONS IN TRANSPLANT RECIPIENTS

Risk Factor	Organism	Prophylactic Antibiotics	Examination(s)[a]
Travel to or residence in area with known risk of fungal infection	*Coccidioides, Histoplasma, Blastomyces*	Consider imidazoles	Chest radiography, antigen testing, serology
Latent viruses	HSV, VZV, EBV, CMV	Acyclovir after hematopoietic stem cell transplantation to prevent HSV and VZV; ganciclovir to prevent CMV in some settings	Serologic test for HSV, VZV, CMV, HHV-6, EBV, KSHV
Latent fungi and parasites	*Pneumocystis jiroveci, Toxoplasma gondii*	Trimethoprim-sulfamethoxazole (dapsone or atovaquone)	Serology for *Toxoplasma*
History of exposure to tuberculosis or latent tuberculosis	*Mycobacterium tuberculosis*	Isoniazid if recent conversion for positive chest imaging and/or no previous treatment	Chest imaging; PPD and/or cell-based assay

[a]Serologic examination, PPD testing, and interferon assays may be less reliable after transplantation.

Note: CMV, cytomegalovirus; EBV, Epstein-Barr virus; HHV-6, human herpesvirus type 6; HSV, herpes simplex virus; KSHV, Kaposi's sarcoma–associated herpesvirus; PPD, purified protein derivative; VZV, varicella-zoster virus.

with intracellular bacteria, mycobacteria, nocardiae, fungi, viruses, and parasites). The high mortality rates associated with *Legionella pneumophila* infection (Chap. 141) led to the closing of renal transplant units in hospitals with endemic legionellosis.

About 50% of all renal transplant recipients presenting with fever 1–4 months after transplantation have evidence of CMV disease; CMV itself accounts for the fever in more than two-thirds of cases and thus is the predominant pathogen during this period. CMV infection (Chap. 175) may also present as arthralgias, myalgias, or organ-specific symptoms. During this period, this infection may represent primary disease (in the case of a seronegative recipient of a kidney from a seropositive donor) or may represent reactivation disease or superinfection. Patients may have atypical lymphocytosis. Unlike immunocompetent patients, however, they often do not have lymphadenopathy or splenomegaly. Therefore, clinical suspicion and laboratory confirmation are necessary for diagnosis. The clinical syndrome may be accompanied by bone marrow suppression (particularly leukopenia). CMV also causes glomerulopathy and is associated with an increased incidence of other opportunistic infections. Because of the frequency and severity of disease, a considerable effort has been made to prevent and treat CMV infection in renal transplant recipients. An immune globulin preparation enriched with antibodies to CMV was used by many centers in the past in an effort to protect the group at highest risk for severe infection (seronegative recipients of seropositive kidneys). However, with the development of highly effective oral antiviral agents, CMV immune globulin is no longer used. Ganciclovir (valganciclovir) is beneficial when prophylaxis is indicated and for the treatment of serious CMV disease. One study showed a significant (50%) reduction in CMV disease and rejection at 6 months among patients who received prophylactic valacyclovir (an acyclovir congener) for the first 90 days after renal transplantation. Acyclovir (valacyclovir) is less efficacious but also less toxic than ganciclovir (valganciclovir). The availability of valganciclovir and valacyclovir has allowed most centers to move to oral prophylaxis for transplant recipients. Additional oral prophylactic agents, such as maribavir, are in clinical study.

Infection with the other herpes-group viruses may become evident within 6 months after transplantation or later. Early after transplantation, HSV may cause either oral or anogenital lesions that are usually responsive to acyclovir. Large ulcerating lesions in the anogenital area may lead to bladder and rectal dysfunction as well as predisposing to bacterial infection. VZV may cause fatal disseminated infection in nonimmune kidney transplant recipients, but in immune patients reactivation zoster usually does not disseminate outside the dermatome; thus disseminated VZV infection is a less fearsome complication in kidney transplantation than in hematopoietic stem cell transplantation. HHV-6 reactivation may take place and (although usually asymptomatic) may be associated with fever, rash, marrow suppression, or encephalitis.

EBV disease is more serious; it may present as an extranodal proliferation of B cells that invade the CNS, nasopharynx, liver, small bowel, heart, and other organs, including the transplanted kidney. The disease is diagnosed by the finding of a mass of proliferating EBV-positive B cells. The incidence of EBV-LPD is higher among patients who acquire EBV infection from the donor and among patients given high doses of cyclosporine, FK506, glucocorticoids, and anti–T cell antibodies. Disease may regress once immunocompetence is restored. KSHV infection can be transmitted with the donor kidney although it more often represents latent infection of the recipient. Kaposi's sarcoma often appears within 1 year after transplantation, although the range of onset is wide (1 month to ~20 years). Avoidance of immunosuppressive agents that inhibit calcineurin has been associated with less outgrowth of EBV and less CMV replication. The use of rapamycin (sirolimus) has led to regression of Kaposi's sarcoma.

The papovaviruses BK virus and JC virus (polyomavirus hominis types 1 and 2) have been cultured from the urine of kidney transplant recipients (as they have from that of HSCT recipients) in the setting of profound immunosuppression. High levels of BK virus replication detected by PCR in urine and blood are predictive of pathology, particularly in the setting of renal transplantation. Excretion of BK virus and BK viremia are associated with the development of ureteral strictures, polyomavirus-associated nephropathy (1–10% of renal transplant recipients), and (less commonly) generalized vasculopathy. Timely reduction of immunosuppression is critical and can reduce rates of graft loss related to polyomavirus-associated nephropathy from 90% to 10–30%. A possible role for treatment with cidofovir (given by the IV route and by bladder instillation), leflunomide, quinolones, and (most recently) lactoferrin has been reported, but the efficacy of these agents has not been substantiated through adequate clinical study. JC virus is associated with rare cases of progressive multifocal leukoencephalopathy. Adenoviruses may persist with continued immunosuppression in these patients, but disseminated disease like that which occurs in HSCT recipients is much less common.

Kidney transplant recipients are also subject to infections with other intracellular organisms. These patients may develop pulmonary infections with *Nocardia*, *Aspergillus*, and *Mucor* as well as infections with other pathogens in which the T cell/macrophage axis plays an important role. In patients without IV catheters, *L. monocytogenes* is a common cause of bacteremia ≥1 month after renal transplantation and should be seriously considered in renal transplant recipients presenting with fever and headache. Kidney transplant recipients may develop *Salmonella* bacteremia, which can lead to endovascular infections and require prolonged therapy. Pulmonary infections with *Pneumocystis* are common unless the patient is maintained on TMP-SMX prophylaxis. *Nocardia* infection (Chap. 155) may present in the skin, bones, and lungs or in the CNS, where it usually takes the form of single or multiple brain abscesses. Nocardiosis generally occurs ≥1 month after transplantation and may follow immunosuppressive treatment for an episode of rejection. Pulmonary findings are nonspecific: localized disease with or without cavities is most common, but the disease may disseminate. The diagnosis is made by culture of the organism from sputum or from the involved nodule. As with *Pneumocystis*, prophylaxis with TMP-SMX is often efficacious in the prevention of disease. The occurrence of *Nocardia* infections >2 years after transplantation suggests that a long-term prophylactic regimen may be justified.

Toxoplasmosis can occur in seropositive patients but is less common than in other transplant settings, usually developing in the first few months after kidney transplantation. Again, TMP-SMX is helpful in prevention. In endemic areas, histoplasmosis, coccidioidomycosis, and blastomycosis may cause pulmonary infiltrates or disseminated disease.

Late Infections Late infections (>6 months after kidney transplantation) may involve the CNS and include CMV retinitis as well as other CNS manifestations of CMV disease. Patients (particularly those whose immunosuppression has been increased) are at risk for subacute meningitis due to *Cryptococcus neoformans*. Cryptococcal disease may present in an insidious manner (sometimes as a skin infection before the development of clear CNS findings). *Listeria* meningitis may have an acute presentation and requires prompt therapy to avoid a fatal outcome.

Patients who continue to take glucocorticoids are predisposed to ongoing infection. "Transplant elbow" is a recurrent bacterial infection in and around the elbow that is thought to result from a combination of poor tensile strength of the skin of steroid-treated patients and steroid-induced proximal myopathy that requires patients to push themselves up with their elbows to get out of chairs. Bouts of cellulitis (usually caused by *S. aureus*) recur until patients are provided with elbow protection.

Kidney transplant recipients are susceptible to invasive fungal infections, including those due to *Aspergillus* and *Rhizopus*, which may present as superficial lesions before dissemination. Mycobacterial infection (particularly that with *Mycobacterium marinum*) can be diagnosed by skin examination. Infection with *Prototheca wickerhamii* (an achlorophyllic alga) has been diagnosed by skin biopsy. Warts caused by human papillomaviruses (HPVs) are a late consequence of persistent immunosuppression; imiquimod or other forms of local therapy are usually satisfactory.

Although BK virus replication and virus-associated disease can be detected far earlier, the median time to clinical diagnosis of polyomavirus-associated nephropathy is ~300 days, qualifying it as a late-onset disease. With establishment of better screening procedures (e.g., blood PCR), it is likely that this disease will be detected earlier (see "Middle-Period Infections," above).

HEART TRANSPLANTATION

Early Infections Sternal wound infection and mediastinitis are early complications of heart transplantation. An indolent course is common, with fever or a mildly elevated white blood cell count preceding the development of site tenderness or drainage. Clinical suspicion based on evidence of sternal instability and failure to heal may lead to the diagnosis. Common microbial residents of the skin (e.g., *S. aureus*, including methicillin-resistant strains, and *Staphylococcus epidermidis*) as well as gram-negative organisms (e.g., *Pseudomonas aeruginosa*) and fungi (e.g., *Candida*) are often involved. In rare cases, mediastinitis in heart transplant recipients can also be due to *Mycoplasma hominis* (Chap. 168). Since this organism requires an anaerobic environment for growth and may be difficult to see on conventional medium, the laboratory should be alerted that *M. hominis* infection is suspected. *M. hominis* mediastinitis has been cured with a combination of surgical debridement (sometimes requiring muscle-flap placement) and the administration of clindamycin and tetracycline. Organisms associated with mediastinitis may be cultured from accompanying pericardial fluid.

Middle-Period Infections *T. gondii* (Chap. 207) residing in the heart of a seropositive donor may be transmitted to a seronegative recipient. Thus serologic screening for *T. gondii* infection is important before and in the months after cardiac transplantation. Rarely, active disease can be introduced at the time of transplantation. The overall incidence of toxoplasmosis is so high in the setting of heart transplantation that some prophylaxis is always warranted. Although alternatives are available, the most frequently used agent is TMP-SMX, which prevents infection with *Pneumocystis* as well as with *Nocardia* and several other bacterial pathogens. CMV also has been transmitted by heart transplantation. CNS infections can be caused by *Toxoplasma*, *Nocardia*, and *Aspergillus*. *L. monocytogenes* meningitis should be considered in heart transplant recipients with fever and headache.

CMV infection is associated with poor outcomes after heart transplantation. The virus is usually cultivable 1–2 months after transplantation, causes early signs and laboratory abnormalities (usually fever and atypical lymphocytosis or leukopenia and thrombocytopenia) at 2–3 months, and can produce severe disease (e.g., pneumonia) at 3–4 months. Seropositive recipients usually develop cultivable virus faster than patients whose primary CMV infection is a consequence of transplantation. Between 40 and 70% of patients develop symptomatic CMV disease in the form of (1) CMV pneumonia, the most likely form to be fatal; (2) CMV esophagitis and gastritis, sometimes accompanied by abdominal pain with or without ulcerations and bleeding; and (3) the CMV syndrome, consisting of CMV in the blood along with fever, leukopenia, thrombocytopenia, and hepatic enzyme abnormalities. Ganciclovir is efficacious in the treatment of CMV infection; prophylaxis with ganciclovir or possibly with other antiviral agents, as described for renal transplantation, may reduce the overall incidence of CMV-related disease. When prophylaxis is stopped, late-onset disease may occur. In fact, because of the expanded use of prophylaxis, this scenario is increasingly common, particularly in patients with ongoing GVHD.

Late Infections EBV infection usually presents as a lymphoma-like proliferation of B cells late after heart transplantation, particularly in patients maintained on intense immunosuppressive therapy. A subset of heart and heart-lung transplant recipients may develop early fulminant EBV-LPD (within 2 months). Treatment includes the reduction of immunosuppression (if possible), the use of glucocorticoid and calcineurin inhibitor–sparing regimens, and the consideration of therapy with anti–B cell antibodies (rituximab and possibly others). Immunomodulatory and antiviral agents continue to be studied, and aggressive chemotherapy is a last resort, as discussed earlier for HSCT recipients. KSHV-associated disease, including Kaposi's sarcoma and primary effusion lymphoma, has been reported in heart transplant recipients. Treatment with rapamycin (sirolimus) may prevent both rejection and outgrowth of KSHV-infected cells. Antitumor therapy is discussed in Chap. 81. Prophylaxis for *Pneumocystis* infection is required for these patients (see "Lung Transplantation, Late Infections," below).

LUNG TRANSPLANTATION

Early Infections It is not surprising that lung transplant recipients are predisposed to the development of pneumonia. The combination of ischemia and the resulting mucosal damage, together with accompanying denervation and lack of lymphatic drainage, probably contributes to the high rate of pneumonia (66% in one series). The prophylactic use of high doses of broad-spectrum antibiotics for the first 3–4 days after surgery may decrease the incidence of pneumonia. Gram-negative pathogens (Enterobacteriaceae and *Pseudomonas* species) are troublesome in the first 2 weeks after surgery (the period of maximal vulnerability). Pneumonia can also be caused by *Candida* (possibly as a result of colonization of the donor lung), *Aspergillus*, and *Cryptococcus*.

Mediastinitis may occur at an even higher rate among lung transplant recipients than among heart transplant recipients and most commonly develops within 2 weeks of surgery. In the absence of prophylaxis, pneumonitis due to CMV (which may be transmitted as a consequence of transplantation) usually presents between 2 weeks and 3 months after surgery, with primary disease occurring later than reactivation disease.

Middle-Period Infections The incidence of CMV infection, either reactivated or primary, is 75–100% if either the donor or the recipient is seropositive for CMV. CMV-induced disease appears to be most severe in recipients of lung and heart-lung transplants. Whether this severity relates to the mismatch in lung antigen-presenting and host immune cells or is attributable to other (nonimmunologic) factors is not known. More than half of lung transplant recipients with symptomatic

CMV disease have pneumonia. Difficulty in distinguishing the radiographic picture of CMV infection from other infections and organ rejection further complicates therapy. CMV can also cause bronchiolitis obliterans in lung transplants. The development of pneumonitis related to HSV has led to the prophylactic use of acyclovir. Such prophylaxis may also decrease rates of CMV disease, but ganciclovir is more active against CMV and is also active against HSV. The prophylaxis of CMV infection with IV ganciclovir—or increasingly with valganciclovir, the oral alternative—is recommended for lung transplant recipients. Antiviral alternatives are discussed in the earlier section on hematopoietic stem cell transplantation. Although the overall incidence of serious disease is decreased during prophylaxis, late disease may occur when prophylaxis is stopped—a pattern observed increasingly in recent years. With recovery from peritransplantation complications and, in many cases, a decrease in immunosuppression, the recipient is often better equipped to combat late infection.

Late Infections The incidence of *Pneumocystis* infection (which may present with a paucity of findings) is high among lung and heart-lung transplant recipients. Some form of prophylaxis for *Pneumocystis* pneumonia is indicated in all organ transplant situations (Table 126-5). Prophylaxis with TMP-SMX for 12 months after transplantation may be sufficient to prevent *Pneumocystis* disease in patients whose degree of immunosuppression is not increased.

As in other transplant recipients, infection with EBV may cause either a mononucleosis-like syndrome or EBV-LPD. The tendency of the B cell blasts to present in the lung appears to be greater after lung transplantation than after the transplantation of other organs. Reduction of immunosuppression and switching of regimens, as discussed in earlier sections, causes remission in some cases, but airway compression can be fatal and more rapid intervention may therefore become necessary. The approach to EBV-LPD is similar to that described in other sections.

LIVER TRANSPLANTATION

Early Infections As in other transplantation settings, early bacterial infections are a major problem after liver transplantation. Many centers administer systemic broad-spectrum antibiotics for the first 24 h or sometimes longer after surgery, even in the absence of documented infection. However, despite prophylaxis, infectious complications are common and are correlated with the duration of the surgical procedure and the type of biliary drainage. An operation lasting >12 h is associated with an increased likelihood of infection. Patients who have a choledochojejunostomy with drainage of the biliary duct to a Roux-en-Y jejunal bowel loop have more fungal infections than those whose bile is drained via a choledochocholedochostomy with anastomosis of the donor common bile duct to the recipient common bile duct.

Peritonitis and intraabdominal abscesses are common complications of liver transplantation. Bacterial peritonitis or localized abscesses may result from biliary leaks. Early leaks are even more common (incidence, ~17%) with live-donor liver transplants (LDLTs). Peritonitis in liver transplant recipients is often polymicrobial, commonly involving enterococci, aerobic gram-negative bacteria, staphylococci, anaerobes, *Candida*, or other invasive fungi. Only one-third of patients with intraabdominal abscesses have bacteremia. Abscesses within the first month after surgery may occur not only in and around the liver but also in the spleen, pericolic area, and pelvis. Treatment includes antibiotic administration and drainage as necessary.

Liver transplant patients have a high incidence of fungal infections, and the occurrence of fungal (often candidal) infection correlates with preoperative use of glucocorticoids, long duration of treatment with antibacterial agents, and posttransplantation use of immunosuppressive agents.

Middle-Period Infections The development of postsurgical biliary stricture predisposes patients to cholangitis. The incidence of strictures is increased in LDLT (~17% of liver transplant recipients); therefore, cholangitis is also more common among these patients. Transplant recipients who develop cholangitis may have high spiking fevers and rigors but often lack the characteristic signs and symptoms of classic cholangitis, including abdominal pain and jaundice. Although these findings may suggest graft rejection, rejection is typically accompanied by marked elevation of liver function enzymes. In contrast, in cholangitis in transplant recipients, results of liver function tests (with the possible exception of alkaline phosphatase levels) are often within the normal range. Definitive diagnosis of cholangitis in liver transplant recipients requires documentation of bacteremia or demonstration of aggregated neutrophils in bile duct biopsy specimens. Unfortunately, invasive studies of the biliary tract (either T-tube cholangiography or endoscopic retrograde cholangiopancreatography) may themselves lead to cholangitis. For this reason, many clinicians recommend an empirical trial of therapy with antibiotics covering gram-negative organisms and anaerobes before these procedures are undertaken as well as antibiotic coverage if they are eventually performed.

Reactivation of viral hepatitis is a common complication of liver transplantation (Chap. 298). Recurrent hepatitis B and C infections, for which transplantation may be performed, are problematic. To prevent hepatitis B virus reinfection, prophylaxis with an optimal antiviral agent or combination of agents (lamivudine, adefovir, entecavir) and hepatitis B immune globulin is currently recommended, although the optimal dose, route, and duration of therapy remain controversial. Success in preventing reinfection with hepatitis B virus has increased in recent years; in contrast, reinfection of the graft with hepatitis C virus occurs in all patients, with a variable time frame. Studies of aggressive pretransplantation treatment of selected recipients with antiviral agents and prophylactic/preemptive regimens are ongoing. However, early initiation of treatment for histologically documented disease with a combination of ribavirin and pegylated interferon has produced sustained responses at rates in the range of 25–40%.

As in other transplantation settings, reactivation disease with herpes-group viruses is common (Table 126-3). Herpesviruses can be transmitted in donor organs. Although CMV hepatitis occurs in ~4% of liver transplant recipients, it is usually not so severe as to require retransplantation. Without prophylaxis, CMV disease develops in the majority of seronegative recipients of organs from CMV-positive donors, but fatality rates are lower among liver transplant recipients than among lung or heart-lung transplant recipients. Disease due to CMV can also be associated with the vanishing bile duct syndrome after liver transplantation. Patients respond to treatment with ganciclovir; prophylaxis with oral forms of ganciclovir or high-dose acyclovir may decrease the frequency of disease. A role for HHV-6 reactivation in posttransplantation fever and leukopenia has been proposed, although the more severe sequelae described in hematopoietic stem cell transplantation are unusual. HHV-6 and HHV-7 appear to exacerbate CMV disease in this setting. EBV-LPD after liver transplantation shows a propensity for involvement of the liver, and such disease may be of donor origin. See previous sections for discussion of EBV infections in solid organ transplantation.

PANCREAS TRANSPLANTATION

Transplantation of the pancreas can be complicated by early bacterial and yeast infections. Most pancreatic transplants are drained into the bowel, whereas the remaining transplants (~20%) are drained into the bladder. A cuff of duodenum is used in the anastomosis between the pancreatic graft and either the gut or the bladder. Bowel drainage poses a risk of early abdominal and allograft infections with enteric bacteria and yeasts. These infections often result in loss of the graft. Bladder drainage causes a high rate of urinary tract infection and sterile cystitis; however, infection can usually be cured with appropriate antimicrobial agents. In both procedures, prophylactic antimicrobial agents are commonly used at the time of surgery. An alternative method—the transplantation of islet cells only—may eliminate the problems characteristically posed by wound and urinary tract sepsis in pancreatic transplant recipients.

Issues related to the development of CMV infection, EBV-LPD, and infections with opportunistic pathogens in patients receiving a pancreatic transplant are similar to those in other SOT recipients.

MISCELLANEOUS INFECTIONS IN SOLID ORGAN TRANSPLANTATION

Indwelling IV Catheter Infections The prolonged use of indwelling IV catheters for administration of medications, blood products, and nutrition is common in diverse transplantation settings and poses a risk of local and bloodstream infections. Significant insertion-site infection is most commonly caused by *S. aureus*. Bloodstream infection most frequently develops within a week of catheter placement or in patients who become neutropenic. Coagulase-negative staphylococci are the most common isolates from the blood. For further discussion of differential diagnosis and therapeutic options, see Chap. 82.

Tuberculosis The incidence of tuberculosis occurring within the first 12 months after solid organ transplantation is greater than that observed after hematopoietic stem cell transplantation (0.23–0.79%) and ranges broadly worldwide (1.2–15%), reflecting the prevalences of tuberculosis in local populations. Lesions suggesting prior tuberculosis on chest x-ray, older age, diabetes, chronic liver disease, GVHD, and intense immunosuppression are predictive of tuberculosis reactivation and development of disseminated disease in a host with latent disease. Tuberculosis has rarely been transmitted from the donor organ. In contrast to the low mortality rate among HSCT recipients, mortality rates among SOT patients are reported to be as high as 30%. Vigilance is indicated, as the presentation of disease is often extrapulmonary (gastrointestinal, genitourinary, central nervous, endocrine, musculoskeletal, laryngeal) and atypical, sometimes manifesting as a fever of unknown origin. A careful history and a direct evaluation of both the recipient and the donor prior to transplantation are optimal. Skin testing of the recipient with PPD may be unreliable because of chronic disease and/or immunosuppression, but newer cell-based assays that measure interferon and/or cytokine production may prove more sensitive in the future. Isoniazid toxicity has not been a significant problem except in the setting of liver transplantation. Therefore, appropriate prophylaxis should proceed. An assessment of the need to treat latent disease should include careful consideration of the possibility of a false-negative test result. Pending final confirmation of suspected tuberculosis, aggressive multidrug treatment in accordance with the guidelines of the Centers for Disease Control and Prevention (CDC), the Infectious Diseases Society of America, and the American Thoracic Society is indicated because of the high mortality rates among these patients. Altered drug metabolism (e.g., upon co-administration of rifampin and certain immunosuppressive agents) can be managed with careful monitoring of drug levels and appropriate dose adjustment. Close follow-up of hepatic enzymes is warranted, particularly during treatment with isoniazid, pyrazinamide, and/or rifampin. Drug-resistant tuberculosis is especially problematic in these individuals (Chap. 158).

Virus-Associated Malignancies In addition to malignancy associated with gammaherpesvirus infection (EBV, KSHV) and simple warts (HPV), other tumors that are virus-associated or suspected of being virus-associated are more likely to develop in transplant recipients, particularly those who require long-term immunosuppression, than in the general population. The interval to tumor development is usually >1 year. Transplant recipients develop nonmelanoma skin or lip cancers that, in contrast to de novo skin cancers, have a high ratio of squamous cells to basal cells. HPV may play a major role in these lesions. Cervical and vulvar carcinomas, quite clearly associated with HPV, develop with increased frequency in female transplant recipients. Among renal transplant recipients, rates of melanoma are modestly increased and rates of cancers of the kidney and bladder are increased.

TABLE 126-6 VACCINATION FOR HEMATOPOIETIC STEM CELL TRANSPLANT (HSCT) OR SOLID ORGAN TRANSPLANT (SOT) RECIPIENTS

	Type of Transplantation	
Vaccine	**HSCT**	**SOT**[a]
Streptococcus pneumoniae, Haemophilus influenzae, Neisseria meningitidis	Immunize after transplantation (optimal timing not established) Use Prevnar Preimmunize donor (graft)[b] See CDC recommendations	Immunize before transplantation and every 5 years for Pneumovax (others not established) See CDC recommendations
Seasonal influenza	Vaccinate in the fall Vaccinate close contacts	Vaccinate in the fall Vaccinate close contacts
Poliomyelitis	Administer inactivated vaccine	Administer inactivated vaccine
Measles/mumps/rubella	Immunize 24 months after transplantation if patient does not have graft-versus-host disease	Immunize before transplantation with attenuated vaccine
Tetanus, diphtheria	Reimmunize after transplantation with primary series See CDC recommendations	Immunize before transplantation; give boosters at 10 years or as required; primary series not required
Hepatitis B and A	Reimmunize after transplantation See CDC recommendations	Immunize before transplantation as appropriate
Human papillomavirus	Recommendations pending	Recommendations pending

[a]Immunizations should be given before transplantation whenever possible.
[b]Studies indicate that it is possible to "immunize the graft" before transplantation.

VACCINATION OF TRANSPLANT RECIPIENTS

In addition to receiving antibiotic prophylaxis, transplant recipients should be vaccinated against likely pathogens (Table 126-6). In the case of HSCT recipients, optimal responses cannot be achieved until after immune reconstitution, despite previous immunization of both donor and recipient. Recipients of allogeneic HSCTs must be reimmunized if they are to be protected against pathogens. The situation is less clear-cut in the case of autologous transplantation. T and B cells in the peripheral blood may reconstitute the immune response if they are transferred in adequate numbers. However, cancer patients (particularly those with Hodgkin's disease, in whom vaccination has been extensively studied) who are undergoing chemotherapy do not respond normally to immunization, and titers of antibodies to infectious agents fall more rapidly than in healthy individuals. Therefore, even immunosuppressed patients who have not had HSCTs may need booster vaccine injections. If memory cells are specifically eliminated as part of a stem cell "cleanup" procedure, it will be necessary to reimmunize the recipient with a new primary series. Optimal times for immunizations of different transplant populations are being evaluated. Yearly immunization of household and other contacts (including health care personnel) against influenza benefits the patient by preventing local spread.

In the absence of compelling data as to optimal timing, it is reasonable to administer the pneumococcal and *H. influenzae* type b conjugate vaccines to both autologous and allogeneic HSCT recipients beginning 12 months after transplantation. A series that includes both the 7-valent pneumococcal conjugate vaccine and the 23-valent Pneumovax is now recommended (following CDC guidelines). The pneumococcal and *H. influenzae* type b vaccines are particularly important for patients who have undergone splenectomy. In addition, diphtheria, tetanus, acellular pertussis, and inactivated polio vaccines can all be given at these same intervals (12 months and, as required, 24 months after transplantation). *Neisseria meningitidis* polysaccharide (a new conjugate vaccine) is now available and will probably be recommended in the future. Some authorities recommend a new primary series for tetanus/diphtheria/pertussis and inactivated polio vaccine beginning 12 months after transplantation. Because of the risk of spread, household contacts of HSCT recipients (or of patients immunosuppressed as a result of chemotherapy) should receive only inactivated polio vaccine. Live-virus measles/mumps/rubella vaccine can be given to autologous HSCT recipients 24 months after transplantation and to most allogeneic HSCT recipients at the same point if they are not receiving maintenance therapy with immunosuppressive drugs and do not have ongoing GVHD. The risk of spread from a household contact is lower for MMR vaccine than for polio vaccine. Neither patients nor their household contacts should be vaccinated with vaccinia unless they have been exposed to the smallpox virus. Among patients who have active GVHD and/or are taking high maintenance doses of glucocorticoids, it may be prudent to avoid all live-virus vaccines. Vaccination to prevent hepatitis B and hepatitis A also seems advisable.

In the case of SOT recipients, administration of all the usual vaccines and of the indicated booster doses should be completed before immunosuppression, if possible, to maximize responses. For patients taking immunosuppressive agents, the administration of pneumococcal vaccine should be repeated every 5 years. No data are available for the meningococcal vaccine, but it is probably reasonable to administer it along with the pneumococcal vaccine. *H. influenzae* conjugate vaccine is safe and should be efficacious in this population; therefore, its administration before transplantation is recommended. Booster doses of this vaccine are not recommended for adults. SOT recipients who continue to receive immunosuppressive drugs should not receive live-virus vaccines. A person in this group who is exposed to measles should be given immune globulin. Similarly, an immunocompromised patient who is seronegative for varicella and who comes into contact with a person who has chickenpox should be given varicella-zoster immune globulin as soon as possible (and certainly within 96 h) or, if this is not possible, should be started immediately on a 10- to 14-day course of acyclovir therapy. Upon the discontinuation of treatment, clinical disease may still occur in a small number of patients; thus vigilance is indicated. Rapid re-treatment should limit the symptoms of disease. Household contacts of transplant recipients can receive live attenuated VZV vaccine, but vaccinees should avoid direct contact with the patient if a rash develops. Virus-like particle (VLP) vaccines (not live attenuated) have recently been licensed for the prevention of infection with several HPV serotypes most commonly implicated in cervical and anal carcinomas and in anogenital and laryngeal warts. For example, the tetravalent vaccine contains HPV serotypes 6, 11, 16, and 18. At present, no information is available about the safety, immunogenicity, or efficacy of this vaccine in transplant recipients.

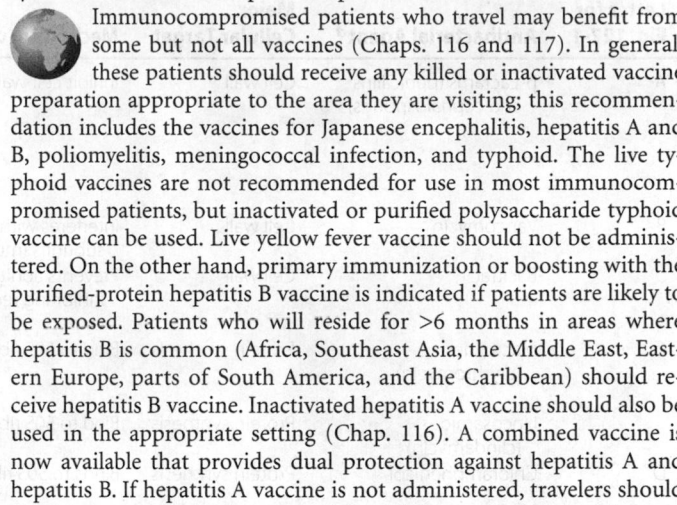

Immunocompromised patients who travel may benefit from some but not all vaccines (Chaps. 116 and 117). In general, these patients should receive any killed or inactivated vaccine preparation appropriate to the area they are visiting; this recommendation includes the vaccines for Japanese encephalitis, hepatitis A and B, poliomyelitis, meningococcal infection, and typhoid. The live typhoid vaccines are not recommended for use in most immunocompromised patients, but inactivated or purified polysaccharide typhoid vaccine can be used. Live yellow fever vaccine should not be administered. On the other hand, primary immunization or boosting with the purified-protein hepatitis B vaccine is indicated if patients are likely to be exposed. Patients who will reside for >6 months in areas where hepatitis B is common (Africa, Southeast Asia, the Middle East, Eastern Europe, parts of South America, and the Caribbean) should receive hepatitis B vaccine. Inactivated hepatitis A vaccine should also be used in the appropriate setting (Chap. 116). A combined vaccine is now available that provides dual protection against hepatitis A and hepatitis B. If hepatitis A vaccine is not administered, travelers should consider receiving passive protection with immune globulin (the dose depending on the duration of travel in the high-risk area).

FURTHER READINGS

Cornely OA et al: Posaconazole vs. fluconazole or itraconazole prophylaxis in patients with neutropenia. N Engl J Med 356:348, 2007

Dykewicz CA: Cytomegalovirus infection after liver transplantation: Summary of the guidelines for preventing opportunistic infections among hematopoietic stem cell transplant recipients. Clin Infect Dis 33:139, 2001

Hirsch HH, Suthanthiran M: The natural history, risk factors and outcomes of polyomavirus BK–associated nephropathy after renal transplantation. Nat Clin Pract Nephrol 2:240, 2006

Kotton CN et al: Prevention of infection in adult travelers after solid organ transplantation. Am J Transplant 5:8, 2004

Munoz P et al: *Mycobacterium tuberculosis* infection in recipients of solid organ transplants. Clin Infect Dis 40:581, 2005

Zerr DM et al: Clinical outcomes of human herpesvirus 6 reactivation after hematopoietic stem cell transplantation. Clin Infect Dis 40:932, 2005

SECTION 4 APPROACH TO THERAPY FOR BACTERIAL DISEASES

127 Treatment and Prophylaxis of Bacterial Infections

Gordon L. Archer, Ronald E. Polk

The development of vaccines and drugs that prevent and cure bacterial infections was one of the twentieth century's major contributions to human longevity and quality of life. Antibacterial agents are among the most commonly prescribed drugs of any kind worldwide. Used appropriately, these drugs are lifesaving. However, their indiscriminate use drives up the cost of health care, leads to a plethora of side effects and drug interactions, and fosters the emergence of bacterial resistance, rendering previously valuable drugs useless. The rational use of antibacterial agents depends on an understanding of (1) the drugs' mechanisms of action, spectrum of activity, pharmacokinetics, pharmacodynamics, toxicities, and interactions; (2) mechanisms underlying bacterial resistance; and (3) strategies that can be used by clinicians to limit resistance. In addition, patient-associated parameters, such as infection site, other drugs being taken, allergies, and immune and excretory status, are critically important to appropriate therapeutic decisions. This chapter provides specific data required for making an informed choice of antibacterial agent.

MECHANISMS OF ACTION

Antibacterial agents, like all antimicrobial drugs, are directed against unique targets not present in mammalian cells. The goal is to limit toxicity to the host and maximize chemotherapeutic activity affecting invading microbes only. *Bactericidal drugs* kill the bacteria that are within their spectrum of activity; *bacteriostatic drugs* only inhibit bacterial growth. While bacteriostatic activity is adequate for the treatment of most infections, bactericidal activity may be necessary for cure in patients with altered immune systems (e.g., neutropenia), protected infectious foci (e.g., endocarditis or meningitis), or specific infections (e.g., complicated *Staphylococcus aureus* bacteremia). The mechanisms of action of the antibacterial agents to be discussed in this section are summarized in **Table 127-1** and are depicted in **Fig. 127-1**.

TABLE 127-1 MECHANISMS OF ACTION OF AND RESISTANCE TO MAJOR CLASSES OF ANTIBACTERIAL AGENTS

Letter for Fig. 127-1	Antibacterial Agent[a]	Major Cellular Target	Mechanism of Action	Major Mechanisms of Resistance
A	β-Lactams (penicillins and cephalosporins)	Cell wall	Inhibit cell-wall cross-linking	1. Drug inactivation (β-lactamase) 2. Insensitivity of target (altered penicillin-binding proteins) 3. Decreased permeability (altered gram-negative outer-membrane porins) 4. Active efflux
B	Vancomycin	Cell wall	Interferes with addition of new cell-wall subunits (muramyl pentapeptides)	Alteration of target (substitution of terminal amino acid of peptidoglycan subunit)
	Bacitracin	Cell wall	Prevents addition of cell-wall subunits by inhibiting recycling of membrane lipid carrier	Not defined
C	Macrolides (erythromycin)	Protein synthesis	Bind to 50S ribosomal subunit	1. Alteration of target (ribosomal methylation and mutation of 23S rRNA) 2. Active efflux
	Lincosamides (clindamycin)	Protein synthesis	Bind to 50S ribosomal subunit	Alteration of target (ribosomal methylation)
D	Chloramphenicol	Protein synthesis	Binds to 50S ribosomal subunit	1. Drug inactivation (chloramphenicol acetyltransferase) 2. Active efflux
E	Tetracycline	Protein synthesis	Binds to 30S ribosomal subunit	1. Decreased intracellular drug accumulation (active efflux) 2. Insensitivity of target
F	Aminoglycosides (gentamicin)	Protein synthesis	Bind to 30S ribosomal subunit	1. Drug inactivation (aminoglycoside-modifying enzyme) 2. Decreased permeability through gram-negative outer membrane 3. Active efflux
G	Mupirocin	Protein synthesis	Inhibits isoleucine tRNA synthetase	Mutation of gene for target protein or acquisition of new gene for drug-insensitive target
H	Quinupristin/dalfopristin (Synercid)	Protein synthesis	Binds to 50S ribosomal subunit	1. Alteration of target (ribosomal methylation: dalfopristin) 2. Active efflux (quinupristin) 3. Drug inactivation (quinupristin and dalfopristin)
I	Linezolid	Protein synthesis	Bind to 50S ribosomal subunit	Alteration of target (mutation of 23S rRNA)
J	Sulfonamides and trimethoprim	Cell metabolism	Competitively inhibit enzymes involved in two steps of folic acid biosynthesis	Production of insensitive targets [dihydropteroate synthetase (sulfonamides) and dihydrofolate reductase (trimethoprim)] that bypass metabolic block
K	Rifampin	Nucleic acid synthesis	Inhibits DNA-dependent RNA polymerase	Insensitivity of target (mutation of polymerase gene)
L	Metronidazole	Nucleic acid synthesis	Intracellularly generates short-lived reactive intermediates that damage DNA by electron transfer system	Not defined
M	Quinolones (ciprofloxacin)	DNA synthesis	Inhibit DNA gyrase (A subunit) and topoisomerase IV	1. Insensitivity of target (mutation of gyrase genes) 2. Decreased intracellular drug accumulation (active efflux)
	Novobiocin	DNA synthesis	Inhibits DNA gyrase (B subunit)	Not defined
N	Polymyxins (polymyxin B)	Cell membrane	Disrupt membrane permeability by charge alteration	Not defined
	Gramicidin	Cell membrane	Forms pores	Not defined
O	Daptomycin	Cell membrane	Forms channels that disrupt membrane potential	Not defined

[a]Compounds in parentheses are major representatives for the class.

INHIBITION OF CELL-WALL SYNTHESIS

One major difference between bacterial and mammalian cells is the presence in bacteria of a rigid wall external to the cell membrane. The wall protects bacterial cells from osmotic rupture, which would result from the cell's usual marked hyperosmolarity (by up to 20 atm) relative to the host environment. The structure conferring cell-wall rigidity and resistance to osmotic lysis in both gram-positive and gram-negative bacteria is peptidoglycan, a large, covalently linked sacculus that surrounds the bacterium. In gram-positive bacteria, peptidoglycan is the only layered structure external to the cell membrane and is thick (20–80 nm); in gram-negative bacteria, there is an outer membrane external to a very thin (1-nm) peptidoglycan layer.

Chemotherapeutic agents directed at any stage of the synthesis, export, assembly, or cross-linking of peptidoglycan lead to inhibition of bacterial cell growth and, in most cases, to cell death. Peptidoglycan is composed of (1) a backbone of two alternating sugars, *N*-acetylglucosamine and *N*-acetylmuramic acid; (2) a chain of four amino acids that extends down from the backbone (stem peptides); and (3) a peptide bridge that cross-links the peptide chains. Peptidoglycan is formed by the addition of subunits (a sugar with its five attached amino acids) that are assembled in the cytoplasm and transported through the cytoplasmic membrane to the cell surface. Subsequent cross-linking is driven by cleavage of the terminal stem-peptide amino acid.

Virtually all the antibiotics that inhibit bacterial cell-wall synthesis are bactericidal. That is, they eventually result in the cell's death due to osmotic lysis. However, much of the loss of cell-wall integrity following treatment with cell wall–active agents is due to the bacteria's own

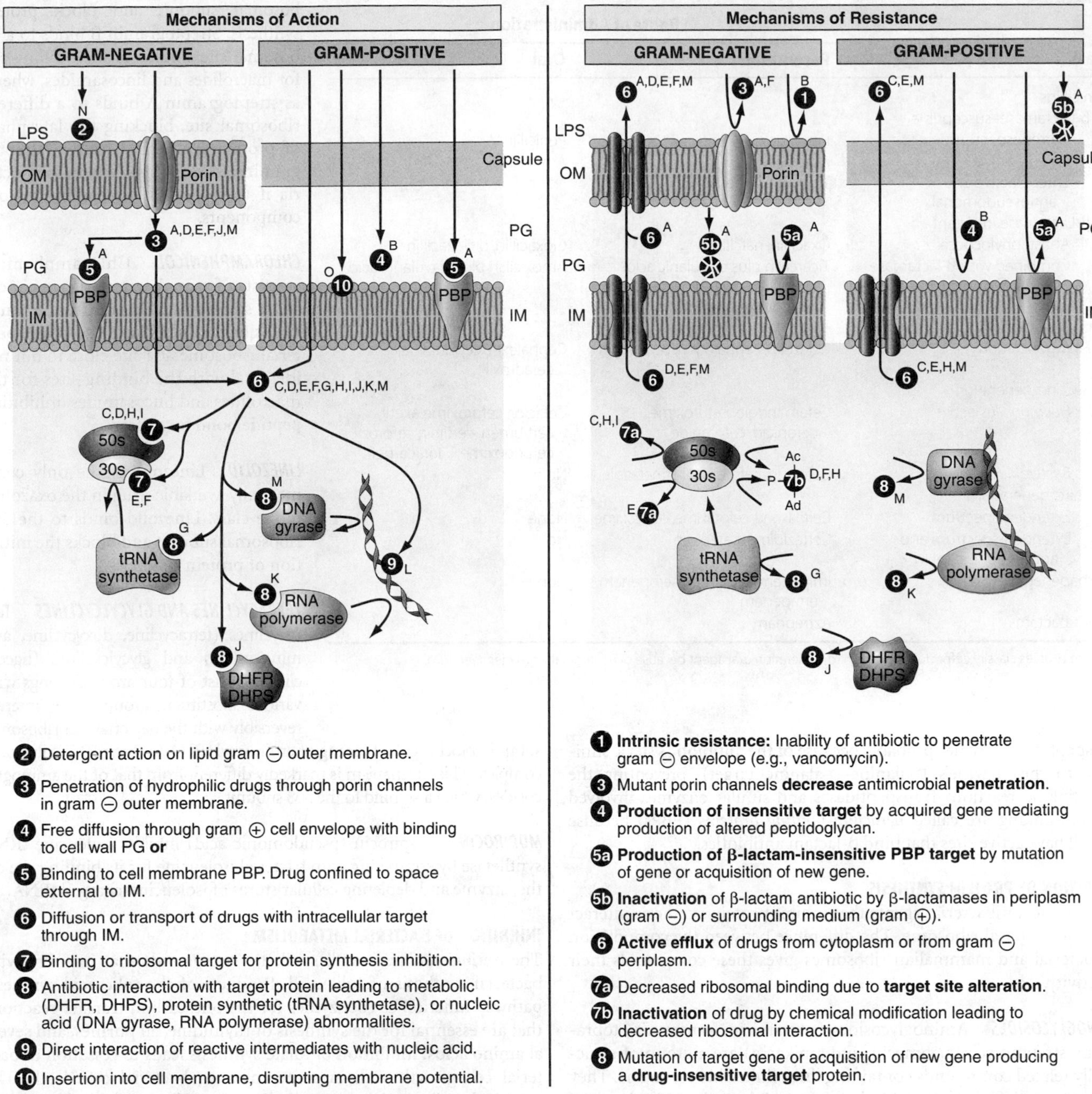
Mechanisms of Action
GRAM-NEGATIVE
GRAM-POSITIVE
LPS
OM
Porin
Capsule
PG
IM
PBP
50s
30s
DNA gyrase
tRNA synthetase
RNA polymerase
DHFR DHPS
Mechanisms of Resistance
GRAM-NEGATIVE
GRAM-POSITIVE
Ac
P
Ad
2 Detergent action on lipid gram ⊖ outer membrane.
3 Penetration of hydrophilic drugs through porin channels in gram ⊖ outer membrane.
4 Free diffusion through gram ⊕ cell envelope with binding to cell wall PG or
5 Binding to cell membrane PBP. Drug confined to space external to IM.
6 Diffusion or transport of drugs with intracellular target through IM.
7 Binding to ribosomal target for protein synthesis inhibition.
8 Antibiotic interaction with target protein leading to metabolic (DHFR, DHPS), protein synthetic (tRNA synthetase), or nucleic acid (DNA gyrase, RNA polymerase) abnormalities.
9 Direct interaction of reactive intermediates with nucleic acid.
10 Insertion into cell membrane, disrupting membrane potential.
1 Intrinsic resistance: Inability of antibiotic to penetrate gram ⊖ envelope (e.g., vancomycin).
3 Mutant porin channels decrease antimicrobial penetration.
4 Production of insensitive target by acquired gene mediating production of altered peptidoglycan.
5a Production of β-lactam-insensitive PBP target by mutation of gene or acquisition of new gene.
5b Inactivation of β-lactam antibiotic by β-lactamases in periplasm (gram ⊖) or surrounding medium (gram ⊕).
6 Active efflux of drugs from cytoplasm or from gram ⊖ periplasm.
7a Decreased ribosomal binding due to target site alteration.
7b Inactivation of drug by chemical modification leading to decreased ribosomal interaction.
8 Mutation of target gene or acquisition of new gene producing a drug-insensitive target protein.

FIGURE 127-1 Mechanisms of action of and resistance to antibacterial agents. Black lines trace the routes of drug interaction with bacterial cells, from entry to target site. The letters in each figure indicate specific antibacterial agents or classes of agents, as shown in Table 127-1. The numbers correspond to mechanisms listed beneath each panel. 50s and 30s, large and small ribosome subunits; Ac, acetylation; Ad, adenylation; DHFR, dihydrofolate reductase; DHPS, dihydropteroate synthetase; IM, inner (cytoplasmic) membrane; LPS, lipopolysaccharide; OM, outer membrane; P, phosphorylation; PBP, penicillin-binding protein; PG, peptidoglycan.

cell-wall remodeling enzymes (autolysins) that cleave peptidoglycan bonds in the normal course of cell growth. In the presence of antibacterial agents that inhibit cell-wall growth, autolysis proceeds without normal cell-wall repair; weakness and eventual cellular lysis occur.

Antibacterial agents act to inhibit cell-wall synthesis in several ways, as described below.

BACITRACIN Bacitracin, a cyclic peptide antibiotic, inhibits the conversion to its active form of the lipid carrier that moves the water-soluble cytoplasmic peptidoglycan subunits through the cell membrane to the cell exterior.

GLYCOPEPTIDES Glycopeptides (vancomycin and teicoplanin) are high-molecular-weight antibiotics that bind to the terminal D-alanine–D-alanine component of the stem peptide while the subunits are external to the cell membrane but still linked to the lipid carrier. This binding sterically inhibits the addition of subunits to the peptidoglycan backbone.

β-LACTAM ANTIBIOTICS β-Lactam antibiotics (penicillins, cephalosporins, carbapenems, and monobactams; Table 127-2) are characterized by a four-membered β-lactam ring and prevent the cross-linking reaction called *transpeptidation*. The energy for attaching a peptide cross-bridge from the stem peptide of one peptidoglycan subunit to another is derived from the cleavage of a terminal D-alanine residue from the subunit stem peptide. The cross-bridge amino acid is then attached to the penultimate D-alanine by transpeptidase enzymes. The β-lactam ring of the antibiotic forms an irreversible covalent acyl bond with the

TABLE 127-2 CLASSIFICATION OF β-LACTAM ANTIBIOTICS

	Route of Administration	
Class	**Parenteral**	**Oral**
Penicillins		
β-Lactamase–susceptible		
Narrow-spectrum	Penicillin G	Penicillin V
Enteric-active	Ampicillin	Amoxicillin, ampicillin
Enteric-active and antipseudomonal	Ticarcillin, piperacillin	None
β-Lactamase–resistant		
Antistaphylococcal	Oxacillin, nafcillin	Cloxacillin, dicloxacillin
Combined with β-lactamase inhibitors	Ticarcillin plus clavulanic acid, ampicillin plus sulbactam, piperacillin plus tazobactam	Amoxicillin plus clavulanic acid
Cephalosporins		
First-generation	Cefazolin, cephalothin, cephapirin	Cephalexin, cephradine, cefadroxil
Second-generation		
Haemophilus-active	Cefamandole, cefuroxime, cefonicid, ceforanide	Cefaclor, cefuroxime axetil, ceftibuten, cefdinir, cefprozil, cefpodoxime,[a] loracarbef
Bacteroides-active	Cefoxitin, cefotetan, cefmetazole	None
Third-generation		
Extended-spectrum	Ceftriaxone, cefotaxime, ceftizoxime	None
Extended-spectrum and antipseudomonal	Ceftazidime, cefepime	None
Carbapenems	Imipenem-cilastatin, meropenem, ertapenem	None
Monobactams	Aztreonam	None

[a]Some sources classify cefpodoxime as a third-generation oral agent because of a marginally broader spectrum.

transpeptidase enzyme (probably because of the antibiotic's steric similarity to the enzyme's D-alanine–D-alanine target), preventing the cross-linking reaction. Transpeptidases and similar enzymes involved in cross-linking are called *penicillin-binding proteins* (PBPs) because they all have active sites that bind β-lactam antibiotics.

INHIBITION OF PROTEIN SYNTHESIS

Most of the antibacterial agents that inhibit protein synthesis interact with the bacterial ribosome. The difference between the composition of bacterial and mammalian ribosomes gives these compounds their selectivity.

AMINOGLYCOSIDES Aminoglycosides (gentamicin, kanamycin, tobramycin, streptomycin, neomycin, and amikacin) are a group of structurally related compounds containing three linked hexose sugars. They exert a bactericidal effect by binding irreversibly to the 30S subunit of the bacterial ribosome and blocking initiation of protein synthesis. Uptake of aminoglycosides and their penetration through the cell membrane constitute an aerobic, energy-dependent process. Thus, aminoglycoside activity is markedly reduced in an anaerobic environment. *Spectinomycin*, an aminocyclitol antibiotic, also acts on the 30S ribosomal subunit but has a different mechanism of action from the aminoglycosides and is bacteriostatic rather than bactericidal.

MACROLIDES, KETOLIDES, AND LINCOSAMIDES *Macrolide antibiotics* (erythromycin, clarithromycin, and azithromycin) consist of a large lactone ring to which sugars are attached. *Ketolide antibiotics*, including telithromycin, replace the cladinose sugar on the macrolactone ring with a ketone group. These drugs bind specifically to the 50S portion of the bacterial ribosome and inhibit protein chain elongation. Although structurally unrelated to the macrolides, *lincosamides* (clindamycin and lincomycin) bind to a site on the 50S ribosome nearly identical to the binding site for macrolides.

STREPTOGRAMINS Streptogramins [quinupristin (streptogramin B) and dalfopristin (streptogramin A)], which are supplied as a combination in Synercid, are peptide macrolactones that also bind to the 50S ribosomal subunit and block protein synthesis. Streptogramin B binds to a ribosomal site similar to the binding site for macrolides and lincosamides, whereas streptogramin A binds to a different ribosomal site, blocking the late phase of protein synthesis. The two streptogramins act synergistically to kill bacteria if the strain is susceptible to both components.

CHLORAMPHENICOL Chloramphenicol consists of a single aromatic ring and a short side chain. This antibiotic binds reversibly to the 50S portion of the bacterial ribosome at a site close to but not identical with the binding sites for the macrolides and lincosamides, inhibiting peptide bond formation.

LINEZOLID Linezolid is the only commercially available drug in the oxazolidinone class. Linezolid binds to the 50S ribosomal subunit and blocks the initiation of protein synthesis.

TETRACYCLINES AND GLYCYLCYCLINES Tetracyclines (tetracycline, doxycycline, and minocycline) and glycylcyclines (tigecycline) consist of four aromatic rings with various substituent groups. They interact reversibly with the bacterial 30S ribosomal subunit, blocking the binding of aminoacyl tRNA to the mRNA-ribosome complex. This mechanism is markedly different from that of the aminoglycosides, which also bind to the 30S subunit.

MUPIROCIN Mupirocin (pseudomonic acid) inhibits isoleucine tRNA synthetase by competing with bacterial isoleucine for its binding site on the enzyme and depleting cellular stores of isoleucine-charged tRNA.

INHIBITION OF BACTERIAL METABOLISM

The *antimetabolites* are all synthetic compounds that interfere with bacterial synthesis of folic acid. Products of the folic acid synthesis pathway function as coenzymes for the one-carbon transfer reactions that are essential for the synthesis of thymidine, all purines, and several amino acids. Inhibition of folate synthesis leads to cessation of bacterial cell growth and, in some cases, to bacterial cell death. The principal antibacterial antimetabolites are sulfonamides (sulfisoxazole, sulfadiazine, and sulfamethoxazole) and trimethoprim.

SULFONAMIDES Sulfonamides are structural analogues of *p*-aminobenzoic acid (PABA), one of the three structural components of folic acid (the other two being pteridine and glutamate). The first step in the synthesis of folic acid is the addition of PABA to pteridine by the enzyme dihydropteroic acid synthetase. Sulfonamides compete with PABA as substrates for the enzyme. The selective effect of sulfonamides is due to the fact that bacteria synthesize folic acid, while mammalian cells cannot synthesize the cofactor and must use exogenous supplies. However, the activity of sulfonamides can be greatly reduced by the presence of excess PABA or by the exogenous addition of end products of one-carbon transfer reactions (e.g., thymidine and purines). High concentrations of the latter substances may be present in some infections as a result of tissue and white cell breakdown, compromising sulfonamide activity.

TRIMETHOPRIM Trimethoprim is a diaminopyrimidine, a structural analogue of the pteridine moiety of folic acid. Trimethoprim is a competitive inhibitor of dihydrofolate reductase; this enzyme is responsible for reduction of dihydrofolic acid to tetrahydrofolic acid—the essential final component in the folic acid synthesis pathway. Like that of the sulfonamides, the activity of trimethoprim is compromised in the presence of exogenous thymine or thymidine.

INHIBITION OF NUCLEIC ACID SYNTHESIS OR ACTIVITY

Numerous antibacterial compounds have disparate effects on nucleic acids.

QUINOLONES The quinolones, including nalidixic acid and its fluorinated derivatives (ciprofloxacin, levofloxacin, and moxifloxacin), are synthetic compounds that inhibit the activity of the A subunit of the bacterial enzyme DNA gyrase as well as topoisomerase IV. DNA gyrase and topoisomerases are responsible for negative supercoiling of DNA—an essential conformation for DNA replication in the intact cell. Inhibition of the activity of DNA gyrase and topoisomerase IV is lethal to bacterial cells. The antibiotic *novobiocin* also interferes with the activity of DNA gyrase, but it interferes with the B subunit.

RIFAMPIN Rifampin, used primarily against *Mycobacterium tuberculosis,* is also active against a variety of other bacteria. Rifampin binds tightly to the B subunit of bacterial DNA-dependent RNA polymerase, thus inhibiting transcription of DNA into RNA. Mammalian-cell RNA polymerase is not sensitive to this compound.

NITROFURANTOIN Nitrofurantoin, a synthetic compound, causes DNA damage. The nitrofurans, compounds containing a single five-membered ring, are reduced by a bacterial enzyme to highly reactive, short-lived intermediates that are thought to cause DNA strand breakage, either directly or indirectly.

METRONIDAZOLE Metronidazole, a synthetic imidazole, is active only against anaerobic bacteria and protozoa. The reduction of metronidazole's nitro group by the bacterial anaerobic electron-transport system produces a transient series of reactive intermediates that are thought to cause DNA damage.

ALTERATION OF CELL-MEMBRANE PERMEABILITY

POLYMYXINS The polymyxins [polymyxin B and colistin (polymyxin E)] are cyclic, basic polypeptides. They behave as cationic, surface-active compounds that disrupt the permeability of both the outer and the cytoplasmic membranes of gram-negative bacteria.

GRAMICIDIN A Gramicidin A is a polypeptide of 15 amino acids that acts as an ionophore, forming pores or channels in lipid bilayers.

DAPTOMYCIN Insertion of daptomycin, a new bactericidal lipopeptide antibiotic, into the cell membrane of gram-positive bacteria forms a channel that causes depolarization of the membrane by efflux of intracellular ions, resulting in cell death.

MECHANISMS OF RESISTANCE

Some bacteria exhibit *intrinsic resistance* to certain classes of antibacterial agents (e.g., obligate anaerobic bacteria to aminoglycosides and gram-negative bacteria to vancomycin). In addition, bacteria that are ordinarily susceptible to antibacterial agents can acquire resistance. *Acquired resistance* is a major limitation to effective antibacterial chemotherapy. Resistance can develop by mutation of resident genes or by acquisition of new genes. New genes mediating resistance are usually spread from cell to cell by way of mobile genetic elements such as plasmids, transposons, and bacteriophages. The resistant bacterial populations flourish in areas of high antimicrobial use, where they enjoy a selective advantage over susceptible populations.

The major mechanisms used by bacteria to resist the action of antimicrobial agents are inactivation of the compound, alteration or overproduction of the antibacterial target through mutation of the target protein's gene, acquisition of a new gene that encodes a drug-insensitive target, decreased permeability of the cell envelope to the agent, failure to convert an inactive prodrug to its active derivative, and active efflux of the compound from the periplasm or interior of the cell. Specific mechanisms of bacterial resistance to the major antibacterial agents are outlined below, summarized in Table 127-1, and depicted in Fig. 127-1.

β-LACTAM ANTIBIOTICS

Bacteria develop resistance to β-lactam antibiotics by a variety of mechanisms. Most common is the destruction of the drug by β-lactamases. The β-lactamases of gram-negative bacteria are confined to the periplasm, between the inner and outer membranes, while gram-positive bacteria secrete their β-lactamases into the surrounding medium. These enzymes have a higher affinity for the antibiotic than the antibiotic has for its target. Binding results in hydrolysis of the β-lactam ring. Genes encoding β-lactamases have been found in both chromosomal and extrachromosomal locations and in both gram-positive and gram-negative bacteria; these genes are often on mobile genetic elements. Many "advanced-generation" β-lactam antibiotics, such as ceftriaxone and cefepime, are stable in the presence of plasmid-mediated β-lactamases and are active against bacteria resistant to earlier-generation β-lactam antibiotics. However, extended-spectrum β-lactamases (ESBLs), either acquired on mobile genetic elements by gram-negative bacteria (e.g., *Klebsiella pneumoniae* and *Escherichia coli*) or present as stable chromosomal genes in other gram-negative species (e.g., *Enterobacter* spp.), have broad substrate specificity, hydrolyzing virtually all penicillins and cephalosporins. One strategy that has been devised for circumventing resistance mediated by β-lactamases is to combine the β-lactam agent with an inhibitor that avidly binds the inactivating enzyme, preventing its attack on the antibiotic. Unfortunately, the inhibitors (e.g., clavulanic acid, sulbactam, and tazobactam) do not bind all chromosomal β-lactamases (e.g., that of *Enterobacter*) and thus cannot be depended on to prevent the inactivation of β-lactam antibiotics by such enzymes. No β-lactam antibiotic or inhibitor has been produced that can resist all of the many β-lactamases that have been identified.

A second mechanism of bacterial resistance to β-lactam antibiotics is an alteration in PBP targets so that the PBPs have a markedly reduced affinity for the drug. While this alteration may occur by mutation of existing genes, the acquisition of new PBP genes (as in staphylococcal resistance to methicillin) or of new pieces of PBP genes (as in streptococcal, gonococcal, and meningococcal resistance to penicillin) is more important.

A final resistance mechanism is the coupling, in gram-negative bacteria, of a decrease in outer-membrane permeability with rapid efflux of the antibiotic from the periplasm to the cell exterior. Mutations of genes encoding outer-membrane protein channels called *porins* decrease the entry of β-lactam antibiotics into the cell, while additional proteins form channels that actively pump β-lactams out of the cell. Resistance of Enterobacteriaceae to some cephalosporins and resistance of *Pseudomonas* spp. to cephalosporins and piperacillin are the best examples of this mechanism.

VANCOMYCIN

Clinically important resistance to vancomycin was first described among enterococci in France in 1988. Vancomycin-resistant enterococci (VRE) have subsequently become disseminated worldwide. The genes encoding resistance are carried on plasmids that can transfer themselves from cell to cell and on transposons that can jump from plasmids to chromosomes. Resistance is mediated by enzymes that substitute D-lactate for D-alanine on the peptidoglycan stem peptide so that there is no longer an appropriate target for vancomycin binding. This alteration does not appear to affect cell-wall integrity, however. This type of acquired vancomycin resistance was confined for 14 years to enterococci—more specifically, to *Enterococcus faecium* rather than the more common pathogen *E. faecalis*. However, since 2002, *S. aureus* isolates that are highly resistant to vancomycin have been recovered from four patients in the United States. All of the isolates contain *vanA*, the gene that mediates vancomycin resistance in enterococci. In addition, since 1996, a few isolates of both *S. aureus* and *Staphylococcus epidermidis* that display a four- to eightfold reduction in susceptibility to vancomycin have been found worldwide, and many more isolates may contain subpopulations with reduced vancomycin susceptibility. These isolates have not acquired the genes that mediate vancomycin resistance in enterococci but are mutant bacteria with markedly thickened cell walls. These mutants were apparently selected in patients who were undergoing prolonged vancomycin therapy. The failure of vancomycin therapy in some patients infected with *S. aureus* or *S. epidermidis* strains exhibiting only intermediate susceptibility to this drug is thought to have resulted from this resistance.

AMINOGLYCOSIDES

The most common aminoglycoside resistance mechanism is inactivation of the antibiotic. Aminoglycoside-modifying enzymes, usually encoded on plasmids, transfer phosphate, adenyl, or acetyl residues from intracellular molecules to hydroxyl or amino side groups on the antibiotic. The modified antibiotic is less active because of diminished binding to its ribosomal target. Modifying enzymes that can inactivate any of the available aminoglycosides have been found in both gram-positive and gram-negative bacteria. A second aminoglycoside resistance mechanism, which has been identified predominantly in clinical isolates of *Pseudomonas aeruginosa*, is decreased antibiotic uptake, presumably due to alterations in the bacterial outer membrane.

MACROLIDES, KETOLIDES, LINCOSAMIDES, AND STREPTOGRAMINS

Resistance in gram-positive bacteria, which are the usual target organisms for macrolides, ketolides, lincosamides, and streptogramins, can be due to the production of an enzyme—most commonly plasmid-encoded—that methylates ribosomal RNA, interfering with binding of the antibiotics to their target. Methylation mediates resistance to erythromycin, clarithromycin, azithromycin, clindamycin, and streptogramin B. Resistance to streptogramin B converts quinupristin/dalfopristin from a bactericidal to a bacteriostatic antibiotic. Streptococci can also actively cause the efflux of macrolides, and staphylococci can cause the efflux of macrolides, clindamycin, and streptogramin A. Ketolides such as telithromycin retain activity against most isolates of *Streptococcus pneumoniae* that are resistant to macrolides. In addition, staphylococci can inactivate streptogramin A by acetylation and streptogramin B by either acetylation or hydrolysis. Finally, mutations in 23S ribosomal RNA that alter the binding of macrolides to their targets have been found in both staphylococci and streptococci.

CHLORAMPHENICOL

Most bacteria resistant to chloramphenicol produce a plasmid-encoded enzyme, chloramphenicol acetyltransferase, that inactivates the compound by acetylation.

TETRACYCLINES AND TIGECYCLINE

The most common mechanism of tetracycline resistance in gram-negative bacteria is a plasmid-encoded active-efflux pump that is inserted into the cytoplasmic membrane and extrudes antibiotic from the cell. Resistance in gram-positive bacteria is due either to active efflux or to ribosomal alterations that diminish binding of the antibiotic to its target. Genes involved in ribosomal protection are found on mobile genetic elements. A new parenteral tetracycline derivative (a glycylcycline), tigecycline, is active against tetracycline-resistant bacteria because it is not removed by efflux and can bind to altered ribosomes.

MUPIROCIN

Although the topical compound mupirocin was introduced into clinical use relatively recently, resistance is already becoming widespread in some areas. The mechanism appears to be either mutation of the target isoleucine tRNA synthetase so that it is no longer inhibited by the antibiotic or plasmid-encoded production of a form of the target enzyme that binds mupirocin poorly.

TRIMETHOPRIM AND SULFONAMIDES

The most prevalent mechanism of resistance to trimethoprim and the sulfonamides in both gram-positive and gram-negative bacteria is the acquisition of plasmid-encoded genes that produce a new, drug-insensitive target—specifically, an insensitive dihydrofolate reductase for trimethoprim and an altered dihydropteroate synthetase for sulfonamides.

QUINOLONES

The most common mechanism of resistance to quinolones is the development of one or more mutations in target DNA gyrases and topoisomerase IV that prevent the antibacterial agent from interfering with the enzymes' activity. Some gram-negative bacteria develop mutations that both decrease outer-membrane porin permeability and cause active drug efflux from the cytoplasm. Mutations that result in active quinolone efflux are also found in gram-positive bacteria.

RIFAMPIN

Bacteria rapidly become resistant to rifampin by developing mutations in the B subunit of RNA polymerase that render the enzyme unable to bind the antibiotic. The rapid selection of resistant mutants is the major limitation to the use of this antibiotic against otherwise-susceptible staphylococci and requires that the drug be used in combination with another antistaphylococcal agent.

LINEZOLID

Enterococci, streptococci, and staphylococci become resistant to linezolid in vitro by mutation of the 23S rRNA binding site. Clinical isolates of *E. faecium* and *E. faecalis* acquire resistance to linezolid readily by this mechanism, often during therapy, but linezolid-resistant staphylococcal and streptococcal isolates are rare.

MULTIPLE ANTIBIOTIC RESISTANCE

The acquisition by one bacterium of resistance to multiple antibacterial agents is becoming increasingly common. The two major mechanisms are the acquisition of multiple unrelated resistance genes and the development of mutations in a single gene or gene complex that mediate resistance to a series of unrelated compounds. The construction of multiresistant strains by acquisition of multiple genes occurs by sequential steps of gene transfer and environmental selection in areas of high-level antimicrobial use. In contrast, mutations in a single gene can conceivably be selected in a single step. Bacteria that are multiresistant by virtue of the acquisition of new genes include hospital-associated strains of gram-negative bacteria, enterococci, and staphylococci and community-acquired strains of salmonellae, gonococci, and pneumococci. Mutations that confer resistance to multiple unrelated antimicrobial agents occur in the genes encoding outer-membrane porins and efflux proteins of gram-negative bacteria. These mutations decrease bacterial intracellular and periplasmic accumulation of β-lactams, quinolones, tetracyclines, chloramphenicol, and aminoglycosides. Multiresistant bacterial isolates pose increasing problems in U.S. hospitals; strains resistant to all available antibacterial chemotherapy have already been identified.

PHARMACOKINETICS OF ANTIBIOTICS

The *pharmacokinetic profile* of an antibacterial agent refers to concentrations in serum and tissue versus time and reflects the processes of absorption, distribution, metabolism, and excretion. Important characteristics include peak and trough serum concentrations and mathematically derived parameters such as half-life, clearance, and distribution volume. Pharmacokinetic information is useful for estimating the appropriate antibacterial dose and frequency of administration, for adjusting dosages in patients with impaired excretory capacity, and for comparing one drug with another. In contrast, the *pharmacodynamic profile* of an antibiotic refers to the relationship between the pharmacokinetics of the antibiotic and its minimal inhibitory concentrations (MICs) for bacteria (see "Principles of Antibacterial Chemotherapy," below). **For further discussion of basic pharmacokinetic principles, see Chap. 5.**

ABSORPTION

Antibiotic *absorption* refers to the rate and extent of a drug's systemic bioavailability after oral, IM, or IV administration.

Oral Administration Most patients with infection are treated with oral antibacterial agents in the outpatient setting. Advantages of oral therapy over parenteral therapy include lower cost, generally fewer adverse effects (including complications of indwelling lines), and greater acceptance by patients. The percentage of an orally administered antibacterial agent that is absorbed (i.e., its *bioavailability*) ranges from as little as 10–20% (erythromycin and penicillin G) to nearly 100% [amoxicillin, clindamycin, metronidazole, doxycycline, trimethoprim-sulfamethoxazole (TMP-SMX), linezolid, and most fluoroquinolones]. These differences in bioavailability are not clinically important as long as drug concentrations at the site of infection are sufficient to inhibit or kill the pathogen. However, therapeutic efficacy may be compromised when absorption is reduced as a result of physiologic or pathologic conditions (such as the presence of food for some drugs or the shunting of blood away from the gastrointestinal tract in patients with hypotension), drug interactions (such as that of quinolones and metal cations), or noncompliance. The oral route is usually used for patients with relatively mild infections in whom absorption is not thought to be compromised by the preceding conditions. In addition, the oral route can often be used in more severely ill patients after they have responded to parenteral therapy.

Intramuscular Administration Although the IM route of administration usually results in 100% bioavailability, it is not as widely used in the United States as the oral and IV routes, in part because of the pain often associated with IM injections and the relative ease of IV access in the hospitalized patient. IM injection may be suitable for specific indications requiring an "immediate" and reliable effect (e.g., with long-acting forms of penicillin, including benzathine and procaine, and with single doses of ceftriaxone for acute otitis media or uncomplicated gonococcal infection).

Intravenous Administration The IV route is appropriate when oral antibacterial agents are not effective against a particular pathogen, when bioavailability is uncertain, or when larger doses are required than are feasible with the oral route. After IV administration, bioavailability is 100%; serum concentrations are maximal at the end of the infusion. For many patients in whom long-term antimicrobial therapy is required and oral therapy is not feasible, outpatient parenteral antibiotic therapy (OPAT), including the use of convenient portable pumps, may be cost-effective and safe. Alternatively, some oral antibacterial drugs (e.g., fluoroquinolones) are sufficiently active against Enterobacteriaceae to provide potency equal to that of parenteral therapy; oral use of such drugs may allow the patient to return home from the hospital earlier or to avoid hospitalization entirely.

DISTRIBUTION

To be effective, concentrations of an antibacterial agent must exceed the pathogen's MIC. Serum antibiotic concentrations usually exceed the MIC for susceptible bacteria, but since most infections are extravascular, the antibiotic must also distribute to the site of the infection. Concentrations of most antibacterial agents in interstitial fluid are similar to free-drug concentrations in serum. However, when the infection is located in a "protected" site where penetration is poor, such as cerebrospinal fluid (CSF), the eye, the prostate, or infected cardiac vegetations, high parenteral doses or local administration for prolonged periods may be required for cure. In addition, even though an antibacterial agent may penetrate to the site of infection, its activity may be antagonized by factors in the local environment, such as an unfavorable pH or inactivation by cellular degradation products. For example, since the activity of aminoglycosides is reduced at acidic pH, the acidic environment in many infected tissues may be partly responsible for the relatively poor efficacy of aminoglycoside monotherapy. In addition, the abscess milieu reduces the penetration and local activity of many antibacterial compounds, so that surgical drainage may be required for cure.

Most bacteria that cause human infections are located extracellularly. Intracellular pathogens such as *Legionella*, *Chlamydia*, *Brucella*, and *Salmonella* may persist or cause relapse if the antibacterial agent does not enter the cell. In general, β-lactams, vancomycin, and aminoglycosides penetrate cells poorly, whereas macrolides, ketolides, tetracyclines, metronidazole, chloramphenicol, rifampin, TMP-SMX, and quinolones penetrate cells well.

METABOLISM AND ELIMINATION

Like other drugs, antibacterial agents are disposed of by hepatic elimination (metabolism or biliary elimination), by renal excretion of the unchanged or metabolized form, or by a combination of the two processes. For most of the antibacterial drugs, metabolism leads to loss of in vitro activity, although some agents, such as cefotaxime, rifampin, and clarithromycin, have bioactive metabolites that may contribute to their overall efficacy.

The most practical application of information on the mode of excretion of an antibacterial agent is in adjusting dosage when elimination capability is impaired (Table 127-3). Direct, nonidiosyncratic toxicity from antibacterial drugs may result from failure to reduce the dosage given to patients with impaired elimination. For agents that are primarily cleared intact by glomerular filtration, drug clearance is correlated with creatinine clearance, and estimates of the latter can be used to guide dosage. For drugs whose elimination is primarily hepatic, no simple marker is useful for dosage adjustment in patients with liver disease. However, in patients with severe hepatic disease, residual metabolic capability is usually sufficient to preclude accumulation and toxic effects.

PRINCIPLES OF ANTIBACTERIAL CHEMOTHERAPY

The choice of an antibacterial compound for a particular patient and a specific infection involves more than just a knowledge of the agent's pharmacokinetic profile and in vitro activity. The basic tenets of chemotherapy, to be elaborated below, include the following: When appropriate, material containing the infecting organism(s) should be obtained before the start of treatment so that presumptive identifica-

TABLE 127-3 ANTIBACTERIAL DRUG DOSE ADJUSTMENTS IN PATIENTS WITH RENAL IMPAIRMENT

Antibiotic	Major Route of Excretion	Dosage Adjustment with Renal Impairment
Aminoglycosides	Renal	Yes
Azithromycin	Biliary	No
Cefazolin	Renal	Yes
Cefepime	Renal	Yes
Ceftazidime	Renal	Yes
Ceftriaxone	Renal/biliary	Modest reduction in severe renal impairment
Ciprofloxacin	Renal/biliary	Only in severe renal insufficiency
Clarithromycin	Renal/biliary	Only in severe renal insufficiency
Daptomycin	Renal	Yes
Erythromycin	Biliary	Only when given in high IV doses
Levofloxacin	Renal	Yes
Linezolid	Metabolism	No
Metronidazole	Biliary	No
Nafcillin	Biliary	No
Penicillin G	Renal	Yes (when given in high IV doses)
Piperacillin	Renal	Only with Cl_{cr} of <40 mL/min
Quinupristin/dalfopristin	Metabolism	No
Ticarcillin	Renal	Yes
Tigecycline	Biliary	No
TMP-SMX	Renal/biliary	Only in severe renal insufficiency
Vancomycin	Renal	Yes

Abbreviations: Cl_{cr}, creatinine clearance rate; TMP-SMX, trimethoprim-sulfamethoxazole.

tion can be made by microscopic examination of stained specimens and the organism can be grown for definitive identification and susceptibility testing. Awareness of local susceptibility patterns is useful when the patient is treated empirically. Once the organism is identified and its susceptibility to antibacterial agents is determined, the regimen with the narrowest effective spectrum should be chosen. The choice of antibacterial agent is guided by the pharmacokinetic and adverse-reaction profile of active compounds, the site of infection, the immune status of the host, and evidence of efficacy from well-performed clinical trials. If all other factors are equal, the least expensive antibacterial regimen should be chosen.

SUSCEPTIBILITY OF BACTERIA TO ANTIBACTERIAL DRUGS IN VITRO

Determination of the susceptibility of the patient's infecting organism to a panel of appropriate antibacterial agents is an essential first step in devising a chemotherapeutic regimen. Susceptibility testing is designed to estimate the susceptibility of a bacterial isolate to an antibacterial drug under standardized conditions. These conditions favor rapidly growing aerobic or facultative organisms and assess bacteriostasis only. Specialized testing is required for the assessment of bactericidal antimicrobial activity; for the detection of resistance among such fastidious organisms as obligate anaerobes, *Haemophilus* spp., and pneumococci; and for the determination of resistance phenotypes with variable expression, such as resistance to methicillin or oxacillin among staphylococci. Antimicrobial susceptibility testing is important when susceptibility is unpredictable, most often as a result of increasing acquired resistance among bacteria infecting hospitalized patients.

PHARMACODYNAMICS: RELATIONSHIP OF PHARMACOKINETICS AND IN VITRO SUSCEPTIBILITY TO CLINICAL RESPONSE

Bacteria have often been considered *susceptible* to an antibacterial drug if the achievable peak serum concentration exceeds the MIC by approximately fourfold. The *breakpoint* is the concentration of the antibiotic that separates susceptible from resistant bacteria (Fig. 127-2). When a majority of the isolates of a given bacterial species are inhibited at concentrations below the breakpoint, the species is considered to be within the spectrum of the antibiotic.

The pharmacodynamic profile of an antibiotic refers to the quantitative relationships between the time course of antibiotic concentrations in serum and tissue, in vitro susceptibility (MIC), and microbial response (inhibition of growth or rate of killing). Three pharmacodynamic parameters quantify these relationships: the ratio of the area under the plasma concentration vs. time curve to MIC (AUC/MIC), the ratio of the maximal serum concentration to the MIC (C_{max}/MIC), and the time during a dosing interval that plasma concentrations exceed the MIC (t > MIC). The pharmacodynamic profile of an antibiotic class is characterized as either *concentration dependent* (fluoroquinolones, aminoglycosides), such that an increase in antibiotic concentration leads to a more rapid rate of bacterial death, or *time dependent* (β-lactams), such that the reduction in bacterial density is proportional to the time that concentrations exceed the MIC. For concentration-dependent antibiotics, the C_{max}/MIC or AUC/MIC ratio correlates best with the reduction in microbial density in vitro and in animal investigations. Dosing strategies attempt to maximize these ratios by the administration of a large dose relative to the MIC for anticipated pathogens, often at long intervals (relative to the serum half-life). Once-daily dosing of aminoglycoside antibiotics is the most practical consequence of these relationships. In contrast, dosage strategies for time-dependent antibiotics emphasize the administration of doses sufficient to maintain serum concentrations above the MIC for a critical portion of the dose interval. Response to β-lactam antibiotics, measured as the decline in bacterial density at the site of infection, is maximal when serum and tissue concentrations are maintained above the MIC for 30–50% of the dose interval. For example, the use of high-dose amoxicillin (90–100 mg/kg per day) in the treatment of acute otitis media increases not only the penetration of amoxicillin into the inner ear but also the duration of time that concentrations exceed the MIC for pneumococci. This approach provides effective therapy in most patients, including those whose pneumococcal isolates are penicillin resistant. The clinical implications of these pharmacodynamic relationships are in the early stages of investigation; their elucidation should eventually result in more rational antibacterial dosage regimens. Table 127-4 summarizes the pharmacodynamic properties of the major antibiotic classes.

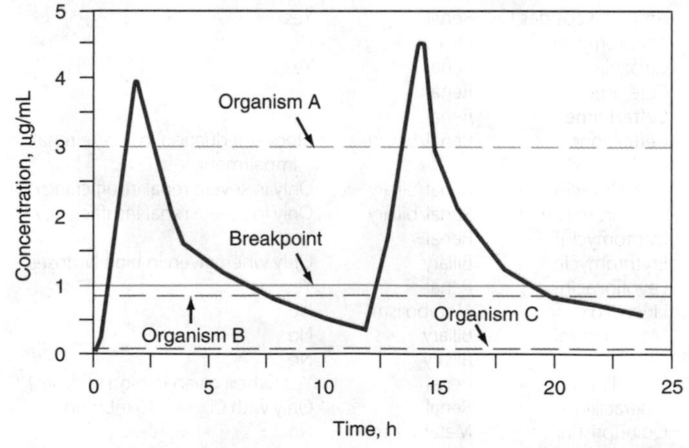

FIGURE 127-2 Relationship between pharmacokinetics of an antibiotic and susceptibility. Organism A is resistant, organism B is moderately susceptible, and organism C is very susceptible. Pharmacodynamic indices include the ratio of the peak serum concentration to MIC (C_{max}/MIC), the ratio of the area under the serum concentration vs. time curve to MIC (AUC/MIC), and the time that serum concentrations exceed the MIC (t > MIC).

TABLE 127-4 PHARMACODYNAMIC INDICES OF MAJOR ANTIMICROBIAL CLASSES

Parameter Predicting Response	Drug or Drug Class
Time above the MIC	Penicillins, cephalosporins, carbapenems, aztreonam
24-h AUC/MIC	Aminoglycosides, fluoroquinolones, tetracyclines, vancomycin, macrolides, clindamycin, quinupristin/dalfopristin, tigecycline, daptomycin
Peak to MIC	Aminoglycosides, fluoroquinolones

Abbreviations: MIC, minimal inhibitory concentration; AUC, area under the concentration curve.

STATUS OF THE HOST

Various host factors must be considered in the devising of antibacterial chemotherapy. The host's antibacterial *immune function* is of importance, particularly as it relates to opsonophagocytic function. Since the major host defense against acute, overwhelming bacterial infection is the polymorphonuclear leukocyte, patients with neutropenia must be treated aggressively and empirically with bactericidal drugs for suspected infection (Chap. 82). Likewise, patients who have deficient humoral immunity (e.g., those with chronic lymphocytic leukemia and multiple myeloma) and individuals with surgical or functional asplenia (e.g., those with sickle cell disease) should be treated empirically for infections with encapsulated organisms, especially the pneumococcus.

Pregnancy increases the risk of toxicity of certain antibacterial drugs for the mother (e.g., hepatic toxicity of tetracycline), affects drug disposition and pharmacokinetics, and—because of the risk of fetal toxicity—severely limits the choice of agents for treating infections. Certain antibacterial agents are contraindicated in pregnancy either because their safety has not been established (categories B and C) or because they are known to be toxic (categories D and X). Table 127-5 summarizes drug safety in pregnancy.

In patients with *concomitant viral infections*, the incidence of adverse reactions to antibacterial drugs may be unusually high. For example, persons with infectious mononucleosis and those infected with HIV experi-

TABLE 127-5 ANTIBACTERIAL DRUGS IN PREGNANCY

Antibacterial Drug	Toxicity in Pregnancy	Recommendation
Aminoglycosides	Possible 8th-nerve toxicity	Caution[a]
Chloramphenicol	Gray syndrome in newborn	Caution at term
Fluoroquinolones	Arthropathy in immature animals	Caution
Clarithromycin	Teratogenicity in animals	Contraindicated
Ertapenem	Decreased weight in animals	Caution
Erythromycin estolate	Cholestatic hepatitis	Contraindicated
Imipenem/cilastatin	Toxicity in some pregnant animals	Caution
Linezolid	Embryonic and fetal toxicity in rats	Caution
Meropenem	Unknown	Caution
Metronidazole	None known, but carcinogenic in rats	Caution
Nitrofurantoin	Hemolytic anemia in newborns	Caution; contraindicated at term
Quinupristin/dalfopristin	Unknown	Caution
Sulfonamides	Hemolysis in newborn with G6PD[b] deficiency; kernicterus in newborn	Caution; contraindicated at term
Tetracyclines/tigecycline	Tooth discoloration, inhibition of bone growth in fetus; hepatotoxicity	Contraindicated
Vancomycin	Unknown	Caution

[a]Use only for strong clinical indication in the absence of a suitable alternative.
[b]G6PD, glucose-6-phosphate dehydrogenase.

ence skin reactions more often to penicillins and folic acid synthesis inhibitors such as TMP-SMX, respectively.

In addition, the patient's age, sex, racial heritage, genetic background, and excretory status all determine the incidence and type of side effects that can be expected with certain antibacterial agents.

SITE OF INFECTION

The location of the infected site may play a major role in the choice and dose of antimicrobial drug. Patients with suspected *meningitis* should receive drugs that can cross the blood-CSF barrier; in addition, because of the relative paucity of phagocytes and opsonins at the site of infection, the agents should be bactericidal. Chloramphenicol, an older drug but occasionally useful in the treatment of meningitis, is bactericidal for common organisms causing meningitis (i.e., meningococci, pneumococci, and *Haemophilus influenzae*, but *not* enteric gram-negative bacilli), is highly lipid-soluble, and enters the CSF well. However, β-lactam drugs, the mainstay of therapy for most of these infections, do not normally reach high levels in CSF. Their efficacy is based on the increased permeability of the blood-brain and blood-CSF barriers to hydrophilic molecules during inflammation and the extreme susceptibility of most infectious organisms to even small amounts of β-lactam drug.

The vegetation, which is the major site of infection in *bacterial endocarditis*, is also a focus that is protected from normal host-defense mechanisms. Antibacterial therapy needs to be bactericidal, with the selected agent administered parenterally over a long period and at a dose that produces serum levels at least eight times higher than the minimal bactericidal concentration (MBC) for the infecting organism. Likewise, *osteomyelitis* involves a site that is resistant to opsonophagocytic removal of infecting bacteria; furthermore, avascular bone (sequestrum) represents a foreign body that thwarts normal host-defense mechanisms. *Chronic prostatitis* is exceedingly difficult to cure because most antibiotics do not penetrate through the capillaries serving the prostate, especially when acute inflammation is absent. *Intraocular infections*, especially endophthalmitis, are difficult to treat because retinal capillaries lacking fenestration hinder drug penetration into the vitreous from blood. Inflammation does little to disrupt this barrier. Thus, direct injection into the vitreous is necessary in many cases. Antibiotic penetration into *abscesses* is usually poor, and local conditions (e.g., low pH or the presence of enzymes that hydrolyze the drug) may further antagonize antibacterial activity.

In contrast, *urinary tract infections* (UTIs), when confined to the bladder, are relatively easy to cure, in part because of the higher concentration of most antibiotics in urine than in blood. Since blood is the usual reference fluid in defining susceptibility (Fig. 127-2), even organisms found to be resistant to achievable serum concentrations may be susceptible to achievable urine concentrations. For drugs that are used only for the treatment of UTIs, such as the urinary tract antiseptics nitrofurantoin and methenamine salts, achievable urine concentrations are used to determine susceptibility. Nitrofurantoin is often active against VRE and is a less expensive alternative to linezolid for the treatment of lower UTIs.

COMBINATION CHEMOTHERAPY

One of the tenets of antibacterial chemotherapy is that if the infecting bacterium has been identified, the most specific chemotherapy possible should be used. The use of a single agent with a narrow spectrum of activity against the pathogen diminishes the alteration of normal flora and thus limits the overgrowth of resistant nosocomial organisms (e.g., *Candida albicans*, enterococci, *Clostridium difficile*, or methicillin-resistant staphylococci), avoids the potential toxicity of multiple-drug regimens, and reduces cost. However, certain circumstances call for the use of more than one antibacterial agent. These are summarized below.

1. *Prevention of the emergence of resistant mutants.* Spontaneous mutations occur at a detectable frequency in certain genes encoding the target proteins for some antibacterial agents. The use of these agents can eliminate the susceptible population, select out resistant mutants at the site of infection, and result in the failure of chemotherapy. Resistant mutants are usually selected when the MIC of the antibacterial agent for the infecting bacterium is close to achievable levels in serum or tissues and/or when the site of infection limits the access or activity of the agent. Among the most common examples are rifampin for staphylococci, imipenem for *Pseudomonas*, and fluoroquinolones for staphylococci and *Pseudomonas*. Small-colony variants of staphylococci resistant to aminoglycosides also emerge during monotherapy with these antibiotics. A second antibacterial agent with a mechanism of action different from that of the first is added to prevent the emergence of these resistant mutants (e.g., imipenem plus an aminoglycoside or a fluoroquinolone for systemic *Pseudomonas* infections). However, since resistant mutants have emerged following combination chemotherapy, this approach clearly is not uniformly successful.
2. *Synergistic or additive activity.* Synergistic or additive activity involves a lowering of the MIC or MBC of each or all of the drugs tested in combination against a specific bacterium. In *synergy*, each agent is more active when combined with a second drug than it would be alone, and the drugs' combined activity is therefore greater than the sum of the individual activities of each drug. In an *additive relationship*, the combined activity of the drugs is equal to the sum of their individual activities. Among the best examples of a synergistic or additive effect, confirmed both in vitro and by animal studies, are the enhanced bactericidal activities of certain β-lactam/aminoglycoside combinations against enterococci, viridans streptococci, and *P. aeruginosa*. The synergistic or additive activity of these combinations has also been demonstrated against selected isolates of enteric gram-negative bacteria and staphylococci. The combination of trimethoprim and sulfamethoxazole has synergistic or additive activity against many enteric gram-negative bacteria. Most other antimicrobial combinations display indifferent activity (i.e., the combination is *no better* than the more active of the two agents alone), and some combinations (e.g., penicillin plus tetracycline against pneumococci) may be antagonistic (i.e., the combination is *worse* than either drug alone).

3. *Therapy directed against multiple potential pathogens.* For certain infections, either a mixture of pathogens is suspected or the patient is desperately ill with an as-yet-unidentified infection (see "Empirical Therapy," below). In these situations, the most important of the likely infecting bacteria must be covered by therapy until culture and susceptibility results become available. Examples of the former infections are intraabdominal or brain abscesses and infections of limbs in diabetic patients with microvascular disease. The latter situations include fevers in neutropenic patients, acute pneumonia from aspiration of oral flora by hospitalized patients, and septic shock or sepsis syndrome.

EMPIRICAL THERAPY

In many situations, antibacterial therapy is begun before a specific bacterial pathogen has been identified. The choice of agent is guided by the results of studies identifying the usual pathogens at that site or in that clinical setting, by pharmacodynamic considerations, and by the resistance profile of the expected pathogens in a particular hospital or geographic area. Situations in which empirical therapy is appropriate include the following:

1. *Life-threatening infection.* Any suspected bacterial infection in a patient with a life-threatening illness should be treated presumptively. Therapy is usually begun with more than one agent and is later tailored to a specific pathogen if one is eventually identified. Early therapy with an effective antimicrobial regimen has consistently been demonstrated to improve survival rates.
2. *Treatment of community-acquired infections.* In many situations, it is appropriate to treat non-life-threatening infections without obtaining cultures. These situations include outpatient infections such as community-acquired upper and lower respiratory tract infections, cystitis, cellulitis or local wound infection, urethritis, and prostatitis. However, if any of these infections recurs or fails to respond to initial therapy, every effort should be made to obtain cultures to guide re-treatment.

CHOICE OF ANTIBACTERIAL THERAPY

Infections for which specific antibacterial agents are among the drugs of choice are detailed in Table 127-6. No attempt has been made to include all of the potential situations in which antibacterial agents may be used. A more detailed discussion of specific bacteria and infections that they cause can be found elsewhere in this volume.

The choice of antibacterial therapy increasingly involves an assessment of the acquired resistance of major microbial pathogens to the antimicrobial agents available to treat them. Resistance rates are dynamic (Table 127-6), both increasing and decreasing in response to the environmental pressure applied by antimicrobial use. For example, a threefold increase in fluoroquinolone use in the community between 1995 and 2002 was associated with increasing rates of quinolone resistance in community-acquired strains of *S. pneumoniae*, *E. coli*, *Neisseria gonorrhoeae*, and *K. pneumoniae*. Fluoroquinolone resistance has also emerged rapidly among nosocomial isolates of *S. aureus* and *Pseudomonas* spp. as hospital use of this drug class has increased. In contrast, staphylococcal resistance to tetracyclines has decreased as the use of these antibiotics has declined. It is important to note that, in many cases, wide variations in worldwide antimicrobial-resistance trends may not be reflected in the values recorded at U.S. hospitals (e.g., for fluoroquinolone resistance in *N. gonorrhoeae*). Therefore, the most important factor in choosing initial therapy for an infection in which the susceptibility of the specific pathogen(s) is not known is information on local resistance rates. This information can be obtained from local clinical microbiology laboratories, state health departments, or publications of the Centers for Disease Control and Prevention (e.g., *Emerging Infectious Diseases* and *Morbidity and Mortality Weekly Report*).

ADVERSE REACTIONS

Adverse drug reactions are frequently classified by mechanism as either *dose-related* ("toxic") or *unpredictable*. Unpredictable reactions are either idiosyncratic or allergic. Dose-related reactions include aminoglycoside-induced nephrotoxicity, linezolid-induced thrombocytopenia, penicillin-induced seizures, and vancomycin-induced anaphylactoid reactions. Many of these reactions can be avoided by reducing dosage in patients with impaired renal function, limiting the duration of therapy, or reducing the rate of administration. Adverse reactions to antibacterial agents are a common cause of morbidity, requiring alteration in therapy and additional expense, and they occasionally result in death. The elderly, often those with the more severe infections, may be especially prone to certain adverse reactions. The most clinically relevant adverse reactions to common antibacterial drugs are listed in Table 127-7. **For further discussion of adverse drug reactions, see Chap. 5.**

DRUG INTERACTIONS

Antimicrobial drugs are a common cause of drug-drug interactions. Table 127-8 lists the most common and best-documented interactions of antibacterial agents with other drugs and characterizes the clinical relevance of these interactions. Coadministration of drugs paired in the tables does not necessarily result in clinically important adverse consequences. Recognition of the potential for an interaction before the administration of an antibacterial agent is crucial to the rational use of these drugs, since adverse consequences can often be prevented if the interaction is anticipated. Table 127-8 is intended only to heighten awareness of the potential for an interaction. Additional sources should be consulted to identify appropriate options. **For further discussion of drug interactions, see Chap. 5.**

MACROLIDES AND KETOLIDES

Erythromycin, clarithromycin, and telithromycin inhibit CYP3A4, the hepatic P450 enzyme that metabolizes many drugs, including cyclosporine, certain statins (lovastatin, simvastatin), theophylline, carbamazepine, warfarin, certain antineoplastic agents (e.g., vincristine, irinotecan), and ergot alkaloids. In ~10% of patients receiving digoxin, concentrations increase significantly when erythromycin or telithromycin is coadministered, and this increase may lead to digoxin toxicity. Azithromycin has little effect on the metabolism of other drugs. Many drugs (e.g., azole antifungal drugs, diltiazem, verapamil, and nefazodone) can also increase absorption or inhibit erythromycin metabolism. These effects are associated with prolongation of the QT interval and a fivefold increase in mortality rate. This example serves as a reminder that the true significance of drug-drug interactions may be subtle yet profound and that close attention to the evolving safety literature is important.

QUINUPRISTIN/DALFOPRISTIN

Quinupristin/dalfopristin is an inhibitor of CYP3A4. Its interactions with other drugs should be similar to those of erythromycin.

LINEZOLID

Linezolid is a monoamine oxidase inhibitor. Its concomitant administration with sympathomimetics (e.g., phenylpropanolamine) and with foods with high concentrations of tyramine should be avoided. Many case reports describe serotonin syndrome following coadministration of linezolid with selective serotonin reuptake inhibitors.

TETRACYCLINES

The most important interaction involving tetracyclines is reduced absorption when these drugs are coadministered with divalent and trivalent cations, such as antacids, iron compounds, or dairy products. Food also adversely affects absorption of most tetracyclines. Inducers of hepatic isoenzymes, such as phenytoin and rifampin, increase the clearance of doxycycline; although the clinical significance of this effect is unknown, use of an alternative antibiotic may be appropriate.

SULFONAMIDES

Sulfonamides, including TMP-SMX, increase the hypoprothrombinemic effect of warfarin by inhibition of its metabolism or by protein-binding displacement.

TABLE 127-6 INFECTIONS FOR WHICH SPECIFIC ANTIBACTERIAL AGENTS ARE AMONG THE DRUGS OF CHOICE

Agent	Infections	Common Pathogen(s) (Resistance Rate, %)[a]
Penicillin G	Syphilis, yaws, leptospirosis, groups A and B streptococcal infections, pneumococcal infections, actinomycosis, oral and periodontal infections, meningococcal meningitis and meningococcemia, viridans streptococcal endocarditis, clostridial myonecrosis, tetanus, anthrax, rat-bite fever, *Pasteurella multocida* infections, and erysipeloid (*Erysipelothrix rhusiopathiae*)	*Neisseria meningitidis*[b] (intermediate,[c] 15–30; resistant, 0; geographic variation) Viridans streptococci (intermediate, 15–30; resistant, 5–10) *Streptococcus pneumoniae* (intermediate, 23; resistant, 17)
Ampicillin, amoxicillin	Salmonellosis, acute otitis media, *Haemophilus influenzae* meningitis and epiglottitis, *Listeria monocytogenes* meningitis, *Enterococcus faecalis* UTI	*Escherichia coli* (37) *H. influenzae* (35) *Salmonella* spp.[b] (30–50; geographic variation) *Enterococcus* spp. (24)
Nafcillin, oxacillin	*Staphylococcus aureus* (non-MRSA) bacteremia and endocarditis	*S. aureus* (46; MRSA) *Staphylococcus epidermidis* (78; MRSE)
Piperacillin plus tazobactam	Intraabdominal infections (facultative enteric gram-negative bacilli plus obligate anaerobes); infections caused by mixed flora (aspiration pneumonia, diabetic foot ulcers); infections caused by *Pseudomonas aeruginosa*	*P. aeruginosa* (6)
Cefazolin	*E. coli* UTI, surgical prophylaxis, *S. aureus* (non-MRSA) bacteremia and endocarditis	*E. coli* (7) *S. aureus* (46; MRSA)
Cefoxitin, cefotetan	Intraabdominal infections and pelvic inflammatory disease	*Bacteroides fragilis* (12)
Ceftriaxone	Gonococcal infections, pneumococcal meningitis, viridans streptococcal endocarditis, salmonellosis and typhoid fever, hospital-acquired infections caused by nonpseudomonal facultative gram-negative enteric bacilli	*S. pneumoniae* (intermediate, 16; resistant, 0) *E. coli* and *Klebsiella pneumoniae* (1; ESBL producers)
Ceftazidime, cefepime	Hospital-acquired infections caused by facultative gram-negative enteric bacilli and *Pseudomonas*	*P. aeruginosa* (16) (See ceftriaxone for ESBL producers)
Imipenem, meropenem	Intraabdominal infections, hospital-acquired infections (non-MRSA), infections caused by *Enterobacter* spp. and ESBL-producing gram-negative bacilli	*P. aeruginosa* (6) *Acinetobacter* spp. (35)
Aztreonam	Hospital-acquired infections caused by facultative gram-negative bacilli and *Pseudomonas* in penicillin-allergic patients	*P. aeruginosa* (16)
Vancomycin	Bacteremia, endocarditis, and other serious infections due to MRSA; pneumococcal meningitis; antibiotic-associated pseudomembranous colitis[d]	*Enterococcus* spp. (24)
Daptomycin	VRE infections; MRSA bacteremia	UNK
Gentamicin, amikacin, tobramycin	Combined with a penicillin for staphylococcal, enterococcal, or viridans streptococcal endocarditis; combined with a β-lactam antibiotic for gram-negative bacteremia; pyelonephritis	Gentamicin: *E. coli* (6) *P. aeruginosa* (17) *Acinetobacter* spp. (32)
Erythromycin, clarithromycin, azithromycin	*Legionella*, *Campylobacter*, and *Mycoplasma* infections; CAP; group A streptococcal pharyngitis in penicillin-allergic patients; bacillary angiomatosis (*Bartonella henselae*); gastric infections due to *Helicobacter pylori*; *Mycobacterium avium-intracellulare* infections	*S. pneumoniae* (28) *Streptococcus pyogenes*[b] (0–10; geographic variation) *H. pylori*[b] (2–20; geographic variation)
Clindamycin	Severe, invasive group A streptococcal infections; infections caused by obligate anaerobes; infections caused by susceptible staphylococci	*S. aureus* (nosocomial = 58; CA-MRSA = 10[b])
Doxycycline, minocycline	Acute bacterial exacerbations of chronic bronchitis, granuloma inguinale, brucellosis (with streptomycin), tularemia, glanders, melioidosis, spirochetal infections caused by *Borrelia* (Lyme disease and relapsing fever; doxycycline), infections caused by *Vibrio vulnificus*, some *Aeromonas* infections, infections due to *Stenotrophomonas* (minocycline), plague, ehrlichiosis, chlamydial infections (doxycycline), granulomatous skin infections due to *Mycobacterium marinum* (minocycline), rickettsial infections, mild CAP, skin and soft tissue infections caused by gram-positive cocci (CA-MRSA infections, leptospirosis, syphilis, actinomycosis in the penicillin-allergic patient)	*S. pneumoniae* (17) MRSA (5)
Trimethoprim-sulfamethoxazole	Community-acquired UTI; *S. aureus* skin and soft tissue infections (CA-MRSA)	*E. coli* (19) MRSA (3)
Sulfonamides	Nocardial infections, leprosy (dapsone, a sulfone), and toxoplasmosis (sulfadiazine)	UNK
Ciprofloxacin, levofloxacin, moxifloxacin	CAP (levofloxacin and moxifloxacin); UTI; bacterial gastroenteritis; hospital-acquired gram-negative enteric infections; *Pseudomonas* infections (ciprofloxacin and levofloxacin)	*S. pneumoniae* (1) *E. coli* (13) *P. aeruginosa* (23) *Salmonella* spp. (10–50; geographic variation) *Neisseria gonorrhoeae*[b] (0–5, non–West Coast U.S.; 10–15, California and Hawaii; 20–70, Asia, England, Wales)
Rifampin	Staphylococcal foreign body infections, in combination with other antistaphylococcal agents; *Legionella* pneumonia	Staphylococci rapidly develop resistance during rifampin monotherapy.
Metronidazole	Obligate anaerobic gram-negative bacteria (*Bacteroides* spp.): abscess in lung, brain, or abdomen; bacterial vaginosis; antibiotic-associated *Clostridium difficile* disease	UNK
Linezolid	VRE; staphylococcal skin and soft tissue infection (CA-MRSA)	UNK
Polymyxin E (colistin)	Hospital-acquired infection due to gram-negative bacilli resistant to all other chemotherapy: *P. aeruginosa*, *Acinetobacter* spp., *Stenotrophomonas maltophilia*	UNK
Quinupristin/dalfopristin	VRE	Vancomycin-resistant *E. faecalis*[b] (100) Vancomycin-resistant *E. faecium* (10)
Mupirocin	Topical application to nares to eradicate *S. aureus* carriage	UNK

[a]Unless otherwise noted, resistance rates are based on all isolates tested in 2005 in the clinical microbiology laboratory at Virginia Commonwealth University Medical Center. The rates are consistent with those reported by the National Nosocomial Infections Surveillance System (Am J Infect Control 32:470, 2004).
[b]Data from recent literature sources.
[c]Intermediate resistance.
[d]Drug is given orally for this indication.

Abbreviations: CA-MRSA, community-acquired methicillin-resistant *S. aureus*; CAP, community-acquired pneumonia; MRSA, methicillin-resistant *S. aureus*; MRSE, methicillin-resistant *S. epidermidis*; UTI, urinary tract infection; VRE, vancomycin-resistant enterococci; ESBL, extended-spectrum β-lactamase; UNK, resistance rates unknown.

TABLE 127-7 MOST CLINICALLY RELEVANT ADVERSE REACTIONS TO COMMON ANTIBACTERIAL DRUGS

Drug	Adverse Event	Comments
β-Lactams	Allergies in ~1–4% of treatment courses	Cephalosporins cause allergy in 2–4% of penicillin-allergic patients. Aztreonam is safe in β-lactam–allergic patients.
	Nonallergic skin reactions	Ampicillin "rash" is common among patients with Epstein-Barr virus infection.
	Diarrhea, including *Clostridium difficile* colitis (Chap. 123)	—
Vancomycin	Anaphylactoid reaction ("red man syndrome")	Give as a 1- to 2-h infusion.
	Nephrotoxicity, ototoxicity, allergy, neutropenia	Rare
Aminoglycosides	Nephrotoxicity (generally reversible)	Greatest with prolonged therapy in the elderly or with preexisting renal insufficiency. Monitor serum creatinine every 2–3 days.
	Ototoxicity (often irreversible)	Risk factors similar to those for nephrotoxicity; both vestibular and hearing toxicities
Macrolides/ ketolides	Gastrointestinal distress	Most common with erythromycin
	Ototoxicity	High-dose IV erythromycin
	Cardiac toxicity	QTc prolongation and torsades de pointes, especially when inhibitors of erythromycin metabolism are given simultaneously
	Hepatic toxicity (telithromycin)	Warning added to prescribing information (July 2006)
	Respiratory failure in patients with myasthenia gravis (telithromycin)	Warning added to prescribing information (July 2006)
Clindamycin	Diarrhea, including *C. difficile* colitis	—
Sulfonamides	Allergic reactions	Rashes (more common in HIV-infected patients); serious dermal reactions, including erythema multiforme, Stevens-Johnson syndrome, toxic epidermal necrolysis
	Hematologic reactions	Uncommon; include agranulocytosis and granulocytopenia (more common in HIV-infected patients), hemolytic and megaloblastic anemia, thrombocytopenia
	Renal insufficiency	Crystalluria with sulfadiazine therapy
Fluoroquinolones	Diarrhea, including *C. difficile* colitis	—
	Contraindicated for general use in patients <18 years old and pregnant women	Appear safe in treatment of pulmonary infections in children with cystic fibrosis
	Central nervous system adverse effects (e.g., insomnia)	—
	Miscellaneous: allergies, tendon rupture, dysglycemias, QTc prolongation	Rare
Rifampin	Hepatotoxicity	Rare
	Orange discoloration of urine and body fluids	Common
	Miscellaneous: flu-like symptoms, hemolysis, renal insufficiency	Uncommon; usually related to intermittent administration
Metronidazole	Metallic taste	Common
Tetracyclines/ glycylcyclines	Gastrointestinal distress	Up to 20% with tigecycline
	Esophageal ulceration	Doxycycline (take in A.M. with fluids)
Linezolid	Myelosuppression	Follows long-term treatment
	Ocular and peripheral neuritis	Follow long-term treatment
Daptomycin	Distal muscle pain or weakness	Weekly creatine phosphokinase measurements, especially in patients also receiving statins

FLUOROQUINOLONES

There are two clinically important drug interactions involving fluoroquinolones. First, like tetracyclines, all fluoroquinolones are chelated by divalent and trivalent cations, with a consequential significant reduction in absorption. Second, ciprofloxacin inhibits the hepatic enzyme that metabolizes theophylline. Scattered case reports suggest that quinolones can also potentiate the effects of warfarin, but this effect has not been observed in most controlled trials.

RIFAMPIN

Rifampin is an excellent inducer of many cytochrome P450 enzymes and increases the hepatic clearance of a large number of drugs, including the following (with the indicated predictable outcomes): HIV-1 protease inhibitors (loss of viral suppression), oral contraceptives (pregnancy), warfarin (decreased prothrombin times), cyclosporine and prednisone (organ rejection or exacerbations of any underlying inflammatory condition), and verapamil and diltiazem (increased dosage requirements). Before rifampin is prescribed for any patient, a review of concomitant drug therapy is essential.

METRONIDAZOLE

Metronidazole can cause a disulfiram-like syndrome when alcohol is ingested. Thus, patients taking metronidazole should be instructed to avoid alcohol. Inhibition of the metabolism of warfarin by metronidazole leads to significant rises in prothrombin times.

PROPHYLAXIS OF BACTERIAL INFECTIONS

Antibacterial agents are occasionally indicated for use in patients who have no evidence of infection but who have been or are expected to be exposed to bacterial pathogens under circumstances that constitute a major risk of infection. The basic tenets of antimicrobial prophylaxis are as follows: (1) The risk or potential severity of infection should outweigh the risk of side effects from the antibacterial agent. (2) The antibacterial agent should be given for the shortest period necessary to prevent target infections. (3) The antibacterial agent should be given before the expected period of risk (e.g., within 1 h of incision before elective surgery) or as soon as possible after contact with an infected individual (e.g., prophylaxis for meningococcal meningitis).

Table 127-9 lists the major indications for antibacterial prophylaxis in adults. The table includes only those indications that are widely accepted, supported by well-designed studies, or recommended by expert panels. Prophylaxis is also used but is less widely accepted for recurrent cellulitis in conjunction with lymphedema, recurrent pneumococcal meningitis in conjunction with deficiencies in humoral immunity or CSF leaks, traveler's diarrhea, gram-negative sepsis in conjunction with neutropenia, and spontaneous bacterial peritonitis in conjunction with ascites. The use of antibacterial agents in children to prevent rheumatic fever and otitis media under certain circumstances is also common practice.

The major use of antibacterial prophylaxis is to prevent infections following surgical procedures. Antibacterial agents are administered just before the surgical procedure—and, for long operations, during the procedure as well—to ensure high drug concentrations in serum and tissues during surgery. The objective is to eradicate bacteria originating from the air of the operating suite, the skin of the surgical team, or the patient's own flora that may contaminate the wound. In all but colorectal surgical procedures, prophylaxis

TABLE 127-8 INTERACTIONS OF ANTIBACTERIAL AGENTS WITH OTHER DRUGS

Antibiotic	Interacts with	Potential Consequence (Clinical Significance[a])
Erythromycin/clarithromycin/ telithromycin	Theophylline	Theophylline toxicity (1)
	Carbamazepine	CNS depression (1)
	Digoxin	Digoxin toxicity (2)
	Triazolam/midazolam	CNS depression (2)
	Ergotamine	Ergotism (1)
	Warfarin	Bleeding (2)
	Cyclosporine/tacrolimus	Nephrotoxicity (1)
	Cisapride	Cardiac arrhythmias (1)
	Statins[b]	Rhabdomyolysis (2)
	Valproate	Valproate toxicity (2)
	Vincristine/vinblastine	Excess neurotoxicity (2)
Quinupristin/dalfopristin	Similar to erythromycin[c]	
Fluoroquinolones	Theophylline	Theophylline toxicity (2)[d]
	Antacids/sucralfate/iron	Subtherapeutic antibiotic levels (1)
Tetracycline	Antacids/sucralfate/iron	Subtherapeutic antibiotic levels (1)
Trimethoprim-sulfamethoxazole	Phenytoin	Phenytoin toxicity (2)
	Oral hypoglycemics	Hypoglycemia (2)
	Warfarin	Bleeding (1)
	Digoxin	Digoxin toxicity (2)
Metronidazole	Ethanol	Disulfiram-like reactions (2)
	Fluorouracil	Bone marrow suppression (1)
	Warfarin	Bleeding (2)
Rifampin	Warfarin	Clot formation (1)
	Oral contraceptives	Pregnancy (1)
	Cyclosporine/tacrolimus	Rejection (1)
	HIV-1 protease inhibitors	Increased viral load, resistance (1)
	Nonnucleoside reverse-transcriptase inhibitors	Increased viral load, resistance (1)
	Glucocorticoids	Loss of steroid effect (1)
	Methadone	Narcotic withdrawal symptoms (1)
	Digoxin	Subtherapeutic digoxin levels (1)
	Itraconazole	Subtherapeutic itraconazole levels (1)
	Phenytoin	Loss of seizure control (1)
	Statins	Hypercholesterolemia (1)
	Diltiazem	Subtherapeutic diltiazem levels (1)
	Verapamil	Subtherapeutic verapamil levels (1)

[a]1 = a well-documented interaction with clinically important consequences; 2 = an interaction of uncertain frequency but of potential clinical importance.
[b]Lovastatin and simvastatin are most affected; pravastatin and atorvastatin are less prone to clinically important effects.
[c]The macrolide antibiotics and quinupristin/dalfopristin inhibit the same human metabolic enzyme, CYP3A4, and similar interactions are anticipated.
[d]Ciprofloxacin only. Levofloxacin and moxifloxacin do not inhibit theophylline metabolism.
Note: New interactions are commonly reported after marketing. Consult the most recent prescribing information for updates.
Abbreviation: CNS, central nervous system.

is predominantly directed against staphylococci and cefazolin is the drug most commonly recommended. Prophylaxis is intended to prevent wound infection or infection of implanted devices, not all infections that may occur during the postoperative period (e.g., UTIs or pneumonia). Prolonged prophylaxis (beyond 24 h) merely alters the normal flora and favors infections with organisms resistant to the antibacterial agents used. A focus on appropriate surgical prophylaxis by the Centers for Medicare and Medicaid Services, coupled with national efforts by surgical societies, appears to be having a favorable impact on the appropriate use of antimicrobial drugs in the surgical setting, although additional improvements are needed.

DURATION OF THERAPY AND TREATMENT FAILURE

Until recently, there was little incentive to establish the most appropriate duration of treatment; patients were instructed to take a 7- or 10-day course of treatment for most common infections. A number of recent investigations have evaluated shorter durations of therapy, especially in patients with community-acquired pneumonia. Table 127-10 lists common bacterial infections for which treatment duration guidelines have been established or for which there is sufficient clinical experience to establish treatment durations. The ultimate test of cure for a bacterial infection is the absence of relapse when therapy is discontinued. *Relapse* is defined as a recurrence of infection with the identical organism that caused the first infection. In general, therefore, the duration of therapy should be long enough to prevent relapse yet not excessive. Extension of therapy beyond the limit of effectiveness may increase the medication's side effects and encourage the selection of resistant bacteria. The art of treating bacterial infections lies in the ability to determine the appropriate duration of therapy for infections that are not covered by established guidelines. Re-treatment of infections for which therapy has failed usually requires a prolonged course (>4 weeks) with combinations of antibacterial agents.

MECHANISMS TO OPTIMIZE ANTIMICROBIAL USE

Antibiotic use is often not "rational," and it is easy to understand why. The diagnosis of bacterial infection is often uncertain, and patients may expect or demand antimicrobial agents in this tenuous situation. There is a bewildering array of drugs, each with claims of superiority over the competition. The rates of resistance for many bacterial pathogens are ever-changing, and even experts may not agree on the clinical significance of resistance in some pathogens. Investigations consistently report that ~50% of antibiotic use is in some way "inappropriate." Aside from the monetary cost of using unnecessary or overly expensive antibiotics, there are the more serious costs associated with excess morbidity from superinfections such as *C. difficile* disease, adverse drug reactions, drug interactions, and selection of resistant organisms. Although these costs are not yet well quantified, they add substantially to the overall costs of medical care.

At a time when fewer new antimicrobial drugs are entering the worldwide market than in the past, much has been written about the continued rise in rates of resistant microorganisms and its causes. The message seems clear: the use of existing and new antimicrobial agents must be more judicious and infection control more effective if we are to slow or reverse trends in resistance. The phrase *antimicrobial stewardship* is used to describe the new attitude toward antibacterial agents that must be adopted to preserve their usefulness. Appropriate stewardship requires that these drugs be used only when necessary, at the most appropriate dosage, and for the most appropriate duration. Increasing attention is being given to the relationships between differences in antibiotic consumption and differences in rates of resistance in different countries. While some newer antibacterial drugs undeniably represent important advances in therapy, many offer no advantage over older, less expensive agents. With rare exceptions, newer drugs are usually found to be no more effective than the comparison antibiotic in controlled trials, despite the "high prevalence of resistance" often touted to market the advantage of the new antibiotic over older therapies.

The following suggestions are intended to provide guidance through the antibiotic maze. First, objective evaluation of the merits of newer and older drugs is available. Online references such as the Johns Hopkins website (*hopkins-abxguide.org*) offer current and practical information regarding antimicrobial drugs and treatment regimens. Evidence-based practice guidelines for most infections are available from the Infectious Diseases

TABLE 127-9 PROPHYLAXIS OF BACTERIAL INFECTIONS IN ADULTS

Condition	Antibacterial Agent	Timing or Duration of Prophylaxis
Nonsurgical		
Cardiac lesions susceptible to bacterial endocarditis	Amoxicillin[a]	Before and after procedures causing bacteremia
Recurrent *S. aureus* infections	Mupirocin	5 days (intranasal)
Contact with patient with meningococcal meningitis	Rifampin Fluoroquinolone	2 days Single dose
Bite wounds[b]	Penicillin V or amoxicillin/clavulanic acid	3–5 days
Recurrent cystitis	Trimethoprim-sulfamethoxazole or a fluoroquinolone or nitrofurantoin	3 times per week for up to 1 year or after sexual intercourse
Surgical		
Clean (cardiac, vascular, neurologic, or orthopedic surgery)	Cefazolin (vancomycin)[c]	Before and during procedure
Ocular	Topical combinations and subconjunctival cefazolin	During and at end of procedure
Clean-contaminated (head and neck, high-risk gastroduodenal or biliary tract surgery; high-risk cesarean section; hysterectomy)	Cefazolin (or clindamycin for head and neck)	Before and during procedure
Clean-contaminated (vaginal or abdominal hysterectomy)	Cefazolin or cefoxitin or cefotetan	Before and during procedure
Clean-contaminated (high-risk genitourinary surgery)	Fluoroquinolone	Before and during procedure
Clean-contaminated (colorectal surgery or appendectomy)	Cefoxitin or cefotetan (add oral neomycin + erythromycin for colorectal)	Before and during procedure
Dirty[b] (ruptured viscus)	Cefoxitin or cefotetan ± gentamicin, clindamycin + gentamicin, or another appropriate regimen directed at anaerobes and gram-negative aerobes	Before and for 3–5 days after procedure
Dirty[b] (traumatic wound)	Cefazolin	Before and for 3–5 days after trauma

[a]Gentamicin should be added to the amoxicillin regimen for high-risk gastrointestinal and genitourinary procedures; vancomycin should be used in penicillin-allergic patients.

[b]In these cases, use of antibacterial agents actually constitutes treatment of infection rather than prophylaxis.

[c]Vancomycin is recommended only in institutions that have a high incidence of infection with methicillin-resistant staphylococci.

Society of America (*www.idsociety.org*). Second, clinicians should become comfortable using a few drugs recommended by independent experts and professional organizations and should resist the temptation to use a new drug unless the merits are clear. A new antibacterial agent with a "broader spectrum and greater potency" or a "higher serum concentration-to-MIC ratio" will not necessarily be more clinically efficacious. Third, clinicians should become familiar with local bacterial susceptibility profiles. It may not be necessary to use a new drug with "improved activity against *P. aeruginosa*" if that pathogen is rarely encountered or if it retains full susceptibility to older drugs. Fourth, a skeptical attitude toward manufacturers' claims is still appropriate. For example, rising rates of penicillin resistance in *S. pneumoniae* have been used to promote the use of broader-spectrum drugs, notably the fluoroquinolones. However, except in patients with meningitis, amoxicillin is still effective for infections caused by these "penicillin-resistant" strains. Finally, with regard to inpatient treatment with antibacterial drugs, a number of efforts to improve use are under study. The strategy of antibiotic "cycling" or rotation has not proved effective, but other strategies, such as heterogeneity or diversity of antibiotic use, may hold promise. Adoption of other evidence-based strategies to improve antimicrobial use may be the best way to retain the utility of existing compounds. For example, appropriate empirical treatment of the seriously ill patient with one or more broad-spectrum agents is important for improving survival rates, but therapy may often be simplified by switching to a narrower-spectrum agent or even an oral drug once the results of cultures and susceptibility tests become available. While there is an understandable temptation not to alter effective therapy, switching to a more specific agent once the patient's clinical condition has improved does not compromise outcome. A promising and active area of research includes the use of shorter courses of antimicrobial therapy. Many antibiotics that once were given for 7–10 days can be given for 3–5 days with no loss of efficacy and no increase in relapse rates (Table 127-10). Adoption of new guidelines for shorter-course therapy will not undermine the care of patients, many unnecessary complications and expenses will be avoided, and the useful life of these valuable drugs will perhaps be extended.

TABLE 127-10 DURATION OF THERAPY FOR BACTERIAL INFECTIONS

Duration of Therapy	Infections
Single dose	Gonococcal urethritis, streptococcal pharyngitis (penicillin G benzathine), primary and secondary syphilis (penicillin G benzathine)
3 days	Cystitis in young women, community- or travel-acquired diarrhea
3–10 days	Community-acquired pneumonia (3–5 days), community-acquired meningitis (pneumococcal or meningococcal), antibiotic-associated diarrhea (10 days), *Giardia* enteritis, cellulitis, epididymitis
2 weeks	*Helicobacter pylori*–associated peptic ulcer, neurosyphilis (penicillin IV), penicillin-susceptible viridans streptococcal endocarditis (penicillin plus aminoglycoside), disseminated gonococcal infection with arthritis, acute pyelonephritis, uncomplicated *S. aureus* catheter-associated bacteremia
3 weeks	Lyme disease, septic arthritis (nongonococcal)
4 weeks	Acute and chronic prostatitis, infective endocarditis (penicillin-resistant streptococcal)
>4 weeks	Acute and chronic osteomyelitis, *S. aureus* endocarditis, foreign-body infections (prosthetic-valve and joint infections), relapsing pseudomembranous colitis

FURTHER READINGS

Bartlett JG, Perl TM: The new *Clostridium difficile*—What does it mean? N Engl J Med 353:2503, 2005

Cosgrove SE, Carmeli Y: The impact of antimicrobial resistance on health and economic outcomes. Clin Infect Dis 36:1433, 2003

Fishman N: Antimicrobial stewardship. Am J Med 119:S53, 2006

Gruchalla RS, Pirmohamed M: Antibiotic allergy. N Engl J Med 354:601, 2006

Jacoby GA, Munoz-Price LS: The new β-lactamases. N Engl J Med 352:380, 2005

Kollef M: Appropriate empirical antibacterial therapy for nosocomial infections: Getting it right the first time. Drugs 63:2157, 2003

Nahum GG et al: Antibiotic use in pregnancy and lactation: What is and is not known about teratogenic and toxic risks. Obstet Gynecol 107:1120, 2006

Peterson LR: Penicillins for treatment of pneumococcal pneumonia: Does in vitro resistance really matter? Clin Infect Dis 42:224, 2006

Polk HC Jr: Continuing refinements in surgical antibiotic prophylaxis. Arch Surg 140:1066, 2005

Ray WA et al: Oral erythromycin and the risk of sudden death from cardiac causes. N Engl J Med 351:1089, 2004

128 Pneumococcal Infections

Daniel M. Musher

Streptococcus pneumoniae (the pneumococcus) was recognized as a major cause of pneumonia in the 1880s. Although the name *Diplococcus pneumoniae* was originally assigned to the pneumococcus, the organism was renamed *Streptococcus pneumoniae* because, like other streptococci, it grows in chains in liquid medium. Widespread vaccination has reduced the incidence of pneumococcal infection, but this organism remains the principal bacterial cause of otitis media, acute purulent rhinosinusitis, pneumonia, and meningitis.

MICROBIOLOGY

Pneumococci are identified in the clinical laboratory as catalase-negative, gram-positive cocci that grow in pairs or chains and cause α-hemolysis on blood agar. More than 98% of pneumococcal isolates are susceptible to ethylhydrocupreine (optochin), and virtually all pneumococcal colonies are dissolved by bile salts.

Peptidoglycan and teichoic acid are the principal constituents of the pneumococcal cell wall, whose integrity depends on the presence of numerous peptide side chains cross-linked by the activity of enzymes such as trans- and carboxypeptidases. β-Lactam antibiotics inactivate these enzymes by covalently binding their active site. Unique to *S. pneumoniae* and present in all strains is C-substance ("cell-wall" substance), a polysaccharide consisting of teichoic acid with a phosphorylcholine residue. Surface-exposed choline residues serve as a site of attachment for potential virulence factors, such as pneumococcal surface protein A (PspA) and pneumococcal surface adhesin A (PsaA), which may prevent phagocytosis. Except for strains that cause conjunctivitis, nearly every clinical isolate of *S. pneumoniae* has a polysaccharide capsule, a structure that renders the bacteria virulent by preventing phagocytosis. All strains produce pneumolysin, a toxin that may cause many of the manifestations of pneumococcal infection.

There are 90 serologically distinct capsules of *S. pneumoniae.* Serotyping remains clinically relevant because the activity of available vaccines is based on stimulating antibody to specific capsular polysaccharides.

EPIDEMIOLOGY

S. pneumoniae colonizes the nasopharynx and, on any single occasion, can be isolated from 5–10% of healthy adults and from 20–40% of healthy children. Once adults are colonized, organisms are likely to persist for 4–6 weeks but may be present for as long as 6 months. Pneumococci spread from one individual to another by direct or droplet transmission as a result of close contact; transmission may be enhanced by crowding or poor ventilation. Day-care centers have been a site of spread, especially of penicillin-resistant strains of serotypes 6B, 14, 19F, and 23F. Outbreaks of pneumococcal disease occur among adults in crowded living conditions—e.g., in military barracks, prisons, and shelters for the homeless—as well as among susceptible populations in settings such as nursing homes. The risk of pneumococcal pneumonia is generally not increased by contact in schools or workplaces (including hospitals).

The incidence data provided below were obtained before widespread administration of pneumococcal conjugate vaccine to infants and children. (For the impact of widespread vaccination, see "Vaccination," below.) In the absence of vaccination (which alters natural history), invasive pneumococcal disease is, by far, most prevalent among children <2 years old. The incidence is low among older children and adults <65 years of age but then rises in older adults. The fatality rate is also highest at the extremes of age. One surveillance study in the late 1980s found incidences of pneumococcal bacteremia among infants, young adults, and persons ≥70 years of age to be 160, 5, and 70 cases per 100,000 population, respectively. Most cases of pneumococcal bacteremia in adults are due to pneumonia, and there are 3–4 cases of nonbacteremic pneumonia for every bacteremic case. Thus an estimated 20 cases of pneumococcal pneumonia per 100,000 young adults and 280 cases per 100,000 persons over the age of 70 occur annually. The disease is more frequent among men than among women. The incidence of pneumococcal bacteremia among adults exhibits a distinct midwinter peak and a striking dip in summer; in children, the incidence is relatively constant throughout the year except for a marked dip in midsummer. For reasons that are unclear but probably multifactorial, Native Americans, Native Alaskans, and African Americans are more susceptible to invasive pneumococcal disease than are Caucasians. Natives of the Pacific Rim region are likewise more susceptible.

PATHOGENETIC MECHANISMS

Infection results when pneumococci colonizing the nasopharynx are carried into anatomically contiguous areas (e.g., the eustachian tubes, the nasal sinuses) and bacterial clearance is hindered (e.g., by mucosal edema due to allergy or viral infection). Clearly, the resistance of pneumococci to phagocytosis is central to their capacity to cause infection. Pneumonia ensues when organisms are inhaled or aspirated into the bronchioles or alveoli and are not cleared—especially, for example, if mucus production is increased and/or ciliary action is damaged by viral infection or by cigarette smoke or other toxic substances. Viral infection may also inhibit clearance by upregulating pneumocyte receptors that bind pneumococci.

In normally sterile sites, such as the sinuses or the lungs, pneumococci activate complement, stimulating the production of cytokines that attract polymorphonuclear leukocytes (PMNs). The polysaccharide capsule, however, renders the pneumococci resistant to phagocytosis. In the absence of anticapsular antibody, a large bacterial inoculum and/or a compromise of phagocytic function allows the initiation of infection. Infection of the meninges, joints, bones, and peritoneal cavity may result from pneumococcal spread through the bloodstream, usually from a respiratory tract focus of infection. Unencapsulated pneumococci virtually never cause invasive disease, although they can cause conjunctivitis.

Symptoms of disease are largely attributable to the inflammatory response, which may cause pain by increasing pressure (as in sinusitis or otitis media) or may interfere with vital bodily functions by preventing oxygenation of blood (as in pneumonia) or by inhibiting blood flow (as in vasculitis due to meningitis). Cell-wall constituents of *S. pneumoniae*, especially peptidoglycan, activate complement by the alternative pathway; the reaction between cell-wall structures and antibody (present in all humans) also activates the classic complement pathway. The result is the release of C5a, a potent attractant for PMNs, into the surrounding medium. Peptidoglycan can also directly stimulate the release of proinflammatory cytokines such as interleukin (IL) 1β, tumor necrosis factor (TNF) α, and IL-6. All pneumococci generate pneumolysin, a toxin that damages ciliary cells and PMNs and also activates the classic complement pathway. Injection of pneumolysin into the lungs of experimental animals produces the histologic features of pneumonia; in mice, immunization with this substance or challenge with genetically engineered mutants that do not produce it is associated with a significant reduction in virulence.

HOST DEFENSE MECHANISMS

Mechanisms of host defense may be nonimmunologic or immunologic. Immunologic mechanisms may be natural (innate) or specific (humoral).

Nonimmunologic Mechanisms Nonimmunologic mechanisms that protect against pneumonia include filtration of air as it passes through the nasopharynx, the glottal reflex, laryngeal closure, the cough reflex, clearance of organisms from the lower airways by ciliated cells, and ingestion by pulmonary macrophages and PMNs of small bacterial inocula that manage to reach alveolar spaces. Respiratory virus infection, chronic pulmonary disease, or heart failure compromises these mechanisms, predisposing to the development of pneumococcal pneumonia.

Immunologic Mechanisms • ***INNATE IMMUNITY*** Innate immune mechanisms participate in clearance of pneumococci from the nasopharynx as well as in phagocytosis by PMNs and macrophages via the microbial pattern recognition receptor Toll-like receptor 2 (TLR2).

HUMORAL IMMUNITY Immunologically specific humoral mechanisms provide the best protection against pneumococcal infection. Most healthy adults have antibody to constituents of *S. pneumoniae*, such as PspA, PsaA, and the cell wall; however, there is no convincing evidence for an opsonic role of these antibodies, especially at their usual concentrations. Most healthy adults lack IgG antibody to the majority of pneumococcal capsular polysaccharides. Antibody appears after colonization, infection, or vaccination. In the first few weeks after colonization, nonspecific mechanisms probably protect the host from infection. Thereafter, newly developed anticapsular antibody provides a high degree of specific protection. Adults who are at risk of aspirating pharyngeal contents and/or who have diminished mechanisms of lower airway clearance are at risk of developing pneumonia before antibody is produced. Persons with a diminished capacity to form antibody probably remain susceptible as long as they are colonized.

The risk of serious pneumococcal infection is greatly increased in persons with conditions that compromise IgG synthesis and/or the phagocytic function of PMNs and macrophages. Most patients hospitalized for pneumococcal pneumonia have one or more of these conditions (Table 128-1). Once a pneumococcal infection has been initiated, the absence of a spleen predisposes to fulminant disease. The liver can remove opsonized (antibody-coated) pneumococci from the circulation; in the absence of antibody, however, only the slow passage of blood through the splenic sinuses and prolonged contact with reticuloendothelial cells in the cords of Billroth can result in bacterial clearance. Patients without spleens tend to develop overwhelming pneumococcal disease that rapidly progresses to death.

TABLE 128-1 CONDITIONS THAT COMMONLY PREDISPOSE TO PNEUMOCOCCAL INFECTION

Increased risk of exposure	Defective complement function
Day-care centers	Defective bacterial clearance[a]
Military training camps	Congenital asplenia, hyposplenia
Prisons	Splenectomy
Shelters for the homeless	Sickle cell disease
Respiratory infection, inflammation	Multifactorial conditions
Influenza, other viral respiratory infections	Infancy and aging
	Chronic disease
Air pollution	Prior hospitalization
Allergies	Alcoholism
Cigarette smoking	Malnutrition
Chronic obstructive pulmonary disease	HIV infection
	Chronic lung disease
Other causes of chronic pulmonary inflammation or obstruction	Glucocorticoid treatment
	Cirrhosis of the liver
	Renal insufficiency
Anatomical disruption of meninges (dural tear)	Diabetes mellitus
	Anemia
Defective antibody formation	Coronary artery disease
Common variable hypogammaglobulinemia	Fatigue, stress, and/or exposure to cold
Selective IgG subclass deficiency	
Multiple myeloma	
Chronic lymphocytic leukemia	
Lymphoma	

[a]The absence of a spleen predisposes to more fulminant infection (see text).

TABLE 128-2 MOST COMMON INFECTIONS CAUSED BY *STREPTOCOCCUS PNEUMONIAE* IN ADULTS

Site	Infections
Respiratory tract	Otitis media Acute sinusitis Tracheobronchitis Pneumonia Empyema
Central nervous system	Meningitis Brain abscess
Cardiac	Endocarditis Pericarditis
Soft tissue/skeletal	Septic arthritis Osteomyelitis Cellulitis
Other	Peritonitis Endometritis Primary bacteremia

SPECIFIC INFECTIONS CAUSED BY *S. PNEUMONIAE*

S. pneumoniae causes infections of the middle ear, sinuses, trachea, bronchi, and lungs (Table 128-2) by direct spread from the nasopharyngeal site of colonization. Infections of the central nervous system (CNS), heart valves, bones, joints, and peritoneal cavity usually arise by hematogenous spread. Peritoneal infection may also result from ascent via the fallopian tubes. The CNS may also be infected by drainage from nasopharyngeal lymphatics or veins or by contiguous spread of organisms (e.g., through a tear in the dura). Primary pneumococcal bacteremia—i.e., the presence of pneumococci in the blood with no apparent source—occurs commonly in children <2 years of age and accounts for a small percentage of all cases of pneumococcal bacteremia in adults; if no therapy is given, a source and/or a secondary site of infection may become apparent. Pleural infection results either from direct extension of pneumonia to the visceral pleura or from hematogenous bacterial spread from a pulmonary or extrapulmonary focus to the pleural space; the route usually cannot be determined in any individual case. Infections listed after meningitis in Table 128-2 are uncommon or rare.

Otitis Media and Sinusitis Otitis media and acute rhinosinusitis are similar in terms of pathogenesis. Bacteria are trapped in a normally sterile site when drainage is impaired, often as a result of viral infection, allergies, or exposure to pollutants (including cigarette smoke). In both disease states, *S. pneumoniae* is the most common or second most common isolate (after nontypable *Haemophilus influenzae*) from cultures of the infected site.

Pneumonia The distinctive symptoms and signs of pneumonia, whether due to the pneumococcus or to other bacteria, are (1) cough and sputum production, which reflect bacterial proliferation and the resulting inflammatory response in the alveoli; (2) fever; and (3) radiographic detection of an infiltrate.

PREDISPOSING CONDITIONS Pneumococcal pneumonia is most common at the extremes of age. Despite the undisputed role of *S. pneumoniae* as a major pathogenic bacterium for humans, the great majority of adults with pneumococcal pneumonia have underlying diseases that predispose them to infection. Otherwise-healthy military recruits involved in outbreaks of infection may be an exception to this rule; however, many of these individuals have been under extreme physical and/or psychological stress and/or have had an antecedent viral-type illness that may have reduced their normal host resistance. Infections with respiratory viruses, especially influenza virus, predispose to pneumococcal pneumonia. Other common predisposing conditions are alcoholism, malnutrition, chronic pulmonary disease of any kind (including asthma), cigarette smoking, HIV infection, diabetes mellitus, cirrhosis of the liver, anemia, prior hospitalization for any reason, renal insufficiency, and coronary artery disease (with or without recognized congestive heart failure). In elderly subjects, the predisposition is generally multifactorial.

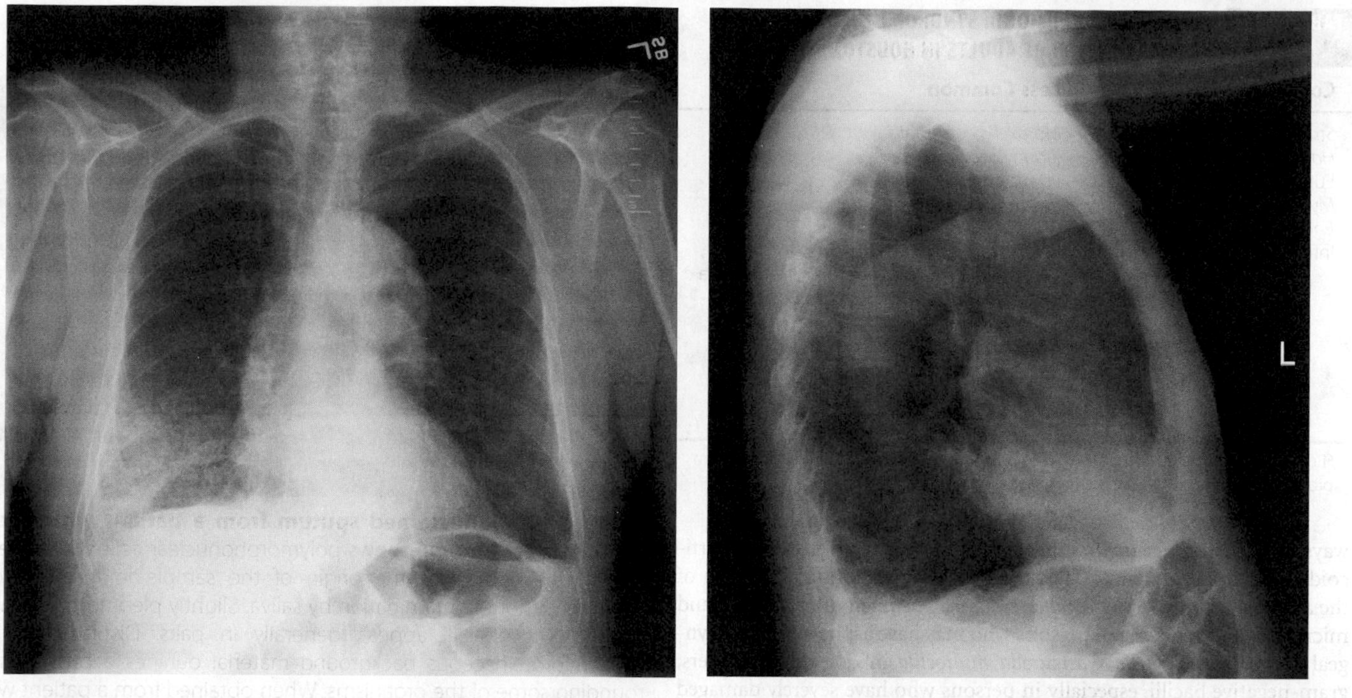

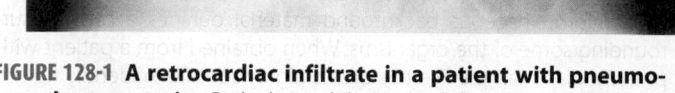

FIGURE 128-1 A retrocardiac infiltrate in a patient with pneumococcal pneumonia. Right-lower-lobe consolidation is apparent in posterior-anterior **(*left*)** and lateral **(*right*)** views of the chest.

PRESENTING SYMPTOMS Patients often present with a clear exacerbation of a preexisting respiratory condition. They may have felt unwell for several days, with coryza or a nonproductive cough and low-grade fever, but they feel distinctly worse at the time of onset of pneumonia. Coughing, often productive of purulent sputum, becomes prominent. The temperature may rise to 38.9°–39.4°C (102°–103°F), although a substantial proportion of patients are afebrile at admission. In a small proportion of cases, the onset of disease follows a hyperacute pattern in which the patient suddenly has a single episode of shaking chills followed by sustained fever and a cough productive of blood-tinged sputum. In the elderly, the onset of disease may be especially insidious and may not suggest pneumonia at all. Such persons may have minimal cough, no sputum production, and no fever, instead appearing tired or confused. Nausea and vomiting or diarrhea occurs in up to 20% of cases of pneumococcal pneumonia. Symptoms of a new cardiac arrhythmia, myocardial ischemia, or an actual infarction occur in 10% of patients at a veterans' hospital who are admitted for pneumonia, and these manifestations may even predominate. The pneumonia may precipitate cardiogenic or noncardiogenic pulmonary edema. Pleuritic chest pain may result from extension of the inflammatory process to the visceral pleura; persistence of this pain, especially after the first day or two of treatment, raises concern about empyema (see "Complications," below). Clearly, the range of symptoms is sufficiently broad that no characteristic presentation distinguishes pneumococcal pneumonia from other types of bacterial pneumonia or from some types of nonbacterial pneumonia.

PHYSICAL FINDINGS Patients with pneumococcal pneumonia usually appear ill and have a grayish, anxious appearance that differs from that of persons with viral or mycoplasmal pneumonia. Temperature, pulse, and respiratory rate are typically elevated. Elderly patients may have only a slight temperature elevation or may be afebrile. Hypothermia may be documented instead of fever and is associated with increased morbidity and mortality. Pleuritic chest pain may cause diminished respiratory excursion (splinting) on the affected side. Dullness to percussion is noted in about half of cases, and vocal fremitus is increased over the area of consolidation. Breath sounds may be bronchial or tubular, and crackles are heard in most cases if enough air is being moved to generate them. Flatness to percussion at the lung base, absent fremitus, and lack of the expected degree of diaphragmatic motion suggest the presence of pleural fluid, which raises the possibility of empyema. The finding of a heart murmur—certainly if new—raises concern about endocarditis, a rare but serious complication. Hypoxia or the generalized response to pneumonia may cause the patient to be confused, but the appearance of confusion should also raise concern about meningitis. Obtundation or neck stiffness should lead to an immediate consideration of this complication.

RADIOGRAPHIC FINDINGS In patients sick enough to be hospitalized, pneumococcal pneumonia is limited to one lung segment in one-fourth of cases and to one lobe in another one-fourth, with multilobar disease in the remaining one-half. Air-space consolidation is the predominant finding and is detected in 80% of cases (Fig. 128-1). Air bronchogram (visualization of the air-filled bronchus against a background of alveolar consolidation) is evident in fewer than half of cases and is more common in bacteremic than in nonbacteremic disease. Rarely, pneumococcal pneumonia leads to a lung abscess. Although some pleural fluid may actually be present in half of cases, ≤20% of patients have a sufficient volume of fluid to allow aspiration, and in only a minority of these patients is empyema documented.

GENERAL LABORATORY FINDINGS Anemia (hemoglobin level, <10 g/dL) is documented in 25% of cases. The peripheral-blood white blood cell (WBC) count exceeds 12,000/μL in the great majority of patients with pneumococcal pneumonia. A low WBC count (<6000/μL) is found in 5–10% of persons hospitalized for pneumococcal pneumonia and is strongly associated with fatal disease. The serum bilirubin level is modestly elevated in one-third of cases; hypoxia, inflammatory changes in the liver, and breakdown of red blood cells in the lung are all thought to contribute to this increase. A serum albumin level of <2.5 g/dL in 30% of cases may indicate predisposing malnutrition or may be the result of sepsis. About 20% of patients have serum sodium concentrations of ≤130 meq/L, and another 20% have serum creatinine concentrations of ≥2 mg/dL. Abnormalities of pleural fluid in empyema are reviewed in Chap. 251.

DIFFERENTIAL DIAGNOSIS *S. pneumoniae* is the most common cause of so-called community-acquired pneumonia, but patients who present with this syndrome may actually have infection due to a broad array of microorganisms. The extensive list includes (but is not limited to) the following: *H. influenzae* or *Moraxella catarrhalis* in persons with little to predispose them other than chronic or acute inflammation of the air-

TABLE 128-3 CAUSES OF A PNEUMONIA SYNDROME LEADING TO HOSPITALIZATION OF ADULTS IN HOUSTON, TEXAS[a]

Common	Less Common
Streptococcus pneumoniae	*Moraxella catarrhalis*
Haemophilus influenzae	*Staphylococcus aureus*
Lung cancer	Pulmonary infarction
Mycobacterium tuberculosis	*Klebsiella pneumoniae*
Pneumocystis	*Cryptococcus, Histoplasma*
Influenza (seasonal)	Respiratory syncytial virus
	Microaerophilic and anaerobic mouth flora
	Pseudomonas aeruginosa
	Legionella species
	Nontuberculous mycobacteria
	Chlamydia pneumoniae
	Nocardia species
	Hamman-Rich syndrome, others

[a]Pneumonia was defined as a syndrome consisting of fever, increased cough, sputum production, and an abnormal pulmonary shadow on chest x-ray.

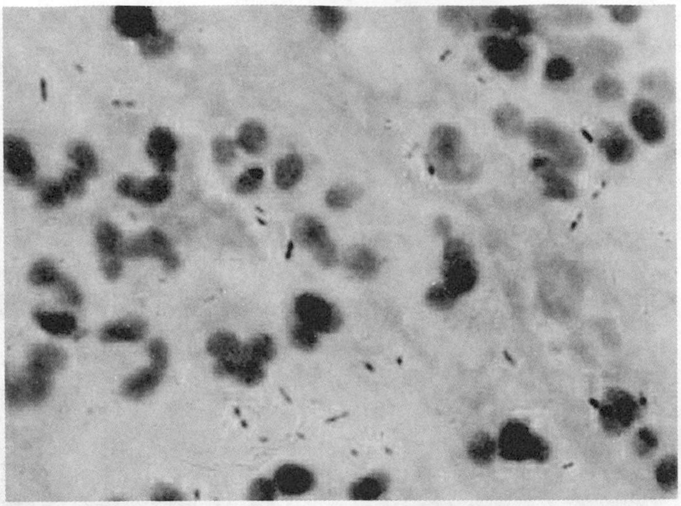

FIGURE 128-2 Gram-stained sputum from a patient with pneumococcal pneumonia shows polymorphonuclear cells with no epithelial cells, indicating the origin of the sample in inflammatory exudate without contamination by saliva. Slightly pleomorphic gram-positive coccobacilli appear, generally in pairs. Displacement of stained proteinaceous background material outlines a capsule surrounding some of the organisms. When obtained from a patient with pneumonia, a sample like this one is highly specific in identifying the pneumococcus as the etiologic agent.

ways; *Staphylococcus aureus,* especially in persons who take glucocorticoids, who have influenza, or who have major anatomic disruption of the airways; *Streptococcus pyogenes*; *Neisseria meningitidis*; anaerobic and microaerophilic bacteria in persons who may have aspirated oropharyngeal contents; *Legionella*; *Pasteurella multocida* in dog or cat owners; gram-negative bacilli, especially in persons who have severely damaged lungs and are taking glucocorticoids; viruses, especially influenza virus (in season), adenovirus, or respiratory syncytial virus; *Mycobacterium tuberculosis*; fungi, including *Pneumocystis* (depending on epidemiologic factors and HIV infection status); *Mycoplasma*; *Chlamydia pneumoniae*, especially in older adults; and *Chlamydia psittaci* in bird owners. Many older men with lung cancer present with pneumonia, as do persons who have acute-onset inflammatory pulmonary conditions of uncertain etiology or those with pulmonary embolus and infarction. The breadth of this list vividly illustrates the deficiency of empirical therapy for community-acquired pneumonia (Table 128-3). Many of these diseases require evaluation, and the increasing availability of specific therapy makes a precise etiologic diagnosis desirable.

DIAGNOSTIC MICROBIOLOGY In patients with community-acquired pneumonia, a pneumococcal etiology is strongly suggested by the microscopic demonstration of large numbers of PMNs and slightly elongated gram-positive cocci in pairs and chains in the sputum. A sample such as the one shown in Fig. 128-2 is highly specific for pneumococcal infection of the lower airways. In the absence of such microscopic findings, the identification of pneumococci by culture is less specific, possibly reflecting colonization of the upper airways. Prior treatment with antibiotics can rapidly clear pneumococci from sputum. These factors need to be considered when sputum cultures from patients who appear to have pneumococcal pneumonia are said to yield only "normal mouth flora" and when the medical literature describes what appear to be poor results of sputum culture. A study of sputum Gram's stain and culture in patients with proven (bacteremic) pneumococcal pneumonia showed that about half of patients could not provide a sputum sample, provided a sample of poor quality, or had received antibiotics for >18 h; results in the remaining cases showed >80% sensitivity of microscopic examination of a Gram-stained sputum sample and 90% sensitivity of a sputum culture. Blood cultures yield *S. pneumoniae* in ~25% of patients hospitalized for pneumococcal pneumonia.

COMPLICATIONS Empyema is the most common complication of pneumococcal pneumonia, occurring in ~2% of cases. Some fluid appears in the pleural space in a substantial proportion of cases of pneumococcal pneumonia, but this parapneumonic effusion usually reflects an inflammatory response to infection that has been contained within the lung, and its presence is self-limited. When bacteria reach the pleural space—either hematogenously or as a result of contiguous spread, possibly across lymphatics of the visceral pleura—empyema results. The finding of frank pus, bacteria (by microscopic examination), or fluid with a pH of ≤7.1 indicates the need for aggressive and complete drainage, preferably by prompt insertion of a chest tube, with verification by CT that fluid has been removed. Failure to drain most or all of the fluid indicates the need for additional treatment, including placement of other tube(s) (thoracostomy) or thoracotomy. Empyema is likely if fluid is present and fever and leukocytosis (even low-grade) persist after 4–5 days of appropriate antibiotic treatment for pneumococcal pneumonia. At this stage, thoracotomy is often needed for cure. Aggressive drainage is likely to reduce morbidity and mortality from empyema (Chap. 257).

Meningitis Except during outbreaks of meningococcal infection, *S. pneumoniae* is the most common cause of bacterial meningitis in adults. Because of the remarkable success of *H. influenzae* type b vaccine, *S. pneumoniae* now predominates among cases in infants and toddlers as well (but not among those in newborns); nevertheless, the incidence of pneumococcal meningitis among children has been dramatically reduced by use of the pediatric pneumococcal conjugate vaccine (see "Vaccination," below).

No distinctive clinical or laboratory features differentiate pneumococcal meningitis from other bacterial meningitides. Patients note the sudden onset of fever, headache, and stiffness or pain in the neck. Without treatment, there is a progression over 24–48 h to confusion and then obtundation. On physical examination, the patient looks acutely ill and has a rigid neck. In such cases, lumbar puncture should not be delayed for CT of the head unless papilledema or focal neurologic signs are evident. Typical findings in cerebrospinal fluid (CSF) consist of an increased WBC count (500–10,000 cells/μL) with ≥85% PMNs, an elevated protein level (100–500 mg/dL), and a decreased glucose level (<30 mg/dL). If antibiotics have not been given, large numbers of pneumococci are seen in Gram-stained CSF in virtually all cases, and specific therapy can be administered, although, because of its similar appearance, *Listeria* may be misidentified as the pneumococcus. If an effective antibiotic has already been given, the number of bacteria may be greatly decreased and microscopic examination of a Gram-stained specimen may yield negative results. In this situation, immunologic methods may detect pneumococcal capsule in the CSF in up to two-thirds of cases.

Other Syndromes The appearance of pneumococcal infection at other, ordinarily sterile body sites indicates hematogenous spread, usually during frank pneumonia or, in a small proportion of cases, from an inapparent focus of infection. A case of pneumococcal endocarditis is seen every few years at large tertiary-care hospitals. Purulent pericarditis, occurring as a separate entity or together with endocarditis, is even rarer. The name *Austrian's syndrome* is given to the concurrence of pneumococcal pneumonia, endocarditis, and meningitis. Septic arthritis can arise spontaneously in a natural or prosthetic joint or as a complication of rheumatoid arthritis. Osteomyelitis in adults tends to involve vertebral bones. Pneumococcal peritonitis occurs by one of three pathogenetic pathways: (1) hematogenous spread when ascites or other preexisting peritoneal disease is present; (2) local spread from a perforated viscus (usually appendicitis or perforated ulcer); or (3) transit via the fallopian tubes. Salpingitis may be recognized with or without accompanying peritonitis. Epidural and brain abscesses arise as a complication of sinusitis or mastoiditis. Cellulitis is also uncommon, developing most often in persons who have connective tissue diseases or HIV infection. The appearance of any of these unusual pneumococcal infections may suggest that tests for HIV infection should be undertaken. Finally, for reasons that are unclear, unencapsulated (but not encapsulated) pneumococci may cause sporadic or epidemic conjunctivitis.

℞ PNEUMOCOCCAL INFECTIONS

ANTIBIOTIC SUSCEPTIBILITY β-Lactam antibiotics, the cornerstone of therapy for serious pneumococcal infection, bind covalently to the active site and thereby block the action of enzymes (endo-, trans-, and carboxypeptidases) needed for cell-wall synthesis. Because these enzymes were identified by their reaction with radiolabeled penicillin, they are called *penicillin-binding proteins*. Until the late 1970s, virtually all clinical isolates of *S. pneumoniae* were susceptible to penicillin (i.e., were inhibited in vitro by concentrations of <0.06 μg/mL). Since then, an increasing number of isolates have shown some degree of resistance to penicillin. Resistance results when spontaneous mutation or acquisition of new genetic material alters penicillin-binding proteins in a manner that reduces their affinity for penicillin, thereby necessitating a higher concentration of penicillin for their saturation. The genetic information that renders pneumococci resistant to penicillin is acquired from oral streptococci and is transmitted along with genes that convey resistance to other antibiotics as well. Selection of antibiotic-resistant strains worldwide—especially in countries where antibiotics are available without prescription and in loci of high antibiotic use, such as day-care centers—greatly contributes to the prevalence of multidrug resistance.

At present, ~20% of pneumococcal isolates in the United States exhibit intermediate resistance to penicillin [minimal inhibitory concentration (MIC) 0.1–1.0 μg/mL], and 15% are resistant (MIC ≥2.0 μg/mL; **Fig. 128-3**). The rate of resistance is lower in countries that, by tradition, are conservative in their antibiotic use (e.g., Holland and Germany) and higher in countries where usage is more liberal (e.g., France). In Hong Kong and Korea, resistance rates approach 80%. These definitions of resistance, however, were based on drug levels achievable in CSF during treatment of meningitis, whereas levels reached in the bloodstream, lungs, and sinuses are actually much higher. Thus the MIC needs to be interpreted in light of the infection being treated. Pneumonia caused by a penicillin-resistant strain is likely to respond to conventional doses of β-lactam antibiotics, whereas meningitis may not. The recently revised definition of amoxicillin resistance (susceptible, MIC ≤2 μg/mL; intermediately resistant, MIC = 4 μg/mL; and resistant, MIC ≥8 μg/mL) is based on susceptibility to serum levels, with the assumption that no physician would knowingly treat meningitis with this oral medication. Pneumonia due to a pneumococcal strain with intermediate amoxicillin resistance is still likely to respond to treatment with this drug, whereas that due to a resistant strain may not. On the assumption that antibiotic concentrations in middle-ear fluid or sinus cavities approach those in serum, similar inferences can be made about the treatment of otitis or sinusitis.

Penicillin-susceptible pneumococci are susceptible to all commonly used cephalosporins. Penicillin-intermediate strains tend to be resistant to all first- and many second-generation cephalosporins (of which cefuroxime retains the best efficacy), but most are susceptible to certain third-generation cephalosporins, including cefotaxime, ceftriaxone, cefepime, and the oral cefpodoxime. One-half of highly penicillin-resistant pneumococci are also resistant to cefotaxime, ceftriaxone, and cefepime, and nearly all are resistant to cefpodoxime. Just as in the case of penicillin, susceptibility to cefotaxime and ceftriaxone is defined on the basis of achievable CSF levels. Thus pneumonia caused by intermediately resistant strains (MIC = 2 μg/mL) still responds well to usual doses of these drugs, and pneumonia due to a resistant organism (MIC ≥4 μg/mL) is likely to respond. Meningitis due to intermediately resistant strains may not respond, and meningitis due to a resistant strain is likely not to respond to treatment with cefotaxime or ceftriaxone.

About one-quarter of all pneumococcal isolates in the United States are resistant to erythromycin and the newer macrolides, including azithromycin and clarithromycin, with much higher rates of resistance among penicillin-resistant strains. This resistance will certainly affect empirical therapy for bronchitis, sinusitis, and pneumonia. In the United States, the majority of macrolide-resistant pneumococci bear the so-called M phenotype (erythromycin MIC = 1–8 μg/mL) and are susceptible to clindamycin. In this case, resistance is mediated by an efflux pump mechanism; to some extent, M-type resistance can be overcome by clinically achievable levels of macrolides. In Europe, most macrolide resistance is due to a mutation in *ermB*, which confers high-level resistance not only to macrolides but also to clindamycin; >90% of pneumococcal isolates in the United States are susceptible to clindamycin. Rates of doxycycline resistance are similar to those observed for macrolides. One-third of pneumococcal isolates are resistant to trimethoprim-sulfamethoxazole. The newer fluoroquinolones remain effective against pneumococci; the rate of resistance is generally <2–3% in the United States but is higher elsewhere and may be much higher in closed environments where these drugs are heavily prescribed, such as nursing homes and assisted-living facilities. Ketolides (such as telithromycin) appear to be uniformly effective against pneumococci, as does vancomycin.

ANTIBIOTIC REGIMENS Otitis Media **(Table 128-4)** Current treatment recommendations for otitis media are based on the following points:

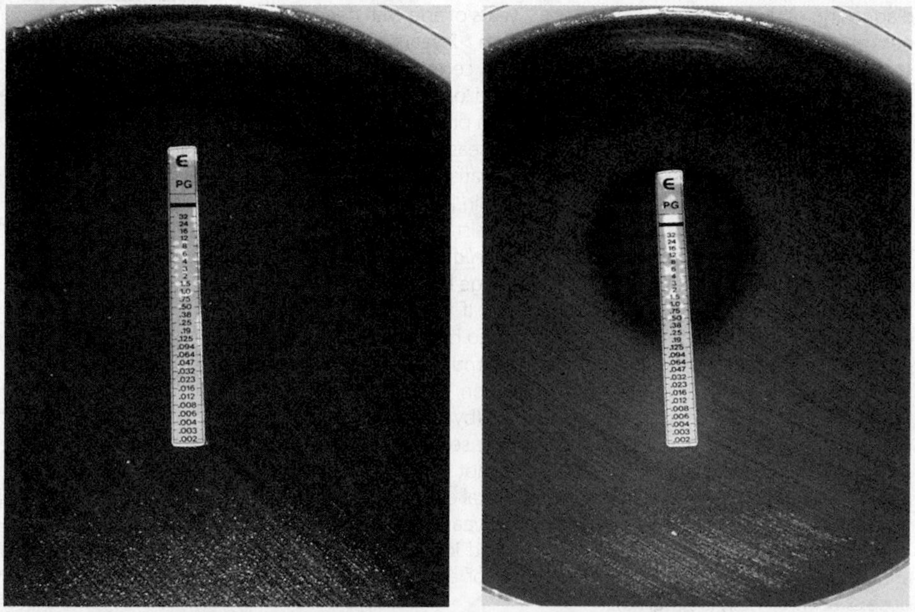

FIGURE 128-3 The e-strip method currently used by most laboratories to determine the susceptibility of *S. pneumoniae* to antibiotics. After the plate is streaked with a suspension of pneumococci, a strip impregnated with graded concentrations of the antibiotic under study (penicillin in the example shown) is placed on the surface, and the plate is incubated overnight at 37°C. The organism on the left is inhibited by a penicillin concentration of 0.016 μg/mL and is fully susceptible to this drug. The organism on the right is inhibited only by a penicillin concentration of 0.25 μg/mL and is intermediately resistant to this agent.

TABLE 128-4 REGIMENS FOR THE TREATMENT OF PNEUMOCOCCAL OTITIS MEDIA OR SINUSITIS[a]

Regimen	Drug, Dose	Duration	Comments
First-line	Amoxicillin, 1 g q8h[b]	Otitis: 3–5 days after clinical response, not to exceed 7 days total (see text) Sinusitis: 7–10 days after clinical response, not to exceed 2 weeks total	If this regimen fails, try a second-line regimen.
Second-line	Amoxicillin, 1 g q8h, plus clavulanic acid, 125 mg q8h[c] *or* Fluoroquinolone[d] *or* Telithromycin, 800 mg/d	Same as above	If this regimen fails, try the third-line regimen.
Third-line	Ceftriaxone, 1 g qd	Otitis: 3–5 days Sinusitis: Longer	If this regimen fails, consider complications. Consult an otolaryngologist and/or infectious disease specialist.

[a]Except as noted, doses are for adults. Treatment for otitis media or sinusitis is empirical, since aspiration of the involved area to establish an etiologic diagnosis is rarely undertaken, except under the conditions of a research protocol.
[b]Dose for infants and toddlers: 80–90 mg/kg per day in 2 or 3 divided doses.
[c]Give half as amoxicillin alone (500 mg) and half as amoxicillin (500 mg)/clavulanic acid (125 mg).
[d]Moxifloxacin, 400 mg/d; or levofloxacin, 500 mg/d.

(1) Acute otitis media is the most common diagnosis leading to an antibiotic prescription in the United States. (2) The diagnosis is often based on inadequate evidence for true middle-ear infection. (3) In proven cases, *S. pneumoniae* and *H. influenzae* are the most likely causes. (4) Because penetration into a closed space may be reduced, high serum levels of an effective antibiotic are required to treat otitis caused by intermediately or fully resistant pneumococci. (5) *S. pneumoniae* is more likely than *Haemophilus* and much more likely than *Moraxella* to cause progression to serious complications without specific therapy. (6) Antibiotics that are effective against pneumococci and yet resist β-lactamases tend to be very expensive compared with amoxicillin.

As a result of these considerations, the American Academies of Pediatrics and Family Practice recommend that clinicians apply due diligence in diagnosing otitis. In children 6 months to 2 years of age with nonsevere illness and an uncertain diagnosis and in children >2 years of age with nonsevere illness (even if the diagnosis seems certain), symptom-based therapy and observation may be used instead of antimicrobial therapy. When parents of children with otitis are given a prescription for an antibiotic but are instructed not to fill it unless the disease progresses, no antibiotic is given in many cases, yet rates of patient satisfaction are high. If otitis media is clearly diagnosed, high-dose amoxicillin is recommended (Table 128-4). If this regimen fails, highly penicillin-resistant pneumococci or β-lactamase-producing *Haemophilus* or *Moraxella* may be responsible; amoxicillin may be given at the same total dosage but with one-half of the dose in the form of amoxicillin/clavulanic acid. If this regimen fails, three doses of ceftriaxone at daily intervals are likely to be curative. A quinolone or ketolide may also be tried in adults. Patients must be monitored closely for a response. An otolaryngology consultation is recommended if all these treatments fail. Despite the detection (by molecular analysis) of pneumococcal DNA in middle-ear fluid, chronic serous otitis ("glue ear") is probably not due to active infection and does not require antibiotic therapy. Treatment for otitis is recommended for a total of 10 days in children <2 years of age but for only 5 days in children ≥2 years old who do not have complicated infections. A recent study reported identical rates of clinical and bacteriologic cure with a 10-day course of amoxicillin and a single dose of azithromycin (30 mg/kg).

Acute Sinusitis Just as the pathogenesis and microbial etiology of acute rhinosinusitis are similar to those of otitis media, so are the principles of diagnosis and treatment. The diagnosis is often empirical, and the less rigorously it is made, the more irrelevant antibiotics are likely to be. The estimated efficacy rate for amoxicillin/clavulanic acid, fluoroquinolones, and ceftriaxone (available for parenteral use only) is 90–92%, as opposed to 83–88% for amoxicillin, trimethoprim-sulfamethoxazole, and oral second- or third-generation cephalosporins and 71–81% for macrolides and doxycycline. Treatment should be given for longer periods than are recommended for otitis media (perhaps 10–14 days), but the optimal duration is uncertain.

Pneumonia (Table 128-5) This section will deal primarily with the treatment of pneumococcal pneumonia. The broader issue of empirical therapy for community-acquired pneumonia is covered elsewhere (Chap. 251). Unless epidemiologic, clinical, and radiologic findings strongly favor another etiology, empirical therapy for pneumonia must include an agent that will be effective against *S. pneumoniae*, which remains the most likely causative agent of community-acquired pneumonia.

Outpatient Therapy Amoxicillin (1 g three times daily) effectively treats virtually all cases of pneumococcal pneumonia. Neither cefuroxime nor cefpodoxime offers any advantages over amoxicillin, and they are far more expensive. Telithromycin is likely to be equally effective. Moxifloxacin is also highly likely to be effective in the United States except in patients who come from a closed population where these drugs are used widely or who have themselves been treated recently with a quinolone. Clindamycin is effective in 90% of cases and doxycycline, azithromycin, or clarithromycin in 80%. Treatment failure resulting in bacteremic disease due to macrolide-resistant isolates has been amply documented in patients treated empirically with azithromycin. As noted above, rates of resistance to all these antibiotics are lower in some countries and much higher in others; high-dose amoxicillin remains the best option worldwide.

Inpatient Therapy Pneumococcal pneumonia is readily treatable with β-lactam antibiotics. The conventional dosages shown in Table 128-5 are acceptable against intermediately resistant strains and against many or

TABLE 128-5 REGIMENS FOR THE TREATMENT OF PNEUMOCOCCAL PNEUMONIA IN ADULTS[a]

Route, Drug	Dose, Schedule[b]
Oral Therapy	
Amoxicillin	1 g q8h
Quinolone, e.g., levofloxacin	500 mg q24h
Telithromycin	800 mg q24h
Parenteral Therapy	
Penicillin[c]	3–4 mU q4h
Ampicillin	1–2 g q6h
Ceftriaxone	1 g q12–24h
Cefotaxime	1–2 g q6–8h
Quinolone, e.g., gatifloxacin	400 mg q24h
Imipenem	500 mg q6h
Vancomycin[d]	500 mg q6h

[a]These regimens are recommended for treatment after a presumptive diagnosis of pneumococcal pneumonia is made on the basis of examination of a Gram-stained sputum sample or as a replacement for broader spectrum empirical therapy after a diagnosis of pneumococcal pneumonia is proven by culture. When a valid sputum specimen cannot be obtained, concern about other likely pathogens should prompt the selection of more all-inclusive therapeutic regimens. Readers are referred to guidelines for empirical treatment of community-acquired pneumonia.
[b]Therapy should continue for 5 days after defervescence, not to exceed 7–10 days total. A switch from parenteral to oral drug administration may be made as soon as the patient can tolerate oral medications.
[c]This regimen is listed more for historic than for practical reasons. The spectrum is overly narrow, although perfectly acceptable if a Gram-stained sputum specimen shows only pneumococci. However, the need for frequent administration, mandated by the short half-life of penicillin, renders this regimen impractical.
[d]Not proven to be effective by the extensive clinical experience that applies to the other regimens.

most fully resistant isolates. Recommended agents include ceftriaxone and cefotaxime. Ampicillin is also widely used, usually in the form of ampicillin/sulbactam. The likely efficacy of newer quinolones such as moxifloxacin, macrolides such as azithromycin, and clindamycin is discussed above. On the basis of in vitro considerations, vancomycin is likely to be uniformly effective against pneumococci; this drug or a quinolone should be used together with a third-generation cephalosporin for initial therapy in a patient who is likely to be infected with a highly antibiotic-resistant strain. Patients who have had a severe allergic reaction to penicillins or cephalosporins may be treated with a carbapenem (e.g., imipenem-cilastatin), a quinolone, or vancomycin. The failure of a patient to respond promptly should at least prompt consideration of drug resistance. Evidence for loculated infections (such as empyema) and/or other causes of fever should be sought and addressed appropriately.

Duration of Therapy The optimal duration of treatment for pneumococcal pneumonia is uncertain. Pneumococci begin to disappear from the sputum within several hours after the first dose of an effective antibiotic, and a single dose of procaine penicillin, which produces an effective antimicrobial level for 24 h, was curative in otherwise-healthy young adults in an era when all isolates were susceptible. Early in the antibiotic era, most physicians treated pneumococcal pneumonia for 5–7 days. In the absence of data suggesting a need for longer treatment, younger physicians tend to treat the infection for 10–14 days. In the opinion of this author, a few days of close observation and parenteral therapy followed by an oral antibiotic—with the entire course of treatment continuing for no more than 5 days after the patient becomes afebrile—may be the best approach for treating pneumococcal pneumonia, even in the presence of bacteremia. Cases with a second focus of infection (e.g., empyema or septic arthritis) require longer therapy.

Meningitis (Table 128-6) Pneumococcal meningitis should be treated initially with ceftriaxone plus vancomycin. Equivalent doses of cefotaxime or cefepime may be used in place of ceftriaxone. The cephalosporin will be effective against most—but not all—isolates and will readily penetrate the blood-brain barrier; all isolates will be susceptible to vancomycin, but this drug has a somewhat unpredictable capacity to cross the blood-brain barrier. If the isolate is shown to be susceptible or intermediately resistant, treatment can be continued with ceftriaxone, and vancomycin can be discontinued. If the organism is resistant, treatment with both drugs should be continued. A very few studies of experimental animals suggest benefits of the addition of rifampin, but in vitro studies indicate antagonism between this drug and ceftriaxone or vancomycin; in the absence of data to support the practice in humans, this author does not recommend that rifampin be added. Imipenem may be used in place of the cephalosporin in patients who have had life-threatening allergic reactions to β-lactam antibiotics. The total duration of therapy for pneumococcal meningitis is 10 days. A recent study demonstrated clear benefit from the addition of glucocorticoids (Chap. 376).

Endocarditis Pneumococcal endocarditis is associated with rapid destruction of heart valves. Pending results of susceptibility studies, treatment should be initiated with ceftriaxone or cefotaxime; if the prevalence of highly resistant strains increases, it might be prudent to add vancomycin until results of susceptibility studies are available. In vitro, aminoglycosides are somewhat synergistic and rifampin or quinolones are antagonistic with β-lactams against pneumococci; there is no clear evidence from in vivo studies that adding any of these antibiotics to the regimen is beneficial.

TABLE 128-6 TREATMENT OF PNEUMOCOCCAL MENINGITIS

Circumstance	Appropriate Course[a]
Diagnosis of pneumococcal meningitis; antibiotic susceptibility unknown	Treat with ceftriaxone, 2 g q12h, plus vancomycin, 500 mg q6h, until antibiotic susceptibility of organism is known.
Susceptibility results available	Continue treatment with ceftriaxone alone if organism is susceptible or intermediate; continue both ceftriaxone and vancomycin if organism is resistant.
Life-threatening penicillin allergy	Treat with imipenem, 500 mg q6h, rather than a β-lactam antibiotic.

[a]Treatment should be administered for 5–7 days after defervescence or for a total of 10 days.

TABLE 128-7 PROTECTIVE EFFICACY OF POLYVALENT PNEUMOCOCCAL POLYSACCHARIDE VACCINE[a]

		Years since Last Vaccination		
Age, Years	No. of Subject Pairs	<3	3–5	>5
<55	125	93	89	85
55–64	149	88	82	75
65–74	213	80	71	58
75–84	188	67	53	32
≥85	133	46	22	−13

[a]Results of a case-control study involving all cases of invasive pneumococcal disease in Connecticut during 7 years (1984–1990). Vaccinated subjects were matched with controls, and the rate of invasive pneumococcal disease was related to age and time since vaccination. The data, showing protective efficacy, suggest that, within 5 years of vaccination, protection rates decline with age—i.e., from ~90% in persons <65 years of age to <50% in persons ≥85 years old. Protection also declines with increasing time from vaccination to infection, and this decline is more prominent in older patients.
Source: Data adapted from ED Shapiro et al: N Engl J Med 325:1453, 1991; with permission.

OTHER THERAPEUTIC MODALITIES Addition of drotrecogin, an activated protein C preparation, may be beneficial in treating patients with severe pneumococcal sepsis. Glucocorticoids and agents that block the action of TNF-α, IL-1, or platelet-activating factor have conferred no benefit.

PREVENTION

Capsular Polysaccharide Vaccine The pneumococcal capsular polysaccharide vaccine administered to adults since the early 1980s contains 25 μg per dose of capsular polysaccharide from each of the 23 most prevalent serotypes of *S. pneumoniae.* Vaccination stimulates antibody to most serotypes in most recipients. One case-control study showed a protection rate of 85% lasting ≥5 years in adults <55 years old (Table 128-7). The level and duration of protection decreased with advancing age. Other studies have suggested an overall protection rate in the adult population of 50–70%. In high-risk subgroups (e.g., debilitated elderly persons and individuals with severe chronic lung disease), vaccine has not been shown conclusively to be effective. Persons who most need the vaccine because of poor IgG responses (e.g., those with lymphoma or AIDS) are likely not to respond at all. Nevertheless, the Advisory Committee on Immunization Practices of the Centers for Disease Control and Prevention has broadened its recommendations for pneumococcal vaccination to include all persons >2 years of age who are at substantially increased risk of developing pneumococcal infection and/or having a serious complication of such an infection. Perhaps most in need of vaccination are persons with anatomic or functional asplenia, who are at risk for overwhelming, life-threatening infections. Others who might fall within these recommendations are persons who (1) are over the age of 65; (2) have a CSF leak, diabetes mellitus, alcoholism, cirrhosis, chronic renal insufficiency, chronic pulmonary disease, or advanced cardiovascular disease; (3) have an immunocompromising condition associated with increased risk of pneumococcal disease (e.g., multiple myeloma, lymphoma, Hodgkin's disease, HIV infection, organ transplantation, or chronic glucocorticoid use); (4) are genetically at increased risk (e.g., Native Americans and Native Alaskans); or (5) live in environments where outbreaks are particularly likely to occur (e.g., nursing homes).

Recommendations regarding revaccination seem somewhat inconsistent. A single revaccination is advocated for persons over the age of 65 if >5 years have elapsed since the first vaccination. Since antibody levels decline and there is no anamnestic response, it seems more reasonable simply to recommend revaccination at 5-year intervals, especially in persons over the age of 65, who tend to have almost no adverse reaction to vaccination, and in splenectomized patients, who are most in need.

Protein-Conjugate Pneumococcal Vaccine Pneumococcal polysaccharide vaccine is not useful in children <2 years of age, whose immune system does not respond well to polysaccharide antigens. Conjugating

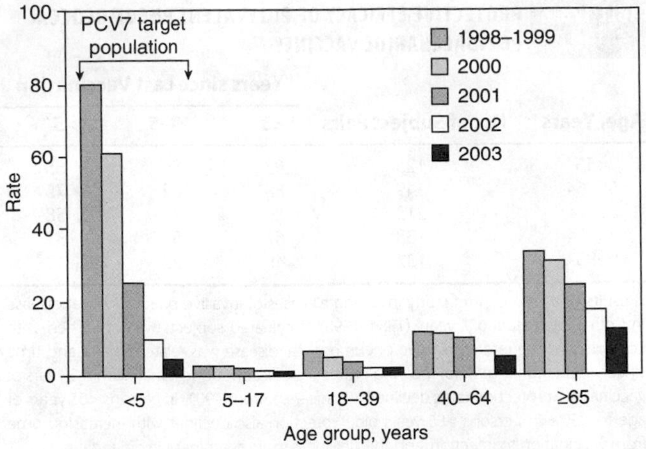

FIGURE 128-4 The rate of invasive pneumococcal disease per 100,000 population (*vertical axis*) is presented for each year since 2000 (*bars*) for different age groups (*horizontal axis*). Invasive pneumococcal disease is more common at the extremes of age. The incidence in all age groups has fallen steadily during the past 5 years. The observed reductions reflect direct effects and indirect ("herd") effects of widespread use of the 7-valent pneumococcal protein-conjugate vaccine (PCV7; see text). *(Adapted from Centers for Disease Control and Prevention, MMWR 54:893, 2005.)*

the polysaccharide to a protein yields an immunogen that is effective in infants and young children. Initial studies of a protein-conjugate pneumococcal vaccine consisting of capsular material from the seven serotypes most likely to cause disease in children (Prevnar) showed a 98% reduction in rates of bacteremia and meningitis and a 67% reduction in rates of otitis media due to vaccine serotypes. Since it was marketed in 2000, widespread use of this vaccine has caused a dramatic decline in the incidence of invasive pneumococcal disease among infants and children (Fig. 128-4). Colonization rates have also greatly decreased. In an Alaskan village, rates of carriage of vaccine strains decreased in children from 55% to 10% and in adults from 15% to 5%. Studies of protein conjugate vaccines that contain antigen from more than seven common infecting serotypes are nearing completion, with favorable results.

The incidence of invasive pneumococcal disease has also declined among unvaccinated children and among adults, to whom this vaccine is not even offered (Fig. 128-4). This decrease illustrates the "herd effect"—i.e., the impact of widespread vaccination on unvaccinated members of the population—and is probably attributable to the effects of the conjugate vaccine on nasopharyngeal carriage of vaccine serotypes. Another effect of the widespread use of this vaccine is the decreasing proportion of all pneumococcal disease that is due to antibiotic-resistant isolates, a trend that reflects the targeting of antibiotic-resistant strains by the vaccine. An unwanted effect of vaccination has been an increase in infections caused by serotypes that are not included in the vaccine (*replacement serotypes*), which, in fact, are increasingly expressing antibiotic resistance. Still, as noted above, the overall incidence of pneumococcal disease in all segments of the population has steadily declined. For further information, the reader is referred to the American Academy of Pediatrics *Red Book Online* (*http://aapredbook.aappublications.org*).

FURTHER READINGS

American Academy of Pediatrics and American Academy of Family Physicians Clinical Practice Guideline: Diagnosis and management of acute otitis media. Pediatrics 113:1451, 2004

Centers for Disease Control and Prevention: Direct and indirect effects of routine vaccination of children with 7-valent conjugate vaccine on incidence of invasive pneumococcal disease—United States 1998-2003. MMWR 54:893, 2005

Fedson DS, Musher DM: Pneumococcal vaccine, in *Vaccines*, 4th ed, SA Plotkin, EA Mortimer Jr (eds). Philadelphia, Saunders, 2003

Karlowsky JA et al: Factors associated with relative rates of antimicrobial resistance among *Streptococcus pneumoniae* in the United States: Results from the TRUST Surveillance Program (1998-2002). Clin Infect Dis 36:963, 2003

Lexau CA et al: Changing epidemiology of invasive pneumococcal disease among older adults in the era of pediatric pneumococcal conjugate vaccine. JAMA 294:2043, 2005

Mandell LA et al: Update of practice guidelines for the management of community-acquired pneumonia in immunocompetent adults. Clin Infect Dis 37:1405, 2003

Musher DM: Pneumococcal vaccine—direct and indirect ("herd") effects (editorial). N Engl J Med 354:1522, 2006

———: *Streptococcus pneumoniae*, in *Principles and Practice of Infectious Diseases*, 6th ed, GL Mandell et al (eds). New York, Churchill Livingstone, 2004

——— et al: A fresh look at the definition of susceptibility of *Streptococcus pneumoniae* to beta-lactam antibiotics. Arch Intern Med 161:2538, 2001

Tuomanen EI et al (eds): *The Pneumococcus*. Washington, DC, ASM Press, 2004

129 Staphylococcal Infections

Franklin D. Lowy

Staphylococcus aureus, the most virulent of the many staphylococcal species, has demonstrated its versatility by remaining a major cause of morbidity and mortality despite the availability of numerous effective antistaphylococcal antibiotics. *S. aureus* is a pluripotent pathogen, causing disease through both toxin-mediated and non-toxin-mediated mechanisms. This organism is responsible for both nosocomial and community-based infections that range from relatively minor skin and soft tissue infections to life-threatening systemic infections.

The "other" staphylococci, collectively designated *coagulase-negative staphylococci* (CoNS), are considerably less virulent than *S. aureus* but remain important pathogens in infections associated with prosthetic devices.

MICROBIOLOGY AND TAXONOMY

Staphylococci, gram-positive cocci in the family Micrococcaceae, form grapelike clusters on Gram's stain (Fig. 129-1). These organisms are catalase-positive (unlike streptococcal species), nonmotile, aerobic, and facultatively anaerobic. They are capable of prolonged survival on environmental surfaces in varying conditions.

More than 30 staphylococcal species are pathogenic. A simple strategy for identification of the more clinically important species is outlined in Fig. 129-2. Automated diagnostic systems, kits for biochemical characterization, and DNA-based assays are available for distinguishing among species. With few exceptions, *S. aureus* is distinguished from other staphylococcal species by its production of coagulase, a surface enzyme that converts fibrinogen to fibrin. Latex kits designed to detect both protein A and clumping factor also distinguish *S. aureus* from other staphylococcal species. *S. aureus* ferments mannitol, is positive for protein A, and produces DNAse. On blood agar plates, *S. aureus* tends to form golden β-hemolytic colonies; in contrast, CoNS produce small white nonhemolytic colonies.

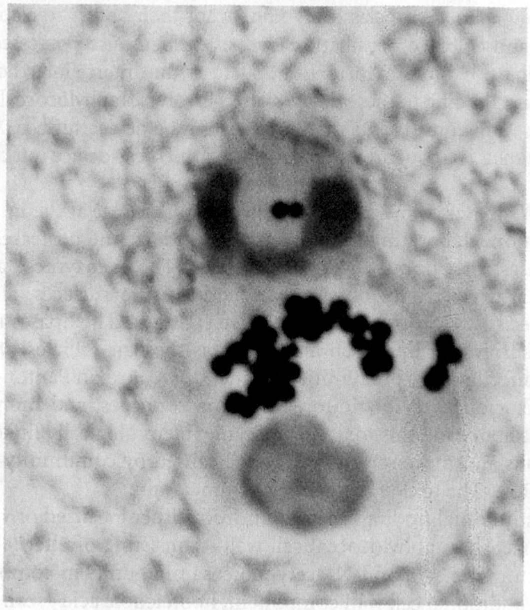

FIGURE 129-1 Gram's stain of *S. aureus* in a sputum sample with polymorphonuclear leukocytes. *(Reprinted with permission from FD Lowy: Staphylococcus aureus infections. N Engl J Med 339:520, 1998. © 1998 Massachusetts Medical Society. All rights reserved.)*

Determining whether multiple isolates (especially of CoNS) from a particular patient are the same or different is often an important factor in distinguishing contaminants from genuine pathogens. Determining whether multiple isolates from different patients are the same or different is relevant when there is concern that a nosocomial outbreak may have been due to a common point source (e.g., a contaminated medical instrument). Biochemical tests, often performed in conjunction with antimicrobial susceptibility testing, have been used as a relatively simple means of distinguishing among staphylococcal species or strains. More discriminating molecular typing methods, such as pulsed-field gel electrophoresis and sequence-based techniques, have also been used for this purpose.

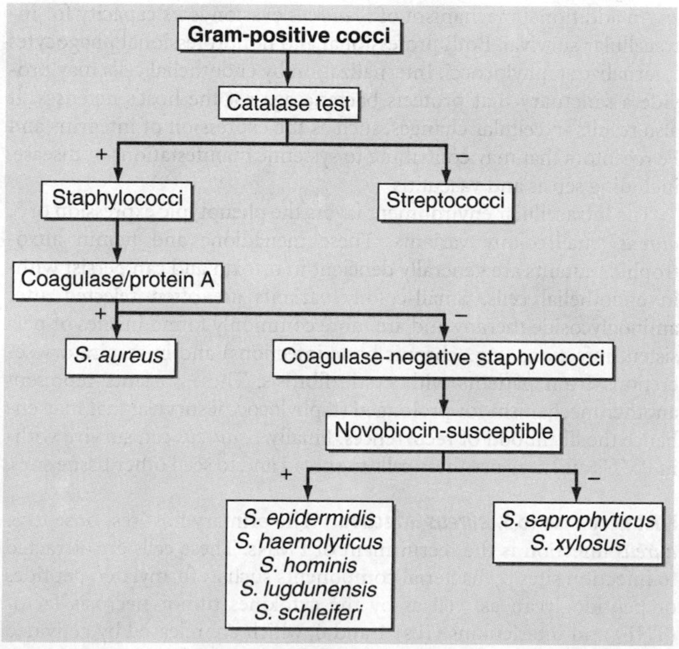

FIGURE 129-2 Biochemical characterization of staphylococci: algorithm of biochemical tests used to discriminate among the clinically important staphylococci. Additional tests are necessary to identify all of the different species.

S. AUREUS INFECTIONS

EPIDEMIOLOGY

S. aureus is a part of the normal human flora; ~25–50% of healthy persons may be persistently or transiently colonized. The rate of colonization is higher among insulin-dependent diabetics, HIV-infected patients, patients undergoing hemodialysis, and individuals with skin damage. The anterior nares are the most frequent site of human colonization, although the skin (especially when damaged), vagina, axilla, perineum, and oropharynx may also be colonized. These colonization sites serve as a reservoir of strains for future infections, and persons colonized with *S. aureus* are at greater risk of subsequent infection than are uncolonized individuals.

Overall, *S. aureus* is a leading cause of nosocomial infections. It is the most common cause of surgical wound infections and is second only to CoNS as a cause of primary bacteremia. Increasingly, nosocomial isolates are resistant to multiple drugs. In the community, *S. aureus* remains an important cause of skin and soft tissue infections, respiratory infections, and (among injection drug users) infective endocarditis. The increasing prevalence of home infusion therapy is another cause of community-acquired staphylococcal infections.

Most individuals who develop *S. aureus* infections are infected with their own colonizing strains. However, *S. aureus* may also be acquired from other people or from environmental exposures. Transmission most frequently results from transient colonization of the hands of hospital personnel, who then transfer strains from one patient to another. Spread of staphylococci in aerosols of respiratory or nasal secretions from heavily colonized individuals has also been reported.

In the past 10 years, numerous outbreaks of community-based infection caused by methicillin-resistant *S. aureus* (MRSA) in individuals with no prior medical exposure have been reported. These outbreaks have taken place in both rural and urban settings in widely separated regions throughout the world. The reports document a dramatic change in the epidemiology of MRSA infections. The outbreaks have occurred among such diverse groups as prisoners, athletes, Native Americans, and drug users. Risk factors common to these outbreaks include poor hygienic conditions, close contact, contaminated material, and damaged skin. The community-associated infections have been caused by a limited number of MRSA strains. In the United States, strain USA300 has been the predominant clone and is also responsible for an increasing number of nosocomial infections. Of concern has been the apparent capacity of community-acquired MRSA strains to cause serious disease in immunocompetent individuals. This ability may be due to the presence of different toxin-producing genes in these strains.

PATHOGENESIS

General Concepts *S. aureus* is a pyogenic pathogen known for its capacity to induce abscess formation at sites of both local and metastatic infections. This classic pathologic response to *S. aureus* defines the framework within which the infection will progress. The bacteria elicit an inflammatory response characterized by an initial intense polymorphonuclear leukocyte (PMN) response and the subsequent infiltration of macrophages and fibroblasts. Either the host cellular response (including the deposition of fibrin and collagen) contains the infection, or infection spreads to the adjoining tissue or the bloodstream.

In toxin-mediated staphylococcal disease, infection is not invariably present. For example, once toxin has been elaborated into food, staphylococcal food poisoning can develop in the absence of viable bacteria. In staphylococcal toxic shock syndrome (TSS), conditions allowing toxin elaboration at colonization sites (e.g., the presence of a superabsorbent tampon) suffice for initiation of clinical illness.

The *S. aureus* Genome The entire genome has been sequenced for numerous strains of *S. aureus*. Among the interesting revelations are (1) a high degree of nucleotide sequence similarity among the different strains; (2) acquisition of a relatively large amount of genetic information by horizontal transfer from other bacterial species; and (3) the presence of unique "pathogenicity" or "genomic" islands—mobile genetic elements that contain clusters of enterotoxin and exotoxin genes or antimicrobial resistance determinants. Among the genes in these islands are those carrying *mecA*, the gene responsible for methicillin resistance. Methicillin resistance–containing islands have been designated *staphylococcal cassette chromosome mecs* (SCC*mecs*) and range in size from ~20 to 60 kb. To date, five SCC*mecs* have been identified. Type 4 and type 5 SCC*mecs* have been associated with community-acquired MRSA strains.

A limited number of MRSA clones have been responsible for most community and hospital-associated infections worldwide. A comparison of these strains with those from earlier outbreaks (e.g., the phage 80/81 strains from the 1950s) has revealed preservation of the nucleotide sequence over time. This observation suggests that these strains possess determinants facilitating survival and spread.

Regulation of Virulence Gene Expression In both toxin-mediated and non-toxin-mediated diseases due to *S. aureus*, the expression of virulence determinants associated with infection depends on a series of regulatory genes [e.g., accessory gene regulator (*agr*) and staphylococcal accessory regulator (*sar*)] that coordinately control the expression of many virulence genes. The regulatory gene *agr* is part of a quorum-sensing signal transduction pathway that senses and responds to bacterial density. Staphylococcal surface proteins are synthesized during the bacterial exponential growth phase in vitro. In contrast, many secreted proteins, such as α toxin, the enterotoxins, and assorted enzymes, are released during the postexponential growth phase.

It has been hypothesized that these regulatory genes serve a similar function in vivo. Successful invasion requires the sequential expression of these different bacterial elements. Bacterial adhesins are needed to initiate colonization of host tissue surfaces. The subsequent release of various enzymes enables the colony to obtain nutritional support and permits bacteria to spread to adjacent tissues. Studies with mutant strains in which these regulatory genes are inactivated show reduced virulence in several animal models of *S. aureus* infection.

Pathogenesis of Invasive *S. aureus* Infection Staphylococci are opportunists. For these organisms to invade the host and cause infection, some or all of the following steps are necessary: inoculation and local colonization of tissue surfaces, invasion, evasion of the host response, and metastatic spread. The initiation of staphylococcal infection requires a breach in cutaneous or mucosal barriers. Colonizing strains or strains transferred from other individuals are inoculated into damaged skin, a wound, or the bloodstream.

Recurrences of *S. aureus* infections are common, apparently because of the capacity of these pathogens to survive, to persist in a quiescent state in various tissues, and then to cause recrudescent infections when suitable conditions arise.

NASAL COLONIZATION The anterior nares is the principal site of staphylococcal colonization in humans. Colonization appears to involve the attachment of *S. aureus* to both nasal mucin and keratinized epithelial cells of the anterior nares. Other factors that may contribute to colonization include the influence of other resident nasal flora and their bacterial density, nasal mucosal damage (e.g., that resulting from inhalational drug use), and the antimicrobial properties of nasal secretions.

INOCULATION AND COLONIZATION OF TISSUE SURFACES Staphylococci may be introduced into tissue as a result of minor abrasions, administration of medications such as insulin, or establishment of IV access with catheters. After their introduction into a tissue site, bacteria replicate and colonize the host tissue surface. A family of structurally related *S. aureus* surface proteins referred to as MSCRAMMs (microbial surface components recognizing adhesive matrix molecules) plays an important role as a mediator of adherence to these sites. MSCRAMMs such as clumping factor and collagen-binding protein enable the bacteria to colonize different tissue surfaces; these proteins contribute to the pathogenesis of invasive infections such as endocarditis and arthritis by facilitating the adherence of *S. aureus* to surfaces with exposed fibrinogen or collagen.

Although CoNS are classically known for their ability to elaborate a biofilm and colonize prosthetic devices, *S. aureus* also possesses genes responsible for biofilm formation, such as the intercellular adhesion (*ica*) locus. Binding to these devices often involves staphylococcal adherence to serum constituents that have coated the device surface. As a result, *S. aureus* is frequently isolated from biomedical-device infections.

INVASION After colonization, staphylococci replicate at the initial site of infection, elaborating enzymes that include serine proteases, hyaluronidases, thermonucleases, and lipases. These enzymes facilitate bacterial survival and local spread across tissue surfaces, although their precise role in infections is not well defined. The lipases may facilitate survival in lipid-rich areas such as the hair follicles, where *S. aureus* infections are often initiated. The *S. aureus* toxin Panton-Valentine leukocidin is cytolytic to PMNs, macrophages, and monocytes. Strains elaborating this toxin have been epidemiologically linked with cutaneous and more serious infections caused by community-associated MRSA. The toxin's biologic role is uncertain.

Constitutional findings may result from either localized or systemic infections. The staphylococcal cell wall—consisting of alternating N-acetyl muramic acid and N-acetyl glucosamine units in combination with an additional cell wall component, lipoteichoic acid—can initiate an inflammatory response that includes the sepsis syndrome. Staphylococcal α toxin, which causes pore formation in various eukaryotic cells, can also initiate an inflammatory response with findings suggestive of sepsis.

EVASION OF HOST DEFENSE MECHANISMS Evasion of host defense mechanisms is critical to invasion. Staphylococci possess an antiphagocytic polysaccharide microcapsule. Most human *S. aureus* infections are due to capsular types 5 and 8. The *S. aureus* capsule also plays a role in the induction of abscess formation. The capsular polysaccharides are characterized by a zwitterionic charge pattern (the presence of both negatively and positively charged molecules) that is critical to abscess formation. Protein A, an MSCRAMM unique to *S. aureus*, acts as an Fc receptor. It binds the Fc portion of IgG subclasses 1, 2, and 4, preventing opsonophagocytosis by PMNs. Both chemotaxis inhibitory protein of staphylococci (CHIPS, a secreted protein) and extracellular adherence protein (EAP, a surface protein) interfere with PMN migration to infection sites. The arginine catabolic mobile element (ACME), a cluster of genes unique to the USA300 clone, also may facilitate evasion.

An additional mechanism of *S. aureus* evasion is its capacity for intracellular survival. Both professional and nonprofessional phagocytes internalize staphylococci. Internalization by endothelial cells may provide a sanctuary that protects bacteria against the host's defenses. It also results in cellular changes, such as the expression of integrins and Fc receptors that may contribute to systemic manifestations of disease, including sepsis and vasculitis.

The intracellular environment favors the phenotypic expression of *S. aureus* small-colony variants. These menadione and hemin auxotrophic mutants are generally deficient in α toxin and can persist within endothelial cells. Small-colony variants are often selected after aminoglycoside therapy and are more commonly found in sites of persistent infections (e.g., chronic bone infections) and in respiratory secretions from patients with cystic fibrosis. These variants represent another mechanism for prolonged staphylococcal survival that may enhance the likelihood of recurrences. Finally, *S. aureus* can survive within PMNs and may use these cells to spread and to seed other tissue sites.

Host Response to *S. aureus* Infection The primary host response to *S. aureus* infection is the recruitment of PMNs. These cells are attracted to infection sites by bacterial components such as formylated peptides or peptidoglycan as well as by the cytokines tumor necrosis factor (TNF) and interleukins (ILs) 1 and 6, which are released by activated macrophages and endothelial cells.

Although most individuals have antistaphylococcal antibodies, it is not clear that the antibody levels are qualitatively or quantitatively sufficient to protect against infection. Anticapsular and anti-MSCRAMM antibodies facilitate opsonization in vitro and have been protective against infection in several animal models.

Groups at Increased Risk of Infection Some diseases appear to entail multiple risk factors for *S. aureus* infection; diabetes, for example, combines an increased rate of *S. aureus* colonization and the use of injectable insulin with the possibility of impaired leukocyte function. Individuals with congenital or acquired qualitative or quantitative PMN defects are at increased risk of *S. aureus* infections; these include neutropenic patients (e.g., those receiving chemotherapeutic agents), individuals with defective intracellular staphylococcal killing (e.g., chronic granulomatous disease), and persons with Job's syndrome or Chédiak-Higashi syndrome. Other groups at risk include individuals with skin abnormalities and those with prosthetic devices.

Pathogenesis of Toxin-Mediated Disease *S. aureus* produces three types of toxin: cytotoxins, pyrogenic-toxin superantigens, and exfoliative toxins. Both epidemiologic and animal data suggest that antitoxin antibodies are protective against illness in TSS, staphylococcal food poisoning, and staphylococcal scalded-skin syndrome (SSSS). Illness develops after toxin synthesis and absorption and the subsequent toxin-initiated host response.

ENTEROTOXIN AND TOXIC SHOCK SYNDROME TOXIN 1 (TSST-1) The pyrogenic toxin superantigens are a family of small-molecular-size, structurally similar proteins that are responsible for two diseases: TSS and food poisoning. TSS results from the ability of enterotoxins and TSST-1 to function as T cell mitogens. In the normal process of antigen presentation, the antigen is first processed within the cell, and peptides are then presented in the major histocompatibility complex (MHC) class II groove, initiating a measured T cell response. In contrast, enterotoxins bind directly to the invariant region of MHC—outside the MHC class II groove. The enterotoxins can then bind T cell receptors via the vβ chain, resulting in a dramatic overexpansion of T cell clones (up to 20% of the total T cell population).

The consequence of this T cell expansion is a "cytokine storm," with the release of inflammatory mediators that include interferon (IFN) γ, IL-1, IL-6, TNF-α, and TNF-β. The resulting multisystem disease produces a constellation of findings that mimic those in endotoxin shock; however, the pathogenic mechanisms differ. It has been hypothesized that a contributing factor to TSS is the release of endotoxin from the gastrointestinal tract, which may synergistically enhance the toxin's effects.

A different region of the enterotoxin molecule is responsible for the symptoms of food poisoning. The enterotoxins are heat stable and can survive conditions that kill the bacteria. Illness results from the ingestion of preformed toxin. As a result, the incubation period is short (1–6 h). The toxin stimulates the vagus nerve and the vomiting center of the brain. It also appears to stimulate intestinal peristaltic activity.

EXFOLIATIVE TOXINS AND THE STAPHYLOCOCCAL SCALDED-SKIN SYNDROME The exfoliative toxins are responsible for SSSS. The toxins that produce disease in humans are of two serotypes: ETA and ETB. These toxins disrupt the desmosomes that link adjoining cells. Although the mechanism of this disruption remains uncertain, studies suggest that the toxins possess serine protease activity, which—through undefined mechanisms—triggers exfoliation. The result is a split in the epidermis at the granular level, and this event is responsible for the superficial desquamation of the skin that typifies this illness.

DIAGNOSIS

Staphylococcal infections are readily diagnosed by Gram's stain (Fig. 129-1) and microscopic examination of abscess contents or of infected tissue. Routine culture of infected material usually yields positive results, and blood cultures are sometimes positive even when infections are localized to extravascular sites. Polymerase chain reaction (PCR)–based assays have been applied to the rapid diagnosis of *S. aureus* infection and are increasingly used in clinical microbiology laboratories.

TABLE 129-1 COMMON ILLNESSES CAUSED BY *STAPHYLOCOCCUS AUREUS*

Skin and Soft Tissue Infections
Folliculitis
Furuncle, carbuncle
Cellulitis
Impetigo
Mastitis
Surgical wound infections
Hidradenitis suppurativa
Musculoskeletal Infections
Septic arthritis
Osteomyelitis
Pyomyositis
Psoas abscess
Respiratory Tract Infections
Ventilator-associated or nosocomial pneumonia
Septic pulmonary emboli
Postviral pneumonia (e.g., influenza)
Empyema
Bacteremia and Its Complications
Sepsis, septic shock
Metastatic foci of infection (kidney, joints, bone, lung)
Infective endocarditis
Infective Endocarditis
Injection drug use–associated
Native-valve
Prosthetic-valve
Nosocomial
Device-Related Infections (e.g., intravascular catheters, prosthetic joints)
Toxin-Mediated Illnesses
Toxic shock syndrome
Food poisoning
Staphylococcal scalded-skin syndrome
Invasive Infections Associated with Community-Acquired MRSA
Necrotizing fasciitis
Waterhouse-Friderichsen syndrome
Necrotizing pneumonia
Purpura fulminans

To date, serologic assays have not proved useful for the diagnosis of staphylococcal infections. Determining whether patients with documented *S. aureus* bacteremia also have infective endocarditis or a metastatic focus of infection remains a diagnostic challenge (see "Bacteremia, Sepsis, and Infective Endocarditis," below).

CLINICAL SYNDROMES
(Table 129-1)

Skin and Soft Tissue Infections *S. aureus* causes a variety of cutaneous infections. Common predisposing factors include skin disease, skin damage (e.g., insect bites, minor trauma), injections (e.g., in diabetes, injection drug use), and poor personal hygiene. These infections are characterized by the formation of pus-containing blisters, which often begin in hair follicles and spread to adjoining tissues. *Folliculitis* is a superficial infection that involves the hair follicle, with a central area of purulence (pus) surrounded by induration and erythema. *Furuncles* (boils) are more extensive, painful lesions that tend to occur in hairy, moist regions of the body and extend from the hair follicle to become a true abscess with an area of central purulence. *Carbuncles* are most often located in the lower neck and are even more severe and painful, resulting from the coalescence of other lesions that extend to a deeper layer of the subcutaneous tissue. In general, furuncles and carbuncles are readily apparent, with pus often expressible or discharging from the abscess.

Mastitis develops in 1–3% of nursing mothers. The infection, which generally presents within 2–3 weeks after delivery, is characterized by findings that range from cellulitis to abscess formation. Systemic signs, such as fever and chills, are often present in more severe cases.

Other cutaneous *S. aureus* infections include impetigo, cellulitis, and hidradenitis suppurativa (recurrent follicular infections in regions such as the axilla). *S. aureus* is one of the most common causes of surgical wound infection.

It should be noted that many of these syndromes may also be due to group A streptococci or, less commonly, to other streptococcal species.

Musculoskeletal Infections *S. aureus* is among the most common causes of bone infections—both those resulting from hematogenous dissemination and those arising from contiguous spread from a soft tissue site.

Hematogenous osteomyelitis in children most often involves the long bones. Infections present as fever and bone pain or with a child's reluctance to bear weight. The white blood cell count and erythrocyte sedimentation rate are often elevated. Blood cultures are positive in ~50% of cases. When necessary, bone biopsies for culture and histopathologic examination are usually diagnostic. Routine x-rays may be normal for up to 14 days after the onset of symptoms. ^{99m}Tc-phosphonate scanning often detects early evidence of infection. MRI is more sensitive than other techniques in establishing a radiologic diagnosis.

In adults, hematogenous osteomyelitis involving the long bones is less common. However, *vertebral osteomyelitis* is among the more common clinical presentations. Vertebral bone infections are most often seen in patients with endocarditis, those undergoing hemodialysis, diabetics, and injection drug users. These infections may present as intense back pain and fever but may also be clinically occult, presenting as chronic back pain and low-grade fever. *S. aureus* is the most common cause of epidural abscess, a complication that can result in neurologic compromise. Patients complain of difficulty voiding or walking and of radicular pain in addition to the symptoms associated with their osteomyelitis. Surgical intervention in this setting often constitutes a medical emergency. MRI most reliably establishes the diagnosis (Fig. 129-3).

Bone infections that result from contiguous spread tend to develop from soft tissue infections, such as those associated with diabetic or vascular ulcers, surgery, or trauma. Exposure of bone, a draining fistulous tract, failure to heal, or continued drainage suggests involvement of underlying bone. Bone involvement is established by bone culture and histopathologic examination (revealing, for example, evidence of PMN infiltration). Contamination of culture material from adjacent tissue can make the diagnosis of osteomyelitis difficult in the absence of pathologic confirmation. In addition, it is sometimes hard to distinguish radiologically between osteomyelitis and overlying soft tissue infection with underlying osteitis.

In both children and adults, *S. aureus* is the most common cause of *septic arthritis* in native joints. This infection is rapidly progressive and may be associated with extensive joint destruction if left untreated. It presents as intense pain on motion of the affected joint, swelling, and fever. Aspiration of the joint reveals turbid fluid, with >50,000 PMNs/μL and gram-positive cocci in clusters on Gram's stain (Fig. 129-1). In adults, arthritis may result from trauma, surgery, or hematogenous dissemination. The most commonly involved joints include the knees, shoulders, hips, and phalanges. Infection frequently develops in joints previously damaged by osteoarthritis or rheumatoid arthritis. Iatrogenic infections resulting from aspiration or injection of agents into the joint also occur. In these settings, the patient experiences increased pain and swelling in the involved joint in association with fever.

Pyomyositis is an unusual infection of skeletal muscles that is seen primarily in tropical climates but also occurs in immunocompromised and HIV-infected patients. Pyomyositis presents as fever, swelling, and pain overlying the involved muscle. Aspiration of fluid from the involved tissue reveals pus. Although a history of trauma may be associated with the infection, its pathogenesis is poorly understood.

Respiratory Tract Infections Respiratory tract infections caused by *S. aureus* occur in selected clinical settings. *S. aureus* is a cause of serious infections in newborns and infants; these infections present as shortness of breath, fever, and respiratory failure. Chest x-ray may reveal pneumatoceles (shaggy, thin-walled cavities). Pneumothorax and empyema are recognized complications of this infection.

In adults, nosocomial *S. aureus* pulmonary infections are commonly seen in intubated patients in intensive care units. The clinical presentation is no different from that encountered in pulmonary infections of other bacterial etiologies. Patients produce increased volumes of purulent sputum and develop respiratory distress, fever, and new pulmonary infiltrates. Distinguishing bacterial pneumonia from respiratory failure of other causes or new pulmonary infiltrates in critically ill patients is often difficult and relies on a constellation of clinical, radiologic, and laboratory findings.

Community-acquired respiratory tract infections due to *S. aureus* most commonly follow viral infections or septic pulmonary emboli (e.g., in injection drug users). Influenza is the most common cause of the former type of presentation. Patients may present with fever, bloody sputum production, and midlung-field pneumatoceles or multiple, patchy pulmonary infiltrates. Diagnosis is made by sputum Gram's stain and culture. Blood cultures, although useful, are usually negative.

Bacteremia, Sepsis, and Infective Endocarditis *S. aureus* bacteremia may be complicated by sepsis, endocarditis, vasculitis, or metastatic seeding (establishment of suppurative collections at other tissue sites). The frequency of metastatic seeding during bacteremia has been estimated to be as high as 31%. Among the more commonly seeded tissue sites are bones, joints, kidneys, and lungs.

Recognition of these complications by clinical and laboratory diagnostic methods alone is often difficult. Comorbid conditions that are frequently seen in association with *S. aureus* bacteremia and that increase the risk of complications include diabetes, HIV infection, and renal insufficiency. Other host factors associated with an increased risk of complications include presentation with community-acquired *S. aureus* bacteremia (except in injection drug users), lack of an identifiable primary focus, and the presence of prosthetic devices or material.

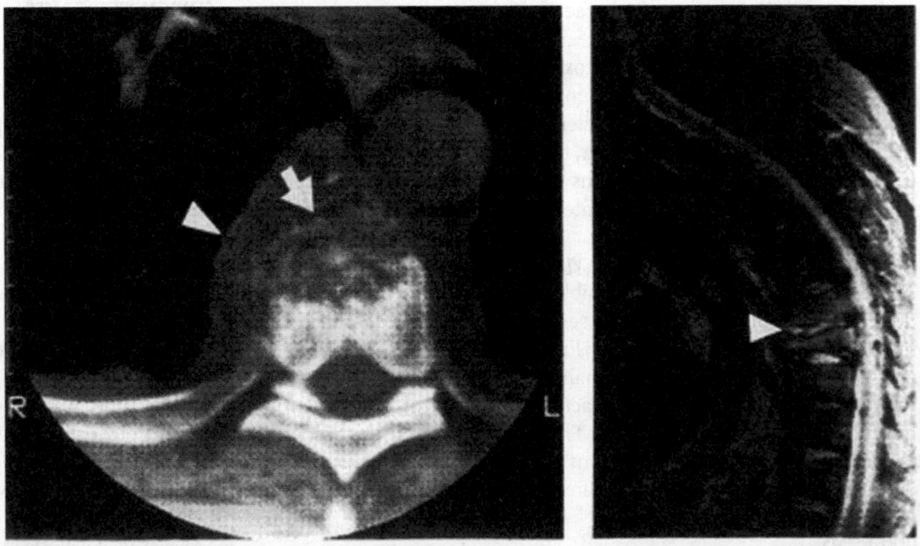

A B

FIGURE 129-3 ***S. aureus* vertebral osteomyelitis involving the thoracic disk between T8 and T9 in a 63-year-old man. *A.*** The lower end plate is damaged (*arrow*), and there is an adjacent paraspinal mass (*arrowhead*). ***B.*** Sagittal T2-weighted magnetic resonance image of the spine, illustrating anterior wedging of the body of T8. *(Reprinted with permission from MA Artinian et al: Images in clinical medicine. Vertebral osteomyelitis. N Engl J Med 329:399, 1993. © 1993 Massachusetts Medical Society. All rights reserved.)*

Clinically, *S. aureus* sepsis presents in a manner similar to that documented for sepsis due to other bacteria. The well-described progression of hemodynamic changes—beginning with respiratory alkalosis and clinical findings of hypotension and fever—is commonly seen. The microbiologic diagnosis is established by positive blood cultures.

The overall incidence of *S. aureus* endocarditis has increased over the past 20 years. *S. aureus* is now the leading cause of endocarditis worldwide, accounting for 25–35% of cases. This increase is due, at least in part, to the increased use of intravascular devices; transesophageal echocardiography (TEE) studies found an infective endocarditis incidence of 25% among patients with *S. aureus* bacteremia and intravascular catheters. Other factors associated with an increased risk of endocarditis are injection drug use, hemodialysis, the presence of intravascular prosthetic devices, and immunosuppression. Despite the availability of effective antibiotics, mortality rates from these infections continue to range from 20 to 40%, depending on both the host and the nature of the infection. Complications of *S. aureus* endocarditis include cardiac valvular insufficiency, peripheral emboli, metastatic seeding, and central nervous system (CNS) involvement.

S. aureus is now a leading cause of endocarditis in many countries. *S. aureus* endocarditis is encountered in four clinical settings: (1) right-sided endocarditis in association with injection drug use, (2) left-sided native-valve endocarditis, (3) prosthetic-valve endocarditis, and (4) nosocomial endocarditis. In each of these settings, the diagnosis is established by recognition of clinical stigmata suggestive of endocarditis. These findings include cardiac manifestations, such as new or changing cardiac valvular murmurs; cutaneous evidence, such as vasculitic lesions, Osler's nodes, or Janeway lesions; evidence of right- or left-sided embolic disease; and a history suggesting a risk for *S. aureus* bacteremia. In the absence of antecedent antibiotic therapy, blood cultures are almost uniformly positive. Transthoracic echocardiography, while less sensitive than TEE, is less invasive and often establishes the presence of valvular vegetations.

Acute right-sided tricuspid valvular *S. aureus* endocarditis is most often seen in injection drug users. The classic presentation includes a high fever, a toxic clinical appearance, pleuritic chest pain, and the production of purulent (sometimes bloody) sputum. Chest x-rays reveal evidence of septic pulmonary emboli (small, peripheral, circular lesions that may cavitate with time). A high percentage of affected patients have no history of antecedent valvular damage. At the outset of their illness, patients may present with fever alone, without cardiac or other localizing findings. As a result, a high index of clinical suspicion is essential to the diagnosis.

Individuals with antecedent cardiac valvular damage more commonly present with left-sided native-valve endocarditis involving the previously affected valve. These patients tend to be older than those with right-sided endocarditis, their prognosis is worse, and their incidence of complications (including peripheral emboli, cardiac decompensation, and metastatic seeding) is higher.

S. aureus is one of the more common causes of prosthetic-valve endocarditis. This infection is especially fulminant in the early postoperative period and is associated with a high mortality rate. In most instances, medical therapy alone is not sufficient and urgent valve replacement is necessary. Patients are prone to develop valvular insufficiency or myocardial abscesses originating from the region of valve implantation.

The increased frequency of nosocomial endocarditis (15–30% of cases, depending on the series) reflects in part the increased use of intravascular devices. This form of endocarditis is most commonly caused by *S. aureus*. Because patients often are critically ill, are receiving antibiotics for various other indications, and have comorbid conditions, the diagnosis is not easily recognized.

Urinary Tract Infections Urinary tract infections (UTIs) are infrequently caused by *S. aureus*. In contrast with that of most other urinary pathogens, the presence of *S. aureus* in the urine suggests hematogenous dissemination. Ascending *S. aureus* infections occasionally result from instrumentation of the genitourinary tract.

Prosthetic Device–Related Infections *S. aureus* accounts for a large proportion of prosthetic device–related infections. These infections often involve intravascular catheters, prosthetic valves, orthopedic devices, peritoneal or intraventricular catheters, left-ventricular-assist devices, and vascular grafts. In contrast with the more indolent presentation of CoNS infections, *S. aureus* device-related infections often present more acutely, with both localized and systemic manifestations. The latter infections also tend to progress more rapidly. It is relatively common for a pyogenic collection to be present at the device site. Aspiration of these collections and performance of blood cultures are important components in establishing a diagnosis. *S. aureus* infections tend to occur more commonly soon after implantation unless the device is used for access (e.g., intravascular or hemodialysis catheters). In the latter instance, infections can occur at any time. As in most prosthetic-device infections, successful therapy usually involves removal of the device. Left in place, the device is a potential nidus for either persistent or recurrent infections.

Infections Associated with Community-Acquired MRSA The many unusual clinical presentations encountered in patients with community-associated MRSA infections include necrotizing fasciitis, necrotizing pneumonia, and sepsis with Waterhouse-Friderichsen syndrome or purpura fulminans. These life-threatening infections reflect the increased virulence of MRSA strains.

Toxin-Mediated Diseases • ***TOXIC SHOCK SYNDROME*** TSS was first recognized as a disease in children in 1978. The disease gained attention in the early 1980s, when a nationwide outbreak occurred among young, otherwise healthy, menstruating women. Epidemiologic investigation demonstrated that these cases were associated with menstruation and the use of a highly absorbent tampon that had recently been introduced to the market. Subsequent studies established the role of TSST-1 in these illnesses. Withdrawal of the tampon from the market resulted in a rapid decline in the incidence of this disease. However, menstrual and nonmenstrual cases continue to be reported.

The clinical presentation is similar in menstrual and nonmenstrual TSS, although the nature of the risk clearly differs. Evidence of clinical *S. aureus* infection is not a prerequisite. TSS results from the elaboration of an enterotoxin or the structurally related enterotoxin-like TSST-1. More than 90% of menstrual cases are caused by TSST-1, whereas a high percentage of nonmenstrual cases are caused by enterotoxins.

TSS begins with relatively nonspecific flulike symptoms. In menstrual cases, the onset usually comes 2 or 3 days after the start of menstruation. Patients present with fever, hypotension, and erythroderma of variable intensity. Mucosal involvement is common (e.g., conjunctival hyperemia). The illness can rapidly progress to symptoms that include vomiting, diarrhea, confusion, myalgias, and abdominal pain. These symptoms reflect the multisystemic nature of the disease, with involvement of the liver, kidneys, gastrointestinal tract, and/or CNS. Desquamation of the skin occurs during convalescence, usually 1–2 weeks after the onset of illness. Laboratory findings may include azotemia, leukocytosis, hypoalbuminemia, thrombocytopenia, and liver function abnormalities.

Diagnosis of TSS still depends on a constellation of findings rather than one specific finding (Table 129-2). Part of the case definition is the absence of laboratory evidence of other illnesses that are often included in the differential (e.g., Rocky Mountain spotted fever, rubeola, leptospirosis). Other diagnoses to be considered are drug toxicities, viral exanthems, sepsis, and Kawasaki disease. Illness occurs only in persons who lack antibody to TSST-1. Recurrences are possible if antibody fails to develop after the illness.

FOOD POISONING *S. aureus* is among the most common causes of food-borne outbreaks of infection in the United States. *S. aureus* food poisoning results from the inoculation of toxin-producing *S. aureus* into food by colonized food handlers. Toxin is then elaborated in such growth-promoting food as custards, potato salad, or processed meats. Even if the bacteria are killed by warming, the heat-stable toxin is not

TABLE 129-2 CASE DEFINITION OF *S. AUREUS* TOXIC SHOCK SYNDROME

1. Fever: temperature of ≥38.9°C (≥102°F)
2. Hypotension: systolic blood pressure of ≤90 mmHg, or orthostatic hypotension (orthostatic drop in diastolic blood pressure by ≥15 mmHg, orthostatic syncope, or orthostatic dizziness)
3. Diffuse macular rash with subsequent desquamation in 1 to 2 weeks after onset (including the palms and soles)
4. Multisystem involvement
   a. Hepatic: bilirubin or aminotransferase levels ≥2 times normal
   b. Hematologic: platelet count ≤100,000/μL
   c. Renal: blood urea nitrogen or serum creatinine level ≥2 times the normal upper limit
   d. Mucous membranes: vaginal, oropharyngeal, or conjunctival hyperemia
   e. Gastrointestinal: vomiting or diarrhea at onset of illness
   f. Muscular: severe myalgias or serum creatine phosphokinase level ≥2 times the upper limit
   g. Central nervous system: disorientation or alteration in consciousness without focal neurologic signs and in the absence of fever and hypotension
5. Negative serologic or other tests for measles, leptospirosis, and Rocky Mountain spotted fever as well as negative blood or cerebrospinal fluid cultures for organisms other than *S. aureus*

Source: M Wharton et al: Case definitions for public health surveillance. MMWR 39:1, 1990; with permission.

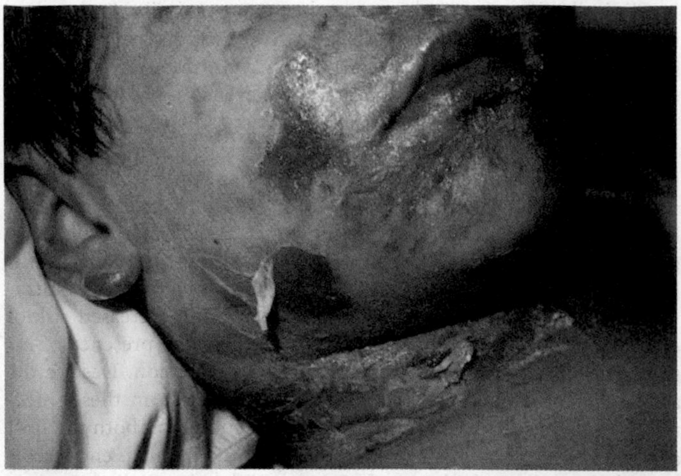

FIGURE 129-4 Evidence of staphylococcal scalded-skin syndrome in a 6-year-old boy. Nikolsky's sign, with separation of the superficial layer of the outer epidermal layer, is visible. *(Reprinted with permission from LA Schenfeld et al: Images in clinical medicine. Staphylococcal scalded skin syndrome. N Engl J Med 342:1178, 2000. © 2000 Massachusetts Medical Society. All rights reserved.)*

destroyed. The onset of illness is rapid, occurring within 1–6 h of ingestion. The illness is characterized by nausea and vomiting, although diarrhea, hypotension, and dehydration may also occur. The differential diagnosis includes diarrhea of other etiologies, especially that caused by similar toxins (e.g., the toxins elaborated by *Bacillus cereus*). The rapidity of onset, the absence of fever, and the epidemic nature of the presentation arouse suspicion of food poisoning. Symptoms generally resolve within 8–10 h. The diagnosis can be established by the demonstration of bacteria or the documentation of enterotoxin in the implicated food. Treatment is entirely supportive.

STAPHYLOCOCCAL SCALDED-SKIN SYNDROME SSSS most often affects newborns and children. The illness may vary from localized blister formation to exfoliation of much of the skin surface. The skin is usually fragile and often tender, with thin-walled, fluid-filled bullae. Gentle pressure results in rupture of the lesions, leaving denuded underlying skin (Nikolsky's sign; **Fig. 129-4**). The mucous membranes are usually spared. In more generalized infection, there are often constitutional symptoms, including fever, lethargy, and irritability with poor feeding. Significant amounts of fluid can be lost in more extensive cases. Illness usually follows localized infection at one of a number of possible sites. SSSS is much less common among adults but can follow infections caused by exfoliative toxin–producing strains.

PREVENTION

Prevention of the spread of *S. aureus* infections in the hospital setting involves hand washing and careful attention to appropriate isolation procedures. Through strict isolation practices, some Scandinavian countries have been remarkably successful at preventing the introduction and dissemination of MRSA in hospitals. Other countries, such as the United States and Great Britain, have been less successful.

The use of topical antimicrobial agents (e.g., mupirocin) to eliminate nasal colonization with *S. aureus* and to prevent subsequent infection has been investigated in a number of clinical settings. Elimination of nasal carriage of *S. aureus* has reduced the incidence of infections among patients undergoing hemodialysis and peritoneal dialysis. The prophylactic efficacy of topical mupirocin applied to the nares has been extensively investigated. While mupirocin eliminates nasal colonization with *S. aureus*, clinical trials to date have failed to demonstrate a subsequent reduction in the incidence of staphylococcal infections.

A capsular polysaccharide–protein conjugate vaccine and antibodies to the ligand-binding domains of several MSCRAMMs (e.g., clumping factor) are under investigation. While in vivo studies have been promising in either preventing or reducing the incidence of infections, none of these vaccines has yet been successful for either prophylaxis or therapy.

COAGULASE-NEGATIVE STAPHYLOCOCCAL INFECTIONS

CoNS, although considerably less virulent than *S. aureus*, are among the most common causes of prosthetic-device infections. Approximately half of the identified CoNS species have been associated with human infections. Of these species, *S. epidermidis* is the most common human pathogen overall; this component of the normal human flora is found on the skin (where it is the most abundant bacterial species) as well as in the oropharynx and vagina. *S. saprophyticus*, a novobiocin-resistant species, is a pathogen in UTIs.

PATHOGENESIS

Among CoNS, *S. epidermidis* is the species most commonly associated with prosthetic-device infections. Infection is a two-step process, with initial adhesion to the device followed by colonization. *S. epidermidis* is uniquely adapted to colonize these devices by its capacity to elaborate the extracellular polysaccharide (glycocalyx or slime) that facilitates formation of a protective biofilm on the device surface.

Implanted prosthetic material is often coated with host serum or tissue constituents such as fibrinogen or fibronectin. These molecules serve as potential bridging ligands, facilitating bacterial attachment to the device surface. A number of surface-associated proteins, such as autolysin (AtlE), fibrinogen-binding protein, and accumulation-associated protein (AAP), may play a role in attachment to either modified or unmodified prosthetic surfaces. The polysaccharide intercellular adhesin facilitates subsequent staphylococcal colonization and accumulation on the device surface. In *S. epidermidis*, *ica* genes are more commonly found in strains associated with device infections than in strains associated with colonization of mucosal surfaces. Biofilm appears to act as a barrier protecting bacteria from host defense mechanisms as well as from antibiotics, while providing a suitable environment for bacterial survival. Poly-γ-DL-glutamic acid is secreted by *S. epidermidis* and promotes protection against neutrophil phagocytosis.

Two additional staphylococcal species, *S. lugdunensis* and *S. schleiferi*, produce more serious infections (native-valve endocarditis and osteomyelitis) than do other CoNS. The basis for this enhanced virulence is not known, although both species appear to share more virulence determinants with *S. aureus* (e.g., clumping factor and lipase) than do other CoNS.

The capacity of *S. saprophyticus* to cause UTIs in young women appears to be related to its enhanced capacity to adhere to uroepithelial cells. A 160-kDa hemagglutinin/adhesin may contribute to this affinity.

DIAGNOSIS

While the detection of CoNS at sites of infection or in the bloodstream is not difficult by standard microbiologic culture methods, interpretation of these results is frequently problematic. Since these organisms are present in large numbers on the skin, they often contaminate cultures. It has been estimated that only 10–25% of blood cultures positive for CoNS reflect true bacteremia. Similar problems arise with cultures of other sites. Among the clinical findings suggestive of true bacteremia are fever, evidence of local infection (e.g., erythema or purulent drainage at the IV catheter site), leukocytosis, and systemic signs of sepsis. Laboratory findings suggestive of true bacteremia include multiple isolations of the same strain (i.e., the same species with the same antibiogram or a closely related DNA fingerprint) from separate cultures, growth of the strain within 48 h, and bacterial growth in both aerobic and anaerobic bottles.

CLINICAL SYNDROMES

CoNS cause diverse prosthetic device–related infections, including those that involve prosthetic cardiac valves and joints, vascular grafts, intravascular devices, and CNS shunts. In all of these settings, the clinical presentation is similar. The signs of localized infection are often subtle, the rate of disease progression is slow, and the systemic findings are often limited. Signs of infection, such as purulent drainage, pain at the site, or loosening of prosthetic implants, are sometimes evident. Fever is frequently but not always present, and there may be mild leukocytosis.

Infections that are not associated with prosthetic devices are infrequent, although native-valve endocarditis due to CoNS has accounted for ~5% of cases in some reviews. *S. lugdunensis* appears to be a more aggressive pathogen in this setting, causing greater mortality and rapid valvular destruction with abscess formation.

Rx STAPHYLOCOCCAL INFECTIONS

GENERAL PRINCIPLES OF THERAPY Surgical incision and drainage of all suppurative collections constitute the most important therapeutic intervention for staphylococcal infections. The emergence of MRSA in the community has increased the importance of culturing all collections in order to identify pathogens and to determine antimicrobial susceptibility. Prosthetic-device infections are unlikely to be successfully managed unless the device is removed. In the limited number of situations in which removal is not possible or the infection is due to CoNS, an initial attempt at medical therapy without device removal may be warranted. Because of the well-recognized risk of complications associated with *S. aureus* bacteremia, therapy is generally prolonged (4–8 weeks) unless the patient is identified as being one of the small percentage of individuals who are at low risk for complications—e.g., immunocompetent patients and patients whose *S. aureus* infection is associated with a removable focus (such as an IV catheter) and whose device is promptly removed.

DURATION OF ANTIMICROBIAL THERAPY Debate continues regarding the duration of therapy for bacteremic *S. aureus* infections. No carefully controlled, prospective study has addressed this question. A meta-analysis reviewing studies relevant to this issue concluded that insufficient information was available to determine which patients were candidates for short-course therapy (2 weeks rather than 4–8 weeks).

Among the findings associated with an increased risk of complicated bacteremia are persistently positive blood cultures 48–96 h after institution of therapy, acquisition of the infection in the community, a removable focus of infection (i.e., an intravascular catheter) that is not removed, and cutaneous or embolic manifestations of infection. In those immunocompetent patients for whom short-course therapy is planned, TEE to rule out endocarditis is warranted since neither clinical nor laboratory findings are adequate to detect cardiac involvement. In addition, an aggressive radiologic investigation to identify potential metastatic collections is indicated. All symptomatic sites must be carefully evaluated.

CHOICE OF ANTIMICROBIAL AGENTS The choice of antimicrobial agents to treat both coagulase-positive staphylococcal and CoNS infections has become increasingly problematic because of the prevalence of multidrug-resistant strains. Data collected by the Centers for Disease Control and Prevention from intensive care units in the United States (1988–1998) show a dramatic increase in the number of isolates susceptible only to vancomycin. This trend is especially apparent with CoNS: >80% of nosocomial isolates are resistant to methicillin, and these MRSA strains are usually resistant to most other antibiotics as well. Because the selection of antimicrobial agents for the treatment of *S. aureus* infections is similar to that for CoNS infections, treatment options for these pathogens are discussed together and are summarized in **Table 129-3**.

As a result of the widespread dissemination of plasmids containing the enzyme penicillinase, few strains of staphylococci (<5%) remain susceptible to penicillin. However, against susceptible strains, penicillin remains the drug of choice. Penicillin-resistant isolates are treated with semisynthetic penicillinase-resistant penicillins (SPRPs), such as oxacillin or nafcillin. Methicillin, the first of the SPRPs, is now used infrequently. Cephalosporins are alternative therapeutic agents for these infections. Second- and third-generation cephalosporins do not have a therapeutic advantage over first-generation cephalosporins for the treatment of staphylococcal infections. The carbapenem imipenem has excellent activity against methicillin-sensitive *S. aureus* (MSSA) but not MRSA.

The isolation of MRSA was reported within 1 year of the introduction of methicillin. The prevalence of MRSA has since increased steadily. In many hospitals, 40–50% of *S. aureus* isolates are now resistant to methicillin. Resistance to methicillin indicates resistance to all SPRPs as well as all cephalosporins. Many MRSA isolates are also resistant to other antimicrobial families, including aminoglycosides, quinolones, and macrolides.

Production of a novel penicillin-binding protein (PBP 2a or 2′) is responsible for methicillin resistance. This protein is synthesized by the *mecA* gene, which (as stated above) is part of a large mobile genetic element—a pathogenicity or genomic island—called SCC*mec*. It is hypothesized that acquisition of this genetic material resulted from horizontal transfer from a related staphylococcal species, such as *S. sciuri*. Phenotypic expression of methicillin resistance may be constitutive (i.e., expressed in all organisms in a population) or heterogeneous (i.e., displayed by only a proportion of the total organism population). Detection of methicillin resistance in the clinical microbiology laboratory can be difficult if the strain expresses heterogeneous resistance. Therefore, susceptibility studies are routinely performed at reduced temperatures (≤35°C for 24 h), with increased concentrations of salt in the medium to enhance the expression of resistance. In addition to PCR-based techniques, a number of rapid methods for the detection of methicillin resistance have been developed.

Vancomycin remains the drug of choice for the treatment of MRSA infections. Because it is less bactericidal than the β-lactams, it should be used only after careful consideration in patients with a history of β-lactam allergies. In 1997, an *S. aureus* strain with reduced susceptibility to vancomycin (VISA) was reported from Japan. Subsequently, additional clinical isolates of VISA were reported from geographically disparate locations. These strains were all resistant to methicillin and many other antimicrobial agents. The VISA strains appear to evolve (under vancomycin selective pressure) from strains that are susceptible to vancomycin but are heterogeneous, with a small proportion of the bacterial population expressing the resistance phenotype. The mechanism of VISA resistance is due to an abnormal cell wall. Vancomycin is trapped by the abnormal peptidoglycan cross-linking and is unable to gain access to its target site.

In 2002, the first clinical isolate of fully vancomycin-resistant *S. aureus* was reported. Resistance in this and three subsequently reported clinical isolates was due to the presence of *vanA*, the gene responsible for expression of vancomycin resistance in enterococci. This observation suggested that resistance was acquired as a result of horizontal conjugal transfer from a vancomycin-resistant strain of *Enterococcus faecalis*. Several patients had both MRSA and vancomycin-resistant enterococci cultured from infection sites. The isolates remained susceptible to chloramphenicol, linezolid, minocycline, quinupristin/dalfopristin, and trimethoprim-sulfamethoxazole (TMP-SMX). The *vanA* gene is responsible for the synthesis of the dipeptide D-Ala-D-Lac in place of D-Ala-D-Ala. Vancomycin cannot bind to the altered peptide.

Alternatives to the β-lactams and vancomycin have less antistaphylococcal activity. Although the quinolones have reasonable in vitro activity against staphylococci, the frequency of fluoroquinolone resistance has in-

TABLE 129-3 ANTIMICROBIAL THERAPY FOR SERIOUS STAPHYLOCOCCAL INFECTIONS[a]

Sensitivity/ Resistance of Isolate	Drug of Choice	Alternative(s)	Comments
Sensitive to penicillin	Penicillin G (4 mU q4h)	Nafcillin (2 g q4h) or oxacillin (2 g q4h), cefazolin (2 g q8h), vancomycin (1 g q12h[b])	Fewer than 5% of isolates are sensitive to penicillin.
Sensitive to methicillin	Nafcillin or oxacillin (2 g q4h)	Cefazolin (2 g q8h[b]), vancomycin (1 g q12h[b])	Patients with penicillin allergy can be treated with a cephalosporin if the allergy does not involve an anaphylactic or accelerated reaction; vancomycin is the alternative. Desensitization to β-lactams may be indicated in selected cases of serious infection where maximal bactericidal activity is needed (e.g., prosthetic-valve endocarditis[d]). Type A β-lactamase may rapidly hydrolyze cefazolin and reduce its efficacy in endocarditis.
Resistant to methicillin	Vancomycin (1 g q12h[b])	TMP-SMX (TMP, 5 mg/kg q12h[b]), minocycline or doxycycline(100 mg PO q12h[b]), ciprofloxacin (400 mg q12h[b]), levofloxacin (500 mg q24h[b]), quinupristin/dalfopristin (7.5 mg/kg q8h), linezolid (600 mg q12h *except*: 400 mg q12h for uncomplicated skin infections); daptomycin (4–6 mg/kg q24h[b, c]) for bacteremia, endocarditis, and complicated skin infections; tigecycline (100 mg IV once, then 50 mg q12h) for skin and soft tissue infections; investigational drugs: oritavancin, dalbavancin, telavancin	Sensitivity testing is necessary before an alternative drug is used. Adjunctive drugs (those that should be used only in combination with other antimicrobial agents) include gentamicin (1 mg/kg q8h[b]), rifampin (300 mg PO q8h), and fusidic acid (500 mg q8h; not readily available in the United States). Quinupristin/dalfopristin is bactericidal against methicillin-resistant isolates unless the strain is resistant to erythromycin or clindamycin. The newer quinolones may retain in vitro activity against ciprofloxacin-resistant isolates; resistance may develop during therapy. The efficacy of adjunctive therapy is not well established in many settings. Both linezolid and quinupristin/dalfopristin have had in vitro activity against most VISA and VRSA strains. See footnote for treatment of prosthetic-valve endocarditis.[d]
Resistant to methicillin with intermediate or complete resistance to vancomycin[e]	Uncertain	Same as for methicillin-resistant strains; check antibiotic susceptibilities	Same as for methicillin-resistant strains; check antibiotic susceptibilities.
Not yet known (i.e., empirical therapy)	Vancomycin (1 g q12h)	—	Empirical therapy is given when the susceptibility of the isolate is not known. Vancomycin with or without an aminoglycoside is recommended for suspected community- or hospital-acquired *S. aureus* infections because of the increased frequency of methicillin-resistant strains in the community.

[a]Recommended dosages are for adults with normal renal and hepatic function. The route of administration is intravenous unless otherwise indicated.
[b]The dosage must be adjusted in patients with reduced creatinine clearance.
[c]Daptomycin cannot be used for pneumonia.
[d]For the treatment of prosthetic-valve endocarditis, the addition of gentamicin (1 mg/kg q8h) and rifampin (300 mg PO q8h) is recommended, with adjustment of the gentamicin dosage if the creatinine clearance rate is reduced.
[e]Vancomycin-resistant *S. aureus* isolates from clinical infections have been reported.
Source: Modified with permission of the *New England Journal of Medicine* (Lowy, 1998).
Note: TMP-SMX, trimethoprim-sulfamethoxazole; VISA, vancomycin-intermediate *S. aureus*; VRSA, vancomycin-resistant *S. aureus*.

creased progressively, especially among methicillin-resistant isolates. MSSA strains have remained more susceptible to the fluoroquinolones than have methicillin-resistant strains. Of particular concern in MRSA is the possible emergence of quinolone resistance during therapy. Resistance to the quinolones is most commonly chromosomal and results from mutations of the topoisomerase IV or DNA gyrase genes, although multidrug efflux pumps may also contribute. While the newer quinolones exhibit increased in vitro activity against staphylococci, it is uncertain whether this increase translates into enhanced in vivo activity. Other antibiotics, such as minocycline and TMP-SMX, have been successfully used to treat MRSA infections in the face of vancomycin toxicity or intolerance.

Among the newer antistaphylococcal agents, the parenteral streptogramin quinupristin/dalfopristin displays bactericidal activity against all staphylococci, including VISA strains. This drug has been used successfully to treat serious MRSA infections. In cases of erythromycin or clindamycin resistance, quinupristin/dalfopristin is bacteriostatic against staphylococci.

Linezolid—the first member of a new drug family, the oxazolidinones—is bacteriostatic against staphylococci, has been well tolerated, and offers the advantage of comparable bioavailability after oral or parenteral administration. Cross-resistance with other inhibitors of protein synthesis has not been reported. Resistance to linezolid, although limited, has been reported. The efficacy of linezolid in the treatment of deep-seated infections such as osteomyelitis has not yet been established. There are insufficient data on the efficacy of either quinupristin/dalfopristin or linezolid for the treatment of infective endocarditis. Daptomycin, a new parenteral bactericidal agent with antistaphylococcal activity, is approved for the treatment of bacteremias (including right-sided endocarditis) and complicated skin infections. It is not effective in respiratory infections. This drug has a novel mechanism of action: it disrupts the cytoplasmic membrane. Staphylococcal resistance to daptomycin has been reported. Tigecycline, a broad-spectrum minocycline analogue, has bacteriostatic activity against MRSA and is approved for use in skin and soft tissue infections as well as intraabdominal infections caused by *S. aureus*. A number of additional antistaphylococcal agents (e.g., dalbavancin, oritavancin, and ceftobiprole) are undergoing clinical trials.

Combinations of antistaphylococcal agents are sometimes used to enhance bactericidal activity in the treatment of serious infections such as endocarditis or osteomyelitis. In selected instances (e.g., right-sided endocarditis), drug combinations are also used to shorten the duration of therapy. Among the antimicrobial agents used in combinations are rifampin, aminoglycosides (e.g., gentamicin), and fusidic acid (which is not readily available in the United States). While these agents are not effective singly because of the frequent emergence of resistance, they have proved useful in combination with other agents because of their bactericidal activity against staphylococci.

In vitro studies have demonstrated synergy against staphylococci with the following combinations: (1) β-lactams and aminoglycosides; (2) vancomycin and gentamicin; (3) vancomycin, gentamicin, and rifampin (against CoNS); and (4) vancomycin and rifampin. In several instances, these in vitro observations have been supported by studies in the experimental animal model of endocarditis. There is limited information on combinations including newer agents such as daptomycin and tigecycline.

ANTIMICROBIAL THERAPY FOR SELECTED SETTINGS For uncomplicated skin and soft tissue infections, the use of oral antistaphylococcal agents is usually successful. For other infections, parenteral therapy is indicated.

S. aureus endocarditis is usually an acute, life-threatening infection. Thus prompt collection of blood for cultures must be followed immediately by empirical antimicrobial therapy. For *S. aureus* native-valve endocarditis, a combination of antimicrobial agents is often used. In a large prospective study, an SPRP combined with an aminoglycoside did not alter clinical outcome but did reduce the duration of *S. aureus* bacteremia. As a result, many clinicians begin therapy for life-threatening infections with a 3- to 5-day course of a β-lactam and an aminoglycoside (gentamicin, 1 mg/kg IV every 8 h). If a MRSA strain is isolated, vancomycin (30 mg/kg every 24 h, given in two equal doses up to a total of 2 g) is recommended. Patients are generally treated for 6 weeks.

In prosthetic-valve endocarditis, surgery in addition to antibiotic therapy is often necessary. The combination of a β-lactam agent—or, if the isolate is β-lactam-resistant, vancomycin (30 mg/kg every 24 h, given in two equal doses up to a total of 2 g)—with an aminoglycoside (gentamicin, 1 mg/kg IV every 8 h) and rifampin (300 mg orally or IV every 8 h) is recommended. This combination is used to avoid the possible emergence of rifampin resistance during therapy if only two drugs are used.

For hematogenous osteomyelitis or septic arthritis in children, a 4-week course of therapy is usually adequate. In adults, treatment is often more prolonged. For chronic forms of osteomyelitis, surgical debridement is necessary in combination with antimicrobial therapy. For joint infections, a critical component of therapy is the repeated aspiration or arthroscopy of the affected joint to prevent damage from leukocytes. The combination of rifampin with ciprofloxacin has been used successfully to treat prosthetic-joint infections, especially when the device cannot be removed. The efficacy of this combination may reflect enhanced activity against staphylococci in biofilms as well as the attainment of effective intracellular concentrations.

The choice of empirical therapy for staphylococcal infections depends in part on susceptibility data for the local geographic area. Increasingly, vancomycin (in combination with an aminoglycoside or rifampin for serious infections) is the drug of choice for both community- and hospital-acquired infections.

The increase in community-based MRSA skin and soft tissue infections has drawn attention to the need for initiation of appropriate empirical therapy. Oral agents that have been effective against these isolates include clindamycin, TMP-SMX, doxycycline, and linezolid. The antimicrobial susceptibility of isolates in different geographic regions has varied.

THERAPY FOR TOXIC SHOCK SYNDROME Supportive therapy with reversal of hypotension is the mainstay of therapy for TSS. Both fluids and pressors may be necessary. Tampons or other packing material should be promptly removed. The role of antibiotics is less clear. Some investigators recommend a combination of clindamycin and a semisynthetic penicillin. Clindamycin is advocated because, as a protein synthesis inhibitor, it reduces toxin synthesis in vitro. A semisynthetic penicillin is suggested to eliminate any potential focus of infection as well as to eradicate persistent carriage that might increase the likelihood of recurrent illness. Anecdotal reports document the successful use of IV immunoglobulin to treat TSS. The role of glucocorticoids in the treatment of this disease is uncertain at present.

THERAPY FOR OTHER TOXIN-MEDIATED DISEASES Therapy for staphylococcal food poisoning is entirely supportive. For SSSS, antistaphylococcal therapy targets the primary site of infection.

FURTHER READINGS

DIEP BA et al: Complete genome sequence of USA300, an epidemic clone of community-acquired meticillin-resistant *Staphylococcus aureus*. Lancet 367:731, 2006

FOWLER VG JR et al: *Staphylococcus aureus* endocarditis: A consequence of medical progress. JAMA 293:3012, 2005

——— et al: Role of echocardiography in evaluation of patients with *Staphylococcus aureus* bacteremia: Experience in 103 patients. J Am Coll Cardiol 30:1072, 1997

FRIDKIN SK et al: Methicillin-resistant *Staphylococcus aureus* disease in three communities. N Engl J Med 352:1436, 2005

GRUNDMANN H et al: Emergence and resurgence of meticillin-resistant *Staphylococcus aureus* as a public-health threat. Lancet 368:874, 2006

LOWY FD: Antimicrobial resistance: The example of *Staphylococcus aureus*. J Clin Invest 111:1265, 2003

MCCORMICK JK et al: Toxic shock syndrome and bacterial superantigens: An update. Annu Rev Microbiol 55:77, 2001

MORAN GJ et al: Methicillin-resistant *S. aureus* infections among patients in the emergency department. N Engl J Med 355:666, 2006

MYLOTTE JM, TAYARA A: *Staphylococcus aureus* bacteremia: Predictors of 30-day mortality in a large cohort. Clin Infect Dis 31:1170, 2000

SEYBOLD U et al: Emergence of community-associated methicillin-resistant *Staphylococcus aureus* USA300 genotype as a major cause of health care–associated blood stream infections. Clin Infect Dis 42:647, 2006

130 Streptococcal and Enterococcal Infections

Michael R. Wessels

Many varieties of streptococci are found as part of the normal flora colonizing the human respiratory, gastrointestinal, and genitourinary tracts. Several species are important causes of human disease. Group A *Streptococcus* (GAS, *S. pyogenes*) is responsible for streptococcal pharyngitis, one of the most common bacterial infections of school-age children, and for the postinfectious syndromes of acute rheumatic fever (ARF) and poststreptococcal glomerulonephritis (PSGN). Group B *Streptococcus* (GBS, *S. agalactiae*) is the leading cause of bacterial sepsis and meningitis in newborns and a major cause of endometritis and fever in parturient women. Enterococci are important causes of urinary tract infection, nosocomial bacteremia, and endocarditis. Viridans streptococci are the most common cause of bacterial endocarditis.

Streptococci are gram-positive, spherical to ovoid bacteria that characteristically form chains when grown in liquid media. Most streptococci that cause human infections are facultative anaerobes, although some are strict anaerobes. Streptococci are relatively fastidious organisms, requiring enriched media for growth in the laboratory. Clinicians and clinical microbiologists identify streptococci by several classification systems, including hemolytic pattern, Lancefield group, species name, and common or trivial name. Many streptococci associated with human infection produce a zone of complete (β) hemolysis around the bacterial colony when cultured on blood agar. The β-hemolytic streptococci can be classified by the Lancefield system, a serologic grouping based on the reaction of specific antisera with bacterial cell-wall carbohydrate antigens. With rare exceptions, organisms belonging to Lancefield groups A, B, C, and G are all β-hemolytic, and each is associated with characteristic patterns of human infection. Other streptococci produce a zone of partial (α) hemolysis, often imparting a greenish appearance to the agar. These α-hemolytic streptococci are further identified by biochemical testing and include *S. pneumoniae* (Chap. 128), an important cause of pneumonia, meningitis, and other infections, and several species referred to collectively as the *viridans streptococci*, which are part of the normal oral flora and are important agents of subacute bacterial endocarditis. Finally, some streptococci are nonhemolytic, a pattern sometimes called *γ hemolysis*. The classification of the major streptococcal groups causing human infections is outlined in Table 130-1. Among the organisms classified serologically as group D streptococci, the enterococci are now considered a separate genus on the basis of DNA homology studies. Thus species previously designated as *S. faecalis* and *S. faecium* have been renamed *Enterococcus faecalis* and *E. faecium*, respectively.

TABLE 130-1 CLASSIFICATION OF STREPTOCOCCI

Lancefield Group	Representative Species	Hemolytic Pattern	Typical Infections
A	*S. pyogenes*	β	Pharyngitis, impetigo, cellulitis, scarlet fever
B	*S. agalactiae*	β	Neonatal sepsis and meningitis, puerperal infection, urinary tract infection, diabetic ulcer infection, endocarditis
C, G	*S. dysgalactiae* subsp. *equisimilis*	β	Cellulitis, bacteremia, endocarditis
D	Enterococci: *E. faecalis; E. faecium*	Usually nonhemolytic	Urinary tract infection, nosocomial bacteremia, endocarditis
	Nonenterococci: *S. bovis*	Usually nonhemolytic	Bacteremia, endocarditis
Variable or nongroupable	Viridans streptococci: *S. sanguis; S. mitis*	α	Endocarditis, dental abscess, brain abscess
	Intermedius or *milleri* group: *S. intermedius, S. anginosus, S. constellatus*	Variable	Brain abscess, visceral abscess
	Anaerobic streptococci: *Peptostreptococcus magnus*	Usually nonhemolytic	Sinusitis, pneumonia, empyema, brain abscess, liver abscess

GROUP A STREPTOCOCCI

Lancefield's group A consists of a single species, *S. pyogenes*. As its species name implies, this organism is associated with a variety of suppurative infections. In addition, GAS can trigger the postinfectious syndromes of ARF (which is uniquely associated with *S. pyogenes* infection; Chap. 315) and PSGN (Chap. 277).

Worldwide, GAS infections and their postinfectious sequelae (primarily ARF and rheumatic heart disease) account for an estimated 500,000 deaths per year. Although data are incomplete, the incidence of all forms of GAS infection and that of rheumatic heart disease are thought to be tenfold higher in resource-limited countries than in developed countries (Fig. 130-1).

PATHOGENESIS

GAS elaborates a number of cell-surface components and extracellular products important in both the pathogenesis of infection and the human immune response. The cell wall contains a carbohydrate antigen that may be released by acid treatment. The reaction of such acid extracts with group A–specific antiserum is the basis for definitive identification of a streptococcal strain as *S. pyogenes*. The major surface protein of GAS is M protein, which occurs in more than 100 antigenically distinct types and is the basis for the serotyping of strains with specific antisera. The M protein molecules are fibrillar structures anchored in the cell wall of the organism that extend as hairlike projections away from the cell surface. The amino acid sequence of the distal or amino-terminal portion of the M protein molecule is quite variable, accounting for the antigenic variation of the different M types, while more proximal regions of the protein are relatively conserved. A newer technique for assignment of M type to GAS isolates uses the polymerase chain reaction to amplify the variable region of the M protein gene. DNA sequence analysis of the amplified gene segment can be compared with an extensive database [developed at the Centers for Disease Control and Prevention (CDC)] for assignment of M type. This method eliminates the need for typing sera, which are available in only a few reference laboratories. The presence of M protein on a GAS isolate correlates with its capacity to resist phagocytic killing in fresh human blood. This phenomenon appears to be due, at least in part, to the binding of plasma fibrinogen to M protein molecules on the streptococcal surface, which interferes with complement activation and deposition of opsonic complement fragments on the bacterial cell. This resistance to phagocytosis may be overcome by M protein–specific antibodies; thus individuals with antibodies to a given M type acquired as a result of prior infection are protected against subsequent infection with organisms of the same M type but not against that with different M types.

GAS also elaborates, to varying degrees, a polysaccharide capsule composed of hyaluronic acid. The production of large amounts of capsule by certain strains lends a characteristic mucoid appearance to the colonies. The capsular polysaccharide plays an important role in protecting GAS from ingestion and killing by phagocytes. In contrast to M protein, the hyaluronic acid capsule is a weak immunogen, and antibodies to hyaluronate have not been shown to be important in protective immunity. The presumed explanation is the apparent structural identity between streptococcal hyaluronic acid and the hyaluronic acid of mammalian connective tissues. The capsular polysaccharide may also play a role in GAS colonization of the pharynx by binding to CD44, a hyaluronic acid–binding protein expressed on human pharyngeal epithelial cells.

GAS produces a large number of extracellular products that may be important in local and systemic toxicity and in the spread of infection through tissues. These products include streptolysins S and O, toxins that damage cell membranes and account for the hemolysis produced by the organisms; streptokinase; DNases; protease; and pyrogenic exotoxins A, B, and C. The pyrogenic exotoxins, previously known as erythrogenic toxins, cause the rash of scarlet fever. Since the mid-1980s, pyrogenic exotoxin–producing strains of GAS have been linked to unusually severe invasive infections, including necrotizing fasciitis and the streptococcal toxic shock syndrome. Several extracellular

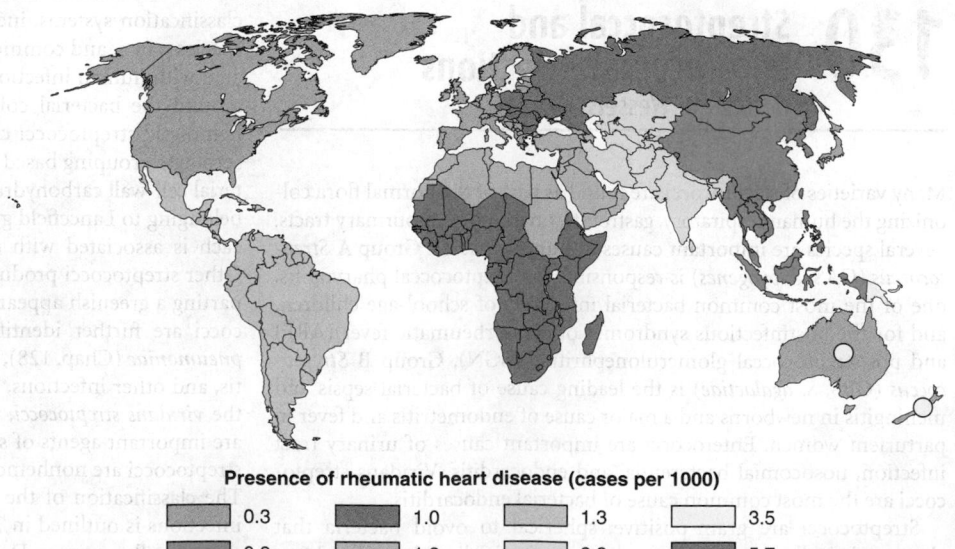

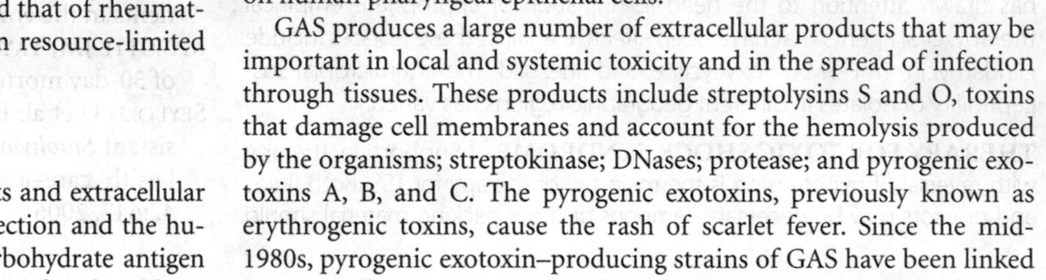

FIGURE 130-1 Prevalence of rheumatic heart disease in children 5–14 years old. The circles within Australia and New Zealand represent indigenous populations (and also Pacific Islanders in New Zealand). *(From Carapetis et al, 2005, with permission.)*

products stimulate specific antibody responses useful for serodiagnosis of recent streptococcal infection. Tests for these antibodies are used primarily for detection of preceding streptococcal infection in cases of suspected ARF or PSGN.

CLINICAL MANIFESTATIONS

Pharyngitis Although seen in patients of all ages, GAS pharyngitis is one of the most common bacterial infections of childhood, accounting for 20–40% of all cases of exudative pharyngitis in children; it is rare among those under the age of 3. Younger children may manifest streptococcal infection with a syndrome of fever, malaise, and lymphadenopathy without exudative pharyngitis. Infection is acquired through contact with another individual carrying the organism. Respiratory droplets are the usual mechanism of spread, although other routes, including food-borne outbreaks, have been well described.

The incubation period is 1–4 days. Symptoms include sore throat, fever and chills, malaise, and sometimes abdominal complaints and vomiting, particularly in children. Both symptoms and signs are quite variable, ranging from mild throat discomfort with minimal physical findings to high fever and severe sore throat associated with intense erythema and swelling of the pharyngeal mucosa and the presence of purulent exudate over the posterior pharyngeal wall and tonsillar pillars. Enlarged, tender anterior cervical lymph nodes commonly accompany exudative pharyngitis.

The differential diagnosis of streptococcal pharyngitis includes the many other bacterial and viral etiologies (Table 130-2). Streptococcal infection is an unlikely cause when symptoms and signs suggestive of viral infection are prominent (conjunctivitis, coryza, cough, hoarseness, or discrete ulcerative lesions of the buccal or pharyngeal mucosa). Because of the range of clinical presentations of streptococcal pharyngitis and the large number of other agents that can produce the same clinical picture, diagnosis of streptococcal pharyngitis on clinical grounds alone is not reliable.

The throat culture remains the diagnostic gold standard. Culture of a throat specimen that is properly collected (i.e., by vigorous rubbing of a sterile swab over both tonsillar pillars) and properly processed is the most sensitive and specific means of definitive diagnosis. A rapid diagnostic kit for latex agglutination or enzyme immunoassay of swab specimens is a useful adjunct to throat culture. While precise figures on sensitivity and specificity vary, rapid diagnostic kits generally are >95% specific. Thus a positive result can be relied upon for definitive diagnosis and eliminates the need for throat culture. However, because rapid diagnostic tests are less sensitive than throat culture (relative sensitivity in comparative studies, 55–90%), a negative result should be confirmed by throat culture.

TABLE 130-2 INFECTIOUS ETIOLOGIES OF ACUTE PHARYNGITIS

Organism	Associated Clinical Syndrome(s)
Viruses	
Rhinovirus	Common cold
Coronavirus	Common cold
Adenovirus	Pharyngoconjunctival fever
Influenza virus	Influenza
Parainfluenza virus	Cold, croup
Coxsackievirus	Herpangina, hand-foot-and-mouth disease
Herpes simplex virus	Gingivostomatitis (primary infection)
Epstein-Barr virus	Infectious mononucleosis
Cytomegalovirus	Mononucleosis-like syndrome
HIV	Acute (primary) infection syndrome
Bacteria	
Group A streptococci	Pharyngitis, scarlet fever
Group C or G streptococci	Pharyngitis
Mixed anaerobes	Vincent's angina
Arcanobacterium haemolyticum	Pharyngitis, scarlatiniform rash
Neisseria gonorrhoeae	Pharyngitis
Treponema pallidum	Secondary syphilis
Francisella tularensis	Pharyngeal tularemia
Corynebacterium diphtheriae	Diphtheria
Yersinia enterocolitica	Pharyngitis, enterocolitis
Yersinia pestis	Plague
Chlamydiae	
Chlamydia pneumoniae	Bronchitis, pneumonia
Chlamydia psittaci	Psittacosis
Mycoplasmas	
Mycoplasma pneumoniae	Bronchitis, pneumonia

TABLE 130-3 TREATMENT OF GROUP A STREPTOCOCCAL INFECTIONS

Infection	Treatment[a]
Pharyngitis	Benzathine penicillin G, 1.2 mU IM; *or* penicillin V, 250 mg PO tid or 500 mg PO bid × 10 days (Children <27 kg: Benzathine penicillin G, 600,000 units IM; *or* penicillin V, 250 mg PO bid or tid × 10 days)
Impetigo	Same as pharyngitis
Erysipelas/cellulitis	Severe: Penicillin G, 1–2 mU IV q4h Mild to moderate: Procaine penicillin, 1.2 mU IM bid
Necrotizing fasciitis/myositis	Surgical debridement; *plus* penicillin G, 2–4 mU IV q4h; *plus* clindamycin,[b] 600–900 mg q8h
Pneumonia/empyema	Penicillin G, 2–4 mU IV q4h; *plus* drainage of empyema
Streptococcal toxic shock syndrome	Penicillin G, 2–4 mU IV q4h; *plus* clindamycin,[b] 600–900 mg q8h; *plus* intravenous immunoglobulin,[b] 2 g/kg as a single dose

[a]Penicillin allergy: Erythromycin (10 mg/kg PO qid up to a maximum of 250 mg per dose) may be substituted for oral penicillin. Alternative agents for parenteral therapy include first-generation cephalosporins—if the nature of the allergy is not an immediate hypersensitivity reaction (anaphylaxis or urticaria) or another potentially life-threatening manifestation (e.g., severe rash and fever)—or vancomycin.
[b]Efficacy unproven, but recommended by several experts. See text for discussion.

℞ GAS PHARYNGITIS

In the usual course of uncomplicated streptococcal pharyngitis, symptoms resolve after 3–5 days. The course is shortened little by treatment, which is given primarily to prevent suppurative complications and ARF. Prevention of ARF depends on eradication of the organism from the pharynx, not simply on resolution of symptoms, and requires 10 days of penicillin treatment (**Table 130-3**). Erythromycin may be substituted for penicillin in cases of penicillin allergy. Once-daily azithromycin is a more convenient but expensive alternative; a 5-day course is approved, but only limited data support equivalent efficacy to a standard 10-day course.

Resistance to erythromycin and other macrolides is common among isolates from several countries, including Spain, Italy, Finland, Japan, and Korea. Macrolide resistance may be becoming more prevalent elsewhere with the increasing use of this class of antibiotics. In areas with resistance rates exceeding 5–10%, macrolides should be avoided unless results of susceptibility testing are known. Follow-up culture after treatment is no longer routinely recommended but may be warranted in selected cases, such as those involving patients or families with frequent streptococcal infections or those occurring in situations in which the risk of ARF is thought to be high (e.g., when cases of ARF have recently been reported in the community).

COMPLICATIONS Suppurative complications of streptococcal pharyngitis have become uncommon with the widespread use of antibiotics for most symptomatic cases. These complications result from the spread of infection from the pharyngeal mucosa to deeper tissues by direct extension or by the hematogenous or lymphatic route and may include cervical lymphadenitis, peritonsillar or retropharyngeal abscess, sinusitis, otitis media, meningitis, bacteremia, endocarditis, and pneumonia. Local complications, such as peritonsillar or parapharyngeal abscess formation, should be considered in a patient with unusually severe or prolonged symptoms or localized pain associated with high fever and a toxic appearance. Nonsuppurative complications include ARF (Chap. 315) and PSGN (Chap. 277), both of which are thought to result from immune responses to streptococcal infection.

Penicillin treatment of streptococcal pharyngitis has been shown to reduce the likelihood of ARF but not that of PSGN.

Bacteriologic Treatment Failure and the Asymptomatic Carrier State Surveillance cultures have shown that up to 20% of individuals in certain populations may have asymptomatic pharyngeal colonization with GAS. There are no definitive guidelines for management of these asymptomatic carriers or of asymptomatic patients who still have a positive throat culture after a full course of treatment for symptomatic pharyngitis. A reasonable course of action is to give a single 10-day course of penicillin for symptomatic pharyngitis and, if positive cultures persist, not to re-treat unless symptoms recur. Studies of the natural history of streptococcal carriage and infection have shown that the risk both of developing ARF and of transmitting infection to others is substantially lower among asymptomatic carriers than among individuals with symptomatic pharyngitis. Therefore, overly aggressive attempts to eradicate carriage probably are not justified under most circumstances. An exception is the situation in which an asymptomatic carrier is a potential source of infection to others. Outbreaks of food-borne infection and nosocomial puerperal infection have been traced to asymptomatic carriers who may harbor the organisms in the throat, vagina, or anus or on the skin.

℞ ASYMPTOMATIC PHARYNGEAL COLONIZATION WITH GAS

When a carrier is transmitting infection to others, attempts to eradicate carriage are warranted. Data are limited on the best regimen to clear GAS after penicillin alone has failed. The combination of penicillin V (500 mg four times daily for 10 days) and rifampin (600 mg twice daily for the last 4 days) has been used to eliminate pharyngeal carriage. A 10-day course of oral vancomycin (250 mg four times daily) and rifampin (600 mg twice daily) has eradicated rectal colonization.

Scarlet Fever Scarlet fever consists of streptococcal infection, usually pharyngitis, accompanied by a characteristic rash (Fig. 130-2). The rash arises from the effects of one of three toxins, currently designated streptococcal pyrogenic exotoxins A, B, and C and previously known as erythrogenic or scarlet fever toxins. In the past, scarlet fever was thought to reflect infection of an individual lacking toxin-specific immunity with a toxin-producing strain of GAS. Susceptibility to scarlet fever was correlated with results of the Dick test, in which a small amount of erythrogenic toxin injected intradermally produced local erythema in susceptible individuals but elicited no reaction in those with specific immunity. Subsequent studies have suggested that development of the scarlet fever rash may reflect a hypersensitivity reaction requiring prior exposure to the toxin. For reasons that are not clear, scarlet fever has become less common in recent years, although strains of GAS that produce pyrogenic exotoxins continue to be prevalent in the population.

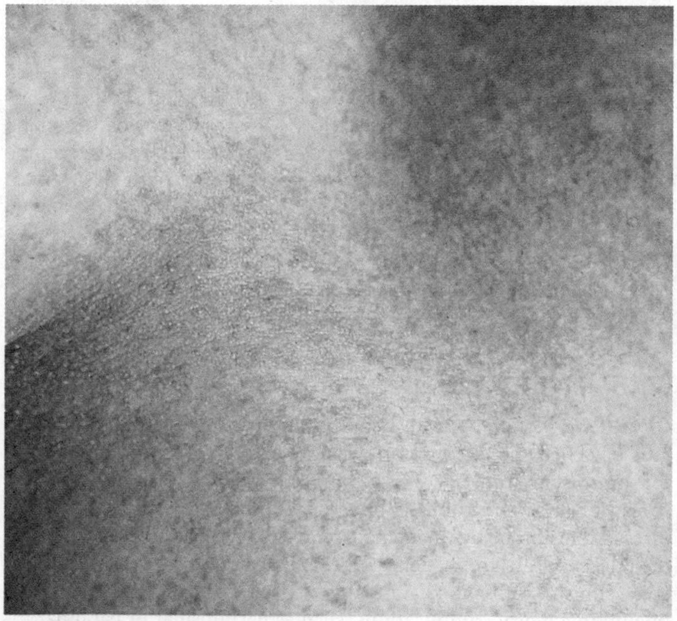

FIGURE 130-2 Scarlet fever exanthem. Finely punctate erythema has become confluent (scarlatiniform); petechiae can occur and have a linear configuration within the exanthem in body folds (Pastia's lines). *(From Fitzpatrick, Johnson, Wolff: Color Atlas and Synopsis of Clinical Dermatology, 4th ed, New York, McGraw-Hill, 2001, with permission.)*

The symptoms of scarlet fever are the same as those of pharyngitis alone. The rash typically begins on the first or second day of illness over the upper trunk, spreading to involve the extremities but sparing the palms and soles. The rash is made up of minute papules, giving a characteristic "sandpaper" feel to the skin. Associated findings include circumoral pallor, "strawberry tongue" (enlarged papillae on a coated tongue, which later may become denuded), and accentuation of the rash in skin folds (Pastia's lines). Subsidence of the rash in 6–9 days is followed after several days by desquamation of the palms and soles. The differential diagnosis of scarlet fever includes other causes of fever and generalized rash, such as measles and other viral exanthems, Kawasaki disease, toxic shock syndrome, and systemic allergic reactions (e.g., drug eruptions).

Skin and Soft Tissue Infections GAS—and occasionally other streptococcal species—causes a variety of infections involving the skin, subcutaneous tissues, muscles, and fascia. While several clinical syndromes offer a useful means for classification of these infections, not all cases fit exactly into one category. The classic syndromes are general guides to predicting the level of tissue involvement in a particular patient, the probable clinical course, and the likelihood that surgical intervention or aggressive life support will be required.

IMPETIGO (PYODERMA) Impetigo, a superficial infection of the skin, is caused primarily by GAS and occasionally by other streptococci or *Staphylococcus aureus*. Impetigo is seen most often in young children, tends to occur during warmer months, and is more common in semitropical or tropical climates than in cooler regions. Infection is more common among children living under conditions of poor hygiene. Prospective studies have shown that colonization of unbroken skin with GAS precedes clinical infection. Minor trauma, such as a scratch or an insect bite, may then serve to inoculate organisms into the skin. Impetigo is best prevented, therefore, by attention to adequate hygiene. The usual sites of involvement are the face (particularly around the nose and mouth) and the legs, although lesions may occur at other locations. Individual lesions begin as red papules, which evolve quickly into vesicular and then pustular lesions that break down and coalesce to form characteristic honeycomb-like crusts (Fig. 130-3). Lesions are generally not painful, and patients do not appear ill. Fever is not a feature of impetigo and, if present, suggests either infection extending to deeper tissues or another diagnosis.

The classic presentation of impetigo usually poses little diagnostic difficulty. Cultures of impetiginous lesions often yield *S. aureus* as well as GAS. In almost all cases, streptococci are isolated initially and staphylococci appear later, presumably as secondary colonizing flora. In the past, penicillin was nearly always effective against these infections. However, an increasing frequency of penicillin treatment failure suggests that *S. aureus* may have become more prominent as a cause of impetigo. *Bullous impetigo* due to *S. aureus* is distinguished from typical streptococcal infection by more extensive, bullous lesions that break down and leave thin paper-like crusts instead of the thick amber crusts of streptococcal impetigo. Other skin lesions that may be confused with impetigo include herpetic lesions—either those of orolabial herpes simplex or those of chickenpox or zoster. Herpetic lesions can generally be distinguished by their appearance as more discrete, grouped vesicles and by a positive Tzanck test. In difficult cases, cultures of vesicular fluid should yield GAS in impetigo and the responsible virus in *Herpesvirus* infections.

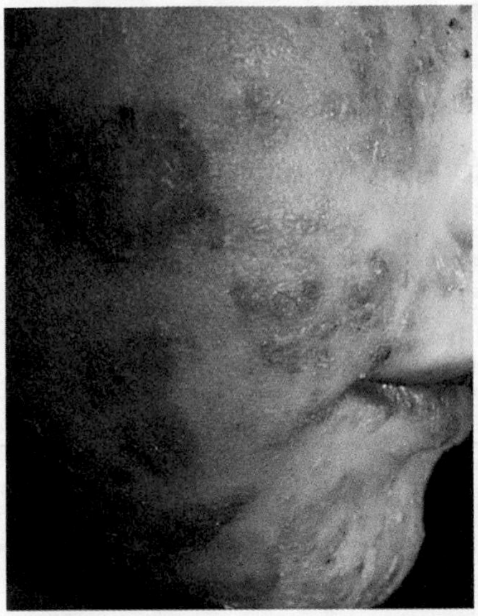

FIGURE 130-3 Impetigo contagiosa is a superficial streptococcal or *Staphylococcus aureus* infection consisting of honey-colored crusts and erythematous weeping erosions. Occasionally, bullous lesions may be seen. *(Courtesy of Mary Spraker, MD; with permission.)*

Rx STREPTOCOCCAL IMPETIGO

Treatment of streptococcal impetigo is the same as that for streptococcal pharyngitis. In view of evidence that *S. aureus* has become a relatively frequent cause of impetigo, empirical regimens should cover both streptococci and *S. aureus*. For example, either dicloxacillin or cephalexin can be given at a dose of 250 mg four times daily for 10 days. Topical mupirocin ointment is also effective. ARF is not a sequela to streptococcal skin infections, although PSGN may follow either skin or throat infection. The reason for this difference is not known. One hypothesis is that the immune response necessary for development of ARF occurs only after infection of the pharyngeal mucosa. In addition, the strains of GAS that cause pharyngitis are generally of different M protein types than those associated with skin infections; thus the strains that cause pharyngitis may have rheumatogenic potential, while the skin-infecting strains may not.

CELLULITIS Inoculation of organisms into the skin may lead to *cellulitis*: infection involving the skin and subcutaneous tissues. The portal of entry may be a traumatic or surgical wound, an insect bite, or any other break in skin integrity. Often, no entry site is apparent.

One form of streptococcal cellulitis, *erysipelas*, is characterized by a bright red appearance of the involved skin, which forms a plateau sharply demarcated from surrounding normal skin (Fig. 130-4). The lesion is warm to the touch, may be tender, and appears shiny and swollen. The skin often has a *peau d'orange* texture, which is thought to reflect involvement of superficial lymphatics; superficial blebs or bullae may form, usually 2–3 days after onset. The lesion typically develops over a few hours and is associated with fever and chills. Erysipelas tends to occur on the malar area of the face (often with extension over the bridge of the nose to the contralateral malar region) and the lower extremities. After one episode, recurrence at the same site—sometimes years later—is not uncommon.

Classic cases of erysipelas, with typical features, are almost always due to β-hemolytic streptococci, usually GAS and occasionally group C or G. Often, however, the appearance of streptococcal cellulitis is not sufficiently distinctive to permit a specific diagnosis on clinical grounds. The area involved may not be typical for erysipelas, the lesion may be less intensely red than usual and may fade into surrounding skin, and/or the patient may appear only mildly ill. In such cases, it is prudent to broaden the spectrum of empirical antimicrobial therapy to include other pathogens, particularly *S. aureus*, that can produce cellulitis with the same appearance. Staphylococcal infection should be suspected if cellulitis develops around a wound or an ulcer.

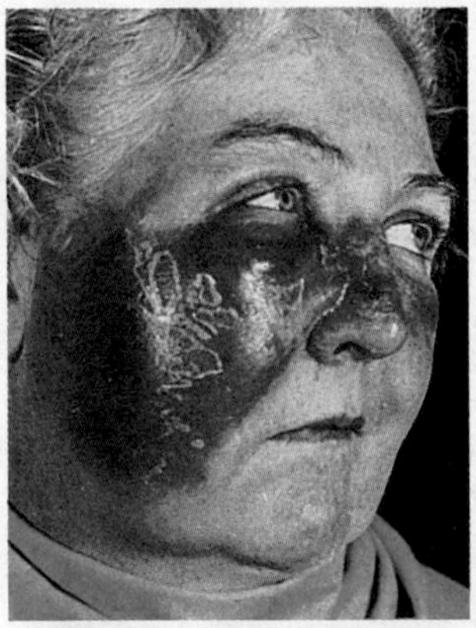

FIGURE 130-4 Erysipelas is a streptococcal infection of the superficial dermis and consists of well-demarcated, erythematous, edematous, warm plaques.

Streptococcal cellulitis tends to develop at anatomic sites in which normal lymphatic drainage has been disrupted, such as sites of prior cellulitis, the arm ipsilateral to a mastectomy and axillary lymph node dissection, a lower extremity previously involved in deep venous thrombosis or chronic lymphedema, or the leg from which a saphenous vein has been harvested for coronary artery bypass grafting. The organism may enter via a dermal breach some distance from the eventual site of clinical cellulitis. For example, some patients with recurrent leg cellulitis following saphenous vein removal stop having recurrent episodes only after treatment of tinea pedis on the affected extremity. Fissures in the skin presumably serve as a portal of entry for streptococci, which then produce infection more proximally in the leg at the site of previous injury. Streptococcal cellulitis may also involve recent surgical wounds. GAS is among the few bacterial pathogens that typically produce signs of wound infection and surrounding cellulitis within the first 24 h after surgery. These wound infections are usually associated with a thin exudate and may spread rapidly, either as cellulitis in the skin and subcutaneous tissue or as a deeper tissue infection (see below). Streptococcal wound infection or localized cellulitis may also be associated with *lymphangitis*, manifested by red streaks extending proximally along superficial lymphatics from the infection site.

Rx STREPTOCOCCAL CELLULITIS

See Table 130-3 and Chap. 119.

Deep Soft-Tissue Infections *Necrotizing fasciitis* (*hemolytic streptococcal gangrene*) involves the superficial and/or deep fascia investing the muscles of an extremity or the trunk. The source of the infection is either the skin, with organisms introduced into tissue through trauma (sometimes trivial), or the bowel flora, with organisms released during abdominal surgery or from an occult enteric source, such as a diverticular or appendiceal abscess. The inoculation site may be inapparent and is often some distance from the site of clinical involvement; e.g., the introduction of organisms via minor trauma to the hand may be associated with clinical infection of the tissues overlying the shoulder or chest. Cases associated with the bowel flora are usually polymicrobial, involving a mixture of anaerobic bacteria (such as *Bacteroides fragilis* or anaerobic streptococci) and facultative organisms (usually gram-negative bacilli). Cases unrelated to contamination from bowel organisms are most commonly caused by GAS alone or in combination with other organisms (most often *S. aureus*). Overall, GAS is implicated in ~60% of cases of necrotizing fasciitis. The onset of symptoms is usually quite acute and is marked by severe pain at the site of involvement, malaise, fever, chills, and a toxic appearance. The physical findings, particularly early on, may not be striking, with only minimal erythema of the overlying skin. Pain and tenderness are usually severe. In contrast, in more superficial cellulitis, the skin appearance is more abnormal, but pain and tenderness are only mild or moderate. As the infection progresses (often over several hours), the severity and extent of symptoms worsen, and skin changes become more evident, with the appearance of dusky or mottled erythema and edema. The marked tenderness of the involved area may evolve into anesthesia as the spreading inflammatory process produces infarction of cutaneous nerves.

Although myositis is more commonly due to *S. aureus* infection, GAS occasionally produces abscesses in skeletal muscles (*streptococcal myositis*), with little or no involvement of the surrounding fascia or overlying skin. The presentation is usually subacute, but a fulminant form has been described in association with severe systemic toxicity, bacteremia, and a high mortality rate. The fulminant form may reflect the same basic disease process seen in necrotizing fasciitis, but with the necrotizing inflammatory process extending into the muscles themselves rather than remaining limited to the fascial layers.

Rx DEEP SOFT-TISSUE INFECTIONS

Once necrotizing fasciitis is suspected, early surgical exploration is both diagnostically and therapeutically indicated. Surgery reveals necrosis and inflammatory fluid tracking along the fascial planes above and between muscle groups, without involvement of the muscles themselves. The process usually extends beyond the area of clinical involvement, and extensive debridement is required. Drainage and debridement are central to the management of necrotizing fasciitis; antibiotic treatment is a useful adjunct (Table 130-3), but surgery is life-saving.

Treatment for streptococcal myositis consists of surgical drainage—usually by an open procedure that permits evaluation of the extent of infection and ensures adequate debridement of involved tissues—and high-dose penicillin (Table 130-3).

Pneumonia and Empyema GAS is an occasional cause of pneumonia, generally in previously healthy individuals. The onset of symptoms may be abrupt or gradual. Pleuritic chest pain, fever, chills, and dyspnea are the characteristic manifestations. Cough is usually present but may not be prominent. Approximately one-half of patients with GAS pneumonia have an accompanying pleural effusion. In contrast to the sterile parapneumonic effusions typical of pneumococcal pneumonia, those complicating streptococcal pneumonia are almost always infected. The empyema fluid is usually visible by chest radiography on initial presentation, and its volume may increase rapidly. These pleural collections should be drained early, as they tend to become loculated rapidly, resulting in a chronic fibrotic reaction that may require thoracotomy for removal.

Bacteremia, Puerperal Sepsis, and Streptococcal Toxic Shock Syndrome GAS bacteremia is usually associated with an identifiable local infection. Bacteremia occurs rarely with otherwise uncomplicated pharyngitis, occasionally with cellulitis or pneumonia, and relatively frequently with necrotizing fasciitis. Bacteremia without an identified source raises the possibility of endocarditis, an occult abscess, or osteomyelitis. A variety of focal infections may arise secondarily from streptococcal bacteremia, including endocarditis, meningitis, septic arthritis, osteomyelitis, peritonitis, and visceral abscesses.

GAS is occasionally implicated in infectious complications of childbirth, usually endometritis and associated bacteremia. In the preantibiotic era, puerperal sepsis was commonly caused by GAS; currently, it is more often caused by GBS. Several nosocomial outbreaks of puerperal GAS infection have been traced to an asymptomatic carrier, usually someone present at delivery. The site of carriage may be the skin, throat, anus, or vagina.

Beginning in the late 1980s, several reports described patients with GAS infections associated with shock and multisystem organ failure. This syndrome was called the streptococcal toxic shock syndrome (TSS) because it shares certain features with staphylococcal TSS. In 1993, a case definition for streptococcal TSS was formulated (Table 130-4). The general features of the illness include fever, hypotension, renal impairment, and respiratory distress syndrome. Various types of rash have been described, but rash usually does not develop. Laboratory abnormalities include a marked shift to the left in the white blood cell differential, with many immature granulocytes; hypocalcemia; hypoalbuminemia; and thrombocytopenia, which usually becomes more pronounced on the second or third day of illness. In contrast to patients with staphylococcal TSS, the majority with streptococcal TSS are bacteremic. The most common associated infection is a soft tissue infection—necrotizing fasciitis, myositis, or cellulitis—although a variety of other associated local infections have been described, including pneumonia, peritonitis, osteomyelitis, and myometritis. Streptococcal TSS is associated with a mortality rate of ≥30%, with most deaths secondary to shock and respiratory failure. Because of its rapidly progressive and lethal course, early recognition of the syndrome is essential. Patients should receive aggressive supportive care (fluid resuscitation, pressors, and mechanical ventilation) in addition to antimicrobial therapy and, in cases associated with necrotizing fasciitis, surgical debridement. Exactly why certain patients develop this fulminant syndrome is not known. Early studies of the streptococcal strains isolated from these patients demonstrated a strong association with the production of pyrogenic exotoxin A. This association has been inconsistent in subsequent case series. Pyrogenic exotoxin A and several other streptococcal exotoxins act as superantigens to trigger release of inflammatory cytokines from T lymphocytes. Fever, shock, and organ dysfunction in streptococcal TSS may reflect, in part, the systemic effects of superantigen-mediated cytokine release.

TABLE 130-4 PROPOSED CASE DEFINITION FOR THE STREPTOCOCCAL TOXIC SHOCK SYNDROME[a]

I. Isolation of group A streptococci (*Streptococcus pyogenes*)
  A. From a normally sterile site
  B. From a nonsterile site
II. Clinical signs of severity
  A. Hypotension *and*
  B. ≥2 of the following signs
    1. Renal impairment
    2. Coagulopathy
    3. Liver function impairment
    4. Adult respiratory distress syndrome
    5. A generalized erythematous macular rash that may desquamate
    6. Soft tissue necrosis, including necrotizing fasciitis or myositis; *or* gangrene

[a]An illness fulfilling criteria IA, IIA, and IIB is defined as a *definite* case. An illness fulfilling criteria IB, IIA, and IIB is defined as a *probable* case if no other etiology for the illness is identified.

Source: Modified from Working Group on Severe Streptococcal Infections: JAMA 269:390, 1993.

Rx STREPTOCOCCAL TOXIC SHOCK SYNDROME

In light of the possible role of pyrogenic exotoxins or other streptococcal toxins in streptococcal TSS, treatment with clindamycin has been advocated by some authorities (Table 130-3), who argue that, through its direct action on protein synthesis, clindamycin is more effective in rapidly terminating toxin production than penicillin—a cell-wall agent. Support for this view comes from studies of an experimental model of streptococcal myositis, in which mice given clindamycin had a higher rate of survival than those given penicillin. Comparable data on the treatment of human infections are not available. Although clindamycin resistance in GAS is uncommon (<2% among U.S. isolates), it has been documented. Thus, if clindamycin is used for initial treatment of a critically ill patient, penicillin should be given as well until the antibiotic susceptibility of the streptococcal isolate is known.

Intravenous immunoglobulin has been used as adjunctive therapy for streptococcal TSS (Table 130-3). Pooled immunoglobulin preparations contain antibodies capable of neutralizing the effects of streptococcal toxins. Anecdotal reports and case series have suggested favorable clinical responses to intravenous immunoglobulin, but no prospective controlled trials have been reported.

Prevention No vaccine against GAS is commercially available. A formulation that consists of recombinant peptides containing epitopes of 26 M-protein types has undergone phase I and II testing in volunteers.

Early results indicate that the vaccine is well tolerated and elicits type-specific antibody responses.

Household contacts of individuals with invasive GAS infection (e.g., bacteremia, necrotizing fasciitis, or streptococcal TSS) are at greater risk of invasive infection than the general population. Asymptomatic pharyngeal colonization with GAS has been detected in up to 25% of persons with >4 h/d of same-room exposure to an index case. However, antibiotic prophylaxis is not routinely recommended for contacts of patients with invasive disease since such an approach (if effective) would require treatment of hundreds of contacts to prevent a single case.

STREPTOCOCCI OF GROUPS C AND G

Group C and group G streptococci are β-hemolytic bacteria that occasionally cause human infections similar to those caused by GAS. Strains that form small colonies on blood agar (<0.5 mm) are generally members of the *S. milleri* (*S. intermedius, S. anginosus*) group (see "Viridans Streptococci," below). Large-colony group C and G streptococci of human origin are now considered a single species, *S. dysgalactiae* subsp. *equisimilis*. They have been associated with pharyngitis, cellulitis and soft-tissue infections, pneumonia, bacteremia, endocarditis, and septic arthritis. Puerperal sepsis, meningitis, epidural abscess, intraabdominal abscess, urinary tract infection, and neonatal sepsis have also been reported. Group C or G streptococcal bacteremia most often affects elderly or chronically ill patients and, in the absence of obvious local infection, is likely to reflect endocarditis. Septic arthritis, sometimes involving multiple joints, may complicate endocarditis or develop in its absence. Distinct streptococcal species of Lancefield group C cause infections in domesticated animals, especially horses and cattle; some human infections are acquired through contact with animals or consumption of unpasteurized milk. These zoonotic organisms include *S. equi* subsp. *zooepidemicus* and *S. equi* subsp. *equi*.

Rx GROUP C OR G STREPTOCOCCAL INFECTION

Penicillin is the drug of choice for treatment of group C or G streptococcal infections. Antibiotic treatment is the same as for similar syndromes due to GAS (Table 130-3). Patients with bacteremia or septic arthritis should receive intravenous penicillin (2–4 mU every 4 h). All group C and G streptococci are sensitive to penicillin; nearly all are inhibited in vitro by concentrations of ≤0.03 μg/mL. Occasional isolates exhibit tolerance: although inhibited by low concentrations of penicillin, they are killed only by significantly higher concentrations. The clinical significance of tolerance is unknown. Because of the poor clinical response of some patients to penicillin alone, the addition of gentamicin (1 mg/kg every 8 h for patients with normal renal function) is recommended by some authorities for treatment of endocarditis or septic arthritis due to group C or G streptococci; however, combination therapy has not been shown to be superior to penicillin treatment alone. Patients with joint infections often require repeated aspiration or open drainage and debridement for cure; the response to treatment may be slow, particularly in debilitated patients and those with involvement of multiple joints. Infection of prosthetic joints almost always requires prosthesis removal in addition to antibiotic therapy.

GROUP B STREPTOCOCCI

Identified first as a cause of mastitis in cows, streptococci belonging to Lancefield's group B have since been recognized as a major cause of sepsis and meningitis in human neonates. GBS is also a frequent cause of peripartum fever in women and an occasional cause of serious infection in nonpregnant adults. Since the widespread institution of prenatal screening for GBS in the 1990s, the incidence of neonatal infection per 1000 live births has fallen from ~2–3 cases to ~1 case. During the same period, GBS infection in adults with underlying chronic illnesses has become more common; adults now account for a larger proportion of invasive GBS infections than do newborns. Lancefield group B consists of a single species, *S. agalactiae*, which is definitively identified with specific antiserum to the group B cell wall–associated carbohydrate antigen. A streptococcal isolate can be classified presumptively as GBS on the basis of biochemical tests, including hydrolysis of sodium hippurate (in which 99% of isolates are positive), hydrolysis of bile esculin agar (in which 99–100% are negative), bacitracin susceptibility (in which 92% are resistant), and production of CAMP factor (in which 98–100% are positive). CAMP factor is a phospholipase produced by GBS that causes synergistic hemolysis with β lysin produced by certain strains of *S. aureus*. Its presence can be demonstrated by cross-streaking of the test isolate and an appropriate staphylococcal strain on a blood agar plate. GBS organisms causing human infections are encapsulated by one of nine antigenically distinct polysaccharides. The capsular polysaccharide is an important virulence factor. Antibodies to the capsular polysaccharide afford protection against GBS of the same (but not of a different) capsular type.

INFECTION IN NEONATES

Two general types of GBS infection in infants are defined by the age of the patient at presentation. *Early-onset infections* occur within the first week of life, with a median age of 20 h at onset. Approximately half of these infants have signs of GBS disease at birth. The infection is acquired during or shortly before birth from the colonized maternal genital tract. Surveillance studies have shown that 5–40% of women are vaginal or rectal carriers of GBS. Approximately 50% of infants delivered vaginally by carrier mothers become colonized, although only 1–2% of those colonized develop clinically evident infection. Prematurity and maternal risk factors (prolonged labor, obstetric complications, and maternal fever) are often involved. The presentation of early-onset infection is the same as that of other forms of neonatal sepsis. Typical findings include respiratory distress, lethargy, and hypotension. Essentially all infants with early-onset disease are bacteremic, one-third to one-half have pneumonia and/or respiratory distress syndrome, and one-third have meningitis.

Late-onset infections occur in infants 1 week to 3 months old (mean age at onset, 3–4 weeks). The infecting organism may be acquired during delivery (as in early-onset cases) or during later contact with a colonized mother, nursery personnel, or another source. Meningitis is the most common manifestation of late-onset infection and in most cases is associated with a strain of capsular type III. Infants present with fever, lethargy or irritability, poor feeding, and seizures. The various other types of late-onset infection include bacteremia without an identified source, osteomyelitis, septic arthritis, and facial cellulitis associated with submandibular or preauricular adenitis.

Rx GROUP B STREPTOCOCCAL INFECTION IN NEONATES

Penicillin is the agent of choice for all GBS infections. Empirical broad-spectrum therapy for suspected bacterial sepsis, consisting of ampicillin and gentamicin, is generally administered until culture results become available. If cultures yield GBS, many pediatricians continue to administer gentamicin, along with ampicillin or penicillin, for a few days until clinical improvement becomes evident. Infants with bacteremia or soft-tissue infection should receive penicillin at a dosage of 200,000 units/kg per day in divided doses; those with meningitis should receive 400,000 units/kg per day. Meningitis should be treated for at least 14 days because of the risk of relapse with shorter courses.

Prevention The incidence of GBS infection is unusually high among infants of women with risk factors: preterm delivery, early rupture of membranes (>24 h before delivery), prolonged labor, fever, or chorioamnionitis. Because the usual source of the organisms infecting a neonate is the mother's birth canal, efforts have been made to prevent GBS infections by the identification of high-risk carrier mothers and their treatment with various forms of antibiotic or immunoprophylaxis. Prophylactic administration of ampicillin or penicillin to such patients during delivery reduces the risk of infection in the newborn. This approach has been hampered by logistical difficulties in identifying colonized women before delivery; the results of vaginal cultures early in pregnancy are poor predictors of carrier status at delivery. The CDC recommends screening for anogenital colonization at 35–37 weeks of pregnancy by a swab culture of the lower vagina and anorectum; intrapartum chemoprophylaxis is recommended for culture-positive women and for women who, regardless of culture status, have previously given birth to an infant with GBS infection or have a history of GBS bacteriuria during pregnancy. Women whose culture status is unknown and who develop premature labor (<37 weeks), prolonged rupture of membranes (>18 h), or intrapartum fever should also receive intrapartum chemoprophylaxis. The recommended regimen for chemoprophylaxis is 5 million units of penicillin G followed by 2.5 million units every 4 h until delivery. Cefazolin is an alternative for women with a history of penicillin allergy who are thought not to be at high risk for anaphylaxis. For women with a history of immediate hypersensitivity, clindamycin or erythromycin may be substituted, but only if the colonizing isolate has been demonstrated to be susceptible. If susceptibility testing results are not available or indicate resistance, vancomycin should be used in this situation.

Treatment of all pregnant women who are colonized or have risk factors for neonatal infection will result in exposure of 15–25% of pregnant women and newborns to antibiotics, with the attendant risks of allergic reactions and selection for resistant organisms. Although still in the developmental stages, a GBS vaccine may ultimately offer a better solution to prevention. Because transplacental passage of maternal antibodies produces protective antibody levels in newborns, efforts are under way to develop a vaccine against GBS that can be given to childbearing-age women before or during pregnancy. Results of phase 1 clinical trials of GBS capsular polysaccharide–protein conjugate vaccines suggest that a multivalent conjugate vaccine would be safe and highly immunogenic.

INFECTION IN ADULTS

The majority of GBS infections in otherwise healthy adults are related to pregnancy and parturition. Peripartum fever, the most common manifestation, is sometimes accompanied by symptoms and signs of endometritis or chorioamnionitis (abdominal distention and uterine or adnexal tenderness). Blood and vaginal swab cultures are often positive. Bacteremia is usually transitory but occasionally results in meningitis or endocarditis. Infections in adults that are not associated with the peripartum period generally involve individuals who are elderly or have an underlying chronic illness, such as diabetes mellitus or a malignancy. Among the infections that develop with some frequency in adults are cellulitis and soft tissue infection (including infected diabetic skin ulcers), urinary tract infection, pneumonia, endocarditis, and septic arthritis. Other reported infections include meningitis, osteomyelitis, and intraabdominal or pelvic abscesses. Relapse or recurrence of invasive infection weeks to months after a first episode is documented in ~4% of cases.

℞ GROUP B STREPTOCOCCAL INFECTION IN ADULTS

GBS is less sensitive to penicillin than GAS, requiring somewhat higher doses. Adults with serious localized infections (pneumonia, pyelonephritis, abscess) should receive doses of ~12 million units of penicillin G daily; patients with endocarditis or meningitis should receive 18–24 million units per day in divided doses. Vancomycin is an acceptable alternative for penicillin-allergic patients.

ENTEROCOCCI AND NONENTEROCOCCAL GROUP D STREPTOCOCCI

ENTEROCOCCI

Lancefield group D includes the enterococci—organisms now classified in a separate genus from other streptococci—and nonenterococcal group D streptococci. Enterococci are distinguished from nonenterococcal group D streptococci by their ability to grow in the presence of 6.5% sodium chloride and by the results of other biochemical tests. The enterococcal species that are significant pathogens for humans are *E. faecalis* and *E. faecium*. Less commonly, similar infections are caused by *E. casseliflavus*, *E. durans*, *E. gallinarum*, or other enterococcal species. These organisms tend to affect patients who are elderly or debilitated, whose mucosal or epithelial barriers have been disrupted, or whose normal flora has been altered by antibiotic treatment. Urinary tract infections due to enterococci are quite common, particularly among patients who have received antibiotic treatment or undergone urinary tract instrumentation. Enterococci are a common cause of nosocomial bacteremia in patients with intravascular catheters and account for 10–20% of cases of bacterial endocarditis on both native and prosthetic valves. The presentation of enterococcal endocarditis is usually subacute but may be acute, with rapidly progressive valve destruction. Enterococci are frequently cultured from bile and are involved in infectious complications of biliary surgery and in liver abscesses. Moreover, enterococci are often isolated from polymicrobial infections arising from the bowel flora (e.g., intraabdominal abscesses), from abdominal surgical wounds, and from diabetic foot ulcers. While such mixed infections are frequently cured by antimicrobials not active against enterococci, specific therapy directed against enterococci is warranted when these organisms predominate or are isolated from blood cultures.

℞ ENTEROCOCCAL INFECTION

Unlike streptococci, enterococci are not reliably killed by penicillin or ampicillin alone at concentrations achieved clinically in the blood or tissues. Ampicillin reaches sufficiently high urinary concentrations to constitute adequate monotherapy for uncomplicated urinary tract infections. Because in vitro testing has shown evidence of synergistic killing of most enterococcal strains by the combination of penicillin or ampicillin with an aminoglycoside, combined therapy is recommended for enterococcal endocarditis and meningitis; the regimen is penicillin (3–4 million units every 4 h) or ampicillin (2 g every 4 h) plus moderate-dose gentamicin (1 mg/kg every 8 h for patients with normal renal function). Enterococcal endocarditis should be treated for at least 4 weeks and for 6 weeks if symptoms have been present for ≥3 months or if the infection involves a prosthetic valve. For nonendocarditis bacteremia and other serious enterococcal infections, it is not known whether the efficacy of a single β-lactam agent is improved by the addition of gentamicin, but many infectious disease specialists use combination therapy for such infections, especially in critically ill patients. Vancomycin, in combination with gentamicin, may be substituted for penicillin in allergic patients. Enterococci are resistant to all cephalosporins.

Antimicrobial susceptibility testing should be performed routinely on enterococcal isolates from serious infections, with therapy adjusted according to the results (**Table 130-5**). Most enterococci are resistant to streptomycin, which should not be used unless in vitro testing indicates susceptibility. Although less widespread than streptomycin resistance, high-level resistance to gentamicin—with a minimum inhibitory concen-

TABLE 130-5 TREATMENT OPTIONS FOR ANTIBIOTIC-RESISTANT ENTEROCOCCAL INFECTIONS

Resistance Pattern	Recommended Therapy
β-Lactamase production	Gentamicin plus ampicillin/sulbactam, amoxicillin/clavulanate, imipenem, or vancomycin
β-Lactam resistance, but no β-lactamase production	Gentamicin plus vancomycin
High-level gentamicin resistance	Streptomycin-sensitive isolate: Streptomycin plus ampicillin or vancomycin
	Streptomycin-resistant isolate: No proven therapy (continuous-infusion ampicillin, prolonged treatment)
Vancomycin resistance	Ampicillin plus gentamicin
Vancomycin and β-lactam resistance	No uniformly bactericidal drugs; linezolid (all enterococci) or quinupristin/dalfopristin (*E. faecium* only)

tration (MIC) of >2000 μg/mL—is common. Gentamicin-resistant enterococci should be tested for streptomycin susceptibility, which they occasionally exhibit. If the isolate is resistant to all aminoglycosides, treatment with penicillin or ampicillin alone may be successful. Prolonged administration (i.e., for at least 6 weeks) of high-dose ampicillin (e.g., 12 g/d) is recommended for endocarditis due to these highly resistant enterococci.

Enterococci may be resistant to penicillins via two distinct mechanisms. The first is β-lactamase production (mediating resistance to penicillin and ampicillin), which has been reported for *E. faecalis* isolates from several locations in the United States and other countries. Because the amount of β-lactamase produced may be insufficient for detection by routine antibiotic susceptibility testing, isolates from serious infections should be screened specifically for β-lactamase production with a chromogenic cephalosporin or another method. For the treatment of β-lactamase–producing strains, vancomycin, ampicillin/sulbactam, amoxicillin/clavulanate, imipenem, or meropenem may be used in combination with gentamicin.

The second mechanism of penicillin resistance is not mediated by β-lactamase and may be due to altered penicillin-binding proteins. This intrinsic penicillin resistance is common among *E. faecium* isolates, which routinely are more resistant to β-lactam antibiotics than are isolates of *E. faecalis*. Moderately resistant enterococci (MICs of penicillin and ampicillin, 16–64 μg/mL) may be susceptible to high-dose penicillin or ampicillin plus gentamicin, but strains with MICs of ≥200 μg/mL must be considered resistant to clinically achievable levels of β-lactam antibiotics, including imipenem and meropenem. Vancomycin plus gentamicin is the recommended regimen for infections due to enterococci with high-level intrinsic resistance to β-lactams.

Vancomycin-resistant enterococci (VRE), first reported from clinical sources in the late 1980s, have become common in many hospitals. Three major vancomycin resistance phenotypes have been described: VanA, VanB, and VanC. The VanA phenotype is associated with high-level resistance to vancomycin and to teicoplanin, a related glycopeptide antibiotic not currently available in the United States. VanB and VanC strains are resistant to vancomycin but susceptible to teicoplanin, although teicoplanin resistance may develop during treatment in VanB strains. For enterococci resistant to both vancomycin and β-lactams, no established therapies provide uniformly bactericidal activity. Two newer agents active against VRE are quinupristin/dalfopristin and linezolid, which were approved for use in the United States in 1999 and 2000, respectively. Quinupristin/dalfopristin is a streptogramin combination with in vitro bacteriostatic activity against *E. faecium*, including VRE, but not against *E. faecalis* or other enterococcal species. Disadvantages of quinupristin/dalfopristin are its limited spectrum of activity against enterococcal species and its relatively frequent side effects of phlebitis and myalgia. Linezolid is an oxazolidinone antibiotic with good bacteriostatic activity against nearly all enterococci, including VRE. Limited clinical experience suggests that linezolid is at least as efficacious as quinupristin/dalfopristin, and linezolid is usually preferred because of its broader activity against all enterococci and the availability of both parenteral and oral formulations. Bone marrow toxicity (especially thrombocytopenia) and peripheral neuropathy are potential side effects. Two other antibiotics are active in vitro against VRE (both *E. faecalis* and *E. faecium*), although neither had been approved for treatment of these infections as of May 2006: daptomycin, a cyclic lipopeptide, and tigecycline, a glycylcycline related to tetracycline.

OTHER GROUP D STREPTOCOCCI

The main nonenterococcal group D streptococcal species that causes human infections is *S. bovis*. *S. bovis* endocarditis is often associated with neoplasms of the gastrointestinal tract—most frequently, a colon carcinoma or polyp—but is also reported in association with other bowel lesions. When occult gastrointestinal lesions are carefully sought, abnormalities are found in ≥60% of patients with *S. bovis* endocarditis. In contrast to the enterococci, nonenterococcal group D streptococci like *S. bovis* are reliably killed by penicillin as a single agent, and penicillin is the agent of choice for *S. bovis* infections.

VIRIDANS AND OTHER STREPTOCOCCI

VIRIDANS STREPTOCOCCI

Consisting of multiple species of α-hemolytic streptococci, the viridans streptococci are a heterogeneous group of organisms that are important agents of bacterial endocarditis (Chap. 118). Several species of viridans streptococci, including *S. salivarius*, *S. mitis*, *S. sanguis*, and *S. mutans*, are part of the normal flora of the mouth, where they live in close association with the teeth and gingiva. Some species contribute to the development of dental caries.

Previously known as *S. morbillorum*, *Gemella morbillorum* has been placed in a separate genus, along with *G. haemolysans*, on the basis of genetic-relatedness studies. These species resemble viridans streptococci with respect to habitat in the human host and associated infections.

The transient viridans streptococcal bacteremia induced by eating, tooth-brushing, flossing, and other sources of minor trauma, together with adherence to biologic surfaces, is thought to account for the predilection of these organisms to cause endocarditis (see Fig. 118-1). Viridans streptococci are also isolated, often as part of a mixed flora, from sites of sinusitis, brain abscess, and liver abscess.

Viridans streptococcal bacteremia occurs relatively frequently in neutropenic patients, particularly after bone marrow transplantation or high-dose chemotherapy for cancer. Some of these patients develop a sepsis syndrome with high fever and shock. Risk factors for viridans streptococcal bacteremia include chemotherapy with high-dose cytosine arabinoside, prior treatment with trimethoprim-sulfamethoxazole or a fluoroquinolone, treatment with antacids or histamine antagonists, mucositis, and profound neutropenia.

The *S. milleri* group (also referred to as the *S. intermedius* or *S. anginosus* group) includes three species that cause human disease: *S. intermedius*, *S. anginosus*, and *S. constellatus*. These organisms are often considered viridans streptococci, although they differ somewhat from other viridans streptococci in both their hemolytic pattern (they may be α-, β-, or nonhemolytic) and the disease syndromes they cause. This group commonly produces suppurative infections, particularly abscesses of brain and abdominal viscera, and infections related to the oral cavity or respiratory tract, such as peritonsillar abscess, lung abscess, and empyema.

℞ INFECTION WITH VIRIDANS STREPTOCOCCI

Isolates from neutropenic patients with bacteremia are often resistant to penicillin; thus these patients should be treated presumptively with vancomycin until the results of susceptibility testing become available. Viridans streptococci isolated in other clinical settings usually are sensitive to penicillin.

ABIOTROPHIA SPECIES (NUTRITIONALLY VARIANT STREPTOCOCCI)

Occasional isolates cultured from the blood of patients with endocarditis fail to grow when subcultured on solid media. These *nutritionally variant streptococci* require supplemental thiol compounds or active forms of vitamin B_6 (pyridoxal or pyridoxamine) for growth in the laboratory. The nutritionally variant streptococci are generally grouped with the viridans streptococci because they cause similar types of infections. However, they have been reclassified on the basis of 16S ribosomal RNA sequence comparisons into a separate genus, *Abiotrophia*, with two species: *A. defectivus* and *A. adjacens*.

℞ INFECTION WITH NUTRITIONALLY VARIANT STREPTOCOCCI

Treatment failure and relapse appear to be more common in cases of endocarditis due to nutritionally variant streptococci than in those due to the usual viridans streptococci. Thus the addition of gentamicin (1 mg/kg every 8 h for patients with normal renal function) to the penicillin regimen is recommended for endocarditis due to the nutritionally variant organisms.

OTHER STREPTOCOCCI

S. suis is an important pathogen in swine and has been reported to cause meningitis in humans, usually in individuals with occupational exposure to pigs. Strains of *S. suis* associated with human infections have generally reacted with Lancefield group R typing serum and sometimes with group D typing serum as well. Isolates may be α- or β-hemolytic and are sensitive to penicillin. *S. iniae*, a pathogen of fish, has been associated with infections in humans who have handled live or freshly killed fish. Cellulitis of the hand is the most common form of human infection, although bacteremia and endocarditis have been reported. *Anaerobic streptococci*, or *peptostreptococci*, are part of the normal flora of the oral cavity, bowel, and vagina. **Infections caused by the anaerobic streptococci are discussed in Chap. 157.**

FURTHER READINGS

BISNO AL et al: Practice guidelines for the diagnosis and management of group A streptococcal pharyngitis. Clin Infect Dis 35:113, 2002

———, STEVENS DL: Streptococcal infections of skin and soft tissues. N Engl J Med 334:240, 1996

CARAPETIS JR et al: The global burden of group A streptococcal diseases. Lancet Infect Dis 5:685, 2005

CENTERS FOR DISEASE CONTROL AND PREVENTION: Prevention of perinatal group B streptococcal disease. MMWR 51(RR-11):1, 2002

GASSAS A et al: Predictors of viridans streptococcal shock syndrome in bacteremic children with cancer and stem-cell transplant recipients. J Clin Oncol 22:1222, 2004

GIBBS RS et al: Perinatal infections due to group B streptococci. Obstet Gynecol 104:1062, 2004

JACKSON LA et al: Risk factors for group B streptococcal disease in adults. Ann Intern Med 123:415, 1995

KAUFFMAN CA: Therapeutic and preventative options for the management of vancomycin-resistant enterococcal infections. J Antimicrob Chemother 51(Suppl3):iii23, 2003

KAUL R et al: Intravenous immunoglobulin therapy for streptococcal toxic shock syndrome—a comparative observational study. The Canadian Streptococcal Study Group. Clin Infect Dis 28:800, 1999

THE PREVENTION OF INVASIVE GROUP A STREPTOCOCCAL INFECTIONS WORKSHOP PARTICIPANTS: Prevention of invasive group A streptococcal disease among household contacts of case patients and among postpartum and postsurgical patients: Recommendations from the Centers for Disease Control and Prevention. Clin Infect Dis 35:950, 2002

131 Diphtheria and Other Infections Caused by Corynebacteria and Related Species

William R. Bishai, John R. Murphy

DIPHTHERIA

Diphtheria is a nasopharyngeal and skin infection caused by *Corynebacterium diphtheriae*. Toxigenic strains of *C. diphtheriae* produce a protein toxin that causes systemic toxicity, myocarditis, and polyneuropathy. The toxin is associated with the formation of pseudomembranes in the pharynx during respiratory diphtheria. While toxigenic strains most frequently cause pharyngeal diphtheria, nontoxigenic strains commonly cause cutaneous disease. In the United States and Europe, diphtheria has been controlled in recent years with effective vaccination, although sporadic outbreaks have occurred. Diphtheria is still common in the Caribbean, Latin America, and the Indian subcontinent, where mass immunization programs are not enforced. Large epidemics have occurred in the independent states formerly encompassed by the Soviet Union. Additional outbreaks have been reported in Algeria, China, and Ecuador.

ETIOLOGY

C. diphtheriae is a gram-positive, unencapsulated, nonmotile, nonsporulating bacillus. *C. diphtheriae* organisms have a characteristic club-shaped bacillary appearance and typically form clusters of parallel rays (palisades) that are referred to as *Chinese characters*. In the specific laboratory media recommended for the cultivation of *C. diphtheriae*, tellurite, colistin, or nalidixic acid is responsible for selective isolation of the organism in the presence of other autochthonous pharyngeal microbes. Human isolates of *C. diphtheriae* may display nontoxigenic (*tox*$^-$) or toxigenic (*tox*$^+$) phenotypes. Corynebacteriophage beta carries the structural gene (*tox*) encoding diphtheria toxin, and a family of closely related corynebacteriophages are responsible for toxigenic conversion of *tox*$^-$ *C. diphtheriae* to the *tox*$^+$ phenotype. Moreover, lysogenic conversion from a nontoxigenic to a toxigenic phenotype has been shown to occur in situ. Growth of toxigenic strains of *C. diphtheriae* under iron-limiting conditions leads to the optimal expression of diphtheria toxin, and these conditions are believed to be a mechanism of pathogenesis during human infection.

EPIDEMIOLOGY

C. diphtheriae is transmitted via the aerosol route, primarily during close contact. There are no significant reservoirs other than humans. The incubation period for respiratory diphtheria is 2–5 days; however, disease can develop as long as 10 days after exposure. Before the vaccine era, most individuals over the age of 10 were immune to *C. diphtheriae*; infants were protected by maternal IgG antibodies but became susceptible after ~6 months of age. Thus, the disease was seen primarily in children and nonimmune young adults. In temperate regions, respiratory diphtheria occurs year-round but is most common during winter months.

The development of diphtheria antitoxin and diphtheria toxoid vaccine led to the near-elimination of diphtheria in Western countries. The annual peak incidence rate was 191 cases per 100,000 population in the United States in 1921; in contrast, since 1980, the annual figure for the United States as a whole has been <5 cases. Nevertheless, pockets of colonization have persisted in North America, particularly in South Dakota, Ontario, and Washington state. Immunity induced by vaccination during childhood gradually decreases in adulthood. An estimated 30% of men 60–69 years old have antitoxin titers below the protective level. In addition to older age and lack of vaccination, risk factors for diphtheria outbreaks include alcoholism, low socioeconomic status, crowded living conditions, and Native American ethnic background. An outbreak that occurred in Seattle in 1972–1982 included 1100 cases, primarily manifesting as cutaneous disease. During the 1990s in the states of the former Soviet Union, a much larger diphtheria epidemic caused >150,000 cases and >5000 deaths. Clonally related toxigenic *C. diphtheriae* strains of the ET8 complex were associated with this outbreak. Given that the ET8 complex expressed a toxin against which the prevalent diphtheria toxoid vaccine was effective, the epidemic was attributed to failure of the public health infrastructure to effectively vaccinate the population. Beginning in 1998, the epidemic was controlled by mass vaccination programs. During the epidemic, the incidence rate was high among individuals from >15 years of age up to 50 years of age. Socioeconomic instability, migration, deteriorating public health programs, frequent vaccine shortages, delays in implementation of vaccination and of treatment in response to cases, and lack of public education and awareness were contributing factors in that outbreak.

Cutaneous diphtheria is usually a secondary infection that follows a primary skin lesion due to trauma, allergy, or autoimmunity. Most often, isolates from cases of cutaneous disease lack the *tox* gene and therefore do not express diphtheria toxin. In tropical regions, cutaneous diphtheria is more common than respiratory diphtheria. In contrast to respiratory disease, cutaneous diphtheria is not a reportable disease in United States.

Nontoxigenic strains of *C. diphtheriae* have also been associated with pharyngitis in Europe. Outbreaks have occurred among homosexual men and IV drug users.

PATHOGENESIS AND IMMUNOLOGY

Diphtheria toxin, produced by toxigenic strains of *C. diphtheriae*, is the primary virulence factor in clinical disease. The toxin is synthesized in precursor form; is released as a 535-amino-acid, single-chain protein; and has an LD_{50} of ~100 ng/kg of body weight. The toxin is produced in the pseudomembranous lesion and is taken up into the bloodstream, through which it is distributed to all organ systems. Once bound to its cell surface receptor (a heparin-binding, epidermal growth factor–like precursor), the toxin is internalized by receptor-mediated endocytosis and enters the cytosol from an acidified early endosomal compartment. In vitro, the toxin may be separated into two chains after digestion with serine proteases: the N-terminal A fragment and the C-terminal B fragment. Delivery of the A fragment into the eukaryotic cell cytosol results in irreversible inhibition of protein synthesis by NAD+-dependent ADP ribosylation of elongation factor 2. The eventual result is the death of the cell.

In 1926, Ramon at the Institut Pasteur found that formalinization of diphtheria toxin resulted in the production of diphtheria toxoid, which was nontoxic but highly immunogenic. Subsequent studies showed that immunization with diphtheria toxoid elicited antibodies that neutralized the toxin and prevented most manifestations of diphtheria. In the 1930s, mass immunization of children and susceptible adults commenced in the United States and Europe.

Individuals with an antitoxin titer of >0.01 unit/mL are at low risk of diphtheria disease. In populations where a majority of individuals have protective antitoxin titers, the carrier rate for toxigenic strains of *C. diphtheriae* decreases and the overall risk of diphtheria among susceptible individuals is reduced. Nevertheless, individuals with nonprotective titers may contract diphtheria through either travel or exposure to individuals who have recently returned from regions where the disease is endemic.

Characteristic pathologic findings of diphtheria include mucosal ulcers with a pseudomembranous coating composed of an inner band of fibrin and a luminal band of neutrophils. Initially white and firmly adherent, in advanced diphtheria the pseudomembranes turn gray and even green or black as necrosis progresses. Mucosal ulcers result from toxin-induced necrosis of the epithelium accompanied by edema, hyperemia, and vascular congestion of the submucosal base. A fibrinosuppurative exudate from the ulcer develops into the pseudomembrane. Ulcers and pseudomembranes in severe respiratory diphtheria may extend from the pharynx into medium-sized bronchial airways. Expanding and sloughing membranes may result in fatal airway obstruction.

APPROACH TO THE PATIENT: Diphtheria

Although diphtheria is rare in the United States and other developed countries, this diagnosis should be considered in patients who have severe pharyngitis, particularly with difficulty swallowing, respiratory compromise, or signs of systemic disease including myocarditis or generalized weakness. In the differential diagnosis, the leading causes of pharyngitis that should be considered are respiratory viruses (rhinoviruses, influenza viruses, parainfluenza viruses, coronaviruses, and adenoviruses; ~25% of cases), group A streptococci (15–30%), group C streptococci (~5%), atypical bacteria such as *Mycoplasma pneumoniae* and *Chlamydophila pneumoniae* (15–20% in some series), and other viruses such as herpes simplex virus (~4%) and Epstein-Barr virus (EBV; <1% in infectious mononucleosis). Less common causes are acute HIV infection, infection with *Neisseria gonorrhoeae*, fusobacterial infection (e.g., Lemierre syndrome), and thrush due to *Candida albicans* or other *Candida* species. The presence of a pharyngeal pseudomembrane or an extensive exudate should prompt consideration of diphtheria (Fig. 131-1).

CLINICAL MANIFESTATIONS

Respiratory Diphtheria The clinical diagnosis of diphtheria is based on the constellation of sore throat; adherent tonsillar, pharyngeal, or nasal pseudomembranous lesions; and low-grade fever. In addition, diagnosis requires the isolation of *C. diphtheriae* or the histopathologic isolation of compatible gram-positive organisms. The Centers for Disease Control and Prevention (CDC) recognizes confirmed respiratory diphtheria (laboratory proven or epidemiologically linked to a culture-confirmed case) and probable respiratory diphtheria (clinically compatible but not laboratory proven or epidemiologically linked). Carriers are defined as individuals who have positive cultures for *C. diphtheriae* and either are asymptomatic or have symptoms but lack pseudomembranes. Most patients seek medical care for initial manifestations of sore throat and fever. Occasionally, weakness, dysphagia, headache, and voice change are the initial manifestations. Neck edema and difficulty breathing are seen in more advanced cases and carry a poor prognosis.

The systemic manifestations of diphtheria stem from the effects of diphtheria toxin and include weakness as a result of neurotoxicity and cardiac arrhythmias or congestive heart failure due to myocarditis. The pseudomembranous lesion is most often located in the tonsillopharyngeal region. Less commonly, the lesions are detected in the larynx, nares, and trachea or bronchial passages. Large pseudomembranes are associated with severe disease and a poor prognosis. A few patients develop massive swelling of the tonsils and present with "bull-neck" diph-

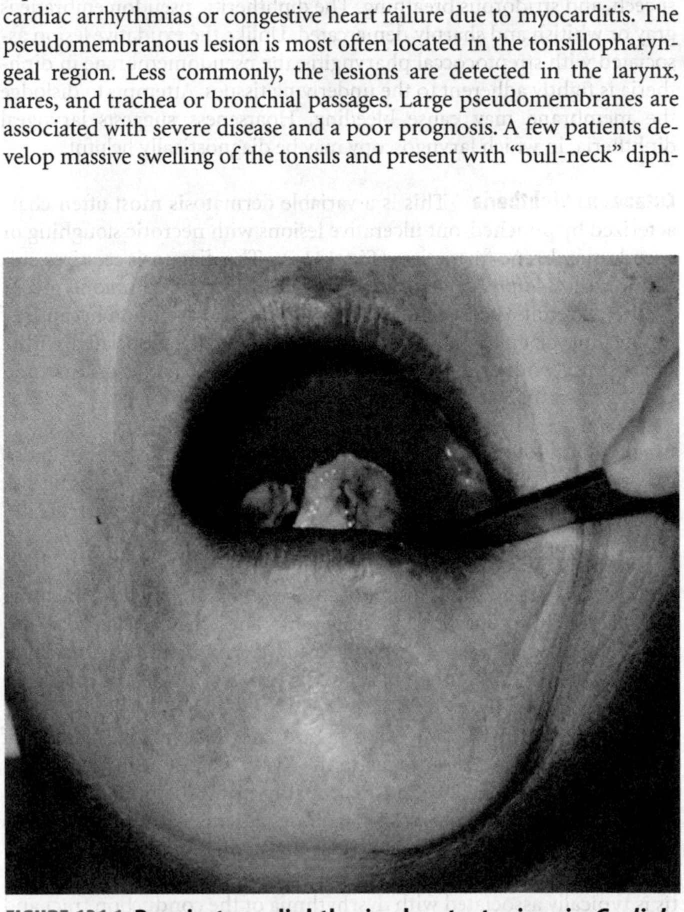

FIGURE 131-1 Respiratory diphtheria due to toxigenic *C. diphtheriae* producing exudative pharyngitis in a 47-year-old woman with neck edema and a pseudomembrane extending from the uvula to the pharyngeal wall. The characteristic white pseudomembrane is caused by diphtheria toxin–mediated necrosis of the respiratory epithelial layer, producing fibrinous coagulative exudate. Submucosal edema adds to airway narrowing. The pharyngitis is acute in onset, and respiratory obstruction from the pseudomembrane may occur in severe cases. Inoculation of pseudomembrane fragments or submembranous swabs onto Löffler's or tellurite selective medium reveals *C. diphtheriae*. *(Photograph by P. Strebel, MD, used by permission. From Kadirova et al.)*

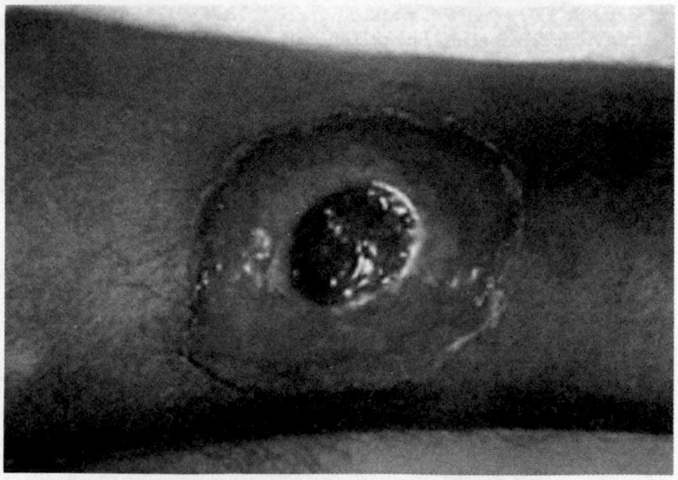

FIGURE 131-2 Cutaneous diphtheria due to nontoxigenic *C. diphtheriae* on the lower extremity. *(From the Centers for Disease Control and Prevention.)*

theria, which results from massive edema of the submandibular and paratracheal region and is further characterized by foul breath, thick speech, and stridorous breathing. The diphtheritic pseudomembrane is gray or whitish and sharply demarcated. Unlike the exudative lesion associated with streptococcal pharyngitis, the pseudomembrane in diphtheria is tightly adherent to the underlying tissues. Attempts to dislodge the membrane may cause bleeding. Hoarseness suggests laryngeal diphtheria, in which laryngoscopy may be diagnostically helpful.

Cutaneous Diphtheria This is a variable dermatosis most often characterized by punched-out ulcerative lesions with necrotic sloughing or pseudomembrane formation (Fig. 131-2). The diagnosis requires cultivation of *C. diphtheriae* from lesions, which most commonly occur on the extremities. Patients usually seek medical attention because of nonhealing or enlarging skin ulcers, which may be associated with a preexisting wound or dermatoses such as eczema, psoriasis, and venous stasis disease. The lesions rarely exceed 5 cm.

Other Clinical Manifestations *C. diphtheriae* causes rare cases of endocarditis and septic arthritis, most often in patients with preexisting risk factors such as cardiac valvular disease, injection drug use, or cirrhosis.

COMPLICATIONS

Airway obstruction poses a significant early risk in patients presenting with advanced diphtheria. Pseudomembranes may slough and obstruct the airway or may advance to the larynx or into the tracheobronchial tree. Children are particularly prone to obstruction because of their small airways.

Polyneuropathy and myocarditis are late toxic manifestations of diphtheria. During the outbreak in the Kyrgyz Republic in 1995, myocarditis was seen in 22% and neuropathy in 5% of hospitalized patients. The mortality rate was 7% among patients with myocarditis as opposed to 2% among those without myocardial manifestations. The median time to death in hospitalized patients was 4.5 days. Myocarditis is typically associated with dysrhythmia of the conduction tract and dilated cardiomyopathy.

Neurologic manifestations may appear during the first or second week of illness, typically beginning with dysphagia and nasal dysarthria and progressing to other signs of cranial nerve involvement, including weakness of the tongue and facial numbness. Ciliary paralysis, which is typical, manifests as blurred vision due to paralysis of pupillary accommodation, with a preserved light reflex. Cranial neuropathy may be followed by respiratory and abdominal muscle weakness requiring artificial ventilation. Several weeks later—sometimes as cranial neuropathy is improving—a generalized sensorimotor polyneuropathy may appear, with prominent autonomic manifestations (including hypotension) in some cases. The clinical syndrome and the findings on lumbar puncture of raised levels of protein without pleocytosis in cerebrospinal fluid resemble Guillain-Barré syndrome (Chap. 380). Pathologically, diphtheria neuropathy is a noninflammatory demyelinating disorder mediated by the exotoxin. Gradual improvement is the rule in patients who survive the acute phase.

Other complications of diphtheria include pneumonia, renal failure, encephalitis, cerebral infarction, and pulmonary embolism. Serum sickness can result from treatment with diphtheria antitoxin (see "Diphtheria Treatment," below).

DIAGNOSIS

The diagnosis of diphtheria is based on clinical signs and symptoms plus laboratory confirmation. Respiratory diphtheria should be considered in patients with sore throat, pharyngeal exudates, and fever. Other symptoms may include hoarseness, stridor, or palatal paralysis. The presence of a pseudomembrane should prompt consideration of diphtheria. Once a clinical diagnosis of diphtheria is made, diphtheria antitoxin should be administered as soon as possible.

Laboratory diagnosis is based either on cultivation of *C. diphtheriae* or toxigenic *C. ulcerans* from the site of infection or on the demonstration of local lesions with characteristic histopathology. *C. pseudodiphtheriticum*, a nontoxigenic organism, is a common component of the normal throat flora and does not pose a significant risk. Throat samples should be submitted to the laboratory for culture with the notation that diphtheria is being considered. This information should prompt cultivation on special selective medium and subsequent biochemical testing to differentiate *C. diphtheriae* from other nasopharyngeal commensal corynebacteria. All laboratory isolates of *C. diphtheriae*, including nontoxigenic strains, should be submitted to the CDC.

A diagnosis of cutaneous diphtheria requires laboratory confirmation since the lesions are not characteristic and are clinically indistinguishable from other dermatoses. Diphtheritic ulcers occasionally—but not consistently—have a punched-out appearance (Fig. 131-2). Patients in whom cutaneous diphtheria is identified should have the nasopharynx cultured for *C. diphtheriae*. The laboratory media for cutaneous diphtheria are the same as those used for respiratory diphtheria: Löffler's or Tinsdale's selective medium in addition to nonselective medium such as blood agar. As has been mentioned, respiratory diphtheria remains a notifiable disease in the United States, whereas cutaneous diphtheria is not.

℞ DIPHTHERIA

DIPHTHERIA ANTITOXIN Prompt administration of diphtheria antitoxin is critical in the management of respiratory diphtheria. The antitoxin—a horse antiserum—is effective in reducing the extent of local disease as well as the risk of complications of myocarditis and neuropathy. Rapid institution of antitoxin therapy is also associated with a significant reduction in mortality risk. Because diphtheria antitoxin cannot neutralize cell-bound toxin, prompt initiation is important. This product, which is no longer made commercially in the United States, is available from the CDC under an investigational new drug protocol and may be obtained by calling the Bacterial Vaccine Preventable Disease Branch of the National Immunization Program at 404-639-8257 between 8:00 A.M. and 4:30 P.M. U.S. Eastern time or at 770-488-7100 at other hours; the relevant website is *http://www.cdc.gov/nip/vaccine/dat/default.htm*. The current protocol for the use of antitoxin includes a test dose to rule out immediate-type hypersensitivity. Patients who exhibit hypersensitivity require desensitization before a full therapeutic dose of antitoxin is administered.

ANTIMICROBIAL THERAPY Antibiotics are used in the management of diphtheria primarily to prevent transmission to other susceptible contacts. Recommended options for the treatment of patients with respiratory diphtheria are as follows: (1) procaine penicillin G at a dosage of 600,000 units (for children, 12,500–25,000 U/kg) IM every 12 h until the patient can swallow comfortably, after which oral penicillin V is given at 125–250 mg four times daily to complete a 14-day course; or (2) erythromycin at a dosage of 500 mg IV every 6 h (for children, 40–50 mg/kg per day IV in two or four divided doses) until the patient can swallow comfortably, after which 500 mg is given PO four times daily to complete a 14-day course.

A clinical study in Vietnam found that penicillin was associated with a more rapid resolution of fever and a lower rate of bacterial resistance than erythromycin; however, relapses were more common with penicillin. Erythromycin therapy targets protein synthesis and thus offers the presumed benefit of stopping toxin synthesis more quickly than a cell wall–active β-lactam agent. Alternative agents for patients who are allergic to penicillin or cannot take erythromycin include rifampin and clindamycin. Eradication of *C. diphtheriae* should be documented at least 1 day after antimicrobial therapy is complete. A repeat throat culture 2 weeks later is recommended. For patients in whom the organism is not eradicated after a 14-day course of erythromycin or penicillin, an additional 10-day course followed by repeat culture is recommended.

Cutaneous diphtheria should be treated as described above for respiratory disease. Individuals infected with toxigenic strains should receive antitoxin. It is important to treat the underlying cause of the dermatoses in addition to the superinfection with *C. diphtheriae*.

Patients who recover from respiratory or cutaneous diphtheria should have antitoxin levels measured. If diphtheria antitoxin has been administered, this test should be performed 6 months later. Patients who recover from respiratory or cutaneous diphtheria should receive the appropriate vaccine (see "Prevention," below) to ensure the development of protective antibody titers, which does not occur in all cases.

MANAGEMENT Patients in whom diphtheria is suspected should be hospitalized in respiratory isolation rooms, with close monitoring of cardiac and respiratory function. A cardiac workup is recommended to assess the possibility of myocarditis. In patients with extensive pseudomembranes, consultation with an anesthesiologist or an ear, nose, and throat specialist is recommended because of the possibility that tracheostomy or intubation will be required. In some settings, pseudomembranes can be removed surgically. Treatment with glucocorticoids has not been shown to reduce the risk of myocarditis or polyneuropathy.

PROGNOSIS

Fatal pseudomembranous diphtheria typically occurs in patients with nonprotective antibody titers and in unimmunized patients. The pseudomembrane may increase in size from the time it is first noted. Risk factors for death include bullneck diphtheria; myocarditis with ventricular tachycardia; atrial fibrillation; complete heart block; an age of >60 years or <6 months; alcoholism; extensive pseudomembrane elongation; and laryngeal, tracheal, or bronchial involvement. Another important predictor of fatal outcome is the interval between local disease development and antitoxin administration. Cutaneous diphtheria has a low mortality rate and is rarely associated with myocarditis or peripheral neuropathy.

PREVENTION

Vaccination Sustained campaigns for vaccination of children and adequate boosting vaccination of adults are responsible for the exceedingly low incidence of diphtheria in most developed nations. At present, diphtheria toxoid vaccine is coadministered with tetanus (with or without acellular pertussis) vaccine. DTaP (full-level diphtheria and tetanus toxoids and acellular pertussis vaccine, adsorbed) is the currently recommended vaccine for children up to the age of 7; DTaP replaced DTP (diphtheria and tetanus toxoids and whole-cell pertussis vaccine) in 1997. Tdap is a tetanus toxoid, reduced diphtheria toxoid, and acellular pertussis vaccine formulated for adolescents and adults. Tdap was licensed for use in the United States in 2005 and is the recommended booster vaccine for children 11–12 years old and the recommended catch-up vaccine for children 7–10 and 13–18 years old. As of 2006, it is recommended that (1) adults 19–64 years old receive a single dose of Tdap if their last dose of Td (tetanus and reduced-dose diphtheria toxoids, adsorbed) was >10 years earlier and (2) intervals of <10 years be implemented for Tdap vaccination of health care workers, adults anticipating contact with infants, and adults not previously vaccinated for pertussis. Adults who have received acellular pertussis vaccines should continue to receive decennial Td booster vaccinations. The vaccination schedule is detailed in Chap. 116.

Prophylaxis of Contacts Close contacts of diphtheria cases should undergo throat culture to determine whether they are carriers. After samples for throat culture are obtained, antimicrobial prophylaxis should be considered for all close contacts, even those who are culture-negative. The options are 7–10 days of oral erythromycin or one dose of IM benzathine penicillin G (1.2 million units for persons ≥6 years old or 600,000 units for children <6 years old).

Contacts of diphtheria cases who have an uncertain immunization status should receive the appropriate diphtheria toxoid–containing vaccine. Tdap (rather than Td) is now recommended as the booster vaccine of choice for adults who have not recently received an acellular pertussis–containing vaccine. Carriers of *C. diphtheriae* in the community should be treated and vaccinated when identified.

NONDIPHTHERIAL CORYNEBACTERIA AND RELATED SPECIES

Nondiphtherial corynebacteria, which are also referred to as *diphtheroids* or *coryneforms*, are a widely diverse collection of bacteria that are taxonomically lumped together on the basis of their 16S rDNA signature nucleotides. The diversity of this group is exemplified by the wide range in guanine-plus-cytosine content (45–70%). Although frequently considered colonizers or contaminants, the nondiphtherial corynebacteria have been associated with invasive disease, particularly in immunocompromised patients. Specifically, for example, these organisms have been implicated in bacteremia, particularly in association with catheterization, endocarditis, prosthetic valve infection, meningitis, neurosurgical shunt infection, brain abscess, peritonitis (often in the setting of chronic ambulatory peritoneal dialysis), osteomyelitis, septic arthritis, urinary tract infection, empyema, and pneumonia. Patients infected with nondiphtherial corynebacteria usually have significant medical comorbidity or immunosuppression. Several of these organisms, including *C. jeikeium* and *C. urealyticum*, are associated with resistance to multiple antibiotics. The related organism *Rhodococcus equi* is associated with necrotizing pneumonia and granulomatous infection, particularly in immunocompromised individuals. Other related species that can cause infections in humans are *Actinomyces* (formerly *Corynebacterium*) *pyogenes* and *Arcanobacterium* (formerly *Corynebacterium*) *haemolyticum*.

MICROBIOLOGY AND LABORATORY DIAGNOSIS

These organisms are non-acid-fast, catalase-positive, aerobic or facultatively anaerobic bacilli. Their colonial morphologies vary widely; some species are small and α-hemolytic (similar to lactobacilli), whereas others form large white colonies (similar to yeasts). Many nondiphtherial coryneforms require special medium (e.g., Löffler's, Tinsdale's, or telluride medium) for growth.

EPIDEMIOLOGY

Humans are the natural reservoirs for several nondiphtherial coryneforms, including *C. xerosis*, *C. pseudodiphtheriticum*, *C. striatum*, *C. minutissimum*, *C. jeikeium*, *C. urealyticum*, and *A. haemolyticum*. Animal reservoirs are responsible for carriage of *A. pyogenes*, *C. ulcerans*, and *C. pseudotuberculosis*. Soil is the natural reservoir for *R. equi*.

C. pseudodiphtheriticum is part of the normal flora of the human pharynx and skin. *C. xerosis* is found on the skin, nasopharynx, and conjunctiva; *C. auris* in the external auditory canal; and *C. striatum* in the anterior nares and on the skin. *C. jeikeium* and *C. urealyticum* are found in the axilla, groin, and perineum, particularly in hospitalized patients. *C. ulcerans* and *C. pseudotuberculosis* infections have been associated with the consumption of raw milk from infected cattle.

Specific Nondiphtherial Coryneforms • ***C. ulcerans*** This organism causes a diphtheria-like illness and produces both diphtheria toxin and a dermonecrotic toxin. *C. ulcerans* is a commensal in horses and cattle and has been isolated from cow's milk. The organism causes exudative pharyngitis, primarily during summer months, in rural areas, and among individuals exposed to cattle. In contrast to diphtheria, *C. ulcerans* infection is considered a zoonosis, and person-to-person transmission has not been firmly established. Nevertheless, treatment with antitoxin and antibiotics should be initiated when respiratory *C. ulcerans* is identified, and a contact investigation (including throat cultures to determine the need for antimicrobial prophylaxis and vaccination with the appropriate diphtheria toxoid–containing vaccine for unimmunized human contacts) should be conducted. The organism grows on Löffler's, Tinsdale's, and telluride media as well as blood agar. In addition to exudative pharyngitis, cutaneous disease due to *C. ulcerans* has been reported. *C. ulcerans* is susceptible to a wide panel of antibiotics. Erythromycin and macrolides appear to be the first-line agents.

C. pseudotuberculosis (ovis) Infections caused by *C. pseudotuberculosis* are rare and are reported almost exclusively from Australia. *C. pseudotuberculosis* causes suppurative granulomatous lymphadenitis and an eosinophilic pneumonia syndrome among individuals who handle horses, cattle, goats, and deer or who drink unpasteurized milk. The organism is an important veterinary pathogen, causing suppurative lymphadenitis, abscesses, and pneumonia, but is rarely a human pathogen. Successful treatment with erythromycin or tetracycline has been reported, with surgery also performed when indicated.

C. jeikeium (GROUP JK) After a 1976 survey of diseases caused by nondiphtherial corynebacteria, CDC Group JK was recognized as an important opportunistic pathogen among neutropenic patients and later emerged in HIV-infected patients as an AIDS-associated opportunistic infection. This led to the organism's reclassification as a separate species, *C. jeikeium*. The predominant syndrome associated with *C. jeikeium* is sepsis, which can occur in conjunction with pneumonia, endocarditis, meningitis, osteomyelitis, or epidural abscess. Risk factors for *C. jeikeium* infection include hematologic malignancy, neutropenia from comorbid conditions, prolonged hospitalization, exposure to multiple antibiotics, and skin disruption. There is evidence that *C. jeikeium* is part of the normal flora of the inguinal, axillary, genital, and perirectal areas in hospitalized patients.

Broad-spectrum antimicrobial therapy appears to select for colonization. Originally described in the United States, *C. jeikeium* has also been reported in Europe. The gram-positive coccobacilli, which slightly resemble streptococci, grow as small, gray to white, glistening, nonhemolytic colonies on blood agar. *C. jeikeium* lacks urease and nitrate reductase and does not ferment most carbohydrates. It is resistant to most antibiotics tested except for vancomycin. Effective therapy involves removal of the source of infection, be it a catheter, a prosthetic joint, or a prosthetic valve. There have been efforts to prevent *C. jeikeium* infection by use of antibacterial soap in the care of high-risk patients in intensive care settings.

C. urealyticum (GROUP D2) Identified as a urease-positive nondiphtherial *Corynebacterium* in 1972, *C. urealyticum* is an opportunistic cause of sepsis and urinary tract infection. This organism appears to be the etiologic agent of a severe urinary tract syndrome known as *alkaline-encrusted cystitis*: a chronic inflammatory bladder infection associated with deposition of ammonium magnesium phosphate on the surface and walls of ulcerating lesions in the bladder. In addition, *C. urealyticum* has been associated with pneumonia, peritonitis, endocarditis, osteomyelitis, and wound infection. It is similar to *C. jeikeium* in its resistance to most antibiotics except vancomycin, which has been used successfully in the treatment of severe infections.

C. minutissimum *Erythrasma* is a cutaneous infection producing reddish-brown, macular, scaly, pruritic intertriginous patches. The dermatologic presentation under the Wood's lamp is of coral-red fluorescence. *C. minutissimum* appears to be a common cause of erythrasma, although there is evidence for a polymicrobial etiology in certain settings. In addition, this fluorescent microbe has been associated with bacteremia in patients with hematologic malignancy. Erythrasma responds to topical erythromycin, clarithromycin, clindamycin, or fusidic acid, although more severe infections may require oral macrolide therapy.

Other Nondiphtherial Corynebacteria *C. xerosis* is a human commensal found in the conjunctiva, nasopharynx, and skin. This nontoxigenic organism is occasionally identified as a source of invasive infection in immunocompromised or postoperative patients and prosthetic joint recipients. *C. striatum* is found in the anterior nares and on the skin, face, and upper torso of normal individuals. Also nontoxigenic, this organism has been associated with invasive opportunistic infections in severely ill or immunocompromised patients. *C. amycolatum* is a new species isolated from human skin and is identified on the basis of a unique 16S ribosomal RNA sequence associated with opportunistic infection. *C. glucuronolyticum* is a new nonlipophilic species that causes male genitourinary tract infections such as prostatitis and urethritis. These infections may be successfully treated with a wide variety of antibacterial agents, including β-lactams, rifampin, aminoglycosides, or vancomycin; however, the organism appears to be resistant to fluoroquinolones, macrolides, and tetracyclines. *C. imitans* has been identified in Eastern Europe as a nontoxigenic cause of pharyngitis. *C. auris* has been isolated from children with otitis media and is susceptible to fluoroquinolones, rifampin, tetracycline, and vancomycin but resistant to penicillin G and variably susceptible to macrolides. *C. pseudodiphtheriticum* (*C. hofmannii*) is a nontoxigenic component of the normal human flora. Human infections—particularly endocarditis of either prosthetic or native valves and invasive pneumonia—have been identified only rarely. Although *C. pseudodiphtheriticum* may be isolated from the nasopharynx of patients with suspected diphtheria, it is part of the normal flora and does not produce diphtheria toxin. *C. propinquum*, a close relative of *C. pseudodiphtheriticum*, is part of CDC Group ANF-3 and is isolated from human respiratory tract specimens and blood. *C. afermentans* subspecies *lipophilum* belongs to CDC Group ANF-1 and has been isolated from human blood and abscess infections. *C. accolens* has been isolated from wound drainage, throat swabs, and sputum and is typically identified as a satellite of staphylococcal organisms; it has been associated with endocarditis. *C. bovis* is a veterinary commensal that has not been clearly identified as a cause of human disease. *C. aquaticum* is a water-associated organism that is occasionally isolated from patients using medical devices (e.g., for chronic ambulatory peritoneal dialysis or venous access).

Rhodococcus *Rhodococcus* species are phylogenetically related to the corynebacteria. These gram-positive coccobacilli have been associated with tuberculosis-like infections in humans with granulomatous pathology. Although *R. equi* is best known, other species have been identified, including *R.* (also *Gordonia*) *bronchialis*, *R.* (also *Tsukamurella*) *aurantiacus*, *R. luteus*, *R. erythropolis*, *R. rhodochrous*, and *R. rubropertinctus*. *R. equi* has been recognized as a cause of pneumonia in horses since the 1920s; it causes related infections in cattle, sheep, and swine. *R. equi* is found in soil as an environmental microbe. The organisms vary in length; appear as spherical to long, curved, clubbed rods; and produce large, irregular mucoid colonies. *R. equi* does not ferment carbohydrates or liquefy gelatin and is often acid fast. An intracellular pathogen of macrophages, *R. equi* can cause granulomatous necrosis and caseation. The organism has been identified most commonly in pulmonary infections, but infections of brain, bone, and skin have also been reported. Most commonly, *R. equi* disease manifests as nodular cavitary pneumonia of the upper lobe—a picture similar to that seen in tuberculosis or nocardiosis. Most patients are immunocompromised, often with HIV infection. Subcutaneous nodular lesions have also been identified. The involvement of *R. equi* should be considered in any patient presenting with a tuberculosis-like syndrome. Infection due to *R. equi* has been treated successfully with antibiotics that penetrate intracellularly, including macrolides, clindamycin, rifampin, and trimethoprim-sulfamethoxazole. β-Lactam antibiotics have not been useful. The organism is routinely susceptible to vancomycin, which is considered the drug of choice.

Actinomyces pyogenes A cause of seasonal leg ulcers in humans in rural Thailand, *A. pyogenes* is a well-known pathogen of cattle, sheep, goats, and pigs. A few human cases of sepsis, endocarditis, septic arthritis, pneumonia, meningitis, and empyema have been reported.

The agent is susceptible to β-lactams, tetracycline, aminoglycosides, and fluoroquinolones.

Arcanobacterium haemolyticum *A. haemolyticum* was identified as an agent of wound infections in U.S. soldiers in the South Pacific during World War II. This organism appears to be a commensal of the human nasopharynx and skin but has been implicated as a cause of pharyngitis and chronic skin ulcers. In contrast to the much more common pharyngitis caused by *Streptococcus pyogenes*, *A. haemolyticum* pharyngitis is associated with a scarlatiniform rash on the trunk and proximal extremities in about half of cases; this illness is occasionally confused with toxic shock syndrome. Because *A. haemolyticum* pharyngitis primarily affects teenagers, it has been postulated that the rash-pharyngitis syndrome may represent copathogenicity or synergy with EBV or opportunistic secondary infection complicating EBV infection. *A. haemolyticum* has also been reported as a cause of bacteremia, soft tissue infection, osteomyelitis, and cavitary pneumonia, predominantly in the setting of underlying diabetes mellitus. The organism is susceptible to β-lactams, macrolides, fluoroquinolones, clindamycin, vancomycin, and doxycycline. Penicillin resistance has been reported.

FURTHER READINGS

Centers for Disease Control and Prevention: Availability of diphtheria antitoxin through an investigational new drug protocol. MMWR 53:413, 2004

———: Vaccine preventable deaths and the Global Immunization Vision and Strategy, 2006–2015. MMWR 55:511, 2006

Dittmann S et al: Successful control of epidemic diphtheria in the states of the former Union of Soviet Socialist Republics: Lessons learned. J Infect Dis 181(Suppl 1):S10, 2000

Holmes RK: Biology and molecular epidemiology of diphtheria toxin and the tox gene. J Infect Dis 181(Suppl 1):S156, 2000

Kadirova R et al: Clinical characteristics and management of 676 hospitalized diphtheria cases, Kyrgyz Republic, 1995. J Infect Dis 181(Suppl 1):S110, 2000

Kretsinger K et al: Preventing tetanus, diphtheria, and pertussis among adults: Use of tetanus toxoid, reduced diphtheria toxoid, and acellular pertussis vaccine; recommendations of the Advisory Committee on Immunization Practices (ACIP) and recommendation of ACIP, supported by the Healthcare Infection Control Practices Advisory Committee (HICPAC), for use of Tdap among health-care personnel. MMWR Recomm Rep 55(RR-17):1, 2006

MacGregor RR: *Corynebacterium diphtheriae*, in *Principles and Practice of Infectious Diseases*, 6th ed, GL Mandell et al (eds). Philadelphia, Elsevier Churchill Livingstone, 2005, pp 2457–2465

McNeil SA et al: Comparison of the safety and immunogenicity of concomitant and sequential administration of an adult formulation tetanus and diphtheria toxoids adsorbed combined with acellular pertussis (Tdap) vaccine and trivalent inactivated influenza vaccine in adults. Vaccine 25:3464, 2007; Epub 2007 Jan 9.

Meyer DK, Reboli AC: Other coryneform bacteria and *Rhodococcus*, in *Principles and Practice of Infectious Diseases*, 6th ed, GL Mandell et al (eds). Philadelphia, Elsevier Churchill Livingstone, 2005, pp 2465–2478

Pichichero ME et al: Combined tetanus, diphtheria, and 5-component pertussis vaccine for use in adolescents and adults. JAMA 293:3003, 2005

132 Infections Caused by *Listeria monocytogenes*

Elizabeth L. Hohmann, Daniel A. Portnoy

Listeria monocytogenes is a food-borne pathogen that can cause serious infections, particularly in pregnant women and immunocompromised individuals. A ubiquitous saprophytic environmental bacterium, *L. monocytogenes* is also a pathogen with a broad host range. Humans are probably accidental hosts for this microorganism. *L. monocytogenes* is of interest not only to clinicians but also to basic scientists as a model intracellular pathogen that is used to study basic mechanisms of microbial pathogenesis and host immunity.

MICROBIOLOGY

L. monocytogenes is a facultatively anaerobic, nonsporulating, gram-positive rod that grows over a broad temperature range, including refrigeration temperatures. This organism is motile during growth at low temperatures but much less so at 37°C. The vast majority of cases of human listerial disease can be traced to serotypes 1/2a, 1/2b, and 4. *L. monocytogenes* is weakly β-hemolytic on blood agar, and (as detailed below) its β-hemolysin is an essential determinant of its pathogenicity.

PATHOGENESIS

Infections with *L. monocytogenes* follow ingestion of contaminated food that contains the bacteria at high concentrations. The conversion from environmental saprophyte to a pathogen involves the coordinate regulation of bacterial determinants of pathogenesis that mediate entry into cells, intracellular growth, and cell-to-cell spread. One essential determinant of *L. monocytogenes* pathogenesis is the transcriptional activator PrfA, which activates the majority of genes required for cell entry and intracellular parasitism. Many of the organism's pathogenic strategies can be examined experimentally in tissue culture models of infection; such a model is presented in Fig. 132-1. Like other enteric

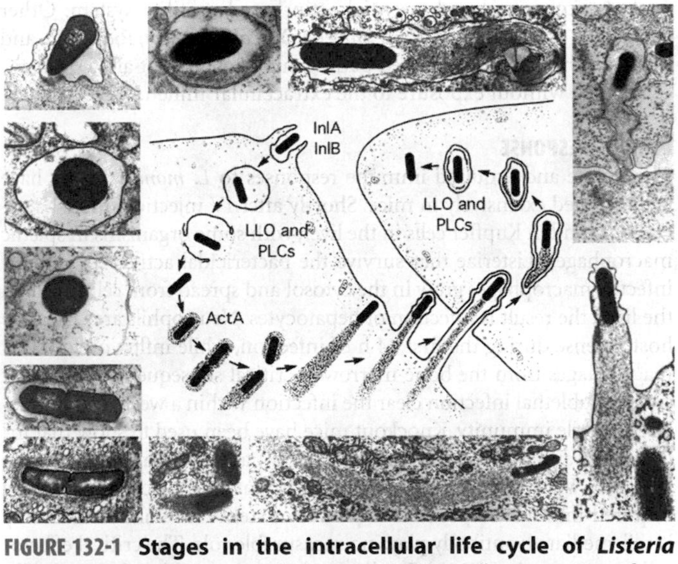

FIGURE 132-1 Stages in the intracellular life cycle of *Listeria monocytogenes*. The central diagram depicts cell entry, escape from a vacuole, actin nucleation, actin-based motility, and cell-to-cell spread. Surrounding the diagram are representative electron micrographs from which it was derived. ActA, surface protein mediating nucleation of host actin filaments to propel bacteria intra- and intercellularly; LLO, listeriolysin O; PLCs, phospholipases C; Inl, internalin. See text for further details. *(Adapted with permission from LG Tilney and DA Portnoy: Actin filaments and the growth, movement, and spread of the intracellular bacterial parasite, Listeria monocytogenes. J Cell Biol 109:1597, 1989. © Rockefeller University Press.)*

pathogens, *L. monocytogenes* induces its own internalization by cells that are not normally phagocytic. Its entry into cells is mediated by host surface proteins classified as internalins. Internalin-mediated entry is important in the crossing of intestinal, blood-brain, and fetoplacental barriers, although how *L. monocytogenes* traffics from the intestine to the brain or fetus is only beginning to be investigated. In a pregnant guinea pig model of infection, *L. monocytogenes* was shown to traffic from maternal organs to the placenta; surprisingly, however, it also trafficked from the placenta back to maternal organs.

Perhaps the most important determinant of the pathogenesis of *L. monocytogenes* is its β-hemolysin, listeriolysin O (LLO). LLO is a pore-forming, cholesterol-dependent cytolysin. (Related cytolysins include streptolysin O, pneumolysin, and perfringolysin O, all of which are produced by extracellular pathogens.) LLO is largely responsible for mediating the rupture of the phagosomal membrane that forms after phagocytosis of *L. monocytogenes.* LLO probably acts by inserting itself into an acidifying phagosome, thereby preventing the vesicle's maturation. In addition, LLO acts as a translocation pore for one or both of the *L. monocytogenes* phospholipases that also contribute to vacuolar lysis. LLO synthesis and activity are controlled at multiple levels to ensure that its lytic activity is limited to acidic vacuoles and does not affect the cytosol. Mutations in LLO that influence its synthesis, cytosolic half-life, or pH optimum cause premature toxicity to infected cells. There is an inverse relationship between toxicity and virulence—i.e., the more cytotoxic the strain, the less virulent it is in animals.

Once in the cytosol, *L. monocytogenes* grows rapidly, with intracellular doubling times equivalent to those in rich media. One of the PrfA-regulated genes encodes a hexose-phosphate transporter that facilitates the growth of cytosolic bacteria on phosphorylated glucose derivatives of host origin.

Shortly after exposure to the mammalian-cell cytosol, *L. monocytogenes* produces ActA, another PrfA-regulated surface protein that mediates the nucleation of host actin filaments to propel the bacteria intra- and intercellularly. ActA mimics host proteins of the Wiskott-Aldrich syndrome protein (WASP) family by promoting the actin nucleation properties of the Arp2/3 complex. Thus, *L. monocytogenes* can enter the cytosol of almost any eukaryotic cell or cell extract and can exploit a conserved and essential actin-based motility system. Other pathogens as diverse as certain *Shigella*, *Mycobacterium*, *Rickettsia*, and *Burkholderia* spp. use a related pathogenic strategy that allows cell-to-cell spread without exposure to the extracellular milieu.

IMMUNE RESPONSE

The innate and acquired immune responses to *L. monocytogenes* have been studied extensively in mice. Shortly after IV injection, most bacteria are found in Kupffer cells in the liver, with some organisms in splenic macrophages. Listeriae that survive the bactericidal activity of initially infected macrophages grow in the cytosol and spread from cell to cell. In the liver, the result is infection of hepatocytes. Neutrophils are crucial to host defense during the first 24 h of infection, while influx of activated macrophages from the bone marrow is critical subsequently. Mice that survive sublethal infection clear the infection within a week, with consequent sterile immunity. Knockout mice have been used to show that interferon γ and tumor necrosis factor (TNF) are essential in controlling infection. While innate immunity is sufficient to control infection, the acquired immune response is required for sterile immunity. Immunity is cell-mediated; antibody plays no measurable role. The critical effector cells are cytotoxic (CD8+) T cells that recognize and lyse infected cells. The bacteria grow and spread from cell to cell. The host recognizes and lyses infected cells, and extracellular bacteria are killed by circulating activated phagocytes. A hallmark of the *L. monocytogenes* model is that killed vaccines do not provide protective immunity. The explanation for this fundamental observation is multifactorial, involving the generation of appropriate cytokines and the compartmentalization of bacterial proteins for antigen processing and presentation.

EPIDEMIOLOGY

L. monocytogenes usually enters the body via the gastrointestinal tract in foods. Listeriosis is most often sporadic, although outbreaks do occur. Recent annual incidences in the United States range from 2 to 9 cases per 1 million population. No epidemiologic or clinical evidence supports human-to-human transmission (other than vertical transmission from mother to fetus) or waterborne infection. In line with its survival and multiplication at refrigeration temperatures, *L. monocytogenes* is commonly found in processed and unprocessed foods of animal and plant origin, especially soft cheeses, delicatessen meats, hot dogs, milk, and cold salads. Because food supplies are increasingly centralized and normal hosts tolerate the organism well, outbreaks may not be immediately apparent; pulsed-field gel electrophoresis has proved useful in linking cases to specific foods. FoodNet, an active U.S. surveillance program, has demonstrated decreases in listeriosis incidence, although recent data from some European countries show a stable or increased number of cases, perhaps because of enhanced active surveillance. The U.S. Food and Drug Administration has a zero-tolerance policy for *L. monocytogenes* in ready-to-eat foods.

DIAGNOSIS

Symptoms of listerial infection overlap greatly with those of other infectious diseases. Timely diagnosis requires that the illness be considered in groups at risk: pregnant women; elderly persons; neonates; individuals immunocompromised by organ transplants, cancer, or treatment with TNF antagonists or glucocorticoids; and patients with a variety of chronic medical conditions, including alcoholism, diabetes, renal disease, rheumatologic illness, and iron overload. Meningitis in older adults (especially with parenchymal brain involvement or subcortical brain abscess) or a local outbreak of culture-negative febrile gastroenteritis should trigger consideration of *L. monocytogenes* infection. Listeriosis occasionally affects healthy, young, nonpregnant individuals. HIV-infected patients are at risk; however, listeriosis seems to be prevented by trimethoprim-sulfamethoxazole (TMP-SMX) prophylaxis targeting other AIDS-related infections. The diagnosis is typically made by culture of blood, cerebrospinal fluid (CSF), or amniotic fluid. *L. monocytogenes* may be confused with "diphtheroids" or pneumococci in gram-stained CSF or may be gram-variable and confused with *Haemophilus* spp. Serologic tests and polymerase chain reaction assays are not clinically useful diagnostic tools at present.

CLINICAL MANIFESTATIONS

Listerial infections present as several clinical syndromes, of which meningitis and septicemia are most common. Monocytosis is seen in infected rabbits but is not a hallmark of human infection.

Gastroenteritis Appreciated only since the outbreaks of the late 1980s, listerial gastroenteritis typically develops within 48 h of ingestion of a large inoculum of bacteria in contaminated foods such as milk, deli meats, and salads. Attack rates are high (50–100%). *L. monocytogenes* is neither sought nor found in routine fecal cultures, but its involvement should be considered in outbreaks when cultures for other likely pathogens are negative. Manifestations include fever, diarrhea, headache, and constitutional symptoms. The largest reported outbreak occurred in an Italian school system and included 1566 individuals; ~20% of patients were hospitalized, but only one person had a positive blood culture. Isolated gastrointestinal illness does not require antibiotic treatment. Surveillance studies show that 0.1–5% of healthy asymptomatic adults may have stool cultures positive for the organism.

Bacteremia *L. monocytogenes* septicemia presents with fever, chills, and myalgias/arthralgias and cannot be differentiated from septicemia involving other organisms. Meningeal symptoms, focal neurologic findings, or mental status changes may suggest the diagnosis. Bacteremia is documented in 70–90% of cancer patients with listeriosis. A nonspecific flulike illness with fever is a common presentation in pregnant women. Endocarditis of prosthetic and native valves is an uncommon complication, with reported fatality rates of 35–50% in case series. A lumbar puncture is often prudent, although not necessary, in pregnant women without central nervous system (CNS) symptoms.

Meningitis *L. monocytogenes* causes ~5–10% of all cases of community-acquired bacterial meningitis in adults in the United States. Case-fatality rates are reported to be 15–26% and do not appear to have changed over time. This diagnosis should be considered in all older or chronically ill adults with "aseptic" meningitis. The presentation is more frequently subacute (with illness developing over several days) than in meningitis of other bacterial etiologies, and nuchal rigidity and meningeal signs are less common. Photophobia is infrequent. Focal findings and seizures are common in some but not all series. The CSF profile in listerial meningitis most often shows white blood cell (WBC) counts in the range of 100–5000/μL (rarely higher); 75% of patients have WBC counts below 1000/μL, usually with a neutrophil predominance more modest than that in other bacterial meningitides. Low glucose levels and positive results on Gram's staining are found ~30–40% of the time.

Meningoencephalitis and Focal CNS Infection *L. monocytogenes* can directly invade the brain parenchyma, producing either cerebritis or focal abscess. Approximately 10% of cases of CNS infection are macroscopic abscesses resulting from bacteremic seeding; the affected patients often have positive blood cultures. Concurrent meningitis can exist, but the CSF may appear normal. Abscesses can be misdiagnosed as metastatic or primary tumors and, in rare instances, occur in the cerebellum and the spinal cord. Invasion of the brainstem results in a characteristic severe rhombencephalitis, usually in otherwise healthy older adults. The presentation may be biphasic, with a prodrome of fever and headache followed by asymmetric cranial nerve deficits, cerebellar signs, and hemiparetic and hemisensory deficits. Respiratory failure can occur. The subacute course and the often minimally abnormal CSF findings may delay the diagnosis, which may be suggested by MRI images showing ring-enhancing lesions after gadolinium contrast and hyperintense lesions on diffusion-weighted imaging. MRI is superior to CT for the diagnosis of these infections.

Other Focal Infections Focal infections of visceral organs; the eye; the pleural, peritoneal and pericardial spaces; and the bones and joints have all been reported.

Infection in Pregnancy and Neonatal Infection Listeriosis in pregnancy is a severe and important infection. The usual presentation is a nonspecific acute or subacute febrile illness with myalgias, arthralgias, backache, and headache. Pregnant women with listeriosis are usually bacteremic. This syndrome should prompt blood cultures, especially in the absence of another reasonable explanation. Involvement of the CNS is rare in the absence of other risk factors. Preterm delivery is a common complication, and the diagnosis may be made only postpartum. As many as 70–90% of fetuses from infected women can become infected. Prepartum treatment of bacteremic women enhances the chances of delivery of a healthy infant. Women usually do well after delivery: maternal deaths are very rare, even when the diagnosis is made late in pregnancy or postpartum. Overall mortality rates for fetuses infected in utero approach 50% in some series; among live-born neonates treated with antibiotics, mortality rates are much lower (~20%). *Granulomatosis infantiseptica* is an overwhelming listerial fetal infection with miliary microabscesses and granulomas, most often in the skin, liver, and spleen. Less severe neonatal infection acquired in utero presents at birth. "Late-onset" neonatal illness typically develops ~10 days after delivery but can occur up to a month postpartum. Mothers of infants with late-onset disease are not ill.

Rx INFECTIONS CAUSED BY *LISTERIA MONOCYTOGENES*

No clinical trials have compared antimicrobial agents for the treatment of *L. monocytogenes* infections. Data obtained in studies conducted in vitro and in animals as well as observational clinical data indicate that ampicillin is the drug of choice, although penicillin is also highly active. Adults should receive IV ampicillin at high doses (2 g every 4 h), and most experts recommend the addition of gentamicin for synergy (1.0–1.7 mg/kg every 8 h). TMP-SMX, given IV, is the best alternative for the penicillin-allergic patient (15–20 mg of TMP/kg per day in divided doses every 6–8 h). The dosages recommended cover CNS infection and bacteremia (see below for duration); dosages must be reduced for patients with renal insufficiency. One small nonrandomized study supports a combination of ampicillin and TMP-SMX. Case reports document success with vancomycin, tetracycline, and erythromycin, although there are also reports of clinical failure with all three agents. Imipenem and the newer quinolones are possible alternative agents that have been efficacious in animal models, but clinical experience is very limited. Cephalosporins are *not* effective and should not be used. Neonates should receive ampicillin and gentamicin at doses based on weight.

The duration of therapy depends on the syndrome: 2 weeks for bacteremia, 3 weeks for meningitis, 6–8 weeks for brain abscess/encephalitis, and 4–6 weeks for endocarditis in both neonates and adults. Early-onset neonatal disease may be more severe and should be treated for >2 weeks.

COMPLICATIONS AND PROGNOSIS

About 50–70% of individuals who are promptly diagnosed and treated recover fully, but permanent neurologic sequelae are common in patients with brain abscess or rhombencephalitis. Of 100 live-born treated neonates in one series, 60% recovered fully, 24% died, and 13% had long-term neurologic or other complications.

PREVENTION

Healthy persons should take standard precautions to prevent foodborne illness: fully cooking meats, washing fresh vegetables, carefully cleaning utensils, and avoiding unpasteurized dairy products. In addition, persons at risk for listeriosis, including pregnant women, should avoid soft cheeses (although hard cheeses and yogurt are not problematic) and should avoid or thoroughly reheat ready-to-eat and delicatessen foods, even though the absolute risk they pose is relatively low.

FURTHER READINGS

BAKARDJIEV AI et al: *Listeria monocytogenes* traffics from maternal organs to the placenta and back. PLoS Pathog 2:e66, 2006

BORTOLUSSI R, MAILMAN TM: Listeriosis, in *Infectious Disease of the Fetus and Newborn Infant*, 6th ed, S Remington et al (eds). Philadelphia, Elsevier Saunders, 2005, p 465

HAMON M et al: *Listeria monocytogenes*: A multifaceted model. Nat Rev Microbiol 4:423, 2006

MYLONAKIS E et al: Listeriosis during pregnancy: A case series and review of 222 cases. Medicine (Baltimore) 81:260, 2002

OOI ST, LORBER B: Gastroenteritis due to *Listeria monocytogenes*. Clin Infect Dis 40:1327, 2005

PORTNOY DA (section ed): The listeriae, in *Gram-Positive Pathogens*, 2d edition, VA Fischetti et al (eds). Washington, DC, ASM Press, 2006, Section 4

TWETEN RK: Cholesterol-dependent cytolysins, a family of versatile pore-forming toxins. Infect Immun 73:6199, 2005

www.cdc.gov/foodnet/

133 Tetanus

Elias Abrutyn†

DEFINITION

Tetanus is a neurologic disorder, characterized by increased muscle tone and spasms, that is caused by tetanospasmin, a powerful protein toxin elaborated by *Clostridium tetani*. Tetanus occurs in several clinical forms, including generalized, neonatal, and localized disease.

ETIOLOGIC AGENT

C. tetani is an anaerobic, motile, gram-positive rod that forms an oval, colorless, terminal spore and thus assumes a shape resembling a tennis racket or drumstick. The organism is found worldwide in soil, in the inanimate environment, in animal feces, and occasionally in human feces. Spores may survive for years in some environments and are resistant to various disinfectants and to boiling for 20 min. Vegetative cells, however, are easily inactivated and are susceptible to several antibiotics, including metronidazole and penicillin.

Tetanospasmin is formed in vegetative cells under plasmid control. With autolysis, the single-chain toxin is released and cleaved to form a heterodimer consisting of a heavy chain (100 kDa), which mediates binding to and entry into nerve cells, and a light chain (50 kDa), which blocks neurotransmitter release. The genome of *C. tetani* has been sequenced. The amino acid structures of the two most powerful toxins known, botulinum toxin and tetanus toxin, are partially homologous.

EPIDEMIOLOGY

Tetanus occurs sporadically and almost always affects unimmunized persons; partially immunized persons and fully immunized individuals who fail to maintain adequate immunity with booster doses of vaccine may be affected as well.

Although tetanus is entirely preventable by immunization, the burden of disease worldwide is great. Tetanus is a notifiable disease in many countries, but reporting is known to be inaccurate and incomplete, particularly in developing countries. As a result, the World Health Organization considers the number of reported cases to be an underestimate and periodically undertakes case/death estimates to assess the burden of disease. In 2002 (the last year for which data are available), the *estimated* number of tetanus-related deaths in all age groups was 213,000, of which 180,000 (85%) were attributable to neonatal tetanus. In contrast, only 18,781 tetanus cases in total and 11,762 neonatal cases were actually *reported* for that year.

Tetanus is common in areas where soil is cultivated, in rural areas, in warm climates, during summer months, and among males. In countries without a comprehensive immunization program, tetanus occurs predominantly in neonates and other young children. It is noteworthy that international programs to eliminate neonatal tetanus have been in place for some time. In the United States and other nations with successful immunization programs, neonatal tetanus is rare (only three cases were reported in the United States during 1990–2004), and the disease affects other age groups (Fig. 133-1) and groups inadequately covered by immunization (such as nonwhites). The success of immunization in the United States is depicted in Fig. 133-2. Since 1976, fewer than 100 cases have been reported yearly. At present, the risk of tetanus in this country is highest among the elderly. A large-scale national serologic survey performed in 1988–1994 showed that 72% of Americans ≥6 years old had protective antibody levels. In contrast, only 30% of persons >70 years old were protected.

In the United States, most cases of tetanus follow an acute injury (puncture wound, laceration, abrasion, or other trauma). Tetanus may be acquired indoors or during outdoor activities (e.g., farming, gardening). The implicated injury may be major but can be so trivial that medical attention is not sought. In some cases, no injury or portal of entry can be identified. The disease may complicate chronic conditions such as skin ulcers, abscesses, and gangrene. Tetanus has also been associated with burns, frostbite, middle-ear infection, surgery, abortion, childbirth, body piercing, and drug abuse (notably "skin popping"). Recurrent tetanus has been reported.

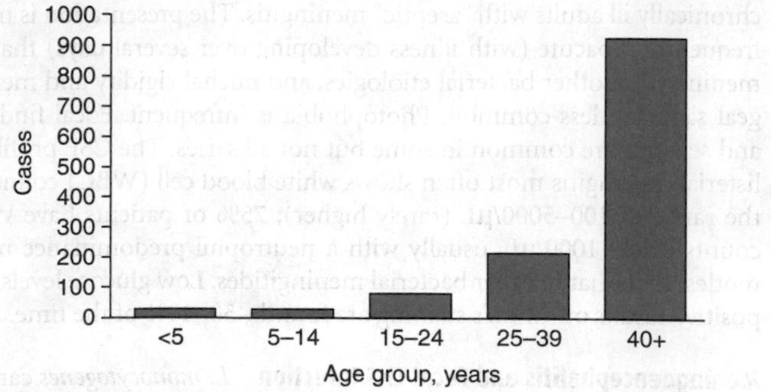

FIGURE 133-1 Tetanus: reported cases in the United States, by age group, 1980–2003; N = 1277. *(From Centers for Disease Control and Prevention, National Immunization Program. Tetanus and Tetanus Toxoid: Epidemiology and Prevention of Vaccine-Preventable Diseases. www.cdc.gov/nip/ed/vpd2006/Slides/chap06-tetanus9.ppt. Revised January 2006. Accessed 1/30/2007.)*

PATHOGENESIS

Contamination of wounds with spores of *C. tetani* is probably a frequent occurrence. Germination and toxin production, however, take place only in wounds with low oxidation-reduction potential, such as those with devitalized tissue, foreign bodies, or active infection. *C. tetani* does not itself evoke inflammation, and the portal of entry retains a benign appearance unless coinfection with other organisms is present.

Toxin released in the wound binds to peripheral motor neuron terminals, enters the axon, and is transported to the nerve-cell body in the brainstem and spinal cord by retrograde intraneuronal transport. The toxin then migrates across the synapse to presynaptic terminals, where it blocks release of the inhibitory neurotransmitters glycine and γ-aminobutyric acid (GABA) from vesicles (see Fig. 134-1). The blocking of neurotransmitter release by tetanospasmin, a zinc metalloprotease, involves cleavage of synaptobrevin, a protein essential to proper function of the synaptic vesicle release apparatus. With diminished inhibition, the resting firing rate of the α motor neuron increases, producing rigidity. With lessened activity of reflexes that limit polysynaptic spread of impulses (a glycinergic activity), agonists and antagonists may be recruited rather than inhibited, with the consequent production of

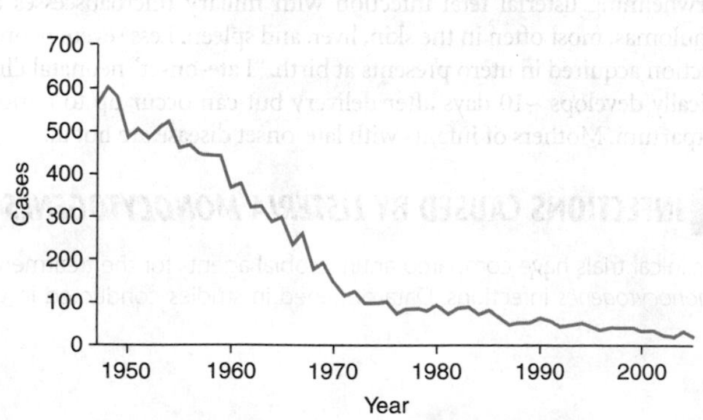

FIGURE 133-2 Impact of tetanus immunization in the United States, 1947–2005 (2005, provisional total). Tetanus vaccine became part of the routine childhood immunization schedule in the late 1940s. *(From Centers for Disease Control and Prevention, National Immunization Program. Tetanus and Tetanus Toxoid: Epidemiology and Prevention of Vaccine-Preventable Diseases. www.cdc.gov/nip/ed/vpd2006/Slides/chap06-tetanus9.ppt. Revised January 2006. Accessed 1/30/2007.)*

†Deceased. A contributor to HPIM since the 12th edition, Dr. Abrutyn passed away on February 22, 2007.

spasms. Toxin may also affect preganglionic sympathetic neurons in the lateral gray matter of the spinal cord and parasympathetic centers. Loss of inhibition of preganglionic sympathetic neurons may produce sympathetic hyperactivity and high circulating catecholamine levels. Tetanospasmin, like botulinum toxin, may block neurotransmitter release at the neuromuscular junction and produce weakness or paralysis, but this effect is clinically evident only in cephalic tetanus. Recovery requires sprouting of new nerve terminals.

In local tetanus, only the nerves supplying the affected muscles are involved. Generalized tetanus occurs when toxin released in the wound enters the lymphatics and bloodstream and is spread widely to distant nerve terminals; the blood-brain barrier blocks direct entry into the central nervous system. If it is assumed that intraneuronal transport times are equal for all nerves, short nerves are affected before long nerves: this fact explains the sequential involvement of nerves of the head, trunk, and extremities in generalized tetanus.

CLINICAL MANIFESTATIONS

Generalized tetanus, the most common form of the disease, is characterized by increased muscle tone and generalized spasms. The median time of onset after injury is 7 days; 15% of cases occur within 3 days and 10% after 14 days.

Typically, the patient first notices increased tone in the masseter muscles (trismus, or lockjaw). Dysphagia or stiffness or pain in the neck, shoulder, and back muscles appears concurrently or soon thereafter. The subsequent involvement of other muscles produces a rigid abdomen and stiff proximal limb muscles; the hands and feet are relatively spared. Sustained contraction of the facial muscles results in a grimace or sneer (risus sardonicus), and contraction of the back muscles produces an arched back (opisthotonos). Some patients develop paroxysmal, violent, painful, generalized muscle spasms that may cause cyanosis and threaten ventilation. These spasms occur repetitively and may be spontaneous or provoked by even the slightest stimulation. A constant threat during generalized spasms is reduced ventilation or apnea or laryngospasm. The severity of illness may be mild (muscle rigidity and few or no spasms), moderate (trismus, dysphagia, rigidity, and spasms), or severe (frequent explosive paroxysms). The patient may be febrile, although many patients have no fever; mentation is unimpaired. Deep tendon reflexes may be increased. Dysphagia or ileus may preclude oral feeding.

Autonomic dysfunction commonly complicates severe cases and is characterized by labile or sustained hypertension, tachycardia, dysrhythmia, hyperpyrexia, profuse sweating, peripheral vasoconstriction, and increased plasma and urinary catecholamine levels. Periods of bradycardia and hypotension may also be documented. Sudden cardiac arrest sometimes occurs, but its basis is unknown. Other complications include aspiration pneumonia, fractures, muscle rupture, deep-vein thrombophlebitis, pulmonary emboli, decubitus ulcer, and rhabdomyolysis.

Neonatal tetanus usually occurs as the generalized form and is usually fatal if left untreated. It develops in children born to inadequately immunized mothers, frequently after unsterile treatment of the umbilical cord stump. Its onset generally comes during the first 2 weeks of life.

Local tetanus is an uncommon form in which manifestations are restricted to muscles near the wound. The prognosis is excellent. *Cephalic tetanus*, a rare form of local tetanus, follows head injury or ear infection and involves one or more facial cranial nerves. The incubation period is a few days and mortality is high.

DIAGNOSIS

The diagnosis of tetanus is based entirely on clinical findings. Tetanus is unlikely if a reliable history indicates the completion of a primary vaccination series and the receipt of appropriate booster doses. Wounds should be cultured in suspected cases. However, *C. tetani* can be isolated from wounds of patients without tetanus and frequently cannot be recovered from wounds of those with tetanus. The leukocyte count may be elevated. Cerebrospinal fluid examination yields normal results. Electromyograms may show continuous discharge of motor units and shortening or absence of the silent interval normally seen after an action potential. Nonspecific changes may be evident on the electrocardiogram. Muscle enzyme levels may be raised. Serum antitoxin levels of ≥0.1 IU/mL (as measured by enzyme-linked immunosorbent assay) are considered protective and make tetanus unlikely, although cases in patients with protective antitoxin levels have been reported.

The differential diagnosis includes conditions also producing trismus, such as alveolar abscess, strychnine poisoning, dystonic drug reactions (e.g., phenothiazines and metoclopramide), and hypocalcemic tetany. In addition, meningitis/encephalitis, rabies, and an acute intra-abdominal process (because of the rigid abdomen) might be considered. Markedly increased tone in central muscles (face, neck, chest, back, and abdomen), with superimposed generalized spasms and relative sparing of the hands and feet, strongly suggests tetanus.

℞ TETANUS

GENERAL MEASURES The goals of therapy are to eliminate the source of toxin, neutralize unbound toxin, and prevent muscle spasms while monitoring the patient's condition and providing support—especially respiratory support—until recovery. Patients should be admitted to a quiet room in an intensive care unit, where observation and cardiopulmonary monitoring can be maintained continuously but stimulation can be minimized. Protection of the airway is vital. Wounds should be explored, carefully cleansed, and thoroughly debrided.

ANTIBIOTIC THERAPY Although of unproven value, antibiotic therapy is administered to eradicate vegetative cells—the source of toxin. The use of penicillin (10–12 million units IV, given daily for 10 days) has been recommended, but metronidazole (500 mg every 6 h or 1 g every 12 h) is preferred by some experts on the basis of this drug's excellent antimicrobial activity and the absence of the GABA-antagonistic activity seen with penicillin. The drug of choice remains unclear: one nonrandomized clinical trial found a survival benefit with metronidazole, but another study failed to find a difference among benzathine penicillin, benzyl penicillin, and metronidazole. Clindamycin and erythromycin are alternatives for the treatment of penicillin-allergic patients. Additional specific antimicrobial therapy should be given for active infection with other organisms.

ANTITOXIN Given to neutralize circulating toxin and unbound toxin in the wound, antitoxin effectively lowers mortality; toxin already bound to neural tissue is unaffected. Human tetanus immune globulin (TIG) is the preparation of choice and should be given promptly. The dose is 3000–6000 units IM, usually in divided doses because the volume is large. The optimal dose is not known, however, and results from one study indicated that a 500-unit dose was as effective as higher doses. Pooled IVIg may be an alternative to TIG, but the specific antitoxin concentration in this formulation is not standardized. The value of administering antitoxin before wound manipulation or of injecting a dose proximal to the wound or infiltrating the wound is unclear. Additional doses are unnecessary because the half-life of antitoxin is long. Antibody does not penetrate the blood-brain barrier. Intrathecal administration should be considered experimental. Equine tetanus antitoxin (TAT) is not available in the United States but is used elsewhere. It is cheaper than human antitoxin, but the half-life is shorter and its administration commonly elicits a hypersensitivity reaction and serum sickness.

CONTROL OF MUSCLE SPASMS Many agents, alone and in combination, have been used to treat the muscle spasms of tetanus, which are painful and can threaten ventilation by causing laryngospasm or sustained contraction of ventilatory muscles.

In some developing countries, cost, availability, and the ability to provide ventilatory support are important factors in the choice of therapy. The ideal therapeutic regimen would abolish spasmodic activity without causing oversedation and hypoventilation. Diazepam, a benzodiazepine and GABA agonist, is in wide use. The dose is titrated, and large doses (≥250 mg/d) may be required. Lorazepam, with a longer duration of action, and midazolam, with a short half-life, are other options. Barbiturates and chlorpromazine are considered second-line agents. Therapeutic paralysis with a nondepolarizing neuromuscular blocking agent and mechanical ventilation may be used for spasms unresponsive to medication or spasms that threaten ventilation. However, prolonged paralysis after discontinuation of therapy has been described. Other agents include propofol, which is expensive; dantrolene and intrathecal baclofen, which may allow shortening of the duration of therapeutic paralysis; succinylcholine, which has been associated with hyperkalemia; and magnesium sulfate. A recent double-blind, randomized, placebo-controlled clinical trial of magnesium sulfate in severe tetanus did not find a reduction in the need for ventilation or in mortality rate; however, use of midazolam and pipecuronium for treatment of muscle spasms and of verapamil for treatment of cardiovascular instability was reduced.

RESPIRATORY CARE Intubation or tracheostomy, with or without mechanical ventilation, may be required for hypoventilation due to oversedation or laryngospasm or for the avoidance of aspiration by patients with trismus, disordered swallowing, or dysphagia. The need for these procedures should be anticipated, and they should be undertaken electively and early.

AUTONOMIC DYSFUNCTION The optimal therapy for sympathetic overactivity has not been defined. Agents that have been considered include labetalol (an α- and β-adrenergic blocking agent that is recommended by some experts but that reportedly has caused sudden death), esmolol administered by continuous infusion (a beta blocker whose short half-life may be advantageous in the event of severe hypertension from unopposed α-adrenergic activity), clonidine (a central-acting antiadrenergic drug), verapamil, and morphine sulfate. Parenteral magnesium sulfate and continuous spinal or epidural anesthesia have been used but may be more difficult to administer and monitor. The relative efficacy of these modalities has yet to be determined. Hypotension or bradycardia may require volume expansion, use of vasopressors or chronotropic agents, or pacemaker insertion.

VACCINE Patients recovering from tetanus should be actively immunized (see below) because immunity is not induced by the small amount of toxin required to produce disease.

ADDITIONAL MEASURES Like all patients receiving ventilatory support, patients with tetanus require attention to hydration; nutrition; physiotherapy; prophylactic anticoagulation; bowel, bladder, and renal function; decubitus ulcer prevention; and treatment of intercurrent infection.

PREVENTION

Active Immunization All partially immunized and unimmunized adults should receive vaccine, as should those recovering from tetanus. The primary series for adults consists of three doses: the first and second doses are given 4–8 weeks apart, and the third dose is given 6–12 months after the second. A booster dose is required every 10 years and may be given at mid-decade ages—35, 45, and so on. Combined tetanus and diphtheria toxoid, adsorbed (Td, for adult use)—rather than single-antigen tetanus toxoid—is preferred for persons >7 years of age. Adsorbed vaccine is preferred because it produces more persistent antibody titers than fluid vaccine. Two combined tetanus/diphtheria/attenuated pertussis vaccines have recently been approved: one (ADACEL) for adults 19–64 years of age and the other (BOOSTRIX) for adolescents 11–18 years of age. The Advisory Committee on Immunization Practices has recommended a single dose of Tdap (ADACEL) for adults 19–64 years old who have not received Tdap.

Wound Management Proper wound management requires consideration of the need for (1) passive immunization with TIG and (2) active immunization with vaccine (Tdap or Td; Table 133-1). The dose of TIG for passive immunization of persons with wounds of average severity (250 units IM) produces a protective serum antibody level for at least 4–6 weeks; the appropriate dose of TAT, an equine-derived product, is 3000–6000 units. Vaccine and antibody should be administered at separate sites with separate syringes.

Neonatal Tetanus Preventive measures include maternal vaccination, even during pregnancy; efforts to increase the proportion of births that take place in the hospital; and the provision of training for nonmedical birth attendants.

TABLE 133-1 GUIDE TO TETANUS PROPHYLAXIS AND ROUTINE WOUND MANAGEMENT

History of Adsorbed Tetanus Toxoid (Doses)	Clean Minor Wound		All Other Wounds[a]	
	Tdap or Td[b]	TIG	Tdap or Td[b]	TIG
Unknown or <3	Yes	No	Yes	Yes
≥3	No[c]	No	No[d]	No

[a]Such as, but not limited to, wounds contaminated with dirt, feces, soil, and saliva; puncture wounds; avulsions; and wounds from missile or crushing injuries, burns, and frostbite.
[b]Tdap is preferred to Td for adults 19–64 years old who have never received Tdap. Td is preferred for adults who have received Tdap previously and is used when Tdap is not available. Td is also recommended for persons >64 years old. If TT and TIG are both used, TT adsorbed rather than TT for booster use only (fluid vaccine) should be used.
[c]Yes, if ≥10 years have elapsed since the last TT-containing vaccine dose.
[d]Yes, if ≥5 years have elapsed since the last TT-containing vaccine dose.
Note: Tdap, tetanus toxoid, reduced diphtheria toxoid, and acellular pertussis vaccine, adsorbed; DT, diphtheria and tetanus vaccine; DTP, diphtheria, tetanus, and pertussis vaccine; Td, tetanus-diphtheria toxoid, adsorbed; TIG, tetanus immune globulin; TT, tetanus toxoid.
Source: Modified from Centers for Disease Control and Prevention, 2006.

PROGNOSIS

The application of methods to monitor and support oxygenation has markedly improved the prognosis in tetanus. Mortality rates as low as 10% have been reported from units accustomed to handling such cases. In the United States in 2003, there were 20 cases and 2 deaths; no cases were in patients <18 years old, and 19 cases were ascribed to inadequate immunization. The outcome is poor in neonates and the elderly and in patients with a short incubation period, a short interval from the onset of symptoms to admission, or a short period from the onset of symptoms to the first spasm (period of onset). Outcome is also related to the extent of prior vaccination.

The course of tetanus extends over 4–6 weeks, and patients may require prolonged ventilator support. Increased tone and minor spasms can last for months, but recovery is usually complete.

FURTHER READINGS

Abrutyn E, Berlin JA: Intrathecal therapy of tetanus: A meta-analysis. JAMA 266:2262, 1991

Ahmadsyah I, Salim A: Treatment of tetanus: An open study to compare the efficacy of procaine penicillin and metronidazole. BMJ 291:648, 1985

Bleck TP: *Clostridium tetani* (tetanus), in *Principles and Practice of Infectious Diseases,* 5th ed, GL Mandell et al (eds). New York, Churchill Livingstone, 2000, pp 2537–2543

Centers for Disease Control and Prevention: Preventing tetanus, diphtheria, and pertussis among adults: Use of tetanus toxoid, reduced diphtheria toxoid and acellular pertussis vaccine: Recommendations of the Advisory Committee on Immunization Practices (ACIP) and recommendation of ACIP, supported by the Healthcare Infection Control Practices Advisory Committee (HICPAC), for use of Tdap among health-care personnel. MMWR 55(RR17):1, 2006

Centers for Disease Control and Prevention: Tetanus—Puerto Rico, 2002. MMWR 51:613, 2002

———: Tetanus surveillance—United States, 1998–2000. Surveillance summaries, June 20, 2003. MMWR 52(SS-3):1, 2003

Cook TM et al: Tetanus: A review of the literature. Br J Anaesth 87:477, 2001

Hsu SS et al: Tetanus in the emergency department: A current review. J Emerg Med 20:357, 2001

McQuillan CM et al: Serologic immunity to diphtheria and tetanus in the United States. Ann Intern Med 136:660, 2002

Thwaites CL et al: Magnesium sulphate for the treatment of severe tetanus: A randomized controlled trial. Lancet 368:1436, 2006

134 Botulism

Elias Abrutyn†

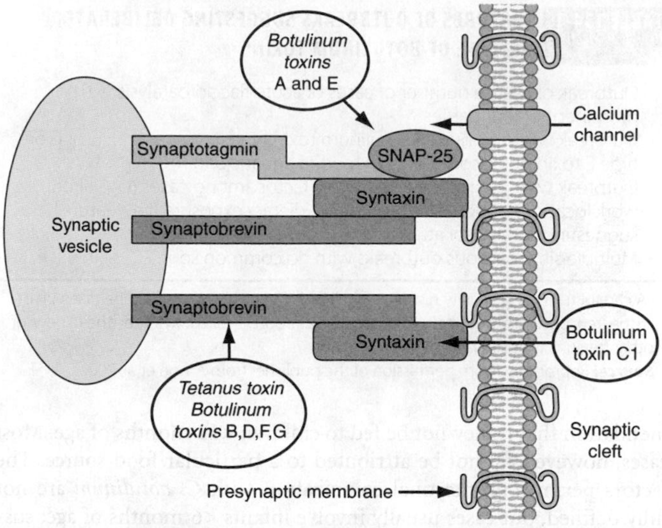

FIGURE 134-1 The synaptic vesicle release apparatus and the sites of action of botulinum toxins. Toxin acts to block neurotransmitter release from the synaptic vesicle into the synaptic cleft. The site of action of tetanus toxin is also shown. *[From TP Bleck et al: In WM Scheld et al (eds): Infections of the Central Nervous System, 2d ed. New York, Raven Press, 1997; with permission.]*

DEFINITION

Botulism is a paralytic disease caused by potent protein neurotoxins elaborated by *Clostridium botulinum*. Illness begins with cranial nerve involvement and proceeds caudally to involve the extremities. Cases may be classified as (1) *food-borne botulism*, from ingestion of preformed toxin in food contaminated with *C. botulinum*; (2) *wound botulism*, from toxin produced in wounds contaminated with the organism; and (3) *intestinal botulism*, from ingestion of spores and production of toxin in the intestine of infants (infant botulism) or adults. Botulinum toxin, because of its extraordinary potency, has long been considered a threat as an agent of bioterrorism or biologic warfare that could be acquired by inhalation or ingestion (Chap. 214). Iatrogenic botulism can follow cosmetic or therapeutic use of toxin.

ETIOLOGIC AGENT

C. botulinum, a species encompassing a heterogeneous group of anaerobic gram-positive organisms that form subterminal spores, is found in soil and marine environments throughout the world and elaborates the most potent bacterial toxin known. Organisms of types A through G have been distinguished by the antigenic specificities of their toxins; a classification system based on physiologic characteristics has also been described. Rare strains of other clostridial species—*C. butyricum* and *C. baratii*—have been found to produce toxin. *C. botulinum* strains with proteolytic activity can digest food and produce a spoiled appearance; nonproteolytic types leave the appearance of food unchanged.

Of the eight distinct toxin types described (A, B, C_1, C_2, D, E, F, and G), all except C_2 are neurotoxins; C_2 is a cytotoxin of unknown clinical significance. Botulinum neurotoxin, whether ingested, inhaled, or produced in the intestine or a wound, enters the vascular system and is transported to peripheral cholinergic nerve terminals, including neuromuscular junctions, postganglionic parasympathetic nerve endings, and peripheral ganglia. The central nervous system is not involved. Steps in neurotoxin activity include binding, internalization in endocytic vesicles, translocation to the cytosol, and proteolysis resulting in a blockage of the release of the neurotransmitter acetylcholine (Fig. 134-1). Cure follows sprouting of new nerve terminals.

Toxin types A, B, E, and (rarely) F cause disease in humans; type G (from *C. argentinense*) has been associated with sudden death, but not with neuroparalytic illness, in a few patients in Switzerland; and types C and D cause disease in animals.

EPIDEMIOLOGY

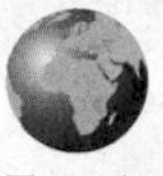

Human botulism occurs worldwide. In the United States, the geographic distribution of cases by toxin type parallels the distribution of organism types found in the environment. Type A predominates west of the Rocky Mountains; type B is generally distributed but is more common in the East; and type E is found in the Pacific Northwest, Alaska, and the Great Lakes area.

Food-borne botulism in the United States is associated primarily with home-canned food (particularly vegetables, fruit, and condiments) and less commonly with meat and fish. Type E outbreaks are frequently associated with fish products. Commercial products occasionally cause outbreaks, some of which are attributable to improper handling after purchase. Outbreaks in restaurants, schools, and private homes have been traced to uncommon sources (commercial potpies, beef stew, turkey loaf, sautéed onions, baked potatoes, preserved green olives, bamboo shoots, and chopped garlic in oil). Food-borne botulism can occur when (1) food to be preserved is contaminated with spores, (2) preservation does not inactivate the spores but kills other putrefactive bacteria that might inhibit growth of *C. botulinum* and provides anaerobic conditions at a pH and temperature that allow germination and toxin production, and (3) food is not heated to a temperature that destroys toxin before being eaten.

CLINICAL MANIFESTATIONS

Food-Borne Botulism After ingestion of food containing toxin, illness varies from a mild condition for which no medical advice is sought to very severe disease that can result in death within 24 h. The incubation period is usually 18–36 h but, depending on toxin dose, can range from a few hours to several days. Symmetric descending paralysis is characteristic and can lead to respiratory failure and death. Cranial nerve involvement, which almost always marks the onset of symptoms, usually produces diplopia, dysarthria, dysphonia, and/or dysphagia. Weakness progresses, often rapidly, from the head to involve the neck, arms, thorax, and legs; occasionally, weakness is asymmetric. Nausea, vomiting, and abdominal pain may precede or follow the onset of paralysis. Dizziness, blurred vision, dry mouth, and very dry, occasionally sore throat are common. Patients are generally alert and oriented, but they may be drowsy, agitated, and anxious. Typically, they have no fever. Ptosis is frequent; the pupillary reflexes may be depressed, and fixed or dilated pupils are noted in half of patients. The gag reflex may be suppressed, and deep tendon reflexes may be normal or decreased. Sensory findings are usually absent. Paralytic ileus, severe constipation, and urinary retention are common.

Wound Botulism Wound botulism occurs when the spores contaminating a wound germinate and form vegetative organisms that produce toxin. This rare condition resembles food-borne illness except that the incubation period is longer, averaging about 10 days, and gastrointestinal symptoms are lacking. Wound botulism has been documented after traumatic injury involving contamination with soil; in injection drug users, for whom black-tar heroin use has been identified as a risk factor; and after cesarean delivery. The illness has occurred even after antibiotics have been given to prevent wound infection. When present, fever is probably attributable to concurrent infection with other bacteria. The wound may appear benign.

Intestinal Botulism In intestinal botulism, toxin is produced in and absorbed from the intestine after the germination of ingested spores. Intestinal botulism in infants (infant botulism) is the most common form of botulism. The severity ranges from mild illness with failure to thrive to fulminant severe paralysis with respiratory failure. Infant botulism may be one cause of sudden infant death. The identification of contaminated honey as one source of spores has led to the recom-

†Deceased. A contributor to HPIM since the 12th edition, Dr. Abrutyn passed away on February 22, 2007.

TABLE 134-1 FEATURES OF OUTBREAKS SUGGESTING DELIBERATE RELEASE OF BOTULINUM TOXIN[a]

- Outbreak of a large number of cases of acute flaccid paralysis with prominent bulbar palsies
- Outbreak with an unusual botulinum toxin type (i.e., type C, D, F, or G or type E toxin not associated with food of aquatic origin)
- Outbreak with a common geographic factor among cases (e.g., airport, work location) but without a common dietary exposure (i.e., features suggesting an aerosol attack)
- Multiple simultaneous outbreaks with no common source

[a]A careful travel and activity history, as well as a dietary history, should be taken in any suspected botulism outbreak. Patients should also be asked whether they know of other persons with similar symptoms.

Source: Reproduced with permission of the publisher from Arnon et al, 2002.

mendation that honey not be fed to children <12 months of age. Most cases, however, cannot be attributed to a particular food source. The factors permitting intestinal colonization with *C. botulinum* are not fully defined, but cases usually involve infants <6 months of age; susceptibility may decrease as the normal intestinal flora develops. Intestinal botulism involving adults is uncommon. The patient may have a history of gastrointestinal disease, gastrointestinal surgery, or recent antibiotic therapy. Toxin and organisms may be identified in the stool.

Bioterrorism and Biologic Warfare (See also Chap. 214) Botulinum toxin could be dispersed as an aerosol (producing inhalational botulism) or as a contaminant in material to be ingested (producing food-borne botulism). Inhalational botulism resembles food-borne illness, but gastrointestinal symptoms are absent. Botulism follows adsorption of toxin from mucosal surfaces (gut, lung) and wounds, but the toxin does not penetrate intact skin. As a toxin-mediated illness, botulism is noncommunicable, and standard isolation precautions are sufficient. Features suggestive of an outbreak due to deliberate release of botulinum toxin are shown in Table 134-1.

DIAGNOSIS

A diagnosis of botulism must be considered in patients with symmetric descending paralysis who are afebrile and mentally intact. The bulbar musculature is involved initially, but sensory findings are absent and, early on, deep tendon reflexes remain intact. The differential diagnosis of botulism and distinguishing features are listed in Table 134-2. Depending on season and other epidemiologic factors, West Nile virus infection may also be a consideration.

The demonstration of toxin in serum by bioassay in mice is definitive, but this test may give negative results, particularly in wound and infant botulism. It is performed only by specific laboratories, which can be identified through regional public health authorities. Other assays are being developed and remain experimental. The demonstration of *C. botulinum* or its toxin in vomitus, gastric fluid, or stool is strongly suggestive of the diagnosis because intestinal carriage is rare. Isolation of the organism from food without toxin is insufficient grounds for the diagnosis. Wound cultures yielding the organism are suggestive of botulism. The edrophonium chloride (Tensilon) test for myasthenia gravis may be falsely positive in botulism but is usually less dramatically positive than in the former condition. Nerve conduction velocity is normal, but compound muscle action potentials on routine nerve stimulation studies are decreased with a supramaximal stimulus, and facilitation is evident after repetitive stimulation at high frequency. Single-fiber electromyography may be helpful. The white blood cell count and erythrocyte sedimentation rate are normal.

TABLE 134-2 SELECTED MIMICS THAT MAY LEAD TO MISDIAGNOSIS OF BOTULISM

Condition	Features Distinguishing Condition from Botulism
Common Misdiagnoses	
Guillain-Barré syndrome[a] and its variants, especially Miller-Fisher variant	History of antecedent infection; paresthesias; often ascending paralysis; early areflexia; eventual CSF protein increase; EMG findings
Myasthenia gravis[a]	Recurrent paralysis; EMG findings; sustained response to anticholinesterase
Stroke[a]	Paralysis often asymmetric; abnormal CNS image
Intoxication with depressants (e.g., acute alcohol intoxication), organophosphates, carbon monoxide, or nerve gas	History of exposure; excessive drug levels detected in body fluids
Lambert-Eaton syndrome	Increased strength with sustained contraction; evidence of lung carcinoma; EMG findings similar to botulism
Tick paralysis	Paresthesias; ascending paralysis; tick attached to skin
Other Misdiagnoses	
Poliomyelitis	Antecedent febrile illness; asymmetric paralysis; CSF pleocytosis
CNS infections, especially of the brainstem	Mental status changes; CSF and EEG abnormalities
CNS tumor	Paralysis often asymmetric; abnormal CNS image
Streptococcal pharyngitis[b]	Absence of bulbar palsies; positive rapid antigen test result or throat culture
Psychiatric illness[a]	Normal EMG in conversion paralysis
Viral syndrome[a]	Absence of bulbar palsies and flaccid paralysis
Inflammatory myopathy[a]	Elevated creatine kinase level
Diabetic complications[a]	Sensory neuropathy; few cranial nerve palsies
Hyperemesis gravidarum[a]	Absence of bulbar palsies and acute flaccid paralysis
Hypothyroidism[a]	Abnormal thyroid function tests
Laryngeal trauma[a]	Absence of flaccid paralysis; dysphonia without flaccid paralysis
Overexertion[a]	Absence of bulbar palsies and acute flaccid paralysis

[a]Misdiagnoses made in a large outbreak of botulism (St. Louis ME et al: Botulism from chopped garlic: Delayed recognition of a major outbreak. Ann Intern Med 108:363, 1988).
[b]Pharyngeal erythema can occur in botulism.

Note: CNS, central nervous system; CSF, cerebrospinal fluid; EEG, electroencephalogram; EMG, electromyogram.

Source: Reproduced with permission of the publisher from Arnon et al, 2002.

Rx BOTULISM

Patients should be hospitalized and monitored closely, both clinically and by spirometry, pulse oximetry, and measurement of arterial blood gases for incipient respiratory failure. Intubation and mechanical ventilation should be strongly considered when the vital capacity is <30% of predicted, especially when paralysis is progressing rapidly and hypoxemia with absolute or relative hypercarbia is documented (Chap. 263). Serial measurements of the maximal static inspiratory pressure may be useful in predicting respiratory failure.

In food-borne illness, equine antitoxin should be administered as soon as possible after specimens are obtained for laboratory analysis. Treatment should not await laboratory analyses, which may take days. The previous trivalent antitoxin preparation (types A, B, and E) is no longer available. Instead, a bivalent preparation containing toxin types A and B and an investigational monovalent type E preparation can be obtained. The bivalent preparation is administered routinely; monovalent type E antitoxin is given in addition when exposure to type E toxin is suspected (after seafood ingestion, for example). In the United States, antitoxin as well as help with clinical management and laboratory confirmation are available at *any* time from state health departments or from the Centers for Disease Control and Prevention (CDC; emergency number, 770-488-7100). A limited supply of an investigational heptavalent antitoxin (types A through G) is maintained by the U.S. military for emergency use.

After testing for hypersensitivity to horse serum, antitoxin is given as recommended by the CDC; repeated doses are not considered necessary. Anaphylaxis and serum sickness are risks inherent in use of the equine product, and desensitization of allergic patients may be required. If there is no ileus, cathartics and enemas may be used to purge the gut of toxin; emetics or gastric lavage can also be used if the time since ingestion is brief (only a few hours). Neither the use of antibiotics to eliminate an intestinal source of possible continued toxin production nor the administration of guanidine hydrochloride and other drugs to reverse paralysis is of proven value.

Treatment of infant botulism requires supportive care and administration of human botulism immune globulin, which can be obtained by calling the California Department of Health Services at 510-231-7600 or by following the instructions at *www.infantbotulism.org*. Neither equine antitoxin nor antibiotics have been shown to be beneficial. In wound botulism, equine antitoxin is administered. The wound should be thoroughly explored and debrided, and an antibiotic such as penicillin should be given to eradicate *C. botulinum* from the site, even though the benefit of this therapy is unproven. Results of wound cultures should guide the use of other antibiotics.

Botulinum toxins are being employed for a variety of cosmetic and therapeutic purposes, and new uses are being evaluated. Generalized botulism-like weakness complicating therapy (iatrogenic botulism) has been reported but is rare.

PROGNOSIS

Type A disease is generally more severe than type B, and mortality rates from botulism are higher among patients above age 60 than among younger patients. With improved respiratory and intensive care, the case-fatality rate in food-borne illness has been reduced to ~7.5% and is low in infant botulism as well. Artificial respiratory support may be required for months in severe cases. Some patients experience residual weakness and autonomic dysfunction for as long as a year after disease onset.

PREVENTION

A pentavalent vaccine (types A through E) is available for use in highly exposed individuals. Spores are highly resistant to heat but can be inactivated by exposure to high temperature (116–121°C) and pressure, as in steam sterilizers or pressure cookers used in accordance with the manufacturer's instructions. Toxin is heat-labile and can be inactivated by exposure to a temperature of 85°C for 5 min. Newly identified cases should be reported immediately to public health authorities.

FURTHER READINGS

Arnon SS et al: Human botulism immune globulin for the treatment of infant botulism. N Engl J Med 354:462, 2006

——— et al: Botulinum toxin as a biological weapon, in *Bioterrorism: Guidelines for Medical and Public Health Management*, DA Henderson et al (eds). Chicago, AMA Press, 2002, pp 141–165

Cawthorne A et al: Botulism and preserved green olives. Emerg Infect Dis 11:781, 2005

Caya JG et al: *Clostridium botulinum* and the clinical laboratorian: A detailed review of botulism, including biological warfare ramifications of botulinum toxin. Arch Pathol Lab Med 128:653, 2004

Centers for Disease Control and Prevention: Botulism from home-canned bamboo shoots—Nan Province, Thailand. MMWR 55:389, 2006

Chertow DS et al: Botulism in 4 adults following cosmetic injections with an unlicensed highly concentrated botulinum preparation. JAMA 206:2476, 2006

Cooper JG et al: *Clostridium botulinum*: An increasing complication of heroin misuse. Eur J Emerg Med 12:251, 2005

Gupta A et al: Adult botulism type F in the United States, 1981-2002. Neurology 65:1694, 2005

Lindström M, Korkeala H: Laboratory diagnostics of botulism. Clin Microbiol Rev 19:298, 2006

Montecucco C, Molgo J: Botulinal neurotoxins: Revival of an old killer. Curr Opin Pharmacol 5:274, 2005

Sobel J: Botulism. Clin Infect Dis 41:1167, 2005

135 Gas Gangrene and Other Clostridial Infections

Dennis L. Kasper, Lawrence C. Madoff

DEFINITION

Bacteria of the genus *Clostridium* are gram-positive, spore-forming, obligate anaerobes that are ubiquitous in nature. There are >60 recognized species of clostridia, many of which are generally considered saprophytic. Some of these species are pathogenic for humans and animals, particularly under conditions of lowered oxidation-reduction potential. Infections associated with these organisms range from localized wound contamination to overwhelming systemic disease. The four major disease categories for which clostridia are responsible are intestinal disorders, suppurative deep-tissue infections, skin and soft tissue infections, and bacteremias. Toxins play a major role in some of these syndromes. Colitis caused by *C. difficile* is discussed in Chap. 123.

ETIOLOGY

In humans, clostridia normally reside in the gastrointestinal tract and in the female genital tract, although they occasionally are isolated from the skin or the mouth. Of the known clostridial species, at least 30 have been isolated from human infections. Like several other pathogenic anaerobic bacterial species, clostridia are quite aerotolerant, but they do not grow on artificial media in the presence of oxygen. Clostridia characteristically produce abundant gas in artificial media and form subterminal endospores. *C. perfringens*, one of the most clinically important species, is encapsulated and nonmotile and rarely sporulates in artificial media; the spores can usually be destroyed by boiling. *C. tetani* and *C. botulinum* are discussed in detail in Chaps. 133 and 134, respectively.

Clostridia are present in the normal colonic flora at concentrations of 10^9–10^{10}/g. Of the ≥30 species that normally colonize humans, *C. ramosum* is the most abundant and is followed in frequency by *C. perfringens*. These organisms are universally present in soil at concentrations of up to 10^4/g. *C. perfringens* strains are classified (on the basis of their production of several lethal toxins) into five types, designated A through E. Type A predominates in fecal flora of humans as well as in soil, whereas the habitats of types B through E are thought to be the intestinal tracts of other animals. Although clostridia are gram-positive organisms, many species may appear to be gram-negative in clinical specimens or stationary-phase cultures. Therefore, the results of Gram's staining of cultures or clinical material should be interpreted with great care.

C. perfringens is the most common of the clostridial species isolated from tissue infections and bacteremias; next in frequency are *C. novyi* and *C. septicum*. In the category of enteric infections, *C. difficile* is an important cause of antibiotic-associated colitis, and *C. perfringens* is associated with food poisoning (type A) and enteritis necroticans (type C).

PATHOGENESIS

Despite the isolation of clostridial species from many serious traumatic wounds, the prevalence of severe infections due to these organisms is low. Two factors that appear to be essential to the development of severe disease are tissue necrosis and a low oxidation-reduction potential. *C. perfringens* requires ~14 amino acids and at least 6 additional growth factors for optimal growth. These nutrients are not found in appreciable concentrations in normal body fluids but are present in necrotic tissue. When *C. perfringens* grows in necrotic tissue, a zone of tissue damage due to the toxins elaborated by the organism allows progressive growth. In contrast, when only a few bacteria leak into the bloodstream from a small defect in the intestinal wall, the organisms do not have the opportunity to multiply rapidly because blood as a medium for growth is relatively deficient in certain amino acids and growth factors. Therefore, in a patient without tissue necrosis, bacteremia is usually benign.

C. perfringens possesses at least 17 possible virulence factors, including 12 active tissue toxins and enterotoxins. The enterotoxins include four major lethal toxins: α, β, ε, and ι. The α toxin is a phospholipase C (lecithinase) that splits lecithin into phosphorylcholine and diglyceride. It has been associated with gas gangrene and is known to be hemolytic, to destroy platelets and polymorphonuclear leukocytes (PMNs), and to cause widespread capillary damage. When injected IV, it causes massive intravascular hemolysis and damages liver mitochondria. The α toxin may be important in the initiation of muscle infections that can progress to gas gangrene. Experimentally, the higher the concentration of α toxin in the culture fluid, the smaller the dose of *C. perfringens* required to produce infection. The protective effect of antiserum is directly proportional to its content of α antitoxin. Studies suggest that θ toxin, a thiol-activated cytolysin that is also called *perfringolysin O* and is related to other cholesterol-dependent cytolysins such as listeriolysin and streptolysin O, may play an important role in pathogenesis by promoting vascular leukostasis, endothelial cell injury, and regional tissue hypoxia. The resulting perfusion defects extend the anaerobic environment and contribute to rapidly advancing tissue destruction. A characteristic pathologic finding in gas gangrene is the near absence of PMNs despite extensive tissue destruction. Experimental data indicate that both α and θ toxins are essential in the leukocyte aggregation that occurs at the margins of tissue injury instead of the expected infiltration of these cells into the area of damage. Genetically altered strains induce less leukocyte aggregation when α toxin is absent and none when θ toxin is missing. The other major toxins—β, ε, and ι—are known to increase capillary permeability.

CLINICAL MANIFESTATIONS

Intestinal Disorders • ***FOOD POISONING*** *C. perfringens*, primarily type A, is the second or third most common cause of food poisoning in the United States (Chap. 122). The responsible toxin is thought to be a cytotoxin produced by >75% of strains isolated from cases of food-borne disease. The cytotoxin binds to a receptor on the small-bowel brush border and induces a calcium ion–dependent alteration in permeability. The associated loss of ions alters intracellular metabolism, resulting in cell death. Outbreaks generally have resulted from problems in the cooling and storage of food cooked in bulk. The food sources primarily involved are meat, meat products, and poultry. Generally, the implicated meats have been cooked, allowed to cool, and then recooked the following day, often in a stew or hash. Strains of *C. perfringens* that contaminate meat manage to survive initial cooking. During reheating, the organisms sporulate and germinate. The disease is associated with an attack rate that is often as high as 70%. Symptoms of food poisoning from type A strains develop 8–24 h after ingestion of foods heavily contaminated with the organism. The primary symptoms include epigastric pain, nausea, and watery diarrhea usually lasting 12–24 h. Fever and vomiting are uncommon. Molecular methods including ribotyping and pulsed-field gel electrophoresis have been used to detect fecal cytotoxin in outbreaks of food poisoning caused by *C. perfringens*.

C. perfringens has also been implicated in a more severe form of diarrhea than that of classic food poisoning. This more severe disease tends to occur in the elderly and has been associated with antibiotic use in hospitalized populations. In this form of disease, diarrhea is generally more profuse, of longer duration, and accompanied by abdominal pain. Blood and mucus have been detected in the feces of the affected patients. In one hospital-based study of a cluster of cases, widespread environmental contamination with *C. perfringens* spores was documented.

ENTERITIS NECROTICANS Necrotizing enteritis (enteritis necroticans, or *pigbel*) is caused by β toxin produced by type C strains of *C. perfringens* following ingestion of a high-protein meal in conjunction with trypsin inhibitors (e.g., in sweet potatoes) by a susceptible host who has limited intestinal proteolytic activity. This disease has been reported among children and adults in New Guinea. A similar disease, *darmbrand*, was epidemic in Germany after World War II. Clinical features of pigbel include acute abdominal pain, bloody diarrhea, vomiting, shock, and peritonitis; 40% of patients die. Pathologic studies reveal an acute ulcerative process of the bowel restricted to the small intestine. The mucosa is lifted off the submucosa, with the formation of large denuded areas. Pseudomembranes composed of sloughed epithelium are common, and gas may dissect into the submucosa. The source of the organisms may be the patient's own intestinal flora; cultures of ingested pork have failed to yield the organism. Antibodies to the β toxin of *C. perfringens* have been of considerable benefit in changing the course of established disease. In a large-scale trial, children immunized with *C. perfringens* β toxoid were protected.

NEUTROPENIC ENTEROCOLITIS (TYPHLITIS) See Chaps. 82 and 157.

Suppurative Deep-Tissue Infections Clostridia are frequently recovered from various suppurative conditions in conjunction with other anaerobic and aerobic bacteria but can also be the only organisms isolated. These suppurative conditions, which exist with severe local inflammation but usually without the characteristic systemic signs induced by clostridial toxins, include intraabdominal sepsis, empyema, pelvic abscess, subcutaneous abscess, frostbite with gas gangrene, infection of a stump in an amputee, brain abscess, prostatic abscess, perianal abscess, conjunctivitis, infection of a renal cell carcinoma, and infection of an aortic graft.

Clostridia are isolated from approximately two-thirds of patients with intraabdominal infections resulting from intestinal perforation. *C. ramosum*, *C. perfringens*, and *C. bifermentans* are the most commonly isolated species. The presence of clostridial species does not affect the clinical presentation or outcome of these infections (Chap. 157).

An association has been made between malignancy and the isolation of *C. septicum* in the absence of a grossly contaminated deep traumatic wound; in this situation, *C. septicum* may cause spontaneous nontraumatic myonecrosis (Fig. 135-1). A major site for such a malignancy is the gastrointestinal tract, particularly the colon. An association with leukemia or with other solid tumors has also been noted, and one case of fatal myonecrosis has been reported in a patient with ovarian cancer. Some of these patients present with *C. septicum* bacteremia; these cases have a fulminant clinical course (discussed below). Others develop localized suppurative infection in the abdomen or the abdominal wall without bacteremia. Presumably, this infection arises from a silent perforation that leads to intraabdominal abscess formation.

Clostridia have been isolated from suppurative infections of the female genital tract, particularly tuboovarian and pelvic abscesses. The major species involved has been *C. perfringens*. Most of these suppurative infections are mild, with no evidence of uterine gangrene. *C. perfringens* has been isolated from as many as 20% of diseased gallbladders at surgery. One clinical syndrome, *emphysematous cholecystitis*, is caused by clostridial species at least 50% of the time. In this syndrome, gas forms in the biliary radicles and the wall of the gallbladder. Emphysematous cholecystitis is seen most often in diabetic patients. Although the mortality rate in this entity is higher than in more common forms of cholecystitis, there is no evidence of myonecrosis.

Clostridia are among the many organisms found in empyema fluid or isolated by transtracheal aspiration from patients with lung abscesses. There is no unique clinical clue to the presence of clostridia (as opposed to other organisms) in these infections. *C. perfringens* has been reported as a cause of empyema arising from aspiration pneumonia, pulmonary emboli, and infarction. However, the majority of cases of clostridial empyema are secondary to trauma.

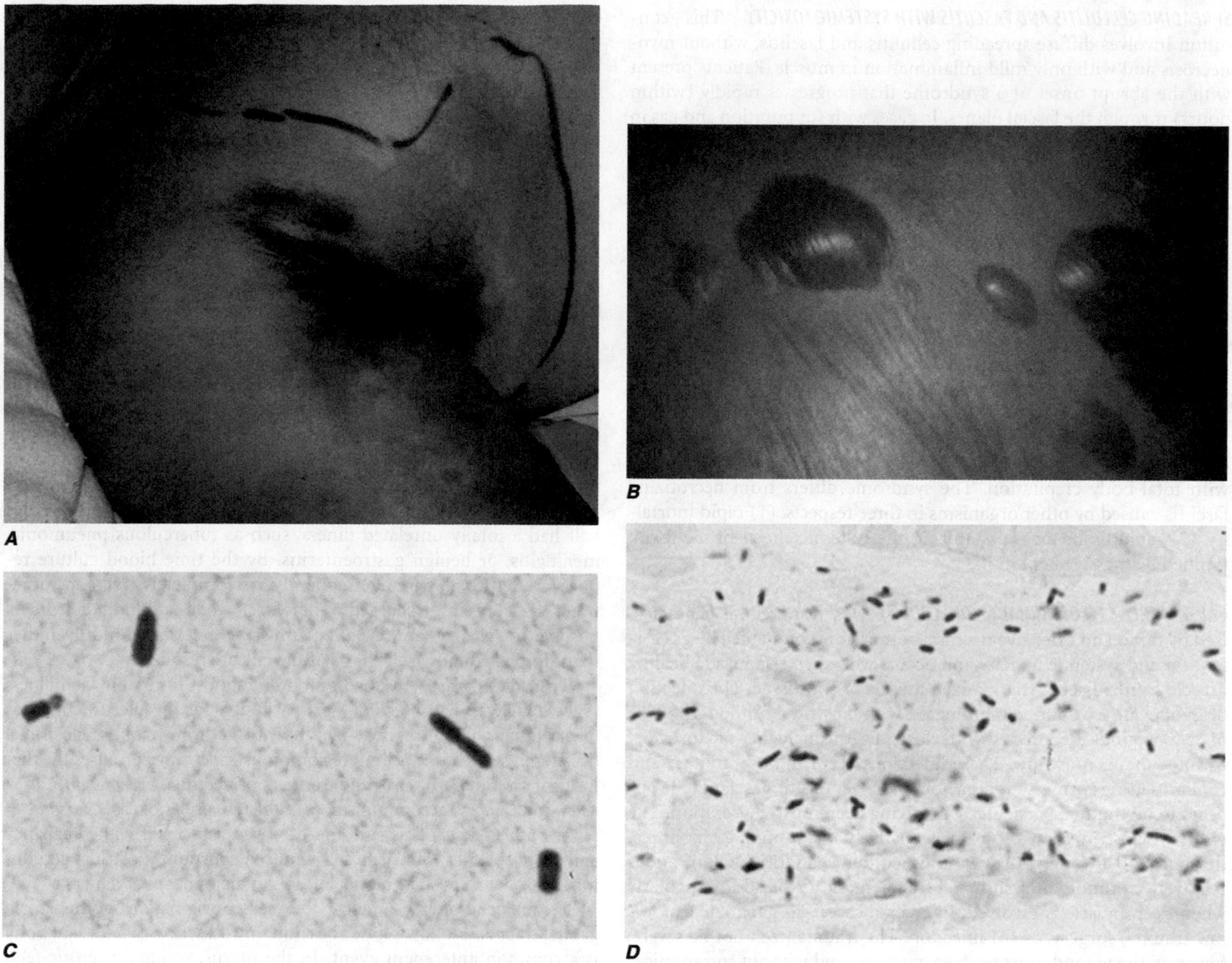

FIGURE 135-1 Spontaneous nontraumatic clostridial myonecrosis (gas gangrene). A man in his 50s presented with severe pain in the right upper extremity. Over several hours, he developed progressive swelling and discoloration in that extremity (***A***), with hemorrhagic ecchymoses and bullae (***B***). Gram's stain of aspirate from bullous lesions revealed gram-positive bacilli (***C***). The patient underwent amputation of the extremity. Tissue Gram's stain (***D***) also showed gram-positive bacilli, and surgical cultures grew *C. septicum.* Subsequent evaluation of the patient led to the diagnosis of invasive colonic carcinoma. *(Images used with permission of Stephen Calderwood, MD, and www.idimages.org.)*

Skin and Soft Tissue Infections Various categories of traumatic wound infections due to clostridia have been described: simple contamination, anaerobic cellulitis, fasciitis with or without systemic manifestations, and anaerobic myonecrosis.

SIMPLE CONTAMINATION Clostridia are cultured most often from wounds in the absence of clinical signs of sepsis. As many as 30% of battle wounds are contaminated by clostridia without signs of suppuration, and 16% of penetrating abdominal wounds yield clostridia on culture despite treatment with cephalothin and kanamycin. In cases of trauma, clostridia are isolated with equal frequency from suppurative and well-healing wounds. Thus the diagnosis of clostridial infection should be based on clinical rather than bacteriologic criteria.

LOCALIZED INFECTION OF THE SKIN AND SOFT TISSUE WITHOUT SYSTEMIC SIGNS This condition, originally referred to as *anaerobic cellulitis*, is a localized infection involving the skin and soft tissue and is due to clostridia alone or with other bacteria. There are no systemic signs of toxicity, although the infection may invade locally, producing necrosis. These infections tend to be relatively indolent, spreading slowly to contiguous areas. Localized infections are relatively free of pain and edema. Perhaps because of the lack of edema, gas that is limited to the wound and the immediately surrounding tissue may be more evident than in gas gangrene. In these localized infections, gas is never found intramuscularly. Cellulitis, perirectal abscesses, and diabetic foot ulcers are typical infections from which clostridial species can be isolated. If inadequately treated, these localized infections advance by extension through subcutaneous tissue and fascial planes into muscle and may produce severe systemic disease with signs of toxemia.

A localized form of suppurative myositis has been described in heroin addicts. These patients develop local pain and tenderness in discrete areas (particularly the thigh and forearm), with the subsequent appearance of fluctuance and crepitance that require surgical drainage. The unusual aspect of these infections is that they remain localized without systemic signs of toxicity. Moreover, the affected local areas are not necessarily sites of trauma or heroin injection. Pathologic examination reveals subcutaneous abscesses, purulent myositis, and fasciitis from which clostridia are recovered in pure culture; on occasion, mixed infections involving aerobes and anaerobes are found. Wound botulism has been reported in association with the injection of black tar heroin.

SPREADING CELLULITIS AND FASCIITIS WITH SYSTEMIC TOXICITY This condition involves diffuse spreading cellulitis and fasciitis, without myonecrosis and with only mild inflammation in muscle. Patients present with the abrupt onset of a syndrome that progresses rapidly (within hours) through the fascial planes. In cases with suppuration and gas in soft tissues as well as overwhelming toxemia, the infection is rapidly fatal. On physical examination there is subcutaneous crepitation but little localized pain. Surgery is of no proven value because there are no discretely involved tissues amenable to resection, as may be the case in myonecrosis. However, in rapidly advancing fasciitis, incision of the affected area is still the cornerstone of therapy. The initial local lesion may be quite innocuous and arises from an area involved by tumor or other infection and not by injury. The systemic toxic effects include hemolysis and injury of capillary membranes. Usually, this infection is fatal within 48 h, despite intensive therapy involving antitoxin and exchange transfusion. This syndrome is seen most commonly in patients with carcinoma, especially of the sigmoid or the cecum. Presumably, the tumor invades the fascia, and colonic contents leak into the abdominal wall. Patients present with extreme toxicity and occasionally with total-body crepitation. The syndrome differs from necrotizing fasciitis caused by other organisms in three respects: (1) rapid mortality, (2) rapid tissue invasion, and (3) the systemic effects of the toxin, typified by massive hemolysis.

GAS GANGRENE (CLOSTRIDIAL MYONECROSIS) Gas gangrene is characterized by rapid and extensive necrosis of muscle accompanied by gas formation and systemic toxicity and occurs when bacteria invade healthy muscle from adjacent traumatized muscle or soft tissue. The infection originates in a wound contaminated with clostridia. Although >30% of deep wounds are infected with clostridia, the incidence of clostridial myonecrosis is quite low. These infections occur in both military and civilian settings. An essential factor in the genesis of gas gangrene appears to be trauma, particularly involving deep muscle laceration. The entity of clostridial myonecrosis is relatively uncommon after simple, through-and-through bullet wounds without shattering of bone and is relatively common after shrapnel fragmentation wounds, particularly when deep muscle is involved. In civilian cases, gas gangrene can follow trauma, surgery, or IM injection. The trauma need not be severe; however, the wound must be deep, necrotic, and without communication to the surface. Indeed, seeding of muscle tissue by *C. septicum* from a gastrointestinal source—often a malignancy—may lead to spontaneous nontraumatic clostridial myonecrosis (Fig. 135-1).

The incubation period of gas gangrene is usually short: almost always <3 days and frequently <24 h. Some 80% of cases are caused by *C. perfringens,* while *C. novyi, C. septicum,* and *C. histolyticum* cause most of the remaining cases. Typically, gas gangrene begins with the sudden onset of pain in the region of the wound, which helps to differentiate it from spreading cellulitis. Once established, the pain increases steadily in severity but remains localized to the infected area and spreads only if the infection spreads. Soon after pain develops, local swelling and edema—accompanied by a thin, often hemorrhagic exudate—appear. Patients frequently develop marked tachycardia, but elevation in temperature may be only minimal. Gas usually is not obvious at this early stage and may be completely absent. Frothiness of the wound exudate may be noted. The skin is tense, white, often marbled with blue, and cooler than normal. The symptoms progress rapidly; swelling, edema, and toxemia increase, and a profuse serous discharge, which may have a peculiar sweetish smell, appears. Gram's staining of the wound exudate shows many gram-positive rods with relatively few inflammatory cells (Fig. 135-1C).

At surgery, muscle may appear pale because of the intensity of edema, but it does not contract when probed with a scalpel. When dissected, the muscle is beefy red and nonviable and can progress to become black, friable, and gangrenous. It is important to establish a diagnosis early, preferably by frozen-section biopsy of muscle.

Despite hypotension, renal failure, and (often) body crepitation, patients with myonecrosis frequently have a heightened awareness of their surroundings until just before death, when they lapse into toxic delirium and coma. In untreated cases, as the local wounds progress, the skin becomes bronzed; bullae appear, become filled with dark red fluid, and are accompanied by dark patches of cutaneous gangrene. Gas appears in later phases but may not be as obvious as in anaerobic cellulitis. Jaundice is rare in wound gas gangrene (in contrast to uterine infections) and, when it does appear, is almost invariably associated with hemoglobinuria, hemoglobinemia, and septicemia. Cases of clostridial myonecrosis without a history of trauma have been reported. These patients have bullous lesions and crepitation of the skin; they present with a rapidly worsening course that includes myonecrosis, especially of the extremities.

Bacteremia and Clostridial Sepsis The relatively common entity of transient clostridial bacteremia can arise in any hospitalized patient but is most common with a predisposing focus in the gastrointestinal tract, biliary tract, or uterus. Fever frequently resolves within 24–48 h without therapy. Despite the finding of clostridial bacteremia following septic abortions and the frequent isolation of clostridia from the lochia, most of the patients involved do not have evidence of sepsis. In one series of 60 patients with clostridial bacteremia, half had an infected site that could be associated with the bacteremia, while the other half had a totally unrelated illness, such as tuberculous pneumonia, meningitis, or benign gastroenteritis. By the time blood culture reports are returned, patients frequently are completely well and sometimes have been discharged. Therefore, when a blood culture is positive for clostridia, the patient must be assessed clinically rather than simply treated on the basis of the culture result.

Clostridial sepsis is an uncommon but almost invariably fatal illness following clostridial infection—primarily that of the uterus, colon, or biliary tract. This entity must be differentiated from transient clostridial bacteremia, which is much more common. *C. perfringens* causes the majority of cases of both sepsis and transient bacteremia. *C. septicum, C. sordellii,* and *C. novyi* account for most of the remainder of cases. *C. sordellii* sepsis with toxic shock syndrome has been associated with pregnancy and more recently with medically induced abortion. Clostridia account for 1–2.5% of all positive blood cultures in major hospital centers.

The majority of cases of clostridial sepsis originate from the female genital tract and follow septic abortion. Introduction of a foreign body is a common antecedent event. In the uterus, residual necrotic fetal and placental tissues and traumatized endometrium may allow the growth of clostridia. Only a small fraction of cases of septic abortion (1%) are followed by serious sepsis. In these instances, sepsis, fever, and chills begin 1–3 days after the attempted abortion. The initial signs are malaise, headache, severe myalgias, abdominal pain, nausea, vomiting, and occasionally diarrhea. Frequently, a bloody or brown vaginal discharge is noted. Patients may rapidly develop oliguria, hypotension, jaundice, and hemoglobinuria. The hemolysis, which is secondary to *C. perfringens* α toxin, causes a characteristic bronzing of the skin. As in myonecrosis, the mental status of severely ill patients is characterized by increased alertness and apprehension. Local examination of the pelvis reveals foul cervical discharge, occasionally with gas. Frequently, laceration marks around the cervix or perforation of the cervical segment is evident. If the infection involves the myometrium or has spread to the adnexa, extreme tenderness, guarding, and an adnexal mass may be found.

Laboratory studies in patients with sepsis reveal an elevated white blood cell count and may show pink, hemoglobin-tinged plasma. Anemia is proportional to the degree of hemolysis, and the hematocrit may be extremely low. Platelet counts may be reduced, and there is often evidence of disseminated intravascular coagulation (DIC). Oliguria or anuria, increasingly refractory hypotension, and hemorrhage and bruising may develop.

Clostridia may enter the bloodstream from the gastrointestinal or biliary tract. This occurrence is associated with ulcerative lesions or obstruction of the small or large intestine, necrotic or infiltrating malignancy, bowel surgery, or various abdominal catastrophes. The patient may present with an acute febrile illness, with chills and fever but no other signs of localized infection. Intravascular hemolysis occurs in

TABLE 135-1 TREATMENT OF CLOSTRIDIAL INFECTIONS[a]

Condition	Antibiotic Treatment	Penicillin Allergy	Adjunctive Treatment/Note
Contamination	None	—	—
Gas gangrene	Penicillin, 3–4 million units IV q4h, *plus* Clindamycin, 600 mg IV q6h	Chloramphenicol, metronidazole, imipenem, doxycycline (see text)[b]	Surgical debridement with wide excision is essential. Consider hyperbaric oxygen.
Clostridial sepsis	Penicillin, 3–4 million units IV q4h, *plus* Clindamycin, 600 mg IV q6h	Chloramphenicol, metronidazole, imipenem, doxycycline (see text)[b]	Transient bacteremia may be clinically insignificant.
Suppurative deep-tissue infections (e.g., abdominal wall, gynecologic)	Penicillin, 3–4 million units IV q4h, *plus* Gentamicin, 5 mg/kg IV q24h, *or* A third-generation cephalosporin (e.g., ceftriaxone, 2 g IV q12h)	As above, plus gentamicin or a quinolone	Empirical therapy should be given. Therapy should be based on Gram's stain and culture results when available.

[a]Treatment recommendations for *C. difficile* colitis, tetanus, and botulism are found in Chaps. 123, 133, and 134, respectively.
[b]Perform sensitivity testing; consider desensitization.

as many as half of such cases. Biliary or gastrointestinal symptoms, if present, may be the only clue to the etiology. Positive blood cultures provide the definitive clue to the diagnosis.

Patients with malignant disease can also develop rapidly fatal clostridial sepsis, particularly from a gastrointestinal focus. The most common species in this setting is *C. septicum*. Characteristic signs and symptoms include fever, tachycardia, hypotension, abdominal pain or tenderness, nausea, vomiting, and (preterminally) coma. The tachycardia may be out of proportion to the fever. Only ~20–30% of patients develop hemolysis. A striking feature of this syndrome is the rapidity of death, which frequently occurs in <12 h.

DIAGNOSIS

The diagnosis of clostridial disease, in association with positive cultures, must be based primarily on clinical findings. Because of the presence of clostridia in many wounds, their mere isolation from any site, including the blood, does not necessarily indicate severe disease. Smears of wound exudates, uterine scrapings, or cervical discharge may show abundant large gram-positive rods as well as other organisms. Cultures should be placed in selective media and incubated anaerobically for identification of clostridia. The diagnosis of clostridial myonecrosis can be established by frozen-section biopsy of muscle.

The urine of patients with severe clostridial sepsis may contain protein and casts, and some patients may develop severe uremia. Profound alterations of circulating erythrocytes are seen in severely toxemic patients. Patients have hemolytic anemia, which develops extremely rapidly, along with hemoglobinemia, hemoglobinuria, and elevated levels of serum bilirubin. Spherocytosis, increased osmotic and mechanical red blood cell fragility, erythrophagocytosis, and methemoglobinemia have been described. DIC may develop in patients with severe infection. In patients with severe sepsis, Wright's or Gram's staining of a smear of peripheral blood or buffy coat may demonstrate clostridia.

X-ray examination sometimes provides an important clue to the diagnosis by revealing gas in muscles, subcutaneous tissue, or the uterus. However, the finding of gas is not pathognomonic for clostridial infection. Other anaerobic bacteria, frequently mixed with aerobic organisms, may produce gas.

Rx CLOSTRIDIAL INFECTIONS

(Table 135-1) Traumatic wounds should be thoroughly cleansed and debrided. Traditionally, the antibiotic of choice for severe clostridial infection has been penicillin G (20 million units per day in adults). Penicillin G treatment of gas gangrene has become more controversial because of increasing resistance to this drug and data obtained from animal models of infection. In a mouse model of gas gangrene, antibiotics inhibiting toxin synthesis appeared to be preferable to cell wall–active drugs; clindamycin treatment enhanced survival more than therapy with penicillin; and the combination of clindamycin and penicillin was superior to penicillin alone. For severe clostridial sepsis, clindamycin may be used at a dose of 600 mg every 6 h in combination with high-dose penicillin (3–4 million units every 4 h). Although no clinical trials validate this choice, it is gaining acceptance in the infectious disease community.

In cases of penicillin sensitivity or allergy, other antibiotics should be considered, but all should be tested for in vitro activity because of the occasional isolation of resistant strains. Clostridia are frequently, but not universally, susceptible in vitro to cefoxitin, carbenicillin, chloramphenicol, clindamycin, metronidazole, doxycycline, imipenem, minocycline, tetracycline, third-generation cephalosporins, and vancomycin. For severe clostridial infections, sensitivity testing should be done before an antimicrobial agent with unpredictable activity is used. Simple contamination of a wound with clostridia should not be treated with antibiotics. Localized skin and soft tissue infection can be managed by debridement rather than with systemic antibiotics. Drugs are required when the process extends into adjacent tissue or when fever and systemic signs of sepsis are present. Surgery is a mainstay of therapy for gas gangrene. Amputation is often required for rapidly spreading infection involving a limb, as the process frequently fails to respond to antibiotics. Hysterectomy is required for uterine myonecrosis. Abdominal wall myonecrosis usually continues despite initial aggressive surgery and antibiotic therapy and requires repeated surgical debridement of all involved muscle.

Suppurative infections should be treated with antibiotics. Frequently, broad-spectrum antibiotics must be used because of the mixed flora involved in these infections. Aminoglycosides can be used for the aerobic gram-negative bacteria involved in mixed infections.

The use of a polyvalent gas gangrene antitoxin is still recommended by some authorities. At present, no such antitoxin is produced in the United States, and most centers have discontinued its use in the management of patients with suspected gas gangrene or clostridial postabortion sepsis because of questionable efficacy and the substantial risk of hypersensitivity to horse serum, from which the antitoxin is derived.

The use of hyperbaric oxygen in the treatment of gas gangrene is also controversial. Studies in humans are not well designed to answer questions on efficacy, but several knowledgeable authors believe that hyperbaric oxygen therapy has contributed to dramatic clinical improvement. Such therapy may, however, be associated with untoward effects due to oxygen toxicity and high atmospheric pressure. Some centers without hyperbaric chambers have reported acceptable mortality rates; thus expert surgical and medical management and control of complications are probably the most important factors in the treatment of gas gangrene. Fasciotomy should not be delayed for hyperbaric oxygen therapy.

ACKNOWLEDGMENTS

The authors acknowledge the contributions of Dori F. Zaleznik, MD, to this chapter in earlier editions.

FURTHER READINGS

BORRIELLO SP: Clostridial disease of the gut. Clin Infect Dis 20:S242, 1995

CENTERS FOR DISEASE CONTROL AND PREVENTION: *Clostridium sordellii* toxic shock syndrome after medical abortion with mifepristone and intravaginal misoprostol—United States and Canada, 2001–2005. MMWR 54:724, 2005

LORBER B: Gas gangrene and other *Clostridium*-associated diseases, in *Principles and Practice of Infectious Diseases*, 6th ed, GL Mandell et al (eds). Philadelphia, Elsevier Churchill Livingstone, 2005, pp 2828–2838

MURRAY-LILLIBRIDGE K et al: Epidemiological findings and medical, legal, and public health challenges of an investigation of severe soft tissue infections and deaths among injecting drug users—Ireland, 2000. Epidemiol Infect 134:894, 2006

PRINSSEN HM et al: *Clostridium septicum* myonecrosis and ovarian cancer: A case report and review of literature. Gynecol Oncol 72:116, 1999

ROOD JI: Virulence genes of *Clostridium perfringens*. Annu Rev Microbiol 52:333, 1998

STEVENS DL, BRYANT AE: The role of clostridial toxins in the pathogenesis of gas gangrene. Clin Infect Dis 35:S93, 2002

WANG C et al: Hyperbaric oxygen for treating wounds: A systematic review of the literature. Arch Surg 138:272, 2003

SECTION 6 DISEASES CAUSED BY GRAM-NEGATIVE BACTERIA

136 Meningococcal Infections

Lee M. Wetzler

DEFINITION

Neisseria meningitidis is the etiologic agent of two life-threatening diseases: meningococcal meningitis and fulminant meningococcemia. More rarely, meningococci cause pneumonia, septic arthritis, pericarditis, urethritis, and conjunctivitis. Most cases are potentially preventable by vaccination.

ETIOLOGIC AGENT

Meningococci are gram-negative aerobic diplococci. Unlike the other neisseriae, they have a polysaccharide capsule. They are transmitted among humans—their only known habitat—via respiratory secretions. Colonization of the nasopharynx or pharynx is much more common than invasive disease.

MICROBIOLOGY AND CLASSIFICATION

On the basis of genome sequencing, *N. meningitidis* is categorized as a β-proteobacterium related to *Bordetella*, *Burkholderia*, *Kingella*, and *Methylomonas* and—more distantly—to *Vibrio*, *Haemophilus*, and *Escherichia coli*. Meningococci are traditionally classified by serologic typing systems based on structural differences in capsule (serogroup), major outer-membrane protein (OMP) porin (PorB, serotype), minor porin (PorA, serosubtype), and lipooligosaccharide (LOS, immunotype). Thus, for example, the meningococcal strain designation B:2b:P1.5:L3,7,9 reflects the serogroup (B), serotype (2b), serosubtype (P1.5), and immunotype (L3,7,9). Meningococci are also differentiated from the other Neisseriaceae by their pattern of sugar fermentation. *N. gonorrhoeae* ferments only glucose; *N. meningitidis* ferments glucose and maltose; and *N. lactamica* ferments glucose, maltose, and lactose.

Meningococci are classified into serogroups according to the antigenicity of their capsular polysaccharides, which reflects structural differences in these carbohydrates. Five serogroups (A, B, C, Y, and W-135; see below) are responsible for >90% of cases of meningococcal disease worldwide. One limitation of serogroup classification based on polysaccharide capsular structure is that the genes for capsule biosynthesis can be transferred from one strain to another, with consequent changes in the capsule structure of the recipient strain and therefore in its serogroup. Meningococcal serotypes and subtypes are defined by antigenic differences in specific OMPs. Thus, other methods for tracking meningococcal strains have become increasingly useful. Multilocus enzyme electrophoresis classifies bacteria into electrophoretic types (ETs), and variations in ET are not based on antigenic variations or alterations in outer-membrane component structures. Other techniques for establishing strain identity or nonidentity—i.e., pulsed-field gel electrophoresis of large DNA fragments and amplification of bacterial genomic sequences by polymerase chain reaction (PCR)—are based on the genetic makeup of the strain. These techniques are used for identification of the strains associated with outbreaks of disease. For example, the virulent III-1 clonal complex of serogroup A was first recognized in Nepal in 1983–1984; it spread to Mecca, then to sub-Saharan Africa, and subsequently to temperate Africa. The serogroup B ET-5 complex was first identified in Norway in the 1970s and later caused outbreaks in Europe, Cuba, and South and North America (most recently, in the Pacific Northwest). Serogroup C ET-24 (the ET-37 complex) has caused sporadic cases and outbreaks in Canada and the United States; in some analyses, it has been associated with high rates of mortality and morbidity.

EPIDEMIOLOGY

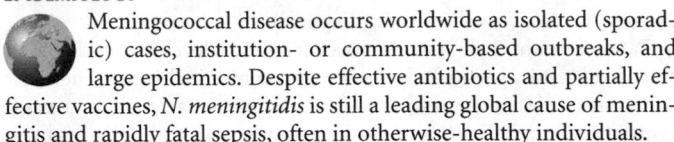

Meningococcal disease occurs worldwide as isolated (sporadic) cases, institution- or community-based outbreaks, and large epidemics. Despite effective antibiotics and partially effective vaccines, *N. meningitidis* is still a leading global cause of meningitis and rapidly fatal sepsis, often in otherwise-healthy individuals.

N. meningitidis is unique among the major bacterial agents of meningitis in that it causes epidemic as well as endemic (sporadic) disease. In all, 300,000–500,000 cases of meningococcal disease occur worldwide each year—numbers that frequently are increased by large epidemics. The annual incidence of meningococcal disease is 1–2 cases per 100,000 population for sporadic disease, 5–10 cases per 100,000 for hypersporadic disease (localized outbreaks and case clusters), and 10–>1000 cases per 100,000 for pandemic and epidemic disease (e.g., serogroup A epidemics).

Serogroup A strains, which caused most of the large epidemics of meningococcal disease during the first half of the twentieth century, are now associated with recurring epidemics in sub-Saharan Africa (the African meningitis belt) and other locales in the developing world. In the largest meningococcal epidemic recorded, >300,000 cases and 30,000 deaths due to serogroup A *N. meningitidis* occurred in sub-Saharan Africa in 1996–1997. Serogroups B and C cause most cases of sporadic and epidemic meningococcal disease in industrialized countries. Since 1980, large serogroup B epidemics and/or outbreaks of serogroup A or C meningococcal disease have also occurred in Europe, the United States, Canada, China, Nepal, Mongolia, New Zealand, Cuba, Brazil, Chile, Saudi Arabia, and South Africa. In the United States and Canada during the 1990s, serogroup B was the most common cause of sporadic disease, while serogroup C was a more frequent cause of outbreaks. Serogroup Y has recently been isolated from almost one-third of cases of meningococcal disease in the United States. In general, patients with serogroup Y disease are older and more likely to be African American or to have a chronic underlying illness than are patients with disease caused by other serogroups. Serogroups Y and W-135 are isolated more often than the other serogroups from patients with pneumonia. In 2000, 2001, and 2002, worldwide epidemics of serogroup W-135 meningococcal disease occurred in association with the Muslim pilgrimage to Mecca (the Hajj) and in the meningitis belt of sub-Saharan Africa.

In the United States, the attack rate for sporadic meningococcal disease is ~1 case per 100,000 persons per year. Disease attack rates are highest among infants 3–9 months of age (10–15 cases per 100,000 infants per year). Attack rates are higher among children than among adults, and there is a second peak of incidence among teenagers, in whom outbreaks have often been tied to residence in barracks, dormitories, or other crowded conditions. This observation has prompted the recommendation that meningococcal polysaccharide-based vaccines (see below) be administered to incoming college freshmen to prevent outbreaks at colleges. Although the age-specific incidence is much lower among adults (<1 case per 100,000 persons per year), one-third to one-half of all cases of sporadic meningococcal disease occur in individuals ≥18 years of age. Peak disease incidence coincides with the winter peak of respiratory viral illnesses. During epidemics, disease incidence increases disproportionately among teenagers and young adults. In sub-Saharan Africa, epidemic outbreaks occur with the dry season and the coming of the dry dusty winds of the harmattan.

Meningococcal disease occurs more commonly among the household contacts of primary cases than in the general population. The secondary attack rate is 400–1000 per 100,000 household members. School-based clusters of cases have also been described; the attack rate among school contacts of cases has been estimated at 2–4 cases per 100,000 exposed individuals. In outbreaks on college campuses, attack rates have been highest among students living in dormitories. Most secondary cases occur within 2 weeks of the primary case, although some cases may develop as long as several months later. Secondary cases account for <2% of all cases reported each year in the United States.

Meningococcal colonization of the nasopharynx (asymptomatic carriage) can persist for months. In nonepidemic periods, ~10% of healthy individuals are colonized, as are up to 30% of persons living in relatively crowded conditions (e.g., in military barracks or college dormitories). Factors that predispose individuals to colonization with *N. meningitidis* include residence in the same household with a person who has meningococcal disease or is a carrier, household or institutional crowding, active or passive exposure to tobacco smoke, and a recent history of a viral upper respiratory infection. These factors have also been associated with an increased risk of meningococcal disease.

PATHOGENESIS

(Fig. 136-1) Meningococci that colonize the upper respiratory tract are internalized by nonciliated mucosal cells and may traverse them to enter the submucosa, from which they can make their way into the bloodstream. While meningococcal colonization of healthy humans is common, bloodstream infection is an infrequent event that is not essential for the organisms' survival and spread. The production of human disease has no obvious evolutionary advantage for either pathogen or host. Although some strains of *N. meningitidis* are thought to cause more severe disease in humans than do other strains, the basis for this difference is not understood. Meningococci may undergo important phenotypic changes when they adapt to growth in vivo; presumed virulence traits include the antiphagocytic capsular polysaccharide, an ability to sialylate LOS so that it mimics host-cell carbohydrate moieties and inhibits complement deposition, the secretion of IgA protease, and mechanisms for iron acquisition. However, there is little evidence that alteration in meningococcal components, putative toxins, or other secreted substances affects virulence. Moreover, the ET-5 strain of serogroup B *N. meningitidis* has been associated with high case-fatality rates in some populations but not in others. These points suggest that host factors, as opposed to bacterial components, are the main mediators of immune resistance and disease pathogenesis.

A meningococcal organism that enters the bloodstream from the nasopharynx and survives host defenses generally has one of two fates. If multiplication occurs slowly, the bacteria eventually may seed local sites, such as the meninges and/or (rarely) the joints or the pericardium. More rapid multiplication in the bloodstream is associated with the clinical features of meningococcemia [i.e., petechiae, purpura, disseminated intravascular coagulation (DIC), and shock], which usually causes symptoms before local sites become infected. Thus, compartmentalization of bacterial growth and host inflammation either in the blood or at a local site (usually the meninges) can occur.

Outer-Membrane Components Associated with Virulence Meningococcal strains are characterized by the expression of capsular polysaccharide and other outer-membrane structures, including LOS (endotoxin). Outer-membrane blebbing, meningococcal autolysis, molecular mimicry, genome plasticity, horizontal DNA exchange, and phase and/or antigenic variation are all important in meningococcal virulence.

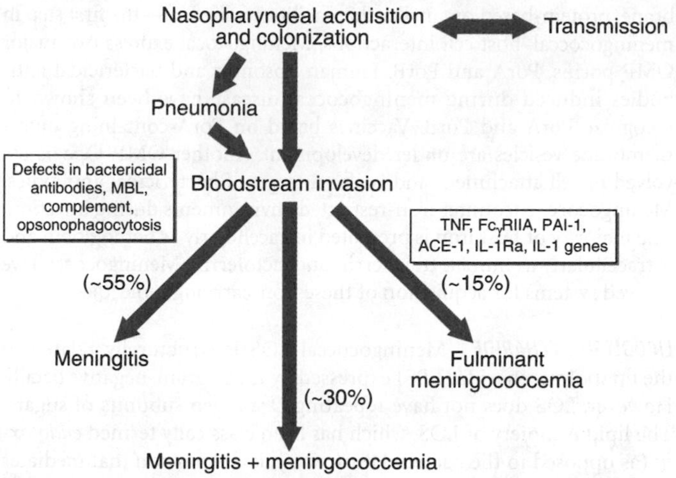

FIGURE 136-1 Meningococcal disease pathogenesis, susceptibility, and severity. After human-to-human transmission, environmental factors (smoking, co-infections), polymorphisms in innate immunity or other genes, and absence of mucosal antibodies may confer susceptibility to meningococcal invasion from the nasopharynx into the bloodstream. In individuals who lack bactericidal antibodies, terminal or alternative pathway complement-deficiency states and other genetic polymorphisms may influence the severity of the ensuing host response and the clinical presentation. Although each of these gene associations has been reported, most of them require confirmation in different ethnic groups. MBL, mannose-binding lectin; TNF, tumor necrosis factor; FcγRIIA, FCγRIIA R131 allele; PAI-1, plasminogen activator inhibitor 1; ACE-1, angiotensin-converting enzyme 1; IL, interleukin; IL-1Ra, interleukin 1 receptor antagonist.

CAPSULE The polysaccharide capsule is a major—if not *the* major—virulence factor of *N. meningitidis*. As stated above, meningococci isolated from the blood or cerebrospinal fluid (CSF) of patients with invasive meningococcal disease most often express capsules of serogroups A, B, C, Y, and W-135. Isolates from asymptomatic nasopharyngeal carriers are nongroupable or express B, Y, X, Z, or 29E capsular serogroups. Capsules impart antiphagocytic and antibactericidal properties to the meningococcus and thus enhance meningococcal survival during invasion of the bloodstream or CSF. Capsules also provide protective properties (e.g., preventing desiccation and phagocytic killing) and antiadherent properties; these properties promote meningococcal transmission, spread, and survival externally and within intracellular compartments such as phagocytic vacuoles.

Except in serogroup A, the major meningococcal capsular polysaccharides associated with invasive disease are composed of polymers of sialic acid (*N*-acetyl neuraminic acid, NANA) derivatives. The serogroup B capsule is composed of (α2→8)-linked NANA, the serogroup C capsule of (α2→9)-linked NANA, the serogroup Y capsule of alternating D-glucose and NANA, and the serogroup W-135 capsule of D-galactose and NANA. The differences in sialic acid capsule composition are derived from the distinct polysialyltransferases encoded by the fourth gene of the capsule biosynthesis operon, which is also used as a basis for capsule-specific PCR diagnosis. A four-gene operon encoding the capsule transport apparatus (ctr) is conserved among different serogroups and is also used in PCR diagnosis. The serogroup A capsule is composed of repeating units of (α)-linked *N*-acetyl-mannosamine-1-phosphate and is encoded by a four-gene biosynthesis cassette unique for this serogroup.

OUTER-MEMBRANE PROTEINS Meningococci isolated from sites of colonization or invasive disease are piliated. Pili are complex outer-membrane, protein-based organelles that facilitate adhesion—the first step in meningococcal–host cell interactions. Meningococci express two major OMP porins, PorA and PorB. Human opsonins and bactericidal antibodies induced during meningococcal disease have been shown to recognize PorA and PorB. Vaccines based on PorA-containing outer-membrane vesicles are under development. Another OMP, Opc, is involved in cell attachment and is also a target of bactericidal antibodies. Meningococci encounter iron-restricted environments during infection. The majority of host iron is presented intracellularly as hemoglobin and extracellularly as human transferrin and lactoferrin. Meningococci have evolved systems for acquisition of these iron-carrying molecules.

LIPOOLIGOSACCHARIDE Meningococcal LOS is structurally related to the lipopolysaccharide (LPS) expressed by many gram-negative bacilli. However, LOS does not have repeating O-antigen subunits of sugars. The lipid A moiety of LOS, which has been classically termed *endotoxin* (as opposed to the bacterial exotoxins), is the portion that mediates the induction of inflammatory cytokines often seen in disease. The effect of lipid A is due to an interaction with the innate immune receptor Toll-like receptor 4 (TLR4) in association with the membrane protein MD2. TLR4 and MD2 are found mainly on macrophages/monocytes, dendritic cells, and other phagocytes.

Rates of morbidity and mortality associated with meningococcal bacteremia and meningitis have been directly correlated with the amount of circulating meningococcal endotoxin. Whether this measure is an indication of overall bacterial load or is a direct pathogenic mechanism of disease is debatable. The ability of signaling through TLR4 by the lipid A moiety of LOS to induce production of inflammatory and proinflammatory cytokines from various immune cells suggests a direct relationship. However, other meningococcal outer-membrane components—e.g., meningococcal porins and lipoproteins (including the H8 lipoprotein)—induce immune cell activation via other TLRs, especially TLR2. A recently derived LOS$^-$ meningococcal mutant was still able to induce significant production of proinflammatory cytokines [especially tumor necrosis factor α (TNF-α), interleukin (IL) 6, and IL-1β] by macrophages and cytokines. This observation suggests a potential role for these components in induction of meningococcal sepsis.

Other Virulence Mechanisms The outer-membrane components of *N. meningitidis* (e.g., pili, LOS, Opa proteins, Opc, capsule) vary in expression or structure at high frequencies (10^{-2}–10^{-4} per cell per generation). Variation is the result of genetic switches that turn expression of a component on or off, regulate the amount of a component, or alter the structure of a component. Genetic events leading to phase and structural variation allow immune escape and create variability in the structures that are important in pathogenesis (on and off expression of attachment ligands, protection against serum killing, invasion determinants). The serogroup B capsule provides an example of how meningococci downregulate the human immune response through the expression of host-like antigens. The (α2→8)-linked polysialic acid capsule of serogroup B meningococci is identical to structures on the human neural cell adhesion molecule N-CAM. Meningococci are also characterized by frequent vesiculation (blebbing) of the outer membrane, and the amount of blebbing may vary between strains. Blebs may contribute to the rapid initiation of the inflammatory and clotting cascades. They may also be related to the natural autolysis of meningococci that results in DNA release and facilitates genetic transformation.

Association of Virulence Mechanisms with Specific Meningococcal Infections Specific disease manifestations of meningococcal infections have specific virulence and pathogenic mechanisms, as described below for fulminant meningococcemia and meningitis.

Fulminant Meningococcemia • ***PURPURA FULMINANS*** Fulminant meningococcemia is perhaps the most rapidly lethal form of septic shock experienced by humans. It differs from most other forms of septic shock by the prominence of hemorrhagic skin lesions (petechiae, purpura; see Fig. 52-5) and the consistent development of DIC.

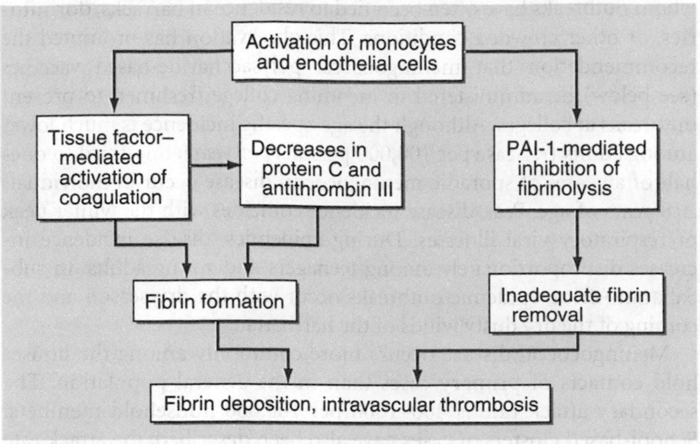

FIGURE 136-2 The pathogenesis of fibrin deposition in patients with fulminant meningococcemia. PAI-1, plasminogen activator inhibitor 1. (*Adapted from M Levi et al: Eur J Clin Invest 27:3, 1997.*)

The dominant proinflammatory molecule in the meningococcal cell wall is the endotoxin or LOS, and the outer membrane that contains it is poorly tethered to the underlying peptidoglycan. This structural peculiarity seems to account for the fact that meningococci shed LOS-containing membrane blebs as they grow. The bacteria can multiply to very high concentrations in the blood. The concentrations of endotoxin detected in the blood of patients with fulminant meningococcemia are 10- to 1000-fold higher than those found in the blood of patients with bacteremia due to other gram-negative bacteria. The bacteria and endotoxin-containing blebs stimulate monocytes, neutrophils, and endothelial cells, which then release cytokines and other mediators that can activate many distant targets, including other leukocytes, platelets, and endothelial cells. In addition, meningococci can invade the vascular endothelium. When activated, the endothelium produces molecules that can be procoagulant as well as adhesive for leukocytes.

Patients with fulminant meningococcemia usually have extremely high blood levels of both proinflammatory mediators—i.e., TNF-α, IL-1, interferon γ (IFN-γ), and IL-8—and anti-inflammatory mediators—i.e., IL-1 receptor antagonist (IL-1Ra), soluble IL-1 receptors, soluble TNF-α receptors, and IL-10. The plasma of patients with meningococcal shock can decrease the responses of normal leukocytes to stimuli such as LOS; the implication is that anti-inflammatory mediators predominate in the blood late in infection.

Procoagulant, antifibrinolytic forces are also active in the blood of patients with fulminant meningococcemia (Fig. 136-2). Monocytes express large amounts of tissue factor. Fibrinopeptide A and thrombin-antithrombin levels are high, reflecting active clotting, while antithrombin and fibrinogen levels are low. Although the tissue factor–regulated ("extrinsic") arm of coagulation predominates, the contact system (factors XII and XI, prekallikrein, high-molecular-weight kininogen) is also activated. Striking deficiencies of antithrombin and proteins C and S can occur; studies have found a strong negative correlation between protein C activity and both the size of purpuric skin lesions and the mortality rate. Plasminogen levels are decreased, while plasmin-antiplasmin complexes and plasminogen activator inhibitor 1 (PAI-1) levels in the blood are very high. PAI-1 levels have been correlated with mortality risk.

Fibrin deposition is therefore favored both by the procoagulant tendency (promoted through activation of tissue factor and deficiencies of proteins C and S and antithrombin) and by an antifibrinolytic tendency (favored by excessive PAI-1). Both platelets and leukocytes doubtless contribute to the formation of microthrombi and to the vascular injury that ensues. Thrombosis of small to mid-sized arteries can produce peripheral necrosis and gangrene, necessitating limb or digit amputation.

MENINGITIS Meningococcal bacteremia can result in the seeding of the meninges, pericardium, and large joints. Up to one-third of patients with meningococcal disease present with meningitis or other closed-space infections without signs of sepsis. How meningococci traverse the blood-brain barrier and enter the CSF or reach other closed sites is unclear. Meningococci have been shown to invade endothelial cells both experimentally and in vivo. The choroid plexus is also a potential site of meningococcal entry into the CSF. Meningococcal pili may bind CD46, a complement-regulatory protein that is expressed by the choroid plexus and meningeal epithelia. Upon meningococcal entry into the CSF, a vigorous local inflammatory response ensues, probably triggered by endotoxin-containing meningococcal membranes. Both bacterial growth and the inflammatory response occur within the CSF, where levels of endotoxin, IL-6, TNF-α, IL-1β, IL-1Ra, and IL-10 exceed the concentrations found in plasma by 100- to 1000-fold. The inflammatory response is largely confined to the subarachnoid space and contiguous structures. The inflammatory cytokines TNF-α and IL-1 released in meningococcal bacteremia may also enhance the permeability of the blood-brain barrier. Meningitis and other closed-space infections (e.g., arthritis, pericarditis) are the result of bacterial survival and multiplication at these sites. For example, meningitis and its sequelae are due to the induction of local inflammatory cytokines and other mediators (e.g., nitric oxide), leukocyte infiltration across the blood-brain barrier, breakdown of the blood-brain barrier with edema, release of metalloproteases, induction of cellular apoptosis, coagulation of vessels, and ischemia.

Patients who develop meningitis without meningococcemia may be individuals in whom meningococci do not grow rapidly in or have been cleared from the blood; may have antibodies or phagocytes that slow meningococcal growth; or may lack the (unknown) factors that allow *N. meningitidis* to multiply rapidly in vivo. If disease is recognized early, the prognosis of patients with meningococcal meningitis is substantially better than that of patients with fulminant meningococcemia.

HOST DEFENSE MECHANISMS

Preventing meningococcal growth in blood requires bactericidal and opsonic antibodies, complement, and phagocytes (Fig. 136-3). The major bactericidal antibodies are IgM and IgG, which (except for serogroup B) bind to the capsular polysaccharide. Immunity to meningococci is therefore serogroup specific. Antibodies to other surface (subcapsular) antigens may confer cross-serogroup protection. PorA, PorB, Opc, and LOS appear to be major targets of cross-reactivity and of serogroup B bactericidal antibodies. Infants are protected from meningococcal disease during the first months of life by passively transferred maternal IgG antibodies. As maternal antibody levels wane, the attack rate increases, peaking at 3–9 months of age. Disease incidence declines as protective antibodies are induced by colonization with nonpathogenic bacteria that have cross-reactive antigens. In addition to *N. lactamica*, which frequently colonizes young children, some enteric bacteria have antigens that cross-react with those of meningococci. One theory relates the occurrence of some cases of meningococcal disease to the presence of high levels of IgA antibodies to meningococci, since these antibodies can block the bactericidal activity of IgM.

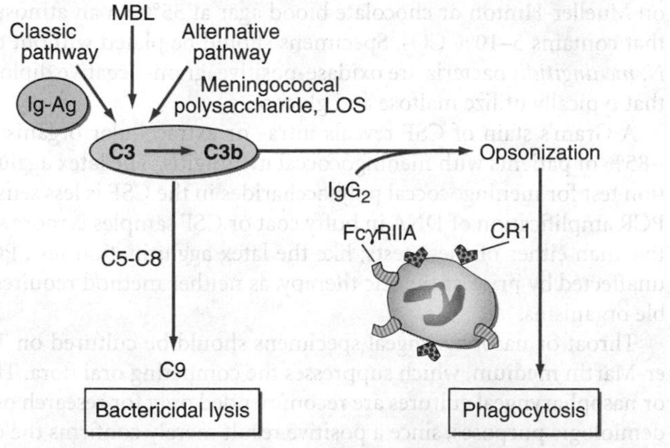

FIGURE 136-3 Protection from meningococcal disease involves both antimeningococcal immunoglobulins and complement. Activation of complement by antimeningococcal IgM or IgG promotes bacterial lysis via the membrane attack complex (C5–C9), while C3b [produced by alternative, mannose-binding lectin (MBL), or classic pathway activation] and antimeningococcal IgG_2 cooperate to produce effective opsonophagocytosis. A neutrophil defect in binding IgG_2 (the FcγRIIA R131 allele) has been associated with more severe meningococcal disease. CR1, complement receptor 1; LOS, lipooligosaccharide.

Complement is required for bactericidal activity and for efficient opsonophagocytosis. Individuals deficient in any of the late complement components (C5–C9) cannot assemble the membrane-attack complex (MAC) needed to kill *Neisseria.* Although the incidence of meningococcal disease is higher among those with late-complement-component deficiencies, these persons typically develop less severe disease than complement-sufficient individuals, do so at an older age, and tend to have disease due to uncommon serogroups (W-135, X, Y, Z, and 29E). Although only one-half of individuals with known late-complement-component deficiency ever experience meningococcal disease, some affected persons have several episodes. Deficiency of each of the terminal complement components is inherited in an autosomal recessive fashion. Properdin deficiency, in contrast, is X-linked; some affected males develop overwhelming meningococcal disease, an observation indicating that the alternative complement pathway is also needed for antimeningococcal host defense. Disease onset in properdin-deficient individuals typically occurs in the teens or twenties. There is also recent evidence that inherited differences in the mannose-binding lectin (MBL) pathway of complement activation may influence the risk of acquiring meningococcal disease in childhood. Alleles that decrease MBL synthesis have been associated with increased risk in the few studies reported to date.

Activation of the classic pathway of complement by antigen-antibody complexes or of the alternative pathway by LOS or capsular polysaccharide is important for producing and maintaining C3b (Fig. 136-3). Without C3b, neither bactericidal lysis nor phagocytosis can proceed effectively. When C3b is generated, meningococcal growth is probably checked by the MAC's bactericidal activity (induction of bacterial lysis) and by robust phagocytosis and opsonophagocytic killing of the bacterium due to complement deposition. Most IgG antibodies to the meningococcal polysaccharide are of the IgG_2 isotype; a phagocytic cell defect (the FcγRIIA R131 allele) that impairs the phagocytosis of IgG_2-coated particles has been associated with more severe meningococcal disease. This allele has also been associated with a more severe clinical course in patients with late-complement-component deficiency; thus effective phagocytosis may contribute to the relatively mild meningococcal disease usually observed in these individuals.

The results of studies of gene polymorphism–disease associations are summarized in Figs. 136-1 and 136-3. In individuals who lack bactericidal antibodies, protection from acquiring meningococcal bacteremia may be provided, at least in part, by innate immune mechanisms such as the MBL pathway for activating complement, complement factor C4b, and the TLR4 pathway for LOS recognition. Other genes may influence meningococcal survival in vivo [FcγIIA (CD32)], while still others seem to regulate the host inflammatory (IL-1β, IL-1Ra, TNF-α, angiotensin-converting enzyme) and clotting (PAI-1) responses to invading meningococci. Although many of these associations await confirmation in other populations of patients, in sum they point to important genetic influences on the acquisition and severity of meningococcal disease. This conclusion is supported by the overrepresentation of ABO blood group nonsecretors among patients with meningococcal disease and by the striking variability in meningococcal disease incidence among different racial groups.

CLINICAL MANIFESTATIONS

Upper Respiratory Tract Infections Although many patients who develop meningococcal meningitis or meningococcemia report having had throat soreness or other upper respiratory symptoms during the preceding week, it is uncertain whether these symptoms are due to infection with meningococci. Meningococcal pharyngitis is rarely diagnosed. Adult patients with *N. meningitidis* bacteremia more often have clinically apparent disease of the respiratory tract (pneumonia, sinusitis, tracheobronchitis, conjunctivitis) than do younger patients.

Meningococcemia Patients with meningococcal disease may have both meningococcemia and meningitis. These conditions have a wide clinical spectrum, with many overlapping features.

Approximately 10–30% of patients with meningococcal disease have meningococcemia without clinically apparent meningitis. Although meningococcal bacteremia may occasionally be transient and asymptomatic, in most individuals it is associated with fever, chills, nausea, vomiting, and myalgias. Prostration is common. The most distinctive feature is rash. Erythematous macules rapidly become petechial and, in severe cases, purpuric (see Fig. 52-5). Although the lesions are typically found on the trunk and lower extremities, they may also occur on the face, arms, and mucous membranes. The petechiae may coalesce into hemorrhagic bullae or may undergo necrosis and ulcerate. Patients with severe coagulopathy may develop ischemic extremities or digits, often with a sharp line of demarcation between normal and ischemic tissue.

In many patients with fulminant meningococcemia, the CSF may be normal and the CSF culture negative. Indeed, the absence of meningitis in a patient with meningococcemia is a poor prognostic sign; it suggests that the bacteria have multiplied so rapidly in the blood that meningeal seeding has not yet occurred or had time to elicit inflammation in the CSF. Most of these patients also lack evidence of an acute-phase response; i.e., the erythrocyte sedimentation rate is normal, and the C-reactive protein concentration in blood is low.

The *Waterhouse-Friderichsen syndrome* is a dramatic example of DIC-induced microthrombosis, hemorrhage, and tissue injury. Although overt adrenal failure is infrequently documented in patients with fulminant meningococcemia, patients may have partial adrenal insufficiency and be unable to mount the normal hypercortisolemic response to severe stress or cosyntropin stimulation. Almost all patients who die from fulminant meningococcemia have adrenal hemorrhages at autopsy.

Chronic meningococcemia (Fig. 136-4) is a rare syndrome of episodic fever, rash, and arthralgias that can last for weeks to months. The rash may be maculopapular; it is occasionally petechial. Splenomegaly may develop. If untreated or if treated with glucocorticoids, chronic meningococcemia may evolve into meningitis, fulminant meningococcemia, or (rarely) endocarditis.

Meningitis (See also Chap. 376) Common presenting symptoms of patients with meningococcal meningitis include nausea and vomiting, headache, neck stiffness, lethargy, and confusion. The symptoms and signs of meningococcal meningitis cannot be distinguished from those elicited by other meningeal pathogens. Many patients with meningococcal meningitis have concurrent meningococcemia, however, and petechial or purpuric skin lesions (see Fig. 52-5) may suggest the correct diagnosis. CSF findings are consistent with those of purulent meningitis: hypoglycorrhachia, an elevated protein concentration, and a neutrophilic leukocytosis. A Gram's stain of CSF is usually positive (see "Diagnosis," below); when this finding is unaccompanied by CSF leukocytosis, the prognosis for normal recovery is often poor.

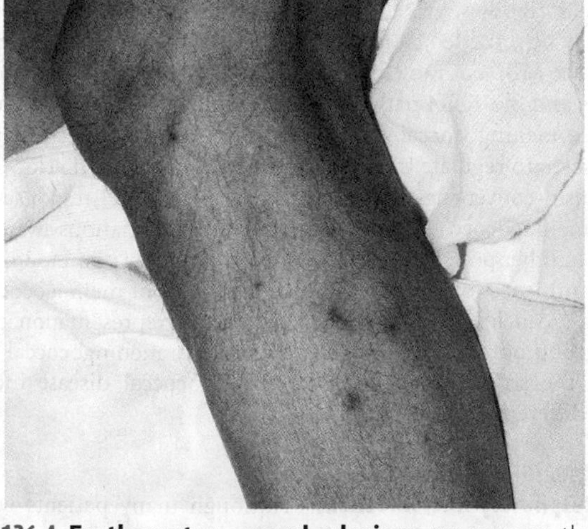

FIGURE 136-4 Erythematous papular lesions are seen on the leg of this patient with chronic meningococcemia. (*Courtesy of Kenneth M. Kaye, MD, and Elaine T. Kaye, MD; with permission*).

Other Manifestations Arthritis occurs in ~10% of patients with meningococcal disease. When arthritis develops during the first few days of the patient's illness, it usually reflects direct meningococcal invasion of the joint. Arthritis that begins later in the course is thought to be due to immune complex deposition. Primary meningococcal pneumonia occurs principally in adults, often in military populations, and is often due to serogroup Y. While meningococcal pericarditis is occasionally seen, endocarditis due to *N. meningitidis* is now exceedingly rare. Primary meningococcal conjunctivitis can be complicated by meningococcemia; systemic therapy is therefore warranted when this condition is diagnosed. Meningococcal urethritis has been reported in individuals who practice oral sex.

Complications Patients with meningococcal meningitis may develop cranial nerve palsies, cortical venous thrombophlebitis, and cerebral edema. Children may develop subdural effusions. Permanent sequelae can include mental retardation, deafness, and hemiparesis. The major long-term morbidity of fulminant meningococcemia is the loss of skin, limbs, or digits that results from ischemic necrosis and infarction.

DIAGNOSIS

Few clinical clues help the physician distinguish the patient with early meningococcal disease from patients with other acute systemic infections. The most useful clinical finding is the petechial or purpuric rash (see Fig. 52-5), but it must be differentiated from the petechial lesions seen with gonococcemia (see Fig. 137-2), Rocky Mountain spotted fever (see Fig. 167-1), hypersensitivity vasculitis (see Fig. 52-4), endemic typhus, and some viral infections. In one case series, one-half of the adults with meningococcal bacteremia had neither meningitis nor a rash.

The definitive diagnosis is established by recovering *N. meningitidis*, its antigens, or its DNA from normally sterile body fluids (e.g., blood, CSF, or synovial fluid) or from skin lesions. Meningococci grow best on Mueller-Hinton or chocolate blood agar at 35°C in an atmosphere that contains 5–10% CO_2. Specimens should be plated without delay. *N. meningitidis* bacteria are oxidase-positive, gram-negative diplococci that typically utilize maltose and glucose.

A Gram's stain of CSF reveals intra- or extracellular organisms in ~85% of patients with meningococcal meningitis. The latex agglutination test for meningococcal polysaccharides in the CSF is less sensitive. PCR amplification of DNA in buffy coat or CSF samples is more sensitive than either of these tests; like the latex agglutination test, PCR is unaffected by prior antibiotic therapy, as neither method requires viable organisms.

Throat or nasopharyngeal specimens should be cultured on Thayer-Martin medium, which suppresses the competing oral flora. Throat or nasopharyngeal cultures are recommended only for research or epidemiologic purposes, since a positive result merely confirms the carrier state and does not establish the existence of systemic disease.

℞ MENINGOCOCCAL INFECTIONS

(Table 136-1) A third-generation cephalosporin, such as cefotaxime or ceftriaxone, is preferred for initial therapy. One of these cephalosporins in combination with other agents may cover other bacteria (such as *Streptococcus pneumoniae* and *Haemophilus influenzae*) that can cause the same syndromes (Chap. 376). Penicillin G remains an acceptable alternative for

TABLE 136-1 ANTIBIOTIC TREATMENT, CHEMOPROPHYLAXIS, AND VACCINATIONS FOR INVASIVE MENINGOCOCCAL DISEASE
Antibiotic Treatment[a]
1. Ceftriaxone 2 g IV q12h (100 mg/kg per day) or cefotaxime 2 g IV q4h
2. For penicillin-sensitive *N. meningitidis*: Penicillin G 18–24 million units per day in divided doses q4h (250,000 units/kg per day)
3. Chloramphenicol 75–100 mg/kg per day in divided doses q6h
4. Meropenem 1.0 g (children, 40 mg) IV q8h
5. In an outbreak setting in developing countries: Long-acting chloramphenicol in oil suspension (Tifomycin), single dose
Adults: 3.0 g (6 mL)
Children 1–15 years old: 100 mg/kg
Children <1 year old: 50 mg/kg
Chemoprophylaxis[b]
Rifampin (oral)
Adults: 600 mg bid for 2 days
Children ≥1 month old: 10 mg/kg bid for 2 days
Children <1 month old: 5 mg/kg bid for 2 days
Ciprofloxacin (oral)
Adults: 500 mg, 1 dose
Ofloxacin (oral)
Adults: 400 mg, 1 dose
Ceftriaxone (IM)
Adults: 250 mg, 1 dose
Children <15 years old: 125 mg, 1 dose
Azithromycin (oral)
500 mg, 1 dose
Vaccination[c]
A, C, Y, W-135 vaccine (Memomune, Aventis Pasteur) or A, C vaccine
Single 0.5-mL subcutaneous injection
New C; A, C; and A, C, Y, W-135 meningococcal conjugate vaccines[d]

[a]Patients with meningococcal meningitis should receive antimicrobial therapy for at least 5 days.
[b]Use is recommended for close contacts of cases or if ceftriaxone is not used for primary treatment.
[c]At present, use is generally limited to the control of epidemics and to individuals with increased risk of meningococcal disease. Vaccine efficacy wanes after 3–5 years, and vaccine is not effective in recipients <2 years of age.
[d]These vaccines appear to provide immunity in young children, a prolonged immune response, and herd immunity (decreased transmission and colonization).

confirmed invasive meningococcal disease in most countries. However, the prevalence of meningococci with reduced susceptibility to penicillin has been increasing, and high-level penicillin resistance has been reported. Other options include meropenem. In the patient who is allergic to β-lactam drugs, chloramphenicol is a suitable alternative; chloramphenicol-resistant meningococci have been reported from Vietnam and France. The newer fluoroquinolones gatifloxacin, moxifloxacin, and gemifloxacin have excellent in vitro activity against *N. meningitidis*, with measurable central nervous system (CNS) penetration, and appear promising in animal models. Patients with meningococcal meningitis should be given antimicrobial therapy for at least 5 days. While glucocorticoid therapy for meningitis in adults is controversial, many experts administer dexamethasone, beginning if possible before antibiotic therapy is initiated; the schedule is 10 mg IV given 15–20 min before the first antibiotic dose and then every 6 h for 4 days. The data regarding steroid use to diminish CNS inflammation are strongest for *H. influenzae* and *S. pneumoniae* meningitis, especially in children.

Patients with fulminant meningococcemia often experience diffuse leakage of fluid into extravascular spaces, shock, and multiple-organ dysfunction (Chaps. 264 and 265). Myocardial depression may be prominent. Supportive therapy, although never studied in randomized, placebo-controlled trials, is recommended. Standard measures include vigorous fluid resuscitation (often requiring several liters over the first 24 h), elective ventilation, and pressors. Some authorities recommend early hemodialysis or hemofiltration. Fresh-frozen plasma is often given to patients who are bleeding extensively or who have severely deranged clotting parameters. Many European experts have administered antithrombin III to such patients. Patients with fulminant meningococcemia in whom shock persists despite vigorous fluid resuscitation should receive supplemental glucocorticoid treatment (hydrocortisone, 1 mg/kg every 6 h) pending tests of adrenal reserve.

Although it has not been formally tested in patients with fulminant meningococcemia, activated protein C (drotrecogin alfa, Xigris) is approved for use in patients with severe sepsis and dysfunction of more than one organ (APACHE II score > 25). Because of the pathophysiology, patients with meningococcemia may represent a group most likely to benefit from administration of activated protein C. The recommended dose is 24 μg/kg per hour, given as a continuous IV infusion for 96 h. Drotrecogin alfa is contraindicated when the peripheral-blood platelet count is <50,000/μL, however, and when there is active bleeding or a high risk of bleeding. Clotting parameters should be monitored closely while the drug is being infused; its administration should be discontinued 4–6 h before the performance of an invasive procedure. Drotrecogin alfa should not be used in patients with meningitis pending further evidence that it does not induce intracranial bleeding when the meninges are inflamed.

PROGNOSIS

When patients are first evaluated, the clinical features most strongly associated with a fatal outcome are shock, a purpuric or ecchymotic rash, a low or normal blood leukocyte count, an age of ≥60 years, and coma. The absence of meningitis, the presence of thrombocytopenia, low blood concentrations of antithrombin or proteins S and C, high blood levels of PAI-1, and a low erythrocyte sedimentation rate (or C-reactive protein level) have also been associated with increased mortality risk from meningococcal disease. It is possible that when meningitis symptoms are lacking, the patient may delay seeking medical therapy; this scenario could account for the increased mortality risk in asymptomatic meningitis. In contrast, the receipt of antibiotics before hospital admission has been associated with lower mortality rates in some studies.

PREVENTION

Meningococcal Polysaccharide Vaccines A single injection of quadrivalent meningococcal polysaccharide vaccine (serogroups A, C, W-135, and Y) immunizes ~80–95% of immunocompetent adults (Table 136-1). Children ≥3 months of age can be vaccinated to prevent serogroup A disease, but multiple doses are required; the vaccine is otherwise ineffective in children <2 years old. The duration of vaccine-induced immunity in adults is probably <5 years. There is currently no vaccine for serogroup B; its polysaccharide is a sialic acid homopolymer that is poorly immunogenic in humans. In addition to individuals with late-complement-component or properdin deficiency, persons with sickle cell anemia, asplenia, or splenectomy should receive the quadrivalent vaccine. Vaccination is also recommended for military recruits, pilgrims on the Hajj, and individuals traveling to sub-Saharan Africa during the dry months (June to December) or to other areas with epidemic meningococcal disease. The Advisory Committee on Immunization Practices of the Centers for Disease Control and Prevention (CDC) recommends vaccination of incoming college freshmen who will live in dormitories. In general, the vaccine should be given only to persons >2 years of age.

New meningococcal capsular oligosaccharide and polysaccharide conjugate vaccines (C; A and C; A, C, Y, and W-135) are being developed; some are currently undergoing clinical trials, and some are now in use in Europe and Canada. These vaccines are based on the approach used for the highly successful *H. influenzae* type b conjugate vaccines. Covalent linkage of the polysaccharide to a carrier protein converts the polysaccharide to a thymus-dependent antigen enhancing IgG anticapsular antibodies and memory B cells. Because levels of antibody in mucosal secretions are much higher after the administration of a conjugate vaccine than after vaccination with an unconjugated preparation, a major benefit of these vaccines may be the introduction of herd immunity. Memory response to meningococcal polysaccharide also appears to be an important effect of the conjugate vaccines. Meningococcal conjugate vaccines are not yet licensed in the United States. However, in the United Kingdom, serogroup C conjugate vaccines introduced in 2000 have had a marked impact on the incidence of serogroup C disease in the population vaccinated. If conjugate meningococcal vaccines prove to be capable of providing durable antibody or memory responses (particularly in infants and young children), their integration into the routine childhood immunization schedule would appear warranted. Vaccines for serogroup B meningococcal disease remain elusive; none of the group B vaccines studied in clinical trials has proven to be broadly effective, but these products have a role in the control of serogroup B epidemics. The identification of new meningococcal protective antigens and the development of better meningococcal vaccines are areas of continued research and hold promise for the prevention of diseases due to *N. meningitidis*.

In one new approach, *reverse vaccinology*, the sequenced genome of *N. meningitidis* is used to identify previously unrecognized OMPs that are common to all meningococcal strains and serogroups and that may be universal vaccinogen candidates. Thus far, a few promising candidates have been identified and are ready to undergo clinical trials.

Screening tests for complement-component deficiency should be conducted in patients who have a family history of meningococcal or disseminated gonococcal disease, especially in areas without epidemic or endemic meningococcal disease; in patients who have a recurrence; in patients whose first case occurs at ≥15 years of age; in patients with cases caused by serogroups other than A, B, or C; and in family members of patients found to have a complement deficiency.

Antimicrobial Chemoprophylaxis The attack rate for meningococcal disease among household or other close contacts of cases is >400-fold greater than that in the population as a whole. Close contacts of cases should receive chemoprophylaxis with rifampin, ciprofloxacin, ofloxacin, or azithromycin (Table 136-1). A single IM injection of ceftriaxone is also effective. Close contacts include persons who live in the same household, day-care center contacts, and anyone directly exposed to a patient's oral secretions. Casual contacts are not at increased risk. Chemoprophylaxis should be administered as soon as possible after the case is identified. Patients with meningococcal disease who have been treated with antibiotics other than ceftriaxone need some type of prophylaxis in order to eliminate meningococcal colonization in the oropharynx.

Isolation Precautions The CDC recommends that patients with meningococcal disease who are hospitalized be placed in respiratory isolation for the first 24 h.

Outbreak Control An organization- or community-based outbreak of meningococcal disease is defined as the occurrence of three or more cases within ≤3 months in persons who have a common affiliation or reside in the same area but who are not close contacts of one another; in addition, the primary disease attack rate must exceed 10 cases per 100,000 persons, and the case strains of *N. meningitidis* must be of the same molecular type. Mass vaccination should be considered when such outbreaks occur, and mass chemoprophylaxis may be used to control school- or other institution-based outbreaks. Consultation with public health authorities is recommended when such campaigns are contemplated.

ACKNOWLEDGMENT

The substantial contributions of David S. Stephens, MD, and Robert S. Munford, MD, to this chapter in previous editions are gratefully acknowledged.

FURTHER READINGS

BILUKHA O et al: Use of meningococcal vaccines in the United States. Pediatr Infect Dis J 26:371, 2007

GARDNER P: Clinical practice. Prevention of meningococcal disease. N Engl J Med 355:1466, 2006 (Erratum: N Engl J Med 356:536, 2007)

GIULIANI MM et al: A universal vaccine for serogroup B meningococcus. Proc Natl Acad Sci USA 103:10834, 2006

SCHNEIDER MC et al: Interactions between *Neisseria meningitidis* and the complement system. Trends Microbiol 15:233, 2007

SMIRNOVA I et al: Assay of locus-specific genetic load implicates rare Toll-like receptor 4 mutations in meningococcal susceptibility. Proc Natl Acad Sci USA 100:6075, 2003

SNAPE MD et al: Meningococcal polysaccharide-protein conjugate vaccines. Lancet Infect Dis 5:21, 2005

SNYDER LA et al: The majority of genes in the pathogenic *Neisseria* species are present in non-pathogenic *Neisseria lactamica*, including those designated as 'virulence genes.' BMC Genomics 7:128, 2006

STEPHENS DS et al: Epidemic meningitis, meningococcaemia, and *Neisseria meningitidis*. Lancet 369:2196, 2007

THOMPSON MJ et al: Clinical recognition of meningococcal disease in children and adolescents. Lancet 367:397, 2006

ZIMMER SM et al: Serogroup B meningococcal vaccines. Curr Opin Invest Drugs 7:733, 2006

137 Gonococcal Infections

Sanjay Ram, Peter A. Rice

DEFINITION

Gonorrhea is a sexually transmitted infection (STI) of epithelium and commonly manifests as cervicitis, urethritis, proctitis, and conjunctivitis. If untreated, infections at these sites can lead to local complications such as endometritis, salpingitis, tuboovarian abscess, bartholinitis, peritonitis, and perihepatitis in female patients; periurethritis and epididymitis in male patients; and ophthalmia neonatorum in newborns. Disseminated gonococcemia is an uncommon event whose manifestations include skin lesions, tenosynovitis, arthritis, and (in rare cases) endocarditis or meningitis.

MICROBIOLOGY

Neisseria gonorrhoeae is a gram-negative, nonmotile, non-spore-forming organism that grows singly and in pairs (i.e., as monococci and diplococci, respectively). Exclusively a human pathogen, the gonococcus contains, on average, three genome copies per coccal unit; this polyploidy permits a high level of antigenic variation and the survival of the organism in its host. Gonococci, like all other *Neisseria* species, are oxidase positive. They are distinguished from other neisseriae by their ability to grow on selective media and to utilize glucose but not maltose, sucrose, or lactose.

EPIDEMIOLOGY

The incidence of gonorrhea has declined significantly in the United States, but there were still ~325,000 newly reported cases in 2006. Gonorrhea remains a major public health problem worldwide, is a significant cause of morbidity in developing countries, and may play a role in enhancing transmission of HIV.

Gonorrhea predominantly affects young, nonwhite, unmarried, less educated members of urban populations. The number of reported cases probably represents half of the true number of cases—a discrepancy resulting from underreporting, self-treatment, and nonspecific treatment without a laboratory-proven diagnosis. The number of reported cases of gonorrhea in the United States rose from ~250,000 in the early 1960s to a high of 1.01 million in 1978. The peak recorded incidence of gonorrhea in modern times was reported in 1975, with 468 cases per 100,000 population in the United States. This peak was attributable to the interaction of several variables, including improved accuracy of diagnosis, changes in patterns of contraceptive use, and changes in sexual behavior. The incidence of the disease has since gradually declined and is currently estimated at 120 cases per 100,000, a figure that is still the highest among industrialized countries. A further decline in the overall incidence of gonorrhea in the United States over the past two decades may reflect increased condom use resulting from public health efforts to curtail HIV transmission. At present, the attack rate in the United States is highest among 15- to 19-year-old women and 20- to 24-year-old men; 40% of all reported cases occur in the preceding two groups together. From the standpoint of ethnicity, rates are highest among African Americans and lowest among persons of Asian or Pacific Island descent.

The incidence of gonorrhea is higher in developing countries than in industrialized nations. The exact incidence of any of the STIs is difficult to ascertain in developing countries because of limited surveillance and variable diagnostic criteria. Studies in Africa have clearly demonstrated that nonulcerative STIs such as gonorrhea (in addition to ulcerative STIs) are an independent risk factor for the transmission of HIV (Chap. 182).

Gonorrhea is transmitted from males to females more efficiently than in the opposite direction. The rate of transmission to a woman during a single unprotected sexual encounter with an infected man is ~40–60%. Oropharyngeal gonorrhea occurs in ~20% of women who practice fellatio with infected partners. Transmission in either direction by cunnilingus is rare.

In any population, there exists a small minority of individuals who have high rates of new-partner acquisition. These "core-group members" or "high-frequency transmitters" are vital in sustaining STI transmission at the population level. Another instrumental factor in sustaining gonorrhea in the population is the large number of infected individuals who are asymptomatic or have minor symptoms that are ignored. These persons, unlike symptomatic individuals, may not cease sexual activity and therefore continue to transmit the infection. This situation underscores the importance of contact tracing and empirical treatment of the sex partners of index cases.

PATHOGENESIS, IMMUNOLOGY, AND ANTIMICROBIAL RESISTANCE

Outer-Membrane Proteins

PILI Fresh clinical isolates of *N. gonorrhoeae* initially form piliated (fimbriated) colonies distinguishable on translucent agar. Pilus expression is rapidly switched off with unselected subculture because of rearrangements in pilus genes. This change is a basis for antigenic variation of gonococci. Piliated strains adhere better to cells derived from human mucosal surfaces and are more virulent in organ culture models and human inoculation experiments than nonpiliated variants. In a fallopian tube explant model, pili mediate gonococcal attachment to nonciliated columnar epithelial cells. This event initiates gonococcal phagocytosis and transport through these cells to intercellular spaces near the basement membrane or directly into the subepithelial tissue. CD46 (membrane cofactor protein) is present on urogenital epithelial cells in both men and women and has been determined to be a receptor for PilC; this subunit is located at the tip of the pilus molecule and is critical in mediating adherence. Pili are also essential for genetic competence and transformation of *N. gonorrhoeae*, which permit horizontal transfer of genetic material between different gonococcal lineages in vivo.

OPACITY-ASSOCIATED PROTEIN Another gonococcal surface protein that is important in adherence to epithelial cells is opacity-associated protein (Opa, formerly called protein II). Opa contributes to intergonococcal adhesion, which is responsible for the opaque nature of gonococcal colonies on translucent agar and the organism's adherence to a variety of eukaryotic cells, including polymorphonuclear leukocytes (PMNs). Certain Opa variants promote invasion of epithelial cells, and this effect has been linked with the ability of Opa to bind vitronectin, glycosaminoglycans, and several members of the carcinoembryonic antigen–related cell adhesion molecule (CEACAM) receptor family. *N. gonorrhoeae* Opa proteins that bind CEACAM 1, which is expressed by primary CD4+ T lymphocytes, suppress the activation and proliferation of these lymphocytes. This phenomenon may serve to explain the transient decrease in CD4+ T lymphocyte counts associated with gonococcal infection.

PORIN Porin (previously designated protein I) is the most abundant gonococcal surface protein, accounting for >50% of the organism's total outer-membrane protein. Porin molecules exist as trimers that provide anion-transporting aqueous channels through the otherwise-hydrophobic outer membrane. Porin shows stable interstrain antigenic variation and forms the basis for gonococcal serotyping. Two main serotypes have been identified: PorB.1A strains are often associated with disseminated gonococcal infection (DGI), while PorB.1B strains usually cause local genital infections only. DGI strains are generally resistant to the killing action of normal human serum and do not incite a significant local inflammatory response; therefore, they may not cause symptoms at genital sites. These characteristics may be related to the ability of PorB.1A strains to bind to complement-inhibitory molecules, resulting in a diminished inflammatory response. Porin can translocate to the cytoplasmic membrane of host cells—a process that could initiate gonococcal endocytosis and invasion.

OTHER OUTER-MEMBRANE PROTEINS Other notable outer-membrane proteins include H.8, a lipoprotein that is present in high concentration on the surface of all gonococcal strains and is an excellent target for antibody-based diagnostic testing. Transferrin-binding proteins (Tbp1 and Tbp2) and lactoferrin-binding protein are required for scavenging iron from transferrin and lactoferrin in vivo. Transferrin and iron have been shown to enhance the attachment of iron-deprived *N. gonorrhoeae* to human endometrial cells. IgA1 protease is produced by *N. gonorrhoeae* and may protect the organism from the action of mucosal IgA.

Lipooligosaccharide

Gonococcal lipooligosaccharide (LOS) consists of a lipid A and a core oligosaccharide that lacks the repeating O-carbohydrate antigenic side chain seen in other gram-negative bacteria (Chap. 114). Gonococcal LOS possesses marked endotoxic activity and contributes to the local cytotoxic effect in a fallopian tube model. LOS core sugars undergo a high degree of phase variation under different conditions of growth; this variation reflects genetic regulation and expression of glycotransferase genes that dictate the carbohydrate structure of LOS. These phenotypic changes may affect interactions of *N. gonorrhoeae* with elements of the humoral immune system (antibodies and complement) and may also influence direct binding of organisms to both professional phagocytes and nonprofessional phagocytes (epithelial cells). For example, gonococci that are sialylated at their LOS sites bind complement factor H and inhibit the alternative pathway of complement. LOS sialylation may also decrease nonopsonic Opa-mediated association with neutrophils and inhibit the oxidative burst in PMNs. The unsialylated terminal lactosamine residue of LOS binds to an asialoglycoprotein receptor on male epithelial cells, which facilitates binding and subsequent gonococcal invasion of these cells.

Host Factors

In addition to gonococcal structures that interact with epithelial cells, host factors seem to be important in mediating entry of gonococci into nonphagocytic cells. Activation of phosphatidylcholine-specific phospholipase C and acidic sphingomyelinase by *N. gonorrhoeae*, which results in the release of diacylglycerol and ceramide, is a requirement for the entry of *N. gonorrhoeae* into epithelial cells. Ceramide accumulation within cells leads to apoptosis, which may disrupt epithelial integrity and facilitate entry of gonococci into subepithelial tissue. Release of chemotactic factors as a result of complement activation contributes to inflammation, as does the toxic effect of LOS in provoking the release of inflammatory cytokines.

The importance of humoral immunity in host defenses against neisserial infections is best illustrated by the predisposition of persons deficient in terminal complement components (C5 through C9) to recurrent bacteremic gonococcal infections and to recurrent meningococcal meningitis or meningococcemia. Gonococcal porin induces T cell–proliferative responses in persons with urogenital gonococcal disease. A significant increase in porin-specific interleukin (IL) 4–producing CD4+ as well as CD8+ T lymphocytes is seen in individuals with mucosal gonococcal disease. A portion of these lymphocytes that show a porin-specific T_H2-type response could traffic to mucosal surfaces and play a role in immune protection against the disease. Few data clearly indicate that protective immunity is acquired from a previous gonococcal infection, although bactericidal and opsonophagocytic antibodies to porin and LOS may offer partial protection. On the other hand, women who are infected and acquire high levels of antibody to another outer-membrane protein, Rmp (reduction modifiable protein, formerly called protein III), may be especially likely to become reinfected with *N. gonorrhoeae* because Rmp antibodies block the effect of bactericidal antibodies to porin and LOS. Rmp shows little, if any, interstrain antigenic variation; therefore, Rmp antibodies potentially may block antibody-mediated killing of all gonococci. The mechanism of blocking has not been fully characterized, but Rmp antibodies noncompetitively inhibit binding of porin and LOS antibodies because of the proximity of these structures in the gonococcal outer membrane. In male volunteers who have no history of gonorrhea, the net effect of these events may influence the outcome of experimental challenge with *N. gonorrhoeae*. Because Rmp bears extensive homology to enterobacterial OmpA and meningococcal class 4 proteins, it is possible that these blocking antibodies result from prior exposure to cross-reacting proteins from these species and also play a role in first-time infection with *N. gonorrhoeae*.

Gonococcal Resistance to Antimicrobial Agents It is no surprise that *N. gonorrhoeae*, with its remarkable capacity to alter its antigenic structure and adapt to changes in the microenvironment, has become resistant to numerous antibiotics. The first effective agents against gonorrhea were the sulfonamides, which were introduced in the 1930s and became ineffective within a decade. Penicillin was then employed as the drug of choice for the treatment of gonorrhea. By 1965, 42% of gonococcal isolates had developed low-level resistance to penicillin G. Resistance due to the production of penicillinase arose later.

Gonococci become fully resistant to antibiotics either by chromosomal mutations or by acquisition of R factors (plasmids). Two types of chromosomal mutations have been described. The first type, which is drug specific, is a single-step mutation leading to high-level resistance. The second type involves mutations at several chromosomal loci that combine to determine the level as well as the pattern of resistance. Strains with mutations in chromosomal genes were first observed in the late 1950s. As recently as 2004, chromosomal mutations accounted for resistance to penicillin, tetracycline, or both in ~12% of strains surveyed in the United States.

β-Lactamase (penicillinase)–producing strains of *N. gonorrhoeae* (PPNG) carrying plasmids with the Pc^r determinant had rapidly spread worldwide by the early 1980s. *N. gonorrhoeae* strains with plasmid-borne tetracycline resistance (TRNG) can mobilize some β-lactamase plasmids, and PPNG and TRNG occur together, sometimes along with strains exhibiting chromosomally mediated resistance (CMRNG). Penicillin, ampicillin, and tetracycline are no longer reliable for the treatment of gonorrhea and should not be used. Third-generation cephalosporins have remained highly effective as single-dose therapy for gonorrhea. Even though the minimal inhibitory concentrations (MICs) of ceftriaxone for certain strains may reach 0.015–0.125 mg/L (higher than the MICs of 0.0001–0.008 mg/L for fully susceptible strains), these levels are greatly exceeded in the blood, the urethra, and the cervix when the routinely recommended ceftriaxone and cefixime regimens are administered (see below). These regimens almost always result in an effective cure.

Quinolone-containing regimens were also recommended for treatment of gonococcal infections; the fluoroquinolones offered the advantage of antichlamydial activity when administered for 7 days. However, quinolone-resistant *N. gonorrhoeae* (QRNG) appeared soon after these agents were first used to treat gonorrhea; in the United States, quinolone-containing regimens are no longer routinely recommended for the treatment of gonorrhea.

QRNG is particularly common in the Pacific Islands (including Hawaii) and Asia, where, in certain areas, all gonococcal strains are now resistant to quinolones. At present, QRNG is also common in parts of Europe and the Middle East. In the United States, QRNG has been identified in midwestern and eastern areas as well as in states on the Pacific coast, where resistant strains were first seen. Alterations in DNA gyrase and topoisomerase IV have been implicated as mechanisms of fluoroquinolone resistance.

Resistance to spectinomycin, which has been used in the past as an alternative agent, has been reported. Since this agent is usually not associated with resistance to other antibiotics, spectinomycin can be reserved for use against multiresistant strains of *N. gonorrhoeae*. Nevertheless, outbreaks caused by strains resistant to spectinomycin have been documented in Korea and England when the drug has been used for primary treatment of gonorrhea.

CLINICAL MANIFESTATIONS

Gonococcal Infections in Males Acute urethritis is the most common clinical manifestation of gonorrhea in males. The usual incubation period after exposure is 2–7 days, although the interval can be longer and some men remain asymptomatic. Strains of the PorB.1A serotype tend to cause a greater proportion of cases of mild and asymptomatic urethritis than do PorB.1B strains. Urethral discharge and dysuria, usually without urinary frequency or urgency, are the major symptoms. The discharge initially is scant and mucoid but becomes profuse and purulent within a day or two. Gram's stain of the urethral discharge may reveal PMNs and gram-negative intracellular monococci and diplococci (Fig. 137-1). The clinical manifestations of gonococcal urethritis are usually more severe and overt than those of nongonococcal urethritis, including urethritis caused by *Chlamydia trachomatis* (Chap. 169); however, exceptions are common, and it is often impossible to differentiate the causes of urethritis on clinical grounds alone. The majority of cases of urethritis seen in the United States today are not caused by *N. gonorrhoeae* and/or *C. trachomatis*. Although a number of other organisms may be responsible, most cases do not have a specific etiologic agent identified.

Most symptomatic men with gonorrhea seek treatment and cease to be infectious. The remaining men, who are largely asymptomatic, accumulate in number over time and constitute about two-thirds of all infected men at any point in time. Together with men incubating the organism (who shed the organism but are asymptomatic), they serve as the source of spread of infection. Before the antibiotic era, symptoms of urethritis persisted for ~8 weeks. Epididymitis is now an uncommon complication, and gonococcal prostatitis occurs rarely, if at all. Other unusual local complications of gonococcal urethritis include edema of the penis due to dorsal lymphangitis or thrombophlebitis, submucous inflammatory "soft" infiltration of the urethral wall, periurethral abscess or fistulae, inflammation or abscess of Cowper's gland, and seminal vesiculitis. Balanitis may develop in uncircumcised men.

Gonococcal Infections in Females • ***GONOCOCCAL CERVICITIS*** Mucopurulent cervicitis is the most common STI diagnosis in American women and may be caused by *N. gonorrhoeae*, *C. trachomatis*, and oth-

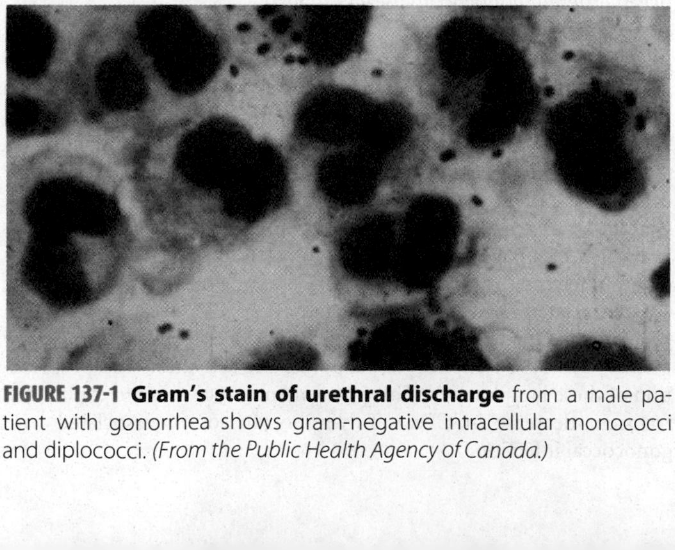

FIGURE 137-1 Gram's stain of urethral discharge from a male patient with gonorrhea shows gram-negative intracellular monococci and diplococci. *(From the Public Health Agency of Canada.)*

er organisms. Cervicitis may coexist with candidal or trichomonal vaginitis. *N. gonorrhoeae* primarily infects the columnar epithelium of the cervical os. Bartholin's glands occasionally become infected.

Women infected with *N. gonorrhoeae* usually develop symptoms. However, the women who either remain asymptomatic or have only minor symptoms may delay in seeking medical attention. These minor symptoms may include scant vaginal discharge issuing from the inflamed cervix (without vaginitis or vaginosis per se) and dysuria (often without urgency or frequency) that may be associated with gonococcal urethritis. Although the incubation period of gonorrhea is less well defined in women than in men, symptoms usually develop within 10 days of infection and are more acute and intense than those of chlamydial cervicitis.

The physical examination may reveal a mucopurulent discharge (mucopus) issuing from the cervical os. Because Gram's stain is not sensitive for the diagnosis of gonorrhea in women, specimens should be submitted for culture or a nonculture assay (see below). Edematous and friable cervical ectopy as well as endocervical bleeding induced by gentle swabbing are more often seen in chlamydial infection. Gonococcal infection may extend deep enough to produce dyspareunia and lower abdominal or back pain. In such cases, it is imperative to consider a diagnosis of pelvic inflammatory disease (PID) and to administer treatment for that disease (Chaps. 124 and 169).

N. gonorrhoeae may be recovered from the urethra and rectum of women with cervicitis, but these are rarely the only infected sites. Urethritis in women may produce symptoms of internal dysuria, which is often attributed to "cystitis." Pyuria in the absence of bacteriuria seen on Gram's stain of unspun urine, accompanied by urine cultures that fail to yield $>10^5$ colonies of bacteria usually associated with urinary tract infection, signifies the possibility of urethritis due to *C. trachomatis*. Urethral infection with *N. gonorrhoeae* may also occur in this context, but in this instance urethral cultures are usually positive.

GONOCOCCAL VAGINITIS The vaginal mucosa of healthy women is lined by stratified squamous epithelium and is rarely infected by *N. gonorrhoeae*. However, gonococcal vaginitis can occur in anestrogenic women (e.g., prepubertal girls and postmenopausal women), in whom the vaginal stratified squamous epithelium is often thinned down to the basilar layer, which can be infected by *N. gonorrhoeae*. The intense inflammation of the vagina makes the physical (speculum and bimanual) examination extremely painful. The vaginal mucosa is red and edematous, and an abundant purulent discharge is present. Infection in the urethra and in Skene's and Bartholin's glands often accompanies gonococcal vaginitis. Inflamed cervical erosion or abscesses in nabothian cysts may also occur. Coexisting cervicitis may result in pus in the cervical os.

Anorectal Gonorrhea Because the female anatomy permits the spread of cervical exudate to the rectum, *N. gonorrhoeae* is sometimes recovered from the rectum of women with uncomplicated gonococcal cervicitis. The rectum is the sole site of infection in only 5% of women with gonorrhea. Such women are usually asymptomatic but occasionally have acute proctitis manifested by anorectal pain or pruritus, tenesmus, purulent rectal discharge, and rectal bleeding. Among men who have sex with men (MSM), the frequency of gonococcal infection, including rectal infection, fell by ≥90% throughout the United States in the early 1980s, but a resurgence of gonorrhea among MSM has been documented in several cities since the 1990s. Gonococcal isolates from the rectum of MSM tend to be more resistant to antimicrobial agents than are gonococcal isolates from other sites. Gonococcal isolates with a mutation in *mtrR* (multiple transferable resistance repressor) or in the promoter region of the gene that encodes for this transcriptional repressor develop increased resistance to antimicrobial hydrophobic agents such as bile acids and fatty acids in feces and thus are found with increased frequency in MSM. This situation may have been responsible for higher rates of failure of treatment for rectal gonorrhea with older regimens consisting of penicillin or tetracyclines.

Pharyngeal Gonorrhea Pharyngeal gonorrhea is usually mild or asymptomatic, although symptomatic pharyngitis does occasionally occur with cervical lymphadenitis. The mode of acquisition is oral-genital sexual exposure, with fellatio being a more efficient means of transmission than cunnilingus. Most cases resolve spontaneously, and transmission from the pharynx to sexual contacts is rare. Pharyngeal infection almost always coexists with genital infection. Swabs from the pharynx should be plated directly onto gonococcal selective media. Pharyngeal colonization with *Neisseria meningitidis* needs to be differentiated from that with other *Neisseria* species.

Ocular Gonorrhea in Adults Ocular gonorrhea in an adult usually results from autoinoculation from an infected genital site. As in genital infection, the manifestations range from severe to occasionally mild or asymptomatic disease. The variability in clinical manifestations may be attributable to differences in the ability of the infecting strain to elicit an inflammatory response. Infection may result in a markedly swollen eyelid, severe hyperemia and chemosis, and a profuse purulent discharge. The massively inflamed conjunctiva may be draped over the cornea and limbus. Lytic enzymes from the infiltrating PMNs occasionally cause corneal ulceration and rarely cause perforation.

Prompt recognition and treatment of this condition are of paramount importance. Gram's stain and culture of the purulent discharge establish the diagnosis. Genital cultures should also be performed.

Gonorrhea in Pregnant Women, Neonates, and Children Gonorrhea in pregnancy can have serious consequences for both the mother and the infant. Recognition of gonorrhea early in pregnancy also identifies a population at risk for other STIs, particularly chlamydial infection and syphilis. The risks of salpingitis and PID—conditions associated with a high rate of fetal loss—are highest during the first trimester. Pharyngeal infection, most often asymptomatic, may be more common during pregnancy because of altered sexual practices. Prolonged rupture of the membranes, premature delivery, chorioamnionitis, funisitis (infection of the umbilical cord stump), and sepsis in the infant (with *N. gonorrhoeae* detected in the newborn's gastric aspirate during delivery) are common complications of maternal gonococcal infection at term. Other microorganisms and conditions, including *Mycoplasma hominis*, *Ureaplasma urealyticum*, *C. trachomatis*, and bacterial vaginosis, have been associated with similar complications.

The most common form of gonorrhea in neonates is ophthalmia neonatorum, which results from exposure to infected cervical secretions during parturition. Ocular neonatal instillation of a prophylactic agent (e.g., 1% silver nitrate eyedrops or ophthalmic preparations containing erythromycin or tetracycline) prevents ophthalmia neonatorum but is not effective for its treatment, which requires systemic antibiotics. The clinical manifestations are acute and usually begin 2–5 days after birth. An initial nonspecific conjunctivitis with a serosanguineous discharge is followed by tense edema of both eyelids, chemosis, and a profuse, thick, purulent discharge. Corneal ulcerations that result in nebulae or perforation may lead to anterior synechiae, anterior staphyloma, panophthalmitis, and blindness. Infections described at other mucosal sites in infants, including vaginitis, rhinitis, and anorectal infection, are likely to be asymptomatic. Pharyngeal colonization has been demonstrated in 35% of infants with gonococcal ophthalmia, and coughing is the most prominent symptom in these cases. Septic arthritis (see below) is the most common manifestation of systemic infection or DGI in the newborn. The onset usually comes at 3–21 days of age, and polyarticular involvement is common. Sepsis, meningitis, and pneumonia are seen in rare instances.

Any STI in children beyond the neonatal period raises the possibility of sexual abuse. Gonococcal vulvovaginitis is the most common manifestation of gonococcal infection in children beyond infancy. Anorectal and pharyngeal infections are common in these children and are frequently asymptomatic. The urethra, Bartholin's and Skene's glands, and the upper genital tract are rarely involved. All children with gonococcal infection should also be evaluated for chlamydial infection, syphilis, and possibly HIV infection.

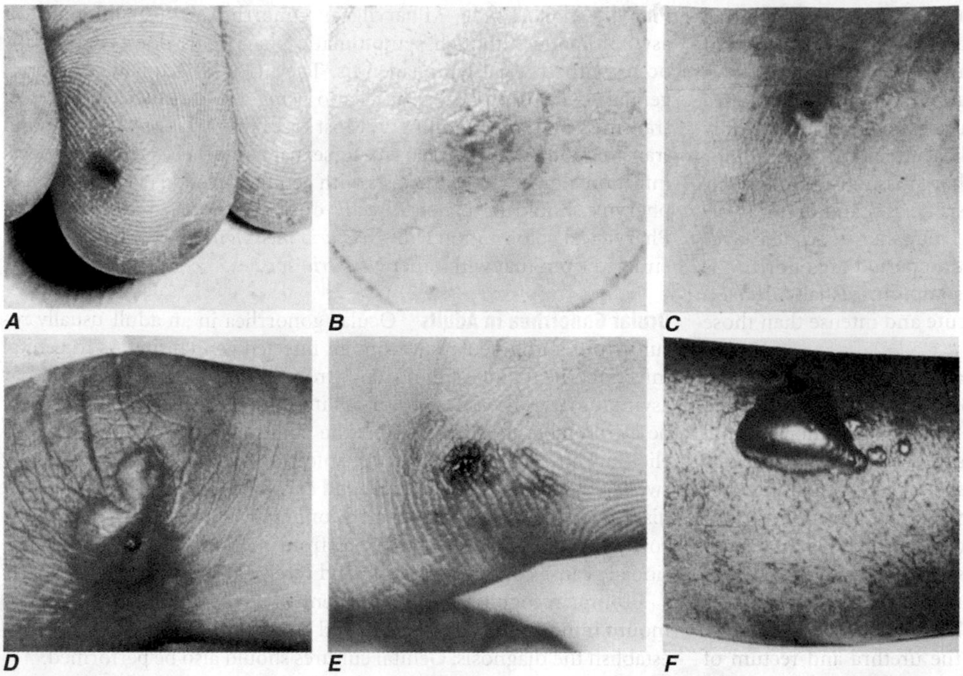

FIGURE 137-2 Characteristic skin lesions in patients with proven gonococcal bacteremia. The lesions are in various stages of evolution. ***A.*** Very early petechia on finger. ***B.*** Early papular lesion, 7 mm in diameter, on lower leg. ***C.*** Pustule with central eschar resulting from early petechial lesion. ***D.*** Pustular lesion on finger. ***E.*** Mature lesion with central necrosis (black) on hemorrhagic base. ***F.*** Bullae on anterior tibial surface. *(Reprinted with permission from KK Holmes et al: Disseminated gonococcal infection. Ann Intern Med 74:979, 1971.)*

Gonococcal Arthritis (DGI) DGI or gonococcal arthritis results from gonococcal bacteremia. In the 1970s, DGI occurred in ~0.5–3% of persons with untreated gonococcal mucosal infection. The lower incidence of DGI at present is probably attributable to a decline in the prevalence of particular strains that are likely to disseminate. DGI strains resist the bactericidal action of human serum and generally do not incite inflammation at genital sites, probably because of limited generation of chemotactic factors. Strains recovered from DGI cases in the 1970s were often of the PorB.1A serotype, were highly susceptible to penicillin, and had special growth requirements (i.e., the AHU auxotype) that made the organism more fastidious and more difficult to isolate.

Menstruation is a risk factor for dissemination, and approximately two-thirds of cases of DGI are in women. In about half of affected women, symptoms of DGI begin within 7 days of onset of menses. Complement deficiencies, especially of the components involved in the assembly of the membrane attack complex (C5 through C9), predispose to neisserial bacteremia, and persons with more than one episode of DGI should be screened with an assay for total hemolytic complement activity.

The clinical manifestations of DGI have sometimes been classified into two stages: a bacteremic stage, which is less common today, and a joint-localized stage with suppurative arthritis. A clear-cut progression usually is not evident. Patients in the bacteremic stage have higher temperatures, and their fever is more frequently accompanied by chills. Painful joints are common and often occur in conjunction with tenosynovitis and skin lesions. Polyarthralgias usually include the knees, elbows, and more distal joints; the axial skeleton is generally spared. Skin lesions are seen in ~75% of patients and include papules and pustules, often with a hemorrhagic component (Fig. 137-2). Other manifestations of noninfectious dermatitis, such as nodular lesions, urticaria, and erythema multiforme, have been described. These lesions are usually on the extremities and number between 5 and 40. The differential diagnosis of the bacteremic stage of DGI includes reactive arthritis, acute rheumatoid arthritis, sarcoidosis, erythema nodosum, drug-induced arthritis, and viral infections (e.g., hepatitis B and acute HIV infection). The distribution of joint symptoms in reactive arthritis differs from that in DGI (Fig. 137-3), as do the skin and genital manifestations (Chap. 318).

Suppurative arthritis involves one or two joints, most often (in decreasing order of frequency) the knees, wrists, ankles, and elbows; other joints are occasionally involved. Most patients who develop gonococcal septic arthritis do so without prior polyarthralgias or skin lesions; in the absence of symptomatic genital infection, this disease cannot be distinguished from septic arthritis caused by other pathogens. The differential diagnosis of acute arthritis in young adults is discussed in Chap. 328. Rarely, osteomyelitis complicates septic arthritis involving small joints of the hand.

Gonococcal endocarditis, although rare today, was a relatively common complication of DGI in the preantibiotic era, causing about one-quarter of reported cases of endocarditis. Another unusual complication of DGI is meningitis.

Gonococcal Infections in HIV-Infected Persons The association between gonorrhea and the acquisition of HIV has been demonstrated in several well-controlled studies, mainly in Kenya and Zaire. The nonulcerative STIs enhance the transmission of HIV by three- to fivefold, possibly because of increased viral shedding by persons with urethritis or cervicitis (Chap. 182). HIV has been detected by polymerase chain reaction (PCR) more commonly in ejaculates from HIV-positive men with gonococcal urethritis than in those from HIV-positive men with nongonococcal urethritis. PCR positivity diminishes twofold after appropriate therapy for urethritis. Not only does gonorrhea enhance the transmission of HIV; it may also increase the individual's risk for acquisition of HIV. A proposed mechanism is the significantly greater number of CD4+ T

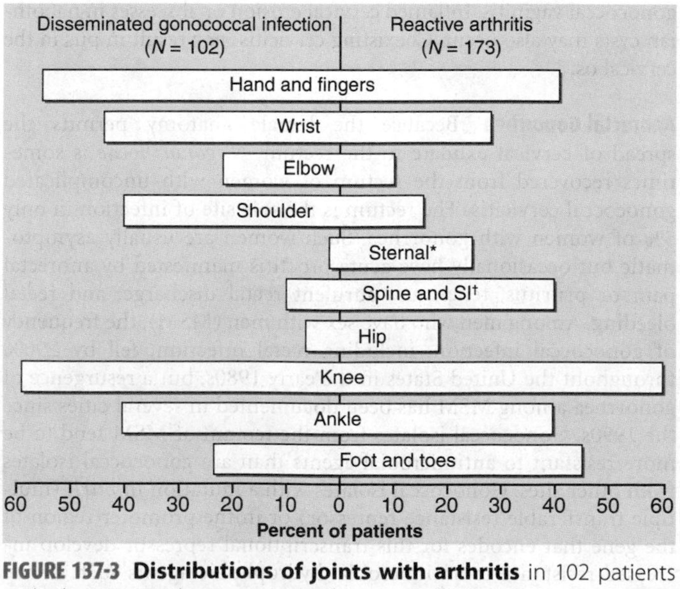

FIGURE 137-3 Distributions of joints with arthritis in 102 patients with disseminated gonococcal infection and 173 patients with reactive arthritis. *Includes the sternoclavicular joints. †SI, sacroiliac joint. *(Reprinted with permission from M Kousa et al: Frequent association of chlamydial infection with Reiter's syndrome. Sex Transm Dis 5:57, 1978.)*

lymphocytes and dendritic cells that can be infected by HIV in endocervical secretions of women with nonulcerative STIs than in those of women with ulcerative STIs.

LABORATORY DIAGNOSIS

A rapid diagnosis of gonococcal infection in men may be obtained by Gram's staining of urethral exudates (Fig. 137-1). The detection of gram-negative intracellular monococci and diplococci is usually highly specific and sensitive in diagnosing gonococcal urethritis in symptomatic males but is only ~50% sensitive in diagnosing gonococcal cervicitis. Samples should be collected with Dacron or rayon swabs. Part of the sample should be inoculated onto a plate of modified Thayer-Martin or other gonococcal selective medium for culture. It is important to process all samples immediately because gonococci do not tolerate drying. If plates cannot be incubated immediately, they can be held safely for several hours at room temperature in candle extinction jars prior to incubation. If processing is to occur within 6 h, transport of specimens may be facilitated by the use of nonnutritive swab transport systems such as Stuart or Amies medium. For longer holding periods (e.g., when specimens for culture are to be mailed), culture media with self-contained CO_2-generating systems (such as the JEMBEC or Gono-Pak systems) may be used. Specimens should also be obtained for the diagnosis of chlamydial infection.

PMNs are often seen in the endocervix on a Gram's stain, and an abnormally increased number (≥30 PMNs per field in five 1000× oil-immersion microscopic fields) establishes the presence of an inflammatory discharge. Unfortunately, the presence or absence of gram-negative intracellular monococci or diplococci in cervical smears does not accurately predict which patients have gonorrhea, and the diagnosis in this setting should be made by culture or another suitable nonculture diagnostic method. The sensitivity of a single endocervical culture is ~80–90%. If a history of rectal sex is elicited, a rectal wall swab (uncontaminated with feces) should be cultured. A presumptive diagnosis of gonorrhea cannot be made on the basis of gram-negative diplococci in smears from the pharynx, where other *Neisseria* species are components of the normal flora.

Nucleic acid probe tests are sometimes substituted for culture for the direct detection of *N. gonorrhoeae* in urogenital specimens. A common assay employs a nonisotopic chemiluminescent DNA probe that hybridizes specifically with gonococcal 16S ribosomal RNA; this assay is as sensitive as conventional culture techniques. A disadvantage of non-culture-based assays is that *N. gonorrhoeae* cannot be grown from the transport systems. Thus a culture-confirmatory test and formal antimicrobial susceptibility testing, if needed, cannot be performed. Nucleic acid amplification tests (NAATs), including Roche Amplicor, Gen-Probe APTIMA Combo2 (which also detects *Chlamydia*), and BD ProbeTec ET, offer an advantage: urine samples can be tested with a sensitivity similar to that obtained when urethral or cervical swab samples are assessed by culture and other non-NAATs.

Because of the legal implications, the preferred method for the diagnosis of gonococcal infection in children is a standardized culture. Two positive NAATs, each targeting a different nucleic acid sequence, may be substituted for culture of the cervix or the urethra as legal evidence of infection; however, cervical specimens are not recommended for prepubertal girls. Nonculture tests for gonococcal infection have not been approved by the U.S. Food and Drug Administration for use with specimens obtained from the pharynx and rectum of infected children. Cultures should be obtained from the pharynx and anus of both girls and boys, the vagina of girls, and the urethra of boys. For boys with a urethral discharge, a meatal specimen of the discharge is adequate for culture. Presumptive colonies of *N. gonorrhoeae* should be identified definitively by at least two independent methods.

Blood should be cultured in suspected cases of DGI. The use of Isolator blood culture tubes may enhance the yield. The probability of positive blood cultures decreases after 48 h of illness. Synovial fluid should be inoculated into blood culture broth medium and plated onto chocolate agar rather than selective medium because this fluid is not likely to be contaminated with commensal bacteria. Gonococci are infrequently recovered from early joint effusions containing <20,000 leukocytes/μL but may be recovered from effusions containing >80,000 leukocytes/μL. The organisms are seldom recovered from blood and synovial fluid of the same patient.

Rx GONOCOCCAL INFECTIONS

Treatment failure can lead to continued transmission and the emergence of antibiotic resistance. The importance of adequate treatment with a regimen that the patient will adhere to cannot be overemphasized. Thus highly effective single-dose regimens have been developed for uncomplicated gonococcal infections. The updated 2006 treatment guidelines for gonococcal infections from the Centers for Disease Control and Prevention are summarized in **Table 137-1**; the recommendations for uncomplicated gonorrhea apply to HIV-infected as well as HIV-uninfected patients.

Single-dose regimens of the third-generation cephalosporins ceftriaxone (given IM) and cefixime (given orally) are the mainstays of therapy for uncomplicated gonococcal infection of the urethra, cervix, rectum, or pharynx. Quinolone-containing regimens are no longer recommended in the United States as first-line treatment because of widespread resistance to these agents.

Because co-infection with *C. trachomatis* occurs frequently, initial treatment regimens must also incorporate an agent (e.g., azithromycin or doxycycline) that is effective against chlamydial infection. Pregnant women with gonorrhea, who should not take doxycycline, should receive concurrent treatment with a macrolide antibiotic for possible chlamydial infection. A single 1-g dose of azithromycin, which is effective therapy for uncomplicated chlamydial infections, results in an unacceptably low cure rate (93%) for gonococcal infections and should not be used alone. Spectinomycin has been an alternative regimen for the treatment of uncomplicated gonococcal infections in penicillin-allergic persons. However, spectinomycin is not available in the United States at this time. A single 2-g dose of azithromycin is effective against sensitive strains, but this drug is expensive, causes gastrointestinal distress, and is not recommended for routine or first-line treatment of gonorrhea.

Persons with uncomplicated infections who receive a recommended regimen do not need a test of cure. Cultures for *N. gonorrhoeae* should be performed if symptoms persist after therapy with an established regimen, and any gonococci isolated should be tested for antimicrobial susceptibility.

Symptomatic gonococcal pharyngitis is more difficult to eradicate than genital infection. Persons who cannot tolerate cephalosporins and those in whom quinolones are contraindicated may be treated with spectinomycin if it is available, but this agent results in a cure rate of ≤52%. Persons given spectinomycin should have a pharyngeal sample cultured 3–5 days after treatment as a test of cure. A single 2-g dose of azithromycin may be used in areas where rates of resistance to azithromycin are low.

Treatments for gonococcal epididymitis and PID are discussed in Chap. 124. Ocular gonococcal infections in older children and adults should be managed with a single dose of ceftriaxone combined with saline irrigation of the conjunctivae (both undertaken expeditiously), and patients should undergo a careful ophthalmologic evaluation that includes a slit-lamp examination.

DGI may require higher dosages and longer durations of therapy (Table 137-1). Hospitalization is indicated if the diagnosis is uncertain, if the patient has localized joint disease that requires aspiration, or if the patient cannot be relied on to comply with treatment. Open drainage is necessary only occasionally—e.g., for management of hip infections that may be difficult to drain percutaneously. Nonsteroidal anti-inflammatory agents may be indicated to alleviate pain and hasten improvement of affected joints. Gonococcal meningitis and endocarditis should be treated in the hospital with high-dose IV ceftriaxone (1–2 g every 12 h); therapy should continue for 10–14 days for meningitis and for at least 4 weeks for endocarditis. All persons who experience more than one episode of DGI should be evaluated for complement deficiency.

PREVENTION AND CONTROL

Condoms, if properly used, provide effective protection against the transmission and acquisition of gonorrhea as well as other infec-

TABLE 137-1 RECOMMENDED TREATMENT FOR GONOCOCCAL INFECTIONS: 2006 GUIDELINES OF THE CENTERS FOR DISEASE CONTROL AND PREVENTION (UPDATED IN 2007)

Diagnosis	Treatment of Choice
Uncomplicated gonococcal infection of the cervix, urethra, pharynx, or rectum[a]	
First-line regimens	Ceftriaxone (125 mg IM, single dose)
	or
	Cefixime (400 mg PO, single dose)
	plus
	Treatment for *Chlamydia* if chlamydial infection is not ruled out:
	Azithromycin (1 g PO, single dose)
	or
	Doxycycline (100 mg PO bid for 7 days)
Alternative regimens	Ceftizoxime (500 mg IM, single dose)
	or
	Cefotaxime (500 mg IM, single dose)
	or
	Spectinomycin (2 g IM, single dose)[b,c]
	or
	Cefotetan (1 g IM, single dose) plus probenecid (1 g PO, single dose)[b]
	or
	Cefoxitin (2 g IM, single dose) plus probenecid (1 g PO, single dose)[b]
Epididymitis	See Chap. 124
Pelvic inflammatory disease	See Chap. 124
Gonococcal conjunctivitis in an adult	Ceftriaxone (1 g IM, single dose)[d]
Ophthalmia neonatorum[e]	Ceftriaxone (25–50 mg/kg IV, single dose, not to exceed 125 mg)
Disseminated gonococcal infection[f]	
Initial therapy[g]	
Patient tolerant of β-lactam drugs	Ceftriaxone (1 g IM or IV q24h; recommended)
	or
	Cefotaxime (1 g IV q8h)
	or
	Ceftizoxime (1 g IV q8h)
Patients allergic to β-lactam drugs	Spectinomycin (2 g IM q12h)[c]
Continuation therapy	Cefixime (400 mg PO bid)
Meningitis or endocarditis	See text[h]

[a]True failure of treatment with a recommended regimen is rare and should prompt an evaluation for reinfection or consideration of an alternative diagnosis.
[b]Spectinomycin, cefotetan, and cefoxitin, which are alternative agents, currently are unavailable or in short supply in the United States.
[c]Spectinomycin may be ineffective for the treatment of pharyngeal gonorrhea.
[d]Plus lavage of the infected eye with saline solution (once).
[e]Prophylactic regimens are discussed in the text.
[f]Hospitalization is indicated if the diagnosis is uncertain, if the patient has frank arthritis with an effusion, or if the patient cannot be relied on to adhere to treatment.
[g]All initial regimens should be continued for 24–48 h after clinical improvement begins, at which time therapy may be switched to one of the continuation regimens to complete a full week of antimicrobial treatment. Treatment for chlamydial infection (as above) should be given if this infection has not been ruled out.
[h]Hospitalization is indicated to exclude suspected meningitis or endocarditis.

tions that are transmitted to and from genital mucosal surfaces. Spermicidal preparations used with a diaphragm or cervical sponges impregnated with nonoxynol 9 offer some protection against gonorrhea and chlamydial infection. However, the frequent use of preparations that contain nonoxynol 9 is associated with mucosal disruption that paradoxically may enhance the risk of HIV infection in the event of exposure. All patients should be instructed to refer sex partners for evaluation and treatment. All sex partners of persons with gonorrhea should be evaluated and treated for *N. gonorrhoeae* and *C. trachomatis* infections if their last contact with the patient took place within 60 days before the onset of symptoms or the diagnosis of infection in the patient. If the patient's last sexual encounter was >60 days before onset of symptoms or diagnosis, the patient's most recent sex partner should be treated. Partner-delivered medications or prescriptions for medications to treat gonorrhea and chlamydial infection diminish the likelihood of reinfection (or relapse) in the infected patient. In states where it is legal, this approach is an option for partner management. Patients should be instructed to abstain from sexual intercourse until therapy is completed and until they and their sex partners no longer have symptoms. Greater emphasis must be placed on prevention by public health education, individual patient counseling, and behavior modification. Sexually active persons, especially adolescents, should be offered screening for STIs. For males, a NAAT on urine or a urethral swab may be used for screening. Preventing the spread of gonorrhea may help reduce the transmission of HIV. No effective vaccine for gonorrhea is yet available, but efforts to test several candidates are under way.

ACKNOWLEDGMENTS

The authors acknowledge the contributions of Dr. King K. Holmes and Dr. Stephen A. Morse to the chapter on this subject in earlier editions.

FURTHER READINGS

Centers for Disease Control and Prevention: Gonococcal Isolate Surveillance Project (GISP); *www.cdc.gov/std/GISP/*

———: Update to CDC's sexually transmitted disease treatment guidelines 2006: Fluoroquinolones no longer recommended for treatment of gonococcal infections. MMWR 56(14):332, 2007

Gaydos CA: Nucleic acid amplification tests for gonorrhea and *Chlamydia*: Practice and applications. Infect Dis Clin North Am 19:367, 2005

Golden MR et al: Effect of expedited treatment of sex partners on recurrent or persistent gonorrhea or chlamydial infections. N Engl J Med 352:676, 2005

Hook EW III, Holmes KK: Gonococcal infections. Ann Intern Med 102:229, 1985

Laga M et al: Non-ulcerative sexually transmitted diseases as risk factors for HIV-1 transmission in women: Results from a cohort study. AIDS 7:95, 1993

O'Brien JP et al: Disseminated gonococcal infection: A prospective analysis of 49 patients and a review of pathophysiology and immune mechanisms. Medicine (Baltimore) 62:395, 1983

138 *Moraxella* Infections

Daniel M. Musher

MORAXELLA CATARRHALIS

The gram-negative coccus *Moraxella catarrhalis* is a component of the normal bacterial flora of the upper airways and has been increasingly recognized as a cause of otitis media, sinusitis, and bronchopulmonary infection. Over the past several decades, this organism has been variously designated as *Micrococcus catarrhalis*, *Neisseria catarrhalis*, and *Branhamella catarrhalis*.

BACTERIOLOGY AND IMMUNITY

On Gram's staining, *M. catarrhalis* organisms appear as gram-negative cocci, sometimes occurring in pairs and having the side-by-side kidney-bean configuration of *Neisseria* (Fig. 138-1). These cocci tend to retain crystal violet during the decolorizing step and may be confused with *Staphylococcus aureus*. *Moraxella* colonies grow well on blood or chocolate agar but may be overlooked because of their resemblance to the *Neisseria* spp. that are major components of the normal pharyngeal flora. *Moraxella* is readily distinguishable from *Neisseria* spp. by biochemical tests.

Strains of *M. catarrhalis* show a surprising degree of homogeneity in terms of their outer-membrane proteins. Antibody to some of these proteins is generally present in serum of children >4 years old; however, colonizing or disease-causing isolates may survive in serum despite this naturally present antibody and complement. Bactericidal antibody emerges after natural infection and may be directed against one or more conserved outer-membrane proteins—a property of potential value in vaccine development. The presence of certain outer-membrane proteins is associated with virulence in mice, and antibody to these proteins may be protective. Antibody to lipooligosaccharide may also provide some degree of protection. These and other bacterial constituents are under investigation for use as vaccines.

EPIDEMIOLOGY

With repeated cultures and the use of selective media, *M. catarrhalis* can be isolated from the upper respiratory tract or saliva of >50% of healthy children and 3–7% of healthy adults. When conventional microbiologic techniques are used, *Moraxella* can be isolated from sputum of ~10% of persons who have chronic bronchitis and ~25% of those who have bronchiectasis in the absence of acute infection. Investigators in both the northern and southern hemispheres have reported a striking seasonal variation in the isolation of this organism from clinical specimens, with a peak in late winter/early spring and a nadir in late summer/early fall. Direct contact has not been shown to contribute to community-acquired infection, but nosocomial spread of infection has been documented occasionally.

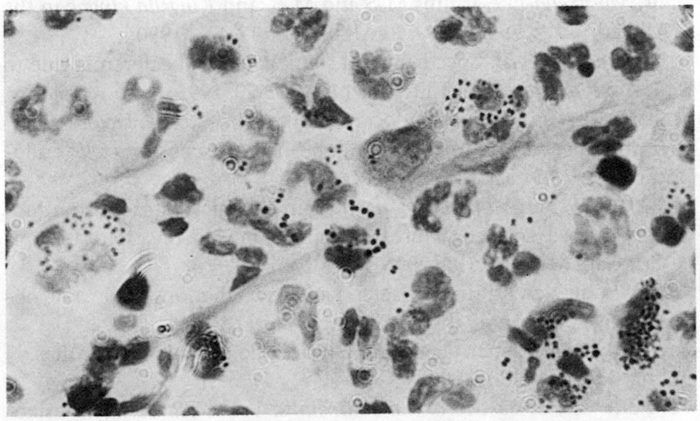

FIGURE 138-1 Gram-stained sputum from a patient with acute purulent tracheobronchitis. Many polymorphonuclear neutrophils and a few macrophages are seen along with many gram-negative cocci (*Moraxella catarrhalis*), a few of which appear as pairs. Nearly all organisms are cell associated and probably have been taken up by phagocytes, consistent with the notion that *Moraxella* is a lower-grade pathogen than organisms that are found extracellularly in sputum specimens (e.g., *Streptococcus pneumoniae*).

CLINICAL MANIFESTATIONS

Otitis Media and Sinusitis *M. catarrhalis* is the third most common bacterial isolate from middle-ear fluid of children with otitis media, being surpassed only by *Streptococcus pneumoniae* and nontypable *Haemophilus influenzae*. This organism is also a prominent isolate from sinus cavities in acute and chronic sinusitis.

Purulent Tracheobronchitis and Pneumonia *M. catarrhalis* causes acute exacerbations of chronic bronchitis (increased production and/or purulence of sputum, which may be accompanied by fever and leukocytosis) and pneumonia. Acquisition of a new bacterial strain is often responsible. The great majority of infected persons are >50 years old and have a long history of cigarette smoking and underlying chronic obstructive pulmonary disease (COPD); many have lung cancer as well. In one study, 76% of affected persons had COPD (severe in many cases), and one-third of those with COPD had lung cancer; most patients also had clinical evidence of malnutrition. In one extensive series of cases, *M. catarrhalis* pneumonia did not occur in otherwise-healthy hosts. Recent prospective studies implicate this organism in ~10% of exacerbations of chronic bronchitis.

Symptoms of *M. catarrhalis* infection have been regarded as modest in severity. Both cough and the amount and purulence of sputum are usually increased above baseline. Chills are reported in one-quarter of patients, pleuritic pain in one-third, and malaise in 40%. Most patients have peak temperatures of <38.3°C (<101°F), and peripheral white blood cell counts are <10,000/μL in nearly one-quarter of cases. Microscopic examination of a high-quality sputum specimen after Gram's staining regularly reveals profuse organisms, and quantitative culture yields ~2 × 10^8 colony-forming units per milliliter. The radiologic appearance is variable; in one study, 43% of subjects had segmental or lobar infiltrates, and the remainder had a mixed pattern of subsegmental, segmental, interstitial, and diffuse involvement. These clinical, laboratory, and radiographic findings do not differ from those of pneumococcal or *Haemophilus* pneumonia in an older patient population. However, a far lesser degree of bloodstream invasion occurs in *M. catarrhalis* infection; in one series, none of 25 patients with *M. catarrhalis* pneumonia had bacteremia. Nevertheless, pneumonia due to *M. catarrhalis* is a marker for severe underlying disease: nearly half of patients die within 3 months of onset.

Other Syndromes Local extension causing empyema is very uncommon, and—as might be inferred from the low rate of bacteremia—metastatic complications of *M. catarrhalis* pneumonia, such as septic arthritis, are exceedingly rare. As of 1995, 58 cases of bacteremic infection due to *M. catarrhalis* had been reported, mainly in children <10 years old or adults >60 years old; most of these patients had severe underlying lung disease and/or were immunocompromised. The syndromes reported have included bacteremia with no apparent focus, pneumonia, endocarditis, and meningitis. A petechial or purpuric rash, reminiscent of that observed in meningococcal sepsis and associated with disseminated intravascular coagulation, has been described in a few cases.

DIAGNOSIS

Microscopic examination of Gram-stained sputum yields characteristic findings (Fig. 138-1). The presence of many polymorphonuclear leukocytes without epithelial cells indicates that the sputum sample is of good quality; since most patients with *Moraxella* infection have chronic lung disease, it is usually not difficult to obtain an acceptable specimen. Large numbers of *Moraxella* organisms are seen as gram-negative cocci, often lining up side by side and thus resembling pairs of kidneys.

TABLE 138-1 THERAPY FOR INFECTION CAUSED BY *MORAXELLA CATARRHALIS*

Drug(s)	Dose and Duration
Oral Therapy for Lower Respiratory Infection[a]	
Trimethoprim-sulfamethoxazole	160/800 mg qd for 5–7 days
Doxycycline	200 mg/d for 5–7 days
Azithromycin	500 mg/d for 5 days
Telithromycin	800 mg/d for 5–7 days
Amoxicillin/clavulanic acid	500 mg tid for 7 days
Ciprofloxacin	500 mg bid for 5 days
Cefuroxime	250–500 mg bid for 10 days
Cefpodoxime	200 mg bid for 10–14 days
Parenteral Therapy for Lower Respiratory Infection in Hospitalized Patients[b]	
Ampicillin/sulbactam	1.5/0.5 g q6h
Ceftriaxone	1 g/d
Cefotaxime	1 g q8h
Azithromycin	500 mg/d

[a]The same dosages apply for sinusitis, but some authorities treat for 10 days with macrolides, tetracyclines, and quinolones and for 14 days with β-lactam agents.
[b]After the patient's condition has stabilized, the regimen may be changed to oral medications at the indicated doses and durations.

℞ *MORAXELLA* INFECTIONS

M. catarrhalis is widely susceptible to most antibiotics used to treat lower respiratory tract infection **(Table 138-1)**. Penicillin resistance first appeared in isolated strains in the mid-1970s and is now found in 94% of clinical isolates. This resistance is mediated by two closely related β-lactamases, BRO-1 and BRO-2. These enzymes are active against penicillin, ampicillin, and amoxicillin but less so against cephalosporins, especially third-generation cephalosporins; they also bind avidly to clavulanic acid and sulbactam. Thus a β-lactam/β-lactamase inhibitor combination such as amoxicillin/clavulanate offers excellent treatment. Second- and third-generation cephalosporins are effective alternatives. Isolates in the United States are also nearly uniformly susceptible to fluoroquinolones, newer macrolides, ketolides, and doxycycline; ~90% are susceptible to trimethoprim-sulfamethoxazole. A 5-day course of therapy has been shown to cure respiratory infection, although a longer course is required in sinusitis.

Treatment of sinusitis or otitis media is empirical, as appropriate specimens are usually obtained only in research studies. In the treatment of pneumonia during the period between the identification of gram-negative cocci in a Gram-stained specimen and the final identification of the organisms by culture, the severity of the condition and the potential presence of other infecting organisms should guide antibiotic selection. For example, an exacerbation of bronchitis caused by *M. catarrhalis* might be treated with doxycycline or an advanced macrolide. However, the microscopic identification of this organism in a patient with pneumonia may still lead to a preference for initial therapy (at least until culture results become available) with ampicillin/sulbactam, a third-generation cephalosporin, or a quinolone because of the possibility that resistant pneumococci are also present but have been overlooked by Gram's stain.

OTHER *MORAXELLA* SPECIES

Other *Moraxella* species are occasional causes of a wide range of infections, including bronchitis, pneumonia, empyema, endocarditis, meningitis, conjunctivitis, endophthalmitis, urinary tract infection, septic arthritis, and wound infection. In a report on all *Moraxella* isolates submitted to the Centers for Disease Control and Prevention between 1953 and 1980, certain clinical associations were apparent (Table 138-2). *M. osloensis* and *M. nonliquefaciens*, the most commonly isolated species, were cultured from various normally sterile body sites, including blood, cerebrospinal fluid, and joints. *M. osloensis* was the *Moraxella* species most frequently isolated from blood; *M. nonliquefaciens* tended to be isolated from the ears, nose, or throat (47%) or the sputum (8%) and has since been implicated as a cause of conjunctivitis and keratitis. *M. urethralis* was isolated most often from urine and the genital tract and probably represents the *Moraxella* species implicated previously in urethritis. More than half of isolates of *M. phenylpyruvica* and *M. atlantae* were obtained from normally sterile sites. One study found *Moraxella* spp., including *M. catarrhalis*, in 35% of infected cat-bite wounds and in 10% of infected dog-bite wounds. The clinical features of infections due to *Moraxella* spp. other than *M. catarrhalis* and the nature of the hosts in which they occur have not been fully characterized.

TABLE 138-2 *MORAXELLA* SPECIES OTHER THAN *M. CATARRHALIS*

Moraxella Species	Number of Isolates	Common Sites/ Clinical Association	Number (Percent) for Each Site
M. osloensis[a]	199	Blood	44 (22)
		CSF	18 (9)
		Urine	17 (9)
		Respiratory tract	24 (12)
M. nonliquefaciens	356	Blood	27 (8)
		CSF	6 (2)
		Respiratory tract	196 (55)
M. canis	74	Dog-bite wound	53 (72)
M-6	47	Blood, bone	15 (32)
M. lacunata	33	Conjunctivitis, keratitis	23 (70)
M. urethralis	28	Urine	16 (57)
		Genital tract	3 (11)
M. phenylpyruvica	73	Blood	19 (26)
		CSF	8 (11)
		Urine	12 (16)
M. atlantae	44	Blood	20 (45)
		CSF	5 (11)

[a]Some of these isolates would now be distinguished as a new species, *Moraxella lincolnii*.
Note: CSF, cerebrospinal fluid.
Source: Adapted from a summary of CDC experience (Graham et al).

FURTHER READINGS

GRAHAM DR et al: Infections caused by *Moraxella*, *Moraxella urethralis*, *Moraxella*-like groups M-5 and M-6, and *Kingella kingae* in the United States, 1953–1980. Rev Infect Dis 12:423, 1990

IOANNIDIS JPA et al: Spectrum and significance of bacteremia due to *Moraxella catarrhalis*. Clin Infect Dis 21:390, 1995

MAAYAN H et al: Infective endocarditis due to *Moraxella lacunata*: Report of 4 patients and review of published cases of *Moraxella* endocarditis. Scand J Infect Dis 36:878, 2005

MURPHY TF et al: *Moraxella catarrhalis* in chronic obstructive pulmonary disease: Burden of disease and immune response. Am J Respir Crit Care Med 172:195, 2005

SETHI S et al: New strains of bacteria and exacerbations of chronic obstructive pulmonary disease. N Engl J Med 347:465, 2002

TALAN DA et al: Bacteriologic analysis of infected dog and cat bites. N Engl J Med 340:85, 1999

VERDUIN CM et al: *Moraxella catarrhalis*: From emerging to established pathogen. Clin Microbiol Rev 15:125, 2002

139 *Haemophilus* Infections

Timothy F. Murphy

HAEMOPHILUS INFLUENZAE

MICROBIOLOGY

Haemophilus influenzae was first recognized in 1892 by Pfeiffer, who erroneously concluded that the bacterium was the cause of influenza. The bacterium is a small (1- by 0.3-μm) gram-negative organism of variable shape; hence, it is often described as a pleomorphic coccobacillus. In clinical specimens such as cerebrospinal fluid (CSF) and sputum, it frequently stains only faintly with phenosafranin and therefore can easily be overlooked.

H. influenzae grows both aerobically and anaerobically. Its aerobic growth requires two factors: hemin (X factor) and nicotinamide adenine dinucleotide (V factor). These requirements are used in the clinical laboratory to identify the bacterium. Caution must be used to distinguish *H. influenzae* from *H. haemolyticus*, a respiratory tract commensal that has identical growth requirements. *H. haemolyticus* has classically been distinguished from *H. influenzae* by hemolysis on horse blood agar. However, a significant proportion of isolates of *H. haemolyticus* have recently been recognized as nonhemolytic. Analysis of 16S ribosomal sequences is one reliable method to distinguish these two species.

Six major serotypes of *H. influenzae* have been identified; designated *a* through *f*, they are based on antigenically distinct polysaccharide capsules. In addition, some strains lack a polysaccharide capsule and are referred to as *nontypable* strains. Type b and nontypable strains are the most relevant strains clinically (Table 139-1), although encapsulated strains other than type b can cause disease. *H. influenzae* was the first free-living organism to have its entire genome sequenced.

The antigenically distinct type b capsule is a linear polymer composed of ribosyl-ribitol phosphate. Strains of *H. influenzae* type b (Hib) cause disease primarily in infants and children <6 years of age. Nontypable strains are primarily mucosal pathogens but occasionally cause invasive disease.

EPIDEMIOLOGY AND TRANSMISSION

H. influenzae, an exclusively human pathogen, is spread by airborne droplets or by direct contact with secretions or fomites. Nontypable strains colonize the upper respiratory tract of up to three-fourths of healthy adults. Colonization with nontypable *H. influenzae* is a dynamic process; new strains are acquired and other strains are replaced periodically.

The widespread use of Hib conjugate vaccines in many industrialized countries has resulted in striking decreases in the rate of nasopharyngeal colonization by Hib and in the incidence of Hib infection (Fig. 139-1). However, the majority of the world's children remain unimmunized. Worldwide, invasive Hib disease occurs predominantly in unimmunized children and in those who have not completed the primary immunization series.

TABLE 139-1 CHARACTERISTICS OF TYPE b AND NONTYPABLE STRAINS OF *HAEMOPHILUS INFLUENZAE*

Feature	Type b Strains	Nontypable Strains
Capsule	Ribosyl-ribitol phosphate	Unencapsulated
Pathogenesis	Invasive infections due to hematogenous spread	Mucosal infections due to contiguous spread
Clinical manifestations	Meningitis and invasive infections in incompletely immunized infants and children	Otitis media in infants and children; lower respiratory tract infections in adults with chronic bronchitis
Evolutionary history	Basically clonal	Genetically diverse
Vaccine	Highly effective conjugate vaccines	None available; under development

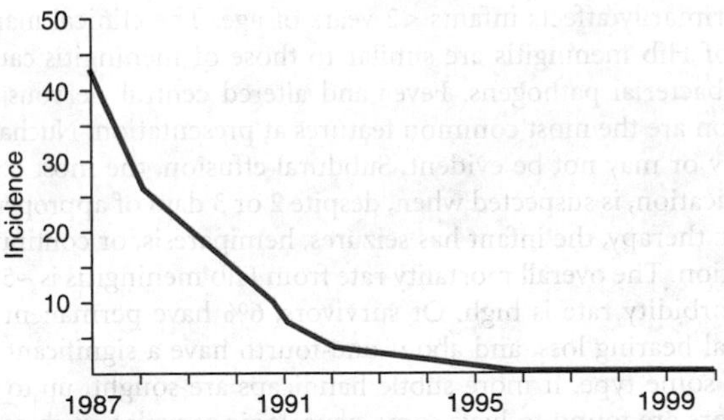

FIGURE 139-1 Estimated incidence (rate per 100,000) of invasive disease due to *Haemophilus influenzae* type b among children <5 years of age: 1987–2000. *(Data from the Centers for Disease Control and Prevention.)*

Certain groups have a higher incidence of invasive Hib disease than the general population. The incidence of meningitis due to Hib has been three to four times higher among black children than among white children in several studies. In some Native American groups, the incidence of invasive Hib disease is 10 times higher than that in the general population. Although this increased incidence has not yet been accounted for, several factors may be relevant, including age at exposure to the bacterium, socioeconomic conditions, and genetic differences in the ability to mount an immune response.

PATHOGENESIS

Hib strains cause systemic disease by invasion and hematogenous spread from the respiratory tract to distant sites such as the meninges, bones, and joints. The type b polysaccharide capsule is an important virulence factor affecting the bacterium's ability to avoid opsonization and cause systemic disease.

Nontypable strains cause disease by local invasion of mucosal surfaces. Otitis media results when bacteria reach the middle ear by way of the eustachian tube. Adults with chronic bronchitis experience recurrent lower respiratory tract infection due to nontypable strains. In addition, persistent nontypable *H. influenzae* colonization of the lower airways of adults with chronic obstructive pulmonary disease (COPD) contributes to the airway inflammation that is a hallmark of the disease. The incidence of invasive disease caused by nontypable strains is low.

IMMUNE RESPONSE

Antibody to the capsule is important in protection from infection by Hib strains. The level of (maternally acquired) serum antibody to the capsular polysaccharide, which is a polymer of polyribitol ribose phosphate (PRP), declines from birth to 6 months of age and, in the absence of vaccination, remains low until ~2 or 3 years of age. The age at the antibody nadir correlates with that of the peak incidence of type b disease. Antibody to PRP then appears partly as a result of exposure to Hib or cross-reacting antigens. Systemic Hib disease is unusual after the age of 6 years because of the presence of protective antibody. Vaccines in which PRP is conjugated to protein carrier molecules have been developed and are now used widely. These vaccines generate an antibody response to PRP in infants and effectively prevent invasive infections in infants and children.

Since nontypable strains lack a capsule, the immune response to infection is directed at noncapsular antigens. These antigens have generated considerable interest as immune targets and potential vaccine components. The human immune response to nontypable strains appears to be strain-specific, accounting in part for the propensity of these strains to cause recurrent otitis media and recurrent exacerbations of chronic bronchitis in immunocompetent hosts.

CLINICAL MANIFESTATIONS

Hib The most serious manifestation of infection with Hib is *meningitis* (Chap. 376). The age of peak incidence varies somewhat among populations, depending in part on the use of vaccine, but this infection primarily affects infants <2 years of age. The clinical manifestations of Hib meningitis are similar to those of meningitis caused by other bacterial pathogens. Fever and altered central nervous system function are the most common features at presentation. Nuchal rigidity may or may not be evident. Subdural effusion, the most common complication, is suspected when, despite 2 or 3 days of appropriate antibiotic therapy, the infant has seizures, hemiparesis, or continued obtundation. The overall mortality rate from Hib meningitis is ~5%, and the morbidity rate is high. Of survivors, 6% have permanent sensorineural hearing loss, and about one-fourth have a significant handicap of some type. If more subtle handicaps are sought, up to half of survivors are found to have some neurologic sequelae, such as partial hearing loss and delayed language development.

Epiglottitis (Chap. 31) is a life-threatening Hib infection involving cellulitis of the epiglottis and supraglottic tissues. It can lead to acute upper airway obstruction. Its unique epidemiologic features are its occurrence in an older age group (2–7 years old) than other Hib infections and its absence among Navajo Indians and Alaskan Eskimos. Sore throat and fever rapidly progress to dysphagia, drooling, and airway obstruction. Epiglottitis also occurs in adults.

Cellulitis (Chap. 119) due to Hib occurs in young children. The most common location is on the head or neck, and the involved area sometimes takes on a characteristic bluish-red color. Most patients have bacteremia, and 10% have an additional focus of infection.

Hib causes *pneumonia* in infants. The infection is clinically indistinguishable from other types of bacterial pneumonia (e.g., pneumococcal pneumonia) except that Hib is more likely to involve the pleura.

Several less common invasive conditions can be important clinical manifestations of Hib infection in children. These include osteomyelitis, septic arthritis, pericarditis, orbital cellulitis, endophthalmitis, urinary tract infection, abscesses, and bacteremia without an identifiable focus. As has been mentioned, Hib infections are unusual among patients >6 years old.

Nontypable *H. influenzae* Nontypable *H. influenzae* is a common cause of community-acquired bacterial pneumonia in adults. Nontypable *H. influenzae* pneumonia is especially common among patients with COPD or AIDS. The clinical features of *H. influenzae* pneumonia are similar to those of other types of bacterial pneumonia (including pneumococcal pneumonia). Patients present with fever, cough, and purulent sputum, usually of several days' duration. Chest radiography reveals alveolar infiltrates in a patchy or lobar distribution. Gram-stained sputum contains a predominance of small, pleomorphic, coccobacillary gram-negative bacteria.

Exacerbations of COPD caused by nontypable *H. influenzae* are characterized by increased cough, sputum production, and shortness of breath. Fever is low-grade, and no infiltrates are evident on chest x-ray.

Nontypable *H. influenzae* is one of the three most common causes of childhood otitis media (the other two being *Streptococcus pneumoniae* and *Moraxella catarrhalis*) (Chap. 31). Infants are febrile and irritable, while older children report ear pain. Symptoms of viral upper respiratory infection often precede otitis media. The diagnosis is made by pneumatic otoscopy. An etiologic diagnosis, although not routinely sought, can be established by tympanocentesis and culture of middle-ear fluid. The increasing use of pneumococcal polysaccharide conjugate vaccines in infants is resulting in a relative increase in the proportion of otitis media cases that are caused by *H. influenzae*.

Nontypable *H. influenzae* also causes puerperal sepsis and is an important cause of neonatal bacteremia. These nontypable strains, which are closely related to *H. haemolyticus*, tend to be of biotype IV and cause invasive disease after colonizing the female genital tract.

Nontypable *H. influenzae* causes sinusitis (Chap. 31) in adults and children. In addition, the bacterium is a less common cause of various invasive infections that are reported primarily as small-series descriptions and case reports. These infections include empyema, adult epiglottitis, pericarditis, cellulitis, septic arthritis, osteomyelitis, endocarditis, cholecystitis, intraabdominal infections, urinary tract infections, mastoiditis, aortic graft infection, and bacteremia without a detectable focus.

DIAGNOSIS

The most reliable method for establishing a diagnosis of Hib infection is recovery of the organism in culture. The CSF of a patient in whom meningitis is suspected should be subjected to Gram's staining and culture. The presence of gram-negative coccobacilli in Gram-stained CSF is strong evidence for Hib meningitis. Recovery of the organism from CSF confirms the diagnosis. Cultures of other normally sterile body fluids, such as blood, joint fluid, pleural fluid, pericardial fluid, and subdural effusion, are confirmatory in other infections.

Detection of PRP is an important adjunct to culture in rapid diagnosis of Hib meningitis. Immunoelectrophoresis, latex agglutination, coagglutination, and enzyme-linked immunosorbent assay are effective in detecting PRP. These assays are particularly helpful when patients have received prior antimicrobial therapy and thus are especially likely to have negative cultures.

Before the early 1980s, nontypable strains of *H. influenzae* were frequently misidentified as Hib because of their autoagglutination when serotypes were determined in agglutination assays. Since nontypable *H. influenzae* is primarily a mucosal pathogen, it is a component of a mixed flora; this situation makes etiologic diagnosis challenging. Nontypable *H. influenzae* infection is strongly suggested by the predominance of gram-negative coccobacilli among abundant polymorphonuclear leukocytes in a Gram-stained sputum specimen from a patient in whom pneumonia or tracheobronchitis is suspected. A sputum culture is helpful when interpreted along with the results of Gram's staining. Although bacteremia is detectable in a small proportion of patients with pneumonia due to nontypable *H. influenzae*, most such patients have negative blood cultures.

A diagnosis of otitis media is based on the detection by pneumatic otoscopy of fluid in the middle ear. An etiologic diagnosis requires tympanocentesis but is not routinely sought. An invasive procedure is also required to determine the etiology of sinusitis; thus, treatment is often empirical once the diagnosis is suspected in light of clinical symptoms and sinus radiographs.

Rx *HAEMOPHILUS INFLUENZAE*

Initial therapy for meningitis due to Hib should consist of a cephalosporin such as ceftriaxone or cefotaxime. For children, the dosage of ceftriaxone is 75–100 mg/kg daily given in two doses 12 h apart. The pediatric dosage of cefotaxime is 200 mg/kg daily given in four doses 6 h apart. Adult dosages are 2 g every 12 h for ceftriaxone and 2 g every 4–6 h for cefotaxime. An alternative regimen for initial therapy is ampicillin (200–300 mg/kg daily in four divided doses) plus chloramphenicol (75–100 mg/kg daily in four divided doses). Therapy should continue for a total of 1–2 weeks.

Administration of glucocorticoids to patients with Hib meningitis reduces the incidence of neurologic sequelae. The presumed mechanism is reduction of the inflammation induced by bacterial cell-wall mediators of inflammation when cells are killed by antimicrobial agents. Dexamethasone (0.6 mg/kg per day intravenously in four divided doses for 2 days) is recommended for the treatment of Hib meningitis in children >2 months of age.

Invasive infections other than meningitis are treated with the same antimicrobial agents. For epiglottitis, the dosage of ceftriaxone is 50 mg/kg daily, and the dosage of cefotaxime is 150 mg/kg daily, given in three divided doses 8 h apart. Epiglottitis constitutes a medical emergency, and maintenance of an airway is critical. The duration of therapy is determined by the clinical response. A course of 1–2 weeks is usually appropriate.

Many infections caused by nontypable strains of *H. influenzae*, such as otitis media, sinusitis, and exacerbations of COPD, can be treated with oral antimicrobial agents. Approximately 20–35% of nontypable strains produce β-lactamase (with the exact proportion depending on geographic location), and these strains are resistant to ampicillin. Several agents have excellent activity against nontypable *H. influenzae*, including amoxicillin/clavulanic acid, various extended-spectrum cephalosporins, the macrolides azithromycin and clarithromycin, and the new ketolide telithromycin. Fluoroquinolones are highly active against *H. influenzae* and are useful in adults with exacerbations of COPD. However, fluoroquinolones are not currently recommended for the treatment of children or pregnant women because of possible effects on articular cartilage.

In addition to β-lactamase production, alteration of penicillin-binding proteins—a second mechanism of ampicillin resistance—has been detected in isolates of *H. influenzae*. Although rare in the United States, these β-lactamase-negative ampicillin-resistant strains are increasing in prevalence in Europe and Japan. Continued monitoring of the evolving antimicrobial susceptibility patterns of *H. influenzae* will be important.

PREVENTION

Vaccination (See also Chap. 116) The development of conjugate vaccines that prevent invasive infections with Hib in infants and children has been a dramatic success. Three such vaccines are licensed in the United States. In addition to eliciting protective antibody, these vaccines prevent disease by reducing rates of pharyngeal colonization with Hib.

The widespread use of conjugate vaccines has dramatically reduced the incidence of Hib disease in developed countries. Even though the manufacture of Hib vaccines is costly, vaccination is cost-effective. The Global Alliance for Vaccines and Immunizations has recognized the underuse of Hib conjugate vaccines. The disease burden has been reduced in developing countries that have implemented routine vaccination (e.g., The Gambia, Chile). An important obstacle to more widespread vaccination is the lack of data on the epidemiology and burden of Hib disease in many developing countries.

All children should be immunized with an Hib conjugate vaccine, receiving the first dose at $\sim$2 months of age, the rest of the primary series at 2–6 months of age, and a booster dose at 12–15 months of age. Specific recommendations vary for the different conjugate vaccines. The reader is referred to the recommendations of the American Academy of Pediatrics (Chap. 116 and *www.cispimmunize.org*). Currently, no vaccines are available for the prevention of disease caused by nontypable *H. influenzae*.

Chemoprophylaxis The risk of secondary disease is greater than normal among household contacts of patients with Hib disease. Therefore, all children and adults (except pregnant women) in households with at least one incompletely immunized contact <4 years of age should receive prophylaxis with oral rifampin. When two or more cases of invasive Hib disease have occurred within 60 days at a child-care facility attended by incompletely vaccinated children, administration of rifampin to all attendees and personnel is indicated, as is recommended for household contacts. Chemoprophylaxis is not indicated in nursery and child-care contacts of a single index case. The reader is referred to the recommendations of the American Academy of Pediatrics.

HAEMOPHILUS INFLUENZAE BIOGROUP AEGYPTIUS

H. influenzae biogroup aegyptius was formerly called *Haemophilus aegyptius* because of phenotypic characteristics distinct from those of *H. influenzae*. However, later studies involving DNA hybridization and DNA transformation demonstrated that *H. aegyptius* and *H. influenzae* are members of the same species.

H. influenzae biogroup aegyptius has long been associated with conjunctivitis. Moreover, this strain is now known to be the cause of Brazilian purpuric fever (BPF), which was first recognized in 1984 in the rural Brazilian town of Promissão. The sharing of many phenotypic and genotypic characteristics by the various strains of *H. influenzae* biogroup aegyptius that cause BPF indicates that these strains represent a clone of *H. influenzae* that has acquired specific virulence factors, several of which are associated with a pathogenicity island. The age of peak incidence of BPF is 1–4 years, with a range of 3 months to 8 years. The illness can occur sporadically or in outbreaks. Typically, after an episode of purulent conjunctivitis, high fever occurs in association with vomiting and abdominal pain. Within 12–48 h after onset, the patient develops petechiae, purpura, and peripheral necrosis and experiences vascular collapse. The characteristic laboratory features are thrombocytopenia, prolonged prothrombin time, uniformly unrevealing CSF findings, and blood cultures positive for *H. influenzae* biogroup aegyptius. Initial reports cited high mortality (70%), but subsequent studies have indicated that milder forms of the illness exist. Most patients have resolved or resolving purulent conjunctivitis, and culture of the conjunctiva is positive in approximately one-third of cases. BPF has been seen in several towns in Brazil and on two occasions in Australia.

HAEMOPHILUS DUCREYI

Haemophilus ducreyi is the etiologic agent of chancroid (Chap. 124), a sexually transmitted disease characterized by genital ulceration and inguinal adenitis. *H. ducreyi* poses a significant health problem in developing countries. Although this infection is less common in the United States, its incidence has increased dramatically in the past several years. In addition to being a cause of morbidity in itself, chancroid is associated with HIV infection because of the role played by genital ulceration in HIV transmission.

MICROBIOLOGY

H. ducreyi is a highly fastidious coccobacillary gram-negative bacterium whose growth requires X factor (hemin). Although, in light of this requirement, the bacterium has been classified in the genus *Haemophilus*, DNA homology and chemotaxonomic studies have established substantial differences between *H. ducreyi* and other *Haemophilus* species. Taxonomic reclassification of the organism is likely in the future but awaits further study.

The histology of the genital ulcer of chancroid is characterized by perivascular and interstitial infiltrates of macrophages and of CD4+ and CD8+ T lymphocytes. The appearance is consistent with a delayed-type hypersensitivity, cell-mediated immune response. The presence of CD4+ T cells and macrophages in the ulcer may explain, in part, the facilitation of HIV transmission in patients with chancroid.

EPIDEMIOLOGY AND PREVALENCE

Chancroid is a common cause of genital ulcers in developing countries. In the United States, chancroid is now endemic in some regions, and several large outbreaks have occurred since 1981. Recurring epidemiologic themes have been apparent in these outbreaks: (1) transmission has been predominantly heterosexual; (2) males have outnumbered females by ratios of 3:1 to 25:1; (3) prostitutes have been important in transmission of the infection; and (4) chancroid has been strongly associated with illicit drug use.

CLINICAL MANIFESTATIONS

Infection is acquired as the result of a break in the epithelium during sexual contact with an infected individual. After an incubation period of 4–7 days, the initial lesion—a papule with surrounding erythema—appears. In 2 or 3 days, the papule evolves into a pustule, which spontaneously ruptures and forms a sharply circumscribed ulcer that is generally not indurated (Fig. 139-2). The ulcers are painful and bleed easily; little or no inflammation of the surrounding skin is evident. Approximately half of patients develop enlarged, tender inguinal lymph nodes, which frequently become fluctuant and spontaneously rupture. Patients usually seek medical care after 1–3 weeks of painful symptoms.

The presentation of chancroid does not usually include all of the typical clinical features and is sometimes atypical. Multiple ulcers can coalesce to form giant ulcers. Ulcers can appear and then resolve, with inguinal adenitis (Fig. 139-2) and suppuration following 1–3 weeks later; this clinical picture can be confused with that of lymphogranuloma venereum (Chap. 169). Multiple small ulcers can resemble folliculitis. Other differential diagnostic considerations include the various infections causing genital ulceration, such as primary syphilis, condyloma latum of secondary syphilis, genital herpes, and donovanosis. In rare cases chancroid lesions become secondarily infected with bacteria; the result is extensive inflammation.

DIAGNOSIS

Clinical diagnosis of chancroid is often inaccurate, and laboratory confirmation should be attempted in suspected cases. Gram's staining

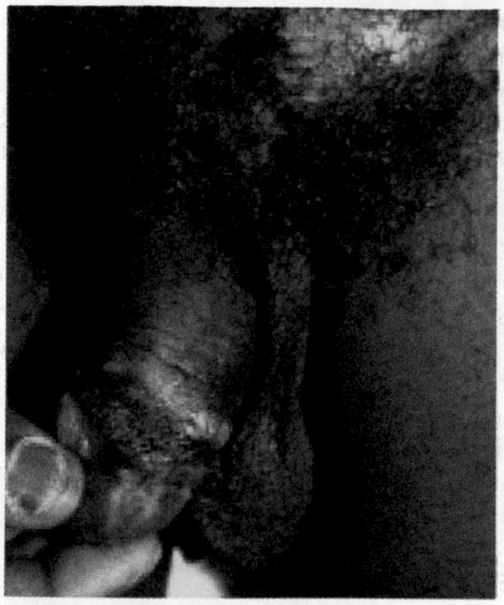

FIGURE 139-2 Chancroid with characteristic penile ulcers and associated left inguinal adenitis (bubo).

of a swab of the lesion may reveal a predominance of characteristic gram-negative coccobacilli, but the presence of other bacteria often makes it difficult to interpret this result. An accurate diagnosis of chancroid relies on culture of *H. ducreyi* from the lesion. In addition, aspiration and culture of suppurative lymph nodes should be considered. Since the organism can be difficult to grow, the use of selective and supplemented media is necessary. A multiplex polymerase chain reaction assay has been developed for simultaneous amplification of DNA targets from *H. ducreyi*, *Treponema pallidum*, and herpes simplex virus types 1 and 2. When this assay becomes commercially available, it will be a useful diagnostic tool with which to identify the etiology of genital ulcers.

Rx HAEMOPHILUS DUCREYI

The treatment regimen recommended by the Centers for Disease Control and Prevention is a single 1-g oral dose of azithromycin. Alternative regimens include ceftriaxone (250 mg intramuscularly in a single dose), ciprofloxacin (500 mg orally bid for 3 days), or erythromycin base (500 mg orally tid for 7 days). Isolates from patients who do not respond promptly to treatment should be tested for antimicrobial susceptibility. In patients with HIV infection, healing may be slow and longer courses of treatment may be necessary. Clinical treatment failure in HIV-seropositive patients may reflect co-infection, especially with herpes simplex virus. Contacts of patients with chancroid should be identified and treated, whether or not symptoms are present, if they had sexual contact with the patient during the 10 days preceding the patient's onset of symptoms.

FURTHER READINGS

Bong CT et al: *Haemophilus ducreyi*: Clinical features, epidemiology, and prospects for disease control. Microbes Infect 4:1141, 2002

Casey JR, Pichichero ME: Changes in frequency and pathogens causing acute otitis media in 1995–2003. Pediatr Infect Dis J 23:824, 2004

Committee on Infectious Diseases: *Haemophilus influenzae* infections, in *2003 Red Book, Report of the Committee on Infectious Diseases*, 26th ed, LK Pickering et al (eds). Elk Grove Village, IL, American Academy of Pediatrics, 2003

Dominguez SR, Daum RS: Toward global *Haemophilus influenzae* type b immunization. Clin Infect Dis 37:1600, 2003

Heilmann KP et al: Decreasing prevalence of beta-lactamase production among respiratory tract isolates of *Haemophilus influenzae* in the United States. Antimicrob Agents Chemother 49:2561, 2005

Kelly DF et al: *Haemophilus influenzae* type b conjugate vaccines. Immunology 113:163, 2004

Liebowitz E et al: *Haemophilus influenzae*: A significant pathogen in acute otitis media. Pediatr Infect Dis J 23:1142, 2004

McGillivary G et al: Cloning and sequencing of a genomic island found in the Brazilian purpuric fever clone of *Haemophilus influenzae* biogroup aegyptius. Infect Immun 73:1927, 2005

Murphy TF: Respiratory infections caused by non-typeable *Haemophilus influenzae.* Curr Opin Infect Dis 16:129, 2003

——— et al: Persistent colonization by *Haemophilus influenzae* in chronic obstructive pulmonary disease. Am J Respir Crit Care Med 170:266, 2004

Sethi S et al: Strain-specific immune response to *Haemophilus influenzae* in chronic obstructive pulmonary disease. Am J Respir Crit Care Med 169:448, 2004

140 Infections Due to the HACEK Group and Miscellaneous Gram-Negative Bacteria

Tamar F. Barlam, Dennis L. Kasper

THE HACEK GROUP

HACEK organisms are a group of fastidious, slow-growing, gram-negative bacteria whose growth requires an atmosphere of carbon dioxide. Species belonging to this group include several *Haemophilus* species, *Actinobacillus actinomycetemcomitans*, *Cardiobacterium hominis*, *Eikenella corrodens*, and *Kingella kingae*. HACEK bacteria normally reside in the oral cavity and have been associated with local infections in the mouth. They are also known to cause severe systemic infections—most often bacterial endocarditis, which can develop on either native or prosthetic valves (Chap. 118).

HACEK ENDOCARDITIS

In large series, up to 3% of cases of infective endocarditis are attributable to HACEK organisms, most often *A. actinomycetemcomitans*, *Haemophilus* species, and *C. hominis*. The clinical course of HACEK endocarditis tends to be subacute; however, embolization is common. The overall prevalence of major emboli associated with HACEK endocarditis ranges from 28 to 71% in different series. On echocardiography, valvular vegetations are seen in up to 85% of patients. The vegetations are frequently large, although vegetation size has not been directly correlated with the risk of embolization. Cultures of blood from patients with suspected HACEK endocarditis may require up to 30 days to become positive, and the microbiology laboratory should be alerted when a HACEK organism is being considered. However, most cultures that ultimately yield a HACEK organism become positive within the first week, especially with improved culture systems such as BACTEC. In addition, polymerase chain reaction techniques are facilitating the diagnosis of HACEK infections. Because of the organisms' slow growth, antimicrobial testing may be difficult, and β-lactamase production may not be detected. E-test methodology may increase the accuracy of susceptibility testing.

***Haemophilus* Species** *Haemophilus* species are differentiated by their in vitro growth requirements for X factor (hemin) and V factor (nicotinamide adenine dinucleotide). *H. aphrophilus* requires only X factor for growth, while species designated *para-* require only V factor. *H. aphrophilus* and *H. parainfluenzae* are the most common *Haemophilus* species isolated from cases of HACEK endocarditis; *H. paraphrophilus* is less common. Invasive infection typically occurs in patients with a history of cardiac valvular disease, often in the setting of a recent dental procedure. Sixty percent of these patients have been ill for <2 months before presentation, and 19–50% develop congestive heart failure. Mortality rates as high as 30–50% have been reported in older series; however, more recent studies have documented mortality rates of <5%. *H. aphrophilus* also causes invasive bone and joint infections, and *H. parainfluenzae* has been isolated from other infections such as meningitis; brain, dental, and liver abscess; pneumonia; and septicemia.

Actinobacillus actinomycetemcomitans *A. actinomycetemcomitans* can be isolated from soft tissue infections and abscesses in association with *Actinomyces israelii*. Typically, patients who develop endocarditis with *A. actinomycetemcomitans* have severe periodontal disease or have recently undergone dental procedures in the setting of underlying cardiac valvular damage. The disease is insidious; patients may be sick for several months before diagnosis. Frequent complications include embolic phenomena, congestive heart failure, and renal failure. *A. actinomycetemcomitans* has been isolated from patients with brain abscess, meningitis, endophthalmitis, parotitis, osteomyelitis, urinary tract infection, pneumonia, and empyema, among other infections.

Cardiobacterium hominis *C. hominis* primarily causes endocarditis in patients with underlying valvular heart disease or with prosthetic valves. This organism most frequently affects the aortic valve. Many patients have signs and symptoms of long-standing infection before diagnosis, with evidence of arterial embolization, vasculitis, cerebrovascular accidents, immune complex glomerulonephritis, or arthritis at presentation. Embolization, mycotic aneurysms, and congestive heart failure are common complications.

Eikenella corrodens *E. corrodens* is most frequently recovered from sites of infection in conjunction with other bacterial species. Clinical sources of *E. corrodens* include sites of human bite wounds (clenched-fist injuries), endocarditis, soft tissue infections, osteomyelitis, respiratory infections, chorioamnionitis, gynecologic infections associated with intrauterine devices, meningitis and brain abscesses, and visceral abscesses.

Kingella kingae Because of improved microbiologic methodology, isolation of *K. kingae* is increasingly common. Inoculation of clinical specimens (e.g., synovial fluid) into aerobic blood culture bottles enhances recovery of this organism. In recent series, *K. kingae* has been the third most common cause of septic arthritis in children <24 months of age; staphylococcal and streptococcal species remain most prevalent. Invasive *K. kingae* infections with bacteremia are associated with upper respiratory tract infections and stomatitis. Both *K. kingae* colonization and primary herpes—a major cause of stomatitis—peak in children 6–48 months of age. *K. kingae* bacteremia can present with a petechial rash similar to that seen in *Neisseria meningitidis* sepsis.

Infective endocarditis, unlike other infections with *K. kingae*, occurs in older children and adults. The majority of patients have preexisting valvular disease. There is a high incidence of complications, including arterial emboli, cerebrovascular accidents, tricuspid insufficiency, and congestive heart failure with cardiovascular collapse.

Rx ENDOCARDITIS CAUSED BY HACEK ORGANISMS

See **Table 140-1**. Native-valve endocarditis should be treated for 4 weeks with antibiotics, whereas prosthetic-valve endocarditis requires 6 weeks of therapy. The cure rates for HACEK prosthetic-valve endocarditis appear to be high. Unlike prosthetic-valve endocarditis caused by other gram-negative organisms, HACEK endocarditis is often cured with antibiotic treatment alone—i.e., without surgical intervention.

OTHER GRAM-NEGATIVE BACTERIA

Achromobacter xylosoxidans *A. xylosoxidans* (previously *Alcaligenes xylosoxidans*) is probably part of the endogenous intestinal flora and has been isolated from water sources. Immunocompromised hosts, including patients with cancer and post-chemotherapy neutropenia, cirrhosis, and chronic renal failure, are at increased risk. Nosocomial outbreaks of *A. xylosoxidans* infection have been attributed to contaminated fluids, and clinical illness has been associated with isolates from many sites, including blood (often in the setting of intravascular devices). Community-acquired bacteremia with *A. xylosoxidans* usually occurs in the setting of pneumonia. Metastatic skin lesions are present in one-fifth of cases. The reported mortality rate is 67%—a figure similar to rates for other bacteremic gram-negative pneumonias.

Rx *ACHROMOBACTER XYLOSOXIDANS* INFECTIONS

Treatment is based on in vitro susceptibility testing of all clinically relevant isolates.

***Aeromonas* Species** More than 85% of *Aeromonas* infections are caused by *A. hydrophila*, *A. caviae*, and *A. veronii* biovar *sobria*. *Aeromonas* proliferates in potable and fresh water and in soil. It remains controversial whether *Aeromonas* is a cause of bacterial gastroenteritis; asymptomatic colonization of the intestinal tract with *Aeromonas* occurs frequently. However, rare cases of hemolytic-uremic syndrome following bloody diarrhea have been shown to be secondary to the presence of *Aeromonas*.

Aeromonas causes sepsis and bacteremia in infants with multiple medical problems and in immunocompromised hosts, particularly those with cancer or hepatobiliary disease. *Aeromonas* infection and sepsis can occur in patients with trauma (including severe trauma with myonecrosis) and in burn patients exposed to *Aeromonas* by environmental (freshwater or soil) contamination of their wounds. Reported mortality rates range from 25% among immunocompromised adults with sepsis to >90% among patients with myonecrosis. *Aeromonas* can produce ecthyma gangrenosum (hemorrhagic vesicles sur-

TABLE 140-1 TREATMENT OF ENDOCARDITIS CAUSED BY HACEK GROUP ORGANISMS[a]

Organism	Initial Therapy	Alternative Agents	Comments
Haemophilus species, *Actinobacillus actinomycetemcomitans*	Ceftriaxone (2 g/d)	Ampicillin/sulbactam (3 g of ampicillin q6h) **or** fluoroquinolones[b]	Ampicillin ± an aminoglycoside can be used if the organism does not produce β-lactamase.[c]
Cardiobacterium hominis	Penicillin (16–18 mU/d in 6 divided doses) or ampicillin (2 g q4h)	Ceftriaxone (2 g/d) **or** ampicillin/sulbactam (3 g of ampicillin q6h)	An aminoglycoside (gentamicin, 3 mg/kg per day in 3 divided doses) may be added, but its value has not been proven. The organism is usually pansensitive, but high-level penicillin resistance has been reported.
Eikenella corrodens	Ampicillin (2 g q4h)	Ceftriaxone (2 g/d) **or** fluoroquinolones[b]	The organism is typically resistant to clindamycin, metronidazole, and aminoglycosides.
Kingella kingae	Ceftriaxone (2 g/d) or ampicillin/sulbactam (3 g of ampicillin q6h)	Fluoroquinolones[b]	The prevalence of β-lactamase-producing strains is increasing. Efficacy for invasive infections is best demonstrated for first-line treatments.

[a]Susceptibility testing should be performed in all cases to guide therapy.
[b]Fluoroquinolones are not recommended for treatment of children <17 years of age.
[c]European guidelines for endocarditis recommend the addition of gentamicin (3 mg/kg per day in 3 divided doses for 2–4 weeks).

rounded by a rim of erythema with central necrosis and ulceration) resembling the lesions seen in *Pseudomonas aeruginosa* infection. *Aeromonas* causes nosocomial infections related to catheters, surgical incisions, or use of leeches. Other manifestations include meningitis, peritonitis, pneumonia, and ocular infections.

Rx *AEROMONAS* INFECTIONS

Aeromonas species are generally susceptible to fluoroquinolones (e.g., ciprofloxacin at a dosage of 500 mg every 12 h PO or 400 mg every 12 h IV), trimethoprim-sulfamethoxazole (TMP-SMX; trimethoprim dosage, 10 mg/kg per day in 3 or 4 divided doses), third-generation cephalosporins, and aminoglycosides. Because *Aeromonas* can produce various β-lactamases, including carbapenemases, susceptibility testing must be used to guide therapy.

***Capnocytophaga* Species** This genus of fastidious, fusiform, gram-negative coccobacilli is facultatively anaerobic and requires an atmosphere enriched in carbon dioxide for optimal growth. *C. ochracea*, *C. gingivalis*, and *C. sputigena* have been associated with sepsis in immunocompromised hosts, particularly neutropenic patients with hematologic malignancy, and probably play a role in localized juvenile periodontitis in the immunocompetent host. These species have been isolated from many other sites as well, usually as part of a polymicrobial infection.

C. canimorsus and *C. cynodegmi* are endogenous to the canine mouth (**Chap. e14**). Patients infected with these species frequently have a history of dog bites or of exposure to dogs without scratches or bites. Asplenia, glucocorticoid therapy, and alcohol abuse are predisposing conditions that can be associated with fulminant infections. *C. canimorsus* causes a wide range of infections, including severe sepsis with shock and disseminated intravascular coagulation, meningitis, endocarditis, cellulitis, and septic arthritis.

Rx *CAPNOCYTOPHAGA* INFECTIONS

Because of increasing β-lactamase production, clindamycin (600–900 mg every 6–8 h) or drug combinations including a penicillin derivative plus a β-lactamase inhibitor—such as ampicillin/sulbactam (1.5–3.0 g of ampicillin every 6 h)—are currently recommended for empirical treatment of infections caused by *C. ochracea*, *C. gingivalis*, and *C. sputigena*. Infections with *C. canimorsus* should be treated with penicillin (12–18 million units every 4 h). This regimen or ampicillin/sulbactam should be given prophylactically to asplenic patients sustaining dog-bite injuries. *C. canimorsus* is also susceptible to clindamycin, imipenem, fluoroquinolones, and third-generation cephalosporins.

***Chryseobacterium* Species (Formerly *Flavobacterium*)** *C. meningosepticum* is an important cause of nosocomial infections, including outbreaks due to contaminated fluids (e.g., disinfectants and aerosolized antibiotics) and sporadic infections due to indwelling devices, feeding tubes, and other fluid-associated apparatuses. Patients with nosocomial *C. meningosepticum* infection usually have underlying immunosuppression (e.g., related to malignancy). *C. meningosepticum* has been reported to cause meningitis (primarily in neonates), sepsis, endocarditis, bacteremia, soft tissue infections, and pneumonia. *C. indologenes* has caused bacteremia, sepsis, and pneumonia, typically in immunocompromised patients with indwelling devices.

Rx *CHRYSEOBACTERIUM* INFECTIONS

Chryseobacteria are often susceptible to fluoroquinolones, TMP-SMX, imipenem, and third- or fourth-generation cephalosporins, but susceptibility testing should be performed.

Pasteurella multocida *P. multocida* is a bipolar-staining, gram-negative coccobacillus that colonizes the respiratory and gastrointestinal tracts of domestic animals; oropharyngeal colonization rates are 70–90% in cats and 50–65% in dogs. *P. multocida* can be transmitted to humans through bites or scratches, via the respiratory tract from contact with contaminated dust or infectious droplets, or via deposition of the organism on injured skin or mucosal surfaces during licking. Most human infections affect skin and soft tissue; almost two-thirds of these infections are caused by cats. Patients at the extremes of age or with serious underlying disorders (e.g., cirrhosis) are at increased risk for systemic manifestations, including meningitis, peritonitis, osteomyelitis, endocarditis, and septic shock, but cases have also occurred in healthy individuals. If inhaled, *P. multocida* can cause acute respiratory tract infection, particularly in patients with underlying sinus and pulmonary disease.

Rx *PASTEURELLA MULTOCIDA* INFECTIONS

P. multocida is susceptible to penicillin, ampicillin, ampicillin/sulbactam, second- and third-generation cephalosporins, tetracyclines, and fluoroquinolones. β-lactamase-producing strains have been reported.

MISCELLANEOUS ORGANISMS

Agrobacterium radiobacter (tumefaciens) has usually been associated with infection in the presence of medical devices, including intravascular catheter–related infections, prosthetic-joint and prosthetic-valve infections, and peritonitis caused by dialysis catheters. Most cases occur in immunocompromised hosts, especially individuals with malignancy or HIV infection. Strains are usually susceptible to fluoroquinolones, third-generation cephalosporins, imipenem, TMP-SMX, and aminoglycosides.

Chromobacterium violaceum, although rarely a human pathogen, reportedly has been responsible for life-threatening infections with severe sepsis and metastatic abscesses, particularly in children with defective neutrophil function (e.g., those with chronic granulomatous disease). *C. violaceum* is generally susceptible to ciprofloxacin (500 mg every 12 h PO or 400 mg every 12 h IV), TMP-SMX, and gentamicin.

Plesiomonas shigelloides is a freshwater organism that causes acute diarrhea (Chap. 122) and occasionally serious extraintestinal disease, most commonly in immunocompromised hosts. *Ochrobactrum anthropi* causes infections related to central venous catheters in compromised hosts; other invasive infections have been described. Other organisms include *Weeksella* species; various CDC groups, such as EF4 and Ve-2; *Flavimonas* species; *Sphingobacterium* species; *Protomonas* species; *Oligella urethralis*; and *Shewanella putrefaciens*. The reader is advised to consult subspecialty texts and references for further guidance on these organisms.

FURTHER READINGS

Brouqui P, Raoult D: Endocarditis due to rare and fastidious bacteria. Clin Microbiol Rev 14:177, 2001

Chometon S et al: Specific real-time polymerase chain reaction places *Kingella kingae* as the most common cause of osteoarticular infections in young children. Pediatr Infect Dis J 26:377, 2007

Elliott TSJ et al: Guidelines for the antibiotic treatment of endocarditis in adults: Report of the Working Party of the British Society for Antimicrobial Chemotherapy. J Antimicrob Chemother 54:971, 2004

Goldberg MH, Katz J: Infective endocarditis caused by fastidious oro-pharyngeal HACEK micro-organisms. J Oral Maxillofac Surg 64:969, 2006

Jolivet-Gougeon A et al: Antimicrobial treatment of *Capnocytophaga* infections. Int J Antimicrob Agents 29:367, 2007

Huang ST et al: Clinical characteristics of invasive *Haemophilus aphrophilus* infections. J Microbiol Immunol Infect 38:271, 2005

Martino R et al: Bacteremia caused by *Capnocytophaga* species in patients with neutropenia and cancer: Results of a multicenter study. Clin Infect Dis 33:E20, 2001

Paturel L et al: *Actinobacillus actinomycetemcomitans* endocarditis. Clin Microbiol Infect 10:98, 2004

Shie SS et al: Characteristics of *Achromobacter xylosoxidans* bacteremia in northern Taiwan. J Microbiol Immunol Infect 38:277, 2005

Udaka T et al: *Eikenella corrodens* in head and neck infections. J Infect 54:343, 2007

141 *Legionella* Infection

Miguel Sabria, Victor L. Yu

Legionellosis refers to the two clinical syndromes caused by bacteria of the genus *Legionella. Pontiac fever* is an acute, febrile, self-limited illness that has been serologically linked to *Legionella* species, whereas *Legionnaires' disease* is the designation for pneumonia caused by these species. Legionnaires' disease was first recognized in 1976, when an outbreak of pneumonia took place at a hotel in Philadelphia during the American Legion Convention. The causative agent proved to be a newly discovered bacterium, *Legionella pneumophila*, that was isolated from lung specimens obtained from the victims at autopsy.

MICROBIOLOGY

The family Legionellaceae comprises more than 49 species with more than 64 serogroups. The species *L. pneumophila* causes 80–90% of human infections and includes at least 16 serogroups; serogroups 1, 4, and 6 are most commonly implicated in human infections. To date, 18 species other than *L. pneumophila* have been associated with human infections, among which *L. micdadei* (Pittsburgh pneumonia agent), *L. bozemanii, L. dumoffii*, and *L. longbeachae* are the most common.

Members of the Legionellaceae are aerobic gram-negative bacilli that do not grow on routine microbiologic media. Buffered charcoal yeast extract (BCYE) agar is the medium used to grow *Legionella*. Antibiotics added to the medium suppress the growth of competing flora from nonsterile sites, and dyes color the colonies and assist in identification.

The direct fluorescent antibody (DFA) test can definitively identify a number of individual species. In the case of *L. pneumophila*, the serogroup-specific antigen and antibodies detected by immunofluorescence are directed primarily at the lipopolysaccharide, a prominent outer-membrane component. Both polyclonal and monoclonal DFA reagents are commercially available. The monoclonal reagent is less cross-reactive but is specific for *L. pneumophila*.

ECOLOGY AND TRANSMISSION

The natural habitats for *L. pneumophila* are aquatic bodies, including lakes and streams. *L. longbeachae* has been isolated from soil. Legionellae can survive under a wide range of environmental conditions; for example, the organisms can live for years in refrigerated water samples. Natural bodies of water contain only small numbers of legionellae. However, once the organisms enter human-constructed aquatic reservoirs (such as water-distribution systems), they can grow and proliferate. Factors known to enhance colonization by and amplification of legionellae include warm temperatures (25°–42°C), stagnation, and scale and sediment. *L. pneumophila* can form microcolonies within biofilms; its eradication from water-distribution systems requires disinfectants that can penetrate the biofilm. The presence of symbiotic microorganisms, including algae, amebas, ciliated protozoa, and other water-dwelling bacteria, promotes the growth of *L. pneumophila*. Legionellae can invade and multiply within free-living protozoa.

The source of *Legionella* is water. Community-acquired Legionnaires' disease has been linked to colonization of residential and industrial water supplies. Potable-water distribution systems in hospitals, long-term-care facilities, hotels, and large buildings have been implicated. Sporadic community-acquired cases have been linked to residential water systems.

Cooling towers and evaporative condensers have been overestimated as sources of *Legionella*. Early investigations that implicated cooling towers antedated the discovery that the organism could also exist in potable-water distribution systems. It is now known that, in many outbreaks attributed to cooling towers, cases of Legionnaires' disease continued to occur despite disinfection of the cooling towers; the potable water supply was the actual source. Koch's postulates have never been fulfilled for cooling tower–associated outbreaks as they have been for hospital-acquired Legionnaires' disease. Nevertheless, cooling towers are occasionally identified in community-acquired outbreaks.

L. longbeachae infections have been linked to potting soil.

Multiple modes of transmission of *Legionella* to humans exist, including aerosolization, aspiration, and direct instillation into the lungs during respiratory tract manipulations. Aspiration is now known to be the predominant mode of transmission, but it is unclear whether *Legionella* enters the lungs via oropharyngeal colonization or directly via the drinking of contaminated water. Oropharyngeal colonization has been demonstrated in patients undergoing transplantation. Nasogastric tubes have been linked to hospital-acquired Legionnaires' disease; microaspiration of contaminated water was the hypothesized mode of transmission. Surgery with general anesthesia is a known risk factor that is consistent with aspiration. Especially compelling is the reported 30% incidence of postoperative *Legionella* pneumonia among patients undergoing head and neck surgery at a hospital with a contaminated water supply; aspiration is a recognized sequela in such cases. Studies of patients with hospital-acquired Legionnaires' disease have shown that these individuals underwent endotracheal intubation significantly more often and for a significantly longer duration than patients with hospital-acquired pneumonia of other etiologies.

Aerosolization of *Legionella* by devices filled with tap water, including whirlpools, nebulizers, and humidifiers, has been implicated. An ultrasonic mist machine in the produce section of a grocery store was the source in a community outbreak. Pontiac fever has been linked to *Legionella*-containing aerosols from water-using machinery, a cooling tower, air-conditioners, and whirlpools.

EPIDEMIOLOGY

The incidence of Legionnaires' disease depends on the degree of contamination of the aquatic reservoir, the immune status of the persons exposed to water from that reservoir, the intensity of exposure, and the availability of specialized laboratory tests on which the correct diagnosis can be based.

Numerous prospective studies have ranked *Legionella* among the top four microbial causes of community-acquired pneumonia (with *Streptococcus pneumoniae, Haemophilus influenzae*, and *Chlamydophila pneumoniae* usually ranked first, second, and third, respectively), accounting for 2–9% of cases. On the basis of a multihospital study of community-acquired pneumonia in Ohio, the Centers for Disease Control and Prevention (CDC) estimated that as many as 18,000 cases of sporadic community-acquired Legionnaires' disease occur annually in the United States and that only 3% of these cases are correctly diagnosed. *Legionella* is responsible for 10–50% of cases of nosocomial pneumonia when a hospital's water system is colonized with the organisms. The incidence of hospital-acquired Legionnaires' disease depends on the degree of contamination of the water system as defined by the rate of positivity of distal water sites (not as defined quantitatively by the number of colony-forming units per milliliter).

Risk factors for Legionnaires' disease include cigarette smoking; chronic lung disease; advanced age; prior hospitalization, with discharge within 10 days before onset of pneumonia symptoms; and immunosuppression. Immunosuppressive conditions that predispose to Legionnaires' disease include transplantation, HIV infection, and treatment with glucocorticoids or tumor necrosis factor α. However, in a large prospective study of community-acquired pneumonia, 28% of patients with Legionnaires' disease did not have these classic risk factors. Surgery is a prominent predisposing factor in hospital-acquired infection, with transplant recipients at highest risk. Hospital-acquired cases are now being recognized among neonates and immunosuppressed children.

Pontiac fever occurs in epidemics. The high attack rate (>90%) reflects airborne transmission.

PATHOGENESIS AND IMMUNITY

Legionella enters the lungs through aspiration or direct inhalation. Attachment to host cells is mediated by bacterial type IV pili, heat-shock proteins, and the major outer-membrane protein. *Legionella* binds to complement CR1 and CR3 integrin receptors on the surface of the host cell. Because the organisms possess pili that may mediate adherence to respiratory tract epithelial cells, conditions that impair mucociliary clearance, including cigarette smoking, lung disease, or alcoholism, predispose to Legionnaires' disease.

Cell-mediated immunity is the primary mechanism of host defense against *Legionella*, as it is against other intracellular pathogens. Thus Legionnaires' disease is more common and its manifestations are more severe among patients with depressed cell-mediated immunity. The disease also occurs with unusual frequency among patients with hairy cell leukemia, which is characterized by monocyte deficiency and dysfunction.

Alveolar macrophages readily phagocytose *Legionella*. The attachment of the bacteria to phagocytes is mediated via Fc receptors and complement receptors, which attach to the bacterial major outer-membrane protein. Binding to these receptors promotes phagocytosis but fails to trigger an oxidative burst. The *L. pneumophila* phagosome resists acidification and evades fusion with late endocytic compartments and lysosomes. Although many legionellae are killed, some proliferate intracellularly until the cells rupture; the bacteria are then phagocytosed again by newly recruited phagocytes, and the cycle begins anew.

The role of neutrophils in immunity appears to be minimal: neutropenic patients are not predisposed to Legionnaires' disease. Although *L. pneumophila* is susceptible to oxygen-dependent microbiologic systems in vitro, it resists killing by neutrophils.

The humoral immune system is active against *Legionella*. Type-specific IgM and IgG antibodies are measurable within weeks of infection. In vitro, antibodies promote killing of *Legionella* by phagocytes (neutrophils, monocytes, and alveolar macrophages). Immunized animals develop a specific antibody response, with subsequent resistance to *Legionella* challenge. However, antibodies neither enhance lysis by complement nor inhibit intracellular multiplication within phagocytes.

Some *L. pneumophila* strains are clearly more virulent than others, although the precise factors mediating virulence remain uncertain. For example, although multiple strains may colonize water-distribution systems, only a few cause disease in patients exposed to water from these systems. At least one surface epitope of *L. pneumophila* serogroup 1 is associated with virulence. Monoclonal antibody subtype mAb2 has been linked to virulence. *L. pneumophila* serogroup 6 is more commonly involved in hospital-acquired Legionnaires' disease and is more likely to be associated with a poor outcome.

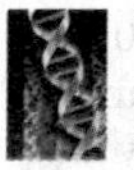

The genome of *L. pneumophila* has been sequenced. A broad range of membrane transporters within the genome are thought to optimize the use of nutrients in water and soil. Genes responsible for establishment of an intracellular growth site in human alveolar macrophages and replication in symbiotic microorganisms have been identified.

CLINICAL AND LABORATORY FEATURES

Pontiac Fever Pontiac fever is an acute, self-limiting, flu-like illness with an incubation period of 24–48 h. Pneumonia does not develop. Malaise, fatigue, and myalgias are the most common symptoms, occurring in 97% of cases. Fever (usually with chills) develops in 80–90% of cases and headache in 80%. Other symptoms (seen in <50% of cases) include arthralgias, nausea, cough, abdominal pain, and diarrhea. Modest leukocytosis with a neutrophilic predominance is sometimes detected. Without antibiotic therapy, complete recovery takes place in only a few days; a few patients may experience lassitude for many weeks thereafter. The diagnosis is established by antibody seroconversion.

Legionnaires' Disease (Pneumonia) Legionnaires' disease is often included in the differential diagnosis of "atypical pneumonia," along with infection due to *C. pneumoniae, Chlamydophila psittaci, Mycoplasma pneumoniae, Coxiella burnetii*, and some viruses. The clinical similarities among these types of pneumonia include a relatively nonproductive cough and a low incidence of grossly purulent sputum. However, the clinical manifestations of Legionnaires' disease are usually more severe than those of most "atypical" pneumonias, and the course and prognosis of *Legionella* pneumonia more closely resemble those of bacteremic pneumococcal pneumonia than those of pneumonia due to other "atypical" pathogens. Patients with community-acquired Legionnaires' disease are significantly more likely than patients with pneumonia of other etiologies to be admitted to an intensive care unit on presentation.

The incubation period for Legionnaires' disease is usually 2–10 days, although longer incubation periods have been documented. The symptoms and signs may range from a mild cough and a slight fever to stupor with widespread pulmonary infiltrates and multisystem failure. Nonspecific symptoms—malaise, fatigue, anorexia, and headache—are seen early in the illness. Myalgias and arthralgias are uncommon but are prominent in a few patients. Upper respiratory symptoms, including coryza, are rare.

The mild cough of Legionnaires' disease is only slightly productive. Sometimes the sputum is streaked with blood. Chest pain—either pleuritic or nonpleuritic—can be a prominent feature and, when coupled with hemoptysis, can lead to an incorrect diagnosis of pulmonary embolism. Shortness of breath is reported by one-third to one-half of patients.

Gastrointestinal difficulties are often pronounced; abdominal pain, nausea, and vomiting affect 10–20% of patients. Diarrhea (watery rather than bloody) is reported in 25–50% of cases. The most common neurologic abnormalities are confusion or changes in mental status; however, the multitudinous neurologic symptoms reported range from headache and lethargy to encephalopathy.

Patients with Legionnaires' disease virtually always have fever. Temperatures in excess of 40.5°C (104.9°F) were recorded in 20% of the cases in one series. Relative bradycardia has been overemphasized as a useful diagnostic finding; it occurs primarily in older patients with severe pneumonia. Chest examination reveals rales early in the course and evidence of consolidations as the disease progresses. Abdominal examination may reveal generalized or local tenderness.

Although the clinical manifestations often considered classic for Legionnaires' disease (Table 141-1) may suggest the diagnosis, prospective comparative studies have shown that clinical manifestations are generally nonspecific and that Legionnaires' disease is not readily distinguishable from pneumonia of other etiologies. In a review of 13 studies of community-acquired pneumonia, clinical manifestations that occurred significantly more often in Legionnaires' disease included diarrhea, neurologic findings (including confusion), and a temperature of >39°C. Hyponatremia, elevated values in liver function tests, and hematuria also occurred more frequently in Legionnaires' disease. Other laboratory abnormalities include creatine phosphokinase elevation, hypophosphatemia, serum creatinine elevation, and proteinuria.

Extrapulmonary Legionellosis Since the portal of entry for *Legionella* is the lung in virtually all cases, extrapulmonary manifestations usually result from bloodborne dissemination from the lung. In a prospective survey of patients with Legionnaires' disease diagnosed by isolation of the organism from sputum, *Legionella* was isolated from the blood by a special culture method in 38% of cases.

Legionella has been identified in lymph nodes, spleen, liver, or kidneys in autopsied cases. The most common extrapulmonary site of legionellosis is the heart; numerous reports have described myocarditis, pericarditis, postcardiotomy syndrome, and prosthetic-valve endocarditis. Most cases have been hospital-acquired. In some patients without overt evidence of pneumonia, the organisms may gain entry through a postoperative sternal wound exposed to contaminated tap water or

TABLE 141-1 CLINICAL CLUES SUGGESTIVE OF LEGIONNAIRES' DISEASE

Diarrhea
High fever (>40°C; >104°F)
Numerous neutrophils but no organisms revealed by Gram's staining of respiratory secretions
Hyponatremia (serum sodium level <131 mg/dL)
Failure to respond to β-lactam drugs (penicillins or cephalosporins) and aminoglycoside antibiotics
Occurrence of illness in an environment in which the potable water supply is known to be contaminated with *Legionella*
Onset of symptoms within 10 days after discharge from the hospital

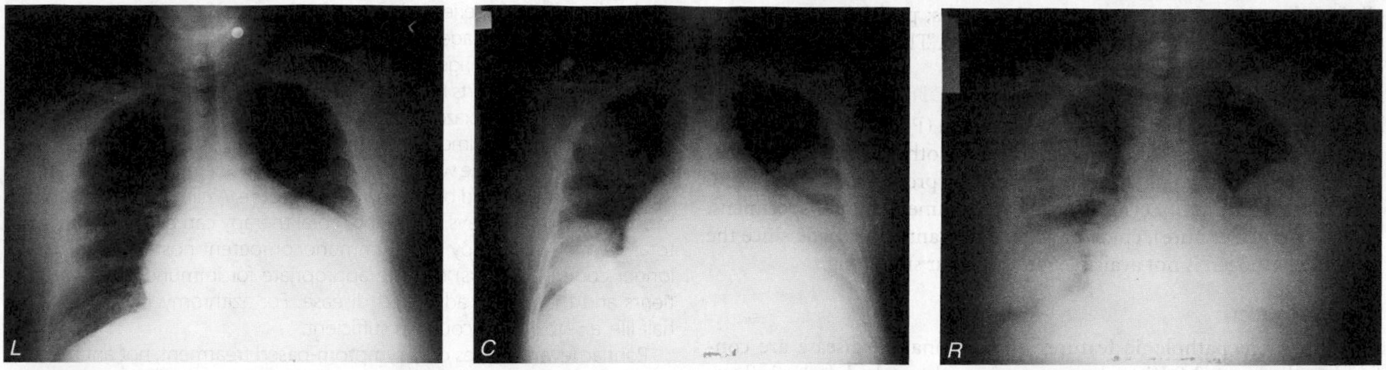

FIGURE 141-1 Chest radiographic findings in a 52-year-old man who presented with pneumonia subsequently diagnosed as Legionnaires' disease. The patient was a cigarette smoker with chronic obstructive pulmonary disease and alcoholic cardiomyopathy; he had received glucocorticoids. *L. pneumophila* was identified by DFA staining and culture of sputum. ***Left:*** Baseline chest radiograph showing long-standing cardiomegaly. ***Center:*** Admission chest radiograph showing new rounded opacities. ***Right:*** Chest radiograph taken 3 days after admission, during treatment with erythromycin.

through a mediastinal-tube insertion site. Sinusitis, peritonitis, pyelonephritis, skin and soft tissue infection, septic arthritis, and pancreatitis have been seen predominantly in immunosuppressed patients.

Chest Radiography Virtually all patients with Legionnaires' disease have abnormal chest radiographs showing pulmonary infiltrates at the time of clinical presentation. In a few cases of hospital-acquired disease, fever and respiratory tract symptoms have preceded the radiographic appearance of the infiltrate. Findings on chest radiography are useful for assessing the severity of illness in that they identify multilobar involvement and permit monitoring of disease progression. However, these findings are nonspecific and do not serve to distinguish Legionnaires' disease from pneumonias of other etiologies. Pleural effusion is evident in 28–63% of patients on hospital admission. In immunosuppressed patients, especially those receiving glucocorticoids, distinctive rounded nodular opacities may be seen; these lesions may expand and cavitate (Fig. 141-1). Likewise, abscesses can occur in immunosuppressed hosts. The progression of infiltrates and pleural effusion on chest radiography despite appropriate antibiotic therapy within the first week is common, and radiographic improvement lags behind clinical improvement by several days. Complete clearing of infiltrates requires 1–4 months.

DIAGNOSIS

Because clinical manifestations are nonspecific, the diagnosis of Legionnaires' disease requires special microbiologic tests (Table 141-2). The sensitivity of bronchoscopy specimens is approximately the same as that of sputum samples for culture on selective media; if sputum is not available, bronchoscopy specimens may yield the organism. Bronchoalveolar lavage fluid gives higher yields than bronchial wash specimens. Thoracentesis should be performed if pleural effusion is found, and the fluid should be evaluated by DFA staining, culture, and the antigen assay designed for use with urine (see "Urinary Antigen," below).

TABLE 141-2 UTILITY OF SPECIAL LABORATORY TESTS FOR THE DIAGNOSIS OF LEGIONNAIRES' DISEASE

Test	Sensitivity, %	Specificity, %
Culture		
Sputum[a]	80	100
Transtracheal aspirate	90	100
Direct fluorescent antibody staining of sputum	50–70	96–99
Urinary antigen testing[b]	70	100
Antibody serology[c]	40–60	96–99

[a]Use of multiple selective media with dyes.
[b]Serogroup 1 only.
[c]IgG and IgM testing of both acute- and convalescent-phase sera. A single titer of ≥1:256 is considered presumptive, while fourfold seroconversion is considered definitive.

Staining Gram's staining of material from normally sterile sites, such as pleural fluid or lung tissue, occasionally suggests the diagnosis; efforts to detect *Legionella* in sputum by Gram's staining typically reveal numerous leukocytes but no organisms. When they are visualized, the organisms appear as small, pleomorphic, faint, gram-negative bacilli. *L. micdadei* organisms can be detected as weakly or partially acid-fast bacilli in clinical specimens. Modified acid-fast staining substitutes 1% sulfuric acid for the traditional 3% hydrochloric acid; the less aggressive decolorizer increases the yield of *L. micdadei*. *Legionella*-infected patients have occasionally been treated empirically with antituberculosis medications because of false-positive acid-fast smears.

The DFA test is rapid and highly specific but is less sensitive than culture because large numbers of organisms are required for microscopic visualization. This test is more likely to be positive in advanced than in early disease.

Culture The definitive method for diagnosis of *Legionella* infection is isolation of the organism from respiratory secretions or other specimens. Multiple selective BCYE media containing dyes are required for maximal sensitivity. Colonies grow slowly, requiring 3–5 days to become grossly visible. When culture plates are overgrown with other microflora, pretreatment of the specimen with acid or heat can markedly improve the yield. *L. pneumophila* is often isolated from sputum that is not grossly or microscopically purulent; sputum containing more than 25 epithelial cells per high-power field (a finding that classically suggests contamination) may still yield *L. pneumophila*.

Antibody Detection Antibody testing of both acute- and convalescent-phase sera is necessary. A fourfold rise in titer is diagnostic; 12 weeks are often required for the detection of an antibody response. A single titer of 1:128 in a patient with pneumonia constitutes circumstantial evidence for Legionnaires' disease. Serology is of use primarily in epidemiologic studies. The specificity of serology for *Legionella* species other than *L. pneumophila* is uncertain; there is cross-reactivity with *Legionella* spp. and some gram-negative bacilli.

Urinary Antigen The assay for *Legionella* soluble antigen in urine is rapid, relatively inexpensive, easy to perform, second only to culture in terms of sensitivity, and highly specific. Several enzyme immunoassays and a rapid immunochromatographic assay are commercially available. Like the urinary antigen assay, the rapid immunochromatographic assay is relatively inexpensive and easy to perform. The use of urinary antigen testing in every clinical laboratory is recommended. The urinary antigen test is available only for *L. pneumophila* serogroup 1, which causes ~80% of *Legionella* infections. Cross-reactivity with other *L. pneumophila* serogroups and other *Legionella* species has been detected in up to 22% of urine samples from patients with culture-proven cases. Antigen in urine is detectable 3 days after the onset of clinical disease and disappears over 2 months; positivity can be prolonged when patients receive glucocorticoids. The test is not affected by antibiotic administration.

Molecular Methods Polymerase chain reaction (PCR) with DNA probes is theoretically more sensitive and specific than other methods. A molecular probe is undergoing evaluation. PCR has proven somewhat useful in the identification of *Legionella* from environmental water specimens. In PCR (unlike culture), epidemiologic links cannot be made since the infecting pathogen is not available for molecular subtyping.

PATHOLOGY

The consistent pathologic features of Legionnaires' disease are confined to the lungs. Multifocal pneumonia, with patchy lobular inflammation and extensive multilobar consolidation, has been observed. Visible abscesses with central necrosis were seen in 20% of autopsied cases in one study. On histologic examination, fibrinopurulent pneumonia with intensive alveolitis and bronchiolitis is evident. The DFA stain is not only specific but also the most sensitive option for visualization of the organism in tissues. Polyvalent but not monoclonal DFA stain can be used for formalinized specimens. Culture is the preferred method for diagnosis based on clinical specimens.

℞ *LEGIONELLA* INFECTION

Because *Legionella* is an intracellular pathogen, antibiotics that can reach intracellular concentrations exceeding the minimal inhibitory concentration are most likely to be clinically efficacious. The dosages for various drugs used in the treatment of *Legionella* infection are listed in **Table 141-3**.

The newer macrolides (especially azithromycin) and respiratory tract quinolones are now the antibiotics of choice and are effective as monotherapy. Compared with erythromycin, the newer macrolides have superior in vitro activity, display greater intracellular activity, reach higher concentrations in respiratory secretions and in lung tissue, and have fewer adverse effects. The pharmacokinetics of the newer macrolides and quinolones also allow once- or twice-daily dosing. Quinolones are the preferred antibiotics for transplant recipients because both macrolides and rifampin interact pharmacologically with cyclosporine and tacrolimus. Retrospective uncontrolled studies have shown that complications of pneumonia are fewer and clinical response is more rapid in patients receiving quinolones than in those receiving macrolides. Ketolides (telithromycin) are highly active in vitro and in intracellular models, but clinical experience is less extensive than that with macrolides and quinolones. Alternative agents include tetracycline and its analogues doxycycline and minocycline. Tigecycline is active in vitro but clinical experience is lacking. Anecdotal reports have described both successes and failures with trimethoprim-sulfamethoxazole, imipenem, and clindamycin. For severely ill patients with extensive pulmonary infiltrates, a two-drug combination of a newer macrolide or a quinolone with rifampin can be considered for initial treatment.

Initial therapy should be given by the IV route. A clinical response usually occurs within 3–5 days, after which oral therapy can be substituted. The total duration of therapy in the immunocompetent host is 10–14 days; a longer course (3 weeks) may be appropriate for immunosuppressed patients and those with advanced disease. For azithromycin, with its long half-life, a 5- to 10-day course is sufficient.

Pontiac fever requires only symptom-based treatment, not antimicrobial therapy.

TABLE 141-3 ANTIBIOTIC THERAPY FOR *LEGIONELLA* INFECTION

Antimicrobial Agent	Dosage[a]
Macrolides	
Azithromycin	500 mg[b] PO or IV[c] q24h
Clarithromycin	500 mg PO or IV[c] q12h
Quinolones	
Levofloxacin	750 mg IV q24h 500 mg[b] PO q24h
Ciprofloxacin	400 mg IV q8h 750 mg PO q12h
Moxifloxacin	400 mg[b] PO q24h
Ketolide	
Telithromycin	800 mg PO q24h
Tetracyclines	
Doxycycline	100 mg[b] PO or IV q12h
Minocycline	100 mg[b] PO or IV q12h
Tetracycline	500 mg PO or IV q6h
Tigecycline	100-mg IV load, then 50 mg IV q12h[d]
Others	
Trimethoprim-sulfamethoxazole	160/800 mg IV q8h 160/800 mg PO q12h
Rifampin[e]	100–600 mg PO or IV q12h

[a]Dosages are derived from clinical experience.
[b]The authors recommend doubling the first dose.
[c]The IV formulation is not available in some countries.
[d]Undergoing evaluation.
[e]Rifampin should be used only in combination with a macrolide or a quinolone.

PROGNOSIS

Mortality rates for Legionnaires' disease vary with the patient's underlying disease and its severity, the patient's immune status, the severity of pneumonia, and the timing of administration of appropriate antimicrobial therapy. Mortality rates are highest (80%) among immunosuppressed patients who do not receive appropriate antimicrobial therapy early in the course of illness. With appropriate and timely antibiotic treatment, mortality rates from community-acquired Legionnaires' disease among immunocompetent patients range from 0 to 11%; without treatment, the figure may be as high as 31%. In a study of survivors of an outbreak of community-acquired Legionnaires' disease, sequelae of fatigue, neurologic symptoms, and weakness were found in 63–75% of patients 17 months after receipt of antibiotics.

PREVENTION

Routine environmental culture of hospital water supplies is recommended as an approach to the prevention of hospital-acquired Legionnaires' disease. Guidelines mandating this proactive approach have been adopted in Denmark, France, Germany, Italy, the Netherlands, and Taiwan. The CDC has thus far avoided this issue, but routine-culture guidelines from U.S. health departments have been adopted in Pittsburgh (PA), New York, and Maryland. Positive cultures from the water supply mandate the use of specialized laboratory tests (especially culture on selective media and the urinary antigen test) for patients with hospital-acquired pneumonia. Studies have shown that neither a high degree of outward cleanliness of the water system nor routine application of maintenance measures decreases the frequency or intensity of *Legionella* contamination. Thus, engineering guidelines and building codes, although routinely advocated as preventive measures, have little impact on the presence of *Legionella*.

Disinfection of the water supply is now feasible. Two methods have proven reliable and cost-effective. The superheat-and-flush method requires heating of the water so that the distal-outlet temperature is 70–80°C and flushing of the distal outlets with hot water for at least 30 min. This method is ideal for emergency situations. A commercial copper and silver ionization method has proved effective in numerous hospitals. Carbon dioxide and monochloramine are undergoing evaluation, and preliminary results are promising. Tap water filters have been effective for high-risk patient areas, such as transplantation units. Hyperchlorination is no longer recommended because of its expense, carcinogenicity, corrosive effects on piping, and unreliable efficacy.

FURTHER READINGS

Greenberg D et al: Problem pathogens: Paediatric legionellosis—implications for improved diagnosis. Lancet Infect Dis 6:529, 2006

Lettinga KD et al: Health-related quality of life and posttraumatic stress disorder among survivors of an outbreak of Legionnaires' disease. Clin Infect Dis 35:11, 2002

Modol J et al: Hospital-acquired Legionnaires' disease in a university hospital: Impact of the copper-silver ionization system. Clin Infect Dis 44:263, 2007

MUDER R, YU VL: Infection due to *Legionella* species other than *L. pneumophila*. Clin Infect Dis 35:990, 2002

MULAZIMOGLU L, YU VL: Can Legionnaires' disease be diagnosed by clinical criteria? A critical review. Chest 120:1049, 2001

PEDRO-BOTET ML et al: Legionnaires' disease contracted from patient homes: The coming of the third plague? Eur J Clin Microbiol Infect Dis 21:699, 2002

ROIG J, PEDRO-BOTET ML: *Legionella* spp: Community acquired and nosocomial infections. Curr Opin Infect Dis 16:45, 2003

SABRIA M et al: Fluoroquinolones vs macrolides in the treatment of Legionnaires' disease. Chest 128:1401, 2005

———, YU VL: Hospital-acquired legionellosis: Solutions for preventable infection. Lancet Infect Dis 2:368, 2002

SQUIER CL et al: A proactive approach to prevention of healthcare-acquired Legionnaires' disease: The Allegheny County (Pittsburgh) experience. Am J Infect Control 33:360, 2005

TUBACH F et al: Emergence of *L. pneumophila* pneumonia in patients receiving tumor necrosis factor-α antagonists. Clin Infect Dis 43:e95, 2006

142 Pertussis and Other *Bordetella* Infections

Scott A. Halperin

Pertussis is an acute infection of the respiratory tract caused by *Bordetella pertussis*. The name *pertussis* means "violent cough," which aptly describes the most consistent and prominent feature of the illness. The inspiratory sound made at the end of an episode of paroxysmal coughing gives rise to the common name for the illness, "whooping cough"; however, this feature is variable: it is uncommon among infants ≤6 months of age and is frequently absent in older children and adults. The Chinese name for pertussis is "the 100-day cough," which accurately describes the clinical course of the illness. The identification of *B. pertussis* was first reported by Bordet and Gengou in 1906, and vaccines were produced over the following two decades.

MICROBIOLOGY

Of the nine identified species in the genus *Bordetella*, only three are of major medical significance. *B. pertussis* infects only humans and is the most important *Bordetella* species causing human disease. *B. parapertussis* causes an illness in humans that is similar to pertussis but is typically milder; co-infections with *B. parapertussis* and *B. pertussis* have been documented. *B. bronchiseptica* is an important pathogen of domestic animals that causes kennel cough in dogs, atrophic rhinitis and pneumonia in pigs, and pneumonia in cats. Both respiratory infection and opportunistic infection are occasionally reported in humans. Two additional species, *B. hinzii* and *B. holmesii*, are unusual causes of bacteremia; both have been isolated from patients with sepsis, most often from those who are immunocompromised.

Bordetella species are gram-negative pleomorphic aerobic bacilli that share common genotypic characteristics. *B. pertussis* and *B. parapertussis* are the most similar of the species, but *B. parapertussis* does not express the gene coding for pertussis toxin. *B. pertussis* is a slow-growing fastidious organism that requires selective medium and forms small glistening bifurcated colonies. Suspicious colonies are presumptively identified as *B. pertussis* by direct fluorescent antibody testing or by agglutination with species-specific antiserum. *B. pertussis* is further differentiated from other *Bordetella* species by biochemical and motility characteristics.

B. pertussis produces a wide array of toxins and biologically active products that are important in its pathogenesis and in immunity. Most of these virulence factors are under the control of a single genetic locus that regulates their production, resulting in antigenic modulation and phase variation. Although these processes occur both in vitro and in vivo, their importance in the pathobiology of the organism is unknown; they may play a role in intracellular persistence and person-to-person spread. The organism's most important virulence factor is *pertussis toxin*, which is composed of a B oligomer–binding subunit and an enzymatically active A protomer that ADP-ribosylates a guanine nucleotide-binding regulatory protein (G protein) in target cells, producing a variety of biologic effects. Pertussis toxin has important mitogenic activity, affects the circulation of lymphocytes, and serves as an adhesin for bacterial binding to respiratory ciliated cells. Other important virulence factors and adhesins are *filamentous hemagglutinin*, a component of the cell wall, and *pertactin*, an outer-membrane protein. *Fimbriae*, bacterial appendages that play a role in bacterial attachment, are the major antigens against which agglutinating antibodies are directed. These agglutinating antibodies have historically been the primary means of serotyping *B. pertussis* strains. Other virulence factors include tracheal cytotoxin, which causes respiratory epithelial damage; adenylate cyclase toxin, which impairs host immune-cell function; dermonecrotic toxin, which may contribute to respiratory mucosal damage; and lipooligosaccharide, which has properties similar to those of other gram-negative bacterial endotoxins.

EPIDEMIOLOGY

Pertussis is a highly communicable disease, with attack rates of 80–100% among unimmunized household contacts and 20% within households in well-immunized populations. The infection has a worldwide distribution, with cyclical outbreaks every 3–5 years (a pattern that has persisted despite widespread immunization). Pertussis occurs in all months; however, in North America, its activity peaks in summer and autumn.

In developing countries, pertussis remains an important cause of infant morbidity and death. The reported incidence of pertussis worldwide has decreased as a result of improved vaccine coverage. However, coverage rates are still <50% in many developing nations (Fig. 142-1); the World Health Organization (WHO) estimates that 90% of the burden of pertussis is in the developing world. In addition, overreporting of immunization coverage and underreporting of disease result in substantial underestimation of the global burden of pertussis (Fig. 142-2). The WHO estimates that more than 17.6 million people worldwide were infected by *B. pertussis* in 2003, with 279,000 deaths from pertussis among children.

Before the institution of widespread immunization programs in the developed world, pertussis was one of the most common infectious causes of morbidity and death. In the United States before the 1940s, between 115,000 and 270,000 cases of pertussis were reported annually, with an average yearly rate of 150 cases per 100,000 population. With universal childhood immunization, the number of reported cases fell by >95%, and mortality rates decreased even more dramatically. Only 1010 cases of pertussis were reported in 1976. Since that time, however, rates have slowly increased. In 2003, more than 11,600 cases of pertussis were reported in the United States.

Although thought of as a disease of childhood, pertussis can affect people of all ages and is increasingly being identified as a cause of prolonged coughing illness in adolescents and adults. In unimmunized populations, pertussis incidence peaks during the preschool years, and well over half of children have the disease before reaching adulthood. In highly immunized populations such as those in North America, the peak incidence is among infants <1 year of age who have not completed the three-dose primary immunization series. Recent trends, however, show an increasing incidence of pertussis among adolescents and adults. In the United States between 2001 and 2003, 23% of patients were <1 year of age, 33% were adolescents, and 23% were adults. The figures for adolescents and adults are probably underestimates because

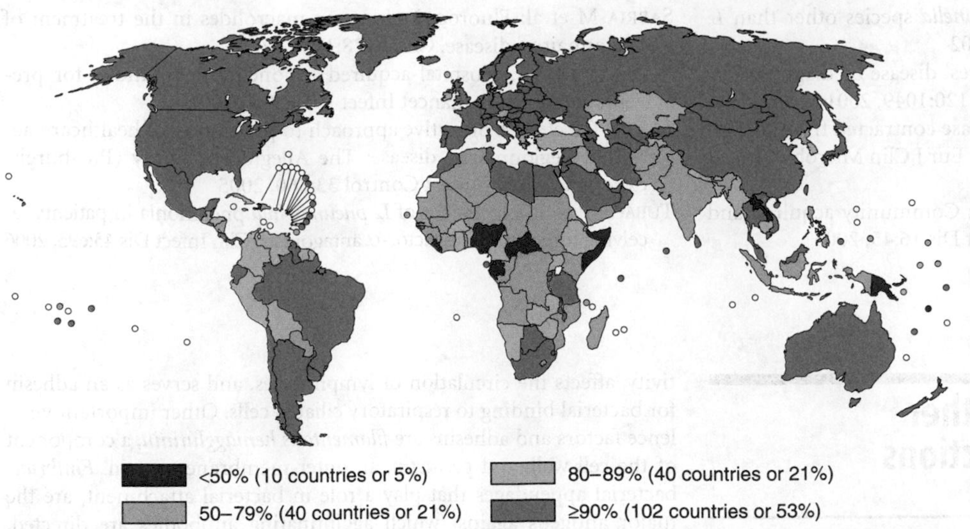

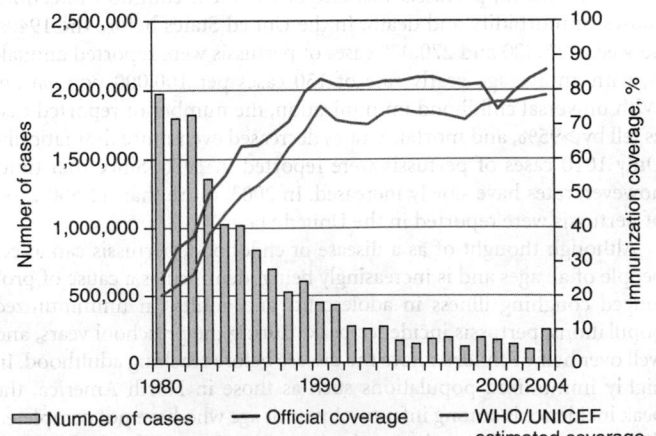

FIGURE 142-1 Immunization coverage with DTP3 vaccines (diphtheria toxoid, tetanus toxoid, and pertussis, 3 doses) in infants, 2004. *(Reprinted with permission of the World Health Organization. Source: WHO/IVB database, 2005. This map does not imply the expression of any opinion whatsoever on the part of the World Health Organization concerning the legal status of any country, territory, city, or area of its authorities or concerning the delimitation of its frontiers or boundaries.)*

of a greater degree of underrecognition and underreporting in these age groups. A number of studies of prolonged coughing illness suggest that pertussis may be the etiologic agent in 12–30% of adults with cough that does not improve within 2 weeks. In one study of the efficacy of an acellular pertussis vaccine in adolescents and adults, the incidence of pertussis in the placebo group was 3.7–4.5 cases per 1000 person-years. Although this prospective cohort study yielded a lower estimate than the studies of cough illness, its results still translate to 600,000–800,000 cases of pertussis annually among adults in the United States. Severe morbidity and high mortality rates, however, are restricted almost entirely to infants. In Canada, there were 10 deaths from pertussis between 1991 and 1998; all those who died were infants ≤6 months of age. Although school-age children are the source of infection for most households, adults are the likely source for high-risk infants and may serve as the reservoir of infection between epidemic years.

PATHOGENESIS

Infection with *B. pertussis* is initiated by attachment of the organism to the ciliated epithelial cells of the nasopharynx. Attachment is mediated by surface adhesins (e.g., pertactin and filamentous hemagglutinin), which bind to the integrin family of cell-surface proteins, probably in conjunction with pertussis toxin. The role of fimbriae in adhesion and in maintenance of infection has not been fully delineated. At the site of attachment, the organism multiplies, producing a variety of other toxins that cause local mucosal damage (tracheal cytotoxin, dermonecrotic toxin). Impairment of host defense by *B. pertussis* is mediated by pertussis toxin and adenylate cyclase toxin. There is local cellular invasion, with intracellular bacterial persistence; however, systemic dissemination does not occur. Systemic manifestations (lymphocytosis) result from the effects of the toxins.

The pathogenesis of the clinical manifestations of pertussis is poorly understood. It is not known what causes the hallmark paroxysmal cough. A pivotal role for pertussis toxin has been proposed. Proponents of this position point to the efficacy of preventing clinical symptoms with a vaccine containing only pertussis toxoid. Detractors counter that pertussis toxin is not the critical factor because paroxysmal cough also occurs in patients infected with *B. parapertussis*, which does not produce pertussis toxin. It is thought that neurologic events in pertussis, such as seizures and encephalopathy, are due to hypoxia from coughing paroxysms or apnea rather than to the effects of specific bacterial products. *B. pertussis* pneumonia, which occurs in up to 10% of infants with pertussis, is usually a diffuse bilateral primary infection. In older children and adults with pertussis, pneumonia is often due to secondary bacterial infection with streptococci or staphylococci.

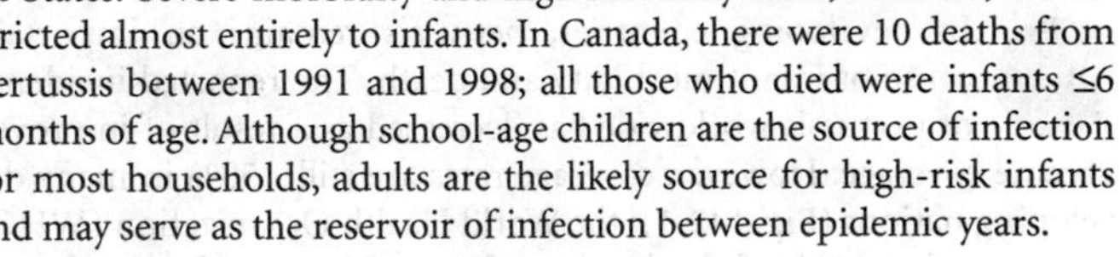

FIGURE 142-2 Global annual reported pertussis incidence and rate of coverage with DTP3 (diphtheria toxoid, tetanus toxoid, and pertussis vaccine, 3 doses), 1980–2004. *(Reprinted with permission of the World Health Organization. Source: WHO/IVB database, 2005.)*

IMMUNITY

Both humoral and cell-mediated immunity are thought to be important in pertussis. Antibodies to pertussis toxin, filamentous hemagglutinin, pertactin, and fimbriae are all protective in animal models. Pertussis agglutinins were correlated with protection in early studies of whole-cell pertussis vaccines. Serologic correlates of protection conferred by acellular pertussis vaccines have not been established, although antibody to pertactin, fimbriae, and (to a lesser degree) pertussis toxin correlated best with protection in two efficacy trials. The duration of immunity after whole-cell pertussis vaccination is short-lived, with little protection remaining after 10–12 years. After a three-dose infant primary series of acellular pertussis vaccine, protection persists for at least 5–6 years; the duration of immunity after a four- or five-dose schedule is not yet known. Although immunity after natural infection has been said to be lifelong, seroepidemiologic evidence suggests that it may not be and that subsequent episodes of clinical pertussis are prevented by intermittent subclinical infection.

CLINICAL MANIFESTATIONS

Pertussis is a prolonged coughing illness with clinical manifestations that vary by age (Table 142-1). Although not uncommon among adolescents and adults, classic pertussis is most often seen in preschool and school-age children. After an incubation period averaging 7–10 days, an illness develops that is indistinguishable from the common cold and is characterized by coryza, lacrimation, mild cough, low-grade fever, and malaise. After 1–2 weeks, this *catarrhal phase* evolves into the *paroxysmal phase*: the cough becomes more frequent and spasmodic with repetitive bursts of 5–10 coughs, often within a single expiration. Posttussive vomiting is frequent, with a mucous plug occasionally expelled at the end of an episode. The episode may be terminated by an audible whoop, which occurs upon rapid inspiration against a closed glottis at the end of a paroxysm. During a spasm, there may be impressive neck-vein distension, bulging eyes, tongue protrusion, and cyanosis. Paroxysms may be precipitated by noise, eating, or physical contact. Between

TABLE 142-1 CLINICAL FEATURES OF PERTUSSIS, BY AGE GROUP AND DIAGNOSTIC STATUS

	Percentage of Patients		
	Adolescents and Adults		
Feature	Laboratory Confirmation	No Laboratory Confirmation	Children
Cough	95–100	95–100	95–100
Prolonged	60–80	60–80	60–95
Paroxysmal	60–90	50–90	80–95
Sleep-disturbing	50–80	50–80	90–100
Whoop	10–40	5–30	40–80
Posttussive vomiting	20–50	5–30	80–90

attacks, the patient's appearance is normal but increasing fatigue is evident. The frequency of paroxysmal episodes varies widely, from several per hour to 5–10 per day. Episodes are often worse at night and interfere with sleep. Weight loss is not uncommon as a result of the illness's interference with eating. Most complications occur during the paroxysmal stage. Fever is uncommon and suggests bacterial superinfection.

After 2–4 weeks, the coughing episodes become less frequent and less severe—changes heralding the onset of the *convalescent phase.* This phase can last 1–3 months and is characterized by gradual resolution of coughing episodes. For 6–12 months, intercurrent viral infections may be associated with a recrudescence of paroxysmal cough.

Not all individuals who develop pertussis have classic disease. The clinical manifestations in adolescents and adults are more often atypical. In a German study of pertussis in adults, more than two-thirds had paroxysmal cough and more than one-third had whoop. Adult illness in North America differs from this experience: the cough may be severe and prolonged but is less frequently paroxysmal, and a whoop is uncommon. Vomiting with cough is the best predictor of pertussis as the cause of prolonged cough in adults. Other predictive features are a cough at night and exposure to other individuals with a prolonged coughing illness.

COMPLICATIONS

Complications are frequently associated with pertussis and are more common among infants than among older children or adults. Subconjunctival hemorrhages, abdominal and inguinal hernias, pneumothoraces, and facial and truncal petechiae can result from increased intrathoracic pressure generated by severe fits of coughing. Weight loss can follow decreased caloric intake. In a series of more than 1100 children <2 years of age who were hospitalized with pertussis, 27.1% had apnea, 9.4% had pneumonia, 2.6% had seizures, and 0.4% had encephalopathy; 10 children (0.9%) died. Pneumonia is reported in <5% of adolescents and adults and increases in frequency after 50 years of age. In contrast to the primary *B. pertussis* pneumonia that develops in infants, pneumonia in adolescents and adults with pertussis is usually caused by a secondary infection with encapsulated organisms such as *Streptococcus pneumoniae* or *Haemophilus influenzae.* Pneumothorax, severe weight loss, inguinal hernia, rib fracture, carotid artery aneurysm, and cough syncope have all been reported in adolescents and adults with pertussis.

DIAGNOSIS

If the classic symptoms of pertussis are present, clinical diagnosis is not difficult. However, particularly in older children and adults, it is difficult to differentiate infections caused by *B. pertussis* and *B. parapertussis* from other respiratory tract infections on clinical grounds. Therefore, laboratory confirmation should be attempted in all cases. Lymphocytosis—an absolute lymphocyte count of $>10 \times 10^9$/L—is common among young children (in whom it is unusual with other infections) but not among adolescents and adults. Culture of nasopharyngeal secretions remains the gold standard of diagnosis, although DNA detection by polymerase chain reaction (PCR) is replacing culture in many laboratories because of increased sensitivity and quicker results. The best specimen is collected by nasopharyngeal aspiration, in which a fine flexible plastic catheter attached to a 10-mL syringe is passed into the nasopharynx and withdrawn while gentle suction is applied. Since *B. pertussis* is highly sensitive to drying, secretions for culture should be inoculated without delay onto appropriate medium (Bordet-Gengou or Regan-Lowe), or the catheter should be flushed with a phosphate-buffered saline solution for culture and/or PCR. An alternative to the aspirate is a Dacron or rayon nasopharyngeal swab; again, inoculation of culture plates should be immediate or an appropriate transport medium (e.g., Regan-Lowe charcoal medium) should be used. Results of PCR can be available within hours; cultures become positive by day 5 of incubation. *B. pertussis* and *B. parapertussis* can be differentiated by agglutination with specific antisera or by direct immunofluorescence.

Nasopharyngeal cultures in untreated pertussis remain positive for a mean of 3 weeks after the onset of illness; these cultures become negative within 5 days of the institution of appropriate antimicrobial therapy. The duration of a positive PCR in untreated pertussis or after therapy is not known but exceeds that of positive cultures. Since much of the period during which the organism can be recovered from the nasopharynx falls into the catarrhal phase, when the etiology of the infection is not suspected, there is only a small window of opportunity for culture-proven diagnosis. Cultures from infants and young children are more frequently positive than those from older children and adults; this difference may reflect earlier presentation of the former age group for medical care. Direct fluorescent antibody tests of nasopharyngeal secretions for direct diagnosis may still be available in some laboratories but should not be used because of poor sensitivity and specificity.

As a result of the difficulties with laboratory diagnosis of pertussis in adolescents, adults, and patients who have been symptomatic for >4 weeks, increasing attention is being given to serologic diagnosis. Enzyme immunoassays detecting IgA and IgG antibodies to pertussis toxin, filamentous hemagglutinin, pertactin, and fimbriae have been developed and assessed for reproducibility. Two- or fourfold increases in antibody titer are suggestive of pertussis, although cross-reactivity of some antigens (such as filamentous hemagglutinin and pertactin) among *Bordetella* species makes it difficult to depend diagnostically on seroconversion involving a single type of antibody. Late presentation for medical care and prior immunization also complicate serologic diagnosis because the first sample obtained may in fact be a convalescent-phase specimen. Criteria for serologic diagnosis based on a single serum specimen compared with established population values are gaining acceptance, and serology will likely become more widely available for the diagnosis of pertussis.

DIFFERENTIAL DIAGNOSIS

A child presenting with paroxysmal cough, posttussive vomiting, and whoop is likely to have an infection caused by *B. pertussis* or *B. parapertussis*; lymphocytosis increases the likelihood of a *B. pertussis* etiology. Viruses such as respiratory syncytial virus and adenovirus have been isolated from patients with clinical pertussis but probably represent co-infection. In adolescents and adults, who often do not have paroxysmal cough or whoop, the differential diagnosis of a prolonged coughing illness is more extensive. Pertussis should be suspected in anyone with a cough that does not improve within 14 days, a paroxysmal cough of any duration, or any respiratory symptoms after contact with a laboratory-confirmed case of pertussis. Other etiologies to consider include infections caused by *Mycoplasma pneumoniae*, *Chlamydia pneumoniae*, adenovirus, influenza virus, and other respiratory viruses. Use of angiotensin-converting enzyme (ACE) inhibitors, reactive airway disease, and gastroesophageal reflux disease are well-described noninfectious causes of prolonged cough in adults.

Rx PERTUSSIS

ANTIBIOTICS The purpose of antibiotic therapy for pertussis is to eradicate the infecting bacteria from the nasopharynx; therapy does not substantially alter the clinical course unless given early in the catarrhal

TABLE 142-2 ANTIMICROBIAL THERAPY FOR PERTUSSIS

Drug	Adult Daily Dose	Frequency	Duration (Days)	Comments
Erythromycin estolate	1–2 g	3 divided doses	7–14	Frequent gastrointestinal side effects
Clarithromycin	500 mg	2 divided doses	7	
Azithromycin	500 mg on day 1, 250 mg subsequently	1 daily dose	5	
Trimethoprim-sulfamethoxazole	160 mg of trimethoprim, 800 mg of sulfamethoxazole	2 divided doses	14	For patients allergic to macrolides; data on effectiveness limited

phase. Macrolide antibiotics are the drugs of choice for treatment of pertussis **(Table 142-2)**; macrolide-resistant *B. pertussis* strains have been reported but are rare. Trimethoprim-sulfamethoxazole is recommended as an alternative for individuals allergic to macrolides.

SUPPORTIVE CARE Young infants have the highest rates of complication and death from pertussis; therefore, most infants (and older children with severe disease) should be hospitalized. A quiet environment may decrease the stimulation that can trigger paroxysmal episodes. Use of β-adrenergic agonists and/or glucocorticoids has been advocated by some authorities but has not been proven to be effective. Cough suppressants are not effective and play no role in the management of pertussis.

INFECTION CONTROL MEASURES Hospitalized patients with pertussis should be placed in respiratory isolation, with the use of precautions appropriate for pathogens spread by large respiratory droplets. Isolation should continue for 5 days after initiation of erythromycin therapy or for 3 weeks (i.e., until nasopharyngeal cultures are consistently negative) when the patient cannot tolerate antimicrobial therapy.

PREVENTION

Chemoprophylaxis Because the risk of transmission of *B. pertussis* within households is high, chemoprophylaxis is widely recommended for household contacts of pertussis cases. The effectiveness of chemoprophylaxis, although unproven, is supported by several epidemiologic studies of institutional and community outbreaks. In the only randomized placebo-controlled study, erythromycin estolate (50 mg/kg per day in three divided doses; maximum dose, 1 g/d) was effective in reducing the incidence of bacteriologically confirmed pertussis by 67%; however, there was no decrease in the incidence of clinical disease. Despite these disappointing results, many authorities continue to recommend chemoprophylaxis, particularly in households with members at high risk of severe disease (children <1 year of age). Data are not available on use of the newer macrolides for chemoprophylaxis, but these drugs are commonly used because of their increased tolerability and their effectiveness.

Immunization (See also Chap. 116) The mainstay of pertussis prevention is active immunization. Pertussis vaccine, now available for >80 years, became widely used in North America after 1940; the reported number of pertussis cases has since fallen by >90%. Whole-cell pertussis vaccines are prepared through the heating, chemical inactivation, and purification of whole *B. pertussis* organisms. Although effective (average efficacy estimate, 85%; range for different products, 30–100%), whole-cell pertussis vaccines are associated with adverse events—both common (fever; injection-site pain, erythema, and swelling; irritability) and uncommon (febrile seizures, hypotonic hyporesponsive episodes). Alleged associations of whole-cell pertussis vaccine with encephalopathy, sudden infant death syndrome, and autism, although not substantiated, have spawned an active anti-immunization lobby. The development of acellular pertussis vaccines, which are effective but less reactogenic, has greatly alleviated concerns about the inclusion of pertussis vaccine in the combined infant immunization series. Although whole-cell vaccines are still used extensively in the developing world, acellular pertussis vaccines are used exclusively for childhood immunization in much of the developed world. In North America, acellular pertussis vaccines are given as a three-dose primary series at 2, 4, and 6 months of age, with a reinforcing dose at 15–18 months of age and a booster dose at 4–6 years of age.

Although a wide variety of acellular pertussis vaccines were developed, only a few are still widely marketed; all contain pertussis toxoid and filamentous hemagglutinin. One acellular pertussis vaccine also contains pertactin, and another contains pertactin and two types of fimbriae. In light of analyses of phase 3 efficacy studies, most experts have concluded that two-component acellular pertussis vaccines are more effective than monocomponent vaccines and that the addition of pertactin increases efficacy still more. The further addition of fimbriae appears to enhance protective efficacy against milder disease. In two studies, protection conferred by pertussis vaccines correlated best with the production of antibody to pertactin, fimbriae, and pertussis toxin.

The development of acellular pertussis vaccines has sparked interest in the potential for pertussis control in adolescents and adults and in the possibility that pertussis control in those groups will enhance the protection of infants too young to be immunized. Whole-cell pertussis vaccine is contraindicated in individuals ≥7 years of age because of their poor toleration of possible adverse events. However, adult formulations of acellular pertussis vaccines have been shown to be safe, immunogenic, and efficacious in clinical trials in adolescents and adults and are now recommended for routine immunization of these groups in several countries, including the United States.

FURTHER READINGS

De Serres G et al: Morbidity of pertussis in adolescents and adults. J Infect Dis 182:174, 2000

Halperin SA et al: A randomized, placebo-controlled trial of erythromycin estolate chemoprophylaxis for household contacts of children with culture-positive *Bordetella pertussis* infection. Pediatrics 104:e42, 1999

——— et al: Epidemiological features of pertussis in hospitalized patients in Canada, 1991–1997: Report of the Immunization Monitoring Program—Active (IMPACT). Clin Infect Dis 28:1238, 1999

Lee GM et al: Pertussis in adolescents and adults: Should we vaccinate? Pediatrics 115:1675, 2005

Mattoo S, Cherry JD: Molecular pathogenesis, epidemiology, and clinical manifestations of respiratory infections due to *Bordetella pertussis* and other *Bordetella* subspecies. Clin Microbiol Rev 18:326, 2005

Riffelmann M et al: Pertussis PCR Consensus Group. Nucleic acid amplification tests for diagnosis of *Bordetella* infections. J Clin Microbiol 43:4925, 2005

Skowronski DM et al: The changing age and seasonal profile of pertussis in Canada. J Infect Dis 185:1448, 2002

Tan T et al: Epidemiology of pertussis. Pediatr Infect Dis J 24(Suppl):S10, 2005

Ward JI et al: APERT Study Group. Efficacy of an acellular pertussis vaccine among adolescents and adults. N Engl J Med 353:1555, 2005

Yih WK et al: The increasing incidence of pertussis in Massachusetts adolescents and adults, 1989–1998. J Infect Dis 182:1409, 2000

143 Diseases Caused by Gram-Negative Enteric Bacilli

Thomas A. Russo, James R. Johnson

GENERAL FEATURES AND PRINCIPLES

EPIDEMIOLOGY

Escherichia coli, Klebsiella, Proteus, Enterobacter, Serratia, Citrobacter, Morganella, Providencia, Edwardsiella, and *Acinetobacter* are components of the normal animal and human colonic flora and/or of the flora of a variety of environmental habitats, including long-term-care facilities (LTCFs) and hospitals. As a result, except for certain pathotypes of intestinal pathogenic *E. coli*, these genera are global pathogens. In healthy humans, *E. coli* is the predominant species of gram-negative bacilli (GNB) in the colonic flora. GNB (primarily *E. coli, Klebsiella,* and *Proteus*) only transiently colonize the oropharynx and skin of healthy individuals. In contrast, in LTCF and hospital settings, a variety of GNB emerge as the dominant flora of both mucosal and skin surfaces, particularly in association with antimicrobial use, severe illness, and extended length of stay. This colonization may lead to subsequent infection; for example, oropharyngeal colonization may lead to pneumonia.

STRUCTURE AND FUNCTION

GNB possess an extracytoplasmic outer membrane, a feature shared generally among gram-negative bacteria. This outer membrane consists of a lipid bilayer with associated proteins, lipoproteins, and polysaccharides [capsule, lipopolysaccharide (LPS)]. The outer membrane interfaces with the bacterial environment, including the human host. A variety of components of the outer membrane are critical determinants in pathogenesis and antimicrobial resistance.

PATHOGENESIS

Multiple bacterial virulence factors are required for the pathogenesis of infections caused by GNB. Possession of specialized virulence genes defines pathogens and enables them to infect the host efficiently. It is becoming clear that hosts and their cognate pathogens have been co-adapting throughout evolutionary history, and it has been speculated that infection is just one point on the spectrum of evolved relationships between microbes and hosts. At one end of this spectrum is a commensal/symbiotic interaction (e.g., mitochondria—formerly bacteria—within eukaryotic cells); at the other end is a lethal outcome, producing a "dead-end relationship" (e.g., Ebola virus). During the host-pathogen "chess match" over time, various and redundant strategies have emerged in both the pathogens and their hosts that enable these partners to maintain their coexistence (Table 143-1).

Extraintestinal pathogenic strains of *E. coli* (ExPEC) and the other genera discussed in this chapter cause infection outside the bowel. All are extracellular pathogens and therefore share certain pathogenic features. Innate immunity (including the activities of complement, antimicrobial peptides, and professional phagocytes) and humoral immunity are the principal host-defense components. Both susceptibility to and severity of infection are increased with dysfunction or deficiencies of these components (Chap. 113). In contrast, the virulence traits of intestinal pathogenic *E. coli*—i.e., the distinctive strains that can cause diarrheal disease—are for the most part different from those of extraintestinal pathogenic *E. coli* and other GNB that cause extraintestinal infections. This difference reflects site-specific differences in host environments and defense mechanisms.

A given extraintestinal pathogen usually possesses multiple adhesins for binding to a variety of host cells (e.g., in *E. coli*: type 1 fimbriae, Sfa/Foc fimbriae, P pili). Nutrient acquisition (e.g., of iron via siderophores) requires many genes that are necessary but not sufficient for pathogenesis. The ability to resist the bactericidal activity of complement and phagocytes in the absence of antibody (e.g., as conferred by capsule or O antigen of LPS) is one of the defining traits of an extracellular pathogen. Tissue damage (e.g., as mediated by hemolysin in the case of *E. coli*) may facilitate spread. Without doubt, many important virulence genes await identification, and our understanding of many aspects of the pathogenesis of infections due to GNB is in its infancy (Chap. 114).

The ability to induce septic shock is another defining feature of these genera. GNB are the most common causes of this potentially lethal syndrome. The lipid A moiety of LPS (via interaction with host Toll-like receptor 4) and probably other bacterial factors as well stimulate a proinflammatory host response that, if overly exuberant, results in shock (Chap. 265).

Many antigenic variants (serotypes) exist in most genera of GNB. For example, there are >150 O-specific antigens and >80 capsular antigens in *E. coli*. This antigenic variability, which permits immune evasion and allows recurrent infection by different strains of the same species, has impeded vaccine development (Chap. 116).

INFECTIOUS SYNDROMES

Although certain strains of *E. coli* have evolved to be strictly intestinal pathogens, causing gastroenteritis by a variety of unique pathogenic mechanisms, extraintestinal infections are the predominant presentation of disease caused by enteric GNB. Depending on both the host and the pathogen, nearly every organ or body cavity can be infected with GNB. *E. coli* and—to a lesser degree—*Klebsiella* and *Proteus* account for most extraintestinal infections due to GNB and are the most virulent pathogens of this group. However, the other genera are becoming increasingly important, particularly among LTCF residents and hospitalized patients. This expanding role is due in large part to the intrinsic or acquired antimicrobial resistance of these organisms and the increasing number of individuals with alterations or disruptions of host defenses. The mortality rate is significant in many GNB infections and correlates with the severity of illness. Especially problematic are pneumonia and bacteremia (arising from any source) when complicated by organ failure (severe sepsis) and/or shock; associated mortality rates are 20–50%.

DIAGNOSIS

Isolation of GNB from ordinarily sterile anatomic sites almost always implies infection, whereas their isolation from nonsterile sites, particularly from open soft-tissue wounds and the respiratory tract, requires clinical correlation to differentiate colonization from infection. Tentative laboratory identification based on lactose fermentation and indole

TABLE 143-1 INTERACTIONS OF EXTRAINTESTINAL PATHOGENIC *E. COLI* WITH THE HUMAN HOST: A PARADIGM FOR EXTRACELLULAR, EXTRAINTESTINAL GRAM-NEGATIVE BACTERIAL PATHOGENS

Bacterial Goal	Host Obstacle	Bacterial Solution
Extraintestinal attachment	Flow of urine, mucociliary blanket	Multiple adhesins (e.g., type 1 fimbriae, Sfa/Foc, P pili)
Nutrient acquisition for growth	Nutrient sequestration (e.g., iron via intracellular storage and extracellular scavenging via lactoferrin and transferrin)	Cellular lysis (e.g., hemolysin); multiple mechanisms for competing for extracellular iron (e.g., siderophores) and other nutrients
Initial avoidance of host bactericidal activity	Complement, phagocytic cells, antimicrobial peptides	Capsular polysaccharide, lipopolysaccharide
Transmission	?	Irritant tissue damage resulting in increased excretion (e.g., toxins such as hemolysin)
Late avoidance of host bactericidal activity	Acquired immunity (e.g., specific antibodies), treatment with antibiotics	? Cell entry, acquisition of antimicrobial resistance

production (described for each genus below), which usually is possible before final identification of the organism and determination of its antimicrobial susceptibilities, may guide empirical antimicrobial therapy.

Rx INFECTIONS CAUSED BY GRAM-NEGATIVE ENTERIC BACILLI

(See also Chap. 127) Accumulating evidence indicates that initiation of appropriate empirical antimicrobial therapy early in the course of GNB infections (particularly serious infections) leads to improved outcomes. Familiarity with evolving patterns of antimicrobial resistance in enteric GNB is necessary in the selection of appropriate empirical therapy. The antimicrobial resistance profiles of GNB vary by species, geographic location, regional antimicrobial use, and hospital site [e.g., intensive care units (ICUs) versus wards]. At present, the most reliably active agents against enteric GNB are the carbapenems (e.g., imipenem), the aminoglycoside amikacin, the fourth-generation cephalosporin cefepime, and piperacillin-tazobactam.

β-Lactamases, which inactivate β-lactam agents, are the most important mediators of resistance to these drugs in GNB. Decreased permeability and/or active efflux of β-lactam agents, although less common, may occur alone or in combination with β-lactamase-mediated resistance. *Broad-spectrum* β-lactamases, which mediate resistance to many penicillins and first-generation cephalosporins, are frequently expressed in enteric GNB. These enzymes are inhibited by agents such as clavulanate. *Extended-spectrum* β-lactamases (ESBLs) confer resistance to the same drugs as broad-spectrum β-lactamases as well as to third-generation cephalosporins, aztreonam, and (in some instances) fourth-generation cephalosporins.

The acquisition of ESBL-encoding genes via transferable plasmids is increasing in GNB worldwide, with rates varying greatly even among hospitals in a given region. To date, ESBLs are most prevalent in *Klebsiella pneumoniae*, *K. oxytoca*, and *E. coli* but also occur (and are probably underrecognized) in *Enterobacter*, *Citrobacter*, *Proteus*, *Serratia*, and other enteric GNB. At present, the regional prevalence of ESBL-producing GNB declines in rank order as follows: Latin America > Western Pacific > Europe > United States and Canada. ESBL-producing GNB are most prevalent in hospitals (ICUs > wards) but recently have emerged in the community. Hospital outbreaks due to ESBL-producing strains have been associated with extensive use of third-generation cephalosporins, particularly ceftazidime. The carbapenems are the most reliably active β-lactam agents against ESBL-expressing strains. GNB that express ESBLs may also possess porin mutations that result in decreased uptake of cephalosporins and β-lactam/β-lactamase inhibitor combinations. Thus, ESBL-producing isolates should be considered resistant to all penicillins, cephalosporins, and aztreonam.

AmpC β-lactamases confer resistance to the same substrates as ESBLs plus the cephamycins, a subset of the second-generation cephalosporins. AmpC enzymes resist inhibition by β-lactamase inhibitors. Constitutive chromosomal AmpC β-lactamases are present in nearly all strains of *Enterobacter*, *Serratia*, *Citrobacter*, *Proteus vulgaris*, *Providencia*, *Morganella*, and *Acinetobacter*, resulting in resistance to aminopenicillins, cefazolin, and cefoxitin. In addition, some strains of *E. coli*, *K. pneumoniae*, and other Enterobacteriaceae have acquired plasmids containing AmpC β-lactamase genes. The fourth-generation cephalosporin cefepime is stable to AmpC β-lactamases and is an appropriate treatment option if the concomitant presence of an ESBL can be excluded.

Carbapenemases confer resistance to the same drugs as ESBLs plus cephamycins and carbapenems. At present, carbapenemase-producing enteric GNB are uncommon. In the United States, strains of *Klebsiella* and *Enterobacter* that possess carbapenemases on transferable plasmids and exhibit resistance to fluoroquinolones and aminoglycosides have been found. Tigecycline (a glycylcycline, a new antimicrobial class) and the polymyxins (agents of last resort, given their potential toxicities) are the most active drugs in vitro, but their clinical efficacy has not been demonstrated.

Resistance to fluoroquinolones usually is due to alterations of the target site (DNA gyrase and/or topoisomerase IV), with or without decreased permeability, active efflux, or protection of the target site. Resistance to fluoroquinolones is increasingly prevalent among GNB; 20–80% of ESBL-producing enteric GNB are also resistant to fluoroquinolones. At present, this drug class should be considered unreliable as empirical therapy for infections due to GNB in critically ill patients.

Not all clinical laboratories screen for ESBLs, screening protocols are limited, and no recommended tests identify AmpC β-lactamases or carbapenemases. For these reasons, these resistance mechanisms are underreported, and it is important to assess the clinical response to treatment in addition to in vitro susceptibility data.

Given the increasing prevalence of multidrug resistance in enteric GNB, it is reasonable—pending susceptibility results—to combine agents for empirical treatment of GNB infections in critically ill patients. Although supporting clinical evidence is limited, combination therapy may increase antimicrobial efficacy and/or diminish the emergence of resistance in some circumstances. In addition, drainage of abscesses and removal of infected foreign bodies are often required for cure.

GNB are commonly involved in polymicrobial infections, in which the role of each specific pathogen is uncertain (Chap. 157). Although some GNB are more pathogenic than others, it is usually prudent, if possible, to design an antimicrobial regimen active against all of the GNB identified, since each is capable of pathogenicity in its own right.

PREVENTION

(See also Chap. 125) Diligent adherence to hand-hygiene protocols by health care personnel and avoidance of inappropriate antimicrobial use are key measures in preventing infection and the further development of antimicrobial resistance. Likewise, avoidance of the use of indwelling devices that predispose to infections due to GNB (e.g., urinary and intravascular catheters, endotracheal tubes) decreases infection risk.

ESCHERICHIA COLI INFECTIONS

COMMENSAL STRAINS

For the most part, commensal *E. coli* variants, which constitute the bulk of the normal facultative intestinal flora in most humans, confer benefits to the host (e.g., resistance to colonization with pathogenic organisms). These strains generally lack the specialized virulence traits that enable extraintestinal and intestinal pathogenic *E. coli* strains to cause disease outside and within the gastrointestinal tract, respectively. However, even commensal *E. coli* strains can be involved in extraintestinal infections in the presence of an aggravating factor, such as a foreign body (e.g., a urinary catheter), host compromise (e.g., local anatomic or functional abnormalities such as urinary or biliary tract obstruction or systemic immunocompromise), or an inoculum that is large or contains a mixture of bacterial species (e.g., fecal contamination of the peritoneal cavity).

EXTRAINTESTINAL PATHOGENIC (ExPEC) STRAINS

The majority of *E. coli* isolates from symptomatic infections of the urinary tract, bloodstream, cerebrospinal fluid, respiratory tract, and peritoneum (spontaneous bacterial peritonitis) can be differentiated from commensal and intestinal pathogenic strains of *E. coli* by virtue of their distinctive virulence factor profiles (Tables 143-1 and 143-2) and phylogenetic background. ExPEC strains can also cause surgical wound infection, osteomyelitis, and myositis, but the number of cases evaluated to date is too small for a reliable assessment of proportions.

Like commensal *E. coli* (but in contrast to intestinal pathogenic *E. coli*), ExPEC strains are often found in the normal intestinal flora and do not cause gastroenteritis in humans. Although acquisition of an ExPEC strain by the host is a prerequisite for ExPEC infection, it is not the rate-limiting step, which instead is entry of an ExPEC strain from its site of colonization (e.g., the colon, vagina, or oropharynx) into a normally sterile extraintestinal site (e.g., the urinary tract, peritoneal cavity, or lungs). ExPEC strains have acquired genes encoding diverse extraintestinal virulence factors that enable the bacteria to cause infections outside the gastrointestinal tract in both normal and compromised hosts (Table 143-1). These virulence genes are, for the most part, distinct from those that enable intestinal pathogenic strains to cause diarrheal disease. All age groups, all types of hosts, and nearly all organs and anatomic sites are susceptible to infection by ExPEC. Previously healthy hosts infected with ExPEC can become severely ill or die; however, adverse outcomes are more prevalent in the presence of comorbid illnesses and host defense abnormalities. *E. coli* is the most

TABLE 143-2 INTESTINAL PATHOGENIC *E. COLI*

Pathotype[a]	Epidemiology	Clinical Syndrome[b]	Defining Molecular Trait	Responsible Genetic Element[c]
STEC	Food, water, person-to-person; all ages, industrialized countries	Hemorrhagic colitis, hemolytic-uremic syndrome	Shiga toxin	Lambda-like Stx1- or Stx2-encoding bacteriophage
ETEC	Food, water; young children in and travelers to developing countries	Traveler's diarrhea	Heat-stable and -labile enterotoxins, colonization factors	Virulence plasmid(s)
EPEC	Person-to-person; young children and neonates in developing countries	Watery diarrhea	Localized adherence, attaching and effacing lesion on intestinal epithelium	EPEC adherence factor plasmid pathogenicity island (locus for enterocyte effacement)
EIEC	Food, water; children in and travelers to developing countries	Dysentery	Invasion of colonic epithelial cells, intracellular multiplication, cell-to-cell spread	Multiple genes contained primarily in large virulence plasmid
EAEC	? Food, water; children in and travelers to developing countries; all ages, industrialized countries	Traveler's diarrhea, acute diarrhea, persistent diarrhea	Aggregative/diffuse adherence, virulence factors regulated by AggR	Chromosomal or plasmid-associated adherence and toxin genes

[a]STEC, Shiga toxin–producing *E. coli*; ETEC, enterotoxigenic *E. coli*; EPEC, enteropathogenic *E. coli*; EIEC, enteroinvasive *E. coli*; EAEC, enteroaggregative *E. coli*.
[b]Classic syndromes; see text for details on spectrum of disease.
[c]Pathogenesis is multigenic, including genes in addition to those listed.

common enteric gram-negative species to cause extraintestinal infection in ambulatory, LTCF, and hospital settings. The diversity and the medical and economic impact of ExPEC infections are evident from consideration of the following specific syndromes.

Extraintestinal Infectious Syndromes • ***URINARY TRACT INFECTION (UTI)*** The urinary tract is the site most frequently infected by ExPEC. An exceedingly common infection among ambulatory patients, UTI accounts for 1% of ambulatory care visits in the United States and is second only to lower respiratory tract infection among infections responsible for hospitalization. UTIs are best considered by clinical syndrome (e.g., uncomplicated cystitis, pyelonephritis, and catheter-associated UTIs) and within the context of specific hosts (e.g., premenopausal women, compromised hosts; Chap. 282). *E. coli* is the single most common pathogen for all UTI syndrome/host group combinations. Each year in the United States, *E. coli* causes 85–95% of an estimated 6–8 million episodes of uncomplicated cystitis in premenopausal women, with an estimated $1 billion in direct health care costs. Furthermore, 20% of women with an initial cystitis episode develop frequent recurrences (from 0.3 to >20 per year).

Uncomplicated cystitis, the most common acute UTI syndrome, is characterized by dysuria, frequency, and suprapubic pain. Fever and/or back pain suggests progression to pyelonephritis. Fever may take 5–7 days to resolve completely in appropriately treated patients with pyelonephritis. Persistently elevated or increasing fever and neutrophil counts should prompt evaluation for intrarenal or perinephric abscess and/or obstruction. Renal parenchymal damage and loss of renal function during pyelonephritis occur primarily with urinary obstruction. Pregnant women are at unusually high risk for developing pyelonephritis, which can adversely affect the outcome of pregnancy. As a result, prenatal screening for and treatment of asymptomatic bacteriuria are standard. Prostatic infection is a potential complication of UTI in men. The diagnosis and treatment of UTI, as detailed in Chap. 282, should be tailored to the individual host, the nature and site of infection, and local patterns of antimicrobial susceptibility.

ABDOMINAL AND PELVIC INFECTION The abdomen/pelvis is the second most common site of extraintestinal infection due to *E. coli*. A wide variety of clinical syndromes occur in this location, including acute peritonitis secondary to fecal contamination, spontaneous bacterial peritonitis, dialysis-associated peritonitis, diverticulitis, appendicitis, intraperitoneal or visceral abscesses (hepatic, pancreatic, splenic), infected pancreatic pseudocysts, and septic cholangitis and/or cholecystitis. In intraabdominal infections, *E. coli* can be isolated either alone or (as is often the case) along with other facultative and/or anaerobic members of the intestinal flora (Chap. 121).

PNEUMONIA *E. coli* is not usually considered a cause of pneumonia (Chap. 251). Indeed, enteric GNB account for only 2–5% of cases of community-acquired pneumonia (CAP), in part because these organisms only transiently colonize the oropharynx of a minority of healthy individuals. However, rates of oral colonization with *E. coli* and other GNB increase with the severity of illness and with antibiotic use. Thus, GNB are a common cause of pneumonia among residents of LTCFs and are the most common cause (60–70% of cases) of hospital-acquired pneumonia (Chap. 125), particularly among postoperative and intensive care patients. Pulmonary infection is usually acquired by small-volume aspiration but occasionally occurs via hematogenous spread, in which case multifocal nodular infiltrates can be seen. Tissue necrosis, probably due to cytotoxins produced by GNB, is common. Despite significant institutional variation, *E. coli* is generally the third or fourth most commonly isolated gram-negative bacillus in hospital-acquired pneumonia, accounting for 5–8% of episodes in both U.S.-based and European-based studies. Regardless of the host, pneumonia due to enteric GNB is a serious disease, with high crude and attributable mortality rates (20–60% and 10–20%, respectively).

MENINGITIS (See also Chap. 376) *E. coli* is one of the two leading causes of neonatal meningitis (the other being group B *Streptococcus*). Most of the responsible strains possess the K1 capsular antigen. After the first month of life, *E. coli* meningitis is uncommon, occurring predominantly in the setting of disruption of the meninges from craniotomy or trauma or in the presence of cirrhosis. In patients with cirrhosis, the meninges are presumably seeded as a result of poor hepatic clearance of portal vein bacteremia.

CELLULITIS/MUSCULOSKELETAL INFECTION *E. coli* contributes frequently to infection of decubitus ulcers and occasionally to infection of ulcers and wounds of the lower extremity in diabetic patients and other hosts with neurovascular compromise. Osteomyelitis secondary to contiguous spread can occur in these settings. In addition, *E. coli* occasionally causes cellulitis or infections of burn sites or surgical wounds, particularly when the infection originates close to the perineum. Hematogenously acquired osteomyelitis, particularly of vertebral bodies, is more commonly caused by *E. coli* than is generally appreciated; this organism accounts for up to 10% of cases in some series (Chap. 120). *E. coli* occasionally causes orthopedic device–associated infection or septic arthritis and rarely causes hematogenous myositis. Upper-leg myositis or fasciitis due to *E. coli* should prompt an evaluation for an abdominal source with contiguous spread.

ENDOVASCULAR INFECTION Despite being one of the most common causes of bacteremia, *E. coli* rarely seeds native or prosthetic heart valves. When the organism does seed native valves, it usually does so in the setting of prior valve disease. *E. coli* infections of aneurysms and vascular grafts are quite uncommon.

MISCELLANEOUS INFECTIONS *E. coli* can cause infection in nearly every organ and anatomic site. It occasionally causes postoperative mediastinitis or complicated sinusitis and uncommonly causes endophthalmitis or brain abscess.

BACTEREMIA *E. coli* bacteremia can arise from primary infection at any extraintestinal site. In addition, primary *E. coli* bacteremia can arise from percutaneous intravascular devices or transrectal prostate biopsy or can result from the increased intestinal mucosal permeability seen in neonates and in the settings of neutropenia and chemotherapy-induced mucositis, trauma, and burns. Roughly equal proportions of *E. coli* bacteremia cases originate in the community and in the hospital. In most studies, *E. coli* and *Staphylococcus aureus* are the two most common blood isolates of clinical significance; *E. coli*, which is isolated in 17–37% of cases, is the gram-negative bacillus most often isolated from the blood in the ambulatory setting and in most LTCF and hospital settings. Isolation of *E. coli* from the blood is almost always clinically significant and typically is accompanied by the sepsis syndrome, severe sepsis (sepsis-induced dysfunction of at least one organ or system), or septic shock (Chap. 265). Calculations based on a conservative estimate for the proportional contribution of *E. coli* to severe sepsis (i.e., 17% of all cases) translate into an estimated 40,000 deaths among the affected patients in the United States in 2001.

The urinary tract is the most common source of *E. coli* bacteremia, accounting for one-half to two-thirds of episodes. Bacteremia from a urinary tract source is particularly common in patients with pyelonephritis, urinary tract obstruction, or instrumentation in the presence of infected urine. The abdomen is the second most common source, accounting for 25% of episodes. Although biliary obstruction (stones, tumor) and overt bowel disruption are responsible for many of these cases, some abdominal sources (e.g., abscesses) are remarkably silent clinically and require identification via imaging studies (e.g., CT). Therefore, the physician should be cautious in designating the urinary tract as the source of *E. coli* bacteremia in the absence of characteristic signs and symptoms of UTI. Soft tissue, bone, pulmonary, and intravascular catheter infections are other sources of *E. coli* bacteremia.

Diagnosis Strains of *E. coli* that cause extraintestinal infections usually grow both aerobically and anaerobically within 24 h on standard diagnostic media and are easily identified by the clinical microbiology laboratory according to routine biochemical criteria. More than 90% of ExPEC strains are rapid lactose fermenters and are indole positive.

℞ EXTRAINTESTINAL *E. COLI* INFECTIONS

In the past, most *E. coli* isolates were highly susceptible to a broad range of antimicrobial agents. Unfortunately, this situation has changed. In general, the frequency of ampicillin resistance precludes its empirical use, even in community-acquired infections. The prevalence of resistance to first-generation cephalosporins and trimethoprim-sulfamethoxazole (TMP-SMX) is increasing among community-acquired strains in the United States (with current rates of 10–40%) and is even higher outside North America. Until recently, TMP-SMX was the drug of choice for the treatment of uncomplicated cystitis in many locales. Although continued empirical use of TMP-SMX will predictably result in ever-diminishing cure rates, a wholesale switch to alternative agents (e.g., fluoroquinolones) will just as predictably accelerate the widespread emergence of resistance to these antimicrobial classes, as is already occurring in some areas. Resistance to fluoroquinolones has increased steadily over the last decade; in 2002–2005, prevalence rates were 5–20% in North America and even higher in other regions. The prevalence of resistance is higher in settings where fluoroquinolone prophylaxis is used extensively (e.g., in patients with leukemia, transplant recipients, and patients with cirrhosis) and among isolates from LTCFs and hospitals. Among quinolone-resistant strains, a significant (30–40%) prevalence of co-resistance to amoxicillin/clavulanic acid and piperacillin has been reported. The prevalence of co-resistance to more advanced cephalosporins (second-, third-, and fourth-generation), monobactams (e.g., aztreonam), piperacillin-tazobactam, and the non-amikacin aminoglycosides is increasing but is still generally <10%. Carbapenems (e.g., imipenem) and amikacin are the most predictably active agents. Although relevant clinical experience is limited, tigecycline and polymyxin B (the agent of last resort because of its potential toxicities) are highly active in vitro.

INTESTINAL PATHOGENIC STRAINS

Certain strains of *E. coli* are capable of causing diarrheal disease. Other important intestinal pathogens are discussed in Chaps. 122, 135, and 146–149. At least in the industrialized world, intestinal pathogenic strains of *E. coli* are rarely encountered in the fecal flora of healthy persons and instead appear to be essentially obligate pathogens. These strains have evolved a special ability to cause enteritis, enterocolitis, and colitis when ingested in sufficient quantities by a naive host. At least five distinct pathotypes of intestinal pathogenic *E. coli* exist: (1) Shiga toxin–producing *E. coli* (STEC)/enterohemorrhagic *E. coli* (EHEC), (2) enterotoxigenic *E. coli* (ETEC), (3) enteropathogenic *E. coli* (EPEC), (4) enteroinvasive *E. coli* (EIEC), and (5) enteroaggregative *E. coli* (EAEC). Diffusely adherent *E. coli* (DAEC) and cytodetaching *E. coli* are additional putative pathotypes. Transmission occurs predominantly via contaminated food and water for ETEC, STEC, EIEC, and probably EAEC and by person-to-person spread for EPEC (and occasionally STEC/EHEC). Gastric acidity confers some protection against infection; therefore, persons with decreased stomach acid levels are especially susceptible. Humans are the major reservoir (except for STEC/EHEC); host range appears to be dictated by species-specific attachment factors. Although there is some overlap, each pathotype possesses a unique combination of virulence traits that results in a distinctive intestinal pathogenic mechanism (Table 143-2). These strains are largely incapable of causing disease outside the intestinal tract. Except in the case of STEC/EHEC and perhaps EAEC, disease due to this group of pathogens occurs primarily in developing countries.

Shiga Toxin–Producing and Enterohemorrhagic *E. coli* STEC/EHEC strains constitute an emerging group of pathogens that can cause hemorrhagic colitis and the hemolytic-uremic syndrome (HUS). Several large outbreaks resulting from the consumption of undercooked ground beef and other foods (e.g., fresh spinach) have received significant media attention. O157:H7 is the most prominent serotype, but serogroups O6, O26, O55, O91, O103, O111, O113, and OX3 have also been associated with these syndromes. The ability of STEC/EHEC to produce Shiga toxin (Stx2 and/or Stx1) or related toxins is a critical factor in the expression of clinical disease. *Shigella dysenteriae* strains that produce the closely related Shiga toxin Stx can cause the same syndrome. Stx2 appears to be more important than Stx1 in the development of HUS. All Shiga toxins studied to date are multimers composing one enzymatically active A subunit and five identical B subunits that mediate binding to globoceramides. The A subunit cleaves an adenine from the host cell's 28S rRNA, thereby irreversibly inhibiting ribosomal function. Therefore, Shiga toxins belong to the class of toxins known as *ribosome-inactivating proteins*.

Additional factors, such as acid tolerance and adherence, are necessary for full pathogenicity among STEC strains. Most disease-causing isolates possess the genomic locus for enterocyte effacement (LEE). This pathogenicity island was first described in EPEC strains and contains genes that mediate adherence to intestinal epithelial cells. EHEC strains make up the subgroup of STEC strains that possess stx_1 and/or stx_2 as well as LEE.

Domesticated ruminant animals, particularly cattle and young calves, serve as the major reservoir for STEC/EHEC. Ground beef—the most common food source of STEC/EHEC strains—is often contaminated during processing. Furthermore, manure from cattle or other animals that is used as fertilizer can contaminate produce (potatoes, lettuce, spinach, sprouts, fallen apples), and fecal runoff from this source can contaminate water. It is estimated that $<10^3$ CFU of STEC/

EHEC can cause disease. Therefore, not only can low levels of food or environmental contamination (e.g., in water swallowed while swimming) result in disease, but person-to-person transmission (e.g., at day-care centers and in institutions) is an important route for secondary spread. Laboratory-associated infections also take place. Illness due to this group of pathogens occurs both as outbreaks and as sporadic cases, with a peak incidence in the summer months.

In contrast to other intestinal pathotypes, STEC/EHEC causes infections more frequently in industrialized countries than in developing regions. O157:H7 strains are the fourth most commonly reported cause of bacterial diarrhea in the United States (after *Campylobacter*, *Salmonella*, and *Shigella*). Colonization of the colon and perhaps the ileum results in symptoms after an incubation period of 3 or 4 days. Colonic edema and an initial secretory diarrhea may develop into the STEC/EHEC hallmark syndrome of grossly bloody diarrhea (as detected by history or examination) in >90% of cases. Significant abdominal pain and fecal leukocytes are common (70% of cases), whereas fever is not; a lack of fever often results in diagnostic consideration of noninfectious conditions (e.g., intussusception and inflammatory or ischemic bowel disease). Occasionally, infections caused by *Clostridium difficile*, *Campylobacter*, and *Salmonella* present in a similar fashion. STEC/EHEC disease is usually self-limited, lasting 5–10 days. This infection can be complicated by HUS, which occurs 2–14 days after diarrhea in 2–8% of cases and most often affects very young or elderly patients. It is estimated that >50% of all cases of HUS in the United States are caused by STEC/EHEC. This complication is probably mediated by the systemic translocation of Shiga toxins. Erythrocytes may serve as carriers of Stx to endothelial cells located in the small vessels of the kidney and brain. The subsequent development of thrombotic microangiopathy (perhaps with direct toxin-mediated effects on various nonendothelial cells) commonly produces some combination of fever, thrombocytopenia, renal failure, and encephalopathy. Although the mortality rate with dialysis support is <10%, residual renal and neurologic dysfunction may persist.

Enterotoxigenic *E. coli* In tropical or developing countries, ETEC is a major cause of endemic diarrhea. After weaning, children in these locales commonly experience several episodes of ETEC infection during the first 3 years of life. The incidence of disease diminishes with age, a pattern that correlates with the development of mucosal immunity to colonization factors (i.e., adhesins). In industrialized countries, infection usually follows travel to endemic areas. ETEC is the most common agent of traveler's diarrhea, causing 25–75% of cases. The incidence of infection is decreased by prudent avoidance of potentially contaminated fluids and foods (Chap. 117). ETEC infection is uncommon in the United States, but outbreaks secondary to consumption of food products imported from endemic areas have occurred. A large inoculum (10^6–10^{10} CFU) is needed to produce disease. After ingestion of contaminated water or food (particularly items that are poorly cooked, unpeeled, or unrefrigerated), colonization factor–mediated intestinal adherence occurs over 12–72 h.

Disease is mediated primarily by a heat-labile toxin (LT-1) and/or a heat-stable toxin (STa) that causes net fluid secretion via activation of adenylate cyclase (LT-1) and/or guanylate cyclase (STa) in the jejunum and ileum. The result is watery diarrhea accompanied by cramps. LT-1 consists of an A and a B subunit and is structurally and functionally similar to cholera toxin. Strong binding of the B subunit to the GM_1 ganglioside on intestinal epithelial cells leads to the intracellular translocation of the A subunit, which functions as an ADP-ribosyltransferase. Mature STa is an 18- or 19-amino-acid secreted peptide whose biologic activity is mediated by binding to the guanylate cyclase C found in the brush-border membrane of enterocytes; this binding results in increased intracellular concentrations of cyclic GMP. Characteristically absent are histopathologic changes within the small bowel; mucus, blood, and inflammatory cells in stool; and fever. The disease spectrum ranges from a mild illness to a life-threatening cholera-like syndrome. Although symptoms are usually self-limited (typically lasting for 3 days), infection may result in significant morbidity and mortality when access to health care is limited and when small and/or undernourished children are affected.

Enteropathogenic *E. coli* EPEC causes disease primarily in young children, including neonates. The first *E. coli* pathotype recognized as an agent of diarrheal disease, EPEC was responsible for outbreaks of infantile diarrhea (including some outbreaks in hospital nurseries) in industrialized countries in the 1940s and 1950s. At present, EPEC infection is an uncommon cause of diarrhea in developed countries but is an important cause of diarrhea (both sporadic and epidemic) among infants in developing countries. Breast-feeding diminishes the incidence of EPEC infection. Rapid person-to-person spread may occur. Upon colonization of the small bowel, symptoms develop after a brief incubation period (1 or 2 days). Initial localized adherence leads to a characteristic effacement of microvilli, with the formation of cuplike, actin-rich pedestals. The actual mechanism(s) of diarrhea production are an area of ongoing investigation. Diarrheal stool often contains mucus but not blood. Although usually self-limited (lasting 5–15 days), EPEC diarrhea may persist for weeks.

Enteroinvasive *E. coli* EIEC, a relatively uncommon cause of diarrhea, is rarely identified in the United States, although a few food-related outbreaks have been described. In developing countries, sporadic disease is infrequently recognized in children and travelers. EIEC shares many genetic and clinical features with *Shigella*; however, unlike *Shigella*, EIEC produces disease only at a large inoculum (10^8–10^{10} CFU), with onset generally following an incubation period of 1–3 days. Initially, enterotoxins are believed to induce secretory small-bowel diarrhea. Subsequently, colonization and invasion of the colonic mucosa, followed by replication therein and cell-to-cell spread, result in the development of inflammatory colitis characterized by fever, abdominal pain, tenesmus, and scant stool containing mucus, blood, and inflammatory cells. Symptoms are usually self-limited (7–10 days).

Enteroaggregative and Diffusely Adherent *E. coli* EAEC has been described primarily in developing countries and in young children. However, a recent study indicates that it may be a relatively common cause of diarrhea in all age groups in industrialized countries. EAEC has also been recognized increasingly as an important cause of traveler's diarrhea. A large inoculum is required for infection, which manifests as watery, sometimes prolonged diarrhea. In vitro, the organisms exhibit a diffuse or "stacked-brick" pattern of adherence to epithelial cells. Virulence factors that probably contribute to disease are regulated in part by the transcriptional activator AggR and include the aggregative adherence fimbriae (AAF/I-III) and the enterotoxins Pet, EAST-1, Shet1, and Shet2. Some but not all strains of DAEC are capable of causing diarrheal disease, primarily in children 2–6 years of age in some developing countries. The Afa/Dr adhesins may contribute to the pathogenesis of infection.

Diagnosis A practical approach to the evaluation of diarrhea is to distinguish noninflammatory from inflammatory cases (Chap. 122). ETEC, EPEC, and DAEC are uncommon causes of noninflammatory diarrhea in the United States; EAEC has recently been described as a cause of diarrhea in this country. The diagnosis of these infections requires specialized assays that are not routinely available and whose use is rarely indicated since the diseases are self-limited. ETEC causes the majority and EAEC a minority of cases of noninflammatory traveler's diarrhea. Definitive diagnosis generally is not necessary. Empirical antimicrobial (or symptom-based) treatment, along with rehydration therapy, is a reasonable approach. If diarrhea persists despite treatment, *Giardia* or *Cryptosporidium* (or, in immunocompromised hosts, certain other microbial agents) should be sought. The diagnosis of infection with EIEC, a rare cause of inflammatory diarrhea in the United States, also requires specialized assays. However, evaluation for STEC/EHEC infection, particularly when bloody diarrhea is reported or observed, is appropriate. Although screening for *E. coli* strains that do not ferment sorbitol, with subsequent serotyping for O157, is the most common method currently used to detect STEC/EHEC, testing for Shiga toxins or toxin genes is more sensitive, specific, and rapid. The latter approach offers another advantage as well: it detects both non-O157 STEC/EHEC and sorbitol-fermenting strains of O157:H7, which otherwise are difficult to identify. DNA-based, enzyme-linked immunosorbent, and cytotoxicity assays are in various stages of development and are likely to emerge as the diagnostic standards.

℞ INTESTINAL *E. COLI* INFECTIONS

The mainstay of treatment for all diarrheal syndromes is replacement of water and electrolytes (Chap. 122). The use of prophylactic antibiotics to prevent traveler's diarrhea generally should be discouraged, especially in light of high rates of antimicrobial resistance. However, in selected patients (e.g., those who cannot afford a brief illness or have an increased susceptibility to infection), the use of rifaximin, which is nonabsorbable and well tolerated, is reasonable. When stools are free of mucus and blood, early patient-initiated treatment of traveler's diarrhea with a quinolone or azithromycin decreases the duration of illness, and the use of loperamide may halt symptoms within a few hours (Chap. 122). Although dysentery caused by EIEC is self-limited, treatment hastens the resolution of symptoms, particularly in severe cases. Antimicrobial therapy for STEC/EHEC infection (the presence of which is suggested by bloody diarrhea without fever) should be avoided, since antibiotics may increase the incidence of HUS (possibly via increased production/release of Stx).

KLEBSIELLA INFECTIONS

K. pneumoniae is the most important *Klebsiella* species from a medical standpoint, causing community-acquired, LTCF-acquired, and nosocomial infections. *K. oxytoca* is primarily a pathogen in LTCF and hospital settings. The *K. pneumoniae* subspecies *rhinoscleromatis* and *ozaenae* are usually isolated from patients in tropical climates. *Klebsiella* species are broadly prevalent in the environment and colonize mucosal surfaces of mammals. In healthy humans, *K. pneumoniae* colonization rates are 5–35% in the colon and 1–5% in the oropharynx; the skin is usually colonized only transiently. In LTCFs and hospitals, colonization occurs with *K. oxytoca* as well, and carriage rates are significant among both staff and patients. Person-to-person spread is the predominant mode of acquisition. Classically, *Klebsiella* is associated with CAP, primarily among alcoholics. However, most *Klebsiella* infections now occur in LTCFs and hospitals. *Klebsiella* causes a spectrum of extraintestinal infections similar to that caused by *E. coli*. However, extraintestinal infections due to *Klebsiella* occur at a lower incidence at all sites except the respiratory tract, possibly because of differences in colonization rates and site-specific virulence traits. Antibiotic-resistant strains have been responsible for a number of outbreaks of nosocomial infection in ICUs and neonatal nurseries. The most common clinical syndromes are pneumonia, UTI, abdominal infection, surgical site infection, soft tissue infection, and subsequent bacteremia. *K. pneumoniae* subspecies *rhinoscleromatis* is the causative agent of rhinoscleroma—a granulomatous, slowly progressive (over months to years) infection of the upper respiratory mucosa that causes necrosis and occasional obstruction of the nasal passages. *K. pneumoniae* subspecies *ozaenae* has been implicated in chronic atrophic rhinitis and in rare cases of invasive disease in compromised hosts.

INFECTIOUS SYNDROMES

Pneumonia *K. pneumoniae* causes only a small proportion of cases of CAP (Chap. 251). CAP due to *K. pneumoniae* occurs primarily in hosts with underlying conditions (e.g., alcoholism, diabetes, or chronic lung disease). As in all pneumonias due to enteric GNB, production of purulent sputum and evidence of airspace disease are typically encountered. Presentation with earlier, less extensive infection is more common than the classically described lobar infiltrate with a bulging fissure. Pulmonary necrosis, pleural effusion, and empyema can occur with disease progression. Pulmonary infection is especially common among residents of LTCFs and hospitalized patients because of increased rates of oropharyngeal colonization. Mechanical ventilation is an important risk factor.

UTI *K. pneumoniae* accounts for only 1–2% of UTI episodes among otherwise healthy adults but for 5–17% of episodes of complicated UTI, including infections associated with indwelling bladder catheters.

Abdominal Infection *Klebsiella* causes a spectrum of abdominal infections similar to that caused by *E. coli* but is less frequently isolated from these infections. Recently, however, the incidence of hepatic abscesses caused by *Klebsiella* (the majority due to strains with the K1 capsular serotype) has increased in Taiwan and elsewhere. Diabetes appears to be an important risk factor. Associated bacteremia is common, resulting in metastatic complications (e.g., endophthalmitis and pulmonary, renal, and CNS abscesses).

Other Infections *Klebsiella* cellulitis or soft tissue infection most frequently affects devitalized tissue (e.g., decubitus and diabetic ulcers, burn sites) and immunocompromised hosts. *Klebsiella* causes some cases of surgical site infection, hematogenously derived endophthalmitis (especially that associated with hepatic abscess), and nosocomial sinusitis as well as occasional cases of osteomyelitis contiguous to soft tissue infection, temperate myositis, and meningitis (in the neonatal period or after neurosurgery).

Bacteremia *Klebsiella* infection at any site can produce bacteremia. Infections of the urinary tract, respiratory tract, and abdomen (especially hepatic abscess) each account for 15–30% of *Klebsiella* bacteremias. Intravascular device–related infections account for another 5–15% of episodes and surgical site and miscellaneous infections for the rest. *Klebsiella* is a cause of sepsis in neonates and of bacteremia in neutropenic patients. Like enteric GNB in general, *Klebsiella* rarely causes endocarditis or endovascular infection.

DIAGNOSIS

Klebsiellae are readily isolated and identified in the laboratory. These organisms usually ferment lactose, although the subspecies *rhinoscleromatis* and *ozaenae* are nonfermenters and are indole negative.

℞ *KLEBSIELLA* INFECTIONS

K. pneumoniae and *K. oxytoca* have antibiotic resistance profiles that are largely similar. These species are intrinsically resistant to ampicillin and ticarcillin. Data from the National Nosocomial Infections Surveillance System (NNIS) indicated that 20.6% of ICU patients were infected with strains resistant to third-generation cephalosporins in 2003—a 47% increase over figures for 1998–2002. Even higher rates have been reported outside North America. This increasing resistance is mediated primarily by plasmid-encoded ESBLs. In addition, these plasmids usually encode resistance to aminoglycosides, tetracyclines, and TMP-SMX. Resistance to β-lactam/β-lactamase inhibitor combinations and second-generation cephalosporins independent of ESBL-containing plasmids has also been described with increasing frequency. The prevalence of quinolone resistance is 15–20% overall and 50% in ESBL-containing strains. Given both the undesirability of treating the latter strains with penicillins or cephalosporins and the quinolone resistance often associated with ESBLs, empirical treatment of serious or health care–associated *Klebsiella* infections with amikacin, carbapenems, or tigecycline (to which resistance rates are generally <10% in North America) is prudent. However, clinical experience with tigecycline is limited, and this approach assumes the continued low prevalence of carbapenemases. Polymyxin B can be considered for use against highly resistant strains but is an agent of last resort because of its potential toxicities.

PROTEUS INFECTIONS

P. mirabilis causes 90% of *Proteus* infections, which occur in the community, LTCFs, and hospitals. *P. vulgaris* and *P. penneri* are associated primarily with infections acquired in LTCFs or hospitals. *Proteus* species are part of the colonic flora of a wide variety of mammals, birds, fish, and reptiles. The ability of these GNB to generate histamine from contaminated fish has implicated them in the pathogenesis of scombroid (fish) poisoning (Chap. 391). *P. mirabilis* colonizes healthy humans (prevalence, 50%), whereas *P. vulgaris* and *P. penneri* are isolated primarily from individuals with underlying disease. The urinary tract is by far the most common site of *Proteus* infection, with adhesins, flagella, IgA protease, and urease representing the principal urovirulence factors. *Proteus* less commonly causes infection at a variety of other extraintestinal sites.

INFECTIOUS SYNDROMES

UTI Most *Proteus* infections arise from the urinary tract. *P. mirabilis* causes only 1–2% of cases of UTI in healthy women, and *Proteus* species collectively cause only 5% of cases of hospital-acquired UTI. However, *Proteus* is responsible for 10–15% of cases of complicated UTI, primarily those associated with catheterization; in the setting of long-term catheterization, the prevalence of *Proteus* UTI is 20–45%. This high prevalence is due in part to bacterial production of urease, which hydrolyzes urea to ammonia and results in alkalization of the urine. Alkalization of urine, in turn, leads to precipitation of organic and inorganic compounds, with the formation of struvite and carbonate-apatite crystals, the formation of biofilms on catheters, and/or the development of calculi. *Proteus* becomes associated with the stones and biofilms; thereafter, it usually can be eradicated only by the removal of the stones or the catheter. Over time, staghorn calculi may form and lead to obstruction and renal failure. Thus, urine samples with unexplained alkalinity should be cultured for *Proteus*, and identification of a *Proteus* species should prompt an evaluation for urolithiasis.

Other Infections *Proteus* occasionally causes pneumonia (primarily in LTCF residents or hospitalized patients), nosocomial sinusitis, intraabdominal abscesses, biliary tract infection, surgical site infection, soft tissue infection (especially decubitus and diabetic ulcers), and osteomyelitis (primarily contiguous); in rare cases, it causes temperate myositis. In addition, *Proteus* occasionally causes neonatal meningitis (with the umbilicus often implicated as the source); this disease is often complicated by the development of a cerebral abscess. Otogenic brain abscess also occurs.

Bacteremia The majority of *Proteus* bacteremias originate from the urinary tract; however, any of the less common sites of infection as well as intravascular devices are also potential sources. Endovascular infection is rare. *Proteus* species are occasional agents of sepsis in neonates and of bacteremia in neutropenic patients.

DIAGNOSIS

Proteus is readily isolated and identified in the laboratory. Most strains are lactose negative, produce H_2S, and demonstrate characteristic swarming motility on agar plates. *P. mirabilis* is indole negative, whereas *P. vulgaris* and *P. penneri* are indole positive.

℞ *PROTEUS* INFECTIONS

P. mirabilis is usually susceptible to most antimicrobial agents except tetracycline, polymyxin B, and tigecycline. Resistance to ampicillin and first-generation cephalosporins has been acquired by 10–50% of strains. Overall, 10–15% of *P. mirabilis* isolates are resistant to quinolones; 5% of isolates in the United States now produce ESBLs. *P. vulgaris* and *P. penneri* exhibit more extensive drug resistance than does *P. mirabilis*. Resistance to ampicillin and first-generation cephalosporins is the rule, and 30–40% of isolates are resistant to quinolones. Derepression of an inducible chromosomal AmpC β-lactamase (not present in *P. mirabilis*) occurs in up to 30% of isolates. Imipenem, fourth-generation cephalosporins (e.g., cefepime), amikacin, and TMP-SMX display excellent activity against *Proteus* species (90–100% of isolates susceptible).

ENTEROBACTER INFECTIONS

E. cloacae and *E. aerogenes* are responsible for most *Enterobacter* infections (65–75% and 15–25%, respectively); *E. sakazakii* and *E. gergoviae* are less commonly isolated (1% and <1% of *Enterobacter* isolates, respectively). Enterobacters cause primarily hospital-acquired and other health care–related infections. The organisms are widely prevalent in foods, environmental sources (including equipment at health care facilities), and a wide variety of animals. Few healthy humans are colonized, but the percentage increases significantly in the setting of LTCF residence or hospitalization. Although colonization is an important prelude to infection, direct introduction via IV lines (e.g., contaminated IV fluids or pressure monitors) also occurs. Significant antibiotic resistance has developed in *Enterobacter* species and has contributed to the emergence of the organisms as prominent nosocomial pathogens. Individuals who have previously received antibiotic treatment, have comorbid disease, and are being treated in ICUs are at greatest risk for infection. *Enterobacter* causes a spectrum of extraintestinal infections similar to that described for other GNB.

INFECTIOUS SYNDROMES

Pneumonia, UTI (particularly catheter-related), intravascular device–related infection, surgical site infection, and abdominal infection (primarily postoperative or related to devices such as biliary stents) are the most common syndromes encountered. Nosocomial sinusitis, meningitis related to neurosurgical procedures (including use of pressure monitors), osteomyelitis, and endophthalmitis after eye surgery are less frequent. *E. sakazakii* is associated with neonatal meningitis/sepsis (particularly in premature infants); contaminated formula has been implicated as a source of this infection, which is often complicated by brain abscess or ventriculitis. Bacteremia can result from infection at any of these sites. In *Enterobacter* bacteremia of unclear origin, the contamination of IV fluids or medications, blood components or plasma derivatives, catheter-flushing fluids, pressure monitors, and dialysis equipment should be considered, particularly in an outbreak setting. *Enterobacter* can also cause bacteremia in neutropenic patients. *Enterobacter* endocarditis is rare, occurring primarily in association with illicit IV drug use or prosthetic valves.

DIAGNOSIS

Enterobacter is readily isolated and identified in the laboratory. Most strains are lactose positive and indole negative.

℞ *ENTEROBACTER* INFECTIONS

Significant antimicrobial resistance exists among *Enterobacter* strains. Ampicillin and the first- and second-generation cephalosporins have little or no activity. The extensive use of third-generation cephalosporins has resulted in the selection of strains that are derepressed for production of AmpC β-lactamase, which confers resistance to third-generation cephalosporins, monobactams (e.g., aztreonam), and (frequently) β-lactam/β-lactamase inhibitor combinations. Resistance may emerge during therapy; in one study, the emergence of resistance was documented in 20% of patients. Resistance should be considered a possibility when clinical deterioration follows initial improvement, and third-generation cephalosporins should be avoided in the treatment of serious *Enterobacter* infections. NNIS data for 2003 identified resistance to third-generation cephalosporins in 31% of ICU isolates. Cefepime is stable, even in the presence of AmpC β-lactamases; thus, it is a suitable option for treatment of *Enterobacter* infections in the absence of a coexistent ESBL. However, the prevalence of ESBL production in *Enterobacter* (particularly in *E. cloacae*) has been increasing and is now 5–30%. Such strains are challenging to treat. Fortunately, in the United States, imipenem, amikacin, and quinolones have generally retained excellent activity (90–99% of isolates susceptible). Although clinical experience is limited, tigecycline is highly active in vitro.

SERRATIA INFECTIONS

S. marcescens causes the majority of *Serratia* infections (>90%), and *S. liquefaciens* is isolated occasionally. Serratiae are found primarily in the environment (including in health care institutions), particularly in moist foci. Although serratiae have been isolated from a variety of animals, healthy humans are rarely colonized. In LTCFs or hospitals, reservoirs for the organisms include health care personnel, food, milk (neonatal units), sinks, respiratory equipment, pressure monitors, IV solutions, multiply accessed medication vials, blood products (e.g., platelets), lotions, irrigation solutions, and even disinfectants. Infection results from either direct inoculation (e.g., via IV fluid) or colonization (primarily of the respiratory tract) and subsequent infection. Sporadic infection is most common, but epidemics and common-source outbreaks occasionally occur. The spectrum of extraintestinal infections caused by *Serratia* is similar to that for other GNB. *Serratia* species account for 1–3% of hospital-acquired infections.

INFECTIOUS SYNDROMES

The respiratory tract, the genitourinary tract, intravascular devices, and surgical wounds are the most common sites of *Serratia* infection and sources of *Serratia* bacteremia. Soft tissue infections (including myositis), osteomyelitis, abdominal and biliary tract infection (post-procedural), contact lens–associated keratitis, endophthalmitis, septic arthritis (primarily from intraarticular injections), and infusion-related bacteremias occur less commonly. Serratiae are uncommon causes of neonatal or postsurgical meningitis and of bacteremia in neutropenic patients. Endocarditis is rare.

DIAGNOSIS

Serratiae are readily cultured and identified by the laboratory and are usually lactose and indole negative. Some *S. marcescens* strains are red-pigmented.

Rx *SERRATIA* INFECTIONS

Most *Serratia* strains (>80%) are resistant to ampicillin, first-generation cephalosporins, and polymyxin B. Derepression of inducible chromosomal AmpC β-lactamases may be preexistent or may develop during therapy. Both in the United States and globally, the prevalence of ESBL-producing isolates is <5%. In general, >90% of *Serratia* isolates are susceptible to other GNB-appropriate antibiotics.

CITROBACTER INFECTIONS

C. freundii and *C. koseri* cause most human *Citrobacter* infections, which are epidemiologically and clinically similar to *Enterobacter* infections. *Citrobacter* species are commonly present in water, food, soil, and certain animals. *Citrobacter* is part of the normal fecal flora in a minority of healthy humans, but colonization rates increase in LTCFs and hospitals—the settings in which nearly all infections occur. *Citrobacter* species account for 1–2% of nosocomial infections. The affected hosts are usually immunocompromised or have comorbid disease. *Citrobacter* causes extraintestinal infections similar to those described for other GNB.

INFECTIOUS SYNDROMES

The urinary tract accounts for 40–50% of *Citrobacter* infections. Less commonly involved sites include the biliary tree (particularly with stones or obstruction), the respiratory tract, surgical sites, soft tissue (e.g., decubitus ulcers), the peritoneum, and intravascular devices. Osteomyelitis (usually from a contiguous focus), neurosurgery-related infection, and myositis occur rarely. *Citrobacter* (particularly *C. koseri*) also uncommonly causes neonatal meningitis, with brain abscess complicating 50–80% of cases. Bacteremia is most often due to UTI, biliary or abdominal infection, or intravascular device infection. *Citrobacter* uncommonly causes bacteremia in neutropenic patients. Endocarditis and endovascular infections are rare.

DIAGNOSIS

Citrobacter species are readily isolated and identified; 35–50% of isolates are lactose positive. *C. freundii* is indole negative, whereas *C. koseri* is indole positive.

Rx *CITROBACTER* INFECTIONS

C. freundii is more resistant to antibiotics than is *C. koseri*. Ampicillin and the first- and second-generation cephalosporins display poor activity. *Citrobacter* species possess inducible AmpC β-lactamases; derepression may be preexistent or may develop during therapy. Resistance to antipseudomonal penicillins, aztreonam, quinolones, gentamicin, and third-generation cephalosporins is variable but increasing. Combination with β-lactamase inhibitors usually does not increase the susceptibility of *Citrobacter* to β-lactam agents. The prevalence of ESBL-producing isolates is <5%. Imipenem, amikacin, cefepime, tigecycline (with which there is limited clinical experience), and polymyxin B (the agent of last resort because of potential toxicities) are most active, with >90% of strains susceptible.

MORGANELLA AND *PROVIDENCIA* INFECTIONS

M. morganii, *P. stuartii*, and (less frequently) *P. rettgeri* are the members of their respective genera that cause human infections. In terms of epidemiologic associations, pathogenic properties, and clinical manifestations, these organisms are largely similar to *Proteus* species; however, *Morganella* and *Providencia* occur almost exclusively among LTCF residents; to a lesser degree, they affect hospitalized patients.

INFECTIOUS SYNDROMES

These species are primarily urinary tract pathogens, causing UTIs that are most often associated with long-term (>30-day) catheterization. Such infections often lead to biofilm formation and catheter encrustation (sometimes causing catheter obstruction) or to the development of struvite bladder or renal stones (sometimes causing renal obstruction and serving as foci for relapse). Other, less common infectious syndromes include surgical site infection, soft tissue infection (primarily involving decubitus and diabetic ulcers), burn site infection, pneumonia (particularly ventilator-associated), intravascular device infection, and intraabdominal infection. Rarely, the other extraintestinal infections described for GNB also occur. Bacteremia is uncommon; although any infected site can serve as the source, the urinary tract accounts for most cases, and the next most common sources are surgical sites and soft tissues.

DIAGNOSIS

M. morganii and *Providencia* are readily isolated and identified. Nearly all isolates are indole positive but are unable to ferment lactose.

Rx *MORGANELLA* AND *PROVIDENCIA* INFECTIONS

Morganella and *Providencia* may be extensively resistant to antibiotics. Most isolates are resistant to ampicillin, first-generation cephalosporins, tigecycline, and polymyxin B; 40% are resistant to quinolones. *Morganella* and *Providencia* possess inducible AmpC β-lactamases; derepression may be preexistent or may develop during therapy. Resistance to antipseudomonal penicillins, aztreonam, gentamicin, TMP-SMX, and the second- and third-generation cephalosporins is emerging but variable. The β-lactamase inhibitor tazobactam increases susceptibility to β-lactam agents, but sulbactam and clavulanic acid do not. Imipenem, amikacin, and cefepime are the most active agents (>90% of isolates susceptible). Removal of an infected catheter or stone may be critical for eradication of UTI.

EDWARDSIELLA INFECTIONS

E. tarda is the only member of the genus *Edwardsiella* that is associated with human disease. This organism is found predominantly in freshwater and marine environments and among the animals associated with these settings. Human acquisition occurs primarily during interaction with these reservoirs. *E. tarda* infection is rare in the United States; recently reported cases are mostly from Southeast Asia. This pathogen shares clinical features with both *Salmonella* species and *Vibrio vulnificus*.

INFECTIOUS SYNDROMES

Gastroenteritis is the predominant infectious syndrome (50–80% of infections). Self-limiting watery diarrhea is most common, but severe colitis also occurs. The most common extraintestinal infection is wound infection due to direct inoculation, which is often associated with freshwater-, marine-, or snake-related injuries. Other infectious syndromes result from invasion of the gastrointestinal tract and subsequent bacteremia. Most afflicted hosts have comorbidities (e.g., hepatobiliary disease or iron overload, cancer, or diabetes mellitus). A primary bacteremic syndrome, sometimes complicated by meningitis, has a 40% case-fatality rate. Visceral (primarily hepatic) and intraperitoneal abscesses also occur.

DIAGNOSIS

Although *E. tarda* can readily be isolated and identified, most laboratories do not routinely seek to identify it in stool samples.

℞ *EDWARDSIELLA* INFECTIONS

E. tarda is susceptible to most antimicrobial agents appropriate for use against GNB. Gastroenteritis is generally self-limiting, but treatment with a quinolone may hasten resolution. In the setting of severe sepsis, quinolones, third- or fourth-generation cephalosporins, imipenem, and amikacin—either alone or in combination—are the safest choices pending susceptibility information.

ACINETOBACTER INFECTIONS

The *A. baumannii-calcoaceticus* complex is responsible for most *Acinetobacter* infections. *Acinetobacter* is highly prevalent in the environment, being found in most water and soil samples. Whereas *Acinetobacter* has only occasionally been cultured from the moist skin of healthy humans, colonization of the skin and the respiratory and gastrointestinal tracts is common among residents of LTCFs and hospitalized patients. It is not surprising that the overwhelming majority of *Acinetobacter* infections are acquired in LTCFs and hospitals, where the sources for acquisition include health care personnel, medical equipment, food, and the environment. The spectrum of extraintestinal infections caused by *Acinetobacter* is similar to that caused by other GNB. *Acinetobacter* species account for 1–3% of hospital-acquired infections and primarily affect immunocompromised hosts and patients with comorbid disease, especially patients in ICUs. In some centers, the incidence of *Acinetobacter* infections, particularly those due to antibiotic-resistant strains, is increasing significantly. Both sporadic and epidemic infections occur, usually after the first week of hospitalization. Until recently, *A. baumannii* was best known as an agent of nosocomial infections. However, *A. baumannii* can also cause severe community-acquired pneumonia and diverse infections following battlefield injuries.

INFECTIOUS SYNDROMES

The respiratory tract (particularly in mechanically ventilated patients) and intravascular devices are the favored sites of infection. *A. baumannii* uncommonly causes severe CAP, usually in compromised hosts (e.g., alcoholic patients), with the preponderance of cases reported from warm, humid geographic locales. Infections of the catheterized urinary tract, postoperative sites, burn sites, biliary stents, and sinuses (with tube-related ostial obstruction) are less common, as are neurosurgical infections, which may be associated with devices such as pressure monitors. Infections of soft tissue and bone have been common among soldiers with battlefield injuries. Uncommon infections include ophthalmic infection and peritonitis associated with continuous ambulatory peritoneal dialysis. The respiratory tract and intravascular devices are the most common sources of bacteremia.

DIAGNOSIS

On Gram's stain, *Acinetobacter* organisms usually appear as short GNB or coccobacilli. They are strictly aerobic, nonfermenting, and oxidase negative and are readily isolated and identified.

℞ *ACINETOBACTER* INFECTIONS

Many strains of *Acinetobacter* are extensively resistant to antimicrobial agents. Empirical combination therapy is prudent pending susceptibility studies. Ampicillin, aztreonam, and the first- and second-generation cephalosporins exhibit little or no activity. The prevalences of resistance to antipseudomonal penicillins, quinolones, third-generation cephalosporins, and gentamicin are 20–90%. Ampicillin/sulbactam, rifampin, tetracyclines, imipenem/cilastatin, tigecycline, and amikacin are often active; however, resistance to all of these agents has been reported. Colistin and polymyxin B have been used with some success against extensively resistant isolates but probably should be considered a last resort because of their potential toxicities.

INFECTIONS CAUSED BY MISCELLANEOUS GENERA

Species of *Hafnia, Kluyvera, Cedecea, Pantoea, Ewingella, and Photorhabdus* are occasionally isolated from diverse clinical specimens, including blood, sputum, cerebrospinal fluid, joint fluid, bile, and wounds. These organisms are rare and usually opportunistic human pathogens.

FURTHER READINGS

DRUDY D et al: *Enterobacter sakazakii*: An emerging pathogen in powdered infant formula. Clin Infect Dis 42:996, 2006

FANG CT et al: *Klebsiella pneumoniae* genotype K1: An emerging pathogen that causes septic ocular or central nervous system complications from pyogenic liver abscess. Clin Infect Dis 45:284, 2007

FOURNIER PE, RICHET H: The epidemiology and control of *Acinetobacter baumannii* in health care facilities. Clin Infect Dis 44:1577, 2007

HEJAZI A, FALKINER FR: *Serratia marcescens*. J Med Microbiol 46:903, 1997

KAPER J et al: Pathogenic *Escherichia coli*. Nat Rev Microbiol 2:123, 2004

KIM B et al: Bacteraemia due to the tribe Proteeae: A review of 132 cases during a decade (1991-2000). Scand J Infect Dis 35:98, 2003

PATERSON DL: Resistance in gram-negative bacteria: Enterobacteriaceae. Am J Infect Control 34:S20, 2006

RUSSO TA, JOHNSON JR: Medical and economic impact of extraintestinal infections due to *Escherichia coli*: Focus on an increasingly important endemic problem. Microbes Infect 5:449, 2003

SCOTT P et al: An outbreak of multidrug-resistant *Acinetobacter baumannii-calcoaceticus* complex infection in the US military health care system associated with military operations in Iraq. Clin Infect Dis 44:1577, 2007

SHIH CC et al: Bacteremia due to *Citrobacter* species: Significance of primary intraabdominal infection. Clin Infect Dis 23:543, 1996

SLAVEN EM et al: Myonecrosis caused by *Edwardsiella tarda:* A case report and case series of extraintestinal *E. tarda* infections. Clin Infect Dis 32:1430, 2001

144 *Helicobacter pylori* Infections

John C. Atherton, Martin J. Blaser

DEFINITION

Helicobacter pylori, which persistently colonizes the stomachs of ~50% of the world's human population, is the main risk factor for peptic ulceration (Chap. 287) as well as for gastric adenocarcinoma and gastric MALT (mucosa-associated lymphoid tissue) lymphoma (Chap. 87). Treatment for *H. pylori* has revolutionized the management of peptic ulcer disease, providing a permanent cure in many cases. The prevention of *H. pylori* colonization could potentially represent primary prevention of gastric malignancy and peptic ulceration. However, controversial but increasing evidence indicates that *H. pylori* may in fact offer some protection against recently emergent diseases—most notably gastroesophageal reflux disease (GERD) and its complications (e.g., esophageal adenocarcinoma). Thus, clearance of *H. pylori* from human populations may not be without negative repercussions.

ETIOLOGIC AGENT

H. pylori is a gram-negative bacillus that has naturally colonized humans for at least tens of thousands of years. It is noninvasive and lives in gastric mucus, with a small proportion of the bacteria adherent to the mucosa. Its spiral shape and flagella render *H. pylori* motile in the mucus environment. This organism has several acid-resistance mechanisms, most notably a highly expressed urease that catalyzes urea hydrolysis to produce buffering ammonia. *H. pylori* is microaerophilic (requiring low levels of oxygen), is slow-growing, and requires complex growth media in vitro. Publication of several complete genomic sequences of *H. pylori* since 1997 has led to significant advances in the understanding of the organism's biology.

A very small proportion of gastric *Helicobacter* infections are due to species other than *H. pylori*, which probably are acquired most often as zoonoses. Whether these non-*pylori* gastric helicobacters cause disease remains controversial. In immunocompromised hosts, several nongastric (intestinal) *Helicobacter* species can cause disease with clinical features resembling those of *Campylobacter* infections; these species are covered in Chap. 148.

EPIDEMIOLOGY

The prevalence of *H. pylori* among adults is ~30% in the United States and other developed countries as opposed to >80% in most developing countries. In the United States, prevalence varies with age: ~50% of 60-year-old persons and ~20% of 30-year-old persons are colonized. *H. pylori* is usually acquired in childhood. The age association is due mostly to a birth-cohort effect whereby current 60-year-olds were more commonly colonized as children than current 30-year-olds. Spontaneous acquisition or loss of *H. pylori* in adulthood is uncommon. Other strong risk factors for *H. pylori* colonization are markers of crowding and poor hygiene in childhood. The very low incidence among children in developed countries at present is probably due, at least in part, to improved living standards and increased use of antibiotics.

Humans are the only important reservoir of *H. pylori*. Children may acquire the organism from their parents (more often from the mother) or from other children. Whether transmission usually takes place by the fecal-oral or the oral-oral route is unknown, but *H. pylori* is easily cultured from vomitus and gastroesophageal refluxate and is less easily cultured from stool.

PATHOLOGY AND PATHOGENESIS

H. pylori colonization induces a tissue response in the stomach; termed *chronic superficial gastritis*, this response includes infiltration of the mucosa by both mononuclear and polymorphonuclear cells. (The term *gastritis* should be used specifically to describe histologic features; it has also been used to describe endoscopic appearances and even symptoms, which do not correlate with microscopic findings or even with the presence of *H. pylori*.) Although *H. pylori* is capable of numerous adaptations that prevent excessive stimulation of the immune system, colonization is accompanied by a considerable persistent immune response, including the production of both local and systemic antibodies as well as cell-mediated responses. However, these responses are ineffective in clearing the bacterium. This inefficient clearing appears to be due in part to *H. pylori*'s downregulation of the immune system, which fosters its own persistence.

Most *H. pylori*–colonized persons do not develop clinical sequelae. That some persons develop overt disease whereas others do not is related to a combination of factors: bacterial strain differences, host susceptibility to disease, and environmental factors. Several *H. pylori* virulence factors are more common among strains that are associated with disease than among those that are not. The *cag* pathogenicity island (PaI) is a group of genes that encodes a secretion system through which a specific protein, CagA, is translocated into epithelial cells. CagA affects host cell signal transduction, inducing proliferative and cytoskeletal changes. The secretion system also induces a proinflammatory cytokine response, which results in enhanced inflammation. Patients with peptic ulcer disease or gastric adenocarcinoma are more likely than persons without these conditions to be colonized by *cag* PaI-positive strains. The secreted *H. pylori* protein VacA occurs in several forms. Strains with the more active forms are more commonly isolated from patients with peptic ulcer disease or gastric carcinoma than from persons without these conditions. BabA and SabA, adhesins expressed by only some strains, are associated with increased gastric inflammation and with increased risk of peptic ulceration and gastric adenocarcinoma. Other *H. pylori* factors that may affect disease risk are still being described.

The best-characterized host determinants of disease are genetic polymorphisms leading to enhanced *H. pylori*–stimulated secretion of proinflammatory cytokines such as interleukin 1β. *H. pylori*–positive individuals with these polymorphisms are at increased risk of hypochlorhydria and gastric adenocarcinoma. In addition, environmental cofactors are important in pathogenesis. Smoking increases the risks of ulcers and cancer in *H. pylori*–positive individuals. Diets high in salt and preserved foods increase cancer risk, whereas diets high in antioxidants and vitamin C are protective.

The pattern of gastric inflammation is associated with disease risk: antral-predominant gastritis is most closely linked with duodenal ulceration, whereas pangastritis is linked with gastric ulceration and adenocarcinoma. This difference probably explains why patients with duodenal ulceration rarely develop gastric adenocarcinoma later in life, despite being colonized by *H. pylori*.

How gastric colonization causes duodenal ulceration is now becoming clearer. *H. pylori*–induced gastritis diminishes the number of somatostatin-producing D cells. Since somatostatin inhibits gastrin release, gastrin levels are higher than in *H. pylori*–negative persons. These increased gastrin levels lead to increased meal-stimulated acid secretion in the gastric corpus, which is only mildly inflamed in antral-predominant gastritis. In turn, increased acid secretion eventually induces protective gastric metaplasia in the duodenum; the duodenum can then become colonized by *H. pylori*, inflamed, and ulcerated.

The pathogenesis of gastric ulceration and that of gastric adenocarcinoma are less well understood, although both conditions arise in association with pan- or corpus-predominant gastritis. The hormonal changes described above still occur, but the inflamed acid-producing gastric corpus produces less acid, with consequent relative hypochlorhydria, despite the hypergastrinemia. Gastric ulcers usually occur at the junction of antral and corpus-type mucosa, and this region is particularly inflamed. Gastric cancer probably stems from progressive DNA damage and the survival of abnormal epithelial cell clones. The DNA damage is thought to be due principally to reactive oxygen and nitrogen species arising from inflammatory cells and perhaps from other bacteria that survive in hypochlorhydric stomachs. Longitudinal analyses of gastric biopsy specimens taken years apart from the same patient show that the common *intestinal* type of gastric adenocarcinoma follows the stepwise changes from simple gastritis to gastric atrophy, intestinal metaplasia,

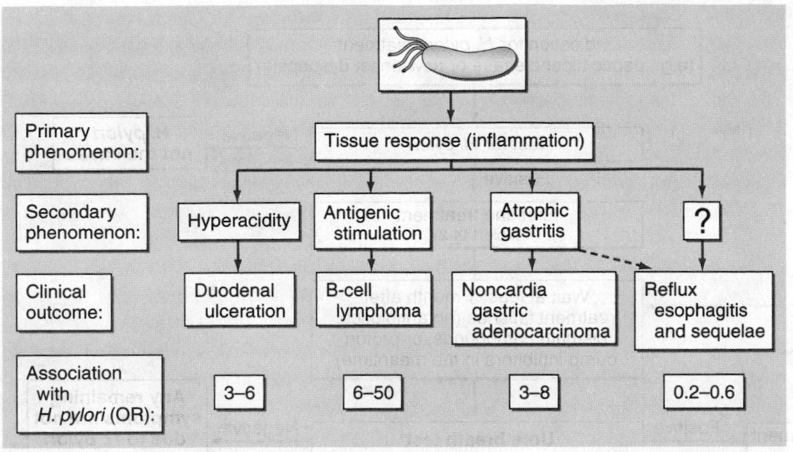

FIGURE 144-1 Schematic of the relationships between colonization with *Helicobacter pylori* and diseases of the upper gastrointestinal tract among persons in developed countries. Essentially all persons colonized with *H. pylori* develop a host response, which is generally termed *chronic gastritis.* The nature of the interaction of the host with the particular bacterial population determines the clinical outcome. *H. pylori* colonization increases the lifetime risk of peptic ulcer disease, noncardia gastric cancer, and B cell non-Hodgkin's gastric lymphoma [odds ratios (ORs) for all, >3]. In contrast, a growing body of evidence indicates that *H. pylori* colonization (especially with *cagA*$^+$ strains) protects against adenocarcinoma of the esophagus (and the sometimes related gastric cardia) and premalignant lesions such as Barrett's esophagus (OR, <1). While the incidences of peptic ulcer disease (cases not due to nonsteroidal anti-inflammatory drugs) and noncardia gastric cancer are declining in developed countries, the incidence of adenocarcinoma of the esophagus is rapidly increasing. *[Adapted from Blaser MJ: Hypothesis: The changing relationships of Helicobacter pylori and humans: Implications for health and disease. J Infect Dis 179:1523, 1999, with permission.]*

and dysplasia. A second, *diffuse* type of gastric adenocarcinoma may arise directly from simple chronic gastritis.

CLINICAL MANIFESTATIONS

Essentially all *H. pylori*–colonized persons have gastric tissue responses, but fewer than 15% develop associated illnesses such as peptic ulceration, gastric adenocarcinoma, or gastric lymphoma (Fig. 144-1).

Worldwide, >80% of duodenal ulcers and >60% of gastric ulcers are related to *H. pylori* colonization (Chap. 287), although the proportion of ulcers due to aspirin and nonsteroidal anti-inflammatory drugs (NSAIDs) is increasing, especially in developed countries. The main lines of evidence for an ulcer-promoting role for *H. pylori* are (1) that the presence of the organism is a risk factor for the development of ulcers, (2) that non-NSAID-induced ulcers rarely develop in the absence of *H. pylori*, (3) that eradication of *H. pylori* markedly reduces rates of ulcer relapse, and (4) that experimental *H. pylori* infection of gerbils causes gastric ulceration.

Prospective nested case-control studies have shown that *H. pylori* colonization is a risk factor for adenocarcinomas of the distal (noncardia) stomach (Chap. 87). Long-term experimental infection of gerbils also may result in gastric adenocarcinoma. Moreover, the presence of *H. pylori* is strongly associated with primary gastric lymphoma, although this condition is less common. Many low-grade gastric B cell lymphomas arising from MALT are driven by T cell stimulation, which in turn is driven by *H. pylori* antigen stimulation; *H. pylori* antigen–driven tumors may regress either fully or partially after *H. pylori* eradication.

Many patients have upper gastrointestinal symptoms but have normal results in upper gastrointestinal endoscopy (so-called functional or nonulcer dyspepsia; Chap. 287). Because *H. pylori* is common, some of these patients will be positive for the organism. *H. pylori* eradication leads to symptom resolution only a little (<10%) more commonly than does placebo treatment. Whether such patients have peptic ulcers in remission at the time of endoscopy or whether a small subgroup of patients with true functional dyspepsia respond to *H. pylori* treatment is unclear.

Much interest has focused on a possible protective role for *H. pylori* against GERD (Chap. 286) and adenocarcinoma of the esophagus and gastric cardia (Chap. 87). The main lines of evidence for this role are (1) that there is a temporal relationship between a falling prevalence of *H. pylori* colonization and a rising incidence of these conditions, and (2) that, in most studies, the prevalence of *H. pylori* colonization (especially with proinflammatory *cagA*$^+$ strains) is significantly lower among patients with these esophageal diseases than among control subjects. The mechanism underlying this protective effect appears to include *H. pylori*–induced hypochlorhydria. Since, at the individual level, GERD symptoms may decrease, worsen, or remain unchanged after treatment targeting *H. pylori*, concerns about GERD should not affect decisions about *H. pylori* treatment when a definite indication exists.

H. pylori has an increasingly recognized role in other gastric pathologies. It may be one initial precipitant of autoimmune gastritis and pernicious anemia and also may predispose some patients to iron deficiency through hypochlorhydria and reduced iron absorption. In addition, several extragastrointestinal pathologies have been linked with *H. pylori* colonization, although evidence of causality is less strong. Several small studies have documented improvement or resolution of idiopathic thrombocytopenic purpura after treatment for *H. pylori* colonization. A potentially important but even more controversial association is with ischemic heart disease and cerebrovascular disease. However, the strength of these associations is reduced if confounding factors are taken into account, and most authorities consider the associations to be noncausal.

DIAGNOSIS

Tests for *H. pylori* can be divided into two groups: invasive tests, which require upper gastrointestinal endoscopy and are based on the analysis of gastric biopsy specimens, and noninvasive tests (Table 144-1). Endoscopy often is not performed in the initial management of young dyspeptic patients without "alarm" symptoms but is commonly used to exclude malignancy in older patients. If endoscopy is performed, the most convenient biopsy-based test is the biopsy urease test, in

TABLE 144-1 TESTS COMMONLY USED TO DETECT *HELICOBACTER PYLORI*

Test	Advantages	Disadvantages
Invasive (Based on Endoscopic Biopsy)		
Biopsy urease test	Quick, simple	Some commercial tests not fully sensitive before 24 h
Histology	May give additional histologic information	Sensitivity dependent on experience and use of special stains
Culture	Permits determination of antibiotic susceptibility	Sensitivity dependent on experience
Noninvasive		
Serology	Inexpensive and convenient	Cannot be used for early follow-up; some commercial kits inaccurate
^{13}C or ^{14}C urea breath test	Inexpensive and simpler than endoscopy; useful for follow-up after treatment	Low-dose irradiation in ^{14}C test (although ^{14}C is rarely used)
Stool antigen test	Inexpensive and convenient; useful for follow-up after treatment; may be useful in children	New test; role not fully established; appears less accurate than urea breath test, particularly when used to assess treatment success

which one large or two small antral biopsy specimens are placed into a gel containing urea and an indicator. The presence of *H. pylori* urease elicits a color change, which often occurs within minutes but can require up to 24 h. Histologic examination of biopsy specimens for *H. pylori* is also accurate, provided that a special stain (e.g., a modified Giemsa or silver stain) permitting optimal visualization of the organism is used. If biopsy specimens are obtained from both antrum and corpus, histologic study yields additional information, including the degree and pattern of inflammation, atrophy, metaplasia, and dysplasia. Microbiologic culture is most specific but may be insensitive because of difficulty with *H. pylori* isolation. Once the organism is cultured, its identity as *H. pylori* can be confirmed by its typical appearance on Gram's stain and its positive reactions in oxidase, catalase, and urease tests. Moreover, the organism's susceptibility to antibiotics can be determined; this information can be clinically useful in difficult cases. The occasional biopsy specimens containing the less common non-*pylori* gastric helicobacters give only weakly positive results in the biopsy urease test. Positive identification of these bacteria requires visualization of the characteristic long, tight spirals in histologic sections.

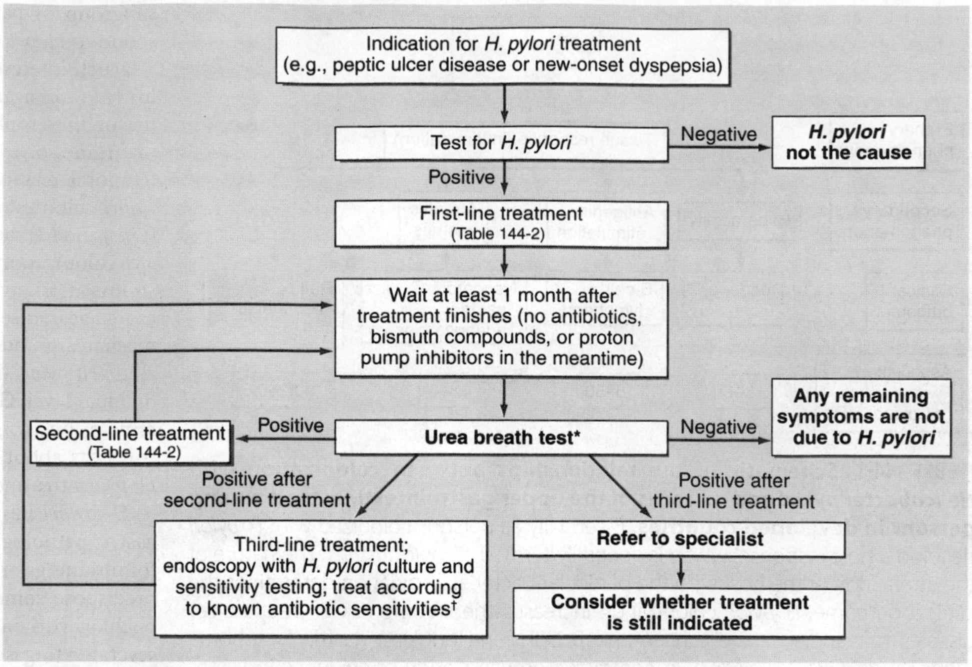

FIGURE 144-2 Algorithm for the management of *Helicobacter pylori* infection. *Occasionally, an endoscopy and a biopsy-based test are used instead of a urea breath test in follow-up after treatment. The main indication for these invasive tests is gastric ulceration; in this condition, as opposed to duodenal ulceration, it is important to check healing and to exclude underlying gastric adenocarcinoma. †Some authorities now use empirical third-line regimens, several of which have been described.

Noninvasive *H. pylori* testing is the norm if gastric cancer does not need to be excluded by endoscopy. The most consistently accurate test is the urea breath test. In this simple test, the patient drinks a labeled urea solution and then blows into a tube. The urea is labeled with either the nonradioactive isotope ^{13}C or a minute dose of the radioactive isotope ^{14}C. If *H. pylori* urease is present, the urea is hydrolyzed and labeled carbon dioxide is detected in breath samples. The stool antigen test, another simple assay, is more convenient and potentially less expensive than the urea breath test but has been slightly less accurate in some comparative studies. The simplest tests for ascertaining *H. pylori* status are serologic assays measuring specific IgG levels in serum by enzyme-linked immunosorbent assay or immunoblot. The best of these tests are as accurate as other diagnostic methods, but many commercial tests—especially rapid office tests—do not perform well.

The urea breath test, the stool antigen test, and biopsy-based tests can all be used to assess the success of treatment (Fig. 144-2). However, because these tests are dependent on *H. pylori* load, their use <4 weeks after treatment may lead to false-negative results. Furthermore, these tests are unreliable if performed within 4 weeks of intercurrent treatment with antibiotics or bismuth compounds or within 2 weeks of the discontinuation of proton pump inhibitor (PPI) treatment. In the assessment of treatment success, noninvasive tests are normally preferred; however, after gastric ulceration, endoscopy should be repeated to ensure healing and to exclude gastric carcinoma by further histologic sampling. Serologic tests are not used to monitor treatment success, as the gradual drop in titer of *H. pylori*–specific antibodies is too slow to be of practical use.

℞ *H. PYLORI* INFECTIONS

The most clear-cut indications for treatment are *H. pylori*–related duodenal or gastric ulceration or low-grade gastric B cell lymphoma. *H. pylori* should be eradicated in patients with documented ulcer disease, whether or not the ulcers are currently active, to reduce the likelihood of relapse (Fig. 144-2). Many guidelines now recommend *H. pylori* treatment in uninvestigated simple dyspepsia following noninvasive diagnosis; others also recommend treatment in functional dyspepsia, in case the patient is one of the perhaps 5–10% to benefit (beyond placebo effects) from such treatment. People with a strong family history of gastric cancer should be treated to eradicate *H. pylori* in the hope that their risk will be reduced. For several reasons, widespread community screening for and treatment of *H. pylori* as primary prophylaxis for gastric cancer and peptic ulcers are not currently recommended. To begin with, it is unclear whether treatment for *H. pylori* reduces the risk of cancer from that in persons who have never acquired the organism. The largest study to date (performed in China) showed no such risk reduction during the 7 years of follow-up. Moreover, treatment has side effects that can be severe in rare cases. Antibiotic resistance may arise in *H. pylori* or other incidentally carried bacteria. Otherwise healthy people may become anxious, especially if treatment is unsuccessful. Finally, it is possible that treatment for *H. pylori* will provoke or exacerbate GERD.

Although *H. pylori* is susceptible to a wide range of antibiotics in vitro, monotherapy has been disappointing in vivo, probably because of inadequate antibiotic delivery to the colonization niche. Failure of monotherapy has prompted the development of multidrug regimens, the most successful of which are triple and quadruple combinations that produce *H. pylori* eradication rates of >90% in many trials and >75% in clinical practice. Current regimens consist of a PPI or ranitidine bismuth citrate and two or three antimicrobial agents given for 7–14 days **(Table 144-2)**.

The two most important factors in successful *H. pylori* treatment are the patient's close compliance with the regimen and the use of drugs to which *H. pylori* has not acquired resistance. Treatment failure following minor lapses in compliance is common and often leads to acquired resistance to metronidazole or clarithromycin. To stress the importance of compliance, written instructions should be given to the patient, and minor side effects of the regimen should be explained. Resistance to metronidazole and clarithromycin is of growing concern. Clarithromycin resistance is less prevalent but, if present, usually results in treatment failure. Metronidazole-resistant strains of *H. pylori* are more common, but these strains still may be cleared by metronidazole-containing regimens. Assessment of antibiotic susceptibilities before treatment would be optimal but is not usually undertaken because endoscopy and mucosal biopsy are necessary to obtain *H. pylori* for culture and because most microbiology laboratories are inexperienced in *H. pylori* culture. In the absence of susceptibility information, a

TABLE 144-2 RECOMMENDED TREATMENT REGIMENS FOR *HELICOBACTER PYLORI*

Regimen, Duration	Drug 1	Drug 2	Drug 3	Drug 4
First-Line Treatment				
Regimen 1: OCA (7–14 days)[a]	Omeprazole[b] (20 mg bid)	Clarithromycin (500 mg bid)	Amoxicillin (1 g bid)	—
Regimen 2: OCM (7–14 days)	Omeprazole[b] (20 mg bid)	Clarithromycin (500 mg bid)	Metronidazole (500 mg bid)	—
Second-Line Treatment[c]				
Regimen 3: OBTM (14 days)[d]	Omeprazole[b] (20 mg bid)	Bismuth subsalicylate (2 tabs qid)	Tetracycline HCl (500 mg qid)	Metronidazole (500 mg tid)

[a]Meta-analyses show that a 14-day course of therapy is slightly superior to a 7-day course. However, the success rate for 7-day therapy is so high in northern Europe (>80%) that 7-day treatment is recommended in most guidelines.
[b]Omeprazole may be replaced with any proton pump inhibitor at an equivalent dosage or, in Regimens 1 and 2, with ranitidine bismuth citrate (400 mg).
[c]An alternative to this second-line therapy is to culture *H. pylori* and to be guided by antibiotic susceptibility data. Patients in whom second-line therapy fails should undergo endoscopy for *H. pylori* culture and antibiotic susceptibility testing.
[d]Data supporting this regimen come mainly from Europe and are based on the use of bismuth subcitrate and metronidazole (400 mg tid).

history of the patient's antibiotic use should be obtained, and, even if only distant exposure is identified (e.g., previous metronidazole consumption for giardiasis or trichomoniasis), use of the agent should be avoided if possible. If initial *H. pylori* treatment fails, two strategies are commonly used (Fig. 144-2). One is re-treatment with a quadruple-drug regimen (Table 144-2). The second is endoscopy, biopsy, and culture plus treatment based on documented antibiotic sensitivities. If re-treatment fails, susceptibility testing should usually be performed, although empirical third-line therapies have been described.

Clearance of non-*pylori* gastric helicobacters can follow the use of bismuth compounds alone or of triple-drug regimens. However, in the absence of trials, it is unclear whether this outcome represents successful treatment or natural clearance of the bacterium.

PREVENTION

Carriage of *H. pylori* has considerable public health significance in developed countries, where it is associated with peptic ulcer disease and gastric adenocarcinoma, and in developing countries, where gastric adenocarcinoma is an even more common cause of cancer death late in life. However, given that *H. pylori* has coevolved with its human host over millennia, preventing or eliminating colonization on a population basis may have distinct disadvantages. For example, absence of *H. pylori* has been reported to increase the risk of diarrheal diseases and of GERD and its complications, including esophageal adenocarcinoma. Recently, we have speculated that the disappearance of *H. pylori* is associated with an increased risk of other emerging diseases reflecting aspects of the current Western lifestyle, such as asthma, obesity, and type 2 diabetes mellitus. If mass prevention were contemplated, vaccination would be the most obvious method, and experimental immunization of animals has given promising results. However, in the United States and other developed countries, rates of *H. pylori* carriage, peptic ulceration, and gastric adenocarcinoma are falling, while rates of esophageal reflux disease and its sequelae are increasing. Thus, prevention of colonization in these countries may be unnecessary or even unwise.

FURTHER READINGS

BLASER MJ: Who are we? Indigenous microbes and the ecology of human diseases. EMBO Rep 7:956, 2006

BLASER MJ, ATHERTON JC: *Helicobacter pylori* persistence: Biology and disease. J Clin Invest 113:321, 2004

CHEN Y, BLASER MJ: Inverse associations of *Helicobacter pylori* with asthma and allergies. Arch Intern Med 167:821, 2007

FRANCO AT et al: Activation of beta-catenin by carcinogenic *Helicobacter pylori*. Proc Natl Acad Sci USA 102:10646, 2005

HANSSON LE et al: The risk of stomach cancer in patients with gastric or duodenal ulcer disease. N Engl J Med 335:242, 1996

KAMANGAR F et al: Opposing risks of gastric cardia and noncardia gastric adenocarcinomas associated with *Helicobacter pylori* seropositivity. J Natl Cancer Inst 98:1445, 2006

MARSHALL BJ, WARREN JR: Unidentified curved bacilli in the stomach of patients with gastritis and peptic ulceration. Lancet 1:1311, 1984

ODENBREIT S et al: Translocation of *Helicobacter pylori* CagA into gastric epithelial cells by type IV secretion. Science 287:1497, 2000

PARSONNET J et al: *Helicobacter pylori* infection and gastric lymphoma. N Engl J Med 330:1267, 1994

RIEDER G et al: *Helicobacter pylori* cag-type IV secretion system facilitates corpus colonization to induce precancerous conditions in Mongolian gerbils. Gastroenterology 128:1229, 2005

TOMB JF et al: The complete genome sequence of the gastric pathogen *Helicobacter pylori*. Nature 388:539, 1997

WONG BC et al: *Helicobacter pylori* eradication to prevent gastric cancer in a high-risk region of China: A randomized controlled trial. JAMA 291:187, 2004

145 Infections Due to *Pseudomonas* Species and Related Organisms

Reuben Ramphal

The pseudomonads are a heterogeneous group of gram-negative bacteria that have in common an inability to ferment lactose. Once classified in the genus *Pseudomonas*, the members of this group are now assigned to three medically important genera—*Pseudomonas, Burkholderia,* and *Stenotrophomonas*—whose biologic behaviors encompass both similarities and marked differences and whose genetic makeups differ in many respects. The pathogenicity of most pseudomonads is based on opportunism; the exceptions are the organisms that cause melioidosis (*B. pseudomallei*) and glanders (*B. mallei*).

P. aeruginosa, the major pathogen of the group, is mainly associated with infections in hospitalized patients and in patients with cystic fibrosis (CF; Chap. 253). Cytotoxic chemotherapy, mechanical ventilation, and broad-spectrum antibiotic therapy probably paved the way for increasing colonization and infection by *P. aeruginosa*. Since the implementation of these advances in medical therapy, most conditions predisposing to *P. aeruginosa* infections have involved host compromise and/or broad-spectrum antibiotic use. Other members of the genus *Pseudomonas*—*P. putida, P. fluorescens,* and *P. stutzeri*—infect humans infrequently.

The genus *Burkholderia* comprises >40 species, of which *B. cepacia* is most frequently encountered in Western countries. Like *P. aeruginosa, B. cepacia* is both a nosocomial pathogen and a cause of infection in CF. The other medically important members of this genus are *B. pseudomallei* and *B. mallei,* which, as mentioned above, cause melioidosis and glanders, respectively.

The genus *Stenotrophomonas* contains one species of medical significance, *S. maltophilia* (previously classified in the genera *Pseudomonas* and *Xanthomonas*). This organism is strictly an opportunist that "overgrows" in the setting of potent broad-spectrum antibiotic use.

PSEUDOMONAS AERUGINOSA

EPIDEMIOLOGY

P. aeruginosa is found in most moist environments. Soil, plants, vegetables, tap water, and countertops can all be reservoirs for this microbe, which has simple nutritional needs. Given the ubiquity of *P. aeruginosa*, contact with the organism obviously is not sufficient for colonization or infection. Clinical and experimental observations suggest that *P. aeruginosa* infection often occurs concomitantly with host defense compromise, mucosal trauma, physiologic derangement, and antibiotic-mediated suppression of normal flora. Thus, it comes as no surprise that the majority of *P. aeruginosa* infections occur in intensive care units (ICUs), where these factors frequently converge. It is believed that the organism is initially acquired from environmental sources, but patient-to-patient spread also occurs in clinics and families.

Burn patients once appeared to be unusually susceptible to *P. aeruginosa*. For example, in 1959–1963, *Pseudomonas* burn-wound sepsis was the principal cause of death in 60% of burn patients at the U.S. Army Institute of Surgical Research. For reasons that are unclear, however, *P. aeruginosa* infection in burn patients is no longer the major problem that it was during the 1950s and 1960s. Similarly, in the 1960s, *P. aeruginosa* appeared as a common pathogen in patients receiving cytotoxic chemotherapy at many institutions in the United States, subsequently diminishing in importance. Despite this subsidence, *P. aeruginosa* remains one of the most feared pathogens in this population because of its high mortality rate.

Moreover, in the Far East and some parts of Latin America, *P. aeruginosa* continues to be the most common cause of gram-negative bacteremia in neutropenic patients.

In contrast to the trends for burn patients and neutropenic patients in the United States, the incidence of *P. aeruginosa* infections among patients with CF has not changed. *P. aeruginosa* remains the most common contributing factor to respiratory failure in CF and is responsible for the majority of deaths among CF patients.

LABORATORY FEATURES

P. aeruginosa is a nonfastidious, motile gram-negative rod that grows on most common laboratory media, including blood and MacConkey agars. It is easily identified in the laboratory on primary-isolation agar plates by pigment production that confers a yellow to dark green or even bluish appearance. Colonies have a shiny "gun-metal" appearance and a characteristic fruity odor. Two of the identifying biochemical characteristics of *P. aeruginosa* are an inability to ferment lactose on MacConkey agar and a positive reaction in the oxidase test. Most strains are identified on the basis of these readily detectable laboratory features even before extensive biochemical testing is done. Some isolates from CF patients are easily identified by their mucoid appearance, which is due to the production of large amounts of the mucoid exopolysaccharide alginate.

PATHOGENESIS

Unraveling the mechanisms underlying disease caused by *P. aeruginosa* has proven challenging. Of the common gram-negative bacteria, no other species produces such a large number of putative virulence factors (Table 145-1). Yet *P. aeruginosa* rarely initiates an infectious process in the absence of host injury or compromise, and few of its putative virulence factors have been shown definitively to be involved in disease in humans. Despite its metabolic versatility and possession of multiple colonizing factors, *P. aeruginosa* exhibits no competitive advantage over enteric bacteria in the human gut; neither is it a normal inhabitant of the human gastrointestinal tract, despite the host's continuous environmental exposure to the organism.

TABLE 145-1 MAIN PUTATIVE VIRULENCE FACTORS OF *PSEUDOMONAS AERUGINOSA*

Substance/ Organelle	Function	Virulence in Animal Disease
Pili	Adhesion to cells	?
Flagella	Adhesion, motility, inflammation	Yes
Lipopolysaccharide	Antiphagocytic activity, inflammation	Yes
Type III secretion system	Cytotoxic activity (ExoU)	Yes
Proteases	Proteolytic activity, cytotoxicity	?
Phospholipases	Cytotoxicity	?
Exotoxin A	Cytotoxicity	?

Acute *P. aeruginosa* Infections • ***MOTILITY AND COLONIZATION*** A general tenet of bacterial pathogenesis is that most bacteria must adhere to surfaces or colonize a host niche in order to initiate disease. Most pathogens examined thus far possess adherence factors called *adhesins*. *P. aeruginosa* is no exception. Among its many adhesins are its pili, which demonstrate adhesive properties for a variety of cells and adhere best to injured cell surfaces. In the organism's flagellum, the flagellin molecule binds to cells, and the flagellar cap attaches to mucins through the recognition of glycan chains. Nonflagellated *P. aeruginosa* mutants are less virulent or avirulent in some animal models; however, it is unclear whether this decreased virulence is due to the loss of adhesion or to the loss of other flagellar functions. Other *P. aeruginosa* adhesins include the outer core of the lipopolysaccharide (LPS) molecule, which binds to the cystic fibrosis transmembrane conductance regulator (CFTR) and aids in internalization of the organism, and the alginate coat of mucoid strains, which enhances adhesion to cells and mucins. In addition, membrane proteins and lectins have been proposed as colonization factors. It appears that the deletion of any given adhesin is not sufficient to abrogate the ability of *P. aeruginosa* to colonize surfaces.

EVASION OF HOST DEFENSES The transition from bacterial colonization to disease requires the evasion of host defenses by a substantial number of bacteria. *P. aeruginosa* appears to be well equipped for evasion. Attached bacteria inject four known toxins (ExoS, ExoU, ExoT, and ExoY) via a type III secretion system that allows the bacteria to evade phagocytic cells either by cytotoxicity or by inhibition of phagocytosis. Mutants with defects in this system fail to disseminate in some animal models of infection. Secreted toxins such as exotoxin A and leukocidin have the potential to kill phagocytic cells, and multiple secreted elastases may degrade host effector molecules released in response to infection.

TISSUE INJURY Among gram-negative bacteria, *P. aeruginosa* probably produces the largest number of substances that are toxic to cells and thus may injure tissues. The type III toxins are capable of tissue injury. However, their delivery requires the adherence of the organism to cells. Thus, the effects of these toxins are likely to be local or to depend on the presence of vast numbers of bacteria. On the other hand, secreted diffusible toxins can act freely wherever they come into contact with cells. Exotoxin A, four different elastases, at least two phospholipases, rhamnolipids, pyocyanin, and hydrocyanic acid are all produced by this organism and are all capable of inducing host injury.

INFLAMMATORY COMPONENTS The inflammatory response to many products of *P. aeruginosa* is arguably the most important factor in disease causation. For example, injurious inflammatory responses to the lipid A component of the LPSs and to the flagellin are mediated through the Toll-like receptor (TLR) system (principally TLR4 and TLR5). These inflammatory responses are required for successful defense against *P. aeruginosa* (i.e., in their absence, animals are defenseless against *P. aeruginosa* infection), but florid responses are likely to result in disease. When the sepsis syndrome and septic shock develop in *P. aeruginosa* infection, they are probably the result of the host response to one or both of these substances. Another layer of complexity is added by the possibility that injury to cells by many of the described factors may cause cell death and the release of cellular components (e.g., heat-shock proteins) that may activate the TLR system.

Chronic *P. aeruginosa* Infections Chronic infection due to *P. aeruginosa* occurs mainly in the lungs in the setting of structural pulmonary diseases. The classic example is CF; others include bronchiectasis and chronic relapsing panbronchiolitis, a disease seen in Japan and some Pacific Islands. Hallmarks of these illnesses are altered mucociliary clearance leading to mucus stasis and mucus accumulation in the lungs. There is probably a common factor that selects for *P. aeruginosa* colonization in these lung diseases—perhaps the adhesiveness of *P. aeruginosa* for mucus, a phenomenon that is not noted for most other common gram-negative bacteria, and/or the ability of *P. aeruginosa* to evade host defenses in mucus. Furthermore, *P. aeruginosa* seems to change in ways that allow its prolonged survival in the lung without an early fatal outcome for the host. The strains found in CF patients exhibit minimal production of virulence factors. Some strains even lose the ability to produce pili and flagella, and most become complement-sensitive because of the loss of the O side chain of their LPS molecules. An example of the impact of these changes is found in the organism's discontinuation of the production of flagellin (probably its most strongly proinflammatory molecule) when it encounters purulent mucus. This response probably dampens the host's response, allowing the organism to survive in mucus. *P. aeruginosa* is also believed to lose the ability to secrete many of its injectable toxins during growth in mucus. Although the alginate coat is thought to play a role in the organism's survival, alginate is not essential, since nonmucoid strains are commonly found in chronic lung diseases other than CF. In short, virulence in chronic infections may be mediated mainly by the attenuated host inflammatory response, which slowly injures the lungs over decades.

CLINICAL MANIFESTATIONS

P. aeruginosa causes infections at almost all sites in the body. The infections encountered most commonly in hospitalized patients are described below.

Bacteremia Crude mortality rates exceeding 50% have been reported among patients with *P. aeruginosa* bacteremia. Consequently, this clinical entity has been much feared, and its management has been attempted with the use of multiple antibiotics. Recent publications report attributable mortality rates of 28–44%, with the precise figure depending on the adequacy of treatment and the seriousness of the underlying disease. In the past, the patient with *P. aeruginosa* bacteremia classically was neutropenic or had a burn injury. Today, however, a minority of patients in these categories have bacteremic *P. aeruginosa* infections. Rather, *P. aeruginosa* bacteremia is seen most often in patients on ICUs.

The clinical presentation of *P. aeruginosa* bacteremia rarely differs from that of sepsis in general (Chap. 264). Patients are usually febrile, but those who are most severely ill may be in shock or even hypothermic. The only point differentiating this entity from gram-negative sepsis of other causes may be the distinctive skin lesions (ecthyma gangrenosum) of *Pseudomonas* infection, which occur almost exclusively in markedly neutropenic patients and patients with AIDS. These small or large, painful, reddish, maculopapular lesions have a geographic margin; they are initially pink, then darken to purple, and finally become black and necrotic (Fig. 145-1). Histopathologic studies indicate that the lesions are due to vascular invasion and are teeming with bacteria. Although similar lesions may occur in aspergillosis and mucormycosis, their presence suggests *P. aeruginosa* bacteremia as the most likely diagnosis.

℞ BACTEREMIA

(Table 145-2) Antimicrobial treatment of *P. aeruginosa* bacteremia has been controversial. Before 1971, the outcome of *Pseudomonas* bacteremia in febrile neutropenic patients treated with the available agents—gentamicin and the polymyxins—was dismal. Studies published around that time

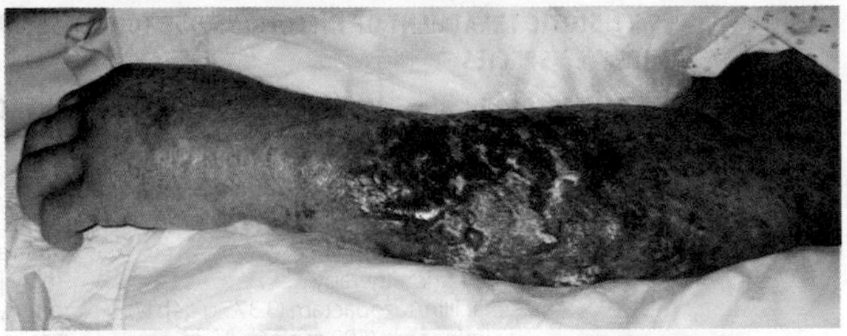

FIGURE 145-1 Ecthyma gangrenosum in a neutropenic patient 3 days after onset.

indicated that treatment with carbenicillin, with or without an aminoglycoside, significantly improved outcome. Concurrently, several retrospective analyses suggested that the use of two agents that were synergistic against gram-negative pathogens in vitro resulted in better outcomes in neutropenic patients. Thus, combination therapy became the standard of care—first for *P. aeruginosa* bacteremia in febrile neutropenic patients and then for all *P. aeruginosa* infections in neutropenic or nonneutropenic patients.

With the introduction of newer antipseudomonal drugs, a number of studies have revisited the choice between combination treatment and monotherapy for *Pseudomonas* bacteremia. Although the majority of experts still favor combination therapy, most of these observational studies indicate that a single modern antipseudomonal β-lactam agent to which the isolate is sensitive is as efficacious as a combination. Even in patients at greatest risk of early death from *P. aeruginosa* bacteremia (i.e., those with fever and neutropenia), empirical antipseudomonal monotherapy is deemed to be as efficacious as empirical combination therapy by the practice guidelines of the Infectious Diseases Society of America. One firm conclusion is that monotherapy with an aminoglycoside is not optimal.

There are, of course, institutions and countries where rates of susceptibility of *P. aeruginosa* to first-line antibiotics are <80%. When a septic patient with a high probability of *P. aeruginosa* infection is encountered in such settings, empirical combination therapy should be administered until the pathogen is identified and susceptibility data become available. Thereafter, whether one or two agents should be continued remains a matter of individual preference.

Acute Pneumonia Respiratory infections are the most common of all infections caused by *P. aeruginosa*. This organism appears first or second on most lists of the causes of ventilator-associated pneumonia (VAP). However, much debate centers on the actual role of *P. aeruginosa* in VAP. Many of the relevant data are based on cultures of sputum or endotracheal tube aspirates and may represent nonpathogenic colonization of the tracheobronchial tree, biofilms on the endotracheal tube, or simple tracheobronchitis.

Older reports of *P. aeruginosa* pneumonia described patients with an acute clinical syndrome of fever, chills, cough, and necrotizing pneumonia indistinguishable from other gram-negative bacterial pneumonias. The traditional accounts described a fulminant infection, with cyanosis, tachypnea, copious sputum, and systemic toxicity. Chest radiographs demonstrated bilateral pneumonia, often with nodular densities with or without cavities. This picture is now remarkably rare. Today, the typical patient is using a ventilator, has a slowly progressive infiltrate, and has been colonized with *P. aeruginosa* for days. While some cases may progress rapidly over 48–72 h, they are the exceptions. Nodular densities are not commonly seen. However, infiltrates may go on to necrosis. Necrotizing pneumonia has also been seen in the community (e.g., after inhalation of hot-tub water contaminated with *P. aeruginosa*). The typical patient has fever, leukocytosis, and purulent sputum, and the chest radiograph shows a new infiltrate or the expansion of a preexisting infiltrate. Chest examination generally detects rales or dullness. Of course, such findings are quite common among ventilated patients in the ICU. A sputum Gram's stain showing mainly polymorphonuclear leukocytes (PMNs) in conjunction with a culture positive for *P. aeruginosa* in this setting suggests a diagnosis of acute *P. aeruginosa* pneumonia. The emerging consensus is that an in-

TABLE 145-2 ANTIBIOTIC TREATMENT OF INFECTIONS DUE TO *PSEUDOMONAS AERUGINOSA* AND RELATED SPECIES

Infection	Antibiotics and Dosages	Other Considerations
Bacteremia		
Nonneutropenic host	Monotherapy: Ceftazidime (2 g q8h IV) or cefepime (2 g q12h IV) Combination therapy: Piperacillin/tazobactam (3.375 g q4h IV) or imipenem (500 mg q6h IV) or meropenem (1 g q8h IV) *plus* Amikacin (7.5 mg/kg q12h or 15 mg/kg q24h IV)	Add an aminoglycoside for patients in shock and in regions or hospitals where rates of resistance to the primary β-lactam agents are high. Tobramycin may be used instead of amikacin (susceptibility permitting).
Neutropenic host	Cefepime (2 g q8h IV) or all other agents in above dosages	
Endocarditis	Antibiotic regimens as for bacteremia for 6–8 weeks	Resistance during therapy is common. Surgery is required for relapse.
Pneumonia	Drugs and dosages as for bacteremia, except that the available carbapenems should not be the primary drugs because of high rates of resistance during therapy	IDSA guidelines recommend the addition of an aminoglycoside or ciprofloxacin. The duration of therapy is 10–14 days.
Bone infection, malignant otitis externa	Cefepime or ceftazidime at the same dosages as for bacteremia; aminoglycosides not a necessary component of therapy; ciprofloxacin (500–750 mg q12h PO) may be used	Duration of therapy varies with the drug used (e.g., 6 weeks for a β-lactam agent; at least 3 months for oral therapy except in puncture-wound osteomyelitis, for which the duration should be 2–4 weeks).
Central nervous system infection	Ceftazidime or cefepime (2 g q8h IV) or meropenem (1 g q8h IV)	Abscesses or other closed-space infections may require drainage. The duration of therapy is ≥2 weeks.
Eye infection		
Keratitis/ulcer	Topical therapy with tobramycin/ciprofloxacin/levofloxacin eyedrops	Use maximal strengths available or compounded by pharmacy.
Endophthalmitis	Ceftazidime or cefepime as for central nervous system infection *plus* Topical therapy	
Urinary tract infection	Ciprofloxacin (500 mg q12h PO) or levofloxacin (750 mg q24h) or any aminoglycoside (total daily dose given once daily)	Relapse may occur if an obstruction or a foreign body is present.
Multidrug-resistant *P. aeruginosa* infection	Colistin (100 mg q12h IV) for the shortest possible period to obtain a clinical response	Doses used have varied. Dosage adjustment is required in renal failure. Inhaled colistin may be added for pneumonia (100 mg q12h).
Stenotrophomonas maltophilia infection	TMP-SMX (1600/320 mg q12h IV for 14 days) Ticarcillin/clavulanate (3.1 g q4h IV for 14 days)	Resistance to all agents is increasing. Levofloxacin may be an alternative, but there is little published clinical experience with this agent.
Burkholderia cepacia infection	Meropenem (1 g q8h IV for 14 days) TMP-SMX (1600/320 mg q12h IV for 14 days)	Resistance to both agents is increasing. Do not use them in combination because of possible antagonism.
Melioidosis, glanders	Ceftazidime (2 g q6h for 2 weeks) or meropenem (1 g q8h for 2 weeks) or imipenem (500 mg q6h for 2 weeks) *followed by* TMP-SMX (1600/320 mg q12h PO for 3 months)	See "Further Readings" for more details on therapy and alternative agents.

Note: IDSA, Infectious Diseases Society of America; TMP-SMX, trimethoprim-sulfamethoxazole.

vasive procedure (e.g., bronchoalveolar lavage or protected-brush sampling of the distal airways) should be used to obtain samples for quantitative lung cultures in order to substantiate the occurrence of *P. aeruginosa* pneumonia and prevent antibiotic overuse.

℞ ACUTE PNEUMONIA

(Table 145-2) The results of therapy for *P. aeruginosa* pneumonia have been unsatisfactory. Reports suggest mortality rates of 40–80%, but how many of these deaths are attributable to underlying disease remains unknown. The drugs of choice for *P. aeruginosa* pneumonia are similar to those given for bacteremia. A potent antipseudomonal β-lactam drug is the mainstay of therapy. Failure rates were high when aminoglycosides were used as single agents, possibly because of binding to airway secretions. Thus a strong case cannot be made for the inclusion of the aminoglycoside component in regimens used against fully susceptible organisms, especially given the evidence that aminoglycosides are not optimally active in the lungs at concentrations normally reached after IV administration. Nonetheless, aminoglycosides are commonly used in clinical practice. Some experts suggest the combination of a β-lactam agent and an antipseudomonal fluoroquinolone instead.

Chronic Respiratory Tract Infections *P. aeruginosa* is responsible for chronic infections of the airways associated with a number of underlying or predisposing conditions—most commonly CF in Caucasian populations (Chap. 253). A state of chronic colonization beginning early in childhood is seen in some Asian populations with chronic or diffuse panbronchiolitis, a disease of unknown etiology. *P. aeruginosa* is one of the organisms that colonizes damaged bronchi in bronchiectasis, a disease secondary to multiple causes in which profound structural abnormalities of the airways result in mucus stasis.

℞ CHRONIC RESPIRATORY TRACT INFECTIONS

Optimal management of chronic *P. aeruginosa* lung infection has not been determined, but it is customary to treat these patients on the basis of bacterial sensitivity. Patients respond clinically to antipseudomonal therapy, but the organism is rarely eradicated. Since eradication is unlikely, the aim of treatment for chronic infection is to quell exacerbations of inflammation. The regimens used are similar to those used for pneumonia, but an aminoglycoside is almost always added because resistance is common in chronic disease. It may be most appropriate to use an inhaled aminoglycoside preparation in order to maximize airway drug levels.

Endovascular Infections Infective endocarditis due to *P. aeruginosa* is seen mainly in IV drug users whose native valves are involved. This organism has also been reported to cause prosthetic valve endocarditis. Sites of prior native-valve injury due to the injection of foreign material such as talc or fibers probably serve as niduses for bacterial attachment to the heart valve. The manifestations of *P. aeruginosa* endocarditis resemble those of other forms of acute endocarditis in IV drug users except that the disease is more indolent than *Staphylococcus aureus* endocarditis. While most disease involves the right side of the heart, left-sided involvement is not rare and multivalvular disease is common. Fever is a common manifestation, as is pulmonary involvement (due to septic emboli to the lungs). Hence, patients may also experience chest pain and hemoptysis. Involvement of the left side of the heart may lead to signs of cardiac failure, systemic emboli, and local cardiac involvement with sinus of Valsalva abscesses and conduction defects. Skin manifestations are rare in this disease, and ecthyma gangrenosum is not seen. The diagnosis is based on positive blood cultures along with clinical signs of endocarditis.

℞ ENDOVASCULAR INFECTIONS

(Table 145-2) It has been customary to use synergistic antibiotic combinations in treating *P. aeruginosa* endocarditis because of the development of resistance during therapy with a single antipseudomonal β-lactam agent. Which combination therapy is preferable is unclear, as all combinations have failed. Cases of *P. aeruginosa* endocarditis that relapse during or fail to respond to therapy are often caused by resistant organisms and may require surgical therapy. Other considerations for valve replacement are similar to those in other forms of endocarditis (Chap. 118).

Bone and Joint Infections Although *P. aeruginosa* is an infrequent cause of bone and joint infections, *Pseudomonas* bacteremia or infective endocarditis caused by the injection of contaminated illicit drugs has been well documented to result in vertebral osteomyelitis and sternoclavicular joint arthritis. The clinical presentation of vertebral *P. aeruginosa* osteomyelitis is more indolent than that of staphylococcal osteomyelitis. The duration of symptoms in IV drug users with vertebral osteomyelitis due to *P. aeruginosa* varies from weeks to months. Fever is not uniformly present; when present, it tends to be low grade. There may be mild tenderness at the site of involvement. Blood cultures are usually negative unless there is concomitant endocarditis. The erythrocyte sedimentation rate (ESR) is generally elevated. Vertebral osteomyelitis due to *P. aeruginosa* has also been reported in the elderly, in whom it originates from urinary tract infections (UTIs). The infection generally involves the lumbosacral area because of a shared venous drainage (Batson's plexus) between the lumbosacral spine and the pelvis. Sternoclavicular septic arthritis due to *P. aeruginosa* is seen almost exclusively in IV drug users. This disease may occur with or without endocarditis, and a primary site of infection often is not found. Plain radiographs show joint or bone involvement. Treatment of these forms of disease is generally successful.

Pseudomonas osteomyelitis of the foot most often follows puncture wounds through sneakers and mostly affects children. The main manifestation is pain in the foot, sometimes with superficial cellulitis around the puncture wound and tenderness on deep palpation of the wound. Multiple joints or bones of the foot may be involved. Systemic symptoms are generally absent, and blood cultures are usually negative. Radiographs may or may not be abnormal, but the bone scan is usually positive, as are MRI studies. Needle aspiration usually yields a diagnosis. Prompt surgery, with exploration of the nail puncture tract and debridement of the involved bones and cartilage, is generally recommended in addition to antibiotic therapy.

Central Nervous System (CNS) Infections CNS infections due to *P. aeruginosa* are relatively rare. Involvement of the CNS is almost always secondary to a surgical procedure or head trauma. The entity seen most often is postoperative or posttraumatic meningitis. Subdural or epidural infection occasionally results from contamination of these areas. Embolic disease arising from endocarditis in IV drug users and leading to brain abscesses has also been described. The cerebrospinal fluid (CSF) profile of *P. aeruginosa* meningitis is no different from that of pyogenic meningitis of any other etiology.

℞ CENTRAL NERVOUS SYSTEM INFECTIONS

(Table 145-2) Treatment of *Pseudomonas* meningitis is difficult; little information has been published, and no controlled trials in humans have been undertaken. However, the general principles involved in the treatment of meningitis apply, including the need for high doses of bactericidal antibiotics to attain high drug levels in the CSF. The agent with which there is the most published experience in *P. aeruginosa* meningitis is ceftazidime, but other antipseudomonal β-lactam drugs that reach high CSF concentrations, such as cefepime and meropenem, have also been used successfully. Other forms of *P. aeruginosa* CNS infection, such as brain abscesses and epidural and subdural empyema, generally require surgical drainage in addition to antibiotic therapy.

Eye Infections Eye infections due to *P. aeruginosa* occur mainly as a result of direct inoculation into the tissue during trauma or surface injury by contact lenses. Keratitis and corneal ulcers are the most common types of eye disease and are often associated with contact lenses (especially the extended-wear variety). Keratitis can be slowly or rapidly progressive, but the classic description is disease progressing over 48 h to involve the entire cornea, with opacification and sometimes perforation. *P. aeruginosa* keratitis should be considered a medical emergency because of the rapidity with which it can progress to loss of sight. *P. aeruginosa* endophthalmitis secondary to bacteremia is the most devastating of *P. aeruginosa* eye infections. The disease is fulminant, with severe pain, chemosis, decreased visual acuity, anterior uveitis, vitreous involvement, and panophthalmitis.

℞ EYE INFECTIONS

(Table 145-2) The usual therapy for keratitis is the administration of topical antibiotics. Therapy for endophthalmitis includes the use of high-dose local and systemic antibiotics (to achieve higher drug concentrations in the eye) and vitrectomy.

Ear Infections *P. aeruginosa* infections of the ears vary from mild swimmer's ear to serious life-threatening infections with neurologic sequelae. Swimmer's ear is common among children and results from infection of moist macerated skin of the external ear canal. Most cases resolve with treatment, but some patients develop chronic drainage. Swimmer's ear is managed with topical antibiotic agents (otic solutions). The most serious form of *Pseudomonas* infection involving the ear has been given various names: two of these designations, malignant otitis externa and necrotizing otitis externa, are now used for the same entity. This disease was originally described in elderly diabetic patients, in whom the majority of cases still occur. However, it has also been described in patients with AIDS and in elderly patients without underlying diabetes or immunocompromise. The usual presenting symptoms are decreased hearing and ear pain, which may be severe and lancinating. The pinna is usually painful, and the external canal may be tender. The ear canal almost always shows signs of inflammation, with granulation tissue and exudate. Tenderness anterior to the tragus may extend as far as the temporomandibular joint and mastoid process. A small minority of patients have systemic symptoms. Patients in whom the diagnosis is made late may present with cranial nerve palsies or even with cavernous venous sinus thrombosis. The ESR is invariably elevated (≥100 mm/h). The diagnosis is made on clinical grounds in severe cases; however, the "gold standard" is a positive technetium-99 bone scan in a patient with otitis externa due to *P. aeruginosa*. In diabetic patients, a positive bone scan constitutes presumptive evidence for this diagnosis and should prompt biopsy or empirical therapy.

℞ EAR INFECTIONS

(Table 145-2) Given the infection of the ear cartilage, sometimes with mastoid or petrous ridge involvement, patients with malignant (necrotizing) otitis externa are treated as for osteomyelitis.

Urinary Tract Infections UTIs due to *P. aeruginosa* generally occur as a complication of a foreign body in the urinary tract, an obstruction in the genitourinary system, or urinary tract instrumentation or surgery.

However, UTIs caused by *P. aeruginosa* have been described in pediatric outpatients without stones or evident obstruction.

℞ URINARY TRACT INFECTIONS

(Table 145-2) Most *P. aeruginosa* UTIs are considered complicated infections that must be treated longer than uncomplicated cystitis. In general, a 7- to 10-day course of treatment suffices, with up to 2 weeks of therapy in cases of pyelonephritis. Urinary catheters, stents, or stones should be removed to prevent relapse, which is common and may be due not to resistance but rather to factors such as a foreign body that has been left in place or an ongoing obstruction.

Skin and Soft Tissue Infections Besides pyoderma gangrenosum in neutropenic patients (an entity described earlier in this chapter), folliculitis and other papular or vesicular lesions due to *P. aeruginosa* have been extensively described and are collectively referred to as *dermatitis*. Multiple outbreaks have been linked to whirlpools, spas, and swimming pools. To prevent such outbreaks, the growth of *P. aeruginosa* in the home and in recreational environments must be controlled by proper chlorination of water. Most cases of hot-tub folliculitis are self-limited, requiring only the avoidance of exposure to the contaminated source of water.

Toe-web infections occur especially often in the tropics, and the "green nail syndrome" is caused by *P. aeruginosa* paronychia, which results from frequent submersion of the hands in water. In the latter entity, the green discoloration results from diffusion of pyocyanin into the nail bed. *P. aeruginosa* remains a prominent cause of burn wound infections in some parts of the world. Its management is best left to specialists in burn wound care.

Infections in Febrile Neutropenic Patients In febrile neutropenia, *P. aeruginosa* has historically been the organism against which empirical coverage is always essential. In the 1960s and early 1970s, *P. aeruginosa* infection occurred commonly in febrile neutropenic patients, with high associated mortality rates. Although in Western countries these infections are now less common, their importance has not diminished because of persistently high mortality rates. In other parts of the world as well, *P. aeruginosa* continues to be a significant problem in febrile neutropenia, causing a larger proportion of infections in febrile neutropenic patients than any other single organism. For example, *P. aeruginosa* was responsible for 28% of documented infections in 499 febrile neutropenic patients in one study from the Indian subcontinent and for 31% of these infections in another. In a large study of infections in leukemia patients from Japan, *P. aeruginosa* was the most frequently documented cause of bacterial infection. In studies performed in North America, northern Europe, and Australia, the incidence of *P. aeruginosa* bacteremia in febrile neutropenia was quite variable. In a review of 97 reports published in 1987–1994, the incidence was reported to be 1–2.5% among febrile neutropenic patients given empirical therapy and 5–12% among microbiologically documented infections. The most common clinical syndromes encountered were bacteremia, pneumonia, and soft tissue infections manifesting mainly as ecthyma gangrenosum.

℞ INFECTIONS IN FEBRILE NEUTROPENIC PATIENTS

(Table 145-2) Compared with rates three decades ago, improved rates of response to antibiotic therapy have been reported in many studies. A study of 127 patients demonstrated a reduction in the mortality rate from 71% to 25% with the introduction of ceftazidime and imipenem. Since neutrophils—the normal host defenses against this organism—are absent in febrile neutropenic patients, maximal doses of antipseudomonal β-lactam antibiotics should be used for the management of *P. aeruginosa* bacteremia in this setting.

Infections in Patients with AIDS Both community- and hospital-acquired *P. aeruginosa* infections were documented in patients with AIDS before the advent of antiretroviral therapy. Since the introduction of protease inhibitors, *P. aeruginosa* infections in AIDS patients have been seen less frequently but still occur, particularly in the form of sinusitis. The clinical presentation of *Pseudomonas* infection (especially pneumonia and bacteremia) in AIDS patients is remarkable in that, although the illness may appear not to be severe, the infection may nonetheless be fatal. Patients with bacteremia may have only a low-grade fever and may present with ecthyma gangrenosum. Bacteremia may herald underlying disease at another site (often pneumonia or sinusitis). Pneumonia, with or without bacteremia, is perhaps the most common type of *P. aeruginosa* infection in AIDS patients. Patients with AIDS and *P. aeruginosa* pneumonia exhibit the classic clinical signs and symptoms of pneumonia, such as fever, productive cough, and chest pain. The infection may be lobar or multilobar and shows no predisposition for any particular location. The most striking feature is the high frequency of cavitary disease.

℞ INFECTIONS IN AIDS PATIENTS

Therapy for any of these conditions in AIDS patients is no different from that in other patients. However, relapse is the rule unless the patient's CD4+ T cell count rises to >50/μL or suppressive antibiotic therapy is given. In attempts to achieve cures and prevent relapses, therapy tends to be more prolonged than that in the immunocompetent patient.

Multidrug-Resistant Infections (Table 145-2) *P. aeruginosa* is notorious for antibiotic resistance. During three decades, the impact of resistance was minimized by the rapid development of potent antipseudomonal agents. However, the situation has recently changed, with the worldwide selection of strains carrying determinants that mediate resistance to β-lactams, fluoroquinolones, and aminoglycosides. This situation has been compounded by the lack of development of new classes of antipseudomonal drugs for nearly two decades. Physicians now resort to drugs such as colistin and polymyxin, which were discarded decades ago. These alternative approaches to the management of multiresistant *P. aeruginosa* infections were first used some time ago in CF patients, who receive colistin (polymyxin E) IV and by aerosol despite its renal toxicity. Colistin is rapidly becoming the last-resort agent of choice, even in non-CF patients infected with multiresistant *P. aeruginosa*.

The clinical outcome of multidrug-resistant *P. aeruginosa* infections treated with colistin is difficult to judge from case reports, especially given the many drugs used in the complicated management of these patients. Although earlier reports described marginal efficacy and serious nephrotoxicity and neurotoxicity, recent reports have been more encouraging. Because colistin shows synergy with other antimicrobial agents in vitro, it may be possible to reduce the dosage—and thus the toxicity—of this drug when it is combined with drugs such as rifampin and β-lactams; however, no studies in humans or animals support this approach at this time.

OTHER PSEUDOMONADS

Stenotrophomonas maltophilia

S. maltophilia is the only potential human pathogen among a genus of ubiquitous organisms found in the rhizosphere (i.e., the soil that surrounds the roots of plants). The organism is an opportunist that is acquired from the environment but is even more limited than *P. aeruginosa* in its ability to colonize patients or cause infections. Immunocompromise is not sufficient to permit these events; rather, major perturbations of the human flora are usually necessary for the establishment of *S. maltophilia*. Accordingly, most cases of human infection occur in the setting of very broad-spectrum antibiotic therapy with agents such as advanced cephalosporins and carbapenems, which eradicate the normal flora and other pathogens. The remarkable ability of *S. maltophilia* to resist virtually all classes of antibiotics is attributable to the possession of antibiotic efflux pumps and of two β-lactamases (L1 and L2) that mediate β-lactam resistance, including that to carbapenems. Fortunately, the virulence of *S. maltophilia* appears to be limited.

Although a serine protease is present in some strains, virulence is probably a result of the host's inflammatory response to components of the organism such as LPS and flagellin. *S. maltophilia* is most commonly found in the respiratory tract of ventilated patients, where the distinction between its roles as a colonizer and as a pathogen is often difficult to make. However, *S. maltophilia* does cause pneumonia and bacteremia in such patients, and these infections have led to septic shock. Also common is central venous line–associated infection (with or without bacteremia), which has been reported most often in patients with cancer. *S. maltophilia* is a rare cause of ecthyma gangrenosum in neutropenic patients. It has been isolated from ~5% of CF patients but is not believed to be a significant pathogen in this setting.

℞ S. MALTOPHILIA

The intrinsic resistance of *S. maltophilia* to most antibiotics renders infection difficult to treat. The antibiotics to which it is most often (although not uniformly) susceptible are trimethoprim-sulfamethoxazole (TMP-SMX), ticarcillin/clavulanate, and levofloxacin (Table 145-2). Consequently, a combination of TMP-SMX and ticarcillin/clavulanate is recommended for initial therapy. Catheters must be removed in the treatment of bacteremia to hasten cure and prevent relapses. The treatment of VAP due to *S. maltophilia* is much more difficult than that of bacteremia, with the frequent development of resistance during therapy.

Burkholderia cepacia

B. cepacia gained notoriety as the cause of a rapidly fatal syndrome of respiratory distress and septicemia (the cepacia syndrome) in CF patients. Previously, it had been recognized as an antibiotic-resistant nosocomial pathogen (then designated *P. cepacia*) in ICU patients. Patients with chronic granulomatous disease are also predisposed to *B. cepacia* lung disease. The organism has been reclassified into nine subgroups, only some of which are common in CF. *B. cepacia* is an environmental organism that inhabits moist environments and is found in the rhizosphere. This organism possesses multiple virulence factors that may play roles in disease as well as colonizing factors that are capable of binding to lung mucus—an ability that may explain the predilection of *B. cepacia* for the lungs in CF. *B. cepacia* secretes elastase and possesses components of an injectable toxin-secretion system like that of *P. aeruginosa*; its LPS is among the most potent of all LPSs in stimulating an inflammatory response in the lungs and may be the cause of the lung disease seen in the cepacia syndrome. The organism can penetrate epithelial surfaces by virtue of motility and inhibition of host innate immune defenses. Besides infecting the lungs in CF, *B. cepacia* appears as an airway colonizer during broad-spectrum antibiotic therapy and is a cause of VAP, catheter-associated infections, and wound infections.

℞ B. CEPACIA

B. cepacia is intrinsically resistant to many antibiotics. Therefore, treatment must be tailored according to sensitivities. TMP-SMX, meropenem, and doxycycline are the most effective agents in vitro and may be started as first-line agents (Table 145-2). Some strains are susceptible to third-generation cephalosporins and fluoroquinolones, and these agents may be used against isolates known to be susceptible. Combination therapy for serious pulmonary infection (e.g., in CF) is suggested for multidrug-resistant strains; the combination of meropenem and TMP-SMX may be antagonistic, however. Resistance to all agents used has been reported during therapy.

Burkholderia pseudomallei

B. pseudomallei is the causative agent of melioidosis, a disease of humans and animals that is geographically restricted to Southeast Asia and northern Australia, with occasional cases in countries such as India and China. This organism may be isolated from individuals returning directly from these endemic regions and from military personnel who have served in endemic regions and then returned home after stops in Europe. Symptoms of this illness may develop only at a later date because of the organism's ability to cause latent infections. *B. pseudomallei* is found in soil and water. Humans and animals are infected by inoculation, inhalation, or ingestion; only rarely is the organism transmitted from person to person. Humans are not colonized without being infected. Among the pseudomonads, *B. pseudomallei* is perhaps the most virulent. Host compromise is not an essential prerequisite for disease, although many patients have common underlying medical diseases (e.g., diabetes or renal failure). *B. pseudomallei* is a facultative intracellular organism whose replication in PMNs and macrophages may be aided by the possession of a polysaccharide capsule. The organism also possesses elements of a type III secretion system that plays a role in its intracellular survival. During infection, there is a florid inflammatory response whose role in disease is unclear.

B. pseudomallei causes a wide spectrum of disease, ranging from asymptomatic infection to abscesses, pneumonia, and disseminated disease. It is a significant cause of fatal community-acquired pneumonia and septicemia in endemic areas, with mortality rates as high as 44% reported in Thailand. Acute pulmonary infections are the most commonly diagnosed form of melioidosis. Pneumonia may be asymptomatic (with routine chest radiographs showing mainly upper-lobe infiltrates) or may present as severe necrotizing disease. *B. pseudomallei* also causes chronic pulmonary infections with systemic manifestations that mimic those of tuberculosis, including chronic cough, fever, hemoptysis, night sweats, and cavitary lung disease. Besides pneumonia, the other principal form of *B. pseudomallei* disease is skin ulceration with associated lymphangitis and regional lymphadenopathy. Spread from the lungs or skin, which is most often documented in debilitated individuals, gives rise to septicemic forms of melioidosis that carry a high mortality rate.

℞ B. PSEUDOMALLEI

B. pseudomallei is susceptible to advanced penicillins and cephalosporins and to carbapenems. Treatment is divided into two stages: an intensive 2-week phase of therapy with ceftazidime or a carbapenem followed by at least 12 weeks of oral TMP-SMX to eradicate the organism and prevent relapse. The recognition of this bacterium as a potential agent of biologic warfare has stimulated interest in the development of a vaccine.

Burkholderia mallei

B. mallei causes the equine disease glanders in Africa, Asia, and South America. The organism was eradicated from Europe and North America decades ago. The last case seen in the United States occurred in 2001 in a laboratory worker; before that, *B. mallei* had last been seen in this country in 1949. In contrast to the other organisms discussed in this chapter, *B. mallei* is not an environmental organism and does not persist outside its equine hosts. Consequently, *B. mallei* infection is an occupational risk for handlers of horses, equine butchers, and veterinarians in areas of the world where it still exists. The polysaccharide capsule is a critical virulence determinant; diabetics are thought to be more susceptible to infection by this organism. The organism is transmitted from animals to humans by inoculation into the skin, where it causes local infection with nodules and lymphadenitis. Regional lymphadenopathy is common. Respiratory secretions from infected horses are extremely infectious. Inhalation results in clinical signs of typical pneumonia but may also cause an acute febrile illness with ulceration of the trachea. The organism may disseminate from the skin or lungs to cause septicemia with signs of sepsis. The septicemic form is frequently associated with shock and a high mortality rate. The infection may also enter a chronic phase and present as disseminated abscesses. *B. mallei* infection may present as early as 1–2 days after inhalation or (in cutaneous disease) may not become evident for months.

℞ B. MALLEI

The antibiotic susceptibility pattern of *B. mallei* is similar to that of *B. pseudomallei*; in addition, the organism is susceptible to the newer macrolides azithromycin and clarithromycin. *B. mallei* infection should be treated with the same drugs and for the same duration as melioidosis.

FURTHER READINGS

CHASTRE J et al: Comparison of 8 vs 15 days of antibiotic therapy for ventilator-associated pneumonia in adults: A randomized trial. JAMA 290:2588, 2003

CURRIE BJ: *Burkholderia pseudomallei* and *Burkholderia mallei*: Melioidosis and glanders, in *Principles and Practice of Infectious Diseases*, 6th ed, GL Mandell et al (eds). Philadelphia, Elsevier Churchill Livingstone, 2005, pp 2622–2632

JOHNSON MP, RAMPHAL R: Malignant external otitis: Report on therapy with ceftazidime and review of therapy and prognosis. Rev Infect Dis 12:173, 1990

KALLEL H et al: Colistin as a salvage therapy for nosocomial infections caused by multidrug-resistant bacteria in the ICU. Int J Antimicrob Agents 28:366, 2006

LODISE TP JR et al: Predictors of 30-day mortality among patients with *Pseudomonas aeruginosa* bloodstream infections: Impact of delayed appropriate antibiotic selection. Antimicrob Agents Chemother 51:3510, 2007

MASCHMEYER G, GÖBEL UB: *Stenotrophomonas maltophilia* and *Burkholderia cepacia*, in *Principles and Practice of Infectious Diseases*, 6th ed, GL Mandell et al (eds). Philadelphia, Elsevier Churchill Livingstone, 2005, pp 2616–2622

MENDELSON MH et al: *Pseudomonas aeruginosa* bacteremia in AIDS. Clin Infect Dis: 886, 1994

MICEK ST et al: *Pseudomonas aeruginosa* bloodstream infection: Importance of appropriate antibiotic therapy. Antimicrob Agents Chemother 49:1306, 2005

OBRITSCH MD et al: Nosocomial infections due to multidrug resistant *Pseudomonas aeruginosa:* Epidemiology and treatment options. Pharmacotherapy 25:1353, 2006

PIER GB, RAMPHAL R et al: *Pseudomonas aeruginosa*, in *Principles and Practice of Infectious Diseases*, 6th ed, GL Mandell et al (eds). Philadelphia, Elsevier Churchill Livingstone, 2005, pp 2587–2615

146 Salmonellosis

David A. Pegues, Samuel I. Miller

Bacteria of the genus *Salmonella* are highly adapted for growth in both humans and animals and cause a wide spectrum of disease. The growth of serotypes *S.* Typhi and *S.* Paratyphi is restricted to human hosts, in whom these organisms cause enteric (typhoid) fever. The remaining serotypes (nontyphoidal *Salmonella*, or NTS) can colonize the gastrointestinal tracts of a broad range of animals, including mammals, reptiles, birds, and insects. More than 200 serotypes are pathogenic to humans, in whom they often cause gastroenteritis and can be associated with localized infections and/or bacteremia.

ETIOLOGY

This large genus of gram-negative bacilli within the family Enterobacteriaceae consists of two species: *S. choleraesuis*, which contains six subspecies, and *S. bongori. S. choleraesuis* subspecies I contains almost all the serotypes pathogenic for humans. Because the designation *S. choleraesuis* refers to both a species and a serotype, the species designation *S. enterica* has been recommended and widely adopted. According to the current *Salmonella* nomenclature system, the full taxonomic designation *Salmonella enterica* subspecies *enterica* serotype Typhimurium can be shortened to *Salmonella* serotype Typhimurium or simply *Salmonella* Typhimurium.

Members of the seven *Salmonella* subspecies are classified into >2400 serotypes (serovars) according to the somatic O antigen [lipopolysaccharide (LPS) cell-wall components], the surface Vi antigen (restricted to *S.* Typhi and *S.* Paratyphi C), and the flagellar H antigen. For simplicity, most *Salmonella* serotypes are named for the city where they were identified, and the serotype is often used as the species designation.

Salmonellae are gram-negative, non-spore-forming, facultatively anaerobic bacilli that measure 2–3 by 0.4–0.6 μm. The initial identification of salmonellae in the clinical microbiology laboratory is based on growth characteristics. Salmonellae, like other Enterobacteriaceae, produce acid on glucose fermentation, reduce nitrates, and do not produce cytochrome oxidase. In addition, all salmonellae except *S.* Gallinarum-Pullorum are motile by means of peritrichous flagella, and all but *S.* Typhi produce gas (H_2S) on sugar fermentation. Notably, only 1% of clinical isolates ferment lactose; a high level of suspicion must be maintained to detect these rare clinical lactose-fermenting isolates.

Although serotyping of all surface antigens can be used for formal identification, most laboratories perform a few simple agglutination reactions that define specific O-antigen serogroups, designated A, B, C_1, C_2, D, and E. Strains in these six serogroups cause ~99% of *Salmonella* infections in humans and warm-blooded animals. Molecular typing methods, including pulsed-field gel electrophoresis, are used in epidemiologic investigations to differentiate *Salmonella* strains of a common serotype.

PATHOGENESIS

All *Salmonella* infections begin with ingestion of organisms in contaminated food or water. The infectious dose is 10^3–10^6 colony-forming units. Conditions that decrease either stomach acidity (an age of <1 year, antacid ingestion, or achlorhydric disease) or intestinal integrity (inflammatory bowel disease, prior gastrointestinal surgery, or alteration of the intestinal flora by antibiotic administration) increase susceptibility to *Salmonella* infection.

Once salmonellae reach the small intestine, they penetrate the mucous layer of the gut and traverse the intestinal layer through phagocytic microfold (M) cells that reside within Peyer's patches. Salmonellae can trigger the formation of membrane ruffles in normally nonphagocytic epithelial cells. These ruffles reach out and enclose adherent bacteria within large vesicles by a process referred to as *bacteria-mediated endocytosis* (BME). BME is dependent on the direct delivery of *Salmonella* proteins into the cytoplasm of epithelial cells by a specialized bacterial secretion system (*type III secretion*). These bacterial proteins mediate alterations in the actin cytoskeleton that are required for *Salmonella* uptake.

After crossing the epithelial layer of the small intestine, *S.* Typhi and *S.* Paratyphi, which cause enteric (typhoid) fever, are phagocytosed by macrophages. These salmonellae survive the antimicrobial environment of the macrophage by sensing environmental signals that trigger alterations in regulatory systems of the phagocytosed bacteria. For example, PhoP/PhoQ (the best-characterized regulatory system) triggers the expression of outer-membrane proteins and mediates modifications in LPS so that the altered bacterial surface can resist microbicidal activities and potentially alter host cell signaling. In addition, salmonellae encode a second type III secretion system that directly delivers bacterial proteins across the phagosome membrane into the macrophage cytoplasm. This secretion system functions to remodel the *Salmonella*-containing vacuole, promoting bacterial survival and replication.

Once phagocytosed, salmonellae disseminate throughout the body in macrophages via the lymphatics and colonize reticuloendothelial tissues (liver, spleen, lymph nodes, and bone marrow). Patients have relatively few or no signs and symptoms during this initial incubation stage. Signs and symptoms, including fever and abdominal pain, probably result from secretion of cytokines by macrophages and epithelial cells in response to bacterial products that are recognized by innate immune receptors when a critical number of organisms have replicated. Over time, the development of hepatosplenomegaly is likely to be related to the recruitment of mononuclear cells and the development of a specific acquired cell-mediated immune response to *S. typhi* colonization. The recruitment of additional mononuclear cells and lymphocytes to Peyer's patches during the several weeks after initial colonization/infection can result in marked enlargement and necrosis of the Peyer's patches, which may be mediated by bacterial products that promote cell death as well as the inflammatory response.

In contrast to enteric fever, which is characterized by an infiltration of mononuclear cells into the small-bowel mucosa, NTS gastroenteritis is characterized by massive polymorphonuclear leukocyte (PMN) infiltration into both the large- and small-bowel mucosa. This response appears to depend on the induction of interleukin (IL) 8, a strong neutrophil chemotactic factor, which is secreted by intestinal cells as a result of *Salmonella* colonization and translocation of bacterial proteins into host cell cytoplasm. The degranulation and release of toxic substances by neutrophils may result in damage to the intestinal mucosa, causing the inflammatory diarrhea observed with nontyphoidal gastroenteritis.

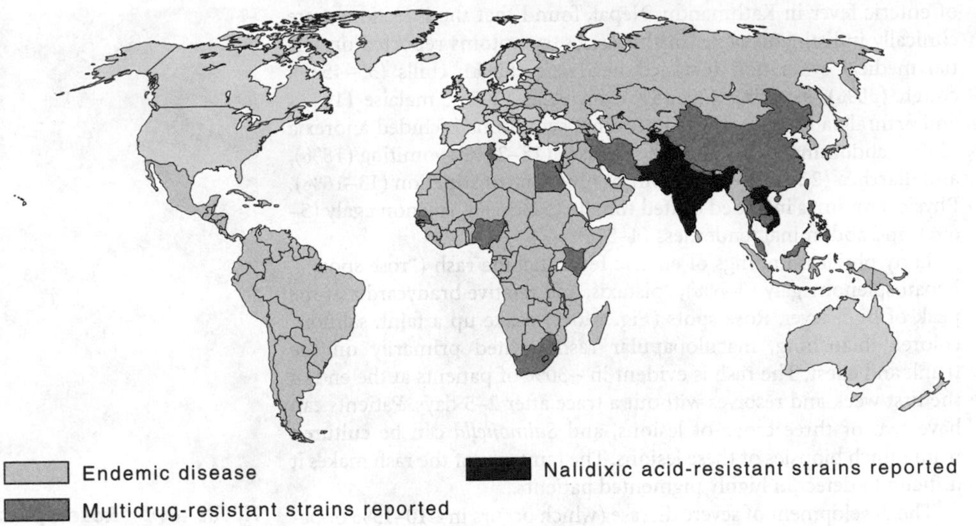

FIGURE 146-1 Global distribution of resistance to *S.* Typhi, 1990–2002. *(Reprinted with permission from Parry CM et al: Typhoid fever. N Engl J Med 347:1770, 2002. © 2002 Massachusetts Medical Society. All rights reserved.)*

ENTERIC (TYPHOID) FEVER

Typhoid fever is a systemic disease characterized by fever and abdominal pain and caused by dissemination of *S.* Typhi or *S.* Paratyphi. The disease was initially called *typhoid fever* because of its clinical similarity to typhus. However, in the early 1800s, typhoid fever was clearly defined pathologically as a unique illness on the basis of its association with enlarged Peyer's patches and mesenteric lymph nodes. In 1869, given the anatomic site of infection, the term *enteric fever* was proposed as an alternative designation to distinguish typhoid fever from typhus. However, to this day, the two designations are used interchangeably.

EPIDEMIOLOGY

In contrast to other *Salmonella* serotypes, the etiologic agents of enteric fever—*S.* Typhi and *S.* Paratyphi serotypes A, B, and C—have no known hosts other than humans. Most commonly, food-borne or waterborne transmission results from fecal contamination by ill or asymptomatic chronic carriers. Sexual transmission between male partners has been described. Health care workers occasionally acquire enteric fever after exposure to infected patients or during processing of clinical specimens and cultures.

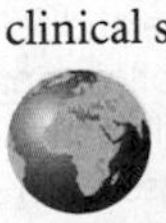

With improvements in food handling and water/sewage treatment, enteric fever has become rare in developed nations. Worldwide, however, there were an estimated 22 million cases of enteric fever, with 200,000 deaths, in 2002. The incidence is highest (>100 cases per 100,000 population per year) in south-central and Southeast Asia; medium (10–100 cases per 100,000) in the rest of Asia, Africa, Latin America, and Oceania (excluding Australia and New Zealand); and low in other parts of the world. A high incidence of enteric fever correlates with poor sanitation and lack of access to clean drinking water. In endemic regions, enteric fever is more common in urban than rural areas and among young children and adolescents. Risk factors include contaminated water or ice, flooding, food and drinks purchased from street vendors, raw fruits and vegetables grown in fields fertilized with sewage, ill household contacts, lack of hand washing and toilet access, and evidence of prior *Helicobacter pylori* infection (an association probably related to chronically reduced gastric acidity). It is estimated that there is one case of paratyphoid fever for every four cases of typhoid fever, but the incidence of infection associated with *S.* Paratyphi A appears to be increasing, especially in India.

Multidrug-resistant (MDR) strains of *S.* Typhi emerged in 1989 in China and Southeast Asia and have since disseminated widely (Fig. 146-1). These strains contain plasmids encoding resistance to chloramphenicol, ampicillin, and trimethoprim—antibiotics long used to treat enteric fever. With the increased use of fluoroquinolones to treat MDR enteric fever, strains of *S.* Typhi and *S.* Paratyphi with reduced susceptibility to ciprofloxacin [minimal inhibitory concentration (MIC), 0.125–1.0 μg/mL] have emerged in India and Vietnam and have been associated with clinical treatment failure. Testing of isolates for resistance to the first-generation quinolone nalidixic acid detects most but not all strains with reduced susceptibility to ciprofloxacin.

The incidence of enteric fever among U.S. travelers is estimated at 3–30 cases per 100,000. Of 1393 cases reported to the Centers for Disease Control and Prevention (CDC) in 1994–1999, 74% were associated with recent international travel, most commonly to India (30%), Pakistan (13%), Mexico (12%), Bangladesh (8%), the Philippines (8%), and Haiti (5%). Likewise, of 356 cases reported in the United States in 2003, ~74% occurred in persons who reported international travel during the preceding 6 weeks. Only 4% of travelers diagnosed with enteric fever gave a history of *S.* Typhi vaccination within the previous 5 years. Increased rates of MDR *S.* Typhi and *S.* Paratyphi have been reported among travelers. In 1996–1997, 80% of U.S. travelers with enteric fever acquired in Vietnam were infected with MDR *S.* Typhi strains. Of the 25–30% of reported cases of enteric fever in the United States that are domestically acquired, the majority are sporadic, but 7% have occurred in recognized outbreaks linked to contaminated food products and previously unrecognized chronic carriers. An increasing proportion of cases (currently ~80%) are associated with foreign-born U.S. residents visiting friends and relatives in their native countries.

CLINICAL COURSE

Enteric fever is a misnomer, in that the hallmark features of this disease—fever and abdominal pain—are variable. While fever is documented at presentation in >75% of cases, abdominal pain is reported in only 30–40%. Thus, a high index of suspicion for this potentially fatal systemic illness is necessary when a person presents with fever and a history of recent travel to a developing country.

The incubation period for *S.* Typhi averages 10–14 days but ranges from 3 to 21 days, with the duration likely reflecting the inoculum size and the host's health and immune status. The most prominent symptom is prolonged fever (38.8°–40.5°C; 101.8°–104.9°F), which can continue for up to 4 weeks if untreated. *S.* Paratyphi A is thought to cause milder disease than *S.* Typhi, with predominantly gastrointestinal symptoms. However, a prospective study of 669 consecutive cases of enteric fever in Kathmandu, Nepal, found that the infections were clinically indistinguishable. In this series, symptoms reported on initial medical evaluation included headache (80%), chills (35–45%), cough (30%), sweating (20–25%), myalgias (20%), malaise (10%), and arthralgia (2–4%). Gastrointestinal symptoms included anorexia (55%), abdominal pain (30–40%), nausea (18–24%), vomiting (18%), and diarrhea (22–28%) more commonly than constipation (13–16%). Physical findings included coated tongue (51–56%), splenomegaly (5–6%), and abdominal tenderness (4–5%).

Early physical findings of enteric fever include rash ("rose spots"), hepatosplenomegaly (3–6%), epistaxis, and relative bradycardia at the peak of high fever. Rose spots (Fig. 146-2) make up a faint, salmon-colored, blanching, maculopapular rash located primarily on the trunk and chest. The rash is evident in ~30% of patients at the end of the first week and resolves without a trace after 2–5 days. Patients can have two or three crops of lesions, and *Salmonella* can be cultured from punch biopsies of these lesions. The faintness of the rash makes it difficult to detect in highly pigmented patients.

The development of severe disease (which occurs in ~10–15% of patients) depends on host factors (immunosuppression, antacid therapy, previous exposure, and vaccination), strain virulence and inoculum, and choice of antibiotic therapy. Gastrointestinal bleeding (10–20%) and intestinal perforation (1–3%) most commonly occur in the third and fourth weeks of illness and result from hyperplasia, ulceration, and necrosis of the ileocecal Peyer's patches at the initial site of *Salmonella* infiltration. Both complications are life-threatening and require immediate fluid resuscitation and surgical intervention, with broadened antibiotic coverage for polymicrobial peritonitis (Chap. 121) and treatment of gastrointestinal hemorrhages, including bowel resection. Neurologic manifestations occur in 2–40% of patients and include meningitis, Guillain-Barré syndrome, neuritis, and neuropsychiatric symptoms (described as "muttering delirium" or "coma vigil"), with picking at bedclothes or imaginary objects.

Rare complications whose incidences are reduced by prompt antibiotic treatment include disseminated intravascular coagulation, hematophagocytic syndrome, pancreatitis, hepatic and splenic abscesses and granulomas, endocarditis, pericarditis, myocarditis, orchitis, hepatitis, glomerulonephritis, pyelonephritis and hemolytic uremic syndrome, severe pneumonia, arthritis, osteomyelitis, and parotitis. Up to 10% of patients develop mild relapse, usually within 2–3 weeks of fever resolution and in association with the same strain type and susceptibility profile.

Up to 10% of untreated patients with typhoid fever excrete *S.* Typhi in the feces for up to 3 months, and 1–4% develop chronic asymptomatic carriage, shedding *S.* Typhi in either urine or stool for >1 year. Chronic carriage is more common among women, infants, and persons with biliary abnormalities or concurrent bladder infection with *Schistosoma haematobium*. The anatomic abnormalities associated with the latter conditions presumably allow prolonged colonization.

DIAGNOSIS

Since the clinical presentation of enteric fever is relatively nonspecific, the diagnosis needs to be considered in any febrile traveler returning from a developing country, especially the Indian subcontinent, the Philippines, or Latin America. Other diagnoses that should be considered in these travelers include malaria, hepatitis, bacterial enteritis, dengue fever, rickettsial infections, leptospirosis, amebic liver abscesses, and acute HIV infection (Chap. 117). Other than a positive culture, no specific laboratory test is diagnostic for enteric fever. In 15–25% of cases, leukopenia and neutropenia are detectable. Leukocytosis is more common among children, during the first 10 days of illness, and in cases complicated by intestinal perforation or secondary infection. Other nonspecific laboratory findings include moderately elevated liver function tests and muscle enzyme levels.

The definitive diagnosis of enteric fever requires the isolation of *S.* Typhi or *S.* Paratyphi from blood, bone marrow, other sterile sites, rose spots, stool, or intestinal secretions. The yield of blood cultures is quite variable; sensitivity is as high as 90% during the first week of infection and decreases to 50% by the third week. A low yield in infected patients is related to low numbers of salmonellae (<15 organisms/mL) and/or to recent antibiotic treatment. Since almost all *S.* Typhi organisms in blood are associated with the mononuclear-cell/platelet fraction, centrifugation of blood and culture of the buffy coat can substantially reduce the time to isolation of the organism but does not increase sensitivity.

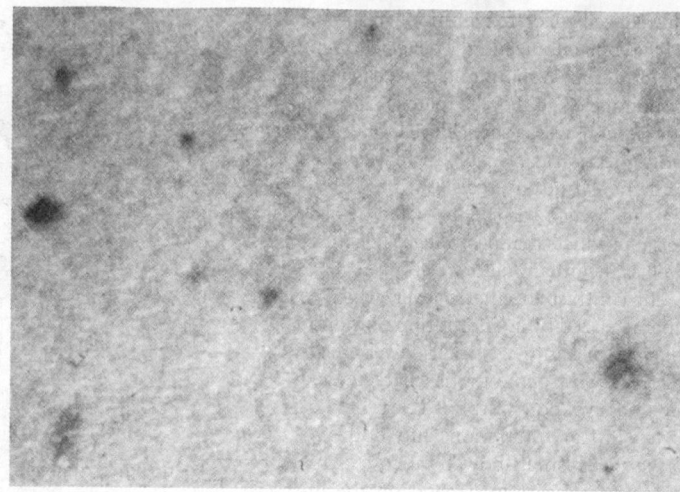

FIGURE 146-2 "Rose spots," the rash of enteric fever due to *S.* Typhi or *S.* Paratyphi.

Unlike blood culture, bone marrow culture remains highly (90%) sensitive despite ≤5 days of antibiotic therapy. Culture of intestinal secretions (best obtained by a noninvasive duodenal string test) can be positive despite a negative bone marrow culture. If blood, bone marrow, and intestinal secretions are all cultured, the yield is >90%. Stool cultures, while negative in 60–70% of cases during the first week, can become positive during the third week of infection in untreated patients.

Several serologic tests, including the classic Widal test for "febrile agglutinins," are available. None of these tests is sufficiently sensitive or specific to replace culture-based methods for the diagnosis of enteric fever in developed countries. Polymerase chain reaction and DNA probe assays to detect *S.* Typhi in blood are being developed.

Rx ENTERIC (TYPHOID) FEVER

Prompt administration of appropriate antibiotic therapy prevents severe complications of enteric fever and results in a case-fatality rate of <1%. The initial choice of antibiotics depends on the susceptibility of the *S.* Typhi and *S.* Paratyphi strains in the area of residence or travel (**Table 146-1**). For treatment of drug-susceptible typhoid fever, fluoroquinolones are the most effective class of agents, with cure rates of ~98% and relapse and fecal carriage rates of <2%. Experience is most extensive with ciprofloxacin. Short-course ofloxacin therapy is similarly successful against infection caused by nalidixic acid–susceptible strains. However, the increased incidence of nalidixic acid–resistant (NAR) *S.* Typhi in Asia, which is probably related to the widespread availability of fluoroquinolones over the counter, is now limiting the use of this drug class for empirical therapy. Patients infected with NAR *S.* Typhi strains should be treated with ceftriaxone, azithromycin, or high-dose ciprofloxacin. However, high-dose fluoroquinolone therapy for NAR enteric fever has been associated with delayed resolution of fever and high rates of fecal carriage during convalescence.

Ceftriaxone, cefotaxime, and (oral) cefixime are effective for treatment of MDR enteric fever, including NAR and fluoroquinolone-resistant strains. These agents clear fever in ~1 week, with failure rates of ~5–10%, fecal carriage rates of <3%, and relapse rates of 3–6%. Oral azithromycin results in defervescence in 4–6 days, with rates of relapse and convalescent stool carriage of <3%. Despite efficient in vitro killing of *Salmonella*, first- and second-generation cephalosporins as well as aminoglycosides are ineffective in treating clinical infections.

Patients with persistent vomiting, diarrhea, and/or abdominal distension should be hospitalized and given supportive therapy as well as a pa-

TABLE 146-1 ANTIBIOTIC THERAPY FOR ENTERIC FEVER IN ADULTS

Indication	Agent	Dosage (Route)	Duration, Days
Empirical Treatment			
	Ceftriaxone[a]	1–2 g/d (IV)	7–14
	Azithromycin	1 g/d (PO)	5
Fully Susceptible			
	Ciprofloxacin[b] (first line)	500 mg bid (PO) or 400 mg q12h (IV)	5–7
	Amoxicillin (second line)	1 g tid (PO) or 2 g q6h (IV)	14
	Chloramphenicol	25 mg/kg tid (PO or IV)	14–21
	Trimethoprim-sulfamethoxazole	160/800 mg bid (PO)	14
Multidrug-Resistant			
	Ciprofloxacin	500 mg bid (PO) or 400 mg q12h (IV)	5–7
	Ceftriaxone	2–3 g/d (IV)	7–14
	Azithromycin	1 g/d (PO)[c]	5
Nalidixic Acid–Resistant			
	Ceftriaxone	1–2 g/d (IV)	7–14
	Azithromycin	1 g/d (PO)	5
	High-dose ciprofloxacin	750 mg bid (PO) or 400 mg q8h (IV)	10–14

[a]Or another third-generation cephalosporin [e.g., cefotaxime, 2 g q8h (IV), or cefixime, 400 mg bid (PO)].
[b]Or ofloxacin, 400 mg bid (PO) for 2–5 days.
[c]Or 1 g on day 1 followed by 500 mg/d PO for 6 days.

renteral third-generation cephalosporin or fluoroquinolone, depending on the susceptibility profile. Therapy should be administered for at least 10 days or for 5 days after fever resolution.

In a randomized, prospective, double-blind study of critically ill patients with enteric fever (i.e., those with shock and obtundation) in Indonesia in the early 1980s, the administration of dexamethasone (3-mg initial dose followed by eight doses of 1 mg/kg every 6 h) with chloramphenicol was associated with a substantially lower mortality rate than treatment with chloramphenicol alone (10% vs 55%). Although this study has not been repeated in the "post-chloramphenicol era," severe enteric fever remains one of the few indications for glucocorticoid treatment of an acute bacterial infection.

The 1–5% of patients who develop chronic carriage of *Salmonella* can be treated for 4–6 weeks with an appropriate oral antibiotic. Treatment with oral amoxicillin, trimethoprim-sulfamethoxazole (TMP-SMX), ciprofloxacin, or norfloxacin is ~80% effective in eradicating chronic carriage of susceptible organisms. However, in cases of anatomic abnormality (e.g., biliary or kidney stones), eradication often requires both antibiotic therapy and surgical correction.

PREVENTION AND CONTROL

Theoretically, it is possible to eliminate the salmonellae that cause enteric fever since they survive only in human hosts and are spread by contaminated food and water. However, given the high prevalence of the disease in developing countries that lack adequate sewage disposal and water treatment, this goal is currently unrealistic. Thus, travelers to developing countries should be advised to monitor their food and water intake carefully and to consider vaccination.

Two typhoid vaccines are commercially available: (1) Ty21a, an oral live attenuated *S.* Typhi vaccine (given on days 1, 3, 5, and 7, with a booster every 5 years); and (2) Vi CPS, a parenteral vaccine consisting of purified Vi polysaccharide from the bacterial capsule (given in 1 dose, with a booster every 2 years). The old parenteral whole-cell typhoid/paratyphoid A and B vaccine is no longer licensed, largely because of significant side effects (see below). An acetone-killed whole-cell vaccine is available only for use by the U.S. military. The minimal age for vaccination is 6 years for Ty21a and 2 years for Vi CPS. Currently, there is no licensed vaccine for paratyphoid fever.

A large-scale meta-analysis of vaccine trials comparing whole-cell vaccine, Ty21a, and Vi CPS in populations in endemic areas indicates that, while all three vaccines are similarly effective for the first year, the 3-year cumulative efficacy of the whole-cell vaccine (73%) exceeds that of both Ty21a (51%) and Vi CPS (55%). In addition, the heat-killed whole-cell vaccine maintains its efficacy for 5 years, whereas Ty21a and Vi CPS maintain their efficacy for 4 and 2 years, respectively. However, the whole-cell vaccine is associated with a much higher incidence of side effects (especially fever: 16% vs 1–2%) than the other two vaccines.

Vi CPS typhoid vaccine is poorly immunogenic in children <5 years of age because of T cell–independent properties. In the recently developed Vi-rEPA vaccine, Vi is bound to a nontoxic recombinant protein that is identical to *Pseudomonas aeruginosa* exotoxin A. In 2- to 4-year-olds, two injections of Vi-rEPA induced higher T-cell responses and higher levels of serum IgG antibody to Vi than did Vi CPS in 5- to 14-year-olds. In a two-dose trial in 2- to 5-year-old children in Vietnam, Vi-rEPA provided 91% efficacy at 27 months and 88% efficacy at 43 months and was very well tolerated. Similar results were obtained in a trial in Cambodia. This vaccine is not yet commercially available in the United States. At least three new live vaccines are in clinical development and may prove more efficacious and longer-lasting than previous live vaccines.

Although data on typhoid vaccines in travelers are limited, some evidence suggests that efficacy rates may be substantially lower than those for local populations in endemic areas. Both the CDC and the World Health Organization recommend typhoid vaccination for travelers to typhoid-endemic countries. Recent analyses from the CDC found that 16% of travel-associated cases occurred among persons who stayed at their travel destination for ≤2 weeks. Thus, vaccination should be strongly considered even for persons planning short-term travel to high-risk areas such as the Indian subcontinent. In the United States, persons who have intimate or household contact with a chronic carrier or laboratory workers who frequently deal with *S.* Typhi also should receive typhoid vaccine.

Enteric fever is a notifiable disease in the United States. Individual health departments have their own guidelines for allowing ill or colonized food handlers or health care workers to return to their jobs. The reporting system enables public health departments to identify potential source patients and to treat chronic carriers in order to prevent further outbreaks. In addition, since 1–4% of patients with *S.* Typhi infection become chronic carriers, it is important to monitor patients (especially child-care providers and food handlers) for chronic carriage and to treat this condition if indicated.

NONTYPHOIDAL SALMONELLOSIS

EPIDEMIOLOGY

During 1996–1999, there were an estimated 1.4 million cases of nontyphoidal salmonellosis in the United States, resulting in 168,000 physician office visits, 15,000 hospitalizations, and 400 deaths annually. In 2004, the incidence of NTS infection in this country was 14.7 per 100,000 persons—the highest rate among the nine food-borne enteric pathogens under active surveillance. Five serotypes accounted for 57% of U.S. infections in 2004: Typhimurium (20%), Enteritidis (15%), Newport (10%), Javiana (7%), and Heidelberg (5%).

The incidence of nontyphoidal salmonellosis is highest during the rainy season in tropical climates and during the warmer months in temperate climates, coinciding with the peak in food-borne outbreaks. Rates of morbidity and mortality associated with NTS are highest among the elderly, infants, and immunocompromised individuals, including those with hemoglobinopathies, HIV infection, or infections that cause blockade of the reticuloendothelial system (e.g., bartonellosis, malaria, schistosomiasis, and histoplasmosis).

Unlike *S.* Typhi and *S.* Paratyphi, whose only reservoir is humans, NTS can be acquired from multiple animal reservoirs. Transmission is most commonly associated with animal food products, especially eggs, poultry, undercooked ground meat, and dairy products and fresh produce contaminated with animal waste.

S. Enteritidis infection associated with chicken eggs emerged as a major cause of foodborne disease during the 1980s and 1990s. *S.* Enteritidis infection of the ovaries and upper oviduct tissue of hens results in contamination of egg contents before shell deposition. Infection is spread to egg-laying hens from breeding flocks and through contact with rodents and manure. Of the 360 outbreaks of *S.* Enteritidis with a confirmed source that were reported to the CDC in 1985–1998, 279 (78%) were associated with raw or undercooked eggs. After peaking at 3.9 cases per 100,000 U.S. population in 1995, the incidence of *S.* Enteritidis infection declined dramatically to 1.98 per 100,000 in 1999; this decrease probably reflected improved on-farm control measures, refrigeration, and education of consumers and food-service workers. Transmission via contaminated eggs can be prevented by cooking eggs until the yolk is solidified and through pasteurization of egg products.

Centralization of food processing and widespread food distribution have contributed to the increased incidence of NTS in developing countries. Manufactured foods to which recent *Salmonella* outbreaks have been traced include pasteurized milk, infant formula, powdered milk products, and various processed foods. Large outbreaks have also been linked to fresh produce, including alfalfa sprouts, cantaloupe, fresh-squeezed orange juice, and tomatoes; these items become contaminated by manure or water at a single site and then are widely distributed.

An estimated 6% of sporadic *Salmonella* infections in the United States are attributed to contact with reptiles and amphibians, especially iguanas, snakes, turtles, and lizards. Reptile-associated *Salmonella* infection more commonly leads to hospitalization and more frequently involves infants than do other *Salmonella* infections. Other pets, including African hedgehogs, snakes, birds, rodents, baby chicks, ducklings, dogs, and cats, are also potential sources of NTS.

Increasing antibiotic resistance in NTS species is a global problem and has been linked to the widespread use of antimicrobial agents in food animals and especially in animal feed. In the early 1990s, *S.* Typhimurium definitive phage type 104 (DT104), characterized by resistance to ≥5 antibiotics (ampicillin, chloramphenicol, streptomycin, sulfonamides, and tetracyclines; R-type ACSSuT), emerged worldwide. From 1979–1980 to 2001, the prevalence of *S.* Typhimurium ACSSuT increased in the United States from 0.6% to 7% of all NTS isolates, and most (65%) of these ACSSuT isolates were phage type DT104. Acquisition is associated with exposure to ill farm animals and to various meat products, including uncooked or undercooked ground beef. In an analysis of U.S. surveillance data for 1996–2001, antibiotic-resistant NTS strains, especially *S.* Typhimurium DT104, were associated with an increased risk of bloodstream infection and hospitalization. NAR and trimethoprim-resistant DT104 strains are emerging, especially in the United Kingdom.

Because of increased resistance to conventional antibiotics such as ampicillin and TMP-SMX, extended-spectrum cephalosporins and fluoroquinolones have emerged as the agents of choice for the treatment of MDR NTS infections. With the increased use of these agents, the CDC reported that the prevalence of ceftriaxone-resistant NTS strains rose from 0 in 1995 to 0.5% in 1998. Of the ceftriaxone-resistant isolates, 77% were from children <18 years of age, in whom ceftriaxone is the antibiotic of choice for treatment of invasive infection. These strains contained plasmid-encoded AmpC β-lactamases that were probably acquired by horizontal genetic transfer from *Escherichia coli* strains in food-producing animals—an event linked to the widespread use of the veterinary cephalosporin ceftiofur.

Resistance to nalidixic acid and fluoroquinolones also has begun to emerge and is most commonly associated with point mutations in the DNA gyrase genes *gyrA* and *gyrB*. Nalidixic acid resistance is a good predictor of reduced susceptibility to clinically useful fluoroquinolones. From 1994–1995 to 2000, the rate of NAR NTS isolates in the United States increased fivefold (from 0.5% to 2.5%). In Denmark, infection with NAR *S.* Typhimurium DT104 has been linked to swine and associated with a threefold higher risk of invasive disease or death within 90 days. In Taiwan in 2000, a strain of ciprofloxacin-resistant (MIC, ≥4 μg/mL) *S.* Choleraesuis caused a large outbreak of invasive infections that was linked to the use of enrofloxacin in swine feed.

CLINICAL MANIFESTATIONS

Gastroenteritis Infection with NTS most often results in gastroenteritis indistinguishable from that caused by other enteric pathogens. Nausea, vomiting, and diarrhea occur 6–48 h after the ingestion of contaminated food or water. Patients often experience abdominal cramping and fever (38–39°C; 100.5–102.2°F). Diarrheal stools are usually loose, nonbloody, and of moderate volume. However, large-volume watery stools, bloody stools, or symptoms of dysentery may occur. Rarely, NTS causes pseudoappendicitis or an illness that mimics inflammatory bowel disease.

Gastroenteritis caused by NTS is usually self-limited. Diarrhea resolves within 3–7 days and fever within 72 h. Stool cultures remain positive for 4–5 weeks after infection and—in rare cases of chronic carriage (<1%)—for >1 year. Antibiotic treatment usually is not recommended and in some studies has prolonged fecal carriage. Neonates, the elderly, and immunosuppressed patients (e.g., transplant recipients, HIV-infected persons) with NTS gastroenteritis are especially susceptible to dehydration and dissemination and may require hospitalization and antibiotic therapy. Acute NTS gastroenteritis was associated with a threefold increased risk of dyspepsia and irritable bowel syndrome at 1 year in a recent study from Spain.

Bacteremia and Endovascular Infections Up to 5% of patients with NTS gastroenteritis develop bacteremia; of these, 5–10% develop localized infections. Bacteremia and metastatic infection are most common with *S.* Choleraesuis and *S.* Dublin and among infants, the elderly, and immunocompromised patients. NTS endovascular infection should be suspected in high-grade bacteremia, especially with preexisting valvular heart disease, atherosclerotic vascular disease, prosthetic vascular graft, or aortic aneurysm. Arteritis should be suspected in elderly patients with prolonged fever and back, chest, or abdominal pain developing after an episode of gastroenteritis. Endocarditis and arteritis are rare (<1% of cases) but are associated with potentially fatal complications, including valve perforation, endomyocardial abscess, infected mural thrombus, pericarditis, mycotic aneurysms, aneurysm rupture, aortoenteric fistula, and vertebral osteomyelitis.

Localized Infections • ***INTRAABDOMINAL INFECTIONS*** Intraabdominal infections due to NTS are rare and usually manifest as hepatic or splenic abscesses or as cholecystitis. Risk factors include hepatobiliary anatomic abnormalities (e.g., gallstones), abdominal malignancy, and sickle cell disease (especially with splenic abscesses). Eradication of the infection often requires surgical correction of abnormalities and percutaneous drainage of abscesses.

CENTRAL NERVOUS SYSTEM INFECTIONS Meningitis most commonly develops in infants 1–4 months of age. It often results in severe sequelae (including seizures, hydrocephalus, brain infarction, and mental retardation) with death in up to 60% of cases. Other rare central nervous system infections include ventriculitis, subdural empyema, and brain abscesses.

PULMONARY INFECTIONS NTS pulmonary infections usually present as lobar pneumonia, and complications include lung abscess, empyema, and bronchopleural fistula formation. The majority of cases occur in patients with lung cancer, structural lung disease, sickle cell disease, or glucocorticoid use.

URINARY AND GENITAL TRACT INFECTIONS Urinary tract infections caused by NTS present as either cystitis or pyelonephritis. Risk factors include malignancy, urolithiasis, structural abnormalities, HIV infection, and renal transplantation. NTS genital infections are rare and include ovarian and testicular abscesses, prostatitis, and epididymitis. Like other focal infections, both genital and urinary tract infections can be complicated by abscess formation.

BONE, JOINT, AND SOFT TISSUE INFECTIONS *Salmonella* osteomyelitis most commonly affects the femur, tibia, humerus, or lumbar vertebrae and is most often seen in association with sickle cell disease, hemoglobinopathies, or preexisting bone disease (e.g., fractures). Prolonged antibiotic treatment is recommended to decrease the risk of relapse and chronic osteomyelitis. Septic arthritis occurs in the same patient population as osteomyelitis and usually involves the knee, hip, or shoulder joints. Reactive arthritis (Reiter's syndrome) can follow NTS gastroenteritis and is seen most frequently in persons with the HLA-B27 histocompatibility antigen. NTS rarely can cause soft tissue infections, usually at sites of local trauma in immunosuppressed patients.

DIAGNOSIS

The diagnosis of NTS infection is based on the isolation of the organism from freshly passed stool or from blood or another ordinarily sterile body fluid. All salmonellae isolated in clinical laboratories should be sent to local public health departments for serotyping. Blood cultures should be done whenever a patient has prolonged or recurrent fever. Endovascular infection should be suspected if there is high-grade bacteremia (>50% of three or more blood cultures positive). Echocardiography, computed tomography, and indium-labeled white cell scanning are used to identify localized infection. When another localized infection is suspected, joint fluid, abscess drainage, or cerebrospinal fluid should be cultured, as clinically indicated.

TABLE 146-2 ANTIBIOTIC THERAPY FOR NONTYPHOIDAL *SALMONELLA* INFECTION IN ADULTS

Indication	Agent	Dosage (Route)	Duration, Days
Preemptive Treatment[a]			
	Ciprofloxacin[b]	500 mg bid (PO)	2–3
Severe Gastroenteritis[c]			
	Ciprofloxacin	500 mg bid (PO) or 400 mg q12h (IV)	3–7
	Trimethoprim-sulfamethoxazole	160/800 mg bid (PO)	
	Amoxicillin	1 g tid (PO)	
	Ceftriaxone	1–2 g/d (IV)	
Bacteremia			
	Ceftriaxone[d]	2 g/d (IV)	7–14
	Ciprofloxacin	400 mg q12h (IV), then 500 mg bid (PO)	
Endocarditis or Arteritis			
	Ceftriaxone	2 g/d (IV)	42
	Ciprofloxacin	400 mg q8h (IV), then 750 mg bid (PO)	
	Ampicillin	2 g q4h (IV)	
Meningitis			
	Ceftriaxone	2 g q12 h (IV)	14–21
	Ampicillin	2 g q4h (IV)	
Other Localized Infection			
	Ceftriaxone	2 g/d (IV)	14–28
	Ciprofloxacin	500 mg bid (PO) or 400 mg q12h (IV)	
	Ampicillin	2 g q6h (IV)	

[a]Consider for neonates; persons >50 years of age with possible atherosclerotic vascular disease; and patients with immunosuppression, endovascular graft, or joint prosthesis.
[b]Or ofloxacin, 400 mg bid (PO).
[c]Consider on an individualized basis for patients with severe diarrhea and high fever who require hospitalization.
[d]Or cefotaxime, 2 g q8h (IV).

Rx NONTYPHOIDAL SALMONELLOSIS

Antibiotics should not be used routinely to treat uncomplicated NTS gastroenteritis. The symptoms are usually self-limited, and the duration of fever and diarrhea is not significantly decreased by antibiotic therapy. In addition, antibiotic treatment has been associated with increased rates of relapse and prolonged gastrointestinal carriage. Dehydration secondary to diarrhea should be treated with fluid and electrolyte replacement.

Preemptive antibiotic treatment **(Table 146-2)** should be considered for patients at increased risk for invasive NTS infection, including neonates (probably up to 3 months of age); persons >50 years of age with suspected atherosclerosis; and patients with immunosuppression, cardiac valvular or endovascular abnormalities, or significant joint disease. Treatment should consist of an oral or IV antibiotic administered for 48–72 h or until the patient becomes afebrile. Immunocompromised persons may require up to 7–14 days of therapy. The <1% of persons who develop chronic carriage of NTS should receive a prolonged antibiotic course, as described above for chronic carriage of *S.* Typhi.

Because of the increasing prevalence of antibiotic resistance, empirical therapy for life-threatening NTS bacteremia or focal NTS infection should include a third-generation cephalosporin or a fluoroquinolone (Table 146-2). If the bacteremia is low-grade (<50% of blood cultures positive), the patient should be treated for 7–14 days. Patients with AIDS and NTS bacteremia should receive 1–2 weeks of IV antibiotic therapy followed by 4 weeks of oral therapy with a fluoroquinolone. Patients whose infections relapse after this regimen should receive long-term suppressive therapy with a fluoroquinolone or TMP-SMX, as indicated by bacterial sensitivities.

If the patient has endocarditis or arteritis, treatment for 6 weeks with an IV β-lactam antibiotic (such as ceftriaxone or ampicillin) is indicated. IV ciprofloxacin followed by prolonged oral therapy is an option, but published experience is limited. Early surgical resection of infected aneurysms or other infected endovascular sites is recommended. Patients with infected prosthetic vascular grafts that cannot be resected have been maintained successfully on chronic suppressive oral therapy. For extraintestinal nonvascular infections, a 2- to 4-week course of antibiotic therapy (depending on the infection site) is usually recommended. In chronic osteomyelitis, abscess, or urinary or hepatobiliary infection associated with anatomic abnormalities, surgical resection or drainage may be required in addition to prolonged antibiotic therapy for eradication of infection.

PREVENTION AND CONTROL

Despite widespread efforts to prevent or reduce bacterial contamination of animal-derived food products and to improve food-safety education and training, recent declines in the incidence of NTS in the United States have been modest compared with those of other food-borne pathogens. This observation probably reflects the complex epidemiology of NTS. Identifying effective risk-reduction strategies requires monitoring of every step of food production, from handling of raw animal or plant products to preparation of finished foods. Contaminated food can be made safe for consumption by pasteurization, irradiation, or proper cooking. All cases of NTS infection should be reported to local public health departments, since tracking and monitoring of these cases can identify the source(s) of infection and help authorities anticipate large outbreaks. Lastly, the prudent use of antimicrobial agents in both humans and animals is needed to limit the emergence of MDR *Salmonella*.

FURTHER READINGS

COHEN JI et al: Extra-intestinal manifestations of *Salmonella* infections. Medicine 66:349, 1987

GLYNN MK et al: Emergence of multidrug-resistant *Salmonella enterica* serotype *typhimurium* DT104 infections in the United States. N Engl J Med 338:1333, 1998

HOFFMAN SL et al: Reduction in mortality in chloramphenicol-treated severe typhoid fever by high-dose dexamethasone. N Engl J Med 310:82, 1984

LIN FY et al: The efficacy of a *Salmonella typhi* Vi conjugate vaccine in two-to-five-year-old children. N Engl J Med 344:1263, 2001

MASKEY AP et al: *Salmonella* enteric serovar Paratyphi A and *S. enterica* serovar Typhi cause indistinguishable clinical syndromes in Kathmandu, Nepal. Clin Infect Dis 42:1247, 2006

OHL ME, MILLER SI: *Salmonella*: A model for bacterial pathogenesis. Annu Rev Med 52:259, 2001

STEINBERG EB et al: Typhoid fever in travelers: Who should be targeted for prevention. Clin Infect Dis 39:186, 2004

SU LH et al: Antimicrobial resistance in nontyphoid *Salmonella* serotypes: A global challenge. Clin Infect Dis 39:546, 2004

VARMA JK et al: Antimicrobial-resistant nontyphoidal *Salmonella* is associated with excess bloodstream infections and hospitalizations. J Infect Dis 191:554, 2005

147 Shigellosis

Philippe Sansonetti, Jean Bergounioux

The discovery of *Shigella* as the etiologic agent of dysentery—a clinical syndrome of fever, intestinal cramps, and frequent passage of small, bloody, mucopurulent stools—is attributed to the Japanese microbiologist Kiyoshi Shiga, who isolated the Shiga bacillus (now known as *Shigella dysenteriae* type 1) from patients' stools in 1897 during a large and devastating dysentery epidemic. *Shigella* cannot be distinguished from *Escherichia coli* by DNA hybridization and remains a separate species only on historical and clinical grounds.

DEFINITION

Shigella is a non-spore-forming, gram-negative bacterium that, unlike *E. coli*, is nonmotile and does not produce gas from sugars, decarboxylate lysine, or hydrolyze arginine. Some serovars produce indole, and occasional strains utilize sodium acetate. *S. dysenteriae*, *S. flexneri*, *S. boydii*, and *S. sonnei* (serogroups A, B, C, and D, respectively) can be differentiated on the basis of biochemical and serologic characteristics. Genome sequencing of *E. coli* K12, *S. flexneri* 2a, *S. sonnei*, *S. dysenteriae* type 1, and *S. boydii* has revealed that these species have ~93% of genes in common. The three major genomic "signatures" of *Shigella* are (1) a 215-kb virulence plasmid that carries most of the genes required for pathogenicity (particularly invasive capacity); (2) the lack or alteration of genetic sequences encoding products (e.g., lysine decarboxylase) that, if expressed, would attenuate pathogenicity; and (3) in *S. dysenteriae* type 1, the presence of genes encoding Shiga toxin, a potent cytotoxin.

EPIDEMIOLOGY

The human intestinal tract represents the major reservoir of *Shigella*, which is also found (albeit rarely) in the higher primates. Because excretion of shigellae is greatest in the acute phase of disease, the bacteria are transmitted most efficiently by the fecal-oral route. Most cases of shigellosis are caused by person-to-person transmission, although some outbreaks reflect contamination of water or food. *Shigella* can also be transmitted by flies and, given its capacity to survive in foodstuffs, can be a significant cause of food-borne infection. The high-level infectivity of *Shigella* is reflected by the very small inoculum required for experimental infection of volunteers [100 colony-forming units (CFU)], by the very high attack rates during outbreaks in day care centers (33–73%), and by the high rates of secondary cases among family members of sick children (26–33%). Shigellosis can also be transmitted sexually.

In a review published under the auspices of the World Health Organization (WHO), the total annual number of cases in 1966–1997 was estimated at 165 million, and 69% of these cases occurred in children <5 years of age. In this review, the annual number of deaths was calculated to range between 500,000 and 1.1 million. More recent data (2000–2004) from six Asian countries (Bangladesh, China, Pakistan, Indonesia, Vietnam, and Thailand) indicate that even though the incidence of shigellosis remains stable, mortality rates associated with this disease may have decreased significantly, possibly as a result of improved nutritional standards. However, extensive and essentially uncontrolled use of antibiotics has increased the risk of emergence of multidrug-resistant *Shigella* strains.

Throughout history, *Shigella* epidemics have often occurred in settings of human crowding under poor hygienic conditions—e.g., among soldiers in campaigning armies, inhabitants of besieged cities, groups on pilgrimages, and refugees in camps. Epidemics follow a cyclic pattern in areas such as the Indian subcontinent and sub-Saharan Africa. These devastating epidemics, which are most often caused by *S. dysenteriae* type 1, are characterized by high attack rates and high mortality rates. In Bangladesh, for instance, an epidemic caused by *S. dysenteriae* type 1 was associated with a 42% increase in mortality rates among children 1–4 years of age. Apart from these epidemics, shigellosis is essentially an endemic disease, with 99% of cases occurring in the developing world and particularly high prevalences in the most impoverished areas, where personal and general hygiene is substandard. *S. flexneri* isolates predominate in less well-developed areas, whereas *S. sonnei* is more prevalent in economically emerging regions and in the industrialized world.

An often-overlooked complication of shigellosis is the short- and long-term impairment of the nutritional status of infected children in endemic areas. Combined with anorexia, the exudative enteropathy resulting from mucosal abrasions contributes to rapid exacerbation of the patient's nutritional status. Shigellosis is thus a major contributor to stunted growth among children in developing countries.

PATHOGENESIS AND PATHOLOGY

Shigella infection occurs through oral contamination. Direct fecal-oral transmission predominates since the organism is not well adapted to survive in the environment. Resistance to low-pH conditions allows shigellae to survive passage through the gastric barrier, an ability that may explain in part why a small inoculum (as few as 100 CFU) is sufficient to cause infection.

The watery diarrhea that usually precedes the dysenteric syndrome is attributable to active secretion and abnormal water reabsorption, a secretory effect at the jejunal level described in experimentally infected rhesus monkeys. This initial purge is probably due to the combined action of an enterotoxin (ShET-1) and mucosal inflammation. The dysenteric syndrome, manifested by bloody and mucopurulent stools, reflects invasion of the mucosa.

The pathogenesis of *Shigella* is essentially determined by a large virulence plasmid of 214 kb comprising ~100 genes, of which 25 encode a type III secretion system that inserts into the membrane of the host cell to allow effectors to transit from the bacterial cytoplasm to the cell cytoplasm (Fig. 147-1). Bacteria are thereby able to invade intestinal epithelial cells by inducing their own uptake after the initial crossing of the epithelial barrier through M cells (the specialized translocating epithelial cells in the follicle-associated epithelium that covers mucosal lymphoid nodules). The organisms induce apoptosis of subepithelial resident macrophages. Once inside the cytoplasm of intestinal epithelial cells, *Shigella* effectors trigger the cytoskeletal rearrangements necessary to direct uptake of the organism into the epithelial cell. The *Shigella*-containing vacuole is then quickly lysed, releasing bacteria into the cytosol.

Intracellular shigellae next use cytoskeletal components to propel themselves inside the infected cell; when the moving organism and the

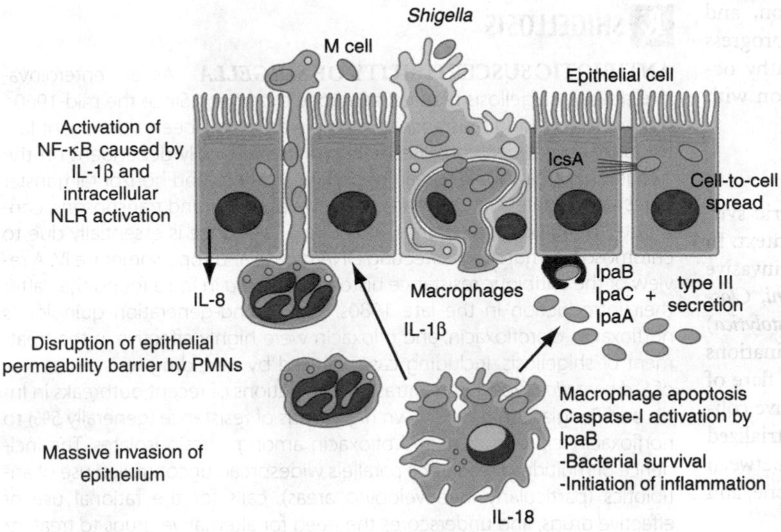

FIGURE 147-1 Invasive strategy of *Shigella flexneri*. IL, interleukin; NLR, nod-like receptor; PMN, polymorphonuclear leukocyte.

host cell membrane come into contact, cellular protrusions form and are engulfed by neighboring cells. This series of events permits bacterial cell-to-cell spread that is protected from immune effector mechanisms.

Cytokines released by a growing number of infected intestinal epithelial cells attract increased numbers of immune cells [particularly polymorphonuclear leukocytes (PMNs)] to the infected site, thus further destabilizing the epithelial barrier, exacerbating inflammation, and leading to the acute colitis that characterizes shigellosis. Recent evidence indicates that some of the type III secretion system–injected effectors can control the extent of inflammation, thus facilitating bacterial survival.

Shiga toxin produced by *S. dysenteriae* type 1 increases disease severity. Shiga toxin and Shiga-like toxins belong to a group of A1-B5 protein toxins whose B subunit binds to the cell surface and whose catalytic A subunit expresses an RNA N-glycosidase on 28S ribosomal RNA. These events lead to inhibition of binding of the amino-acyl-tRNA to the 60S ribosomal subunit and thus to a general shutoff of cell protein biosynthesis. Shiga toxins are translocated from the bowel into the circulation. After binding to the receptor globotriaosylceramide on target cells in the kidney, toxin is internalized by receptor-mediated endocytosis and interacts with the subcellular machinery to inhibit protein synthesis. The consequent pathophysiologic changes may result in hemolytic-uremic syndrome (HUS; see below).

CLINICAL MANIFESTATIONS

The presentation and severity of shigellosis depend to some extent on the infecting species but even more on the age and the immunologic and nutritional status of the host. Poverty and a poor hygienic environment are strongly related to the number and severity of diarrheal episodes, especially in children <5 years old.

Shigellosis typically evolves through four phases: incubation, watery diarrhea, dysentery, and the postinfectious phase. The incubation period usually lasts 1–4 days but may be as long as 8 days. Typical initial manifestations are transient fever, limited watery diarrhea, malaise, and anorexia. Signs and symptoms may range from mild abdominal discomfort to severe cramps, diarrhea, fever, vomiting, and tenesmus. The manifestations are usually exacerbated in children, with temperatures up to 40°–41°C and more severe anorexia and watery diarrhea. Unlike most diarrheal syndromes, dysenteric syndromes do not have dehydration as a major feature. This initial phase may represent the only clinical manifestation of shigellosis, especially in developed countries. Otherwise, dysentery follows within hours or days and is characterized by small volumes of bloody mucopurulent stools with increased tenesmus and abdominal cramps. At this stage, *Shigella* produces acute colitis involving mainly the distal colon and the rectum. Endoscopy demonstrates an edematous and hemorrhagic mucosa, with ulcerations and possibly overlying exudates resembling pseudomembranes. The extent of the lesions correlates with the number and frequency of stools and with the degree of protein loss by exudative mechanisms. Most episodes are self-limited and resolve without treatment in 1 week. With appropriate treatment, recovery takes place within a few days to a week, with no sequelae.

Acute life-threatening complications are seen most often in children <5 years of age, particularly affecting malnourished children in developing countries. Risk factors for death include nonbloody diarrhea, moderate to severe dehydration, bacteremia, absence of fever, abdominal tenderness, and rectal prolapse. Major complications are predominantly intestinal (e.g., toxic megacolon, intestinal perforations, rectal prolapse) or metabolic (e.g., hypoglycemia, hyponatremia, dehydration). Bacteremia is rare and is reported most frequently in severely malnourished children, HIV-infected patients, and patients with defects in innate immunity. Alterations of consciousness, including seizures, delirium, and coma, may occur, especially in children <5 years old, and are associated with a poor prognosis; fever and severe metabolic alterations are more often the major causes of altered consciousness than is meningitis or the Ekiri syndrome (toxic encephalopathy associated with bizarre posturing, cerebral edema, and fatty degeneration of viscera), which has been reported in Japanese children. Pneumonia, vaginitis, and keratoconjunctivitis due to *Shigella* are rarely reported. In the absence of serious malnutrition, severe and very unusual clinical manifestations, such as meningitis, may be linked to disorders of immune function and require relevant investigations.

Two complications of particular importance are toxic megacolon and HUS. Toxic megacolon is a consequence of severe inflammation extending to the colonic smooth-muscle layer and causing paralysis and dilatation. The patient presents with abdominal distention and tenderness, with or without signs of localized or generalized peritonitis. The abdominal x-ray characteristically shows marked dilatation of the transverse colon (with the greatest distention in the ascending and descending colons); thumbprinting caused by mucosal inflammatory edema; and loss of the normal haustral pattern associated with pseudopolyps, often extending into the lumen. Pneumatosis coli is an occasional finding. If perforation occurs, radiographic signs of pneumoperitoneum may be apparent. Predisposing factors (e.g., hypokalemia and use of opioids, anticholinergics, loperamide, psyllium seeds, and antidepressants) should be sought.

Shiga toxin produced by *S. dysenteriae* type 1 has been linked to HUS in developing countries but rarely in industrialized countries. HUS is an early complication that most often develops after several days of diarrhea. Clinical examination shows pallor, asthenia, and irritability and, in some cases, bleeding of the nose and gums, oliguria, and increasing edema. HUS is a nonimmune (Coombs test–negative) hemolytic anemia defined by a diagnostic triad: microangiopathic hemolytic anemia [hemoglobin level typically <80 g/L (<8 g/dL)], thrombocytopenia (mild to moderate in severity; typically <60,000 platelets/μL), and acute renal failure due to thrombosis of the glomerular capillaries (with markedly elevated creatinine levels). Anemia is severe, with fragmented red blood cells (schizocytes) in the peripheral smear, high serum concentrations of lactate dehydrogenase and free circulating hemoglobin, and elevated reticulocyte counts. Acute renal failure occurs in 55–70% of cases; however, renal function recovers in most of these cases (up to 70% in various series). Leukemoid reactions, with leukocyte counts of 50,000/μL, are sometimes noted in association with HUS.

The postinfectious immunologic complication known as reactive arthritis (Reiter's syndrome) can develop weeks or months after shigellosis, especially in patients expressing the histocompatibility antigen HLA-B27. About 3% of patients infected with *S. flexneri* later develop Reiter's syndrome, with arthritis, ocular inflammation, and urethritis—a condition that can last for months or years and progress to difficult-to-treat chronic arthritis. Postinfectious arthropathy occurs only after infection with *S. flexneri* and not after infection with the other *Shigella* serotypes.

LABORATORY DIAGNOSIS

The differential diagnosis in patients with a dysenteric syndrome depends on the clinical and environmental context. In developing areas, infectious diarrhea caused by other invasive pathogenic bacteria (*Salmonella enteritidis, Campylobacter jejuni, Clostridium difficile, Yersinia enterocolitica*) or parasites (*Entamoeba histolytica*) should be considered. Only bacteriologic and parasitologic examinations of stool can truly differentiate among these pathogens. A first flare of inflammatory bowel disease, such as Crohn's disease or ulcerative colitis (Chap. 289), should be considered in patients in industrialized countries. Despite similar symptoms, anamnesis discriminates between shigellosis, which usually follows recent travel in an endemic zone, and these other conditions.

Microscopic examination of stool smears shows the presence of erythrophagocytic trophozoites with very few PMNs in *E. histolytica* infection, whereas bacterial enteroinvasive infections (particularly shigellosis) are characterized by high PMN counts in each microscopic field. However, because shigellosis often manifests only as watery diarrhea, systematic attempts to isolate *Shigella* are necessary.

The "gold standard" for the diagnosis of *Shigella* infection remains the isolation and identification of the pathogen from fecal material. One major difficulty, particularly in endemic areas where laboratory facilities are not immediately available, is the fragility of *Shigella* and its common disappearance during transport, especially with rapid changes in temperature and pH. In the absence of a reliable enrichment medium, buffered glycerol saline or Cary-Blair medium can be used as a holding medium, but prompt inoculation onto isolation medium is essential. The probability of isolation is higher if the portion of stools that contains bloody and/or mucopurulent material is directly sampled. Rectal swabs can be used as they offer the highest rate of successful isolation during the acute phase of disease. Blood cultures are positive in <5% of cases and should be done only when a patient presents with a clinical picture of severe sepsis.

In addition to quick processing, the use of several media increases the likelihood of successful isolation: a nonselective medium such as bromocresol-purple agar lactose; a low-selectivity medium such as MacConkey or eosin-methylene blue; and a high-selectivity medium such as Hektoen, *Salmonella-Shigella*, or xylose-lysine-deoxycholate agar. After incubation on these media for 12–18 h at 37°C, shigellae appear as non-lactose-fermenting colonies that measure 0.5–1 mm in diameter and have a convex, translucent, smooth surface. Suspected colonies on nonselective or low-selectivity medium can be subcultured on a high-selectivity medium before being specifically identified or can be identified directly by standard commercial systems on the basis of four major characteristics: glucose positivity (usually without production of gas), lactose negativity, H_2S negativity, and lack of motility. The four *Shigella* serogroups (A–D) can then be differentiated by additional characteristics. This approach adds time and difficulty to the identification process, however; thus, after presumptive diagnosis, the use of serologic methods—e.g., slide agglutination, with group- and then type-specific antisera—should be considered. Group-specific antisera are widely available; in contrast, because of the large number of serotypes and sub-serotypes that must be considered, type-specific antisera are rare and more expensive and are often restricted to reference laboratories.

℞ SHIGELLOSIS

ANTIBIOTIC SUSCEPTIBILITY OF *SHIGELLA* As an enteroinvasive disease, shigellosis requires antibiotic treatment. Since the mid-1960s, however, increasing resistance to multiple drugs has been a dominant factor in treatment decisions. Resistance rates are highly dependent on the geographic area. Clonal spread of particular strains and horizontal transfer of resistance determinants, particularly via plasmids and transposons, contribute to multidrug resistance. Quinolone resistance is essentially due to chromosomal mutations affecting DNA gyrase and topoisomerase IV. A review of the antibiotic resistance history of *Shigella* in India found that, after their introduction in the late 1980s, the second-generation quinolones norfloxacin, ciprofloxacin, and ofloxacin were highly effective in the treatment of shigellosis, including cases caused by multidrug-resistant strains of *S. dysenteriae* type 1. In contrast, investigations of recent outbreaks in India and Bangladesh have shown high levels of resistance (generally 5%) to norfloxacin, ciprofloxacin, and ofloxacin among certain isolates. The incidence of multidrug resistance parallels widespread uncontrolled use of antibiotics (particularly in developing areas), calls for the rational use of effective drugs, and underscores the need for alternative drugs to treat infections caused by resistant strains.

ANTIBIOTIC TREATMENT OF SHIGELLOSIS (Table 147-1) Because of the ready transmissibility of *Shigella*, current public health recommendations in the United States are that every case be treated with antibiotics. Ciprofloxacin is recommended as first-line treatment. A number of other drugs have been tested and shown to be effective, including ceftriaxone, azithromycin, pivmecillinam, and some fifth-generation quinolones. While infections caused by non-*dysenteriae Shigella* in immunocompetent individuals are routinely treated with a 3-day course of antibiotics, it is recommended that *S. dysenteriae* infections be treated for 5 days and that *Shigella* infections in immunocompromised patients be treated for 7–10 days.

Treatment for shigellosis must be adapted to the clinical context, with the recognition that the most fragile patients are children <5 years old, who represent two-thirds of all cases worldwide. There are few data on the use of quinolones in children. The half-life of ciprofloxacin is longer in infants than in older individuals. The ciprofloxacin dose generally recommended for children is 30 mg/kg per day in two divided doses. Adults living in areas with high hygienic standards are likely to develop milder, shorter-duration disease, whereas infants in endemic areas can develop severe, sometimes fatal dysentery. In the former setting, treatment will remain minimal and bacteriologic proof of infection will often come after symptoms have resolved; in the latter setting, more aggressive measures, possibly including resuscitation, may be required.

REHYDRATION AND NUTRITION *Shigella* infection rarely causes significant dehydration. Cases requiring aggressive rehydration (particularly in industrialized countries) are uncommon. In developing countries, malnu-

TABLE 147-1 RECOMMENDED ANTIMICROBIAL THERAPY FOR SHIGELLOSIS

Antimicrobial Agent	Treatment Schedule: In Children	Treatment Schedule: In Adults	Limitations
First line			
Ciprofloxacin	15 mg/kg 2 times per day for 3 days, PO	500 mg	
Second line			
Pivmecillinam	20 mg/kg 4 times per day for 5 days, PO	100 mg	Cost No pediatric formulation Frequent administration Resistance emerging
Ceftriaxone	50–100 mg/kg Once a day IM for 2–5 days	–	Efficacy not validated Must be injected
Azithromycin	6–20 mg/kg Once a day for 1–5 days, PO	1–1.5 g	Cost Efficacy not validated MIC near serum concentration Resistance emerges rapidly and spreads to other bacteria

Source: WHO Library Cataloguing-in-Publication Data: Guidelines for the control of shigellosis, including epidemics due to *Shigella dysenteriae* type 1 (*www.searo.who.int/LinkFiles/CAH_Publications_shigella.pdf*).

trition remains the primary indicator for diarrhea-related death, highlighting the importance of nutrition in early management. Rehydration should be oral unless the patient is comatose or presents in shock. Because of the improved effectiveness of reduced-osmolarity oral rehydration solution (especially for children with acute noncholera diarrhea), the WHO and UNICEF now recommend a standard solution of 245 mOsm/L (sodium, 75 mmol/L; chloride, 65 mmol/L; glucose (anhydrous), 75 mmol/L; potassium, 20 mmol/L; citrate, 10 mmol/L). In shigellosis, as in acute infectious diarrhea of most etiologies (including cholera), the coupled transport of sodium to glucose or other solutes is largely unaffected, and oral rehydration therapy represents the easiest and most efficient form of rehydration, especially in severe cases.

Nutrition should be started as soon as possible after completion of initial rehydration. Early refeeding is safe, well tolerated, and clinically beneficial. Because breast-feeding reduces diarrheal losses and the need for oral rehydration in infants, it should be maintained in the absence of contraindications (e.g., maternal HIV infection).

NONSPECIFIC, SYMPTOM-BASED THERAPY Antimotility agents have been implicated in prolonged fever in volunteers with shigellosis. These agents are suspected of increasing the risk of toxic megacolon and are thought to have been responsible for HUS in children infected by Shiga toxin–producing strains of *E. coli*. For safety reasons, it is better to avoid antimotility agents in bloody diarrhea.

TREATMENT OF COMPLICATIONS There is no consensus regarding the best treatment for toxic megacolon. The patient should be assessed frequently by both medical and surgical teams. Anemia, dehydration, and electrolyte deficits (particularly hypokalemia) may aggravate colonic atony and should be actively treated. Nasogastric aspiration helps to deflate the colon. Parenteral nutrition has not been proved to be beneficial. Fever persisting beyond 48–72 h raises the possibility of local perforation or abscess. Most studies recommend colectomy if, after 48–72 h, colonic distention persists. However, some physicians recommend continuation of medical therapy for up to 7 days if the patient seems to be improving clinically despite persistent megacolon without free perforation. Intestinal perforation, either isolated or complicating toxic megacolon, requires surgical treatment and intensive medical support.

Rectal prolapse must be treated as soon as possible. With the health care provider using surgical gloves or a soft warm wet cloth and the patient in the knee-chest position, the prolapsed rectum is gently pushed back into place. If edema of the rectal mucosa is evident (rendering reintegration difficult), it can be osmotically reduced by applying gauze impregnated with a warm solution of saturated magnesium sulfate. Rectal prolapse often relapses but usually resolves along with the resolution of dysentery.

HUS must be treated by water restriction, including discontinuation of oral rehydration solution and potassium-rich alimentation. Hemofiltration is usually required.

PREVENTION

Hand washing after defecation or handling of children's feces and before handling of food is recommended. However, this protocol entails an average of 32 hand washes per day, with consumption of 20 L of water. If soap is too costly, ash or mud can be used, but access to water remains essential. Stool precautions, together with a cleaning protocol for medical staff as well as for patients, have proven useful in limiting the spread of infection during *Shigella* outbreaks. Ideally, patients should have a negative stool culture before their infection is considered cured. Recurrences are rare if treatment and prevention are correctly implemented.

Although several live attenuated oral and subunit parenteral vaccine candidates have been produced and are undergoing clinical trials, no vaccine against shigellosis is currently available. Especially given the rapid progression of antibiotic resistance in *Shigella*, a vaccine is urgently needed.

FURTHER READINGS

Bennish ML, Wojtyniak BJ: Mortality due to shigellosis: Community and hospital data. Rev Infect Dis 13(Suppl 4):S245, 1991

Cossart P, Sansonetti PJ: Bacterial invasion: The paradigms of enteroinvasive pathogens. Science 304:242, 2004

Kotloff KL et al: Overview of live vaccine strategies against *Shigella*, in *New Generation Vaccines*, 3d ed, MM Levine et al (eds). London, Informa Healthcare, 2004, pp 723–735

——— et al: Global burden of *Shigella* infections: Implications for vaccine development and implementation of control strategies. Bull World Health Organ 77:651, 1999

Niyogi SK: Shigellosis. J Microbiol 43:133, 2005

Phalipon A, Sansonetti PJ: Shigella's ways of manipulating the host intestinal innate and adaptive immune system: A tool box for survival? Immunol Cell Biol 85:119, 2007

von Seidlein L et al: A multicentre study of *Shigella* diarrhoea in six Asian countries: Disease burden, clinical manifestations, and microbiology. PLoS Med 3(9):e353, 2006

World Health Organization: Guidelines for the control of shigellosis, including epidemics due to *Shigella dysenteriae* type 1. WHO Library Cataloguing-in-Publication Data (*www.searo.who.int/LinkFiles/CAH_Publications_shigella.pdf*)

148 Infections Due to *Campylobacter* and Related Species

Martin J. Blaser

DEFINITION

Bacteria of the genus *Campylobacter* and of the related genera *Arcobacter* and *Helicobacter* (Chap. 144) cause a variety of inflammatory conditions. Although acute diarrheal illnesses are most common, these organisms may cause infections in virtually all parts of the body, especially in compromised hosts, and these infections may have late nonsuppurative sequelae. The designation *Campylobacter* comes from the Greek for "curved rod" and refers to the organism's vibrio-like morphology.

ETIOLOGY

Campylobacters are motile, non-spore-forming, curved, gram-negative rods. Originally known as *Vibrio fetus*, these bacilli were reclassified as a new genus in 1973, after their dissimilarity to other vibrios was recognized. More than 15 species have since been identified. These species are currently divided into three genera: *Campylobacter*, *Arcobacter*, and *Helicobacter*. Not all of the species are pathogens of humans. The human pathogens fall into two major groups: those that primarily cause diarrheal disease and those that cause extraintestinal infection. The principal diarrheal pathogen is *C. jejuni*, which accounts for 80–90% of all cases of recognized illness due to campylobacters and related genera. Other organisms that cause diarrheal disease include *C. coli*, *C. upsaliensis*, *C. lari*, *C. hyointestinalis*, *C. fetus*, *A. butzleri*, *A. cryaerophilus*, *H. cinaedi*, and *H. fennelliae*. The two *Helicobacter* species causing diarrheal disease, *H. cinaedi* and *H. fennelliae*, are intestinal rather than gastric organisms; in terms of the clinical features of the illnesses they cause, these species most closely resemble *Campylobacter* rather than *H. pylori* (Chap. 144) and thus are considered in this chapter.

The major species causing extraintestinal illnesses is *C. fetus*. However, any of the diarrheal agents listed above may cause systemic or localized infection as well. Neither aerobes nor strict anaerobes, these microaerophilic organisms are adapted for survival in the gastrointestinal mucous layer. This chapter focuses on *C. jejuni* and *C. fetus* as the major pathogens in and prototypes for their groups. The key features of infection are listed by species (excluding *C. jejuni*, described in detail in the text below) in **Table 148-1**.

TABLE 148-1 CLINICAL FEATURES ASSOCIATED WITH INFECTION DUE TO "ATYPICAL" *CAMPYLOBACTER* AND RELATED SPECIES IMPLICATED AS CAUSES OF HUMAN ILLNESS

Species	Common Clinical Features	Less Common Clinical Features	Additional Information
Campylobacter coli	Fever, diarrhea, abdominal pain	Bacteremia[a]	Clinically indistinguishable from *C. jejuni*
Campylobacter fetus	Bacteremia,[a] sepsis, meningitis, vascular infections	Diarrhea, relapsing fevers	Not usually isolated from media containing cephalothin or incubated at 42°C
Campylobacter upsaliensis	Watery diarrhea, low-grade fever, abdominal pain	Bacteremia, abscesses	Difficult to isolate because of cephalothin susceptibility
Campylobacter lari	Abdominal pain, diarrhea	Colitis, appendicitis	Seagulls frequently colonized; organism often transmitted to humans via contaminated water
Campylobacter hyointestinalis	Watery or bloody diarrhea, vomiting, abdominal pain	Bacteremia	Causes proliferative enteritis in swine
Helicobacter fennelliae	Chronic mild diarrhea, abdominal cramps, proctitis	Bacteremia[a]	Best treated with fluoroquinolones
Helicobacter cinaedi	Chronic mild diarrhea, abdominal cramps, proctitis	Bacteremia[a]	Best treated with fluoroquinolones; identified in healthy hamsters
Campylobacter jejuni subspecies *doylei*	Diarrhea	Chronic gastritis, bacteremia[b]	Uncertain role as human pathogen
Arcobacter cryaerophilus	Diarrhea	Bacteremia	Cultured under aerobic conditions
Arcobacter butzleri	Fever, diarrhea, abdominal pain, nausea	Bacteremia, appendicitis	Cultured under aerobic conditions; enzootic in nonhuman primates
Campylobacter sputorum	Pulmonary, perianal, groin, and axillary abscesses	Bacteremia	Three clinically relevant biovars: *C. sputorum* subspecies *sputorum*, *C. sputorum* subspecies *bubulus*, and *Campylobacter mucosalis*

[a]In immunocompromised hosts, especially HIV-infected persons.
[b]In children.

Source: Adapted from BM Allos, MJ Blaser: *Campylobacter jejuni* and the expanding spectrum of related infections. Clin Infect Dis 20:1092, 1995.

EPIDEMIOLOGY

Campylobacters are found in the gastrointestinal tract of many animals used for food (including poultry, cattle, sheep, and swine) and many household pets (including birds, dogs, and cats). These microorganisms usually do not cause illness in their animal hosts. In most cases, campylobacters are transmitted to humans in raw or undercooked food products or through direct contact with infected animals. In the United States and other developed countries, ingestion of contaminated poultry that has not been sufficiently cooked is the most common mode of acquisition (30–70% of cases). Other modes include ingestion of raw (unpasteurized) milk or untreated water, contact with infected household pets, travel to developing countries (campylobacters being among the leading causes of traveler's diarrhea; Chaps. 117 and 122), oral-anal sexual contact, and (occasionally) contact with an index case who is incontinent of stool.

Campylobacter infections are common. Several studies indicate that, in the United States, diarrheal disease due to campylobacters is more common than that due to *Salmonella* and *Shigella* combined. Infections occur throughout the year, but their incidence peaks during summer and early autumn. Persons of all ages are affected; however, attack rates for *C. jejuni* are highest among young children and young adults, while those for *C. fetus* are highest at the extremes of age. Systemic infections due to *C. fetus* (and to other *Campylobacter* and related species) are most common among compromised hosts. Persons at increased risk include those with AIDS, hypogammaglobulinemia, neoplasia, liver disease, diabetes mellitus, and generalized atherosclerosis as well as neonates and pregnant women. However, apparently healthy nonpregnant persons occasionally develop transient *Campylobacter* bacteremia as part of a gastrointestinal illness.

In developing countries, *C. jejuni* infections are hyperendemic, with the highest rates among children <2 years old. Infection rates fall with age, as does the illness-to-infection ratio. These observations suggest that frequent exposure to *C. jejuni* leads to the acquisition of immunity.

PATHOLOGY AND PATHOGENESIS

Many *C. jejuni* infections are subclinical, especially in hosts in developing countries who have had multiple prior infections and thus are partially immune. Most illnesses occur within 2–4 days (range, 1–7 days) of exposure to the organism in food or water. The sites of tissue injury include the jejunum, ileum, and colon. Biopsies show an acute nonspecific inflammatory reaction, with neutrophils, monocytes, and eosinophils in the lamina propria, as well as damage to the epithelium, including loss of mucus, glandular degeneration, and crypt abscesses. Biopsy findings may be consistent with Crohn's disease or ulcerative colitis, but these "idiopathic" chronic inflammatory diseases should not be diagnosed unless infectious colitis, *specifically including* that due to infection with *Campylobacter* species and related organisms, has been ruled out.

The high frequency of *C. jejuni* infections and their severity and recurrence among hypogammaglobulinemic patients suggest that antibodies are important in protective immunity. The pathogenesis of infection is uncertain. Both the motility of the strain and its capacity to adhere to host tissues appear to favor disease, but classic enterotoxins and cytotoxins (although described and including cytolethal distending toxin, or CDT) appear not to play substantial roles in tissue injury or disease production. The organisms have been visualized in the epithelium, albeit in low numbers. The documentation of a significant tissue response and occasionally of *C. jejuni* bacteremia further suggests that tissue invasion is clinically significant, and in vitro studies are consistent with this pathogenetic feature.

The pathogenesis of *C. fetus* infections is better defined. Virtually all clinical isolates of *C. fetus* possess a proteinaceous capsule-like structure (an S-layer) that renders the organisms resistant to complement-mediated killing and opsonization. As a result, *C. fetus* can cause bacteremia and can seed sites beyond the intestinal tract. The ability of the organism to switch the S-layer proteins expressed—a phenomenon that results in antigenic variability—may contribute to the chronicity and high rate of recurrence of *C. fetus* infections in compromised hosts.

CLINICAL MANIFESTATIONS

The clinical features of infections due to *Campylobacter* and the related *Arcobacter* and intestinal *Helicobacter* species causing enteric disease appear to be highly similar. *C. jejuni* can be considered the prototype, in part because it is by far the most common enteric pathogen. A prodrome of fever, headache, myalgia, and/or malaise often occurs 12–48 h before the onset of diarrheal symptoms. The most common signs and symptoms of the intestinal phase are diarrhea, abdominal pain, and fever. The degree of diarrhea varies from several loose stools to grossly bloody stools; most patients presenting for medical attention have ≥10 bowel movements on the worst day of illness. Abdominal pain usually consists of cramping and may be the most prominent symptom. Pain is usually generalized but may become localized; *C. jejuni* infection may cause pseudoappendicitis. Fever may be the only initial manifestation of *C. jejuni* infection, a situation mimicking the early stages of typhoid fever. Febrile young children may develop convulsions. *Campylobacter* enteritis is generally self-limited; however, symptoms persist for >1 week in 10–20% of patients seeking medical attention, and clinical relapses occur in 5–10% of untreated patients.

C. fetus may cause a diarrheal illness similar to that due to *C. jejuni*, especially in normal hosts. This organism may also cause either intermittent diarrhea or nonspecific abdominal pain without localizing signs. Sequelae are uncommon, and the outcome is benign. *C. fetus* may also cause a prolonged relapsing systemic illness (with fever, chills, and myalgias) that has no obvious primary source; this manifestation is especially common among compromised hosts. Secondary seeding of an organ (e.g., meninges, brain, bone, urinary tract, or soft tissue) complicates the course, which may be fulminant. *C. fetus* infections have a tropism for vascular sites: endocarditis, mycotic aneurysm, and septic thrombophlebitis may all occur. Infection during pregnancy often leads to fetal death. A variety of *Campylobacter* species and *H. cinaedi* can cause recurrent cellulitis with fever and bacteremia in immunocompromised hosts.

COMPLICATIONS

Except in infection with *C. fetus*, bacteremia is uncommon, developing most often in immunocompromised hosts and at the extremes of age. Three patterns of extraintestinal infection have been noted: (1) transient bacteremia in a normal host with enteritis (benign course, no specific treatment needed); (2) sustained bacteremia or focal infection in a normal host (bacteremia originating from enteritis, with patients responding well to antimicrobial therapy); and (3) sustained bacteremia or focal infection in a compromised host. Enteritis may not be clinically apparent. Antimicrobial therapy, possibly prolonged, is necessary for suppression or cure of the infection.

Campylobacter, *Arcobacter*, and intestinal *Helicobacter* infections in patients with AIDS or hypogammaglobulinemia may be severe, persistent, and extraintestinal; relapse after cessation of therapy is common. Hypogammaglobulinemic patients may also develop osteomyelitis and an erysipelas-like rash or cellulitis.

Local suppurative complications of infection include cholecystitis, pancreatitis, and cystitis; distant complications include meningitis, endocarditis, arthritis, peritonitis, cellulitis, and septic abortion. All these complications are rare, except in immunocompromised hosts. Hepatitis, interstitial nephritis, and the hemolytic-uremic syndrome occasionally complicate acute infection. Reactive arthritis and other rheumatologic complaints may develop several weeks after infection, especially in persons with the HLA-B27 phenotype. Guillain-Barré syndrome (or its Miller Fisher or cranial polyneuropathy variant) follows *Campylobacter* infections uncommonly—i.e., in 1 of every 1000–2000 cases or, for certain *C. jejuni* serotypes (such as O19), in 1 of every 100–200 cases. Despite the low frequency of this complication, it is now estimated that *Campylobacter* infections, because of their high incidence, may trigger 20–40% of all cases of Guillain-Barré syndrome. Immunoproliferative small-intestinal disease (*alpha chain disease*), a form of lymphoma that originates in small-intestinal mucosa-associated lymphoid tissue, has been associated with *C. jejuni*; antimicrobial therapy has led to marked clinical improvement.

DIAGNOSIS

In patients with *Campylobacter* enteritis, peripheral leukocyte counts reflect the severity of the inflammatory process. However, stools from nearly all *Campylobacter*-infected patients presenting for medical attention in the United States contain leukocytes or erythrocytes. Fecal smears should be treated with Gram's or Wright's stain and examined in all suspected cases. When the diagnosis of *Campylobacter* enteritis is suspected on the basis of findings indicating inflammatory diarrhea (fever, fecal leukocytes), clinicians can ask the laboratory to attempt the visualization of organisms with characteristic vibrioid morphology by direct microscopic examination of stools with Gram's staining or to use phase-contrast or dark-field microscopy to identify the organisms' characteristic "darting" motility. Confirmation of the diagnosis of *Campylobacter* infection is based on identification of an isolate from cultures of stool, blood, or another site. *Campylobacter*-specific media should be used to culture stools from all patients with inflammatory or bloody diarrhea. Since all *Campylobacter* species are fastidious, they will not be isolated unless selective media or other selective techniques are used. Not all media are equally useful for isolation of the broad array of campylobacters; therefore, failure to isolate campylobacters from stool does not entirely rule out their presence. The detection of the organisms in stool almost always implies infection; there is a brief period of postconvalescent fecal carriage and no commensalism in humans. In contrast, *C. sputorum* and related organisms found in the oral cavity are commensals with rare pathogenic significance. Because of low levels of metabolic activity in standard blood culture media, *Campylobacter* bacteremia may be difficult to detect unless laboratorians are looking for low-positive results in quantitative assays.

DIFFERENTIAL DIAGNOSIS

The symptoms of *Campylobacter* enteritis are not sufficiently unusual to distinguish this illness from that due to *Salmonella*, *Shigella*, *Yersinia*, and other pathogens. The combination of fever and fecal leukocytes or erythrocytes is indicative of inflammatory diarrhea, and definitive diagnosis is based on culture or demonstration of the characteristic organisms on stained fecal smears. Similarly, extraintestinal *Campylobacter* illness is diagnosed by culture. Infection due to *Campylobacter* should be suspected in the setting of septic abortion, and that due to *C. fetus* should be suspected specifically in the setting of septic thrombophlebitis. It is important to reiterate that (1) the presentation of *Campylobacter* enteritis may mimic that of ulcerative colitis or Crohn's disease, (2) *Campylobacter* enteritis is much more common than either of the latter (especially among young adults), and (3) biopsy may not distinguish among these entities. Thus a diagnosis of inflammatory bowel disease should not be made until *Campylobacter* infection has been ruled out, especially in persons with a history of foreign travel, significant animal contact, immunodeficiency, or exposure incurring a high risk of transmission.

Rx INFECTIONS DUE TO *CAMPYLOBACTER* AND RELATED SPECIES

Fluid and electrolyte replacement is central to the treatment of diarrheal illnesses (Chap. 122). Even among patients presenting for medical attention with *Campylobacter* enteritis, not all clearly benefit from specific antimicrobial therapy. Indications for therapy include high fever, bloody diarrhea, severe diarrhea, persistence for >1 week, and worsening of symptoms. A 5- to 7-day course of erythromycin (250 mg orally four times daily or—for children—30–50 mg/kg per day, in divided doses) is the regimen of choice. Both clinical trials and in vitro susceptibility testing indicate that other macrolides, including clarithromycin and azithromycin, also are useful therapeutic agents. An alternative regimen for adults is ciprofloxacin (500 mg orally twice daily) or another fluoroquinolone for 5–7 days, but resistance to this class of agents as well as to tetracyclines has been increasing. Patients infected with antibiotic-resistant strains are at increased risk of adverse outcomes. Use of antimotility agents, which may prolong the duration of symptoms and have been associated with toxic megacolon and with death, is not recommended.

For systemic infections, treatment with gentamicin (1.7 mg/kg IV every 8 h after a loading dose of 2 mg/kg), imipenem (500 mg IV every 6 h), or chloramphenicol (50 mg/kg IV each day in three or four divided doses) should be started empirically, but susceptibility testing should then be performed. Ciprofloxacin and amoxicillin/clavulanate are alternative agents for susceptible strains. In the absence of immunocompromise or endovascular infections, therapy should be administered for 14 days. For immunocompromised patients with systemic infections due to *C. fetus* and for patients with endovascular infections, prolonged therapy (for up to 4 weeks) is usually necessary. For recurrent infections in immunocompromised hosts, lifelong therapy/prophylaxis is sometimes necessary.

PROGNOSIS

Nearly all patients recover fully from *Campylobacter* enteritis, either spontaneously or after antimicrobial therapy. Volume depletion probably contributes to the few deaths that are reported. As stated above, occasional patients develop reactive arthritis or Guillain-Barré syndrome or its variants. Systemic infection with *C. fetus* is much more often fatal than that due to related species; this higher mortality rate reflects in part the population affected. Prognosis depends on the rapidity with which appropriate therapy is begun. Otherwise-healthy hosts usually survive *C. fetus* infections without sequelae. Compromised hosts often have recurrent and/or life-threatening infections due to a variety of *Campylobacter* species.

FURTHER READINGS

HELMS M et al: Adverse health events associated with antimicrobial drug resistance in *Campylobacter* species: A registry-based cohort study. J Infect Dis 191:1050, 2005

LANG DR et al (eds): Development of Guillain-Barré syndrome following *Campylobacter* infection. J Infect Dis 176(Suppl 2):S91, 1997

LECUIT M et al: Immunoproliferative small intestinal disease associated with *Campylobacter jejuni*. N Engl J Med 350:239, 2004

MEAD PS et al: Food-related illness and death in the United States. Emerg Infect Dis 5:607, 1999

NACHAMKIN I, BLASER MJ (eds): *Campylobacter jejuni*, 2d ed. Washington, American Society for Microbiology, 2000

SMITH KE et al: Quinolone-resistant *Campylobacter jejuni* infections in Minnesota, 1992–1998. Investigation Team. N Engl J Med 340:1525, 1999

149 Cholera and Other Vibrioses

Matthew K. Waldor, Gerald T. Keusch

Members of the genus *Vibrio* cause a number of important infectious syndromes. Classic among them is cholera, a devastating diarrheal disease caused by *V. cholerae* that has been responsible for seven global pandemics and much suffering over the past two centuries. Epidemic cholera remains a significant public health concern in the developing world today. Other vibrioses caused by other *Vibrio* species include syndromes of diarrhea, soft tissue infection, or primary sepsis. All *Vibrio* species are highly motile, facultatively anaerobic, curved gram-negative rods with one or more flagella. In nature, vibrios most commonly reside in tidal rivers and bays under conditions of moderate salinity. They proliferate in the summer months when water temperatures exceed 20°C. As might be expected, the illnesses they cause also increase in frequency during the warm months.

CHOLERA

DEFINITION

Cholera is an acute diarrheal disease that can, in a matter of hours, result in profound, rapidly progressive dehydration and death. Accordingly, cholera gravis (the severe form of cholera) is a much-feared disease, particularly in its epidemic presentation. Fortunately, prompt aggressive fluid repletion and supportive care can obviate the high mortality that cholera has historically wrought. While the term *cholera* has occasionally been applied to any severely dehydrating secretory diarrheal illness, whether infectious in etiology or not, it has generally referred to disease caused by *V. cholerae* serogroup O1. In 1992, however, a new serogroup (O139) that causes epidemic cholera emerged on the Indian subcontinent and has since killed thousands of people.

MICROBIOLOGY AND EPIDEMIOLOGY

The species *V. cholerae* comprises a host of organisms classified on the basis of the carbohydrate determinants of their lipopolysaccharide (LPS) O antigens. Some 200 serogroups have now been recognized. They are divided into those that agglutinate in antisera to the O1 group antigen (*V. cholerae* O1) and those that do not (non-O1 *V. cholerae*). Although some non-O1 *V. cholerae* serogroups have occasionally caused sporadic outbreaks of diarrhea, serogroup O1 was, until the emergence of serogroup O139, the exclusive cause of epidemic cholera. Two biotypes of *V. cholerae* O1, classical and El Tor, are distinguished. Each biotype is further subdivided into two serotypes, termed *Inaba* and *Ogawa*.

The natural habitat of *V. cholerae* is coastal salt water and brackish estuaries, where the organism lives in close relation to plankton. Humans become infected incidentally but, once infected, can act as vehicles for spread. Ingestion of water contaminated by human feces is the most common means of acquisition of *V. cholerae*. Consumption of contaminated food can also contribute to spread. There is no known animal reservoir. While the infectious dose is relatively high, it is markedly reduced in hypochlorhydric persons, in those using antacids, and when gastric acidity is buffered by a meal. Cholera is predominantly a pediatric disease in endemic areas, but it affects adults and children equally when newly introduced into a population. Children <2 years of age are less likely to develop severe cholera than are older children, perhaps because of passive immunity acquired from breast milk. In endemic areas, the disease is more common in the summer and fall months. For unexplained reasons, susceptibility to cholera is significantly influenced by ABO blood group status; persons with type O blood are at greatest risk, while those with type AB are at least risk.

Cholera is native to the Ganges delta in the Indian subcontinent. Since 1817, seven global pandemics have occurred. The current (seventh) pandemic—the first due to the El Tor biotype—began in Indonesia in 1961 and spread throughout Asia as *V. cholerae* El Tor displaced the endemic classical strain. In the early 1970s, El Tor cholera erupted in Africa, causing major epidemics before becoming a persistent endemic problem. Currently, >90% of cholera cases reported annually to the World Health Organization (WHO) are from Africa (Fig. 149-1). In the period 2000–2004, the annual worldwide number of cholera cases reported to the WHO remained stable at ~100,000. This number is certainly a significant underestimate, as several nations with endemic cholera do not report cholera cases to the WHO.

The recent history of cholera has been punctuated by severe outbreaks. Such outbreaks are often precipitated by war or other circumstances that lead to the breakdown of public health measures. Such was the case in the camps for Rwandan refugees set up in 1994 around Goma, Zaire.

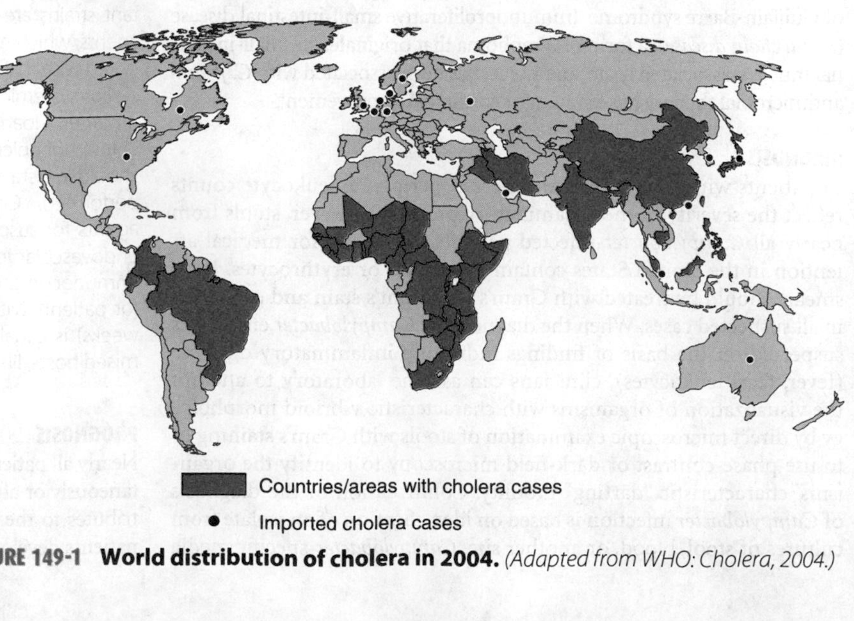

FIGURE 149-1 World distribution of cholera in 2004. *(Adapted from WHO: Cholera, 2004.)*

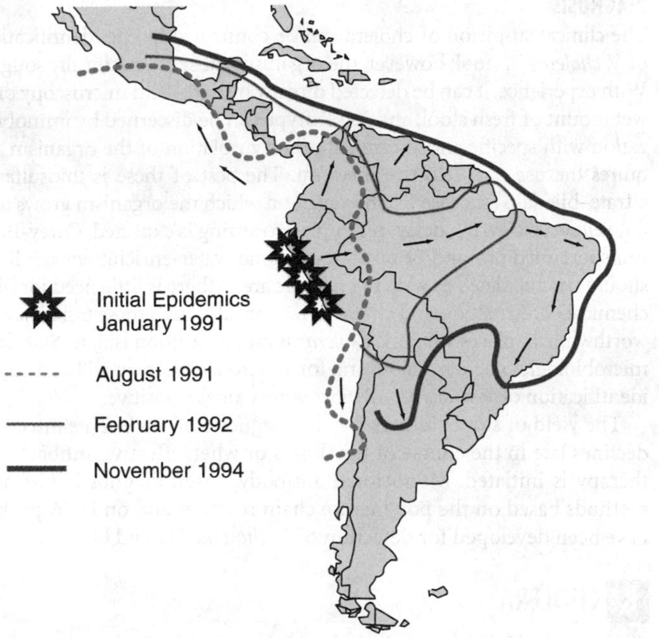

FIGURE 149-2 Spread of *Vibrio cholerae* O1 in the Americas, 1991–1994. *(Courtesy of Dr. Robert V. Tauxe, Centers for Disease Control and Prevention, Atlanta; with permission.)*

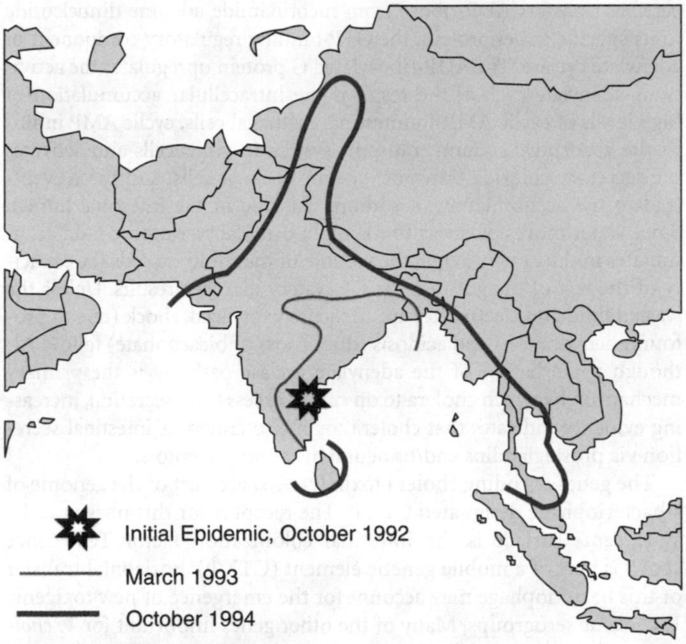

FIGURE 149-3 Spread of *Vibrio cholerae* O139 in the Indian subcontinent and elsewhere in Asia, 1992–1994. *(Courtesy of Dr. Robert V. Tauxe, CDC, Atlanta; with permission.)*

Since 1973, sporadic endemic infections due to *V. cholerae* O1 strains related to the seventh-pandemic strain have been recognized along the U.S. Gulf Coast of Louisiana and Texas. These infections are typically associated with the consumption of contaminated, locally harvested shellfish. Occasionally, cases in U.S. locations remote from the Gulf Coast have been linked to shipped-in Gulf Coast seafood.

It was not until 1991 that the current cholera pandemic reached Latin America. Beginning along the Peruvian coast in January 1991, the disease spread in an explosive epidemic to virtually all of South and Central America and to Mexico (Fig. 149-2). About 400,000 cases were reported in the first year of the outbreak, and >1 million had been reported by the end of 1994. While the cumulative mortality rate has been <1%, the mortality rate approached 30% in the communities first affected, where a lack of familiarity with the disease led initially to the deployment of ineffective treatment. Intensive education of health care providers and of the community at large has enhanced awareness of the disease and its appropriate management and has greatly diminished mortality. As it did in Africa two decades earlier, the epidemic El Tor strain proved capable of establishing itself in inland waters rather than in its classic niche of coastal salt waters; the organism has already become endemic in many of the Latin American countries into which it was recently introduced. Cases linked to the Latin American epidemic have occurred (via importation of contaminated seafood) in the United States. Although secondary spread of this strain has not taken place in the United States, these events underscore the need for vigilance among health care professionals, even in locations remote from an epidemic.

In October 1992, a large-scale outbreak of clinical cholera occurred in southeastern India. The etiologic agent proved to be of a novel *V. cholerae* serogroup. This strain spread rapidly up and down the coast of the Bay of Bengal, reaching Bangladesh in December 1992. There alone, it caused more than 100,000 cases of cholera in the first 3 months of 1993. It subsequently spread across the Indian subcontinent and to neighboring countries, affecting Pakistan, Nepal, western China, Thailand, and Malaysia by the end of 1994 (Fig. 149-3). The organism has since been designated *V. cholerae* O139 Bengal in recognition of its novel O antigen and its geographic origin. The clinical manifestations and epidemiologic features of the disease caused by *V. cholerae* O139 Bengal are indistinguishable from those of O1 cholera. Immunity to the latter, however, is not protective against the former. Because naturally acquired immunity to *V. cholerae* O1 does not cross-protect against *V. cholerae* O139 Bengal, vaccines being developed against the former are unlikely to be effective against the latter.

Some authorities believed that the emergence of *V. cholerae* O139 signaled the beginning of the eighth global cholera pandemic. Indeed, just as O1 El Tor replaced the classical biotype that preceded it, O139 Bengal in 1993 rapidly replaced O1 El Tor as the most common environmental isolate and the predominant cause of clinical cholera in the areas in which it had appeared. However, by the beginning of 1994, O1 El Tor had resumed its dominance in Bangladesh. *V. cholerae* O139 has not spread outside of Asia, and currently, in most regions of Southeast Asia, *V. cholerae* O1 remains dominant.

PATHOGENESIS

In the final analysis, cholera is a toxin-mediated disease. Its characteristic watery diarrhea is due to the action of cholera toxin, a potent protein enterotoxin elaborated by the organism after it colonizes the small intestine. For *V. cholerae* to colonize the small intestine and produce cholera toxin, it must first recognize, contend with, and traverse several hostile environments. The first of these is the acidic milieu of the stomach. To elude the bactericidal effects of gastric acidity, *V. cholerae* relies, at least in part, on a relatively large inoculum size (compared to that needed for colonization by *Shigella*, for instance). The organism must next traverse the mucous layer lining the small bowel. *V. cholerae* chemotaxis and motility and the action of a variety of proteases may allow the organism to traverse this gel covering the intestinal epithelium. The toxin-coregulated pilus (TCP), so named because its synthesis is regulated in parallel with that of cholera toxin, is essential for *V. cholerae* intestinal colonization. Cholera toxin, TCP, and several other virulence factors are coordinately regulated by ToxR. This protein modulates the expression of virulence genes in response to environmental signals via a cascade of regulatory proteins. Additional regulatory processes, including bacterial responses to the density of the bacterial population (in a phenomenon known as *quorum sensing*), control the virulence of *V. cholerae*.

Once established in the human small bowel, the organism produces cholera toxin, which consists of a monomeric enzymatic moiety (the A subunit) and a pentameric binding moiety (the B subunit). The B pentamer binds to G_{M1} ganglioside, a glycolipid on the surface of epithelial cells that serves as the toxin receptor and makes possible the delivery of the A subunit to its cytosolic target. The activated A subunit (A_1) irreversibly transfers ADP-ribose from nicotinamide adenine dinucleotide to its specific target protein, the GTP-binding regulatory component of adenylate cyclase. The ADP-ribosylated G protein upregulates the activity of adenylate cyclase; the result is the intracellular accumulation of high levels of cyclic AMP. In intestinal epithelial cells, cyclic AMP inhibits the absorptive sodium transport system in villus cells and activates the secretory chloride transport system in crypt cells, and these events lead to the accumulation of sodium chloride in the intestinal lumen. Since water moves passively to maintain osmolality, isotonic fluid accumulates in the lumen. When the volume of that fluid exceeds the capacity of the rest of the gut to resorb it, watery diarrhea results. Unless the wasted fluid and electrolytes are adequately replaced, shock (due to profound dehydration) and acidosis (due to loss of bicarbonate) follow. Although perturbation of the adenylate cyclase pathway is the primary mechanism by which cholera toxin causes excess fluid secretion, increasing evidence indicates that cholera toxin also enhances intestinal secretion via prostaglandins and/or neural histamine receptors.

The genes encoding cholera toxin (*ctxAB*) are part of the genome of a bacteriophage designated CTXΦ. The receptor for this phage on the *V. cholerae* surface is the intestinal colonization factor TCP. Since *ctxAB* is part of a mobile genetic element (CTXΦ), horizontal transfer of this bacteriophage may account for the emergence of new toxigenic *V. cholerae* serogroups. Many of the other genes important for *V. cholerae* pathogenicity, including the genes encoding the biosynthesis of TCP, those encoding accessory colonization factors, and those regulating virulence gene expression, are clustered together in the *V. cholerae* pathogenicity island. Similar clustering of virulence genes is found in other bacterial pathogens. It is believed that pathogenicity islands are acquired by horizontal gene transfer.

V. cholerae O139 Bengal is closely related to the O1 El Tor strains of the seventh pandemic and seems to have arisen from them by horizontal gene transfer. It shares the virulence attributes and general pathogenic mechanisms of O1 vibrios. *V. cholerae* O139 Bengal is in fact virtually identical to the seventh-pandemic strains of *V. cholerae* O1 El Tor except for two important differences: production of the novel O139 LPS and of an immunologically related O-antigen polysaccharide capsule. Encapsulation is not a feature of O1 strains and may explain the resistance of O139 strains to human serum in vitro as well as the occasional development of O139 bacteremia.

CLINICAL MANIFESTATIONS

After a 24- to 48-h incubation period, cholera begins with the sudden onset of painless watery diarrhea that may quickly become voluminous and is often followed shortly by vomiting. In severe cases, stool volume can exceed 250 mL/kg in the first 24 h. If fluids and electrolytes are not replaced, hypovolemic shock and death ensue. Fever is usually absent. Muscle cramps due to electrolyte disturbances are common. The stool has a characteristic appearance: a nonbilious, gray, slightly cloudy fluid with flecks of mucus, no blood, and a somewhat sweet, inoffensive odor. It has been called "rice-water" stool because of its resemblance to the water in which rice has been washed. Clinical symptoms parallel volume contraction: At losses of 3–5% of normal body weight, thirst develops; at 5–8%, postural hypotension, weakness, tachycardia, and decreased skin turgor are documented; and at >10%, oliguria, weak or absent pulses, sunken eyes (and, in infants, sunken fontanelles), wrinkled ("washerwoman") skin, somnolence, and coma are characteristic. Complications derive exclusively from the effects of volume and electrolyte depletion and include renal failure due to acute tubular necrosis. Thus, if the patient is adequately treated with fluid and electrolytes, complications are averted and the process is self-limited, resolving in a few days.

Laboratory data usually reveal an elevated hematocrit (due to hemoconcentration) in nonanemic patients; mild neutrophilic leukocytosis; elevated levels of blood urea nitrogen and creatinine consistent with prerenal azotemia; normal sodium, potassium, and chloride levels; a markedly reduced bicarbonate level (<15 mmol/L); and an elevated anion gap (due to increases in serum lactate, protein, and phosphate). Arterial pH is usually low (~7.2).

DIAGNOSIS

The clinical suspicion of cholera can be confirmed by the identification of *V. cholerae* in stool; however, the organism must be specifically sought. With experience, it can be detected directly by dark-field microscopy on a wet mount of fresh stool, and its serotype can be discerned by immobilization with specific antiserum. Laboratory isolation of the organism requires the use of a selective medium. The best of these is thiosulfate–citrate–bile salts–sucrose (TCBS) agar, on which the organism grows as a flat yellow colony. If a delay in sample processing is expected, Carey-Blair transport medium and/or alkaline-peptone water-enrichment medium should be inoculated as well. In endemic areas, there is little need for biochemical confirmation and characterization, although these tasks may be worthwhile in places where *V. cholerae* is an uncommon isolate. Standard microbiologic biochemical testing for Enterobacteriaceae will suffice for identification of *V. cholerae*. All vibrios are oxidase-positive.

The yield of stool cultures for the diagnosis of *V. cholerae* infection declines late in the course of the illness or when effective antibacterial therapy is initiated. Monoclonal antibody–based diagnostic kits and methods based on the polymerase chain reaction and on DNA probes have been developed for detection of *V. cholerae* O1 and O139.

℞ CHOLERA

Cholera is simple to treat; only the rapid and adequate replacement of fluids, electrolytes, and base is required. The mortality rate for appropriately treated disease is usually <1%. However, analysis of a large outbreak of cholera among airline travelers from an endemic country to the United States revealed frequent misdiagnoses by U.S. health professionals and poor appreciation on their part of the principles of management. Fluid replacement may be given orally, but oral rehydration is not always feasible in the presence of significant vomiting. Oral rehydration takes advantage of the hexose-Na^+ cotransport mechanism to move Na^+ across the gut mucosa together with an actively transported molecule such as glucose. For the sake of simplicity, the WHO advises routine use of a single solution of oral rehydration salts (ORS) for diarrheal disease rather than encouraging attempts to choose among multiple formulations according to etiology **(Table 149-1)**. If available, rice-based ORS is considered superior to standard ORS in the treatment of cholera.

For initial management of severely dehydrated patients, IV fluid replacement is preferable. Because profound acidosis (pH < 7.2) is common in this group, Ringer's lactate is the best choice among commercial products **(Table 149-2)**. It must be used with additional potassium supplements, preferably given by mouth. The total fluid deficit in severely dehydrated patients (≥10% of body weight) can be replaced safely within the first 4 h of therapy, half within the first hour. Thereafter, oral therapy can usually be initiated, with the goal of maintaining fluid intake equal to fluid output. However, patients with continued large-volume diarrhea may require prolonged IV treatment to keep up with gastrointestinal fluid losses. Severe hypokalemia can develop but will respond to potassium given either IV or orally. In the absence of adequate staff to monitor the patient's progress, the oral route of rehydration and potassium replacement is safer than the IV route.

Although not necessary for cure, the use of an antibiotic to which the organism is susceptible diminishes the duration and volume of fluid loss and

TABLE 149-1 COMPOSITION OF WORLD HEALTH ORGANIZATION ORAL REHYDRATION SOLUTION (ORS)[a,b]

Constituent	Concentration, mmol/L
Na^+	75
K^+	20
Cl^-	65
Citrate[c]	10
Glucose	75

[a]Contains (per package, to be added to 1 L of drinking water): NaCl, 2.6 g; $Na_3C_6H_5O_7 \cdot 2H_2O$, 2.9 g; KCl, 1.5 g; and glucose, 15 g.

[b]If prepackaged ORS is unavailable, a simple homemade alternative can be prepared by combining 5 g NaCl (about 1 level teaspoon) with either 50 g precooked rice cereal or 40 g sucrose in 1 L of drinking water. In that case, potassium must be supplied separately (e.g., in orange juice or coconut water).

[c]10 mmol citrate per liter, which supplies 30 mmol HCO_3^-/L.

TABLE 149-2 ELECTROLYTE COMPOSITION OF CHOLERA STOOL AND OF INTRAVENOUS REHYDRATION SOLUTION

	Concentration, mmol/L			
Substance	**Na^+**	**K^+**	**Cl^-**	**Base**
Stool				
Adult	135	15	90	30
Child	100	25	90	30
Ringer's lactate	130	4[a]	109	28

[a]Potassium supplements, preferably administered by mouth, are required to replace the usual potassium losses from stool.

hastens clearance of the organism from the stool. Single-dose tetracycline (2 g) or doxycycline (300 mg) is effective in adults but is not recommended for children <8 years of age because of possible deposition in bone and developing teeth. Emerging drug resistance is an ever-present concern. For adults with cholera in areas where tetracycline resistance is prevalent, ciprofloxacin [either in a single dose (30 mg/kg, not to exceed a total dose of 1 g) or in a short course (15 mg/kg bid for 3 days, not to exceed a total daily dose of 1 g)], erythromycin (a total of 40 mg/kg daily in three divided doses for 3 days), or a single 1-g dose of azithromycin is a clinically effective substitute. These drugs are highly effective in reducing total stool output and are significantly better than trimethoprim-sulfamethoxazole. For children, furazolidone has been the recommended agent and trimethoprim-sulfamethoxazole the second choice. Because of cost and/or toxicity issues related to the other drugs, erythromycin is a good choice for pediatric cholera.

PREVENTION

Provision of safe water and facilities for sanitary disposal of feces, improved nutrition, and attention to food preparation and storage in the household can significantly reduce the incidence of cholera.

Much effort has been devoted to the development of an effective cholera vaccine over the past two decades, with a particular focus on oral vaccine strains. Traditional killed cholera vaccine given intramuscularly provides little protection to nonimmune subjects and predictably causes adverse effects, including pain at the injection site, malaise, and fever. The vaccine's limited efficacy is due, at least in part, to its failure to induce a local immune response at the intestinal mucosal surface.

Two types of oral cholera vaccines have been developed. The first is a killed whole-cell (WC) vaccine. Two formulations of the killed WC vaccine have been prepared: one that also contains the nontoxic B subunit of cholera toxin (WC/BS) and one composed solely of killed bacteria. In field trials in Bangladesh, both of the killed vaccines offered significant protection from cholera compared with placebo for the first 6 months after vaccination, with protection rates of ~58% for WC and 85% for WC/BS. Protective efficacy rates for both vaccines declined to ~50% by 3 years after vaccine administration. Immunity was relatively sustained in persons vaccinated at an age of >5 years but was not well sustained in younger vaccinees. The WC/BS vaccine proved effective in a trial conducted in a sub-Saharan African population with a high prevalence of HIV infection. Killed oral vaccines also confer herd protection to unvaccinated individuals living in proximity to vaccinated individuals. Serious consideration should be given to the administration of the WC/BS vaccine in high-risk environments such as refugee camps. The WC/BS vaccine is available in Europe but not in the United States.

The second approach is a live attenuated vaccine strain developed, for example, by the isolation or creation of mutants lacking the genes encoding cholera toxin. Strain CVD 103-HgR, an oral live cholera vaccine licensed for immunization of travelers in Europe, is derived from a classical biotype strain of *V. cholerae* and contains a deletion of the cholera toxin A subunit gene. This strain has been extensively tested in volunteers; a single dose yielded a high degree of protection against experimental challenge with classical *V. cholerae* strains, with almost no side effects. Protective efficacy was not as great against challenge with El Tor *V. cholerae*. Unfortunately, in a large field trial in Indonesian children, this vaccine failed to induce protection against clinical cholera. Other live attenuated vaccine candidate strains have been prepared from El Tor and O139 *V. cholerae* and are now undergoing clinical trials. Because of the minimal efficacy of existing parenteral vaccines, cholera immunization is recommended for U.S. travelers only if it is mandated by the countries they plan to visit.

OTHER *VIBRIO* SPECIES

The genus *Vibrio* includes several human pathogens that do not cause cholera. Abundant in coastal waters throughout the world, noncholera vibrios can reach high concentrations in the tissues of filter-feeding mollusks. As a result, human infection commonly follows the ingestion of seawater or of raw or undercooked shellfish (Table 149-3). Most noncholera vibrios can be cultured on blood or MacConkey agar, which contains enough salt to support the growth of these halophilic species. In the microbiology laboratory, the species of noncholera vibrios are distinguished by standard biochemical tests. The most important of these organisms are *V. parahaemolyticus* and *V. vulnificus*.

The two major types of syndromes for which these species are responsible are gastrointestinal illness (due to *V. parahaemolyticus*, non-O1 *V. cholerae*, *V. mimicus*, *V. fluvialis*, *V. hollisae*, and *V. furnissii*) and soft tissue infections (due to *V. vulnificus*, *V. alginolyticus*, and *V. damselae*). *V. vulnificus* is also a cause of primary sepsis in some compromised individuals. *V. parahaemolyticus* causes rare cases of wound infection and otitis and very rare cases of sepsis.

SPECIES ASSOCIATED PRIMARILY WITH GASTROINTESTINAL ILLNESS

V. parahaemolyticus Widespread in marine environments, *V. parahaemolyticus* grows in saline concentrations up to 8–10%. This species was originally implicated in enteritis in Japan in 1953, accounting for 24% of reported cases in one study—a rate that presumably was due to the common practice of eating raw seafood in that country. *V. parahaemolyticus* has since been identified as a significant intestinal pathogen in many regions of the world. In the United States, common-source outbreaks of diarrhea caused by this organism have been linked to the consumption of undercooked or improperly handled seafood or of other foods contaminated by seawater. Since the mid-1990s, the incidence of *V. parahaemolyticus* infections has increased in several countries, including the United States. Serotypes O3:K6, O4:K68, and O1:K-untypable, which are genetically related to one another, account for this increase. The enteropathogenicity of *V. parahaemolyticus* is closely linked to its ability to cause hemolysis on Wagatsuma agar (i.e., the *Kanagawa phenomenon*). Although the mechanism by which the organism causes diarrhea remains unclear, the genome sequence of *V. parahaemolyticus* contains a pathogenicity island—a cluster of likely virulence-associated genes. *V. parahaemolyticus* should be considered

TABLE 149-3 FEATURES OF SELECTED NONCHOLERA VIBRIOSES

Organism	Vehicle or Activity	Host at Risk	Syndrome
V. parahaemolyticus	Shellfish, seawater	Normal	Gastroenteritis
	Seawater	Normal	Wound infection
Non-O1 *V. cholerae*	Shellfish, travel	Normal	Gastroenteritis
	Seawater	Normal	Wound infection, otitis media
V. vulnificus	Shellfish	Immunosuppressed[a]	Sepsis, secondary cellulitis
	Seawater	Normal	Wound infection, cellulitis
V. alginolyticus	Seawater	Normal	Wound infection, cellulitis, otitis
	Seawater	Burned, other immunosuppressed	Sepsis

[a]Especially with liver disease or hemochromatosis.

Source: Table 161-3 in *Harrison's Principles of Internal Medicine*, 14th edition.

a possible etiologic agent in all cases of diarrhea that can be linked epidemiologically to seafood consumption or to the sea itself.

Infections with *V. parahaemolyticus* can result in two distinct gastrointestinal presentations. The more common of the two presentations (including nearly all cases in North America) is characterized by watery diarrhea, usually occurring in conjunction with abdominal cramps, nausea, and vomiting and accompanied in ~25% of cases by fever and chills. After an incubation period of 4 h to 4 days, symptoms develop and persist for a median of 3 days. Dysentery, the less common presentation, is characterized by severe abdominal cramps, nausea, vomiting, and bloody or mucoid stools.

Most cases of *V. parahaemolyticus*–associated gastrointestinal illness, regardless of the presentation, are self-limited and require neither antimicrobial treatment nor hospitalization. Deaths are extremely rare. Severe infections are associated with underlying diseases, including diabetes, preexisting liver disease, iron-overload states, or immunosuppression. The occasional severe case should be treated with fluid replacement and antibiotics, as described above for cholera.

Non-01 *V. cholerae* The heterogeneous non-O1 *V. cholerae* organisms cannot be distinguished from *V. cholerae* O1 by routine biochemical tests but do not agglutinate in O1 antiserum. Non-O1 strains have caused several well-studied food-borne outbreaks of gastroenteritis and have also been responsible for sporadic cases of otitis media, wound infection, and bacteremia. Like other vibrios, non-O1 *V. cholerae* organisms are widely distributed in marine environments. In most instances, recognized cases in the United States have been associated with the consumption of raw oysters or with recent travel, typically to Mexico. The broad clinical spectrum of diarrheal illness caused by these organisms is probably due to the group's heterogeneous virulence attributes. *V. cholerae* O139 Bengal, although technically a non-O1 vibrio, is not grouped with these pathogens because it can cause epidemic cholera.

In the United States, about half of all non-O1 *V. cholerae* isolates are from stool samples. The typical incubation period for gastroenteritis due to these organisms is <2 days, and the illness lasts for ~2–7 days. Patients' stools may be copious and watery or may be partly formed, less voluminous, and bloody or mucoid. Diarrhea can result in severe dehydration. Many cases include abdominal cramps, nausea, vomiting, and fever. Like those with cholera, patients who are seriously dehydrated should receive oral or IV fluids; the value of antibiotics is not clear.

Extraintestinal infections due to non-O1 *V. cholerae* commonly follow occupational or recreational exposure to seawater. Around 10% of non-O1 *V. cholerae* isolates come from cases of wound infection, 10% from cases of otitis media, and 20% from cases of bacteremia (which is particularly likely to develop in patients with liver disease). Extraintestinal infections should be treated with antibiotics. Information to guide antibiotic selection and dosing is limited, but most strains are sensitive in vitro to tetracycline, ciprofloxacin, and third-generation cephalosporins.

SPECIES ASSOCIATED PRIMARILY WITH SOFT TISSUE INFECTION OR BACTEREMIA

(See also Chap. 119)

V. vulnificus *V. vulnificus* is the most common cause of severe vibrio infections in the United States. Like most vibrios, this organism proliferates in the warm summer months and requires a saline environment for growth. In this country, infections in humans typically occur in coastal states between May and October and most commonly affect men >40 years of age. *V. vulnificus* has been linked to two distinct syndromes: primary sepsis, which usually occurs in patients with underlying liver disease, and primary wound infection, which generally affects people without underlying disease. Some authors have suggested that *V. vulnificus* also causes gastroenteritis independent of other clinical manifestations. *V. vulnificus* is endowed with a number of virulence attributes, including a capsule that confers resistance to phagocytosis and to the bactericidal activity of human serum as well as a cytolysin. Measured as the 50% lethal dose in mice, the organism's virulence is considerably increased under conditions of iron overload; this observation is consistent with the propensity of *V. vulnificus* to infect patients who have hemochromatosis.

Primary sepsis most often develops in patients who have cirrhosis or hemochromatosis. However, *V. vulnificus* bacteremia can also affect individuals who have hematopoietic disorders or chronic renal insufficiency, those who are using immunosuppressive medications or alcohol, or (in rare instances) those who have no known underlying disease. After a median incubation period of 16 h, the patient develops malaise, chills, fever, and prostration. One-third of patients develop hypotension, which is often apparent at admission. Cutaneous manifestations develop in most cases (usually within 36 h of onset) and characteristically involve the extremities (the lower more often than the upper). In a common sequence, erythematous patches are followed by ecchymoses, vesicles, and bullae. In fact, sepsis and bullous skin lesions suggest the diagnosis in appropriate settings. Necrosis and sloughing may also be evident. Laboratory studies reveal leukopenia more often than leukocytosis, thrombocytopenia, or elevated levels of fibrin split products. *V. vulnificus* can be cultured from blood or cutaneous lesions. The mortality rate approaches 50%, with most deaths due to uncontrolled sepsis. Accordingly, prompt treatment is critical and should include empirical antibiotic administration, aggressive debridement, and general supportive care. *V. vulnificus* is sensitive in vitro to a number of antibiotics, including tetracycline, fluoroquinolones, and third-generation cephalosporins. Data from animal models suggest that either a fluoroquinolone or the combination of minocycline and cefotaxime should be used in the treatment of *V. vulnificus* septicemia.

V. vulnificus can infect either a fresh or an old wound that comes into contact with seawater; the patient may or may not have underlying disease. After a short incubation period (4 h to 4 days; mean, 12 h), the disease begins with swelling, erythema, and (in many cases) intense pain around the wound. These signs and symptoms are followed by cellulitis, which spreads rapidly and is sometimes accompanied by vesicular, bullous, or necrotic lesions. Metastatic events are uncommon. Most patients have a fever and leukocytosis. *V. vulnificus* can be cultured from skin lesions and occasionally from the blood. Prompt antibiotic therapy and debridement are usually curative.

V. alginolyticus First identified as a pathogen of humans in 1973, *V. alginolyticus* occasionally causes eye, ear, and wound infections. This species is the most salt-tolerant of the vibrios and can grow in salt concentrations of >10%. Most clinical isolates come from superinfected wounds that presumably become contaminated at the beach. Although severity varies, *V. alginolyticus* infection tends not to be serious and generally responds well to antibiotic therapy and drainage. A few cases of otitis externa, otitis media, and conjunctivitis due to this pathogen have been described. Tetracycline treatment usually results in cure. *V. alginolyticus* is a rare cause of bacteremia in immunocompromised hosts.

ACKNOWLEDGMENT

The authors gratefully acknowledge the valuable contributions of Dr. Robert Deresiewicz, a coauthor of this chapter for the 14th edition.

FURTHER READINGS

LUCAS MES et al: Effectiveness of mass oral cholera vaccination in Beira, Mozambique. N Engl J Med 352:757, 2005

SACK DA et al: Cholera. Lancet 363:223, 2004

SAHA D et al: Single-dose azithromycin for the treatment of cholera in adults. N Engl J Med 354:2452, 2006

TANG HJ et al: In vitro and in vivo activities of newer fluoroquinolones against *Vibrio vulnificus*. Antimicrob Agents Chemother 46:3580, 2002

WORLD HEALTH ORGANIZATION: *The Treatment of Diarrhoea: A Manual for Physicians and Other Senior Health Workers*. Geneva, World Health Organization, 2005 (*www.who.int/child-adolescent-health/New_Publications/CHILD_HEALTH/ISBN_92_4_159318_0.pdf*)

———: Cholera, 2004. Wkly Epidemiol Rec 80:261, 2005 (*www.who.int/wer*)

150 Brucellosis

Michael J. Corbel, Nicholas J. Beeching

DEFINITION

Brucellosis is a bacterial zoonosis transmitted directly or indirectly to humans from infected animals, predominantly domesticated ruminants and swine. The disease is known colloquially as *undulant fever* because of its remittent character. Its distribution is worldwide apart from the few countries where it has been eradicated from the animal reservoir. Although brucellosis commonly presents as an acute febrile illness, its clinical manifestations vary widely, and definitive signs indicative of the diagnosis may be lacking. Thus the clinical diagnosis usually must be supported by the results of bacteriologic and/or serologic tests.

ETIOLOGIC AGENTS

Human brucellosis is caused by strains of *Brucella*, a bacterial genus that has been suggested, on genetic grounds, to comprise a single species, *Brucella melitensis*, with a number of biologic variants that exhibit particular host preferences. Recently, this view has been challenged on the basis of detailed differences in chromosomal structure and host preference. The traditional classification into nomen species is now favored both because of these differences and because this classification scheme closely reflects the epidemiologic patterns of the infection. The nomen system recognizes *B. melitensis*, which is the commonest cause of symptomatic disease in humans and for which the main sources are sheep, goats, and camels; *B. abortus*, which is usually acquired from cattle or buffalo: *B. suis*, which generally is acquired from swine but has one variant enzootic in reindeer and caribou and another in rodents; and *B. canis*, which is acquired most often from dogs. *B. ovis*, which causes reproductive disease in sheep, and *B. neotomae*, which is specific for desert rodents, have not been clearly implicated in human disease. Other brucellae have been isolated from marine mammals, and two new nomen species, *B. cetaceae* and *B. pinnipediae*, have been proposed. At least one case of laboratory-acquired human disease due to one of these proposed species has been described, and apparent cases of natural infection have been reported. As infections in marine mammals seem widespread, more cases of zoonotic infection may be identified.

All brucellae are small, gram-negative, unencapsulated, nonsporulating rods or coccobacilli. They grow aerobically on peptone-based medium incubated at 37° C; the growth of some types is improved by supplementary CO_2. In vivo, brucellae behave as facultative intracellular parasites. The organisms are sensitive to sunlight, ionizing radiation, and moderate heat; they are killed by boiling and pasteurization but are resistant to freezing and drying. Their resistance to drying renders brucellae stable in aerosol form, facilitating airborne transmission. The organisms can survive for up to 2 months in soft cheeses made from goat's or sheep's milk; for at least 6 weeks in dry soil contaminated with infected urine, vaginal discharge, or placental or fetal tissues; and for at least 6 months in damp soil or liquid manure kept under cool dark conditions. Brucellae are easily killed by a wide range of common disinfectants used under optimal conditions but are likely to be much more resistant at low temperatures or in the presence of heavy organic contamination.

EPIDEMIOLOGY

Brucellosis is a zoonosis whose occurrence is closely related to its prevalence in domesticated animals. The true global prevalence of human brucellosis is unknown because of the imprecision of diagnosis and the inadequacy of reporting and surveillance systems in many countries. Even in developed countries, the true incidence may be 10–20 times higher than the reported figures. Bovine brucellosis has been the target of control programs in many parts of the world and has been eradicated from the cattle populations of Australia, New Zealand, Bulgaria, Canada, Cyprus, Great Britain (including the Channel Islands), Japan, Luxembourg, Romania, the Scandinavian countries, Switzerland, and the Czech and Slovak Republics. Its incidence has been reduced to a low level in the United States and most Western European countries, with a varied picture in other parts of the world. There is evidence of a resurgence in Eastern Europe following economic changes in recent years, and new outbreaks have also occurred in Ireland. Efforts to eradicate *B. melitensis* infection from sheep and goat populations have been much less successful. These efforts have relied heavily on vaccination programs, which have tended to fluctuate with changing economic and political conditions. In some countries (e.g., Israel), *B. melitensis* has caused serious outbreaks in cattle. Infections with *B. melitensis* still pose a major public health problem in Mediterranean countries; in western, central, and southern Asia; and in parts of Africa and South and Central America.

Human brucellosis is usually associated with occupational or domestic exposure to infected animals or their products. Farmers, shepherds, goatherds, veterinarians, and employees in slaughterhouses and meat-processing plants in endemic areas are occupationally exposed to infection. Family members of individuals involved in animal husbandry may be at risk, although it is often difficult to differentiate food-borne infection from environmental contamination under these circumstances. Laboratory workers who handle cultures or infected samples are also at risk. Travelers and urban dwellers usually acquire the infection through consumption of contaminated foods. In countries that have eradicated the disease, new cases are most commonly acquired abroad. Dairy products, especially soft cheeses, unpasteurized milk, and ice cream, are the most frequently implicated sources of infection; raw meat and bone marrow may be sources under exceptional circumstances. Infections acquired through cosmetic treatments using materials of fetal origin have been reported. Person-to-person transmission is extremely rare, as is transfer of infection by blood or tissue donation. Although brucellosis is a chronic intracellular infection, there is no evidence for increased prevalence or severity among individuals with HIV infection or with immunodeficiency or immunosuppression of other etiologies.

Brucellosis may be acquired by ingestion, inhalation, or mucosal or percutaneous exposure. Accidental injection of the live vaccine strains of *B. abortus* (19 and RB51) and *B. melitensis* (Rev 1) can cause disease. *B. melitensis* and *B. suis* have been developed as biological weapons by several countries and could be exploited for bioterrorism (Chap. 214). This possibility should be borne in mind in the event of sudden unexplained outbreaks.

IMMUNITY AND PATHOGENESIS

Exposure to brucellosis elicits both humoral and cell-mediated immune responses. The mechanisms of protective immunity against human brucellosis are presumed to be similar to those documented in laboratory animals. The response to infection and its outcome are influenced by the virulence, phase, and species of the infecting strain. Differences have been reported between *B. abortus* and *B. suis* in the modes of cellular entry and subsequent compartmentalization and processing. Antibodies promote clearance of extracellular brucellae by bactericidal action and by facilitation of phagocytosis by polymorphonuclear and mononuclear phagocytes; however, antibodies alone cannot eradicate infection. Organisms taken up by macrophages and other cells can establish persistent intracellular infections. The key target cell is the macrophage, and bacterial mechanisms for suppressing intracellular killing and apoptosis result in very large intracellular populations. Opsonized bacteria are actively phagocytosed by neutrophilic granulocytes and by monocytes. In these and other cells, initial attachment takes place via specific receptors, including Fc, C3, fibronectin, and mannose-binding proteins. Opsonized—but not unopsonized—bacteria trigger an oxidative burst inside phagocytes. Unopsonized bacteria are internalized via similar receptors but at much lower efficiency. Smooth strains enter host cells via lipid rafts. Smooth lipopolysaccharide (LPS), β-cyclic glucan, and possibly an invasion-attachment protein (IalB) are involved in this process. Tumor necrosis factor α (TNF-α) produced early in the course of infection stimulates cytotoxic lymphocytes and activates macrophages, which can kill intracellular brucellae (probably mainly through production of reactive oxygen and nitrogen intermediates) and may clear infection. However, virulent *Brucella* cells can suppress the TNF-α response, and control of infection in this situation depends on macrophage activation and interferon γ (IFN-γ) responses. Cytokines such as interleukin (IL) 12 promote production of IFN-γ, which drives T_H1-type responses and stimulates macrophage activation. Inflammatory cytokines, including IL-4, IL-6, and IL-10, downregulate the protective response. As in other types of intracellular infection, it is assumed that initial replication of brucellae takes place within cells of the lymph nodes draining the point of entry. Subsequent hematogenous spread may result in chronic localizing infection at almost any site, although the reticuloendothelial system, musculoskeletal tissues, and genitourinary system are most frequently targeted. Both acute and chronic inflammatory responses develop in brucellosis, and the local tissue response may include granuloma formation with or without necrosis and caseation. Abscesses may also develop, especially in chronic localized infection.

The determinants of pathogenicity of *Brucella* have not been fully characterized, and the mechanisms underlying the manifestations of brucellosis are incompletely understood. The organism's survival strategy is centered on processes that permit survival within monocytic cells. The smooth *Brucella* LPS, which has an unusual O-chain and core-lipid composition, has relatively low endotoxin activity and plays a key role in pyrogenicity and in resistance to phagocytosis and serum killing in the nonimmune host. LPS is believed also to play a key role in suppressing phagosome-lysosome fusion and diverting the internalized bacteria into vacuoles located in endoplasmic reticulum, where intracellular replication takes place. Specific exotoxins have not been isolated, but a type IV secretion system (VirB) that regulates intracellular survival and trafficking has been identified. In *B. abortus* this system can be activated extracellularly, but in *B. suis* it is activated (by low pH) only during intracellular growth. Brucellae then produce acid-stable proteins that facilitate the organisms' survival in phagosomes and may enhance their resistance to reactive oxygen intermediates. Virulent brucellae are resistant to defensins and produce a Cu-Zn superoxide dismutase that increases their resistance to reactive oxygen intermediates.

CLINICAL FEATURES

Brucellosis almost invariably causes fever, which may be associated with profuse sweats, especially at night. In endemic areas, brucellosis may be difficult to distinguish from the many other causes of fever. However, two features recognized in the nineteenth century distinguish brucellosis from other tropical fevers, such as typhoid and malaria. (1) Left untreated, the fever of brucellosis shows an undulating pattern that persists for weeks before the commencement of an afebrile period that may be followed by relapse. (2) The fever of brucellosis is associated with musculoskeletal symptoms and signs in about one-half of all patients.

The clinical syndromes caused by the different nomen species are similar, although *B. melitensis* tends to be associated with a more acute and aggressive presentation and *B. suis* with focal abscess induction. *B. abortus* infections may be more insidious in onset and more likely to become chronic.

The incubation period varies from 1 week to several months, and the onset of fever and other symptoms may be abrupt or insidious. In addition to experiencing fever and sweats, patients become increasingly apathetic and fatigued; lose appetite and weight; and have nonspecific myalgia, headache, and chills. Overall, the presentation of brucellosis often fits one of three patterns: febrile illness that resembles typhoid but is less severe; fever and acute monoarthritis, typically of the hip or knee, in a young child; and long-lasting fever, misery, and low-back or hip pain in an older man. In an endemic area (e.g., much of the Middle East), a patient with fever and difficulty walking into the clinic would be regarded as having brucellosis until it was proved otherwise.

Diagnostic clues in the patient's history include travel to an endemic area, employment in a diagnostic microbiology laboratory, consumption of unpasteurized milk products (including soft cheeses), contact with animals, and—in an endemic setting—a history of similar illness in the family (documented in almost 50% of cases).

TABLE 150-1 RADIOLOGY OF THE SPINE: DIFFERENTIATION OF BRUCELLOSIS FROM TUBERCULOSIS

	Brucellosis	Tuberculosis
Site	Lumbar and others	Dorsolumbar
Vertebrae	Multiple or contiguous	Contiguous
Diskitis	Late	Early
Body	Intact until late	Morphology lost early
Canal compression	Rare	Common
Epiphysitis	Anterosuperior (Pom's sign)	General: upper and lower disk regions, central, subperiosteal
Osteophyte	Anterolateral (parrot beak)	Unusual
Deformity	Wedging uncommon	Anterior wedge, gibbus
Recovery	Sclerosis, whole body	Variable
Paravertebral abscess	Small, well-localized	Common and discrete loss, transverse process
Psoas abscess	Rare	More likely

Focal features are present in the majority of patients. The most common are musculoskeletal pain and physical findings in the peripheral and axial skeleton (~40% of cases). Osteomyelitis more commonly involves the lumbar and low thoracic vertebrae than the cervical and high thoracic spine. Individual joints that are most commonly affected by septic arthritis are the knee, hip, sacroiliac, shoulder, and sternoclavicular joints; the pattern may be one of monoarthritis or polyarthritis. Osteomyelitis may also accompany septic arthritis.

In addition to the usual causes of vertebral osteomyelitis or septic arthritis, the most important differential diagnosis is tuberculosis. This point influences the therapeutic approach as well as the prognosis, given that several antimicrobial agents used to treat brucellosis are also used to treat tuberculosis. Septic arthritis in brucellosis progresses slowly, starting with small pericapsular erosions. In the vertebrae, anterior erosions of the superior end plate are typically the first features to become evident, with eventual involvement and sclerosis of the whole vertebra. Anterior osteophytes eventually develop, but vertebral destruction or impingement on the spinal cord is rare and usually suggests tuberculosis (Table 150-1).

Other systems may be involved in a manner that resembles typhoid. About one-quarter of patients have a dry cough, usually with few changes visible on the chest x-ray, although pneumonia, empyema, intrathoracic adenopathy, or lung abscess can occur. One-quarter of patients have hepatosplenomegaly, and 10–20% have significant lymphadenopathy; the differential diagnosis includes glandular fever–like illness such as that caused by Epstein-Barr virus, *Toxoplasma*, and cytomegalovirus; HIV infection; or tuberculosis. Up to 10% of men have acute epididymoorchitis, which must be distinguished from mumps and from surgical problems such as torsion. Prostatitis, inflammation of the seminal vesicles, salpingitis, and pyelonephritis all occur. There is an increased incidence of fetal loss among infected pregnant women, although teratogenicity has not been described and the tendency to cause abortions is much less pronounced in humans than in farm animals.

Neurologic involvement is common, with depression and lethargy whose severity may not be truly appreciated by either the patient or the physician until after treatment. A small proportion of patients develop lymphocytic meningoencephalitis that mimics neurotuberculosis or noninfectious conditions and that may be complicated by intracerebral abscess, a variety of cranial nerve deficits, or ruptured mycotic aneurysms.

Endocarditis occurs in ~1% of cases, most often affecting the aortic valve (natural or prosthetic). Any site in the body may be involved in metastatic abscess formation or inflammation; the female breast and the thyroid gland are affected particularly often. Nonspecific maculo-

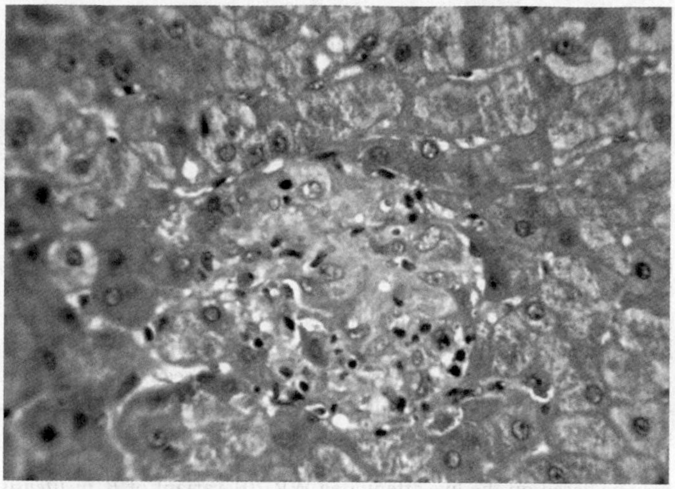

FIGURE 150-1 Liver biopsy specimen from a patient with brucellosis shows a noncaseating granuloma. *[From Mandell's Atlas of Infectious Diseases, Vol II, in DL Stevens (ed): Skin, Soft Tissue, Bone and Joint Infections, Fig. 5-9; with permission.]*

papular rashes and other skin manifestations are uncommon and are rarely noticed by the patient even if they are present.

DIAGNOSIS

Because the clinical picture of brucellosis is not distinctive, the diagnosis must be based on a history of potential exposure, a presentation consistent with the disease, and supporting laboratory findings. Results of routine biochemical assays are usually within normal limits, although serum levels of hepatic enzymes and bilirubin may be elevated. Peripheral leukocyte counts are usually normal or low, with relative lymphocytosis. Mild anemia may be documented. Thrombocytopenia and disseminated intravascular coagulation with raised levels of fibrinogen degradation products can develop. The erythrocyte sedimentation rate and C-reactive protein levels are often normal but may be raised.

In body fluids such as cerebrospinal fluid (CSF) or joint fluid, lymphocytosis and low glucose levels are the norm. Elevated CSF levels of adenosine deaminase cannot be used to distinguish tubercular meningitis, as they may also be found in brucellosis. Biopsied samples of tissues such as lymph node or liver may show noncaseating granulomas (Fig. 150-1) without acid/alcohol-fast bacilli. The radiologic features of bony disease develop late and are much more subtle than those of tuberculosis or septic arthritis of other etiologies, with less bone and joint destruction. Isotope scanning is more sensitive than plain x-ray and continues to give positive results long after successful treatment.

Isolation of brucellae from blood, CSF, bone marrow, or joint fluid or from a tissue aspirate or biopsy sample is definitive, and attempts at isolation are usually successful in 50–70% of cases. Duplicate cultures should be incubated for up to 6 weeks (in air and 10% CO_2, respectively). Concentration and lysis of buffy coat cells before culture may increase the isolation rate. Cultures in modern nonradiometric or similar signaling systems (e.g., Bactec) usually become positive within 7–10 days but should be maintained for at least 3 weeks before the results are declared negative. All cultures should be handled under containment conditions appropriate for dangerous pathogens. *Brucella* spp. may be misidentified as *Agrobacterium, Ochrobactrum*, or *Psychrobacter (Moraxella) phenylpyruvicus* by the gallery identification strips commonly used in the diagnostic laboratory.

The peripheral blood–based polymerase chain reaction (PCR) has enormous potential to detect bacteremia, to predict relapse, and to exclude "chronic brucellosis." PCR is probably more sensitive and is certainly quicker than blood culture, and it does not carry the attendant biohazard risk posed by culture. Nucleic acid amplification techniques are now quite widely used, although no single standardized procedure has been adopted. Primers for the spacer region between the genes encoding the 16S and 23S ribosomal RNAs (*rrs-rrl*), the outer membrane protein Omp2, the insertion sequence *IS711*, and protein BCSP31 are sensitive and specific. Blood and other tissues are the most suitable samples for analysis.

Serologic examination often provides the only positive laboratory findings in brucellosis. In acute infection, IgM antibodies appear early and are followed by IgG and IgA. All these antibodies are active in agglutination tests, whether performed by tube, plate, or microagglutination methods. The majority of patients have detectable agglutinins at this stage. As the disease progresses, IgM levels decline, and the avidity and subclass distribution of IgG and IgA change. The result is reduced or undetectable agglutinin titers. However, the antibodies are detectable by alternative tests, including the complement fixation test, Coombs' antiglobulin test, and enzyme-linked immunosorbent assay. There is no clear cutoff value for a diagnostic titer. Rather, serology results must be interpreted in the context of exposure history and clinical presentation. In endemic areas or in settings of potential occupational exposure, agglutinin titers of 1:320–1:640 or higher are considered diagnostic; in nonendemic areas, a titer of ≥1:160 is considered significant. Repetition of tests after 2–4 weeks may demonstrate a rising titer.

In most centers, the standard agglutination test (SAT) is still the mainstay of serologic diagnosis, although some investigators rely on the rose bengal test, which has not been fully validated for human diagnostic use. Dipstick assays for anti-*Brucella* IgM are useful for the diagnosis of acute infection but are less sensitive for infection with symptoms of several months' duration. In an endemic setting, >90% of patients with acute bacteremia have SAT titers of at least 1:320.

Antibody to the *Brucella* LPS O chain—the dominant antigen—is detected by all the conventional tests that employ smooth *B. abortus* cells as antigen. Since *B. abortus* cross-reacts with *B. melitensis* and *B. suis*, there is no advantage in replicating the tests with these antigens. Cross-reactions also occur with the O chains of some other gram-negative bacteria, including *Escherichia coli* O157, *Francisella tularensis, Salmonella enterica* group N, *Stenotrophomonas maltophilia*, and *Vibrio cholerae*. Cross-reactions do not occur with the cell-surface antigens of rough *Brucella* strains such as *B. canis* or *B. ovis*; serologic tests for these nomen species must employ an antigen prepared from either one. Most protein antigens are shared by all *Brucella* strains, and some are also common to *Ochrobactrum* species. Immunoblotting against protein extracts has been advocated as a differential test, but no validated procedure is yet available.

Rx BRUCELLOSIS

The broad aims of antimicrobial therapy are to treat current infection and relieve its symptoms and to prevent relapse. Focal disease presentations may require specific intervention in addition to more prolonged and tailored antibiotic therapy. In addition, tuberculosis must always be excluded, or—to prevent the emergence of resistance—therapy must be tailored to specifically exclude drugs active against tuberculosis (e.g., rifampin used alone) or to include a full antituberculous regimen.

Early experience with streptomycin monotherapy showed that relapse was common; thus dual therapy with tetracyclines became the norm. This is still the most effective combination, but alternatives may be used, with the options depending on local or national policy about the use of rifampin for the treatment of nonmycobacterial infection. Antimicrobial efficacy can usually be predicted by in vitro testing; however, the use of fluoroquinolones remains controversial despite the good in vitro activity and white cell penetration of most agents of this class. Low intravacuolar pH is probably a factor in the poor performance of these drugs.

For adults with acute nonfocal brucellosis (duration, <1 month), a 6-week course of therapy incorporating at least two antimicrobial agents is required. Complex or focal disease necessitates ≥3 months of therapy. Adherence to the therapeutic regimen is very important, and poor compliance underlies almost all cases of apparent treatment failure; such failure is rarely due to the emergence of drug resistance, although increasing resistance to trimethoprim-sulfamethoxazole (TMP-SMX) has been reported at one center. There is good retrospective evidence that a 3-week course of two agents is as effective as a 6-week course for treatment and prevention of relapse in children, but this point has not yet been proven in prospective studies.

The "gold standard" for the treatment of brucellosis in adults is IM streptomycin (0.75–1 g daily for 14–21 days) together with doxycycline (100 mg twice daily for 6 weeks). In both clinical trials and observational studies, relapse follows such treatment in 5–10% of patients. The usual alternative regimen (and the current World Health Organization recommendation) is rifampin (600–900 mg/d) plus doxycycline (100 mg twice daily) for 6 weeks. The relapse/failure rate is ~10% in trial conditions but rises to >20% in many nontrial situations, possibly because doxycycline levels are reduced and clearance rates increased by concomitant rifampin administration. Patients who cannot tolerate or receive tetracyclines (children, pregnant women) can be given high-dose TMP-SMX instead (2 or 3 standard-strength tablets twice daily for adults, depending on weight).

Evidence is beginning to accumulate that other aminoglycosides can be substituted for streptomycin—e.g., netilmicin or gentamicin given at a dosage of 5–6 mg/kg per day for at least 2 weeks. (Shorter courses have been associated with high failure rates in adults.) A 5- to 7-day course of therapy with gentamicin (and a 3-week course of TMP-SMX) is probably adequate for children with uncomplicated disease. Early experience with fluoroquinolone monotherapy was disappointing, but high-dose ofloxacin (400 mg twice daily) or ciprofloxacin (500 mg twice daily), given together with rifampin for 6 weeks, may become accepted as an alternative to the other 6-week regimens for adults.

Significant neurologic disease due to *Brucella* requires prolonged treatment (i.e., for 3–6 months), usually with ceftriaxone supplementation of a standard regimen. *Brucella* endocarditis is treated with at least three drugs (an aminoglycoside, a tetracycline, and rifampin), and many experts add ceftriaxone and/or a fluoroquinolone to reduce the need for valve replacement. Treatment is usually given for at least 6 months, and clinical endpoints for its discontinuation are often difficult to define. Surgery is still required for the majority of cases of infection of prosthetic heart valves and prosthetic joints.

There is no evidence base to guide prophylaxis after exposure to brucellae (e.g., in the laboratory), inadvertent immunization with live vaccine intended for use in animals, or deliberately released brucellae. Most authorities recommend the administration of rifampin plus doxycycline for 3 weeks after a low-risk exposure (e.g., a nonspecific laboratory accident) and for 6 weeks after a major exposure to aerosol or injected material. However, such regimens are poorly tolerated, and doxycycline monotherapy of the same duration may be substituted.

PROGNOSIS AND FOLLOW-UP

Relapse occurs in up to 30% of poorly compliant patients. Thus patients should ideally be followed clinically for up to 2 years to detect relapse, which responds to a prolonged course of the same therapy used originally. The general well-being and the body weight of the patient are more useful guides than serology to lack of relapse. IgG antibody levels detected by the SAT and its variants can remain in the diagnostic range for >2 years after successful treatment. Complement fixation titers usually fall to normal within 1 year of cure. Immunity is not solid; patients can be reinfected after repeated exposures. Fewer than 1% of patients die of brucellosis. When the outcome is fatal, death is usually a consequence of cardiac involvement; more rarely, it results from severe neurologic disease. Despite the low mortality rate, recovery from brucellosis is slow, and the illness can cause prolonged inactivity, with consequent domestic and economic losses.

The existence of a prolonged chronic brucellosis state after successful treatment remains controversial. Evaluation of patients in whom this state is considered (often those with work-related exposure to brucellae) includes careful exclusion of malingering, nonspecific chronic fatigue syndromes, and other causes of excessive sweating, such as alcohol abuse and obesity. In the future, the availability of more sensitive assays to detect *Brucella* antigen or DNA may help to identify patients with ongoing infection.

PREVENTION

Vaccines based on live attenuated *Brucella* strains, such as *B. abortus* strain 19BA or 104M, have been used in some countries to protect high-risk populations but have displayed only short-term efficacy and high reactogenicity. Subunit vaccines have been developed but are of uncertain value and cannot be recommended at present. Research in this area has been stimulated by interest in biodefense (Chap. 214) and may eventually yield new products, some of which may be based on the live attenuated WR 201 variant of *B. melitensis* strain 16M. The mainstay of veterinary prevention is a national commitment to testing and slaughter of infected herds/flocks (with compensation for owners), control of animal movement, and active immunization of animals. These measures are usually sufficient to control human disease as well. In their absence, pasteurization of all milk products before consumption is sufficient to prevent nonoccupational animal-to-human transmission. All cases of brucellosis in animals and humans should be reported to the appropriate public health authorities.

FURTHER READINGS

ALMUNEEF M, MEMISH ZA: Prevalence of brucella antibodies after acute brucellosis. J Chemother 15:148, 2003

CORBEL MJ, BANAI M: Genus *Brucella* Meyer and Shaw 1920,173[AL], in *Bergey's Manual of Systematic Bacteriology*, 2d ed, vol 2: *The Proteobacteria*, DJ Bruner et al (eds). New York, Springer, 2006, pp 370–386

HASANJANI ROUSHAN MR et al: Efficacy of gentamicin and doxycycline versus streptomycin plus doxycycline in the treatment of brucellosis in humans. Clin Infect Dis 42:1075, 2006

KHAN MY et al: Brucellosis in pregnant women. Clin Infect Dis 32:1172, 2000

MALEY MW et al: Prevention of laboratory-acquired brucellosis: Significant side effects of prophylaxis. Clin Infect Dis 42:433, 2006

MEMISH Z et al: *Brucella* bacteraemia: Clinical and laboratory observations in 160 patients. J Infect 40:59, 2000

NAVARRO E et al: Use of real time quantitative polymerase chain reaction to monitor the evolution of *Brucella melitensis* DNA load during therapy and post-therapy follow-up in patients with brucellosis. Clin Infect Dis 42:1266, 2006

PAPPAS G et al: New approaches to the antibiotic therapy of brucellosis. Int J Antimicrob Agents 26:101, 2005

——— et al: Brucellosis. N Engl J Med 352:2325, 2005

SALTOGLU N et al: Efficacy of rifampicin plus doxycycline versus rifampicin plus quinolone in the treatment of brucellosis. Saudi Med J 23:921, 2002

151 Tularemia

Richard F. Jacobs, Gordon E. Schutze

DEFINITION

Tularemia is a zoonosis caused by *Francisella tularensis*. Humans of any age, sex, or race are universally susceptible to this systemic infection. Tularemia is primarily a disease of wild animals and persists in contaminated environments, ectoparasites, and animal carriers. Human infection is incidental and usually results from interaction with biting or blood-sucking insects, contact with wild or domestic animals, ingestion of contaminated water or food, or inhalation of infective aerosols.

Tularemia is common in Arkansas, Oklahoma, and Missouri, where >50% of the cases in the United States occur. Increasing numbers of cases have been reported from the Scandinavian countries, eastern Europe, and Siberia. The illness is characterized by various clinical syndromes, the most common of which consists of an ulcerative lesion at the site of inoculation, with regional lymphadenopathy and lymphadenitis. Systemic manifestations, including pneumonia, typhoidal tularemia, and fever without localizing findings, pose a greater diagnostic challenge.

ETIOLOGY AND EPIDEMIOLOGY

With rare exceptions, tularemia is the only disease produced by *F. tularensis*—a small (0.2 μm by 0.2–0.7 μm), gram-negative, pleomorphic, nonmotile, non-spore-forming bacillus. Bipolar staining results in a coccoid appearance. The organism is a thinly encapsulated, nonpiliated strict aerobe that invades host cells. In nature, *F. tularensis* is a hardy organism that persists for weeks or months in mud, water, and decaying animal carcasses. Dozens of biting and blood-sucking insects, especially ticks and tabanid flies, serve as vectors. Ticks and wild rabbits are the source for most of the human cases in the endemic areas of the southeastern and Rocky Mountain states. In Utah, Nevada, and California, tabanid flies are the most common vectors. Animal reservoirs include wild rabbits, squirrels, birds, sheep, beavers, muskrats, and domestic dogs and cats. Person-to-person transmission is rare or nonexistent. Tularemia is more common among men than among women.

The two main biovars of *F. tularensis*—*tularensis* (type A) and *holarctica* (type B)—are both found in the United States. Type A produces more serious disease in humans; without treatment, the associated fatality rate is ~5%. Type B produces a milder, often subclinical infection that is usually contracted from water or marine mammals. Although all strains appear serologically identical, individual strains may possess varying degrees of virulence. Currently, there are four proposed subspecies among which 16S RNA analyses show ≥ 99.8% similarity. *F. tularensis* does not produce an exotoxin, but an endotoxin similar to that of other gram-negative bacilli has been identified. The progression of illness depends on the organism's virulence, the inoculum size, the portal of entry, and the host's immune status.

Ticks pass *F. tularensis* to their offspring transovarially. The organism is found in tick feces but not in large quantities in tick salivary glands. In the United States, the disease is carried by *Dermacentor andersoni* (Rocky Mountain wood tick), *D. variabilis* (American dog tick), *D. occidentalis* (Pacific coast dog tick), and *Amblyomma americanum* (Lone Star tick). *F. tularensis* is transmitted frequently during blood meals taken by embedded ticks after hours of attachment. It is the taking of a blood meal through a fecally contaminated field that transmits the organism. Transmission of the organism by ticks and tabanid flies takes place mainly in the spring and summer. However, continued transmission in the winter by trapped or hunted animals has been documented. The organism is extremely infectious. Biosafety level 2 is recommended for clinical laboratory work with material whose contamination with *F. tularensis* is suspected, and biosafety level 3 is required for culture of the organism in large quantities. Issues related to the intentional spread of tularemia through ingestion or inhalation are discussed in Chap. 214.

PATHOGENESIS AND PATHOLOGY

The most common portal of entry for human infection is through skin or mucous membranes, either directly—through the bite of ticks, other arthropods, or other animals—or via inapparent abrasions. Inhalation or ingestion of *F. tularensis* also can result in infection. Although $>10^8$ organisms are usually required to produce infection via the oral route (oropharyngeal or gastrointestinal tularemia), fewer than 50 organisms will result in infection when injected into the skin (ulceroglandular/glandular tularemia) or inhaled (tularemia pneumonia). After inoculation into the skin, the organism multiplies locally; within 2–5 days (range, 1–10 days), it produces an erythematous, tender, or pruritic papule. The papule rapidly enlarges and forms an ulcer with a black base (chancriform lesion). The bacteria spread to regional lymph nodes, producing lymphadenopathy (buboes), and, with bacteremia, may spread to distant organs.

Tularemia is characterized by mononuclear cell infiltration with pyogranulomatous pathology. The histopathologic findings can be quite similar to those in tuberculosis, although tularemia develops more rapidly. As a facultatively intracellular bacterium, *F. tularensis* can parasitize both phagocytic and nonphagocytic host cells and can survive intracellularly for prolonged periods. In the acute phase of infection, the primary organs affected (skin, lymph nodes, liver, and spleen) include areas of focal necrosis, initially surrounded by polymorphonuclear leukocytes (PMNs). Subsequently, granulomas form, with epithelioid cells, lymphocytes, and multinucleated giant cells surrounded by areas of necrosis. These areas may resemble caseation necrosis but later coalesce to form abscesses.

Conjunctival inoculation can result in infection of the eye, with regional lymph node enlargement (preauricular lymphadenopathy, Parinaud's complex). Aerosolization and inhalation or hematogenous spread of organisms can result in pneumonia. In the lung, an inflammatory reaction develops, including foci of alveolar necrosis and cell infiltration (initially polymorphonuclear and later mononuclear) with granulomas. Chest roentgenograms usually reveal bilateral patchy infiltrates rather than large areas of consolidation. Pleural effusions are common and may contain blood. Lymphadenopathy occurs in regions draining infected organs. Therefore, in pulmonary infection, mediastinal adenopathy may be evident, whereas patients with oropharyngeal tularemia develop cervical lymphadenopathy. In gastrointestinal or typhoidal tularemia, mesenteric lymphadenopathy may follow the ingestion of large numbers of organisms. (The term *typhoidal tularemia* may be used to describe severe bacteremic disease, irrespective of the mode of transmission or portal of entry.) Meningitis has been reported as a primary or secondary manifestation of bacteremia. Patients may also present with fever and no localizing signs.

IMMUNOLOGY

Infection with *F. tularensis* stimulates the host to produce antibodies. However, this antibody response probably plays only a minor role in the containment of infection. In contrast, cell-mediated immunity, which develops over 2–4 weeks, plays a major role in containment and eradication. Macrophages, once activated, can kill *F. tularensis*. Recovery from infection generally renders the patient resistant to reinfection; this point is not completely understood.

Immunospecific protection against tularemia can be afforded either by natural infection or by vaccination with live attenuated strains of *F. tularensis*. Killed vaccines, on the other hand, induce no protection against virulent *F. tularensis*. After natural infection or vaccination, serum antibodies to surface-exposed carbohydrate antigens predominate, whereas T cell determinants are located on membrane proteins beneath the bacterial capsule. T cell responses are thought to be due to priming by the organism. The anamnestic T cell response to *F. tularensis* seems to involve a multitude of microbial proteins, each with a distinct set of T cell determinants. A predominant role for CD4+ T cells is supported by the results of experiments in mice, which indicated that resistance to infection was restricted at the level of the major histocompatibility complex (MHC) class II determinants. Humans primed to *F. tularensis* (like those primed to *Mycobacterium tuberculosis*) show a T_H1-like response. T cell proliferation is associated with the production of interleukin (IL) 2 and interferon γ but with little or no production of IL-4. Recent evidence indicates that the percentage of γδ T cells expressing tumor necrosis factor α is decreased during the first 7–40 days after infection. This decrease may reflect the modulation of an inflammatory response. Investigations of neutrophils in tularemia suggest that PMNs are needed for defense against primary infection. PMNs may restrict the growth of *F. tularensis* before the organism becomes intracellular.

CLINICAL MANIFESTATIONS

Tularemia often starts with a sudden onset of fever, chills, headache, and generalized myalgias and arthralgias (Table 151-1). This onset takes place when the organism penetrates the skin, is ingested, or is inhaled. An incubation period of 2–10 days is followed by the formation of an ulcer at the site of penetration, with local inflammation. The ulcer may persist for several months as organisms are transported via the lymphatics to the re-

TABLE 151-1 CLINICAL PRESENTATION OF TULAREMIA

Sign or Symptom	Rate of Occurrence, % Children	Adults
Lymphadenopathy	96	65
Fever (≥38.3°C or ≥101°F)	87	21
Ulcer/eschar/papule	45	51
Myalgias/arthralgias	39	2
Headache	9	5
Cough	9	5
Pharyngitis	43	—
Diarrhea	43	—

Source: Adapted from RF Jacobs, JP Narain: Tularemia in adults and children: A changing presentation. *Pediatrics* 76:818, 1985; with permission.

gional lymph nodes. These nodes enlarge and may become necrotic and suppurative. If the organism enters the bloodstream, widespread dissemination as well as signs and symptoms of endotoxemia may result.

In the United States, most patients with tularemia (75–85%) acquire the infection by inoculation of the skin. In adults, the most common localized form is inguinal/femoral lymphadenopathy; in children, it is cervical lymphadenopathy. About 20% of patients develop a generalized maculopapular rash, which occasionally becomes pustular. Erythema nodosum occurs infrequently. The clinical manifestations of tularemia have been divided into various syndromes, which are listed in Table 151-2.

Ulceroglandular/Glandular Tularemia These two forms of tularemia account for ~75–85% of cases. The predominant form in children involves cervical or posterior auricular lymphadenopathy and is usually related to tick bites on the head and neck. In adults, the most common form is inguinal/femoral lymphadenopathy resulting from insect and tick exposures on the lower limbs. In cases related to wild game, the usual portal of entry for *F. tularensis* is either an injury sustained while skinning or cleaning an animal carcass or a bite (usually on the hand). Epitrochlear lymphadenopathy/lymphadenitis is common in patients with bite-related injuries.

In ulceroglandular tularemia, the ulcer is erythematous, indurated, and nonhealing, with a punched-out appearance that lasts 1–3 weeks. The papule may begin as an erythematous lesion that is tender or pruritic; it evolves over several days into an ulcer with sharply demarcated edges and a yellow exudate. The ulcer gradually develops a black base, and simultaneously the regional lymph nodes become tender and severely enlarged (Fig. 151-1). The affected lymph nodes may become fluctuant and drain spontaneously, but usually the condition resolves with effective treatment. Late suppuration of lymph nodes has been described in up to 25% of patients with ulceroglandular/glandular tularemia. Examination of material taken from these late fluctuant nodes after successful antimicrobial treatment reveals sterile necrotic tissue. In 5–10% of patients, the skin lesion may be inapparent, with lymphadenopathy plus systemic signs and symptoms the only physical findings (*glandular tularemia*). Conversely, a tick or deerfly bite on the trunk may result in an ulcer without evident lymphadenopathy.

TABLE 151-2 CLINICAL SYNDROMES OF TULAREMIA

Syndrome	Rate of Occurrence, % Children	Adults
Ulceroglandular	45	51
Glandular	25	12
Pulmonary (pneumonia)	14	18
Oropharyngeal	4	—
Oculoglandular	2	—
Typhoidal	2	12
Unclassified	6	11

Source: Adapted from RF Jacobs, JP Narain: Tularemia in adults and children: A changing presentation. *Pediatrics* 76:818, 1985; with permission.

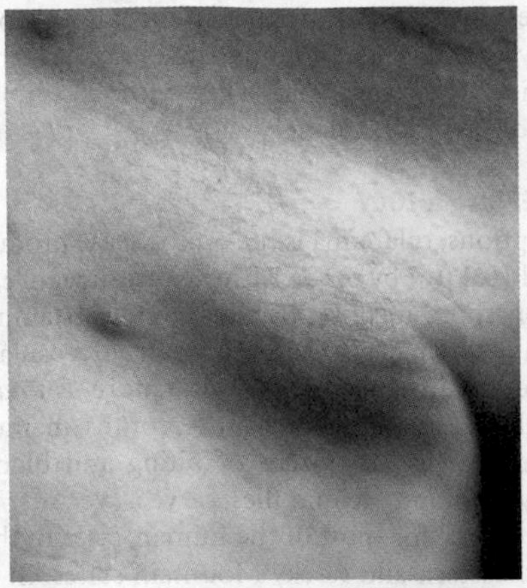

FIGURE 151-1 An 8-year-old boy with inguinal lymphadenitis and associated tick-bite site characteristic of ulceroglandular tularemia.

Oculoglandular Tularemia In ~1% of patients, the portal of entry for *F. tularensis* is the conjunctiva. Usually, the organism reaches the conjunctiva through contact with contaminated fingers. The inflamed conjunctiva is painful, with numerous yellowish nodules and pinpoint ulcers. Purulent conjunctivitis with regional lymphadenopathy (preauricular, submandibular, or cervical) is evident. Because of debilitating pain, the patient may seek medical attention before regional lymphadenopathy develops. Painful preauricular lymphadenopathy is unique to tularemia and distinguishes it from cat-scratch disease, tuberculosis, sporotrichosis, and syphilis. Corneal perforation may occur.

Oropharyngeal and Gastrointestinal Tularemia Rarely, tularemia follows ingestion of contaminated undercooked meat, oral inoculation of *F. tularensis* from the hands in association with the skinning and cleaning of animal carcasses, or consumption of contaminated food or water. Oral inoculation may result in acute, exudative, or membranous pharyngitis associated with cervical lymphadenopathy or in ulcerative intestinal lesions associated with mesenteric lymphadenopathy, diarrhea, abdominal pain, nausea, vomiting, and gastrointestinal bleeding. Infected tonsils become enlarged and develop a yellowish-white pseudomembrane, which can be confused with that of diphtheria. The clinical severity of gastrointestinal tularemia varies from mild, unexplained, persistent diarrhea with no other symptoms to a fulminant, fatal disease. In fatal cases, the extensive intestinal ulceration found at autopsy suggests an enormous inoculum.

Pulmonary Tularemia Tularemia pneumonia presents as variable parenchymal infiltrates that are unresponsive to treatment with β-lactam antibiotics. Tularemia must be considered in the differential diagnosis of atypical pneumonia in a patient with a history of travel to an endemic area. The disease can result from inhalation of an infectious aerosol or can spread to the lungs and pleura after bloodstream dissemination. Inhalation-related pneumonia has been described in laboratory workers after exposure to contaminated materials and is associated with a relatively high mortality rate. Exposure to *F. tularensis* in aerosols from live domestic animals or dead wildlife (including birds) has been reported to cause pneumonia. Hematogenous dissemination to the lungs occurs in 10–15% of cases of ulceroglandular tularemia and in about half of cases of typhoidal tularemia. Previously, tularemia pneumonia was thought to be a disease of older patients, but as many as 10–15% of children with clinical manifestations of tularemia have parenchymal infiltrates detected by chest roentgenography. Patients with pneumonia usually have a nonproductive cough and may have dyspnea or pleuritic chest pain. Roentgenograms of the chest usually reveal bilateral patchy infiltrates (described as ovoid or lobar densities), lobar parenchymal infiltrates, and cavitary lesions. Pleural effusions may have a predominance of mononuclear leukocytes or PMNs and sometimes red blood cells. Empyema may develop. Blood cultures may be positive for *F. tularensis*.

Typhoidal Tularemia The typhoidal presentation is now considered rare in the United States. The source of infection in typhoidal tularemia is usually associated with pharyngeal and/or gastrointestinal inoculation or bacteremic disease. Fever usually develops without apparent skin lesions or lymphadenopathy. Some patients have cervical and mesenteric lymphadenopathy. In the absence of a history of possible contact with a vector, diagnosis can be extremely difficult. Blood cultures may be positive and patients may present with classic sepsis or septic shock in this acute systemic form of the infection. Typhoidal tularemia is usually associated with a huge inoculum or with a preexisting compromising condition. High continuous fevers, signs of endotoxemia, and severe headache are common. The patient may be delirious and may develop prostration and shock. If presumptive antibiotic therapy in culture-negative cases does not include an aminoglycoside, the mortality rate can approach 30%.

TABLE 151-3 TULAREMIA: DIFFERENTIAL DIAGNOSIS, BY CLINICAL DISEASE CATEGORY

Glandular	Oropharyngeal	Typhoidal	Pneumonia
Pyogenic bacterial infection[a]	Group A streptococcal pharyngitis	Typhoid fever	*Mycoplasma pneumoniae* pneumonia
Nontuberculous mycobacterial infection	*Arcanobacterium haemolyticum* pharyngitis	Other *Salmonella* bacteremias	*Chlamydophila pneumoniae* pneumonia
Sporotrichosis	Diphtheria	Rocky Mountain spotted fever	Psittacosis
Tuberculosis	Infectious mononucleosis	Human monocytotropic ehrlichiosis	*Legionella pneumophila* pneumonia
Syphilis	Various viral infections[b]	Human granulocytotropic ehrlichiosis	Q fever
Anthrax		Infectious mononucleosis	Histoplasmosis
Rat-bite fever		Brucellosis	Blastomycosis
Scrub typhus		Toxoplasmosis	Coccidioidomycosis
Plague		Tuberculosis	Various viral infections[d]
Lymphogranuloma venereum		Sarcoidosis	
Cat-scratch disease		Malignancy[c]	

[a]*Staphylococcus aureus, Streptococcus pyogenes.*
[b]Adenovirus, enteroviruses, parainfluenza virus, influenza virus A and B, respiratory syncytial virus.
[c]Hematologic and reticuloendothelial malignancies.
[d]Influenza virus A and B, parainfluenza virus, respiratory syncytial virus, adenovirus, enteroviruses, hantavirus.

Other Manifestations *F. tularensis* infection has been associated with meningitis, pericarditis, hepatitis, peritonitis, endocarditis, osteomyelitis, and sepsis and septic shock with rhabdomyolysis and acute renal failure. In the rare cases of tularemia meningitis, a predominantly lymphocytic response is demonstrated in cerebrospinal fluid.

DIFFERENTIAL DIAGNOSIS

When patients in endemic areas present with fever, chronic ulcerative skin lesions, and large tender lymph nodes (Fig. 151-1), a diagnosis of tularemia should be made presumptively, and confirmatory diagnostic testing and appropriate therapy should be undertaken. When the possibility of tularemia is considered in a nonendemic area, an attempt should be made to identify contact with a potential animal vector. The level of suspicion should be especially high in hunters, trappers, game wardens, veterinarians, laboratory workers, and individuals exposed to an insect or another animal vector. However, up to 40% of patients with tularemia have no known history of epidemiologic contact with an animal vector.

The characteristic presentation of ulceroglandular tularemia does not pose a diagnostic problem, but a less classic progression of regional lymphadenopathy or glandular tularemia must be differentiated from other diseases (Table 151-3). The skin lesion of tularemia may resemble those seen in various other diseases but is generally accompanied by more impressive regional lymphadenopathy. In children, the differentiation of tularemia from cat-scratch disease is made more difficult by the chronic papulovesicular lesion associated with *Bartonella henselae* infection (Chap. 153). Oropharyngeal tularemia can resemble and must be differentiated from pharyngitis due to other bacteria or viruses. Tularemia pneumonia may resemble any atypical pneumonia. Typhoidal tularemia may resemble a variety of other infections.

LABORATORY DIAGNOSIS

Direct microscopic examination of polychromatically stained tissue smears or clinical specimens reveals *F. tularensis* organisms, singly and in groups, both intra- and extracellularly. Gram's staining of clinical or biopsy material is of little value, as the small, weakly staining, gram-negative, nonmotile, non-spore-forming bacteria are difficult to distinguish from the background. An indirect fluorescent antibody test with commercially available antisera can be useful, although false-positive results due to *Legionella* spp. have been reported.

The diagnosis of tularemia is most frequently confirmed by agglutination testing. Microagglutination and tube agglutination are the techniques most commonly used to detect antibody to *F. tularensis*. In the standard tube agglutination test, a single titer of ≥1:160 is interpreted as a presumptive positive result. A fourfold increase in titer between paired serum samples collected 2–3 weeks apart is considered diagnostic. False-negative serologic responses are obtained early in infection; up to 30% of patients infected for 3 weeks have sera that test negative. Late in infection, titers into the thousands are common, and titers of 1:20–1:80 may persist for years. Enzyme-linked immunosorbent assays have proved useful for the detection of both antibodies and antigens. Analysis of urine for *F. tularensis* antigen has yielded promising results in clinical trials, but facilities for this type of analysis are not widely available. A skin test for delayed hypersensitivity to *F. tularensis* turns positive during the first week of illness and remains positive for years. The skin-test antigen, which is not commercially available, can boost titers of agglutinating antibody.

Culture and isolation of *F. tularensis* are difficult. In one study, the organism was isolated in only 10% of more than 1000 human cases, 84% of which were confirmed by serology. The medium of choice is cysteine-glucose-blood agar. *F. tularensis* can be isolated directly from infected ulcer scrapings, lymph-node biopsy specimens, gastric washings, sputum, and blood cultures. Colonies are blue-gray, round, smooth, and slightly mucoid. On media containing blood, a small zone of α hemolysis usually surrounds the colony. Slide agglutination tests or direct fluorescent antibody tests with commercially available antisera can be applied directly to culture suspensions for identification. Most clinical laboratories will not attempt to culture *F. tularensis* because of the infectivity of the organism from the culture media. Although tularemia is not spread from person to person, the organism can be inhaled from culture plates and infect unsuspecting laboratory workers. In most clinical laboratories, biosafety level 2 practices are recommended to handle clinical specimens thought to contain *F. tularensis*.

A variety of polymerase chain reaction (PCR) methods have been used to detect *F. tularensis* DNA in multiple clinical specimens. The majority of these methods target the genes encoding the outer-membrane proteins (e.g., *fopA* or *tul4*). A 16S rDNA sequence identification PCR is helpful when the patient's clinical information does not lead the clinician to suspect a diagnosis of tularemia.

℞ TULAREMIA

F. tularensis cannot be subjected to standardized antimicrobial susceptibility testing because the organism will not grow on the media used. A wide variety of antibiotics, including all β-lactam antibiotics and the newer cephalosporins, are ineffective for the treatment of tularemia. Several studies indicated that third-generation cephalosporins were active against *F. tularensis* in vitro, but clinical case reports suggested a nearly universal failure rate of ceftriaxone in pediatric patients with tularemia. Although in vitro data indicate that imipenem may be active, therapy with imipenem, sulfanilamides, and macrolides is not presently recommended because of the lack of relevant clinical data. Fluoroquinolones have shown promise in terms of their relatively low toxicity and their potential for oral administration. With intracellular activity, fluoroquinolones have been used for successful treatment of tularemia and are candidates for primary or alternative therapy, pending clinical trials. The use of these agents should also be considered when patients are allergic or intolerant to other treatments. When used, ciprofloxacin should be given for a total of 10 days. Chloramphenicol and tetracycline have been used successfully for treatment of the acute stages of tularemia but have been associated with higher relapse rates (up to 20%) than conventionally used agents. Oral chloramphenicol is no longer available in the United States.

Gentamicin is considered the drug of choice for both adults and children. The dosage for adults is 5 mg/kg daily in two divided doses. The dosage for children is 2.5 mg/kg tid or 5 mg/kg bid. Gentamicin therapy is typically continued for 7–10 days; however, in mild to moderate cases of tularemia in which the patient becomes afebrile within the first 48–72 h of gentamicin treatment, a 5- to 7-day course has been successful.

If available (shortages have been reported over the past several years), streptomycin given intramuscularly also is effective. The dosage for adults is 2 g/d in two divided doses. For children, the dosage is 30 mg/kg daily in two divided doses (maximal daily dose, 2 g). After a clinical response is demonstrated at 3–5 days, the dose can be reduced to 10–15 mg/kg daily in two divided doses. The total duration of streptomycin therapy in both adults and children is usually 10 days.

Virtually all strains of *F. tularensis* are susceptible to streptomycin and gentamicin. In successfully treated patients, defervescence usually occurs within 2 days, but skin lesions and lymph nodes may take 1–2 weeks to heal. When therapy is not initiated within the first several days of illness, defervescence may be delayed. Relapses are uncommon with streptomycin or gentamicin therapy. Late lymph-node suppuration, however, occurs in ~40% of children, regardless of the treatment received. These nodes have typically been found to contain sterile necrotic tissue without evidence of active infection. Patients with fluctuant nodes should receive several days of antibiotic therapy before drainage to minimize the risk to hospital personnel. Unlike streptomycin and gentamicin, tobramycin is ineffective in the treatment of tularemia and should not be used.

PROGNOSIS

If tularemia goes untreated, symptoms usually last 1–4 weeks but may continue for months. The mortality rate from severe untreated infection (including all cases of untreated tularemia pneumonia and typhoidal tularemia) can be as high as 30%. However, the overall mortality rate for untreated tularemia is <8%. Mortality is <1% with appropriate treatment. Poor outcomes are often associated with long delays in diagnosis and treatment. Lifelong immunity usually follows tularemia.

PREVENTION

The prevention of tularemia is based on avoidance of exposure to biting and blood-sucking insects, especially ticks and deerflies. A vaccine made from live attenuated *F. tularensis* was developed in the United States and found to be effective. Because of difficulty with standardization, however, the vaccine is not currently licensed in the United States or Europe. A live attenuated vaccine is still available in some parts of the former Soviet Union. Prophylaxis of tularemia has not proved effective in patients with embedded ticks or insect bites. However, in patients who are known to have been exposed to large quantities of organisms (e.g., in the laboratory) and who have incubating infection with *F. tularensis*, early treatment can prevent the development of significant clinical disease.

FURTHER READINGS

BARNS SM et al: Detection of diverse new *Francisella*-like bacteria in environmental samples. Appl Environ Microbiol 71:5494, 2005

CENTERS FOR DISEASE CONTROL AND PREVENTION: Tularemia—United States, 1990–2000. MMWR 51:181, 2002

DE LA PUENTE-REDONDO VA et al: Comparison of different PCR approaches for typing of *Francisella tularensis* strains. J Clin Microbiol 38:1016, 2000

DENNIS DT et al: Tularemia as a biological weapon: Medical and public health management. JAMA 285:2763, 2001

ELIASSON H et al: The 2000 tularemia outbreak: A case-control study of risk factors in disease-endemic and emergent areas, Sweden. Emerg Infect Dis 8:956, 2002

IKÄHEIMO I et al: In vitro antibiotic susceptibility of *Francisella tularensis* isolated from humans and animals. J Antimicrob Chemother 46:287, 2000

JOHANSSON A et al: In vitro susceptibility to quinolones of *Francisella tularensis* subspecies *tularensis*. Scand J Infect Dis 34:327, 2002

PETERSEN JM et al: Methods for the enhanced recovery of *Francisella tularensis* cultures. Appl Environ Microbiol 70:3733, 2004

TARNVIK A et al: Tularemia in Europe: An epidemiological overview. Scand J Infect Dis 36:350, 2004

VERSAGE JL et al: Development of a multitarget real-time TaqMan PCR assay for enhanced detection of *Francisella tularensis* in complex specimens. J Clin Microbiol 41:5492, 2003

152 Plague and Other *Yersinia* Infections

David T. Dennis, Grant L. Campbell

PLAGUE

DEFINITION

Plague is an acute febrile disease caused by infection with *Yersinia pestis*. Human cases are infrequent and are curable with antibiotics. Plague is, however, one of the most virulent and potentially lethal bacterial diseases known, and fatality rates remain high among patients who are not treated in the early stages of infection. Plague occurs in widely scattered foci in Asia, Africa, and the Americas (Fig. 152-1), where its usual hosts are various wild rodents and human-associated rats. Infection is transmitted to humans typically by flea bite and infrequently by direct contact with infected animal tissues or by airborne droplet. The principal clinical forms of plague are bubonic, septicemic, and pneumonic. Although most cases are now sporadic, occurring singly or in small clusters, the potential for outbreaks and epidemic spread remains. Because of its virulence and transmissibility, *Y. pestis* is considered an important potential agent of biological terrorism that requires special countermeasures to protect the public's health (Chap. 214).

ETIOLOGIC AGENT

Y. pestis is a gram-negative coccobacillus in the family Enterobacteriaceae. Genomic analysis suggests that it has only recently evolved from *Y. pseudotuberculosis*. *Y. pestis* is microaerophilic, nonmotile, nonsporulating, oxidase and urease negative, and biochemically unreactive. The organism is nonfastidious and infective for laboratory rodents. It grows well, if slowly, on routinely used microbiologic media (e.g., sheep blood agar, brain-heart infusion broth, and MacConkey agar). *Y. pestis* can multiply within a wide range of temperatures (–2°C to 45°C) and pH values (5.0–9.6), but optimal growth occurs at 28°C and at pH ~7.4. When stained with a polychromatic stain (e.g., Wayson or Giemsa), *Y. pestis* isolated from clinical specimens exhibits a characteristic bipolar appearance, resembling closed safety pins. The bacterium is nonencapsulated but, when grown at ≥30°C, produces a plasmid-expressed envelope glycoprotein, fraction 1 (F1) antigen—a virulence factor that serves as the principal immunodiagnostic marker of infection.

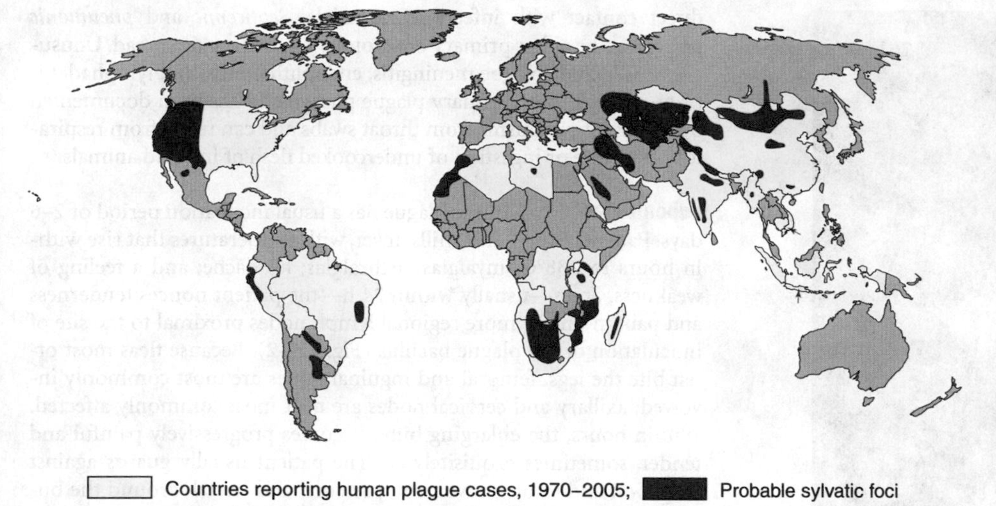

FIGURE 152-1 Approximate global distribution of *Yersinia pestis*. *(Compiled from WHO, CDC, and country sources.)*

EPIDEMIOLOGY

Y. pestis is maintained in well-established "silent" enzootic cycles involving relatively resistant wild rodents and their fleas in remote, lightly populated areas of Asia, Africa, and the Americas and in limited rural foci in extreme southeastern Europe near the Caspian Sea (Fig. 152-1). Humans and mammals other than rodents are incidental hosts. Outbreaks (epizootics) of plague in susceptible rodent populations may result in widespread rodent die-offs, an avid search by their fleas for new hosts, and an increased risk of spread of infection to humans. In the United States, the principal epizootic hosts are various ground squirrels, prairie dogs, and chipmunks; various burrowing rodents act as reservoir hosts in natural areas elsewhere in the world. *Y. pestis* occasionally spills over from wild rodents to rat species that inhabit cultivated fields and adjacent homes, villages, and towns. The organism can then be transported from towns to cities by these highly adaptable rats and their fleas.

Plague in populated areas is most likely to develop when sanitation is poor and rats are numerous—especially the common black or roof rat (*Rattus rattus*), its close relatives, and the larger brown sewer or Norway rat (*R. norvegicus*). The cosmopolitan oriental rat flea *Xenopsylla cheopis* and (in southern Africa and Brazil) the related species *X. brasiliensis* are efficient vectors of the plague bacillus from rat to rat and from rats to humans. *Y. pestis* multiplies to enormous numbers in the foregut (proventriculus) of these fleas, resulting in a bolus of organisms and clotted blood that blocks the passage of subsequent blood meals. This blockage occurs at temperatures of ≤28°C and depends on a single protease expressed by the plasminogen activator (*pla*) gene of a 9.5-kb plasmid of *Y. pestis*. Regurgitation by a "blocked" flea while it feeds facilitates transmission of the plague bacillus to the new host. Except for large outbreaks of pneumonic plague in Manchuria in the early part of the twentieth century, person-to-person respiratory transmission of plague has since occurred only sporadically and has been limited to clusters of close, direct contacts of pneumonic plague patients, such as household members and caregivers.

International health regulations require that national authorities immediately report plague cases to the World Health Organization (WHO). During 1989–2003, a total of 38,359 human cases of plague were reported to the WHO from 25 countries (a mean of 2557 cases per year). The reported case-fatality rate was 7%. More than 80% (31,273) of the total number of cases were reported from Africa, ~14% (5449) from Asia, and the rest (1637) from the Americas.

In the United States, 5–10 human plague cases typically are reported each year. Most cases occur in New Mexico, Arizona, Colorado, and California (*http://www.cdc.gov/ncidod/dvbid/plague/plagwest.htm*). The most common modes of transmission are flea bite and direct contact with infected animals, especially exposure to an infected domestic cat. The overall case-fatality rate is ~10%. Most cases of plague occur in the summer months, when rodents and their fleas are most active. The disease is acquired often in the environs of the patient's residential property and less often during work or recreation in natural areas remote from the patient's place of residence. The arid Native American reservations of New Mexico and Arizona are active plague foci, and Native Americans account for a disproportionately high percentage of plague cases.

Plague can be transmitted during the skinning and handling of carcasses of wild animals such as rabbits and hares, prairie dogs, wildcats, and coyotes. Such direct inoculation of mammal-adapted organisms expressing the F1 antigen is associated with primary septicemia and high mortality rates. Pharyngeal plague can result from the ingestion of undercooked contaminated meat; outbreaks of pharyngeal plague have been reported among persons eating undercooked camel and goat meat. Plague can also be acquired by inhalation of infective respiratory droplets and perhaps by manual transfer of infected fluids to the mouth during the handling of infected animal tissues.

Carnivores, including dogs and cats, can become infected with *Y. pestis* by eating infected rodents and possibly by being bitten by infective fleas. Although clinical plague commonly develops in infected cats, it rarely does so in infected dogs. Both dogs and cats may transport infected fleas from rodent-infested areas to the home environment.

PATHOGENESIS AND PATHOLOGY

Y. pestis is highly invasive and pathogenic. The mechanisms by which the organism causes disease are incompletely understood, but both chromosome- and plasmid-encoded gene products as well as altered cell-mediated immune responses are involved. Three plasmids encode for a variety of known or presumed virulence factors, including the F1 envelope antigen and various *Yersinia* outer-membrane proteins, which confer bacterial resistance to phagocytosis; the V antigen, which is essential for virulence and suppresses the synthesis of various proinflammatory cytokines (e.g., interferon γ and tumor necrosis factor α); pesticin, which interferes with iron uptake; a protease that activates plasminogen and degrades serum complement and is thought to enhance dissemination of *Y. pestis* following inoculation of the skin; a coagulase; and a fibrinolysin. A chromosomally encoded lipopolysaccharide endotoxin is important in sepsis, playing a role in triggering the systemic inflammatory response syndrome and its complications.

Y. pestis organisms inoculated through the skin or mucous membranes are typically carried to regional lymph nodes via lymphatic channels, although direct bloodstream inoculation and dissemination may take place. Mononuclear phagocytes, which can phagocytize *Y. pestis* organisms without destroying them, may play a role in dissemination of the infection to distant sites. Plague can involve almost any organ, and untreated plague generally results in widespread and massive tissue destruction. In the early stages, infected lymph nodes (*buboes*, Fig. 152-2) are characterized by edema and congestion without inflammatory infiltrates or apparent vascular injury. Fully developed buboes contain huge numbers of infectious plague organisms and show distorted or obliterated lymph node architecture with loss of vascular integrity, hemorrhage, necrosis, infiltration of polymorphonuclear neutrophils (PMNs), and extensive serosanguineous effusion. The effusion typically involves perinodal tissues. If several adjacent lymph nodes are involved, a boggy edematous mass can result.

Primary septicemic plague consists of sepsis in the absence of a bubo; secondary septicemic plague is a complication of bubonic or pneumonic plague that occurs when local host defenses are breached. In fatal septicemic plague, multifocal hepatic and splenic necrosis is com-

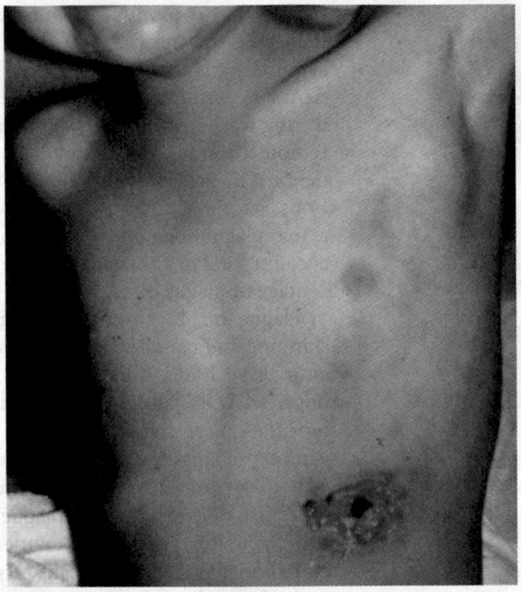

FIGURE 152-2 Plague patient in the southwestern United States with a left axillary bubo and an unusual plague ulcer and eschar at the site of the infective flea bite.

mon. Diffuse interstitial myocarditis with cardiac dilatation is sometimes found. If disseminated intravascular coagulation (DIC) ensues, vascular necrosis may lead to widespread cutaneous, mucosal, and serosal ecchymoses and petechiae. Acral ischemia and resulting gangrene sometimes develop.

Primary plague pneumonia generally begins as a lobular process and then extends by confluence, becoming lobar and then multilobar (Fig. 152-3). Plague organisms are typically most numerous in the alveoli. Secondary plague pneumonia begins more diffusely, with organisms at first most numerous in the interstitium. In advanced cases of both primary and secondary plague pneumonia, affected lung tissue is characterized by edema, hemorrhagic necrosis, and infiltration by neutrophilic leukocytes.

CLINICAL MANIFESTATIONS

Plague is characterized by a rapid onset of fever and other systemic manifestations of gram-negative bacterial infection. If it is not quickly and correctly treated, plague can follow a toxic course, resulting in shock, multiple-organ failure, and death. In humans, the three principal forms of plague are bubonic, septicemic, and pneumonic. *Bubonic* plague, accounting in the United States for ~75% of cases, is almost always caused by the bite of an infected flea but occasionally results from direct contact with infectious materials. *Septicemic* and *pneumonic* plague can be either primary or secondary to metastatic spread. Unusual forms include plague meningitis, endophthalmitis, and lymphadenitis at multiple sites. Primary plague pharyngitis has been documented by culture of organisms from throat swabs and can result from respiratory exposure or ingestion of undercooked flesh of infected animals.

Bubonic Plague Bubonic plague has a usual incubation period of 2–6 days. Patients experience chills; fever, with temperatures that rise within hours to ≥38°C; myalgias; arthralgias; headache; and a feeling of weakness. Soon—usually within 24 h—the patient notices tenderness and pain in one or more regional lymph nodes proximal to the site of inoculation of the plague bacillus (Fig. 152-2). Because fleas most often bite the legs, femoral and inguinal nodes are most commonly involved; axillary and cervical nodes are next most commonly affected. Within hours, the enlarging bubo becomes progressively painful and tender, sometimes exquisitely so. The patient usually guards against palpation and limits movement, pressure, and stretch around the bubo. The surrounding tissue often becomes edematous, sometimes markedly so, and the overlying skin may be erythematous, warm, and tense. Inspection of the skin surrounding or distal to the bubo sometimes reveals the site of a flea bite marked by a papule, pustule, or ulcer. The ulcer may be covered by an eschar (Fig. 152-2). A list of lymphadenitic conditions that could be confused with bubonic plague includes *Staphylococcus aureus* and group A β-hemolytic streptococcal infections, cat-scratch disease, tularemia, and—in filariasis-endemic areas—acute filarial lymphadenitis. The bubo of plague is distinguishable from lymphadenitis of most other causes, however, by its rapid onset, its extreme tenderness, the accompanying signs of toxemia, and the absence of cellulitis or obvious ascending lymphangitis. The pain and swelling of bubonic plague can be confused with a strangulated hernia or trauma.

Treated in the uncomplicated state with an appropriate antibiotic, bubonic plague usually responds quickly, with resolution of fever and alleviation of other systemic manifestations over 2–5 days. Buboes often remain enlarged and tender for a week or more after the initiation of treatment and can become fluctuant. Without effective antimicrobial treatment, patients with typical bubonic plague manifest an increasingly toxic state of fever, tachycardia, lethargy leading to prostration, agitation and confusion, and (occasionally) convulsions and delirium. Secondary plague sepsis may result in an alarmingly rapid and refractory cascade of DIC, bleeding, shock, and organ failure.

Septicemic Plague Primary septicemia, which accounts for ~20% of cases in the United States, develops in the absence of a detectable bubo. The diagnosis often is not suspected until preliminary blood culture results are reported to be positive by the laboratory. *Y. pestis*, however, can also be cultured from the blood of most patients with

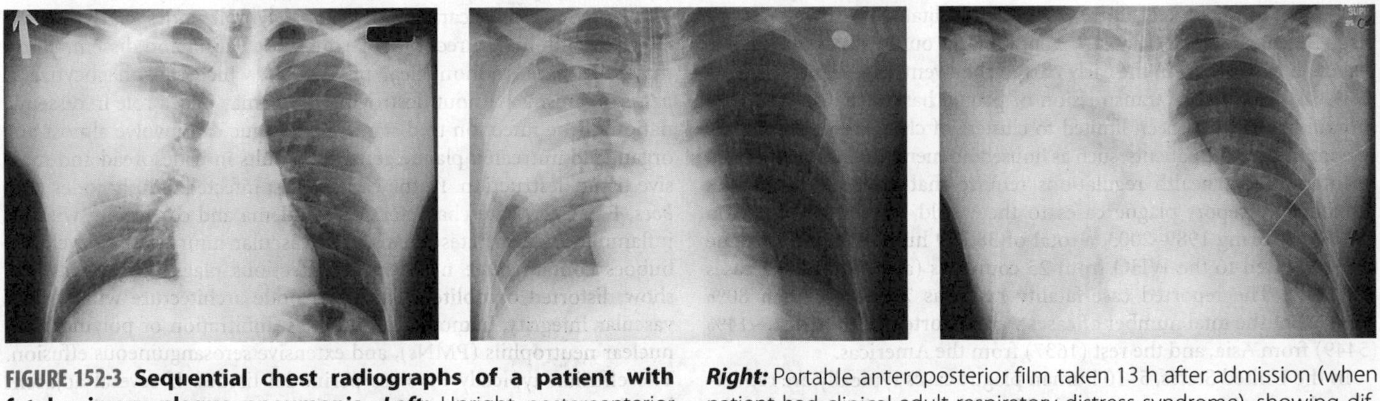

FIGURE 152-3 Sequential chest radiographs of a patient with fatal primary plague pneumonia. *Left:* Upright posteroanterior film taken at admission to hospital emergency department on third day of illness, showing segmental consolidation of right upper lobe. ***Center:*** Portable anteroposterior film taken 8 h after admission, showing extension of pneumonia to right middle and right lower lobes. ***Right:*** Portable anteroposterior film taken 13 h after admission (when patient had clinical adult respiratory distress syndrome), showing diffuse infiltration throughout right lung and patchy infiltration of left lower lung. A cavity later developed at the site of initial right-upper-lobe consolidation.

bubonic plague, and bacteremia must be distinguished from septicemia, in which the patient is desperately ill and requires aggressive care. Septic patients often present with gastrointestinal symptoms of nausea, vomiting, diarrhea, and abdominal pain, which may confound the correct diagnosis. In the United States in 1947–2001, 55 cases of primary septicemic plague with 13 deaths were reported, for a case-fatality rate of 24%. Petechiae, ecchymoses, bleeding from puncture wounds and orifices, and gangrene of acral parts are manifestations of DIC; refractory hypotension, renal shutdown, obtundation, and other signs of shock are preterminal events. Adult respiratory distress syndrome (ARDS) can occur at any stage of septicemic plague. The differential diagnosis of septicemic plague includes sepsis of other gram-negative bacterial etiology, meningococcemia, and acute severe viral infections such as hantavirus illness.

Pneumonic Plague Pneumonic plague is the most life-threatening form of the disease. Primary pneumonic plague accounts for ~5% of plague cases in the United States. The incubation period for primary pneumonic plague is usually 3–5 days (range, 1–7 days). The onset is most often sudden, with chills, fever, headache, myalgias, weakness, and dizziness. Pulmonary signs, including tachypnea and dyspnea, cough, sputum production, and chest pain, typically arise on the second day of illness and may be accompanied by hemoptysis, increasing respiratory distress, cardiopulmonary insufficiency, and circulatory collapse. In primary plague pneumonia, the sputum is most often watery or mucoid, frothy, and blood-tinged, but it may become frankly bloody. Pulmonary signs in primary pneumonic plague may indicate involvement of a single lobe in the early stage, with rapidly developing segmental consolidation before bronchopneumonic spread to other lobes of the same and opposite lungs (Fig. 152-3). Liquefaction necrosis and cavitation may occur early in areas of consolidation and may or may not leave significant residual scarring.

Secondary plague pneumonia, which occurs in 10–15% of bubonic plague cases in the United States, typically manifests first as diffuse interstitial pneumonitis in which sputum production is scant; because the sputum is more likely to be inspissated and tenacious in character than the sputum found in primary pneumonia, it may be less infectious. In the United States in 1947–2001, 46 cases of secondary pneumonic plague and 8 cases of primary pneumonic plague were described, with no known transmission to contacts and an overall case-fatality rate of 41%.

Plague Meningitis Meningitis is an unusual manifestation of plague. In the United States, there were 17 meningitis cases among the 409 evaluable plague cases reported during 1947–2005. All cases of meningitis were complications of bubonic plague, and all but three patients survived. Although meningitis may be a part of the initial presentation of plague, its onset is often delayed and is a manifestation of insufficient treatment. Recent cases in the United States have occurred in association with treatment of bubonic plague with tetracyclines, which are bacteriostatic against *Y. pestis*. Chronic relapsing meningeal plague over periods of weeks or even months was described in the preantibiotic era. The affected patients typically present with fever, headache, meningismus, and neutrophilic pleocytosis.

Plague Pharyngitis Plague pharyngitis presents as fever, sore throat, cervical lymphadenitis, and headache and is often indistinguishable clinically from pharyngitis and tonsillitis of other infectious etiologies, especially streptococcal pharyngitis. Plague pharyngitis can be difficult to distinguish from cervical bubonic plague arising from an infective flea bite on the head and neck region.

LABORATORY FINDINGS AND DIAGNOSIS

A high index of clinical suspicion and a thorough clinical and epidemiologic examination are required for timely diagnosis and treatment. When the diagnosis of plague is delayed or missed, a high case-fatality rate results; infected travelers who seek medical care after they have left endemic areas (peripatetic plague cases) are at especially high risk. When the diagnosis of plague is being considered, close communication between clinicians and the diagnostic laboratory and between the diagnostic laboratory and a qualified reference laboratory is essential. Tests for plague are highly reliable when conducted by laboratory personnel experienced with *Y. pestis*, but such expertise is usually limited to selected reference laboratories, including state health department laboratories in some plague-endemic states and the CDC plague laboratory (Fort Collins, CO; tel. 970-221-6400).

When plague is suspected, specimens should be collected promptly for laboratory studies, chest roentgenograms should be obtained, and specific antimicrobial therapy should be initiated pending confirmation. Appropriate diagnostic specimens for smear and culture include blood from all patients; lymph node aspirates from those with buboes; sputum samples, pharyngeal swabs, and lower respiratory secretions from those with suspected pneumonic plague; and cerebrospinal fluid (CSF) from those with meningeal signs. Since early buboes are often exquisitely tender and are seldom fluctuant or necrotic, they usually require aspiration under local anesthesia after the injection of 1–2 mL of normal saline (sterile but nonbacteriostatic) into the bubo with a 20- to 22-gauge needle. Typically, aspiration produces a scant amount of serosanguineous fluid.

Patients with plague typically have white blood cell (WBC) counts of 10,000–25,000/μL, with a predominance of PMNs and a left shift. Leukemoid reactions, with WBC counts as high as 100,000/μL, can occur. Modest thrombocytopenia is usually present, and fibrin-fibrinogen split products are often detected, even in patients without frank DIC. In plague pneumonia, stained respiratory secretions usually contain PMNs and characteristic bipolar-staining bacilli. In *Y. pestis* septicemia, visualization of the characteristic bacilli in a routine blood smear or a buffy-coat smear is an uncommon but grave prognostic sign (Fig. 152-4). In patients with plague meningitis, PMN pleocytosis is typical, and the bacilli are usually visible in stained CSF smears.

A variety of appropriate culture media (including brain-heart infusion broth, sheep blood agar, and MacConkey agar) should be inoculated with a portion of each specimen. Moreover, for each specimen, at least one smear should be examined immediately with Wayson or Giemsa stain and at least one with Gram's stain; a smear should also be submitted to a reference laboratory for direct fluorescent antibody testing, antigen-capture enzyme-linked immunosorbent assay (ELISA), polymerase chain reaction (PCR) analysis, or testing by another rapid detection method (e.g., immunochromatographic hand-held assay). An acute-phase serum specimen should be tested for antibody to *Y. pestis*; whenever possible, a convalescent-phase serum specimen collected 3–4 weeks later should also be tested. When a patient dies and plague is suspected, appropriate autopsy tissues for culture, direct fluorescent antibody testing, and immunohistochemical staining include buboes, all solid organs (especially liver, spleen, and lung), and bone marrow. If culture of such specimens is to be attempted, they should be sent to the laboratory either fresh or frozen on dry ice, not in preservatives or fixatives. If necessary, Cary-Blair or a similar medium can be used to transport *Y. pestis*–infected tissues.

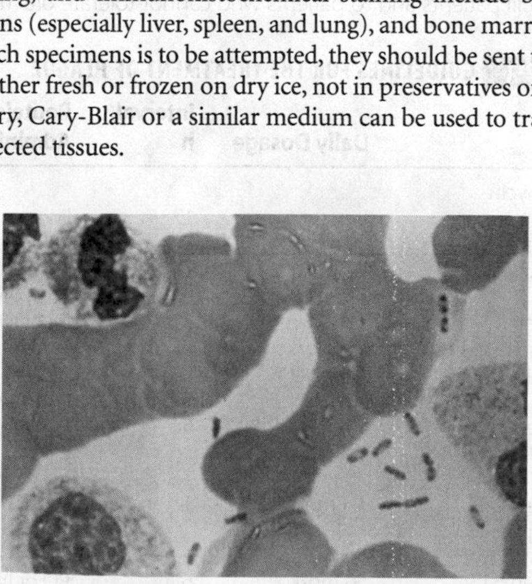

FIGURE 152-4 Peripheral blood smear from a patient with fatal plague septicemia and shock, showing characteristic bipolar-staining *Y. pestis* bacilli (Wright's stain, oil immersion).

Laboratory confirmation of plague depends on the isolation of *Y. pestis* from cultures of body fluids or tissues. Cultures of three blood samples taken over a 45-min period before treatment usually result in isolation of the bacterium. *Y. pestis* strains are readily distinguished from those of the closely related species *Y. pseudotuberculosis* by differences in biochemical profile, temperature-dependent susceptibility to lysis by a *Y. pestis*–specific bacteriophage, and motility. Automated bacteriologic test systems can be used to assist in the identification of isolates as *Y. pestis*, but *Y. pestis* can be misidentified (e.g., as *Y. pseudotuberculosis*) or overlooked if these systems are improperly programmed.

In the absence of *Y. pestis* isolation, plague cases can be confirmed either by the demonstration of seroconversion (a fourfold or greater titer rise) to *Y. pestis* F1 antigen in passive hemagglutination tests of acute- and convalescent-phase serum specimens or by detection of an antibody titer of >128 in a single serum sample from a patient with a plague-compatible illness who has not received plague vaccine. The specificity of a positive passive-hemagglutination test requires confirmation with the F1 antigen hemagglutination-inhibition test. A few plague patients seroconvert to F1 antigen as early as 5 days after the onset of illness; most seroconvert 1–2 weeks after onset; a few seroconvert >3 weeks after onset; and a few (<5%) fail to seroconvert at all. Early, specific antibiotic treatment may delay seroconversion by several weeks. After seroconversion, positive serologic titers diminish gradually over months to years. ELISAs for IgM and IgG antibodies to *Y. pestis* are replacing hemagglutination tests in some laboratories. Other new test methods include those mentioned above: antigen-capture ELISAs, PCR, and immunochromatographic hand-held assays for rapid identification of *Y. pestis* in aspirates, sputum, and other infected body fluids or tissues. The hand-held assays can be used at the bedside in the remote rural settings where most plague cases occur and could prove important in responding to bioterrorism (Chap. 214).

℞ PLAGUE

Left untreated, plague is fatal in >50% of bubonic cases and in nearly all septicemic and pneumonic cases. The overall mortality rate for plague cases in the United States since 1950 has been ~14%; deaths are almost always due to delays in seeking treatment, misdiagnosis, delays in the institution of treatment, or incorrect treatment. Rapid diagnosis and appropriate antimicrobial therapy are essential.

Guidelines for the treatment of plague are given in **Table 152-1**. Although streptomycin is the drug of choice, gentamicin is increasingly used for the treatment of plague in the United States because of its ready availability; it is probably as effective as streptomycin and less toxic. Alternative antibiotics include the tetracyclines and chloramphenicol; these agents are usually given orally with initial loading doses but may be given intravenously to critically ill patients and to patients who cannot tolerate oral medication. Doxycycline is considered the tetracycline of choice. Penicillins, cephalosporins, and macrolides are suboptimal and should not be used. Trimethoprim-sulfamethoxazole (TMP-SMX) has been used successfully to treat bubonic plague but is not considered a first-line agent. Chloramphenicol may be indicated for the treatment of plague meningitis, pleuritis, endophthalmitis, and myocarditis because of its superior tissue penetration; it is used alone or in combination with streptomycin or another first-line agent. In general, antimicrobial treatment should be continued for 7–10 days or for at least 3 days after the patient has become afebrile and has made a clinical recovery. Patients initially given IV antibiotics may be switched to oral regimens upon clinical improvement. Such improvement is usually evident 2–3 days after the start of treatment, even though fever may continue for several days. National bioterrorism-response protocols propose gentamicin, ciprofloxacin, and doxycycline as antimicrobial agents of first choice for treatment and postexposure prophylaxis in the event of an attack using *Y. pestis* (Chap. 214).

Complications of sepsis require intensive monitoring and close physiologic support, as outlined elsewhere (Chaps. 110 and 265). Buboes may require surgical drainage. Abscessed nodes can cause recurrent fever in patients who have apparently recovered; the cause may be occult if intrathoracic or intraabdominal nodes are involved. Although *Y. pestis* is considered to be genetically stable, a multidrug-resistant strain was isolated from a plague patient in Madagascar. This strain exhibited resistance (mediated by a transferable plasmid) to principal first-line antibiotics used for treatment and prophylaxis of plague.

TABLE 152-1 GUIDELINES FOR THE TREATMENT OF PLAGUE

Drug	Daily Dosage	Interval, h	Route(s) of Administration
Streptomycin			
Adults	2 g	12	IM
Children	30 mg/kg	12	IM
Gentamicin			
Adults	3–5 mg/kg[a]	8	IM or IV
Children	6.0–7.5 mg/kg	8	IM or IV
Infants/neonates	7.5 mg/kg	8	IM or IV
Tetracycline			
Adults	2 g	6	PO or IV
Children ≥8 y	25–50 mg/kg	6	PO or IV
Doxycycline			
Adults	200 mg	12 or 24	PO or IV
Children ≥8 y	4.4 mg/kg	12 or 24	PO or IV
Chloramphenicol			
Adults	50 mg/kg[b]	6	PO or IV
Children ≥1 y	50 mg/kg[b]	6	PO or IV

[a]Dosage should be reduced to 3 mg/kg daily as soon as clinically indicated.
[b]For meningitis, up to 100 (mg/kg)/d initially.

PREVENTION AND CONTROL

Persons at greatest risk for plague in the United States are individuals who live, work, and participate in outdoor recreational activities in areas of those western states in which plague is enzootic. Surveillance, education, and environmental management are the cornerstones of prevention and control. Personal protective measures include the avoidance of areas with known epizootic plague (in which warning signs may be posted) and of sick or dead animals; the use of repellents, insecticides, and protective clothing when at risk of exposure to rodents' fleas; and the wearing of gloves when handling animal carcasses. Short-term antibiotic prophylaxis (Table 152-2) is recommended for persons known to have had close contact with a patient with suspected or confirmed pneumonic plague. The recommended duration of postexposure prophylaxis is 5 days. Patients in whom respiratory plague is suspected should be managed under isolation, with use of respiratory-droplet precautions until pneumonia has been ruled out or until 48 h of effective antimicrobial therapy has been administered, after which standard infection-control precautions are adequate. Masks that block droplets are considered to be protective against respiratory transmission of plague and would be expected to be an important tool to prevent secondary plague spread in the event of bioterrorism (Chap. 214).

Rodent food (garbage, pet food) and habitats (brush piles, junk heaps, woodpiles) should be eliminated in residential and occupational environments; buildings and food stores should be rodent-proofed. The con-

TABLE 152-2 GUIDELINES FOR PLAGUE PROPHYLAXIS

Drug	Daily Dosage	Interval, h	Route of Administration
Tetracycline			
Adults	1–2 g	6 or 12	PO
Children ≥8 y	25–50 mg/kg	6 or 12	PO
Doxycycline			
Adults	100–200 mg	12 or 24	PO
Children ≥8 y	2–4 mg/kg	12 or 24	PO
Trimethoprim-sulfamethoxazole			
Adults	320 mg[a]	12	PO
Children ≥2 mo	8 mg/kg[a]	12	PO
Ciprofloxacin[b]			
Adults	1 g	12	PO
Children	40 mg/kg	12	PO

[a]Trimethoprim component.
[b]Recommended as an alternative to doxycycline in bioterrorism-response plans.

trol of fleas with insecticides is a key public health measure in situations where epizootic plague activity places humans at high risk; this effort includes dusting and spraying of rodent burrows, rodent runs, and other sites where rodents and their fleas are found. In plague-endemic areas of the western United States, persons should keep their dogs and cats free of fleas and restrained. The decision to control plague by killing rodents should be left to public health authorities, and such a program should be carried out only in conjunction with effective flea control. Killing of rodents has no lasting benefit without environmental sanitation.

The previously used killed, whole-cell plague vaccine is no longer available in the United States. New and improved vaccines that use recombinant F1 and V antigens to induce protective antibodies are undergoing clinical trials. In the United States, the indications for use of these newer vaccines would probably be similar to those for the previously available killed vaccine, which was mostly limited to protecting laboratory personnel who routinely worked with *Y. pestis* and some persons whose vocations brought them into regular contact with wild rodents and their fleas in areas with enzootic or epizootic plague. In addition, a vaccine might be useful in protecting selected persons at risk from biowarfare or bioterrorism.

OTHER *YERSINIA* INFECTIONS

DEFINITION

Yersiniosis is an uncommon bacterial zoonosis caused primarily by infection with either of two enteropathogenic *Yersinia* species: *Y. enterocolitica* or *Y. pseudotuberculosis*. Reservoir hosts of these bacteria include swine and other wild and domestic animals, and transmission to humans is predominantly via the oral route. Both sporadic cases and common-source outbreaks occur. The most frequent acute clinical manifestations are (1) enteritis or enterocolitis with self-limited diarrhea (especially with *Y. enterocolitica*) and (2) mesenteric adenitis and terminal ileitis (especially with *Y. pseudotuberculosis*), which can be confused with acute appendicitis. Septicemia and metastatic focal infections are less common. Yersiniosis can be complicated by nonsuppurative, extraintestinal, inflammatory sequelae—e.g., reactive arthritis (Chap. 318) and erythema nodosum (Chap. 18). Other nonplague *Yersinia* species, including *Y. intermedia*, *Y. frederiksenii*, and *Y. kristensenii*, have been associated with enteritis or enterocolitis in humans (particularly immunocompromised adults), but little is known about their pathogenicity, public health importance, or clinical management.

ETIOLOGIC AGENTS

Y. enterocolitica and *Y. pseudotuberculosis* are pleomorphic gram-negative bacilli in the family Enterobacteriaceae. These organisms can multiply within a wide temperature range (–1°C to 45°C). Pathogenic *Y. enterocolitica* isolates are most commonly identified by biotyping based on biochemical profiles and serotyping according to somatic O and H antigens. Six biotypes and >60 serotypes of *Y. enterocolitica* are recognized. A separate serotyping system for *Y. pseudotuberculosis* (also based on somatic antigens) has distinguished six major serotypes (I–VI) and their subtypes.

EPIDEMIOLOGY

Yersinia enterocolitica *Y. enterocolitica* is distributed worldwide and has been isolated from soil, fresh water, contaminated foodstuffs (e.g., meat, milk, and vegetables), and a wide variety of wild and domestic animals. Many serotypes isolated from environmental sources, however, evidently are not human pathogens. Most human infections have been caused by *Y. enterocolitica* serotypes O:3; O:5,27; O:8; and O:9. These serotypes are primarily associated with wild and domestic mammals. The recognized incidence of these infections and their sequelae is highest in Scandinavia and some other northern European countries, but reliable population-based estimates of incidence are unavailable.

All age groups are susceptible to *Y. enterocolitica* infections, but the majority of cases of enterocolitis are in children 1–4 years old. These infections show a modest predilection for males. Mesenteric adenitis and terminal ileitis are most common among older children and young adults. Risk factors for *Y. enterocolitica* septicemia and metastatic focal infections include chronic liver disease, malignancy, diabetes mellitus, immunosuppressive therapy, HIV disease, alcoholism, malnutrition, advanced age, iron overload (see "Pathogenesis and Pathology," below), and hemolytic anemias (including the thalassemias). The nonsuppurative sequelae of yersiniosis are most common among adults. HLA-B27 is expressed in 70–80% of patients who develop reactive arthritis associated with yersiniosis. HLA-B27 is not a risk factor for *Yersinia*-induced erythema nodosum; females with this condition outnumber males by 2 to 1.

Among *Y. enterocolitica* strains isolated from patients in recent decades, serotypes O:3 and O:9 have predominated in Europe, while serotype O:3 has predominated in Canada, Japan, and the United States. The apparent incidence of *Yersinia*-induced nonsuppurative sequelae reportedly is 10–30% in Scandinavia and much lower in most other countries, including the United States.

Common-source outbreaks of *Y. enterocolitica* enteritis have been traced to such vehicles as raw milk, contaminated pasteurized milk, and foods prepared with contaminated fresh water. Because *Y. enterocolitica* commonly colonizes the gastrointestinal tracts of swine, sporadic human cases and outbreaks of yersiniosis have also been associated with the preparation or ingestion of raw pork products (e.g., chitterlings). In some cases of yersiniosis, circumstantial evidence suggests transmission via contact with dogs and cats or their feces. Several nosocomial outbreaks of *Y. enterocolitica* infection have been described; fecal-oral transmission from person to person was suspected. Fecal-oral transmission among family members may also explain occasional secondary cases in households. In a prospective study of 50 children with *Y. enterocolitica* enteritis, fecal excretion of the organism persisted for an average of 27 days (range, 4–79 days) after the cessation of symptoms. A chronic carrier state, however, has not been demonstrated. *Y. enterocolitica* is a rare but often lethal cause of transfusion-associated septicemia. The explanation is that blood donors occasionally have transient, occult *Y. enterocolitica* bacteremia and that this organism can slowly multiply to high concentrations in blood refrigerated for at least 10 days.

Yersinia pseudotuberculosis The ecology of *Y. pseudotuberculosis* seems to parallel that of *Y. enterocolitica* closely. *Y. pseudotuberculosis* is also widespread in wild and domestic animals and is isolated from many environmental sources. Swine appear to be an important reservoir for pathogenic strains. Although human infections appear to be relatively rare, large common-source epidemics can occur.

PATHOGENESIS AND PATHOLOGY

With rare exceptions (e.g., transmission via contaminated blood products or direct cutaneous inoculation), the enteropathogenic yersiniae are thought to enter the host via the oral route. The incubation period averages 5 days (range, 1–11 days). Studies of animals have shown that the organisms initially invade the ileal epithelium, then are translocated via M cells into the lamina propria, and finally enter Peyer's patches, where they replicate. They subsequently drain into the mesenteric lymph nodes, which undergo hyperplasia and from which the bacteria can be disseminated. The mesenteric lymph nodes can become intensely swollen and matted and are occasionally detected on physical examination as a tender right-lower-quadrant mass. Intestinal inflammation (most commonly of the distal ileum and less commonly of the ascending colon) develops and may be accompanied by mucosal ulcerations and by the shedding of PMNs and red blood cells into the intestinal lumen. In relatively severe cases, thrombosis of mesenteric blood vessels, intestinal hemorrhage, and necrosis can occur. In patients with enteropathogenic yersinial infections who undergo exploratory laparotomy, the appendix usually is histologically normal or shows only lymphoid hyperplasia, but frank suppuration is sometimes evident.

A plasmid of ~70 kb is essential for virulence of the enteropathogenic yersiniae because it encodes at least six *Yersinia* outer-membrane proteins, which confer a variety of pathogenic properties—e.g., cytotoxicity; resistance to phagocytosis by PMNs; and the ability to cause monocyte apoptosis (programmed cell death), to suppress the host's expression of tumor necrosis factor α, and to interfere with platelet aggregation and host complement activation. A chromosomal gene (*inv*) encodes for the surface protein invasin, which is necessary for yersinial invasion of nonphagocytic host cells (e.g., epithelial cells) in vitro and which facilitates the translocation of bacteria across the intestinal epithelium. Both *Y. enterocolitica* and *Y. pseudotuberculosis* can express at least one protein superantigen that selectively stimulates the proliferation of T cells. Many strains of *Y. enterocolitica* produce a heat-stable enterotoxin that is similar to *Escherichia coli* enterotoxin. The cell walls of *Y. enterocolitica* and *Y. pseudotuberculosis* contain a lipopolysaccharide (endotoxin). Some *Yersinia* strains are unable to synthesize bacterial iron chelators called *siderophores*. However, they can exploit host-chelated iron stores and the drug deferoxamine (a siderophore produced by *Streptomyces pilosus*). Therefore, iron overload (e.g., caused by hemodialysis or multiple transfusions) and deferoxamine therapy appear to be independent risk factors for *Y. enterocolitica* bacteremia, especially that involving serotypes O:3 and O:9, and to a lesser degree for *Y. pseudotuberculosis* bacteremia.

Immunogenetic factors and cell-mediated immune responses are clearly involved in the pathogenesis of reactive arthritis following infection with the enteropathogenic yersiniae. As noted above, most patients with *Yersinia*-induced reactive arthritis express HLA-B27. In addition, *Y. pseudotuberculosis* shares at least one cross-reactive epitope with HLA-B27, and *Y. enterocolitica* infection alters the expression of serologic HLA-B27 epitopes on lymphocytes and monocytes. In patients with reactive arthritis following *Y. enterocolitica* infection, yersinial antigens are commonly detectable in synovial fluid cells in the apparent absence of whole organisms. Thus, it is unknown whether the arthritis results from occult bacterial persistence through self-tolerance of HLA-B27 with a failure of cross-reactive immune responses to yersiniae, from an immune response to common antigenic determinants shared by the bacteria and host HLA-B27 (i.e., molecular mimicry), or from other mechanisms. The pathogenesis of *Yersinia*-induced erythema nodosum is obscure.

In some assays, patients with Graves' disease have an increased prevalence of serum antibodies to *Y. enterocolitica*, and the immunoglobulins of patients recovering from *Y. enterocolitica* infections react with the human thyroid-stimulating hormone receptor. However, a link between *Y. enterocolitica* infection and the subsequent development of autoimmune thyroiditis has not been convincingly demonstrated. Similarly, the hypothesis that the nonplague yersinioses can trigger ulcerative colitis or Crohn's disease remains intriguing but unproven.

CLINICAL MANIFESTATIONS

Yersinia enterocolitica The principal clinical manifestations of *Y. enterocolitica* infection are enteritis, enterocolitis, mesenteric adenitis, and terminal ileitis. Less common manifestations include exudative pharyngitis, septicemia, metastatic focal infections, reactive polyarthritis, and erythema nodosum. When age groups are combined, the most common presentation of *Y. enterocolitica* infection is acute diarrhea from enteritis or enterocolitis. Low-grade fever and cramping abdominal pain occur in most cases, nausea and vomiting in 15–40%, hematochezia in up to 30%, and a generalized maculopapular skin rash in a few cases. Diarrhea persists for an average of 2 weeks (range, 1 day to many months), during which the frequency of bowel movements diminishes. Uncommonly, enteritis or enterocolitis can be complicated by severe abdominal pain and high fever. Rare (and sometimes fatal) complications include diffuse inflammation, ulceration, hemorrhage, and necrosis of the small bowel and colon; intestinal perforation; peritonitis; ascending cholangitis; mesenteric vein thrombosis; diverticulitis; toxic megacolon; and ileocecal intussusception.

The syndrome of mesenteric adenitis and terminal ileitis without diarrhea is easily confused with appendicitis. Low-grade fever and right-lower-quadrant pain, tenderness, guarding, and rebound tenderness are common. During six recognized common-source outbreaks in the United States, 10% of 444 patients with symptomatic undiagnosed *Y. enterocolitica* infections underwent laparotomy for suspected appendicitis; surgical incisions became infected with *Y. enterocolitica* in a few of these cases.

Acute pharyngitis and pharyngotonsillitis, with or without cervical adenitis or intestinal illness, are less common but potentially lethal manifestations of *Y. enterocolitica* infection, particularly in adults. *Y. enterocolitica* septicemia generally presents as a severe illness with fever and leukocytosis, often with abdominal pain and jaundice and without localized signs of infection. Metastatic focal *Y. enterocolitica* infections can occur with or without clinically apparent bacteremia and can affect almost any organ system. Examples include abscess formation (e.g., in liver, spleen, kidney, lung, skeletal muscle, lymph node, or cutaneous tissue), osteomyelitis, meningitis, peritonitis, urinary tract infection, pneumonia, empyema, endocarditis, pericarditis, mycotic aneurysm, septic arthritis, suppurative conjunctivitis, panophthalmitis, Parinaud's oculoglandular syndrome, and cutaneous pustules or bullae.

In Scandinavia, the incidence of reactive arthritis following *Y. enterocolitica* infection among adults is estimated to be at least 10%. About 80% of these patients have prior symptoms such as fever, diarrhea, or abdominal pain. Typically, these symptoms precede the arthritis by 1 week and are of short duration. The most commonly affected joints are the knees and ankles, but other joints can be involved. Typically, multiple (two to eight) joints become involved sequentially and asymmetrically over a period of a few days to 2 weeks, after which no additional joints are affected. Monarticular arthritis occurs less commonly. In two-thirds of cases, the acute arthritis remits spontaneously within 1–3 months. Chronic joint disease is documented in a minority of cases. A few HLA-B27-positive patients with *Y. enterocolitica*–induced arthritis have subsequent ankylosing spondylitis, but this development is best explained by the fact that HLA-B27 is a major risk factor for each of these diseases. Mild, self-limited myocarditis accompanies ~10% of cases of *Yersinia*-induced arthritis and can occur independently. Typical manifestations include cardiac murmurs and transient electrocardiographic abnormalities, such as prolongation of the PR interval and nonspecific ST-segment and T-wave changes. The syndrome of *Yersinia*-induced arthritis and carditis can be confused with acute rheumatic fever. In Scandinavia, erythema nodosum occurs in 15–20% of patients with yersiniosis, usually within a few days to 3 weeks after the onset of intestinal illness. Lesions typically are located on the lower extremities and resolve within 1 month. Less commonly reported nonsuppurative sequelae of *Y. enterocolitica* infections include reactive uveitis, iritis, conjunctivitis, urethritis, and glomerulonephritis. The complete triad of Reiter's syndrome (arthritis, conjunctivitis, and urethritis) is seen in 5–10% of patients with *Yersinia*-induced arthritis.

Yersinia pseudotuberculosis The most common clinical presentation of *Y. pseudotuberculosis* infection is fever and abdominal pain caused by mesenteric adenitis; diarrheal illness is less common than in *Y. enterocolitica* infection. Systemic manifestations, including septicemia, focal infections, reactive arthritis, and erythema nodosum, are generally similar to those associated with *Y. enterocolitica* infection. In addition, *Y. pseudotuberculosis* has been associated with a scarlet fever–like syndrome, acute interstitial nephritis, and hemolytic-uremic syndrome.

LABORATORY FINDINGS AND DIAGNOSIS

Results of routine laboratory tests in most patients with yersiniosis are nonspecific. Leukocyte counts are usually normal or slightly elevated, often with a modest left shift. Standard microbiologic methods are sufficient to isolate *Y. enterocolitica* and *Y. pseudotuberculosis* from otherwise-sterile sites, such as blood, CSF, lymph node tissue, and peritoneal fluid, and from abscesses. Isolation of these organisms from feces is impeded by their slow growth and the overgrowth of normal fecal flora on culture media routinely used to select for enteric bacteria. The yield from feces and other grossly contaminated specimens can be increased by the use of *Yersinia*-selective [e.g., cefsulodin-Irgasan-novobiocin (CIN)] agar and by cold enrichment. Because bacteriologic procedures designed to isolate yersiniae from feces are not considered cost-effective, many laboratories undertake them by special request only.

The results of serologic tests can be used to support a diagnosis of yersiniosis. Agglutination tests or ELISAs are used most commonly; immunoblotting has also been used. The existence of multiple serotypes makes routine serologic tests laborious; thus these tests are generally conducted only in research laboratories or large commercial laboratories. Since these tests are experimental and are neither standardized nor well validated, and since some strains of *Yersinia* cross-react with other bacteria (e.g., *Brucella*, *Salmonella*, *Vibrio*, and *Borrelia*) and with serum from some patients with thyroiditis, results should be interpreted with caution. In typical uncomplicated cases of yersiniosis, agglutinin titers begin to rise within the first week of illness, peak in the second week, and then gradually diminish and return to normal within 3–6 months, although agglutinating antibody may remain detectable for several years in some cases. Because an initial serum specimen is often collected ≥1 week after the onset of illness, when agglutinin titers are already high, it is usually impossible to document a fourfold or greater rise in titer between paired specimens (although a fourfold or greater fall in titer may be found). Immunohistochemical techniques and PCR tests to detect yersinial antigens and DNA, respectively, in clinical specimens are experimental at this time.

In patients with *Yersinia*-induced reactive arthritis, synovial fluid is sterile and the leukocyte count ranges from a few hundred to 60,000/μL, with a majority of PMNs. The erythrocyte sedimentation rate is often >100 mm/h. Rheumatoid factor and antinuclear antibodies are usually absent. The diagnosis of *Yersinia*-induced reactive arthritis or other nonsuppurative inflammatory sequelae can be difficult, especially when triggering infections are asymptomatic or clinically mild or occur several weeks before the diagnosis is attempted. Because the isolation of a pathogenic *Yersinia* strain from feces is the most specific diagnostic test in such cases, it should be attempted. Since culture is of limited sensitivity in this clinical setting, a high index of suspicion and positive results of serologic tests for *Y. enterocolitica* or *Y. pseudotuberculosis* are usually required for diagnosis.

℞ OTHER *YERSINIA* INFECTIONS

The effectiveness of antimicrobial agents in the treatment of yersinial enteritis, enterocolitis, mesenteric adenitis, or terminal ileitis has not been established. These conditions are usually self-limited, and their treatment is symptom-based and supportive. In uncomplicated cases, diarrhea should be treated with fluid and electrolyte replacement, with the route of delivery dependent on clinical severity. Enteric precautions are advisable for patients hospitalized with yersinial diarrhea. In general, antimicrobial treatment should be reserved for patients with septicemia, metastatic focal infections, or immunosuppression and enterocolitis. Controlled clinical comparisons of antimicrobial agents in the treatment of severe cases of yersiniosis have not yet been conducted. In such cases, drug selection should ultimately be guided by clinical response and bacterial sensitivity patterns. Clinical isolates of *Y. enterocolitica* and *Y. pseudotuberculosis* are usually susceptible in vitro to aminoglycosides, third-generation cephalosporins, chloramphenicol, quinolones, tetracyclines, and TMP-SMX. In laboratory animals infected with enteropathogenic yersiniae, the fluoroquinolones have exerted the strongest bactericidal effects in vivo; clinical experience with these drugs against these pathogens in humans is promising but limited. Because they produce β-lactamases, isolates typically are resistant to penicillin, ampicillin, carbenicillin, and first-generation and most second-generation cephalosporins. Optimal dosages and durations of therapy have not been established. Mortality rates from *Y. enterocolitica* septicemia are ~10% despite treatment. Focal extraintestinal infections may require at least 3 weeks of therapy. No role for antimicrobial agents in the management of the nonsuppurative inflammatory manifestations of yersiniosis has been established. Patients with reactive arthritis may benefit from treatment with nonsteroidal anti-inflammatory drugs, intraarticular steroid injections, and physical therapy.

PREVENTION AND CONTROL

The importance of safe food-handling and food-preparation practices in the prevention of yersiniosis cannot be overemphasized. Caution is particularly warranted in the case of pork and other animal products. The consumption of raw or undercooked meats, especially pork, should be avoided. Increased efforts to prevent the spread of enteric pathogens in household, pet-care, day-care, and hospital settings and in the food industry would be likely to decrease the incidence of yersiniosis. Current regulations of the U.S. Food and Drug Administration require visual inspection of packed red cell units before transfusion, with the discarding of units in which bacterial contamination is suspected on the basis of darkening (reflecting decreased oxygen saturation and hemolysis). Since the risk is minimal, more specific measures to further decrease the likelihood of transfusion of *Y. enterocolitica*–contaminated blood products (e.g., limiting the period for which red cells can be stored before transfusion) have not been widely implemented.

Yersiniosis is not routinely reportable to public health authorities in most jurisdictions. However, clinicians who suspect a common-source outbreak (e.g., because they have documented a familial case cluster) or some other public health threat (e.g., because they have found *Y. enterocolitica* bacteremia in a recent blood donor) should consult promptly with local public health officials.

FURTHER READINGS

ABDEL-HAQ NM et al: Antibiotic susceptibilities of *Yersinia enterocolitica* recovered from children over a 12-year period. Int J Antimicrob Agents 27:449, 2006

DAS R et al: Study of proinflammatory responses induced by *Yersinia pestis* in human monocytes using cDNA arrays. Genes Immun 8:308, 2007

EISEN RJ et al: Human plague in the southwestern United States, 1957–2004: Spatial models of elevated risk of human exposure to *Yersinia pestis*. J Med Entomol 44:530, 2007

GRAHEK-OGDEN D: Outbreak of *Yersinia enterocolitica* serogroup O:9 infection and processed pork, Norway. Emerg Infect Dis 13:754, 2007

PERDIKOGIANNI C et al: *Yersinia enterocolitica* infection mimicking surgical conditions. Pediatr Surg Int 22:589, 2006

PRENTICE MB, RAHALISON L: Plague. Lancet 369:1196, 2007

153 *Bartonella* Infections, Including Cat-Scratch Disease

David H. Spach, Emily Darby

Bartonella species are gram-negative bacteria that can cause an array of infectious diseases, including cat-scratch disease (CSD), bacillary angiomatosis, bacteremia, culture-negative endocarditis, trench fever, and bartonellosis (Table 153-1). Three *Bartonella* species play a major role in causing human disease: *B. bacilliformis*, *B. quintana*, and *B. henselae*. Recent advances in molecular diagnostics have expanded the list of diseases known to be caused by *Bartonella* species.

CAT-SCRATCH DISEASE

DEFINITION AND ETIOLOGY

CSD is typically a self-limited illness characterized by regional lymphadenopathy lasting weeks to months. *B. henselae* is the primary caus-

TABLE 153-1 MAJOR DISEASES CAUSED BY *BARTONELLA* SPECIES

Disease	Organism	Risk Factor
Cat-scratch disease	*B. henselae*	Cat scratch or bite
Bacillary angiomatosis	*B. quintana, B. henselae*	Cat scratch or bite
Bacillary peliosis	*B. henselae*	Cat scratch or bite
Trench fever	*B. quintana*	Homelessness, body louse infestation, alcoholism
Endocarditis	*B. quintana, B. henselae, B. elizabethae*	As for cat-scratch disease and trench fever
Bartonellosis	*B. bacilliformis*	Sandfly bite

ative agent. Infrequently, patients with CSD develop disseminated *B. henselae* infection.

EPIDEMIOLOGY

CSD has a global distribution. In the United States, the annual incidence is ~4–9 cases per 100,000 persons, with ~40% of cases involving adults. Cats are the primary host for *B. henselae* and transmit the infection to humans via a scratch, bite, or lick. In cats (particularly kittens), the incidence of asymptomatic *B. henselae* bacteremia is high. The cat flea (*Ctenocephalides felis*) serves as the vector for transmission between animals. Rarely, CSD occurs after exposure to dogs.

CLINICAL PRESENTATION

The initial clinical manifestation—the primary inoculation lesion—consists of a 0.5- to 1-cm papule, vesicle, or nodule that appears at the site where *B. henselae* is introduced and persists for ~1–3 weeks. Adenopathy typically develops 2–3 weeks after the initial scratch or bite (range, 3–50 days). Unilateral solitary or regional lymphadenopathy (Fig. 153-1) occurs in more than 90% of patients; its location corresponds with the route of lymphatic drainage. Lymph nodes are tender, firm, and mobile, and ~10% suppurate; overlying erythema is occasionally present. Nonspecific systemic symptoms, such as fever, anorexia, headache, myalgias, malaise, and abdominal pain, are variably present at this stage. Lymphadenopathy usually resolves within 3 months.

Atypical presentations of CSD are described in up to one-quarter of cases. Parinaud's oculoglandular syndrome is a frequently reported atypical presentation that follows inoculation of bacteria onto the conjunctiva or eyelid. Patients develop unilateral manifestations that may include conjunctivitis, granulomatous lesions, and preauricular lymphadenopathy. Systemic spread of *B. henselae* may occur independent of lymphadenopathy or may follow the more typical manifestations of the disease. Disseminated disease most often involves the nervous system, visceral organs, or bone. Patients with neuroretinitis generally present with sudden, painless loss of vision. Most ocular abnormalities caused by CSD usually resolve within several months without residual damage; however, some patients have long-lasting visual deficits. Other rare complications include encephalitis, peripheral nerve abnormalities, myelitis, facial palsy, and granulomatous hepatitis or splenitis.

PATHOLOGY

Early in the course of CSD, histologic examination of lymph nodes reveals follicular hyperplasia and arteriolar proliferation. Cortical granulomas, with occasional multinucleated giant cells, neutrophilic infiltrates, and coalescing microabscesses (stellate microabscesses), appear within weeks; the granulomas are surrounded by histiocytes and peripheral lymphocytes. Warthin-Starry stain may reveal typical clusters of pleomorphic gram-negative organisms within areas of necrosis, blood vessel walls, or erythrocytes.

DIAGNOSIS

A suspected diagnosis of CSD is usually based on a typical clinical presentation in conjunction with a history of recent cat exposure. Results of routine laboratory studies are generally normal. The differential diagnosis most often includes lymphoma, mycobacterial infection, and soft tissue infection caused by methicillin-resistant *Staphylococcus aureus*. Not only can CSD overlap clinically with lymphoma and mycobacterial infection; it can also occur in conjunction with these diseases. Serologic tests for antibody to *B. henselae* can support the clinical diagnosis but do not have optimal sensitivity and specificity. Accordingly, in most instances, lymph node biopsy or aspiration is required to rule out other diseases and establish the diagnosis. In this situation, polymerase chain reaction (PCR) analysis of the tissue sample is generally preferred. Cultures of lymph node tissue are rarely positive.

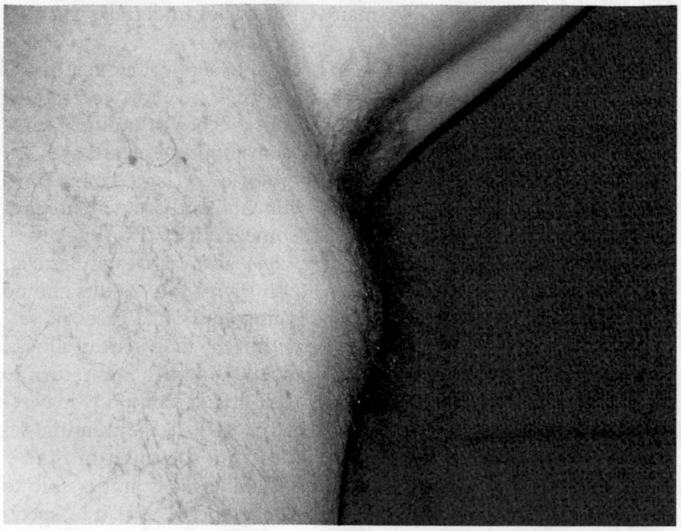

FIGURE 153-1 Characteristic regional (axillary) lymphadenopathy in a patient with cat-scratch disease.

Rx CAT-SCRATCH DISEASE

(Table 153-2) In most cases of typical CSD, illness eventually resolves without therapy. Studies of antimicrobial treatment for CSD in immunocompetent patients have demonstrated only modest benefit. Some experts advocate reassurance and supportive care for management of lymphadenopathy in immunocompetent patients, whereas others recommend treatment with azithromycin to expedite resolution of lymphadenopathy. Antimicrobial therapy is uniformly recommended for immunosuppressed patients with CSD. Most clinicians treat atypical manifestations of CSD, but there are few data to guide the management of atypical disease.

BARTONELLA INFECTIONS IN HIV-INFECTED PERSONS

B. henselae and *B. quintana* can cause a broad spectrum of disease in HIV-infected individuals, including bacillary angiomatosis, peliosis hepatis, osteomyelitis, unexplained fever, bacteremia, and endocarditis. Bacillary angiomatosis is the most common of these manifestations (Chap. 182). Regardless of the manifestations, serologic tests may help support the diagnosis. (See below for a full discussion of all these specific conditions.)

Rx *BARTONELLA* INFECTIONS IN HIV-INFECTED PERSONS

As detailed below, antibiotic therapy (Table 153-2) is strongly recommended for all HIV-infected patients with *Bartonella* infections. Indeed, visceral disease may be progressive and fatal without appropriate antibiotic therapy. Relapses of *Bartonella* infections in HIV-infected persons are common, particularly after relatively short antibiotic courses.

BACILLARY ANGIOMATOSIS AND PELIOSIS HEPATIS

ETIOLOGY AND EPIDEMIOLOGY

Bacillary angiomatosis and peliosis hepatis occur primarily in HIV-infected persons whose CD4+ T cell counts are <100/μL. Earlier studies suggested that ~1 in 1000 HIV-infected persons developed bacillary angiomatosis; however, this incidence has declined in recent years, probably

TABLE 153-2 TREATMENT OF ADULTS WITH DISEASE CAUSED BY *BARTONELLA* SPECIES[a]

Disease	Treatment
Cat-scratch disease	
Lymphadenopathy	Consider azithromycin (500 mg PO on day 1, then 250 mg PO qd for 4 days)
Retinitis	Doxycycline (100 mg PO bid for 4–6 weeks) *plus* Rifampin (300 mg PO bid for 4–6 weeks)
Bacillary angiomatosis	Erythromycin (500 mg PO qid for 3 months) *or* Doxycycline (100 mg PO bid for 3 months)
Bacillary peliosis	Erythromycin (500 mg PO qid for 4 months) *or* Doxycycline (100 mg PO bid for 4 months)
Bartonella endocarditis	
Suspected	Gentamicin (3 mg/kg qd IV for 14 days) *plus* ceftriaxone (2 g IV qd for 6 weeks) *with or without* Doxycycline (100 mg PO bid for 6 weeks)
Confirmed	Gentamicin (3 mg/kg qd IV for 14 days) *plus* Doxycycline (100 mg PO bid for 6 weeks)
Trench fever	Doxycycline (200 mg PO qd for 4 weeks) *plus* Gentamicin (3 mg/kg qd IV for 14 days)
Bartonellosis	
Oroya fever	Chloramphenicol (500 mg PO or IV qid for 14 days) *plus* a β-lactam agent *or* Ciprofloxacin (500 mg bid for 10 days)
Verruga peruana	Rifampin (10 mg/kg qd PO for 14 days) *or* Streptomycin (15–20 mg/kg qd IM for 10 days)

[a]Based on recommendations from Rolain et al, 2004.

as a result of effective antiretroviral therapy and the consequent decrease in the number of patients with advanced immunodeficiency. Cutaneous bacillary angiomatosis is caused by *B. henselae* or *B. quintana*, subcutaneous nodules and lytic bone predominantly by *B. quintana*, and bacillary peliosis by *B. henselae*. Risk factors for *B. henselae* infection consist of contact with cats or fleas, whereas *B. quintana* infections are associated with low income, homelessness, and louse infestation.

CLINICAL PRESENTATION

Patients with bacillary angiomatosis most often present with painless cutaneous lesions, but other manifestations include subcutaneous masses or nodules (Fig. 153-2), superficial ulcerated plaques, and verrucous growths. The cutaneous lesions may be single or multiple and may vary in color from tan to red to deep purple. The differential diagnosis of cutaneous bacillary angiomatosis includes Kaposi's sarcoma, pyogenic granuloma, and subcutaneous tumors. Painful osseous lesions may develop beneath the cutaneous lesions. Bacillary angiomatosis may rarely involve the oropharynx, lungs, heart, intestines, lymph nodes, muscle, or brain. Patients with bacillary peliosis usually present with nonspecific systemic symptoms, with or without cutaneous involvement. Radiographic studies of osseous bacillary angiomatosis typically demonstrate lytic bone lesions on plain films and focal uptake of technetium on bone scans. Imaging of patients with peliosis hepatis generally reveals hypodense regions in the liver. In patients with advanced immunodeficiency, *B. henselae* and *B. quintana* can cause unexplained fever. In addition, *B. henselae* or *B. quintana* is occasionally identified as the cause of endocarditis in HIV-infected persons.

PATHOLOGY

Histologic examination of bacillary angiomatosis lesions demonstrates lobular proliferation of blood vessels lined by enlarged endothelial cells with a mixed infiltrate of neutrophils and lymphocytes. Examination of bacillary peliosis tissue reveals small blood-filled cystic lesions partially lined by endothelial cells and generally surrounded by a fibromyxoid

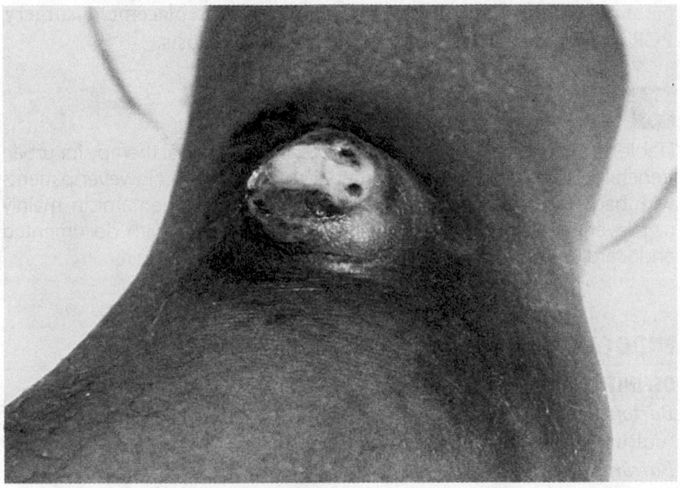

FIGURE 153-2 Nodular lesion of bacillary angiomatosis with superficial ulceration in an AIDS patient with advanced immunodeficiency.

stroma containing a mixture of inflammatory cells, dilated capillaries, and clumps of granular material. Warthin-Starry stain may reveal bacilli.

DIAGNOSIS

The diagnosis of bacillary angiomatosis is ideally based on histologic findings (see "Pathology," above).

℞ BACILLARY ANGIOMATOSIS AND PELIOSIS HEPATIS

(Table 153-2) As stated above, prolonged therapy with oral erythromycin or doxycycline is recommended for both bacillary angiomatosis and peliosis hepatis.

TRENCH FEVER

DEFINITION AND ETIOLOGY

Trench fever, a febrile illness caused by *B. quintana*, was initially described in World War I, during which the disease developed in an estimated 1 million soldiers on the western and eastern European fronts. In modern times, *B. quintana* infection has resurfaced as "urban trench fever."

EPIDEMIOLOGY

Available data suggest that *B. quintana* has a global distribution, and cases of trench fever have now been reported sporadically throughout the world. Risk factors associated with urban trench fever include poverty, homelessness, and alcoholism. Multiple studies have established the body louse as the principal vector for transmitting *B. quintana* to humans. No animal reservoirs have been identified.

CLINICAL PRESENTATION

Reports of classic trench fever in World War I described an incubation period of 5–20 days followed by one of four patterns of illness: (1) a solitary episode of fever; (2) a brief febrile period typically lasting <1 week; (3) febrile episodes lasting ~5 days interspersed with asymptomatic intervals of ~5 days ("quintan fever"); and (4) a persistent and debilitating febrile illness, often lasting >1 month. Despite the seriousness of the illness, mortality rates are low. In modern-day cases, patients have presented with nonspecific and inconsistent clinical symptoms that have included fever, headache, weight loss, and leg pain. Many patients in contemporary case series have been diagnosed with chronic bacteremia (often asymptomatic), and occasional patients have been diagnosed with culture-negative endocarditis (see below).

DIAGNOSIS

The diagnosis of urban trench fever is most often made on the basis of serologic studies or by isolating *B. quintana* from blood cultures. In patients with endocarditis who require valve replacement surgery, PCR testing of valve tissue can establish the diagnosis.

℞ TRENCH FEVER

(Table 153-2) Relatively few data exist regarding optimal therapy for urban trench fever. Mild cases can be treated with doxycycline. However, patients with bacteremia should receive both doxycycline and gentamicin, mainly to prevent the development of endocarditis. Patients with documented endocarditis also should receive doxycycline plus gentamicin.

ENDOCARDITIS

DEFINITION AND ETIOLOGY

Bartonella species have now been established as an important cause of "culture-negative" endocarditis. Although reports have identified five *Bartonella* species as causes of infective endocarditis in humans, >95% of cases have involved either *B. quintana* or *B. henselae.*

EPIDEMIOLOGY

Sporadic cases of *Bartonella*-associated endocarditis have been reported in multiple regions of the world. Most cases have involved adults, and most have affected native heart valves. Identified risk factors for *B. quintana* endocarditis consist of homelessness and infestation with body lice, whereas exposure to cats and previous valvular heart disease are associated with *B. henselae* endocarditis.

CLINICAL PRESENTATION

Clinical findings in *Bartonella* endocarditis resemble the typical findings in subacute bacterial endocarditis. Because blood cultures usually have no evident growth in the first 7–10 days, *Bartonella* endocarditis often is initially diagnosed as culture-negative endocarditis.

DIAGNOSIS

The diagnosis of endocarditis is based on clinical, laboratory, and echocardiographic findings. The identification of *Bartonella* as the specific pathogen causing endocarditis can prove challenging, especially since only ~25% of patients with *Bartonella* endocarditis have *Bartonella* isolated from blood cultures. The yield of blood cultures is enhanced by extended incubation (for 4–6 weeks). In patients from whose blood cultures *Bartonella* is not isolated, the diagnosis is usually based on either a strongly positive serologic test or evidence (most often obtained with a PCR-based method) of *Bartonella* in cardiac valve tissue.

℞ ENDOCARDITIS

(Table 153-2) For "culture-negative" endocarditis in which *Bartonella* is the suspected cause, empirical treatment consists of ceftriaxone plus gentamicin, with or without doxycycline. For confirmed *Bartonella* endocarditis, treatment consists of doxycycline plus gentamicin. If gentamicin cannot be used, rifampin should be considered as a substitute.

BARTONELLOSIS (CARRIÓN'S DISEASE)

DEFINITION AND ETIOLOGY

Bartonellosis, or Carrión's disease, is caused by *B. bacilliformis*. The disease is characterized by two distinct phases: (1) an acute febrile hematic phase, known as Oroya fever; and (2) an eruptive phase manifested by cutaneous lesions, known as verruga peruana. In 1885, Daniel Carrión, a Peruvian medical student, established the common source of the two phases of this illness by inoculating himself with material from a verruga peruana lesion and subsequently developing fatal Oroya fever.

EPIDEMIOLOGY

Bartonellosis occurs endemically in certain regions of South America. It has been reported predominantly in river valleys of the Andes Mountains in Peru as well as in some localized regions of Colombia and Ecuador. The sandfly *Lutzomyia verrucarum* serves as the vector for *B. bacilliformis* and transmits the organism to humans via a bite on the skin. Most patients with acute bartonellosis are immunologically naïve, and most cases involve tourists and transient workers. In contrast, the eruptive phase of bartonellosis most often occurs among the native population in the Andes.

CLINICAL PRESENTATION

The clinical manifestations of acute bartonellosis typically begin ~3 weeks after inoculation of *B. bacilliformis* and include fever, malaise, changes in mental status, hepatomegaly, lymphadenopathy, and profound macrocytic anemia. Patients are typically bacteremic with *B. bacilliformis* at this phase. Without antimicrobial therapy, the mortality rate exceeds 40%; infections with other pathogens and noninfectious complications contribute to this high mortality rate. Treatment with chloramphenicol during the acute phase decreases, but does not eliminate, the risk of developing eruptive bartonellosis. Only ~5% of persons with eruptive cutaneous verrugas recall having experienced an acute febrile illness in the preceding 3 months. The cutaneous verrugas typically manifest as reddish-purple pruritic papules or nodules and may resemble the cutaneous lesions of bacillary angiomatosis. Untreated, the lesions can persist for years.

DIAGNOSIS

The diagnosis of acute bartonellosis can reliably be made by detection of intraerythrocytic organisms in a Wright-Giemsa-stained thin blood smear. In addition, most patients have positive blood cultures, but 2–3 weeks are typically required for the organism's isolation. For patients with cutaneous verrugas in the eruptive phase, biopsy should be performed. Histopathologic examination characteristically shows intense proliferation of newly formed capillaries and marked endothelial hyperplasia. The yield of blood smear and blood culture is markedly lower among patients in the eruptive phase. The utility of serologic tests is high for patients in both phases.

℞ BARTONELLOSIS

(Table 153-2) Use of chloramphenicol plus a second antimicrobial agent (generally a β-lactam) is generally recommended to provide effective treatment of *B. bacilliformis* and to cover any likely concomitant secondary bacterial infection. Treatment with ciprofloxacin, streptomycin, tetracycline, and erythromycin is also effective. Rifampin or streptomycin should be used to treat chronic bartonellosis.

FURTHER READINGS

Foucault C et al: *Bartonella quintana* characteristics and clinical management. Emerg Infect Dis 12:217, 2006

Hansmann Y et al: Diagnosis of cat scratch disease with detection of *Bartonella henselae* by PCR: A study of patients with lymph node enlargement. J Clin Microbiol 43:3800, 2005

Houpikian P, Raoult D: Blood culture–negative endocarditis in a reference center: Etiologic diagnosis of 348 cases. Medicine (Baltimore) 84:162, 2005

Maguina C et al: Bartonellosis (Carrión's disease) in the modern era. Clin Infect Dis 33:772, 2001

Mohle-Boetani JC et al: Bacillary angiomatosis and bacillary peliosis in patients infected with human immunodeficiency virus: Clinical characteristics in a case-control study. Clin Infect Dis 22:794, 1996

Ohl ME, Spach DH: *Bartonella quintana* and urban trench fever. Clin Infect Dis 31:131, 2000

Rolain JM et al: Lymph node biopsy specimens and diagnosis of cat scratch disease. Emerg Infect Dis 12:1338, 2006

Rolain JM et al: Recommendations for treatment of human infections caused by *Bartonella* species. Antimicrob Agents Chemother 48:1921, 2004

Spach DH, Koehler JE: *Bartonella*-associated infections. Infect Dis Clin North Am 12:137, 1998

154 Donovanosis

Gavin Hart

Donovanosis is a chronic, progressively destructive bacterial infection of the genital region that is generally regarded as sexually transmitted (see "Epidemiology," below). The disease has been known by many other names, the most common of which are *granuloma inguinale* and *granuloma venereum.*

ETIOLOGY

Donovanosis is caused by *Klebsiella granulomatis* (formerly known as *Calymmatobacterium granulomatis*), an intracellular, gram-negative, pleomorphic, encapsulated (when mature) bacterium measuring 1.5 by 0.7 μm. *K. granulomatis* shares many morphologic and serologic characteristics and >99% homology at the nucleotide level with *Klebsiella* species that are pathogenic to humans. Polymerase chain reaction (PCR) amplification of the *phoE* gene shows it to be closely related to that in *Klebsiella pneumoniae, K. rhinoscleromatis,* and *K. ozaenae.* Electron microscopy shows typical gram-negative morphology and a large capsule but no flagella. Filiform or vesicular protrusions occur on a corrugated cell wall.

EPIDEMIOLOGY

Donovanosis is endemic among Aborigines in central Australia as well as in Papua New Guinea, southeastern India, southern Africa, Vietnam, the Caribbean, Brazil, and Argentina. In the first half of the twentieth century, the disease was endemic in parts of the United States (with an estimated 5000–10,000 cases in 1947); small epidemics still occur in this country and in other developed countries. The decline in the United States to fewer than 20 reported cases annually in the past decade has probably resulted from lower transmission rates due to earlier presentation for increasingly effective antibiotic therapy. More than 70% of cases involve persons 20–40 years of age.

The infection is predominantly sexually transmitted, but extragenital skin lesions can follow transmission from concurrent genital lesions via the fingers or through other nonsexual contact, and autoinoculation may produce new lesions from contact with adjacent skin ("kissing" lesions). Infants born to infected mothers have acquired infection at birth.

CLINICAL MANIFESTATIONS

The incubation period is usually 1–4 weeks but may extend to 1 year. Skin lesions have been detected in infants 6 weeks to 6 months after birth. The disease begins as one or more subcutaneous nodules that erode through the skin to produce clean, granulomatous, sharply defined, usually painless lesions (Fig. 154-1). These lesions, which bleed readily on contact, slowly enlarge. The genitalia are involved in 90% of cases, the inguinal region in 10%, and the anal region in 5–10%. Genital swelling, particularly of the labia, is a common feature and occasionally progresses to pseudoelephantiasis. Phimosis and paraphimosis are common local complications, and progressive erosion of affected tissues may completely destroy the penis or other organs. Less common clinical variants include a hypertrophic form (cauliflower- or wartlike lesions), a necrotic form (destructive lesions with foul-smelling exudate, often resembling amebiasis), and a sclerotic or cicatricial form, which has a dry base with extensive scar tissue. Tissue destruction may be greater in patients co-infected with HIV than in those without HIV infection.

Extragenital lesions occur in at least 6% of cases. Oral donovanosis, the most common extragenital manifestation, presents as pain or bleeding in the mouth, lesions on the lips, or extensive swelling of the gums and palate. Donovanosis may affect most bones, and sometimes many bones are affected at the same time; the tibia is involved in >50% of such cases. Bony lesions are associated with constitutional symptoms (weight loss, fever, night sweats, and malaise) and are usually found in women. More than 50% of women with donovanosis have primary lesions on the cervix. Prompt pelvic examinations and early diagnosis are likely to substantially decrease the morbidity and mortality (likely outcomes in misdiagnosed spinal lesions) associated with extragenital donovanosis in women.

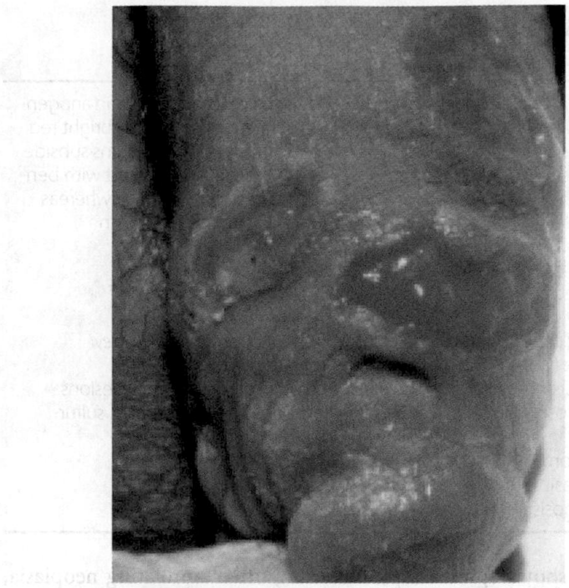

FIGURE 154-1 Multiple granulomatous lesions of the penis in a patient with donovanosis.

DIAGNOSIS

Laboratory Diagnosis The preferred diagnostic method involves demonstration of typical intracellular Donovan bodies within large mononuclear cells visualized in smears prepared from lesions (Fig. 154-2) or biopsy specimens. With typical beefy lesions, a small piece of tissue is removed with forceps and scalpel, and a crush impression of the deep surface is made on a glass slide. The smear is air-dried, heat-fixed, and stained with Giemsa, Leishman's, or Wright's stain. For dry, flat, or necrotic lesions, a punch-biopsy specimen should be obtained from the advancing edge. This specimen can be used to prepare a smear or embedded for histologic examination (with a silver stain). Histologic ex-

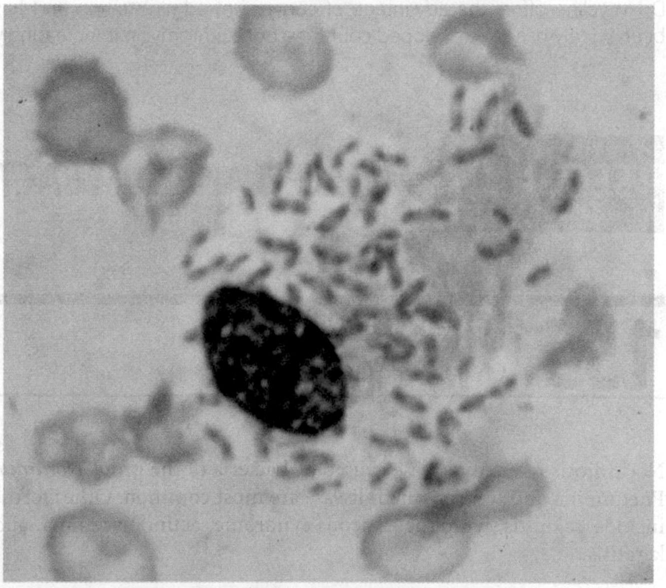

FIGURE 154-2 The typical appearance of Donovan bodies is seen in a large mononuclear cell (20–90 μm in diameter; Giemsa stain; original magnification, ×1000). The host cell nucleus is usually oval, eccentric, and vesicular or pyknotic. The causative organisms appear as bipolar-staining (closed safety-pin) forms that measure 1–1.5 μm in length and 0.5–0.7 μm in diameter and are contained in cytoplasmic vacuoles.

TABLE 154-1 DIFFERENTIAL DIAGNOSIS OF DONOVANOSIS

Disease (Chapter)	Distinguishing Features
Secondary syphilis: condylomata lata (162)	White or pale moist plaques in anogenital region (as opposed to bright red donovanosis lesions); lesions subside within 1 week of treatment with benzathine penicillin, 2.4 mU (whereas donovanosis lesions remain unchanged)
Squamous cell carcinoma (83)	Histologic appearance
Penile amebiasis (202)	Microscopic identification of *Entamoeba histolytica*
Chancroid: pseudogranuloma inguinale (139)	Culture of *Haemophilus ducreyi*
Tuberculosis (158)	Histologic features of bony lesions
Actinomycosis (156)	Microscopic identification of sulfur granules
Rhinoscleroma (143)	Histologic features
Leishmaniasis (205)	Histologic features
Histoplasmosis (192)	Histologic features

amination shows epithelial proliferation, often simulating neoplasia, with a heavy inflammatory infiltrate of plasma cells, some neutrophils, and few if any lymphocytes. *K. granulomatis* has never been grown on artificial solid media but has been cultured in chicken embryonic yolk sacs, on human monocytes, and on human epithelial (HEp-2) cells. A diagnostic PCR test has been developed and incorporated into a colorimetric detection system for *K. granulomatis*. A serologic test, based on indirect immunofluorescence, is more useful in confirming the diagnosis in cases with long-standing lesions than in early disease.

Differential Diagnosis The differential diagnosis of donovanosis is summarized in Table 154-1. Syphilis and donovanosis frequently coexist because syphilis is usually highly prevalent in areas where donovanosis is endemic; thus positive syphilis serology does not exclude a diagnosis of donovanosis. Genital ulcers are a risk factor for HIV acquisition in developing countries, and patients with donovanosis should be tested for HIV infection.

℞ DONOVANOSIS

Table 154-2 shows the most effective regimens for treating donovanosis. Doxycycline offers the advantage of convenient administration and has been widely used in developed countries, but azithromycin is increasingly being used as first-choice therapy. Extensive lesions have been cured with oral azithromycin at a dosage of 500 mg/d, but the more convenient dose of 1 g weekly is also effective. Although chloramphenicol is the drug of choice in some developing countries, it is unlikely to be acceptable in developed countries because of bone marrow toxicity. Penicillin is not effective for treating donovanosis. Patients should be examined weekly, and therapy should be continued until lesions have healed (3–5 weeks, except in severe cases). If antibiotic therapy is stopped earlier, lesions often continue to heal, but the relapse rate is higher. If the lesions are unchanged after 2 weeks of treatment, an alternative antibiotic regimen should be used.

The treatment regimens listed in Table 154-2—perhaps with increased duration—are usually adequate in HIV-infected patients without immunosuppression, but an increasing failure rate has been reported in immunosuppressed patients, for whom daily administration of azithromycin is recommended if other regimens fail to elicit a response.

TABLE 154-2 THE MOST EFFECTIVE ANTIBIOTIC REGIMENS FOR TREATMENT OF DONOVANOSIS[a]

Antibiotic	Oral Dosage
Azithromycin	1 g weekly or 500 mg/d
Erythromycin	500 mg qid
Tetracycline	500 mg qid
Doxycycline	100 mg bid
Trimethoprim-sulfamethoxazole	1 double-strength tablet[b] bid
Chloramphenicol	500 mg tid

[a]Patients should be examined weekly, and therapy should be continued until lesions have healed (3–5 weeks, except in severe cases).
[b]160 mg/800 mg.

FURTHER READINGS

See www.stdservices.on.net/std/donovanosis/Default.htm for an illustrated lecture and a comprehensive bibliography on donovanosis.

HART G: Donovanosis (granuloma inguinale), in *Atlas of Infectious Diseases*, vol V: *Sexually Transmitted Diseases*, MF Rein (ed). Philadelphia, Churchill Livingstone, 1996, pp 17.1–17.10

———: Donovanosis. Clin Infect Dis 25:24, 1997

O'FARRELL N: Donovanosis. Sex Transm Infect 78:452, 2002

SARDANA K, SEHGAL V: Genital ulcer disease and human immunodeficiency virus: A focus. Int J Dermatol 44:391, 2005

WU JJ et al: Selected sexually transmitted diseases and their relationship to HIV. Clin Dermatol 22:499, 2004

SECTION 7 MISCELLANEOUS BACTERIAL INFECTIONS

155 Nocardiosis

Gregory A. Filice

Nocardiosis refers to disease caused by bacteria of the genus *Nocardia*. Pneumonia and disseminated disease are most common. Other forms include cellulitis, lymphocutaneous syndrome, actinomycetoma, and keratitis.

MICROBIOLOGY

Nocardiae are saprophytic aerobic actinomycetes and are common worldwide in soil, where they contribute to decay of organic matter. Nocardial taxonomy is complex and incompletely understood. As taxonomy continues to evolve, any nocardiae isolated from a human should be considered potential pathogens.

Nocardia asteroides, which is most commonly isolated from clinical material and associated with invasive disease, is actually a species complex. Six other *Nocardia* species [*N. brasiliensis*, *N. otitidiscaviarum* (formerly *N. caviae*), *N. farcinica*, *N. nova*, *N. transvalensis*, and *N. pseudobrasiliensis*] have been firmly established as human pathogens, and at least 11 additional species have been associated with human disease.

N. farcinica is a less common human pathogen than *N. asteroides* but is more virulent and prone to dissemination. *N. pseudobrasiliensis* is most often associated with invasive disease, and *N. brasiliensis* is usually associated with disease limited to the skin. *N. transvalensis* is generally associated with pulmonary or systemic disease in immunosuppressed patients or with actinomycetoma, an indolent, slowly progressive disease of skin and underlying tissues with nodular swellings and draining sinuses.

EPIDEMIOLOGY

Approximately 1100 cases of nocardial infection are diagnosed annually in the United States, 85% of them pulmonary and/or systemic.

The annual incidence is ~0.375 cases per 100,000 persons. The disease is more common among adults than among children and among males than among females. Nearly all cases are sporadic, but outbreaks have been associated with contamination of the hospital environment, solutions, or drug injection equipment. Person-to-person spread is not well documented. There is no known seasonality.

The risk of pulmonary or disseminated disease is greater than usual among persons with deficient cell-mediated immunity, especially that associated with lymphoma, transplantation, glucocorticoid therapy, or AIDS. The incidence is ~140-fold greater among patients with AIDS and ~340-fold greater among bone marrow transplant recipients than in general populations. In AIDS, nocardiosis usually affects persons with <250 CD4+ T lymphocytes/μL. Nocardiosis has also been associated with pulmonary alveolar proteinosis, tuberculosis and other mycobacterial diseases, chronic granulomatous disease, interleukin 12 deficiency, and treatment with monoclonal antibodies to tumor necrosis factor. Any child with nocardiosis and no known cause of immunosuppression should undergo tests to determine the adequacy of the phagocytic respiratory burst.

Actinomycetoma associated with *N. brasiliensis*, *N. asteroides*, *N. otitidiscaviarum*, and *N. transvalensis* occurs mainly in tropical and subtropical regions, especially those of Mexico, Central and South America, Africa, and India. The most important risk factor is frequent contact with soil or vegetable matter.

PATHOLOGY AND PATHOGENESIS

Pneumonia and disseminated disease are both thought to follow inhalation of fragmented bacterial mycelia. The characteristic histologic feature of nocardiosis is an abscess with extensive neutrophil infiltration and prominent necrosis. Granulation tissue usually surrounds the lesions, but extensive fibrosis or encapsulation is uncommon. Actinomycetoma is characterized by suppurative inflammation with sinus tract formation. Granules—microcolonies composed of dense masses of bacterial filaments extending radially from a central core—are occasionally observed in histologic preparations. They are frequently found in discharges from lesions of actinomycetoma but almost never from lesions in other forms of nocardiosis. Infrequently, nocardiae and other indolent pathogens, including fungi or mycobacteria, are isolated from the same patient.

Nocardiae have evolved a number of properties that enable them to survive within phagocytes, including neutralization of oxidants, prevention of phagosome-lysosome fusion, and prevention of phagosome acidification. Neutrophils phagocytose the organisms and limit their growth but do not kill them efficiently. Cell-mediated immunity is important for definitive control and elimination of nocardiae.

CLINICAL MANIFESTATIONS

Respiratory Tract Disease Pneumonia, the most common form of nocardial disease in the respiratory tract, is typically subacute; symptoms have usually been present for days or weeks at presentation. The onset is occasionally more acute in immunosuppressed patients. Cough is prominent and produces small amounts of thick, purulent sputum that is not malodorous. Fever, anorexia, weight loss, and malaise are common; dyspnea, pleuritic pain, and hemoptysis are less common. Remissions and exacerbations over several weeks are frequent. Roentgenographic patterns vary, but some are highly suggestive of nocardial pneumonia. Infiltrates vary in size and are typically of at least moderate density. Single or multiple nodules are common (Figs. 155-1 and 155-2), sometimes suggesting tumor metastases. Infiltrates and nodules tend to cavitate (Fig. 155-2). Empyema is present in one-third of cases.

Nocardiosis may spread directly from the lungs to adjacent tissues. Pericarditis, mediastinitis, and the superior vena cava syndrome have all been reported. Nocardial laryngitis, tracheitis, and bronchitis are much less common than pneumonia. In the major airways, disease often presents as a nodular or granulomatous mass. A few cases of sinusitis have been reported.

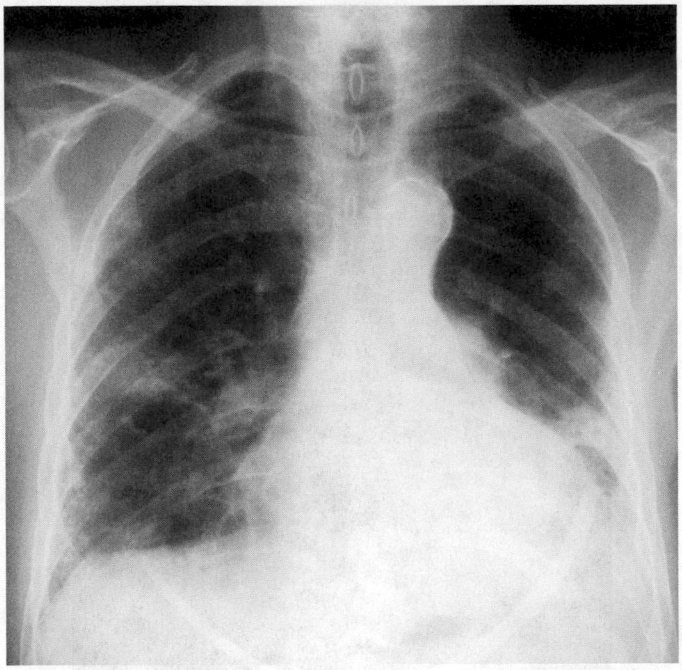

FIGURE 155-1 Nocardial pneumonia. Discrete nodular infiltrates are present in midlung fields on both sides.

Nocardiae are sometimes isolated from respiratory secretions of patients without apparent nocardial disease. These patients usually have chronic pulmonary disease with airway or parenchymal abnormalities and do not necessarily require treatment for nocardiosis (see "Diagnosis," below).

Extrapulmonary Disease In half of all cases of pulmonary nocardiosis, disease appears outside the lungs. In one-fifth of cases of disseminated disease, lung disease is not apparent. The most common site of dissemination is the brain. Other common sites include the skin and supporting structures, kidneys, bone, and muscle, but almost any organ can be involved. Peritonitis and epididymo-orchitis have been reported recently. Nocardiae have been recovered from blood in a few cases of pneumonia, disseminated disease, or central venous catheter

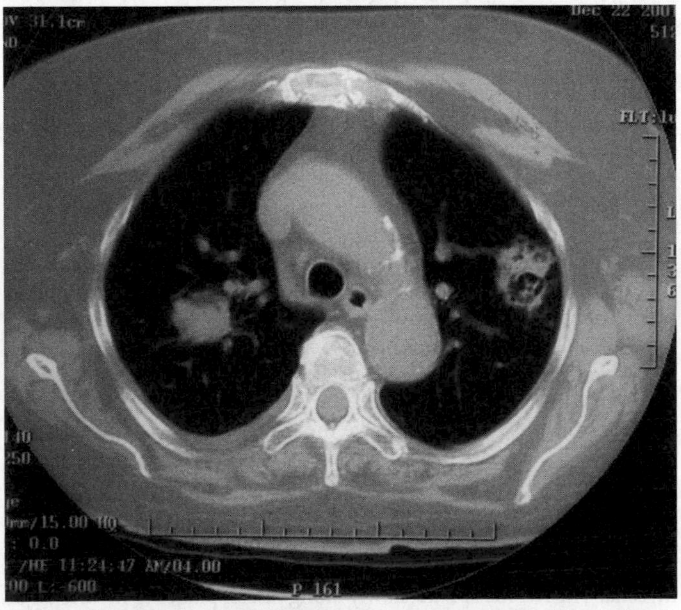

FIGURE 155-2 Nocardial pneumonia. A CT scan shows bilateral nodules, with cavitation in the nodule in the left lung.

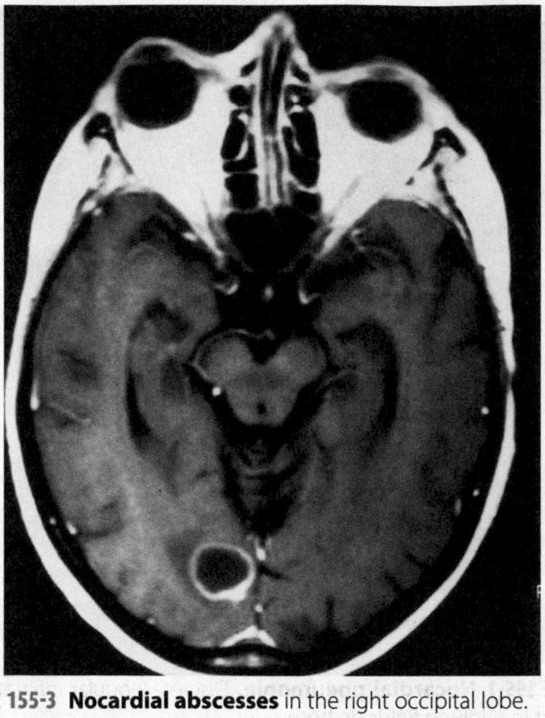

FIGURE 155-3 Nocardial abscesses in the right occipital lobe.

infection. Nocardial endocarditis occurs rarely and can affect either native or prosthetic valves.

The typical manifestation of extrapulmonary dissemination is a subacute abscess. A minority of abscesses outside the lungs or central nervous system (CNS) form fistulae and discharge small amounts of pus. In CNS infections, brain abscesses are usually supratentorial, are often multiloculated, and may be single or multiple (Fig. 155-3). Brain abscesses tend to burrow into the ventricles or extend out into the subarachnoid space. The symptoms and signs are somewhat more indolent than those of other types of bacterial brain abscess. Meningitis is uncommon and is usually due to spread from a nearby brain abscess. Nocardiae are not easily recovered from cerebrospinal fluid (CSF).

Disease following Transcutaneous Inoculation Disease that follows transcutaneous nocardial inoculation usually takes one of three forms: cellulitis, lymphocutaneous syndrome, or actinomycetoma.

Cellulitis generally begins 1–3 weeks after a recognized breach of the skin, often with soil contamination. Subacute cellulitis, with pain, swelling, erythema, and warmth, develops over days to weeks. The lesions are usually firm and not fluctuant. Disease may progress to involve underlying muscles, tendons, bones, or joints. Dissemination is rare. *N. brasiliensis* is the most common isolate, but *N. asteroides* is often isolated from people living in cooler climates.

Lymphocutaneous disease usually begins as a pyodermatous lesion at the site of inoculation, with central ulceration and purulent or honey-colored drainage. Subcutaneous nodules often appear along lymphatics that drain the primary lesion. The lymphangitic form closely resembles lymphocutaneous sporotrichosis (Chap. 199). Most cases of the lymphocutaneous syndrome are associated with *N. brasiliensis*.

Actinomycetoma (Fig. 155-4) usually begins with a nodular swelling, sometimes at a site of local trauma. Lesions typically develop on the feet or hands but may involve the posterior part of the neck, the upper back, the head, and other sites. The nodule eventually breaks down, and a fistula appears. This fistula is typically followed by others. The fistulae tend to come and go, with new ones forming as old ones disappear. The discharge is serous or purulent, may be bloody, and often contains 0.1- to 2-mm white granules consisting of masses of mycelia. The lesions spread slowly along fascial planes to involve adjacent areas of skin, subcutaneous tissue, and bone. Over months or years, there may be extensive deformation of the affected part. Lesions

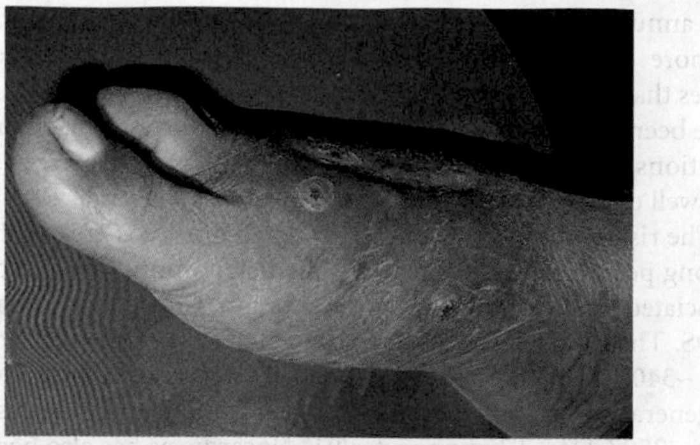

FIGURE 155-4 Nocardial actinomycetoma illustrating common features including swelling, multiple sinus tracts, and involvement of the foot. *(Image provided by Amor Khachemoune and Ronald O. Perelman, New York University School of Medicine.)*

involving soft tissues are only mildly painful; those affecting bones or joints are more so. Systemic symptoms are absent or minimal. Infection rarely disseminates from actinomycetoma, and lesions on the hands and feet usually cause only local disability. Lesions on the head, neck, and trunk can invade locally to involve deep organs, with consequent severe disability or death.

Eye Infections *Nocardia* species (particularly *N. asteroides*) are uncommon causes of subacute keratitis, usually following eye trauma. Nocardial endophthalmitis can develop after eye surgery. In one series, nocardiae accounted for more than half of culture-proved cases of endophthalmitis after cataract surgery. Endophthalmitis can also occur during disseminated disease. Nocardial infection of lachrymal glands has been reported.

DIAGNOSIS

The first step in diagnosis is examination of sputum or pus for crooked, branching, beaded, gram-positive filaments 1 μm wide and up to 50 μm long (Fig. 155-5). Most nocardiae are acid-fast in direct smears if a weak acid is used for decolorization (e.g., in the modified Kinyoun, Ziehl-Neelsen, and Fite-Faraco methods). The organisms often take up silver stains. Nocardiae grow relatively slowly; colonies may take up to 2 weeks to appear and may not develop their characteristic appearance for up to 4 weeks. Several blood culture systems support nocardial growth. Yield in manual systems is enhanced when blood cultures are incubated aerobically for up to 4 weeks and when blind subcultures are performed. Nocardial growth is so different from that of more common pathogens that the laboratory should be alerted when

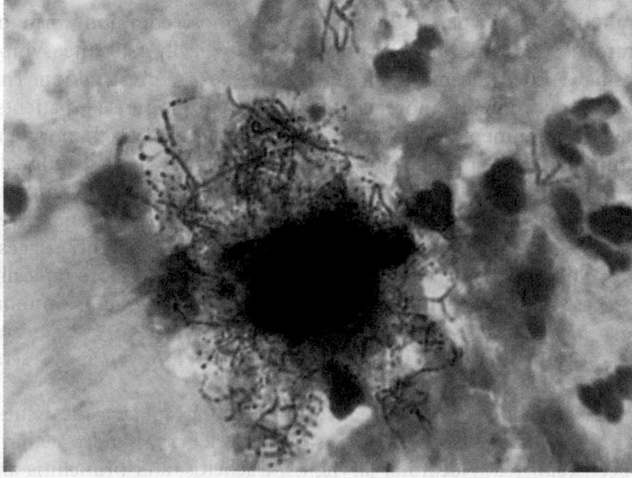

FIGURE 155-5 Gram-stained sputum from a patient with nocardial pneumonia. *(Image provided by Charles Cartwright and Susan Nelson, Hennepin County Medical Center, Minneapolis, MN.)*

nocardiosis is suspected in order to maximize the likelihood of isolation. Since nocardiae are among the few aerobic microorganisms that use paraffin as a carbon source, paraffin baiting can be used to isolate the organisms from mixed cultures.

In nocardial pneumonia, sputum smears are often negative. Unless the diagnosis can be made in smear-negative cases by sampling lesions in more accessible sites, bronchoscopy or lung aspiration is usually necessary. Transtracheal aspiration should be avoided, as it frequently leads to nocardial cellulitis in tissues around the puncture wound.

To evaluate the possibility of dissemination in patients with nocardial pneumonia, a careful history should be obtained and a thorough physical examination performed. Suggestive symptoms or signs should be pursued with further diagnostic tests. CT or MRI of the head, with and without contrast material, should be undertaken if signs or symptoms suggest brain involvement. Some authorities recommend brain imaging in all cases of pulmonary or disseminated disease.

When clinically indicated, CSF or urine should be concentrated and then cultured. In actinomycetoma, granules should be sought in the discharge. Suspect particles should be washed in saline, examined microscopically, and cultured.

Isolation of nocardiae from sputum or blood occasionally represents colonization, transient infection, or contamination. In typical cases of respiratory tract colonization, Gram-stained specimens are negative and cultures are only intermittently positive. A positive sputum culture in an immunosuppressed patient usually reflects disease. When nocardiae are isolated from an immunocompetent patient without apparent nocardial disease, the patient should be observed carefully without treatment. A patient with a host-defense defect that increases the risk of nocardiosis should usually receive antimicrobial treatment.

Nocardia species are difficult to differentiate from one another with standard biochemical tests. The Clinical and Laboratory Standards Institute has published a broth microdilution method for nocardiae, but experience with nocardiae and quality-control testing are required for reliable results. Isolates from patients with systemic or severe disease should be sent to a reference laboratory for definitive identification and susceptibility testing.

Several presumptive diagnostic tests for nocardial infection have been studied, including tests for antibodies, nocardial metabolites, and nocardial DNA. None is ready for clinical use at this time.

Rx NOCARDIOSIS

Sulfonamides are the drugs of choice for nocardiosis **(Table 155-1)**. The combination of sulfamethoxazole (SMX) and trimethoprim (TMP) is probably equivalent to sulfonamides; some authorities believe that the combination may in fact be more effective, but it also poses a modestly greater risk of hematologic toxicity. At the outset, 10–20 mg of TMP per kg and 50–100 mg of SMX per kg should be given each day in two divided doses. Later, the daily doses can be decreased to as little as 5 mg/kg and 25 mg/kg, respectively. In difficult cases, sulfonamide levels should be measured and dosages adjusted to keep serum concentrations between 100 and 150 μg/mL. In persons with sulfonamide allergies, desensitization usually allows continuation of therapy with these effective and inexpensive drugs.

Minocycline is the best-established alternative oral drug and should be given in doses of 100–200 mg twice a day. Other tetracyclines are usually ineffective. Linezolid appears to be active in vitro and has been effective in a few clinical cases. *N. nova* infections can be treated with erythromycin (500–750 mg four times a day) and/or ampicillin (1 g four times a day), but other *Nocardia* species are often resistant to both drugs. Amoxicillin (500 mg) combined with clavulanic acid (125 mg), given three times a day, has been effective in a few cases but should be avoided in cases due to *N. nova*, in which clavulanate induces β-lactamase production. Ofloxacin (400 mg twice a day) and clarithromycin (500 mg twice a day) have each been successful in a few cases.

Amikacin, the best-established parenteral drug, is given in doses of 5–7.5 mg/kg every 12 h. Serum levels should be monitored during prolonged therapy in patients with diminished renal function and in the elderly. Newer β-lactam antibiotics, including cefotaxime, ceftizoxime, ceftriaxone, and imipenem, are usually effective. These agents may be less effective in some cases caused by *N. farcinica*.

In vitro, *N. farcinica* differs from most nocardiae in that it is resistant to cephalosporins in most cases and to imipenem in one-fifth of cases. *N. pseudobrasiliensis* often exhibits resistance to minocycline or amoxicillin/clavulanic acid and susceptibility to ciprofloxacin or clarithromycin. *N. transvalensis* displays increased resistance to many antimicrobial agents, including amikacin, tobramycin, cefotaxime, ceftriaxone, and amoxicillin/clavulanic acid. *N. nova* isolates appear to be susceptible to ampicillin and erythromycin in vitro but also produce β-lactamase constitutively or in the presence of a β-lactam drug.

Use of SMX and TMP in high-risk populations to prevent *Pneumocystis* disease or urinary tract infections appears to reduce the risk of nocardiosis as well. However, the incidence of nocardiosis is low enough that prophylaxis of this disease is not recommended.

In patients with nocardiosis who need immunosuppressive therapy for an underlying disease or prevention of transplant rejection, such therapy should be continued. In many cases, two or more antimicrobial agents have been used to treat nocardiosis, often in combinations including drugs that are usually effective by themselves, like a sulfonamide or minocycline. Whether such combination therapy is better than monotherapy is not known, and it certainly increases the risk of toxicity. In treating patients with severe disease, some experts begin with a combination including TMP-SMX, amikacin, and ceftriaxone or imipenem. If combination therapy is used initially, a single drug should be used after clinical improvement, which usually occurs within the first week or two of treatment.

Surgical management of nocardial disease is similar to that of other bacterial diseases. Brain abscesses should be aspirated, drained, or excised if the diagnosis is unclear, if an abscess is large and accessible, or if an abscess fails to respond to chemotherapy. Small or inaccessible brain abscesses should be treated medically; clinical improvement should be noticeable within 1–2 weeks. Brain imaging should be repeated to document the resolution of lesions, although abatement on images often lags behind clinical improvement.

Antimicrobial therapy usually suffices for nocardial actinomycetoma. In deep or extensive cases, drainage or excision of heavily involved tissue may facilitate healing, but structure and function should be preserved whenever possible.

Nocardial infections tend to relapse (particularly in patients with chronic gran-

TABLE 155-1 TREATMENT FOR NOCARDIOSIS

Disease	Duration	Drugs (Daily Dose)[a]
Pulmonary or systemic		Systemic therapy
Intact host defenses	6–12 mo	Oral
Deficient host defenses	12 mo[b]	1. Trimethoprim (10–20 mg/kg) and sulfamethoxazole (50–100 mg/kg)
CNS disease	12 mo[c]	
Cellulitis, lymphocutaneous syndrome	2 mo	2. Minocycline (200–400 mg)
		3. Linezolid (1200 mg)
Osteomyelitis, arthritis, laryngitis, sinusitis	4 mo	Parenteral
		1. Amikacin (10–15 mg/kg)
Actinomycetoma	6–12 mo after clinical cure	2. Cefotaxime (6 g), ceftizoxime (6 g), ceftriaxone (1–2 g), imipenem (2 g)
Keratitis	Topical: Until apparent cure	1. Sulfonamide drops
		2. Amikacin drops
	Systemic: Until 2–4 mo after apparent cure	Drugs for systemic therapy as listed above

[a]For each category, choices are numbered in order of preference.
[b]In some patients with AIDS or chronic granulomatous disease, therapy for pulmonary or systemic disease must be continued indefinitely.
[c]If all apparent CNS disease has been excised, the duration of therapy may be reduced to 6 months.

ulomatous disease), and long courses of antimicrobial therapy are necessary. If disease is unusually extensive, if the patient is immunosuppressed, or if the response to therapy is slow, the recommendations in Table 155-1 should be exceeded.

The mortality rate for pulmonary or disseminated nocardiosis outside the CNS should be <5%. CNS disease carries a higher mortality rate. Patients should be followed carefully for at least 6 months after therapy has ended.

FURTHER READINGS

BROWN-ELLIOTT BA et al: Clinical and laboratory features of the *Nocardia* spp. based on current molecular taxonomy. Clin Microbiol Rev 19:259, 2006

CHOUCIÑO C et al: Nocardial infections in bone marrow transplant recipients. Clin Infect Dis 23:1012, 1996

FABRE S et al: Primary cutaneous *Nocardia otitidiscaviarum* infection in a patient with rheumatoid arthritis treated with infliximab. J Rheumatol 32:2432, 2005

FILICE GA: Nocardiosis in persons with human immunodeficiency virus infection, transplant recipients, and large, geographically defined populations. J Lab Clin Med 145:156, 2005

LALITHA P et al: Postcataract endophthalmitis in South India incidence and outcome. Ophthalmology 112:1884, 2005

PALMER DL et al: Diagnostic and therapeutic considerations in *Nocardia asteroides* infection. Medicine 53:391, 1974

POONWAN N et al: Characterization of clinical isolates of pathogenic *Nocardia* strains and related actinomycetes in Thailand from 1996 to 2003. Mycopathologia 159:361, 2005

ROUTH JC et al: Epididymo-orchitis and testicular abscess due to *Nocardia asteroides* complex. Urology 65:591, 2005

RUPPRECHT TA, PFISTER HW: Clinical experience with linezolid for the treatment of central nervous system infections. Eur J Neurol 12:536, 2005

UTTAMCHANDANI RB et al: Nocardiosis in 30 patients with advanced human immunodeficiency virus infection: Clinical features and outcome. Clin Infect Dis 18:348, 1994

156 Actinomycosis

Thomas A. Russo

Actinomycosis is an indolent, slowly progressive infection caused by anaerobic or microaerophilic bacteria, primarily of the genus *Actinomyces*, that colonize the mouth, colon, and vagina. Mucosal disruption may lead to infection at virtually any site in the body. In vivo growth of actinomycetes usually results in the formation of characteristic clumps called *grains* or *sulfur granules*. The clinical presentations of actinomycosis are myriad. Common in the preantibiotic era, actinomycosis has diminished in incidence, as has its timely recognition. Actinomycosis has been called the most misdiagnosed disease, and it has been said that no disease is so often missed by experienced clinicians. Thus this entity remains a diagnostic challenge.

Three clinical presentations that should prompt consideration of this unique infection are (1) the combination of chronicity, progression across tissue boundaries, and mass-like features (mimicking malignancy, with which it is often confused); (2) the development of a sinus tract, which may spontaneously resolve and recur; and (3) a refractory or relapsing infection after a short course of therapy, since cure of established actinomycosis requires prolonged treatment. An awareness of the full spectrum of the disease will expedite its diagnosis and treatment and will minimize the unnecessary surgical interventions, morbidity, and mortality that are reported all too often.

ETIOLOGIC AGENTS

Actinomycosis is most commonly caused by *A. israelii. A. naeslundii, A. odontolyticus, A. viscosus, A. meyeri, A. gerencseriae*, and *Propionibacterium propionicum* are established but less common causes. Most if not all actinomycotic infections are polymicrobial. *Actinobacillus actinomycetemcomitans, Eikenella corrodens*, Enterobacteriaceae, and species of *Fusobacterium, Bacteroides, Capnocytophaga, Staphylococcus*, and *Streptococcus* are commonly isolated with actinomycetes in various combinations, depending on the site of infection. The contribution of these other species to the pathogenesis of actinomycosis is uncertain.

Comparative 16S rRNA gene sequencing has led to the identification of an ever-expanding list of *Actinomyces* spp., presently numbered at 92. Increasing data support *A. europaeus, A. neuii, A. radingae, A. graevenitzii, A. turicensis, A. cardiffensis, A. houstonensis, A. hongkongensis*, and *A. funkei* as additional causes of human actinomycosis.

EPIDEMIOLOGY

Actinomycosis has no geographic boundaries and occurs throughout life, with a peak incidence in the middle decades. Males have a threefold higher incidence than females, possibly because of poorer dental hygiene and/or more frequent trauma. Factors that have probably contributed to the decrease in actinomycosis incidence since the advent of antibiotics include improved dental hygiene and the initiation of antimicrobial treatment before the disease develops fully. Individuals who do not seek or have access to health care are undoubtedly at higher risk.

PATHOGENESIS AND PATHOLOGY

The etiologic agents of actinomycosis are members of the normal oral flora and are often cultured from the bronchi, the gastrointestinal tract, and the female genital tract. The critical step in the development of actinomycosis is disruption of the mucosal barrier. Local infection may ensue. Once established, actinomycosis spreads contiguously in a slow progressive manner, ignoring tissue planes. Although acute inflammation may initially develop at the infection site, the hallmark of actinomycosis is the characteristic chronic, indolent phase manifested by lesions that usually appear as single or multiple indurations. Central necrosis consisting of neutrophils and sulfur granules develops and is virtually diagnostic. The fibrotic walls of the mass are typically described as "wooden." The responsible bacterial and/or host factors have not been identified. Over time, sinus tracts to the skin, adjacent organs, or bone may develop. In rare instances, distant hematogenous seeding may occur. As mentioned above, these unique features of actinomycosis mimic malignancy, with which it is often confused.

Foreign bodies appear to facilitate infection. This association most frequently involves intrauterine contraceptive devices (IUCDs). An increasing number of reports have described an association of actinomycosis with HIV infection, transplantation, and radio- or chemotherapy. Ulcerative mucosal infections (e.g., by herpes simplex virus or cytomegalovirus) and abnormalities in host defenses may facilitate the development of actinomycosis in the latter settings.

CLINICAL MANIFESTATIONS

Oral-Cervicofacial Disease Actinomycosis occurs most frequently at an oral, cervical, or facial site, usually as a soft tissue swelling, abscess, or mass lesion that is often mistaken for a neoplasm. The angle of the jaw is generally involved, but a diagnosis of actinomycosis should be considered with any mass lesion or relapsing infection in the head and neck (Chap. 31). Otitis, sinusitis, and canaliculitis also can develop. Pain, fever, and leukocytosis are variably reported. Contiguous extension to the cranium, cervical spine, or thorax is a potential sequela.

Thoracic Disease Thoracic actinomycosis usually follows an indolent progressive course, with involvement of the pulmonary parenchyma and/or the pleural space. Chest pain, fever, and weight loss are common. A cough, when present, is variably productive. The usual radiographic finding is either a mass lesion or pneumonia. On computed

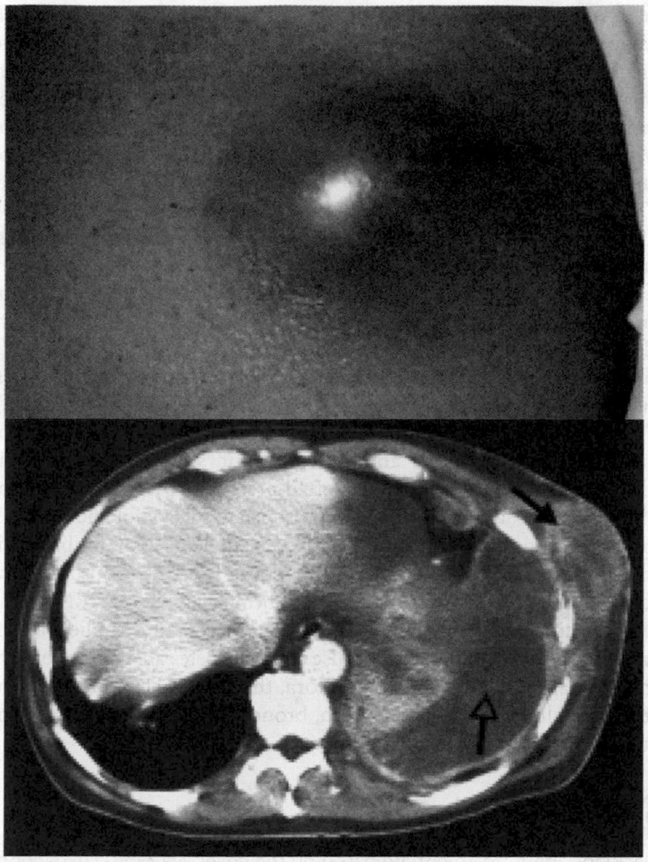

FIGURE 156-1 Thoracic actinomycosis. *Top:* A chest wall mass from extension of pulmonary infection. ***Bottom:*** Pulmonary infection is complicated by empyema (*open arrow*) and extension to the chest wall (*closed arrow*). (*Courtesy of Dr. C. B. Hsiao, Division of Infectious Diseases, Department of Medicine, State University of New York at Buffalo; with permission.*)

tomography (CT), central areas of low attenuation and ringlike rim enhancement may be seen. Cavitary disease or hilar adenopathy may develop. More than 50% of cases include pleural thickening, effusion, or empyema (Fig. 156-1). Rarely, pulmonary nodules or endobronchial lesions occur. Pulmonary lesions suggestive of actinomycosis may cross fissures or pleura; may involve the mediastinum, contiguous bone, or chest wall; or may be associated with a sinus tract. In the absence of these findings, thoracic actinomycosis is usually mistaken for a neoplasm or for pneumonia due to more usual causes.

Mediastinal infection is uncommon, usually arising from thoracic extension but rarely resulting from perforation of the esophagus, from trauma, or from head and neck or abdominal disease. The structures within the mediastinum and the heart can be involved in various combinations; consequently, the possible presentations are diverse. Primary endocarditis and isolated disease of the breast have been described.

Abdominal Disease Abdominal actinomycosis poses a great diagnostic challenge. Months or years usually pass from the inciting event (e.g., appendicitis, diverticulitis, peptic ulcer disease, foreign-body perforation, bowel surgery, or ascension from IUCD-associated pelvic disease) to clinical recognition. Because of the flow of peritoneal fluid and/or the direct extension of primary disease, virtually any abdominal organ, region, or space can be involved. The disease usually presents as an abscess, a mass, or a mixed lesion that is often fixed to underlying tissue and mistaken for a tumor. On CT, enhancement is most often heterogeneous and adjacent bowel is thickened. Sinus tracts to the abdominal wall, to the perianal region, or between the bowel and other organs may develop and mimic inflammatory bowel disease (Chap. 289). Recurrent disease or a wound or fistula that fails to heal suggests actinomycosis.

Hepatic infection usually presents as one or more abscesses or masses (Fig. 156-2). Isolated disease presumably develops via hematogenous seeding from cryptic foci. Imaging and percutaneous techniques have resulted in improved diagnosis and treatment.

All levels of the urogenital tract can be infected. Renal disease usually presents as pyelonephritis and/or renal and perinephric abscess. Bladder involvement, usually due to extension of pelvic disease, may result in ureteral obstruction or fistulas to bowel, skin, or uterus. *Actinomyces* can be detected in urine with appropriate stains and cultures.

Pelvic Disease Actinomycotic involvement of the pelvis occurs most commonly in association with an IUCD. When an IUCD is in place or has recently been removed, pelvic symptoms should prompt consideration of actinomycosis. The risk, although not quantified, appears small. The disease rarely develops when the IUCD has been in place for <1 year, but the risk increases with time. Actinomycosis can also present months after IUCD removal. Symptoms are typically indolent; fever, weight loss, abdominal pain, and abnormal vaginal bleeding or discharge are the most common. The earliest stage of disease—often endometritis—commonly progresses to pelvic masses or a tuboovarian abscess (Fig. 156-3). Unfortunately, because the diagnosis is often

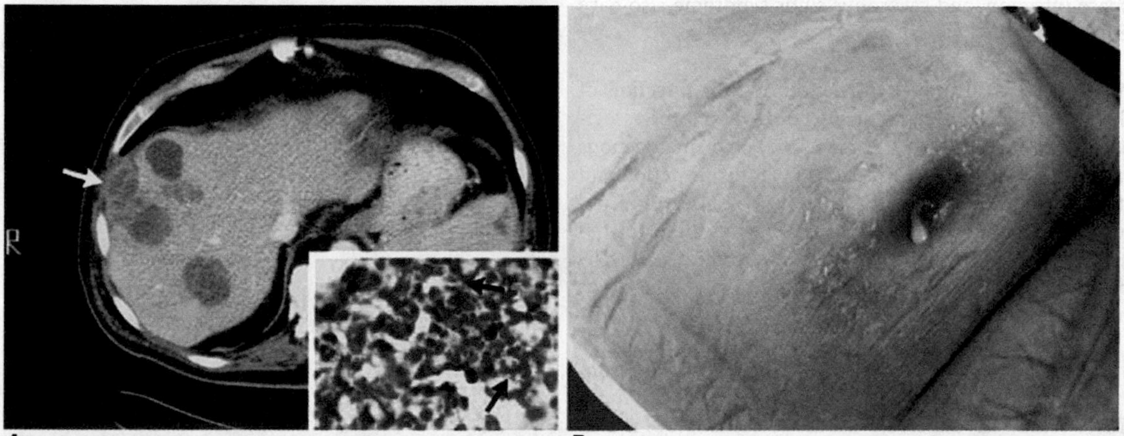

A B

FIGURE 156-2 Hepatic-splenic actinomycosis. *A.* Computed tomogram showing multiple hepatic abscesses and a small splenic lesion due to *A. israelii.* Arrow indicates extension outside the liver. ***Inset:*** Gram's stain of abscess fluid demonstrating beaded filamentous gram-positive rods. ***B.*** Subsequent formation of a sinus tract. (*Reprinted with permission from Saad M: Actinomyces hepatic abscess with cutaneous fistula. N Engl J Med 353:e16, 2005. © 2005 Massachusetts Medical Society. All rights reserved.*)

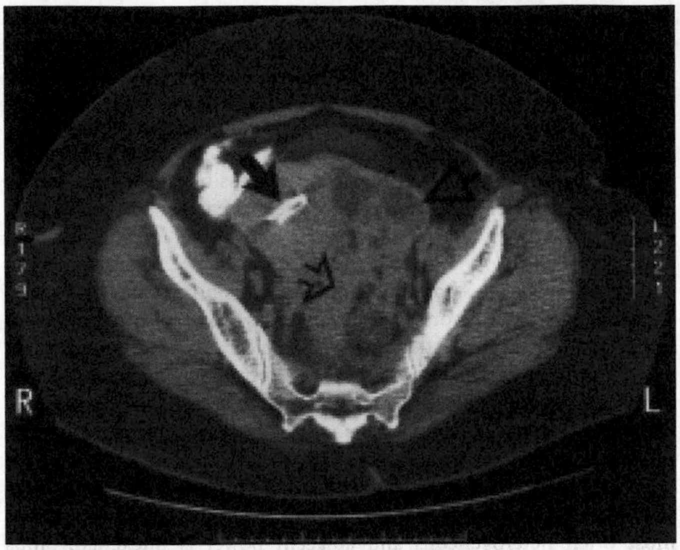

FIGURE 156-3 Computed tomogram showing pelvic actinomycosis associated with an intrauterine contraceptive device. The device is encased by endometrial fibrosis (*solid arrow*); also visible are paraendometrial fibrosis (*open triangular arrowhead*) and an area of suppuration (*open arrow*).

delayed, a "frozen pelvis" mimicking malignancy or endometriosis can develop by the time of recognition.

An unresolved issue is whether screening of cervical or endometrial specimens for *Actinomyces*-like organisms (ALOs) can predict or prevent IUCD-associated disease. Although the risk appears small, the consequences of infection are significant. Therefore, until more quantitative data become available, it seems prudent to remove the IUCD in the presence of symptoms that cannot be accounted for, regardless of whether ALOs or immunofluorescence-positive organisms are detected, and—if advanced disease is excluded—to initiate a 14-day course of empirical treatment for possible early pelvic actinomycosis. The detection of ALOs or immunofluorescence-positive organisms in the absence of symptoms warrants education of the patient and close follow-up but not removal of the IUCD unless a suitable contraceptive alternative is agreed on.

Central Nervous System Disease Actinomycosis of the central nervous system (CNS) is rare. Single or multiple brain abscesses are most common. An abscess usually appears on CT as a ring-enhancing lesion with a thick wall that may be irregular or nodular. Meningitis, epidural or subdural space infection, and cavernous sinus syndrome also have been described.

Musculoskeletal and Soft Tissue Infection Actinomycotic infection of bone is usually due to adjacent soft-tissue infection but may be associated with trauma (e.g., fracture of the mandible) or hematogenous spread. Because of slow disease progression, new bone formation and bone destruction are seen concomitantly. Infection of an extremity is uncommon and is usually a result of trauma. Skin, subcutaneous tissue, muscle, and bone (with periostitis or acute or chronic osteomyelitis) are involved alone or in various combinations. Cutaneous sinus tracts frequently develop.

Disseminated Disease Hematogenous dissemination of disease from any location rarely results in multiple-organ involvement. The lungs and liver are most commonly affected, with the presentation of multiple nodules mimicking disseminated malignancy. The clinical presentation may be surprisingly indolent given the extent of disease.

DIAGNOSIS

The diagnosis of actinomycosis is rarely considered. All too often, the first mention of actinomycosis is by the pathologist after extensive surgery. Since medical therapy alone is often sufficient for cure, the challenge for the clinician is to consider the possibility of actinomycosis, to diagnose it in the least invasive fashion, and to avoid unnecessary surgery. The clinical and radiographic presentations that suggest actinomycosis are discussed above. Aspirations and biopsies (with or without CT or ultrasound guidance) are being used successfully to obtain clinical material for diagnosis, although surgery may be required. The diagnosis is most commonly made by microscopic identification of sulfur granules (an in vivo matrix of bacteria, calcium phosphate, and host material) in pus or tissues. Occasionally, these granules are identified grossly from draining sinus tracts or pus. Although sulfur granules are a defining characteristic of actinomycosis, granules are also found in mycetoma (Chaps. 155 and 199) and botryomycosis (a chronic suppurative bacterial infection of soft tissue or, in rare cases, visceral tissue that produces clumps of bacteria resembling granules). These entities can easily be differentiated from actinomycosis with appropriate histopathologic and microbiologic studies. Microbiologic identification of actinomycetes is often precluded by prior antimicrobial therapy or failure to perform appropriate microbiologic cultures. For optimal yield, the avoidance of even a single dose of antibiotics is mandatory. Primary isolation usually requires 5–7 days but may take as long as 2–4 weeks. Although not routinely used, 16S rRNA gene amplification and sequencing have been successfully applied to increase diagnostic sensitivity. Because actinomycetes are components of the normal oral and genital-tract flora, their identification in the absence of sulfur granules in sputum, bronchial washings, and cervicovaginal secretions is of little significance.

Rx ACTINOMYCOSIS

Decisions about treatment are based on the collective clinical experience of the past 50 years. Actinomycosis requires prolonged treatment with high doses of antimicrobial agents. The need for intensive treatment is presumably due to the drugs' poor penetration of the thick-walled masses common in this infection and/or the sulfur granules themselves. Although therapy must be individualized, the intravenous administration of 18–24 million units of penicillin daily for 2–6 weeks, followed by oral therapy with penicillin or amoxicillin (total duration, 6–12 months), is a reasonable

TABLE 156-1 APPROPRIATE AND INAPPROPRIATE ANTIBIOTIC THERAPY FOR ACTINOMYCOSIS[a]

Category	Agent
Extensive successful clinical experience[b]	Penicillin: 18–24 mU/d IV q4h, 1–2 g/d PO q6h
	Erythromycin: 2–4 g/d IV q6h, 1–2 g/d PO q6h
	Tetracycline: 1–2 g/d PO q6h
	Doxycycline: 200 mg/d IV or PO q12–24h
	Minocycline: 200 mg/d IV or PO q12h
	Clindamycin: 2.7 g/d IV q8h, 1.2–1.8 g/d PO q6–8h
Anecdotal successful clinical experience	Ceftriaxone
	Ceftizoxime
	Imipenem
	Piperacillin-tazobactam
Agents that should be avoided	Metronidazole
	Aminoglycosides
	Oxacillin
	Dicloxacillin
	Cephalexin
Agents predicted to be efficacious on the basis of in vitro activity	Moxifloxacin
	Vancomycin
	Linezolid
	Quinupristin-dalfopristin

[a]Additional coverage for concomitant "companion" bacteria may be required.
[b]Controlled evaluations have not been performed. Dose and duration require individualization depending on the host, site, and extent of infection. As a general rule, a maximal parenteral antimicrobial dose for 2–6 weeks followed by oral therapy, for a total duration of 6–12 months, is required for serious infections and bulky disease, whereas a shorter course may suffice for less extensive disease, particularly in the oral-cervicofacial region.

guideline for serious infections and bulky disease. Less extensive disease, particularly that involving the oral-cervicofacial region, may be cured with a shorter course. If therapy is extended beyond the resolution of measurable disease, the risk of relapse—a clinical hallmark of this infection—will be minimized; CT and magnetic resonance imaging (MRI) are generally the most sensitive and objective techniques by which to accomplish this goal. A similar approach is reasonable for immunocompromised patients, although refractory disease has been described in HIV-infected individuals. Suitable alternative antimicrobial agents and those deemed unreliable are listed in **Table 156-1**. Although the role played by "companion" microbes in actinomycosis is unclear, many isolates are pathogens in their own right, and a regimen covering these organisms during the initial treatment course is reasonable.

Combined medical-surgical therapy is still advocated by some authorities. However, an increasing body of literature now supports an initial attempt at cure with medical therapy alone, even in extensive disease. CT and MRI should be used to monitor the response to therapy. In most cases, either surgery can be avoided or a less extensive procedure can be used. This approach is particularly valuable in sparing critical organs, such as the bladder or the reproductive organs in women of child-bearing age. For a well-defined abscess, percutaneous drainage in combination with medical therapy is a reasonable approach. When a critical location is involved (e.g., the epidural space, the CNS) or when suitable medical therapy fails, surgical intervention may be appropriate.

FURTHER READINGS

CLARRIDGE JE III, ZHANG Q: Genotypic diversity of clinical *Actinomyces* species: Phenotype, source, and disease correlation among genospecies. J Clin Microbiol 40:3442, 2002

COLMEGNA I et al: Disseminated *Actinomyces meyeri* infection resembling lung cancer with brain metastases. Am J Med Sci 326:152, 2003

KAYIKCIOGLU F et al: *Actinomyces* infection in the female genital tract. Eur J Obstet Gynecol Reprod Biol 118:77, 2005

LECOUVET F et al: The etiologic diagnosis of infectious discitis is improved by amplification-based DNA analysis. Arthritis Rheum 50:2985, 2004

PULVERER G et al: Human cervicofacial actinomycoses: Microbiologic data for 1997 cases. Clin Infect Dis 37:490, 2003

RUSSO TA: Actinomycosis, in *Principles and Practice of Infectious Diseases*, 6th ed, GL Mandell et al (eds). New York, Churchill Livingstone, 2005, pp 2924–2934

157 Infections Due to Mixed Anaerobic Organisms

Dennis L. Kasper, Ronit Cohen-Poradosu

DEFINITIONS

Anaerobic bacteria are organisms that require reduced oxygen tension for growth, failing to grow on the surface of solid media in 10% CO_2 in air. (In contrast, *microaerophilic bacteria* can grow in an atmosphere of 10% CO_2 in air or under anaerobic or aerobic conditions, although they grow best in the presence of only a small amount of atmospheric oxygen, and *facultative bacteria* can grow in the presence or absence of air.) This chapter describes infections caused by nonsporulating anaerobic bacteria. In general, anaerobes associated with human infections are relatively aerotolerant. They can survive for as long as 72 h in the presence of oxygen, although generally they do not multiply in this environment. A far smaller number of pathogenic anaerobic bacteria (which are also part of the normal flora) die after brief contact with oxygen, even in low concentrations.

The nonsporulating anaerobic bacteria exist as components of the normal flora on the mucosal surfaces of humans and animals. The major reservoirs of these bacteria are the mouth, lower gastrointestinal (GI) tract, skin, and female genital tract (**Table 157-1**). Among the constituents of the oral flora, anaerobes are the predominant commensal organisms, ranging in concentration from 10^9/mL in saliva to 10^{12}/mL in gingival scrapings. In the oral cavity, the ratio of anaerobic to aerobic bacteria ranges from 1:1 on the surface of a tooth to 1000:1 in the gingival crevices. Anaerobic bacteria are not found in appreciable numbers in the normal upper intestine until the distal ileum. In the colon, the proportion of anaerobes increases significantly, as does the overall bacterial count. In the colon, for example, there are 10^{11}–10^{12} organisms per gram of stool, and >99% of these organisms are anaerobic, with an anaerobe-to-aerobe ratio of ~1000:1. In the female genital tract, there are ~10^9 organisms per milliliter of secretions, with an anaerobe-to-aerobe ratio of ~10:1.

TABLE 157-1 ANAEROBIC HUMAN FLORA: AN OVERVIEW

Anatomic Site	Total Bacteria[a]	Aerobic/Anaerobic Ratio	Potential Pathogens
Oral cavity			
Saliva	10^8–10^9	1:1	*Fusobacterium nucleatum, Prevotella melaninogenica, Prevotella oralis* group, *Bacteroides ureolyticus* group, *Peptostreptococcus* spp.
Tooth surface	10^{10}–10^{11}	1:1	
Gingival crevices	10^{11}–10^{12}	10^3:1	
Gastrointestinal tract			
Stomach	0–10^5	1:1	
Jejunum/ileum	10^4–10^7	1:1	
Terminal ileum and colon	10^{11}–10^{12}	10^3:1	*Bacteroides* spp. (principally members of the *B. fragilis* group), *Prevotella* spp., *Clostridium* spp., *Peptostreptococcus* spp.
Female genital tract	10^7–10^9	10:1	*Peptostreptococcus* spp., *Bacteroides* spp., *Prevotella bivia*

[a]Per gram or milliliter.

Anaerobes play a key role in maintaining the balance between the host and its colonizing organisms. Hundreds of species of anaerobic bacteria have been identified as part of the normal flora of humans. Identification of as many as 500 anaerobic species in fecal specimens reflects the diversity of the anaerobic flora. Despite the complex array of bacteria in the normal flora, relatively few species are isolated commonly from human infection. Anaerobic infections occur when the harmonious relationship between the host and the bacteria is disrupted. Any site in the body is susceptible to infection with these indigenous organisms when a mucosal barrier or the skin is compromised by surgery, trauma, tumor, ischemia, or necrosis, all of which can reduce local tissue redox potentials. Because the sites that are colonized by anaerobes contain many species of bacteria, disruption of anatomic barriers allows the penetration of many organisms, resulting in mixed infections involving multiple species of anaerobes combined with facultative or microaerophilic organisms. Such mixed infections are seen in the head and neck (chronic sinusitis, chronic otitis media, Ludwig's angina, and periodontal abscesses). Brain abscesses and subdural empyema are the most common anaerobic infections of the central nervous system (CNS). Anaerobes are responsible for pleuropulmonary diseases such as aspiration pneumonia, necrotizing pneumonia, lung abscess, and empyema.

These organisms also play an important role in various intraabdominal infections, such as peritonitis and intraabdominal and hepatic abscesses (Chap. 121). They are isolated frequently in female genital tract infections, such as salpingitis, pelvic peritonitis, tuboovarian abscess, vulvovaginal abscess, septic abortion, and endometritis (Chap. 124). Anaerobic bacteria are also found often in infections of the skin, soft tissues, and bones and in bacteremia.

ETIOLOGY

The taxonomic classification of anaerobes is rapidly evolving, with frequent changes in nomenclature based on newly discovered relationships among bacterial species. The major anaerobic gram-positive cocci that produce disease are *Peptostreptococcus* spp. The major species of this genus that are involved in infections are *Peptostreptococcus micros, P. magnus, P. asaccharolyticus, P. anaerobius,* and *P. prevotii.* Clostridia (Chap. 135) are gram-positive rods that are isolated from wounds, abscesses, sites of abdominal infection, and blood. The principal anaerobic gram-negative bacilli found in human infections are the *Bacteroides fragilis* group as well as *Fusobacterium, Prevotella,* and *Porphyromonas* spp. Other members of the Bacteroidaceae family include *Bilophila wadsworthia,* an organism that has been isolated from infected sites and has been reported to cause serious infections. Gram-positive anaerobic non-spore-forming bacilli are uncommon as etiologic agents of human infection. *Propionibacterium acnes,* a rare cause of foreign-body infections, is one of the few nonclostridial gram-positive rods associated with infections.

The *B. fragilis* group contains the anaerobic pathogens most frequently isolated from clinical infections. Members of this group are part of the normal bowel flora; they include several distinct species, such as *B. fragilis, B. thetaiotaomicron, B. vulgatus, B. uniformis, B. ovatus,* and *Parabacteroides distasonis. B. fragilis* is the most important clinical isolate. However, in cultures of commensal fecal flora, *B. fragilis* is isolated in lower numbers than some of the other *Bacteroides* spp.

A second major group of phenotypically similar organisms is part of the indigenous oral flora. Thus these organisms are found at infected sites that can be seeded with oral microflora. Many of these species are pigment-producing bacteria belonging to two distinct genera, *Prevotella* and *Porphyromonas*; these genera comprise several pathogenic species, including *Porphyromonas gingivalis, Porphyromonas asaccharolytica,* and *Prevotella oralis. Porphyromonas* and *Prevotella* spp. cause localized infections that can spread contiguously.

In female genital tract infections, organisms normally colonizing the vagina (e.g., *Prevotella bivia* and *Prevotella disiens*) are the most frequent isolates, although *B. fragilis* is not uncommon. The *Fusobacterium* species *F. necrophorum, F. nucleatum,* and *F. varium,* which reside primarily in the oral cavity and the GI tract, are also isolated from clinical infections, including necrotizing pneumonia and abscesses. The skin flora contains anaerobic bacteria as well: *Propionibacterium* (mainly *P. acnes*) and peptostreptococci.

Infections caused by anaerobic bacteria most frequently are due to more than one organism. These polymicrobial infections may be caused by one or several anaerobic species or by a combination of anaerobic organisms and microaerophilic or facultative bacteria acting synergistically.

APPROACH TO THE PATIENT: Infections Due to Mixed Anaerobic Organisms

The physician must consider several points when approaching the patient with presumptive infection due to anaerobic bacteria.

1. Most of the organisms colonizing mucosal sites are harmless commensals; very few cause disease. When these organisms do cause disease, it often occurs in proximity to the mucosal site they colonize.
2. For anaerobes to cause tissue infection, they must spread beyond the normal mucosal barriers.
3. Conditions favoring the propagation of these bacteria, particularly a lowered oxidation-reduction potential, are necessary. These conditions exist at sites of trauma, tissue destruction, compromised vascular supply, and complications of preexisting infection, which produce necrosis.
4. There is a complex array of infecting flora. For example, as many as 12 types of organisms can be isolated from a suppurative site.
5. Anaerobic organisms tend to be found in abscess cavities or in necrotic tissue. The failure of an abscess to yield organisms on routine culture is a clue that the abscess is likely to contain anaerobic bacteria. Often smears of this "sterile pus" are found to be teeming with bacteria when Gram's stain is applied. Malodorous pus suggests anaerobic infection. Although some facultative organisms (e.g., *Staphylococcus aureus*) are also capable of causing abscesses, abscesses in organs or deeper body tissues should call to mind anaerobic infection.
6. Gas is found in many anaerobic infections of deep tissues but is not diagnostic because it can be produced by aerobic bacteria as well.
7. Although a putrid-smelling infection site or discharge is considered diagnostic for anaerobic infection, this manifestation usually develops late in the course and is present in only 30–50% of cases.
8. Some species (the best example being the *B. fragilis* group) require specific therapy. However, many synergistic infections can be cured with antibiotics directed at some but not all of the organisms involved. Antibiotic therapy, combined with debridement and drainage, disrupts the interdependent relationship among the bacteria, and some species that are resistant to the antibiotic do not survive without the co-infecting organisms.
9. Manifestations of severe sepsis and disseminated intravascular coagulation (DIC) are unusual in patients with purely anaerobic infection.

EPIDEMIOLOGY

Difficulties in the performance of appropriate cultures, contamination of cultures by aerobic bacteria or components of the normal flora, and the lack of readily available, reliable culture techniques have made it impossible to obtain accurate data on incidence or prevalence. However, anaerobic infections are encountered frequently in hospitals with active surgical, trauma, and obstetric and gynecologic services. Depending on the institution, anaerobic bacteria account for 0.5–12% of all cases of bacteremia.

PATHOGENESIS

Anaerobic bacterial infections usually occur when an anatomic barrier becomes disrupted and constituents of the local flora enter a site that was previously sterile. Because of the specific growth requirements of anaerobic organisms and their presence as commensals on mucosal surfaces, conditions must arise that allow these organisms to penetrate mucosal barriers and enter tissue with a lowered oxidation-reduction potential. Therefore, tissue ischemia, trauma, surgery, perforated viscus, shock, and aspiration provide environments conducive to the proliferation of anaerobes. In the case of a perforated viscus, hundreds of species of anaerobic bacteria are spilled into the peritoneal cavity, but many of these organisms are unable to survive because the highly vascularized tissue provides a sufficiently high redox potential. The entry of oxygen into the environment results in the selection of the more aerotolerant anaerobic organisms.

The ability of an organism to adhere to host tissues is important to the establishment of infection. Some oral species adhere to crevicular epithelium in the oral cavity. *Prevotella melaninogenica* actually attaches to other microorganisms; *P. gingivalis* is a common isolate in periodontal disease. These organisms have fimbriae that facilitate attachment. Some *Bacteroides* strains appear to be piliated, a characteristic that may account for their ability to adhere.

The most extensively studied virulence factor of the nonsporulating anaerobes is the capsular polysaccharide complex of *B. fragilis*. This organism is unique among anaerobes in its potential for virulence during growth at normally sterile sites. Although it constitutes only 0.5–1% of the normal colonic flora, *B. fragilis* is the anaerobe most commonly isolated from intraabdominal infections and bacteremia. One polysaccharide of *B. fragilis* possesses distinct biologic properties, such as the ability (owing to a unique zwitterionic motif of charged sugars) to promote abscess formation. Intraabdominal abscess induction is related to the capacity of the polysaccharide to stimulate the release of cytokines and chemokines—in particular, interleukin (IL) 8, IL-17, and tumor necrosis factor (TNF) α—from resident peritoneal cells. The release of cytokines and chemokines results in the chemotaxis of polymorphonuclear neutrophils (PMNs) into the peritoneum, where they adhere to mesothelial cells induced by TNF-α to upregulate their expression of intercellular adhesion molecule 1 (ICAM-1). PMNs adherent to ICAM-1-expressing cells probably represent the nidus for an abscess. Prophylactic or therapeutic administration of the polysaccharide to experimental animals confers protection against abscess induction after challenge with intestinal microorganisms capable of inducing abscesses. This protection is mediated by T cells controlling cytokine release; IL-10 appears to be the cytokine primarily responsible for downregulating the tissue response of abscess formation. Although abscesses constitute a host response that localizes and contains infecting bacteria, abscess formation in patients with sepsis often results in severe and chronic illness that requires surgical drainage in combination with antimicrobial therapy.

Anaerobic bacteria produce a number of exoproteins that are capable of enhancing the organisms' virulence. The collagenase produced by *P. gingivalis* may enhance tissue destruction. An enterotoxin has been identified in *B. fragilis* strains associated with diarrheal disease in animals and young children. Anaerobic gram-negative bacteria such as *B. fragilis* possess lipopolysaccharides (LPSs, endotoxins) that are 100–1000 times less biologically potent than endotoxins associated with aerobic gram-negative bacteria. This relative biologic inactivity may account for the lower frequency of DIC and purpura in *Bacteroides* bacteremia than in facultative and aerobic gram-negative bacillary bacteremia. An exception is the LPS from *Fusobacterium*, which may account for the severity of Lemierre's syndrome.

CLINICAL MANIFESTATIONS

Anaerobic Infections of the Mouth, Head, and Neck (See also Chap. 31) Anaerobic bacteria are commonly involved in infections of the mouth, head, and neck. The predominant isolates are components of the normal flora of the upper airways—mainly the *Bacteroides oralis* group, pigmented *Prevotella* spp., *P. asaccharolytica*, *Fusobacterium* spp., peptostreptococci, and microaerophilic streptococci.

Soft tissue infections of the oral-facial area may or may not be odontogenic. Odontogenic infections—primarily dental caries and periodontal disease—are common and have both local consequences (especially tooth loss) and the potential for life-threatening spread to the deep fascial spaces of the head and neck. Infections of the mouth can arise from either the supragingival or the subgingival dental plaque composed of bacteria colonizing the tooth surface. Supragingival plaque formation begins with the adherence of gram-positive bacteria to the tooth surface. This form of plaque is influenced by salivary and dietary components, oral hygiene, and local host factors. Supragingival plaque can lead to dental caries and, with further invasion, to pulpitis (endodontic infection) that can further perforate the alveolar bone, causing periapical abscess. Subgingival plaque is associated with periodontal infections (e.g., gingivitis, periodontitis, and periodontal abscess) that can further disseminate to adjacent structures such as the mandible, causing osteomyelitis of the maxillary sinuses. Periodontitis may also result in spreading infection that can involve adjacent bone or soft tissues.

NECROTIZING ULCERATIVE GINGIVITIS Gingivitis may become a necrotizing infection (trench mouth, Vincent's stomatitis). The onset of disease is usually sudden and is associated with tender bleeding gums, foul breath, and a bad taste. The gingival mucosa, especially the papillae between the teeth, becomes ulcerated and may be covered by a gray exudate, which is removable with gentle pressure. Patients may become systemically ill, developing fever, cervical lymphadenopathy, and leukocytosis. Occasionally, ulcerative gingivitis can spread to the buccal mucosa, the teeth, and the mandible or maxilla, resulting in widespread destruction of bone and soft tissue. This infection is termed *acute necrotizing ulcerative mucositis* (cancrum oris, noma). It destroys tissue rapidly, causing the teeth to fall out and large areas of bone—or even the whole mandible—to be sloughed. A strong putrid odor is frequently detected, although the lesions are not painful. The gangrenous lesions eventually heal, leaving large disfiguring defects. This infection most commonly follows a debilitating illness or affects severely malnourished children. It has been known to complicate leukemia or to develop in individuals with a genetic deficiency of catalase.

ACUTE NECROTIZING INFECTIONS OF THE PHARYNX These infections usually occur in association with ulcerative gingivitis. Symptoms include an extremely sore throat, foul breath, and a bad taste accompanied by fever and a sensation of choking. Examination of the pharynx demonstrates that the tonsillar pillars are swollen, red, ulcerated, and covered with a grayish membrane that peels easily. Lymphadenopathy and leukocytosis are common. The disease may last for only a few days or, if not treated, may persist for weeks. Lesions begin unilaterally but may spread to the other side of the pharynx or the larynx. Aspiration of the infected material by the patient can result in lung abscesses.

PERIPHARYNGEAL SPACE INFECTIONS These infections arise from the spread of organisms from the upper airways to potential spaces formed by the fascial planes of the head and neck. The etiology is typically polymicrobial and represents the normal flora of the mucosa of the originating site.

Peritonsillar abscess (*quinsy*) is a complication of acute tonsillitis caused mainly by a mixed flora containing anaerobes and group A *Streptococcus*. In submandibular space infection (*Ludwig's angina*), 80% of cases are caused by infection of the tissues surrounding the second and third molar teeth. This infection results in marked local swelling of tissues, with pain, trismus, and superior and posterior displacement of the tongue. Submandibular swelling of the neck can impair swallowing and cause respiratory obstruction. In some cases, tracheotomy may be life-saving. *Cervicofacial actinomycosis* (Chap. 156) is caused by a branching, gram-positive, non-spore-forming, strict/facultative anaerobe that is a part of the normal oral flora. This chronic disease is characterized by abscesses, draining sinus tracts, fistula, bone destruction, and fibrosis. It can easily be mistaken for malignancy or granulomatous disease. Actinomycosis less frequently involves the thorax, abdomen, pelvis, and CNS.

SINUSITIS AND OTITIS Anaerobic bacteria have been implicated in chronic sinusitis but play little role in acute sinusitis. In chronic sinusitis, anaerobic bacteria are found in 0–52% of cases, depending on the method used to collect specimens. In one study, cultures of samples from patients with chronic sinusitis and patients with an acute exacerbation of chronic sinusitis yielded aerobes only in 25% and 27% of cases, respectively; anaerobes only in 34% and 37%; and mixed organisms in 41% and 37%. The predominant aerobic bacteria were Enterobacteriaceae and *S. aureus* in both groups; in addition, *Streptococcus pneumoniae* was commonly isolated from the acute-exacerbation group. The predominant anaerobic bacteria in both groups were *Peptostreptococcus* spp., *Fusobacterium* spp., anaerobic gram-negative bacilli, and *P. acnes*.

Anaerobic bacteria are much more easily implicated in chronic suppurative otitis media than in acute otitis media. Purulent exudate from chronically draining ears has been found to contain anaerobes, particularly *Bacteroides* spp., in up to 50% of cases. *B. fragilis* has been isolated from up to 28% of patients with chronic otitis media.

COMPLICATIONS OF ANAEROBIC HEAD AND NECK INFECTIONS Contiguous craniad spread of these infections may result in osteomyelitis of the skull or mandible or in intracranial infections such as brain abscess and subdural empyema. Caudal spread can produce mediastinitis or pleuropulmonary infection. Hematogenous complications may also result from anaerobic infections of the head and neck. Bacteremia, which occasionally is polymicrobial, can lead to endocarditis or other distant infections. Lemierre's syndrome, which has been uncommon in the antimicrobial era, is an acute oropharyngeal infection with secondary septic thrombophlebitis of the internal jugular vein and frequent metastasis, most commonly to the lung. *F. necrophorum* is the usual cause. This infection typically begins with pharyngitis, which is followed by local invasion in the lateral pharyngeal space with resultant internal jugular vein thrombophlebitis. A typical clinical triad seen in recent series is pharyngitis, a tender/swollen neck, and noncavitating pulmonary infiltrates.

CNS Infections CNS infections associated with anaerobic bacteria are brain abscess (Chap. 376), epidural abscess, and subdural empyema. Anaerobic meningitis is rare and is usually related to parameningeal collection or shunt infection. If optimal bacteriologic techniques are employed, as many as 85% of brain abscesses yield anaerobic bacteria, which usually originate from otolaryngeal infection. Commonly isolated are peptostreptococci, *Fusobacterium* spp., *Bacteroides* spp., and *Prevotella* spp. Facultative or microaerophilic streptococci and coliforms are often part of a mixed infecting flora in brain abscesses.

Pleuropulmonary Infections Anaerobic pleuropulmonary infections result from the aspiration of oropharyngeal contents, often in the context of an altered state of consciousness or an absent gag reflex. Four clinical syndromes are associated with anaerobic pleuropulmonary infection produced by aspiration: simple aspiration pneumonia, necrotizing pneumonia, lung abscess, and empyema.

ASPIRATION PNEUMONITIS Bacterial aspiration pneumonitis must be distinguished from two other clinical syndromes associated with aspiration that are not of bacterial etiology. One syndrome results from aspiration of solids, usually food. Obstruction of major airways typically results in atelectasis and moderate nonspecific inflammation. Therapy consists of removal of the foreign body.

The second aspiration syndrome is more easily confused with bacterial aspiration. *Mendelson's syndrome,* a chemical pneumonitis, results from regurgitation of stomach contents and aspiration of chemical material, usually acidic gastric juices. Pulmonary inflammation—including the destruction of the alveolar lining, with transudation of fluid into the alveolar space—occurs with remarkable rapidity. Typically this syndrome develops within hours, often following anesthesia when the gag reflex is depressed. The patient becomes tachypneic, hypoxic, and febrile. The leukocyte count may rise, and the chest x-ray may evolve suddenly from normal to a complete bilateral "whiteout" within 8–24 h. Sputum production is minimal. The pulmonary signs and symptoms can resolve quickly with symptom-based therapy or can culminate in respiratory failure, with the subsequent development of bacterial superinfection over a period of days. Antibiotic therapy is not indicated unless bacterial infection supervenes.

In contrast to these syndromes, bacterial aspiration pneumonia develops over a period of several days or weeks rather than hours. It is seen in patients who are hospitalized and have a depressed gag reflex, impaired swallowing, or a tracheal or nasogastric tube; elderly patients; and patients with transiently impaired consciousness in the wake of seizures, cerebrovascular accidents, or alcoholic blackouts. Patients who enter the hospital with this syndrome typically have been ill for several days and generally report low-grade fever, malaise, and sputum production. In some patients, weight loss and anemia reflect a more chronic process. Usually the history reveals factors predisposing to aspiration, such as alcohol overdose or residence in a nursing home. Examination sometimes yields evidence of periodontal disease. Sputum characteristically is not malodorous unless the process has been under way for at least a week. A mixed bacterial flora with many PMNs is evident on Gram's staining of sputum. Expectorated sputum is unreliable for anaerobic cultures because of inevitable contamination by normal oral flora. Reliable specimens for culture can be obtained by transtracheal or transthoracic aspiration—techniques that are rarely used at present. Culture of protected-brush specimens or bronchoalveolar lavage fluid obtained by bronchoscopy is controversial.

Chest x-rays show consolidation in dependent pulmonary segments: in the basilar segments of the lower lobes if the patient has aspirated while upright and in either the posterior segment of the upper lobe (usually on the right side) or the superior segment of the lower lobe if the patient has aspirated while supine. The organisms isolated from the lungs reflect the pharyngeal flora; pigmented and nonpigmented *Prevotella* spp., *Peptostreptococcus* spp., *Bacteroides* spp., *Fusobacterium* spp., and anaerobic cocci are the most common isolates. The patient who aspirates in the hospital may also have a mixed infection involving enteric gram-negative rods. In a study on the microbiology of severe aspiration pneumonia in institutionalized elderly patients, gram-negative bacilli were cultured in 49% of cases (with an anaerobe also recovered in 14% of this group), anaerobes in 16%, and *S. aureus* in 12%.

NECROTIZING PNEUMONITIS This form of anaerobic pneumonitis is characterized by numerous small abscesses that spread to involve several pulmonary segments. The process can be indolent or fulminating. This syndrome is less common than either aspiration pneumonia or lung abscess and includes features of both types of infection.

ANAEROBIC LUNG ABSCESSES These abscesses result from subacute anaerobic pulmonary infection. The clinical syndrome typically involves a history of constitutional signs and symptoms (including malaise, weight loss, fever, night sweats, and foul-smelling sputum), perhaps over a period of weeks (Chap. 251). Patients who develop lung abscesses characteristically have dental infection and periodontitis, but lung abscesses in edentulous patients have been reported. Abscess cavities may be single or multiple and generally occur in dependent pulmonary segments (Fig. 157-1). Anaerobic abscesses must be distinguished from lesions associated with tuberculosis, neoplasia, and other conditions. Oral anaerobes predominate and are found in 60–80% of cases. There is also an important role for microaerophilic streptococci such as *S. milleri*. *S. aureus* and enteric gram-negative bacilli may be found as well. Septic pulmonary emboli may originate from intraabdominal or female genital tract infections and can produce anaerobic pneumonia.

EMPYEMA Empyema is a manifestation of long-standing anaerobic pulmonary infection. The clinical presentation, which includes foul-smelling sputum, resembles that of other anaerobic pulmonary infections. Patients may report pleuritic chest pain and marked chest-wall tenderness.

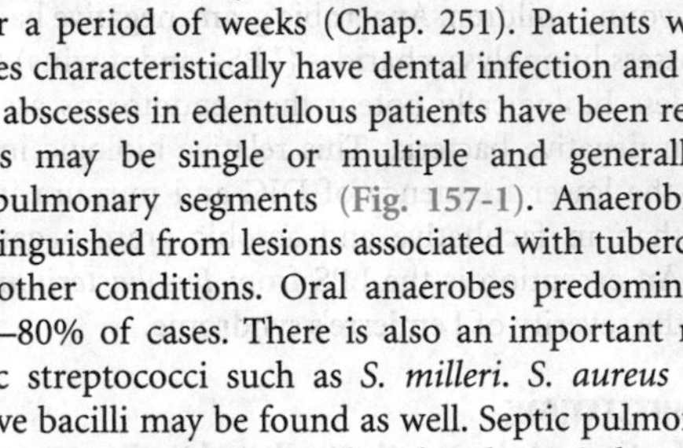

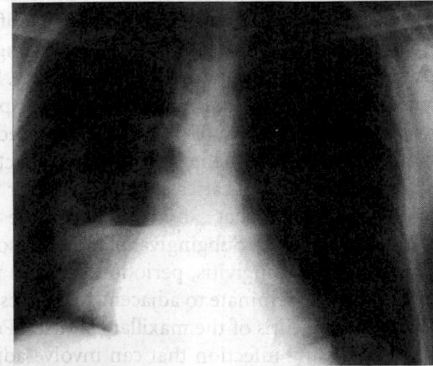

FIGURE 157-1 Chest radiograph of right-lower-lobe lung abscess in a 60-year-old alcoholic patient. *[From GL Mandell (ed): Atlas of Infectious Diseases, Vol VI. Philadelphia, Current Medicine Inc, Churchill Livingstone, 1996; with permission.]*

Empyema may be masked by overlying pneumonitis and should be considered especially in cases of persistent fever despite antibiotic therapy. Diligent physical examination and the use of ultrasound to localize a loculated empyema are important diagnostic tools. The collection of a foul-smelling exudate by thoracentesis is typical. Cultures of infected pleural fluid yield an average of 3.5 anaerobes and 0.6 facultative or aerobic bacterial species. Drainage is required. Defervescence, a return to a feeling of well-being, and resolution of the process may require several months.

Extension from a subdiaphragmatic infection may also result in anaerobic empyema.

Intraabdominal Infections Intraabdominal infections—mainly peritonitis and abscesses—are usually polymicrobial and represent the normal intestinal (especially colonic) flora. These infections usually follow a breach in the mucosal barrier occurring as a result of appendicitis, diverticulitis, neoplasm, inflammatory bowel disease, surgery, or trauma. On average, four to six species are isolated per specimen submitted to the microbiology laboratory, with a predominance of coliforms, anaerobes, and enterococci. The most common isolates are *Escherichia coli* and *B. fragilis.* Disease originating from proximal-bowel perforation reflects the flora of this site, with a predominance of aerobic and anaerobic gram-positive bacteria and *Candida*.

Enterotoxigenic *B. fragilis* has been associated with watery diarrhea in a few young children and adults. In case-control studies of children with undiagnosed diarrheal disease, enterotoxigenic *B. fragilis* was isolated from significantly more children with diarrhea than children in the control group. Neutropenic enterocolitis (typhlitis) has been associated with anaerobic infection of the cecum but—in the setting of neutropenia (Chap. 82)—may involve the entire bowel. Patients usually present with fever; abdominal pain, tenderness, and distention; and watery diarrhea. The bowel wall is edematous with hemorrhage and necrosis. The primary pathogen is thought by some authorities to be *Clostridium septicum*, but other clostridia and mixed anaerobic infections have also been implicated. More than 50% of patients developing early clinical signs can benefit from antibiotic therapy and bowel rest. Surgery is sometimes required to remove gangrenous bowel. See Chap. 121 for a complete discussion of intraabdominal infections.

Pelvic Infections The vagina of a healthy woman is one of the major reservoirs of anaerobic and aerobic bacteria. In the normal flora of the female genital tract, anaerobes outnumber aerobes by a ratio of ~10:1 and include anaerobic gram-positive cocci and *Bacteroides* spp. Anaerobes are isolated from most women with genital tract infections that are not caused by a sexually transmitted pathogen. The major anaerobic pathogens are *B. fragilis, P. bivia, P. disiens, P. melaninogenica*, anaerobic cocci, and *Clostridium* spp. Anaerobes are frequently encountered in tuboovarian abscess, septic abortion, pelvic abscess, endometritis, and postoperative wound infection, particularly following hysterectomy. Although these infections are often of mixed etiology, involving both anaerobes and coliforms, pure anaerobic infections without coliform or other facultative bacterial species occur more often in pelvic than in intraabdominal sites and are characterized by drainage of foul-smelling pus or blood from the uterus, generalized uterine or local pelvic tenderness, and continued fever and chills. Suppurative thrombophlebitis of the pelvic veins may complicate the infections and lead to repeated episodes of septic pulmonary emboli.

Anaerobic bacteria have been thought to be contributing factors in the etiology of bacterial vaginosis. This syndrome of unknown etiology is characterized by a profuse malodorous discharge and a change in the bacterial ecology that results in replacement of the *Lactobacillus*-dominated normal flora with an overgrowth of bacterial species including *Gardnerella vaginalis, Prevotella* spp., *Mobiluncus* spp., peptostreptococci, and genital mycoplasmas. A study based on 16S rRNA identification found other anaerobes that were predominant in cases but not in controls: *Atopobium, Leptotrichia, Megasphaera*, and *Eggerthella.* Anaerobic bacteria are thought to play a role in the etiology of pelvic inflammatory disease (Chap. 124), and several investigations have shown an association between bacterial vaginosis and the development of pelvic inflammatory disease.

Pelvic infections due to *Actinomyces* spp. have been associated with the use of intrauterine devices (Chap. 156).

Skin and Soft Tissue Infections Injury to skin, bone, or soft tissue by trauma, ischemia, or surgery creates a suitable environment for anaerobic infections. These infections are most frequently found in sites prone to contamination with feces or with upper airway secretions—e.g., wounds associated with intestinal surgery, decubitus ulcers, or human bites. Deep soft-tissue infections associated with anaerobic bacteria are crepitant cellulitis, synergistic cellulitis, gangrene, and necrotizing fasciitis (Chaps. 119 and 135). Moreover, these organisms have been isolated from cutaneous abscesses, rectal abscesses, and axillary sweat gland infections (hidradenitis suppurativa). Anaerobes are frequently cultured from foot ulcers of diabetic patients.

These soft tissue or skin infections are usually polymicrobial. A mean of 4.8 bacterial species are isolated, with an anaerobe-to-aerobe ratio of ~3:2. The most frequently isolated organisms include *Bacteroides* spp., peptostreptococci, enterococci, clostridia, and *Proteus* spp. The involvement of anaerobes in these types of infections is associated with a higher frequency of fever, foul-smelling lesions, gas in the tissues, and visible foot ulcer.

Anaerobic bacterial synergistic gangrene (*Meleney's gangrene*), a rare infection of the superficial fascia, is characterized by exquisite pain, redness, and swelling followed by induration. Erythema surrounds a central zone of necrosis. A granulating ulcer forms at the original center as necrosis and erythema extend outward. Symptoms are limited to pain; fever is not typical. These infections usually involve a combination of *Peptostreptococcus* spp. and *S. aureus*; the usual site of infection is an abdominal surgical wound or the area surrounding an ulcer on an extremity. Treatment includes surgical removal of necrotic tissue and antimicrobial administration.

Necrotizing fasciitis, a rapidly spreading destructive disease of the fascia, is usually attributed to group A streptococci (Chap. 130) but can also be a mixed infection involving anaerobes and aerobes, usually after surgeries and in patients with diabetes or peripheral vascular disease. The most frequently isolated anaerobes in these infections are *Peptostreptococcus* and *Bacteroides* spp. Gas may be found in the tissues. Similarly, myonecrosis can be associated with mixed anaerobic infection. *Fournier's gangrene* consists of cellulitis involving the scrotum, perineum, and anterior abdominal wall, with mixed anaerobic organisms spreading along deep external fascial planes and causing extensive loss of skin.

Bone and Joint Infections Although actinomycosis (Chap. 156) accounts on a worldwide basis for most anaerobic infections in bone, organisms including peptostreptococci or microaerophilic cocci, *Bacteroides* spp., *Fusobacterium* spp., and *Clostridium* spp. can also be involved. These infections frequently arise adjacent to soft tissue infections. Hematogenous seeding of bone is uncommon. *Prevotella* and *Porphyromonas* spp. are detected in infections involving the maxilla and mandible, whereas *Clostridium* spp. have been reported as anaerobic pathogens in cases of osteomyelitis of the long bones following fracture or trauma. Fusobacteria have been isolated in pure culture from sites of osteomyelitis adjacent to the perinasal sinuses. Peptostreptococci and microaerophilic cocci have been reported as significant pathogens in infections involving the skull, mastoid, and prosthetic implants placed in bone. In patients with osteomyelitis (Chap. 120), the most reliable culture specimen is a bone biopsy sample free of normal uninfected skin and subcutaneous tissue. In patients with anaerobic osteomyelitis, a mixed flora is frequently isolated from a bone biopsy specimen.

In cases of anaerobic septic arthritis, the most common isolates are *Fusobacterium* spp. Most of the patients involved have uncontrolled peritonsillar infections progressing to septic cervical venous thrombophlebitis (Lemierre's syndrome) and resulting in hematogenous dissemination with a predilection for the joints. Unlike anaerobic osteomyelitis, anaerobic pyoarthritis in most cases is not polymicrobial and may be acquired hematogenously. Anaerobes are important pathogens in infections involving prosthetic joints; in these infections, the causative organisms (such as *Peptostreptococcus* spp. and *P. acnes*) are part of the normal skin flora.

Bacteremia Transient bacteremia is a well-known event in healthy people whose anatomic mucosal barriers have been injured (e.g., during dental extractions or dental scaling). These bacteremic episodes, which are often due to anaerobes, have no pathologic consequences. However, anaerobic bacteria are found in cultures of blood from clinically ill patients when proper culture techniques are used. Anaerobes have accounted for 0.5–12% of all bacteremias, depending on the institution. *B. fragilis* is the single most common anaerobic isolate from the bloodstream, accounting for 60–80% of anaerobic bacteremias.

In recent years, the rate of isolation of anaerobic bacteria from blood cultures has been decreasing. Studies from the 1970s and early 1980s found that 10–15% of positive blood cultures yielded anaerobes, while more recent surveys have found rates as low as 4%. This change may be related to the administration of antibiotic prophylaxis before intestinal surgery, the earlier recognition of localized infections, and the empirical use of broad-spectrum antibiotics for presumed infection. However, anaerobic bacteremia may be reemerging. Comparing two periods (1993–1996 and 2001–2004), investigators at the Mayo Clinics found a 74% increase in the incidence of anaerobic bacteremias per 100,000 patient-days; this finding contrasts with a 45% decrease in incidence from 1977 to 1988 at the same institution.

Once the organism in the blood has been identified, both the portal of bloodstream entry and the underlying problem that probably led to seeding of the bloodstream can often be deduced from an understanding of the organism's normal site of residence. For example, mixed anaerobic bacteremia including *B. fragilis* usually implies colonic pathology with mucosal disruption from neoplasia, diverticulitis, or some other inflammatory lesion. The initial manifestations are determined by the portal of entry and reflect the localized condition. When bloodstream invasion occurs, patients can become extremely ill, with rigors and hectic fevers. The clinical picture may be quite similar to that seen in sepsis involving aerobic gram-negative bacilli. Although complications of anaerobic bacteremia (e.g., septic thrombophlebitis and septic shock) have been reported, their incidence in association with anaerobic bacteremia is low. Anaerobic bacteremia is potentially fatal and requires rapid diagnosis and appropriate therapy. The mortality rate appears to increase with the age of the patient (with reported rates of >66% among patients >60 years old), with the isolation of multiple species from the bloodstream, and with the failure to surgically remove a focus of infection.

Endocarditis and Pericarditis (See also Chap. 118) Endocarditis due to anaerobes is uncommon. However, anaerobic streptococci, which are often classified incorrectly, are responsible for this disease more frequently than is generally appreciated. Gram-negative anaerobes are unusual causes of endocarditis. Signs and symptoms of anaerobic endocarditis are similar to those of endocarditis due to facultative organisms. Mortality rates of 21–43% have been reported for anaerobic endocarditis.

Anaerobes, particularly *B. fragilis* and *Peptostreptococcus* spp., are uncommonly found in infected pericardial fluids. Anaerobic pericarditis is associated with a mortality rate of >50%.

DIAGNOSIS

There are three critical steps in the diagnosis of anaerobic infection: (1) proper specimen collection; (2) rapid transport of the specimens to the microbiology laboratory, preferably in anaerobic transport media; and (3) proper handling of the specimens by the laboratory. Specimens must be collected by meticulous sampling of infected sites, with avoidance of contamination by the normal flora. When such contamination is likely, the specimen is unacceptable. Examples of specimens unacceptable for anaerobic culture include sputum collected by expectoration or nasal tracheal suction, bronchoscopy specimens, samples collected directly through the vaginal vault, urine collected by voiding, and feces. Specimens appropriate for anaerobic culture include sterile body fluids such as blood, pleural fluid, peritoneal fluid, cerebrospinal fluid, and aspirates or biopsies from normally sterile sites.

Because even brief exposure to oxygen may kill some anaerobic organisms and result in failure to isolate them in the laboratory, air must be expelled from the syringe used to aspirate the abscess cavity, and the needle must be capped with a sterile rubber stopper. It is also important to remember that prior antibiotic therapy reduces cultivability of these bacteria. Specimens can be injected into transport bottles containing a reduced medium or taken immediately in syringes to the laboratory for direct culture on anaerobic media. In general, swabs should not be used. If a swab must be used, it should be placed in a reduced semisolid carrying medium before transport to the laboratory. Delays in transport may lead to a failure to isolate anaerobes due to exposure to oxygen or overgrowth of facultative organisms, which may eliminate or obscure any anaerobes that are present. All clinical specimens from suspected anaerobic infections should be Gram-stained and examined for organisms with characteristic morphology. It is not unusual for organisms to be observed on Gram's staining but not isolated in culture. If purulent materials are found to be sterile or organisms are seen on Gram's staining but do not grow in the culture, the involvement of anaerobes should be suspected.

Because of the time and difficulty involved in the isolation of anaerobic bacteria, diagnosis of anaerobic infections must frequently be based on presumptive evidence. Certain sites with lowered oxidation-reduction potential (e.g., avascular necrotic tissues) favor the diagnosis of an anaerobic infection. When infections occur in proximity to mucosal surfaces normally harboring an anaerobic flora, such as the GI tract, female genital tract, or oropharynx, anaerobes should be considered as potential etiologic agents. A foul odor is often indicative of anaerobes, which produce certain organic acids as they proliferate in necrotic tissue. Although these odors are nearly pathognomonic for anaerobic infection, the absence of odor does not exclude an anaerobic etiology. Because anaerobes often coexist with other bacteria to cause mixed or synergistic infection, Gram's staining of exudate frequently reveals numerous pleomorphic cocci and bacilli suggestive of anaerobes. Sometimes these organisms have morphologic characteristics associated with specific species.

The presence of gas in tissues is highly suggestive, but not diagnostic, of anaerobic infection. When cultures of obviously infected sites yield no growth, streptococci only, or a single aerobic species (such as *E. coli*) and Gram's staining reveals a mixed flora, the implication is that the anaerobic microorganisms failed to grow because of inadequate transport and/or culture techniques. Failure of an infection to respond to antibiotics that are not active against anaerobes (e.g., aminoglycosides and—in some circumstances—penicillin, cephalosporins, or tetracyclines) suggests an anaerobic etiology.

℞ ANAEROBIC INFECTIONS

Successful therapy for anaerobic infections requires the administration of a combination of appropriate antibiotics, surgical resection, debridement of devitalized tissues, and drainage either by surgery or percutaneously (guided by an imaging technique such as CT, MRI, or ultrasound). Perforations must be closed promptly, closed spaces drained, tissue compartments decompressed, and an adequate blood supply established. Abscess cavities should be drained as soon as fluctuation or localization occurs.

ANTIBIOTIC THERAPY AND RESISTANCE Decisions about the treatment of anaerobic infections with antibiotics are usually based on known resistance patterns in certain species, on the likelihood of encountering a given species in the case at hand, and on Gram's stain findings. Antibiotics active against clinically relevant anaerobes can be grouped into four categories on the basis of their predicted activity (**Table 157-2**). (Nearly all the drugs listed have toxic side effects, which are described in detail in Chap. 127.) In many infections, anaerobes are mixed with coliforms and other facultative organisms. The best therapeutic regimens, therefore, are usually those active against both aerobic and anaerobic bac-

TABLE 157-2 ANTIMICROBIAL THERAPY FOR INFECTIONS INVOLVING COMMONLY ENCOUNTERED ANAEROBIC GRAM-NEGATIVE RODS

Category 1 (<2% Resistance)	Category 2 (<15% Resistance)	Category 3 (Variable Resistance)	Category 4 (Resistance)
Carbapenems (imipenem, meropenem) Metronidazole[a] β-Lactam/β-lactamase inhibitor combination (ampicillin/sulbactam, ticarcillin/clavulanic acid, piperacillin/tazobactam) Chloramphenicol[b]	Cephamycins Clindamycin High-dose antipseudomonal penicillins	Penicillin Cephalosporins Tetracycline Vancomycin Erythromycin Tigecycline Newer quinolones (moxifloxacin, gatifloxacin)	Aminoglycosides Monobactams Trimethoprim-sulfamethoxazole

[a]Usually needs to be given in combination with aerobic bacterial coverage. For infections originating below the diaphragm, aerobic gram-negative coverage is essential. For infections from an oral source, aerobic gram-positive coverage is added. Metronidazole also is not active against *Actinomyces, Propionibacterium*, or other gram-positive non-spore-forming bacilli (e.g., *Eubacterium, Bifidobacterium*) and is unreliable against peptostreptococci.
[b]Chloramphenicol is probably not as effective as other category 1 antimicrobials in treating anaerobic infections.

teria. The choice of empirical antibiotics for the anaerobes in mixed infections can nearly always be made reliably, since patterns of antimicrobial susceptibility are usually predictable (Chap. 127 and Table 157-2).

Antibiotic susceptibility testing of anaerobic bacteria has been difficult and controversial. Owing to the slow growth rate of many anaerobes, the lack of standardized testing methods and of clinically relevant standards for resistance, and the generally good results obtained with empirical therapy, there has been limited interest in testing these organisms for antibiotic susceptibility. However, a recent study of antibiotic-treated patients with *Bacteroides* isolates from blood found mortality rates of 45% among those whose isolates were deemed resistant to the agent used and 16% among those whose isolates were deemed sensitive. These figures suggest that in vitro susceptibility testing should be performed for *Bacteroides* isolates from hospitalized patients with bacteremia and that the results of this testing should guide treatment. In general, cure rates of >80% can be attained among *Bacteroides*-infected patients with appropriate antimicrobial therapy and drainage. Of the drugs active against most clinically relevant anaerobes, metronidazole, β-lactam/β-lactamase inhibitor combinations, and carbapenems are preferred.

Antibiotic resistance in anaerobic bacteria is an increasing problem. Nearly all organisms in the *B. fragilis* group (>97%) are resistant to penicillin G. The cephamycins (cefoxitin and cefotetan) are more active against this group, but resistance rates between 8% and 14% were observed between 1987 and 2000. Rates of resistance to β-lactam agents among anaerobes other than *Bacteroides* are lower but highly variable. β-Lactam/β-lactamase inhibitor combinations such as ampicillin/sulbactam, ticarcillin/clavulanic acid, and piperacillin/tazobactam are usually a good option. Metronidazole is active against gram-negative anaerobes, including the *B. fragilis* group; resistance is rare but has been reported. Resistance to metronidazole is more common among gram-positive anaerobes, including *P. acnes, Actinomyces* spp., lactobacilli, and anaerobic streptococci. In the United States, rates of clindamycin resistance among isolates of the *B. fragilis* group increased from 3% in 1982 to 16% in 1996 and 26% in 2000, with figures as high as 44% in some series. Rates of resistance to clindamycin among non-*Bacteroides* anaerobes are much lower (<10%).

If a patient fails to respond to one of the category 1 or category 2 drugs (Table 157-2), consideration should be given to alternative therapy and to determination of the resistance patterns among *Bacteroides* isolates. Although in vitro resistance of *Bacteroides* spp. to chloramphenicol has not been reported, this drug may not be as effective as other category 1 drugs. Newer available options include tigecycline, the first glycylcycline to be approved by the U.S. Food and Drug Administration. Tigecycline is active against some anaerobic bacteria, including *Peptostreptococcus* spp., *Propionibacterium* spp., *Prevotella* spp., *Fusobacterium* spp., and most *Bacteroides* spp. Its efficacy for treatment of intraabdominal infections was comparable to that of imipenem in two phase 2 clinical trials. Data from in vitro susceptibility studies and clinical trials suggest that the newer fluoroquinolones (e.g., moxifloxacin, gatifloxacin, and gemifloxacin) will be useful in the treatment of mixed aerobic-anaerobic infections. However, these drugs exhibit relatively weak in vitro activity against many *Bacteroides* spp. other than *B. fragilis*, including *B. thetaiotaomicron, B. vulgatus*, and *B. uniformis*.

TREATMENT OF INFECTIONS AT SPECIFIC SITES In clinical situations, specific regimens must be tailored to the initial site of infection. The duration of therapy also depends on the infection site; the reader is referred to specific chapters on sites of infection for recommendations.

β-Lactamase production has been reported in anaerobic strains that are usually isolated from infections originating above the diaphragm. Up to 60% of clinical isolates classified as *Prevotella* or *Porphyromonas* spp., non–*B. fragilis* species of *Bacteroides*, or *Fusobacterium* spp. reportedly produce β-lactamase. The clinical significance of resistance in these organisms has been suggested by studies showing clindamycin to be superior to penicillin (which for many years was considered the therapeutic "gold standard") for the treatment of lung abscesses. Presumably, the success of clindamycin is attributable to a broader spectrum of activity against oral anaerobes; thus, a combination of penicillin and metronidazole or another antibiotic combination that is active against both oral anaerobes and aerobes is likely to be as effective as clindamycin. Bronchoscopy in lung abscess is indicated only to rule out airway obstruction and does not enhance drainage; in any event, it should be delayed until the antimicrobial regimen has begun to affect the disease process so that the procedure does not spread the infection. Surgery is almost never indicated because of the danger of spilling the abscess contents into the lungs.

Although many oral anaerobic infections and most cases of anaerobic pneumonia still respond to penicillin therapy, some infections due to oral organisms fail to respond to this drug, and in these cases the use of a drug that is effective against penicillin-resistant anaerobes is recommended (Table 157-2). Life-threatening infections involving the anaerobic flora of the mouth, such as space infections of the head and neck, should be treated empirically as if penicillin-resistant anaerobes are involved. Less serious infections involving the oral microflora can be treated with penicillin alone; metronidazole can be added (or clindamycin can be substituted) if the patient responds poorly to penicillin therapy. Combinations of antibiotics used to treat mixed infections of oral origin must include drugs active against the gram-positive aerobic flora of the mouth.

Chloramphenicol has been used successfully against anaerobic CNS infections at doses of 30–60 mg/kg per day, with the exact dose depending on the severity of illness. However, penicillin G and metronidazole also cross the blood-brain barrier and are bactericidal for many anaerobic organisms (Chap. 376).

Anaerobic infections arising below the diaphragm (e.g., colonic and intraabdominal infections) must be treated specifically with agents active against *Bacteroides* spp. (Table 157-2). In intraabdominal sepsis (Chap. 121), the use of antibiotics effective against penicillin-resistant anaerobes has clearly reduced the incidence of postoperative infections and serious infectious complications. Specifically, a drug from category 1 (Table 157-2) must be included for broad-spectrum coverage. Recommended doses for commonly used category 1 drugs are given in **Table 157-3**. Therapy for intraabdominal sepsis must also include drugs active against the gram-neg-

TABLE 157-3 DOSES AND SCHEDULES FOR TREATMENT OF SERIOUS INFECTIONS DUE TO COMMONLY ENCOUNTERED ANAEROBIC GRAM-NEGATIVE RODS

First-Line Therapy	Dose	Schedule[a]
Metronidazole[b]	500 mg	q6h
Ticarcillin/clavulanic acid	3.1 g	q4h
Piperacillin/tazobactam	3.375 g	q6h
Imipenem	0.5 g	q6h
Meropenem	1.0 g	q8h

[a]See disease-specific chapters for recommendations on duration of therapy.
[b]Should generally be used in conjunction with drugs active against aerobic or facultative organisms.
Note: All drugs are given by the IV route.

ative aerobic flora of the bowel. If the involvement of gram-positive bacteria such as enterococci is suspected, either ampicillin or vancomycin should be added. A meta-analysis of 40 randomized or quasi-randomized controlled trials of 16 antibiotic regimens for secondary peritonitis showed equivalent clinical success for all regimens.

Cases of anaerobic osteomyelitis in which a mixed flora is isolated from a bone biopsy specimen should be treated with a regimen that covers all the isolates. When an anaerobic organism is recognized as a major or sole pathogen infecting a joint, the duration of treatment should be similar to that used for arthritis caused by aerobic bacteria (Chap. 328). Therapy includes the management of underlying disease states, the administration of appropriate antimicrobial agents, temporary joint immobilization, percutaneous drainage of effusions, and (usually) the removal of infected protheses or internal fixation devices. Surgical drainage and debridement procedures such as sequestrectomy are essential for the removal of necrotic tissue that can sustain anaerobic infections.

The outcome of anaerobic bacteremia is significantly better in patients either initially given or switched to appropriate therapy based on known antibiotic susceptibilities.

FAILURE OF THERAPY Anaerobic infections that fail to respond to treatment or that relapse should be reassessed. Consideration should be given to additional surgical drainage or debridement. Superinfections with resistant gram-negative facultative or aerobic bacteria should be ruled out. The possibility of drug resistance must be entertained; if resistance is involved, repeated cultures may yield the pathogenic organism.

SUPPORTIVE MEASURES Other supportive measures in the management of anaerobic infections include careful attention to fluid and electrolyte balance (since extensive local edema may lead to hypoalbuminemia), hemodynamic support for septic shock, immobilization of infected extremities, maintenance of adequate nutrition during chronic infections by parenteral hyperalimentation, relief of pain, and anticoagulation with heparin for thrombophlebitis. For patients with severe anaerobic infections of soft tissues, hyperbaric oxygen therapy is advocated by some experts, but its value has not been proven in controlled trials.

FURTHER READINGS

ALDRIDGE KE et al: Bacteremia due to *Bacteroides fragilis* group: Distribution of species, beta-lactamase production and antimicrobial susceptibility patterns. Antimicrob Agents Chemother 47:148, 2003

KURIYAMA T et al: Antimicrobial susceptibility of 800 anaerobic isolates from patients with dentoalveolar infection to 13 oral antibiotics. Oral Microbiol Immunol 22:285, 2007

LASSMAN B et al: Reemergence of anaerobic bacteremia. Clin Infect Dis 44:895, 2007

MAZMANIAN SK et al: The love-hate relationship between bacterial polysaccharides and the immune system. Nat Rev Immunol 6:849, 2006

SALONEN JH et al: Clinical significance and outcome of anaerobic bacteremia. Clin Infect Dis 26:1413, 1998

SNYDMAN DR et al: National survey on the susceptibility of *Bacteroides fragilis* group: Report and analysis of trends in the United States from 1997 to 2004. Antimicrob Agents Chemother 51:1649, 2007

SOLOMKIN JS et al: Guidelines for the selection of anti-infective agents for complicated intra-abdominal infections. Clin Infect Dis 37:997, 2003

TZIANABOS AO et al: Anaerobic infections: General concepts, in *Principles and Practice of Infectious Diseases*, 6th ed, GL Mandell et al (eds). Philadelphia, Elsevier Churchill Livingstone, 2005, pp 2810–2816

SECTION 8 MYCOBACTERIAL DISEASES

158 Tuberculosis

Mario C. Raviglione, Richard J. O'Brien

Tuberculosis, one of the oldest diseases known to affect humans, is a major cause of death worldwide. This disease, which is caused by bacteria of the *Mycobacterium tuberculosis* complex, usually affects the lungs, although other organs are involved in up to one-third of cases. If properly treated, tuberculosis caused by drug-susceptible strains is curable in virtually all cases. If untreated, the disease may be fatal within 5 years in 50–65% of cases. Transmission usually takes place through the airborne spread of droplet nuclei produced by patients with infectious pulmonary tuberculosis.

ETIOLOGIC AGENT

Mycobacteria belong to the family Mycobacteriaceae and the order Actinomycetales. Of the pathogenic species belonging to the *M. tuberculosis* complex, the most common and important agent of human disease is *M. tuberculosis*. The complex includes *M. bovis* (the bovine tubercle bacillus—characteristically resistant to pyrazinamide, once an important cause of tuberculosis transmitted by unpasteurized milk, and currently the cause of a small percentage of cases worldwide), *M. caprae* (related to *M. bovis*), *M. africanum* (isolated from cases in West, Central, and East Africa), *M. microti* (the "vole" bacillus, a less virulent and rarely encountered organism), *M. pinnipedii* (a bacillus infecting seals and sea lions in the southern hemisphere and recently isolated from humans), and *M. canettii* (a rare isolate from East African cases that produces unusual smooth colonies on solid media and is considered closely related to a supposed progenitor type).

M. tuberculosis is a rod-shaped, non-spore-forming, thin aerobic bacterium measuring 0.5 μm by 3 μm. Mycobacteria, including *M. tuberculosis*, are often neutral on Gram's staining. However, once stained, the bacilli cannot be decolorized by acid alcohol; this characteristic justifies their classification as acid-fast bacilli (AFB; **Fig. 158-1**). Acid fastness is due mainly to the organisms' high content of mycolic acids, long-chain cross-linked fatty acids, and other cell-wall lipids. Microorganisms other than mycobacteria that display some acid fastness include species of *Nocardia* and *Rhodococcus*, *Legionella micdadei*, and the protozoa *Isospora* and *Cryptosporidium*. In the mycobacterial cell wall, lipids (e.g., mycolic acids) are linked to underlying arabinogalactan and peptidoglycan. This structure confers very low permeability of the cell wall, thus reducing the effectiveness of most antibiotics. Another molecule in the mycobacterial cell wall, lipoarabinomannan, is involved in the pathogen-host interaction and facilitates the survival of *M. tuberculosis* within macrophages. The complete genome sequence of *M. tuberculosis* comprises 4043 genes encoding 3993 proteins and 50 genes encoding RNAs; its high guanine-plus-cytosine content (65.6%) is indicative of an aerobic lifestyle. A large proportion of genes are devoted to the production of enzymes involved in cell wall metabolism.

EPIDEMIOLOGY

More than 5 million new cases of tuberculosis (all forms, both pulmonary and extrapulmonary) were reported to the World Health Organization (WHO) in 2005; >90% of cases were reported from developing countries. However, because of insufficient case detection and incomplete notification, reported cases represent only ~60% of total estimated cases. The WHO estimated that 8.8 million new cases of tuberculosis occurred worldwide in 2005, 95% of them in developing countries of Asia (4.9 million), Africa (2.6 million), the Middle East

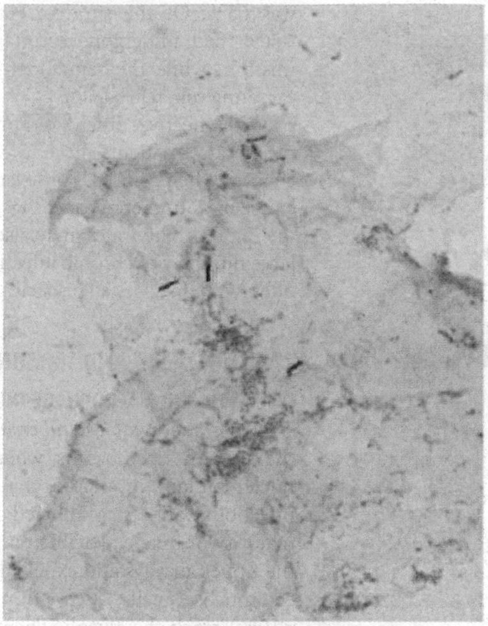

FIGURE 158-1 Acid-fast bacillus smear showing *M. tuberculosis* bacilli. *(Courtesy of the CDC, Atlanta.)*

(0.6 million), and Latin America (0.4 million). It is further estimated that 1.6 million deaths from tuberculosis occurred in 2005, 95% of them in developing countries. Estimates of tuberculosis incidence rates (per 100,000 population) and numbers of tuberculosis-related deaths in 2005 are depicted in Fig. 158-2 and Fig. 158-3, respectively.

During the late 1980s and early 1990s, numbers of reported cases of tuberculosis increased in industrialized countries. These increases were related largely to immigration from countries with a high prevalence of tuberculosis; infection with HIV; social problems, such as increased urban poverty, homelessness, and drug abuse; and dismantling of tuberculosis services. During the past few years, numbers of reported cases have begun to decline again or stabilized in industrialized nations. In the United States, with the implementation of stronger control programs, the decrease resumed in 1993. In 2005, 14,097 cases of tuberculosis (4.8 cases per 100,000 population) were reported to the Centers for Disease Control and Prevention (CDC).

In the United States, tuberculosis is uncommon among young adults of European descent, who have only rarely been exposed to *M. tuberculosis* infection during recent decades. In contrast, because of a high risk in the past, the prevalence of *M. tuberculosis* infection is relatively high among elderly Caucasians, who remain at increased risk of developing active tuberculosis. Tuberculosis in the United States is also a disease of young adult members of the HIV-infected, immigrant, and disadvantaged/marginalized populations. Similarly, in Europe, tuberculosis has reemerged as an important public health problem, mainly as a result of cases among immigrants from high-prevalence countries.

Recent data on trends indicate that in 2005 tuberculosis incidence was stable or falling in most regions; the result is a small decline globally from figures in previous years. This global reduction is due largely to an apparent peaking in sub-Saharan Africa, where incidence had risen steeply since the 1980s as a result of the HIV epidemic and the paucity of health services. In eastern Europe, incidence increased during the 1990s because of deterioration in socioeconomic conditions and the health care infrastructure; however, after peaking in 2001, incidence has recently stabilized.

FROM EXPOSURE TO INFECTION

M. tuberculosis is most commonly transmitted from a person with infectious pulmonary tuberculosis to others by droplet nuclei, which are aerosolized by coughing, sneezing, or speaking. The tiny droplets dry rapidly; the smallest (<5–10 μm in diameter) may remain suspended in the air for several hours and may reach the terminal air passages when inhaled. There may be as many as 3000 infectious nuclei per cough. Other routes of transmission of tubercle bacilli (e.g., through the skin or the placenta) are uncommon and of no epidemiologic significance.

The probability of contact with a person who has an infectious form of tuberculosis, the intimacy and duration of that contact, the degree of infectiousness of the case, and the shared environment in which the contact takes place are all important determinants of the likelihood of transmission. Several studies of close-contact situations have clearly demonstrated that tuberculosis patients whose sputum contains AFB visible by microscopy are the most likely to transmit the infection. The most infectious patients have cavitary pulmonary disease or, much less commonly, laryngeal tuberculosis and produce sputum containing as many as 10^5–10^7 AFB/mL. Patients with sputum smear–negative/culture-positive tuberculosis are less infectious, and those with culture-negative pulmonary disease and extrapulmonary tuberculosis are essentially noninfectious. Because persons with both HIV infection and tuberculosis are less likely to have cavitations, they may be less infectious than persons without HIV co-infection. Crowding in poorly ventilated rooms is one of the most important factors in the transmission of tubercle bacilli, since it increases the intensity of contact with a case.

In short, the risk of acquiring *M. tuberculosis* infection is determined mainly by exogenous factors. Because of delays in seeking care and in making a diagnosis, it is estimated that, in high-prevalence settings, up to 20 contacts may be infected by each AFB-positive case before the index case is found to have tuberculosis.

FROM INFECTION TO DISEASE

Unlike the risk of acquiring infection with *M. tuberculosis*, the risk of developing disease after being infected depends largely on endogenous fac-

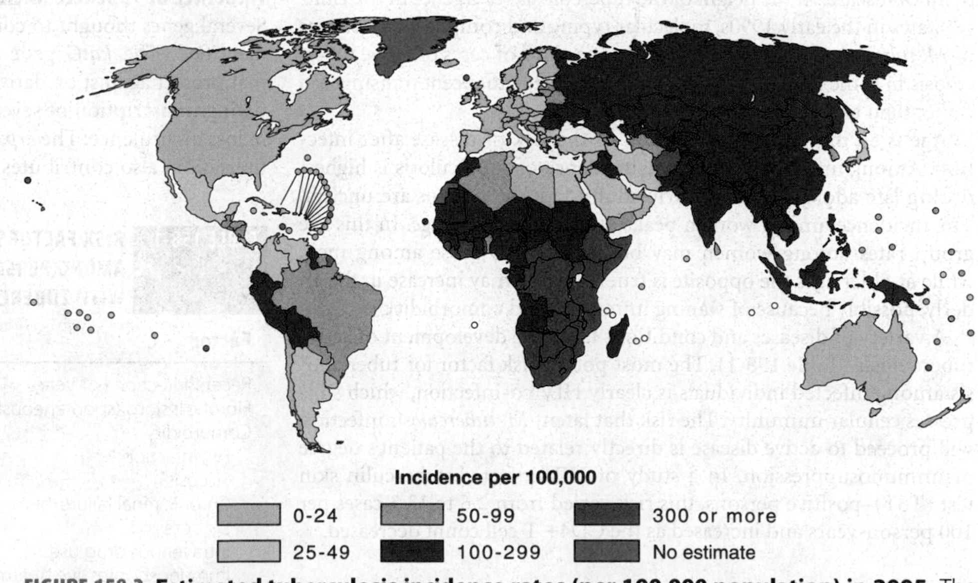

FIGURE 158-2 Estimated tuberculosis incidence rates (per 100,000 population) in 2005. The designations employed and the presentation of material on this map do not imply the expression of any opinion whatsoever on the part of the WHO concerning the legal status of any country, territory, city, or area or of its authorities or concerning the delimitation of its frontiers or boundaries. White lines on maps represent approximate border lines for which there may not yet be full agreement. *(Courtesy of the Stop TB Department, WHO; with permission.)*

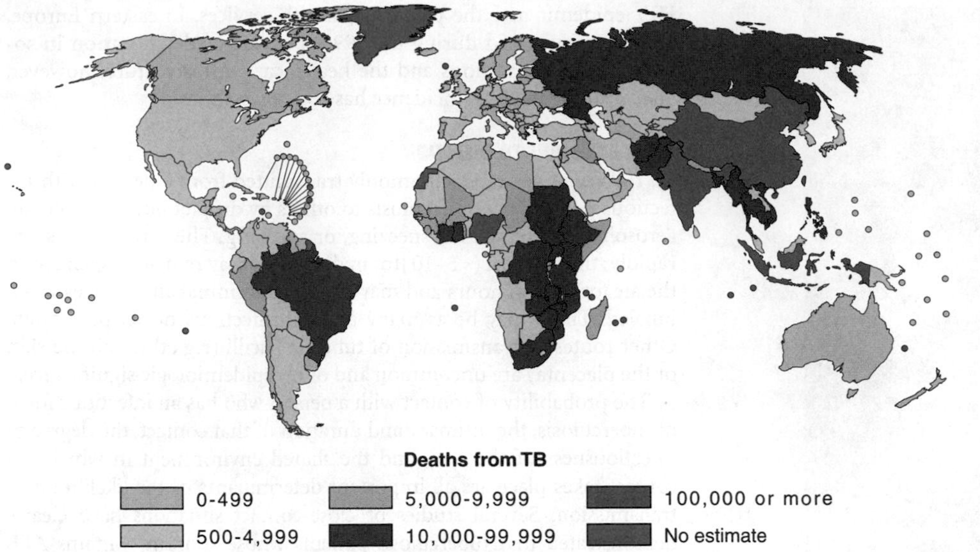

FIGURE 158-3 Estimated numbers of tuberculosis-related deaths in 2005. *(See also disclaimer in Fig. 158-2. Courtesy of the Stop TB Department, WHO; with permission.)*

tors, such as the individual's innate immunologic and nonimmunologic defenses and level of function of cell-mediated immunity (CMI). Clinical illness directly following infection is classified as *primary tuberculosis* and is common among children up to 4 years of age and among immunocompromised persons. Although primary tuberculosis may be severe and disseminated, it is not generally associated with high-level transmissibility. When infection is acquired later in life, the chance is greater that the mature immune system will contain it at least temporarily. The majority of infected individuals who ultimately develop tuberculosis do so within the first year or two after infection. Dormant bacilli, however, may persist for years before reactivating to produce *secondary* (or *postprimary*) *tuberculosis*, which, because of frequent cavitation, is more often infectious than is primary disease. Overall, it is estimated that up to 10% of infected persons will eventually develop active tuberculosis in their lifetime. The risk is much higher among HIV-infected persons. Reinfection of a previously infected individual, which is common in areas with high rates of tuberculosis transmission, may also favor the development of disease. At the height of the tuberculosis resurgence in the United States in the early 1990s, molecular typing and comparison of strains of *M. tuberculosis* suggested that up to one-third of cases of active tuberculosis in some inner-city communities were due to recent transmission rather than to reactivation of latent infection.

Age is an important determinant of the risk of disease after infection. Among infected persons, the incidence of tuberculosis is highest during late adolescence and early adulthood; the reasons are unclear. The incidence among women peaks at 25–34 years of age. In this age group rates among women may be higher than those among men, while at older ages the opposite is true. The risk may increase in the elderly, possibly because of waning immunity and comorbidity.

A variety of diseases and conditions favor the development of active tuberculosis (Table 158-1). The most potent risk factor for tuberculosis among infected individuals is clearly HIV co-infection, which suppresses cellular immunity. The risk that latent *M. tuberculosis* infection will proceed to active disease is directly related to the patient's degree of immunosuppression. In a study of HIV-infected, tuberculin skin test (TST)–positive persons, this risk varied from 2.6 to 13.3 cases per 100 person-years and increased as the CD4+ T cell count decreased.

NATURAL HISTORY OF DISEASE

Studies conducted in various countries before the advent of chemotherapy showed that untreated tuberculosis is often fatal. About one-third of patients died within 1 year after diagnosis, and one-half died within 5 years. The 5-year mortality rate among sputum smear–positive cases was 65%. Of the survivors at 5 years, ~60% had undergone spontaneous remission, while the remainder were still excreting tubercle bacilli.

With effective, timely, and proper chemotherapy, patients have a very high chance of being cured. However, improper use of antituberculosis drugs, while reducing mortality rates, may also result in large numbers of chronic infectious cases, often with drug-resistant bacilli.

PATHOGENESIS AND IMMUNITY

INFECTION AND MACROPHAGE INVASION

The interaction of *M. tuberculosis* with the human host begins when droplet nuclei containing microorganisms from infectious patients are inhaled. While the majority of inhaled bacilli are trapped in the upper airways and expelled by ciliated mucosal cells, a fraction (usually <10%) reach the alveoli. There, alveolar macrophages that have not yet been activated phagocytize the bacilli. Invasion of macrophages by mycobacteria results largely from binding of the bacterial cell wall with a variety of macrophage cell-surface molecules, including complement receptors, mannose receptor, immunoglobulin GFcγ receptor, and type A scavenger receptors. Phagocytosis is enhanced by complement activation leading to opsonization of bacilli with C3 activation products such as C3b. After a phagosome forms, the survival of *M. tuberculosis* within it seems to depend on reduced acidification due to lack of accumulation of vesicular proton-adenosine triphosphatase. A complex series of events is probably generated by the bacterial cell-wall glycolipid lipoarabinomannan (LAM). LAM inhibits the intracellular increase of Ca^{2+}. Thus the Ca^{2+}/calmodulin pathway (leading to phagosome-lysosome fusion) is impaired, and the bacilli may survive within the phagosomes. If the bacilli are successful in arresting phagosome maturation, then replication begins and the macrophage eventually ruptures and releases its bacillary contents.

VIRULENCE OF TUBERCLE BACILLI

Several genes thought to confer virulence to *M. tuberculosis* have been identified. The *katG* gene encodes for catalase/peroxidase enzymes that protect against oxidative stress; *rpoV* is the main sigma factor initiating transcription of several genes. Defects in these two genes result in loss of virulence. The *erp* gene, encoding a protein required for multiplication, also contributes to virulence. Strains of the Beijing/W ge-

TABLE 158-1 RISK FACTORS FOR ACTIVE TUBERCULOSIS AMONG PERSONS WHO HAVE BEEN INFECTED WITH TUBERCLE BACILLI

Factor	Relative Risk/Odds[a]
Recent infection (<1 year)	12.9
Fibrotic lesions (spontaneously healed)	2–20
Comorbidity	
HIV infection	100
Silicosis	30
Chronic renal failure/hemodialysis	10–25
Diabetes	2–4
Intravenous drug use	10–30
Immunosuppressive treatment	10
Gastrectomy	2–5
Jejunoileal bypass	30–60
Posttransplantation period (renal, cardiac)	20–70
Malnutrition and severe underweight	2

[a]Old infection = 1.

notype family have been identified in outbreak conditions in a variety of settings worldwide and have been associated with higher mortality rates and occasionally with multidrug resistance.

INNATE RESISTANCE TO INFECTION

Several observations suggest that genetic factors play a key role in innate nonimmune resistance to infection with *M. tuberculosis* and the development of disease. The existence of this resistance, which is polygenic in nature, is suggested by the differing degrees of susceptibility to tuberculosis in different populations. In mice, a gene called *Nramp1* (natural resistance–associated macrophage protein 1) plays a regulatory role in resistance/susceptibility to mycobacteria. The human homologue NRAMP1, which maps to chromosome 2q, may play a role in determining susceptibility to tuberculosis, as is suggested by a study among West Africans. Polymorphisms in multiple genes, such as those encoding for histocompatibility leukocyte antigen (HLA), interferon γ (IFN-γ), T cell growth factor β (TGF-β), interleukin (IL) 10, mannose-binding protein, IFN-γ receptor, Toll-like receptor (TLR) 2, vitamin D receptor, and IL-1, have been associated with susceptibility to tuberculosis.

THE HOST RESPONSE

In the initial stage of host-bacterium interaction, either fusion between phagosomes and lysosomes occurs, preventing bacillary survival, or the bacilli begin to multiply, ultimately killing the macrophage. A variety of chemoattractants that are released after cell lysis (e.g., complement components, bacterial molecules, and cytokines) recruit additional immature monocyte-derived macrophages, including dendritic cells, which migrate to the draining lymph nodes and present mycobacterial antigens to T lymphocytes. At this point, the development of CMI and humoral immunity begins. These initial stages of infection are usually asymptomatic.

About 2–4 weeks after infection, two host responses to *M. tuberculosis* develop: a macrophage-activating CMI response and a tissue-damaging response. The *macrophage-activating response* is a T cell–mediated phenomenon resulting in the activation of macrophages that are capable of killing and digesting tubercle bacilli. The *tissue-damaging response* is the result of a delayed-type hypersensitivity (DTH) reaction to various bacillary antigens; it destroys unactivated macrophages that contain multiplying bacilli but also causes caseous necrosis of the involved tissues (see below). Although both of these responses can inhibit mycobacterial growth, it is the balance between the two that determines the form of tuberculosis that will develop subsequently.

GRANULOMA FORMATION

With the development of specific immunity and the accumulation of large numbers of activated macrophages at the site of the primary lesion, granulomatous lesions (tubercles) are formed. These lesions consist of accumulations of lymphocytes and activated macrophages that evolve toward epithelioid and giant cell morphologies. Initially, the tissue-damaging response can limit mycobacterial growth within macrophages. As stated above, this response, mediated by various bacterial products, not only destroys macrophages but also produces early solid necrosis in the center of the tubercle. Although *M. tuberculosis* can survive, its growth is inhibited within this necrotic environment by low oxygen tension and low pH. At this point, some lesions may heal by fibrosis, with subsequent calcification, whereas inflammation and necrosis occur in other lesions.

THE MACROPHAGE-ACTIVATING RESPONSE

CMI is critical at this early stage. In the majority of infected individuals, local macrophages are activated when bacillary antigens processed by macrophages stimulate T lymphocytes to release a variety of lymphokines. These activated macrophages aggregate around the lesion's center and effectively neutralize tubercle bacilli without causing further tissue destruction. In the central part of the lesion, the necrotic material resembles soft cheese (*caseous necrosis*)—a phenomenon that may also be observed in other conditions, such as neoplasms. Even when healing takes place, viable bacilli may remain dormant within macrophages or in the necrotic material for many years. These "healed" lesions in the lung parenchyma and hilar lymph nodes may later undergo calcification.

THE DELAYED-TYPE HYPERSENSITIVITY REACTION

In a minority of cases, the macrophage-activating response is weak, and mycobacterial growth can be inhibited only by intensified DTH reactions, which lead to lung tissue destruction. The lesion tends to enlarge further, and the surrounding tissue is progressively damaged. At the center of the lesion, the caseous material liquefies. Bronchial walls as well as blood vessels are invaded and destroyed, and cavities are formed. The liquefied caseous material, containing large numbers of bacilli, is drained through bronchi. Within the cavity, tubercle bacilli multiply, spill into the airways, and are discharged into the environment through expiratory maneuvers such as coughing and talking. In the early stages of infection, bacilli are usually transported by macrophages to regional lymph nodes, from which they gain access to the bloodstream and disseminate widely throughout the body. The resulting lesions may undergo the same evolution as those in the lungs, although most tend to heal. In young children with poor natural immunity, hematogenous dissemination may result in fatal miliary tuberculosis or tuberculous meningitis.

ROLE OF MACROPHAGES AND MONOCYTES

While CMI confers partial protection against *M. tuberculosis*, humoral immunity plays a less well-defined role in protection (although evidence is accumulating on the existence of LAM antibodies, which may prevent dissemination of infection in children). In the case of CMI, two types of cells are essential: macrophages, which directly phagocytize tubercle bacilli, and T cells (mainly CD4+ T lymphocytes), which induce protection through the production of cytokines, especially IFN-γ. After infection with *M. tuberculosis*, alveolar macrophages secrete various cytokines responsible for a number of events (e.g., the formation of granulomas) as well as systemic effects (e.g., fever and weight loss). Monocytes and macrophages attracted to the site are key components of the immune response. Their primary mechanism is probably related to production of nitric oxide, which has antimycobacterial activity and increases synthesis of cytokines such as tumor necrosis factor α (TNF-α) and IL-1, which in turn regulate release of reactive nitrogen intermediates. In addition, macrophages can undergo apoptosis—a defensive mechanism to prevent release of cytokines and bacilli via their sequestration in the apoptotic cell.

ROLE OF T LYMPHOCYTES

Alveolar macrophages, monocytes, and dendritic cells are also critical in processing and presenting antigens to T lymphocytes, primarily CD4+ and CD8+ T cells; the result is the activation and proliferation of CD4+ T lymphocytes, which are crucial to the host's defense against *M. tuberculosis*. Qualitative and quantitative defects of CD4+ T cells explain the inability of HIV-infected individuals to contain mycobacterial proliferation. Activated CD4+ T lymphocytes can differentiate into cytokine-producing T_H1 or T_H2 cells. T_H1 cells produce IFN-γ—an activator of macrophages and monocytes—and IL-2. T_H2 cells produce IL-4, IL-5, IL-10, and IL-13 and also may promote humoral immunity. The interplay of these various cytokines and their cross-regulation determine the host's response. The role of cytokines in promoting intracellular killing of mycobacteria, however, has not been entirely elucidated. IFN-γ may induce the generation of reactive nitrogen intermediates and regulate genes involved in bactericidal effects. TNF-α also seems to be important.

Observations made originally in transgenic knockout mice and more recently in humans suggest that other T cell subsets, especially CD8+ T cells, may play an important role. CD8+ T cells have been associated with protective activities via cytotoxic responses and lysis of infected cells as well as with production of IFN-γ and TNF-α. Finally, natural killer cells act as co-regulators of CD8+ T cell lytic activities, and $\gamma\delta$ T cells are increasingly thought to be involved in protective responses in humans.

MYCOBACTERIAL LIPIDS AND PROTEINS

Lipids have been involved in mycobacterial recognition by the innate immune system, and lipoproteins (such as 19-kDa lipoprotein) have been proven to trigger potent signals through TLRs present in blood dendritic cells. *M. tuberculosis* possesses various protein antigens. Some are present in the cytoplasm and cell wall; others are secreted. That the latter are more important in eliciting a T lymphocyte response is suggested by experiments documenting the appearance of protective immunity in animals after immunization with live, protein-secreting mycobacteria. Among the antigens that may play a protective role are the 30-kDa (or 85B) and ESAT-6 antigens. Protective immunity is probably the result of reactivity to many different mycobacterial antigens.

SKIN TEST REACTIVITY

Coincident with the appearance of immunity, DTH to *M. tuberculosis* develops. This reactivity is the basis of the TST, which is used primarily for the detection of *M. tuberculosis* infection in persons without symptoms. The cellular mechanisms responsible for TST reactivity are related mainly to previously sensitized CD4+ T lymphocytes, which are attracted to the skin-test site. There, they proliferate and produce cytokines. While DTH is associated with protective immunity (TST-positive persons being less susceptible to a new *M. tuberculosis* infection than TST-negative persons), it by no means guarantees protection against reactivation. In fact, cases of active tuberculosis are often accompanied by strongly positive skin-test reactions. There is also evidence of reinfection with a new strain of *M. tuberculosis* in patients previously treated for active disease. This evidence underscores the fact that previous latent or active tuberculosis may not confer fully protective immunity.

CLINICAL MANIFESTATIONS

Tuberculosis is classified as pulmonary, extrapulmonary, or both. Before the advent of HIV infection, ~80% of all new cases of tuberculosis were limited to the lungs. However, up to two-thirds of HIV-infected patients with tuberculosis may have both pulmonary and extrapulmonary disease or extrapulmonary disease alone.

PULMONARY TUBERCULOSIS

Pulmonary tuberculosis can be categorized as primary or postprimary (secondary).

Primary Disease Primary pulmonary tuberculosis occurs soon after the initial infection with tubercle bacilli. In areas of high tuberculosis transmission, this form of disease is often seen in children. Because most inspired air is distributed to the middle and lower lung zones, these areas of the lungs are most commonly involved in primary tuberculosis. The lesion forming after infection is usually peripheral and accompanied in more than half of cases by hilar or paratracheal lymphadenopathy, which may not be detectable on chest radiography. In the majority of cases, the lesion heals spontaneously and may later be evident as a small calcified nodule (*Ghon lesion*).

In children and in persons with impaired immunity (e.g., those with malnutrition or HIV infection), primary pulmonary tuberculosis may progress rapidly to clinical illness. The initial lesion increases in size and can evolve in different ways. Pleural effusion, which is found in up to two-thirds of cases, results from the penetration of bacilli into the pleural space from an adjacent subpleural focus. In severe cases, the primary site rapidly enlarges, its central portion undergoes necrosis, and cavitation develops (*progressive primary tuberculosis*). Tuberculosis in young children is almost invariably accompanied by hilar or mediastinal lymphadenopathy due to the spread of bacilli from the lung parenchyma through lymphatic vessels. Enlarged lymph nodes may compress bronchi, causing obstruction and subsequent segmental or lobar collapse. Partial obstruction may cause obstructive emphysema, and bronchiectasis may also develop. Hematogenous dissemination, which is common and often asymptomatic, may result in the most severe manifestations of primary *M. tuberculosis* infection. Bacilli reach the bloodstream from the pulmonary lesion or the lymph nodes and disseminate into various organs, where they may produce granulomatous lesions. Although healing frequently takes place, immunocompromised persons (e.g., patients with HIV infection) may develop miliary tuberculosis and/or tuberculous meningitis.

Postprimary Disease Also called *adult-type, reactivation,* or *secondary tuberculosis*, postprimary disease results from endogenous reactivation of latent infection and is usually localized to the apical and posterior segments of the upper lobes, where the substantially higher mean oxygen tension (compared with that in the lower zones) favors mycobacterial growth. In addition, the superior segments of the lower lobes are frequently involved. The extent of lung parenchymal involvement varies greatly, from small infiltrates to extensive cavitary disease. With cavity formation, liquefied necrotic contents are ultimately discharged into the airways, resulting in satellite lesions within the lungs that may in turn undergo cavitation (Figs. 158-4 and 158-5). Massive involvement of pulmonary segments or lobes, with coalescence of lesions, produces tuberculous pneumonia. While up to one-third of untreated patients reportedly succumb to severe pulmonary tuberculosis within a few weeks or months after onset (the classical "galloping consumption" of the past), others undergo a process of spontaneous remission or proceed along a chronic, progressively debilitating course ("consumption"). Under these circumstances, some pulmonary lesions become fibrotic and may later calcify, but cavities persist in other parts of the lungs. Individuals with such chronic disease continue to discharge tubercle bacilli into the environment. Most patients respond to treatment, with defervescence, decreasing cough, weight gain, and a general improvement in well-being within several weeks.

Early in the course of disease, symptoms and signs are often nonspecific and insidious, consisting mainly of fever and night sweats, weight loss, anorexia, general malaise, and weakness. However, in the majority of cases, cough eventually develops—often initially nonproductive and subsequently accompanied by the production of purulent sputum, sometimes with blood streaking. Massive hemoptysis may ensue as a consequence of the erosion of a blood vessel in the wall of a cavity. Hemoptysis, however, may also result from rupture of a dilated vessel in a cavity (*Rasmussen's aneurysm*) or from aspergilloma formation in an old cavity. Pleuritic chest pain sometimes develops in patients with subpleural parenchymal lesions. Extensive disease may produce dyspnea and, in rare instances, adult respiratory distress syndrome (ARDS).

Physical findings are of limited use in pulmonary tuberculosis. Many patients have no abnormalities detectable by chest examina-

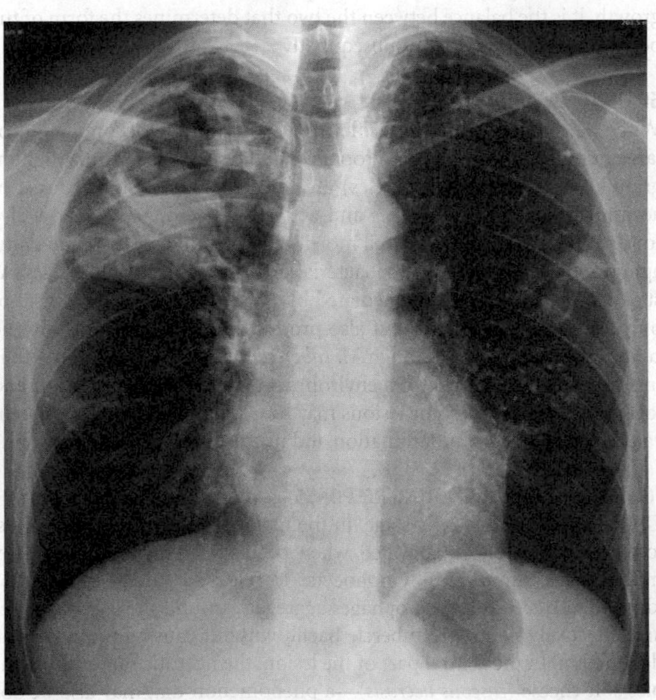

FIGURE 158-4 Chest radiograph showing a right upper-lobe infiltrate and a cavity with an air-fluid level in a patient with active tuberculosis. *(Courtesy of Dr. Andrea Gori, Department of Infectious Diseases, S. Paolo University Hospital, Milan, Italy; with permission.)*

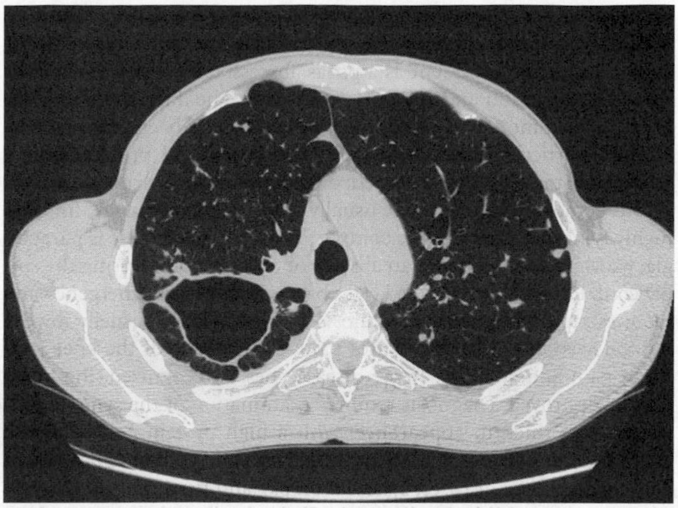

FIGURE 158-5 CT scan showing a large cavity in the right lung of a patient with active tuberculosis. *(Courtesy of Dr. Enrico Girardi, National Institute for Infectious Diseases, Spallanzani Hospital, Rome, Italy; with permission.)*

tion, whereas others have detectable rales in the involved areas during inspiration, especially after coughing. Occasionally, rhonchi due to partial bronchial obstruction and classic amphoric breath sounds in areas with large cavities may be heard. Systemic features include fever (often low-grade and intermittent) in up to 80% of cases and wasting. Absence of fever, however, does not exclude tuberculosis. In some cases, pallor and finger clubbing develop. The most common hematologic findings are mild anemia and leukocytosis. Hyponatremia due to the syndrome of inappropriate secretion of antidiuretic hormone (SIADH) has also been reported.

EXTRAPULMONARY TUBERCULOSIS

In order of frequency, the extrapulmonary sites most commonly involved in tuberculosis are the lymph nodes, pleura, genitourinary tract, bones and joints, meninges, peritoneum, and pericardium. However, virtually all organ systems may be affected. As a result of hematogenous dissemination in HIV-infected individuals, extrapulmonary tuberculosis is seen more commonly today than in the past.

Lymph-Node Tuberculosis (Tuberculous Lymphadenitis) The most common presentation of extrapulmonary tuberculosis (>40% of cases in the United States in recent series), lymph-node disease is particularly frequent among HIV-infected patients. In the United States, children and women (particularly non-Caucasians) also seem to be especially susceptible. Once caused mainly by *M. bovis*, tuberculous lymphadenitis is today due largely to *M. tuberculosis*. Lymph-node tuberculosis presents as painless swelling of the lymph nodes, most commonly at posterior cervical and supraclavicular sites (a condition historically referred to as *scrofula*). Lymph nodes are usually discrete and nontender in early disease but may be inflamed and have a fistulous tract draining caseous material. Associated pulmonary disease is seen in >40% of cases. Systemic symptoms are usually limited to HIV-infected patients. The diagnosis is established only by fine-needle aspiration or surgical biopsy. AFB are seen in up to 50% of cases, cultures are positive in 70–80%, and histologic examination shows granulomatous lesions. Among HIV-infected patients, granulomas usually are not seen. Differential diagnosis includes a variety of infectious conditions, neoplastic diseases such as lymphomas or metastatic carcinomas, and rare disorders like Kikuchi disease (necrotizing histiocytic lymphadenitis), Kimura's disease, and Castleman's disease.

Pleural Tuberculosis Involvement of the pleura, which accounts for ~20% of extrapulmonary cases in the United States, is common in primary tuberculosis and may result from either contiguous spread of parenchymal inflammation or, as in many cases of pleurisy accompanying postprimary disease, actual penetration by tubercle bacilli into the pleural space. Depending on the extent of reactivity, the effusion may be small, remain unnoticed, and resolve spontaneously or may be sufficiently large to cause symptoms such as fever, pleuritic chest pain, and dyspnea. Physical findings are those of pleural effusion: dullness to percussion and absence of breath sounds. A chest radiograph reveals the effusion and, in up to one-third of cases, also shows a parenchymal lesion. Thoracentesis is required to ascertain the nature of the effusion and to differentiate it from manifestations of other etiologies. The fluid is straw-colored and at times hemorrhagic; it is an exudate with a protein concentration >50% of that in serum (usually ~4–6 g/dL), a normal to low glucose concentration, a pH of ~7.3 (occasionally <7.2), and detectable white blood cells (usually 500–6000/μL). Neutrophils may predominate in the early stage, while mononuclear cells are the typical finding later. Mesothelial cells are generally rare or absent. AFB are seen on direct smear in only 10–25% of cases, but cultures may be positive for *M. tuberculosis* in 25–75% of cases; positive cultures are more common among postprimary cases. Determination of the pleural concentration of adenosine deaminase (ADA) is a useful screening test: tuberculosis is virtually excluded if the value is very low. Needle biopsy of the pleura is often required for diagnosis and reveals granulomas and/or yields a positive culture in up to 80% of cases. This form of pleural tuberculosis responds well to chemotherapy and may resolve spontaneously. The usefulness of glucocorticoid administration is doubtful.

Tuberculous empyema is a less common complication of pulmonary tuberculosis. It is usually the result of the rupture of a cavity, with spillage of a large number of organisms into the pleural space. This process may create a bronchopleural fistula with evident air in the pleural space. A chest radiograph shows hydropneumothorax with an air-fluid level. The pleural fluid is purulent and thick and contains large numbers of lymphocytes. Acid-fast smears and mycobacterial cultures are often positive. Surgical drainage is usually required as an adjunct to chemotherapy. Tuberculous empyema may result in severe pleural fibrosis and restrictive lung disease. Removal of the thickened visceral pleura (decortication) is occasionally necessary to improve lung function.

Tuberculosis of the Upper Airways Nearly always a complication of advanced cavitary pulmonary tuberculosis, tuberculosis of the upper airways may involve the larynx, pharynx, and epiglottis. Symptoms include hoarseness, dysphonia, and dysphagia in addition to chronic productive cough. Findings depend on the site of involvement, and ulcerations may be seen on laryngoscopy. Acid-fast smear of the sputum is often positive, but biopsy may be necessary in some cases to establish the diagnosis. Carcinoma of the larynx may have similar features but is usually painless.

Genitourinary Tuberculosis Genitourinary tuberculosis, which accounts for ~15% of all extrapulmonary cases in the United States, may involve any portion of the genitourinary tract. Local symptoms predominate, and up to one-third of patients may concomitantly have pulmonary disease. Urinary frequency, dysuria, nocturia, hematuria, and flank or abdominal pain are common presentations. However, patients may be asymptomatic and the disease discovered only after severe destructive lesions of the kidneys have developed. Urinalysis gives abnormal results in 90% of cases, revealing pyuria and hematuria. The documentation of culture-negative pyuria in acidic urine raises the suspicion of tuberculosis. Intravenous pyelography, abdominal CT, or MRI (Fig. 158-6) may show deformities and obstructions, and calcifications and ureteral strictures are suggestive findings. Culture of three morning urine specimens yields a definitive diagnosis in nearly 90% of cases. Severe ureteral strictures may lead to hydronephrosis and renal damage.

Genital tuberculosis is diagnosed more commonly in female than in male patients. In female patients, it affects the fallopian tubes and the endometrium and may cause infertility, pelvic pain, and menstrual abnormalities. Diagnosis requires biopsy or culture of specimens obtained by dilatation and curettage. In male patients, tuberculosis

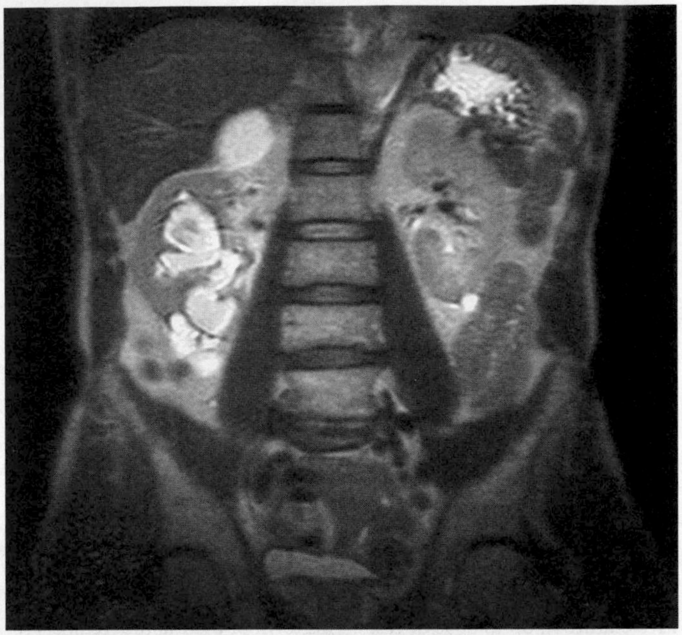

FIGURE 158-6 MRI of culture-confirmed renal tuberculosis. T2-weighted coronary plane: coronal sections showing several renal lesions in both the cortical and the medullary tissues of the right kidney. *(Courtesy of Dr. Alberto Matteelli, Department of Infectious Diseases, University of Brescia, Italy; with permission.)*

preferentially affects the epididymis, producing a slightly tender mass that may drain externally through a fistulous tract; orchitis and prostatitis may also develop. In almost half of cases of genitourinary tuberculosis, urinary tract disease is also present. Genitourinary tuberculosis responds well to chemotherapy.

Skeletal Tuberculosis In the United States, tuberculosis of the bones and joints is responsible for ~10% of extrapulmonary cases. In bone and joint disease, pathogenesis is related to reactivation of hematogenous foci or to spread from adjacent paravertebral lymph nodes. Weight-bearing joints (the spine in 40% of cases, the hips in 13%, and the knees in 10%) are most commonly affected. Spinal tuberculosis (Pott's disease or tuberculous spondylitis; Fig. 158-7) often involves two or more adjacent vertebral bodies. While the upper thoracic spine is the most common site of spinal tuberculosis in children, the lower thoracic and upper lumbar vertebrae are usually affected in adults. From the anterior superior or inferior angle of the vertebral body, the lesion slowly reaches the adjacent body, later affecting the intervertebral disk. With advanced disease, collapse of vertebral bodies results in kyphosis (*gibbus*). A paravertebral "cold" abscess may also form. In the upper spine, this abscess may track to and penetrate the chest wall, presenting as a soft tissue mass; in the lower spine, it may reach the inguinal ligaments or present as a psoas abscess. CT or MRI reveals the characteristic lesion and suggests its etiology. The differential diagnosis includes tumors and other infections. Pyogenic bacterial osteomyelitis, in particular, involves the disk very early and produces rapid sclerosis. Aspiration of the abscess or bone biopsy confirms the tuberculous etiology, as cultures are usually positive and histologic findings highly typical. A catastrophic complication of Pott's disease is paraplegia, which is usually due to an abscess or a lesion compressing the spinal cord. Paraparesis due to a large abscess is a medical emergency and requires rapid drainage. Tuberculosis of the hip joints, usually involving the head of the femur, causes pain; tuberculosis of the knee produces pain and swelling. If the disease goes unrecognized, the joints may be destroyed. Diagnosis requires examination of the synovial fluid, which is thick in appearance, with a high protein concentration and a variable cell count. Although synovial fluid culture is positive in a high percentage of cases, synovial biopsy and tissue culture may be necessary to establish the diagnosis. Skeletal tuberculosis responds to chemotherapy, but severe cases may require surgery.

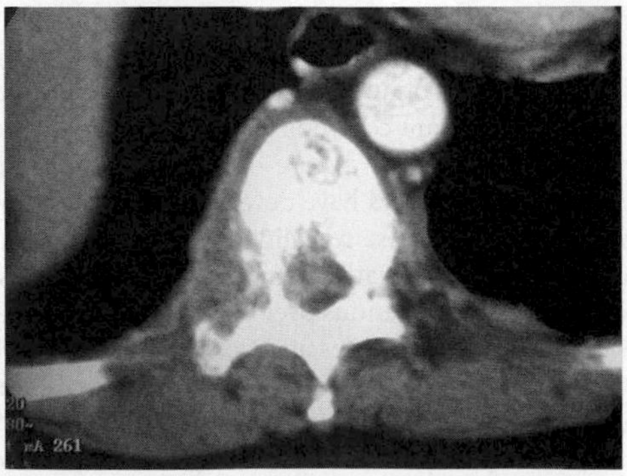

FIGURE 158-7 CT scan demonstrating destruction of the right pedicle of T10 due to Pott's disease. The patient, a 70-year-old Asian woman, presented with back pain and weight loss and had biopsy-proven tuberculosis. *(Courtesy of Charles L. Daley, M.D., University of California, San Francisco; with permission.)*

Tuberculous Meningitis and Tuberculoma Tuberculosis of the central nervous system (CNS) accounts for ~5% of extrapulmonary cases in the United States. It is seen most often in young children but also develops in adults, especially those infected with HIV. Tuberculous meningitis results from the hematogenous spread of primary or postprimary pulmonary disease or from the rupture of a subependymal tubercle into the subarachnoid space. In more than half of cases, evidence of old pulmonary lesions or a miliary pattern is found on chest radiography. The disease often presents subtly as headache and slight mental changes after a prodrome of weeks of low-grade fever, malaise, anorexia, and irritability. If not recognized, tuberculous meningitis may evolve acutely with severe headache, confusion, lethargy, altered sensorium, and neck rigidity. Typically, the disease evolves over 1–2 weeks, a course longer than that of bacterial meningitis. Paresis of cranial nerves (ocular nerves in particular) is a frequent finding, and the involvement of cerebral arteries may produce focal ischemia. The ultimate evolution is toward coma, with hydrocephalus and intracranial hypertension.

Lumbar puncture is the cornerstone of diagnosis. In general, examination of the cerebrospinal fluid (CSF) reveals a high leukocyte count (up to 1000/μL), usually with a predominance of lymphocytes but sometimes with a predominance of neutrophils in the early stage; a protein content of 1–8 g/L (100–800 mg/dL); and a low glucose concentration. However, any of these three parameters can be within the normal range. AFB are seen on direct smear of CSF sediment in up to one-third of cases, but repeated lumbar punctures increase the yield. Culture of CSF is diagnostic in up to 80% of cases and remains the gold standard. Polymerase chain reaction (PCR) has a sensitivity of up to 80%, but rates of false-positivity reach 10%. The ADA concentration may be a sensitive test but has low specificity. Imaging studies (CT and MRI) may show hydrocephalus and abnormal enhancement of basal cisterns or ependyma.

If unrecognized, tuberculous meningitis is uniformly fatal. This disease responds to chemotherapy; however, neurologic sequelae are documented in 25% of treated cases, in most of which the diagnosis has been delayed. Clinical trials have demonstrated that patients given adjunctive glucocorticoids may experience faster resolution of CSF abnormalities and elevated CSF pressure. In a recent study, adjunctive dexamethasone (0.4 mg/kg per day given IV and tapering by 0.1 mg/kg per week until the fourth week, when 0.1 mg/kg per day was administered; followed by 4 mg/d given by mouth and tapering by 1 mg per week until the fourth week, when 1 mg/d was administered) significantly enhanced the chances of survival among persons >14 years of age but did not reduce the frequency of neurologic sequelae.

Tuberculoma, an uncommon manifestation of CNS tuberculosis, presents as one or more space-occupying lesions and usually causes seizures and focal signs. CT or MRI reveals contrast-enhanced ring lesions, but biopsy is necessary to establish the diagnosis.

Gastrointestinal Tuberculosis Gastrointestinal tuberculosis is uncommon, making up 3.5% of extrapulmonary cases in the United States. Various pathogenetic mechanisms are involved: swallowing of sputum with direct seeding, hematogenous spread, or (largely in developing areas) ingestion of milk from cows affected by bovine tuberculosis. Although any portion of the gastrointestinal tract may be affected, the terminal ileum and the cecum are the sites most commonly involved. Abdominal pain (at times similar to that associated with appendicitis) and swelling, obstruction, hematochezia, and a palpable mass in the abdomen are common findings at presentation. Fever, weight loss, anorexia, and night sweats are also common. With intestinal-wall involvement, ulcerations and fistulae may simulate Crohn's disease; the differential diagnosis with this entity is always difficult. Anal fistulae should prompt an evaluation for rectal tuberculosis. As surgery is required in most cases, the diagnosis can be established by histologic examination and culture of specimens obtained intraoperatively.

Tuberculous peritonitis follows either the direct spread of tubercle bacilli from ruptured lymph nodes and intraabdominal organs (e.g., genital tuberculosis in women) or hematogenous seeding. Nonspecific abdominal pain, fever, and ascites should raise the suspicion of tuberculous peritonitis. The coexistence of cirrhosis (Chap. 301) in patients with tuberculous peritonitis complicates the diagnosis. In tuberculous peritonitis, paracentesis reveals an exudative fluid with a high protein content and leukocytosis that is usually lymphocytic (although neutrophils occasionally predominate). The yield of direct smear and culture is relatively low; culture of a large volume of ascitic fluid can increase the yield, but peritoneal biopsy (with a specimen best obtained by laparoscopy) is often needed to establish the diagnosis.

Pericardial Tuberculosis (Tuberculous Pericarditis) Due to direct progression of a primary focus within the pericardium, to reactivation of a latent focus, or to rupture of an adjacent subcarinal lymph node, pericardial tuberculosis has often been a disease of the elderly in countries with low tuberculosis prevalence but also develops frequently in HIV-infected patients. Case-fatality rates are as high as 40% in some series. The onset may be subacute, although an acute presentation, with dyspnea, fever, dull retrosternal pain, and a pericardial friction rub, is possible. An effusion eventually develops in many cases; cardiovascular symptoms and signs of cardiac tamponade may ultimately appear (Chap. 232). In the presence of effusion, tuberculosis must be suspected if the patient belongs to a high-risk population (HIV-infected, originating in a high-prevalence country); if there is evidence of previous tuberculosis in other organs; or if echocardiography, CT, or MRI shows effusion and thickness across the pericardial space. A definitive diagnosis can be obtained by pericardiocentesis under echocardiographic guidance. The pericardial fluid must be submitted for biochemical, cytologic, and microbiologic study. The effusion is exudative in nature, with a high count of leukocytes (predominantly mononuclear cells). Hemorrhagic effusion is frequent. Direct smear examination is very rarely positive. Culture of pericardial fluid reveals *M. tuberculosis* in up to two-thirds of cases, while pericardial biopsy has a higher yield. High levels of ADA and IFN-γ may also suggest a tuberculous etiology.

Without treatment, pericardial tuberculosis is usually fatal. Even with treatment, complications may develop, including chronic constrictive pericarditis with thickening of the pericardium, fibrosis, and sometimes calcification, which may be visible on a chest radiograph. A course of glucocorticoid treatment (e.g., prednisone, 20–60 mg/d for up to 6 weeks) is useful in the management of acute disease, reducing effusion, facilitating hemodynamic recovery, and thus decreasing mortality rates. Progression to chronic constrictive pericarditis, however, seems unaffected by such therapy.

Miliary or Disseminated Tuberculosis Miliary tuberculosis is due to hematogenous spread of tubercle bacilli. Although in children it is often the consequence of primary infection, in adults it may be due to either recent infection or reactivation of old disseminated foci. The lesions are usually yellowish granulomas 1–2 mm in diameter that resemble millet seeds (thus the term *miliary*, coined by nineteenth-century pathologists).

Clinical manifestations are nonspecific and protean, depending on the predominant site of involvement. Fever, night sweats, anorexia, weakness, and weight loss are presenting symptoms in the majority of cases. At times patients have a cough and other respiratory symptoms due to pulmonary involvement as well as abdominal symptoms. Physical findings include hepatomegaly, splenomegaly, and lymphadenopathy. Eye examination may reveal choroidal tubercles, which are pathognomonic of miliary tuberculosis, in up to 30% of cases. Meningismus occurs in <10% of cases.

A high index of suspicion is required for the diagnosis of miliary tuberculosis. Frequently, chest radiography reveals a miliary reticulonodular pattern (more easily seen on underpenetrated film), although no radiographic abnormality may be evident early in the course and among HIV-infected patients. Other radiologic findings include large infiltrates, interstitial infiltrates (especially in HIV-infected patients), and pleural effusion. Sputum smear microscopy is negative in 80% of cases. Various hematologic abnormalities may be seen, including anemia with leukopenia, lymphopenia, neutrophilic leukocytosis and leukemoid reactions, and polycythemia. Disseminated intravascular coagulation has been reported. Elevation of alkaline phosphatase levels and other abnormal values in liver function tests are detected in patients with severe hepatic involvement. The TST may be negative in up to half of cases, but reactivity may be restored during chemotherapy. Bronchoalveolar lavage and transbronchial biopsy are more likely to provide bacteriologic confirmation, and granulomas are evident in liver or bone-marrow biopsy specimens from many patients. If it goes unrecognized, miliary tuberculosis is lethal; with proper early treatment, however, it is amenable to cure. Glucocorticoid therapy has not proved beneficial.

A rare presentation seen in the elderly is *cryptic miliary tuberculosis*, which has a chronic course characterized by mild intermittent fever, anemia, and—ultimately—meningeal involvement preceding death. An acute septicemic form, *nonreactive miliary tuberculosis*, occurs very rarely and is due to massive hematogenous dissemination of tubercle bacilli. Pancytopenia is common in this form of disease, which is rapidly fatal. At postmortem examination, multiple necrotic but nongranulomatous ("nonreactive") lesions are detected.

Less Common Extrapulmonary Forms Tuberculosis may cause chorioretinitis, uveitis, panophthalmitis, and painful hypersensitivity-related phlyctenular conjunctivitis. Tuberculous otitis is rare and presents as hearing loss, otorrhea, and tympanic membrane perforation. In the nasopharynx, tuberculosis may simulate Wegener's granulomatosis. Cutaneous manifestations of tuberculosis include primary infection due to direct inoculation, abscesses and chronic ulcers, scrofuloderma, lupus vulgaris (a smoldering disease with nodules, plaques, and fissures), miliary lesions, and erythema nodosum. Adrenal tuberculosis is a manifestation of disseminated disease presenting rarely as adrenal insufficiency. Finally, congenital tuberculosis results from transplacental spread of tubercle bacilli to the fetus or from ingestion of contaminated amniotic fluid. This rare disease affects the liver, spleen, lymph nodes, and various other organs.

HIV-ASSOCIATED TUBERCULOSIS

(See also Chap. 182) Tuberculosis is one of the most common diseases among HIV-infected persons worldwide. In some African countries, the rate of HIV infection among tuberculosis patients reaches 70–80% in certain urban settings. A person with a positive TST who acquires HIV infection has a 3–13% annual risk of developing active tuberculosis. A new tuberculosis infection acquired by an HIV-infected individual may evolve to active disease in a matter of weeks rather than months or years.

Tuberculosis can appear at any stage of HIV infection, and its presentation varies with the stage. When CMI is only partially compromised, pulmonary tuberculosis presents in a typical manner (Figs. 158-4 and 158-5), with upper-lobe infiltrates and cavitation and without significant lymphadenopathy or pleural effusion. In late stages of HIV infection, a primary tuberculosis–like pattern, with diffuse interstitial or miliary infiltrates, little or no cavitation, and intrathoracic lymphadenopathy, is more common. Overall, sputum smears may be positive less frequently among tuberculosis patients with HIV infection than among those without; thus, the diagnosis of tuberculosis may be unusually difficult, especially in view of the variety of HIV-related pulmonary conditions mimicking tuberculosis.

Extrapulmonary tuberculosis is common among HIV-infected patients. In various series, extrapulmonary tuberculosis—alone or in association with pulmonary disease—has been documented in 40–60% of all cases in HIV–co-infected individuals. The most common forms are lymphatic, disseminated, pleural, and pericardial. Mycobacteremia and meningitis are also frequent, particularly in advanced HIV disease.

The diagnosis of tuberculosis in HIV-infected patients may be difficult not only because of the increased frequency of sputum-smear negativity (up to 40% in culture-proven pulmonary cases) but also because of atypical radiographic findings, a lack of classic granuloma formation in the late stages, and a negative TST. Delays in treatment may prove fatal. Recommendations for the prevention and treatment of tuberculosis in HIV-infected individuals are provided below.

DIAGNOSIS OF TUBERCULOSIS

The key to the diagnosis of tuberculosis is a high index of suspicion. Diagnosis is not difficult with a high-risk patient—e.g., a homeless alcoholic who presents with typical symptoms and a classic chest radiograph showing upper-lobe infiltrates with cavities (Fig. 158-4). On the other hand, the diagnosis can easily be missed in an elderly nursing home resident or a teenager with a focal infiltrate.

Often, the diagnosis is first entertained when the chest radiograph of a patient being evaluated for respiratory symptoms is abnormal. If the patient has no complicating medical conditions that cause immunosuppression, the chest radiograph may show typical upper-lobe infiltrates with cavitation (Fig. 158-4). The longer the delay between the onset of symptoms and the diagnosis, the more likely is the finding of cavitary disease. In contrast, immunosuppressed patients, including those with HIV infection, may have "atypical" findings on chest radiography—e.g., lower-zone infiltrates without cavity formation.

AFB MICROSCOPY

A presumptive diagnosis is commonly based on the finding of AFB on microscopic examination of a diagnostic specimen, such as a smear of expectorated sputum or of tissue (e.g., a lymph node biopsy). Although rapid and inexpensive, AFB microscopy has relatively low sensitivity (40–60%) in confirmed cases of pulmonary tuberculosis. Most modern laboratories processing large numbers of diagnostic specimens use auramine-rhodamine staining and fluorescence microscopy. The more traditional method—light microscopy of specimens stained with Kinyoun or Ziehl-Neelsen basic fuchsin dyes—is satisfactory, although more time-consuming. For patients with suspected pulmonary tuberculosis, three sputum specimens, preferably collected early in the morning, should be submitted to the laboratory for AFB smear and mycobacterial culture. If tissue is obtained, it is critical that the portion of the specimen intended for culture not be put in formaldehyde. The use of AFB microscopy on urine or gastric lavage fluid is limited by the presence of commensal mycobacteria that can cause false-positive results.

MYCOBACTERIAL CULTURE

Definitive diagnosis depends on the isolation and identification of *M. tuberculosis* from a clinical specimen or the identification of specific sequences of DNA in a nucleic acid amplification test (see below). Specimens may be inoculated onto egg- or agar-based medium (e.g., Löwenstein-Jensen or Middlebrook 7H10) and incubated at 37°C (under 5% CO_2 for Middlebrook medium). Because most species of mycobacteria, including *M. tuberculosis*, grow slowly, 4–8 weeks may be required before growth is detected. Although *M. tuberculosis* may be presumptively identified on the basis of growth time and colony pigmentation and morphology, a variety of biochemical tests have traditionally been used to speciate mycobacterial isolates. In modern, well-equipped laboratories, the use of broth-based culture for isolation and speciation by molecular methods or high-pressure liquid chromatography of mycolic acids has replaced isolation on solid media and identification by biochemical tests. These new methods have decreased the time required for bacteriologic confirmation to 2–3 weeks.

NUCLEIC ACID AMPLIFICATION

Several test systems based on amplification of mycobacterial nucleic acid are available. These systems permit the diagnosis of tuberculosis in as little as several hours, with high specificity and sensitivity approaching that of culture. These tests are most useful for the rapid confirmation of tuberculosis in persons with AFB-positive specimens but also have utility for the diagnosis of AFB-negative pulmonary and extrapulmonary tuberculosis.

DRUG SUSCEPTIBILITY TESTING

In general, the initial isolate of *M. tuberculosis* should be tested for susceptibility to isoniazid, rifampin, and ethambutol. In addition, expanded susceptibility testing is mandatory when resistance to one or more of these drugs is found or the patient either fails to respond to initial therapy or has a relapse after the completion of treatment (see "Treatment Failure and Relapse," below). Susceptibility testing may be conducted directly (with the clinical specimen) or indirectly (with mycobacterial cultures) on solid or liquid medium. Results are obtained most rapidly by direct susceptibility testing on liquid medium, with an average reporting time of 3 weeks. With indirect testing on solid medium, results may be unavailable for ≥8 weeks. Molecular methods for the rapid identification of genetic mutations known to be associated with resistance to rifampin and isoniazid have been developed but are not marketed in the United States.

RADIOGRAPHIC PROCEDURES

As noted above, the initial suspicion of pulmonary tuberculosis is often based on abnormal chest radiographic findings in a patient with respiratory symptoms. Although the "classic" picture is that of upper-lobe disease with infiltrates and cavities (Fig. 158-4), virtually any radiographic pattern—from a normal film or a solitary pulmonary nodule to diffuse alveolar infiltrates in a patient with ARDS—may be seen. In the era of AIDS, no radiographic pattern can be considered pathognomonic. CT (Fig. 158-5) may be useful in interpreting questionable findings on plain chest radiography and may be helpful in diagnosing some forms of extrapulmonary tuberculosis [e.g., Pott's disease (Fig. 158-7)]. MRI is useful in the diagnosis of intracranial tuberculosis.

ADDITIONAL DIAGNOSTIC PROCEDURES

Other diagnostic tests may be used when pulmonary tuberculosis is suspected. Sputum induction by ultrasonic nebulization of hypertonic saline may be useful for patients who cannot produce a sputum specimen spontaneously. Frequently, patients with radiographic abnormalities that are consistent with other diagnoses (e.g., bronchogenic carcinoma) undergo fiberoptic bronchoscopy with bronchial brushings and endobronchial or transbronchial biopsy of the lesion. Bronchoalveolar lavage of a lung segment containing an abnormality may also be performed. In all cases, it is essential that specimens be submitted for AFB smear and mycobacterial culture. For the diagnosis of primary pulmonary tuberculosis in children, who often do not expectorate sputum, specimens from early-morning gastric lavage may yield positive cultures.

Invasive diagnostic procedures are indicated for patients with suspected extrapulmonary tuberculosis. In addition to testing of specimens from involved sites (e.g., CSF for tuberculous meningitis, pleural fluid and biopsy samples for pleural disease), biopsy and culture of bone marrow and liver tissue have a good diagnostic yield in disseminated (miliary) tuberculosis, particularly in HIV-infected patients, who also have a high frequency of positive blood cultures.

In some cases, cultures are negative but a clinical diagnosis of tuberculosis is supported by consistent epidemiologic evidence (e.g., a history of close contact with an infectious patient), a positive TST, and a compatible clinical and radiographic response to treatment. In the United States and other industrialized countries with low rates of tuberculosis, some patients with limited abnormalities on chest radiographs and sputum positive for AFB are infected with nontuberculous mycobacteria, most commonly organisms of the *M. avium* complex (MAC) or *M. kansasii* (Chap. 160). Factors favoring the diagnosis of nontuberculous mycobacterial disease over tuberculosis include an absence of risk factors for tuberculosis, a negative TST, and underlying chronic pulmonary disease.

Patients with HIV-associated tuberculosis pose several diagnostic problems (see "HIV-Associated Tuberculosis," above). Moreover, HIV-infected patients with sputum culture–positive, AFB-positive tuberculosis may present with a normal chest radiograph. With the advent of highly active antiretroviral therapy, the occurrence of disseminated MAC disease that can be confused with tuberculosis has become much less common.

SEROLOGIC AND OTHER DIAGNOSTIC TESTS FOR ACTIVE TUBERCULOSIS

A number of serologic tests based on detection of antibodies to a variety of mycobacterial antigens are marketed in developing countries but not in the United States. Careful independent assessments of these tests suggest that they are not useful as diagnostic aids, especially in persons with a low probability of tuberculosis. Various methods aimed at detection of mycobacterial antigens in diagnostic specimens are being investigated but are limited at present by low sensitivity. Determination of ADA levels in pleural fluid may be useful in the diagnosis of pleural tuberculosis; the utility of this test in the diagnosis of other forms of extrapulmonary tuberculosis (e.g., pericardial, peritoneal, and meningeal) is less clear.

DIAGNOSIS OF LATENT *M. TUBERCULOSIS* INFECTION

Tuberculin Skin Testing In 1891, Robert Koch discovered that components of *M. tuberculosis* in a concentrated liquid culture medium, subsequently named "old tuberculin" (OT), were capable of eliciting a skin reaction when injected subcutaneously into patients with tuberculosis. In 1932, Seibert and Munday purified this product by ammonium sulfate precipitation to produce an active protein fraction known as *tuberculin purified protein derivative (PPD)*. In 1941, PPD-S, developed by Seibert and Glenn, was chosen as the international standard. Later, the WHO and UNICEF sponsored large-scale production of a master batch of PPD (RT23) and made it available for general use. The greatest limitation of PPD is its lack of mycobacterial species specificity, a property due to the large number of proteins in this product that are highly conserved in the various species. In addition, subjectivity of the skin-reaction interpretation, deterioration of the product, and batch-to-batch variations limit the usefulness of PPD.

Skin testing with tuberculin-PPD (TST) is most widely used in screening for latent *M. tuberculosis* infection (LTBI). The test is of limited value in the diagnosis of active tuberculosis because of its relatively low sensitivity and specificity and its inability to discriminate between latent infection and active disease. False-negative reactions are common in immunosuppressed patients and in those with overwhelming tuberculosis. False-positive reactions may be caused by infections with nontuberculous mycobacteria (Chap. 160) and by bacille Calmette-Guérin (BCG) vaccination.

IFN-γ Release Assays (IGRAs) Recently, two in vitro assays that measure T cell release of IFN-γ in response to stimulation with the highly tuberculosis-specific antigens ESAT-6 and CFP-10 have become commercially available. QuantiFERON-TB Gold® (Cellestis Ltd., Carnegie, Australia) is a whole-blood enzyme-linked immunosorbent assay (ELISA) for measurement of IFN-γ, and T-SPOT.TB® (Oxford Immunotec, Oxford, UK) is an enzyme-linked immunospot (ELISpot) assay.

IGRAs are more specific than the TST as a result of less cross-reactivity due to BCG vaccination and sensitization by nontuberculous mycobacteria. IGRAs also appear to be at least as sensitive as the TST for active tuberculosis (used as a surrogate for LTBI). Although diagnostic sensitivity for LTBI cannot be directly estimated because of the absence of a gold standard, these tests have shown better correlation than the TST with exposure to *M. tuberculosis* in contact investigations in low-incidence settings.

Other potential advantages of IGRAs include logistical convenience, the need for fewer patient visits to complete testing, the avoidance of unreliable and somewhat subjective measurements such as skin induration, and the ability to perform serial testing without inducing the boosting phenomenon (a spurious TST conversion due to boosting of reactivity on subsequent TSTs among BCG-vaccinated persons and those infected with other mycobacteria). Because of the high specificity and other potential advantages, IGRAs are likely to replace the TST for LTBI diagnosis in low-incidence, high-income settings where cross-reactivity due to BCG might adversely impact the interpretation and utility of the TST. Direct comparative studies in routine practice thus far suggest that the ELISpot has a lower rate of indeterminate results and probably a higher degree of diagnostic sensitivity than the whole-blood ELISA. Further studies are under way to assess the performance of these tests in contact investigations and in persons with suspected tuberculosis disease, health care workers, HIV-infected individuals, persons with iatrogenic immunosuppression, and children.

℞ TUBERCULOSIS

The two aims of tuberculosis treatment are to interrupt tuberculosis transmission by rendering patients noninfectious and to prevent morbidity and death by curing patients with tuberculosis. Chemotherapy for tuberculosis became possible with the discovery of streptomycin in the mid-1940s. Randomized clinical trials clearly indicated that the administration of streptomycin to patients with chronic tuberculosis reduced mortality rates and led to cure in the majority of cases. However, monotherapy with streptomycin was frequently associated with the development of resistance to this drug and the attendant failure of treatment. With the discovery of para-aminosalicylic acid (PAS) and isoniazid, it became axiomatic that cure of tuberculosis required the concomitant administration of at least two agents to which the organism was susceptible. Furthermore, early clinical trials demonstrated that a long period of treatment—i.e., 12–24 months—was required to prevent recurrence.

The introduction of rifampin in the early 1970s heralded the era of effective short-course chemotherapy, with a treatment duration of <12 months. The discovery that pyrazinamide, which was first used in the 1950s, augmented the potency of isoniazid/rifampin regimens led to the use of a 6-month course of this triple-drug regimen as standard therapy.

DRUGS Four major drugs are considered the first-line agents for the treatment of tuberculosis: isoniazid, rifampin, pyrazinamide, and ethambutol **(Table 158-2)**. These drugs are well absorbed after oral administration, with peak serum levels at 2–4 h and nearly complete elimination within 24 h. These agents are recommended on the basis of their bactericidal activity (i.e., their ability to rapidly reduce the number of viable organisms and render patients noninfectious), their sterilizing activity (i.e., their ability to kill all bacilli and thus sterilize the affected tissues, measured in terms of the ability to prevent relapses), and their low rate of induction of drug resistance. Rifapentine and rifabutin, two drugs related to rifampin, are also available in the United States and are useful for selected patients. **For a detailed discussion of the drugs used for the treatment of tuberculosis, see Chap. 161.**

Because of a lower degree of efficacy and a higher degree of intolerability and toxicity, six classes of second-line drugs are generally used only for the treatment of patients with tuberculosis resistant to first-line drugs. Included in this group are the injectable aminoglycosides streptomycin (formerly a first-line agent), kanamycin, and amikacin; the injectable polypeptide capreomycin; the oral agents ethionamide, cycloserine, and PAS; and the fluoroquinolone antibiotics. Of the quinolones, third-generation agents are preferred: levofloxacin, gatifloxacin (no longer marketed in the United States), and moxifloxacin. Amithiozone (thiacetazone) is still used in some developing countries but is associated with severe and sometimes even fatal skin reactions among HIV-infected patients. Other drugs of unproven efficacy that have been used in the treatment of patients with resistance to most of the first- and second-line agents include clofazimine, amoxicillin/clavulanic acid, and linezolid.

TABLE 158-2 RECOMMENDED DOSAGE[a] FOR INITIAL TREATMENT OF TUBERCULOSIS IN ADULTS[b]

Drug	Dosage: Daily Dose	Dosage: Thrice-Weekly Dose[c]
Isoniazid	5 mg/kg, max 300 mg	15 mg/kg, max 900 mg
Rifampin	10 mg/kg, max 600 mg	10 mg/kg, max 600 mg
Pyrazinamide	20–25 mg/kg, max 2 g	30–40 mg/kg, max 3 g
Ethambutol[d]	15–20 mg/kg	25–30 mg/kg

[a]The duration of treatment for individual drugs varies by regimen, as detailed in Table 158-3.
[b]Dosages for children are similar, except that some authorities recommend higher doses of isoniazid (10–15 mg/kg daily; 20–30 mg/kg intermittent) and rifampin (10–20 mg/kg).
[c]Dosages for twice-weekly administration are the same for isoniazid and rifampin but are higher for pyrazinamide (50 mg/kg, with a maximum of 4 g/d) and ethambutol (40–50 mg/d).
[d]In certain settings, streptomycin (15 mg/kg daily, with a maximum dose of 1 g; or 25–30 mg/kg thrice weekly, with a maximum dose of 1.5 g) can replace ethambutol in the initial phase of treatment. However, streptomycin is no longer considered a first-line drug by the ATS, the IDSA, or the CDC.
Source: Based on recommendations of the American Thoracic Society, the Infectious Diseases Society of America, and the Centers for Disease Control and Prevention.

REGIMENS Standard short-course regimens are divided into an initial, or bactericidal, phase and a continuation, or sterilizing, phase. During the initial phase, the majority of the tubercle bacilli are killed, symptoms resolve, and usually the patient becomes noninfectious. The continuation phase is required to eliminate persisting mycobacteria and prevent relapse.

The treatment regimen of choice for virtually all forms of tuberculosis in both adults and children consists of a 2-month initial phase of isoniazid, rifampin, pyrazinamide, and ethambutol followed by a 4-month continuation phase of isoniazid and rifampin (**Table 158-3**). Treatment may be given daily throughout the course or intermittently (either three times weekly throughout the course or twice weekly after an initial phase of daily therapy, although the twice-weekly option is not recommended by the WHO). A continuation phase of once-weekly rifapentine and isoniazid is equally effective for HIV-seronegative patients with noncavitary pulmonary tuberculosis who have negative sputum cultures at 2 months. Intermittent treatment is especially useful for patients whose therapy is being directly observed (see below). Patients with cavitary pulmonary tuberculosis and delayed sputum-culture conversion (i.e., those who remain culture-positive at 2 months) should have the continuation phase extended by 3 months, for a total course of 9 months. For patients with sputum culture–negative pulmonary tuberculosis, the duration of treatment may be reduced to a total of 4 months. To prevent isoniazid-related neuropathy, pyridoxine (10–25 mg/d) should be added to the regimen given to persons at high risk of vitamin B6 deficiency (e.g., alcoholics; malnourished persons; pregnant and lactating women; and patients with conditions such as chronic renal failure, diabetes, and HIV infection, which are also associated with neuropathy). A full course of therapy (completion of treatment) is defined more accurately by the total number of doses taken than by the duration of treatment. Specific recommendations on the required numbers of doses for each of the various treatment regimens have been published jointly by the American Thoracic Society, the Infectious Diseases Society of America, and the CDC. In some developing countries where the ability to ensure compliance with treatment is limited, a continuation-phase regimen of daily isoniazid and ethambutol for 6 months is acceptable. However, this regimen is associated with a higher rate of relapse and failure, especially among HIV-infected patients.

Lack of adherence to treatment is recognized worldwide as the most important impediment to cure. Moreover, the tubercle bacilli infecting patients who do not adhere to the prescribed regimen are likely to become drug resistant. Both patient- and provider-related factors may affect compliance. Patient-related factors include a lack of belief that the illness is significant and/or that treatment will have a beneficial effect; the existence of concomitant medical conditions (notably substance abuse); lack of social support; and poverty, with attendant joblessness and homelessness. Provider-related factors that may promote compliance include the education and encouragement of patients, the offering of convenient clinic hours, and the provision of incentives and enablers such as meals and travel vouchers.

In addition to specific measures addressing noncompliance, two other strategic approaches are used: direct observation of treatment and provision of fixed-drug-combination (FDC) products. Because it is difficult to predict which patients will adhere to the recommended treatment, all patients should have their therapy directly supervised, especially during the initial phase. In the United States, personnel to supervise therapy are usually available through tuberculosis control programs of local public health departments. Supervision increases the proportion of patients completing treatment and greatly lessens the chances of relapse and acquired drug resistance. FDC products (e.g., isoniazid/rifampin, isoniazid/rifampin/pyrazinamide, and isoniazid/rifampin/pyrazinamide/ethambutol) are available

TABLE 158-3 RECOMMENDED ANTITUBERCULOSIS TREATMENT REGIMENS

Indication	Initial Phase: Duration, Months	Initial Phase: Drugs	Continuation Phase: Duration, Months	Continuation Phase: Drugs
New smear- or culture-positive cases	2	HRZE[a,b]	4	HR[a,c,d]
New culture-negative cases	2	HRZE[a]	2	HR[a]
Pregnancy	2	HRE[e]	7	HR
Failure and relapse[f]	—	—	—	—
Resistance (or intolerance) to H	Throughout (6)	RZE[g]		
Resistance to H + R	Throughout (12–18)	ZEQ + S (or another injectable agent[h])		
Resistance to all first-line drugs	Throughout (24)	1 injectable agent[h] + 3 of these 4: ethionamide, cycloserine, Q, PAS		
Standardized re-treatment (susceptibility testing unavailable)	3	HRZES[i]	5	HRE
Drug intolerance to R	Throughout (12)[j]	HZE		
Drug intolerance to Z	2	HRE	7	HR

[a]All drugs can be given daily or intermittently (three times weekly throughout or twice weekly after 2–8 weeks of daily therapy during the initial phase).
[b]Streptomycin can be used in place of ethambutol but is no longer considered to be a first-line drug by ATS/IDSA/CDC.
[c]The continuation phase should be extended to 7 months for patients with cavitary pulmonary tuberculosis who remain sputum culture–positive after the initial phase of treatment.
[d]HIV-negative patients with noncavitary pulmonary tuberculosis who have negative sputum AFB smears after the initial phase of treatment can be given once-weekly rifapentine/isoniazid in the continuation phase.
[e]The 6-month regimen with pyrazinamide can probably be used safely during pregnancy and is recommended by the WHO and the International Union Against Tuberculosis and Lung Disease. If pyrazinamide is not included in the initial treatment regimen, the minimum duration of therapy is 9 months.
[f]Regimen is tailored according to the results of drug susceptibility tests.
[g]A fluoroquinolone may strengthen the regimen for patients with extensive disease.
[h]Amikacin, kanamycin, or capreomycin. All these agents should be discontinued after 2–6 months, depending upon tolerance and response.
[i]Streptomycin should be discontinued after 2 months. This regimen is less effective for patients in whom treatment has failed, who have an increased probability of rifampin-resistant disease. In such cases, the re-treatment regimen might include second-line drugs chosen in light of the likely pattern of drug resistance.
[j]Streptomycin for the initial 2 months or a fluoroquinolone might strengthen the regimen for patients with extensive disease.
Abbreviations: H, isoniazid; R, rifampin; Z, pyrazinamide; E, ethambutol; S, streptomycin; Q, a quinolone antibiotic; PAS, para-aminosalicylic acid.

(except, in the United States, for the four-drug FDC) and are strongly recommended as a means of minimizing the likelihood of prescription error and of the development of drug resistance as the result of monotherapy. In some formulations of these combination products, the bioavailability of rifampin has been found to be substandard. In North America and Europe, regulatory authorities ensure that combination products are of good quality; however, this type of quality assurance cannot be assumed to take place in less affluent countries. Alternative regimens for patients who exhibit drug intolerance or adverse reactions are listed in Table 158-3. However, severe side effects prompting discontinuation of any of the first-line drugs and use of these alternative regimens are uncommon.

MONITORING TREATMENT RESPONSE AND DRUG TOXICITY

Bacteriologic evaluation is the preferred method of monitoring the response to treatment for tuberculosis. Patients with pulmonary disease should have their sputum examined monthly until cultures become negative. With the recommended regimen, >80% of patients will have negative sputum cultures at the end of the second month of treatment. By the end of the third month, virtually all patients should be culture-negative. In some patients, especially those with extensive cavitary disease and large numbers of organisms, AFB smear conversion may lag behind culture conversion. This phenomenon is presumably due to the expectoration and microscopic visualization of dead bacilli. As noted above, patients with cavitary disease who do not achieve sputum culture conversion by 2 months require extended treatment. When a patient's sputum cultures remain positive at ≥3 months, treatment failure and drug resistance or poor adherence with the regimen should be suspected (see below). A sputum specimen should be collected by the end of treatment to document cure. If mycobacterial cultures are not practical, then monitoring by AFB smear examination should be undertaken at 2, 5, and 6 months. Smears that are positive after 5 months of treatment in a patient known to be adherent are indicative of treatment failure.

Bacteriologic monitoring of patients with extrapulmonary tuberculosis is more difficult and often not feasible. In these cases, the response to treatment must be assessed clinically and radiographically.

Monitoring of the response to treatment during chemotherapy by serial chest radiographs is not recommended, as radiographic changes may lag behind bacteriologic response and are not highly sensitive. After the completion of treatment, neither sputum examination nor chest radiography is recommended for routine follow-up purposes. However, a chest radiograph obtained at the end of treatment may be useful for comparative purposes should the patient develop symptoms of recurrent tuberculosis months or years later. Patients should be instructed to report promptly for medical assessment should they develop any such symptoms.

During treatment, patients should be monitored for drug toxicity (see Table 161-3). The most common adverse reaction of significance is hepatitis. Patients should be carefully educated about the signs and symptoms of drug-induced hepatitis (e.g., dark urine, loss of appetite) and should be instructed to discontinue treatment promptly and see their health care provider should these symptoms occur. Although biochemical monitoring is not routinely recommended, all adult patients should undergo baseline assessment of liver function (e.g., measurement of serum levels of hepatic aminotransferases and serum bilirubin). Older patients, those with concomitant diseases, those with a history of hepatic disease (especially hepatitis C), and those using alcohol daily should be monitored especially closely (i.e., monthly), with repeated measurements of aminotransferases, during the initial phase of treatment. Up to 20% of patients have small increases in aspartate aminotransferase (up to three times the upper limit of normal) that are not accompanied by symptoms and are of no consequence. For patients with symptomatic hepatitis and those with marked (five- to sixfold) elevations in serum levels of aspartate aminotransferase, treatment should be stopped and drugs reintroduced one at a time after liver function has returned to normal.

Hypersensitivity reactions usually require the discontinuation of all drugs and rechallenge to determine which agent is the culprit. Because of the variety of regimens available, it is usually not necessary—although it is possible—to desensitize patients. Hyperuricemia and arthralgia caused by pyrazinamide can usually be managed by the administration of acetylsalicylic acid; however, pyrazinamide treatment should be stopped if the patient develops gouty arthritis. Individuals who develop autoimmune thrombocytopenia secondary to rifampin therapy should not receive the drug thereafter. Similarly, the occurrence of optic neuritis with ethambutol is an indication for permanent discontinuation of this drug. Other common manifestations of drug intolerance, such as pruritus and gastrointestinal upset, can generally be managed without the interruption of therapy.

TREATMENT FAILURE AND RELAPSE As stated above, treatment failure should be suspected when a patient's sputum cultures remain positive after 3 months or when AFB smears remain positive after 5 months. In the management of such patients, it is imperative that the current isolate be tested for susceptibility to first- and second-line agents. When the results of susceptibility testing are expected to become available within a few weeks, changes in the regimen can be postponed until that time. However, if the patient's clinical condition is deteriorating, an earlier change in regimen may be indicated. A cardinal rule in the latter situation is always to add more than one drug at a time to a failing regimen: at least two and preferably three drugs that have never been used and to which the bacilli are likely to be susceptible should be added. The patient may continue to take isoniazid and rifampin along with these new agents pending the results of susceptibility tests.

The mycobacterial strains infecting patients who experience a relapse after apparently successful treatment are less likely to have acquired drug resistance (see below) than are strains from patients in whom treatment has failed. However, if the regimen administered initially does not contain rifampin, the probability of isoniazid resistance is high. Acquired resistance is uncommon among strains from patients who relapse after completing a standard short-course regimen. However, it is prudent to begin the treatment of all patients who have relapsed with all four first-line drugs plus streptomycin, pending the results of susceptibility testing. In less affluent countries and other settings where facilities for culture and drug susceptibility testing are not available, a standard regimen should be used in all instances of relapse and treatment failure (Table 158-3).

DRUG-RESISTANT TUBERCULOSIS Strains of *M. tuberculosis* resistant to individual drugs arise by spontaneous point mutations in the mycobacterial genome, which occur at low but predictable rates. Because there is no cross-resistance among the commonly used drugs, the probability that a strain will be resistant to two drugs is the product of the probabilities of resistance to each drug and thus is low. The development of drug-resistant tuberculosis is invariably the result of monotherapy—i.e., the failure of the health care provider to prescribe at least two drugs to which tubercle bacilli are susceptible or of the patient to take properly prescribed therapy.

Drug-resistant tuberculosis may be either primary or acquired. Primary drug resistance is that in a strain infecting a patient who has not previously been treated. Acquired resistance develops during treatment with an inappropriate regimen. In North America and Europe, rates of primary resistance are generally low, and isoniazid resistance is most common. In the United States, while primary isoniazid resistance was stable at ~7–8% between 1993 and 2002, the rate of primary multidrug-resistant (MDR) tuberculosis (defined as tuberculosis due to a strain resistant at least to isoniazid and rifampin) declined from 2.5% to 1%. Resistance rates are higher among foreign-born and HIV-infected patients. Worldwide, MDR tuberculosis is a serious problem in some regions, especially in the former Soviet Union and parts of Asia (**Fig. 158-8**). As noted above, drug-resistant tuberculosis can be prevented by adherence to the principles of sound therapy: the inclusion of at least two bactericidal drugs to which the organism is susceptible, the use of FDC products, and the verification that patients complete the prescribed course.

Although the 6-month regimen described in Table 158-3 is generally effective for patients with initial isoniazid-resistant disease, it is prudent to include ethambutol and pyrazinamide for the full 6 months. In such cases, isoniazid probably does not contribute to a successful outcome and should be omitted. MDR tuberculosis is more difficult to manage than is disease caused by a drug-susceptible organism, especially because resistance to other first-line drugs as well as to isoniazid and rifampin is common. For strains resistant to isoniazid and rifampin, combinations of a fluoroquinolone, ethambutol, pyrazinamide, and streptomycin (or, for strains resistant to streptomycin as well, another injectable agent such as amikacin or kanamycin), given for 18–24 months and for at least 9 months after sputum culture conversion, may be effective. For patients with bacilli resistant to all of the first-line agents, cure may be attained with a combi-

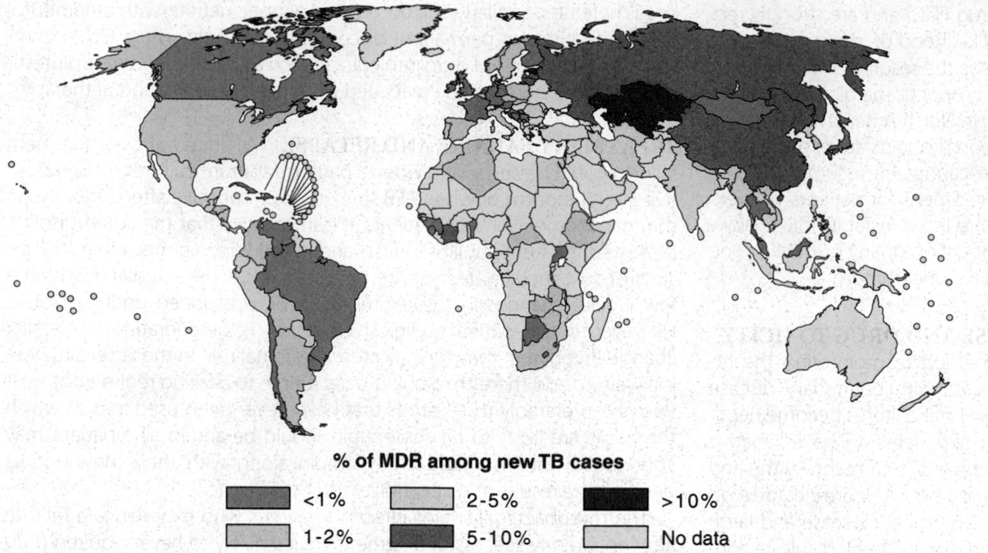

FIGURE 158-8 Percentage of new tuberculosis cases exhibiting multidrug resistance in all countries surveyed by the WHO/Union Global Drug Resistance Surveillance Project during 1994–2005. *(See also disclaimer in Fig. 158-2. Courtesy of the Stop TB Department, WHO; with permission.)*

nation of four second-line drugs, including one injectable agent (Table 158-3). The optimal duration of treatment in this situation is not known; however, a duration of 24 months is recommended. MDR strains of *M. tuberculosis* that are also resistant to at least the fluoroquinolones and one or more of the injectable drugs amikacin, kanamycin, or capreomycin [extensive drug-resistant (XDR) strains] have fewer treatment options and a much poorer prognosis. For patients with localized disease and sufficient pulmonary reserve, lobectomy or pneumonectomy may be helpful. Because the management of patients with MDR and XDR tuberculosis is complicated by both social and medical factors, care of these patients should be restricted to those tuberculosis control programs with resources and capacity and to specialized centers.

HIV-ASSOCIATED TUBERCULOSIS In general, the standard treatment regimens are equally efficacious in HIV-negative and HIV-positive patients. However, adverse drug effects may be more pronounced in HIV-infected patients. Since these effects may include serious or even fatal skin reactions to amithiozone (thiacetazone), this drug, which has been used in place of ethambutol in developing countries, is no longer recommended by the WHO.

Three important considerations are relevant to tuberculosis treatment in HIV-infected patients: an increased frequency of paradoxical reactions, drug interactions between antiretroviral therapy and rifamycins, and development of rifampin monoresistance with widely spaced intermittent treatment. Exacerbations in symptoms, signs, and laboratory or radiographic manifestations of tuberculosis—termed the *immune reconstitution inflammatory syndrome* (IRIS)—have been associated with the administration of antiretroviral regimens. IRIS is more common among patients with advanced immunosuppression and extrapulmonary tuberculosis. The presumed pathogenesis of IRIS is an immune response that is elicited by antigens released as bacilli are killed during effective chemotherapy and that is temporally associated with improving immune function. The first priority in the management of a possible case of IRIS is to ensure that the clinical syndrome does not represent a failure of tuberculosis treatment or the development of another infection. Mild paradoxical reactions can be managed with symptom-based treatment. Glucocorticoids have been used for more severe reactions, although their use in this setting has not been formally evaluated in clinical trials.

Most HIV-infected tuberculosis patients are candidates for antiretroviral therapy, although the optimal timing of this treatment is not known. Rifampin, a potent inducer of enzymes of the cytochrome P450 system, lowers serum levels of many HIV protease inhibitors and some nonnucleoside reverse transcriptase inhibitors—essential drugs used in antiretroviral regimens. In such cases, rifabutin, which has much less enzyme-inducing activity, has been recommended in place of rifampin. However, dosage adjustment for rifabutin and/or the antiretroviral drugs may be necessary. Because recommendations are frequently updated, consultation of the CDC website is advised (*www.cdc.gov/tb/TB_HIV_Drugs/default.htm*).

Several clinical trials of HIV-associated tuberculosis have found that patients with advanced immunosuppression (CD4+ T cell counts of <100/μL) are prone to treatment failure and relapse with rifampin-resistant organisms when treated with "highly intermittent" (i.e., once- or twice-weekly) rifamycin-containing regimens. Consequently, it is recommended that these patients receive daily or thrice-weekly therapy for the entire course.

SPECIAL CLINICAL SITUATIONS

Although comparative clinical trials of treatment for extrapulmonary tuberculosis are limited, the available evidence indicates that most forms of disease can be treated with the 6-month regimen recommended for patients with pulmonary disease. The American Academy of Pediatrics recommends that children with bone and joint tuberculosis, tuberculous meningitis, or miliary tuberculosis receive 9–12 months of treatment.

Treatment for tuberculosis may be complicated by underlying medical problems that require special consideration (see Table 161-1). As a rule, patients with chronic renal failure should not receive aminoglycosides and should receive ethambutol only if serum levels can be monitored. Isoniazid, rifampin, and pyrazinamide may be given in the usual doses in cases of mild to moderate renal failure, but the dosages of isoniazid and pyrazinamide should be reduced for all patients with severe renal failure except those undergoing hemodialysis. Patients with hepatic disease pose a special problem because of the hepatotoxicity of isoniazid, rifampin, and pyrazinamide. Patients with severe hepatic disease may be treated with ethambutol, streptomycin, and possibly another drug (e.g., a fluoroquinolone); if required, isoniazid and rifampin may be administered under close supervision. The use of pyrazinamide by patients with liver failure should be avoided. Silicotuberculosis necessitates the extension of therapy by at least 2 months.

The regimen of choice for pregnant women (Tables 161-1 and 158-3) is 9 months of treatment with isoniazid and rifampin supplemented by ethambutol for the first 2 months. Although the WHO has recommended routine use of pyrazinamide in pregnant women, this drug has not been recommended in the United States because of insufficient data documenting its safety in pregnancy. Streptomycin is contraindicated because it is known to cause eighth-cranial-nerve damage in the fetus. Treatment for tuberculosis is not a contraindication to breast-feeding; most of the drugs administered will be present in small quantities in breast milk, albeit at concentrations far too low to provide any therapeutic or prophylactic benefit to the child.

Medical consultation on difficult-to-manage cases is provided by the CDC Regional Training and Medical Consultation Centers (*http://www.cdc.gov/tb/rtmcc.htm*).

PREVENTION

By far the best way to prevent tuberculosis is to diagnose and isolate infectious cases rapidly and administer appropriate treatment until patients are rendered noninfectious and the disease is cured. Additional strategies include BCG vaccination and treatment of persons with latent tuberculosis infection who are at high risk of developing active disease.

BCG VACCINATION

BCG was derived from an attenuated strain of *M. bovis* and first administered to humans in 1921. Many BCG vaccines are available worldwide; all are derived from the original strain, but the vaccines vary in efficacy, ranging from 80% to nil in randomized, placebo-controlled trials. A similar range of efficacy was found in recent observational studies (case-control, historic cohort, and cross-sectional) in areas where infants are vaccinated at birth. These studies also found higher rates of efficacy in the protection of infants and young children from relatively serious forms of tuberculosis, such as tuberculous meningitis and miliary tuberculosis.

BCG vaccine is safe and rarely causes serious complications. The local tissue response begins 2–3 weeks after vaccination, with scar formation and healing within 3 months. Side effects—most commonly, ulceration at the vaccination site and regional lymphadenitis—occur in 1–10% of vaccinated persons. Some vaccine strains have caused osteomyelitis in ~1 case per million doses administered. Disseminated BCG infection and death have occurred in 1–10 cases per 10 million doses administered, although this problem is restricted almost exclusively to persons with impaired immunity, such as children with severe combined immunodeficiency syndrome or adults with HIV infection. BCG vaccination induces TST reactivity, which tends to wane with time. The presence or size of TST reactions after vaccination does not predict the degree of protection afforded.

BCG vaccine is recommended for routine use at birth in countries with high tuberculosis prevalence. However, because of the low risk of transmission of tuberculosis in the United States, the unreliable protection afforded by BCG, and its impact on the TST, the vaccine has never been recommended for general use in the United States. The CDC has recommended that HIV-infected adults and children not receive BCG vaccine, although the WHO has recommended that asymptomatic HIV-infected children residing in tuberculosis-endemic areas receive BCG.

Rx LATENT TUBERCULOSIS INFECTION

Treatment of selected persons with LTBI aims at preventing active disease. This intervention (formerly called *preventive chemotherapy* or *chemoprophylaxis*) is based on the results of a large number of randomized, placebo-controlled clinical trials demonstrating that a 6- to 12-month course of isoniazid reduces the risk of active tuberculosis in infected people by up to 90%. Analysis of available data indicates that the optimal duration of treatment is 9–10 months. In the absence of reinfection, the protective effect is believed to be lifelong. Clinical trials have shown that isoniazid reduces rates of tuberculosis among TST-positive persons with HIV infection. Studies in HIV-infected patients have also demonstrated the effectiveness of shorter courses of rifampin-based treatment.

In most cases, candidates for treatment of LTBI **(Table 158-4)** are identified by the TST of persons in defined high-risk groups. For skin testing, 5 tuberculin units of polysorbate-stabilized PPD should be injected intradermally into the volar surface of the forearm (Mantoux method). Multipuncture tests are not recommended. Reactions are read at 48–72 h as the transverse diameter (in millimeters) of induration; the diameter of erythema is not considered. In some persons, TST reactivity wanes with time but can be recalled by a second skin test administered ≥1 week after the first (i.e., two-step testing). For persons periodically undergoing the TST, such as health care workers and individuals admitted to long-term-care institutions, initial two-step testing may preclude subsequent misclassification of persons with boosted reactions as TST converters.

The cutoff for a positive TST (and thus for treatment) is related both to the probability that the reaction represents true infection and to the likelihood that the individual, if truly infected, will develop tuberculosis (Table 158-4). Thus, positive reactions for close contacts of infectious cases, persons with HIV infection, persons receiving drugs that suppress the immune system, and previously untreated persons whose chest radiograph is consistent with healed tuberculosis are defined as an area of induration ≥5 mm in diameter. A 10-mm cutoff is used to define positive reactions in most other at-risk persons. For persons with a very low risk of developing tuberculosis if infected, a cutoff of 15 mm is used. (Except for employment purposes where longitudinal screening is anticipated, the TST is not indicated for these low-risk persons.) Treatment should be considered for persons from tuberculosis-endemic countries who have a history of BCG vaccination. A positive reaction in an IGRA is not based on the degree of response—i.e., the level of IFN-γ induced.

Some TST-negative individuals are also candidates for treatment. Infants and children who have come into contact with infectious cases should be treated and should have a repeat skin test 2 or 3 months after contact ment. HIV-infected persons who have been exposed to an infectious tuberculosis patient should receive treatment regardless of the TST result.

TABLE 158-4 TUBERCULIN REACTION SIZE AND TREATMENT OF LATENT TUBERCULOSIS INFECTION

Risk Group	Tuberculin Reaction Size, mm
HIV-infected persons or persons receiving immunosuppressive therapy	≥5
Close contacts of tuberculosis patients	≥5[a]
Persons with fibrotic lesions on chest radiography	≥5
Recently infected persons (≤2 years)	≥10
Persons with high-risk medical conditions[b]	≥10
Low-risk persons[c]	≥15

[a]Tuberculin-negative contacts, especially children, should receive prophylaxis for 2–3 months after contact ends and should then undergo repeat TST. Those whose results remain negative should discontinue prophylaxis. HIV-infected contacts should receive a full course of treatment regardless of TST results.

[b]Includes diabetes mellitus, some hematologic and reticuloendothelial diseases, injection drug use (with HIV seronegativity), end-stage renal disease, and clinical situations associated with rapid weight loss.

[c]Except for employment purposes where longitudinal TST screening is anticipated, TST is not indicated for these low-risk persons. A decision to treat should be based on individual risk/benefit considerations.

Isoniazid is administered at a daily dose of 5 mg/kg (up to 300 mg/d) for 9 months **(Table 158-5)**. On the basis of cost-benefit analyses, a 6-month period of treatment has been recommended in the past and may be considered for HIV-negative adults with normal chest radiographs when financial considerations are important. When supervised treatment is desirable and feasible, isoniazid may be given at a dose of 15 mg/kg (up to 900 mg) twice weekly. An alternative regimen for adults is 4 months of daily rifampin. A 3-month regimen of isoniazid and rifampin is recommended in the United Kingdom for both adults and children. A previously recommended regimen of 2 months of rifampin and pyrazinamide has been associated with serious and fatal hepatotoxicity and now is generally not recommended. The rifampin regimen should be considered for persons who are likely to have been infected with an isoniazid-resistant strain.

Isoniazid should not be given to persons with active liver disease. All persons at increased risk of hepatotoxicity (e.g., those abusing alcohol daily and those with a history of liver disease) should undergo baseline and then monthly assessment of liver function. All patients should be carefully educated about hepatitis and instructed to discontinue use of the drug immediately should any symptoms develop. Moreover, patients should be seen and questioned monthly during therapy about adverse reactions and should be given no more than 1 month's supply of drug at each visit.

It may be more difficult to ensure compliance when treating persons with latent infection than when treating those with active tuberculosis. If family members of active cases are being treated, compliance and monitoring may be easier. When feasible, twice-weekly supervised therapy may increase the likelihood of completion. As in active cases, the provision of incentives may also be helpful.

PRINCIPLES OF TUBERCULOSIS CONTROL

The highest priority in any tuberculosis control program is the prompt detection of cases and the provision of short-course chemotherapy to all tuberculosis patients under proper case-management conditions, including directly observed therapy. In addition, in low-prevalence countries with adequate resources, screening of high-risk groups (such as immigrants from high-prevalence countries, migratory workers, prisoners, the homeless, substance abusers, and HIV-seropositive persons) is recommended. TST-positive high-risk persons should be treated for latent infection. Contact investigation is an important component of efficient tuberculosis control. In the United States, a great deal of attention has been given to the transmission of tuberculosis (particularly in association with HIV infection) in institutional settings such as hospitals, homeless shelters, and prisons. Measures to limit such transmission include respiratory isolation of persons with

TABLE 158-5 REVISED DRUG REGIMENS FOR TREATMENT OF LATENT TUBERCULOSIS INFECTION (LTBI) IN ADULTS

Drug	Interval and Duration	Comments[a]	Rating[b] (Evidence[c]) HIV-Negative	Rating[b] (Evidence[c]) HIV-Infected
Isoniazid	Daily for 9 months[d,e]	In HIV-infected persons, isoniazid may be administered concurrently with nucleoside reverse transcriptase inhibitors, protease inhibitors, or nonnucleoside reverse transcriptase inhibitors (NNRTIs).	A (II)	A (II)
	Twice weekly for 9 months[d,e]	Directly observed therapy (DOT) must be used with twice-weekly dosing.	B (II)	B (II)
	Daily for 6 months[e]	Regimen is not indicated for HIV-infected persons, those with fibrotic lesions on chest radiographs, or children.	B (I)	C (I)
	Twice weekly for 6 months[e]	DOT must be used with twice-weekly dosing.	B (II)	C (I)
Rifampin[f]	Daily for 4 months	Regimen is used for contacts of patients with isoniazid-resistant, rifampin-susceptible tuberculosis. In HIV-infected persons, most protease inhibitors and delavirdine should not be administered concurrently with rifampin. Rifabutin, with appropriate dose adjustments, can be used with protease inhibitors (saquinavir should be augmented with ritonavir) and NNRTIs (except delavirdine). Clinicians should consult web-based updates for the latest specific recommendations.	B (II)	B (III)
Rifampin plus pyrazinamide (RZ)	Daily for 2 months	Regimen generally should not be offered for treatment of LTBI in either HIV-infected or HIV-negative persons.	D (II)	D (II)
	Twice weekly for 2–3 months		D (III)	D (III)

[a]Interactions with HIV-related drugs are updated frequently and are available at *http://www.aidsinfo.nih.gov/guidelines*.

[b]Strength of the recommendation: A. Both strong evidence of efficacy and substantial clinical benefit support recommendation for use. Should always be offered. B. Moderate evidence for efficacy or strong evidence for efficacy but only limited clinical benefit supports recommendation for use. Should generally be offered. C. Evidence for efficacy is insufficient to support a recommendation for or against use, or evidence for efficacy might not outweigh adverse consequences (e.g., drug toxicity, drug interactions) or cost of the treatment or alternative approaches. Optional. D. Moderate evidence for lack of efficacy or for adverse outcome supports a recommendation against use. Should generally not be offered. E. Good evidence for lack of efficacy or for adverse outcome supports a recommendation against use. Should never be offered.

[c]Quality of evidence supporting the recommendation: I. Evidence from at least one properly randomized controlled trial. II. Evidence from at least one well-designed clinical trial without randomization, from cohort or case-controlled analytic studies (preferably from more than one center), from multiple time-series studies, or from dramatic results in uncontrolled experiments. III. Evidence from opinions of respected authorities based on clinical experience, descriptive studies, or reports of expert committees.

[d]Recommended regimen for persons aged <18 years.

[e]Recommended regimen for pregnant women.

[f]The substitution of rifapentine for rifampin is not recommended because rifapentine's safety and effectiveness have not been established for patients with LTBI.

Source: Adapted from CDC: Targeted tuberculin testing and treatment of latent tuberculosis infection. MMWR 49(RR-6), 2000

suspected tuberculosis until they are proven to be noninfectious (i.e., by sputum AFB smear negativity), proper ventilation in rooms of patients with infectious tuberculosis, use of ultraviolet irradiation in areas of increased risk of tuberculosis transmission, and periodic screening of personnel who may come into contact with known or unsuspected cases of tuberculosis. In the past, radiographic surveys, especially those conducted with portable equipment and miniature films, were advocated for case finding. Today, however, the prevalence of tuberculosis in industrialized countries is sufficiently low that "mass miniature radiography" is not cost-effective.

In high-prevalence countries, many tuberculosis control programs have made good progress in reducing morbidity and mortality during the past decade by adopting and implementing the DOTS strategy promoted by the WHO. This strategy consists of: (1) political commitment with increased and sustained financing; (2) case detection through quality-assured bacteriology (starting with microscopic examination of sputum from patients with cough of >2–3 weeks' duration); (3) administration of standardized treatment, with supervision and patient support; (4) an effective drug supply and management system; and (5) a monitoring and evaluation system, with impact measurement (including assessment of treatment outcomes—e.g., cure, completion of treatment without bacteriologic proof of cure, death, treatment failure, and default—in all cases registered and notified). In 2006, the WHO indicated that, while DOTS remains the essential component of any control strategy, additional steps must be undertaken to reach the 2015 tuberculosis control targets set within the United Nations Millennium Development Goals. Thus, a new "Stop TB Strategy" with six components has been promoted: (1) Pursue high-quality DOTS expansion and enhancement. (2) Address HIV-associated tuberculosis, MDR tuberculosis, and other special challenges. (3) Contribute to health system strengthening. (4) Engage all care providers. (5) Empower people with tuberculosis and communities. (6) Enable and promote research. As part of the fourth component, new evidence-based International Standards for Tuberculosis Care, focused on diagnosis, treatment, and public health responsibilities, have recently been introduced for wide adoption by medical and professional societies, academic institutions, and all practitioners worldwide.

FURTHER READINGS

AMERICAN THORACIC SOCIETY, CENTERS FOR DISEASE CONTROL AND PREVENTION: Targeted tuberculin testing and treatment of latent tuberculosis infection. Am J Respir Crit Care Med 161:S221, 2000

AMERICAN THORACIC SOCIETY, INFECTIOUS DISEASES SOCIETY OF AMERICA, CENTERS FOR DISEASE CONTROL AND PREVENTION: Treatment of tuberculosis. Am J Respir Crit Care Med 167:603, 2003

CENTERS FOR DISEASE CONTROL AND PREVENTION: Control of tuberculosis in the United States: Recommendations from the American Thoracic Society, CDC, and the Infectious Diseases Society of America. MMWR 54:RR1, 2005

HOPEWELL PC et al: International standards for tuberculosis care. Lancet Infect Dis 6:710, 2006

PAI M et al: New tools and emerging technologies for the diagnosis of tuberculosis. Part I: Latent tuberculosis. Part II: Active tuberculosis and drug resistance. Expert Rev Mol Diagn 6:413, 2006

RAVIGLIONE MC, SMITH IM: XDR tuberculosis—Implications for global public health. N Engl J Med 356:656, 2007

———, UPLEKAR M: WHO's new Stop TB Strategy. Lancet 367:952, 2006

REID A et al: Towards universal access to HIV prevention, treatment, care and support: The role of tuberculosis/HIV collaboration. Lancet Infect Dis 6:483, 2006

WORLD HEALTH ORGANIZATION: Guidelines for the programmatic management of drug-resistant tuberculosis. Geneva, WHO, 2006

159 Leprosy (Hansen's Disease)

Robert H. Gelber

Leprosy, first described in ancient Indian texts from the sixth century B.C., is a nonfatal, chronic infectious disease caused by *Mycobacterium leprae*, whose clinical manifestations are largely confined to the skin, peripheral nervous system, upper respiratory tract, eyes, and testes. The unique tropism of *M. leprae* for peripheral nerves (from large nerve trunks to microscopic dermal nerves) and certain immunologically mediated reactional states are the major causes of morbidity in leprosy. The propensity of the disease, when untreated, to result in characteristic deformities and the recognition in most cultures that the disease is communicable from person to person have resulted historically in a profound social stigma. Today, with early diagnosis and the institution of appropriate and effective antimicrobial therapy, patients can lead productive lives in the community, and deformities and other visible manifestations can largely be prevented.

ETIOLOGY

M. leprae is an obligate intracellular bacillus (0.3–1 μm wide and 1–8 μm long) that is confined to humans, armadillos in certain locales, and sphagnum moss. The organism is acid-fast, indistinguishable microscopically from other mycobacteria, and ideally detected in tissue sections by a modified Fite stain. Strain variability has been documented in this organism. *M. leprae* produces no known toxins and is well adapted to penetrate and reside within macrophages, yet it may survive outside the body for months. In untreated patients, only ~1% of *M. leprae* organisms are viable. The morphologic index (MI), a measure of the number of acid-fast bacilli (AFB) in skin scrapings that stain uniformly bright, correlates with viability. The bacteriologic index (BI), a logarithmic-scaled measure of the density of *M. leprae* in the dermis, may be as high as 4–6+ in untreated patients, falling by 1 unit per year during effective therapy; the rate of decrease is independent of the relative potency of effective antimicrobial therapy. A rising MI or BI suggests relapse and perhaps—if the patient is being treated—drug resistance. The latter possibility can be confirmed or excluded in the mouse model.

As a result of reductive evolution, almost half of the *M. leprae* genome contains nonfunctional genes; only 1605 genes encode for proteins, and 1439 genes are shared with *Mycobacterium tuberculosis*. In contrast, *M. tuberculosis* uses 91% of its genome to encode for 4000 proteins. Among the lost genes in *M. leprae* are those for catabolic and respiratory pathways; transport systems; purine, methionine, and glutamine synthesis; and nitrogen regulation. The genome of *M. leprae* provides a metabolic rationale for its obligate intracellular existence and reliance on host biochemical support, a template for targets of drug development, and ultimately a pathway to cultivation. The finding of strain variability among *M. leprae* isolates has provided a powerful tool with which to address anew the organism's epidemiology and pathobiology and to determine whether relapse represents reactivation or reinfection. The bacterium's complex cell wall contains large amounts of an *M. leprae*–specific phenolic glycolipid (PGL-1), which is detected in serologic tests. The unique trisaccharide of *M. leprae* binds to the basal lamina of Schwann cells; this interaction is probably relevant to the fact that *M. leprae* is the only bacterium to invade peripheral nerves.

Although it was the first bacterium to be etiologically associated with human disease, *M. leprae* remains one of the few bacterial species that still has not been cultivated on artificial medium or tissue culture. The multiplication of *M. leprae* in mouse footpads (albeit limited, with a doubling time of ~2 weeks) has provided a means to evaluate antimicrobial agents, monitor clinical trials, and screen vaccines. *M. leprae* grows best in cooler tissues (the skin, peripheral nerves, anterior chamber of the eye, upper respiratory tract, and testes), sparing warmer areas of the skin (the axilla, groin, scalp, and midline of the back).

EPIDEMIOLOGY

Demographics Leprosy is almost exclusively a disease of the developing world, affecting areas of Asia, Africa, Latin America, and the Pacific (Fig. 159-1). While Africa has the highest disease prevalence, Asia has the most cases. More than 80% of the world's cases occur in a few countries: India, China, Myanmar, Indonesia, Brazil, Nigeria, Madagascar, and Nepal. Within endemic locales, the distribution of leprosy is quite uneven, with areas of high prevalence bordering on areas with little or no disease. In Brazil the majority of cases occur in the Amazon basin and two western states, while in Mexico leprosy is mostly confined to the Pacific coast. Except as imported cases, leprosy is largely absent from the United States, Canada, and northwestern Europe. In the United States, ~4000 persons have leprosy and 100–200 new cases are reported annually, most of them in California, Texas, New York, and Hawaii among immigrants from Mexico, Southeast Asia, the Philippines, and the Caribbean. The comparative genomics of single-nucleotide polymorphisms support the likelihood that four distinct strains exist, having originated in East Africa or Central Asia. A mutation spread to Europe and subsequently underwent two separate mutations that were then followed by spread to West Africa and the Americas.

The global prevalence of leprosy is difficult to assess, given that many of the locales with high prevalence lack a significant medical or public health infrastructure. Estimates range from 0.6 to 8 million affected individuals. The lower estimate includes only persons who have not completed chemotherapy, excluding those who may be physically or psychologically damaged from leprosy and who may yet relapse or develop immune-mediated reactions. The higher figure includes patients whose infections probably are already cured and many who have no leprosy-related deformity or disability. Although the figures on the worldwide prevalence of leprosy are debatable, it is not falling; there are an estimated 600,000 new cases annually, 60% of them in India.

Leprosy is associated with poverty and rural residence. It appears not to be associated with AIDS, perhaps because of leprosy's long in-

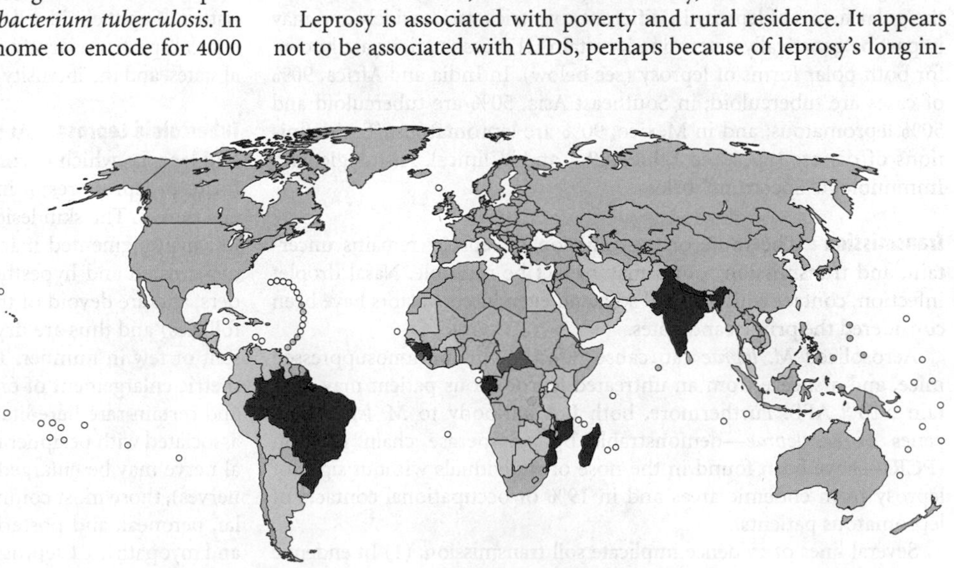

FIGURE 159-1 Estimated prevalence of leprosy at the turn of the millennium. Because data on leprosy prevalence in many endemic countries are unreliable, global prevalence is difficult to assess with any great degree of accuracy; however, it is not falling (see text). *(Courtesy of Patrick J. Brennan, Ph.D., with permission; www.cvmbs.colostate.edu/microbiology/leprosy/globalleprosy3.html.)*

TABLE 159-1 CLINICAL, BACTERIOLOGIC, PATHOLOGIC, AND IMMUNOLOGIC SPECTRUM OF LEPROSY

Feature	Tuberculoid (TT, BT) Leprosy	Borderline (BB, BL) Leprosy	Lepromatous (LL) Leprosy
Skin lesions	One or a few sharply defined annular asymmetric macules or plaques with a tendency toward central clearing, elevated borders	Intermediate between BT and LL type lesions; ill-defined plaques with an occasional sharp margin; few or many in number	Symmetric, poorly marginated, multiple infiltrated nodules and plaques or diffuse infiltration; xanthoma-like or dermatofibroma papules; leonine facies and eyebrow alopecia
Nerve lesions	Skin lesions anesthetic early; nerve near lesions sometimes enlarged; nerve abscesses most common in BT	Hypesthetic or anesthetic skin lesions; nerve trunk palsies, at times symmetric	Hypesthesia a late sign; nerve palsies variable; acral, distal, symmetric anesthesia common
Acid-fast bacilli (BI[a])	0–1+	3–5+	4–6+
Lymphocytes	2+	1+	0–1+
Macrophage differentiation	Epithelioid	Epithelioid in BB; usually undifferentiated, but may have foamy changes in BL	Foamy change the rule; may be undifferentiated in early lesions
Langhans' giant cells	1–3+	—	—
Lepromin skin test	+++	—	—
Lymphocyte transformation test	Generally positive	1–10%	1–2%
CD4+/CD8+ T-cell ratio in lesions	1.2	BB (NT); BL: 0.48	0.50
M. leprae PGL-1 antibodies	60%	85%	95%

[a]See text.

Abbreviations: BB, mid-borderline; BL, borderline lepromatous; BT, borderline tuberculoid; TT, polar tuberculoid; LL, polar lepromatous; BI, bacteriologic index; NT, not tested; PGL-1, phenolic glycolipid 1.

cubation period. Most people appear to be naturally immune to leprosy and do not develop disease manifestations after exposure. The time of peak onset is in the second and third decades of life. The most severe lepromatous form of leprosy is twice as common among men as among women and is rarely encountered in children. The frequency of the polar forms of leprosy in different countries varies widely and may in part be genetically determined; certain HLA associations are known for both polar forms of leprosy (see below). In India and Africa, 90% of cases are tuberculoid; in Southeast Asia, 50% are tuberculoid and 50% lepromatous; and in Mexico, 90% are lepromatous. (For definitions of disease types, see Table 159-1 and "Clinical, Histologic, and Immunologic Spectrum," below.)

Transmission The route of transmission of leprosy remains uncertain, and transmission routes may in fact be multiple. Nasal droplet infection, contact with infected soil, and even insect vectors have been considered the prime candidates.

Aerosolized *M. leprae* can cause infection in immunosuppressed mice, and a sneeze from an untreated lepromatous patient may contain $>10^{10}$ AFB. Furthermore, both IgA antibody to *M. leprae* and genes of *M. leprae*—demonstrable by polymerase chain reaction (PCR)—have been found in the nose of individuals without signs of leprosy from endemic areas and in 19% of occupational contacts of lepromatous patients.

Several lines of evidence implicate soil transmission. (1) In endemic countries such as India, leprosy is primarily a rural and not an urban disease. (2) *M. leprae* products reside in soil in endemic locales. (3) Direct dermal inoculation (e.g., during tattooing) may transmit *M. leprae*, and common sites of leprosy in children are the buttocks and thighs, suggesting that microinoculation of infected soil may transmit the disease.

Evidence for insect vectors of leprosy includes the demonstration that bedbugs and mosquitoes in the vicinity of leprosaria regularly harbor *M. leprae* and that experimentally infected mosquitoes can transmit infection to mice. Skin-to-skin contact is generally not considered an important route of transmission.

In endemic countries, ~50% of leprosy patients have a history of intimate contact with an infected person (often a household member), while, for unknown reasons, leprosy patients in nonendemic locales can identify such contact only 10% of the time. Moreover, household contact with an infected lepromatous case carries an eventual risk of disease acquisition of ~10% in endemic areas as opposed to only 1% in nonendemic locales. Contact with a tuberculoid case carries a very low risk. Physicians and nurses caring for leprosy patients and the co-workers of these patients are not at risk for leprosy.

M. leprae causes disease primarily in humans. However, in Texas and Louisiana, 15% of nine-banded armadillos are infected, and armadillo contact occasionally results in human disease. Armadillos develop disseminated infection after IV inoculation of live *M. leprae.*

CLINICAL, HISTOLOGIC, AND IMMUNOLOGIC SPECTRUM

The incubation period prior to manifestation of clinical disease can vary between 2 and 40 years, although it is generally 5–7 years in duration. Leprosy presents as a spectrum of clinical manifestations that have bacteriologic, pathologic, and immunologic counterparts. The spectrum from polar tuberculoid (TT) to borderline tuberculoid (BT) to mid-borderline (BB, which is rarely encountered) to borderline lepromatous (BL) to polar lepromatous (LL) disease is associated with an evolution from asymmetric localized macules and plaques to nodular and indurated symmetric generalized skin manifestations, an increasing bacterial load, and loss of *M. leprae*–specific cellular immunity (Table 159-1). Distinguishing dermatopathologic characteristics include the number of lymphocytes, giant cells, and AFB as well as the nature of epithelioid cell differentiation. Where a patient presents on the clinical spectrum largely determines prognosis, complications, reactional states, and the intensity of antimicrobial therapy required.

Tuberculoid Leprosy At the less severe end of the spectrum is tuberculoid leprosy, which encompasses TT and BT disease. In general, these forms of leprosy result in symptoms confined to the skin and peripheral nerves. The skin lesions of tuberculoid leprosy consist of one or a few hypopigmented macules or plaques (Fig. 159-2) that are sharply demarcated and hypesthetic, often have erythematous or raised borders, and are devoid of the normal skin organs (sweat glands and hair follicles) and thus are dry, scaly, and anhidrotic. AFB are generally absent or few in number. Tuberculoid leprosy patients may have asymmetric enlargement of one or a few peripheral nerves. Indeed, leprosy and certain rare hereditary neuropathies are the only human diseases associated with peripheral-nerve enlargement. Although any peripheral nerve may be enlarged (including small digital and supraclavicular nerves), those most commonly affected are the ulnar, posterior auricular, peroneal, and posterior tibial nerves, with associated hypesthesia and myopathy. TT leprosy is the most common form of the disease encountered in India and Africa but is virtually absent in Southeast Asia, where BT leprosy is frequent.

In tuberculoid leprosy, T cells breach the perineurium, and destruction of Schwann cells and axons may be evident, resulting in fibrosis of the epineurium, replacement of the endoneurium with epithelial granulomas, and occasionally caseous necrosis. Such invasion and destruction of nerves in the dermis by T cells are pathognomonic for leprosy.

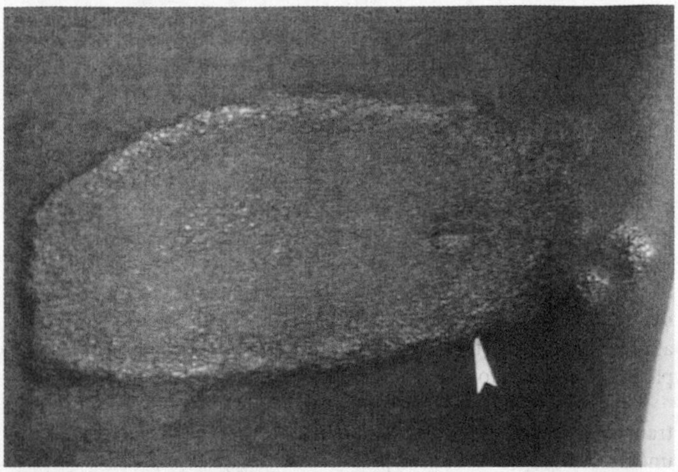

FIGURE 159-2 Tuberculoid (TT) leprosy: a well-defined, hypopigmented, anesthetic macule with anhidrosis and a raised granular margin *(arrowhead)*.

Circulating lymphocytes from patients with tuberculoid leprosy readily recognize *M. leprae* and its constituent proteins, patients have positive lepromin skin tests (see "Diagnosis," below), and—owing to a type 1 cytokine pattern in tuberculoid tissues—strong T cell and macrophage activation results in a localized infection. In tuberculoid leprosy tissue, there is a 2:1 predominance of helper CD4+ over CD8+ T lymphocytes. Tuberculoid tissues are rich in the mRNAs of the proinflammatory T_H1 family of cytokines: interleukin (IL) 2, interferon γ (IFN-γ), and IL-12; in contrast, IL-4, IL-5, and IL-10 mRNAs are scarce.

Lepromatous Leprosy Lepromatous leprosy patients present with symmetrically distributed skin nodules (Fig. 159-3), raised plaques, or diffuse dermal infiltration, which, when on the face, results in leonine facies. Late manifestations include loss of eyebrows (initially the lateral margins only) and eyelashes, pendulous earlobes, and dry scaling skin, particularly on the feet. In LL leprosy, bacilli are numerous in the skin (as many as 10^9/g), where they are often found in large clumps (*globi*), and in peripheral nerves, where they initially invade Schwann cells, resulting in foamy degenerative myelination and axonal degeneration and later in Wallerian degeneration. In addition, bacilli are plentiful in circulating blood and in all organ systems except the lungs and the central nervous system. Nevertheless, patients are afebrile, and there is no evidence of major organ system

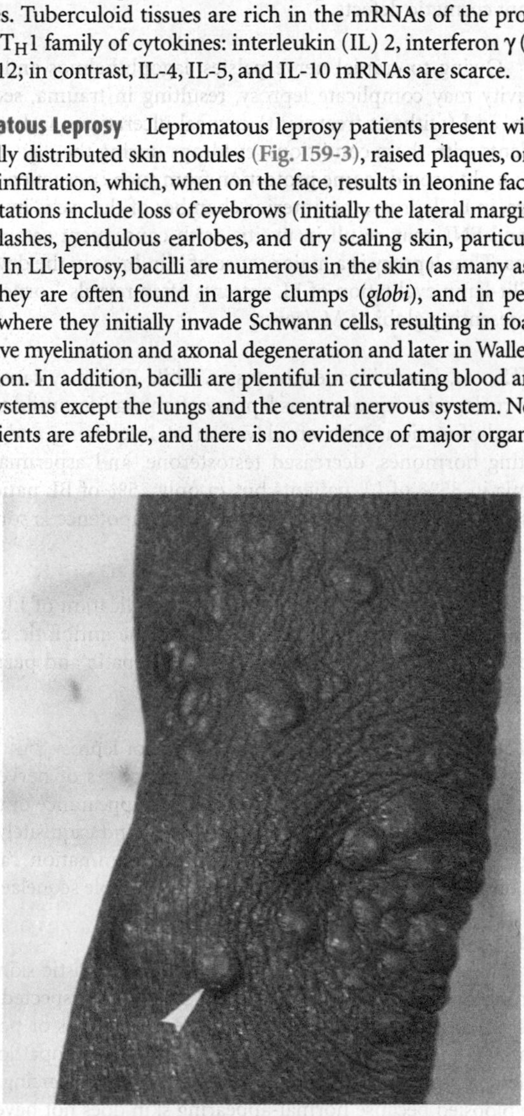

FIGURE 159-3 Lepromatous (LL) leprosy: advanced nodular lesions.

dysfunction. Found almost exclusively in western Mexico and the Caribbean is a form of lepromatous leprosy without visible skin lesions but with diffuse dermal infiltration and a demonstrably thickened dermis, termed *diffuse lepromatosis*. In lepromatous leprosy, nerve enlargement and damage tend to be symmetric, result from actual bacillary invasion, and are more insidious but ultimately more extensive than in tuberculoid leprosy. Patients with LL leprosy have acral, distal, symmetric peripheral neuropathy and a tendency toward symmetric nerve-trunk enlargement. They may also have signs and symptoms related to involvement of the upper respiratory tract, the anterior chamber of the eye, and the testes.

In untreated LL patients, lymphocytes regularly fail to recognize either *M. leprae* or its protein constituents, and lepromin skin tests are negative (see "Diagnosis," below). This loss of protective cellular immunity appears to be antigen-specific, as patients are not unusually susceptible to opportunistic infections, cancer, or AIDS and maintain delayed-type hypersensitivity to *Candida*, *Trichophyton*, mumps, tetanus toxoid, and even purified protein derivative of tuberculin. At times, *M. leprae*–specific anergy is reversible with effective chemotherapy. In LL tissues, there is a 2:1 ratio of CD8+ to CD4+ T lymphocytes. LL patients have a predominant T_H2 response and hyperglobulinemia, and LL tissues demonstrate a T_H2 cytokine profile, being rich in mRNAs for IL-4, IL-5, and IL-10 and poor in those for IL-2, IFN-γ, and IL-12. It appears that cytokines mediate a protective tissue response in leprosy, as injection of IFN-γ or IL-2 into lepromatous lesions causes a loss of AFB and histopathologic conversion toward a tuberculoid pattern. Macrophages of lepromatous leprosy patients appear to be functionally intact; circulating monocytes exhibit normal microbicidal function and responsiveness to IFN-γ.

Reactional States Lepra reactions comprise several common immunologically mediated inflammatory states that cause considerable morbidity. Some of these reactions precede diagnosis and the institution of effective antimicrobial therapy; indeed, these reactions may precipitate presentation for medical attention and diagnosis. Other reactions occur after the initiation of appropriate chemotherapy and may cause patients to perceive that their leprosy is worsening and to lose confidence in conventional therapy. Only by warning patients of the potential for these reactions and describing their manifestations can physicians treating leprosy patients ensure continued credibility.

TYPE 1 LEPRA REACTIONS (DOWNGRADING AND REVERSAL REACTIONS) Type 1 lepra reactions occur in almost half of patients with borderline forms of leprosy but not in patients with pure lepromatous disease. Manifestations include classic signs of inflammation within previously involved macules, papules, and plaques and, on occasion, the appearance of new skin lesions, neuritis, and (less commonly) fever—generally low-grade. The nerve trunk most commonly involved in this process is the ulnar nerve at the elbow, which may be painful and exquisitely tender. If patients with affected nerves are not treated promptly with glucocorticoids (see below), irreversible nerve damage may result in as little as 24 h. The most dramatic manifestation is footdrop, which occurs when the peroneal nerve is involved.

When type 1 lepra reactions precede the initiation of appropriate antimicrobial therapy, they are termed *downgrading reactions*, and the case becomes histologically more lepromatous; when they occur after the initiation of therapy, they are termed *reversal reactions*, and the case becomes more tuberculoid. Reversal reactions often occur in the first months or years after the initiation of therapy but may also develop several years thereafter.

Edema is the most characteristic microscopic feature of type 1 lepra lesions, whose diagnosis is primarily clinical. Reversal reactions are typified by a T_H1 cytokine profile, with an influx of CD4+ helper cells and increased levels of IFN-γ and IL-2. In addition, type 1 reactions are associated with large numbers of T cells bearing γ/δ receptors—a unique feature of leprosy.

TYPE 2 LEPRA REACTIONS: ERYTHEMA NODOSUM LEPROSUM Erythema nodosum leprosum (ENL) (Fig. 159-4) occurs exclusively in patients near

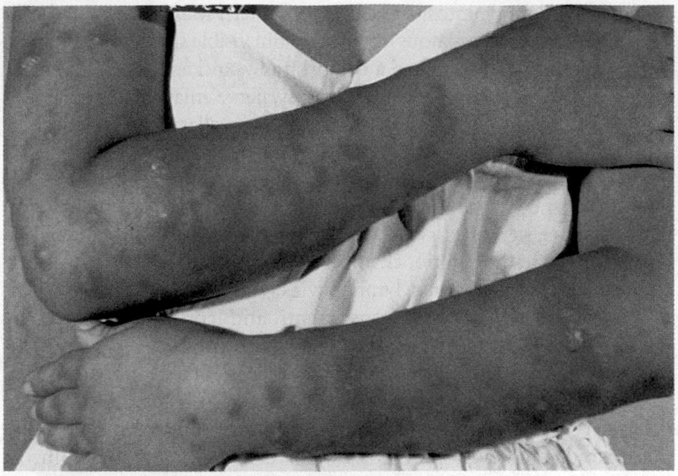

FIGURE 159-4 Moderately severe skin lesions of erythema nodosum leprosum (ENL), some with postulation and ulceration.

the lepromatous end of the leprosy spectrum (BL-LL), affecting nearly 50% of this group. Although ENL may precede leprosy diagnosis and initiation of therapy (sometimes, in fact, prompting the diagnosis), in 90% of cases it follows the institution of chemotherapy, generally within 2 years. The most common features of ENL are crops of painful erythematous papules that resolve spontaneously in a few days to a week but may recur; malaise; and fever that can be profound. However, patients may also experience symptoms of neuritis, lymphadenitis, uveitis, orchitis, and glomerulonephritis and may develop anemia, leukocytosis, and abnormal liver function tests (particularly increased aminotransferase levels). Individual patients may have either a single bout of ENL or chronic recurrent manifestations. Bouts may be either mild or severe and generalized; in rare instances, ENL results in death.

Skin biopsy of ENL papules reveals vasculitis or panniculitis, sometimes with many lymphocytes but characteristically with polymorphonuclear leukocytes as well.

Elevated levels of circulating tumor necrosis factor (TNF) have been demonstrated in ENL; thus, TNF may play a central role in the pathobiology of this syndrome. ENL is thought to be a consequence of immune complex deposition, given its T_H2 cytokine profile and its high levels of IL-6 and IL-8. However, in ENL tissue, the presence of HLA-DR framework antigen of epidermal cells—considered a marker for a delayed-type hypersensitivity response—and evidence of higher levels of IL-2 and IFN-γ than are usually seen in polar lepromatous disease suggest an alternative mechanism.

LUCIO'S PHENOMENON Lucio's phenomenon is an unusual reaction seen exclusively in patients from the Caribbean and Mexico who have the diffuse lepromatosis form of lepromatous leprosy, most often those who are untreated. Patients with this reaction develop recurrent crops of large, sharply marginated, ulcerative lesions—particularly on the lower extremities—that may be generalized and, when so, are frequently fatal as a result of secondary infection and consequent septic bacteremia. Histologically, the lesions are characterized by ischemic necrosis of the epidermis and superficial dermis, heavy parasitism of endothelial cells with AFB, and endothelial proliferation and thrombus formation in the larger vessels of the deeper dermis. Like ENL, the Lucio phenomenon is probably mediated by immune complexes.

Complications • ***THE EXTREMITIES*** Complications of the extremities in leprosy patients are primarily a consequence of neuropathy leading to insensitivity and myopathy. Insensitivity affects fine touch, pain, and heat receptors but generally spares position and vibration appreciation. The most commonly affected nerve trunk is the ulnar nerve at the elbow, whose involvement results in clawing of the fourth and fifth fingers, loss of dorsal interosseous musculature in the affected hand, and loss of sensation in these distributions. Median nerve involvement in leprosy impairs thumb opposition and grasp; radial nerve dysfunction, although rare in leprosy, leads to wristdrop. Tendon transfers can restore hand function but should not be performed until 6 months after the initiation of antimicrobial therapy and the conclusion of episodes of acute neuritis.

Plantar ulceration, particularly at the metatarsal heads, is probably the most frequent complication of leprous neuropathy. Therapy requires careful debridement; administration of appropriate antibiotics; avoidance of weight-bearing until ulcerations are healed, with slowly progressive ambulation thereafter; and wearing of special shoes to prevent recurrence.

Footdrop as a result of peroneal nerve palsy should be treated with a simple nonmetallic brace within the shoe or with surgical correction attained by tendon transfers. Although uncommon, Charcot's joints, particularly of the foot and ankle, may result from leprosy.

The loss of distal digits in leprosy is a consequence of insensitivity, trauma, secondary infection, and—in lepromatous patients—a poorly understood and sometimes profound osteolytic process. Conscientious protection of the extremities during cooking and work and the early institution of therapy have substantially reduced the frequency and severity of distal digit loss in recent times.

THE NOSE In lepromatous leprosy, bacillary invasion of the nasal mucosa can result in chronic nasal congestion and epistaxis. Saline nose drops may relieve these symptoms. Long-untreated LL leprosy may further result in destruction of the nasal cartilage, with consequent saddle-nose deformity or anosmia (more common in the preantibiotic era than at present). Nasal reconstructive procedures can ameliorate significant cosmetic defects.

THE EYE Owing to cranial nerve palsies, lagophthalmos and corneal insensitivity may complicate leprosy, resulting in trauma, secondary infection, and (without treatment) corneal ulcerations and opacities. For patients with these conditions, eyedrops during the day and ointments at night provide some protection from such consequences. Furthermore, in LL leprosy, the anterior chamber of the eye is invaded by bacilli, and ENL may result in uveitis, with consequent cataracts and glaucoma. Thus leprosy is a major cause of blindness in the developing world. Slit-lamp evaluation of LL patients often reveals "corneal beading," representing globi of *M. leprae*.

THE TESTES *M. leprae* invades the testes, while ENL may cause orchitis. Thus males with lepromatous leprosy often manifest mild to severe testicular dysfunction, with an elevation of luteinizing and follicle-stimulating hormones, decreased testosterone, and aspermia or hypospermia in 85% of LL patients but in only 25% of BL patients. LL patients may become impotent and infertile. Impotence is sometimes responsive to testosterone replacement.

AMYLOIDOSIS Secondary amyloidosis is a complication of LL leprosy and ENL that is encountered infrequently in the antibiotic era. This complication may result in abnormalities of hepatic and particularly renal function.

NERVE ABSCESSES Patients with various forms of leprosy, but particularly those with the BT form, may develop abscesses of nerves (most commonly the ulnar) with an adjacent cellulitic appearance of the skin. In such conditions, the affected nerve is swollen and exquisitely tender. Although glucocorticoids may reduce signs of inflammation, rapid surgical decompression is necessary to prevent irreversible sequelae.

DIAGNOSIS

Leprosy most commonly presents with both characteristic skin lesions and skin histopathology. Thus the disease should be suspected when a patient from an endemic area has suggestive skin lesions or peripheral neuropathy. The diagnosis should be confirmed by histopathology. In tuberculoid leprosy, lesional areas—preferably the advancing edge—must be biopsied because normal-appearing skin does not have pathologic features. In lepromatous leprosy, nodules, plaques, and indurated areas are optimal biopsy sites, but biopsies of normal-appearing skin are also generally diagnostic. Lepromatous leprosy is associated with diffuse hyperglobulinemia, which may result in false-positive serologic tests (e.g., VDRL, RA, ANA) and therefore may cause diagnostic confusion. On occasion, tuberculoid lesions may not (1) appear typical, (2) be hypesthetic, and (3) contain granulomas but only nonspecific lymphocytic infiltrates. In such instances, two of these three characteristics are considered sufficient for a diagnosis. It is preferable to overdiagnose leprosy rather than to allow a patient to remain untreated.

IgM antibodies to PGL-1 are found in 95% of untreated lepromatous leprosy patients; the titer decreases with effective therapy. However, in tuberculoid leprosy—the form of disease most often associated with diagnostic uncertainty owing to the absence or paucity of AFB—patients have significant antibodies to PGL-1 only 60% of the time; moreover, in endemic locales, exposed individuals without clinical leprosy may harbor antibodies to PGL-1. Thus PGL-1 serology is of little diagnostic utility in tuberculoid leprosy. Heat-killed *M. leprae* (lepromin) has been used as a skin test reagent. It generally elicits a reaction in tuberculoid leprosy patients, may do so in individuals without leprosy, and gives negative results in lepromatous leprosy patients; consequently, it is likewise of little diagnostic value. Unfortunately, PCR of the skin for *M. leprae*, although positive in LL and BL leprosy, yields negative results in 50% of tuberculoid leprosy cases, again offering little diagnostic assistance.

Included in the differential diagnosis of lesions that resemble leprosy are sarcoidosis, leishmaniasis, lupus vulgaris, dermatofibroma, histiocytoma, lymphoma, syphilis, yaws, granuloma annulare, and various other disorders causing hypopigmentation (notably pityriasis alba, tinea, and vitiligo). Sarcoidosis may result in perineural inflammation, but actual granuloma formation within dermal nerves is pathognomonic for leprosy. In lepromatous leprosy, sputum specimens may be loaded with AFB—a finding that can be inappropriately interpreted as representing pulmonary tuberculosis.

Rx LEPROSY

ANTIMICROBIAL THERAPY **Active Agents** Established agents used to treat leprosy include dapsone (50–100 mg/d), clofazimine (50–100 mg/d, 100 mg three times weekly, or 300 mg monthly), and rifampin (600 mg daily or monthly). Of these drugs, only rifampin is bactericidal. The sulfones (folate antagonists), the foremost of which is dapsone, were the first antimicrobial agents found to be effective for the treatment of leprosy and are still the mainstay of therapy. With sulfone treatment, skin lesions resolve and numbers of viable bacilli in the skin are reduced. Although primarily bacteriostatic, dapsone monotherapy results in only a 2.5% resistance-related relapse rate; after ≥18 years of therapy and subsequent discontinuation, only another 10% of patients relapse, developing new, usually asymptomatic, shiny, "histoid" nodules. Dapsone is generally safe and inexpensive. Individuals with glucose-6-phosphate dehydrogenase deficiency who are treated with dapsone may develop severe hemolysis; those without this deficiency also have reduced red cell survival and a hemoglobin decrease averaging 1 g/dL. Dapsone's usefulness is limited occasionally by allergic dermatitis and rarely by the sulfone syndrome (including high fever, anemia, exfoliative dermatitis, and a mononucleosis-type blood picture). It must be remembered that rifampin induces microsomal enzymes, necessitating increased doses of medications such as glucocorticoids and oral birth control regimens. Clofazimine is often cosmetically unacceptable to light-skinned leprosy patients because it causes a red-black skin discoloration that accumulates, particularly in lesional areas, and makes the patient's diagnosis obvious to members of the community.

Other antimicrobial agents active against *M. leprae* in animal models and at the usual daily doses used in clinical trials include ethionamide/prothionamide; the aminoglycosides streptomycin, kanamycin, and amikacin (but not gentamicin or tobramycin); minocycline; clarithromycin; and several fluoroquinolones, particularly ofloxacin. Next to rifampin, minocycline, clarithromycin, and ofloxacin appear to be most bactericidal for *M. leprae*, but these drugs have not been used extensively in leprosy control programs. Most recently, rifapentine and moxifloxacin have been found to be especially potent against *M. leprae*. In preliminary clinical trials, moxifloxacin has been matched in potency only by rifampin.

Choice of Regimens Antimicrobial therapy for leprosy must be individualized, depending on the clinical/pathologic form of the disease encountered. Tuberculoid leprosy, which is associated with a low bacterial burden and a protective cellular immune response, is the easiest form to treat and can be reliably cured with a finite course of chemotherapy. In contrast, lepromatous leprosy may have a higher bacillary load than any other human bacterial disease, and the absence of a salutary T cell repertoire requires prolonged or even lifelong chemotherapy. Hence, careful classification of disease prior to therapy is important.

In developed countries, clinical experience with leprosy classification is limited; fortunately, however, the resources needed for skin biopsy are highly accessible and pathologic interpretation is readily available. In developing countries, clinical expertise is greater but is now waning substantially as the care of leprosy patients is integrated into general health services. In addition, access to dermatopathology services is often limited. In such instances, skin smears may prove useful, but in many locales access to the resources needed for their preparation and interpretation may also be unavailable. Use of skin smears is no longer encouraged by the World Health Organization (WHO) and is often replaced by mere counting of lesions, which, together with the lack of histopathology, may negatively affect decisions about chemotherapy, increase the potential for reactions, and worsen the ultimate prognosis.

A reasoned approach to the treatment of leprosy is confounded by these and several other issues:

1. Even without therapy, TT leprosy may heal spontaneously, and prolonged dapsone monotherapy (even for LL leprosy) is generally curative in 80% of cases.
2. In tuberculoid disease, there are often no bacilli found in the skin prior to therapy, and thus there is no objective measure of therapeutic success. Furthermore, despite adequate treatment, TT and particularly BT lesions often resolve little or incompletely, while relapse and late type 1 lepra reactions can be difficult to distinguish.
3. LL leprosy patients commonly harbor viable persistent *M. leprae* organisms after prolonged intensive therapy; the propensity of these organisms to initiate clinical relapse is unclear. Because relapse in LL patients after discontinuation of rifampin-containing regimens usually begins only after 7–10 years, follow-up over the very long term is necessary to assess ultimate clinical outcomes.
4. Even though primary dapsone resistance is exceedingly rare and multidrug therapy is generally recommended (at least for lepromatous leprosy), there is a paucity of information from experimental animals and clinical trials on the optimal combination of antimicrobial agents, dosing schedule, or duration of therapy.

In 1982, the WHO made recommendations for "the chemotherapy of leprosy for control programs." These recommendations came on the heels of the demonstration of the relative success of long-term dapsone monotherapy and in the context of concerns about dapsone resistance. Other complicating considerations included the limited resources available for leprosy care in the very areas where it is most prevalent and the frustration and discouragement of patients and program managers with the previous requirement for lifelong therapy for many leprosy patients. The WHO delineated for the first time a finite duration of therapy for all forms of leprosy and—given the prohibitive cost of daily rifampin treatment in developing countries—encouraged the monthly administration of this agent as part of a multidrug regimen.

Over the ensuing years, these WHO recommendations have been broadly implemented, and the duration of therapy required, particularly for lepromatous leprosy, has been progressively shortened. For treatment purposes, the WHO classifies patients as *paucibacillary* or *multibacillary*. Previously, patients without demonstrable AFB in the dermis were classified as paucibacillary and those with AFB as multibacillary. Currently, owing to the perceived unreliability of skin smears in the field, patients are classified as multibacillary if they have six or more skin lesions and as paucibacillary if they have fewer. The WHO recommends that paucibacillary adults be treated with 100 mg of dapsone daily and 600 mg of rifampin monthly (supervised) for 6 months **(Table 159-2)**. For patients with single-lesion paucibacillary leprosy, the WHO recommends as an alternative a single dose of rifampin (600 mg), ofloxacin (400 mg), and minocycline (100 mg). Multibacillary adults should be treated with 100 mg of dapsone plus 50 mg of clofazimine daily (unsupervised) and with 600 mg of rifampin plus 300 mg of clofazimine monthly (supervised). Originally, the WHO recommended that lepromatous patients be treated for 2 years or until smears became nega-

TABLE 159-2 ANTIMICROBIAL REGIMENS RECOMMENDED FOR THE TREATMENT OF LEPROSY IN ADULTS

Form of Leprosy	More Intensive Regimen	WHO Recommended Regimen (1982)
Tuberculoid (paucibacillary)	Dapsone (100 mg/d) for 5 years	Dapsone (100 mg/d, unsupervised) *plus* rifampin (600 mg/month, supervised) for 6 months
Lepromatous (multibacillary)	Rifampin (600 mg/d) for 3 years *plus* dapsone (100 mg/d) indefinitely	Dapsone (100 mg/d) *plus* clofazimine (50 mg/d), unsupervised; *and* rifampin (600 mg) *plus* clofazimine (300 mg) monthly (supervised) for 1–2 years

Note: See text for discussion and comparison of WHO recommendations and more intensive approach as well as alternative WHO regimen for single-lesion paucibacillary leprosy.

tive (generally in ~5 years); subsequently, the acceptable course was reduced to 1 year—a change that remains especially controversial in the absence of supporting clinical trials.

Several factors have caused many authorities to question the WHO recommendations and to favor a more intensive approach. Among these factors are—for multibacillary patients—a high (double-digit) relapse rate in three locales (reaching 20–40% in one locale, with the rate directly related to the initial bacterial burden) and—for paucibacillary patients—demonstrable lesional activity for years in fully half of patients after the completion of therapy. The more intensive approach (Table 159-2) calls for tuberculoid leprosy to be treated with dapsone (100 mg/d) for 5 years and for lepromatous leprosy to be treated with rifampin (600 mg/d) for 3 years and with dapsone (100 mg/d) throughout life.

On effective antimicrobial therapy, new skin lesions and signs and symptoms of peripheral neuropathy cease appearing. Nodules and plaques of lepromatous leprosy noticeably flatten in 1–2 months and resolve in 1 year or a few years, while tuberculoid skin lesions may disappear, improve, or remain relatively unchanged. Although the peripheral neuropathy of leprosy may improve somewhat in the first few months of therapy, rarely is it significantly ameliorated by treatment.

THERAPY FOR REACTIONS **Type 1** Type 1 lepra reactions are best treated with glucocorticoids (e.g., prednisone, initially at doses of 40–60 mg/d). As the inflammation subsides, the glucocorticoid dose can be tapered, but steroid therapy must be continued for at least 3 months lest recurrence supervene. Because of the myriad toxicities of prolonged glucocorticoid therapy, the indications for its initiation are strictly limited to lesions whose intense inflammation poses a threat of ulceration; lesions at cosmetically important sites, such as the face; and cases in which neuritis is present. Mild to moderate lepra reactions that do not meet these criteria should be tolerated and glucocorticoid treatment withheld. Thalidomide is ineffective against type 1 lepra reactions. Clofazimine (200–300 mg/d) is of questionable benefit but in any event is far less efficacious than glucocorticoids.

Type 2 Treatment of ENL must be individualized. If ENL is mild (i.e., without fever or other organ involvement, with occasional crops of only a few skin papules), it may be treated with antipyretics alone. However, in cases with many skin lesions, fever, malaise, and other tissue involvement, brief courses (1–2 weeks) of glucocorticoids (initially 40–60 mg/d) are often effective. With or without therapy, individual inflamed papules last for >1 week. Successful therapy is defined by the cessation of skin lesion development and the disappearance of other systemic signs and symptoms. If, despite two courses of glucocorticoid therapy, ENL appears to be recurring and persisting, treatment with thalidomide (100–300 mg nightly) should be initiated, with the dose depending on the initial severity of the reaction. Because even a single dose of thalidomide administered early in pregnancy may result in severe birth defects, including phocomelia, the use of this drug in the United States for the treatment of fertile female patients is tightly regulated and requires informed consent, prior pregnancy testing, and maintenance of birth control measures. Although the mechanism of thalidomide's dramatic action against ENL is not entirely clear, the drug's efficacy is probably attributable to its reduction of TNF levels and IgM synthesis and its slowing of polymorphonuclear leukocyte migration. After the reaction is controlled, lower doses of thalidomide (50–200 mg nightly) are effective in preventing relapses of ENL. Clofazimine in high doses (300 mg nightly) has some efficacy against ENL, but its use permits only a modest reduction of the glucocorticoid dose necessary for ENL control.

Lucio's Phenomenon Neither glucocorticoids nor thalidomide is effective against this syndrome. Optimal wound care and therapy for bacteremia are indicated. Ulcers tend to be chronic and heal poorly. In severe cases, exchange transfusion may prove useful.

PREVENTION AND CONTROL

Vaccination at birth with bacille Calmette-Guérin (BCG) has proved variably effective in preventing leprosy: the results have ranged from total inefficacy to 80% efficacy. The addition of heat-killed *M. leprae* to BCG does not increase vaccine efficacy. Because whole mycobacteria contain large amounts of lipids and carbohydrates that have proven in vitro to be immunosuppressive for lymphocytes and macrophages, *M. leprae* proteins may prove to be superior vaccines. Data from a mouse model support this possibility.

Chemoprophylaxis with dapsone may reduce the number of cases of tuberculoid leprosy but not of lepromatous leprosy and hence is not recommended, even for household contacts. Because leprosy transmission appears to require close prolonged household contact, hospitalized patients need not be isolated.

In 1992, the WHO—on the basis of that organization's treatment recommendations—launched a landmark campaign to eliminate leprosy as a public health problem by the year 2000 (goal, <1 case per 10,000 population). The campaign mobilized and energized nongovernmental organizations and national health services to treat leprosy with multiple drugs and to clean up outdated registries. In these respects, the effort has proven hugely successful, with >6 million patients completing therapy. However, the target of leprosy elimination has not yet been reached. In fact, the success of the WHO campaign in reducing the number of cases worldwide has been largely attributable to the redefinition of what constitutes a case of leprosy. Formerly calculated by disease prevalence, the case count is now limited to those not yet treated with multiple drugs. In each of the 23 countries with the largest number of leprosy cases, the annual incidence of leprosy is stable or actually rising. Furthermore, after the completion of therapy, when a patient is no longer considered to represent a "case," half of all patients continue to manifest disease activity for years; relapse rates (at least for multibacillary patients) are unacceptably high; disabilities and deformities go unchecked; and the social stigma of the disease persists.

During most of the twentieth century, nongovernmental organizations, particularly Christian missionaries, provided a medical infrastructure devoted to the care and treatment of leprosy patients—the envy of those with other medical priorities in the developing world. With the public perception that leprosy is near eradication, resources for patient care are rapidly being diverted, and the burden of patient care is being transferred to nonexistent or overloaded national health services and to health workers who lack the tools and skills needed for disease diagnosis, classification, and nuanced therapy (particularly in cases of reactional neuritis). Thus the prerequisites for a salutary outcome increasingly go unmet.

FURTHER READINGS

COLE ST et al: Massive gene decay in the leprosy bacillus. Nature 409:1007, 2001

GELBER RH: The chemotherapy of leprosy: Lessons learned, some forgotten, current status and future prospects. Malaysian Journal of Dermatology 18:10, 2005

——— et al: The relapse rate in MB leprosy patients treated with 2-years of WHO-MDT is not low. Int J Lepr Other Mycobact Dis 72:493, 2004

LOCKWOOD D: Leprosy elimination—a virtual phenomenon or a reality? BMJ 324:1516, 2002

MODLIN RL, REA TH: Immunology of leprosy granulomas. Springer Semin Immunopathol 10:359, 1998

MONET M et al: On the origin of leprosy. Science 308:1040, 2005

RIDLEY DS: Histological classification and the immunological spectrum of leprosy. Bull World Health Organ 51:451, 1974

SHEPARD CC: The experimental disease that follows injection of human leprosy bacilli into foot pads of mice. J Exp Med 112:445, 1960

WARWICK JB, LOCKWOOD D: Leprosy. Lancet 363:1209, 2004

WHO EXPERT COMMITTEE ON LEPROSY: Seventh Report. WHO Tech Rep Ser No. 874. Geneva, World Health Organization, 1998

160 Nontuberculous Mycobacteria

C. Fordham von Reyn

The designation *nontuberculous mycobacteria* (NTM) encompasses the mycobacterial species other than organisms of the *Mycobacterium tuberculosis* complex and *M. leprae.* The NTM are distributed widely in the environment, are typically acquired from environmental sources, and therefore are also referred to as *environmental mycobacteria.* Most species are less virulent for humans than *M. tuberculosis.* Thus symptomatic infections are often associated with local or generalized defects in host defenses. Because isolation of NTM from a clinical specimen may represent true infection, colonization, or environmental contamination, strict criteria are required to assess the clinical significance of a positive culture. Although the >90 species of NTM have been associated with a wide variety of infections, most infections are due to a relatively limited number of species that cause characteristic patterns of disease (Table 160-1).

MICROBIOLOGY

Like *M. tuberculosis,* NTM organisms are acid-fast bacilli (AFB), resisting decolorization after staining. NTM have conventionally been characterized by the time required for clinical specimens to yield visible growth on solid media. Rapidly growing NTM species, such as *M. abscessus, M. fortuitum,* and *M. chelonae,* appear within 7 days. These organisms grow on standard microbiologic media and thus may be reported even when the clinician has not explicitly requested cultures for mycobacteria. Slow-growing species, in contrast, often take 2–3 weeks to grow on solid media and require special mycobacterial media such as Lowenstein-Jensen or Middlebrook. Accordingly, slow-growing NTM species are usually isolated only when the clinician specifically requests cultures for mycobacteria. Representative slow-growing species include *M. avium, M. kansasii, M. ulcerans,* and *M. marinum.* The automated broth culture systems now used in many laboratories may permit isolation of slow-growing NTM organisms within 10–14 days.

Further classification based on colony pigmentation (Runyon classification) has been replaced by the use of DNA probes for identification of common species such as *M. avium, M. intracellulare, M. gordonae* (which is rarely pathogenic), and *M. kansasii.* Less common species may be identified rapidly on the basis of fatty acid composition or DNA sequencing. Molecular strain typing ("fingerprinting") based on analysis of polymorphisms among large restriction fragments can be used to determine whether two or more isolates are genotypically and, by implication, epidemiologically related. This technique has been useful for identifying common-source outbreaks of infection or contamination.

Antibiotic susceptibility testing should be performed for rapidly growing NTM species. However, susceptibility testing of slow-growing species is of limited value: testing methods are not well standardized, and the relevance of the results to outcome is uncertain since patients are usually treated with multiple-drug regimens. As discussed later in this chapter, testing of *M. avium* or *M. kansasii* for susceptibility to specific drugs may be useful in certain situations.

DISTRIBUTION

NTM have a waxy, hydrophobic, triple-layered cell wall that renders them unusually resistant to varied physical conditions and chemical agents (including disinfectants such as chlorine at concentrations used in drinking water). These organisms can make use of a wide variety of carbon and nitrogen sources and can survive in nutrient-poor environments. Thus they are widely distributed in water, biofilms, and soil as well as in numerous animal species. Optimal growth temperatures vary and may influence distribution. For example, *M. avium* and *M. intracellulare* are often isolated from potable hot-water sources, whereas *M. marinum* is found in the cooler water of fish tanks. Most species of NTM are obligate aerobes and grow best at acid pH. Soil and natural water samples from most regions of the world contain numerous species of NTM, which are as common in northern regions (e.g., Finland) as they are in more temperate areas (e.g., the southern United States).

EPIDEMIOLOGY

Asymptomatic infections with NTM are common in humans and are probably acquired most often from childhood contact with soil, water, and possibly animals. Studies with skin-test agents derived from NTM indicate that 30–40% of adults in the northern and southern United States have had prior unrecognized or asymptomatic infection with NTM—most often with organisms of the *M. avium* complex (MAC). Since latent infection is not a recognized characteristic of NTM, most symptomatic infections are thought to represent recent exposure. Molecular methods have identified clusters of infections and pseudoinfections associated with potable water as well as nosocomial infections

TABLE 160-1 MAIN SPECIES OF NONTUBERCULOUS MYCOBACTERIA (NTM) AND PATTERNS OF DISEASE

Species	Growth on Solid Media	Environmental Reservoir	Patterns of Disease[a]			
			Cutaneous	Pulmonary	Disseminated	Other
M. avium	Slow	Hot water systems, natural water, soil	–	++	+++	Lymphadenitis
M. intracellulare	Slow	Hot water systems, natural water, soil	–	+++	+	Lymphadenitis
M. kansasii	Slow	Potable and natural water	–	+++	++	–
M. abscessus, *M. chelonae,* *M. fortuitum*	Rapid	Potable and natural water, soil	++	+	–	Sporotrichoid spread
M. marinum	Slow	Fish tanks, salt water	++	–	–	Sporotrichoid spread
M. ulcerans	Slow	Natural water	++	–	–	"Buruli ulcer," osteomyelitis

[a]Symbols indicate relative prevalence among NTM infections of the indicated species and pattern of disease: +++, most common; ++, common; +, reported but uncommon; –, rare or not reported.

related to clinical procedures such as endoscopy and surgery. Environmental exposures are assumed to cause most symptomatic infections; however, this point has been difficult to document by molecular methods, presumably because there are many potential exposures (some of which are sporadic) and because a specific NTM species may be present only transiently or in low numbers in any given source.

PATHOGENESIS

NTM may be acquired through cutaneous, respiratory, gastrointestinal, or (rarely) parenteral exposure. Organisms are ingested by host macrophages and may survive within these cells to replicate and cause symptomatic infection. Disease manifestations in immunocompetent hosts are due to host cellular immune responses and the formation of granulomas. Intracellular killing of mycobacteria, with ultimate control of infection, requires the action of cellular immune mechanisms including proliferation of CD4+ T lymphocytes and elaboration of interferon γ (IFN-γ) and interleukin 12. Deficiencies in CD4+ T cell function due to HIV infection, anti–tumor necrosis factor (TNF) therapy, and inherited deficiencies in the production of or response to IFN-γ are associated with disseminated NTM infection (Chap. 182).

The cellular immune response to NTM may be evident in tuberculin skin testing or newer interferon-γ release assays (IGRAs). Tuberculin skin testing with *M. tuberculosis* purified protein derivative may elicit small reactions with some NTM and larger reactions (comparable to those in tuberculosis) among immunocompetent individuals infected with *M. marinum* or *M. kansasii*. IGRAs that employ *M. tuberculosis*–specific antigens (ESAT-6, CFP-10) are negative in most NTM infections but may be positive with *M. marinum* or *M. kansasii.*

There is no convincing evidence that NTM can establish latent infection with subsequent clinical reactivation—a pattern characteristic of *M. tuberculosis*. Asymptomatic infection with NTM in a healthy host may induce beneficial immunity; persons with skin-test reactivity to NTM antigens (e.g., *M. intracellulare*) are at decreased risk for the subsequent development of tuberculosis. Likewise, immunization with bacille Calmette-Guérin (BCG) from *M. bovis* provides protection against childhood cervical adenitis due to NTM.

CLINICAL SYNDROMES

Cutaneous Disease NTM can cause a variety of cutaneous disease syndromes when inoculated directly from an environmental source into an area of open or diseased skin or into a surgical wound. These organisms are also associated with localized or disseminated cutaneous disease in immunosuppressed patients. *M. abscessus*, *M. fortuitum*, *M. chelonae*, *M. marinum*, and *M. ulcerans* are the most commonly involved species. Cutaneous disease may be nodular or ulcerating, sometimes with reddish-blue discoloration and typically with minimal drainage. Lesions may be single, or the infection may spread proximally up the lymphatics, producing additional nodules (sporotrichoid spread). In compromised hosts, disseminated lesions may appear as a result of bacteremic spread. Clinical suspicion of NTM infection is based on chronicity, the absence of bacterial growth on routine culture, and the failure to respond to standard antibacterial therapy. Biopsies often reveal granuloma formation, and acid-fast stains may be positive.

Pulmonary Disease NTM species cause chronic progressive pulmonary infection both in normal hosts and in those with underlying pulmonary disease or immunosuppression. The clinical features may resemble slowly progressive pulmonary tuberculosis, which is often the initial diagnosis in patients with positive AFB smears. Among patients born in the United States, pulmonary disease due to AFB is more likely to be due to NTM than to *M. tuberculosis*.

The diagnosis of pulmonary infection with NTM is complicated by the variability in clinical and radiologic manifestations, the frequent presence of significant prior pulmonary disease, and the fact that isolation of NTM from the sputum may represent harmless colonization of the lower respiratory tract. The diagnosis should be based on specific, validated criteria that emphasize a compatible clinical syndrome, characteristic findings on chest x-ray or CT, and repeated isolation of NTM from the sputum or growth of NTM from a lung biopsy (Table 160-2).

TABLE 160-2 ATS/IDSA CRITERIA FOR THE DIAGNOSIS OF PULMONARY DISEASE DUE TO NONTUBERCULOUS MYCOBACTERIA[a]

Category	Requirement
Clinical	Pulmonary symptoms (e.g., chronic cough) and appropriate exclusion of other diagnoses
Radiologic	Chest x-ray: nodular or cavitary opacities *or*
	High-resolution CT: multifocal bronchiectasis with multiple small nodules
Bacteriologic	Sputum: ≥2 positive cultures *or*
	Bronchial wash or lavage: ≥1 positive culture *or*
	Lung biopsy: granulomatous inflammation or positive stain for acid-fast bacilli plus ≥1 positive culture (of biopsy, sputum, or bronchial wash sample)

[a]Diagnosis requires the fulfillment of clinical criteria plus one radiologic criterion and one bacteriologic criterion. ATS, American Thoracic Society; IDSA, Infectious Diseases Society of America.
Source: Griffith et al, 2007.

In immunocompetent hosts, infection may result in the onset of chronic cough, dyspnea, and fatigue; fever is unusual. Pathologic and radiologic manifestations of pulmonary infection due to NTM include the formation of solitary or multiple nodules, chronic pneumonitis, bronchiectasis, cavity formation, or a combination of these features. In some patients with NTM pulmonary disease, CT shows a characteristic pattern of small cylindrical bronchiectasis and multiple small (<5-mm) nodules and fibrosis. Compared with patients who have tuberculosis, those who have lung disease caused by NTM are more likely to have bilateral and midzone infiltrates and less likely to have pleural effusions. Patients with characteristic radiologic findings and negative results of routine sputum cultures for mycobacteria should have bronchoscopy and transbronchial biopsy performed in an attempt to identify granulomas and AFB. In patients with chronic pulmonary disease, the superimposition of infection with NTM may not be associated with easily recognizable changes in symptoms or radiologic features.

Together, MAC organisms (especially *M. intracellulare*) are the most common cause of pulmonary disease due to NTM in developed countries; next in frequency are *M. kansasii* (United States, Europe, South Africa), *M. abscessus* (United States), *M. xenopi* (Europe, Canada), and *M. malmoense* (United Kingdom, northern Europe). However, isolation of NTM from the sputum must be considered in the context of clinical manifestations. For example, NTM (most prominently, MAC organisms; less commonly, *M. abscessus*) can be cultured from 13% of cystic fibrosis patients in the United States (Chap. 253); however, not all of these patients appear to have invasive NTM disease. Although invasive disease should be strongly suspected when the same NTM species is isolated on multiple occasions from a patient with lung disease, even persistent organisms may represent colonization or slowly progressive disease apparent only on long-term follow-up. Additional laboratory tests (e.g., immunologic assessments) are of no value in the diagnosis.

Although treatment should be considered in patients who meet the clinical, radiologic, and microbiologic criteria for NTM disease (Table 160-2), several other factors require consideration. For example, whereas species such as *M. kansasii* are usually pathogenic and a single isolate may be significant, species such as *M. gordonae* are rarely pathogenic, even when isolated repeatedly. In addition, in some patients with true invasive disease, infection may progress so slowly that it is unlikely to have much impact on longevity determined by age or comorbid illness. Since therapy for NTM requires prolonged administration of multiple drugs and is associated with significant side effects, the decision to institute treatment in patients with noncavitary disease who do not have clearly progressive pulmonary disease should be made with careful deliberation after a period of clinical and radiologic follow-up.

Disseminated Disease Patients with impaired cellular immunity—most notably, patients with advanced HIV disease (Chap. 182), immunosuppressed recipients of solid-organ or hematopoietic stem-cell transplants (Chap. 126), and patients receiving anti-TNF therapy—are susceptible to disseminated disease due to NTM. Other predisposing conditions include treatment with glucocorticoids, lymphoma and leukemia (especially hairy cell leukemia), and heritable disorders of IFN-γ production and function. *M. avium* and *M. kansasii* are the species most commonly isolated in disseminated disease, but numerous other organisms (e.g., *M. genavense, M. haemophilum*) have also been recovered.

Patients with disseminated infection present with fever, weight loss, and fatigue and sometimes with hepatosplenomegaly or lymphadenopathy. Chest radiographs are typically normal in infection with *M. avium* (although they may show a miliary pattern) but are usually abnormal with *M. kansasii.* Laboratory studies may demonstrate anemia and an elevated level of alkaline phosphatase in serum. Disseminated disease is characterized by the widespread presence of foamy macrophages with AFB, which may be demonstrated in biopsy samples of bone marrow, intestine, or liver. Granulomas are typically absent in patients with impaired cellular immunity. In most cases, the diagnosis can be established by one or two sets of mycobacterial blood cultures, which will be positive for the etiologic mycobacteria in 2–3 weeks. Treatment requires long-term administration of a multiple-drug antimycobacterial regimen and attempts to ameliorate the defect in cellular immunity [e.g., institution of antiretroviral therapy (ART) and discontinuation of glucocorticoid administration].

Other Disease NTM have been associated with disease at numerous other anatomic locations, including ocular infections, mastoiditis, sinusitis, mastitis, catheter site infections, endocarditis, meningitis, peritonitis, appendicitis, pericarditis, pyelonephritis, prostatitis, tenosynovitis, bursitis, septic arthritis, osteomyelitis, and lymphadenitis (especially in children). Accumulating data support an association between infection with *M. avium* subspecies *paratuberculosis* and Crohn's disease.

ORGANISMS

M. AVIUM COMPLEX

Pulmonary Disease MAC organisms (*M. avium, M. intracellulare*, and genetically related unnamed species) are more common than *M. tuberculosis* as a cause of mycobacterial pulmonary disease among persons born in the United States. Epidemiologic data support a marked increase in the incidence of MAC infection over the past two to three decades. Two patterns of MAC disease are recognized: one form is typically the primary basis for a diagnosis of pulmonary disease and is often nodular/bronchiectatic, whereas the other form develops as a secondary complication of underlying pulmonary disease and is sometimes fibrocavitary (Table 160-3). The description of subtle defects in cellular immune responses and body morphotype in patients with primary disease raises the possibility of an as-yet-undefined immune defect predisposing to MAC infection. Patients with secondary disease include those with chronic obstructive pulmonary disease, prior tuberculosis, cystic fibrosis, or pulmonary alveolar proteinosis. The sources of infection have not been identified.

CLINICAL FEATURES AND DIAGNOSIS Symptoms and diagnostic studies are described above (see "Clinical Syndromes"). CT identifies characteristic cylindrical bronchiectasis with nodule formation, documents the extent of disease, and establishes a baseline for possible treatment. Standard diagnostic criteria should be applied (Table 160-2). Isolates from patients with prolonged prior macrolide exposure or prior treatment failure should be tested for susceptibility to clarithromycin.

TABLE 160-3 TYPICAL FEATURES OF PRIMARY AND SECONDARY PULMONARY DISEASE DUE TO THE *M. AVIUM* COMPLEX

Feature	Primary	Secondary
Age	>50 years	30–70 (mean, 60) years
Sex	F > M	M > F
Underlying disease	None definitively identified; subtle defect in cellular immunity postulated	Chronic obstructive pulmonary disease, cystic fibrosis, prior tuberculosis, alveolar proteinosis
Radiologic features	Typically nodular (<5 mm)/ bronchiectatic (cylindrical) with midzone involvement	Sometimes fibrocavitary; infiltrates or nodules in some cases

℞ MAC PULMONARY DISEASE

Treatment should be initiated in most patients with secondary MAC pulmonary disease. For patients with primary MAC pulmonary disease, decisions about treatment must be made on an individual basis. A period of observation before consideration of treatment may be useful when there is no evidence of a progressive pulmonary process and when the patient's age or underlying disease is likely to be the critical determinant of survival over the next few years.

Recommended treatment for MAC pulmonary disease includes two drugs: daily clarithromycin (or daily or thrice-weekly azithromycin) and ethambutol. Some authorities recommend a three-drug regimen including these two agents plus rifampin, although there are no comparative data for two- versus three-drug regimens and concomitant administration of rifampin lowers serum levels of clarithromycin **(Table 160-4)**. For seriously ill patients with advanced disease, a four-drug regimen including the three drugs listed above as well as streptomycin or amikacin for the first 2 months should be considered. In many cases, treatment may serve only to halt the progression of radiologic findings; in some cases, symptoms and radiologic findings improve. The response to treatment is best in patients whose isolates have the lowest minimum inhibitory concentrations of clarithromycin. As many as 30% of patients treated with standard drugs at standard doses cannot tolerate therapy, generally because of gastrointestinal side effects. Rifabutin appears to have the highest rate of side effects. Stepwise introduction of drugs at 1-week intervals, starting with half the usual dose, may improve tolerance. In many cases, final doses need to be reduced or drugs eliminated or replaced with alternatives. Gatifloxacin and

TABLE 160-4 REGIMENS FOR PREVENTION AND TREATMENT OF DISEASE DUE TO THE *M. AVIUM* COMPLEX

Category	Regimen	Indication and Duration
Pulmonary Disease		
Treatment	Clarithromycin (250–500 mg bid[a]) or azithromycin (250 mg daily or thrice weekly[b]) ***plus*** Ethambutol (15 mg/kg qd)[c]	Treat when patient meets ATS/IDSA criteria (Table 160-2) and has secondary MAC disease or has primary MAC disease plus indication for treatment (see text). Treat for 18 months or until 12 months after conversion of sputum culture.
Disseminated Disease		
Treatment	Clarithromycin (500 mg PO bid) or azithromycin (500 mg daily[b]) ***plus*** Ethambutol (15 mg/kg qd[d])	Treat when MAC blood culture is positive or MAC is isolated from ordinarily sterile site. Continue with secondary prevention.
Prevention	Azithromycin (1200 mg PO weekly[b]) or clarithromycin (500 mg PO bid)	Treat when CD4+ T cell count is <50/μL. Discontinue if CD4+ T cell count exceeds 100/μL for >3 months during antiretroviral therapy.

[a]Give 250 mg of clarithromycin bid if the patient weighs <50 kg.
[b]Azithromycin is preferred to clarithromycin in pregnancy.
[c]An intermittent three-drug regimen with concomitant rifampin, rather than a daily two-drug regimen, is recommended in the current ATS/IDSA guidelines (Griffith et al, 2007) but not by this author; a four-drug regimen including streptomycin may be indicated in severe cases.
[d]Concomitant rifabutin (150–300 mg/d) may protect against the development of clarithromycin resistance and be associated with a modest clinical benefit but can cause interactions with antiretroviral therapy.

moxifloxacin exhibit in vitro activity against many strains but have not been studied for the treatment of pulmonary disease due to MAC.

For patients with positive sputum cultures who receive a macrolide-containing regimen, treatment should be continued for at least 12 months after cultures revert to negative; the typical duration is 18 months. The duration of therapy with other regimens may need to be extended to 24 months. Approximately 20% of patients experience treatment failure or relapse; some apparent treatment failures may actually represent reinfection. Surgical resection is an option for patients with localized disease who are intolerant of or unresponsive to multiple-drug therapy; however, this approach is associated with postoperative complications in as many as 20% of patients and should be undertaken only by surgeons who have considerable experience with this intervention.

Hot-Tub Lung Hot-tub lung is a form of hypersensitivity pneumonitis due to NTM, most commonly MAC organisms. Affected individuals present with cough, fever, and dyspnea after repeated exposure to indoor hot tubs contaminated with MAC. Some patients are hypoxemic. The chest x-ray shows diffuse nodular infiltrates, and high-resolution CT may also demonstrate ground-glass infiltrates. MAC organisms can be isolated from expectorated sputum or lung tissue, and biopsy specimens display centrilobular and bronchocentric granuloma formation. Resolution typically follows avoidance of exposure and/or treatment with glucocorticoids. Most patients do not appear to require specific antimicrobial therapy.

Disseminated Disease Disseminated MAC disease occurs principally among patients with immunosuppression (including those with advanced HIV disease) who live in developed countries but are not receiving ART. Almost all cases occur at CD4+ T cell counts of <100/µL, and the risk is ~20% per year for untreated patients with CD4+ T cell counts of <50/µL. The risk of disease is essentially eliminated for recipients of ART who have an increase in CD4+ T cell count to >100/µL that is maintained for 3 months. Most cases are due to *M. avium*, and molecular studies indicate that as many as 25% of disseminated infections involve more than one strain. Strains causing bacteremia differ genetically from those typically isolated from respiratory sources or the environment. Molecular techniques have documented nosocomial acquisition from potable hot water and have demonstrated common genotypes among isolates from humans and those from peat used in potting soil. Epidemiologic studies have demonstrated an increased risk associated with consumption of untreated spring water and of raw or partially cooked fish or shellfish and a decreased risk associated with showering. Overall, sources of acquisition appear to be diverse and exposure is probably unavoidable; at this time, no specific behavioral changes can be recommended for at-risk patients.

CLINICAL FEATURES AND DIAGNOSIS Disseminated MAC infection in AIDS is associated with fever, weakness, and weight loss and usually presents as a wasting syndrome in patients who are not receiving ART or chemoprophylaxis for *M. avium* (Chap. 182). Untreated disease shortens the survival period of patients with advanced AIDS by 4–5 months. Laboratory findings may include anemia, hypoalbuminemia, and elevated serum levels of alkaline phosphatase and lactate dehydrogenase. HIV-infected patients with prior disseminated MAC infection or unrecognized or subclinical MAC infection may experience an immune reconstitution syndrome when they start to receive ART (Chap. 182). This syndrome presents 1–12 weeks after the institution of ART and often manifests as localized (or generalized) culture-positive lymphadenitis with blood cultures negative for *M. avium*.

℞ DISSEMINATED MAC DISEASE

Disseminated MAC disease requires treatment with the combination of clarithromycin and ethambutol, with or without rifabutin (Table 160-4), along with ART for HIV. Antimycobacterial treatment should be continued for at least 12 months and until the CD4+ T cell count has been >100/µL for at least 6 months. The immune reconstitution syndrome should be treated with initiation or continuation of the same antimycobacterial regimen.

PREVENTION Chemoprophylaxis is highly effective for the prevention of disseminated MAC infection in AIDS (Table 160-4). Weekly azithromycin administration should be instituted when the CD4+ T cell count is <50/µL or when a patient with HIV infection has had an AIDS-defining opportunistic infection (e.g., *Pneumocystis* infection). Chemoprophylaxis may be discontinued when the CD4+ T cell count has been >100/µL for >3 months.

M. KANSASII

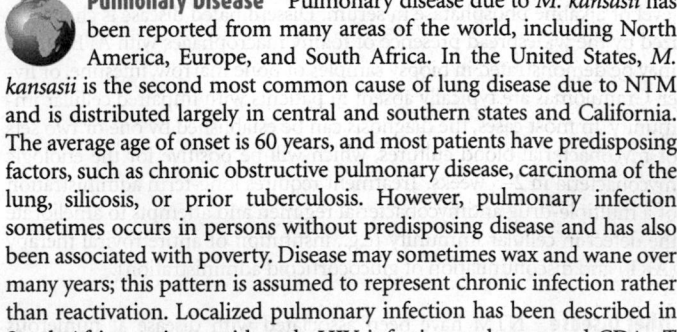

Pulmonary Disease Pulmonary disease due to *M. kansasii* has been reported from many areas of the world, including North America, Europe, and South Africa. In the United States, *M. kansasii* is the second most common cause of lung disease due to NTM and is distributed largely in central and southern states and California. The average age of onset is 60 years, and most patients have predisposing factors, such as chronic obstructive pulmonary disease, carcinoma of the lung, silicosis, or prior tuberculosis. However, pulmonary infection sometimes occurs in persons without predisposing disease and has also been associated with poverty. Disease may sometimes wax and wane over many years; this pattern is assumed to represent chronic infection rather than reactivation. Localized pulmonary infection has been described in South African miners with early HIV infection and preserved CD4+ T cell counts. The source of infection has not been identified, although *M. kansasii* has been isolated from both potable and natural water sources.

CLINICAL FEATURES AND DIAGNOSIS *M. kansasii* is the most pathogenic nontuberculous mycobacterial species affecting the lung, and the clinical features of *M. kansasii* disease resemble those of tuberculosis. Most cases include cough and sputum production; 30% include frank hemoptysis. Systemic signs and symptoms, including fever, night sweats, and weight loss, are reported by as many as 50% of patients. However, symptoms may be subtle or absent in patients with underlying malignancy. Chest radiographs show cavitation in 50% of patients, pleural scarring in 40%, and infiltrates in 30%; abnormalities are most prominent in the apices. Clinical and radiographic effects progress in the absence of treatment.

Sputum samples should be obtained for AFB staining and mycobacterial culture. The isolation of *M. kansasii* sometimes represents colonization; the diagnostic criteria in Table 160-2 are useful when multiple sputum samples can be obtained. However, the growth of *M. kansasii* from even a single sputum culture should be considered to have potential clinical significance, especially in HIV-positive patients. Testing of *M. kansasii* isolates for susceptibility to rifampin is recommended.

℞ *M. KANSASII* PULMONARY DISEASE

For rifampin-susceptible strains of *M. kansasii*, the recommended regimen is daily rifampin (600 mg), isoniazid (300 mg), and ethambutol (15 mg/kg). Sputum cultures almost always become negative by 4 months; patients should be treated for at least 12 months after the last positive culture. Resistance to rifampin may develop, in which case clarithromycin or azithromycin may be substituted.

Disseminated Disease Disseminated *M. kansasii* disease occurs principally among patients with advanced AIDS and CD4+ T cell counts of <100/µL. It has also been reported in patients with leukemia, lymphoma, or solid-organ transplantation.

CLINICAL FEATURES AND DIAGNOSIS Symptoms are similar to those reported for disseminated MAC infection, although in disseminated *M. kansasii* infection cough is more common and chest radiographs more often demonstrate alveolar or interstitial infiltrates or cavities. An immune reconstitution syndrome may follow the institution of ART in HIV-infected patients, manifesting as cervical or mediastinal lymphadenitis (Chap. 182).

The diagnosis is established by the isolation of *M. kansasii* from a normally sterile parenchymal site or from blood. In one series of cases, concurrent disseminated infection with a second NTM species (most often *M. avium*) was found in one-third of patients. The isolation of *M. kansasii* from sputum from a patient with advanced HIV disease suggests disseminated infection and is an indication for mycobacterial blood culture.

℞ *M. KANSASII* DISSEMINATED DISEASE

Treatment of disseminated *M. kansasii* disease is the same as that for pulmonary disease due to this organism. Patients with AIDS should receive an ART regimen that is compatible with a rifamycin (rifampin or rifabutin). Untreated disease is associated with shortened survival, and the response to treatment is good in patients who do not have rapidly progressive HIV infection. HIV-positive patients who experience clearing of systemic symptoms and have positive cultures with sustained recovery of the CD4+ T cell count can probably have treatment discontinued (as described above for *M. avium* infection). There is no recommended prophylactic regimen, although the azithromycin regimen given to prevent disseminated *M. avium* infection may also be effective in preventing disseminated *M. kansasii* infection.

M. ABSCESSUS, M. CHELONAE, AND *M. FORTUITUM*

Three rapidly growing NTM species are prominent in reports of human infection and colonization: *M. abscessus, M. chelonae,* and *M. fortuitum.* These organisms are acquired from water, soil, or nosocomial sources. The most common clinical manifestation of infection is disseminated cutaneous disease in patients who have defects in cellular immunity or are receiving glucocorticoid therapy. Immunocompetent hosts can develop localized cutaneous infection in surgical or traumatic wounds, from contaminated injections, or after body piercing. Cutaneous lesions are cellulitic or nodular; are typically erythematous, indurated, and tender; and may progress to ulceration and purulent drainage. Proximal sporotrichoid spread has also been reported. Pulmonary infection (usually due to *M. abscessus*) is the next most common manifestation and occurs principally in patients with underlying lung disease, such as cystic fibrosis.

The rapidly growing NTM species may be isolated from clinical specimens submitted for routine microbiologic testing. However, reliable evaluation requires inoculation onto special mycobacterial media and an extended incubation period. Because rapidly growing NTM species are also common laboratory contaminants, numerous false alarms in the form of pseudoepidemics have been reported.

℞ *M. ABSCESSUS, M. CHELONAE,* AND *M. FORTUITUM* INFECTIONS

Treatment varies with the patient group and with the species of rapidly growing NTM. Susceptibility tests should be performed and used to guide antibiotic selection. All three species are usually susceptible to clarithromycin and amikacin; *M. abscessus* and *M. fortuitum* are also susceptible to cefoxitin and imipenem. Other agents that may be active include doxycycline and fluoroquinolones. Patients with localized cutaneous disease may respond to a single active agent (e.g., clarithromycin at a dosage of 500 mg twice daily by mouth for ≥2 weeks). Up to 6 months of therapy may be optimal for bacteremic or disseminated cutaneous disease, and a second agent should be added on the basis of susceptibility tests. Pulmonary disease due to *M. fortuitum* or *M. chelonae* should be treated with two active agents (usually including clarithromycin) until sputum cultures have been negative for 12 months. Pulmonary disease due to *M. abscessus* is especially difficult to treat since prolonged therapy is necessary and the most active drugs require parenteral administration and carry a significant risk of toxicity with prolonged use. The most potent regimen is typically IV amikacin (10–15 mg/kg daily) and IV cefoxitin (3 g every 6 h) or imipenem (500 mg every 6–12 h) with oral clarithromycin (500 mg twice daily). Expert consultation should be sought for management of this chronic, often incurable pulmonary infection.

M. MARINUM

M. marinum is widely distributed in water and causes chronic cutaneous infection when an open cutaneous lesion is exposed to a colonized water source. Most infections are due to hand or upper-extremity exposure to fish tanks, and some are due to shellfish or marine exposures. Swimming pools are no longer a common source of infection because of current chlorination standards. *M. marinum* grows optimally at 30°C—a lower temperature than is optimal for most pathogenic mycobacteria. After a median incubation period of 21 days (≥30 days in 35% of cases), a granulomatous or ulcerating skin lesion develops at the site of entry, with subsequent sporotrichoid spread in many cases. In some patients, especially those with serious underlying disease and those receiving immunosuppressive therapy, infection may extend to deeper structures, producing tenosynovitis or osteomyelitis. The diagnosis is established by mycobacterial culture of a biopsied lesion or by demonstration of granulomas or AFB in a biopsy sample from a patient with a compatible exposure history.

℞ *M. MARINUM* INFECTIONS

Treatment consists of the combination of clarithromycin and ethambutol; the regimen is given for 1–2 months after resolution of lesions—typically 3–4 months in total. Surgical debridement may be necessary in extensive or deep disease; however, routine incision and drainage are not helpful. Rifampin should be added in cases of osteomyelitis. Persons with occupational or avocational exposure to fish tanks or salt water should wear waterproof gloves to prevent infection of open cutaneous lesions.

M. ULCERANS

M. ulcerans causes cutaneous infection (Buruli ulcer) in endemic regions of Central and West Africa, Central and South America, Malaysia, Indonesia, Papua New Guinea, and Australia. The organism is closely related to *M. marinum*, has a similar temperature for optimal growth, and has been isolated from natural bodies of water. Most cases of human infection occur on the bare arms or legs of children or young adults living near rivers, lakes, or swamps. Transmission is thought to result from minor trauma or the bite of an aquatic insect. The initial lesion is a small painless nodule that progresses to a deep ulcer. The ulcer expands, resulting in sloughing of skin and subcutaneous tissue; osteomyelitis may also occur. Stellate scarring and deforming contractures may result from extensive necrosis.

Biopsy analyses demonstrate extracellular AFB in early lesions, with a limited inflammatory reaction. Tissue destruction extends beyond the area of demonstrable bacterial infection and has been attributed to a unique mycobacterial toxin, mycolactone.

℞ *M. ULCERANS* INFECTIONS

Antimicrobial therapy has not yet been shown to be beneficial, although rifampin, dapsone, clarithromycin, streptomycin, and amikacin display in vitro activity against *M. ulcerans*. Surgical treatment is of primary importance, and skin grafting may be required. Immunization with BCG reduces the risk of disease by ~50%.

OTHER NTM SPECIES

Numerous other NTM species have been associated with human disease, although they may represent contaminants in clinical specimens. Species and sites of possible infection include *M. celatum* (lung, lymph nodes), *M. genavense* (disseminated), *M. gordonae* (skin, contaminant), *M. haemophilum* (skin, disseminated), *M. malmoense* (lung), *M. simiae* (lung, disseminated), *M. scrofulaceum* (lymphadenitis), *M. szulgai* (skin, lung), and *M. xenopi* (lung, disseminated).

FURTHER READINGS

DOUCETTE K, FISHMAN JA: Nontuberculous mycobacterial infection in hematopoietic stem cell and solid organ transplant recipients. Clin Infect Dis 38:1428, 2004

GRIFFITH DE et al: An official ATS/IDSA statement: Diagnosis, treatment and prevention of nontuberculous mycobacterial diseases. Am J Respir Crit Care Med 175:367, 2007

HANAK V et al: Hot tub lung: Presenting features and clinical course of 21 patients. Respir Med 100:610, 2006

KOBASHI Y et al: Relationship between clinical efficacy of treatment of pulmonary *Mycobacterium avium* complex disease and drug-sensitivity testing of *M. avium* complex isolates. J Infect Chemother 12:195, 2006

PHILLIPS M, VON REYN CF: Nosocomial infections due to nontuberculous mycobacteria. Clin Infect Dis 33:1363, 2001

REED C et al: Environmental risk factors for infection with *Mycobacterium avium* complex. Am J Epidemiol 164:32, 2006

VON REYN CF et al: Skin test reactions to *Mycobacterium tuberculosis* purified protein derivative and *Mycobacterium avium* sensitin among health care workers and medical students in the United States. Int J Tuberc Lung Dis 5:1122, 2001

161 Antimycobacterial Agents

Richard J. Wallace, Jr., David E. Griffith

The physician is greatly challenged to provide optimal therapy for mycobacterial illnesses because of the increase in both drug-susceptible and multidrug-resistant tuberculosis; the increasing number of pathogenic nontuberculous mycobacteria (NTM); drug-related toxicities and drug-drug interactions (especially in patients who have AIDS, with their complex antiretroviral drug regimens); and the plethora of new antibiotics with antimycobacterial potential. This chapter reviews the therapeutic agents used for treatment of tuberculosis, leprosy (Hansen's disease), and diseases caused by NTM, including the *Mycobacterium avium* complex (MAC), *M. kansasii*, the rapidly growing mycobacteria, and *M. marinum*. The use of first-line antimycobacterial agents in patients with renal or hepatic disease and in pregnant women is summarized in Table 161-1. The effects of antimycobacterial agents on the levels, activity, and toxicity of other commonly used drugs are summarized in Table 161-2. The reader is referred to the other chapters in this section for a more complete discussion of therapy for specific mycobacterial diseases.

TUBERCULOSIS

Drugs used to treat tuberculosis have been classified into first-line and second-line agents. *First-line essential* antituberculous agents are the most effective and are a necessary component of any short-course therapeutic regimen. The four drugs in this category are rifampin, isoniazid, ethambutol, and pyrazinamide. The *first-line supplemental* agents, which are highly effective with acceptable toxicity, include rifabutin, rifapentine, and streptomycin. *Second-line* antituberculous drugs are clinically much less effective than first-line agents and elicit severe reactions much more frequently. These drugs are rarely used in therapy and then only by caregivers experienced with their use. The older agents include para-aminosalicylic acid (PAS), ethionamide, cycloserine, amikacin, and capreomycin. Favorable experience in patients with tuberculosis resistant to or intolerant of first-line drugs suggests that the fluoroquinolones levofloxacin and moxifloxacin are important additions to multidrug antituberculous regimens; thus these agents have now been added to the list of second-line drugs.

FIRST-LINE ESSENTIAL ANTITUBERCULOUS DRUGS

Rifampin Rifampin, a semisynthetic derivative of *Streptomyces mediterranei*, is considered the most important and potent antituberculous agent. It is also active against a wide spectrum of other organisms, including some gram-positive and gram-negative bacteria, *Legionella* spp., *M. kansasii*, and *M. marinum*.

MECHANISM OF ACTION Rifampin has both intracellular and extracellular bactericidal activity. It blocks RNA synthesis by specifically binding and inhibiting DNA-dependent RNA polymerase. Susceptible strains of *M. tuberculosis* as well as *M. kansasii* and *M. marinum* are inhibited by ≤1 μg/mL.

PHARMACOLOGY Rifampin is a fat-soluble complex macrocyclic antibiotic that is absorbed readily after either PO or IV administration. Serum levels of 10–20 μg/mL follow a standard adult oral dose of 600 mg. Rifampin distributes well throughout most body tissues, including inflamed meninges. The fact that rifampin turns body fluids (urine, saliva, sputum, tears) a red-orange color makes it simple and inexpensive to check on patients' compliance with therapy. Rifampin is excreted primarily through the bile and the enterohepatic circulation, while 30–40% of a dose is excreted via the kidneys. The drug is administered three times weekly, twice weekly, or daily at a dose of 600 mg for adults (10 mg/kg) and 10–20 mg/kg for children. As mentioned above, rifampin is also available for IV administration.

ADVERSE EFFECTS (Table 161-3) Rifampin is generally well tolerated; the most common adverse event is gastrointestinal upset. This drug rarely causes hepatocellular injury when given alone; however, hepatitis is more common when rifampin is given in combination with isoniazid or pyrazinamide. Other adverse effects of rifampin include rash (0.8%), hemolytic anemia (<1%), thrombocytopenia, and immunosuppression of unknown clinical importance. Rifampin is a potent inducer of the hepatic microsomal enzymes and thereby decreases the half-life of a number of drugs, including digoxin, warfarin, prednisone, cyclosporine, methadone, oral contraceptives, clarithromycin, the HIV protease inhibitors, the HIV nonnucleoside reverse transcriptase inhibitors, and quinidine (Table 161-2). The dose of rifampin generally does not require reduction in patients with

TABLE 161-1 USE OF FIRST-LINE ANTIMYCOBACTERIAL AGENTS IN PATIENTS WITH RENAL OR HEPATIC DISEASE AND IN PREGNANT WOMEN

	Use in Indicated Circumstances			
		Renal Disease: Creatinine Clearance Rate		
Agent	Severe Hepatic Disease	<60 but >30 mL/min	≤30 mL/min	Pregnancy[a]
Azithromycin	No change	No change	?Decrease dose	No evidence of risk (B)
Clarithromycin	No change	No change	Decrease dose	Risk cannot be ruled out (C)
Ethambutol	No change	No change	No change	Risk cannot be ruled out (C)
Isoniazid	Avoid use or monitor carefully	No change	No change	Risk cannot be ruled out (C)
Pyrazinamide	Avoid use or monitor carefully	No change	Decrease dose[b]	Risk cannot be ruled out (C)[c]
Rifabutin	No change	No change	No change	No evidence of risk (B)
Rifampin	Avoid use or monitor carefully	No change	No change	Risk cannot be ruled out (C)
Rifapentine	Avoid use or monitor carefully	No change	No change	Risk cannot be ruled out (C)
Streptomycin	No change	Decrease dose	Decrease dose and frequency	Definite evidence of risk (D)

[a]Based on Food and Drug Administration pregnancy categories of A–D, X.
[b]Prudent but not absolutely necessary.
[c]Use in pregnancy is recommended by international organizations outside the United States.

TABLE 161-2 EFFECTS OF MAJOR ANTIMYCOBACTERIAL AGENTS ON LEVELS/ACTIVITY/TOXICITY OF OTHER COMMONLY USED DRUGS[a]

Rifampin/rifabutin[b]	Isoniazid
Acetaminophen (↓)	Alcohol (↑ in risk of hepatitis)
Antiarrhythmics (↓)	Carbamazepine (↑)
Anticonvulsants (↓)	Diphenylhydantoin (↑)
Azole antifungals (↓)	Enflurane (↑ in risk of renal failure)
Barbiturates (↓)	Warfarin (↑)
β Blockers (↓)	**Clarithromycin**
Calcium channel blockers (↓)	Astemizole (↑)
Chloramphenicol (↓)	Carbamazepine (↑)
Clarithromycin (↓)	Digoxin (↑)
Cyclosporine (↓)	Rifabutin (↑)
Dapsone (↓)	Ritonavir (↓)
Delavirdine (↓)	Terfenadine (↑)
Diazepam (↓)	Zidovudine (↓)
Digoxin (↓)	
Doxycycline (↓)	
Fluoroquinolones (↓)	
Glucocorticoids (↓)	
Halothane (↓)	
Hormonal contraceptives (↓)	
Narcotics (↓)	
NNRTIs[c] (↓)	
Oral hypoglycemics (↓)	
Probenecid (↓)	
Protease inhibitors (↓)	
Quinidine (↓)	
Theophylline (↓)	
Tricyclic antidepressants (↓)	
Warfarin (↓)	
Zidovudine (↓)	

[a]The following antimycobacterial agents have no or minimal effects on other drugs: amikacin, azithromycin, capreomycin, ethambutol, streptomycin, pyrazinamide.
[b]Rifabutin, which induces the cytochrome P450 system, has the same effects (↓) as rifampin but to a lesser degree. All drugs whose half-life is decreased by rifampin induction of hepatic microsomal enzymes may be subject to the same effect when coadministered with rifabutin; however, this point has not yet been studied.
[c]NNRTIs, nonnucleoside reverse transcriptase inhibitors.

renal failure, especially those receiving intermittent rifampin treatment (Table 161-1).

RESISTANCE Acquired resistance to rifampin results from spontaneous point mutations that alter the β subunit of the RNA polymerase (*rpoB*) gene. Studies have shown that 96% of rifampin-resistant strains have a missense mutation within a 91-bp central core region of the gene. Rifampin-resistant strains of *M. leprae* have similar mutations that alter a single serine residue (Ser-425) in the same core region of the *rpoB* gene. Intrinsic resistance to rifampin is relatively common among most species of rapidly growing and slowly growing NTM; the mechanisms underlying this resistance have yet to be determined.

Isoniazid After rifampin, isoniazid is considered the best antituberculous drug available. Isoniazid should be included in all tuberculosis treatment regimens unless the organism is resistant. This agent is inexpensive, readily synthesized, available worldwide, highly selective for mycobacteria, and well tolerated, with only 5% of patients exhibiting adverse effects.

MECHANISM OF ACTION Isoniazid is the hydrazide of isonicotinic acid, a small, water-soluble molecule that easily penetrates the cell. Its mechanism of action involves inhibition of mycolic acid cell-wall synthesis via oxygen-dependent pathways such as the catalase-peroxidase reaction. Isoniazid is bacteriostatic against resting bacilli and bactericidal against rapidly multiplying organisms, both extracellularly and intracellularly. The minimal inhibitory concentrations (MICs) of isoniazid for wild-type (untreated) strains of *M. tuberculosis* are <0.1 μg/mL, while those for *M. kansasii* are usually 0.5–2.0 μg/mL. The MICs of this drug for other NTM are often higher.

PHARMACOLOGY Both oral and IM preparations of isoniazid are readily absorbed. The standard adult daily oral dose of 300 mg produces peak serum levels of 3–5 μg/mL. Isoniazid diffuses well throughout the body and reaches therapeutic concentrations in serum, cerebrospinal fluid (CSF), and infected tissue, including caseous granulomas. Isoniazid is metabolized in the liver via acetylation and hydrolysis; its metabolites are excreted into the urine. The rate of acetylation is genetically controlled. The recommended daily dose for the treatment of tuberculosis in the United States is 5 mg/kg for adults and 10–20 mg/kg for children, with a maximal daily dose of 300 mg for both groups. (Tuberculosis organizations outside the United States have recommended 5 mg/kg daily for both groups.) For intermittent therapy (usually directly observed), a maximal dose of 900 mg twice or thrice weekly is used. Isoniazid does not require dosage adjustment in patients with renal insufficiency or with end-stage renal disease requiring chronic hemodialysis. Although not approved by the U.S. Food and Drug Administration (FDA), IV isoniazid can be given in an urgent situation.

TABLE 161-3 MONITORING SIDE EFFECTS OF COMMON ANTITUBERCULOUS DRUGS

Drug	Side Effect	Management
Rifampin	Rash	Observe patient/stop drug if significant
	Liver dysfunction	Monitor AST/limit alcohol consumption/monitor for hepatitis symptoms
	Flulike syndrome	Administer at least twice weekly/limit dose to 10 mg/kg (adults)
	Red-orange urine	Reassure patient
	Drug interactions	Consider monitoring levels of other drugs affected by rifampin, especially with contraceptives, anticoagulants, and digoxin/avoid use with protease inhibitors
	Fever, chills	Stop drug
Isoniazid	Hepatitis	Monitor AST/limit alcohol consumption/monitor for hepatitis symptoms/educate patient/stop drug at first symptoms of hepatitis (nausea, vomiting, anorexia, flulike syndrome)
	Peripheral neuritis	Administer vitamin B_6
	Optic neuritis	Administer vitamin B_6/stop drug
	Seizures	Administer vitamin B_6
Pyrazinamide	Hepatitis	Monitor AST/limit daily dosage to 15–30 mg/kg/discontinue with signs or symptoms of hepatitis
	Hyperuricemia	Monitor uric acid level only in cases of gout or renal failure
Ethambutol	Optic neuritis	Use 25 mg/kg daily only for first 2 months (except in drug-resistant tuberculosis), then use lower daily dose (15 mg/kg) when possible/monitor visual acuity (eye chart) and red-green color vision (Ishihara Color Book) at baseline and with any visual complaint/educate patient/stop drug at first change in vision, get ophthalmologic evaluation
Streptomycin, amikacin, capreomycin	Ototoxicity, renal toxicity	Limit dose and duration of therapy as much as possible/avoid daily therapy in patients >50 years old/monitor BUN and serum creatinine levels and possibly conduct audiometry before and as needed during therapy/question patient regularly about tinnitus, dizziness, vertigo, and decreased hearing/measure serum drug levels if possible/educate patient/stop drug at first development of adverse effect (usually tinnitus)

Note: AST, aspartate aminotransferase; BUN, blood urea nitrogen.

ADVERSE EFFECTS (Table 161-3) The two most important adverse effects of isoniazid therapy are hepatotoxicity and peripheral neuropathy. Other adverse reactions are either rare or less significant and include rash (2%), fever (1.2%), anemia, acne, arthritic symptoms, a systemic lupus erythematosus–like syndrome, optic atrophy, seizures, and psychiatric symptoms. Isoniazid-associated hepatotoxicity includes asymptomatic transient elevation in aminotransferase levels (20%), symptomatic hepatitis (<1%), and fulminant hepatitis with hepatic failure (<<0.01%). Isoniazid-associated hepatitis is idiosyncratic and increases in incidence with age, daily alcohol consumption, concomitant rifampin administration, and active hepatitis B infection as well as in women who are pregnant or in the immediate postpartum period (up to 3 months after delivery). Appropriate clinical monitoring of patients receiving isoniazid includes at least monthly questioning about hepatitis-related symptoms and filling of prescriptions for no more than 1 month's worth of medication. Clinical monitoring is essential for all patients since discontinuation of the drug at the onset of hepatitis symptoms reduces the risk of progression to fatal hepatitis. The Centers for Disease Control and Prevention (CDC) and the American Thoracic Society (ATS) recommend that serum concentrations of alanine aminotransferase (ALT) be determined at baseline in patients with liver disorders or HIV infection, in women who are pregnant or in the immediate postpartum period (3 months), in persons with a history of liver disease (e.g., hepatitis B or C, alcoholic hepatitis, or cirrhosis), in persons who use alcohol regularly, and in other individuals at risk for chronic liver disease who are receiving isoniazid for treatment of latent tuberculosis. Baseline testing is no longer routinely indicated in persons >35 years of age. Routine laboratory monitoring during isoniazid treatment is indicated for patients whose baseline liver function tests yield abnormal results and for persons at risk for hepatic disease, including the groups just mentioned. Measurement of the ALT level is mandatory whenever a patient notices the onset of symptoms suggestive of isoniazid-associated hepatitis (e.g., fever, anorexia, nausea, vomiting, and/or a flulike syndrome including fever and myalgias), and treatment should be discontinued until the relationship between therapy and symptoms is ascertained. The CDC and the ATS recommend that isoniazid should be discontinued whenever (1) an asymptomatic elevation of the ALT level exceeds five times the upper limit of normal or (2) the ALT is three times the upper limit of normal in conjunction with hepatitis symptoms or jaundice. Peripheral neuritis associated with isoniazid is uncommon and probably relates to interference with pyridoxine (vitamin B_6) metabolism. The risk of isoniazid-related neurotoxicity is greatest for patients with preexisting disorders that also pose a risk of neuropathy, such as diabetes, alcohol abuse, or malnutrition. In these patients, the prophylactic administration of 25–50 mg of pyridoxine daily should be considered.

RESISTANCE The molecular sites of isoniazid resistance have been detailed. Most isoniazid-resistant strains have amino acid changes in either the catalase-peroxidase gene (*katG*) or the promoter of a two-gene locus known as *inhA*. Missense mutations or deletion of *katG* is also associated with reduced catalase and peroxidase activity. Rates of primary isoniazid resistance in untreated patients are much higher in many foreign-born populations than in populations born in the United States.

Ethambutol A derivative of ethylenediamine, ethambutol is a water-soluble compound that is active only against mycobacteria. Susceptible species include *M. tuberculosis, M. marinum, M. kansasii*, and MAC organisms. Among first-line drugs, ethambutol is the least potent against *M. tuberculosis*. It is used most often with rifampin for treatment of tuberculosis in patients who cannot tolerate isoniazid or who are thought or known to be infected with isoniazid-resistant organisms.

MECHANISM OF ACTION Ethambutol at standard doses is bacteriostatic against *M. tuberculosis*. Its primary mechanism of action appears to be inhibition of an arabinosyltransferase that mediates the polymerization of arabinose into arabinogalactan within the cell wall.

PHARMACOLOGY After oral administration, 75–80% of a dose of ethambutol is absorbed from the gastrointestinal tract. Peak serum levels of 2–4 μg/mL are achieved 2–4 h after the standard adult daily dose of 15 mg/kg. The drug's distribution throughout the body is adequate except in the CSF, where it reaches only low levels. However, ethambutol can reach CSF levels up to 50% as high as peak plasma levels when administered at a daily dosage of 25 mg/kg (which may be given in one daily dose) for the first 2 months, with subsequent reduction to 15 mg/kg. In cases of drug-resistant tuberculosis or where retreatment is necessary, the higher dose may be given for the duration. For intermittent therapy, the dosage is 50 mg/kg twice weekly or 30 mg/kg thrice weekly. The dosage must be lowered for patients with renal insufficiency (a creatinine clearance rate of <50 mL/min) to prevent drug accumulation and toxicity.

ADVERSE EFFECTS (Table 161-3) Ethambutol is usually well tolerated. Retrobulbar optic neuritis is the most serious adverse effect; axial or central neuritis—the only form reported in patients taking doses of <30 mg/kg—involves the papillomacular bundle of fibers and results in reduced visual acuity, central scotoma, and loss of ability to see green. Symptoms of ocular toxicity typically develop several months after initiation of therapy, but rapid-onset optic neuritis has been reported. The risk of optic neuritis depends on the dose and duration of therapy: this reaction develops in 5% of patients receiving a daily dose of 25 mg/kg but in fewer than 1% of patients given a daily dose of 15 mg/kg. Patients taking the lower dose should be tested for visual acuity and red-green color discrimination at baseline and whenever there is a subjective change in vision. Patients taking the higher dose should be tested at baseline, monthly thereafter, and whenever there is a subjective change in vision. Intermittent (three times weekly) administration of ethambutol at 25 mg/kg per dose appears to be better tolerated than daily administration of 15 mg/kg, especially in elderly populations being treated for MAC infection. Optic neuritis with associated visual loss is usually reversible, but recovery may take >6 months.

Other adverse effects of ethambutol are infrequent. Hyperuricemia occurs but is usually asymptomatic. Peripheral sensory neuropathy occurs in rare instances. Optic neuritis is rare at the low dose in children; however, the use of ethambutol in very young children is problematic because visual complications are difficult to monitor.

RESISTANCE Ethambutol resistance in *M. tuberculosis* most commonly relates to missense mutations in the *embB* gene that encodes for arabinosyltransferase. Such mutations have been found in 70% of resistant strains and involve amino acid replacements at position 306 or 406 in ~90% of cases. Species of NTM that are intrinsically resistant to ethambutol have variant amino acids in this region of the gene, while susceptible species have the same amino acid sequences as *M. tuberculosis*.

Pyrazinamide A derivative of nicotinic acid, pyrazinamide is an important bactericidal drug used in short-course therapy for tuberculosis.

MECHANISM OF ACTION Pyrazinamide is similar to isoniazid in its narrow spectrum of antibacterial activity, which essentially includes only *M. tuberculosis*. The drug is bactericidal to slowly metabolizing organisms located within the acidic environment of the phagocyte or caseous granuloma; it is active only at a pH of <6.0. Pyrazinamide is considered a prodrug and is converted by the tubercle bacillus to the active form pyrazinoic acid. The target for this compound is thought to be a fatty acid synthase gene (*fasI*). Susceptible strains of *M. tuberculosis* are inhibited by 20 μg/mL.

PHARMACOLOGY Pyrazinamide is well absorbed after oral administration, with a plasma concentration range of 20–60 μg/mL 1–2 h after oral ingestion of the currently recommended adult daily dose of 15–30 mg/kg (maximum, 2 g/d). The drug is well distributed throughout the body. Levels in CSF are excellent, reaching 50–100% of levels in serum. The serum half-life of the drug is 9–11 h. Pyrazinamide is metabolized by at least two major pathways and one minor pathway in the liver; its several metabolites include pyrazinoic acid, 5-hydroxypyrazinamide, and 5-hydroxypyrazinoic acid. Pyrazinamide is not available in a parenteral formulation.

ADVERSE EFFECTS (Table 161-3) At the high dosages used in the past, hepatotoxicity was a prominent complication of pyrazinamide therapy. However, at the currently recommended dosages, the frequency of hepatotoxicity is no higher than that for concomitant isoniazid and rifampin therapy. Although pyrazinamide is recommended by international tuberculosis organizations for routine use in pregnancy, it is not recommended in the United States because of inadequate teratogenicity data (Table 161-1). The combination of rifampin/pyrazinamide once recommended for treatment of latent tuberculosis has recently been shown to be associated with an unacceptably high rate of hepatitis. Hyperuricemia is a common adverse effect of pyrazinamide therapy; the incidence is probably reduced by concurrent rifampin therapy. Clinical gout is seen only rarely. Polyarthralgias are encountered fairly commonly but are not related to the hyperuricemia.

RESISTANCE Resistance to pyrazinamide is associated with loss of pyrazinamidase activity such that pyrazinamide is no longer converted to pyrazinoic acid. More than 90% of isolates with MICs of >100 μg/mL have mutations in the *pncA* gene, which encodes for pyrazinamidase. All strains of *M. bovis* are naturally resistant to pyrazinamide and have a point substitution within the *pncA* gene.

FIRST-LINE SUPPLEMENTAL DRUGS

Streptomycin An aminoglycoside isolated from *Streptomyces griseus*, streptomycin is available for IM and IV administration only. In the United States, it is the least-used first-line supplemental drug for tuberculosis because of its toxicity, the difficulty in obtaining adequate CSF levels, and the inconvenience of parenteral administration. In developing countries, however, streptomycin is frequently used because of its low cost. The drug is active against untreated strains of *M. tuberculosis*, *M. kansasii*, and *M. marinum* and against some strains of MAC organisms at achievable serum levels.

MECHANISM OF ACTION Streptomycin inhibits protein synthesis by disruption of ribosomal function.

PHARMACOLOGY Serum levels of streptomycin peak at 25–40 μg/mL after a 1.0-g dose. Streptomycin is bactericidal for rapidly dividing extracellular mycobacteria but is ineffective in the acidic environment within the macrophage. It diffuses poorly into the meninges and, in patients with meningitis, reaches CSF levels that are only 20% of serum levels.

The usual adult dose of streptomycin for a 70-kg patient under age 50 is 0.5–1.0 g (10–15 mg/kg) given IM daily or five times per week; the pediatric dose is 20–40 mg/kg daily, with a maximum of 1 g/d. Because streptomycin is eliminated almost exclusively by the kidneys, the dosage must be lowered and the frequency of administration reduced (to only two or three times per week) in most patients >50 years of age and in any patient with renal impairment (Table 161-1) or reduced body weight. Streptomycin can be given IV, although this approach is not approved by the FDA.

ADVERSE EFFECTS (Table 161-3) Adverse reactions to streptomycin therapy occur in 10–20% of recipients. Ototoxicity and renal toxicity are the most common and the most serious. Renal toxicity, usually manifested as nonoliguric renal failure, is less common with streptomycin than with other frequently used aminoglycosides, such as gentamicin. Ototoxicity involves both hearing loss and vestibular dysfunction. The latter is more common and includes loss of balance, vertigo, and tinnitus. Patients receiving streptomycin must be monitored carefully for these adverse effects. Less serious reactions include perioral paresthesia, eosinophilia, rash, and drug fever.

RESISTANCE In two-thirds of streptomycin-resistant strains of *M. tuberculosis*, mutations have been identified in one of two targets: a 16S rRNA gene (*rrs*) or the gene encoding ribosomal protein S12 (*rpsL*). Both targets are believed to be involved in streptomycin ribosomal binding. No mutational change has been identified in the other one-third of resistant isolates. Strains of *M. tuberculosis* resistant to streptomycin are not cross-resistant to capreomycin or amikacin.

Rifabutin Rifabutin, a semisynthetic rifamycin spiropiperidyl derivative, shares many characteristics with rifampin, including activity against *M. tuberculosis*. Rifabutin is also active against some strains of rifampin-resistant *M. tuberculosis* and is more active than rifampin against the *M. avium* complex and other NTM. To date, rifabutin has been most useful in the prophylaxis of disseminated MAC infection and in the treatment of drug-resistant tuberculosis. Rifabutin is recommended in place of rifampin for the treatment of HIV-positive individuals who are also taking protease inhibitors because its effect on these agents is less pronounced (Table 161-2).

MECHANISM OF ACTION In *Escherichia coli* and *Bacillus subtilis*, rifabutin inhibits DNA-dependent RNA polymerase in the same manner as rifampin. Its mode of action against mycobacteria is believed to be the same.

PHARMACOLOGY The pharmacology of rifabutin is dramatically different from that of rifampin. Rifabutin is readily absorbed after a single oral dose of 300 mg and reaches peak serum levels (0.35 μg/mL) in 2–4 h. This lipophilic drug distributes best to tissues: tissue levels are 5–10 times higher than plasma levels. CSF concentrations are 30–70% of plasma levels in HIV-infected patients who have meningitis. The drug's slow clearance via hepatic metabolism and renal excretion results in a mean serum half-life of 45 h, which is much longer than the 3- to 5-h half-life of rifampin. Clarithromycin (but not azithromycin) and fluconazole appear to block the hepatic metabolism of rifabutin, with consequent increases in serum levels. Adjustment of dosage is usually unnecessary in elderly patients and in patients with reduced hepatic or renal function (Table 161-1).

ADVERSE EFFECTS The majority of rifabutin's adverse effects are dose related. These events occur most frequently in patients receiving >300 mg/d. The most common symptoms are gastrointestinal; other reactions include rash, headache, asthenia, chest pain, myalgia, and insomnia. Like those taking rifampin, most patients taking rifabutin have discolored (orange to tan) urine and other body fluids. Less common adverse reactions include fever, chills, a flulike syndrome, anterior uveitis, hepatitis, *Clostridium difficile*–associated diarrhea, a diffuse polymyalgia syndrome, and a yellow skin discoloration ("pseudojaundice"). Laboratory abnormalities include neutropenia, leukopenia, thrombocytopenia, and increased levels of liver enzymes. Rifabutin induces hepatic cytochrome P450 enzymes but does so much less strongly than rifampin.

RESISTANCE Resistance to rifabutin is attributable to the same mechanism as that to rifampin—i.e., mutations involving the *rpoB* gene. However, of the 14 mutant *rpoB* alleles that confer resistance to rifampin, only 9 confer high-level resistance to rifabutin; the remaining 5 result in only small changes in rifabutin MICs, which remain at ≤0.5 μg/mL. Thus rifabutin inhibits about one-quarter of rifampin-resistant strains of *M. tuberculosis*.

Rifapentine A semisynthetic cyclopentyl rifamycin antibiotic, rifapentine received accelerated approval from the FDA for the treatment of tuberculosis. It is the first new drug approved for tuberculosis in the United States in 30 years. While similar to rifampin, rifapentine is lipophilic and longer acting—characteristics that enhance patient compliance; the drug can be administered at a dose of 600 mg once or twice weekly. Rifapentine has not yet been approved for the treatment of patients with HIV disease because rifapentine/rifampin monoresistance frequently develops in HIV-positive patients receiving isoniazid plus once-weekly rifapentine.

MECHANISM OF ACTION Rifapentine exerts its bactericidal effect by inhibiting DNA-dependent RNA polymerase in susceptible bacteria. The MICs of rifapentine for rifampin-susceptible strains of *M. tuberculosis* range from 0.03 to 0.12 μg/mL.

PHARMACOLOGY After oral administration, rifapentine reaches peak serum concentrations in 5–6 h and achieves a steady state in 10 days. The half-life of rifapentine and its active metabolite 25-desacetyl rifapentine is ~13 h. The administered dose is excreted via the liver (70%).

ADVERSE EFFECTS Rifapentine's adverse-event pattern is similar to that of rifampin. Rifapentine induces the hepatic cytochrome P450 enzymes CYP3A4 and 2C8/9. Current induction studies suggest that its potential for drug-drug interaction may be lower than that of rifampin but greater than that of rifabutin. Drugs potentially affected by concomitant administration of rifapentine are listed under "Rifampin/rifabutin" in Table 161-2. Rifapentine is in category C for use in pregnancy (Table 161-1) because of its teratogenesis in rats and rabbits.

RESISTANCE Strains of *M. tuberculosis* resistant to rifapentine, rifampin, and rifabutin all involve spontaneous point mutations in the *rpoB* gene. All strains resistant to rifampin are also resistant to rifapentine.

SECOND-LINE ANTITUBERCULOUS DRUGS

Second-line and/or newer antituberculosis agents are used either when tuberculosis is drug resistant or when first-line supplemental drugs are not available. The more important second-line drugs are discussed below in their general (descending) order of usefulness.

Quinolones The mode of action of the fluorinated quinolones presumably is the prevention of DNA synthesis through the inhibition of DNA gyrase. Ofloxacin, levofloxacin, ciprofloxacin, and moxifloxacin are active against many mycobacteria, including *M. tuberculosis, M. leprae, M. marinum, M. kansasii*, and *M. fortuitum*. Levofloxacin and moxifloxacin are the most active quinolones against *M. tuberculosis*. Recent studies suggest that use of moxifloxacin may reduce the duration of therapy for drug-susceptible tuberculosis. These drugs are well absorbed orally, reach high serum levels, and distribute well to body tissues and fluids. While not approved for antituberculous therapy in the United States, ofloxacin—used in combination with isoniazid and rifampin for the treatment of pulmonary tuberculosis—has been as active and safe as ethambutol in initial trials. Adverse effects are relatively uncommon, occurring in 0.5–10% of cases and consisting mostly of benign reactions such as gastrointestinal intolerance, rashes, dizziness, and headache. The quinolones are rapidly becoming some of the most important and effective drugs for the treatment of patients who have resistant tuberculosis or are intolerant to first-line essential drugs. Some experts would classify the quinolones, especially moxifloxacin, as first-line supplemental agents. The quinolones can also be administered IV.

Mycobacterial resistance to the fluoroquinolones develops rapidly. Its molecular basis is complex; only some strains exhibit missense mutations in the A subunit (*gyrA* gene) of DNA gyrase. Fluoroquinolone-resistant tuberculosis is a source of growing concern. Because of their broad spectrum and the ease with which mutational resistance develops, antituberculous therapy with quinolones should be reserved (pending the results of ongoing studies) for patients with multidrug-resistant disease and for those who cannot tolerate first-line drugs.

Capreomycin Capreomycin, a complex cyclic polypeptide antibiotic derived from *Streptomyces capreolus*, is similar to streptomycin in terms of dosing, mechanism of action, pharmacology, and toxicity. It is administered only by the IM route in doses of 10–15 mg/kg daily or five times per week (maximal daily dose, 1 g), with peak blood levels of 20–40 μg/mL. After 2–4 months, the dosage should be reduced to 1 g two or three times a week. Cross-resistance to kanamycin and amikacin—but not to streptomycin—is common. After streptomycin, capreomycin is the injectable drug of choice for tuberculosis.

Amikacin This well-known aminoglycoside is bactericidal to extracellular organisms. Amikacin is active against *M. tuberculosis* and several of the nontuberculous species, including the rapidly growing mycobacteria, *M. kansasii, M. leprae*, and the *M. avium* complex. The usual adult dosage is 7–10 mg/kg IM or IV three to five times per week (generally no more than 500–750 mg/d). Resistance relates to a single A → G base-pair change at position 1408 in the 16S ribosomal RNA gene.

Ethionamide Like isoniazid and pyrazinamide, ethionamide is a derivative of isonicotinic acid. This agent is bacteriostatic against metabolizing *M. tuberculosis* and some NTM. It is most useful in the treatment of multidrug-resistant tuberculosis. However, its use is severely limited by its toxicity and frequent side effects, which include intense gastrointestinal intolerance (anorexia, vomiting, and dysgeusia), serious neurologic reactions, reversible hepatitis (5% of cases), hypersensitivity reactions, and hypothyroidism.

Para-Aminosalicylic Acid PAS as a calcium or sodium salt inhibits the growth of *M. tuberculosis* by impairing folate synthesis. It is rarely indicated for the treatment of tuberculosis because of its low level of antituberculous activity and its high level of gastrointestinal toxicity (manifesting as nausea, vomiting, and diarrhea). Enteric-coated PAS granules (4 g every 8 h) may be better tolerated than other formulations and produce higher therapeutic blood levels. The drug has a short half-life (1 h), and 80% of the dose is excreted in the urine.

Cycloserine Cycloserine (D-4-amino-3-isoxazolidinone) is produced by *Streptomyces orchidaceus* and is active against a broad spectrum of bacteria, including *M. tuberculosis*. Cycloserine is well absorbed after oral administration and is widely distributed throughout body fluids, including the CSF. Serious side effects limit the use of this drug and include psychosis (with suicide in some cases), seizures, peripheral neuropathy, headaches, somnolence, and allergic reactions. Cycloserine should not be given to patients with epilepsy, active alcohol abuse, severe renal insufficiency, or a history of depression or psychosis.

NEWER ANTITUBERCULOUS DRUGS

A number of drugs are being evaluated for their antituberculous activity. This group includes newer rifamycins, fluoroquinolones, oxazolidinones (linezolid; see below), nitroimidazopyrans, and diarylquinolines. Although it is not clear how many of the new agents will prove to be clinically useful, there are currently more antituberculosis drugs in development than at any previous time.

Linezolid Linezolid is one of a new class of gram-positive-active antimicrobial agents called oxazolidinones that inhibit protein synthesis by binding to the 70S ribosomal initiation complex. Linezolid has very low MICs against both drug-susceptible and drug-resistant *M. tuberculosis* in vitro and has been used successfully as a component of multidrug regimens in a small number of patients with drug-resistant tuberculosis. This agent is available in IV and oral forms. Linezolid is associated with frequent, severe adverse events, including bone marrow suppression (which appears to be dose dependent and reversible) and peripheral neuropathy (which appears to be neither dose dependent nor reversible).

LEPROSY (HANSEN'S DISEASE)

Therapy for leprosy remains difficult, especially in developing countries. Obstacles include the long courses of drug therapy required, the high cost and limited availability of most drugs, the frequency of adverse drug reactions, the difficulty of determining a treatment endpoint, and (given that *M. leprae* still cannot be grown in vitro) the difficulty of conducting susceptibility testing. While many drugs are active against *M. leprae*, efficacy in the treatment of leprosy has been established only for dapsone, rifampin, clofazimine, and ethionamide; because of its potentially severe side effects, the WHO no longer recommends ethionamide for the treatment of leprosy. Initiation of multidrug treatment has reduced the problem of acquired drug resistance seen previously with dapsone monotherapy.

Rifampin Rifampin is considered the most active agent for the treatment of leprosy. Its worldwide use is limited only by its cost. This drug is highly bactericidal against *M. leprae* and reduces the number of viable bacilli in patients' tissues faster than any other available agent. Rifampin must be combined with other antileprosy drugs to forestall resistance. For cost reasons, the drug dose of 600 mg is given once a month (supervised) outside the United States, but this dose is given daily in the United States. For details on pharmacology, adverse events, and resistance, see relevant sections under "Tuberculosis."

Dapsone Dapsone (4,4′-diaminodiphenylsulfone) inhibits bacterial folic acid synthesis. It is now considered the second most active drug (after rifampin) in the treatment of leprosy because of its ready availability, low cost, and low toxicity and the susceptibility of untreated strains of *M. leprae* to low concentrations.

PHARMACOLOGY Dapsone is well absorbed orally and distributes well throughout the body. The usual daily dosage is 100 mg for adults and 0.9–1.4 mg/kg for children. Plasma concentrations peak within 1–3 h. The median elimination half-life is 22 h. Dapsone is cleared by acetylation in the liver. The drug is 70% bound to plasma protein. Usual daily doses produce serum concentrations of 10–15 μg/mL, which far exceed the MIC for *M. leprae* (0.01–0.001 μg/mL).

ADVERSE EFFECTS Hemolysis and methemoglobinemia are common untoward reactions to dapsone. Patients should be screened for glucose-6-phosphate dehydrogenase deficiency to prevent serious drug-induced hemolysis. However, most patients tolerate dapsone therapy well with adequate clinical and laboratory supervision. Other side effects include gastrointestinal intolerance, headache, pruritus, peripheral neuropathies, nephrotic syndrome, fever, and rash.

Clofazimine A phenazine iminoquinone dye, clofazimine is weakly bactericidal against *M. leprae*. It is useful in treating dapsone-resistant leprosy and may lessen the severity of erythema nodosum leprosum (ENL). Clofazimine's mode of action is not well understood. Its serum half-life is ~60–70 days; only a small proportion of the dose is excreted daily into the urine or bile. Bactericidal activity is very slow and is evident for ~50 days after administration. The usual adult dosage is 50–100 mg/d, 100 mg three times a week, or (for treatment of ENL) 300 mg/d. Untoward effects include skin discoloration and, less commonly, gastrointestinal intolerance.

Other Agents A number of other drugs exhibit significant activity against *M. leprae*, but clinical experience with these agents is lacking. Thalidomide is now approved by the FDA for treatment of ENL. This drug is sedating and extremely teratogenic and should *never* be taken by anyone who is or may become pregnant. Physicians wishing to prescribe thalidomide must register with the System for Thalidomide Education and Prescribing Safety (S.T.E.P.S.) at 1-888-423-5436 (Celgene Corporation). The newer macrolide antibiotics (particularly clarithromycin), minocycline (a long-acting tetracycline), and a number of fluoroquinolones (including ofloxacin, sparfloxacin, and pefloxacin) have shown promising bactericidal activity against *M. leprae*. For the most minor form of leprosy, the WHO now suggests the use of single-dose rifampin/ofloxacin/minocycline (ROM).

NONTUBERCULOUS MYCOBACTERIA

Although less pathogenic than *M. tuberculosis*, NTM can cause pulmonary, skin, bone, joint, lymph node, and soft tissue infection as well as disseminated disease in immunocompromised hosts, including patients with AIDS. MAC organisms and *M. kansasii* are the two most common causes of NTM pulmonary infection. Up to 40% of AIDS patients with CD4+ T cell counts of <50/μL develop disseminated disease due to *M. avium* unless they are receiving specific *M. avium* prophylaxis.

Clarithromycin Clarithromycin (6-*O*-methylerythromycin) is a newer macrolide that is similar to erythromycin in its mechanism of action. It is well absorbed with or without meals but may elicit gastrointestinal intolerance. Clarithromycin distributes well into body tissues and fluids and is highly concentrated in macrophages. The drug is metabolized in the liver, with ~30% of a given dose excreted in the urine. The dosage should be reduced if the creatinine clearance rate is ≤30 mL/min. Like erythromycin, clarithromycin binds with plasma proteins (65–70%) and can raise the levels of drugs such as theophylline and carbamazepine. Serum levels of clarithromycin are reduced by rifampin and, to a lesser degree, by rifabutin; clarithromycin increases serum levels of rifabutin and some antihistamines (e.g., terfenadine), thus potentially increasing their toxicity. The drug is also highly active not only against MAC organisms but also against almost all other NTM, including *M. marinum, M. kansasii, M. haemophilum, M. genavense, M. xenopi, M. abscessus*, and *M. chelonae*. Recent studies have shown that most members of the *M. fortuitum* group are resistant to macrolides on the basis of chromosomal *erm* genes. Standard antimycobacterial doses have been 500 mg twice daily or, in the case of MAC pulmonary disease, three times weekly. The more common side effects of high doses include nausea, vomiting, and (occasionally) abnormal liver function tests. A bitter taste is common even with routine doses. Most gastrointestinal side effects can be minimized by reducing the dose or using slow-release formulations. Clarithromycin is teratogenic in laboratory animals and is in category C for use in pregnancy (Table 161-1). Resistance results from point mutations involving adenine at position 2058 or 2059 in the 23S ribosomal RNA gene macrolide binding site and is a major concern for all slowly growing species and the rapid growers *M. chelonae* and *M. abscessus*, which have only a single copy of the ribosomal genes.

Azithromycin Azithromycin is a macrolide that belongs to the family of azalides. This drug reaches much lower serum levels than clarithromycin (usually ≤0.5 μg/mL), but its high tissue and macrophage concentrations and longer half-life suggest the feasibility of intermittent therapy. Azithromycin is involved in few drug interactions since it does not affect the cytochrome P450 system. The usual doses are 250–500 mg three times weekly (MAC therapy) or 1200 mg once a week (prophylaxis for disseminated *M. avium*). No alteration in dose is required in renal failure. The most common side effects are gastrointestinal symptoms and reversible hearing loss. Resistance to azithromycin develops by the same mechanism as that to clarithromycin, with cross-resistance between the two macrolides.

Therapy for Specific NTM Infections • ***MAC ORGANISMS*** The treatment of MAC lung disease involves the use of two or three drugs administered either daily or three times per week. Given the potential for drug-related toxicity and the remaining uncertainties about the optimal regimen and schedule, treatment frequently needs to be individualized.

Therapy for MAC lung disease in the adult patient with nodular disease and bronchiectasis usually involves the administration of clarithromycin (500 mg morning and night), ethambutol (25 mg/kg), and rifampin (600 mg) on a Monday–Wednesday–Friday schedule. For patients with upper-lobe cavitary disease, daily therapy is usually recommended. Therapy is generally continued until cultures have been negative for 12 months.

For disseminated disease in AIDS, daily administration of one of the newer macrolides (clarithromycin or azithromycin) and ethambutol (15 mg/kg) is considered an essential component of any treatment regimen, with rifabutin (300 mg) a commonly used third drug. Other alternative drugs include streptomycin and amikacin. Clofazimine appears to increase mortality risk and should be avoided. For prophylaxis of disseminated MAC disease, rifabutin (300 mg/d), clarithromycin (500 mg twice daily), and azithromycin (1200 mg once weekly) have all been effective in controlled or comparative clinical trials. Once-weekly azithromycin is the drug most often used.

M. KANSASII *M. kansasii* is usually susceptible to most antituberculous drugs except for pyrazinamide. Current ATS recommendations for the treatment of *M. kansasii* pulmonary disease are daily isoniazid (300 mg), rifampin (600 mg), and ethambutol (15 mg/kg); this regimen is continued until 12 months after the last positive sputum culture. In patients taking protease inhibitors, rifabutin (150 mg/d) or clarithromycin

(500 mg twice daily) should be substituted for rifampin. The potential advantages of the highly active rifabutin and the newer macrolides in immunocompetent patients have not been studied.

RAPIDLY GROWING MYCOBACTERIA The *M. fortuitum* group, *M. abscessus*, and *M. chelonae* account for >80% of cases of clinical disease due to rapidly growing mycobacteria. These organisms are resistant to antituberculous agents other than amikacin but are variably susceptible to several traditional antibiotics. Clarithromycin has dramatically changed the approach to therapy for infections with rapidly growing mycobacteria, since it inhibits most species. Other drugs with good activity include amikacin, cefoxitin, doxycycline, imipenem, the fluorinated quinolones, sulfonamides, and linezolid.

M. MARINUM *M. marinum*, a cause of posttraumatic localized skin infection, is typically susceptible to minocycline, rifampin, ethambutol, clarithromycin, and trimethoprim-sulfamethoxazole and is resistant to isoniazid.

FURTHER READINGS

American Thoracic Society: Targeted tuberculin testing and treatment of latent tuberculosis infection. Am J Respir Crit Care Med 161:S221, 2000

———/Centers for Disease Control and Prevention/Infectious Diseases Society of America: Treatment of tuberculosis. Am J Respir Crit Care Med 167:603, 2003

Bock NN et al: A prospective, randomized, double-blind study of the tolerability of rifapentine 600, 900, and 1,200 mg plus isoniazid in the continuation phase of tuberculosis treatment. Am J Respir Crit Care Med 165:1526, 2002

Burman WJ et al: Moxifloxacin versus ethambutol in the first 2 months of treatment for pulmonary tuberculosis. Am J Respir Crit Care Med 174:331, 2006

Griffith DE et al: An official ATS/IDSA statement: Diagnosis, treatment, and prevention of nontuberculous mycobacterial diseases. Am J Respir Crit Care Med 175:367, 2007

Jasmer RM et al: Short-course rifampin and pyrazinamide compared with isoniazid for latent tuberculosis infection: A multicenter clinical trial. Ann Intern Med 137:640, 2002

Musser JM: Antimicrobial agent resistance in mycobacteria: Molecular genetic insights. Clin Microbiol Rev 8:496, 1995

Saukkonen JJ et al: An official ATS statement: Hepatotoxicity of antituberculosis therapy. Am J Respir Crit Care Med 174:935, 2006

WHO Expert Committee on Leprosy: Seventh Report. Geneva, World Health Organization, 1998, Technical Report Series, No. 874

SECTION 9 SPIROCHETAL DISEASES

162 Syphilis

Sheila A. Lukehart

DEFINITION

Syphilis, a chronic systemic infection caused by *Treponema pallidum* subspecies *pallidum*, is usually sexually transmitted and is characterized by episodes of active disease interrupted by periods of latency. After an incubation period averaging 2–6 weeks, a primary lesion appears, often associated with regional lymphadenopathy. The secondary stage, associated with generalized mucocutaneous lesions and generalized lymphadenopathy, is followed by a latent period of subclinical infection lasting years or decades. In about one-third of untreated cases, the tertiary stage appears, characterized by progressive destructive mucocutaneous, musculoskeletal, or parenchymal lesions; aortitis; or symptomatic central nervous system (CNS) disease.

ETIOLOGY

The Spirochaetales include three genera that are pathogenic for humans and for a variety of other animals: *Leptospira*, which causes human leptospirosis (Chap. 164); *Borrelia*, which causes relapsing fever and Lyme disease (Chaps. 165 and 166); and *Treponema*, which causes the diseases known as treponematoses (see also Chap. 163). The genus *Treponema* includes *T. pallidum* subspecies *pallidum*, which causes venereal syphilis; *T. pallidum* subspecies *pertenue*, which causes yaws; *T. pallidum* subspecies *endemicum*, which causes endemic syphilis or bejel; and *T. carateum*, which causes pinta. Until recently, the subspecies were distinguished primarily by the clinical syndromes they produce. Researchers have now identified molecular signatures that can differentiate the three subspecies of *T. pallidum* by culture-independent, polymerase chain reaction (PCR)–based methods. Other *Treponema* species found in the human mouth, genital mucosa, and gastrointestinal tract have been associated with disease (e.g., periodontitis), but their role as primary etiologic agents is unclear.

T. pallidum subspecies *pallidum* (referred to hereafter simply as *T. pallidum*), a thin spiral organism, has a cell body surrounded by a trilaminar cytoplasmic membrane, a delicate peptidoglycan layer providing some structural rigidity, and a lipid-rich outer membrane containing relatively few integral membrane proteins. Endoflagella wind around the cell body in the periplasmic space and are responsible for motility.

T. pallidum cannot be cultured in vitro, and little was known about its metabolism until the genome was sequenced in 1998. This spirochete possesses severely limited metabolic capabilities, lacking the genes required for de novo synthesis of most amino acids, nucleotides, and lipids. In addition, *T. pallidum* lacks genes encoding the enzymes of the Krebs cycle and oxidative phosphorylation. To compensate, the organism contains numerous genes predicted to code for transporters of amino acids, carbohydrates, and cations. In addition, genome analyses and other studies have revealed the existence of a 12-member gene family (called *tpr*) that bears similarities to variable outer-membrane antigens of other spirochetes. One member, TprK, has discrete variable (V) regions that are targets of the humoral immune response. Data suggest that sequence variation occurs in TprK during infection and that this variation is a mechanism for immune invasion.

The only known natural host for *T. pallidum* is the human host. *T. pallidum* can infect many mammals, but only humans, higher apes, and a few laboratory animals regularly develop syphilitic lesions. Virulent strains of *T. pallidum* are grown in rabbits.

EPIDEMIOLOGY

Nearly all cases of syphilis are acquired by sexual contact with infectious lesions (i.e., the chancre, mucous patch, skin rash, or condylomata lata). Less common modes of transmission include nonsexual personal contact, infection in utero, blood transfusion, and organ transplantation.

SYPHILIS IN THE UNITED STATES

With the advent of penicillin therapy, the total number of cases of syphilis reported annually in the United States declined significantly to a low of 31,575 in 2000—a 95% decrease from 1943. In 2005, 33,278 cases were reported. Surveillance of the number of new cases of primary and secondary (infectious) syphilis, which is a better indicator of disease activity, has revealed multiple cycles of 7–10 years, each with a rapid rise and fall in incidence. The current increase in infectious syphilis (to 8724 cases in 2005) began in the western United States in 1997 and has particularly affected men who have sex with men (MSM), many of whom are co-infected with HIV. This outbreak has spread to large cities on the west coast of North America and to major cities elsewhere in the United States. It has been suggested that the regular fluctuation in syphilis rates is due to herd immunity in susceptible populations. Although there are no data to suggest that persons treated for syphilis possess significant resistance to reinfection, it has been recognized for many years that persons with untreated syphilis are refractory to symptomatic reinfection.

The populations at highest risk for acquiring syphilis have changed over time, with outbreaks among MSM in the late 1970s and early 1980s as well as at present. The epidemic that peaked in 1990 predominantly involved African-American heterosexual men and women and occurred largely in urban areas, where infectious syphilis was correlated significantly with the exchange of sex for crack cocaine. Since 1996, syphilis rates have declined among African Americans but remain higher than those for other racial/ethnic groups. Foci of syphilis still exist in a small number of counties in the southern United States.

The incidence of congenital syphilis roughly parallels that of infectious syphilis in females. The number of reported cases of congenital syphilis among infants ≤1 year of age fell to a low of 107 cases in 1978, when infectious syphilis was most prevalent among homosexual and bisexual men, and then rose dramatically from 1986 to 1991 during the epidemic in African-American women. In 2005, 329 cases were reported. It is important to note that the case definition for congenital syphilis was broadened in 1989 and now includes all live or stillborn infants delivered to women with untreated or inadequately treated syphilis.

One-third to one-half of individuals named as sexual contacts of persons with infectious syphilis become infected. Many sexual contacts will already have developed manifestations of syphilis when they are first seen, and ~30% of apparently uninfected contacts who are examined within 30 days of exposure actually have incubating infection and will later develop infectious syphilis if not treated. Thus, identification and treatment of all recently exposed sexual contacts are important aspects of syphilis control. Also important is the identification of infected persons by serologic testing of pregnant women, persons admitted to hospitals, and military inductees. Routine premarital serologic testing for syphilis is controversial because of low yield.

GLOBAL SYPHILIS

Syphilis remains a significant health problem globally, with an estimated 12 million new infections per year. The regions that are most affected include sub-Saharan Africa, South America, and Southeast Asia (Fig. 162-1). Some African studies have shown antenatal syphilis seropositivity rates as high as 30%, and congenital syphilis has been reported to account for up to 50% of stillbirths. Large increases in syphilis have occurred in the independent states of the former Soviet Union, and higher numbers of cases have recently been reported in European countries.

NATURAL COURSE AND PATHOGENESIS OF UNTREATED SYPHILIS

T. pallidum rapidly penetrates intact mucous membranes or microscopic abrasions in skin and within a few hours enters the lymphatics and blood to produce systemic infection and metastatic foci long before the appearance of a primary lesion. Blood from a patient with incubating or early syphilis is infectious. The generation time of *T. pallidum* during early active disease in vivo is estimated to be ~30 h, and the incubation period of syphilis is inversely proportional to the number of organisms inoculated. The 50% infectious dose for intradermal inoculation in humans has been calculated to be 57 organisms, and the treponeme concentration generally reaches 10^7/g of tissue before a clinical lesion appears. The median incubation period in humans (~21 days) suggests an average inoculum of 500–1000 infectious organisms for naturally acquired disease; the incubation period rarely exceeds 6 weeks.

The primary lesion appears at the site of inoculation, usually persists for 4–6 weeks, and then heals spontaneously. Histopathologic examination shows perivascular infiltration, chiefly by CD4+ and CD8+ T lymphocytes, plasma cells, and macrophages, with capillary endothelial proliferation and subsequent obliteration of small blood vessels. The cellular infiltration displays a T_H1-type cytokine profile consistent with the activation of macrophages. Phagocytosis of opsonized organisms by activated macrophages ultimately causes their destruction, resulting in spontaneous resolution of the chancre.

The generalized parenchymal, constitutional, and mucocutaneous manifestations of secondary syphilis usually appear ~6–8 weeks after the chancre heals. Approximately 15% of patients with secondary syphilis still have persisting or healing chancres, and the stages may overlap more frequently in persons with concurrent HIV infection. In other patients, secondary lesions may appear several months after the chancre has healed, and some patients may enter the latent stage without ever recognizing secondary lesions. The histopathologic features of secondary maculopapular skin lesions are hyperkeratosis of the epidermis; capillary proliferation with endothelial swelling in the superficial corium; and dermal papillae with transmigration of polymorphonuclear leukocytes and, in the deeper corium, perivascular infiltration by CD8+ T lymphocytes, CD4+ T lymphocytes, macrophages, and plasma cells. Treponemes are found in many tissues, including the aqueous humor of the eye and the cerebrospinal fluid (CSF). Invasion of the CNS by *T. pallidum* occurs during the first weeks or months of infection, and CSF abnormalities are detected in as many as 40% of patients during the secondary stage. Clinical hepatitis and immune complex–induced membranous glomerulonephritis are relatively rare but recognized manifestations of secondary syphilis; liver function tests may yield abnormal results in up to one-quarter of patients with early syphilis. Generalized nontender lymphadenopathy is noted in 85% of patients with secondary syphilis. The paradoxical appearance of secondary manifestations despite high titers of antibody (including immobilizing antibody) to *T. pallidum* is unexplained but may result from antigenic variation or changes in expression of surface antigens. Secondary lesions subside within 2–6 weeks, and the infection enters the latent stage, which is detectable only by serologic testing. In the preantibiotic era, up to 25% of untreated patients experienced at least one generalized or localized mucocutaneous relapse, usually during the first

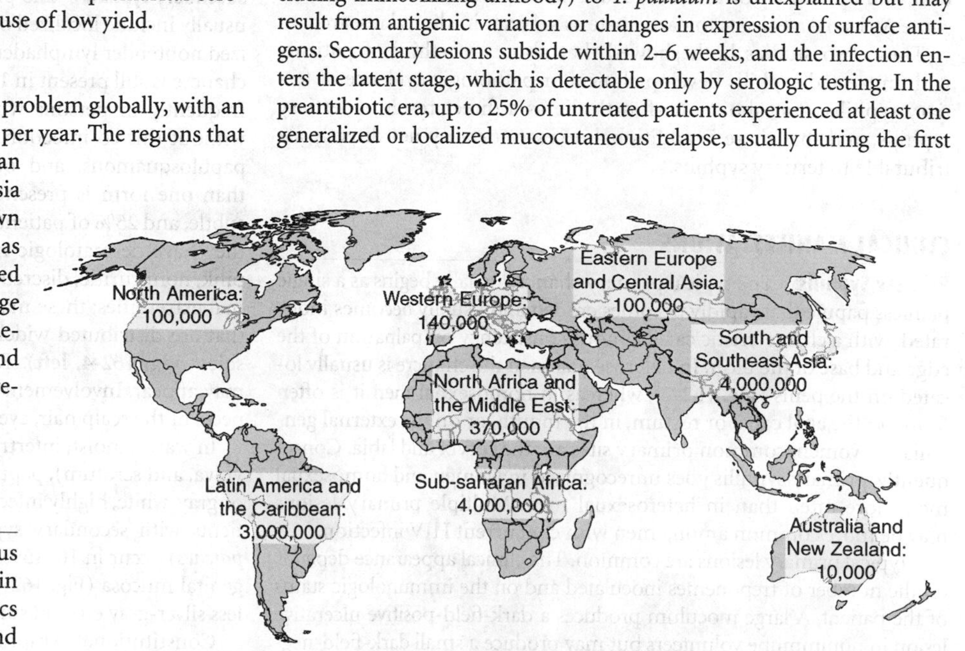

FIGURE 162-1 Estimated annual new cases of syphilis among adults, 1999. *(Courtesy of the World Health Organization.)*

year. Therefore, identification and examination of sexual contacts are most important for patients with syphilis of <1 year's duration. Recurrent generalized rash is now rare.

About one-third of patients with untreated latent syphilis developed clinically apparent tertiary disease in the preantibiotic era. In industrialized countries today, specific treatment for early and latent syphilis and coincidental therapy have nearly eliminated tertiary disease except for cases of neurosyphilis in HIV-infected persons. In the past, the most common types of tertiary disease were the gumma (a usually benign granulomatous lesion), cardiovascular syphilis (usually involving the vasa vasorum of the ascending aorta and resulting in aneurysm), and symptomatic neurosyphilis (tabes dorsalis and paresis). Asymptomatic CNS involvement, however, is still demonstrable in up to 25% of patients with late latent syphilis. The factors that contribute to the development and progression of tertiary disease are unknown.

The course of untreated syphilis was studied retrospectively in a group of nearly 2000 patients with primary or secondary disease diagnosed clinically (the Oslo Study, 1891–1951) and was assessed prospectively in 431 African-American men with seropositive latent syphilis of ≥3 years' duration (the notorious Tuskegee Study, 1932–1972). In the Oslo Study, 24% of patients developed relapsing secondary lesions within 4 years, and 28% eventually developed one or more manifestations of tertiary syphilis. Cardiovascular syphilis, including aortitis, was detected in 10% of patients, none of whom had been infected before age 15; 7% of patients developed symptomatic neurosyphilis, and 16% developed benign tertiary syphilis (gummas of the skin, mucous membranes, and skeleton). Syphilis was the primary cause of death in 15% of men and 8% of women. Cardiovascular syphilis was documented in 35% of men and 22% of women who eventually came to autopsy. In general, serious late complications were nearly twice as common among men as among women.

The Tuskegee Study showed that the death rate among untreated African-American men with syphilis (25–50 years old) was 17% higher than that among uninfected subjects and that 30% of all deaths were attributable to cardiovascular or CNS syphilis. By far the most important factor in increased mortality was cardiovascular syphilis. Anatomic evidence of aortitis was found in 40–60% of autopsied subjects with syphilis (vs. 15% of control subjects), whereas CNS syphilis was found in only 4%. Rates of hypertension were also higher among the infected subjects. The ethical issues eventually raised by this study, begun in the preantibiotic era but continuing into the early 1970s, had a major influence on the development of current guidelines for human medical experimentation, and the history of the study may still contribute to a reluctance of some African Americans to participate as subjects in clinical research.

These two studies both showed that about one-third of patients with untreated syphilis develop clinical or pathologic evidence of tertiary syphilis, that about one-fourth die as a direct result of tertiary syphilis, and that there is additional excess mortality not directly attributable to tertiary syphilis.

CLINICAL MANIFESTATIONS

Primary Syphilis The typical primary chancre usually begins as a single painless papule that rapidly becomes eroded and usually becomes indurated, with a characteristic cartilaginous consistency on palpation of the edge and base of the ulcer. In heterosexual men the chancre is usually located on the penis (Fig. 162-2), whereas in homosexual men it is often found in the anal canal or rectum, in the mouth, or on the external genitalia. In women, common primary sites are the cervix and labia. Consequently, primary syphilis goes unrecognized in women and homosexual men more often than in heterosexual men. Multiple primary lesions may be more common among men with concurrent HIV infection.

Atypical primary lesions are common. The clinical appearance depends on the number of treponemes inoculated and on the immunologic status of the patient. A large inoculum produces a dark-field-positive ulcerative lesion in nonimmune volunteers but may produce a small dark-field-negative papule, an asymptomatic but seropositive latent infection, or no response at all in some individuals with a history of syphilis. A small

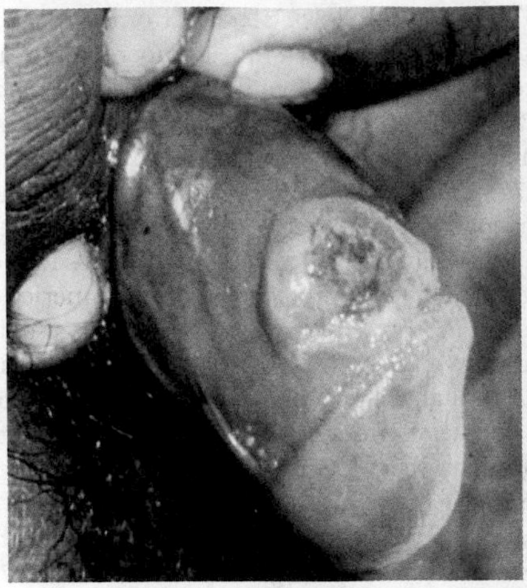

FIGURE 162-2 Primary syphilis with a firm, nontender chancre.

inoculum may produce only a papular lesion, even in nonimmune individuals. Therefore, syphilis should be considered even in the evaluation of trivial or atypical dark-field-negative genital lesions. The genital lesions that most commonly must be differentiated from those of primary syphilis include those caused by herpes simplex virus infection (Chap. 172), chancroid (Chap. 139), traumatic injury, and donovanosis (Chap. 154). *Primary genital herpes* may produce inguinal adenopathy, but the nodes are tender and the lesions consist of multiple painful vesicles, which later ulcerate and are often accompanied by systemic symptoms, including fever. *Recurrent genital herpes* typically begins with a unilateral cluster of painful vesicles, usually without associated adenopathy. *Chancroid* produces painful, superficial, exudative, nonindurated ulcers, more often multiple than in syphilis (see Fig. 139-2); adenopathy is common, can be either unilateral or bilateral, is tender, and may be suppurative. *Donovanosis*, which is rare in the United States and Europe, is usually seen as a granulomatous ulcer that, although painless, is friable.

Regional (usually inguinal) lymphadenopathy accompanies the primary syphilitic lesion, appearing within 1 week of lesion onset. The nodes are firm, nonsuppurative, and painless. Inguinal lymphadenopathy is bilateral and may occur with anal as well as with external genital chancres. The chancre generally heals within 4–6 weeks (range, 2–12 weeks), but lymphadenopathy may persist for months.

Secondary Syphilis The protean manifestations of the secondary stage usually include localized or diffuse mucocutaneous lesions and generalized nontender lymphadenopathy. As stated above, the healing primary chancre is still present in 15% of cases, and the stages may overlap more frequently in persons with concurrent HIV infection than in those without this co-infection. The skin rash consists of macular, papular, papulosquamous, and occasionally pustular syphilides; often more than one form is present simultaneously. The eruption may be very subtle, and 25% of patients with a discernible rash may be unaware that they have dermatologic manifestations. Initial lesions are pale red or pink, nonpruritic, discrete macules distributed on the trunk and proximal extremities; these macules progress to papular lesions (Fig. 162-3) that are distributed widely and that frequently involve the palms and soles (Fig. 162-4, left). Rarely, severe necrotic lesions (*lues maligna*) may appear. Involvement of the hair follicles may result in patchy alopecia of the scalp hair, eyebrows, or beard in up to 5% of cases.

In warm, moist, intertriginous areas (commonly the perianal region, vulva, and scrotum), papules can enlarge to produce broad, moist, pink or gray-white, highly infectious lesions (*condylomata lata*) in 10% of patients with secondary syphilis. Superficial mucosal erosions (*mucous patches*) occur in 10–15% of patients and commonly involve the oral or genital mucosa (Fig. 162-4, right). The typical mucous patch is a painless silver-gray erosion surrounded by a red periphery.

Constitutional symptoms that may accompany or precede secondary syphilis include sore throat (15–30%), fever (5–8%), weight loss (2–20%), malaise (25%), anorexia (2–10%), headache (10%), and

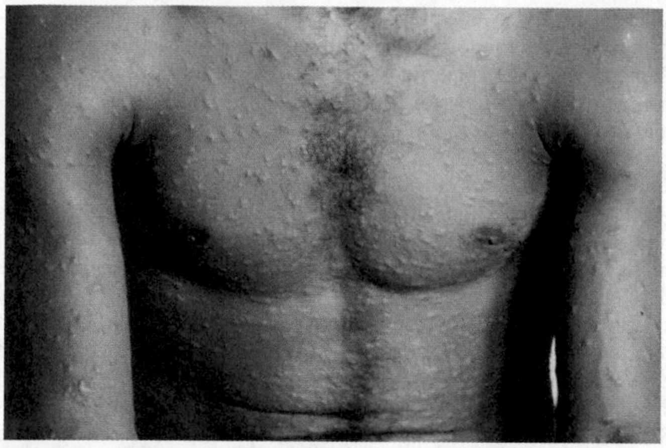

FIGURE 162-3 Secondary syphilis: the papulosquamous truncal eruption.

meningismus (5%). *Acute meningitis* occurs in only 1–2% of cases, but cell and protein concentrations in CSF are increased in ≥30% of cases. *T. pallidum* has been recovered from CSF during primary and secondary syphilis in 30% of cases; this finding is often but not always associated with other CSF abnormalities.

Less common complications of secondary syphilis include hepatitis, nephropathy, gastrointestinal involvement (hypertrophic gastritis, patchy proctitis, or a rectosigmoid mass), arthritis, and periostitis. Ocular findings that suggest secondary syphilis include pupillary abnormalities and optic neuritis as well as the classic iritis or uveitis. The diagnosis of secondary syphilis is often considered in the affected patients only after they fail to respond to steroid therapy. Anterior uveitis has been reported in 5–10% of patients with secondary syphilis, and *T. pallidum* has been demonstrated in the aqueous humor from such patients. Hepatic involvement is common in syphilis; although it is usually asymptomatic, up to 25% of patients may have abnormal liver function tests. Frank *syphilitic hepatitis* is distinguished by an unusually high serum level of alkaline phosphatase and by a nonspecific histologic appearance that is unlike that of viral hepatitis and includes moderate inflammation with polymorphonuclear leukocytes and lymphocytes, some hepatocellular damage, and no cholestasis. *Renal involvement* usually results from immune complex deposition and produces proteinuria associated with an acute nephrotic syndrome (or rarely with hemorrhagic glomerulonephritis). Like those of primary syphilis, the manifestations of the secondary stage resolve spontaneously, usually within 1–6 months.

Latent Syphilis Positive serologic tests for syphilis, together with a normal CSF examination and the absence of clinical manifestations of syphilis, indicate a diagnosis of latent syphilis. The diagnosis is often suspected on the basis of a history of primary or secondary lesions, a history of exposure to syphilis, or the delivery of an infant with congenital syphilis. A previous negative serologic test or a history of lesions or exposure may help establish the duration of latent infection, which is an important factor in the selection of appropriate therapy. *Early latent* syphilis is limited to the first year after infection, whereas *late latent* syphilis is defined as that of ≥1 year's (or unknown) duration. *T. pallidum* may still seed the bloodstream intermittently during the latent stage, and pregnant women with latent syphilis may infect the fetus in utero. Moreover, syphilis has been transmitted through blood transfusion or organ donation from patients with latent syphilis. It was previously thought that untreated late latent syphilis had three possible outcomes: (1) persistent lifelong infection; (2) development of late syphilis; or (3) spontaneous cure, with reversion of serologic tests to negative. It is now apparent, however, that the more sensitive treponemal antibody tests rarely, if ever, become negative without treatment. Although progression to clinically evident late syphilis is very rare today, the occurrence of spontaneous cure is in doubt.

Involvement of the CNS Traditionally, neurosyphilis has been considered a late manifestation of syphilis, but this view is inaccurate. CNS syphilis represents a continuum encompassing early invasion (usually within the first weeks or months of infection), months to years of asymptomatic involvement, and, in some cases, development of early or late neurologic manifestations.

ASYMPTOMATIC NEUROSYPHILIS The diagnosis of asymptomatic neurosyphilis is made in patients who lack neurologic symptoms and signs but who have CSF abnormalities including mononuclear pleocytosis, increased protein concentrations, or a reactive Venereal Disease Research Laboratory (VDRL) slide test. Such abnormalities are found in up to one-quarter of patients with untreated latent syphilis, and these patients are at risk for development of neurologic complications. In primary and secondary syphilis, such abnormalities may be found in up to 40% of untreated patients, and *T. pallidum* can be isolated from CSF of 30% of patients even in the absence of other CSF abnormalities. Although the therapeutic implications of these findings in early syphilis are uncertain, it seems appropriate to conclude that even patients with early syphilis who have such findings do indeed have asymptomatic neurosyphilis and should be treated for neurosyphilis. In patients with untreated asymptomatic neurosyphilis, the overall cumulative probability of progression to clinical neurosyphilis is ~20% in the first 10 years but increases with time; the likelihood is highest among patients with the greatest degree of pleocytosis or protein elevation. Patients with untreated latent syphilis and normal CSF probably run no risk of subsequent neurosyphilis. In one study, neurosyphilis was associated with a rapid plasma reagin (RPR) titer of ≥1:32, regardless of clinical stage or HIV infection status.

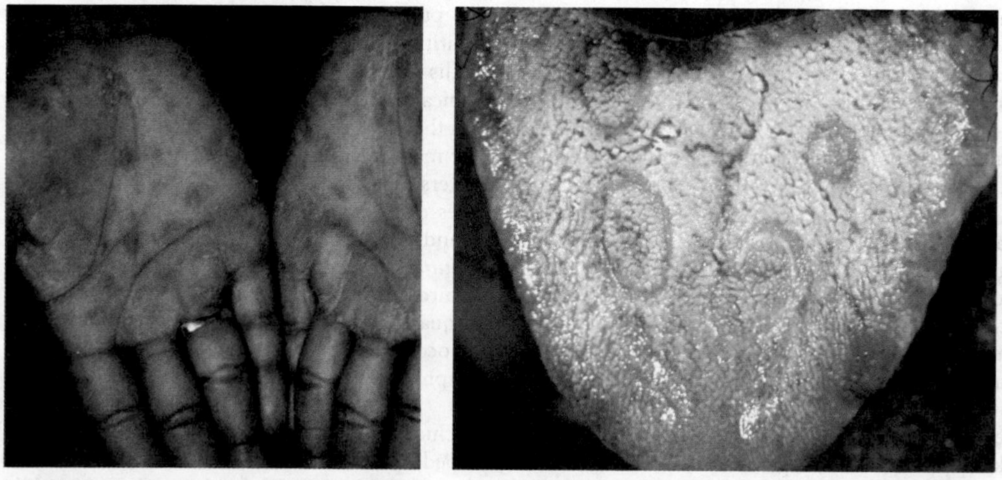

FIGURE 162-4 Secondary syphilis. ***Left:*** Papules on the palms. ***Right:*** Mucous patches on the tongue. *(Courtesy of Ron Roddy; with permission.)*

SYMPTOMATIC NEUROSYPHILIS Although mixed features are common, the major clinical categories of symptomatic neurosyphilis include meningeal, meningovascular, and parenchymatous syphilis. The last category includes general paresis and tabes dorsalis. The onset of symptoms usually comes <1 year after infection for meningeal syphilis, at 5–10 years for meningovascular syphilis, at 20 years for general paresis, and at 25–30 years for tabes dorsalis. However, symptomatic neurosyphilis, particularly in the antibiotic era, often presents not as a classic picture but rather as mixed and subtle or incomplete syndromes.

Meningeal syphilis may involve either the brain or the spinal cord, and patients may present with headache, nausea, vomiting, neck stiffness, cranial nerve involvement, seizures, and changes in mental status. This condition may be concurrent with or may follow the secondary stage. Patients presenting with uveitis or iritis frequently have meningeal syphilis.

Meningovascular syphilis reflects diffuse inflammation of the pia and arachnoid together with evidence of focal or widespread arterial involvement of small, medium, or large vessels. The most common presentation is a stroke syndrome involving the middle cerebral artery of a relatively young adult. However, unlike the usual thrombotic or embolic stroke syndrome of sudden onset, meningovascular syphilis often becomes manifest after a subacute encephalitic prodrome (with headaches, vertigo, insomnia, and psychological abnormalities), which is followed by a gradually progressive vascular syndrome.

The manifestations of *general paresis* reflect widespread late parenchymal damage and include abnormalities corresponding to the mnemonic *paresis:* *p*ersonality, *a*ffect, *r*eflexes (hyperactive), *e*ye (e.g., Argyll Robertson pupils), *s*ensorium (illusions, delusions, hallucinations), *i*ntellect (a decrease in recent memory and in the capacity for orientation, calculations, judgment, and insight), and *s*peech. *Tabes dorsalis* is a late manifestation of syphilis that presents as symptoms and signs of demyelination of the posterior columns, dorsal roots, and dorsal root ganglia. Symptoms include ataxic wide-based gait and footslap; paresthesia; bladder disturbances; impotence; areflexia; and loss of position, deep pain, and temperature sensations. Trophic joint degeneration (Charcot's joints) and perforating ulceration of the feet can result from loss of pain sensation. The small, irregular Argyll Robertson pupil, a feature of both tabes dorsalis and paresis, reacts to accommodation but not to light. *Optic atrophy* also occurs frequently in association with tabes.

Other Manifestations of Late Syphilis The slowly progressive inflammatory disease leading to tertiary manifestations begins early during the pathogenesis of syphilis, although these manifestations may not become clinically apparent for years. Early syphilitic aortitis becomes evident soon after secondary lesions subside, and treponemes that trigger the development of gummas may have seeded the tissue years earlier.

CARDIOVASCULAR SYPHILIS Cardiovascular manifestations, usually appearing 10–40 years after infection, are attributable to endarteritis obliterans of the vasa vasorum, which provide the blood supply to large vessels. This condition results in uncomplicated aortitis, aortic regurgitation, saccular aneurysm (usually of the ascending aorta), or coronary ostial stenosis. In the preantibiotic era, symptomatic cardiovascular complications developed in ~10% of persons with late untreated syphilis, although syphilitic aortitis was demonstrated at autopsy in about one-half of African-American men with untreated syphilis. Today, this form of late syphilis is rarely seen in the developed world.

Linear calcification of the ascending aorta on chest x-ray films suggests asymptomatic syphilitic aortitis, as arteriosclerosis seldom produces this sign. Syphilitic aneurysms—usually saccular, occasionally fusiform—do not lead to dissection. Only 1 in 10 aortic aneurysms of syphilitic origin involves the abdominal aorta.

LATE BENIGN SYPHILIS (GUMMA) Gummas are usually solitary lesions ranging from microscopic to several centimeters in diameter. Histologic examination shows a granulomatous inflammation, with a central area of necrosis due to endarteritis obliterans. Although rarely demonstrated microscopically, *T. pallidum* has reportedly been recovered from these lesions, and penicillin treatment results in rapid resolution, confirming the treponemal stimulus for the inflammation. Common sites include the skin and skeletal system; however, any organ may be involved. Gummas of the skin produce indolent, painless, indurated nodular or ulcerative lesions that may resemble other chronic granulomatous conditions, including tuberculosis, sarcoidosis, leprosy, and deep fungal infections. Skeletal gummas most frequently involve the long bones, although any bone may be affected. Radiographic abnormalities with advanced gummas of bone include periostitis or destructive or sclerosing osteitis. Upper respiratory gummas can lead to perforation of the nasal septum or palate.

Congenital Syphilis Transmission of *T. pallidum* from a syphilitic woman to her fetus across the placenta may occur at any stage of pregnancy, but fetal damage generally does not occur until after the fourth month of gestation, when fetal immunologic competence begins to develop. This timing suggests that the pathogenesis of congenital syphilis depends on the host immune response rather than on a direct toxic effect of *T. pallidum*. The risk of fetal infection during untreated early maternal syphilis is ~75–95%, decreasing to ~35% for maternal syphilis of >2 years' duration. Adequate treatment of the mother before the 16th week of pregnancy should prevent fetal damage, and treatment of the mother before the third trimester should adequately treat the infected fetus. Untreated maternal infection may result in a rate of fetal loss of up to 40% (with stillbirth more common than abortion because of the late onset of fetal pathology), prematurity, neonatal death, or nonfatal congenital syphilis. Among infants born alive, only fulminant congenital syphilis is clinically apparent at birth, and these babies have a very poor prognosis. The most common clinical problem is the healthy-appearing baby born to a mother with a positive serologic test. Routine serologic testing in early pregnancy is considered cost-effective in virtually all populations, even in areas with a low prenatal prevalence of syphilis. Where the prevalence of syphilis is high or when the patient is at high risk of reinfection, serologic testing should be repeated in the third trimester and at delivery. Neonatal congenital syphilis must be differentiated from other generalized congenital infections, including rubella, cytomegalovirus or herpes simplex virus infection, and toxoplasmosis, as well as from erythroblastosis fetalis.

The manifestations of congenital syphilis can be divided into three types according to their timing: (1) early manifestations, which appear within the first 2 years of life (often at 2–10 weeks of age), are infectious, and resemble the manifestations of severe secondary syphilis in the adult; (2) late manifestations, which appear after 2 years and are noninfectious; and (3) residual stigmata. The earliest sign of congenital syphilis (appearing 2–6 weeks after birth) is usually rhinitis, or "snuffles" (23%), which is soon followed by other mucocutaneous lesions (35–41%). These may include bullae (syphilitic pemphigus), vesicles, superficial desquamation, petechiae, and (later) papulosquamous lesions, mucous patches, and condylomata lata. The most common early manifestations are bone changes (61%), including osteochondritis, osteitis, and periostitis detectable by x-ray examination of long bones; hepatosplenomegaly (50%); lymphadenopathy (32%); anemia (34%); jaundice (30%); thrombocytopenia; and leukocytosis. CNS invasion by *T. pallidum* is detectable in 22% of infected neonates. Neonatal death is usually due to pulmonary hemorrhage, secondary bacterial infection, or severe hepatitis.

Late congenital syphilis (untreated after 2 years of age) is subclinical in 60% of cases; the clinical spectrum in the remainder of cases differs in certain respects from that of acquired late syphilis in the adult. For example, cardiovascular manifestations rarely develop in late congenital syphilis, whereas interstitial keratitis is much more common and occurs between the ages of 5 and 25. Other manifestations include eighth-nerve deafness and recurrent arthropathy. Bilateral knee effusions are known as *Clutton's joints*. Asymptomatic neurosyphilis is present in about one-third of untreated patients, and clinical neurosyphilis occurs in one-quarter of untreated individuals >6 years old. Gummatous periostitis occurs between the ages of 5 and 20 and, as in nonvenereal endemic syphilis, tends to cause destructive lesions of the palate and nasal septum.

Classic stigmata include *Hutchinson's teeth* (centrally notched, widely spaced, peg-shaped upper central incisors), "mulberry" molars (sixth-year molars with multiple, poorly developed cusps), saddle nose, and saber shins.

LABORATORY EXAMINATIONS

Demonstration of the Organism *T. pallidum* cannot be detected by culture. Historically, dark-field microscopy and immunofluorescence antibody staining have been used to identify this spirochete in samples from moist lesions such as chancres or condylomata lata, but these tests are rarely available today outside of research laboratories. More sensitive PCR tests have been developed but are not commercially available.

T. pallidum can be found in tissue with appropriate silver stains, but these results should be interpreted with caution because artifacts resembling *T. pallidum* are often seen. Tissue treponemes can be demonstrated more reliably in research laboratories by PCR or by immunofluorescence or immunohistochemical methods using specific monoclonal or polyclonal antibodies to *T. pallidum*.

Serologic Tests for Syphilis There are two types of serologic test for syphilis: nontreponemal and treponemal. Both are reactive in persons with any treponemal infection, including yaws, pinta, and endemic syphilis.

The most widely used nontreponemal antibody tests for syphilis are the RPR and VDRL tests, which measure IgG and IgM directed against a cardiolipin-lecithin-cholesterol antigen complex. The RPR test is easier to perform and uses unheated serum; it is the test of choice for rapid serologic diagnosis in a clinical setting and can be automated. The VDRL test remains the standard for examining CSF.

The RPR and VDRL tests are used for screening or for quantitation of serum antibody. The titer reflects disease activity, rising during the evolution of early syphilis and often exceeding 1:32 in secondary syphilis. A persistent fall by two dilutions (fourfold) or more after treatment of early syphilis is considered an adequate response to therapy. VDRL titers do not correspond directly to RPR titers, and sequential quantitative testing (as for response to therapy) must employ a single test.

The treponemal tests measure antibodies to native or recombinant *T. pallidum* antigens. These include the fluorescent treponemal antibody–absorbed (FTA-ABS) test and several agglutination assays. The microhemagglutination assay for *T. pallidum* (MHA-TP) has been replaced by the Serodia TP-PA test (Fujirebio, Tokyo), which is more sensitive for primary syphilis. The *T. pallidum* hemagglutination test (TPHA) is widely used in Europe but is not available in the United States. When used to confirm positive nontreponemal test results, treponemal tests have a very high positive predictive value for diagnosis of syphilis. In a screening setting, however, these tests give false-positive results at rates as high as 1–2%. New enzyme-linked immunosorbent assays have also been approved as confirmatory tests.

Considerable interest has recently been focused on point-of-care immunochromatographic strip tests that can be used in the field or in resource-poor settings.

The relative sensitivities of the standard tests for untreated syphilis are shown in Table 162-1. All tests may be nonreactive in early primary syphilis, although the treponemal tests have slightly higher sensitivity during this stage. All tests are reactive during secondary syphilis. (Fewer than 1% of patients with secondary syphilis have a VDRL test that is nonreactive or weakly reactive with undiluted serum but is positive at higher serum dilutions—the *prozone phenomenon*.) Whereas nontreponemal test titers will decline or the tests will become nonreactive after therapy for early syphilis, treponemal tests often remain reactive after therapy and are not helpful in determining infection status of persons with past syphilis.

For practical purposes, most clinicians need to be familiar with the three uses of serologic tests for syphilis: (1) screening or diagnostic purposes (RPR or VDRL), (2) quantitative measurement of antibody to assess clinical syphilis activity or to monitor response to therapy (RPR or VDRL), and (3) confirmation of a syphilis diagnosis in a patient with a reactive RPR or VDRL test (FTA-ABS or Serodia TP-PA).

IgM testing is not useful for adult syphilis. Moreover, no commercially available IgM test is recommended for evaluation of infants with suspected congenital syphilis.

TABLE 162-1 SENSITIVITY OF SERODIAGNOSTIC TESTS IN UNTREATED SYPHILIS

	Mean Percentage Positive (Range) at Indicated Stage of Disease[b]			
Test[a]	**Primary**	**Secondary**	**Latent**	**Tertiary**
VDRL, RPR	78 (74–87)	100	95 (88–100)	71 (37–94)
FTA-ABS	84 (70–100)	100	100	96
TP-PA[c]	89	100	100	NA

[a]The specificity for each of these tests is 94–99%.
[b]In CDC studies.
[c]Limited numbers of sera have been evaluated by TP-PA.
Source: Modified from SA Larsen et al: Clin Microbiol Rev 8:1, 1995; and V Pope et al: J Clin Microbiol 38:2543, 2000.

False-Positive Serologic Tests for Syphilis The lipid antigens of nontreponemal tests are found in human tissues, and the tests may be reactive (usually with titers ≤1:8) in persons without treponemal infection. Among patients selected on the basis of risk factors, clinical suspicion, or history of exposure, <1% of reactive tests are falsely positive. Modern VDRL and RPR tests are 97–99% specific, and false-positive reactions are largely limited to persons with autoimmune conditions or injection drug use. The prevalence of false-positive results increases with advancing age, approaching 10% among persons >70 years old. In a patient with a false-positive nontreponemal test, syphilis is excluded by a nonreactive treponemal test.

Evaluation for Neurosyphilis Involvement of the CNS is detected by examination of CSF for pleocytosis (>5 white blood cells/mm^3), increased protein concentration (>45 mg/dL), or VDRL reactivity. CSF abnormalities can be demonstrated in up to 40% of cases of primary or secondary syphilis and in 25% of cases of latent syphilis. In older asymptomatic seropositive individuals, the yield of lumbar puncture is relatively low. *T. pallidum* has been recovered by CSF inoculation into rabbits from up to 30% of patients with primary or secondary syphilis but rarely from those with latent syphilis. The presence of *T. pallidum* in CSF is often associated with other CSF abnormalities; however, organisms can be recovered from patients with otherwise-normal CSF. Before the advent of penicillin, the risk of developing clinical neurosyphilis was roughly proportional to the intensity of CSF changes. CSF examination is recommended by the Centers for Disease Control and Prevention (CDC) in the evaluation of any seropositive patient with neurologic or ophthalmic signs and symptoms, patients with other late syphilis, cases of suspected treatment failure, and HIV-infected patients with untreated late latent syphilis or syphilis of unknown duration. The possibility of asymptomatic neurosyphilis in some patients with early disease is not addressed by these recommendations. Because standard therapy with penicillin G benzathine fails to result in treponemicidal drug levels in the CSF, some experts also advise lumbar puncture in early syphilis, particularly in patients with HIV infection or with nontreponemal test titers of ≥1:32.

The CSF VDRL test is highly specific but is insensitive and may be nonreactive even in cases of symptomatic neurosyphilis. The degree of sensitivity is highest in meningovascular syphilis and paresis and is lower in asymptomatic neurosyphilis and tabes dorsalis. The unabsorbed FTA test on CSF is reactive far more often than the CSF VDRL test in all stages of syphilis, but FTA reactivity may reflect passive transfer of serum antibody into the CSF. A nonreactive CSF FTA test, however, may be used to rule out neurosyphilis.

Evaluation for Syphilis in HIV-Infected Patients Because persons at highest risk for syphilis are also at increased risk for HIV infection, these two infections frequently coexist. There is evidence that syphilis and other genital-ulcer diseases may be important risk factors for the acquisition and transmission of HIV infection.

The manifestations of syphilis may be altered in patients with concurrent HIV infection, and multiple cases of neurologic relapse after standard therapy have been reported in HIV-infected patients. *T. pallidum* has been isolated from the CSF of several patients after penicillin G benzathine therapy for early syphilis. A multicenter U.S. study of early syphilis found similar clinical responses to therapy in persons with and without concurrent HIV infection, although the study lacked sufficient statistical power to exclude an effect of HIV and 41% of subjects were lost to follow-up. Serologically defined treatment failure was more common among HIV-infected patients than among those without this co-infection. This investigation confirmed the high rate of CNS invasion in early syphilis and the persistence of *T. pallidum* after standard therapy: 11 of 43 HIV-infected patients and 21 of 88 HIV-uninfected patients had *T. pallidum* detectable in CSF before therapy; 7 of the 35 patients who underwent lumbar puncture after therapy (some HIV-infected and others uninfected) still had *T. pallidum* detectable in CSF.

There is no clear evidence that the sensitivity of serologic tests for syphilis differs in HIV-infected versus HIV-uninfected patients. Rates of decline of serologic titers appear to be slower in HIV-infected individuals. The clinical significance of this observation is unclear.

Persons with newly diagnosed HIV infection should be tested for syphilis; conversely, all patients with newly diagnosed syphilis should be tested for HIV infection. Some authorities, persuaded by reports of persistent *T. pallidum* in CSF of HIV-infected persons after standard therapy for early syphilis, recommend CSF examination for evidence of neurosyphilis for all co-infected patients, regardless of the stage of syphilis, with treatment for neurosyphilis if CSF abnormalities are found. Others believe that standard therapy is sufficient for all cases of early syphilis, without CSF examination. Serologic testing after treatment is important for all patients with syphilis, particularly for those also infected with HIV.

TABLE 162-2 RECOMMENDATIONS FOR THE TREATMENT OF SYPHILIS[a]

Stage of Syphilis	Patients without Penicillin Allergy	Patients with Confirmed Penicillin Allergy
Primary, secondary, or early latent	Penicillin G benzathine (single dose of 2.4 mU IM)	Tetracycline hydrochloride (500 mg PO qid) or doxycycline (100 mg PO bid) for 2 weeks
Late latent (or latent of uncertain duration), cardiovascular, or benign tertiary	Lumbar puncture CSF normal: Penicillin G benzathine (2.4 mU IM weekly for 3 weeks) CSF abnormal: Treat as neurosyphilis	Lumbar puncture CSF normal and patient not infected with HIV: Tetracycline hydrochloride (500 mg PO qid) or doxycycline (100 mg PO bid) for 4 weeks CSF normal and patient infected with HIV: Desensitization and treatment with penicillin if compliance cannot be ensured CSF abnormal: Treat as neurosyphilis
Neurosyphilis (asymptomatic or symptomatic)	Aqueous penicillin G (18–24 mU/d IV, given as 3–4 mU q4h or continuous infusion) for 10–14 days *or* Aqueous penicillin G procaine (2.4 mU/d IM) plus oral probenecid (500 mg qid), both for 10–14 days	Desensitization and treatment with penicillin
Syphilis in pregnancy	According to stage	Desensitization and treatment with penicillin

[a]See text for full discussion of indications for lumbar puncture and syphilis therapy in HIV-infected individuals.
Abbreviations: mU, million units; CSF, cerebrospinal fluid.
Source: These recommendations are based on those issued by the Centers for Disease Control and Prevention in 2006.

℞ SYPHILIS

TREATMENT OF ACQUIRED SYPHILIS The CDC's 2006 guidelines for the treatment of syphilis are summarized in **Table 162-2** and are discussed below. Penicillin G is the drug of choice for all stages of syphilis. *T. pallidum* is killed by very low concentrations of penicillin G, although a long period of exposure to penicillin is required because of the unusually slow rate of multiplication of the organism. The efficacy of penicillin against syphilis remains undiminished after 60 years of use. Other antibiotics effective in syphilis include the tetracyclines, erythromycin, and the cephalosporins. Aminoglycosides and spectinomycin inhibit *T. pallidum* only in very large doses, and the sulfonamides and the quinolones are inactive. Azithromycin has shown significant promise as an effective oral agent against *T. pallidum*; however, recent studies have documented clinical failures associated with a mutation in the 23S rRNA gene known to confer macrolide resistance. Strains harboring this mutation are present in >50% of recent isolates from Seattle and San Francisco. In contrast, an ongoing trial of single-dose azithromycin for early syphilis in Madagascar and several eastern U.S. sites has not documented clinical failures. Thus, the prevalence of resistant strains varies by geographic location. In all cases, careful follow-up should be assured for any patient treated for syphilis with azithromycin.

Early Syphilis Patients and Their Contacts Penicillin G benzathine is the most widely used agent for the treatment of early syphilis; a single dose of 2.4 million units is recommended. Preventive treatment is also recommended for individuals who have been exposed to infectious syphilis within the previous 3 months. *The regimens recommended for prevention are the same as those recommended for early syphilis*.

Penicillin G benzathine cures >95% of cases of early syphilis. Clinical relapse can follow treatment with penicillin G benzathine in patients with both HIV infection and early syphilis. Because the risk of neurologic relapse may be higher in HIV-infected patients, some experts recommend examination of CSF from HIV-seropositive individuals with syphilis at any stage, particularly if the RPR or VDRL titer is ≥1:32. Therapy appropriate for neurosyphilis should be given if there is any evidence of CNS syphilis.

Late Latent and Late Syphilis If CSF abnormalities are found, the patient should be treated for neurosyphilis. If CSF is normal, the recommended treatment is penicillin G benzathine (7.2 million units total; Table 162-2). The clinical response to treatment for benign tertiary syphilis is usually impressive. However, responses to therapy for cardiovascular syphilis are not dramatic because aortic aneurysm and aortic regurgitation cannot be reversed by antibiotic treatment.

Penicillin-Allergic Patients For penicillin-allergic patients with syphilis, a 2-week (early syphilis) or 4-week (late or late latent syphilis) course of therapy with doxycycline or tetracycline is recommended. These regimens appear to be effective in early syphilis but have not been tested for late or late latent syphilis, and compliance may be problematic. Limited studies suggest that ceftriaxone (1 g/d, given IM or IV, for 8–10 days) is effective for early syphilis. These nonpenicillin regimens have not been carefully evaluated in HIV-infected individuals and should be used with caution. If compliance and follow-up cannot be ensured, penicillin-allergic HIV-infected persons with late latent or late syphilis should be desensitized and treated with penicillin.

Neurosyphilis Penicillin G benzathine, given in total doses of up to 7.2 million units, does not produce detectable concentrations of penicillin G in CSF and should not be used for treatment of neurosyphilis. Asymptomatic neurosyphilis may relapse following treatment with benzathine penicillin, and the risk of relapse may be higher in HIV-infected patients. Administration of IV aqueous crystalline penicillin G in recommended doses is thought to ensure treponemicidal concentrations of penicillin G in CSF. The clinical response to penicillin therapy for meningeal syphilis is dramatic, but treatment of neurosyphilis with existing parenchymal damage may only arrest disease progression.

Some recent publications have reported neurologic relapse even after high-dose IV penicillin therapy for neurosyphilis in HIV-infected patients. No alternative therapies have been explored, but careful follow-up is essential, and re-treatment is warranted in such patients.

No data support the use of antibiotics other than penicillin G for the treatment of neurosyphilis. In patients with penicillin allergy demonstrated by skin testing, desensitization and treatment with penicillin is the recommended course.

Management of Syphilis in Pregnancy Every pregnant woman should undergo a nontreponemal test at her first prenatal visit and, if at high risk

TABLE 162-3 RECOMMENDED FOLLOW-UP EVALUATION AFTER THERAPY FOR SYPHILIS

Stage of Syphilis	Tests to Perform	When to Perform	Re-Treatment[a] Considered If:
Primary or secondary	Quantitative RPR or VDRL[b]	HIV-uninfected: 6 and 12 months HIV-infected: 3, 6, 9, 12, and 24 months	1. Titer increases by fourfold *or* 2. Titer fails to decline by fourfold or test fails to become nonreactive by 6 months *or* 3. Clinical signs persist or recur
Latent or late	Quantitative RPR or VDRL[b]	HIV-uninfected: 6, 12, and 24 months HIV-infected: 6, 12, 18, and 24 months	1. Titer increases by fourfold *or* 2. Initial titer of ≥1:32 fails to decline by fourfold by 6 months *or* 3. New clinical signs develop
Neurosyphilis (asymptomatic or symptomatic)	1. If CSF pleocytosis was documented initially, repeat CSF exam. 2. Monitor decline in CSF protein and CSF-VDRL. (Note: Rate of decline may be slow.) 3. Quantitative serum RPR or VDRL.[b]	1. Every 6 months until CSF cell count is normal 2. Until normal 3. 6, 12, 18, and 24 months	1. CSF cell count has not decreased at 6 months *or* 2. CSF is not normal after 2 years

[a]Try to distinguish between reinfection and treatment failure. If no clear evidence of reinfection exists, perform CSF examination. If CSF is normal, treat as for late latent syphilis (Table 162-2). If CSF is abnormal, treat as for neurosyphilis (Table 162-2).
[b]VDRL and RPR titers cannot be compared; use the same test for each follow-up sample.

of exposure, again in the third trimester and at delivery. In the untreated pregnant patient with presumed syphilis, expeditious treatment appropriate to the stage of the disease is essential. Patients should be warned of the risk of a Jarisch-Herxheimer reaction, which may be associated with mild premature contractions but rarely results in premature delivery.

Penicillin is the only recommended agent for the treatment of syphilis in pregnancy. If the patient has a documented penicillin allergy, desensitization and penicillin therapy should be undertaken according to the CDC's 2006 treatment guidelines. After treatment, a quantitative nontreponemal test should be repeated monthly throughout pregnancy to assess therapeutic efficacy. Treated women whose antibody titers rise by fourfold or who do not show a fourfold decrease in titer over a 3-month period should be re-treated.

EVALUATION AND MANAGEMENT OF CONGENITAL SYPHILIS Whether or not they are infected, newborn infants of mothers with reactive serologic tests may themselves have reactive tests because of transplacental transfer of maternal IgG antibody. For asymptomatic infants born to women treated adequately with penicillin during the first or second trimester of pregnancy, monthly quantitative nontreponemal tests may be performed to monitor for appropriate reduction in antibody titers. Rising or persistent titers indicate infection, and the infant should be treated. Detection of neonatal IgM antibody may be useful, but no commercially available test is currently recommended.

An infant should be treated at birth if the treatment status of the seropositive mother is unknown; if the mother has received inadequate or nonpenicillin therapy or has received penicillin therapy in the third trimester; or if the infant may be difficult to follow. The CSF should be examined to obtain baseline values before treatment. Penicillin is the only recommended drug for the treatment of syphilis in infants. Specific recommendations for the treatment of infants and older children are included in the CDC's 2006 guidelines.

JARISCH-HERXHEIMER REACTION A dramatic though usually mild reaction consisting of fever, chills, myalgias, headache, tachycardia, increased respiratory rate, increased circulating neutrophil count, and vasodilation with mild hypotension may follow the initiation of treatment for syphilis. This reaction is thought to be a response to lipoproteins released by dying *T. pallidum* organisms. The Jarisch-Herxheimer reaction occurs in ~50% of patients with primary syphilis, 90% of those with secondary syphilis, and a lower proportion of persons with later-stage disease. Defervescence takes place within 12–24 h. In patients with secondary syphilis, erythema and edema of the mucocutaneous lesions may increase. Patients should be warned to expect such symptoms, which can be managed with symptom-based treatment. Steroid and other anti-inflammatory therapy is not required for this mild transient reaction.

FOLLOW-UP EVALUATION OF RESPONSES TO THERAPY Efficacy of treatment should be assessed by monitoring of the quantitative VDRL or RPR titer **(Table 162-3)**. More frequent serologic examination is recommended for patients concurrently infected with HIV. Because the FTA-ABS and agglutination tests remain positive in most patients treated for seropositive syphilis, these tests are not useful in following the response to therapy. After successful treatment of seropositive first-episode primary or secondary syphilis, the VDRL or RPR titer progressively declines, becoming negative by 12 months in 40–75% of seropositive primary cases and in 20–40% of secondary cases. Patients with a history of syphilis have less rapid declines in titer and are less likely to become VDRL- or RPR-negative. Re-treatment should be considered if serologic responses are not adequate or if clinical signs persist or recur. Because it is difficult to differentiate treatment failure from reinfection, the CSF should be examined, with treatment for neurosyphilis if CSF is abnormal and treatment for late latent syphilis if CSF is normal.

Patients treated for late latent syphilis frequently have low initial VDRL or RPR titers and may not have a fourfold decline after therapy with penicillin. Re-treatment is not warranted unless the titer rises or signs and symptoms of syphilis appear. Because treponemal tests may remain positive despite treatment for seropositive syphilis, these tests are not useful in following the response to therapy.

The activity of neurosyphilis correlates best with CSF pleocytosis, and this measure provides the most sensitive index of response to treatment. An elevated CSF cell count falls to normal in 3–12 months in adequately treated HIV-uninfected patients. The persistence of mild pleocytosis in HIV-infected patients may be due to the presence of HIV in CSF; this scenario may be difficult to distinguish from treatment failure. Elevated levels of CSF protein fall more slowly, and the CSF VDRL titer declines gradually over a period of several years.

IMMUNITY TO SYPHILIS

The rate of development of acquired resistance to *T. pallidum* after natural or experimental infection is related to the size of the antigenic stimulus, which depends on both the size of the infecting inoculum and the duration of infection before treatment. The role of serum antibody in conferring immunity to syphilis remains undefined, although antibodies have been implicated in strain-specific immunity. Cellular immunity is considered to be of major importance in immunity and in the healing of early lesions. The cellular infiltration, predominantly T lymphocytes and macrophages, produces a T_H1 cytokine milieu consistent with the clearance of organisms by activated macrophages. Specific antibody enhances phagocytosis and is required for macrophage-mediated killing of *T. pallidum*. Recent studies indicate that sequence variation of TprK occurs during *T. pallidum* infection. This observation suggests a role for antigenic variation in the persistence of infection and in susceptibility to reinfection with another strain. No likely vaccine candidate antigens have been identified to date.

FURTHER READINGS

Centers for Disease Control and Prevention: 2006 Sexually transmitted diseases treatment guidelines. MMWR 55:22, 2006

Centurion-Lara A et al: Gene conversion: A mechanism for generation of heterogeneity in the *tprK* gene of *Treponema pallidum* during infection. Mol Microbiol 52:1579, 2004

Grassly NC et al: Host immunity and synchronized epidemics of syphilis across the United States. Nature 433:417, 2005

Lukehart SA et al: Macrolide resistance in *Treponema pallidum* in the United States and Ireland. N Engl J Med 351:154, 2004

Marra CM et al: Cerebrospinal fluid abnormalities in patients with syphilis: Association with clinical and laboratory features. J Infect Dis 189:369, 2004

——— et al: Normalization of cerebrospinal fluid abnormalities after neurosyphilis therapy: Does HIV status matter? Clin Infect Dis 38:1001, 2004

Michelow IC et al: Central nervous system infection in congenital syphilis. N Engl J Med 346:1792, 2002

Peeling R et al: Avoiding HIV and dying of syphilis. Lancet 364:1561, 2004

Rolfs RT et al: A randomized trial of enhanced therapy for early syphilis in patients with and without human immunodeficiency virus infection. N Engl J Med 337:307, 1997

163 Endemic Treponematoses

Sheila A. Lukehart

The endemic, or nonvenereal, treponematoses are bacterial infections caused by close relatives of *Treponema pallidum* subspecies *pallidum*, the etiologic agent of venereal syphilis (Chap. 162). Yaws, pinta, and endemic syphilis are distinguished from venereal syphilis by mode of transmission, age of acquisition, geographic distribution, and clinical features. These infections are limited to rural areas of developing nations and are seen in developed countries only in recent immigrants from endemic regions. Our "knowledge" about the endemic treponematoses is based on observations of health care workers who have visited endemic areas; virtually no well-designed studies of the natural history, diagnosis, or treatment of these infections have been conducted. The treponemal infections are compared and contrasted in Table 163-1.

EPIDEMIOLOGY

The endemic treponematoses are chronic diseases transmitted by direct contact during childhood and, like syphilis, can cause severe late manifestations years after initial infection. In a World Health Organization (WHO)–sponsored mass eradication campaign from 1952 to 1969, more than 160 million people in Africa, Asia, and South America were examined for treponemal infections, and more than 50 million cases, contacts, and latent infections were treated. This campaign reduced the prevalence of active yaws from >20% to <1% in many areas. In recent decades, lack of focused surveillance and diversion of resources have resulted in a resurgence of these infections in some regions. The estimated geographic distribution of the endemic treponematoses in the 1990s is shown in Fig. 163-1. The most recent WHO estimate (1997) suggested that there are 460,000 new cases per year and a prevalence of 3 million infected persons. Areas of resurgent yaws morbidity include West Africa (Ivory Coast, Ghana, Togo, Benin), the Central African Republic, Nigeria, and rural Democratic Republic of Congo (formerly Zaire). The prevalence of endemic syphilis is estimated to be >10% in some regions of Mali, Niger, Burkina Faso, and Senegal. In Asia and the Pacific Islands, recent reports suggest active outbreaks of yaws in Papua New Guinea, East Timor, Vanuatu, Laos, Kampuchea, and Indonesia. India renewed its focus on yaws eradication in 1996 and reported no cases in 2004. In the Americas, foci of yaws persist in Haiti and other Caribbean islands, Peru, Colombia, Ecuador, Brazil, Guyana, and Surinam. Pinta is limited to Central America and northern South America, where it is found rarely and only in remote villages.

MICROBIOLOGY

The etiologic agents of the endemic treponematoses are *T. pallidum* subspecies *pertenue* (yaws), *T. pallidum* subspecies *endemicum* (endemic syphilis), and *T. carateum* (pinta). These little-studied organisms are morphologically identical to *T. pallidum* subspecies *pallidum*, and no antigenic differences among them have been identified to date. A controversy has existed about whether the pathogenic treponemes are truly different organisms. Three of the four organisms are classified as subspecies of *T. pallidum*; the fourth (*T. carateum*) remains a separate species simply because no organisms have been available for genetic studies. Molecular signatures that can differentiate the causative agents of venereal syphilis, yaws, and bejel have been identified by polymerase chain reaction amplification of *tpr* genes and restriction digestion. Whether these genetic differences are related to the distinct clinical courses of these diseases has not been determined.

CLINICAL FEATURES

All of the treponemal infections are chronic and are characterized by defined disease stages, with a localized primary lesion, disseminated secondary lesions, periods of latency, and possible late lesions. Primary and secondary stages are more frequently overlapping in yaws and endemic syphilis, and the late manifestations of pinta are very mild relative to the destructive lesions of the other treponematoses. The current preference is to divide the clinical course of the endemic treponematoses into "early" and "late" stages.

TABLE 163-1 COMPARISON OF THE TREPONEMES AND ASSOCIATED DISEASES

Feature	Venereal Syphilis	Yaws	Endemic Syphilis	Pinta
Organism	*T. pallidum* subsp. *pallidum*	*T. pallidum* subsp. *pertenue*	*T. pallidum* subsp. *endemicum*	*T. carateum*
Mode of transmission	Sexual, transplacental	Skin-to-skin	Household contacts: mouth-to-mouth or via shared drinking/eating utensils	Skin-to-skin
Usual age of acquisition	Adulthood	Early childhood	Early childhood	Late childhood
Primary lesion	Cutaneous ulcer (chancre)	Papilloma, often ulcerative	Rarely seen	Nonulcerating papule with satellites, pruritic
Location	Genital, oral, anal	Extremities	Oral	Extremities, face
Secondary lesions	Mucocutaneous lesions; condylomata lata	Cutaneous papulosquamous lesions; osteoperiostitis	Florid mucocutaneous lesions (mucous patch, split papule, condyloma latum); osteoperiostitis	Pintides, pigmented, pruritic
Infectious relapses	~25%	Common	Unknown	None
Late complications	Gummas, cardiovascular and CNS involvement[a]	Destructive gummas of skin, bone, cartilage	Destructive gummas of skin, bone, cartilage	Nondestructive, dyschromic, achromic macules

[a]CNS involvement in the endemic treponematoses has been postulated by some investigators (see text).

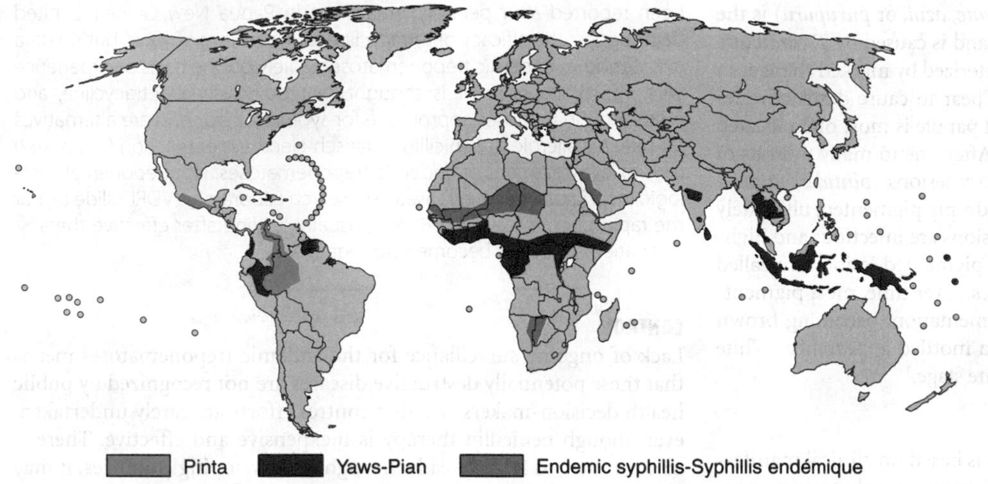

FIGURE 163-1 Geographic distribution of endemic treponematoses in the 1990s. *(Courtesy of the World Health Organization.)*

The major clinical features differing between venereal syphilis and the nonvenereal infections are the apparent lack of congenital transmission and of central nervous system (CNS) involvement in the nonvenereal infections. It is not known whether these distinctions are entirely accurate. Because of the high degree of genetic relatedness among the organisms, there is little biologic reason to think that *T. pallidum* subspecies *endemicum* and *T. pallidum* subspecies *pertenue* would be unable to cross the blood-brain barrier or to invade the placenta. These organisms are like *T. pallidum* subspecies *pallidum* in that they can disseminate from the site of primary infection and can persist for decades. The lack of recognized congenital infection may be due to the fact that childhood infections are in the latent stage (low bacterial load) before girls reach sexual maturity. Neurologic involvement may go unrecognized because of the lack of trained medical personnel in endemic regions, the delay of many years between infection and possible CNS manifestations, or a low rate of symptomatic CNS disease. Some published evidence supports congenital transmission as well as cardiovascular, ophthalmologic, and CNS involvement in yaws. Although the reported studies have been small, have failed to control for other causes of CNS abnormalities, have not included specific treponemal serologic tests, and have not analyzed the response to therapy, it may be erroneous to accept unquestioningly the frequently repeated belief that these organisms fail to cause such manifestations.

Yaws Also known as *pian*, *framboesia*, or *bouba*, yaws is caused by *T. pallidum* subspecies *pertenue* and is characterized by the development of one or several primary lesions ("mother yaw"), which is followed by the appearance of multiple disseminated skin lesions. All early skin lesions are infectious and may persist for many months; cutaneous relapses are common during the first 5 years. Late manifestations, affecting 10% of untreated persons, are destructive and can involve skin, bone, and joints.

The infection is transmitted by direct contact with infectious lesions, often during play or group sleeping, and may be enhanced by disruption of the skin by insect bites or abrasions. After an average of 3–4 weeks, the first lesion begins as a papule—usually on an extremity—and then enlarges (particularly during moist warm weather) to become papillomatous or "raspberry-like" (thus the name "framboesia") (Fig. 163-2). Regional lymphadenopathy develops, and the lesion usually heals within 6 months; dissemination is thought to occur during the early weeks of infection. A generalized secondary eruption, accompanied by generalized lymphadenopathy, appears either concurrent with or following the primary lesion, may take several forms (macular, papular, or papillomatous), and may become secondarily infected with other bacteria. Painful papillomatous lesions on the soles of the feet result in a painful crablike gait ("crab yaws"), and periostitis may result in nocturnal bone pain and polydactylitis. Late yaws is manifested by gummas of the skin and long bone, hyperkeratoses of the palms and soles, osteitis and periostitis, and hydrarthrosis. The late gummatous lesions are characteristically extensive. Destruction of the nose, maxilla, palate, and pharynx is termed *gangosa* and is similar to the destructive lesions seen in leprosy and leishmaniasis.

Endemic Syphilis Endemic syphilis, also called *bejel*, *siti*, *dichuchwa*, *njovera*, or *skerljevo*, is caused by *T. pallidum* subspecies *endemicum*. The early lesions are localized primarily to the mucocutaneous and mucosal surfaces, and the infection may be transmitted by direct contact, by kissing, or by sharing drinking and eating utensils. A role for insects in transmission has been suggested but is unproven. The initial lesion, usually an intraoral papule (Fig. 163-2), often goes unrecognized and is followed by mucous patches on the oral mucosa and mucocutaneous lesions resembling the condylomata lata of secondary syphilis. This eruption may last for months or even years, and treponemes can readily be demonstrated in early lesions. Periostitis and regional lymphadenopathy are common. After a variable period of latency, late manifestations may appear, including osseous and cutaneous gummas. Destructive gummas, osteitis, and gangosa are more common in endemic syphilis than in late yaws.

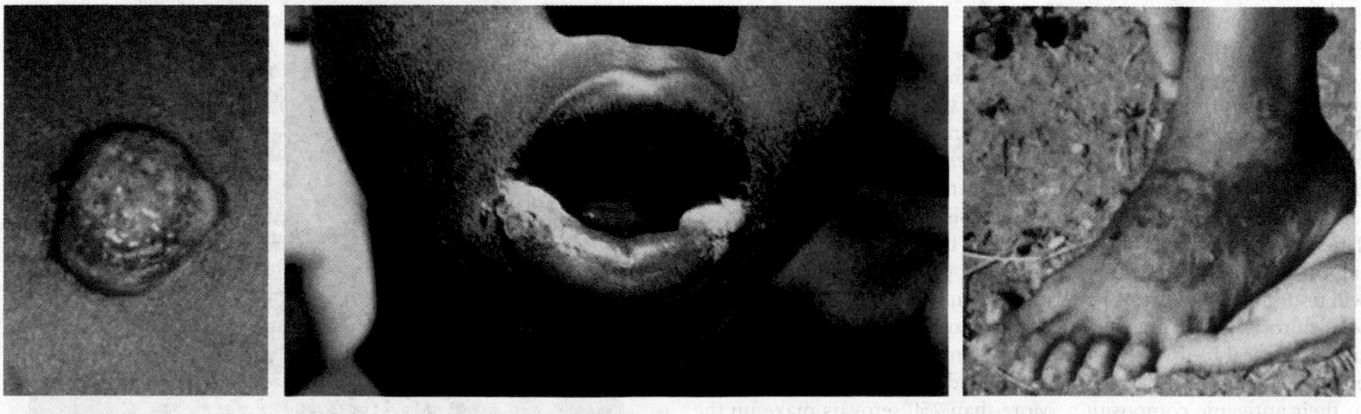

FIGURE 163-2 Clinical manifestations of endemic treponematoses. *Left:* Papillomatous primary lesion of yaws. ***Center:*** Split papules of early endemic syphilis. ***Right:*** Pigmented macules of pinta. *(From PL Perine et al. Handbook of Endemic Treponematoses, Geneva, World Health Organization, 1984.)*

Pinta Pinta (also called *mal del pinto, carate, azul,* or *purupuru*) is the most benign of the treponemal infections and is caused by *T. carateum*. This disease has three stages that are characterized by marked changes in skin color (Fig. 163-2), but it does not appear to cause destructive lesions or to involve other tissues. The initial papule is most often located on the extremities or face and is pruritic. After one to many months of infection, numerous disseminated secondary lesions (*pintides*) appear. These lesions are initially red but become deeply pigmented, ultimately turning a dark slate blue. The secondary lesions are infectious and highly pruritic and may persist for years. Late pigmented lesions are called *dyschromic macules* and contain treponemes. Over time, most pigmented lesions show varying degrees of depigmentation, becoming brown and eventually white and giving the skin a mottled appearance. White achromic lesions are characteristic of the late stage.

DIAGNOSIS

Diagnosis of the endemic treponematoses is based on clinical manifestations and, when available, dark-field microscopy and serologic testing. The same tests that are used for venereal syphilis (Chap. 162) become reactive during all treponemal infections, and there is no serologic test that can discriminate among the different infections. The nonvenereal treponemal infections should be considered in the evaluation of a reactive syphilis serology in any person who has emigrated from an endemic area.

Rx ENDEMIC TREPONEMATOSES

The recommended therapy for patients and their contacts is benzathine penicillin (1.2 million units IM for adults; 600,000 units for children <10 years old). This dose is half of that recommended for early venereal syphilis, and no controlled efficacy studies have been conducted. Definitive evidence of resistance to penicillin is lacking, although relapsing lesions have been reported after penicillin treatment in Papua New Guinea. Limited data suggest the efficacy of tetracycline for treatment of yaws, but no data exist for other endemic treponematoses. Solely on the basis of experience with venereal syphilis, it is thought that doxycycline, tetracycline, and erythromycin (at doses appropriate for syphilis; Chap. 162) are alternatives for patients allergic to penicillin. A Jarisch-Herxheimer reaction (Chap. 162) may follow treatment of endemic treponematoses. Nontreponemal serologic titers [in the Venereal Disease Research Laboratory (VDRL) slide test or the rapid plasma reagin (RPR) test] usually decline after effective therapy, but patients may not become seronegative.

CONTROL

Lack of ongoing surveillance for the endemic treponematoses means that these potentially destructive diseases are not recognized by public health decision-makers and that control efforts are rarely undertaken, even though penicillin therapy is inexpensive and effective. There is concern that, as HIV spreads throughout developing countries, it may markedly affect the manifestations and transmission of the endemic treponematoses.

FURTHER READINGS

Antal GM et al: The endemic treponematoses. Microbes Infect 4:83, 2002

Bora D et al: Yaws and its eradication in India—a brief review. J Commun Dis 37:1, 2005

Centurion-Lara A et al: Molecular differentiation of *Treponema pallidum* subspecies. J Clin Microbiol 44:3377, 2006

Engelkens HJH et al: Nonvenereal treponematoses in tropical countries. Clin Dermatol 17:143, 1999

Walker SL et al: Yaws—a review of the last 50 years. Int J Dermatol 39:258, 2000

164 Leptospirosis

Peter Speelman, Rudy Hartskeerl

Leptospirosis is an emerging infectious disease of global importance, as illustrated by recent large outbreaks in Asia, Central and South America, and the United States. The disease is caused by pathogenic leptospires and is characterized by a broad spectrum of clinical manifestations, varying from inapparent infection to fulminant, fatal disease. In its mild form, leptospirosis may present as an influenza-like illness with headache and myalgias. Severe leptospirosis, characterized by jaundice, renal dysfunction, and hemorrhagic diathesis, is referred to as *Weil's syndrome*.

ETIOLOGIC AGENTS

Leptospires are spirochetes belonging to the order Spirochaetales and the family Leptospiraceae. Traditionally, the genus *Leptospira* comprised two species: the pathogenic *L. interrogans* and the free-living *L. biflexa*; the current designations are *L. interrogans sensu lato* and *L. biflexa sensu lato*, respectively. Seventeen genomospecies of pathogenic leptospires are now recognized on the basis of their DNA relatedness. The genome sequences of two strains have been published, and reporting of the genomes of other strains is in progress. This information will undoubtedly lead to a better understanding of the pathogenesis of leptospirosis. However, for clinical and epidemiologic reasons, it is still more practical to use a classification system based on serologic differences. The pathogenic leptospires are divided into serovars according to their antigenic composition. More than 250 serovars make up the 26 serogroups.

Leptospires are coiled, thin, highly motile organisms with hooked ends and two periplasmic flagella that permit burrowing into tissue (Fig. 164-1). These organisms are 6–20 μm long and ~0.1 μm wide. They stain poorly but can be seen microscopically by dark-field examination and after silver impregnation staining. Leptospires require special media and conditions for growth; it may take weeks for cultures to become positive.

EPIDEMIOLOGY

Leptospirosis is an important zoonosis with a worldwide distribution, affecting at least 160 mammalian species. Rodents, especially rats, are the most important reservoir, although other wild mammals as well as domestic and farm animals may also harbor leptospires. These microorganisms establish a symbiotic relationship

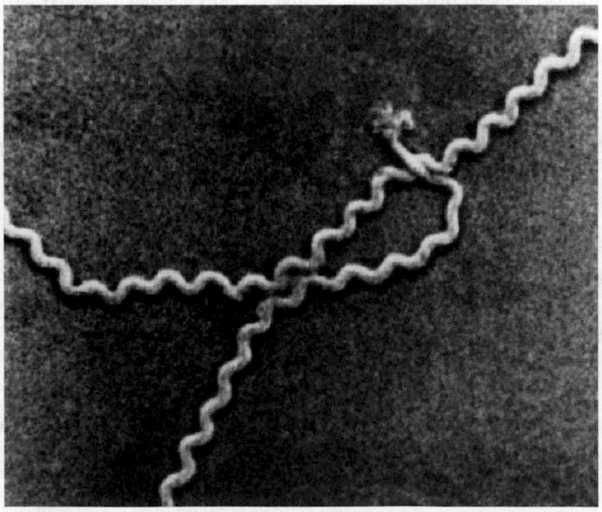

FIGURE 164-1 Scanning electron micrograph of leptospires.

with their host and can persist in the renal tubules for years. Some serovars are generally associated with particular animals (e.g., Icterohaemorrhagiae and Copenhageni with rats, Grippotyphosa with voles, Hardjo with cattle, Canicola with dogs, and Pomona with pigs) but may occur in other animals as well.

In most countries, leptospirosis in humans is an underestimated problem. This infection occurs most commonly in the tropics because the climate as well as the sometimes-poor hygienic conditions favor the pathogen's survival and distribution. Most cases occur in men, with a peak incidence during the summer and fall in Western countries and during the rainy season in the tropics. Transmission of leptospires to humans may follow direct contact with urine, blood, or tissue from an infected animal or exposure to a contaminated environment; human-to-human transmission is rare. Since leptospires are excreted in the urine and can survive in water for many months, water is an important vehicle in their transmission. Epidemics of leptospirosis may result from exposure to flood waters contaminated by urine from infected animals, as has been reported from Nicaragua.

Reliable data on morbidity and mortality from leptospirosis have gradually started to appear. In 1999, more than 500,000 cases were reported from China, with case-fatality rates ranging from 0.9 to 7.9%. In Brazil, more than 28,000 cases were reported in the same year. Although humans are commonly infected with leptospires, only a minority become symptomatic or develop severe leptospirosis. In an ongoing cohort study in Brazil, 5% of the persons studied have been infected, whereas the incidence of severe leptospirosis is 9.5 per 100,000 cases.

In the United States, the 40–120 cases reported annually to the Centers for Disease Control and Prevention (CDC) surely represent a significant underestimation of the total number. Certain occupational groups are at especially high risk; included are veterinarians, agricultural workers, sewage workers, slaughterhouse employees, and workers in the fishing industry. Such individuals may acquire leptospirosis through direct exposure to or contact with contaminated water and soil. Leptospirosis has also been recognized in deteriorating inner cities and suburbs where rat populations are expanding. One report described leptospirosis in urban residents of Baltimore who were sporadically exposed to rat urine.

Recreational exposure and domestic-animal contact are also prominent sources of leptospirosis. Recreational water activities, such as canoeing, windsurfing, swimming, and waterskiing, place persons at risk. Several outbreaks have followed sporting events. For example, a large outbreak occurred in 1998 among athletes after a triathlon in Illinois. Ingestion of one or more swallows of lake water was a prominent risk factor for illness. Heavy rains that preceded the triathlon, with consequent agricultural runoff, are likely to have increased the level of leptospiral contamination in the lake water. In 2000, 80 participants contracted leptospirosis during an Eco-Challenge multisport endurance race in Malaysian Borneo. Swimming in the Segama River was an independent risk factor for infection.

In a study in the Netherlands, 14% of patients with confirmed leptospirosis had acquired the infection while traveling in tropical countries, most often in Southeast Asia. Transmission via laboratory accidents has been reported but is rare. Leptospirosis develops occasionally after unanticipated immersion in contaminated water (e.g., in an automobile accident) and rarely after an animal bite.

PATHOGENESIS

The pathogenesis of leptospirosis is incompletely understood. Leptospires enter the host through abrasions in the skin or through intact mucous membranes, especially the conjunctiva and the lining of the oro- and nasopharynx. Drinking of contaminated water may introduce leptospires through the mouth, throat, or esophagus. After entry of the organisms, leptospiremia develops, with subsequent spread to all organs. Multiplication takes place in blood and in tissues, and leptospires can be isolated from blood and cerebrospinal fluid (CSF) during the first 4–10 days of illness. CSF examination during this period documents pleocytosis in the majority of instances, but only a minority of patients develop symptoms and signs of meningitis at this point. All forms of leptospires can damage the wall of small blood vessels; this damage leads to vasculitis with leakage and extravasation of cells, including hemorrhages. The most important known pathogenic properties of leptospires are adhesion to cell surfaces and cellular toxicity.

Vasculitis is responsible for the most important manifestations of the disease. Although leptospires mainly infect the kidneys and liver, any organ may be affected. In the kidney, leptospires migrate to the interstitium, renal tubules, and tubular lumen, causing interstitial nephritis and tubular necrosis. Hypovolemia due to dehydration or altered capillary permeability may contribute to the development of renal failure. In the liver, centrilobular necrosis with proliferation of Kupffer cells may be found. However, severe hepatocellular necrosis is not a feature of leptospirosis. Pulmonary involvement is the result of hemorrhage and not of inflammation. Invasion of skeletal muscle by leptospires results in swelling, vacuolation of the myofibrils, and focal necrosis. In severe leptospirosis, vasculitis may ultimately impair the microcirculation and increase capillary permeability, resulting in fluid leakage and hypovolemia.

When antibodies are formed, leptospires are eliminated from all sites in the host except the eye, the proximal renal tubules, and perhaps the brain, where they may persist for weeks or months. The persistence of leptospires in the aqueous humor occasionally causes chronic or recurrent uveitis. The systemic immune response is effective in eliminating the organism but may also produce symptomatic inflammatory reactions. A rise in antibody titer coincides with the development of meningitis; this association suggests that an immunologic mechanism is responsible.

After the start of antimicrobial treatment for leptospirosis, a Jarisch-Herxheimer reaction similar to that seen in other spirochetal diseases may develop. Although frequently described in older publications, this reaction seems to be a rare event in leptospirosis and is certainly less frequent in this infection than in other spirochetal diseases.

CLINICAL MANIFESTATIONS

(Fig. 164-2) Many *Leptospira*-infected persons remain asymptomatic. Serologic evidence of past inapparent infection is frequently found in persons who have been exposed to leptospires but have not become ill. In symptomatic cases of leptospirosis, clinical manifestations vary from mild to serious or even fatal. More than 90% of symptomatic persons have the relatively mild and usually anicteric form of leptospirosis, with or without meningitis. Severe leptospirosis with profound jaundice (Weil's syndrome) develops in 5–10% of infected individuals. The idea that distinct clinical syndromes are associated with specific serogroups has been refuted, although some serovars tend to cause more severe disease than others.

The incubation period is usually 1–2 weeks but ranges from 2 to 20 days (Fig. 164-2). Typically, an acute leptospiremic phase is followed by an immune leptospiruric phase. The distinction between the first and second phases is not always clear, and milder cases do not always include the second phase.

Anicteric Leptospirosis Leptospirosis may present as an acute influenza-like illness, with fever, chills, severe headache, nausea, vomiting, and myalgias. Muscle pain, which especially affects the calves, back, and abdomen, is an important feature of leptospiral infection. Less common features include sore throat and rash. The patient usually has an intense headache (frontal or retroorbital) and sometimes develops photophobia. Mental confusion may be evident. Pulmonary involvement, manifested in most cases by cough and chest pain and in a few cases by hemoptysis, is not uncommon.

The most common finding on physical examination is fever with conjunctival suffusion. Less common findings include muscle tenderness, lymphadenopathy, pharyngeal injection, rash, hepatomegaly, and splenomegaly. The rash may be macular, maculopapular, erythematous, urticarial, or hemorrhagic. Mild jaundice may be present.

Most patients become asymptomatic within 1 week. After an interval of 1–3 days, the illness recurs in a number of cases. The start of this second (immune) phase coincides with the development of antibodies. Symptoms are more variable than during the first (leptospiremic) phase. Usually the symptoms last for only a few days, but occasionally they per-

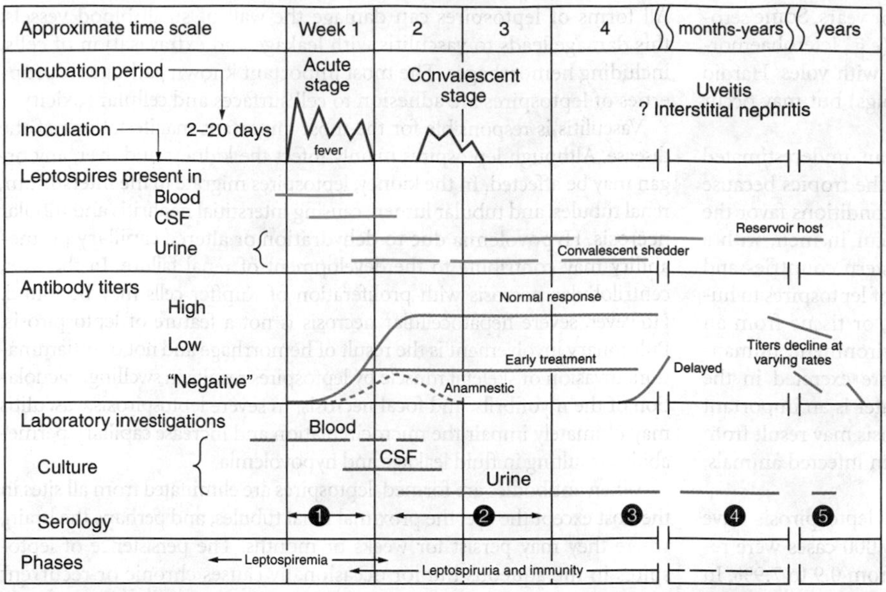

FIGURE 164-2 Biphasic nature of leptospirosis and relevant investigations at different stages of disease. Specimens 1 and 2 for serology are acute-phase serum samples; specimen 3 is a convalescent-phase serum sample that may facilitate detection of a delayed immune response; and specimens 4 and 5 are follow-up serum samples that can provide epidemiologic information, such as the presumptive infecting serogroup. *[Reprinted as adapted by Levett (from Turner LH: Leptospirosis. BMJ 1:231, 1969) with permission from the American Society for Microbiology and the BMJ Publishing Group.]*

sist for weeks. Often the fever is less pronounced and the myalgias are less severe than in the leptospiremic phase. An important event during the immune phase is the development of aseptic meningitis. Although no more than 15% of all patients have symptoms and signs of meningitis, many patients have CSF pleocytosis. Meningeal symptoms usually disappear within a few days but may persist for weeks. Similarly, pleocytosis generally disappears within 2 weeks but occasionally persists for months. Aseptic meningitis is more common among children than among adults. Iritis, iridocyclitis, and chorioretinitis—late complications that may persist for years—can become apparent as early as the third week but often present several months after the initial illness. One epidemic of uveitis among patients with leptospirosis has been reported. Mortality rates in anicteric leptospirosis are low, although death as a result of pulmonary hemorrhage occurred in 2.4% of cases in a Chinese outbreak.

Severe Leptospirosis (Weil's Syndrome) Weil's syndrome, the most severe form of leptospirosis, is characterized by jaundice, renal dysfunction, and hemorrhagic diathesis; by pulmonary involvement in many cases; and by mortality rates of 5–15%. In Europe, this syndrome is frequently but not exclusively associated with infection due to serovar Icterohaemorrhagiae/Copenhageni. The onset of illness is no different from that of less severe leptospirosis; however, after 4–9 days, jaundice as well as renal and vascular dysfunction generally develop. Although some degree of defervescence may be noted after the first week of illness, a biphasic disease pattern like that seen in anicteric leptospirosis is lacking. The jaundice of Weil's syndrome, which can be profound and give an orange cast to the skin, is usually not associated with severe hepatic necrosis. Death is rarely due to liver failure. Hepatomegaly and tenderness in the right upper quadrant are usually detected. Splenomegaly is found in 20% of cases.

Renal failure may develop, often during the second week of illness. Hypovolemia and decreased renal perfusion contribute to the development of acute tubular necrosis with oliguria or anuria. Dialysis is sometimes required, although a fair number of cases can be managed without dialysis. Renal function may be completely regained.

Pulmonary involvement occurs frequently; in some clusters of cases, it is a major manifestation, resulting in cough, dyspnea, chest pain, and blood-stained sputum and sometimes in hemoptysis or even respiratory failure. Hemorrhagic manifestations are seen in Weil's syndrome: epistaxis, petechiae, purpura, and ecchymoses are found commonly, while severe gastrointestinal bleeding and adrenal or subarachnoid hemorrhage are detected rarely.

Rhabdomyolysis, hemolysis, myocarditis, pericarditis, congestive heart failure, cardiogenic shock, adult respiratory distress syndrome, necrotizing pancreatitis, and multiorgan failure have all been described during severe leptospirosis.

LABORATORY AND RADIOLOGIC FINDINGS

(Fig. 164-2) The kidneys are invariably involved in leptospirosis. Related findings range from urinary sediment changes (leukocytes, erythrocytes, and hyaline or granular casts) and mild proteinuria in anicteric leptospirosis to renal failure and azotemia in severe disease.

The erythrocyte sedimentation rate is usually elevated. In anicteric leptospirosis, peripheral leukocyte counts range from 3000 to 26,000/μL, with a left shift; in Weil's syndrome, leukocytosis is often marked. Mild thrombocytopenia occurs in up to 50% of patients and is associated with renal failure.

In contrast to patients with acute viral hepatitis, those with leptospirosis typically have elevated serum levels of bilirubin and alkaline phosphatase as well as mild increases (up to 200 U/L) in serum levels of aminotransferases. In Weil's syndrome, the prothrombin time may be prolonged but can be corrected with vitamin K. Levels of creatine phosphokinase, which are elevated in up to 50% of patients with leptospirosis during the first week of illness, may help to differentiate this infection from viral hepatitis.

When a meningeal reaction develops, polymorphonuclear leukocytes predominate initially and the number of mononuclear cells increases later. The protein concentration in the CSF may be elevated; CSF glucose levels are normal.

In severe leptospirosis, pulmonary radiographic abnormalities are more common than would be expected on the basis of physical examination. These abnormalities most frequently develop 3–9 days after the onset of illness. The most common radiographic finding is a patchy alveolar pattern that corresponds to scattered alveolar hemorrhage. Radiographic abnormalities most often affect the lower lobes in the periphery of the lung fields.

DIAGNOSIS

(Fig. 164-2) A definite diagnosis of leptospirosis is based either on isolation of the organism from the patient or on seroconversion or a rise in antibody titer in the microscopic agglutination test (MAT). In the United States, the MAT is performed only at the CDC. In cases with strong clinical evidence of infection, a single antibody titer of 1:200–1:800 (depending on whether the case occurs in a low- or high-endemic area) in the MAT is required. Preferably, a fourfold or greater rise in titer is detected between acute- and convalescent-phase serum specimens. Antibodies generally do not reach detectable levels until the second week of illness. The antibody response can be affected by early treatment.

The MAT, which uses a battery of live leptospiral strains, and the enzyme-linked immunosorbent assay (ELISA), which uses a broadly reacting antigen, are the standard serologic procedures. These tests usually are available only in specialized laboratories and are used for determination of the antibody titer and for tentative identification of the serogroup—and in some cases the serovar—involved (thus the importance of using antigens representative of the serovars prevalent in the particular geographic area). Since cross-reactions occur frequently, however, it is often impossible to identify the infecting serogroup or serovar. Serologic testing cannot be used as the basis for a decision about whether to start treatment.

In addition to the MAT and the ELISA, various rapid tests with diagnostic value (some of them commercially available) have been developed. These rapid tests, which mainly apply lateral flow, (latex) agglutination, or ELISA methodology, have reasonable sensitivity and specificity; variation in reported data probably reflects differences in test interpretation, (re)exposure risks, and serovar distribution and the use of biased serum panels. These methods do not require culture or MAT facilities. However, in endemic areas, pooled serum samples from the local population are required as positive and negative controls. Polymerase chain reaction techniques have been developed but so far have not found widespread use outside research and reference laboratories.

Leptospires can be isolated from blood and/or CSF during the first 10 days of illness and from urine for several weeks beginning at ~1 week. Cultures most often become positive after 2–4 weeks, with a range of 1 week to 6 months. Sometimes urine cultures remain positive for months or years after the start of illness. For isolation of leptospires from body fluids or tissues, Ellinghausen-McCullough-Johnson-Harris (EMJH) medium is useful; other possibilities are Fletcher medium and Korthof medium. Specimens can be mailed to a reference laboratory for culture, since leptospires remain viable in anticoagulated blood (heparin, EDTA, or citrate) for up to 11 days at room temperature. Isolation of leptospires is important since it is the only way the infecting serovar can be correctly identified. Dark-field examination of blood or urine frequently results in misdiagnosis and should not be used.

DIFFERENTIAL DIAGNOSIS

Leptospirosis should be differentiated from other febrile illnesses associated with headache and muscle pain, such as dengue, malaria, enteric fever, viral hepatitis, *Hantavirus* infections, and rickettsial diseases. In light of the strong similarity in epidemiology and clinical presentation between leptospirosis and *Hantavirus* infections and given the reported occurrence of dual infections, it is advisable to conduct serologic testing for *Hantavirus* in cases of suspected leptospirosis. When patients have a flulike disease with disproportionately severe myalgia or aseptic meningitis, a diagnosis of leptospirosis should be considered.

Rx LEPTOSPIROSIS

Although a review of antibiotics for the treatment of leptospirosis concluded that there is insufficient evidence to provide clear guidelines for practice, the outcomes of the randomized clinical trials included in this review suggest that penicillin and doxycycline may be useful agents. Accordingly, these are the most commonly used antibiotics. Treatment should be initiated as early as possible; nevertheless, contrary to previous reports, treatment started after the first 4 days of illness is still effective. In milder cases, oral treatment with tetracycline, doxycycline, ampicillin, or amoxicillin should be considered. For severe cases of leptospirosis, intravenous administration of penicillin G, amoxicillin, ampicillin, or erythromycin is recommended **(Table 164-1)**. One comparative trial of the efficacy of ceftriaxone and penicillin for the treatment of severe leptospirosis found no significant differences between the two drugs in terms of complications or mortality rates. Another open-label randomized study compared parenteral cefotaxime, penicillin G, and doxycycline for the treatment of suspected severe leptospirosis. Among 264 patients with leptospirosis confirmed by serologic testing or culture, the mortality rate was 5%. There were no significant differences between antibiotics with regard to associated mortality, defervescence, or time to resolution of abnormal laboratory findings. Thus doxycycline, cefotaxime, or ceftriaxone is a satisfactory alternative to penicillin G for the treatment of severe leptospirosis.

In rare cases, a Jarisch-Herxheimer reaction develops within hours after the start of antimicrobial therapy (see "Pathogenesis" above). Although so far the only effective mode of management is supportive, the role of antibodies to tumor necrosis factor in the treatment of this reaction deserves further study. A beneficial effect of the use of such antibodies for the modulation of the reaction has been demonstrated in patients with louse-borne relapsing fever. Patients with severe leptospirosis and renal failure may require dialysis. Those with Weil's syndrome may need transfusions of whole blood and/or platelets. Intensive care may be necessary.

TABLE 164-1 TREATMENT AND CHEMOPROPHYLAXIS OF LEPTOSPIROSIS

Purpose of Drug Administration	Regimen
Treatment	
Mild leptospirosis	Doxycycline, 100 mg orally bid *or* Ampicillin, 500–750 mg orally qid *or* Amoxicillin, 500 mg orally qid
Moderate/severe leptospirosis	Penicillin G, 1.5 million units IV qid *or* Ampicillin, 1 g IV qid *or* Amoxicillin, 1 g IV qid *or* Ceftriaxone, 1 g IV once daily *or* Cefotaxime, 1 g IV qid *or* Erythromycin, 500 mg IV qid
Chemoprophylaxis	Doxycycline, 200 mg orally once a week

Note: All regimens used for treatment are administered for 7 days.

PROGNOSIS

Most patients with leptospirosis recover. Mortality rates are highest among patients who are elderly and those who have Weil's syndrome. Leptospirosis during pregnancy is associated with high rates of fetal mortality. Long-term follow-up of patients with renal failure and hepatic dysfunction has documented good recovery of renal and hepatic function.

PREVENTION

Individuals who may be exposed to leptospires through their occupations or their involvement in recreational water activities should be informed about the risks. Measures for controlling leptospirosis include avoidance of exposure to urine and tissues from infected animals, vaccination of animals, and rodent control. The animal vaccine used in a given area should contain the serovars known to be present in that area. Unfortunately, some vaccinated animals still excrete leptospires in their urine. Vaccination of humans against a specific serovar prevalent in an area has been undertaken in some European and Asian countries and has proved effective. Although a large-scale trial of vaccine in humans has been reported from Cuba, no conclusions can be drawn about efficacy and adverse reactions because of insufficient details on study design. Chemoprophylaxis with doxycycline (200 mg once a week) has appeared to be efficacious to some extent but is indicated only in rare instances of sustained short-term exposure (Table 164-1).

FURTHER READINGS

BHARTI AR et al: Leptospirosis: A zoonotic disease of global importance. Lancet Infect Dis 3:757, 2003

GUIDUGLI F et al: Antibiotics for leptospirosis. Cochrane Database Syst Rev 2:CD001306, 2000

LEVETT PN: Leptospirosis. Clin Microbiol Rev 14:296, 2001

MORGAN J et al: Outbreak of leptospirosis among triathlon participants and community residents in Springfield, Illinois, 1998. Clin Infect Dis 34:1593, 2002

PANAPHUT T et al: Ceftriaxone compared with sodium penicillin G for treatment of severe leptospirosis. Clin Infect Dis 36:1507, 2003

SEHGAL SC et al: Randomized controlled trial of doxycycline prophylaxis against leptospirosis in an endemic area. Int J Antimicrob Agents 13:249, 2000

SEJVAR J et al: Leptospirosis in "Eco-Challenge" athletes, Malaysian Borneo, 2000. Emerg Infect Dis 9:702, 2003

SUPPUTAMONGKOL Y et al: An open, randomized, controlled trial of penicillin, doxycycline, and cefotaxime for patients with severe leptospirosis. Clin Infect Dis 39:1417, 2004

VINETZ JM: Leptospirosis. Curr Opin Infect Dis 14:527, 2001

WORLD HEALTH ORGANIZATION/INTERNATIONAL LEPTOSPIROSIS SOCIETY: *Human Leptospirosis: Guidance for Diagnosis, Surveillance and Control.* Geneva, World Health Organization, 2003, 109 pp

165 Relapsing Fever

David T. Dennis

DEFINITION

The term *relapsing fever* describes two distinct diseases. *Tick-borne (endemic)* relapsing fever (TBRF) is a zoonosis that is transmitted principally from rodents to humans by the bite of various soft ticks. *Louse-borne (epidemic)* relapsing fever (LBRF) is a disease of humans that is transmitted from one person to another by the body louse. Both diseases are characterized by recurrent acute episodes of spirochetemia and fever alternating with variable periods of remission.

ETIOLOGY

Relapsing fever is caused by infection with spirochetal gram-negative bacteria of the genus *Borrelia* (family Spirochaetaceae). The borreliae are helical in shape and average 0.2–0.5 μm in width and 5–20 μm in length. They comprise an outer membrane, an intermediate peptidoglycan layer, and an inner cytoplasmic membrane, which encloses the protoplasmic cylinder. A variable number of periplasmic flagella are situated beneath the outer membrane. Relapsing-fever borreliae are slow-growing and microaerophilic; they grow best at 30°–35°C in Barbour-Stoenner-Kelly (BSK II) medium.

B. recurrentis is the only species that causes LBRF. Most of the various species of *Borrelia* that cause TBRF are named after the species of *Ornithodoros* tick responsible for their transmission. In North America, TBRF is caused mostly by *B. hermsii* and only occasionally by *B. turicatae*; *B. duttoni* is the most common cause of TBRF in sub-Saharan Africa, an area of high endemicity. Borreliae are unique among bacteria in having a genome composed of a linear chromosome and a series of linear and circular plasmids. The sequences of both the flagellin and the 16S ribosomal RNA genes are homogeneous among LBRF strains; in contrast, there is considerable heterogeneity of these genes between Old World and New World TBRF strains. A unique process of DNA rearrangement within *vmp* genes located on linear plasmids results in extensive variation in the expression of the surface antigens in relapsing fever borreliae. These *vmp* genes encode variable major proteins (VMPs) found on the spirochete's outer-membrane surface. The antigenic variation generated by sequential expression of previously silent *vmp* genes allows the borreliae to intermittently escape the immune response of the host and results in the febrile spirochetemic relapses that are characteristic of infection with these organisms.

EPIDEMIOLOGY

Louse-Borne Relapsing Fever Body lice (*Pediculus humanus* var. *corporis*) become infected with *B. recurrentis* by feeding on spirochetemic humans, the only reservoirs of infection. In lice, *B. recurrentis* spirochetes are found almost exclusively in the hemolymph; humans acquire infection when body lice are crushed and their infective fluids enter breaks in the skin, typically abrasions caused by scratching of pruritic louse bites. Spirochetes are *not* transmitted directly by the bite of a louse (anterior station transmission) but may possibly be transmitted in a manner similar to epidemic typhus by percutaneous inoculation of louse feces (posterior station transmission). Lice have a life span of only a few weeks, feed at frequent intervals, and survive only a few days off the human host. Typically, body lice reside in seams of clothing and bedclothes, where they deposit their eggs (nits). Head lice have not been shown to be vectors of LBRF.

LBRF has severely affected military and civilian populations disrupted by war and other disasters. Historically, the disease has been most common among slum dwellers, prisoners, and others living in impoverished, overcrowded, and unhygienic conditions. In the first half of the twentieth century, during periods of war and famine, both LBRF and louse-borne typhus were epidemic in Eastern Europe, the Balkans, and the former Soviet Union. The global distribution and incidence of LBRF have been substantially reduced by improvements in standards of living, sanitation, and hygiene; LBRF is now an important disease only in northeastern Africa, especially the highlands of Ethiopia, where an estimated 10,000 cases occur annually. LBRF has repeatedly spilled out of Ethiopia into populations of displaced persons in neighboring Somalia and Sudan.

Short-term visitors to endemic areas are at almost no risk of LBRF. Persons who have close contact with LBRF-affected populations (such as relief workers) can acquire the disease from lice or by direct contact with contaminated blood.

Tick-Borne Relapsing Fever Argasid ticks of the genus *Ornithodoros* transmit TBRF through their saliva and excreta when they take blood meals. Ticks typically become infected with TBRF borreliae as part of a zoonotic cycle when they feed on spirochetemic rodents and lagomorphs; the exception is *O. moubata*, a tick species that is thought to acquire *B. duttoni* only by feeding on infected humans. Ticks transmit TBRF borreliae vertically from one stage to the next; in some species, infection is transmitted transovarially over several generations. Soft ticks are hardy and can survive for as long as 10 years with only an occasional blood meal. These ticks feed painlessly, relatively quickly (for 20–45 min), and usually at night while hosts are sleeping. Thus patients with TBRF are often unaware of tick exposures.

TBRF borreliae are widely distributed throughout the world. Human infection with these organisms is generally underrecognized and underreported. TBRF is most highly endemic in sub-Saharan Africa but is also found in countries of the Mediterranean littoral, Middle Eastern states, southern Russia, the Indian subcontinent, Central Asia, and China and rarely in North, Central, and South America. The disease typically occurs sporadically or in small—often familial—clusters. Infected soft ticks may cause repeated infections among persons living or sleeping in the same dwelling. In sub-Saharan Africa, *O. moubata*, the vector of *B. duttoni*, infests native huts and rest houses, hiding in crevices of floors and walls during the day and emerging at night to feed on sleeping inhabitants.

In the United States, TBRF occurs west of the Mississippi River, especially in forested mountainous areas of far western states, where *B. hermsii* is the causative agent. Less commonly, persons become infected with *B. turicatae* after exposures in tick-infested caves in semidesert areas of the Southwest. On average, ~35 cases of TBRF are reported annually in the United States. *B. hermsii* infections most often occur during spring and summer months among persons sleeping in rustic mountain cabins and vacation homes and occasionally in permanent residences and in outdoor settings. The vertebrate reservoirs of infection are chipmunks and other rodents that nest in foundations, wall spaces, and attics of these dwellings. Outbreaks caused by *B. hermsii* have taken place among persons staying in cabins along the north rim of the Grand Canyon and in the mountains of California, Idaho, and Colorado. In North America, most recent cases have been reported from Washington, California, Colorado, Idaho, Oregon, and British Columbia.

PATHOGENESIS AND PATHOLOGY

In humans, relapsing-fever borreliae pass through the skin or mucous membranes, multiply in the blood, and circulate in great numbers during febrile periods. The organisms have also been found in the liver, spleen, bone marrow, and central nervous system (CNS) and may be sequestered at these sites during periods of remission. The severity of disease is positively correlated with spirochete density in the blood. Even though the pathophysiologic manifestations of the disease resemble responses to endotoxin, and although plasma from some patients with relapsing fever coagulates *Limulus* amebocyte lysates, borreliae and other spirochetes have not been shown to express a true lipopolysaccharide (endotoxin) molecule. Infection with *B. recurrentis* has been shown, however, to activate protein mediators of inflammation, such as Hageman factor (factor XII), prekallikrein, and proteins of the complement system; furthermore, a spirochetal heat-stable pyrogenic factor stimulates mononuclear phagocytes to express increased amounts of leukocyte pyrogen and thromboplastin.

The treatment of relapsing fever with antibiotics may provoke a Jarisch-Herxheimer reaction (see "Rx: Relapsing Fever," below). In patients with LBRF, this reaction has been associated with a release of various cytokines into the plasma, including interleukin 6, interleukin 8, C-reactive protein, and large amounts of tumor necrosis factor α (TNF-α). Pretreatment of LBRF patients with antibody to TNF-α suppresses Jarisch-Herxheimer reactions and reduces plasma concentrations of certain cytokines.

Death due to TBRF is rare. In contrast, fatality rates of 20% have been recorded during outbreaks of LBRF in malnourished and stressed populations. Relapsing fever in pregnancy can result in abortion, stillbirth, and fatal neonatal infections. Autopsies of patients with relapsing fever most often reveal hepatosplenomegaly and variable edema and swelling of other organs, including brain, lungs, and kidneys. On microscopic examination, the spleen is congested and contains multiple microabscesses composed of mononuclear cells that replace the white pulp, the myocardium displays diffuse histiocytic inflammation and interstitial edema, and the liver has areas of midzonal necrosis. Petechial hemorrhages are commonly evident over the surfaces of the meninges, pleura, heart, spleen, liver, kidneys, and mesentery. Subcapsular and parenchymal hemorrhagic infarcts of the spleen, heart, liver, and brain are sometimes grossly visible.

CLINICAL MANIFESTATIONS

The clinical manifestations of LBRF and TBRF are similar. The common signs and symptoms of TBRF, as documented in North America, are listed in Table 165-1. The mean incubation period is 7 days (range, 2–18 days), and the onset of illness is sudden, with fever, headache, shaking chills, sweats, myalgias, and arthralgias. The arthralgia of relapsing fever can be severe, involving small and large joints, but there is no evidence of arthritis. Dizziness, nausea, and vomiting are common. Sleep may be difficult and is sometimes accompanied by disturbing dreams. The patient is coherent but withdrawn, thirsty, and uninterested in food and other outside stimuli. The fever is high from the first, with the temperature usually reaching ≥40°C (≥104°F) and then becoming irregular in pattern. High fever is sometimes accompanied by delirium. Patients are usually tachycardic and mildly tachypneic and become prostrate as the disease progresses. Some patients have meningismus. The conjunctivae are often injected, and photophobia is common. The sclerae may become icteric, particularly in the later stages of illness. The mucous membranes may be dry, and patients are often dehydrated. Scattered petechiae develop on the trunk, extremities, and mucous membranes in one-third or more of patients with LBRF but in a smaller proportion of patients with TBRF. A nonproductive cough is common, but chest sounds are usually normal; pleuritic pain and an accompanying pleuritic rub are sometimes noted. Cardiac findings are compatible with a high-output state; tachycardia and summation gallop are common. Tender enlargement of the spleen and liver frequently occurs in the acute phase of illness.

TABLE 165-1 MANIFESTATIONS OF TICK-BORNE RELAPSING FEVER ACQUIRED IN THE NORTHWESTERN UNITED STATES AND SOUTHWESTERN BRITISH COLUMBIA

Sign or Symptom	%	Sign or Symptom	%
Headache	94	Photophobia	25
Myalgia	92	Neck pain	24
Chills	88	Rash	18
Nausea	76	Dysuria	13
Arthralgia	73	Jaundice	10
Vomiting	71	Hepatomegaly	10
Abdominal pain	44	Splenomegaly	6
Confusion	38	Conjunctival injection	5
Dry cough	27	Eschar	2
Eye pain	26	Meningitis	2
Diarrhea	25	Nuchal rigidity	2
Dizziness	25		

Source: From a review of 182 cases reported in the period 1980–1995 (Dworkin et al.).

Epistaxis and blood-tinged sputum are common complications, and gastrointestinal and CNS hemorrhage can occur. Because of bleeding, outbreaks of LBRF have been initially confused with viral hemorrhagic fever. Other complications of variable incidence include iridocyclitis, optic neuritis, lymphocytic meningitis, coma, isolated cranial-nerve palsy, pneumonitis, myocarditis, and splenic rupture. Acute respiratory distress syndrome is becoming increasingly recognized as a complication of TBRF in the United States. However, life-threatening complications are unusual in otherwise healthy persons given supportive care, especially if the illness is diagnosed and treated early. Children generally have a milder course of illness than adults.

Without treatment, symptoms intensify over 2–7 days (average, 5 days in LBRF and 3 days in TBRF), ending in a spontaneous crisis that coincides with the disappearance of spirochetes from the circulation. The crisis comprises two phases over several hours: a *chill phase*, characterized by rigors, rising temperature, and hypermetabolism, and a *flush phase* of falling temperature, diaphoresis, and a decreased effective circulating blood volume. The pathophysiologic events associated with this crisis are magnified when precipitated by antibiotic treatment and are indistinguishable from the Jarisch-Herxheimer reaction of treated syphilis (see "Rx: Relapsing Fever," below). The crisis is followed by a period of exhaustion, sleep, and an uneventful recovery. Orthostatic hypotension is typical in the early recovery phase. Not uncommonly, in the first week of convalescence, the patient experiences 1 or 2 days of mild fever unassociated with detectable spirochetemia. In untreated patients, spirochetemia and symptoms may recur after a period of several days or weeks (average interval to first relapse, 9 days in LBRF and 7 days in TBRF). Only one or two relapses characteristically occur in untreated patients with LBRF, whereas as many as 10 (average, three) can occur in untreated patients with TBRF. In most cases, the illness becomes shorter and milder and the afebrile intervals longer with each relapse. Because of the great antigenic variation among *Borrelia* strains, infection confers only partial immunity, and repeated infections of the same individual have been recorded.

DIFFERENTIAL DIAGNOSIS AND LABORATORY FINDINGS

Diseases that should be considered in the differential diagnosis of relapsing fever or that may complicate relapsing fever include typhus fever, typhoid fever, nontyphoidal salmonellosis, malaria, dengue and other arboviral illnesses, tuberculosis, leptospirosis, and viral hemorrhagic fevers. In the United States, the geographic distribution of Colorado tick fever (Chap. 189) overlaps that of TBRF, and the two diseases have similar manifestations early in their courses.

The diagnosis of relapsing fever is confirmed most easily by the detection of spirochetes in blood, bone marrow aspirates, or cerebrospinal fluid. Motile spirochetes can be seen when specimens are examined by dark-field microscopy. Fixed organisms are clearly visible in Wright-, Giemsa-, or acridine orange–stained preparations of thin or dehemoglobinized thick smears of peripheral blood or buffy-coat preparations (Fig. 165-1). Organisms are most numerous in specimens taken during periods of high temperature preceding the crisis; smears of peripheral blood are positive in ≥70% of patients with LBRF and in a lower percentage of patients with TBRF. In reference laboratories, relapsing-fever spirochetes are cultured from blood by the inoculation of BSK II medium or by the intraperitoneal inoculation of immature laboratory mice. Serum antibodies to *Borrelia* can be detected by enzyme immunoassays, indirect fluorescent antibody (IFA) assay, and Western immunoblotting using whole-cell sonicates as antigen; however, these tests are unstandardized and are subject to insensitivity and cross-reactivity with other spirochetal agents, including *B. burgdorferi* (the agent of Lyme disease) and *Treponema pallidum*. The Western immunoblot test employing species-specific recombinant glycerophosphodiester phosphodiesterase (GlpQ) as antigen is more sensitive and specific than the whole-cell sonicate IFA test or the enzyme-linked immunosorbent assay.

Other laboratory findings in relapsing fever are nonspecific. The leukocyte count is normal or moderately elevated, with an unremarkable cell differential. Serum bilirubin levels are generally only slightly

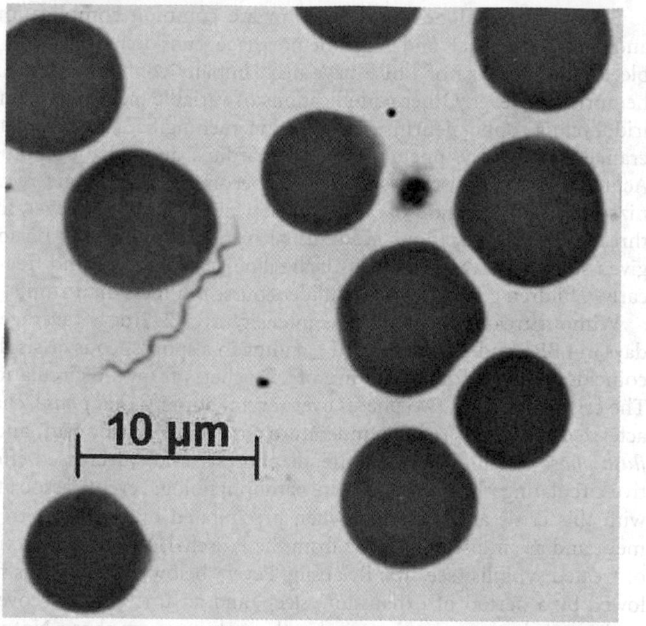

FIGURE 165-1 Photomicrograph of tick-borne relapsing fever spirochete (*B. hermsii*) in a Wright-Giemsa-stained peripheral blood film.

elevated. Thrombocytopenia commonly occurs in relapsing-fever patients during the acute phase of the illness; platelet counts rebound during early convalescence. Prothrombin and partial thromboplastin times are often moderately prolonged during acute illness, as are standardized bleeding times. Fibrinogen concentrations in the blood are normal, and fibrinolysis is mild or absent. Results of the Rumpel-Leede tourniquet test for capillary fragility are negative, despite the presence of petechiae.

℞ RELAPSING FEVER

Relapsing-fever borreliae are exquisitely sensitive to antibiotics. Treatment with doxycycline (or another tetracycline), erythromycin, or chloramphenicol produces rapid clearance of spirochetes and a remission of symptoms (**Table 165-2**). The response to a single dose of penicillin may be delayed and incomplete. Although a single dose of doxycycline (or another tetracycline), erythromycin, or chloramphenicol is highly effective in the treatment of LBRF, less is known about the efficacy of single-dose treatment of TBRF. Empirical treatment of TBRF for 7 days is therefore recommended to reduce the risk of persisting or relapsing borreliosis. For children <8 years of age and for pregnant women, erythromycin or penicillin may be preferred, given the potential adverse effects of tetracyclines.

Treatment of LBRF with a rapidly acting antibiotic regularly precipitates a Jarisch-Herxheimer-like reaction within 1–4 h of the first dose. This reaction, which occurs in >50% of treated TBRF patients in North America, tends to be more severe when the patient has LBRF rather than TBRF and when high numbers of spirochetes are circulating in the bloodstream. In the chill phase of the reaction, rigors and rising fever are accompanied by an increasing metabolic rate, alveolar hyperventilation, high cardiac output, increasing peripheral vascular resistance, and decreased pulmonary arterial pressure. The body temperature commonly rises to ≥41°C (≥105.8°F). This high fever is accompanied often by agitation and confusion and sometimes by delirium. Fever can be partially controlled by the use of a cooling blanket and ice packs and by sponging of the patient with tepid water and alcohol. The chill phase terminates after 10–30 min, giving way to a flush phase characterized by a fall in body temperature, drenching sweats, and sometimes (more commonly in LBRF) a potentially dangerous fall in systemic arterial pressure and rise in pulmonary arterial pressure. Although cardiac output is maintained at high levels, the effective circulating blood volume decreases as peripheral vascular resistance falls. Vital signs must be monitored carefully during this period of the reaction, which usually lasts ≤8 h. Clinical and electrocardiographic evidence of myocarditis and myocardial dysfunction includes a prolonged QT_C interval, a third heart sound (S_3), elevated central venous pressure, arterial hypotension, and rare pulmonary congestion. The use of delayed-release IM penicillin may prolong or delay the clearance of spirochetes and thereby attenuate the accompanying Jarisch-Herxheimer reaction, but this response is not predictable; furthermore, single-dose penicillin treatment sometimes results in relapse of spirochetemia and symptoms. Glucocorticoids and nonsteroidal anti-inflammatory agents do not prevent or significantly modify the cardiopulmonary disturbances of the Jarisch-Herxheimer reaction, although hydrocortisone and acetaminophen given at the same time as antibiotics reduce peak body temperature. Although pretreatment with antibody to TNF-α may moderate the Jarisch-Herxheimer reaction in treated patients with LBRF, its use in LBRF is impractical and its use in TBRF (whose treatment is typically associated with a relatively mild Jarisch-Herxheimer reaction) is not warranted. Close monitoring of fluid balance, arterial and venous pressures, and myocardial function is advised in supportive management of the Jarisch-Herxheimer reaction in patients with LBRF.

The management of patients with relapsing fever–induced myocardial dysfunction requires caution in the administration of IV fluids and, in some cases, use of short-term inotropic therapy. The inability of heparin to control bleeding in LBRF suggests that disseminated intravascular coagulation is not important in its causation. Vitamin K and other soluble vitamins are sometimes given to counter dietary deficiencies in patients with LBRF. Because postural hypotension is often pronounced during the acute phase of relapsing fever and in the early stage of recovery, patients should be assisted when arising from bed.

Untreated LBRF has a high case-fatality rate, especially among persons in otherwise poor health, such as those in famine-affected populations. The fatality rate among treated persons is usually <5%. In general, TBRF is a milder disease than LBRF: the spontaneous crisis and the Jarisch-Herxheimer reactions are less pronounced and the case-fatality rates are lower for TBRF than for LBRF.

TABLE 165-2 ANTIBIOTIC TREATMENT OF LOUSE-BORNE AND TICK-BORNE RELAPSING FEVER IN ADULTS

Medication	Louse-Borne Relapsing Fever (Single Dose)	Tick-Borne Relapsing Fever (7-Day Schedule)
Oral		
Erythromycin	500 mg	500 mg q6h
Tetracycline	500 mg	500 mg q6h
Doxycycline	100 mg	100 mg q12h
Chloramphenicol	500 mg	500 mg q6h
Parenteral[a]		
Erythromycin	500 mg	500 mg q6h
Tetracycline	250 mg	250 mg q6h
Doxycycline	100 mg	100 mg q12h
Chloramphenicol	500 mg	500 mg q6h
Penicillin G (procaine)	600,000 IU	600,000 IU daily

[a]For tick-borne relapsing fever, parenteral therapy is used only until oral treatment is tolerated.

PREVENTION AND CONTROL

LBRF is best prevented by addressing socioeconomic circumstances that promote louse infestation (crowding, poverty, homelessness), by applying hygienic practices that reduce numbers of body lice (washing clothes, drying clothes in direct sunlight, changing clothes at frequent intervals), and by delousing. In infested situations like those in refugee camps, individuals, their clothes, and their bedding should be deloused with appropriate acaricides, such as 0.5% permethrin dust. Impregnation of clothing with liquid permethrin, a residual acaricide, can provide long-term protection against infestation. Spread of infection can be controlled by early case detection and treatment of infected persons and close contacts. In outbreaks of fever that involve louse-infested populations, empirical single-dose treatment with doxycycline will be effective against typhus as well as LBRF. *B. recurrentis* has a fragile life cycle and is eradicable.

In TBRF-endemic areas, risk of exposure can be reduced by avoiding rodent- and tick-infested dwellings and infested natural sites and by applying control measures. Access of rodents to foundation spaces, attics, and other harborages in dwellings, outbuildings, and their surroundings should be eliminated. Rodents and rodent nests should be removed from infested buildings. Tick harborages can be chemically treated by pest-control specialists using various acaricides, such as carbaryl, diazinon, chlorpyrifos, pyrethrins, and malathion. Persons who enter tick-infested sites can protect themselves by wearing clothing that denies ticks access to the skin, by applying repellents to exposed skin and to clothing, and by applying an acaricide containing permethrin to clothing. Reporting of suspected cases of relapsing fever to public health authorities is important so that an epidemiologic investigation and control measures can be initiated promptly. Prompt diagnosis and treatment of relapsing fever in pregnant women is important in avoiding the potentially severe consequences of fetal or neonatal infection.

FURTHER READINGS

CUTLER SJ et al: *Borrelia recurrentis* characterization and comparison with relapsing fever, Lyme-associated, and other *Borrelia* spp. Int J Syst Bacteriol 47:958, 1997

DAI Q et al: Antigenic variation by *Borrelia hermsii* occurs through recombination between extragenic repetitive elements on linear plasmids. Mol Microbiol 60:1329, 2006

DWORKIN MS et al: Tick-borne relapsing fever in North America. Med Clin North Am 86:417, 2002

GOODMAN JL et al (eds): *Tick-Borne Diseases of Humans.* Washington, DC, ASM Press, 2005

LONDONO D et al: Cardiac apoptosis in severe relapsing fever borreliosis. Infect Immun 73:7669, 2005

PAROLA P, RAOULT D: Ticks and tickborne bacterial diseases in humans: An emerging infectious threat. Clin Infect Dis 32:897, 2001

PAUL WS et al: Outbreak of tick-borne relapsing fever at the north rim of the Grand Canyon: Evidence for effectiveness of preventive measures. Am J Trop Med Hyg 66:71, 2002

PORCELLA SF et al: Serodiagnosis of louse-borne relapsing fever with glycerophosphodiester phosphodiesterase (GlpQ) from *Borrelia recurrentis.* J Clin Microbiol 38:3561, 2000

TAL H et al: Postexposure treatment with doxycycline for the prevention of tick-borne relapsing fever. N Engl J Med 355:148, 2006

VIAL L et al: Incidence of tick-borne relapsing fever in west Africa: Longitudinal study. Lancet 368:37, 2006

166 Lyme Borreliosis

Allen C. Steere

DEFINITION

Lyme borreliosis is caused by a spirochete, *Borrelia burgdorferi sensu lato*, that is transmitted by ticks of the *Ixodes ricinus* complex. The infection usually begins with a characteristic expanding skin lesion, erythema migrans (EM; stage 1, localized infection). After several days or weeks, the spirochete may spread to many different sites (stage 2, disseminated infection). Possible manifestations of disseminated infection include secondary annular skin lesions, meningitis, cranial neuritis, radiculoneuritis, peripheral neuritis, carditis, atrioventricular nodal block, or migratory musculoskeletal pain. Months or years later (usually after periods of latent infection), intermittent or chronic arthritis, chronic encephalopathy or polyneuropathy, or acrodermatitis may develop (stage 3, persistent infection). Most patients experience early symptoms of the illness during the summer, but the infection may not become symptomatic until it progresses to stage 2 or 3.

Lyme disease was recognized as a separate entity in 1976 because of geographic clustering of children in Lyme, Connecticut, who were thought to have juvenile rheumatoid arthritis. It became apparent that Lyme disease was a multisystem illness that affected primarily the skin, nervous system, heart, and joints. Epidemiologic studies of patients with EM implicated certain *Ixodes* ticks as vectors of the disease. Early in the twentieth century, EM had been described in Europe and attributed to *I. ricinus* tick bites. In 1982, a previously unrecognized spirochete, now called *Borrelia burgdorferi*, was recovered from *Ixodes scapularis* ticks and then from patients with Lyme disease. The entity is now called Lyme disease or Lyme borreliosis.

ETIOLOGIC AGENT

B. burgdorferi, the causative agent of Lyme disease, is a fastidious, microaerophilic bacterium. The spirochete's genome is quite small (~1.5 Mb) and consists of a highly unusual linear chromosome of 950 kb as well as 9 circular and 12 linear plasmids. The most remarkable aspect of the *B. burgdorferi* genome is that there are sequences for more than 100 known or predicted lipoproteins—a larger number than in any other organism. The spirochete has few proteins with biosynthetic activity and depends on its host for most of its nutritional requirements. It has no sequences for recognizable toxins.

Currently, 13 closely related borrelial species are collectively referred to as *Borrelia burgdorferi sensu lato* (*B. burgdorferi* in the general sense). The human infection Lyme borreliosis is caused primarily by three pathogenic genospecies: *B. burgdorferi sensu stricto* (*B. burgdorferi* in the strict sense, hereafter referred to as *B. burgdorferi*), *Borrelia garinii*, and *Borrelia afzelii*. *B. burgdorferi* is the sole cause of the infection in the United States; all three genospecies are found in Europe, and the latter two species occur in Asia.

EPIDEMIOLOGY

The 13 known genospecies of *B. burgdorferi sensu lato* live in nature in enzootic cycles involving 14 different species of ticks that are part of the *I. ricinus* complex. *I. scapularis* (Fig. 392-1) is the principal vector in the northeastern United States from Maine to Virginia and in the midwestern states of Wisconsin and Minnesota. *I. pacificus* is the vector in the western states of California and Oregon. The disease is acquired throughout Europe (from Great Britain to Scandinavia to European Russia), where *I. ricinus* is the vector, and in Asian Russia, China, and Japan, where *I. persulcatus* is the vector. These ticks may transmit other diseases as well. In the United States, *I. scapularis* also transmits babesiosis and human anaplasmosis; in Europe and Asia, *I. ricinus* and *I. persulcatus* also transmit tick-borne encephalitis.

Ticks of the *I. ricinus* complex have larval, nymphal, and adult stages. They require a blood meal at each stage. The risk of infection in a given area depends largely on the density of these ticks as well as their feeding habits and animal hosts, which have evolved differently in different locations. For *I. scapularis* in the northeastern United States, the white-footed mouse and certain other rodents are the preferred hosts of the immature larvae and nymphs. It is critical that both of the tick's immature stages feed on the same host, because the life cycle of the spirochete depends on horizontal transmission: in early summer from infected nymphs to mice and in late summer from infected mice to larvae, which then molt to become the infected nymphs that will begin the cycle again the following year. It is the tiny nymphal tick that is primarily responsible for transmission of the disease to humans during the early summer months. White-tailed deer, which are not involved in the life cycle of the spirochete, are the preferred host for the adult stage of *I. scapularis* and seem to be critical to the tick's survival.

Lyme disease is now the most common vector-borne infection in the United States and Europe. Since surveillance was begun by the Centers for Disease Control and Prevention (CDC) in 1982, the number of cases in the United States has increased dramatically. More than 20,000 new cases are now reported each summer. In Europe, the highest reported frequencies of the disease are in the middle of the continent and in Scandinavia.

PATHOGENESIS AND IMMUNITY

To maintain its complex enzootic cycle, *B. burgdorferi* must adapt to two markedly different environments: the tick and the mammalian host. The spirochete expresses outer-surface protein A (OspA) in the midgut of the tick, whereas OspC is upregulated as the organism travels to the tick's salivary gland. There, OspC binds a tick salivary-gland protein (Salp15), which is required for infection of the mammalian host. The tick must usually be attached for at least 24 h for transmission of *B. burgdorferi*.

After injection into the human skin, *B. burgdorferi* may migrate outward, producing EM, and may spread hematogenously or in the lymph to other organs. The only known virulence factors of *B. burgdorferi* are surface proteins that allow the spirochete to attach to mammalian proteins, integrins, glycosaminoglycans, or glycoproteins. For example, spread through the skin and other tissue matrices may be facilitated by the binding of human plasminogen and its activators to the surface of the spirochete. Some *Borrelia* strains bind complement regulator–acquiring surface proteins (FHL-1/reconectin, or factor H), which help to protect spirochetes from complement-mediated lysis. Dissemination of the organism in the blood is facilitated by binding to the fibrinogen receptor on activated platelets ($\alpha_{IIb}\beta_3$) and the vitronectin receptor ($\alpha_v\beta_3$) on endothelial cells. Spirochetal decorin-binding proteins A and B bind decorin, a glycosaminoglycan on collagen fibrils; this binding may explain why the organism is commonly aligned with collagen fibrils in the extracellular matrix in the heart, nervous system, or joints.

To control and eradicate *B. burgdorferi*, the host mounts both innate and adaptive immune responses, resulting in macrophage- and antibody-mediated killing of the spirochete. As part of the innate immune response, complement may lyse the spirochete in the skin. Chemokines released by constituent cells in the skin lead to the recruitment of neutrophils and macrophages; the latter release potent proinflammatory cytokines. The purpose of the adaptive immune response appears to be the production of specific antibodies, which opsonize the organism—a step necessary for optimal spirochetal killing. Histologic examination of all affected tissues reveals an infiltration of lymphocytes, macrophages, and plasma cells with some degree of vascular damage (including mild vasculitis or hypervascular occlusion). These findings suggest that the spirochete may have been present in or around blood vessels.

Despite the innate and adaptive immune responses, *B. burgdorferi* may sometimes survive in certain sites, such as collagen bundles in synovial tissue. The ability of the spirochete to downregulate the expression of surface-exposed protein antigens and, in the case of the VlsE lipoprotein, the ability to change amino acid sequences in the protein are important mechanisms of immune evasion. However, in the battle between *B. burgdorferi* survival factors and host immune responses, spirochetes do not seem to be able to survive indefinitely against the immune responses of normal human patients. Moreover, the organisms do not have mechanisms that help to protect them from antibiotic therapy. For example, *B. burgdorferi* has only been seen extracellularly in affected tissues; it has not been shown to "hide out" in intracellular locations, thereby evading antibiotic exposure.

CLINICAL MANIFESTATIONS

Early Infection: Stage 1 (Localized Infection) Because of the small size of nymphal ixodid ticks, most patients do not remember the preceding tick bite. After an incubation period of 3–32 days, EM, which occurs at the site of the tick bite, usually begins as a red macule or papule that expands slowly to form a large annular lesion (Fig. 166-1). As the lesion increases in size, it often develops a bright red outer border and partial central clearing. The center of the lesion sometimes becomes intensely erythematous and indurated, vesicular, or necrotic. In other instances, the expanding lesion remains an even, intense red; several red rings are found within an outside ring; or the central area turns blue before the lesion clears. Although EM can be located anywhere, the thigh, groin, and axilla are particularly common sites. The lesion is warm but not often painful. Approximately 20% of patients do not exhibit this characteristic skin manifestation.

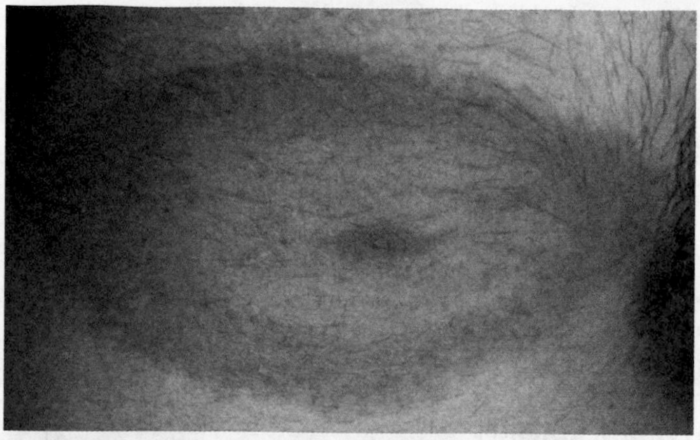

FIGURE 166-1 A classic erythema migrans lesion (9 cm in diameter) is shown near the right axilla. The lesion has partial central clearing, a bright red outer border, and a target center. *(Courtesy of Vijay K. Sikand, MD; with permission.)*

Early Infection: Stage 2 (Disseminated Infection) In cases in the United States, *B. burgdorferi* often spreads hematogenously to many sites within days or weeks after the onset of EM. In these cases, patients may develop secondary annular skin lesions similar in appearance to the initial lesion. Skin involvement is commonly accompanied by severe headache, mild stiffness of the neck, fever, chills, migratory musculoskeletal pain, arthralgias, and profound malaise and fatigue. Less common manifestations include generalized lymphadenopathy or splenomegaly, hepatitis, sore throat, nonproductive cough, conjunctivitis, iritis, or testicular swelling. Except for fatigue and lethargy, which are often constant, the early signs and symptoms of Lyme disease are typically intermittent and changing. Even in untreated patients, the early symptoms usually become less severe or disappear within several weeks. In ~15% of patients, the infection presents with these nonspecific systemic symptoms.

Symptoms suggestive of meningeal irritation may develop early in Lyme disease when EM is present but usually are not associated with cerebrospinal fluid (CSF) pleocytosis or an objective neurologic deficit. After several weeks or months, ~15% of untreated patients develop frank neurologic abnormalities, including meningitis, subtle encephalitic signs, cranial neuritis (including bilateral facial palsy), motor or sensory radiculoneuropathy, peripheral neuropathy, mononeuritis multiplex, cerebellar ataxia, or myelitis—alone or in various combinations. In the United States, the usual pattern consists of fluctuating symptoms of meningitis accompanied by facial palsy and peripheral radiculoneuropathy. Lymphocytic pleocytosis (~100 cells/μL) is found in CSF, often along with elevated protein levels and normal or slightly low glucose concentrations. In Europe and Asia, the first neurologic sign is characteristically radicular pain, which is followed by the development of CSF pleocytosis (called meningopolyneuritis, or *Bannwarth's syndrome*); meningeal or encephalitic signs are frequently absent. In children, the optic nerve may be affected because of inflammation or increased intracranial pressure, which may lead to blindness. These early neurologic abnormalities usually resolve completely within months, but in rare cases chronic neurologic disease may occur later.

Within several weeks after the onset of illness, ~8% of patients develop cardiac involvement. The most common abnormality is a fluctuating degree of atrioventricular block (first-degree, Wenckebach, or complete heart block). Some patients have more diffuse cardiac involvement, including electrocardiographic changes indicative of acute myopericarditis, left ventricular dysfunction evident on radionuclide scans, or (in rare cases) cardiomegaly or pancarditis. Cardiac involvement usually lasts for only a few weeks but may recur. Chronic cardiomyopathy caused by *B. burgdorferi* has been reported in Europe.

During this stage, musculoskeletal pain is common. The typical pattern consists of migratory pain in joints, tendons, bursae, muscles, or bones (usually without joint swelling) lasting for hours or days and affecting one or two locations at a time.

Late Infection: Stage 3 (Persistent Infection) Months after the onset of infection, ~60% of patients in the United States who have received no antibiotic treatment develop frank arthritis. The typical pattern comprises intermittent attacks of oligoarticular arthritis in large joints (especially the knees), lasting for weeks or months in a given joint. A few small joints or periarticular sites may also be affected, primarily during early attacks. The number of patients who continue to have recurrent attacks decreases each year. However, in a small percentage of cases, involvement of large joints—usually one or both knees—becomes chronic and may lead to erosion of cartilage and bone.

White cell counts in joint fluid range from 500–110,000/μL (average, 25,000/μL); most of these cells are polymorphonuclear leukocytes. Tests for rheumatoid factor or antinuclear antibodies usually give negative results. Examination of synovial biopsy samples reveals fibrin deposits, villous hypertrophy, vascular proliferation, microangiopathic lesions, and a heavy infiltration of lymphocytes and plasma cells.

Although most patients with Lyme arthritis respond well to antibiotic therapy, a small percentage have persistent arthritis for months or even for several years after the apparent eradication of spirochetes from the joints by antibiotic therapy. Compared with antibiotic-responsive patients, those with antibiotic-refractory arthritis have a higher frequency of certain class II major histocompatibility complex molecules (particularly HLA-DRBI*0401 or -*0101 molecules) that bind an epitope of OspA ($OspA_{163-175}$), and they often exhibit T cell recognition of this epitope. In addition, these patients have significantly higher levels of proinflammatory chemokines and cytokines in joint fluid (especially CXCL9 and interferon γ) than do antibiotic-responsive patients; these higher levels persist during the postantibiotic period, when polymerase chain reaction (PCR) results for *B. burgdorferi* DNA are uniformly negative. It has been postulated that, in these genetically susceptible individuals, *B. burgdorferi* may trigger autoimmunity within the proinflammatory milieu of the joints.

Although less common, chronic neurologic involvement may also become apparent months to several years after the onset of infection, sometimes following long periods of latent infection. The most common form of chronic central nervous system involvement is subtle encephalopathy affecting memory, mood, or sleep, and the most common form of peripheral neuropathy is an axonal polyneuropathy manifested as either distal paresthesia or spinal radicular pain. Patients with encephalopathy frequently have evidence of memory impairment in neuropsychological tests and abnormal results in CSF analyses. In cases of polyneuropathy, electromyography generally shows extensive abnormalities of proximal and distal nerve segments. Encephalomyelitis or leukoencephalitis, a rare manifestation of Lyme borreliosis associated primarily with *B. garinii* infection in Europe, is a severe neurologic disorder that may include spastic paraparesis, upper motor-neuron bladder dysfunction, and, rarely, lesions in the periventricular white matter.

Acrodermatitis chronica atrophicans, the late skin manifestation of the disorder, has been associated primarily with *B. afzelii* infection in Europe and Asia. It has been observed especially often in elderly women. The skin lesions, which are usually found on the acral surface of an arm or leg, begin insidiously with reddish-violaceous discoloration; they become sclerotic or atrophic over a period of years.

The basic patterns of Lyme borreliosis are similar worldwide, but there are regional variations, primarily between the illness found in America, which is caused exclusively by *B. burgdorferi*, and that found in Europe, which is caused primarily by *B. afzelii* and *B. garinii*. With each of the *Borrelia* spp., the infection usually begins with EM. However, *B. burgdorferi* often disseminates widely; it is particularly arthritogenic, and it may cause antibiotic-refractory arthritis. *B. garinii* typically disseminates less widely, but it is especially neurotropic and may cause borrelial encephalomyelitis. *B. afzelii* often infects only the skin but may persist in that site, where it may cause several different dermatoborrelioses, including acrodermatitis chronica atrophicans.

DIAGNOSIS

The culture of *B. burgdorferi* in Barbour-Stoenner-Kelly (BSK) medium permits definitive diagnosis, but this method has been used primarily in research studies. Moreover, with a few exceptions, positive cultures have been obtained only early in the illness—particularly from biopsy samples of EM skin lesions, less often from plasma samples, and occasionally from CSF samples. Later in the infection, PCR is greatly superior to culture for the detection of *B. burgdorferi* DNA in joint fluid—the major use for PCR testing in Lyme disease. However, the sensitivity of PCR determinations in CSF from patients with neuroborreliosis has been much lower. There seems to be little if any role for PCR in the detection of *B. burgdorferi* DNA in blood or urine samples. Moreover, this procedure, which must be carefully controlled to prevent contamination, is not routinely available.

Because of the problems associated with direct detection of *B. burgdorferi*, Lyme disease is usually diagnosed by the recognition of a characteristic clinical picture with serologic confirmation. Although serologic testing may yield negative results during the first several weeks of infection, most patients have a positive antibody response to *B. burgdorferi* after that time. The limitation of serologic tests is that they do not clearly distinguish between active and inactive infection. Patients with previous Lyme disease—particularly in cases progressing to late stages—often remain seropositive for years, even after adequate antibiotic treatment. In addition, ~10% of patients are seropositive because of asymptomatic infection. If these individuals subsequently develop another illness, the positive serologic test for Lyme disease may cause diagnostic confusion. According to an algorithm published by the American College of Physicians (Table 166-1), serologic testing for Lyme disease is recommended only for patients with at least an intermediate pretest probability of Lyme disease, such as those with oligoarticular arthritis. It should not be used as a screening procedure in patients with pain or fatigue syndromes. In such patients, the probability of a false-positive serologic result is higher than that of a true-positive result.

For serologic analysis of Lyme disease in the United States, the CDC recommends a two-step approach in which samples are first tested by enzyme-linked immunosorbent assay (ELISA) and equivocal or positive results are then tested by Western blotting. During the first month of infection, both IgM and IgG responses to the spirochete should be determined, preferably in both acute- and convalescent-phase serum samples. Approximately 20–30% of patients have a positive response detectable in acute-phase samples, whereas ~70–80% have a positive response during convalescence (2–4 weeks later). After 1 month of infection (by which time most patients with active Lyme disease have disseminated infection), the sensitivity and specificity of the IgG response to the spirochete are both very high—in the range of 95–99%—as determined by the two-test approach of ELISA and Western blot. At this point and thereafter, a single test (that for IgG) is usually sufficient. In persons with illness of >1

TABLE 166-1 ALGORITHM FOR TESTING FOR AND TREATING LYME DISEASE

Pretest Probability	Example	Recommendation
High	Patients with erythema migrans	Empirical antibiotic treatment without serologic testing
Intermediate	Patients with oligoarticular arthritis	Serologic testing and antibiotic treatment if test results are positive
Low	Patients with nonspecific symptoms (myalgias, arthralgias, fatigue)	Neither serologic testing nor antibiotic treatment

Source: Adapted from the recommendations of the American College of Physicians (G Nichol et al: Ann Intern Med 128:37, 1998, with permission).

month's duration, a positive IgM test result alone is likely to be false-positive and therefore should not be used to support the diagnosis.

According to current criteria adopted by the CDC, an IgM Western blot is considered positive if two of the following three bands are present: 23, 39, and 41 kDa. However, the combination of the 23- and 41-kDa bands may still represent a false-positive result. An IgG blot is considered positive if 5 of the following 10 bands are present: 18, 23, 28, 30, 39, 41, 45, 58, 66, and 93 kDa. In European cases, there is less expansion of the antibody response, and no single set of criteria for the interpretation of immunoblots results in high levels of sensitivity and specificity in all countries.

Several second-generation tests that use recombinant spirochetal proteins or synthetic peptides have shown promising results. For example, an IgG ELISA employing a 26-mer peptide from invariant region 6 (IR_6) of the VlsE lipoprotein has a sensitivity and a specificity similar to those achieved with the IgM and IgG two-test approach using sonicated whole spirochetes. However, the IR_6 ELISA has a limitation similar to that affecting standard serology, in that a positive test result does not distinguish clearly between active and past infection. The IR_6 ELISA may be of value with regard to European as well as American strains of the spirochete.

DIFFERENTIAL DIAGNOSIS

Classic EM is a slowly expanding erythema, often with partial central clearing. If the lesion expands little, it may represent the red papule of an uninfected tick bite. If the lesion expands rapidly, it may represent cellulitis (e.g., streptococcal cellulitis) or an allergic reaction, perhaps to tick saliva. Patients with secondary annular lesions may be thought to have erythema multiforme, but neither the development of blistering mucosal lesions nor the involvement of the palms or soles is a feature of *B. burgdorferi* infection. In the southeastern United States, an EM-like skin lesion, sometimes with mild systemic symptoms, may be associated with *Amblyomma americanum* tick bites, but the cause of this illness has not yet been identified.

In the United States, *I. scapularis* ticks may transmit not only *B. burgdorferi* but also *Babesia microti*, a red blood cell parasite (Chap. 204), or *Anaplasma phagocytophilum*, the agent of human granulocytotropic anaplasmosis (formerly human granulocytotropic ehrlichiosis; Chap. 167). Although babesiosis and anaplasmosis are most often asymptomatic, infection with any of these three agents may cause nonspecific systemic symptoms, and co-infected patients may have more severe or persistent symptoms than patients infected with a single agent. Standard blood counts may yield clues regarding the presence of co-infection. Anaplasmosis may cause leukopenia or thrombocytopenia, and babesiosis may cause thrombocytopenia or (in severe cases) hemolytic anemia. IgM serologic responses may confuse the diagnosis. For example, *A. phagocytophilum* may elicit a positive IgM response to *B. burgdorferi*. The frequency of co-infection in different studies has been variable. In one prospective study, 4% of patients with EM had evidence of co-infection.

Facial palsy caused by *B. burgdorferi*, which occurs in the early disseminated phase of the infection (often in July, August, or September), is usually recognized by its association with EM. However, in rare cases, facial palsy without EM may be the presenting manifestation of Lyme disease. In such cases, both the IgM and the IgG responses to the spirochete are usually positive. The most common infectious agents that cause facial palsy are herpes simplex virus type 1 (Bell's palsy; Chap. 172) and varicella-zoster virus (Ramsay Hunt syndrome; Chap. 173).

Later in the infection, oligoarticular Lyme arthritis most resembles reactive arthritis in an adult or the pauciarticular form of juvenile rheumatoid arthritis in a child. Patients with Lyme arthritis usually have the highest IgG antibody responses seen in the infection, with reactivity to many spirochetal proteins.

The most common problem in diagnosis is to mistake Lyme disease for chronic fatigue syndrome (Chap. 384) or fibromyalgia (Chap. 329). This difficulty is compounded by the fact that a small percentage of patients do in fact develop these chronic pain or fatigue syndromes in association with or soon after Lyme disease. Compared with Lyme disease, chronic fatigue syndrome or fibromyalgia tends to produce more generalized and disabling symptoms, including marked fatigue, severe headache, diffuse musculoskeletal pain, multiple symmetric tender points in characteristic locations, pain and stiffness in many joints, diffuse dysesthesia, difficulty with concentration, and sleep disturbances. Patients with chronic fatigue syndrome or fibromyalgia lack evidence of joint inflammation; they have normal results in neurologic tests; and they usually have a greater degree of anxiety and depression than patients with chronic neuroborreliosis.

℞ LYME BORRELIOSIS

As outlined in the algorithm in **Fig. 166-2**, the various manifestations of Lyme disease can usually be treated successfully with orally administered antibiotics; the exceptions are objective neurologic abnormalities and third-degree atrioventricular heart block, which are generally treated with IV antibiotics. For early Lyme disease, doxycycline is effective in men and in nonpregnant women. An advantage of this regimen is that it is also effective against *A. phagocytophilum*, which is transmitted by the same tick that transmits the Lyme disease agent. Amoxicillin, cefuroxime axetil, and erythromycin or its congeners are second-, third-, and fourth-choice alternatives, respectively. In children, amoxicillin is effective (not more than 2 g/d); in cases of penicillin allergy, cefuroxime axetil or erythromycin may be used. In contrast to second- or third-generation cephalosporin antibiotics, first-generation cephalosporins, such as cephalexin, are not effective. For patients with infection localized to the skin, a 14-day course of therapy is generally sufficient; in contrast, for patients with disseminated infection, a 21-day course is recommended. Approximately 15% of patients experience a Jarisch-Herxheimer-like reaction during the first 24 h of therapy. In multicenter studies, >90% of patients whose early Lyme disease was treated with these regimens had satisfactory outcomes. Although some pa-

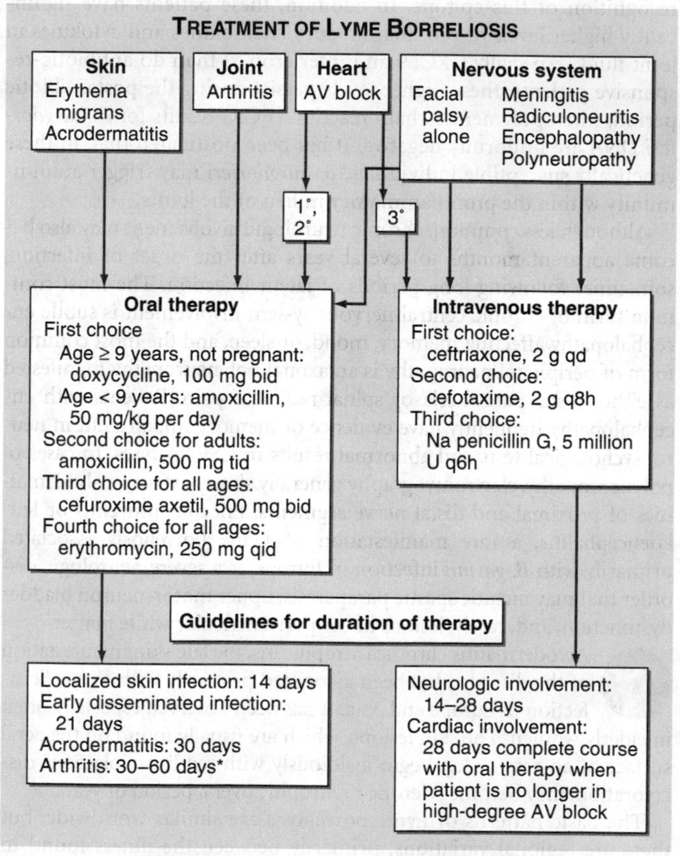

FIGURE 166-2 Algorithm for the treatment of the various acute or chronic manifestations of Lyme borreliosis. AV, atrioventricular. *For Lyme arthritis, IV ceftriaxone (2 g given once a day for 14–28 days) is also effective and is necessary for a small percentage of patients; however, compared with oral treatment, this regimen is less convenient to administer, has more side effects, and is more expensive.

tients reported symptoms after treatment, objective evidence of persistent infection or relapse was rare, and re-treatment was usually unnecessary.

Oral administration of doxycycline or amoxicillin for 30 days is recommended for the initial treatment of Lyme arthritis in patients who do not have concomitant neurologic involvement. Among patients with arthritis who do not respond to oral antibiotics, re-treatment with IV ceftriaxone for 28 days is appropriate. In patients with arthritis in whom joint inflammation persists for months or even several years after both oral and IV antibiotics, despite a negative PCR result for *B. burgdorferi* DNA in joint fluid, treatment with anti-inflammatory agents or synovectomy may be successful.

For objective neurologic abnormalities (with the possible exception of facial palsy alone), parenteral antibiotic therapy is indicated. IV ceftriaxone, given for 14–28 days, is most commonly used for this purpose, but IV cefotaxime or IV penicillin G for the same duration may also be effective. In patients with high-degree atrioventricular block or a PR interval > 0.3 s, IV therapy for at least part of the course and cardiac monitoring are recommended, but the insertion of a permanent pacemaker is not necessary.

It is unclear how and whether asymptomatic infection should be treated, but patients with such infection are often given a course of oral antibiotics. Because maternal-fetal transmission of *B. burgdorferi* seems to occur rarely (if at all), standard therapy for the manifestations of the illness is recommended for pregnant women. Long-term persistence of *B. burgdorferi* has not been documented in any large series of patients after treatment with currently recommended regimens. Therefore, there is no indication for multiple, repeated antibiotic courses in the treatment of Lyme disease.

After appropriately treated Lyme disease, a small percentage of patients continue to have subjective symptoms, primarily musculoskeletal pain, neurocognitive difficulties, or fatigue. This *chronic Lyme disease* or *post–Lyme syndrome* is a disabling condition that is similar to chronic fatigue syndrome or fibromyalgia. In a large study, one group of patients with post–Lyme syndrome received IV ceftriaxone for 30 days followed by oral doxycycline for 60 days, while another group received IV and oral placebo preparations for the same durations. No significant differences were found between groups in the numbers of patients reporting that their symptoms had improved, become worse, or stayed the same. Such patients are best treated for the relief of symptoms rather than with prolonged courses of antibiotics.

The risk of infection with *B. burgdorferi* after a recognized tick bite is so low that antibiotic prophylaxis is not routinely indicated. However, if an attached, engorged *I. scapularis* nymph is found or if follow-up is anticipated to be difficult, a single 200-mg dose of doxycycline, which usually prevents Lyme disease when given within 72 h after the tick bite, may be administered.

PROGNOSIS

The response to treatment is best early in the disease. Later treatment of Lyme borreliosis is still effective, but the period of convalescence may be longer. Eventually, most patients recover with minimal or no residual deficits.

REINFECTION

Reinfection may occur after EM when patients are treated with antimicrobial agents. In such cases, the immune response is not adequate to provide protection from subsequent infection. However, patients who develop an expanded immune response to the spirochete over a period of months (such as those with Lyme arthritis) have protective immunity for a period of years and do not acquire the infection again.

PREVENTION

Protective measures for the prevention of Lyme disease may include the avoidance of tick-infested areas, the use of repellents and acaricides, tick checks, and modification of landscapes in or near residential areas. Although a vaccine for Lyme disease used to be available, the manufacturer has discontinued its production. Therefore, no vaccine is now commercially available for the prevention of this infection.

FURTHER READINGS

BACON RM et al: Serodiagnosis of Lyme disease by kinetic immunosorbent assay using recombinant VlsE1 or peptide antigens of *Borrelia burgdorferi* compared with 2-tiered testing using whole-cell lysates. J Infect Dis 187:1187, 2003

KLEMPNER MS et al: Two controlled trials of antibiotic treatment in patients with persistent symptoms and a history of Lyme disease. N Engl J Med 345:85, 2001

NADELMAN RB et al: Prophylaxis with single-dose doxycycline for the prevention of Lyme disease after *Ixodes scapularis* tick bite. N Engl J Med 345:79, 2001

STEERE AC: Lyme disease. N Engl J Med 345:115, 2001

_____, ANGELIS SM: Therapy for Lyme arthritis: Strategies for the treatment of antibiotic-refractory arthritis. Arthritis Rheum 54:3079, 2006

_____ et al: Antibiotic-refractory Lyme arthritis is associated with HLA-DR molecules that bind a *Borrelia burgdorferi* peptide. J Exp Med 203:961, 2006

_____ et al: The emergence of Lyme disease. J Clin Invest 113:1093, 2004

WORMSER GP et al: The clinical assessment, treatment and prevention of Lyme disease, anaplasmosis, and babesiosis: Clinical practice guidelines of the Infectious Diseases Society of America. Clin Infect Dis 43:1089, 2006

SECTION 10 DISEASES CAUSED BY RICKETTSIAE, MYCOPLASMAS, AND CHLAMYDIAE

167 Rickettsial Diseases

David H. Walker, J. Stephen Dumler, Thomas Marrie

The rickettsiae are a heterogeneous group of small, obligately intracellular, gram-negative coccobacilli and short bacilli, most of which are transmitted by a tick, mite, flea, or louse vector. Except for louse-borne typhus, humans are incidental hosts. Among rickettsiae, *Coxiella burnetii, Rickettsia prowazekii,* and *R. typhi* have the well-documented ability to survive for an extended period outside the reservoir or vector and to be extremely infectious: inhalation of a single *Coxiella* microorganism can cause pneumonia. High infectivity and severe illness after inhalation make *R. prowazekii, R. rickettsii, R. typhi, R. conorii,* and *C. burnetii* bioterrorism threats.

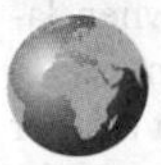

Clinical infections with rickettsiae can be classified according to (1) the taxonomy and diverse microbial characteristics of the agents, which belong to six genera (*Rickettsia, Orientia, Ehrlichia, Anaplasma, Neorickettsia,* and *Coxiella*); (2) epidemiology; or (3) clinical manifestations. The clinical manifestations of all the acute presentations are similar during the first 5 days: fever, headache, and myalgias with or without nausea, vomiting, and cough. As the course progresses, clinical manifestations—including occurrence of a macular, maculopapular, or vesicular rash; eschar; pneumonitis; and meningoencephalitis—vary from one disease to another. Given the 12 etiologic agents with varied mechanisms of transmission, geographic distribu-

TABLE 167-1 FEATURES OF SELECTED RICKETTSIAL INFECTIONS

Disease	Organism	Transmission	Geographic Range	Incubation Period (Days)	Duration (Days)	Rash (%)	Eschar (%)	Lymphadenopathy[a]
Rocky Mountain spotted fever	*Rickettsia rickettsii*	Tick bite: *Dermacentor andersoni*	United States	2–14	10–20	90	<1	+
		D. variabilis	United States					
		Amblyomma cajennense, A. aureolatum	Central/South America					
		Rhipicephalus sanguineus	Mexico, United States					
Mediterranean spotted fever[b]	*R. conorii*	Tick bite: *R. sanguineus, R. pumilio*	Southern Europe, Africa, Middle East, Central Asia	5–7	7–14	97	50	+
African tick-bite fever	*R. africae*	Tick bite: *A. hebraeum, A. variegatum*	Sub-Saharan Africa, West Indies	4–10	?	50	90	++++
Rickettsialpox	*R. akari*	Mite bite: *Liponyssoides sanguineus*	United States, Ukraine, Croatia	10–17	3–11	100	90	+++
Flea-borne spotted fever	*R. felis*	Flea (mechanism undetermined): *Ctenocephalides felis*	North and South America, Europe	8–16	8–16	80	15	—
Epidemic typhus	*R. prowazekii*	Louse feces: *Pediculus humanus corporis*, fleas and lice of flying squirrels, or recrudescence	Worldwide	7–14	10–18	80	None	—
Tick-borne lymphadenopathy	*R. slovaca*	Tick bite: *Dermacentor marginatus, D. reticularis*	Europe	7–9	17–180	5	100	++++
Murine typhus	*R. typhi*	Flea feces: *Xenopsylla cheopis, C. felis*, others	Worldwide	8–16	8–16	80	None	—
Human monocytotropic ehrlichiosis	*Ehrlichia chaffeensis*	Tick bite: *Amblyomma americanum, D. variabilis*	United States	1–21	3–21	36	None	++
Human granulocytotropic anaplasmosis	*Anaplasma phagocytophilum*	Tick bite: *Ixodes scapularis, I. ricinus, I. pacificus*	United States, Europe, Asia	1–21	3–14	Rare	None	—
Scrub typhus	*Orientia tsutsugamushi*	Mite bite: *Leptotrombidium deliense*, others	Asia, Australia, New Guinea, Pacific Islands	9–18	6–21	50	35	+++
Q fever	*Coxiella burnetii*	Inhalation of aerosols of infected parturition material (sheep, dogs, others), ingestion of infected milk or milk products	Worldwide	3–30	5–57	<1	None	—

[a]++++, severe; +++, marked; ++, moderate; +, present in a small portion of cases; —, not a noted feature.
[b]Eschar is usually present at the bite site.

tions, and associated disease manifestations, the consideration of rickettsial diseases as a single entity poses complex challenges (Table 167-1).

Establishing the etiologic diagnosis of rickettsioses is very difficult during the acute stage of illness, and definitive diagnosis usually requires the examination of paired serum samples after convalescence. Heightened clinical suspicion is based on epidemiologic data, history of exposure to vectors or reservoir animals, travel to endemic locations, clinical manifestations (sometimes including rash or eschar), and characteristic laboratory findings [including thrombocytopenia, normal or low white blood cell (WBC) counts, elevated hepatic enzyme levels, and hyponatremia]. Such suspicion should prompt empirical treatment. Doxycycline is the drug of choice for most of these infections. Only one agent, *C. burnetii*, has been documented to cause chronic illness. One other, *R. prowazekii*, causes recrudescent illness (Brill-Zinsser disease) when latent infection is reactivated years after resolution of the acute illness.

Rickettsial infections dominated by fever may resolve without further clinical evolution. However, after nonspecific early manifestations, the illnesses can also evolve along one or more of several principal clinical lines: (1) development of a macular or maculopapular rash; (2) development of an eschar at the site of tick or mite feeding; (3) development of a vesicular rash (often in rickettsialpox and African tick-bite fever); (4) development of pneumonitis with chest radiographic opacities and/or rales [Q fever and severe cases of Rocky Mountain spotted fever (RMSF), Mediterranean spotted fever (MSF), louse-borne typhus, human monocytotropic ehrlichiosis (HME), human granulocytotropic anaplasmosis (HGA), scrub typhus, and murine typhus]; (5) development of meningoencephalitis [louse-borne typhus and severe cases of RMSF, scrub typhus, HME, murine typhus, MSF, and (rarely) Q fever]; and (6) progressive hypotension and multiorgan failure as seen with sepsis or toxic shock syndrome (RMSF, MSF, louse-borne typhus, murine typhus, scrub typhus, HME, and HGA).

Epidemiologic clues to the transmission of a particular pathogen include (1) environmental exposure to ticks, fleas, or mites during the season of activity of the vector species for the disease in the appropriate geographic region (spotted fever and typhus group rickettsioses, scrub typhus, ehrlichioses, anaplasmosis); (2) travel to or residence in an endemic geographic region during the incubation period (Table 167-1); (3) exposure to parturient ruminants, cats, and dogs (Q fever); (4) exposure to flying squirrels (*R. prowazekii* infection); and (5) history of previous louse-borne typhus (recrudescent typhus).

Clinical laboratory findings, such as thrombocytopenia (particularly in spotted fever and typhus rickettsioses, ehrlichioses, anaplasmosis, and scrub typhus), normal or low WBC counts, mild to moderate serum elevations of hepatic aminotransferases, and hyponatremia suggest some common pathophysiologic mechanisms.

Application of these clinical, epidemiologic, and laboratory principles requires a consideration of the possibility of a rickettsial diagnosis and a knowledge of the individual diseases.

TICK-, MITE-, LOUSE-, AND FLEA-BORNE RICKETTSIOSES

These diseases, caused by organisms of the genera *Rickettsia* and *Orientia* in the family Rickettsiaceae, result from endothelial infection and increased vascular permeability. Pathogenic rickettsial species are very closely related, have small genomes (as a result of reductive evolution, which eliminated genes for biosynthesis of intracellularly available molecules), and are traditionally separated into typhus and spotted fever groups on the basis of lipopolysaccharide antigens. Some diseases and their agents (e.g., *R. africae*, *R. parkeri*, and *R. sibirica*) are too similar to require separate descriptions. Indeed, the similarities among MSF (*R. conorii*, all strains), North Asian tick typhus (*R. sibirica*), Japanese spotted fever (*R. japonica*), and Flinders Island spotted fever (*R. honei*) far outweigh the minor variations. The Rickettsiaceae that cause life-threatening infections are, in order of decreasing case-fatality rate, *R. rickettsii* (RMSF); *R. prowazekii* (louse-borne typhus); *Orientia tsutsugamushi* (scrub typhus); *R. conorii* (MSF); *R. typhi* (murine typhus); and, in rare cases, other spotted fever group organisms. Some agents (e.g., *R. africae*, *R. akari*, *R. slovaca*, *R. honei*, *R. felis*, *R. aeschlimannii*, and *R. parkeri*) have never been documented to cause a fatal illness.

ROCKY MOUNTAIN SPOTTED FEVER

RMSF occurs in 48 states (with the highest prevalence in the south-central and southeastern states) as well as in Canada, Mexico, and Central and South America. The infection is transmitted by *Dermacentor variabilis*, the American dog tick, in the eastern two-thirds of the United States and California; by *D. andersoni*, the Rocky Mountain wood tick, in the western United States; by *Rhipicephalus sanguineus* in Mexico and Arizona; and by *Amblyomma cajennense* in Central and South America. Maintained principally by transovarian transmission from one generation of ticks to the next, *R. rickettsii* can be acquired by uninfected ticks through the ingestion of a blood meal from rickettsemic small mammals.

Humans become infected during tick season (in the Northern Hemisphere, from May to September), although some cases occur in winter. The mortality rate was 20–25% in the preantibiotic era and remains at ~3–5% principally because of delayed diagnosis and treatment. The case-fatality ratio increases with each decade of life above age 20.

Pathogenesis *R. rickettsii* organisms are inoculated into the dermis along with secretions of the tick's salivary glands after ≥6 h of feeding. The rickettsiae spread lymphohematogenously throughout the body and infect numerous foci of contiguous endothelial cells. The dose-dependent incubation period is ~1 week (range, 2–14 days). Occlusive thrombosis and ischemic necrosis are not the fundamental pathologic basis for tissue and organ injury. Instead, increased vascular permeability, with resulting edema, hypovolemia, and ischemia, is responsible. Consumption of platelets results in thrombocytopenia in 32–52% of patients, but disseminated intravascular coagulation with hypofibrinogenemia is rare. Activation of platelets, generation of thrombin, and activation of the fibrinolytic system all appear to be homeostatic physiologic responses to endothelial injury.

Clinical Manifestations Early in the illness, when medical attention usually is first sought, RMSF is difficult to distinguish from many self-limiting viral illnesses. Fever, headache, malaise, myalgia, nausea, vomiting, and anorexia are the most common symptoms during the first 3 days. The patient becomes progressively more ill as vascular infection and injury advance. In one large series, only one-third of patients were diagnosed with presumptive RMSF early in the clinical course and treated appropriately as outpatients. In the tertiary care setting, RMSF is all too often recognized only when late severe manifestations, developing at the end of the first week or during the second week of illness in patients without appropriate treatment, prompt return to a physician or hospital and admission to an intensive care unit.

The progressive nature of the infection is clearly manifested in the skin. Rash is evident in only 14% of patients on the first day of illness and in only 49% during the first 3 days. Macules (1–5 mm) appear first on the wrists and ankles and then on the remainder of the extremities and the trunk. Later, more severe vascular damage results in frank hemorrhage at the center of the maculopapule, producing a petechia that does not disappear upon compression (Fig. 167-1). This sequence of events is sometimes delayed or aborted by effective treatment. However, the rash is a variable manifestation, appearing on day 6 or later in 20% of cases and not appearing at all in 9–16% of cases. Petechiae occur in 41–59% of cases, appearing on or after day 6 in 74% of cases that include a rash. Involvement of the palms and soles, often considered diagnostically important, usually develops relatively late in the course (after day 5 in 43% of cases) and does not develop at all in 18–64% of cases.

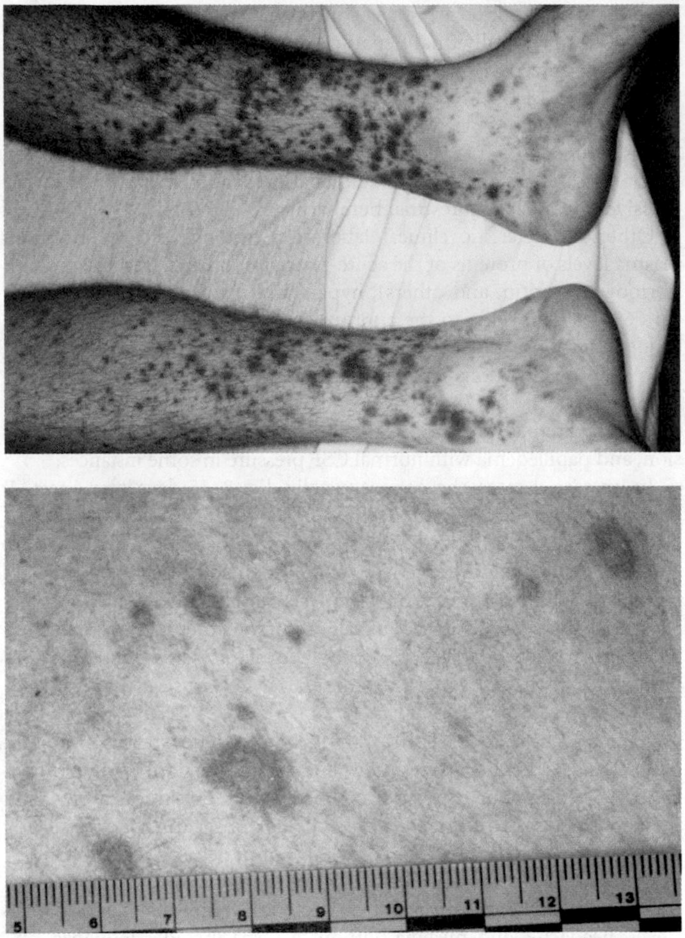

FIGURE 167-1 ***Top:*** **Petechial lesions of Rocky Mountain spotted fever** on the lower legs and soles of a young, previously healthy patient. ***Bottom:*** **Close-up of lesions** from the same patient. *(Photos courtesy of Dr. Lindsey Baden; with permission.)*

Hypovolemia leads to prerenal azotemia and (in 17% of cases) hypotension. Infection of the pulmonary microcirculation leads to noncardiogenic pulmonary edema; 12% of patients have severe respiratory disease, and 8% require mechanical ventilation. Cardiac involvement manifests as dysrhythmia in 7–16% of cases.

Besides the preceding respiratory failure, central nervous system (CNS) involvement is the other important determinant of the outcome of RMSF. Encephalitis, presenting as confusion or lethargy, is apparent in 26–28% of cases. Progressively severe encephalitis manifests as stupor or delirium in 21–26% of cases, as ataxia in 18%, as coma in 10%, and as seizures in 8%. Numerous focal neurologic deficits have been reported. Meningoencephalitis results in cerebrospinal fluid (CSF) pleocytosis in 34–38% of cases; usually there are 10–100 cells/μL and a mononuclear predominance, but occasionally there are >100 cells/μL and a polymorphonuclear predominance. The CSF protein concentration is increased in 30–35% of cases, but the CSF glucose concentration is usually normal.

Renal failure, often reversible with rehydration, is caused by acute tubular necrosis in severe cases with shock. Hepatic injury with increased serum aminotransferase concentrations (38% of cases) is due to focal death of individual hepatocytes without hepatic failure. Jaundice is recognized in 9% of cases and an elevated serum bilirubin concentration in 18–30%.

Life-threatening bleeding is rare. Anemia develops in 30% of cases and is severe enough to require transfusions in 11%. Blood is detected in the stools or vomitus of 10% of patients, and death has followed massive upper gastrointestinal hemorrhage.

Other characteristic clinical laboratory findings include increased plasma levels of proteins of the acute-phase response (C-reactive protein, fibrinogen, ferritin, and others), hypoalbuminemia, and hyponatremia (in 56% of cases) due to the appropriate secretion of antidiuretic hormone in response to the hypovolemic state. Myositis occurs occasionally, with marked elevations in serum creatine kinase levels and multifocal rhabdomyonecrosis. Ocular involvement includes conjunctivitis in 30% of cases and retinal vein engorgement, flame hemorrhages, arterial occlusion, and papilledema with normal CSF pressure in some instances.

In untreated cases, the patient usually dies 8–15 days after onset. A rare presentation, fulminant RMSF, is fatal within 5 days after onset. This fulminant presentation is seen most often in black males with glucose-6-phosphate dehydrogenase (G6PD) deficiency and may be related to an undefined effect of hemolysis on the rickettsial infection. Although survivors of RMSF usually return to their previous state of health, permanent sequelae, including neurologic deficits and gangrene necessitating amputation of extremities, may follow severe illness.

Diagnosis The diagnosis of RMSF during the acute stage is more difficult than is generally appreciated. The most important epidemiologic factor is a history of exposure to a potentially tick-infested environment within the 12 days preceding disease onset during a season of possible tick activity. However, only 60% of patients actually recall being bitten by a tick during the incubation period.

The differential diagnosis for early clinical manifestations of RMSF (fever, headache, and myalgia without a rash) includes influenza, enteroviral infection, infectious mononucleosis, viral hepatitis, leptospirosis, typhoid fever, gram-negative or gram-positive bacterial sepsis, HME, HGA, murine typhus, sylvatic flying-squirrel typhus, and rickettsialpox. Enterocolitis may be suggested by nausea, vomiting, and abdominal pain; prominence of abdominal tenderness has resulted in exploratory laparotomy. CNS involvement may masquerade as bacterial or viral meningoencephalitis. Cough, pulmonary signs, and chest radiographic opacities may lead to a diagnostic consideration of bronchitis or pneumonia.

At presentation during the first 3 days of illness, only 3% of patients exhibit the classic triad of fever, rash, and history of tick exposure. When a rash appears, a diagnosis of RMSF should certainly be considered. However, many illnesses considered in the differential diagnosis may also be associated with a rash, including rubeola, rubella, meningococcemia, disseminated gonococcal infection, secondary syphilis, toxic shock syndrome, drug hypersensitivity, idiopathic thrombocytopenic purpura, thrombotic thrombocytopenic purpura, Kawasaki syndrome, and immune complex vasculitis. Conversely, any person in an endemic area with a provisional diagnosis of one of the above illnesses may have RMSF. Thus, if a viral infection is suspected during RMSF season in an endemic area, it should always be kept in mind that RMSF can mimic viral infection early in the course; if the illness worsens over the next couple of days after initial presentation, the patient should return for reevaluation.

The most common serologic test for confirmation of the diagnosis is the indirect immunofluorescence assay. Not until 7–10 days after onset is a diagnostic titer of ≥1:64 usually detectable. The sensitivity and specificity of the indirect immunofluorescence assay are 94–100% and 100%, respectively. It is important to understand that serologic tests for RMSF are usually negative at the time of presentation for medical care and that treatment should not be delayed while a positive serologic result is awaited.

The only diagnostic test that is useful during the acute illness is immunohistologic examination of a cutaneous biopsy sample from a rash lesion for *R. rickettsii*. Examination of a 3-mm punch biopsy from such a lesion is 70% sensitive and 100% specific. Polymerase chain reaction (PCR) amplification and detection of *R. rickettsii* DNA in peripheral blood is a relatively insensitive approach except when the patient is already in the preterminal state. Rickettsiae are present in large quantities in heavily infected foci of endothelial cells but in relatively low quantities in the circulation. Cultivation of rickettsiae in cell culture is feasible but is seldom undertaken because of biohazard concerns.

Rx ROCKY MOUNTAIN SPOTTED FEVER

The drug of choice for the treatment of both children and adults with RMSF is doxycycline, except when the patient is pregnant or allergic to this drug (see below). Because of the severity of RMSF, immediate empirical administration of doxycycline should be strongly considered for any patient with a consistent clinical presentation in the appropriate epidemiologic setting. Doxycycline is administered orally (or, in the presence of coma or vomiting, intravenously) at 200 mg/d in two divided doses. For children with suspected RMSF, up to five courses of doxycycline may be administered with minimal risk of dental staining. Other regimens include oral tetracycline (25–50 mg/kg per day) in four divided doses. Treatment with chloramphenicol is advised only for patients who are pregnant or allergic to doxycycline. The antirickettsial drug should be administered until the patient has been afebrile and improving clinically for 2–3 days. β-Lactam antibiotics, erythromycin, and aminoglycosides have no role in the treatment of RMSF, and sulfa-containing drugs are likely to exacerbate this infection. There is little clinical experience with fluoroquinolones, clarithromycin, and azithromycin, which are not recommended. The most seriously ill patients are managed in intensive care units, with careful administration of fluids to achieve optimal tissue perfusion without precipitating noncardiogenic pulmonary edema. In some severely ill patients, hypoxemia requires intubation and mechanical ventilation; oliguric or anuric acute renal failure requires hemodialysis; seizures necessitate the use of antiseizure medication; anemia or severe hemorrhage necessitates transfusions of packed red blood cells; or bleeding with severe thrombocytopenia requires platelet transfusions. Heparin is not a useful component of treatment, and there is no evidence that glucocorticoids affect outcome.

Prevention Avoidance of tick bites is the only available preventive approach. Use of protective clothing and tick repellents, inspection of the body once or twice a day, and removal of ticks before they inoculate rickettsiae reduce the risk of infection.

MEDITERRANEAN SPOTTED FEVER (BOUTONNEUSE FEVER), AFRICAN TICK-BITE FEVER, AND OTHER TICK-BORNE SPOTTED FEVERS

R. conorii is prevalent in southern Europe, Africa, and southwestern and south-central Asia. Regional names for the disease caused by this organism include Mediterranean spotted fever, Kenya tick typhus, Indian tick typhus, Israeli spotted fever, and Astrakhan spotted fever. The disease is characterized by high fever, rash, and—in most geographic locales—an inoculation eschar (*tâche noire*) at the site of the tick bite. A severe form of the disease (mortality rate, 50%) occurs in patients with diabetes, alcoholism, or heart failure.

African tick-bite fever, caused by *R. africae*, occurs in rural areas of sub-Saharan Africa and in the Caribbean islands and is transmitted by *Amblyomma hebraeum* and *A. variegatum* ticks. The average incubation period is 7 days. The mild illness consists of headache, fever, eschar, and regional lymphadenopathy. *Amblyomma* ticks often feed in groups, with the consequent development of multiple eschars. Rash may be vesicular, sparse, or absent altogether. Because of tourism in sub-Saharan Africa, African tick-bite fever is the most frequently imported rickettsiosis in Europe and North America. A similar disease caused by the very closely related *R. parkeri* is transmitted by *A. maculatum* in the United States and *A. triste* in South America.

R. japonica causes *Japanese spotted fever*, which also occurs in Korea. A similar disease in northern Asia is caused by *R. sibirica*. *Queensland tick typhus* due to *R. australis* is transmitted by *Ixodes holocyclus*. *Flinders Island spotted fever*, found on the island for which it is named as well as in other parts of Tasmania, in mainland Australia, and in southeastern Asia, is caused by *R. honei*. In Europe, patients infected with *R. slovaca* after a wintertime *Dermacentor* tick bite manifest an afebrile illness with an eschar (usually on the scalp) and regional lymphadenopathy.

Diagnosis Diagnosis of these tick-borne spotted fevers is based on clinical and epidemiologic findings and is confirmed by serology, immunohistochemical demonstration of rickettsiae in skin biopsy specimens, cell-culture isolation of rickettsiae, or PCR of skin biopsy or blood samples. The serologic identification of the etiologic species requires knowledge of all the potential agents as well as expensive, laborious cross-adsorption of the patient's serum. In an endemic area, patients presenting with fever, rash, and/or a skin lesion consisting of a black necrotic area or a crust surrounded by erythema should be considered to have one of these rickettsial spotted fevers.

℞ TICK-BORNE SPOTTED FEVERS

Successful therapeutic agents include doxycycline (100 mg bid orally for 1–5 days), ciprofloxacin (750 mg bid orally for 5 days), and chloramphenicol (500 mg qid orally for 7–10 days). Pregnant patients may be treated with josamycin (3 g/d orally for 5 days). Data on the efficacy of treatment of mildly ill children with clarithromycin or azithromycin should not be extrapolated to adults or to patients with moderate or severe illness.

RICKETTSIALPOX

R. akari infects mice and their mites (*Liponyssoides sanguineus*), which maintain the organisms by transovarian transmission.

Epidemiology Rickettsialpox is recognized principally in New York City, but cases have also been reported in other urban and rural locations in the United States and in Ukraine, Croatia, and Turkey. Investigation of eschars suspected of representing bioterrorism-associated cutaneous anthrax has revealed that rickettsialpox occurs more frequently than previously realized.

Clinical Manifestations A papule forms at the site of the mite's feeding, develops a central vesicle, and becomes a 1- to 2.5-cm painless black crusted eschar surrounded by an erythematous halo (Fig. 167-2). Enlargement of the regional lymph nodes draining the eschar suggests initial lymphogenous spread. After an incubation period of 10–17 days, during which the eschar and regional lymphadenopathy frequently go unnoticed, onset is marked by malaise, chills, fever, headache, and myalgia. A macular rash appears 2–6 days after onset and evolves sequentially into papules, vesicles, and crusts that heal without scarring (Fig. 167-3). The rash may remain macular or maculopapular. Some patients develop nausea, vomiting, abdominal pain, cough, conjunctivitis, or photophobia. If untreated, fever lasts 6–10 days.

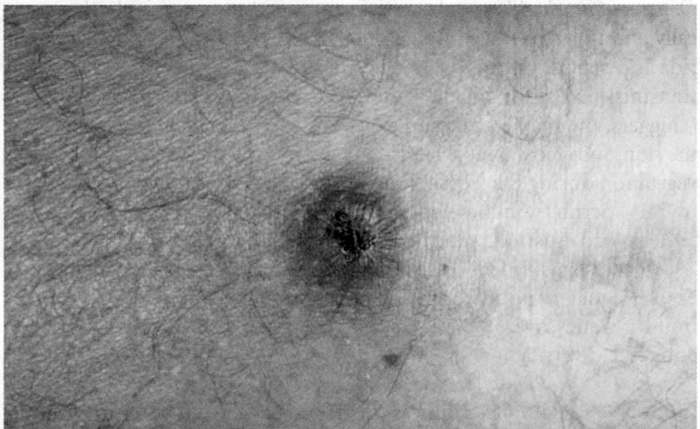

FIGURE 167-2 Eschar at the site of the mite bite in a patient with rickettsialpox. *(Reprinted from A Krusell et al: Emerg Infect Dis 8:727, 2002. Photo obtained by Dr. Kenneth Kaye.)*

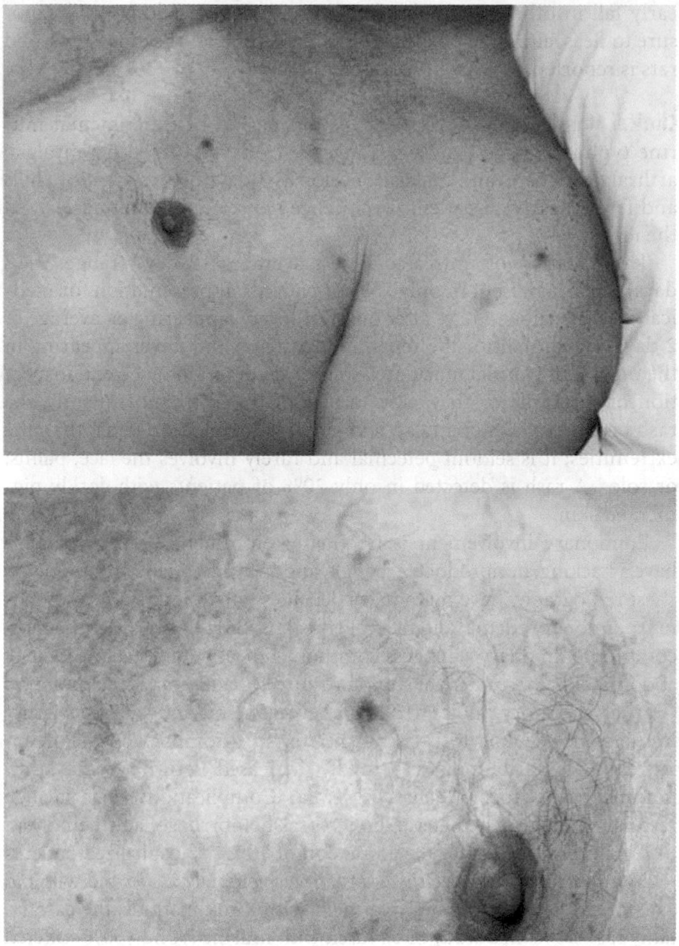

FIGURE 167-3 ***Top:*** **Papulovesicular lesions on the trunk of the patient with rickettsialpox** shown in Fig. 167-2. ***Bottom:*** **Close-up of lesions** from the same patient. *(Reprinted from A Krusell et al: Emerg Infect Dis 8:727, 2002. Photos obtained by Dr. Kenneth Kaye.)*

Diagnosis and Treatment Clinical, epidemiologic, and convalescent serologic data establish the diagnosis of a spotted fever group rickettsiosis that is seldom pursued further. Doxycycline is the drug of choice for treatment.

FLEA-BORNE SPOTTED FEVER

An emerging rickettsiosis caused by *R. felis* probably occurs worldwide. Maintained transovarially in the geographically widespread cat flea *Ctenocephalides felis*, the infection has been described as moderately severe, with fever, rash, headache, and CNS and gastrointestinal symptoms.

ENDEMIC MURINE TYPHUS

Epidemiology *R. typhi* is maintained in mammalian host/flea cycles, with rats (*Rattus rattus* and *R. norvegicus*) and the Oriental rat flea (*Xenopsylla cheopis*) as the classic zoonotic niche. Fleas acquire *R. typhi* from rickettsemic rats and carry the organism throughout their life span. Nonimmune rats and humans are infected when rickettsia-laden flea feces contaminate pruritic bite lesions; less frequently, the flea bite transmits the organisms. Transmission also may occur via inhalation of aerosolized rickettsiae from flea feces. Infected rats appear healthy, although they are rickettsemic for ~2 weeks.

Murine typhus occurs mainly in southern Texas and southern California, where the classic rat/flea cycle is absent and an opossum/cat flea (*C. felis*) cycle is prominent. Globally, endemic typhus occurs year-round, mainly in warm (often coastal) areas throughout the tropics and subtropics, where it is highly prevalent though often unrecognized. The incidence peaks from April through June in southern Texas and during the warm months of summer and early fall in other geographic locations. Patients seldom recall exposure to fleas, although exposure to animals such as cats, opossums, and rats is reported in nearly 40% of cases.

Clinical Manifestations The incubation period of experimental murine typhus averages 11 days (range, 8–16 days). Headache, myalgia, arthralgia, nausea, and malaise develop 1–3 days before onset of chills and fever. Nearly all patients experience nausea and vomiting early in the illness.

The duration of untreated illness averages 12 days (range, 9–18 days). Rash is present in only 13% of patients at presentation for medical care (usually ~4 days after onset of fever), appearing an average of 2 days later in half of the remaining patients and never appearing in the others. The initial macular rash is often detected by careful inspection of the axilla or the inner surface of the arm. Subsequently, the rash becomes maculopapular, involving the trunk more often than the extremities; it is seldom petechial and rarely involves the face, palms, or soles. A rash is detected in only 20% of patients with darkly pigmented skin.

Pulmonary involvement is frequently prominent; 35% of patients have a hacking, nonproductive cough, and 23% of patients who undergo chest radiography have pulmonary densities due to interstitial pneumonia, pulmonary edema, and pleural effusions. Bibasilar rales are the most common pulmonary sign. Less common clinical manifestations include abdominal pain, confusion, stupor, seizures, ataxia, coma, and jaundice. Clinical laboratory studies frequently reveal anemia and leukopenia early in the course, leukocytosis late in the course, thrombocytopenia, hyponatremia, hypoalbuminemia, mildly increased serum hepatic aminotransferases, and prerenal azotemia. Complications may include respiratory failure, hematemesis, cerebral hemorrhage, and hemolysis. Severe illness necessitates the admission of 10% of hospitalized patients to an intensive care unit. Greater severity is generally associated with old age, underlying disease, and treatment with a sulfonamide; the case-fatality rate is 1%. In a study of children with murine typhus, 50% suffered only nocturnal fevers, feeling well enough for active daytime play.

Diagnosis and Treatment Cultivation, PCR, or cross-adsorption serologic studies of acute- and convalescent-phase sera can provide a specific diagnosis, and an immunohistochemical method for identification of typhus group-specific antigens has been developed. Nevertheless, most patients are treated empirically with doxycycline (100 mg bid orally for 7–15 days) on the basis of clinical suspicion. Serologic methods are usually used when laboratory confirmation of the diagnosis is sought.

EPIDEMIC (LOUSE-BORNE) TYPHUS

The human body louse (*Pediculus humanus corporis*) lives in clothing under poor hygienic conditions and usually in impoverished cold areas. Lice acquire *R. prowazekii* when they ingest blood from a rickettsemic patient. The rickettsiae multiply in the midgut epithelial cells of the louse and are shed in the louse's feces. The infected louse leaves a febrile person and deposits infected feces on its subsequent host during its blood meal; the patient autoinoculates the organisms by scratching. The louse is killed by the rickettsiae and does not pass *R. prowazekii* to its offspring.

Epidemic typhus haunts regions afflicted by wars and disasters. An outbreak involved 100,000 people in refugee camps in Burundi in 1997. A small focus occurred in Russia in 1998; sporadic cases have been reported from Algeria, and frequent outbreaks have occurred in Peru. Eastern flying-squirrels (*Glaucomys volans*) and their lice and fleas maintain *R. prowazekii* in a zoonotic cycle. The fleas transmit the infection sporadically to humans.

Brill-Zinsser disease is a recrudescent illness occurring years after acute epidemic typhus, probably as a result of waning immunity. Typhus infection remains latent for years; its reactivation results in sporadic cases of disease in louse-free populations or in epidemics in louse-infested populations.

Rickettsiae are potential agents of bioterrorism (Chap. 214). Infections with *R. prowazekii* and *R. rickettsii* have high case-fatality ratios. These organisms cause difficult-to-diagnose diseases, are highly infectious when inhaled as aerosols, and have been selected for resistance to tetracycline or chloramphenicol in the laboratory.

Clinical Manifestations After an incubation period of ~1 week, the onset of illness is abrupt, with prostration, severe headache, and fever rising rapidly to 38.8°–40.0°C (102°–104°F). Cough is prominent, occurring in 70% of patients. Myalgias are usually severe. In the outbreak in Burundi, the disease was referred to as sutama ("crouching"), a designation reflecting the posture of patients attempting to alleviate the pain. A rash begins on the upper trunk, usually on the fifth day, and then becomes generalized, involving the entire body except the face, palms, and soles. Initially, this rash is macular; without treatment, it becomes maculopapular, petechial, and confluent. The rash often is not detected on black skin; 60% of African patients have spotless epidemic typhus. Photophobia, with considerable conjunctival injection and eye pain, is frequent. The tongue may be dry, brown, and furred. Confusion and coma are common. Skin necrosis and gangrene of the digits as well as interstitial pneumonia may occur in severe cases. Untreated disease is fatal in 7–40% of cases, with outcome depending primarily on the condition of the host. Patients with untreated infections develop renal insufficiency and multiorgan involvement in which neurologic manifestations are frequently prominent. Overall, 12% of patients with epidemic typhus have neurologic involvement. Infection associated with North American flying squirrels is a milder illness; whether this milder disease is due to host factors (e.g., better health status) or attenuated virulence is unknown.

Diagnosis and Treatment Epidemic typhus is sometimes misdiagnosed as typhoid fever in tropical countries (Chap. 146). The means even for serologic studies are often unavailable in settings of louse-borne typhus. Epidemics may be recognized by the serologic or immunohistochemical diagnosis of a single case or by detection of *R. prowazekii* in a louse found on a patient. Cross-adsorption indirect fluorescent antibody (IFA) studies can distinguish *R. prowazekii* and *R. typhi* infections. Doxycycline (200 mg/d, given in two divided doses) is administered orally or—if the patient is comatose or vomiting—intravenously. Although under epidemic conditions a single 200-mg dose has proved effective, treatment is generally continued until 2–3 days after defervescence. Pregnant patients should be evaluated individually and treated with either chloramphenicol early in pregnancy or, if necessary, doxycycline late in pregnancy.

Prevention Prevention of epidemic typhus involves control of body lice. Clothes should be changed regularly, and insecticides should be used every 6 weeks to control the louse population.

SCRUB TYPHUS

O. tsutsugamushi differs substantially from *Rickettsia* species both genetically and in terms of cell wall composition (i.e., it lacks lipopolysaccharide and peptidoglycan). *O. tsutsugamushi* is maintained by transovarian transmission in trombiculid mites. After hatching, infected larval mites (chiggers, the only stage that feeds on a host) inoculate organisms into the skin. Infected chiggers are found particularly in areas of heavy scrub vegetation during the wet season, when mites lay eggs.

Scrub typhus is endemic in eastern and southern Asia, northern Australia, and islands of the western Pacific and Indian Oceans. Infections are prevalent in these regions; in some areas, >3% of the population is infected or reinfected each month. Immunity wanes over 1–3 years, and the organism exhibits remarkable antigenic diversity.

Clinical Manifestations Illness varies from mild and self-limiting to fatal. After an incubation period of 6–21 days, onset is characterized by fever, headache, myalgia, cough, and gastrointestinal symptoms. Some patients recover spontaneously after a few days. The classic case description includes an eschar where the chigger feeds, regional lymphadenopathy, and a maculopapular rash—signs that are seldom seen in indigenous patients. Fewer than 50% of Westerners develop an eschar, and fewer than 40% develop a rash (on day 4–6 of illness). Severe cases typically include encephalitis and interstitial pneumonia due to vascular injury. The case-fatality rate for untreated classic cases is 7% but would probably be lower if all mild cases were diagnosed.

Diagnosis and Treatment Serologic assays (IFA, indirect immunoperoxidase, and enzyme immunoassays) are the mainstays of laboratory diagnosis. Patients are treated with doxycycline (100 mg bid orally for 7–15 days) or chloramphenicol (500 mg qid orally for 7–15 days).

Some cases of scrub typhus in Thailand are caused by doxycycline- or chloramphenicol-resistant strains that are susceptible to rifampin. Azithromycin and clarithromycin have been used successfully in a few patients.

EHRLICHIOSES AND ANAPLASMOSIS

Ehrlichioses are acute febrile infections caused by members of the family Anaplasmataceae, which is made up of obligately intracellular organisms transmitted by ticks and contains four genera: *Ehrlichia*, *Anaplasma*, *Wolbachia*, and *Neorickettsia*. The bacteria reside in vertebrate reservoirs and target vacuoles of hematopoietic cells (Fig. 167-4). Two *Ehrlichia* species and one *Anaplasma* species cause human infections that can be severe and frequent. *E. chaffeensis*, the agent of HME, infects predominantly mononuclear phagocytic cells. *E. ewingii* and *A. phagocytophilum* infect neutrophils.

Ehrlichia and *Anaplasma* are maintained by horizontal tick-mammal-tick transmission, and humans are only inadvertently infected. Wolbachiae are associated with human diseases caused by filariae, since they are important for filarial viability and pathogenicity; antibiotic treatment targeting wolbachiae is a strategy for the control of filariasis. Neorickettsiae parasitize flukes that in turn parasitize aquatic snails, fish, and insects. Only a single human neorickettsiosis has been described: sennetsu fever, an infectious mononucleosis–like illness that was first identified in 1953. Transmission is probably due to the ingestion of raw fish containing *N. sennetsu*–infected flukes.

HUMAN MONOCYTOTROPIC EHRLICHIOSIS

Epidemiology More than 2657 cases of *E. chaffeensis* infection had been reported to the Centers for Disease Control and Prevention (CDC) as of September 2006. However, active prospective surveillance has demonstrated an incidence as high as 414 cases per 100,000 population in some regions of the United States. Most *E. chaffeensis* infections are identified in the south-central, southeastern, and mid-Atlantic states, but cases have also been recognized in California. All life stages of the Lone Star tick *(A. americanum)* vector feed on white-tailed deer—a major reservoir host. Subclinically infected dogs and coyotes also serve as reservoirs. Tick bites and exposures are reported by patients, frequently in rural areas and especially in May through July. The median age of HME patients is 53 years; however, severe and fatal infections in children are also well recognized. Of patients with HME, 61% are male.

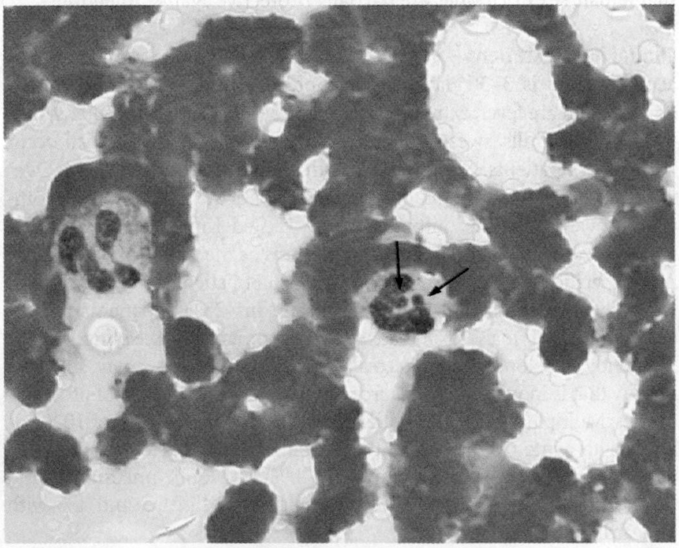

FIGURE 167-4 Peripheral blood smear from a patient with human granulocytotropic anaplasmosis. A neutrophil contains two morulae (vacuoles filled with *A. phagocytophilum*). *(Photo courtesy of Dr. J. Stephen Dumler.)*

Clinical Manifestations *E. chaffeensis* disseminates hematogenously from the dermal blood pool created by the feeding tick. After a median incubation period of 8 days, illness develops. Clinical manifestations are undifferentiated and include fever (97% of cases), headache (80%), myalgia (57%), and malaise (82%). Less frequently observed are nausea, vomiting, and diarrhea (23–64%); cough (26%); rash (31% overall, 6% at presentation); and confusion (19%). HME can be severe: 62% of patients with documented cases are hospitalized, and ~3% die. Severe complications include toxic shock–like or septic shock–like syndromes, adult respiratory distress syndrome, cardiac failure, hepatitis, meningoencephalitis, hemorrhage, and—in immunocompromised patients—overwhelming infection. Laboratory findings are valuable in the differential diagnosis of HME; 62% of patients have leukopenia (initially lymphopenia, later neutropenia), 71% have thrombocytopenia, and 83% have elevated serum levels of hepatic aminotransferases. Despite low blood cell counts, the bone marrow is hypercellular, and noncaseating granulomas may be present. Vasculitis is not a component of HME.

Diagnosis Because HME can be fatal, empirical antibiotic therapy based on clinical diagnosis is required. This diagnosis is suggested by fever with a known tick exposure during the preceding 3 weeks, thrombocytopenia and/or leukopenia, and increased serum aminotransferase activities. Morulae are infrequently demonstrated on peripheral blood smears. Active HME can be confirmed by PCR amplification of *E. chaffeensis* nucleic acids in blood obtained before the start of doxycycline therapy. Retrospective serodiagnosis requires a consistent clinical picture and a fourfold increase in *E. chaffeensis* antibody titer (to ≥1:64 in paired sera obtained ~3 weeks apart). Separate specific diagnostic tests are necessary for HME and HGA.

EHRLICHIOSIS EWINGII

Ehrlichia ewingii, originally a neutrophil pathogen causing febrile lameness in dogs, resembles *E. chaffeensis* in its tick vector (*A. americanum*) and vertebrate reservoirs (white-tailed deer and dogs). *E. ewingii* illness is similar to but less severe than HME. The majority of cases have occurred in immunocompromised patients. No specific diagnostic test for ehrlichiosis ewingii is readily available.

Rx EHRLICHIOSES

Doxycycline is effective for HME and ehrlichiosis ewingii. Therapy with doxycycline (100 mg given orally or intravenously twice daily) or tetracycline (250–500 mg given orally every 6 h) lowers hospitalization rates and shortens fever duration. *E. chaffeensis* is not susceptible to chloramphenicol in vitro, and the use of this drug is controversial. While a few reports document *E. chaffeensis* persistence in humans, this finding is rare; most infections are cured by short courses of doxycycline (continuing for 3–5 days after defervescence). Although poorly studied, rifampin may be suitable when doxycycline is contraindicated.

Prevention HME and ehrlichiosis ewingii are prevented by the avoidance of ticks in endemic areas. The use of protective clothing and tick repellents, careful postexposure tick searches, and prompt removal of attached ticks markedly diminish infection risk.

HUMAN GRANULOCYTOTROPIC ANAPLASMOSIS

Epidemiology As of September 2006, 3257 cases of HGA had been reported to the CDC, most in the upper midwestern and northeastern

United States; the case distribution is similar to that for Lyme disease because of the shared *I. scapularis* tick vector. White-footed mice and white-tailed deer in the United States and red deer in Europe are natural reservoirs for *A. phagocytophilum*. HGA incidence peaks in May through July, but the disease can occur throughout the year with exposure to *Ixodes* ticks. HGA often affects males (57%) and older persons (median age, 51 years).

Clinical Manifestations Seroprevalence rates are high in endemic regions; thus it seems likely that most individuals develop subclinical infections. The incubation period for HGA is 4–8 days, after which the disease manifests as fever (93% of cases), myalgia (77%), headache (76%), and malaise (94%). A minority of patients develop nausea, vomiting, or diarrhea (16–38%); cough (19%); or confusion (17%). Rash (6%) is almost invariably concurrent erythema migrans attributable to Lyme disease. Most patients develop thrombocytopenia (71%) and/or leukopenia (49%) with increased serum hepatic aminotransferase activities (71%).

Severe complications occur most often in the elderly and include adult respiratory distress syndrome, a toxic shock–like syndrome, and life-threatening opportunistic infections. Meningoencephalitis has not been conclusively documented with HGA, but brachial plexopathy and demyelinating polyneuropathy are reported. For HGA, 7% of patients require intensive care, and the case-fatality rate is 0.5%. Neither vasculitis nor granulomas are components of HGA. While co-infections with *Borrelia burgdorferi* and *Babesia microti* [transmitted by the same tick vector(s)] occur, there is little evidence of comorbidity or persistence.

Diagnosis HGA should be included in the differential diagnosis of influenza-like illnesses during seasons with *Ixodes* tick activity (May through December), especially with tick bite or exposure. Concurrent thrombocytopenia, leukopenia, or elevation in serum alanine or aspartate aminotransferase further increases the likelihood of HGA. Many HGA patients develop Lyme disease antibodies in the absence of clinical findings consistent with that diagnosis. Thus, HGA should be considered in the differential diagnosis of atypical severe Lyme disease presentations. Peripheral blood film examination for neutrophil morulae can yield a diagnosis in 20–75% of infections. PCR testing of blood from patients with active disease before doxycycline therapy is sensitive and specific. Serodiagnosis is retrospective, requiring a fourfold increase in *A. phagocytophilum* antibody titer (to ≥1:80) in paired serum samples obtained 1 month apart. In regions where seroprevalence is high, a single acute-phase titer may be misleading.

Rx HUMAN GRANULOCYTOTROPIC ANAPLASMOSIS

No prospective studies of therapy for HGA have been conducted. However, doxycycline (100 mg by mouth twice daily) is effective. Rifampin therapy is associated with improvement of HGA in pregnant women and children. Most treated patients defervesce within 24–48 h.

Prevention HGA prevention requires tick avoidance. Transmission can be documented as few as 4 h after a tick bite.

Q FEVER

Q fever results from infection with *C. burnetii*, which can exist as a highly infectious phase I form within humans or as an avirulent phase II form. This organism forms spores that allow its survival in harsh environments. *Coxiella* escapes intracellular killing in macrophages by inhibiting the final phagosome maturation step (cathepsin fusion) and adapts to the acidic phagolysosome.

Q fever encompasses two broad clinical syndromes: acute and chronic infection. The host's immune response (rather than the infecting strain) most likely determines whether chronic Q fever develops. *C. burnetii* survives in monocytes from patients with chronic Q fever but not in those from patients with acute Q fever or from uninfected persons. Impairment of the bactericidal activity of the *C. burnetii*–infected monocyte seems to be due to overproduction of interleukin 10. The CD4+/CD8+ ratio is decreased in Q fever endocarditis. Very few organisms and a strong cellular response are observed in patients with acute Q fever, while many organisms and a moderate cellular response are seen in chronic Q fever. Immunologic control of *C. burnetii* is T cell–dependent, but 80–90% of bone marrow aspirates obtained after recovery from Q fever contain *C. burnetii* DNA.

Epidemiology Q fever is a zoonosis. The primary sources of human infection are infected cattle, sheep, and goats. However, cats, rabbits, pigeons, and dogs have also transmitted *C. burnetii* to humans. The wildlife reservoir includes ticks. In the infected female mammal, *C. burnetii* localizes to the uterus and the mammary glands. Infection is reactivated during pregnancy. High concentrations of *C. burnetii* are found in the placenta. At the time of parturition, *C. burnetii* organisms are released into the air, and infection follows inhalation of aerosolized organisms by a susceptible host. Soil is contaminated during parturition, and *C. burnetii* aerosols can be generated months later during windstorms. Individuals up to 18 km from the source have been infected. *C. burnetii* is a potential agent of bioterrorism.

Persons at risk for Q fever include abattoir workers, veterinarians, and other individuals who have contact with infected animals, particularly newborn animals or products of conception. The organism is shed in milk for weeks to months after parturition. The ingestion of contaminated milk in some geographic areas probably represents a major route of transmission to humans, although the experimental evidence on this point is contradictory. In rare instances, human-to-human transmission has followed labor and childbirth in an infected woman, autopsy of an infected individual, or blood transfusion. Some evidence suggests that *C. burnetii* can be sexually transmitted among humans. Nevertheless, the vast majority of Q fever cases result from inhalation of contaminated aerosols.

Infections due to *C. burnetii* occur in most geographic locations except New Zealand and Antarctica. The primary manifestations of acute Q fever vary with the area. For example, the primary manifestation is pneumonia in Nova Scotia (Canada) but is granulomatous hepatitis in Marseille (France). These differences may reflect the route of infection—i.e., the ingestion of contaminated milk for hepatitis and inhalation of contaminated aerosols for pneumonia.

Young age seems to be protective against infection with *C. burnetii*. In a large outbreak in Switzerland, symptomatic infection occurred five times more often among persons >15 years of age than among those <15 years old. In many outbreaks, men are affected more commonly than women. In France, despite similar occupational exposure of the sexes, the male-to-female ratio is 2.45:1; this difference reflects the fact that female sex hormones are partially protective against infection.

Clinical Manifestations • ***ACUTE Q FEVER*** The incubation period for acute Q fever is 3–30 days. The symptoms are nonspecific; common among them are fever, extreme fatigue, and severe headache. Other symptoms include chills, sweats, nausea, vomiting, and diarrhea, which occur in 5–20% of patients. Cough develops in about half of patients with Q fever pneumonia. Neurologic manifestations of acute Q fever are uncommon; however, in one outbreak in the United Kingdom, 23% of 102 patients had neurologic signs and symptoms as the major manifestation. A nonspecific rash may be evident in 4–18% of patients. The WBC count is usually normal. Thrombocytopenia occurs in ~25% of patients, and reactive thrombocytosis (with platelet counts sometimes exceeding $10^6/\mu L$) frequently develops during recovery. Chest radiography may show an opacity that is indistinguishable from that seen in pneumonia of other etiologies. Multiple rounded opacities are common. In one study of 1070 patients with acute Q fever in southern France, 40% of patients presented with hepatitis, 17% with pneumonia, 20% with both pneumonia and hepatitis, 14% with isolated fever, 2% with CNS disease, and 1% with pericarditis and myocarditis.

Acute Q fever occasionally complicates pregnancy. In one series, Q fever in pregnancy resulted in premature birth in 35% of cases, and 43% of pregnancies ended in abortion or neonatal death. In Halifax, Nova Scotia, a current or previous neonatal death was three times more likely among women seropositive for *C. burnetii* than among seronegative women. Up to 70% of cases of Q fever in children are asymptomatic. Only a few cases of Q fever endocarditis have been reported in children.

In Australia and the United Kingdom, a fatigue state lasting 5–10 years has followed Q fever in 8–15% of cases. Low levels of *C. burnetii* DNA have been detected in the affected patients 0.75–5 years after infection. Patients who develop Q fever fatigue syndrome have a higher frequency of carriage of HLA-DRB1*11 and of the 2/2 genotype of the interferon γ intron 1 microsatellite.

Patients with acute Q fever and lesions of native heart valves, prosthetic heart valves, or prosthetic intravascular material should undergo serologic monitoring every 4 months for 2 years. If the phase I IgG titer is >1:800, further investigation is warranted. Some authorities recommend that patients with valvulopathy and acute Q fever receive doxycycline and hydroxychloroquine for 12 months to prevent chronic Q fever.

CHRONIC Q FEVER Chronic Q fever, which almost always implies endocarditis, usually occurs in patients with previous valvular heart disease, immunosuppression, or chronic renal insufficiency. Fever is usually absent or low grade. Patients may have nonspecific symptoms for up to 1 year before diagnosis. Valvular vegetations are detected in only 12% of patients by transthoracic echocardiography, but the rate of detection may be higher with transesophageal echocardiography. The vegetations in chronic Q fever endocarditis differ from those in bacterial endocarditis, manifesting as endothelialized nodules on the valves. A high index of suspicion is necessary for a correct diagnosis. The disease should be suspected in all patients with culture-negative endocarditis. In addition, all patients with valvular heart disease and an unexplained purpuric eruption, renal insufficiency, stroke, and/or progressive heart failure should be tested for *C. burnetii* infection. Patients with chronic Q fever have hepatomegaly and/or splenomegaly, which, in combination with rheumatoid factor, elevated erythrocyte sedimentation rate, high C-reactive protein level, and/or increased γ-globulin concentrations (up to 60–70 g/L), suggests this diagnosis. Other manifestations of chronic Q fever include infection of vascular prostheses, aneurysms, and bone as well as chronic sternal wound infection. Unusual manifestations include chronic thrombocytopenia, mixed cryoglobulinemia, and livedo reticularis.

Diagnosis Isolation of *C. burnetii* from buffy-coat blood samples or tissue specimens by a shell-vial technique is seldom attempted because of biohazard concerns. PCR detects *C. burnetii* DNA in tissues, including paraffin-embedded tissues. Serology is the most commonly used diagnostic tool. Indirect immunofluorescence is sensitive and specific and is the method of choice. Rheumatoid factor should be adsorbed from the specimen before testing. An IgG titer of ≥1:800 to phase I antigen is suggestive of chronic Q fever. In chronic infection, the antibody titer to phase I antigen is usually much higher than that to phase II antigen; the reverse is true in acute infection, in which a fourfold rise in titer may be demonstrated between acute- and convalescent-phase serum samples.

Rx Q FEVER

Treatment of acute Q fever with doxycycline (100 mg twice daily for 14 days) is usually successful. Quinolones are also effective. When Q fever is diagnosed in a pregnant woman, treatment with trimethoprim-sulfamethoxazole is recommended for the duration of the pregnancy.

The treatment of chronic Q fever is difficult and requires careful follow-up. Addition of hydroxychloroquine (to alkalinize the phagolysosome) renders doxycycline bactericidal against *C. burnetii,* and this combination is currently the favored regimen. Treatment with doxycycline (100 mg bid) and hydroxychloroquine (200 mg tid; plasma concentration maintained at 0.8–1.2 μg/mL) for 18 months is superior to a regimen of doxycycline and ofloxacin. Optimal management of Q fever endocarditis entails determination of the minimal inhibitory concentration (MIC) of doxycycline for the patient's isolate and measurement of serum doxycycline levels. A serum level–to–doxycycline MIC ratio of ≥1 is associated with a rapid decline in phase I antibodies. Patients treated with this regimen must be advised about photosensitivity and retinal toxicity risks. The doxycycline-hydroxychloroquine regimen was successful in one patient with HIV infection and Q fever endocarditis. The Jarisch-Herxheimer reaction occasionally complicates the treatment of chronic Q fever.

Treatment of *C. burnetii*–infected aortic aneurysms is the same as that for Q fever endocarditis. Surgical intervention is often required.

If doxycycline-hydroxychloroquine cannot be used, the regimen should include at least two antibiotics active against *C. burnetii*. Rifampin (300 mg once daily) combined with doxycycline (100 mg twice daily) or ciprofloxacin (750 mg twice daily) has been used successfully. The optimal duration of antibiotic therapy for chronic Q fever remains undetermined. The authors recommend at least 3 years of treatment, with discontinuation only if the phase I IgA antibody titer is ≤1:50 and the IgG phase I titer is ≤1:200.

THERAPY WITH BIOLOGIC MODIFYING AGENTS Interferon γ was successful in the treatment of a 3-year-old boy with prolonged fever, abdominal pain, and thrombocytopenia due to *C. burnetii* that was not eradicated with conventional antibiotic therapy. Many patients with granulomatous hepatitis due to Q fever have a prolonged febrile illness that is unresponsive to antibiotics. For these individuals, treatment with prednisone (0.5 mg/kg) has resulted in defervescence within 2–15 days. After defervescence, the glucocorticoid dose is tapered over the next month.

Prevention A whole-cell vaccine (Q-Vax) licensed in Australia effectively prevents Q fever in abattoir workers. Before administration of the vaccine, skin testing with intradermal diluted *C. burnetii* vaccine is performed, serologic testing is undertaken, and a history of possible Q fever is sought. Vaccine is given only to patients with no history of Q fever and negative results in serologic and skin tests.

Good animal-husbandry practices are important in preventing widespread contamination of the environment by *C. burnetii*. These practices include isolating aborting animals for up to 14 days, raising feed bunks to prevent contamination of feed by excreta, destroying aborted materials (i.e., burning and burying fetal membranes and stillborn animals), and wearing masks and gloves when handling aborted materials. Only seronegative pregnant animals should be used in research settings, and only seronegative animals should be permitted in petting zoos.

ACKNOWLEDGMENT
The contributions of Didier Raoult, MD, to this chapter in previous editions are gratefully acknowledged.

FURTHER READINGS

BLANCO JR et al (eds): *Century of Rickettsiology: Emerging, Reemerging Rickettsioses, Molecular Diagnostics, and Emerging Veterinary Rickettsioses.* Malden, MA, Blackwell Scientific, 2006

CHAPMAN AS et al: Diagnosis and management of tickborne rickettsial diseases: Rocky Mountain spotted fever, ehrlichioses, and anaplasmosis—United States. MMWR 55:1, 2006

DUMLER JS: *Anaplasma* and *Ehrlichia* infection. Ann NY Acad Sci 1063:361, 2005

MCQUISTON JH et al: National surveillance and the epidemiology of Q fever in the United States, 1978–2004. Am J Trop Med Hyg 75:36, 2006

RAOULT D et al: Q fever 1985–1998. Clinical and epidemiologic features of 1,383 infections. Medicine (Baltimore) 79:109, 2000

WALKER DH: Rickettsiae and rickettsial infections: The current state of knowledge. Clin Infect Dis 45(Suppl1):539, 2007

168 Infections Due to Mycoplasmas

William M. McCormack

Mycoplasmas, the smallest free-living organisms known, are prokaryotes that are bounded only by a plasma membrane. Their lack of a cell wall is associated with cellular pleomorphism and resistance to cell wall–active antimicrobial agents, such as penicillins and cephalosporins. The organisms' small genome limits biosynthesis and explains the difficulties encountered with in vitro cultivation. Mycoplasmas typically colonize mucosal surfaces of the respiratory and urogenital tracts of many animal species. Of the 17 species of mycoplasmas recovered from humans, most are commensals. *Mycoplasma pneumoniae* causes upper and lower respiratory tract infections. *M. genitalium* and ureaplasmas are established causes of urethritis and have been implicated in other genital conditions. *M. hominis* and ureaplasmas are part of the complex microbial flora of bacterial vaginosis (Chap. 124). The two biovars of *Ureaplasma*, previously classified together as *U. urealyticum*, have recently been separated into two species: *U. parvum* and *U. urealyticum*.

MECHANISMS OF PATHOGENICITY

Adherence of mycoplasmas to the surface of the host cell is necessary for colonization and infection. Some pathogenic mycoplasmas are flask-shaped, with specialized tips that enhance adherence. *M. pneumoniae* adheres via a network of interactive adhesins and accessory proteins and produces hydrogen peroxide, which may cause injury to host cells. *M. hominis* metabolizes arginine, with the production of potentially cytotoxic amounts of ammonia. Ureaplasmas have been placed in a separate genus because of their unique urease activity; the metabolism of urea also produces ammonia. *M. pneumoniae* may evoke IgM autoantibodies that agglutinate human erythrocytes at 4°C. These cold agglutinins can cause anemia and other complications.

MYCOPLASMA PNEUMONIAE

Epidemiology *M. pneumoniae* causes upper and lower respiratory tract symptoms in all age groups, with the highest attack rates in 5- to 20-year-olds. Infection with *M. pneumoniae* is acquired by inhalation of aerosols. The incubation period is 2–3 weeks, considerably longer than that of most other respiratory infections. Although epidemics have taken place in closed populations, such as those at schools and military installations, most cases occur sporadically or in families. Cases in families typically occur serially and are separated by 2- to 3-week intervals. Infections in adults are often the result of contact with children.

Infection with *M. pneumoniae* occurs worldwide and year round, with epidemics every few years. Some studies have noted an increase in the number of cases during the autumn months in temperate climates. Although pneumonia is the classic presentation, nonpneumonic infection is considerably more common. In very young children, most infections result only in upper respiratory symptoms, whereas children >5 years of age and adults may have bronchitis and pneumonia.

Clinical Presentation After the prolonged incubation period, fever and constitutional symptoms develop along with headache and cough, both of which can be prominent and distressing. Symptoms typically progress less rapidly than those of viral respiratory tract infections. In the minority (perhaps 5–10%) of infected individuals who develop tracheobronchitis or pneumonia, cough becomes more prominent. Sputum, if produced at all, is usually white and may be tinged with blood. The temperature seldom rises above 38.9°–39.4°C (102°–103°F). Shaking chills, myalgias, and gastrointestinal symptoms (e.g., nausea, vomiting, and diarrhea) are unusual. Chest muscle soreness may result from frequent and prolonged coughing, but true pleuritic pain is uncommon.

Pharyngeal injection is often noted. Cervical lymph node enlargement is unusual. Ear pain due to bullous myringitis (blisters on the tympanic membrane) is a unique but uncommon manifestation. As in other "atypical" pneumonias, findings on auscultation of the lung may be normal or nearly normal despite striking radiographic abnormalities. Pleural effusions develop in <20% of patients.

M. pneumoniae infection may be particularly severe in patients who have sickle cell disease and other hemoglobin S–related hemoglobinopathies. The functional asplenia seen in sickle cell disease may contribute to severe disease as it does in pneumococcal infection. Severe respiratory distress and large pleural effusions may occur.

Extrapulmonary Manifestations A broad array of extrapulmonary abnormalities have been associated with *M. pneumoniae* infection (Table 168-1). Although these events are unusual, they complicate other respiratory diseases even more rarely and often provide the only clue that an otherwise-unremarkable respiratory infection may be mycoplasmal. Erythema multiforme (Stevens-Johnson syndrome; see Fig. 52-9) typically occurs in young male patients with *M. pneumoniae* infection. Digital necrosis has been seen in patients with sickle cell disease who develop very high titers of cold agglutinins. Arthralgias are not unusual in patients who have mycoplasmal pneumonia; mycoplasmal arthritis is rare except in patients who have hypogammaglobulinemia.

The pathogenesis of the extrapulmonary manifestations of *M. pneumoniae* infection is controversial. Occasional reports have described the identification of *M. pneumoniae* or its nucleic acids in involved tissues. The fact that most attempts at detection have yielded negative results, however, suggests that these extrapulmonary complications have an immunologic basis.

Diagnosis Most infections with *M. pneumoniae* are not diagnosed, as they are indistinguishable from upper and lower respiratory tract infections caused by myriad other viral and bacterial pathogens. When the diagnosis is suspected, it is usually because illness is prolonged or extrapulmonary manifestations develop. The white blood cell count is generally somewhat elevated, with few immature cells. Gram's staining of sputum shows leukocytes without a predominance of any bacterial morphologic type. Since *M. pneumoniae* lacks a cell wall, it cannot be detected on Gram's stain. In patients who have pneumonia, the chest radiograph may show reticulonodular or interstitial infiltration, primarily in the lower lobes. As in other "atypical" pneumonias, radiographic abnormalities may be more prominent than would be predicted by auscultation of the chest.

M. pneumoniae can be grown on artificial media, but the process is exacting, requires special media, and takes upwards of 2 weeks. Thus, mycoplasmal cultures do not provide timely information to aid in patient management. The same, unfortunately, is true of serologic diagnosis. Specific antibodies can be detected by enzyme-linked immunoassays, indirect immunofluorescence, or complement fixation but do not develop early enough to guide decisions regarding treatment. As with most serologic tests, examination of paired acute- and convalescent-phase serum specimens is required for good sensitivity and specificity.

TABLE 168-1 EXTRAPULMONARY MANIFESTATIONS OF *MYCOPLASMA PNEUMONIAE* INFECTION

System	Manifestations
Dermatologic	Erythema multiforme Maculopapular exanthems Vesicular exanthems Erythema nodosum Urticaria
Cardiovascular	Myocarditis Pericarditis
Neurologic	Encephalitis Aseptic meningitis Cerebellar ataxia Guillain-Barré syndrome Transverse myelitis Polyradiculopathy
Rheumatologic	Arthralgias Arthritis Juvenile-onset spondyloarthropathy
Hematologic	Hemolytic anemia Coagulopathies

Cold agglutinins are nonspecific but develop within the first 7–10 days in more than half of patients with *M. pneumoniae* pneumonia and may be detectable when the patient presents to a health care provider. In a patient with a compatible clinical picture, a cold agglutinin titer of ≥1:32 supports the diagnosis of mycoplasmal pneumonia. Cold agglutinin determinations are readily available from diagnostic laboratories. The test can also be performed at the bedside by the addition of 1 mL of the patient's blood to a tube containing anticoagulant (e.g., a tube used to collect blood for determination of prothrombin activity). Before cooling, the nonaggregated red blood cells coat the sides of the inverted tube. The blood is cooled to 4°C when the tube is placed in an ice bath for 3–5 min or in a standard refrigerator. In a positive test, clumps of red blood cells can be observed when the tube is inverted. Rewarming of the sample to 37°C in an incubator or by exposure to body heat should reverse the agglutination. A positive "bedside" cold agglutinin test is equivalent to a laboratory titer of ≥1:64.

The lack of sensitive, specific, and timely diagnostic tests has prompted the development of a variety of antigen detection tests (e.g., nucleic acid amplification) that do not involve serology or the cultivation of live organisms. Since many viral and bacterial infections result in clinical presentations similar to that caused by *M. pneumoniae*, examination of specimens for single antigens is unlikely to be useful. Multiplex nucleic acid amplification tests that examine a single throat swab or sputum sample for the most likely causative microorganisms have been developed. Such tests may provide more precise etiologic diagnosis of upper and lower respiratory tract infections.

℞ PNEUMONIA CAUSED BY *M. PNEUMONIAE*

Pneumonia due to *M. pneumoniae* is usually self-limited and is seldom life-threatening. Effective antimicrobial agents do shorten the duration of illness and, by reducing coughing, may conceivably render the patient less infectious. Although symptoms are alleviated by antimicrobial treatment, the organism usually is not eradicated. Cultures positive for *M. pneumoniae* may persist for months despite clinically effective antimicrobial therapy. The beneficial effects, if any, of such treatment on extrapulmonary manifestations of *M. pneumoniae* infection are unknown.

Because most mycoplasmal infections are not specifically diagnosed, management is directed at one of two syndromes: upper respiratory tract infection or community-acquired pneumonia. Upper respiratory infections, whether caused by viruses or by *M. pneumoniae*, do not require antimicrobial treatment. Community-acquired pneumonia (Chap. 251) may be caused by bacteria such as *Streptococcus pneumoniae* and *Haemophilus influenzae* or by "atypical" agents such as *Chlamydophila pneumoniae*, *Legionella pneumophila*, and *M. pneumoniae*. Recommended treatment regimens are detailed in **Tables 168-2** and **168-3**. Treatment of documented *M. pneumoniae* pneumonia is usually continued for 14–21 days.

GENITAL MYCOPLASMAS (See also Chap. 124)

Epidemiology *M. hominis*, *U. urealyticum*, and *U. parvum* are the most prevalent genital mycoplasmas. Infants may become colonized with these organisms during passage through a colonized birth canal.

TABLE 168-2 ORAL ANTIMICROBIAL AGENTS FOR THE TREATMENT OF AMBULATORY PATIENTS WITH COMMUNITY-ACQUIRED PNEUMONIA

Agent	Dose and Schedule
Doxycycline	100 mg bid
Erythromycin	500 mg qid
Clarithromycin	500 mg bid
Azithromycin	500 mg qd
Levofloxacin	750 mg qd
Moxifloxacin	400 mg qd
Gemifloxacin	320 mg qd

Note: Treatment of documented *M. pneumoniae* pneumonia is usually continued for 14–21 days.

TABLE 168-3 ANTIMICROBIAL AGENTS FOR THE TREATMENT OF HOSPITALIZED PATIENTS WITH COMMUNITY-ACQUIRED PNEUMONIA

1. Intravenous ceftriaxone (1.0 g/d) *or*
   Intravenous cefotaxime (1.0 g q8h) *or*
   Intravenous ampicillin/sulbactam (1.5–3.0 g q6h)
   plus
   Intravenous or oral erythromycin (500 mg qid) *or*
   Intravenous or oral azithromycin (500 mg qd) *or*
   Oral clarithromycin (500 mg bid)
2. Intravenous or oral levofloxacin (750 mg qd)
3. Intravenous or oral moxifloxacin (400 mg qd)

Note: Treatment of documented *M. pneumoniae* pneumonia is usually continued for 14–21 days.

Neonatal colonization tends not to persist. Only ~10% of prepubertal girls and even fewer prepubertal boys are colonized with ureaplasmas. After puberty, colonization occurs mainly as a result of sexual activity. Among adults, disadvantaged populations have higher colonization rates. Ureaplasmas can be cultured from the vaginas of ~80% of women cared for in public clinics and about half of women cared for by private obstetricians and gynecologists. Similarly, vaginal *M. hominis* is found in ~50% of women attending public clinics and in ~20% of private patients. Men have somewhat lower rates of genital colonization than women. In short, *U. urealyticum*, *U. parvum*, and *M. hominis* are frequently detected in genital specimens from healthy, sexually experienced adults. Evaluation of the role of these organisms in human disease must take into account their high prevalence among healthy people.

M. fermentans colonizes both the respiratory and genital tracts in >20% of adults. There is no convincing evidence that *M. fermentans* causes human disease. *M. genitalium* is a fastidious organism that is difficult to cultivate. Polymerase chain reaction (PCR) studies have identified the organism more successfully.

Association with Human Disease • ***NONGONOCOCCAL URETHRITIS (NGU)*** Although *Chlamydia trachomatis* is the organism most firmly implicated in the etiology of NGU, there is no doubt that sexually transmitted ureaplasmas and *M. genitalium* also cause some cases. The ubiquity of ureaplasmas among men who do not have urethritis and the difficulty of identifying *M. genitalium* do not allow precise estimation of the proportion of cases of NGU caused by each of these mycoplasmas.

EPIDIDYMITIS AND PROSTATITIS Ureaplasmas may be an occasional cause of epididymitis. *M. hominis* has not been implicated in this disease. Neither organism has been convincingly associated with prostatitis.

PELVIC INFLAMMATORY DISEASE (PID) *M. hominis* and ureaplasmas are prominent components of the complex microbial flora of bacterial vaginosis. Since bacterial vaginosis is associated with PID, it is difficult to determine whether these organisms play an independent role in this condition. Although *M. genitalium* is not associated with bacterial vaginosis, preliminary studies have linked it to cervicitis, PID, and tubal factor infertility in women who are not infected with either *Neisseria gonorrhoeae* or *C. trachomatis*.

DISORDERS OF REPRODUCTION Ureaplasmas have been considered as causes of involuntary infertility in both men and women, but there is no convincing evidence for such an association. These organisms have been associated with chorioamnionitis and preterm birth. Given the close association of ureaplasmas with bacterial vaginosis, a condition that is strongly associated with chorioamnionitis and preterm birth, it is difficult to define an independent role for ureaplasmas in these conditions. In infants of very low birth weight, ureaplasmas have been shown to cause pneumonia and long-term respiratory dysfunction. *M. hominis* can cause postpartum fever, which has been associated with isolation of this organism from blood and its occasional dissemination to joints, resulting in septic arthritis.

EXTRAGENITAL INFECTIONS Sexually acquired reactive arthritis and Reiter's syndrome may be triggered by ureaplasmas, although *C. trachomatis* is the usual triggering agent. Patients who have hypogammaglobulinemia may develop chronic arthritis due to ureaplasmas and some other mycoplasmal species. *M. hominis* has been identified in patients with post-thoracotomy sternal wound infection and in rare instances of prosthetic heart valve and prosthetic joint infection.

Diagnosis There is seldom any reason to examine specimens from the lower genital tract (vagina, male urethra) for mycoplasmas. The ubiquity of the organisms among healthy individuals makes a positive result uninterpretable. The organisms should be sought only in specimens from normally sterile areas, such as joint fluid with evidence of inflammation and cultures negative for conventional microorganisms.

M. hominis can replicate in many routine blood culture media without changing the appearance of the media. Although the organism forms nonhemolytic pinpoint colonies on blood agar, it cannot be visualized in gram-stained smears of these colonies. Neither ureaplasmas nor *M. genitalium* will grow in ordinary microbiologic media.

Microbiologic diagnosis of genital mycoplasmal infection requires specially prepared media and is beyond the capability of all but reference and research laboratories. Nucleic acid amplification tests such as PCR have been developed.

℞ GENITAL MYCOPLASMAS

Ureaplasmas, *M. genitalium*, and *M. hominis* are usually susceptible to tetracyclines (e.g., doxycycline). Infections caused by tetracycline-resistant ureaplasmas can be treated with erythromycin, while those due to tetracycline-resistant strains of *M. hominis* respond to treatment with clindamycin. As noted above, a specific microbiologic diagnosis of mycoplasmal infection is seldom made. Appropriate treatment provides antimicrobial coverage for the organisms that cause the particular syndrome. Accordingly, NGU is treated with doxycycline (100 mg orally twice a day for 7 days) or azithromycin (1.0 g as a single oral dose) to provide activity against *C. trachomatis, U. urealyticum, U. parvum*, and *M. genitalium*. Recommended regimens for the treatment of PID provide antimicrobial activity against gonococci, chlamydiae, and anaerobes as well as genital mycoplasmas.

FURTHER READINGS

ALEXANDER ER et al: Pneumonia due to *Mycoplasma pneumoniae*. N Engl J Med 275:131, 1966

MANDELL LA et al: Update of practice guidelines for the management of community-acquired pneumonia in immunocompetent adults. Clin Infect Dis 37:1405, 2003

MOROZUMI M et al: Simultaneous detection of pathogens in clinical samples from patients with community-acquired pneumonia by real-time PCR with pathogen-specific molecular beacon probes. J Clin Microbiol 44:1440, 2006

MURRAY HW et al: The protean manifestations of *Mycoplasma pneumoniae* in adults. Am J Med 58:229, 1975

TAYLOR SN: *Mycoplasma genitalium*. Curr Infect Dis Rep 7:453, 2005

WAITES KB et al: Mycoplasmas and ureaplasmas as neonatal pathogens. Clin Microbiol Rev 18:757, 2005

169 Chlamydial Infections

Walter E. Stamm

Three chlamydial species cause human infections: *Chlamydia trachomatis, Chlamydophila psittaci*, and *Chlamydophila pneumoniae. C. psittaci* is widely distributed in nature, producing genital, conjunctival, intestinal, or respiratory infections in many mammalian and avian species. Genital infections with *C. psittaci* have been well characterized in several species and cause abortion and infertility. Although mammalian strains of *C. psittaci* are not known to infect humans, avian strains occasionally do so, causing pneumonia and the systemic illness known as *psittacosis. C. pneumoniae* is a fastidious chlamydial species that appears to be a common cause of upper respiratory tract infection and pneumonia, primarily in children and young adults, and is a cause of recurrent respiratory infections in older adults. Studies have also linked *C. pneumoniae* infection to atherosclerotic cardiovascular disease and perhaps to asthma. No animal reservoir has been identified for *C. pneumoniae*; it appears to be an exclusively human pathogen spread via the respiratory route through close personal contact. *C. trachomatis* is also an exclusively human pathogen and was identified as the cause of trachoma in the 1940s. Since then, *C. trachomatis* has been recognized as a major cause of sexually transmitted and perinatal infection.

Chlamydiae are obligate intracellular bacteria that are classified in their own order, Chlamydiales (Fig. 169-1). They possess both DNA and RNA, have a cell wall and ribosomes similar to those of gram-negative bacteria, and are inhibited by antibiotics such as tetracycline. A unique feature of all chlamydiae is their complex reproductive cycle (Fig. 169-2). Two forms of the microorganism—the extracellular elementary body (EB) and the intracellular reticulate body (RB)—participate in this cycle. The EB is adapted for extracellular survival and is the infective form transmitted from one person to another. EBs attach to susceptible target cells (usually columnar or transitional epithelial cells) and enter the cells inside a phagosome. Within 8 h of cell entry, the EBs reorganize into RBs, which are adapted to intracellular survival and multiplication. They undergo binary fission, eventually producing numerous replicates contained within the intracellular membrane-bound "inclusion body," which occupies much of the infected host cell. Chlamydial inclusions resist lysosomal fusion until late in the developmental cycle. After 24 h, the RBs condense and form EBs still

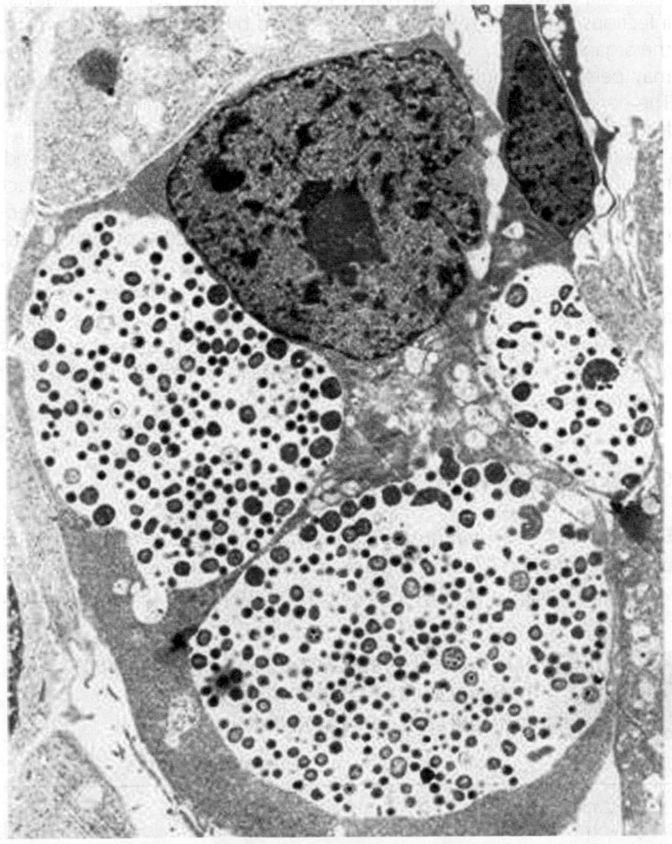

FIGURE 169-1 Chlamydial intracellular inclusions filled with smaller dense elementary bodies and larger reticulate bodies.

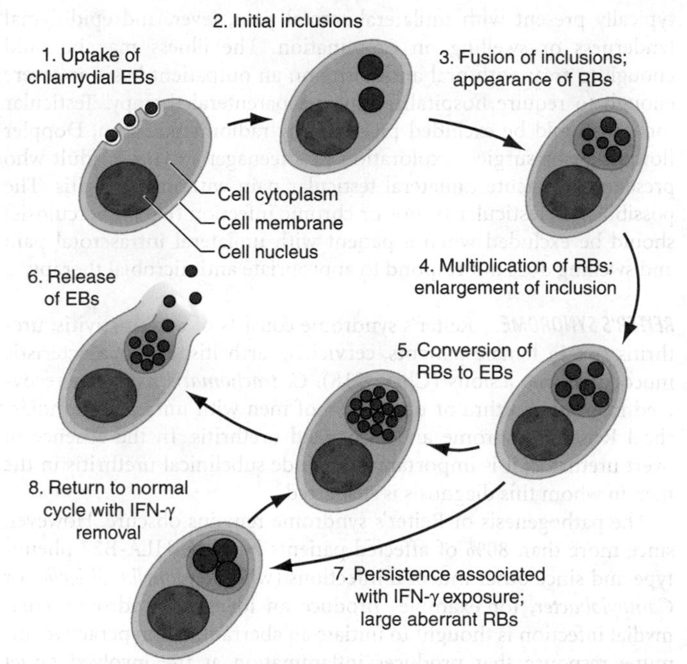

FIGURE 169-2 Chlamydial life cycle. EBs, elementary bodies; RBs, reticulate bodies; IFN-γ, interferon γ.

contained within the inclusion. The inclusion then lyses, releasing EBs from the cell to initiate infection of adjacent cells or transmission to another person. Under some conditions [e.g., exposure to interferon γ (IFN-γ) or antibiotics], an altered life cycle is induced in which large, metabolically inactive RBs persist but do not replicate. Removal of the IFN-γ or antibiotics is followed by restoration of the normal life cycle.

Studies with monoclonal antibodies and nucleotide sequencing of the major outer-membrane protein have delineated at least 20 serotypes of *C. trachomatis*. According to the classification of Wang and Grayston, strains associated with trachoma are generally of the A, B, Ba, and C serovars, while serovars D through K are largely associated with sexually transmitted and perinatally acquired infections. Serovars L_1, L_2, and L_3 produce lymphogranuloma venereum (LGV) and hemorrhagic proctocolitis. The LGV strains exhibit unique biologic behavior in that they are more invasive than the other serovars, produce disease in lymphatic tissue, grow readily in cell culture systems and macrophages, and are lethal when inoculated intracerebrally into mice and monkeys. Non-LGV strains of *C. trachomatis* characteristically produce infections involving the superficial columnar epithelium of the eye, genitalia, and respiratory tract.

C. trachomatis is an infrequent cause of endocarditis, peritonitis, pleuritis, and possibly periappendicitis and occasionally causes respiratory infections in older children and adults. Some immunosuppressed patients with pneumonia have had either serologic or cultural evidence of *C. trachomatis* infection, but more data are necessary to define a pathogenic role for this organism in these patients.

C. TRACHOMATIS INFECTIONS

GENITAL INFECTIONS

Genital infections caused by *C. trachomatis* represent the most common bacterial sexually transmitted infections (STIs) in the United States (Chap. 124). An estimated 4 million cases occur each year. In adults, the clinical spectrum of sexually transmitted *C. trachomatis* infections parallels that of gonococcal infections. Both infections have been associated with urethritis, proctitis, and conjunctivitis in both sexes; with epididymitis in men; and with mucopurulent cervicitis (MPC), acute salpingitis, bartholinitis, and the Fitz-Hugh–Curtis syndrome (perihepatitis) in women. Moreover, both infections can be associated with septic arthritis. In general, however, chlamydial infections produce fewer symptoms and signs than gonococcal infections at the same anatomic site; in fact, chlamydial infections are often totally asymptomatic. Increasing evidence suggests that many chlamydial infections of the genital tract, especially in women, persist for months without producing symptoms. Simultaneous infection with *C. trachomatis* often occurs in women with cervical gonococcal infection and in heterosexual men with gonococcal urethritis.

Epidemiology Infections due to *C. trachomatis* have been reportable in the United States since 1985, and national incidence data show steadily rising numbers of reported infections, probably reflecting both increased testing and increased reporting more than increasing incidence. Most testing to date has focused on women, and thus the reported incidence is severalfold greater among women than among men; this difference likely represents a surveillance artifact.

The age of peak incidence of genital *C. trachomatis* infections, as of other STIs, is the late teens and early twenties. The prevalence of chlamydial urethral infection among young men is at least 3–5% for those seen in general medical settings or in urban high schools and is >10% for asymptomatic soldiers undergoing routine physical examination; 15–20% of heterosexual men seen in sexually transmitted disease (STD) clinics may be positive for *C. trachomatis*. In areas where chlamydial control programs have been implemented, the overall prevalence may be markedly reduced. In short, the prevalence among men varies widely with the population group studied and with the geographic locale. With the newer, more sensitive nucleic acid amplification tests (NAATs), such as polymerase chain reaction (PCR) and transcription-mediated amplification (TMA), prevalences in most populations have been 10–30% higher than those measured with older, less sensitive tests.

The prevalence of cervical infection among women is ~5% for asymptomatic college students and prenatal patients in the United States, >10% for women seen in family planning clinics, and >20% for women seen in STD clinics. As in men, the prevalence of genital *C. trachomatis* infections varies substantially by geographic locale, with the highest rates in the southeastern United States. However, substantial prevalences (~8%) of asymptomatic chlamydial infection have been demonstrated among young female military recruits from all parts of the United States. In this country, the prevalence of *C. trachomatis* in the cervix of pregnant women is 5–10 times higher than that of *Neisseria gonorrhoeae*. The prevalence of genital infection with either agent is highest among individuals who are between the ages of 18 and 24, single, and non-Caucasian (e.g., African-American or Latino). Recurrent chlamydial infections occur frequently in these same risk groups and are often acquired from untreated sexual partners. Use of oral contraceptive pills and the presence of cervical ectopy also confer an increased risk of chlamydial infection. The proportion of infections that are asymptomatic appears to be higher for *C. trachomatis* than for *N. gonorrhoeae*, and symptomatic *C. trachomatis* infections are clinically less severe. Mild or asymptomatic chlamydial infections of the fallopian tubes nonetheless cause ongoing tubal damage and infertility. Furthermore, because the total number of *C. trachomatis* infections exceeds the total number of *N. gonorrhoeae* infections in industrialized countries, the total morbidity caused by *C. trachomatis* genital infections in these countries exceeds that caused by *N. gonorrhoeae*. The prevalence of *C. trachomatis* is higher than that of *N. gonorrhoeae* in industrialized countries, in part because measures such as treatment of sex partners and routine cultures for case detection in asymptomatic individuals have been applied much longer and more effectively to the control of gonorrhea than to the control of *C. trachomatis* infection.

Pathogenesis *C. trachomatis* preferentially infects the columnar epithelium of the eye and the respiratory and genital tracts. The infection induces an immune response but often persists for months or years in the absence of antimicrobial therapy. Serious sequelae often occur in association with repeated or persistent infections. The precise mechanism through which repeated or persistent infection elicits an inflammatory response that leads to tubal scarring and damage in the female upper genital tract is not yet clear. One antigen, the chlamydial 60-kDa heat-shock protein, may be involved in inducing a pathologic immune response or may elicit antibodies that cross-react with human heat-shock proteins. Several complete chlamydial genomes have been sequenced, and genetic studies may soon offer further insights into the pathogenic mechanisms of *C. trachomatis.*

Clinical Manifestations • ***NONGONOCOCCAL AND POSTGONOCOCCAL URETHRITIS*** Nongonococcal urethritis (NGU) is a diagnosis of exclusion that is applied to men with symptoms and/or signs of urethritis who do not have gonorrhea. Postgonococcal urethritis (PGU) refers to NGU developing in men 2–3 weeks after treatment of gonococcal urethritis with single doses of agents such as penicillins or cephalosporins that lack antimicrobial activity against chlamydiae. Since current treatment regimens for gonorrhea include tetracycline, doxycycline, or azithromycin for possible concomitant chlamydial infection, both the incidence of PGU and the causative role of chlamydiae in this syndrome have declined. *C. trachomatis* causes 20–40% of cases of NGU in heterosexual men but is less commonly isolated from homosexual men with this syndrome. The cause of most of the remaining cases of NGU is uncertain; considerable evidence suggests that *Ureaplasma urealyticum* and *Mycoplasma genitalium* cause many cases of NGU, while *Trichomonas vaginalis* and herpes simplex virus (HSV) cause some cases.

NGU is diagnosed by documentation of a leukocytic urethral exudate and by exclusion of gonorrhea by Gram's staining or culture. *C. trachomatis* urethritis is generally less severe than gonococcal urethritis, although in an individual patient these two forms of urethritis cannot be reliably differentiated solely on clinical grounds. Symptoms include urethral discharge (often whitish and mucoid rather than frankly purulent), dysuria, and urethral itching. Physical examination may reveal meatal erythema and tenderness and a urethral exudate that is often demonstrable only by stripping of the urethra.

At least one-third of males with *C. trachomatis* urethral infection have no demonstrable signs or symptoms of urethritis. Use of NAATs on first-void urine specimens to diagnose chlamydial infections in men has facilitated broader-based testing for asymptomatic infection in males. As a result, asymptomatic chlamydial urethritis has been demonstrated in 5–10% of sexually active adolescent males screened in school-based clinics or community centers. Such patients generally have first-glass pyuria (≥15 leukocytes per 400× microscopic field in the sediment of first-void urine), a positive leukocyte esterase test, or an increased number of leukocytes on a Gram-stained smear prepared from a urogenital swab inserted 1–2 cm into the anterior urethra. For the enumeration of leukocytes, the smear is first scanned at low power to identify areas of the slide containing the highest concentration of leukocytes. These areas are then examined under oil immersion (1000×). An average of four or more leukocytes in at least three of five 1000× oil-immersion fields is indicative of urethritis and correlates with the recovery of *C. trachomatis.* To differentiate between true urethritis and functional symptoms among symptomatic patients or to make a presumptive diagnosis of *C. trachomatis* infection in "high-risk" but asymptomatic men (e.g., male patients in STD clinics, sex partners of women with nongonococcal salpingitis or MPC, fathers of children with inclusion conjunctivitis), the examination of an endourethral specimen for increased leukocytes is useful if specific diagnostic tests for chlamydiae are not available. Alternatively, urethritis can be assayed noninvasively by examination of a first-void urine sample for pyuria, either by microscopy or by the leukocyte esterase test. Urine (or a urethral swab) can also be directly tested for chlamydiae or gonococci by DNA amplification methods, as described below.

EPIDIDYMITIS *C. trachomatis* is the foremost cause of epididymitis in sexually active heterosexual men <35 years of age, accounting for ~70% of cases. *N. gonorrhoeae* causes most of the remaining cases, and some men have simultaneous infections with both pathogens, usually accompanied by asymptomatic urethritis as defined above. In homosexual men, sexually transmitted coliform infection acquired via insertive rectal intercourse may cause epididymitis. Coliform bacteria and *Pseudomonas aeruginosa*, usually detected in association with preceding urologic instrumentation or surgery, are the most common causes of epididymitis in men over 35. Men with chlamydial epididymitis typically present with unilateral scrotal pain, fever, and epididymal tenderness or swelling on examination. The illness may be mild enough to treat with oral antibiotics on an outpatient basis or severe enough to require hospitalization and parenteral therapy. Testicular torsion should be excluded promptly by radionuclide scan, Doppler flow study, or surgical exploration in a teenager or young adult who presents with acute unilateral testicular pain without urethritis. The possibility of testicular tumor or chronic infection (e.g., tuberculosis) should be excluded when a patient with unilateral intrascrotal pain and swelling does not respond to appropriate antimicrobial therapy.

REITER'S SYNDROME Reiter's syndrome consists of conjunctivitis, urethritis (or, in female patients, cervicitis), arthritis, and characteristic mucocutaneous lesions (Chap. 318). *C. trachomatis* has been recovered from the urethra of up to 70% of men with untreated nondiarrheal Reiter's syndrome and associated urethritis. In the absence of overt urethritis, it is important to exclude subclinical urethritis in the men in whom this diagnosis is suspected.

The pathogenesis of Reiter's syndrome remains obscure. However, since more than 80% of affected patients have the HLA-B27 phenotype and since other mucosal infections (with *Salmonella*, *Shigella*, or *Campylobacter*, for example) produce an identical syndrome, chlamydial infection is thought to initiate an aberrant and hyperactive immune response that produces inflammation at the involved target organs in these genetically predisposed individuals. Evidence of exaggerated cell-mediated and humoral immune responses to chlamydial antigens in Reiter's syndrome supports this hypothesis. The presumptive demonstration of chlamydial EBs and chlamydial DNA in the joint fluid and synovial tissue of patients with Reiter's syndrome suggests that chlamydiae may actually spread from genital to joint tissues in these patients, perhaps in macrophages.

PROCTITIS *C. trachomatis* strains of either the genital immunotypes D through K or the LGV immunotypes cause proctitis in homosexual men who practice receptive anorectal intercourse. In the United States, the vast majority of cases are due to immunotypes D through K and present either as asymptomatic infection or as mild proctitis not unlike gonococcal proctitis. These infections may develop in heterosexual women as well. Patients present with mild rectal pain, mucous discharge, tenesmus, and (occasionally) bleeding. Nearly all have neutrophils in Gram-stained rectal samples. Anoscopy in these non-LGV cases of chlamydial proctitis reveals mild, patchy mucosal friability and mucopurulent discharge, and the disease process is limited to the distal rectum. LGV strains produce more severe ulcerative proctitis or proctocolitis that can be confused clinically with HSV proctitis (severe rectal pain, rectal bleeding, discharge, and tenesmus) and that histologically resembles Crohn's disease in that giant cell formation and granulomas can be seen (Chap. 289). In the United States, these cases of LGV proctitis occur almost exclusively in homosexual men, many of whom are positive for HIV.

MUCOPURULENT CERVICITIS Although many women with *C. trachomatis* infection of the cervix have no symptoms or signs, a careful speculum examination reveals evidence of MPC in 30–50% of cases. As is discussed more fully in Chap. 124, MPC is associated with yellow mucopurulent endocervical discharge and with ≥20 neutrophils per 1000× microscopic field within strands of cervical mucus on a thinly smeared, Gram-stained preparation of endocervical exudate. Other characteristic findings include edema of the zone of cervical ectopy and a propensity of the mucosa to bleed on minor trauma—e.g., when specimens are collected with a swab. A Pap smear shows increased numbers of neutrophils as well as a characteristic pattern of mononuclear inflammatory cells, including plasma cells, transformed lymphocytes, and histiocytes. Cervical biopsy shows a predominantly mononuclear cell infiltrate of the subepithelial stroma, often with follicular cervicitis.

PELVIC INFLAMMATORY DISEASE (See also Chap. 124) In the United States, *C. trachomatis* has been identified in the fallopian tubes or endometrium of up to 50% of women with pelvic inflammatory disease

(PID), and its role as an important etiologic agent in this syndrome is well accepted. PID occurs via ascending intraluminal spread of *C. trachomatis* from the lower genital tract. MPC is thus followed by endometritis, endosalpingitis, and finally pelvic peritonitis. Evidence of MPC is usually found in women with laparoscopically verified salpingitis. Similarly, endometritis, demonstrated by endometrial biopsy showing plasma cell infiltration of the endometrial epithelium, is documented in most women with laparoscopically verified chlamydial (or gonococcal) salpingitis. Chlamydial endometritis can also occur in the absence of clinical evidence of salpingitis: ~40–50% of women with MPC have plasma cell endometritis. Histologic evidence of endometritis has been correlated with an "endometritis syndrome" consisting of vaginal bleeding, lower abdominal pain, and uterine tenderness in the absence of adnexal tenderness. Chlamydial salpingitis produces milder symptoms than does gonococcal salpingitis and may be associated with less marked adnexal tenderness. Thus mild adnexal or uterine tenderness in sexually active women with cervicitis suggests PID.

Infertility associated with fallopian-tube scarring has been strongly linked to antecedent *C. trachomatis* infection in serologic studies. Since many infertile women with tubal scarring and antichlamydial antibody have no history of PID, it appears that subclinical tubal infection ("silent salpingitis") may produce scarring. Studies in animals and humans with salpingitis and tubal scarring suggest the continuing presence of persistent, slowly replicating chlamydial infection in tubal tissue. While the pathogenesis of *C. trachomatis*–induced tubal scarring remains poorly understood, antibodies to the chlamydial 60-kDa heat-shock protein have been correlated with tubal infertility, ectopic pregnancy, and Fitz-Hugh–Curtis syndrome (see below). Thus this antigen may initiate an immune-mediated process that ultimately damages the fallopian tube. Host genetic susceptibility, as defined by HLA type, may also play an important role.

Perihepatitis, or the Fitz-Hugh–Curtis syndrome, was originally described as a complication of gonococcal PID. The syndrome should be suspected whenever a young, sexually active woman presents with an illness resembling cholecystitis (fever and right-upper-quadrant pain of subacute or acute onset). Symptoms and signs of salpingitis may be minimal. Cultural and/or serologic evidence of *C. trachomatis* infection is found in three-quarters of women with this syndrome.

URETHRAL SYNDROME IN WOMEN In the absence of infection with uropathogens such as coliforms or *Staphylococcus saprophyticus*, *C. trachomatis* is the pathogen most commonly isolated from college women with dysuria, frequency, and pyuria (Chap. 282). This organism can also be isolated from the urethra of women without symptoms of urethritis, and up to 25% of female STD clinic patients with chlamydial urogenital infection have cultures positive for *C. trachomatis* from the urethra only.

INFECTION IN PREGNANCY AND THE NEONATAL PERIOD Studies in the United States have demonstrated that 5–25% of pregnant women have *C. trachomatis* infections of the cervix. In these studies, approximately one-half to two-thirds of children exposed during birth have acquired *C. trachomatis* infection. Roughly half of the infected infants (25% of the group exposed) have developed clinical evidence of inclusion conjunctivitis. In addition to infecting the eye, *C. trachomatis* has been isolated frequently and persistently from the nasopharynx, rectum, and vagina of such infants, occasionally for >1 year in the absence of treatment. Pneumonia develops in 10% of children infected perinatally, and otitis media may in some cases result from perinatally acquired chlamydial infection.

Neonatal chlamydial conjunctivitis has an acute onset 5–14 days after birth and often produces a profuse mucopurulent discharge. However, it is impossible to differentiate chlamydial conjunctivitis from other forms of neonatal conjunctivitis (such as that due to *N. gonorrhoeae*, *Haemophilus influenzae*, *Streptococcus pneumoniae*, or HSV) on clinical grounds; thus laboratory diagnosis is required. Inclusions within epithelial cells are often detected in Giemsa-stained conjunctival smears, but these smears are considerably less sensitive than cultures, antigen detection tests, or NAATs for chlamydiae. Gram-stained smears may show gonococci or occasional small gram-negative coccobacilli in *Haemophilus* conjunctivitis, but smears should be accompanied by cultures for these agents.

C. trachomatis causes a distinctive pneumonia syndrome in infants. Epidemiologic studies have linked chlamydial pulmonary infection in infants with increased occurrence of subacute lung disease (bronchitis, asthma, wheezing) in later childhood.

Lymphogranuloma Venereum • ***DEFINITION*** LGV is an STI caused by *C. trachomatis* strains of the L_1, L_2, and L_3 serovars. In the United States, most cases are caused by L_2 organisms. Classically, acute LGV is characterized by a transient primary genital lesion followed by multilocular suppurative regional lymphadenopathy. However, patients exposed via insertive rectal intercourse usually develop hemorrhagic proctitis with regional lymphadenitis. Acute LGV is almost always associated with systemic symptoms such as fever and leukocytosis but is rarely associated with systemic complications such as meningoencephalitis. Without treatment, late complications that develop after a period of years include genital elephantiasis due to lymphatic involvement; strictures; and fistulas of the penis, urethra, and rectum.

EPIDEMIOLOGY LGV is usually sexually transmitted, but occasional transmission by nonsexual personal contact, fomites, or laboratory accidents has been documented. Laboratory work involving the creation of aerosols of LGV organisms (e.g., sonication, homogenization) must be conducted only with appropriate measures for biologic containment.

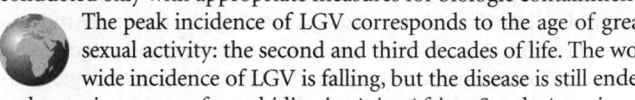

The peak incidence of LGV corresponds to the age of greatest sexual activity: the second and third decades of life. The worldwide incidence of LGV is falling, but the disease is still endemic and a major cause of morbidity in Asia, Africa, South America, and parts of the Caribbean. In the Bahamas, an apparent outbreak of LGV was described in association with a concurrent increase in heterosexual infection with HIV. For more than a decade, however, the reported incidence of LGV in the United States has been only 0.1 case per 100,000 persons. Recently, clusters of LGV cases have been described in the United States and in Western Europe, largely among men having sex with men. These cases have usually presented as hemorrhagic proctocolitis in HIV-positive men. More widespread use of NAATs for identification of rectal infections may have enhanced case recognition.

The frequency of infection following exposure is believed to be much lower for LGV than for gonorrhea and syphilis. Early manifestations are recognized more often in men than in women, who usually present with late complications. In the United States, where the reported male-to-female ratio of cases is 3.4:1, most cases involve homosexually active men and persons returning from abroad (travelers, sailors, and military personnel). The main reservoir of infection, although it has not been directly demonstrated, is presumed to be asymptomatically infected individuals.

CLINICAL MANIFESTATIONS A *primary genital lesion* develops 3 days to 3 weeks after exposure. It is a small, painless vesicle or nonindurated ulcer or papule located on the penis in men and on the labia, posterior vagina, or fourchette in women. The primary lesion is noticed by fewer than one-third of men with LGV and only rarely by women. It heals in a few days without scarring and, even when noticed, is usually recognized as LGV only in retrospect. LGV strains of *C. trachomatis* have occasionally been recovered from genital ulcers and from the urethra of men and the endocervix of women who present with inguinal adenopathy; these areas may be the primary site of infection in some cases.

Primary anal or *rectal infection* develops after receptive anorectal intercourse. In women, rectal infection with LGV (or non-LGV) strains of *C. trachomatis* presumably can also arise by the contiguous spread of infected secretions along the perineum (as in rectal gonococcal infections in women) or perhaps by spread to the rectum via the pelvic lymphatics.

From the site of the primary urethral, genital, anal, or rectal infection, the organism spreads via the regional lymphatics. Penile, vulvar, or anal infection can lead to inguinal and femoral lymphadenitis. Rectal infection produces hypogastric and deep iliac lymphadenitis. Upper vaginal or cervical infection results in enlargement of the obturator and iliac nodes.

The most common presenting picture in heterosexual men is the *inguinal syndrome*, which is characterized by painful inguinal lymphadenopathy beginning 2–6 weeks after presumed exposure; in rare instances, the onset comes after a few months. The inguinal adenopathy is unilateral in two-thirds of cases, and palpable enlargement of the iliac and femoral nodes is often evident on the same side as the enlarged inguinal nodes. The nodes are initially discrete, but progressive periadenitis results in a matted mass of nodes that becomes fluctuant and suppurative. The overlying skin becomes fixed, inflamed, and thin and finally develops multiple draining fistulas. Extensive enlargement of chains of inguinal nodes above and below the inguinal ligament ("the sign of the groove") is not specific and, although not uncommon, is documented in only a minority of cases. On histologic examination, infected nodes are initially found to have characteristic small stellate abscesses surrounded by histiocytes. These abscesses coalesce to form large, necrotic, suppurative foci. Spontaneous healing usually takes place after several months; inguinal scars or granulomatous masses of various sizes persist for life. Massive pelvic lymphadenopathy may lead to exploratory laparotomy.

As NAATs for *C. trachomatis* are being used more often, increasing numbers of cases of LGV proctitis are being recognized in homosexual men. Such patients present with anorectal pain and mucopurulent, bloody rectal discharge. Although these patients may report diarrhea, they are often referring not to diarrhea but rather to frequent, painful, unsuccessful attempts at defecation (tenesmus). Sigmoidoscopy reveals ulcerative proctitis or proctocolitis, with purulent exudate and mucosal bleeding. The histopathologic findings in the rectal mucosa include granulomas with giant cells, crypt abscesses, and extensive inflammation. These clinical, sigmoidoscopic, and histopathologic findings may closely resemble those of Crohn's disease of the rectum.

Constitutional symptoms are common during the stage of regional lymphadenopathy and, in cases of proctitis, may include fever, chills, headache, meningismus, anorexia, myalgias, and arthralgias. These findings in the presence of lymphadenopathy are sometimes mistakenly interpreted as malignant lymphoma. Other systemic complications are infrequent but include arthritis with sterile effusion, aseptic meningitis, meningoencephalitis, conjunctivitis, hepatitis, and erythema nodosum. Chlamydiae have been recovered from the cerebrospinal fluid and in one case were isolated from the blood of a patient with severe constitutional symptoms—a result indicating the dissemination of infection. Laboratory-acquired infections suspected of being due to the inhalation of aerosols have been associated with mediastinal lymphadenitis, pneumonitis, and pleural effusion.

Complications of untreated anorectal infection include perirectal abscess; fistula in ano; and rectovaginal, rectovesical, and ischiorectal fistulas. Secondary bacterial infection probably contributes to these complications. Rectal stricture is a late complication of anorectal infection and usually develops 2–6 cm from the anal orifice—i.e., at a site within reach on digital rectal examination. Proximal extension of the stricture for several centimeters may lead to a mistaken clinical and radiographic diagnosis of carcinoma.

A small percentage of cases of LGV in men present as chronic progressive infiltrative, ulcerative, or fistular lesions of the penis, urethra, or scrotum. Associated lymphatic obstruction may produce elephantiasis. When urethral stricture occurs, it usually involves the posterior urethra and causes incontinence or difficulty with urination.

Approach to the Diagnosis and Treatment of *C. trachomatis* Genital Infections Four types of laboratory procedure are available to confirm *C. trachomatis* infection: direct microscopic examination of tissue scrapings for typical intracytoplasmic inclusions or EBs; isolation of the organism in cell culture; demonstration of chlamydial antigens by immunologic detection or demonstration of chlamydial genes in NAATs; and detection of antibody in serum or in local secretions.

Except in conjunctivitis, direct microscopic examination of Giemsa-stained cell scrapings for typical inclusions has an unacceptably low degree of sensitivity, and false-positive interpretations by inexperienced observers are also common. Even for conjunctivitis, this approach has been replaced by direct fluorescent antibody staining of conjunctival smears to identify chlamydial EBs with specific monoclonal antibodies (see below) or, where available, NAATs.

Cell culture techniques for isolation of *C. trachomatis* are available only in large medical centers. In addition to limited availability, other disadvantages of cell culture include its low and variable level of sensitivity (40–80%), its requirement for rigorous transport conditions, and its high cost and technically demanding nature. Therefore, nonculture alternatives involving antigen detection or nucleic acid amplification have been developed. In the direct immunofluorescent antibody (DFA) slide test, potentially infected genital or ocular secretions are smeared onto a slide, fixed, and stained with fluorescein-conjugated monoclonal antibody specific for chlamydial antigens. The observation of fluorescing EBs confirms the diagnosis. Enzyme-linked immunosorbent assay (ELISA) techniques for the detection of chlamydial antigens provide another alternative to culture. The reported sensitivity and specificity of these tests for genital infections (as compared with culture) have been 60–80% and 97–99%, respectively, in high-risk populations. More recently, NAATs have been developed for chlamydial diagnosis using PCR, ligase chain reaction (LCR), TMA, and other techniques. These tests are quite clearly the most sensitive and specific chlamydial diagnostic methods available; they are also the most expensive. Because of their very high analytic sensitivity, NAATs allow the use of novel specimens: these tests can detect chlamydial genes in first-void urine samples or patient-collected vaginal swabs with a high degree of sensitivity and specificity. The use of urine specimens and patient-collected vaginal swabs rather than conventional urethral and cervical swabs is particularly appealing for public-health chlamydial screening programs because of the ease of sample collection and transport, even in community-based settings. These tests have also facilitated population-based studies of chlamydial infections.

Serologic tests are of limited usefulness in the diagnosis of most chlamydial oculogenital infections. The complement fixation test with heat-stable, genus-specific antigen has been used with some success to diagnose LGV but is insensitive in infections due to non-LGV strains of *C. trachomatis*. The microimmunofluorescence (micro-IF) test with *C. trachomatis* antigens is more sensitive but is generally available only in research laboratories. The test measures antibodies by serovar specificity and by immunoglobulin class (IgM, IgG, IgA, secretory IgA) in both serum and local secretions. Cross-reacting antibodies to *C. pneumoniae* may sometimes be problematic. Serologic diagnosis by the micro-IF test may be useful in infant pneumonia (in which high-titer IgM antibody and/or fourfold rises in titer are often demonstrated), in chlamydial salpingitis (especially Fitz-Hugh–Curtis syndrome), and in LGV. In all of these more invasive syndromes, high antibody levels are present.

Table 169-1 summarizes the diagnostic tests of choice for patients with suspected *C. trachomatis* infection. It is clear that, in most settings and for most purposes, sensitivity and specificity will be greatest with NAATs. For patients to whom medicolegal considerations may apply (victims of sexual or child abuse), cultures or NAATs should always be used. In men with suspected urethritis, application of NAATs to a first-void urine specimen offers a sensitive and noninvasive diagnostic method other than the use of urethral swabs. For the diagnosis of urogenital (cervical or urethral) infections in women, testing of a first-void urine specimen by nucleic acid amplification methods is about as sensitive as testing of a cervical swab. Patient-collected vaginal swabs analyzed by NAAT have also been used successfully and with equal sensitivity and specificity. Since chlamydial diagnostic testing has become more widely available and is now more sensitive and specific than in the past, its use for specific diagnosis in patients with suspected chlamydial syndromes (e.g., MPC, NGU, and PID) and their partners should be promoted. High priority should also be given to the screening of asymptomatic high-risk women who would not otherwise receive treatment for presumptive chlamydial infection, especially those seen in high-risk settings (e.g., STD clinics or abortion clinics) and those with a high-risk profile (e.g., sexually active and ≤ 21 years of age, new sex partner within the preceding 2 months, or more than one current sex partner). Similar screening programs should be used to detect and treat asymptomatic urethritis in high-risk adolescent males. Where implemented, screening programs of this type have generally been associated with reductions in the prevalence of chlamydial infection and of its complications, such as PID, ectopic pregnancy, and infertility.

TABLE 169-1 DIAGNOSTIC TESTS FOR SEXUALLY TRANSMITTED AND PERINATAL *CHLAMYDIA TRACHOMATIS* INFECTION

Infection	Suggestive Signs/Symptoms	Presumptive Diagnosis[a]	Confirmatory Test of Choice
Men			
NGU, PGU	Discharge, dysuria	Gram's stain with >4 neutrophils per oil-immersion field; no gonococci	Urine or urethral NAAT for *C. trachomatis*
Epididymitis	Unilateral intrascrotal swelling, pain, tenderness; fever; NGU	Gram's stain with >4 neutrophils per oil-immersion field; no gonococci; urinalysis with pyuria	Urine or urethral NAAT for *C. trachomatis*
Women			
Cervicitis	Mucopurulent cervical discharge, bleeding and edema of the zone of cervical ectopy	Cervical Gram's stain with ≥20 neutrophils per oil-immersion field in cervical mucus	Urine, cervical, or vaginal NAAT for *C. trachomatis*
Salpingitis	Lower abdominal pain, cervical motion tenderness, adnexal tenderness or masses	*C. trachomatis* always potentially present in salpingitis	Urine, cervical, or vaginal NAAT for *C. trachomatis*
Urethritis	Dysuria and frequency without hematuria	MPC; sterile pyuria; negative routine urine culture	Urine or urethral NAAT for *C. trachomatis*
Adults of Either Sex			
Proctitis	Rectal pain, discharge, tenesmus, bleeding; history of receptive anorectal intercourse	Negative gonococcal culture and Gram's stain; at least 1 neutrophil per oil-immersion field in rectal Gram's stain	Rectal NAAT for *C. trachomatis* or culture
Reiter's syndrome	NGU, arthritis, conjunctivitis, typical skin lesions	Gram's stain with >4 neutrophils per oil-immersion field; lack of gonococci indicative of NGU	Urine or urethral NAAT for *C. trachomatis*
LGV	Regional adenopathy, primary lesion, proctitis, systemic symptoms	None	Culture of LGV strain from node or rectum, occasionally from urethra or cervix; NAAT for *C. trachomatis* from these sites; LGV CF titer, ≥1:64; micro-IF titer, ≥1:512
Neonates			
Conjunctivitis	Purulent conjunctival discharge 6–18 days after delivery	Negative culture and Gram's stain for gonococci, *Haemophilus* spp., pneumococci, staphylococci	Conjunctival NAAT for *C. trachomatis*; FA-stained scraping of conjunctival material
Infant pneumonia	Afebrile, staccato cough, diffuse rales, bilateral hyperinflation, interstitial infiltrates	None	Chlamydial culture or NAAT of sputum, pharynx, eye, rectum; micro-IF antibody to *C. trachomatis*—fourfold change in IgG or IgM antibody titer

[a]A presumptive diagnosis of chlamydial infection is often made in the syndromes listed when gonococci are not found. A positive test for *Neisseria gonorrhoeae* does not exclude the involvement of *C. trachomatis*, which often is present in patients with gonorrhea.

Note: CF, complement-fixing; FA, fluorescent antibody; LGV, lymphogranuloma venereum; micro-IF, microimmunofluorescence; MPC, mucopurulent cervicitis; NAAT, nucleic acid amplification test; NGU, nongonococcal urethritis; PGU, postgonococcal urethritis.

Rx *C. TRACHOMATIS* GENITAL AND PERINATAL INFECTIONS

Until the introduction of azithromycin, chlamydial infections could not be eradicated by single-dose or short-term antimicrobial regimens, and most uncomplicated genital infections in adults were treated with a 7-day course of doxycycline or tetracycline. A 2-week course is recommended for complicated chlamydial infections (e.g., PID, epididymitis) and at least a 3-week course of doxycycline (100 mg orally bid) or erythromycin base (500 mg orally qid) for LGV. Failure of treatment with a tetracycline in genital infections usually indicates poor compliance or reinfection rather than the involvement of a drug-resistant strain. To date, clinically significant drug resistance has not been observed in *C. trachomatis* infection.

Therapy for *C. trachomatis* urethritis is more efficacious than therapy for nonchlamydial NGU. *C. trachomatis* is eradicated from the urethra in nearly all cases by treatment with tetracycline hydrochloride (500 mg qid for 7 days) or doxycycline (100 mg by mouth bid for 7 days).

Eradication of *C. trachomatis* from the cervix by tetracycline and doxycycline, with doses and durations similar to those specified above for urethritis, has been demonstrated. Azithromycin (a single oral 1-g dose) is the regimen of choice for pregnant women with *C. trachomatis* infection. However, amoxicillin (500 mg tid for 7 days) can also be given to pregnant women. Tetracycline hydrochloride (500 mg qid) or doxycycline (100 mg bid) for 14 days produces clinical and microbiologic cure of epididymitis and PID associated with *C. trachomatis* infection, but in this situation a tetracycline should always be used together with a drug that is highly effective against gonorrhea.

Azithromycin is highly active against *C. trachomatis*; exhibits prolonged bioavailability; is concentrated intracellularly; and has, for the first time, made it possible to use single-dose therapy for chlamydial infection. In comparative trials, a 1-g single dose of azithromycin has been as effective as 7 days of doxycycline therapy for uncomplicated chlamydial infection. Azithromycin causes fewer adverse gastrointestinal reactions than do older macrolides such as erythromycin. The single-dose regimen of azithromycin has great appeal for the treatment of patients with uncomplicated chlamydial infection (especially those without symptoms and those with a likelihood of poor compliance) and of sexual partners of infected patients. These advantages must be weighed against the considerably greater cost of azithromycin. Whenever possible, the single 1-g dose should be given as directly observed therapy. Although not approved by the U.S. Food and Drug Administration for the treatment of pregnant women, the 1-g single-dose regimen of azithromycin appears to be safe and effective for this purpose.

Of the fluoroquinolones, ofloxacin (300 mg by mouth bid for 7 days) and levofloxacin (500 mg/d by mouth for 7 days) are as effective as doxycycline for the treatment of chlamydial infection and appear to be safe and well tolerated. These drugs cannot be used in pregnancy.

TREATMENT OF SEX PARTNERS The continued high prevalence of chlamydial infections in most parts of the United States is due primarily to the failure to diagnose—and therefore treat—patients with symptomatic or asymptomatic infection and their sex partners. *C. trachomatis* urethral or cervical infection has been well documented in a high proportion of the sex partners of patients with NGU, epididymitis, Reiter's syndrome, salpingitis, or endocervicitis. If possible, confirmatory laboratory tests for *Chlamydia* should be undertaken in these individuals, but even those without positive tests or evidence of clinical disease who have recently been exposed to proven or possible chlamydial infection (e.g., NGU) should be offered therapy. A novel approach is the use of partner-delivered therapy, in which the infected patient receives treatment and is also provided with single-dose azithromycin to give to his or her sex partner(s).

TREATMENT OF NEONATES AND INFANTS In neonates with conjunctivitis or infants with pneumonia, erythromycin ethylsuccinate or estolate can be given orally at a dosage of 50 mg/kg per day, preferably in four divided doses, for 2 weeks. Careful attention must be given to compliance with therapy—a frequent problem. Relapses of eye infection are common after treatment with topical erythromycin or tetracycline ophthalmic ointment and may also follow oral erythromycin therapy. Thus follow-up cultures should be performed after treatment. Both parents should be examined for *C. trachomatis* infection and, if diagnostic testing is not readily available, should be treated with doxycycline or azithromycin.

Prevention Efforts to develop a vaccine for chlamydial infection have not yet been successful. Early diagnosis and treatment shorten the duration of the infectious period and therefore constitute primary prevention of chlamydial infection. By the early 1990s, one of the 10 regions of the United States (Region X, the Pacific Northwest) had formally undertaken a chlamydial control program involving widespread screening of women attending family planning clinics. In women meeting the criteria for high risk, ~500,000 tests per year were conducted at 150 such clinics throughout the region. Within 5 years, the prevalence of chlamydial infection had been reduced by >30% in this population. However, the chlamydial prevalence in Region X has since leveled off and even begun to increase once again. Thus, further study of chlamydial screening programs and their impact on *Chlamydia*-associated reproductive sequelae is needed. While most regions of the United States have now initiated screening programs, some family planning and STD clinics still do not offer chlamydial testing. The availability of highly sensitive and specific diagnostic tests that can be done with urine specimens and of single-dose therapy makes it feasible to mount an effective chlamydial control program nationwide, with screening of high-risk persons both in traditional health care settings and in novel community- and school-based settings.

TRACHOMA AND ADULT INCLUSION CONJUNCTIVITIS

Definition *Trachoma* is a chronic conjunctivitis associated with infection by *C. trachomatis* serovar A, B, Ba, or C. It has been responsible for an estimated 20 million cases of blindness throughout the world and remains an important cause of preventable blindness. *Inclusion conjunctivitis* is an acute ocular infection caused by sexually transmitted *C. trachomatis* strains (usually serovars D through K) in adults exposed to infected genital secretions and in their newborn offspring.

Epidemiology In trachoma-endemic areas where the classic eye disease is seen, *C. trachomatis* is transmitted from eye to eye via hands, flies, towels, and other fomites; serovar A, B, Ba, or C is usually involved. The worldwide incidence and severity of trachoma have decreased dramatically during the past 35 years, mainly as a result of improving hygienic and economic conditions. However, endemic trachoma is still the major cause of preventable blindness in northern Africa, sub-Saharan Africa, the Middle East, and parts of Asia. Transmission occurs primarily through close personal contact, particularly among young children in rural communities with limited water supplies. In endemic areas, trachoma is associated with repeated exposure and reinfection, but the infection can also become chronic and persistent. Acute relapse of old trachoma occasionally follows treatment with cortisone eye ointment or develops in very old persons who were exposed in their youth.

Clinical Manifestations Both endemic trachoma and adult inclusion conjunctivitis present initially as a conjunctivitis characterized by small lymphoid follicles in the conjunctiva. In regions with hyperendemic classic blinding trachoma, the disease usually starts insidiously before the age of 2 years. Reinfection is common and probably contributes to the pathogenesis of trachoma. Studies using PCR techniques indicate that chlamydial DNA is often present in the ocular secretions of patients with trachoma, even in the absence of positive cultures. Thus persistent infection may be more common than was previously thought.

The cornea becomes involved, with inflammatory leukocytic infiltrations and superficial vascularization (pannus formation). As the inflammation continues, conjunctival scarring eventually distorts the eyelids, causing them to turn inward so that the inturned lashes constantly abrade the eyeball (trichiasis and entropion); eventually the corneal epithelium is abraded and may ulcerate, with subsequent corneal scarring and blindness. Destruction of the conjunctival goblet cells, lacrimal ducts, and lacrimal gland may produce a "dry-eye" syndrome, with resultant corneal opacity due to drying (xerosis) or secondary bacterial corneal ulcers.

Communities with blinding trachoma often experience seasonal epidemics of conjunctivitis due to *H. influenzae* that contribute to the intensity of the inflammatory process. In such areas the active infectious process usually resolves spontaneously in affected persons at 10–15 years of age, but the conjunctival scars continue to shrink, producing trichiasis and entropion and subsequent corneal scarring in adults. In areas with milder and less prevalent disease, the process may be much slower, with active disease continuing into adulthood; blindness is rare in these cases.

Eye infection with genital *C. trachomatis* strains in sexually active young adults presents as the acute onset of unilateral follicular conjunctivitis and preauricular lymphadenopathy similar to that seen in acute adenovirus or herpesvirus conjunctivitis. If untreated, the disease may persist for 6 weeks to 2 years. It is frequently associated with corneal inflammation in the form of discrete opacities ("infiltrates"), punctate epithelial erosions, and minor degrees of superficial corneal vascularization. Very rarely, conjunctival scarring and eyelid distortion occur, particularly in patients treated for many months with topical glucocorticoids. Recurrent eye infections develop most often in patients whose sexual consorts are not treated with antimicrobial agents.

Diagnosis The clinical diagnosis of classic trachoma can be made if two of the following signs are present: (1) lymphoid follicles on the upper tarsal conjunctiva; (2) typical conjunctival scarring; (3) vascular pannus; or (4) limbal follicles or their sequelae, Herbert's pits. The clinical diagnosis of endemic trachoma should be confirmed by laboratory tests in children with more marked degrees of inflammation. Intracytoplasmic chlamydial inclusions are found in 10–60% of Giemsa-stained conjunctival smears in such populations, but chlamydial NAATs are more sensitive and are often positive when smears or cultures are negative. Follicular conjunctivitis in adult Europeans or Americans living in trachomatous regions is rarely due to trachoma.

℞ ADULT INCLUSION CONJUNCTIVITIS

Adult inclusion conjunctivitis responds well to treatment with the same regimens used for treatment of uncomplicated genital infections—namely, azithromycin (a 1-g single oral dose) or doxycycline (100 mg bid for 7 days). Simultaneous treatment of all sexual consorts of the patient is also necessary to prevent ocular reinfection and to avoid chlamydial genital disease. Topical antibiotic treatment is not required for patients who receive systemic antibiotics.

Prevention Efforts to develop a trachoma vaccine have not yet been successful. General hygienic measures associated with improved living standards are effective in the elimination of endemic trachoma. An adequate water supply for personal cleanliness may be a critical factor. In some areas the reduction of numbers of flies in the household is important. The key elements of the World Health Organization's Global Campaign to Eliminate Trachoma are encompassed in the S-A-F-E strategy: *s*urgery for deformed eyelids; periodic mass treatment with *a*zithromycin; *f*ace washing; and *e*nvironmental improvements. Mass treatment of entire villages with single-dose azithromycin has been associated with marked declines in chlamydial infection and eye disease.

C. PSITTACI INFECTIONS

Definition Psittacosis is primarily an infectious disease of birds and mammals that is caused by *C. psittaci*. Transmission of infection from birds to humans results in a febrile illness characterized by pneumonitis and systemic manifestations. Inapparent infections or mild influenza-like illnesses may also occur. The term *ornithosis* is sometimes applied to infections contracted from birds other than parrots or parakeets, but *psittacosis* is the preferred generic term for all forms of the disease.

Epidemiology Almost any avian species can harbor *C. psittaci*. Psittacine birds (parrots, parakeets, budgerigars) are most commonly infected, but human cases have been traced to contact with pigeons, ducks, turkeys, chickens, and many other birds. Psittacosis may be considered an occupational disease of pet-shop owners, poultry workers, pigeon fanciers, taxidermists, veterinarians, and zoo attendants. Incidence has increased during the past 25 years, with cases and outbreaks occurring primarily among employees of poultry-processing plants. It is suspected that many cases go undiagnosed and unreported.

C. psittaci is present in nasal secretions, excreta, tissues, and feathers of infected birds. Although the disease can be fatal, infected birds frequently show only minor evidence of illness, such as ruffled feathers, lethargy, and anorexia. Asymptomatic avian carriers are common, and complete recovery may be followed by continued shedding of the organism for many months.

Psittacosis is almost always transmitted to humans by the respiratory route. On rare occasions the disease may be acquired from the bite of a pet bird. Prolonged contact is not essential for transmission of the disease; spending a few minutes in an environment previously occupied by an infected bird has resulted in human infection. In one outbreak, gardening rather than direct exposure to birds was associated with infection. A psittacosis-like agent has been transmitted among hospital personnel, with severe and sometimes fatal infections. There is evidence that these "human" strains are more virulent than avian organisms. There is no record of infection acquired by the ingestion of poultry products.

Pathogenesis The psittacosis agent gains entrance to the body through the upper respiratory tract, spreads via the bloodstream, and eventually localizes in the pulmonary alveoli and in the reticuloendothelial cells of the spleen and liver. Invasion of the lung probably takes place by way of the bloodstream rather than by direct extension from the upper air passages. A lymphocytic inflammatory response occurs on both the interstitial and the respiratory surfaces of the alveoli as well as in the perivascular spaces. The alveolar walls and interstitial tissues of the lung are thickened, edematous, necrotic, and occasionally hemorrhagic. Histologic examination of the affected areas reveals alveolar spaces filled with fluid, erythrocytes, and lymphocytes. The picture is not pathognomonic for psittacosis unless macrophages containing characteristic cytoplasmic inclusion bodies (Levinthal-Coles-Lillie bodies) are identified. The respiratory epithelium of the bronchi and bronchioles usually remains intact.

Clinical Manifestations The clinical manifestations and course of psittacosis are extremely variable. After an incubation period of 7–14 days or longer, the disease may start abruptly with shaking chills and fever, with temperatures ranging as high as 40.5°C (105°F); however, the onset is often gradual, with fever increasing over 3–4 days. Headache is almost always prominent, is usually diffuse and excruciating, and is often the chief complaint.

Many patients present with a dry hacking cough that is usually nonproductive, but small amounts of mucoid or bloody sputum may be raised as the disease progresses. Cough may begin early in the course of the disease or as late as 5 days after the onset of fever. Chest pain, pleurisy with effusion, or a friction rub may all occur but are rare. Pericarditis and myocarditis have been reported. Most patients have a normal or slightly increased respiratory rate; marked dyspnea with cyanosis occurs only in severe psittacosis with extensive pulmonary involvement. In psittacosis, as in mycoplasmal pneumonias, the physical signs of pneumonitis tend to be less prominent than symptoms and x-ray findings would suggest. The initial examination may reveal fine sibilant rales, or clinical evidence of pneumonia may be completely lacking. Rales usually become audible and more numerous as the illness progresses. Signs of frank pulmonary consolidation are usually absent. Symptoms of upper respiratory tract infection are not prominent, although mild sore throat, pharyngitis, and cervical adenopathy are often documented; on occasion, the last may be the only manifestation of illness. Epistaxis is encountered early in the course of nearly one-fourth of cases. Photophobia is also common.

Patients often report generalized myalgia, and spasm and stiffness of the muscles of the back and neck may lead to an erroneous diagnosis of meningitis. Lethargy, mental depression, agitation, insomnia, and disorientation have been prominent features of the illness in some epidemics but not in others; delirium and stupor develop near the end of the first week in severe cases. Occasional patients are comatose when first seen; the diagnosis of psittacosis may be elusive in these cases. Gastrointestinal manifestations such as abdominal pain, nausea, vomiting, or diarrhea are noted in some cases; constipation and abdominal distention sometimes occur as late complications. Icterus, the result of severe hepatic involvement, is a rare and ominous finding. A faint macular rash (Horder's spots) resembling the rose spots of typhoid fever has been described.

Patients without cough or other clinical evidence of respiratory involvement present with fever of unknown origin (Chap. 19). The pulse rate is slow in relation to the fever. When splenomegaly is noted in a patient with acute pneumonitis, psittacosis should be considered; the reported incidence of splenomegaly in this disease ranges from 10 to 70%. Nontender hepatic enlargement also occurs, but jaundice is rare. Thrombophlebitis is not unusual during convalescence; indeed, pulmonary infarction is sometimes a late complication and may be fatal.

In untreated cases of psittacosis, sustained or mildly remittent fever persists for 10 days to 3 weeks or occasionally for as long as 3 months. Over this period, the respiratory manifestations gradually abate. Psittacosis contracted from parrots or parakeets is more likely to be a severe, prolonged illness than infection acquired from pigeons or barnyard fowl. Relapses occur but are rare. Occasional patients develop endocarditis, and *C. psittaci* infection should be considered in cases of culture-negative endocarditis. Secondary bacterial infections are uncommon. Immunity to reinfection is probably permanent.

Laboratory Findings The chest x-ray in psittacosis is nonspecific and may show pneumonic lesions that are usually patchy in appearance but can be hazy, diffuse, homogeneous, lobar, atelectatic, wedge-shaped, nodular, or miliary. The white blood cell count is normal or moderately decreased in the acute phase of the disease but may rise in convalescence. The erythrocyte sedimentation rate frequently is not elevated. Transient proteinuria is common. The cerebrospinal fluid sometimes contains a few mononuclear cells but is otherwise normal. Despite hepatomegaly, the results of liver function tests are generally normal or only mildly elevated.

The diagnosis can be confirmed only by isolation of the causative microorganism or by serologic studies. The agent is present in the blood during the acute phase of the disease and in the bronchial secretions for weeks or sometimes years after infection, but it is difficult to isolate. Further, the organism is hazardous to work with in the laboratory, and most clinical laboratories do not offer culture for *C. psittaci*. Thus psittacosis is most readily diagnosed by the demonstration of a rising titer of complement fixation antibody in the serum of a patient with a compatible clinical syndrome. Both an acute-phase and a convalescent-phase specimen should always be tested. *C. trachomatis*, *C. psittaci*, and *C. pneumoniae* all share a genus-specific "group" antigen, which is the basis of the complement fixation test. Thus acute infections with *C. trachomatis* or *C. pneumoniae* can also produce titer rises in this test. However, these three species have different major outer-membrane proteins that are the principal antigens in the micro-IF test. If there is doubt as to the interpretation of the complement fixation test, the micro-IF test can be used to differentiate among these antigens. The prompt initiation of treatment with tetracycline has been shown to delay an antibody rise in convalescence for several weeks or months.

Differential Diagnosis A history of exposure to birds may be the only clinical basis for differentiating psittacosis from a variety of infectious and noninfectious febrile disorders. The list of pulmonary diseases that may be confused with psittacosis includes *Mycoplasma* pneumonia, *C. pneumoniae* pneumonia, legionellosis, viral pneumonia, Q fever, coccidioidomycosis, tuberculosis, enterovirus infection, carcinoma of the lung with bronchial obstruction, and common bacterial pneumonias. In the early stages, before pneumonitis appears, psittacosis may be mistaken for influenza, typhoid fever, miliary tuberculosis, or infectious mononucleosis.

℞ *C. PSITTACI* INFECTIONS

The tetracyclines are consistently effective in the treatment of psittacosis. Defervescence and alleviation of symptoms usually take place within 24–48 h after the institution of therapy with 2 g daily in four divided doses. To avoid relapse, treatment should probably be continued for at least 7–14 days after defervescence. Doxycycline (100 mg by mouth bid) can also be used. In severe cases, hospitalization and pulmonary intensive care may be indicated. Sulfonamides are not active against *C. psittaci*. Erythromycin can be used in patients allergic to or intolerant of tetracyclines. Limited data from studies in vitro and in animal models suggest that azithromycin and some fluoroquinolones are active against *C. psittaci*.

C. PNEUMONIAE INFECTIONS

Definition *C. pneumoniae* can be distinguished from the other two chlamydial species causing human infections on the basis of DNA hybridization and EB morphology. Although *C. pneumoniae* can be grown in a variety of cell cultures, it is considerably more difficult to culture than other chlamydiae, especially from clinical specimens. HL cells appear to be the most effective cell line for isolation of *C. pneumoniae*.

Epidemiology Knowledge of the epidemiology of *C. pneumoniae* infections comes primarily from serologic studies. Infections begin to occur in late childhood, achieve peak incidence in early adulthood, and continue throughout adult life.

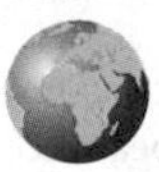

Seroprevalence in the many adult populations that have been tested throughout the world exceeds 40%—a figure suggesting that *C. pneumoniae* infections are ubiquitous. Secondary episodes (reinfections) appear to occur commonly in older adults throughout life. *C. pneumoniae* also produces epidemics of pneumonia and respiratory illness, especially in close residential quarters such as military barracks. The incidence of infections outside of epidemics remains poorly defined. The organism appears to be transmitted from person to person, probably primarily in schools and family units.

Pathogenesis Little is known about the pathogenesis of *C. pneumoniae* infection. The infection begins in the upper respiratory tract and in many persons is a long-lived asymptomatic condition of the upper respiratory mucosal surfaces. However, evidence of replication within vascular endothelium and synovial membranes of joints shows that, in at least some individuals, the organism is transported to distant sites, perhaps within macrophages. A *C. pneumoniae* outer-membrane protein may induce host immune responses whose cross-reaction with human proteins results in an autoimmune reaction.

Clinical Manifestations The clinical spectrum of *C. pneumoniae* infection includes acute pharyngitis, sinusitis, bronchitis, and pneumonitis, primarily in young adults. The clinical manifestations of primary infection appear to be more severe and prolonged than those of reinfection. The pneumonitis resembles that of *Mycoplasma* pneumonia in that leukocytosis is frequently lacking and patients often have prominent antecedent upper respiratory tract symptoms, fever, nonproductive cough, mild to moderate illness, minimal findings on chest auscultation, and small segmental infiltrates on chest x-ray. In elderly patients, pneumonia due to *C. pneumoniae* can be especially severe and may necessitate hospitalization and respiratory support.

Epidemiologic studies have demonstrated an association between serologic evidence of *C. pneumoniae* infection and atherosclerotic disease of the coronary and other arteries. In addition, *C. pneumoniae* has been identified in atherosclerotic plaques by electron microscopy, DNA hybridization, and immunocytochemistry. The organism has also been recovered in culture from atheromatous plaque—a result indicating the presence of viable replicating bacteria in vessels. Evidence from animal models supports the hypothesis that *C. pneumoniae* infection of the upper respiratory tract is followed by recovery of the organism from atheromatous lesions in the aorta and that the infection accelerates the process of atherosclerosis, especially in hypercholesterolemic animals. Antimicrobial treatment of the infected animals reverses the increased risk of atherosclerosis. In humans, two small trials in patients with unstable angina or recent myocardial infarction suggested that antibiotics reduce subsequent untoward cardiac events. However, larger trials have not demonstrated that various antibiotic regimens affect the risk of these events.

Diagnosis Diagnosis of *C. pneumoniae* infection is difficult because cell culture techniques are not available for routine clinical use and nonculture tests using antigen detection methods or DNA probes have not been developed for commercial use. Acute- and convalescent-phase sera can be tested for chlamydial complement fixation antibody to make a retrospective diagnosis. However, this test does not distinguish *C. pneumoniae* infection from infection due to *C. trachomatis* or *C. psittaci*.

℞ *C. PNEUMONIAE* INFECTIONS

Although few controlled trials of treatment have been reported, *C. pneumoniae* is inhibited in vitro by erythromycin, tetracycline, azithromycin, clarithromycin, gatifloxacin, and gemifloxacin. Recommended therapy consists of 2 g/d of either tetracycline or erythromycin for 10–14 days. Other macrolides (e.g., azithromycin) and some fluoroquinolones (e.g., levofloxacin and gatifloxacin) also appear to be effective.

FURTHER READINGS

ADIMORA AA: Treatment of uncomplicated genital *Chlamydia trachomatis* infections in adults. Clin Infect Dis 35(Suppl 2):S183, 2002

CASSELL JA et al: Trends in sexually transmitted infections in general practice 1990–2000: Population based study using data from the UK general practice research database. BMJ 332:332, 2006

CHIDAMBARAN JD et al: Effect of a single mass antibiotic distribution on the prevalence of infectious trachoma. JAMA 295:1142, 2006

GOLDEN MR et al: Effect of expedited treatment of sex partners on recurrent or persistent gonorrhea or chlamydial infection. N Engl J Med 352:676, 2005

GRAYSTON JT et al: Azithromycin for the secondary prevention of coronary events. N Engl J Med 352:1637, 2005

———: Infections caused by *Chlamydia pneumoniae*, strain TWAR. Clin Infect Dis 15:757, 1992

HOLMES KK, STAMM WE: Lower genital tract infections in women: Cystitis, urethritis, vulvovaginitis, and cervicitis, in *Sexually Transmitted Diseases*, 4th ed, KK Holmes et al (eds). New York, McGraw-Hill, 2008

SOLOMON AW et al: Mass treatment with single-dose azithromycin for trachoma. N Engl J Med 351:1962, 2004

STAMM WE: *Chlamydia* screening: Expanding the scope. Ann Intern Med 141:570, 2004

———: *Chlamydia trachomatis*: The persistent pathogen. Sex Transm Dis 13:684, 2001

———: *Chlamydia trachomatis* infections in adults, in *Sexually Transmitted Diseases*, 4th ed, KK Holmes et al (eds). New York, McGraw-Hill, 2008

SECTION 11 VIRAL DISEASES: GENERAL CONSIDERATIONS

170 Medical Virology

Fred Wang, Elliott Kieff

DEFINING A VIRUS

Viruses consist of a nucleic acid surrounded by one or more proteins. Some viruses also have an outer-membrane envelope. Viruses are obligate intracellular parasites: they can replicate only within cells since their nucleic acids do not encode the many enzymes necessary for protein, carbohydrate, or lipid metabolism and for the generation of high-energy phosphates. Typically, viral nucleic acids encode proteins necessary for replicating and packaging their nucleic acids within the biochemical milieu of host cells.

Viruses differ from viroids, prions, and virusoids. *Virusoids* are nucleic acids that depend on helper viruses to package their nucleic acids into virus-like particles. *Viroids* are naked, cyclical, mostly double-stranded, small RNAs. Viroids appear to be restricted to plants, spread from cell to cell, and are replicated by cellular RNA polymerase II. *Prions* (Chap. 378) are abnormal protein molecules that can spread. These molecules reproduce by changing the structure of their normal cellular protein counterparts. Prions have been implicated in neurodegenerative conditions such as Creutzfeldt-Jakob disease, Gerstmann-Straüssler disease, kuru, and human bovine spongiform encephalopathy ("mad cow disease").

VIRAL STRUCTURE

Viruses have from a few to several hundred genes. These genes may be in a single-strand or double-strand DNA genome or in a single-strand sense, a single-strand or segmented antisense, or a double-strand segmented RNA genome. Sense-strand RNA genomes can be translated directly into protein. Sense and antisense genomes are also referred to as *positive-strand* and *negative-strand genomes*, respectively. The viral nucleic acid is usually associated with one or more virus-encoded nucleoproteins in the core of the viral particle. The viral nucleic acid and nucleoproteins are almost always enclosed in a protein shell called a *capsid*. Because of the limited genetic complexity of viruses, their capsids are usually composed of multimers of identical capsomeres. Capsomeres are in turn composed of one or a few proteins. Capsids have icosahedral or helical symmetry. Icosahedral structures approximate spheres but have two-, three-, and fivefold axes of symmetry, while helical structures have only a twofold axis of symmetry. The entire structural unit of nucleic acid, nucleoprotein(s), and capsid is called a *nucleocapsid*.

Many human viruses are simply composed of a core and a capsid. For these viruses, the outer surface of the capsid mediates contact with uninfected cells. Other viruses are more complex and have an outer lipid-containing envelope derived from virus-modified membranes of the infected cell. The piece of infected-cell membrane that becomes the viral envelope has usually been modified during infection by the insertion of virus-encoded glycoproteins, which usually mediate contact of enveloped viruses with uninfected cells. Matrix or tegument proteins fill the space between the nucleocapsid and the envelope in many enveloped viruses. In general, enveloped viruses are sensitive to lipid solvents and nonionic detergents that can dissolve the envelope, while viruses that consist only of nucleocapsids are somewhat resistant. A schematic diagram for large and complex herpesviruses is shown in Fig. 170-1. Prototypical pathogenic human viruses are listed in Table 170-1. The relative sizes and structures of typical pathogenic human viruses are shown in Fig. 170-2.

TAXONOMY OF PATHOGENIC HUMAN VIRUSES

As is apparent from Table 170-1 and Fig. 170-2, the classification of viruses into orders and families is based on nucleic acid composition, nucleocapsid size and symmetry, and presence or absence of an envelope. Viruses of a single family have similar types of genomes and are often morphologically indistinguishable in electron micrographs. Further subclassification into genera depends on similarities in epidemiology and biologic effects and on the degree of colinear nucleic acid sequence homology.

Most human viruses have a common name related to their pathologic effects or the circumstances of their discovery. Formal species names have been assigned by the International Committee on Taxonomy of Viruses. The formal designation consists of the name of the host followed by the family or genus of the virus and a number. This dual terminology has created a confusing situation in which viruses are referred to and referenced by either name—e.g., varicella-zoster virus (VZV) or human herpesvirus (HHV) 3.

VIRAL INFECTION IN VITRO

STAGES OF VIRAL INFECTION AT THE CELLULAR LEVEL

Viral Interactions with the Cell Surface and Cell Entry Viral infection is initiated by adsorption of the virus to the cell surface. Adsorption results from the molecular interaction of viral surface proteins with receptors on the cell's plasma membrane (see Table 114-1). For example, a poliovirus capsid protein binds to a cell plasma-membrane protein of the immunoglobulin superfamily type. A rhinovirus capsid protein binds to intercellular adhesion molecule 1. An echovirus capsid protein binds to an integrin. The influenza A virus envelope hemagglutinin protein binds to sialic acid. The HIV envelope glycoprotein binds to CD4 and then engages one of several chemokine receptors that function as coreceptors for the virus. Herpes simplex virus (HSV) envelope glycoproteins bind to heparan sulfate on cell surfaces and then engage one of several immunoglobulin superfamily or tumor necrosis factor (TNF) receptors. Epstein-Barr virus (EBV) glycoprotein gp350 binds to the B lymphocyte complement receptor CD21 and then engages major histocompatibility complex (MHC) class II molecules as a coreceptor. Adsorption characteristically proceeds almost as well at 4°C as at 37°C. Adsorbed virus can still be neutralized by antibody. Adsorption frequently initiates changes in virion surface proteins that

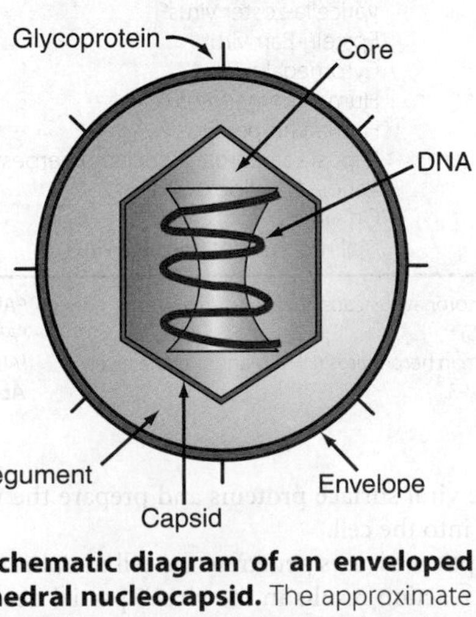

FIGURE 170-1 Schematic diagram of an enveloped herpesvirus with an icosahedral nucleocapsid. The approximate respective dimensions of the nucleocapsid and the enveloped particles are 110 and 180 nm. The capsid is composed of 162 capsomeres: 150 with sixfold and 12 with fivefold axes of symmetry.

TABLE 170-1 VIRUS FAMILIES PATHOGENIC FOR HUMANS

Family	Representative Viruses	Type of RNA/DNA	Lipid Envelope
RNA Viruses			
Picornaviridae	Poliovirus Coxsackievirus Echovirus Enterovirus Rhinovirus Hepatitis A virus	(+) RNA	No
Caliciviridae	Norwalk agent Hepatitis E virus	(+) RNA	No
Togaviridae	Rubella virus Eastern equine encephalitis virus Western equine encephalitis virus	(+) RNA	Yes
Flaviviridae	Yellow fever virus Dengue virus St. Louis encephalitis virus West Nile virus Hepatitis C virus Hepatitis G virus	(+) RNA	Yes
Coronaviridae	Coronaviruses[a]	(+) RNA	Yes
Rhabdoviridae	Rabies virus Vesicular stomatitis virus	(–) RNA	Yes
Filoviridae	Marburg virus Ebola virus	(–) RNA	Yes
Paramyxoviridae	Parainfluenza virus Respiratory syncytial virus Newcastle disease virus Mumps virus Rubeola (measles) virus	(–) RNA	Yes
Orthomyxoviridae	Influenza A, B, and C viruses	(–) RNA, 8 segments	Yes
Bunyaviridae	Hantavirus California encephalitis virus Sandfly fever virus	(–) RNA, 3 circular segments	Yes
Arenaviridae	Lymphocytic choriomeningitis virus Lassa fever virus South American hemorrhagic fever virus	(–) RNA, 2 circular segments	Yes
Reoviridae	Rotavirus Reovirus Colorado tick fever virus	ds RNA, 10–12 segments	No
Retroviridae	Human T-lymphotropic virus types I and II Human immunodeficiency virus types 1 and 2	(+) RNA, 2 identical segments	Yes
DNA Viruses			
Hepadnaviridae	Hepatitis B virus	ds DNA with ss portions	Yes
Parvoviridae	Parvovirus B19	ss DNA	No
Papovaviridae	Human papillomaviruses JC virus BK virus	ds DNA	No
Adenoviridae	Human adenoviruses	ds DNA	No
Herpesviridae	Herpes simplex virus types 1 and 2[b] Varicella-zoster virus[c] Epstein-Barr virus[d] Cytomegalovirus[e] Human herpesvirus 6 Human herpesvirus 7 Kaposi's sarcoma–associated herpesvirus[f]	ds DNA	Yes
Poxviridae	Variola (smallpox) virus Orf virus Molluscum contagiosum virus	ds DNA	Yes

[a]Including the coronavirus causing severe acute respiratory syndrome (SARS).
[b]Also called human herpesvirus (HHV) 1 and 2, respectively.
[c]Also called HHV-3.
[d]Also called HHV-4.
[e]Also called HHV-5.
[f]Also called HHV-8.
Abbreviations: ds, double-strand; ss, single-strand.

destabilize the viral surface proteins and prepare the way for the next stage of entry into the cell.

After adsorption, viruses penetrate the cell membrane by fusing with it. The fusion reaction results in the virus's partial decomposition. The virus becomes insensitive to neutralizing antibody as it penetrates, becomes uncoated, and enters the cytoplasm. Penetration and uncoating result in viral nucleocapsid or nucleoprotein entry into the cytoplasm. Penetration and uncoating as well as subsequent steps in viral replication depend on the cell's energy metabolism and on biochemical changes in the cell's plasma membrane and cytoskeleton. Therefore, penetration proceeds slowly at temperatures <37°C. Interaction of viral surface proteins with cell receptors can induce receptor aggregation at the site of adsorption. Receptor aggregation can trigger signaling events within the cytoplasm and changes in the plasma membrane. The cell frequently misperceives that the receptor has encountered its "normal ligand." Aggregated receptor may be internalized with the attached virus in an endocytic process. Viral endocytosis may proceed through clathrin-coated pits. Endocytosis is important in the entry of viruses as diverse as picornaviruses, influenza viruses, HIV, adenoviruses, and herpesviruses. In many cases, entry of the virus into the cytoplasm depends on acidification of the viral endosome.

Influenza virus provides a well-studied example of the effect of low pH on viral penetration. Influenza hemagglutinin mediates adsorption, receptor aggregation, and endocytosis. In low-pH endosomes, changes in the conformation of the hemagglutinin expose amphipathic domains that interact chemically with the cell membrane and initiate fusion of the viral and cellular membranes. (The HIV envelope glycoprotein undergoes similar conformational changes after interaction with CD4 and chemokine receptors.) For influenza virus, the M2 membrane protein also plays a key role in the uncoating of the viral envelope by providing an ion channel in the envelope. The fusion of viral proteins with cell membranes is a crucial step in viral infection, resulting in the mixture of viral envelope lipids and proteins with cell membrane lipids and proteins and (in this case) in the penetration of the influenza nucleocapsid into the cytoplasm. Viral glycoproteins other than the protein that mediates initial adsorption may be critical in mediating envelope fusion with cell membranes, which involves hydrophobic interactions. The hydrophobic interactions required for fusion can be susceptible to chemical inhibition or blockade.

Viral Gene Expression and Replication

After uncoating and release of viral nucleoprotein into the cytoplasm, the viral genome is transported to a site for expression and replication. In order to produce infectious progeny, viruses must (1) produce proteins necessary to replicate their nucleic acid, (2) produce structural proteins, and (3) assemble the nucleic acid and proteins into progeny virions. Different viruses use different strategies and gene repertoires to accomplish these goals. DNA viruses, except for poxviruses, replicate their nucleic acid and assemble into nucleocapsid complexes in the cell

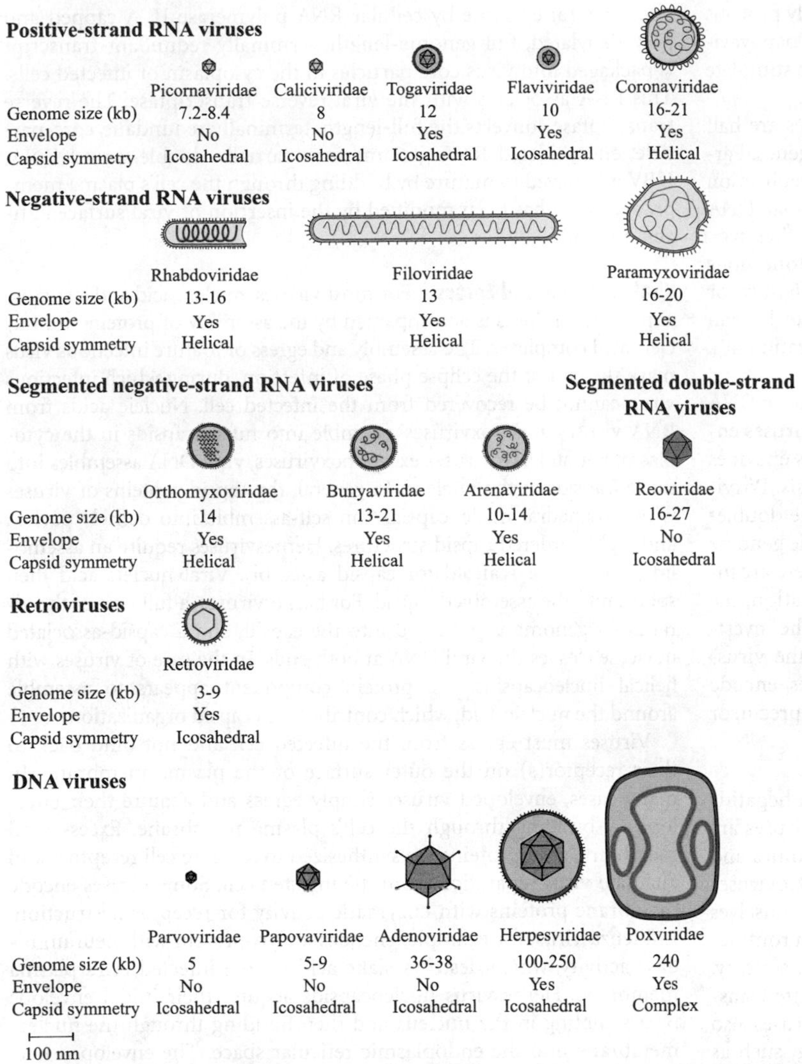

FIGURE 170-2 Schematic diagrams of the major virus families including species that infect humans. The viruses are grouped by genome type and are drawn approximately to scale. Prototype viruses of each family that cause human disease are listed in Table 170-1.

nucleus. RNA viruses, except for influenza viruses, transcribe and replicate their nucleic acid and assemble entirely in the cytoplasm. Thus, the replication strategies of DNA and RNA viruses are presented separately below. Positive-strand and negative-strand RNA viruses are discussed separately. Medically important viruses of each group are used for illustrative purposes.

POSITIVE-STRAND RNA VIRUSES Medically important positive-strand RNA viruses include picornaviruses, flaviviruses, togaviruses, caliciviruses, and coronaviruses. Genomic RNA from positive-strand RNA viruses is released into the cytoplasm without associated enzymes. Cell ribosomes recognize and associate with an internal ribosome entry sequence in the viral genomic RNA and translate a polyprotein that is a fusion of many or all of the viral proteins. The viral RNA polymerase and other viral proteins are cleaved from the polyprotein by protease components of the polyprotein. Antigenomic RNA is then transcribed from the genomic RNA template. Positive-strand genomes and mRNAs are next transcribed from the antigenomic RNA by the viral RNA polymerase. Positive-strand genomic RNA is encapsidated in the cytoplasm.

NEGATIVE-STRAND RNA VIRUSES Medically important negative-strand RNA viruses include rhabdoviruses, filoviruses, paramyxoviruses, myxoviruses, and bunyaviruses. Negative-strand RNA virus genomes are released into the cytoplasm with an associated RNA polymerase and one or more accessory proteins. Some of these genomes are segmented. Except for influenza viruses, negative-strand RNA viruses replicate entirely in the cytoplasm. The viral RNA polymerase transcribes messenger RNAs (mRNAs) as well as full-length antigenomic RNA, which is the template for replication of genomic RNA. These mRNAs encode for the viral RNA polymerase and accessory factors as well as for viral structural proteins. Influenza virus is an unusual negative-strand RNA virus that transcribes its mRNAs and antigenomic RNAs in the cell's nucleus. All negative-strand RNA viruses, including influenza viruses, assemble in the cytoplasm.

DOUBLE-STRAND SEGMENTED RNA VIRUSES These viruses, which are taxonomically grouped in the reovirus family, have 10–12 RNA segments that make up their genome. The medically important viruses in this group are rotaviruses and Colorado tick fever virus. Reovirus virions include an RNA polymerase complex. Reoviruses replicate and assemble in the cytoplasm.

DNA VIRUSES Medically important DNA viruses include parvoviruses, papovaviruses [e.g., human papillomaviruses (HPVs) and polyomaviruses], adenoviruses, herpesviruses, and poxviruses. Other than poxviruses, most DNA virus genomes must get to the cell's nucleus for transcription by cellular RNA polymerase II. For example, after receptor binding and fusion, herpesvirus nucleocapsids are released into the cytoplasm along with tegument proteins. The complex is then transported along microtubules to nuclear pores, and the DNA is released into the nucleus.

Transcriptional regulation and mRNA processing for nuclear DNA viruses depend on both viral and cellular proteins. For HSVs, a virus tegument protein activates transcription of viral immediate-early genes, a class of genes expressed immediately after infection. Transcription of immediate-early genes requires the viral tegument protein and preexisting cellular transcription factors. One of the key preexisting cellular factors for HSV-1 immediate-early gene transcription is docked in the cytoplasm in neurons. Nuclear absence of this cell factor important for viral gene transcription may explain why HSV-1 goes into a latent state in neurons and how lytic infection is activated by signaling in a latently infected cell.

DNA virus gene transcription is usually regulated and proceeds in an organized cascade. Transcription and expression of adenovirus and herpesvirus immediate-early genes turn on the promoters for early genes, whereas poxvirus virions carry all the factors necessary for early-gene transcription. Smaller DNA viruses are not as dependent on transactivators encoded from the viral genome for early-gene transcription. Most early genes encode proteins that are necessary for viral DNA synthesis and for the turn-on of late-gene transcription. Late genes encode mostly viral structural proteins or viral proteins necessary for the assembly and egress of the virus from the infected cell. Late-gene transcription is continuously dependent on DNA replication. Therefore, inhibitors of DNA replication also stop late-gene transcription.

Each DNA virus family uses unique mechanisms for replicating its DNA. Herpesvirus DNAs are linear in the virion but circularize in the infected cell. In lytic virus infection, circular herpesvirus genomes are replicated into linear concatemers through a "rolling-circle" mechanism. Herpesviruses encode a DNA polymerase and at least six other viral proteins necessary for viral DNA replication; these viruses also encode several enzymes that increase the pool of precursor deoxynucleotide triphosphates. Adenovirus genomes are linear in the virion and are replicated into complementary linear copies by a virus-encoded DNA polymerase and an initiator protein complex. The double-strand circular papovavirus genomes are replicated into progeny circular DNA molecules by cellular DNA replication enzymes. Two viral early proteins contribute to viral DNA replication and to the persistence of papovavirus DNA in latently infected cells. Early papovavirus proteins stimulate cells to remain in cycle, thus facilitating viral DNA replication.

Parvoviruses are the smallest DNA viruses: their genomes are half the size of the papovavirus genomes and include only two genes. Parvoviruses have negative single-strand DNA genomes. The replication of autonomous parvoviruses, such as B19, depends on cellular DNA replication and requires the virus-encoded Rep protein. Other parvoviruses, such as adeno-associated virus (AAV), are not autonomous and require helper viruses of the adenovirus or herpesvirus family for their replication. AAV has been touted as a potentially safe human gene therapy vector because its Rep protein causes its integration at a single chromosomal site.

Poxviruses are the largest DNA viruses and are unique among DNA viruses in replicating and assembling in the cytoplasm. Poxviruses encode transcription factors and an RNA polymerase as well as enzymes for RNA capping and polyadenylation and for DNA synthesis. Poxvirus DNA also has a unique structure. The two strands of the double-strand linear DNA are covalently linked at the ends so that the genome is also a covalently closed single-strand circle. In addition, there are inverted repeats at the ends of the DNA. During DNA replication, the genome is cleaved within the terminal inverted repeat, and the inverted repeats self-prime complementary-strand synthesis by the virus-encoded DNA polymerase. Like herpesviruses, poxviruses encode several enzymes that increase deoxynucleotide triphosphate precursor levels and thus facilitate viral DNA synthesis.

VIRUSES WITH BOTH RNA AND DNA GENOMES Retroviruses and hepatitis B virus (HBV) are not purely RNA or DNA viruses. Retroviruses are enveloped RNA viruses with two identical sense-strand genomes and associated reverse transcriptase and integrase enzymes. Retroviruses differ from all other viruses in that they reverse-transcribe themselves into partially duplicated double-strand DNA copies and then routinely integrate into the host genome as part of their replication strategy. Cellular RNA polymerase II and transcription factors regulate transcription from the integrated provirus genome. Some retroviruses also encode for regulators of transcription and RNA processing, such as Tax and Rex in human T-lymphotropic virus (HTLV) types I and II and Tat and Rev in HIV-1 and HIV-2. HIV genomes also encode for the additional accessory proteins Vpr, Vpu, and Vif, which are important for efficient infection and immune escape. Full-length proviral transcripts are made from a promoter in the viral terminal repeat and serve as both genomic RNAs that will be packaged in the nucleocapsids and mRNAs that encode for the viral Gag protein, polymerase/integrase protein, and envelope glycoprotein. The Gag protein includes a protease that cleaves it into several components, including a viral matrix protein that coats the viral RNA. Viral RNA polymerase/integrase, matrix protein, and cellular tRNA are key components of the viral nucleocapsid. The HIV Gag protease has been an important target for inhibition of HIV replication. Remnants and even complete copies of simple retroviral DNA in the human genome indicate that there may be replication-competent simple human retroviruses. However, replication has not been documented or associated with any disease. Integrated retroviral DNAs are also present in other animal species, such as pigs. These porcine retroviruses are a potential cause for concern in xenotransplantation because retroviral replication could cause disease in humans. Since the retroviral DNA is integrated into the porcine genome, special pathogen-free breeding practices cannot cleanse the donor herd of retroviral infection.

HBV is unique because virion DNA expression in infected cells results in the packaging of reverse transcriptase and genomic RNA in the virion. The genomic RNA is then copied into an incomplete double-strand circular DNA genome before the virion matures and is released from the infected cell. On entry of HBV into the cytoplasm of an infected cell, the virion reverse transcriptase/DNA polymerase completes DNA synthesis, and the covalently closed circular genome resides in the nucleus. Viral mRNAs are transcribed from the closed circular viral episome by cellular RNA polymerase II. A capped and polyadenylated, full-genome-length, terminally redundant transcript is packaged into virus core particles in the cytoplasm of infected cells. This RNA associates with the viral reverse transcriptase. The reverse transcriptase converts the full-length, terminally redundant, core-particle, encapsidated RNA genome into partially double-strand DNA. HBV is believed to mature by budding through the cell's plasma membrane, which has been modified by the insertion of viral surface antigen protein.

Viral Assembly and Egress For most viruses, nucleic acid and structural protein synthesis is accompanied by the assembly of protein and nucleic acid complexes. The assembly and egress of mature infectious virus mark the end of the eclipse phase of infection, during which infectious virus cannot be recovered from the infected cell. Nucleic acids from RNA viruses and poxviruses assemble into nucleocapsids in the cytoplasm. For all DNA viruses except poxviruses, viral DNA assembles into nucleocapsids in the nucleus. In general, the capsid proteins of viruses with icosahedral nucleocapsids can self-assemble into densely packed and highly ordered capsid structures. Herpesviruses require an assemblin protein as a scaffold for capsid assembly. Viral nucleic acid then spools into the assembled capsid. For herpesviruses, a full unit of the viral DNA genome is packaged into the capsid, and a capsid-associated nuclease cleaves the viral DNA at both ends. In the case of viruses with helical nucleocapsids, the protein component appears to assemble around the nucleic acid, which contributes to capsid organization.

Viruses must egress from the infected cell and not bind back to their receptor(s) on the outer surface of the plasma membrane. In many cases, enveloped viruses simply egress and acquire their envelope by budding through the cell's plasma membrane. Excess viral membrane glycoproteins are synthesized to saturate cell receptors and facilitate virus separation from the infected cell. Some viruses encode membrane proteins with enzymatic activity for receptor destruction. Influenza virus, for example, encodes a glycoprotein with neuraminidase activity, which destroys sialic acid on the infected cell's plasma membrane. Herpesvirus nucleocapsids acquire their initial envelope by assembling in the nucleus and then budding through the nuclear membrane into the endoplasmic reticular space. The enveloped herpesvirus is then released from the cell either by maturation in cytoplasmic vesicles, which fuse with the plasma membrane and release the virus by exocytosis, or by "de-envelopment" into the cytoplasm and "re-envelopment" at the Golgi or plasma membrane. In most instances, nonenveloped viruses appear to depend on the death and dissolution of the infected cell for their release.

FIDELITY OF VIRAL REPLICATION

Hundreds or thousands of progeny may be produced from a single virus-infected cell. Many particles partially assemble and never mature into virions. Many mature-appearing virions are imperfect and have only incomplete or nonfunctional genomes. Despite the inefficiency of assembly, a typical virus-infected cell releases 10–1000 infectious progeny. Some of these progeny may contain genomes that differ from those of the virus that infected the cell. Smaller, "defective" virus genomes have been noted with the replication of many RNA and DNA viruses. Virions with defective genomes can be produced in large numbers through packaging of incompletely synthesized nucleic acid. Adenovirus packaging is notoriously inefficient, and a high ratio of particle to infectious virus may limit the amount of recombinant adenovirus that can be administered for gene therapy. Mutant viral genomes are also produced and can be of medical significance. In general, viral nucleic acid replication is more error-prone than cellular nucleic acid replication. RNA polymerases and reverse transcriptases are significantly more error-prone than DNA polymerases. Mutant viruses can be virulent and may preferentially cause disease through evasion of the host immune response or through resistance to antiviral drugs. Persistent hepatitis C virus (HCV) infection is due in part to genome mutation and persistent immune escape. Viral nucleic acids can also mutate by recombination or reassortment between two related viruses in a single infected cell. While this occurrence is unusual under most circumstances of natural infection, the changes can be substantial and can significantly alter virulence or epidemiology. Reassortment of an avian or mammalian influenza A hemagglutinin gene into a human influenza background is believed to play a role in the emergence of new epidemic influenza A strains.

VIRAL GENES NOT REQUIRED FOR VIRAL REPLICATION

Viruses frequently have genes encoding proteins that are not directly involved in replication or packaging of the viral nucleic acid, in virion assembly, or in regulation of the transcription of viral genes involved in those processes. Most of these proteins fall into five classes: (1) proteins that directly or indirectly alter cell growth; (2) proteins that inhibit cellular RNA or protein synthesis so that viral mRNA can be efficiently transcribed or translated; (3) proteins that promote cell survival or inhibit apoptosis so that progeny virus can mature and escape from the infected cell; (4) proteins that inhibit the host interferon response; and (5) proteins that downregulate host inflammatory or immune responses so that virus infection can proceed in an infected person to the extent consistent with the survival of the virus and its efficient transmission to a new host. More complex viruses of the poxvirus or herpesvirus family encode many proteins that serve these functions. Some of these viral proteins have motifs similar to those of cell proteins, while others are quite novel. Virology has increasingly focused on these more sophisticated strategies evolved by viruses to permit the establishment of long-term infection in humans and other animals. These strategies often provide unique insights into the control of cell growth, cell survival, macromolecular synthesis, proteolytic processing, immune or inflammatory suppression, immune resistance, cytokine mimicry, or cytokine blockade.

HOST RANGE

The concept of host range was originally based on the cell types in which a virus replicated in tissue culture. For the most part, the host range is limited by specific cell-surface proteins required for viral adsorption or penetration—i.e., to the cell types that express receptors or coreceptors for a specific virus. Another common basis for host-range limitation is the degree of transcriptional activity from viral promoters in different cell types. Most DNA viruses depend not only on cellular RNA polymerase II and the basal components of the cellular transcription complex but also on activated components and transcriptional accessory factors, both of which differ among differentiated tissues, among cells at various phases of the cell cycle, and between resting and cycling cells.

The importance of host range factors is illustrated by the identification of determinants that prevent certain animal viruses from infecting humans. The SARS coronavirus and the influenza virus strain from the 1918 pandemic are believed to have originated from animal viruses in which minor genetic mutations resulted in more efficient human infection or enhanced transmission among humans.

VIRAL CYTOPATHIC EFFECTS AND INHIBITORS OF APOPTOSIS

The replication of almost all viruses has adverse effects on the infected cell, inhibiting cellular synthesis of DNA, RNA, or proteins. This inhibitory effect probably stems from the viruses' need to prevent or limit nonspecific, innate host resistance factors, including interferon (IFN). Most commonly, viruses specifically inhibit host protein synthesis by attacking a component of the translational initiation complex—frequently, a component that is not required for efficient translation of viral RNAs. Poliovirus protease 2A, for example, cleaves a cellular component of the complex that ordinarily facilitates translation of cell mRNAs by interacting with their cap structure. Poliovirus RNA is efficiently translated without a cap since it has an internal ribosome entry sequence. Influenza virus inhibits the processing of mRNA by snatching cap structures from nascent cell RNAs and using them as primers in the synthesis of viral mRNA. HSV has a virion tegument protein that inhibits cellular mRNA translation.

Apoptosis is the expected consequence of virus-induced inhibition of cellular macromolecular synthesis and viral nucleic acid replication. While the induction of apoptosis may be important for the release of some viruses (particularly nonenveloped viruses), many viruses have acquired genes or parts of genes that enable them to forestall infected-cell apoptosis. This delay may be advantageous in allowing the completion of viral replication. Adenoviruses and herpesviruses encode analogues of the cellular Bc12 protein, which blocks mitochondrial enhancement of proapoptotic stimuli. Poxviruses and some herpesviruses encode caspase inhibitors. Many viruses, including HPVs and adenoviruses, encode proteins that inhibit p53 or its downstream proapoptotic effects.

VIRAL INFECTION IN VIVO

TRANSMISSION

The capsid and envelope of a virus protect its genome and permit its efficient transmission from cell to cell and to prospective hosts. Most common viral infections are spread by direct contact, by ingestion of contaminated water or food, or by inhalation of aerosolized particles. In all these situations, infection begins on an epithelial or mucosal surface and spreads along it or from it to deeper tissues. Infection may then spread through the body via the bloodstream, lymphatics, or neural circuits. Parenteral inoculation can also transmit some viral infections among humans or from animals (including insects) to humans.

Some viruses are transmitted only between humans. The dependence of smallpox and poliovirus infections on interhuman transmission makes it feasible to eliminate these viruses from human circulation by mass vaccination. In contrast, herpesviruses survive over time by establishing persistent infection in humans for decades, with eventual reactivation and infection of new and naïve generations.

Animals are important reservoirs and vectors for transmission of viruses causing human disease. Herpes B, monkeypox, and viral hemorrhagic fevers are examples of zoonotic infections caused by direct contact with animals or transmission from animals through other vectors. These infections may not be sustainable among humans alone because of the lack of efficient interhuman transmission. SARS resulted when an animal coronavirus apparently gained access to the human population concomitant with a mutation that enhanced its pathogenicity and spread in humans. Avian influenza viruses have drawn increased public attention because of their potential to undergo genetic changes and contribute to human disease.

PRIMARY INFECTION

The first (primary) episode of viral infection usually lasts from several days to several weeks. During this period, the concentration of virus at sites of infection rises and then falls, usually to unmeasurable levels. The rate at which the intensity of viral infection rises and falls at a given site depends on the accessibility of that organ or tissue to both the virus and systemic immune effectors, the intrinsic ability of the virus to replicate at that site, and endogenous nonspecific and specific resistance. Typically, infections with enterovirus, mumps virus, measles virus, rubella virus, rotavirus, influenza virus, AAV, adenovirus, HSV, and VZV are cleared from almost all sites within 3–4 weeks. Some of these viruses are especially proficient in altering or evading the innate and acquired immune responses; thus primary infection with AAV, EBV, or cytomegalovirus (CMV) can last for several months. Characteristically, primary infections due to HBV, HCV, hepatitis D virus (HDV), HIV, HPV, and molluscum contagiosum virus extend beyond several weeks. For some of these viruses (e.g., HPV, HBV, HCV, HDV, and molluscum contagiosum virus), the primary phase of infection is almost indistinguishable from the persistent phase.

Disease manifestations usually arise as a consequence of viral replication and the resultant inflammatory response at a specific site but do not necessarily correlate with levels of replication at that site. For example, the clinical manifestations of limited infection with poliovirus, enterovirus, rabies virus, measles virus, mumps virus, or HSV in neural cells are severe relative to the level of viral replication at mucosal surfaces. Similarly, significant morbidity may accompany in utero fetal infection with rubella virus or CMV.

Primary infections are cleared by nonspecific innate and specific adaptive immune responses. Thereafter, an immunocompetent host is usually immune to the disease manifestations of reinfection by the same virus. Immunity frequently does not prevent transient surface colonization on reexposure, persistent colonization, or even limited deep infection.

PERSISTENT AND LATENT INFECTIONS

Relatively few viruses cause persistent or latent infections. HBV, HCV, rabies virus, measles virus, HIV, HTLV, HPV, HHV, and some poxviruses are notable exceptions. The mechanisms for persistent infection vary widely. HCV RNA polymerase and HIV reverse transcriptase have high mutation rates, and the generation of variant genomes that evade the host immune response facilitates persistent infection. HIV is also directly immunosuppressive, depleting CD4+ T lymphocytes and compromising CD8+ cytotoxic T cell immune responsiveness. Moreover, HIV encodes a Nef protein that downmodulates MHC class I expression, rendering HIV-infected cells partially resistant to immune CD8+ cytolysis.

In contrast, DNA viruses have much lower mutation rates. Their persistence in human populations can be due to their ability to establish latent infection and to reactivate from latency. In this instance, *latency* is defined as a state of infection in which the virus is not replicating. Viral genes associated with lytic infection are not expressed, and infectious virus is not made. The complete viral genome is present and may be replicated by cellular DNA polymerase in conjunction with the cell genome replication. HPVs establish latent infection in basal epithelial cells, which replicate. Some of the progeny cells provide a stable supply of latently infected basal cells, while others go on to squamous differentiation and, in the process, become permissive for lytic viral infection. For herpesviruses, latent infection is established in nonreplicating neural cells (HSV and VZV) or in replicating cells of hematopoietic lineages [EBV and probably CMV, HHV-6, HHV-7, and Kaposi's sarcoma–associated herpesvirus (KSHV, also known as HHV-8)]. In their latent stage, HPV and herpesvirus genomes are largely hidden from the normal immune response. It is still not fully understood how partially latent and reactivated HPV and herpesvirus infections escape immediate and effective immune responses in highly immune hosts. HPV, HSV, and VZV may be somewhat protected because they replicate in middle and upper layers of the squamous epithelium—sites not routinely visited by immune and inflammatory cells. HSV and CMV are also known to encode proteins that downregulate MHC class I expression and antigenic peptide presentation on infected cells, thereby enabling these cells to escape CD8+ T lymphocyte cytotoxicity.

Like other poxviruses, molluscum contagiosum virus cannot establish latent infection but rather causes persistent infection in hypertrophic lesions that last for months or years. This virus encodes a chemokine homologue that probably blocks inflammatory responses and an MHC class I analogue that may block cytotoxic T lymphocyte attack.

PERSISTENT VIRAL INFECTIONS AND CANCER

Persistent viral infection is estimated to be the root cause of as many as 20% of human malignancies. For the most part, cancer is an accidental and highly unusual or long-term effect of infection with oncogenic human viruses. In these malignancies, viral infection is a critical and ultimately determinative early step, forcing infected cells to enter the cell cycle and enhancing their survival. An unusual virus-infected cell undergoes the subsequent genetic changes that permit the enhanced autonomous growth and survival characteristic of a malignant cell.

Most hepatocellular carcinoma is now believed to be caused by chronic inflammatory, immune, and regenerative responses to HBV or HCV infection. Epidemiologic data firmly link HBV and HCV infections to hepatocellular carcinoma. These infections elicit repetitive cycles of virus-induced liver injury followed by tissue repair and regeneration. Over decades, chronic virus infection, repetitive tissue regeneration, and acquired chromosomal changes can result in enhanced cell proliferation and survival and eventually in hepatocellular carcinoma. In rare instances, HBV DNA integrates into cellular DNA—an event that probably contributes to the development of some tumors.

Almost all cervical carcinoma is caused by persistent infection with "high-risk" genital HPV strains. Whereas HBV and HCV infections stimulate cell growth indirectly in response to virus-induced injury, proteins E6 and E7 of HPV type 16 or 18 can directly affect cell growth by causing the loss of p53 and RB, two cell proteins with tumor-suppressive function. These viral proteins can also increase genomic instability. However, like HBV and HCV infections, HPV infection alone is not sufficient for carcinogenesis. Cervical carcinoma is inevitably associated with persistent HPV infection and integration of the HPV genome into chromosomal DNA. Integrations that result in overexpression of E6 and E7 from HPV type 16 or 18 can cause profound changes in cell growth and survival, and subsequent chromosomal changes accumulating over ensuing cycles of cell growth can lead to malignant conversion and cervical carcinoma.

EBV infection and expression of the latent-infection viral proteins can immortalize B lymphocyte growth in tissue culture. In most humans, the immune response to the strongly antigenic EBV latent-infection proteins prevents uncontrolled B cell lymphoproliferation. However, when humans are immunosuppressed by posttransplantation medications, HIV infection, or genetic immunodeficiencies, EBV-induced B cell malignancies can emerge.

EBV infection also plays a role in the long-term development of certain B lymphocyte and epithelial cell malignancies. Persistent EBV infection and expression of the EBV oncogene LMP1 in latently infected epithelial cells appear to be critical early steps in the evolution of anaplastic nasopharyngeal carcinoma, a common malignancy in Chinese and North African populations. As in other virus-associated malignancies, genomic instability and chromosomal abnormalities contribute to the development of EBV-associated nasopharyngeal carcinomas. High-level LMP1 expression in Reed-Sternberg cells is also a hallmark of many cases of Hodgkin's disease. LMP1-induced nuclear factor κB (NF-κB) activity may rescue and prolong the survival of defective B cells that are normally eliminated by apoptosis, thereby allowing the acquisition of other genetic changes leading to malignant Reed-Sternberg cells.

The HTLV-I Tax and Rex proteins appear to be critical to the initiation of cutaneous adult T cell lymphoma/leukemias that may occur long after primary HTLV-I infection. Tax-induced NF-κB activation may contribute to cytokine production, infected cell survival, and eventual outgrowth of malignant cells.

Molecular data confirm the presence of KSHV DNA in all Kaposi's tumors, including those associated with HIV infection, transplantation, and familial transmission. KSHV infection is also etiologically implicated in pleural-effusion lymphomas and multicentric Castleman's disease, which are more common among HIV-infected than among HIV-uninfected people. Several KSHV proteins that can be expressed in latently infected cells, such as v-cyclin, v-interferon regulatory factor (v-IRF), and latency-associated nuclear antigen (LANA), are implicated in increased cell proliferation and survival.

Evidence supporting a causal role of viral infection in these malignancies includes (1) epidemiologic data, (2) the presence of viral DNA in all tumor cells, (3) the ability of the viruses to transform human cells in culture, (4) the results of in vitro assays for transforming effects of specific viral genes on cell growth or survival, and (5) pathologic data indicating the expression of transforming viral genes in premalignant or malignant cells in vivo. Virus-related malignancies provide an opportunity to expand our understanding of the biologic mechanisms important in the development of cancer; they also offer unique opportunities for the development of vaccines and therapeutics that could prevent or specifically treat cancers associated with virus infection. Widespread immunization against hepatitis B has resulted in a decreased prevalence of HBV-associated hepatitis and will likely prevent most HBV-related liver cancers. Studies of an HPV vaccine have shown reduced rates of colonization with high-risk HPV strains and a decreased risk of cervical cancer. The successful use of in vitro–expanded EBV-specific T cell populations to treat or prevent EBV-associated posttransplantation lymphoproliferative disease demonstrates the potential of immunotherapy against virus-associated cancers.

RESISTANCE TO VIRAL INFECTIONS

Resistance to viral infections is initially provided by factors that are not virus-specific. Physical protection is afforded by the cornified layers of the skin and by mucous secretions that continuously sweep over mucosal surfaces. Once the first cell is infected, IFNs are induced and confer resistance to virus replication. Viral infection may also trigger the release of other cytokines from infected cells; these cytokines may be chemotactic to inflammatory and immune cells. Viral protein epitopes expressed on the cell surface in the context of MHC class I and II proteins stimulate the expansion of T cell populations with T cell receptors that can recognize the virus-encoded peptides. Cytokines, inflammatory agents, and antigens released by virus-induced cell death further attract inflammatory cells, dendritic cells, granulocytes, natural killer (NK) cells, and B lymphocytes to the sites of initial infection and to draining lymph nodes. IFNs and NK cells are particularly important in containing viral infection for the first several days. Granulocytes and macrophages are also important in the phagocytosis and degradation of viruses, especially after an initial antibody response.

By 7–10 days after infection, virus-specific antibody responses, virus-specific HLA class II–restricted CD4+ helper T lymphocyte responses, and virus-specific HLA class I–restricted CD8+ cytotoxic T lymphocyte responses have developed. These responses, whose magnitude typically increases over the second and third weeks of infection, are important in rapid recovery. Also between the second and third weeks, the antibody type usually changes from IgM to IgG; IgG or IgA antibody can then be detected at infected mucosal surfaces. Antibody may directly neutralize virus by binding to its surface and preventing its adsorption or penetration. Complement usually enhances antibody-mediated virus neutralization. Antibody and complement can also lyse virus-infected cells that express viral proteins on their surface. A cell infected with a replicating enveloped virus usually expresses the virus-envelope glycoproteins on the cell plasma membrane. Specific antibodies can bind to the glycoproteins, fix complement, and lyse the infected cell.

Antibody and CD4+/CD8+ T lymphocyte responses tend to persist for several months after primary infection. Antibody-producing lymphocytes persist in small numbers as memory cells and begin to proliferate rapidly in response to a second infection, providing an early barrier to reinfection with the same virus. Immunologic memory for T cell responses appears to be shorter-lived. Redevelopment of T cell immunity may take longer than secondary antibody responses, particularly when many years have elapsed between primary infection and reexposure. However, persistent infections or frequent reactivations from latency can result in sustained high-level T cell responses. For example, EBV and CMV typically induce high-level CD4+ and CD8+ T cell responses that are sustained for decades after primary infection.

Some viruses have genes that alter innate and acquired host defenses. Adenoviruses encode small RNAs that inhibit IFN-induced, PKR-mediated shutoff of infected-cell protein synthesis. Furthermore, adenovirus E1A can directly inhibit IFN-mediated changes in cell gene transcription. Moreover, adenovirus E3 proteins prevent TNF-induced cytolysis and block HLA class I antigen synthesis by the infected cell. HSV ICP47 and CMV US11 block class I antigen presentation. EBV encodes an interleukin (IL) 10 homologue that inhibits NK and T cell responses. Vaccinia virus encodes a soluble receptor for IFN-α and binding proteins for IFN-γ, IL-1, IL-18, and TNF, which inhibit host innate and adaptive immune responses. Vaccinia virus also encodes a caspase inhibitor that inhibits the ability of CD8+ cytotoxic cells to kill virus-infected cells. Some poxviruses and herpesviruses also encode chemokine-binding proteins that inhibit cellular inflammatory responses. The adoption of these strategies by viruses highlights the importance of the corresponding host resistance factors in containing viral infection and the importance of redundancy in host resistance.

The host inflammatory and immune response to viral infection does not come without a price. This response contributes to the symptoms, signs, and other pathophysiologic manifestations of viral infection. Inflammation at sites of viral infection can subvert an effective immune response and induce tissue death and dysfunction. Moreover, immune responses to viral infection could, in principle, result in immune attack upon cross-reactive epitopes on normal cells, with consequent autoimmunity. While such effects have been demonstrated in experimental models, their role in the autoimmune manifestations of primary or recurrent human viral infections is uncertain.

INTERFERONS

All human cells can synthesize IFN-α or -β in response to viral infection. These IFN responses are usually induced by the presence of double-strand viral RNA, which can be made by both RNA and DNA viruses and sensed by double-strand RNA binding proteins in the cell cytoplasm, such as PKR and RIG-I. IFN-γ is not highly related to IFN-α or -β and is produced mainly by NK cells and by immune T lymphocytes responding to IL-12. IFN-α and -β bind to the IFN-α receptor, while IFN-γ binds to a different but related receptor. Both receptors signal through receptor-associated JAK kinases and other cytoplasmic proteins, including "STAT" proteins. STAT proteins are tyrosine-phosphorylated by JAK kinases, translocate to the nucleus, and activate promoters for specific cell genes. Three types of antiviral effects are induced by IFN at the transcriptional level. The first effect is attributable to the induction of 2′-5′ oligo(A) synthetases, which require double-strand RNA for their activation. Activated synthetase polymerizes oligo(A) and thereby activates RNAse L, which in turn degrades single-strand RNA. The second effect takes place through the induction of PKR, a serine and threonine kinase that is also activated by double-strand RNA. PKR phosphorylates and negatively regulates the translational initiation factor eIF2-α, shutting down protein synthesis in the infected cell. A third effect is initiated through the induction of Mx proteins, a family of GTPases that is particularly important in inhibiting the replication of influenza virus and vesicular stomatitis virus (VSV). These IFN effects are mostly directed against the infected cell, causing both viral and cellular dysfunction and thereby limiting viral replication.

DIAGNOSTIC VIROLOGY

A wide variety of methods are now used to diagnose viral infection. Serology and viral isolation in tissue culture remain important standards. Acute- and convalescent-phase sera with rising titers of antibody to virus-specific antigens and a shift from IgM to IgG antibodies are generally accepted as diagnostic of acute viral infection. Serologic diagnosis is based on a >4-fold rise in IgG antibody concentration when acute- and convalescent-phase serum samples are analyzed at the same time.

Immunofluorescence, hemadsorption, and hemagglutination assays for antiviral antibodies are labor-intensive and are being replaced by enzyme-linked immunosorbent assays (ELISAs). ELISAs generally use specific viral proteins that are most frequently targeted by the antibody response. The proteins are purified from virus-infected cells or produced by recombinant DNA technology and are attached to a solid phase, where they can be incubated with serum, washed to eliminate nonspecific antibodies, and allowed to react with an enzyme-linked reagent to detect human IgG or IgM antibody specifically adhering to the viral antigen. The amount of antibody can then be quantitated by the intensity of a color reaction mediated by the linked enzyme. ELISAs can be sensitive and automated. Western blots can confirm the presence of antibody to multiple specific viral proteins simultaneously. The proteins are separated by size and transferred to an inert membrane, where they are incubated with serum antibodies. Western blots have an internal specificity control, since the level of reactivity for viral proteins can be compared with that for cellular proteins in the same sample. Western blots require individual evaluation and are inherently difficult to quantitate or automate.

Virus isolation in tissue culture depends on infection of susceptible cells and amplification by replication in infected cells. Virus growth in cell cultures can frequently be identified by its effects on cell morphology under light microscopy. For example, HSV produces a typical cytopathic effect in rabbit kidney cells within 3 days. Other viral cytopathic effects may not be as diagnostically useful. Identification usually requires confirmation by staining with virus-specific monoclonal antibodies. The efficiency and speed of virus identification can be enhanced by combining short-term culture with immune detection. In assays with "shell vials" of tissue culture cells growing on a coverslip, viral infection can be detected by staining of the culture with a monoclonal antibody to a specific viral protein expressed early in viral replication. Thus, virus-infected cells can be detected within hours or days of inoculation; several rounds of infection would be required to produce a visible cytopathic effect.

Virus isolation in tissue culture also depends on the collection of specimens from the appropriate site and the rapid transport of these specimens in the appropriate medium to the virology laboratory. Rapid transport maintains viral viability and limits bacterial and fungal overgrowth. Enveloped viruses are generally much more sensitive to freezing and thawing than nonenveloped viruses. The most appropriate site for culture depends on the pathogenesis of the virus in question. Nasopharyngeal, tracheal, or endobronchial aspirates are most appropriate for the identification of respiratory viruses. Sputum cultures generally are less appropriate because bacterial contamination and viscosity threaten tissue-culture cell viability. Aspirates of vesicular fluid are useful for isolation of HSV and VZV. Nasopharyngeal aspirates and stool specimens may be useful when the patient has fever and a rash and an enteroviral infection is suspected. Adenoviruses can be cultured from the urine of patients with hemorrhagic cystitis. CMV can frequently be isolated from cultures of urine or buffy coat. Biopsy material can be effectively cultured when viruses infect major organs, as in HSV encephalitis or adenovirus pneumonia.

Virus isolation does not necessarily establish disease causality. Viruses can persistently or intermittently colonize normal human mucosal surfaces. Saliva can be positive for herpesviruses, and normal urine samples can be positive for CMV. Isolations from blood, cerebrospinal fluid (CSF), or tissue are more often diagnostic of significant viral infection.

Another method aimed at increasing the speed of viral diagnosis is direct testing for antigen or cytopathic effects. Virus-infected cells from the patient may be detected by staining with virus-specific monoclonal antibodies; e.g., epithelial cells obtained by nasopharyngeal aspiration can be stained with a variety of monoclonal antibodies to respiratory viruses.

Nucleic acid amplification techniques bring speed, sensitivity, and specificity to diagnostic virology. The ability to directly amplify minute amounts of viral nucleic acids present in specimens means that detection no longer depends on viable virus and its replication. For example, amplification and detection of HSV nucleic acids in the CSF of patients with HSV encephalitis is a more sensitive detection method than culture of virus from CSF. The extreme sensitivity of these tests can be a problem, since subclinical infection or contamination can lead to false-positive results. Detection of viral nucleic acids does not necessarily indicate virus-induced disease.

Measurement of the amount of viral RNA or DNA in peripheral blood is an important means of determining which patients are at increased risk for virus-induced disease and of evaluating clinical responses to antiviral chemotherapy. Nucleic acid technologies for RNA quantification are routinely used in AIDS patients to evaluate responses to antiviral agents and to detect virus resistance or noncompliance with therapy. Viral-load measurements are also useful for evaluating the treatment of patients with HBV and HCV infections. Nucleic acid testing or direct staining with CMV-specific monoclonal antibodies to quantitate virus-infected cells in the peripheral blood (CMV antigenemia) is useful for identifying immunosuppressed patients who may be at risk for CMV-induced disease.

DRUG TREATMENT FOR VIRAL INFECTIONS

Multiple steps in the viral life cycle can be effectively targeted by antiviral drugs. Nucleoside and nonnucleoside reverse transcriptase inhibitors prevent synthesis of the HIV provirus, while protease inhibitors block maturation of the HIV polyprotein after infection of the cell. Enfuvirtide is a small peptide derived from HIV gp41 that acts before infection by preventing a conformational change required for virus fusion. Integrase inhibitors are now in clinical testing. Amantadine and rimantadine inhibit the influenza M2 protein, preventing release of viral RNA early during infection, whereas zanamivir and oseltamivir inhibit the influenza neuraminidase, which is necessary for the efficient release of mature virions from infected cells.

Virus genomes can evolve resistance to drugs by mutation and selection, by recombination with a drug-resistant virus, or (in the case of influenza virus and other multicomponent RNA virus genomes) by reassortment. The emergence of drug-resistant strains can limit therapeutic efficacy. As with antibacterial therapy, excessive and inappropriate use of antiviral therapy can select for the emergence of drug-resistant strains. HIV genotyping is a rapid method for identifying drug-resistant viruses. Resistance to reverse transcriptase or protease inhibitors has been associated with specific mutations in the reverse transcriptase or protease genes. Identification of these mutations by polymerase chain reaction amplification and nucleic acid sequencing can be clinically useful for determining which antiviral agents may still be effective. Drug resistance in herpesviruses is a more unusual problem.

IMMUNIZATION FOR THE PREVENTION OF VIRAL INFECTIONS

Viral vaccines are among the outstanding accomplishments of medical science. Smallpox has been eradicated except as a potential weapon of biological warfare or bioterrorism (Chap. 214). Poliovirus eradication may soon follow. Measles can be contained or eliminated. Excess mortality due to influenza virus epidemics can be prevented, and the threat of influenza pandemics can be decreased by contemporary killed or live attenuated influenza vaccines. Mumps, rubella, and chickenpox are well controlled by childhood vaccination in the developed world. Reimmunization of mature adults can be used to control herpes zoster. New rotavirus vaccines are entering the market. Widespread HBV vaccination has dramatically lowered the frequency of acute and chronic hepatitis and is expected to lead to a dramatic decrease in the incidence of hepatocellular carcinoma. Use of purified proteins, genetically engineered live-virus vaccines, and recombinant DNA–based strategies will make it possible to immunize against severe infections with other viruses. The development of effective vaccines against HIV and HCV is complicated by the high mutation rate of RNA polymerase and reverse transcriptase, the evolutionary and individual divergence of HIV and HCV genomes, and repeated high-level exposure in some populations. Concerns about the use of smallpox and other viruses as weapons necessitate maintenance of immunity to agents that are not naturally encountered.

VIRUSES AS NOVEL THERAPEUTIC TOOLS OR AGENTS

Viruses are being experimentally developed for the delivery of biotherapeutics or novel vaccines. Foreign genes can be inserted into viral nucleic acids, and the recombinant virus vectors can be used to infect the patient or the patient's cells ex vivo. Retroviruses integrate into the cell genome and have been used to functionally replace the abnormal gene in T cells of patients with severe combined immunodeficiency, thereby restoring immune function. Recombinant adenovirus, AAV, and retroviruses are being explored for use in diseases due to single-gene defects, such as cystic fibrosis and hemophilia. Recombinant poxviruses and adenoviruses are also being used experimentally as vaccine vectors. Viral vectors are being tested experimentally for expressing cytokines that can enhance immunity against tumor cells or for expressing proteins that can increase the sensitivity of tumor cells to chemotherapy. Live HSV is now being used experimentally to kill glioblastoma cells after injections into tumors.

For improved safety, nonreplicating viruses are frequently employed in clinical trial settings. Potential adverse events associated with virus-mediated gene transfer include the induction of inflammatory and antiviral immune responses. Integration is useful for permanent gene therapy, but integrations can induce disease by enhancing or interrupting the expression of important cellular genes.

FURTHER READINGS

FINLAY BB, MCFADDEN G: Anti-immunology: Evasion of the host immune system by bacterial and viral pathogens. Cell 124:767, 2006

HILLEMAN MR: Strategies and mechanisms for host and pathogen survival in acute and persistent viral infections. Proc Natl Acad Sci USA 101(Suppl 2):14560, 2004

KNIPE DM et al (eds): *Fields Virology*, 6th ed. New York, Lippincott Williams & Wilkins, 2006

MUNGER K et al: Viral carcinogenesis and genomic instability. EXS 96:179, 2006

171 Antiviral Chemotherapy, Excluding Antiretroviral Drugs

Lindsey R. Baden, Raphael Dolin

The field of antiviral therapy—both the number of antiviral drugs and our understanding of their optimal use—continues to lag behind the field of antibacterial drug treatment, in which >70 years of experience have now been accumulated, but significant progress has been made in recent years on new drugs for several viral infections.

The development of antiviral drugs poses several challenges. Viruses replicate intracellularly and often employ host cell enzymes, macromolecules, and organelles for synthesis of viral particles. Therefore, useful antiviral compounds must discriminate between host and viral functions with a high degree of specificity; agents without such selectivity are likely to be too toxic for clinical use.

The development of laboratory assays to assist clinicians in the appropriate use of antiviral drugs is also in its early stages. Phenotypic and genotypic assays for resistance to antiviral drugs are becoming more widely available, and correlations of laboratory results with clinical outcomes in various settings are beginning to be defined. Of particular note has been the development of highly sensitive and specific methods that measure the concentration of virus in blood (*virus load*) and permit direct assessment of the antiviral effect of a given drug regimen in that compartment in the host. Virus load measurements have been useful in recognizing the risk of disease progression in patients with certain viral infections and in identifying patients to whom antiviral chemotherapy might be of greatest benefit. Like any in vitro laboratory test, these tests yield results that are highly dependent on (and likely to vary with) the laboratory techniques employed.

Information regarding the pharmacokinetics of some antiviral drugs, particularly in diverse clinical settings, is limited. Assays to measure the concentrations of these drugs, especially of their active moieties within cells, are primarily research procedures and are not widely available to clinicians. Thus, there are relatively few guidelines for adjusting dosages of antiviral agents to maximize antiviral activity and minimize toxicity. Consequently, clinical use of antiviral drugs must be accompanied by particular vigilance with regard to unanticipated adverse effects.

Like that of other infections, the course of viral infections is profoundly affected by an interplay of the pathogen with a complex set of host defenses. The presence or absence of preexisting immunity, the ability to mount humoral and/or cell-mediated immune responses, and the stimulation of innate immunity are important determinants of the outcome of viral infections. The state of the host's defenses needs to be considered when antiviral agents are used or evaluated.

As with any therapy, the optimal use of antiviral compounds requires a specific and timely diagnosis. For some viral infections, such as herpes zoster, the clinical manifestations are so characteristic that a diagnosis can be made on clinical grounds alone. For other viral infections, such as influenza A, epidemiologic information (e.g., the documentation of a community-wide outbreak) can be used to make a presumptive diagnosis with a high degree of accuracy. However, for most other viral infections, including herpes simplex encephalitis, cytomegaloviral infections other than retinitis, and enteroviral infections, diagnosis on clinical grounds alone cannot be accomplished with certainty. For such infections, rapid viral diagnostic techniques are of great importance. Considerable progress has been made in recent years in the development of such tests, which are now widely available for a number of viral infections.

Despite these complexities, the efficacy of a number of antiviral compounds has been clearly established in rigorously conducted and controlled studies. As summarized in Table 171-1, this chapter reviews the antiviral drugs that are currently approved or are likely to be considered for approval in the near future for use against viral infections other than those caused by HIV. Antiretroviral drugs are reviewed in Chap. 182.

TABLE 171-1 ANTIVIRAL CHEMOTHERAPY AND CHEMOPROPHYLAXIS

Infection	Drug	Route	Dosage	Comment
Influenza A and B				
Prophylaxis	Oseltamivir	Oral	Adults: 75 mg/d Children ≥1 yr: 30–75 mg/d, depending on weight	Prophylaxis must continue for the duration of the outbreak and can be administered simultaneously with inactivated vaccine. Unless the sensitivity of isolates is known, neither amantadine nor rimantadine is currently recommended for prophylaxis or therapy because of the high rate of resistance in influenza A/H3N2 viruses since the 2005–2006 season.
	Zanamivir	Inhaled orally	Adults and children ≥5 yrs: 10 mg/d	
	Amantadine[a] or rimantadine[a]	Oral	Adults: 200 mg/d Children 1–9 yrs: 5 mg/kg per day (maximum, 150 mg/d)	
Treatment	Oseltamivir	Oral	Adults: 75 mg bid for 5 days Children 1–12 yrs: 30–75 mg bid for 5 days	When started within 2 days of onset, zanamivir and oseltamivir reduce symptoms by 1.0–1.5 and 1.3 days, respectively, in uncomplicated disease. Zanamivir may exacerbate bronchospasm in patients with asthma. Oseltamivir's side effects of nausea and vomiting can be reduced in frequency by drug administration with food. Amantadine and rimantadine are similarly effective in uncomplicated influenza caused by sensitive viruses. None of the listed drugs has been thoroughly studied in complicated cases (e.g., pneumonia).
	Zanamivir	Inhaled orally	Adults and children ≥7 yrs: 10 mg bid for 5 days	
	Amantadine[a]	Oral	Adults: 100 qd or bid Children 1–9 yrs: 5 mg/kg per day (maximum, 150 mg/d) for 5–7 days	
	Rimantadine[a]	Oral	100 qd or bid for 5–7 days in adults	
RSV infection	Ribavirin	Small-particle aerosol	Administered continuously from reservoir containing 20 mg/mL for 3–6 days	Ribavirin is used for treatment of infants and young children hospitalized with RSV pneumonia and bronchiolitis.
CMV retinitis in immunocompromised host (AIDS)	Ganciclovir	IV	5 mg/kg bid for 14–21 days; then 5 mg/kg per day as maintenance dose	Ganciclovir, valganciclovir, foscarnet, and cidofovir are approved for treatment of CMV retinitis in patients with AIDS. They are also used for colitis, pneumonia, or "wasting" syndrome associated with CMV and for prevention of CMV disease in transplant recipients.
		Oral	1 g tid as maintenance dose	
	Valganciclovir	Oral	900 mg bid for 21 days; then 900 mg/d as maintenance dose	Valganciclovir has largely supplanted oral ganciclovir and is frequently used in place of IV ganciclovir.

(continued)

TABLE 171-1 ANTIVIRAL CHEMOTHERAPY AND CHEMOPROPHYLAXIS (CONTINUED)

Infection	Drug	Route	Dosage	Comment
CMV retinitis *(continued)*	Foscarnet	IV	60 mg/kg q8h for 14–21 days; then 90–120 mg/kg per day as maintenance dose	Foscarnet is not myelosuppressive and is active against acyclovir- and ganciclovir-resistant herpesviruses.
	Cidofovir	IV	5 mg/kg once weekly for 2 weeks, then once every other week; given with probenecid and hydration	
	Fomivirsen	Intravitreal	330 mg on day 1 and day 15, followed by 330 mg monthly as maintenance	Fomivirsen has reduced the rate of progression of CMV retinitis in patients in whom other regimens have failed or have not been well tolerated. The major form of toxicity is ocular inflammation.
Varicella				
Immunocompetent host	Acyclovir	Oral	20 mg/kg (maximum, 800 mg) 4 or 5 times daily for 5 days	Treatment confers modest clinical benefit when administered within 24 h of rash onset.
Immunocompromised host	Acyclovir	IV	10 mg/kg q8h for 7 days	A change to oral valacyclovir can be considered once fever has subsided if there is no evidence of visceral involvement.
Herpes simplex encephalitis	Acyclovir	IV	10 mg/kg q8h for 14–21 days	Results are optimal when therapy is initiated early. Some authorities recommend treatment for 21 days to prevent relapses.
Neonatal herpes simplex	Acyclovir	IV	10 mg/kg q8h for 14–21 days	Serious morbidity is common despite therapy. Prolonged oral administration of acyclovir after initial IV therapy has been suggested because of long-term sequelae associated with cutaneous recurrences of HSV infection.
Genital herpes simplex				
Primary (treatment)		IV	5 mg/kg q8h for 5–10 days	The IV route is preferred for infections severe enough to warrant hospitalization or with neurologic complications.
		Oral	200 mg 5 times daily for 10 days	The oral route is preferred for patients whose condition does not warrant hospitalization. Adequate hydration must be maintained.
	Acyclovir	Topical	5% ointment; 4–6 applications daily for 7–10 days	Topical use—largely supplemented by oral therapy—may obviate systemic administration to pregnant women. Systemic symptoms and untreated areas are not affected.
	Valacyclovir	Oral	1 g bid for 10 days	Valacyclovir appears to be as effective as acyclovir but can be administered less frequently.
	Famciclovir	Oral	250 mg tid for 5–10 days[b]	Famciclovir appears to be similar in effectiveness to acyclovir.
Recurrent (treatment)	Acyclovir Famciclovir Valacyclovir	Oral Oral Oral	200 mg 5 times daily for 5 days 1000 mg bid for 1 day 500 mg bid for 3 days	Clinical effect is modest and is enhanced if therapy is initiated early. Treatment does not affect recurrence rates.
Recurrent (suppression)	Acyclovir Valacyclovir Famciclovir	Oral Oral Oral	400 mg bid for ≥12 months 500–1000 mg/d 125–250 mg bid	Suppressive therapy is recommended only for patients with at least 6–10 recurrences per year. "Breakthrough" occasionally takes place, and asymptomatic shedding of virus occurs. The need for suppressive therapy should be reevaluated after 1 year. Suppression with valacyclovir reduces transmission of genital HSV among discordant couples.
Mucocutaneous herpes simplex in immunocompromised host				
Treatment	Acyclovir	IV Oral Topical	5 mg/kg q8h for 7 days 400 mg 5 times daily for 10 days 5% ointment; 4–6 applications daily for 7 days or until healed	The choice of the IV or oral route depends on the severity of infection and the patient's ability to take oral medication. Oral or IV treatment has supplanted topical therapy except for small, easily accessible lesions. Foscarnet is used for acyclovir-resistant viruses.
	Valacyclovir Famciclovir	Oral Oral	1 g tid for 7 days[b] 500 mg bid for 4 days[c]	
Prevention of recurrence during intense immunosuppression	Acyclovir Valacyclovir Famciclovir	Oral IV Oral Oral	200 mg bid 5 mg/kg q12h 1 g tid[b] 500 mg bid[b]	Treatment is administered during periods when intense immunosuppression is expected—e.g., during antitumor chemotherapy or after transplantation—and is usually continued for 2–3 months.
Herpes simplex orolabialis (recurrent)	Penciclovir	Topical	1.0% cream applied q2h during waking hours for 4 days	Treatment shortens healing time and symptoms by 0.5–1.0 day (compared with placebo).
	Valacyclovir	Oral	2 g q12h for 1 day	Therapy begun at the earliest symptom reduces disease duration by 1 day.
	Famciclovir[b]	Oral	500 mg tid for 5 days	Therapy begun 48 h after UV light exposure decreases time to healing by 2 days.
	Docosonal[d]	Topical	10% cream 5 times daily until healed	Application at initial symptoms reduces healing time by 1 day.
Herpes simplex keratitis	Trifluridine	Topical	1 drop of 1% ophthalmic solution q2h while awake (maximum, 9 drops daily)	Therapy should be undertaken in consultation with an ophthalmologist.
	Vidarabine	Topical	0.5-in. ribbon of 3% ophthalmic ointment 5 times daily	

(continued)

TABLE 171-1 ANTIVIRAL CHEMOTHERAPY AND CHEMOPROPHYLAXIS (CONTINUED)

Infection	Drug	Route	Dosage	Comment
Herpes zoster				
Immunocompetent host	Valacyclovir	Oral	1 g tid for 7 days	Valacyclovir may be more effective than acyclovir for pain relief; otherwise, it has a similar effect on cutaneous lesions and should be given within 72 h of rash onset.
	Famciclovir	Oral	500 mg q8h for 7 days	The duration of postherpetic neuralgia is shorter than with placebo. Famciclovir showed overall efficacy similar to that of acyclovir in a comparative trial. It should be given ≤72 h after rash onset.
	Acyclovir	Oral	800 mg 5 times daily for 7–10 days	Acyclovir causes faster resolution of skin lesions than placebo and provides some relief of acute symptoms if given within 72 h of rash onset. Combined with tapering doses of prednisone, acyclovir improves quality-of-life outcomes.
Immunocompromised host	Acyclovir	IV Oral	10 mg/kg q8h for 7 days 800 mg 5 times daily for 7 days	Effectiveness in localized zoster is most marked when treatment is given early. Foscarnet may be used for VZV infections that are resistant to acyclovir.
	Famciclovir	Oral	500 mg tid for 10 days[b]	
Herpes zoster ophthalmicus	Acyclovir	Oral	600 mg 5 times daily for 10 days	Treatment reduces ocular complications, including ocular keratitis and uveitis.
Condyloma acuminatum	IFN-α2b	Intralesional	1 million units per wart (maximum of 5) thrice weekly for 3 weeks	Intralesional treatment frequently results in regression of warts, but lesions often recur. Parenteral administration may be useful if lesions are numerous.
	IFN-αn3	Intralesional	250,000 units per wart (maximum of 10) twice weekly for up to 8 weeks	
Chronic hepatitis B	IFN-α2b	SC	5 million units daily or 10 million units thrice weekly for 16–24 weeks	HBeAg and DNA are eliminated in 33–37% of cases. Histopathologic improvement is also seen.
	Pegylated IFN-α2a	SC	180 μg weekly for 48 weeks	HBeAg and DNA are eliminated in 32–43% of recipients.
	Lamivudine	Oral	100 mg/d for 12–18 months; 150 mg bid as part of therapy for HIV infection	The efficacy of lamivudine is similar to that of IFN, but lamivudine is better tolerated. Resistance develops in 24% of recipients when lamivudine is used as monotherapy for 1 year.
	Adefovir dipivoxil	Oral	10 mg/d for 48 months	A return of ALT levels to normal is documented in 48–72% of recipients and improved liver histopathology in 53–64%. Adefovir is effective in lamivudine-resistant hepatitis B. Renal function should be monitored.
	Entecavir	Oral	0.5 mg/d for 48 weeks (1 mg/d if HBV is resistant to lamivudine)	Normalization of ALT is seen in 68–78% of recipients and loss of HBeAg in 21%. Entecavir is active against lamivudine-resistant HBV.
	Telbivudine	Oral	600 mg/d for 52 weeks	Reduction of HBV DNA by >5 $\log_{10}$ copies/mL along with either normalization of ALT or loss of serum HBeAg is seen in 75% of recipients. Myopathy may occur.
Chronic hepatitis C	IFN-α2a or IFN-α2b	SC	3 million units thrice weekly for 12–18 months	A return of ALT levels to normal is documented in 54% of recipients but is sustained in only 28%. Improvement in liver histopathology is seen.
	IFN-α2b/ ribavirin	SC (IFN)/oral (ribavirin)	3 million units thrice weekly (IFN)/1000–1200 mg daily (ribavirin) for 6–12 months	Combination therapy results in sustained responses in up to 40–50% of all recipients.
	Pegylated IFN-α2b	SC	1 μg/kg weekly for 12–24 months	The slower clearance of pegylated IFNs than of standard IFNs permits once-weekly administration. The pegylated formulations appear to be superior to standard IFNs in tolerability and efficacy, both as monotherapy and in combination with ribavirin. Sustained virologic responses were seen in 42–46% of genotype 1 patients and in 76–82% of those infected with genotype 2 or 3.
	Pegylated IFN-α2a	SC	180 μg weekly for 12–24 months	
	Pegylated IFN-α2b/ ribavirin	SC (IFN)/oral (ribavirin)	1.5 μg/kg weekly (IFN)/800–1200 mg daily (ribavirin)[d] for 24–48 weeks	
	Pegylated IFN-α2a/ ribavirin	SC (IFN)/oral (ribavirin)	180 μg weekly (IFN)/800–1200 mg daily (ribavirin) for 24–48 weeks	
	IFN-alfacon	SC	9–15 μg thrice weekly for 6–12 months	Doses of 9 and 15 μg are equivalent to IFN-α2a and IFN-α2b doses of 3 million and 5 million units, respectively.
Chronic hepatitis D	IFN-α2a or IFN-α2b	SC	9 million units thrice weekly for 12 months	The overall efficacy and the optimal regimen and duration of therapy have not been established. Responses usually are not sustained when therapy is stopped.

[a]Influenza A only. Unless isolate sensitivity is known, not recommended for prophylaxis or therapy since 2005–2006 because of high rates of resistance in influenza A/H3N2 viruses.

[b]Not approved for this indication by the U.S. Food and Drug Administration (FDA).

[c]Approved by the FDA for treatment of HIV-infected individuals.

[d]Active ingredient: benzyl alcohol. Available without prescription.

Abbreviations: ALT, alanine aminotransferase; CMV, cytomegalovirus; HBeAg, hepatitis B e antigen; HBV, hepatitis B virus; HSV, herpes simplex virus; IFN, interferon; RSV, respiratory syncytial virus; UV, ultraviolet; VZV, varicella-zoster virus.

ZANAMIVIR AND OSELTAMIVIR

Zanamivir and oseltamivir are inhibitors of the influenza viral neuraminidase enzyme, which is essential for release of the virus from infected cells and for its subsequent spread throughout the respiratory tract of the infected host. The enzyme cleaves terminal sialic acid residues and thus destroys the cellular receptors to which the viral hemagglutinin attaches. Zanamivir and oseltamivir are sialic acid transition-state analogues and are highly active and specific inhibitors of the neuraminidases of both influenza A and B viruses. The antineuraminidase activity of the two drugs is similar, although zanamivir has somewhat greater in vitro activity against influenza B. Both zanamivir and oseltamivir act through competitive and reversible inhibition of the active site of influenza A and B viral neuraminidases and have relatively little effect on mammalian cell enzymes.

Oseltamivir phosphate is an ethyl ester prodrug that is converted to oseltamivir carboxylate by esterases in the liver. Orally administered oseltamivir has a bioavailability of >60% and a plasma half-life of 7–9 h. The drug is excreted unmetabolized, primarily by the kidneys. Zanamivir has low oral bioavailability and is administered orally via a hand-held inhaler. By this route, ~15% of the dose is deposited in the lower respiratory tract, and low plasma levels of the drug are detected.

Orally inhaled zanamivir is generally well tolerated, although exacerbations of asthma may occur. The toxicities most frequently encountered with orally administered oseltamivir are nausea, gastrointestinal discomfort, and (less commonly) vomiting. Gastrointestinal discomfort is usually transient and is less likely if the drug is administered with food. Recently, neuropsychiatric events (delirium, self-injury) have been reported in children who have been taking oseltamivir, primarily in Japan.

Inhaled zanamivir and orally administered oseltamivir have been effective in the treatment of naturally occurring influenza A or B in otherwise-healthy adults. In placebo-controlled studies, illness has been shortened by 1.0–1.5 days of therapy with either of these drugs when treatment is administered within 2 days of onset. A recent meta-analysis of clinical studies of oseltamivir suggests that treatment may reduce the likelihood of certain respiratory tract complications of influenza. Once-daily inhaled zanamivir or once-daily orally administered oseltamivir provides effective prophylaxis against laboratory-documented influenza A– and influenza B–associated illness.

The emergence of viruses resistant to zanamivir or oseltamivir occurs but appears to be less frequent than the emergence of resistance to the adamantanes in clinical studies carried out thus far. In one pediatric study, 5.5% of patients treated with oseltamivir developed resistant isolates. A somewhat higher rate of resistance was noted in a recent pediatric study of oseltamivir from Japan. Resistance to the neuraminidase inhibitors may develop by changes in the viral neuraminidase enzyme, by changes in the hemagglutinin that make it more resistant to the actions of the neuraminidase, or by both mechanisms. Some isolates that are resistant to oseltamivir may remain sensitive to zanamivir. Since the mechanisms of action of the neuraminidase inhibitors differ from those of the adamantanes (see below), zanamivir and oseltamivir are active against strains of influenza A virus that are resistant to amantadine and rimantadine.

Zanamivir and oseltamivir have been approved by the U.S. Food and Drug Administration (FDA) for treatment of influenza in adults and in children (those ≥7 years old for zanamivir and those ≥1 year old for oseltamivir) who have been symptomatic for ≤2 days. Oseltamivir is approved for prophylaxis of influenza in individuals ≥1 year of age and zanamivir for those ≥5 years of age (Table 171-1).

AMANTADINE AND RIMANTADINE

Amantadine and the closely related compound rimantadine are primary symmetric amines that display antiviral activity limited to influenza A viruses. Amantadine and rimantadine have been shown to be efficacious in the prophylaxis and treatment of influenza A infections in humans for >40 years. High frequencies of resistance to these drugs were noted among influenza A/H3N2 viruses in the 2005–2006 influenza season and continue to be seen up to the present (2006–2007). Therefore, these agents are no longer recommended unless the sensitivity of the individual influenza A isolate is known, in which case their use may be considered. Amantadine and rimantadine act through inhibition of the ion channel function of the influenza A M2 matrix protein, on which appropriate uncoating of the virus depends. A substitution of a single amino acid at critical sites in the M2 protein can result in a virus that is resistant to amantadine and rimantadine.

Amantadine and rimantadine have been shown to be effective in the prophylaxis of influenza A in large-scale studies of young adults and in less extensive studies of children and elderly persons. In such studies, efficacy rates of 55–80% in the prevention of influenza-like illness were noted, and even higher rates were reported when virus-specific attack rates were calculated. Amantadine and rimantadine have also been found to be effective in the treatment of influenza A infection in studies involving predominantly young adults and, to a lesser extent, children. Administration of these compounds within 24–72 h after the onset of illness has resulted in a reduction of the duration of signs and symptoms by ~50% from that in placebo recipients. The effect on signs and symptoms of illness is superior to that of commonly used antipyretic-analgesic agents. Only anecdotal reports are available concerning the efficacy of amantadine or rimantadine in the prevention or treatment of complications of influenza (e.g., pneumonia).

Amantadine and rimantadine are available only in oral formulations and are ordinarily administered to adults once or twice daily, with a dosage of 100–200 mg/d. Despite their structural similarities, the two compounds have different pharmacokinetics. Amantadine is not metabolized and is excreted almost entirely by the kidney, with a half-life of 12–17 h and peak plasma concentrations of 0.4 μg/mL. In contrast, rimantadine is extensively metabolized to hydroxylated derivatives and has a half-life of 30 h. Only 30–40% of an orally administered dose of rimantadine is recovered in the urine. The peak plasma levels of rimantadine are approximately half those of amantadine, but rimantadine is concentrated in respiratory secretions to a greater extent than amantadine. For prophylaxis, the compounds must be administered daily for the period at risk (i.e., the peak duration of the outbreak). For therapy, amantadine or rimantadine is generally administered for 5–7 days.

Although these compounds are generally well tolerated, 5–10% of amantadine recipients experience mild central nervous system side effects consisting primarily of dizziness, anxiety, insomnia, and difficulty in concentrating. These effects are rapidly reversible upon cessation of the drug's administration. At a dose of 200 mg/d, rimantadine is better tolerated than amantadine; in a large-scale study of young adults, adverse effects were no more frequent among rimantadine recipients than among placebo recipients. Seizures and worsening of congestive heart failure have also been reported in patients treated with amantadine, although a causal relationship has not been established. The dosage of amantadine should be reduced to 100 mg/d in patients with renal insufficiency [i.e., a creatinine clearance rate (Cr_{Cl}) of <50 mL/min] and in the elderly. A rimantadine dose of 100 mg/d should be used for patients with a Cr_{Cl} of <10 mL/min and in the elderly.

RIBAVIRIN

Ribavirin is a synthetic nucleoside analogue that inhibits a wide range of RNA and DNA viruses. The mechanism of action of ribavirin is not completely defined and may be different for different groups of viruses. Ribavirin-5′-monophosphate blocks the conversion of inosine-5′-monophosphate to xanthosine-5′-monophosphate and interferes with the synthesis of guanine nucleotides as well as that of both RNA and DNA. Ribavirin-5′-monophosphate also inhibits capping of virus-specific messenger RNA in certain viral systems. In studies demonstrating the effectiveness of ribavirin in the treatment of respiratory syncytial virus (RSV) infection in infants, the compound was administered as a small-particle aerosol. In infants with RSV infection who were given ribavirin by continuous aerosol for 3–6 days, illness and lower respiratory tract signs resolved more rapidly and arterial oxygen desaturation was less pronounced than in placebo-treated groups. In addition, ribavirin has had a beneficial clinical effect in infants with RSV infection who require mechanical ventilation. Aerosolized ribavirin has also been administered to older children and adults with severe RSV and parainfluenza virus infections (including immunosuppressed patients) and to older children and adults with influenza A or B infection, but the benefit of this treatment, if any, is unclear. In RSV infections in immunosuppressed patients, ribavirin is often given in combination with immunoglobulins.

Orally administered ribavirin has not been effective in the treatment of influenza A virus infections. IV or oral ribavirin has reduced mortality rates among patients with Lassa fever; it has been particularly effective in this regard when given within the first 6 days of illness. IV ribavirin has been reported to be of clinical benefit in the treatment of hemorrhagic fever with renal syndrome caused by Hantaan virus and as therapy for Argentinian hemorrhagic fever. Moreover, oral ribavirin has been recommended for the treatment and prophylaxis of Congo-Crimean hemorrhagic fever. An open-label trial suggested that oral ribavirin may be beneficial in the treatment of Nipah virus encephalitis. Use of IV ribavirin in patients with hantavirus pulmonary syndrome in the United States has not been associated with clear-cut benefits. Oral administration of ribavirin reduces serum aminotransferase levels in patients with chronic hepatitis C virus (HCV) infection; since it appears not to reduce serum HCV RNA levels, the mechanism of this effect is unclear. The drug provides added benefit when given by mouth in doses of 800–1200 mg/d in combination with interferon (IFN) α2b or α2a (see below), and the ribavirin/IFN combination has been approved for the treatment of patients with chronic HCV infection.

Large doses of ribavirin (800–1000 mg/d PO) have been associated with reversible hematopoietic toxicity. This effect has not been observed with aerosolized ribavirin, apparently because little drug is absorbed systemically. Aerosolized administration of ribavirin is generally well tolerated but occasionally is associated with bronchospasm, rash, or conjunctival irritation. Aerosolized ribavirin has been approved for treatment of RSV infection in infants and should be administered under close supervision—particularly in the setting of mechanical ventilation, where precipitation of the drug is possible. Health care workers exposed to the drug have experienced minor toxicity, including eye and respiratory tract irritation. Because ribavirin is mutagenic, teratogenic, and embryotoxic, its use is generally contraindicated in pregnancy. Its administration as an aerosol poses a risk to pregnant health care workers.

ANTIVIRAL DRUGS ACTIVE AGAINST HERPESVIRUS INFECTIONS

ACYCLOVIR AND VALACYCLOVIR

Acyclovir is a highly potent and selective inhibitor of the replication of certain herpesviruses, including herpes simplex virus (HSV) types 1 and 2, varicella-zoster virus (VZV), and Epstein-Barr virus (EBV). It is relatively ineffective in the treatment of human cytomegalovirus (CMV) infections; however, some studies have indicated its effectiveness in the prevention of CMV-associated disease in immunosuppressed patients. Valacyclovir, the L-valyl ester of acyclovir, is converted almost entirely to acyclovir by intestinal and hepatic hydrolysis after oral administration. Valacyclovir has pharmacokinetic advantages over orally administered acyclovir: it exhibits significantly greater oral bioavailability, results in higher blood levels, and can be given less frequently than acyclovir (two or three rather than five times daily).

The high degree of selectivity of acyclovir is related to its mechanism of action, which requires that the compound first be phosphorylated to acyclovir monophosphate. This phosphorylation occurs efficiently in herpesvirus-infected cells by means of a virus-coded thymidine kinase. In uninfected mammalian cells, little phosphorylation of acyclovir occurs, and the drug is therefore concentrated in herpesvirus-infected cells. Acyclovir monophosphate is subsequently converted by host cell kinases to a triphosphate that is a potent inhibitor of virus-induced DNA polymerase but has relatively little effect on host-cell DNA polymerase. Acyclovir triphosphate can also be incorporated into viral DNA, with early chain termination.

Acyclovir is available in IV, oral, and topical forms, while valacyclovir is available in an oral formulation. IV acyclovir is markedly effective in the treatment of mucocutaneous HSV infections in immunocompromised hosts, in whom it reduces time to healing, duration of pain, and virus shedding. When administered prophylactically during periods of intense immunosuppression (e.g., related to chemotherapy for leukemia or transplantation) and before the development of lesions, IV acyclovir reduces the frequency of HSV-associated disease. After prophylaxis is discontinued, HSV lesions recur. IV acyclovir is also effective in the treatment of HSV encephalitis; two comparative trials have indicated that acyclovir is more effective than vidarabine for this indication (see below).

Because VZV is generally less sensitive to acyclovir than is HSV, higher doses of acyclovir must be used to treat VZV infections. In immunocompromised patients with herpes zoster, IV acyclovir reduces the frequency of cutaneous dissemination and visceral complications and—in one comparative trial—was more effective than vidarabine. Acyclovir, administered at doses of 800 mg PO five times a day, had a modest beneficial effect on localized herpes zoster lesions in both immunocompromised and immunocompetent patients. Combination of acyclovir with a tapering regimen of prednisone appeared to be more effective than acyclovir alone in terms of quality-of-life outcomes in immunocompetent patients over age 50 with herpes zoster. A comparative study of acyclovir (800 mg PO five times daily) and valacyclovir (1 g PO tid) in immunocompetent patients with herpes zoster indicated that the latter drug may be more effective in eliciting the resolution of zoster-associated pain. Orally administered acyclovir (600 mg five times a day) reduced complications of herpes zoster ophthalmicus in a placebo-controlled trial.

In chickenpox, a modest overall clinical benefit is attained when oral acyclovir therapy is begun within 24 h of the onset of rash in otherwise-healthy children (20 mg/kg, up to a maximum of 800 mg, four times a day) or adults (800 mg five times a day). IV acyclovir has also been reported to be effective in the treatment of immunocompromised children with chickenpox.

The most widespread use of acyclovir is in the treatment of genital HSV infections. IV or oral acyclovir or oral valacyclovir has shortened the duration of symptoms, reduced virus shedding, and accelerated healing when employed for the treatment of primary genital HSV infections. Oral acyclovir and valacyclovir have also had a modest effect in treatment of recurrent genital HSV infections. However, the failure of treatment of either primary or recurrent disease to reduce the frequency of subsequent recurrences has indicated that acyclovir is ineffective in eliminating latent infection. Chronic oral administration of acyclovir for ≥1–6 years or of valacyclovir for ≥1 year has reduced the frequency of recurrences markedly during therapy; once the drug is discontinued, lesions recur. In one study, suppressive therapy with valacyclovir (500 mg once daily for 8 months) reduced transmission of HSV-2 genital infections among discordant couples by 50%. A modest effect on herpes labialis (i.e., a reduction of disease duration by 1 day) was seen when valacyclovir was administered upon detection of the first symptom of a lesion at a dose of 2 g every 12 h for 1 day. In AIDS patients, chronic or intermittent administration of acyclovir has been associated with the development of HSV and VZV strains resistant to the action of the drug and with clinical failures. The most common mechanism of resistance is a deficiency of the virus-induced thymidine kinase. Patients with HSV or VZV infections resistant to acyclovir have frequently responded to foscarnet.

With the availability of the oral and IV forms, there are few indications for topical acyclovir, although treatment with this formulation has been modestly beneficial in primary genital HSV infections and in mucocutaneous HSV infections in immunocompromised hosts.

Overall, acyclovir is remarkably well tolerated and is generally free of toxicity. The most frequently encountered form of toxicity is renal dysfunction because of drug crystallization, particularly after rapid IV administration or with inadequate hydration. Central nervous system changes, including lethargy and tremors, are occasionally reported, primarily in immunosuppressed patients. However, whether these changes are related to acyclovir, to concurrent administration of other therapy, or to underlying infection remains unclear. Acyclovir is excreted primarily unmetabolized by the kidney via both glomerular filtration and tubular secretion. Approximately 15% of a dose of acyclovir is metabolized to 9-[(carboxymethoxy)methyl]guanine or other minor metabolites. Reduction in dosage is indicated in patients with a Cr_{Cl} of <50 mL/min. The half-life of acyclovir is ~3 h in normal adults, and the peak plasma concentration after a 1-h infusion of a dose of 5 mg/kg is 9.8 μg/mL. Approximately 22% of an orally administered acyclovir dose is absorbed, and peak plasma concentrations of 0.3–0.9 μg/mL are attained after administration of a 200-mg dose. Acyclovir penetrates relatively well into the cerebrospinal fluid (CSF), with concentrations approaching half of those found in plasma.

Acyclovir causes chromosomal breakage at high doses, but its administration to pregnant women has not been associated with fetal abnormalities. Nonetheless, the potential risks and benefits of acyclovir should be carefully assessed before the drug is used in pregnancy.

Valacyclovir exhibits three to five times greater bioavailability than acyclovir. The concentration-time curve for valacyclovir, given as 1 g PO three times daily, is similar to that for acyclovir, given as 5 mg/kg IV every 8 h. The safety profiles of valacyclovir and acyclovir are similar, although thrombotic thrombocytopenic purpura/hemolytic-uremic syndrome has been reported in immunocompromised patients who have received high doses of valacyclovir (8 g/d). Valacyclovir is approved for the treatment of herpes zoster, of initial and recurrent episodes of genital HSV infections in immunocompetent adults, and of herpes labialis as well as for suppressive treatment of genital herpes. Although it has not been extensively studied in other clinical settings involving HSV or VZV infections, many consultants use valacyclovir rather than oral acyclovir in settings where the latter has been approved because of valacyclovir's superior pharmacokinetics and more convenient dosing schedule.

CIDOFOVIR

Cidofovir is a phosphonate nucleotide analogue of cytosine. Its major use is in CMV infections, particularly retinitis, but it is active against a broad range of herpesviruses, including HSV, human herpesvirus (HHV) type 6, HHV-8, and certain other DNA viruses such as polyomaviruses, papillomaviruses, adenoviruses, and poxviruses, including variola (smallpox) and vaccinia. Cidofovir does not require initial phosphorylation by virus-induced kinases; the drug is phosphorylated by host cell enzymes to cidofovir diphosphate, which is a competitive inhibitor of viral DNA polymerases and, to a lesser extent, of host cell DNA polymerases. Incorporation of cidofovir diphosphate slows or terminates nascent DNA chain elongation. Cidofovir is active against HSV isolates that are resistant to acyclovir because of absent or altered thymidine kinase and against CMV isolates that are resistant to ganciclovir because of UL97 phosphotransferase mutations. Cidofovir is usually active against foscarnet-resistant CMV, although cross-resistance to foscarnet as well as to ganciclovir has been described.

Cidofovir has poor oral availability and is administered IV. It is excreted primarily by the kidney and has a plasma half-life of 2.6 h. Cidofovir diphosphate's intracellular half-life of >48 h is the basis for the recommended dosing regimen of 5 mg/kg once a week for the initial 2 weeks and then 5 mg/kg every other week. The major toxic effect of cidofovir is proximal renal tubular injury, as manifested by elevated serum creatinine levels and proteinuria. The risk of nephrotoxicity can be reduced by vigorous saline hydration and by concomitant oral administration of probenecid. Neutropenia, rashes, and gastrointestinal tolerance may also occur.

IV cidofovir has been approved for the treatment of CMV retinitis in AIDS patients who are intolerant of ganciclovir or foscarnet or in whom those drugs have failed. In a controlled study, a maintenance dosage of 5 mg/kg per week administered to AIDS patients reduced the progression of CMV retinitis from that seen at 3 mg/kg. IV cidofovir has been reported anecdotally to be effective for treatment of acyclovir-resistant mucocutaneous HSV infections. Likewise, topically administered cidofovir is reportedly beneficial against these infections in HIV-infected patients; it is also being studied for the treatment of anogenital warts. Anecdotal use of IV cidofovir has been described in disseminated adenoviral infections in immunosuppressed patients, but its efficacy, if any, is not known. An ophthalmic formulation is being studied as treatment for adenoviral keratoconjunctivitis. Intravitreal cidofovir has been used to treat CMV retinitis but has been associated with significant toxicity.

FOMIVIRSEN

Fomivirsen is the first antisense oligonucleotide approved by the FDA for therapy in humans. This phosphorothioate oligonucleotide, 21 nucleotides in length, inhibits CMV replication through interaction with CMV messenger RNA. Fomivirsen is complementary to messenger transcripts of the major immediate early region 2 (IE2) of CMV, which codes for proteins regulating viral gene expression. In addition to its antisense mechanism of action, fomivirsen may exert activity against CMV through inhibition of viral adsorption to cells as well as direct inhibition of viral replication. Because of its different mechanism of action, fomivirsen is active against CMV isolates that are resistant to nucleoside or nucleotide analogues, such as ganciclovir, foscarnet, or cidofovir.

Fomivirsen has been approved for intravitreal administration in the treatment of CMV retinitis in AIDS patients who have failed to respond to other treatments or cannot tolerate them. Injections of 330 mg for two doses 2 weeks apart, followed by maintenance doses of 330 mg monthly, significantly reduce the rate of progression of CMV retinitis. The major toxicity is ocular inflammation, including vitritis and iritis, which usually responds to topically administered glucocorticoids.

GANCICLOVIR AND VALGANCICLOVIR

An analogue of acyclovir, ganciclovir is active against HSV and VZV and is markedly more active than acyclovir against CMV. Ganciclovir triphosphate inhibits CMV DNA polymerase and can be incorporated into CMV DNA, whose elongation it eventually terminates. In HSV- and VZV-infected cells, ganciclovir is phosphorylated by virus-encoded thymidine kinases; in CMV-infected cells, it is phosphorylated by a viral kinase encoded by the UL97 gene. Ganciclovir triphosphate is present in tenfold higher concentrations in CMV-infected cells than in uninfected cells. Ganciclovir is approved for the treatment of CMV retinitis in immunosuppressed patients and for the prevention of CMV disease in transplant recipients. It is widely used for the treatment of other CMV-associated syndromes, including pneumonia, esophagogastrointestinal infections, hepatitis, and "wasting" illness.

Ganciclovir is available for IV or oral administration. Because its oral bioavailability is low (5–9%), relatively large doses (1 g three times daily) must be administered by this route. Oral ganciclovir has largely been supplanted by valganciclovir, which is the L-valyl ester of ganciclovir. Valganciclovir is well absorbed orally, with a bioavailability of 60%, and is rapidly hydrolyzed to ganciclovir in the intestine and liver. The area under the curve for a 900-mg dose of valganciclovir is equivalent to that for 5 mg/kg of ganciclovir given IV, although peak serum concentrations are ~40% lower for valganciclovir. The serum half-life is 3.5 h after IV administration of ganciclovir and 4.0 h after PO administration of valganciclovir. Ganciclovir is excreted primarily by the kidneys in an unmetabolized form, and its dosage should be reduced in cases of renal failure. The most commonly employed dosage for initial IV therapy is 5 mg/kg every 12 h for 14–21 days; this regimen is followed by an IV maintenance dose of 5 mg/kg per day or five times per week. For oral therapy with valganciclovir, the dose is 900 mg twice daily for 21 days followed by 900 mg once a day for maintenance, with dose adjustment in patients with renal dysfunction. Intraocular ganciclovir, given by either intravitreal injection or intraocular implantation, has also been used to treat CMV retinitis.

Ganciclovir is effective as prophylaxis against CMV-associated disease in organ and bone marrow transplant recipients. Oral ganciclovir administered prophylactically to AIDS patients with CD4+ T cell counts of <100/μL has provided protection against the development of CMV retinitis. However, the long-term benefits of this approach to prophylaxis in AIDS patients have not been established, and most experts do not recommend the use of oral ganciclovir for this purpose. As already mentioned, valganciclovir has supplanted oral ganciclovir in settings where oral prophylaxis or therapy is considered.

The administration of ganciclovir has been associated with profound bone marrow suppression, particularly neutropenia, which significantly limits the drug's use in many patients. Bone marrow toxicity is potentiated in the setting of renal dysfunction and when other bone marrow suppressants, such as zidovudine, are used concomitantly.

Resistance has been noted in CMV isolates obtained after therapy with ganciclovir, especially in patients with AIDS. Such resistance may develop through a mutation in either the viral UL97 gene or the viral DNA polymerase. Ganciclovir-resistant isolates are usually sensitive to foscarnet (see below) or cidofovir (see above).

FAMCICLOVIR AND PENCICLOVIR

Famciclovir is the diacetyl 6-deoxyester of the guanosine analogue penciclovir. Famciclovir is well absorbed orally, has a bioavailability of 77%, and is rapidly converted to penciclovir by deacetylation and oxidation in the intestine and liver. Penciclovir's spectrum of activity and mechanism of action are similar to those of acyclovir. Thus, penciclovir is usually not active against acyclovir-resistant viruses. However, some acyclovir-resistant viruses with altered thymidine kinase or DNA polymerase substrate specificity may be sensitive to penciclovir. This drug is phosphorylated initially by a virus-encoded thymidine kinase and subsequently by cellular kinases to penciclovir triphosphate, which inhibits HSV-1, HSV-2, VZV, and EBV as well as hepatitis B virus (HBV). The serum half-life of penciclovir is 2 h, but the intracellular half-life of penciclovir triphosphate is 7–20 h—markedly longer than that of acyclovir triphosphate. The latter is the basis for the less frequent (twice-daily) dosing schedule for famciclovir than for acyclovir. Penciclovir is eliminated primarily in the urine by both glomerular filtration and tubular secretion. The usually recommended dosage interval should be adjusted for renal insufficiency.

Clinical trials involving immunocompetent adults with herpes zoster showed that famciclovir was superior to placebo in eliciting the resolution of skin lesions and virus shedding and in shortening the duration of postherpetic neuralgia; moreover, administered at 500 mg every 8 h, famciclovir was at least as effective as acyclovir administered at a dose of 800 mg PO five times daily. Famciclovir was also effective in the treatment of herpes zoster in immunosuppressed patients. Clinical trials have demonstrated its effectiveness in the suppression of genital HSV infections for up to 1 year and in the treatment of initial and recurrent episodes of genital herpes. Famciclovir is effective as therapy for mucocutaneous HSV infections in HIV-infected patients. Application of a 1% penciclovir cream reduces the duration of signs and symptoms of herpes labialis in immunocompetent patients (by 0.5–1.0 day) and has been approved for that purpose by the FDA. Famciclovir is generally well tolerated, with occasional headache, nausea, and diarrhea reported in frequencies similar to those among placebo recipients. The administration of high doses of famciclovir for 2 years was associated with an increased incidence of mammary adenocarcinomas in female rats, but the clinical significance of this effect is unknown.

FOSCARNET

Foscarnet (phosphonoformic acid) is a pyrophosphate-containing compound that potently inhibits herpesviruses, including CMV. This drug inhibits DNA polymerases at the pyrophosphate binding site at concentrations that have relatively little effect on cellular polymerases. Foscarnet does not require phosphorylation to exert its antiviral activity and is therefore active against HSV and VZV isolates that are resistant to acyclovir because of deficiencies in thymidine kinase as well as against most ganciclovir-resistant strains of CMV. Foscarnet also inhibits the reverse transcriptase of HIV and is active against HIV in vivo.

Foscarnet is poorly soluble and must be administered IV via an infusion pump in a dilute solution over 1–2 h. The plasma half-life of foscarnet is 3–5 h and increases with decreasing renal function, since the drug is eliminated primarily by the kidneys. It has been estimated that 10–28% of a dose may be deposited in bone, where it can persist for months. The most common initial dosage of foscarnet—60 mg/kg every 8 h for 14–21 days—is followed by a maintenance dose of 90–120 mg/kg once a day.

Foscarnet is approved for the treatment of CMV retinitis in patients with AIDS and of acyclovir-resistant mucocutaneous HSV infections. In a comparative clinical trial, the drug appeared to be about as efficacious as ganciclovir against CMV retinitis but was associated with a longer survival period, possibly because of its activity against HIV. Intraocular foscarnet has been used to treat CMV retinitis. Foscarnet has also been employed to treat acyclovir-resistant HSV and VZV infections as well as ganciclovir-resistant CMV infections, although resistance to foscarnet has been reported in CMV isolates obtained during therapy. Foscarnet has also been used to treat HHV-6 infections in immunosuppressed patients.

The major form of toxicity associated with foscarnet is renal impairment. Thus renal function should be monitored closely, particularly during the initial phase of therapy. Since foscarnet binds divalent metal ions, hypocalcemia, hypomagnesemia, hypokalemia, and hypo- or hyperphosphatemia can develop. Saline hydration and slow infusion appear to protect the patient against nephrotoxicity and electrolyte disturbances. Although hematologic abnormalities have been documented (most commonly anemia), foscarnet is not generally myelosuppressive and may be administered concomitantly with myelosuppressive medications such as zidovudine.

TRIFLURIDINE

Trifluridine is a pyrimidine nucleoside active against HSV-1, HSV-2, and CMV. Trifluridine monophosphate irreversibly inhibits thymidylate synthetase, and trifluridine triphosphate inhibits viral and, to a lesser extent, cellular DNA polymerases. Because of systemic toxicity, its use is limited to topical therapy. Trifluridine is approved for treatment of HSV keratitis, for which trials have shown that it is more effective than topical idoxuridine but similar in efficacy to topical vidarabine. The drug has benefited some patients with HSV keratitis who have failed to respond to idoxuridine or vidarabine. Topical application of trifluridine to sites of acyclovir-resistant HSV mucocutaneous infections has also been beneficial in some cases.

VIDARABINE

Vidarabine is a purine nucleoside analogue with activity against HSV-1, HSV-2, VZV, and EBV. Vidarabine inhibits viral DNA synthesis through its 5′-triphosphorylated metabolite, although its precise molecular mechanisms of action are not completely understood. IV-administered vidarabine has been shown to be effective in the treatment of herpes simplex encephalitis, mucocutaneous HSV infections, herpes zoster in immunocompromised patients, and neonatal HSV infections. Its use has been supplanted by that of IV acyclovir, which is more effective and easier to administer. Production of the IV preparation has been discontinued by the manufacturer, but vidarabine is available as an ophthalmic ointment, which is effective in the treatment of HSV keratitis.

ANTIVIRAL DRUGS ACTIVE AGAINST HEPATITIS VIRUSES

LAMIVUDINE

Lamivudine is a pyrimidine nucleoside analogue that is used primarily in combination therapy against HIV infection (Chap. 182). It is also active against HBV through inhibition of the viral DNA polymerase and has been approved for the treatment of chronic HBV infection. At doses of 100 mg/d for 1 year, lamivudine is well tolerated and results in suppression of HBV DNA levels, normalization of serum aminotransferase levels in 50–70% of patients, and reduction of hepatic inflammation and fibrosis in 50–60% of patients. Loss of hepatitis B e antigen (HBeAg) occurs in 30% of patients. Resistance to lamivudine develops in 24% of patients treated for 1 year and is associated with changes in the YMDD motif of HBV DNA polymerase. This is an important limitation of monotherapy with the drug. Lamivudine is being evaluated as a component of combination regimens (with IFNs and other nucleoside or nucleotide analogues listed below) for the treatment of hepatitis B. Lamivudine appears to be useful in the prevention or suppression of HBV infection associated with liver transplantation.

ADEFOVIR

Adefovir dipivoxil is an acyclic nucleotide analogue of adenosine monophosphate that has activity against HBV, HIV, HSV, and CMV. It is phosphorylated by cellular kinases to the active triphosphate moiety, which is a competitive inhibitor of HBV DNA polymerase and results in chain termination after incorporation into nascent viral DNA. Adefovir is administered orally and is eliminated primarily by the kidneys, with a plasma half-life of 7.5 h. In clinical studies, therapy with adefovir at a dose of 10 mg/d for 48 weeks resulted in normalization of alanine aminotransferase (ALT) levels in 48–72% of patients and improved liver histology in 53–64%; it also resulted in a 3.6-$\log_{10}$ reduction in the number of HBV DNA copies per milliliter of plasma. Adefovir was effective in treatment-naive patients as well as in those infected with lamivudine-resistant HBV. Resistance to adefovir appears to develop less readily than that to lamivudine, but adefovir resistance rates of 15–18% have been reported after 192 weeks of treatment. This agent is generally well tolerated. Significant nephrotoxicity attributable to adefovir is uncommon at the dose employed in the treatment of HBV infections (10 mg/d) but is a treatment-limiting adverse effect at the higher doses used in therapy for HIV infections (30–120 mg/d). In any case, renal function should be monitored in patients taking adefovir, even at the lower dose. Adefovir is approved only for treatment of chronic HBV infection.

TENOFOVIR

Tenofovir disoproxil fumarate is a nucleotide analogue of adenosine monophosphate with activity against both retroviruses and hepadnaviruses. In patients co-infected with HIV and HBV, tenofovir reduces HBV loads by 3–4 $\log_{10}$ copies/mL at 24 weeks and is effective against lamivudine-resistant HBV. The drug is approved only for treatment of HIV infection, but its use should be considered in patients co-infected with HIV and HBV. For a more detailed discussion of tenofovir, see Chap. 182.

ENTECAVIR

Entecavir is a cyclopentyl guanosine analogue that inhibits HBV through inhibition of HBV DNA polymerase by entecavir triphosphate and is also active against HIV. In vitro, entecavir is more potent than lamivudine or adefovir against HBV and is also effective against lamivudine-resistant HBV. Administration of entecavir at a dose of 0.5 mg/d PO for 48 weeks results in a reduction of HBV DNA by 5.0–6.9 $\log_{10}$ copies/mL, normalization of ALT values in 68–78% of recipients, and loss of HBeAg in 21%. Entecavir is highly bioavailable but should be taken on an empty stomach since food interferes with its absorption. The drug is eliminated primarily in unchanged form by the kidneys, and its dosage should be adjusted for patients with Cr_{Cl} values of <50 mg/min. Overall, entecavir is well tolerated. Resistance to entecavir has not been observed during the treatment of naïve patients; however, resistance was noted in 7–10% of lamivudine-refractory patients at 48 weeks of treatment with entecavir. Entecavir-resistant strains appear to be sensitive to adefovir. As with other anti-HBV treatments, exacerbation of hepatitis may occur when entecavir therapy is stopped. Entecavir is approved for treatment of chronic hepatitis B in adults.

TELBIVUDINE

Telbivudine is the β-L enantiomer of thymidine and is a potent inhibitor of HBV. Its active form is telbivudine triphosphate, which inhibits HBV DNA polymerase but has little or no activity against human DNA polymerase. Administration of telbivudine at a dose of 600 mg/d PO for 52 weeks to patients with chronic hepatitis B resulted in reduction of HBV DNA by >5 $\log_{10}$ copies/mL along with either loss of serum HBeAg or normalization of ALT in 75% of recipients. After 2 years of therapy, resistance to telbivudine was noted in isolates from 8.6–21.6% of patients. Telbivudine-resistant HBV is usually resistant to lamivudine as well but is generally susceptible to adefovir.

Telbivudine is eliminated primarily by the kidneys, and the dosage should be reduced in patients with a Cl_{Cr} value of <50 mL/min. Telbivudine is generally well tolerated, but increases in serum creatinine kinases and clinically evident myopathy have been observed. As with other anti-HBV drugs, hepatitis may be exacerbated in patients who have discontinued telbivudine therapy. Telbivudine has been approved for treatment of adults with chronic hepatitis B who have evidence of viral replication and either persistent elevation in serum aminotransferases or histologically active disease.

INTERFERONS

IFNs are cytokines that exhibit a broad spectrum of antiviral activities as well as immunomodulating and antiproliferative properties. IFNs are not available for oral administration but must be given IM, SC, or IV. Early studies with human leukocyte IFN demonstrated an effect in the prophylaxis of experimentally induced rhinovirus infections in humans and in the treatment of VZV infections in immunosuppressed patients. DNA recombinant technology has made available highly purified α, β, and γ IFNs that have been evaluated in a variety of viral infections. Results of such trials have confirmed the effectiveness of intranasally administered IFN in the prophylaxis of rhinovirus infections, although its use has been associated with nasal mucosal irritation. Studies have also demonstrated a beneficial effect of intralesionally or systemically administered IFNs on genital warts. The effect of systemic administration consists primarily of a reduction in the size of the warts, and this mode of therapy may be useful in persons who have numerous warts that cannot easily be treated by individual intralesional injections. However, lesions frequently recur after either intralesional or systemic IFN therapy is discontinued.

IFNs have undergone extensive study in the treatment of chronic HBV infection. The administration of IFN-α2b (5 million units daily or 10 million units three times a week for 16–24 weeks) to patients with stable chronic HBV infection resulted in loss of markers of HBV replication, such as HBeAg and HBV DNA, in 33–37% of cases; 8% of patients also became negative for hepatitis B surface antigen. In >80% of patients who lose HBeAg and HBV DNA markers, serum aminotransferases return to normal levels, and both short- and long-term improvements in liver histopathology have been described. Predictors of a favorable response to therapy include low pretherapy levels of HBV DNA, high pretherapy serum levels of ALT, a short duration of chronic HBV infection, and active inflammation in liver histopathology. Poor responses are seen in immunosuppressed patients, including those with HIV infection. A longer duration of therapy (12–24 months) is recommended for HBeAg-negative chronic hepatitis B. Adverse effects of the above doses of IFN are common and include fever, chills, myalgia, fatigue, neurotoxicity (primarily manifested as somnolence, depression, anxiety, and confusion), and leukopenia. Approximately 25% of patients receiving a daily dose of 5 million units require dose reduction, but <5% require discontinuation of therapy. Pegylated IFNs, which are covalently linked with monomethoxy polyethylene glycol, have a markedly reduced clearance rate. Therefore, they can be administered less frequently, are better tolerated, and may be more effective in some settings than standard IFNs (see discussion of hepatitis C below). Pegylated IFN-α2a is approved for the treatment of patients with chronic hepatitis B who are either positive or negative for HBeAg (Table 171-1).

Several IFN preparations, including IFN-α2a, IFN-α2b, IFN-alfacon-1, and IFN-αm1 (lymphoblastoid), have been studied as therapy for chronic HCV infections. A variety of monotherapy regimens have been employed, of which the most common is IFN-α2b or -α2a at 3 million units three times per week for 12–18 months. The addition of oral ribavirin to IFN-α2b—either as initial therapy or after failure of IFN therapy alone—results in significantly higher rates of sustained virologic and/or serum ALT responses (40–50%) than are obtained with monotherapy. Comparative studies indicate that pegylated IFN-α2b or -α2a therapy is more effective than standard IFN treatment against chronic HCV infection. The combination of SC pegylated IFN and oral ribavirin is more convenient and appears to be the most effective regimen for treatment of chronic hepatitis C. With this combination regimen, sustained virologic responses were seen in 42–46% of patients with genotype 1 infection and in 76–82% of patients with genotype 2 or 3 infection. Ribavirin appears to have a small antiviral effect in HCV infection but may also be working through an immunomodulatory effect in combination with IFN. Optimal results with ribavirin appear to be associated with weight-based dosing. Prognostic factors for a favorable response include an age of <45 years, a short duration of infection, low levels of HCV RNA, and infection with HCV genotypes other than 1. IFN-alfacon, a synthetic "consensus" α interferon, appears to produce response rates similar to those elicited by IFN-α2a or -α2b alone and is also approved in the United States for the treatment of chronic hepatitis C.

The efficacy of IFN-α treatment for chronic hepatitis D remains unestablished. Anecdotal reports suggested that doses ranging from 5 million units daily to 9 million units three times per week for 12 months elicit biochemical and virologic responses. Results from small controlled trials have been inconsistent, and observed responses have not generally been sustained. Limited experience has been published with the use of pegylated IFN-α2b for treatment of hepatitis D, but some consultants prefer this agent for this indication because of its pharmacologic advantages over standard IFN.

FURTHER READINGS

BEUTNER KR et al: Valaciclovir compared with acyclovir for improved therapy for herpes zoster in immunocompetent adults. Antimicrob Agents Chemother 39:1546, 1995

COUCH RB: Drug therapy: Prevention and treatment of influenza. N Engl J Med 343:1778, 2000

CRUMPACKER CS: Ganciclovir. N Engl J Med 335:721, 1996

DOLIN R et al: A controlled trial of amantadine and rimantadine in the prophylaxis of influenza A infection. N Engl J Med 307:580, 1982

FIELD JJ, HOOFNAGLE JH: Mechanism of action of interferon and ribavirin in treatment of hepatitis C. Nature 436:967, 2005

GISH RG et al: Safety and antiviral activity of emtricitabine (FTC) for the treatment of chronic hepatitis B infection: A two-year study. J Hepatol 43:60, 2005

HALL CB et al: Aerosolized ribavirin treatment of infants with respiratory syncytial viral infection: A randomized double-blind study. N Engl J Med 308:1443, 1983

HAYDEN FG: Antiviral drugs (other than antiretrovirals), in *Principles and Practice of Infectious Diseases*, 6th ed, JE Bennett et al (eds). Philadelphia, Elsevier Churchill Livingstone, 2005, pp 514–551

LAI CL et al: Entecavir versus lamivudine for patients with HBeAg-negative chronic hepatitis B. N Engl J Med 354:186, 2006

LALEZARI JP et al: Randomized controlled study of the safety and efficacy of IV cidofovir for the treatment of relapsing cytomegalovirus retinitis in patients with AIDS. J AIDS 17:339, 1998

LOK AS et al: Management of hepatitis B: 2000—summary of a workshop. Gastroenterology 120:1828, 2001

MARTIN DF et al: A controlled trial of valganciclovir as induction therapy for cytomegalovirus retinitis. N Engl J Med 346:1119, 2002

National Institutes of Health Consensus Development Conference Statement: Management of hepatitis C. September 12, 2002 (available at *www.niaid.nih.gov*)

TREANOR JJ et al: Efficacy and safety in treating acute influenza: A randomized controlled trial. U.S. Oral Neuraminidase Study Group. JAMA 283:1016, 2000

SECTION 12 INFECTIONS DUE TO DNA VIRUSES

172 Herpes Simplex Viruses

Lawrence Corey

DEFINITION

Herpes simplex viruses (HSV-1, HSV-2; *Herpesvirus hominis*) produce a variety of infections involving mucocutaneous surfaces, the central nervous system (CNS), and—on occasion—visceral organs. Prompt recognition and treatment reduce the morbidity and mortality associated with HSV infections.

ETIOLOGIC AGENT

The genome of HSV is a linear, double-strand DNA molecule (molecular weight, ~100×10^6 units) that encodes >90 transcription units with 84 identified proteins. The genomic structures of the two HSV subtypes are similar. The overall genomic sequence homology between HSV-1 and HSV-2 is ~50%, while the proteome homology is >80%. The homologous sequences are distributed over the entire genome map, and most of the polypeptides specified by one viral type are antigenically related to polypeptides of the other viral type. Many type-specific regions unique to HSV-1 and HSV-2 proteins do exist, however, and a number of them appear to be important in host immunity. These type-specific regions have been used to develop serologic assays that distinguish between the two viral subtypes. Either restriction endonuclease analysis of viral DNA or DNA sequencing can be used to distinguish between the two subtypes and among strains of each subtype. The variability of nucleotide sequences from clinical strains of HSV-1 and HSV-2 is such that HSV isolates obtained from two individuals can be differentiated by restriction enzyme patterns or genomic sequences. Moreover, epidemiologically related sources, such as sexual partners, mother-infant pairs, or persons involved in a common-source outbreak, can be inferred from such patterns.

The viral genome is packaged in a regular icosahedral protein shell (capsid) composed of 162 capsomeres (see Fig. 170-1). The outer covering of the virus is a lipid-containing membrane (envelope) acquired as the DNA-containing capsid buds through the inner nuclear membrane of the host cell. Between the capsid and lipid bilayer of the envelope is the tegument. Viral replication has both nuclear and cytoplasmic phases. Attachment and fusion of the viral envelope and the cell membrane involve several ubiquitous heparin-like surface receptors. Replication is highly regulated. After fusion and entry, the nucleocapsid enters the cytoplasm and several viral proteins are released from the virion. Some of these viral proteins shut off host protein synthesis (by increasing cellular RNA degradation), while others "turn on" the transcription of early genes of HSV replication. These early gene products, designated *α genes*, are required for synthesis of the subsequent polypeptide group, the β polypeptides, many of which are regulatory proteins and enzymes required for DNA replication. Most current antiviral drugs interfere with β proteins, such as the viral DNA polymerase enzyme. The third (γ) class of HSV genes requires viral DNA replication for expression and constitutes most of the structural proteins specified by the virus.

After replication of the viral genome and synthesis of structural proteins, nucleocapsids are assembled in the nucleus of the cell. Envelopment occurs as the nucleocapsids bud through the inner nuclear membrane into the perinuclear space. In some cells, viral replication in the nucleus forms two types of inclusion bodies: type A basophilic Feulgen-positive bodies that contain viral DNA and eosinophilic inclusion bodies that are devoid of viral nucleic acid or protein and represent a "scar" of viral infection. Enveloped virions are then transported via the endoplasmic reticulum and the Golgi apparatus to the cell surface.

HSV infection of some neuronal cells does not result in cell death. Instead, viral genomes are maintained by the cell in a repressed state compatible with survival and normal activities of the cell, a condition called *latency*. Latency is associated with transcription of only a limited number of virus-encoded proteins. Subsequently, the viral genome may become activated; its activation results in the normal pattern of regulated viral gene expression, viral replication, and viral release. The release of HSV from the neuron and its subsequent entry into epithelial cells result in viral replication in these cells, destruction of the cells, and the subsequent reappearance of virus on mucosal surfaces. This process is termed *reactivation*. Whereas infectious virus is rarely recovered from sensory or autonomic nervous system ganglia dissected from cadavers, maintenance and growth of the neural cells (as "explants") in tissue culture result in production of infectious virions and in subsequent permissive infection of susceptible cells (*cocultivation*). The mechanisms by which latency is established, maintained, or broken are incompletely understood. Two RNA "latency-associated" transcripts that overlap the immediate early (α) gene products, called *ICP-O*, are found in abundance in the nuclei of latently infected neurons. Deletion mutants of this region that can become latent have been made. However, the efficiency of their later reactivation is reduced; thus, these latency-associated transcripts may play a role in maintaining rather than in establishing latency. Recent studies suggest that HSV-specific micro-RNAs in these and other regions of the viral genome may play an important role in virus maintenance in and release from neurons. CD8+ T cells have been found in ganglia of experimental animals and humans and appear to influence the process of reactivation, possibly by inducing antiviral factors such as interferon (IFN) γ. At present, strategies to interrupt latency or to maintain molecular latency in neurons are not available. In experimental animals, ultraviolet light, systemic and local immunosuppression, and trauma to the skin or ganglia are associated with reactivation.

PATHOGENESIS

Exposure to HSV at mucosal surfaces or abraded skin sites permits entry of the virus and initiation of its replication in cells of the epidermis and dermis. HSV infections are usually acquired subclinically. Whether clinical or subclinical, HSV acquisition is associated with sufficient viral replication to permit infection of either sensory or autonomic nerve endings. On entry into the neuronal cell, the virus—or, more likely, the nucleocapsid—is transported intra-axonally to the nerve cell bodies in ganglia. In humans, the transit interval from inoculation of virus in peripheral tissue to spread to the ganglia is unknown. During the initial phase of infection, viral replication occurs in ganglia and contiguous neural tissue. Virus then spreads to other mucocutaneous surfaces through centrifugal migration of infectious virions via peripheral sensory nerves. This mode of spread helps explain the large surface area involved, the high frequency of new lesions distant from the initial crop of vesicles that is characteristic in patients with primary genital or oral-labial HSV infection, and the ability to recover virus from neural tissue distant from neurons innervating the inoculation site. Contiguous spread of locally inoculated virus also may take place and allow further mucosal extension of disease. Recent studies have demonstrated HSV viremia—another mechanism for extension of infection throughout the body—in ~30–40% of persons with primary HSV-2 infection. Latent infection with both viral subtypes in both sensory and autonomic ganglia has been demonstrated.

Analysis of the DNA from sequential isolates of HSV or from isolates from multiple infected ganglia in any one individual has revealed similar, if not identical, restriction endonuclease or DNA sequence patterns in most persons. Occasionally (most frequently in immunocompromised persons), multiple strains of the same viral subtype are detected in one individual. As exposure to mucosal shedding is relatively common during a person's lifetime, these data suggest that exogenous infection with different strains of the same subtype is possible.

IMMUNITY

Host responses influence the acquisition of HSV disease, the severity of infection, resistance to the development of latency, the maintenance of latency, and the frequency of recurrences. Both antibody-mediated and cell-mediated reactions are clinically important. Immunocompromised patients with defects in cell-mediated immunity experience more severe and more extensive HSV infections than those with deficits in humoral immunity, such as agammaglobulinemia. Experimental ablation of lymphocytes indicates that T cells play a major role in preventing lethal disseminated disease, although antibodies help reduce virus titers in neural tissue. Some of the clinical manifestations of HSV appear to be related to the host immune response (e.g., stromal opacities associated with recurrent herpetic keratitis). The surface viral glycoproteins have been shown to be targets of antibodies that mediate neutralization and immune-mediated cytolysis (antibody-dependent cell-mediated cytotoxicity). Monoclonal antibodies specific for each of the known viral glycoproteins have, in experimental infections, conferred protection against subsequent neurologic disease or ganglionic latency. In humans, however, subunit glycoprotein vaccines have been only partially successful in reducing acquisition of infection. Multiple cell populations, including natural killer cells, macrophages, and a variety of T lymphocytes, play a role in host defenses against HSV infections, as do lymphokines generated by T lymphocytes. In animals, passive transfer of primed lymphocytes confers protection from subsequent challenge. Maximal protection usually requires the activation of multiple T cell subpopulations, including cytotoxic T cells and T cells responsible for delayed hypersensitivity. The latter cells may confer protection by the antigen-stimulated release of lymphokines (e.g., IFNs), which in turn have a direct antiviral effect and both activate and enhance a variety of specific and nonspecific effector cells. Increasing evidence suggests that HSV-specific CD8+ T cell responses are critical for clearance of virus from lesions. In addition, immunosuppressed patients with frequent and prolonged HSV lesions have fewer functional CD8+ T cells directed at HSV. The HSV virion contains a variety of genes that are directed at the inhibition of host responses. These include gene no. 12 (*US-12*), which can bind to the cellular transporter-activating protein TAP-1 and reduce the ability of this protein to bind HSV peptides to human leukocyte antigen (HLA) class I, thereby reducing recognition of viral proteins by cytotoxic T cells of the host. This effect can be overcome by the addition of IFN-γ, but this reversal requires 24–48 h; thus, the virus has time to replicate and invade other host cells. To date, the immunodominant T cell responses appear to be type-specific. Entry of infectious HSV-1 and HSV-2 inhibits several signaling pathways of both CD4+ and CD8+ T cells, leading to their functional impairment in killing and influencing the spectrum of their cytokine secretion.

EPIDEMIOLOGY

Seroepidemiologic studies have documented HSV infections worldwide. Serologic assays with whole-virus antigen preparations, such as complement fixation, neutralization, indirect immunofluorescence, passive hemagglutination, radioimmunoassay, and enzyme-linked immunosorbent assay, are useful for differentiating uninfected (seronegative) persons from those with past HSV-1 or HSV-2 infection, but they do not reliably distinguish between the two viral subtypes. Serologic assays that identify antibodies to type-specific surface proteins (epitopes) of the two viral subtypes have been developed and can distinguish reliably between the human antibody responses to HSV-1 and HSV-2. The most commonly used assays are those that measure antibodies to glycoprotein G of HSV-1 (gG1) and HSV-2 (gG2). A Western blot assay that can detect several HSV type-specific proteins can also be used.

Infection with HSV-1 is acquired more frequently and earlier than infection with HSV-2. More than 90% of adults have antibodies to

HSV-1 by the fifth decade of life. In populations of low socioeconomic status, most persons acquire HSV-1 infection before the third decade of life.

Antibodies to HSV-2 are not detected routinely until puberty. Antibody prevalence rates correlate with past sexual activity and vary greatly among different population groups. There is some evidence that the prevalence of HSV-2 has decreased slightly over the past 5 years in the United States. Serosurveys indicate that 15–20% of the U.S. population has antibodies to HSV-2. In most routine obstetric and family planning clinics, 25% of women have HSV-2 antibodies, although only 10% of those who are seropositive for HSV-2 report a history of genital lesions. As many as 50% of heterosexual adults attending sexually transmitted disease clinics have antibodies to HSV-2.

A wide variety of serologic surveys have indicated a similar or even higher seroprevalence of HSV-2 in most parts of Central America, South America, and Africa. There is an epidemiologic synergy between HSV-2 and HIV-1. HSV-2 infection is associated with a two- to fourfold increase in HIV-1 acquisition. In addition, HSV-2 is reactivated and transmitted more frequently in persons co-infected with HIV-1 and HSV-2 than in persons not infected with HIV-1. Thus, most areas of the world with a high HIV-1 prevalence also have a high HSV-2 prevalence. In Africa, HSV-2 seroprevalence has ranged from 40% to 70% in obstetric and other sexually experienced populations. Antibody prevalence rates average ~5–10% higher among women than among men.

Several studies suggest that many cases of "asymptomatic" genital HSV-2 infection are, in fact, simply unrecognized: when "asymptomatic" seropositive persons are shown pictures of genital lesions, >60% subsequently identify episodes of symptomatic reactivation. Most important, these asymptomatic seropositive persons with reactivation shed virus on mucosal surfaces almost as frequently as those with symptomatic disease. The large reservoir of unidentified carriers of HSV-2 and the frequent asymptomatic reactivation of the virus from the genital tract have fostered the continued spread of genital herpes throughout the world. HSV-2 infection is an independent risk factor for the acquisition and transmission of infection with HIV-1. Among co-infected persons, HIV-1 virions can be shed from herpetic lesions of the genital region. This shedding may facilitate the spread of HIV through sexual contact.

HSV infections occur throughout the year. Transmission can result from contact with persons who have active ulcerative lesions or with persons who have no clinical manifestations of infection but who are shedding HSV from mucocutaneous surfaces. Studies using the polymerase chain reaction (PCR) have shown that HSV reactivation on genital skin and mucosal surfaces is much more common than previously recognized. Among immunocompetent adults, HSV-2 can be cultured from the genital tract on 2–10% of days tested, and HSV DNA can be detected on 20–30% of days by PCR. Corresponding figures for HSV-1 in oral secretions are similar. Rates of shedding are highest during the initial years after acquisition, with viral shedding occurring on as many as 30–50% of days during this period. Immunosuppressed patients shed HSV from mucosal sites at an even higher frequency (20–80% of days). Reactivation rates vary widely among individuals. Among HIV-positive patients, a low CD4+ T cell count and a heavy viral load are associated with increased rates of HSV reactivation. (Daily antiviral chemotherapy for HSV-2 can markedly reduce shedding rates, as measured by PCR.) These high rates of mucocutaneous reactivation suggest that exposure to HSV from sexual or other close contact (kissing, sharing of glasses or silverware) is common and help explain the continuing spread and high seroprevalence of HSV infections worldwide.

CLINICAL SPECTRUM

HSV has been isolated from nearly all visceral and mucocutaneous sites. The clinical manifestations and course of HSV infection depend on the anatomic site involved, the age and immune status of the host, and the antigenic type of the virus. Primary HSV infections (i.e., first infections with either HSV-1 or HSV-2 in which the host lacks HSV antibodies in acute-phase serum) are frequently accompanied by systemic signs and symptoms. Compared with recurrent episodes, primary infections, which involve both mucosal and extramucosal sites, are characterized by a longer duration of symptoms and virus isolation from lesions. The incubation period ranges from 1 to 26 days (median, 6–8 days). Both viral subtypes can cause genital and oral-facial infections, and the infections caused by the two subtypes are clinically indistinguishable. However, the frequency of reactivation of infection is influenced by anatomic site and virus type. Genital HSV-2 infection is twice as likely to reactivate and recurs 8–10 times more frequently than genital HSV-1 infection. Conversely, oral-labial HSV-1 infection recurs more frequently than oral-labial HSV-2 infection. Asymptomatic shedding rates follow the same pattern.

Oral-Facial Infections Gingivostomatitis and pharyngitis are the most common clinical manifestations of first-episode HSV-1 infection, while recurrent herpes labialis is the most common clinical manifestation of reactivation HSV-1 infection. HSV pharyngitis and gingivostomatitis usually result from primary infection and are most commonly seen among children and young adults. Clinical symptoms and signs, which include fever, malaise, myalgias, inability to eat, irritability, and cervical adenopathy, may last 3–14 days. Lesions may involve the hard and soft palate, gingiva, tongue, lip, and facial area. HSV-1 or HSV-2 infection of the pharynx usually results in exudative or ulcerative lesions of the posterior pharynx and/or tonsillar pillars. Lesions of the tongue, buccal mucosa, or gingiva may occur later in the course in one-third of cases. Fever lasting 2–7 days and cervical adenopathy are common. It can be difficult to differentiate HSV pharyngitis clinically from bacterial pharyngitis, *Mycoplasma pneumoniae* infections, and pharyngeal ulcerations of noninfectious etiologies (e.g., Stevens-Johnson syndrome). No substantial evidence suggests that reactivation of oral-labial HSV infection is associated with symptomatic recurrent pharyngitis.

Reactivation of HSV from the trigeminal ganglia may be associated with asymptomatic virus excretion in the saliva, development of intraoral mucosal ulcerations, or herpetic ulcerations on the vermilion border of the lip or external facial skin. About 50–70% of seropositive patients undergoing trigeminal nerve-root decompression and 10–15% of those undergoing dental extraction develop oral-labial HSV infection a median of 3 days after these procedures. Clinical differentiation of intraoral mucosal ulcerations due to HSV from aphthous, traumatic, or drug-induced ulcerations is difficult.

In immunosuppressed patients, HSV infection may extend into mucosal and deep cutaneous layers. Friability, necrosis, bleeding, severe pain, and inability to eat or drink may result. The lesions of HSV mucositis are clinically similar to mucosal lesions caused by cytotoxic drug therapy, trauma, or fungal or bacterial infections. Persistent ulcerative HSV infections are among the most common infections in patients with AIDS. HSV and *Candida* infections often occur concurrently. Systemic antiviral therapy speeds the rate of healing and relieves the pain of mucosal HSV infections in immunosuppressed patients. The frequency of HSV reactivation during the early phases of transplantation or induction chemotherapy is high (50–90%), and prophylactic systemic antiviral agents such as IV acyclovir, penciclovir, or the oral congeners of these drugs are used to reduce reactivation rates. Patients with atopic eczema may also develop severe oral-facial HSV infections (*eczema herpeticum*), which may rapidly involve extensive areas of skin and occasionally disseminate to visceral organs. Extensive eczema herpeticum has resolved promptly with the administration of IV acyclovir. Erythema multiforme may also be associated with HSV infections (see Fig. 52-9); some evidence suggests that HSV infection is the precipitating event in ~75% of cases of cutaneous erythema multiforme. HSV antigen has been demonstrated both in circulatory immune complexes and in skin lesion biopsy samples from these cases. Patients with severe HSV-associated erythema multiforme are candidates for chronic suppressive oral antiviral therapy.

HSV-1 and varicella-zoster virus (VZV) have been implicated in the etiology of Bell's palsy (flaccid paralysis of the mandibular portion of

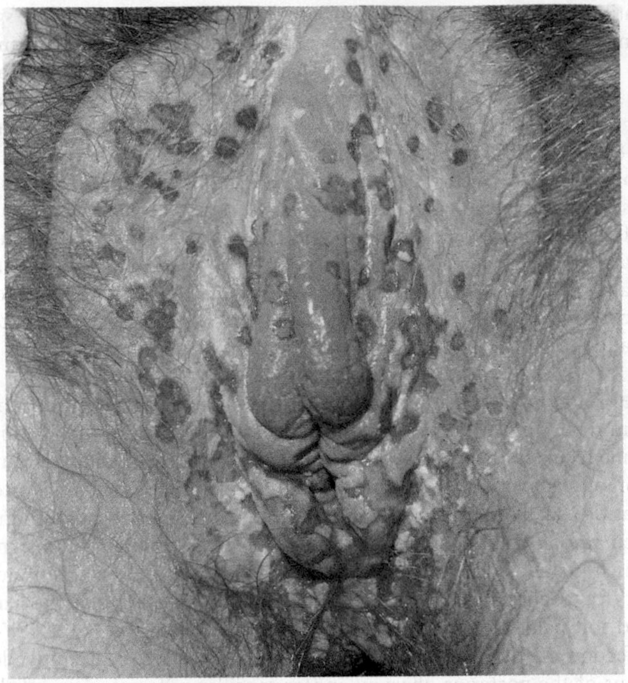

FIGURE 172-1 Genital herpes: primary vulvar infection. Multiple, extremely painful, punched-out, confluent, shallow ulcers on the edematous vulva and perineum. Micturition is often very painful. Associated inguinal lymphadenopathy is common. *(Reprinted with permission from K Wolff, RA Johnson, D Summond: Fitzpatrick's Color Atlas and Synopsis of Clinical Dermatology, 5th ed.)*

the facial nerve). Although uniform recommendations for treatment of this entity are not available, recent evidence suggests that antiviral chemotherapy in conjunction with a short course of glucocorticoids may result in improved outcomes.

Genital Infections First-episode primary genital herpes is characterized by fever, headache, malaise, and myalgias. Pain, itching, dysuria, vaginal and urethral discharge, and tender inguinal lymphadenopathy are the predominant local symptoms. Widely spaced bilateral lesions of the external genitalia are characteristic (Fig. 172-1). Lesions may be present in varying stages, including vesicles, pustules, or painful erythematous ulcers. The cervix and urethra are involved in >80% of women with first-episode infections. First episodes of genital herpes in patients who have had prior HSV-1 infection are associated with systemic symptoms in a few patients and with faster healing than primary genital herpes. The clinical courses of acute first-episode genital herpes are similar for HSV-1 and HSV-2 infection. However, the recurrence rates of genital disease differ with the viral subtype: the 12-month recurrence rates among patients with first-episode HSV-2 and HSV-1 infections are ~90% and ~55%, respectively (median number of recurrences, 4 and <1, respectively). Recurrence rates for genital HSV-2 infections vary greatly among individuals and over time within the same individual. HSV has been isolated from the urethra and urine of men and women without external genital lesions. A clear mucoid discharge and dysuria are characteristics of symptomatic HSV urethritis. HSV has been isolated from the urethra of 5% of women with the dysuria-frequency syndrome. Occasionally, HSV genital tract disease is manifested by endometritis and salpingitis in women and by prostatitis in men. About 15% of cases of HSV-2 acquisition are associated with nonlesional clinical syndromes, such as aseptic meningitis, cervicitis, or urethritis. A more complete discussion of the differential diagnosis of genital herpes is presented in Chap. 124.

Both HSV-1 and HSV-2 can cause symptomatic or asymptomatic rectal and perianal infections. HSV proctitis is usually associated with rectal intercourse. However, subclinical perianal shedding of HSV is detected in women and men who report no rectal intercourse. This phenomenon is due to the establishment of latency in the sacral dermatome from prior genital tract infection, with subsequent reactivation in epithelial cells in the perianal region. Such reactivations are often subclinical. Symptoms of HSV proctitis include anorectal pain, anorectal discharge, tenesmus, and constipation. Sigmoidoscopy reveals ulcerative lesions of the distal 10 cm of the rectal mucosa. Rectal biopsies show mucosal ulceration, necrosis, polymorphonuclear and lymphocytic infiltration of the lamina propria, and (in occasional cases) multinucleated intranuclear inclusion–bearing cells. Perianal herpetic lesions are also found in immunosuppressed patients receiving cytotoxic therapy. Extensive perianal herpetic lesions and/or HSV proctitis is common among patients with HIV infection.

Herpetic Whitlow Herpetic whitlow—HSV infection of the finger—may occur as a complication of primary oral or genital herpes by inoculation of virus through a break in the epidermal surface or by direct introduction of virus into the hand through occupational or some other type of exposure. Clinical signs and symptoms include abrupt-onset edema, erythema, and localized tenderness of the infected finger. Vesicular or pustular lesions of the fingertip that are indistinguishable from lesions of pyogenic bacterial infection are seen. Fever, lymphadenitis, and epitrochlear and axillary lymphadenopathy are common. The infection may recur. Prompt diagnosis (to avoid unnecessary and potentially exacerbating surgical therapy and/or transmission) is essential. Antiviral chemotherapy is usually recommended (see below).

Herpes Gladiatorum HSV may infect almost any area of skin. Mucocutaneous HSV infections of the thorax, ears, face, and hands have been described among wrestlers. Transmission of these infections is facilitated by trauma to the skin sustained during wrestling. Several recent outbreaks have illustrated the importance of prompt diagnosis and therapy to contain the spread of this infection.

Eye Infections HSV infection of the eye is the most common cause of corneal blindness in the United States. HSV keratitis presents as an acute onset of pain, blurred vision, chemosis, conjunctivitis, and characteristic dendritic lesions of the cornea. Use of topical glucocorticoids may exacerbate symptoms and lead to involvement of deep structures of the eye. Debridement, topical antiviral treatment, and/or IFN therapy hastens healing. However, recurrences are common, and the deeper structures of the eye may sustain immunopathologic injury. Stromal keratitis due to HSV appears to be related to T cell–dependent destruction of deep corneal tissue. An HSV-1 epitope that is autoreactive with T cell–targeting corneal antigens has been postulated to be a factor in this infection. Chorioretinitis, usually a manifestation of disseminated HSV infection, may occur in neonates or in patients with HIV infection. HSV and VZV can cause acute necrotizing retinitis as an uncommon but severe manifestation.

Central and Peripheral Nervous System Infections HSV accounts for 10–20% of all cases of sporadic viral encephalitis in the United States. The estimated incidence is ~2.3 cases per 1 million persons per year. Cases are distributed throughout the year, and the age distribution appears to be biphasic, with peaks at 5–30 and >50 years of age. HSV-1 causes >95% of cases.

The pathogenesis of HSV encephalitis varies. In children and young adults, primary HSV infection may result in encephalitis; presumably, exogenously acquired virus enters the CNS by neurotropic spread from the periphery via the olfactory bulb. However, most adults with HSV encephalitis have clinical or serologic evidence of mucocutaneous HSV-1 infection before the onset of CNS symptoms. In ~25% of the cases examined, the HSV-1 strains from the oropharynx and brain tissue of the same patient differ; thus some cases may result from reinfection with another strain of HSV-1 that reaches the CNS. Two theories have been proposed to explain the development of actively replicating HSV in localized areas of the CNS in persons whose ganglionic and CNS isolates are similar. Reactivation of latent HSV-1 infection in trigeminal or autonomic nerve roots may be associated with extension of virus into the CNS via nerves innervating the middle cranial fossa. HSV DNA has been demonstrated by DNA hybridization in brain tissue obtained at autopsy—even from healthy adults. Thus, reactivation of long-standing latent CNS infection may be another mechanism for the development of HSV encephalitis.

Recent studies have identified genetic polymorphisms in two separate genes among children with HSV encephalitis. Peripheral-blood mononuclear cells from these children appear to secrete reduced levels of IFN in response to HSV; if confirmed, this observation suggests that sporadic HSV encephalitis may be related to a variety of host genetic determinants.

The clinical hallmark of HSV encephalitis has been the acute onset of fever and focal neurologic symptoms and signs, especially in the temporal lobe (Fig. 172-2). Clinical differentiation of HSV encephalitis from other viral encephalitides, focal infections, or noninfectious processes is difficult. Elevated cerebrospinal fluid (CSF) protein levels, leukocytosis (predominantly lymphocytes), and red blood cell counts due to hemorrhagic necrosis are common. While brain biopsy has been the gold standard for defining HSV encephalitis, the high sensitivity and specificity of HSV DNA detection by PCR in CSF has largely replaced biopsy for defining HSV CNS infection. Although titers of antibody to HSV in CSF and serum increase in most cases of HSV encephalitis, they rarely do so earlier than 10 days into the illness and therefore, while useful retrospectively, are generally not helpful in establishing an early clinical diagnosis. Demonstration of HSV antigen, HSV DNA, or HSV replication in brain tissue obtained by biopsy is highly sensitive and has a low complication rate; examination of such tissue also provides the best opportunity to identify alternative, potentially treatable causes of encephalitis. Antiviral chemotherapy with acyclovir reduces the rate of death from HSV encephalitis. Even with therapy, however, neurologic sequelae are common, especially in persons >50 years of age. Most authorities recommend the administration of IV acyclovir to patients with presumed HSV encephalitis until the diagnosis is confirmed or an alternative diagnosis is made. Among proven cases of HSV encephalitis, IV therapy is usually recommended until HSV DNA levels in CSF are substantially reduced or nearly undetectable.

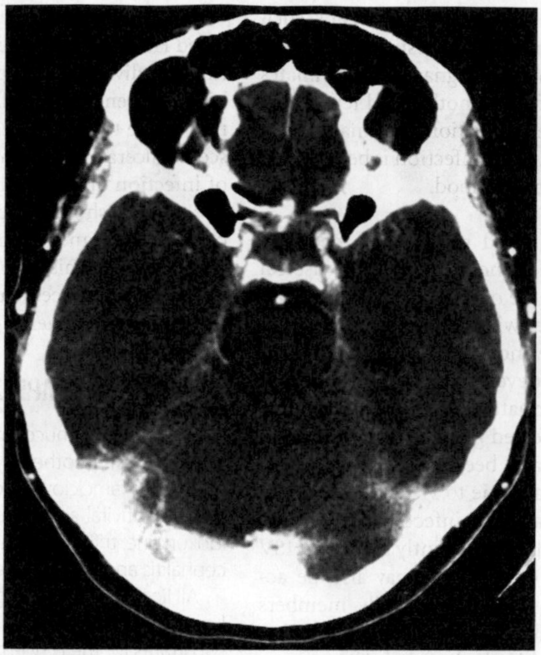

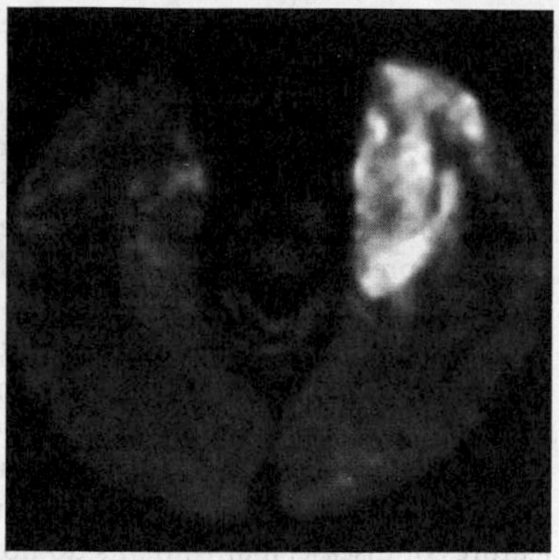

FIGURE 172-2 CT and diffusion-weighted MRI scans of the brain of a patient with left-temporal-lobe HSV encephalitis.

HSV DNA has been detected in CSF from 3–15% of persons presenting to the hospital with aseptic meningitis. HSV meningitis, which is usually seen in association with primary genital HSV infection, is an acute, self-limited disease manifested by headache, fever, and mild photophobia and lasting 2–7 days. Lymphocytic pleocytosis in the CSF is characteristic. Neurologic sequelae of HSV meningitis are rare. HSV is the most commonly identified cause of recurrent lymphocytic meningitis (Mollaret's meningitis). Demonstration of HSV antibodies in CSF or persistence of HSV DNA in CSF can establish the diagnosis. For persons with frequent recurrences of HSV meningitis, antiviral therapy has reduced the occurrence of such episodes.

Autonomic nervous system dysfunction, especially of the sacral region, has been reported in association with both HSV and VZV infections. Numbness, tingling of the buttocks or perineal areas, urinary retention, constipation, CSF pleocytosis, and (in males) impotence may occur. Symptoms appear to resolve slowly over days or weeks. Occasionally, hypoesthesia and/or weakness of the lower extremities persists for many months. Rarely, transverse myelitis, manifested by a rapidly progressive symmetric paralysis of the lower extremities or Guillain-Barré syndrome, follows HSV infection. Similarly, peripheral nervous system involvement (Bell's palsy) or cranial polyneuritis may be related to reactivation of HSV-1 infection. Transitory hypoesthesia of the area of skin innervated by the trigeminal nerve and vestibular system dysfunction as measured by electronystagmography are the predominant signs of disease. Whether antiviral chemotherapy can abort these signs or reduce their frequency and severity is not yet known.

Visceral Infections HSV infection of visceral organs usually results from viremia, and multiple-organ involvement is common. Occasionally, however, the clinical manifestations of HSV infection involve only the esophagus, lung, or liver. HSV esophagitis may result from direct extension of oral-pharyngeal HSV infection into the esophagus or may occur de novo by reactivation and spread of HSV to the esophageal mucosa via the vagus nerve. The predominant symptoms of HSV esophagitis are odynophagia, dysphagia, substernal pain, and weight loss. Multiple oval ulcerations appear on an erythematous base with or without a patchy white pseudomembrane. The distal esophagus is most commonly involved. With extensive disease, diffuse friability may spread to the entire esophagus. Neither endoscopic nor barium examination can reliably differentiate HSV esophagitis from *Candida* esophagitis or from esophageal ulcerations due to thermal injury, radiation, or corrosives. Endoscopically obtained secretions for cytologic examination and culture or DNA detection by PCR provide the most useful material for diagnosis. Systemic antiviral chemotherapy usually reduces symptoms and heals esophageal ulcerations.

HSV pneumonitis is uncommon except in severely immunosuppressed patients and may result from extension of herpetic tracheobronchitis into lung parenchyma. Focal necrotizing pneumonitis usually ensues. Hematogenous dissemination of virus from sites of oral or genital mucocutaneous disease may also occur, producing bilateral interstitial pneumonitis. Bacterial, fungal, and parasitic pathogens are commonly present in HSV pneumonitis. The mortality rate from untreated HSV pneumonia in immunosuppressed patients is high (>80%). HSV has also been isolated from the lower respiratory tract of persons with adult respiratory distress syndrome and prolonged intubation. The role of lower respiratory tract HSV infection in overall rates of morbidity and mortality associated with these conditions is unclear.

HSV is an uncommon cause of hepatitis in immunocompetent patients. HSV infection of the liver is associated with fever, abrupt elevations of bilirubin and serum aminotransferase levels, and leukopenia (<4000 white blood cells/μL). Disseminated intravascular coagulation may also develop.

Other reported complications of HSV infection include monarticular arthritis, adrenal necrosis, idiopathic thrombocytopenia, and glomerulonephritis. Disseminated HSV infection in immunocompetent patients is rare. In immunocompromised, burned, or malnourished patients, HSV occasionally disseminates to other visceral organs, such as the adrenal glands, pancreas, small and large intestines, and bone marrow. Rarely, primary HSV infection in pregnancy disseminates and may be associated with the death of both mother and fetus. This uncommon event is usually related to the acquisition of primary infection in the third trimester. Disseminated HSV infection is best detected by the presence of HSV DNA in plasma or blood.

Neonatal HSV Infections Of all HSV-infected populations, neonates (infants younger than 6 weeks) have the highest frequency of visceral and/or CNS infection. Without therapy, the overall rate of death from neonatal herpes is 65%; <10% of neonates with CNS infection develop normally. Although skin lesions are the most commonly recognized features of disease, many infants do not develop lesions at all or do so only well into the course of disease. Neonatal infection is usually acquired perinatally from contact with infected genital secretions at delivery. Congenitally infected infants have been reported. In most series, 30% of neonatal HSV infections are due to HSV-1 and 70% to HSV-2. The risk of developing neonatal HSV infection is 10 times higher for an infant born to a mother who has recently acquired HSV than for other infants. Neonatal HSV-1 infections may also be acquired through postnatal contact with immediate family members who have symptomatic or asymptomatic oral-labial HSV-1 infection or through nosocomial transmission within the hospital. All neonates with presumed neonatal herpes should be treated with IV acyclovir. Antiviral chemotherapy with high-dose IV acyclovir (60 mg/kg per day) has reduced the mortality rate from neonatal herpes to ~15%. However, morbidity, especially among infants with HSV-2 infection involving the CNS, is still very high.

DIAGNOSIS

Both clinical and laboratory criteria are useful for diagnosing HSV infections. A clinical diagnosis can be made accurately when characteristic multiple vesicular lesions on an erythematous base are present. However, herpetic ulcerations may resemble skin ulcerations of other etiologies. Mucosal HSV infections may also present as urethritis or pharyngitis without cutaneous lesions. Thus, laboratory studies to confirm the diagnosis and to guide therapy are recommended. While staining of scrapings from the base of the lesions with Wright's, Giemsa's (Tzanck preparation), or Papanicolaou's stain to detect giant cells or intranuclear inclusions of *Herpesvirus* infection is a well-described procedure, few clinicians are skilled in these techniques, the sensitivity of staining is low (<30% for mucosal swabs), and these cytologic methods do not differentiate between HSV and VZV infections.

HSV infection is best confirmed in the laboratory by detection of virus, viral antigen, or viral DNA in scrapings from lesions. HSV DNA detection by PCR, when available, is the most sensitive laboratory technique. HSV causes a discernible cytopathic effect in a variety of cell culture systems, and this effect can be identified within 48–96 h after inoculation. Spin-amplified culture with subsequent staining for HSV antigen has shortened the time needed to identify HSV to <24 h. The sensitivity of all detection methods depends on the stage of the lesions (with higher sensitivity in vesicular than in ulcerative lesions), on whether the patient has a first or a recurrent episode of the disease (with higher sensitivity in first than in recurrent episodes), and on whether the sample is from an immunosuppressed or an immunocompetent patient (with more antigen or DNA in immunosuppressed patients). Laboratory confirmation permits subtyping of the virus; information on subtype may be useful epidemiologically and may help to predict the frequency of reactivation after first-episode oral-labial or genital HSV infection.

Acute- and convalescent-phase serum can be useful in demonstrating seroconversion during primary HSV-1 or HSV-2 infection. However, few available tests report titers, and increases in index values do not reflect first episodes in all patients. Serologic assays based on type-specific proteins should be used to identify asymptomatic carriers of HSV-1 or HSV-2 infection. No reliable IgM method for defining acute HSV infection is available.

Several studies have shown that persons with previously unrecognized HSV-2 infection can be taught to identify symptomatic reactivations. Individuals seropositive for HSV-2 should be told about the high frequency of subclinical reactivation in mucosal surfaces that are not visible to the eye (e.g., cervix, urethra, perianal skin) or in microscopic ulcerations that may not be clinically symptomatic. Transmission of infection during such episodes is well established. HSV-2-seropositive persons should be educated about the high likelihood of subclinical shedding and the role condoms (male or female) may play in reducing transmission. Antiviral therapy with valacyclovir (500 mg once daily) has been shown to reduce the transmission of HSV-2 between sexual partners.

℞ HERPES SIMPLEX VIRUS INFECTIONS

Many aspects of mucocutaneous and visceral HSV infections are amenable to antiviral chemotherapy. For mucocutaneous infections, acyclovir and its congeners famciclovir and valacyclovir have been the mainstays of therapy. Several antiviral agents are available for topical use in HSV eye infections: idoxuridine, trifluorothymidine, topical vidarabine, and cidofovir. For HSV encephalitis and neonatal herpes, IV acyclovir is the treatment of choice.

All licensed antiviral agents for use against HSV inhibit the viral DNA polymerase. One class of drugs, typified by the drug acyclovir, is made up of substrates for the HSV enzyme thymidine kinase (TK). Acyclovir, ganciclovir, famciclovir, and valacyclovir are all selectively phosphorylated to the monophosphate form in virus-infected cells. Cellular enzymes convert the monophosphate form of the drug to the triphosphate, which is then incorporated into the viral DNA chain.

Acyclovir is the agent most frequently used for the treatment of HSV infections and is available in IV, oral, and topical formulations. Valacyclovir, the valyl ester of acyclovir, offers greater bioavailability than acyclovir and thus can be administered less frequently. Famciclovir, the oral formulation of penciclovir, is clinically effective in the treatment of a variety of HSV-1 and HSV-2 infections. Ganciclovir is active against both HSV-1 and HSV-2; however, it is more toxic than acyclovir, valacyclovir, and famciclovir and generally is not recommended for the treatment of HSV infections. Anecdotal case reports suggest that ganciclovir may also be less effective than acyclovir for treatment of HSV infections.

All three recommended compounds—acyclovir, valacyclovir, and famciclovir—have proved effective in shortening the duration of symptoms and lesions of mucocutaneous HSV infections in both immunocompromised and immunocompetent patients **(Table 172-1)**. IV and oral formulations prevent reactivation of HSV in seropositive immunocompromised patients during induction chemotherapy or in the period immediately after bone marrow or solid organ transplantation. Chronic daily suppressive therapy reduces the frequency of reactivation disease among patients with frequent genital or oral-labial herpes. Only valacyclovir has been subjected to clinical trials that demonstrated reduced transmission of HSV-2 infection between sexual partners.

IV acyclovir (30 mg/kg per day, given as a 10-mg/kg infusion over 1 h at 8-h intervals) is effective in reducing rates of death and morbidity from HSV encephalitis. Early initiation of therapy is a critical factor in outcome. The major side effect associated with IV acyclovir is transient renal insufficiency, usually due to crystallization of the compound in the renal parenchyma. This adverse reaction can be avoided if the medication is given slowly over 1 h and the patient is well hydrated. Because CSF levels of acyclovir average only 30–50% of plasma levels, the dosage of acyclovir used for treatment of CNS infection (30 mg/kg per day) is double that used for treatment of mucocutaneous or visceral disease (15 mg/kg per day). Even higher doses of IV acyclovir are used for neonatal HSV infection (60 mg/kg per day in three divided doses).

Among immunocompetent patients, recent studies have shown the effectiveness of short-course, high-dose oral therapy to reduce the signs and symptoms of oral and genital HSV infection. These regimens include valacyclovir (for 1–3 days) for oral-labial HSV and acyclovir (2 days), valacyclovir (3 days), or famciclovir (1 or 2 days) for recurrent-episode genital herpes (Table 172-1). These short-course regimens are less expensive and more convenient but should be reserved for immunocompetent hosts.

SUPPRESSION OF MUCOCUTANEOUS HERPES Recognition of the high frequency of subclinical reactivation provides a well-accepted rationale for the use of daily antiviral therapy to suppress reactivations of HSV, especially in persons with frequent clinical reactivations (e.g., those with recently acquired genital HSV infection). Immunosuppressed persons, including those with HIV infection, may also benefit from daily antiviral therapy. Recent studies have shown the efficacy of daily acyclovir and valacyclovir in reducing the frequency of HSV reactivations among HIV-positive persons. Regimens used include acyclovir (400 mg three times daily), famciclovir (500 mg twice daily), and valacyclovir (1 g twice daily); valacyclovir at a dose of 4 g daily was associated with thrombotic thrombocytopenic purpura in one study of HIV-infected persons. In addition, daily treatment of HSV-2 reduces the titer of HIV RNA in plasma (0.5-log reduction) and in genital mucosa (0.33-log reduction).

REDUCED HSV TRANSMISSION TO SEXUAL PARTNERS Once-daily valacyclovir (500 mg) has been shown to reduce transmission of HSV-2 between sexual partners. Transmission rates are higher from males to females and among persons with frequent HSV-2 reactivation. Serologic screening can be used to identify at-risk couples. Daily valacyclovir appears more effective at reducing subclinical shedding than daily famciclovir.

ACYCLOVIR RESISTANCE Acyclovir-resistant strains of HSV have been identified. Most of these strains have an altered substrate specificity for phosphorylating acyclovir. Thus, cross-resistance to famciclovir and valacyclovir is usually found. Occasionally, an isolate with altered TK specificity arises and is sensitive to famciclovir but not to acyclovir. In some patients infected with TK-deficient virus, higher doses of acyclovir are associated with clearing of lesions. In others, clinical disease progresses despite high-dose therapy. Almost all clinically significant acyclovir resistance has been seen in immunocompromised patients, and HSV-2 isolates are more often resistant than HSV-1 strains. A study by the Centers for Disease Control and Prevention indicated that ~5% of HSV-2 isolates from HIV-positive persons exhibit some degree of in vitro resistance to acyclovir. Of HSV-2 isolates from immunocompetent patients attending sexually transmitted disease clinics, <0.5% show reduced in vitro sensitivity to acyclovir. The lack of appreciable change in the frequency of detection of such isolates in the past 20 years probably reflects the reduced transmission of TK-deficient mutants. Isolation of HSV from lesions persisting despite adequate dosages and blood levels of acyclovir should raise the suspicion of acyclovir resistance. Therapy with the antiviral drug foscarnet is useful in acyclovir-resistant cases (Chap. 171). Because of its toxicity and cost, this drug is usually reserved for patients with extensive mucocutaneous infections. Cidofovir is a nucleotide analogue and exists as a phosphonate or monophosphate form. Most TK-deficient strains of HSV are sensitive to cidofovir. Cidofovir ointment speeds healing of acyclovir-resistant lesions. No well-controlled trials of systemic cidofovir have been reported. True TK-negative variants of HSV appear to have a reduced capacity to spread because of altered neurovirulence—a feature important in the relatively infrequent presence of such strains in immunocompetent populations, even with increasing use of antiviral drugs.

TABLE 172-1 ANTIVIRAL CHEMOTHERAPY FOR HSV INFECTION

I. Mucocutaneous HSV infections

A. Infections in immunosuppressed patients

1. *Acute symptomatic first or recurrent episodes:* IV acyclovir (5 mg/kg q8h) or oral acyclovir (400 mg qid), famciclovir (500 mg bid or tid), or valacyclovir (500 mg bid) is effective. Treatment duration may vary from 7 to 14 days.
2. *Suppression of reactivation disease (genital or oral-labial):* IV acyclovir (5 mg/kg q8h) or oral valacyclovir (500 mg bid) or acyclovir (400–800 mg 3–5 times per day) prevents recurrences during the 30-day period immediately after transplantation. Longer-term HSV suppression is often used for persons with continued immunosuppression. In bone marrow and renal transplant recipients, oral valacyclovir (2 g/d) is also effective in reducing cytomegalovirus infection. Oral valacyclovir at a dose of 4 g/d has been associated with thrombotic thrombocytopenic purpura after extended use in HIV-positive persons. In HIV-infected persons, oral acyclovir (400–800 mg bid), valacyclovir (500 mg bid), or famciclovir (500 mg bid) is effective in reducing clinical and subclinical reactivations of HSV-1 and HSV-2.

B. Infections in immunocompetent patients

1. *Genital herpes*
   - a. *First episodes:* Oral acyclovir (200 mg 5 times per day or 400 mg tid), valacyclovir (1 g bid), or famciclovir (250 mg bid) for 7–14 days is effective. IV acyclovir (5 mg/kg q8h for 5 days) is given for severe disease or neurologic complications such as aseptic meningitis.
   - b. *Symptomatic recurrent genital herpes:* Short-course (1- to 3-day) regimens are preferred because of low cost and convenience. Oral acyclovir (800 mg tid for 2 days), valacyclovir (500 mg bid for 3 days), or famciclovir (750 or 1000 mg bid for 1 day, a 1500-mg single dose, or 500 mg stat followed by 250 mg q12h for 3 days) effectively shortens lesion duration. Other options include oral acyclovir (200 mg 5 times per day), valacyclovir (500 mg bid), and famciclovir (125 mg bid for 5 days).
   - c. *Suppression of recurrent genital herpes:* Oral acyclovir (200-mg capsules tid or qid, 400 mg bid, or 800 mg qd), famciclovir (250 mg bid), or valacyclovir (500 mg daily) is effective. Patients with >9 episodes per year should take oral valacyclovir at a dosage of 1 g daily or 500 mg bid.
2. *Oral-labial HSV infections*
   - a. *First episode:* Oral acyclovir (200 mg) is given 4 or 5 times per day; an oral acyclovir suspension can be used (600 mg/m^2 qid). Oral famciclovir (250 mg bid) or valacyclovir (1 g bid) has been used clinically.
   - b. *Recurrent episodes:* If initiated at the onset of the prodrome, single-dose or 1-day therapy effectively reduces pain and speeds healing. Regimens include oral famciclovir (a 1500 mg single dose or 750 mg bid for 1 day) or valacyclovir (a 2-g single dose or 2 g bid for 1 day). Self-initiated therapy with 6-times-daily topical penciclovir cream effectively speeds healing of oral-labial HSV. Topical acyclovir cream has also been shown to speed healing.
   - c. *Suppression of reactivation of oral-labial HSV:* If started before exposure and continued for the duration of exposure (usually 5–10 days), oral acyclovir (400 mg bid) prevents reactivation of recurrent oral-labial HSV infection associated with severe sun exposure.
3. *Surgical prophylaxis of oral or genital HSV infection:* Several surgical procedures, such as laser skin resurfacing, trigeminal nerve-root decompression, and lumbar disk surgery, have been associated with HSV reactivation. IV acyclovir (5 mg/kg q8h) or oral acyclovir (800 mg bid), valacyclovir (500 mg bid), or famciclovir (250 mg bid) effectively reduces reactivation. Therapy should be initiated 48 h before surgery and continued for 3–7 days.
4. *Herpetic whitlow:* Oral acyclovir (200 mg) is given 5 times daily for 7–10 days.
5. *HSV proctitis:* Oral acyclovir (400 mg 5 times per day) is useful in shortening the course of infection. In immunosuppressed patients or in patients with severe infection, IV acyclovir (5 mg/kg q8h) may be useful.
6. *Herpetic eye infections:* In acute keratitis, topical trifluorothymidine, vidarabine, idoxuridine, acyclovir, penciclovir, and interferon are all beneficial. Debridement may be required. Topical steroids may worsen disease.

II. CNS HSV infections

- A. *HSV encephalitis:* IV acyclovir (10 mg/kg q8h; 30 mg/kg per day) is given for 10 days or until HSV DNA is no longer detected in CSF.
- B. *HSV aseptic meningitis:* No studies of systemic antiviral chemotherapy exist. If therapy is to be given, IV acyclovir (15–30 mg/kg per day) should be used.
- C. *Autonomic radiculopathy:* No studies are available. Most authorities recommend a trial of IV acyclovir.

III. Neonatal HSV infections: Oral acyclovir (60 mg/kg per day, divided into 3 doses) is given. The recommended duration of treatment is 21 days. Monitoring for relapse should be undertaken, and some authorities recommend continued suppression with oral acyclovir suspension for 3–4 months.

IV. Visceral HSV infections

- A. *HSV esophagitis:* IV acyclovir (15 mg/kg per day). In some patients with milder forms of immunosuppression, oral therapy with valacyclovir or famciclovir is effective.
- B. *HSV pneumonitis:* No controlled studies exist. IV acyclovir (15 mg/kg per day) should be considered.

V. Disseminated HSV infections: No controlled studies exist. IV acyclovir (5 mg/kg q8h) should be tried. Adjustments for renal insufficiency may be needed. No definite evidence indicates that therapy will decrease the risk of death.

VI. Erythema multiforme associated with HSV: Anecdotal observations suggest that oral acyclovir (400 mg bid or tid) or valacyclovir (500 mg bid) will suppress erythema multiforme.

VII. Infections due to acyclovir-resistant HSV: IV foscarnet (40 mg/kg IV q8h) should be given until lesions heal. The optimal duration of therapy and the usefulness of its continuation to suppress lesions are unclear. Some patients may benefit from cutaneous application of trifluorothymidine or 5% cidofovir gel.

PREVENTION

The success of efforts to control HSV disease on a population basis through suppressive antiviral chemotherapy and/or educational programs will be limited.

Barrier forms of contraception (especially condoms) decrease the likelihood of transmission of HSV infection, particularly during periods of asymptomatic viral excretion. When lesions are present, HSV infection may be transmitted by skin-to-skin contact despite the use of a condom. Nevertheless, the available data suggest that consistent condom use is an effective means of reducing the risk of genital HSV-2 transmission. Chronic daily antiviral therapy with valacyclovir can also be partially effective in reducing acquisition of HSV-2, especially among susceptible women. There are no comparative efficacy studies of valacyclovir versus condom use. Most authorities suggest both approaches. The need for a vaccine to prevent acquisition of HSV infection is great, especially in light of the role HSV-2 plays in enhancing the acquisition and transmission of HIV-1.

A substantial portion of neonatal HSV cases could be prevented by reducing the acquisition of HSV by women in the third trimester of pregnancy. Identification of women susceptible to HSV acquisition in pregnancy through serologic screening, with a focus on counseling against unprotected oral or genital sex, is receiving increasing attention. Neonatal HSV infection can result from either the acquisition of maternal infection near term or the reactivation of infection at delivery in the already-infected mother. Thus strategies for reducing neonatal HSV are complex. Some authorities have recommended that antiviral therapy with acyclovir or valacyclovir be given to HSV-2-infected women in late pregnancy as a means of reducing reactivation of HSV-2 at term. Data are not available to support the efficacy of this approach. Moreover, the high treatment-to-prevention ratio makes this a dubious public health approach, even though it can reduce the frequency of HSV-associated cesarean delivery.

FURTHER READINGS

Brown ZA et al: Effect of serologic status and cesarean delivery on transmission rates of herpes simplex virus from mother to infant. JAMA 289:203, 2003

Chilukuri S, Rosen T: Management of acyclovir-resistant herpes simplex virus. Dermatol Clin 21:311, 2003

Corey L et al: The effects of herpes simplex virus-2 on HIV-1 acquisition and transmission: A review of two overlapping epidemics. J AIDS 35:435, 2004

Kimberlin DW et al: Safety and efficacy of high-dose intravenous acyclovir in the management of neonatal herpes simplex virus infections. Pediatrics 108:230, 2001

Wald A et al: The relationship between condom use and herpes simplex virus acquisition. Ann Intern Med 143:707, 2005

Whitley RJ et al: Herpes simplex encephalitis: Adolescents and adults. Antiviral Res 71:141, 2006

173 Varicella-Zoster Virus Infections

Richard J. Whitley

DEFINITION

Varicella-zoster virus (VZV) causes two distinct clinical entities: varicella (chickenpox) and herpes zoster (shingles). Chickenpox, a ubiquitous and extremely contagious infection, is usually a benign illness of childhood characterized by an exanthematous vesicular rash. With reactivation of latent VZV (which is most common after the sixth decade of life), herpes zoster presents as a dermatomal vesicular rash, usually associated with severe pain.

ETIOLOGY

A clinical association between varicella and herpes zoster has been recognized for nearly 100 years. Early in the twentieth century, similarities in the histopathologic features of skin lesions resulting from varicella and herpes zoster were demonstrated. Viral isolates from patients with chickenpox and herpes zoster produced similar alterations in tissue culture—specifically, the appearance of eosinophilic intranuclear inclusions and multinucleated giant cells. These results suggested that the viruses were biologically similar. Restriction endonuclease analyses of viral DNA from a patient with chickenpox who subsequently developed herpes zoster verified the molecular identity of the two viruses responsible for these different clinical presentations.

VZV is a member of the family Herpesviridae, sharing with other members such structural characteristics as a lipid envelope surrounding a nucleocapsid with icosahedral symmetry, a total diameter of ~180–200 nm, and centrally located double-stranded DNA that is ~125,000 bp in length.

PATHOGENESIS AND PATHOLOGY

Primary Infection Transmission occurs readily by the respiratory route; the subsequent localized replication of the virus at an undefined site (presumably the nasopharynx) leads to seeding of the reticuloendothelial system and ultimately to the development of viremia. Viremia in patients with chickenpox is reflected in the diffuse and scattered nature of the skin lesions and can be verified in selected cases by the recovery of VZV from the blood or routinely by the detection of viral DNA in either blood or lesions by polymerase chain reaction (PCR). Vesicles involve the corium and dermis, with degenerative changes characterized by ballooning, the presence of multinucleated giant cells, and eosinophilic intranuclear inclusions. Infection may involve localized blood vessels of the skin, resulting in necrosis and epidermal hemorrhage. With the evolution of disease, the vesicular fluid becomes cloudy because of the recruitment of polymorphonuclear leukocytes and the presence of degenerated cells and fibrin. Ultimately, the vesicles either rupture and release their fluid (which includes infectious virus) or are gradually reabsorbed.

Recurrent Infection The mechanism of reactivation of VZV that results in herpes zoster is unknown. Presumably, the virus infects dorsal root ganglia during chickenpox, where it remains latent until reactivated. Histopathologic examination of representative dorsal root ganglia during active herpes zoster demonstrates hemorrhage, edema, and lymphocytic infiltration.

Active replication of VZV in other organs, such as the lung or the brain, can occur during either chickenpox or herpes zoster but is uncommon in the immunocompetent host. Pulmonary involvement is characterized by interstitial pneumonitis, multinucleated giant cell formation, intranuclear inclusions, and pulmonary hemorrhage. Central nervous system (CNS) infection leads to histopathologic evidence of perivascular cuffing similar to that encountered in measles and other viral encephalitides. Focal hemorrhagic necrosis of the brain, characteristic of herpes simplex virus (HSV) encephalitis, is uncommon in VZV infection.

EPIDEMIOLOGY AND CLINICAL MANIFESTATIONS

Chickenpox Humans are the only known reservoir for VZV. Chickenpox is highly contagious, with an attack rate of at least 90% among susceptible (seronegative) individuals. Persons of both sexes and all races are infected equally often. The virus is endemic in the population at large; however, it becomes epidemic among susceptible individuals during seasonal peaks—namely, late winter and early spring in the temperate zone. Historically, children 5–9 years old are most commonly affected and account for 50% of all cases. Most other cases involve children 1–4 and 10–14 years old. Approximately 10% of the population of the United States over the age of 15 is susceptible to infection. VZV vaccination during the second year of life is dramatically changing the epidemiology of infection. As a consequence, the annualized incidence of chickenpox is decreasing significantly.

The incubation period of chickenpox ranges from 10 to 21 days but is usually 14–17 days. Secondary attack rates in susceptible siblings within a household are 70–90%. Patients are infectious ~48 h before onset of the vesicular rash, during the period of vesicle formation (which generally lasts 4–5 days), and until all vesicles are crusted.

Clinically, chickenpox presents as a rash, low-grade fever, and malaise, although a few patients develop a prodrome 1–2 days before onset of the exanthem. In the immunocompetent patient, chickenpox is usually a benign illness associated with lassitude and with body temperatures of 37.8°–39.4°C (100°–103°F) of 3–5 days' duration. The skin lesions—the hallmark of the infection—include maculopapules, vesicles, and scabs in various stages of evolution (Fig. 173-1). These lesions, which evolve from maculopapules to vesicles over hours to days, appear on the trunk and face and rapidly spread to involve other areas of the body. Most are small and have an erythematous base with a diameter of 5–10 mm. Successive crops appear over a 2- to 4-day period. Lesions can also be found on the mucosa of the pharynx and/or the vagina. Their severity varies from one person to another. Some individuals have very few lesions, while others have as many as 2000. Younger children tend to have fewer vesicles than older individuals. Secondary and tertiary cases within families are associated with a relatively large number of vesicles. Immunocompromised patients—both children and adults, particularly those with leukemia—have lesions (often with a hemorrhagic base) that are more numerous and take longer to heal than those of immunocompetent patients. Immunocompromised individuals are also at greater risk for visceral complications, which occur in 30–50% of cases and are fatal 15% of the time in the absence of antiviral therapy.

The most common infectious complication of varicella is secondary bacterial superinfection of the skin, which is usually caused by *Streptococcus pyogenes* or *Staphylococcus aureus*, including strains that are methicillin resistant. Skin infection results from excoriation of lesions after scratching. Gram's staining of skin lesions should help clarify the etiology of unusually erythematous and pustulated lesions.

The most common extracutaneous site of involvement in children is the CNS. The syndrome of acute cerebellar ataxia and meningeal inflammation generally appears ~21 days after onset of the rash and rarely develops in the preeruptive phase. The cerebrospinal fluid (CSF) contains lymphocytes and elevated levels of protein. CNS involvement

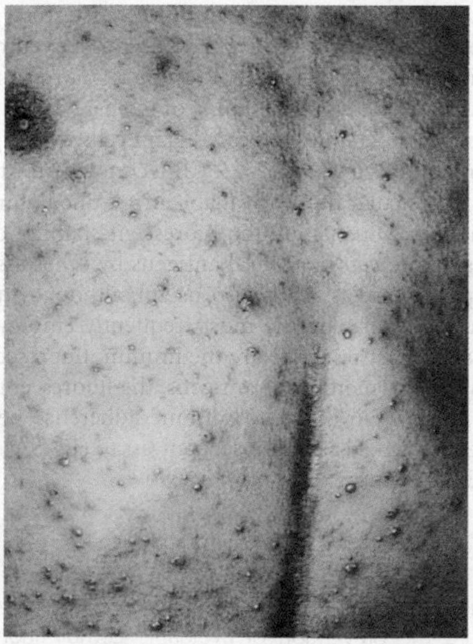

FIGURE 173-1 Numerous varicella lesions at various stages of evolution: vesicles on an erythematous base, umbilical vesicles, and crusts.

is a benign complication of VZV infection in children and generally does not require hospitalization. Aseptic meningitis, encephalitis, transverse myelitis, Guillain-Barré syndrome, and Reye's syndrome can also occur. Encephalitis is reported in 0.1–0.2% of children with chickenpox. Other than supportive care, no specific therapy is available for patients with CNS involvement.

Varicella pneumonia, the most serious complication following chickenpox, develops more commonly in adults (up to 20% of cases) than in children and is particularly severe in pregnant women. Pneumonia due to VZV usually has its onset 3–5 days into the illness and is associated with tachypnea, cough, dyspnea, and fever. Cyanosis, pleuritic chest pain, and hemoptysis are common. Roentgenographic evidence of disease consists of nodular infiltrates and interstitial pneumonitis. Resolution of pneumonitis parallels improvement of the skin rash; however, patients may have persistent fever and compromised pulmonary function for weeks.

Other complications of chickenpox include myocarditis, corneal lesions, nephritis, arthritis, bleeding diatheses, acute glomerulonephritis, and hepatitis. Hepatic involvement, distinct from Reye's syndrome and usually asymptomatic, is common in chickenpox and is generally characterized by elevated levels of liver enzymes, particularly aspartate and alanine aminotransferases.

Perinatal varicella is associated with a high mortality rate when maternal disease develops within 5 days before delivery or within 48 h thereafter. Because the newborn does not receive protective transplacental antibodies and has an immature immune system, the illness may be unusually severe. The reported mortality rate is as high as 30% in this group. *Congenital varicella*, with clinical manifestations of limb hypoplasia, cicatricial skin lesions, and microcephaly at birth, is extremely uncommon.

Herpes Zoster Herpes zoster (also called shingles) is a sporadic disease that results from reactivation of latent VZV from dorsal root ganglia. Most patients have no history of recent exposure to other individuals with VZV infection. Herpes zoster occurs at all ages, but its incidence is highest (5–10 cases per 1000 persons) among individuals in the sixth decade of life and beyond. Recent data suggest that 1.2 million cases occur annually in the United States. Recurrent herpes zoster is exceedingly rare except in immunocompromised hosts, especially those with AIDS.

Herpes zoster is characterized by a unilateral vesicular eruption within a dermatome, often associated with severe pain. The dermatomes from T3 to L3 are most frequently involved. If the ophthalmic branch of the trigeminal nerve is involved, *zoster ophthalmicus* results. The factors responsible for the reactivation of VZV are not known. In children, reactivation is usually benign; in adults, it can be debilitating. The continuum of pain from onset to resolution is known as *zoster-associated pain*. The onset of disease is heralded by pain within the dermatome, which may precede lesions by 48–72 h; an erythematous maculopapular rash evolves rapidly into vesicular lesions (Fig. 173-2). In the normal host, these lesions may remain few in number and continue to form for only 3–5 days. The total duration of disease is generally 7–10 days; however, it may take as long as 2–4 weeks for the skin to return to normal. Patients with herpes zoster can transmit infection to seronegative individuals, with consequent chickenpox. In a few patients, characteristic localization of pain to a dermatome with serologic evidence of herpes zoster has been reported in the absence of skin lesions. When branches of the trigeminal nerve are involved, lesions may appear on the face, in the mouth, in the eye, or on the tongue. Zoster ophthalmicus is usually a debilitating condition that can result in blindness in the absence of antiviral therapy. In the *Ramsay Hunt syndrome*, pain and vesicles appear in the external auditory canal, and patients lose their sense of taste in the anterior two-thirds of the tongue while developing ipsilateral facial palsy. The geniculate ganglion of the sensory branch of the facial nerve is involved.

In both normal and immunocompromised hosts, the most debilitating complication of herpes zoster is pain associated with acute neuritis and postherpetic neuralgia. Postherpetic neuralgia is uncommon in young individuals; however, at least 50% of zoster patients over age

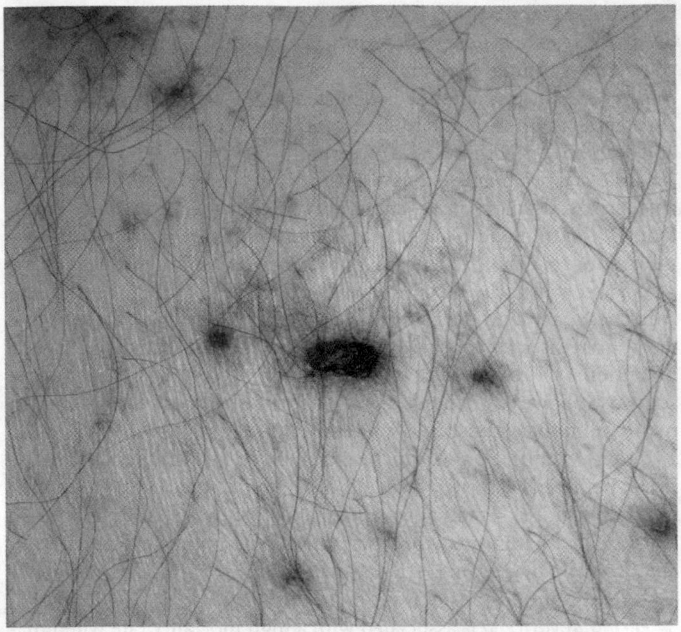

FIGURE 173-2 Close-up of lesions of disseminated zoster. Note lesions at different stages of evolution, including pustules and crusting. (*Photo courtesy of Lindsey Baden; with permission.*)

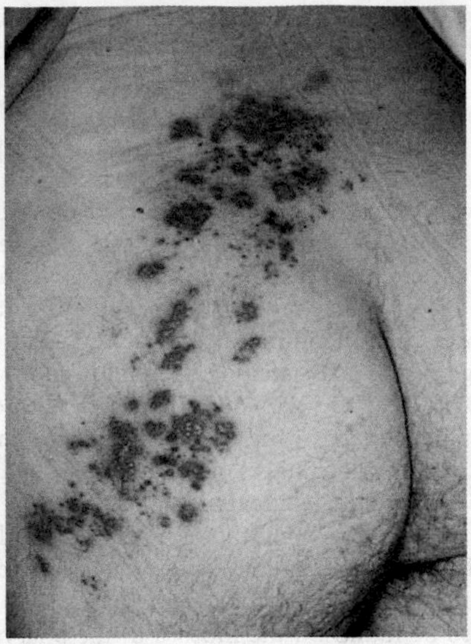

FIGURE 173-3 Herpes zoster is seen in this HIV-infected patient as hemorrhagic vesicles and pustules on an erythematous base grouped in a dermatomal distribution.

50 report some degree of pain in the involved dermatome months after the resolution of cutaneous disease. Changes in sensation in the dermatome, resulting in either hypo- or hyperesthesia, are common.

CNS involvement may follow localized herpes zoster. Many patients without signs of meningeal irritation have CSF pleocytosis and moderately elevated levels of CSF protein. Symptomatic meningoencephalitis is characterized by headache, fever, photophobia, meningitis, and vomiting. A rare manifestation of CNS involvement is granulomatous angiitis with contralateral hemiplegia, which can be diagnosed by cerebral arteriography. Other neurologic manifestations include transverse myelitis with or without motor paralysis.

Like chickenpox, herpes zoster is more severe in immunocompromised than immunocompetent individuals. Lesions continue to form for >1 week, and scabbing is not complete in most cases until 3 weeks into the illness. Patients with Hodgkin's disease and non-Hodgkin's lymphoma are at greatest risk for progressive herpes zoster. Cutaneous dissemination (Fig. 173-3) develops in ~40% of these patients. Among patients with cutaneous dissemination, the risk of pneumonitis, meningoencephalitis, hepatitis, and other serious complications is increased by 5–10%. However, even in immunocompromised patients, disseminated zoster is rarely fatal.

Recipients of hematopoietic stem cell transplants are at particularly high risk of VZV infection. Of all cases of posttransplantation VZV infection, 30% occur within 1 year (50% of these within 9 months); 45% of the patients involved have cutaneous or visceral dissemination. The mortality rate in this situation is 10%. Postherpetic neuralgia, scarring, and bacterial superinfection are especially common in VZV infections occurring within 9 months of transplantation. Among infected patients, concomitant graft-versus-host disease increases the chance of dissemination and/or death.

DIFFERENTIAL DIAGNOSIS

The diagnosis of chickenpox is not difficult. The characteristic rash and a history of recent exposure should lead to a prompt diagnosis. Other viral infections that can mimic chickenpox include disseminated HSV infection in patients with atopic dermatitis and the disseminated vesiculopapular lesions sometimes associated with coxsackievirus infection, echovirus infection, or atypical measles. However, these rashes are more commonly morbilliform with a hemorrhagic component rather than vesicular or vesiculopustular. Rickettsialpox (Chap. 167) can be confused with chickenpox; however, rickettsialpox can be distinguished easily by detection of the "herald spot" at the site of the mite bite and the development of a more pronounced headache. Serologic testing is also useful in differentiating rickettsialpox from varicella and can confirm susceptibility in adults unsure of their chickenpox history. Concern about smallpox has recently increased because of the threat of bioterrorism (Chap. 214). The lesions of smallpox are larger than those of chickenpox and are all at the same stage of evolution at any given time.

Unilateral vesicular lesions in a dermatomal pattern should lead rapidly to the diagnosis of herpes zoster, although the occurrence of shingles without a rash has been reported. Both HSV infections and coxsackievirus infections can cause dermatomal vesicular lesions. Supportive diagnostic virology and fluorescent staining of skin scrapings with monoclonal antibodies are helpful in ensuring the proper diagnosis. In the prodromal stage of herpes zoster, the diagnosis can be exceedingly difficult and may be made only after lesions have appeared or by retrospective serologic assessment.

LABORATORY FINDINGS

Unequivocal confirmation of the diagnosis is possible only through the isolation of VZV in susceptible tissue-culture cell lines, the demonstration of either seroconversion or a fourfold or greater rise in antibody titer between convalescent- and acute-phase serum specimens, or the detection of VZV DNA by PCR. A rapid impression can be obtained by a Tzanck smear, with scraping of the base of the lesions in an attempt to demonstrate multinucleated giant cells, although the sensitivity of this method is low (~60%). PCR technology for the detection of viral DNA in vesicular fluid is available in a limited number of diagnostic laboratories. Direct immunofluorescent staining of cells from the lesion base or detection of viral antigens by other assays (such as the immunoperoxidase assay) is also useful, although these tests are not commercially available. The most frequently employed serologic tools for assessing host response are the immunofluorescent detection of antibodies to VZV membrane antigens, the fluorescent antibody to membrane antigen (FAMA) test, immune adherence hemagglutination, and enzyme-linked immunosorbent assay (ELISA). The FAMA test and the ELISA appear to be most sensitive.

Rx VARICELLA-ZOSTER VIRUS INFECTION

Medical management of chickenpox in the immunologically normal host is directed toward the prevention of avoidable complications. Obviously, good hygiene includes daily bathing and soaks. Secondary bacterial infection of the skin can be avoided by meticulous skin care, particularly with close cropping of fingernails. Pruritus can be decreased with topical dressings or the administration of antipruritic drugs. Tepid water baths and wet compresses are better than drying lotions for the relief of itching. Administration of aspirin to children with chickenpox should be avoided because of the association of aspirin derivatives with the development of Reye's syndrome. Acyclovir therapy (800 mg by mouth five times daily for 5–7 days) is recommended for adolescents and adults with chickenpox of ≤24 h duration. Likewise, acyclovir therapy may be of benefit to children <12 years of age if initiated early in the disease (<24 h) at a dose of 20 mg/kg every 6 h. The second-generation antiherpetic drugs valacyclovir and famciclovir are probably as efficacious or more so; however, no controlled clinical trials comparing these drugs have been reported. The advantages (i.e., pharmacokinetics) of the second-generation agents are described in Chap. 171.

Aluminum acetate soaks for the management of herpes zoster can be both soothing and cleansing. Patients with herpes zoster benefit from oral antiviral therapy, as evidenced by accelerated healing of lesions and resolution of zoster-associated pain with acyclovir, valacyclovir, or famciclovir. Acyclovir, now off patent, is administered at a dosage of 800 mg five times daily for 7–10 days. Famciclovir, the prodrug of penciclovir, is at least as effective as acyclovir and perhaps more so. One study showed twofold faster resolution of postherpetic neuralgia in famciclovir-treated patients with zoster than in recipients of placebo. The dose is 500 mg by mouth three times daily for 7 days. Valacyclovir, the prodrug of acyclovir, accelerates healing and resolution of zoster-associated pain more promptly than acyclovir. The dose is 1 g by mouth three times daily for 5–7 days. Compared with acyclovir, both famciclovir and valacyclovir offer the advantage of less frequent administration.

In severely immunocompromised hosts (e.g., transplant recipients, patients with lymphoproliferative malignancies), both chickenpox and herpes zoster (including disseminated disease) should be treated, at least at the outset, with intravenous acyclovir, which reduces the occurrence of visceral complications but has no effect on healing of skin lesions or pain. The dose is 10–12.5 mg/kg every 8 h for 7 days. For low-risk immunocompromised hosts, oral therapy with valacyclovir or famciclovir appears beneficial. Concomitant with the administration of intravenous acyclovir, it is desirable to wean these patients from immunosuppressive treatment.

Patients with varicella pneumonia may require removal of bronchial secretions and ventilatory support. Persons with zoster ophthalmicus should be referred immediately to an ophthalmologist. Therapy for this condition consists of the administration of analgesics for severe pain and the use of atropine. Acyclovir, valacyclovir, and famciclovir all accelerate healing.

The management of acute neuritis and/or postherpetic neuralgia can be particularly difficult. In addition to the judicious use of analgesics, ranging from nonnarcotics to narcotic derivatives, drugs such as gabapentin, pregabalin, amitriptyline hydrochloride, lidocaine patches, and fluphenazine hydrochloride are reportedly beneficial for pain relief. In one study, glucocorticoid therapy administered early in the course of localized herpes zoster significantly accelerated such quality-of-life improvements as a return to usual activity and termination of analgesia. The dose of prednisone administered orally was 60 mg/d on days 1–7, 30 mg/d on days 8–14, and 15 mg/d on days 15–21. This regimen is appropriate only for relatively healthy elderly persons with moderate or severe pain at presentation. Patients with osteoporosis, diabetes mellitus, glycosuria, or hypertension may not be appropriate candidates. Glucocorticoids should not be used without concomitant antiviral therapy.

PREVENTION

Three methods are used for the prevention of VZV infections. First, a live attenuated varicella vaccine (Oka) is recommended for all children >1 year of age (up to 12 years of age) who have not had chickenpox and for adults known to be seronegative for VZV. Two doses are recommended for all children: the first at 12–15 months of age and the second at ~4–6 years of age. VZV-seronegative persons >13 years of age should receive two doses of vaccine at least 1 month apart. The vaccine is both safe and efficacious. Breakthrough cases are mild and may result in spread of the vaccine virus to susceptible contacts. The universal vaccination of children is resulting in a decreased incidence of chickenpox in sentinel communities. Furthermore, inactivation of the vaccine virus significantly decreases the occurrence of herpes zoster after hematopoietic stem-cell transplantation. After administration of a vaccine with 18 times the viral content of the Oka vaccine to individuals >60 years of age, the incidence of shingles was found to decrease by 51%, the burden of illness by 61%, and the incidence of postherpetic neuralgia by 66%. The Advisory Committee on Immunization Practices has therefore recommended that persons in this age group be offered this vaccine in order to reduce the frequency of shingles and the severity of postherpetic neuralgia.

TABLE 173-1 RECOMMENDATIONS FOR VZIG ADMINISTRATION

Exposure Criteria

1. Exposure to person with chickenpox or zoster
   a. Household: residence in the same household
   b. Playmate: face-to-face indoor play
   c. Hospital
      Varicella: same 2- to 4-bed room or adjacent beds in large ward, face-to-face contact with infectious staff member or patient, visit by a person deemed contagious
      Zoster: intimate contact (e.g., touching or hugging) with a person deemed contagious
   d. Newborn infant: onset of varicella in the mother ≤5 days before delivery or ≤48 h after delivery; VZIG not indicated if the mother has zoster
2. Patient should receive VZIG as soon as possible but not >96 h after exposure

Candidates (Provided They Have Significant Exposure) Include:

1. Immunocompromised susceptible children without a history of varicella or varicella immunization
2. Susceptible pregnant women
3. Newborn infants whose mother had onset of chickenpox within 5 days before or within 48 h after delivery
4. Hospitalized premature infant (≥28 weeks of gestation) whose mother lacks a reliable history of chickenpox or serologic evidence of protection against varicella
5. Hospitalized premature infant (<28 weeks of gestation or ≤1000-g birth weight), regardless of maternal history of varicella or varicella-zoster virus serologic status

A second approach is to administer varicella-zoster immune globulin (VZIG) to individuals who are susceptible, are at high risk for developing complications of varicella, and have had a significant exposure. This product should be given within 96 h (preferably within 72 h) of the exposure. Indications for administration of VZIG appear in Table 173-1. Unfortunately, the availability of this product in the future will be limited at best.

Lastly, antiviral therapy can be given as prophylaxis to individuals at high risk who are ineligible for vaccine or who are beyond the 96-h window after direct contact. While the initial studies have used acyclovir, similar benefit can be anticipated with either valacyclovir or famciclovir. Therapy is instituted 7 days after intense exposure. At this time, the host is midway into the incubation period. This approach significantly decreases disease severity, if not totally preventing disease.

FURTHER READINGS

ARVIN A: Aging, immunity, and the varicella-zoster virus. N Engl J Med 352:2266, 2005

GNANN JW, WHITLEY RJ: Herpes zoster. N Engl J Med 347:340, 2002

IZURIETA HS et al: Postlicensure effectiveness of varicella vaccine during an outbreak in a child care center. JAMA 278:1495, 1997

NGUYEN HQ et al: Decline in mortality due to varicella after implementation of varicella vaccination in the United States. N Engl J Med 352:450, 2005

OXMAN MN et al: A vaccine to prevent herpes zoster and postherpetic neuralgia in older adults. N Engl J Med 352:2271, 2005

ROWBOTHAM M et al: Gabapentin for the treatment of postherpetic neuralgia. A randomized controlled trial. JAMA 280:1837, 1998

SEWARD JF et al: Contagiousness of varicella in vaccinated cases: A household contact study. JAMA 292:704, 2004

——— et al: Varicella disease after introduction of varicella vaccine in the United States, 1995-2000. JAMA 28:606, 2002

174 Epstein-Barr Virus Infections, Including Infectious Mononucleosis

Jeffrey I. Cohen

DEFINITION

Epstein-Barr virus (EBV) is the cause of heterophile-positive infectious mononucleosis (IM), which is characterized by fever, sore throat, lymphadenopathy, and atypical lymphocytosis. EBV is also associated with several human tumors, including nasopharyngeal carcinoma, Burkitt's lymphoma, Hodgkin's disease, and (in patients with immunodeficiencies) B cell lymphoma. The virus, a member of the family Herpesviridae, consists of a linear DNA core surrounded by a nucleocapsid and an envelope that contains glycoproteins. The two types of EBV that are widely prevalent in nature are not distinguishable by conventional serologic tests.

EPIDEMIOLOGY

EBV infections occur worldwide. These infections are most common in early childhood, with a second peak during late adolescence. By adulthood, more than 90% of individuals have been infected and have antibodies to the virus. IM is usually a disease of young adults. In lower socioeconomic groups and in areas of the world with lower standards of hygiene (e.g., developing countries), EBV tends to infect children at an early age, and symptomatic IM is uncommon. In areas with higher standards of hygiene, infection with EBV is often delayed until adulthood, and IM is more prevalent.

EBV is spread by contact with oral secretions. The virus is frequently transmitted from asymptomatic adults to infants and among young adults by transfer of saliva during kissing. Transmission by less intimate contact is rare. EBV has been transmitted by blood transfusion and by bone marrow transplantation. More than 90% of asymptomatic seropositive individuals shed the virus in oropharyngeal secretions. Shedding is increased in immunocompromised patients and those with IM.

PATHOGENESIS

EBV is transmitted by salivary secretions. The virus infects the epithelium of the oropharynx and the salivary glands and is shed from these cells. While B cells may become infected after contact with epithelial cells, studies suggest that lymphocytes in the tonsillar crypts can be infected directly. The virus then spreads through the bloodstream. The proliferation and expansion of EBV-infected B cells along with reactive T cells during IM result in enlargement of lymphoid tissue. Polyclonal activation of B cells leads to the production of antibodies to host-cell and viral proteins. During the acute phase of IM, up to 1 in every 100 B cells in the peripheral blood is infected by EBV; after recovery, 1–50 in every 1 million B cells is infected. During IM, there is an inverted CD4+/CD8+ T cell ratio. The percentage of CD4+ T cells decreases, while there are large clonal expansions of CD8+ T cells; up to 40% of CD8+ T cells are directed against EBV antigens during acute infection. Data suggest that memory B cells, not epithelial cells, are the reservoir for EBV in the body. When patients are treated with acyclovir, shedding of EBV from the oropharynx stops but the virus persists in B cells.

The EBV receptor (CD21) on the surface of B cells is also the receptor for the C3d component of complement. EBV infection of epithelial cells results in viral replication and production of virions. When B cells are infected by EBV in vitro, they become transformed and can proliferate indefinitely. During latent infection of B cells, only the EBV nuclear antigens (EBNAs), latent membrane proteins (LMPs), and small EBV RNAs are expressed in vitro. EBV-transformed B cells secrete immunoglobulin; only a small fraction of cells produce virus.

Cellular immunity is more important than humoral immunity in controlling EBV infection. In the initial phase of infection, suppressor T cells, natural killer cells, and nonspecific cytotoxic T cells are important in controlling the proliferation of EBV-infected B cells. Levels of markers of T cell activation and serum interferon (IFN) γ are elevated. Later in infection, HLA-restricted cytotoxic T cells that recognize EBNAs and LMPs and destroy EBV-infected cells are generated. Studies have shown that one of the late genes expressed during EBV replication, *BCRF1*, is a homologue of interleukin 10 and can inhibit the production of IFN-γ by mononuclear cells in vitro.

If T cell immunity is compromised, EBV-infected B cells may begin to proliferate. When EBV is associated with lymphoma, virus-induced proliferation is but one step in a multistep process of neoplastic transformation. In many EBV-containing tumors, LMP-1 mimics members of the tumor necrosis factor receptor family (e.g., CD40), transmitting growth-proliferating signals.

CLINICAL MANIFESTATIONS

Signs and Symptoms Most EBV infections in infants and young children either are asymptomatic or present as mild pharyngitis with or without tonsillitis. In contrast, up to 75% of infections in adolescents present as IM. IM in the elderly presents relatively often as nonspecific symptoms, including prolonged fever, fatigue, myalgia, and malaise. In contrast, pharyngitis, lymphadenopathy, splenomegaly, and atypical lymphocytes are relatively rare in elderly patients.

The incubation period for IM in young adults is ~4–6 weeks. A prodrome of fatigue, malaise, and myalgia may last for 1–2 weeks before the onset of fever, sore throat, and lymphadenopathy. Fever is usually low-grade and is most common in the first 2 weeks of the illness; however, it may persist for >1 month. Common signs and symptoms are listed along with their frequencies in Table 174-1. Lymphadenopathy and pharyngitis are most prominent during the first 2 weeks of the illness, while splenomegaly is more prominent during the second and third weeks. Lymphadenopathy most often affects the posterior cervical nodes but may be generalized. Enlarged lymph nodes are frequently tender and symmetric but are not fixed in place. Pharyngitis, often the most prominent sign, can be accompanied by enlargement of the tonsils with an exudate resembling that of streptococcal pharyngitis. A morbilliform or papular rash, usually on the arms or trunk, develops in ~5% of cases (Fig. 174-1). Most patients treated with ampicillin develop a macular rash; this rash is not predictive of future adverse reactions to penicillins. Erythema nodosum and erythema multiforme have also been described (Chap. 54). Most patients have symptoms for 2–4 weeks, but malaise and difficulty concentrating can persist for months.

Laboratory Findings The white blood cell count is usually elevated and peaks at 10,000–20,000/μL during the second or third week of illness. Lymphocytosis is usually demonstrable, with >10% atypical lymphocytes. The latter cells are enlarged lymphocytes that have abundant cytoplasm, vacuoles, and indentations of the cell membrane (Fig. 174-2). CD8+ cells predominate among the atypical lympho-

TABLE 174-1 SIGNS AND SYMPTOMS OF INFECTIOUS MONONUCLEOSIS

Manifestation	Median Percentage of Patients (Range)
Symptoms	
Sore throat	75 (50–87)
Malaise	47 (42–76)
Headache	38 (22–67)
Abdominal pain, nausea, or vomiting	17 (5–25)
Chills	10 (9–11)
Signs	
Lymphadenopathy	95 (83–100)
Fever	93 (60–100)
Pharyngitis or tonsillitis	82 (68–90)
Splenomegaly	51 (43–64)
Hepatomegaly	11 (6–15)
Rash	10 (0–25)
Periorbital edema	13 (2–34)
Palatal enanthem	7 (3–13)
Jaundice	5 (2–10)

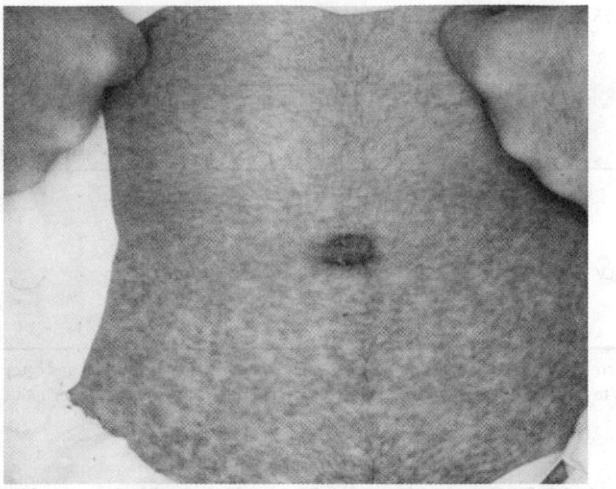

FIGURE 174-1 Rash in a patient with infectious mononucleosis due to Epstein-Barr virus. *(Courtesy of Maria Turner, MD; with permission.)*

cytes. Low-grade neutropenia and thrombocytopenia are common during the first month of illness. Liver function is abnormal in >90% of cases. Serum levels of aminotransferases and alkaline phosphatase are usually mildly elevated. The serum concentration of bilirubin is elevated in ~40% of cases.

Complications Most cases of IM are self-limited. Deaths are very rare and most often are due to central nervous system (CNS) complications, splenic rupture, upper airway obstruction, or bacterial superinfection.

When CNS complications develop, they usually do so during the first 2 weeks of EBV infection; in some patients, especially children, they are the only clinical manifestations of IM. Heterophile antibodies and atypical lymphocytes may be absent. Meningitis and encephalitis are the most common neurologic abnormalities, and patients may present with headache, meningismus, or cerebellar ataxia. Acute hemiplegia and psychosis have also been described. The cerebrospinal fluid (CSF) contains mainly lymphocytes, with occasional atypical lymphocytes. Most cases resolve without neurologic sequelae. Acute EBV infection has also been associated with cranial nerve palsies (especially those involving cranial nerve VII), Guillain-Barré syndrome, acute transverse myelitis, and peripheral neuritis.

Autoimmune hemolytic anemia occurs in ~2% of cases during the first 2 weeks. In most cases, the anemia is Coombs-positive, with cold agglutinins directed against the i red blood cell antigen. Most patients with hemolysis have mild anemia that lasts for 1–2 months, but some patients have severe disease with hemoglobinuria and jaundice. Nonspecific antibody responses may also include rheumatoid factor, antinuclear antibodies, anti–smooth muscle antibodies, antiplatelet antibodies, and cryoglobulins. IM has been associated with red-cell aplasia, severe granulocytopenia, thrombocytopenia, pancytopenia, and hemophagocytic syndrome. The spleen ruptures in <0.5% of cases. Splenic rupture is more common among male than female patients and may manifest as abdominal pain, referred shoulder pain, or hemodynamic compromise.

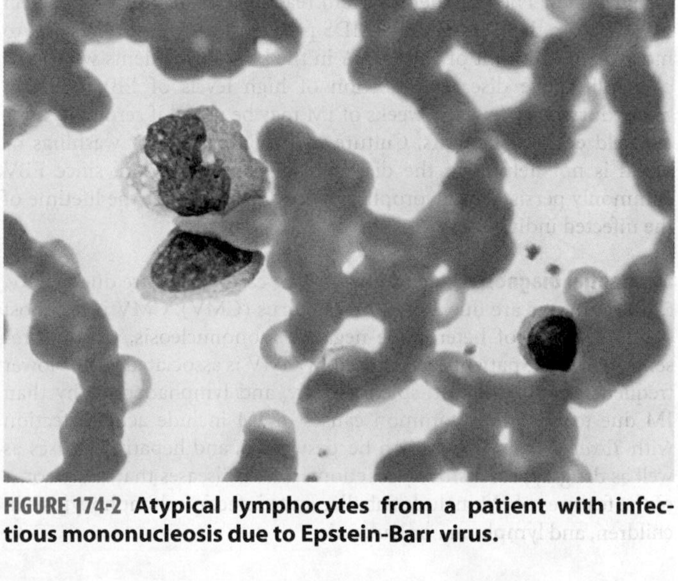

FIGURE 174-2 Atypical lymphocytes from a patient with infectious mononucleosis due to Epstein-Barr virus.

Hypertrophy of lymphoid tissue in the tonsils or adenoids can result in upper airway obstruction, as can inflammation and edema of the epiglottis, pharynx, or uvula. About 10% of patients with IM develop streptococcal pharyngitis after their initial sore throat resolves.

Other rare complications associated with acute EBV infection include hepatitis (which can be fulminant), myocarditis or pericarditis with electrocardiographic changes, pneumonia with pleural effusion, interstitial nephritis, genital ulcerations, and vasculitis.

EBV-Associated Diseases Other Than IM EBV-associated lymphoproliferative disease has been described in patients with congenital or acquired immunodeficiency, including those with severe combined immunodeficiency, patients with AIDS, and recipients of bone marrow or organ transplants who are receiving immunosuppressive drugs (especially cyclosporine). Proliferating EBV-infected B cells infiltrate lymph nodes and multiple organs, and patients present with fever and lymphadenopathy or gastrointestinal symptoms. Pathologic studies show B cell hyperplasia or poly- or monoclonal lymphoma. The X-linked lymphoproliferative syndrome (Duncan's disease) is a recessive disorder of young boys who have a normal response to childhood infections but develop fatal lymphoproliferative disorders after infection with EBV. The protein associated with this syndrome (SAP) binds to a protein that mediates interactions of B and T cells. Most patients with this syndrome die of acute IM. Others develop hypogammaglobulinemia, malignant B cell lymphomas, aplastic anemia, or agranulocytosis. IM has also proved fatal to some patients with no obvious preexisting immune abnormality.

Oral hairy leukoplakia (Fig. 174-3) is an early manifestation of infection with HIV in adults (Chap. 182). Most patients present with raised, white corrugated lesions on the tongue (and occasionally on the buccal mucosa) that contain EBV DNA. Children infected with HIV can develop lymphoid interstitial pneumonitis; EBV DNA is often found in lung tissue from these patients.

Patients with chronic fatigue syndrome may have titers of antibody to EBV that are elevated but are not significantly different from those in healthy EBV-seropositive adults. While some patients have malaise and fatigue that persist for weeks or months after IM, persistent EBV infection is not a cause of chronic fatigue syndrome. Chronic active EBV infection is very rare and is distinct from chronic fatigue syndrome. The affected patients have an illness lasting >6 months, with elevated levels of EBV DNA in the blood, very high titers of antibody to EBV, and evidence of organ involvement, including hepatospleno-

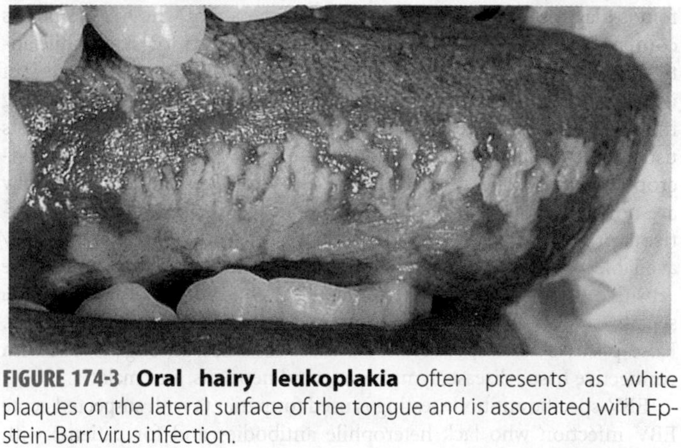

FIGURE 174-3 Oral hairy leukoplakia often presents as white plaques on the lateral surface of the tongue and is associated with Epstein-Barr virus infection.

megaly, lymphadenopathy, and pneumonitis, uveitis, or neurologic disease.

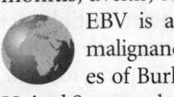

EBV is associated with several malignancies. About 15% of cases of Burkitt's lymphoma in the United States and ~90% of those in Africa are associated with EBV (Chap. 105). African patients with Burkitt's lymphoma have high levels of antibody to EBV, and their tumor tissue usually contains viral DNA. Malaria infection in Africa may impair cellular immunity to EBV and induce polyclonal B cell activation with an expansion of EBV-infected B cells. These changes may enhance the proliferation of B cells, increasing the likelihood of a *c-myc* translocation—the hallmark of Burkitt's lymphoma. EBV-containing Burkitt's lymphoma also occurs in patients with AIDS.

TABLE 174-2 SEROLOGIC FEATURES OF EBV-ASSOCIATED DISEASES

Condition	Result in Indicated Test[a]					
		Anti-VCA		Anti-EA		
	Heterophile	IgM	IgG	EA-D	EA-R	Anti-EBNA
Acute infectious mononucleosis	+	+	++	+	−	−
Convalescence	±	−	+	−	±	+
Past infection	−	−	+	−	−	+
Reactivation with immunodeficiency	−	−	++	+	+	±
Burkitt's lymphoma	−	−	+++	±	++	+
Nasopharyngeal carcinoma	−	−	+++	++	±	+

[a]VCA, viral capsid antigen; EA, early antigen; EA-D antibody, antibody to early antigen in diffuse pattern in nucleus and cytoplasm of infected cells; EA-R antibody, antibody to early antigen restricted to the cytoplasm; and EBNA, Epstein-Barr nuclear antigen.
Source: Adapted from Okano, 1988.

Anaplastic nasopharyngeal carcinoma is uniformly associated with EBV; the affected tissues contain viral DNA and antigens. Patients with nasopharyngeal carcinoma often have elevated titers of antibody to EBV (Chap. 84). High levels of EBV plasma DNA before treatment or detectable levels of EBV DNA after radiation therapy correlate with lower rates of overall survival and relapse-free survival among patients with nasopharyngeal carcinoma.

EBV has been associated with Hodgkin's disease, especially the mixed-cellularity type (Chap. 105). Patients with Hodgkin's disease often have elevated titers of antibody to EBV. In about half of cases, viral DNA and antigens are found in Reed-Sternberg cells. The risk of EBV-positive Hodgkin's disease is significantly increased in young adults after EBV-seropositive IM. About 50% of non-Hodgkin's lymphomas in patients with AIDS are EBV-positive.

In some cases, EBV DNA has been detected in tumors from immunocompetent patients with tonsillar carcinoma, angioimmunoblastic lymphadenopathy, angiocentric nasal NK/T cell immunoproliferative lesions, T cell lymphoma, thymoma, gastric carcinoma, and CNS lymphoma. Studies have demonstrated viral DNA in leiomyosarcomas from AIDS patients and in smooth-muscle tumors from organ transplant recipients. Virtually all CNS lymphomas in AIDS patients are associated with EBV. While serologic studies have found higher levels of antibodies to EBV before the onset of multiple sclerosis in persons ≥25 years old, other studies (including measurement of EBV antibody titers in the CSF) are needed to ascertain a possible causal relationship.

DIAGNOSIS

Serologic Testing The heterophile test is used for the diagnosis of IM in children and adults (Table 174-2). In the test for this antibody, human serum is absorbed with guinea pig kidney, and the heterophile titer is defined as the greatest serum dilution that agglutinates sheep, horse, or cow erythrocytes. Although heterophile antibody binds to certain animal erythrocytes, it does not interact with EBV proteins. A titer of ≥40-fold is diagnostic of acute EBV infection in a patient who has symptoms compatible with IM and atypical lymphocytes. Tests for heterophile antibodies are positive in 40% of patients with IM during the first week of illness and in 80–90% during the third week. Therefore, repeated testing may be necessary, especially if the initial test is performed early. Tests usually remain positive for 3 months after the onset of illness, but heterophile antibodies can persist for up to 1 year. These antibodies usually are not detectable in children <5 years of age, in the elderly, or in patients presenting with symptoms not typical of IM. The commercially available monospot test for heterophile antibodies is somewhat more sensitive than the classic heterophile test. The monospot test is ~75% sensitive and ~90% specific compared with EBV-specific serologies. False-positive monospot results are more common among persons with connective tissue disease, lymphoma, viral hepatitis, and malaria.

EBV-specific antibody testing is used for patients with suspected acute EBV infection who lack heterophile antibodies and for patients with atypical infections (Table 174-2). Titers of IgM and IgG antibodies to viral capsid antigen (VCA) are elevated in the serum of more than 90% of patients at the onset of disease. IgM antibody to VCA is most useful for the diagnosis of acute IM because it is present at elevated titers only during the first 2–3 months of the disease; in contrast, IgG antibody to VCA is usually not useful for diagnosis of IM but is often used to assess past exposure to EBV because it persists for life. Seroconversion to EBNA positivity is also useful for the diagnosis of acute infection with EBV. Antibodies to EBNA become detectable relatively late (3–6 weeks after the onset of symptoms) in nearly all cases of acute EBV infection and persist for the lifetime of the patient. These antibodies may be lacking in immunodeficient patients and in those with chronic active EBV infection.

Titers of other antibodies may also be elevated in IM; however, these elevations are less useful for diagnosis. Antibodies to early antigens (EAs) are found either in a diffuse pattern in the nucleus and cytoplasm of infected cells (EA-D antibody) or restricted to the cytoplasm (EA-R antibody). These antibodies are detectable 3–4 weeks after the onset of symptoms in patients with IM. About 70% of individuals with IM have EA-D antibodies during the illness; the presence of EA-D antibodies is especially likely in patients with relatively severe disease. These antibodies usually persist for only 3–6 months. Levels of EA-D antibodies are also elevated in patients with nasopharyngeal carcinoma or chronic active EBV infection. EA-R antibodies are only occasionally detected in patients with IM but are often found at elevated titers in patients with African Burkitt's lymphoma or chronic active EBV infection. IgA antibodies to EBV antigens have proved useful for the identification of patients with nasopharyngeal carcinoma and of persons at high risk for the disease.

Other Studies Detection of EBV DNA, RNA, or proteins has been valuable in demonstrating the association of the virus with various malignancies. The polymerase chain reaction has been used to detect EBV DNA in the CSF of some AIDS patients with lymphomas and to monitor the amount of EBV DNA in the blood of patients with lymphoproliferative disease. Detection of high levels of EBV DNA in blood during the first few weeks of IM may be useful if serologic studies yield equivocal results. Culture of EBV from throat washings or blood is not helpful in the diagnosis of acute infection, since EBV commonly persists in the oropharynx and in B cells for the lifetime of the infected individual.

Differential Diagnosis Whereas ~90% of cases of IM are due to EBV, 5–10% of cases are due to cytomegalovirus (CMV). CMV is the most common cause of heterophile-negative mononucleosis, usually presenting in older patients. IM caused by CMV is associated with a lower frequency of sore throat, splenomegaly, and lymphadenopathy than IM due to EBV. Less common causes of IM include acute infection with *Toxoplasma*, HIV, human herpesvirus 6, and hepatitis viruses as well as drug hypersensitivity reactions. Other diseases that share some of the features of IM include rubella, acute infectious lymphocytosis in children, and lymphoma or leukemia.

TABLE 174-3 TREATMENT OPTIONS FOR POSTTRANSPLANTATION EBV LYMPHOPROLIFERATIVE DISEASE

1. Reduction of immunosuppression, when possible
2. Excision of localized lesions
3. Interferon α
4. Monoclonal antibody to CD20 (rituximab)
5. Radiation therapy (especially for CNS lesions)
6. For stem cell transplant recipients: donor lymphocyte infusions or donor EBV-specific cytotoxic T cell infusions[a]
7. For solid organ transplant recipients: autologous or HLA-matched, EBV-specific, cytotoxic T cell infusions[a]
8. Cytotoxic chemotherapy

[a]Infused T cells must be HLA matched; lymphoproliferative lesions are usually of donor origin for stem cell transplant recipients and of recipient origin for solid organ transplant recipients.

Rx EBV-ASSOCIATED DISEASE

Therapy for IM consists of supportive measures, with rest and analgesia. Excessive physical activity during the first month should be avoided to reduce the possibility of splenic rupture, which necessitates splenectomy. Glucocorticoid therapy is not indicated for uncomplicated IM and in fact may predispose to bacterial superinfection. Prednisone (40–60 mg/d for 2–3 days, with subsequent tapering of the dose over 1–2 weeks) has been used for the prevention of airway obstruction in patients with severe tonsillar hypertrophy, for autoimmune hemolytic anemia, and for severe thrombocytopenia. Glucocorticoids have also been administered to a few selected patients with severe malaise and fever and to patients with severe CNS or cardiac disease. Acyclovir has had no significant clinical impact on IM in controlled trials. In one study, the combination of acyclovir and prednisolone had no significant effect on the duration of symptoms of IM.

Acyclovir, at a dosage of 400–800 mg five times daily, has been effective for the treatment of oral hairy leukoplakia (despite common relapses). The posttransplantation EBV lymphoproliferative syndrome (Chap. 126) generally does not respond to antiviral therapy. When possible, therapy should be directed toward reduction of immunosuppression **(Table 174-3)**. IFN α or antibody to CD20 has been effective in some cases. Infusions of donor lymphocytes are often effective for stem cell transplant recipients, although graft-versus-host disease can occur. Infusions of EBV-specific cytotoxic T cells have been used to prevent EBV lymphoproliferative disease in high-risk settings as well as to treat the disease. Infusion of autologous EBV-specific cytotoxic T lymphocytes has shown promise in small studies of patients with nasopharyngeal carcinoma and Hodgkin's disease. Treatment of two cases of X-linked lymphoproliferative syndrome with antibody to CD20 resulted in a successful outcome of what otherwise would probably have been fatal acute EBV infection.

PREVENTION

The isolation of patients with IM is unnecessary. Vaccines directed against the major EBV glycoprotein have been effective in animal studies and are undergoing clinical trials.

FURTHER READINGS

AUWAERTER PG: Infectious mononucleosis in middle age. JAMA 281:454, 1999

BOLLARD CM et al: Cytotoxic T lymphocyte therapy for Epstein-Barr virus positive Hodgkin's disease. J Exp Med 200:1623, 2004

CHOQUET S et al: Efficacy and safety of rituximab in B-cell post-transplant lymphoproliferative disorders: Results of a prospective multicenter phase 2 study. Blood 107:3053, 2006

COHEN JI: Epstein-Barr virus infection. N Engl J Med 343:481, 2000

FAFI-KREMER S et al: Long term shedding of infectious Epstein-Barr virus after infectious mononucleosis. J Infect Dis 191:985, 2005

HAQUE T et al: Allogeneic cytotoxic T-cell therapy for EBV-positive posttransplantation lymphoproliferative disease: results of a phase 2 multicenter clinical trial. Blood 110:1123, 2007

MILNONE MC et al: Treatment of primary Epstein-Barr virus infection in patients with X-linked lymphoproliferative disease using B-cell-directed therapy. Blood 105:994, 2005

TORRE D, TAMBINI R: Acyclovir for treatment of infectious mononucleosis: A meta-analysis. Scand J Infect Dis 31:543, 1999

WILLIAMS H, CRAWFORD DH: Epstein-Barr virus: The impact of scientific advances on clinical practice. Blood 107:862, 2006

175 Cytomegalovirus and Human Herpesvirus Types 6, 7, and 8

Martin S. Hirsch

CYTOMEGALOVIRUS

DEFINITION

Cytomegalovirus (CMV), which was initially isolated from patients with congenital cytomegalic inclusion disease, is now recognized as an important pathogen in all age groups. In addition to inducing severe birth defects, CMV causes a wide spectrum of disorders in older children and adults, ranging from an asymptomatic, subclinical infection to a mononucleosis syndrome in healthy individuals to disseminated disease in immunocompromised patients. Human CMV is one of several related species-specific viruses that cause similar diseases in various animals. All are associated with the production of characteristic enlarged cells—hence the name *cytomegalovirus*.

CMV, a β-herpesvirus, has double-strand DNA, four species of mRNA, a protein capsid, and a lipoprotein envelope. Like other herpesviruses, CMV demonstrates icosahedral symmetry, replicates in the cell nucleus, and can cause either a lytic and productive or a latent infection. CMV can be distinguished from other herpesviruses by certain biologic properties, such as host range and type of cytopathology. Viral replication is associated with production of large intranuclear inclusions and smaller cytoplasmic inclusions. CMV appears to replicate in a variety of cell types in vivo; in tissue culture it grows preferentially in fibroblasts. Although there is little evidence that CMV is oncogenic in vivo, it does transform fibroblasts in rare instances, and genomic transforming fragments have been identified.

EPIDEMIOLOGY

CMV has a worldwide distribution. Of newborns in the United States, ~1% are infected with CMV; the percentage is higher in many less-developed countries. Communal living and poor personal hygiene facilitate early spread. Perinatal and early childhood infections are common. CMV may be present in breast milk, saliva, feces, and urine. Transmission has occurred among young children in day-care centers and has been traced from infected toddler to pregnant mother to developing fetus. When an infected child introduces CMV into a household, 50% of susceptible family members seroconvert within 6 months.

CMV is not readily spread by casual contact but rather requires repeated or prolonged intimate exposure for transmission. In late adolescence and young adulthood, CMV is often transmitted sexually, and asymptomatic carriage in semen or cervical secretions is common. Antibody to CMV is present at detectable levels in a high proportion of sexually active men and women, who may harbor several strains simultaneously. Transfusion of whole blood or certain blood products containing viable leukocytes may transmit CMV, with a frequency of 0.14–10% per unit transfused.

Once infected, an individual generally carries CMV for life. The infection usually remains silent. However, CMV reactivation syndromes develop frequently when T lymphocyte–mediated immunity is compromised—for example, after organ transplantation or in association with lymphoid neoplasms and certain acquired immunodeficiencies (in particular, HIV infection; Chap. 182). Most primary CMV infections in organ transplant recipients (Chap. 126) result from transmission in the graft itself. In CMV-seropositive transplant recipients, infection results from reactivation of latent virus or, less commonly, from reinfection by a new strain. CMV infection may be associated with coronary artery stenosis following heart transplantation or coronary angioplasty, but this association requires further validation.

TABLE 175-1 CMV DISEASE IN THE IMMUNOCOMPROMISED HOST

Population	Risk Factors	Principal Syndromes	Treatment	Prevention
Fetus	Primary maternal infection/early pregnancy	Cytomegalic inclusion disease	None (?ganciclovir)	Avoidance of exposure or maternal treatment with CMV immunoglobulin during pregnancy
Organ transplant recipient	Serostatus of donor and recipient; immunosuppressive regimen; degree of rejection	Febrile leukopenia; pneumonia; gastrointestinal disease	Ganciclovir or valganciclovir	Donor matching; prophylaxis or preemptive therapy with ganciclovir or valganciclovir
Bone marrow transplant recipient	Graft-vs.-host disease; older age; seropositive recipient; viremia	Pneumonia; gastrointestinal disease	Ganciclovir plus CMV immunoglobulin	Donor matching; prophylaxis or preemptive therapy with ganciclovir or valganciclovir
Person with AIDS	<100 CD4+ T cells per microliter; CMV seropositivity	Retinitis; gastrointestinal disease; neurologic disease	Ganciclovir, valganciclovir, foscarnet, or cidofovir	Oral valganciclovir

PATHOGENESIS

Congenital CMV infection can result from either primary or reactivation infection of the mother. However, clinical disease in the fetus or newborn is almost exclusively related to primary maternal infection (Table 175-1). The factors determining the severity of congenital infection are unknown; a deficient capacity to produce precipitating antibodies and to mount T cell responses to CMV is associated with relatively severe disease.

Primary infection in late childhood or adulthood is often associated with a vigorous T lymphocyte response that may contribute to the development of a mononucleosis syndrome similar to that observed after Epstein-Barr virus (EBV) infection (Chap. 174). The hallmark of such infection is the appearance of atypical lymphocytes in the peripheral blood; these cells are predominantly activated CD8+ T lymphocytes. Polyclonal activation of B cells by CMV contributes to the development of rheumatoid factors and other autoantibodies during mononucleosis.

Once acquired, CMV persists indefinitely in host tissues. The sites of persistent infection probably include multiple cell types and various organs. Transmission via blood transfusion or organ transplantation is due to silent infections in these tissues. Autopsy studies suggest that salivary glands and bowel may be sites of latent infection.

If the host's T cell responses become compromised by disease or by iatrogenic immunosuppression, latent virus can be reactivated to cause a variety of syndromes. Chronic antigenic stimulation in the presence of immunosuppression (for example, after tissue transplantation) appears to be an ideal setting for CMV activation and CMV-induced disease. Certain particularly potent suppressants of T cell immunity (e.g., antithymocyte globulin) are associated with a high rate of clinical CMV syndromes, which may follow either primary or reactivation infection. CMV may itself contribute to further T lymphocyte hyporesponsiveness, which often precedes superinfection with other opportunistic pathogens, such as *Pneumocystis*. CMV and *Pneumocystis* are frequently found together in immunosuppressed patients with severe interstitial pneumonia.

PATHOLOGY

Cytomegalic cells in vivo (presumed to be infected epithelial cells) are two to four times larger than surrounding cells and often contain an 8- to 10-μm intranuclear inclusion that is eccentrically placed and is surrounded by a clear halo, producing an "owl's eye" appearance. Smaller granular cytoplasmic inclusions are demonstrated occasionally. Cytomegalic cells are found in a wide variety of organs, including the salivary gland, lung, liver, kidney, intestine, pancreas, adrenal gland, and central nervous system.

The cellular inflammatory response to infection consists of plasma cells, lymphocytes, and monocyte-macrophages. Granulomatous reactions occasionally develop, particularly in the liver. Immunopathologic reactions may contribute to CMV disease. Immune complexes have been detected in infected infants, sometimes in association with CMV-related glomerulopathies. Immune-complex glomerulopathy has also been observed in some CMV-infected patients after renal transplantation.

CLINICAL MANIFESTATIONS

Congenital CMV Infection Fetal infections range from inapparent to severe and disseminated. Cytomegalic inclusion disease develops in ~5% of infected fetuses and is seen almost exclusively in infants born to mothers who develop primary infections during pregnancy. Petechiae, hepatosplenomegaly, and jaundice are the most common presenting features (60–80% of cases). Microcephaly with or without cerebral calcifications, intrauterine growth retardation, and prematurity are reported in 30–50% of cases. Inguinal hernias and chorioretinitis are less common. Laboratory abnormalities include elevated alanine aminotransferase levels, thrombocytopenia, conjugated hyperbilirubinemia, hemolysis, and elevated cerebrospinal fluid protein levels. The prognosis for severely infected infants is poor; the mortality rate is 20–30%, and few survivors escape intellectual or hearing difficulties later in childhood. The differential diagnosis of cytomegalic inclusion disease in infants includes syphilis, rubella, toxoplasmosis, infection with herpes simplex virus or enterovirus, and bacterial sepsis.

Most congenital CMV infections are clinically inapparent at birth. Of asymptomatically infected infants, 5–25% develop significant psychomotor, hearing, ocular, or dental abnormalities over the next several years.

Perinatal CMV Infection The newborn may acquire CMV at delivery by passage through an infected birth canal or by postnatal contact with infected breast milk or other maternal secretions. Of infants who are breast-fed for >1 month by seropositive mothers, 40–60% become infected. Iatrogenic transmission can result from neonatal blood transfusion; screening of blood products before transfusion into low-birth-weight seronegative infants or seronegative pregnant women decreases risk.

The great majority of infants infected at or after delivery remain asymptomatic. However, protracted interstitial pneumonitis has been associated with perinatally acquired CMV infection, particularly in premature infants, and occasionally has been accompanied by infection with *Chlamydia trachomatis*, *Pneumocystis*, or *Ureaplasma urealyticum*. Poor weight gain, adenopathy, rash, hepatitis, anemia, and atypical lymphocytosis may also be found, and CMV excretion often persists for months or years.

CMV Mononucleosis The most common clinical manifestation of CMV infection in normal hosts beyond the neonatal period is a heterophile antibody–negative mononucleosis syndrome, which may develop spontaneously or follow transfusion of leukocyte-containing blood products. Although the syndrome occurs at all ages, it most often involves sexually active young adults. With incubation periods of 20–60 days, the illness generally lasts for 2–6 weeks. Prolonged high fevers, sometimes with chills, profound fatigue, and malaise, characterize this disorder. Myalgias, headache, and splenomegaly are common, but in CMV (as opposed to EBV) mononucleosis, exudative pharyngitis and cervical lymphadenopathy are rare. Occasional patients develop rubelliform rashes, often after exposure to ampicillin or certain other antibiotics. Less common are interstitial or segmental pneumonia, myocarditis, pleuritis, arthritis, and encephalitis. In rare cases, Guillain-Barré syndrome complicates CMV mononucleosis. The characteristic laboratory abnormality is relative lymphocytosis in peripheral blood, with >10% atypical lymphocytes. Total leukocyte counts may be low, normal, or markedly elevated. Although significant jaundice is uncommon, serum aminotransferase and alkaline phosphatase levels are often moderately elevated. Heterophile antibodies are absent; however, transient immunologic abnormalities are common and may include the presence of cryoglobulins, rheumatoid factors, cold agglutinins, and antinuclear antibodies. Hemolytic anemia, thrombocytopenia, and granulocytopenia complicate recovery in rare instances.

Most patients recover without sequelae, although postviral asthenia may persist for months. The excretion of CMV in urine, genital secretions, and/or saliva often continues for months or years. Rarely, CMV infection is fatal in immunocompetent hosts; survivors can have recurrent episodes of fever and malaise, sometimes associated with autonomic nervous system dysfunction (e.g., attacks of sweating or flushing).

CMV Infection in the Immunocompromised Host (Table 175-1) CMV appears to be the most common and important viral pathogen complicating organ transplantation (Chap. 126). In recipients of kidney, heart, lung, and liver transplants, CMV induces a variety of syndromes, including fever and leukopenia, hepatitis, pneumonitis, esophagitis, gastritis, colitis, and retinitis. CMV disease may be an independent risk factor for both graft loss and death. The period of maximal risk is between 1 and 4 months after transplantation, although retinitis may be a later complication. Disease likelihood and viral replication levels generally are greater after primary infection than after reactivation. In addition, molecular studies indicate that seropositive transplant recipients are susceptible to reinfection with donor-derived, genotypically variant CMV, and such infection often results in disease. Reactivation infection, although common, is less likely than primary infection to be important clinically. The risk of clinical disease is related to various factors, such as the degree of immunosuppression; the use of antibodies to T cell receptors; and co-infection with other pathogens. The transplanted organ is particularly vulnerable as a target for CMV infection; thus, there is a tendency for CMV hepatitis to follow liver transplantation and for CMV pneumonitis to follow lung transplantation.

CMV pneumonia occurs in 15–20% of bone marrow transplant recipients; the case-fatality rate is 84–88%, although the risk of severe disease may be reduced by prophylaxis or preemptive therapy with antiviral drugs. The risk is greatest 5–13 weeks after transplantation, and identified risk factors include certain types of immunosuppressive therapy, acute graft-versus-host disease, older age, viremia, and pretransplantation seropositivity.

CMV is an important pathogen in patients with advanced HIV infection (Chap. 182), in whom it often causes retinitis or disseminated disease, particularly when peripheral-blood CD4+ T cell counts fall below 50–100/μL. As treatment for underlying HIV infection has improved, the incidence of serious CMV infections (e.g., retinitis) has decreased. However, during the first few weeks after institution of highly active antiretroviral therapy, acute flare-ups of CMV retinitis may occur secondary to an immune reconstitution inflammatory syndrome.

Syndromes produced by CMV in immunocompromised hosts often begin with prolonged fever, malaise, anorexia, fatigue, night sweats, and arthralgias or myalgias. Liver function abnormalities, leukopenia, thrombocytopenia, and atypical lymphocytosis may be observed during these episodes. The development of tachypnea, hypoxia, and unproductive cough signals respiratory involvement. Radiologic examination of

the lung often shows bilateral interstitial or reticulonodular infiltrates that begin in the periphery of the lower lobes and spread centrally and superiorly; localized segmental, nodular, or alveolar patterns are less common. The differential diagnosis includes *Pneumocystis* infection; other viral, bacterial, or fungal infections; pulmonary hemorrhage; and injury secondary to irradiation or to treatment with cytotoxic drugs.

Gastrointestinal CMV involvement may be localized or extensive and almost exclusively affects compromised hosts. Ulcers of the esophagus, stomach, small intestine, or colon may result in bleeding or perforation. CMV infection may lead to exacerbations of underlying ulcerative colitis. Hepatitis occurs frequently, particularly after liver transplantation, and acalculous cholecystitis and adrenalitis have been described.

CMV rarely causes meningoencephalitis in otherwise-healthy individuals. Two forms of CMV encephalitis are seen in patients with AIDS. One resembles HIV encephalitis and presents as progressive dementia; the other is a ventriculoencephalitis characterized by cranial-nerve deficits, nystagmus, disorientation, lethargy, and ventriculomegaly. In immunocompromised patients, CMV can also cause subacute progressive polyradiculopathy, which is often reversible if recognized and treated promptly.

CMV retinitis is an important cause of blindness in immunocompromised patients, particularly patients with advanced AIDS (Chap. 182). Early lesions consist of small, opaque, white areas of granular retinal necrosis that spread in a centrifugal manner and are later accompanied by hemorrhages, vessel sheathing, and retinal edema (Fig. 175-1). CMV retinopathy must be distinguished from that due to other conditions, including toxoplasmosis, candidiasis, and herpes simplex virus infection.

Fatal CMV infections are often associated with persistent viremia and the involvement of multiple organ systems. Progressive pulmonary infiltrates, pancytopenia, hyperamylasemia, and hypotension are characteristic features that are frequently found in conjunction with a terminal bacterial, fungal, or protozoan superinfection. Extensive adrenal necrosis with CMV inclusions is often documented at autopsy, as is CMV involvement of many other organs.

DIAGNOSIS

The diagnosis of CMV infection usually cannot be made reliably on clinical grounds alone. Isolation of CMV or detection of its antigens or DNA in appropriate clinical specimens is the preferred approach. Virus excretion or viremia is readily detected by culture of appropriate specimens on human fibroblast monolayers. If CMV titers are high, as is common in congenital disseminated infection and in patients with AIDS, characteristic cytopathic effects may be detected within a few days. However, in some situations (e.g., CMV mononucleosis), viral titers are low, and cytopathic effects may take several weeks to appear. Many laboratories expedite diagnosis with an overnight tissue-culture

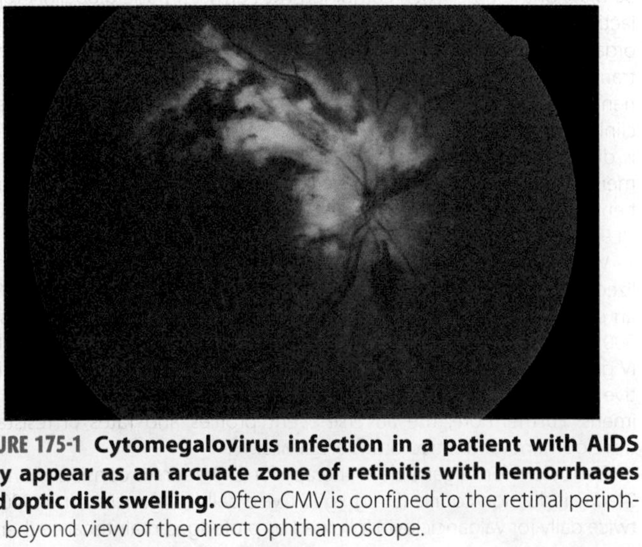

FIGURE 175-1 Cytomegalovirus infection in a patient with AIDS may appear as an arcuate zone of retinitis with hemorrhages and optic disk swelling. Often CMV is confined to the retinal periphery, beyond view of the direct ophthalmoscope.

method (shell vial assay) involving centrifugation and an immunocytochemical detection technique employing monoclonal antibodies to an immediate-early CMV antigen. Isolation of virus from urine or saliva does not, by itself, constitute proof of acute infection, since excretion from these sites may continue for months or years after illness. Detection of viremia is a better predictor of acute infection.

Detection of CMV antigens (pp65) in peripheral-blood leukocytes or of CMV DNA in blood or tissues may hasten diagnosis. Such assays may yield a positive result several days earlier than culture methods. The most sensitive way to detect CMV in blood or other fluids may be by amplifying CMV DNA by polymerase chain reaction (PCR). PCR detection of CMV DNA in blood may predict the risk for disease progression, and PCR detection of CMV DNA in cerebrospinal fluid is useful in the diagnosis of CMV encephalitis or polyradiculopathy.

A variety of serologic assays detect increases in titers of antibody to CMV antigens. An increased antibody level may not be detectable for up to 4 weeks after primary infection, and titers often remain high for years after infection. For this reason, single-sample antibody determinations are of no value in assessing the acuteness of infection. Detection of CMV-specific IgM is sometimes useful in the diagnosis of recent or active infection; circulating rheumatoid factors may result in occasional false-positive IgM tests.

Rx CYTOMEGALOVIRUS INFECTION

Several measures are useful for the prevention of CMV infection in high-risk patients. The use of blood from seronegative donors or of blood that has been frozen, thawed, and deglycerolized greatly decreases the rate of transfusion-associated transmission. Matching of organ or bone marrow transplants by CMV serology, with exclusive use of organs from seronegative donors in seronegative recipients, reduces rates of primary infection after transplantation. Both live attenuated and CMV subunit vaccines have been evaluated, but neither is close to approval for general use.

CMV immune or hyperimmune globulin has been reported (1) to reduce rates of CMV-associated syndromes and of fungal or parasitic superinfections among seronegative renal transplant recipients and (2) to prevent congenital CMV infection in infants of women with primary infection during pregnancy. Studies in bone marrow transplant recipients have produced conflicting results. Prophylactic acyclovir or valacyclovir may reduce rates of CMV infection and disease in certain seronegative renal transplant recipients, although neither drug is effective in the treatment of active CMV disease.

Ganciclovir is a guanosine derivative that has considerably more activity against CMV than its congener acyclovir. After intracellular conversion by a viral phosphotransferase encoded by CMV gene region UL97, ganciclovir triphosphate is a selective inhibitor of CMV DNA polymerase. Several clinical studies have indicated response rates of 70–90% among patients with AIDS who are given ganciclovir for the treatment of CMV retinitis or colitis. In bone marrow transplant recipients with CMV pneumonia, ganciclovir is less effective when given alone, but it elicits a favorable clinical response 50–70% of the time when combined with CMV immune globulin. Prophylactic or suppressive ganciclovir may be useful in high-risk bone marrow or organ transplant recipients (e.g., those who are CMV-seropositive before transplantation or who are CMV culture–positive afterward). In many patients with AIDS, persistently low CD4+ T cell counts, and CMV disease, clinical and virologic relapses occur promptly if treatment with ganciclovir is discontinued. Therefore, prolonged maintenance regimens are recommended for such patients. Resistance to ganciclovir is common among patients treated for >3 months and is usually related to mutations in the CMV UL97 gene.

Valganciclovir is an orally bioavailable prodrug that is rapidly metabolized to ganciclovir in intestinal tissues and the liver. Approximately 60% of an oral dose of valganciclovir is absorbed. An oral valganciclovir dose of 900 mg results in ganciclovir blood levels similar to those obtained with an IV ganciclovir dose of 5 mg/kg. Oral valganciclovir appears to be as effective as IV ganciclovir for both CMV retinitis induction and maintenance regimens. Furthermore, the adverse-event profiles and rates of resistance development for the two drugs are similar.

Ganciclovir or valganciclovir therapy for CMV retinitis consists of a 14- to 21-day induction course (5 mg/kg IV twice daily for ganciclovir or 900 mg twice daily for valganciclovir) followed by prolonged maintenance therapy. For parenteral maintenance, the ganciclovir dose is 5 mg/kg daily or 6 mg/kg 5 days per week; for oral maintenance, 900 mg of valganciclovir once daily is recommended. Peripheral-blood neutropenia develops in 16–29% of treated patients but may be ameliorated by granulocyte colony-stimulating factor or granulocyte-macrophage colony-stimulating factor. Discontinuation of maintenance therapy should be considered in patients with AIDS who, while receiving antiretroviral therapy, have a sustained (>6-month) increase in CD4+ T cell counts to >100–150/μL.

Ganciclovir may also be administered via a slow-release pellet sutured into the eye. Although this intraocular device provides good local protection, contralateral eye disease and disseminated disease are not affected, and early retinal detachment is possible. A combination of intraocular and systemic therapy may be better than the intraocular implant alone.

Foscarnet (sodium phosphonoformate) inhibits CMV DNA polymerase. Because this agent does not require phosphorylation to be active, it is also effective against most ganciclovir-resistant isolates. Foscarnet is less well tolerated than ganciclovir and causes considerable toxicity, including renal dysfunction, hypomagnesemia, hypokalemia, hypocalcemia, genital ulcers, dysuria, nausea, and paresthesia. Moreover, foscarnet administration requires the use of an infusion pump and close clinical monitoring. With aggressive hydration and dose adjustments for renal dysfunction, the toxicity of foscarnet can be reduced. The use of foscarnet should be avoided when a saline load cannot be tolerated (e.g., in cardiomyopathy). The approved induction regimen is 60 mg/kg every 8 h for 2 weeks, although 90 mg/kg every 12 h is equally effective and no more toxic. Maintenance infusions should deliver 90–120 mg/kg once daily. No oral preparation is available. Foscarnet-resistant virus may emerge during extended therapy.

Cidofovir is a nucleotide analogue with a long intracellular half-life that allows intermittent IV administration. Induction regimens of 5 mg/kg weekly for 2 weeks are followed by maintenance regimens of 3–5 mg/kg every 2 weeks. Cidofovir can cause severe nephrotoxicity through dose-dependent proximal tubular cell injury; however, this adverse effect can be tempered somewhat by saline hydration and probenecid.

It is not clear whether universal prophylaxis or preemptive therapy is the preferable approach in CMV-seropositive immunocompromised hosts. Both ganciclovir and valganciclovir have been used successfully for prophylaxis and preemptive therapy in transplant recipients. For patients with advanced HIV infection (CD4+ T cell counts of <50/μL), some authorities have advocated prophylaxis with oral ganciclovir or valganciclovir. However, side effects, lack of proven benefit, possible induction of viral resistance, and high cost have precluded the wide acceptance of this practice. Preemptive ganciclovir or valganciclovir therapy based on detection of CMV viremia by either antigenemia or PCR techniques is under study.

HUMAN HERPESVIRUS TYPES 6, 7, AND 8

Human herpesvirus (HHV) type 6 was first isolated in 1986 from peripheral-blood leukocytes of six persons with various lymphoproliferative disorders. The virus has a worldwide distribution, and two genetically distinct variants (HHV-6A and HHV-6B) are now recognized. HHV-6 appears to be transmitted by saliva and possibly by genital secretions.

Infection with HHV-6 frequently occurs during infancy as maternal antibody wanes. The peak age of acquisition is 9–21 months; by 24 months, seropositivity rates approach 80%. Older siblings appear to serve as a source of transmission. Congenital infection may also occur. Most infected children develop symptoms (fever, fussiness, and diarrhea). A minority develop exanthem subitum (roseola infantum), a common illness characterized by fever with subsequent rash. Approximately 10–20% of febrile seizures without rash during infancy are caused by HHV-6.

In older age groups, HHV-6 has been associated with mononucleosis syndromes, focal encephalitis, and (in immunocompromised hosts) pneumonitis and disseminated disease. In transplant recipients, HHV-6 infection may be associated with similar syndromes and with graft dysfunction. High plasma loads of HHV-6 DNA in stem cell transplant recipients are associated with allelic-mismatched donors, use of steroids, delayed monocyte and platelet engraftment, development of limbic encephalitis, and increased all-cause mortality. Like many other viruses, HHV-6 has been implicated in the pathogenesis of multiple sclerosis, although further study is needed to distinguish between association and etiology.

HHV-7 was isolated in 1990 from T lymphocytes from the peripheral blood of a healthy 26-year-old man. The virus is frequently acquired during childhood, albeit at a later age than HHV-6. HHV-7 is commonly present in saliva, which is presumed to be the principal source of infection; breast milk can also carry the virus. Viremia can be associated with either primary or reactivation infection. The most common clinical manifestations of childhood HHV-7 infections are fever and seizures. Some children present with respiratory or gastrointestinal signs and symptoms. An association has been made between HHV-7 and pityriasis rosea, but evidence is insufficient to indicate a causal relationship.

HHV-6, HHV-7, and CMV infections may cluster in transplant recipients, making it difficult to sort out the roles of the various agents in individual clinical syndromes. HHV-6 and HHV-7 appear to be susceptible to ganciclovir and foscarnet, although definitive evidence of clinical responses is lacking.

Unique herpesvirus-like DNA sequences were reported during 1994 and 1995 in tissues derived from Kaposi's sarcoma (KS) and body cavity–based lymphoma occurring in patients with AIDS. The virus from which these sequences were derived is designated HHV-8 or Kaposi's sarcoma–associated herpesvirus (KSHV). HHV-8, which infects certain B lymphocytes and endothelium-derived spindle cells, appears to be causally related not only to KS but also to a subgroup of AIDS-related B cell body cavity–based lymphomas (primary effusion lymphomas) and to multicentric Castleman's disease, a lymphoproliferative disorder of B cells. Initial suggestions that HHV-8 is associated with primary pulmonary hypertension have not been confirmed by subsequent studies.

Unlike other herpesvirus infections, HHV-8 infection is much more common in some geographic areas (e.g., central and southern Africa) than in others (North America, Asia, northern Europe). In high-prevalence areas, infection occurs in childhood, seropositivity is associated with having a seropositive mother or (to a lesser extent) older sibling, and HHV-8 may be transmitted in saliva. In low-prevalence areas, infections typically occur in adults, probably with sexual transmission. Concurrent epidemics of HIV-1 and HHV-8 infections among certain populations (e.g., homosexual and bisexual men) in the late 1970s and early 1980s appear to have resulted in the frequent association of AIDS and KS. Transmission of HHV-8 may also be associated with organ transplantation and injection drug use.

Primary HHV-8 infection in immunocompetent children may manifest as fever and maculopapular rash. Among individuals with intact immunity, chronic asymptomatic infection is the rule, and neoplastic disorders generally develop only after subsequent immunocompromise. Immunocompromised persons with primary infection may present with fever, splenomegaly, lymphoid hyperplasia, pancytopenia, or rapid-onset KS. Quantitative analysis of HHV-8 DNA suggests a predominance of latently infected cells in KS lesions and frequent lytic replication in multicentric Castleman's disease.

Effective antiretroviral therapy for HIV-infected individuals has led to a marked reduction in rates of KS among persons dually infected with HHV-8 and HIV in resource-rich areas. HHV-8 itself is susceptible in vitro to ganciclovir, foscarnet, and cidofovir, although clinical evidence for benefit of these agents is lacking.

FURTHER READINGS

ASAHI-OZAKI Y et al: Quantitative analysis of Kaposi sarcoma–associated herpesvirus (KSHV) in KSHV-associated diseases. J Infect Dis 193:773, 2006

CANNON MJ et al: Blood-borne and sexual transmission of human herpesvirus 8 in women with or at risk for human immunodeficiency virus infection. N Engl J Med 344:637, 2001

HALL CB et al: Characteristics and acquisition of human herpesvirus (HHV)-7 infections in relation to infection with HHV-6. J Infect Dis 193:1063, 2006

HEINEMAN TC et al: A phase 1 study of 4 live, recombinant human cytomegalovirus Towne/Toledo chimeric vaccines. J Infect Dis 193:1350, 2006

KALIL AC et al: Meta-analysis: The efficacy of strategies to prevent organ disease by cytomegalovirus in solid organ transplant recipients. Ann Intern Med 143:870, 2005

MARTIN DF et al: A controlled trial of valganciclovir as induction therapy for cytomegalovirus retinitis. N Engl J Med 346:1119, 2002

MBULAITEYE S et al: Molecular evidence for mother-to-child transmission of Kaposi sarcoma–associated herpesvirus in Uganda and K1 gene evolution within the host. J Infect Dis 193:1250, 2006

NIGRO G et al: Passive immunization during pregnancy for congenital cytomegalovirus infection. N Engl J Med 353:1350, 2005

OGATA M et al: Human herpesvirus 6 DNA in plasma after allogeneic stem cell transplantation: Incidence and clinical significance. J Infect Dis 193:68, 2006

ZERR DM et al: A population-based study of primary human herpesvirus 6 infection. N Engl J Med 352:768, 2005

176 Molluscum Contagiosum, Monkeypox, and Other Poxviruses, Excluding Smallpox Virus

Fred Wang

The poxvirus family includes a large number of related DNA viruses that infect various vertebrate hosts. The poxviruses responsible for infections in humans, along with the main manifestations of these infections, are listed in Table 176-1. Infections with orthopoxviruses—e.g., smallpox (variola major) virus (Chap. 214) or the zoonotic monkeypox virus—can result in systemic, potentially lethal human disease. Other poxvirus infections cause primarily localized skin disease in humans.

TABLE 176-1 POXVIRUSES AND HUMAN INFECTIONS

Genus	Species	Human Disease
Orthopoxvirus	Variola[a]	Smallpox, systemic
	Monkeypox	Smallpox-like, systemic
	Vaccinia	Local pox lesion, occasionally systemic
	Cowpox	Local pox lesions
Molluscipoxvirus	Molluscum contagiosum	Molluscum contagiosum, multiple cutaneous lesions
Parapoxvirus	Orf	Contagious pustular dermatitis, local pox lesions
	Pseudocowpox	Milker's nodule, local pox lesions
Yatapoxvirus	Tanapox	Local pox lesions

[a]See Chap. 214.

MOLLUSCUM CONTAGIOSUM

Molluscum contagiosum virus is an obligate human pathogen that causes distinctive proliferative skin lesions. These lesions measure 2–5 mm in diameter and are pearly, flesh-colored, and umbilicated, with a characteristic dimple at the center (Fig. 176-1). A relative lack of inflammation and necrosis distinguishes these proliferative lesions from other poxvirus lesions. Lesions may be found—singly or in clusters—anywhere on the body except on the palms and soles and may be associated with an eczematous rash.

Molluscum contagiosum is the most common human disease resulting from poxvirus infection and is transmitted by close contact, including sexual intercourse. Swimming pools are a common vector for transmission. Atopy and compromise of skin integrity increase the risk of

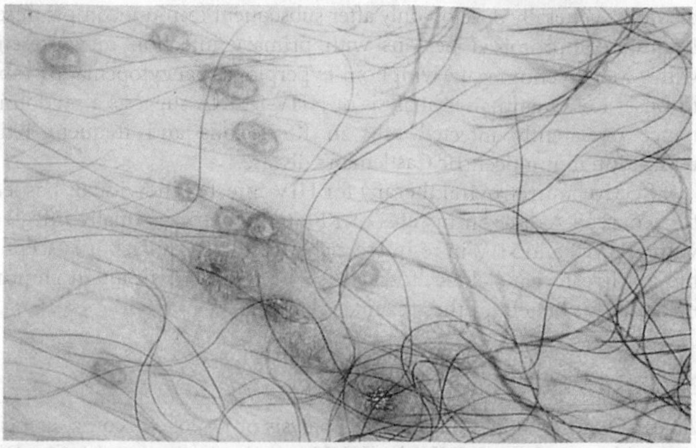

FIGURE 176-1 Molluscum contagiosum is a cutaneous poxvirus infection characterized by multiple umbilicated flesh-colored or hypopigmented papules.

infection. The incubation period ranges from 2 weeks to 6 months, with an average of 2–7 weeks. In most cases, the disease is self-limited and regresses spontaneously after 3–4 months in immunocompetent hosts. There are no systemic complications, but skin lesions may persist for 3–5 years. Molluscum contagiosum develops especially often in association with advanced HIV infection; the prevalence is 5–18% among HIV-infected patients (Chap. 182). The disease is often more generalized, severe, and persistent in AIDS patients than in other groups, frequently involving the face and upper body. Paradoxically, rates of molluscum contagiosum are reportedly elevated among patients receiving antiretroviral therapy. Moreover, the disease can be exacerbated in the immune reconstitution inflammatory syndrome (IRIS) associated with the initiation of antiretroviral therapy. Extensive molluscum contagiosum has also been reported in conjunction with other types of immunodeficiency.

The diagnosis of molluscum contagiosum is typically made by its clinical presentation and can be confirmed by histologic demonstration of the cytoplasmic eosinophilic inclusions, or ***molluscum bodies***, that are characteristic of poxvirus replication. Molluscum contagiosum virus cannot be propagated in vitro, but electron microscopy and molecular studies can be used for its identification.

There is no specific systemic treatment for molluscum contagiosum, but a variety of techniques for physical ablation have been used. Cidofovir displays in vitro activity against many poxviruses, including smallpox virus and molluscum contagiosum virus, and case reports suggest that parenteral or topical cidofovir may have some efficacy in the treatment of recalcitrant molluscum contagiosum in immunosuppressed hosts.

MONKEYPOX

Although monkeypox virus was named after the animal from which it was originally isolated, rodents are the primary viral reservoir.

Human infections with monkeypox virus typically occur in Africa when humans come into direct contact with infected animals. Human disease is rare and is characterized by a systemic illness and a vesicular rash similar to those of variola. The clinical presentation of monkeypox can be confused with that of the more common varicella-zoster virus infection (Chap. 173). Compared with the lesions of this herpesvirus infection, monkeypox lesions tend to be more uniform (i.e., in the same stage of development), diffuse, and peripheral in distribution. Lymphadenopathy is a prominent feature of monkeypox infection.

The first outbreak of human monkeypox infection in the Western Hemisphere occurred in the midwestern United States during May and June 2003, when more than 70 cases were reported, of which 35 were laboratory confirmed. The outbreak was linked to contact with pet prairie dogs that had become infected while being housed with rodents imported from Ghana. Patients presented most frequently with fever, rash, and lymphadenopathy ~12 days after exposure. The median durations of fever and rash were 8 and 12 days, respectively. Of the nine patients who were hospitalized, five were judged to be severely ill, but there were no deaths. Smallpox vaccination can provide cross-reactive immunity to monkeypox infection; nevertheless, there were no significant clinical differences between vaccinated and unvaccinated individuals in this outbreak. Additional studies of people exposed in the outbreak detected subclinical infection in a few vaccinated individuals—an observation suggesting the possibility of long-term vaccine protection. The risk of human disease from animal orthopoxvirus infections may increase as smallpox immunity wanes in the general population and the popularity of exotic animals as household pets grows.

OTHER ZOONOTIC POXVIRUS INFECTIONS

Orf virus and *pseudocowpox* virus are parapoxviruses that naturally infect sheep and cattle. Direct contact with infected animals can result in human infections, typically on the hands, with the development of a nodular, highly vascular proliferative lesion that may ulcerate. Human orf virus infection is also called *ecthyma contagiosum*, and human pseudocowpox virus infection causes "milker's nodules."

Zoonotic infection with *cowpox* virus causes painful hemorrhagic lesions, mostly on the hands or face, with fever or flulike symptoms and lymphadenitis. Lesions generally resolve in 6–8 weeks. Human infection with *tanapox* virus occurs after contact with infected monkeys. In most cases, a febrile prodrome is followed by eruption of a single nodular lesion on the exposed area, but multiple lesions have also been reported. The lesions are relatively large, often break down to form an ulcer, and resolve in 5–6 weeks.

FURTHER READINGS

CENTERS FOR DISEASE CONTROL AND PREVENTION: Update: Multistate outbreak of monkeypox—Illinois, Indiana, Kansas, Missouri, Ohio, and Wisconsin, 2003. MMWR 52:642, 2003

DHAR AD et al: Tanapox infection in a college student. N Engl J Med 350:361, 2004

HAMMARLUND E et al: Multiple diagnostic techniques identify previously vaccinated individuals with protective immunity against monkeypox. Nat Med 11:1005, 2005

HUHN GD et al: Clinical characteristics of human monkeypox, and risk factors for severe disease. Clin Infect Dis 41:1742, 2005

REED KD et al: The detection of monkeypox in humans in the Western Hemisphere. N Engl J Med 350:342, 2004

177 Parvovirus Infections

Kevin E. Brown

Parvoviruses, members of the family Parvoviridae, are small (diameter, ~22 nm), nonenveloped, icosahedral-shaped viruses with a linear single-stranded DNA genome of ~5000 nucleotides. These viruses are dependent on either rapidly dividing host cells or helper viruses for replication. At least four types of parvovirus infect humans: parvovirus B19, adeno-associated viruses (AAVs), the recently described PARV4/5 virus, and human bocavirus (HBoV). To date, only B19 has been shown definitively to be a human pathogen.

PARVOVIRUS B19

DEFINITION

B19 is the type member of the genus *Erythrovirus*. On the basis of viral sequence, B19 is divided into three genotypes (designated 1, 2, and 3), but only a single B19 antigenic type has been described. Genotypes 2 and 3 are detected relatively infrequently in Europe and the United States.

EPIDEMIOLOGY

B19 exclusively infects humans, and infection is endemic in virtually all parts of the world. Transmission occurs predominantly via the respiratory route and is followed by the onset of rash and arthralgia. By the age of 15 years, ~ 50% of children have detectable IgG; this figure rises to >90% among the elderly. In pregnant women, the estimated annual seroconversion rate is ~1%. Within households, secondary infection rates approach 50%.

Detection of high-titer B19 in blood is not unusual (see "Pathogenesis," below). Transmission can occur as a result of transfusion, most commonly of pooled components. To reduce the risk of transmission, plasma pools are screened by nucleic acid amplification technology, and high-titer pools are discarded. B19 is resistant to both heat and solvent-detergent inactivation.

PATHOGENESIS

B19 replicates primarily in erythroid progenitors. This specificity is due in part to the limited tissue distribution of the B19 receptor, blood group P antigen (globoside). Infection leads to high-titer viremia, with $>10^{12}$ virus particles/mL detectable in the blood at the apex (Fig. 177-1), and virus-induced cytotoxicity results in cessation of red cell production. In immunocompetent individuals, viremia and arrest of erythropoiesis are transient and resolve as the IgM and IgG antibody response is mounted. In individuals with normal erythropoiesis, there is only a minimal drop in hemoglobin levels; however, in those with increased erythropoiesis (especially with hemolytic anemia), this cessation of red cell production can induce a transient crisis with severe anemia (Fig. 177-1). Similarly, if an individual (or, after maternal infection, a fetus) does not mount a neutralizing antibody response and halt the lytic infection, erythroid production is compromised and chronic anemia develops (Fig. 177-1).

The immune-mediated phase of illness, which begins 2–3 weeks after infection as the IgM response peaks, manifests as the rash of fifth disease together with arthralgia and/or frank arthritis. Low-level B19 DNA can be detected by polymerase chain reaction (PCR) in blood and tissues for months to years after acute infection.

The B19 receptor is found in a variety of other cells and tissues, including megakaryocytes, endothelial cells, placenta, myocardium, and liver. Infection of these tissues by B19 may be responsible for some of the more unusual presentations of the infection. Rare individuals who lack P antigen are naturally resistant to B19 infection.

CLINICAL MANIFESTATIONS

Erythema Infectiosum Most B19 infections are asymptomatic. The main manifestation of symptomatic B19 infection is erythema infectiosum, also known as *fifth disease* or *slapped-cheek disease* (Fig. 177-2). Infection begins with a minor febrile prodrome ~7–10 days after exposure, and the classic facial rash develops several days later. The rash may spread to the extremities in a lacy reticular pattern. However, its intensity and distribution vary, and the B19-induced rash is difficult to distinguish from other viral exanthems. Adults may not exhibit the "slapped-cheek" phenomenon.

Polyarthropathy Syndrome Although uncommon among children, arthropathy occurs in ~50% of adults and is more common among women than among men. The distribution of the affected joints is often symmetrical, with arthralgia affecting the small joints of the hands

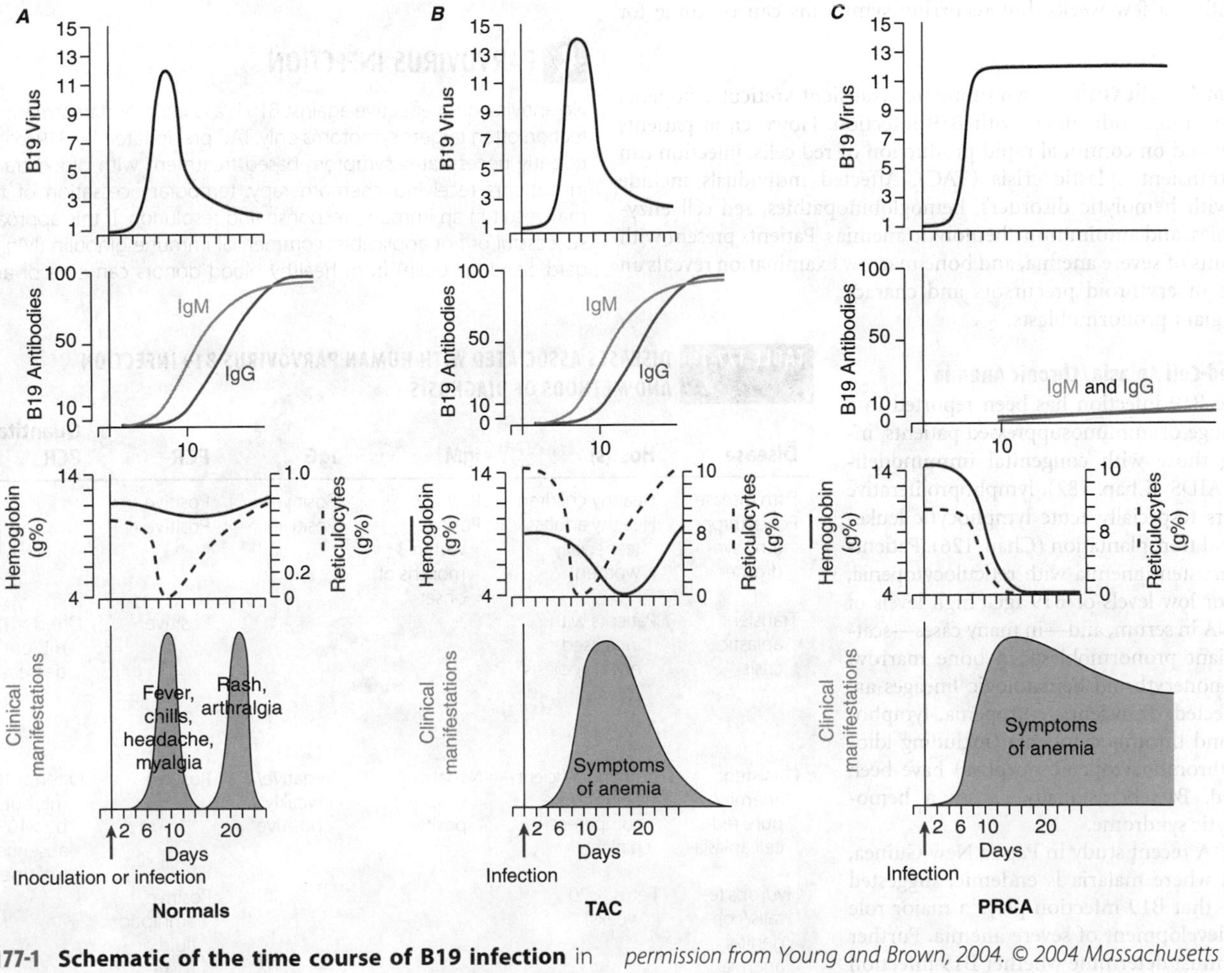

FIGURE 177-1 Schematic of the time course of B19 infection in (***A***) normals (erythema infectiosum), (***B***) transient aplastic crisis (TAC), and (***C***) chronic anemia/pure red-cell aplasia (PRCA). *(Reprinted with permission from Young and Brown, 2004. © 2004 Massachusetts Medical Society. All rights reserved.)*

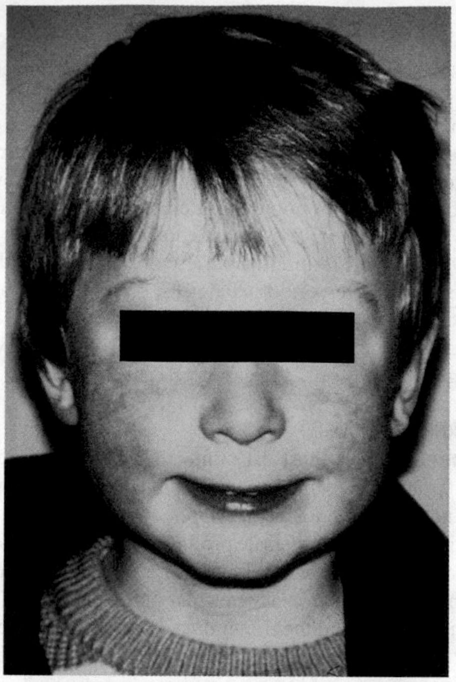

FIGURE 177-2 Child with erythema infectiosum, or fifth disease, showing typical "slapped-cheek" appearance. *(Courtesy of Bernard Cohen, Virus Reference Department, Health Protection Agency, London; with permission.)*

and occasionally the ankles, knees, and wrists. Resolution usually occurs within a few weeks, but recurring symptoms can continue for months.

Transient Aplastic Crisis Asymptomatic transient reticulocytopenia occurs in most individuals with B19 infection. However, in patients who depend on continual rapid production of red cells, infection can cause transient aplastic crisis (TAC). Affected individuals include those with hemolytic disorders, hemoglobinopathies, red cell enzymopathies, and autoimmune hemolytic anemias. Patients present with symptoms of severe anemia, and bone marrow examination reveals an absence of erythroid precursors and characteristic giant pronormoblasts.

Pure Red-Cell Aplasia/Chronic Anemia
Chronic B19 infection has been reported in a wide range of immunosuppressed patients, including those with congenital immunodeficiency, AIDS (Chap. 182), lymphoproliferative disorders (especially acute lymphocytic leukemia), and transplantation (Chap. 126). Patients have persistent anemia with reticulocytopenia, absent or low levels of B19 IgG, high levels of B19 DNA in serum, and—in many cases—scattered giant pronormoblasts in bone marrow. Rarely, nonerythroid hematologic lineages are also affected. Transient neutropenia, lymphopenia, and thrombocytopenia (including idiopathic thrombocytopenic purpura) have been observed. B19 occasionally causes a hemophagocytic syndrome.

A recent study in Papua New Guinea, where malaria is endemic, suggested that B19 infection plays a major role in the development of severe anemia. Further studies must determine whether B19 infection contributes to severe anemia in other malarial regions.

Hydrops Fetalis B19 infection during pregnancy can lead to hydrops fetalis and/or fetal loss. The risk of transplacental fetal infection is ~30%, and the risk of fetal loss (predominantly early in the second trimester) is ~9%. The risk of congenital infection is <1%. Although B19 does not appear to be teratogenic, anecdotal cases of eye damage and CNS abnormalities have been reported. Cases of congenital anemia have also been described. B19 probably causes 10–20% of all cases of nonimmune hydrops.

Unusual Manifestations Hepatitis, vasculitis, myocarditis, glomerulosclerosis, and central nervous system (CNS) disease have all been reported. However, B19 DNA can be detected by PCR for years in many tissues; this finding is of no known clinical significance, but its interpretation may cause confusion regarding B19 disease association.

DIAGNOSIS

Diagnosis of B19 infection in immunocompetent individuals is generally based on detection of B19 IgM antibodies (Table 177-1). IgM can be detected at the time of rash in erythema infectiosum and by the third day of TAC in patients with hematologic disorders; these antibodies remain detectable for ~3 months. B19 IgG is detectable by the seventh day of illness and persists throughout life. Detection of B19 DNA should be used for the diagnosis of early TAC or chronic anemia. Although B19 levels fall rapidly with the development of the immune response, DNA can be detectable by PCR for months or even years after infection, even in healthy individuals; therefore, quantitative PCR should be used. In acute infection at the height of viremia, $>10^{12}$ B19 DNA genome equivalents (ge)/mL of serum can be detected; however, titers fall rapidly within 2 days. Patients with aplastic crisis or B19-induced chronic anemia generally have $>10^5$ B19 DNA ge/mL.

Rx PARVOVIRUS INFECTION

No antiviral drug effective against B19 is available, and treatment of B19 infection often targets symptoms only. TAC precipitated by B19 infection frequently necessitates symptom-based treatment with blood transfusions. In patients receiving chemotherapy, temporary cessation of treatment may result in an immune response and resolution. If this approach is unsuccessful or not applicable, commercial immune globulin (IVIg; Gammagard, Sandoglobulin) from healthy blood donors can cure or ameliorate

TABLE 177-1 DISEASES ASSOCIATED WITH HUMAN PARVOVIRUS B19 INFECTION AND METHODS OF DIAGNOSIS

Disease	Host(s)	IgM	IgG	PCR	Quantitative PCR
Fifth disease	Healthy children	Positive	Positive	Positive	
Polyarthropathy syndrome	Healthy adults (especially women)	Positive within 3 months of onset	Positive	Positive	
Transient aplastic crisis	Patients with increased erythropoiesis			Positive	Often > 10^{12} ge/mL, but rapidly decreases
Persistent anemia/pure red-cell aplasia	Immunodeficient or immunocompetent patients	Negative/weakly positive	Negative/weakly positive	Positive	Often > 10^{12} ge/mL, but should be $>10^6$ in the absence of treatment
Hydrops fetalis/congenital anemia	Fetus (<20 weeks)			Positive amniotic fluid or tissue	

Note: ge, genome equivalents; PCR, polymerase chain reaction.

persistent B19 infection in immunosuppressed patients. Generally, the dose used is 400 mg/kg daily for 5–10 days. Like patients with TAC, immunosuppressed patients with persistent B19 infection should be considered infectious. Administration of IVIg is not beneficial for erythema infectiosum or B19-associated polyarthropathy. Intrauterine blood transfusion can prevent fetal loss in some cases of fetal hydrops.

PREVENTION

No vaccine has been approved for the prevention of B19 infection. A vaccine based on virus-like particles expressed in insect cells is under development; the results of phase 1 trials were promising.

OTHER PARVOVIRUSES

ADENO-ASSOCIATED VIRUSES

Antibody studies indicate that AAV infections are common in childhood, but AAVs have not been associated with any disease and are considered nonpathogenic. Most of the interest in AAVs is related to their potential use as vectors for gene therapy.

PARV4/5

The PARV4 viral sequence was initially detected in a patient with an acute viral syndrome. Similar sequences, including the related PARV5 sequence, have been detected in pooled plasma collections. The DNA sequence of PARV4/5 is distinctly different from that of all other parvoviruses, and this virus cannot be classified within the current *Parvovirus* genus. Preliminary serologic studies indicate that PARV4/5 infection is common in childhood, but no association with disease has been shown.

HUMAN BOCAVIRUS

Animal bocaviruses are associated with mild respiratory symptoms and enteritis in young animals. HBoV was recently identified in the respiratory tract of young children with lower respiratory tract infections. However, its contribution to pathogenesis is unknown, and HBoV sequences are often found in the presence of other pathogens. The relation of HBoV and PARV4/5 viruses to the commonly observed fecal parvoviruses also remains to be established.

FURTHER READINGS

ALLANDER T et al: Cloning of a human parvovirus by molecular screening of respiratory tract samples. Proc Natl Acad Sci USA 102:12891, 2005

BROWN KE, YOUNG NS: Parvovirus B19, in NS Young et al (eds). *Clinical Hematology*. Philadelphia, Mosby Elsevier, 2006, pp 981–991

——— et al: Resistance to parvovirus B19 infection due to lack of virus receptor (erythrocyte P antigen). N Engl J Med 330:1192, 1994

——— et al: Erythrocyte P antigen: Cellular receptor for B19 parvovirus. Science 262:114, 1993

FRYER JF et al: Novel parvovirus and related variant in human plasma. Emerg Infect Dis 12:151, 2006

KERR JR et al: *Parvoviruses*. London, Hodder Arnold, 2006

KURTZMAN GJ et al: Chronic bone marrow failure due to persistent B19 parvovirus infection. N Engl J Med 317:287, 1987

WILDIG J et al: Parvovirus B19 infection contributes to severe anemia in young children in Papua New Guinea. J Infect Dis 194:146, 2006

YOUNG NS, BROWN KE: Parvovirus B19. N Engl J Med 350:586, 2004

178 Human Papillomavirus Infections

Richard C. Reichman

DEFINITION

Human papillomaviruses (HPVs) selectively infect the epithelium of skin and mucous membranes. These infections may be asymptomatic, produce warts, or be associated with a variety of both benign and malignant neoplasias.

ETIOLOGIC AGENT

Papillomaviruses are members of the family Papillomaviridae. They are nonenveloped, measure 50–55 nm in diameter, have icosahedral capsids composed of 72 capsomeres, and contain a double-strand circular DNA genome of ~7900 base pairs. The genomic organization of all papillomaviruses is similar and consists of an early (E) region, a late (L) region, and a noncoding upstream regulatory region (URR). Oncogenic HPV types can immortalize human keratinocytes, and this activity has been mapped to products of early genes E6 and E7. E6 protein facilitates the degradation of the p53 tumor-suppressor protein, and E7 protein binds the retinoblastoma gene product and related proteins. The E1 and E2 proteins modulate viral DNA replication and regulate gene expression. The L1 gene codes for the major capsid protein, which makes up 80% of the virion mass. L2 codes for a minor capsid protein. Type-specific conformational antigenic determinants are located on the virion surface. Papillomavirus types are distinguished from one another by the degree of nucleic acid sequence homology. Distinct types share <90% of their DNA sequences in L1. More than 100 HPV types are recognized, and individual types are associated with specific clinical manifestations. For example, HPV-1 causes plantar warts, HPV-6 causes anogenital warts, and HPV-16 infection can produce cervical dysplasia and invasive cervical cancer. HPVs are species-specific and have not been propagated in tissue culture or in common experimental animals. However, some HPV types have been produced in human tissues implanted in immunodeficient mice.

EPIDEMIOLOGY

There are few good studies of the incidence or prevalence of human warts in well-defined populations. Common warts (*verruca vulgaris*) are found in as many as 25% of some groups and are most prevalent among young children. Plantar warts (*verruca plantaris*) are also widely prevalent; they occur most often among adolescents and young adults. Anogenital warts (*condyloma acuminatum*) represent one of the most common sexually transmitted diseases in the United States. HPV infection of the uterine cervix produces the squamous cell abnormalities most frequently detected on Papanicolaou smears.

Most anogenital HPV infections are transmitted through direct contact with infectious lesions. However, lesion characteristics that are associated with transmission, including appearance, have not been defined, and individuals without obvious disease may transmit infection. Close personal contact is also assumed to play a role in the transmission of most cutaneous warts; the importance of fomites in this setting is not clear. Minor trauma at the site of inoculation may facilitate transmission. Recurrent respiratory papillomatosis in young children is an uncommon disease that is acquired from the infected maternal genital tract. In adults, orogenital sexual contact may transmit the disease.

According to a consensus panel gathered by the World Health Organization, a large body of epidemiologic and biologic data has established that some HPV infections cause cervical cancer. For example, >95% of cervical cancers contain HPV DNA of oncogenic (high-risk) types, such as 16, 18, 31, 33, and 45. HPV DNA is also present in the precursor lesions of cervical cancer (cervical intraepithelial neoplasias). Such lesions containing DNA of oncogenic types are more likely to progress than those associated with low-risk HPV types, such as 6 and 11. HPV DNA is transcribed in tumor tissues, and many epidemiologic studies have confirmed a strong relationship between HPV infection (with or without cofactors) and the development of cervical cancer. Definitive proof of the causative role of high-risk HPV types in the pathogenesis of high-grade cervical dysplasia has been provided by the results of recently conducted trials of HPV vaccines. However, it is important to realize that most cervical HPV infections, including those caused by high-risk types, are self-limited. Infection with high-risk HPV types has also been associated with squamous cell carcinomas and dysplasias of the penis, anus, vagina, and vulva. In patients with *epidermodysplasia verruciformis* (see "Clinical Manifestations," below), squamous cell cancers develop frequently at sites infected with specific HPV types, including 5 and 8.

CLINICAL MANIFESTATIONS

The clinical manifestations of HPV infection depend on the location of lesions and the type of virus. Common warts usually occur on the hands as flesh-colored to brown, exophytic, and hyperkeratotic papules. Plantar warts may be quite painful; they can be differentiated from calluses by paring of the surface to reveal thrombosed capillaries. Flat warts (*verruca plana*) are most common among children and occur on the face, neck, chest, and flexor surfaces of the forearms and legs.

Anogenital warts develop on the skin and mucosal surfaces of external genitalia and perianal areas (Fig. 178-1). Among circumcised men, warts are most commonly found on the penile shaft. Lesions frequently occur at the urethral meatus and may extend proximally. Receptive anal intercourse predisposes both men and women to the development of perianal warts, but such lesions occasionally develop without such a history. In women, warts appear first at the posterior introitus and adjacent labia. They then spread to other parts of the vulva and commonly involve the vagina and cervix. In both sexes, external warts suggest the presence of internal lesions; however, internal lesions may be present without external warts, particularly in women. The differential diagnosis of anogenital warts includes condylomata lata of secondary syphilis, molluscum contagiosum, hirsutoid papillomatosis (pearly penile papules), fibroepitheliomas, and a variety of benign and malignant mucocutaneous neoplasms. Respiratory papillomatosis in young children, which may be life-threatening, presents as hoarseness, stridor, or respiratory distress. The disease in adults is usually milder.

Immunosuppressed patients, particularly those undergoing organ transplantation, often develop pityriasis versicolor–like lesions, from which DNA of several HPV types has been extracted. Occasionally, such lesions appear to undergo malignant transformation. Patients infected with HIV are often infected with uncommon HPV types, frequently have severe clinical manifestations of HPV infection, and are at high risk for cervical and anal dysplasia as well as for invasive cancer. HPV disease in patients with HIV infection may be associated with multiple HPV types, is difficult to treat, and often recurs (Chap. 182).

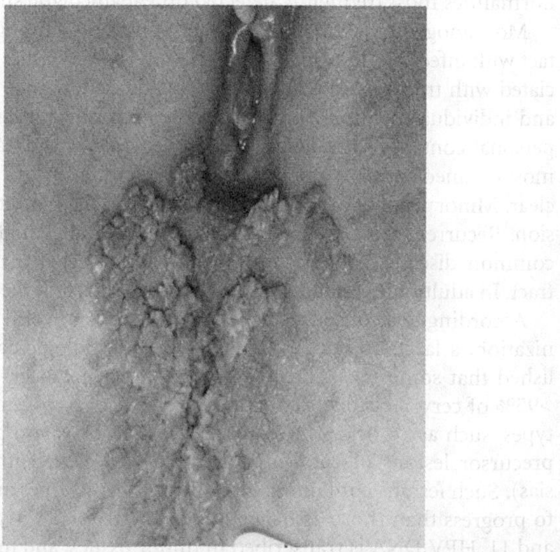

FIGURE 178-1 Anogenital warts are lesions produced by human papillomavirus and in this patient are seen as multiple verrucous papules coalescing into plaques.

Epidermodysplasia verruciformis is a rare autosomal recessive disease characterized by an inability to control HPV infection. Patients are often infected with unique HPV types (i.e., types that affect only this group) and frequently develop cutaneous squamous cell malignancies, particularly in sun-exposed areas. The lesions resemble flat warts or macules similar to those of pityriasis versicolor.

The complications of warts include itching and occasionally bleeding. In rare cases, warts become secondarily infected with bacteria or fungi. Large masses of warts may cause mechanical problems, such as obstruction of the birth canal or the urinary tract. Dysplasias of the uterine cervix are generally asymptomatic until frank carcinoma develops. Patients with anogenital HPV disease may develop serious psychological symptoms due to anxiety and depression over this condition.

PATHOGENESIS

The incubation period of HPV disease is usually 3–4 months (range, 1 month to 2 years). All types of squamous epithelium can be infected by HPV, and the gross and histologic appearances of individual lesions vary with the site of infection and the type of virus. The replication of HPV begins with the infection of basal cells. As cellular differentiation proceeds, HPV DNA replicates and is transcribed. Ultimately, virions are assembled in the nucleus and released when keratinocytes are shed. This process is associated with proliferation of all epidermal layers except the basal layer and produces acanthosis, parakeratosis, and hyperkeratosis. Koilocytes—large round cells with pyknotic nuclei—appear in the granular layer. Histologically normal epithelium may contain HPV DNA, and residual DNA after treatment can be associated with recurrent disease.

Episomal HPV DNA is present in the nuclei of infected cells in benign lesions caused by HPV. However, in severe dysplasias and cancers, HPV DNA is generally integrated, with disruption of the E1/E2 open reading frames. This disruption leads to upregulation of E6 and E7 and subsequent interference with cellular tumor-suppressor proteins. Expression of E6 and E7 proteins of oncogenic HPV types is necessary for the development and maintenance of the transformed state in both cervical cancers and cell lines derived from these tumors.

Host defense responses to HPV infection remain incompletely understood. However, several studies of recently developed HPV vaccines have demonstrated that production of high titers of type-specific neutralizing antibodies by vaccinated individuals is associated with type-specific protection from HPV infection and disease. Because patients with defects in cell-mediated immune responses (including transplant recipients and patients with HIV infection) frequently develop severe HPV disease, such responses are probably important for the control of established virus replication and disease. Histologic studies demonstrating an epidermal lymphomonocytic infiltrate in resolving warts suggest that local immunity may be of particular importance in the resolution of disease. HPV infection also elicits a detectable serologic response in many patients. Using HPV virus-like particles (VLPs) as antigens, type-specific antibodies can be found in sera of about two-thirds of patients with anogenital infection. Antibodies to E-region proteins, most notably E7, have been detected among patients with cervical carcinoma.

DIAGNOSIS

Most warts that are visible to the naked eye can be diagnosed correctly by history and physical examination alone. The use of a colposcope is invaluable in assessing vaginal and cervical lesions and is helpful in the diagnosis of oral and cutaneous HPV disease as well. Application of 3–5% solutions of acetic acid may aid in the visualization of lesions, although the sensitivity and specificity of this procedure are unknown. Papanicolaou smears prepared from cervical or anal scrapings often show cytologic evidence of HPV infection. Persistent or atypical lesions should be biopsied and examined by routine histologic methods. The most sensitive and specific methods of virologic diagnosis use techniques such as the polymerase chain reaction or the hybrid capture assay to detect HPV nucleic acids and to identify specific virus types. Such tests may be useful in the diagnosis and management of cervical HPV disease, although their utility may vary according to the preva-

TABLE 178-1 TREATMENT OF EXTERNAL, EXOPHYTIC ANOGENITAL WARTS

I. Administered by provider
  A. Cryotherapy with liquid nitrogen or cryoprobe weekly
  B. Podophyllin resin, 10–25% weekly for up to 4 weeks
  C. Trichloroacetic acid or bichloroacetic acid, 80–90% weekly
  D. Surgical excision
  E. Other regimens
    1. Intralesionally administered interferon
    2. Laser surgery
II. Administered by patient
  A. Podofilox, 0.5% solution or gel twice daily for 3 days, followed by 4 days without therapy. This cycle may be repeated four times.
  B. Imiquimod, 5% cream 3 times per week for up to 16 weeks

Source: Modified from Centers for Disease Control and Prevention: MMWR 55(RR-11):1, 2006 (*www.cdc.gov/mmwr/preview/mmwrhtml/rr5511a1/htm*).

lence of disease and the availability of traditional cytologic and histologic testing. Serologic techniques to diagnose HPV infection are not helpful in individual cases and are not widely available.

℞ HUMAN PAPILLOMAVIRUS INFECTIONS

(Table 178-1) Decisions regarding the initiation of therapy should be made with the recognition that currently available modes of treatment are not completely effective and some have significant side effects. In addition, treatment may be expensive, and many HPV lesions resolve spontaneously. Frequently used therapies include cryosurgery, application of caustic agents, electrodesiccation, surgical excision, and ablation with a laser. Topical antimetabolites such as 5-fluorouracil have also been used. Both failure and recurrence have been well documented with all of these methods of treatment. Cryosurgery is the initial treatment of choice for condyloma acuminatum. Topically applied podophyllum preparations as well as podofilox may also be used. Various interferon preparations have been employed with modest success in the treatment of respiratory papillomatosis and condyloma acuminatum. A topically applied interferon inducer, imiquimod, is also of benefit in the treatment of condyloma acuminatum. The diagnosis and management of anogenital dysplasias and of internal anogenital warts require special skills and resources, and patients with such lesions should be referred to a qualified specialist.

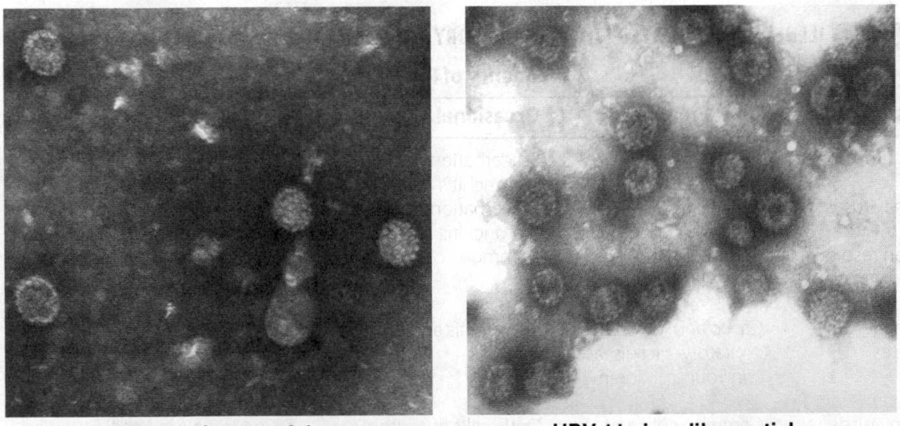

FIGURE 178-2 HPV-11 virus-like particles produced in insect cells (***right***) are morphologically and antigenically indistinguishable from wild-type HPV-11 particles (***left***). *(Images courtesy of Drs. William Bonnez and Robert C. Rose; with permission.)*

PREVENTION

Recently developed HPV VLP vaccines dramatically reduce rates of infection and disease produced by the HPV types in the vaccines. These products are directed against virus types that cause anogenital tract disease and are derived from expression of the major capsid protein (L1) gene in tissue culture. When expressed using appropriate vectors and tissue culture systems, L1 self-assembles into a VLP that cannot be distinguished morphologically or antigenically from its wild-type counterpart (Fig. 178-2) but that contains no viral nucleic acid. Currently, one quadrivalent product (Gardasil, Merck) containing HPV types 6, 11, 16, and 18 has been licensed in the United States and recommended by the Centers for Disease Control and Prevention for administration to girls and young women 9–26 years of age. Another product (Cervarix, GlaxoSmithKline) contains HPV types 16 and 18 and is likely to be available in the near future. HPV types 6 and 11 cause 90% of anogenital warts, whereas types 16 and 18 are responsible for 70% of cervical cancers. Because 30% of cervical cancers are caused by HPV types not contained in the vaccines, no changes in cervical cancer screening programs are currently recommended. Barrier methods of contraception may also be helpful in preventing transmission of condyloma acuminatum and other anogenital HPV-associated diseases.

FURTHER READINGS

BONNEZ W, REICHMAN RC: Papillomaviruses, in *Principles and Practice of Infectious Diseases*, 6th ed, GL Mandell et al (eds). Churchill Livingstone, New York, 2005, pp 1841–1856

CENTERS FOR DISEASE CONTROL AND PREVENTION: Sexually transmitted diseases treatment guidelines, 2006. MMWR 55(RR-11):1, 2006 (*www.cdc.gov/mmwr/preview/mmwrhtml/rr5511a1.htm*)

HARPER DM et al: Sustained efficacy up to 4.5 years of a bivalent L1 virus-like particle vaccine against human papillomavirus types 16 and 18: Follow-up from a randomised control trial. Lancet 367:1247, 2006

LUQUE AE et al: Prevalence of human papillomavirus (HPV) genotypes and relation to cervical cytology among HIV-1 infected women in Rochester, New York. J Infect Dis 194:428, 2006

VILLA LL et al: High sustained efficacy of a prophylactic quadrivalent human papillomavirus types 6/11/16/18 L1 virus-like particle vaccine through 5 years of follow-up. Br J Cancer 11:1459, 2006

179 Common Viral Respiratory Infections and Severe Acute Respiratory Syndrome (SARS)

Raphael Dolin

GENERAL CONSIDERATIONS

Acute viral respiratory illnesses are among the most common of human diseases, accounting for one-half or more of all acute illnesses. The incidence of acute respiratory disease in the United States is 3–5.6 cases per person per year. The rates are highest among children <1 year old (6.1–8.3 cases per year) and remain high until age 6, when a progressive decrease begins. Adults have 3–4 cases per person per year. Morbidity from acute respiratory illnesses accounts for 30–50% of time lost from work by adults and for 60–80% of time lost from school by children. The use of antibacterial agents to treat viral respiratory infections represents a major source of abuse of that category of drugs.

It has been estimated that two-thirds to three-fourths of cases of acute respiratory illnesses are caused by viruses. More than 200 antigenically distinct viruses from 10 genera have been reported to cause acute respiratory illness, and it is likely that additional agents will be described in the future. The vast majority of these viral infections involve the upper respiratory tract, but lower respiratory tract disease can also develop, particularly in younger age groups, in the elderly, and in certain epidemiologic settings.

The illnesses caused by respiratory viruses traditionally have been divided into multiple distinct syndromes, such as the "common cold," pharyngitis, croup (laryngotracheobronchitis), tracheitis, bronchiolitis, bronchitis, and pneumonia. Each of these general categories of illness has a certain epidemiologic and clinical profile; for example, croup occurs exclusively in very young children and has a characteristic clinical course. Some types of respiratory illness are more likely to be associated with certain viruses (e.g., the common cold with rhinoviruses), while others occupy characteristic epidemiologic niches (e.g., adenovirus infections in military recruits). The syndromes most commonly associated with infections with the major respiratory virus groups are summarized in Table 179-1. Most respiratory viruses clearly have the potential to cause more than one type of respiratory illness, and features of several types of illness may be found in the same patient. Moreover, the clinical illnesses induced by these viruses are rarely sufficiently distinctive to permit an etiologic diagnosis on clinical grounds alone, although the epidemiologic setting increases the likelihood that one group of viruses rather than another is involved. In general, laboratory methods must be relied on to establish a specific viral diagnosis.

This chapter reviews viral infections caused by six of the major groups of respiratory viruses: rhinoviruses, coronaviruses, respiratory syncytial viruses, metapneumoviruses, parainfluenza viruses, and adenoviruses. The extraordinary outbreaks of lower respiratory tract disease associated with coronaviruses (severe acute respiratory syndrome, or SARS) in 2002–2003 are also discussed. **Influenza viruses, which are a major cause of death as well as morbidity, are reviewed in Chap. 180. Herpesviruses, which occasionally cause pharyngitis and which also cause lower respiratory tract disease in immunosuppressed patients, are reviewed in Chap. 172. Enteroviruses, which account for occasional respiratory illnesses during the summer months, are reviewed in Chap. 184.**

RHINOVIRUS INFECTIONS

ETIOLOGIC AGENT

Rhinoviruses are members of the Picornaviridae family, small (15–30 nm) nonenveloped viruses that contain a single-stranded RNA genome. In contrast to other members of the picornavirus family, such as enteroviruses, rhinoviruses are acid-labile and are almost completely inactivated at pH ≤ 3. Rhinoviruses grow preferentially at 33°–34°C (the temperature of the human nasal passages) rather than at 37°C (the temperature of the lower respiratory tract). Of the 102 recognized serotypes of rhinovirus, 91 use intercellular adhesion molecule 1 (ICAM-1) as a cellular receptor and constitute the "major" receptor group, 10 use the low-density lipoprotein receptor and constitute the "minor" receptor group, and 1 uses decay-accelerating factor.

EPIDEMIOLOGY

Rhinoviruses are a prominent cause of the common cold and have been detected in up to 50% of common cold–like illnesses by tissue culture and polymerase chain reaction (PCR) techniques. Overall rates of rhinovirus infection are higher among infants and young children

TABLE 179-1 ILLNESSES ASSOCIATED WITH RESPIRATORY VIRUSES

	Frequency of Respiratory Syndromes		
Virus	**Most Frequent**	**Occasional**	**Infrequent**
Rhinoviruses	Common cold	Exacerbation of chronic bronchitis and asthma	Pneumonia in children
Coronaviruses[a]	Common cold	Exacerbation of chronic bronchitis and asthma	Pneumonia and bronchiolitis
Human respiratory syncytial virus	Pneumonia and bronchiolitis in young children	Common cold in adults	Pneumonia in elderly and immunosuppressed patients
Parainfluenza viruses	Croup and lower respiratory tract disease in young children	Pharyngitis and common cold	Tracheobronchitis in adults; lower respiratory tract disease in immunosuppressed patients
Adenoviruses	Common cold and pharyngitis in children	Outbreaks of acute respiratory disease in military recruits[b]	Pneumonia in children; lower respiratory tract and disseminated disease in immunosuppressed patients
Influenza A viruses	Influenza[c]	Pneumonia and excess mortality in high-risk patients	Pneumonia in healthy individuals
Influenza B viruses	Influenza[c]	Rhinitis or pharyngitis alone	Pneumonia
Enteroviruses	Acute undifferentiated febrile illnesses[d]	Rhinitis or pharyngitis alone	Pneumonia
Herpes simplex viruses	Gingivostomatitis in children; pharyngotonsillitis in adults	Tracheitis and pneumonia in immunocompromised patients	Disseminated infection in immunocompromised patients
Human metapneumoviruses[e]	Lower respiratory tract disease in children	Upper respiratory tract illness in adults	Pneumonia in elderly and immunosuppressed patients

[a]SARS-associated coronavirus (SARS-CoV) caused epidemics of pneumonia from November 2002 to July 2003 (see text).
[b]Serotypes 4 and 7.
[c]Fever, cough, myalgia, malaise.
[d]May or may not have a respiratory component.
[e]Newly recognized human metapneumoviruses cause upper and lower respiratory tract illnesses; their relative frequency is under investigation.

and decrease with increasing age. Rhinovirus infections occur throughout the year, with seasonal peaks in early fall and spring in temperate climates. These infections are most often introduced into families by preschool or grade-school children <6 years old. Of initial illnesses in family settings, 25–70% are followed by secondary cases, with the highest attack rates among the youngest siblings at home. Attack rates also increase with family size.

Rhinoviruses appear to spread through direct contact with infected secretions, usually respiratory droplets. In some studies of volunteers, transmission was most efficient by hand-to-hand contact, with subsequent self-inoculation of the conjunctival or nasal mucosa. Other studies demonstrated transmission by large- or small-particle aerosol. Virus can be recovered from plastic surfaces inoculated 1–3 h previously; this observation suggests that environmental surfaces contribute to transmission. In studies of married couples in which neither partner had detectable serum antibody, transmission was associated with prolonged contact (≥122 h) during a 7-day period. Transmission was infrequent unless (1) virus was recoverable from the donor's hands and nasal mucosa, (2) at least 1000 $TCID_{50}$ of virus was present in nasal washes from the donor, and (3) the donor was at least moderately symptomatic with the "cold." Despite anecdotal observations, exposure to cold temperatures, fatigue, and sleep deprivation have not been associated with increased rates of rhinovirus-induced illness in volunteers, although some studies have suggested that psychologically defined "stress" may contribute to development of symptoms.

Infection with rhinoviruses is worldwide in distribution. By adulthood, nearly all individuals have neutralizing antibodies to multiple serotypes, although the prevalence of antibody to any one serotype varies widely. Multiple serotypes circulate simultaneously, and generally no single serotype or group of serotypes has been more prevalent than the others.

PATHOGENESIS

Rhinoviruses infect cells through attachment to specific cellular receptors; as mentioned above, most serotypes attach to ICAM-1, while a few use the low-density lipoprotein receptor. Relatively limited information is available on the histopathology and pathogenesis of acute rhinovirus infections in humans. Examination of biopsy specimens obtained during experimentally induced and naturally occurring illness indicates that the nasal mucosa is edematous, is often hyperemic, and—during acute illness—is covered by a mucoid discharge. There is a mild infiltrate with inflammatory cells, including neutrophils, lymphocytes, plasma cells, and eosinophils. Mucus-secreting glands in the submucosa appear hyperactive; the nasal turbinates are engorged, a condition that may lead to obstruction of nearby openings of sinus cavities. Several mediators—e.g., bradykinin; lysylbradykinin; prostaglandins; histamine; interleukins 1β, 6, and 8; and tumor necrosis factor α—have been linked to the development of signs and symptoms in rhinovirus-induced colds.

The incubation period for rhinovirus illness is short, generally 1–2 days. Virus shedding coincides with the onset of illness or may begin shortly before symptoms develop. The mechanisms of immunity to rhinovirus are not well worked out. In some studies, the presence of homotypic antibody has been associated with significantly reduced rates of subsequent infection and illness, but data conflict regarding the relative importance of serum and local antibody in protection from rhinovirus infection.

CLINICAL MANIFESTATIONS

The most common clinical manifestations of rhinovirus infections are those of the common cold. Illness usually begins with rhinorrhea and sneezing accompanied by nasal congestion. The throat is frequently sore, and in some cases sore throat is the initial complaint. Systemic signs and symptoms, such as malaise and headache, are mild or absent, and fever is unusual. Illness generally lasts for 4–9 days and resolves spontaneously without sequelae. In children, bronchitis, bronchiolitis, and bronchopneumonia have been reported; nevertheless, it appears that rhinoviruses are not major causes of lower respiratory tract disease in children. Rhinoviruses may cause exacerbations of asthma and chronic pulmonary disease in adults. The vast majority of rhinovirus infections resolve without sequelae, but complications related to obstruction of the eustachian tubes or sinus ostia, including otitis media or acute sinusitis, can develop. In immunosuppressed patients, particularly bone marrow transplant recipients, severe and even fatal pneumonias have been associated with rhinovirus infections.

DIAGNOSIS

Although rhinoviruses are the most frequently recognized cause of the common cold, similar illnesses are caused by a variety of other viruses, and a specific viral etiologic diagnosis cannot be made on clinical grounds alone. Rather, rhinovirus infection is diagnosed by isolation of the virus from nasal washes or nasal secretions in tissue culture. In practice, this procedure is rarely undertaken because of the benign, self-limited nature of the illness. In most settings, detection of rhinovirus RNA by PCR is more sensitive than that by tissue culture; however, PCR for rhinoviruses is largely a research procedure. Given the many serotypes of rhinovirus, diagnosis by serum antibody tests is currently impractical. Likewise, common laboratory tests, such as white blood cell count and erythrocyte sedimentation rate, are not helpful.

Rx RHINOVIRUS INFECTIONS

Because rhinovirus infections are generally mild and self-limited, treatment is not usually necessary. Therapy in the form of first-generation antihistamines and nonsteroidal anti-inflammatory drugs may be beneficial in patients with particularly pronounced symptoms, and an oral decongestant may be added if nasal obstruction is particularly troublesome. Reduction of activity is prudent in instances of significant discomfort or fatigability. Antibacterial agents should be used only if bacterial complications such as otitis media or sinusitis develop. Specific antiviral therapy is not available.

PREVENTION

Intranasal application of interferon sprays has been effective in the prophylaxis of rhinovirus infections but is also associated with local irritation of the nasal mucosa. Studies of the prevention of rhinovirus infection by administration of antibodies to ICAM-1 or by the soluble purified receptors themselves have yielded disappointing results. Experimental vaccines to certain rhinovirus serotypes have been generated, but their usefulness is questionable because of the myriad serotypes and the uncertainty about mechanisms of immunity. Thorough hand washing, environmental decontamination, and protection against autoinoculation may help to reduce rates of transmission of infection.

CORONAVIRUS INFECTIONS, INCLUDING SARS

ETIOLOGIC AGENT

Coronaviruses are pleomorphic, single-stranded RNA viruses that measure 100–160 nm in diameter. The name derives from the crownlike appearance produced by the club-shaped projections that stud the viral envelope. Coronaviruses infect a wide variety of animal species and have been divided into three antigenic groups. Previously recognized coronaviruses that infect humans fell into two of these groups (serogroups I and II), which include human isolates HCoV-229E and HCoV-OC43, respectively. The coronavirus associated with SARS (SARS-CoV) was first believed to represent a novel group but now is considered to be a distantly related member of group II (Fig. 179-1). To date, the SARS-CoV strains that have been fully sequenced have shown only minimal variation.

In general, human coronaviruses have been difficult to cultivate in vitro, and some strains grow only in human tracheal organ cultures rather than in tissue culture. SARS-CoV is an exception whose ready growth in African green monkey kidney (Vero E6) cells greatly facilitates its study.

EPIDEMIOLOGY

Generally, human coronavirus infections are present throughout the world. Seroprevalence studies of strains HCoV-229E and HCoV-OC43 have demonstrated that serum antibodies are acquired early in life and increase in prevalence with advancing age, so that >80% of adult populations have antibodies as measured by enzyme-linked immunosorbent assay (ELISA). Overall, coronaviruses account for

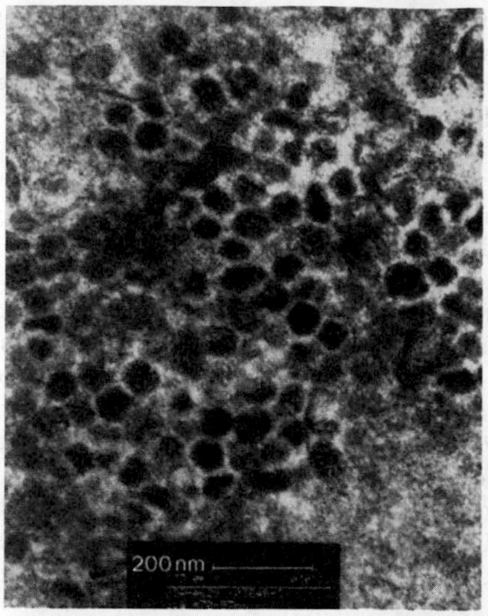

FIGURE 179-1 Electron micrograph of SARS-associated coronavirus (SARS-CoV) isolated in fetal rhesus kidney tissue culture from a lung biopsy sample from a patient with SARS. Viral particles are 55–90 mm in diameter. [*Reprinted with permission from Elsevier (JSM Peiris et al., Lancet 361:1319, 2003).*]

10–35% of common colds, depending on the season. Coronavirus infections appear to be particularly prevalent in late fall, winter, and early spring—times when rhinovirus infections are less common.

An extraordinary outbreak of the coronavirus-associated illness known as SARS occurred in 2002–2003. The outbreak apparently began in southern China and eventually resulted in 8096 recognized cases in 28 countries in Asia, Europe, and North and South America; ~90% of cases occurred in China and Hong Kong. The natural reservoir of SARS-CoV appears to be the horseshoe bat, and the outbreak may have originated from human contact with infected semidomesticated animals such as the palm civet. In most cases, however, the infection was transmitted from human to human. Case-fatality rates varied among the outbreaks, with an overall figure of ~9.5%. The disease appeared to be somewhat milder in cases in the United States and was clearly less severe among children. The outbreak ceased in 2003; 17 cases were detected in 2004, mostly in laboratory-associated settings, and no cases were reported in 2005–2006.

The mechanisms of transmission of SARS are incompletely understood. Clusters of cases suggest that spread may occur by both large and small aerosols and perhaps by the fecal-oral route as well. The outbreak of illness in a large apartment complex in Hong Kong suggested that environmental sources, such as sewage or water, may also play a role in transmission. Some ill individuals ("super-spreaders") appeared to be hyperinfectious and were capable of transmitting infection to 10–40 contacts, although most infections resulted in spread either to no one or to three or fewer individuals.

PATHOGENESIS

Coronaviruses that cause the common cold (e.g., strains HCoV-229E and HCoV-OC43) infect ciliated epithelial cells in the nasopharynx via the aminopeptidase N receptor (group I) or a sialic acid receptor (group II). Viral replication leads to damage of ciliated cells and induction of chemokines and interleukins, with consequent common-cold symptoms similar to those induced by rhinoviruses.

SARS-CoV infects cells of the respiratory tract via the angiotensin-converting enzyme 2 receptor. The result is a systemic illness in which virus is also found in the bloodstream, in the urine, and (for up to 2 months) in the stool. Virus persists in the respiratory tract for 2–3 weeks, and titers peak ~10 days after the onset of systemic illness. Pulmonary pathology consists of hyaline membrane formation, desquamation of pneumocytes in alveolar spaces, and an interstitial infiltrate made up of lymphocytes and mononuclear cells. Giant cells are frequently seen, and coronavirus particles have been detected in type II pneumocytes. Elevated levels of proinflammatory cytokines and chemokines have been detected in sera from patients with SARS.

CLINICAL MANIFESTATIONS

After an incubation period that generally lasts 2–7 days (range, 1–14 days), SARS usually begins as a systemic illness marked by the onset of fever, which is often accompanied by malaise, headache, and myalgias and is followed in 1–2 days by a nonproductive cough and dyspnea. Approximately 25% of patients have diarrhea. Chest x-rays can show a variety of infiltrates, including patchy areas of consolidation—most frequently in peripheral and lower lung fields—or interstitial infiltrates, which can progress to diffuse involvement (Fig. 179-2).

In severe cases, respiratory function may worsen during the second week of illness and progress to frank adult respiratory distress syndrome (ARDS) accompanied by multiorgan dysfunction. Risk factors for severe disease include an age of >50 years and comorbidities such as cardiovascular disease, diabetes, or hepatitis. Illness in pregnant women may be particularly severe, but SARS-CoV infection appears to be milder in children than in adults.

The clinical features of common colds caused by human coronaviruses are similar to those of illness caused by rhinoviruses. In studies of volunteers, the mean incubation period of colds induced by coronaviruses (3 days) is somewhat longer than that of illness caused by rhinoviruses, and the duration of illness is somewhat shorter (mean, 6–7 days). In some studies, the amount of nasal discharge was greater in colds induced by coronaviruses than in those induced by rhinoviruses. Coronaviruses other than SARS-CoV have been recovered occasionally from infants with pneumonia and from military recruits with lower respiratory tract disease and have been associated with worsening of chronic bronchitis. Two novel coronaviruses, HCoV-NL63 (group I) and HCoV-HKU1 (group II), have recently been isolated from patients hospitalized with acute respiratory illness. Their role as causes of human respiratory disease remains to be determined.

LABORATORY FINDINGS AND DIAGNOSIS

Laboratory abnormalities in SARS include lymphopenia, which is present in ~50% of cases and which mostly affects CD4+ T cells but also involves CD8+ T cells and NK cells. Total white blood cell counts

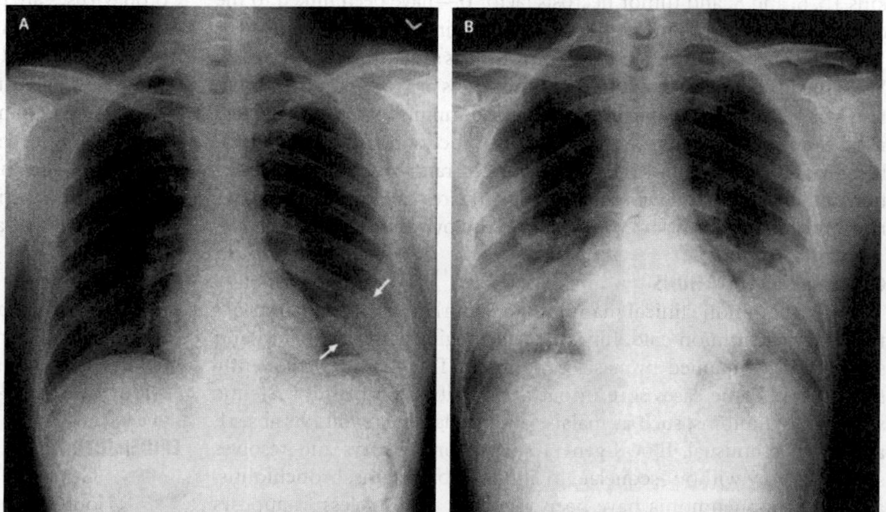

FIGURE 179-2 Chest x-rays of a 46-year-old man with SARS. The left lower lung infiltrate seen initially (***A***) progressed to multiple bilateral opacities (***B***). (*Reprinted with permission from N Lee et al. © 2003 Massachusetts Medical Society.*)

are normal or slightly low, and thrombocytopenia may develop as the illness progresses. Elevated serum levels of aminotransferases, creatine kinase, and lactate dehydrogenase have been reported.

A rapid diagnosis of SARS-CoV infection can be made by reverse-transcriptase PCR (RT-PCR) of respiratory tract samples and plasma early in illness and of urine and stool later on. SARS-CoV can also be grown from respiratory tract samples by inoculation into Vero E6 tissue culture cells, in which a cytopathic effect is seen within days. RT-PCR appears to be more sensitive than tissue culture, but only around one-third of cases are positive by PCR at initial presentation. Serum antibodies can be detected by ELISA or immunofluorescence, and nearly all patients develop detectable serum antibodies within 28 days after the onset of illness.

Laboratory diagnosis of coronavirus-induced colds is rarely required. Coronaviruses that cause those illnesses are frequently difficult to cultivate in vitro but can be detected in clinical samples by ELISA or immunofluorescence assays or by RT-PCR for viral RNA. These research procedures can be used to detect coronaviruses in unusual clinical settings.

Rx CORONAVIRUS INFECTIONS

There is no specific therapy of established efficacy for SARS. Although ribavirin has frequently been used, it has little if any activity against SARS-CoV in vitro, and no beneficial effect on the course of illness has been demonstrated. Because of suggestions that immunopathology may contribute to the disease, glucocorticoids have also been widely used, but their benefit, if any, is likewise unestablished. Supportive care to maintain pulmonary and other organ system functions remains the mainstay of therapy.

The approach to the treatment of common colds caused by coronaviruses is similar to that discussed above for rhinovirus-induced illnesses.

PREVENTION

The recognition of SARS led to a worldwide mobilization of public health resources to apply infection-control practices to contain the disease. Case definitions were established, travel advisories were proposed, and quarantines were imposed in certain locales. As of this writing, no additional cases of SARS have been reported since 2004. However, it remains unknown whether the disappearance of cases is a result of control measures, whether it is part of a seasonal or otherwise unexplained epidemiologic pattern of SARS, or when or whether SARS might reemerge. The U.S. Centers for Disease Control and Prevention and the World Health Organization maintain recommendations for surveillance and assessment of potential cases of SARS (*www.cdc.gov/ncidod/sars/*). The frequent transmission of the disease to health care workers makes it mandatory that strict infection-control practices be employed by health care facilities to prevent airborne, droplet, and contact transmission from any suspected cases of SARS. Health care workers who enter areas in which patients with SARS may be present should don gowns, gloves, and eye and respiratory protective equipment (e.g., an N95 filtering facepiece respirator certified by the National Institute for Occupational Safety and Health).

Vaccines have been developed against several animal coronaviruses but not against known human coronaviruses. The emergence of SARS-CoV has stimulated interest in the development of vaccines against such agents.

HUMAN RESPIRATORY SYNCYTIAL VIRUS INFECTIONS

ETIOLOGIC AGENT

Human respiratory syncytial virus, previously referred to as RSV and now designated HRSV, is a member of the Paramyxoviridae family (genus *Pneumovirus*). HRSV, an enveloped virus ~150–350 nm in diameter, is so named because its replication in vitro leads to the fusion of neighboring cells into large multinucleated syncytia. The single-stranded RNA genome codes for 11 virus-specific proteins. Viral RNA is contained in a helical nucleocapsid surrounded by a lipid envelope bearing two glycoproteins: the G protein, by which the virus attaches to cells, and the F (fusion) protein, which facilitates entry of the virus into the cell by fusing host and viral membranes. HRSV was once considered to be of a single antigenic type, but two distinct subgroups (A and B) and multiple subtypes within each subgroup have now been described. Antigenic diversity is reflected by differences in the G protein, while the F protein is highly conserved. Both antigenic groups can circulate simultaneously in outbreaks, although there are typically alternating patterns in which one subgroup predominates over 1- to 2-year periods. Infections with group B viruses may be somewhat milder than those with group A viruses.

EPIDEMIOLOGY

HRSV is a major respiratory pathogen of young children and the foremost cause of lower respiratory disease in infants. Infection with HRSV is seen throughout the world in annual epidemics that occur in late fall, winter, or spring and last up to 5 months. The virus is rarely encountered during the summer. Rates of illness are highest among infants 1–6 months of age, peaking at 2–3 months of age. The attack rates among susceptible infants and children are extraordinarily high, approaching 100% in settings such as day-care centers where large numbers of susceptible infants are present. By age 2, virtually all children will have been infected with HRSV. HRSV accounts for 20–25% of hospital admissions of young infants and children for pneumonia and for up to 75% of cases of bronchiolitis in this age group. It has been estimated that more than half of infants who are at risk will become infected during an HRSV epidemic.

In older children and adults, reinfection with HRSV is frequent but disease is milder than in infancy. A common cold–like syndrome is the illness most commonly associated with HRSV infection in adults. Severe lower respiratory tract disease with pneumonitis can occur in elderly (often institutionalized) adults and in patients with immunocompromising disorders or treatment, including recipients of stem cell and solid-organ transplants. HRSV is also an important nosocomial pathogen; during an outbreak, it can infect pediatric patients and up to 25–50% of the staff on pediatric wards. The spread of HRSV among families is efficient: up to 40% of siblings may become infected when the virus is introduced into the family setting.

HRSV is transmitted primarily by close contact with contaminated fingers or fomites and by self-inoculation of the conjunctiva or anterior nares. Virus may also be spread by coarse aerosols produced by coughing or sneezing, but it is inefficiently spread by fine-particle aerosols. The incubation period is ~4–6 days, and virus shedding may last for ≥2 weeks in children and for shorter periods in adults. In immunosuppressed patients, shedding can continue for weeks.

PATHOGENESIS

Little is known about the histopathology of minor HRSV infection. Severe bronchiolitis or pneumonia is characterized by necrosis of the bronchiolar epithelium and a peribronchiolar infiltrate of lymphocytes and mononuclear cells. Interalveolar thickening and filling of alveolar spaces with fluid can also be found. The correlates of protective immunity to HRSV are incompletely understood. Because reinfection occurs frequently and is often associated with illness, the immunity that develops after single episodes of infection clearly is not complete or long-lasting. However, the cumulative effect of multiple reinfections is to temper subsequent disease and to provide some temporary measure of protection against infection. Studies of experimentally induced disease in healthy volunteers indicate that the presence of nasal IgA neutralizing antibody correlates more closely with protection than does the presence of serum antibody. Studies in infants, however, suggest that maternally acquired antibody provides some protection from lower respiratory tract disease, although illness can be severe even in infants who have moderate levels of maternally derived serum antibody. The relatively severe disease observed in immunosuppressed patients and experimental animal models indicates that cell-mediated immunity is an important mechanism of host defense against HRSV. Evidence suggests that class I MHC-restricted cytotoxic T cells may be particularly important in this regard.

CLINICAL MANIFESTATIONS

HRSV infection leads to a wide spectrum of respiratory illnesses. In infants, 25–40% of infections result in lower respiratory tract involvement, including pneumonia, bronchiolitis, and tracheobronchitis. In this age group, illness begins most frequently with rhinorrhea, low-grade fever, and mild systemic symptoms, often accompanied by cough and wheezing. Most patients recover gradually over 1–2 weeks. In more severe illness, tachypnea and dyspnea develop, and eventually frank hypoxia, cyanosis, and apnea can ensue. Physical examination may reveal diffuse wheezing, rhonchi, and rales. Chest radiography shows hyperexpansion, peribronchial thickening, and variable infiltrates ranging from diffuse interstitial infiltrates to segmental or lobar consolidation. Illness may be particularly severe in children born prematurely and in those with congenital cardiac disease, bronchopulmonary dysplasia, nephrotic syndrome, or immunosuppression. One study documented a 37% mortality rate among infants with HRSV pneumonia and congenital cardiac disease.

In adults, the most common symptoms of HRSV infection are those of the common cold, with rhinorrhea, sore throat, and cough. Illness is occasionally associated with moderate systemic symptoms such as malaise, headache, and fever. HRSV has also been reported to cause lower respiratory tract disease with fever in adults, including severe pneumonia in the elderly—particularly in nursing-home residents, among whom its impact can rival that of influenza. HRSV pneumonia can be a significant cause of morbidity and death among patients undergoing stem cell and solid-organ transplantation, where case-fatality rates of 20–80% have been reported. Sinusitis, otitis media, and worsening of chronic obstructive and reactive airway disease have also been associated with HRSV infection.

LABORATORY FINDINGS AND DIAGNOSIS

The diagnosis of HRSV infection can be suspected on the basis of a suggestive epidemiologic setting—that is, severe illness among infants during an outbreak of HRSV in the community. Infections in older children and adults cannot be differentiated with certainty from those caused by other respiratory viruses. The specific diagnosis is established by detection of HRSV in respiratory secretions, such as sputum, throat swabs, or nasopharyngeal washes. Virus can be isolated in tissue culture and is identified specifically by immunofluorescence, ELISA, or other immunologic techniques. Rapid viral diagnosis is available by immunofluorescence techniques or ELISA of nasopharyngeal washes, aspirates, and (less satisfactorily) nasopharyngeal swabs. With specimens from children, these techniques have sensitivities and specificities of 80–95%; they are somewhat less sensitive with specimens from adults. Serologic diagnosis may be made by comparison of acute- and convalescent-phase serum specimens by ELISA or by neutralization or complement-fixation tests. These tests may be useful in older children and adults but are less sensitive in children <4 months of age.

℞ HUMAN RESPIRATORY SYNCYTIAL VIRUS INFECTIONS

Treatment of upper respiratory tract HRSV infection is aimed primarily at the alleviation of symptoms and is similar to that for other viral infections of the upper respiratory tract. For lower respiratory tract infections, respiratory therapy, including hydration, suctioning of secretions, and administration of humidified oxygen and antibronchospastic agents, is given as needed. In severe hypoxia, intubation and ventilatory assistance may be required. Studies of infants with HRSV infection who were given aerosolized ribavirin, a nucleoside analogue active in vitro against HRSV, demonstrated a modest beneficial effect on the resolution of lower respiratory tract illness, including alleviation of blood-gas abnormalities. The American Academy of Pediatrics recommends that treatment with aerosolized ribavirin "may be considered" for infants who are severely ill or who are at high risk for complications of HRSV infection; included are premature infants and those with bronchopulmonary dysplasia, congenital heart disease, or immunosuppression. The efficacy of ribavirin against HRSV pneumonia in older children and adults, including those with immunosuppression, has not been established. Administration of standard immunoglobulin, immunoglobulin with high titers of antibody to HRSV (RSVIg), or chimeric mouse-human monoclonal IgG antibody to HRSV (palivizumab) has not been found to be beneficial in the treatment of HRSV pneumonia. Combined therapy with aerosolized ribavirin and palivizumab is being evaluated in immunosuppressed patients with HRSV pneumonia.

PREVENTION

Monthly administration of RSVIg or palivizumab has been approved as prophylaxis against HRSV for children <2 years of age who have bronchopulmonary dysplasia or cyanotic heart disease or who were born prematurely. Considerable interest exists in the development of vaccines against HRSV. Inactivated whole-virus vaccines have been ineffective; in one study, they actually potentiated disease in infants. Other approaches include immunization with purified F and G surface glycoproteins of HRSV or generation of stable, live attenuated virus vaccines. In settings such as pediatric wards where rates of transmission are high, barrier methods for the protection of hands and conjunctivae may be useful in reducing the spread of virus.

HUMAN METAPNEUMOVIRUS INFECTIONS

ETIOLOGIC AGENT

Human metapneumovirus (HMPV) is a recently described viral respiratory pathogen that has been assigned to the Paramyxoviridae family (genus *Metapneumovirus*). Its morphology and genomic organization are similar to those of avian metapneumoviruses, which are recognized respiratory pathogens of turkeys. HMPV particles may be spherical, filamentous, or pleomorphic in shape and measure 150–600 nm in diameter. Particles contain 15-nm projections from the surface that are similar in appearance to those of other Paramyxoviridae. The single-stranded RNA genome codes for nine proteins that, except for the absence of nonstructural proteins, generally correspond to those of HRSV. There is only one antigenic type; two closely related genetic subgroups (A and B) have been described.

EPIDEMIOLOGY

HMPV infections are worldwide in distribution, are most frequent during the winter, and occur early in life, so that serum antibodies to the virus are present in nearly all children by the age of 5. HMPV infections have been detected in older age groups, including elderly adults, and in both immunocompetent and immunosuppressed hosts. To date, studies indicate that HMPV infections account for 4% of respiratory tract illnesses requiring hospitalization of children, 12% of outpatient lower respiratory illnesses, and 2–4% of acute respiratory illnesses in ambulatory adults and elderly patients. HMPV has been detected in a few cases of SARS, but its role (if any) in these illnesses has not been established. Assessment of the overall significance of HMPV infections awaits the conduct of large-scale epidemiologic studies.

CLINICAL MANIFESTATIONS

The spectrum of clinical illnesses associated with HMPV is similar to that associated with HRSV and includes both upper and lower respiratory tract illnesses, such as bronchiolitis, croup, and pneumonia. Reinfection with HMPV is common in older children and adults and has manifestations ranging from subclinical infections to common cold syndromes and occasionally pneumonia, which is seen primarily in elderly patients and those with cardiopulmonary diseases. Serious HMPV infections occur in immunocompromised patients, including those with neoplasia and stem cell transplants.

DIAGNOSIS

HMPV can be detected in nasal aspirates and respiratory secretions by PCR or by growth in rhesus monkey kidney (LLC-MK2) tissue cultures. Rapid immunodetection methods are under development. A serologic diagnosis can be made by ELISA, which uses HMPV-infected tissue culture lysates as sources of antigens.

℞ HUMAN METAPNEUMOVIRUS INFECTIONS

Treatment for HMPV infections is primarily supportive and symptom-based. Ribavirin and RSVIg are both active against HMPV in vitro, but their efficacy in vivo is unknown.

PREVENTION

Vaccines against HMPV are in the early stages of development.

PARAINFLUENZA VIRUS INFECTIONS

ETIOLOGIC AGENT

Parainfluenza viruses belong to the Paramyxoviridae family (genera *Respirovirus* and *Rubulavirus*). They are 150–200 nm in diameter, are enveloped, and contain a single-stranded RNA genome. The envelope is studded with two glycoproteins: one possesses both hemagglutinin and neuraminidase activity, and the other contains fusion activity. The viral RNA genome is enclosed in a helical nucleocapsid and codes for six structural and several accessory proteins. There are four distinct serotypes of parainfluenza virus, all of which share certain antigens with other members of the Paramyxoviridae family, including mumps and Newcastle disease viruses.

EPIDEMIOLOGY

Parainfluenza viruses are distributed throughout the world; infection with type 4 (subtypes 4A and 4B) has been reported less widely, probably because type 4 is more difficult to grow in tissue culture. Infection is acquired in early childhood, so that by 5 years of age most children have antibodies to serotypes 1, 2, and 3. Types 1 and 2 cause epidemics during the fall, often occurring in an alternate-year pattern. Type 3 infection has been detected during all seasons of the year, but epidemics have occurred annually in the spring.

The contribution of parainfluenza infections to respiratory disease varies with both the location and the year. In studies conducted in the United States, parainfluenza virus infections have accounted for 4.3–22% of respiratory illnesses in children. In adults, parainfluenza infections are generally mild and account for <10% of respiratory illnesses. The major importance of parainfluenza viruses is as a cause of respiratory illness in young children, in whom they rank second only to HRSV as causes of lower respiratory tract illness. Parainfluenza virus type 1 is the most frequent cause of croup (laryngotracheobronchitis) in children, while serotype 2 causes similar, although generally less severe, disease. Type 3 is an important cause of bronchiolitis and pneumonia in infants, while illnesses associated with type 4 have generally been mild. Unlike types 1 and 2, type 3 frequently causes illness during the first month of life, when passively acquired maternal antibody is still present. Parainfluenza viruses are spread through infected respiratory secretions, primarily by person-to-person contact and/or by large droplets. The incubation period has varied from 3 to 6 days in experimental infections but may be somewhat shorter for naturally occurring disease in children.

PATHOGENESIS

Immunity to parainfluenza viruses is incompletely understood, but evidence suggests that immunity to infections with serotypes 1 and 2 is mediated by local IgA antibodies in the respiratory tract. Passively acquired serum neutralizing antibodies also confer some protection against infection with types 1, 2, and (to a lesser degree) 3. Studies in experimental animal models and in immunosuppressed patients suggest that T cell–mediated immunity may also be important in parainfluenza virus infections.

CLINICAL MANIFESTATIONS

Parainfluenza virus infections occur most frequently among children, in whom initial infection with serotype 1, 2, or 3 is associated with an acute febrile illness 50–80% of the time. Children may present with coryza, sore throat, hoarseness, and cough that may or may not be croupy. In severe croup, fever persists, with worsening coryza and sore throat. A brassy or barking cough may progress to frank stridor. Most children recover over the next 1 or 2 days, although progressive airway obstruction and hypoxia ensue occasionally. If bronchiolitis or pneumonia develops, progressive cough accompanied by wheezing, tachypnea, and intercostal retractions may occur. In this setting, sputum production increases modestly. Physical examination shows nasopharyngeal discharge and oropharyngeal injection, along with rhonchi, wheezes, or coarse breath sounds. Chest x-rays can show air trapping and occasionally interstitial infiltrates.

In older children and adults, parainfluenza infections tend to be milder, presenting most frequently as a common cold or as hoarseness, with or without cough. Lower respiratory tract involvement in older children and adults is uncommon, but tracheobronchitis in adults has been reported. Severe, prolonged, and even fatal parainfluenza infection has been reported in children and adults with severe immunosuppression, including stem cell and solid-organ transplant recipients.

LABORATORY FINDINGS AND DIAGNOSIS

The clinical syndromes caused by parainfluenza viruses (with the possible exception of croup in young children) are not sufficiently distinctive to be diagnosed on clinical grounds alone. A specific diagnosis is established by detection of virus in respiratory tract secretions, throat swabs, or nasopharyngeal washings. Viral growth in tissue culture is detected either by hemagglutination or by a cytopathic effect. Rapid viral diagnosis may be made by identification of parainfluenza antigens in exfoliated cells from the respiratory tract with immunofluorescence or ELISA, although these techniques appear to be less sensitive than tissue culture. Highly specific and sensitive PCR assays have also been developed. Serologic diagnosis can be established by hemagglutination inhibition, complement-fixation, or neutralization tests of acute- and convalescent-phase specimens. However, since frequent heterotypic responses occur among the parainfluenza serotypes, the serotype causing illness often cannot be identified by serologic techniques alone.

Acute epiglottitis caused by *Haemophilus influenzae* type b must be differentiated from viral croup. Influenza A virus is also a common cause of croup during epidemic periods.

Rx PARAINFLUENZA VIRUS INFECTIONS

For upper respiratory tract illness, symptoms can be treated as discussed for other viral respiratory tract illnesses. If complications such as sinusitis, otitis, or superimposed bacterial bronchitis develop, appropriate antibacterial antibiotics should be administered. Mild cases of croup should be treated with bed rest and moist air generated by vaporizers. More severe cases require hospitalization and close observation for the development of respiratory distress. If acute respiratory distress develops, humidified oxygen and intermittent racemic epinephrine are usually administered. Aerosolized or systemically administered glucocorticoids are beneficial; the latter have a more profound effect. No specific antiviral therapy is available, although ribavirin is active against parainfluenza viruses in vitro and anecdotal reports describe its use clinically, particularly in immunosuppressed patients.

PREVENTION

Vaccines against parainfluenza viruses are under development.

ADENOVIRUS INFECTIONS

ETIOLOGIC AGENT

Adenoviruses are complex DNA viruses that measure 70–80 nm in diameter. Human adenoviruses belong to the genus *Mastadenovirus*, which includes 51 serotypes. Adenoviruses have a characteristic morphology consisting of an icosahedral shell composed of 20 equilateral triangular faces and 12 vertices. The protein coat (capsid) consists of hexon subunits with group-specific and type-specific antigenic determinants and penton subunits at each vertex primarily containing group-specific antigens. A fiber with a knob at the end projects from each penton; this fiber contains type-specific and some group-specific antigens. Human adenoviruses have been divided into six subgenera (A through F) on the basis of the homology of DNA genomes and other properties. The adenovirus genome is a linear double-stranded DNA that codes for structural and nonstructural polypeptides. The replicative cycle of adenovirus may result either in lytic infection of cells or in the establishment of a latent infection (primarily involving lymphoid cells). Some adenovirus types can induce oncogenic transformation, and tumor formation has been observed in rodents; however, despite intensive investigation, adenoviruses have not been associated with tumors in humans.

EPIDEMIOLOGY

Adenovirus infections most frequently affect infants and children. Infections occur throughout the year but are most common from fall to spring. Adenoviruses account for ~10% of acute respiratory infections in children but for <2% of respiratory illnesses in civilian adults. Nearly 100% of adults have serum antibody to multiple serotypes—a finding indicating that infection is common in childhood. Types 1, 2, 3, and 5 are the most frequent isolates from children. Certain adenovirus serotypes—particularly 4 and 7 but also 3, 14, and 21—are associated with outbreaks of acute respiratory disease in military recruits in winter and spring. Adenovirus infection can be transmitted by inhalation of aerosolized virus, by inoculation of virus into conjunctival sacs, and probably by the fecal-oral route as well. Type-specific antibody generally develops after infection and is associated with protection, albeit incomplete, against infection with the same serotype.

CLINICAL MANIFESTATIONS

In children, adenoviruses cause a variety of clinical syndromes. The most common is an acute upper respiratory tract infection, with prominent rhinitis. On occasion, lower respiratory tract disease, including bronchiolitis and pneumonia, also develops. Adenoviruses, particularly types 3 and 7, cause pharyngoconjunctival fever, a characteristic acute febrile illness of children that occurs in outbreaks, most often in summer camps. The syndrome is marked by bilateral conjunctivitis in which the bulbar and palpebral conjunctivae have a granular appearance. Low-grade fever is frequently present for the first 3 to 5 days, and rhinitis, sore throat, and cervical adenopathy develop. The illness generally lasts for 1–2 weeks and resolves spontaneously. Febrile pharyngitis without conjunctivitis has also been associated with adenovirus infection. Adenoviruses have been isolated from cases of whooping cough with or without *Bordetella pertussis*; the significance of adenovirus in that disease is unknown.

In adults, the most frequently reported illness has been acute respiratory disease caused by adenovirus types 4 and 7 in military recruits. This illness is marked by a prominent sore throat and the gradual onset of fever, which often reaches 39°C (102.2°F) on the second or third day of illness. Cough is almost always present, and coryza and regional lymphadenopathy are frequently seen. Physical examination may show pharyngeal edema, injection, and tonsillar enlargement with little or no exudate. If pneumonia has developed, auscultation and x-ray of the chest may indicate areas of patchy infiltration.

Adenoviruses have been associated with a number of non–respiratory tract diseases, including acute diarrheal illness caused by types 40 and 41 in young children and hemorrhagic cystitis caused by types 11 and 21. Epidemic keratoconjunctivitis, caused most frequently by types 8, 19, and 37, has been associated with contaminated common sources such as ophthalmic solutions and roller towels. Adenoviruses have also been implicated in disseminated disease and pneumonia in immunosuppressed patients, including recipients of solid-organ or stem cell transplants. In stem cell transplant recipients, adenovirus infections have manifested as pneumonia, hepatitis, nephritis, colitis, encephalitis, and hemorrhagic cystitis. In solid-organ transplant recipients, adenovirus infection may involve the organ transplanted (e.g., hepatitis in liver transplants, nephritis in renal transplants) but can disseminate to other organs as well. In patients with AIDS, high-numbered and intermediate adenovirus serotypes have been isolated, usually in the setting of low CD4+ T cell counts, but their isolation often has not been clearly linked to disease manifestations. Adenovirus nucleic acids have been detected in myocardial cells from patients with "idiopathic" myocardiopathies, and adenoviruses have been suggested as causative agents in some cases.

LABORATORY FINDINGS AND DIAGNOSIS

Adenovirus infection should be suspected in the epidemiologic setting of acute respiratory disease in military recruits and in certain of the clinical syndromes (such as pharyngoconjunctival fever or epidemic keratoconjunctivitis) in which outbreaks of characteristic illnesses occur. In most cases, however, illnesses caused by adenovirus infection cannot be differentiated from those caused by a number of other viral respiratory agents and *Mycoplasma pneumoniae*. A definitive diagnosis of adenovirus infection is established by detection of the virus in tissue culture (as evidenced by cytopathic changes) and by specific identification with immunofluorescence or other immunologic techniques. Rapid viral diagnosis can be established by immunofluorescence or ELISA of nasopharyngeal aspirates, conjunctival or respiratory secretions, urine, or stool. Highly sensitive and specific PCR assays and nucleic acid hybridization are also available. Adenovirus types 40 and 41, which have been associated with diarrheal disease in children, require special tissue-culture cells for isolation, and these serotypes are most commonly detected by direct ELISA of stool. Serum antibody rises can be demonstrated by complement-fixation or neutralization tests, ELISA, radioimmunoassay, or (for those adenoviruses that hemagglutinate red cells) hemagglutination inhibition tests.

Rx ADENOVIRUS INFECTIONS

Only symptom-based treatment and supportive therapy are available for adenovirus infections, and clinically useful antiviral therapy has not been established. Ribavirin and cidofovir have activity in vitro against certain adenoviruses. Retrospective studies and anecdotes describe the use of these agents in disseminated adenovirus infections, but definitive efficacy data from controlled studies are not available.

PREVENTION

Live vaccines have been developed against adenovirus types 4 and 7 and have been used to control illness among military recruits. These vaccines consist of live, unattenuated virus administered in enteric-coated capsules. Infection of the gastrointestinal tract with types 4 and 7 does not cause disease but stimulates local and systemic antibodies that are protective against subsequent acute respiratory disease due to those serotypes. This vaccine has not been produced since 1999, and outbreaks of acute respiratory illness caused by adenovirus types 4 and 7 have emerged again among military recruits. Therefore, a program to redevelop type 4 and 7 vaccines is under way. Adenoviruses are also being studied as live-virus vectors for the delivery of vaccine antigens and for gene therapy.

FURTHER READINGS

American Academy of Pediatrics: Diagnosis and management of bronchiolitis. Pediatrics 118:1774, 2006

Chanock RM et al: Serious respiratory tract disease caused by respiratory syncytial virus: Prospects for improved therapy and effective immunization. Pediatrics 90:137, 1992

Christian MD et al: Severe acute respiratory syndrome. Clin Infect Dis 38:1420, 2004

Graham BS et al: Respiratory syncytial virus immunobiology and pathogenesis. Virology 297:1, 2002

Gwaltney JM: Rhinoviruses, in *Principles and Practice of Infectious Diseases*, 6th ed, GF Mandell et al (eds). Philadelphia, Elsevier, 2005, pp 2185–2193

Lee N et al: A major outbreak of severe acute respiratory syndrome in Hong Kong. N Engl J Med 348:1986, 2003

Peiris JS et al: Severe acute respiratory syndrome. Nat Med 10:S88, 2004

Peret T et al: Characterization of human metapneumoviruses isolated from patients in North America. J Infect Dis 185:1660, 2002

Stockton J et al: Human metapneumovirus as a cause of community-acquired respiratory illness. Emerg Infect Dis 8:897, 2002

Wright PF: Parainfluenza viruses, in *Viral Infections of the Respiratory Tract*, R Dolin, PF Wright (eds). New York, Marcel Dekker, 1999

180 Influenza

Raphael Dolin

DEFINITION

Influenza is an acute respiratory illness caused by infection with influenza viruses. The illness affects the upper and/or lower respiratory tract and is often accompanied by systemic signs and symptoms such as fever, headache, myalgia, and weakness. Outbreaks of illness of variable extent and severity occur nearly every winter. Such outbreaks result in significant morbidity in the general population and in increased mortality rates among certain high-risk patients, mainly as a result of pulmonary complications.

ETIOLOGIC AGENT

Influenza viruses are members of the Orthomyxoviridae family, of which influenza A, B, and C viruses constitute three separate genera. The designation of influenza viruses as type A, B, or C is based on antigenic characteristics of the nucleoprotein (NP) and matrix (M) protein antigens. Influenza A viruses are further subdivided (subtyped) on the basis of the surface hemagglutinin (H) and neuraminidase (N) antigens (see below); individual strains are designated according to the site of origin, isolate number, year of isolation, and subtype—for example, influenza A/Hiroshima/52/2005 (H3N2). Influenza A has 16 distinct H subtypes and 9 distinct N subtypes, of which only H1, H2, H3, N1, and N2 have been associated with epidemics of disease in humans. Influenza B and C viruses are similarly designated, but H and N antigens from these viruses do not receive subtype designations, since intratypic variations in influenza B antigens are less extensive than those in influenza A viruses and may not occur with influenza C virus.

Influenza A and B viruses are major human pathogens and the most extensively studied of the Orthomyxoviridae. Type A and type B viruses are morphologically similar. The virions are irregularly shaped spherical particles, measure 80–120 nm in diameter, and have a lipid envelope from the surface of which the H and N glycoproteins project (Fig. 180-1). The hemagglutinin is the site by which the virus binds to sialic acid cell receptors, whereas the neuraminidase degrades the receptor and plays a role in the release of the virus from infected cells after replication has taken place. Influenza viruses enter cells by receptor-mediated endocytosis, forming a virus-containing endosome. The viral hemagglutinin mediates fusion of the endosomal membrane with the virus envelope, and viral nucleocapsids are subsequently released into the cytoplasm. Immune responses to the H antigen are the major determinants of protection against infection with influenza virus, while those to the N antigen limit viral spread and contribute to reduction of the infection. The lipid envelope of influenza A virus also contains the M proteins M1 and M2, which are involved in stabilization of the lipid envelope and in virus assembly. The virion also contains the NP antigen, which is associated with the viral genome, as well as three polymerase (P) proteins that are essential for transcription and synthesis of viral RNA. Two nonstructural proteins function as an interferon antagonist and posttranscriptional regulator (NS1) and a nuclear export factor (NS2 or NEP).

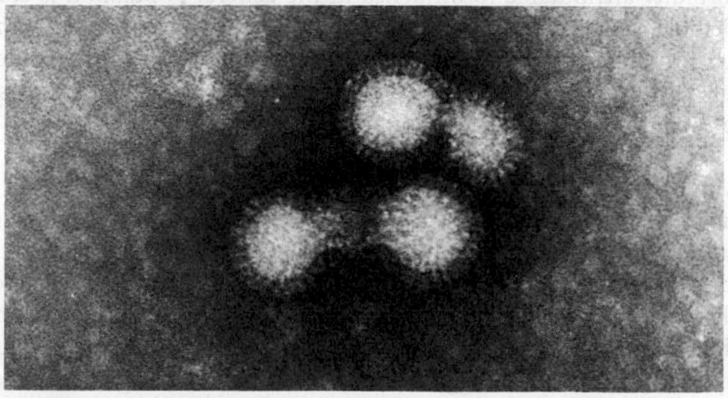

FIGURE 180-1 An electron micrograph of influenza A virus (× 40,000).

TABLE 180-1 EMERGENCE OF ANTIGENIC SUBTYPES OF INFLUENZA A VIRUS ASSOCIATED WITH PANDEMIC OR EPIDEMIC DISEASE

Years	Subtype	Extent of Outbreak
1889–90	H2N8[a]	Severe pandemic
1900–03	H3N8[a]	?Moderate epidemic
1918–19	H1N1[b] (formerly HswN1)	Severe pandemic
1933–35	H1N1[b] (formerly H0N1)	Mild epidemic
1946–47	H1N1	Mild epidemic
1957–58	H2N2	Severe pandemic
1968–69	H3N2	Moderate pandemic
1977–78[c]	H1N1	Mild pandemic

[a]As determined by retrospective serologic survey of individuals alive during those years ("seroarcheology").
[b]Hemagglutinins formerly designated as Hsw and H0 are now classified as variants of H1.
[c]From this time until the present (2006–2007), viruses of the H1N1 and H3N2 subtypes have circulated either in alternating years or concurrently.

The genomes of influenza A and B viruses consist of eight single-stranded RNA segments, which code for the structural and nonstructural proteins. Because the genome is segmented, the opportunity for gene reassortment during infection is high; reassortment often occurs during infection of cells with more than one influenza A virus.

EPIDEMIOLOGY

Influenza outbreaks are recorded virtually every year, although their extent and severity vary widely. Localized outbreaks take place at variable intervals, usually every 1–3 years. Global pandemics have occurred at variable intervals, but much less frequently than interpandemic outbreaks (Table 180-1). The most recent pandemic occurred in 1977—some 30 years ago as of this writing; because of this relatively long interval, concern exists that the next pandemic may be imminent.

Influenza A Virus • *ANTIGENIC VARIATION AND INFLUENZA OUTBREAKS*

The most extensive and severe outbreaks are caused by influenza A viruses, in part because of the remarkable propensity of the H and N antigens of these viruses to undergo periodic antigenic variation. Major antigenic variations, called *antigenic shifts*, may be associated with pandemics and are restricted to influenza A viruses. Minor variations are called *antigenic drifts*. These types of antigenic variation may involve the hemagglutinin alone or both the hemagglutinin and the neuraminidase. An example of an antigenic shift involving both the hemagglutinin and the neuraminidase is that of 1957, when the predominant influenza A virus subtype shifted from H1N1 to H2N2; this shift resulted in a severe pandemic, with an estimated 70,000 excess deaths (i.e., deaths in excess of the number expected without an influenza epidemic) in the United States alone. In 1968, an antigenic shift involving only the hemagglutinin occurred (H2N2 to H3N2); the subsequent pandemic was less severe than that of 1957. In 1977, an H1N1 virus emerged and caused a pandemic that primarily affected younger individuals (i.e., those born after 1957). As can be seen in Table 180-1, H1N1 viruses circulated from 1918 to 1956; thus, individuals born prior to 1957 would be expected to have some degree of immunity to H1N1 viruses. During most outbreaks of influenza A, a single subtype has circulated at a time. However, since 1977, H1N1 and H3N2 viruses have circulated simultaneously, resulting in outbreaks of varying severity. In some outbreaks, influenza B viruses have also circulated simultaneously with influenza A viruses.

AVIAN INFLUENZA In 1997, human cases of influenza caused by avian influenza viruses (A/H5N1) were detected in Hong Kong during an extensive outbreak of influenza in poultry. Between that time and January 2007, 261 cases of avian influenza in humans were reported in 10 countries in Asia and the Middle East. Nearly all of these cases were associated with contact with infected poultry. Efficient person-to-person transmission has not been observed to date. Mortality rates have been high (60%), and clinical manifestations have differed somewhat from those associated with "typical" outbreaks of influenza (see below). Transmission of avian influenza A/H7N7 viruses from infected poultry to humans has been observed in The Netherlands, resulting predominantly in cases of conjunctivitis and some respiratory illnesses. Infection with avian A/H9N2 viruses along with mild respiratory illness has been reported in children in Hong Kong. Because of the absence of widespread immunity to the H5, H7, and H9 viruses, concern has been raised that avian-to-human transmission may be the basis for the emergence of pandemic strains.

The origin of actual pandemic influenza A virus strains has now been partially elucidated with molecular virologic techniques. It appears that the pandemic strains of 1957 and 1968 resulted from a genetic reassortment between human viruses and avian viruses with novel surface glycoproteins (H2N2, H3). The influenza virus responsible for the most severe pandemic of modern times (1918–1919) appears to have represented an adaptation of an avian virus to efficient infection of humans. Close molecular surveillance of the avian viruses currently infecting humans is being conducted to provide early detection of possible pandemic strains.

FEATURES OF PANDEMIC AND INTERPANDEMIC INFLUENZA A Pandemics provide the most dramatic evidence of the impact of influenza A. However, illnesses occurring between pandemics (interpandemic disease) account for extensive mortality and morbidity, albeit over a longer period. In the United States, influenza was associated with at least 19,000 excess deaths per season in 1976–1990 and with 36,000 excess deaths per season in 1990–1999. On average, there were 226,000 influenza-associated hospitalizations per year in this country in 1979–2001.

Influenza A viruses that circulate between pandemics demonstrate antigenic drifts in the H antigen. These antigenic drifts result from point mutations involving the RNA segment that codes for the hemagglutinin, which occur most frequently in five hypervariable regions. Epidemiologically significant strains—that is, those with the potential to cause widespread outbreaks—exhibit changes in amino acids in at least two of the major antigenic sites in the hemagglutinin molecule. Since two point mutations are unlikely to occur simultaneously, it is believed that antigenic drifts result from point mutations occurring sequentially during the spread of virus from person to person. Antigenic drifts have been reported nearly annually since 1977 for H1N1 viruses and since 1968 for H3N2 viruses.

Influenza A epidemics begin abruptly, peak over a 2- to 3-week period, generally last for 2–3 months, and often subside almost as rapidly as they began. The first indication of influenza activity in a community is an increase in the number of children with febrile respiratory illnesses who present for medical attention. This increase is followed by increases in rates of influenza-like illnesses among adults and eventually by an increase in hospital admissions for patients with pneumonia, worsening of congestive heart failure, and exacerbations of chronic pulmonary disease. Rates of absence from work and school also rise at this time. An increase in the number of deaths caused by pneumonia and influenza is generally a late observation in an outbreak. Attack rates have been highly variable from outbreak to outbreak but most commonly are in the range of 10–20% of the general population. During the pandemic of 1957, it was estimated that the attack rate of clinical influenza exceeded 50% in urban populations and that an additional 25% or more of individuals in these populations may have been subclinically infected with influenza A virus. Among institutionalized populations and in semiclosed settings with many susceptible individuals, even higher attack rates have been reported.

Epidemics of influenza A occur almost exclusively during the winter months in the temperate zones of the northern and southern hemispheres. In those locations, it is highly unusual to detect influenza A virus at other times, although rises in serum antibody titer or even outbreaks have been noted rarely during warm-weather months. In contrast, influenza virus infections occur throughout the year in the tropics. Where or how influenza A virus persists between outbreaks in temperate zones is unknown. It is possible that influenza A viruses are maintained in the human population on a worldwide basis by person-to-person transmission and that large population clusters support a low level of interepidemic transmission. Alternatively, human strains may persist in animal reservoirs. Convincing evidence to support either explanation is not available. In the modern era, rapid transportation may contribute to the transmission of viruses among widespread geographic locales.

The factors that result in the inception and termination of outbreaks of influenza A are incompletely understood. A major determinant of the extent and severity of an outbreak is the level of immunity in the population at risk. With the emergence of an antigenically novel influenza virus to which little or no immunity is present in a community, extensive outbreaks may occur. When the absence of immunity is worldwide, epidemic disease may spread around the globe, resulting in a pandemic. Such pandemic waves can continue for several years, until immunity in the population reaches a high level. In the years following pandemic influenza, antigenic drifts among influenza viruses result in outbreaks of variable severity in populations with high levels of immunity to the pandemic strain that circulated earlier. This situation persists until another antigenically novel pandemic strain emerges. On the other hand, outbreaks sometimes end despite the persistence of a large pool of susceptible individuals in the population. It has been suggested that certain influenza A viruses, such as recently circulating A/H1N1 strains, may be intrinsically less virulent and cause less severe disease than other variants, even in immunologically virgin subjects. If so, then other (undefined) factors besides the level of preexisting immunity must play a role in the epidemiology of influenza.

Influenza B and C Viruses Influenza B virus causes outbreaks that are generally less extensive and are associated with less severe disease than those caused by influenza A virus. The hemagglutinin and neuraminidase of influenza B virus undergo less frequent and less extensive variation than those of influenza A viruses; this characteristic may account, in part, for the lesser extent of disease. Influenza B outbreaks are seen most frequently in schools and military camps, although outbreaks in institutions in which elderly individuals reside have also been noted on occasion. The most serious complication of influenza B virus infection is Reye's syndrome (Chap. 303).

In contrast to influenza A and B viruses, influenza C virus appears to be a relatively minor cause of disease in humans. It has been associated with common cold–like symptoms and occasionally with lower respiratory tract illness. Serum antibody to this virus is widely prevalent and indicates that asymptomatic infection may be common.

Influenza-Associated Morbidity and Mortality The morbidity and mortality caused by influenza outbreaks continue to be substantial. Most individuals who die in this setting have underlying diseases that place them at high risk for complications of influenza. Excess hospitalizations for groups of adults and children with high-risk medical conditions ranged from 56 to 1900 per 100,000 during outbreaks of influenza in 1973–1993. The most prominent high-risk conditions are chronic cardiac and pulmonary diseases and old age. Mortality rates among individuals with chronic metabolic or renal disease or certain immunosuppressive diseases have also been elevated, albeit lower than those among patients with chronic cardiopulmonary diseases. The morbidity attributable to influenza in the general population is considerable. It is estimated that interpandemic outbreaks of influenza currently incur annual costs of more than $12 billion in the United States. If a pandemic were to occur, it is estimated that annual costs would range from $71 to $167 billion for attack rates of 15–35%.

PATHOGENESIS AND IMMUNITY

The initial event in influenza is infection of the respiratory epithelium with influenza virus acquired from respiratory secretions of acutely infected individuals. In all likelihood, the virus is transmitted via aerosols generated by coughs and sneezes, although hand-to-hand contact, other personal contact, and even fomite transmission may take place. Experimental evidence suggests that infection by a small-particle aerosol (particle diameter, <10 μm) is more efficient than that by larger droplets. Initially, viral infection involves the ciliated columnar epithelial cells, but it may also involve other respiratory tract cells, including alveolar cells, mucous gland cells, and macrophages. In infected cells, virus replicates within 4–6 h, after which infectious virus is released to infect adjacent or nearby cells. In this way, infection spreads from a few foci to a large number of respiratory cells over several hours. In experimentally induced infection, the incubation period of illness has ranged from 18 to 72 h, depending on the size of the viral inoculum. Histopathologic study reveals degenerative changes, including granulation, vacuolization, swelling, and pyknotic nuclei, in infected ciliated cells. The cells eventually become necrotic and desquamate; in some areas, previously columnar epithelium is replaced by flattened and metaplastic epithelial cells. The severity of illness is correlated with the quantity of virus shed in secretions; thus, the degree of viral replication itself may be an important factor in pathogenesis. Despite the frequent development of systemic signs and symptoms such as fever, headache, and myalgias, influenza virus has only rarely been detected in extrapulmonary sites (including the bloodstream). Evidence suggests that the pathogenesis of systemic symptoms in influenza may be related to the induction of certain cytokines, particularly tumor necrosis factor α, interferon α, interleukin 6, and interleukin 8, in respiratory secretions and in the bloodstream.

The host response to influenza infections involves a complex interplay of humoral antibody, local antibody, cell-mediated immunity, interferon, and other host defenses. Serum antibody responses, which can be detected by the second week after primary infection, are measured by a variety of techniques: hemagglutination inhibition (HI), complement fixation (CF), neutralization, enzyme-linked immunosorbent assay (ELISA), and antineuraminidase antibody assay. Antibodies to the hemagglutinin appear to be the most important mediators of immunity; in several studies, HI titers of ≥40 have been associated with protection from infection. Secretory antibodies produced in the respiratory tract are predominantly of the IgA class and also play a major role in protection against infection. Secretory antibody neutralization titers of ≥ 4 have also been associated with protection. A variety of cell-mediated immune responses, both antigen-specific and antigen-nonspecific, can be detected early after infection and depend on the prior immune status of the host. These responses include T cell proliferative, T cell cytotoxic, and natural killer cell activity. In humans, CD8+ HLA class I–restricted cytotoxic T lymphocytes (CTLs) are directed at conserved regions of internal proteins (NP, M, and polymerases) as well as against the surface proteins (H and N). Interferons can be detected in respiratory secretions shortly after the shedding of virus has begun, and rises in interferon titers coincide with decreases in virus shedding.

The host defense factors responsible for cessation of virus shedding and resolution of illness have not been defined specifically. Virus shedding generally stops within 2–5 days after symptoms first appear, at a time when serum and local antibody responses often are not detectable by conventional techniques (although antibody rises may be detected earlier by use of highly sensitive techniques, particularly in individuals with previous immunity to the virus). It has been suggested that interferon, cell-mediated immune responses, and/or nonspecific inflammatory responses all contribute to the resolution of illness. CTL responses may be particularly important in this regard.

CLINICAL MANIFESTATIONS

Influenza has most frequently been described as an illness characterized by the abrupt onset of systemic symptoms, such as headache, feverishness, chills, myalgia, or malaise, and accompanying respiratory tract signs, particularly cough and sore throat. In many cases, the onset is so abrupt that patients can recall the precise time they became ill. However, the spectrum of clinical presentations is wide, ranging from a mild, afebrile respiratory illness similar to the common cold (with either a gradual or an abrupt onset) to severe prostration with relatively few respiratory signs and symptoms. In most of the cases that come to a physician's attention, the patient has a fever, with temperatures of 38°–41°C (100.4°–105.8°F). A rapid temperature rise within the first 24 h of illness is generally followed by gradual defervescence over 2–3 days, although, on occasion, fever may last as long as 1 week. Patients report a feverish feeling and chilliness, but true rigors are rare. Headache, either generalized or frontal, is often particularly troublesome. Myalgias may involve any part of the body but are most common in the legs and lumbosacral area. Arthralgias may also develop.

Respiratory symptoms often become more prominent as systemic symptoms subside. Many patients have a sore throat or persistent cough, which may last for ≥ 1 week and which is often accompanied by substernal discomfort. Ocular signs and symptoms include pain on motion of the eyes, photophobia, and burning of the eyes.

Physical findings are usually minimal in uncomplicated influenza. Early in the illness, the patient appears flushed, and the skin is hot and dry, although diaphoresis and mottled extremities are sometimes evident, particularly in older patients. Examination of the pharynx may yield surprisingly unremarkable results despite a severe sore throat, but injection of the mucous membranes and postnasal discharge are apparent in some cases. Mild cervical lymphadenopathy may be noted, especially in younger individuals. The results of chest examination are largely negative in uncomplicated influenza, although rhonchi, wheezes, and scattered rales have been reported with variable frequency in different outbreaks. Frank dyspnea, hyperpnea, cyanosis, diffuse rales, and signs of consolidation are indicative of pulmonary complications. Patients with apparently uncomplicated influenza have been reported to have a variety of mild ventilatory defects and increased alveolar-capillary diffusion gradients; thus, subclinical pulmonary involvement may be more common than is appreciated.

In uncomplicated influenza, the acute illness generally resolves over 2–5 days, and most patients have largely recovered in 1 week, although cough may persist 1–2 weeks longer. In a significant minority (particularly the elderly), however, symptoms of weakness or lassitude (postinfluenzal asthenia) may persist for several weeks and may prove troublesome for persons who wish to resume their full level of activity promptly. The pathogenetic basis for this asthenia is unknown, although pulmonary function abnormalities may persist for several weeks after uncomplicated influenza.

COMPLICATIONS

Complications of influenza occur most frequently in patients >64 years old and in those with certain chronic disorders, including cardiac or pulmonary diseases, diabetes mellitus, hemoglobinopathies, renal dysfunction, and immunosuppression. Pregnancy in the second or third trimester also predisposes to complications with influenza. Children <2 years old (especially infants) are also at high risk for complications.

Pulmonary Complications

PNEUMONIA The most significant complication of influenza is pneumonia: "primary" influenza viral pneumonia, secondary bacterial pneumonia, or mixed viral and bacterial pneumonia.

PRIMARY INFLUENZA VIRAL PNEUMONIA Primary influenza viral pneumonia is the least common but most severe of the pneumonic complications. It presents as acute influenza that does not resolve but instead progresses relentlessly, with persistent fever, dyspnea, and eventual cyanosis. Sputum production is generally scanty, but the sputum can contain blood. Few physical signs may be evident early in the illness. In more advanced cases, diffuse rales may be noted, and chest x-ray findings consistent with diffuse interstitial infiltrates and/or acute respiratory distress syndrome may be present. In such cases, arterial blood-gas determinations show marked hypoxia. Viral cultures of respiratory secretions and lung parenchyma, especially if samples are taken early in illness, yield high titers of virus. In fatal cases of primary viral pneumonia, histopathologic examination reveals a marked inflammatory reaction in the alveolar septa, with edema and infiltration by lymphocytes, macrophages, occasional plasma cells, and variable numbers of neutrophils. Fibrin thrombi in alveolar capillaries, along with necrosis and hemorrhage, have also been noted. Eosinophilic hyaline membranes can be found lining alveoli and alveolar ducts.

Primary influenza viral pneumonia has a predilection for individuals with cardiac disease, particularly those with mitral stenosis, but has also been reported in otherwise-healthy young adults as well as in older individuals with chronic pulmonary disorders. In some epidemics of influenza (notably those of 1918 and 1957), pregnancy increased the risk of primary influenza pneumonia. Subsequent epidemics of influenza have been associated with increased rates of hospitalization among pregnant women.

SECONDARY BACTERIAL PNEUMONIA Secondary bacterial pneumonia follows acute influenza. Improvement of the patient's condition over 2–3 days is followed by a reappearance of fever along with clinical signs and symptoms of bacterial pneumonia, including cough, production of purulent sputum, and physical and x-ray signs of consolidation. The most common bacterial pathogens in this setting are *Streptococcus pneumoniae, Staphylococcus aureus,* and *Haemophilus influenzae*—organisms that can colonize the nasopharynx and that cause infection in the wake of changes in bronchopulmonary defenses. The etiology can often be determined by Gram's staining and culture of an appropriately obtained sputum specimen. Secondary bacterial pneumonia occurs most frequently in high-risk individuals with chronic pulmonary and cardiac disease and in elderly individuals. Patients with secondary bacterial pneumonia often respond to antibiotic therapy when it is instituted promptly.

MIXED VIRAL AND BACTERIAL PNEUMONIA Perhaps the most common pneumonic complications during outbreaks of influenza have mixed features of viral and bacterial pneumonia. Patients may experience a gradual progression of their acute illness or may show transient improvement followed by clinical exacerbation, with eventual manifestation of the clinical features of bacterial pneumonia. Sputum cultures may contain both influenza A virus and one of the bacterial pathogens described above. Patchy infiltrates or areas of consolidation may be detected by physical examination and chest x-ray. Patients with mixed viral and bacterial pneumonia generally have less widespread involvement of the lung than those with primary viral pneumonia, and their bacterial infections may respond to appropriate antibacterial drugs. Mixed viral and bacterial pneumonia occurs primarily in patients with chronic cardiovascular and pulmonary diseases.

OTHER PULMONARY COMPLICATIONS Other pulmonary complications associated with influenza include worsening of chronic obstructive pulmonary disease and exacerbation of chronic bronchitis and asthma. In children, influenza infection may present as croup. Sinusitis as well as otitis media (the latter occurring particularly often in children) may also be associated with influenza.

Extrapulmonary Complications In addition to the pulmonary complications of influenza, a number of extrapulmonary complications may occur. These include *Reye's syndrome* (Chap. 303), a serious complication in children that is associated with influenza B and to a lesser extent with influenza A virus infection as well as with varicella-zoster virus infection. An epidemiologic association between Reye's syndrome and aspirin therapy for the antecedent viral infection has been noted, and the syndrome's incidence has decreased markedly with widespread warnings regarding aspirin use by children with acute viral respiratory infections.

Myositis, rhabdomyolysis, and myoglobinuria are occasional complications of influenza infection. Although myalgias are exceedingly common in influenza, true myositis is rare. Patients with acute myositis have exquisite tenderness of the affected muscles, most commonly in the legs, and may not be able to tolerate even the slightest pressure, such as the touch of bedsheets. In the most severe cases, there is frank swelling and bogginess of muscles. Serum levels of creatine phosphokinase and aldolase are markedly elevated, and an occasional patient develops renal failure from myoglobinuria. The pathogenesis of influenza-associated myositis is also unclear, although the presence of influenza virus in affected muscles has been reported.

Myocarditis and pericarditis were reported in association with influenza virus infection during the 1918–1919 pandemic; these reports were based largely on histopathologic findings, and these complications have been reported only infrequently since that time. Electrocardiographic changes during acute influenza are common among patients who have cardiac disease but have been ascribed most often to exacerbations of the underlying cardiac disease rather than to direct involvement of the myocardium with influenza virus.

Central nervous system (CNS) diseases, including encephalitis, transverse myelitis, and Guillain-Barré syndrome, have been reported during influenza. The etiologic relationship of influenza virus to such CNS illnesses remains uncertain. Toxic shock syndrome associated with *S. aureus* or group A streptococcal infection following acute influenza infection has also been reported (Chaps. 129 and 130).

In addition to complications involving the specific organ systems described above, influenza outbreaks include a number of cases in which elderly and other high-risk individuals develop influenza and subsequently experience a gradual deterioration of underlying cardiovascular, pulmonary, or renal function—changes that occasionally are irreversible and lead to death. These deaths contribute to the overall excess mortality associated with influenza A outbreaks.

Complications of Avian Influenza Cases of influenza caused by avian A/H5N1 virus are reportedly associated with high rates of pneumonia (>50%) and extrapulmonary manifestations such as diarrhea and CNS involvement. Deaths have been associated with multisystem dysfunction, including cardiac and renal failure.

LABORATORY FINDINGS AND DIAGNOSIS

During acute influenza, virus may be detected in throat swabs, nasopharyngeal washes, or sputum. The virus can be isolated by use of tissue culture—or, less commonly, chick embryos—within 48–72 h after inoculation. Most commonly, the laboratory diagnosis is established with rapid viral tests that detect viral nucleoprotein or neuraminidase by means of immunologic or enzymatic techniques that are highly sensitive and 60–90% as specific as tissue culture. Viral nucleic acids can also be detected in clinical samples by reverse transcriptase polymerase chain reaction. The type of the infecting influenza virus (A or B) may be determined by either immunofluorescence or HI techniques, and the hemagglutinin subtype of influenza A virus (H1, H2, or H3) may be identified by HI with use of subtype-specific antisera. Serologic methods for diagnosis require comparison of antibody titers in sera obtained during the acute illness with those in sera obtained 10–14 days after the onset of illness and are useful primarily in retrospect. Fourfold or greater titer rises as detected by HI or CF or significant rises as measured by ELISA are diagnostic of acute infection. CF tests are generally less sensitive than other serologic techniques, but, as they detect type-specific antigens, they may be particularly useful when subtype-specific reagents are not available.

Other laboratory tests generally are not helpful in the specific diagnosis of influenza virus infection. Leukocyte counts are variable, frequently being low early in illness and normal or slightly elevated later. Severe leukopenia has been described in overwhelming viral or bacterial infection, while leukocytosis with >15,000 cells/μL raises the suspicion of secondary bacterial infection.

DIFFERENTIAL DIAGNOSIS

During a community-wide outbreak, a clinical diagnosis of influenza can be made with a high degree of certainty in patients who present to a physician's office with the typical febrile respiratory illness described above. In the absence of an outbreak (i.e., in sporadic or isolated cases), influenza may be difficult to differentiate on clinical grounds alone from an acute respiratory illness caused by any of a variety of respiratory viruses or by *Mycoplasma pneumoniae.* Severe streptococcal pharyngitis or early bacterial pneumonia may mimic acute influenza, although bacterial pneumonias generally do not run a self-limited course. Purulent sputum in which a bacterial pathogen can be detected by Gram's staining is an important diagnostic feature in bacterial pneumonia.

TABLE 180-2 ANTIVIRAL MEDICATIONS FOR TREATMENT AND PROPHYLAXIS OF INFLUENZA

	Age Group (years)		
Antiviral Drug	**Children (≤12)**	**13–64**	**≥65**
Oseltamivir			
Treatment, influenza A and B	Age 1–12, dose varies by weight[a]	75 mg PO bid	75 mg PO bid
Prophylaxis, influenza A and B	Age 1–12, dose varies by weight[b]	75 PO qd	75 mg PO qd
Zanamivir			
Treatment, influenza A and B	Age 7–12, 10 mg bid by inhalation	10 mg bid by inhalation	10 mg bid by inhalation
Prophylaxis, influenza A and B	Age 5–12, 10 mg qd by inhalation	10 mg qd by inhalation	10 mg qd by inhalation
Amantadine[c]			
Treatment, influenza A	Age 1–9, 5 mg/kg in 2 divided doses, up to 150 mg/d	Age ≥10, 100 mg PO bid	≤100 mg/d
Prophylaxis, influenza A	Age 1–9, 5 mg/kg in 2 divided doses, up to 150 mg/d	Age ≥10, 100 mg PO bid	≤100 mg/d
Rimantadine[c]			
Treatment, influenza A	Not approved	100 mg PO bid	100–200 mg/d
Prophylaxis, influenza A	Age 1–9, 5 mg/kg in 2 divided doses, up to 150 mg/d	Age ≥10, 100 mg PO bid	100–200 mg/d

[a]<15 kg: 30 mg bid; >15–23 kg: 45 mg bid; >23–40 kg: 60 mg bid; >40 kg: 75 mg bid.
[b]<15 kg: 30 mg qd; >15–23 kg: 45 mg qd; >23–40 kg: 60 mg qd; >40 kg: 75 mg qd.
[c]Amantadine and rimantadine are not currently recommended (2006–2007) because of widespread resistance in influenza A/H3N2 viruses. Their use may be reconsidered if viral susceptibility is reestablished.

℞ INFLUENZA

In uncomplicated cases of influenza, symptom-based therapy with acetaminophen for the relief of headache, myalgia, and fever may be considered, but the use of salicylates should be avoided in children <18 years of age because of the possible association of salicylates with Reye's syndrome. Since cough is ordinarily self-limited, treatment with cough suppressants generally is not indicated, although codeine-containing compounds may be employed if the cough is particularly troublesome. Patients should be advised to rest and maintain hydration during acute illness and to return to full activity only gradually after illness has resolved, especially if it has been severe.

Specific antiviral therapy is available for influenza (**Table 180-2**): the neuraminidase inhibitors zanamivir and oseltamivir for both influenza A and influenza B and the adamantane agents amantadine and rimantadine for influenza A (Chap. 171) In 2005–2006, resistance to amantadine was reported in >90% of A/H3N2 viral isolates; thus amantadine and rimantadine are no longer recommended, but their use may be reconsidered if sensitivity becomes reestablished.

Oseltamivir (administered orally at a dose of 75 mg twice a day for 5 days) or zanamivir (which must be given by an oral inhalation device; 10 mg twice a day for 5 days) reduces the duration of signs and symptoms of influenza by 1–1.5 days if treatment is started within 2 days of the onset of illness. Zanamivir may exacerbate bronchospasm in asthmatic patients, and oseltamivir has been associated with nausea and vomiting, whose frequency can be reduced by administration of the drug with food. Oseltamivir has also been associated with neuropsychiatric side effects in children.

If begun within 48 h of the onset of illness due to sensitive influenza A virus strains, treatment with amantadine or rimantadine reduces the duration of systemic and respiratory symptoms of influenza by ~50%. Of individuals who receive amantadine, 5–10% experience mild CNS side effects, primarily jitteriness, anxiety, insomnia, or difficulty concentrating. These side effects disappear promptly upon cessation of therapy. Rimantadine appears to be equally efficacious and is associated with less frequent CNS side effects than is amantadine. In adults, the usual dose of amantadine or rimantadine is 200 mg/d for 3–7 days. Since both drugs are excreted via the kidney, the dose should be reduced to ≤100 mg/d in elderly patients and in patients with renal insufficiency. Resistant viruses emerge frequently during treatment with amantadine or rimantadine and can be transmitted among family members. Development of resistance to zanamivir or oseltamivir appears to be less common but can occur. Ribavirin is a nucleoside analogue with activity against influenza A and B viruses in vitro. It has been reported to be variably effective against influenza when administered as an aerosol but ineffective when administered orally. Its efficacy in the treatment of influenza A or B is unestablished.

Studies demonstrating the therapeutic efficacy of antiviral compounds in influenza have primarily involved young adults with uncomplicated disease. A meta-analysis of studies with oseltamivir suggests that treatment may reduce the likelihood of some lower respiratory tract complications of influenza. However, it is not known whether antiviral agents are themselves effective in the treatment of influenza pneumonia or of other complications of influenza. Therapy for primary influenza pneumonia is directed at maintaining oxygenation and is most appropriately undertaken in an intensive care unit, with aggressive respiratory and hemodynamic support as needed. Bypass membrane oxygenators have been employed in this setting with variable results. When an acute respiratory distress syndrome develops, fluids must be administered cautiously, with close monitoring of blood gases and hemodynamic function.

Antibacterial drugs should be reserved for the treatment of bacterial complications of acute influenza, such as secondary bacterial pneumonia. The choice of antibiotics should be guided by Gram's staining and culture of appropriate specimens of respiratory secretions, such as sputum or transtracheal aspirates. If the etiology of a case of bacterial pneumonia is unclear from an examination of respiratory secretions, empirical antibiotics effective against the most common bacterial pathogens in this setting (*S. pneumoniae*, *S. aureus*, and *H. influenzae*) should be selected (Chaps. 128, 129, and 139).

PROPHYLAXIS

Inactivated and live attenuated vaccines against influenza are available, and their use represents the major public health measure for prevention of influenza. The vast majority of currently used vaccines are inactivated ("killed") preparations derived from influenza A and B viruses that circulated during the previous influenza season. If the vaccine virus and the currently circulating viruses are closely related, 50–80% protection against influenza would be expected from inactivated vaccines. The available inactivated vaccines have been highly purified and are associated with few reactions. Up to 5% of individuals experience low-grade fever and mild systemic symptoms 8–24 h after vaccination, and up to one-third develop mild redness or tenderness at the vaccination site. Since the vaccine is produced in eggs, individuals with true hypersensitivity to egg products either should be desensitized or should not be vaccinated. Although the 1976 swine influenza vaccine appears to have been associated with an increased frequency of Guillain-Barré syndrome, influenza vaccines administered since 1976 generally have not been. Possible exceptions were noted during the 1992–1993 and 1993–1994 influenza seasons, when there may have been an excess risk of Guillain-Barré syndrome of slightly more than 1 case per million vaccine recipients. However, the overall health risk following influenza outweighs the potential risk associated with vaccination.

The U.S. Public Health Service recommends the administration of inactivated influenza vaccine to individuals who, because of age or underlying disease, are at increased risk for complications of influenza and to the contacts of these individuals (**Table 180-3**). Inactivated vaccines may be administered safely to immunocompromised patients. Influenza vaccination is not associated with exacerbations of chronic nervous-system diseases such as multiple sclerosis. Vaccine should be administered early in the autumn before influenza outbreaks occur and should then be given annually to maintain immunity against the most current influenza virus strains.

TABLE 180-3 PERSONS FOR WHOM ANNUAL INFLUENZA VACCINATION IS RECOMMENDED

Children 6–59 months old
Women who will be pregnant during the influenza season
Persons ≥50 years old
Children and adolescents (6 months to 18 years old) who are receiving long-term aspirin therapy and therefore may be at risk for developing Reye's syndrome after influenza
Adults and children who have chronic disorders of the pulmonary or cardiovascular systems, including asthma[a]
Adults and children who have required regular medical follow-up or hospitalization during the preceding year because of chronic metabolic diseases (including diabetes mellitus), renal dysfunction, hemoglobinopathies, or immunodeficiency (including immunodeficiency caused by medications or by HIV)
Adults and children who have any condition (e.g., cognitive dysfunction, spinal cord injuries, seizure disorders, or other neuromuscular disorders) that can compromise respiratory function or the handling of respiratory secretions or can increase the risk of aspiration
Residents of nursing homes and other chronic-care facilities that house persons of any age who have chronic medical conditions
Persons who live with or care for persons at high risk for influenza-related complications, including healthy household contacts of and caregivers for children from birth through 59 months of age
Health care workers

[a]Hypertension itself is not considered a chronic disorder for which influenza vaccination is recommended.

Source: Centers for Disease Control and Prevention: Prevention and control of influenza: Recommendations of the Advisory Committee on Immunization Practices (ACIP). MMWR 55(RR-11):1, 2006.

A live attenuated influenza vaccine that is administered by intranasal spray is also available. The vaccine is generated by reassortment between currently circulating strains of influenza A and B virus and a cold-adapted, attenuated master strain. The cold-adapted vaccine is well tolerated and highly efficacious (92% protective) in young children; in one study, it provided protection against a circulating influenza virus that had drifted antigenically away from the vaccine strain. Live attenuated vaccine is approved for use in healthy persons 5–49 years of age.

Antiviral drugs may also be used as chemoprophylaxis against influenza (Table 180-2). Chemoprophylaxis with oseltamivir (75 mg/d by mouth) or zanamivir (10 mg/d inhaled) has been 84–89% efficacious against influenza A and B. Chemoprophylaxis with amantadine or rimantadine is no longer recommended because of reports of widespread resistance to these drugs. In earlier studies with sensitive viruses, prophylaxis with amantadine or rimantadine (100–200 mg/d) was 70–100% effective against illness associated with influenza A. Chemoprophylaxis is most likely to be used for high-risk individuals who have not received influenza vaccine or in a situation where the vaccines previously administered are relatively ineffective because of antigenic changes in the circulating virus. During an outbreak, antiviral chemoprophylaxis can be administered simultaneously with inactivated vaccine, since the drugs do not interfere with an immune response to the vaccine. In fact, there is evidence that the protective effects of chemoprophylaxis and inactivated vaccine may be additive. However, concurrent administration of chemoprophylaxis and the live attenuated vaccine may interfere with the immune response to the latter. Antiviral drugs should not be administered until at least 2 weeks after administration of live vaccine, and vaccination with live vaccine should not begin until at least 48 h after antiviral drug administration has been stopped. Chemoprophylaxis may also be employed to control nosocomial outbreaks of influenza. For that purpose, prophylaxis should be instituted promptly when influenza activity is detected and must be continued daily for the duration of the outbreak.

FURTHER READINGS

Beigel JH et al: Avian influenza A (H5N1) infection in humans. N Engl J Med 353:1374, 2005

Belshe RB et al: The efficacy of live attenuated, cold adapted trivalent, intranasal influenza vaccine in children. N Engl J Med 38:1405, 1998

Centers for Disease Control and Prevention: Prevention and control of influenza. MMWR 55(RR–11):1, 2006

Cooper NJ et al: Effectiveness of neuraminidase inhibitors in treatment and prevention of influenza A and B: Systematic review and meta-analysis of randomized controlled trials. BMJ 326:1235, 2003

Dolin R: Interpandemic as well as pandemic disease. N Engl J Med 353:2535, 2005

Hayden FG et al: Use of the selective oral neuraminidase inhibitor oseltamivir to prevent influenza. N Engl J Med 341:1336, 1999

Meltzer MI et al: The economic impact of pandemic influenza in the United States: Priorities for intervention. Emerg Infect Dis 5:659, 1999

MIST [Management of Influenza in the Southern Hemisphere Trialists] Study Group: Randomized trial of efficacy and safety of inhaled zanamivir in treatment of influenza A and B infections. Lancet 352:1871, 1998

Neuzil KM et al: Influenza-associated morbidity and mortality in young and middle-aged women. JAMA 281:901, 1999

Simonsen L et al: Pandemic vs epidemic mortality: A pattern of changing age distribution. J Infect Dis 178:53, 1998

Treanor JJ: Influenza virus, in *Principles and Practice of Infectious Diseases*, 6th ed, GL Mandell et al (eds). Philadelphia, Elsevier, 2005, pp 2201–2203

SECTION 14 INFECTIONS DUE TO HUMAN IMMUNODEFICIENCY VIRUS AND OTHER HUMAN RETROVIRUSES

181 The Human Retroviruses

Dan L. Longo, Anthony S. Fauci

The retroviruses, which make up a large family (Retroviridae), infect mainly vertebrates. These viruses have a unique replication cycle whereby their genetic information is encoded by RNA rather than DNA. Retroviruses contain an RNA-dependent DNA polymerase (a reverse transcriptase) that directs the synthesis of a DNA form of the viral genome after infection of a host cell. The designation *retrovirus* denotes that information in the form of RNA is transcribed into DNA in the host cell—a sequence that overturned a central dogma of molecular biology: that information passes unidirectionally from DNA to RNA to protein. The observation that RNA was the source of genetic information in the causative agents of certain animal tumors led to a number of paradigm-shifting biologic insights regarding not only the direction of genetic information passage but also the viral etiology of certain cancers and the concept of oncogenes as normal host genes scavenged and altered by a viral vector.

The family Retroviridae includes three subfamilies (Table 181-1): Oncovirinae, of which human T cell lymphotropic virus (HTLV) type I is the most important in humans; Lentivirinae, of which HIV is the

TABLE 181-1 CLASSIFICATION OF RETROVIRUSES: THE FAMILY RETROVIRIDAE

Subfamily, Group[a]	Example(s)	Feature
Oncovirinae (oncogenic viruses)		
Avian leukosis	Rous sarcoma virus	Contains *src* oncogene
Mammalian C-type	Abelson leukemia virus	Contains *abl* oncogene
B-type	Murine mammary tumor virus	Can be endogenous or exogenous
D-type	Mason-Pfizer monkey virus	—
HTLV-BLV	HTLV-I	Causes T-cell lymphoma and neurologic disease
Lentivirinae (slow viruses)	HIV-1, HIV-2	Cause AIDS
	Visna virus	Causes lung and brain diseases in sheep
	Feline immunodeficiency virus	Causes immunodeficiency in cats
Spumavirinae (foamy viruses)	Simian foamy virus, human foamy virus	Cause no known disease

[a]The Oncovirinae were originally grouped into types A–D on the basis of morphologic features (size, core location, budding) under electron microscopy; however, this system has been replaced by groupings based on relationships of genome structure and sequence.

Note: HTLV, human T cell lymphotropic virus; BLV, bovine leukemia virus.

most important in humans; and Spumavirinae, the "foamy" viruses, named for the pathologic appearance of infected cells. A number of spumaviruses have been isolated from humans; however, they are not associated with any known disease and therefore are not discussed further in this chapter.

The wide variety of interactions of a retrovirus with its host range from completely benign events (e.g., silent carriage of endogenous retroviral sequences in the germ-line genome of many animal species) to rapidly fatal infections (e.g., exogenous infection with an oncogenic virus such as Rous sarcoma virus in chickens). The ability of retroviruses to acquire and alter the structure and function of host cell sequences has revolutionized our understanding of molecular carcinogenesis. The viruses can insert into the germ-line genome of the host cell and behave as a transposable or movable genetic element. They can activate or inactivate genes near the site of integration into the genome. They can rapidly alter their own genome by recombination and mutation under selective environmental stimuli.

Most human viral diseases occur as a consequence of either tissue destruction by the virus itself or the host's response to the virus. Although these mechanisms are operative in retroviral infections, retroviruses have additional mechanisms of inducing disease, including the malignant transformation of an infected cell and the induction of an immunodeficiency state that leads to opportunistic diseases (infections and neoplasms; Chap. 182).

STRUCTURE AND LIFE CYCLE

Despite the wide range of biologic consequences of retroviral infection, all retroviruses are similar in structure, genome organization, and mode of replication. Retroviruses are 70–130 nm in diameter and have a lipid-containing envelope surrounding an icosahedral capsid with a dense inner core. The core contains two identical copies of the single-strand RNA genome. The RNA molecules are 8–10 kb long and are complexed with reverse transcriptase and tRNA. Other viral proteins, such as integrase, are also components of the virion particle. The RNA has features usually found in mRNA: a cap site at the 5′ end of the molecule, which is important in the initiation of mRNA translation, and a polyadenylation site at the 3′ end, which influences mRNA turnover (i.e., messages with shorter polyA tails turn over faster than messages with longer polyA tails). However, the retroviral RNA is not translated; instead it is transcribed into DNA. The DNA form of the retroviral genome is called a *provirus*.

The replication cycle of retroviruses proceeds in two phases (Fig. 181-1). In the first phase, the virus enters the cytoplasm after binding to a specific cell-surface receptor; the viral RNA and reverse transcriptase synthesize a double-strand DNA version of the RNA template; and the provirus moves into the nucleus and integrates into the host cell genome. This proviral integration is permanent. Although some animal retroviruses integrate into a single specific site of the host genome in every infected cell, the four known human retroviruses (HTLV-I, HTLV-II, HIV-1, and HIV-2) integrate randomly. This first phase of replication depends entirely on gene products in the virus. The second phase includes the synthesis and processing of viral genomes, mRNAs, and proteins using host cell machinery, often under the influence of viral gene products. Virions are assembled and released from the cell by budding from the membrane; host cell membrane proteins are frequently incorporated into the envelope of the virus. Proviral integration occurs during the S-phase of the cell cycle; thus, in general, nondividing cells are resistant to retroviral infection. Only the lentiviruses are able to infect nondividing cells. Once a host cell is infected, it is infected for the life of the cell.

Retroviral genomes include both coding and noncoding sequences (Fig. 181-2). In general, noncoding sequences are important recognition signals for DNA or RNA synthesis or processing events and are located in the 5′ and 3′ terminal regions of the genome. All retroviral genomes are terminally redundant, containing identical sequences called *long terminal repeats* (LTRs). The ends of the retroviral RNA genome differ slightly in sequence from the integrated retroviral DNA. In the latter, the LTR sequences are repeated in both the 5′ and the 3′ terminus of the virus. The LTRs contain sequences involved in initiating the expression of the viral proteins, the integration of the provirus, and the polyadenylation of viral RNAs. The primer binding site, which is critical for the initiation of reverse transcription, and the viral packaging sequences are located outside the LTR sequences. The coding regions include the *gag* (group-specific antigen, core protein), *pol* (RNA-dependent DNA polymerase), and *env* (envelope) genes. The *gag* gene encodes a precursor polyprotein that is cleaved to form three to five capsid proteins; a fraction of the Gag precursor proteins also contain a protease responsible for cleaving the Gag and Pol polyproteins. A Gag-Pol polyprotein gives rise to the protease that is responsible for cleaving the Gag-Pol polyprotein. The *pol* gene encodes three proteins: the reverse transcriptase, the integrase, and the protease. The reverse transcriptase functions to copy the viral RNA into the double-strand DNA provirus, which inserts itself into the host cell DNA via the action of integrase. The protease functions to cleave the Gag-Pol polyprotein into smaller protein products. The *env* gene encodes the envelope glycoproteins: one protein that binds to specific surface receptors and determines what cell types can be infected and a smaller transmembrane protein that anchors the complex to the envelope. Figure 181-3 shows how the retroviral gene products make up the virus structure.

HTLVs have a region between *env* and the 3′ LTR that encodes at least two proteins in overlapping reading frames: Tax, a 40-kDa protein that does not bind to DNA but induces the expression of host cell transcription factors that alter host cell gene expression; and Rex, a 27-kDa protein that regulates the expression of viral mRNAs. These two proteins are produced from messages that are similar but that are spliced differently from overlapping but distinct exons.

The lentiviruses in general, and HIV-1 and -2 in particular, contain a larger genome than other pathogenic retroviruses. They contain an untranslated region between *pol* and *env* that encodes portions of several proteins, varying with the reading frame into which the mRNA is spliced. Tat is a 14-kDa protein that augments the expression of virus from the LTR. The Rev protein of HIV-1, similar to the Rex protein of HTLV, regulates RNA splicing and/or RNA transport. The Nef protein downregulates CD4, the cellular receptor for HIV; alters host T cell activation pathways; and enhances viral infectivity. The Vif protein is necessary for the proper assembly of the HIV nucleoprotein core in

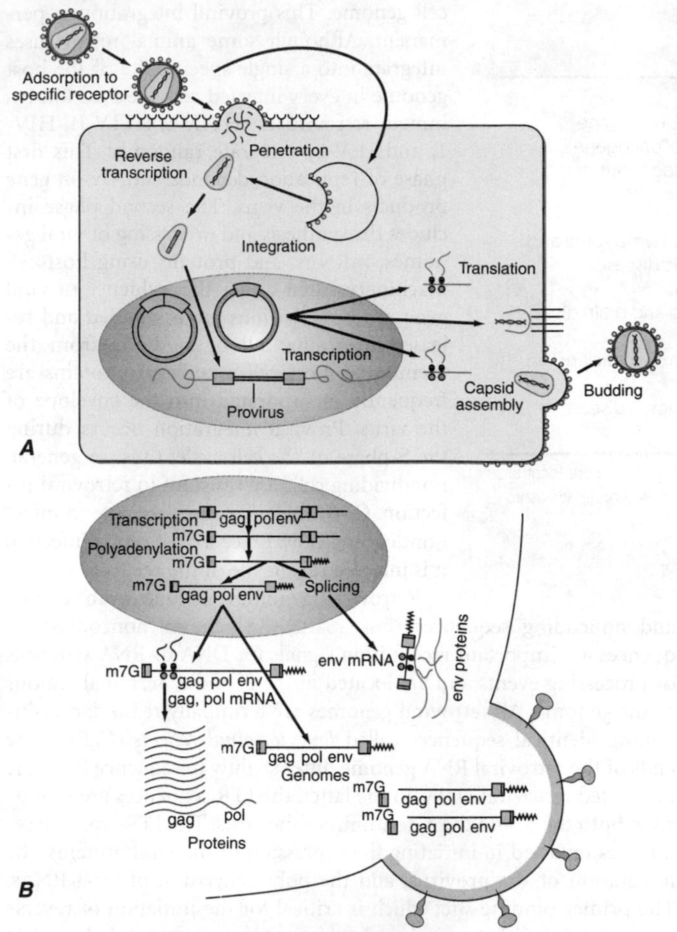

FIGURE 181-1 The life cycle of retroviruses. *A.* Overview of virus replication. The retrovirus enters a target cell by binding to a specific cell-surface receptor; once the virus is internalized, its RNA is released from the nucleocapsid and is reverse-transcribed into proviral DNA. The provirus is inserted into the genome and then transcribed into RNA; the RNA is translated; and virions assemble and are extruded from the cell membrane by budding. ***B.*** Overview of retroviral gene expression. The provirus is transcribed, capped, and polyadenylated. Viral RNA molecules then have one of three fates: they are exported to the cytoplasm, where they are packaged as the viral RNA in infectious viral particles; they are spliced to form the message for the envelope polyprotein; or they are translated into Gag and Pol proteins. Most of the messages for the Pol protein fail to initiate Pol translation because of a stop codon before its initiation; however, in a fraction of the messages, the stop codon is missed and the Pol proteins are translated. *[Modified from JM Coffin, in BN Fields, DM Knipe (eds): Fields Virology. New York, Raven, 1990; with permission.]*

many types of cells; without Vif, proviral DNA is not efficiently produced in these infected cells. In addition, the Vif protein targets APOBEC (apolipoprotein B mRNA-editing enzyme catalytic polypeptide, a cytidine deaminase that mutates the viral sequence) for proteasomal degradation, thus blocking its virus-suppressing effect. Vpr, Vpu (HIV-1 only), and Vpx (HIV-2 only) are viral proteins encoded by translation of the same message in different reading frames. As noted above, oncogenic retroviruses depend on cell proliferation for their replication; lentiviruses can infect nondividing cells, largely through effects mediated by Vpr. Vpr facilitates transport of the provirus into the nucleus and can induce other cellular changes, such as G_2 growth arrest and differentiation of some target cells. Vpx is structurally related to Vpr, but its functions are not fully defined. Vpu promotes the degradation of CD4 in the endoplasmic reticulum and stimulates the release of virions from infected cells.

Retroviruses can be either exogenously acquired by infection with a virion capable of replication or transmitted in the germ line as endogenous virus. Endogenous retroviruses are often replication-defective. The human genome contains endogenous retroviral sequences, but there are no known replication-competent endogenous retroviruses in humans.

In general, viruses that contain only the *gag*, *pol*, and *env* genes either are not pathogenic or take a long time to induce disease; these observations indicate the importance of the other regulatory genes in viral disease pathogenesis. The pathogenesis of neoplastic transformation by retroviruses relies on the chance integration of the provirus at a spot in the genome that will result in the expression of a cellular gene (proto-oncogene) that becomes transforming by virtue of its unregulated expression. For example, avian leukosis virus causes B cell leukemia by inducing the expression of *myc*. Some retroviruses possess captured and altered cellular genes near their integration site, and these viral oncogenes are capable of transforming the infected host cell. Viruses that have oncogenes often have lost a portion of their genome that is required for replication. Such viruses need helper viruses to reproduce, a feature that may explain why these acute transforming retroviruses are rare in nature. All human retroviruses identified to date are exogenous and are not acutely transforming (i.e., they lack a transforming oncogene).

These remarkable properties of retroviruses have led to experimental efforts to use them as vectors to insert specific genes into particular cell types, a process known as *gene therapy* or *gene transfer*. The process could be used to repair a genetic defect or to introduce a new property that could be used therapeutically; for example, a gene (e.g., thymidine kinase) that would make a tumor cell susceptible to killing by a drug (e.g., ganciclovir) could be inserted. One source of concern about the use of retroviral vectors in humans is that replication-competent viruses might rescue endogenous retroviral replication, with unpredictable results. This concern is not merely hypothetical: the detection of proteins encoded by endogenous retroviral sequences on the surface of cancer cells implies that the genetic events leading to the cancer were able to activate the synthesis of these usually silent genes.

HUMAN T CELL LYMPHOTROPIC VIRUS

HTLV-I was isolated in 1980 from a T cell lymphoma cell line from a patient originally thought to have cutaneous T cell lymphoma. Later it became clear that the patient had a distinct form of lymphoma (originally reported in Japan) called *adult T cell leukemia/lymphoma* (ATL). Serologic data have determined that HTLV-I is the cause of at least two important diseases: ATL and tropical spastic paraparesis, also called *HTLV-I-associated myelopathy* (HAM). HTLV-I may also play a role in infective dermatitis and uveitis syndromes.

Two years after the isolation of HTLV-I, HTLV-II was isolated from a patient with an unusual form of hairy cell leukemia that affected T cells. Although early epidemiologic studies of HTLV-II failed to reveal a consistent disease association, more recent studies suggest an association of HTLV-II with human disease (see "Associated Diseases" under "Features of HTLV-II Infection," below), particularly among injection drug users.

BIOLOGY AND MOLECULAR BIOLOGY

Because the biology of HTLV-I and that of HTLV-II are similar, the following discussion will focus on HTLV-I.

The human glucose transporter protein 1 (GLUT-1) functions as a receptor for HTLV-1, probably acting together with neuropilin-1 (NRP1). Generally, only T cells are productively infected, but infection of B cells and other cell types is occasionally detected. The most common outcome of HTLV-I infection is latent carriage of randomly integrated provirus in CD4+ T cells. HTLV-I does not contain an oncogene and does not insert into a unique site in the genome. Indeed, most infected cells express no viral gene products. The only viral gene product that is routinely expressed in tumor cells transformed by HTLV-I in vivo is *tax*, and even *tax* is not expressed in the tumor cells of many ATL patients. Cells transformed in vitro, by contrast, actively transcribe HTLV-I RNA and produce infectious virions. Most HTLV-I-transformed cell lines are the result of the infection of a normal host T cell in vitro. It is difficult to establish cell lines derived from authentic ATL cells.

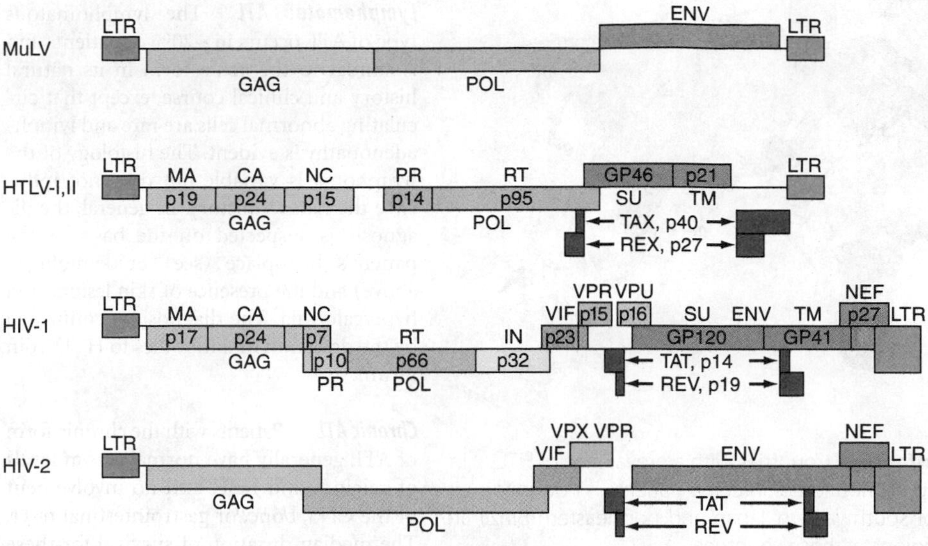

FIGURE 181-2 Genomic structure of retroviruses. The murine leukemia virus MuLV has the typical three structural genes: *gag*, *pol*, and *env*. The *gag* region gives rise to three proteins: matrix (MA), capsid (CA), and nucleic acid–binding (NC) proteins. The *pol* region encodes both a protease (PR) responsible for cleaving the viral polyproteins and a reverse transcriptase (RT). In addition, HIV *pol* encodes an integrase (IN). The *env* region encodes a surface protein (SU) and a small transmembrane protein (TM). The human retroviruses have additional gene products translated in each of the three possible reading frames. HTLV-I and HTLV-II have *tax* and *rex* genes with exons on either side of the *env* gene. HIV-1 and HIV-2 have six accessory gene products: *tat, rev, vif, nef, vpr*, and either *vpu* (in HIV-1) or *vpx* (in HIV-2). The genes for these proteins are located mainly between the *pol* and *env* genes. LTR, long terminal repeat.

Although *tax* does not itself bind to DNA, it does induce the expression of a wide range of host cell gene products, including transcription factors (especially c-rel/NF-κB, ets-1 and -2, and members of the fos/jun family), cytokines [e.g., interleukin (IL) 2, granulocyte-macrophage colony-stimulating factor, and tumor necrosis factor (TNF)], and membrane proteins and receptors [major histocompatibility (MHC) molecules and IL-2 receptor α]. The genes activated by *tax* are generally controlled by transcription factors of the c-rel/NF-κB and cyclic AMP response element binding (CREB) protein families. It is unclear how this induction of host gene expression leads to neoplastic transformation; *tax* can interfere with G_1 and mitotic cell-cycle checkpoints, block apoptosis, inhibit DNA repair, and promote antigen-independent T cell proliferation. Induction of a cytokine-autocrine loop has been proposed; however, IL-2 is not the crucial cytokine. The involvement of IL-4, IL-7, and IL-15 has been proposed.

In light of the irregular expression of *tax* in ATL cells, it has been suggested that *tax* is important in the early phases of transformation but is not essential for the maintenance of the transformed state. As is clear from the epidemiology of HTLV-I infection, transformation of an infected cell is a rare event and may depend on heterogeneous second, third, or fourth genetic hits. No consistent chromosomal abnormalities have been described in ATL; however, individual cases with p53 mutations and translocations involving the T cell receptor genes on chromosome 14 have been reported. *Tax* may repress certain DNA repair enzymes, permitting the accumulation of genetic damage that would normally be repaired. However, the molecular pathogenesis of HTLV-I-induced neoplasia is not fully understood.

FEATURES OF HTLV-I INFECTION

Epidemiology HTLV-I infection is transmitted in at least three ways: from mother to child, especially via breast milk; through sexual activity, more commonly from men to women; and through the blood—via contaminated transfusions or contaminated needles. The virus is most commonly transmitted perinatally. Compared with HIV, which can be transmitted in cell-free form, HTLV-I is less infectious, and its transmission usually requires cell-to-cell contact.

HTLV-I is endemic in southwestern Japan and Okinawa, where >1 million persons are infected. Antibodies to HTLV-I are present in the serum of up to 35% of Okinawans, 10% of residents of the Japanese island of Kyushu, and <1% of persons in nonendemic regions of Japan. Despite this high prevalence of infection, only ~500 cases of ATL are diagnosed in this area each year. Clusters of infection have been noted in other areas of the Orient, such as Taiwan; in the Caribbean basin, including northeastern South America; in northwestern South America; in central and southern Africa; in Italy, Israel, Iran, and Papua New Guinea; in the Arctic; and in the southeastern part of the United States (Fig. 181-4). An estimated 15–20 million persons have HTLV-I infection worldwide.

A progressive spastic or ataxic myelopathy developing in an individual who is HTLV-I positive (i.e., who has serum antibodies to HTLV-I) is likely to be due to direct infection of the nervous system with the virus; a similar disorder may result from infection with HIV or HTLV-II. In rare instances, patients with HAM are seronegative but have detectable antibody to HTLV-I in the cerebrospinal fluid (CSF).

The cumulative lifetime risk of developing ATL is 3% among HTLV-I-infected patients, with a threefold greater risk among men than among women; a similar cumulative risk is projected for HAM (4%), but with women more commonly affected than men. The distribution of the two diseases overlaps the distribution of HTLV-I, with >95% of affected patients showing serologic evidence of HTLV-I infection. The latency period between infection and the emergence of disease is 20–30 years for ATL. For HAM, the median latency period is ~3.3 years (range, 4 months to 30 years). The development of ATL is rare among persons

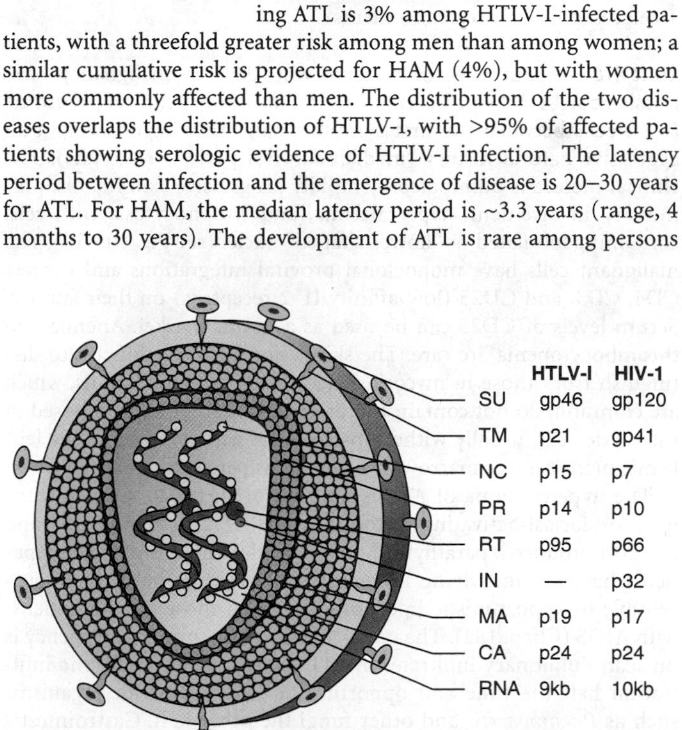

FIGURE 181-3 Schematic structure of human retroviruses. The surface glycoprotein (SU) is responsible for binding to receptors of host cells. The transmembrane protein (TM) anchors SU to the virus. NC is a nucleic acid–binding protein found in association with the viral RNA. A protease (PR) cleaves the polyproteins encoded by the *gag*, *pol*, and *env* genes into their functional components. RT is reverse transcriptase, and IN is an integrase present in some retroviruses (e.g., HIV-1) that facilitates insertion of the provirus into the host genome. The matrix protein (MA) is a Gag protein closely associated with the lipid of the envelope. The capsid protein (CA) forms the major internal structure of the virus, the core shell.

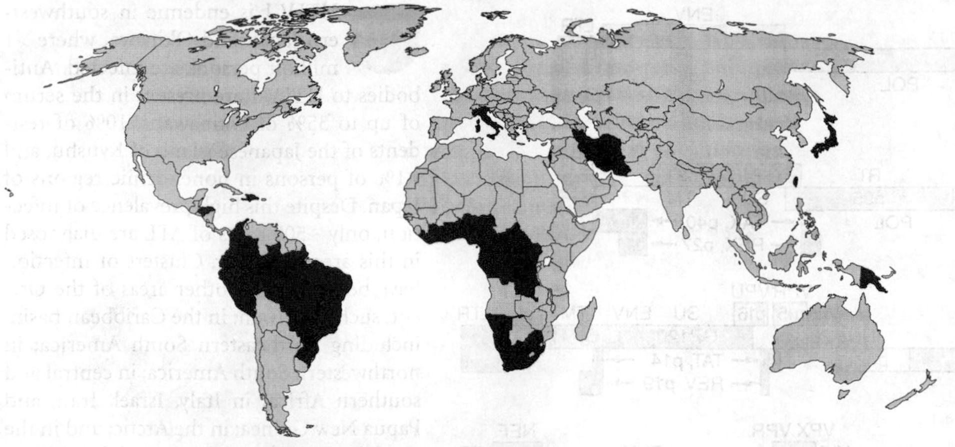

FIGURE 181-4 Global distribution of HTLV-I infection. Countries with a prevalence of HTLV-I infection of 1–5% are shaded darkly. Note that the distribution of infected patients is not uniform in endemic countries. For example, the people of southwestern Japan and northeastern Brazil are more commonly affected than those in other regions of those countries.

infected by blood products; however, ~20% of patients with HAM acquire HTLV-I from contaminated blood. ATL is more common among perinatally infected individuals, whereas HAM is more common among persons infected via sexual transmission.

Associated Diseases • ***ATL*** Four clinical types of HTLV-I-induced neoplasia have been described: acute, lymphomatous, chronic, and smoldering. All of these tumors are monoclonal proliferations of CD4+ post-thymic T cells with clonal proviral integrations and clonal T cell receptor gene rearrangements.

Acute ATL About 60% of patients who develop malignancy have classic acute ATL, which is characterized by a short clinical prodrome (~2 weeks between the first symptoms and the diagnosis) and an aggressive natural history (median survival period, 6 months). The clinical picture is dominated by rapidly progressive skin lesions, pulmonary involvement, hypercalcemia, and lymphocytosis with cells containing lobulated or "flower-shaped" nuclei (see Fig. 105-10). The malignant cells have monoclonal proviral integrations and express CD4, CD3, and CD25 (low-affinity IL-2 receptors) on their surface. Serum levels of CD25 can be used as a tumor marker. Anemia and thrombocytopenia are rare. The skin lesions may be difficult to distinguish from those in mycosis fungoides. Lytic bone lesions, which are common, do not contain tumor cells but rather are composed of osteolytic cells, usually without osteoblastic activity. Despite the leukemic picture, bone marrow involvement is patchy in most cases.

The hypercalcemia of ATL is multifactorial; the tumor cells produce osteoclast-activating factors (TNF-α, IL-1, lymphotoxin) and can also produce a parathyroid hormone–like molecule. Affected patients have an underlying immunodeficiency that makes them susceptible to opportunistic infections similar to those seen in patients with AIDS (Chap. 182). The pathogenesis of the immunodeficiency is unclear. Pulmonary infiltrates in ATL patients reflect leukemic infiltration half the time and opportunistic infections with organisms such as *Pneumocystis* and other fungi the other half. Gastrointestinal symptoms are nearly always related to opportunistic infection. *Strongyloides stercoralis* is a gastrointestinal parasite that has a pattern of endemic distribution similar to that of HTLV-I. HTLV-I-infected persons also infected with this parasite may develop ATL more often or more rapidly than those without *Strongyloides* infections. Serum concentrations of lactate dehydrogenase (LDH) and alkaline phosphatase are often elevated in ATL. About 10% of patients have leptomeningeal involvement leading to weakness, altered mental status, paresthesia, and/or headache. Unlike other forms of central nervous system (CNS) lymphoma, ATL may be accompanied by normal CSF protein levels. The diagnosis depends on finding ATL cells in the CSF (Chap. 105).

Lymphomatous ATL The lymphomatous type of ATL occurs in ~20% of patients and is similar to the acute form in its natural history and clinical course, except that circulating abnormal cells are rare and lymphadenopathy is evident. The histology of the lymphoma is variable but does not influence the natural history. In general, the diagnosis is suspected on the basis of the patient's birthplace (see "Epidemiology," above) and the presence of skin lesions and hypercalcemia. The diagnosis is confirmed by the detection of antibodies to HTLV-I in serum.

Chronic ATL Patients with the chronic form of ATL generally have normal serum levels of calcium and LDH and no involvement of the CNS, bone, or gastrointestinal tract. The median duration of survival for these patients is 2 years. In some cases, chronic ATL progresses to the acute form of the disease.

Smoldering ATL Fewer than 5% of patients have the smoldering form of ATL. In this form, the malignant cells have monoclonal proviral integration; <5% of peripheral blood cells exhibit typical morphologic abnormalities; hypercalcemia, adenopathy, and hepatosplenomegaly do not develop; the CNS, the bones, and the gastrointestinal tract are not involved; and skin lesions and pulmonary lesions may be present. The median survival period of this small subset of patients appears to be ≥5 years.

HAM (TROPICAL SPASTIC PARAPARESIS) In contrast to ATL, in which there is a slight predominance of male patients, HAM affects females disproportionately. HAM resembles multiple sclerosis in certain ways (Chap. 375). The onset is insidious. Symptoms include weakness or stiffness in one or both legs, back pain, and urinary incontinence. Sensory changes are usually mild, but peripheral neuropathy may develop. The disease generally takes the form of slowly progressive and unremitting thoracic myelopathy; one-third of patients are bedridden within 10 years of diagnosis, and one-half are unable to walk unassisted by this point. Patients display spastic paraparesis or paraplegia with hyperreflexia, ankle clonus, and extensor plantar responses. Cognitive function is usually spared; cranial nerve abnormalities are unusual.

MRI reveals lesions in both the white matter and the paraventricular regions of the brain as well as in the spinal cord. Pathologic examination of the spinal cord shows symmetric degeneration of the lateral columns, including the corticospinal tracts; some cases involve the posterior columns as well. The spinal meninges and cord parenchyma contain an inflammatory infiltrate with myelin destruction.

HTLV-I is not usually found in cells of the CNS but may be detected in a small population of lymphocytes present in the CSF. In general, HTLV-I replication is greater in HAM than in ATL, and patients with HAM have a stronger immune response to the virus. Antibodies to HTLV-I are present in the serum and appear to be produced in the CSF of HAM patients, where titers are often higher than in the serum. The pathophysiology of HAM may involve the induction of autoimmune destruction of neural cells by T cells with specificity for viral components such as Tax or Env proteins. One theory is that susceptibility to HAM may be related to the presence of human leukocyte antigen (HLA) alleles capable of presenting viral antigens in a fashion that leads to autoimmunity. Insufficient data are available to confirm an HLA association. However, antibodies in the sera of HAM patients have been shown to bind a neuron-specific antigen [heteronuclear ribonuclear protein A1 (hnRNP A1)] and to interfere with neurotransmission in vitro.

It is unclear what factors influence whether HTLV-I infection will cause disease and, if it does, whether it will induce a neoplasm (ATL) or an autoimmune disorder (HAM). Differences in viral strains, the susceptibility of particular MHC haplotypes, the route of HTLV-I infection, the viral load, and the nature of the HTLV-I-related immune response are putative factors, but few definitive data are available.

OTHER PUTATIVE HTLV-I-RELATED DISEASES In areas where HTLV-I is endemic, diverse inflammatory and autoimmune diseases have been attributed to the virus, including uveitis, dermatitis, pneumonitis, rheumatoid arthritis, and polymyositis. However, a causal relationship between HTLV-I and these illnesses has not been established.

Prevention Women in endemic areas should not breast-feed their children, and blood donors should be screened for serum antibodies to HTLV-I. As in the prevention of HIV infection, the practice of safe sex and the avoidance of needle sharing are important.

℞ HTLV-I INFECTION

For the small number of patients who develop HTLV-I-related disease, therapies are not curative. In patients with the acute and lymphomatous types of ATL, the disease progresses rapidly. Hypercalcemia is generally controlled by glucocorticoid administration and cytotoxic therapy directed against the neoplasm. The tumor is highly responsive to combination chemotherapy that is employed against other forms of lymphoma; however, patients are susceptible to overwhelming bacterial and opportunistic infections, and ATL relapses within 4–10 months after remission in most cases. The combination of interferon α and zidovudine may extend survival. Because viral replication is not clearly associated with ATL progression, zidovudine is probably effective through its cytotoxic effects (as a chain-terminating thymidine analogue) rather than its antiviral effects. An experimental approach using an yttrium 90–labeled or toxin-conjugated antibody to the IL-2 receptor appears promising but is not widely available. Patients with the chronic or smoldering form of ATL may be managed with an expectant approach: treat any infections, and watch and wait for signs of progression to acute disease.

Patients with HAM may obtain some benefit from the use of glucocorticoids to reduce inflammation. Antiretroviral regimens have not been effective. In one study, danazol (200 mg three times daily) produced significant neurologic improvement in five of six treated patients, with resolution of urinary incontinence in two cases, decreased spasticity in three, and restoration of the ability to walk after confinement to a wheelchair in two. Physical therapy and rehabilitation are important components of management.

FEATURES OF HTLV-II INFECTION

Epidemiology HTLV-II is endemic in certain Native American tribes and in Africa. It is generally considered to be a New World virus that was brought from Asia to the Americas 10,000–40,000 years ago during the migration of infected populations across the Bering land bridge. The mode of transmission of HTLV-II is probably the same as that of HTLV-I (see above). HTLV-II may be less readily transmitted sexually than HTLV-I.

Studies of large cohorts of injection drug users with serologic assays that reliably distinguish HTLV-I from HTLV-II indicated that the vast majority of HTLV-positive cohort members were infected with HTLV-II. The seroprevalence of HTLV in a cohort of 7841 injection drug users from drug treatment centers in Baltimore, Chicago, Los Angeles, New Jersey (Asbury Park and Trenton), New York City (Brooklyn and Harlem), Philadelphia, and San Antonio was 20.9%, with >97% of cases due to HTLV-II. The seroprevalence of HTLV-II was higher in the Southwest and the Midwest than in the Northeast. In contrast, the seroprevalence of HIV-1 was higher in the Northeast than in the Southwest or the Midwest. Approximately 3% of the cohort members were infected with both HTLV-II and HIV-1. The seroprevalence of HTLV-II increased linearly with age. Women were significantly more likely to be infected with HTLV-II than were men; the virus is thought to be more efficiently transmitted from male to female than from female to male.

Associated Diseases Although HTLV-II was isolated from a patient with a T cell variant of hairy cell leukemia, this virus has not been consistently associated with a particular disease and in fact has been thought of as "a virus searching for a disease." However, evidence is accumulating that HTLV-II may play a role in certain neurologic, hematologic, and dermatologic diseases. These data require confirmation, particularly in light of the previous confusion regarding the relative prevalences of HTLV-I and HTLV-II among injection drug users.

Prevention Avoidance of needle sharing, adherence to safe-sex practices, screening of blood (by assays for HTLV-I, which also detect HTLV-II), and avoidance of breast-feeding by infected women are important principles in the prevention of spread of HTLV-II.

HUMAN IMMUNODEFICIENCY VIRUS

HIV-1 and HIV-2 are members of the lentivirus subfamily of Retroviridae and are the only lentiviruses known to infect humans. The lentiviruses are slow-acting by comparison with viruses that cause acute infection (e.g., influenza virus) but not by comparison with other retroviruses. The features of acute primary infection with HIV resemble those of more classic acute infections. The characteristic chronicity of HIV disease is consistent with the designation *lentivirus*. For a detailed discussion of HIV, see Chap. 182.

FURTHER READINGS

GHEZ D et al: Neuropilin-1 is involved in human T-cell lymphotropic virus type 1 entry. J Virol 80:6844, 2006

KASHANCHI F, BRADY JN: Transcriptional and post-transcriptional gene regulation of HTLV-1. Oncogene 24:5938, 2005

LEE SM et al: HTLV-1 induced molecular mimicry in neurological disease. Curr Top Microbiol Immunol 296:125, 2005

MANEL N et al: HTLV-I tropism and envelope receptor. Oncogene 24:6016, 2005

MATSUOKA M, JEANG KT: Human T-cell leukaemia virus type 1 (HTLV-1) infectivity and cellular transformation. Nat Rev Cancer 7:270, 2007

PELOPONESE JM et al: Modulation of nuclear factor-κB by human T cell leukemia virus type 1 Tax protein. Immunol Res 34:1, 2006

PROIETTI FA et al: Global epidemiology of HTLV-I infection and associated diseases. Oncogene 24:6058, 2005

TAYLOR GP, MATSUOKA M: Natural history of adult T-cell leukemia/lymphoma and approaches to therapy. Oncogene 24:6047, 2005

182 Human Immunodeficiency Virus Disease: AIDS and Related Disorders

Anthony S. Fauci, H. Clifford Lane

AIDS was first recognized in the United States in the summer of 1981, when the U.S. Centers for Disease Control and Prevention (CDC) reported the unexplained occurrence of *Pneumocystis jiroveci* (formerly *P. carinii*) pneumonia in five previously healthy homosexual men in Los Angeles and of Kaposi's sarcoma (KS) with or without *P. jiroveci* pneumonia in 26 previously healthy homosexual men in New York and Los Angeles. Within months, the disease became recognized in male and female injection drug users (IDUs) and soon thereafter in recipients of blood transfusions and in hemophiliacs. As the epidemiologic pattern of the disease unfolded, it became clear that an infectious agent transmissible by sexual (homosexual and heterosexual) contact and blood or blood products was the most likely etiologic cause of the epidemic.

In 1983, human immunodeficiency virus (HIV) was isolated from a patient with lymphadenopathy, and by 1984 it was demonstrated clearly to be the causative agent of AIDS. In 1985, a sensitive enzyme-linked immunosorbent assay (ELISA) was developed, which led to an appreciation of the scope and evolution of the HIV epidemic at first in the United States and other developed nations and ultimately among developing nations throughout the world (see below). The staggering worldwide evolution of the HIV pandemic has been matched by an explosion of information in the areas of HIV virology, pathogenesis (both immunologic and virologic), treatment of HIV disease, treatment and prophylaxis of the opportunistic diseases associated with HIV infection, prevention of infection, and vaccine development. The information flow related to HIV disease is enormous and continues to expand, and it has become almost impossible for the health care generalist to stay abreast of the literature. The purpose of this chapter is to present the most current information available on the scope of the epidemic; on its pathogenesis, treatment, and prevention; and on prospects for vaccine development. Above all, the aim is to provide a solid scientific basis and practical clinical guidelines for a state-of-the-art approach to the HIV-infected patient.

DEFINITION

The current CDC classification system for HIV-infected adolescents and adults categorizes persons on the basis of clinical conditions associated with HIV infection and CD4+ T lymphocyte counts. The system is based on three ranges of CD4+ T lymphocyte counts and three clinical categories and is represented by a matrix of nine mutually exclusive categories (Tables 182-1 and 182-2). Using this system, any HIV-infected individual with a CD4+ T cell count of <200/μL has AIDS by definition, regardless of the presence of symptoms or opportunistic diseases (Table 182-1). Once individuals have had a clinical condition in category B, their disease classification cannot be reverted back to category A, even if the condition resolves; the same holds true for category C in relation to category B.

The definition of AIDS is indeed complex and comprehensive and was established not for the practical care of patients, but for surveillance purposes. Thus, the clinician should not focus on whether or not the patient fulfills the strict definition of AIDS, but should view HIV disease as a spectrum ranging from primary infection, with or without the acute syndrome, to the asymptomatic stage, to advanced disease (see below).

ETIOLOGIC AGENT

The etiologic agent of AIDS is HIV, which belongs to the family of human retroviruses (Retroviridae) and the subfamily of lentiviruses (Chap. 181). Nononcogenic lentiviruses cause disease in other animal species, including sheep, horses, goats, cattle, cats, and monkeys. The four recognized human retroviruses belong to two distinct groups: the human T lymphotropic viruses (HTLV)-I and HTLV-II, which are transforming retroviruses; and the human immunodeficiency viruses, HIV-1 and HIV-2, which cause cytopathic effects either directly or indirectly (see below and Chap. 181). The most common cause of HIV disease throughout the world, and certainly in the United States, is HIV-1, which comprises several subtypes with different geographic distributions (see below). HIV-2 was first identified in 1986 in West African patients and was originally confined to West Africa. However, a number of cases that can be traced to West Africa or to sexual contacts with West Africans have been identified throughout the world. Both HIV-1 and HIV-2 are zoonotic infections. The *Pan troglodytes troglodytes* species of chimpanzees has been established as the natural reservoir of HIV-1 and the most likely source of original human infection. HIV-2 is more closely related phylogenetically to the simian immunodeficiency virus (SIV) found in sooty mangabeys than it is to HIV-1. The taxonomic relationship among primate lentiviruses is shown in Fig. 182-1.

TABLE 182-1 1993 REVISED CLASSIFICATION SYSTEM FOR HIV INFECTION AND EXPANDED AIDS SURVEILLANCE CASE DEFINITION FOR ADOLESCENTS AND ADULTS[a]

	Clinical Categories		
CD4+ T Cell Categories	A Asymptomatic, Acute (Primary) HIV or PGL[b]	B Symptomatic, Not A or C Conditions	C AIDS-Indicator Conditions
>500/μL	A1	B1	C1
200–499/μL	A2	B2	C2
<200/μL	A3	B3	C3

[a]The shaded areas indicate the expanded AIDS surveillance case definition.
[b]PGL, progressive generalized lymphadenopathy.
Source: MMWR 42(No. RR-17), December 18, 1992.

TABLE 182-2 CLINICAL CATEGORIES OF HIV INFECTION

Category A: Consists of one or more of the conditions listed below in an adolescent or adult (>13 years) with documented HIV infection. Conditions listed in categories B and C must not have occurred.
- Asymptomatic HIV infection
- Persistent generalized lymphadenopathy
- Acute (primary) HIV infection with accompanying illness or history of acute HIV infection

Category B: Consists of symptomatic conditions in an HIV-infected adolescent or adult that are not included among conditions listed in clinical category C and that meet at least one of the following criteria: (1) The conditions are attributed to HIV infection or are indicative of a defect in cell-mediated immunity; or (2) the conditions are considered by physicians to have a clinical course or to require management that is complicated by HIV infection. Examples include, but are not limited to, the following:
- Bacillary angiomatosis
- Candidiasis, oropharyngeal (thrush)
- Candidiasis, vulvovaginal; persistent, frequent, or poorly responsive to therapy
- Cervical dysplasia (moderate or severe)/cervical carcinoma in situ
- Constitutional symptoms, such as fever (38.5°C) or diarrhea lasting >1 month
- Hairy leukoplakia, oral
- Herpes zoster (shingles), involving at least two distinct episodes or more than one dermatome
- Idiopathic thrombocytopenic purpura
- Listeriosis
- Pelvic inflammatory disease, particularly if complicated by tuboovarian abscess
- Peripheral neuropathy

Category C: Conditions listed in the AIDS surveillance case definition.
- Candidiasis of bronchi, trachea, or lungs
- Candidiasis, esophageal
- Cervical cancer, invasive[a]
- Coccidioidomycosis, disseminated or extrapulmonary
- Cryptococcosis, extrapulmonary
- Cryptosporidiosis, chronic intestinal (>1 month's duration)
- Cytomegalovirus disease (other than liver, spleen, or nodes)
- Cytomegalovirus retinitis (with loss of vision)
- Encephalopathy, HIV-related
- Herpes simplex: chronic ulcer(s) (>1 month's duration); or bronchitis, pneumonia, or esophagitis
- Histoplasmosis, disseminated or extrapulmonary
- Isosporiasis, chronic intestinal (>1 month's duration)
- Kaposi's sarcoma
- Lymphoma, Burkitt's (or equivalent term)
- Lymphoma, primary, of brain
- *Mycobacterium avium* complex or *M. kansasii*, disseminated or extrapulmonary
- *Mycobacterium tuberculosis*, any site (pulmonary[a] or extrapulmonary)
- *Mycobacterium*, other species or unidentified species, disseminated or extrapulmonary
- *Pneumocystis jiroveci* pneumonia
- Pneumonia, recurrent[a]
- Progressive multifocal leukoencephalopathy
- *Salmonella* septicemia, recurrent
- Toxoplasmosis of brain
- Wasting syndrome due to HIV

[a]Added in the 1993 expansion of the AIDS surveillance case definition.
Source: MMWR 42(No. RR-17), December 18, 1992.

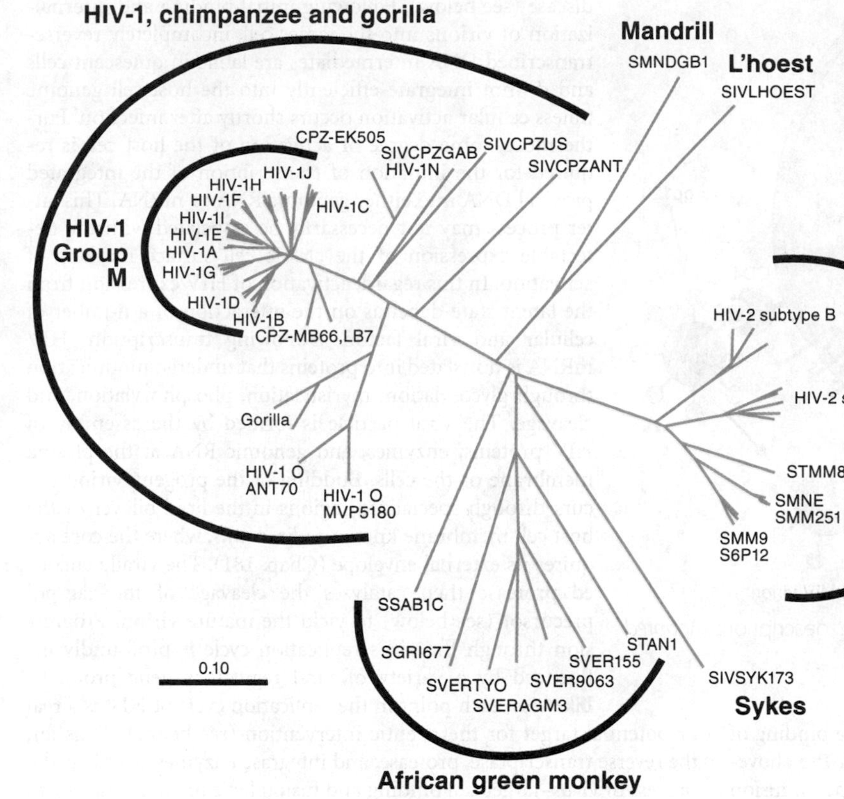

FIGURE 182-1 A phylogenetic tree, based on the complete genomes of primate immunodeficiency viruses. The scale at the bottom (0.10) indicates a 10% difference at the nucleotide level. *(Prepared by Brian Foley, PhD, of the HIV Sequence Database, Theoretical Biology and Biophysics Group, Los Alamos National Laboratory.)*

MORPHOLOGY OF HIV

Electron microscopy shows that the HIV virion is an icosahedral structure (Fig. 182-2*A*) containing numerous external spikes formed by the two major envelope proteins, the external gp120 and the transmembrane gp41. The virion buds from the surface of the infected cell and incorporates a variety of host proteins, including major histocompatibility complex (MHC) class I and II antigens (Chap. 309), into its lipid bilayer. The structure of HIV-1 is schematically diagrammed in Fig. 182-2*B* (Chap. 181).

REPLICATION CYCLE OF HIV

HIV is an RNA virus whose hallmark is the reverse transcription of its genomic RNA to DNA by the enzyme *reverse transcriptase*. The replication cycle of HIV begins with the high-affinity binding of the gp120 protein via a portion of its V1 region near the N terminus to its receptor on the host cell surface, the CD4 molecule (Fig. 182-3). The CD4 molecule is a 55-kDa protein found predominantly on a subset of T lymphocytes that are responsible for helper function in the immune system (Chap. 308). It is also expressed on the surface of monocytes/macrophages and dendritic/Langerhans cells. Once gp120 binds to CD4, the gp120 undergoes a conformational change that facilitates binding to one of a group of co-receptors. The two major co-receptors for HIV-1 are CCR5 and CXCR4. Both receptors belong to the family of seven-transmembrane-domain G protein–coupled cellular receptors, and the use of one or the other or both receptors by the virus for entry into the cell is an important determinant of the cellular tropism of the virus (see below for details). Certain dendritic cells express a diversity of C-type lectin receptors on their surface, one of which is called *DC-SIGN*, that also bind with high affinity to the HIV gp120 envelope protein, allowing the dendritic cell to facilitate the binding of virus to the CD4+ T cell upon

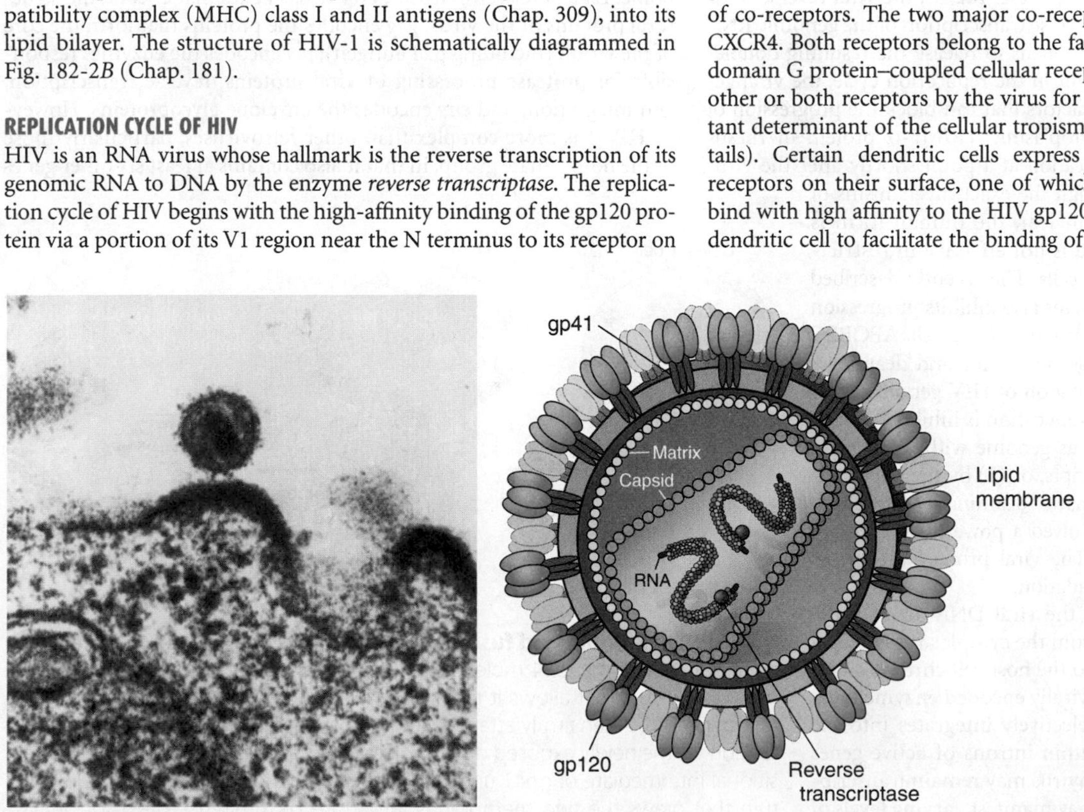

FIGURE 182-2 *A.* Electron micrograph of HIV. Figure illustrates a typical virion following budding from the surface of a CD4+ T lymphocyte, together with two additional incomplete virions in the process of budding from the cell membrane. ***B.*** Structure of HIV-1, including the gp120 outer membrane, gp41 transmembrane components of the envelope, genomic RNA, enzyme reverse transcriptase, p18(17) inner membrane (matrix), and p24 core protein (capsid) (copyright by George V. Kelvin). *(Adapted from RC Gallo: Sci Am 256:46, 1987.)*

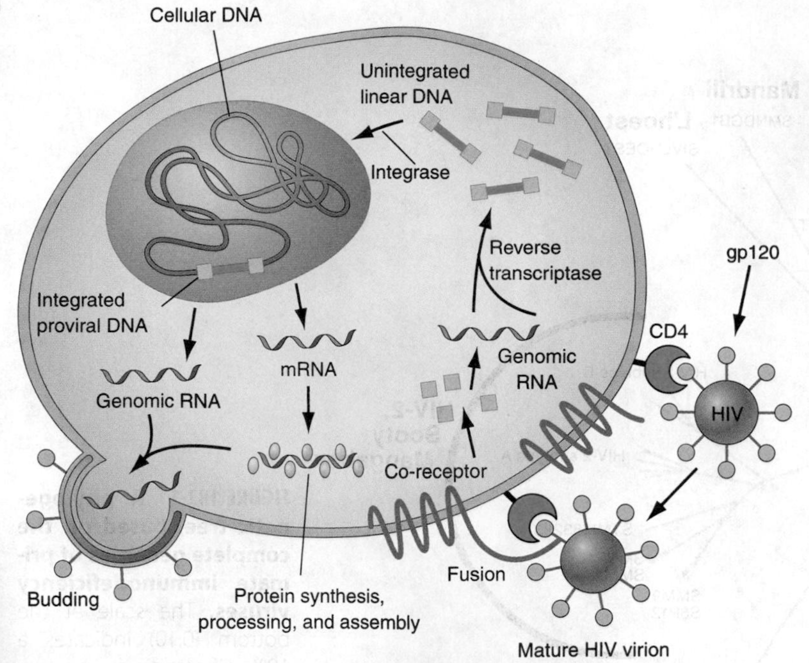

FIGURE 182-3 The replication cycle of HIV. See text for description. *(Adapted from Fauci, 1996.)*

Cellular activation plays an important role in the replication cycle of HIV and is critical to the pathogenesis of HIV disease (see below). Following initial binding and internalization of virions into the target cell, incompletely reverse-transcribed DNA intermediates are labile in quiescent cells and do not integrate efficiently into the host cell genome unless cellular activation occurs shortly after infection. Furthermore, some degree of activation of the host cell is required for the initiation of transcription of the integrated proviral DNA into either genomic RNA or mRNA. This latter process may not necessarily be associated with the detectable expression of the classic cell surface markers of activation. In this regard, activation of HIV expression from the latent state depends on the interaction of a number of cellular and viral factors. Following transcription, HIV mRNA is translated into proteins that undergo modification through glycosylation, myristylation, phosphorylation, and cleavage. The viral particle is formed by the assembly of HIV proteins, enzymes, and genomic RNA at the plasma membrane of the cells. Budding of the progeny virion occurs through specialized regions in the lipid bilayer of the host cell membrane known as *lipid rafts*, where the core acquires its external envelope (Chap. 181). The virally encoded protease then catalyzes the cleavage of the gag-pol precursor (see below) to yield the mature virion. Progression through the virus replication cycle is profoundly influenced by a variety of viral regulatory gene products. Likewise, each point in the replication cycle of HIV is a real or potential target for therapeutic intervention (see below). Thus far, the reverse transcriptase, protease, and integrase enzymes as well as the process of virus–target cell binding and fusion have proven clinically to be susceptible to pharmacologic disruption (see below). Inhibitors of the maturation process of virions during the latter phase of the replication cycle are currently being evaluated in clinical trials.

engagement of dendritic cells with CD4+ T cells. Following binding of the envelope protein to the CD4 molecule associated with the above-mentioned conformational change in the viral envelope gp120, fusion with the host cell membrane occurs via the newly exposed gp41 molecule penetrating the plasma membrane of the target cell and then coiling upon itself to bring the virion and target cell together. Following fusion, the preintegration complex, composed of viral RNA and viral enzymes and surrounded by a capsid protein coat, is released into the cytoplasm of the target cell (Fig. 182-4). As the preintegration complex traverses the cytoplasm to reach the nucleus (Fig. 182-3), the viral reverse transcriptase enzyme catalyzes the reverse transcription of the genomic RNA into DNA, and the protein coat opens to release the resulting double-stranded HIV-DNA. At this point in the replication cycle, the viral genome is vulnerable to cellular factors that can block the progression of infection. In particular, the cytoplasmic TRIM5-α protein in rhesus macaque cells blocks SIV replication at a point shortly after the virus fuses with the host cell. Although the exact mechanisms of action of TRIM5-α remain unclear, the human form is inhibited by cyclophilin A and is not effective in restricting HIV replication in human cells. The recently described APOBEC family of cellular proteins also inhibits progression of virus infection after virus has entered the cell. APOBEC proteins bind to nascent reverse transcripts and deaminate viral cytidine, causing hypermutation of HIV genomes. It is still not clear whether (1) viral replication is inhibited by the binding of APOBEC to the virus genome with subsequent accumulation of reverse transcripts, or (2) by the hypermutations caused by the enzymatic deaminase activity of APOBEC proteins. HIV has evolved a powerful strategy to protect itself from APOBEC. The viral protein Vif targets APOBEC for proteasomal degradation.

With activation of the cell, the viral DNA accesses the nuclear pore and is exported from the cytoplasm to the nucleus, where it is integrated into the host cell chromosomes through the action of another virally encoded enzyme, *integrase.* HIV provirus (DNA) selectively integrates into the nuclear DNA preferentially within introns of active genes and regional hotspots. This provirus may remain transcriptionally inactive (latent) or it may manifest varying levels of gene expression, up to active production of virus.

HIV GENOME

Figure 182-5 illustrates schematically the arrangement of the HIV genome. Like other retroviruses, HIV-1 has genes that encode the structural proteins of the virus: *gag* encodes the proteins that form the core of the virion (including p24 antigen); *pol* encodes the enzymes responsible for protease processing of viral proteins, reverse transcription, and integration; and *env* encodes the envelope glycoproteins. However, HIV-1 is more complex than other retroviruses, particularly those of the nonprimate group, in that it also contains at least six other genes

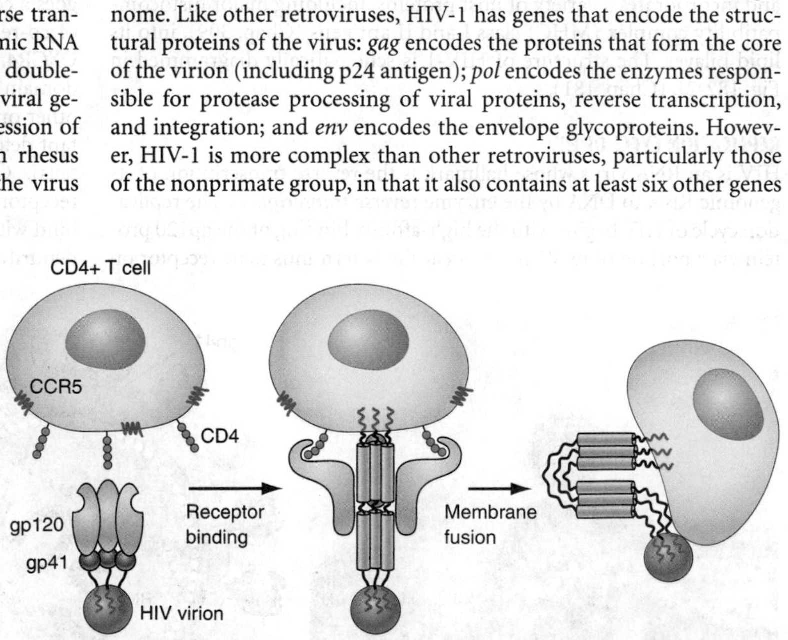

FIGURE 182-4 Binding and fusion of HIV-1 with its target cell. HIV-1 binds to its target cell via the CD4 molecule, leading to a conformational change in the gp120 molecule that allows it to bind to the co-receptor CCR5 (for R5-using viruses). The virus then firmly attaches to the host cell membrane in a coiled-spring fashion via the newly exposed gp41 molecule. Virus-cell fusion occurs as the transitional intermediate of gp41 undergoes further changes to form a hairpin structure that draws the two membranes into close proximity (see text for details). *(Adapted from D Montefiori, JP Moore: Science 283:336, 1999; with permission.)*

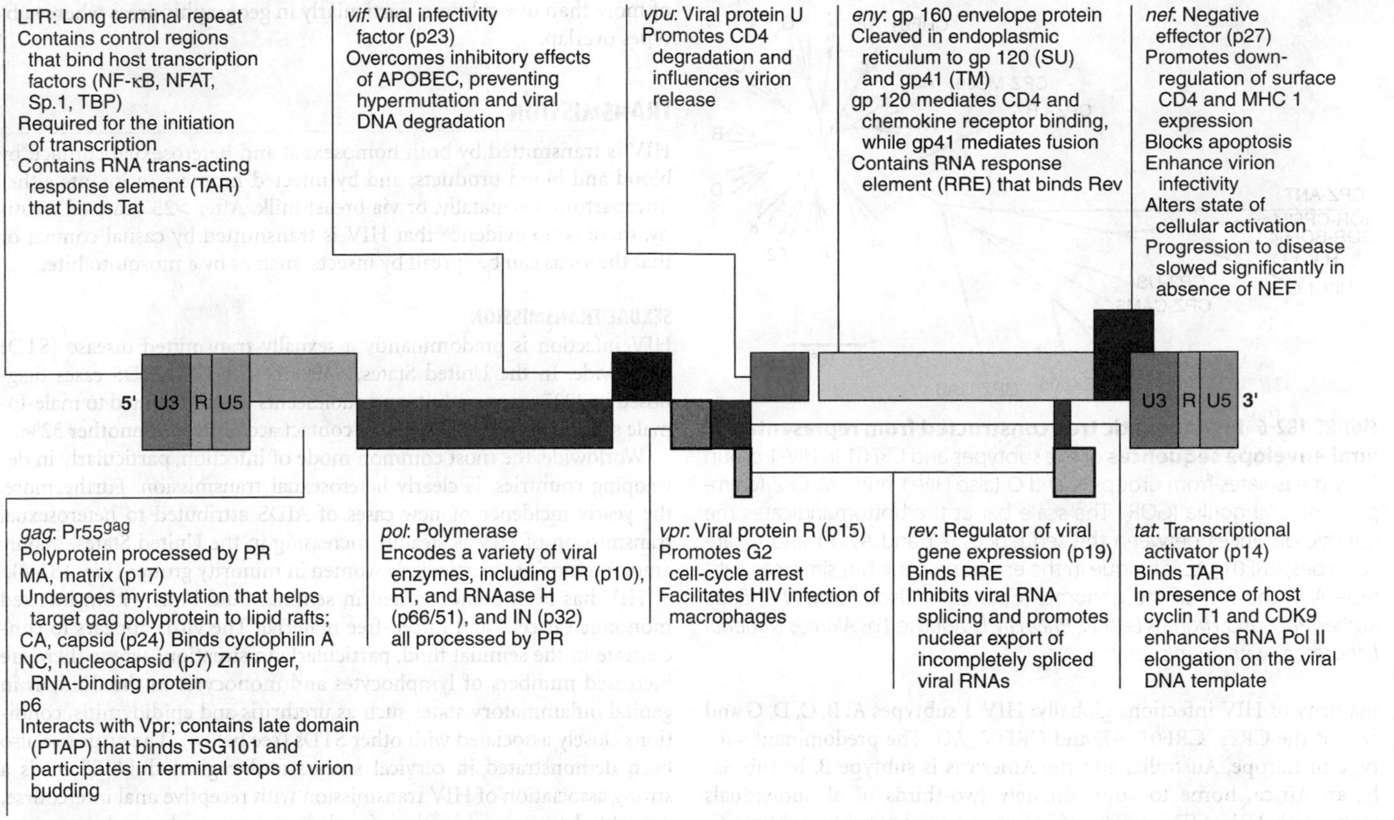
LTR: Long terminal repeat
Contains control regions that bind host transcription factors (NF-κB, NFAT, Sp.1, TBP)
Required for the initiation of transcription
Contains RNA trans-acting response element (TAR) that binds Tat
vif: Viral infectivity factor (p23)
Overcomes inhibitory effects of APOBEC, preventing hypermutation and viral DNA degradation
vpu: Viral protein U
Promotes CD4 degradation and influences virion release
eny: gp 160 envelope protein
Cleaved in endoplasmic reticulum to gp 120 (SU) and gp41 (TM)
gp 120 mediates CD4 and chemokine receptor binding, while gp41 mediates fusion
Contains RNA response element (RRE) that binds Rev
nef: Negative effector (p27)
Promotes down-regulation of surface CD4 and MHC 1 expression
Blocks apoptosis
Enhance virion infectivity
Alters state of cellular activation
Progression to disease slowed significantly in absence of NEF
5'
U3
R
U5
U3
R
U5
3'
gag: Pr55gag
Polyprotein processed by PR
MA, matrix (p17)
Undergoes myristylation that helps target gag polyprotein to lipid rafts;
CA, capsid (p24) Binds cyclophilin A
NC, nucleocapsid (p7) Zn finger, RNA-binding protein
p6
Interacts with Vpr; contains late domain (PTAP) that binds TSG101 and participates in terminal stops of virion budding
pol: Polymerase
Encodes a variety of viral enzymes, including PR (p10), RT, and RNAase H (p66/51), and IN (p32) all processed by PR
vpr: Viral protein R (p15)
Promotes G2 cell-cycle arrest
Facilitates HIV infection of macrophages
rev: Regulator of viral gene expression (p19)
Binds RRE
Inhibits viral RNA splicing and promotes nuclear export of incompletely spliced viral RNAs
tat: Transcriptional activator (p14)
Binds TAR
In presence of host cyclin T1 and CDK9 enhances RNA Pol II elongation on the viral DNA template

FIGURE 182-5 Organization of the genome of the HIV provirus together with a summary description of its nine genes encoding 15 proteins. *(Adapted from Greene and Peterlin.)*

(*tat, rev, nef, vif, vpr*, and *vpu*), which code for proteins involved in the modification of the host cell to enhance virus growth and the regulation of viral gene expression (Chap. 181). Several of these proteins are thought to play a role in the pathogenesis of HIV disease; their various functions are listed in Fig. 182-5. Flanking these genes are the long terminal repeats (LTRs), which contain regulatory elements involved in gene expression (Fig. 182-5). The major difference between the genomes of HIV-1 and HIV-2 is the fact that HIV-2 lacks the *vpu* gene and has a *vpx* gene not contained in HIV-1.

MOLECULAR HETEROGENEITY OF HIV-1

Molecular analyses of HIV isolates reveal varying levels of sequence diversity over all regions of the viral genome. For example, the degree of difference in the coding sequences of the viral envelope protein ranges from a few percent (very close, between isolates from the same infected individual) to 50% (extreme diversity, between isolates from the different groups of HIV-1, M, N, and O; see below). The changes tend to cluster in hypervariable regions. HIV can evolve by several means, including simple base substitution, insertions and deletions, recombination, and gain and loss of glycosylation sites. HIV sequence diversity arises directly from the limited fidelity of the reverse transcriptase. The balance of immune pressure and functional constraints on proteins influences the regional level of variation within proteins. For example, Envelope, which is exposed on the surface of the virion and is under immune selective pressure from both antibodies and cytolytic T lymphocytes, is extremely variable, with clusters of mutations in hypervariable domains. In contrast, Reverse Transcriptase, with important enzymatic functions, is relatively conserved, particularly around the active site. The extraordinary variability of HIV-1 is in marked contrast to the relative stability of HTLV-I and -II.

There are three groups of HIV-1: group M (major), which is responsible for most of the infections in the world; group O (outlier), a relatively rare viral form found originally in Cameroon, Gabon, and France; and group N, first identified in a Cameroonian woman with AIDS; only a few cases of the latter have been identified. Among primate lentiviruses, HIV-1 is most closely related to viruses isolated from chimpanzees and gorillas. The chimpanzee subspecies *Pan troglodytes troglodytes* has been established to be the natural reservoir of the HIV-1 M and N groups. The HIV-1 O group is most closely related to viruses found in Cameroonian gorillas. The M group comprises nine subtypes, or *clades*, designated A, B, C, D, F, G, H, J, and K, as well as a growing number of major and minor circulating recombinant forms (CRFs). CRFs are generated by infection of an individual with two subtypes that then recombine and create a virus with a selective advantage. These CRFs range from highly prevalent forms such as the AE virus, CRF01_AE, which is predominant in southeast Asia and often referred to simply as E, despite the fact that the parental E virus has never been found, and CRF02_AG from west and central Africa, to a large number of CRFs that are relatively rare. The subtypes and CRFs create the major lineages of the M group of HIV-1. The picture has been complicated somewhat when it was found that some subtypes are not equidistant from one another, while others contained sequences so diverse that they could not properly be considered to be the same subtype. Thus, the term *sub-subtype* was introduced, and subtypes A and F are now subdivided into A1 and A2, F1 and F2. It has also been argued that subtypes B and D are really too close to be separate subtypes and should be considered sub-subtypes; it was decided, however, not to increase the confusion by renaming the clades (Fig. 182-6).

The global patterns of HIV-1 variation likely result from accidents of viral trafficking. Subtype B viruses, which now differ by up to 17% in their *env* coding sequences, are the overwhelmingly predominant viruses seen in the United States, Canada, certain countries in South America, western Europe, and Australia. Other subtypes are also present in these countries to varying degrees. It is thought that, purely by chance, subtype B was seeded into the United States in the late 1970s, thereby establishing an overwhelming founder effect. Subtype C viruses (of the M group) are the most common form worldwide; many countries have co-circulating viral subtypes that are giving rise to new CRFs. Figure 182-7 schematically diagrams the worldwide distribution of HIV-1 subtypes by region. Seven strains account for the

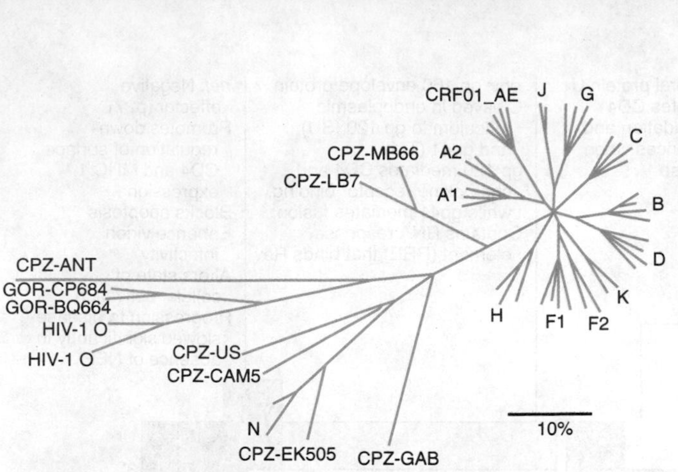

FIGURE 182-6 Phylogenetic tree constructed from representative viral envelope sequences of the subtypes and CRF01 in HIV-1 group M, some isolates from groups N and O (also HIV-1 human), CPZ (chimpanzee), and gorilla (GOR). The scale bar at the bottom indicates the genetic distances between the sequences. A1 and A2, F1 and F2 are subtypes; CRF01_AE is unique in the envelope gene but similar to subtype A in the rest of the genome. *(Courtesy of Brian Foley, PhD, Bette Korber, PhD, and Thomas Leitner, PhD, HIV Database, Los Alamos National Laboratory; with permission.)*

majority of HIV infections globally: HIV-1 subtypes A, B, C, D, G and two of the CRFs, CRF01_AE and CRF02_AG. The predominant subtype in Europe, Australia, and the Americas is subtype B. In sub-Saharan Africa, home to approximately two-thirds of all individuals living with HIV/AIDS, >50% of infections are caused by subtype C, with smaller proportions of infections caused by subtype A, subtype G, CRF02_AG, and other subtypes and recombinants. In Asia, HIV-1 isolates of the CRF01_AE lineage and subtypes C and B predominate. CRF01_AE accounts for most infections in south and southeast Asia, while subtype C is prevalent in India (see "HIV Infection and AIDS Worldwide," below). Sequence analyses of HIV-1 isolates from infected individuals indicate that recombination among viruses of different clades likely occurs as a result of infection of an individual with viruses of more than one subtype, particularly in geographic areas where subtypes overlap.

TRANSMISSION

HIV is transmitted by both homosexual and heterosexual contact; by blood and blood products; and by infected mothers to infants either intrapartum, perinatally, or via breast milk. After >25 years of scrutiny, there is no evidence that HIV is transmitted by casual contact or that the virus can be spread by insects, such as by a mosquito bite.

SEXUAL TRANSMISSION

HIV infection is predominantly a sexually transmitted disease (STD) worldwide. In the United States, ~49% of the HIV/AIDS cases diagnosed in 2005 among adults and adolescents were attributed to male-to-male sexual contact. Heterosexual contact accounted for another 32%.

Worldwide, the most common mode of infection, particularly in developing countries, is clearly heterosexual transmission. Furthermore, the yearly incidence of new cases of AIDS attributed to heterosexual transmission of HIV is steadily increasing in the United States, mainly among minorities, particularly women in minority groups (Fig. 182-8).

HIV has been demonstrated in seminal fluid both within infected mononuclear cells and in cell-free material. The virus appears to concentrate in the seminal fluid, particularly in situations where there are increased numbers of lymphocytes and monocytes in the fluid, as in genital inflammatory states such as urethritis and epididymitis, conditions closely associated with other STDs (see below). The virus has also been demonstrated in cervical smears and vaginal fluid. There is a strong association of HIV transmission with receptive anal intercourse, probably because only a thin, fragile rectal mucosal membrane separates the deposited semen from potentially susceptible cells in and beneath the mucosa and trauma may be associated with anal intercourse. Anal douching and sexual practices that traumatize the rectal mucosa also increase the likelihood of infection. It is likely that anal intercourse provides at least two modalities of infection: (1) direct inoculation into blood in cases of traumatic tears in the mucosa; and (2) infection of susceptible target cells, such as Langerhans cells, in the mucosal layer in the absence of trauma (see below). Although the vaginal mucosa is sev-

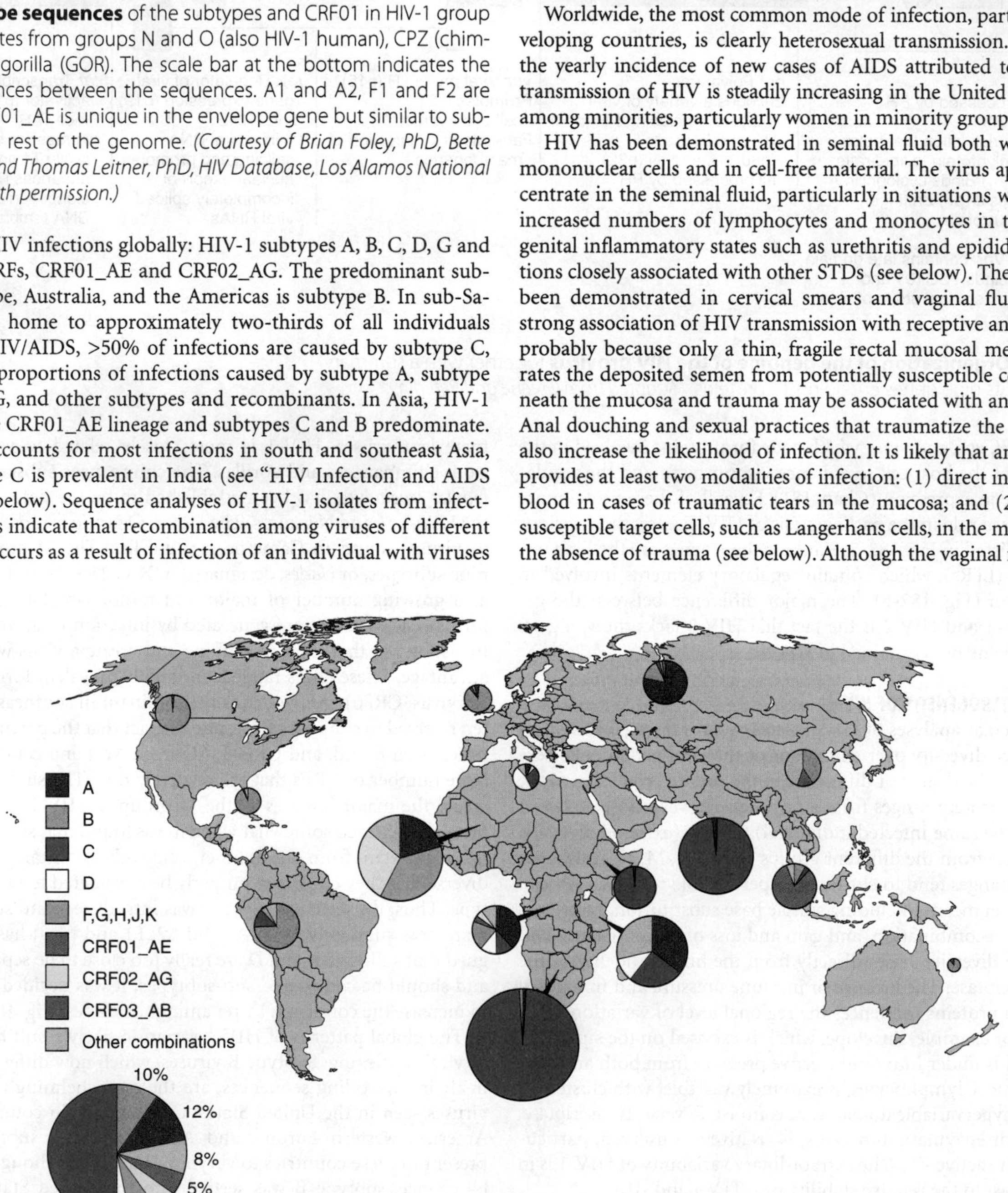

FIGURE 182-7 Geographic distribution of HIV-1 subtypes and recombinants. The prevalence of HIV-1 genetic subtypes varies by geographic region. The proportions of subtypes in different regions are indicated by pie charts. *(From J Hemelaar et al: AIDS 20:W13, 2006.)*

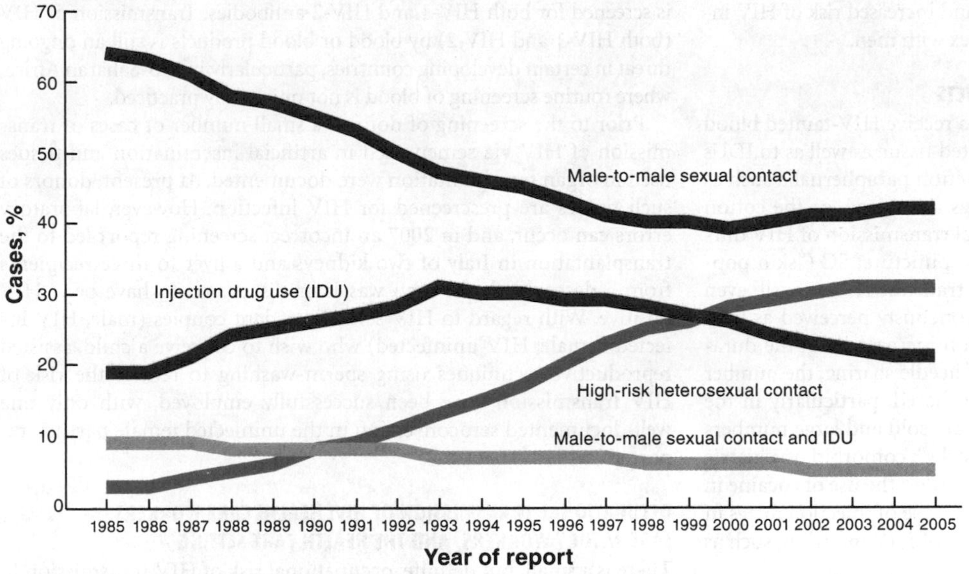

FIGURE 182-8 AIDS cases among U.S. adults and adolescents by exposure category and year of diagnosis. The proportion of AIDS cases attributed to heterosexual contact with a person known to have or at high risk for HIV infection (high-risk heterosexual) increased from 3% in 1985 to 31% in 2005. *[From The Centers for Disease Control and Prevention (CDC).]*

eral layers thicker than the rectal mucosa and less likely to be traumatized during intercourse, it is clear that the virus can be transmitted to either partner through vaginal intercourse. Studies in the United States and Europe have found that male-to-female HIV transmission is usually more efficient than female-to-male transmission, but small numbers of HIV-positive female index partners limit conclusive sex-specific estimates of transmission probabilities per sex act. The differences in reported transmission rates between men and women may be due in part to the prolonged exposure to infected seminal fluid of the vaginal and cervical mucosa, as well as the endometrium (when semen enters through the cervical os). By comparison, the penis and urethral orifice are exposed relatively briefly to infected vaginal fluid. Among various cofactors examined in studies of heterosexual HIV transmission, the presence of other sexually transmitted diseases (STDs; see below) has been strongly associated with HIV transmission. In this regard, there is a close association between genital ulcerations and transmission, from the standpoints of both susceptibility to infection and infectivity. Infections with microorganisms such as *Treponema pallidum* (Chap. 162), *Haemophilus ducreyi* (Chap. 139), and herpes simplex virus (HSV; Chap. 172) are important causes of genital ulcerations linked to transmission of HIV. In addition, pathogens responsible for nonulcerative inflammatory STDs such as those caused by *Chlamydia trachomatis* (Chap. 169), *Neisseria gonorrhoeae* (Chap. 137), and *Trichomonas vaginalis* (Chap. 208) are also associated with an increased risk of transmission of HIV infection. Bacterial vaginosis, an infection related to sexual behavior, but not strictly an STD, may also be linked to an increased risk of transmission of HIV infection. Several studies suggest that treating other STDs and genital tract syndromes may help prevent transmission of HIV. This effect is most prominent in populations in which the prevalence of HIV infection is relatively low. In studies conducted in Uganda, the chief predictor of heterosexual transmission of HIV was the level of plasma viremia. In a cohort of couples in which one partner was HIV-infected and one was initially uninfected, the mean serum HIV RNA level was significantly higher among HIV-infected subjects whose partners seroconverted than among those whose partners did not seroconvert. In fact transmission was rare when the infected partner had a plasma level of <1500 copies of HIV RNA per milliliter. The rate of HIV transmission per coital act was highest during the early stage of HIV infection when plasma HIV RNA levels are highest and in advanced disease as the viral set point increases (Fig. 182-9).

A number of studies have indicated that male *circumcision* is associated with a lower risk of HIV infection among men. This difference may be due to increased susceptibility of uncircumcised men to ulcerative STDs, as well as other factors such as microtrauma to the foreskin and glans penis. In addition, the highly vascularized inner foreskin tissue contains a high density of Langerhans cells as well as increased numbers of CD4+ T cells, macrophages, and other cellular targets for HIV. Finally, the moist environment under the foreskin may promote the presence or persistence of microbial flora that, via inflammatory changes, may lead to even higher concentrations of target cells for HIV in the foreskin. In some studies the use of oral contraceptives was associated with an increase in incidence of HIV infection over and above that which might be expected by not using a condom for birth control. This phenomenon may be due to drug-induced changes in the cervical mucosa, rendering it more vulnerable to penetration by the virus. Adolescent girls might also be more susceptible to infection upon exposure due to the properties of an immature genital tract with increased cervical ectopy or exposed columnar epithelium.

Oral sex is a much less efficient mode of transmission of HIV than is receptive anal intercourse. A number of studies have reported that the incidence of transmission of infection by oral sex among couples discordant for HIV was extremely low. However, there have been reports of documented HIV transmission resulting solely from receptive fellatio and insertive cunnilingus. Therefore, the assumption that receptive oral sex is completely safe is not warranted. The association of alcohol consumption and illicit drug use with unsafe sexual behavior, both homosexual and heterosexual, leads to an increased risk of sexual transmission of HIV. Methamphetamine ("crystal meth," "tina") and other so-called club drugs (e.g., ecstasy, ketamine, and gamma hydroxybutyrate), sometimes taken in conjunction with sildenafil (Viagra) or related drugs have

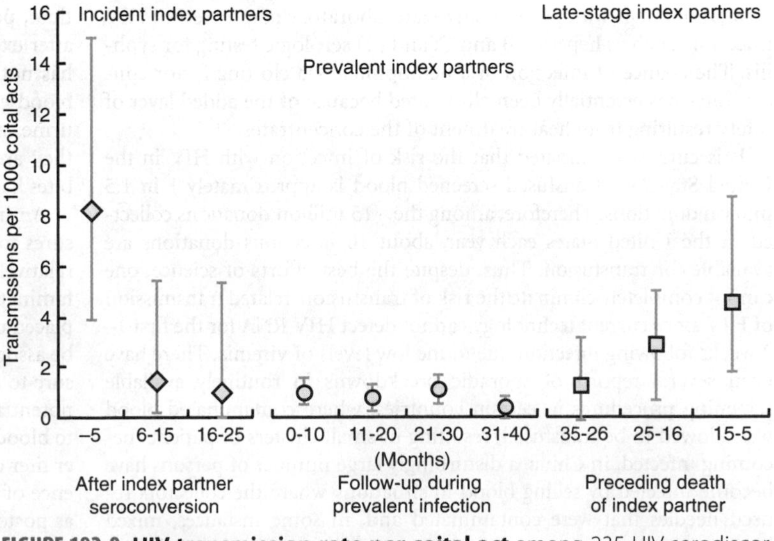

FIGURE 182-9 HIV transmission rate per coital act among 235 HIV serodiscordant couples in Uganda, and 95% confidence intervals, by follow-up interval. The risk of HIV transmission was highest during early-stage and late-stage infection. *(From Wawer et al.)*

been associated with risky sexual practices and increased risk of HIV infection, particularly among men who have sex with men.

TRANSMISSION BY BLOOD AND BLOOD PRODUCTS

HIV can be transmitted to individuals who receive HIV-tainted blood transfusions, blood products, or transplanted tissue as well as to IDUs who are exposed to HIV while sharing injection paraphernalia such as needles, syringes, the water in which drugs are mixed, or the cotton through which drugs are filtered. Parenteral transmission of HIV during injection drug use does not require IV puncture; SC ("skin popping") or IM ("muscling") injections can transmit HIV as well, even though these behaviors are sometimes erroneously perceived as low-risk. Among IDUs, the risk of HIV infection increases with the duration of injection drug use; the frequency of needle sharing; the number of partners with whom paraphernalia are shared, particularly in the setting of "shooting galleries" where drugs are sold and large numbers of IDUs may share a limited number of "works"; comorbid psychiatric conditions such as antisocial personality disorder; the use of cocaine in injectable form or smoked as "crack"; and the use of injection drugs in a geographic location with a high prevalence of HIV infection, such as certain inner-city areas in the United States.

The first transfusion-associated cases of AIDS were reported in 1982, and by the end of 2005, >9300 individuals in the United States who survived the illness for which they received HIV-contaminated blood transfusions, blood components, or transplanted tissue had developed AIDS. Virtually all these cases were due to HIV infection prior to the spring of 1985, when mandatory testing of donated blood for HIV-1 was initiated. It is estimated that 90–100% of individuals who were exposed to HIV-contaminated products became infected. Transfusions of whole blood, packed red blood cells, platelets, leukocytes, and plasma are all capable of transmitting HIV infection. In contrast, hyperimmune γ globulin, hepatitis B immune globulin, plasma-derived hepatitis B vaccine, and Rh_0 immune globulin have not been associated with transmission of HIV infection. The procedures involved in processing these products either inactivate or remove the virus.

In addition to the above, an estimated 8000–10,000 individuals in the United States with hemophilia or other clotting disorders were infected with HIV by receipt of HIV-contaminated fresh-frozen plasma or concentrates of clotting factors; by the end of 2005, >5400 of these individuals had developed AIDS. Currently, in the United States and in most developed countries, the following measures have made the risk of transmission of HIV infection by transfused blood or blood products extremely small: (1) the screening of all blood for HIV nucleic acid, p24 antigen, and/or anti-HIV antibodies; (2) the self-deferral of donors on the basis of risk behavior; (3) the screening out of HIV-negative individuals with positive surrogate laboratory parameters of HIV infection, such as hepatitis B and C; and (4) serologic testing for syphilis. The chance of infection of a hemophiliac via clotting factor concentrates has essentially been eliminated because of the added layer of safety resulting from heat treatment of the concentrates.

It is currently estimated that the risk of infection with HIV in the United States via transfused screened blood is approximately 1 in 1.5 million donations. Therefore, among the ~15 million donations collected in the United States each year, about 10 infectious donations are available for transfusion. Thus, despite the best efforts of science, one cannot completely eliminate the risk of transfusion-related transmission of HIV since current technology cannot detect HIV RNA for the first 1–2 weeks following infection due to the low levels of viremia. There have been several reports of sporadic breakdowns in routinely available screening procedures in certain countries, where contaminated blood was allowed to be transfused, resulting in small clusters of patients becoming infected. In China, a disturbingly large number of persons have become infected by selling blood in situations where the collectors reused needles that were contaminated and, in some instances, mixed blood products from a number of individuals, separated the plasma, and reinfused red blood cells back into individual donors.

There have been no reported cases of transmission of HIV-2 in the United States via donated blood or tissues, and, currently, donated blood is screened for both HIV-1 and HIV-2 antibodies. Transmission of HIV (both HIV-1 and HIV-2) by blood or blood products is still an ongoing threat in certain developing countries, particularly in sub-Saharan Africa, where routine screening of blood is not universally practiced.

Prior to the screening of donors, a small number of cases of transmission of HIV via semen used in artificial insemination and tissues used in organ transplantation were documented. At present, donors of such tissues are prescreened for HIV infection. However, laboratory errors can occur, and in 2007 an incorrect screening report led to the transplantation in Italy of two kidneys and a liver to three recipients from a deceased donor who was later discovered to have been HIV positive. With regard to HIV sero-discordant couples (male, HIV infected; female, HIV-uninfected) who wish to conceive a child, assisted reproductive techniques using sperm-washing to reduce the risk of HIV transmission have been successfully employed, with only one well-documented seroconversion in the uninfected female partner, reported in 1990.

OCCUPATIONAL TRANSMISSION OF HIV: HEALTH CARE WORKERS, LABORATORY WORKERS, AND THE HEALTH CARE SETTING

There is a small, but definite, occupational risk of HIV transmission to health care workers and laboratory personnel and potentially others who work with HIV-containing materials, particularly when sharp objects are used. An estimated 600,000–800,000 health care workers are stuck with needles or other sharp medical instruments in the United States each year.

Exposures that place a health care worker at potential risk of HIV infection are percutaneous injuries (e.g., a needle stick or cut with a sharp object) or contact of mucous membrane or nonintact skin (e.g., exposed skin that is chapped, abraded, or afflicted with dermatitis) with blood, tissue, or other potentially infectious body fluids. Large, multi-institutional studies have indicated that the risk of HIV transmission following skin puncture from a needle or a sharp object that was contaminated with blood from a person with documented HIV infection is ~0.3% and after a mucous membrane exposure it is 0.09% (see "HIV and the Health Care Worker," below). HIV transmission after non-intact skin exposure has been documented, but the average risk for transmission by this route has not been precisely determined; however, it is estimated to be less than the risk for mucous membrane exposure. Transmission of HIV through intact skin has not been documented.

In addition to blood and visibly bloody body fluids, semen and vaginal secretions are also considered potentially infectious but have not been implicated in occupational transmission from patients to health care workers. The following fluids are also considered potentially infectious: cerebrospinal fluid, synovial fluid, pleural fluid, peritoneal fluid, pericardial fluid, and amniotic fluid. The risk for transmission after exposure to fluids or tissues other than HIV-infected blood also has not been quantified but is probably considerably lower than for blood exposures. Feces, nasal secretions, saliva, sputum, sweat, tears, urine, and vomitus are not considered potentially infectious unless they are visibly bloody. Rare cases of HIV transmission via human bites have been reported, but not after an occupational exposure.

An increased risk for HIV infection following percutaneous exposures to HIV-infected blood is associated with exposures involving a relatively large quantity of blood, as in the case of a device visibly contaminated with the patient's blood, a procedure that involves a needle placed directly in a vein or artery, or a deep injury. Factors that might be associated with mucocutaneous transmission of HIV include exposure to an unusually large volume of blood, prolonged contact, and a potential portal of entry. In addition, the risk increases for exposures to blood from patients with advanced-stage disease, owing to the higher titer of HIV in the blood as well as to other factors, such as the presence of more virulent strains of virus. The use of antiretroviral drugs as postexposure prophylaxis decreases the risk of infection compared to historic controls in occupationally exposed health care workers (see "HIV and the Health Care Worker," below). The risk of hepatitis B virus (HBV) infection following a similar type of exposure is ~6–30% in nonimmune individuals; if a susceptible worker is exposed to HBV, postexposure prophylaxis with hepatitis B immune globulin and initiation of HBV vaccine is >90% effective in preventing HBV infection. The risk of hepatitis C virus (HCV) infection following percutaneous injury is ~1.8% (Chap. 298).

Since the beginning of the HIV epidemic, there have been at least three reported instances in which transmission of infection from a health care worker to patients seemed highly probable. One cluster of infections involved an HIV-infected dentist in Florida who apparently infected as many as six of his patients, most likely through contaminated instruments. Another case involved an HIV-infected orthopedic surgeon in France who apparently infected a patient during placement of a total hip prosthesis. A third case involved the apparent transmission of HIV from an HIV-infected nurse to a surgical patient in France. Breaches in infection control and the reuse of contaminated syringes have also resulted in the transmission of HIV from patient to patient in hospitals, nursing homes, and outpatient settings. For example, in the only report of HIV transmission from patient to patient during a surgical procedure, four patients in Australia were apparently infected by an HIV-negative general surgeon during routine outpatient surgery. Although the mechanism of transmission was not definitively identified, a failure on the part of the surgeon to sterilize instruments properly following prior surgery on an HIV-infected patient was considered a likely explanation for this outbreak. Three patients (two in hospitals in the United States and one in the Netherlands) undergoing nuclear medicine procedures were reported to have inadvertently received IV injections of blood or other material from patients infected with HIV. Hemodialysis centers have also been implicated in several reported HIV transmission incidents.

The most dramatic reports involved transmission of HIV to 8000–10,000 children in Romanian orphanages in the 1980s. Other large incidents occurred in hospitals in Russia and Libya in the late 1980s and late 1990s, respectively. Each of these incidents received considerable attention and likely was related to reuse of contaminated needles and/or administration of contaminated blood products. Despite the small number of documented cases, the risk of HIV transmission involving health care workers (infected or not) to patients is extremely low in developed countries; in fact, too low to be measured accurately. In this regard, several epidemiologic studies have been performed tracing thousands of patients of HIV-infected dentists, physicians, surgeons, obstetricians, and gynecologists, and no other cases of HIV infection that could be linked to the health care providers were identified. The very rare occurrence of transmission of HIV as well as HBV and HCV to and from health care workers in the workplace underscores the importance of the use of universal precautions when caring for all patients (see below and Chap. 125).

MATERNAL-FETAL/INFANT TRANSMISSION

HIV infection can be transmitted from an infected mother to her fetus during pregnancy, during delivery, or by breast-feeding. This is an extremely important form of transmission of HIV infection in certain developing countries, where the proportion of infected women to infected men is ~1:1. Virologic analysis of aborted fetuses indicate that HIV can be transmitted to the fetus as early as the first and second trimester of pregnancy. However, maternal transmission to the fetus occurs most commonly in the perinatal period. Two studies performed in Rwanda and the former Zaire indicated that the relative proportions of mother-to-child transmissions were 23–30% before birth, 50–65% during birth, and 12–20% via breast-feeding.

In the absence of prophylactic antiretroviral therapy to the mother during pregnancy, labor, and delivery, and to the fetus following birth (see below), the probability of transmission of HIV from mother to infant/fetus ranges from 15–25% in industrialized countries and from 25–35% in developing countries. These differences may relate to the adequacy of prenatal care as well as to the stage of HIV disease and the general health of the mother during pregnancy. Higher rates of transmission have been reported to be associated with many factors, the best documented of which is the presence of high maternal levels of plasma viremia. In one study of 552 singleton pregnancies in the United States, the rate of mother-to-baby transmission was 0% among women with <1000 copies of HIV RNA per milliliter of blood, 16.6% among women with 1000–10,000 copies/mL, 21.3% among women with 10,001–50,000 copies/mL, 30.9% among women with 50,001–100,000 copies/mL, and 40.6% among women with >100,000 copies/mL. However, there may not be a lower "threshold" below which transmission never occurs, since other studies have reported transmission by women with viral RNA levels <50 copies/mL. Low maternal CD4+ T cell counts have also been associated with higher rates of transmission; however, since low CD4+ T cell counts are often associated with high levels of plasma viremia, in one study using multivariate analysis including plasma viral load and CD4+ T cell count, only the level of plasma HIV RNA was significant. Increased mother-to-child transmission is also correlated with closer HLA match between mother and child. A prolonged interval between membrane rupture and delivery is another well-documented risk factor for transmission. Other conditions that are potential risk factors, but which have not been consistently demonstrated, are the presence of chorioamnionitis at delivery; STDs during pregnancy; hard drug use during pregnancy; cigarette smoking; preterm delivery; and obstetrical procedures such as amniocentesis, amnioscopy, fetal scalp electrodes, and episiotomy. In a study conducted in the United States and France, zidovudine treatment of HIV-infected pregnant women from the beginning of the second trimester through delivery and of the infant for 6 weeks following birth dramatically decreased the rate of intrapartum and perinatal transmission of HIV infection from 22.6% in the untreated group to <5%. The rate of mother-to-child transmission is approaching 1% or less in pregnant women who are receiving combination antiretroviral therapy for their HIV infection. Such treatment, combined with cesarean section delivery, has rendered mother-to-child transmission of HIV an unusual event in the United States and other developed nations. In developed countries, current recommendations to reduce perinatal transmission of HIV include universal voluntary HIV testing and counseling of pregnant women, antiretroviral prophylaxis with one or more drugs in cases in which the mother does not require therapy for her HIV infection, combination therapy for women who do require therapy, obstetric management that attempts to minimize exposure of the infant to maternal blood and genital secretions, and avoidance of breast-feeding. It is recommended that the choice of antiretroviral therapy for pregnant women should be based on the same considerations used for women who are not pregnant, with discussion of the recognized and unknown risks and benefits of such therapy during pregnancy (see below under "Treatment"). This approach has led to a remarkable decrease in the number of infants infected with HIV through mother-to-child transmission in the United States, from an estimated peak of 1750 HIV-infected infants born each year during the early to mid-1990s to 280–370 infants in 2000, and a dramatic decrease in reported AIDS cases among children (Fig. 182-10). Certain studies have demonstrated that truncated regimens of zidovudine alone or in combination with lamivudine given to the mother during the last few weeks of pregnancy or even only during labor and delivery, and to the infant for a week or less, significantly reduced transmission to the infant compared to placebo. Short-course prophylactic antiretroviral (ARV) regimens, such as a single dose of nevirapine given to the mother at the onset of labor and a single dose to the infant within 72 h of birth, are of particular relevance to low- to mid-income nations because of the low cost and the fact that in these regions perinatal care is often not available and pregnant women are often seen by a health care provider for the first time at or near the time of delivery. Indeed, short-course ARV regimens have now been used for several years in developing nations for the prevention of mother-to-child transmission. It is estimated that the successful implementation of such regimens has saved as many as 1000 babies per day from becoming infected with HIV, the vast majority of whom are in sub-Saharan Africa. Given that combination ARV therapy is now increasingly available to individuals in developing countries due to the lower cost of drugs and programs that are making drugs available to these regions of the world, combinations of drugs are being used more frequently, where available, to treat HIV-infected pregnant women who require therapy notwithstanding their pregnancy. This has had the

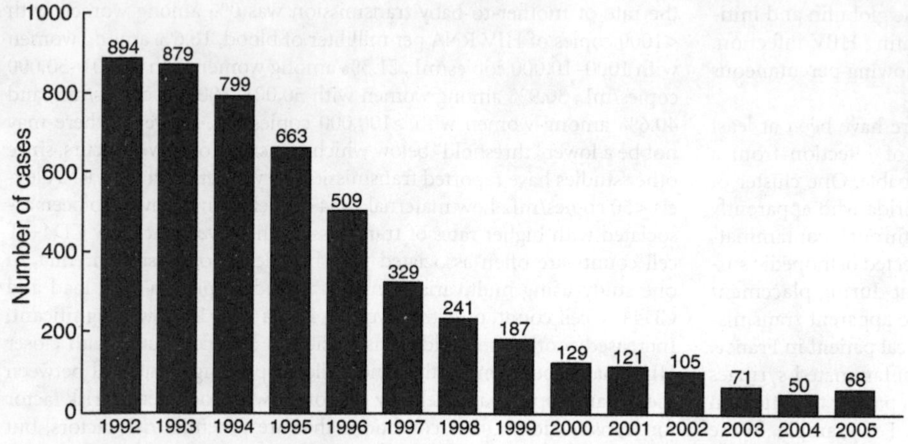

FIGURE 182-10 Estimated numbers of AIDS cases in children <13 years of age, by year of diagnosis, 1992–2005, 50 states and the District of Columbia. *(From CDC.)*

effect of benefitting the women, blocking HIV transmission to the fetus, and protecting against subsequent transmission by breast-feeding (see below).

Breast-feeding is an important modality of transmission of HIV infection in developing countries, particularly where mothers continue to breast-feed for prolonged periods. The risk factors for mother-to-child transmission of HIV via breast-feeding are not fully understood; factors that increase the likelihood of transmission include detectable levels of HIV in breast milk, the presence of mastitis, low maternal CD4+ T cell counts, and maternal vitamin A deficiency. The risk of HIV infection via breast-feeding is highest in the early months of breast-feeding. In addition, exclusive breast-feeding has been reported to carry a lower risk of HIV transmission than mixed feeding. Certainly in developed countries, breast-feeding by an infected mother should be avoided. However, there is disagreement regarding recommendations for breast-feeding in certain developing countries, where breast milk is the only source of adequate nutrition as well as immunity against potentially serious infections for the infant. The optimal approach to prevent transmission by infected mothers who choose to breast-feed would be to provide continual treatment to the infected mother. This approach has become more feasible as ARV therapy becomes more widely available in developing countries. Despite progress in this regard, ARV therapy is currently available to only ~25% of persons in developing nations who require it. Therefore, alternative approaches to block transmission by breast-feeding are being tested. In this regard, studies are being conducted to determine whether intermittent administration of nevirapine, which has a relatively long half-life, to uninfected babies born of infected mothers decreases the incidence of infection via breast-feeding.

TRANSMISSION BY OTHER BODY FLUIDS

Although HIV can be isolated typically in low titers from saliva of a small proportion of infected individuals, there is no convincing evidence that saliva can transmit HIV infection, either through kissing or through other exposures, such as occupationally to health care workers. Saliva contains endogenous antiviral factors; among these factors, HIV-specific immunoglobulins of IgA, IgG, and IgM isotypes are detected readily in salivary secretions of infected individuals. It has been suggested that large glycoproteins such as mucins and thrombospondin-1 sequester HIV into aggregates for clearance by the host. In addition, a number of soluble salivary factors inhibit HIV to various degrees in vitro, probably by targeting host cell receptors rather than the virus itself. Perhaps the best-studied of these, secretory leukocyte protease inhibitor (SLPI), blocks HIV infection in several cell culture systems, and it is found in saliva at levels that approximate those required for inhibition of HIV in vitro. In this regard, higher salivary levels of SLPI in breast-fed infants were associated with a decreased risk of HIV transmission through breast milk. It has also been suggested that submandibular saliva reduces HIV infectivity by stripping gp120 from the surface of virions, and that saliva-mediated disruption and lysis of HIV-infected cells occurs because of the hypotonicity of oral secretions. There have been outlier cases of suspected transmission by saliva, but these have probably been blood-to-blood transmissions. Transmission of HIV by a human bite can occur but is a rare event; at least four cases of such transmission have been reported. In addition, a most unusual form of HIV transmission from infected children to mothers in the former Soviet Union has been identified. In those cases, the children (infected through transfusion) were said to have bleeding sores in the mouth, and the mothers were said to have lacerations and abrasions on and around the nipples of the breast resulting from trauma from the children's teeth. Breast-feeding had been continued until the children were older than is usual in other developed countries.

Although virus can be identified, if not isolated, from virtually any body fluid, there is no evidence that HIV transmission can occur as a result of exposure to tears, sweat, and urine. However, there have been isolated cases of transmission of HIV infection by body fluids that may or may not have been contaminated with blood. Most of these situations occurred in the setting of a close relative providing intensive nursing care for an HIV-infected person without observing universal precautions, underscoring the importance of observing such precautions in the handling of body fluids and wastes from HIV-infected individuals (see below).

EPIDEMIOLOGY

HIV INFECTION AND AIDS WORLDWIDE

HIV infection/AIDS is a global pandemic, with cases reported from virtually every country. At the end of 2007, 33.2 million individuals were living with HIV infection (range: 30.6–36.1 million) according to the Joint United Nations Programme on HIV/AIDS (UNAIDS). More than 95% of people living with HIV/AIDS reside in low- and middle-income countries; ~50% are female, and 2.5 million are children <15 years. The global distribution of these cases is illustrated in **Fig. 182-11**.

In 2007, there were an estimated 2.5 million new cases of HIV infection worldwide, including 420,000 in children <15 years. In 2007, global AIDS deaths totaled 2.1 million (including 330,000 children <15 years). UNAIDS estimates that global HIV prevalence has been level since 2001. HIV incidence likely peaked in the late 1990s at >3 million new infections per year (**Fig. 182-12**). Recent reductions in global HIV incidence likely reflect natural trends in the pandemic as well as the results of prevention programs resulting in behavior change.

The HIV epidemic has occurred in "waves" in different regions of the world, each wave having somewhat different characteristics depending on the demographics of the country and region in question and the timing of the introduction of HIV into the population. Although the AIDS epidemic was first recognized in the United States and shortly thereafter in Western Europe, it very likely began in sub-Saharan Africa (see above), which has been particularly devastated by the epidemic. More than two-thirds of all people with HIV infection (~22.5 million) live in that region, even though sub-Saharan Africa is home to just 10–11% of the world's population (Fig. 182-11). Within the region, southern Africa is worst-affected. In eight southern African countries, available seroprevalence data indicate that >15% of the adult population aged 15–49 is HIV-infected. In addition, among high-risk individuals (e.g., commercial sex workers, patients attending STD clinics) who live in urban areas of sub-Saharan Africa, seroprevalence is now >50% in some countries. According to projections of the

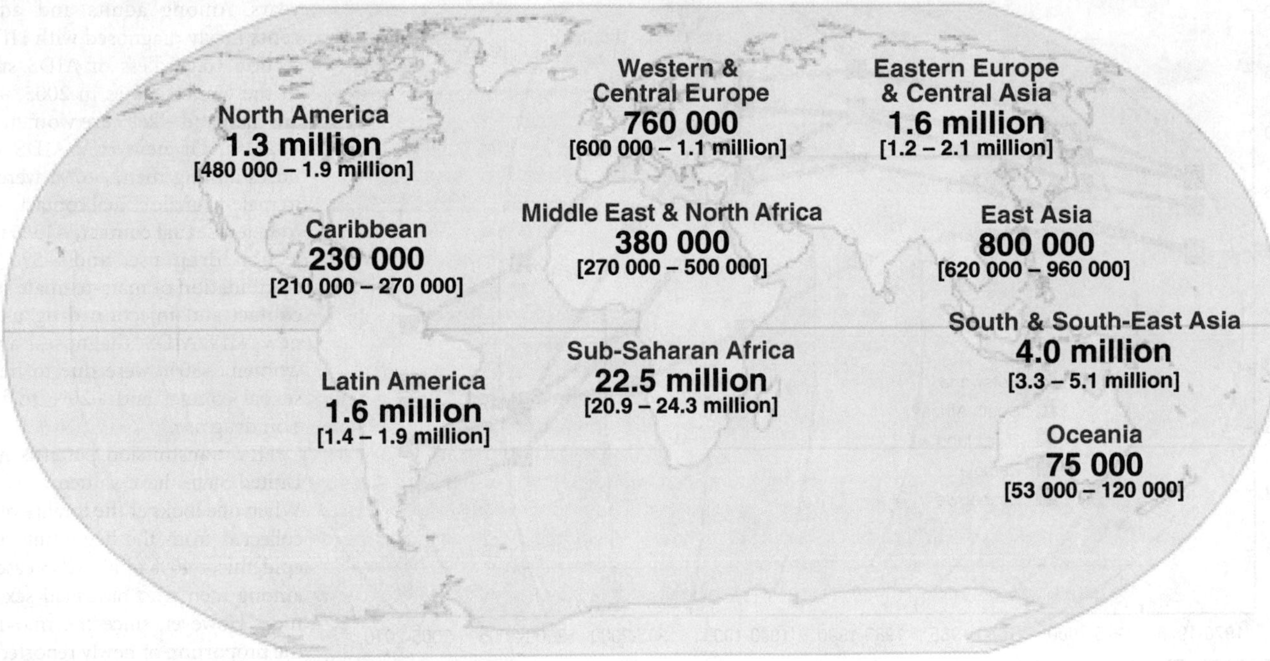

FIGURE 182-11 Estimated number of adults and children living with HIV infection as of December, 2007. Total: 33.2 (30.6–36.1) million. *[From United Nations AIDS Program (UNAIDS).]*

United Nations Population Division, life expectancies in several highly affected countries could drop to <40 years, well below what they would have been without HIV/AIDS and below levels reached in the pre-AIDS era (Fig. 182-13).

In Asia, an estimated 4.9 million people were living with HIV at the end of 2007. National HIV prevalence is highest in southeast Asia, with wide variation in trends between different countries. The epidemic in Asia lagged temporally behind that in Africa; however, the populations of many Asian nations are so large (especially India and China) that even low national HIV prevalence rates result in large numbers of people living with HIV. Encouragingly, HIV prevalence has declined in Myanmar, Cambodia and in Thailand; however, HIV prevalence continues to increase in other countries such as Indonesia and Vietnam.

The epidemic is expanding in Eastern Europe and Central Asia, where ~1.6 million people were living with HIV at the end of 2007. Ninety percent of new HIV infections reported in 2007 occurred in two countries, the Russian Federation and Ukraine. Driven initially by injection drug use and increasingly by heterosexual transmission, the number of new infections in this region has increased dramatically over the past decade.

Approximately 1.8 million people are living with HIV/AIDS in Latin America and the Caribbean. Brazil is home to the largest number of HIV-infected people in the region. However, the epidemic has been slowed in that country due to successful treatment and prevention efforts. The Caribbean region has the highest regional adult seroprevalence rate after Africa, due in large part to the huge case load in Haiti. Approximately 2.1 million people are living with HIV/AIDS in North America and in Western and Central Europe.

The major mode of HIV transmission worldwide is unquestionably heterosexual sex; this is particularly true, and has been so since the beginning of the epidemic, in developing countries, where the numbers of infected men and women are approximately equal. The epidemic in most developed countries was first introduced among men who have sex with men and, to a greater or lesser degree (depending on the individual country), among IDUs. In this regard, the total numbers of AIDS cases in those countries still reflect a high proportion of cases among these high-risk groups. However, in most developed countries, including the United States (see above and below), there has been a gradual shift toward heterosexual transmission (Fig. 182-8).

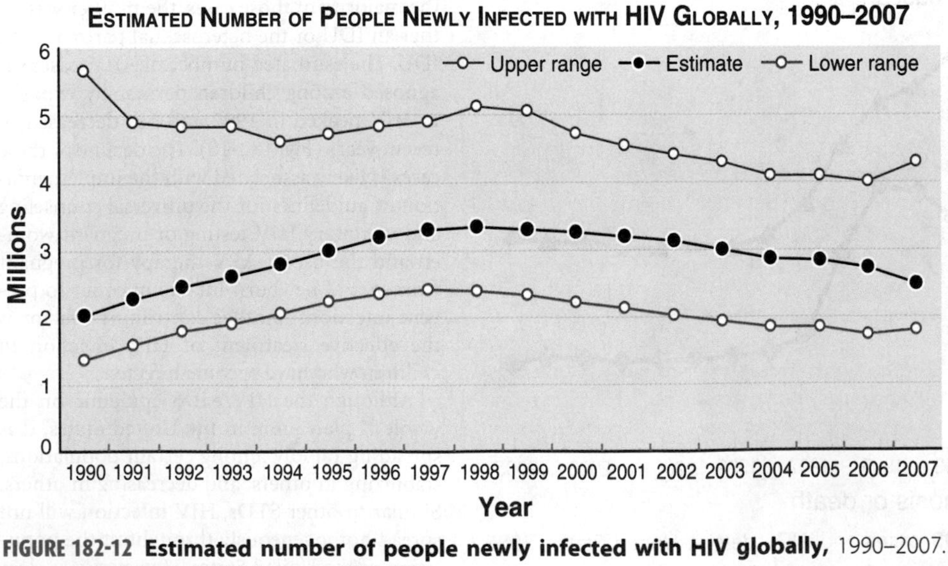

FIGURE 182-12 Estimated number of people newly infected with HIV globally, 1990–2007. *[From United Nations AIDS Program (UNAIDS).]*

AIDS IN THE UNITED STATES

AIDS has had—and will continue to have—an extraordinary public health impact in the United States. As of January 1, 2006, an estimated 984,155 cases of AIDS had been diagnosed in the United States and dependent areas, and ~550,394 AIDS-related deaths had occurred. AIDS cases have been reported in all 50 states, the District of Columbia; and in U.S. dependencies, possessions, and associated nations. An estimated 1.1 million individuals in the United States are living with HIV infection, one-quarter of whom are unaware of their infection. The estimated

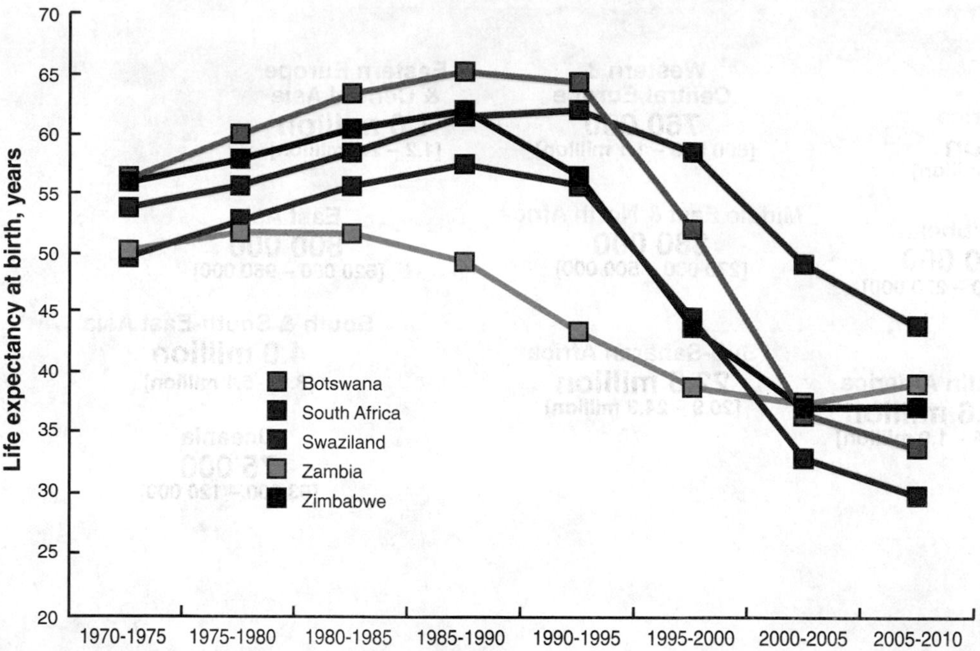

FIGURE 182-13 The impact of HIV/AIDS on life expectancy in five Sub-Saharan African countries, 1970–2010. *[From United Nations AIDS Program (UNAIDS).]*

years. Among adults and adolescents newly diagnosed with HIV infection (regardless of AIDS status) in the United States in 2005, ~74% are men and ~26% are women (Fig. 182-15). Of new HIV/AIDS diagnoses among men, ~67% were due to male-to-male sexual contact, ~15% to heterosexual contact, ~13% to injection drug use, and ~5% to a combination of male-to-male sexual contact and injection drug use. Of new HIV/AIDS diagnoses among women, ~80% were due to heterosexual contact and ~20% to injection drug use.

HIV transmission patterns in the United States have shifted over time. When one looks at the totality of data collected from the beginning of the epidemic, ~46% of all AIDS cases are among men who have had sex with men. However, since the mid-1980s the proportion of newly reported cases of AIDS in this population has declined from ~64% of cases diagnosed in 1985 to ~42% of cases diagnosed in 2005 (Fig. 182-8). Meanwhile, the proportion of new AIDS cases attributed to heterosexual contact has increased dramatically, from 3% in 1985 to 31% in 2005. The share of AIDS diagnoses due to injection drug use was 19% in 1985, peaked at 31% in 1993, and was 21% in 2005. Women are increasingly affected: the proportion of AIDS cases among female adults and adolescents (age >13 years) increased from 7% in 1985 to 27% in 2005.

HIV infection and AIDS have disproportionately affected minority populations in the United States. Among those diagnosed with HIV (regardless of AIDS status) in 2005, 49% percent were African Americans, a group that comprises only 13% of the U.S. population (Fig. 182-16). An estimated 3% of black men and 1% of black women in their thirties are living with HIV infection. HIV/AIDS ranked ninth among all causes of mortality in the United States in 2004 among those aged 35–64 years, but among African Americans it ranked third.

As of January 1, 2006, an estimated 9112 cases of AIDS in children <13 years old had been diagnosed, and ~54% of these children have died. Approximately 93% of these children were born to mothers who were HIV-infected or who were at risk for HIV infection and, in the majority of those cases, the mother was either an IDU or the heterosexual partner of an IDU. The estimated number of AIDS cases diagnosed among children perinatally exposed to HIV peaked in 1992 and has decreased in recent years (Fig. 182-10). The decline of these cases is likely associated with the implementation of guidelines for the universal counseling and voluntary HIV testing of pregnant women and the use of ARV therapy for pregnant women and newborn infants in order to prevent infection. Another contributing factor is the effective treatment of HIV infection in children who have become infected.

Although the HIV/AIDS epidemic on the whole is plateauing in the United States, it is spreading rapidly among certain populations, stabilizing in others, and decreasing in others. Similar to other STDs, HIV infection will not spread homogeneously throughout the population of the United States. However, it is clear

HIV seroprevalence rate among adults aged 15–49 years in the United States is ~0.6%. Prevalence is highest among young adults in their late twenties and thirties and among minorities.

The number of AIDS cases and deaths rose steadily through the 1980s; AIDS cases peaked in 1993 and deaths in 1995 (Fig. 182-14). Since then, the annual numbers of AIDS-related deaths in the United States have fallen ~70%. This trend is due to several factors, including the improved prophylaxis and treatment of opportunistic infections, the growing experience among the health professions in caring for HIV-infected individuals, improved access to health care, and a decrease in new infections due to saturational effects and prevention efforts. However, the most influential factor clearly has been the increased use of potent ARV drugs, generally administered in a combination of three or four agents (see below).

Approximately 40,000 individuals are newly infected each year in the United States, a figure that has remained stable for at least 15

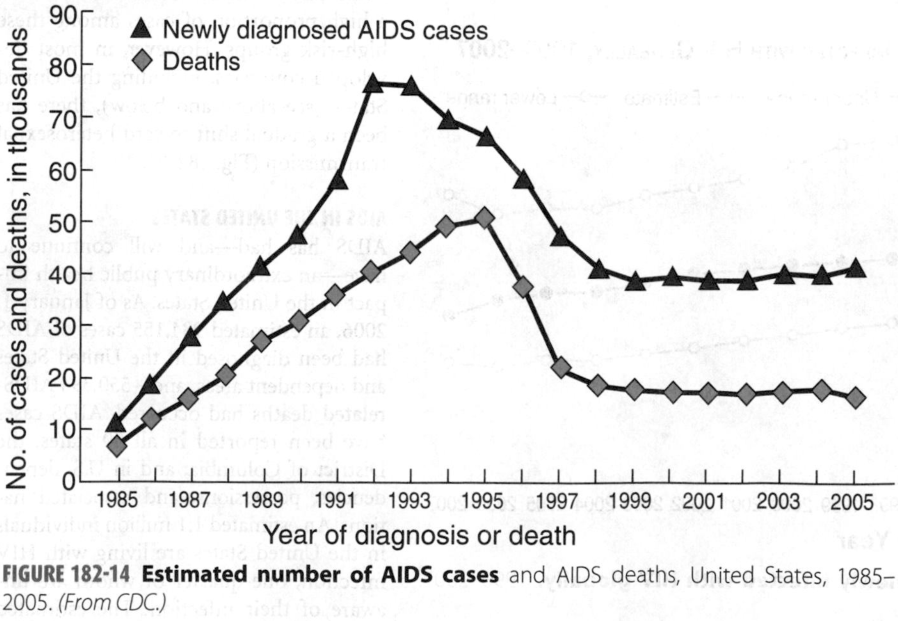

FIGURE 182-14 Estimated number of AIDS cases and AIDS deaths, United States, 1985–2005. *(From CDC.)*

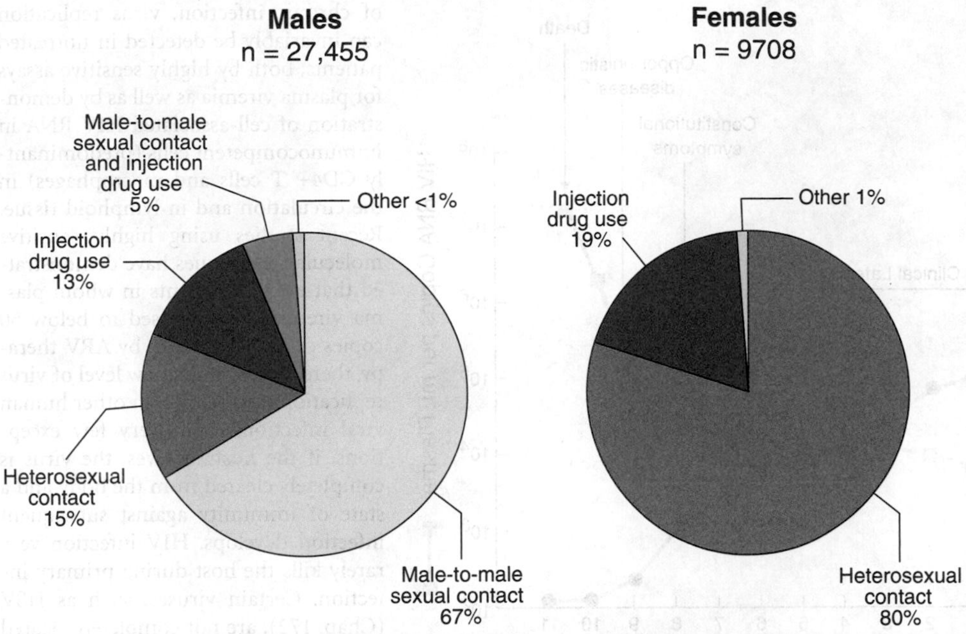

FIGURE 182-15 Transmission categories of adults and adolescents with HIV/AIDS diagnosed during 2005 in the United States. Estimates based on data from 33 states with long-term, confidential, name-based HIV infection reporting. Data include persons with a diagnosis of HIV infection regardless of AIDS status at diagnosis. *(From CDC.)*

that anyone who practices high-risk behavior is at risk for HIV infection. In addition, recent increases in infections and AIDS cases among young men who have sex with men and among heterosexuals (particularly sexual partners of IDUs, women, and adolescents) as well as the spread in pockets of poverty in both urban and rural regions (particularly among underserved minority populations in the southern United States with inadequate access to health care) testify to the fact that the epidemic of HIV infection in the United States remains a public health problem of major proportions.

PATHOPHYSIOLOGY AND PATHOGENESIS

The hallmark of HIV disease is a profound immunodeficiency resulting primarily from a progressive quantitative and qualitative deficiency of the subset of T lymphocytes referred to as *helper T cells.* This subset of T cells is defined phenotypically by the presence on its surface of the CD4 molecule (Chap. 308), which serves as the primary cellular receptor for HIV. A co-receptor must also be present together with CD4 for efficient fusion and entry of HIV-1 into its target cells (Figs. 182-3 and 182-4). HIV uses two major co-receptors for fusion and entry; these co-receptors are also the primary receptors for certain chemoattractive cytokines termed *chemokines* and belong to the seven-transmembrane-domain G protein–coupled family of receptors. CCR5 and CXCR4 are the major co-receptors used by HIV (see above and below). A number of mechanisms responsible for cellular depletion and/or immune dysfunction of CD4+ T cells have been demonstrated in vitro; these include direct infection and destruction of these cells by HIV and immune clearance of infected cells, as well as indirect effects such as immune exhaustion due to aberrant cellular activation and activation-induced cell death (see below). Patients with CD4+ T cell levels below certain thresholds (see below) are at high risk of developing a variety of opportunistic diseases, particularly the infections and neoplasms that are AIDS-defining illnesses. Some features of AIDS, such as Kaposi's sarcoma and neurologic abnormalities (see below), cannot be explained completely by the immunodeficiency caused by HIV infection, since these complications may occur prior to the development of severe immunologic impairment.

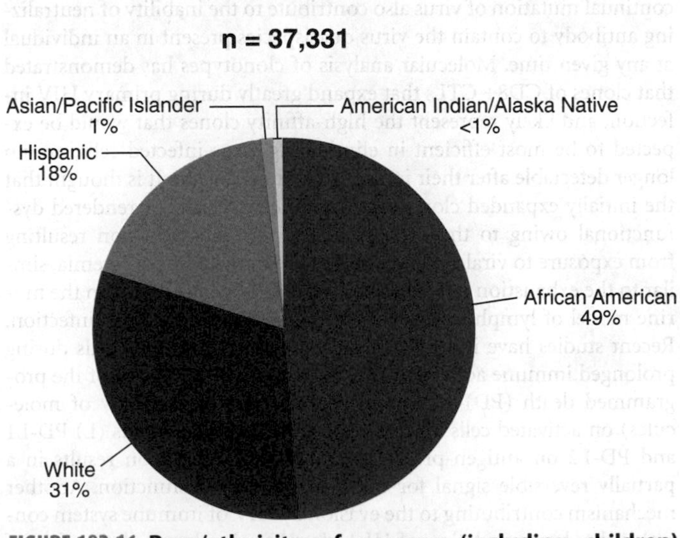

FIGURE 182-16 Race/ethnicity of persons (including children) with HIV/AIDS diagnosed during 2005 in the United States. Estimates based on data from 33 states with long-term, confidential, name-based HIV infection reporting. Data include persons with a diagnosis of HIV infection regardless of AIDS status at diagnosis. *(From CDC.)*

The combination of viral pathogenic and immunopathogenic events that occurs during the course of HIV disease from the moment of initial (primary) infection through the development of advanced-stage disease is complex and varied. It is important to appreciate that the pathogenic mechanisms of HIV disease are multifactorial and multiphasic and are different at different stages of the disease. Therefore, it is essential to consider the typical clinical course of an untreated HIV-infected individual in order to more fully appreciate these pathogenic events (Fig. 182-17).

PRIMARY HIV INFECTION, INITIAL VIREMIA, AND DISSEMINATION OF VIRUS

The events associated with primary HIV infection are likely critical determinants of the subsequent course of HIV disease. In particular, the early dissemination of virus to lymphoid organs, particularly the gut-associated lymphoid tissue (GALT), is a major factor in the establishment of a chronic and persistent infection (see below). The initial infection of susceptible cells may vary somewhat with the route of infection. Virus that enters directly into the bloodstream via infected blood or blood products (i.e., transfusions, use of contaminated needles for injecting drugs, sharp-object injuries, maternal-to-fetal transmission either intrapartum or perinatally, or sexual intercourse where there is enough trauma to cause bleeding) is likely cleared from the circulation to the spleen and other lymphoid organs, where primary focal infections begin, followed by wider dissemination throughout other lymphoid tissues, particularly the GALT, leading to a burst of viremia. Dendritic cells play an important role in the initiation of HIV infection. These cells express a diversity of C-type lectin receptors on their surface, one of which is called *DC-SIGN* (see above). DC-SIGN binds with high affinity to the HIV envelope gp120 and can retain infectious particles for days in vitro. In this regard, dendritic cells can trap HIV and mediate the efficient transinfection of CD4+ T cells. In addition, DC-SIGN may also facilitate CD4-mediated infection of dendritic cells. These mechanisms likely op-

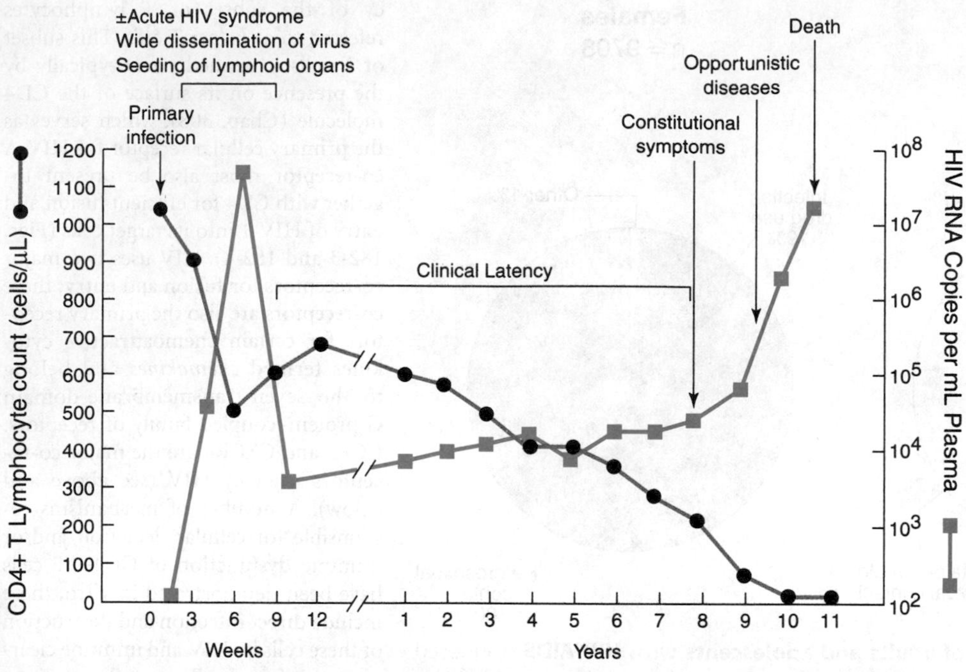

FIGURE 182-17 Typical course of an untreated HIV-infected individual. See text for detailed description. *[From G Pantaleo et al: N Engl J Med 328(5):327, 1993. Copyright 1993 Massachusetts Medical Society. All rights reserved.]*

erate in humans when HIV enters "locally" (as opposed to directly into the blood) and encounters mucosal dendritic cells via the vagina, rectum, or urethra during intercourse or via the upper gastrointestinal tract from swallowed infected breast milk or rarely semen or vaginal fluid. In primary HIV infection, virus replication in CD4+ T cells intensifies prior to the initiation of an HIV-specific immune response (see below, Fig.182-17), with a burst of viremia resulting from the rapid replication of virus in susceptible cells in lymphoid organs (particularly the GALT), with subsequent dissemination of virus to the brain and other tissues. Of note, animal studies have demonstrated that a significant percentage of CD4+ T cells (particularly memory cells) in the GALT is depleted early after SIV infection, via either direct infection of cells or bystander cell killing. The repopulation of such cells may be extremely problematic, even after initiation of ARV therapy. Individuals who experience the "acute HIV syndrome," which occurs to varying degrees in ~50% of individuals with primary infection, have high levels of viremia measured in millions of copies of HIV RNA per milliliter that last for several weeks (see below). Acute mononucleosis-like symptoms are well correlated with the presence of viremia. Virtually all patients develop some degree of viremia during primary infection, which contributes to virus dissemination throughout the lymphoid tissue (see above), even though they may remain asymptomatic or not recall experiencing symptoms. It appears that the initial level of plasma viremia in primary HIV infection does not necessarily determine the rate of disease progression; however, the set point of the level of steady-state plasma viremia after ~1 year does seem to correlate with the slope of disease progression (see below).

ESTABLISHMENT OF CHRONIC AND PERSISTENT INFECTION

Persistent Virus Replication HIV infection is unique among human viral infections. Despite the robust cellular and humoral immune responses that are mounted following primary infection (see below), once infection has been established the virus succeeds in escaping immune-mediated clearance (see below), paradoxically seems to thrive on immune activation, and is never eliminated completely from the body. Rather, a chronic infection develops that persists with varying degrees of continual virus replication in the untreated patient for a median of ~10 years before the patient becomes clinically ill (see below). It is this establishment of a chronic, persistent infection that is the hallmark of HIV disease. Throughout the often protracted course of chronic infection, virus replication can invariably be detected in untreated patients, both by highly sensitive assays for plasma viremia as well as by demonstration of cell-associated HIV RNA in immunocompetent cells (predominantly CD4+ T cells and macrophages) in the circulation and in lymphoid tissue. Recent studies using highly sensitive molecular techniques have demonstrated that even in patients in whom plasma viremia is suppressed to below 50 copies of HIV RNA/mL by ARV therapy, there is a continual low level of virus replication (see below). In other human viral infections, with very few exceptions, if the host survives, the virus is completely cleared from the body and a state of immunity against subsequent infection develops. HIV infection very rarely kills the host during primary infection. Certain viruses, such as HSV (Chap. 172), are not completely cleared from the body after infection but instead enter a latent state; in these cases, clinical latency is accompanied by microbiologic latency. This is not the case with HIV infection as described above. Chronicity associated with persistent virus replication can also be seen in certain cases of HBV and HCV infections (Chap. 300); however, in these infections the immune system is not a target of the virus.

Evasion of Immune System Control Inherent to the establishment of chronicity of HIV infection is the ability of the virus to evade elimination and control by the immune system. There are a number of mechanisms whereby the virus accomplishes this evasion. Paramount among these is the establishment of a sustained level of replication associated with the generation of viral diversity via mutation and recombination, thus providing a means to evade control and elimination by the immune system. The selection of mutants that escape control by CD8+ cytolytic T lymphocytes (CTLs) is critical to the propagation and progression of HIV infection. The high rate of virus replication and the continual mutation of virus also contribute to the inability of neutralizing antibody to contain the virus quasispecies present in an individual at any given time. Molecular analysis of clonotypes has demonstrated that clones of CD8+ CTLs that expand greatly during primary HIV infection, and likely represent the high-affinity clones that would be expected to be most efficient in eliminating virus-infected cells, are no longer detectable after their initial burst of expansion. It is thought that the initially expanded clones may have been deleted or rendered dysfunctional owing to the overwhelming immune activation resulting from exposure to viral antigens during the initial burst of viremia, similar to the exhaustion of CD8+ CTLs that has been reported in the murine model of lymphocytic choriomeningitis virus (LCMV) infection. Recent studies have indicated that exhaustion of effector cells during prolonged immune activation is associated with expression of the programmed death (PD)-1 molecule (of the B7-CD28 family of molecules) on activated cells and its interaction with its ligands (L) PD-L1 and PD-L2 on antigen-presenting cells. This interaction results in a partially reversible signal for cell death and/or dysfunction. Another mechanism contributing to the evasion by HIV of immune system control is the downregulation of HLA class I molecules on the surface of HIV-infected cells by the Nef protein of HIV, resulting in the lack of ability of the CD8+ CTL to recognize and kill the infected target cell. Although this downregulation of HLA class I molecules would favor elimination of HIV-infected cells by natural killer (NK) cells, this latter mechanism does not seem to remove HIV-infected cells effectively (see below). The principal targets of neutralizing antibodies against HIV are the envelope proteins gp120 and gp41. HIV employs three mechanisms to evade neutralizing responses: hypervariability in the primary sequence of the envelope, extensive glycosylation of the envelope, and conformational masking of neutralizing epitopes.

CD4+ T cell help is essential for the integrity of antigen-specific immune responses, both humoral and cell-mediated. HIV preferentially infects activated CD4+ T cells including HIV-specific CD4+ T cells, and so this loss of viral-specific helper T cell responses has profound negative consequences for the immunologic control of HIV replication. Furthermore, this loss occurs early in the course of infection, and animal studies indicate that 40–70% of all memory CD4+ T cells in the GALT are eliminated during acute infection. Another means of escape of HIV-infected cells from elimination by CD8+ CTLs is the sequestration of infected cells in immunologically privileged sites such as the central nervous system (CNS).

Finally, the escape of HIV from elimination during primary infection allows the formation of a pool of latently infected cells that cannot be eliminated by virus-specific CTLs (see below). Thus, despite a potent immune response and the marked downregulation of virus replication following primary HIV infection, HIV succeeds in establishing a state of chronic infection with a variable degree of persistent virus replication. In most cases, during this period patients make the clinical transition from acute primary infection to variable periods of clinical latency or smoldering disease activity(see below).

Reservoirs of HIV-Infected Cells: Obstacle to the Eradication of Virus There exists in virtually all HIV-infected individuals a pool of latently infected, resting CD4+ T cells that serves as at least one component of the persistent reservoir of virus. Such cells manifest postintegration latency in that the HIV provirus integrates into the genome of the cell and can remain in this state until an activation signal drives the expression of HIV transcripts and ultimately replication-competent virus. This form of latency is to be distinguished from preintegration latency, in which HIV enters a resting CD4+ T cell and, in the absence of an activation signal, only a limited degree of reverse transcription of the HIV genome occurs. This period of preintegration latency may last hours to days, and if no activation signal is delivered to the cell, the proviral DNA loses its capacity to initiate a productive infection. If these cells do become activated, reverse transcription proceeds to completion and the virus continues along its replication cycle (see above and Fig. 182-18). The pool of cells that are in the postintegration state of latency is established early during the course of primary HIV infection. Despite the suppression of plasma viremia to <50 copies of HIV RNA per milliliter by potent combinations of several ARV drugs administered over several years, this pool of latently infected cells persists and can give rise to replication-competent virus. Modeling studies built on projections of decay curves (see below) have estimated that in such a setting of prolonged suppression, it would require from 7–70 years for the pool of latently infected cells to be completely eliminated. Furthermore, the reservoir of latently infected cells is replenished during minor detectable rebounds of virus replication that may occur intermittently, during the low levels of persistent virus replication that goes undetectable (see below) (Fig. 182-18), even in patients who for the most part are treated successfully, and certainly during major rebounds of viremia in patients whose therapy is interrupted for a period of weeks or longer. Over the past several years attempts have been made to eliminate HIV in the latent viral reservoir using agents that stimulate resting CD4+ T cells during the course of antiretroviral therapy; however, such attempts have been unsuccessful. As more sophisticated techniques become available for measuring extremely low levels of virus replication, it is becoming clear that virus replication continually occurs at very low levels in a substantial proportion of individuals whose viral load is "undetectable" by the standard assays of plasma viremia (see above and below). Thus, although a small pool of truly resting, latently infected cells exists at any given point in time, this pool is continually being activated and replenished by ongoing low levels of virus replication. Reservoirs of HIV infected

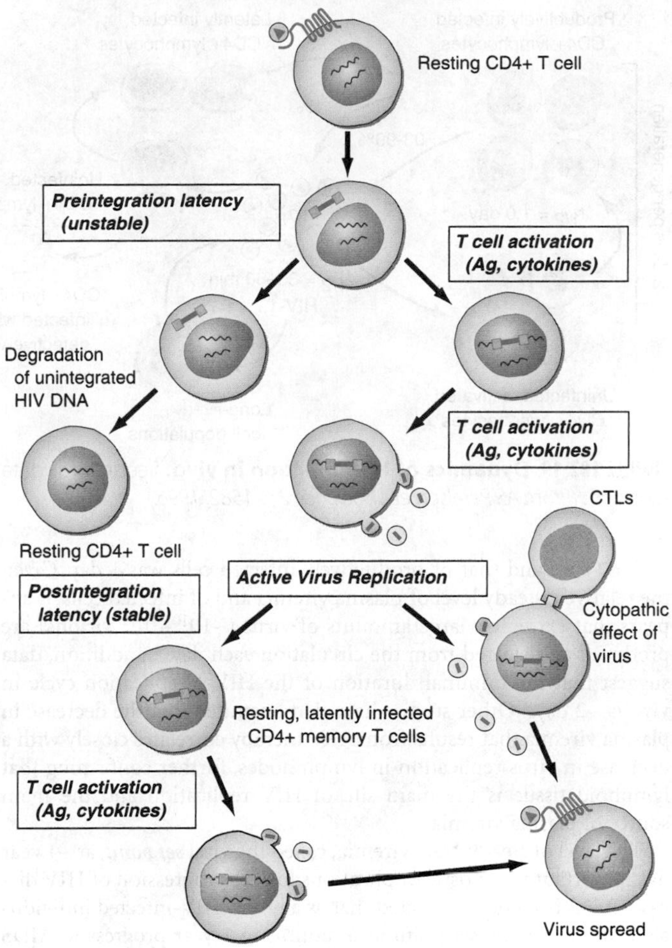

FIGURE 182-18 Generation of latently infected, resting CD4+ T cells in HIV-infected individuals. See text for details. Ag, antigen; CTLs, cytolytic T lymphocytes. *(Courtesy of TW Chun; with permission.)*

cells, latent or otherwise, can exist in a number of compartments including the lymphoid tissue, peripheral blood, and the CNS (likely in cells of the monocyte/macrophage lineage) as well as in other unidentified locations. Thus, this persistent reservoir of infected cells at various stages of latency and/or low levels of persistent virus replication are major obstacles to any goal of eradication of virus from infected individuals, despite the favorable clinical outcomes that have resulted from ARV therapy (see below).

Viral Dynamics The dynamics of viral production and turnover have been quantified using mathematical modeling in the setting of the administration of reverse transcriptase and protease inhibitors to HIV-infected individuals in clinical studies. Treatment with these drugs resulted in a precipitous decline in the level of plasma viremia, which typically fell by well over 90% within 2 weeks. The number of CD4+ T cells in the blood increased concurrently, which suggested that the killing of CD4+ T cells was linked directly to the levels of replicating virus. However, a significant component of the early rise in CD4+ T cell numbers following the initiation of therapy may be due to the redistribution of cells into the peripheral blood from other body compartments as a consequence of therapy-related diminution in viremia-associated immune system activation. It was determined on the basis of modeling the kinetics of viral decline and the emergence of resistant mutants during therapy that 93–99% of the circulating virus originated from recently infected, rapidly turning over CD4+ T cells and that ~1–7% of circulating virus originated from longer-lived cells, likely monocytes/macrophages. A negligible amount of circulating virus originated from the pool of latently infected cells (see above) (Fig. 182-19). It was also determined that the half-life of a circulating virion was

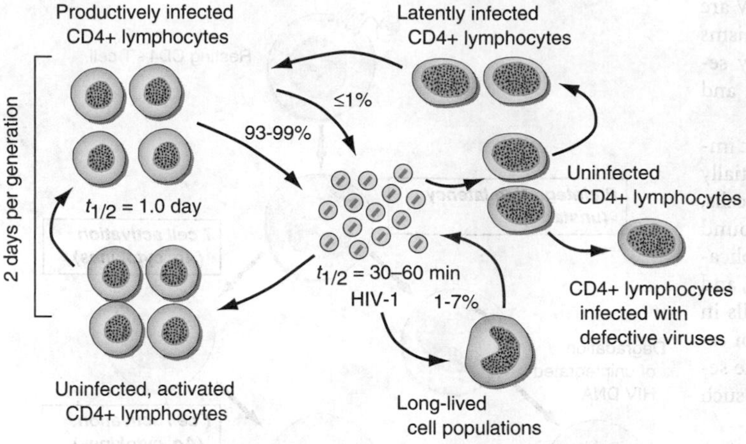

FIGURE 182-19 Dynamics of HIV infection in vivo. See text for detailed description. *(From AS Perelson et al: Science 271:1582, 1996.)*

~30–60 min and that of productively infected cells was 1 day. Given the relatively steady level of plasma viremia and of infected cells, it appears that extremely large amounts of virus (~10^{10}–10^{11} virions) are produced and cleared from the circulation each day. In addition, data suggest that the minimal duration of the HIV-1 replication cycle in vivo is ~2 days. Other studies have demonstrated that the decrease in plasma viremia that results from ARV therapy correlates closely with a decrease in virus replication in lymph nodes, further confirming that lymphoid tissue is the main site of HIV replication and the main source of plasma viremia.

The level of steady-state viremia, called the viral *set point*, at ~1 year has important prognostic implications for the progression of HIV disease. It has been demonstrated that as a group HIV-infected individuals who have a low set point at 6 months to 1 year progress to AIDS much more slowly than individuals whose set point is very high at that time (Fig. 182-20). Levels of viremia generally increase as disease progresses. Measurement of the level of viremia is critical in guiding therapeutic decisions in HIV-infected individuals (see below).

Clinical Latency versus Microbiologic Latency With the exception of long-term nonprogressors (see below), the level of CD4+ T cells in the blood decreases progressively in HIV-infected individuals. The decline in CD4+ T cells may be gradual or abrupt, the latter usually reflecting a significant spike in the level of plasma viremia. Most patients are relatively asymptomatic while this progressive decline is taking place (see below) and are often described as being in a state of *clinical latency*. However, this term is misleading; it does not mean disease latency, since progression, although slow in many cases, is generally relentless during this period. Furthermore, clinical latency should not be confused with microbiologic latency, since some level of virus replication invariably occurs during this period of clinical latency. Even in those rare patients who have <50 copies of HIV RNA per milliliter in the absence of therapy, there is virtually always some degree of ongoing virus replication.

ADVANCED HIV DISEASE

In untreated patients or in patients in whom therapy has not adequately controlled virus replication (see below), after a variable period, usually measured in years, the CD4+ T cell count falls below a critical level (<200/μL) and the patient becomes highly susceptible to opportunistic disease (Fig. 182-17). For this reason, the CDC case definition of AIDS includes all HIV-infected individuals with CD4+ T cell counts below this level (Table 182-1). Patients may experience constitutional signs and symptoms or may develop an opportunistic disease abruptly without any prior symptoms, although the latter scenario is unusual. The depletion of CD4+ T cells continues to be progressive and unrelenting in this phase. It is not uncommon for CD4+ T cell counts in the untreated patient to drop as low as 10/μL or even to zero. In countries where ARV therapy and prophylaxis and treatment for opportunistic infections are readily accessible to such patients, survival is increased dramatically even with this level of advanced disease. In contrast, untreated patients who progress to this severest form of immunodeficiency usually succumb to opportunistic infections or neoplasms (see below).

LONG-TERM SURVIVORS AND LONG-TERM NONPROGRESSORS

The prognosis for HIV-infected individuals who have access to health care and ARV therapy has improved greatly since the beginning of the epidemic. The median time from primary HIV infection to the development of AIDS in untreated individuals in the developed world is ~10 years. This period has been markedly extended by the wide availability of combinations of ARV drugs in the developed world, and increasingly in low- to mid-income countries; the full extent of this benefit is yet to be realized (see below). It is important to distinguish between the terms *long-term survivor* and *long-term nonprogressor*. Long-term nonprogressors are by definition long-term survivors; however, the reverse is not always true. The definitions of these categories are empirical and continue to change as more data are collected from prospective cohort studies. Predictions from one study that antedated the availability of effective ARV therapy estimated that ~13% of homosexual/bisexual men who were infected at an early age may remain free of clinical AIDS for >20 years. Originally, individuals were considered to be long-term survivors if they remained alive for 10–15 years after initial infection. Currently, individuals are considered to be long-term survivors if they remain alive for ≥20 years after initial infection. In most such individuals the disease has progressed, in that they have significant immunodeficiency, and many have experienced opportunistic diseases. Some of these individuals have CD4+ T cell counts that have decreased to ≤200/μL but have remained stable at that level for years. The mechanisms of this stabilization are not entirely clear but may relate to the beneficial effects of ARV therapy and prophylaxis against opportunistic infections. In addition, a number of viral and/or host determinants likely contribute to the long-term survival of these individuals. Quantitative and qualitative aspects of the HIV-specific immune response, as well as recognized and unrecognized genetic factors (see below), may also contribute to the long-term survival of these individuals.

Definitions of long-term nonprogressors have varied considerably over the years, and so such individuals constitute a heterogeneous

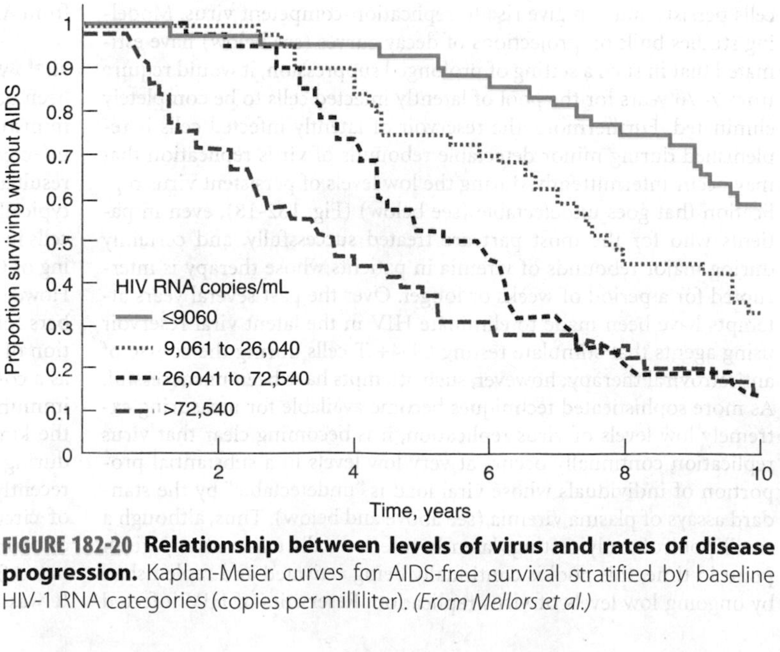

FIGURE 182-20 Relationship between levels of virus and rates of disease progression. Kaplan-Meier curves for AIDS-free survival stratified by baseline HIV-1 RNA categories (copies per milliliter). *(From Mellors et al.)*

group. Originally, individuals considered to be long-term nonprogressors were those who had been infected with HIV for a long period (≥10 years), whose CD4+ T cell counts were in the normal range and remained stable over years, and who had not received ARV therapy. Such patients had relatively low, but usually detectable, levels of plasma viremia, generally normal immune function according to commonly measured parameters (skin tests, in vitro lymphocyte responses to various mitogens and antigens), and normal-appearing lymphoid tissue architecture as determined on lymph node biopsy. In general, long-term nonprogressors manifested robust HIV-specific immune responses, both humoral (neutralizing antibodies) and cell-mediated (HIV-specific CTLs). However, this may also be true of some individuals early in the course of disease who ultimately progress to advanced disease. No qualitative abnormalities in the virus were detected in most of these patients. However, a small subset of patients did have defective virus; in particular, in one cohort of five long-term nonprogressors, the virus had a defect in the *nef* gene. In another report, a blood donor in Australia who was HIV-infected and a group of seven individuals who were infected by blood or blood products from that donor remained free of HIV-related disease and maintained normal and stable CD4+ T cell counts for several years after infection. Sequence analysis of viruses isolated from the donor and recipients revealed similar deletions in the *nef* gene and the region of overlap of *nef* and the U3 region of the HIV LTR (Fig. 182-5). The vast majority of these originally reported long-term nonprogressors have now gone on to progressive disease. More recently, cohorts of rare long-term nonprogressors have been described who have been infected for 20 years with normal CD4+ T cell counts and who typically maintain plasma viral RNA <50 copies per milliliter without ARV therapy. When these more stringent definitions based predominantly on levels of plasma viremia are applied, very strong associations with HLA B*5701 or HLA B*2705 alleles have been found. In addition, the HIV-specific CD8+ T cell response in these patients is highly focused on B5701-restricted peptides, suggesting that the B5701 molecule plays a direct role in restriction of virus replication in these individuals, although the precise mechanisms of this effect remain unclear.

A number of other host genetic factors exert more modest effects on restriction of HIV replication, yet they also may be associated with slower progression of disease (see "Genetic Factors in HIV Pathogenesis," below). The precise role of host factors in long-term nonprogression remains unclear. There is no single genetic determinant for nonprogression. However, several genetic variants and mutations have been demonstrated to result in a delay in the progression of HIV disease. These include heterozygosity for the *CCR5*-Δ32 deletion, heterozygosity for the *CCR2*-64I mutation, homozygosity for the *SDF1*-3′A mutation, and heterozygosity for the *RANTES*-28G mutation (see "Genetic Factors in HIV Pathogenesis," below). Since CCR5 is the major co-receptor for R5 or macrophage-tropic strains of HIV and since individuals who are homozygous for the *CCR5*-Δ32 deletion are, with rare exceptions, protected against HIV infection, the potential mechanism for slow progression in heterozygotes is clear. In addition, certain single nucleotide polymorphisms in the *CCR5* promoter have been shown to be associated with slower progression of disease. The reason for the slowing of progression of HIV disease in individuals who are heterozygous for the *CCR2*-64I mutation is less clear; however, it has been demonstrated that CXCR4 can dimerize with the CCR2-64I mutant but not with wild-type CCR2. This dimerization may reduce the amount of CXCR4 on the cell surface and as a result inhibit infection with X4 viruses. Homozygosity for the *SDF1*-3′ A mutation may upregulate the *SDF1* gene enabling SDF-1, which is the natural ligand for CXCR4, to compete more effectively with X4 virus for the CXCR4 coreceptor. The *RANTES*-28G mutation increases RANTES (CCL5) expression, which is the natural ligand for CCR5 and may thus inhibit infection with R5 viruses. The gene *CCL3L1* codes for MIP1αP and has an influence on both susceptibility to infection and disease progression based upon the gene copy number in the individual. Finally, maximal HLA heterozygosity of class I loci (A, B, and C) has been shown to be associated with delayed progression of HIV disease. Although most long-term nonprogressors have robust HIV-specific immune responses as well as competent CD8+ T cell suppressors of HIV replication, it is unclear whether these factors are directly responsible for the state of nonprogression. A substantial proportion of HIV-infected individuals manifest comparable immune responses early in the course of their disease and still experience disease progression. As noted above, long-term nonprogressors likely represent a heterogeneous group. It has recently been reported in some cohorts that individuals co-infected with HIV and *GB virus C* (GBV-C) have lower mortality than HIV-infected individuals without GBV-C infection. The precise mechanisms of this apparent beneficial effect are unclear at present.

LYMPHOID ORGANS AND HIV PATHOGENESIS

Regardless of the portal of entry of HIV, lymphoid tissues are the major anatomic sites for the establishment and propagation of HIV infection (see above). Despite the use of measurements of plasma viremia to determine the level of disease activity, virus replication occurs mainly in lymphoid tissue and not in blood; indeed, the level of plasma viremia directly reflects virus production in lymphoid tissue.

Some patients experience progressive generalized lymphadenopathy (see below) early in the course of the infection; others experience varying degrees of transient lymphadenopathy. Lymphadenopathy reflects the cellular activation and immune response to the virus in the lymphoid tissue, which is generally characterized by follicular or germinal center hyperplasia. Lymphoid tissue involvement is a common denominator of virtually all patients with HIV infection, even those without easily detectable lymphadenopathy.

Simultaneous examinations of lymph tissue and peripheral blood in patients and monkeys during various stages of HIV and SIV infection, respectively, have led to substantial insight into the pathogenesis of HIV disease. In most of the original human studies, peripheral lymph nodes have been used predominantly as the source of lymphoid tissue. More recent studies in monkeys and humans have focused on the GALT, where the earliest burst of virus replication occurs associated with marked depletion of CD4+ T cells (see below). In detailed studies in peripheral lymph node tissue, using a combination of polymerase chain reaction (PCR) techniques for HIV DNA and HIV RNA in tissue and HIV RNA in plasma, in situ hybridization for HIV RNA, and light and electron microscopy, the following picture has emerged. During acute HIV infection high levels of plasma viremia at first originating from virus replication in the GALT occurs with dissemination of virus to peripheral lymphoid tissue where extensive viral replication in individual cells is demonstrated. A profound degree of cellular activation occurs (see below) and is reflected in follicular or germinal center hyperplasia. At this time copious amounts of extracellular virions (both infectious and defective) are trapped on the processes of the follicular dendritic cells (FDCs) in the germinal centers of the lymph nodes. Virions that have bound complement components on their surfaces attach to the surface of FDCs via interactions with complement receptors and likely via Fc receptors that bind to antibodies that are attached to the virions. In situ hybridization reveals expression of virus in individual cells of the paracortical area and, to a lesser extent, the germinal center (Fig. 182-21). The persistence of trapped virus after the transition from acute to chronic infection likely reflects a steady state whereby trapped virus turns over and is replaced by fresh virions, which are continually produced to a greater or lesser degree in individual patients. The trapped virus, either as whole virion or shed envelope, serves as a continual activator of CD4+ T cells, thus driving further virus replication.

During early-stage HIV disease, the architecture of the germinal centers is generally preserved and may even be hyperplastic owing to in situ proliferation of cells (mostly B lymphocytes) and recruitment to the lymph nodes of a number of cell types (B cells, CD4+ and CD8+ T cells). Electron-microscopic studies have demonstrated a fine network of FDCs with many long, fingerlike processes that envelop virtually every lymphocyte in the germinal center. Extracellular virions can be seen attached to the processes, yet the FDCs appear to be relatively healthy. The trapping of antigen is a physiologically normal function

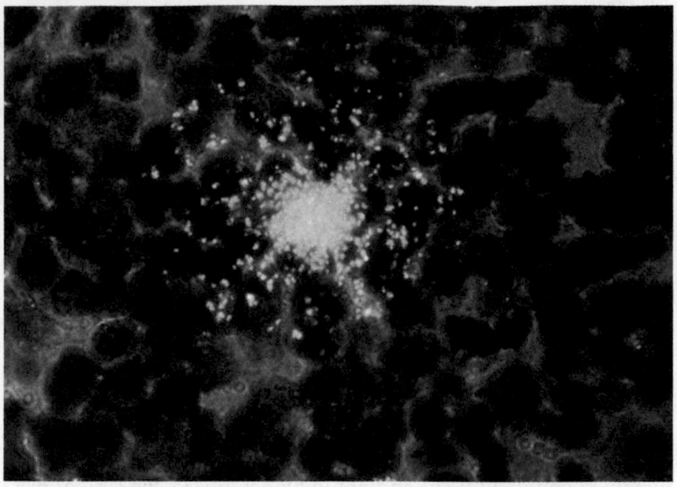

FIGURE 182-21 HIV in the lymph node of an HIV-infected individual. An individual cell infected with HIV shown expressing HIV RNA by in situ hybridization using a radiolabeled molecular probe. Original ×500. *(Adapted from G Pantaleo et al: Nature 362:355, 1993.)*

for the FDCs, which present antigen to B cells and contribute to the generation of B cell memory. However, in the case of HIV, the trapped virions serve as a persistent source of cellular activation, resulting in the secretion of proinflammatory cytokines such as interleukin (IL)-1β, tumor necrosis factor (TNF)-α, and IL-6, which can upregulate virus replication in infected cells (see below). Furthermore, although trapped virus is coated by neutralizing antibodies, it has been demonstrated that certain of these virions remain infectious for CD4+ T cells while attached to the processes of the FDCs. CD4+ T cells that migrate into the germinal center to provide help to B cells in the generation of an HIV-specific immune response are susceptible to infection by these trapped virions. Thus, in HIV infection, a normal physiologic function of the immune system, which contributes to the clearance of virus as well as to the generation of a specific immune response, can also have deleterious consequences.

As the disease progresses, the architecture of the germinal centers begins to show disruption, and the trapping efficiency of the lymphoid tissue diminishes. Electron microscopy reveals swollen organelles, and the FDCs begin to undergo cell death. The mechanisms of FDC death remain unclear; there is no indication by electron microscopy of copious virus replication or budding of virions off the cell in great quantities. This process of FDC death is accompanied by the deposition of collagen, leading to irreparable damage to the germinal centers. As the disease progresses to an advanced stage, there is complete disruption of the architecture of the germinal centers, accompanied by dissolution of the FDC network and massive dropout of FDCs. At this point, the lymph nodes are "burnt out." This destruction of lymphoid tissue compounds the immunodeficiency of HIV disease and contributes both to the inability to control HIV replication (leading usually to high levels of plasma viremia in the untreated or inadequately treated patient) and to the inability to mount adequate immune responses against opportunistic pathogens. The events from primary infection to the ultimate destruction of the immune system are illustrated in Fig. 182-22. Recently, nonhuman primate studies and some human studies have examined GALT at various stages of HIV disease. It is noteworthy that prior to infection approximately half of all CD4+ T cells in the jejunum express the HIV cellular co-receptor CCR5, rendering them highly susceptible to infection. Within the GALT, the basal level of activation combined with virus-mediated cellular activation results in the infection and elimination of an estimated 50–90% of CD4+ T cells in the gut. The extent of this early damage to GALT, which comprises a major component of lymphoid tissue in the body, plays a role in determining the potential for immunologic recovery of the memory cell subset.

CELLULAR ACTIVATION AND HIV PATHOGENESIS

Activation of the immune system is an essential component of an appropriate immune response to a foreign antigen. The immune system is normally in a state of homeostasis, awaiting perturbation by foreign antigenic stimuli. Once the immune response deals with and clears the antigen, the system returns to relative quiescence (Chap. 308). In HIV infection, however, the immune system is chronically activated, providing the cell substrates necessary for persistent virus replication throughout the course of HIV disease, particularly in the untreated patient (see above) and to variable degrees even in certain patients receiving ARV

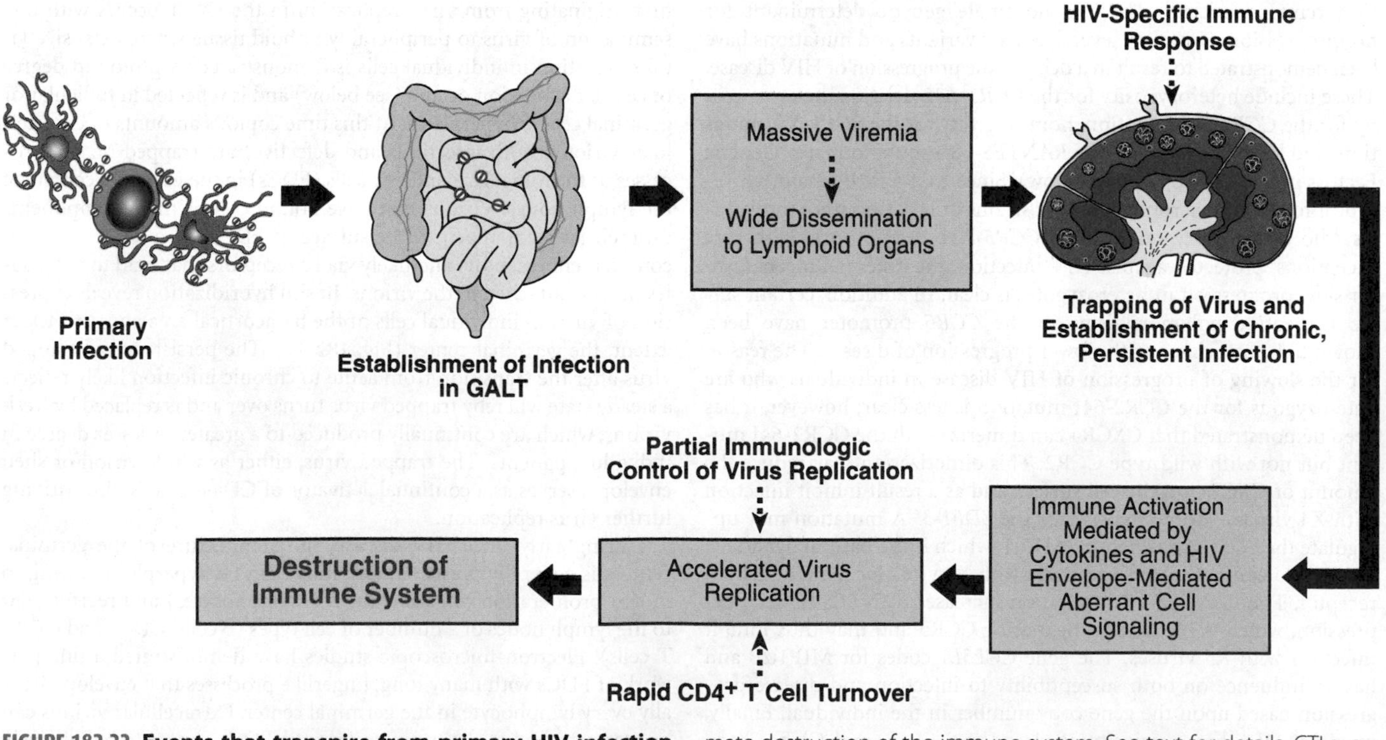

FIGURE 182-22 Events that transpire from primary HIV infection through the establishment of chronic persistent infection to the ultimate destruction of the immune system. See text for details. CTLs, cytolytic T lymphocytes; GALT, gut-associated lymphoid tissue.

therapy whose level of plasma viremia is suppressed to below the level of detection by standard assays (see below). Aberrant immune activation is the hallmark of HIV infection and is a critical component of the pathogenesis of HIV disease. This activated state is reflected by hyperactivation of B cells leading to hypergammaglobulinemia; spontaneous lymphocyte proliferation; activation of monocytes; expression of activation markers on CD4+ and CD8+ T cells; increased activation-associated cellular apoptosis; lymph node hyperplasia, particularly early in the course of disease (see above); increased secretion of proinflammatory cytokines (see below); elevated levels of neopterin, β_2-microglobulin, acid-labile interferon, and soluble IL-2 receptors; and autoimmune phenomena (see below). Even in the absence of direct infection of a target cell, HIV envelope proteins can interact with cellular receptors (CD4 molecules and chemokine receptors) to deliver potent activation signals resulting in calcium flux, the phosphorylation of certain proteins involved in signal transduction, co-localization of cytoplasmic proteins including those involved in cell trafficking, immune dysfunction, and, under certain circumstances, apoptosis (see below). The secretion of certain proinflammatory and immunoregulatory cytokines is both a consequence of the aberrant immune activation associated with HIV infection and a mechanism of propagation of the process of aberrant cellular activation (see below).

In addition to endogenous factors such as cytokines, a number of exogenous factors such as other microbes that are associated with heightened cellular activation can enhance HIV replication and thus may have important effects on HIV pathogenesis. Co-infection in vivo or in vitro with a range of viruses, such as HSV types 1 and 2, cytomegalovirus (CMV), human herpesvirus (HHV) 6, Epstein-Barr virus (EBV), HBV, adenovirus, and HTLV-I have been shown to upregulate HIV expression. Other microbes, such as *Mycoplasma*, have been reported to contribute to the induction of HIV expression. In addition, infestation with nematodes has been shown to be associated with a heightened state of immune activation that facilitates HIV replication; in certain studies deworming of the infected host has resulted in a decrease in plasma viremia. Two diseases of extraordinary global health significance, malaria and tuberculosis (TB), have been shown to increase HIV viral load in dually infected individuals. Globally, *Mycobacterium tuberculosis* is probably the most common opportunistic infection in HIV-infected individuals (see below and Chap. 158). In addition to the fact that HIV-infected individuals are more likely to develop active TB after exposure, it has been demonstrated that active TB can accelerate the course of HIV infection. It has also been shown that levels of plasma viremia are greatly elevated in HIV-infected individuals with active TB, compared to pre-TB levels and levels of viremia after successful treatment of the active TB. In vitro studies demonstrated that virus replication was markedly enhanced in lymphocytes of HIV-infected individuals who were skin test–positive for purified protein derivative (PPD) when PPD antigen was added to culture, resulting in cellular activation. Confirmatory evidence that antigen-induced activation was a major contributor to the accelerated viremia in HIV-infected individuals with active TB was provided by studies in which HIV-infected individuals were immunized with common recall antigens such as tetanus toxoid, influenza, or pneumococcal polysaccharide. Under these circumstances, a transient elevation of plasma viremia accompanied the cellular activation induced by the immunization. A greater degree of induction of virus was seen in those individuals with early-stage as opposed to advanced stage HIV disease (i.e., in those with more competent immune systems), and the degree of virus induction correlated with the level of immune system activation. The situation is similar in the interaction between HIV and malaria parasites (Chap. 203). Acute infection of HIV-infected individuals with *Plasmodium falciparum* increases HIV viral load and the increased viral load is reversed by effective malaria treatment

Persistent immune activation may have several deleterious consequences. From a virologic standpoint, although quiescent CD4+ T cells can be infected with HIV, reverse transcription, integration, and virus spread are much more efficient in activated cells. Furthermore, cellular activation induces expression of virus in cells latently infected with HIV (see above). From an immunologic standpoint, chronic exposure of the immune system to a particular antigen over an extended period may ultimately lead to an inability to sustain an adequate immune response to the antigen in question. In many chronic viral infections, including HIV infection, persistent viremia is associated with "functional exhaustion" and apoptosis of virus-specific T cells. It has been demonstrated that this phenomenon may be mediated, at least in part, by the engagement of PD-1, which is highly expressed on the majority of HIV-specific T cells, with its ligands (PD-L1 and PD-L2) on antigen-presenting cells and epithelial cells, resulting in either T cell death or anergy (see above). Furthermore, the ability of the immune system to respond to a broad spectrum of antigens may be compromised if immunocompetent cells are maintained in a state of chronic activation. In addition, activation of the immune system may favor the elimination of cells via programmed cell death (apoptosis) (see below) as well as the secretion of certain cytokines that can induce HIV expression (see below).

The deleterious effects of chronic immune activation on the progression of HIV disease are well established. As in most conditions of persistent antigen exposure, the host must maintain sufficient activation of antigen (HIV)-specific responses but must also prevent excessive activation and potential immune-mediated damage to tissues. Certain studies suggest that normal immunosuppressive mechanisms that act to keep hyperimmune activation in check, particularly CD4+, FoxP3+, CD25+ regulatory T cells (T-regs), may be dysfunctional or depleted in the context of advanced HIV disease.

Apoptosis *Apoptosis* is a form of programmed cell death that is a normal mechanism for the elimination of effete cells in organogenesis as well as in the cellular proliferation that occurs during a normal immune response (Chap. 308). Apoptosis is strictly dependent on cellular activation, and the aberrant cellular activation associated with HIV disease (see above) is correlated with a heightened state of apoptosis. It has been hypothesized that, in HIV infection, sequential activation signals delivered to CD4+ T cells induce apoptosis. Cross-linking of the CD4 molecule by gp120 or gp120/anti-gp120 complexes delivers the first of two signals required for apoptosis. The second signal supposedly leading to cell death is delivered via the T cell receptor by antigen. According to this hypothesis, direct infection of CD4+ T cells is not required for apoptosis to occur, although it has been demonstrated that alterations in tyrosine kinase activity of HIV-infected cells may induce the cell to undergo apoptosis. HIV can trigger both Fas-dependent and Fas-independent pathways of apoptosis. Mechanisms involved in this process include upregulation of Fas and Fas ligand, upregulation of caspase-1 and caspase-6, downregulation of the antiapoptotic Bcl-2 protein, and activation of cyclin-dependent kinases. Certain viral gene products have been associated with enhanced susceptibility to apoptosis including Env, Tat, and Vpr. In contrast, Nef has been shown to possess antiapoptotic properties. A number of studies, including those examining lymphoid tissue, have demonstrated that the rate of apoptosis is elevated in HIV infection and that apoptosis is seen in "bystander" cells such as CD8+ T cells and B cells as well as in CD4+ T cells. The intensity of apoptosis correlates with the general state of activation of the immune system and not with the stage of disease or with viral burden. It is likely that apoptosis of immunocompetent cells contributes to the immune abnormalities in HIV disease; however, this is probably a nonspecific mechanism that merely reflects the aberrant state of immune activation.

Autoimmune Phenomena The autoimmune phenomena that are common in HIV-infected individuals reflect, at least in part, chronic immune system activation as well as molecular mimicry by viral components. Although these phenomena usually occur in the absence of autoimmune disease, a wide spectrum of clinical manifestations that may be associated with autoimmunity have been described (see below). Autoimmune phenomena include antibodies to lymphocytes and, less commonly, to platelets and neutrophils. Antiplatelet antibodies have some clinical relevance, in that they may contribute to the thrombocytopenia of HIV disease (see below). Antibodies to nuclear and cytoplasmic components of cells have been reported, as have antibodies to cardiolipin; CD4 molecules; CD43 molecules, C1q-A; variable regions of the T cell receptor α, β, and γ chains; Fas; denatured collagen; and IL-2. In addition, autoantibodies to a range of serum proteins, including albumin, immunoglobulin, and thyroglobulin, have been reported. There is antigenic cross-reactivity between HIV viral proteins (gp120 and gp41) and MHC class II determinants, and anti-MHC class II antibodies have been reported in HIV infection. These antibodies could potentially lead to the elimination of MHC class II–bearing cells via antibody-dependent cellular cytotoxicity (ADCC), although this has not been clearly demonstrated to occur (Chap. 308). In addition, regions of homology exist between HIV envelope glycoproteins and IL-2 as well as MHC class I molecules. With the widespread use of effective antiretroviral therapy, an *immune reconstitution inflammatory syndrome* (IRIS) has become increasingly more common. IRIS is an autoimmune-like phenomenon characterized by a paradoxical deterioration of clinical condition, which is usually compartmentalized to a particular organ system, in individuals in whom ARV therapy has recently been initiated. It is associated with a decrease in viral load and at least partial recovery of immune competence, usually associated with increases in CD4+ T cell counts. The immunopathogenesis is felt to be related to an increase in immune response against the presence of residual antigens that are usually microbial and is commonly seen with underlying *Mycobacterium tuberculosis* and cryptococcosis. This syndrome is discussed in more detail below.

THE CYTOKINE NETWORK IN HIV PATHOGENESIS

The immune system is homeostatically regulated by a complex network of immunoregulatory cytokines, which are pleiotropic and redundant and operate in an autocrine and paracrine manner. They are expressed continuously, even during periods of apparent quiescence of the immune system. On perturbation of the immune system by antigenic challenge, the expression of cytokines increases to varying degrees (Chap. 308). Cytokines that are important components of this immunoregulatory network have been demonstrated to play a major role in the regulation of HIV expression in vitro. Potent modulation of HIV expression has been demonstrated either by manipulating endogenous cytokines or by adding exogenous cytokines to culture. Cytokines that induce HIV expression in one or more of these systems include IL-1, IL-2, IL-3, IL-6, IL-12, TNF-α, TNF-β, macrophage colony-stimulating factor (M-CSF), and granulocyte-macrophage colony-stimulating factor (GM-CSF). Among these cytokines, the most consistent and potent inducers of HIV expression are the *proinflammatory cytokines* TNF-α, IL-1β, and IL-6. Interferon (IFN)-α and -β suppress HIV replication, whereas transforming growth factor (TGF) β, IL-4, IL-10, and IFN-γ can either induce or suppress HIV expression, depending on the system involved. The *CC-chemokines* RANTES (CCL5), macrophage inflammatory protein (MIP)-1α (CCL3), and MIP-1β (CCL4) (Chap. 308) inhibit infection by and spread of R5 HIV-1 strains, while *stromal cell–derived factor* (SDF) 1 inhibits infection by and spread of X4 strains (see below). The alpha defensin family of cytokines has been shown to inhibit both R5 and X4 viruses, and other soluble factors that have not yet been fully characterized have also been shown to suppress HIV replication.

The molecular mechanisms of HIV regulation are best understood for TNF-α, which activates NF-κB proteins that function as transcriptional activators of HIV expression. The HIV-inducing effect of IL-1β is thought to occur at the level of viral transcription in an NF-κB-independent manner. IL-6, GM-CSF, and IFN-γ regulate HIV expression mainly by posttranscriptional mechanisms. Elevated levels of TNF-α and IL-6 have been demonstrated in plasma and cerebrospinal fluid (CSF), and increased expression of TNF-α, IL-1β, IFN-γ, and IL-6 has been demonstrated in the lymph nodes of HIV-infected individuals. The mechanisms whereby the CC-chemokines RANTES (CCL5), MIP-1α (CCL3), and MIP-1β (CCL4) inhibit infection of R5 strains of HIV or SDF-1 blocks X4 strains of HIV involve blocking of the binding of the virus to its co-receptors, the CC-chemokine receptor CCR5 and the CXC-chemokine receptor CXCR4, respectively (see above and below). However, several CC-chemokines, including but not limited to CCL3, -4, and -5, induce intracellular signals that actually enhance infection by X4 strains of virus at both the entry and postentry levels. The mechanisms whereby other less well characterized factors (see above) inhibit HIV replication are not completely understood.

Blocking of endogenous HIV-inducing cytokines or addition of inhibitors of HIV-suppressor cytokines in cultures of peripheral blood and lymph node mononuclear cells from HIV-infected individuals has demonstrated that HIV replication is controlled tightly by endogenous cytokines that act synergistically and in an autocrine and paracrine manner, similar to their physiologic function in the regulation of the immune system. Indeed, the net level of virus replication in an HIV-infected individual reflects at least in part a balance between inductive and suppressive host factors, mediated mainly by cytokines.

LYMPHOCYTE TURNOVER IN HIV INFECTION

The immune systems of patients with HIV infection are characterized by a profound increase in lymphocyte turnover that is immediately reduced with effective ARV therapy. Studies utilizing in vivo or in vitro labelling of lymphocytes in the S-phase of the cell cycle have demonstrated a tight correlation between the degree of lymphocyte turnover and plasma levels of HIV RNA. This increase in turnover is seen in CD4+ and CD8+ T lymphocytes as well as B lymphocytes and can be observed in peripheral blood and lymphoid tissue. Mathematical models derived from these data suggest that one can view the lymphoid pool as consisting of dynamically distinct subpopulations of cells that are differentially affected by HIV infection. A major consequence of HIV infection appears to be a shift in cells from a more quiescent pool to a pool with a higher turnover rate. It is likely that a consequence of a higher rate of turnover is a higher rate of cell death. The role of the thymus in adult human T cell homeostasis and HIV pathogenesis is an area of controversy. While some data point to an important role for the thymus in maintaining T cell numbers and suggest that impairment of thymic function may be responsible for the declines in CD4+ T cells seen in the setting of HIV infection, other studies have concluded that the thymus plays a minor role in HIV pathogenesis. Among the data supporting an important role for the thymus are those that demonstrate an increase in the levels of T cell receptor excision circles (TRECs) following initiation of ARV therapy. TRECs are a byproduct of T cell development and represent episomal fragments of DNA that are excised during T cell receptor gene rearrangement (Chap. 308). Levels of TRECs will be the net result of changes in thymic output together with changes in T cell turnover. An increase in thymic output and/or a decrease in T cell turnover will lead to an increase in levels of TRECs. While it is clear that levels of TRECs increase following initiation of ARV therapy, it is not clear whether this is a consequence of increased thymic output or decreased T cell turnover.

THE ROLE OF CO-RECEPTORS IN HIV PATHOGENESIS

As mentioned above, HIV-1 utilizes two major co-receptors along with CD4 to bind to, fuse with, and enter target cells; these co-receptors are CCR5 and CXCR4, which are also receptors for certain endogenous chemokines. Strains of HIV that utilize CCR5 as a co-receptor are referred to as *R5 viruses*. Strains of HIV that utilize CXCR4 are referred to as *X4 viruses*. Many virus strains are *dual tropic* in that they utilize both CCR5 and CXCR4; these are referred to as *R5X4 viruses*.

The natural chemokine ligands for the major HIV co-receptors can readily block entry of HIV. For example, the CC-chemokines RANTES (CCL5), MIP-1α (CCL3), and MIP-1β (CCL4), which are the natural ligands for CCR5, block entry of R5 viruses, whereas SDF-1, the natural ligand for CXCR4, blocks entry of X4 viruses. The mechanism of inhibition of viral entry is a steric inhibition of binding that is not dependent on signal transduction (Fig. 182-23).

The transmitting virus is almost invariably an R5 virus that predominates during the early stages of HIV disease. In ~40% of HIV-infected individuals, there is a transition to a predominantly X4 virus that is associated with a relatively rapid progression of disease. However, at least 60% of infected individuals progress in their disease while maintaining predominance of an R5 virus. It should be pointed out

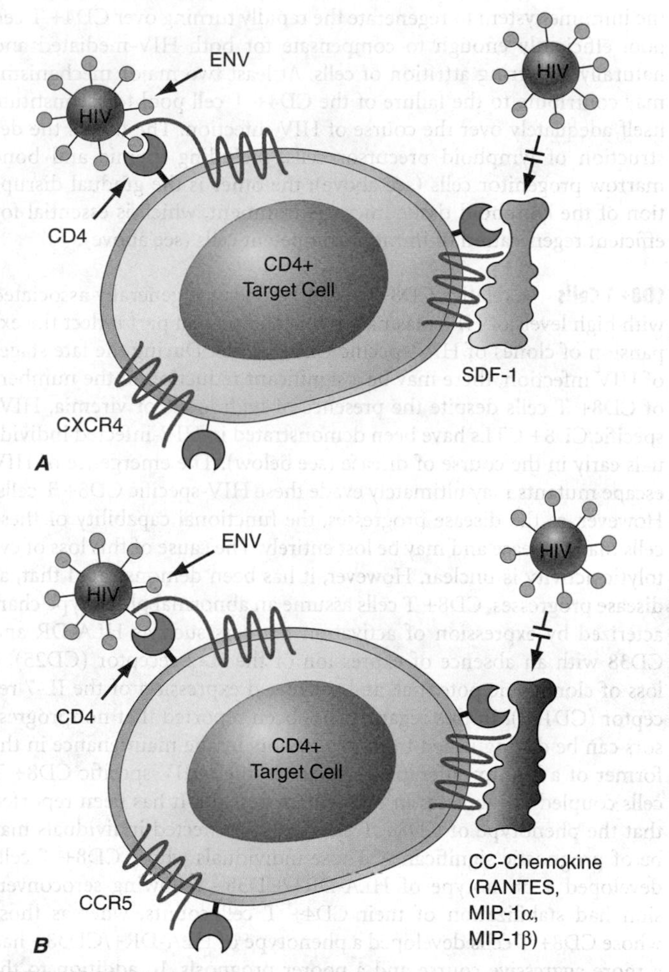

FIGURE 182-23 Model for the role of co-receptors CXCR4 and CCR5 in the efficient binding and entry of X4 (***A***) and R5 (***B***) strains of HIV-1, respectively, into CD4+ target cells. Blocking of this initial event in the virus life cycle can be accomplished by inhibition of binding to the co-receptor by the normal ligand for the receptor in question. The ligand for CXCR4 is stromal cell–derived factor (SDF-1); the ligands for CCR5 are RANTES, MIP-1α, and MIP-1β.

that clade C viruses, unlike other subgroups, almost never switch from CCR5 tropism to CXCR4 tropism; the reason for this difference is unclear. Other chemokine receptor family members may function as co-receptors for HIV and SIV entry, but to a much lesser extent than do CCR5 and CXCR4; these include CCR3, BOB/GPR15, CXCR6 (Bonzo/STRL33/TYMSTR), CCR2, CCR8, CX_3CR1(V28), and GPR1.

The basis for the tropism of different envelope glycoproteins for either CCR5 or CXCR4 relates to the ability of the HIV envelope, including the third variable region (V3 loop) of gp120, to interact with these co-receptors. In this regard, binding of gp120 to CD4 induces a conformational change in gp120 that increases its affinity for CCR5 (see above). Finally, R5 viruses are more efficient in infecting monocytes/macrophages and microglial cells of the brain (see "Neuropathogenesis," below).

CELLULAR TARGETS OF HIV

Although the CD4+ T lymphocytes and CD4+ cells of monocyte lineage are the principal targets of HIV, virtually any cell that expresses the CD4 molecule together with co-receptor molecules (see above and below) can potentially be infected with HIV. Circulating dendritic cells have been reported to express low levels of CD4 and, depending on their stage of maturation, these cells can be infected with HIV (see below). Epidermal Langerhans cells express CD4 and have been infected by HIV in vivo. In vitro, HIV has been reported also to infect a wide range of cells and cell lines that express low levels of CD4, no detectable CD4, or only CD4 mRNA; among these are FDCs, megakaryocytes, eosinophils, astrocytes, oligodendrocytes, microglial cells, CD8+ T cells, B cells, and NK cells as well as a variety of organ-specific cells. Since the only cells that have been shown unequivocally to be infected with HIV and to support replication of the virus are CD4+ T lymphocytes and cells of monocyte/macrophage lineage, the relevance of the in vitro infection of these other cell types is questionable.

Of potentially important clinical relevance is the demonstration that thymic precursor cells, which were assumed to be negative for CD3, CD4, and CD8 molecules, actually do express low levels of CD4 and can be infected with HIV in vitro. In addition, human thymic epithelial cells transplanted into an immunodeficient mouse can be infected with HIV by direct inoculation of virus into the thymus. Since these cells may play a role in the normal regeneration of CD4+ T cells, it is possible that their infection and depletion contribute, at least in part, to the impaired ability of the CD4+ T cell pool to completely reconstitute itself in certain infected individuals in whom ARV therapy has suppressed viral replication to <50 copies of HIV RNA per milliliter (see below). In addition, CD34+ monocyte precursor cells have been shown to be infected in vivo in patients with advanced HIV disease. It is likely that these cells express low levels of CD4, and therefore it is not essential to invoke CD4-independent mechanisms to explain the infection.

ABNORMALITIES OF MONONUCLEAR CELLS

CD4+ T Cells The range of T cell abnormalities in advanced HIV infection is broad. The defects are both quantitative and qualitative and affect virtually every limb of the immune system (see below), indicating the critical dependence of the integrity of the immune system on the inducer/helper function of CD4+ T cells. In advanced HIV disease, most of the observed immune defects can ultimately be explained by the quantitative depletion of CD4+ T cells. However, T cell dysfunction (see below) can be demonstrated in patients early in the course of infection, even when the CD4+ T cell count is in the low-normal range. The degree and spectrum of dysfunctions increase as the disease progresses. One of the first abnormalities to be detected is a defect in response to remote recall antigens, such as tetanus toxoid and influenza, at a time when mononuclear cells can still respond normally to mitogenic stimulation. Indeed, defects of central memory cells are a critical component of HIV immunopathogenesis. The progressive loss of antigen-specific CD4+ T cells has important implications for the control of HIV infection. In this regard, there is a correlation between the maintenance of HIV-specific CD4+ T cell proliferative responses and improved control of infection. Essentially every T cell function has been reported to be abnormal at some stage of HIV infection. These abnormalities include defective T cell cloning and colony-forming efficiencies, impaired expression of IL-2 receptors, defective IL-2 production, reduced expression of the IL-7 receptor (CD127), and decreased IFN-γ production in response to antigens. The proportion of CD4+ T cells that express CD28, which is a major co-stimulatory molecule necessary for the normal activation of T cells, is reduced during HIV infection. Cells lacking expression of CD28 do not respond normally to activation signals and may express markers of terminal activation including HLA-DR, CD38, and CD45RO. CD4+ T cells from HIV-infected individuals express abnormally low levels of CD40 ligand, which may contribute to the dysregulation of B cell function observed in HIV disease. As mentioned above (see "Cellular Activation and HIV Pathogenesis"), a subset of CD4+ T cells referred to as *T regulatory cells*, or T-regs, may be involved in dampening aberrant immune activation that propagates HIV replication. The presence of these T-reg cells correlates with lower viral loads and higher CD4+/CD8+ T cell ratios. A loss of this T-reg capability with advanced disease may be detrimental to the control of virus replication.

It is difficult to explain completely the profound immunodeficiency noted in HIV-infected individuals solely on the basis of direct infection and quantitative depletion of CD4+ T cells. This is particularly apparent during the early stages of HIV disease, when CD4+ T cell numbers may be only marginally decreased. In this regard, it is likely that CD4+ T cell dysfunction results from a combination of depletion

TABLE 182-3 MECHANISMS OF CD4+ T CELL DYSFUNCTION AND DEPLETION

Direct Mechanisms	Indirect Mechanisms
Loss of plasma membrane integrity due to viral budding	Aberrant intracellular signaling events
Accumulation of unintegrated viral DNA	Autoimmunity
Interference with cellular RNA processing	Innocent bystander killing of viral antigen–coated cells
Intracellular gp120-CD4 autofusion events	Apoptosis
Syncytia formation	Inhibition of lymphopoiesis
	Activation-induced cell death
	Elimination of HIV-infected cells by virus-specific immune responses

of cells due to direct infection of the cell and a number of virus-related but indirect effects on the cell (Table 182-3). Indeed, it has been demonstrated that patients with high levels of plasma viremia have a variety of subtle abnormalities of CD4+ T cell function, particularly involving aberrancies in signal transduction pathways. These abnormalities could be due either to aberrant activation induced by the cascade of cytokines that are expressed in viremic patients or by the direct effect of virus on the cell. In this regard, certain of these abnormalities can be reproduced by exposing CD4+ T cells of normal individuals to oligomeric HIV envelope proteins in vitro (see below).

Single-cell killing and the formation of syncytia between infected and uninfected cells have been demonstrated clearly in vitro, although there is little evidence that this process occurs in vivo. Cytopathicity in an infected cell in vitro may result from a number of mechanisms, including copious budding of virions from the cell surface with resulting disruption of the integrity of the cell membrane; interference with cellular RNA processing or the accumulation of high levels of heterodisperse RNA molecules; disruption of cellular protein synthesis owing to high levels of viral RNA; accumulation of high levels of unintegrated viral DNA in the cell cytoplasm; induction of aberrant patterns of protein tyrosine phosphorylation; and the interaction between HIV gp120 and CD4 intracellularly. Strain differences in single-cell killing are determined largely by gp120 sequences, which supports the importance of the viral envelope in this process. Humoral and cellular immune responses to HIV may contribute to protective immunity by eliminating virus and virus-infected cells (see below). However, since the main targets of HIV infection are immunocompetent cells, these responses may contribute to immune cell depletion and immunologic dysfunction by eliminating both infected cells and "innocent bystander" cells. Soluble viral proteins, particularly gp120, can bind with high affinity to the CD4 molecules on uninfected T cells and monocytes; in addition, virus and/or viral proteins can bind to dendritic cells or FDCs. HIV-specific antibody can recognize these bound molecules and potentially collaborate in the elimination of the cells by ADCC.

Nonpolymorphic determinants of MHC class I products share a degree of homology with gp120 and gp41 proteins of HIV. Such similarities may lead to the generation of autoantibodies to self-MHC determinants. Anti-HLA-DR antibodies have been demonstrated in the sera of HIV-infected individuals (see "Autoimmune Phenomena," above). These antibodies could contribute to the elimination of HLA-DR–expressing cells by ADCC; in addition, it has been suggested that these antibodies may inhibit certain T cell functions that involve HLA-DR molecules.

HIV envelope glycoproteins gp120 and gp160 manifest high-affinity binding to CD4 as well as to various chemokine receptors (see above). Intracellular signals transduced by gp120 through both CD4 and CCR5/CXCR4 have been associated with a number of immunopathogenic processes including anergy, apoptosis, and abnormalities of cell trafficking. The molecular mechanisms responsible for these abnormalities include dysregulation of the T cell receptor–phosphoinositide pathway, p56lck activation, phosphorylation of focal adhesion kinase, activation of the MAP kinase and ras signaling pathways, and downregulation of the co-stimulatory molecules CD40 ligand and CD80.

Finally, the inexorable decline in CD4+ T cell counts that occurs in most HIV-infected individuals may result in part from the inability of the immune system to regenerate the rapidly turning over CD4+ T cell pool efficiently enough to compensate for both HIV-mediated and naturally occurring attrition of cells. At least two major mechanisms may contribute to the failure of the CD4+ T cell pool to reconstitute itself adequately over the course of HIV infection. The first is the destruction of lymphoid precursor cells, including thymic and bone marrow progenitor cells (see above); the other is the gradual disruption of the lymphoid tissue microenvironment, which is essential for efficient regeneration of immunocompetent cells (see above).

CD8+ T Cells A relative CD8+ T lymphocytosis is generally associated with high levels of HIV plasma viremia and may in part reflect the expansion of clones of HIV-specific CD8+ CTLs. During the late stages of HIV infection, there may be a significant reduction in the numbers of CD8+ T cells despite the presence of high levels of viremia. HIV-specific CD8+ CTLs have been demonstrated in HIV-infected individuals early in the course of disease (see below). The emergence of HIV escape mutants may ultimately evade these HIV-specific CD8+ T cells. However, as the disease progresses, the functional capability of these cells may decrease and may be lost entirely. The cause of this loss of cytolytic activity is unclear. However, it has been demonstrated that, as disease progresses, CD8+ T cells assume an abnormal phenotype characterized by expression of activation markers such as HLA-DR and CD38 with an absence of expression of the IL-2 receptor (CD25), a loss of clonogenic potential, and a reduced expression of the IL-7 receptor (CD127). In this regard, it has been reported that nonprogressors can be distinguished from progressors by the maintenance in the former of a high proliferative capacity of their HIV-specific CD8+ T cells coupled to increases in perforin expression. It has been reported that the phenotype of CD8+ T cells in HIV-infected individuals may be of prognostic significance. Those individuals whose CD8+ T cells developed a phenotype of HLA-DR+/CD38– following seroconversion had stabilization of their CD4+ T cell counts, whereas those whose CD8+ T cells developed a phenotype of HLA-DR+/CD38+ had a more aggressive course and a poorer prognosis. In addition to the defects in HIV-specific CTLs, functional defects in other MHC-restricted CTLs, such as those directed against influenza and CMV, have been demonstrated. CD8+ T cells secrete a variety of soluble factors that inhibit HIV replication including the CC-chemokines RANTES (CCL5), MIP-1α (CCL3), and MIP-1β (CCL4) as well as one or more as yet poorly identified factors (see above). The presence of high levels of HIV viremia in vivo as well as exposure of CD8+ T cells in vitro to HIV envelope, both of which are associated with aberrant immune activation, has been shown to be associated with a variety of cellular functional abnormalities. Furthermore, since the integrity of CD8+ T cell function depends in part on adequate inductive signals from CD4+ T cells, the defect in CD8+ CTLs is likely compounded by the quantitative loss and qualitative dysfunction of CD4+ T cells. Finally, as mentioned above, certain cell surface negative regulatory molecules such as CTLA-4 and PD-1 are upregulated on activated T cells, and engagement of these molecules with their ligands may play a role in the exhaustion and death of CD8+, HIV-specific T cells.

B Cells The predominant defect in B cells from HIV-infected individuals is one of aberrant cellular activation, which is reflected by spontaneous proliferation and immunoglobulin secretion and by increased spontaneous secretion of TNF-α and IL-6. In addition, B cells from HIV viremic patients manifest a decreased capacity to mount a proliferative response to ligation of the B cell antigen receptor (surface IgM) at the same time as they are capable of robust differentiation in response to a variety of stimuli. B cells from HIV-infected individuals manifest enhanced spontaneous in vitro transformation with EBV, a process that is likely due to defective T cell immune surveillance. The in vivo counterpart of this phenomenon is an increase in the incidence of EBV-related B cell lymphomas in HIV-infected individuals. Untransformed B cells cannot be infected with HIV. However, HIV or its products can activate B cells directly; portions of the HIV gp41 envelope protein have been reported to induce polyclonal B cell activation. In addition, it has been reported that products of the VH_3 genes on the surface of B cells can serve as a receptor for HIV. B cells from patients with high levels of viremia bind virions to their surface via the CD21 complement receptor. It is likely that in vivo activation of B cells by replication-competent or -defective virus as well as viral products during the viremic state account at least in part for the spontaneous activation of these cells noted ex vivo. B cell subpopulations from HIV-infected individuals undergo a number of changes over the course of HIV disease, including the attrition of memory B cells; the appearance of mature, activated B cells defined by reduced expression of CD21, increased expression of activation markers, increased secretion of immunoglobulins, and increased susceptibility to Fas-mediated apoptosis; and the appearance of immature B cells associated with CD4+ T cell lymphopenia. Cognate B cell–CD4+ T cell interactions are abnormal in viremic HIV-infected individuals in that B cells respond poorly to CD4+ T cell help and CD4+ T cells receive inadequate co-stimulatory signals from activated B cells. In vivo, the aberrant activated state of B cells manifests itself by hypergammaglobulinemia and by the presence of circulating immune complexes and autoantibodies (see above). HIV-infected individuals respond poorly to primary and secondary immunizations with protein and polysaccharide antigens. Using immunization with influenza vaccine it has been demonstrated that there is a memory B cell defect in HIV-infected individuals, particularly those with high levels of HIV viremia. Taken together, these B cell defects are likely responsible in part for the increase in certain bacterial infections seen in advanced HIV disease in adults, as well as for the important role of bacterial infections in the morbidity and mortality of HIV-infected children, who cannot mount an adequate humoral response to common bacterial pathogens. The absolute number of circulating B cells may be depressed in HIV infection; this phenomenon likely reflects increased activation-induced apoptosis as well as a redistribution of cells out of the circulation and into the lymphoid tissue—phenomena that are associated with ongoing viral replication.

Monocytes/Macrophages Circulating monocytes are generally normal in number in HIV-infected individuals. Monocytes express the CD4 molecule and several co-receptors for HIV on their surface, including CCR5, CXCR4, and CCR3, and thus are targets of HIV infection. The degree of cytopathicity of HIV for cells of the monocyte lineage is low, and HIV can replicate extensively in cells of the monocyte lineage with relatively little cytopathic effect. Hence, monocyte-lineage cells may play a role in the dissemination of HIV in the body and can serve as reservoirs of HIV infection, thus representing an obstacle to the eradication of HIV by ARV drugs. In vivo infection of circulating monocytes is difficult to demonstrate; however, infection of tissue macrophages and macrophage-lineage cells in the brain (infiltrating macrophages or resident microglial cells) and lung (pulmonary alveolar macrophages) can be demonstrated easily. Tissue macrophages are an important source of HIV during the inflammatory response associated with opportunistic infections. Infection of monocyte precursors in the bone marrow may directly or indirectly be responsible for certain of the hematologic abnormalities in HIV-infected individuals. A number of abnormalities of circulating monocytes have been reported in HIV-infected individuals, including decreased secretion of IL-1 and IL-12; increased secretion of IL-10; defects in antigen presentation and induction of T cell responses due to decreased MHC class II expression; and abnormalities of Fc receptor function, C3 receptor–mediated clearance, oxidative burst responses, and certain cytotoxic functions such as ADCC, possibly related to low levels of expression of Fc and complement receptors. Exposure of monocytes to viral proteins such as gp120 and Tat, as well as to certain cytokines, can cause abnormal activation, and this may play a role in cellular dysfunction (see above).

Dendritic and Langerhans Cells Dendritic cells may play an important role in the initiation of HIV infection by virtue of the ability of HIV to bind to cell surface C-type lectin receptors, particularly DC-SIGN (see above). This allows efficient presentation of virus to CD4+ T cell targets that become infected; complexes of infected CD4+ T cells and dendritic cells provide an optimal microenvironment for virus replication. There has been considerable disagreement regarding the HIV infectibility and hence the depletion as well as the dysfunction of dendritic cells themselves. Depending on their state of maturation, dendritic cells express varying levels of CD4 as well as several chemokine receptors. In this regard, it appears that the ability of a dendritic cell to become infected depends in part on its state of maturation. Mature dendritic cells have been demonstrated to be infectable by both R5 and X4 isolates of HIV-1. Immature tissue dendritic cells have been less well studied in their native state. Even in those dendritic cells in which infection occurs, the efficiency of infection and level of productivity of infection is quite low compared to CD4+ T cells.

Natural Killer Cells The role of NK cells is to provide immunosurveillance against virus-infected cells, certain tumor cells, and allogeneic cells (Chap. 308). Functional abnormalities in NK cells have been observed throughout the course of HIV disease, and the severity of these abnormalities increases as disease progresses. HIV infection of target cells downregulates HLA-A and -B, but not HLA-C and -D molecules; this may explain in part the relative inability of NK cells to kill HIV-infected target cells. Most studies report that NK cells are normal in number; however, patients with high levels of virus replication manifest an abnormal representation of a functionally defective CD56–/CD16+ NK cell subset. This abnormal subset of NK cells manifests an increased expression of inhibitory NK cell receptors (iNKRs) and a substantial decrease in expression of natural cytotoxicity receptors (NCRs) and shows a markedly impaired lytic activity. The overrepresentation of this abnormal subset of NK cells may explain in part the observed defects in NK cell function in HIV-infected individuals. NK cells also serve as important sources of HIV-inhibitory CC-chemokines. NK cells isolated from HIV-infected individuals constitutively produce high levels of MIP-1α (CCL3), MIP-1β (CCL4), and RANTES (CCL5). In addition, high levels of these chemokines are seen when NK cells are stimulated with IL-2 or IL-15 or when CD16 is cross-linked or during the process of lytic killing of target cells. HIV-infected patients with high levels of plasma viremia manifest a decreased ability, compared to HIV-infected individuals who are aviremic, of their NK cells to block HIV replication in vitro in assays of both cell contact and supernatant-mediated suppression of virus. Finally, NK cell–dendritic cell interactions are important for normal immune function. NK cells and dendritic cells reciprocally modulate each other's activation and maturation. These interactions are markedly impaired in HIV-infected individuals with high levels of plasma viremia.

GENETIC FACTORS IN HIV PATHOGENESIS

MHC Genes Several reports have described MHC alleles and other host factors that may influence the pathogenesis and course of HIV disease. These include associations with transmission and with the type of clinical course, such as slow or rapid rates of progression to AIDS (Table 182-4). For example, researchers recently employed a whole-genome association strategy to identify two independently acting groups of polymorphisms associated with HLA loci B and C, which explained 15% of the variation in viral load among individuals during the asymptomatic period of infection. A number of mechanisms have been proposed whereby MHC-encoded molecules might predispose an individual either to rapid progression or to nonprogression to AIDS. These proposed mechanisms include the ability to present certain immunodominant HIV T helper or CTL epitopes, leading to a relatively protective immune response against HIV and hence to a slower rate of disease progression. In contrast, certain MHC class I or class II alleles might predispose an individual to an immunopathogenic response against viral epitopes in certain tissues, such as the CNS or lungs, or against certain HIV-infected cell types, such as macrophages or dendritic cells/Langerhans cells. In addition, certain rare MHC class I and class II alleles might facilitate rapid recognition of HIV-infected cells from the infecting partner in primary HIV infection and promote rejection of these cells by alloreactive responses.

Similarly, common MHC alleles could lead to less effective removal of HIV-infected allogeneic cells. In this regard, it has been demonstrated that allele sharing at HLA-B loci is associated with increased risk of transmission of HIV infection between heterosexual Zambian couples discordant for HIV. It has been clearly demonstrated that maximal *HLA* heterozygosity for class I loci (A, B, and C) is associated with a delayed onset of AIDS among HIV-infected individuals, whereas homozygosity for these loci was associated with a more rapid progression to AIDS and death. This observation is likely due to the fact that individuals who are heterozygous at *HLA* loci are able to present a greater variety of antigenic peptides to cytotoxic T lymphocytes than are homozygotes, resulting in a more effective immune response against a number of pathogens including HIV. Of particular note is the fact that the HLA class I alleles B*35 and Cw*04 were consistently associated with rapid development of AIDS. Other data have indicated that transporter associated with antigen-processing (TAP) genes play a role in determining the outcome of HIV infection. HLA profiles that reflect certain combinations of MHC-encoded TAP and class I and class II genes are strongly associated with different rates of progression to AIDS. A recent finding of genetic association with HIV disease progression has highlighted the role for NK cells in HIV disease. A single nucleotide polymorphism (SNP) in the killer immunoglobulin-like receptor (KIR) gene was shown to be strongly associated with rapid progression to AIDS. However, when the KIR3 DS1 SNP was present with HLA-B Bw4-80I, the resultant phenotype was delayed progression to AIDS, even though this HLA-B allele alone has no effect on HIV disease progression. Furthermore, the KIR3 DS1/HLA-B Bw4-80I-carrying individuals had a significantly reduced viral load, beginning early in the course of infection, and protection against opportunistic infections during the later stages of the disease. This observation points to the potential role of NK cells in the maintenance of the viral set point, and strongly suggests that HLA-B Bw4-80I serves

TABLE 182-4 HOST GENETIC FACTORS THAT INFLUENCE RISK OF TRANSMISSION AND RATES OF DISEASE PROGRESSION TO AIDS

	MHC Genes	
	HLA Class I[a]	**HLA Class II[a]**
Disease progression		
Rapid	**A23, A24,** *A26, A28, A29, A31, B7 supertype,* **B*08,** *B14, B21,* **B22,** *B25,* **B35,** *B37, B38,* **B53,** *B44, B49,* **C4, C7,** *C8, C16,* **homozygosity for class I alleles**	**DRB1*01, DRB1*03,** *DRB1*05, DRB1*11*
Slow	*A10, A19, A*30,* **A32,** *B14, B16, B17, B18,* **B27,** *B*39, B51,* **B57,** *B58, C8,* **heterozygosity for class I alleles**	*DRB1*03, DRB1*13*
Transmission		
Increased risk	*A2, B21, B35, Cw4,* **allele sharing between HIV donor and recipient**	*DRB1*05, DRB1*06, DRB1*13*
Reduced risk	*A2/A6802 supertype, A11, B18, B52, B57, B58, C2*	

Factor	**Association**
Chemokine and Chemokine Receptor Genes	
CCR5	Homozygous defect involving a 32-bp deletion corresponding to the second extracellular loop of the receptor results in loss of surface expression, and consequently, resistance to infection; heterozygous defect appears to result in partial protection against transmission and disease progression. Several single nucleotide polymorphisms (SNPs) in the *CCR5* promoter have been identified that along with the CCR2-64I polymorphism define nine human haplogroups (HHA to HHE, HHF*1, HHF*2, HHG*1 and HHG*2). Homozygosity for the HHE haplotype is associated with an increased risk of transmission and an accelerated rate of disease progression.
CCR2	Heterozygosity for the CCR2-64I polymorphism is associated with a slower rate of disease progression, and in one study this effect was found to be more prominent in African Americans.
CX3CR1	Mutations 249I and 280M are associated with a rapid rate of disease progression to AIDS in a French-Caucasian cohort. Inconsistent effects were detected in other cohorts.
CCL3L1 (MIP-1αP)	The copy number of *CCL3L1* varies within and among populations (range 0–10 copies per diploid genome). A copy number lower than the average gene dose found in a population is associated with an increased risk of acquiring HIV and a more rapid rate of disease progression to AIDS.
CCL5 (RANTES)	SNPs in the promoter, intron, and 3′-untranslated region can influence transcription and protein production, and consequently, affect risk of acquiring HIV and rates of disease progression. For example, a haplotype defined by two promoter SNPs (-471A/-96C) is associated with a faster rate of disease progression in European Americans. However, the -471A/-96G haplotype is found mostly in populations from East Asia, and this haplotype was associated with a slow rate of disease progression in a Japanese cohort.
CCL2 (MCP-1)	The *MCP-1 -2578G* allele results in increased transcription, protein production, and monocyte recruitment. Homozygosity for the *MCP-1 -2578G* allele is associated with an enhanced risk of developing HIV-1-associated dementia and a rapid disease course.
CXCL12 (SDF-1)	The *SDF-1* 3′A SNP in the 3′ untranslated region was initially reported to be associated with a slower disease rate of progression in a large U.S.-based cohort, but the results in other cohorts suggest an opposite effect.
Cytokine Genes	
IL-10	Individuals carrying the *IL-10*-592A promoter allele were at increased risk for HIV infection and, once infected, progressed more rapidly than did homozygotes for the alternative *IL-10-5′*-592 C/C genotype.
IL-4	The *IL-4*-589T results in higher levels of IL-4 production in vivo, resulting in downregulation of *CCR5*. However, the effects of this polymorphism on disease progression are inconsistent.
IL-6	A single report showed that possession of the IL-6 promoter polymorphism (-174G) is associated with an increased risk of developing Kaposi sarcoma in HIV-1-positive individuals.
TNF-α	A single report showed that the SNP *TNF-α*-238A, but not the -308A allele correlates with a higher frequency of lipodystrophy.
Other Genes	
APOBEC3G	The 186R allele is associated with a decline in CD4 T cells and an accelerated rate of progression to AIDS in African Americans.
VDR	Homozygosity for the vitamin D receptor gene polymorphism B (VDR-BB) correlates with a rapid progression to AIDS.
MBL2	Conflicting effects have been reported for MBL variants.
Gene-Gene Interactions	
KIR gene with *HLA-B*	In the absence of *HLA-B* Bw4-80I, *KIR3DS1* is strongly associated with rapid progression to AIDS. This effect is reversed by the presence of *HLA-B* Bw4-80I. Individuals carrying both genes have a delayed progression to AIDS; in the absence of *KIR3DS1*, *HLA-B* Bw4-80I has no effect on disease progression.
CCL3L1 and *CCR5*	Based on possession of a low or high copy number of *CCL3L1* ($CCL3L1^{low}$ or $CCL3L1^{high}$) and a detrimental or nondetrimental ($CCR5^{det}$ or $CCR5^{nondet}$) *CCR5* genotype, variations in these two genes segregate into four genetic risk groups (GRGs). In HIV-infected adults followed in a U.S.-based cohort, an association for a low, moderate, and high risk of acquiring HIV or progressing rapidly to AIDS and death was detected in those possessing a $CCL3L1^{high}/CCR5^{nondet}$, $CCL3L1^{high}/CCR5^{det}$ or $CCL3L1^{low}/CCR5^{nondet}$, and $CCL3L1^{low}/CCR5^{det}$ GRG, respectively.

[a]For MHC genes, bold denotes alleles that in multiple reports have been shown to have consistent effects in different cohorts, whereas italic denotes alleles that have been show to have effects in a few cohorts. HH, human haplogroup.

Sources: Sunil K. Ahuja, MD, and adapted from HA Stephens: Trends Immunol 26(1):41, 2005; M Carrington, SJ O'Brien: Annu Rev Med 54:535 2003; Epub 2001 Dec 3; RA Kaslow et al: J Infect Dis. 191 [Suppl 1]:S68, 2005; A Telenti, G Bleiber: Future Virol 1:55, 2006.

as the ligand activating the KIR, resulting in the death of the target cell. These gene-gene interactions between KIR and MHC genes are illustrated in Table 182-4.

Chemokine Receptors The most dramatic example of a genetic factor influencing HIV infection and/or pathogenesis relates to the gene that codes for the HIV cellular co-receptor CCR5. Rare individuals have been reported who had repetitive sexual exposure to HIV in high-risk situations but remained uninfected. The peripheral blood mononuclear cells of two such individuals were found to be highly resistant to infection in vitro with R5 strains of HIV-1 but were readily infected with X4 strains. Genetic analysis revealed that these two individuals inherited a homozygous defect in the gene that codes for CCR5, the cellular co-receptor for R5 strains of HIV-1. The defective *CCR5* allele contained a 32-bp deletion corresponding to the second extracellular loop of the receptor (Δ*32* allele). The encoded protein was severely truncated and the receptor was nonfunctional, explaining the refractoriness to infection with R5 strains of HIV-1. Population studies revealed that ~1% of the Caucasian population of western European ancestry possessed the homozygous defect. Up to 20% of individuals of European descent were found to be heterozygous for the *CCR5* Δ*32* allele. Of note, cohort studies of hundreds of DNA samples originating from western and central Africa and Far East Asia indicate that the *CCR5* Δ*32* allele is either absent or extremely rare in these populations. A number of studies found that the frequency of *CCR5* Δ*32* allele was enriched in exposed, uninfected individuals. Furthermore, in a cohort of 1400 HIV-1–infected Caucasian individuals, no subject homozygous for the mutation was found, strongly supporting the concept that the homozygous defect confers protection against infection. This finding is particularly compelling in light of the fact that transmitting viruses are strongly biased toward R5 strains of HIV-1 (see above). Of note, several individuals have been identified who were homozygous for the *CCR5* Δ*32* defect who in fact did become infected with HIV. These individuals were found to have an X4 strain of HIV that was associated in some cases with an accelerated course of disease. In some studies, HIV-infected individuals who are heterozygous for the *CCR5* Δ*32* allele had a slower rate of disease progression. Slow progression of HIV disease is also seen in individuals who are heterozygous for the *CCR2-64I* polymorphism. This *CCR2-64I* allele–associated effect could be due to its linkage with SNPs in the *CCR5* promoter that are known to influence disease progression rates and/or due to dimerization of CXCR4 with the mutated *CCR2-64I* resulting in a decreased expression of CXCR4 on the cell surface.

A number of SNPs in the *CCR5* promoter have been associated with varied rates of disease progression. The promoter SNPs along the *CCR5* Δ*32* and CCR2-V64I alleles define nine *CCR5* human haplogroups (HH)designated as HHA through HHE, and HHG*1, HHG*2, HHF*1 and HHF*2 (Table 182-4). Studies have shown that homozygosity for the HHE haplotype is associated with an increased risk of acquiring HIV and progressing rapidly to AIDS. Pairing of the HHC and the *CCR5* Δ*32*-containing HHG*2 haplotype is associated with a slower rate of disease progression and reduced risk of acquiring HIV.

Chemokines The varied distribution of the copy number of *CCL3L1* and *RANTES* polymorphisms provides some striking examples of the effect of chemokine genes on HIV pathogenesis. The *CCL3L1* gene encodes MIP-1αP, the most potent agonist of CCR5 and HIV-suppressive chemokine for R5 strains of HIV-1. This gene is present in a range of copy numbers in and among different racial groups. Individuals with fewer than average copy numbers for their racial group showed both an increased susceptibility to infection with HIV and a faster rate of progression to AIDS. When the interaction of this gene with the different *CCR5* alleles was examined, individuals with a low *CCL3L1* gene dose and certain *CCR5* alleles, which have a detrimental effect on disease progression, were shown to have a significantly greater risk of transmission and faster disease progression rates. SNPs have been identified in the gene that encodes for CCL5 (*RANTES*), another potent agonist of CCR5 and an R5 HIV-suppressive chemokine. Some of these SNPs correlate with either an increased or decreased *CCL5* gene transcription and this is thought to underlie the disease associations detected. For example, the *CCL5* -96G SNP upregulates *CCL5* gene transcription and is associated with delayed progression to AIDS in a Japanese cohort; the prevalence of this allele is very low in other populations. The opposite effects are observed for an intronic *CCL5* SNP designated as In1.1C. This SNP is associated with decreased *CCL5* gene transcription and correlates strongly with a rapid progression rate to AIDS. Other SNPs that decrease *CCL5* gene transcription are associated with a higher rate of HIV infection. The results of these genotype-phenotype studies with *CCL3L1* and *CCL5* genes reinforce the central role for R5 viruses in the establishment of HIV infection.

Additional associations for other chemokines have been noted. CCL2 is a one of the most potent chemokines that attracts and activates mononuclear phagocytes (MP). In a U.S. population-based study, homozygosity for the *CCL2* (*MCP-1*) -2578G allele was associated with a 50% reduction in the risk of acquiring HIV-1. However, once HIV-1 infection was established, this same *CCL2* genotype was associated with accelerated disease progression and a 4.5-fold increased risk of HIV-associated dementia. Possession of the *CCL2* -2578G allele is associated with increased CCL2 serum levels and recruitment of MPs to inflamed tissues. Since recruitment of MPs to the CNS and the activation status of MPs in the CNS is thought to be a key determinant of HIV-associated dementia, these association studies implicate a central role for CCL2 in the pathogenesis of HIV-related CNS disease.

Cytokines In addition to the chemokine receptors and chemokines, polymorphisms in cytokine genes have also been found to influence intersubject differences in susceptibility to HIV/AIDS. Individuals who carry a certain allele (-592A) of the IL-10 promoter are at increased risk of infection and, once infected, progress more rapidly than homozygotes for the alternative genotype. The mechanism of this effect is felt to be a downregulation of the inhibitory cytokine IL-10 resulting in facilitation of HIV replication. The SNP, IL-4 -589T, increases IL-4 production. This allele associates with a slower progression to AIDS, presumably through the downregulation of CCR5 by higher and more sustained levels of IL-4. However, the effects of this IL-4 polymorphism on disease progression are inconsistent in different studies.

Other Genes Additional genes such as those involved in innate immunity, lipid metabolism, and cell cycle have also been found to be associated with altered HIV/AIDS susceptibility. For example, a histidine-arginine change at position 186 in the gene that encodes APOBEC3G is found at a higher frequency in individuals of African descent and is associated with more rapid disease progression rates. Homozygosity for the vitamin D receptor form B correlates with rapid progression to AIDS. The mechanism is thought to relate to the known effects of vitamin D on immune modulation.

The effects of some genes [e.g., *CX3CR1*, *CXCL12 (SDF-1)*, *IL-4*, *IL-6*, *TNF-α*, and *MBL2*] on HIV pathogenesis are either from a single cohort or the findings are inconsistent in different cohorts. Nevertheless, there is growing appreciation that the evolutionary histories of human populations have had a significant impact on the distribution of variation of some genes that are thought to play a key role in HIV-1/AIDS pathogenesis, and that this might be responsible, in part, for the heterogeneous nature of the epidemiology of the HIV-1 pandemic.

NEUROPATHOGENESIS

While there has been a remarkable decrease in the incidence of HIV encephalopathy among those with access to treatment in the era of effective ARV therapy, HIV-infected individuals can still experience a variety of neurologic abnormalities due either to opportunistic infections and neoplasms or to direct effects of HIV or its products (see below). With regard to the latter, HIV has been demonstrated in the brain and CSF of infected individuals with and without neuropsychiatric abnormalities. The main cell types that are infected in the brain in vivo are the perivascular macrophages and the microglial cells; monocytes that have already been infected in the blood can migrate into the brain, where they then reside as macrophages, or macrophages can be directly infected within the brain. The precise mechanisms whereby HIV enters the brain are unclear; however, they are thought to relate, at least in part, to the ability of virus-infected and immune-activated macrophages to induce adhesion molecules such as E-selectin and vascular cell adhesion molecule-1 (VCAM-1) on brain endothelium. Other studies have demonstrated that HIV gp120 enhances the expression of intercellular adhesion molecule-1 (ICAM-1) in glial cells; this effect may facilitate entry of HIV-infected cells into the CNS and may promote syncytia formation. Virus isolates from the brain are preferentially R5 strains as opposed to X4 strains (see above); in this regard, HIV-infected individuals who are heterozygous for *CCR5-Δ32* appear to be relatively protected against the development of HIV encephalopathy compared to wild-type individuals. Distinct HIV envelope sequences are associated with the clinical expression of the AIDS dementia complex (see below). There is no convincing evidence that brain cells other than those of monocyte/macrophage lineage can be productively infected in vivo. Astrocytes have been reported to be susceptible to HIV infection in vitro despite the fact that they do not express detectable levels of cell-surface CD4 or the main HIV co-receptors. Nonetheless, they do not support active virus replication. There is no convincing evidence that oligodendrocytes or neurons can be infected with HIV (see below).

HIV-infected individuals may manifest white matter lesions as well as neuronal loss. Given the absence of evidence of HIV infection of neurons either in vivo or in vitro, it is highly unlikely that direct infection of these cells accounts for their loss. Rather, the HIV-mediated effects on neurons and oligodendrocytes are thought to involve indirect pathways whereby viral proteins, particularly gp120 and Tat, trigger the release of endogenous neurotoxins from macrophages and to a lesser extent from astrocytes. In addition, it has been demonstrated that both HIV-1 Nef and Tat can induce chemotaxis of leukocytes, including monocytes, into the CNS. Neurotoxins can be released from monocytes as a consequence of infection and/or immune activation. Monocyte-derived neurotoxic factors have been reported to kill neurons via the *N*-methyl-D-aspartate (NMDA) receptor. In addition, HIV gp120 shed by virus-infected monocytes could cause neurotoxicity by antagonizing the function of vasoactive intestinal peptide (VIP), by elevating intracellular calcium levels, and by decreasing nerve growth factor levels in the cerebral cortex. A variety of monocyte-derived cytokines can contribute directly or indirectly to the neurotoxic effects in HIV infection; these include TNF-α, IL-1, IL-6, TGF-β, IFN-γ, platelet-activating factor, and endothelin. Furthermore, among the CC-chemokines, elevated levels of monocyte chemotactic protein (MCP)1 in the brain and CSF have been shown to correlate best with the presence and degree of HIV encephalopathy. In addition, infection and/or activation of monocyte-lineage cells can result in increased production of eicosanoids, nitric oxide, and quinolinic acid, which may contribute to neurotoxicity. Astrocytes may play diverse roles in HIV neuropathogenesis. Reactive gliosis or astrocytosis has been demonstrated in the brains of HIV-infected individuals, and TNF-α and IL-6 have been shown to induce astrocyte proliferation. In addition, astrocyte-derived IL-6 can induce HIV expression in infected cells in vitro. Furthermore, it has been suggested that astrocytes may downregulate macrophage-produced neurotoxins. It has been reported that HIV-infected individuals with the E4 allele for apolipoprotein E (apo E) are at increased risk for AIDS encephalopathy and peripheral neuropathy. The likelihood that HIV or its products are involved in neuropathogenesis is supported by the observation that neuropsychiatric abnormalities may undergo remarkable and rapid improvement upon the initiation of ARV therapy.

It has also been suggested that the CNS may serve as a relatively sequestered site for a reservoir of latently infected cells and for the slow, continual replication of HIV that might be a barrier for the eradication of virus by ARV therapy (see "Reservoirs of HIV-Infected Cells: Obstacle to the Eradication of Virus," above).

PATHOGENESIS OF KAPOSI'S SARCOMA

There are at least four distinct epidemiologic forms of KS: (1) the classic form that occurs in older men of predominantly Mediterranean or eastern European Jewish backgrounds with no recognized contributing factors; (2) the equatorial African form that occurs in all ages, also without any recognized precipitating factors; (3) the form associated with organ transplantation and its attendant iatrogenic immunosuppressed state; and (4) the form associated with HIV-1 infection. In the latter two forms, KS is an opportunistic disease; in HIV-infected individuals, unlike typical opportunistic infections, its occurrence is not strictly related to the level of depression of CD4+ T cell counts (see below). The pathogenesis of KS is complex; fundamentally, it is an angioproliferative disease that is not a true neoplastic sarcoma, at least not in its early stages. It is a manifestation of excessive proliferation of spindle cells that are believed to be of vascular origin and have features in common with endothelial and smooth-muscle cells. In HIV disease the development of KS is dependent on the interplay of a variety of factors including HIV-1 itself, human herpes virus 8 (HHV-8), immune activation, and cytokine secretion. A number of epidemiologic and virologic studies have clearly linked HHV-8, which is also referred to as *Kaposi's sarcoma–associated herpesvirus* (KSHV), to KS not only in HIV-infected individuals but also in individuals with the other forms of KS. HHV-8 is a γ-herpesvirus related to EBV and herpesvirus saimiri. It encodes a homologue to human IL-6 and in addition to KS has been implicated in the pathogenesis of body cavity lymphoma, multiple myeloma, and monoclonal gammopathy of undetermined significance. Sequences of HHV-8 are found universally in the lesions of KS, and patients with KS are virtually all seropositive for HHV-8. HHV-8 DNA sequences can be found in the B cells of 30–50% of patients with KS and 7% of patients with AIDS without clinically apparent KS.

Between 1 and 2% of eligible blood donors are positive for antibodies to HHV-8, while the prevalence of HHV-8 seropositivity in HIV-infected men is 30–35%. The prevalence in HIV-infected women is ~4%. This finding is reflective of the lower incidence of KS in women. It has been debated whether HHV-8 is actually the transforming agent in KS; the bulk of the cells in the tumor lesions of KS are not neoplastic cells. However, it has been demonstrated that endothelial cells can be transformed in vitro by HHV-8. In this regard, HHV-8 possesses a number of genes including homologues of the IL-8 receptor, Bcl-2, and cyclin D, which can potentially transform the host cell. Despite the complexity of the pathogenic events associated with the development of KS in HIV-infected individuals, HHV-8 is the etiologic agent of this disease. The initiation and/or propagation of KS requires an activated state and is mediated, at least in part, by cytokines. A number of factors, including TNF-α, IL-1β, IL-6, GM-CSF, basic fibroblast growth factor, and oncostatin M, function in an autocrine and paracrine manner to sustain the growth and chemotaxis of the KS spindle cells. In this regard, KSHV-derived IL-6 has been demonstrated to induce proliferation of lymphoma cells and to inhibit the cytostatic effects of INF-α on KSHV-infected lymphoma cells.

IMMUNE RESPONSE TO HIV

As detailed above and below, following the initial burst of viremia during primary infection, HIV-infected individuals mount robust immune responses that in most cases substantially curtail the levels of plasma viremia and likely contribute to delaying the ultimate development of clinically apparent disease for a median of 10 years in untreated individuals. This immune response contains elements of both humoral and cell-mediated immunity involving both innate and adaptive immune responses (**Table 182-5**; **Fig. 182-24**). It is directed against multiple antigenic determinants of the HIV virion as well as against viral proteins expressed on the surface of infected cells. Ironically, those CD4+ T cells with T cell receptors specific for HIV are theoretically those CD4+ T cells most likely to be activated and thus to serve as early targets for productive HIV infection and the cell death or dysfunction associated with infection. Thus, an early consequence of HIV infection is interference with and decrease of the helper cell population needed to generate an effective immune response.

Although a great deal of investigation has been directed toward delineating and better understanding the components of this immune

TABLE 182-5 ELEMENTS OF THE IMMUNE RESPONSE TO HIV

- Humoral immunity
  - Binding antibodies
  - Neutralizing antibodies
    - Type specific
    - Group specific
  - Antibodies participating in antibody-dependent cellular cytotoxicity (ADCC)
    - Protective
    - Pathogenic (bystander killing)
  - Enhancing antibodies
  - Complement
- Cell-mediated immunity
  - Helper CD4+ T lymphocytes
  - Class I MHC–restricted cytotoxic CD8+ T lymphocytes
  - CD8+ T cell–mediated inhibition (noncytolytic)
  - ADCC
  - Natural killer cells

response, it remains unclear which immunologic effector mechanisms are most important in delaying progression of infection and which, if any, play a role in the pathogenesis of HIV disease. This lack of knowledge has also hampered the ability to develop an effective vaccine for HIV disease.

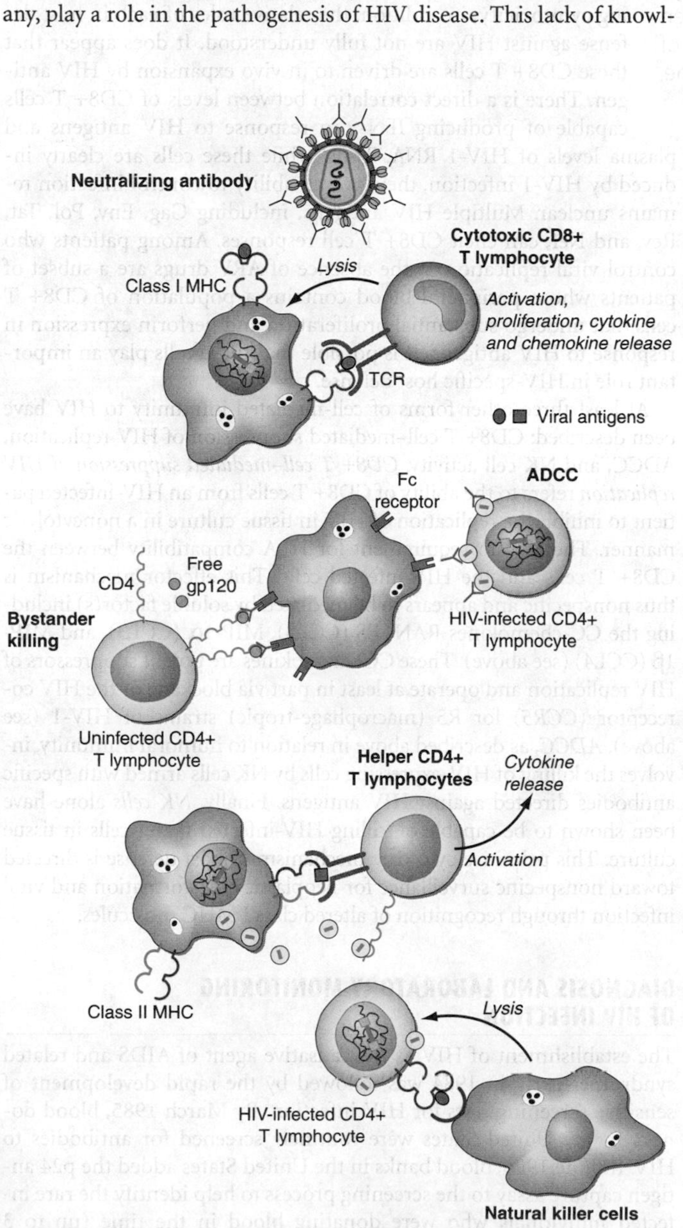

FIGURE 182-24 Schematic representation of the different immunologic effector mechanisms thought to be active in the setting of HIV infection. Detailed descriptions are given in the text. TCR, T cell receptor; ADCC, antibody-dependent cellular cytotoxicity; MHC, major histocompatibility complex.

HUMORAL IMMUNE RESPONSE

Antibodies to HIV usually appear within 6 weeks and almost invariably within 12 weeks of primary infection (Fig. 182-25); rare exceptions are individuals who have defects in the ability to produce HIV-specific antibodies. Detection of these antibodies forms the basis of most diagnostic screening tests for HIV infection. The appearance of HIV-binding antibodies detected by ELISA and Western blot assays occurs prior to the appearance of neutralizing antibodies; the latter generally appear following the initial decreases in plasma viremia, which is more closely related to the appearance of HIV-specific CD8+ T lymphocytes. The first antibodies detected are those directed against the structural or gag proteins of HIV, p24 and p17, and the gag precursor p55. The development of antibodies to p24 is associated with a decrease in the serum levels of free p24 antigen. Antibodies to the gag proteins are followed by the appearance of antibodies to the envelope proteins (gp160, gp120, p88, and gp41) and to the products of the *pol* gene (p31, p51, and p66). In addition, one may see antibodies to the low-molecular-weight regulatory proteins encoded by the HIV genes *vpr*, *vpu*, *vif*, *rev*, *tat*, and *nef*. On rare occasion, levels of HIV-specific antibodies may decline during treatment of acute HIV infection.

While antibodies to multiple antigens of HIV are produced, the precise functional significance of these different antibodies is unclear. The only viral proteins that elicit neutralizing antibodies are the envelope proteins gp120 and gp41. As noted above, the envelope of HIV consists of an outer envelope glycoprotein with a molecular mass of 120 kDa and a transmembrane glycoprotein with a molecular mass of 41 kDa. These are initially synthesized as a 160-kDa precursor that is cleaved by cellular proteases. Most of the antienvelope antibodies are directed either toward an epitope in the gp41 region comprising amino acids 579–613 or toward a hypervariable region in the gp120 molecule, known as the *V3 loop region*, comprising amino acids 303–338. This V3 region is a major site for the development of mutations that lead to variants of HIV that are not well recognized by the immune system.

Antibodies directed toward the envelope proteins of HIV have been characterized both as being protective and as possibly contributing to the pathogenesis of HIV disease. Among the protective antibodies are those that function to neutralize HIV directly and prevent the spread of infection to additional cells, as well as those that participate in ADCC. Within the first 6 months of infection neutralizing antibodies appear; however, the virus quickly escapes these neutralizing antibodies. One of the principal mechanisms of immune escape is the addition of N-linked glycosylation sites. The added carbohydrate moieties interfere with envelope recognition by these initial antibodies. The hyperglycosylation of the envelope protein has been termed the *glycan shield*. Neutralizing antibodies appear to be of two forms, type-specific and group-specific. *Type-specific neutralizing antibodies* are generally directed to the V3 loop region. These antibodies neutralize only viruses of a given strain and are present in low titer in most infected individuals. *Group-specific neutralizing antibodies* are capable of neutralizing a wide variety of HIV isolates. At least two forms of group-specific antibodies have been identified: those binding to amino acids 423–437 of gp120, which lie close to the CD4 binding site, and those binding to amino acids 728–745 of gp41, which lie proximal to the viral membrane. The other major class of protective antibodies are those that participate in ADCC, which is actually a form of cell-mediated immunity (Chap. 308) in which NK cells that bear Fc receptors are armed with specific anti-HIV antibodies that bind to the NK cells via their Fc portion. These armed NK cells then bind to and destroy cells expressing HIV antigens. Antibodies to both gp120 and gp41 have been shown to participate in ADCC-mediated killing of HIV-infected cells. The levels of antienvelope antibodies capable of mediating ADCC are highest in the earlier stages of HIV infection. In vitro, IL-2 can augment ADCC-mediated killing.

In addition to playing a role in host defense, HIV-specific antibodies have also been implicated in disease pathogenesis. Antibodies di-

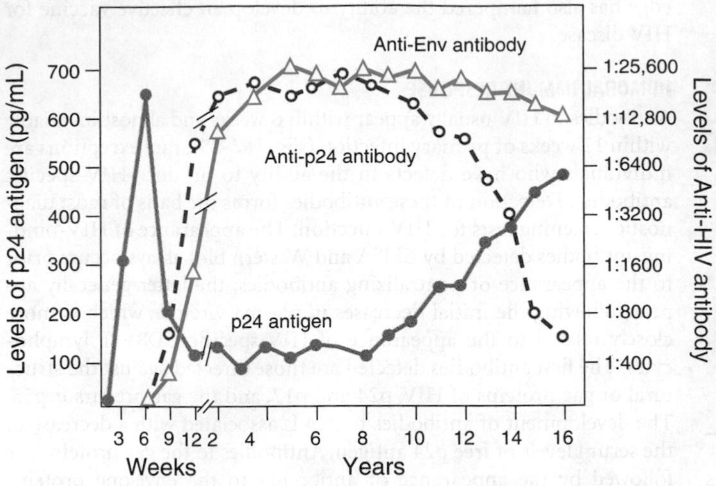

FIGURE 182-25 Relationship between antigenemia and the development of antibodies to HIV. Antibodies to HIV proteins are generally seen 6–12 weeks following infection and 3–6 weeks after the development of plasma viremia. Late in the course of illness, antibody levels to p24 decline, generally in association with a rising titer of p24 antigen.

rected to gp41, when present in low titer, have been shown in vitro to be capable of facilitating infection of cells through an Fc receptor–mediated mechanism known as *antibody enhancement.* Thus, the same regions of the envelope protein of HIV that give rise to antibodies capable of mediating ADCC also elicit the production of antibodies that can facilitate infection of cells in vitro. In addition, it has been postulated that anti-gp120 antibodies that participate in the ADCC killing of HIV-infected cells might also kill uninfected CD4+ T cells if the uninfected cells had bound free gp120, a phenomenon referred to as *bystander killing.* One of the most primitive components of the humoral immune system is the complement system (Chap. 308). This element of innate immunity consists of ~30 proteins that are found circulating in blood or associated with cell membranes. While HIV alone is capable of directly activating the complement cascade, the resulting lysis is weak due to the presence of host cell regulatory proteins captured in the virion envelope during budding. It is possible that complement-opsonized HIV virions have increased infectivity in a manner analogous to antibody-mediated enhancement.

CELLULAR IMMUNE RESPONSE

Given the fact that T cell–mediated immunity is known to play a major role in host defense against most viral infections (Chap. 308), it is generally thought to be an important component of the host immune response to HIV. T cell immunity can be divided into two major categories, mediated respectively by the *helper/inducer CD4+ T cells* and the *cytotoxic/immunoregulatory CD8+ T cells.*

HIV-specific CD4+ T cells can be detected in the majority of HIV-infected patients through the use of flow cytometry to measure intracellular cytokine production in response to MHC class II tetramers pulsed with HIV peptides or through lymphocyte proliferation assays utilizing HIV antigens such as p24. HIV-specific CD4+ T cells may be preferential targets of HIV infection by HIV-infected antigen-presenting cells during the generation of an immune response to HIV (see above). However, they also are likely to undergo clonal expansions in response to HIV antigens and thus survive as a population of cells. No clear correlations exist between levels of HIV-specific CD4+ T lymphocytes and plasma HIV RNA levels; however, in the setting of high viral loads, CD4+ T cell responses to HIV antigens appear to shift from one of proliferation and IL-2 production to one of IFN-γ production. Thus, while a reverse correlation exists between the level of p24-specific proliferation and levels of plasma HIV viremia, the nature of the causal relationship between these parameters is unclear.

MHC class I–restricted, HIV-specific CD8+ T cells have been identified in the peripheral blood of patients with HIV-1 infection. These cells include CTLs that produce perforins and T cells that can be induced by HIV antigens to express an array of cytokines such as IFN-γ. CTLs have been identified in the peripheral blood of patients within weeks of HIV infection. These CD8+ T lymphocytes, through their HIV-specific antigen receptors, bind to and cause the lytic destruction of target cells bearing autologous MHC class I molecules associated with HIV antigens. Two types of CTL activity can be demonstrated in the peripheral blood or lymph node mononuclear cells of HIV-infected individuals. The first type directly lyses appropriate target cells in culture without prior in vitro stimulation (*spontaneous CTL activity*). The other type of CTL activity reflects the *precursor frequency of CTLs* (CTLp); this type of CTL activity can be demonstrated by stimulation of CD8+ T cells in vitro with a mitogen such as phytohemagglutinin or anti-CD3 antibody.

In addition to CTLs, CD8+ T cells capable of being induced by HIV antigens to express cytokines such as IFN-γ also appear in the setting of HIV-1 infection. It is not clear whether these are the same or different effector pools compared to those cells mediating cytotoxicity; in addition, the relative roles of each in host defense against HIV are not fully understood. It does appear that these CD8+ T cells are driven to in vivo expansion by HIV antigen. There is a direct correlation between levels of CD8+ T cells capable of producing IFN-γ in response to HIV antigens and plasma levels of HIV-1 RNA. Thus, while these cells are clearly induced by HIV-1 infection, their overall ability to control infection remains unclear. Multiple HIV antigens, including Gag, Env, Pol, Tat, Rev, and Nef, can elicit CD8+ T cell responses. Among patients who control viral replication in the absence of ARV drugs are a subset of patients whose peripheral blood contains a population of CD8+ T cells that undergo substantial proliferation and perforin expression in response to HIV antigens. It is possible that these cells play an important role in HIV-specific host defense.

At least three other forms of cell-mediated immunity to HIV have been described: CD8+ T cell–mediated suppression of HIV replication, ADCC, and NK cell activity. *CD8+ T cell–mediated suppression of HIV replication* refers to the ability of CD8+ T cells from an HIV-infected patient to inhibit the replication of HIV in tissue culture in a noncytolytic manner. There is no requirement for HLA compatibility between the CD8+ T cells and the HIV-infected cells. This effector mechanism is thus nonspecific and appears to be mediated by soluble factor(s) including the CC-chemokines RANTES (CCL5), MIP-1α (CCL3), and MIP-1β (CCL4) (see above). These CC-chemokines are potent suppressors of HIV replication and operate at least in part via blockade of the HIV coreceptor (*CCR5*) for R5 (macrophage-tropic) strains of HIV-1 (see above). *ADCC*, as described above in relation to humoral immunity, involves the killing of HIV-expressing cells by NK cells armed with specific antibodies directed against HIV antigens. Finally, *NK cells* alone have been shown to be capable of killing HIV-infected target cells in tissue culture. This primitive cytotoxic mechanism of host defense is directed toward nonspecific surveillance for neoplastic transformation and viral infection through recognition of altered class I MHC molecules.

DIAGNOSIS AND LABORATORY MONITORING OF HIV INFECTION

The establishment of HIV as the causative agent of AIDS and related syndromes early in 1984 was followed by the rapid development of sensitive screening tests for HIV infection. By March 1985, blood donors in the United States were routinely screened for antibodies to HIV. In June 1996, blood banks in the United States added the p24 antigen capture assay to the screening process to help identify the rare infected individuals who were donating blood in the time (up to 3 months) between infection and the development of antibodies. In 2002 the ability to detect early infection with HIV was further enhanced by the licensure of nucleic acid testing (NAT) as a routine part of blood donor screening. These refinements decreased the interval between infection and detection (window period) from 22 days for

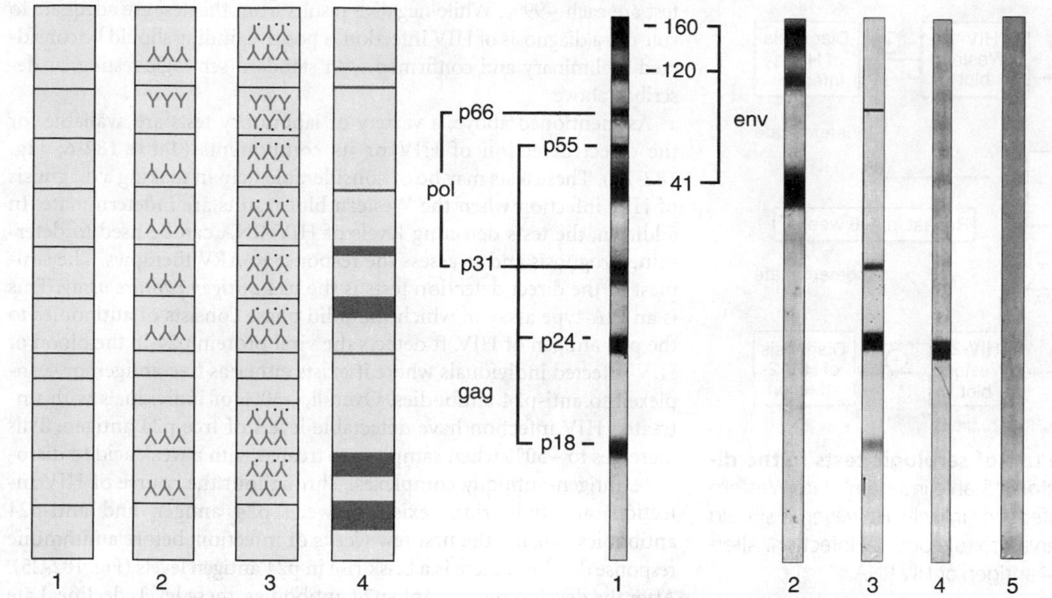

A
1. Virus digested: digest separated into components by molecular weight
2. Proteins transferred to filter paper: reaction with test serum
3. Enzyme-conjugated antihuman antibody added
4. Substrate added and color noted

B
1. Positive HIV-1 infection
2. gp 160 immunization
3. Indeterminate (HIV-2 infection)
4. Indeterminate (cross-reacting antibody to p24)
5. Negative

FIGURE 182-26 Western blot assay for detection of antibodies to HIV. *A.* Schematic representation of how a Western blot is performed. ***B.*** Examples of patterns of Western blot reactivity. In each instance the Western blot strip contains antigens to HIV-1. The sera from the patient immunized to the HIV-1 envelope contains only antibodies to the HIV-1 envelope proteins. The sera from the patient with HIV-2 infection cross-reacts with both *reverse transcriptase* and *gag* gene products of HIV-1.

antibody testing to 16 days with p24 antigen testing and subsequently to 12 days with nucleic acid testing. The development of sensitive assays for monitoring levels of plasma viremia ushered in a new era of being able to monitor the progression of HIV disease more closely. Utilization of these tests, coupled with the measurement of levels of CD4+ T lymphocytes in peripheral blood, is essential in the management of patients with HIV infection.

DIAGNOSIS OF HIV INFECTION

The CDC has recommended that screening for HIV infection be performed as a matter of routine health care. The diagnosis of HIV infection depends upon the demonstration of antibodies to HIV and/or the direct detection of HIV or one of its components. As noted above, antibodies to HIV generally appear in the circulation 2–12 weeks following infection.

The standard blood screening test for HIV infection is the ELISA, also referred to as an *enzyme immunoassay* (EIA). This solid-phase assay is an extremely good screening test with a sensitivity of >99.5%. Most diagnostic laboratories use a commercial EIA kit that contains antigens from both HIV-1 and HIV-2 and thus are able to detect either. These kits use both natural and recombinant antigens and are continuously updated to increase their sensitivity to newly discovered species, such as group O viruses (Fig. 182-6). The fourth generation EIA tests combine detection of antibodies to HIV with detection of the p24 antigen of HIV. EIA tests are generally scored as positive (highly reactive), negative (nonreactive), or indeterminate (partially reactive). While the EIA is an extremely sensitive test, it is not optimal with regard to specificity. This is particularly true in studies of low-risk individuals, such as volunteer blood donors. In this latter population, only 10% of EIA-positive individuals are subsequently confirmed to have HIV infection. Among the factors associated with false-positive EIA tests are antibodies to class II antigens, autoantibodies, hepatic disease, recent influenza vaccination, and acute viral infections. For these reasons, anyone suspected of having HIV infection based upon a positive or inconclusive EIA result must have the result confirmed with a more specific assay such as the Western blot. One can estimate whether or not an individual has a recent infection with HIV-1 by comparing the results on a standard assay that will score positive for all infected individuals to the results on an assay modified to be less sensitive ("detuned assay") that will score positive only for individuals with established HIV infection. In rare instances, an HIV-infected individual treated early in the course of infection may revert to a negative EIA. This does *not* indicate clearing of infection; rather, it signifies levels of ongoing exposure to virus insufficient to maintain a measurable antibody response. When these individuals have discontinued therapy, viruses and antibodies have reappeared.

The most commonly used confirmatory test is the Western blot (Fig. 182-26). This assay takes advantage of the fact that multiple HIV antigens of different, well-characterized molecular weights elicit the production of specific antibodies. These antigens can be separated on the basis of molecular weight, and antibodies to each component can be detected as discrete bands on the Western blot. A negative Western blot is one in which no bands are present at molecular weights corresponding to HIV gene products. In a patient with a positive or indeterminate EIA and a negative Western blot, one can conclude with certainty that the EIA reactivity was a false positive. On the other hand, a Western blot demonstrating antibodies to products of all three of the major genes of HIV (*gag*, *pol*, and *env*) is conclusive evidence of infection with HIV. Criteria established by the U.S. Food & Drug Administration (FDA) in 1993 for a positive Western blot state that a result is considered positive if antibodies exist to two of the three HIV proteins: p24, gp41, and gp120/160. Using these criteria, ~10% of all blood donors deemed positive for HIV-1 infection lacked an antibody band to the *pol* gene product p31. Some 50% of these blood donors were subsequently found to be false positives. Thus, the absence of the p31 band should increase the suspicion that one may be dealing with a false-positive test result. In this setting it is prudent to obtain additional confirmation with an RNA-based test and/or a follow-up Western blot. By definition, Western blot patterns of reactivity that do not fall into the positive or negative categories are considered "indeterminate." There are two possible explanations for an indeterminate Western blot result. The most likely explanation in a low-risk individual is that the patient being tested has antibodies that cross-react with one of the proteins of HIV. The most common patterns of cross-reactivity are antibodies that react with p24 and/or p55. The least likely explanation in this setting is that the individual is infected with HIV and is in the process of mounting a classic antibody response. In either instance, the Western blot should be repeated in 1 month to determine whether or not the indeterminate pattern is a pattern in evolution.

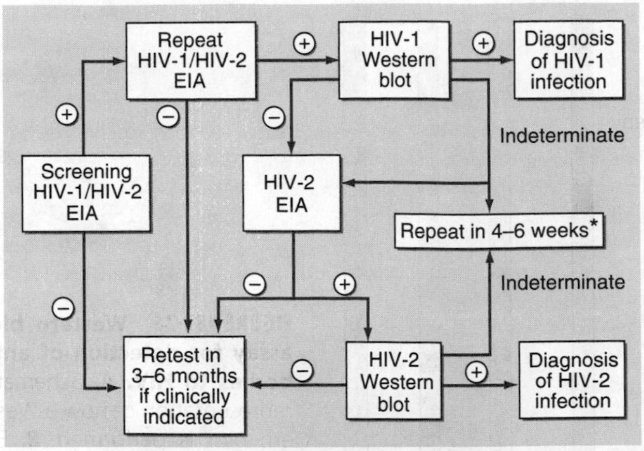

FIGURE 182-27 Algorithm for the use of serologic tests in the diagnosis of HIV-1 or HIV-2 infection. *Stable indeterminate Western blot 4–6 weeks later makes HIV infection unlikely. However, it should be repeated twice at 3-month intervals to rule out HIV infection. Alternatively, one may test for HIV-1 p24 antigen or HIV RNA.

In addition, one may attempt to confirm a diagnosis of HIV infection with the p24 antigen capture assay or one of the tests for HIV RNA (discussed below). While the Western blot is an excellent confirmatory test for HIV infection in patients with a positive or indeterminate EIA, it is a poor screening test. Among individuals with a negative EIA and PCR for HIV, 20–30% may show one or more bands on Western blot. While these bands are usually faint and represent cross-reactivity, their presence creates a situation in which other diagnostic modalities (such as DNA PCR, RNA PCR, the bDNA assay, or p24 antigen capture) must be employed to ensure that the bands do not indicate early HIV infection.

A guideline for the use of these serologic tests in attempting to make a diagnosis of HIV infection is depicted in Fig. 182-27. In patients in whom HIV infection is suspected, the appropriate initial test is the EIA. If the result is negative, unless there is strong reason to suspect early HIV infection (as in a patient exposed within the previous 3 months), the diagnosis is ruled out and retesting should be performed only as clinically indicated. If the EIA is indeterminate or positive, the test should be repeated. If the repeat is negative on two occasions, one can assume that the initial positive reading was due to a technical error in the performance of the assay and that the patient is negative. If the repeat is indeterminate or positive, one should proceed to the HIV-1 Western blot. If the Western blot is positive, the diagnosis is HIV-1 infection. If the Western blot is negative, the EIA can be assumed to have been a false positive for HIV-1 and the diagnosis of HIV-1 infection is ruled out. It would be prudent at this point to perform specific serologic testing for HIV-2 following the same type of algorithm. If the Western blot for HIV-1 is indeterminate, it should be repeated in 4–6 weeks; in addition, one may proceed to a p24 antigen capture assay, HIV-1 RNA assay, or HIV-1 DNA PCR and specific serologic testing for HIV-2. If the p24 and HIV RNA assays are negative and there is no progression in the Western blot, a diagnosis of HIV-1 is ruled out. If either the p24 or HIV-1 RNA assay is positive and/or the HIV-1 Western blot shows progression, a tentative diagnosis of HIV-1 infection can be made and later confirmed with a follow-up Western blot demonstrating a positive pattern. In addition to these standard laboratory-based assays for detecting antibodies to HIV, a series of point-of-care tests are also available. Among the most popular of these is the OraQuick Rapid HIV-1 antibody test that can be run on blood, plasma, or saliva. The sensitivity and specificity of this test are each ~99%. While negative results from this test are adequate to rule out a diagnosis of HIV infection, a positive finding should be considered preliminary and confirmed with standard serologic testing, as described above.

As mentioned above, a variety of laboratory tests are available for the direct detection of HIV or its components (Table 182-6; Fig. 182-28). These tests may be of considerable help in making a diagnosis of HIV infection when the Western blot results are indeterminate. In addition, the tests detecting levels of HIV RNA can be used to determine prognosis and to assess the response to ARV therapies. The simplest of the direct detection tests is the *p24 antigen capture assay*. This is an EIA-type assay in which the solid phase consists of antibodies to the p24 antigen of HIV. It detects the viral protein p24 in the blood of HIV-infected individuals where it exists either as free antigen or complexed to anti-p24 antibodies. Overall, ~30% of individuals with untreated HIV infection have detectable levels of free p24 antigen. This increases to ~50% when samples are treated with a weak acid to dissociate antigen-antibody complexes. Throughout the course of HIV infection, an equilibrium exists between p24 antigen and anti-p24 antibodies. During the first few weeks of infection, before an immune response develops, there is a brisk rise in p24 antigen levels (Fig. 182-25). After the development of anti-p24 antibodies, these levels decline. Late in the course of infection, when circulating levels of virus are high, p24 antigen levels also increase, particularly when detected by techniques involving dissociation of antigen-antibody complexes. The p24 antigen capture assay has its greatest use as a screening test for HIV infection in patients suspected of having the acute HIV syndrome, as high levels of p24 antigen are present prior to the development of antibodies. Its use for routine blood donor screening for HIV infection has been replaced by use of nucleic acid testing. The ability to measure and monitor levels of HIV RNA in the plasma of patients with HIV infection has been of extraordinary value in furthering our understanding of the pathogenesis of HIV infection and in providing a diagnostic tool in settings where measurements of anti-HIV antibodies may be misleading, such as in acute infection and neonatal infection. Three assays are predominantly used for this purpose. They are reverse transcriptase PCR (*RT-PCR*; Amplicor); branched DNA (*bDNA*; VERSANT); and nucleic acid sequence–based amplification (*NASBA*; NucliSens). These tests are of value in making a diagnosis of HIV infection, in establishing initial prognosis, in determining the need for therapy, and for monitoring the effects of therapy. In addition to these three commercially available tests, the *DNA PCR* is also employed by research laboratories for making a diagnosis of HIV infection by amplifying HIV proviral DNA from peripheral blood mononuclear cells. The commercially available RNA detection tests have a sensitivity of 40–80 copies of HIV RNA per milliliter of plasma. Research laboratory–based RNA assays can detect as few as one HIV RNA copy per milliliter, while the DNA PCR tests can detect proviral DNA at a frequency of one copy per 10,000–100,000 cells. Thus, these tests are ex-

TABLE 182-6 CHARACTERISTICS OF TESTS FOR DIRECT DETECTION OF HIV

Test	Technique	Sensitivity[a]	Cost/ Test[b]
Immune complex–dissociated p24 antigen capture assay	Measurement of levels of HIV-1 core protein in an EIA-based format following dissociation of antigen-antibody complexes by weak acid treatment	Positive in 50% of patients; detects down to 15 pg/mL of p24 protein	$1–2
HIV RNA by PCR	PCR amplification of cDNA generated from viral RNA (target amplification)	Reliable to 40 copies/mL of HIV RNA	$75–150
HIV RNA by bDNA	Measurement of levels of particle-associated HIV RNA in a nucleic acid capture assay employing signal amplification	Reliable to 50 copies/mL of HIV RNA	$75–150
HIV RNA by NucliSens	Isothermic nucleic acid amplification with internal controls	Reliable to 80 copies/mL of HIV RNA	$75–150

[a]Sensitivity figures refer to those approved by the US FDA.
[b]Prices may be lower in large volume settings.
Note: EIA, enzyme immunoassay; PCR, polymerase chain reaction.

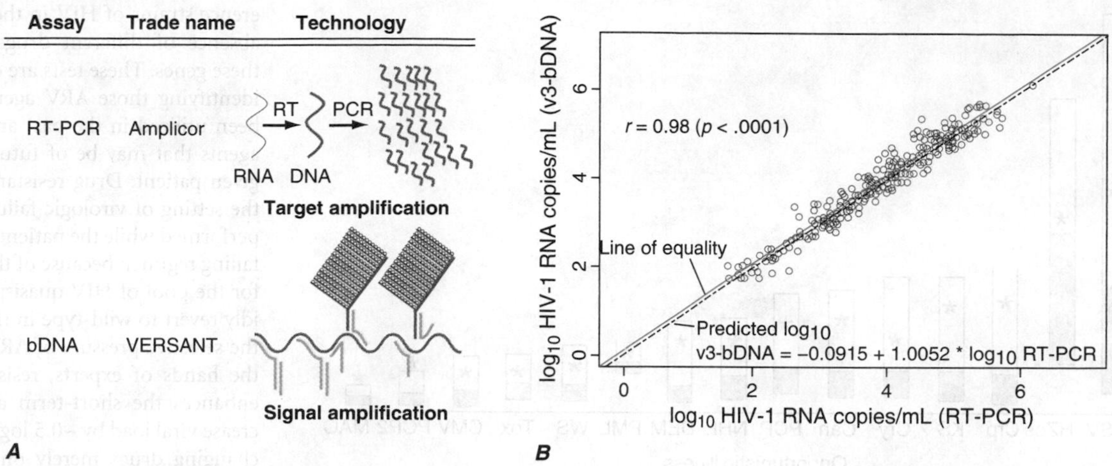

FIGURE 182-28 Comparison of RT-PCR and bDNA assays. ***A.*** Schematic representation of reverse transcriptase–polymerase chain reaction (RT-PCR) and bDNA assays. See text for detailed description. ***B.*** Scatter plot of $\log_{10}$ v3-bDNA versus $\log_{10}$ RT-PCR with the line of equity (solid) and the fitted regression line (hatched). The equation for the fitted regression line is given in the lower-right-hand corner. There is good agreement between the two assays. v3, version 3 of the bDNA assay. *(Adapted from HC Highbarger et al: J Clin Microbiol 37:3612, 1999.)*

tremely sensitive. One frequent consequence of a high degree of sensitivity is some loss of specificity, and false-positive results have been reported with each of these techniques. For this reason, a positive EIA with a confirmatory Western blot remains the "gold standard" for a diagnosis of HIV infection, and the interpretation of other test results must be done with this in mind.

In the RT-PCR technique, following DNase treatment, a cDNA copy is made of all RNA species present in plasma. Insofar as HIV is an RNA virus, this will result in the production of DNA copies of the HIV genome in amounts proportional to the amount of HIV RNA present in plasma. This cDNA is then amplified and characterized using standard PCR techniques, employing primer pairs that can distinguish genomic cDNA from messenger cDNA. The bDNA assay involves the use of a solid-phase nucleic acid capture system and signal amplification through successive nucleic acid hybridizations to detect small quantities of HIV RNA. Both tests can achieve a tenfold increase in sensitivity to 40–50 copies of HIV RNA per milliliter with a preconcentration step in which plasma undergoes ultracentrifugation to pellet the viral particles. The NASBA technique involves the isothermal amplification of a sequence within the gag region of HIV in the presence of internal standards and employs the production of multiple RNA copies through the action of T7-RNA polymerase. The resulting RNA species are quantitated through hybridization with a molecular beacon DNA probe that is quenched in the absence of hybridization. The lower limit of detection for the NucliSens assay is 80 copies/mL.

In addition to being a diagnostic and prognostic tool, RT-PCR is also useful for amplifying defined areas of the HIV genome for sequence analysis and has become an important technique for studies of sequence diversity and microbial resistance to ARV agents. In patients with a positive or indeterminate EIA test and an indeterminate Western blot, and in patients in whom serologic testing may be unreliable (such as patients with hypogammaglobulinemia or advanced HIV disease), these tests for quantitating HIV RNA in plasma provide valuable tools for making a diagnosis of HIV infection; however, they should be used for diagnosis only when standard serologic testing has failed to provide a definitive result.

LABORATORY MONITORING OF PATIENTS WITH HIV INFECTION

The epidemic of HIV infection and AIDS has provided the clinician with new challenges for integrating clinical and laboratory data to effect optimal patient management. The close relationship between clinical manifestations of HIV infection and CD4+ T cell count has made measurement of the latter a routine part of the evaluation of HIV-infected individuals. Determinations of CD4+ T cell counts and measurements of the levels of HIV RNA in serum or plasma provide a powerful set of tools for determining prognosis and monitoring response to therapy.

CD4+ T Cell Counts The CD4+ T cell count is the laboratory test generally accepted as the best indicator of the immediate state of immunologic competence of the patient with HIV infection. This measurement, which can be made directly or calculated as the product of the percent of CD4+ T cells (determined by flow cytometry) and the total lymphocyte count [determined by the white blood cell count (WBC) and the differential percent], has been shown to correlate very well with the level of immunologic competence. Patients with CD4+ T cell counts <200/μL are at high risk of disease from *P. jiroveci*, while patients with CD4+ T cell counts <50/μL are at high risk of disease from CMV, mycobacteria of the *M. avium* complex (MAC) and/or *T. gondii* (Fig. 182-29). Patients with HIV infection should have CD4+ T cell measurements performed at the time of diagnosis and every 3–6 months thereafter. More frequent measurements should be made if a declining trend is noted. According to most guidelines, a CD4 T cell count <350/μL is an indication for consideration of initiating ARV therapy, and a decline in CD4+ T cell count of >25% is an indication for considering a change in therapy. Once the CD4+ T cell count is <200/μL, patients should be placed on a regimen for *P. jiroveci* prophylaxis, and once the count is <50/μL, primary prophylaxis for MAC infection is indicated. As with any laboratory measurement, one may wish to obtain two determinations prior to any significant changes in patient management based upon CD4+ T cell count alone. In patients with hypersplenism or who have undergone splenectomy the CD4+ T cell percentage may be a more reliable indication of immune function than the CD4+ T cell count. A CD4+ T cell percent of 15 is comparable to a CD4+ T cell count of 200/μL.

HIV RNA Determinations Facilitated by highly sensitive techniques for the precise quantitation of small amounts of nucleic acids, the measurement of serum or plasma levels of HIV RNA has become an essential component in the monitoring of patients with HIV infection. As discussed under diagnosis of HIV infection, the two most commonly used techniques are the RT-PCR assay and the bDNA assay. Both assays generate data in the form of number of copies of HIV RNA per milliliter of serum or plasma. Standard assays can detect as few as 40–50 copies of HIV RNA per milliliter of plasma, while research-based assays can detect down to one copy per milliliter. Although earlier versions of the bDNA assay generated values that were ~50% of those of the RT-PCR assay, the more recent versions (version 3 or higher) provide numbers essentially identical to those of the RT-PCR test (Fig. 182-28). While it is common practice to describe levels of HIV RNA

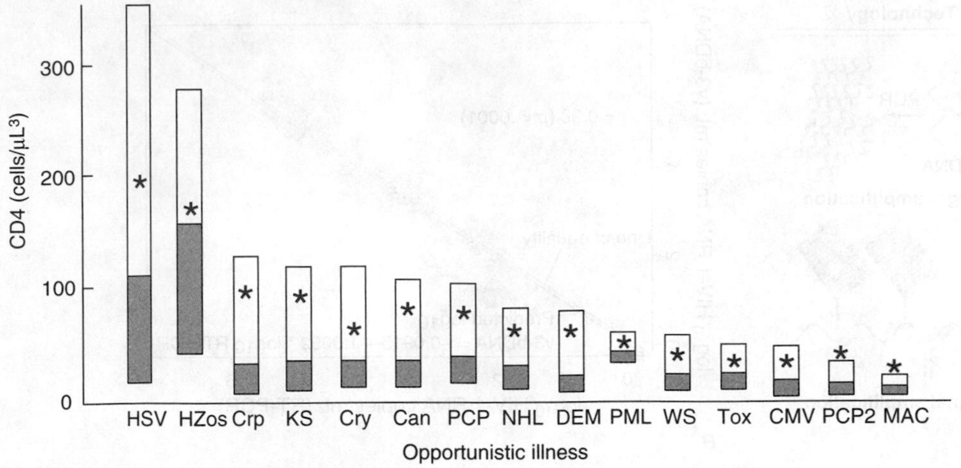

FIGURE 182-29 Relationship between CD4+ T cell counts and the development of opportunistic diseases. Boxplot of the median (line inside the box), first quartile (bottom of the box), third quartile (top of the box), and mean (asterisk) CD4+ lymphocyte count at the time of the development of opportunistic disease. Can, candidal esophagitis; CMV, cytomegalovirus infection; Crp, cryptosporidiosis; Cry, cryptococcal meningitis; DEM, AIDS dementia complex; HSV, herpes simplex virus infection; HZos, herpes zoster; KS, Kaposi's sarcoma; MAC, *Mycobacterium avium* complex bacteremia; NHL, non-Hodgkin's lymphoma; PCP, primary *Pneumocystis jiroveci* pneumonia; PCP2, secondary *P. jiroveci* pneumonia; PML, progressive multifocal leukoencephalopathy; Tox, *Toxoplasma gondii* encephalitis; WS, wasting syndrome. *(From RD Moore, RE Chaisson: Ann Intern Med 124:633, 1996.)*

below these cut-offs as "undetectable," this is a term that should be avoided as it is imprecise and leaves the false impression that the level of virus is 0. By utilizing more sensitive, nested PCR techniques and by studying tissue levels of virus as well as plasma levels, HIV RNA can be detected in virtually every patient with HIV infection. Measurements of changes in HIV RNA levels over time have been of great value in delineating the relationship between levels of virus and rates of disease progression (Fig. 182-20), the rates of viral turnover, the relationship between immune system activation and viral replication, and the time to development of drug resistance. HIV RNA measurements are greatly influenced by the state of activation of the immune system and may fluctuate greatly in the setting of secondary infections or immunization. For these reasons, decisions based upon HIV RNA levels should never be made on a single determination. Measurements of plasma HIV RNA levels should be made at the time of HIV diagnosis and every 3–6 months thereafter in the untreated patient. In general, most guidelines suggest that therapy be considered in patients with >100,000 copies of HIV RNA per milliliter (see below). Following the initiation of therapy or any change in therapy, plasma HIV RNA levels should be monitored approximately every 4 weeks until the effectiveness of the therapeutic regimen is determined by the development of a new steady-state level of HIV RNA. In most instances of effective therapy this will be <50 copies per milliliter. This level of virus is generally achieved within 6 months of the initiation of effective treatment. During therapy, levels of HIV RNA should be monitored every 3–4 months to evaluate the continuing effectiveness of therapy.

HIV Resistance Testing The availability of multiple ARV drugs as treatment options has generated a great deal of interest in the potential for measuring the sensitivity of an individual's HIV virus(es) to different ARV agents. HIV resistance testing can be done through either genotypic or phenotypic measurements. In the genotypic assays, sequence analyses of the HIV genomes obtained from patients are compared to sequences of viruses with known ARV resistance profiles. In the phenotypic assays, the in vivo growth of viral isolates obtained from the patient are compared to the growth of reference strains of the virus in the presence or absence of different ARV drugs. A modification of this phenotypic approach utilizes a comparison of the enzymatic activities of the reverse transcriptase or protease genes obtained by molecular cloning of patients' isolates to the enzymatic activities of genes obtained from reference strains of HIV in the presence or absence of different drugs targeted to these genes. These tests are quite good in identifying those ARV agents that have been utilized in the past and suggesting agents that may be of future value in a given patient. Drug resistance testing in the setting of virologic failure should be performed while the patient is still on the failing regimen because of the propensity for the pool of HIV quasispecies to rapidly revert to wild-type in the absence of the selective pressure of ARV therapy. In the hands of experts, resistance testing enhances the short-term ability to decrease viral load by ~0.5 log compared to changing drugs merely on the basis of drug history. In addition to the use of resistance testing to help in the selection of new drugs in patients with virologic failure, it may also be of value in selecting an initial regimen for treatment of therapy-naïve individuals. This is particularly true in geographic areas with a high level of background resistance.

Co-Receptor Tropism Assays Following the licensure of maraviroc as the first CCR5 antagonist for the treatment of HIV infection (see below), it became necessary to be able to determine whether or not a patient's virus was likely to respond to this treatment. Patients tend to have CCR5-tropic virus (see above) early in the course of infection with a trend toward CXCR4 viruses later in disease. Maraviroc is only effective against CCR5-tropic viruses. Due to the fact that the genotypic determinants of cellular tropism are poorly defined, a phenotypic assay is necessary to determine this property of HIV. Two commercial assays; the Trofile assay (Monogram Biosciences) and the Phenoscript assay (VIRalliance), are available to make this determination. These assays clone the envelope regions of the patient's virus into an indicator virus that is then used to infect target cells expressing either CCR5 or CXCR4 as their co-receptor. These assays take weeks to perform and are expensive.

Other Tests A variety of other laboratory tests have been studied as potential markers of HIV disease activity. Among these are quantitative culture of replication-competent HIV from plasma, peripheral blood mononuclear cells, or resting CD4+ T cells; circulating levels of β_2-microglobulin, soluble IL-2 receptor, IgA, acid-labile endogenous interferon, or TNF-α; and the presence or absence of activation markers such as CD38, HLA-DR, or PD-1 on CD8+ T cells. While these measurements have value as markers of disease activity and help to increase our understanding of the pathogenesis of HIV disease, they do not currently play a major role in the monitoring of patients with HIV infection.

CLINICAL MANIFESTATIONS

The clinical consequences of HIV infection encompass a spectrum ranging from an acute syndrome associated with primary infection to a prolonged asymptomatic state to advanced disease. It is best to regard HIV disease as beginning at the time of primary infection and progressing through various stages. As mentioned above, active virus replication and progressive immunologic impairment occur throughout the course of HIV infection in most patients. With the exception of the rare true long-term nonprogressors (see above), HIV disease in untreated patients inexorably progresses even during the clinically latent stage. However, ARV therapy has had a major impact on blocking or slowing the progression of disease over extended periods of time in a substantial proportion of adequately treated patients (see below).

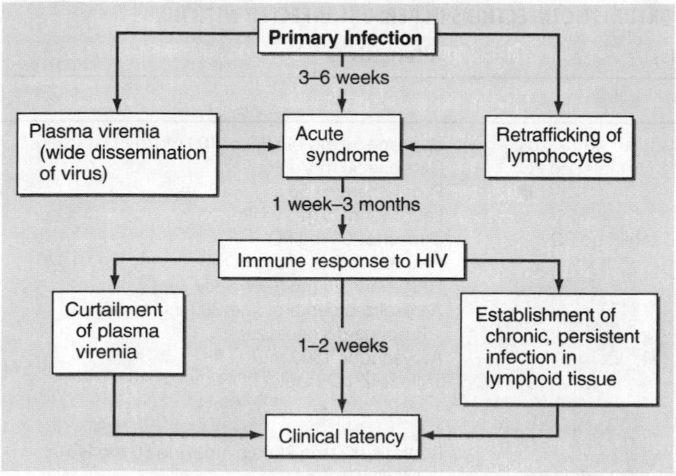

FIGURE 182-30 The acute HIV syndrome. See text for detailed description. *(Adapted from G Pantaleo et al: N Engl J Med 328:327, 1993. Copyright 1993 Massachusetts Medical Society. All rights reserved.)*

THE ACUTE HIV SYNDROME

It is estimated that 50–70% of individuals with HIV infection experience an acute clinical syndrome ~3–6 weeks after primary infection (Fig. 182-30). Varying degrees of clinical severity have been reported, and although it has been suggested that symptomatic seroconversion leading to the seeking of medical attention indicates an increased risk for an accelerated course of disease, there does not appear to be a correlation between the level of the initial burst of viremia in acute HIV infection and the subsequent course of disease. The typical clinical findings in the acute HIV syndrome are listed in Table 182-7; they occur along with a burst of plasma viremia. It has been reported that several symptoms of the acute HIV syndrome (fever, skin rash, pharyngitis, and myalgia) occur less frequently in those infected by injection drug use versus those infected by sexual contact. The syndrome is typical of an acute viral syndrome and has been likened to acute infectious mononucleosis. Symptoms usually persist for one to several weeks and gradually subside as an immune response to HIV develops and the levels of plasma viremia decrease. Opportunistic infections have been reported during this stage of infection, reflecting the immunodeficiency that results from reduced numbers of CD4+ T cells and likely also from the dysfunction of CD4+ T cells owing to viral protein and endogenous cytokine-induced perturbations of cells (see "Mechanisms of CD4+ T Lymphocyte Depletion and Dysfunction," above) associated with the extremely high levels of plasma viremia. A number of immunologic abnormalities accompany the acute HIV syndrome, including multiphasic perturbations of the numbers of circulating lymphocyte subsets. The number of total lymphocytes and T cell subsets (CD4+ and CD8+) are initially reduced. An inversion of the CD4+/CD8+ T cell ratio occurs later because of a rise in the number of CD8+ T cells. In fact, there may be a selective and transient expansion of CD8+ T cell subsets, as determined by T cell receptor analysis (see above). The total circulating CD8+ T cell count may remain elevated or return to normal; however, CD4+ T cell levels usually remain somewhat depressed, although there may be a slight rebound toward normal. Lymphadenopathy occurs in ~70% of individuals with primary HIV infection. Most patients recover spontaneously from this syndrome and many are left with only a mildly depressed CD4+ T cell count that remains stable for a variable period before beginning its progressive decline (see below); in some individuals, the CD4+ T cell count returns to the normal range. Approximately 10% of patients manifest a fulminant course of immunologic and clinical deterioration after primary infection, even after the disappearance of initial symptoms. In most patients, primary infection with or without the acute syndrome is followed by a prolonged period of clinical latency or smoldering low disease activity. A small percentage of HIV-infected individuals treated with ARV drugs during acute infection may revert to a negative EIA test during the time they remain on therapy. They rapidly re-seroconvert with the discontinuation of treatment.

TABLE 182-7 CLINICAL FINDINGS IN THE ACUTE HIV SYNDROME

General	Neurologic
Fever	Meningitis
Pharyngitis	Encephalitis
Lymphadenopathy	Peripheral neuropathy
Headache/retroorbital pain	Myelopathy
Arthralgias/myalgias	Dermatologic
Lethargy/malaise	Erythematous maculopapular rash
Anorexia/weight loss	
Nausea/vomiting/diarrhea	Mucocutaneous ulceration

Source: From B Tindall, DA Cooper: AIDS 5:1, 1991.

THE ASYMPTOMATIC STAGE—CLINICAL LATENCY

Although the length of time from initial infection to the development of clinical disease varies greatly, the median time for untreated patients is ~10 years. As emphasized above, HIV disease with active virus replication is ongoing and progressive during this asymptomatic period. The rate of disease progression is directly correlated with HIV RNA levels. Patients with high levels of HIV RNA in plasma progress to symptomatic disease faster than do patients with low levels of HIV RNA (Fig. 182-20). Some patients referred to as *long-term nonprogressors* show little if any decline in CD4+ T cell counts over extended periods of time. These patients generally have extremely low levels of HIV RNA with a subset, referred to as *elite nonprogressors*, exhibiting HIV RNA levels <50 copies per milliliter. Certain other patients remain entirely asymptomatic despite the fact that their CD4+ T cell counts show a steady progressive decline to extremely low levels. In these patients, the appearance of an opportunistic disease may be the first manifestation of HIV infection. During the asymptomatic period of HIV infection, the average rate of CD4+ T cell decline is ~50/μL per year. When the CD4+ T cell count falls to <200/μL, the resulting state of immunodeficiency is severe enough to place the patient at high risk for opportunistic infection and neoplasms, and hence for clinically apparent disease.

SYMPTOMATIC DISEASE

Symptoms of HIV disease can appear at any time during the course of HIV infection. Generally speaking, the spectrum of illnesses that one observes changes as the CD4+ T cell count declines. The more severe and life-threatening complications of HIV infection occur in patients with CD4+ T cell counts <200/μL. A diagnosis of AIDS is made in anyone with HIV infection and a CD4+ T cell count <200/μL and in anyone with HIV infection who develops one of the HIV-associated diseases considered to be indicative of a severe defect in cell-mediated immunity (category C, Table 182-2). While the causative agents of the secondary infections are characteristically opportunistic organisms such as *P. jiroveci*, atypical mycobacteria, CMV, and other organisms that do not ordinarily cause disease in the absence of a compromised immune system, they also include common bacterial and mycobacterial pathogens. Fewer than 50% of deaths among AIDS patients are as a direct result of an AIDS-defining illness, and the average CD4+ T cell count of an HIV-infected patient at the time of death is just over 300 cells/μL. Similarly, following the widespread use of combination ARV therapy and implementation of guidelines for the prevention of opportunistic infections (Table 182-8), the incidence of secondary infections has decreased dramatically (Fig. 182-31). Overall, the clinical spectrum of HIV disease is constantly changing as patients live longer and new and better approaches to treatment and prophylaxis are developed. In addition to the classic AIDS-defining illnesses, patients with HIV infection also have an increase in serious non-AIDS illnesses, including cardiovascular, renal, and hepatic disease. The physician providing care to a patient with HIV infection must be well versed in general internal medicine as well as HIV-related infectious diseases and new clinical syndromes related to chronic illness and long-term ARV therapy. In general, it should be stressed that a key element of treatment of symptomatic complications of HIV disease, whether they are primary or secondary, is achieving good control of HIV replication through the use of combination ARV therapy and instituting primary and secondary prophylaxis for opportunistic infections as indicated.

TABLE 182-8 NIH/CDC/IDSA 2008 GUIDELINES FOR THE PREVENTION OF OPPORTUNISTIC INFECTIONS IN PERSONS INFECTED WITH HIV

Pathogen	Indications	First Choice(s)	Alternatives
Recommended as Standard of Care for Primary and Secondary Prophylaxis			
Pneumocystis jiroveci	CD4+ T cell count <200/μL or Oropharyngeal candidiasis or Prior bout of PCP	Trimethoprim/sulfamethoxazole (TMP/SMZ), 1 DS tablet qd PO	Dapsone 50 mg bid PO or 100 mg/d PO Dapsone 50 mg/d PO + Pyrimethamine 50 mg/wk PO + Leucovorin 25 mg/wk PO
	May stop prophylaxis if CD4+ T cell count > 200/μL for ≥3 mo	TMP/SMZ, 1 SS tablet qd PO	Dapsone 200 mg PO + Pyrimethamine 75 mg PO + Leucovorin 25 mg PO weekly Aerosolized pentamidine, 300 mg qm via Respirgard II nebulizer Atovaquone 1500 mg/d PO TMP/SMZ 1 DS tablet PO 3×/wk
Mycobacterium tuberculosis			
Isoniazid sensitive	Skin test >5 mm or Prior positive test without treatment or Close contact with case of active pulmonary TB	Isoniazid 300 mg PO + Pyridoxine 50 mg PO qd ×9 mo Isoniazid 900 mg PO + Pyridoxine 100 mg PO 2 ×/wk ×9 mo	Isoniazid 900 mg PO + pyridoxine 50 mg PO 2×/wk × 9 mo Isoniazid 300 mg + rifampin 600 mg (or rifabutin 300 mg) + pyridoxine 50 mg/d ×4 mo
Isoniazid resistant	Same with high probability of exposure to isoniazid-resistant TB	Rifabutin 300 mg or Rifampin 600 mg PO qd ×4 mo	
Multidrug resistant	Same with high probability of exposure to multidrug resistant TB	Consult local public health authorities	
Mycobacterium-avium complex	CD4+ T cell count <50/μL	Azithromycin 1200 mg weekly PO or Clarithromycin 500 mg bid PO	Rifabutin 300 mg/d PO Azithromycin 1200 mg weekly PO + Rifabutin 300 mg/d PO
	Prior documented disseminated disease May stop prophylaxis if CD4+ T cell count > 100/μL for ≥3 mo	Clarithromycin 500 mg bid PO + Ethambutol 15 (mg/kg)/d PO +/− Rifabutin 300 mg/d PO	Azithromycin 500 mg/d PO + Ethambutol 15 (mg/kg)/d PO +/− Rifabutin 300 mg/d PO
Toxoplasma gondii	TOXO IgG antibody and CD4+ T cell count <100/μL	TMP/SMZ 1 DS tablet PO qd	TMP/SMZ 1 DS 3× weekly Dapsone 50 mg/d PO + Pyrimethamine 50 mg weekly PO + Leucovorin 25 mg weekly PO Dapsone 200 mg PO + Pyrimethamine 75 mg PO + Leucovorin 25 mg PO weekly Atovaquone 1500 mg PO +/− Pyrimethamine 25 mg PO + Leucovorin 10 mg PO daily
	Prior toxoplasmic encephalitis and CD4+ T cell count <200	Sulfadiazine 500–1000 mg qid PO + pyrimethamine 25–50 mg/d PO + leucovorin 10–25 mg/d PO	Clindamycin 600 mg q8h PO + Pyrimethamine 25–50 mg/d PO + Leucovorin 10–25 mg/d PO
	May stop prophylaxis if CD4+ T cell count >200/μL for ≥3 months		Atovaquone 750 mg PO q6–12 h +/− Pyrimethamine 25 mg/d + Leucovorin 10 mg/d PO
Varicella zoster virus	Significant exposure to chickenpox or shingles in a patient with no history of immunization or prior exposure to either	Varicella zoster immune globulin 6.25 mL, IM, within 96 h of exposure	
Cryptococcus neoformans	Prior documented disease May stop prophylaxis if CD4+ T cell count >200 for 6 mo and no evidence of active infection	Fluconazole 200 mg/d PO	Itraconazole 200 mg/d PO
Histoplasma capsulatum	Prior documented disease May stop prophylaxis after 1 year if CD4+ T cell count >150 and patient on ARV therapy for ≥6 mo	Itraconazole 200 mg bid PO	Fluconazole 800 mg/d PO
Coccidioides immitis	Prior documented disease or Positive serology and CD4+ T cell count <250 [For this indication prophylaxis can be stopped if CD4+ T cell count ≥250 for 6 mo.]	Fluconazole 400 mg/d PO	Itraconazole 200 mg bid PO
Penicillium marneffei	Prior documented disease May stop secondary prophylaxis in patients on ARVs with CD4+ T cell count >100 for ≥6 mo	Itraconazole 200 mg/d PO	
Salmonella species	Prior bacteremia	Ciprofloxacin 500 mg bid PO for 6 mo or more	
Bartonella	Prior infection May stop if CD4+ T cell count >200 for >3 mo	Doxycycline 200 mg/d Azithromycin 1200 mg weekly PO Clarithromycin 500 mg bid PO	
Cytomegalovirus	Prior end-organ disease May stop prophylaxis if CD4+ T cell count > 100/μL for 6 mo and no evidence of active CMV disease Restart if prior retinitis and CD4+ T cells <100/μL	Ganciclovir, 5–6 mg/kg 5–7 d/wk IV Valganciclovir 900 mg bid PO Foscarnet 90–120 (mg/kg)/d IV Ganciclovir sustained-release implant q6–9mo + Valganciclovir 900 mg bid PO	Cidofovir 5 mg/kg every other week IV + Probenecid Formivirsen 330 μg intravitreal q2–4 wk Valganciclovir 900 mg PO daily Formivirsen, 1 vial injected into the vitreous q2–4wk

(continued)

TABLE 182-8 NIH/CDC/IDSA 2008 GUIDELINES FOR THE PREVENTION OF OPPORTUNISTIC INFECTIONS IN PERSONS INFECTED WITH HIV (CONTINUED)

Pathogen	Indications	First Choice(s)	Alternatives
Immunizations Generally Recommended			
Hepatitis B virus	All susceptible (anti-HBc and anti-HBs negative) patients	Hepatitis B vaccine: 3 doses	
Hepatitis A virus	All susceptible (anti-HAV negative) patients	Hepatitis A vaccine: 2 doses	
Influenza virus	All patients annually	Inactivated trivalent influenza virus vaccine 1 dose yearly	Oseltamivir 75 mg PO qd Rimantadine or amantadine 100 mg PO bid (influenza A only)
Streptococcus pneumoniae	All patients, preferably before CD4+ T cell count ≥200/μL	Pneumococcal vaccine 0.5 mL IM ×1 if CD4+ T cell count >200/μL Reimmunize patients initially immunized at a CD4+ T cell count <100/μL whose CD4+ T cell count then increases to >200/μL	
Human papilloma virus	Girls and women 9–26 years of age	HPV vaccine; 3 doses	
Recommended for Prevention of Severe or Frequent Recurrences			
Herpes simplex	Frequent/severe recurrences	Acyclovir 200 mg tid PO Acyclovir 400 mg bid PO Famciclovir 250 mg bid PO	Valacyclovir 500 mg PO bid
Candida	Frequent/severe recurrences	Fluconazole 100–200 mg/d PO	Itraconazole solution 200 mg/d PO

Note: DS, double strength; SS, single strength; PCP, *Pneumocystis carinii* pneumonia; TB, tuberculosis.

Disease of the Respiratory System Acute bronchitis and sinusitis are prevalent during all stages of HIV infection. The most severe cases tend to occur in patients with lower CD4+ T cell counts. Sinusitis presents as fever, nasal congestion, and headache. The diagnosis is made by CT or MRI. The maxillary sinuses are most commonly involved; however, disease is also frequently seen in the ethmoid, sphenoid, and frontal sinuses. While some patients may improve without antibiotic therapy, radiographic improvement is quicker and more pronounced in patients who have received antimicrobial therapy. It is postulated that this high incidence of sinusitis results from an increased frequency of infection with encapsulated organisms such as *H. influenzae* and *Streptococcus pneumoniae*. In patients with low CD4+ T cell counts one may see mucormycosis infections of the sinuses. In contrast to the course of this infection in other patient populations, mucormycosis of the sinuses in patients with HIV infection may progress more slowly. In this setting aggressive, frequent local debridement in addition to local and systemic amphotericin B may be needed for effective treatment.

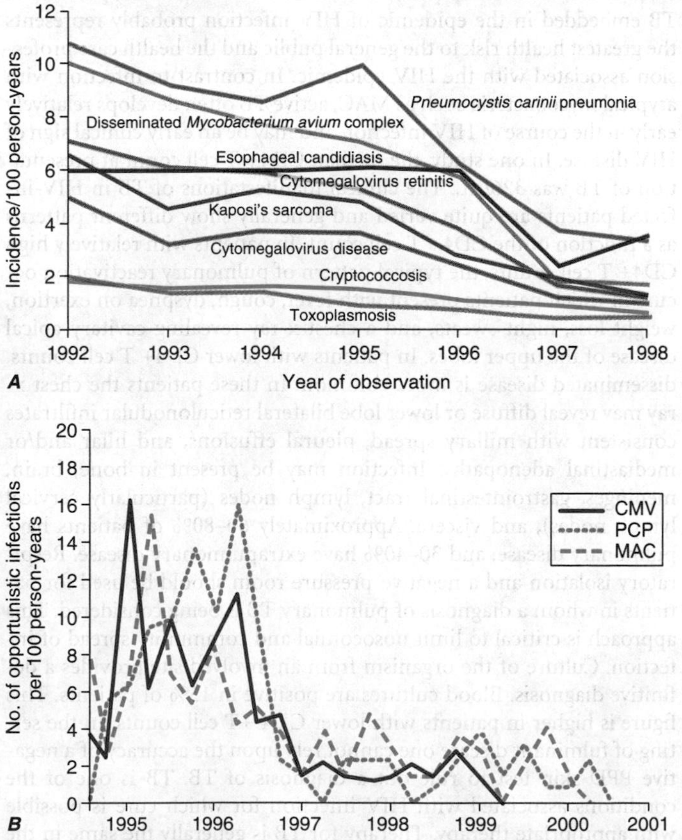

FIGURE 182-31 ***A.*** Decrease in the incidence of opportunistic infections and Kaposi's sarcoma in HIV-infected individuals with CD4+ T cell counts <100/μl from 1992 through 1998. *[Adapted and updated from FJ Palella et al: N Engl J Med 338:853, 1998, and JE Kaplan et al: Clin Infect Dis 30(S1):S5, 2000, with permission.]* ***B.*** Quarterly incidence rates of cytomegalovirus (CMV), *Pneumocystis jiroveci* pneumonia (PCP), and *Mycobacterium avium* complex (MAC) from 1995–2001. *(From FJ Palella et al: AIDS 16:1617, 2002.)*

Pulmonary disease is one of the most frequent complications of HIV infection. The most common manifestation of pulmonary disease is pneumonia. The two most common causes of pneumonia are bacterial infections and the unicellular fungus *P. jiroveci* infection. Other major causes of pulmonary infiltrates include mycobacterial infections, other fungal infections, nonspecific interstitial pneumonitis, KS, and lymphoma.

Pneumonia is seen with an increased frequency in patients with HIV infection; they appear to be particularly prone to infections with encapsulated organisms. *S. pneumoniae* (Chap. 128) and *H. influenzae* (Chap. 139) are responsible for most cases of bacterial pneumonia in patients with AIDS. This may be a consequence of altered B cell function and/or defects in neutrophil function that may be secondary to HIV disease (see above). *S. pneumoniae* (pneumococcal) infection may be the earliest serious infection to occur in patients with HIV disease. This can present as pneumonia, sinusitis, and/or bacteremia. Patients with untreated HIV infection have a sixfold increase in the incidence of pneumococcal pneumonia and a 100-fold increase in the incidence of pneumococcal bacteremia. Pneumococcal disease may be seen in patients with relatively intact immune systems. In one study, the baseline CD4+ T cell count at the time of a first episode of pneumococcal pneumonia was ~300/μL. Of interest is the fact that the inflammatory response to pneumococcal infection appears proportional to the CD4+ T cell count. Due to this high risk of pneumococcal disease, immunization with pneumococcal polysaccharide is one of the generally recommended prophylactic measures for patients with HIV infection. This is likely most effective if given while the CD4+ T cell count is >200/μL. It is less clear whether this intervention is effective when given to patients with more advanced disease and high viral loads.

Pneumocystis pneumonia (PCP), once the hallmark of AIDS, has dramatically declined in incidence following the development of effective prophylactic regimens and the widespread use of combination ARV therapy. It is, however, the single most common cause of pneumonia in patients with HIV infection in the United States and can be identified as a likely etiologic agent in 25% of cases of pneumonia in patients with HIV infection. Approximately 25% of cases of HIV-associated PCP occur in patients who are unaware of their HIV status. The risk of PCP is greatest among those who have experienced a previous bout of PCP and those who have CD4+ T cell counts of <200/μL. Overall, 79% of patients with PCP have CD4+ T cell counts <100/μL and 95% of patients have CD4+ T cell counts <200/μL. Recurrent fever, night sweats, thrush, and unexplained weight loss are also associated with an increased incidence of PCP. For these reasons, it is strongly recommended that all patients with CD4+ T cell counts <200/μL (or a CD4 percentage <15) receive some form of PCP prophylaxis. The incidence of PCP is approaching zero in patients with known HIV infection receiving appropriate ARV therapy and prophylaxis. In the United States, primary PCP is now occurring at a median CD4+ T cell count of 36/μL, while secondary PCP is occurring at a median CD4+ T cell count of 10/μL. Patients with PCP generally present with fever and a cough that is usually nonproductive or productive of only scant amounts of white sputum. They may complain of a characteristic retrosternal chest pain that is worse on inspiration and is described as sharp or burning. HIV-associated PCP may have an indolent course characterized by weeks of vague symptoms and should be included in the differential diagnosis of fever, pulmonary complaints, or unexplained weight loss in any patient with HIV infection and <200 CD4+ T cells/μL. The most common finding on chest x-ray is either a normal film, if the disease is suspected early, or a faint bilateral interstitial infiltrate. The classic finding of a dense perihilar infiltrate is unusual in patients with AIDS. In patients with PCP who have been receiving aerosolized pentamidine for prophylaxis, one may see an x-ray picture of upper lobe cavitary disease, reminiscent of TB. Other less common findings on chest x-ray include lobar infiltrates and pleural effusions. Routine laboratory evaluation is usually of little help in the differential diagnosis of PCP. A mild leukocytosis is common, although this may not be obvious in patients with prior neutropenia. Arterial blood gases may indicate hypoxemia with a decline in Pa_{O_2} and an increase in the arterial-alveolar (a – A) gradient. Arterial blood gas measurements not only aid in making the diagnosis of PCP but also provide important information for staging the severity of the disease and directing treatment (see below). A definitive diagnosis of PCP requires demonstration of the organism in samples obtained from induced sputum, bronchoalveolar lavage, transbronchial biopsy, or open lung biopsy. PCR has been used to detect specific DNA sequences for *P. jiroveci* in clinical specimens where histologic examinations have failed to make a diagnosis.

In addition to pneumonia, a number of other clinical problems have been reported in HIV-infected patients as a result of infection with *P. jiroveci*. Otic involvement may be seen as a primary infection, presenting as a polypoid mass involving the external auditory canal. In patients receiving aerosolized pentamidine for prophylaxis against PCP one may see a variety of extrapulmonary manifestations of *P. jiroveci*. These include ophthalmic lesions of the choroid, a necrotizing vasculitis that resembles Burger's disease, bone marrow hypoplasia, and intestinal obstruction. Other organs that have been involved include lymph nodes, spleen, liver, kidney, pancreas, pericardium, heart, thyroid, and adrenals. Organ infection may be associated with cystic lesions that may appear calcified on CT or ultrasound.

The standard treatment for PCP or disseminated pneumocystosis is trimethoprim/sulfamethoxazole (TMP/SMX). A high incidence of side effects, particularly skin rash and bone marrow suppression, is seen with TMP/SMX in patients with HIV infection. Alternative treatments for mild to moderate PCP include dapsone/trimethoprim and clindamycin/primaquine. Intravenous pentamidine is the treatment of choice for severe disease in the patient unable to tolerate TMP/SMX. For patients with a Pa_{O_2} < 70 mmHg or with an a – A gradient >35 mmHg, adjunct glucocorticoid therapy should be used in addition to specific antimicrobials. Overall, treatment should be for 21 days and followed by secondary prophylaxis. Prophylaxis for PCP is indicated for any HIV-infected individual who has experienced a prior bout of PCP, any patient with a CD4+ T cell count of <200/μL or a CD4 percentage <15, any patient with unexplained fever for >2 weeks, and any patient with a history of oropharyngeal candidiasis. The preferred regimen for prophylaxis is TMP/SMX, one double-strength tablet daily. This regimen also provides protection against toxoplasmosis and some bacterial respiratory pathogens. For patients who cannot tolerate TMP/SMX, alternatives for prophylaxis include dapsone plus pyrimethamine plus leucovorin, aerosolized pentamidine administered by the Respirgard II nebulizer, and atovaquone. Primary or secondary prophylaxis for PCP can be discontinued in those patients treated with combination ARV therapy who maintain good suppression of HIV (<50 copies per milliliter) and CD4+ T cell counts >200/μL for 3–6 months.

M. tuberculosis, once thought to be on its way to extinction in the United States, experienced a resurgence associated with the HIV epidemic (Chap. 158). Worldwide, approximately one-third of all AIDS-related deaths are associated with TB. In the United States ~5% of AIDS patients have active TB. HIV infection increases the risk of developing active TB by a factor of 100. For the patient with untreated HIV infection and a positive PPD skin test, the rate of reactivation TB is 7–10% per year. Untreated TB can accelerate the course of HIV infection. Levels of plasma HIV RNA increase in the setting of active TB and decline in the setting of successful TB treatment. Active TB is most common in patients 25–44 years of age, in African Americans and Hispanics, in patients in New York City and Miami, and in patients in developing countries. In these demographic groups, 20–70% of the new cases of active TB are in patients with HIV infection. The epidemic of TB embedded in the epidemic of HIV infection probably represents the greatest health risk to the general public and the health care profession associated with the HIV epidemic. In contrast to infection with atypical mycobacteria such as MAC, active TB often develops relatively early in the course of HIV infection and may be an early clinical sign of HIV disease. In one study, the median CD4+ T cell count at presentation of TB was 326/μL. The clinical manifestations of TB in HIV-infected patients are quite varied and generally show different patterns as a function of the CD4+ T cell count. In patients with relatively high CD4+ T cell counts, the typical pattern of pulmonary reactivation occurs in which patients present with fever, cough, dyspnea on exertion, weight loss, night sweats, and a chest x-ray revealing cavitary apical disease of the upper lobes. In patients with lower CD4+ T cell counts, disseminated disease is more common. In these patients the chest x-ray may reveal diffuse or lower lobe bilateral reticulonodular infiltrates consistent with miliary spread, pleural effusions, and hilar and/or mediastinal adenopathy. Infection may be present in bone, brain, meninges, gastrointestinal tract, lymph nodes (particularly cervical lymph nodes), and viscera. Approximately 60–80% of patients have pulmonary disease, and 30–40% have extrapulmonary disease. Respiratory isolation and a negative-pressure room should be used for patients in whom a diagnosis of pulmonary TB is being considered. This approach is critical to limit nosocomial and community spread of infection. Culture of the organism from an involved site provides a definitive diagnosis. Blood cultures are positive in 15% of patients. This figure is higher in patients with lower CD4 +T cell counts. In the setting of fulminant disease one cannot rely upon the accuracy of a negative PPD skin test to rule out a diagnosis of TB. TB is one of the conditions associated with HIV infection for which cure is possible with appropriate therapy. Therapy for TB is generally the same in the HIV-infected patient as in the HIV-negative patient (Chap. 158). Due to the possibility of multidrug resistant or extensively drug-resistant TB, drug susceptibility testing should be performed to guide therapy. Due to pharmacokinetic interactions, adjusted doses of rifabutin should be substituted for rifampin in patients receiving the HIV protease inhibitors or nonnucleoside reverse transcriptase inhibitors. Treatment is most effective in programs that involve directly observed therapy. Initiation of ARV therapy and/or anti-TB therapy may be associated with clinical deterioration due to immune reconstitution inflammatory syndrome (IRIS) reactions. These are most common in patients initiating both treatments at the same time, occur several weeks following initiation of therapy, and are seen more frequently in patients with advanced HIV disease. Effective prevention of active TB can be a reality if the health care professional is aggressive in looking for evidence of latent TB by making sure that all patients with HIV infection receive a PPD skin test or evaluation with an interferon-γ release assay. Anergy testing is not of value in this setting. HIV-infected individuals with a skin test reaction of >5 mm, a positive interferon-γ release assay or those who are close household contacts of persons with active TB should receive treatment with 9 months of isoniazid.

Atypical mycobacterial infections are also seen with an increased frequency in patients with HIV infection. Infections with at least 12 different mycobacteria have been reported, including *M. bovis* and representatives of all four Runyon groups. The most common atypical mycobacterial infection is with *M. avium* or *M. intracellulare* species—MAC. Infections with MAC are seen mainly in patients in the United States and are rare in Africa. It has been suggested that prior infection with *M. tuberculosis* decreases the risk of MAC infection. MAC infections probably arise from organisms that are ubiquitous in the environment, including both soil and water. The presumed portals of entry are the respiratory and gastrointestinal tract. MAC infection is a late complication of HIV infection, predominantly occurring in patients with CD4+ T cell counts of <50/μL. The average CD4+ T cell count at the time of diagnosis is 10/μL. The most common presentation is disseminated disease with fever, weight loss, and night sweats. At least 85% of patients with MAC infection are mycobacteremic, and large numbers of organisms can often be demonstrated on bone marrow biopsy. The chest x-ray is abnormal in ~25% of patients, with the most common pattern being that of a bilateral, lower lobe infiltrate suggestive of miliary spread. Alveolar or nodular infiltrates and hilar and/or mediastinal adenopathy can also occur. Other clinical findings include endobronchial lesions, abdominal pain, diarrhea, and lymphadenopathy. The diagnosis is made by the culture of blood or involved tissue. The finding of two consecutive sputum samples positive for MAC is highly suggestive of pulmonary infection. Cultures may take 2 weeks to turn positive. Therapy consists of a macrolide, usually clarithromycin, with ethambutol. Some physicians elect to add a third drug from among rifabutin, ciprofloxacin, or amikacin in patients with extensive disease. Therapy is generally for life; however, with the use of highly active antiretroviral therapy (HAART), it is possible to discontinue therapy in patients with sustained suppression of HIV replication and CD4+ T cell counts >100/μL for 3–6 months. Primary prophylaxis for MAC is indicated in patients with HIV infection and CD4+ T cell counts <50/μL. This may be discontinued in patients in whom HAART induces a sustained suppression of viral replication and increases in CD4+ T cell counts to >100/μL for 3–6 months.

Rhodococcus equi is a gram-positive pleomorphic acid-fast nonspore-forming bacillus that can cause pulmonary and/or disseminated infection in patients with HIV infection. Fever and cough are the most common presenting signs. Radiographically one may see cavitary lesions and consolidation. Blood cultures are often positive. Treatment is based upon antimicrobial sensitivity testing.

Fungal infections of the lung, in addition to PCP, can be seen in patients with AIDS. Patients with pulmonary cryptococcal disease present with fever, cough, dyspnea, and in some cases, hemoptysis. A focal or diffuse interstitial infiltrate is seen on chest x-ray in >90% of patients. In addition, one may see lobar disease, cavitary disease, pleural effusions, and hilar or mediastinal adenopathy. Over half of patients are fungemic, and 90% of patients have concomitant CNS infection. *Coccidioides immitis* is a mold that is endemic in the southwest United States. It can cause a reactivation pulmonary syndrome in patients with HIV infection. Most patients with this condition will have CD4+ T cell counts <250/μL. Patients present with fever, weight loss, cough, and extensive, diffuse reticulonodular infiltrates on chest x-ray. One may also see nodules, cavities, pleural effusions, and hilar adenopathy. While serologic testing is of value in the immunocompetent host, serologies are negative in 25% of HIV-infected patients with coccidioidal infection. Invasive aspergillosis is not an AIDS-defining illness and is generally not seen in patients with AIDS in the absence of neutropenia or administration of glucocorticoids. *Aspergillus* infection may have an unusual presentation in the respiratory tract of patients with AIDS where it gives the appearance of a pseudomembranous tracheobronchitis. Primary pulmonary infection of the lung may be seen with *histoplasmosis.* The most common pulmonary manifestation of histoplasmosis, however, is in the setting of disseminated disease, presumably due to reactivation. In this setting respiratory symptoms are usually minimal, with cough and dyspnea occurring in 10–30% of patients. The chest x-ray is abnormal in ~50% of patients, showing either a diffuse interstitial infiltrate or diffuse small nodules.

Two forms of *idiopathic interstitial pneumonia* have been identified in patients with HIV infection: lymphoid interstitial pneumonitis (LIP) and nonspecific interstitial pneumonitis (NIP). LIP, a common finding in children, is seen in about 1% of adult patients with untreated HIV infection. This disorder is characterized by a benign infiltrate of the lung and is thought to be part of the polyclonal activation of lymphocytes seen in the context of HIV and EBV infections. Transbronchial biopsy is diagnostic in 50% of the cases, with an open-lung biopsy required for diagnosis in the remainder of cases. This condition is generally self-limited and no specific treatment is necessary. Severe cases have been managed with brief courses of glucocorticoids. Although rarely a clinical problem since the use of HAART, evidence of NIP may be seen in up to half of all patients with untreated HIV infection. Histologically, interstitial infiltrates of lymphocytes and plasma cells in a perivascular and peribronchial distribution are present. When symptomatic, patients present with fever and nonproductive cough occasionally accompanied by mild chest discomfort. Chest x-ray is usually normal or may reveal a faint interstitial pattern. Similar to LIP, NIP is a self-limited process for which no therapy is indicated other than appropriate management of the underlying HIV infection. HIV-related pulmonary arterial hypertension (HIV-PAH) is seen in ~0.5% of HIV-infected individuals. Patients may present with an array of symptoms including shortness of breath, fatigue, syncope, chest pain, and signs of right-sided heart failure. Chest x-ray reveals dilated pulmonary vessels and right-sided cardiomegaly with right ventricular hypertrophy seen on electrocardiogram. ARV therapy does not appear to be of clear benefit, and the prognosis is quite poor with a median survival in the range of 2 years.

Neoplastic diseases of the lung including KS and lymphoma are discussed below in the section on malignancies.

Diseases of the Cardiovascular System Heart disease is a relatively common postmortem finding in HIV-infected patients (25–75% in autopsy series). Cardiovascular disease may be seen as a direct consequence of HIV infection or as a consequence of ARV therapy as part of the lipodystrophy syndrome. As a primary consequence of HIV infection, the most common clinically significant finding is a dilated cardiomyopathy associated with congestive heart failure (CHF), referred to as *HIV-associated cardiomyopathy*. This generally occurs as a late complication of HIV infection and, histologically, displays elements of myocarditis. For this reason some have advocated treatment with intravenous immunoglobulin (IVIg). HIV can be directly demonstrated in cardiac tissue in this setting, and there is debate over whether or not it plays a direct role in this condition. Patients present with typical findings of CHF, namely edema and shortness of breath. Patients with HIV infection may also develop cardiomyopathy as side effects of IFN-α or nucleoside analogue therapy. These are reversible once therapy is stopped. KS, cryptococcosis, Chagas' disease, and toxoplasmosis can involve the myocardium, leading to cardiomyopathy. In one series, most patients with HIV infection and a treatable myocarditis were found to have myocarditis associated with toxoplasmosis. Most of these patients also had evidence of CNS toxoplasmosis. Thus, MRI or double-dose contrast CT scan of the brain should be included in the workup of any patient with advanced HIV infection and cardiomyopathy.

A variety of other cardiovascular problems are found in patients with HIV infection. Pericardial effusions may be seen in the setting of advanced HIV infection. Predisposing factors include TB, CHF, mycobacterial infection, cryptococcal infection, pulmonary infection, lymphoma, and KS. While pericarditis is quite rare, in one series 5% of patients with HIV disease had pericardial effusions that were considered to be moderate or severe. Tamponade and death have occurred in association with pericardial KS, presumably owing to acute hemorrhage. Nonbacterial thrombotic endocarditis has been reported and should be considered in patients with unexplained embolic phenomena. Intravenous pentamidine, when given rapidly, can result in hypotension as a consequence of cardiovascular collapse. A high percentage of patients have hypertriglyceridemia and elevations in serum cholesterol, and coronary artery disease has been a relatively frequent finding at autopsy. This problem appears to becoming even more prevalent as a side effect of HAART and in particular in patients with co-infection with HCV. While the clinical significance of these findings has not been precisely defined, recent data suggest a linear relationship between time on HAART and development of ischemic heart disease. In one large series the overall rate of myocardial infarction (MI) was 3.5/1000 years, 28% of these events were fatal, and MI was responsible for 7% of all deaths in the cohort. The risk of MI increased by 26% per year of HAART. This small increase in the risk of death from MI in the setting of HAART has to be balanced against the marked increase in overall survival brought about by HAART. Efforts to decrease the risk of cardiovascular diseases by minimizing the time on HAART were associated with a paradoxical increase in the rate of cardiovascular disease suggesting that the pathogenesis of cardiovascular diseases in the setting of HIV infection is multifactorial, with HIV infection and the resulting immune activation and coagulopathy likely playing a significant role.

Diseases of the Oropharynx and Gastrointestinal System Oropharyngeal and gastrointestinal diseases are common features of HIV infection. They are most frequently due to secondary infections. In addition, oral and gastrointestinal lesions may occur with KS and lymphoma.

Oral lesions, including *thrush*, *hairy leukoplakia*, and *aphthous ulcers* (Fig. 182-32), are particularly common in patients with untreated HIV infection. Thrush, due to *Candida* infection, and oral hairy leukoplakia, presumed due to EBV, are usually indicative of fairly advanced immunologic decline; they generally occur in patients with CD4+ T cell counts of <300/μL. In one study, 59% of patients with oral candidiasis went on to develop AIDS in the next year. Thrush appears as a white, cheesy exudate, often on an erythematous mucosa in the posterior oropharynx. While most commonly seen on the soft palate, early lesions are often found along the gingival border. The diagnosis is made by direct examination of a scraping for pseudohyphal elements. Culturing is of no diagnostic value, as most patients with HIV infection will have a positive throat culture for *Candida* even in the absence of thrush. Oral hairy leukoplakia presents as white, frondlike lesions, generally along the lateral borders of the tongue and sometimes on the adjacent buccal mucosa (Fig. 182-32). Despite its name, oral hairy leukoplakia is not considered a premalignant condition. Lesions are associated with florid replication of EBV. While usually more disconcerting

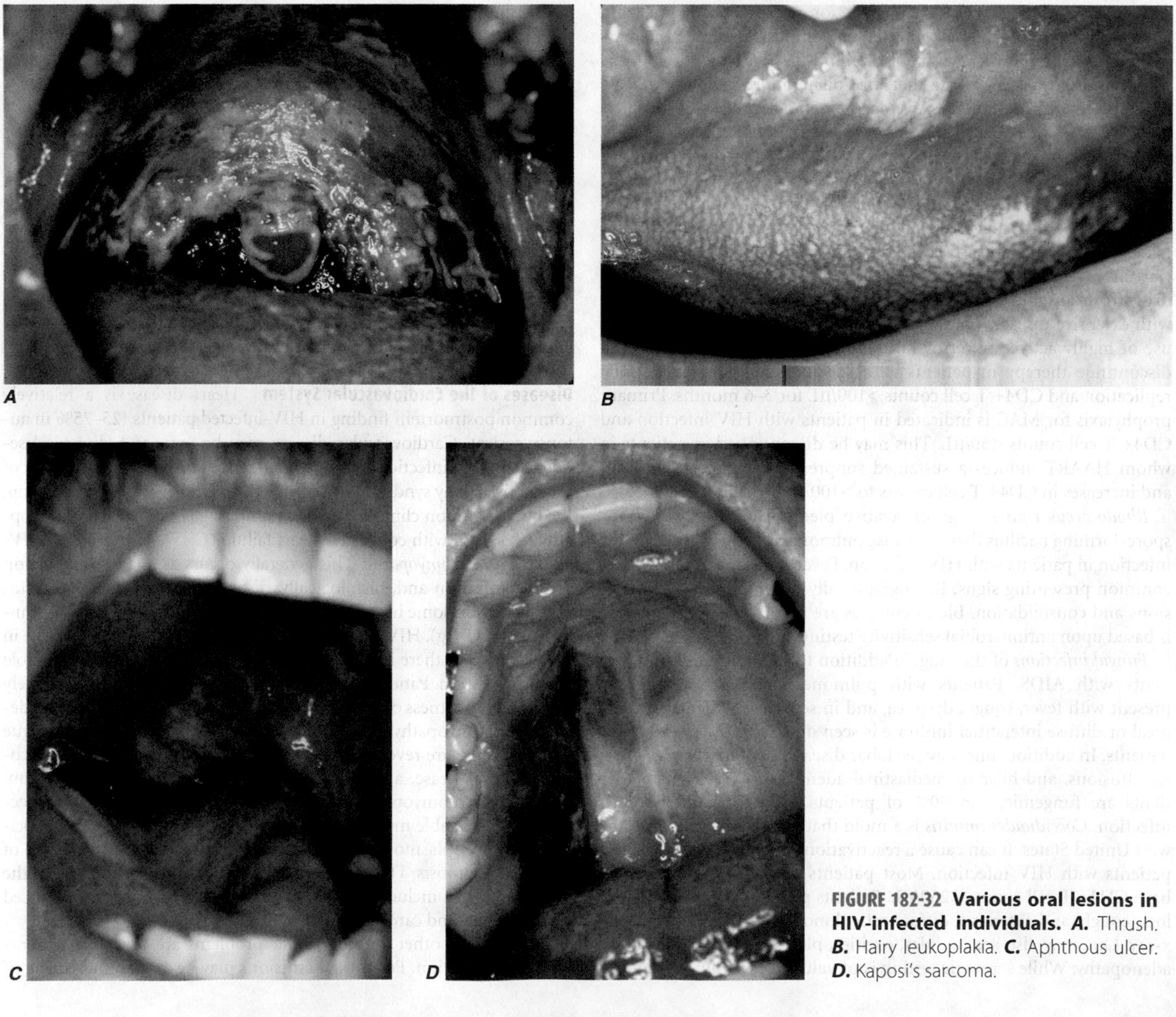

FIGURE 182-32 Various oral lesions in HIV-infected individuals. ***A.*** Thrush. ***B.*** Hairy leukoplakia. ***C.*** Aphthous ulcer. ***D.*** Kaposi's sarcoma.

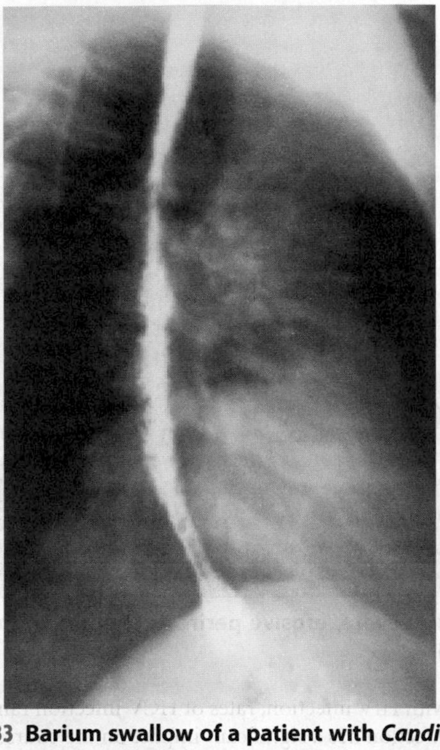

FIGURE 182-33 Barium swallow of a patient with *Candida* esophagitis. The flow of barium along the mucosal surface is grossly irregular.

as a sign of HIV-associated immunodeficiency than a clinical problem in need of treatment, severe cases have been reported to respond to topical podophyllin or systemic therapy with anti-herpesvirus agents. Aphthous ulcers of the posterior oropharynx are also seen with regularity in patients with HIV infection (Fig. 182-32). These lesions are of unknown etiology and can be quite painful and interfere with swallowing. Topical anesthetics provide immediate symptomatic relief of short duration. The fact that thalidomide is an effective treatment for this condition suggests that the pathogenesis may involve the action of tissue-destructive cytokines. Palatal, glossal, or gingival ulcers may also result from cryptococcal disease or histoplasmosis.

Esophagitis (Fig. 182-33) may present with odynophagia and retrosternal pain. Upper endoscopy is generally required to make an accurate diagnosis. Esophagitis may be due to *Candida*, CMV, or HSV. While CMV tends to be associated with a single large ulcer, HSV infection is more often associated with multiple small ulcers. The esophagus may also be the site of KS and lymphoma. Like the oral mucosa, the esophageal mucosa may have large, painful ulcers of unclear etiology that may respond to thalidomide. While achlorhydria is a common problem in patients with HIV infection, other gastric problems are generally rare. Among the conditions involving the stomach are KS and lymphoma. Infections of the small and large intestine leading to diarrhea, abdominal pain, and occasionally fever are among the most significant gastrointestinal problems in HIV-infected patients. They include infections with bacteria, protozoa, and viruses.

Bacteria may be responsible for secondary infections of the gastrointestinal tract. Infections with enteric pathogens such as *Salmonella*, *Shigella*, and *Campylobacter* are more common in homosexual men and are often more severe and more apt to relapse in patients with HIV infection. Patients with untreated HIV have approximately a 20-fold increased risk of infection with *S. typhimurium*. They may present with a variety of nonspecific symptoms including fever, anorexia, fatigue, and malaise of several weeks' duration. Diarrhea is common but may be absent. Diagnosis is made by culture of blood and stool. Long-term therapy with ciprofloxacin is the recommended treatment. HIV-infected patients also have an increased incidence of *S. typhi* infection in areas of the world where typhoid is a problem. *Shigella* spp., particularly *S. flexneri*, can cause severe intestinal disease in HIV-infected individuals. Up to 50% of patients will develop bacteremia. *Campylobacter* infections occur with an increased frequency in patients with HIV infection. While *C. jejuni* is the strain most frequently isolated, infections with many other strains have been reported. Patients usually present with crampy abdominal pain, fever, and bloody diarrhea. Infection may present as proctitis. Stool examination reveals the presence of fecal leukocytes. Systemic infection can occur, with up to 10% of infected patients exhibiting bacteremia. Most strains are sensitive to erythromycin. Abdominal pain and diarrhea may be seen with MAC infection.

Fungal infections may also be a cause of diarrhea in patients with HIV infection. Histoplasmosis, coccidioidomycosis, and penicilliosis have all been identified as a cause of fever and diarrhea in patients with HIV infection. Peritonitis has been seen with *C. immitis*.

Cryptosporidia, microsporidia, and *Isospora belli* (Chap. 208) are the most common opportunistic protozoa that infect the gastrointestinal tract and cause diarrhea in HIV-infected patients. Cryptosporidial infection may present in a variety of ways, ranging from a self-limited or intermittent diarrheal illness in patients in the early stages of HIV infection to a severe, life-threatening diarrhea in severely immunodeficient individuals. In patients with untreated HIV infection and CD4+ T cell counts of <300/μL, the incidence of cryptosporidiosis is ~1% per year. In 75% of cases the diarrhea is accompanied by crampy abdominal pain, and 25% of patients have nausea and/or vomiting. Cryptosporidia may also cause biliary tract disease in the HIV-infected patient, leading to cholecystitis with or without accompanying cholangitis. The diagnosis of cryptosporidial diarrhea is made by stool examination. The diarrhea is noninflammatory, and the characteristic finding is the presence of oocysts that stain with acid-fast dyes. Therapy is predominantly supportive, and marked improvements have been reported in the setting of effective ARV therapy. Treatment with up to 2000 mg/d of nitazoxanide (NTZ) is associated with improvement in symptoms or a decrease in shedding of organisms in about half of patients. Its overall role in the management of this condition remains unclear. Patients can minimize their risk of developing cryptosporidiosis by avoiding contact with human and animal feces and by not drinking untreated water from lakes or rivers.

Microsporidia are small, unicellular, obligate intracellular parasites that reside in the cytoplasm of enteric cells (Chap. 208). The main species causing disease in humans is *Enterocytozoon bieneusi*. The clinical manifestations are similar to those described for cryptosporidia and include abdominal pain and diarrhea. The small size of the organism may make it difficult to detect; however, with the use of chromotrope-based stains, organisms can be identified in stool samples by light microscopy. Definitive diagnosis generally depends on electron-microscopic examination of a stool specimen, intestinal aspirate, or intestinal biopsy specimen. In contrast to cryptosporidia, microsporidia have been noted in a variety of extraintestinal locations, including the eye, muscle, and liver, and have been associated with conjunctivitis and hepatitis. Albendazole, 400 mg bid, has been reported to be of benefit in some patients.

I. belli is a coccidian parasite (Chap. 208) most commonly found as a cause of diarrhea in patients from the Caribbean and Africa. Its cysts appear in the stool as large, acid-fast structures that can be differentiated from those of cryptosporidia on the basis of size, shape, and number of sporocysts. The clinical syndromes of *Isospora* infection are identical to those caused by cryptosporidia. The important distinction is that infection with *Isospora* is generally relatively easy to treat with TMP/SMX. While relapses are common, a thrice-weekly regimen of TMP/SMX appears adequate to prevent recurrence.

CMV colitis was once seen as a consequence of advanced immunodeficiency in 5–10% of patients with AIDS. It is much less common with the advent of HAART. CMV colitis presents as diarrhea, abdominal pain, weight loss, and anorexia. The diarrhea is usually nonbloody, and the diagnosis is achieved through endoscopy and biopsy. Multiple mucosal ulcerations are seen at endoscopy, and biopsies reveal characteristic intranuclear inclusion bodies. Secondary bacteremias may result as a consequence of thinning of the bowel wall. Treatment is with either ganciclovir or foscarnet for 3–6 weeks. Relapses are common, and maintenance therapy is typically necessary in patients whose HIV infection is poorly controlled. Patients with CMV disease of the gastrointestinal tract should be carefully monitored for evidence of CMV retinitis.

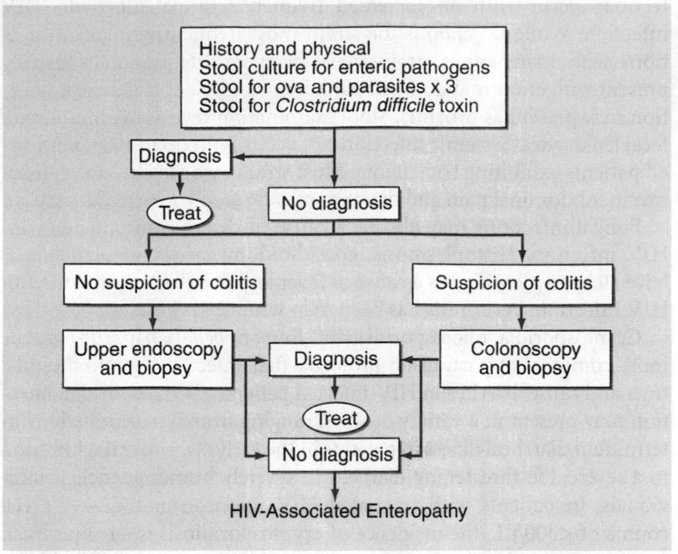

FIGURE 182-34 Algorithm for the evaluation of diarrhea in a patient with HIV infection. HIV-associated enteropathy is a diagnosis of exclusion and can be made only after other, generally treatable, forms of diarrheal illness have been ruled out.

In addition to disease caused by specific secondary infections, patients with HIV infection may also experience a chronic diarrheal syndrome for which no etiologic agent other than HIV can be identified. This entity is referred to as *AIDS enteropathy* or *HIV enteropathy*. It is most likely a direct result of HIV infection in the gastrointestinal tract. Histologic examination of the small bowel in these patients reveals low-grade mucosal atrophy with a decrease in mitotic figures, suggesting a hyporegenerative state. Patients often have decreased or absent small-bowel lactase and malabsorption with accompanying weight loss.

The initial evaluation of a patient with HIV infection and diarrhea should include a set of stool examinations, including culture, examination for ova and parasites, and examination for *Clostridium difficile* toxin. Approximately 50% of the time this workup will demonstrate infection with pathogenic bacteria, mycobacteria, or protozoa. If the initial stool examinations are negative, additional evaluation, including upper and/or lower endoscopy with biopsy, will yield a diagnosis of microsporidial or mycobacterial infection of the small intestine ~30% of the time. In patients for whom this diagnostic evaluation is nonrevealing, a presumptive diagnosis of HIV enteropathy can be made if the diarrhea has persisted for >1 month. An algorithm for the evaluation of diarrhea in patients with HIV infection is given in Fig. 182-34.

Rectal lesions are common in HIV-infected patients, particularly the perirectal ulcers and erosions due to the reactivation of HSV (Fig. 182-35). These may appear quite atypical, as denuded skin without vesicles, and they respond well to treatment with acyclovir, famciclovir, or foscarnet. Other rectal lesions encountered in patients with HIV infection include condylomata acuminata, KS, and intraepithelial neoplasia (see below).

Hepatobiliary Disease Diseases of the hepatobiliary system are a major problem in patients with HIV infection. It has been estimated that approximately one-third of the deaths of patients with HIV infection are in some way related to liver disease. While this is predominantly a reflection of the problems encountered in the setting of co-infection with hepatitis B or C, it is also a reflection of the hepatic injury, ranging from hepatic steatosis to hypersensitivity reactions to immune reconstitution, that can be seen in the context of ARV therapy.

The prevalence of co-infection with HIV and hepatitis viruses varies by geographic region. In the United States, ~90% of HIV-infected individuals have evidence of infection with HBV; 6–14% have chronic HBV infection; 5–50% of patients are co-infected with HCV; and co-infection with hepatitis D, E, and/or G viruses is common. Among IV drug users with HIV infection, rates of HCV infection range from 70–95%. HIV infection has a significant impact on the course of hepatitis virus infection. It is associated with approximately a threefold increase in the development of persistent hepatitis B surface antigenemia. Patients infected with both HBV and HIV have decreased evidence of inflammatory liver disease. The presumption that this is due to the immunosuppressive effects of HIV infection is supported by the observations that this situation can be reversed, and one may see the development of more severe hepatitis following the initiation of effective ARV therapy. In studies of the impact of HIV on HBV infection four- to tenfold increases in liver-related mortality have been noted in patients with HIV and active HBV infection compared to rates in patients with either infection alone. There is a slight increase in overall mortality in HIV-infected individuals who are also hepatitis B surface antigen (HBsAg) positive. IFN-α is less successful as a treatment of HBV in patients with HIV co-infection, and lamivudine, emtricitabine, or adefovir/tenofovir and entecavir alone or in combination are useful in the treatment of hepatitis B in patients with HIV infection. It is important to remember that all the above-mentioned drugs also have activity against HIV and should not be used as single agents in patients with HIV infection, in order to avoid the rapid development of resistant quasispecies of HIV. HCV infection is more severe in the patient with HIV infection; it does not appear to affect overall mortality in HIV-infected individuals when other variables such as age, baseline CD4+ T cell count, and use of HAART are taken into account. In the setting of HIV and HCV co-infection, levels of HCV are approximately tenfold higher than in the HIV-negative patient with HCV infection and there is a tenfold increased risk of death due to liver disease in co-infected patients. Treatment for HCV infection consists of pegylated IFN-α and ribavirin. If a 2-log drop in levels of HCV RNA is not seen within 12 weeks, it is unlikely that therapy will be of value. Hepatitis A virus infection is not seen with an increased frequency in patients with HIV infection. It is recommended that all patients with HIV infection who have not experienced natural infection be immunized with hepatitis A and/or hepatitis B vaccines. Infection with hepatitis G virus, also known as GB virus C, is seen in ~50% of patients with HIV infection. For reasons that are currently unclear there are data to suggest that patients with HIV infection co-infected with this virus have a decreased rate of progression to AIDS.

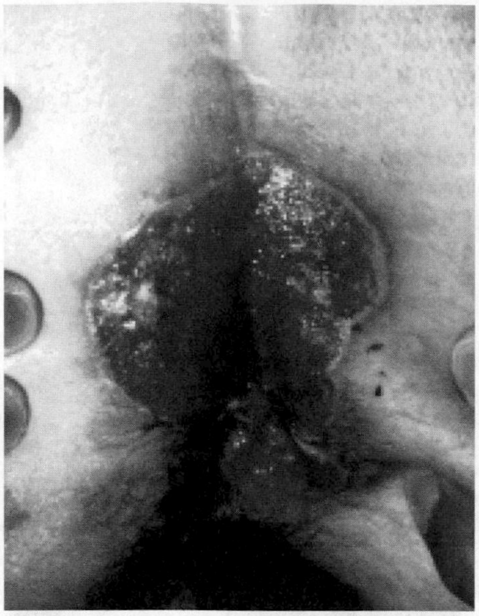

FIGURE 182-35 Severe, erosive perirectal herpes simplex in a patient with AIDS.

A variety of other infections may also involve the liver. Granulomatous hepatitis may be seen as a consequence of mycobacterial or fungal infections, particularly MAC infection. Hepatic masses may be seen in the context of TB, peliosis hepatis, or fungal infection. Among the fungal opportunistic infections *C. immitis* and *Histoplasma capsulatum* are those most likely to involve the liver. Biliary tract disease in the form of papillary stenosis or sclerosing cholangitis has been reported in the context of cryptosporidiosis, CMV infection, and KS.

Many of the drugs used to treat HIV infection are metabolized by the liver and can cause liver injury. Fatal hepatic reactions have been reported with a wide array of ARVs including nucleoside analogues, nonnucleoside analogues, and protease inhibitors. Nucleoside analogues work by inhibiting DNA synthesis. This can result in toxicity to mitochondria, which can lead to disturbances in oxidative metabolism. This may manifest as hepatic steatosis and, in severe cases, lactic acidosis and fulminant liver failure. It is important to be aware of this condition and to watch for it in patients with HIV infection receiving nucleoside analogues. It is reversible if diagnosed early and the offending agent(s) discontinued. Nevirapine has been associated with at times fatal fulminant and cholestatic hepatitis, hepatic necrosis, and hepatic failure. Indinavir may cause mild to moderate elevations in serum bilirubin in 10–15% of patients in a syndrome similar to Gilbert's syndrome. A similar pattern of hepatic injury may be seen with atazanavir. In the patient receiving HAART with an unexplained increase in hepatic transaminases, strong consideration should be given to drug toxicity. *Pancreatic injury* is most commonly a consequence of drug toxicity, notably that secondary to pentamidine or dideoxynucleosides. While up to half of patients in some series have biochemical evidence of pancreatic injury, <5% of patients show any clinical evidence of pancreatitis that is not linked to a drug toxicity.

Diseases of the Kidney and Genitourinary Tract Diseases of the kidney or genitourinary tract may be a direct consequence of HIV infection, due to an opportunistic infection or neoplasm, or related to drug toxicity. *HIV-associated nephropathy* was first described in IDUs and was initially thought to be IDU nephropathy in patients with HIV infection; it is now recognized as a true direct complication of HIV infection. Although the majority of patients have CD4+ T cell counts <200/μL, HIV-associated nephropathy can be an early manifestation of HIV infection and is also seen in children. Over 90% of reported cases have been in African-American or Hispanic individuals; the disease is not only more prevalent in these populations but also more severe and is the third leading cause of end-stage renal failure among African Americans aged 20–64 in the United States. Proteinuria is the hallmark of this disorder. Overall, microalbuminuria is seen in ~20% of untreated HIV-infected patients; significant proteinuria is seen in closer to 2%. Edema and hypertension are rare. Ultrasound examination reveals enlarged, hyperechogenic kidneys. A definitive diagnosis is obtained through renal biopsy. Histologically, focal segmental glomerulosclerosis is present in 80%, and mesangial proliferation in 10–15% of cases. Prior to effective antiretroviral therapy, this disease was characterized by relatively rapid progression to end-stage renal disease and patients with HIV-associated nephropathy should be treated for their HIV infection regardless of CD4+ T cell count. Treatment with angiotensin-converting enzyme (ACE) inhibitors and/or prednisone, 60 mg/d, has also been reported to be of benefit in some cases. The incidence of this disease in patients receiving adequate ARV therapy has not been well defined; however, the impression is that it has decreased in frequency and severity. It is the leading cause of end-stage renal disease in patients with HIV infection.

Among the drugs commonly associated with renal damage in patients with HIV disease are pentamidine, amphotericin, adefovir, cidofovir, tenofovir, and foscarnet. TMP/SMX may compete for tubular secretion with creatinine and cause an increase in the serum creatinine level. Sulfadiazine may crystallize in the kidney and result in an easily reversible form of renal shutdown. One of the most common drug-induced renal complications is indinavir-associated renal calculi. This condition is seen in ~10% of patients receiving this HIV protease inhibitor. It may present with a variety of manifestations, ranging from asymptomatic hematuria to renal colic. Adequate hydration is the mainstay of treatment and prevention for this condition.

Genitourinary tract infections are seen with a high frequency in patients with HIV infection; they present with skin lesions, dysuria, hematuria, and/or pyuria and are managed in the same fashion as in patients without HIV infection. Infections with HSV are covered below under dermatologic disorders. Infections with *T. pallidum*, the etiologic agent of *syphilis*, play an important role in the HIV epidemic (Chap. 181). In HIV-negative individuals, genital syphilitic ulcers as well as the ulcers of chancroid are major predisposing factors for heterosexual transmission of HIV infection. While most HIV-infected individuals with syphilis have a typical presentation, a variety of formerly rare clinical problems may be encountered in the setting of dual infection. Among them are *lues maligna*, an ulcerating lesion of the skin due to a necrotizing vasculitis; unexplained fever; nephrotic syndrome; and neurosyphilis. The most common presentation of syphilis in the HIV-infected patient is that of *condylomata lata*, a form of secondary syphilis. Neurosyphilis may be asymptomatic or may present as acute meningitis, neuroretinitis, deafness, or stroke. The rate of neurosyphilis may be as high as 1% in patients with HIV infection. As a consequence of the immunologic abnormalities seen in the setting of HIV infection, diagnosis of syphilis through standard serologic testing may be challenging. On the one hand, a significant number of patients have false-positive Venereal Disease Research Laboratory (VDRL) tests due to polyclonal B cell activation. On the other hand, the development of a new positive VDRL may be delayed in patients with new infections, and the anti-fluorescent treponema antibody (anti-FTA) test may be negative due to immunodeficiency. Thus, dark-field examination of appropriate specimens should be performed in any patient in whom syphilis is suspected, even if the patient has a negative VDRL. Similarly, any patient with a positive serum VDRL test, neurologic findings, and an abnormal spinal fluid examination should be considered to have neurosyphilis, regardless of the CSF VDRL result. In any setting, patients treated for syphilis need to be carefully monitored to ensure adequate therapy.

Vulvovaginal candidiasis is a common problem in women with HIV infection. Symptoms include pruritus, discomfort, dyspareunia, and dysuria. Vulvar infection may present as a morbilliform rash that may extend to the thighs. Vaginal infection is usually associated with a white discharge, and plaques may be seen along an erythematous vaginal wall. Diagnosis is made by microscopic examination of the discharge for pseudohyphal elements in a 10% potassium hydroxide solution. Mild disease can be treated with topical therapy. More serious disease can be treated with fluconazole. Other causes of vaginitis include *Trichomonas* and mixed bacteria.

Diseases of the Endocrine System and Metabolic Disorders A variety of endocrine and metabolic disorders are seen in the context of HIV infection. Between 33 and 75% of patients with HIV infection receiving HAART develop a syndrome often referred to as *lipodystrophy*, consisting of elevations in plasma triglycerides, total cholesterol, and apolipoprotein B, as well as hyperinsulinemia and hyperglycemia. Many of the patients have been noted to have a characteristic set of body habitus changes associated with fat redistribution, consisting of truncal obesity coupled with peripheral wasting (Fig. 182-36). Truncal obesity is apparent as an increase in abdominal girth related to increases in mesenteric fat, a dorsocervical fat pad ("buffalo hump") reminiscent of patients with Cushing's syndrome, and enlargement of the breasts. The peripheral wasting or lipoatrophy is particularly noticeable in the face and buttocks and by the prominence of the veins in the legs. These changes may develop at any time ranging from ~6 weeks to several years following the initiation of HAART. Approximately 20% of the patients with HIV-associated lipodystrophy meet the criteria for the *metabolic syndrome* as defined by The International Diabetes Federation or The U.S. National Cholesterol Education Program Adult Treatment Panel III. The lipodystrophy syndrome has been reported in association with regimens containing a variety of different drugs, and while initially reported in the setting of protease inhibitor therapy, it appears similar changes can also be induced by potent protease-sparing regimens. It has been suggested that the lipoatrophy changes are particularly severe in patients receiving thymidine analogues. National Cholesterol Education Program (NCEP) guidelines should be followed in the management of these lipid abnor-

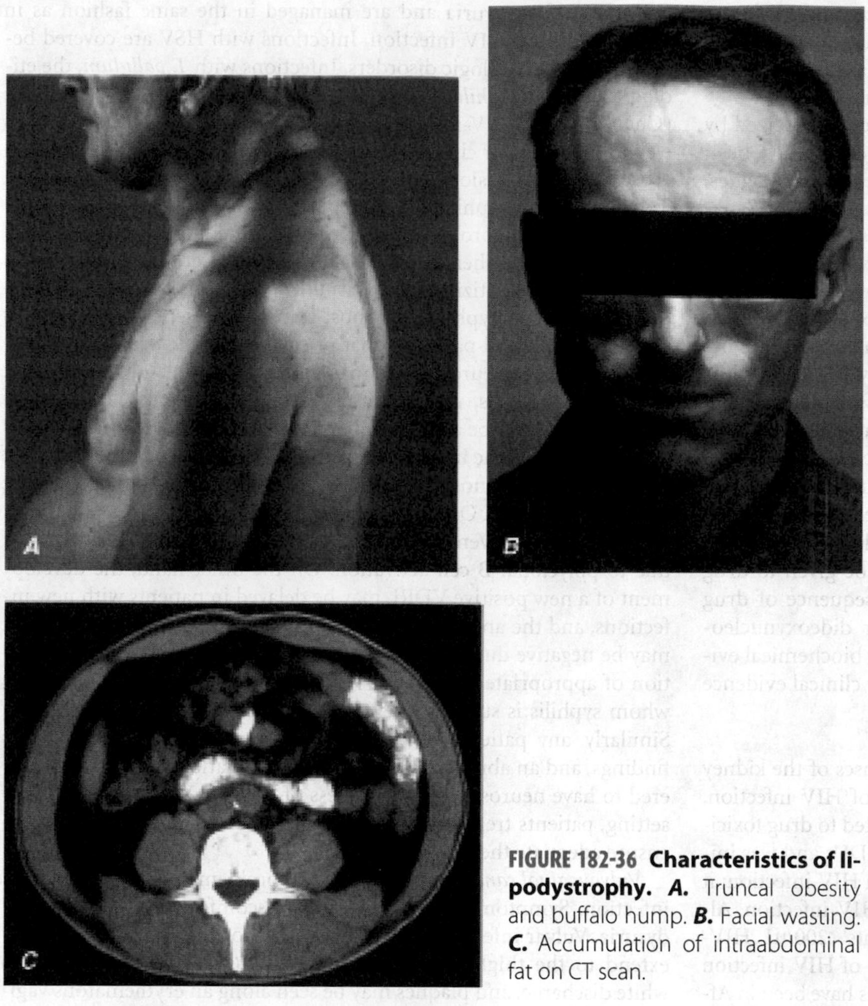

FIGURE 182-36 Characteristics of lipodystrophy. ***A.*** Truncal obesity and buffalo hump. ***B.*** Facial wasting. ***C.*** Accumulation of intraabdominal fat on CT scan.

malities (Chap. 235). Due to concerns regarding drug interactions, the most commonly utilized agents in this setting are gemfibrozil and atorvastatin. In addition to these abnormalities, patients with HIV infection treated with HAART have been found to have an increased incidence of osteonecrosis or avascular necrosis of the hip and shoulders. In a study of asymptomatic patients, 4.4% were found to have evidence of osteonecrosis on MRI. This complication has been associated with the use of lipid-lowering agents, systemic glucocorticoids, or testosterone; bodybuilding exercise; alcohol consumption; and the presence of anticardiolipin antibodies. Osteoporosis has been reported in 7% of women with HIV infection, with 41% of women demonstrating some degree of osteopenia. In addition, lactic acidosis is associated with ARV therapy. This is most commonly seen with nucleoside analogue reverse transcriptase inhibitors and can be fatal (see below).

Patients with advanced HIV disease may develop hyponatremia due to the syndrome of inappropriate antidiuretic hormone (vasopressin) secretion (SIADH) as a consequence of increased free water intake and decreased free water excretion. SIADH is usually seen in conjunction with pulmonary or CNS disease. Low serum sodium may also be due to adrenal insufficiency; concomitant high serum potassium should alert one to this possibility. Adrenal gland disease may be due to mycobacterial infections, CMV disease, cryptococcal disease, histoplasmosis, or ketoconazole toxicity.

Thyroid function may be altered in 10–15% of patients with HIV infection. Both hypo- and hyperthyroidism may be seen. The predominant abnormality is subclinical hypothyroidism. In the setting of HAART up to 10% of patients have been noted to have elevated thyroid-stimulating hormone levels, suggesting that this may be a manifestation of immune reconstitution. Immune-reconstitution Graves' disease may occur as a late (9–48 months) complication of HAART. In advanced HIV disease, infection of the thyroid gland may occur with opportunistic pathogens, including *P. jiroveci*, CMV, mycobacteria, *Toxoplasma gondii*, and *Cryptococcus neoformans.* These infections are generally associated with a nontender, diffuse enlargement of the thyroid gland. Thyroid function is usually normal. Diagnosis is made by fine-needle aspirate or open biopsy.

Advanced HIV disease is associated with *hypogonadism* in ~50% of men. While this is generally a complication of underlying illness, testicular dysfunction may also be a side effect of ganciclovir therapy. In some surveys, up to two-thirds of patients report decreased libido and one-third complain of impotence. Androgen-replacement therapy should be considered in patients with symptomatic hypogonadism. HIV infection does not seem to have a significant effect on the menstrual cycle outside the setting of advanced disease.

Rheumatologic Diseases Immunologic and rheumatologic disorders are common in patients with HIV infection and range from excessive immediate-type hypersensitivity reactions (Chap. 311) to an increase in the incidence of reactive arthritis (Chap. 318) to conditions characterized by a diffuse infiltrative lymphocytosis. The occurrence of these phenomena is an apparent paradox in the setting of the profound immunodeficiency and immunosuppression that characterizes HIV infection.

Drug allergies are the most significant allergic reactions occurring in HIV-infected patients and appear to become more common as the disease progresses. They occur in up to 65% of patients who receive therapy with TMP/SMX for PCP. In general, these drug reactions are characterized by erythematous, morbilliform eruptions that are pruritic, tend to coalesce, and are often associated with fever. Nonetheless, ~33% of patients can be maintained on the offending therapy, and thus these reactions are not an immediate indication to stop the drug. Anaphylaxis is extremely rare in patients with HIV infection, and patients who have a cutaneous reaction during a single course of therapy can still be considered candidates for future treatment or prophylaxis with the same agent. The one exception to this is the nucleoside analogue abacavir, where fatal hypersensitivity reactions have been reported with rechallenge. This hypersensitivity is strongly associated with the HLA-B57 haplotype and a hypersensitivity reaction to abacavir is an absolute contraindication to future therapy. For other agents, including TMP/SMX, desensitization regimens are moderately successful. While the mechanisms underlying these allergic-type reactions remain unknown, patients with HIV infection have been noted to have elevated IgE levels that increase as the CD4+ T cell count declines. The numerous examples of patients with multiple drug reactions suggest that a common pathway is involved.

HIV infection shares many similarities with a variety of autoimmune diseases, including a substantial polyclonal B cell activation that is associated with a high incidence of antiphospholipid antibodies, such as anticardiolipin antibodies, VDRL antibodies, and lupus-like anticoagulants. In addition, HIV-infected individuals have an increased incidence of antinuclear antibodies. Despite these serologic findings, there is no evidence that HIV-infected individuals have an increase in two of the more common autoimmune diseases, i.e., systemic lupus erythematosus and rheumatoid arthritis. In fact, it has been observed that these diseases may be somewhat ameliorated by the concomitant presence of HIV infection, suggesting that an intact CD4+ T cell limb of the immune response plays an integral role in the pathogenesis of these conditions. Similarly, there are anecdotal reports of patients with common variable immunodeficiency (Chap. 310), characterized by hypogammaglobulinemia, who have had a normalization of Ig levels following the development of HIV infection, suggesting a possible role for overactive CD4+ T cell immunity in certain forms of that syndrome. The one autoimmune disease that may occur with an increased frequency in patients with HIV infection is a variant of primary Sjögren's syndrome (Chap. 317). Patients with HIV infection may develop a syndrome consisting of parotid gland enlargement, dry eyes, and dry mouth that is associated with lymphocytic infiltrates of the salivary gland and lung. In contrast to Sjögren's syndrome, in which these infiltrates are composed predominantly of CD4+ T cells, in patients with HIV infection the infiltrates are composed predominantly of CD8+ T cells. In addition, while patients with Sjögren's syndrome are mainly women who have autoantibodies to Ro and La and who frequently have HLA-DR3 or -B8 MHC haplotypes, HIV-infected individuals with this syndrome are usually African-American men who do not have anti-Ro or anti-La and who most often are HLA-DR5. This syndrome appears to be less common with the increased use of effective ARV therapy. The term *diffuse infiltrative lymphocytosis syndrome* (DILS) has been proposed to describe this entity and to distinguish it from Sjögren's syndrome.

Approximately one-third of HIV-infected individuals experience arthralgias; furthermore, 5–10% are diagnosed as having some form of reactive arthritis, such as Reiter's syndrome or psoriatic arthritis (Chap. 318). These syndromes occur with increasing frequency as the competency of the immune system declines. This association may be related to an increase in the number of infections with organisms that may trigger a reactive arthritis with progressive immunodeficiency or to a loss of important regulatory T cells. Reactive arthritides in HIV-infected individuals generally respond well to standard treatment; however, therapy with methotrexate has been associated with an increase in the incidence of opportunistic infections and should be used with caution and only in severe cases.

HIV-infected individuals also experience a variety of joint problems without obvious cause that are referred to generically as *HIV-* or *AIDS-associated arthropathy*. This syndrome is characterized by subacute oligoarticular arthritis developing over a period of 1–6 weeks and lasting 6 weeks to 6 months. It generally involves the large joints, predominantly the knees and ankles, and is nonerosive with only a mild inflammatory response. X-rays of the joint are nonrevealing. Nonsteroidal anti-inflammatory drugs are only marginally helpful; however, relief has been noted with the use of intraarticular glucocorticoids. A second form of arthritis also thought to be secondary to HIV infection is called *painful articular syndrome*. This condition, reported as occurring in as many as 10% of AIDS patients, presents as an acute, severe, sharp pain in the affected joint. It affects primarily the knees, elbows, and shoulders; lasts 2–24 h; and may be severe enough to require narcotic analgesics. The cause of this arthropathy is unclear; however, it is thought to result from a direct effect of HIV on the joint. This condition is reminiscent of the fact that other lentiviruses, in particular the caprine arthritis-encephalitis virus, are capable of directly causing arthritis.

A variety of other immunologic or rheumatologic diseases have been reported in HIV-infected individuals, either de novo or in association with opportunistic infections or drugs. Using the criteria of widespread musculoskeletal pain of at least 3 months' duration and the presence of at least 11 of 18 possible tender points by digital palpation, 11% of an HIV-infected cohort containing 55% IDUs were diagnosed as having *fibromyalgia* (Chap. 329). While the incidence of frank arthritis was less in this population than in other studied populations that consisted predominantly of homosexual men, these data support the concept that there are musculoskeletal problems that occur as a direct result of HIV infection. In addition there have been reports of leukocytoclastic vasculitis in the setting of zidovudine therapy. CNS angiitis and polymyositis have also been reported in HIV-infected individuals. Septic arthritis is surprisingly rare, especially given the increased incidence of staphylococcal bacteremias seen in this population. When septic arthritis has been reported, it has usually been due to *Staphylococcus aureus*, systemic fungal infections with *C. neoformans*, *Sporothrix schenckii*, or *H. capsulatum* or to systemic mycobacterial infection with *M. tuberculosis*, *M. haemophilum*, *M. avium*, or *M. kansasii*.

TABLE 182-9 CHARACTERISTICS OF IMMUNE RECONSTITUTION INFLAMMATORY SYNDROME (IRIS)

- Paradoxical worsening of clinical condition following the initiation of antiretroviral therapy
- Occurs weeks to months following the initiation of antiretroviral therapy
- Most common in patients starting therapy with a CD4+ T cell count under 50/μL who experience a precipitous drop in viral load
- Frequently seen in the setting of tuberculosis
- Can be fatal

As noted above, 4.4% of patients with HIV infection were found to have some evidence of osteonecrosis by MRI during systematic screening of asymptomatic patients. The percentage of patients with symptomatic osteonecrosis has been estimated to be as high as 1%. While this problem was first recognized in the setting of HAART, it has been difficult to establish a cause-and-effect relationship. Alcohol consumption and a history of glucocorticoid use have been particularly associated with this condition in patients with HIV infection.

Immune Reconstitution Inflammatory Syndrome Following the initiation of effective ARV therapy, a paradoxical worsening of preexisting, untreated, or partially treated opportunistic infections may be noted (Table 182-9). These IRISs are particularly common in patients with underlying untreated mycobacterial infections. They are seen in anywhere from 10–50% of patients, depending upon the clinical setting, and are most common in patients starting therapy with CD4+ T cell counts <50 cells/μL who have a precipitous drop in HIV RNA levels following the initiation of HAART. Signs and symptoms may appear anywhere from 2 weeks to 2 years after the initiation of HAART and can include localized lymphadenitis, prolonged fever, pulmonary infiltrates, increased intracranial pressure, uveitis, and Graves' disease. The clinical course can be protracted and severe cases can be fatal. The underlying mechanism appears to be related to a phenomenon similar to type IV hypersensitivity reactions and reflects the immediate improvements in immune function that occur as levels of HIV RNA drop and the immunosuppressive effects of HIV infection are controlled. In severe cases, the use of immunosuppressive drugs such as glucocorticoids may be required to blunt the inflammatory component of these reactions while specific antimicrobial therapy takes effect.

Diseases of the Hematopoietic System Disorders of the hematopoietic system including lymphadenopathy, anemia, leukopenia, and/or thrombocytopenia are common throughout the course of HIV infection and may be the direct result of HIV, manifestations of secondary infections and neoplasms, or side effects of therapy (Table 182-10). Direct histologic examination and culture of lymph node or bone marrow tissue are often diagnostic. A significant percentage of bone marrow aspirates from patients with HIV infection have been reported to contain lymphoid aggregates, the precise significance of which is unknown. Initiation of HAART will lead to reversal of most hematologic complications that are the direct result of HIV infection.

Some patients, otherwise asymptomatic, may develop *persistent generalized lymphadenopathy* as an early clinical manifestation of HIV

TABLE 182-10 CAUSES OF BONE MARROW SUPPRESSION IN PATIENTS WITH HIV INFECTION

HIV infection	Medications
Mycobacterial infections	Zidovudine
Fungal infections	Dapsone
B19 parvovirus infection	Trimethoprim/sulfamethoxazole
Lymphoma	Pyrimethamine
	5-Flucytosine
	Ganciclovir
	Interferon-α
	Trimetrexate
	Foscarnet

infection. This condition is defined as the presence of enlarged lymph nodes (>1 cm) in two or more extrainguinal sites for >3 months without an obvious cause. The lymphadenopathy is due to marked follicular hyperplasia in the node in response to HIV infection. The nodes are generally discrete and freely movable. This feature of HIV disease may be seen at any point in the spectrum of immune dysfunction and is not associated with an increased likelihood of developing AIDS. Paradoxically, a loss in lymphadenopathy or a decrease in lymph node size outside the setting of ARV therapy may be a prognostic marker of disease progression. In patients with CD4+ T cell counts >200/μL, the differential diagnosis of lymphadenopathy includes KS, TB, Castleman's disease, and lymphoma. In patients with more advanced disease, lymphadenopathy may also be due to atypical mycobacterial infection, toxoplasmosis, systemic fungal infection, or bacillary angiomatosis. While indicated in patients with CD4+ T cell counts <200/μL, lymph node biopsy is not indicated in patients with early-stage disease unless there are signs and symptoms of systemic illness, such as fever and weight loss, or unless the nodes begin to enlarge, become fixed, or coalesce. Monoclonal gammopathy of unknown significance (MGUS; Chap. 106), defined as the presence of a serum monoclonal IgG, IgA, or IgM in the absence of a clear cause, has been reported in 3% of patients with HIV infection. The overall clinical significance of this finding in patients with HIV infection is unclear, although it has been associated with other viral infections, non-Hodgkin's lymphoma, and plasma cell malignancy.

Anemia is the most common hematologic abnormality in HIV-infected patients and in the absence of a specific treatable cause is independently associated with a poor prognosis. While generally mild, anemia can be quite severe and require chronic blood transfusions. Among the specific reversible causes of anemia in the setting of HIV infection are drug toxicity, systemic fungal and mycobacterial infections, nutritional deficiencies, and parvovirus B19 infections. Zidovudine may block erythroid maturation, prior to its effects on other marrow elements. A characteristic feature of zidovudine therapy is an elevated mean corpuscular volume (MCV). Another drug used in patients with HIV infection that has a selective effect on the erythroid series is dapsone. This drug can cause a serious hemolytic anemia in patients who are deficient in glucose-6-phosphate dehydrogenase and can create a functional anemia in others through induction of methemoglobinemia. Folate levels are usually normal in HIV-infected individuals; however, vitamin B_{12} levels may be depressed as a consequence of achlorhydria or malabsorption. True autoimmune hemolytic anemia is rare, although ~20% of patients with HIV infection may have a positive direct antiglobulin test as a consequence of polyclonal B cell activation. Infection with parvovirus B19 may also cause anemia. It is important to recognize this possibility given the fact that it responds well to treatment with IVIg. Erythropoietin levels in patients with HIV infection and anemia are generally less than expected given the degree of anemia. Treatment with erythropoietin at doses of 100 μg/kg three times a week may result in an increase in hemoglobulin levels. An exception to this is a subset of patients with zidovudine-associated anemia in whom erythropoietin levels may be quite high.

During the course of HIV infection, neutropenia may be seen in approximately half of patients. In most instances it is mild; however, it can be severe and can put patients at risk of spontaneous bacterial infections. This is most frequently seen in patients with severely advanced HIV disease and in patients receiving any of a number of potentially myelosuppressive therapies. In the setting of neutropenia, diseases that are not commonly seen in HIV-infected patients, such as aspergillosis or mucormycosis, may occur. The potential role of colony-stimulating factors in the management of patients with HIV infection has undergone extensive evaluation. Both granulocyte colony-stimulating factor (G-CSF) and GM-CSF increase neutrophil counts in patients with HIV infection regardless of the cause of the neutropenia. Earlier concerns about the potential of these agents to also increase levels of HIV were not confirmed in controlled clinical trials.

Thrombocytopenia may be an early consequence of HIV infection. Approximately 3% of patients with untreated HIV infection and CD4+ T cell counts ≥400/μL have platelet counts <150,000/μL. For untreated patients with CD4+ T cell counts <400/μL, this incidence increases to 10%. Thrombocytopenia is rarely a serious clinical problem in patients with HIV infection and generally responds well to ARV therapy. Clinically, it resembles the thrombocytopenia seen in patients with idiopathic thrombocytopenic purpura (Chap. 109). Immune complexes containing anti-gp120 antibodies and anti-anti-gp120 antibodies have been noted in the circulation and on the surface of platelets in patients with HIV infection. Patients with HIV infection have also been noted to have a platelet-specific antibody directed toward a 25-kDa component of the surface of the platelet. Other data suggest that the thrombocytopenia in patients with HIV infection may be due to a direct effect of HIV on megakaryocytes. Whatever the cause, it is very clear that the most effective medical approach to this problem has been the use of HAART. For patients with platelet counts <20,000/μL a more aggressive approach combining IVIg or anti-Rh Ig for an immediate response with ARV therapy for a more lasting response is appropriate. Rituximab has been used with some success in otherwise refractory cases. Splenectomy is a rarely needed option and is reserved for patients refractory to medical management. Because of the risk of serious infection with encapsulated organisms, all patients with HIV infection about to undergo splenectomy should be immunized with pneumococcal polysaccharide. It should be noted that, in addition to causing an increase in the platelet count, removal of the spleen will result in an increase in the peripheral blood lymphocyte count, making CD4+ T cell counts unreliable. In this setting, the clinician should rely on the CD4+ T cell percent for making diagnostic decisions with respect to the likelihood of opportunistic infections. A CD4+ T cell percent of 15 is approximately equivalent to a CD4+ T cell count of 200/μL. In patients with early HIV infection, thrombocytopenia has also been reported as a consequence of classic thrombotic thrombocytopenic purpura (Chap. 109). This clinical syndrome, consisting of fever, thrombocytopenia, hemolytic anemia, and neurologic and renal dysfunction, is a rare complication of early HIV infection. As in other settings, the appropriate management is the use of salicylates and plasma exchange. Other causes of thrombocytopenia include lymphoma, mycobacterial infections, and fungal infections.

Approximately 4% of patients with HIV infection experience venous thrombotic events such as deep vein thrombosis or pulmonary embolism. Among the factors associated with clinical thrombosis are age over 45, history of an opportunistic infection, and estrogen use.

Abnormalities of the coagulation cascade including decreased protein S activity, increases in factor VIII, and the presence of anticardiolipin antibodies have been reported in patients with HIV infection. Elevations in D-dimer appear predictive of a poor clinical outcome.

Dermatologic Diseases Dermatologic problems occur in >90% of patients with HIV infection. From the macular, roseola-like rash seen with the acute seroconversion syndrome to extensive end-stage KS, cutaneous manifestations of HIV disease can be seen throughout the course of HIV infection. Among the more common nonneoplastic problems are seborrheic dermatitis, folliculitis, and opportunistic infections. Extrapulmonary pneumocystosis may cause a necrotizing vasculitis. Neoplastic conditions are covered below in the section on malignant diseases.

Seborrheic dermatitis occurs in 3% of the general population and in up to 50% of patients with HIV infection. Seborrheic dermatitis increases in prevalence and severity as the CD4+ T cell count declines. In HIV-infected patients, seborrheic dermatitis may be aggravated by concomitant infection with *Pityrosporum*, a yeastlike fungus; use of topical antifungal agents has been recommended in cases refractory to standard topical treatment.

Folliculitis is among the most prevalent dermatologic disorders in patients with HIV infection and is seen in ~20% of patients. It is more common in patients with CD4+ T cell counts <200 cells/μL. One form of folliculitis, *eosinophilic pustular folliculitis,* is a rare dermatologic condition that is seen with increased frequency in patients with HIV infection. It presents as multiple, urticarial perifollicular papules that may coalesce into plaquelike lesions. Skin biopsy reveals an eosinophilic infiltrate of the hair follicle, which in certain cases has been associated with the presence of a mite. Patients typically have an elevated serum IgE level and may respond to treatment with topical antihelminthics. Pruritus is a common symptom in patients with HIV infection and can lead to prurigo nodularis. Patients with HIV infection have also been reported to develop a severe form of *Norwegian scabies* with hyperkeratotic psoriasiform lesions.

Both *psoriasis* and *ichthyosis*, although they are not reported to be increased in frequency, may be particularly severe when they occur in patients with HIV infection. Preexisting psoriasis may become guttate in appearance and more refractory to treatment in the setting of HIV infection.

Reactivation herpes zoster (*shingles*) is seen in 10–20% of patients with HIV infection. This reactivation syndrome of varicella-zoster virus indicates a modest decline in immune function and may be the first indication of clinical immunodeficiency. In one series, patients who developed shingles did so an average of 5 years after HIV infection. In a cohort of patients with HIV infection and localized zoster, the subsequent rate of the development of AIDS was 1% per month. In that study, AIDS was more likely to develop if the outbreak of zoster was associated with severe pain, extensive skin involvement, or involvement of cranial or cervical dermatomes. The clinical manifestations of reactivation zoster in HIV-infected patients, although indicative of immunologic compromise, are not as severe as those seen in other immunodeficient conditions. Thus, while lesions may extend over several dermatomes and frank cutaneous dissemination may be seen, visceral involvement has not been reported. In contrast to patients without a known underlying immunodeficiency state, patients with HIV infection tend to have recurrences of zoster with a relapse rate of ~20%. Acyclovir or famciclovir is the treatment of choice. Foscarnet may be of value in patients with acyclovir-resistant virus.

Infection with *herpes simplex virus* in HIV-infected individuals is associated with recurrent orolabial, genital, and perianal lesions as part of recurrent reactivation syndromes (Chap. 172). As HIV disease progresses and the CD4+ T cell count declines, these infections become more frequent and severe. Lesions often appear as beefy red, are exquisitely painful, and have a tendency to occur high in the gluteal cleft (Fig. 182-35). Perirectal HSV may be associated with proctitis and anal fissures. HSV should be high in the differential diagnosis of any HIV-infected patient with a poorly healing, painful perirectal lesion. In addition to recurrent mucosal ulcers, recurrent HSV infection in the form of *herpetic whitlow* can be a problem in patients with HIV infection, presenting with painful vesicles or extensive cutaneous erosion. Acyclovir or famciclovir is the treatment of choice in these settings. Of note is the fact that even subclinical reactivation of herpes simplex may be associated with increases in plasma HIV RNA levels. In a cohort of patients from Burkina Faso seropositive for HIV-1 and HSV-2 with CD4+ T cell counts >200 cells/μL, chronic use of valacyclovir was associated with a 0.5 log decrease in HIV viral load. Thus, consideration should be given to chronic suppressive therapy in patients with recurrent outbreaks of herpesvirus.

Diffuse skin eruptions due to *Molluscum contagiosum* may be seen in patients with advanced HIV infection. These flesh-colored, umbilicated lesions may be treated with local therapy. They tend to regress with effective ARV therapy. Similarly, *condyloma acuminatum* lesions may be more severe and more widely distributed in patients with low CD4+ T cell counts. Atypical mycobacterial infections may present as erythematous cutaneous nodules as may fungal infections, *Bartonella*, *Acanthamoeba*, and KS.

The skin of patients with HIV infection is often a target organ for drug reactions (Chap. 56). Although most skin reactions are mild and not necessarily an indication to discontinue therapy, patients may have particularly severe cutaneous reactions, including erythroderma and *Stevens-Johnson syndrome*, as a reaction to drugs, particularly sulfa drugs, the nonnucleoside reverse transcriptase inhibitors, abacavir, amprenavir, darunavir, fosamprenavir, and tipranavir. Similarly, patients with HIV infection are often quite photosensitive and burn easily following exposure to sunlight or as a side effect of radiation therapy (Chap. 57).

TABLE 182-11 NEUROLOGIC DISEASES IN PATIENTS WITH HIV INFECTION

Opportunistic infections	Myelopathy
Toxoplasmosis	Vacuolar myelopathy
Cryptococcosis	Pure sensory ataxia
Progressive multifocal leukoencephalopathy	Paresthesia/dysesthesia
Cytomegalovirus	Peripheral neuropathy
Syphilis	Acute inflammatory demyelinating polyneuropathy (Guillain-Barré syndrome)
Mycobacterium tuberculosis	Chronic inflammatory demyelinating polyneuropathy (CIDP)
HTLV-I infection	Mononeuritis multiplex
Neoplasms	Distal symmetric polyneuropathy
Primary CNS lymphoma	Myopathy
Kaposi's sarcoma	
Result of HIV-1 infection	
Aseptic meningitis	
HIV-associated neurocognitive impairment, including HIV encephalopathy/AIDS dementia complex	

HIV infection and its treatment may be accompanied by cosmetic changes of the skin that are not of great clinical importance but may be troubling to patients. Yellowing of the nails and straightening of the hair, particularly in African-American patients, have been reported as a consequence of HIV infection. Zidovudine therapy has been associated with elongation of the eyelashes and the development of a bluish discoloration to the nails, again more common in African-American patients. Therapy with clofazimine may cause a yellow-orange discoloration of the skin and urine.

Neurologic Diseases Clinical disease of the nervous system accounts for a significant degree of morbidity in a high percentage of patients with HIV infection (Table 182-11). The neurologic problems that occur in HIV-infected individuals may be either primary to the pathogenic processes of HIV infection or secondary to opportunistic infections or neoplasms (see above). Among the more frequent opportunistic diseases that involve the CNS are toxoplasmosis, cryptococcosis, progressive multifocal leukoencephalopathy, and primary CNS lymphoma. Other less common problems include mycobacterial infections; syphilis; and infection with CMV, HTLV-I, *T. cruzi*, or *Acanthamoeba*. Overall, secondary diseases of the CNS occur in approximately one-third of patients with AIDS. These data antedate the widespread use of combination ARV therapy, and this frequency is considerably less in patients receiving effective ARV drugs. Primary processes related to HIV infection of the nervous system are reminiscent of those seen with other lentiviruses, such as the Visna-Maedi virus of sheep.

Neurologic problems directly attributable to HIV occur throughout the course of infection and may be inflammatory, demyelinating, or degenerative in nature. The term *HIV-associated neurocognitive impairment* (HNCI) is used to describe a spectrum of disorders that range from asymptomatic to apparent only through extensive neuropsychiatric testing to clinically severe. The most severe form, the *AIDS dementia complex*, or *HIV encephalopathy*, is considered an AIDS-defining illness. Most HIV-infected patients have some neurologic problem during the course of their disease. As noted in the section on pathogenesis, damage to the CNS may be a direct result of viral infection of the CNS macrophages or glial cells or may be secondary to the release of neurotoxins and potentially toxic cytokines such as IL-1β, TNF-α, IL-6, and TGF-β. It has been reported that HIV-infected individuals with the E4 allele for apo E are at increased risk for AIDS encephalopathy and peripheral neuropathy. Virtually all patients with HIV infection have some degree of nervous system involvement with the virus. This is evidenced by the fact that CSF findings are abnormal in ~90% of patients, even during the asymptomatic phase of HIV infection. CSF abnormalities include pleocytosis (50–65% of patients), detection of viral RNA (~75%), elevated CSF protein (35%), and evidence of intrathecal synthesis of anti-HIV antibodies (90%). It is im-

TABLE 182-12 CLINICAL STAGING OF HIV ENCEPHALOPATHY (AIDS DEMENTIA COMPLEX)

Stage	Definition
Stage 0 (normal)	Normal mental and motor function
Stage 0.5 (equivocal/ subclinical)	Absent, minimal, or equivocal symptoms without impairment of work or capacity to perform activities of daily living. Mild signs (snout response, slowed ocular or extremity movements) may be present. Gait and strength are normal.
Stage 1 (mild)	Able to perform all but the more demanding aspects of work or activities of daily living but with unequivocal evidence (signs or symptoms that may include performance on neuropsychological testing) of functional, intellectual, or motor impairment. Can walk without assistance.
Stage 2 (moderate)	Able to perform basic activities of self-care but cannot work or maintain the more demanding aspects of daily life. Ambulatory, but may require a single prop.
Stage 3 (severe)	Major intellectual incapacity (cannot follow news or personal events, cannot sustain complex conversation, considerable slowing of all output) or motor disability (cannot walk unassisted, usually with slowing and clumsiness of arms as well).
Stage 4 (end-stage)	Nearly vegetative. Intellectual and social comprehension and output are at a rudimentary level. Nearly or absolutely mute. Paraparetic or paraplegic with urinary and fecal incontinence.

Source: Adapted from JJ Sidtis, RW Price, Neurology 40:197, 1990.

portant to point out that evidence of infection of the CNS with HIV does not imply impairment of cognitive function. The neurologic function of an HIV-infected individual should be considered normal unless clinical signs and symptoms suggest otherwise.

Aseptic meningitis may be seen in any but the very late stages of HIV infection. In the setting of acute primary infection patients may experience a syndrome of headache, photophobia, and meningismus. Rarely, an acute encephalopathy due to encephalitis may occur. Cranial nerve involvement may be seen, predominantly cranial nerve VII but occasionally V and/or VIII. CSF findings include a lymphocytic pleocytosis, elevated protein level, and normal glucose level. This syndrome, which cannot be clinically differentiated from other viral meningitides (Chap. 377), usually resolves spontaneously within 2–4 weeks; however, in some patients, signs and symptoms may become chronic. Aseptic meningitis may occur any time in the course of HIV infection; however, it is rare following the development of AIDS. This fact suggests that clinical aseptic meningitis in the context of HIV infection is an immune-mediated disease.

C. neoformans is the leading infectious cause of meningitis in patients with AIDS (Chap. 195). It is the initial AIDS-defining illness in ~2% of patients and generally occurs in patients with CD4+ T cell counts <100/μL. Cryptococcal meningitis is particularly common in patients with AIDS in Africa, occurring in ~20% of patients. Most patients present with a picture of subacute meningoencephalitis with fever, nausea, vomiting, altered mental status, headache, and meningeal signs. The incidence of seizures and focal neurologic deficits is low. The CSF profile may be normal or may show only modest elevations in WBC or protein levels and decreases in glucose. In addition to meningitis, patients may develop cryptococcomas and cranial nerve involvement. Approximately one-third of patients also have pulmonary disease. Uncommon manifestations of cryptococcal infection include skin lesions that resemble *molluscum contagiosum*, lymphadenopathy, palatal and glossal ulcers, arthritis, gastroenteritis, myocarditis, and prostatitis. The prostate gland may serve as a reservoir for smoldering cryptococcal infection. The diagnosis of cryptococcal meningitis is made by identification of organisms in spinal fluid with India ink examination or by the detection of cryptococcal antigen. A biopsy may be needed to make a diagnosis of CNS cryptococcoma. Treatment is with IV amphotericin B, at a dose of 0.7 mg/kg daily, with flucytosine, 25 mg/kg qid for 2 weeks, followed by fluconazole, 400 mg/d PO for 10 weeks, and then fluconazole, 200 mg/d until the CD4+ T cell count has increased to >200 cells/μL for 6 months in response to HAART. Repeated lumbar puncture may be required to manage increased intracranial pressure. Symptoms may recur with initiation of HAART as an immune reconstitution syndrome (see above). Other fungi that may cause meningitis in patients with HIV infection are *C. immitis* and *H. capsulatum*. Meningoencephalitis has also been reported due to *Acanthamoeba* or *Naegleria*.

HIV encephalopathy, also called HIV-associated dementia or AIDS dementia complex, consists of a constellation of signs and symptoms of CNS disease. While this is generally a late complication of HIV infection that progresses slowly over months, it can be seen in patients with CD4+ T cell counts >350 cells/μL. A major feature of this entity is the development of dementia, defined as a decline in cognitive ability from a previous level. It may present as impaired ability to concentrate, increased forgetfulness, difficulty reading, or increased difficulty performing complex tasks. Initially these symptoms may be indistinguishable from findings of situational depression or fatigue. In contrast to "cortical" dementia (such as Alzheimer's disease), aphasia, apraxia, and agnosia are uncommon, leading some investigators to classify HIV encephalopathy as a "subcortical dementia" (see below). In addition to dementia, patients with HIV encephalopathy may also have motor and behavioral abnormalities. Among the motor problems are unsteady gait, poor balance, tremor, and difficulty with rapid alternating movements. Increased tone and deep tendon reflexes may be found in patients with spinal cord involvement. Late stages may be complicated by bowel and/or bladder incontinence. Behavioral problems include apathy and lack of initiative, with progression to a vegetative state in some instances. Some patients develop a state of agitation or mild mania. These changes usually occur without significant changes in level of alertness. This is in contrast to the finding of somnolence in patients with dementia due to toxic/metabolic encephalopathies.

HIV encephalopathy is the initial AIDS-defining illness in ~3% of patients with HIV infection and thus only rarely precedes clinical evidence of immunodeficiency. Clinically significant encephalopathy eventually develops in ~25% of patients with AIDS. As immunologic function declines, the risk and severity of HIV encephalopathy increase. Autopsy series suggest that 80–90% of patients with HIV infection have histologic evidence of CNS involvement. Several classification schemes have been developed for grading HIV encephalopathy; a commonly used clinical staging system is outlined in **Table 182-12**.

The precise cause of HIV encephalopathy remains unclear, although the condition is thought to be a result of a combination of direct effects of HIV on the CNS and associated immune activation. HIV has been found in the brains of patients with HIV encephalopathy by Southern blot, in situ hybridization, PCR, and electron microscopy. Multinucleated giant cells, macrophages, and microglial cells appear to be the main cell types harboring virus in the CNS. Histologically, the major changes are seen in the subcortical areas of the brain and include pallor and gliosis, multinucleated giant cell encephalitis, and vacuolar myelopathy. Less commonly, diffuse or focal spongiform changes occur in the white matter. Areas of the brain involved in motor, language, and judgment are most severely affected.

There are no specific criteria for a diagnosis of HIV encephalopathy, and this syndrome must be differentiated from a number of other diseases that affect the CNS of HIV-infected patients (Table 182-11). The diagnosis of dementia depends upon demonstrating a decline in cognitive function. This can be accomplished objectively with the use of a Mini-Mental Status Examination (MMSE) in patients for whom prior scores are available. For this reason, it is advisable for all patients with a diagnosis of HIV infection to have a baseline MMSE. However, changes in MMSE scores may be absent in patients with mild HIV encephalopathy. Imaging studies of the CNS, by either MRI or CT, often demonstrate evidence of cerebral atrophy (**Fig. 182-37**). MRI may also reveal small areas of increased density on T2-weighted images. Lumbar puncture is an important element of the evaluation of patients with HIV infection and neurologic abnormalities. It is generally most

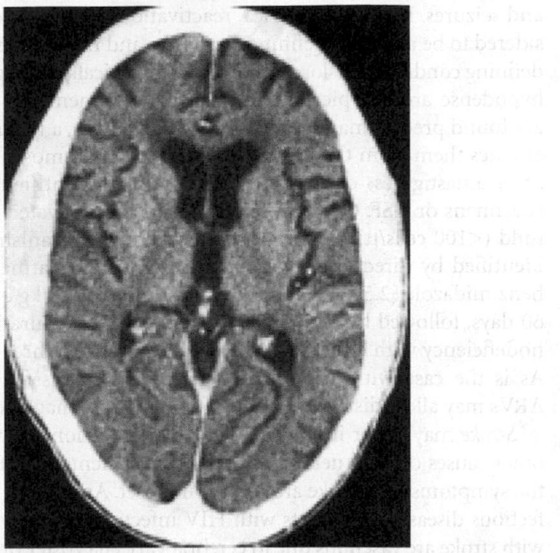

FIGURE 182-37 **AIDS dementia complex.** Postcontrast CT scan through the lateral ventricles of a 47-year-old man with AIDS, altered mental status, and dementia. The lateral and third ventricles and the cerebral sulci are abnormally prominent. Mild white matter hypodensity is also seen adjacent to the frontal horns of the lateral ventricles.

helpful in ruling out or making a diagnosis of opportunistic infections. In HIV encephalopathy, patients may have the nonspecific findings of an increase in CSF cells and protein level. While HIV RNA can often be detected in the spinal fluid and HIV can be cultured from the CSF, this finding is not specific for HIV encephalopathy. There appears to be no correlation between the presence of HIV in the CSF and the presence of HIV encephalopathy. Elevated levels of macrophage chemoattractant protein (MCP-1), β_2-microglobulin, neopterin, and quinolinic acid (a metabolite of tryptophan reported to cause CNS injury) have been noted in the CSF of patients with HIV encephalopathy. These findings suggest that these factors as well as inflammatory cytokines may be involved in the pathogenesis of this syndrome.

Combination ARV therapy is of benefit in patients with HIV encephalopathy. Improvement in neuropsychiatric test scores has been noted for both adult and pediatric patients treated with ARVs. The rapid improvement in cognitive function noted with the initiation of ARV therapy suggests that at least some component of this problem is quickly reversible, again supporting at least a partial role of soluble mediators in the pathogenesis. It should also be noted that these patients have an increased sensitivity to the side effects of neuroleptic drugs. The use of these drugs for symptomatic treatment is associated with an increased risk of extrapyramidal side effects; therefore, patients with HIV encephalopathy who receive these agents must be monitored carefully.

Seizures may be a consequence of opportunistic infections, neoplasms, or HIV encephalopathy (Table 182-13). The seizure threshold is often lower than normal in patients with advanced HIV infection due to the frequent presence of electrolyte abnormalities. Seizures are

TABLE 182-13 CAUSES OF SEIZURES IN PATIENTS WITH HIV INFECTION

Disease	Overall Contribution to First Seizure, %	Fraction of Patients Who Have Seizures, %
HIV encephalopathy	24–47	7–50
Cerebral toxoplasmosis	28	15–40
Cryptococcal meningitis	13	8
Primary central nervous system lymphoma	4	15–30
Progressive multifocal leukoencephalopathy	1	

Source: From DM Holtzman et al: Am J Med 87:173, 1989.

seen in 15–40% of patients with cerebral toxoplasmosis, 15–35% of patients with primary CNS lymphoma, 8% of patients with cryptococcal meningitis, and 7–50% of patients with HIV encephalopathy. Seizures may also be seen in patients with CNS tuberculosis, aseptic meningitis, and progressive multifocal leukoencephalopathy. Seizures may be the presenting clinical symptom of HIV disease. In one study of 100 patients with HIV infection presenting with a first seizure, cerebral mass lesions were the most common cause, responsible for 32 of the 100 new-onset seizures. Of these 32 cases, 28 were due to toxoplasmosis and 4 to lymphoma. HIV encephalopathy accounted for an additional 24 new-onset seizures. Cryptococcal meningitis was the third most common diagnosis, responsible for 13 of the 100 seizures. In 23 cases, no cause could be found, and it is possible that these cases represent a subcategory of HIV encephalopathy. Of these 23 cases, 16 (70%) had two or more seizures, suggesting that anticonvulsant therapy is indicated in all patients with HIV infection and seizures unless a rapidly correctable cause is found. While phenytoin remains the initial treatment of choice, hypersensitivity reactions to this drug have been reported in >10% of patients with AIDS, and therefore the use of phenobarbital or valproic acid must be considered as alternatives.

Patients with HIV infection may present with *focal neurologic deficits* from a variety of causes. The most common causes are toxoplasmosis, progressive multifocal leukoencephalopathy, and CNS lymphoma. Other causes include cryptococcal infections (discussed above; also Chap. 195), stroke, and reactivation Chagas' disease.

Toxoplasmosis has been one of the most common causes of secondary CNS infections in patients with AIDS, but its incidence is decreasing in the era of HAART. It is most common in patients from the Caribbean and from France. Toxoplasmosis is generally a late complication of HIV infection and usually occurs in patients with CD4+ T cell counts <200/μL. Cerebral toxoplasmosis is thought to represent a reactivation syndrome. It is 10 times more common in patients with antibodies to the organism than in patients who are seronegative. Patients diagnosed with HIV infection should be screened for IgG antibodies to *T. gondii* during the time of their initial workup. Those who are seronegative should be counseled about ways to minimize the risk of primary infection including avoiding the consumption of undercooked meat and careful hand washing after contact with soil or changing the cat litter box. The most common clinical presentation of cerebral toxoplasmosis in patients with HIV infection is fever, headache, and focal neurologic deficits. Patients may present with seizure, hemiparesis, or aphasia as a manifestation of these focal deficits or with a picture more influenced by the accompanying cerebral edema and characterized by confusion, dementia, and lethargy, which can progress to coma. The diagnosis is usually suspected on the basis of MRI findings of multiple lesions in multiple locations, although in some cases only a single lesion is seen. Pathologically, these lesions generally exhibit inflammation and central necrosis and, as a result, demonstrate ring enhancement on contrast MRI (Fig. 182-38) or, if MRI is unavailable or contraindicated, on double-dose contrast CT. There is usually evidence of surrounding edema. In addition to toxoplasmosis, the differential diagnosis of single or multiple enhancing mass lesions in the HIV-infected patient includes primary CNS lymphoma (see below) and, less commonly, TB or fungal or bacterial abscesses. The definitive diagnostic procedure is brain biopsy. However, given the morbidity than can accompany this procedure, it is usually reserved for the patient who has failed 2–4 weeks of empirical therapy. If the patient is seronegative for *T. gondii*, the likelihood that a mass lesion is due to toxoplasmosis is <10%. In that setting, one may choose to be more aggressive and perform a brain biopsy sooner. Standard treatment is sulfadiazine and pyrimethamine with leucovorin as needed for a minimum of 4–6 weeks. Alternative therapeutic regimens include clindamycin in combination with pyrimethamine; atovaquone plus pyrimethamine; and azithromycin plus pyrimethamine plus rifabutin. Relapses are common, and it is recommended that patients with a history of prior toxoplasmic encephalitis receive maintenance therapy with sulfadiazine, pyrimethamine, and leucovorin as long as their CD4+ T cell counts remain <200 cells/μL. Patients with CD4+ T

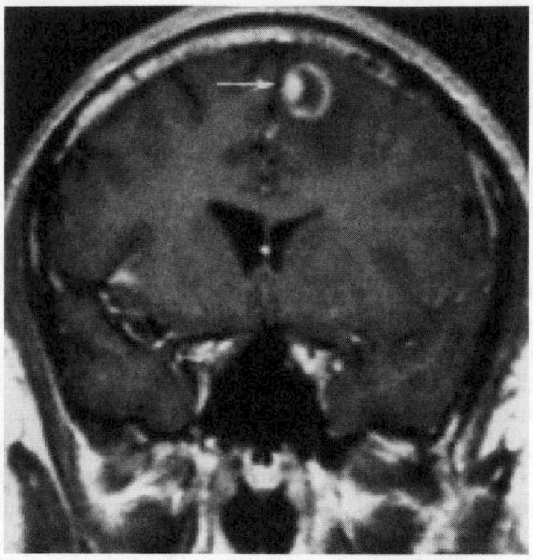

FIGURE 182-38 Central nervous system toxoplasmosis. A coronal postcontrast T1-weighted MR scan demonstrates a peripheral enhancing lesion in the left frontal lobe, associated with an eccentric nodular area of enhancement (*arrow*); this so-called eccentric target sign is typical of toxoplasmosis.

cell counts <100/μL and IgG antibody to *Toxoplasma* should receive primary prophylaxis for toxoplasmosis. Fortunately, the same daily regimen of a single double-strength tablet of TMP/SMX used for *P. jiroveci* prophylaxis provides adequate primary protection against toxoplasmosis. Secondary prophylaxis/maintenance therapy for toxoplasmosis may be discontinued in the setting of effective ARV therapy and increases in CD4+ T cell counts to >200/μL for 6 months.

JC virus, a human polyomavirus that is the etiologic agent of *progressive multifocal leukoencephalopathy* (PML), is an important opportunistic pathogen in patients with AIDS (Chap. 377). While ~70% of the general adult population have antibodies to JC virus, indicative of prior infection, <10% of healthy adults show any evidence of ongoing viral replication. PML is the only known clinical manifestation of JC virus infection. It is a late manifestation of AIDS and is seen in ~4% of patients with AIDS. The lesions of PML begin as small foci of demyelination in subcortical white matter that eventually coalesce. The cerebral hemispheres, cerebellum, and brainstem may all be involved. Patients typically have a protracted course with multifocal neurologic deficits, with or without changes in mental status. Approximately 20% of patients experience seizures. Ataxia, hemiparesis, visual field defects, aphasia, and sensory defects may occur. MRI typically reveals multiple, nonenhancing white matter lesions that may coalesce and have a predilection for the occipital and parietal lobes. The lesions show signal hyperintensity on T2-weighted images and diminished signal on T1-weighted images. The measurement of JC virus DNA levels in CSF has a diagnostic sensitivity of 76% and a specificity of close to 100%. Prior to the availability of potent ARV combination therapy, the majority of patients with PML died within 3–6 months of the onset of symptoms. Paradoxical worsening of PML has been seen with initiation of HAART as an immune reconstitution syndrome. There is no specific treatment for PML; however, a minimal median survival of 18 months and survival of >7 years have been reported in patients with PML treated with HAART for their HIV disease. Unfortunately only ~50% of patients with HIV infection and PML show neurologic improvement with HAART. Studies with other antiviral agents such as cidofovir have failed to show clear benefit. Factors influencing a favorable prognosis for PML in the setting of HIV infection include a CD4+ T cell count >100/μL at baseline and the ability to maintain an HIV viral load of <500 copies per milliliter. Baseline HIV-1 viral load does not have independent predictive value of survival. PML is one of the few opportunistic infections that continues to occur with some frequency despite the widespread use of HAART.

Reactivation American trypanosomiasis may present as acute meningoencephalitis with focal neurologic signs, fever, headache, vomiting, and seizures. In South America, reactivation of *Chagas' disease* is considered to be an AIDS-defining condition and may be the initial AIDS-defining condition. Lesions appear radiographically as single or multiple hypodense areas, typically with ring enhancement and edema. They are found predominantly in the subcortical areas, a feature that differentiates them from the deeper lesions of toxoplasmosis. *Trypanosoma cruzi* amastigotes, or trypanosomes, can be identified from biopsy specimens or CSF. Other CSF findings include elevated protein and a mild (<100 cells/μL) lymphocytic pleocytosis. Organisms can also be identified by direct examination of the blood. Treatment consists of benzimidazole (2.5 mg/kg bid) or nifurtimox (2 mg/kg qid) for at least 60 days, followed by maintenance therapy for the duration of immunodeficiency with either drug at a dose of 5 mg/kg three times a week. As is the case with cerebral toxoplasmosis, successful therapy with ARVs may allow discontinuation of therapy for Chagas' disease.

Stroke may occur in patients with HIV infection. In contrast to the other causes of focal neurologic deficits in patients with HIV infection, the symptoms of a stroke are sudden in onset. Among the secondary infectious diseases in patients with HIV infection that may be associated with stroke are vasculitis due to cerebral varicella zoster or neurosyphilis and septic embolism in association with fungal infection. Other elements of the differential diagnosis of stroke in the patient with HIV infection include atherosclerotic cerebral vascular disease, thrombotic thrombocytopenic purpura, and cocaine or amphetamine use.

Primary CNS lymphoma is discussed below in the section on neoplastic diseases.

Spinal cord disease, or myelopathy, is present in ~20% of patients with AIDS, often as part of HIV encephalopathy. In fact, 90% of the patients with HIV-associated myelopathy have some evidence of dementia, suggesting that similar pathologic processes may be responsible for both conditions. Three main types of spinal cord disease are seen in patients with AIDS. The first of these is a vacuolar myelopathy, as discussed above under HIV encephalopathy. This condition is pathologically similar to subacute combined degeneration of the cord such as occurs with pernicious anemia. Although vitamin B_{12} deficiency can be seen in patients with AIDS as a primary complication of HIV infection, it does not appear to be responsible for the myelopathy seen in the majority of patients. Vacuolar myelopathy is characterized by a subacute onset and often presents with gait disturbances, predominantly ataxia and spasticity; it may progress to include bladder and bowel dysfunction. Physical findings include evidence of increased deep tendon reflexes and extensor plantar responses. The second form of spinal cord disease involves the dorsal columns and presents as a pure sensory ataxia. The third form is also sensory in nature and presents with paresthesias and dysesthesias of the lower extremities. In contrast to the cognitive problems seen in patients with HIV encephalopathy, these spinal cord syndromes do not respond well to ARV drugs, and therapy is mainly supportive.

One important disease of the spinal cord that also involves the peripheral nerves is a *myelopathy* and *polyradiculopathy* seen in association with CMV infection. This entity is generally seen late in the course of HIV infection and is fulminant in onset, with lower extremity and sacral paresthesias, difficulty in walking, areflexia, ascending sensory loss, and urinary retention. The clinical course is rapidly progressive over a period of weeks. CSF examination reveals a predominantly neutrophilic pleocytosis, and CMV DNA can be detected by CSF PCR. Therapy with ganciclovir or foscarnet can lead to rapid improvement, and prompt initiation of foscarnet or ganciclovir therapy is important in minimizing the degree of permanent neurologic damage. Combination therapy with both drugs should be considered in patients who have been previously treated for CMV disease. Other diseases involving the spinal cord in patients with HIV infection include HTLV-I-associated myelopathy (HAM) (Chap. 181), neurosyphilis (Chap. 162), infection with herpes simplex (Chap. 172) or varicella-zoster (Chap. 173), TB (Chap. 158), and lymphoma (Chap. 105).

Peripheral neuropathies are common in patients with HIV infection. They occur at all stages of illness and take a variety of forms. Early in the course of HIV infection, an acute inflammatory demyelinating polyneuropathy resembling Guillain-Barré syndrome may occur (Chap. 381). In other patients, a progressive or relapsing-remitting inflammatory neuropathy resembling chronic inflammatory demyelinating polyneuropathy (CIDP) has been noted. Patients commonly present with progressive weakness, areflexia, and minimal sensory changes. CSF examination often reveals a mononuclear pleocytosis, and peripheral nerve biopsy demonstrates a perivascular infiltrate suggesting an autoimmune etiology. Plasma exchange or IVIg has been tried with variable success. Because of the immunosuppressive effects of glucocorticoids, they should be reserved for severe cases of CIDP refractory to other measures. Another autoimmune peripheral neuropathy seen in patients with AIDS is mononeuritis multiplex (Chaps. 381 and 319) due to a necrotizing arteritis of peripheral nerves. The most common peripheral neuropathy in patients with HIV infection is a *distal sensory polyneuropathy* that may be a direct consequence of HIV infection or a side effect of dideoxynucleoside therapy. Two-thirds of patients with AIDS may be shown by electrophysiologic studies to have some evidence of peripheral nerve disease. Presenting symptoms are usually painful burning sensations in the feet and lower extremities. Findings on examination include a stocking-type sensory loss to pinprick, temperature, and touch sensation and a loss of ankle reflexes. Motor changes are mild and are usually limited to weakness of the intrinsic foot muscles. Response of this condition to ARVs has been variable, perhaps because ARVs are responsible for the problem in some instances. When due to dideoxynucleoside therapy, patients with lower extremity peripheral neuropathy may complain of a sensation that they are walking on ice. Other entities in the differential diagnosis of peripheral neuropathy include diabetes mellitus, vitamin B_{12} deficiency, and side effects from metronidazole or dapsone. For distal symmetric polyneuropathy that fails to resolve following the discontinuation of dideoxynucleosides, therapy is symptomatic; gabapentin, carbamazepine, tricyclics, or analgesics may be effective for dysesthesias. Treatment-naive patients may respond to combination ARV therapy.

Myopathy may complicate the course of HIV infection; causes include HIV infection itself, zidovudine, and the generalized wasting syndrome. HIV-associated myopathy may range in severity from an asymptomatic elevation in creatine kinase levels to a subacute syndrome characterized by proximal muscle weakness and myalgias. Quite pronounced elevations in creatine kinase may occur in asymptomatic patients, particularly after exercise. The clinical significance of this as an isolated laboratory finding is unclear. A variety of both inflammatory and noninflammatory pathologic processes have been noted in patients with more severe myopathy, including myofiber necrosis with inflammatory cells, nemaline rod bodies, cytoplasmic bodies, and mitochondrial abnormalities. Profound muscle wasting, often with muscle pain, may be seen after prolonged zidovudine therapy. This toxic side effect of the drug is dose-dependent and is related to its ability to interfere with the function of mitochondrial polymerases. It is reversible following discontinuation of the drug. Red ragged fibers are a histologic hallmark of zidovudine-induced myopathy.

Ophthalmologic Disease Ophthalmologic problems occur in ~50% of patients with advanced HIV infection. The most common abnormal findings on funduscopic examination are cotton-wool spots. These are hard white spots that appear on the surface of the retina and often have an irregular edge. They represent areas of retinal ischemia secondary to microvascular disease. At times they are associated with small areas of hemorrhage and thus can be difficult to distinguish from CMV retinitis. In contrast to CMV retinitis, however, these lesions are not associated with visual loss and tend to remain stable or improve over time.

One of the most devastating consequences of HIV infection is CMV retinitis. Patients at high risk of CMV retinitis (CD4+ T cell count <100/μL) should undergo an ophthalmologic examination every 3–6 months. The majority of cases of CMV retinitis occur in patients with a CD4+ T cell count <50/μL. Prior to the availability of HAART, this CMV reactivation syndrome was seen in 25–30% of patients with AIDS. CMV retinitis usually presents as a painless, progressive loss of vision. Patients may also complain of blurred vision, "floaters," and scintillations. The disease is usually bilateral, although typically it affects one eye more than the other. The diagnosis is made on clinical grounds by an experienced ophthalmologist. The characteristic retinal appearance is that of perivascular hemorrhage and exudate. In situations where the diagnosis is in doubt due to an atypical presentation or an unexpected lack of response to therapy, vitreous or aqueous humor sampling with molecular diagnostic techniques may be of value. CMV infection of the retina results in a necrotic inflammatory process, and the visual loss that develops is irreversible. CMV retinitis may be complicated by rhegmatogenous retinal detachment as a consequence of retinal atrophy in areas of prior inflammation. Therapy for CMV retinitis consists of oral valganciclovir, IV ganciclovir, or IV foscarnet, with cidofovir as an alternative. Combination therapy with ganciclovir and foscarnet has been shown to be slightly more effective than either ganciclovir or foscarnet alone in the patient with relapsed CMV retinitis. A 3-week induction course is followed by maintenance therapy with oral valganciclovir. If CMV disease is limited to the eye, a ganciclovir-releasing intraocular implant, periodic injections of the antisense nucleic acid preparation fomivirsen, or intravitreal injections of ganciclovir or foscarnet may be considered; some choose to combine intraocular implants with oral valganciclovir. Intravitreal injections of cidofovir are generally avoided due to the increased risk of uveitis and hypotony. Maintenance therapy is continued until the CD4+ T cell count remains >100–150/μL for >6 months. The majority of patients with HIV infection and CMV disease develop some degree of uveitis with the initiation of ARV therapy. The etiology of this is unknown; however, it has been suggested that this may be due to the generation of an enhanced immune response to CMV as an IRIS (see above). In some instances this has required the use of topical glucocorticoids.

Both HSV and varicella zoster virus can cause a rapidly progressing, bilateral necrotizing retinitis referred to as the *acute retinal necrosis syndrome*, or *progressive outer retinal necrosis* (PORN). This syndrome, in contrast to CMV retinitis, is associated with pain, keratitis, and iritis. It is often associated with orolabial HSV or trigeminal zoster. Ophthalmologic examination reveals widespread pale gray peripheral lesions. This condition is often complicated by retinal detachment. It is important to recognize and treat this condition with IV acyclovir as quickly as possible to minimize the loss of vision.

Several other secondary infections may cause ocular problems in HIV-infected patients. *P. jiroveci* can cause a lesion of the choroid that may be detected as an incidental finding on ophthalmologic examination. These lesions are typically bilateral, are from half to twice the disc diameter in size, and appear as slightly elevated yellow-white plaques. They are usually asymptomatic and may be confused with cotton-wool spots. Chorioretinitis due to toxoplasmosis can be seen alone or, more commonly, in association with CNS toxoplasmosis. KS may involve the eyelid or conjunctiva while lymphoma may involve the retina.

Additional Disseminated Infections and Wasting Syndrome Infections with species of the small, gram-negative rickettsia-like organism *Bartonella* (Chap. 153) are seen with increased frequency in patients with HIV infection. While not considered an AIDS-defining illness by the CDC, many experts view infection with *Bartonella* as indicative of a severe defect in cell-mediated immunity. It is usually seen in patients with CD4+ T cell counts <100/μL. Among the clinical manifestations of *Bartonella* infection are bacillary angiomatosis, cat-scratch disease, and trench fever. *Bacillary angiomatosis* is usually due to infection with *B. henselae*. It is characterized by a vascular proliferation that leads to a variety of skin lesions that have been confused with the skin lesions of KS. In contrast to the lesions of KS, the lesions of bacillary angiomatosis generally blanch, are painful, and typically occur in the setting of systemic symptoms. Infection can extend to the lymph nodes, liver (peliosis hepatis), spleen, bone, heart, CNS, respiratory tract, and gastrointestinal tract. *Cat-scratch disease* generally begins with a papule at the site of inoculation. This is followed several weeks later by the development of regional adenopathy and malaise. Infection with *B. quintana* is transmitted by lice and has been associated with case reports of trench fever, endocarditis, adenopathy, and bacillary angiomatosis. The organism is quite difficult to culture, and diagnosis often relies upon identifying the organism in biopsy specimens using the Warthin-Starry or similar stains. Treatment is with either erythromycin or doxycycline for at least 3 months.

Histoplasmosis is an opportunistic infection that is seen most frequently in patients in the Mississippi and Ohio River valleys, Puerto Rico, the Dominican Republic, and South America. These are all areas in which infection with *H. capsulatum* is endemic (Chap. 192). Because of this limited geographic distribution, the percentage of AIDS cases in the United States with histoplasmosis is only ~0.5. Histoplasmosis is generally a late manifestation of HIV infection; however, it may be the initial AIDS-defining condition. In one study, the median CD4+ T cell count for patients with histoplasmosis and AIDS was 33/μL. While disease due to *H. capsulatum* may present as a primary infection of the lung, disseminated disease, presumably due to reactivation, is the most common presentation in HIV-infected patients. Patients usually present with a 4- to 8-week history of fever and weight loss. Hepatosplenomegaly and lymphadenopathy are each seen in about 25% of patients. CNS disease, either meningitis or a mass lesion, is seen in 15% of patients. Bone marrow involvement is common, with thrombocytopenia, neutropenia, and anemia occurring in 33% of patients. Approximately 7% of patients have mucocutaneous lesions consisting of a maculopapular rash and skin or oral ulcers. Respiratory symptoms are usually mild, with chest x-ray showing a diffuse infiltrate or diffuse small nodules in ~50% of cases. Diagnosis is made by culturing the organisms from blood, bone marrow, or tissue. Treatment is typically with amphotericin B, 0.7–1.0 mg/kg daily to a total dose of 1 g followed by maintenance therapy with itraconazole. In the setting of mild infection, it may be appropriate to treat with itraconazole alone.

Following the spread of HIV infection to southeast Asia, disseminated infection with the fungus *Penicillium marneffei* was recognized as a complication of HIV infection and is considered an AIDS-defining condition in those parts of the world where it occurs. *P. marneffei* is the third most common AIDS-defining illness in Thailand, following TB and cryptococcosis. It is more frequently diagnosed in the rainy than the dry season. Clinical features include fever, generalized lymphadenopathy, hepatosplenomegaly, anemia, thrombocytopenia, and papular skin lesions with central umbilication. Treatment is with amphotericin B followed by itraconazole.

Visceral leishmaniasis (Chap. 205) is recognized with increasing frequency in patients with HIV infection who live in or travel to areas endemic for this protozoal infection transmitted by sandflies. The clinical presentation is one of hepatosplenomegaly, fever, and hematologic abnormalities. Lymphadenopathy and other constitutional symptoms may be present. A chronic, relapsing course is seen in two-thirds of co-infected patients. Organisms can be isolated from cultures of bone marrow aspirates. Histologic stains may be negative, and antibody titers are of little help. Patients with HIV infection usually respond well initially to standard therapy with amphotericin B or pentavalent antimony compounds. Eradication of the organism is difficult, however, and relapses are common.

Patients with HIV infection are at increased risk of clinical malaria. This is particularly true for patients from nonendemic areas with presumed primary infection and in patients with lower CD4+ T cell counts. HIV-positive individuals with CD4+ T cell counts <300 cells/μL have a poorer response to malaria treatment than others. Co-infection with malaria is associated with a modest increase in HIV viral load. The risk of malaria may be decreased with TMP/SMX prophylaxis.

Generalized wasting is an AIDS-defining condition; it is defined as involuntary weight loss of >10% associated with intermittent or constant fever and chronic diarrhea or fatigue lasting >30 days in the absence of a defined cause other than HIV infection. It is the initial AIDS-defining condition in ~10% of patients with AIDS in the United States and is an indication for initiation of HAART. A constant feature of this syndrome is severe muscle wasting with scattered myofiber degeneration and occasional evidence of myositis. Glucocorticoids may be of some benefit; however, this approach must be carefully weighed against the risk of compounding the immunodeficiency of HIV infection. Androgenic steroids, growth hormone, and total parenteral nutrition have been used as therapeutic interventions with variable success.

Neoplastic Diseases The neoplastic diseases clearly seen with an increased frequency in patients with HIV infection are KS and non-Hodgkin's lymphoma. In addition, there also appears to be an increased incidence of Hodgkin's disease; multiple myeloma; leukemia; melanoma; and cervical, brain, testicular, oral, lung, and anal cancers. Recent years have witnessed a marked reduction in the incidence of KS (Fig. 182-31) and improvements in the outcomes of HIV-infected patients with non-AIDS-defining malignancies. These changes are primarily due to the use of potent ARV therapy. Rates of non-Hodgkin's lymphoma have declined as well; however, this decline has not been as dramatic as the decline in rates of KS. In contrast, HAART has had little effect on human papilloma virus (HPV)-associated malignancies. As patients with HIV infection live longer, a wider array of cancers are being seen in this population of patients. While some may only reflect known risk factors (i.e., smoking) that are increased in patients with HIV infection, some may be a direct consequence of HIV.

Kaposi's sarcoma is a multicentric neoplasm consisting of multiple vascular nodules appearing in the skin, mucous membranes, and viscera. The course ranges from indolent, with only minor skin or lymph node involvement, to fulminant, with extensive cutaneous and visceral involvement. In the initial period of the AIDS epidemic, KS was a prominent clinical feature of the first cases of AIDS, occurring in 79% of the patients diagnosed in 1981. By 1989 it was seen in only 25% of cases, by 1992 the number had decreased to 9%, and by 1997 the number was <1%. HHV-8 or KSHV has been strongly implicated as a viral cofactor in the pathogenesis of KS (see above).

Clinically, KS has varied presentations and may be seen at any stage of HIV infection, even in the presence of a normal CD4+ T cell count. The initial lesion may be a small, raised reddish-purple nodule on the skin (Fig. 182-39), a discoloration on the oral mucosa (Fig. 182-32*D*), or a swollen lymph node. Lesions often appear in sun-exposed areas, particularly the tip of the nose, and have a propensity to occur in areas of trauma (Koebner phenomenon). Because of the vascular nature of the tumors and the presence of extravasated red blood cells in the lesions, their colors range from reddish to purple to brown and often take the appearance of a bruise, with yellowish discoloration and tattooing. Lesions range in size from a few millimeters to several centimeters in diameter and may be either discrete or confluent. KS lesions most commonly appear as raised macules; however, they can also be papular, particularly in patients with higher CD4+ T cell counts. Confluent lesions may give rise to surrounding lymphedema and may be disfiguring when they involve the face and disabling when they involve the lower extremities or the surfaces of joints. Apart from skin, lymph nodes, gastrointestinal tract, and lung are the organ systems most commonly affected by KS. Lesions have been reported in virtually every organ, including the heart and the CNS. In contrast to most malignancies, in which lymph node involvement implies metastatic spread and a poor prognosis, lymph node involvement may be seen very early in KS and is of no special clinical significance. In fact, some patients

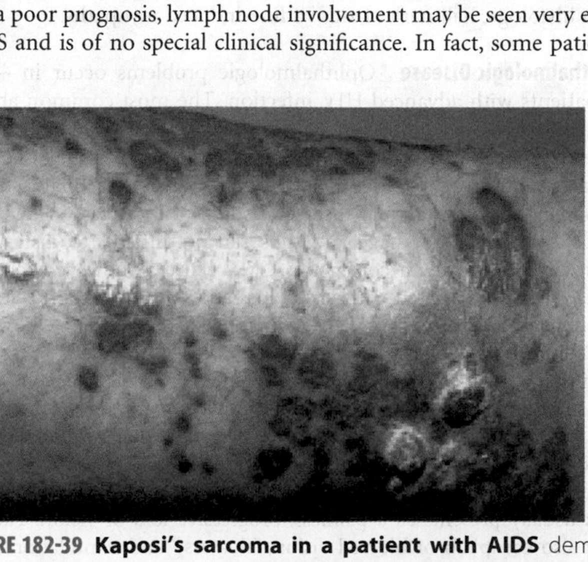

FIGURE 182-39 Kaposi's sarcoma in a patient with AIDS demonstrating patch, plaque, and tumor stages.

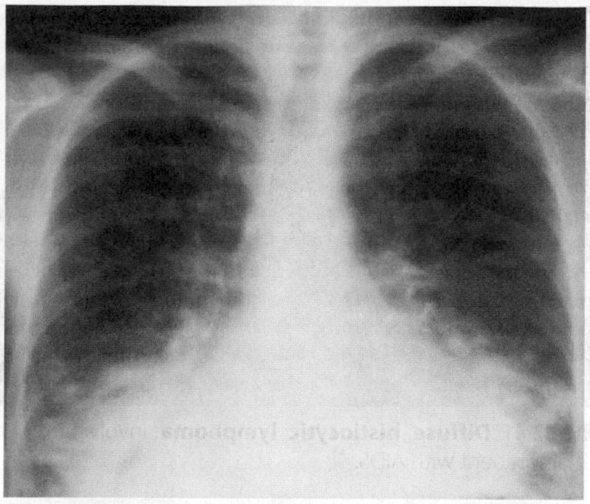

FIGURE 182-40 Chest x-ray of a patient with AIDS and pulmonary Kaposi's sarcoma. The characteristic findings include dense bilateral lower lobe infiltrates obscuring the heart borders and a pleural effusion.

may present with disease limited to the lymph nodes. These are generally patients with relatively intact immune function and thus the patients with the best prognosis. Pulmonary involvement with KS generally presents with shortness of breath. Some 80% of patients with pulmonary KS also have cutaneous lesions. The chest x-ray characteristically shows bilateral lower lobe infiltrates that obscure the margins of the mediastinum and diaphragm (Fig. 182-40). Pleural effusions are seen in 70% of cases of pulmonary KS, a fact that is often helpful in the differential diagnosis. Gastrointestinal involvement is seen in 50% of patients and usually takes one of two forms: (1) mucosal involvement, which may lead to bleeding that can be severe; these patients sometimes also develop symptoms of gastrointestinal obstruction if lesions become large; and (2) biliary tract involvement. KS lesions may infiltrate the gallbladder and biliary tree, leading to a clinical picture of obstructive jaundice similar to that seen with sclerosing cholangitis. Several staging systems have been proposed for KS. One in common use was developed by the National Institute of Allergy and Infectious Diseases AIDS Clinical Trials Group; it distinguishes patients on the basis of tumor extent, immunologic function, and presence or absence of systemic disease (Table 182-14).

A diagnosis of KS is based upon biopsy of a suspicious lesion. Histologically one sees a proliferation of spindle cells and endothelial cells, extravasation of red blood cells, hemosiderin-laden macrophages, and, in early cases, an inflammatory cell infiltrate. Included in the differential diagnosis are lymphoma (particularly for oral lesions), bacillary angiomatosis, and cutaneous mycobacterial infections.

Management of KS (Table 182-15) should be carried out in consultation with an expert since definitive treatment guidelines do not exist.

TABLE 182-14 NATIONAL INSTITUTE OF ALLERGY AND INFECTIOUS DISEASES AIDS CLINICAL TRIALS GROUP TIS STAGING SYSTEM FOR KAPOSI'S SARCOMA

Parameter	Good Risk (Stage 0): All of the Following	Poor Risk (Stage 1): Any of the Following
Tumor (T)	Confined to skin and/or lymph nodes and/or minimal oral disease	Tumor-associated edema or ulceration Extensive oral lesions Gastrointestinal lesions Nonnodal visceral lesions
Immune system (I)	CD4+ T cell count ≥200/μL	CD4+ T cell count <200/μL
Systemic illness (S)	No B symptoms[a] Karnofsky performance status ≥70 No history of opportunistic infection, neurologic disease, lymphoma, or thrush	B symptoms[a] present Karnofsky performance status <70 History of opportunistic infection, neurologic disease, lymphoma, or thrush

[a]Defined as unexplained fever, night sweats, >10% involuntary weight loss, or diarrhea persisting for more than 2 weeks.

TABLE 182-15 MANAGEMENT OF AIDS-ASSOCIATED KAPOSI'S SARCOMA

- Observation and optimization of antiretroviral therapy
- Single or limited number of lesions
  - Radiation
  - Intralesional vinblastine
  - Cryotherapy
- Extensive disease
  - Initial therapy
    - Interferon-α (if CD4+ T cells >150/μL)
    - Liposomal daunorubicin
  - Subsequent therapy
    - Liposomal doxorubicin
    - Paclitaxel
  - Combination chemotherapy with low-dose doxorubicin, bleomycin, and vinblastine (ABV)
  - Radiation treatment

In the majority of cases, effective ARV therapy will go a long way in achieving control. Indeed, spontaneous regressions have been reported in the setting of HAART. For patients in whom tumor persists or in whom control of HIV replication is not possible, a variety of options exist. In some cases, lesions remain quite indolent, and many of these patients can be managed with no specific treatment. Fewer than 10% of AIDS patients with KS die as a consequence of their malignancy, and death from secondary infections is considerably more common. Thus, whenever possible one should avoid treatment regimens that may further suppress the immune system and increase susceptibility to opportunistic infections. Treatment is indicated under two main circumstances. The first is when a single lesion or a limited number of lesions are causing significant discomfort or cosmetic problems, such as with prominent facial lesions, lesions overlying a joint, or lesions in the oropharynx that interfere with swallowing or breathing. Under these circumstances, treatment with localized radiation, intralesional vinblastine, or cryotherapy may be helpful. It should be noted that patients with HIV infection are particularly sensitive to the side effects of radiation therapy. This is especially true with respect to the development of radiation-induced mucositis; doses of radiation directed at mucosal surfaces, particularly in the head and neck region, should be adjusted accordingly. The use of systemic therapy, either IFN-α or chemotherapy, should be considered in patients with a large number of lesions or in patients with visceral involvement. The single most important determinant of response appears to be the CD4+ T cell count. This relationship between response rate and baseline CD4+ T cell count is particularly true for IFN-α. The response rate for patients with CD4+ T cell counts >600/μL is ~80%, while the response rate for patients with counts <150/μL is <10%. In contrast to the other systemic therapies, IFN-α provides an added advantage of having ARV activity; thus, it may be the appropriate first choice for single-agent systemic therapy for early patients with disseminated disease. A variety of chemotherapeutic agents have also been shown to have activity against KS. Three of them, liposomal daunorubicin, liposomal doxorubicin, and paclitaxel, have been approved by the FDA for this indication. Liposomal daunorubicin is approved as first-line therapy for patients with advanced KS. It has fewer side effects than conventional chemotherapy. In contrast, liposomal doxorubicin and paclitaxel are approved only for KS patients who have failed standard chemotherapy. Response rates vary from 23–88%, appear to be comparable to what had been achieved earlier with combination chemotherapy regimens, and are greatly influenced by CD4+ T cell count.

Lymphomas occur with an increased frequency in patients with congenital or acquired T cell immunodeficiencies (Chap. 310). AIDS is no exception; at least 6% of all patients with AIDS develop lymphoma at some time during the course of their illness. This is a 120-fold increase in incidence compared to the general population. In contrast to the situation with KS, primary CNS lymphoma, and most opportunistic infections, the incidence of AIDS-associated systemic lymphomas has not experienced as dramatic a decrease as a consequence of the widespread use of effective ARV therapy. Lymphoma occurs in all risk groups, with the highest incidence in patients with hemophilia and the lowest incidence in patients from the Caribbean or Africa with heterosexually acquired infection. Lymphoma is a late manifestation of HIV infection, generally occurring in patients with CD4+ T cell counts <200/μL. As HIV disease progresses, the risk of lymphoma increases. In contrast to KS, which occurs at a relatively constant rate throughout the course of HIV disease, the attack rate for lymphoma increases exponentially with increasing duration of HIV infection and decreasing level of immunologic function. At 3 years following a diagnosis of HIV infection, the risk of lymphoma is 0.8% per year; by 8 years after infection, it is 2.6% per year. As individuals with HIV infection live longer as a consequence of improved ARV therapy and better treatment and prophylaxis of opportunistic infections, it is anticipated that the incidence of lymphomas may increase.

Three main categories of lymphoma are seen in patients with HIV infection: grade III or IV immunoblastic lymphoma, Burkitt's lymphoma, and primary CNS lymphoma. Approximately 90% of these lymphomas are B cell in phenotype, and half contain EBV DNA. These tumors may be either monoclonal or oligoclonal in nature and are probably in some way related to the pronounced polyclonal B cell activation seen in patients with AIDS.

Immunoblastic lymphomas account for ~60% of the cases of lymphoma in patients with AIDS. These are generally high grade and would have been classified as diffuse histiocytic lymphomas in earlier classification schemes. This tumor is more common in older patients, increasing in incidence from 0% in HIV-infected individuals <1 year old to >3% in those >50. One variant of immunoblastic lymphoma is body cavity lymphoma. This malignancy presents with lymphomatous pleural, pericardial, and/or peritoneal effusions in the absence of discrete nodal or extranodal masses. The tumor cells do not express surface markers for B cells or T cells. HHV-8 DNA sequences have been found in the genomes of the malignant cells from patients with body cavity lymphomas (see above).

Small noncleaved cell lymphoma (*Burkitt's lymphoma*) accounts for ~20% of the cases of lymphoma in patients with AIDS. It is most frequent in patients 10–19 years old and usually demonstrates characteristic c-*myc* translocations from chromosome 8 to chromosomes 14 or 22. Burkitt's lymphoma is not commonly seen in the setting of immunodeficiency other than HIV-associated immunodeficiency, and the incidence of this particular tumor is over 1000-fold higher in the setting of HIV infection than in the general population. In contrast to African Burkitt's lymphoma, where 97% of the cases contain EBV genome, only 50% of HIV-associated Burkitt's lymphomas are EBV-positive.

Primary CNS lymphoma accounts for ~20% of the cases of lymphoma in patients with HIV infection. In contrast to HIV-associated Burkitt's lymphoma, primary CNS lymphomas are usually positive for EBV. In one study, the incidence of Epstein-Barr positivity was 100%. This malignancy does not have a predilection for any particular age group. The median CD4+ T cell count at the time of diagnosis is ~50/μL. Thus, CNS lymphoma generally presents at a later stage of HIV infection than systemic lymphoma. This fact may at least in part explain the poorer prognosis for this subset of patients.

The clinical presentation of lymphoma in patients with HIV infection is quite varied, ranging from focal seizures to rapidly growing mass lesions in the oral mucosa (Fig. 182-41) to persistent unexplained fever. At least 80% of patients present with extranodal disease, and a similar percentage have B-type symptoms of fever, night sweats, or weight loss. Virtually any site in the body may be involved. The most common extranodal site is the CNS, which is involved in approximately one-third of all patients with lymphoma. Approximately 60% of these cases are primary CNS lymphoma. Primary CNS lymphoma generally presents with focal neurologic deficits, including cranial nerve findings, headaches, and/or seizures. MRI or CT generally reveals a limited number (one to three) of 3- to 5-cm lesions (Fig. 182-42). The lesions often show ring enhancement on contrast administration and may occur in any location. Locations that are most commonly involved with CNS lymphoma are deep in the white matter. Contrast enhancement is usually less pronounced than that seen with toxoplasmosis. The main diseases in the differential diagnosis are cerebral toxoplasmosis and cerebral Chagas' disease. In addition to the 20% of lymphomas in HIV-infected individuals that are primary CNS lymphomas, CNS disease is also seen in HIV-infected patients with systemic lymphoma. Approximately 20% of patients with systemic lymphoma have CNS disease in the form of leptomeningeal involvement. This fact underscores the importance of lumbar puncture in the staging evaluation of patients with systemic lymphoma.

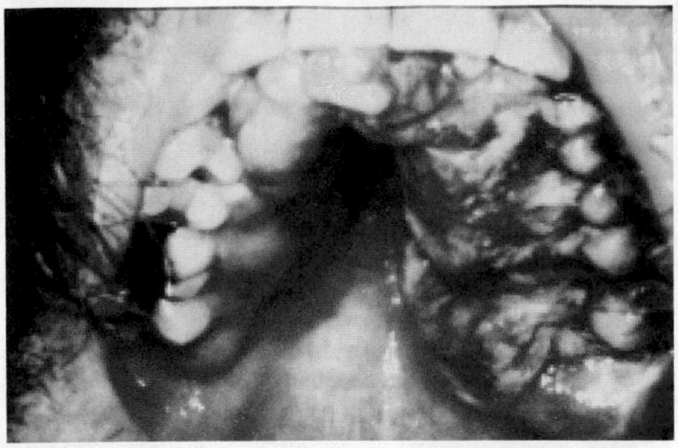

FIGURE 182-41 Diffuse histiocytic lymphoma involving the hard palate of a patient with AIDS.

Systemic lymphoma is seen at earlier stages of HIV infection than primary CNS lymphoma. In one series the mean CD4+ T cell count was 189/μL. In addition to lymph node involvement, systemic lymphoma may commonly involve the gastrointestinal tract, bone marrow, liver, and lung. Gastrointestinal tract involvement is seen in ~25% of patients. Any site in the gastrointestinal tract may be involved, and patients may complain of difficulty swallowing or abdominal pain. The diagnosis is usually suspected on the basis of CT or MRI of the abdomen. Bone marrow involvement is seen in ~20% of patients and may lead to pancytopenia. Liver and lung involvement are each seen in ~10% of patients. Pulmonary disease may present as either a mass lesion, multiple nodules, or an interstitial infiltrate.

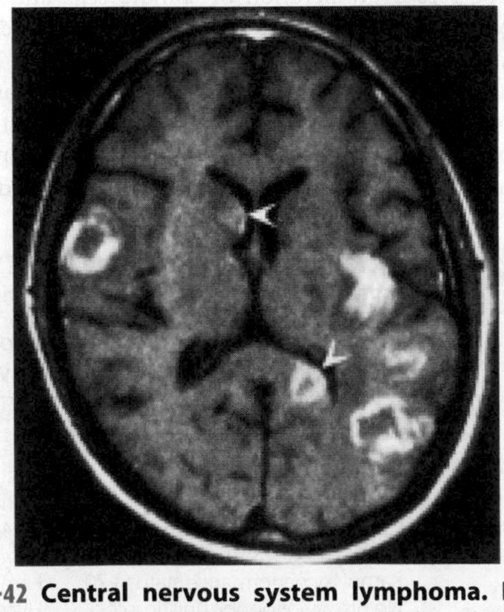

FIGURE 182-42 Central nervous system lymphoma. Postcontrast T1-weighted MR scan in a patient with AIDS, an altered mental status, and hemiparesis. Multiple enhancing lesions, some ring-enhancing, are present. The left Sylvian lesion shows gyral and subcortical enhancement, and the lesions in the caudate and splenium (*arrowheads*) show enhancement of adjacent ependymal surfaces.

Both conventional and unconventional approaches have been employed in an attempt to treat HIV-related lymphomas. Systemic lymphoma is generally treated by the oncologist with combination chemotherapy. Earlier disappointing figures are being replaced with more optimistic results for the treatment of systemic lymphoma following the availability of more effective combination ARV therapy. As in most situations in patients with HIV disease, those with the higher CD4+ T cell counts tend to do better. Response rates as high as 72% with a median survival of 33 months and disease-free intervals up to 9 years have been reported. Treatment of primary CNS lymphoma remains a significant challenge. Treatment is complicated by the fact that this illness usually occurs in patients with advanced HIV disease. Palliative measures such as radiation therapy provide some relief. The prognosis remains poor in this group, with a 2-year survival of 29%.

Multicentric Castleman's disease is an HHV-8 associated lymphoproliferative disorder that is seen with an increased frequency in patients with HIV infection. While not a true malignancy, it shares many features with lymphoma including generalized lymphadenopathy, hepatosplenomegaly, and systemic symptoms of fever, fatigue, and weight loss. Pulmonary symptoms may be seen in ~50% of patients. Kaposi's sarcoma is present in 75–82% of cases. Lymph node biopsies reveal a predominance of interfollicular plasma cells and/or germinal centers with vascularization and an "onion skin" appearance (hyaline vascular). Prior to the availability of HAART, HIV-infected patients with multicentric Castleman's disease had a 15-fold increased risk of developing non-Hodgkin's lymphoma compared to HIV-infected patients in general. Treatment typically involves chemotherapy. Anecdotal reports of success with rituximab suggest that more specific treatment may be successful, although in one series treatment with rituximab was associated with worsening of coexisting KS. The median survival of patients with treated multicentric Castleman's disease pre-HAART was 14 months. This has increased to 4 years in the era of HAART.

Evidence of infection with *human papilloma virus* (HPV), associated with *intraepithelial dysplasia of the cervix* or *anus*, is approximately twice as common in HIV-infected individuals as in the general population and can lead to intraepithelial neoplasia and eventually invasive cancer. In separate studies, HIV-infected men were examined for evidence of anal dysplasia, and Papanicolaou (Pap) smears were found to be abnormal in 20–80%. These changes tend to persist and are generally not affected by HAART, raising the possibility of a subsequent transition to a more malignant condition. While the incidence of an abnormal Pap smear of the cervix is ~5% in otherwise healthy women, the incidence of abnormal cervical smears in women with HIV infection is 30–60%, and *invasive cervical cancer* is included as an AIDS-defining condition. Thus far, however, only small increases in the incidence of cervical or anal cancer have been seen as a consequence of HIV infection. However, given this high rate of dysplasia, a comprehensive gynecologic and rectal examination, including Pap smear, is indicated at the initial evaluation and 6 months later for all patients with HIV infection. If these examinations are negative at both time points, the patient should be followed with yearly evaluations. If an initial or repeat Pap smear shows evidence of severe inflammation with reactive squamous changes, the next Pap smear should be performed at 3 months. If, at any time, a Pap smear shows evidence of squamous intraepithelial lesions, colposcopic examination with biopsies as indicated should be performed. The 2-year survival rate for HIV infected patients with invasive cervical cancer is 64% compared to 79% in non-HIV-infected patients. The most common HPV genotypes in the general population and the genotypes upon which current HPV vaccines are based are 16 and 18. This is not the case in the HIV-infected population where other genotypes such as 56 and 53 predominate. This raises concerns as to the potential effectiveness of the current HPV vaccines for HIV-infected patients.

IDIOPATHIC CD4+ T LYMPHOCYTOPENIA

A syndrome was recognized in 1992 that was characterized by an absolute CD4+ T cell count of <300/μL or <20% of total T cells on a minimum of two occasions at least 6 weeks apart; no evidence of HIV-1, HIV-2, HTLV-I, or HTLV-II on testing; and the absence of any defined immunodeficiency or therapy associated with decreased levels of CD4+ T cells. By mid-1993, ~100 patients had been described. After extensive multicenter investigations, a series of reports were published in early 1993, which together allowed a number of conclusions. Idiopathic CD4+ lymphocytopenia (ICL) is a very rare syndrome, as determined by studies of blood donors and cohorts of HIV-seronegative men who have sex with men. Cases were clearly identified as early as 1983, and cases remarkably similar to ICL had been identified decades ago. The definition of ICL based on CD4+ T cell counts coincided with the ready availability of testing for CD4+ T cells in patients suspected of being immunosuppressed. Although, as a result of immune deficiency, certain patients with ICL develop some of the opportunistic diseases (particularly cryptococcosis) seen in HIV-infected patients, the syndrome is demographically, clinically, and immunologically unlike HIV infection and AIDS. Fewer than half of the reported ICL patients had risk factors for HIV infection, and there were wide geographic and age distributions. The fact that a significant proportion of patients did have risk factors probably reflects a selection bias, in that physicians who take care of HIV-infected patients are more likely to monitor CD4+ T cells. Approximately one-third of the patients are women, compared to 16% of women among HIV-infected individuals in the United States. Many patients with ICL remained clinically stable, and their condition did not deteriorate progressively as is common with seriously immunodeficient HIV-infected patients. Certain patients with ICL even experienced spontaneous reversal of the CD4+ T lymphocytopenia. Immunologic abnormalities in ICL are somewhat different from those of HIV infection. ICL patients often also have decreases in CD8+ T cells and in B cells. Furthermore, immunoglobulin levels were either normal or, more commonly, decreased in patients with ICL, compared to the usual hypergammaglobulinemia of HIV-infected individuals. Finally, virologic studies revealed no evidence of HIV-1, HIV-2, HTLV-I, or HTLV-II or of any other mononuclear cell–tropic virus. Furthermore, there was no epidemiologic evidence to suggest that a transmissible microbe was involved. The cases of ICL were widely dispersed, with no clustering. Close contacts and sexual partners who were studied were clinically well and were serologically, immunologically, and virologically negative for HIV. ICL is a heterogeneous syndrome, and it is highly likely that there is no common cause; however, there may be common causes among subgroups of patients that are currently unrecognized.

Patients who present with laboratory data consistent with ICL should be worked up for underlying diseases that could be responsible for the immune deficiency. If no underlying cause is detected, no specific therapy should be initiated. However, if opportunistic diseases occur, they should be treated appropriately (see above). Depending on the level of the CD4+ T cell count, patients should receive prophylaxis for the commonly encountered opportunistic infections.

Rx AIDS AND RELATED DISORDERS

GENERAL PRINCIPLES OF PATIENT MANAGEMENT The CDC guidelines call for the testing for HIV infection to be a part of routine medical care. It is recommended that the patient be informed of the intention to test as is the case with other routine laboratory determinations and be given the opportunity to "opt out." Such an approach is critical to the goal of identifying as many infected individuals as possible since ~25% of the >1 million individuals in the United States who are HIV-infected are not aware of their status. Under these circumstances of routine testing, although desirable, pretest counseling may not always be built into the testing process. However, no matter how well prepared a patient is for adversity, the discovery of a diagnosis of HIV infection is a devastating event. Thus, physicians should be sensitive to this fact and, where possible, execute some degree of pretest counseling to at least partially prepare the patient should the results demonstrate the presence of HIV infection. Following a diagnosis of HIV infection, the health care provider should be prepared to activate support systems immediately for the newly diagnosed patient. These should include an experienced social worker or nurse who can spend time talking to the person and ensuring that he or she is emotionally stable. Most communities have HIV support centers that can be of great help in these difficult situations.

The treatment of patients with HIV infection requires not only a comprehensive knowledge of the possible disease processes that may occur and up-to-date knowledge of and experience with ARV therapy, but also the ability to deal with the problems of a chronic, potentially life-threatening illness. A comprehensive knowledge of internal medicine is required to deal with the changing spectrum of illness associated with HIV infection. Great advances have been made in the treatment of patients with HIV infection. The appropriate use of potent combination ARV therapy and other treatment and prophylactic interventions is of critical importance in providing each patient with the best opportunity to live a long and healthy life despite the presence of HIV infection. In contrast to the earlier days of this epidemic, a diagnosis of HIV infection need no longer be equated with an inevitably fatal disease. In addition to medical interventions, the health care provider has a responsibility to provide each patient with appropriate counseling and education concerning their disease as part of a comprehensive care plan. Patients must be educated about the potential transmissibility of their infection and about the fact that while health care providers may refer to levels of the virus as "undetectable," this is more a reflection of the sensitivity of the assay being used to measure the virus than a comment on the presence or absence of the virus. It is important for patients to be aware that the virus is still present and capable of being transmitted at all stages of HIV disease. Thus, there need to be frank discussions concerning sexual practices and the sharing of needles. The treating physician must not only be aware of the latest medications available for patients with HIV infection but must also educate patients concerning the natural history of their illness and listen and be sensitive to their fears and concerns. As with other diseases, therapeutic decisions should be made in consultation with the patient, when possible, and with the patient's proxy if the patient is incapable of making decisions. In this regard, it is recommended that all patients with HIV infection, and in particular those with CD4+ T cell counts <200/μL, designate a trusted individual with durable power of attorney to make medical decisions on their behalf, if necessary.

Following a diagnosis of HIV infection, there are several examinations and laboratory studies that should be performed to help determine the extent of disease and provide baseline standards for future reference (**Table 182-16**). In addition to routine chemistry, fasting lipid profile, fasting glucose and hematology screening panels, Pap smear, and chest x-ray, one should also obtain a CD4+ T cell count, two separate plasma HIV RNA levels, an HIV resistance test, an RPR or VDRL test, an anti-*Toxoplasma* antibody titer, and serologies for hepatitis A, B, and C. A PPD test should be done, and a MMSE performed and recorded. Patients should be immunized with pneumococcal polysaccharide and, if seronegative for these viruses, with hepatitis A and hepatitis B vaccines. The status of hepatitis C infection should be determined. In addition, patients should be counseled with regard to sexual practices and needle sharing, and counseling should be offered to those whom the patient knows or suspects may also be infected. Once these baseline activities are performed, short- and long-term medical management strategies should be developed based upon the most recent information available and modified as new information becomes available. The field of HIV medicine is changing rapidly, and it is difficult to remain fully up to date. Fortunately there are a series of excellent sites on the internet that are frequently updated, and they provide the most recent information on a variety of topics, including consensus panel reports on treatment (**Table 182-17**).

TABLE 182-16 INITIAL EVALUATION OF THE PATIENT WITH HIV INFECTION

History and physical examination
Routine chemistry and hematology
Lipid profile and fasting glucose
CD4+ T lymphocyte count
Two plasma HIV RNA levels
HIV resistance testing
RPR test
Anti-*Toxoplasma* antibody titer
PPD skin test
Mini-mental status examination
Serologies for hepatitis A, hepatitis B, and hepatitis C
Immunization with pneumococcal polysaccharide; influenza as indicated
Immunization with hepatitis A and hepatitis B if seronegative
Counseling regarding natural history and transmission
Help contacting others who might be infected

Note: VDRL, Venereal Disease Research Laboratory; PPD, purified protein derivative.

TABLE 182-17 RESOURCES AVAILABLE ON THE WORLD WIDE WEB ON HIV DISEASE

http://www.aidsinfo.nih.gov	AIDS info, a service of the U.S. Department of Health and Human Services, posts federally approved treatment guidelines for HIV and AIDS; provides information on federally funded and privately funded clinical trials and CDC publications and data
http://www.cdcnpin.org	Updates on epidemiologic data from the CDC

Note: CDC, Centers for Disease Control and Prevention.

ANTIRETROVIRAL THERAPY Combination antiretroviral therapy (ART), or highly active antiretroviral therapy (HAART), is the cornerstone of management of patients with HIV infection. Following the initiation of widespread use of HAART in the United States in 1995–1996, marked declines have been noted in the incidence of most AIDS-defining conditions (Fig. 182-31). Suppression of HIV replication is an important component in prolonging life as well as in improving the quality of life in patients with HIV infection. Adequate suppression requires strict adherence to prescribed regimens of ARV drugs. This has been facilitated by the coformulations of ARVs and the development of once-daily regimens. Unfortunately, many of the most important questions related to the treatment of HIV disease currently lack definitive answers. Among them are the questions of when should therapy be started, what is the best initial regimen, when should a given regimen be changed, and what should it be changed to when a change is made. Notwithstanding these uncertainties, the physician and patient must come to a mutually agreeable plan based upon the best available data. In an effort to facilitate this process, the U.S. Department of Health and Human Services has published a series of frequently updated guidelines including the "*Principles of Therapy of HIV Infection*," "*Guidelines for the Use of Antiretroviral Agents in HIV-Infected Adults and Adolescents*," and "*Guidelines for the Prevention of Opportunistic Infections in Persons Infected with Human Immunodeficiency Virus*." At present, an extensive clinical trials network, involving both clinical investigators and patient advocates, is in place attempting to develop improved approaches to therapy. Consortia comprising representatives of academia, industry, independent foundations, and the federal government are involved in the process of drug development, including a wide-ranging series of clinical trials. As a result, new therapies and new therapeutic strategies are continually emerging. New drugs are often available through expanded access programs prior to official licensure. Given the complexity of this field, decisions regarding ARV therapy are best made in consultation with experts. Currently available drugs for the treatment of HIV infection fall into four categories: those that inhibit the viral reverse transcriptase enzyme, those that inhibit the viral protease enzyme, those that inhibit the viral integrase enzyme, and those that interfere with viral entry (**Table 182-18, Fig. 182-43**).

The FDA-approved reverse transcriptase inhibitors include the *nucleoside analogues* zidovudine, didanosine, zalcitabine, stavudine, lamivudine, abacavir, and emtricitabine; the *nucleotide analogue* tenofovir; and the *nonnucleoside reverse transcriptase inhibitors* nevirapine, delavirdine, and efavirenz (Fig. 182-43; Table 182-18). These were the first class of drugs that were licensed for the treatment of HIV infection. They are indicated for this use as part of combination regimens. It should be stressed that none of these drugs should be used as monotherapy for HIV infection due to the relative ease with which drug resistance may develop under such circumstances. Thus, when lamivudine or tenofovir are used to treat hepatitis B infection in the setting of HIV infection, one should ensure that the patient is also on additional ARV medication. The reverse transcriptase inhibitors block the HIV replication cycle at the point of RNA-dependent DNA synthesis, the reverse transcription step. While the nonnucleoside reverse transcriptase inhibitors are quite selective for the HIV-1 reverse transcriptase, the nucleoside and nucleotide analogues inhibit a variety of DNA polymerization reactions in addition to those of the HIV-1 reverse transcriptase. For this reason, serious side effects are more varied with the nucleoside analogues and include mitochondrial damage that can lead to hepatic steatosis and lactic acidosis as

TABLE 182-18 ANTIRETROVIRAL DRUGS USED IN THE TREATMENT OF HIV INFECTION

Drug	Status	Indication	Dose in Combination	Supporting Data	Toxicity
Reverse Transcriptase Inhibitors					
Zidovudine (AZT, azidothymidine, Retrovir, 3′azido-3′-deoxythymidine)	Licensed	Treatment of HIV infection in combination with other antiretroviral agents Prevention of maternal-fetal HIV transmission	200 mg q8h or 300 mg bid	19 vs 1 death in original placebo-controlled trial in 281 patients with AIDS or ARC. Decreased progression to AIDS in patients with CD4+ T cell counts <500/μL, $n = 2051$ In pregnant women with CD4+ T cell count ≥200/μL, AZT PO beginning at weeks 14–34 of gestation plus IV drug during labor and delivery plus PO AZT to infant for 6 wk decreased transmission of HIV by 67.5% (from 25.5% to 8.3%), $n = 363$	Anemia, granulocytopenia, myopathy, lactic acidosis, hepatomegaly with steatosis, headache, nausea
Didanosine (Videx, Videx EC, ddI, dideoxyinosine, 2′,3′-dideoxyinosine)	Licensed	For treatment of HIV infection in combination with other antiretroviral agents	Buffered: Requires 2 tablets to achieve adequate buffering of stomach acid; should be administered on an empty stomach ≥60 kg: 200 mg bid <60 kg: 125 mg bid Enteric coated: ≥60 kg: 400 mg qd < 60 kg: 250 mg qd	Clinically superior to AZT as monotherapy in 913 patients with prior AZT therapy. Clinically superior to AZT and comparable to AZT + ddI and AZT + ddC in 1067 AZT-naive patients with CD4+ T cell counts of 200–500/μL	Pancreatitis, peripheral neuropathy, abnormalities on liver function tests, lactic acidosis, hepatomegaly with steatosis
Zalcitabine (ddC, HIVID, 2′3′-dideoxycytidine)	Licensed Discontinued in 2006	In combination with other antiretroviral agents for the treatment of HIV infection	0.75 mg tid	Clinically inferior to AZT monotherapy as initial treatment. Clinically as good as ddI in advanced patients intolerant to AZT. In combination with AZT, was clinically superior to AZT alone in patients with AIDS or CD4+ T cell count <350/μL	Peripheral neuropathy, pancreatitis, lactic acidosis, hepatomegaly with steatosis, oral ulcers
Stavudine (d4T, Zerit, 2′3′-didehydro-3′-dideoxythymidine)	Licensed	Treatment of HIV-infected patients in combination with other antiretroviral agents	≥60 kg: 40 mg bid <60 kg: 30 mg bid	Superior to AZT with respect to changes in CD4+ T cell counts in 359 patients who had received ≥24 wk of AZT. Following 12 wk of randomization, the CD4+ T cell count had decreased in AZT-treated controls by a mean of 22/μL, while in stavudine-treated patients, it had increased by a mean of 22/μL	Peripheral neuropathy, pancreatitis, lactic acidosis, hepatomegaly with steatosis, ascending neuromuscular weakness, lipodystrophy
Lamivudine (Epivir, 2′3′-dideoxy-3′-thiacytidine, 3TC)	Licensed	In combination with other antiretroviral agents for the treatment of HIV infection	150 mg bid 300 mg qd	Superior to AZT alone with respect to changes in CD4 counts in 495 patients who were zidovudine-naive and 477 patients who were zidovudine-experienced. Overall CD4+ T cell counts for the zidovudine group were at baseline by 24 wk, while in the group treated with zidovudine plus lamivudine, they were 10–50 cells/μL above baseline. 54% decrease in progression to AIDS/death compared to AZT alone	Hepatotoxicity
Emtricitabine (FTC, Emtriva)	Licensed	In combination with other antiretroviral agents for the treatment of HIV infection	200 mg qd	Comparable to d4T in combination with ddI and efavirenz in 571 treatment-naive patients. Similar to 3TC in combination with AZT or d4T + NNRT1 or PI in 440 patients doing well for at least 12 weeks on a 3TC regimen	Hepatotoxicity
Abacavir (Ziagen)	Licensed	For treatment of HIV infection in combination with other antiretroviral agents	300 mg bid	Abacavir + AZT + 3TC equivalent to indinavir + AZT + 3TC with regard to viral load suppression (~60% in each group with <400 HIV RNA copies/mL plasma) and CD4 cell increase (~100/μL in each group) at 24 weeks	Hypersensitivity reaction (can be fatal); fever, rash, nausea, vomiting, malaise or fatigue, and loss of appetite
Tenofovir (Viread)	Licensed	For use in combination with other antiretroviral agents when treatment is indicated	300 mg qd	Reduction of ~0.6 log in HIV-1 RNA levels when added to background regimen in treatment-experienced patients	Potential for renal toxicity

(continued)

TABLE 182-18 ANTIRETROVIRAL DRUGS USED IN THE TREATMENT OF HIV INFECTION (CONTINUED)

Drug	Status	Indication	Dose in Combination	Supporting Data	Toxicity
Delavirdine (Rescriptor)	Licensed	For use in combination with appropriate antiretrovirals when treatment is warranted	400 mg tid	Delavirdine + AZT superior to AZT alone with regard to viral load suppression at 52 weeks	Skin rash, abnormalities in liver function tests
Nevirapine (Viramune)	Licensed	In combination with other antiretroviral agents for treatment of progressive HIV infection	200 mg/d × 14 days then 200 mg bid	Increases in CD4+ T cell count, decrease in HIV RNA when used in combination with nucleosides	Skin rash, hepatotoxicity
Efavirenz (Sustiva)	Licensed	For treatment of HIV infection in combination with other antiretroviral agents	600 mg qhs	Efavirenz + AZT + 3TC comparable to indinavir + AZT + 3TC with regard to viral load suppression (a higher percentage of the efavirenz group achieved viral load <50 copies/mL; however, the discontinuation rate in the indinavir group was unexpectedly high, accounting for most treatment "failures"); CD4 cell increase (~140/μL in each group) at 24 weeks	Rash, dysphoria, elevated liver function tests, drowsiness, abnormal dreams, depression
Etravirine	Expanded access 1-866-889-2074	Pending	Pending	Pending	Rash, headache, dizziness, nausea, diarrhea
Protease Inhibitors					
Saquinavir mesylate (Invirase—hard gel capsule)	Licensed	In combination with other antiretroviral agents when therapy is warranted	1000 mg + 100 mg ritonavir bid	Increases in CD4+ T cell counts, reduction in HIV RNA most pronounced in combination therapy with ddC. 50% reduction in first AIDS-defining event or death in combination with ddC compared to either agent alone	Diarrhea, nausea, headaches, hyperglycemia, fat redistribution, lipid abnormalities
(Fortovase—soft gel capsule)	Licensed Discontinued 2006	For use in combination with other antiretroviral agents when treatment is warranted	1200 mg tid	Reduction in the mortality rate and AIDS-defining events for patients who received hard-gel formulation in combination with ddC	Diarrhea, nausea, abdominal pain, headaches, hyperglycemia, fat redistribution, lipid abnormalities
Ritonavir (Norvir)	Licensed	In combination with other antiretroviral agents for treatment of HIV infection when treatment is warranted	600 mg bid	Reduction in the cumulative incidence of clinical progression or death from 34 to 17% in patients with CD4+ T cell count <100/μL treated for a median of 6 months	Nausea, abdominal pain, hyperglycemia, fat redistribution, lipid abnormalities, may alter levels of many other drugs, including saquinavir
Indinavir sulfate (Crixivan)	Licensed	For treatment of HIV infection in combination with other antiretroviral agents when antiretroviral treatment is warranted	800 mg q8h or 800 mg + 100 mg ritonavir bid or 1000 mg q8h when used with efavirenz or nevirapine	Increase in CD4+ T cell count by 100/μL and 2-log decrease in HIV RNA levels when given in combination with zidovudine and lamivudine. Decrease of 50% in risk of progression to AIDS or death when given with zidovudine and lamivudine compared with zidovudine and lamivudine alone	Nephrolithiasis, indirect hyperbilirubinemia, hyperglycemia, fat redistribution, lipid abnormalities
Nelfinavir mesylate (Viracept)	Licensed	For treatment of HIV infection in combination with other antiretroviral agents when antiretroviral therapy is warranted	750 mg tid or 1250 mg bid	2.0-log decline in HIV RNA when given in combination with stavudine	Diarrhea, loose stools, hyperglycemia, fat redistribution, lipid abnormalities May contain traces of the potential carcinogen/teratogen ethyl methane sulfonate
Amprenavir (Agenerase)	Licensed	In combination with other antiretroviral agents for treatment of HIV infection	1200 mg bid or 600 mg + 100 mg ritonavir bid or 1200 mg + 200 mg ritonavir qd	In treatment-naïve patients, amprenavir + AZT + 3TC superior to AZT + 3TC with regard to viral load suppression (53% vs 11% with <400 HIV RNA copies/mL plasma at 24 weeks). CD4+ T cell responses similar between treatment groups. In treatment-experienced patients, amprenavir + NRTIs similar to indinavir + NRTIs with regard to viral load suppression (43% vs 53% with <400 HIV RNA copies/mL plasma at 24 weeks). CD4+ T cell responses superior in the indinavir + NRTIs group	Nausea, vomiting, diarrhea, rash, oral paresthesias, elevated liver function tests, hyperglycemia, fat redistribution, lipid abnormalities
Fosamprenavir (Lexiva)	Licensed		1400 mg bid or 700 mg + 100 mg ritonavir bid		

(continued)

TABLE 182-18 ANTIRETROVIRAL DRUGS USED IN THE TREATMENT OF HIV INFECTION (CONTINUED)

Drug	Status	Indication	Dose in Combination	Supporting Data	Toxicity
Lopinavir/ritonavir (Kaletra)	Licensed	For treatment of HIV infection in combination with other antiretroviral agents	400 mg/100 mg bid	In treatment-naïve patients, lopinavir/ritonavir + d4T + 3TC superior to nelfinavir+ d4T + 3TC with regard to viral load suppression (79% vs 64% with <400 HIV RNA copies/mL at 40 weeks). CD4+ T cell increases similar in both groups.	Diarrhea, hyperglycemia, fat redistribution, lipid abnormalities
Atazanavir (Reyataz)	Licensed	For treatment of HIV infection in combination with other antiretroviral agents	400 mg qd or 300 mg qd +Ritonavir 100 mg qd when given with efavirenz	Comparable to efavirenz when given in combination with AZT + 3TC in a study of 810 treatment-naive patients. Comparable to nelfinavir when given in combination with d4T + 3TC in a study of 467 treatment-naive patients.	Hyperbilirubinemia, PR prolongation, nausea, vomiting, hyperglycemia, fat maldistribution
Tipranavir (Aptivus)	Licensed	In combination with 200 mg ritonavir for combination therapy in treatment-experienced adults	500 mg + 200 mg ritonavir twice daily	At 24 weeks, patients with prior extensive exposure to ARVs showed a −0.8 log change in HIV RNA levels and a 34 cell increase in CD4+ T cells compound to −0.25 log and 4 cells in the control arm. Inferior to lopinavir/ritonavir in a randomized, controlled trial in naïve patients.	Diarrhea, nausea, fatigue, headache, skin rash, hepatotoxicity, intracranial hemorrhage
Darunavir (Prezista)	Licensed	In combination with 100 mg ritonavir for combination therapy in treatment-experienced adults	600 mg + 100 mg ritonavir twice daily with food	At 24 weeks, patients with prior extensive exposure to antiretrovirals treated with a new combination including darunavir showed a −1.89 log change in HIV RNA levels and a 92 cell increase in CD4+ T cells compared to −0.48 log and 17 cells in the control arm.	Diarrhea, nausea, headache
Entry Inhibitors					
Enfuvirtide (Fuzeon)	Licensed	In combination with other agents in treatment-experienced patients with evidence of HIV-1 replication despite ongoing antiretroviral therapy	90 mg SC bid	In treatment of experienced patients, superior to placebo when added to new optimized background (37% vs 16% with <400 HIV RNA copies/mL at 24 weeks; + 71 vs + 35 CD4+ T cells at 24 weeks)	Local injection reactions, hypersensitivity reactions, increased rate of bacterial pneumonia
Maraviroc (Selzentry)	Licensed	In combination with other antiretroviral agents in treatment experienced adults infected with only CCR5-tropic HIV-1 that is resistant to multiple antiretroviral agents	150–600 mg bid depending upon concomitant medications (see text)	At 24 weeks, among 635 patients with CCR5-tropic virus and HIV-1 RNA >5000 copies/mL despite at least 6 months of prior therapy with at least one agent from 3 of the 4 antiretroviral drug classes, 61% of patients randomized to maraviroc achieved HIV RNA levels <400 copies/mL compared to 28% of patients randomized to placebo	Hepatotoxicity, nasopharyngitis, fever, cough, rash, abdominal pain, dizziness, fever, musculoskeletal symptoms
Integrase Inhibitor					
Raltegravir (Isentress)	Licensed	In combination with other antiretroviral agents in treatment experienced patients with evidence of ongoing HIV-1 replication	400 mg bid	At 24 weeks, among 436 patients with three-class drug resistance, 76% of patients randomized to receive raltegravir achieved HIV RNA levels <400 copies/mL compared to 41% of patients randomized to receive placebo	Nausea, rash

Note: ARC, AIDS-related complex; NRTIs, nonnucleoside reverse transcriptase inhibitors.

well as peripheral neuropathy and pancreatitis. One of the more recently recognized problems that has been encountered with the widespread use of HAART therapy has been a syndrome of hyperlipidemia, glucose intolerance/insulin resistance, and fat redistribution often referred to as *lipodystrophy syndrome* (discussed above under metabolic abnormalities).

Zidovudine (AZT; 3′-azido-2′,3′-dideoxythymidine) was the first drug approved for the treatment of HIV infection and is the prototype nucleoside analogue. These compounds, in which the hydroxyl group in the 3′ position of the ribose moiety is substituted with a hydrogen or other chemical group, act as DNA chain terminators owing to their inability to form a 3′-5′ phosphodiester linkage with another nucleoside. They bind much more avidly to the active site of the RNA-dependent DNA polymerase of HIV (reverse transcriptase) than to the active site of mammalian cell DNA polymerases; this explains their selective effect on HIV replication. Zidovudine also has a relatively high avidity for the DNA polymerase-γ of human mitochondria. This may contribute to the development of the fatty liver and the myopathy sometimes observed in patients taking zidovudine. As with all the nucleoside analogues, the active form of zidovudine is the triphosphate, and the rate of phosphorylation, a thymidine kinase–dependent pathway, may be different in different cells. This may explain why zidovudine is more effective at inhibiting HIV replication in some cells than others. The clinical benefit of zidovudine was clearly established in 1986 in a phase II, randomized, placebo-controlled trial in patients with advanced HIV disease. However, while treatment of patients with early stages of HIV infection with zidovudine monotherapy was associated with increases in CD4+ T cell count, it was not associated with a better overall outcome than waiting until later to treat. Subsequent trials established the ability of this drug to dramatically decrease the incidence of perinatal transmission of HIV from infected mother to infant. Eventually a series of studies demonstrated the superiority of combination ARV regimens over zidovudine alone, and combination therapy (discussed below) remains the standard of treatment today. Among the side effects of zidovudine at the initiation of therapy are fatigue, malaise, nausea, and headache. These side effects often subside over time. Patients on zidovudine may develop a macrocytic anemia, neutropenia, myopathy, cardiomyopathy, and lactic acidosis associated with fatty infiltration of the liver. As with every ARV drug, HIV has the ability to develop resistance to zidovudine. Zidovudine resistance has been reported to occur ~6 months following the initiation of zidovudine monotherapy. More recently, zidovudine-resistant viruses have been noted in patients with acute infection prior to the initiation of therapy, implying that zidovudine-resistant viruses can be transmitted from person to person. Resistance emerges more rapidly in late-stage patients, presumably as a consequence of a greater degree of viral replication and thus a greater opportunity for mutation. A variety of amino acid changes including substitutions, insertions, and deletions have been reported to confer zidovudine resistance (**Fig. 182-44**). One combination preparation, Combivir, consists of zidovudine and lamivudine, while another, Trizivir, consists of zidovudine, lamivudine, and abacavir.

Didanosine (ddI; 2′,3′-dideoxyinosine) was the second drug licensed for the treatment of HIV infection, followed shortly thereafter by zalcitabine. Didanosine is metabolized to dideoxyadenosine in vivo. It is best absorbed on an empty stomach at a high pH. The toxicity profile of didanosine is quite different from that of zidovudine. The most common toxicity is a painful sensory peripheral neuropathy that occurs in ~30% of patients receiving >400 mg/d. It generally resolves with discontinuation of the drug and may not recur if the drug is resumed at a reduced dose. At higher doses than are currently used one may see pancreatitis in ~10% of patients. Pancreatitis associated with didanosine therapy can be fatal. Didanosine should be discontinued if a patient experiences abdominal pain consistent with pancreatitis or if an elevated serum amylase or lipase level is found in association with an edematous pancreas on ultrasound. Didanosine is contraindicated in patients with a prior history of pancreatitis, regardless of etiology. A higher incidence of didanosine-associated toxicities has been seen when it is used in combination with stavudine, hydroxyurea, ribavirin, or tenofovir.

Zalcitabine (ddC; 2′,3′-dideoxycytidine) is rarely used today in the management of patients with HIV infectionand was discontinued from the US market in 2006. Among the nucleoside analogues licensed for the treatment of HIV infection, it is probably the weakest. The main toxicities of ddC are peripheral neuropathy and pancreatitis.

Stavudine (d4T; 2′,3′-didehydro-3′-deoxythymidine) was the fourth drug licensed for the treatment of HIV infection and was discontinued from the US market in 2006. Like zidovudine, stavudine is a thymidine analogue. These two drugs are antagonistic in vitro and in vivo and should not be given together. Stavudine has been associated with a higher incidence of mitochondrial toxicity than the other licensed nucleoside analogues. Peripheral neuropathy, lipoatrophy, lactic acidosis, and hepatic steatosis are the main toxicities of stavudine.

Lamivudine (3TC; 2′,3′-dideoxy-3′-thiacytidine) is the fifth of the nucleoside analogues to be licensed in the United States. In actual practice, lami-

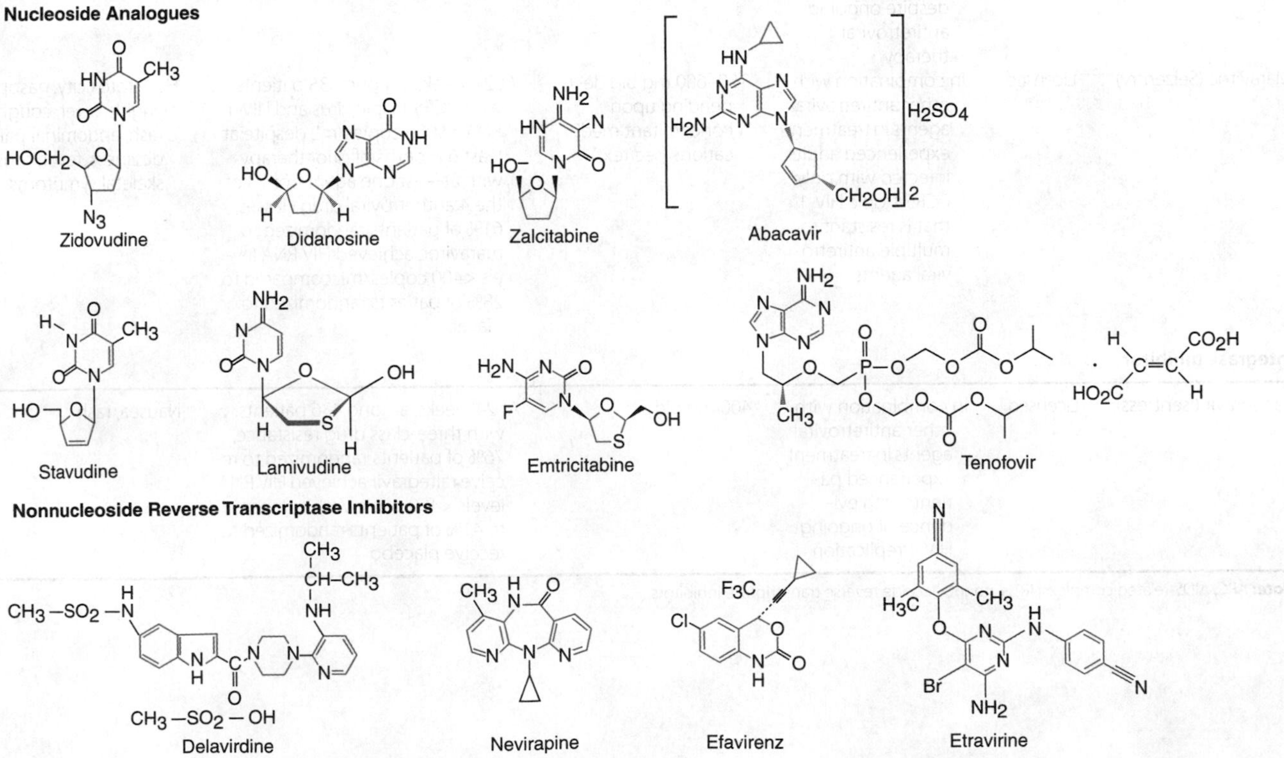

FIGURE 182-43 Molecular structures of antiretroviral agents.

Protease Inhibitors

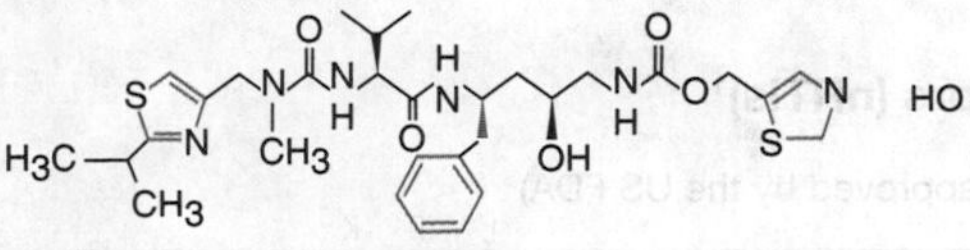

Ritonavir

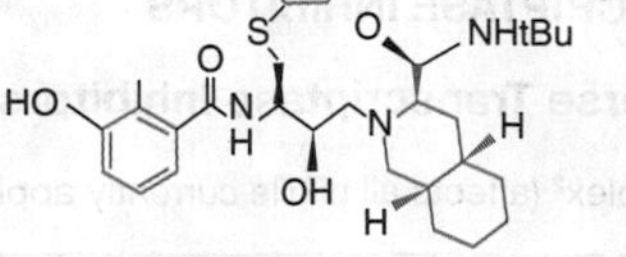

Nelfinavir mesylate

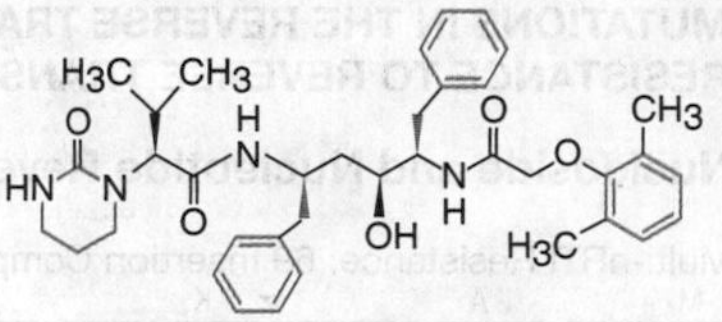

Lopinavir

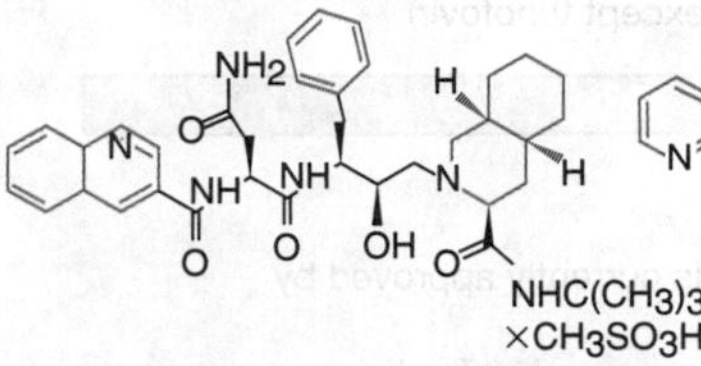

Saquinavir mesylate

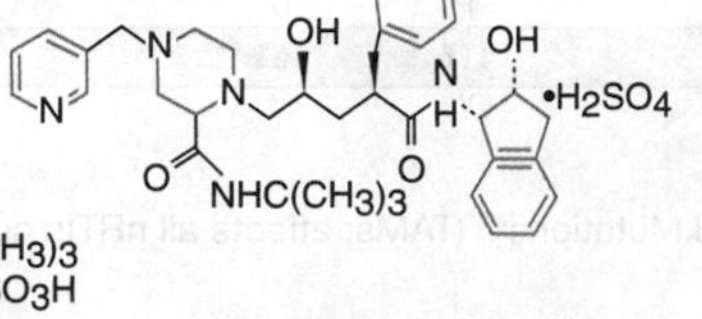

Indinavir sulfate

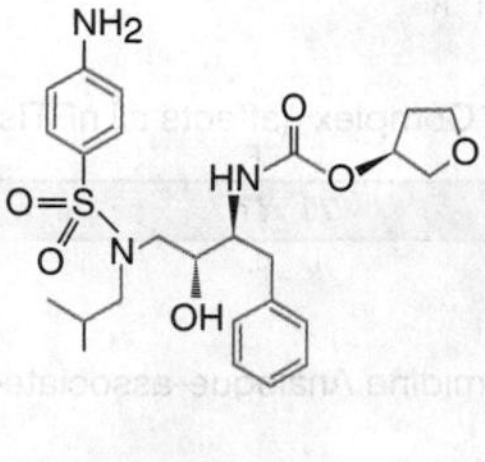

Amprenavir

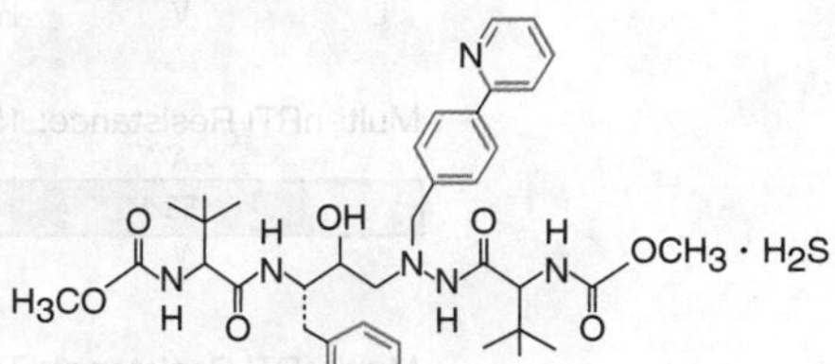

Atazanavir

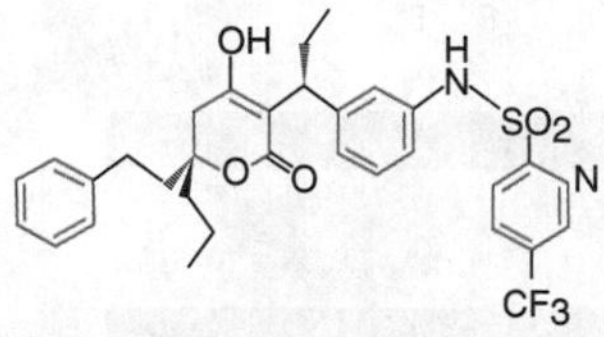

Tipranavir

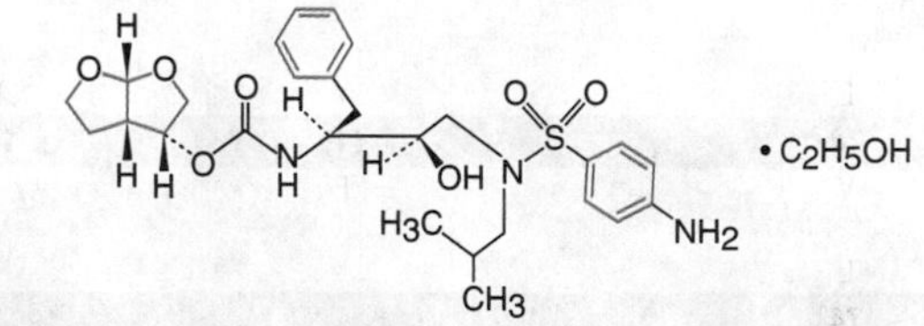

Darunavir

Entry Inhibitors

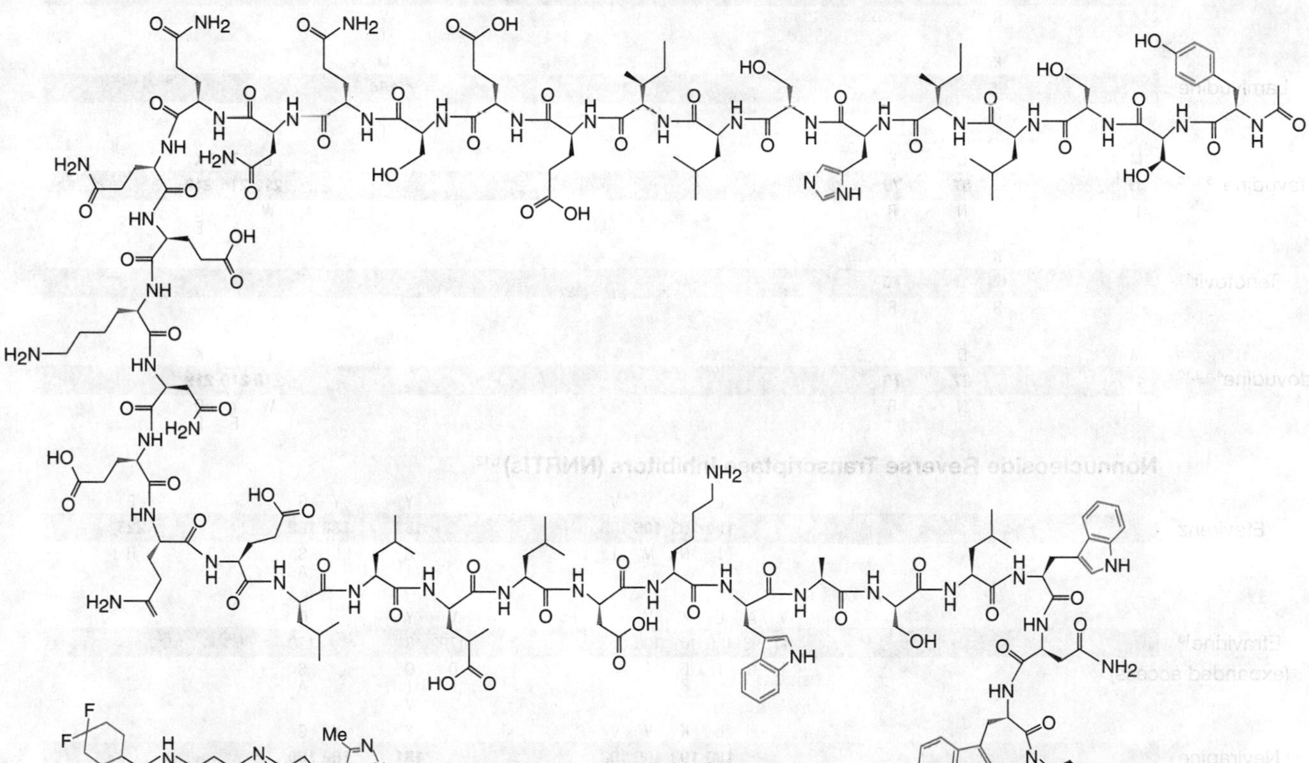

Enfuvirtide

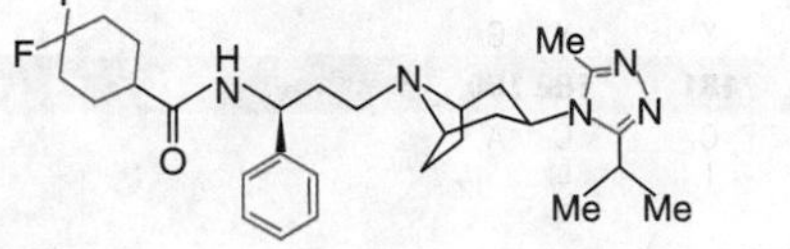

Maraviroc

Integrase Inhibitor

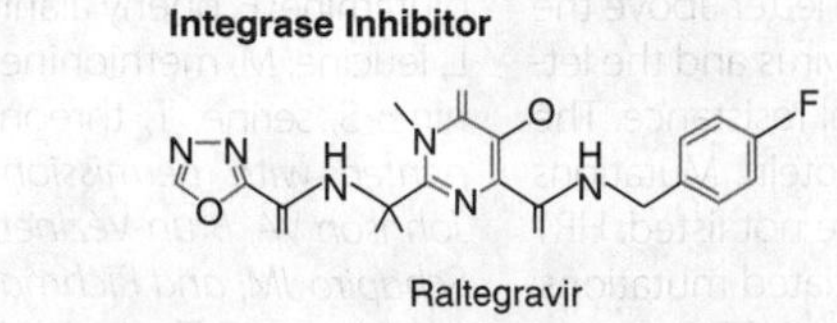

Raltegravir

FIGURE 182-43 (*Continued*)

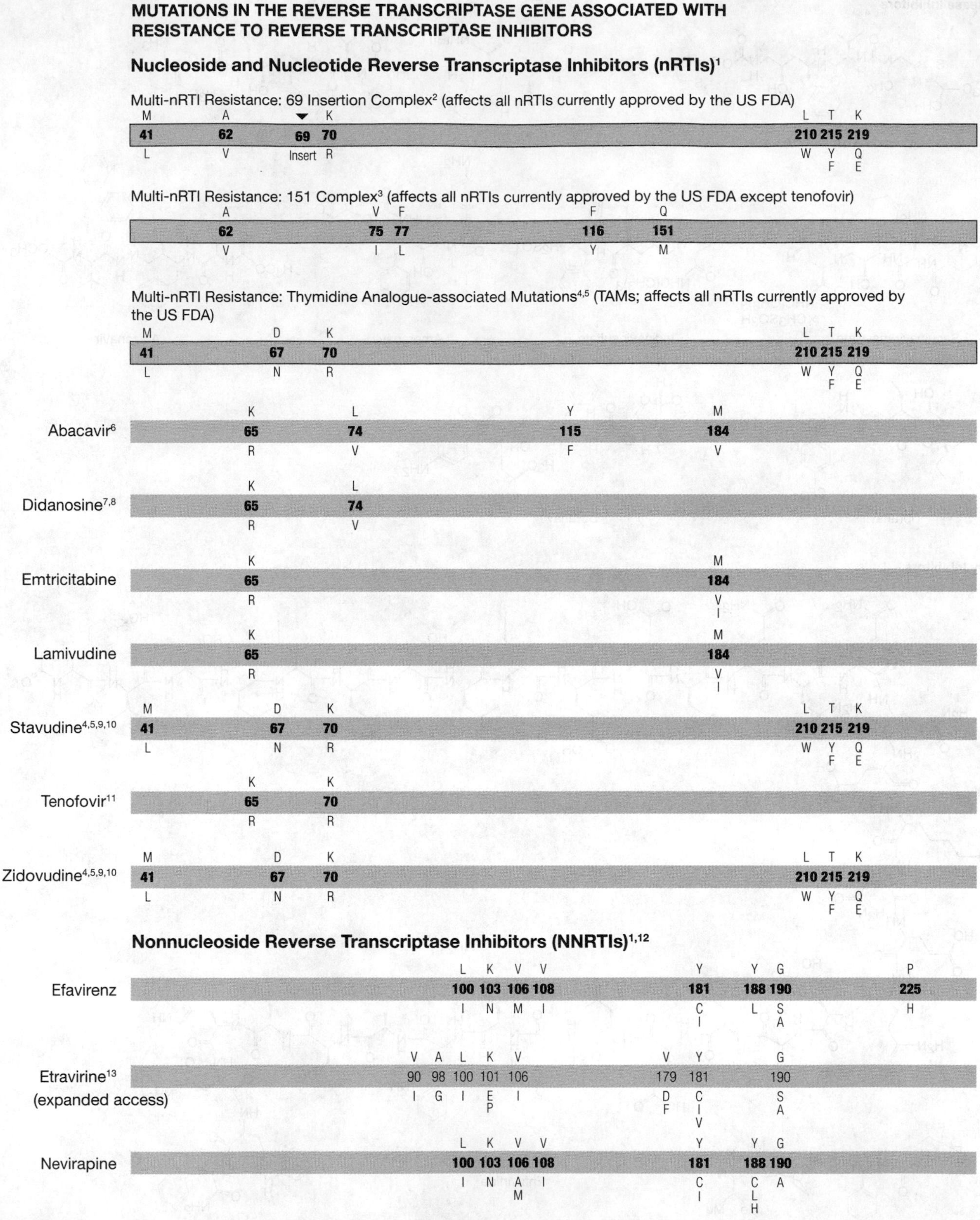

FIGURE 182-44 Amino acid substitutions conferring resistance to antiretroviral drugs. For each amino acid residue, the letter above the bar indicates the amino acid associated with wild-type virus and the letter(s) below indicate the substitution(s) that confer viral resistance. The number shows the position of the mutation in the protein. Mutations selected by protease inhibitors in Gag cleavage sites are not listed. HR1 indicates first heptad repeat; NAMs indicates nRTI-associated mutations; nRTI indicates nucleoside reverse transcriptase inhibitor; NNRTI indicates nonnucleoside reverse transcriptase inhibitor; PI indicates protease inhibitor. Amino acid abbreviations: A, alanine; C, cysteine; D, aspartate; E, glutamine; F, phenylalanine; G, glycine; H, histidine; I, isoleucine; K, lysine; L, leucine; M, methionine; N, asparagine; P, proline; Q, glutamine; R, arginine; S, serine; T, threonine; V, valine; W, tryptophan; Y, tyrosine. *[Reprinted with permission from the International AIDS Society—USA. Johnson VA, Brun-Vézinet F, Clotet B, Günthard HF, Kuritzkes DR, Pillay D, Schapiro JM, and Richman DD. Update of the Drug Resistance Mutations in HIV-1: 2007. Topics in HIV Medicine. 2007; 15(4):119–125. Updated information (and thorough explanatory notes) is available at www.iasusa.org.]*

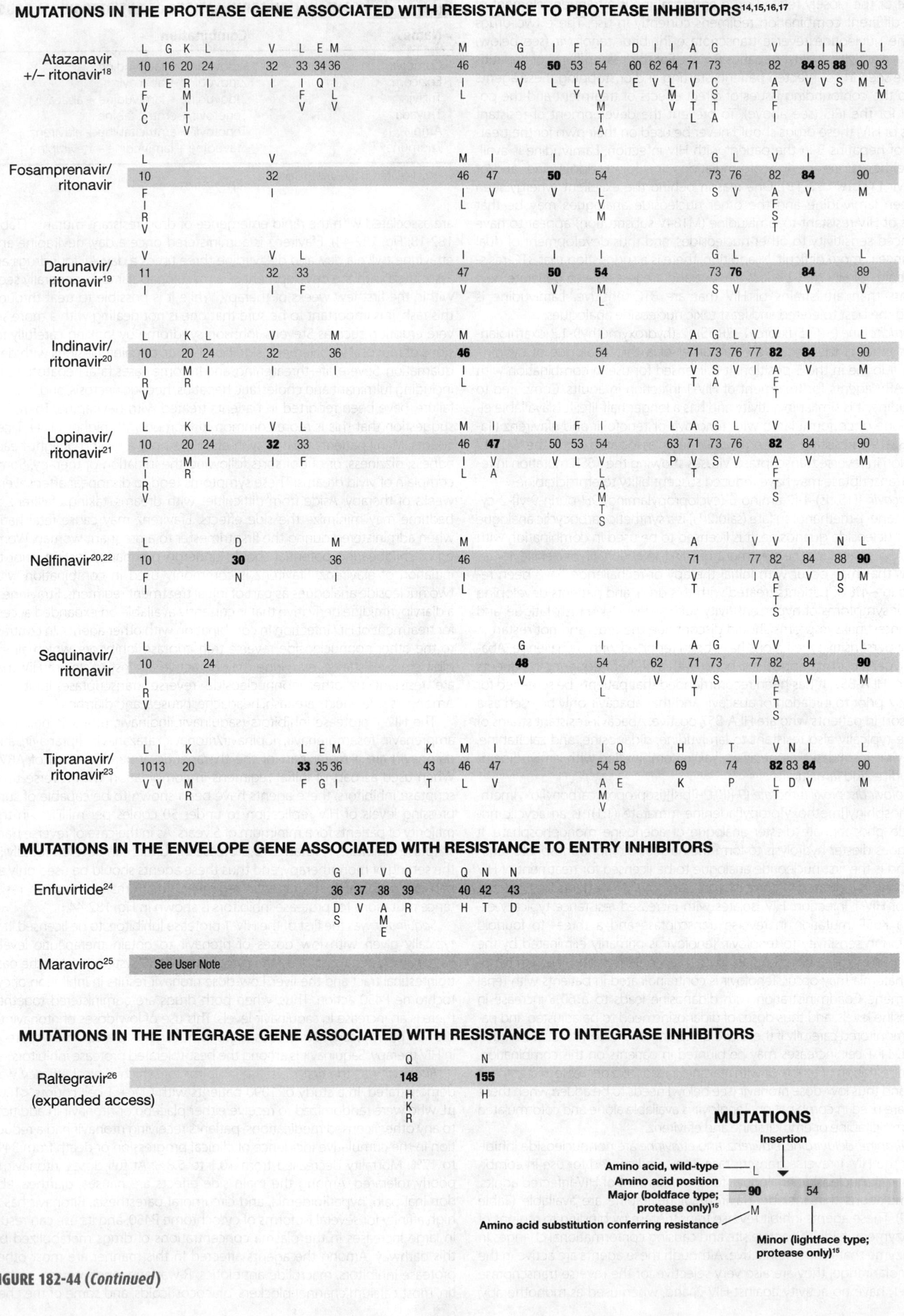
MUTATIONS IN THE PROTEASE GENE ASSOCIATED WITH RESISTANCE TO PROTEASE INHIBITORS[14,15,16,17]
Atazanavir +/– ritonavir[18]
L G K L V L E M M G I F I D I I A G V I I N L I
10 16 20 24 32 33 34 36 46 48 50 53 54 60 62 64 71 73 82 84 85 88 90 93
I F V C / E / R M I T V / I / I / I F V / Q / I L V / I L / V / L / L Y / L V M T A / E / V / L M / V I T / C S T A / A T F I / V / V / S / M / L M
Fosamprenavir/ ritonavir
L V M I I I G L V I L
10 32 46 47 50 54 73 76 82 84 90
F I R V / I / I L / V / V / L V M / S / V / A F S T / V / M
Darunavir/ ritonavir[19]
V V L I I I G L I L
11 32 33 47 50 54 73 76 84 89
I / I / F / V / V / M L / S / V / V / V
Indinavir/ ritonavir[20]
L K L V M M I A G L V V I L
10 20 24 32 36 46 54 71 73 76 77 82 84 90
I R V / M R / I / I / I / I L / V / V T / S A / V / I / A F T / V / M
Lopinavir/ ritonavir[21]
L K L V L M I F I L A G L V I L
10 20 24 32 33 46 47 50 53 54 63 71 73 76 82 84 90
F I R V / M R / I / I / F / I L / V A / V / L / V L A M T S / P / V T / S / V / A F T S / V / M
Nelfinavir[20,22]
L D M M A V V I N L
10 30 36 46 71 77 82 84 88 90
F I / N / I / I L / V T / I / A F T S / V / D S / M
Saquinavir/ ritonavir
L L G I I A G V V I L
10 24 48 54 62 71 73 77 82 84 90
I R V / I / V / V L / V / V T / S / I / A F T S / V / M
Tipranavir/ ritonavir[23]
L L I K L E M K M I I Q H T V N I L
10 13 20 33 35 36 43 46 47 54 58 69 74 82 83 84 90
V / V / M R / F / G / I / T / L / V / A M V / E / K / P / L T / D / V / M
MUTATIONS IN THE ENVELOPE GENE ASSOCIATED WITH RESISTANCE TO ENTRY INHIBITORS
Enfuvirtide[24]
G I V Q Q N N
36 37 38 39 40 42 43
D S / V / A M E / R / H / T / D
Maraviroc[25]
See User Note
MUTATIONS IN THE INTEGRASE GENE ASSOCIATED WITH RESISTANCE TO INTEGRASE INHIBITORS
Raltegravir[26] (expanded access)
Q N
148 155
H K R / H
MUTATIONS
Insertion
Amino acid, wild-type
Amino acid position
Major (boldface type; protease only)[15]
Amino acid substitution conferring resistance
Minor (lightface type; protease only)[15]
L
90 54
M

FIGURE 182-44 *(Continued)*

vudine or the closely related drug emtricitabine is a frequent element of many different combination regimens currently in use. These two drugs and the nucleotide reverse transcriptase inhibitor tenofovir (see below) also have activity against hepatitis B virus. For this reason flares of hepatitis may be seen in co-infected patients starting and or stopping these agents due to the confounding issues of direct effects of treatment and the potential for the IRIS (see above). To prevent the development of resistant strains of HIV, these drugs should never be used on their own for the treatment of hepatitis B in the patient with HIV infection. Lamivudine is available either alone or in coformulations including zidovudine and/or abacavir **(Table 182-19)**. One reason behind the excellent synergy seen between lamivudine and the other nucleoside analogues may be that strains of HIV resistant to lamivudine (M184V substitution) appear to have enhanced sensitivity to other nucleosides, and thus development of dual resistance is more difficult. In addition, there is a suggestion that 3TC-resistant strains of HIV may be less virulent and are less able to generate new mutants than are strains of HIV that are 3TC-sensitive. Lamivudine is among the best tolerated and least toxic nucleoside analogues.

Emtricitabine (FTC; 5-fluoro-1-(2R,5S)-[2-(hydroxymethyl)-1,3-oxathiolan-5-yl]cytosine) is the negative enantiomer of a thio analogue of cytidine with a fluorine in the 5 position. It is licensed for use in combination with other ARV agents for treatment of HIV-1 infection in adults. Compared to lamivudine, it is similar in activity and has a longer half-life. It is available either alone or co-formulated with tenofovir or tenofovir and efavirenz (Table 182-19). Resistance to emtricitabine is associated with the M184V mutation in reverse transcriptase. Viruses showing the K65R mutation in reverse transcriptase may have reduced susceptibility to emtricitabine.

Abacavir {(1S,cis)-4-[2-amino-6-(cyclopropylamino)-9H-purin-9-yl]-2-cyclopentene-1-methanol sulfate (salt)(2:1)} is a synthetic carbocyclic analogue of the nucleoside guanosine. It is licensed to be used in combination with other ARV agents for the treatment of HIV-1 infection. Hypersensitivity reactions that may occur with initial therapy or rechallenge have been reported in ~4% of patients treated with this drug, and patients developing signs or symptoms of hypersensitivity such as fever, skin rash, fatigue, and gastrointestinal symptoms should discontinue the drug and not restart it. Fatal hypersensitivity reactions have been reported with rechallenge. Abacavir hypersensitivity appears to occur with a higher frequency in patients who are HLA-B57. It has been recommended that patients be screened for HLA-B57 prior to initiation of abacavir and that abacavir only be used as a last resort in patients who are HLA-B57 postive. Abacavir-resistant strains of HIV are typically also resistant to lamivudine, didanosine, and zalcitabine. Abacavir is formulated alone as well as in combination with lamivudine or zidovudine and lamivudine.

Tenofovir disoproxil fumarate (9-[(R)-2-[[bis[[(isopropoxycarbonyl)oxy]methoxy]phosphinyl]methoxy]propyl]adenine fumarate (1:1)) is an acyclic nucleoside phosphonate diester analogue of adenosine monophosphate. It undergoes diester hydrolysis to form the nucleoside monophosphate tenofovir and is the first nucleotide analogue to be licensed for treatment of HIV infection. It is indicated in combination with other ARV agents for the treatment of HIV-1 infection. HIV isolates with increased resistance typically express a K65R mutation in reverse transcriptase and a three- to fourfold reduction in sensitivity to tenofovir. Tenofovir is primarily eliminated by the kidneys, and renal impairment including a Fanconi-like syndrome with hypophosphatemia may occur. Tenofovir is contraindicated in patients with renal impairment. Coadministration with didanosine leads to a 60% increase in didanosine levels, and thus doses of didanosine need to be adjusted and patients monitored carefully if these two drugs are used in combination. In addition CD4+ T cell increases may be blunted in patients on this combination. Coadministration of tenofovir with atazanavir leads to a decrease in atazanavir levels and thus low-dose ritonavir (see below) needs to be added when these drugs are used in combination. Tenofovir is available alone and coformulated with emtricitabine or emtricitabine and efavirenz.

Nevirapine, delavirdine, efavirenz, and *etravirine* are nonnucleoside inhibitors of the HIV-1 reverse transcriptase. They are licensed for use in combination with nucleoside analogues for the treatment of HIV-infected adults. Coformulations that include efavirenz or nevirapine are available (Table 182-19). These agents inhibit reverse transcriptase by binding to regions of the enzyme outside the active site and causing conformational changes in the enzyme that render it inactive. Although these agents are active in the nanomolar range, they are also very selective for the reverse transcriptase of HIV-1, have no activity against HIV-2, and, when used as monotherapy, are associated with the rapid emergence of drug-resistant mutants (Table 182-18; Fig. 182-44). Efavirenz is administered once a day, nevirapine and etravirine twice a day, and delavirdine three times a day. All four drugs are associated with the development of a maculopapular rash, generally seen within the first few weeks of therapy. While it is possible to treat through this rash, it is important to be sure that one is not dealing with a more severe eruption such as Stevens-Johnson syndrome by looking carefully for signs of mucosal involvement, significant fever, or painful lesions with desquamation. Severe, life-threatening, and in some cases fatal hepatotoxicity, including fulminant and cholestatic hepatitis, hepatic necrosis, and hepatic failure, have been reported in patients treated with nevirapine. There is a suggestion that this is more common in women with higher CD4+ T cell counts. Many patients treated with efavirenz note a feeling of light-headedness, dizziness, or out of sorts following the initiation of therapy. Some complain of vivid dreams. These symptoms tend to disappear after several weeks of therapy. Aside from difficulties with dreams, taking efavirenz at bedtime may minimize the side effects. Efavirenz may cause fetal harm when administered during the first trimester to a pregnant woman. Women of childbearing potential should undergo pregnancy testing prior to initiation of efavirenz. Efavirenz is commonly used in combination with two nucleoside analogues as part of initial treatment regimens. Etravirine is a diarylpyrimidine derivative that is currently available on expanded access for treatment of HIV infection in combination with other agents. In contrast to the other nonnucleoside reverse transcriptase inhibitors, which all exhibit cross-resistance, etravirine may be active against strains of HIV that are resistant to other nonnucleoside reverse transcriptase inhibitors. Among its side effects are rash, headache, nausea, and diarrhea.

TABLE 182-19 COMBINATION FORMULATIONS OF ANTIRETROVIRAL DRUGS

Name	Combination
Combivir	Zidovudine + lamivudine
Epzicom	Zidovudine + abacavir
Trizivir	Zidovudine + lamivudine + abacavir
Truvada	Tenofovir + emtricitabine
Atripla	Tenofovir + emtricitabine + efavirenz
Triomune[a]	Stavudine + lamivudine + nevirapine

[a]Not licensed in the United States.

The HIV-1 protease inhibitors (saquinavir, indinavir, ritonavir, nelfinavir, amprenavir, fosamprenavir, lopinavir/ritonavir, atazanavir, tipranavir, and darunavir) are a major part of the therapeutic armamentarium of ARVs. When used as part of initial regimens in combination with reverse transcriptase inhibitors, these agents have been shown to be capable of suppressing levels of HIV replication to under 50 copies per milliliter in the majority of patients for a minimum of 5 years. As in the case of reverse transcriptase inhibitors, resistance to protease inhibitors can develop rapidly in the setting of monotherapy, and thus these agents should be used only as part of combination therapeutic regimens. A summary of known resistance mutations for protease inhibitors is shown in Fig. 182-44.

Saquinavir was the first of the HIV-1 protease inhibitors to be licensed. It is typically given with low doses of ritonavir to obtain therapeutic levels. Saquinavir is metabolized by the cytochrome P450 system in both the gastrointestinal tract and the liver. Low-dose ritonavir results in inhibition of cytochrome P450 action. Thus, when both drugs are administered together there is an increase in saquinavir levels. This use of low doses of ritonavir to provide pharmacodynamic boosting of other agents is a common strategy in HIV therapy. Saquinavir is among the best-tolerated protease inhibitors.

Ritonavir was the first protease inhibitor for which clinical efficacy was demonstrated. In a study of 1090 patients with CD4+ T cell counts <100/μL who were randomized to receive either placebo or ritonavir in addition to any other licensed medications, patients receiving ritonavir had a reduction in the cumulative incidence of clinical progression or death from 34% to 17%. Mortality decreased from 10.1 to 5.8%. At full doses, ritonavir is poorly tolerated. Among the main side effects are nausea, diarrhea, abdominal pain, hyperlipidemia, and circumoral paresthesia. Ritonavir has a high affinity for several isoforms of cytochrome P450, and its use can result in large increases in the plasma concentrations of drugs metabolized by this pathway. Among the agents affected in this manner are most other protease inhibitors, macrolide antibiotics, R-warfarin, ondansetron, rifabutin, most calcium channel blockers, glucocorticoids, and some of the chemotherapeutic agents used to treat KS and/or lymphomas. In addition, ritonavir may increase the activity of glucuronyltransferases, thus decreasing the levels of drugs metabolized by this pathway. Overall, great care must be taken when prescribing additional drugs to patients taking protease inhibitors in general and ritonavir in particular. As mentioned above, the pharmacodynamic boosting property of ritonavir, seen with doses as low as 100–200 mg once or twice a day, is often used in the setting of combination ARV therapy for HIV infection to derive more convenient regimens. For example, when given with low-dose ritonavir, saquinavir and indinavir can both be given on twice-a-day schedules and taken with food.

Indinavir was the first protease inhibitor used in combination with dual nucleoside therapy. The combination of zidovudine, lamivudine, and indinavir was the first "triple combination" shown to have a profound effect on HIV replication. The main side effects of indinavir are nephrolithiasis (seen in 4% of patients) and asymptomatic indirect hyperbilirubinemia (seen in 10%). Indinavir is predominantly metabolized by the liver. The dose should be lowered in patients with cirrhosis. Levels of indinavir are decreased during concurrent therapy with rifabutin, efavirenz, or nevirapine and increased during concurrent therapy with ketoconazole, delavirdine, or ritonavir. Dosages should be modified appropriately in these circumstances (Table 182-18).

Nelfinavir was approved in 1997 and *amprenavir* was approved in 1999 for the treatment of adult or pediatric HIV infection when ARV therapy is warranted. As with most of the newer ARV agents, these approvals were based on randomized, controlled trials that demonstrated decreases in plasma HIV RNA levels and increases in CD4+ T cell counts. The presence of the potential carcinogen and teratogen ethyl methanesulfonate in nelfinavir preparations makes it a drug to be avoided in pregnant women. Both nelfinavir and amprenavir have unique resistance profiles. Nelfinavir resistance is associated with a D30N substitution in the protease gene. Viruses harboring this single mutation retain sensitivity to other protease inhibitors. While it has been suggested that for this reason nelfinavir is a good initial protease inhibitor, enthusiasm for its use has waned following the 48-week clinical trials data demonstrating the virologic inferiority of nelfinavir to lopinavir/ritonavir, to fosamprenavir, and to efavirenz. Protease inhibitor resistance typically involves multiple amino acid substitutions and reduced susceptibility across the class. Amprenavir resistance is associated with a unique substitution at amino acid 50 (I50V). Nelfinavir and amprenavir are both associated with gastrointestinal side effects. About 1% of patients receiving amprenavir have experienced severe and life-threatening skin reactions. An additional disadvantage of amprenavir is that the original formulation requires the patient to take 8 large capsules twice a day. Amprenavir has largely been replaced by fosamprenavir (see below).

Fosamprenavir was licensed in 2003 for the treatment of HIV infection in combination with other ARV agents in adults. It is a prodrug of amprenavir that is rapidly converted to amprenavir by cellular phosphatases. It is supplied as a 700-mg tablet. The recommended dosage is 1400 mg bid or 700 mg bid with ritonavir, 100 mg bid, or 1400 mg once a day with ritonavir, 200 mg once a day. As noted above, ritonavir-boosted fosamprenavir has been shown to be comparable to lopinavir/ritonavir and efavirenz in combination regimens.

Lopinavir/ritonavir (Kaletra) is a fixed-dose combination of the protease inhibitors lopinavir (200 mg) and ritonavir (50 mg). It was licensed in 2000 for treatment of HIV-1 infection in adults and children in combination with other agents. A main advantage of this pill is that it combines the pharmacologic enhancement of low-dose ritonavir with a second protease inhibitor in a single capsule. In a randomized, controlled trial, this combination capsule was found to be superior to nelfinavir. Its main complications are gastrointestinal upset and hyperlipidemia.

Atazanavir is an azapeptide inhibitor of the HIV-1 protease that was licensed in 2003. An advantage of atazanavir is that total cholesterol and triglyceride levels do not increase as much with atazanavir as with other protease inhibitors. This coupled with the fact that it can be given on a once-daily schedule has made atazanavir a popular component of initial treatment regimens. Atazanavir is associated with increases in serum bilirubin and prolongations of the ECG PR interval. Atazanavir-resistant isolates emerging in previously treatment-naïve individuals frequently harbor an I50L substitution. This mutation in some instances is associated with increased sensitivity to other protease inhibitors. Atazanavir requires an acidic gastric pH for absorption, and its use in combination with a proton pump inhibitor is contraindicated due to concerns about absorption. Atazanavir is an inhibitor of cytochrome P3A and its use may be associated with increased levels of calcium channel blockers, macrolide antibiotics, HMB-CoA reductase inhibitors, and sildenafil. Levels of atazanavir are lower in the presence of tenofovir or efavirenz. In these settings, levels of atazanavir should be boosted with the use of low-dose ritonavir.

Tipranavir is a non-peptidic HIV protease inhibitor licensed in 2005. It is licensed for use in combination with 200 mg ritonavir and is indicated for combination ARV therapy of HIV-1 infection in treatment-experienced adults or in adults with evidence of HIV-1 strains resistant to multiple protease inhibitors. Tipranavir was found to be inferior to lopinavir/ritonavir in a randomized controlled trial in naïve patients. In that study, at lower doses it was virologically inferior while at higher doses it exhibited a greater degree of hepatotoxicity. The main side effects of tipranavir are gastrointestinal intolerance and skin rash; the latter is seen in ~10% of patients and may be related to the sulfonamide moiety in the molecule. Tipranavir coadministered with ritonavir has also been associated with reports of intracranial hemorrhage as well as reports of clinical hepatitis and hepatic decompensation, including some fatalities in both settings. The risk of hepatotoxicity is increased in patients with hepatitis B or C co-infection.

Darunavir is a non-peptidic HIV protease inhibitor licensed in 2006 to be coadministered with 100 mg of ritonavir and other ARV agents for the treatment of HIV infection in ARV treatment–experienced adults. This indication is based on the fact that the trials leading to licensure of darunavir were carried out in treatment-experienced patients. In these studies 46% of patients achieved a reduction in HIV RNA viral loads to <50 copies per milliliter. Studies are underway in treatment-naïve patients. Skin rash, which may be severe, is seen in 7% of patients and may be related to the sulfonamide moiety contained in the molecule. Gastrointestinal intolerance and headache are the other most frequent side effects.

Entry inhibitors act by interfering with the binding of HIV to its receptor or co-receptor or by interfering with the process of fusion (see above). The first drug in this class to be licensed was the fusion inhibitor *enfuvirtide*, or T-20, followed by the CCR5 antagonist *maraviroc*. A variety of additional small molecules that bind to HIV-1 co-receptors are currently in clinical trials.

Enfuvirtide is a linear 36-amino-acid synthetic peptide with the *N*-terminus acetylated and the *C*-terminus a carboxamide. It is composed of naturally occurring L-amino acid residues and interferes with the fusion of the viral and cellular membranes by binding to the HR1 region in the gp41 subunit of the HIV-1 envelope. This binding interferes with the coil-coil interaction required to approximate the two membranes. Resistant isolates of HIV exhibit amino acid changes in positions 36–45 of gp41. In two independent studies, patients who had persistent viremia despite prior treatment with agents from all three available classes of drugs were randomized to receive an individualized regimen (based upon prior treatment history and resistance profile) with or without enfuvirtide. The change in plasma HIV-1 RNA from baseline was ~1 log greater (–1.53 vs. –0.68) in patients randomized to receive enfuvirtide. Among the drawbacks of this agent are the requirement for twice-a-day injection, the occurrence of injection site reactions in close to 100% of patients, and an increase in bacterial pneumonia in the enfuvirtide-treated patients compared to the patients in the control arm (4.68 vs. 0.61 events per 100 patient years) in the phase III studies.

Maraviroc is a CCR5 antagonist that interferes with HIV binding at the stage of co-receptor engagement. It was licensed in 2007 for treatment of HIV infection in combination with other agents in treatment-experienced patients infected with only CCR5-tropic virus resistant to multiple agents. A co-receptor tropism assay should be performed if one is considering the use of maraviroc to ensure that the potential patient is harboring R5 virus. In phase III trials of treatment-experienced patients randomized to receive optimal therapy plus maraviroc or placebo, 61% of patients randomized to maraviroc achieved HIV RNA levels <400 copies/mL compared to 28% of patients randomized to placebo. An allergic reaction-associated hepatotoxicity has been reported with maraviroc. Among the most common side effects of maraviroc are dizziness due to postural hypotension, cough, fever, colds, rash, muscle and joint pain, and stomach pain. Maraviroc is a substrate of CYP3A and Pgp and the recommend dose varies depending upon concomitant medications. In combination with nucleoside analogues, tipranavir/ritonavir, enfuvirtide and/or nevirapine the dose is 300 mg twice daily. In the presence of CYP3A inhibitors such as most protease inhibitors the dose is 150 mg twice daily and in presence of CYP3A inducers such as efavirenz the dose is 600 mg twice daily.

The newest class of ARV compounds are the *integrase inhibitors*. *Raltegravir* is an inhibitor of the viral enzyme integrase and the first of this class to be approved. It was approved in 2007 for treatment of HIV infection in combination with other agents in treatment experienced patients. Raltegravir exhibits a wide range of activity against HIV-1 and HIV-2 including viruses with multiple resistance mutations to other classes of drugs. As with several other compounds, resistance to raltegravir comes at the expense of replicative fitness. In two phase III studies in which 436 patients with 3-class ARV drug resistance were randomized to an optimized background regimen with raltegravir or placebo, 76% of patients receiving raltegravir achieved HIV RNA levels <400 copies/mL compared to 41% of patients randomized to the placebo arm. In contrast to many other antiretroviral drugs the side effect profile of raltegravir is minimal with similar side effect profiles noted for the raltegravir and placebo groups.

PRINCIPLES OF THERAPY The principles of therapy for HIV infection have been articulated by a panel sponsored by the U.S. Department of Health and Human Services as a working group of the NIH Office of AIDS Research Advisory Council These principles are summarized in **Table 182-20**. As noted in these guidelines, eradication of HIV infection has not yet been possible. Treatment decisions must take into account the fact that one is dealing with a chronic infection. While early therapy is generally the rule in infectious diseases, immediate treatment of every HIV-infected individual upon diagnosis may not be prudent, and therapeutic decisions must take into account the balance between risks and benefits. While it seems reasonable to assume that the complications associated with ARV therapy could be minimized by regimens designed to minimize exposure to the drugs in question, all efforts to do so have paradoxically been associated with an increase in serious adverse events in the patients randomized to intermittent therapy suggesting that some "non-AIDS" associated serious adverse events such as heart attack and stroke may be linked to HIV replication. Thus, unless contraindicated for reasons of toxicity, patients started on ARV therapy should remain on ARV therapy.

At present, a reasonable course of action is to initiate ARV therapy in anyone with the acute HIV syndrome; all pregnant women; patients with symptomatic disease; and patients with asymptomatic disease with CD4+ T cell counts <350/μL (**Table 182-21**). In addition, one may wish to administer a 6-week course of therapy to uninfected individuals immediately following a high-risk exposure to HIV.

Once the decision has been made to initiate therapy, the health care provider must decide which drugs to use as the first regimen. The decision regarding choice of drugs not only will affect the immediate response to therapy but also will have implications regarding options for future therapeutic regimens. The initial regimen is usually the most effective insofar as the virus has yet to develop significant resistance. The two options for initial therapy most commonly in use today are two different three-drug regimens. The first regimen utilizes two nucleoside analogues (one of which is usually lamivudine or emtricitabine) and a nonnucleoside reverse transcriptase inhibitor. The second regimen utilizes two nucleoside analogues and a protease inhibitor. Unfortunately there are no clear data at present on which to base distinctions between these two approaches. Following the initiation of therapy one should expect a 1 log (tenfold) reduction in plasma HIV RNA levels within 1–2 months and eventually a decline in plasma HIV RNA levels to <50 copies per milliliter. During this same time there should be a rise in the CD4+ T cell count of 100–150/μL that is particularly brisk during the first month of therapy. Many clinicians feel that failure to achieve this endpoint is an indication for a change in therapy. Other reasons for a change in therapy include a persistently declining CD4+ T cell count, clinical deterioration, or drug toxicity (**Table 182-22**). As in the case of initiating therapy, changing therapy may have a lasting impact on future therapeutic options. When changing therapy because of treatment failure (clinical progression or worsening laboratory parameters), it is important to attempt to provide a regimen with at least two new active drugs. This decision can be guided by resistance testing (see below). In the patient in whom a change is made for reasons of drug toxicity, a simple replacement of one drug is reasonable. It should be stressed that in attempting to sort out a drug toxicity it may be advisable to hold all therapy for a period of time to distinguish between drug toxicity and disease progression. Drug toxicity will usually begin to show signs of reversal within 1–2 weeks. Prior to changing a treatment regimen because of drug failure, it is important to ensure that the patient has been adherent to the prescribed regimen. As in the case of initial therapy, the simpler the new therapeutic regimen, the easier it is for the patient to be compliant. Plasma HIV RNA levels and CD4+ T lymphocyte counts should be monitored every 3–4 months during therapy and more frequently if one is contemplating a change in regimen or immediately following a change in regimen.

In an attempt to determine an optimal therapeutic regimen, one may attempt to measure ARV drug susceptibility through genotyping or phenotyping of HIV quasispecies and determine adequacy of dosing through measurement of drug levels. Genotyping may be done through dideoxynucleotide sequencing, DNA chip hybridization, or line probe assays. Phe-

TABLE 182-20 PRINCIPLES OF THERAPY OF HIV INFECTION

1. Ongoing HIV replication leads to immune system damage and progression to AIDS.
2. Plasma HIV RNA levels indicate the magnitude of HIV replication and the rate of CD4+ T cell destruction. CD4+ T cell counts indicate the current level of competence of the immune system.
3. Rates of disease progression differ among individuals, and treatment decisions should be individualized based upon plasma HIV RNA levels and CD4+ T cell counts.
4. Maximal suppression of viral replication is a goal of therapy; the greater the suppression the less likely the appearance of drug-resistant quasispecies.
5. The most effective therapeutic strategies involve the simultaneous initiation of combinations of effective anti-HIV drugs with which the patient has not been previously treated and that are not cross-resistant with antiretroviral agents that the patient has already received.
6. The antiretroviral drugs used in combination regimens should be used according to optimum schedules and dosages.
7. The number of available drugs is limited. Any decisions on antiretroviral therapy have a long-term impact on future options for the patient.
8. Women should receive optimal antiretroviral therapy regardless of pregnancy status.
9. The same principles apply to children and adults. The treatment of HIV-infected children involves unique pharmacologic, virologic, and immunologic considerations.
10. Compliance is an important part of ensuring maximal effect from a given regimen. The simpler the regimen, the easier it is for the patient to be compliant.

Source: Modified from *Principles of Therapy of HIV Infection*, USPHS, and the Henry J. Kaiser Family Foundation.

TABLE 182-21 INDICATIONS FOR THE INITIATION OF ANTIRETROVIRAL THERAPY IN PATIENTS WITH HIV INFECTION

I. Acute infection syndrome
II. Chronic infection
  A. Symptomatic disease (including HIV-associated nephropathy)
  B. Asymptomatic diseases
    1. CD4+ T cell count <350/μL[a]
    2. Pregnancy
III. Postexposure prophylaxis

[a]This is an area of controversy. Some experts would wait until the CD4 cell count declines to 200/μL, some would treat everyone with a viral load >100,000 copies/mL, whereas others would treat everyone regardless of CD4+ T cell count.
Source: *Guidelines for the Use of Antiretroviral Agents in HIV-Infected Adults and Adolescents*, USPH.

TABLE 182-22 INDICATIONS FOR CHANGING ANTIRETROVIRAL THERAPY IN PATIENTS WITH HIV INFECTION[a]

Less than a 1-log drop in plasma HIV RNA by 4 weeks following the initiation of therapy
A reproducible significant increase (defined as 3-fold or greater) from the nadir of plasma HIV RNA level not attributable to intercurrent infection, vaccination, or test methodology
Persistently declining CD4+ T cell numbers
Clinical deterioration
Side effects

[a]Generally speaking, a change should involve the initiation of at least 2 drugs felt to be effective in the given patient. The exception to this is when change is being made to manage toxicity, in which case a single substitution is reasonable.
Source: *Guidelines for the Use of Antiretroviral Agents in HIV-Infected Adults and Adolescents*, USPHS.

notypic assays typically measure the enzymatic activity of viral enzymes in the presence or absence of different concentrations of different drugs and have also been used to determine co-receptor tropism. These assays will generally detect quasispecies present at a frequency of ≥10%. The precise role of resistance testing in the management of patients with HIV infection is not yet clear. It is generally recommended that resistance testing be used in selecting initial therapy in settings where the risk of transmission of resistant virus is high (such as the United States and Europe) and in determining new regimens for patients experiencing virologic failure while on therapy. Resistance testing may be of particular value in distinguishing drug-resistant virus from poor patient compliance. Due to the rapid rate at which drug-resistant viruses revert to wild-type, it is recommended that resistant testing performed in the setting of drug failure be carried out while the patient is still on the failing regimen. Measurement of plasma drug levels can also be used to tailor an individual treatment. The inhibitory quotient, defined as the trough blood level/IC50 of the patient's virus, is used by some to determine the adequacy of dosing of a given treatment regimen.

In addition to the licensed medications discussed above, a large number of experimental agents are being evaluated as possible therapies for HIV infection. Therapeutic strategies are being developed that interfere with virtually every step of the replication cycle of the virus (Fig. 182-3). In addition, as more is discovered about the role of the immune system in controlling viral replication, additional strategies, generically referred to as "immune-based therapies," are being developed as a complement to antiviral therapy. Among the antiviral agents in early clinical trials are additional nucleoside and nucleotide analogues, protease inhibitors, fusion inhibitors, receptor and co-receptor antagonists, and integrase inhibitors as well as new anti-viral strategies including antisense nucleic acids and maturation inhibitors. Among the immune-based therapies being evaluated are IFN-α, bone marrow transplantation, adoptive transfer of lymphocytes genetically modified to resist infection or enhance HIV-specific immunity, active immunotherapy with inactivated HIV or its components, IL-2, and IL-7.

HIV AND THE HEALTH CARE WORKER

Health care workers, especially those who deal with large numbers of HIV-infected patients, have a small but definite risk of becoming infected with HIV as a result of professional activities (see "Occupational Transmission of HIV: Health Care Workers, Laboratory Workers, and the Health Care Setting," above). The first case of HIV transmission from a patient to health care worker was reported in 1984. By the end of 2002, 106 health care workers worldwide were documented as having seroconverted to HIV following occupational HIV exposure; another 238 possible occupational seroconversions had been reported. Only three of these cases were reported from sub-Saharan Africa, where HIV is most prevalent. Hence it is likely that the global prevalence of occupationally acquired HIV infection is much higher than has been reported.

In the United States 57 health care workers have become infected with HIV by occupational exposure; 26 have developed AIDS. The individuals who seroconverted include 19 laboratory workers (16 of whom were clinical laboratory workers), 24 nurses, 6 physicians, 2 surgical technicians, 1 dialysis technician, 1 respiratory therapist, 1 health aide, 1 embalmer/morgue technician, and 2 housekeeper/maintenance workers. The exposures included 48 percutaneous (puncture/cut injury), 5 mucocutaneous (mucous membrane and/or skin), 2 both percutaneous and mucocutaneous, and 2 unknown route of exposure. Forty-nine exposures were to HIV-infected blood, three to concentrated virus in a laboratory, one to visibly bloody fluid, and four to an unspecified fluid. As of January 1, 2003, there had been 139 other cases of HIV infection or AIDS among health care workers who have not reported other risk factors for HIV infection and who report a history of exposure to blood, body fluids, or HIV-infected laboratory material, but for whom seroconversion after exposure was not documented. The number of these workers who actually acquired their infection through occupational exposures is not known. Taken together, the data from several large studies suggest that the risk of HIV infection following a percutaneous exposure to HIV-contaminated blood is ~0.3%, and after a mucous membrane exposure, ~0.09%. Although episodes of HIV transmission after nonintact skin exposure have been documented, the average risk for transmission by this route has not been precisely quantified but is estimated to be less than the risk for mucous membrane exposures. The risk for transmission after exposure to fluids or tissues other than HIV-infected blood also has not been quantified but is probably considerably lower than for blood exposures. A seroprevalence survey of 3420 orthopedic surgeons, 75% of whom practiced in an area with a relatively high prevalence of HIV infection and 39% of whom reported percutaneous exposure to patient blood, usually through an accident involving a suture needle, failed to reveal any cases of possible occupational infection, suggesting that the risk of infection with a suture needle may be considerably less than that with a blood-drawing needle.

Most cases of health care worker seroconversion occur as a result of needle-stick injuries. When one considers the circumstances that result in needle-stick injuries, it is immediately obvious that adhering to the standard guidelines for dealing with sharp objects would result in a significant decrease in this type of accident. In one study, 27% of needle-stick injuries resulted from improper disposal of the needle (over half of these were due to recapping the needle), 23% occurred during attempts to start an IV line, 22% occurred during blood drawing, 16% were associated with an IM or SC injection, and 12% were associated with giving an IV infusion.

Clinicians should consider potential occupational exposures to HIV as urgent medical concerns to ensure timely postexposure management and possible administration of postexposure ARV prophylaxis (PEP). Recommendations regarding PEP must take into account that several circumstances determine the risk of transmission of HIV following occupational exposure. In this regard, several factors have been associated with an increased risk for occupational transmission of HIV infection, including deep injury, the presence of visible blood on the instrument causing the exposure, injury with a device that had been placed in the vein or artery of the source patient, terminal illness in the source patient, and lack of postexposure ARV therapy in the exposed health care worker. Other important considerations when considering PEP in the health care worker include known or suspected pregnancy or breastfeeding, the possibility of exposure to drug-resistant virus, and toxicities of PEP regimens. Regardless of the decision to use PEP, the wound should be cleansed immediately and antiseptic applied. If a decision is made to offer PEP, U.S. Public Health Service guidelines recommend (1) a combination of two nucleoside analogue reverse transcriptase inhibitors given for 4 weeks for less severe exposures, or (2) a combination of two nucleoside analogue reverse transcriptase inhibitors plus a third drug given for 4 weeks for more severe exposures. Most clinicians administer the latter regimen in all cases in which a decision is made to treat. Detailed guidelines are available from the *Updated U.S. Public Health Service Guidelines for the Management of Occupational Exposures to HIV and Recommendations for Postexposure Prophylaxis* (CDC, 2005). The report emphasizes the importance of adherence to PEP when it is indicated; follow-up of exposed workers to improve PEP adherences, monitoring for adverse events (including seroconversion), and expert consultation in the management of exposures.

For consultation on the treatment of occupational exposures to HIV and other bloodborne pathogens, the clinician managing the exposed patient can call the National Clinicians' Post-Exposure Prophylaxis Hotline (Pepsine) at 888-HIV-4911 (888-448-4911). This service is available 24 h a day, at no charge (additional information on the Internet is available at *http://www.ucsf.edu/hivcntr*). Pepsine support may be especially useful in challenging situations, such as when drug-resistant HIV strains are suspected or the health care worker is pregnant.

Health care workers can minimize their risk of occupational HIV infection by following the CDC guidelines of July 1991, which include adherence to universal precautions, refraining from direct patient care if one has exudative lesions or weeping dermatitis, and disinfecting and sterilizing reusable devices employed in invasive procedures. The premise of universal precautions is that every specimen should be handled as if it came from someone infected with a bloodborne pathogen. All samples should be double-bagged, gloves should be worn when drawing blood, and spills should be immediately disinfected with bleach.

In attempting to put this small but definite risk to the health care worker in perspective, it is important to point out that ~200 health care workers die each year as a result of occupationally acquired hepatitis B infection. The tragedy in this instance is that these infections and deaths due to HBV could be greatly decreased by more extended use of the HBV vaccine. The risk of HBV infection following a needle-stick injury from a hepatitis antigen–positive patient is much higher than the risk of HIV infection (see "Transmission," above). There are multiple examples of needle-stick injuries where the patient was positive for both HBV and HIV and the health care worker became infected only with HBV. For these reasons, it is advisable, given the high prevalence of HBV infection in HIV-infected individuals, that all health care workers dealing with HIV-infected patients be immunized with the HBV vaccine.

TB is another infection common to HIV-infected patients that can be transmitted to the health care worker. For this reason, all health care workers should know their PPD status, have it checked yearly, and receive 6 months of isoniazid treatment if their skin test converts to positive. In addition, all patients in whom a diagnosis of TB is being entertained should be placed immediately in respiratory isolation, pending results of the diagnostic evaluation. The emergence of drug-resistant organisms, including the extensively drug resistant TB strains that have been identified in Africa, has made TB an increasing problem for health care workers. This is particularly true for the health care worker with preexisting HIV infection.

One of the most charged issues ever to come between health care workers and patients is that of transmission of infection from HIV-infected health care workers to their patients. This is discussed under "Occupational Transmission of HIV: Health Care Workers, Laboratory Workers, and the Health Care Setting," above. Theoretically, the same universal precautions that are used to protect the health care worker from the HIV-infected patient will also protect the patient from the HIV-infected health care worker.

VACCINES

Given that human behavior, especially human sexual behavior, is extremely difficult to change, a critical modality for preventing the spread of HIV infection is the development of a safe and effective vaccine. Historically, vaccines have provided a safe, cost-effective, and efficient means of preventing illness, disability, and death from infectious diseases. Successful vaccines for the most part are predicated on the assumption that the body can mount an adequate immune response to the microbe or virus in question during natural infection, and that the vaccine will mimic the natural response to infection. Even with serious diseases such as smallpox, poliomyelitis, measles, and influenza among others, the body in the vast majority of cases clears the infectious agent and provides protection against future exposure. Unfortunately, this is not the case with HIV infection since the natural immune response to HIV infection is unable to clear the virus from the body and cases of superinfection have been reported. Some of the factors that contribute to the problematic nature of development of a preventive HIV vaccine are the high mutability of the virus, the fact that the infection can be transmitted by cell-free or cell-associated virus, the likely need for the development of effective mucosal immunity, and the fact that it has been difficult to establish the precise correlates of protective immunity to HIV infection. Some HIV-infected individuals are long-term nonprogressors (see above), and a number of individuals have been exposed to HIV multiple times but remain uninfected; these facts suggest that there are elements of an HIV-specific immune response that have the potential to be protective. Early attempts to develop a vaccine with the envelope protein gp120 aimed at inducing neutralizing antibodies in humans were performed based on the induction of neutralizing antibodies in non-human primates. The significance of the laboratory assays were unknown at the time, and the elicited antisera failed to neutralize primary isolates of HIV cultured and tested in fresh peripheral blood mononuclear cells. In this regard, two phase 3 trials were undertaken in the United States and Thailand using soluble gp120, and the vaccines failed to protect human volunteers from HIV infection. It should be pointed out that while the ideal goal of an HIV vaccine is to prevent infection, a vaccine given to an uninfected individual that significantly alters the course of disease or the infectivity of the individual, should that person become infected, could have an impact not only on the individual in question but also on the spread of infection in the community. In this regard, a number of studies in monkeys using vaccines that induce predominantly cellular (T cell) immune responses have not protected the animals against infection but have lowered the initial burst of viremia following acute infection as well as decreased temporarily the viral set point. Since most sexually transmitted HIV infections occur when the transmitting partner is experiencing high levels of viremia such as during the acute phase of HIV infection or during the advanced stage of disease when the viral load is high, such a vaccine, which might limit the initial burst of viremia in primary infection and decrease the established viral set point, could have benefits for the individual as well as for their sexual partners. It is clear that it will take several years of clinical trials to establish the efficacy or lack thereof of a candidate vaccine for HIV.

PREVENTION

Education, counseling, and behavior modification are the cornerstones of an HIV prevention strategy. A major problem in the United States and elsewhere is that many infections are passed on by those who do not know that they are infected. Of the >1 million persons in the United States who are HIV-infected, it is estimated that ~25% do not know their HIV status and thus may be putting others at risk by their own behavior. In this regard, the CDC has recently recommended that HIV testing become part of routine medical care and that all individuals between the ages of 13 and 64 years be informed of the testing and be tested without the need for written informed consent. The individual could "opt out" of testing, but if not, testing would be routinely administered. In addition to identifying individuals who might benefit from ARV therapy, information gathered from such an approach should serve as the basis for behavior-modification programs, both for infected individuals who may be unaware of their HIV status and who could infect others and for uninfected individuals practicing high-risk behavior. The practice of "safer sex" is the most effective way for sexually active uninfected individuals to avoid contracting HIV infection and for infected individuals to avoid spreading infection. Abstinence from sexual relations is the only absolute way to prevent sexual transmission of HIV infection. However, for many individuals this may not be feasible, and there are a number of relatively safe practices that can markedly decrease the chances of transmission of HIV infection. Partners engaged in monogamous sexual relationships who wish to be assured of safety should both be tested for HIV antibody. If both are negative, it must be understood that any divergence from monogamy puts both partners at risk; open discussion of the importance of honesty in such relationships should be encouraged. When the HIV status of either partner is not known, or when one partner is positive, there are a number of options. Use of condoms can markedly decrease the chance of HIV transmission. It should be remembered that condoms are not 100% effective in preventing transmission of HIV infection, and there is an ~10% failure rate of condoms used for contraceptive purposes. Most condom failures result from breakage or improper usage, such as not wearing the condom for the entire period of intercourse. Latex condoms are preferable, since virus has been shown to leak through natural skin condoms. Petroleum-based gels should never be used for lubrication of the condom, since they increase the likelihood of condom rupture. Some men who have sex with men practice fellatio as a "minimal risk" activity compared to anal intercourse. It should be emphasized that receptive fellatio is definitely not safe sex, and although the incidence of transmission via fellatio is considerably less than that of rectal or vaginal intercourse, there has been documentation of transmission of HIV where receptive fellatio was the only sexual act performed (see "Transmission," above). Topical microbicides for vaginal and anal use are being pursued actively as a means by which individuals could avoid infection when the insertive partner cannot be relied on to use a condom. Three clinical trials in South Africa, Uganda, and Kenya have shown that adult male circumcision results in an ~50% reduction in HIV acquisition in the circumcised subject. Clearly, this approach has considerable potential as a preventive strategy for HIV infection and is currently being pursued, particularly in developing nations, as a component of HIV prevention. Kissing is considered safe, although there is a theoretical possibility of transmission via virus in saliva. The low concentration of virus in saliva of infected individuals, as well as the presence in saliva of HIV-inhibitory proteins (see above), lessens any risk of transmission by kissing.

The most effective way to prevent transmission of HIV infection among IDUs is to stop the use of injectable drugs. Unfortunately, that is extremely difficult to accomplish unless the individual enters a treatment program. For those who will not or cannot participate in a drug treatment program and who will continue to inject drugs, the avoidance of sharing of needles and other paraphernalia ("works") is the next best way to avoid transmission of infection. However, the cultural and social factors that contribute to the sharing of paraphernalia are complex and difficult to overcome. In addition, needles and syringes may be in short supply. Under these circumstances, paraphernalia should be cleaned after each usage with a virucidal solution, such as undiluted sodium hypochlorite (household bleach). Data from a number of studies have indicated that programs that provide sterile needles to addicts in exchange for used needles have resulted in a decrease in HIV transmission without increasing the use of injection drugs. It is important for IDUs to be tested for HIV infection and counseled, to avoid transmission to their sexual partners. Secondary and tertiary spread of HIV infection by the heterosexual route within settings of a high level of injection drug use has increased greatly in the United States, particularly among African Americans (see above). Studies are underway to determine the safety and efficacy of preexposure as well as postexposure administration of ARV drugs for the prevention of HIV infection.

Transmission of HIV via transfused blood or blood products has been decreased dramatically by a combination of screening of all blood donors for HIV infection by assays for both HIV antibody and nucleic acid and self-deferral of individuals at risk for HIV infection. In addition, clotting factor concentrates are heat-treated, essentially eliminating the risk to hemophiliacs who require these products. Autologous transfusions are preferable to transfusions from another individual. However, logistic constraints as well as the unpredictability of the need for most transfusions limit the feasibility of this approach. At present the risk of becoming HIV-infected from a contaminated blood transfusion is approximately 1 in 1.5 million donations.

Treatment of an HIV-infected mother with ARV therapy during pregnancy and the infant during the first weeks following birth has proved very effective in dramatically decreasing mother-to-child transmission of HIV. In situations such as that seen in certain developing countries where pregnant women frequently present to a health care system during labor, administration of a short course (as little as a single dose of one drug) of ARV therapy to the mother during labor and to the infant within 48 h of birth has also been successful in decreasing the incidence of mother-to-child transmission of HIV.

HIV can be transmitted via breast milk and colostrum. The avoidance of breast-feeding may not be practical in developing countries, where nutritional concerns override the risk of HIV transmission. However, it is becoming appreciated that 5–15% of infants who were born of HIV-infected mothers and who were fortunate enough not to have been infected intrapartum or peripartum become infected via breast-feeding. Therefore, in developing countries, breast-feeding from an infected mother should be avoided if at all possible. Unfortunately, this is rarely the case, and given the disadvantages of withholding breast-feeding in developing countries (see above), health authorities in most developing countries continue to recommend breast-feeding despite the potential for HIV transmission. Treatment of the infected mother with ARV therapy, in addition to decreasing perinatal mother-to-child transmission, can also decrease transmission by breast-feeding. In developed countries such as the United States, where bottled formula and milk are readily accessible, breast-feeding is absolutely contraindicated when a mother is HIV positive.

FURTHER READINGS

BAILEY RC et al: Male circumcision for HIV prevention in young men in Casuum, Kenya: A randomised controlled trial. Lancet 369:643, 2007

BENSON CA et al: Treating opportunistic infections among HIV-infected adults and adolescents. Recommendations from CDC, the National Institutes of Health, and the HIV Medicine Association/Infectious Diseases Society of America. MMWR 53(RR-15):1, 2004. Updates available at *http://www.aidsinfo.nih.gov*

BRENNER BG et al: High rates of forward transmission events after acute/early HIV-1 infection. J Infect Dis 195:951, 2007

CENTERS FOR DISEASE CONTROL AND PREVENTION: Revised guidelines for HIV counseling, testing, and referral. MMWR Recomm Rep 50(RR-19):1, 2001

———: Updated U.S. Public Health Service guidelines for the management of occupational exposures to HIV and recommendations for postexposure prophylaxis. MMWR Recomm Rep 54(RR-9): 1, 2005

———: HIV/AIDS Surveillance Report, 2005;17 (Revised ed), 2007. Available at *http://www.cdc.gov/hiv/*

———: Revised recommendations for HIV testing of adults, adolescents, and pregnant women in health-care settings. MMWR Recomm Rep 55(RR-14):1, 2006

———: Essential Components of a Comprehensive Strategy to Prevent Domestic HIV, 2006. Available at *http://www.cdc.gov/Hiv/resources/reports/comp_hiv_prev/index.htm*

———; HEALTH RESOURCES AND SERVICES ADMINISTRATION; NATIONAL INSTITUTES OF HEALTH; HIV MEDICINE ASSOCIATION OF THE INFECTIOUS DISEASES SOCIETY OF AMERICA: Incorporating HIV prevention into the medical care of persons living with HIV. MMWR Recomm Rep 52(RR-12):1, 2003

CENTLIVRE M et al: In HIV-1 pathogenesis the die is cast during primary infection. AIDS 21:1, 2007

COHEN MS, PILCHER CD: Amplified HIV transmission and new approaches to HIV prevention. J Infect Dis 191:1391, 2005

COLLINS LS et al: Multicentric Castleman's disease in HIV infection. Int J STD AIDS 17:19, 2006

COREY L: Synergistic copathogens—HIV-1 and HSV-2. N Engl J Med 356:854, 2007

DEEKS SG, WALKER BD: Human immunodeficiency virus controllers: Mechanisms of durable virus control in the absence of antiretroviral therapy. Immunity 27:406, 2007

DEPARTMENT OF HEALTH AND HUMAN SERVICES PANEL ON ANTIRETROVIRAL GUIDELINES FOR ADULTS AND ADOLESCENTS: *Guidelines for the Use of Antiretroviral Agents in HIV-1-Infected Adults and Adolescents*, October 10, 2006. Updates available at *http://www.aidsinfo.nih.gov*

DORAK MT et al: Transmission of HIV-1 and HLA-B allele-sharing within serodiscordant heterosexual Zambian couples. Lancet 363:2137, 2004

DRUMRIGHT L et al: Unprotected anal intercourse and substance use among men who have sex with men with recent HIV infection. J AIDS 43:344, 2006

ESTE JA, TELENTI A: HIV entry inhibitors. Lancet 370:81, 2007

FAUCI AS: Host factors and the pathogenesis of HIV-induced disease. Nature 384:529, 1996

———: The AIDS epidemic—considerations for the 21st century. N Engl J Med 341:1046, 1999

FELLAY J et al: A whole-genome association study of major determinants for host control of HIV-1. Science 317:944, 2007

FREEMAN GJ et al: Reinvigorating exhausted HIV-specific T cells via PD-1–PD-1 ligand blockade. J Exp Med 203:2223, 2006

FREIBERG M et al: The association between hepatitis C infection and prevalent cardiovascular disease among HIV-infected individuals. AIDS 21:193, 2007

GERETTI AM: Epidemiology of antiretroviral drug resistance in drug-naive persons. Curr Opin Infect Dis 20:22, 2007

GONZALEZ-SCARANO F, MARTIN-GARCIA J: The neuropathogenesis of AIDS. Nat Rev Immunol 5:69, 2005

GRAY RH et al: Male circumcision for HIV prevention in men in Rakai, Uganda: A randomised trial. Lancet 369:657, 2007

GREENE WC, PETERLIN BM: Charting HIV's remarkable voyage through the cell: Basic science as a passport to future therapy. Nat Med 8:673, 2002

GUTIERREZ F et al: Osteonecrosis in patients infected with HIV: clinical epidemiology and natural history in a large case series from Spain. J AIDS 42(3):286, 2006

HAMMER SM et al: Treatment for adult HIV infection: 2006 recommendations of the International AIDS Society-USA panel. JAMA 296:827, 2006

HAN Y et al: Experimental approaches to the study of HIV-1 latency. Nat Rev Microbiol 5:95, 2007

HO DD et al: Rapid turnover of plasma virions and CD4 lymphocytes in HIV infection. Nature 373:123, 1995

HOFFMAN RM, CURRIER JS: Management of antiretroviral treatment-related complications. Infect Clin Dis North Am 21:103, 2007

HUANG L et al: Current concepts: Intensive care of patients with HIV Infection. N Engl J Med 355:173, 2006

IZZEDINE H, DERAY G: The nephrologist in the HAART era. AIDS 21:409, 2007

JOHNSTON MI, FAUCI AS: An HIV vaccine: Evolving concepts. N Engl J Med 356:2073, 2007

JOINT UNITED NATIONS PROGRAMME ON HIV/AIDS (UNAIDS): Report on the global AIDS epidemic, 2006

———: AIDS epidemic update, 2007

KAPLAN JE et al: Guidelines for preventing opportunistic infections among HIV-infected persons—2002. Recommendations of the U.S. Public Health Service and the Infectious Diseases Society of America. MMWR Recomm Rep 51(RR-8):1, 2002. Updates available at *http://www.aidsinfo.nih.gov*

KEELE BF et al: Chimpanzee reservoirs of pandemic and nonpandemic HIV-1. Science 313:523, 2006

KERULY JC, MOORE RD: Immune status at presentation to care did not improve among antiretroviral-naive persons from 1990 to 2006. Clin Infect Dis 45:1369, 2007

KOZIEL MJ, PETERS MG: Current concepts: Viral hepatitis in HIV infection. N Engl J Med 356:1445, 2007

LIPMAN M, BREEN R: Immune reconstitution inflammatory syndrome in HIV. Curr Opin Infect Dis 19:20, 2006

LYLES CM et al: Best-evidence interventions: Findings from a systematic review of HIV behavioral interventions for US populations at high risk, 2000–2004. Am J Public Health 97:133, 2007

MANGILI A et al: Risk of cardiovascular disease in a cohort of HIV-infected adults: A study using carotid intima-media thickness and coronary artery calcium score. Clin Infect Dis 43:1482, 2006

MAY MT et al: HIV treatment response and prognosis in Europe and North America in the first decade of highly active antiretroviral therapy: A collaborative analysis. Lancet 368:451, 2006

MELLORS JW et al: Prognosis in HIV-1 infection predicted by the quantity of virus in plasma. Science 272:1167, 1996

MORSE CG, KOVACS JA: Metabolic and skeletal complications of HIV infection: The price of success. JAMA 296:844, 2006

PANTALEO G, FAUCI AS: HIV infection is active and progressive in lymphoid tissue during the clinically latent stage of disease. Nature 362:355, 1993

PALEFSKY JM et al: Anal intraepithelial neoplasia in the highly active antiretroviral therapy era among HIV-positive men who have sex with men. AIDS 19:1407, 2005

PALELLA FJ JR et al: Mortality in the highly active antiretroviral therapy era: Changing causes of death and disease in the HIV Outpatient Study. J AIDS 43(1):27, 2006

PERINATAL HIV GUIDELINES WORKING GROUP: U.S. Public Health Service Task Force recommendations for use of antiretroviral drugs in pregnant HIV-1-infected women for maternal health and interventions to reduce perinatal HIV-1 transmission in the United States, November 2, 2007. Updates available at *http://www.aidsinfo.nih.gov*

SHELBURNE SA et al: Incidence and risk factors for immune reconstitution inflammatory syndrome during highly active antiretroviral therapy. AIDS 19:399, 2005

SILVESTRI G et al: Understanding the benign nature of SIV infection in natural hosts. J Clin Invest 11:3148, 2007

SIMON V et al: HIV/AIDS epidemiology, pathogenesis, prevention, and treatment. Lancet 368:489, 2006

STEPHENS HA: HIV-1 diversity versus HLA class I polymorphism. Trends Immunol 26:41, 2005

U.S. PUBLIC HEALTH SERVICE: Updated U.S. Public Health Service Guidelines for the Management of Occupational Exposures to HBV, HCV, and HIV and Recommendations for Postexposure Prophylaxis. MMWR Recomm Rep 50(RR-11):1, 2001. Updates available at *http://www.aidsinfo.nih.gov*

THE STRATEGIES FOR MANAGEMENT OF ANTIRETROVIRAL THERAPY (SMART) STUDY GROUP: CD4+ count-guided interruption of antiretroviral treatment. N Engl J Med 355(22):2283, 2006

VOLMINK J et al: Antiretrovirals for reducing the risk of mother-to-child transmission of HIV infection. Cochrane Database Syst Rev 1:CD003510, 2007

WALENSKY RP et al: The survival benefits of AIDS treatment in the United States. J Infect Dis 194:11, 2006

WAWER MJ et al: Rates of HIV-1 transmission per coital act, by stage of HIV-1 infection, in Rakai, Uganda. J Infect Dis 191:1403, 2005

WEI X et al: Viral dynamics in human immunodeficiency virus type 1 infection. Nature 373:117, 1995

WELLS CD et al: HIV infection and multidrug-resistant tuberculosis: The perfect storm. J Infect Dis 196(Suppl 1):S86, 2007

ZANCANARO PCQ et al: Cutaneous manifestations of HIV in the era of highly active antiretroviral therapy: An institutional urban clinic experience. J Am Acad Dermatol 54(4):581, 2006

SECTION 15 INFECTIONS DUE TO RNA VIRUSES

183 Viral Gastroenteritis

Umesh D. Parashar, Roger I. Glass

Acute infectious gastroenteritis is a common illness that affects persons of all ages worldwide. It is a leading cause of mortality among children in developing countries, accounting for an estimated 2 million deaths each year, and is responsible for up to 10–12% of all hospitalizations among children in industrialized countries, including the United States. Elderly persons, especially those with debilitating health conditions, are also at risk of severe complications and death from acute gastroenteritis. Among healthy young adults, acute gastroenteritis is rarely fatal but incurs substantial medical and social costs, including those of time lost from work.

Several enteric viruses have been recognized as important etiologic agents of acute infectious gastroenteritis (**Table 183-1**, **Fig. 183-1**). Illness caused by these viruses is characterized by the acute onset of vomiting and/or diarrhea, which may be accompanied by fever, nausea, abdominal cramps, anorexia, and malaise. As shown in **Table 183-2**,

TABLE 183-1 VIRAL CAUSES OF GASTROENTERITIS AMONG HUMANS

Virus	Family	Genome	Primary Age Group at Risk	Clinical Severity	Detection Assays[a]
Group A rotavirus	Reoviridae	Double-strand segmented RNA	Children <5 years	+++	EM, EIA (commercial), PAGE, RT-PCR
Norovirus	Caliciviridae	Positive-sense single-strand RNA	All ages	++	EM, EIA, RT-PCR
Sapovirus	Caliciviridae	Positive-sense single-strand RNA	Children <5 years	+	EM, EIA, RT-PCR
Astrovirus	Astroviridae	Positive-sense single-strand RNA	Children <5 years	+	EM, EIA, RT-PCR
Adenovirus (types 40 and 41)	Adenoviridae	Double-strand DNA	Children <5 years	+/++	EM, EIA (commercial), PCR

[a]EIA, enzyme immunoassay; EM, electron microscopy; PAGE, polyacrylamide gel electrophoresis; PCR, polymerase chain reaction; RT-PCR, reverse-transcriptase PCR.

several features can help distinguish gastroenteritis caused by viruses from that caused by bacterial agents. However, the distinction based on clinical and epidemiologic parameters alone is often difficult, and laboratory tests may be required to confirm the diagnosis.

HUMAN CALICIVIRUSES

Etiologic Agent The Norwalk virus is the prototype strain of a group of nonenveloped, small (27–40 nm), round, icosahedral viruses with relatively amorphous surface features on visualization by electron microscopy. These viruses have been difficult to classify because they have not been adapted to cell culture, they often are shed in low titers for only a few days, and no animal models are available. Molecular cloning and characterization have demonstrated that these viruses have a single, positive-strand RNA genome ~7.5 kb in length and that they possess a single virion-associated protein—similar to that of typical caliciviruses—with a molecular mass of 60 kDa. On the basis of these molecular characteristics, these viruses are presently classified in two genera belonging to the family Caliciviridae: the *noroviruses* and the *sapoviruses* (previously called Norwalk-like viruses and Sapporo-like viruses, respectively).

Epidemiology Infections with the Norwalk and related human caliciviruses are common worldwide, and most adults have antibodies to these viruses. Antibody is acquired at an earlier age in developing countries—a pattern consistent with the presumed fecal-oral mode of transmission. Infections occur year-round, although, in temperate climates, a distinct increase has been noted in cold-weather months. Noroviruses may be the most common infectious agents of mild gastroenteritis in the community and affect all age groups, whereas sapoviruses primarily cause gastroenteritis in children. Noroviruses also cause traveler's diarrhea, and outbreaks have occurred among military personnel deployed to various parts of the world. The etiologic role of noroviruses in moderate and severe gastroenteritis requiring a visit to a physician or hospitalization is still being studied. However, the limited data available indicate that norovirus may be the second most common viral agent (after rotavirus) among young children and the most common agent among older children and adults. Noroviruses are also recognized as the major cause of epidemics of gastroenteritis worldwide. In the United States, >90% of outbreaks of nonbacterial gastroenteritis are caused by noroviruses. Epidemics occur throughout the year, in all age groups, and in a variety of settings.

Virus is transmitted predominantly by the fecal-oral route but is also present in vomitus. Because an inoculum with very few viruses can be infectious, transmission can occur by aerosolization, by contact with contaminated fomites, and by person-to-person contact. Viral shedding and infectivity are greatest during the acute illness, but challenge studies with Norwalk virus in volunteers indicate that viral antigen may be shed by asymptomatically infected persons and also by symptomatic persons before the onset of symptoms and for up to 2 weeks after the resolution of illness. In one study, 11 of 15 norovirus-infected children <2 years of age shed the virus for >2 weeks after onset; this group included 3 infants <6 months of age who shed virus for 42–47 days or even longer.

Pathogenesis The exact sites and cellular receptors for attachment of viral particles have not been determined. Data suggest that carbohydrates that are similar to human histo-blood group antigens and are present on the gastroduodenal epithelium of individuals with the secretor phenotype may serve as ligands for the attachment of Norwalk virus. Additional studies must more fully elucidate norovirus-carbohydrate interactions, including potential strain-specific variations. After the infection of volunteers, reversible lesions are noted in the upper jejunum, with broadening and blunting of the villi, shortening of the microvilli, vacuolization of the lining epithelium, crypt hyperplasia, and infiltration of the lamina propria by polymorphonuclear neutrophils and lymphocytes. The lesions persist for at least 4 days after the resolution of symptoms and are associated with malabsorption of carbohydrates and fats and a decreased level of brush-border enzymes. Adenylate cyclase activity is not altered. No histopathologic changes are seen in the stomach or colon, but gastric motor function is delayed, and this alteration is believed to contribute to the nausea and vomiting that are typical of this illness.

Clinical Manifestations Gastroenteritis caused by Norwalk and related human caliciviruses has a sudden onset, following an average incubation period of 24 h (range, 12–72 h). The illness generally lasts 12–60 h and is characterized by one or more of the following symptoms:

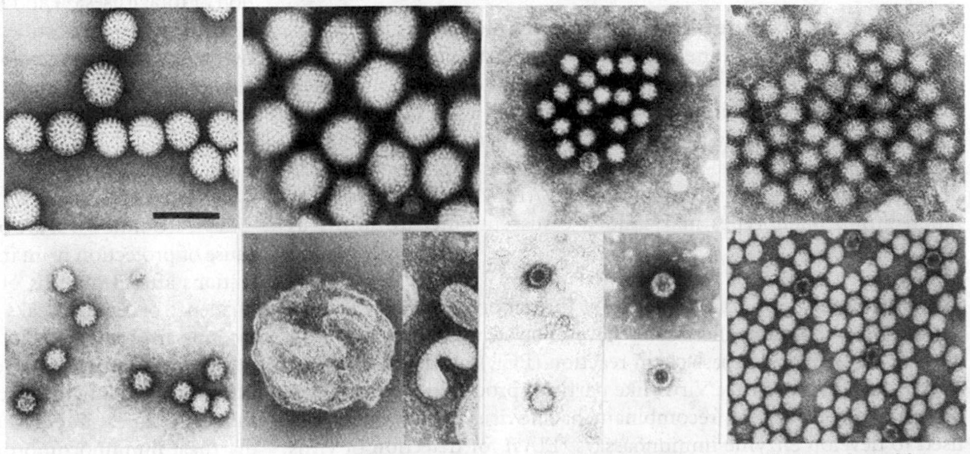

FIGURE 183-1 Viral agents of gastroenteritis. NV, Norwalk-like virus; SV, Sapporo-like virus.

TABLE 183-2 CHARACTERISTICS OF GASTROENTERITIS CAUSED BY VIRAL AND BACTERIAL AGENTS

Feature	Viral Gastroenteritis	Bacterial Gastroenteritis
Setting	Incidence similar in developing and developed countries	More common in settings with poor hygiene and sanitation
Infectious dose	Low (10–100 viral particles) for most agents	High (>10^5 bacteria) for *Escherichia coli, Salmonella, Vibrio*; medium (10^2–10^5 bacteria) for *Campylobacter jejuni*; low (10–100 bacteria) for *Shigella*
Seasonality	In temperate climates, winter seasonality for most agents; year-round occurrence in tropical areas	More common in summer or rainy months, particularly in developing countries with a high disease burden
Incubation period	1–3 days for most agents; can be shorter for norovirus	1–7 days for common agents (e.g., *Campylobacter, E. coli, Shigella, Salmonella*); a few hours for bacteria producing preformed toxins (e.g., *Staphylococcus aureus, Bacillus cereus*)
Reservoir	Primarily humans	Depending on species, human (e.g., *Shigella, Salmonella*), animal (e.g., *Campylobacter, Salmonella, E. coli*), and water (e.g., *Vibrio*) reservoirs exist.
Fever	Common with rotavirus and norovirus; uncommon with other agents	Common with agents causing inflammatory diarrhea (e.g., *Salmonella, Shigella*)
Vomiting	Prominent and can be the only presenting feature, especially in children	Common with bacteria producing preformed toxins; less prominent in diarrhea due to other agents
Diarrhea	Common; nonbloody in almost all cases	Prominent and frequently bloody with agents causing inflammatory diarrhea
Duration	1–3 days for norovirus and sapovirus; 2–8 days for other viruses	1–2 days for bacteria producing preformed toxins; 2–8 days for most other bacteria
Diagnosis	This is often a diagnosis of exclusion in clinical practice. Commercial enzyme immunoassays are available for detection of rotavirus and adenovirus, but identification of other agents is limited to research and public health laboratories.	Fecal examination for leukocytes and blood is helpful in differential diagnosis. Culture of stool specimens, sometimes on special media, can identify several pathogens. Molecular techniques are useful epidemiologic tools but are not routinely used in most laboratories.
Treatment	Supportive therapy to maintain adequate hydration and nutrition should be given. Antibiotics and antimotility agents are contraindicated.	Supportive hydration therapy is adequate for most patients. Antibiotics are recommended for patients with dysentery caused by *Shigella* or *Vibrio cholerae* and for some patients with *Clostridium difficile* colitis.

nausea, vomiting, abdominal cramps, and diarrhea. Vomiting is more prevalent among children, whereas a greater proportion of adults develop diarrhea. Constitutional symptoms are common, including headache, fever, chills, and myalgias. Noroviruses appear to cause more severe illness than sapoviruses, although both illnesses are less severe than that due to rotavirus. The stools are characteristically loose and watery, without blood, mucus, or leukocytes. White cell counts are generally normal; rarely, leukocytosis with relative lymphopenia may be observed. Death is a rare outcome and usually results from severe dehydration in vulnerable persons (e.g., elderly patients with debilitating health conditions).

Immunity Approximately 50% of persons challenged with Norwalk virus become ill and acquire short-term immunity against the infecting strain. Immunity to Norwalk virus appears to correlate inversely with level of antibody; i.e., persons with higher levels of preexisting antibody to Norwalk virus are more susceptible to illness. This observation suggests that some individuals have a genetic predisposition to illness. Recent data indicate that specific ABO, Lewis, and secretor blood group phenotypes may influence susceptibility to norovirus infection.

Diagnosis Cloning and sequencing of the genomes of Norwalk and several other human caliciviruses have allowed the development of assays based on polymerase chain reaction (PCR) for detection of virus in stool and vomitus. Virus-like particles produced by expression of capsid proteins in a recombinant baculovirus vector have been used to develop enzyme immunoassays (EIAs) for detection of virus in stool or a serologic response to a specific viral antigen. These newer diagnostic techniques are considerably more sensitive than previous detection methods, such as electron microscopy, immune electron microscopy, and EIAs based on reagents derived from humans. However, no currently available single assay can detect all human caliciviruses because of their great genetic and antigenic diversity. In addition, the assays are still cumbersome and are available primarily in research laboratories, although they are increasingly being adopted by public health laboratories for routine screening of fecal specimens from patients affected by outbreaks of gastroenteritis. Commercial EIA kits have been developed but are still being evaluated to determine their optimal use for both outbreak-related and sporadic acute gastroenteritis cases.

Rx INFECTIONS WITH NORWALK AND RELATED HUMAN CALICIVIRUSES

The disease is self-limited, and oral rehydration therapy is generally adequate. If severe dehydration develops, IV fluid therapy is indicated. No specific antiviral therapy is available.

Prevention Epidemic prevention relies on situation-specific measures, such as control of contamination of food and water, exclusion of ill food handlers, and reduction of person-to-person spread through good personal hygiene and disinfection of contaminated fomites. The role of immunoprophylaxis is not clear, given the lack of long-term immunity from natural disease and the paradoxical inverse association between the level of immune response and protection from disease.

ROTAVIRUS

Etiologic Agent Rotaviruses are members of the family Reoviridae. The viral genome consists of 11 segments of double-strand RNA that are enclosed in a triple-layered, nonenveloped, icosahedral capsid 75 nm in diameter. Viral protein 6 (VP6), the major structural protein, is the target of commercial immunoassays and determines the group specificity of rotaviruses. There are seven major groups of rotavirus (A through G); human illness is caused primarily by group A and, to a much lesser extent, by groups B and C. Two outer-capsid proteins, VP7 (G-protein) and VP4 (P-protein), determine serotype specificity, induce neutralizing antibodies, and form the basis for binary classification of rotaviruses (G and P types). The segmented genome of rotavirus allows genetic reassortment (i.e., exchange of genome segments between viruses) during co-infection—a property that may play a role in viral evolution and has been utilized in the development of reassortant animal-human rotavirus–based vaccines.

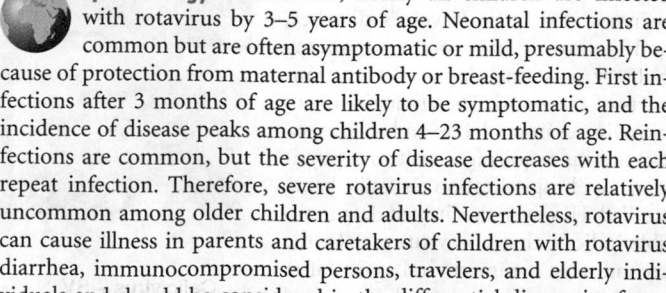

Epidemiology Worldwide, nearly all children are infected with rotavirus by 3–5 years of age. Neonatal infections are common but are often asymptomatic or mild, presumably because of protection from maternal antibody or breast-feeding. First infections after 3 months of age are likely to be symptomatic, and the incidence of disease peaks among children 4–23 months of age. Reinfections are common, but the severity of disease decreases with each repeat infection. Therefore, severe rotavirus infections are relatively uncommon among older children and adults. Nevertheless, rotavirus can cause illness in parents and caretakers of children with rotavirus diarrhea, immunocompromised persons, travelers, and elderly individuals and should be considered in the differential diagnosis of gastroenteritis among adults. In temperate climates, rotavirus disease

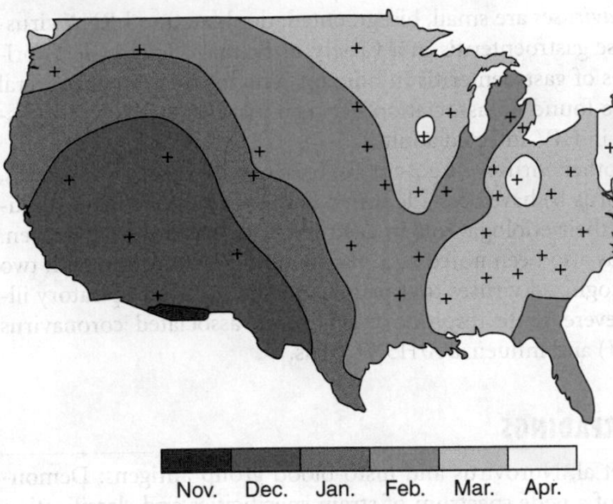

FIGURE 183-2 Time of peak rotavirus activity in the contiguous 48 states: United States, July 1991 to June 1997. Data are from ~90 U.S. laboratories. *(Adapted from TJ Torok et al: Visualizing geographic and temporal trends in rotavirus activity in the United States, 1991 to 1996. National Respiratory and Enteric Virus Surveillance System Collaborating Laboratories. Pediatr Infect Dis J 16:941, 1997.)*

occurs predominantly during the cooler fall and winter months. In the United States, the rotavirus season each year begins in the Southwest during the autumn (October through December) and migrates across the continent, peaking in the Northeast during the spring (March through May) (Fig. 183-2); the reasons for this characteristic pattern are not clear. In tropical settings, rotavirus disease occurs year-round, with less pronounced seasonal peaks.

Rotavirus gastroenteritis is more frequently associated with dehydration than is gastroenteritis caused by other pathogens. Therefore, the proportion of gastroenteritis cases that are attributable to rotavirus increases with increasing severity of illness, ranging from a median of 8% in the community to 18% among outpatients and 40% among hospitalized patients. Each year, rotavirus is estimated to cause ~500,000 childhood deaths worldwide.

During episodes of rotavirus-associated diarrhea, virus is shed in large quantities in stool (10^7–10^{12}/g). Viral shedding detectable by EIA usually subsides within 1 week but may persist for >30 days in immunocompromised individuals. Viral shedding may be detected for longer periods by sensitive molecular assays, such as PCR. The virus is transmitted predominantly through the fecal-oral route. Spread through respiratory secretions, person-to-person contact, or contaminated environmental surfaces has also been postulated to explain the rapid acquisition of antibody in the first 3 years of life, regardless of sanitary conditions.

At least 10 different G serotypes of group A rotavirus have been identified in humans, but only five types (G1 through G4 and G9) are common. While human rotavirus strains that possess a high degree of genetic homology with animal strains have been identified, animal-to-human transmission appears to be uncommon.

Group B rotaviruses have been associated with several large epidemics of severe gastroenteritis among adults in China since 1982 and have recently been identified in India but not in other parts of the world. Group C rotaviruses have been associated with a small proportion of pediatric gastroenteritis cases in several countries worldwide.

Pathogenesis Rotaviruses infect and ultimately destroy mature enterocytes in the villous epithelium of the proximal small intestine. The loss of absorptive villous epithelium, coupled with the proliferation of secretory crypt cells, results in secretory diarrhea. Brush-border enzymes characteristic of differentiated cells are reduced, and this change leads to the accumulation of unmetabolized disaccharides and consequent osmotic diarrhea. Studies in mice indicate that a nonstructural rotavirus protein, NSP4, functions as an enterotoxin and contributes to secretory diarrhea by altering epithelial cell function and permeability. In addition, rotavirus may evoke fluid secretion through activation of the enteric nervous system in the intestinal wall. Recent data indicate that rotavirus antigenemia and viremia are common among children with acute rotavirus infection, although the antigen and RNA levels in serum are substantially lower than those in stool.

Clinical Manifestations The clinical spectrum of rotavirus infection ranges from subclinical infection to severe gastroenteritis leading to life-threatening dehydration. After an incubation period of 1–3 days, the illness has an abrupt onset, with vomiting frequently preceding the onset of diarrhea. Up to one-third of patients may have a temperature of >39°C. The stools are characteristically loose and watery and only infrequently contain red or white cells. Gastrointestinal symptoms generally resolve in 3–7 days.

Respiratory and neurologic features in children with rotavirus infection have been reported, but causal associations have not been proven. Moreover, rotavirus infection has been associated with a variety of other clinical conditions (e.g., sudden infant death syndrome, necrotizing enterocolitis, intussusception, Kawasaki disease, and type 1 diabetes), but no causal relationship has been confirmed with any of these syndromes.

Rotavirus does not appear to be a major opportunistic pathogen in children with HIV infection. In severely immunodeficient children, rotavirus can cause protracted diarrhea with prolonged viral excretion and, in rare instances, can disseminate systemically. Persons who are immunosuppressed for bone marrow transplantation are also at risk for severe or even fatal rotavirus disease.

Immunity Protection against rotavirus disease is correlated with the presence of virus-specific secretory IgA antibodies in the intestine and, to some extent, the serum. Because virus-specific IgA production at the intestinal surface is short-lived, complete protection against disease is only temporary. However, each infection and subsequent reinfection confers progressively greater immunity; thus severe disease is most common among young children with first or second infections. Immunologic memory is believed to be important in the attenuation of disease severity upon reinfection.

Diagnosis Illness caused by rotavirus is difficult to distinguish clinically from that caused by other enteric viruses. Because large quantities of virus are shed in feces, the diagnosis can usually be confirmed by a wide variety of commercially available EIAs or by techniques for detecting viral RNA, such as gel electrophoresis, probe hybridization, or PCR.

Rx ROTAVIRUS INFECTIONS

Rotavirus gastroenteritis can lead to severe dehydration. Thus appropriate treatment should be instituted early. Standard oral rehydration therapy is successful in most children who can take oral fluids, but IV fluid replacement may be required for patients who are severely dehydrated or are unable to tolerate oral therapy because of frequent vomiting. The therapeutic role of probiotics, bismuth subsalicylate, enkephalinase inhibitors, and nitazoxanide has been evaluated in clinical studies but is not clearly defined. Antibiotics and antimotility agents should be avoided. In immunocompromised children with chronic symptomatic rotavirus disease, orally administered immunoglobulins or colostrum may resolve symptoms, but the choice of agents and their doses have not been well studied and are often empirical.

Prevention Efforts to develop rotavirus vaccines were pursued because it was apparent—given the similar rates in less developed and industrialized nations—that improvements in hygiene and sanitation were unlikely to reduce disease incidence. The first rotavirus vaccine licensed in the United States in 1998 was withdrawn from the market within 1 year because it was linked with intussusception, a severe bowel obstruction.

In 2006, promising safety and efficacy results for two new rotavirus vaccines were reported from large clinical trials conducted in North America, Europe, and Latin America. One of these vaccines, a multivalent bovine-human reassortant rotavirus-based preparation, was recommended for routine immunization of all U.S. infants in early 2006. The second vaccine, based on a single attenuated human rotavirus strain, is not licensed in the United States but has been introduced in immunization programs in several countries in Latin America and Europe.

Global Considerations Rotavirus is ubiquitous and infects nearly all children worldwide by 5 years of age. However, compared with rotavirus disease in industrialized countries, that in developing countries occurs at a younger age, is less seasonal, is more often associated with severe outcomes (including death), and is more frequently caused by uncommon rotavirus strains. The different epidemiology of rotavirus disease and the greater prevalence of co-infection with other enteric pathogens, of comorbidities, and of malnutrition in developing countries may adversely affect the performance of rotavirus vaccines. Therefore, before global recommendations for vaccine use can be issued, it is vital to evaluate the efficacy of rotavirus vaccines in resource-poor settings of Africa and Asia. Trials in these areas are under way.

OTHER VIRAL AGENTS OF GASTROENTERITIS

Enteric *adenoviruses* of serotypes 40 and 41 belonging to subgroup F are 70- to 80-nm viruses with double-strand DNA that cause ~2–12% of all diarrhea episodes in young children. Unlike adenoviruses that cause respiratory illness, enteric adenoviruses are difficult to cultivate in cell lines, but they can be detected with commercially available EIAs.

Astroviruses, 28- to 30-nm viruses with a characteristic icosahedral structure, contain a positive-sense, single-strand RNA. At least seven serotypes have been identified, of which serotype 1 is most common. Astroviruses are primarily pediatric pathogens, causing ~2–10% of cases of mild to moderate gastroenteritis in children. The availability of simple immunoassays to detect virus in fecal specimens and of molecular methods to confirm and characterize strains will permit more comprehensive assessment of the etiologic role of these agents.

Toroviruses are 100- to 140-nm, enveloped, positive-strand RNA viruses that are recognized as causes of gastroenteritis in horses (Berne virus) and cattle (Breda virus). Their role as a cause of diarrhea in humans is still unclear, but studies from Canada have demonstrated associations between torovirus excretion and both nosocomial gastroenteritis and necrotizing enterocolitis in neonates. These associations require further evaluation.

Picobirnaviruses are small, bisegmented, double-strand RNA viruses that cause gastroenteritis in a variety of animals. Their role as primary causes of gastroenteritis in humans remains unclear, but several studies have found an association between picobirnaviruses and gastroenteritis in HIV-infected adults.

Several other viruses (e.g., enteroviruses, reoviruses, pestiviruses, and parvovirus B) have been identified in the feces of patients with diarrhea, but their etiologic role in gastroenteritis has not been proven. Diarrhea has also been noted as a manifestation of infection with two recently recognized viruses that primarily cause severe respiratory illness: the severe acute respiratory syndrome–associated coronavirus (SARS-CoV) and influenza A/H5N1 virus.

FURTHER READINGS

HUANG P et al: Norovirus and histo-blood group antigens: Demonstration of a wide spectrum of strain specificities and classification of two major binding groups among multiple binding patterns. J Virol 79:6714, 2005

KO G et al: Noroviruses as a cause of traveler's diarrhea among students from the United States visiting Mexico. J Clin Microbiol 43:6126, 2005

LEUNG WK et al: Enteric involvement of severe acute respiratory syndrome–associated coronavirus infection. Gastroenterology 125:1011, 2003

LODHA A et al: Human torovirus: A new virus associated with neonatal necrotizing enterocolitis. Acta Paediatr 94:1085, 2005

MURATA T et al: Prolonged norovirus shedding in infants <or=6 months of age with gastroenteritis. Pediatr Infect Dis J 26:46, 2007

RAY P et al: Quantitative evaluation of rotaviral antigenemia in children with acute rotaviral diarrhea. J Infect Dis 194:588, 2006

ROSSIGNOL JF et al: Effect of nitazoxanide for treatment of severe rotavirus diarrhoea: Randomised double-blind placebo-controlled trial. Lancet 368:124, 2006

RUIZ-PALACIOS G et al: Safety and efficacy of an attenuated vaccine against severe rotavirus gastroenteritis. N Engl J Med 354:11, 2006

TRAN TH et al: Avian influenza A (H5N1) in 10 patients in Vietnam. N Engl J Med 350:1179, 2004

VESIKARI T et al: Safety and efficacy of a pentavalent human-bovine (WC3) reassortant rotavirus vaccine. N Engl J Med 354:23, 2006

184 Enteroviruses and Reoviruses

Jeffrey I. Cohen

ENTEROVIRUSES

CLASSIFICATION AND CHARACTERIZATION

Enteroviruses are so named because of their ability to multiply in the gastrointestinal tract. Despite their name, these viruses are not a prominent cause of gastroenteritis. Enteroviruses encompass 65 human serotypes: 3 serotypes of poliovirus, 23 serotypes of coxsackievirus A, 6 serotypes of coxsackievirus B, 29 serotypes of echovirus, and enteroviruses 68–71. Enteroviruses 73–102 have recently been identified in humans by molecular techniques, but their clinical features have not been described. Enterovirus surveillance conducted in the United States by the Centers for Disease Control and Prevention (CDC) in 2002–2004 showed that two enteroviruses—echoviruses 9 and 30—accounted for 59% of all enterovirus isolates.

Human enteroviruses contain a single-stranded RNA genome surrounded by an icosahedral capsid comprising four viral proteins. These viruses have no lipid envelope and are stable in acidic environments, including the stomach. They are resistant to inactivation by standard disinfectants (e.g., alcohol, detergents) and can persist for days at room temperature.

PATHOGENESIS AND IMMUNITY

Much of what is known about the pathogenesis of enteroviruses has been derived from studies of poliovirus infection. After ingestion, poliovirus is thought to infect epithelial cells in the mucosa of the gastrointestinal tract and then to spread to and replicate in the submucosal lymphoid tissue of the tonsils and Peyer's patches. The virus next spreads to the regional lymph nodes, a viremic phase ensues, and the virus replicates in organs of the reticuloendothelial system. In some cases, a second viremia occurs and the virus replicates further in various tissues, sometimes causing symptomatic disease.

It is uncertain whether poliovirus reaches the central nervous system (CNS) during viremia or whether it also spreads via peripheral nerves. Since viremia precedes the onset of neurologic disease in humans and in experimentally infected chimpanzees, it has been assumed that the virus enters the CNS via the bloodstream. The poliovirus receptor is a member of the immunoglobulin superfamily. Poliovirus infection is limited to primates, largely because their cells express the viral receptor. Studies demonstrating the poliovirus receptor in the end-plate region of muscle at the neuromuscular junction suggest that, if the virus enters the muscle during viremia, it could travel across the neuromuscular junction up the axon to the anterior horn cells. Studies of monkeys and of transgenic mice expressing the poliovirus receptor show that, after IM injection, poliovirus does not reach the spinal cord if the sciatic nerve is cut. Taken together, these findings suggest that poliovirus can spread directly from muscle to the CNS by neural pathways. Intercellular adhesion molecule 1 (ICAM-1) is a receptor for coxsackieviruses A13, A18, and A21; CAR for coxsackievirus B; VLA-2 integrin for echovirus types 1 and 8; and CD55 for enterovirus 70 and some serotypes of coxsackievirus A and B and echovirus.

Poliovirus can usually be cultured from the blood 3–5 days after infection, before the development of neutralizing antibodies. While viral replication at secondary sites begins to slow 1 week after infection, it continues in the gastrointestinal tract. Poliovirus is shed from the oropharynx for up to 3 weeks after infection and from the gastrointestinal tract for as long as 12 weeks; immunodeficient patients can shed poliovirus for up to 20 years. During replication in the gastrointestinal tract, attenuated oral poliovirus can mutate, reverting to a more neurovirulent phenotype within a few days. The clinical significance of this increased neurovirulence is unknown.

Humoral and secretory immunity in the gastrointestinal tract is important for the control of enterovirus infections. Enteroviruses induce specific IgM, which usually persists for <6 months, and specific IgG, which persists for life. Capsid protein VP1 is the predominant target of neutralizing antibody, which generally confers lifelong protection against subsequent disease caused by the same serotype but does not prevent infection or virus shedding. Enteroviruses also induce cellular immunity, but the significance of this mechanism in limiting infection is uncertain. Patients with impaired cellular immunity are not known to develop unusually severe disease when infected with enteroviruses. In contrast, the severe infections in patients with agammaglobulinemia emphasize the importance of humoral immunity in controlling enterovirus infections. Disseminated enterovirus infections have occurred in stem cell transplant recipients. IgA antibodies are instrumental in reducing poliovirus replication in and shedding from the gastrointestinal tract. Breast milk contains IgA specific for enteroviruses and can protect humans from infection.

EPIDEMIOLOGY

Enteroviruses have a worldwide distribution. More than 50% of nonpoliovirus enterovirus infections and more than 90% of poliovirus infections are subclinical. When symptoms do develop, they are usually nonspecific and occur in conjunction with fever; only a minority of infections are associated with specific clinical syndromes. The incubation period for most enterovirus infections ranges from 2 to 14 days but usually is <1 week.

Enterovirus infection is more common in socioeconomically disadvantaged areas, especially in those where conditions are crowded and in tropical areas where hygiene is poor. Infection is most common among infants and young children; serious illness develops most often during the first few days of life and in older children and adults. In developing countries, where children are infected at an early age, poliovirus infection has less often been associated with paralysis; in countries with better hygiene, older children and adults are more likely to be seronegative, become infected, and develop paralysis. Passively acquired maternal antibody reduces the risk of symptomatic infection in neonates. Young children are the most frequent shedders of enteroviruses and are usually the index cases in family outbreaks. In temperate climates, enterovirus infections occur most often in the summer and fall; no seasonal pattern is apparent in the tropics.

Most enteroviruses are transmitted primarily by the fecal-oral route from fecally contaminated fingers or inanimate objects. Patients are most infectious shortly before and after the onset of symptomatic disease, when virus is present in the stool and throat. The ingestion of virus-contaminated food or water can also cause disease. Certain enteroviruses (such as enterovirus 70, which causes acute hemorrhagic conjunctivitis) can be transmitted by direct inoculation from the fingers to the eye. Airborne transmission is important for some viruses that cause respiratory tract disease, such as coxsackievirus A21. Enteroviruses can be transmitted across the placenta from mother to fetus, causing severe disease in the newborn. The transmission of enteroviruses through blood transfusions or insect bites has not been documented. Nosocomial spread of coxsackievirus and echovirus has taken place in hospital nurseries.

CLINICAL FEATURES

Poliovirus Infection Most infections with poliovirus are asymptomatic. After an incubation period of 3–6 days, ~5% of patients present with a minor illness (abortive poliomyelitis) manifested by fever, malaise, sore throat, anorexia, myalgias, and headache. This condition usually resolves in 3 days. About 1% of patients present with aseptic meningitis (nonparalytic poliomyelitis). Examination of cerebrospinal fluid (CSF) reveals lymphocytic pleocytosis, a normal glucose level, and a normal or slightly elevated protein level; CSF polymorphonuclear leukocytes may be present early. In some patients, especially children, malaise and fever precede the onset of aseptic meningitis.

PARALYTIC POLIOMYELITIS The least common presentation is that of paralytic disease. After one or several days, signs of aseptic meningitis are followed by severe back, neck, and muscle pain and by the rapid or gradual development of motor weakness. In some cases the disease appears to be biphasic, with aseptic meningitis followed first by apparent recovery but then (1–2 days later) by the return of fever and the development of paralysis; this form is more common among children than among adults. Weakness is generally asymmetric, is proximal more than distal, and may involve the legs (most commonly); the arms; or the abdominal, thoracic, or bulbar muscles. Paralysis develops during the febrile phase of the illness and usually does not progress after defervescence. Urinary retention may also occur. Examination reveals weakness, fasciculations, decreased muscle tone, and reduced or absent reflexes in affected areas. Transient hyperreflexia sometimes precedes the loss of reflexes. Patients frequently report sensory symptoms, but objective sensory testing usually yields normal results. Bulbar paralysis may lead to dysphagia, difficulty in handling secretions, or dysphonia. Respiratory insufficiency due to aspiration, involvement of the respiratory center in the medulla, or paralysis of the phrenic or intercostal nerves may develop, and severe medullary involvement may lead to circulatory collapse. Most patients with paralysis recover some function weeks to months after infection. About two-thirds of patients have residual neurologic sequelae.

Paralytic disease is more common among older individuals, pregnant women, and persons exercising strenuously or undergoing trauma at the time of CNS symptoms. Tonsillectomy predisposes to bulbar poliomyelitis, and IM injections increase the risk of paralysis in the involved limb(s).

VACCINE-ASSOCIATED POLIOMYELITIS Until recently, poliomyelitis due to live poliovirus vaccine occurred in the United States. The risk of developing poliomyelitis after oral vaccination is estimated at 1 case per 2.5 million doses. The risk is ~2000 times higher among immunodeficient persons, especially in persons with hypo- or agammaglobulinemia. Before 1997, an average of eight cases of vaccine-associated poliomyelitis occurred—in both vaccinees and their contacts—in the United States each year. With the change in recommendations first to a sequential regimen of inactivated poliovirus vaccine (IPV) and oral poliovirus vaccine (OPV) in 1997 and then to an all-IPV regimen in 2000, the number of cases of vaccine-associated polio declined. From 1997 to 1999, six such cases were reported in the United States; no cases have been reported since 1999.

POSTPOLIO SYNDROME The *postpolio syndrome* presents as a new onset of weakness, fatigue, fasciculations, and pain with additional atrophy of the muscle group involved during the initial paralytic disease 20–40 years earlier. The syndrome is more common among women and with increasing time after acute disease. The onset is usually insidious, and weakness occasionally extends to muscles that were not involved during the initial illness. The prognosis is generally good; progression to further

TABLE 184-1 MANIFESTATIONS COMMONLY ASSOCIATED WITH ENTEROVIRUS SEROTYPES

	Serotype(s) of Indicated Virus	
Manifestation	**Coxsackievirus**	**Echovirus (E) and Enterovirus (Ent)**
Acute hemorrhagic conjunctivitis	A24	E70
Aseptic meningitis	A2, 4, 7, 9, 10; B1-5	E4, 6, 7, 9, 11, 13, 16, 18, 19, 30, 33; Ent70, 71
Encephalitis	A9; B1-5	E3, 4, 6, 9, 11, 25, 30; Ent71
Exanthem	A4, 5, 9, 10, 16; B1, 3-5	E4-7, 9, 11, 16-19, 25, 30; Ent71
Generalized disease of the newborn	B1-5	E4-6, 7, 9, 11, 14, 16, 18, 19
Hand-foot-and-mouth disease	A5, 7, 9, 10, 16; B1, 2, 5	Ent71
Herpangina	A1-10, 16, 22; B1-5	E6, 9, 11, 16, 17, 25; Ent71
Myocarditis, pericarditis	A4, 9, 16; B1-5	E6, 9, 11, 22
Paralysis	A4, 7, 9; B1-5	E2, 4, 6, 9, 11, 30; Ent70, 71
Pleurodynia	A1, 2, 4, 6, 9, 10, 16; B1-6	E1-3, 6, 7, 9, 11, 12, 14, 16, 19, 24, 25, 30
Pneumonia	A9, 16; B1-5	E6, 7, 9, 11, 12, 19, 20, 30; Ent68, 71

weakness is usually slow, with plateau periods of 1–10 years. The postpolio syndrome is thought to be due to progressive dysfunction and loss of motor neurons that compensated for the neurons lost during the original infection and not to persistent or reactivated poliovirus infection.

Other Enteroviruses An estimated 5–10 million cases of symptomatic disease due to enteroviruses other than poliovirus occur in the United States each year. Among neonates, enteroviruses are the most common cause of aseptic meningitis and nonspecific febrile illnesses. Certain clinical syndromes are more likely to be caused by certain serotypes (Table 184-1), but there is much overlap. In 2002–2004, 85% of enterovirus infections were caused by only 9 human serotypes. Echoviruses 9 and 30 accounted for 60% of recognized enterovirus infections.

NONSPECIFIC FEBRILE ILLNESS (SUMMER GRIPPE) The most common clinical manifestation of enterovirus infection is a nonspecific febrile illness. After an incubation period of 3–6 days, patients present with an acute onset of fever, malaise, and headache. Occasional cases are associated with upper respiratory symptoms, and some cases include nausea and vomiting. Symptoms often last for 3–4 days, and most cases resolve in a week. While infections with other respiratory viruses occur more often from late fall to early spring, enterovirus febrile illness frequently occurs in the summer and early fall.

GENERALIZED DISEASE OF THE NEWBORN Most serious enterovirus infections in infants develop during the first week of life, although severe disease can occur up to 3 months of age. Neonates often present with an illness resembling bacterial sepsis, with fever, irritability, and lethargy. Laboratory abnormalities include leukocytosis with a left shift, thrombocytopenia, elevated values in liver function tests, and CSF pleocytosis. The illness can be complicated by myocarditis and hypotension, fulminant hepatitis and disseminated intravascular coagulation, meningitis or meningoencephalitis, or pneumonia. It may be difficult to distinguish neonatal enterovirus infection from bacterial sepsis, although a history of a recent virus-like illness in the mother provides a clue.

ASEPTIC MENINGITIS AND ENCEPHALITIS Enteroviruses are the cause of up to 90% of cases of aseptic meningitis in children and young adults in which an etiologic agent can be identified. Patients with aseptic meningitis typically present with an acute onset of fever, chills, headache, photophobia, and pain on eye movement. Nausea and vomiting are also common. Examination reveals meningismus without localizing neurologic signs; drowsiness or irritability may also be apparent. In some cases, a febrile illness may be reported that remits but returns several days later in conjunction with signs of meningitis. Other systemic manifestations may provide clues to an enteroviral cause, including diarrhea, myalgias, rash, pleurodynia, myocarditis, and herpangina. Examination of the CSF invariably reveals pleocytosis; early in the course, polymorphonuclear leukocytes may be present or even predominant—a finding that raises the possibility of bacterial or other nonviral causes of meningitis. Partially treated bacterial meningitis may be particularly difficult to exclude in some instances. A useful rule is that the CSF cell count in enteroviral meningitis shows a shift to lymphocytic predominance within 24 h of presentation, and the total count generally does not exceed 1000 cells/μL. Additional CSF findings consist of a normal glucose content and a normal or only slightly elevated (by ≤100 mg/dL) level of protein. Enteroviruses and mumps virus may produce a similar picture of meningitis; a low CSF glucose level suggests mumps, whereas a normal CSF glucose level and transient CSF polymorphonuclear pleocytosis suggest enterovirus infection. Enteroviral meningitis is more frequent in summer and fall in temperate climates, while viral meningitis of other etiologies (e.g., mumps) is more common in winter and spring. Symptoms ordinarily resolve within a week, although CSF abnormalities can persist for several weeks. Enteroviral meningitis is often more severe in adults than in children. Neurologic sequelae are rare, and most patients have an excellent prognosis.

Enteroviral encephalitis is much less common than enteroviral aseptic meningitis. Occasional highly inflammatory cases of enteroviral meningitis may be complicated by a mild form of encephalitis that is recognized on the basis of progressive lethargy, disorientation, and sometimes seizures. Less commonly, severe primary encephalitis may develop. An estimated 10–20% of cases of viral encephalitis are due to enteroviruses. Immunocompetent patients generally have a good prognosis.

Patients with hypogammaglobulinemia or agammaglobulinemia or severe combined immunodeficiency may develop chronic meningitis or encephalitis; about half of these patients have a dermatomyositis-like syndrome, with peripheral edema, rash, and myositis. They may also have chronic hepatitis. Patients may develop neurologic disease while receiving gamma globulin replacement therapy. Echoviruses (especially echovirus 11) are the most common pathogens in this situation.

Paralytic disease due to enteroviruses other than poliovirus occurs sporadically and is usually less severe than poliomyelitis. Most cases are due to enterovirus 70 or 71 or to coxsackievirus A7 or A9. Guillain-Barré syndrome is also associated with enterovirus infection. While some studies have suggested a link between enteroviruses and the chronic fatigue syndrome, most recent studies have not demonstrated such an association.

PLEURODYNIA (BORNHOLM DISEASE) Patients with pleurodynia present with an acute onset of fever and spasms of pleuritic chest or upper abdominal pain. Chest pain is more common in adults, and abdominal pain is more common in children. Paroxysms of severe, knifelike pain usually last 15–30 min and are associated with diaphoresis and tachypnea. Fever peaks within an hour after the onset of paroxysms and subsides when pain resolves. The involved muscles are tender to palpation, and a pleural rub may be detected. The white blood cell count and chest x-ray are usually normal. Most cases are due to coxsackievirus B and occur during epidemics. Symptoms resolve in a few days, and recurrences are rare. Treatment includes the administration of nonsteroidal anti-inflammatory agents or the application of heat to the affected muscles.

MYOCARDITIS AND PERICARDITIS Enteroviruses are estimated to cause up to one-third of cases of acute myocarditis. Coxsackievirus B and its RNA have been detected in pericardial fluid and myocardial tissue in some cases of acute myocarditis and pericarditis. Most cases of enteroviral myocarditis or pericarditis occur in newborns, adolescents, or young adults. More than two-thirds of patients are male. Patients often present with an upper respiratory tract infection that is followed by fever, chest pain, dyspnea, arrhythmias, and occasionally heart failure. A pericardial friction rub is documented in half of cases, and the electrocardiogram shows ST-segment elevations or ST- and T-wave abnormalities. Serum levels of myocardial enzymes are often elevated. Neonates commonly have severe disease, while most older children and adults recover completely. Up to 10% of cases progress to chronic dilated cardiomyopathy. Chronic constrictive pericarditis may also be a sequela.

EXANTHEMS Enterovirus infection is the leading cause of exanthems in children in the summer and fall. While exanthems are associated with many enteroviruses, certain types have been linked to specific syndromes. Echoviruses 9 and 16 have frequently been associated with exanthem and fever. Rashes may be discrete (rubelliform) or confluent (morbilliform), beginning on the face and spreading to the trunk and extremities. Echovirus 9 is the most common cause of rubelliform rash. Unlike the rash of rubella, the enteroviral rash occurs in the summer and is not associated with lymphadenopathy. Roseola-like rashes develop after defervescence, with macules and papules on the face and trunk. The Boston exanthem, caused by echovirus 16, is a roseola-like rash that often affects multiple members of a family. A variety of other rashes have been associated with enteroviruses, including erythema multiforme and vesicular, urticarial, petechial, or purpuric lesions. Enanthems also occur, including lesions that resemble the Koplik's spots seen with measles.

HAND-FOOT-AND-MOUTH DISEASE After an incubation period of 4–6 days, patients with hand-foot-and-mouth disease present with fever, anorexia, and malaise; these manifestations are followed by the development of sore throat and vesicles (Fig. 184-1*A*) on the buccal mucosa and often on the tongue and then by the appearance of tender vesicular lesions on the dorsum of the hands, sometimes with involvement of the palms. The vesicles may form bullae and quickly ulcerate. About one-third of patients also have lesions on the palate, uvula, or tonsillar pillars, and one-third have a rash on the feet (including the soles) or on the buttocks. The disease is highly infectious, with attack rates of close to 100% among young children. The lesions usually resolve in 1 week. Most cases are due to coxsackievirus A16 or enterovirus 71.

An epidemic of enterovirus 71 infection in Taiwan in 1998 resulted in thousands of cases of hand-foot-and-mouth disease or herpangina. Severe complications included CNS disease, myocarditis, and pulmonary hemorrhage. About 90% of those who died were children ≤5 years old, and these deaths were associated with pulmonary edema or pulmonary hemorrhage. CNS disease included aseptic meningitis, flaccid paralysis (similar to poliomyelitis), or rhombencephalitis with myoclonus and tremor or ataxia. The mean age of patients with CNS complications was 2.5 years, and MRI in cases with encephalitis usually showed brain-stem lesions. Follow-up of children at 6 months showed persistent dysphagia, cranial nerve palsies, hypoventilation, limb weakness, and atrophy.

HERPANGINA Herpangina is usually caused by coxsackievirus A and presents as acute-onset fever, sore throat, dysphagia, and grayish-white papulovesicular lesions on an erythematous base that ulcerate (Fig. 184-1*B*). The lesions can persist for weeks; are present on the soft palate, anterior pillars of the tonsils, and uvula; and are concentrated in the posterior portion of the mouth. In contrast to herpes stomatitis, enteroviral herpangina is not associated with gingivitis. Acute lymphonodular pharyngitis associated with coxsackievirus A10 presents as white or yellow nodules surrounded by erythema in the posterior oropharynx. The lesions do not ulcerate.

ACUTE HEMORRHAGIC CONJUNCTIVITIS Patients with acute hemorrhagic conjunctivitis present with an acute onset of severe eye pain, blurred vision, photophobia, and watery discharge from the eye. Examination reveals edema, chemosis, and subconjunctival hemorrhage and often shows punctate keratitis and conjunctival follicles as well (Fig. 184-1*C*). Preauricular adenopathy is often found. Epidemics and

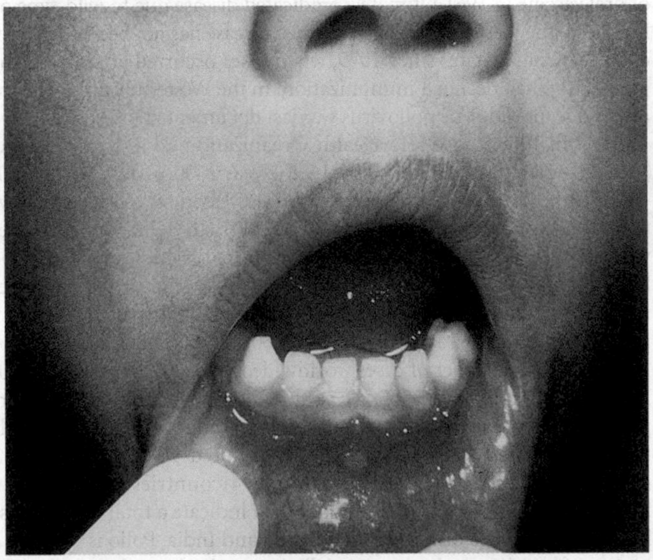

A

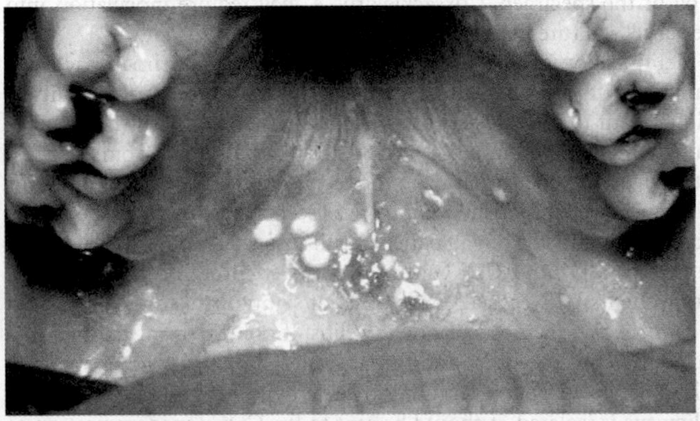

B

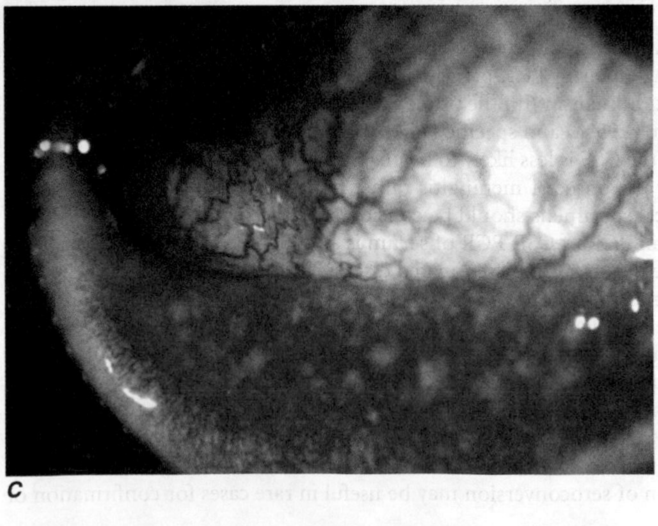

C

FIGURE 184-1 ***A.*** Tender vesicles and erosions in the mouth of a patient with hand-foot-and-mouth disease. ***B.*** Soft-palate lesions of herpangina due to coxsackievirus. ***C.*** Acute hemorrhagic conjunctivitis due to enterovirus 71. *(Images B and C are reprinted with permission from Redbook 2006: Committee on Infectious Diseases, 27th ed. Elk Grove Village, IL: American Academy of Pediatrics.)*

nosocomial spread have been associated with enterovirus 70 and coxsackievirus A24. Systemic symptoms, including headache and fever, develop in 20% of cases, and recovery is usually complete in 10 days. The sudden onset and short duration of the illness help to distinguish acute hemorrhagic conjunctivitis from other ocular infections such as those due to adenovirus and *Chlamydia*. Paralysis has been associated with some cases of acute hemorrhagic conjunctivitis due to enterovirus 70 during epidemics.

OTHER MANIFESTATIONS Enteroviruses are an infrequent cause of childhood pneumonia and the common cold. Coxsackievirus B has been isolated at autopsy from the pancreas of a few children presenting with type 1 diabetes mellitus; however, most attempts to isolate the virus have been unsuccessful. Other diseases that have been associated with enterovirus infection include parotitis, bronchitis, bronchiolitis, croup, infectious lymphocytosis, polymyositis, acute arthritis, and acute nephritis.

DIAGNOSIS

Isolation of enterovirus in cell culture is the traditional diagnostic procedure. While cultures of stool, nasopharyngeal, or throat samples from patients with enterovirus diseases are often positive, isolation of the virus from these sites does not prove that it is directly associated with disease because these sites are frequently colonized for weeks in patients with subclinical infections. Isolation of virus from the throat is more likely to be associated with disease than isolation from the stool since virus is shed for shorter periods from the throat. Cultures of CSF, serum, fluid from body cavities, or tissues are positive less frequently, but a positive result is indicative of disease caused by enterovirus. In some cases, the virus is isolated only from the blood or only from the CSF; therefore, it is important to culture multiple sites. Cultures are more likely to be positive earlier than later in the course of infection. Most human enteroviruses can be detected within a week after inoculation of cell cultures. Cultures may be negative because of the presence of neutralizing antibody, lack of susceptibility of the cells used, or inappropriate handling of the specimen. Coxsackievirus A may require inoculation into special cell-culture lines or into suckling mice.

Identification of the enterovirus serotype is useful primarily for epidemiologic studies and, with a few exceptions, has little clinical utility. It is important to identify serious infections with enterovirus during epidemics and to distinguish the vaccine strain of poliovirus from the other enteroviruses in the throat or in the feces. Stool and throat samples for culture as well as acute- and convalescent-phase serum specimens should be obtained from all patients with suspected poliomyelitis. In the absence of a positive CSF culture, a positive culture of stool obtained within the first 2 weeks after the onset of symptoms is most often used to confirm the diagnosis of poliomyelitis. If poliovirus infection is suspected, two or more fecal and throat swab samples should be obtained at least 1 day apart and cultured for enterovirus as soon as possible. If poliovirus is isolated, it should be sent to the CDC for identification as either wild-type or vaccine virus.

The polymerase chain reaction (PCR) has been used to amplify viral nucleic acid from CSF, serum, urine, throat swabs, and tissues. A single pair of PCR primers can detect >92% of the serotypes that infect humans. With the proper controls, PCR of the CSF is highly sensitive (≥95%) and specific (>80%) and is more rapid than culture. PCR of the CSF is less likely to be positive when patients present ≥3 days after the onset of meningitis rather than earlier; in these cases, PCR of fecal specimens should be considered, although the test is less specific than PCR of CSF. PCR of serum is also highly sensitive and specific in the diagnosis of disseminated disease. PCR may be particularly helpful for the diagnosis and follow-up of enterovirus disease in immunodeficient patients receiving immunoglobulin therapy, whose viral cultures may be negative. Antigen detection and hybridization of enterovirus sequences in human tissues with a specific probe are additional options, but these techniques are generally less sensitive than PCR.

Serologic diagnosis of enterovirus infection is limited by the large number of serotypes and the lack of a common antigen. Demonstration of seroconversion may be useful in rare cases for confirmation of culture results, but serologic testing is usually limited to epidemiologic studies. Serum should be collected and frozen soon after the onset of disease and again ~4 weeks later. Measurement of neutralizing titers is the most accurate method for antibody determination; measurement of complement-fixation titers is usually less sensitive. Titers of virus-specific IgM are elevated in both acute and chronic infection.

℞ ENTEROVIRUS INFECTIONS

Most enterovirus infections are mild and resolve spontaneously; however, intensive supportive care may be needed for cardiac, hepatic, or CNS disease. IV, intrathecal, or intraventricular immunoglobulin has been used with apparent success for the treatment of chronic enterovirus meningoencephalitis and dermatomyositis in patients with hypogammaglobulinemia or agammaglobulinemia. The disease may stabilize or resolve during therapy; however, some patients decline inexorably despite therapy. IV administration of immunoglobulin with high titers of antibody to the infecting virus has been used in some cases of life-threatening infection in neonates, who may not have maternally acquired antibody. In one trial involving neonates with enterovirus infections, immunoglobulin containing very high titers of antibody to the infecting virus reduced rates of viremia; however, the study was too small to show a substantial clinical benefit. The level of enteroviral antibodies varies with the immunoglobulin preparation. For a time, pleconaril was given to patients with severe enterovirus infections on a compassionate-use basis, but this drug is no longer available for this use. Glucocorticoids are contraindicated.

Good hand-washing practices and the use of gowns and gloves are important in limiting nosocomial transmission of enteroviruses during epidemics. Enteric precautions are indicated for 7 days after the onset of enterovirus infections.

PREVENTION AND ERADICATION OF POLIOVIRUS

(See also Chap. 116) After a peak of 57,879 cases of poliomyelitis in the United States in 1952, the introduction of inactivated vaccine in 1955 and of oral vaccine in 1961 ultimately eradicated disease due to wild-type poliovirus in the Western Hemisphere. Such disease has not been documented in the United States since 1979, when cases occurred among religious groups who had declined immunization. In the Western Hemisphere, paralysis due to wild-type poliovirus was last documented in 1991.

In 1988, the World Health Organization adopted a resolution to eradicate poliomyelitis by the year 2000. From 1988 to 2001, the number of cases worldwide decreased by >99%, with fewer than 1000 confirmed cases reported in 2001. In 2002, however, there were ~1900 cases of polio, with ~1500 reported in India. Wild-type poliovirus type 2 has not been detected in the world since 1999. The Americas were certified free of indigenous wild-type poliovirus transmission in 1994, the Western Pacific Region in 2000, and the European Region in 2002. The total number of cases worldwide fell to a nadir of 498 in 2001. However, from 2002 to 2005, 21 countries previously free of polio reported cases imported from 6 polio-endemic countries. By 2006, polio transmission had been reduced or interrupted in most of these 21 countries, and polio was endemic in only 4 countries, with a total of 2000 cases (Table 184-2). Preliminary data indicate a total of 1959 cases in 2006, with ~90% of cases from Nigeria and India. Polio is a source of concern for unimmunized or partially immunized travelers to these regions. Outbreaks of polio in Europe and North America have been traced to cases imported from the Indian subcontinent. Clearly, global eradication of polio is necessary to eliminate the risk of importation of wild-type virus. Outbreaks are thought to have been facilitated by suboptimal rates of vaccination, isolated pockets of unvaccinated children, poor sanitation and crowding, improper vaccine-storage conditions, and a reduced level of response to one of the serotypes in the vaccine. While the global eradication campaign has markedly reduced the number of cases of polio, doubts have been raised as to whether eradication is a realistic goal given the large number of asymptomatic cases and the political instability in developing countries.

Outbreaks of poliomyelitis due to circulating vaccine-derived poliovirus have recently occurred. In Egypt, 30 cases of vaccine-derived polio oc-

TABLE 184-2 LABORATORY-CONFIRMED CASES OF POLIOMYELITIS IN 2006

Country	Type of Transmission	Number of Cases
Nigeria	Endemic	1123[a]
India	Endemic	676
Pakistan	Endemic	40
Afghanistan	Endemic	31
Somalia	Imported	35
Others[b]	Imported	93
Others[c]	Vaccine-derived	2
Total		2000

[a]Of these cases, 1 was vaccine-derived.
[b]Imported cases: Namibia, 19; Bangladesh, 18; Ethiopia, 17; Democratic Republic of the Congo, 13; Niger, 11; Nepal, 5; Angola, 2; Cameroon, 2; Kenya, 2; Indonesia, 2; Chad, 1; Yemen, 1.
[c]Vaccine-derived cases: Myanmar, 1; Cambodia, 1.
Source: World Health Organization.

curred in 1988–1993; in the Dominican Republic and Haiti, 21 cases occurred in 2000–2001; and fewer than 5 cases each occurred in the Philippines (2001), Madagascar (2002), and China (2004). These OPV-derived viruses reverted to a more neurovirulent phenotype after undetected circulation (probably for >2 years). The epidemic in Hispaniola was rapidly terminated after intensive vaccination with OPV. In 2005, a case of vaccine-derived polio occurred in an unvaccinated U.S. woman returning from a visit to Central and South America. In the same year, an unvaccinated immunocompromised infant in Minnesota was found to be shedding vaccine-derived poliovirus; further investigation identified 3 other infants in the same community who were shedding the virus. All 4 infants were asymptomatic. These outbreaks emphasize the need for maintaining high levels of vaccine coverage and continued surveillance for circulating virus.

IPV is used in most industrialized countries and OPV in most developing countries, including those in which polio still is or recently was endemic. After several doses of OPV alone, the seropositivity rate for individual poliovirus serotypes may still be suboptimal for children in developing countries; one or more supplemental doses of IPV can increase the rate of seropositivity for these serotypes. While IM injections of other vaccines (live or attenuated) can be given concurrently with OPV, unnecessary IM injections should be avoided during the first month after vaccination because they increase the risk of vaccine-associated paralysis. Since 1988, an enhanced-potency inactivated poliovirus vaccine has been available in the United States.

OPV and IPV induce antibodies that persist for at least 5 years. Both vaccines induce IgG and IgA antibodies. Compared with recipients of IPV, recipients of OPV shed less virus and less frequently develop reinfection with wild-type virus after exposure to poliovirus. Although IPV is safe and efficacious, OPV offers the advantages of ease of administration, lower cost, and induction of intestinal immunity resulting in a reduction in the risk of community transmission of wild-type virus. Because of progress toward global eradication of polio (with a reduced risk of imported cases) and the continued occurrence of cases of vaccine-associated polio, an all-IPV regimen was recommended in 2000 for childhood poliovirus vaccination in the United States, with vaccine administration at 2, 4, and 6–18 months and 4–6 years of age. The risk of vaccine-associated polio should be discussed before OPV is administered. Recommendations for vaccination of adults are listed in Table 184-3.

There are concerns about discontinuing vaccination in the event that endemic spread of poliovirus is eliminated. Among the reasons for these concerns are that poliovirus is shed from some immunocompromised persons for several years, that vaccine-derived poliovirus can circulate and cause disease, and that wild-type poliovirus is present in a large number of laboratories. A national survey began in October 2002 to encourage laboratories to dispose of all unneeded wild-type poliovirus materials and to identify laboratories that have wild-type poliovirus or specimens that may contain virus.

TABLE 184-3 RECOMMENDATIONS FOR POLIOVIRUS VACCINATION OF ADULTS

1. Most adults in the United States have been vaccinated during childhood and have little risk of exposure to wild-type virus in the United States. Immunization is recommended for those with a higher risk of exposure than the general population, including:
   a. travelers to areas where poliovirus is or may be epidemic or endemic;
   b. members of communities or population groups with disease caused by wild-type polioviruses;
   c. laboratory workers handling specimens that may contain wild-type polioviruses; and
   d. health care workers in close contact with patients who may be excreting wild-type polioviruses.
2. Three doses of IPV are recommended for adults who need to be immunized. The second dose should be given 1–2 months after the first dose; the third dose should be given 6–12 months after the second dose.
3. Adults who are at increased risk of exposure to wild-type poliovirus and who have previously completed primary immunization should receive a single dose of IPV. Adults who did not complete primary immunization should receive the remaining vaccinations with IPV.

Note: IPV, inactivated poliovirus vaccine.
Source: Modified from Pickering LK, ed. Redbook 2006: Committee on Infectious Diseases, 27th ed. Elk Grove Village, IL: American Academy of Pediatrics.

REOVIRUSES

Reoviruses are double-stranded RNA viruses encompassing three serotypes. Serologic studies indicate that most humans are infected with reoviruses during childhood. Most infections either are asymptomatic or cause very mild disease. One outbreak of reovirus infection in children resulted in minor upper respiratory tract symptoms. Reovirus is considered a rare cause of mild gastroenteritis in infants and children. Speculation regarding an association of reovirus type 3 with idiopathic neonatal hepatitis and extrahepatic biliary atresia is based on an elevated prevalence of antibody to reovirus among some of these patients and the detection of viral RNA by PCR in hepatobiliary tissues in some studies.

FURTHER READINGS

Alexander LN et al: Vaccine policy changes and epidemiology of poliomyelitis in the United States. JAMA 292:1696, 2004

Arita I et al: Is polio eradication realistic? Science 312:852, 2006

Centers for Disease Control and Prevention: Enterovirus surveillance—United States, 2002–2004. MMWR 55:153, 2006

———: Resurgence of wild poliovirus type 1 transmission and consequences of importation—21 countries, 2002–2005. MMWR 55:145, 2006

Chang L-Y et al: Transmission and clinical features of enterovirus 71 infections in household contacts in Taiwan. JAMA 291:222, 2004

Jubelt B, Aagre JC: Characteristics and management of postpolio syndrome. JAMA 284:412, 2000

Kew O et al: Vaccine-derived polioviruses and the endgame strategy for global polio eradication. Annu Rev Microbiol 59:587, 2005

Kupilia L et al: Diagnosis of enteroviral meningitis by use of polymerase chain reaction of cerebrospinal fluid, stool, and serum specimens. Clin Infect Dis 40:982, 2005

MacLennan C et al: Failure to clear persistent vaccine-derived neurovirulent poliovirus infection in an immunocompromised man. Lancet 363:1509, 2004

Perez-Velez CM et al: Outbreak of neurologic enterovirus type 71 disease: A diagnostic challenge. Clin Infect Dis 45:950, 2007

Thompson KM, Tebbens RJ: Eradication versus control for poliomyelitis: An economic analysis. Lancet 369:1363, 2007

185 Measles (Rubeola)

Anne Gershon

DEFINITION

Measles (rubeola) is a highly contagious, acute, exanthematous respiratory disease with a characteristic clinical picture and a pathognomonic enanthem: Koplik's spots, an eruption on the buccal mucous membranes (Fig. 185-1).

A successful live attenuated measles vaccine became available in 1963 in the United States and elsewhere, and measles is now an unusual disease in most developed countries where this vaccine is widely used. However, measles continues to occur sporadically in miniepidemics in the United States, and major epidemics in developing nations make this disease a persistent cause of childhood morbidity and mortality.

In 2000, measles was the fifth leading cause of childhood mortality worldwide, with an estimated 777,000 deaths. The incidence of global measles in 2004 is shown in Fig. 185-2.

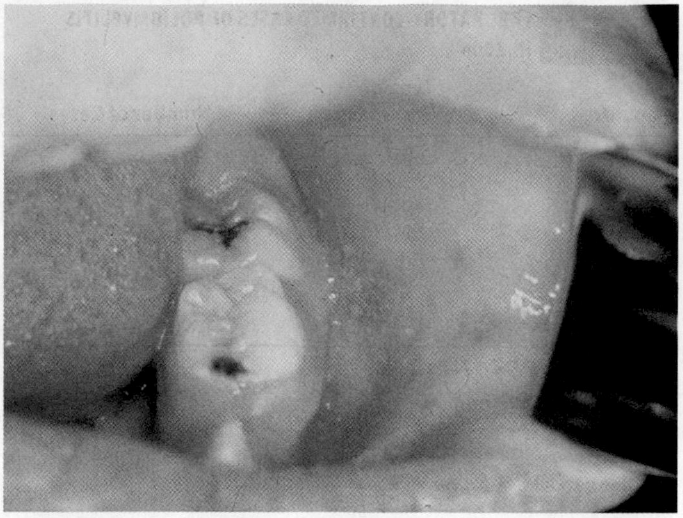

FIGURE 185-1 **Koplik's spots,** which manifest as white or bluish lesions with an erythematous halo on the buccal mucosa, usually occur in the first 2 days of measles symptoms and may briefly overlap the measles exanthem. The presence of the erythematous halo differentiates Koplik's spots from Fordyce's spots (ectopic sebaceous glands), which occur in the mouths of healthy individuals. *(Source: Centers for Disease Control and Prevention. Photo selected by Dr. Kenneth Kaye.)*

ETIOLOGIC AGENT

Measles virus is the only member of the genus *Morbillivirus* that infects humans. Part of the family Paramyxoviridae, it is related to viruses causing similar infections in other mammals: distemper, rinderpest, morbilli, and *peste des petits ruminants*. There is only one antigenic type. Virions—pleomorphic spheres with a diameter of 100–250 nm—consist of six proteins. The inner capsid is composed of RNA and three proteins. The outer envelope consists of a matrix protein bearing short surface-glycoprotein projections or peplomers, one a hemagglutinin (H) and the other a fusion (F) protein. Sequencing of the single-stranded genome makes it possible to distinguish vaccine-type from wild-type virus. The genetic variability of wild-type virus (23 genotypes identified) permits identification of strains endemic within a given locale where measles cases have occurred. The cellular receptors for measles virus are the CD46 and CD150 molecules expressed on many human cells.

EPIDEMIOLOGY

Measles has a worldwide distribution; humans are the only natural hosts, although other primates can be experimentally infected. During the prevaccination era in the United States, measles epidemics took place every 2–5 years. In epidemic years, roughly half a million measles cases occurred; 99% of adults had serologic evidence of previous measles infection. After the live attenuated vaccine became available, the number of cases reported to the Centers for Disease Control and Prevention fell, with a nadir of 1497 cases in 1983. In 1990, after an upsurge to more than 27,000 cases (with 89 deaths), the disease was once more brought under control, mainly through the routine administration of two doses of vaccine. Reasons for the resurgence included failure to immunize young children, especially in inner-city areas; primary vaccine failure (rate, ~5%); and (rarely) waning immunity.

Between 1993 and 1996, fewer than 1000 cases per year were reported in the United States; 309 cases were reported in 1995, 116 in 2001, and only 37 in 2004. Molecular studies indicated interruption of transmission of indigenous measles in 1993. Most cases since have resulted from international importations of the virus by immigrants or U.S. citizens returning from travel abroad. Mortality rates are highest among children <2 years of age and among adults. Patients with impaired cell-mediated immunity are at especially high risk for severe or even fatal measles. The measles-associated mortality rate in the United States is ~0.3%; in developing countries, it frequently exceeds 1% and sometimes approaches 10% because of malnutrition and associated immunodeficiency and HIV infection.

Measles virus is transmitted by respiratory secretions, predominantly through exposure to aerosols but also through direct contact with larger droplets. Patients are contagious from 1 or 2 days before symptom onset until 4 days after the rash appears. Infectivity peaks during the prodromal phase. The mean intervals from infection to symptom onset and rash appearance are 10 and 14 days, respectively.

PATHOGENESIS, IMMUNITY, AND PATHOLOGY

Measles virus invades the respiratory epithelium and spreads via the bloodstream to the reticuloendothelial system, from which it infects

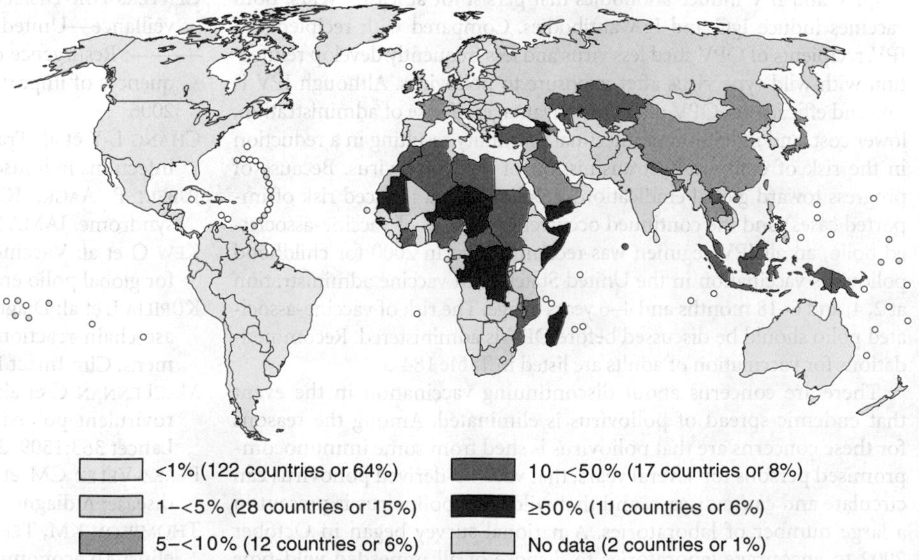

FIGURE 185-2 **Worldwide reported measles incidence rate per 100,000 population, 2004.** *(Source: WHO/IBV database, 2005. This map does not imply the expression of any opinion whatsoever on the part of the World Health Organization concerning the legal status of any country, territory, city, or area of its authorities or concerning the delimitation of its frontiers or boundaries.)*

white blood cells, thereby establishing infection of the skin, respiratory tract, and other organs. Both viremia and viruria develop. Multinucleated giant cells with inclusion bodies in the nucleus and cytoplasm (Warthin-Finkeldey cells) are found in respiratory and lymphoid tissues and are pathognomonic for measles. Direct invasion of T lymphocytes and increased levels of suppressive cytokines (e.g., interleukin 4) may play a role in the temporary depression of cellular immunity that accompanies and transiently follows measles. The major infected cell in the blood is the monocyte. Infection of the entire respiratory tract accounts for the characteristic cough and coryza of measles and for the less frequent manifestations of croup, bronchiolitis, and pneumonia. Generalized damage to the respiratory tract, with loss of cilia, predisposes to secondary bacterial infections such as pneumonia and otitis media.

Specific antibodies are not detectable before the onset of rash. Cellular immunity (consisting of cytotoxic T cells and possibly natural killer cells) plays a prominent role in host defense, and patients who are deficient in cellular immunity are at high risk for severe measles. Children with isolated agammaglobulinemia are not at increased risk. Immune reactions to the virus in the endothelial cells of dermal capillaries play a substantial role in the development of Koplik's spots (the pathognomonic enanthem) and rash; in immunodeficient hosts, measles may be severe despite the absence of these manifestations. Measles antigens have been demonstrated in involved skin during early stages of the illness.

Pathologic changes in measles encephalitis include focal hemorrhage, congestion, and perivascular demyelination. Measles virus is rarely isolated from cerebrospinal fluid (CSF) in cases of encephalitis, which are thought to be due to the interaction of virus-infected cells with local cellular immune factors.

CLINICAL MANIFESTATIONS

Measles begins with a 2- to 4-day respiratory prodrome of malaise, cough, coryza, conjunctivitis with lacrimation, nasal discharge, and increasing fever [with temperatures as high as 40.6°C (105°F), probably reflecting secondary viremia]. At this stage of the illness, in which the rash has not yet developed, influenza may be suspected. Just before rash onset, Koplik's spots appear as 1- to 2-mm blue-white spots on a bright red background (Fig. 185-1). Without adequate illumination for examination, they may be overlooked. Koplik's spots are typically located on the buccal mucosa, alongside the second molars, and may be extensive; they are not associated with any other infectious disease. The spots wane after the onset of rash and soon disappear. The entire buccal and inner labial mucosa may be inflamed, and the lips may be reddened.

The characteristic erythematous, nonpruritic, maculopapular rash of measles begins at the hairline and behind the ears, spreads down the trunk and limbs to include the palms and soles, and often becomes confluent (Fig. 185-3). At this time, the patient is at the most severe point of the illness. By the fourth day, the rash begins to fade in the order in which it appeared. Brownish discoloration of the skin and desquamation may occur later. Fever usually resolves by the fourth or fifth day after the onset of rash; prolonged fever suggests a complication of measles. Lymphadenopathy, diarrhea, vomiting, and splenomegaly are common features. The chest x-ray may be abnormal, even in uncomplicated measles, because of the propensity of measles virus to invade the respiratory tract. The entire illness, which usually lasts ~10 days, tends to be more severe in adults than in children, with higher fever, more prominent rash, and a higher incidence of complications.

Milder forms of the illness with less intense symptoms and a milder rash, termed *modified measles*, may occur in individuals with preexisting partial immunity induced by active or passive vaccination. These patients include infants <1 year of age who retain some proportion of passively acquired maternal antibodies. On occasion, individuals with a history of immunization may develop modified measles.

COMPLICATIONS

The complications of measles (Table 185-1) can be divided into three groups, according to the site involved: the respiratory tract, the central nervous system (CNS), and the gastrointestinal tract. Respiratory tract

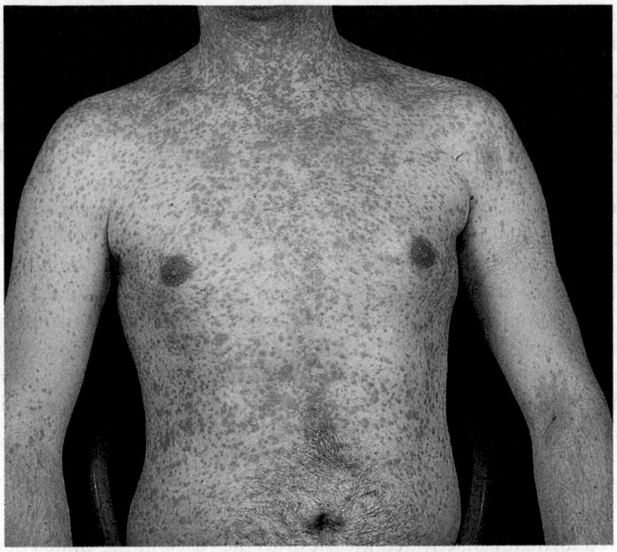

FIGURE 185-3 In measles, discrete erythematous lesions become confluent as the rash spreads downward. *(Reprinted with permission from Fitzpatrick TB et al: Color Atlas & Synopsis of Clinical Dermatology, 4th ed. New York, McGraw-Hill, 2001, p 775.)*

involvement, manifested as laryngitis, croup, or bronchitis, occurs in the majority of cases of uncomplicated measles. In young children, otitis media is the most common complication. Pneumonia is a frequent reason for hospitalization, especially of adults. The pneumonia is of viral origin in the majority of cases, but secondary bacterial infection (most commonly caused by streptococci, pneumococci, or staphylococci) also develops with some frequency. Primary giant-cell (Hecht's) pneumonia is most often documented in immunocompromised and/or malnourished patients.

Encephalographic abnormalities in the absence of symptoms of CNS disease are extremely common in measles. Symptomatic CNS disease may present with fever, headache, drowsiness, coma, and/or seizures. Symptoms usually begin within days after the onset of rash but occasionally appear for the first time several weeks later. About 10% of patients do not survive acute measles encephalitis; a significant percentage of survivors have permanent sequelae (e.g., mental retardation or epilepsy). Most cases appear to result from an immune-mediated response to myelin proteins (postinfectious encephalomyelitis) and not directly from viral infection of the CNS (Chap. 375). Rarely, transverse myelitis follows measles. Immunocompromised patients are at risk for progressive fatal encephalitis 1–6 months after measles; in some cases, even though prior measles has not been recognized, the virus is identified at autopsy. Sub-

TABLE 185-1 COMPLICATIONS OF MEASLES

Complication	Comments
Otitis media	Very common in infants with measles
Pneumonia	May be primary viral pneumonia or bacterial superinfection; frequent reason for hospitalization of adults; measles rash sometimes lacking in immunocompromised patients with measles pneumonia
Croup	Occasionally severe, requiring intubation in infants
Gastroenteritis	Diarrhea can be life threatening in infants
Cervical adenitis	Due to lymphoid hyperplasia as host response to virus; common
Acute encephalitis	May be mild to severe/fatal; occurs in 1 in 1000 cases of measles; cerebral and cerebellar forms; immune-mediated pathogenesis
Subacute sclerosing panencephalitis (SSPE)	In 1 in 100,000 cases of measles, usually when measles occurs in infancy; seen 5–10 years later. In the United States, most children with SSPE were born in another country where measles vaccine is not routinely used.

acute sclerosing panencephalitis (SSPE)—a protracted, chronic, extremely rare form of measles encephalitis—sometimes follows measles and is particularly common among children who have measles before the age of 2 years (Chap. 376). As a result of widespread vaccination, SSPE has virtually disappeared in the United States. Typically, progressive dementia evolves over several months. SSPE is thought to be due to a complex interaction of the host with defective measles virus.

Gastrointestinal complications of measles include gastroenteritis, hepatitis, appendicitis, ileocolitis, and mesenteric adenitis. It is not uncommon to detect high levels of alanine and aspartate aminotransferases in the absence of gastrointestinal signs such as jaundice.

Rare complications include myocarditis, glomerulonephritis, and postinfectious thrombocytopenic purpura. Measles can exacerbate preexisting tuberculosis, presumably through virus-induced depression of cellular immunity. Natural measles and immunization against measles can result in tuberculin skin-test anergy lasting for ~1 month.

ATYPICAL MEASLES

An atypical form of measles has been reported in individuals who received formalin-inactivated measles vaccine (used in the United States in 1963–1967 and in Canada until 1970) and subsequently were exposed to measles virus. After a several-day prodrome of fever, myalgia, and headache, the rash appears (Fig. 185-4); it begins peripherally and can be urticarial, maculopapular, hemorrhagic, and/or vesicular. Fever is high and accompanied by edema of the extremities, interstitial pulmonary infiltrates, hepatitis, and (on occasion) pleural effusion. The differential diagnosis includes Rocky Mountain spotted fever, Henoch-Schönlein purpura, meningococcemia, drug allergy, toxic shock syndrome, and varicella. Despite its severity, the illness is self-limited. Measles virus cannot be isolated from these patients. This disease is believed to be due to hypersensitivity to measles virus induced by the inactivated vaccine. To prevent it, adults who received formalin-inactivated measles vaccine should be immunized with live attenuated measles vaccine. Because inactivated measles vaccine has not been available for >35 years, atypical measles has virtually disappeared.

MEASLES IN THE IMMUNOCOMPROMISED HOST

Patients with defects in cell-mediated immunity are at risk for severe protracted and fatal measles. Included in this category are patients with congenital cellular immune defects or malignancy, recipients of immunosuppressive therapy, or persons infected with HIV. In these patients, measles may not be accompanied by a rash. Complications are primary measles (giant-cell) pneumonia, progressive encephalitis beginning weeks or months after initial infection, and (in HIV-infected patients) progression to AIDS.

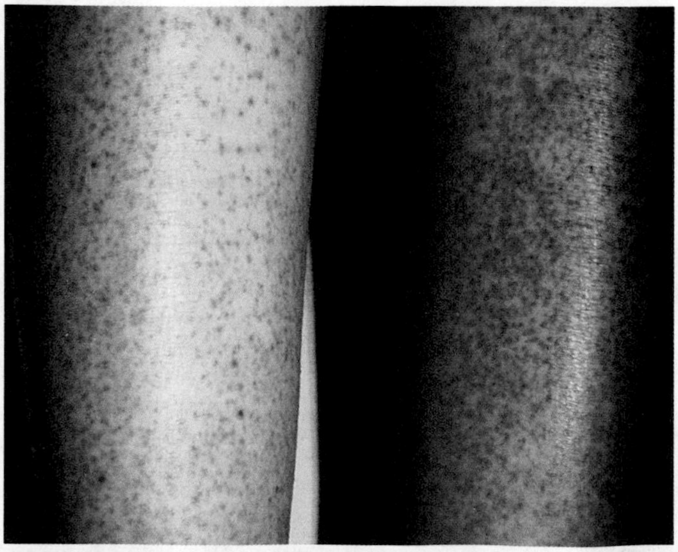

FIGURE 185-4 Petechial lesions in a patient with atypical measles. *(Photo courtesy of Stephen E. Gellis, MD; with permission.)*

MEASLES IN ADULTS

Measles is naturally a disease of childhood and, like many other viral infections, is more severe in adults than in children. About 3% of young adults with measles develop primary viral pneumonia and require hospitalization. Hepatitis and bronchospasm are more common among adults with measles than among children, and the rash is more severe and more confluent in adults. Bacterial superinfection is more common among adults, more than one-third of whom develop respiratory complications such as otitis media, sinusitis, and pneumonia. Adults may develop measles because they were never immunized or (more rarely) because their vaccine-induced immunity has waned. Very low titers of antibody to measles virus have been associated with lack of protection.

LABORATORY FINDINGS

Lymphopenia and neutropenia are common in measles and may be due to invasion of leukocytes by the virus, with subsequent cell death. Leukocytosis may herald a bacterial superinfection. Patients with measles encephalitis usually have an elevated protein concentration in CSF as well as lymphocytosis.

DIAGNOSIS

A specific diagnosis of measles can be made quickly by immunofluorescent staining of a smear of respiratory secretions for measles antigen; monoclonal antibodies conjugated to fluorescein are commercially available. Secretions can be examined microscopically for multinucleated giant cells. Measles virus can be demonstrated by culture or polymerase chain reaction in respiratory secretions or urine. A number of serologic tests are available. A serologic diagnosis by enzyme immunoassay (EIA) cannot necessarily be made rapidly if acute- and convalescent-phase serum specimens are examined. However, EIA measurement of specific IgM permits diagnosis on the basis of an acute-phase serum sample. Specific IgM antibodies are detectable within 1–2 days after rash onset, and the IgG titer rises significantly after 10 days. Atypical measles and SSPE are associated with extremely high levels of measles antibodies in blood and/or CSF.

DIFFERENTIAL DIAGNOSIS

Classic measles—with Koplik's spots, cough, coryza, conjunctivitis, and a rash beginning on the head—is easily diagnosed on clinical grounds. Modified measles is more difficult to diagnose because one or more characteristic signs or symptoms may be lacking. The differential diagnosis of measles includes Kawasaki disease, scarlet fever, infectious mononucleosis, toxoplasmosis, drug eruption, and *Mycoplasma pneumoniae* infection. In the differential diagnosis of measles, attention should be paid to the current epidemiology of the disease in the community and to the patient's history of measles vaccination and foreign travel.

PREVENTION

The development of live attenuated measles vaccine by Enders and colleagues was a milestone in American medicine. This vaccine, used in the United States for the routine immunization of children since 1963, induces seroconversion in ~95% of recipients and probably confers lifelong protection. Waning immunity to measles after immunization is rare. For the past three decades, measles vaccine has been available as the combination vaccine measles-mumps-rubella (MMR); this vaccine should be administered to children at 12–15 months of age. (Vaccination at 12 months is preferred for infants whose mothers were immunized against measles in childhood.) A second dose of MMR vaccine is recommended for school-age children. This two-dose policy was developed in the late 1980s in response to measles outbreaks in the United States. MMR vaccine is likely to be supplanted by MMRV vaccine, which also covers varicella and was licensed by the U.S. Food and Drug Administration in 2005. MMRV vaccine is licensed only for children 1–13 years of age.

Older susceptible persons should be immunized. Individuals should be considered susceptible to measles unless they have documentation of physician-diagnosed measles or of the receipt of two doses of vaccine, have laboratory evidence of measles immunity, or were born before 1957. Rarely, individuals born before 1957 develop measles, and those who are at risk of exposure to measles (e.g., health care workers, teachers, and international travelers) should be tested for measles antibody and immunized if necessary. Approximately 10% of healthy vaccinees develop a fever, with temperatures up to 39.4°C (103°F), 5–7 days after vaccination; this fever lasts 1–5 days and is accompanied by a transient rash. Individuals previously immunized only with killed vaccine are considered susceptible and should receive at least one dose—preferably two doses—of MMR vaccine. Transient adverse reactions in these individuals include fever, malaise, and redness and swelling at the injection site.

Because of the severity of measles in this group and the lack of reported problems following vaccination, children with asymptomatic HIV infection should receive MMR vaccine; those with severe immunosuppression (<15% CD4+ T lymphocytes) should not. A case of fatal measles due to vaccine-type virus was reported in a college student with AIDS in 1998. Measles vaccine is contraindicated for persons with impaired cell-mediated immunity, for pregnant women, and for persons with a history of anaphylaxis due to egg protein or neomycin. Minor illnesses, with or without fever and a history of convulsions, are not contraindications to vaccination. Vaccination should be deferred for 6–11 months after the receipt of immune globulin or of blood products containing antibodies and for at least 3 months after the discontinuation of immunosuppressive treatment. Vaccine failures have been ascribed to faulty vaccine storage, the presence of maternally derived antibodies in infants, and simultaneous administration of measles vaccine and immune globulin.

The only temporally related causal complications of measles vaccination are febrile seizures, which rarely have long-term sequelae; self-limited thrombocytopenia; and rare anaphylaxis. An exhaustive analysis conducted in 2000 by a number of official committees, including those of the American Academy of Pediatrics and the Institute of Medicine, found no causal relationship between MMR vaccination and subsequent development of autism.

Children and adults who are susceptible to measles and are exposed to the disease should receive postexposure prophylaxis. Standard immune globulin, given intramuscularly within 6 days of exposure, can exert a protective or modifying effect. The dose is 0.25 mL/kg for healthy persons and 0.5 mL/kg for immunocompromised persons, with a maximum dose of 15 mL. Immune globulin is particularly strongly indicated for susceptible household contacts, especially those <1 year of age, and for immunocompromised persons. HIV-infected individuals, particularly those with severe immunosuppression, should be given immune globulin after exposure, regardless of their measles immune status and whether or not they are receiving intravenous immune globulin. Vaccination within 72 h of exposure may also provide protection against clinical measles but is contraindicated in immunocompromised patients. Vaccine and immune globulin should not be given concurrently.

℞ MEASLES

Therapy for measles is largely supportive and symptom based. Patients with otitis media and pneumonia should be given standard antibiotics. Patients with encephalitis need supportive care, including observation for increased intracranial pressure. Controlled trials suggest clinical benefit from high doses of vitamin A in severe or potentially severe measles, especially in children <2 years old who are or may be malnourished. On the basis of limited data, a dose of 50,000 IU is used for infants 1–6 months old; 100,000 IU is recommended for infants 7–12 months old and 200,000 IU for children >1 year old. A single dose is administered on two consecutive days. In the United States, vitamin A treatment is recommended for young children hospitalized for measles and for pediatric measles patients with immunodeficiency, clinical evidence of vitamin A deficiency, impaired intestinal absorption, moderate to severe malnutrition, or recent immigration from an area where there is high mortality from measles. Transient vomiting and headache may be associated with the administration of vitamin A. Ribavirin is effective against measles virus in vitro and may be considered for use in immunocompromised individuals.

FURTHER READINGS

CENTERS FOR DISEASE CONTROL AND PREVENTION: Measles, mumps, and rubella—vaccine use and strategies for elimination of measles, rubella, and congenital rubella syndrome and control of mumps. MMWR Morb Mortal Wkly Rep 47:1, 1998

———: Measles—United States, 2004. MMWR Morb Mortal Wkly Rep 54:1229, 2005

D'SOUZA RM, D'SOUZA R: Vitamin A for preventing secondary infections in children with measles—a systematic review. J Trop Pediatr 48:72, 2002

FORNI AL et al: Severe measles pneumonitis in adults: Evaluation of clinical characteristics and therapy with intravenous ribavirin. Clin Infect Dis 19:454, 1994

IMMUNIZATION SAFETY REVIEW COMMITTEE, INSTITUTE OF MEDICINE: *Immunization Safety Review: Measles-Mumps-Rubella Vaccine and Autism*, K Stratton et al (eds). Washington, DC, National Academy of Sciences, 2001 *(www.nap.edu/catalog/10101.html)*

KAPLAN LJ et al: Severe measles in immunocompromised patients. JAMA 267:1237, 1992

STALKUP JR: A review of measles virus. Dermatol Clin 20:209, 2002

YEUNG LF et al: A limited measles outbreak in a highly vaccinated US boarding school. Pediatrics 116:1287, 2005

186 Rubella (German Measles)

Anne Gershon

DEFINITION

Rubella is an acute viral infection of children and adults that characteristically includes rash, fever, and lymphadenopathy and has a broad spectrum of other possible manifestations. However, a high percentage of rubella infections in both children and adults are subclinical. In addition, the illness can resemble a mild attack of measles (rubeola) and can cause arthritis, especially in adults. Rubella was formerly known as *German measles* because it was first distinguished clinically from rubeola in Germany, where it generated much medical interest in the mid-eighteenth and early nineteenth centuries. Rubella during pregnancy can lead to fetal infection, with the production of a significant constellation of malformations (*congenital rubella syndrome*) in a high proportion of infected fetuses. Rubella virus was first isolated in cell culture just before the last pandemic of the disease began in 1962. Since the licensing of rubella vaccine in the United States in 1969, there have been no further epidemics in this country.

ETIOLOGIC AGENT

Rubella virus, a togavirus, is the only member of the *Rubivirus* genus and is closely related to the alphaviruses. Unlike these agents, however, it does not require a vector for transmission. Moreover, there is no RNA sequence homology between rubella virus and the alphaviruses.

The rubella virion is composed of an inner icosahedral capsid of RNA and protein that is surrounded by a lipid-containing envelope with glycoprotein spikes and a diameter of ~60 nm. The structural proteins associated with rubella virus are E1 and E2 (transmembrane envelope glycoproteins) and C (the capsid protein that surrounds the viral RNA). Only one serotype has been identified.

EPIDEMIOLOGY

In the United States during the prevaccine era, rubella was most common in the spring and most often affected school-age children; only 80–90% of adults were immune; and major epidemics occurred every 6–9 years. The most recent epidemic in the United States occurred in 1964–1965, when more than 12 million cases of postnatal rubella and more than 20,000 cases of the congenital rubella syndrome were reported. Although there have been no epidemics since the introduction of live attenuated rubella vaccine in 1969, limited outbreaks have been reported in settings where susceptible individuals come into close contact with one another (e.g., schools and workplaces). Since 2001, the annual incidences of rubella have been the lowest ever recorded in the United States. In 2001–2004, an average of only 14 cases of postnatally acquired rubella were reported annually to the Centers for Disease Control and Prevention (CDC). During these 4 years, only 4 confirmed cases of congenital rubella syndrome were reported. Three of the affected infants were born to women who had immigrated to the United States. Currently, 91% of U.S. residents are estimated to be immune to rubella, and at least 95% of schoolchildren have been immunized. When rubella is reported in the United States, the genotype of the virus is consistent with an imported agent.

Although rubella is no longer considered endemic in the United States, global challenges remain. According to the World Health Organization, 57% of countries included rubella vaccine in their national programs in 2003, but rubella continues to be endemic in many areas of the world.

Whether symptomatic or subclinical, rubella is contagious, albeit less so than measles. Its incubation period is 18 days on average, with a range of 12–23 days. The virus, which is spread in droplets shed in respiratory secretions, infects the respiratory tract and then the bloodstream. In postnatally acquired infections, rubella virus is shed during the prodromal phase of the illness, and shedding from the pharynx can continue for ~1 week after onset. Despite high titers of specific neutralizing antibodies, infants with congenital rubella may excrete rubella virus from the respiratory tract and in the urine until the age of 2 years. This excretion raises important issues related to infection control in hospital and day-care settings. Persons recently immunized with live attenuated rubella vaccine do not transmit the vaccine virus to others, although low titers of rubella virus may be detected transiently in the pharynx.

After an attack of rubella, specific antibodies and cell-mediated immunity develop and probably play a significant role in protection against future disease. Asymptomatic reinfection at the level of the respiratory tract is common upon re-exposure to the virus but is rarely, if ever, associated with viremia.

Rubella virus has been cultured from respiratory secretions during reinfection. Fetal infection may occur during maternal reinfection but is acknowledged to be extremely rare because of the absence of maternal viremia under these circumstances. Viremia following reinfection of individuals immunized against rubella also is rare.

Although the current level of congenital rubella in the United States is exceedingly low, it has been observed that young immigrants to the United States from countries in Latin America and the Caribbean, where rubella vaccine is not routinely given to children, are at increased risk for rubella susceptibility. Because infants with the congenital rubella syndrome have been born to immigrant Hispanic women, increasing efforts have been made to identify and vaccinate such women before they become pregnant.

PATHOGENESIS AND PATHOLOGY

Little is known about the microscopic pathology of postnatally acquired rubella because the disease is invariably self-limited. Like that of measles, the rash of rubella is immunologically mediated; its onset coincides with the development of specific antibodies. Viremia can be demonstrated for ~1 week before and ends within a few days after the onset of rash.

The cause of the damage to cells and organs in congenital rubella is not well understood. Proposed mechanisms of fetal damage include mitotic arrest of cells, tissue necrosis without inflammation, and chromosomal damage. The growth of the fetus may be retarded. Other findings may include decreased numbers of megakaryocytes in the bone marrow, extramedullary hematopoiesis, and interstitial pneumonia.

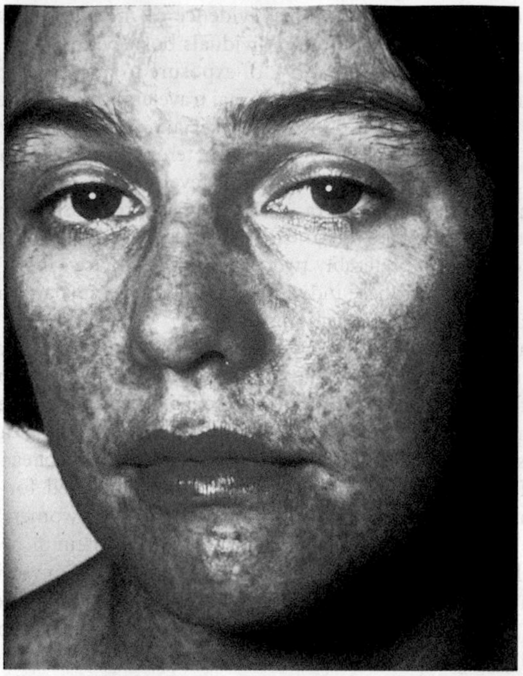

FIGURE 186-1 In rubella, an erythematous exanthem spreads from the hairline downward and clears as it spreads. *(Photo courtesy of Stephen E. Gellis, MD; with permission.)*

CLINICAL MANIFESTATIONS

Postnatally Acquired Rubella Infection acquired after birth usually results in an extremely mild or subclinical illness. A prodromal phase is uncommon in children; adults may have more severe disease, with a brief prodrome of malaise, fever, and anorexia. The foremost symptoms of postnatally acquired rubella include posterior auricular, cervical, and suboccipital lymphadenopathy; fever; and rash. The rash often begins on the face (Fig. 186-1) and spreads down the body. It is maculopapular but not confluent, is sometimes accompanied by mild coryza and conjunctivitis, and generally lasts for 3–5 days. A petechial enanthem on the soft palate, designated *Forschheimer spots*, may occur but is not specific for rubella. Fever may be absent entirely or may be present for only several days in the early phase of the illness.

Complications of postnatally acquired rubella are uncommon; bacterial superinfection is rare. One particularly troublesome complication is seen almost exclusively in women: arthritis, most frequently involving the fingers, wrists, and/or knees. Arthritis develops as the rash is appearing and may take several weeks to resolve. Chronic arthritis resulting from rubella is extremely rare. Rubella virus has been isolated from joint fluid during acute rubella arthritis and from peripheral blood in chronic rubella arthritis.

Another complication of postnatally acquired rubella is hemorrhage due to both thrombocytopenia and vascular damage; this complication occurs in 1 of every 3000 patients. Thrombocytopenia may last for weeks or months; it can have long-term consequences if there is bleeding into organs such as the eye or the brain.

Both children and adults may develop encephalitis after rubella; the incidence is about five times lower than that of encephalitis following measles. Adults are more likely than children to develop encephalitis; the mortality rate from this complication is 20–50%. Mild hepatitis is an unusual complication. Immunosuppressed patients are not at increased risk for rubella as they are for measles.

Congenital Rubella Maternal infection in early pregnancy can lead to fetal infection, with resultant congenital rubella. The classic signs of

TABLE 186-1 CLINICAL PROBLEMS ASSOCIATED WITH THE CONGENITAL RUBELLA SYNDROME

Transient Signs/Symptoms (at Birth Only)	Permanent Signs/Symptoms (Developmental)
Bony abnormalities	Autism
Cloudy cornea	Behavioral disorders
Hemolytic anemia	Congenital heart disease (patent ductus arteriosus, pulmonic stenosis)
Hepatitis	Cryptorchidism
Hepatosplenomegaly	Deafness
Jaundice	Degenerative brain disease
Low birth weight	Diabetes mellitus
Lymphadenopathy	Glaucoma
Meningoencephalitis	Inguinal hernia
Rubella viral pneumonia	Mental retardation
Thrombocytopenic purpura	Microcephaly
	Myopia
	Precocious puberty
	Retinopathy
	Seizures
	Spastic diplegia
	Thyroid disorders

congenital rubella are cataract, heart disease, deafness, and myriad other defects (Table 186-1). The most important factor in the pathogenicity of rubella virus for the fetus is gestational age at the time of infection. Maternal infection during the first trimester leads to fetal infection in ~50% of cases; maternal infection early in the second trimester leads to fetal infection in about one-third of cases. Fetal malformations not only are more common after maternal infection in the first trimester but also tend to be more severe and to involve more organ systems. Whereas a fetus infected in the fourth week of gestation may develop many problems, one infected later (e.g., in the twentieth week) may have isolated deafness as the only symptom.

DIAGNOSIS

Because postnatally acquired rubella is often a mild disease and because many cases are subclinical, diagnosis on clinical grounds can be difficult. Other diseases that may mimic rubella include toxoplasmosis, scarlet fever, modified measles, roseola, fifth disease (erythema infectiosum due to parvovirus B19), and enteroviral infection. Routine laboratory tests usually reveal leukopenia and atypical lymphocytes.

The isolation of rubella virus in cell cultures of throat samples, urine, or other secretions is difficult and expensive but is sometimes undertaken. Polymerase chain reaction (PCR) is also useful for diagnosis. These techniques are particularly useful when congenital rubella is suspected. A laboratory diagnosis may also be made serologically. The most commonly used test is an enzyme-linked immunosorbent assay (ELISA) for IgG and IgM antibodies. Acute rubella is diagnosed by the documentation of a fourfold or greater rise in the titer of IgG antibodies in paired acute- and convalescent-phase serum specimens or by the detection of rubella-specific IgM antibodies in one serum specimen. However, false-negative and false-positive IgM reactions are sometimes obtained. Moreover, true-positive IgM reactions can occur in both primary infection and reinfection. Congenital rubella is diagnosed by the isolation of rubella virus, a positive PCR assay, the detection of IgM antibodies in a single serum sample, and/or the documentation of either the persistence of rubella antibodies in serum beyond 1 year of age or a rising antibody titer anytime during infancy in an unvaccinated child. Biopsied tissues and/or blood and cerebrospinal fluid have also been used for the demonstration of rubella antigens with monoclonal antibodies and for the detection of rubella RNA by in situ hybridization and PCR.

Cases of suspected postnatal or congenital rubella should be reported to the CDC.

PREVENTION

Live attenuated rubella vaccine was licensed in 1969, 7 years after rubella virus was first isolated in culture. This vaccine was developed as a strategy to prevent congenital rubella by ensuring that very few pregnant women would be susceptible and that there would be little circulating wild-type virus. Rubella vaccine induces seroconversion in >95% of recipients. Since its licensure, there have been no major epidemics in the United States, and the number of cases has declined by 98%. The vaccine currently licensed in the United States, RA 27/3, is propagated in human diploid cells and is more immunogenic (particularly with regard to the stimulation of secretory immunity) than previously licensed vaccines. The present vaccination strategy, developed in part when measles was not being adequately controlled, is to immunize all infants at 12–15 months of age with measles-mumps-rubella (MMR) vaccine and to administer a second dose in early childhood. Rubella vaccine may also be administered to anyone who is thought to be susceptible to the infection and is not pregnant; it is particularly important that hospital workers of either sex be immune to rubella so that nosocomial transmission is avoided. Although there has been little change in the prevalence of immunity to rubella among women of childbearing age (~80%), the incidence of congenital rubella is extremely low, with fewer than 10 cases annually. It is likely that, although antibody may be undetectable years after immunization, protection against infection—possibly due to cell-mediated immunity—is the rule. At present, there is little if any evidence of significant waning of clinically important immunity to rubella with time.

On occasion, rubella vaccine may cause arthralgia or arthritis, especially in young women. Very rarely, rubella vaccination results in chronic arthritis; however, even cases of frank arthritis in vaccinees are generally self-limited, lasting only ~1 week.

After investigation of a series of more than 400 women who were inadvertently immunized during pregnancy and who carried their infants to term, the CDC has concluded that vaccine-type rubella virus either does not cause the congenital rubella syndrome at all or does so at an incidence too low to be detected. Nonetheless, rubella vaccine is contraindicated for use in pregnant women, and it is recommended that pregnancy be avoided for at least 3 months after rubella vaccination. It is acceptable for rubella-susceptible children whose mothers also are susceptible to be immunized, as vaccine recipients do not shed rubella virus or transmit it to susceptible individuals. Although it is recommended that rubella vaccine not be given to immunosuppressed persons, the vaccine is given to children infected with HIV. No adverse effects of rubella vaccine have been reported in immunocompromised patients.

℞ RUBELLA

There is no specific therapy for rubella. At one time, immune globulin was used in an effort to prevent congenital rubella when pregnant women became infected. However, because administration of immune globulin did not prevent maternal viremia, this approach was discarded. Symptom-based treatment is given for manifestations such as fever, arthralgia, and arthritis.

FURTHER READINGS

ANDRADE JQ et al: Rubella in pregnancy: Intrauterine transmission and perinatal outcome during a Brazilian epidemic. J Clin Virol 35:285, 2005

BANATVALA JE, BROWN DWG: Rubella. Lancet 363:1127, 2004

CENTERS FOR DISEASE CONTROL AND PREVENTION: Measles, mumps, and rubella—vaccine use and strategies for elimination of measles, rubella, and congenital rubella syndrome and control of mumps. MMWR Morb Mortal Wkly Rep 47:1, 1998

———: Control and prevention of rubella: Evaluation and management of suspected outbreaks, rubella in pregnant women, and surveillance for congenital rubella syndrome. MMWR Morb Mortal Wkly Rep 50:1, 2001

———: Elimination of rubella and congenital rubella syndrome—United States, 1969–2004. MMWR Morb Mortal Wkly Rep 54:279, 2005

———: Imported case of congenital rubella syndrome—New Hampshire, 2005. MMWR Morb Mortal Wkly Rep 54:1160, 2005

DANAVARO-HOLLIDAY MC et al: A large rubella outbreak with spread from the workplace to the community. JAMA 284:2733, 2000

PLOTKIN SA, REEF S: Rubella vaccine, in *Vaccines*, SA Plotkin and WA Orenstein (eds). Philadelphia, Saunders, 2004, pp 389–440

REEF SE et al: The changing epidemiology of rubella in the 1990s: On the verge of elimination and new challenges for control and prevention. JAMA 287:464, 2002

SHERIDAN E: Congenital rubella syndrome: A risk in immigrant populations. Lancet 359:674, 2002

187 Mumps

Anne Gershon

DEFINITION

Mumps is an acute, systemic, communicable viral infection whose most distinctive feature is swelling of one or both parotid glands. Involvement of other salivary glands, the meninges, the pancreas, and the gonads also is common.

ETIOLOGIC AGENT

Mumps virus, a paramyxovirus, is pleomorphic and has a diameter ranging from 100 to 300 nm. The virion is composed of RNA and seven proteins. The RNA is surrounded by an envelope composed of glycoproteins, including a hemagglutinin-neuraminidase (HN), a hemolysis cell fusion antigen (F), and a matrix envelope protein (M). A fourth protein (SH) may also be membrane-associated. There are three internal components: a nucleocapsid protein (NP), a phosphoprotein (P), and a large protein (L). There is only one antigenic type of mumps virus. Polymerase chain reaction (PCR) has detected geographic differences among mumps viruses from different locales.

EPIDEMIOLOGY

After the introduction of mumps vaccine in 1967, the incidence of clinical mumps declined significantly in the United States. In 1968 (before widespread immunization), 185,691 cases of mumps were reported in this country. The 231–277 cases reported annually in 2001–2005 represent a >99% reduction from prevaccine levels. Before widespread vaccination, the incidence of mumps was highest in the winter and spring, with epidemics every 2–5 years. At that time, mumps was principally a disease of childhood, although today >50% of cases occur in young adults. Epidemics tended to occur in confined populations (e.g., in schools and the military services).

The incubation period of mumps generally ranges from 14 to 18 days, with extremes of 7 and 23 days. However, because a contact may be shedding virus before the onset of clinical disease or (like one-third of patients) may have subclinical infection, the incubation period in individual cases is often uncertain. One attack of mumps usually confers lifelong immunity. Long-term immunity is also associated with immunization.

PATHOGENESIS

Mumps virus is transmitted by droplet nuclei, saliva, and fomites. Replication of the virus in the epithelium of the upper respiratory tract leads to viremia, which is followed by infection of glandular tissues and/or the central nervous system (CNS).

Little is known of the pathology of mumps since the disease is rarely fatal. The affected glands contain perivascular and interstitial mononuclear cell infiltrates with prominent edema. Necrosis of acinar and epithelial duct cells is evident in the salivary glands and in the germinal epithelium of the seminiferous tubules.

CLINICAL MANIFESTATIONS

The prodrome of mumps consists of fever, malaise, myalgia, and anorexia. Parotitis, if it develops, usually does so within the next 24 h but may be delayed for as long as a week; it is generally bilateral, although the onset on the two sides may not be synchronous and at times only one side is affected. The submaxillary and sublingual glands are involved less often than the parotid and are almost never involved alone. Swelling of the parotid is accompanied by tenderness and obliteration of the space between the ear lobe and the angle of the mandible (Fig. 187-1). The patient frequently reports an earache and finds it difficult to eat, swallow, or talk. Glandular swelling increases for a few days and then gradually subsides, disappearing within a week. The orifice of Stensen's duct is commonly red and swollen. Presternal pitting edema has been described in ~5% of mumps cases, often in association with submandibular adenitis.

Other than parotitis, orchitis is the most common manifestation of mumps among postpubertal males, developing in ~20% of cases. The testis is painful, tender, and enlarged to several times its normal size; accompanying fever is common. Later, testicular atrophy develops in half of the affected men. Since orchitis is bilateral in <15% of cases, sterility after mumps is rare. Oophoritis in women—far less common than orchitis in men—may cause lower abdominal pain but does not lead to sterility.

Aseptic meningitis, which may develop before, during, after, or in the absence of parotitis, is common in both children and adults. Symptoms include stiff neck, headache, and drowsiness. Pleocytosis of the cerebrospinal fluid (CSF), with up to 1000 cells/μL, may develop in up to 50% of cases of clinical mumps, but clinical signs of meningeal irritation are documented in only 5–25% of cases. Within the first 24 h, polymorphonuclear leukocytes may predominate in CSF, but by the second day nearly all the cells are lymphocytes. The glucose level in CSF may be abnormally low, and this finding may arouse suspicion of bacterial meningitis. Aseptic meningitis due to mumps without parotitis is indistinguishable clinically from that caused by other viruses. Mumps meningitis is almost invariably self-limited, although cranial nerve palsies have occasionally led to permanent sequelae, particularly deafness. More rarely, mumps virus may cause encephalitis, which presents as high fever with marked changes in the level of consciousness and frequently results in permanent sequelae in survivors. Other CNS problems occasionally associated with mumps include cerebellar ataxia, facial palsy, transverse myelitis, Guillain-Barré syndrome, and aqueductal stenosis leading to hydrocephalus.

Mumps pancreatitis, which may present as abdominal pain, is difficult to diagnose because an elevated serum amylase level can be associated with either parotitis or pancreatitis. Other unusual complications of mumps include myocarditis, mastitis, thyroiditis, nephritis, arthritis, and thrombocytopenic purpura. An excessive number of sponta-

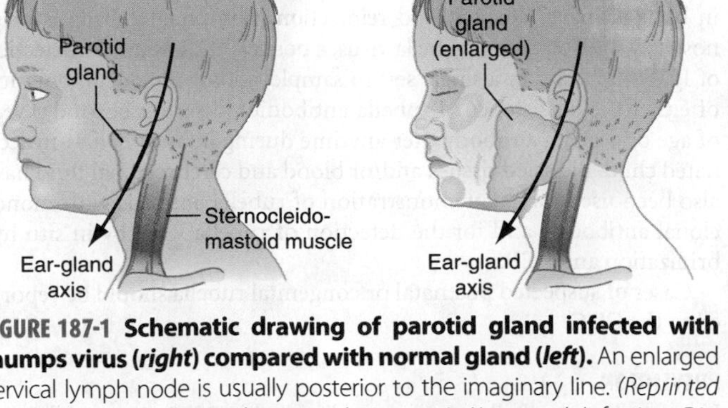

FIGURE 187-1 Schematic drawing of parotid gland infected with mumps virus (*right*) compared with normal gland (*left*). An enlarged cervical lymph node is usually posterior to the imaginary line. *(Reprinted with permission from Gershon A et al: Mumps, in Krugman's Infectious Diseases of Children, 11th ed. Philadelphia, Elsevier, 2004, p 392.)*

TABLE 187-1 DIFFERENTIAL DIAGNOSIS OF PAROTITIS

Etiology	Comments
Systemic Infections	
Mumps	Rare in countries with vaccination programs
Coxsackievirus infection	Particularly likely in children
HIV infection	In HIV-positive children receiving no antiretroviral therapy; additional disease manifestations likely
Parainfluenza virus type 3 infection	Particularly likely in children; associated with acute respiratory tract symptoms
Influenza A virus infection	Seasonal (winter, spring); associated with acute respiratory tract symptoms
Cat-scratch disease	Unusual but described
Epstein-Barr virus infection	Unusual but described
Systemic Noninfectious Causes	
Sarcoidosis	Additional manifestations of disease likely
Sjögren's syndrome	Additional manifestations of disease likely
Uremia	Additional manifestations of disease likely
Diabetes mellitus	Additional manifestations of disease likely
Drugs	Phenylbutazone, thiouracil
Unilateral Parotitis	
Ductal obstruction due to stones or strictures	Unilateral, gradual onset, suppurative
Parotid cyst	Unilateral, gradual onset
Parotid tumor	Unilateral, gradual onset
Acute Suppurative Parotitis	
Staphylococcus aureus, Streptococcus species, and (rarely) gram-negative bacteria, anaerobes	

neous abortions are associated with gestational mumps when the disease occurs during the first trimester. Mumps in pregnancy does not lead to premature birth or fetal malformations.

DIFFERENTIAL DIAGNOSIS

Because of widespread vaccination, mumps is currently a rare disease in the United States. The diagnosis is made easily in patients with acute bilateral parotitis and a history of recent exposure. When parotitis is unilateral or absent or when sites other than the parotid gland are involved, laboratory diagnosis may be required.

The differential diagnosis of parotitis is presented in Table 187-1. Other entities should be considered when manifestations consistent with mumps appear in organs other than the parotid. Testicular torsion may produce a painful scrotal mass resembling that seen in mumps orchitis. Other viruses (e.g., enteroviruses) may cause aseptic meningitis that is clinically indistinguishable from that due to mumps virus.

Myocarditis as a severe but usually self-limited complication of mumps has been described. Molecular diagnostic assays have implicated mumps virus in some cases of endocardial fibroelastosis following myocarditis.

LABORATORY DIAGNOSIS

Mumps virus is readily isolated after inoculation of appropriate clinical specimens into cell cultures. The virus can be identified rapidly in shell vial cultures by immunofluorescence. Mumps virus may be recovered from saliva, throat, and urine during the first few days of illness and from the CSF of patients with mumps meningitis. Shedding of virus in the urine may persist for as long as 2 weeks. PCR also is used to detect mumps virus in clinical specimens. No particular peripheral blood cell count is characteristic of mumps.

Highly sensitive enzyme-linked immunosorbent assays are useful for serologic diagnosis of mumps and for determination of susceptibility to the disease. Acute mumps can be diagnosed either by the examination of acute- and convalescent-phase sera for a significant increase in IgG antibody levels or by the demonstration of specific IgM in one serum specimen. The mumps skin test is no longer used.

PREVENTION

Live attenuated mumps vaccine (Jeryl Lynn strain) induces antibodies that protect the recipient against infection in >95% of cases. Mumps vaccine is usually administered as part of the measles-mumps-rubella (MMR) vaccine at the age of 12–15 months and again at 4–12 years of age. MMR vaccine will probably be supplanted by MMRV vaccine, which also covers varicella. Licensed by the U.S. Food and Drug Administration in 2005, MMRV is licensed for use only in children 1–13 years of age. Vaccination is also recommended for susceptible older children, adolescents, and adults, particularly male adolescents who have not had mumps. For these patients, either MMR or monovalent mumps vaccine may be given; two doses are preferred. Inadvertent immunization of individuals who are already immune is not associated with significant adverse reactions. Mumps vaccine is not recommended for pregnant women, for patients receiving glucocorticoids, or for other immunocompromised hosts. However, children with HIV infection who are not severely immunocompromised can safely be immunized against mumps; MMR vaccine is usually used for this purpose (Chap. 116). Occasionally, febrile reactions and parotitis have been reported soon after mumps vaccination. Allergic reactions after vaccination, such as rash and pruritus, occur uncommonly and are usually mild and self-limited. In the United States, the incidence of encephalitis during the month after mumps vaccination is no greater than the background incidence rate of encephalitis in the population.

Rx MUMPS

Therapy for parotitis and other manifestations of mumps is symptom-based. The administration of analgesics and the application of warm or cold compresses to the parotid area may be helpful. Mumps immune globulin is of no value. Testicular pain may be minimized by the local application of cold compresses and gentle support for the scrotum. Anesthetic blocks also may be used. Neither the administration of glucocorticoids nor incision of the tunica albuginea is of proven value for the treatment of severe orchitis. Anecdotal information on a small number of patients with orchitis suggests that administration of interferon α may be helpful.

FURTHER READINGS

Briss PA et al: Sustained transmission of mumps in a highly vaccinated population: Assessment of primary vaccine failure and waning vaccine-induced immunity. J Infect Dis 169:77, 1994

Centers for Disease Control and Prevention: Mumps epidemic—United Kingdom, 2004–2005. MMWR Morb Mortal Wkly Rep 55:173, 2006

———: Mumps outbreak at a summer camp—New York, 2005. MMWR Morb Mortal Wkly Rep 55:175, 2006

———: Update: Multistate outbreak of mumps—United States, January 1–May 2, 2006. MMWR Morb Mortal Wkly Rep 55:559, 2006

———: Measles, mumps, and rubella—vaccine use and strategies for elimination of measles, rubella, and congenital rubella syndrome and control of mumps. MMWR Morb Mortal Wkly Rep 47:1, 1998

Chaudary S et al: Fulminant mumps myocarditis. Ann Intern Med 110:569, 1989

Davidkin I et al: Etiology of mumps-like illnesses in children and adolescents vaccinated for measles, mumps, and rubella. J Infect Dis 191:719, 2005

Gut JP et al: Symptomatic mumps reinfections. J Med Virol 45:17, 1995

McDonald JC et al: Clinical and epidemiologic features of mumps encephalitis and possible causes of vaccine-related disease. Pediatr Infect Dis J 8:751, 1989

Uchida K et al: Rapid and sensitive detection of mumps virus RNA directly from clinical samples by real-time PCR. J Med Virol 75:470, 2005

188 Rabies and Other Rhabdovirus Infections

Alan C. Jackson, Eric C. Johannsen

RABIES

Rabies is an acute viral disease of the central nervous system (CNS) that is transmitted to humans by infected animals. After a prodromal phase, rabies manifests most often as encephalitis—or less frequently as a paralytic form of the disease—and then progresses to coma and death.

ETIOLOGIC AGENT

Rabies virus is a member of the genus *Lyssavirus* in the family Rhabdoviridae, which includes vesicular stomatitis virus (VSV), a bovine pathogen of significant economic importance that can infect humans (see "Other Rhabdoviruses," below). *Rhabdos*, meaning "rodlike," refers to the distinctive elongated shape of these viruses. Their enveloped virions contain a single-strand, nonsegmented, negative-sense RNA. The rabies virus genome consists of 11,932 nucleotides and encodes five proteins: nucleocapsid, matrix, phosphoprotein, glycoprotein, and an RNA polymerase. Each animal reservoir harbors one or more distinct rabies virus variants that can be distinguished by the sequence of the nucleocapsid gene.

EPIDEMIOLOGY

Rabies is a zoonosis that is generally transmitted to humans by the bite of a rabid animal. Understanding the epizootiology of rabies is essential in evaluating the need for rabies postexposure prophylaxis (PEP; see "Prevention," below). Rabies virus can infect most mammals and is worldwide in distribution.

Historically, dogs were the primary reservoir and vector for rabies, and they remain the major source of transmission to humans in Asia and Africa (see "Global Considerations," below). Coordinated vaccination and surveillance programs have essentially eliminated the rabies reservoir in dogs in North America and Europe and have uncovered previously unsuspected reservoirs in wildlife species. Surveillance data from 2006 identified 6940 confirmed animal cases of rabies in the United States. Only 8% of these cases were in domestic animals, including 318 cases in cats, 82 in cattle, and 79 in dogs. Essentially all infections of domestic animals were the result of "spillover" from wildlife reservoirs, not of transmission from one domestic animal to another. In North America, bats, raccoons, skunks, and foxes have endemic rabies virus infection. The importance of each reservoir varies geographically: rabies in raccoons is endemic on the east coast; rabies in skunks occurs predominantly in the Midwest, with another focus in California; and rabies in foxes is found in parts of Texas, Arizona, and Alaska. Rabies in bats is not geographically restricted.

Because each species harbors one or more specific rabies virus variants (or strains), it is possible to trace the source of a human infection even when there is no known exposure. Since 1990, bats have accounted for most cases of human rabies in the United States, with the majority of the remaining cases due to dog exposures occurring in other countries. The majority of human rabies cases acquired from bats have been associated with a single variant (Ln/Ps) harbored by silver-haired and eastern pipistrelle bats. The implication is that the Ln/Ps variant may have particular attributes that render it capable of readily establishing human infections—e.g., an affinity for specific cell receptors or more efficient initial replication in nonneuronal tissues. A contributing factor may be that rabies virus can be transmitted by minor, seemingly unimportant or unrecognized bat bites. In contrast, bites of terrestrial mammals are more likely to receive medical attention. Fatal cases of rabies have resulted when the significance of a known bat exposure was not appreciated. In circumstances where a bat bite or bat salivary contact with broken skin or mucous membranes cannot be excluded (e.g., when a bat is found in a room with an infant or a sleeping adult), the bat should be tested for rabies and expert consultation sought.

Nonbite exposures only rarely transmit rabies virus infection. Exposures to aerosols in the laboratory or in caves containing millions of bats have resulted in human rabies. Transplanted corneal tissue has been the source of eight cases of human rabies, and strict guidelines for donor screening have been adopted in an effort to eliminate this risk. In 2004, three deaths resulted from transplantation of solid organs and another death from transplantation of a vascular conduit from a donor who was initially thought to have died from an intracranial hemorrhage but was retrospectively diagnosed with rabies. Although all organ donors are screened and tested for infectious risks, routine testing of donors for rabies in the absence of epidemiologic risk has not been recommended. There are no known instances in which health care workers have acquired rabies from infected patients. However, standard universal and respiratory precautions should be observed by care givers because contact of the patients' saliva or neuronal tissue with mucous membranes or nonintact skin could result in transmission.

PATHOGENESIS

The incubation period of rabies (defined as the interval between virus exposure and onset of clinical disease) is usually 1–3 months but in rare cases is as short as 2 weeks or >1 year. During most of the incubation period, rabies virus is thought to be present at or close to the site of inoculation (Fig. 188-1), predominantly in muscle cells. Administration of rabies PEP during this incubation period is critical; the benefit of PEP in preventing disease progression once rabies virus has entered peripheral nerves is limited. Several receptors probably account for the ability of rabies virus to infect both sensory and motor neurons. The virus is known to bind to nicotinic acetylcholine receptors, and acetylcholine receptor blockade inhibits rabies virus attachment. Experimental evidence also supports a role for the neural cell adhesion molecule and the $p75^{NTR}$ neurotrophin receptor as receptors for rabies virus. After entering sensory and motor neurons, rabies virus spreads centripetally at a rate of 100–400 mm/d via fast axonal transport to the spinal cord or brainstem. Once the virus enters the CNS, it spreads rapidly throughout the gray matter via established neuroanatomic connections. There are inflammatory changes, but there are few degenerative changes involving neurons and little evidence of neuronal death. These observations have led to the concept that neuronal dysfunction—rather than neuronal death—is responsible for clinical disease in rabies. The basis for the behavioral changes, including aggression, is not well understood. After CNS infection is established, there is centrifugal spread along peripheral nerves to other tissues, including the salivary glands, liver, muscle, skin, adrenal glands, and heart. Rabies virus replication in acinar cells of the salivary glands results in viral excretion in the saliva of rabid animals.

Pathology studies show mild inflammatory changes in the CNS in rabies, with mononuclear inflammatory infiltration in the leptomeninges, perivascular regions, and parenchyma, including microglial nodules called *Babes nodules*. Degenerative neuronal changes are usually not prominent, and neuronophagia is observed occasionally. The most characteristic pathologic finding in rabies is the *Negri body* (Fig. 188-2). Negri bodies are eosinophilic cytoplasmic inclusions in brain neurons and are composed of randomly oriented rabies virus nucleocapsids embedded in an amorphous substance or matrix. These inclusions occur in a minority of infected cells, are most commonly present in Purkinje cells of the cerebellum and in pyramidal cells in the hippocampus, and are less frequently seen in cortical neurons and in the brainstem. For obscure reasons, Negri bodies are rarely produced in infections caused by laboratory variants of rabies virus, whereas wild, or "street," rabies infection results in Negri bodies in ~80% of cases. Thus, the absence of Negri bodies does not exclude the diagnosis.

CLINICAL MANIFESTATIONS

Rabies has the highest case-fatality rate of any infectious disease. Although the diagnosis of rabies should be considered in any case of unexplained encephalitis or flaccid paralysis accompanied by fever, efforts to prevent the disease are appropriately focused on early identification of

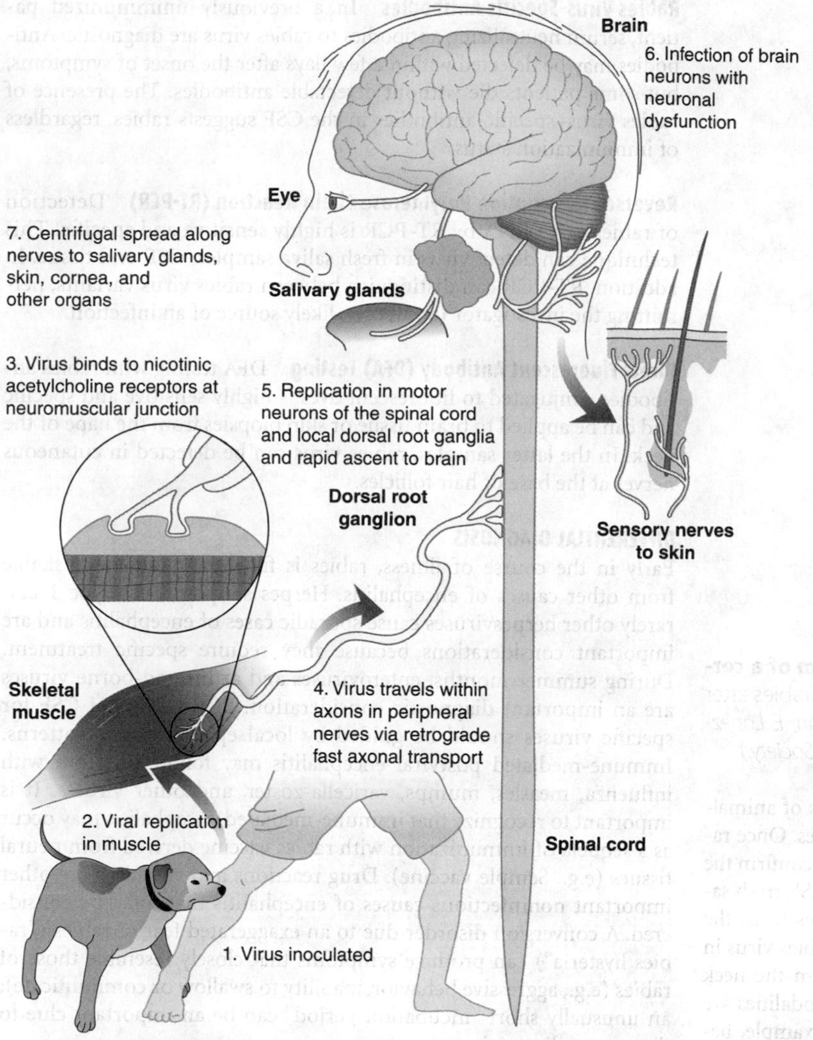
Brain
6. Infection of brain neurons with neuronal dysfunction
Eye
7. Centrifugal spread along nerves to salivary glands, skin, cornea, and other organs
Salivary glands
3. Virus binds to nicotinic acetylcholine receptors at neuromuscular junction
5. Replication in motor neurons of the spinal cord and local dorsal root ganglia and rapid ascent to brain
Dorsal root ganglion
Sensory nerves to skin
Skeletal muscle
4. Virus travels within axons in peripheral nerves via retrograde fast axonal transport
2. Viral replication in muscle
Spinal cord
1. Virus inoculated

FIGURE 188-1 Schematic representation of the pathogenetic events following peripheral inoculation of rabies virus. *(Adapted from Jackson AC: Human disease, in Rabies, edited by AC Jackson and WH Wunner, 2002, Academic Press, San Diego, pp 219-244; with permission.)*

rabies exposure and administration of PEP. After an asymptomatic incubation period, clinical rabies progresses through three general phases: a prodrome, an acute neurologic phase, and coma/death (Table 188-1).

Prodromal Features Clinically apparent rabies infection begins with nonspecific prodromal symptoms, including fever, malaise, headache, nausea, and vomiting. Anxiety or agitation may also occur. Paresthesias, pain, or pruritus near the site of the exposure occurs in 50–80% of patients and suggests rabies. The wound has usually healed by this point, and these symptoms may reflect infection of local dorsal root or cranial sensory ganglia.

Encephalitic Rabies Two acute neurologic forms of rabies are seen in humans: encephalitic (furious) in 80% and paralytic in 20%. Manifestations of encephalitic rabies may be seen in many other viral encephalitides as well. These features include fever, confusion, hallucinations, combativeness, muscle spasms, hyperactivity, and seizures. Autonomic dysfunction is common and may result in hypersalivation, excessive perspiration, gooseflesh, pupillary dilation, and/or priapism. In encephalitic rabies, episodes of hyperexcitability are typically followed by periods of complete lucidity that become shorter as the disease progresses. Rabies encephalitis is most distinguished by early brainstem involvement, which results in the classic symptoms of hydrophobia and aerophobia: involuntary, painful contraction of the diaphragm and accessory respiratory, laryngeal, and pharyngeal muscles in response to swallowing liquids (hydrophobia) or a draft of air (aerophobia). These symptoms are probably due to dysfunction of infected brainstem neurons that normally inhibit inspiratory neurons near the nucleus ambiguus, resulting in exaggerated defense reflexes that protect the respiratory tract. The combination of hypersalivation and pharyngeal dysfunction is also responsible for the classic appearance of "foaming at the mouth" (Fig. 188-3). Brainstem dysfunction progresses rapidly, and coma followed within days by death is the rule unless the course is prolonged by supportive measures. With such measures, late complications can include disturbances of water balance (syndrome of inappropriate antidiuretic hormone secretion or diabetes insipidus), noncardiogenic pulmonary edema, and cardiac arrhythmias due to brainstem dysfunction and/or myocarditis.

Paralytic Rabies For unknown reasons, muscle weakness predominates and cardinal features of encephalitic rabies (hydrophobia, aerophobia, fluctuating consciousness) are lacking in ~20% of rabies cases. Paralytic rabies is characterized by early and prominent muscle weakness, often beginning in the bitten extremity and spreading to produce quadriparesis and facial weakness. Sphincter involvement is common, but sensory involvement is usually mild. Guillain-Barré syndrome is a common misdiagnosis. Transplantation of corneal tissue from donors in whom paralytic rabies was misdiagnosed as Guillain-Barré syndrome has resulted in clinical rabies and death in recipients. Patients with paralytic rabies generally survive a few days longer than is typical in encephalitic rabies, but multiple-organ failure ensues even with aggressive supportive care.

LABORATORY INVESTIGATIONS

During the early clinical stages of rabies, laboratory findings are nonspecific. Complete blood counts are usually normal. Examination of cerebrospinal fluid (CSF) often reveals mild mononuclear cell pleocytosis with a mildly elevated protein level. Severe pleocytosis (>1000 cells/μL) is unusual and should prompt a search for an alternative diagnosis. CT head scans are usually normal in rabies. MRI brain scans sometimes show signal abnormalities in the brainstem or other areas, but these findings are variable and nonspecific. Electroencephalograms show only nonspecific abnormalities. The most important tests in suspected cases of rabies are those that may identify an alternative, potentially treatable diagnosis (see "Differential Diagnosis," below).

DIAGNOSIS

In North America, a diagnosis of rabies often is not considered until relatively late in the clinical course, even with a typical clinical presentation. This diagnosis should be considered in patients presenting with acute encephalitis or with unexplained ascending paralysis, including

TABLE 188-1 PROGRESSION OF RABIES VIRUS INFECTION

Phase	Duration	Signs/Symptoms
Incubation period	1–3 months[a]	None
Prodrome	1–7 days	Fever, malaise, headache, nausea, vomiting, agitation, focal paresthesias, pain
Acute neurologic phase		
Encephalitic (80%)	1–7 days	Fever, confusion, hallucinations, hyperactivity, pharyngeal spasms (hydrophobia/aerophobia), seizures
Paralytic (20%)	2–10 days	Ascending flaccid paralysis
Coma/death	1–14 days	. . .

[a]Typical duration, with a possible range of 2 weeks to >1 year.

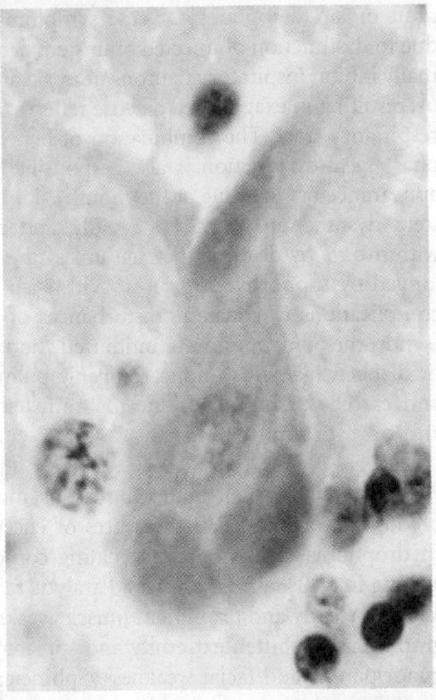

FIGURE 188-2 Three large Negri bodies in the cytoplasm of a cerebellar Purkinje cell from an 8-year-old boy who died of rabies after being bitten by a rabid dog in Mexico. *(From AC Jackson, E Lopez-Corella, N Engl J Med 335:568, 1996. © Massachusetts Medical Society.)*

those in whom Guillain-Barré syndrome is suspected. A lack of animal-bite history or a lack of hydrophobia is not unusual in rabies. Once rabies is suspected, rabies-specific tests should be employed to confirm the diagnosis. Diagnostically useful specimens include serum, CSF, fresh saliva, brain tissue (when available), and skin biopsy samples from the neck. Because skin biopsy relies on the demonstration of rabies virus in cutaneous nerves at the base of hair follicles, samples from the neck should include at least 10 hair follicles. Multiple testing modalities are required to ensure a high negative predictive value. For example, because rabies virus infects immunologically privileged neuronal tissues, serum antibodies often do not develop until very late in the disease.

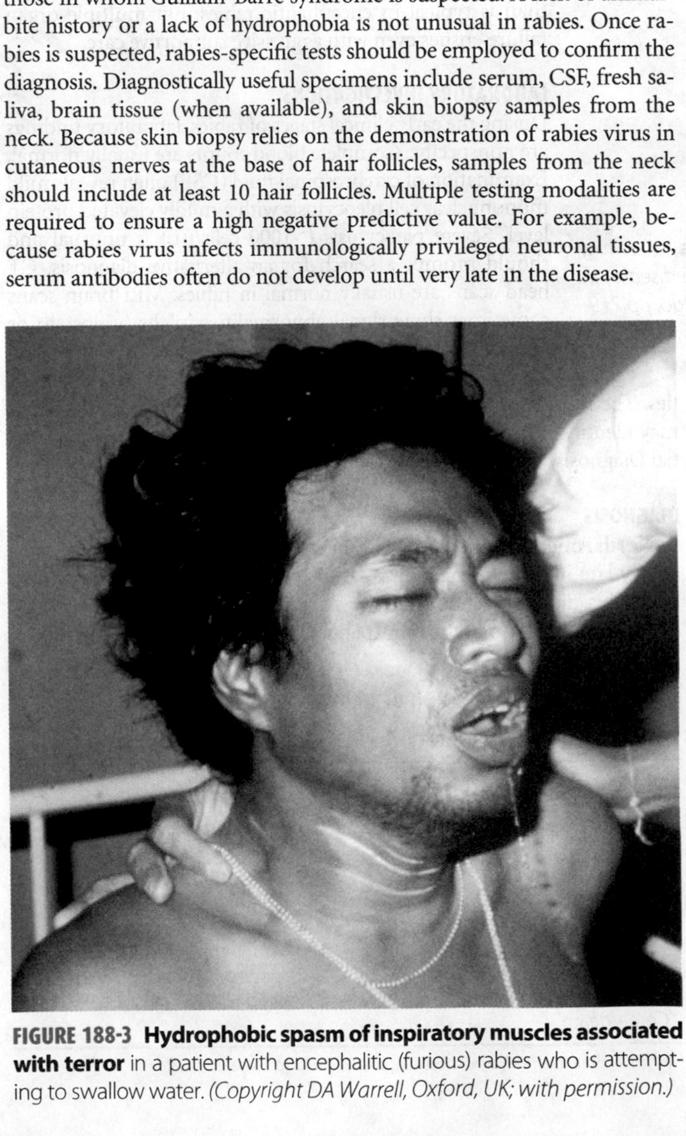

FIGURE 188-3 Hydrophobic spasm of inspiratory muscles associated with terror in a patient with encephalitic (furious) rabies who is attempting to swallow water. *(Copyright DA Warrell, Oxford, UK; with permission.)*

Rabies Virus-Specific Antibodies In a previously unimmunized patient, serum neutralizing antibodies to rabies virus are diagnostic. Antibodies may be detected within a few days after the onset of symptoms, but some patients die without detectable antibodies. The presence of rabies virus–specific antibodies in the CSF suggests rabies, regardless of immunization status.

Reverse Transcription Polymerase Chain Reaction (RT-PCR) Detection of rabies virus RNA by RT-PCR is highly sensitive and specific. This technique can detect virus in fresh saliva samples, CSF, and tissue. In addition, RT-PCR can distinguish between rabies virus variants, permitting the investigator to infer the likely source of an infection.

Direct Fluorescent Antibody (DFA) Testing DFA testing with rabies antibodies conjugated to fluorescent dyes is highly sensitive and specific and can be applied to brain tissue or skin biopsies from the nape of the neck. In the latter samples, rabies virus can be detected in cutaneous nerves at the base of hair follicles.

DIFFERENTIAL DIAGNOSIS

Early in the course of illness, rabies is frequently indistinguishable from other causes of encephalitis. Herpes simplex virus type 1 and rarely other herpesviruses cause sporadic cases of encephalitis and are important considerations because they require specific treatment. During summer months, enteroviruses and arthropod-borne viruses are an important diagnostic consideration. PCR testing of CSF for specific viruses should be guided by local epidemiologic patterns. Immune-mediated postviral encephalitis may follow infection with influenza, measles, mumps, varicella-zoster, and other viruses. It is important to recognize that immune-mediated encephalitis may occur as a sequela of immunization with rabies vaccine derived from neural tissues (e.g., Semple vaccine). Drug reactions and vasculitis are other important noninfectious causes of encephalitis that must be considered. A conversion disorder due to an exaggerated fear of rabies ("rabies hysteria") can produce symptoms that closely resemble those of rabies (e.g., aggressive behavior, inability to swallow or communicate); an unusually short "incubation period" can be an important clue to the correct diagnosis.

As previously mentioned, paralytic rabies may mimic Guillain-Barré syndrome. In these cases, the documentation of fever or bladder dysfunction can suggest the diagnosis of rabies. Conversely, Guillain-Barré syndrome may rarely occur as a complication of rabies vaccination and may be mistaken for paralytic rabies (i.e., vaccine failure).

℞ RABIES

There is no established treatment for rabies. There have been several recent treatment failures of antiviral therapy, ketamine, and therapeutic coma—measures that were used in a healthy survivor who had rabies virus antibodies present at the time of presentation. Expert opinion should be sought before any course of experimental therapy is embarked upon. A palliative approach may be appropriate for some patients.

PROGNOSIS

Rabies is an almost uniformly fatal disease but is almost always preventable with appropriate postexposure therapy during the incubation period (see below). There are only six well-documented cases of survival after symptomatic rabies infection. All but one of the patients involved had received rabies vaccine before disease onset; these patients represented failures of postexposure rabies prophylaxis. Most patients with rabies die within several days, even with aggressive care in a critical care unit.

PREVENTION

Postexposure Prophylaxis Since there is no effective therapy for rabies, it is extremely important to prevent the disease after an animal exposure. Figure 188-4 shows the steps involved in making decisions about rabies PEP. On the basis of the history of the exposure and local epidemiologic information, the physician must decide whether initia-

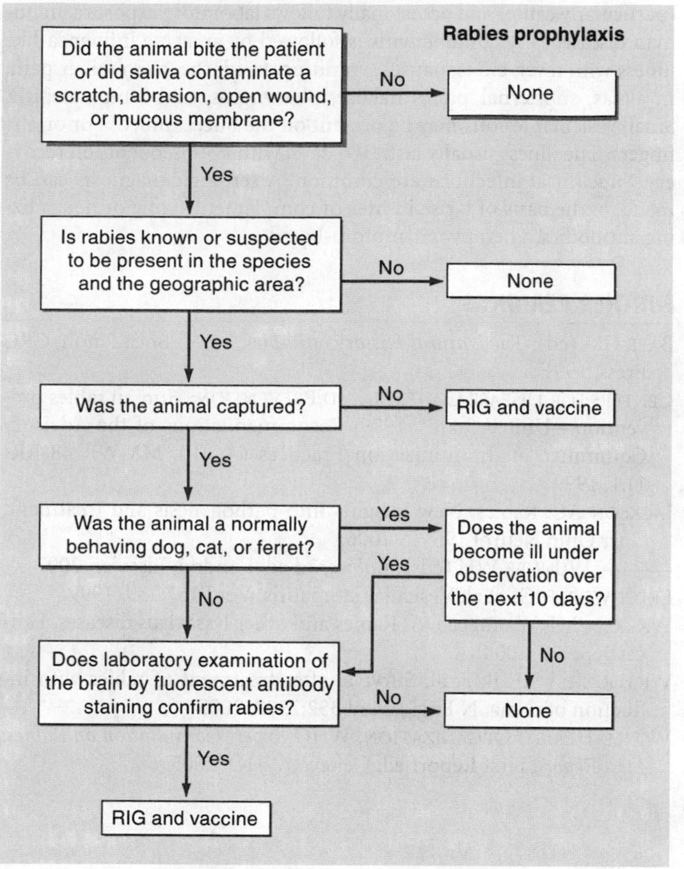

FIGURE 188-4 Algorithm for rabies postexposure prophylaxis. RIG, rabies immune globulin. *[From L Corey, in Harrison's Principles of Internal Medicine, 15th ed. E Braunwald et al (eds): New York, McGraw-Hill, 2001, adapted with permission.]*

tion of PEP is warranted. Healthy dogs, cats, or ferrets may be confined and observed for 10 days. PEP is not necessary if the animal remains healthy. If the animal develops signs of rabies during the observation period, it should be euthanized immediately, and the head should be transported to the laboratory under refrigeration and examined for the presence of rabies virus by DFA testing and viral isolation using cell culture or mouse inoculation. Any animal other than a dog, cat, or ferret should be euthanized immediately and the head submitted for examination. In high-risk exposures and in areas where canine rabies is endemic, rabies prophylaxis should be initiated without waiting for laboratory results. If the laboratory results prove to be negative, it may safely be concluded that the animal's saliva did not contain rabies virus, and immunization should be discontinued. If an animal escapes after an exposure, it must be considered rabid, and PEP must be initiated unless information from public health officials indicates otherwise (i.e., there is no endemic rabies in the area). PEP may be warranted when a person present in the same space as a bat (e.g., a small child or a sleeping adult) cannot reliably rule out contact with an unrecognized bite.

PEP includes local wound care and both active and passive immunization. Local wound care is essential and may decrease the risk of rabies virus infection by as much as 90%. Wound care should not be delayed, even if the initiation of immunization is postponed pending the results of the 10-day observation period. All bite wounds and scratches should be washed thoroughly with soap and water. Devitalized tissues should be debrided, tetanus prophylaxis given, and antibiotic treatment initiated whenever indicated.

All previously unvaccinated persons should be passively immunized with rabies immune globulin (RIG). If RIG is not immediately available, it should be administered no later than 7 days after the first vaccine dose. After day 7, endogenous antibodies are being produced, and passive immunization may actually be counterproductive. If anatomically feasible, the entire dose of RIG (20 IU/kg) should be infused at the site of the bite; otherwise, any RIG remaining after infiltration of the bite site should be administered IM at a distant site. With multiple or large wounds, the RIG preparation may need to be diluted in order to obtain a sufficient volume for adequate infiltration of all wound sites. If the exposure involves a mucous membrane, the entire dose should be administered IM. Rabies vaccine and RIG should never be administered at the same site or with the same syringe. Commercially available RIG in the United States is purified from the serum of hyperimmunized human donors. These human RIG preparations are much better tolerated than are the equine-derived preparations still in use in some countries (see "Global Considerations," below). Serious adverse effects of human RIG are uncommon. Local pain and low-grade fever may occur.

Two purified inactivated rabies vaccines are available for rabies PEP in the United States. They are highly immunogenic and remarkably safe compared with earlier vaccines. Five 1-mL doses of rabies vaccine should be given IM in the deltoid area. (The anterolateral aspect of the thigh is also acceptable in children.) Gluteal injections, which may not always reach muscle, should not be given and have been associated with rare vaccine failures. Ideally, the first dose should be given as soon as possible after exposure; failing that, it should be given without further delay. The four additional doses should be given on days 3, 7, 14, and 28. Pregnancy is not a contraindication for immunization. Glucocorticoids and other immunosuppressive medications may interfere with the development of active immunity and should not be administered during PEP unless they are essential. In several studies, all persons vaccinated with the above schedule developed a serologic response within 2–4 weeks. Routine measurement of serum neutralizing antibody titers is not required, but titers should be measured 2–4 weeks after immunization in immunocompromised persons. Local reactions (pain, erythema, edema, and pruritus) and mild systemic reactions (fever, myalgias, headache, and nausea) are common; anti-inflammatory and antipyretic medications may be used, but immunization should not be discontinued. Systemic allergic reactions are uncommon, but anaphylaxis does occur rarely and can be treated with epinephrine and antihistamines. The risk of rabies development should be carefully considered before the decision is made to discontinue vaccination because of an adverse reaction. Advice and assistance from state health officials or the Centers for Disease Control and Prevention may be helpful in managing adverse reactions to vaccine.

Preexposure Rabies Vaccination Preexposure rabies prophylaxis should be considered for people with an occupational or recreational risk of rabies exposures, including certain travelers to rabies-endemic areas. This primary schedule consists of three doses of rabies vaccine given on days 0, 7, and 21 or 28. Serum neutralizing antibody tests help determine the need for subsequent booster doses. When a previously immunized individual is exposed to rabies, two booster doses of vaccine should be administered on days 0 and 3. Wound care remains critical. RIG should not be administered to previously vaccinated persons.

GLOBAL CONSIDERATIONS

Worldwide, endemic canine rabies is estimated to cause 55,000 human deaths annually. Most of these deaths occur in Asia and Africa, with rural populations and children most frequently affected. Because of this distribution, most of the burden of rabies PEP is borne by those least able to pay. In Latin America, rabies control efforts in dogs have been quite successful in recent years. In Europe and Canada, an epizootic of rabies in red foxes has been partly controlled by widespread use of baits containing rabies vaccine.

In addition to the rabies vaccines discussed above, vaccines grown in either primary cell lines (hamster or dog kidney) or continuous cell lines (Vero cells) are satisfactory and are available in many countries outside the United States. Less expensive vaccines derived from neural tissues have been used in developing countries; however, these vaccines are associated with serious neuroparalytic complications, and their use should be discontinued as soon as possible. Worldwide, >10 million individuals receive postexposure vaccination against rabies each year.

If human RIG is unavailable, purified equine RIG can be used in the same manner at a dose of 40 IU/kg. Before the administration of equine RIG, hypersensitivity should be assessed by intradermal testing with a 1:10 dilution. The incidence of anaphylactic reactions and serum sickness has been low with recent equine RIG products.

OTHER RHABDOVIRUSES

OTHER LYSSAVIRUSES

A growing number of lyssaviruses other than rabies virus have been discovered to infect bat populations throughout the world. Four of these viruses have produced at least one case of human illness indistinguishable from rabies: European bat lyssaviruses 1 and 2, Australian bat lyssavirus, and the Duvenhage virus (in Africa). Mokola virus, a lyssavirus that has been isolated from shrews with an unknown reservoir species, has also produced human illness in Africa.

VESICULAR STOMATITIS VIRUS

Vesicular stomatitis is a viral disease of cattle, horses, pigs, and some wild mammals. VSV is a member of the genus *Vesiculovirus* in the family Rhabdoviridae. Outbreaks of vesicular stomatitis in animals occur sporadically in the southwestern United States. The infection is associated with severe vesiculation and ulceration of oral tissues, teats, and feet and may be clinically indistinguishable from the more dangerous foot-and-mouth disease. Epidemics are usually seasonal and are probably due to arthropod vectors. Direct animal-to-animal spread can also occur, although the virus cannot penetrate intact skin. Transmission to humans usually results from direct contact with infected animals (particularly cattle) and occasionally follows laboratory exposure. In human disease, early conjunctivitis is followed by an acute influenza-like illness with fever, chills, nausea, vomiting, headache, retrobulbar pain, myalgias, substernal pain, malaise, pharyngitis, and lymphadenitis. Small vesicular lesions may be present on the buccal mucosa or on the fingers. The illness usually lasts 3–6 days, with a subsequent full recovery. Subclinical infections are common. A serologic diagnosis can be made on the basis of a rise in titer of complement-fixing or neutralizing antibodies. Therapy is symptom-based.

FURTHER READINGS

BAER GM (ed): *The Natural History of Rabies*, 2d ed. Boca Raton, CRC Press, 1991

CENTERS FOR DISEASE CONTROL AND PREVENTION: Human rabies prevention—United States, 1999: Recommendations of the Advisory Committee on Immunization Practices (ACIP). MMWR 48(RR-1):1, 1999

JACKSON AC: Rabies: New insights into pathogenesis and treatment. Curr Opin Neurol 19:267, 2006

———, WUNNER WH (eds): *Rabies*, 2d ed. London, Elsevier, 2007

LETCHWORTH GJ et al: Vesicular stomatitis. Vet J 157:239, 1999

WARRELL MJ, WARRELL DA: Rabies and other lyssavirus diseases. Lancet 363:959, 2004

WILLOUGHBY RE JR et al: Survival after treatment of rabies with induction of coma. N Engl J Med 352:2508, 2005

WORLD HEALTH ORGANIZATION: *WHO Expert Consultation on Rabies: First Report*. First Report ed. Geneva, WHO, 2005

189 Infections Caused by Arthropod- and Rodent-Borne Viruses

Clarence J. Peters

Some zoonotic viruses are transmitted in nature without regard to humans and only incidentally infect and produce disease in humans; in addition, a few agents are regularly spread among humans by arthropods. Most of these viruses either are maintained by arthropods or chronically infect rodents. Obviously, the mode of transmission is not a rational basis for taxonomic classification. Indeed, zoonotic viruses from at least seven families act as significant human pathogens (Table 189-1). The virus families differ fundamentally from one another in terms of morphology, replication mechanisms, and genetics. Information on a virus's membership in a family or genus is enlightening with regard to maintenance strategies, sensitivity to antiviral agents, and some aspects of pathogenesis but does not necessarily predict which clinical syndromes (if any) the virus will cause in humans.

FAMILIES OF ARTHROPOD- AND RODENT-BORNE VIRUSES (TABLE 189-1)

The Arenaviridae The Arenaviridae are spherical, 110- to 130-nm particles that bud from the cell's plasma membrane and utilize ambisense RNA genomes with two segments for replication. There are two main phylogenetic branches of Arenaviridae: the Old World viruses, such as Lassa fever and lymphocytic choriomeningitis (LCM) viruses, and the New World viruses, including those causing the South American hemorrhagic fevers (HFs). Arenaviruses persist in nature by chronically infecting rodents with a striking one-virus–one-rodent species relationship. These rodent infections result in long-term virus excretion and perhaps in lifelong viremia; vertical infection is common with some arenaviruses. Humans become infected through the inhalation of aerosols containing arenaviruses, which are then deposited in the terminal air passages, and probably also through close contact with rodents and their excreta, which results in the contamination of mucous membranes or breaks in the skin.

The Bunyaviridae The family Bunyaviridae includes four medically significant genera. All of these spherical viruses have three negative-sense RNA segments maturing into 90- to 120-nm particles in the Golgi complex and exiting the cell by exocytosis. Viruses of the genus *Bunyavirus* are largely mosquito-borne and have a viremic vertebrate intermediate host; many are also transovarially transmitted in their specific mosquito host. One serologic group also uses biting midges as vectors. Sandflies or mosquitoes are the vectors for the genus *Phlebovirus* (named after phlebotomus fever or sandfly fever, the best-known disease associated with the genus), while ticks serve as vectors for the genus *Nairovirus*. Viruses of both of these genera are also associated with vertical transmission in the arthropod host and with horizontal spread through viremic vertebrate hosts. The genus *Hantavirus* is unique among the Bunyaviridae in that it is not transmitted by arthropods but is maintained in nature by rodent hosts that chronically shed virus. Like the arenaviruses, the hantaviruses usually display striking virus–rodent species specificity. Hantaviruses do not cause chronic viremia in their rodent hosts and are transmitted only horizontally from rodent to rodent.

Other Families The Flaviviridae are positive-sense, single-strand RNA viruses that form particles of 40–50 nm in the endoplasmic reticulum. The flaviviruses discussed here are from the genus *Flavivirus* and make up two phylogenetically and antigenically distinct divisions transmitted among vertebrates by mosquitoes and ticks, respectively. The mosquito-borne viruses fall into phylogenetic groups that include yellow fever virus, the four dengue viruses, and encephalitis viruses, while the tick-borne group encompasses a geographically varied spectrum of species, some of which are responsible for encephalitis or for hemorrhagic disease with encephalitis. The Reoviridae are double-strand RNA viruses with multisegmented genomes. These 80-nm particles are the only viruses discussed in this chapter that do not have a lipid envelope and thus are insensitive to detergents. The Togaviridae

TABLE 189-1 MAJOR ZOONOTIC VIRUS FAMILIES AND SOME CHARACTERISTICS OF TYPICAL MEMBERS

Family	Genus or Group	Syndrome(s): Typical Viruses	Maintenance Strategy
Arenaviridae	Old World complex	FM, E: Lymphocytic choriomeningitis virus HF: Lassa fever virus	Chronic infection of rodents, often with persistent viremia; vertical transmission common
	New World or Tacaribe complex	HF: South American HF viruses (Machupo, Junin, Guanarito, Sabia)	Chronic infection of rodents, sometimes with persistent viremia; vertical infection may occur
Bunyaviridae	*Bunyavirus*	E: California serogroup viruses (La Crosse, Jamestown Canyon, California encephalitis) FM: Bunyamwera, group C, Tahyna viruses	Mosquito-vertebrate cycle; transovarial transmission in mosquito common
		FM: Oropouche virus	Transmitted by *Culicoides*
	Phlebovirus	FM: Sandfly fever, Toscana viruses FM: Punta Toro virus	Sandfly transmission between vertebrates, with prominent transovarial component in sandfly
		HF, FM, E: Rift Valley fever virus	Mosquito-vertebrate transmission, with transovarial component in mosquito
	Nairovirus	HF: Crimean-Congo HF virus	Tick-vertebrate, with transovarial transmission in tick
	Hantavirus	HF: Hantaan, Dobrava, Puumala viruses	Rodent reservoir; chronic virus shedding, but chronic viremia unknown
		HF: Sin Nombre and related hantaviruses	Sigmodontine rodent reservoir
Filoviridae[a]	*Ebolavirus, Marburgvirus*	HF: Marburg viruses, Ebola viruses (4 species)	Unknown
Flaviviridae	*Flavivirus* (mosquito-borne)	HF: Yellow fever virus FM, HF: Dengue viruses (4 serotypes) E: St. Louis, Japanese, West Nile, and Murray Valley encephalitis viruses; Rocio viruses	Mosquito-vertebrate; transovarial rare
	Flavivirus (tick-borne)	E: Central European tick-borne encephalitis, Russian spring-summer encephalitis, Powassan viruses HF: Omsk HF, Kyasanur Forest disease viruses	Tick-vertebrate
Reoviridae	*Coltivirus*	FM, E: Colorado tick fever virus	Tick-vertebrate
	Orbivirus	FM, E: Orungo, Kemerovo viruses	Arthropod-vertebrate
Rhabdoviridae[b]	*Vesiculovirus*	FM: Vesicular stomatitis virus (Indiana, New Jersey); Chandipura, Piry viruses	Sandfly-vertebrate, with prominent transovarial component in sandfly
Togaviridae	*Alphavirus*	AR: Sindbis, chikungunya, Mayaro, Ross River, Barmah Forest viruses E: Eastern, western, and Venezuelan equine encephalitis viruses	Mosquito-vertebrate

[a]The Filoviridae are discussed in Chap. 190.
[b]The Rhabdoviridae are discussed in Chap. 188.

Note: Abbreviations refer to the disease syndrome most commonly associated with the virus: FM, fever, myalgia; AR, arthritis, rash; E, encephalitis; HF, hemorrhagic fever.

have a single positive-strand RNA genome and bud particles of ~60–70 nm from the plasma membrane. The togaviruses discussed here are all members of the genus *Alphavirus* and are transmitted among vertebrates by mosquitoes in their natural cycle. The Filoviridae and the Rhabdoviridae are discussed in Chaps. 190 and 188, respectively.

PROMINENT FEATURES OF ARTHROPOD- AND RODENT-BORNE VIRUSES

Although this chapter discusses the major features of selected arthropod- and rodent-borne viruses, it does not deal with >500 other distinct recognized zoonotic viruses, about one-fourth of which infect humans. Zoonotic viruses are undergoing genetic evolution, "new" zoonotic viruses are being discovered, and the epidemiology of zoonotic viruses is continuing to evolve through environmental changes affecting vectors, reservoirs, and humans. These zoonotic viruses are most numerous in the tropics but are also found in temperate and frigid climates. Their distribution and seasonal activity may be variable and often depend largely on ecologic conditions such as rainfall and temperature, which in turn affect the density of vectors and reservoirs and the development of infection therein.

Maintenance and Transmission Arthropod-borne viruses infect their vectors after the ingestion of a blood meal from a viremic vertebrate. The vectors then develop chronic, systemic infection as the viruses penetrate the gut and spread throughout the body. The viruses eventually reach the salivary glands during a period that is referred to as *extrinsic incubation* and that typically lasts 1–3 weeks in mosquitoes. At this point, an arthropod is competent to continue the chain of transmission by infecting another vertebrate when a subsequent blood meal is taken. The arthropod generally is unharmed by the infection, and the natural vertebrate partner usually has only transient viremia with no overt disease. An alternative mechanism for virus maintenance in its arthropod host is transovarial transmission, which is common among members of the family Bunyaviridae.

Rodent-borne viruses such as the hantaviruses and arenaviruses are maintained in nature by chronic infection transmitted between rodents. As in arthropod-borne virus cycles, there is usually a high degree of rodent-virus specificity, and there is no overt disease in the reservoir/vector.

Epidemiology The distribution of arthropod- and rodent-borne viruses is restricted by the areas inhabited by their reservoir/vectors and provides an important clue in the differential diagnosis. Table 189-2 shows the approximate geographic distribution of the most important of these viruses. Members of each family, each genus, and even each serologically related group usually occur in each area but may not be pathogenic in all areas or may not be a commonly recognized cause of disease in all areas and so may not be included in the table.

Most of these diseases are acquired in a rural setting; a few have urban vectors. Seoul, sandfly fever, and Oropouche viruses are examples of urban viruses, but the most notable are yellow fever, dengue, and chikungunya viruses. A history of mosquito bite has little diagnostic significance in the individual; a history of tick bite is more diagnostically specific. Rodent exposure is often reported by persons infected with an arenavirus or a hantavirus but again has little specificity. Indeed, aerosols may infect persons who have no recollection of having even seen rodents.

Syndromes Human disease caused by arthropod- and rodent-borne viruses is often subclinical. The spectrum of possible responses to infection is wide, and our knowledge of the outcome of most of these infections is limited. The usual disease syndromes associated with these viruses have been grouped into four categories: fever and myalgia, arthritis and rash, encephalitis, and hemorrhagic fever. Although for the purposes of this discussion most viruses have been placed in a single group, the categories often overlap. For example, West Nile and Venezuelan equine encephalitis viruses are discussed as encephalitis viruses,

TABLE 189-2 GEOGRAPHIC DISTRIBUTION OF SOME IMPORTANT AND COMMONLY ENCOUNTERED HUMAN ZOONOTIC VIRAL DISEASES

Area	Arenaviridae	Bunyaviridae	Flaviviridae	Rhabdoviridae	Togaviridae
North America	Lymphocytic choriomeningitis	La Crosse, Jamestown Canyon, California encephalitis; hantavirus pulmonary syndrome	St. Louis, Powassan, West Nile encephalitis; dengue	Vesicular stomatitis	Eastern, western equine encephalitis
South America	Bolivian, Argentine, Venezuelan, and Brazilian HF; lymphocytic choriomeningitis	Oropouche, group C, Punta Toro infection; hantavirus pulmonary syndrome	Yellow fever, dengue, Rocio virus infection	Vesicular stomatitis, Piry virus infection	Mayaro virus infection, Venezuelan equine encephalitis
Europe	Lymphocytic choriomeningitis	Tahyna, Toscana, sandfly fever; HF with renal syndrome	West Nile, Central European tick-borne, Russian spring-summer encephalitis	—	Sindbis virus infection
Middle East	—	Sandfly fever, Crimean-Congo HF	West Nile encephalitis, dengue	—	—
Eastern Asia	—	Sandfly fever; Hantaan, Seoul virus infection	Dengue; Japanese, Russian spring-summer encephalitis; Omsk HF	Chandipura virus infection	—
Southwestern Asia	—	Sandfly fever, Crimean-Congo HF	West Nile, Japanese encephalitis; dengue; Kyasanur Forest disease	—	Chikungunya virus infection
Southeast Asia	—	Seoul virus infection	Japanese encephalitis, dengue	—	Chikungunya virus infection
Africa	Lassa fever	Bunyamwera virus infection, Rift Valley fever	Yellow fever, dengue	—	Sindbis, chikungunya virus infection
Australia	—	—	Murray Valley encephalitis, dengue	—	Ross River, Barmah Forest virus infection

Note: HF, hemorrhagic fever.

but during epidemics they may cause many cases of milder febrile syndromes and relatively uncommon cases of encephalitis. Similarly, Rift Valley fever virus is best known as a cause of HF, but the attack rates for febrile disease are far higher, and encephalitis is occasionally seen as well. LCM virus is classified as a cause of fever and myalgia because this syndrome is its most common disease manifestation and because, even when central nervous system (CNS) disease occurs, it is usually mild and is preceded by fever and myalgia. Dengue virus infection is considered as a cause of fever and myalgia (dengue fever) because this is by far the most common manifestation worldwide and is the syndrome most likely to be seen in the United States; however, dengue HF is also discussed in the HF section because of its complicated pathogenesis and importance in pediatric practice in certain areas of the world.

Diagnosis Laboratory diagnosis is required in any given case, although epidemics occasionally provide clinical and epidemiologic clues on which an educated guess as to etiology can be based. For most arthropod- and rodent-borne viruses, acute-phase serum samples (collected within 3 or 4 days of onset) have yielded isolates, and paired sera have been used to demonstrate rising antibody titers by a variety of tests. Intensive efforts to develop rapid tests for HF have resulted in an antigen-detection enzyme-linked immunosorbent assay (ELISA) and an IgM-capture ELISA that can provide a diagnosis based on a single serum sample within a few hours and are particularly useful in severe cases. More sensitive reverse-transcription polymerase chain reaction (RT-PCR) tests may yield diagnoses based on samples without detectable antigen and may also provide useful genetic information about the virus. Hantavirus infections differ from others discussed here in that severe acute disease is immunopathologic; patients present with serum IgM that serves as the basis for a sensitive and specific test.

At diagnosis, patients with encephalitis are generally no longer viremic or antigenemic and usually do not have virus in cerebrospinal fluid (CSF). In this situation, the value of serologic methods and RT-PCR is being validated. IgM capture is increasingly being used for the simultaneous testing of serum and CSF. IgG ELISA or classic serology is useful in the evaluation of past exposure to the viruses, many of which circulate in areas with a minimal medical infrastructure and sometimes cause mild or subclinical infection.

The remainder of this chapter offers general descriptions of the broad syndromes caused by arthropod- and rodent-borne viruses. Most of the diseases under consideration have not been studied in detail with modern medical approaches; thus available data may be incomplete or biased.

FEVER AND MYALGIA

Fever and myalgia constitute the syndrome most commonly associated with zoonotic virus infection. Many of the numerous viruses belonging to the families listed in Table 189-1 probably cause this syndrome, but several viruses have been selected for inclusion in the table because of their prominent associations with the syndrome and their biomedical importance.

The syndrome typically begins with the abrupt onset of fever, chills, intense myalgia, and malaise. Patients may also report joint pains, but no true arthritis is detectable. Anorexia is characteristic and may be accompanied by nausea or even vomiting. Headache is common and may be severe, with photophobia and retroorbital pain. Physical findings are minimal and are usually confined to conjunctival injection with pain on palpation of muscles or the epigastrium. The duration of symptoms is quite variable but generally is 2–5 days, with a biphasic course in some instances. The spectrum of disease varies from subclinical to temporarily incapacitating.

Less constant findings include a maculopapular rash. Epistaxis may occur but does not necessarily indicate a bleeding diathesis. A minority of the cases caused by some viruses are known or suspected to include aseptic meningitis, but this diagnosis is difficult to make in remote areas, given the patients' photophobia and myalgia as well as the lack of opportunity to examine the CSF. Although pharyngitis may be noted or radiographic evidence of pulmonary infiltrates found in some cases, these viruses are not primary respiratory pathogens. The differential diagnosis includes anicteric leptospirosis, rickettsial diseases, and the early stages of other syndromes discussed in this chapter. These diseases are often described as "flulike," but the usual absence of cough and coryza makes influenza an unlikely confounder except at the earliest stages.

Complete recovery is generally the outcome in this syndrome, although prolonged asthenia and nonspecific symptoms have been described in some cases, particularly after infection with LCM or dengue virus. Treatment is supportive, with aspirin avoided because of the potential for exacerbated bleeding and Reye's syndrome. Efforts at prevention are best based on vector control, which, however, may be expensive or impossible. For mosquito control, destruction of breeding sites is generally the most economically and environmentally sound approach. Measures taken by the individual to avoid the vector can be valuable. Avoiding the vector's habitat and times of peak activity, using screens or other barriers (e.g., permethrin-impregnated bed nets) to prevent the vector from entering dwellings, judiciously applying arthropod repellents such as diethyltoluamide (DEET) to the skin, and wearing permethrin-impregnated clothing are all possible approaches, depending on the vector and its habits.

LYMPHOCYTIC CHORIOMENINGITIS

LCM is transmitted from the common house mouse (*Mus musculus*) to humans by aerosols of excreta and secreta. LCM virus, an arenavirus, is maintained in the mouse mainly by vertical transmission from infected dams. The vertically infected mouse remains viremic for life, with high concentrations of virus in all tissues. Infected colonies of pet hamsters have also served as a link to humans. LCM virus is widely used in immunology laboratories as a model of T cell function and can silently infect cell cultures and passaged tumor lines, resulting in infections among scientists and animal caretakers. Patients with LCM may have a history of residence in rodent-infested housing or other exposure to rodents. An antibody prevalence of ~5–10% has been reported among adults from the United States, Argentina, and endemic areas of Germany.

LCM differs from the general syndrome of fever and myalgia in that its onset is gradual. Among the conditions occasionally associated with LCM are orchitis, transient alopecia, arthritis, pharyngitis, cough, and maculopapular rash. An estimated one-fourth of patients or fewer experience a febrile phase of 3–6 days and then, after a brief remission, develop renewed fever accompanied by severe headache, nausea and vomiting, and meningeal signs lasting for ~1 week. These patients virtually always recover fully, as do the uncommon patients with clear-cut signs of encephalitis. Recovery may be delayed by transient hydrocephalus.

During the initial febrile phase, leukopenia and thrombocytopenia are common and virus can usually be isolated from blood. During the CNS phase, virus may be found in the CSF, but antibodies are present in blood. The pathogenesis of LCM is thought to resemble that following direct intracranial inoculation of the virus into adult mice; the onset of the immune response leads to T cell–mediated immunopathologic meningitis. During the meningeal phase, CSF mononuclear-cell counts range from the hundreds to the low thousands per microliter, and hypoglycorrhachia is found in one-third of cases. The IgM-capture ELISA of serum and CSF is usually positive; RT-PCR assays have been developed for application to CSF. Recent infections transmitted by organ transplantation did not include evidence of an immune response, followed a fulminant course (not unlike that of Lassa fever), and required immunohistochemistry or RT-PCR for diagnosis.

Infection with LCM virus should be suspected in acutely ill febrile patients with marked leukopenia and thrombocytopenia. In cases of aseptic meningitis, any of the following should suggest LCM: well-marked febrile prodrome, adult age, autumn seasonality, low CSF glucose levels, or CSF mononuclear cell counts of >1000/μL.

In pregnant women, LCM virus infection may lead to fetal invasion with consequent congenital hydrocephalus and chorioretinitis. Since the maternal infection may be mild, consisting of only a short febrile illness, antibodies to the virus should be sought in both the mother and the fetus in suspicious circumstances, particularly TORCH-negative neonatal hydrocephalus. [TORCH is a battery of tests encompassing *t*oxoplasmosis, *o*ther conditions (congenital syphilis and viral infection), *r*ubella, *c*ytomegalovirus infection, and *h*erpes simplex virus infection.]

BUNYAMWERA VIRUS INFECTION

The mosquito-transmitted Bunyamwera serogroup viruses are found on every continent except Australia and Antarctica. Bunyamwera virus and its close relative Ilesha virus commonly cause febrile disease in Africa. Nigari virus, a reassortant of Bunyamwera virus, has recently been identified as an important human pathogen in Africa. Other related viruses are implicated in such disease in Southeast Asia (Batai virus), Europe (Calovo virus), and South America (Wyeomyia virus). In North America, Cache Valley virus has been implicated in febrile human disease and in rare instances of more serious systemic illness; the presence of serum antibodies to this virus may be associated with congenital malformations. In Central America, the closely related Fort Sherman virus causes the fever-myalgia syndrome.

GROUP C VIRUS INFECTION

The group C viruses include at least 11 agents transmitted by mosquitoes in neotropical forests. These agents are among the most common causes of arboviral infection in humans entering American jungles and cause acute febrile disease.

TAHYNA VIRUS INFECTION

This California serogroup virus (see discussion of California encephalitis, below) occurs in central and western Europe, and related viruses are emerging in Russia. The significance of Tahyna virus in human health has been well studied only in the Czech and Slovak Republics; there, the virus was found to be a prominent cause of febrile disease, in some cases causing pharyngitis, pulmonary syndromes, and aseptic meningitis. The potential for arboviruses to be unexpectedly involved in such cases in areas of high mosquito prevalence needs to be kept in mind.

OROPOUCHE FEVER

Oropouche virus is transmitted in Central and South America by a biting midge, *Culicoides paraensis*, which often breeds to high density in cacao husks and other vegetable detritus found in towns and cities. Explosive epidemics involving thousands of cases have been reported from several towns in Brazil and Peru. Rash and aseptic meningitis have been detected in a number of cases.

SANDFLY FEVER

The sandfly *Phlebotomus papatasi* transmits sandfly fever. Female sandflies may be infected by the oral route as they take a blood meal and may transmit the virus to offspring when they lay their eggs after a second blood meal. This prominent transovarial pattern was the first to be recognized among dipterans and complicates virus control. A previous designation for sandfly fever, "3-day fever," instructively describes the brief, debilitating course associated with this essentially benign infection. There is neither a rash nor CNS involvement, and complete recovery is the rule.

Sandfly fever is found in the circum-Mediterranean area, extending to the east through the Balkans into China as well as into the Middle East and southwestern Asia. The vector is found in both rural and urban settings and is known for its small size, which enables it to penetrate standard mosquito screens and netting, and for its short flight range. Epidemics have been described in the wake of natural disasters and wars. In parts of Europe, sandfly populations and virus transmission were greatly reduced by the extensive residual spraying conducted after World War II to control malaria, and the incidence continues to be low. A common pattern of disease in endemic areas consists of high attack rates among travelers and military personnel with little or no disease in the local population, who are protected after childhood infection. More than 30 related phleboviruses are transmitted by sandflies and mosquitoes, but most are of unknown significance in terms of human health.

TOSCANA VIRUS DISEASE

Toscana virus is a *Phlebovirus* (family Bunyaviridae) transmitted primarily by the circum-Mediterranean sandfly *P. perniciosus*. The vertebrate amplifying host, if one exists, is unknown. Toscana virus infection is common during the summer among rural residents and vacationers, particularly in Italy, Spain, and Portugal; a number of cases have been identified in travelers returning to Germany and Scandinavia. The disease may manifest as an uncomplicated febrile illness but is often associated with aseptic meningitis, with virus isolated from the CSF.

PUNTA TORO VIRUS DISEASE

Of the several phleboviruses that are associated with New World sandflies and infect humans, Punta Toro virus is the best known. The disease caused by this virus is clinically similar to but epidemiologically different from that caused by the Naples or Sicilian sandfly fever viruses. Punta Toro virus infections are sporadic and are acquired in the tropical forest, where the vectors rest on tree buttresses. Epidemics have not been reported, but antibody prevalences among inhabitants of villages in the endemic areas indicate a cumulative lifetime exposure rate of >50%.

DENGUE FEVER

All four distinct dengue viruses (dengue 1–4) have *Aedes aegypti* as their principal vector, and all cause a similar clinical syndrome. In rare cases, second infection with a serotype of dengue virus different from that involved in the primary infection leads to dengue HF with severe shock (see below). Sporadic cases are seen in the settings of endemic transmission and epidemic disease. Year-round transmission between latitudes 25°N and 25°S has been established, and seasonal forays of the viruses to points as far north as Philadelphia are thought to have taken place in the United States. Dengue fever is seen in the Caribbean region, including Puerto Rico. With increasing spread of the vector mosquito throughout the tropics and subtropics, large areas of the world have become vulnerable to the introduction of dengue viruses, particularly through air travel by infected humans, and both dengue fever and the related dengue HF are becoming increasingly common. Conditions favorable to dengue transmission exist in the southern United States, and bursts of dengue fever activity are to be expected in this region, particularly along the Mexican border, where water may be stored in containers and *A. aegypti* numbers may therefore be greatest. This mosquito, which is also an efficient vector of the yellow fever and chikungunya viruses, typically breeds near human habitation, using relatively fresh water from sources such as water jars, vases, discarded containers, coconut husks, and old tires. *A. aegypti* usually inhabits dwellings and bites during the day.

After an incubation period of 2–7 days, the typical patient experiences the sudden onset of fever, headache, retroorbital pain, and back pain along with the severe myalgia that gave rise to the colloquial designation "break-bone fever." There is often a macular rash on the first day as well as adenopathy, palatal vesicles, and scleral injection. The illness may last a week, with additional symptoms usually including anorexia, nausea or vomiting, marked cutaneous hypersensitivity, and—near the time of defervescence—a maculopapular rash beginning on the trunk and spreading to the extremities and the face. Epistaxis and scattered petechiae are often noted in uncomplicated dengue, and preexisting gastrointestinal lesions may bleed during the acute illness.

Laboratory findings include leukopenia, thrombocytopenia, and, in many cases, serum aminotransferase elevations. The diagnosis is made by IgM ELISA or paired serology during recovery or by antigen-detection ELISA or RT-PCR during the acute phase. Virus is readily isolated from blood in the acute phase if mosquito inoculation or mosquito cell culture is used.

COLORADO TICK FEVER

Several hundred cases of Colorado tick fever are reported annually in the United States. The infection is acquired between March and November through the bite of an infected *Dermacentor andersoni* tick in mountainous western regions at altitudes of 1200–3000 m (4000–10,000 ft). Small mammals serve as the amplifying host. The most common presentation consists of fever and myalgia; meningoencephalitis is not uncommon, and hemorrhagic disease, pericarditis, myocarditis, orchitis, and pulmonary presentations are also reported. Rash develops in a substantial minority of cases. The disease usually lasts 7–10 days and is often biphasic. The most important differential diagnostic considerations since the beginning of the twentieth century have been Rocky Mountain spotted fever and tularemia. In Colorado, Colorado tick fever is much more common than Rocky Mountain spotted fever.

Infection of erythroblasts and other marrow cells by Colorado tick fever virus results in the appearance and persistence (for several weeks) of erythrocytes containing the virus. This feature, detected in smears stained by immunofluorescence, can be diagnostically helpful. The clinical laboratory detects leukopenia and thrombocytopenia.

ORBIVIRUS INFECTION

The orbiviruses encompass many human and veterinary pathogens. For example, Orungo virus is widely transmitted by mosquitoes in tropical Africa and causes febrile disease in humans. The Kemerovo complex includes the Kemerovo, Lipovnik, and Tribec viruses of Russia and central Europe; these viruses are transmitted by ticks and are associated with febrile and neurologic disease.

ENCEPHALITIS

Arboviral encephalitis is a seasonal disease, commonly occurring in the warmer months. Its incidence varies markedly with time and place, depending on ecologic factors. The causative viruses differ substantially in terms of case-infection ratio (i.e., the ratio of clinical to subclinical infections), mortality rate, and residua (Table 189-3). Humans are not an important amplifier of these viruses.

All the viral encephalitides discussed in this section have a similar pathogenesis as far as is known. An infected arthropod ingests a blood meal from a human and infects the host. The initial period of viremia is thought to originate most commonly from the lymphoid system. Viremia leads to CNS invasion, presumably through infection of olfactory neuroepithelium with passage through the cribriform plate or through infection of brain capillaries and multifocal entry into the CNS. During the viremic phase, there may be little or no recognized disease except in the case of tick-borne flaviviral encephalitis, in which there may be a clearly delineated phase of fever and systemic illness. The disease process in the CNS arises partly from direct neuronal infection and subsequent damage and partly from edema, inflammation, and other indirect effects. The usual pathologic picture is one of focal necrosis of neurons, inflammatory glial nodules, and perivascular lymphoid cuffing; the severity and distribution of these abnormalities vary with the infecting virus. Involved areas display the "luxury perfusion" phenomenon, with normal or increased total blood flow and low oxygen extraction.

The typical patient presents with a prodrome of nonspecific constitutional symptoms, including fever, abdominal pain, vertigo, sore throat, and respiratory symptoms. Headache, meningeal signs, photophobia, and vomiting follow quickly. Involvement of deeper structures may be signaled by lethargy, somnolence, and intellectual deficit (as disclosed by the mental status examination or failure at serial 7 subtraction); more severely affected patients are obviously disoriented and may be comatose. Tremors, loss of abdominal reflexes, cranial nerve palsies, hemiparesis, monoparesis, difficulty in swallowing, and frontal lobe signs are all common. Spinal and motor neuron diseases are documented with West Nile and Japanese encephalitis viruses. Convulsions and focal signs may be evident early or may appear during the course of the disease. Some patients present with an abrupt onset of fever, convulsions, and other signs of CNS involvement. The results of human infection range from no significant symptoms through febrile headache to aseptic meningitis and finally to full-blown encephalitis; the proportions and severity of these manifestations vary with the infecting virus.

The acute encephalitis usually lasts from a few days to as long as 2–3 weeks, but recovery may be slow, with weeks or months required for the return of maximal recoupable function. Difficulty concentrating, fatigability, tremors, and personality changes are common during recovery. The acute illness requires management of a comatose patient who may have intracranial pressure elevations, inappropriate secretion of antidiuretic hormone, respiratory failure, and convulsions. There is no specific therapy for these viral encephalitides. The only practical preventive measures are vector management and personal protection against the arthropod transmitting the virus; for Japanese encephalitis or tick-borne encephalitis, vaccination should be considered in certain circumstances (see relevant sections below).

TABLE 189-3 PROMINENT FEATURES OF ARBOVIRAL ENCEPHALITIS

Virus	Natural Cycle	Incubation Period, Days	Annual No. of Cases	Case-to-Infection Ratio	Age of Cases	Case-Fatality Rate, %	Residua
La Crosse	*Aedes triseriatus*–chipmunk (transovarial component in mosquito also important)	~3–7	70 (U.S.)	<1:1000	<15 years	<0.5	Recurrent seizures in ~10%; severe deficits in rare cases; decreased school performance and behavioral change suspected in small proportion
St. Louis	*Culex tarsalis, C. pipiens, C. quinquefasciatus*–birds	4–21	85, with hundreds to thousands in epidemic years (U.S.)	<1:200	Milder cases in the young; more severe cases in adults >40 years old, particularly the elderly	7	Common in the elderly
Japanese	*Culex tritaeniorhynchus*–birds	5–15	>25,000	1:200–300	All ages; children in highly endemic areas	20–50	Common (approximately half of cases); may be severe
West Nile	*Culex* mosquitoes–birds	3–6	?	Very low	Mainly the elderly	5–10	Uncommon
Central European	*Ixodes ricinus*–rodents, insectivores	7–14	Thousands	1:12	All ages; milder in children	1–5	20%
Russian spring-summer	*I. persulcatus*–rodents, insectivores	7–14	Hundreds	—	All ages; milder in children	20	Approximately half of cases; often severe; limb-girdle paralysis
Powassan	*I. cookei*–wild mammals	~10	~1 (U.S.)	—	All ages; some predilection for children	~10	Common (approximately half of cases)
Eastern equine	*Culiseta melanura*–birds	~5–10	5 (U.S.)	1:40 adult 1:17 child	All ages; predilection for children	50–75	Common
Western equine	*Culex tarsalis*–birds	~5–10	~20 (U.S.)	1:1000 adult 1:50 child 1:1 infant	All ages; predilection for children <2 years old (increased mortality in elderly)	3–7	Common only among infants <1 year old
Venezuelan equine (epidemic)	Unknown (multiple mosquito species and horses in epidemics)	1–5	?	1:250 adult 1:25 child (approximate)	All ages; predilection for children	~10	—

The diagnosis of arboviral encephalitis depends on the careful evaluation of a febrile patient with CNS disease, with rapid identification of treatable herpes simplex encephalitis, ruling out of brain abscess, exclusion of bacterial meningitis by serial CSF examination, and performance of laboratory studies to define the viral etiology. Leptospirosis, neurosyphilis, Lyme disease, cat-scratch fever, and newer viral encephalitides such as Nipah virus infection from Malaysia should be considered. The CSF examination usually shows a modest cell count—in the tens or hundreds or perhaps a few thousand. Early in the process, a significant proportion of these cells may be polymorphonuclear leukocytes, but usually there is a mononuclear cell predominance. CSF glucose levels are usually normal. There are exceptions to this pattern of findings. In eastern equine encephalitis, for example, polymorphonuclear leukocytes may predominate during the first 72 h of disease and hypoglycorrhachia may be detected. In LCM, lymphocyte counts may be in the thousands, and the glucose concentration may be diminished. Experience with imaging studies is still evolving; clearly, however, both CT and MRI may be normal, except for evidence of preexisting conditions, or sometimes may suggest diffuse edema. Several patients with eastern equine encephalitis have had focal abnormalities, and individuals with severe Japanese encephalitis have presented with bilateral thalamic lesions that have often been hemorrhagic. Electroencephalography usually shows diffuse abnormalities and is not directly helpful.

A humoral immune response is usually detectable at or near the onset of disease. Both serum and CSF should be examined for IgM antibodies. Virus generally cannot be isolated from blood or CSF, although Japanese encephalitis virus has been recovered from CSF in severe cases. RT-PCR analysis of CSF may yield positive results. Virus can be obtained from and viral antigen is present in brain tissue, although its distribution may be focal.

CALIFORNIA, LA CROSSE, AND JAMESTOWN CANYON VIRUS ENCEPHALITIS

The isolation of California encephalitis virus established the California serogroup of viruses as a cause of encephalitis, and its use as a diagnostic antigen led to the description of many cases of "California encephalitis." In fact, however, this virus has been implicated in only a few cases of encephalitis, and the serologically related La Crosse virus is the major cause of encephalitis among viruses in the California serogroup. "California encephalitis" due to La Crosse virus infection is most commonly reported from the upper Midwest but is also found in other areas of the central and eastern United States, most often in West Virginia, Tennessee, North Carolina, and Georgia. The serogroup includes 13 other viruses, some of which may also be involved in human disease that is misattributed because of the complexity of the group's serology; these viruses include the Jamestown Canyon, snowshoe hare, Inkoo, and Trivittatus viruses, all of which have *Aedes* mosquitoes as their vector and all of which have a strong element of transovarial transmission in their natural cycles.

The mosquito vector of La Crosse virus is *A. triseriatus*. In addition to a prominent transovarial component of transmission, a mosquito can become infected through feeding on viremic chipmunks and other mammals as well as through venereal transmission from another mosquito. The mosquito breeds in sites such as tree holes and abandoned tires and bites during daylight hours. These habits correlate with the risk factors for human cases: recreation in forested areas, residence at the forest's edge, and the presence of abandoned tires around the home. Intensive environmental modification based on these findings has reduced the incidence of disease in a highly endemic area in the

Midwest. Most cases occur from July through September. The Asian tiger mosquito, *A. albopictus*, efficiently transmits the virus to mice and also transmits the agent transovarially in the laboratory; this aggressive anthropophilic mosquito has the capacity to urbanize, and its possible impact on transmission to humans is of concern.

An antibody prevalence of ≥20% in endemic areas indicates that infection is common, but CNS disease has been recognized primarily in children <15 years of age. The illness varies from a picture of aseptic meningitis accompanied by confusion to severe and occasionally fatal encephalitis. Although there may be prodromal symptoms, the onset of CNS disease is sudden, with fever, headache, and lethargy often joined by nausea and vomiting, convulsions (in one-half of patients), and coma (in one-third of patients). Focal seizures, hemiparesis, tremor, aphasia, chorea, Babinski signs, and other evidence of significant neurologic dysfunction are common, but residua are not. Perhaps 10% of patients have recurrent seizures in the succeeding months. Other serious sequelae are rare, although a decrease in scholastic standing has been reported and mild personality change has occasionally been suggested. Treatment is supportive over a 1- to 2-week acute phase during which status epilepticus, cerebral edema, and inappropriate secretion of antidiuretic hormone are important concerns. Ribavirin has been used in severe cases, and a clinical trial of this drug is under way.

The blood leukocyte count is commonly elevated, sometimes reaching levels of 20,000/μL, and there is usually a left shift. CSF cell counts are typically 30–500/μL with a mononuclear cell predominance (although 25–90% of cells are polymorphonuclear in some cases). The protein level is normal or slightly increased, and the glucose level is normal. Specific virologic diagnosis based on IgM-capture assays of serum and CSF is efficient. The only human anatomic site from which virus has been isolated is the brain.

Jamestown Canyon virus has been implicated in several cases of encephalitis in adults; in these cases, the disease was usually associated with a significant respiratory illness at onset. Human infection with this virus has been documented in New York, Wisconsin, Ohio, Michigan, Ontario, and other areas of North America where the vector mosquito, *A. stimulans*, feeds on its main host, the white-tailed deer.

ST. LOUIS ENCEPHALITIS

St. Louis encephalitis virus is transmitted between *Culex* mosquitoes and birds. This virus causes low-level endemic infection among rural residents of the western and central United States, where *C. tarsalis* is the vector (see "Western Equine Encephalitis," below), but the more urbanized mosquito species *C. pipiens* and *C. quinquefasciatus* have been responsible for epidemics resulting in hundreds or even thousands of cases in cities of the central and eastern United States. Most cases occur in June through October. The urban mosquitoes breed in accumulations of stagnant water and sewage with high organic content and readily bite humans in and around houses at dusk. The elimination of open sewers and trash-filled drainage systems is expensive and may not be possible, but screening of houses and implementation of personal protective measures may be an effective approach for individuals. The rural vector is most active at dusk and outdoors; its bites can be avoided by modification of activities and use of repellents.

Disease severity increases with age: infections that result in aseptic meningitis or mild encephalitis are concentrated in children and young adults, while severe and fatal cases primarily affect the elderly. Infection rates are similar in all age groups; thus the greater susceptibility of older persons to disease is a biologic consequence of aging. The disease has an abrupt onset, sometimes following a prodrome, and begins with fever, lethargy, confusion, and headache. In addition, nuchal rigidity, hypotonia, hyperreflexia, myoclonus, and tremor are common. Severe cases can include cranial nerve palsies, hemiparesis, and convulsions. Patients often report dysuria and may have viral antigen in urine as well as pyuria. The overall mortality rate is generally ~7% but may reach 20% among patients over the age of 60. Recovery is slow. Emotional lability, difficulties in concentration and memory, asthenia, and tremor are commonly prolonged in older patients.

The CSF of patients with St. Louis encephalitis usually contains tens to hundreds of cells, with a lymphocytic predominance and a normal glucose level. Leukocytosis with a left shift is often documented.

JAPANESE ENCEPHALITIS

Japanese encephalitis virus is found throughout Asia, including far eastern Russia, Japan, China, India, Pakistan, and Southeast Asia, and causes occasional epidemics on western Pacific islands. The virus has been detected in the Torres Strait islands, and a human encephalitis case has been identified on the nearby Australian mainland. This flavivirus is particularly common in areas where irrigated rice fields attract the natural avian vertebrate hosts and provide abundant breeding sites for mosquitoes such as *C. tritaeniorhynchus*, which transmit the virus to humans. Additional amplification by pigs, which suffer abortion, and horses, which develop encephalitis, may be significant as well. Vaccination of these additional amplifying hosts may reduce the transmission of the virus. An effective, formalin-inactivated vaccine purified from mouse brain is produced in Japan and licensed for human use in the United States. It is given on days 0, 7, and 30 or—with some sacrifice in serum neutralizing titer—on days 0, 7, and 14. Vaccination is indicated for summer travelers to rural Asia, where the risk of clinical disease may be 0.05–2.1/10,000 per week (Table 116-2). The severe and often fatal disease reported in expatriates must be balanced against the 0.1–1% chance of a late systemic or cutaneous allergic reaction. These reactions are rarely fatal but may be severe and have been known to begin 1–9 days after vaccination, with associated pruritus, urticaria, and angioedema. Live attenuated vaccines are being used in China but are not recommended in the United States at this time.

WEST NILE VIRUS INFECTION

West Nile virus is transmitted among wild birds by *Culex* mosquitoes in Africa, the Middle East, southern Europe, and Asia. It is a common cause of febrile disease without CNS involvement, but it occasionally causes aseptic meningitis and severe encephalitis; these serious infections are particularly common among the elderly. The febrile-myalgic syndrome caused by West Nile virus differs from many others by the frequent appearance of a maculopapular rash concentrated on the trunk and lymphadenopathy. Headache, ocular pain, sore throat, nausea and vomiting, and arthralgia (but not arthritis) are common accompaniments. In addition, the virus has been implicated in severe and fatal hepatic necrosis in Africa.

West Nile virus was introduced into New York City in 1999 and subsequently spread to other areas of the northeastern United States, causing >60 cases of aseptic meningitis or encephalitis among humans as well as die-offs among crows, exotic zoo birds, and other birds. The virus has continued to spread and is now found in almost all states, Canada, and Mexico. *C. pipiens* remains the major vector in the northeastern United States, but several other *Culex* species are also involved, and blue jays compete with crows as amplifiers and lethal targets in other areas of the country. Annually, ~1000–3000 cases of encephalitis with ~100–300 deaths are reported in the United States. The ratio of CNS involvement to infection is thought to be ~1:100; the remainder of patients have subclinical infection or West Nile fever. Encephalitis, sequelae, and death are all more common among the elderly, diabetics, and patients with previous CNS insults. In addition to the more severe motor and cognitive sequelae, milder findings may include tremor, slight abnormalities in motor skills, and loss of executive functions. Intense clinical interest and the availability of laboratory diagnostic methods have made it possible to define a number of unusual clinical features, including chorioretinitis, flaccid paralysis with histologic lesions resembling poliomyelitis, and initial presentation with fever and focal neurologic deficits in the absence of diffuse encephalitis. Immunosuppressed patients may have fulminant courses or develop persistent CNS infection. Virus transmission through both transplantation and blood transfusion has necessitated screening of blood and organ donors by nucleic acid–based tests.

West Nile virus falls into the same phylogenetic group of flaviviruses as St. Louis and Japanese encephalitis viruses, as do Murray Valley and

Rocio viruses. The latter two viruses are both maintained in mosquitoes and birds and produce a clinical picture resembling that of Japanese encephalitis. Murray Valley virus has caused occasional epidemics and sporadic cases in Australia. Rocio virus caused recurrent epidemics in a focal area of Brazil in 1975–1977 and then virtually disappeared.

CENTRAL EUROPEAN TICK-BORNE ENCEPHALITIS AND RUSSIAN SPRING-SUMMER ENCEPHALITIS

A spectrum of tick-borne flaviviruses has been identified across the Eurasian land mass. Many are known mainly as agricultural pathogens (e.g., louping ill virus in the United Kingdom). From Scandinavia to the Urals, central European tick-borne encephalitis is transmitted by *Ixodes ricinus*. Human cases occur between April and October, with a peak in June and July. A related and more virulent virus is that of Russian spring-summer encephalitis, which is associated with *I. persulcatus* and is distributed from Europe across the Urals to the Pacific Ocean. The ticks transmit the disease primarily in the spring and early summer, with a lower rate of transmission later in summer. Small mammals are the vertebrate amplifiers for both viruses. The risk varies by geographic area and can be highly localized within a given area; human cases usually follow outdoor activities or consumption of raw milk from infected goats or other infected animals.

After an incubation period of 7–14 days or perhaps longer, the central European viruses classically result in a febrile-myalgic phase that lasts for 2–4 days and is thought to correlate with viremia. A subsequent remission for several days is followed by the recurrence of fever and the onset of meningeal signs. The CNS phase varies from mild aseptic meningitis, which is more common among younger patients, to severe encephalitis with coma, convulsions, tremors, and motor signs lasting for 7–10 days before improvement begins. Spinal and medullary involvement can lead to typical limb-girdle paralysis and to respiratory paralysis. Most patients recover, only a minority with significant deficits. Infections with the Far Eastern viruses generally run a more abrupt course. The encephalitic syndrome caused by these viruses sometimes begins without a remission and has more severe manifestations than the European syndrome. Mortality is high, and major sequelae—most notably, lower motor neuron paralyses of the proximal muscles of the extremities, trunk, and neck—are common.

In the early stage of the illness, virus may be isolated from the blood. In the CNS phase, IgM antibodies are detectable in serum and/or CSF. Thrombocytopenia sometimes develops during the initial febrile illness, which resembles the early hemorrhagic phase of some other tick-borne flaviviral infections, such as Kyasanur Forest disease. Other tick-borne flaviviruses are less common causes of encephalitis, including louping ill virus in the United Kingdom and Powassan virus.

There is no specific therapy for infection with these viruses. However, effective alum-adjuvanted, formalin-inactivated vaccines are produced in Austria, Germany, and Russia. Two doses of the Austrian vaccine separated by an interval of 1–3 months appear to be effective in the field, and antibody responses are similar when vaccine is given on days 0 and 14. Other vaccines have elicited similar neutralizing antibody titers. Since rare cases of postvaccination Guillain-Barré syndrome have been reported, vaccination should be reserved for persons likely to experience rural exposure in an endemic area during the season of transmission. Cross-neutralization for the central European and Far Eastern strains has been established, but there are no published field studies on cross-protection of formalin-inactivated vaccines. Because 0.2–4% of ticks in endemic areas may be infected, tick bites raise the issue of immunoglobulin prophylaxis. Prompt administration of high-titered specific preparations should probably be undertaken, although no controlled data are available to prove the efficacy of this measure. Immunoglobulin should not be administered late because of the risk of antibody-mediated enhancement.

POWASSAN ENCEPHALITIS

Powassan virus is a member of the tick-borne encephalitis virus complex and is transmitted by *I. cookei* among small mammals in eastern Canada and the United States, where it has been responsible for 20 recognized cases of human disease. Other ticks may transmit the virus in a wider geographic area, and there is some concern that *I. scapularis* (also called *I. dammini*), a competent vector in the laboratory, may become involved as it becomes more prominent in the United States. Patients with Powassan encephalitis (many of whom are children) present in May through December after outdoor exposure and an incubation period thought to be ~1 week. Powassan encephalitis is severe, and sequelae are common.

EASTERN EQUINE ENCEPHALITIS

Eastern equine encephalitis is found primarily within endemic swampy foci along the eastern coast of the United States, with a few inland foci as far removed as Michigan. Human cases present from June through October, when the bird–*Culiseta* mosquito cycle spills over into other mosquito species such as *A. sollicitans* or *A. vexans*, which are more likely to bite mammals. There is concern over the potential role of the introduced anthropophilic mosquito species *A. albopictus*, which has been found to be naturally infected and is an effective vector in the laboratory. Horses are a common target for the virus; contact with unvaccinated horses may be associated with human disease, but horses probably do not play a significant role in amplification of the virus.

Eastern equine encephalitis is one of the most destructive of the arboviral conditions, with a brusque onset, rapid progression, high mortality, and frequent residua. This severity is reflected in the extensive necrotic lesions and polymorphonuclear infiltrates found at postmortem examination of the brain and the acute polymorphonuclear CSF pleocytosis often occurring during the first 1–3 days of disease. In addition, leukocytosis with a left shift is a common feature. A formalin-inactivated vaccine has been used to protect laboratory workers but is not generally available or applicable.

WESTERN EQUINE ENCEPHALITIS

The primary maintenance cycle for western equine encephalitis virus in the United States is between *C. tarsalis* and birds, principally sparrows and finches. Equines and humans become infected, and both species suffer encephalitis without amplifying the virus in nature. St. Louis encephalitis is transmitted in a similar cycle in the same region but causes human disease about a month earlier than the period (July through October) in which western equine encephalitis virus is active. Large epidemics of western equine encephalitis took place in the western and central United States and Canada during the 1930s to 1950s, but in recent years the disease has been uncommon. There were 41 reported cases in the United States in 1987 but only 5 reported cases from 1988 to 2001. This decline in incidence may reflect in part the integrated approach to mosquito management that has been employed in irrigation projects and the increasing use of agricultural pesticides; it almost certainly reflects the increased tendency for humans to be indoors behind closed windows at dusk—the peak period of biting by the major vector.

Western equine encephalitis virus causes a typical diffuse viral encephalitis with an increased attack rate and increased morbidity among the young, particularly children <2 years old. In addition, mortality rates are high among the young and the very elderly. One-third of individuals who have convulsions during the acute illness have subsequent seizure activity. Infants <1 year old—particularly those in the first months of life—are at serious risk of motor and intellectual damage. Twice as many males as females develop clinical encephalitis after 5–9 years of age; this difference may be related to greater outdoor exposure of boys to the vector but is also likely to be due in part to biologic differences. A formalin-inactivated vaccine has been used to protect laboratory workers but is not generally available or applicable.

VENEZUELAN EQUINE ENCEPHALITIS

There are six known types of virus in the Venezuelan equine encephalitis complex. An important distinction is between the *epizootic* viruses (subtypes IAB and IC) and the *enzootic* viruses (subtypes ID to IF and types II to VI). The epizootic viruses have an unknown natural cycle but periodically cause extensive epidemics in equines and humans in the Americas. These epidemics rely on the high-level viremia in horses and mules that results in the infection of several species of mosquitoes, which in turn infect humans and perpetuate virus transmission. Humans also have high-level viremia but probably are not important in virus transmission. Enzootic viruses are found primarily in humid tropical forest habitats and are maintained between *Culex* mosquitoes and rodents; these viruses cause human disease but are not pathogenic for horses and do not cause epizootics.

Epizootics of Venezuelan equine encephalitis occurred repeatedly in Venezuela, Colombia, Ecuador, Peru, and other South American countries at intervals of ≤10 years from the 1930s until 1969, when a massive epizootic spread throughout Central America and Mexico, reaching southern Texas in 1972. Genetic sequencing of the virus from the 1969–1972 outbreak suggested that it originated from residual "un-inactivated" virus in veterinary vaccines. The outbreak was terminated in Texas with the use of a live attenuated vaccine (TC-83) originally developed for human use by the U.S. Army; the epizootic virus was then used for further production of inactivated veterinary vaccines. No further epizootic disease was identified until 1995 and subsequently, when additional epizootics took place in Colombia, Venezuela, and Mexico. The viruses involved in these epizootics as well as previously epizootic subtype IC viruses have been shown to be close phylogenetic relatives of known enzootic subtype ID viruses. This finding suggests that active evolution and selection of epizootic viruses are under way in northern South America.

During epizootics, extensive human infection is the rule, with clinical disease in 10–60% of infected individuals. Most infections result in notable acute febrile disease, while relatively few result in encephalitis. A low rate of CNS invasion is supported by the absence of encephalitis among the many infections resulting from exposure to aerosols in the laboratory or from vaccine accidents. The most recent large epizootic of Venezuelan equine encephalitis occurred in Colombia and Venezuela in 1995; of the >85,000 clinical cases, 4% (with a higher proportion among children than adults) included neurologic symptoms and 300 ended in death.

Enzootic strains of Venezuelan equine encephalitis virus are common causes of acute febrile disease, particularly in areas such as the Florida Everglades and the humid Atlantic coast of Central America. Encephalitis has been documented only in the Florida infections; the three cases were caused by type II enzootic virus, also called *Everglades virus*. All three patients had preexisting cerebral disease. Extrapolation from the rate of genetic change suggests that Everglades virus may have been introduced into Florida <200 years ago and that it is most closely related to the ID subtypes that appear to have given evolutionary rise to the epizootic strains active in South America.

The prevention of epizootic Venezuelan equine encephalitis depends on vaccination of horses with the attenuated TC-83 vaccine or with an inactivated vaccine prepared from that strain. Humans can be protected with similar vaccines, but the use of such products is restricted to laboratory personnel because of reactogenicity and limited availability. In addition, wild-type virus and perhaps TC-83 vaccine may have some degree of fetal pathogenicity. Enzootic viruses are genetically and antigenically different from epizootic viruses, and protection against the former with vaccines prepared from the latter is relatively ineffective.

ARTHRITIS AND RASH

True arthritis is a common accompaniment of several viral diseases, such as rubella (caused by a non-alphavirus togavirus), parvovirus B19 infection, and hepatitis B; it is an occasional accompaniment of infection due to mumps virus, enteroviruses, herpesviruses, and adenoviruses. It is not generally appreciated that the alphaviruses are also common causes of arthritis. In fact, the alphaviruses discussed below all cause acute febrile diseases accompanied by the development of true arthritis and a maculopapular rash. Rheumatic involvement includes arthralgia alone, periarticular swelling, and (less commonly) joint effusions. Most of these diseases are less severe and have fewer articular manifestations in children than in adults. In temperate climates, these are summer diseases. No specific therapy or licensed vaccines exist.

SINDBIS VIRUS INFECTION

Sindbis virus is transmitted among birds by mosquitoes. Infections with the northern European strains of this virus (which cause, for example, Pogosta disease in Finland, Karelian fever in the independent states of the former Soviet Union, and Okelbo disease in Sweden) and with the genetically related southern African strains are particularly likely to result in the arthritis-rash syndrome. Exposure to a rural environment is commonly associated with this infection, which has an incubation period of <1 week.

The disease begins with rash and arthralgia. Constitutional symptoms are not marked, and fever is modest or lacking altogether. The rash, which lasts ~1 week, begins on the trunk, spreads to the extremities, and evolves from macules to papules that often vesiculate. The arthritis of this condition is multiarticular, migratory, and incapacitating, with resolution of the acute phase in a few days. Wrists, ankles, phalangeal joints, knees, elbows, and—to a much lesser extent—proximal and axial joints are involved. Persistence of joint pains and occasionally of arthritis is a major problem and may go on for months or even years despite a lack of deformity.

CHIKUNGUNYA VIRUS INFECTION

It is likely that chikungunya virus ("that which bends up") is of African origin and is maintained among nonhuman primates on that continent by *Aedes* mosquitoes of the subgenus *Stegomyia* in a fashion similar to yellow fever virus. Like yellow fever virus, chikungunya virus is readily transmitted among humans in urban areas by *A. aegypti*. The *A. aegypti*–chikungunya virus transmission cycle has also been introduced into Asia, where it poses a prominent health problem. The disease is endemic in rural areas of Africa, and intermittent epidemics take place in towns and cities of Africa and Asia. In 2004, a massive epidemic in the Indian Ocean region began; it now appears to have been spread totally by travelers. *A. albopictus* was identified as the major vector, and there were multiple exportations to temperate zones and to areas where *A. aegypti* is present. Chikungunya is one more reason (in addition to dengue and yellow fever) that *A. aegypti* must be controlled.

Full-blown disease is most common among adults, in whom the clinical picture may be dramatic. The abrupt onset follows an incubation period of 2–3 days. Fever and severe arthralgia are accompanied by chills and constitutional symptoms such as headache, photophobia, conjunctival injection, anorexia, nausea, and abdominal pain. Migratory polyarthritis mainly affects the small joints of the hands, wrists, ankles, and feet, with lesser involvement of the larger joints. Rash may appear at the outset or several days into the illness; its development often coincides with defervescence, which takes place around day 2 or 3 of disease. The rash is most intense on the trunk and limbs and may desquamate. Petechiae are occasionally seen, and epistaxis is not uncommon, but this virus is not a regular cause of the HF syndrome, even in children. A few patients develop leukopenia. Elevated levels of aspartate aminotransferase (AST) and C-reactive protein have been described, as have mildly decreased platelet counts. Recovery may require weeks. Some older patients continue to experience stiffness, joint pain, and recurrent effusions for several years; this persistence may be especially common in HLA-B27 patients. An investigational live attenuated vaccine has been developed but requires additional testing. It appears to be headed for further development and commercial manufacture stimulated by the Indian Ocean outbreak.

A related virus, O'nyong-nyong, caused a major epidemic of arthritis and rash involving at least 2 million people as it moved across eastern and central Africa in the 1960s. After its mysterious emergence, the virus virtually disappeared, leaving only occasional evidence of its persistence in Kenya until a transient resurgence of epidemic activity in 1997.

MAYARO FEVER

Mayaro virus is maintained in the forests of the Americas by *Haemagogus* mosquitoes and nonhuman primates. It causes a frequently endemic and sometimes epidemic infection of humans and appears to produce a syndrome resembling chikungunya virus infection.

EPIDEMIC POLYARTHRITIS (ROSS RIVER VIRUS INFECTION)

Ross River virus has caused epidemics of distinctive clinical disease in Australia since the beginning of the twentieth century and continues to be responsible for thousands of cases in rural and suburban areas annually. The virus is transmitted by *A. vigilax* and other mosquitoes, and its persistence is thought to involve transovarial transmission. No definitive vertebrate host has been identified, but several mammalian species, including wallabies, have been suggested. Endemic transmission has also been documented in New Guinea, and in 1979 the virus swept through the eastern Pacific Islands, causing hundreds of thousands of illnesses. The virus was carried from island to island by infected humans and was believed to have been transmitted among humans by *A. polynesiensis* and *A. aegypti*.

The incubation period is 7–11 days long, and the onset of illness is sudden, with joint pain usually ushering in the disease. The rash generally develops coincidentally or follows shortly but in some cases precedes joint pains by several days. Constitutional symptoms such as low-grade fever, asthenia, myalgia, headache, and nausea are not prominent and indeed are absent in many cases. Most patients are incapacitated for considerable periods by joint involvement, which interferes with sleeping, walking, and grasping. Wrist, ankle, metacarpophalangeal, interphalangeal, and knee joints are the most commonly involved, although toes, shoulders, and elbows may be affected with some frequency. Periarticular swelling and tenosynovitis are common, and one-third of patients have true arthritis. Only half of all arthritis patients can resume normal activities within 4 weeks, and 10% still must limit their activity at 3 months. Occasional patients are symptomatic for 1–3 years but without progressive arthropathy. Aspirin and nonsteroidal anti-inflammatory drugs are effective for the treatment of symptoms.

Clinical laboratory values are normal or variable in Ross River virus infection. Tests for rheumatoid factor and antinuclear antibodies are negative, and the erythrocyte sedimentation rate is acutely elevated. Joint fluid contains 1000–60,000 mononuclear cells/μL, and Ross River virus antigen is demonstrable in macrophages. IgM antibodies are valuable in the diagnosis of this infection, although they occasionally persist for years. The isolation of the virus from blood by mosquito inoculation or mosquito cell culture is possible early in the illness. Because of the great economic impact of annual epidemics in Australia, an inactivated vaccine is being developed and has been found to be protective in mice.

Perhaps because of the local interest in arboviruses in general and in Ross River virus in particular, other arthritogenic arboviruses have been identified in Australia, including Gan Gan virus, a member of the family Bunyaviridae; Kokobera virus, a flavivirus; and Barmah Forest virus, an alphavirus. The last virus is a common cause of infection and must be differentiated from Ross River virus by specific testing.

HEMORRHAGIC FEVERS

The viral HF syndrome is a constellation of findings based on vascular instability and decreased vascular integrity. An assault, direct or indirect, on the microvasculature leads to increased permeability and (particularly when platelet function is decreased) to actual disruption and local hemorrhage. Blood pressure is decreased, and in severe cases shock supervenes. Cutaneous flushing and conjunctival suffusion are examples of common, observable abnormalities in the control of local circulation. The hemorrhage is inconstant and is in most cases an indication of widespread vascular damage rather than a life-threatening loss of blood volume. Disseminated intravascular coagulation (DIC) is occasionally found in any severely ill patient with HF but is thought to occur regularly only in the early phases of HF with renal syndrome, Crimean-Congo HF, and perhaps some cases of filovirus HF. In some viral HF syndromes, specific organs may be particularly impaired, such as the kidney in HF with renal syndrome, the lung in hantavirus pulmonary syndrome, or the liver in yellow fever, but in all these diseases the generalized circulatory disturbance is critically important.

The pathogenesis of HF is poorly understood and varies among the viruses regularly implicated in the syndrome, which number more than a dozen. In some cases direct damage to the vascular system or even to parenchymal cells of target organs is important, whereas in others soluble mediators are thought to play the major role. The acute phase in most cases of HF is associated with ongoing virus replication and viremia. Exceptions are the hantavirus diseases and dengue HF/dengue shock syndrome (DHF/DSS), in which the immune response plays a major pathogenic role.

The HF syndromes all begin with fever and myalgia, usually of abrupt onset. Within a few days the patient presents for medical attention because of increasing prostration that is often accompanied by severe headache, dizziness, photophobia, hyperesthesia, abdominal or chest pain, anorexia, nausea or vomiting, and other gastrointestinal disturbances. Initial examination often reveals only an acutely ill patient with conjunctival suffusion, tenderness to palpation of muscles or abdomen, and borderline hypotension or postural hypotension, perhaps with tachycardia. Petechiae (often best visualized in the axillae), flushing of the head and thorax, periorbital edema, and proteinuria are common. Levels of AST are usually elevated at presentation or within a day or two thereafter. Hemoconcentration from vascular leakage, which is usually evident, is most marked in hantavirus diseases and in DHF/DSS. The seriously ill patient progresses to more severe symptoms and develops shock and other findings typical of the causative virus. Shock, multifocal bleeding, and CNS involvement (encephalopathy, coma, convulsions) are all poor prognostic signs.

One of the major diagnostic clues is travel to an endemic area within the incubation period for a given syndrome (Table 189-4). Except for Seoul, dengue, and yellow fever virus infections, which have urban vectors, travel to a rural setting is especially suggestive of a diagnosis of HF.

Early recognition is important because of the need for virus-specific therapy and supportive measures, including prompt, atraumatic hospitalization; judicious fluid therapy that takes into account the patient's increased capillary permeability; administration of cardiotonic drugs; use of pressors to maintain blood pressure at levels that will support renal perfusion; treatment of the relatively common secondary bacterial infections; replacement of clotting factors and platelets as indicated; and the usual precautionary measures used in the treatment of patients with hemorrhagic diatheses. DIC should be treated only if clear laboratory evidence of its existence is found and if laboratory monitoring of therapy is feasible; there is no proven benefit of such therapy. The available evidence suggests that HF patients have a decreased cardiac output and will respond poorly to fluid loading as it is often practiced in the treatment of shock associated with bacterial sepsis. Specific therapy is available for several of the HF syndromes. In addition, several diseases considered in the differential diagnosis—malaria, shigellosis, typhoid, leptospirosis, relapsing fever, and rickettsial disease—are treatable and potentially lethal. Strict barrier nursing and other precautions against infection of medical staff and visitors are indicated in HF except that due to hantaviruses, yellow fever, Rift Valley fever, and dengue.

LASSA FEVER

Lassa virus is known to cause endemic and epidemic disease in Nigeria, Sierra Leone, Guinea, and Liberia, although it is probably more widely distributed in West Africa. This virus and its relatives exist elsewhere in Africa, but their health significance is unknown. Like other arenaviruses, Lassa virus is spread to humans by small-particle aerosols from chronically infected rodents and may also be acquired during the capture or eating of these animals. It can be transmitted by close person-to-person contact. The virus is often present in urine during convalescence and is suspected to be present in seminal fluid early in recovery. Nosocomial spread has occurred but is uncommon if proper sterile parenteral techniques are used. Individuals of all ages and both sexes are affected; the incidence of disease is highest in the dry season, but transmission takes place year-round. In countries where Lassa virus is endemic, Lassa fever can be a prominent cause of febrile disease. For example, in one hospital in Sierra Leone, laboratory-confirmed Lassa fever is consistently responsible for one-fifth of ad-

TABLE 189-4 VIRAL HEMORRHAGIC FEVER (HF) SYNDROMES AND THEIR DISTRIBUTION

Disease	Incubation Period, Days	Case-Infection Ratio	Case-Fatality Rate, %	Geographic Range	Target Population
Lassa fever	5–16	Mild infections probably common	15	West Africa	All ages, both sexes
South American HF	7–14	Most infections (more than half) result in disease	15–30	Selected rural areas of Bolivia, Argentina, Venezuela, and Brazil	Bolivia: Men in countryside; all ages, both sexes in villages Argentina: All ages, both sexes; excess exposure and disease in men Venezuela: All ages, both sexes
Rift Valley fever	2–5	~1:100[a]	~50	Sub-Saharan Africa, Madagascar, Egypt	All ages, both sexes; more often diagnosed in men; preexisting liver disease may predispose
Crimean-Congo HF	3–12	≥1:5	15–30	Africa, Middle East, Turkey, Balkans, southern region of former Soviet Union, western China	All ages, both sexes; men more exposed in some settings
HF with renal syndrome	9–35	Hantaan, >1:1.25; Puumala, 1:20	Hantaan, 5–15; Puumala, <1	Worldwide, depending on rodent reservoir	Excess of male patients (partly due to greater exposure); mainly adults
Hantavirus pulmonary syndrome	~7–28	Very high	40–50	Americas	Excess of male patients due to some occupational exposure; mainly adults
Marburg or Ebola HF	3–16	High	25–90	Sub-Saharan Africa	All ages, both sexes; children less exposed
Yellow fever	3–6	1:2–1:20	20	Africa, South America	All ages, both sexes; adults more exposed in jungle setting; preexisting flavivirus immunity may cross-protect
Dengue HF/dengue shock syndrome	2–7	Nonimmune, 1:10,000; heterologous immune, 1:100	<1 with supportive treatment	Tropics and subtropics worldwide	Predominantly children; previous heterologous dengue infection predisposes to HF
Kyasanur Forest/Omsk HF	3–8	Variable	0.5–10	Mysore State, India/western Siberia	Variable

[a]Figure is for HF cases only. Most infections with Rift Valley fever virus result in fever and myalgia rather than HF.

missions to the medical wards. There are probably tens of thousands of Lassa fever cases annually in West Africa alone.

Among the HF agents, only the arenaviruses are typically associated with a gradual onset of illness. The average case of Lassa fever has a gradual onset that gives way to more severe constitutional symptoms and prostration. Bleeding is seen in only ~15–30% of cases. A maculopapular rash is often noted in light-skinned Lassa patients. Effusions are common, and male-dominant pericarditis may develop late. The fetal death rate is 92% in the last trimester, when the maternal mortality rate is also increased from the usual 15–30%; these figures suggest that interruption of the pregnancy of infected women should be considered. White blood cell counts are normal or slightly elevated, and platelet counts are normal or somewhat low. Deafness coincides with clinical improvement in ~20% of cases and is permanent and bilateral in some. Reinfection may occur but has not been associated with severe disease.

High-level viremia or a high serum concentration of AST statistically predicts a fatal outcome. Thus patients with an AST level of >150 IU/mL should be treated with IV ribavirin. This antiviral nucleoside analogue appears to be effective in reducing mortality rates from the levels documented among retrospective controls, and its only major side effect is reversible anemia that usually does not require transfusion. The drug should be given by slow IV infusion in a dose of 32 mg/kg; this dose should be followed by 16 mg/kg every 6 h for 4 days and then by 8 mg/kg every 8 h for 6 days.

SOUTH AMERICAN HF SYNDROMES (ARGENTINE, BOLIVIAN, VENEZUELAN, AND BRAZILIAN)

These diseases are similar to one another clinically, but their epidemiology differs with the habits of their rodent reservoirs and the interactions of these animals with humans. Person-to-person or nosocomial transmission is rare but has occurred.

The basic disease resembles Lassa fever, with two marked differences. First, thrombocytopenia—often marked—is the rule, and bleeding is quite common. Second, CNS dysfunction is much more common than in Lassa fever and is often manifested by marked confusion, tremors of the upper extremities and tongue, and cerebellar signs. Some cases follow a predominantly neurologic course, with a poor prognosis. The clinical laboratory is helpful in diagnosis since thrombocytopenia, leukopenia, and proteinuria are typical findings.

Argentine HF is readily treated with convalescent-phase plasma given within the first 8 days of illness. In the absence of passive antibody therapy, IV ribavirin in the dose recommended for Lassa fever is likely to be effective in all the South American HF syndromes. The transmission of the disease from men convalescing from Argentine HF to their wives suggests the need for counseling of arenavirus HF patients concerning the avoidance of intimate contacts for several weeks after recovery. A safe, effective, live attenuated vaccine exists for Argentine HF. In experimental animals, this vaccine is cross-protective against the Bolivian HF virus.

RIFT VALLEY FEVER

The mosquito-borne Rift Valley fever virus is also a pathogen of domestic animals such as sheep, cattle, and goats. It is maintained in nature by transovarial transmission in floodwater *Aedes* mosquitoes and presumably also has a vertebrate amplifier. Epizootics and epidemics occur when sheep or cattle become infected during particularly heavy rains; developing high-level viremia, these animals infect many species of mosquitoes. Remote sensing via satellite can detect the ecologic changes associated with high rainfall that predict the likelihood of Rift Valley fever transmission; it can also detect the special depressions from which the floodwater *Aedes* mosquito vectors emerge. In addition, the virus is infectious when transmitted by contact with blood or aerosols from domestic animals or their abortuses. The slaughtered meat is not infectious; anaerobic glycolysis in postmortem tissues results in an acidic environment that rapidly inactivates Bunyaviridae such as Rift Valley fever virus and Crimean-Congo HF virus. The natural range of Rift Valley fever virus is confined to sub-Saharan Africa, where its circulation is markedly enhanced by substantial rainfall such as that which occurred during the El Niño phenomenon of 1997; subsequent spread to the Arabian Peninsula caused epidemic disease in 2000. The virus has also been found in Madagascar and has been introduced into Egypt, where it caused major epidemics in 1977–1979, 1993, and subsequently. Neither person-to-person nor nosocomial transmission has been documented.

Rift Valley fever virus is unusual in that it causes several clinical syndromes. Most infections are manifested as the febrile-myalgic syndrome. A small proportion of infections result in HF with especially prominent liver involvement. Renal failure and DIC are also common features. Perhaps 10% of otherwise mild infections lead to retinal vasculitis; funduscopic examination reveals edema, hemorrhages, and infarction, and some patients have permanently impaired vision. A small proportion of cases (<1 in 200) are followed by typical viral encephalitis. One of the complicated syndromes does not appear to predispose to another.

There is no proven therapy for any of the syndromes described above. Both retinal disease and encephalitis occur after the acute febrile syndrome has ended and serum neutralizing antibody has developed—events suggesting that only supportive care need be given. Epidemic disease is best prevented by vaccination of livestock. The established ability of this virus to propagate after an introduction into Egypt suggests that other potentially receptive areas, including the United States, should have a response ready for such an eventuality. It seems likely that this disease, like Venezuelan equine encephalitis, can be controlled only with adequate stocks of an effective live attenuated vaccine, and there are no such global stocks. A formalin-inactivated vaccine confers immunity to humans, but quantities are limited and three injections are required; this vaccine is recommended for exposed laboratory workers and for veterinarians working in sub-Saharan Africa.

CRIMEAN-CONGO HF

This severe HF syndrome has a wide geographic distribution, potentially being found wherever ticks of the genus *Hyalomma* occur. The propensity of these ticks to feed on domestic livestock and certain wild mammals means that veterinary serosurveys are the most effective mechanism for the surveillance of virus circulation in a region. Human infection is acquired via a tick bite or during the crushing of infected ticks. Domestic animals do not become ill but do develop viremia; thus there is danger of infection at the time of slaughter and for a brief interval thereafter (through contact with hides or carcasses). Cases have followed sheep shearing. An epidemic in South Africa was associated with slaughter of tick-infested ostriches. Nosocomial epidemics are common and are usually related to extensive blood exposure or needle sticks.

Although generally similar to other HF syndromes, Crimean-Congo HF causes extensive liver damage, resulting in jaundice in some cases. Clinical laboratory values indicate DIC and show elevations in AST, creatine phosphokinase, and bilirubin. Patients with fatal cases generally have more marked changes, even in the early days of illness, and also develop leukocytosis rather than leukopenia. In addition, thrombocytopenia is more marked and develops earlier in cases with a fatal outcome.

No controlled trials have been performed with IV ribavirin, but clinical experience and retrospective comparison of patients with ominous clinical laboratory values suggest that ribavirin is efficacious and should be given. No human or veterinary vaccines are recommended.

HF WITH RENAL SYNDROME

This disease, the first to be identified as an HF, is widely distributed over Europe and Asia; the major causative viruses and their rodent reservoirs on these two continents are Puumala virus (bank vole, *Clethrionomys glareolus*) and Hantaan virus (striped field mouse, *Apodemus agrarius*), respectively. Other potential causative viruses exist, including Dobrava virus (yellow-necked field mouse, *A. flavicollis*), which causes severe HF with renal syndrome in the Balkans. Seoul virus is associated with the Norway or sewer rat, *Rattus norvegicus*, and has a worldwide distribution through the migration of the rodent; it is associated with mild or moderate HF with renal syndrome in Asia, but in many areas of the world the human disease has been difficult to identify. Most cases occur in rural residents or vacationers; the exception is Seoul virus disease, which may be acquired in an urban or rural setting or from contaminated laboratory rat colonies. Classic Hantaan disease in Korea (Korean HF) and in rural China (epidemic HF) is most common in spring and fall and is related to rodent density and agricultural practices. Human infection is acquired primarily through aerosols of rodent urine, although virus is also present in saliva and feces. Patients with hantavirus diseases are not infectious. HF with renal syndrome is the most important form of HF today, with >100,000 cases of severe disease in Asia annually and milder Puumala infections numbering in the thousands as well.

Severe cases of HF with renal syndrome caused by Hantaan virus evolve in identifiable stages: the febrile stage with myalgia, lasting 3 or 4 days; the hypotensive stage, often associated with shock and lasting from a few hours to 48 h; the oliguric stage with renal failure, lasting 3–10 days; and the polyuric stage with diuresis and hyposthenuria.

The *febrile stage* is initiated by the abrupt onset of fever, headache, severe myalgia, thirst, anorexia, and often nausea and vomiting. Photophobia, retroorbital pain, and pain on ocular movement are common, and the vision may become blurred with ciliary body inflammation. Flushing over the face, the V area of the neck, and the back is characteristic, as are pharyngeal injection, periorbital edema, and conjunctival suffusion. Petechiae often develop in areas of pressure, the conjunctivae, and the axillae. Back pain and tenderness to percussion at the costovertebral angle reflect massive retroperitoneal edema. Laboratory evidence of mild to moderate DIC is present. Other laboratory findings include proteinuria and an active urinary sediment.

The *hypotensive stage* is ushered in by falling blood pressure and sometimes by shock. The relative bradycardia typical of the febrile phase is replaced by tachycardia. Kinin activation is marked. The rising hematocrit reflects increasing vascular leakage. Leukocytosis with a left shift develops, and thrombocytopenia continues. Atypical lymphocytes—which in fact are activated CD8+ (and, to a lesser extent, CD4+) T cells—circulate. Proteinuria is marked, and the urine's specific gravity falls to 1.010. The renal circulation is congested and compromised from local and systemic circulatory changes resulting in necrosis of tubules, particularly at the corticomedullary junction, and oliguria.

During the *oliguric stage*, hemorrhagic tendencies continue, probably in large part because of uremic bleeding defects. The oliguria persists for 3–10 days before the return of renal function marks the onset of the *polyuric stage*, which carries the danger of dehydration and electrolyte abnormalities.

Mild cases of HF with renal syndrome may be much less stereotypical. The presentation may include only fever, gastrointestinal abnormalities, and transient oliguria followed by hyposthenuria.

HF with renal syndrome should be suspected in patients with rural exposure in an endemic area. Prompt recognition of the disease permits rapid hospitalization and expectant management of shock and renal failure. Useful clinical laboratory parameters include leukocytosis, which may be leukemoid and is associated with a left shift; thrombocytopenia; and proteinuria. Mainstays of therapy are the management of shock, reliance on pressors, modest crystalloid infusion, IV use of human serum albumin, and treatment of renal failure with prompt dialysis for the usual indications. Hydration may result in pulmonary edema, and hypertension should be avoided because of the possibility of intracranial hemorrhage. Use of IV ribavirin has reduced mortality and morbidity in severe cases provided treatment is begun within the first 4 days of illness. The case-fatality ratio may be as high as 15% but with proper therapy should be <5%. Sequelae have not been definitively established, but there is a correlation in the United States between chronic hypertensive renal failure and the presence of antibodies to Seoul virus.

Infections with Puumala virus, the most common cause of HF with renal syndrome in Europe, result in a much attenuated picture but the same general presentation. The syndrome may be referred to by its former name, *nephropathia epidemica*. Bleeding manifestations are found in only 10% of cases, hypotension rather than shock is usually seen, and oliguria is present in only about half of patients. The dominant features may be fever, abdominal pain, proteinuria, mild oliguria, and sometimes blurred vision or glaucoma followed by polyuria and hyposthenuria in recovery. The mortality rate is <1%.

The diagnosis is readily made by IgM-capture ELISA, which should be positive at admission or within 24–48 h thereafter. The isolation of virus is difficult, but RT-PCR of a blood clot collected early in the clinical course or of tissues obtained postmortem will give positive results. Such testing is usually undertaken only if definitive identification of the infecting viral species is required or if molecular epidemiologic questions exist.

HANTAVIRUS PULMONARY SYNDROME

Hantavirus pulmonary syndrome was discovered in 1993, but retrospective identification of cases by immunohistochemistry (1978) and serology (1959) support the idea that it is a recently discovered rather than a truly new disease. The causative agents are hantaviruses of a distinct phylogenetic lineage that is associated with the rodent subfamily Sigmodontinae. Sin Nombre virus, which chronically infects the deer mouse (*Peromyscus maniculatus*), is the most important agent of hantavirus pulmonary syndrome in the United States. The disease is also caused by a Sin Nombre virus variant from the white-footed mouse (*P. leucopus*), by Black Creek Canal virus (*Sigmodon hispidus*, the cotton rat), and by Bayou virus (*Oryzomys palustris*, the rice rat). Several other related viruses cause the disease in South America, but Andes virus is unusual in that it, alone among hantaviruses, has been implicated in human-to-human transmission. The disease is linked to rodent exposure and particularly affects rural residents living in dwellings permeable to rodent entry or working at occupations that pose a risk of rodent exposure. Each rodent species has its own particular habits; in the case of the deer mouse, these behaviors include living in and around human habitation.

The disease begins with a prodrome of ~3–4 days (range, 1–11 days) comprising fever, myalgia, malaise, and often gastrointestinal disturbances such as nausea, vomiting, and abdominal pain. Dizziness is common and vertigo occasional. Severe prodromal symptoms bring some individuals to medical attention, but patients are usually recognized as the cardiopulmonary phase begins. Typically, there is slightly lowered blood pressure, tachycardia, tachypnea, mild hypoxemia, and early radiographic signs of pulmonary edema. Physical findings in the chest are often surprisingly scant. The conjunctival and cutaneous signs of vascular involvement seen in other types of HF are absent. During the next few hours, decompensation may progress rapidly to severe hypoxemia and respiratory failure. Most patients surviving the first 48 h of hospitalization are extubated and discharged within a few days, with no apparent residua.

Management during the first few hours after presentation is critical. The goal is to prevent severe hypoxemia by oxygen therapy, with intubation and intensive respiratory management if needed. During this period, hypotension and shock with increasing hematocrit invite aggressive fluid administration, but this intervention should be undertaken with great caution. Because of low cardiac output with myocardial depression and increased pulmonary vascular permeability, shock should be managed expectantly with pressors and modest infusion of fluid guided by the pulmonary capillary wedge pressure. Mild cases can be managed by frequent monitoring and oxygen administration without intubation. Many patients require intubation to manage hypoxemia and also develop shock. Mortality rates remain at ~30–40% even with good management. The antiviral drug ribavirin inhibits the virus in vitro but did not have a marked effect on patients treated in an open-label study.

During the prodrome, the differential diagnosis of hantavirus pulmonary syndrome is difficult, but by the time of presentation or within 24 h thereafter, a number of diagnostically helpful clinical features become apparent. Cough is not usually present at the outset but may develop later. Interstitial edema is evident on the chest x-ray. Later, bilateral alveolar edema with a central distribution develops in the setting of a normal-sized heart; occasionally, the edema is initially unilateral. Pleural effusions are often seen. Thrombocytopenia, circulating atypical lymphocytes, and a left shift (often with leukocytosis) are almost always evident; thrombocytopenia is a particularly important early clue. Hemoconcentration, proteinuria, and hypoalbuminemia should also be sought. Although thrombocytopenia virtually always develops and prolongation of the partial thromboplastin time is the rule, clinical evidence for coagulopathy or laboratory indications of DIC are found in only a minority of cases, usually in severely ill patients. Patients with severe illness also have acidosis and elevated serum levels of lactate. Mildly increased values in renal function tests are common, but patients with severe cases often have markedly elevated concentrations of serum creatinine; some of the viruses other than Sin Nombre virus have been associated with more kidney involvement, but few such cases have been studied. The differential diagnosis includes abdominal surgical conditions and pyelonephritis as well as rickettsial disease, sepsis, meningococcemia, plague, tularemia, influenza, and relapsing fever.

A specific diagnosis is best made by IgM testing of acute-phase serum, which has yielded positive results even in the prodrome. Tests using a Sin Nombre virus antigen detect the related hantaviruses causing the pulmonary syndrome in the Americas. Occasionally, heterologous viruses will react only in the IgG ELISA, but this finding is highly suspicious given the very low seroprevalence of these viruses in normal populations. RT-PCR is usually positive when used to test blood clots obtained in the first 7–9 days of illness as well as tissues; this test is useful in identifying the infecting virus in areas outside the home range of the deer mouse and in atypical cases.

YELLOW FEVER

Yellow fever virus caused major epidemics in the Americas, Africa, and Europe before the discovery of mosquito transmission in 1900 led to its control through attacks on its urban vector, *A. aegypti*. Only then was it found that a jungle cycle also existed in Africa, involving other *Aedes* mosquitoes and monkeys, and that colonization of the New World with *A. aegypti*, originally an African species, had established urban yellow fever as well as an independent sylvatic yellow fever cycle involving *Haemagogus* mosquitoes and New World monkeys in American jungles. Today, urban yellow fever transmission occurs only in some African cities, but the threat exists in the great cities of South America, where reinfestation by *A. aegypti* has taken place and dengue transmission by the same mosquito is common. As late as 1905, New Orleans suffered >3000 cases with 452 deaths from "yellow jack." Despite the existence of a highly effective and safe vaccine, several hundred jungle yellow fever cases occur annually in South America, and thousands of jungle and urban cases occur each year in Africa.

Yellow fever is a typical HF accompanied by prominent hepatic necrosis. A period of viremia, typically lasting 3 or 4 days, is followed by a period of "intoxication." During the latter phase in severe cases, the characteristic jaundice, hemorrhages, black vomit, anuria, and terminal delirium occur, perhaps related in part to extensive hepatic involvement. Blood leukocyte counts may be normal or reduced and are often high in terminal stages. Albuminuria is usually noted and may be marked; as renal function fails in terminal or severe cases, the level of blood urea nitrogen rises proportionately. Abnormalities detected in liver function tests range from modest elevations of AST levels in mild cases to severe derangement.

Urban yellow fever can be prevented by the control of *A. aegypti*. The continuing sylvatic cycle requires vaccination of all visitors to areas of potential transmission. With few exceptions, reactions to vaccine are minimal; immunity is provided within 10 days and lasts for at least 10 years. An egg allergy dictates caution in vaccine administration. Although there are no documented harmful effects of the vaccine on the fetus, pregnant women should be immunized only if they are definitely at risk of yellow fever exposure. Since vaccination has been associated with several cases of encephalitis in children <6 months of age, it should be delayed until after 12 months of age unless the risk of exposure is very high. Rare, serious, multisystemic adverse reactions (occasionally fatal) have been reported, particularly affecting the elderly; nevertheless, the number of deaths of unvaccinated travelers with yellow fever exceeds the number of deaths from vaccination, and a liberal vaccination policy for travelers to involved areas should be pursued. Timely information on changes in yellow fever distribution and yellow fever vaccine requirements can be obtained from Health Information for Travelers, Centers for Disease Control and Prevention, Atlanta, GA 30333; by fax request (404-332-4565; document number 220022); by phone (404-332-4559); or via the Internet (*www.cdc.gov*).

DENGUE HEMORRHAGIC FEVER/DENGUE SHOCK SYNDROME

A syndrome of HF noted in the 1950s among children in the Philippines and Southeast Asia was soon associated with dengue virus infections, particularly those occurring against a background of previous exposure to another dengue-virus serotype. The transient heterotypic protection after dengue virus infection is replaced within several weeks by the potential for heterotypic infection resulting in typical dengue fever (see above) or—uncommonly—in enhanced disease (secondary DHF/DSS). In rare instances, primary dengue infections lead to an HF syndrome, but much less is known about pathogenesis in this situation. In the past 20 years, *A. aegypti* has progressively reinvaded Latin America and other areas, and frequent travel by infected individuals has introduced multiple strains of dengue virus from many geographic areas. Thus the pattern of hyperendemic transmission of multiple dengue serotypes has now been established in the Americas and the Caribbean and has led to the emergence of DHF/DSS as a major problem there as well. Millions of dengue infections, including many thousands of cases of DHF/DSS, occur annually. The severe syndrome is unlikely to be seen in U.S. citizens since few children have the dengue antibodies that can trigger the pathogenetic cascade when a second infection is acquired.

Macrophage/monocyte infection is central to the pathogenesis of dengue fever and to the origin of DHF/DSS. Previous infection with a heterologous dengue-virus serotype may result in the production of nonprotective antiviral antibodies that nevertheless bind to the virion's surface and through interaction with the Fc receptor focus secondary dengue viruses on the target cell, the result being enhanced infection. The host is also primed for a secondary antibody response when viral antigens are released and immune complexes lead to activation of the classic complement pathway, with consequent phlogistic effects. Cross-reactivity at the T cell level results in the release of physiologically active cytokines, including interferon γ and tumor necrosis factor α. The induction of vascular permeability and shock depends on multiple factors, including the following:

1. *Presence of enhancing and nonneutralizing antibodies*—Transplacental maternal antibody may be present in infants <9 months old, or antibody elicited by previous heterologous dengue infection may be present in older individuals. T cell reactivity is also intimately involved.
2. *Age*—Susceptibility to DHF/DSS drops considerably after 12 years of age.
3. *Sex*—Females are more often affected than males.
4. *Race*—Caucasians are more often affected than blacks.
5. *Nutritional status*—Malnutrition is protective.
6. *Sequence of infection*—For example, serotype 1 followed by serotype 2 seems to be more dangerous than serotype 4 followed by serotype 2.
7. *Infecting serotype*—Type 2 is apparently more dangerous than other serotypes.

In addition, there is considerable variation among strains of a given serotype, with Southeast Asian serotype 2 strains having more potential to cause DHF/DSS than others.

Dengue HF is identified by the detection of bleeding tendencies (tourniquet test, petechiae) or overt bleeding in the absence of underlying causes such as preexisting gastrointestinal lesions. Dengue shock syndrome, usually accompanied by hemorrhagic signs, is much more serious and results from increased vascular permeability leading to shock. In mild DHF/DSS, restlessness, lethargy, thrombocytopenia (<100,000/μL), and hemoconcentration are detected 2–5 days after the onset of typical dengue fever, usually at the time of defervescence. The maculopapular rash that often develops in dengue fever may also appear in DHF/DSS. In more severe cases, frank shock is apparent, with low pulse pressure, cyanosis, hepatomegaly, pleural effusions, ascites, and in some cases severe ecchymoses and gastrointestinal bleeding. The period of shock lasts only 1 or 2 days, and most patients respond promptly to close monitoring, oxygen administration, and infusion of crystalloid or—in severe cases—colloid. The case-fatality rates reported vary greatly with case ascertainment and the quality of treatment; however, most DHF/DSS patients respond well to supportive therapy, and the overall mortality rate at an experienced center in the tropics is probably as low as 1%.

A virologic diagnosis can be made by the usual means, although multiple flavivirus infections lead to a broad immune response to several members of the group, and this situation may result in a lack of virus specificity of the IgM and IgG immune responses. A secondary antibody response can be sought with tests against several flavivirus antigens to demonstrate the characteristic wide spectrum of reactivity.

The key to control of both dengue fever and DHF/DSS is the control of *A. aegypti*, which also reduces the risk of urban yellow fever and chikungunya virus circulation. Control efforts have been handicapped by the presence of nondegradable tires and long-lived plastic containers in trash repositories, insecticide resistance, urban poverty, and an inability of the public health community to mobilize the populace to respond to the need to eliminate mosquito breeding sites. Live attenuated dengue vaccines are in the late stages of development and have produced promising results in early tests. Whether vaccines can provide safe, durable immunity to an immunopathologic disease such as DHF/DSS in endemic areas is an issue that will have to be tested, but it is hoped that vaccination will reduce transmission to negligible levels.

KYASANUR FOREST DISEASE AND OMSK HEMORRHAGIC FEVER

See Chap. 189 in *Harrison's Online* (*www.harrisonsonline.com*).

FILOVIRUS HEMORRHAGIC FEVER

See Chap. 190.

FURTHER READINGS

BRUNO P et al: The protean manifestations of hemorrhagic fever with renal syndrome. A retrospective review of 26 cases from Korea. Ann Intern Med 113:385, 1990

CALISHER CH: Medically important arboviruses of the United States and Canada. Clin Microbiol Rev 7:89, 1994

CENTERS FOR DISEASE CONTROL AND PREVENTION: Update: Management of patients with suspected viral hemorrhagic fever—United States. MMWR 44:475, 1995 (*http://www.cdc.gov/mmwr/preview/mmwrhtml/00038033.htm*)

DERESIEWICZ RL et al: Clinical and neuroradiographic manifestations of eastern equine encephalitis. N Engl J Med 336:1867, 1997

ENRIA D et al: Arenaviruses, in *Tropical Infectious Diseases: Principles, Pathogens, & Practice*, RL Guerrant et al (eds). New York, Saunders, 1999, pp 1189–1212

PETERS CJ, KHAN AS: Hantavirus pulmonary syndrome: The new American hemorrhagic fever. Clin Infect Dis 34:1224, 2002

RIVAS F et al: Epidemic Venezuelan equine encephalitis in La Guajira, Colombia, 1995. J Infect Dis 175:828, 1997

SOLOMON SR, VAUGHN DW: Pathogenesis and clinical features of Japanese encephalitis and West Nile virus infections. Curr Top Microbiol Immunol 267:171, 2002

SOLOMON T et al: West Nile encephalitis. BMJ 326:865, 2003

WURTZ R, PALEOLOGOS N: La Crosse encephalitis presenting like herpes simplex encephalitis in an immunocompromised adult. Clin Infect Dis 31:1113, 2000

190 Ebola and Marburg Viruses

Clarence J. Peters

DEFINITION

Both Marburg virus and Ebola virus cause an acute febrile illness associated with high mortality. This illness is characterized by multisystem involvement that begins with the abrupt onset of headache, myalgias, and fever and proceeds to prostration, rash, and shock and often to bleeding manifestations. Epidemics usually begin with a single case acquired from an unknown reservoir in nature and spread mainly through close contact with sick persons or their body fluids, either at home or in the hospital.

ETIOLOGY

The family Filoviridae (Fig. 190-1) comprises two antigenically and genetically distinct genera: *Marburgvirus* and *Ebolavirus*. *Ebolavirus* has four readily distinguishable species named for their original sites of recognition: Zaire, Sudan, Côte d'Ivoire, and Reston. Except for the Reston virus, all the Filoviridae are African viruses that cause severe and often fatal disease in humans. The Reston virus, which has been exported from the Philippines on several occasions, has caused fatal infections in monkeys but only subclinical infections in humans. Different strains of the four Ebola species, isolated over time and space, exhibit remarkable sequence conservation, indicating marked genetic stability in their selective niche.

Typical filovirus particles contain a single linear, negative-sense, single-stranded RNA arranged in a helical nucleocapsid. The virions are 790–970 nm in length; they may also appear in elongated, contorted forms. The lipid envelope confers sensitivity to lipid solvents and common detergents. The viruses are largely destroyed by heat (60°C, 30 min) and by acidity but may persist for weeks in blood at room temperature. The surface glycoprotein self-associates to form the virion surface spikes, which presumably mediate attachment to cells and fusion. The glycoprotein's high sugar content may contribute to its low capacity to elicit neutralizing antibodies. A smaller form of the glycoprotein, bearing many of its antigenic determinants, is produced by in vitro–infected cells and is found in the circulation in human disease; it has been speculated that this circulating soluble protein may suppress the immune response to the virion surface protein or block antiviral effector mechanisms. Both Marburg virus and Ebola virus are biosafety level 4 pathogens because of their high associated mortality rate and aerosol infectivity.

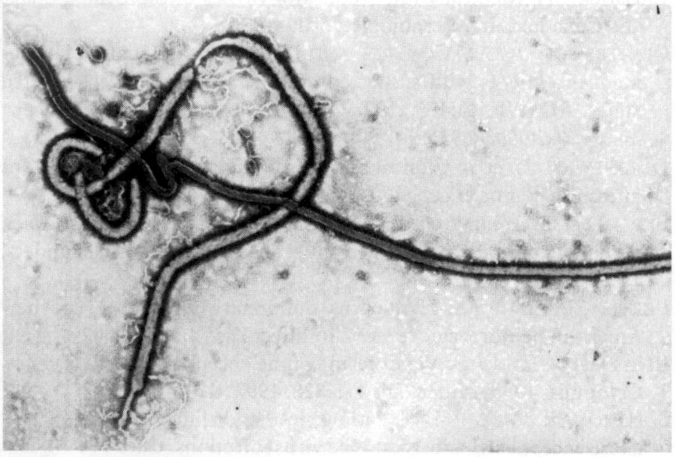

FIGURE 190-1 Ebola virions: diagnostic specimen from the first passage in Vero cells of a blood sample from a patient. Some of the filamentous (negatively stained) virions were fused together, end-to-end, giving the appearance of a "bowl of spaghetti." This image was from the first isolation and visualization of Ebola virus in 1970. *(Courtesy of Fredrick A. Murphy, MD, University of Texas Medical Branch, Galveston, Texas; with permission.)*

EPIDEMIOLOGY

Marburg virus was first identified in Germany in 1967, when infected African green monkeys (*Cercopithecus aethiops*) imported from Uganda transmitted the agent to workers in a vaccine laboratory. Of the 25 human cases acquired from monkeys, seven ended in death. The six secondary cases were associated with close contact or parenteral exposure. Secondary spread to the wife of one patient was documented, and virus was isolated from the husband's semen despite the presence of circulating antibodies. Subsequently, isolated cases of Marburg virus infection have been reported from eastern and southern Africa, with limited spread.

In 1999, repeated transmission of Marburg virus to workers in a gold mine in eastern Democratic Republic of the Congo was documented. The secondary spread of the virus among patients' families was more extensive than previously noted, resembling that of Ebola virus and emphasizing the importance of hygiene and proper barrier nursing in the epidemiology of these viruses in Africa.

In 2004–2005, an alarming, massive Marburg virus epidemic, with >250 cases, occurred in Angola. The epidemiologic features resembled those of the Ebola virus epidemics described below, and the case-fatality rate was 90%. This high figure may have been due in part to poor conditions in African hospitals; however, the virus isolated in this epidemic was slightly different phylogenetically from other known strains and exhibited increased virulence in nonhuman primates.

In 1976, epidemics of severe hemorrhagic fever (550 human cases) occurred simultaneously in Zaire and Sudan, and Ebola virus was found to be the etiologic agent. Later, it was shown that different species of virus (with associated mortality rates of 90% and 50%, respectively) had caused the two epidemics. Both epidemics were associated with interhuman spread (particularly in the hospital setting) and the use of unsterilized needles and syringes—a common practice in developing-country hospitals. The epidemics dwindled as the clinics were closed and as people in the endemic area increasingly shunned affected persons and avoided traditional burial practices.

The Zaire Ebola virus recurred in a major epidemic (317 cases, 88% mortality rate) in the Democratic Republic of the Congo in 1995 and in smaller epidemics in Gabon in 1994–1996. Mortality rates were high, transmission to caregivers and others who had direct contact with body fluids was common, and poor hygiene in hospitals exacerbated spread. In the Congo epidemic, an index case was infected in Kikwit in January 1995. The epidemic smoldered until April, when intense nosocomial transmission forced closure of the hospitals; samples were finally sent to the laboratory for Ebola testing, which yielded positive results within a few hours. International assistance, with barrier nursing instruction and materials, was provided; nosocomial transmission ceased, hospitals reopened, and patients were segregated to prevent intrafamilial spread. The last case was reported in June 1995.

Separate emergences of Ebola virus (Zaire) were detected in Gabon in 1994–2003, usually in association with deep-forest exposure and subsequent familial and nosocomial transmission. Die-offs of nonhuman primates were sometimes documented, and Ebola infection was confirmed in at least some animals. In a 1996 episode, a physician exposed to Ebola-infected patients traveled to South Africa with a fever; a nurse who assisted in a cutdown on the physician developed Ebola hemorrhagic fever and died despite intensive care. The index patient was identified retrospectively on the basis of serum antibodies and virus isolation from semen. No additional cases were detected from care of the primary or secondary case, nor were there any secondary cases following care of an unsuspected Côte d'Ivoire Ebola case in Switzerland. Thus, distant transport of Ebola virus is an established risk, but limited nosocomial spread occurs under proper hygienic conditions.

In 2000–2001, an indolent outbreak of Sudan Ebola virus claimed the lives of 224 (53%) of 425 patients with presumptive cases in Uganda.

Reston Ebola virus was first seen in the United States in 1989, when it caused a fatal, highly transmissible disease among cynomolgus macaques imported from the Philippines and quarantined in Reston, Virginia, pending distribution to biomedical researchers. This and other appearances of the Reston virus have been traced to a single export facility in the Philippines, but no source in nature has been established.

Epidemiologic studies (including a specific search in the Kikwit epidemic) have failed to yield evidence for an important role of airborne particles in human disease. This lack of epidemiologic evidence is surprising and seems to conflict with the viruses' classification as biosafety level 4 pathogens (which is based in part on their aerosol infectivity) and with formal laboratory assessments showing a high degree of aerosol infectivity for monkeys. Sick humans apparently do not usually generate sufficient amounts of infectious aerosols to pose a significant hazard to those around them.

Although numerous die-offs have recently been reported among chimpanzees and gorillas (some even threatening the viability of these endangered species), these animals (like humans) appear to be sentinels for virus activity. Speculation about the true reservoirs has centered on bats, and preliminary evidence indicates that bats may indeed be the reservoirs of filoviruses. This evidence includes the detection of antibodies and reverse-transcriptase polymerase chain reaction (RT-PCR) products in bats, the epidemiologic findings in subterranean gold mines in Durba (Democratic Republic of the Congo) where Marburg transmission has occurred, and reported associations of human antibody production with the handling of bats.

PATHOLOGY AND PATHOGENESIS

In humans and in animal models, Ebola and Marburg viruses replicate well in virtually all cell types, including endothelial cells, macrophages, and parenchymal cells of multiple organs. The earliest involvement—that of the mononuclear phagocyte system—is responsible for initiation of the disease process. Viral replication is associated with cellular necrosis both in vivo and in vitro. Significant findings at the light-microscopic level include liver necrosis with Councilman bodies, intracellular inclusions that correlate with extensive collections of viral nucleocapsids, interstitial pneumonitis, cerebral glial nodules, and small infarcts. Antigen and virions are abundant in fibroblasts, interstitium, and (to a lesser extent) the appendages of the subcutaneous tissues in fatal cases; escape through small breaks in the skin or possibly through sweat glands may occur and, if so, may be correlated with the established epidemiologic risk of close contact with patients and the touching of the deceased. Inflammatory cells are not prominent, even in necrotic areas.

In addition to sustaining direct damage from viral infection, patients infected with Ebola virus (Zaire) have high circulating levels of proinflammatory cytokines, which presumably contribute to the severity of the illness. In fact, the virus interacts intimately with the cellular cytokine system. It is resistant to the antiviral effects of interferon α, although this mediator is amply induced. Viral infection of endothelial cells selectively inhibits the expression of major histocompatibility complex class I molecules and blocks the induction of several genes by the interferons. In addition, glycoprotein expression inhibits αV integrin expression, an effect that has been shown to lead to detachment and subsequent death of endothelial cells in vitro.

Acute infection is associated with high levels of circulating virus and viral antigen. Clinical improvement takes place when viral titers decrease concomitantly with the onset of a virus-specific immune response, as detected by enzyme-linked immunosorbent assay (ELISA) or fluorescent antibody testing. In fatal cases, there is usually little evidence of an antibody response, and there is extensive depletion of spleen and lymph nodes. Recovery is apparently mediated by the cellular immune response: convalescent-phase plasma has little in vitro virus-neutralizing capacity and is not protective in passive transfer experiments in monkey and guinea pig models.

CLINICAL MANIFESTATIONS

After an incubation period of ~7–10 days (range, 3–16 days), the patient abruptly develops fever, severe headache, malaise, myalgia, nausea, and vomiting. Continued fever is joined by diarrhea (often severe), chest pain (accompanied by cough), prostration, and depressed mentation. In light-skinned patients (and less often in dark-skinned individuals), a maculopapular rash appears around day 5–7 and is followed by desquamation. Bleeding may begin about this time and is apparent from any mucosal site and into the skin. In some epidemics, fewer than half of patients have had overt bleeding, and this manifestation has been absent even in some fatal cases. Additional findings include edema of the face, neck, and/or scrotum; hepatomegaly; flushing; conjunctival injection; and pharyngitis. Around 10–12 days after the onset of disease, the sustained fever may break, with improvement and eventual recovery of the patient. Recrudescence of fever may be associated with secondary bacterial infections or possibly with localized virus persistence. Late hepatitis, uveitis, and orchitis have been reported, with isolation of virus from semen or detection of PCR products in vaginal secretions for several weeks.

LABORATORY FINDINGS

Leukopenia is common early on; neutrophilia has its onset later. Platelet counts fall below (sometimes much below) 50,000/μL. Laboratory evidence of disseminated intravascular coagulation is found, but its clinical significance and the need for therapy are controversial. Serum levels of alanine and aspartate aminotransferases (particularly the latter) rise progressively, and jaundice develops in some cases. The serum amylase level may be elevated, and this elevation may be associated with abdominal pain, suggesting pancreatitis. Proteinuria is usual; decreased kidney function is proportional to shock.

DIAGNOSIS

Most patients acutely ill as a result of infection with Ebola or Marburg virus have high concentrations of virus in blood. Antigen-detection ELISA is a sensitive, robust diagnostic modality. Virus isolation and RT-PCR are also effective and provide additional sensitivity in some cases. Patients who are recovering develop IgM and IgG antibodies that are best detected by ELISA but are also reactive in the less specific fluorescent antibody test. Skin biopsies are an extremely useful adjunct in postmortem diagnosis of infection with Ebola virus (and, to a lesser extent, Marburg virus) because of the presence of large amounts of viral antigen, the relatively low risk posed by sample collection, and the lack of cold-chain requirements for formalin-fixed tissues.

℞ EBOLA AND MARBURG VIRUS INFECTIONS

No virus-specific therapy is available, and—given the extensive viral involvement in fatal cases—supportive treatment may not be as useful as was once hoped. However, recent studies in rhesus monkeys have shown improved survival among animals treated with an inhibitor of factor VIIa/tissue factor or with activated protein C. Vigorous treatment of shock should take into account the likelihood of vascular leak in the pulmonary and systemic circulation and of myocardial functional compromise. The membrane fusion mechanism of Ebola virus resembles that of retroviruses, and the identification of "fusogenic" sequences suggests that inhibitors of cell entry may be developed. Despite the poor neutralizing capacity of polyclonal convalescent-phase sera, phage display of immunoglobulin mRNA from convalescent-phase bone marrow has yielded monoclonal antibodies that have in vitro neutralizing capacity and mediate protection in guinea pig models (but, unfortunately, not in monkey models).

PREVENTION

No vaccine or antiviral drug is currently available, but barrier nursing precautions in African hospitals can greatly decrease the spread of the virus beyond the index case and thus prevent epidemics of infection with filoviruses and with other agents as well. An adenovirus-vectored Ebola glycoprotein gene has proved protective in nonhuman primates and is undergoing phase 1 trials in humans.

FURTHER READINGS

FELDMANN H et al: Proceedings of an international symposium on filoviruses. J Infect Dis Suppl, 2007

GEISBERT TW et al: Treatment of Ebola virus infection with a recombinant inhibitor of factor VIIa/tissue factor: A study in rhesus monkeys. Lancet 362:1953, 2003

PETERS CJ, LEDUC JW: An introduction to Ebola: The virus and the disease. J Infect Dis 179(Suppl 1):ix, 1999 (Also available at *www.journals.uchicago.edu/JID/*)

SANCHEZ A et al: Analysis of human peripheral blood samples from fatal and nonfatal cases of Ebola (Sudan) hemorrhagic fever: Cellular responses, virus load, and nitric oxide levels. J Virol 78:10370, 2004

SULLIVAN NT: Accelerated vaccination for Ebola virus haemorrhagic fever in non-human primates. Nature 424:681, 2003

TOWNER JS et al: *Marburgvirus* genomics and association with a large hemorrhagic fever outbreak in Angola. J Virol 80:6497, 2006

SECTION 16 FUNGAL AND ALGAL INFECTIONS

191 Diagnosis and Treatment of Fungal Infections

John E. Edwards, Jr.

TERMINOLOGY AND MICROBIOLOGY

Traditionally, fungal infections have been classified into specific categories based on both anatomic location and epidemiology. The most common general anatomic categories are mucocutaneous and deep organ infection; the most common general epidemiologic categories are endemic and opportunistic. Although *mucocutaneous infections* can cause serious morbidity, they are rarely fatal. *Deep organ infections* also cause severe illness in many cases but, in contrast to mucocutaneous infections, are often fatal. The *endemic mycoses* (e.g., coccidioidomycosis) are infections caused by fungal organisms that are not part of the normal human microbial flora and are acquired from environmental sources. In contrast, *opportunistic mycoses* are caused by organisms (e.g., *Candida* and *Aspergillus*) that frequently are components of the normal human flora and whose ubiquity in nature renders them easily acquired by the immunocompromised host. Opportunistic fungi cause serious infections when the immunologic response of the host becomes ineffective, allowing the organisms to transition from harmless commensals to invasive pathogens. Frequently, the diminished effectiveness of the immune system is a result of advanced modern therapies that coincidentally either unbalance the host's microflora or directly interfere with immunologic responses. Endemic mycoses cause more severe illness in immunocompromised patients than in immunocompetent individuals.

Patients acquire infection with endemic fungi almost exclusively by inhalation. The soil is the natural reservoir for the vast majority of endemic mycoses. The dermatophytic fungi may be acquired by human-to-human transmission, but the majority of infections result from environmental contact. In contrast, the opportunistic fungus *Candida* invades the host from normal sites of colonization, usually the mucous membranes of the gastrointestinal tract. In general, innate immunity is the primary defense mechanism against fungi. Although antibodies are formed during many fungal infections (and even during commensalism), they generally do not constitute the primary mode of defense. Nevertheless, in selected infections, as discussed below, measurement of antibody titers may be a useful diagnostic test.

Three other terms frequently used in clinical discussions of fungal infections are *yeast, mold*, and *dimorphic fungus. Yeasts* are seen as rounded single cells or as budding organisms. *Candida* and *Cryptococcus* are traditionally classified as yeasts. Molds grow as filamentous forms called *hyphae* both at room temperature and when they invade tissue. *Aspergillus, Rhizopus* [the species that causes mucormycosis (zygomycosis)], and fungi commonly infecting the skin to cause ringworm and related cutaneous conditions are classified as molds. Variations occur within this classification of yeasts and molds. For instance, when *Candida* infects tissue, both yeasts and filamentous forms may occur (except with *C. glabrata*, which forms only yeasts in tissue); in contrast, *Cryptococcus* exists only in yeast form. *Dimorphic* is the term used to describe fungi that grow as yeasts or large spherical structures in tissue but as filamentous forms at room temperature in the environment. Classified in this group are the organisms causing blastomycosis, paracoccidioidomycosis, coccidioidomycosis, histoplasmosis, blastomycosis, and sporotrichosis.

The incidence of fungal infections has risen substantially over the past several decades. Opportunistic infections have increased in frequency as a consequence of intentional immunosuppression in organ and stem cell transplantation and many other diseases, the administration of cytotoxic chemotherapy for cancers, and the liberal use of antibacterial agents. The incidence of endemic mycoses has increased in geographic locations where there has been substantial population growth.

DIAGNOSIS

The definitive diagnosis of any fungal infection requires histopathologic identification of the fungus invading tissue, accompanied by evidence of an inflammatory response. The identification of an inflammatory response has been especially important with regard to *Aspergillus* infection. *Aspergillus* is ubiquitous and can float from the air onto biopsy material. Therefore, in rare but important instances, this fungus is an ex vivo contaminant during processing of a specimen for microscopy, with a consequent incorrect diagnosis. The stains most commonly used to identify fungi are periodic acid–Schiff and Gomori methenamine silver. *Candida*, unlike other fungi, is visible on gram-stained tissue smears. Hematoxylin and eosin stain is not sufficient to identify *Candida* in tissue specimens. When positive, an India ink preparation of cerebrospinal fluid (CSF) is diagnostic for cryptococcosis. Most laboratories now use calcofluor white staining coupled with fluorescent microscopy to identify fungi in fluid specimens.

Extensive investigations of the diagnosis of deep organ fungal infections have yielded a variety of tests with different degrees of specificity and sensitivity. The most reliable tests are the detection of antibody to *Coccidioides immitis* and *Histoplasma capsulatum* in serum and CSF, the detection of cryptococcal polysaccharide antigen in serum and CSF, and the detection of *Histoplasma* antigen in urine or serum. The test for galactomannan has been used extensively in Europe and is now approved in the United States for diagnosis of aspergillosis. This test requires additional validation before its true usefulness can be determined. Sources of concern are the incidence of false-negative results and the need for multiple serial tests to reduce this incidence. The β-glucan test for *Candida* is also under evaluation but, like the galactomannan test, requires additional validation. Numerous polymerase chain reaction assays to detect antigens are in the developmental stages, as are nucleic acid hybridization techniques; however, these methods are not currently used on a widespread basis in major medical centers.

Of the fungal organisms, *Candida* is by far most frequently recovered from blood. Although *Candida* species can be detected with any of the automated blood culture systems widely used at present, the lysis-centrifugation technique increases the sensitivity of blood cultures for less common organisms (e.g., *H. capsulatum*) and should be used when disseminated fungal infection is suspected.

Except in the cases of coccidioidomycosis, cryptococcosis, and histoplasmosis, there are no fully validated and widely used tests for serodiagnosis of disseminated fungal infection. Skin tests for the endemic mycoses are no longer available.

PART 7 Infectious Diseases

℞ FUNGAL INFECTIONS

This discussion is intended as a brief overview of general strategies for the use of antifungal agents in the treatment of fungal infections. Details on regimens, schedules, and strategies are discussed in the chapters on specific mycoses that follow in this section.

Since fungal organisms are eukaryotic cells that contain most of the same organelles (with many of the same physiologic functions) as human cells, the identification of drugs that selectively kill or inhibit fungi but are not toxic to human cells has been highly problematic. Far fewer antifungal than antibacterial agents have been introduced into clinical medicine.

AMPHOTERICIN B (AmB) The introduction of AmB in the late 1950s revolutionized the treatment of fungal infections in deep organs. Before AmB became available, cryptococcal meningitis and other disseminated fungal infections were nearly always fatal. For nearly a decade after AmB was introduced, it was the only effective agent for the treatment of life-threatening fungal infections. AmB remains the broadest-spectrum antifungal agent but carries several disadvantages, including significant nephrotoxicity, lack of an oral preparation, and unpleasant side effects (fever, chills, and nausea) during treatment. To circumvent nephrotoxicity and infusion side effects, lipid formulations of AmB were developed and have virtually replaced the original colloidal deoxycholate formulation in clinical use (although the older formulation is still available). The lipid formulations include liposomal AmB (L-AB; 435 mg/kg per day) and AmB lipid complex (ABLC; 5 mg/kg per day). A third preparation, AmB colloidal dispersion (ABCD; 3–4 mg/kg per day), is rarely used because of the high incidence of side effects associated with infusion. (The doses listed are standard doses for adults with invasive infection.)

The lipid formulations of AmB have the disadvantage of being considerably more expensive than the deoxycholate formulation. Experience is still accumulating on the comparative efficacy, toxicity, and advantages of the different formulations for specific clinical fungal infections [e.g., central nervous system (CNS) infection]. Whether there is a clinically significant difference in these drugs with respect to CNS penetration or nephrotoxicity remains controversial. Despite these issues and despite the expense, the lipid formulations are now much more commonly used than AmB deoxycholate in the United States.

AZOLES This class of antifungal drugs offers important advantages over AmB: the azoles cause little or no nephrotoxicity and are available in oral preparations. Early azoles included ketoconazole and miconazole, which have been replaced by newer agents for the treatment of deep organ fungal infections. The azoles' mechanism of action is inhibition of ergosterol synthesis in the fungal cell wall. Unlike AmB, these drugs are considered fungistatic, not -cidal.

Fluconazole Since its introduction, fluconazole has played an extremely important role in the treatment of a wide variety of serious fungal infections. Its major advantages are the availability of both oral and IV formulations, a long half-life, satisfactory penetration of most body fluids (including ocular fluid and CSF), and minimal toxicity (especially relative to AmB). Its disadvantages include (usually reversible) hepatotoxicity and—at high doses—alopecia, muscle weakness, and dry mouth with a metallic taste. Fluconazole is not effective for the treatment of aspergillosis, mucormycosis, or *Scedosporium apiospermum* infections. It is less effective than the newer azoles against *C. glabrata* and *C. krusei*.

Fluconazole has become the agent of choice for the treatment of coccidioidal meningitis, although relapses have followed therapy with this drug. In addition, fluconazole is useful for both consolidation and maintenance therapy for cryptococcal meningitis. This agent has been shown to be as efficacious as AmB in the treatment of candidemia. The effectiveness of fluconazole in candidemia and the drug's relatively minimal toxicity, in conjunction with the inadequacy of diagnostic tests for widespread hematogenously disseminated candidiasis, have led to a change in the paradigm for candidemia management. The standard of care is now to treat all candidemic patients with an antifungal agent and to change all their intravascular lines, if feasible, rather than merely to remove a singular suspect intravascular line and then observe the patient. The usual fluconazole regimen for treatment of candidemia is 400 mg/d given until 2 weeks after the last positive blood culture.

Fluconazole is considered effective as fungal prophylaxis in bone marrow transplant recipients and high-risk liver transplant patients. Its use for prophylaxis in patients with leukemia, in AIDS patients with low CD4+ T cell counts, and in patients on surgical intensive care units remains controversial.

Voriconazole Like fluconazole, voriconazole is available in both oral and IV formulations. Voriconazole has a broader spectrum than fluconazole against *Candida* species (including *C. glabrata* and *C. krusei*) and is active against *Aspergillus*, *Scedosporium*, and *Fusarium*. It is generally considered the first-line drug of choice for treatment of aspergillosis. A few case reports have shown voriconazole to be effective in individual patients with coccidioidomycosis, blastomycosis, and histoplasmosis, but (because of limited data) this agent is not recommended for treatment of the endemic mycoses. Among the disadvantages of voriconazole (compared with fluconazole) are its more numerous interactions with many of the drugs used in patients predisposed to fungal infections. Hepatotoxicity, skin rashes (including photosensitivity), and visual disturbances are relatively common. Voriconazole is also considerably more expensive than fluconazole. Moreover, it is advisable to monitor voriconazole levels in certain patients since (1) this drug is completely metabolized in the liver by CYP2C9, CYP3A4, and CYP2C19; and (2) human genetic variability in CYP2C19 activity exists. Dosages should be reduced accordingly in those patients with liver failure. Dose adjustments for renal insufficiency are not necessary; however, because the IV formulation is prepared in cyclodextrin, it should not be given to patients with severe renal insufficiency.

Itraconazole Itraconazole is available in IV and oral (capsule and suspension) formulations. Varying blood levels among patients taking oral itraconazole reflect a disadvantage compared with the other azoles. Itraconazole is the drug of choice for mild to moderate histoplasmosis and blastomycosis and has often been used for chronic mucocutaneous candidiasis. It has been approved by the U.S. Food and Drug Administration (FDA) for use in febrile neutropenic patients. Itraconazole has also proven useful for the treatment of chronic coccidioidomycosis, sporotrichosis, and *S. apiospermum* infection. The mucocutaneous and cutaneous fungal infections that have been treated successfully with itraconazole include oropharyngeal candidiasis (especially in AIDS patients), tinea versicolor, tinea capitis, and onychomycosis. Disadvantages of itraconazole include its poor penetration into the CSF, the use of cyclodextrin in both the oral suspension and the IV preparation, the variable absorption of the capsules, and the need for monitoring of blood levels in patients taking capsules for disseminated mycoses. In recent years, reported cases of severe congestive heart failure in patients taking itraconazole have been a source of concern. Like the other azoles, itraconazole can cause hepatic toxicity.

Posaconazole Posaconazole is approved by the FDA for prophylaxis of aspergillosis and candidiasis in patients at high risk for developing these infections because of severe immunocompromise. This drug has also been evaluated for the treatment of zygomycosis, fusariosis, aspergillosis, and oropharyngeal candidiasis. The relevant studies of posaconazole in zygomycosis, fusariosis, and aspergillosis have examined salvage therapy. A study of >90 patients whose zygomycosis was refractory to other therapy yielded encouraging results. No trials of posaconazole for the treatment of candidemia have yet been reported. Case reports have described the drug's efficacy in coccidioidomycosis and histoplasmosis. Controlled trials have shown its effectiveness as a prophylactic agent in patients with acute leukemia and in bone marrow transplant recipients. In addition, posaconazole has been found to be effective against fluconazole-resistant *Candida* species. The results of a large-scale study of the use of posaconazole as salvage therapy for aspergillosis have been promising but, as of this writing, have not been published in a peer-reviewed format.

ECHINOCANDINS The echinocandins, including the approved drugs caspofungin, anidulafungin, and micafungin, have added considerably to the antifungal armamentarium. All three of these agents inhibit β-1,3-glucan synthase, which is necessary for cell wall synthesis in fungi and is not a component of human cells. None of these agents is available in an oral formulation. The echinocandins are considered fungicidal for *Candida* and fungistatic for *Aspergillus*. Their greatest use to date is against candidal infections. They offer two advantages: broad-spectrum activity against all *Candida* species and relatively low toxicity. The minimum inhibitory concentrations (MICs) of all the echinocandins are highest against *C. parapsilosis*; it is not clear whether these higher MIC values represent less clinical effectiveness against this species. The echinocandins are among the safest antifungal agents.

In controlled trials, *caspofungin* has been at least as efficacious as AmB for the treatment of candidemia and invasive candidiasis and as efficacious as fluconazole for the treatment of candidal esophagitis. In addition, caspofungin has been efficacious as salvage therapy for aspergillosis. At present, it is used most extensively for the treatment of candidemic patients, especially before the infecting species is precisely identified.

Anidulafungin has been approved by the FDA as therapy for candidemia in nonneutropenic patients and for *Candida* esophagitis, intraabdominal infection, and peritonitis. In controlled trials, anidulafungin has been more efficacious than fluconazole against candidemia and invasive candidiasis and as efficacious as fluconazole against candidal esophagitis. When anidulafungin is used with cyclosporine, tacrolimus, or voriconazole, no dosage adjustment is required for either drug in the combination.

Micafungin has been approved for the treatment of esophageal candidiasis and for prophylaxis in patients receiving stem cell transplants. Studies thus far have shown that coadministration of micafungin and cyclosporine does not require dose adjustments for either drug. When micafungin is given with sirolimus, the AUC rises for sirolimus, usually necessitating a reduction in its dose. In open-label trials, favorable results have been obtained with micafungin for the treatment of deep-seated *Aspergillus* and *Candida* infections.

FLUCYTOSINE (5-FLUOROCYTOSINE) The use of flucytosine has diminished in recent years as newer antifungal drugs have been developed. Flucytosine has a unique mechanism of action based on intrafungal conversion to 5-fluorouracil, which is toxic to the cell. Development of resistance to the compound has limited its use as a single agent. Flucytosine is nearly always used in combination with AmB. Its good penetration into the CSF makes it attractive for use with AmB for treatment of cryptococcal meningitis. Flucytosine has also been recommended for the treatment of candidal meningitis in combination with AmB; comparative trials with AmB alone have not been done. Significant and frequent bone marrow depression is seen with flucytosine when this drug is used with AmB.

GRISEOFULVIN AND TERBINAFINE Historically, griseofulvin has been useful primarily for ringworm infection. This agent is usually given for relatively long periods. Terbinafine has been used primarily for onychomycosis but also for ringworm. In comparative studies, terbinafine has been as effective as itraconazole and more effective than griseofulvin for both conditions.

TOPICAL ANTIFUNGAL AGENTS A detailed discussion of the agents used for the treatment of cutaneous fungal infections and onychomycosis is beyond the scope of this chapter; the reader is referred to the dermatology literature. Many classes of compounds have been used to treat the common fungal infections of the skin. Among the azoles used are clotrimazole, econazole, miconazole, oxiconazole, sulconazole, ketoconazole, tioconazole, butaconazole, and terconazole. In general, topical treatment of vaginal candidiasis has been successful. Since there is considered to be little difference in the efficacy of the various vaginal preparations, the choice of agent is made by the physician and/or the patient on the basis of preference and availability. Fluconazole given orally at 150 mg has the advantage of not requiring repeated intravaginal application. Nystatin is a polyene that has been used for both oropharyngeal thrush and vaginal candidiasis. Useful agents in other classes include ciclopirox olamine, halprogin, terbinafine, naftifine, tolnaftate, and undecylenic acid.

FURTHER READINGS

BATTI Z et al: Review of epidemiology, diagnosis, and treatment of invasive mould infections in allogeneic hematopoietic stem cell transplant recipients. Mycopathologia 162:1, 2006

CHU JH et al: Hospitalizations for endemic mycoses: A population-based national study. Clin Infect Dis 42:822, 2006

DEPAUW BE: Increasing fungal infections in the intensive care unit. Surg Infect (Larchmt) 7(Suppl 2):S93, 2006

DISMUKES WE: Antifungal therapy: Lessons learned over the past 27 years. Clin Infect Dis 42:1289, 2006

ENOCH DA et al: Invasive fungal infections: A review of epidemiology and management options. J Med Microbiol 55:809, 2006

KAUFFMAN CA: Clinical efficacy of new antifungal agents. Curr Opin Microbiol 9:1, 2006

LIPSETT PA: Surgical critical care: Fungal infections in surgical patients. Crit Care Med 34(9 Suppl):S215, 2006

MANDELL GL et al (eds): Mycoses, in *Principles and Practice of Infectious Diseases*, 6th ed. Elsevier Churchill Livingstone, Philadelphia, 2005, pp 2935–3094

WHEAT LJ: Antigen detection, serology, and molecular diagnosis of invasive mycoses in the immunocompromised host. Transpl Infect Dis 8:128, 2006

192 Histoplasmosis

Chadi A. Hage, L. Joseph Wheat

ETIOLOGY

Histoplasma capsulatum, a thermal dimorphic fungus, is the etiologic agent of histoplasmosis. In most endemic areas, *H. capsulatum* var. *capsulatum* is the causative agent; in Africa, *H. capsulatum* var. *duboisii* is also found. Mycelia—the naturally infectious form of *Histoplasma*—have a characteristic appearance, with microconidial and macroconidial forms. Microconidia are oval and are small enough (2–5 μm) to reach the terminal bronchioles and alveoli. Shortly after infecting the host, mycelia transform into the yeasts that are found inside macrophages and other phagocytes. The yeast forms are characteristically small (2–5 μm), with occasional narrow budding. In the laboratory, mycelia are best grown at room temperature, whereas yeasts are grown at 37°C on enriched media.

EPIDEMIOLOGY

Histoplasmosis is the most prevalent endemic mycosis in North America. Although this fungal disease has been reported throughout the world, its endemicity is particularly notable in certain parts of North, Central, and South America; Africa; and Asia. In the United States, the endemic areas spread over the Ohio and Mississippi river valleys. This pattern is related to the humid and acidic nature of the soil in these areas. Soil enriched with bird or bat droppings promotes the growth and sporulation of *Histoplasma*. Disruption of soil containing the organism leads to aerosolization of the microconidia and exposure of humans nearby. Activities associated with high-level exposure include spelunking, excavation, cleaning of chicken coops, demolition and remodeling of old buildings, and cutting of dead trees. Most cases seen outside of highly endemic areas represent imported disease—e.g., cases reported in Europe after travel to the Americas, Africa, or Asia.

PATHOGENESIS AND PATHOLOGY

Infection follows inhalation of microconidia (Fig. 192-1). Once they reach the alveolar spaces, microconidia are rapidly recognized and engulfed by alveolar macrophages. At this point, the microconidia transform into budding yeasts (Fig. 192-2), a process that is integral to the pathogenesis of histoplasmosis and is dependent on the availability of calcium and iron inside the phagocytes. The yeasts are capable of growing and multiplying inside resting macrophages. Neutrophils and then lymphocytes are attracted to the site of infection. Before the development of cellular immunity, yeasts use the phagosomes as a vehicle for translocation to local draining lymph nodes, whence they spread hematogenously throughout the reticuloendothelial system. Adequate cellular immunity develops ~2 weeks after infection. T cells produce interferon γ to assist the macrophages in killing the organism and controlling the progression of disease. Interleukin 12 and tumor necrosis factor α (TNF-α) play an essential role in cellular immunity to *H. capsulatum*. In the immunocompetent host, macrophages, lymphocytes, and epithelial cells eventually organize and form granulo-

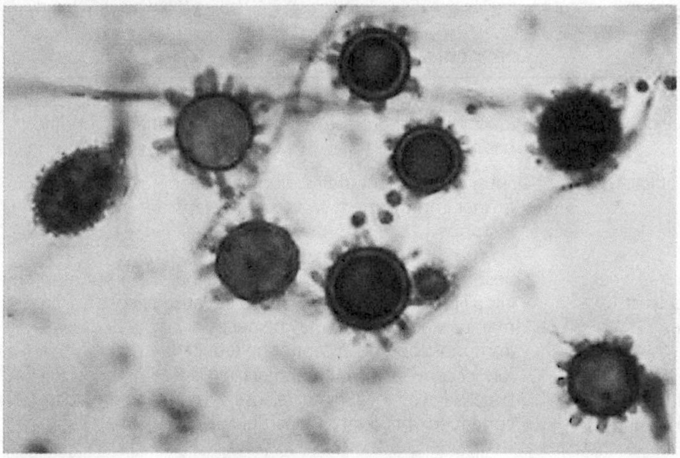

FIGURE 192-1 Spiked spherical conidia of *H. capsulatum* (lactol-phenol cotton blue stain).

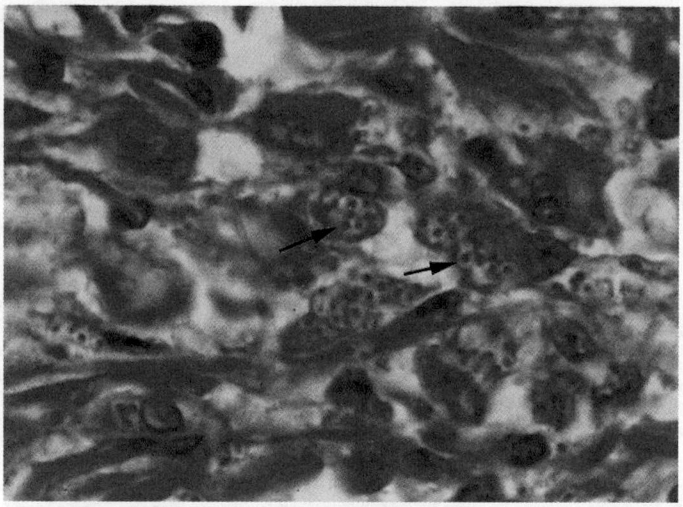

FIGURE 192-3 Intracellular yeasts (*arrows*) of *H. capsulatum* in a liver biopsy specimen (hematoxylin and eosin stain).

mas that contain the organisms. These granulomas typically fibrose and calcify; calcified mediastinal lymph nodes and hepatosplenic calcifications are frequently found in healthy individuals from endemic areas. In immunocompetent hosts, infection with *H. capsulatum* confers some immunity to reinfection. In patients with impaired cellular immunity, the infection is not contained and can disseminate. Progressive disseminated histoplasmosis (PDH) can involve multiple organs, most commonly the bone marrow, spleen, liver (Fig. 192-3), adrenal glands, and mucocutaneous membranes. Unlike latent tuberculosis, latent histoplasmosis is rarely reactivated.

Structural lung disease (e.g., emphysema) impairs the clearance of pulmonary histoplasmosis, and chronic pulmonary disease can result. This chronic process is characterized by progressive inflammation, tissue necrosis, and fibrosis mimicking cavitary tuberculosis.

CLINICAL MANIFESTATIONS

The clinical spectrum of histoplasmosis ranges from asymptomatic infection to life-threatening illness. The attack rate and the extent and severity of the disease depend on the intensity of exposure, the immune status of the exposed individual, and the underlying lung architecture of the host.

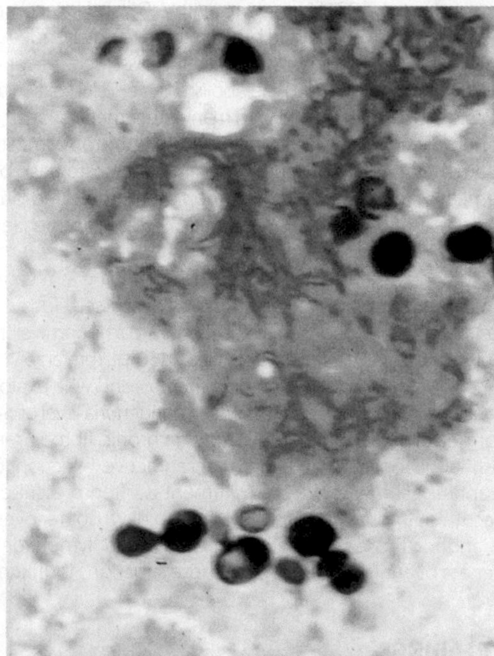

FIGURE 192-2 Small (2–5 μm) narrow budding yeasts of *H. capsulatum* from bronchoalveolar lavage fluid (Grocott's methenamine silver stain).

In immunocompetent individuals with low-level exposure, most *Histoplasma* infections are either asymptomatic or mild and self-limited. Of adults residing in endemic areas, 50–80% have skin-test and/or radiographic evidence of previous infection without clinical manifestations. When symptoms do develop, they usually appear 2–4 weeks after exposure. Heavy exposure leads to a flulike illness with fever, chills, sweats, headache, myalgia, anorexia, cough, dyspnea, and chest pain. Chest radiographs usually show signs of pneumonitis with hilar or mediastinal adenopathy. Pulmonary infiltrates may be focal with light exposure or diffuse with heavy exposure. Rheumatologic symptoms of arthralgia or arthritis, often associated with erythema nodosum, occur in 5–10% of patients with acute histoplasmosis. Pericarditis may also develop. These manifestations represent inflammatory responses to the acute infection rather than its direct effects. Hilar or mediastinal lymph nodes may undergo necrosis and coalesce to form large mediastinal masses that can cause compression of great vessels, proximal airways, and the esophagus. These necrotic lymph nodes also may rupture and create fistulas between mediastinal structures (e.g., bronchoesophageal fistulas).

PDH is typically seen in immunocompromised individuals, who account for ~70% of cases. Common risk factors include AIDS (CD4+ T cell count, <200/μL), extremes of age, and the use of immunosuppressive medications such as prednisone, methotrexate, and anti-TNF-α agents. The spectrum of PDH ranges from an acute, rapidly fatal course—with diffuse interstitial or reticulonodular lung infiltrates causing respiratory failure, shock, coagulopathy, and multiorgan failure—to a more subacute course with a focal organ distribution. Common manifestations include fever and weight loss. Hepatosplenomegaly is also common. Other findings may include meningitis or focal brain lesions, ulcerations of the oral mucosa, gastrointestinal ulcerations, and adrenal insufficiency. Prompt recognition of this devastating illness is of paramount importance in patients with more severe manifestations or with underlying immunosuppression, especially AIDS (Chap. 182).

Chronic cavitary histoplasmosis is seen in smokers who have structural lung disease (e.g., bullous emphysema). This chronic illness is characterized by productive cough, dyspnea, low-grade fever, night sweats, and weight loss. Chest radiographs usually show upper-lobe infiltrates, cavitation, and pleural thickening—findings resembling those of tuberculosis. Without treatment, the course is slowly progressive.

Fibrosing mediastinitis is an uncommon and serious complication of histoplasmosis. In certain patients, acute infection is followed for unknown reasons by progressive fibrosis around the hilar and mediastinal lymph nodes. Involvement may be unilateral or bilateral; bilateral involvement carries a worse prognosis. Major manifestations include superior vena cava syndrome, obstruction of pulmonary vessels, and

TABLE 192-1 RECOMMENDATIONS FOR THE TREATMENT OF HISTOPLASMOSIS

Type of Histoplasmosis	Treatment Recommendations	Comments
Acute pulmonary, moderate to severe illness with diffuse infiltrates and/or hypoxemia	Lipid amphotericin B (3–5 mg/kg per day) ± glucocorticoids for 1–2 weeks; then itraconazole (200 mg twice daily) for 12 weeks. Monitor renal and hepatic function.	Patients with mild cases usually recover without therapy, but itraconazole should be considered if the patient's condition has not improved after 1 month.
Chronic/cavitary pulmonary	Itraconazole (200 mg once or twice daily) for at least 12 months. Monitor hepatic function.	Continue treatment until radiographic findings show no further improvement. Monitor for relapse after treatment is stopped.
Progressive disseminated	Lipid amphotericin B (3–5 mg/kg per day) for 1–2 weeks; then itraconazole (200 mg twice daily) for at least 12 months. Monitor renal and hepatic function.	Liposomal amphotericin B is preferred, but the amphotericin B lipid complex may be used because of cost. Chronic maintenance therapy may be necessary if the degree of immunosuppression cannot be reduced.
Central nervous system	Liposomal amphotericin B (5 mg/kg per day) for 4–6 weeks; then itraconazole (200 mg 2 or 3 times daily) for at least 12 months. Monitor renal and hepatic function.	A longer course of lipid amphotericin B is recommended because of the high risk of relapse. Itraconazole should be continued until cerebrospinal fluid or CT abnormalities clear.

recurrent airway obstruction. Patients may experience recurrent pneumonia, hemoptysis, or respiratory failure. Fibrosing mediastinitis is fatal in up to one-third of cases.

In healed histoplasmosis, calcified mediastinal nodes or lung parenchyma may erode through the walls of the airways and cause hemoptysis. This condition is called *broncholithiasis*.

African histoplasmosis caused by *H. capsulatum* var. *duboisii* is clinically distinct and is characterized by frequent skin and bone involvement.

DIAGNOSIS

Fungal culture remains the gold standard diagnostic test for histoplasmosis. However, culture results may not be known for up to 1 month, and cultures are often negative in less severe cases. Cultures are positive in ~75% of cases of PDH and chronic pulmonary histoplasmosis. Cultures of bronchoalveolar lavage (BAL) fluid are positive in about half of patients with acute pulmonary histoplasmosis causing diffuse infiltrates with hypoxemia. In PDH, the culture yield is highest for BAL fluid, bone marrow aspirate, and blood. Cultures of sputum or bronchial washings are usually positive in chronic pulmonary histoplasmosis. Cultures are typically negative, however, in other forms of histoplasmosis.

Fungal stains of cytopathology or biopsy materials showing structures resembling *Histoplasma* yeasts are helpful in the diagnosis of PDH, yielding positive results in about half of cases. Yeasts can be seen in BAL fluid (Fig. 192-2) from patients with diffuse pulmonary infiltrates, in bone marrow biopsy samples, and in biopsy specimens of other involved organs (e.g., the adrenal glands). Occasionally, yeasts are seen in blood smears from patients with severe PDH. However, staining artifacts and other fungal elements may be misidentified as *Histoplasma* yeasts.

The detection of *Histoplasma* antigen in body fluids is extremely useful in the diagnosis of PDH and acute diffuse pulmonary histoplasmosis. The sensitivity of this technique is >90% for urine and 80% for serum from patients with PDH and ~75% for urine from patients with acute pulmonary histoplasmosis. Antigen can be detected in cerebrospinal fluid from patients with meningitis and in BAL fluid from those with pneumonia. Cross-reactivity occurs with African histoplasmosis, blastomycosis, coccidioidomycosis, paracoccidioidomycosis, and *Penicillium marneffei* infection.

Serologic tests, including immunodiffusion and complement fixation, are especially useful for the diagnosis of self-limited acute pulmonary histoplasmosis; however, at least 1 month is required for the production of antibodies after acute infection. A fourfold rise in antibody titer may be seen in patients with acute pulmonary histoplasmosis. Serologic tests are also useful for the diagnosis of chronic pulmonary histoplasmosis. Limitations of serology, however, include insensitivity early in the course of infection in immunosuppressed patients and the persistence of detectable antibody for several years after infection. Positive results from past infection may lead to a misdiagnosis of active histoplasmosis in a patient with another disease process.

Rx HISTOPLASMOSIS

Treatment recommendations for histoplasmosis are summarized in **Table 192-1**. Treatment is indicated for all patients with PDH or chronic pulmonary histoplasmosis as well as for symptomatic patients with acute pulmonary histoplasmosis causing diffuse infiltrates, especially with hypoxemia. In the vast majority of cases, however, acute pulmonary histoplasmosis resolves without therapy, and treatment is not recommended.

The preferred treatments for histoplasmosis include the lipid formulations of amphotericin B in more severe cases and itraconazole in others. Liposomal amphotericin B has been more effective than the deoxycholate formulation for treatment of PDH in patients with AIDS. The deoxycholate formulation of amphotericin B is an alternative to a lipid formulation in patients who are at a low risk for nephrotoxicity. Posaconazole, voriconazole, and fluconazole are alternatives for patients who cannot take itraconazole.

In severe cases requiring hospitalization, a lipid formulation of amphotericin B is followed by itraconazole. In patients with meningitis, a lipid formulation of amphotericin B should be given for 4–6 weeks before the switch to itraconazole. In immunosuppressed patients, the degree of immunosuppression should be reduced if possible. Antiretroviral treatment improves the outcome of PDH in patients with AIDS and is recommended.

Blood levels of itraconazole should be monitored to ensure adequate drug exposure, and drug interactions should be carefully assessed: itraconazole not only is cleared by cytochrome P450 metabolism but also inhibits cytochrome P450. This profile causes interactions with many other medications.

The duration of treatment for acute pulmonary histoplasmosis is 6–12 weeks, while that for PDH and chronic pulmonary histoplasmosis is ≥1 year. Antigen levels in urine and serum should be monitored during and for at least 1 year after therapy for PDH. Stable or rising antigen levels suggest treatment failure or relapse.

Previously, lifelong itraconazole maintenance therapy was recommended for patients with AIDS once histoplasmosis was diagnosed. Today, however, maintenance therapy is not required for patients who respond well to antiretroviral therapy, with CD4+ T cell counts of at least 150/μL (preferably >250/μL); who complete at least 1 year of itraconazole therapy; and who exhibit neither clinical evidence of active histoplasmosis nor an antigenuria level of >4 ng/mL.

Fibrosing mediastinitis, which represents a chronic fibrotic reaction to past mediastinal histoplasmosis rather than an active infection, does not respond to antifungal therapy. While treatment is often prescribed for patients with acute pulmonary histoplasmosis who have not recovered within 1 month and for those with persistent mediastinal lymphadenopathy, the effectiveness of antifungal therapy in these situations is unknown.

FURTHER READINGS

GOLDMAN M et al: Safety of discontinuation of maintenance therapy for disseminated histoplasmosis after immunologic response to antiretroviral therapy. Clin Infect Dis 38:1485, 2004

GOODWIN R et al: Histoplasmosis in normal hosts. Medicine (Baltimore) 60:231, 1981

JOHNSON PC et al: Safety and efficacy of liposomal amphotericin B compared with conventional amphotericin B for induction therapy of histoplasmosis in patients with AIDS. Ann Intern Med 137:105, 2002

KAUFFMAN CA: Histoplasmosis: A clinical and laboratory update. Clin Microb Rev 20:115, 2007

NEWMAN SL: Cell-mediated immunity to *Histoplasma capsulatum*. Semin Respir Infect 16:102, 2001

VAIL GM et al: Incidence of histoplasmosis following allogeneic bone marrow transplant or solid organ transplant in a hyperendemic area. Transpl Infect Dis 4:148, 2002

WHEAT LJ: Current diagnosis of histoplasmosis. Trends Microbiol 11:488, 2003

———: Histoplasmosis. Experience during outbreaks in Indianapolis and review of the literature. Medicine (Baltimore) 76:339, 1997

———: Improvements in diagnosis of histoplasmosis. Expert Opin Biol Ther 6:1207, 2006

——— et al: Clinical practice guidelines for the management of patients with histoplasmosis: 2007 update by the Infectious Diseases Society of America. Clin Infect Dis 45:807, 2007

——— et al: Pulmonary histoplasmosis syndromes: Recognition, diagnosis, and management. Semin Respir Crit Care Med 25:129, 2004

193 Coccidioidomycosis

Neil M. Ampel

DEFINITION AND ETIOLOGY

Coccidioidomycosis, commonly known as valley fever, is caused by the dimorphic soil-dwelling fungus *Coccidioides*. Genetic analysis has demonstrated the existence of two species, *C. immitis* and *C. posadasii*. These species are indistinguishable with regard to the clinical disease they cause as well as in routine laboratory tests. Thus, the organism will be referred to simply as *Coccidioides* for the remainder of this chapter.

EPIDEMIOLOGY

Coccidioidomycosis is confined to the Western Hemisphere between the latitudes of 40°N and 40°S. In the United States, areas of high endemicity include the southern portion of the San Joaquin Valley of California, the south-central region of Arizona, and the southwestern Rio Grande Valley. However, infection may be acquired in other areas of the southwestern United States, including the southern coastal counties in California, southern Nevada, and southwestern Utah. Outside the United States, coccidioidomycosis is endemic to northern Mexico as well as to localized regions of Central America. In South America, there are endemic foci in Colombia, Venezuela, northeastern Brazil, Paraguay, Bolivia, and north-central Argentina.

The risk of infection is increased by direct exposure to soil harboring *Coccidioides*. Because of difficulty in isolating *Coccidioides* from the soil, the precise characteristics of potentially infectious soil are not known. In general, *Coccidioides* appears to be supported in previously uncultivated desert soil, such as that found in the Lower Sonoran Life Zone. However, several outbreaks have been associated with soil from archaeologic excavations of Amerindian sites both within and outside of the recognized endemic region.

In endemic areas, many cases of *Coccidioides* infection occur without obvious soil or dust exposure. Climatic factors appear to increase the infection rate in these regions. In particular, periods of dryness after rainy seasons have been associated with marked increases in the number of cases.

Recently, the number of cases of symptomatic coccidioidomycosis has increased dramatically in south-central Arizona, where most of the state's population resides. The factors causing this increase have not been fully elucidated; however, an influx of older, susceptible individuals into the region as well as increased construction in previously undeveloped desert appear to be involved.

PATHOGENESIS, PATHOLOGY, AND IMMUNE RESPONSE

On agar media and in the soil, *Coccidioides* exists as a filamentous mold. Within this mycelial structure, individual filaments (*hyphae*) elongate and branch, some growing upward. Cells within the hyphae degenerate, leaving alternating barrel-shaped viable cells called *arthroconidia*. Measuring only ~2 × 5 μm, arthroconidia may become airborne for extended periods. The small size of the arthroconidia also allows them to evade initial mechanical mucosal defenses and reach the alveolus, where infection is initiated in the nonimmune host.

Once in a susceptible host, the arthroconidia enlarge, become rounded, and develop internal septations. The resulting structures, called *spherules* (Fig. 193-1), may attain sizes of 80 μm and are unique to *Coccidioides*. The septations encompass uninuclear elements called *endospores*. Spherules may rupture and release packets of endospores that can themselves develop into spherules, thus propagating infection locally. If returned to artificial media or the soil, the fungus reverts to its mycelial stage.

Clinical observations and data from studies of animals strongly support the critical role of a robust cellular immune response in the host's control of coccidioidomycosis. Necrotizing granulomas containing spherules are typically identified in patients with resolved pulmonary infection. In disseminated disease, granulomas are generally

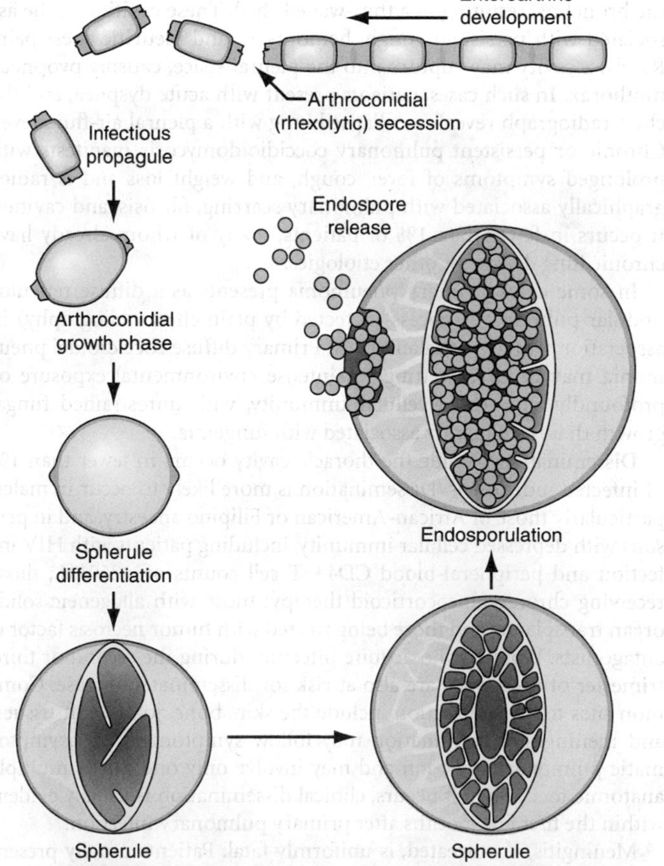

FIGURE 193-1 Life cycle of *Coccidioides*. *(From Kirkland TN, Fierer J: Coccidioidomycosis: A reemerging infectious disease. Emerg Infect Dis 2:192, 1996.)*

poorly formed or do not develop at all, and a polymorphonuclear leukocyte response occurs frequently. In patients who are asymptomatic or in whom the initial pulmonary infection resolves, delayed-type hypersensitivity to coccidioidal antigens is routinely documented.

CLINICAL AND LABORATORY MANIFESTATIONS

Coccidioidomycosis is protean in its manifestations. Of infected individuals, 60% are completely asymptomatic, and the remaining 40% have symptoms that are related principally to pulmonary infection, including fever, cough, and pleuritic chest pain. The risk of symptomatic illness increases with age. Coccidioidomycosis is commonly misdiagnosed as community-acquired bacterial pneumonia.

There are several cutaneous manifestations of primary pulmonary coccidioidomycosis. Toxic erythema consisting of a maculopapular rash has been noted in some cases. Erythema nodosum (typically over the lower extremities) or erythema multiforme (usually in a necklace distribution) may occur; these manifestations are seen particularly often in women. Arthralgias and arthritis may develop. The diagnosis of primary pulmonary coccidioidomycosis is suggested by a history of night sweats or profound fatigue as well as by peripheral-blood eosinophilia or hilar or mediastinal lymphadenopathy on chest radiography. While pleuritic chest pain is common, pleural effusion is less so, occurring in fewer than 10% of cases. Such effusions are invariably associated with a pulmonary infiltrate on the same side. The cellular content of these effusions is mononuclear in nature; *Coccidioides* is rarely grown from effusions.

Although primary pulmonary coccidioidomycosis usually resolves without sequelae, several complications may ensue. Pulmonary nodules are residua of primary pneumonia. Generally single, located in the upper lobes, and ≤4 cm in diameter, nodules are often discovered on a routine chest radiograph in an asymptomatic patient. Calcification is uncommon.

Pulmonary cavities occur when a nodule extrudes its contents into the bronchus, resulting in a thin-walled shell. These cavities can be associated with persistent cough, hemoptysis, and pleuritic chest pain. Rarely, a cavity may rupture into the pleural space, causing pyopneumothorax. In such cases, patients present with acute dyspnea, and the chest radiograph reveals a collapsed lung with a pleural air-fluid level. Chronic or persistent pulmonary coccidioidomycosis manifests with prolonged symptoms of fever, cough, and weight loss and is radiographically associated with pulmonary scarring, fibrosis, and cavities. It occurs in fewer than 1% of patients, many of whom already have chronic lung disease of other etiologies.

In some cases, primary pneumonia presents as a diffuse reticulonodular pulmonary process (detected by plain chest radiography) in association with dyspnea and fever. Primary diffuse coccidioidal pneumonia may occur in settings of intense environmental exposure or profoundly suppressed cellular immunity, with unrestrained fungal growth that is frequently associated with fungemia.

Dissemination outside the thoracic cavity occurs in fewer than 1% of infected individuals. Dissemination is more likely to occur in males, particularly those of African-American or Filipino ancestry, and in persons with depressed cellular immunity, including patients with HIV infection and peripheral-blood CD4+ T cell counts of <250/μL; those receiving chronic glucocorticoid therapy; those with allogeneic solid-organ transplants; and those being treated with tumor necrosis factor α antagonists. Women who acquire infection during the second or third trimester of pregnancy are also at risk for disseminated disease. Common sites for dissemination include the skin, bone, joints, soft tissues, and meninges. Dissemination may follow symptomatic or asymptomatic pulmonary infection and may involve only one site or multiple anatomic foci. When it occurs, clinical dissemination is usually evident within the first few months after primary pulmonary infection.

Meningitis, if untreated, is uniformly fatal. Patients usually present with a persistent headache, which is occasionally accompanied by lethargy and confusion. Nuchal rigidity, if present, is not severe. Examination of cerebrospinal fluid (CSF) demonstrates lymphocytic pleocytosis with profound hypoglycorrhachia and elevated protein levels. CSF eosinophilia is occasionally documented. With or without appropriate therapy, patients may develop hydrocephalus, which presents clinically as a marked decline in mental status, often with gait disturbances.

DIAGNOSIS

As mentioned above, coccidioidomycosis is often misdiagnosed as community-acquired bacterial pneumonia. Serology plays an important role in establishing the diagnosis of coccidioidomycosis. Several techniques are available, including the traditional tube-precipitin (TP) and complement-fixation (CF) assays, immunodiffusion (IDTP and IDCF), and enzyme immunoassay (EIA) to detect IgM and IgG antibodies. TP antibody is found in serum soon after infection and persists for weeks. TP titers are not useful for gauging disease progression, and this antibody is not found in the CSF. Titers of CF antibody generally rise later than do those of TP antibody, and CF antibody usually persists longer. Rising CF titers are associated with clinical progression, and the presence of CF antibody in CSF is an indicator for coccidioidal meningitis.

Because of its commercial availability, the coccidioidal EIA is frequently used as a screening tool for coccidioidal serology. However, the frequent false-positive results obtained with the IgM EIA make this test unreliable. Instead, the traditional TP or IDTP should be used. In addition, while the sensitivity and specificity of the IgG EIA appear to be high when compared with those of the CF and IDCF assays, the optical density obtained in the EIA does not correlate with the serologic titer of either of the latter tests.

Coccidioides grows within 3–7 days at 37°C on a variety of artificial media, including blood agar. Therefore, it is always useful to obtain samples of sputum or other respiratory fluids and tissues for culture in suspected cases of coccidioidomycosis. The clinical laboratory should be alerted to the possibility of this diagnosis, since *Coccidioides* can pose a significant hazard to laboratory workers if it is inadvertently inhaled. *Coccidioides* can also be identified directly. While treatment of samples with potassium hydroxide is rarely fruitful in establishing the diagnosis, examination of sputum or other respiratory fluids after Papanicolaou or Gomori methenamine silver staining reveals spherules in a significant proportion of patients with pulmonary coccidioidomycosis. For fixed tissues (e.g., those obtained from biopsy specimens), spherules with surrounding inflammation can be demonstrated with hematoxylin-eosin or Gomori methenamine silver staining.

℞ COCCIDIOIDOMYCOSIS

(Table 193-1) Currently, there are two main classes of antifungals useful for the treatment of coccidioidomycosis. While once routinely prescribed, amphotericin B in all its formulations is now reserved for only the most severe cases of dissemination and for intrathecal or intraventricular administration to patients with coccidioidal meningitis in whom triazole therapy has failed. The original formulation of amphotericin B, which is dispersed with deoxycholate, is usually administered intravenously in doses of 0.7–1.0 mg/kg either daily or three times per week. The newer lipid-based formulations—amphotericin B lipid complex (ABLC), amphotericin B colloidal dispersion (ABCD), and amphotericin B liposomal complex—appear to offer no therapeutic advantage over the deoxycholate formulation but are associated with less renal toxicity. The lipid dispersions are administered intravenously at doses of 5 mg/kg daily or three times per week.

Triazole antifungals are the principal drugs now used to treat most cases of coccidioidomycosis. Clinical trials have demonstrated the usefulness of both fluconazole and itraconazole, and evidence indicates that itraconazole may be more efficacious against bone and joint disease. Because of its demonstrated penetration into CSF, fluconazole is the azole of choice for the treatment of coccidioidal meningitis. For both drugs, a minimal oral adult dosage of 400 mg/d should be used. The maximal dose of itraconazole is 200 mg three times daily, but higher doses of fluconazole may be given. Two newer triazole antifungals, posaconazole and voriconazole, are now available. However, given the paucity of clinical data, the high cost, and (particularly for voriconazole) the potential toxicity, these agents should be reserved for cases that remain recalcitrant when treated with fluconazole or itraconazole. High-dose triazole therapy may be teratogen-

TABLE 193-1 CLINICAL PRESENTATIONS OF COCCIDIOIDOMYCOSIS, THEIR FREQUENCY, AND RECOMMENDED INITIAL THERAPY FOR THE IMMUNOCOMPETENT HOST

Clinical Presentation	Frequency, %	Recommended Therapy
Asymptomatic	60	None
Primary pneumonia (focal)	40	In most cases, none[a]
Diffuse pneumonia	<1	Amphotericin B followed by prolonged oral triazole therapy
Pulmonary sequelae	5	
Nodule	—	None
Cavity	—	In most cases, none[b]
Chronic pneumonia	—	Prolonged triazole therapy
Disseminated disease	≤1	
Skin, bone, joint, soft tissue	—	Prolonged triazole therapy[c]
Meningitis	—	Life-long triazole therapy[d]

[a]Treatment is indicated for hosts with depressed cellular immunity as well as for those with prolonged symptoms and signs of increased severity, including night sweats for >3 weeks, weight loss of >10%, a complement-fixation titer of >16, and extensive pulmonary involvement on chest radiography.
[b]Treatment (usually the oral triazoles fluconazole and itraconazole) is recommended for persistent symptoms.
[c]In severe cases, some clinicians would use amphotericin B as initial therapy.
[d]Intraventricular or intrathecal amphotericin B is recommended in cases of triazole failure. Hydrocephalus may occur, requiring a CSF shunt.

ic; thus, amphotericin B should be considered as therapy for coccidioidomycosis in pregnant women.

Most patients with focal primary pulmonary coccidioidomycosis require no therapy. Patients for whom antifungal therapy should be considered include those with underlying cellular immunodeficiencies and those with prolonged symptoms and signs of extensive disease. Specific criteria include symptoms persisting for ≥2 months, night sweats occurring for >3 weeks, weight loss of >10%, a serum CF antibody titer of >1:16, and extensive pulmonary involvement apparent on chest radiograph.

Diffuse pulmonary coccidioidomycosis represents a special situation. Because most patients with this form of disease are profoundly hypoxemic and critically ill, many clinicians favor beginning therapy with amphotericin B and switching to an oral triazole once clinical improvement occurs.

The nodules that may follow primary pulmonary coccidioidomycosis do not require treatment. However, nodules are not easily distinguished from pulmonary malignancies by means of radiographic imaging (including positron emission tomography scans). Close clinical follow-up and biopsy may be required to distinguish these two entities. Most pulmonary cavities do not require therapy. Antifungal treatment should be considered in patients with persistent cough, pleuritic chest pain, and hemoptysis. Occasionally, pulmonary coccidioidal cavities become secondarily infected. This development is usually manifested by an air-fluid level within the cavity. Bacterial flora or *Aspergillus* species are commonly involved, and therapy directed at these organisms should be considered. Surgery is rarely required except in cases of persistent hemoptysis or pyopneumothorax. For chronic pulmonary coccidioidomycosis, prolonged antifungal therapy—lasting for at least 1 year—is usually required, with monitoring of symptoms, radiographic changes, sputum cultures, and serologic titers.

Most cases of disseminated coccidioidomycosis require prolonged antifungal therapy. Duration of treatment is based on resolution of the signs and symptoms of the lesion in conjunction with a significant decline in serum CF antibody titer. Such therapy routinely is continued for at least several years. Relapse occurs in 15–30% of individuals once therapy is discontinued.

Coccidioidal meningitis poses a special challenge. While most patients with this form of disease respond to treatment with oral triazoles, 80% experience relapse when therapy is stopped. Thus, life-long therapy is recommended. In cases of triazole failure, intrathecal or intraventricular amphotericin B may be used. Installation requires considerable expertise and should be performed only by an experienced health care provider. Shunting of CSF in addition to appropriate antifungal therapy is required in cases of meningitis complicated by hydrocephalus. It is prudent to obtain expert consultation in all cases of coccidioidal meningitis.

PREVENTION

There are no proven methods to reduce the risk of acquiring coccidioidomycosis among residents of an endemic region. Avoidance of direct contact with uncultivated soil or with visible dust containing soil presumably reduces the risk. Prophylactic antifungal therapy may be useful in patients who have evidence of active or recent coccidioidomycosis and are about to undergo allogeneic solid-organ transplantation. Data on the use of antifungal agents for prophylaxis in other situations are scanty and do not suggest efficacy.

FURTHER READINGS

Bergstrom L et al: Increased risk of coccidioidomycosis in patients treated with tumor necrosis factor alpha antagonists. Arthritis Rheum 50:1959, 2004

Blair JE et al: The prevention of recrudescent coccidioidomycosis after solid organ transplantation. Transplantation 83:1182, 2007

DiCaudo DJ et al: The exanthem of acute pulmonary coccidioidomycosis: Clinical and histopathologic features of 3 cases and review of the literature. Arch Dermatol 142:744, 2006

Drutz DJ, Catanzaro A: Coccidioidomycosis (parts I and II). Am Rev Respir Dis 117:559 and 727, 1978

Fisher MC et al: Molecular and phenotypic description of *Coccidioides posadasii* sp. nov., previously recognized as the non-California population of *Coccidioides immitis*. Mycologia 94:73, 2002

Galgiani JN et al: Coccidioidomycosis. Clin Infect Dis 41:1217, 2005

——— et al: Comparison of oral fluconazole and itraconazole for progressive, nonmeningeal coccidioidomycosis. A randomized, double-blind trial. Mycoses Study Group. Ann Intern Med 133:676, 2000

Park BJ et al: An epidemic of coccidioidomycosis in Arizona associated with climatic changes, 1998–2001. J Infect Dis 191:1981, 2005

Valdivia L et al: Coccidioidomycosis as a common cause of community-acquired pneumonia. Emerg Infect Dis 12:958, 2006

194 Blastomycosis

Stanley W. Chapman, Donna C. Sullivan

Blastomycosis is a systemic pyogranulomatous infection, primarily involving the lungs, that arises after inhalation of the conidia of *Blastomyces dermatitidis*. Pulmonary blastomycosis varies from an asymptomatic infection to acute or chronic pneumonia. Hematogenous dissemination occurs frequently. Extrapulmonary disease of the skin, bones, and genitourinary system is common, but almost any organ can be infected.

ETIOLOGIC AGENT

B. dermatitidis is the asexual state of *Ajellomyces dermatitidis*. Two serotypes have been identified on the basis of the presence or absence of the A antigen. *B. dermatitidis* exhibits thermal dimorphism, growing as the mycelial phase at room temperature and as the yeast phase at 37°C. Primary isolation is most dependable for the mycelial phase incubated at 30°C. Definitive identification usually requires conversion to the yeast phase at 37°C or, more commonly, the use of nucleic acid amplification techniques (e.g., AccuProbe, Gen-Probe, San Diego, CA) that detect mycelial-phase growth. Yeast cells are usually 8–15 μm in diameter, have thick refractile cell walls, are multinucleate, and reproduce by a single, large, broad-based bud.

EPIDEMIOLOGY

Most cases of blastomycosis have been reported in North America. Endemic areas include the southeastern and south-central states bordering the Mississippi and Ohio river basins, the midwestern states and Canadian provinces bordering the Great Lakes, and a small area in New York and Canada along the St. Lawrence River. Outside North America, blastomycosis has been reported most frequently in Africa.

Early studies of endemic cases indicated that middle-aged men with outdoor occupations were at greatest risk. Reported outbreaks, however, do not suggest a predilection according to sex, age, race, occupation, or season. *B. dermatitidis* probably grows as microfoci in the warm, moist soil of wooded areas rich in organic debris. Exposure to soil, whether related to work or recreation, appears to be the common factor associated with infection.

PATHOGENESIS

After inhalation, the conidia of *B. dermatitidis* are susceptible to phagocytosis and killing in the lungs by polymorphonuclear leukocytes, monocytes, and alveolar macrophages. This phagocytic response represents innate immunity and probably explains the high frequency of asymptomatic infections in outbreaks. Conidia that escape phagocytosis rapidly convert to the yeast phase in tissue. The greater resistance of the thick-walled yeast form to phagocytosis and killing probably contributes to infection. This yeast-phase conversion also induces the expression of the 120-kDa glycoprotein BAD-1, which is an adhesin, an essential virulence factor, and the major epitope for humoral and cellular immunity. The primary acquired host defense against *B. dermatitidis* is cellular immunity mediated by antigen-specific T cells and lymphokine-activated macrophages.

TABLE 194-1 TREATMENT OF BLASTOMYCOSIS

Disease	Primary Therapy	Alternative Therapy
Immunocompetent Patient/Life-Threatening Disease		
Pulmonary	AmB,[a] 0.7–1.0 mg/kg qd (total dose: 1.5–2.5 g)	Itraconazole, 200–400 mg/d (once patient's condition has stabilized)
Disseminated		
CNS	AmB, 0.7–1.0 mg/kg qd (total dose: at least 2 g)	Fluconazole, 800 mg/d (if patient is intolerant to full course of AmB)
Non-CNS	AmB, 0.7–1.0 mg/kg qd (total dose: 1.5–2.5 g)	Itraconazole, 200–400 mg/d (once patient's condition has stabilized)
Immunocompetent Patient/Non-Life-Threatening Disease		
Pulmonary or disseminated (non-CNS)	Itraconazole, 200–400 mg/d *or* AmB, 0.5–0.7 mg/kg qd (in patients intolerant to itraconazole or whose disease progresses despite therapy)	Fluconazole, 400–800 mg/d *or* Ketoconazole, 400–800 mg/d
Immunocompromised Patient[b]		
All infections	AmB, 0.7–1.0 mg/kg qd (total dose: 1.5–2.5 g)	Itraconazole, 200–400 mg/d (non-CNS disease, once clinically improved)

[a]In all regimens listed, an AmB lipid formulation (3.0–5.0 mg/kg qd) can be substituted for AmB deoxycholate.
[b]Suppressive therapy with itraconazole may be considered for patients whose immunocompromised state continues. Fluconazole (800 mg/d) may be useful for patients who have CNS disease or are intolerant to itraconazole.
Note: AmB, amphotericin B; CNS, central nervous system.

APPROACH TO THE PATIENT: Blastomycosis

Whether acute or chronic, blastomycosis mimics many other disease processes. For example, acute pulmonary blastomycosis may present with signs and symptoms indistinguishable from those of bacterial pneumonia or influenza. Chronic pulmonary blastomycosis most commonly mimics malignancy or tuberculosis. Skin lesions are often misdiagnosed as basal cell or squamous cell carcinoma, pyoderma gangrenosum, or keratoacanthoma. Laryngeal lesions are frequently mistaken for squamous cell carcinoma. Thus, the clinician must maintain a high index of suspicion and perform a careful histologic evaluation of secretions or biopsy material from patients who live in or have visited regions endemic for blastomycosis.

CLINICAL MANIFESTATIONS

Acute pulmonary infection is usually diagnosed in association with point-source outbreaks and is accompanied by the abrupt onset of fever, chills, pleuritic chest pain, arthralgias, and myalgias. Cough is initially nonproductive but frequently becomes purulent as disease progresses. Chest radiographs usually reveal alveolar infiltrates with consolidation. Pleural effusions and hilar adenopathy are uncommon. Most patients diagnosed with pulmonary blastomycosis have chronic indolent pneumonia with signs and symptoms of fever, weight loss, productive cough, and hemoptysis. The most common radiologic findings are alveolar infiltrates with or without cavitation, mass lesions that mimic bronchogenic carcinoma, and fibronodular infiltrates. Respiratory failure (adult respiratory distress syndrome) associated with miliary disease or diffuse pulmonary infiltrates is more common among immunocompromised patients, especially those in the late stages of AIDS (Chap. 182). Mortality rates are ≥50% among these patients, and most deaths occur within the first few days of therapy.

Skin disease is the most common extrapulmonary manifestation of blastomycosis. Two types of skin lesions occur: verrucous (more common) and ulcerative. Osteomyelitis is associated with as many as one-fourth of *B. dermatitidis* infections. The vertebrae, pelvis, sacrum, skull, ribs, or long bones are most frequently involved. Patients with *B. dermatitidis* osteomyelitis often present with contiguous soft-tissue abscesses or chronic draining sinuses. In men, blastomycosis may involve the prostate and epididymis. Central nervous system (CNS) disease occurs in <5% of immunocompetent patients with blastomycosis. In AIDS patients, however, CNS disease has been reported in ~40% of cases, usually presenting as a brain abscess. Less common forms of CNS disease are cranial or spinal epidural abscess and meningitis.

DIAGNOSIS

Definitive diagnosis of blastomycosis requires growth of the organism from sputum, pus, or biopsy material. A presumptive diagnosis is made by visualization of the characteristic broad-based budding yeast in clinical specimens. Serologic diagnosis of blastomycosis is of limited usefulness because of cross-reactivity with other fungal antigens.

A *Blastomyces* antigen assay that detects antigen in urine and serum is commercially available (Mira Vista Diagnostics, Indianapolis, IN). Antigen detection in urine appears to be more sensitive than serum antigen detection. This antigen test may be useful for monitoring of patients during therapy or for early detection of relapse.

Rx BLASTOMYCOSIS

The Infectious Diseases Society of America has published guidelines for the treatment of blastomycosis. Selection of an appropriate therapeutic regimen must be based on the clinical form and severity of the disease, the immune status of the patient, and the toxicity of the antifungal agent (**Table 194-1**). Although spontaneous cures of acute pulmonary infection have been well documented, there are no criteria by which to distinguish patients whose disease will progress or disseminate. Thus, almost all patients with blastomycosis should be treated.

Itraconazole is the agent of choice for immunocompetent patients with mild to moderate pulmonary or non-CNS extrapulmonary disease.

Therapy is continued for 6–12 months. Amphotericin B is the preferred initial treatment for patients who are severely immunocompromised, who have life-threatening disease or CNS disease, or whose disease progresses during treatment with itraconazole. Although not rigorously studied, lipid formulations of amphotericin B can provide an alternative for patients who cannot tolerate amphotericin B deoxycholate. Most patients with non-CNS disease whose clinical condition improves after an initial course of amphotericin B (usually 2 weeks in duration) can be switched to itraconazole to complete 6–12 months of therapy. Fluconazole, because of its excellent penetration of the CNS, may have a role in the treatment of patients with brain abscess or meningitis after an initial course of amphotericin B.

The newer triazoles voriconazole and posaconazole have not been studied extensively in human cases of blastomycosis. The echinocandins have variable activity against *B. dermatitidis* and have no place in the treatment of blastomycosis.

PROGNOSIS

Clinical and mycologic response rates are 90–95% among compliant immunocompetent patients given itraconazole for mild to moderate pulmonary and extrapulmonary disease without CNS involvement. Bone and joint disease usually requires 12 months of therapy. The <5% of infections that relapse after an initial course of itraconazole usually respond well to a second treatment course.

FURTHER READINGS

Bradsher RW: Blastomycosis, in *Clinical Mycology*, WE Dismukes et al (eds). New York, Oxford University Press, 2003, pp 299–310

——— et al: Blastomycosis. Infect Dis Clin North Am 17:21, 2003

Chapman SW: *Blastomyces dermatitidis*, in *Principles and Practice of Infectious Diseases*, 6th ed, GL Mandell et al (eds). New York, Churchill Livingstone, 2005, pp 3026–3040

———, Sullivan DC: Diagnosis and treatment of blastomycosis, in *Diagnosis and Treatment of Human Mycoses*, D Hospental, M Rinaldi (eds). Totowa, NJ, Humana Press, 2007

——— et al: Practice guidelines for the management of patients with blastomycosis. Clin Infect Dis 30:679, 2000 (updates: *www.idsociety.org*)

Deepe GS et al: Progress in vaccination for histoplasmosis and blastomycosis: Coping with cellular immunity. Med Mycol 43:381, 2005

195 Cryptococcosis

Arturo Casadevall

DEFINITION AND ETIOLOGY

Cryptococcus neoformans, a yeast-like fungus, is the etiologic agent of cryptococcosis. Cryptococcal strains are antigenically and genetically diverse. Both *C. neoformans* and *C. gattii* are pathogenic for humans and can cause cryptococcosis. *C. neoformans* consists of serotypes A and D, and *C. gattii* consists of serotypes B and C. Currently, most authorities further subdivide *C. neoformans* into two varieties: *grubii* (serotype A) and *neoformans* (serotype D). Most clinical microbiology laboratories do not routinely distinguish among cryptococcal species and varieties but rather identify all isolates simply as *C. neoformans*.

EPIDEMIOLOGY

Cryptococcosis was first described in the 1890s but remained relatively rare until the mid-twentieth century, when advances in diagnosis and increases in the number of immunosuppressed individuals markedly raised its reported prevalence. The spectrum of disease caused by *C. neoformans* consists predominantly of meningoencephalitis and pneumonia, but skin and soft tissue infections also occur. Serologic studies have shown that, although cryptococcal *infection* is common among immunocompetent individuals, cryptococcal *disease* (cryptococcosis) is relatively rare in the absence of impaired immunity. Individuals at high risk for cryptococcosis include patients with hematologic malignancies, recipients of solid organ transplants who require ongoing immunosuppressive therapy, persons whose medical conditions necessitate glucocorticoid therapy, and patients with advanced HIV infection and CD4+ T lymphocyte counts of <200/μL. Since the onset of the HIV pandemic in the early 1980s, the overwhelming majority of cryptococcosis cases have occurred in patients with AIDS (Chap. 182). To understand the impact of HIV infection on the epidemiology of cryptococcosis, it is instructive to note that in the early 1990s there were >1000 cases of cryptococcal meningitis each year in New York City—a figure far exceeding that for all cases of bacterial meningitis. With the advent of effective antiretroviral therapy, the incidence of AIDS-related cryptococcosis has been sharply reduced among treated individuals; however, the disease remains distressingly common in regions where antiretroviral therapy is not readily available, such as Africa and Asia, where up to one-third of patients with AIDS have cryptococcosis.

Cryptococcal infection is acquired from the environment. *C. neoformans* and *C. gattii* inhabit different ecologic niches. *C. neoformans* is frequently found in soils contaminated with avian excreta and can easily be recovered from shaded and humid soils contaminated with pigeon droppings. In contrast, *C. gattii* is not found in bird feces. Instead, it inhabits a variety of arboreal species, including several types of eucalyptus tree. *C. neoformans* strains are found throughout the world; however, var. *grubii* (serotype A) strains are far more common than var. *neoformans* (serotype D) strains among both clinical and environmental isolates. The geographic distribution of *C. gattii* was thought to be largely limited to tropical regions until an outbreak of cryptococcosis caused by a new serotype B strain began in Vancouver in 1999. In addition to the different geographic distributions of the two cryptococcal species, individual susceptibility to these species affects epidemiology. Cryptococcosis caused by the *C. neoformans* varieties occurs mostly in individuals with AIDS (Chap. 182) and other forms of impaired immunity. In contrast, *C. gattii*–related disease is not associated with specific immune deficits and often occurs in immunocompetent individuals.

PATHOGENESIS

Cryptococcal infection is acquired by inhalation of aerosolized infectious particles. The exact nature of these particles is not known; the two leading candidate forms are small desiccated yeast cells and basidiospores. Little is known about the pathogenesis of initial infection. Serologic studies have shown that cryptococcal infection is acquired in childhood, but it is not known whether the initial infection is symptomatic. Given serologic documentation that cryptococcal infection is common yet cryptococcal disease is rare, the consensus is that pulmonary defense mechanisms in immunologically intact individuals are highly effective at containing *C. neoformans*. It is not clear whether initial infection leads to a state of immunity or whether most individuals are subject throughout life to frequent and recurrent infections that resolve without clinical disease. However, evidence indicates that some human cryptococcal infections lead to a state of latency in which viable organisms are harbored for prolonged periods, possibly in granulomas. Thus the inhalation of *C. neoformans* can be followed by clearance of the organism or establishment of the latent state. The consequences of prolonged harboring of *C. neoformans* in the lung are not known, but evidence from animal studies indicates that the organism's prolonged presence could alter the immunologic milieu in the lung and predispose to allergic airway disease.

Cryptococcosis usually presents clinically as chronic meningoencephalitis. The mechanisms by which *C. neoformans* undergoes extrapulmonary

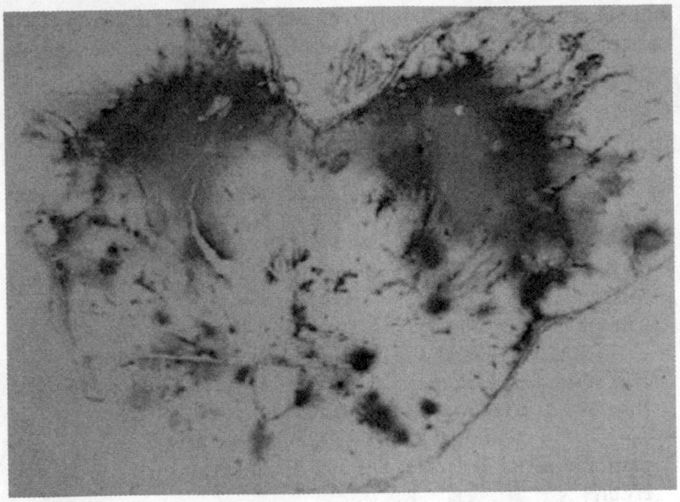

FIGURE 195-1 Cryptococcal antigen in human brain tissue, as revealed by immunohistochemical staining. Brown areas show polysaccharide deposits in the midbrain of a patient who died of cryptococcal meningitis. *(Reprinted with permission from SC Lee et al: Hum Pathol 27:839, 1996.)*

dissemination and enters the central nervous system (CNS) remain poorly understood. There is evidence that yeast cells can migrate directly across the endothelium by a mechanism that may be associated with changes in polysaccharide structure. *C. neoformans* has well-defined virulence factors that include the polysaccharide capsule, the ability to make melanin, and the elaboration of enzymes (e.g., phospholipase and urease) that enhance the survival of fungal cells in tissue. Among these virulence factors, the capsule and melanin production have been most extensively studied. The *C. neoformans* capsule is antiphagocytic, and the capsular polysaccharide has been associated with numerous deleterious effects on host immune function. Cryptococcal infections elicit little or no tissue inflammatory response. The immune dysfunction seen in cryptococcosis has been attributed to the release of copious amounts of capsular polysaccharide into tissues, where it probably interferes with local immune responses (Fig. 195-1). In clinical practice, the cryptococcal polysaccharide is the antigen that is measured as a diagnostic marker of *C. neoformans* infection.

APPROACH TO THE PATIENT: Cryptococcosis

Cryptococcosis should be included in the differential diagnosis when any patient presents with findings suggestive of chronic meningitis. Concern about cryptococcosis is heightened by a history of headache and neurologic symptoms in a patient with an underlying immunosuppressive disorder or state that is associated with an increased incidence of cryptococcosis, such as advanced HIV infection or solid organ transplantation.

CLINICAL MANIFESTATIONS

The clinical manifestations of cryptococcosis reflect the site of fungal infection. *C. neoformans* infection can affect any tissue or organ, but the majority of cases that come to clinical attention involve the CNS and/or the lungs. CNS involvement usually presents as signs and symptoms of chronic meningitis, such as headache, fever, lethargy, sensorium deficits, memory deficits, cranial nerve paresis, vision deficits, and meningismus. Cryptococcal meningitis differs from bacterial meningitis in that many *Cryptococcus*-infected patients present with symptoms of several weeks' duration. In addition, classic characteristics of meningeal irritation, such as meningismus, may be absent in cryptococcal meningitis. Indolent cases can present as subacute dementia. Meningeal cryptococcosis can lead to sudden catastrophic vision loss.

Pulmonary cryptococcosis usually presents as cough, increased sputum production, and chest pain. Patients infected with *C. gattii* can present with granulomatous pulmonary masses known as *cryptococcomas*. Fever develops in a minority of cases. Like CNS disease, pulmonary cryptococcosis can follow an indolent course, and the majority of cases probably do not come to clinical attention. In fact, many cases are discovered incidentally during the workup of an abnormal chest radiograph obtained for other diagnostic purposes. Pulmonary cryptococcosis is often associated with antecedent diseases such as malignancy, diabetes, and tuberculosis.

Skin lesions are common in patients with disseminated cryptococcosis and can be highly variable, including papules, plaques, purpura, vesicles, tumor-like lesions, and rashes. The spectrum of cryptococcosis in HIV-infected patients is so varied and has changed so much since the advent of antiretroviral therapy that a distinction between HIV-related and HIV-unrelated cryptococcosis is no longer pertinent. In patients with AIDS and solid organ transplant recipients, the lesions of cutaneous cryptococcosis often resemble those of molluscum contagiosum (Fig. 195-2; Chap. 182).

DIAGNOSIS

A diagnosis of cryptococcosis requires the demonstration of *C. neoformans* in normally sterile tissues. Visualization of the capsule of fungal cells in cerebrospinal fluid (CSF) mixed with India ink is a useful rapid diagnostic technique. *C. neoformans* cells in India ink have a distinctive appearance because their capsules exclude ink particles. However, the CSF India ink examination may yield negative results in patients with a low fungal burden. This examination should be performed by a trained individual, since leukocytes and fat globules can sometimes be mistaken for fungal cells. Cultures of CSF and blood that are positive for *C. neoformans* are diagnostic for cryptococcosis. In cryptococcal meningitis, CSF examination usually reveals evidence of chronic meningitis with mononuclear cell pleocytosis and increased protein levels. A particularly useful test is cryptococcal antigen (CRAg) detection in CSF and blood. The assay is based on serologic detection of cryptococcal polysaccharide and is both sensitive and specific. A positive cryptococcal antigen test provides strong presumptive evidence for cryptococcosis; however, because the result is often negative in pulmonary cryptococcosis, the test is less useful in the diagnosis of pulmonary disease.

℞ CRYPTOCOCCOSIS

Both the site of infection and the immune status of the host must be considered in the selection of therapy for cryptococcosis. The disease has two

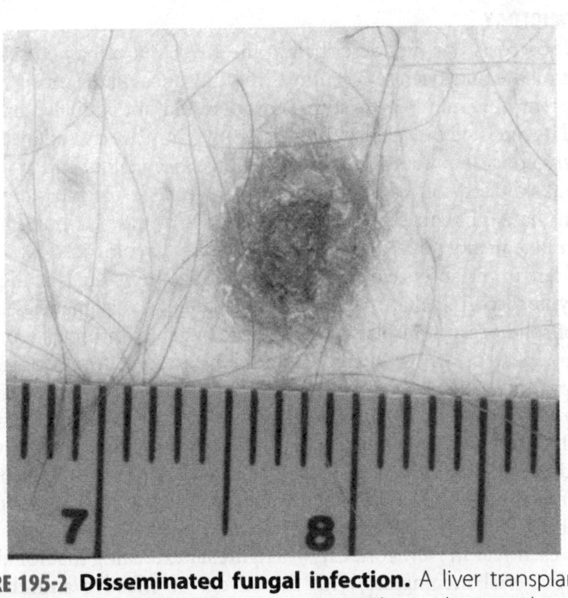

FIGURE 195-2 Disseminated fungal infection. A liver transplant recipient developed six cutaneous lesions similar to the one shown. Biopsy and serum antigen testing demonstrated *Cryptococcus*. Important features of the lesion include a benign-appearing fleshy papule with central umbilication resembling molluscum contagiosum. *(Photo courtesy of Dr. Lindsey Baden; with permission.)*

general patterns of manifestation: (1) pulmonary cryptococcosis, with no evidence of extrapulmonary dissemination; and (2) extrapulmonary (systemic) cryptococcosis, with or without meningoencephalitis. Pulmonary cryptococcosis in an immunocompetent host sometimes resolves without therapy. However, given the propensity of *C. neoformans* to disseminate from the lung, the inability to gauge the host's immune status precisely, and the availability of low-toxicity therapy in the form of fluconazole, the current recommendation is for pulmonary cryptococcosis in an immunocompetent individual to be treated with fluconazole (200–400 mg/d for 3–6 months). Extrapulmonary cryptococcosis without CNS involvement in an immunocompetent host can be treated with the same regimen, although amphotericin B (AmB; 0.5–1.0 mg/kg daily for 4–6 weeks) may be required for more severe cases. In general, extrapulmonary cryptococcosis without CNS involvement requires less intensive therapy—with the caveat that morbidity and death in cryptococcosis are associated with meningeal involvement. Thus the decision to categorize cryptococcosis as "extrapulmonary without CNS involvement" should be made only after careful evaluation of the CSF reveals no evidence of *C. neoformans* infection. For CNS involvement in a host without AIDS or obvious immune impairment, most authorities recommend initial therapy with AmB (0.5–1.0 mg/kg daily) during an induction phase, which is followed by prolonged therapy with fluconazole (400 mg/d) during a consolidation phase. For cryptococcal meningoencephalitis without a concomitant immunosuppressive condition, the recommended regimen is AmB (0.5–1.0 mg/kg) plus flucytosine (100 mg/kg) daily for 6–10 weeks. Alternatively, patients can be treated with AmB (0.5–1.0 mg/kg) plus flucytosine (100 mg/kg) daily for 2 weeks and then with fluconazole (400 mg/d) for at least 10 weeks. Patients with immunosuppression are treated with the same initial regimens except that consolidation therapy with fluconazole is given for a prolonged period to prevent relapse.

Cryptococcosis in patients with HIV infection always requires aggressive therapy and is considered incurable unless immune function improves. Consequently, therapy for cryptococcosis in the setting of AIDS has two phases: induction therapy (intended to reduce the fungal burden and alleviate symptoms) and lifelong maintenance therapy (to prevent a symptomatic clinical relapse). Pulmonary and extrapulmonary cryptococcosis without evidence of CNS involvement can be treated with fluconazole (200–400 mg/d). In patients who have more extensive disease, flucytosine (100 mg/d) may be added to the fluconazole regimen for 10 weeks, with lifelong fluconazole maintenance therapy thereafter. For HIV-infected patients with evidence of CNS involvement, most authorities recommend induction therapy with AmB. An acceptable regimen is AmB (0.7–1.0 mg/kg) plus flucytosine (100 mg) daily for 2 weeks followed by fluconazole (400 mg/d) for at least 10 weeks and then by lifelong maintenance therapy with fluconazole (200 mg/d). Fluconazole (400–800 mg/d) plus flucytosine (150–100 mg/d) for 6–10 weeks followed by fluconazole (200 mg/d) as maintenance therapy can be used as an alternative. Lipid formulations of AmB can be substituted for AmB deoxycholate in patients with renal impairment. Neither caspofungin nor mycofungin is effective against *C. neoformans*, and neither drug has a role in the treatment of cryptococcosis. Cryptococcal meningoencephalitis is often associated with increased intracranial pressure, which is believed to be responsible for damage to the brain and cranial nerves. Appropriate management of CNS cryptococcosis requires careful attention to the management of intracranial pressure, including the reduction of pressure by repeated therapeutic lumbar puncture and the placement of shunts.

In HIV-infected patients with previously treated cryptococcosis who are receiving fluconazole maintenance therapy, it may be possible to discontinue antifungal drug treatment if antiretroviral therapy results in immunologic improvement. However, certain recipients of maintenance therapy who have a history of successfully treated cryptococcosis can develop a troublesome immune reconstitution syndrome when antiretroviral therapy produces a rebound in immunologic function.

PROGNOSIS AND COMPLICATIONS

Even with antifungal therapy, cryptococcosis is associated with high rates of morbidity and death. For the majority of patients with cryptococcosis, the most important prognostic factor is the extent and the duration of the underlying immunologic deficits that predisposed them to develop the disease. Therefore, cryptococcosis is often curable with antifungal therapy in individuals with no apparent immunologic dysfunction, but, in patients with severe immunosuppression (e.g., those with AIDS), the best that can be hoped for is that antifungal therapy will induce remission, which can then be maintained with lifelong suppressive therapy. Before the advent of antiretroviral therapy, the median overall survival period for AIDS patients with cryptococcosis was <1 year. Cryptococcosis in patients with underlying neoplastic disease has a particularly poor prognosis. For CNS cryptococcosis, poor prognostic markers are a positive CSF assay for yeast cells by initial India ink examination (evidence of a heavy fungal burden), high CSF pressure, low CSF glucose levels, low CSF pleocytosis (<2/μL), recovery of yeast cells from extraneural sites, the absence of antibody to *C. neoformans*, a CSF or serum cryptococcal antigen level of ≥1:32, and concomitant glucocorticoid therapy or hematologic malignancy. A response to treatment does not guarantee cure since relapse of cryptococcosis is common even among patients with relatively intact immune systems. Complications of CNS cryptococcosis include cranial nerve deficits, vision loss, and cognitive impairment.

PREVENTION

No vaccine is available for cryptococcosis. In patients at high risk (e.g., those with advanced HIV infection and CD4+ T lymphocyte counts of <200/μL), primary prophylaxis with fluconazole (200 mg/d) is effective in reducing the prevalence of disease. Since antiretroviral therapy raises the CD4+ T lymphocyte count, it constitutes an immunologic form of prophylaxis. However, cryptococcosis in the setting of immune reconstitution has been reported in patients with HIV infection and recipients of solid organ transplants.

FURTHER READINGS

ABERT J et al: A pilot study of the discontinuation of antifungal therapy for disseminated cryptococcal disease in patients with acquired immunodeficiency syndrome, following immunologic response to antiretroviral therapy. J Infect Dis 185:1179, 2002

CHAYAKULKEEREE M, PERFECT JP: Cryptococcosis. Infect Dis Clin North Am 20:507, 2006

LILIANG P et al: Use of ventriculoperitoneal shunts to treat uncontrollable intracranial hypertension in patients who have cryptococcal meningitis without hydrocephalus. Clin Infect Dis 34:E64, 2002

LORTHOLARY O et al: Incidence and risk factors of immune reconstitution inflammatory syndrome complicating HIV-associated cryptococcosis in France. AIDS 19:1043, 2005

MASUR H et al: Guidelines for preventing opportunistic infections among HIV-infected persons—2002. Ann Intern Med 137:435, 2002

SAAG MS et al: Practice guidelines for the management of cryptococcal disease. Clin Infect Dis 30:710, 2000

196 Candidiasis

John E. Edwards, Jr.

The genus *Candida* encompasses more than 150 species, only a few of which cause disease in humans. With rare exceptions, the human pathogens are *C. albicans, C. guilliermondii, C. krusei, C. parapsilosis, C. tropicalis, C. kefyr, C. lusitaniae, C. dubliniensis,* and *C. glabrata.* Ubiquitous in nature, these organisms are found on inanimate objects, in foods, and on animals and are normal commensals of humans. They inhabit the gastrointestinal tract (including the mouth and oropharynx), the female genital tract, and the skin. Although cases of candidiasis have been described since antiquity in debilitated patients, the advent of *Candida* species as common human pathogens dates to the introduction of modern therapeutic approaches that suppress normal host defense mechanisms. Of these relatively recent advances, the most important is the use of antibacterial agents that alter the normal human microbial flora and allow nonbacterial species to become more prevalent in the commensal flora. With the introduction of antifungal agents, the causes of *Candida* infections shifted from an almost complete dominance of *C. albicans* to the common involvement of *C. glabrata* and the other species listed above. The non-*albicans* species now account for approximately half of all cases of candidemia and hematogenously disseminated candidiasis. Recognition of this change is clinically important, since the various species differ in susceptibility to the newer antifungal agents. In developed countries, where medical therapeutics are commonly used, *Candida* species are now among the most common nosocomial pathogens. In the United States, these species are the fourth most common isolates from the blood of hospitalized patients.

Candida is a small, thin-walled, ovoid yeast that measures 4–6 μm in diameter and reproduces by budding. Organisms of this genus occur in three forms in tissue: blastospores, pseudohyphae, and hyphae. *Candida* grows readily on simple medium; lysis centrifugation enhances its recovery from blood. Species are identified by biochemical testing (currently with automated devices) or on special agar.

PATHOGENESIS

In the most serious form of *Candida* infection, the organisms disseminate hematogenously and form microabscesses and small macroabscesses in major organs. Although the exact mechanism is not known, *Candida* probably enters the bloodstream from mucosal surfaces after growing to large numbers as a consequence of bacterial suppression by antibacterial drugs; alternatively, in some instances, the organism may enter from the skin. A change from the blastospore stage to the pseudohyphal and hyphal stages is generally considered integral to the organism's penetration into tissue. However, *C. glabrata* can cause extensive infection even though it does not transform into pseudohyphae or hyphae. Numerous reviews of cases of hematogenously disseminated candidiasis have identified the following predisposing factors or conditions: antibacterial agents, indwelling intravascular catheters, hyperalimentation fluids, indwelling urinary catheters, parenteral glucocorticoids, respirators, neutropenia, abdominal and thoracic surgery, cytotoxic chemotherapy, and immunosuppressive agents for organ transplantation. Patients with severe burns, low-birth-weight neonates, and persons using illicit IV drugs are also susceptible. HIV-infected patients with low CD4+ T cell counts and patients with diabetes are susceptible to mucocutaneous infection, which may eventually develop into the disseminated form when other predisposing factors are encountered. Women who receive antibacterial agents may develop vaginal candidiasis.

Innate immunity is the most important defense mechanism against hematogenously disseminated candidiasis, and the neutrophil is the most important component of this defense. Although many immunocompetent individuals have antibodies to *Candida*, the role of these antibodies in defense against the organism is not clear.

CLINICAL MANIFESTATIONS

Mucocutaneous Candidiasis *Thrush* is characterized by white, adherent, painless, discrete or confluent patches in the mouth, tongue, or esophagus, occasionally with fissuring at the corners of the mouth. This form of *Candida* disease may also occur at points of contact with dentures. Organisms are identifiable in gram-stained scrapings from lesions. The occurrence of thrush in a young, otherwise healthy-appearing person should prompt an investigation for underlying HIV infection. More commonly, thrush is seen as a nonspecific manifestation of severe debilitating illness. Vulvovaginal candidiasis is accompanied by pruritus, pain, and vaginal discharge that is usually thin but may contain whitish "curds" in severe cases.

Other Candida *skin infections* include paronychia, a painful swelling at the nail-skin interface; onychomycosis, a fungal nail infection rarely caused by this genus; intertrigo, an erythematous irritation with redness and pustules in the skin folds; balanitis, an erythematous-pustular infection of the glans penis; erosio interdigitalis blastomycetica, an infection between the digits of the hands or toes; folliculitis, with pustules developing most frequently in the area of the beard; perianal candidiasis, a pruritic, erythematous, pustular infection surrounding the anus; and diaper rash, a common erythematous-pustular perineal infection in infants. Generalized disseminated cutaneous candidiasis, another form of infection that occurs primarily in infants, is characterized by widespread eruptions over the trunk, thorax, and extremities. The diagnostic macronodular lesions of hematogenously disseminated candidiasis (Fig. 196-1) indicate a high probability for dissemination to multiple organs as well as the skin. While the lesions are seen predominantly in immunocompromised patients treated with cytotoxic drugs, they may also develop in patients without neutropenia.

Chronic mucocutaneous candidiasis is a heterogeneous infection of the hair, nails, skin, and mucous membranes that persists despite intermittent therapy. The onset of disease usually comes in infancy or within the first two decades of life but in rare cases can come in later life. The condition may be mild and limited to a specific area of the skin or nails, or it may take a severely disfiguring form (*Candida* granuloma) characterized by exophytic outgrowths on the skin. The condition is usually associated with specific immunologic dysfunction; most frequently reported is a failure of T lymphocytes to proliferate or to stimulate cytokines in response to stimulation by *Candida* antigens in vitro. Approximately half of patients have associated endocrine abnormalities that together are designated the *a*utoimmune *p*olyendocri-

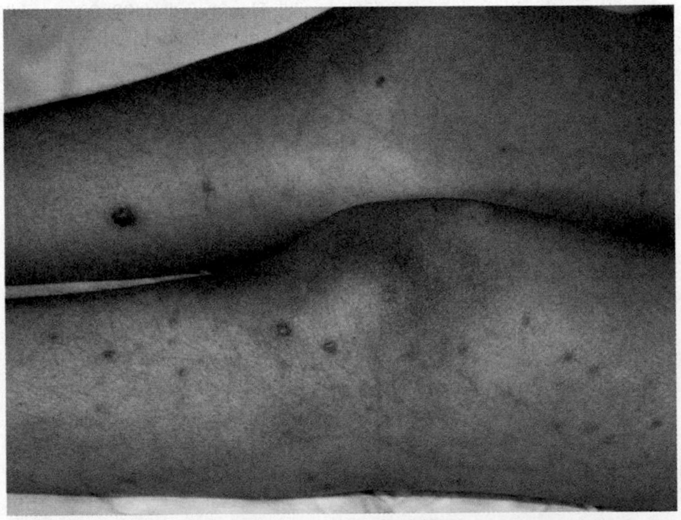

FIGURE 196-1 Macronodular skin lesions associated with hematogenously disseminated candidiasis. *Candida* organisms are usually but not always visible on histopathologic examination. The fungi grow when a portion of the biopsied specimen is cultured. Therefore, for optimal identification, both histopathology and culture should be performed. *(Image courtesy of Dr. Noah Craft and the Victor Newcomer collection at UCLA, archived by Logical Images, Inc.; with permission.)*

nopathy–candidiasis–ectodermal dystrophy (APECED) syndrome. This syndrome is due to mutations in the autoimmune regulator (*AIRE*) gene and is most prevalent among Finns, Iranian Jews, Sardinians, northern Italians, and Swedes. Conditions that usually follow the onset of the disease include hypoparathyroidism, adrenal insufficiency, autoimmune thyroiditis, Graves' disease, chronic active hepatitis, alopecia, juvenile-onset pernicious anemia, malabsorption, and primary hypogonadism. In addition, dental enamel dysplasia, vitiligo, pitted nail dystrophy, and calcification of the tympanic membranes may occur. Patients with chronic mucocutaneous candidiasis rarely develop hematogenously disseminated candidiasis, probably because their neutrophil function remains intact.

Deeply Invasive Candidiasis Deeply invasive *Candida* infections may or may not be due to hematogenous seeding. Deep esophageal infection may result from penetration by organisms from superficial esophageal erosions; joint or deep wound infection from contiguous spread of organisms from the skin; kidney infection from catheter-initiated spread of organisms through the urinary tract; infection of intraabdominal organs and the peritoneum from perforation of the gastrointestinal tract; and gallbladder infection from retrograde migration of organisms from the gastrointestinal tract into the biliary drainage system.

However, far more commonly, deeply invasive candidiasis is a result of hematogenous seeding of various organs as a complication of candidemia. Once the organism gains access to the intravascular compartment (either from the gastrointestinal tract or, less often, from the skin through the site of an indwelling intravascular catheter), it may spread hematogenously to a variety of deep organs. The brain, chorioretina (Fig. 196-2), heart, and kidneys are most commonly infected and the liver and spleen less commonly so (most often in neutropenic patients). In fact, nearly any organ can become involved, including the endocrine glands, pancreas, heart valves (native or prosthetic), skeletal muscle, joints (native or prosthetic), bone, and meninges. *Candida* organisms may also spread hematogenously to the skin and cause classic macronodular lesions (Fig. 196-1). Frequently, painful muscular involvement is also evident beneath the area of affected skin. Chorioretinal involvement and skin involvement are highly significant, since both findings are associated with a very high probability of abscess formation in multiple deep organs as a result of generalized hematogenous seeding. Ocular involvement (Fig. 196-2) may require specific treatment, such as partial vitrectomy to prevent permanent blindness.

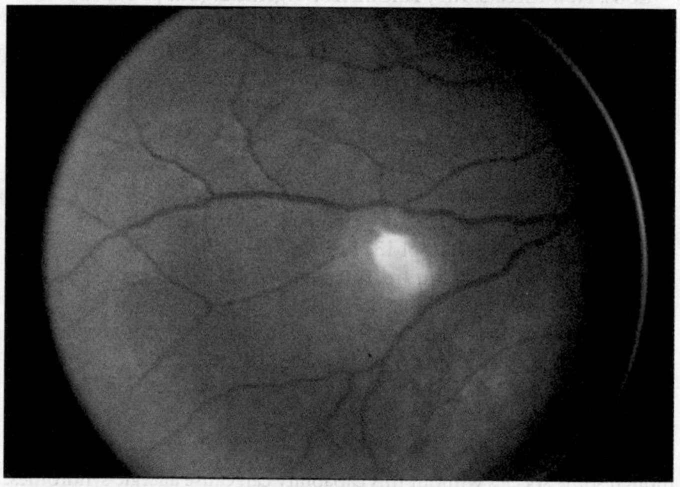

FIGURE 196-2 Hematogenous *Candida* endophthalmitis. A classic off-white lesion projecting from the chorioretina into the vitreous causes the surrounding haze. The lesion is composed primarily of inflammatory cells rather than organisms. Lesions of this type may progress to cause extensive vitreal inflammation and eventual loss of the eye. Partial vitrectomy, combined with IV and possibly intravitreal antifungal therapy, may be helpful in controlling the lesions. *(Image courtesy of Dr. Gary Holland; with permission.)*

TABLE 196-1 TREATMENT OF MUCOCUTANEOUS CANDIDAL INFECTIONS

Disease	Preferred Treatment	Alternatives
Cutaneous	Topical azole	Topical nystatin
Vulvovaginal	Oral fluconazole (150 mg) or azole cream or suppository	Nystatin suppository
Thrush	Clotrimazole troches	Nystatin
Esophageal	Fluconazole tablets (100–200 mg/d) or itraconazole solution (200 mg/d)	Caspofungin, micafungin, or amphotericin B

An ocular examination is indicated for all patients with candidemia, whether or not they have ocular manifestations.

DIAGNOSIS

The diagnosis of *Candida* infection is established by visualization of pseudohyphae or hyphae on wet mount (saline and 10% KOH), tissue Gram's stain, periodic acid–Schiff stain, or methenamine silver stain in the presence of inflammation. Absence of organisms on hematoxylin-eosin staining does not reliably exclude *Candida* infection. The most challenging aspect of diagnosis is determining which patients with *Candida* isolates have hematogenously disseminated candidiasis. For instance, recovery of *Candida* from sputum, urine, or peritoneal catheters may indicate mere colonization rather than deep-seated infection, and *Candida* isolation from the blood of patients with indwelling intravascular catheters may reflect inconsequential seeding of the blood from or growth of the organisms on the catheter. Despite extensive research into both antigen and antibody detection systems, there is currently no widely available and validated diagnostic test to distinguish patients with inconsequential seeding of the blood from those whose positive blood cultures represent hematogenous dissemination to multiple organs. Many studies are under way to establish the utility of the β-glucan test. Meanwhile, the presence of ocular or macronodular skin lesions is highly suggestive of widespread infection of multiple deep organs.

Rx *CANDIDA* INFECTIONS

MUCOCUTANEOUS *CANDIDA* INFECTION The treatment of mucocutaneous candidiasis is summarized in **Table 196-1**.

CANDIDEMIA AND SUSPECTED HEMATOGENOUSLY DISSEMINATED CANDIDIASIS All patients with candidemia are now treated with a systemic antifungal agent. A certain percentage of patients, including many of those who have candidemia associated with an indwelling intravascular catheter, probably have "benign" candidemia rather than deep-organ seeding. However, because there is no reliable way to distinguish benign candidemia from deep-organ infection, and because antifungal drugs less toxic than amphotericin B are available, it has become the standard of practice to treat all patients with candidemia, whether or not there is clinical evidence of deep-organ involvement. In addition, if an indwelling intravascular catheter may be involved, it is best to remove or replace the device whenever possible.

The drugs used for the treatment of candidemia and suspected disseminated candidiasis are listed in **Table 196-2**. Various lipid formulations of amphotericin B, three echinocandins, and the azoles fluconazole and voriconazole are used; no agent within a given class has been clearly identified as superior to the others. Most institutions choose an agent from each class on the basis of their own specific microbial epidemiology, strategies to minimize toxicities, and cost considerations. Unless azole resistance is considered likely, fluconazole is the agent of choice for the treatment of candidemia and suspected disseminated candidiasis in nonneutropenic, hemodynamically stable patients. Initial treatment in the context of likely azole resistance depends, as mentioned above, on the epidemiology of the individual hospital. For example, certain hospitals have a high rate of recovery of *C. glabrata*, while others do not. For hemodynamically unstable or neutropenic patients, initial treatment with broader-spectrum agents is desirable; these drugs include polyenes, echinocandins, or later-generation azoles such as voriconazole. Once the clinical response has been assessed and the pathogen specifically identified, the regimen can be altered

TABLE 196-2 AVAILABLE AGENTS FOR THE TREATMENT OF DISSEMINATED CANDIDIASIS

Agent	Route of Administration	Comment
Amphotericin B deoxycholate	IV only	Being replaced by lipid formulations
Amphotericin B lipid formulations		Not FDA approved as primary therapy, but used commonly because less toxic than amphotericin B deoxycholate; ABCD associated with frequent infusion reactions
Liposomal (AmBisome, Abelcet)	IV only	
Lipid complex (ABLC)	IV only	
Colloidal dispersion (ABCD)	IV only	
Azoles		
Fluconazole	IV and oral	Most commonly used
Voriconazole	IV and oral	Multiple drug interactions
Echinocandins		Broad spectrum against *Candida* species
Caspofungin	IV only	Approved for disseminated candidiasis
Anidulafungin	IV only	Approved for disseminated candidiasis
Micafungin	IV only	Under evaluation for disseminated candidiasis

Note: Although ketoconazole is approved for the treatment of disseminated candidiasis, it has been replaced by the newer agents listed in this table.
Abbreviation: FDA, U.S. Food and Drug Administration.

accordingly. At present, the vast majority of *C. albicans* isolates are sensitive to fluconazole. Isolates of *C. glabrata* and *C. krusei* are less sensitive to fluconazole and more sensitive to polyenes and echinocandins. *C. parapsilosis* is less sensitive to echinocandins in vitro, although the clinical significance of this finding is not known.

Some generalizations about the management of specific *Candida* infections are possible. Recovery of *Candida* from sputum is almost never indicative of underlying pulmonary candidiasis and does not by itself warrant antifungal treatment. Similarly, *Candida* in the urine of a patient with an indwelling bladder catheter may represent colonization only rather than bladder or kidney infection; however, the threshold for systemic treatment is lower in severely ill patients in this category since it is not possible to distinguish colonization from lower or upper urinary tract infection. If the isolate is *C. albicans*, most clinicians use oral fluconazole rather than a bladder washout with amphotericin, which was more commonly used in the past. The significance of the recovery of *Candida* from abdominal drains in postoperative patients is also unclear, but again, the threshold for treatment is generally low because most of the affected patients have been subjected to factors predisposing to disseminated candidiasis.

Removal of the infected valve and long-term antifungal therapy constitute appropriate treatment for *Candida* endocarditis. Although definitive studies are not available, patients usually are treated for weeks with a systemic antifungal agent and then given chronic suppressive therapy for months or years (and sometimes indefinitely) with an oral azole.

Hematogenous *Candida* endophthalmitis is a special problem requiring ophthalmologic consultation. In lesions that are expanding or that threaten the macula, an IV polyene combined with flucytosine has been the regimen of choice. However, as more data on the azoles and echinocandins become available, new strategies may evolve. Of paramount importance is the decision to perform a partial vitrectomy. This procedure debulks the infection and can preserve sight, which may otherwise be lost as a result of vitreal scarring. All patients with candidemia should undergo ophthalmologic examination because of the relatively high frequency of this ocular complication. Not only can this examination detect a developing eye lesion early in its course; in addition, identification of a lesion signifies a probability of ~90% of deep-organ abscesses and may prompt prolongation of therapy for candidemia beyond the recommended 2 weeks after the last positive blood culture.

Although the basis for the consensus is a very small data set, the recommended treatment for *Candida* meningitis is a polyene plus flucytosine. Successful treatment of *Candida*-infected prosthetic material (e.g., an artificial joint) nearly always requires removal of the infected material followed by long-term administration of an antifungal agent selected on the basis of the isolate's sensitivity and the logistics of administration.

PROPHYLAXIS

The use of antifungal agents to prevent *Candida* infections has been controversial, but some general principles have emerged. Most centers administer prophylactic fluconazole (400 mg/d) to recipients of allogeneic stem cell transplants. High-risk liver transplant recipients are also given fluconazole prophylaxis in most centers. The use of prophylaxis for neutropenic patients has varied considerably from center to center; most centers that elect to give prophylaxis to this population use either fluconazole or a comparatively low dose of an IV polyene—either amphotericin B deoxycholate or a lipid formulation of this agent. Some centers have used itraconazole suspension.

Prophylaxis is sometimes given to surgical patients at very high risk. The widespread use of prophylaxis in general surgical or medical intensive care units is not—and should not be—a common practice for three reasons: (1) the incidence of disseminated candidiasis is relatively low, (2) the cost-benefit ratio is suboptimal, and (3) increased resistance with widespread prophylaxis is a valid concern.

Prophylaxis for oropharyngeal or esophageal candidiasis in HIV-infected patients is not recommended unless there are frequent recurrences.

FURTHER READINGS

EDWARDS JE JR: Candidiasis, in *Principles and Practice of Infectious Diseases*, 6th ed, GL Mandell et al (eds). Philadelphia, Elsevier Churchill Livingstone, 2005, pp 2938–2973

KAUFFMAN CA: Clinical efficacy of new antifungal agents. Curr Opin Microbiol 9:1, 2006

MASCHMEYER G: The changing epidemiology of invasive fungal infections: New threats. Int J Antimicrob Agents 27(Suppl 1):3, 2006

OSTROSKY-ZEICHNER L et al: Multicenter clinical evaluation of the (1→3) beta-D-glucan assay as an aid to diagnosis of fungal infections in humans. Clin Infect Dis 41:654, 2005

PAPPAS PG et al: Guidelines for treatment of candidiasis. Clin Infect Dis 38:161, 2004

RUHNKE M: Epidemiology of *Candida albicans* infections and role of non-*Candida-albicans* yeasts. Curr Drug Targets 7:495, 2006

SOBEL JD: Current trends and challenges in candidiasis. Oncology (Williston Park) 18(Suppl 13):7, 2004

SPELLBERG BJ et al: Current treatment strategies for disseminated candidiasis. Clin Infect Dis 42:244, 2006

TORTORANO AM et al: Candidaemia in Europe: Epidemiology and resistance. Int J Antimicrob Agents 27:359, 2006

197 Aspergillosis

David W. Denning

Aspergillosis is the collective term used to describe all disease entities caused by any one of ~35 pathogenic and allergenic species of *Aspergillus*. Only those species that grow at 37°C can cause invasive infection, although some species without this capability can cause allergic syndromes. *A. fumigatus* is responsible for most cases of invasive aspergillosis, almost all cases of chronic aspergillosis, and most allergic syndromes. *A. flavus* is more prevalent in some hospitals and causes a higher proportion of cases of sinus and cutaneous infection and keratitis than *A. fumigatus*. *A. niger* can cause invasive infection but more commonly colonizes the respiratory tract and causes external otitis. *A. terreus* causes only invasive disease, usually with a poor prognosis. *A. nidulans* occasionally causes invasive infection, primarily in patients with chronic granulomatous disease.

EPIDEMIOLOGY AND ECOLOGY

Aspergillus has a worldwide distribution, most commonly growing in decomposing plant materials (i.e., compost) and in bedding. This hyaline (nonpigmented), septate, branching mold produces vast numbers of conidia (spores) on stalks above the surface of mycelial growth. Aspergilli are found in indoor and outdoor air, on surfaces, and in water from surface reservoirs. Daily exposures vary from a few to many millions of conidia; the latter high numbers of conidia are encountered in hay barns and other very dusty environments. The required size of the infecting inoculum is uncertain; however, only intense exposures (e.g., during construction work, handling of moldy bark or hay, or composting) are sufficient to cause disease in healthy immunocompetent individuals. Allergic syndromes may be exacerbated by continuous antigenic exposure arising from sinus or airway colonization or from nail infection. High-efficiency particulate air (HEPA) filtration is often protective against infection; thus HEPA filters should be installed and monitored for efficiency in operating rooms and in hospital environments that house very high-risk patients.

The incubation period of invasive aspergillosis after exposure is highly variable, extending in documented cases from 2 to 90 days. Thus community-acquired acquisition of an infecting strain frequently manifests as invasive infection during hospitalization, although nosocomial acquisition is also common. Outbreaks usually are directly related to a contaminated air source in the hospital.

TABLE 197-1 MAJOR MANIFESTATIONS OF ASPERGILLOSIS

	Major Manifestations in Indicated Type of Disease			
Organ	**Invasive (Acute and Subacute)**	**Chronic**	**Saprophytic**	**Allergic**
Lung	Angioinvasive in neutropenia, non-angioinvasive, granulomatous	Chronic cavitary, chronic fibrosing	Aspergilloma (single), airway colonization	Allergic bronchopulmonary, severe asthma with fungal sensitization, extrinsic allergic alveolitis
Sinus	Acute invasive	Chronic invasive, chronic granulomatous	Maxillary fungal ball	Allergic fungal sinusitis, eosinophilic fungal rhinosinusitis
Brain	Abscess, hemorrhagic infarction, meningitis, mycotic cerebral aneurysm	Granulomatous, meningitis	None	None
Skin	Acute disseminated, locally invasive (trauma, burns, IV access)	External otitis, onychomycosis	None	None
Heart	Endocarditis (native or prosthetic), pericarditis	None	None	None
Eye	Keratitis, endophthalmitis (postoperative and disseminated)	None	None	None described

RISK FACTORS AND PATHOGENESIS

The primary risk factors for invasive aspergillosis are profound neutropenia and glucocorticoid use; risk increases with longer duration of these conditions. Higher doses of glucocorticoids increase the risk of both acquisition of invasive aspergillosis and death from the infection. Neutrophil and/or phagocyte dysfunction is also an important risk factor, as evidenced by aspergillosis in chronic granulomatous disease, advanced HIV infection, and relapsed leukemia. An increasing incidence of invasive aspergillosis in medical intensive care units suggests that, in patients who are not immunocompromised, temporary abrogation of protective responses as a result of glucocorticoid use or a general anti-inflammatory state is a significant risk factor. Many patients have some evidence of prior pulmonary disease—typically, a history of pneumonia or chronic obstructive pulmonary disease. Glucocorticoid use does not appear to predispose to invasive *Aspergillus* sinusitis but probably increases the risk of dissemination after pulmonary infection.

Patients with chronic pulmonary aspergillosis have a wide spectrum of underlying pulmonary disease, often tuberculosis or sarcoidosis. Patients are immunocompetent except that a genetic defect in mannose-binding protein is common, as are some cytokine regulation defects, most of which are consistent with an inability to mount an inflammatory immune (T_H1-like) response. Glucocorticoids accelerate disease progression.

Allergic bronchopulmonary aspergillosis (ABPA) is associated with certain HLA class II types; polymorphisms of interleukin (IL) 4Ra, IL-10, and SPA2 genes; and heterozygosity of the cystic fibrosis transmembrane conductance regulator (*CFTR*) gene. These associations suggest a strong genetic basis for the development of a T_H2-like and "allergic" response to *A. fumigatus*; this response probably is also protective against invasive disease, since high-dose glucocorticoid treatment for exacerbations of ABPA almost never leads to invasive aspergillosis.

CLINICAL FEATURES AND APPROACH TO THE PATIENT

(Table 197-1)

Invasive Pulmonary Aspergillosis Both the frequency of invasive disease and the pace of its progression increase with greater degrees of immunocompromise (Fig. 197-1). Invasive aspergillosis is arbitrarily divided into acute and subacute forms that have courses of ≤1 month and 1–3 months, respectively. More than 80% of cases of invasive aspergillosis involve the lungs. The most common clinical features are no symptoms at all, fever, cough (sometimes productive), nondescript chest discomfort, trivial hemoptysis, and shortness of breath. Although the fever often responds to glucocorticoids, the disease progresses. The keys to early diagnosis in at-risk patients are a high index of suspicion, screening for circulating antigen, and urgent CT of the thorax.

Invasive Sinusitis The sinuses are involved in 5–10% of cases of invasive aspergillosis, especially in patients with leukemia and recipients of hematopoietic stem cell transplants. In addition to fever, the most common features are nasal or facial discomfort, blocked nose, and nasal discharge (sometimes bloody). Direct examination of the interior of the nose reveals dusky or necrotic-looking tissue in any location. CT or MRI of the sinuses is essential but does not distinguish invasive *Aspergillus* sinusitis from pre-existing allergic sinusitis, bacterial sinusitis, or other fungal sinusitis early in the disease process.

Disseminated Aspergillosis In the most severely immunocompromised patients, *Aspergillus* disseminates from the lungs to multiple organs—most often to the brain but also to the skin, thyroid, bone, kidney, liver, gastrointestinal tract, eye, and heart valve. Aside from cutaneous lesions, the most common features are gradual clinical deterioration over 1–3 days, with low-grade fever and features of mild sepsis, and multiple nonspecific abnormalities in laboratory tests. In most cases, at least one localization becomes apparent. Blood cultures are not helpful since they are almost always negative.

Cerebral Aspergillosis Hematogenous dissemination to the brain is a devastating complication of invasive aspergillosis. Single or multiple lesions may develop. In acute disease, hemorrhagic infarction is most typical, and cerebral abscess is common. Rarer manifestations include meningitis, mycotic aneurysm, and cerebral granuloma. Local spread also occurs, resulting in a single abscess. Postoperative infection from cranial sinuses is occasionally recorded and is exacerbated by glucocorticoid use after neurosurgery. The presentation can be either acute or subacute, with mood changes, focal signs, seizures, and decline in mental status. Cerebral granuloma can mimic a primary or secondary tumor. MRI is the most useful immediate investigation; unenhanced CT of the brain is usually nonspecific, and contrast is often contraindicated in the affected patients because of poor renal function.

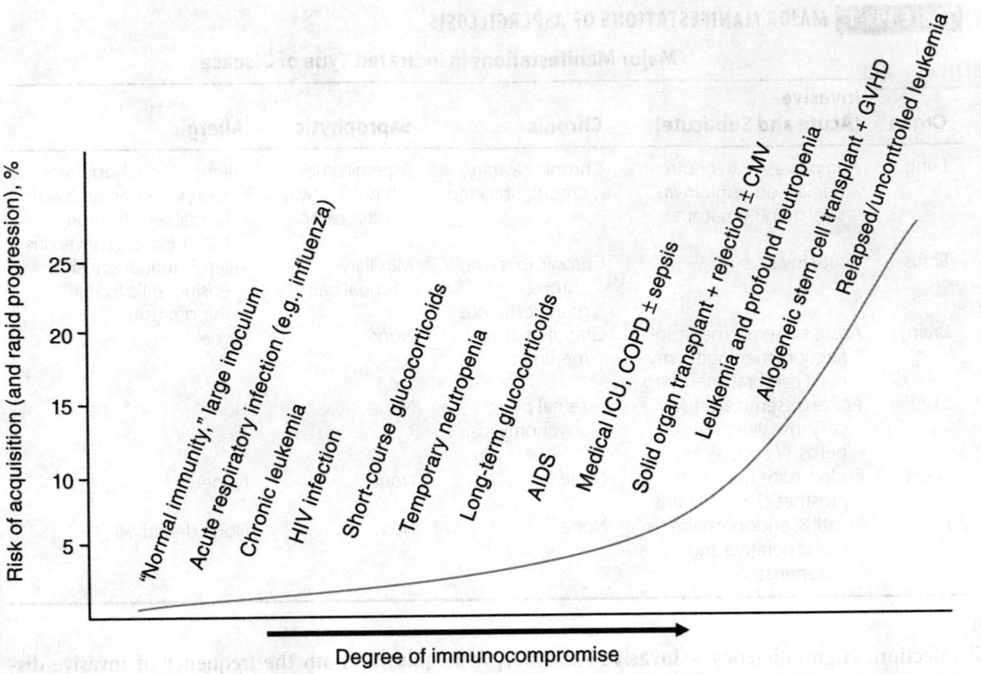

FIGURE 197-1 Invasive aspergillosis: conditions placing patients at elevated risk of acquisition and relatively rapid progression. ICU, intensive care unit; COPD, chronic obstructive pulmonary disease; CMV, cytomegalovirus; GVHD, graft-vs-host disease.

Endocarditis Most cases of *Aspergillus* endocarditis are prosthetic valve infections resulting from contamination during surgery. Native valve disease is reported, especially as a feature of disseminated infection and in persons using illicit IV drugs. Culture-negative endocarditis with large vegetations is the most common presentation, but embolectomy reveals the diagnosis in a few cases.

Cutaneous Aspergillosis Dissemination of *Aspergillus* occasionally results in cutaneous features, usually an erythematous or purplish nontender area that progresses to a necrotic eschar. Direct invasion of the skin occurs in neutropenic patients at the site of IV catheter insertion and in burn patients. Rapidly progressive local aspergillosis of the skin and underlying tissue may follow trauma, and wounds may become infected with *Aspergillus* after surgery.

Chronic Pulmonary Aspergillosis The hallmark of chronic cavitary pulmonary aspergillosis (also called semi-invasive aspergillosis, chronic necrotizing aspergillosis, or complex aspergilloma) (Fig. 197-2) is one or more pulmonary cavities expanding over a period of months or years in association with pulmonary symptoms and systemic manifestations such as fatigue and weight loss. (Pulmonary aspergillosis developing over <3 months is better classified as subacute invasive aspergillosis.) Often mistaken initially for tuberculosis, almost all cases occur in patients with prior pulmonary disease (e.g., tuberculosis, atypical mycobacterial infection, sarcoidosis, ankylosing spondylitis, rheumatoid lung disease, pneumothorax, bullae) or prior lung surgery. The onset is insidious, and systemic features are sometimes more prominent than pulmonary symptoms. Cavities may have a fluid level or a well-formed fungal ball, but pericavitary infiltrates and multiple cavities—with or without pleural thickening—are typical. Antibodies to *Aspergillus* are almost always detectable in blood, usually as precipitating antibody and sometimes at high titers. Some patients have concurrent infections—even without a fungal ball—with atypical mycobacteria and/or other bacterial pathogens, such as *Staphylococcus aureus* or *Pseudomonas aeruginosa*. If untreated, chronic pulmonary aspergillosis typically progresses (sometimes relatively rapidly) to unilateral or upper-lobe fibrosis. This end-stage entity is termed *chronic fibrosing pulmonary aspergillosis*.

Aspergilloma Aspergilloma (fungal ball) occurs in up to 20% of residual chest cavities ≥2 cm in diameter. Some fungal balls remain stable in a single cavity for many years, and 10% resolve spontaneously. However, aspergillomas are often a feature of chronic pulmonary aspergillosis with its associated features. Signs and symptoms associated with single (simple) aspergillomas are minor, including a cough (sometimes productive), hemoptysis, wheezing, and mild fatigue. More significant signs and symptoms are associated with chronic cavitary pulmonary aspergillosis. The vast majority of fungal balls are caused by *A. fumigatus*, but *A. niger* has been implicated, particularly in diabetic patients; aspergillomas due to *A. niger* can lead to oxalosis with renal dysfunction. The most significant complication of aspergilloma is life-threatening hemoptysis, which may be the presenting manifestation.

Chronic Sinusitis Three entities are subsumed under this broad label: sinus aspergilloma, chronic invasive sinusitis, and chronic granulomatous sinusitis. *Sinus aspergilloma* is limited to the maxillary sinus and consists of a chronic saprophytic entity in which the sinus cavity is filled with a fungal ball. This form of disease is associated with prior upper-jaw root canal work and chronic (bacterial) sinusitis. About 90% of CT scans show focal hyperattenuation related to concretions; on MRI scans, the T2-weighted signal is decreased, whereas that of bacterial sinusitis is increased. Removal of the fungal ball is curative. No tissue invasion is demonstrable histologically or radiologically.

In contrast, *chronic invasive sinusitis* is a slowly destructive process that most commonly affects the ethmoid and sphenoid sinuses but can involve any sinus. Patients are usually but not always immunocompro-

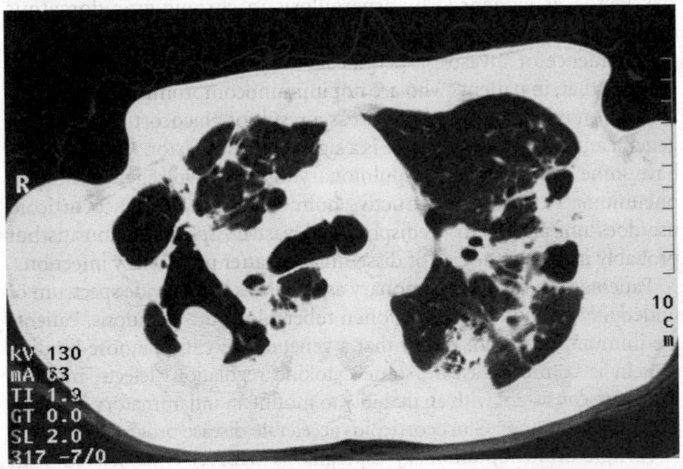

FIGURE 197-2 CT scan image of the chest in a patient with longstanding bilateral chronic cavitary pulmonary aspergillosis. He had a prior history of several bilateral pneumothoraces and required bilateral pleurodesis (1990). CT scan then demonstrated multiple bullae, and sputum cultures grew *A. fumigatus*. The patient had initially weakly and later strongly positive serum *Aspergillus* antibody tests (precipitins). This scan (2003) shows a mixture of thick- and thin-walled cavities in both lungs, with a large cavity containing a probable fungal ball protruding into the large cavity on the right. There is also considerable pleural thickening bilaterally.

mised to some degree (e.g., as a result of diabetes or HIV infection). Imaging of the cranial sinuses shows opacification of one or more sinuses, local bone destruction, and invasion of local structures. The differential diagnosis is wide, as numerous other fungi may cause a similar disease and sphenoid sinusitis is often caused by bacteria. Apart from a history of chronic nasal discharge and blockage, loss of the sense of smell, and persistent headache, the usual presenting features are related to local involvement of critical structures. The orbital apex syndrome (blindness and proptosis) is characteristic. Facial swelling, cavernous sinus thrombosis, carotid artery occlusion, pituitary fossa, and brain and skull base invasion have been described.

Chronic granulomatous sinusitis due to *Aspergillus* is most commonly seen in the Middle East and India and is often caused by *A. flavus.* It typically presents late, with facial swelling and unilateral proptosis. The prominent granulomatous reaction histologically distinguishes this disease from chronic invasive sinusitis, in which tissue necrosis with a low-grade mixed-cell infiltrate is typical.

Allergic Bronchopulmonary Aspergillosis In almost all cases, ABPA represents a hypersensitivity reaction to *A. fumigatus*; rare cases are due to other aspergilli and other fungi. ABPA occurs in ~1% of patients with asthma and in up to 15% of adults with cystic fibrosis, and occasional cases are reported in patients without either of these diseases. Episodes of bronchial obstruction with mucous plugs leading to coughing fits, "pneumonia," consolidation, and breathlessness are typical. Many patients report coughing up thick sputum casts, usually brown or clear. Eosinophilia commonly develops before systemic glucocorticoids are given. The cardinal diagnostic tests include an elevated serum level of total IgE (usually >1000 IU/mL), a positive skin-prick test to *A. fumigatus* extract, or detection of *Aspergillus*-specific IgE and IgG (precipitating) antibodies. Central bronchiectasis is characteristic, but patients may present before it becomes apparent.

Severe Asthma with Fungal Sensitization (SAFS) Many adults with severe asthma do not fulfill the criteria for ABPA and yet are allergic to fungi. Although *A. fumigatus* is a common allergen, numerous other fungi (e.g., *Cladosporium* and *Alternaria* spp.) are implicated by skin-prick testing and/or specific IgE radioallergosorbent (RAST) testing.

Allergic Sinusitis Like the lungs, the sinuses manifest allergic responses to *Aspergillus* and other fungi. The affected patients present with chronic (i.e., perennial) sinusitis typically requiring multiple course of antibiotics that are of only limited benefit. Many of these patients have nasal polyps, and all have congested nasal mucosa and sinuses full of mucoid material. The histologic hallmark of allergic fungal sinusitis is local eosinophilia and the breakdown products of eosinophils, Charcot-Leyden crystals. Removal of abnormal mucus and polyps, with local and occasionally systemic administration of glucocorticoids, usually leads to resolution. Persistent or recurrent signs and symptoms may require more extensive surgery (ethmoidectomy) and possibly local antifungal therapy.

Superficial Aspergillosis *Aspergillus* can cause keratitis and otitis externa. The former may be difficult to diagnose early enough to save the patient's sight. Treatment requires local surgical debridement as well as both systemic and topical antifungal therapy. Otitis externa is a common problem for which local debridement and local application of antifungal agents constitute the most common approach to treatment.

DIAGNOSIS

Several techniques are required to establish the diagnosis of any form of aspergillosis with confidence. Patients with acute invasive aspergillosis have a relatively heavy load of fungus in the affected organ; thus culture, molecular diagnosis, antigen detection, and histopathology usually confirm the diagnosis. However, the pace of progression leaves only a narrow window for making the diagnosis without losing the patient, and some invasive procedures are not possible because of coagulopathy, respiratory compromise, and other factors. Currently, ~40% of cases of invasive aspergillosis are missed clinically and are diagnosed only at autopsy. Histologic examination of affected tissue reveals either infarction, with invasion of blood vessels by many fungal hyphae, or acute necrosis, with limited inflammation and hyphae. *Aspergillus* hyphae are hyaline, narrow, and septate, with branching at 45°; no yeast forms are present in infected tissue. Hyphae can be seen in cytology or microscopy preparations, which therefore provide a rapid means of presumptive diagnosis.

Culture is important in confirming the diagnosis, given that multiple other (rarer) fungi can mimic *Aspergillus* spp. histologically. Bacterial agar is less sensitive than fungal media for culture. Thus, if physicians do not request fungal culture, the diagnosis may be missed. Culture may be falsely positive (e.g., in patients whose airways are colonized by *Aspergillus*) or falsely negative. Only 10–30% of patients with invasive aspergillosis have a positive culture at any time. Molecular diagnostic techniques promise to be both faster and more sensitive than culture.

The *Aspergillus* antigen test relies on detection of galactomannan release from *Aspergillus* spp. during growth. Antigen testing in high-risk patients is best done prospectively, as positive results usually precede clinical or radiologic features by several days. Antigen testing may be falsely positive in patients receiving certain β-lactam/β-lactamase inhibitor antibiotic combinations, such as tazocillin/sulbactam and amoxicillin/clavulanic acid; in these cases, a second test is required for confirmation. Antigen testing and molecular testing on bronchoalveolar lavage fluid and cerebrospinal fluid are useful if performed before antifungal therapy has been given for more than a few days. The sensitivity of antigen detection is reduced by antifungal prophylaxis.

Definitive confirmation of the diagnosis requires (1) a positive culture of a sample taken directly from an ordinarily sterile site (e.g., a brain abscess) or (2) positive results of both histologic testing and culture of a sample taken from an affected organ (e.g., sinuses or skin). Most diagnoses of invasive aspergillosis are inferred from fewer data, including the presence of the *halo sign* on a high-resolution thoracic CT scan, in which a localized ground-glass appearance representing hemorrhagic infarction surrounds a nodule. While a halo sign may be produced by other fungi, *Aspergillus* spp. are by far the most common cause. Halo signs are present for ~7 days early in the course of infection in neutropenic patients and are a good prognostic feature. Thick CT sections can give the false appearance of a halo sign, as can other technical factors. Other common radiologic features of invasive pulmonary aspergillosis include pleural-based infarction or cavitation.

For chronic invasive aspergillosis, *Aspergillus* antibody testing is invaluable although relatively imprecise. Titers fall with successful therapy. Cultures are infrequently positive. Some patients with chronic pulmonary aspergillosis also have elevated titers of total serum IgE and *Aspergillus*-specific IgE.

ABPA and SAFS are diagnosed serologically or with skin-prick tests. Allergic *Aspergillus* sinusitis is usually diagnosed histologically, although precipitating antibodies in blood may also be useful.

Rx ASPERGILLOSIS

Antifungal drugs active against *Aspergillus* include voriconazole, itraconazole, posaconazole, caspofungin, micafungin, and amphotericin B. Initial IV administration is preferred for acute invasive aspergillosis and oral administration for all other disease that requires antifungal therapy. Current recommendations are shown in **Table 197-2.** Voriconazole is the preferred agent for invasive aspergillosis; caspofungin, posaconazole, and lipid-associated amphotericin B are second-line agents. Amphotericin B is not active against *A. terreus* or *A. nidulans.* An infectious disease consultation is advised for patients with invasive disease, given the complexity of management. It is not clear whether combination therapy for acute invasive aspergillosis is beneficial, but it is widely used for very ill patients and for those with a poor prognosis. Commonly used combinations include an azole with either caspofungin or micafungin. The interactions of voriconazole and itraconazole with many drugs must be considered before these agents are prescribed. In addition, the effects of both drugs vary substantially from one patient to another, and many authorities recommend monitoring to ensure that drug concentrations are adequate but not excessive. The duration of therapy for invasive aspergillosis

TABLE 197-2 TREATMENT OF ASPERGILLOSIS

Indication	Primary Treatment	Evidence Level[a]	Precautions	Secondary Treatment	Comments
Invasive[a]	Voriconazole	AI	Drug interactions (especially with rifampin), renal failure (IV only)	Amphotericin B, caspofungin, posaconazole, micafungin	As primary therapy, voriconazole carries 20% more responses than amphotericin B. If azole prophylaxis fails, it is unclear whether a class change is required for therapy.
Prophylaxis	Itraconazole solution, posaconazole	AI	Diarrhea and vomiting with itraconazole, vincristine interaction	Micafungin, aerosolized amphotericin B	Some centers monitor plasma levels of itraconazole.
ABPA	Itraconazole	AI	Some glucocorticoid interactions, including with inhaled formulations	Voriconazole	Long-term therapy is helpful in most patients. Others can discontinue treatment. No evidence indicates whether or not therapy modifies progression to bronchiectasis/fibrosis.
Single aspergilloma	Surgery	BII	Multicavity disease: poor outcome of surgery; medical therapy preferable	Itraconazole, voriconazole, intracavity amphotericin B	Single large cavities with an aspergilloma are best resected.
Chronic pulmonary[b]	Itraconazole	BII	Poor absorption of capsules with proton pump inhibitors or H_2 blockers	Voriconazole, IV amphotericin B	Resistance may emerge during treatment, especially if plasma drug levels are subtherapeutic.

Note: The oral dose is usually 200 mg bid for voriconazole and itraconazole and 400 mg bid for posaconazole. The IV dose of voriconazole is 6 mg/kg twice at 12-h intervals (loading doses) followed by 4 mg/kg q12h. Plasma monitoring is helpful in optimizing the dosage. Caspofungin is given as a single loading dose of 70 mg, followed by 50 mg/d; some authorities use 70 mg/d for patients weighing >80 kg, and lower doses are required with hepatic dysfunction. Micafungin is given as 50 mg/d for prophylaxis and as at least 150 mg/d for treatment; this drug is not yet approved by the U.S. Food and Drug Administration (FDA) for this indication. Amphotericin B deoxycholate is given at a daily dose of 1 mg/kg if tolerated. Several strategies are available for minimizing renal dysfunction. Lipid-associated amphotericin B is given at 3 mg/kg (AmBisome) or 5 mg/kg (Abelcet). Different regimens are available for aerosolized amphotericin B, but none is FDA approved. Other considerations that may alter dose selection or route include age; concomitant medications; renal, hepatic, or intestinal dysfunction; and drug tolerability.

[a]Evidence levels are those used in treatment guidelines (Stevens DA et al: Practice guidelines for diseases caused by *Aspergillus*. Clin Infect Dis 30:696, 2000).

[b]An infectious disease consultation is appropriate for these patients.

varies from ~3 months to several years, depending on the patient's immune status and response to therapy. Relapse occurs if the response is suboptimal and immune reconstitution is not complete.

Itraconazole is the preferred oral agent for chronic and allergic forms of aspergillosis. Voriconazole and posaconazole can be substituted when failure, emergence of resistance, or adverse events occur. An itraconazole dose of 200 mg twice daily is recommended, with monitoring of drug concentrations in the blood. Chronic cavitary pulmonary aspergillosis probably requires life-long therapy, whereas the duration of treatment for other forms of chronic and allergic aspergillosis requires case-by-case evaluation.

Resistance to one or more azoles, although uncommon, may develop during long-term treatment, and a positive culture during antifungal therapy is an indication for susceptibility testing. Glucocorticoids should be used with caution in chronic cavitary pulmonary aspergillosis.

Surgical treatment is important in several forms of aspergillosis, including maxillary fungal ball and single aspergillomas, in which surgery is curative; invasive aspergillosis involving bone, heart valve, sinuses, proximal areas of the lung, and areas impinging on the great vessels; brain abscess; keratitis; and endophthalmitis. In allergic fungal sinusitis, removal of abnormal mucus and polyps, with local and occasionally systemic glucocorticoid treatment, usually leads to resolution. Persistent or recurrent signs and symptoms may require more extensive surgery (ethmoidectomy) and possibly local antifungal therapy. Surgery is problematic in chronic pulmonary aspergillosis, usually resulting in serious complications. Bronchial artery embolization is preferred for problematic hemoptysis.

PROPHYLAXIS

In situations in which moderate or high risk is predicted (e.g., after induction therapy for acute myeloid leukemia), the need for antifungal prophylaxis for superficial and systemic candidiasis and for invasive aspergillosis is generally accepted. Fluconazole is commonly used in these situations but has no activity against *Aspergillus* spp. Itraconazole capsules are ineffective, and itraconazole solution offers only modest efficacy. Posaconazole solution is probably more effective. Some data support the use of IV low-dose micafungin. No prophylactic regimen is completely successful.

OUTCOME

Invasive aspergillosis is curable if immune reconstitution occurs, whereas allergic and chronic forms are not. The mortality rate for invasive aspergillosis is ~50% if the infection is diagnosed and treated but is 100% if the diagnosis is missed. Cerebral aspergillosis, *Aspergillus* endocarditis, and bilateral extensive invasive pulmonary aspergillosis have very poor outcomes, as does invasive infection in patients with late-stage AIDS, patients with relapsed uncontrolled leukemia, and recipients of allogeneic hematopoietic stem cell transplants.

FURTHER READINGS

Clancy CJ et al: Bronchoalveolar lavage galactomannan in diagnosis of invasive aspergillosis among solid-organ transplant recipients. J Clin Microbiol 45:1759, 2007

Camuset J et al: Treatment of chronic pulmonary aspergillosis by voriconazole in nonimmunocompromised patients. Chest 131:1435, 2007

Denning DW et al: The link between fungi and asthma—a summary of the evidence. Eur Respir J 27:615, 2006

Herbrecht R et al: Voriconazole versus amphotericin B for primary therapy of invasive aspergillosis. N Engl J Med 347:408, 2002

Hope WW et al: Laboratory diagnosis of invasive aspergillosis. Lancet Infect Dis 9:609, 2005

——— et al: The invasive and saprophytic syndromes due to *Aspergillus* spp. Med Mycol 43(Suppl 1):S207, 2005

Meersseman W et al: Invasive aspergillosis in the intensive care unit. Clin Infect Dis 45:205, 2007

Moss RB: Pathophysiology and immunology of allergic bronchopulmonary aspergillosis. Med Mycol 43(Suppl1):S203, 2005

Pasqualotto AC, Denning DW: Post-operative aspergillosis. Clin Microbiol Rev 12:1060, 2006

Tekaia F, Latge JP: *Aspergillus fumigatus*: Saprophyte or pathogen? Curr Opin Microbiol 8:385, 2005

198 Mucormycosis

Alan M. Sugar

Mucormycosis (also called *zygomycosis*) is a serious, relatively uncommon invasive fungal infection and one of the most aggressive and lethal invasive mycoses. Physicians caring for patients with diabetes mellitus, immunocompromise (including that following organ transplantation), or iron overload syndromes (particularly those associated with hemodialysis) should be acutely aware of the enhanced susceptibility of these individuals to infection with the Mucorales. Timely diagnosis is critical to survival and minimization of morbidity. Institution of aggressive surgical and medical therapy is critical in maximizing the likelihood of a good outcome. Delay in considering the diagnosis and instituting appropriate therapeutic measures results in increasingly severe disfigurement at best and in death at worst.

ETIOLOGY

Fungi from the order Mucorales are the etiologic agents of mucormycosis. Despite the name of this infection, *Mucor* is not the most common genus recovered from patients. Rather, *Rhizopus* and *Rhizomucor* are the genera usually cultured from tissue samples. Other, less common fungi, including *Absidia*, *Cunninghamella*, *Apophysomyces*, and *Saksenaea*, are increasingly being isolated and, for the most part, cause similar clinical syndromes. Thus, there is no specific clinical feature that permits identification of the precise fungus involved. Submission of appropriate biopsy material to the microbiology laboratory is mandatory to ensure a pathogen's identification.

PATHOGENESIS

Mucorales are found commonly in the environment, and spores of these usually nonpathogenic fungi are likely to be inhaled daily. In the normal human lung, spores are inhibited from germinating into hyphae by alveolar macrophages. However, in diabetic patients, especially those with elevated blood sugar levels and acidemia, the spores germinate, hyphae develop (Fig. 198-1), and the fungi begin an inexorable march throughout the lung tissue, invading blood vessels and surrounding tissues. As blood vessels become involved, thrombosis occurs, tissue necrosis results, and the fungi continue to grow in this devitalized tissue. The use of deferoxamine to treat iron overload is a risk factor for mucormycosis; the siderophore supplies the fungi with iron that enhances their growth.

Spores settle in the upper airways, lower airways, or gastrointestinal tract and can spread beyond the initial site of infection, causing disseminated mucormycosis. Increasingly, patients are presenting with extensive cutaneous involvement after direct implantation of spores into the skin as a result of trauma (e.g., that sustained in a motor vehicle accident). The pathology in all these sites is the same, with blood vessel invasion and tissue necrosis as hallmarks and specific organ dysfunction depending on the location of the infection.

CLINICAL MANIFESTATIONS

The manifestations of mucormycosis depend on the site of infection. Patients with *rhinocerebral mucormycosis* may present with symptoms typical of sinusitis. However, progression of symptoms over several days indicates a more serious process than the more common bacterial or viral sinusitis. As the infection spreads, hypesthesia or numbness of the face overlying the infection may develop. Concomitant symptoms include headache, bloody nasal discharge, and changes in mental status. The black eschar of the palate is widely described as a hallmark of rhinocerebral mucormycosis, but the astute clinician will recognize earlier manifestations of this end-stage lesion reflecting invasion of the palate. These subtler lesions, which may consist of discolored, often hyperemic areas on the palate, will, if untreated, progress rapidly to the commonly recognized black eschar, which indicates angioinvasion and tissue necrosis. Involvement of the orbit (Fig. 198-2) compromises proper ocular-muscle function and normal movement of the eye within the skull, resulting in double vision. If the blood supply to the eye is affected by invasion of the retinal artery, blindness develops, often quite rapidly. Proptosis and ptosis are late findings reflecting a mass lesion within the orbit and cranial nerve involvement, respectively. Progression of the infection into the brain results in the formation of brain abscesses and phlegmon; symptoms and signs depend on the location of these lesions. Cavernous sinus thrombosis is an ominous sign. CT and MRI reveal sinus opacification and destruction of contiguous bone, and brain involvement can be readily appreciated.

Pulmonary mucormycosis presents as severe, progressive, tissue-destructive pneumonia. Neutropenia is a common predisposing factor. A high fever and a critical clinical condition are typical. Cavitation of involved lung develops rapidly, and hematogenous spread beyond the lungs to the brain and other organs may occur.

Gastrointestinal mucormycosis occurs primarily in those patients with protein-calorie malnutrition and usually presents as a perforated viscus. Premortem diagnosis is rare, and most patients with this form of mucormycosis do not survive.

Cutaneous mucormycosis is more common than disease at other sites and develops after traumatic injuries in which wounds are contaminated with dirt. Areas of tissue necrosis enlarge rapidly, involving all layers of the skin and underlying structures.

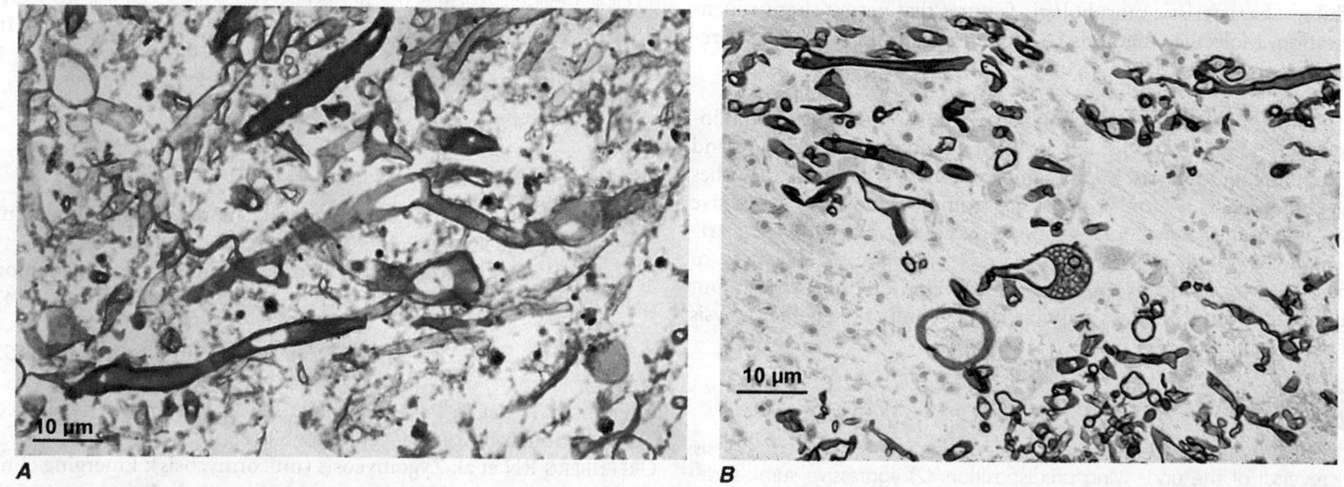

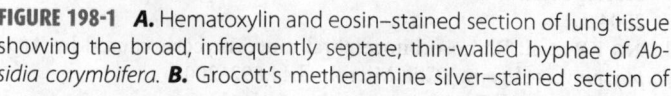

FIGURE 198-1 ***A.*** Hematoxylin and eosin–stained section of lung tissue showing the broad, infrequently septate, thin-walled hyphae of *Absidia corymbifera*. ***B.*** Grocott's methenamine silver–stained section of lung tissue showing typical zygomycete hyphae of *A. corymbifera*. *(Courtesy of David Ellis, PhD, Mycology Unit, Women's and Children's Hospital, Adelaide, Australia; with permission.)*

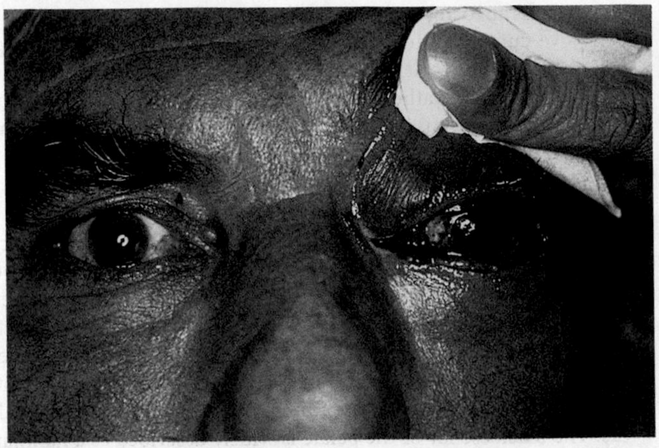

A

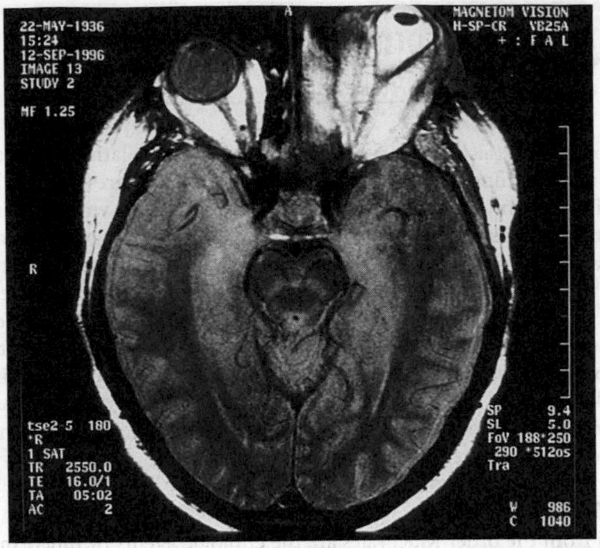

B

FIGURE 198-2 ***A.*** Rhinocerebral zygomycosis caused by *Rhizopus oryzae*, with extensive involvement of the orbit. ***B.*** Associated MRI scan. *(Courtesy of David Ellis, PhD, Mycology Unit, Women's and Children's Hospital, Adelaide, Australia; with permission.)*

DIAGNOSIS

Laboratory Features There are no pathognomonic hematologic changes. The abnormalities that are found reflect underlying predisposing conditions (e.g., diabetic ketoacidosis) and general indications of infection, such as elevated white blood cell counts and acute-phase reactant levels. Blood cultures are virtually always negative.

Microscopic examination and culture of biopsy samples from the involved area are critical in making an accurate diagnosis. As much tissue as possible should be submitted to the microbiology and histopathology laboratories. Swabs are insufficient. These fungi grow rapidly and are usually visible on culture plates within a day or two. Their identification is based on traditional morphologic features. Fixed tissue samples are treated with special stains for fungi; for example, Gomori methenamine silver stains the fungi black against a green background, and periodic acid–Schiff stains the hyphae red. Mucorales appear as broad (diameter, 6–50 μm), usually nonseptate hyphae with branches at right angles; the organisms are often described as ribbon-like. Hyphae cut and viewed on end can deceptively appear yeast-like. The microscopic appearance of the Mucorales is sufficiently different from that of *Aspergillus*, *Fusarium*, and other pathogenic molds (which characteristically appear as narrow, septate hyphae with narrow-angle branching) that a pathologist can readily make a preliminary diagnosis of mucormycosis. Identification of the specific organism requires culture. In the laboratory, each species of Mucorales exhibits characteristic morphologic features that permit specific identification. Molecular methods of speciation are still used only as research tools.

Differential Diagnosis Other fungal infections, including aspergillosis, fusariosis, and scedosporiosis, must be ruled out by culture and histopathologic analysis. Microscopic examination easily distinguishes the etiologic agents of these infections from the Mucorales. Aggressive pyogenic bacterial infections—e.g., those caused by *Pseudomonas*, *Aeromonas*, or *Vibrio* species; *Staphylococcus aureus*; and a variety of anaerobes—occasionally produce similar clinical presentations but can be ruled out by Gram's staining, culture, and microscopic analysis of tissue samples.

Rx MUCORMYCOSIS

Three factors are key to a successful outcome of therapy for mucormycosis: (1) reversal of the underlying predisposition; (2) aggressive surgical debridement; and (3) aggressive antifungal therapy, with early initiation and high drug doses. Failure to undertake all three of these interventions simultaneously has a significant and negative impact on outcome.

Reversal of underlying disease is relatively easy in patients with diabetic ketoacidosis but is more difficult in patients who require continued immunosuppression for control of an underlying disease or after organ transplantation. In all cases, minimization of immunosuppressive medications enhances overall control of the fungal infection.

Aggressive surgical debridement requires the removal of all dead tissue and of tissue that appears to be so severely compromised that its continued viability is in question. Extensive reconstructive surgery may be required once the infection has been cured.

Traditionally, high-dose conventional amphotericin B has been used for the treatment of mucormycosis, but doses have been limited to <1.5 mg/kg per day because of the nearly universal development of nephrotoxicity. Use of lipid formulations at doses of 15–20 mg/kg per day (AmBisome) or 15 mg/kg per day (Abelcet) maximizes the amount of amphotericin B delivered to the tissues as well as the speed of its delivery. At these doses, nephrotoxicity occurs in <50% of patients.

Posaconazole, an experimental triazole antifungal agent, has been shown to be active against mucormycosis in mouse models of infection and in patients who cannot tolerate or do not respond to other antifungal drugs. The precise clinical role for posaconazole in the treatment of mucormycosis is not clear, but this drug may prove to be a valuable alternative to amphotericin B in selected cases. Given the relative rarity of mucormycosis, it is not likely that a randomized study will rigorously compare the roles of the various antifungal agents.

The optimal duration of therapy for mucormycosis is not known precisely. If possible, antifungal administration should be continued for at least 3 months after (1) all clinical abnormalities resolve or stabilize, leaving no clinical evidence of infection at the involved site(s); and (2) scans, x-rays, and laboratory studies yield normal or stable results. Careful follow-up should continue for at least 1 year to confirm that there is no evidence of recurrent infection. With this approach, recurrences should be rare.

FURTHER READINGS

Chayakulkeeree M et al: Zygomycosis: The re-emerging fungal infection. Eur J Clin Microbiol Infect Dis 25:215, 2006

Davari HR et al: Outcome of mucormycosis in liver transplantation: Four cases and a review of literature. Exp Clin Transplant 1:147, 2003

Gonzalez CE et al: Zygomycosis. Infect Dis Clin North Am 16:895, 2002

Greenberg RN et al: Posaconazole as salvage therapy for zygomycosis. Antimicrob Agents Chemother 50:126, 2006

Greenberg RN et al: Zygomycosis (mucormycosis): Emerging clinical importance and new treatments. Curr Opin Infect Dis 17:517, 2004

Liang KP et al: Rhino-orbitocerebral mucormycosis caused by *Apophysomyces elegans*. J Clin Microbiol 44:892, 2006

O'Neill BM et al: Disseminated rhinocerebral mucormycosis: A case report and review of the literature. J Oral Maxillofac Surg 64:326, 2006

Prabhu RM et al: Mucormycosis and entomophthoramycosis: A review of the clinical manifestations, diagnosis and treatment. Clin Microbiol Infect 10(Suppl 1):31, 2004

Roden MM et al: Epidemiology and outcome of zygomycosis: A review of 929 reported cases. Clin Infect Dis 41:634, 2005

Spellberg B et al: Novel perspectives on mucormycosis: Pathophysiology, presentation, and management. Clin Microbiol Rev 18:556, 2005

199 Miscellaneous Mycoses and Algal Infections

Stanley W. Chapman, Donna C. Sullivan

MYCOSES

The clinical spectrum of fungal disease varies from superficial infections of the skin, hair, and nails to life-threatening systemic infections. Superficial infections involve the outermost layers of skin and hair and are associated with little or no inflammation. Cutaneous infections involve deeper layers of the skin, hair follicles, and nails and are accompanied by inflammation. Subcutaneous infections involve the dermis and subcutaneous tissues. Systemic disease involves deep tissue invasion of one or more internal organs and usually follows inhalation of the fungus. In immunocompromised patients, disseminated disease may result from superficial, cutaneous, or subcutaneous fungal infections.

SUPERFICIAL INFECTIONS

Malasseziasis Tinea (pityriasis) versicolor, caused by lipophilic yeasts of the genus *Malassezia,* is the most common superficial skin infection. The clinical presentation usually consists of scaly hypo- or hyperpigmented macular lesions on the chest, back, neck, and arms.

ETIOLOGIC AGENTS *Malassezia* species are components of the human cutaneous flora that are dimorphic, existing in both yeast and mycelial phases. Each phase was originally classified as a separate genus: *Pityrosporum* for the yeast form and *Malassezia* for the mycelial form. The two genera were reclassified in 1986 as a single genus, *Malassezia.* Initially, only one species, *M. furfur,* was recognized, but seven distinct species have since been identified: *M. furfur, M. sympodialis, M. obtusa, M. globosa, M. restricta, M. slooffiae,* and *M. pachydermatis.*

EPIDEMIOLOGY *Malassezia* species can be isolated from sebaceous-rich areas of the skin, most frequently from the chest and the midline of the back. The prevalence of tinea versicolor in susceptible age groups (primarily adolescents and young adults) is low in temperate climates but may reach 40–60% in tropical climates.

PATHOGENESIS The pathogenesis of tinea versicolor is unclear but may involve the conversion of colonizing yeasts into the mycelial form, which then invades the stratum corneum.

CLINICAL MANIFESTATIONS The lesions of tinea versicolor are usually asymptomatic. Most patients seek medical advice for cosmetic reasons. Lesions typically appear as patches of pink or coppery-brown skin but may appear paler than the surrounding skin, especially in dark-skinned individuals. Although some patients report mild pruritus, the lesions do not usually elicit an immune response. Other cutaneous manifestations associated with *Malassezia* species include seborrheic dermatitis, folliculitis, atopic dermatitis, and dandruff.

DIAGNOSIS Tinea versicolor is diagnosed on clinical grounds by the characteristic distribution and appearance of skin lesions. Lesions may fluoresce yellow-green under long-wave UVA (Wood's light). Treatment of skin scrapings with potassium hydroxide (KOH) reveals yeasts and hyphal elements with a "spaghetti and meatballs" appearance.

Rx MALASSEZIASIS

Malassezia species are susceptible to a variety of topical antifungal agents, including 2.5% selenium sulfide shampoo (a 10- to 15-min application followed by rinsing); topical azoles such as clotrimazole, miconazole, econazole, and ketoconazole; terbinafine gel; and ciclopirox cream/solution. The typical treatment duration is 2 weeks. In patients with extensive or persistent lesions, short-course or pulse therapy with oral ketoconazole (a single 400-mg dose), fluconazole (a single 400-mg dose or 150 mg every week for 4 weeks), or itraconazole (200 mg every other day for 7 days) has proved effective.

COMPLICATIONS *M. furfur* is lipophilic and causes catheter-related fungemia in premature neonates and immunocompromised adults receiving IV lipids by central venous catheter. Infection of the lungs is pronounced and frequently results in respiratory failure. *M. pachydermatis,* although not lipophilic, is an increasingly important pathogen in neonatal intensive care units. When its presence is suspected, the microbiology laboratory should be notified because its isolation requires special culture conditions. Catheter-related *Malassezia* infections should be managed with prompt catheter removal and systemic antifungal therapy with amphotericin B or an azole (Table 199-1). Because transmission of both *M. furfur* and *M. pachydermatis* on the hands of health care workers has been documented, a strict hand-washing protocol should be enforced when outbreaks are identified.

PROGNOSIS In general, the prognosis in tinea versicolor is excellent, but the disease recurs in up to 80% of patients within 2 years after cessation of treatment. Early diagnosis and treatment in patients with disseminated infection improve outcome.

Other Superficial Mycoses Tinea nigra is a rare infection of the palms caused by the dematiaceous fungus *Hortaea* (formerly *Exophiala*) *werneckii.* Two types of piedra characterized by nodules of fungal elements on the hair shaft have been reported: black piedra caused by *Piedraia hortae* and white piedra caused by *Trichosporon* species (which may also be associated with other superficial infections as well as with invasive trichosporonosis). *T. beigelii* has historically been the most significant pathogen in the genus *Trichosporon.* Recently proposed revisions in classification and nomenclature are based on analysis of 26S rRNA sequences and use of nonmolecular techniques to differentiate 17 species—only 6 of which cause human disease—and 5 varieties of *Trichosporon.* Under this system, *T. beigelii* will be designated *T. cutaneum.* The other five human pathogens included in this revised classification are *T. asteroides, T. ovoides, T. inkin, T. asahii,* and *T. mucoides.* In addition, four serotypes of *Trichosporon* (serotypes I, II, III, and I-III) have been recognized, of which only serotypes I (*T. cutaneum* and *T. mucoides*) and II (*T. asahii, T. asteroides, T. inkin,* and *T. ovoides*) are pathogenic. Given that this revised nomenclature has not been universally adopted, the previous classification system may remain in use for some time and may be a source of confusion.

T. ovoides is usually associated with white piedra of the scalp, whereas *T. inkin* is primarily associated with white piedra of the groin. *T. ovoides* has also been implicated in summer-type hypersensitivity pneumonitis. The treatment of white piedra requires shaving off all the hair in the affected areas and applying a topical azole for 1–4 months.

CUTANEOUS INFECTIONS

The cutaneous mycoses are caused by *dermatophytes,* which infect keratinized tissues, including skin, hair follicles, and nails. These der-

TABLE 199-1 SYSTEMIC THERAPY FOR MISCELLANEOUS INVASIVE MYCOSES AND THE ALGAL INFECTION PROTOTHECOSIS

Type of Infection	First-Line Therapy	Alternative Therapy
Malasseziasis		
Central venous catheter–related infections	Removal of central venous catheter AmB[a]	In vitro susceptibility studies indicate that azoles may offer a therapeutic alternative.
Trichosporonosis	AmB in combination with voriconazole[b] (300 mg bid)	GM-CSF or IFN-γ may be a useful therapeutic adjunct.
Sporotrichosis		
Cutaneous/ lymphocutaneous	Itraconazole[c] (100–200 mg/d for 3–6 months)	Terbinafine, 500–1000 mg/d
Non-life-threatening pulmonary, osteoarticular, or disseminated disease	Itraconazole (200 mg bid for 12 months)	AmB (lipid formulation) *or* fluconazole (800 mg/d for 12 months) in patients who cannot tolerate AmB or itraconazole
Life-threatening pulmonary or disseminated disease	AmB	Selected patients may be switched to oral itraconazole (200 mg bid for 12 months)
Eumycetoma	Surgery in combination with: Ketoconazole (200–400 mg/d) *or* Voriconazole (600 mg/d) *or* Terbinafine (500 mg/d)	Posaconazole is currently being evaluated.
Dematiaceous fungal infections	Surgical excision or cryosurgery combined with:	. . .
Chromoblastomycosis	Itraconazole (200–600 mg/d), alone or with 5-fluorocytosine (50–100 mg/kg qd in 3 or 4 divided doses)	
Phaeohyphomycosis		
Cutaneous or subcutaneous disease	Itraconazole (200 mg once or twice daily before surgery and to prevent relapse)	
Systemic/CNS	AmB in combination with itraconazole (200 mg bid) or voriconazole (200 mg bid)	
Paracoccidioidomycosis		
Mild to moderate disease	Itraconazole (200–400 mg/d)	. . .
Severe disease	AmB	Selected patients may be switched to itraconazole after an initial course of AmB.
Penicilliosis		
Mild to moderate disease	Itraconazole (200 mg bid for 2 months)	. . .
Severe disease	AmB	Selected patients may be switched to itraconazole (200 mg bid) after an initial course of AmB. The duration of primary treatment is 2 months.
Suppressive therapy for patients with HIV infection or AIDS	Itraconazole (200 mg/d)	
Fusariosis and pseudallescheriasis/ scedosporiosis	IV voriconazole (6 mg/kg q12h for first 24 h, then 4 mg/kg q12h until neutropenia resolves and clinical response is documented)	Selected patients may be switched to oral voriconazole (200 mg bid) after a clinical response and reversal of neutropenia.
Protothecosis	Itraconazole (200 mg/d for 2 months or until lesions resolve)	Disseminated infections should be treated with IV AmB.

[a]Unless otherwise noted, AmB dosages are 0.6–1.0 mg/kg per day of the deoxycholate formulation or 3–5 mg/kg per day of a lipid formulation.
[b]An initial loading dose of voriconazole is recommended on day 1 for both IV therapy (6 mg/kg q12h) and oral therapy (400 mg q12h).
[c]An initial loading dose of itraconazole is recommended for both IV therapy (200 mg bid for 2 days) and oral therapy (200 mg bid for 2 days).
Note: AmB, amphotericin B; CNS, central nervous system; GM-CSF, granulocyte-macrophage colony-stimulating factor; IFN-γ, interferon γ.

matophytic fungi invade the epidermis and elicit an inflammatory reaction, including redness and pruritus. Dermatophytic infections are designated according to the anatomic location of the lesions—e.g., *tinea corporis* (the trunk, shoulders, or limbs), *tinea cruris* (the warm moist areas of the groin, perianal, and perineal areas), *tinea faciei* (the nonhairy areas of the face), *tinea pedis* (the feet), *tinea unguium* (the nails), and *tinea capitis* (the scalp).

ETIOLOGIC AGENTS Three genera of dermatophytes—*Microsporum*, *Trichophyton*, and *Epidermophyton*—are associated with human infections. Members of these genera can be divided into three groups according to their natural reservoir and potential for infection: anthropophilic, zoophilic, and geophilic organisms.

EPIDEMIOLOGY Tinea is common worldwide. It is estimated that more than 8 million office visits to primary care physicians are made annually for tinea-related symptoms.

PATHOGENESIS Dermatophytic fungi release proteolytic enzymes and keratinases into the skin. These exocellular enzymes release nutrients and facilitate dissemination through the stratum corneum. A specific host immune response is directed against the organisms.

CLINICAL MANIFESTATIONS Any dermatophyte can cause tinea corporis, which is commonly called "ringworm" because of the typical appearance of lesions: annular scaly patches with raised, erythematous vesicular borders and central clearing. Tinea faciei, like tinea corporis, can be caused by any dermatophyte. *T. rubrum* and *E. floccosum* are common causes of tinea cruris; similar lesions can be caused by *Candida* infection.

Tinea pedis, the most common clinical dermatophytic infection, usually presents with interdigital cracking, scaling, and maceration. Hyperkeratosis and peeling of the soles of the feet are common, with a scaly red "moccasin-like" appearance in chronic cases. The most common cause of tinea pedis is *T. rubrum*. Clinical lesions similar to those of tinea pedis can be caused by nondermatophytic fungi, yeasts, and bacteria.

Tinea unguium is caused by *T. rubrum*, *T. mentagrophytes*, and *E. floccosum*. The term *onychomycosis* encompasses nail infections due to either dermatophytes or nondermatophytic fungi. Dermatophytes cause 80–90% of cases of onychomycosis. The prevalence of these infections is ~2% among young adults and increases to 20% among individuals 40–60 years of age. Onychomycosis occurs in diabetic patients at the same rate as in the general population but poses a greater risk of bacterial superinfection in diabetes.

Tinea capitis is a common dermatophytic disease of children but is relatively rare among adults. The clinical presentation may vary from a diffuse scaly scalp to scattered areas of scale with or without alopecia. Hair may break off at the scalp ("black-dot ringworm"). Pruritus is not a constant symptom. Inflammatory responses may be minimal or severe, with the formation of a kerion characterized by alopecia, a tender or painful boggy scalp, purulent drainage, and localized lymphadenopathy. *T. tonsurans* is the most common dermatophyte associated with tinea capitis.

DIAGNOSIS Some skin lesions have distinctive characteristics that allow a presumptive diagnosis, and topical therapy is often initiated solely on the basis of the lesions' appearance. However, the ease of obtaining specimens for microscopic examination and culture should encourage definitive diagnosis. Scrapings of skin lesions can be examined as a wet preparation, with a drop of 10% KOH used to dissolve cells and debris. Samples for fungal cultures should be obtained from patients whose history, physical examination, and KOH-treated specimens are inconclusive with regard to the diagnosis of dermatophytic infection. It is recommended that a definitive diagnosis be established in patients before systemic antifungal agents are administered.

℞ CUTANEOUS INFECTIONS

Most tinea infections can be treated with topical agents alone. Many such antifungal agents are widely available as both prescription and over-the-counter products. Topical imidazoles (e.g., clotrimazole, miconazole, econazole, and ketoconazole) are generally well tolerated and efficacious when used twice daily for at least 2 weeks. The allylamines, including terbinafine and naftifine (available in 1% creams or 1% solutions), provide cure rates of ≥75% and require only once-daily application for shorter periods. Tolnaftate powder is best suited for prevention of tinea pedis.

Systemic therapy is indicated for patients who are unresponsive to topical therapy; for those who have infections involving the scalp or bearded areas, who have hyperkeratotic areas on the palms or soles, or who have widespread disease; and for immunocompromised individuals. Once-daily itraconazole (200 mg), terbinafine (250 mg), and griseofulvin (500 mg of the microcrystalline formulation or 375 mg of the ultramicrocrystalline formulation) has proved effective. Treatment should be administered until lesions resolve. For patients with nail disease, itraconazole (200 mg/d) or terbinafine (250 mg/d) is preferred. The duration of therapy is 2–3 months for fingernails and 4–6 months for toenails. Pulse therapy with itraconazole and terbinafine is an option. Relapse of nail disease is common.

COMPLICATIONS Sites of tinea pedis frequently become superinfected with bacteria. Sometimes these infections are serious, especially in diabetic patients, patients who have undergone saphenous-vein harvest for coronary artery bypass grafts, and patients with any significant venous incompetence.

SUBCUTANEOUS INFECTIONS

Fungal infections that primarily involve the dermis and subcutaneous tissue result from implantation of the organism in the skin through trauma. The major subcutaneous mycoses are sporotrichosis, mycetoma, chromoblastomycosis, and phaeohyphomycosis.

Sporotrichosis Sporotrichosis most commonly presents as chronic cutaneous, lymphocutaneous, and/or subcutaneous disease. This infection may also be extracutaneous, occurring at pulmonary, osteoarticular, or disseminated sites.

ETIOLOGIC AGENT Sporotrichosis is caused by the thermally dimorphic fungus *Sporothrix schenckii*, which is found in soil, plants, and moss and on animals. *S. schenckii* exists worldwide but is most common in tropical and warmer temperate regions, such as Mexico and Central and South America.

EPIDEMIOLOGY Sporotrichosis is usually an occupational disease of gardeners, farmers, forestry workers, florists, and horticulturists. There have been well-documented epidemics (e.g., among South African gold miners) as well as scattered outbreaks (e.g., among workers handling sphagnum, hay, and wood). Recent reports indicate that infection can be related to zoonotic spread from cats and armadillos.

PATHOGENESIS Sporotrichosis most often follows inoculation of the organism into the skin.

CLINICAL MANIFESTATIONS The majority of infections with *S. schenckii* present either as fixed cutaneous sporotrichosis or as lymphangitic or lymphocutaneous disease. Fixed cutaneous disease (plaque sporotrichosis) is limited to the site of inoculation. The primary lesion enlarges and may ulcerate and become verrucous. In lymphocutaneous disease, which accounts for ~80% of cases, secondary lesions ascend along the lymphatics that drain the area, producing small painless nodules that erupt, drain, and ulcerate. Other organisms (e.g., nontuberculous mycobacteria, *Nocardia, Leishmania,* and chromoblastomycotic agents) may cause similar lesions. Osteoarticular sporotrichosis is an uncommon complication but may cause granulomatous tenosynovitis and bursitis, particularly in alcoholic patients. Pulmonary sporotrichosis following inhalation of *S. schenckii* conidia has been reported in alcoholic patients with chronic obstructive pulmonary disease. Disseminated disease, including that involving the central nervous system, is most likely to occur in patients who have AIDS or are otherwise immunocompromised.

DIAGNOSIS A definitive diagnosis is made by culture of *S. schenckii* on any of a variety of media. Histopathologic examination of biopsy material may also contribute to the diagnosis, with detection of the characteristic ovoid or cigar-shaped yeast forms.

℞ SPOROTRICHOSIS

Sporotrichosis requires systemic therapy (Table 199-1). Historically, oral therapy with a saturated solution of potassium iodide (SSKI; 5 drops 3 times daily, increasing to 40–50 drops 3 times daily as tolerated) has been successful, but the use of this intervention is often limited by its toxicity. Because it has fewer side effects and is better tolerated, oral itraconazole has replaced SSKI as the treatment of choice for cutaneous and lymphocutaneous sporotrichosis. Terbinafine has also been effective against lymphocutaneous disease, although it has not been approved for this indication by the U.S. Food and Drug Administration. Patients with non-life-threatening pulmonary disease and those with osteoarticular disease should be treated with itraconazole for at least 12 months. Amphotericin B is the preferred agent for patients with life-threatening pulmonary disease or disseminated infection, for patients who cannot tolerate itraconazole, and for patients in whom itraconazole treatment has failed.

COMPLICATIONS Hematogenous dissemination of *S. schenckii* is most common among immunocompromised patients, including those with HIV infection or AIDS. These patients may develop widespread cutaneous ulcers, granulomas, and systemic disease with pulmonary, meningeal, articular, or generalized infection.

PROGNOSIS Success rates of 90–100% have been reported for itraconazole treatment of lymphocutaneous sporotrichosis. A clinical response usually occurs within 4–6 weeks of the start of therapy. Patients who relapse usually respond to a second course of itraconazole.

Mycetoma Mycetoma is a chronic suppurative infection that begins in the subcutaneous tissue and spreads to fascia and bone. Mycetoma due to fungi is called *eumycetoma*, while that caused by actinomycetes is referred to as *actinomycetoma*. Both diseases are characterized by abscesses containing grains composed of large aggregates of filaments (fungal or actinomycete). Traumatic inoculation is responsible for initial infection.

ETIOLOGY AND EPIDEMIOLOGY Mycetomas are common in Mexico, Central America, Venezuela, Brazil, Africa, the Middle East, India, Pakistan, and Bangladesh. The most common cause of eumycetoma worldwide is *Madurella mycetomatis*, while the rare cases that occur in the United States are associated with *Pseudallescheria boydii*. Actinomycetoma, the usual form of mycetoma in Mexico and Central America, is associated with *Nocardia brasiliensis, Streptomyces somaliensis, Actinomadura madurae,* and *Actinomadura pelletieri*.

CLINICAL MANIFESTATIONS Clinically, eumycetoma and actinomycetoma are similar, beginning as small, firm, painless subcutaneous plaques or nodules on the foot or leg and, less frequently, on the arms, torso, and scalp. Patients usually present with draining sinus tracts, subcutaneous abscesses, fibrosis with woody induration, and extension to fascia and bone.

DIAGNOSIS Diagnosis is based on visualization of grains in pus, sinus exudate, or tissue biopsy. Fungal hyphae must be distinguished from the filamentous forms seen in actinomycetoma. Organisms associated with mycetoma, whether fungi or actinomycetes, can be grown on a variety of culture media.

℞ MYCETOMA

The treatment of mycetoma is problematic. A combined medical/surgical approach is the option of choice (Table 199-1). Because actinomycetoma does not respond to antifungal agents, the differentiation between eumycetoma and actinomycetoma is crucial. (For the treatment of actinomycetoma, see Chaps. 155 and 156.) Amphotericin B has not generally been effective for the treatment of eumycetoma. A limited number of patients have responded to long-term azole therapy. Posaconazole, an investigational agent, may have a role in the treatment of eumycetoma in the future.

Dematiaceous Fungal Infections Of the many names applied to infections caused by brown- or black-pigmented soil fungi, *phaeohyphomycosis* and *chromoblastomycosis* are the most widely accepted. Phaeohyphomycosis refers to infections in which the organisms in tissue occur as pigmented yeast-like forms and/or hyphae. Chromoblastomycosis is distinguished by the presence of pigmented sclerotic bodies in tissue.

Chromoblastomycosis is characterized by slow-growing verrucous plaques or nodules, usually on the lower extremities. The most common etiologic agents are *Fonsecaea pedrosoi, F. compacta, Phialophora verrucosa, Rhinocladiella aquaspersa*, and *Cladosporium (Cladophialophora) carrionii*. Most cases affect rural workers living in tropical and subtropical regions, and infection is acquired by traumatic inoculation. Small verrucous papules enlarge slowly but remain painless. Lesions seen in late stages may be superficial or raised purplish irregular plaques; less commonly, they may be nodular, tumorous, verrucous, or cicatricial. In advanced cases, secondary lymphedema, bacterial infections, and keratin necrosis can develop. Although histologic examination of scrapings or biopsy material for characteristic sclerotic bodies can lead to the diagnosis of chromoblastomycosis, culture is required for identification of the causative agent. Treatment is difficult, although many therapeutic interventions have been described (Table 199-1). Results are best when early surgical excision or cryosurgery is used in combination with antifungal therapy. Treatment with itraconazole—either alone or with 5-fluorocytosine—has had some success.

Phaeohyphomycosis presents in four clinical forms: superficial, cutaneous-corneal, subcutaneous, and systemic. *Exophiala jeanselmei, Wangiella dermatitidis*, and *Bipolaris* species are the most common etiologic agents. The route of infection is most likely implantation, with the subsequent formation of an inflammatory cyst. A single inflammatory nondraining cyst located on a proximal limb is the most typical presentation. The diagnosis is usually made by histopathologic detection (in biopsy material) of a fibrous capsule with a granulomatous reaction and a necrotic center. Culture is required to identify specific organisms. Surgical excision of the lesion is essential. Itraconazole treatment reduces the size of large lesions before excision and prevents relapse afterward (Table 199-1). Cerebral phaeohyphomycosis is thought to be due to direct extension from adjacent paranasal sinuses or from a penetrating trauma to the head. Most cases present as a brain abscess with focal neurologic deficits and/or generalized seizures. A review of 101 cases revealed that one-half of patients had no apparent immunocompromising condition. Infections in immunocompromised patients are more likely to disseminate; disseminated infections have been reported in patients with HIV infection, solid-organ transplant recipients, patients with malignancies, and one pregnant woman. Rhinocerebral disease requires surgical drainage along with antifungal therapy. A combination of amphotericin B and itraconazole or voriconazole is recommended.

SYSTEMIC MYCOSES

Paracoccidioidomycosis Often referred to as South American blastomycosis, paracoccidioidomycosis is a systemic disease caused by the dimorphic fungus *Paracoccidioides brasiliensis*. Pulmonary infection follows inhalation of conidia and may disseminate to other organs, producing secondary lesions in the skin, lymph nodes, and adrenal glands. Subclinical infections have been documented in healthy residents of endemic regions. Paracoccidioidomycosis is most common in Venezuela, Colombia, Ecuador, Argentina, and Brazil. Histopathologic examination of clinical specimens may reveal globose yeast cells with multiple buds. Definitive diagnosis relies on culture of the organism. Itraconazole treatment has been effective (Table 199-1). An initial course of amphotericin B may be required in seriously ill patients.

Penicilliosis Caused by the thermally dimorphic fungus *Penicillium marneffei*, penicilliosis is a disease of immunocompromised individuals living in or traveling to Southeast Asia. The primary portal of entry is the lungs, and hematologic dissemination follows. Clinical manifestations are similar to those of disseminated histoplasmosis and include fever, chills, weight loss, anemia, generalized lymphadenopathy, and hepatomegaly. Diffuse papular lesions similar to those of molluscum contagiosum are common in patients with HIV infection or AIDS. Small yeast cells may be seen on histopathologic examination of tissue, but definitive diagnosis depends on culture. Amphotericin B is the treatment of choice for severely ill patients (Table 199-1). Patients who have less severe disease or who have responded to an initial course of amphotericin B may be treated with itraconazole. Primary therapy is usually given for 2 months; in patients with HIV infection or AIDS, suppressive therapy with itraconazole may be useful in preventing relapse.

Fusariosis Fusariosis is an invasive mold infection associated with *Fusarium* species, most commonly *F. solani*. The skin and respiratory tract are the primary portals of entry. Localized skin infections may occur at sites of trauma in immunocompetent hosts. Disease may disseminate from the skin or respiratory tract in immunocompromised patients; 90% of such cases are reported in neutropenic patients with leukemia or recipients of allogeneic bone marrow transplants. The clinical presentation is generally nonspecific, with fever and skin lesions that eventually become necrotic and resemble ecthyma gangrenosum. Clinical, radiographic, and pathologic findings are similar to those in invasive aspergillosis or zygomycosis. Blood cultures are positive in up to 50% of cases, and the presence of a mold in cultured blood from neutropenic patients suggests fusariosis. *Fusarium* species are often resistant to antifungal therapy. High-dose amphotericin B has met with limited success. Therapy with voriconazole (Table 199-1) has been successful in a few patients. Therapy is continued until neutropenia resolves and a clinical response is documented. The prognosis of disseminated infection is related to the reversal of neutropenia and other immunodeficiencies.

Pseudallescheriasis and Scedosporiosis The emerging pathogens *P. boydii, Scedosporium apiospermum* (the asexual form of *P. boydii*), and *S. prolificans* are molds that cause rare sinopulmonary infections in immunocompetent hosts and that may present as fungus balls in the lungs or paranasal sinuses. Severe pneumonia, invasive sinusitis, and hematogenous dissemination (including brain abscess) occur in immunosuppressed hosts, especially bone marrow transplant recipients. The hyphal elements seen in the tissues of patients with *Pseudallescheria* and *Scedosporium* infections resemble those seen in intravascular invasion by *Aspergillus*. The outcome of treatment is poor, and most patients with disseminated disease die. Amphotericin B is not effective in the treatment of pseudallescheriasis or scedosporiosis. A small number of patients have been cured with voriconazole in the same doses listed for fusariosis (Table 199-1). Surgical debridement and drainage of abscesses may also be necessary.

Trichosporonosis *Trichosporon* species, predominantly *T. asahii* and to a lesser extent *T. mucoides*, can cause disseminated trichosporonosis in immunocompromised patients, especially those with profound neutropenia. Unpublished studies describe isolation of *Trichosporon* from pubic sites of white piedra, sputum, skin lesions, and blood. *T. pullulans* (formerly *Monilia pullulans*) is a rare cause of systemic infection. Portals of entry include the skin, gastrointestinal tract, and lungs. The clinical presentation mimics candidiasis. Cultures of blood, skin lesions, or biopsy specimens confirm the diagnosis. *Trichosporon* shares antigens with *Cryptococcus neoformans* and produces positive results in the latex agglutination test. Treatment of *Trichosporon* infections is complicated by resistance to amphotericin B. Mortality rates of >80% have been reported. The azoles, especially voriconazole, have been effective alone or in combination with amphotericin B (Table 199-1). Adjunctive therapy with granulocyte-macrophage colony-stimulating factor or interferon γ may be beneficial. The prognosis, however, is related to the resolution of neutropenia.

ALGAL INFECTIONS

Prototheca, an achlorophyllic alga common in nature, has been associated with rare human infections in Europe, Asia, Oceania, and the United States (particularly the southeastern states). This organism has been isolated from slime flux of trees, industrial ponds, tap water, sewage systems, swimming pools, and soil. Infections with *P. wickerhamii* and *P. zopfii* occur primarily in immunocompromised patients. Protothecosis may present as a cutaneous disease with erythematous nodules, plaques, or superficial ulcers on exposed skin; as olecranon bursitis; or as a systemic infection. Histologic examination of biopsy material may reveal multinucleated giant cells and extra- and intracellular, basophilic to amphiphilic organisms containing endospores. *Prototheca* can be cultured on Sabouraud's agar. The most frequently used therapeutic agent is amphotericin B, which has proved effective even in patients with disseminated protothecosis. Azole antifungal agents such as itraconazole, ketoconazole, and fluconazole have also been used successfully. Surgical excision may play a role in the treatment of localized cutaneous lesions.

FURTHER READINGS

ALY R: Skin, hair, and nail fungal infections. Infect Dis Clin Pract 10:117, 1998

CHAPMAN SW, DANIEL CR III: Cutaneous manifestations of fungal infection. Infect Dis Clin North Am 4:879, 1994

DIGNANI MC et al: Immunomodulation with interferon-gamma and colony-stimulating factors for refractory fungal infections in patients with leukemia. Cancer 104:199, 2005

FLEMING RV, ANAISSIE EJ: Emerging fungal infections, in *Fungal Infections in the Immunocompromised Patient*, JR Wingard, EJ Anaissie (eds). Boca Raton, Taylor & Francis Group, 2005, pp 311–340

——— et al: Emerging and less common fungal pathogens. Infect Dis Clin North Am 16:915, 2002

QUEIROZ-TELLES F et al: Subcutaneous mycoses. Infect Dis Clin North Am 17:59, 2003

SEGAL BH et al: Fungal infections in nontransplant patients with hematologic malignancies. Infect Dis Clin North Am 16:935, 2002

SILVEIRA F, NUCCI M: Emergence of black moulds in fungal disease: Epidemiology and therapy. Curr Opin Infect Dis 14:679, 2001

www.doctorfungus.org

200 *Pneumocystis* Infection

A. George Smulian, Peter D. Walzer

DEFINITION AND DESCRIPTION

Pneumocystis is an opportunistic fungal pulmonary pathogen that is an important cause of pneumonia in the immunocompromised host. Although organisms within the *Pneumocystis* genus are morphologically very similar, they are genetically diverse and host-specific. *P. jirovecii* infects humans, whereas *P. carinii*—the original species described in 1909—infects rats. For clarity, only the genus designation *Pneumocystis* will be used in this chapter.

Developmental stages of the organism include the trophic form, the cyst, and the precyst (an intermediate stage). The life cycle of *Pneumocystis* probably involves sexual and asexual reproduction, although definitive proof awaits the development of a reliable culture system. *Pneumocystis* contains several different antigen groups, the most prominent of which is the 95- to 140-kDa major surface glycoprotein (MSG). MSG plays a central role in the interaction of *Pneumocystis* with its host.

EPIDEMIOLOGY

Serologic surveys have demonstrated that *Pneumocystis* has a worldwide distribution and that most healthy children have been exposed to the organism by 3–4 years of age. Airborne transmission of *Pneumocystis* has been documented in animal studies; person-to-person transmission has been suggested by hospital outbreaks of *Pneumocystis* pneumonia (PcP) and by molecular epidemiologic analysis of isolates. *Pneumocystis* colonization of immunocompetent individuals has been detected by polymerase chain reaction (PCR) techniques.

PATHOGENESIS AND PATHOLOGY

The host factors that predispose to the development of PcP include defects in cellular and humoral immunity. The risk of PcP among HIV-infected patients rises markedly when circulating CD4+ T cell counts fall below 200/μL. Other persons at risk for PcP are patients receiving immunosuppressive agents (particularly glucocorticoids) for cancer and organ transplantation; those receiving biologic agents such as infliximab and etanercept for rheumatoid arthritis and inflammatory bowel disease; children with primary immunodeficiency diseases; and premature malnourished infants.

The principal host effector cells against *Pneumocystis* are alveolar macrophages, which ingest and kill the organism, releasing a variety of inflammatory mediators. Proliferating organisms remain extracellular within the alveolus, attaching tightly to type I cells. Alveolar damage results in increased alveolar-capillary permeability and surfactant abnormalities, including a fall in phospholipids and an increase in surfactant proteins A and D. The host inflammatory response to lung injury leads to increases in levels of interleukin 8 and in neutrophil counts in bronchoalveolar lavage (BAL) fluid. These changes correlate with disease severity.

On lung sections stained with hematoxylin and eosin, the alveoli are filled with a typical foamy, vacuolated exudate. Severe disease may include interstitial edema, fibrosis, and hyaline membrane formation. The host inflammatory changes usually consist of hypertrophy of alveolar type II cells, a typical reparative response, and a mild mononuclear cell interstitial infiltrate. Malnourished infants display an intense plasma cell infiltrate that gave the disease its early name: interstitial plasma cell pneumonia.

CLINICAL FEATURES

Patients with PcP develop dyspnea, fever, and nonproductive cough. HIV-infected patients are usually ill for several weeks and may have relatively subtle manifestations. Symptoms in non-HIV-infected pa-

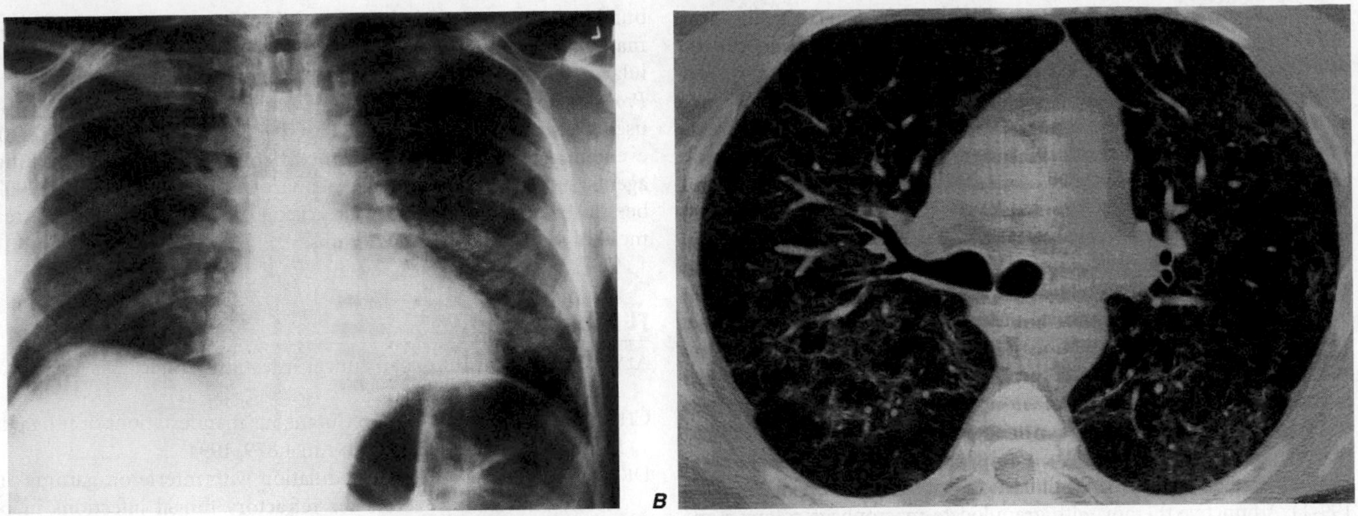

A B

FIGURE 200-1 ***A.*** Chest radiograph depicting diffuse infiltrates in an HIV-infected patient with PcP. ***B.*** High-resolution CT of the lung showing ground-glass opacification in an HIV-infected patient with PcP. *(Courtesy of Dr. Cristopher Meyer, with permission.)*

tients are of shorter duration and often begin after the glucocorticoid dose has been tapered. A high index of suspicion and a thorough history are key factors in early detection.

Physical findings include tachypnea, tachycardia, and cyanosis, but lung auscultation reveals few abnormalities. Reduced arterial oxygen pressure (Pa_{O_2}), increased alveolar-arterial oxygen gradient (PA_{O_2} – Pa_{O_2}), and respiratory alkalosis are evident. Diffusion capacity is reduced, and heightened uptake with nonspecific nuclear imaging techniques (gallium scan) may be noted. Elevated serum concentrations of lactate dehydrogenase, reflecting lung parenchymal damage, have been reported; however, the increase is not specific for PcP.

The classic findings on chest radiography consist of bilateral diffuse infiltrates beginning in the perihilar regions (Fig. 200-1*A*), but various atypical manifestations (nodular densities, cavitary lesions) have also been reported. Pneumothorax occurs, and its management is often difficult. Early in the course of PcP, the chest radiograph may be normal, although high-resolution CT of the lung may reveal ground-glass opacities at this stage (Fig. 200-1*B*).

While *Pneumocystis* usually remains confined to the lungs, cases of disseminated infection have occurred in both HIV-infected and non-HIV-infected patients. Common sites of involvement include the lymph nodes, spleen, liver, and bone marrow.

DIAGNOSIS

Because of the nonspecific nature of the clinical picture, the diagnosis must be based on specific identification of the organism. A definitive diagnosis is made by histopathologic staining. Traditional cell wall stains such as methenamine silver selectively stain the wall of *Pneumocystis* cysts, while reagents such as Wright-Giemsa stain the nuclei of all developmental stages. Immunofluorescence with monoclonal antibodies is more sensitive and specific than histologic staining. DNA amplification by PCR may become part of routine diagnostics but may not distinguish colonization from infection.

The successful diagnosis of PcP depends on the collection of proper specimens. In general, the yield from different diagnostic procedures is higher in HIV-infected patients than in non-HIV-infected patients because of the higher organism burden in the former group. Sputum induction and oral washes have gained popularity as simple, noninvasive techniques; however, these procedures require trained and dedicated personnel. Fiberoptic bronchoscopy with BAL, which provides information about the organism burden, the host inflammatory response, and the presence of other opportunistic infections, continues to be the mainstay of *Pneumocystis* diagnosis. Transbronchial biopsy and open lung biopsy, the most invasive procedures, are used only when a diagnosis cannot be made by BAL.

COURSE AND PROGNOSIS

In the typical case of untreated PcP, progressive respiratory embarrassment leads to death. Therapy is most effective when instituted early, before there is extensive alveolar damage. If examination of induced sputum is nondiagnostic and BAL cannot be performed in a timely manner, empirical therapy for PcP is reasonable. However, this practice does not eliminate the need for a specific etiologic diagnosis. With improved management of HIV and its complications, mortality from PcP is 15–20% at 1 month and 50–55% at 1 year. Rates of early death remain high among patients who require mechanical ventilation (60%) and among non-HIV-infected patients (40%).

Rx *PNEUMOCYSTIS* INFECTION

Trimethoprim-sulfamethoxazole (TMP-SMX), which acts by inhibiting folic acid synthesis, is considered the drug of choice for all forms of PcP (**Table 200-1**). Therapy is continued for 14 days in non-HIV-infected patients and for 21 days in persons infected with HIV. Since HIV-infected patients respond more slowly than non-HIV-infected patients, it is prudent to wait at least 7 days after the initiation of treatment before concluding that therapy has failed. TMP-SMX is well tolerated by non-HIV-infected patients, whereas more than half of HIV-infected patients experience serious adverse reactions.

Several alternative regimens are available for the treatment of mild to moderate cases of PcP (a Pa_{O_2} of >70 mmHg or a PA_{O_2} – Pa_{O_2} of <35 mmHg on breathing room air). TMP plus dapsone and clindamycin plus primaquine are about as effective as TMP-SMX. Dapsone and primaquine should not be administered to patients with glucose-6-phosphate dehydrogenase (G6PD) deficiency. Atovaquone is less effective than TMP-SMX but is better tolerated. Since *Pneumocystis* lacks ergosterol, it is not susceptible to antifungal agents that inhibit ergosterol synthesis.

Alternative regimens that are recommended for the treatment of moderate to severe PcP (a Pa_{O_2} of ≤70 mmHg or a PA_{O_2} – Pa_{O_2} of ≥35 mmHg) are parenteral pentamidine, parenteral clindamycin plus primaquine, or trimetrexate plus leucovorin. Parenteral clindamycin plus primaquine may be more efficacious than pentamidine.

Molecular evidence of resistance to sulfonamides and to atovaquone has emerged among human *Pneumocystis* isolates. Although prior sulfonamide exposure is a risk factor, this resistance has also occurred in HIV-infected patients who have never received sulfonamides. The outcome of therapy appears to be linked more strongly to traditional measures—e.g., high Acute Physiology, Age, and Chronic Health Evaluation III (APACHE III) scores, need for positive-pressure ventilation, delayed intubation, and development of pneumothorax—than to the presence of molecular markers of sulfonamide resistance. HIV-infected patients frequently experience deterioration of respiratory function shortly after receiving anti-*Pneumocystis* drugs. The adjunctive administration of tapering doses of glucocorticoids to HIV-infected patients with moderate to severe PcP can prevent this

TABLE 200-1 TREATMENT OF PNEUMOCYSTOSIS

Drug(s), Dose, Route	Adverse Effects
First Choice[a]	
TMP-SMX (5 mg/kg TMP, 25 mg/kg SMX[b]) q6–8 h PO or IV	Fever, rash, cytopenias, hepatitis, hyperkalemia, GI disturbances
Other Agents[a]	
TMP, 5 mg/kg q6–8h, plus dapsone, 100 mg qd PO	Hemolysis (G6PD deficiency), methemoglobinemia, fever, rash, GI disturbances
Atovaquone, 750 mg bid PO	Rash, fever, GI and hepatic disturbances
Clindamycin, 300–450 mg q6h PO or 600 mg q6–8h IV, plus primaquine, 15–30 mg qd PO	Hemolysis (G6PD deficiency), methemoglobinemia, rash, colitis, neutropenia
Pentamidine, 3–4 mg/kg qd IV	Hypotension, azotemia, cardiac arrhythmias, pancreatitis, dysglycemias, hypocalcemia, neutropenia, hepatitis
Trimetrexate, 45 mg/m^2 qd IV, plus leucovorin,[c] 20 mg/kg q6h PO or IV	Cytopenias, peripheral neuropathy, hepatic disturbances
Adjunctive Agent	
Prednisone, 40 mg bid × 5 d, 40 mg qd × 5 d, 20 mg qd × 11 d; PO or IV	Immunosuppression, peptic ulcer, hyperglycemia, mood changes, hypertension

[a]Therapy is administered for 14 days to non-HIV-infected patients and for 21 days to HIV-infected patients.
[b]Equivalent of 2 double-strength (DS) tablets. (One DS tablet contains 160 mg of TMP and 800 mg of SMX.)
[c]Leucovorin prevents bone marrow toxicity from trimetrexate.
Note: GI, gastrointestinal; G6PD, glucose-6-phosphate dehydrogenase; TMP-SMX, trimethoprim-sulfamethoxazole.

problem and improve the rate of survival (Table 200-1). For maximal benefit, this adjunctive therapy should be started early in the course of the illness. The use of steroids as adjunctive therapy in HIV-infected patients with mild PcP or in non-HIV-infected patients remains to be evaluated.

PREVENTION

Prophylaxis is indicated for HIV-infected patients with CD4+ T cell counts of <200/μL or a history of oropharyngeal candidiasis and for both HIV-infected and non-HIV-infected patients who have recovered from PcP. Prophylaxis may be discontinued in HIV-infected patients once CD4+ T cell counts have risen to >200/μL and remained at that level for ≥3 months. Primary prophylaxis guidelines for immunocompromised hosts not infected with HIV are less clear.

TMP-SMX is the drug of choice for primary and secondary prophylaxis (Table 200-2). This agent also provides protection against toxoplasmosis and some bacterial infections. Alternative regimens are available for individuals intolerant of TMP-SMX (Table 200-2). Although there are no specific recommendations for preventing the spread of *Pneumocystis* in health care facilities, it seems prudent to prevent direct contact between patients with PcP and other susceptible hosts.

TABLE 200-2 PROPHYLAXIS OF PNEUMOCYSTOSIS[a]

Drug(s), Dose, Route	Comments
First Choice	
TMP-SMX, 1 DS tablet or 1 SS tablet qd PO[b]	TMP-SMX can be safely reintroduced in some patients who have experienced mild to moderate side effects.
Other Agents	
Dapsone, 50 mg bid or 100 mg qd PO	—
Dapsone, 50 mg qd PO, plus pyrimethamine, 50 mg weekly PO, plus leucovorin, 25 mg weekly PO	Leucovorin prevents bone marrow toxicity from pyrimethamine.
Dapsone, 200 mg weekly PO, plus pyrimethamine, 75 mg weekly PO, plus leucovorin, 25 mg weekly PO	Leucovorin prevents bone marrow toxicity from pyrimethamine.
Pentamidine, 300 mg monthly via Respirgard II nebulizer	Adverse reactions include cough and bronchospasm.
Atovaquone, 1500 mg qd PO	—
TMP-SMX, 1 DS tablet three times weekly PO	TMP-SMX can be safely reintroduced in some patients who have experienced mild to moderate side effects.

[a]For list of adverse effects, see Table 200-1.
[b]One DS tablet contains 160 mg of TMP and 800 mg of SMX.
Note: DS, double-strength; SS, single-strength; TMP-SMX, trimethoprim-sulfamethoxazole.

FURTHER READINGS

Centers for Disease Control and Prevention: Treating opportunistic infections among HIV-infected adults and adolescents: Recommendations from the CDC, the National Institutes of Health and the HIV Medicine Association/Infectious Diseases Society of America. MMWR 53(RR-15):1, 2004

Daly KR et al: Antibody responses to the *Pneumocystis jirovecii* major surface glycoprotein. Emerg Infect Dis 12:1231, 2006

Festic E et al: Acute respiratory failure due to *Pneumocystis* pneumonia in patients without human immunodeficiency virus infection: Outcome and associated features. Chest 128:573, 2005

Medrano FJ et al: *Pneumocystis jirovecii* in general population. Emerg Infect Dis 11:245, 2005

Miller RF et al: Improved survival for HIV infected patients with severe *Pneumocystis jirovecii* pneumonia is independent of highly active antiretroviral therapy. Thorax 61:716, 2006

Redhead SA et al: *Pneumocystis* and *Trypanosoma cruzi*: Nomenclature and typifications. J Eukaryot Microbiol 53:1, 2006

Thomas CF Jr, Limper AH: *Pneumocystis* pneumonia. N Engl J Med 350:2487, 2004

Zar HJ: Pneumonia in HIV-infected and HIV-uninfected children in developing countries: Epidemiology, clinical features, and management. Curr Opin Pulm Med 10:176, 2004

SECTION 17 PROTOZOAL AND HELMINTHIC INFECTIONS: GENERAL CONSIDERATIONS

201 Agents Used to Treat Parasitic Infections

Thomas A. Moore

Parasitic infections afflict more than half of the world's population and impose a substantial health burden, particularly in underdeveloped nations, where they are most prevalent. The remarkable success of global campaigns aimed at controlling or eliminating ancient scourges such as dracunculiasis and onchocerciasis has been offset by the spread of other diseases such as trypanosomiasis due to crumbling infrastructures in settings of HIV infection, civil war, and unstable government. The reach of some parasitic diseases, including malaria, has expanded over the past few decades as a result of factors such as deforestation, population shifts, global warming, and other climatic events. Despite major efforts at vaccine development and vector control, chemotherapy remains the single most effective means of controlling parasitic infections. However, efforts to combat the spread of some diseases are hindered by the development and spread of drug resistance, the limited introduction of new antiparasitic agents, and the proliferation of counterfeit medications. Significant advances toward the reduction of the burden of parasitic disease have nevertheless been made, and the significant increase in funding of global health initiatives offers promise for the future.

This chapter deals exclusively with the agents used to treat infections due to parasites. Specific treatment recommendations for the parasitic diseases of humans are listed in subsequent chapters. **The pharmacology of the antiparasitic agents is discussed in great detail in Chap. e17.**

Table 201-1 presents a brief overview of each agent (including some drugs that are covered in other chapters), along with its major toxicities, spectrum of activity, and safety for use during pregnancy and lactation. Many of the agents are approved by the U.S. Food and Drug Administration but are considered investigational for the treatment of certain infections; these drugs are marked accordingly in the table. In addition, drugs available only through the Centers for Disease Control and Prevention (CDC) Drug Service (telephone: 404-639-3670 or 404-639-2888; *www.cdc.gov/ncidod/dpd/professional/drug_service.htm*) or only through their manufacturers (whose contact information may be available from the CDC) are specified by footnotes in the table.

TABLE 201-1 OVERVIEW OF AGENTS USED FOR THE TREATMENT OF PARASITIC INFECTIONS

Drugs by Class	Parasitic Infection(s)	Adverse Effects	Major Drug-Drug Interactions	Pregnancy Class[a]	Breast Milk
4-Aminoquinolines					
Amodiaquine	Malaria[b]	Agranulocytosis, hepatotoxicity	No information	Not assigned	No information
Chloroquine	Malaria[b]	*Occasional:* pruritus, nausea, vomiting, headache, hair depigmentation, exfoliative dermatitis, reversible corneal opacity. *Rare:* irreversible retinal injury, nail discoloration, blood dyscrasias	Antacids and kaolin: reduced absorption of chloroquine Ampicillin: bioavailability reduced by chloroquine Cimetidine: increased serum levels of chloroquine Cyclosporine: serum levels increased by chloroquine	Not assigned[c]	Yes
8-Aminoquinolines					
Primaquine	Malaria[b]	*Frequent:* hemolysis in patients with G6PD deficiency. *Occasional:* methemoglobinemia, GI disturbances. *Rare:* CNS symptoms	Quinacrine: potentiated toxicity of primaquine	Contraindicated	No information
Tafenoquine	Malaria[b]	*Frequent:* hemolysis in patients with G6PD deficiency, mild GI upset. *Occasional:* methemoglobinemia, headaches	No information	Not assigned	No information
Aminoalcohols					
Halofantrine	Malaria[b]	*Frequent:* abdominal pain, diarrhea. *Occasional:* ECG disturbances (dose-related prolongation of QTc and PR interval), nausea, pruritus. Contraindicated in persons who have cardiac disease or who have taken mefloquine in the preceding 3 weeks	Concomitant use of agents that prolong QTc interval contraindicated	C	No information
Lumefantrine	Malaria	*Occasional:* nausea, vomiting, diarrhea, abdominal pain, anorexia, headache, dizziness	No major interactions	Not assigned	No information
Aminoglycosides					
Paromomycin	Amebiasis,[b] infection with *Dientamoeba fragilis,* giardiasis, cryptosporidiosis, leishmaniasis	*Frequent:* GI disturbances (oral dosing only). *Occasional:* nephrotoxicity, ototoxicity, vestibular toxicity (parenteral dosing only)	No major interactions	Not assigned[c]	No information

(continued)

TABLE 201-1 OVERVIEW OF AGENTS USED FOR THE TREATMENT OF PARASITIC INFECTIONS (CONTINUED)

Drugs by Class	Parasitic Infection(s)	Adverse Effects	Major Drug-Drug Interactions	Pregnancy Class[a]	Breast Milk
Amphotericin B Amphotericin B deoxycholate Amphotec (InterMune) Amphotericin B lipid complex, ABLC (Abelcet) Amphotericin B, liposomal (AmBisome)	Leishmaniasis,[d] amebic meningoencephalitis	*Frequent:* fever, chills, hypokalemia, hypomagnesemia, nephrotoxicity. *Occasional:* vomiting, dyspnea, hypotension	Antineoplastic agents: renal toxicity, bronchospasm, hypotension Glucocorticoids, ACTH, digitalis: hypokalemia Zidovudine: increased myelo- and nephrotoxicity	B	No information
Antimonials	Leishmaniasis				
Pentavalent antimony[e]		*Frequent:* arthralgias/myalgias, pancreatitis, ECG changes (QT prolongation, T wave flattening or inversion)	No major interactions	Not assigned	Yes
Meglumine antimonate		*Frequent:* arthralgias/myalgias, pancreatitis, ECG changes (QT prolongation, T wave flattening or inversion)	Antiarrhythmics and tricyclic antidepressants: increased risk of cardiotoxicity	Not assigned	No information
Artemisinin and derivatives	Malaria	*Occasional:* neurotoxicity (ataxia, convulsions), nausea, vomiting, anorexia, contact dermatitis		Not assigned	No information
Arteether			No information		
Artemether			No clinically significant interactions		
Artesunate			Mefloquine: levels decreased and clearance accelerated by artesunate		
Dihydroartemisinin			Mefloquine: increased absorption		
Atovaquone	Malaria,[a] babesiosis	*Frequent:* nausea, vomiting. *Occasional:* abdominal pain, headache	Plasma levels decreased by rifampin, tetracycline; bioavailability decreased by metoclopramide	C	No information
Azoles Fluconazole Itraconazole Ketoconazole	Leishmaniasis	*Serious:* hepatotoxicity. *Rare:* exfoliative skin disorders, anaphylaxis	Warfarin, oral hypoglycemics, phenytoin, cyclosporine, theophylline, digoxin, dofetilide, quinidine, carbamazepine, rifabutin, busulfan, docetaxel, vinca alkaloids, pimozide, alprazolam, diazepam, midazolam, triazolam, verapamil, atorvastatin, cerivastatin, lovastatin, simvastatin, tacrolimus, sirolimus, indinavir, ritonavir, saquinavir, alfentanil, buspirone, methylprednisolone, trimetrexate: plasma levels increased by azoles Carbamazepine, phenobarbital, phenytoin, isoniazid, rifabutin, rifampin, antacids, H2-receptor antagonists, proton pump inhibitors, nevirapine: decreased plasma levels of azoles Clarithromycin, erythromycin, indinavir, ritonavir: increased plasma levels of azoles	C	Yes
Benzimidazoles					
Albendazole	Ascariasis, capillariasis, clonorchiasis, cutaneous larva migrans, cysticercosis,[b] echinococcosis,[b] enterobiasis, eosinophilic enterocolitis, gnathostomiasis, hookworm, lymphatic filariasis, microsporidiosis, strongyloidiasis, trichinellosis, trichostrongyliasis, trichuriasis, visceral larva migrans	*Occasional:* nausea, vomiting, abdominal pain, headache, reversible alopecia, elevated aminotransferases. *Rare:* leukopenia, rash	Dexamethasone, praziquantel: plasma level of albendazole sulfoxide increased by ~50%	C	Yes[f]

(continued)

CHAPTER 201 Agents Used to Treat Parasitic Infections

Drugs by Class	Parasitic Infection(s)	Adverse Effects	Major Drug-Drug Interactions	Pregnancy Class[a]	Breast Milk
Mebendazole	Ascariasis,[b] capillariasis, eosinophilic enterocolitis, enterobiasis,[b] hookworm,[b] trichinellosis, trichostrongyliasis, trichuriasis,[b] visceral larva migrans	*Occasional:* diarrhea, abdominal pain, elevated aminotransferases. *Rare:* agranulocytosis, thrombocytopenia, alopecia	Cimetidine: inhibited mebendazole metabolism	C	No information
Thiabendazole	Strongyloidiasis,[b] cutaneous larva migrans,[b] visceral larva migrans[b]	*Frequent:* anorexia, nausea, vomiting, diarrhea, headache, dizziness, asparagus-like urine odor. *Occasional:* drowsiness, giddiness, crystalluria, elevated aminotransferases, psychosis. *Rare:* hepatitis, seizures, angioneurotic edema, Stevens-Johnson syndrome, tinnitus	Theophylline: serum levels increased by thiabendazole	C	No information
Triclabendazole	Fascioliasis, paragonimiasis	*Occasional:* abdominal cramps, diarrhea, biliary colic, transient headache	No information	Not assigned	Yes
Benznidazole	Chagas' disease	*Frequent:* rash, pruritus, nausea, leukopenia, paresthesias	No major interactions	Not assigned	No information
Bithionol[e]	Fascioliasis, paragonimiasis	Diarrhea, abdominal cramps (usually mild and transient)			
Clindamycin	Babesiosis, malaria, toxoplasmosis	*Occasional:* pseudomembranous colitis, abdominal pain, diarrhea, nausea/vomiting. *Rare:* pruritus, skin rashes	No major interactions	B	Yes[f]
Diloxanide furoate	Amebiasis	*Frequent:* flatulence. *Occasional:* nausea, vomiting, diarrhea. *Rare:* pruritus	None reported	Contraindicated	No information
Eflornithine[g] (difluoromethylornithine, DFMO)	Trypanosomiasis	*Frequent:* pancytopenia. *Occasional:* diarrhea, seizures. *Rare:* transient hearing loss	No major interactions	Contraindicated	No information
Emetine and dehydroemetine[e]	Amebiasis, fascioliasis	*Severe:* cardiotoxicity. *Frequent:* pain at injection site. *Occasional:* dizziness, headache, GI symptoms	None reported	X	No information
Folate antagonists					
Dihydrofolate reductase inhibitors					
Pyrimethamine	Malaria,[b] isosporiasis, toxoplasmosis[b]	*Occasional:* folate deficiency. *Rare:* rash, seizures, severe skin reactions (toxic epidermal necrolysis, erythema multiforme, Stevens-Johnson syndrome)	Sulfonamides, proguanil, zidovudine: increased risk of bone marrow suppression when used concomitantly	C	Yes
Proguanil and chlorproguanil	Malaria	*Occasional:* urticaria. *Rare:* hematuria, GI disturbances	No major interactions	C	Yes
Trimethoprim	Cyclosporiasis, isosporiasis	Hyperkalemia, GI upset, mild stomatitis	Methotrexate: reduced clearance Warfarin: effect prolonged Phenytoin: hepatic metabolism increased	C	Yes
Dihydropteroate synthetase inhibitors: sulfonamides Sulfadiazine Sulfamethoxazole Sulfadoxine	Malaria,[b] toxoplasmosis[b]	*Frequent:* GI disturbances, allergic skin reactions, crystalluria. *Rare:* severe skin reactions (toxic epidermal necrolysis, erythema multiforme, Stevens-Johnson syndrome), agranulocytosis, aplastic anemia, hypersensitivity of the respiratory tract, hepatitis, interstitial nephritis, hypoglycemia, aseptic meningitis	Thiazide diuretics: increased risk of thrombocytopenia in elderly patients Warfarin: effect prolonged by sulfonamides Methotrexate: levels increased by sulfonamides Phenytoin: metabolism impaired by sulfonamides Sulfonylureas: effect prolonged by sulfonamides	B	Yes
Dihydropteroate synthetase inhibitors: sulfones					
Dapsone	Leishmaniasis, malaria, toxoplasmosis	*Frequent:* rash, anorexia. *Occasional:* hemolysis, methemoglobinemia, neuropathy, allergic dermatitis, anorexia, nausea, vomiting, tachycardia, headache, insomnia, psychosis, hepatitis. *Rare:* agranulocytosis	Rifampin: lowered plasma levels of dapsone	C	Yes
Fumagillin	Microsporidiosis	*Rare:* neutropenia, thrombocytopenia	None reported	No information	No information

(continued)

TABLE 201-1 OVERVIEW OF AGENTS USED FOR THE TREATMENT OF PARASITIC INFECTIONS (CONTINUED)

Drugs by Class	Parasitic Infection(s)	Adverse Effects	Major Drug-Drug Interactions	Pregnancy Class[a]	Breast Milk
Furazolidone	Giardiasis	*Frequent:* nausea/vomiting, brown urine. *Occasional:* rectal itching, headache. *Rare:* hemolytic anemia, disulfiram-like reactions, MAO-inhibitor interactions	Risk of hypertensive crisis when administered for >5 days with MAO inhibitors	C	No information
Iodoquinol	Amebiasis,[b] balantidiasis, *D. fragilis* infection	*Occasional:* headache, rash, pruritus, thyrotoxicosis, nausea, vomiting, abdominal pain, diarrhea. *Rare:* optic neuritis, peripheral neuropathy, seizures, encephalopathy	No major interactions	C	No information
Ivermectin	Ascariasis, cutaneous larva migrans, gnathostomiasis, loiasis, lymphatic filariases, onchocerciasis,[b] scabies, strongyloidiasis,[b] trichuriasis	*Occasional:* fever, pruritus, headache, myalgias. *Rare:* hypotension	No major interactions	C	Yes[f]
Levamisole	Ascariasis, hookworm	*Frequent:* GI disturbances, dizziness, headache. *Rare:* agranulocytosis, peripheral neuropathy	Alcohol: disulfiram-like effect Warfarin: prolonged prothrombin time	C	No information
Macrolides					
Azithromycin	Babesiosis	*Occasional:* nausea, vomiting, diarrhea, abdominal pain. *Rare:* angioedema, cholestatic jaundice	Cyclosporine and digoxin: levels increased by azithromycin Nelfinavir: increased levels of azithromycin	B	Yes
Spiramycin[g]	Toxoplasmosis	*Occasional:* GI disturbances, transient skin eruptions. *Rare:* thrombocytopenia, QT prolongation in an infant, cholestatic hepatitis	No major interactions	Not assigned[c]	Yes[f]
Mefloquine	Malaria[b]	*Frequent:* lightheadedness, nausea, headache. *Occasional:* confusion; nightmares; insomnia; visual disturbance; transient and clinically silent ECG abnormalities, including sinus bradycardia, sinus arrhythmia, first-degree AV block, prolongation of QTc interval, and abnormal T waves. *Rare:* psychosis, convulsions, hypotension	Administration of halofantrine <3 weeks after mefloquine use may produce fatal QTc prolongation. Mefloquine may lower plasma levels of anticonvulsants. Levels decreased and clearance accelerated by artesunate	C	Yes
Melarsoprol[e]	Trypanosomiasis	*Frequent:* myocardial injury, encephalopathy, peripheral neuropathy, hypertension. *Occasional:* G6PD-induced hemolysis, erythema nodosum leprosum. *Rare:* hypotension	No major interactions	Not assigned	No information
Metrifonate	Schistosomiasis	*Frequent:* abdominal pain, nausea, vomiting, diarrhea, headache, vertigo, bronchospasm. *Rare:* cholinergic symptoms	No major interactions	B	No
Miltefosine	Leishmaniasis	*Frequent:* mild and transient (1–2 days) GI disturbances within first 2 weeks of therapy (resolve after treatment completion); motion sickness. *Occasional:* reversible elevations of creatinine and aminotransferases	No major interactions	Not assigned	No information
Niclosamide	Intestinal cestodes[b]	*Occasional:* nausea, vomiting, dizziness, pruritus	No major interactions	B	No information
Nifurtimox[e]	Chagas' disease	*Frequent:* nausea, vomiting, abdominal pain, insomnia, paresthesias, weakness, tremors. *Rare:* seizures (all are reversible and dose-related)	No major interactions	Not assigned	No information
Nitazoxanide	Cryptosporidiosis,[b] giardiasis[b]	*Occasional:* abdominal pain, diarrhea. *Rare:* vomiting, headache	No major interactions	B	No information
Nitroimidazoles					
Metronidazole	Amebiasis,[b] balantidiasis, dracunculiasis, giardiasis, trichomoniasis,[b] *D. fragilis* infection	*Frequent:* nausea, headache, anorexia, metallic aftertaste. *Occasional:* vomiting, insomnia, vertigo, paresthesias, disulfiram-like effects. *Rare:* seizures, peripheral neuropathy	Warfarin: effect enhanced by metronidazole Disulfiram: psychotic reaction Phenobarbital, phenytoin: accelerate elimination of metronidazole Lithium: serum levels elevated by metronidazole Cimetidine: prolonged half-life of metronidazole	B	Yes

(continued)

TABLE 201-1 OVERVIEW OF AGENTS USED FOR THE TREATMENT OF PARASITIC INFECTIONS (CONTINUED)

Drugs by Class	Parasitic Infection(s)	Adverse Effects	Major Drug-Drug Interactions	Pregnancy Class[a]	Breast Milk
Tinidazole	Amebiasis,[b] giardiasis, trichomoniasis	*Occasional:* nausea, vomiting, metallic taste	See metronidazole	C	Yes
Oxamniquine	Schistosomiasis	*Occasional:* dizziness, drowsiness, headache, orange urine, elevated aminotransferases. *Rare:* seizures	No major interactions	C	No information
Paromomycin	Amebiasis,[b] *D. fragilis* infection, giardiasis, cryptosporidiosis, leishmaniasis	*Frequent:* GI disturbances (oral dosing only). *Occasional:* nephrotoxicity, ototoxicity, vestibular toxicity (parenteral dosing only)	No major interactions	Oral: B Parenteral: not assigned[c]	No information
Pentamidine isethionate	Leishmaniasis, trypanosomiasis	*Frequent:* hypotension, hypoglycemia, pancreatitis, sterile abscesses at IM injection sites, GI disturbances, reversible renal failure. *Occasional:* hepatotoxicity, cardiotoxicity, delirium. *Rare:* anaphylaxis	No major interactions	C	No information
Piperazine and derivatives					
Piperazine	Ascariasis, enterobiasis	*Occasional:* nausea, vomiting, diarrhea, abdominal pain, headache. *Rare:* neurotoxicity, seizures	None reported	C	No information
Diethylcarbamazine[e]	Lymphatic filariasis, loiasis, tropical pulmonary eosinophilia	*Frequent:* dose-related nausea, vomiting. *Rare:* fever, chills, arthralgias, headaches	None reported	Not assigned[c]	No information
Praziquantel	Clonorchiasis,[b] cysticercosis, diphyllobothriasis, hymenolepiasis, taeniasis, opisthorchiasis, intestinal trematodes, paragonimiasis, schistosomiasis[b]	*Frequent:* abdominal pain, diarrhea, dizziness, headache, malaise. *Occasional:* fever, nausea. *Rare:* pruritus, singultus	No major interactions	B	Yes
Pyrantel pamoate	Ascariasis, eosinophilic enterocolitis, enterobiasis,[b] hookworm, trichostrongyliasis	*Occasional:* GI disturbances, headache, dizziness, elevated aminotransferases	No major interactions	C	No information
Quinacrine[g]	Giardiasis[b]	*Frequent:* headache, nausea, vomiting, bitter taste. *Occasional:* yellow-orange discoloration of skin, sclerae, urine; begins after 1 week of treatment and lasts up to 4 months after drug discontinuation. *Rare:* psychosis, exfoliative dermatitis, retinopathy, G6PD-induced hemolysis, exacerbation of psoriasis, disulfiram-like effects	Primaquine: toxicity potentiated by quinacrine	C	No information
Quinine and quinidine	Malaria, babesiosis	*Frequent:* cinchonism (tinnitus, high-tone deafness, headache, dysphoria, nausea, vomiting, abdominal pain, visual disturbances, postural hypotension), hyperinsulinemia resulting in life-threatening hypoglycemia. *Occasional:* deafness, hemolytic anemia, arrhythmias, hypotension due to rapid IV infusion	Carbonic-anhydrase inhibitors, thiazide diuretics: reduced renal elimination of quinidine Amiodarone, cimetidine: increased quinidine levels Nifedipine: decreased quinidine levels; quinidine slows metabolism of nifedipine Phenobarbital, phenytoin, rifampin: accelerated hepatic elimination of quinidine Verapamil: reduced hepatic clearance of quinidine Diltiazem: decreased clearance of quinidine	X	Yes[f]
Quinolones					
Ciprofloxacin	Cyclosporiasis, isosporiasis	*Occasional:* nausea, diarrhea, vomiting, abdominal pain/discomfort, headache, restlessness, rash. *Rare:* myalgias/arthralgias, tendon rupture, CNS symptoms (nervousness, agitation, insomnia, anxiety, nightmares or paranoia); convulsions	Probenecid: increased serum levels of ciprofloxacin Theophylline, warfarin: serum levels increased by ciprofloxacin	C	Yes

(continued)

TABLE 201-1 OVERVIEW OF AGENTS USED FOR THE TREATMENT OF PARASITIC INFECTIONS (CONTINUED)

Drugs by Class	Parasitic Infection(s)	Adverse Effects	Major Drug-Drug Interactions	Pregnancy Class[a]	Breast Milk
Suramin[e]	Trypanosomiasis	*Frequent:* immediate: fever, urticaria, nausea, vomiting, hypotension; delayed (up to 24 h): exfoliative dermatitis, stomatitis, paresthesias, photophobia, renal dysfunction. *Occasional:* nephrotoxicity, adrenal toxicity, optic atrophy, anaphylaxis	No major interactions	Not assigned	No information
Tetracyclines	Balantidiasis, *D. fragilis* infection, malaria; lymphatic filariasis (doxycycline)	*Frequent:* GI disturbances. *Occasional:* photosensitivity dermatitis. *Rare:* exfoliative dermatitis, esophagitis, hepatotoxicity	Warfarin: effect prolonged by tetracyclines	D	Yes

[a]Based on U.S. Food and Drug Administration (FDA) pregnancy categories of A–D, X.
[b]Approved by the FDA for this indication.
[c]Use in pregnancy is recommended by international organizations outside the United States.
[d]Only AmBisome has been approved for this indication.
[e]Available through the Centers for Disease Control and Prevention (CDC).
[f]Not believed to be harmful.
[g]Available through the manufacturer.
Note: ACTH, adrenocorticotropic hormone; AV, atrioventricular; CNS, central nervous system; ECG, electrocardiogram; G6PD, glucose 6-phosphate dehydrogenase; MAO, monoamine oxidase.

FURTHER READINGS

ABRAMOWICZ M (ed): Drugs for parasitic infections. Med Lett Drugs Ther 46:1, 2004

MOORE TA, MCCARTHY JS: Benzimidazoles (albendazole, mebendazole, thiabendazole, triclabendazole), in *Antimicrobial Therapy and Vaccines*, 2d ed, VL Yu et al (eds). Pittsburgh, ESun Technologies, 2005, pp 1021–1036

SHAPIRO TA, GOLDBERG DE: Drugs used in the chemotherapy of protozoal infections: Malaria, in *Goodman and Gilman's The Pharmacological Basis of Therapeutics*, 11th ed, L Brunton et al (eds). New York, McGraw-Hill, 2005, pp 1021–1048

WINSTANLEY P, WARD S: Malaria chemotherapy. Adv Parasitol 61:47, 2006

WORLD HEALTH ORGANIZATION: *Model Prescribing Information: Drugs Used in Parasitic Diseases*, 2d ed. Geneva, WHO, 1995

SECTION 18 PROTOZOAL INFECTIONS

202 Amebiasis and Infection with Free-Living Amebas

Sharon L. Reed

AMEBIASIS

DEFINITION

Amebiasis is an infection with the intestinal protozoan *Entamoeba histolytica*. About 90% of infections are asymptomatic, and the remaining 10% produce a spectrum of clinical syndromes ranging from dysentery to abscesses of the liver or other organs.

LIFE CYCLE AND TRANSMISSION

E. histolytica is acquired by ingestion of viable cysts from fecally contaminated water, food, or hands. Food-borne exposure is most prevalent and is particularly likely when food handlers are shedding cysts or food is being grown with feces-contaminated soil, fertilizer, or water. Besides the drinking of contaminated water, less common means of transmission include oral and anal sexual practices and—in rare instances—direct rectal inoculation through colonic irrigation devices. Motile trophozoites are released from cysts in the small intestine and, in most patients, remain as harmless commensals in the large bowel. After encystation, infectious cysts are shed in the stool and can survive for several weeks in a moist environment. In some patients, the trophozoites invade either the bowel mucosa, causing symptomatic colitis, or the bloodstream, causing distant abscesses of the liver, lungs, or brain. The trophozoites may not encyst in patients with active dysentery, and motile hematophagous trophozoites are frequently present in fresh stools. Trophozoites are rapidly killed by exposure to air or stomach acid, however, and therefore cannot transmit infection.

EPIDEMIOLOGY

About 10% of the world's population is infected with *Entamoeba*, the majority with noninvasive *Entamoeba dispar*. Amebiasis results from infection with *E. histolytica* and is the third most common cause of death from parasitic disease (after schistosomiasis and malaria). The wide spectrum of clinical disease caused by *Entamoeba* is due in part to the differences between these two infecting species. Cysts of *E. histolytica* and *E. dispar* are morphologically identical, but *E. histolytica* has unique isoenzymes, surface antigens, DNA markers, and virulence properties (Table 202-1). Most asymptomatic carriers, including homosexual men and patients with AIDS, harbor *E. dispar* and have self-limited infections. These observations indicate that *E. dispar* is incapable of causing invasive disease, since *Cryptosporidium* and *Isospora belli*, which also cause only self-limited illnesses in immunocompetent people, cause devastating diarrhea in

TABLE 202-1 *E. HISTOLYTICA* AND *E. DISPAR*, COMPARED AND CONTRASTED

Similarities

1. Both species are spread through ingestion of infectious cysts.
2. Cysts of the two species are morphologically identical.
3. Both species colonize the large intestine.

Differences

1. Only *E. histolytica* causes invasive disease.
2. Only *E. histolytica* infections elicit a positive amebic serology.
3. The two species have distinct rRNA sequences.
4. The two species have distinct surface antigens and isoenzyme markers.
5. Gal/GalNAc lectin can be used to differentiate the two species in stool ELISA.

Note: ELISA, enzyme-linked immunosorbent assay; Gal/GalNAc, galactose *N*-acetylgalactosamine. See text.

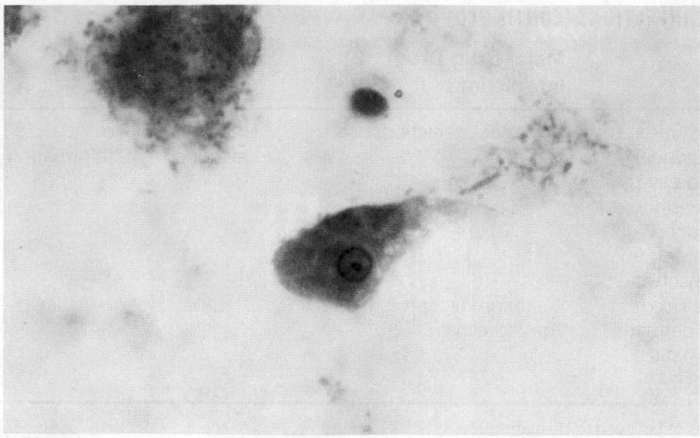

FIGURE 202-1 Trophozoite of *E. histolytica* demonstrating a single nucleus with a central, dot-like nucleolus (trichrome stain).

patients with AIDS. However, host factors play a role as well. In one study, 10% of asymptomatic patients who were colonized with *E. histolytica* went on to develop amebic colitis, while the rest remained asymptomatic and cleared the infection within 1 year.

Areas of highest incidence (due to inadequate sanitation and crowding) include most developing countries in the tropics, particularly Mexico, India, and nations of Central and South America, tropical Asia, and Africa. In a 4-year follow-up study of preschool children in a highly endemic area of Bangladesh, 80% of children had at least one episode of infection with *E. histolytica* and 53% had more than one episode. Naturally acquired immunity did develop but was usually short-lived and correlated with the presence in the stool of secretory IgA antibody to the major adherence lectin galactose *N*-acetylgalactosamine (Gal/GalNAc). The main groups at risk for amebiasis in developed countries are returned travelers, recent immigrants, homosexual men, and inmates of institutions.

PATHOGENESIS AND PATHOLOGY

Both trophozoites (Fig. 202-1) and cysts (Fig. 202-2) are found in the intestinal lumen, but only trophozoites of *E. histolytica* invade tissue. The trophozoite is 20–60 μm in diameter and contains vacuoles and a nucleus with a characteristic central nucleolus. In animals, depletion of intestinal mucus, diffuse inflammation, and disruption of the epithelial barrier occur before trophozoites actually come into contact with the colonic mucosa. Trophozoites attach to colonic mucus and epithelial cells by Gal/GalNAc. The earliest intestinal lesions are microulcerations of the mucosa of the cecum, sigmoid colon, or rectum that release erythrocytes, inflammatory cells, and epithelial cells. Proctoscopy reveals small ulcers with heaped-up margins and normal intervening mucosa. Submucosal extension of ulcerations under viable-appearing surface mucosa causes the classic "flask-shaped" ulcer containing trophozoites at the margins of dead and viable tissues. Although neutrophilic infiltrates may accompany the early lesions in animals, human intestinal infection is marked by a paucity of inflammatory cells, probably in part because of the killing of neutrophils by trophozoites (Fig. 202-3). Treated ulcers characteristically heal with little or no scarring. Occasionally, however, full-thickness necrosis and perforation occur.

Rarely, intestinal infection results in the formation of a mass lesion, or *ameboma*, in the bowel lumen. The overlying mucosa is usually thin and ulcerated, while other layers of the wall are thickened, edematous, and hemorrhagic; this condition results in exuberant formation of granulation tissue with little fibrous-tissue response.

A number of virulence factors have been linked to the ability of *E. histolytica* to invade through the interglandular epithelium. One consists of the extracellular cysteine proteinases that degrade collagen, elastin, IgA, IgG, and the anaphylatoxins C3a and C5a. Other enzymes may disrupt glycoprotein bonds between mucosal epithelial cells in the gut. Amebas can lyse neutrophils, monocytes, lymphocytes, and cells of colonic and hepatic lines. The cytolytic effect of amebas appears to require direct contact with target cells and may be linked to the release of phospholipase A and pore-forming peptides. *E. histolytica* trophozoites also cause apoptosis of human cells.

Liver abscesses are always preceded by intestinal colonization, which may be asymptomatic. Blood vessels may be compromised early by wall lysis and thrombus formation. Trophozoites invade veins to reach the liver through the portal venous system. *E. histolytica* is resistant to complement-mediated lysis—a property critical to survival in the bloodstream. In contrast, *E. dispar* is rapidly lysed by complement and is thus restricted to the bowel lumen. Inoculation of amebas into the portal system of hamsters results in an acute cellular infiltrate consisting predominantly of neutrophils. Later, the neutrophils are lysed by contact with amebas, and the release of neutrophil toxins may contribute to necrosis of hepatocytes. The liver parenchyma is replaced by necrotic material that is surrounded by a thin rim of congested liver tissue. The necrotic contents of a liver abscess are classically described as "anchovy paste," although the fluid is variable in color and is composed of bacteriologically sterile granular debris with few or no cells. Amebas, if seen, tend to be found near the capsule of the abscess.

A study in Bangladeshi schoolchildren revealed that an intestinal IgA response to Gal/GalNAc reduced the risk of new *E. histolytica* infection by 64%. Serum IgG antibody is not protective; titers correlate with the duration of illness rather than with the severity of disease. Indeed, Bangladeshi children with a serum IgG response were more likely than those without such a response to develop new *E. histolytica* infection. Studies of animals suggest that cell-mediated immunity may

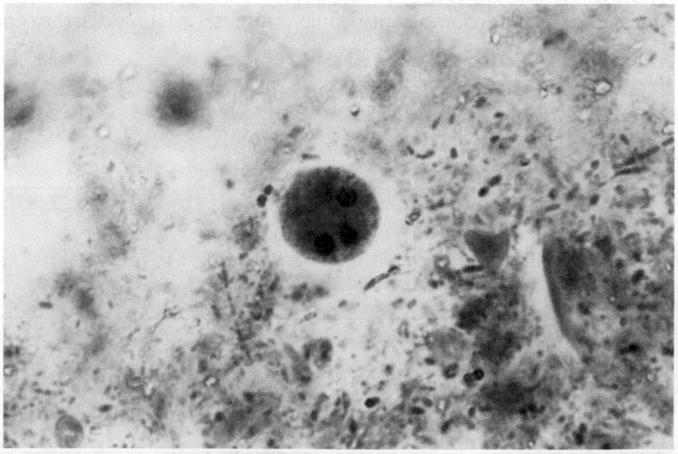

FIGURE 202-2 Cyst of *E. histolytica* showing three of the four nuclei (trichrome stain).

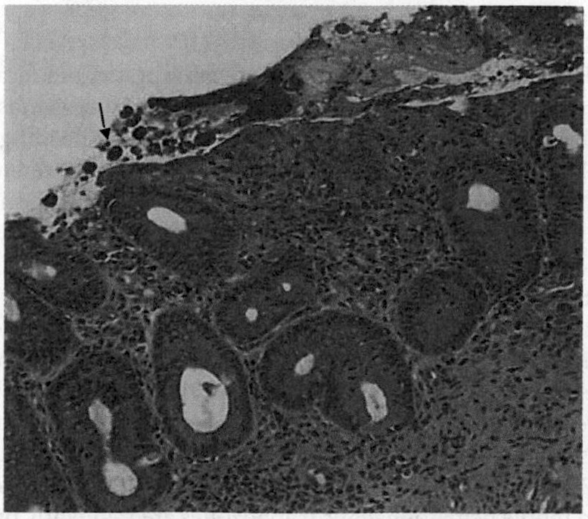

FIGURE 202-3 Pathology of amebic ulcer with colonic invasion. Arrow points to trophozoites (hematoxylin and eosin, 400X).

be important for protection, although patients with AIDS appear not to be predisposed to more severe disease.

CLINICAL SYNDROMES

Intestinal Amebiasis The most common type of amebic infection is asymptomatic cyst passage. Even in highly endemic areas, most patients harbor *E. dispar*.

Symptomatic amebic colitis develops 2–6 weeks after the ingestion of infectious cysts. A gradual onset of lower abdominal pain and mild diarrhea is followed by malaise, weight loss, and diffuse lower abdominal or back pain. Cecal involvement may mimic acute appendicitis. Patients with full-blown dysentery may pass 10–12 stools per day. The stools contain little fecal material and consist mainly of blood and mucus. In contrast to those with bacterial diarrhea, fewer than 40% of patients with amebic dysentery are febrile. Virtually all patients have heme-positive stools.

More fulminant intestinal infection, with severe abdominal pain, high fever, and profuse diarrhea, is rare and occurs predominantly in children. Patients may develop toxic megacolon, in which there is severe bowel dilation with intramural air. Patients receiving glucocorticoids are at risk for severe amebiasis. Uncommonly, patients develop a chronic form of amebic colitis, which can be confused with inflammatory bowel disease. The association between severe amebiasis complications and glucocorticoid therapy emphasizes the importance of excluding amebiasis when inflammatory bowel disease is suspected. An occasional patient presents with only an asymptomatic or tender abdominal mass caused by an ameboma, which is easily confused with cancer on barium studies. A positive serologic test or biopsy can prevent unnecessary surgery in this setting. The syndrome of postamebic colitis—persistent diarrhea following documented cure of amebic colitis—is controversial; no evidence of recurrent amebic infection can be found, and re-treatment usually has no effect.

Amebic Liver Abscess Extraintestinal infection by *E. histolytica* most often involves the liver. Of travelers who develop an amebic liver abscess after leaving an endemic area, 95% do so within 5 months. Young patients with an amebic liver abscess are more likely than older patients to present in the acute phase with prominent symptoms of <10 days' duration. Most patients are febrile and have right-upper-quadrant pain, which may be dull or pleuritic in nature and may radiate to the shoulder. Point tenderness over the liver and right-sided pleural effusion are common. Jaundice is rare. Although the initial site of infection is the colon, fewer than one-third of patients with an amebic abscess have active diarrhea. Older patients from endemic areas are more likely to have a subacute course lasting 6 months, with weight loss and hepatomegaly. About one-third of patients with chronic presentations are febrile. Thus, the clinical diagnosis of an amebic liver abscess may be difficult to establish because the symptoms and signs are often nonspecific. Since 10–15% of patients present only with fever, amebic liver abscess must be considered in the differential diagnosis of fever of unknown origin (Chap. 19).

Complications of Amebic Liver Abscess Pleuropulmonary involvement, which is reported in 20–30% of patients, is the most frequent complication of amebic liver abscess. Manifestations include sterile effusions, contiguous spread from the liver, and rupture into the pleural space. Sterile effusions and contiguous spread usually resolve with medical therapy, but frank rupture into the pleural space requires drainage. A hepatobronchial fistula may cause cough productive of large amounts of necrotic material that may contain amebas. This dramatic complication carries a good prognosis. Abscesses that rupture into the peritoneum may present as an indolent leak or an acute abdomen and require both percutaneous catheter drainage and medical therapy. Rupture into the pericardium, usually from abscesses of the left lobe of the liver, carries the gravest prognosis; it can occur during medical therapy and requires surgical drainage.

Other Extraintestinal Sites The genitourinary tract may become involved by direct extension of amebiasis from the colon or by hematogenous spread of the infection. Painful genital ulcers, characterized by a punched-out appearance and profuse discharge, may develop secondary to extension from either the intestine or the liver. Both these conditions respond well to medical therapy. Cerebral involvement has been reported in fewer than 0.1% of patients in large clinical series. Symptoms and prognosis depend on the size and location of the lesion.

DIAGNOSTIC TESTS

Laboratory Diagnosis Stool examinations, serologic tests, and noninvasive imaging of the liver are the most important procedures in the diagnosis of amebiasis. Fecal findings suggestive of amebic colitis include a positive test for heme, a paucity of neutrophils, and amebic cysts or trophozoites. The definitive diagnosis of amebic colitis is made by the demonstration of hematophagous trophozoites of *E. histolytica* (Fig. 202-1). Because trophozoites are killed rapidly by water, drying, or barium, it is important to examine at least three fresh stool specimens. Examination of a combination of wet mounts, iodine-stained concentrates, and trichrome-stained preparations of fresh stool and concentrates for cysts (Fig. 202-2) or trophozoites (Fig. 202-1) confirms the diagnosis in 75–95% of cases. Cultures of amebas are more sensitive but are not routinely available. If stool examinations are negative, sigmoidoscopy with biopsy of the edge of ulcers may increase the yield, but this procedure is dangerous during fulminant colitis because of the risk of perforation. Trophozoites in a biopsy specimen from a colonic mass confirm the diagnosis of ameboma, but trophozoites are rare in liver aspirates because they are found in the abscess capsule and not in the readily aspirated necrotic center. Accurate diagnosis requires experience, since the trophozoites may be confused with neutrophils and the cysts must be differentiated morphologically from *Entamoeba hartmanni*, *Entamoeba coli*, and *Endolimax nana*, which do not cause clinical disease and do not warrant therapy. Unfortunately, the cysts of *E. histolytica* cannot be distinguished microscopically from those of *E. dispar*. Therefore, the microscopic diagnosis of *E. histolytica* can be made only by the detection of *Entamoeba* trophozoites that have ingested erythrocytes. In terms of sensitivity, stool diagnostic tests based on the detection of the Gal/GalNAc lectin of *E. histolytica* compare favorably with the polymerase chain reaction and with isolation in culture followed by isoenzyme analysis.

Serology is an important addition to the methods used for parasitologic diagnosis of invasive amebiasis. Enzyme-linked immunosorbent assays (ELISAs) and agar gel diffusion assays are positive in more than 90% of patients with colitis, amebomas, or liver abscess. Positive results in conjunction with the appropriate clinical syndrome suggest active disease because serologic findings usually revert to negative within 6–12 months. Even in highly endemic areas such as South Africa, fewer than 10% of asymptomatic individuals have a positive amebic serology. The interpretation of the indirect hemagglutination test is more difficult because titers may remain positive for as long as 10 years.

Up to 10% of patients with acute amebic liver abscess may have negative serologic findings; in suspected cases with an initially negative result, testing should be repeated in a week. In contrast to carriers of *E. dispar*, most asymptomatic carriers of *E. histolytica* develop antibodies. Thus, serologic tests are helpful in assessing the risk of invasive amebiasis in asymptomatic, cyst-passing individuals in nonendemic areas. Serologic tests also should be performed in patients with ulcerative colitis before the institution of glucocorticoid therapy to prevent the development of severe colitis or toxic megacolon owing to unsuspected amebiasis.

Routine hematology and chemistry tests usually are not very helpful in the diagnosis of invasive amebiasis. About three-fourths of patients with an amebic liver abscess have leukocytosis (>10,000 cells/μL); this condition is particularly likely if symptoms are acute or complications have developed. Invasive amebiasis does not elicit eosinophilia. Anemia, if present, is usually multifactorial. Even with large liver abscesses, liver enzyme levels are normal or minimally elevated. The alkaline phosphatase level is most often elevated and may remain so for months. Aminotransferase elevations suggest acute disease or a complication.

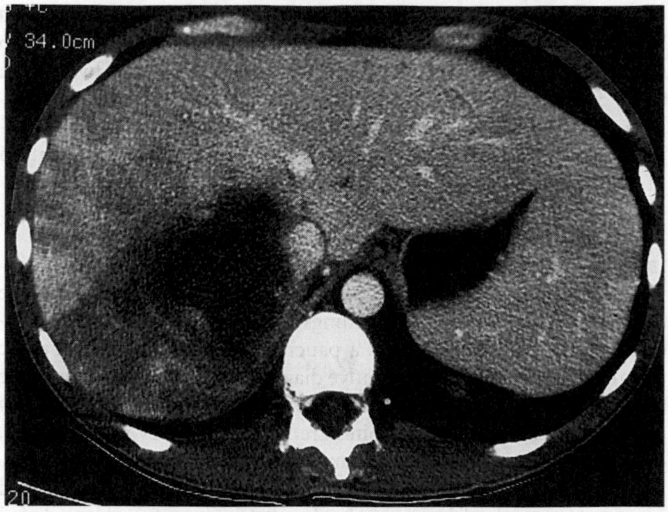

FIGURE 202-4 Abdominal CT scan of a large amebic abscess of the right lobe of the liver. *(Courtesy of the Department of Radiology, UCSD Medical Center, San Diego; with permission.)*

Radiographic Studies Radiographic barium studies are potentially dangerous in acute amebic colitis. Amebomas are usually identified first by a barium enema, but biopsy is necessary for differentiation from carcinoma.

Radiographic techniques such as ultrasonography, CT, and MRI are all useful for detection of the round or oval hypoechoic cyst. More than 80% of patients who have had symptoms for >10 days have a single abscess of the right lobe of the liver (Fig. 202-4). Approximately 50% of patients who have had symptoms for <10 days have multiple abscesses. Findings associated with complications include large abscesses (>10 cm) in the superior part of the right lobe, which may rupture into the pleural space; multiple lesions, which must be differentiated from pyogenic abscesses; and lesions of the left lobe, which may rupture into the pericardium. Because abscesses resolve slowly and may increase in size in patients who are responding clinically to therapy, frequent follow-up ultrasonography may prove confusing. Complete resolution of a liver abscess within 6 months can be anticipated in two-thirds of patients, but 10% may have persistent abnormalities for a year.

DIFFERENTIAL DIAGNOSIS

The differential diagnosis of intestinal amebiasis includes bacterial diarrheas (Chap. 122) caused by *Campylobacter* (Chap. 148); enteroinvasive *Escherichia coli* (Chap. 143); and species of *Shigella* (Chap. 147), *Salmonella* (Chap. 146), and *Vibrio* (Chap. 149). Although the typical patient with amebic colitis has less prominent fever than in these other conditions as well as heme-positive stools with few neutrophils, correct diagnosis requires bacterial cultures, microscopic examination of stools, and amebic serologic testing. As has already been mentioned, amebiasis must be ruled out in any patient thought to have inflammatory bowel disease.

Because of the variety of presenting signs and symptoms, amebic liver abscess can easily be confused with pulmonary or gallbladder disease or with any febrile illness with few localizing signs, such as malaria (Chap. 203) or typhoid fever (Chap. 146). The diagnosis should be considered in members of high-risk groups who have recently traveled outside the United States (Chap. 117) and in inmates of institutions. Once radiographic studies have identified an abscess in the liver, the most important differential diagnosis is between amebic and pyogenic abscess. Patients with pyogenic abscess typically are older and have a history of underlying bowel disease or recent surgery. Amebic serology is helpful, but aspiration of the abscess, with Gram's staining and culture of the material, may be required for differentiation of the two diseases.

℞ AMEBIASIS

INTESTINAL DISEASE (Table 202-2) The drugs used to treat amebiasis can be classified according to their primary site of action. Luminal amebicides are poorly absorbed and reach high concentrations in the bowel, but their activity is limited to cysts and trophozoites close to the mucosa. Only two luminal drugs are available in the United States: iodoquinol and paromomycin. Indications for the use of luminal agents include eradication of cysts in patients with colitis or a liver abscess and treatment of asymptomatic carriers. The majority of asymptomatic individuals who pass cysts are colonized with *E. dispar*, which does not warrant specific therapy. However, it is prudent to treat asymptomatic individuals who pass cysts unless *E. dispar* colonization can be definitively demonstrated by specific antigen-detection tests.

TABLE 202-2 DRUG THERAPY FOR AMEBIASIS

Indication	Therapy
Asymptomatic carriage	Luminal agent: iodoquinol (650-mg tablets), 650 mg tid for 20 days; *or* paromomycin (250-mg tablets), 500 mg tid for 10 days
Acute colitis	Metronidazole (250- or 500-mg tablets), 750 mg PO or IV tid for 5–10 days, *plus* Luminal agent as above
Amebic liver abscess	Metronidazole, 750 mg PO or IV for 5–10 days, *or* Tinidazole, 2 g PO once, *or* Ornidazole,[a] 2 g PO once, *plus* Luminal agent as above

[a]Not available in the United States.

Tissue amebicides reach high concentrations in the blood and tissue after oral or parenteral administration. The development of nitroimidazole compounds, especially metronidazole, was a major advance in the treatment of invasive amebiasis. Patients with amebic colitis should be treated with intravenous or oral metronidazole. Side effects include nausea, vomiting, abdominal discomfort, and a disulfiram-like reaction. Another longer-acting imidazole compound, tinidazole, is also effective and was recently approved in the United States. All patients should also receive a full course of therapy with a luminal agent, since metronidazole does not eradicate cysts. Resistance to metronidazole has been selected in the laboratory but has not been found in clinical isolates. Relapses are not uncommon and probably represent reinfection or failure to eradicate amebas from the bowel because of an inadequate dosage or duration of therapy.

AMEBIC LIVER ABSCESS Metronidazole is the drug of choice for amebic liver abscess. Longer-acting nitroimidazoles (tinidazole and ornidazole) have been effective as single-dose therapy in developing countries. With early diagnosis and therapy, mortality rates from uncomplicated amebic liver abscess are <1%. The second-line therapeutic agents emetine and chloroquine should be avoided if possible because of the potential cardiovascular and gastrointestinal side effects of the former and the higher relapse rates with the latter. There is no evidence that combined therapy with two drugs is more effective than the single-drug regimen. Studies of South Africans with liver abscesses demonstrated that 72% of patients without intestinal symptoms had bowel infection with *E. histolytica*; thus, all treatment regimens should include a luminal agent to eradicate cysts and prevent further transmission. Amebic liver abscess recurs rarely.

ASPIRATION OF LIVER ABSCESSES More than 90% of patients respond dramatically to metronidazole therapy with decreases in both pain and fever within 72 h. Indications for aspiration of liver abscesses are (1) the need to rule out a pyogenic abscess, particularly in patients with multiple lesions; (2) the lack of a clinical response in 3–5 days; (3) the threat of imminent rupture; and (4) the need to prevent rupture of left-lobe abscesses into the pericardium. There is no evidence that aspiration, even of large abscesses (up to 10 cm), accelerates healing. Percutaneous drainage may be successful even if the liver abscess has already ruptured. Surgery should be reserved for instances of bowel perforation and rupture into the pericardium.

PREVENTION

Amebic infection is spread by ingestion of food or water contaminated with cysts. Since an asymptomatic carrier may excrete up to 15 million cysts per day, prevention of infection requires adequate sanitation and

eradication of cyst carriage. In high-risk areas, infection can be minimized by the avoidance of unpeeled fruits and vegetables and the use of bottled water. Because cysts are resistant to readily attainable levels of chlorine, disinfection by iodination (tetraglycine hydroperiodide) is recommended. There is no effective prophylaxis.

INFECTION WITH FREE-LIVING AMEBAS

EPIDEMIOLOGY

Free-living amebas of the genera *Acanthamoeba* and *Naegleria* are distributed throughout the world and have been isolated from a wide variety of fresh and brackish water, including that from lakes, taps, hot springs, swimming pools, and heating and air-conditioning units, and even from the nasal passages of healthy children. Encystation may protect the protozoa from desiccation and food deprivation. The persistence of *Legionella pneumophila* in water supplies may be attributable in part to chronic infection of free-living amebas, particularly *Naegleria*. Free-living amebas of the genus *Balamuthia* have only recently been isolated from soil samples, including a sample from a flowerpot linked to a fatal infection in a child.

NAEGLERIA INFECTIONS

Primary amebic meningoencephalitis caused by *Naegleria fowleri* follows the aspiration of water contaminated with trophozoites or cysts or the inhalation of contaminated dust, leading to invasion of the olfactory neuroepithelium. After an incubation period of 2–15 days, severe headache, high fever, nausea, vomiting, and meningismus develop. Photophobia and palsies of the third, fourth, and sixth cranial nerves are common. Rapid progression to seizures and coma may follow. The prognosis is uniformly poor: most patients die within a week. Only a few survivors, treated with high-dose amphotericin B and rifampin, have been reported. Infection is most common in otherwise-healthy children or young adults, who often report recent swimming in lakes or heated swimming pools.

The diagnosis of *Naegleria* infection should be considered in any patient who has purulent meningitis without evidence of bacteria on Gram's staining, antigen detection assay, and culture. Other laboratory findings resemble those for fulminant bacterial meningitis, with elevated intracranial pressure, high white blood cell counts (up to 20,000/μL), and elevated protein concentrations and low glucose levels in cerebrospinal fluid (CSF). Diagnosis depends on the detection of motile trophozoites in wet mounts of fresh spinal fluid. Antibodies to *Naegleria* spp. have been detected in normal adults; serologic testing is not useful in the diagnosis of acute infection.

ACANTHAMOEBA INFECTIONS

Granulomatous Amebic Encephalitis Infection with *Acanthamoeba* species follows a more indolent course and typically occurs in chronically ill or debilitated patients. Risk factors include lymphoproliferative disorders, chemotherapy, glucocorticoid therapy, lupus erythematosus, and AIDS. Infection usually reaches the central nervous system (CNS) hematogenously from a primary focus in the sinuses, skin, or lungs. In the CNS, the onset is insidious, and the syndrome often mimics a space-occupying lesion. Altered mental status, headache, and stiff neck may be accompanied by focal findings such as cranial nerve palsies, ataxia, and hemiparesis. Cutaneous ulcers or hard nodules containing amebas are frequently detected in AIDS patients with disseminated *Acanthamoeba* infection.

Examination of the CSF for trophozoites may be diagnostically helpful, but lumbar puncture may be contraindicated because of increased intracerebral pressure. CT frequently reveals cortical and subcortical lesions of decreased density consistent with embolic infarcts. In other patients, multiple enhancing lesions with edema may mimic the computed tomographic appearance of toxoplasmosis (Chap. 207). Demonstration of the trophozoites and cysts of *Acanthamoeba* on wet mounts or in biopsy specimens establishes the diagnosis. Culture on nonnutrient agar plates seeded with *E. coli* may also be helpful. Fluorescein-labeled antiserum is available from the Centers for Disease Control and Prevention (CDC) for the detection of protozoa in biopsy specimens. Granulomatous amebic encephalitis in patients with AIDS may have an accelerated course (with survival for only 3–40 days) because of the difficulty these individuals have in forming granulomas. Various antimicrobial agents have been used to treat *Acanthamoeba* infection, including pentamidine, trimethoprim-sulfamethoxazole, and fluconazole, but the infection is almost uniformly fatal.

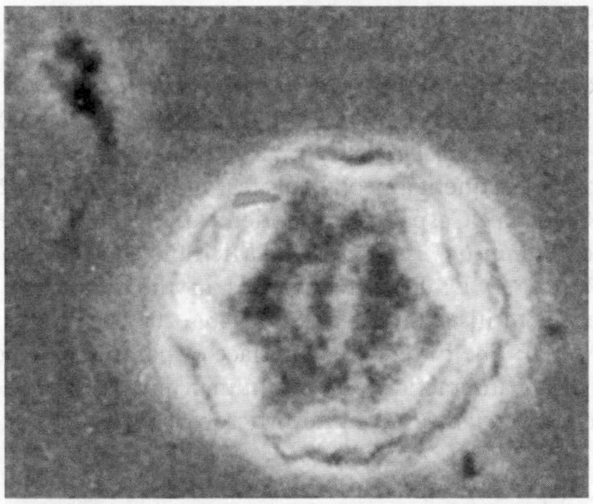

FIGURE 202-5 Double-walled cyst of *Acanthamoeba castellani*, as seen by phase-contrast microscopy. *[From DJ Krogstad et al, in A Balows et al (eds): Manual of Clinical Microbiology, 5th ed. Washington, DC, American Society for Microbiology, 1991.]*

Keratitis The incidence of keratitis caused by *Acanthamoeba* has increased in the past 20 years, in part as a result of improved diagnosis. Earlier infections were associated with trauma to the eye and exposure to contaminated water. At present, most infections are linked to extended-wear contact lenses, and rare cases are associated with laser-assisted in situ keratomileusis (LASIK). Risk factors include the use of homemade saline, the wearing of lenses while swimming, and inadequate disinfection. Since contact lenses presumably cause microscopic trauma, the early corneal findings may be nonspecific. The first symptoms usually include tearing and the painful sensation of a foreign body. Once infection is established, progression is rapid; the characteristic clinical sign is an annular, paracentral corneal ring representing a corneal abscess. Deeper corneal invasion and loss of vision may follow.

The differential diagnosis includes bacterial, mycobacterial, and herpetic infection. The irregular polygonal cysts of *Acanthamoeba* (Fig. 202-5) may be identified in corneal scrapings or biopsy material, and trophozoites can be grown on special media. Cysts are resistant to available drugs, and the results of medical therapy have been disappointing. Some reports have suggested partial responses to propamidine isethionate eyedrops. Severe infections usually require keratoplasty.

BALAMUTHIA INFECTIONS

Balamuthia mandrillaris, a free-living ameba previously referred to as a leptomyxid ameba, is an important etiologic agent of amebic meningoencephalitis in immunocompetent hosts. The course is typically subacute, with focal neurologic signs, fever, seizures, and headaches leading to death within 1 week to several months after onset. Examination of CSF reveals mononuclear or neutrophilic pleocytosis, elevated protein levels, and normal to low glucose concentrations. Multiple hypodense lesions are usually detected with imaging studies. This mixed picture of space-occupying lesions with CSF pleocytosis is suggestive of *Balamuthia*. Detection of an indirect fluorescent antibody response may be helpful in noninvasive diagnosis, but usually a definitive diagnosis is made post-mortem. Fluorescent antibody is available from the CDC. The variety of drugs used to treat the few surviving patients (numbering fewer than five in the United States) include pentamidine, flucytosine, sulfadiazine, and macrolides. The differential diagnosis includes tuberculomas (Chap. 158) and neurocysticercosis (Chap. 213).

DEETZ TR et al: Successful treatment of *Balamuthia* amoebic encephalitis: Presentation of two cases. Clin Infect Dis 37:1304, 2003

HAQUE R et al: *Entamoeba histolytica* infection in children and protection from subsequent amebiasis. Infect Immun 37:1304, 2003

HUSTON CD et al: Caspase-3-dependent killing of host cells by the parasite *Entamoeba histolytica*. Cell Microbiol 2:617, 2000

KUMAR R, LLOYD D: Recent advances in the treatment of *Acanthamoeba* keratitis. Clin Infect Dis 35:434, 2002

PETRI WA et al: The bittersweet interface of parasite and host lectin-carbohydrate interactions during human invasion by the parasite *Entamoeba histolytica*. Annu Rev Microbiol 56:39, 2002

QUE X, REED SL: Cysteine proteinases and the pathogenesis of amebiasis. Clin Microbiol Rev 13:196, 2002

SCHUSTER FL, VISVESVARA GS: Free-living amoebae as opportunistic and non-opportunistic pathogens of humans and animals. Int J Parasitol 345:1001, 2004

SOLAYMANI-MOHAMMADI S et al: Comparison of a stool antigen detection kit and PCR for diagnosis of *Entamoeba histolytica* and *Entamoeba dispar* infections in asymptomatic cyst passers in Iran. J Clin Microbiol 44:2258, 2006

STANLEY SL: Amoebiasis. Lancet 361:1025, 2006

———, REED SL: Microbes and microbial toxins: Paradigms for microbial-mucosal interactions. VI. *Entamoeba histolytica*: Parasite-host interactions. Am J Physiol Gastrointest Liver Physiol 280:G1049, 2001

203 Malaria

Nicholas J. White, Joel G. Breman

Humanity has but three great enemies: Fever, famine and war; of these by far the greatest, by far the most terrible, is fever.

William Osler

Malaria is a protozoan disease transmitted by the bite of infected *Anopheles* mosquitoes. It is the most important of the parasitic diseases of humans, with transmission in 107 countries containing 3 billion people and causing 1–3 million deaths each year. Malaria has now been eliminated from the United States, Canada, Europe, and Russia but, despite enormous control efforts, has resurged in many parts of the tropics. Added to this resurgence are the increasing problems of drug resistance of the parasite and insecticide resistance of the vectors. Occasional local transmission after importation of malaria has occurred recently in several southern and eastern areas of the United States and in Europe, indicating the continual danger to nonmalarious countries. Although there are promising new control and research initiatives, malaria remains today, as it has been for centuries, a heavy burden on tropical communities, a threat to nonendemic countries, and a danger to travelers.

ETIOLOGY AND PATHOGENESIS

Four species of the genus *Plasmodium* cause nearly all malarial infections in humans (although rare infections involve species normally affecting other primates). These are *P. falciparum*, *P. vivax*, *P. ovale*, and *P. malariae* (Table 203-1). Almost all deaths are caused by falciparum malaria. Human infection begins when a female anopheline mosquito inoculates plasmodial *sporozoites* from its salivary gland during a blood meal (Fig. 203-1). These microscopic motile forms of the malarial parasite are carried rapidly via the bloodstream to the liver, where they invade hepatic parenchymal cells and begin a period of asexual reproduction. By this amplification process (known as *intrahepatic* or *preerythrocytic schizogony* or *merogony*), a single sporozoite eventually may produce from 10,000 to >30,000 daughter merozoites. The swollen infected liver cell eventually bursts, discharging motile *merozoites* into the bloodstream. These then invade the red blood cells (RBCs) and multiply six- to twentyfold every 48–72 h. When the parasites reach densities of ~50/μL of blood, the symptomatic stage of the infection begins. In *P. vivax* and *P. ovale* infections, a proportion of the intrahepatic forms do not divide immediately but remain dormant for a period ranging from 3 weeks to a year or longer before reproduction begins. These dormant forms, or *hypnozoites*, are the cause of the relapses that characterize infection with these two species.

After entry into the bloodstream, merozoites rapidly invade erythrocytes and become *trophozoites*. Attachment is mediated via a specific erythrocyte surface receptor. In the case of *P. vivax*, this receptor is related to the Duffy blood-group antigen Fy^a or Fy^b. Most West Africans and people with origins in that region carry the Duffy-negative FyFy phenotype and are therefore resistant to *P. vivax* malaria. During the early stage of intraerythrocytic development, the small "ring forms" of the four parasitic species appear similar under light microscopy. As the trophozoites enlarge, species-specific characteristics become evident, pigment becomes visible, and the parasite assumes an irregular or ameboid shape. By the end of the 48-h intraerythrocytic life cycle (72 h for *P. malariae*), the parasite has consumed nearly all the hemoglobin and grown to occupy most of the RBC. It is now called a *schizont*. Multiple nuclear divisions have taken place (*schizogony* or *merogony*), and the RBC then ruptures to release 6–30 daughter merozoites, each potentially capable of invading a new RBC and repeating the cycle. The disease in human beings is caused by the direct effects of RBC invasion and destruction by the asexual parasite and the host's reaction. After a series of asexual cycles (*P. falciparum*) or immediately after release from the liver (*P. vivax, P. ovale, P. malariae*), some of the para-

TABLE 203-1 CHARACTERISTICS OF *PLASMODIUM* SPECIES INFECTING HUMANS

	Finding for Indicated Species			
Characteristic	***P. falciparum***	***P. vivax***	***P. ovale***	***P. malariae***
Duration of intrahepatic phase (days)	5.5	8	9	15
Number of merozoites released per infected hepatocyte	30,000	10,000	15,000	15,000
Duration of erythrocytic cycle (hours)	48	48	50	72
Red cell preference	Younger cells (but can invade cells of all ages)	Reticulocytes and cells up to 2 weeks old	Reticulocytes	Older cells
Morphology	Usually only ring forms[a]; banana-shaped gametocytes	Irregularly shaped large rings and trophozoites; enlarged erythrocytes; Schüffner's dots	Infected erythrocytes, enlarged and oval with tufted ends; Schüffner's dots	Band or rectangular forms of trophozoites common
Pigment color	Black	Yellow-brown	Dark brown	Brown-black
Ability to cause relapses	No	Yes	Yes	No

[a]Parasitemias of >2% are suggestive of *P. falciparum* infection.

sites develop into morphologically distinct, longer-lived sexual forms (*gametocytes*) that can transmit malaria.

After being ingested in the blood meal of a biting female anopheline mosquito, the male and female gametocytes form a zygote in the insect's midgut. This zygote matures into an ookinete, which penetrates and encysts in the mosquito's gut wall. The resulting oocyst expands by asexual division until it bursts to liberate myriad motile sporozoites, which then migrate in the hemolymph to the salivary gland of the mosquito to await inoculation into another human at the next feeding.

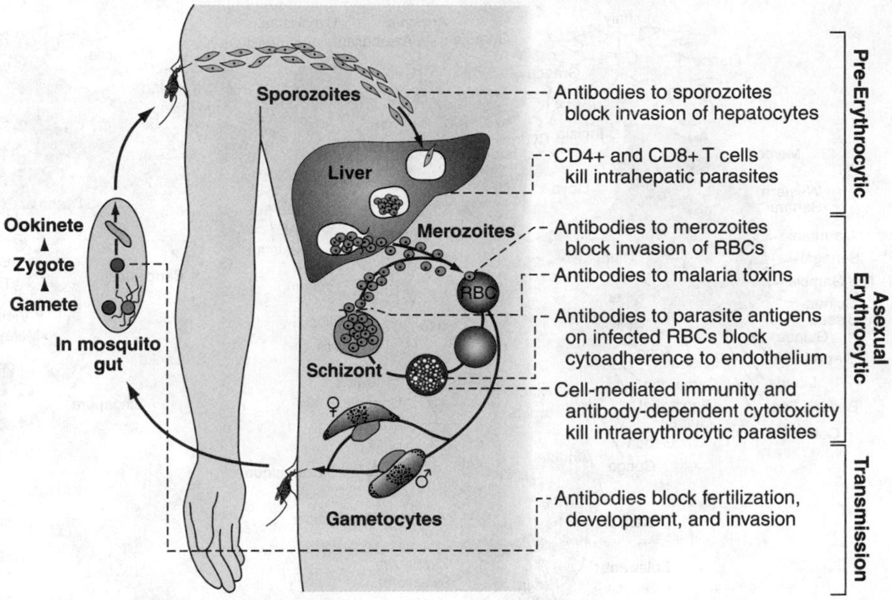

FIGURE 203-1 The malaria transmission cycle from mosquito to human. RBC, red blood cell.

EPIDEMIOLOGY

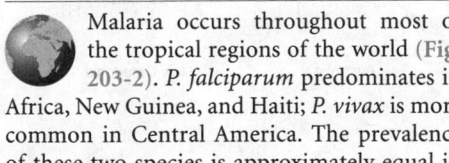

Malaria occurs throughout most of the tropical regions of the world (Fig. 203-2). *P. falciparum* predominates in Africa, New Guinea, and Haiti; *P. vivax* is more common in Central America. The prevalence of these two species is approximately equal in South America, the Indian subcontinent, eastern Asia, and Oceania. *P. malariae* is found in most endemic areas, especially throughout sub-Saharan Africa, but is much less common. *P. ovale* is relatively unusual outside of Africa and, where it is found, comprises <1% of isolates.

The epidemiology of malaria is complex and may vary considerably even within relatively small geographic areas. Endemicity traditionally has been defined in terms of parasitemia rates or palpable-spleen rates in children 2–9 years of age as hypoendemic (<10%), mesoendemic (11–50%), hyperendemic (51–75%), and holoendemic (>75%); however, it is uncommon to use these indices for planning control programs. In holo- and hyperendemic areas (e.g., certain regions of tropical Africa or coastal New Guinea) where there is intense *P. falciparum* transmission, people may sustain more than one infectious mosquito bite per day and are infected repeatedly throughout their lives. In such settings, rates of morbidity and mortality due to malaria are considerable during childhood. Immunity against disease is hard won in these areas, and the burden of disease in young children is high; by adulthood, however, most malarial infections are asymptomatic. Constant, frequent, year-round infection is termed *stable transmission*. In areas where transmission is low, erratic, or focal, full protective immunity is not acquired, and symptomatic disease may occur at all ages. This situation usually exists in hypoendemic areas and is termed *unstable transmission*. Even in stable transmission areas, there is often an increased incidence of symptomatic malaria coinciding with increased mosquito breeding and transmission during the rainy season. Malaria behaves like an epidemic disease in some areas, particularly those with unstable malaria, such as northern India, Sri Lanka, Southeast Asia, Ethiopia, Eritrea, Rwanda, Burundi, southern Africa, and Madagascar. An epidemic can develop when there are changes in environmental, economic, or social conditions, such as heavy rains following drought or migrations (usually of refugees or workers) from a nonmalarious region to an area of high transmission; a breakdown in malaria control and prevention services can intensify epidemic conditions. This situation usually results in considerable mortality among all age groups.

The principal determinants of the epidemiology of malaria are the number (density), the human-biting habits, and the longevity of the anopheline mosquito vectors. Not all of the >400 anophelines can transmit malaria, and those that do vary considerably in their efficiency as malaria vectors. More specifically, the transmission of malaria is directly proportional to the density of the vector, the square of the number of human bites per day per mosquito, and the tenth power of the probability of the mosquito's surviving for 1 day. Mosquito longevity is particularly important, because the portion of the parasite's life cycle that takes place within the mosquito—from gametocyte ingestion to subsequent inoculation (*sporogony*)—lasts 8–30 days, depending on ambient temperature; thus, to transmit malaria, the mosquito must survive for >7 days. In general, at temperatures below 16°–18°C, sporogony is not completed and transmission does not occur, although malaria outbreaks and transmission have recently occurred in the highlands of east Africa—areas (>1500 m) previously free of vectors. The most effective mosquito vectors of malaria are those, such as *Anopheles gambiae* in Africa, which are long-lived, occur in high densities in tropical climates, breed readily, and bite humans in preference to other animals. The entomologic inoculation rate (the number of sporozoite-positive mosquito bites per person per year) is the most common measure of malaria transmission and varies from <1 in some parts of Latin America and Southeast Asia to >300 in parts of tropical Africa.

ERYTHROCYTE CHANGES IN MALARIA

After invading an erythrocyte, the growing malarial parasite progressively consumes and degrades intracellular proteins, principally hemoglobin. The potentially toxic heme is detoxified by polymerization to biologically inert hemozoin (malaria pigment). The parasite also alters the RBC membrane by changing its transport properties, exposing cryptic surface antigens, and inserting new parasite-derived proteins. The RBC becomes more irregular in shape, more antigenic, and less deformable.

In *P. falciparum* infections, membrane protuberances appear on the erythrocyte's surface 12–15 h after the cell's invasion. These "knobs" extrude a high-molecular-weight, antigenically variant, strain-specific erythrocyte membrane adhesive protein (PfEMP1) that mediates attachment to receptors on venular and capillary endothelium—an event termed *cytoadherence*. Several vascular receptors have been identified, of which intercellular adhesion molecule 1 (ICAM-1) is probably the most important in the brain, chondroitin sulfate B in the placenta, and CD36 in most other organs. Thus, the infected erythrocytes stick inside and eventually block capillaries and venules. At the same stage, these *P. falciparum*–infected RBCs may also adhere to uninfected RBCs (to form rosettes) and to other parasitized erythrocytes (agglutination). The processes of cytoadherence, rosetting, and agglutination are central to the pathogenesis of falciparum malaria. They result in the sequestration of RBCs containing mature forms of the parasite in vital organs (particularly the brain), where they interfere with microcirculatory flow and metabolism. Sequestered parasites continue to develop out of reach of the principal host defense mechanism: splenic processing and filtration. As a consequence, only the younger ring forms of the asexual parasites are seen circulating in the peripheral blood in falciparum malaria, and the level of peripheral parasitemia underestimates the true number of par-

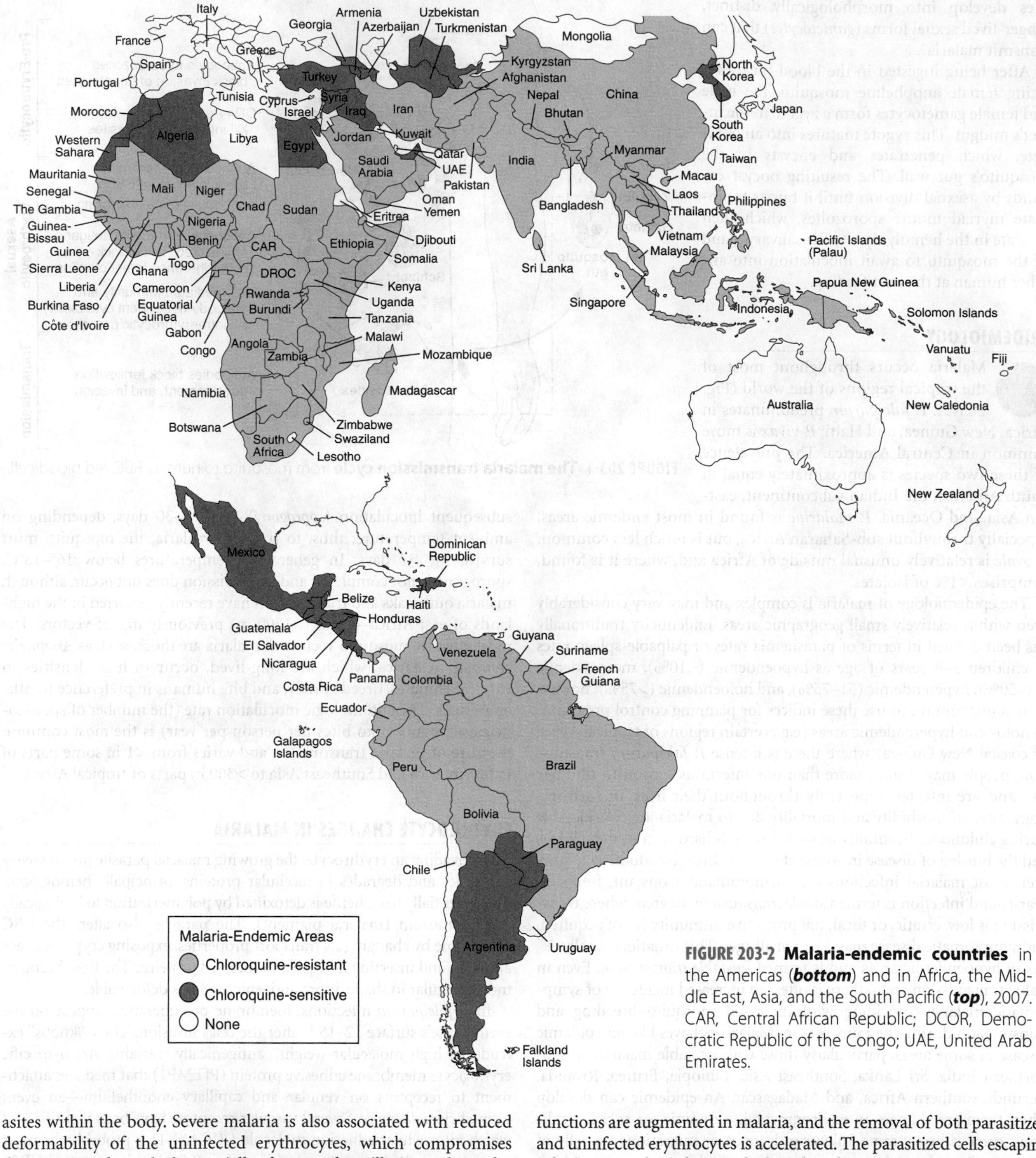

FIGURE 203-2 Malaria-endemic countries in the Americas (***bottom***) and in Africa, the Middle East, Asia, and the South Pacific (***top***), 2007. CAR, Central African Republic; DCOR, Democratic Republic of the Congo; UAE, United Arab Emirates.

asites within the body. Severe malaria is also associated with reduced deformability of the uninfected erythrocytes, which compromises their passage through the partially obstructed capillaries and venules and shortens RBC survival.

In the other three ("benign") malarias, sequestration does not occur, and all stages of the parasite's development are evident on peripheral blood smears. Whereas *P. vivax*, *P. ovale*, and *P. malariae* show a marked predilection for either young RBCs (*P. vivax*, *P. ovale*) or old cells (*P. malariae*) and produce a level of parasitemia that is seldom >2%, *P. falciparum* can invade erythrocytes of all ages and may be associated with very high levels of parasitemia.

HOST RESPONSE

Initially, the host responds to plasmodial infection by activating nonspecific defense mechanisms. Splenic immunologic and filtrative clearance functions are augmented in malaria, and the removal of both parasitized and uninfected erythrocytes is accelerated. The parasitized cells escaping splenic removal are destroyed when the schizont ruptures. The material released induces the activation of macrophages and the release of proinflammatory mononuclear cell–derived cytokines, which cause fever and exert other pathologic effects. Temperatures of ≥40°C damage mature parasites; in untreated infections, the effect of such temperatures is to further synchronize the parasitic cycle, with eventual production of the regular fever spikes and rigors that originally served to characterize the different malarias. These regular fever patterns (tertian, every 2 days; quartan, every 3 days) are seldom seen today in patients who receive prompt and effective antimalarial treatment.

The geographic distributions of sickle cell disease, ovalocytosis, thalassemia, and glucose-6-phosphate dehydrogenase (G6PD) deficiency closely resemble that of malaria before the introduction of control measures. This similarity suggests that these genetic disorders confer protection against death from falciparum malaria. For example, HbA/S heterozygotes (sickle cell trait) have a sixfold reduction in the risk of dying from severe falciparum malaria. This decrease in risk appears to be related to impaired parasite growth at low oxygen tensions. Parasite multiplication in HbA/E heterozygotes is reduced at high parasite densities. In Melanesia, children with α-thalassemia appear to have more frequent malaria (both vivax and falciparum) in the early years of life, and this pattern of infection appears to protect against severe disease. In Melanesian ovalocytosis, rigid erythrocytes resist merozoite invasion, and the intraerythrocytic milieu is hostile.

Nonspecific host defense mechanisms stop the infection's expansion, and the subsequent specific immune response controls the infection. Eventually, exposure to sufficient strains confers protection from high-level parasitemia and disease but not from infection. As a result of this state of infection without illness (*premunition*), asymptomatic parasitemia is common among adults and older children living in regions with stable and intense transmission (i.e., holo- or hyperendemic areas). Immunity is mainly specific for both the species and the strain of infecting malarial parasite. Both humoral immunity and cellular immunity are necessary for protection, but the mechanisms of each are incompletely understood (Fig. 203-1). Immune individuals have a polyclonal increase in serum levels of IgM, IgG, and IgA, although much of this antibody is unrelated to protection. Antibodies to a variety of parasitic antigens presumably act in concert to limit in vivo replication of the parasite. In the case of falciparum malaria, the most important of these antigens is the surface adhesin—the variant protein PfEMP1 mentioned above. Passively transferred IgG from immune adults has been shown to reduce levels of parasitemia in children; although parasitemia in very young infants can occur, passive transfer of maternal antibody contributes to the relative (but not complete) protection of infants from severe malaria in the first months of life. This complex immunity to disease declines when a person lives outside an endemic area for several months or longer.

Several factors retard the development of cellular immunity to malaria. These factors include the absence of major histocompatibility antigens on the surface of infected RBCs, which precludes direct T cell recognition; malaria antigen–specific immune unresponsiveness; and the enormous strain diversity of malarial parasites, along with the ability of the parasites to express variant immunodominant antigens on the erythrocyte surface that change during the period of infection. Parasites may persist in the blood for months (or, in the case of *P. malariae*, for many years) if treatment is not given. The complexity of the immune response in malaria, the sophistication of the parasites' evasion mechanisms, and the lack of a good in vitro correlate with clinical immunity have all slowed progress toward an effective vaccine.

CLINICAL FEATURES

Malaria is a very common cause of fever in tropical countries. The first symptoms of malaria are nonspecific; the lack of a sense of well-being, headache, fatigue, abdominal discomfort, and muscle aches followed by fever are all similar to the symptoms of a minor viral illness. In some instances, a prominence of headache, chest pain, abdominal pain, arthralgia, myalgia, or diarrhea may suggest another diagnosis. Although headache may be severe in malaria, there is no neck stiffness or photophobia resembling that in meningitis. While myalgia may be prominent, it is not usually as severe as in dengue fever, and the muscles are not tender as in leptospirosis or typhus. Nausea, vomiting, and orthostatic hypotension are common. The classic malarial paroxysms, in which fever spikes, chills, and rigors occur at regular intervals, are relatively unusual and suggest infection with *P. vivax* or *P. ovale*. The fever is irregular at first (that of falciparum malaria may never become regular); the temperature of nonimmune individuals and children often rises above 40°C in conjunction with tachycardia and sometimes delirium. Although childhood febrile convulsions may occur with any of the malarias, generalized seizures are specifically associated with falciparum malaria and may herald the development of cerebral disease. Many clinical abnormalities have been described in acute malaria, but most patients with uncomplicated infections have few abnormal physical findings other than fever, malaise, mild anemia, and (in some cases) a palpable spleen. Anemia is common among young children living in areas with stable transmission, particularly where resistance has compromised the efficacy of antimalarial drugs. In nonimmune individuals with acute malaria, the spleen takes several days to become palpable, but splenic enlargement is found in a high proportion of otherwise healthy individuals in malaria-endemic areas and reflects repeated infections. Slight enlargement of the liver is also common, particularly among young children. Mild jaundice is common among adults; it may develop in patients with otherwise uncomplicated falciparum malaria and usually resolves over 1–3 weeks. Malaria is not associated with a rash like those seen in meningococcal septicemia, typhus, enteric fever, viral exanthems, and drug reactions. Petechial hemorrhages in the skin or mucous membranes—features of viral hemorrhagic fevers and leptospirosis—develop only rarely in severe falciparum malaria.

SEVERE FALCIPARUM MALARIA

Appropriately and promptly treated, uncomplicated falciparum malaria (i.e., the patient can swallow medicines and food) carries a mortality rate of ~0.1%. However, once vital-organ dysfunction occurs or the total proportion of erythrocytes infected increases to >2% (a level corresponding to $>10^{12}$ parasites in an adult), mortality risk rises steeply. The major manifestations of severe falciparum malaria are shown in Table 203-2, and features indicating a poor prognosis are listed in Table 203-3.

Cerebral Malaria Coma is a characteristic and ominous feature of falciparum malaria and, despite treatment, is associated with death rates of ~20% among adults and 15% among children. Any obtundation, delirium, or abnormal behavior should be taken very seriously. The onset may be gradual or sudden following a convulsion.

Cerebral malaria manifests as diffuse symmetric encephalopathy; focal neurologic signs are unusual. Although some passive resistance to head flexion may be detected, signs of meningeal irritation are lacking. The eyes may be divergent and a pout reflex is common, but other primitive reflexes are usually absent. The corneal reflexes are preserved, except in deep coma. Muscle tone may be either increased or decreased. The tendon reflexes are variable, and the plantar reflexes may be flexor or extensor; the abdominal and cremasteric reflexes are absent. Flexor or extensor posturing may be seen. Approximately 15% of patients have retinal hemorrhages; with pupillary dilatation and indirect ophthalmoscopy, this figure increases to 30–40%. Other funduscopic abnormalities (Fig. 203-3) include discrete spots of retinal opacification (30–60%), papilledema (8% among children, rare among adults), cotton wool spots (<5%), and decolorization of a retinal vessel or segment of vessel (occasional cases). Convulsions, usually generalized and often repeated, occur in up to 50% of children with cerebral malaria. More covert seizure activity is also common, particularly among children, and may manifest as repetitive tonic-clonic eye movements or even hypersalivation. Whereas adults rarely (i.e., in <3% of cases) suffer neurologic sequelae, ~15% of children surviving cerebral malaria—especially those with hypoglycemia, severe anemia, repeated seizures, and deep coma—have some residual neurologic deficit when they regain consciousness; hemiplegia, cerebral palsy, cortical blindness, deafness, and impaired cognition and learning (all of varying duration) have been reported. Approximately 10% of children surviving cerebral malaria have a persistent language deficit. The incidence of epilepsy is increased and the life expectancy decreased among these children.

Hypoglycemia Hypoglycemia, an important and common complication of severe malaria, is associated with a poor prognosis and is particularly problematic in children and pregnant women. Hypoglycemia in malaria results from a failure of hepatic gluconeogenesis and an increase in the consumption of glucose by both host and, to a much less-

TABLE 203-2 MANIFESTATIONS OF SEVERE FALCIPARUM MALARIA

Signs	Manifestations
Major	
Unarousable coma/cerebral malaria	Failure to localize or respond appropriately to noxious stimuli; coma persisting for >30 min after generalized convulsion
Acidemia/acidosis	Arterial pH <7.25 or plasma bicarbonate level of <15 mmol/L; venous lactate level of >5 mmol/L; manifests as labored deep breathing, often termed "respiratory distress"
Severe normochromic, normocytic anemia	Hematocrit of <15% or hemoglobin level of <50 g/L (<5 g/dL) with parasitemia level of >100,000/μL
Renal failure	Urine output (24 h) of <400 mL in adults or <12 mL/kg in children; no improvement with rehydration; serum creatinine level of >265 μmol/L (>3.0 mg/dL)
Pulmonary edema/adult respiratory distress syndrome	Noncardiogenic pulmonary edema, often aggravated by overhydration
Hypoglycemia	Plasma glucose level of <2.2 mmol/L (<40 mg/dL)
Hypotension/shock	Systolic blood pressure of <50 mmHg in children 1–5 years or <80 mmHg in adults; core/skin temperature difference of >10°C; capillary refill >2 s
Bleeding/disseminated intravascular coagulation	Significant bleeding and hemorrhage from the gums, nose, and gastrointestinal tract and/or evidence of disseminated intravascular coagulation
Convulsions	More than two generalized seizures in 24 h; signs of continued seizure activity sometimes subtle (e.g., tonic-clonic eye movements without limb or face movement)
Hemoglobinuria[a]	Macroscopic black, brown, or red urine; not associated with effects of oxidant drugs and red blood cell enzyme defects (such as G6PD deficiency)
Other	
Impaired consciousness/arousable	Unable to sit or stand without support
Extreme weakness	Prostration; inability to sit unaided[b]
Hyperparasitemia	Parasitemia level of >5% in nonimmune patients (>20% in any patient)
Jaundice	Serum bilirubin level of >50 mmol/L (>3.0 mg/dL) if combined with other evidence of vital-organ dysfunction

[a]Hemoglobinuria may occur in uncomplicated malaria.
[b]In a child who is normally able to sit.
Note: G6PD, glucose-6-phosphate dehydrogenase.

er extent, the malaria parasites. To compound the situation, quinine and quinidine—drugs used for the treatment of severe chloroquine-resistant malaria—are powerful stimulants of pancreatic insulin secretion. Hyperinsulinemic hypoglycemia is especially troublesome in pregnant women receiving quinine treatment. In severe disease, the clinical diagnosis of hypoglycemia is difficult: the usual physical signs (sweating, gooseflesh, tachycardia) are absent, and the neurologic impairment caused by hypoglycemia cannot be distinguished from that caused by malaria.

Acidosis Acidosis, an important cause of death from severe malaria, results from accumulation of organic acids. Hyperlactatemia commonly coexists with hypoglycemia. In adults, coexisting renal impairment often compounds the acidosis; in children, ketoacidosis may also contribute. Other still-unidentified organic acids are major contributors to acidosis. Acidotic breathing, sometimes called respiratory distress, is a sign of poor prognosis. It is often followed by circulatory failure refractory to volume expansion or inotropic drugs and ultimately by respiratory arrest. The plasma concentrations of bicarbonate or lactate are the best biochemical prognosticators in severe malaria. Lactic acidosis is caused by the combination of anaerobic glycolysis in tissues where sequestered parasites interfere with microcirculatory flow, hypovolemia, lactate production by the parasites, and a failure of hepatic and renal lactate clearance. The prognosis of severe acidosis is poor.

TABLE 203-3 FEATURES INDICATING A POOR PROGNOSIS IN SEVERE FALCIPARUM MALARIA

Clinical
- Marked agitation
- Hyperventilation (respiratory distress)
- Hypothermia (<36.5°C)
- Bleeding
- Deep coma
- Repeated convulsions
- Anuria
- Shock

Laboratory
- Biochemistry
  - Hypoglycemia (<2.2 mmol/L)
  - Hyperlactatemia (>5 mmol/L)
  - Acidosis (arterial pH <7.3, serum HCO_3 <15 mmol/L)
  - Elevated serum creatinine (>265 μmol/L)
  - Elevated total bilirubin (>50 μmol/L)
  - Elevated liver enzymes (AST/ALT 3 times upper limit of normal, 5-nucleotidase ↑)
  - Elevated muscle enzymes (CPK ↑, myoglobin ↑)
  - Elevated urate (>600 μmol/L)
- Hematology
  - Leukocytosis (>12,000/μL)
  - Severe anemia (PCV <15%)
  - Coagulopathy
    - Decreased platelet count (<50,000/μL)
    - Prolonged prothrombin time (>3 s)
    - Prolonged partial thromboplastin time
    - Decreased fibrinogen (<200 mg/dL)
- Parasitology
  - Hyperparasitemia
    - Increased mortality at >100,000/μL
    - High mortality at >500,000/μL
    - >20% of parasites identified as pigment-containing trophozoites and schizonts
    - >5% of neutrophils with visible pigment

Note: ALT, alanine aminotransferase; AST, aspartate aminotransferase; CPK, creatine phosphokinase; PCV, packed cell volume.

Noncardiogenic Pulmonary Edema Adults with severe falciparum malaria may develop noncardiogenic pulmonary edema even after several days of antimalarial therapy. The pathogenesis of this variant of the

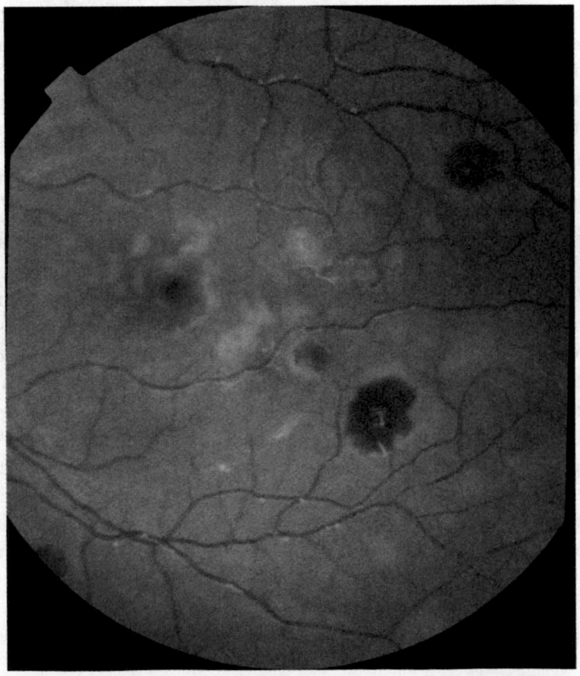

FIGURE 203-3 The eye in cerebral malaria: perimacular whitening and pale-centered retinal hemorrhages. *(Courtesy of N. Beare, T. Taylor, S. Harding, S. Lewallen, and M. Molyneux; with permission.)*

adult respiratory distress syndrome is unclear. The mortality rate is >80%. This condition can be aggravated by overly vigorous administration of IV fluid. Noncardiogenic pulmonary edema can also develop in otherwise uncomplicated vivax malaria, where recovery is usual.

Renal Impairment Renal impairment is common among adults with severe falciparum malaria but rare among children. The pathogenesis of renal failure is unclear but may be related to erythrocyte sequestration interfering with renal microcirculatory flow and metabolism. Clinically and pathologically, this syndrome manifests as acute tubular necrosis, although renal cortical necrosis never develops. Acute renal failure may occur simultaneously with other vital-organ dysfunction (in which case the mortality risk is high) or may progress as other disease manifestations resolve. In survivors, urine flow resumes in a median of 4 days, and serum creatinine levels return to normal in a mean of 17 days (Chap. 273). Early dialysis or hemofiltration considerably enhances the likelihood of a patient's survival, particularly in acute hypercatabolic renal failure.

Hematologic Abnormalities Anemia results from accelerated RBC removal by the spleen, obligatory RBC destruction at parasite schizogony, and ineffective erythropoiesis. In severe malaria, both infected and uninfected RBCs show reduced deformability, which correlates with prognosis and development of anemia. Splenic clearance of all RBCs is increased. In nonimmune individuals and in areas with unstable transmission, anemia can develop rapidly and transfusion is often required. As a consequence of repeated malarial infections, children in many areas of Africa may develop severe anemia resulting from both shortened RBC survival and marked dyserythropoiesis. Anemia is a common consequence of antimalarial drug resistance, which results in repeated or continued infection.

Slight coagulation abnormalities are common in falciparum malaria, and mild thrombocytopenia is usual. Of patients with severe malaria, <5% have significant bleeding with evidence of disseminated intravascular coagulation. Hematemesis from stress ulceration or acute gastric erosions may also occur.

Liver Dysfunction Mild hemolytic jaundice is common in malaria. Severe jaundice is associated with *P. falciparum* infections; is more common among adults than among children; and results from hemolysis, hepatocyte injury, and cholestasis. When accompanied by other vital-organ dysfunction (often renal impairment), liver dysfunction carries a poor prognosis. Hepatic dysfunction contributes to hypoglycemia, lactic acidosis, and impaired drug metabolism. Occasional patients with falciparum malaria may develop deep jaundice (with hemolytic, hepatitic, and cholestatic components) without evidence of other vital-organ dysfunction.

Other Complications Septicemia may complicate severe malaria, particularly in children. In endemic areas, *Salmonella* bacteremia has been associated specifically with *P. falciparum* infections. Chest infections and catheter-induced urinary tract infections are common among patients who are unconscious for >3 days. Aspiration pneumonia may follow generalized convulsions. The frequency of complications of severe falciparum malaria is summarized in Table 203-4.

MALARIA IN PREGNANCY

In heavily endemic (hyper- and holoendemic) areas, falciparum malaria in primi- and secundigravid women is associated with low birth weight (average reduction, ~170 g) and consequently increased infant and childhood mortality. In general, infected mothers in areas of stable transmission remain asymptomatic despite intense accumulation of parasitized erythrocytes in the placental microcirculation. Maternal HIV infection predisposes pregnant women to malaria, predisposes their newborns to congenital malarial infection, and exacerbates the reduction in birth weight associated with malaria.

In areas with unstable transmission of malaria, pregnant women are prone to severe infections and are particularly vulnerable to high-

TABLE 203-4 RELATIVE INCIDENCE OF SEVERE COMPLICATIONS OF FALCIPARUM MALARIA

Complication	Nonpregnant Adults	Pregnant Women	Children
Anemia	+	++	+++
Convulsions	+	+	+++
Hypoglycemia	+	+++	+++
Jaundice	+++	+++	+
Renal failure	+++	+++	–
Pulmonary edema	++	+++	+

Key: –, rare; +, infrequent; ++, frequent; +++, very frequent.

edema. Fetal distress, premature labor, and stillbirth or low birth weight are common results. Fetal death is usual in severe malaria. Congenital malaria occurs in <5% of newborns whose mothers are infected; its frequency and the level of parasitemia are related directly to the parasite density in maternal blood and in the placenta. *P. vivax* malaria in pregnancy is also associated with a reduction in birth weight (average, 110 g), but, in contrast to the situation in falciparum malaria, this effect is more pronounced in multigravid than in primigravid women.

MALARIA IN CHILDREN

Most of the estimated 1–3 million persons who die of falciparum malaria each year are young African children. Convulsions, coma, hypoglycemia, metabolic acidosis, and severe anemia are relatively common among children with severe malaria, whereas deep jaundice, acute renal failure, and acute pulmonary edema are unusual. Severely anemic children may present with labored deep breathing, which in the past has been attributed incorrectly to "anemic congestive cardiac failure" but in fact is usually caused by metabolic acidosis, often compounded by hypovolemia. Evidence is accruing that severe malaria can result in long-term neurocognitive and developmental deficits. In general, children tolerate antimalarial drugs well and respond rapidly to treatment.

TRANSFUSION MALARIA

Malaria can be transmitted by blood transfusion, needle-stick injury, sharing of needles by infected injection drug users, or organ transplantation. The incubation period in these settings is often short because there is no preerythrocytic stage of development. The clinical features and management of these cases are the same as for naturally acquired infections. Radical chemotherapy with primaquine is unnecessary for transfusion-transmitted *P. vivax* and *P. ovale* infections.

CHRONIC COMPLICATIONS OF MALARIA

TROPICAL SPLENOMEGALY (HYPERREACTIVE MALARIAL SPLENOMEGALY)

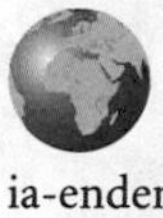

Chronic or repeated malarial infections produce hypergammaglobulinemia; normochromic, normocytic anemia; and, in certain situations, splenomegaly. Some residents of malaria-endemic areas in tropical Africa and Asia exhibit an abnormal immunologic response to repeated infections that is characterized by massive splenomegaly, hepatomegaly, marked elevations in serum titers of IgM and malarial antibody, hepatic sinusoidal lymphocytosis, and (in Africa) peripheral B cell lymphocytosis. This syndrome has been associated with the production of cytotoxic IgM antibodies to CD8+ T lymphocytes, antibodies to CD5+ T lymphocytes, and an increase in the ratio of CD4+ T cells to CD8+ T cells. These events may lead to uninhibited B cell production of IgM and the formation of cryoglobulins (IgM aggregates and immune complexes). This immunologic process stimulates reticuloendothelial hyperplasia and clearance activity and eventually produces splenomegaly. Patients with hyperreactive malarial splenomegaly (HMS) present with an abdominal mass or a dragging sensation in the abdomen and occasional sharp abdominal pains suggesting perisplenitis. Anemia and some degree of pancytopenia are usually evident, and in some cases malarial parasites cannot be found in peripheral-blood smears. Vulnerability to respira-

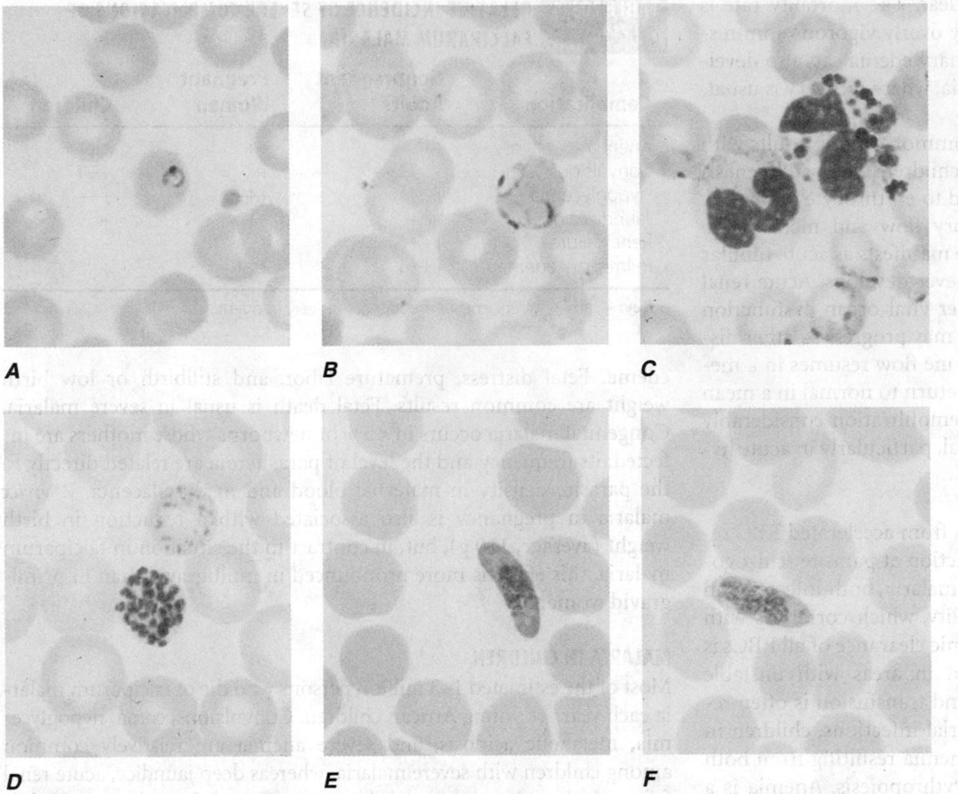

FIGURE 203-4 Thin blood films of *Plasmodium falciparum*. ***A.*** Young trophozoites. ***B.*** Old trophozoites. ***C.*** Pigment in polymorphonuclear cells and trophozoites. ***D.*** Mature schizonts. ***E.*** Female gametocytes. ***F.*** Male gametocytes. *(Reproduced from Bench Aids for the Diagnosis of Malaria Infections, 2d ed, with the permission of the World Health Organization.)*

tory and skin infections is increased; many patients die of overwhelming sepsis. Persons with HMS who are living in endemic areas should receive antimalarial chemoprophylaxis; the results are usually good. In nonendemic areas, antimalarial treatment is advised. In some cases refractory to therapy, clonal lymphoproliferation may develop and then evolve into a malignant lymphoproliferative disorder.

QUARTAN MALARIAL NEPHROPATHY

Chronic or repeated infections with *P. malariae* (and possibly with other malarial species) may cause soluble immune-complex injury to the renal glomeruli, resulting in the nephrotic syndrome. Other unidentified factors must contribute to this process since only a very small proportion of infected patients develop renal disease. The histologic appearance is that of focal or segmental glomerulonephritis with splitting of the capillary basement membrane. Subendothelial dense deposits are seen on electron microscopy, and immunofluorescence reveals deposits of complement and immunoglobulins; in samples of renal tissue from children, *P. malariae* antigens are often visible. A coarse-granular pattern of basement membrane immunofluorescent deposits (predominantly IgG3) with selective proteinuria carries a better prognosis than a fine-granular, predominantly IgG2 pattern with nonselective proteinuria. Quartan nephropathy usually responds poorly to treatment with either antimalarial agents or glucocorticoids and cytotoxic drugs.

BURKITT'S LYMPHOMA AND EPSTEIN-BARR VIRUS INFECTION

It is possible that malaria-related immunosuppression provokes infection with lymphoma viruses. Burkitt's lymphoma is strongly associated with Epstein-Barr virus. The prevalence of this childhood tumor is high in malarious areas of Africa.

DIAGNOSIS

DEMONSTRATION OF THE PARASITE

The diagnosis of malaria rests on the demonstration of asexual forms of the parasite in stained peripheral-blood smears. After a negative blood smear, repeat smears should be made if there is a high degree of suspicion. Of the Romanowsky stains, Giemsa at pH 7.2 is preferred; Wright's, Field's, or Leishman's stain can also be used. Both thin (**Figs. 203-4** and **203-5**; see also **Figs. e18-1** and **e18-2**) and thick (**Figs. 203-6, 203-7, 203-8,** and **203-9**) blood smears should be examined. The thin blood smear should be rapidly air-dried, fixed in anhydrous methanol, and stained; the RBCs in the tail of the film should then be examined under oil immersion (×1000 magnification). The level

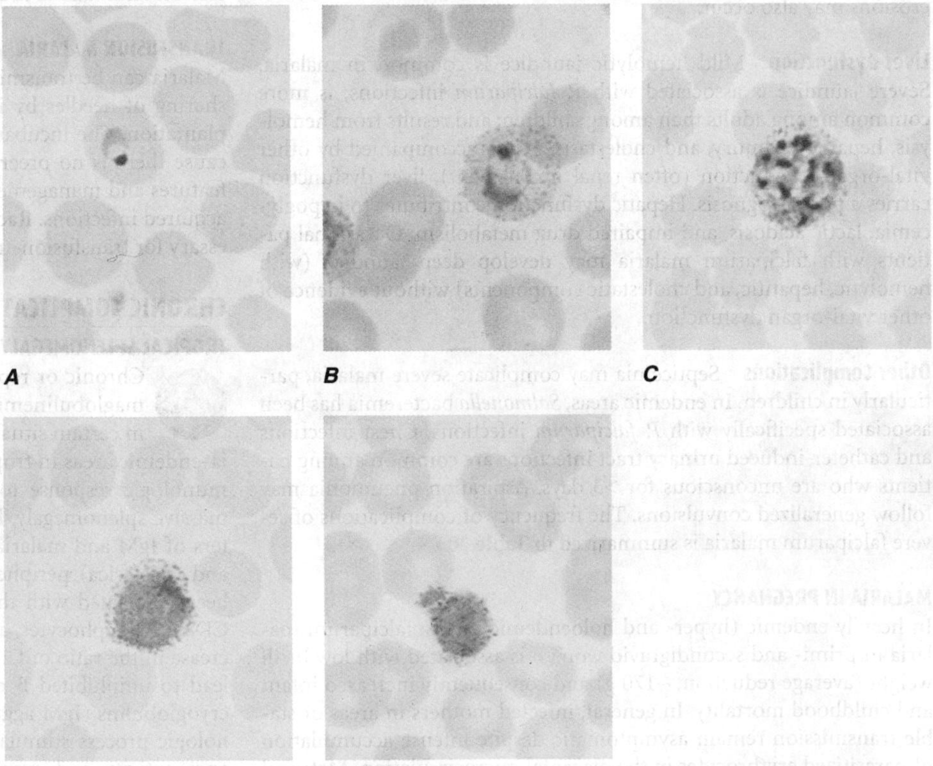

FIGURE 203-5 Thin blood films of *Plasmodium vivax*. ***A.*** Young trophozoites. ***B.*** Old trophozoites. ***C.*** Mature schizonts. ***D.*** Female gametocytes. ***E.*** Male gametocytes. *(Reproduced from Bench Aids for the Diagnosis of Malaria Infections, 2d ed, with the permission of the World Health Organization.)*

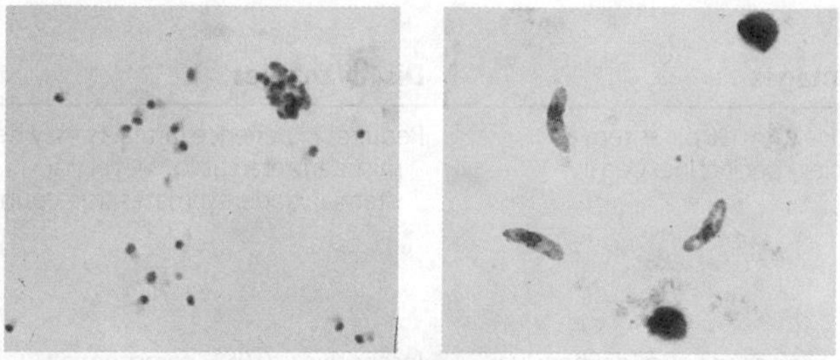

A B

FIGURE 203-6 Thick blood films of *Plasmodium falciparum*. *A.* Trophozoites. ***B.*** Gametocytes. *(Reproduced from Bench Aids for the Diagnosis of Malaria Infections, 2d ed, with the permission of the World Health Organization.)*

of parasitemia is expressed as the number of parasitized erythrocytes per 1000 RBCs. The thick blood film should be of uneven thickness. The smear should be dried thoroughly and stained without fixing. As many layers of erythrocytes overlie one another and are lysed during the staining procedure, the thick film has the advantage of concentrating the parasites (by 40- to 100-fold compared with a thin blood film) and thus increasing diagnostic sensitivity. Both parasites and white blood cells (WBCs) are counted, and the number of parasites per unit volume is calculated from the total leukocyte count. Alternatively, a WBC count of 8000/μL is assumed. This figure is converted to the number of parasitized erythrocytes per microliter. A minimum of 200 WBCs should be counted under oil immersion. Interpretation of blood smear films requires some experience because artifacts are common. Before a thick smear is judged to be negative, 100–200 fields should be examined under oil immersion. In high-transmission areas, the presence of up to 10,000 parasites/μL of blood may be tolerated without symptoms or signs in partially immune individuals. Thus the detection of malaria parasites is sensitive but only poorly specific in identifying malaria as the cause of illness.

Rapid, simple, sensitive, and specific antibody-based diagnostic stick or card tests that detect *P. falciparum*–specific, histidine-rich protein 2 (PfHRP2) or lactate dehydrogenase antigens in finger-prick blood samples have been introduced (Table 203-5). Some of these tests carry a second antibody, which allows falciparum malaria to be distinguished from the less dangerous malarias. PfHRP2-based tests may remain positive for several weeks after acute infection. This feature is a disadvantage in high-transmission areas where infections are frequent but is of value in the diagnosis of severe malaria in patients who have taken antimalarial drugs and cleared peripheral parasitemia (but in whom the PfHRP2 test remains strongly positive).

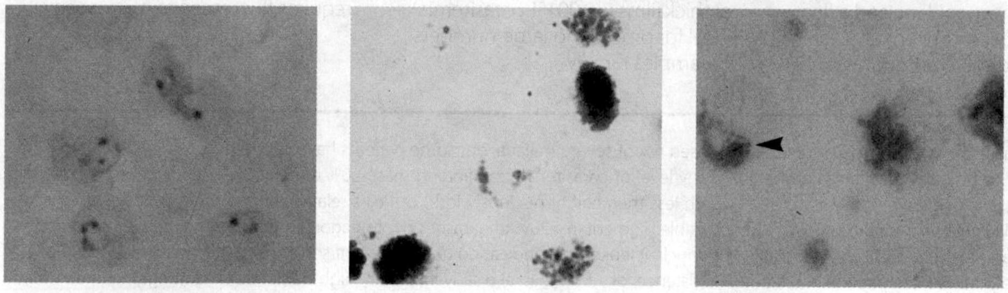

A B C

FIGURE 203-7 Thick blood films of *Plasmodium vivax*. *A.* Trophozoites. ***B.*** Schizonts. ***C.*** Gametocytes. *(Reproduced from Bench Aids for the Diagnosis of Malaria Infections, 2d ed, with the permission of the World Health Organization.)*

The relationship between parasitemia and prognosis is complex; in general, patients with $>10^5$ parasites/μL are at increased risk of dying, but nonimmune patients may die with much lower counts, and partially immune persons may tolerate parasitemia levels many times higher with only minor symptoms. In severe malaria, a poor prognosis is indicated by a predominance of more mature *P. falciparum* parasites (i.e., >20% of parasites with visible pigment) in the peripheral blood film or by the presence of phagocytosed malarial pigment in >5% of neutrophils. In *P. falciparum* infections, gametocytemia peaks 1 week after the peak of asexual parasites. Because the mature gametocytes of *P. falciparum* are not affected by most antimalarial drugs, their persistence does not constitute evidence of drug resistance. Phagocytosed malarial pigment is sometimes seen inside peripheral-blood monocytes or polymorphonuclear leukocytes and may provide a clue to recent infection if malaria parasites are not detectable. After the clearance of the parasites, this intraphagocytic malarial pigment is often evident for several days in the peripheral blood or for longer in bone marrow aspirates or smears of fluid expressed after intradermal puncture. Staining of parasites with the fluorescent dye acridine orange allows more rapid diagnosis of malaria (but not speciation of the infection) in patients with low-level parasitemia.

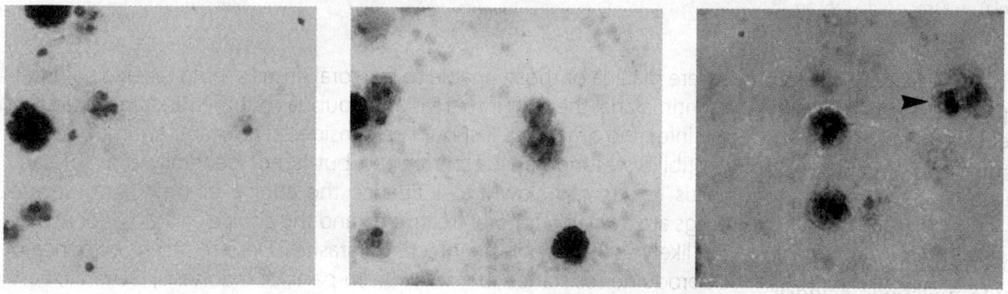

A B C

FIGURE 203-8 Thick blood films of *Plasmodium ovale*. *A.* Trophozoites. ***B.*** Schizonts. ***C.*** Gametocytes. *(Reproduced from Bench Aids for the Diagnosis of Malaria Infections, 2d ed, with the permission of the World Health Organization.)*

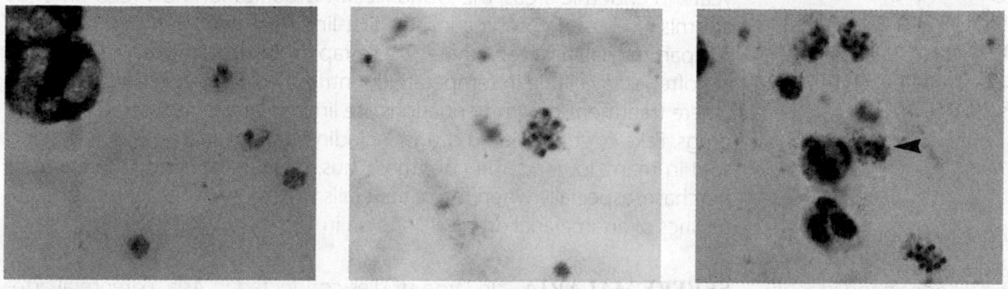

A B C

FIGURE 203-9 Thick blood films of *Plasmodium malariae*. *A.* Trophozoites. ***B.*** Schizonts. ***C.*** Gametocytes. *(Reproduced from Bench Aids for the Diagnosis of Malaria Infections, 2d ed, with the permission of the World Health Organization.)*

LABORATORY FINDINGS

Normochromic, normocytic anemia is usual. The leukocyte count is generally normal, although it may be raised in very severe infections. There is slight monocytosis, lymphopenia, and eosinopenia, with reactive lymphocytosis and eosinophilia in the weeks after the acute infection. The erythrocyte

TABLE 203-5 METHODS FOR THE DIAGNOSIS OF MALARIA[a]

Method	Procedure	Advantages	Disadvantages
Thick blood film[b]	Blood should be uneven in thickness but sufficiently thin to read watch hands through part of the spot. Stain dried, unfixed blood spot with Giemsa, Field's, or other Romanowsky stain. Count number of asexual parasites per 200 WBCs (or per 500 at low densities). Count gametocytes separately.[c]	Sensitive (0.001% parasitemia); species specific; inexpensive	Requires experience (artifacts may be misinterpreted as low-level parasitemia); underestimates true count
Thin blood film[d]	Stain fixed smear with Giemsa, Field's, or other Romanowsky stain. Count number of RBCs containing asexual parasites per 1000 RBCs. In severe malaria, assess stage of parasite development and count neutrophils containing malaria pigment.[e] Count gametocytes separately.[c]	Rapid; species specific; inexpensive; in severe malaria, provides prognostic information[e]	Insensitive (<0.05% parasitemia); uneven distribution of *P. vivax*, as enlarged infected red cells concentrate at leading edge
PfHRP2 dipstick or card test	A drop of blood is placed on the stick or card, which is then immersed in washing solutions. Monoclonal antibody captures the parasite antigen and reads out as a colored band.	Robust and relatively inexpensive; rapid; sensitivity similar to or slightly lower than that of thick films (~0.001% parasitemia)	Detects only *Plasmodium falciparum*; remains positive for weeks after infection[f]; does not quantitate *P. falciparum* parasitemia
Plasmodium LDH dipstick or card test	A drop of blood is placed on the stick or card, which is then immersed in washing solutions. Monoclonal antibodies capture the parasite antigens and read out as colored bands. One band is genus specific (all malarias), and the other is specific for *P. falciparum*.	Rapid; sensitivity similar to or slightly lower than that of thick films for *P. falciparum* (~0.001% parasitemia)	Slightly more difficult preparation than PfHRP2 tests; may miss low-level parasitemia with *P. vivax*, *P. ovale*, and *P. malariae* and does not speciate these organisms; does not quantitate *P. falciparum* parasitemia
Microtube concentration methods with acridine orange staining	Blood is collected in a specialized tube containing acridine orange, anticoagulant, and a float. After centrifugation, which concentrates the parasitized cells around the float, fluorescence microscopy is performed.	Sensitivity similar or superior to that of thick films (~0.001% parasitemia); ideal for processing large numbers of samples rapidly	Does not speciate or quantitate; requires fluorescence microscopy

[a]Malaria cannot be diagnosed clinically with accuracy, but treatment should be started on clinical grounds if the laboratory confirmation is likely to be delayed. In areas of the world where malaria is endemic and transmission is high, low-level asymptomatic parasitemia is common in otherwise-healthy people. Thus malaria may not be the cause of a fever, although in this context the presence of >10,000 parasites/μL (~0.2% parasitemia) *does* indicate that malaria is the cause. Antibody and polymerase chain reaction tests have no role in the diagnosis of malaria.

[b]Asexual parasites/200 WBCs × 40 = parasite count/μL (assumes a WBC count of 8000/μL). See Figs. 203-6 through 203-9.

[c]Gametocytemia may persist for days or weeks after clearance of asexual parasites. Gametocytemia without asexual parasitemia does not indicate active infection.

[d]Parasitized RBCs (%) × hematocrit × 1256 = parasite count/μL. See Figs. 203-3 and 203-4.

[e]The presence of >100,000 parasites/μL (~2% parasitemia) is associated with an increased risk of severe malaria, but some patients have severe malaria with lower counts. At any level of parasitemia, the finding that >50% of parasites are tiny rings (cytoplasm width less than half of nucleus width) carries a relatively good prognosis. The presence of visible pigment in >20% of parasites or of phagocytosed pigment in >5% of polymorphonuclear leukocytes (indicating massive recent schizogony) carries a worse prognosis.

[f]Persistence of PfHRP2 is a disadvantage in high-transmission settings, where many asymptomatic people have positive tests, but can be used to diagnostic advantage in low-transmission settings when a sick patient has received previous unknown treatment (which, in endemic areas, often consists of antimalarial drugs). A positive PfHRP2 test indicates that the illness is falciparum malaria, even if the blood smear is negative.

Note: LDH, lactate dehydrogenase; PfHRP2, *P. falciparum* histidine-rich protein 2; RBCs, red blood cells; WBCs, white blood cells.

sedimentation rate, plasma viscosity, and levels of C-reactive protein and other acute-phase proteins are high. The platelet count is usually reduced to ~10^5/μL. Severe infections may be accompanied by prolonged prothrombin and partial thromboplastin times and by more severe thrombocytopenia. Levels of antithrombin III are reduced even in mild infection. In uncomplicated malaria, plasma concentrations of electrolytes, blood urea nitrogen (BUN), and creatinine are usually normal. Findings in severe malaria may include metabolic acidosis, with low plasma concentrations of glucose, sodium, bicarbonate, calcium, phosphate, and albumin together with elevations in lactate, BUN, creatinine, urate, muscle and liver enzymes, and conjugated and unconjugated bilirubin. Hypergammaglobulinemia is usual in immune and semi-immune subjects. Urinalysis generally gives normal results. In adults and children with cerebral malaria, the mean opening pressure at lumbar puncture is ~160 mm of cerebrospinal fluid (CSF); usually the CSF is normal or has a slightly elevated total protein level [<1.0 g/L (<100 mg/dL)] and cell count (<20/μL).

℞ MALARIA

(Table 203-6) When a patient in or from a malarious area presents with fever, thick and thin blood smears should be prepared and examined immediately to confirm the diagnosis and identify the species of infecting parasite (Figs. 203-4 through 203-9). Repeat blood smears should be performed at least every 12–24 h for 2 days if the first smears are negative and malaria is strongly suspected. Alternatively, a rapid antigen detection card or stick test should be performed. Patients with severe malaria or those unable to take oral drugs should receive parenteral antimalarial therapy. If there is any doubt about the resistance status of the infecting organism, it should be considered resistant. Antimalarial susceptibility testing can be performed but is not generally available and yields results too slowly to influence the choice of treatment. Several drugs are available for oral treatment, and the choice of drug depends on the likely sensitivity of the infecting parasites. Despite recent evidence of chloroquine resistance in *P. vivax* (from parts of Indonesia, Oceania, eastern and southern Asia, and Central and South America), chloroquine remains the treatment of choice for the "benign" human malarias (*P. vivax*, *P. ovale*, *P. malariae*) except in Indonesia and Papua New Guinea, where high levels of resistance are prevalent.

The treatment of falciparum malaria has changed radically in recent years. In endemic areas, the World Health Organization now recommends artemisinin-based combinations as first-line treatment for uncomplicated falciparum malaria everywhere. These rapidly and reliably effective drugs are often unavailable in temperate countries (including the United States), where treatment recommendations are limited by the registered available drugs. Fake or substandard drugs, including antimalarial agents, are being sold in many low-income countries; thus, careful attention is required at purchase, especially when the patient fails to respond as expected. Characteristics of antimalarial drugs are shown in **Table 203-7**.

SEVERE MALARIA In large studies conducted in Asia, parenteral artesunate, a water-soluble artemisinin derivative, has been shown to reduce mortality rates in severe falciparum malaria by 35% from rates obtained with quinine. Artesunate has therefore become the drug of choice. Artesunate is given by the IV route but can also be given by IM injection. Artemether and

TABLE 203-6 REGIMENS FOR THE TREATMENT OF MALARIA

Type of Disease or Treatment	Regimen(s)
Uncomplicated Malaria	
Known chloroquine-sensitive strains of *Plasmodium vivax, P. malariae, P. ovale, P. falciparum*[a]	Chloroquine (10 mg of base/kg stat followed by 5 mg/kg at 12, 24, and 36 h or by 10 mg/kg at 24 h and 5 mg/kg at 48 h) *or* Amodiaquine (10–12 mg of base/kg qd for 3 days)
Radical treatment for *P. vivax* or *P. ovale* infection	In addition to chloroquine or amodiaquine as detailed above, primaquine (0.25 mg of base/kg qd; 0.375–0.5 mg of base/kg qd in Southeast Asia and Oceania) should be given for 14 days to prevent relapse. In mild G6PD deficiency, 0.75 mg of base/kg should be given once weekly for 6 weeks. Primaquine should not be given in severe G6PD deficiency.
Sensitive *P. falciparum* malaria[b]	Artesunate[c] (4 mg/kg qd for 3 days) plus sulfadoxine (25 mg/kg)/pyrimethamine (1.25 mg/kg) as a single dose *or* Artesunate[c] (4 mg/kg qd for 3 days) plus amodiaquine (10 mg of base/kg qd for 3 days)[d]
Multidrug-resistant *P. falciparum* malaria	Either artemether-lumefantrine[c] (1.5/9 mg/kg bid for 3 days with food) or artesunate[c] (4 mg/kg qd for 3 days) *plus* Mefloquine (25 mg of base/kg—either 8 mg/kg qd for 3 days or 15 mg/kg on day 2 and then 10 mg/kg on day 3)[d]
Second-line treatment/treatment of imported malaria	Either artesunate[c] (2 mg/kg qd for 7 days) or quinine (10 mg of salt/kg tid for 7 days) *plus 1 of the following 3:* 1. Tetracycline[e] (4 mg/kg qid for 7 days) 2. Doxycycline[e] (3 mg/kg qd for 7 days) 3. Clindamycin (10 mg/kg bid for 7 days) *or* Atovaquone-proguanil (20/8 mg/kg qd for 3 days with food)
Severe Falciparum Malaria[f]	
	Artesunate[c] (2.4 mg/kg stat IV followed by 2.4 mg/kg at 12 and 24 h and then daily if necessary)[g] *or* Artemether[c] (3.2 mg/kg stat IM followed by 1.6 mg/kg qd) *or* Quinine dihydrochloride (20 mg of salt/kg[h] infused over 4 h, followed by 10 mg of salt/kg infused over 2–8 h q8h[i]) *or* Quinidine (10 mg of base/kg[h] infused over 1–2 h, followed by 1.2 mg of base/kg per hour[i] with electrocardiographic monitoring)

[a]Very few areas now have chloroquine-sensitive malaria (Fig. 203-2).
[b]In areas where the partner drug to artesunate is known to be effective.
[c]Artemisinin derivatives are not registered in the United States and some other temperate countries.
[d]Fixed-dose coformulated combinations are available.
[e]Tetracycline and doxycycline should not be given to pregnant women or to children <8 years of age.
[f]Oral treatment should be substituted as soon as the patient recovers sufficiently to take fluids by mouth.
[g]Artesunate is the drug of choice when available. The data from large studies in Southeast Asia showed a 35% reduction in mortality rate from that with quinine. Severe malaria in children in high-transmission settings has different characteristics; thus trials are ongoing in Africa comparing artesunate with quinine to determine whether there is a survival benefit in African children.
[h]A loading dose should not be given if therapeutic doses of quinine or quinidine have definitely been adminstered in the previous 24 h. Some authorities recommend a lower dose of quinidine.
[i]Infusions can be given in 0.9% saline and 5% or 10% dextrose in water. Infusion rates for quinine and quinidine should be carefully controlled.
Note: G6PD, glucose-6-phosphate dehydrogenase.

the closely related drug artemotil (arteether) are oil-based formulations given by IM injection; they are erratically absorbed and do not confer the same survival benefit as artesunate. A rectal formulation of artesunate has been developed as a community-based prereferral treatment for patients in the rural tropics who cannot take oral medications. Although the artemisinin compounds are safer than quinine and considerably safer than quinidine, only one formulation is available in the United States. IV artesunate has recently been approved by the FDA for emergency use for severe malaria through the Centers for Disease Control and Prevention (CDC) Drug Service (see end of chapter for contact information). The antiarrhythmic quinidine gluconate is as effective as quinine and, as it is more readily available, has replaced quinine for the treatment of malaria in the United States. The administration of quinidine must be closely monitored if dysrhythmias and hypotension are to be avoided. Total plasma levels >8 μg/mL, a QT_c interval >0.6 s, or QRS widening beyond 25% of baseline are indications for slowing infusion rates. If arrhythmia or saline-unresponsive hypotension develops, treatment with this drug should be discontinued. Quinine is safer than quinidine; cardiovascular monitoring is not required except when the recipient has cardiac disease.

Severe falciparum malaria constitutes a medical emergency requiring intensive nursing care and careful management. The patient should be weighed and, if comatose, placed on his or her side or prone. Frequent evaluation of the patient's condition is essential. Ancillary drugs such as high-dose glucocorticoids, urea, heparin, dextran, desferrioxamine, antibody to tumor necrosis factor α, and high-dose phenobarbital (20 mg/kg) have proved either ineffective or harmful in clinical trials and should not be used. In acute renal failure or severe metabolic acidosis, hemofiltration or hemodialysis should be started as early as possible.

Parenteral antimalarial treatment should be started as soon as possible. If artemether, quinine, or quinidine is used, an initial loading dose must be given so that therapeutic concentrations are reached as soon as possible. Both quinine and quinidine will cause dangerous hypotension if injected rapidly; when given IV, they must be administered carefully by rate-controlled infusion only. If this approach is not possible, quinine may be given by deep IM injections into the anterior thigh. The optimal therapeutic range for quinine and quinidine in severe malaria is not known with certainty, but total plasma concentrations of 8–15 mg/L for quinine and 3.5–8.0 mg/L for quinidine are effective and do not cause serious toxicity. The systemic clearance and apparent volume of distribution of these alkaloids are markedly reduced and plasma protein binding is increased in severe malaria, so that the blood concentrations attained with a given dose are higher. If the patient remains seriously ill or in acute renal failure for >2 days, maintenance doses of quinine or quinidine should be reduced by 30–50% to prevent toxic accumulation of the drug. The initial doses should never be reduced. If one of the artemisinin derivatives is given, dose reductions are unnecessary, even in renal failure. Exchange transfusion should be considered for severely ill patients, although the precise indications for this procedure have not been agreed upon. It has been recommended that—if safe and feasible—exchange should be considered for patients with severe malaria, but there is no clear evidence that this measure is beneficial. The role of prophylactic anticonvulsants is uncertain. If respiratory support is not available, then a full loading dose of phenobarbital (20 mg/kg) to prevent convulsions should not be given as it may cause respiratory arrest.

When the patient is unconscious, the blood glucose level should be measured every 4–6 h, and values <2.2 mmol/L (40 mg/dL) should mandate treatment with IV dextrose. All patients treated with IV quinine or quinidine should receive a continuous infusion of 5–10% dextrose. The parasite count and hematocrit level should be measured every 6–12 h. Anemia develops rapidly; if the hematocrit falls to <20%, then whole blood (preferably fresh) or packed cells should be transfused slowly, with careful attention to circulatory status. Renal function should be checked daily. Children presenting with severe anemia and acidotic breathing are often

TABLE 203-7 PROPERTIES OF ANTIMALARIAL DRUGS

Drug(s)	Pharmacokinetic Properties	Antimalarial Activity	Minor Toxicity	Major Toxicity
Quinine, quinidine	Good oral and IM absorption (quinine); *Cl* and V_d reduced, but plasma protein binding (principally to α1 acid glycoprotein) increased (90%) in malaria; quinine $t_{1/2}$: 16 h in malaria, 11 h in healthy persons; quinidine $t_{1/2}$: 13 h in malaria, 8 h in healthy persons	Acts mainly on trophozoite blood stage; kills gametocytes of *P. vivax*, *P. ovale*, and *P. malariae* (but not *P. falciparum*); no action on liver stages	*Common:* "Cinchonism": tinnitus, high-tone hearing loss, nausea, vomiting, dysphoria, postural hypotension; ECG QT_c interval prolongation (quinine usually by <10% but quinidine by up to 25%) *Rare:* Diarrhea, visual disturbance, rashes *Note:* Very bitter taste	*Common:* Hypoglycemia *Rare:* Hypotension, blindness, deafness, cardiac arrhythmias, thrombocytopenia, hemolysis, hemolytic-uremic syndrome, vasculitis, cholestatic hepatitis, neuromuscular paralysis *Note:* Quinidine more cardiotoxic
Chloroquine	Good oral absorption, very rapid IM and SC absorption; complex pharmacokinetics; enormous *Cl* and V_d (unaffected by malaria); blood concentration profile determined by distribution processes in malaria; $t_{1/2}$: 1–2 months	As for quinine but acts slightly earlier in asexual cycle	*Common:* Nausea, dysphoria, pruritus in dark-skinned patients, postural hypotension *Rare:* Accommodation difficulties, keratopathy, rash *Note:* Bitter taste, well tolerated	*Acute:* Hypotensive shock (parenteral), cardiac arrhythmias, neuropsychiatric reactions *Chronic:* Retinopathy (cumulative dose, >100 g), skeletal and cardiac myopathy
Amodiaquine	Good oral absorption; largely converted to active metabolite desethylamodiaquine	As for chloroquine	Nausea (tastes better than chloroquine)	Agranulocytosis; hepatitis, mainly with prophylactic use
Mefloquine	Adequate oral absorption; no parenteral preparation; $t_{1/2}$: 14–20 days (shorter in malaria)	As for quinine	Nausea, giddiness, dysphoria, fuzzy thinking, sleeplessness, nightmares, sense of dissociation	Neuropsychiatric reactions, convulsions, encephalopathy
Tetracycline, doxycycline[a]	Excellent absorption; $t_{1/2}$: 8 h for tetracycline, 18 h for doxycycline	Weak antimalarial activity; should not be used alone for treatment	Gastrointestinal intolerance, deposition in growing bones and teeth, photosensitivity, moniliasis, benign intracranial hypertension	Renal failure in patients with impaired renal function (tetracycline)
Halofantrine[b]	Highly variable absorption related to fat intake; $t_{1/2}$: 1–3 days (active desbutyl metabolite $t_{1/2}$: 3–7 days)	As for quinine	Diarrhea	Cardiac conduction disturbances; atrioventricular block; ECG QT_c interval prolongation; potentially lethal ventricular tachyarrhythmias
Artemisinin and derivatives (artemether, artesunate)	Good oral absorption, slow and variable absorption of IM artemether; artesunate and artemether biotransformed to active metabolite dihydroartemisinin; all drugs eliminated very rapidly; $t_{1/2}$: <1 h	Broader stage specificity and more rapid than other drugs; no action on liver stages; kills all but fully mature gametocytes of *P. falciparum*	Reduction in reticulocyte count (but not anemia)	Anaphylaxis, urticaria, fever
Pyrimethamine	Good oral absorption, variable IM absorption; $t_{1/2}$: 4 days	For blood stages, acts mainly on mature forms; causal prophylactic	Well tolerated	Megaloblastic anemia, pancytopenia, pulmonary infiltration
Proguanil (chloroguanide)	Good oral absorption; biotransformed to active metabolite cycloguanil; $t_{1/2}$: 16 h; biotransformation reduced by oral contraceptive use and in pregnancy	Causal prophylactic; not used alone for treatment	Well tolerated; mouth ulcers and rare alopecia	Megaloblastic anemia in renal failure
Primaquine	Complete oral absorption; active compound not known; $t_{1/2}$: 7 h	Radical cure; eradicates hepatic forms of *P. vivax* and *P. ovale*; kills all stages of gametocyte development of *P. falciparum*	Nausea, vomiting, diarrhea, abdominal pain, hemolysis, methemoglobinemia	Massive hemolysis in subjects with severe G6PD deficiency
Atovaquone	Highly variable absorption related to fat intake; $t_{1/2}$: 30–70 h	Acts mainly on trophozoite blood stage	None identified	None identified
Lumefantrine	Highly variable absorption related to fat intake; $t_{1/2}$: 3–4 days	As for quinine	None identified	None identified

[a]Tetracycline and doxycycline should not be given to pregnant women or to children <8 years of age.

[b]Halofantrine should not be used by patients with long ECG QT_c intervals or known conduction disturbances or by those taking drugs that may affect ventricular repolarization, e.g., quinidine, quinine, mefloquine, chloroquine, neuroleptics, antiarrhythmics, tricyclic antidepressants, terfenadine, or astemizole.

Abbreviations: *Cl*, systemic clearance; V_d, total apparent volume of distribution; IM, intramuscular; SC, subcutaneous; ECG, electrocardiogram; G6PD, glucose-6-phosphate dehydrogenase.

hypovolemic; in this situation, resuscitation with crystalloids or blood is indicated. Accurate assessment is vital. Management of fluid balance is difficult in severe malaria, particularly in adults, because of the thin dividing line between overhydration (leading to pulmonary edema) and underhydration (contributing to renal impairment). If necessary, central venous pressures should be measured and maintained in the low-normal range. As soon as the patient can take fluids, oral therapy should be substituted for parenteral treatment.

UNCOMPLICATED MALARIA Infections due to *P. vivax*, *P. malariae*, and *P. ovale* should be treated with oral chloroquine (total dose, 25 mg of base/kg). In much of the tropics, drug-resistant *P. falciparum* has been increasing in distribution, frequency, and intensity. Chloroquine-resistant *P. falciparum* is now present throughout most of the tropical world, and resistance to sulfadoxine/pyrimethamine is widespread and increasing. It is now accepted that, to prevent resistance, falciparum malaria should be treated with drug combinations and not with single drugs in endemic areas; the same rationale has been applied successfully to the treatment of tuberculosis and HIV/AIDS. This combination strategy is based on simultaneous use of two or more drugs with different modes of action: one is usually an artemisinin derivative (artesunate, artemether, or dihydroartemisinin) given for 3 days, and the other is usually a slower-acting antimalarial to which *P. falciparum* is sensitive. Artemisinin combination regimens now constitute first-line recommended treatment for falciparum malaria. In areas with multidrug-resistant falciparum malaria (parts of Asia and South America), either artemether-lumefantrine or artesunate-mefloquine should be used. Although significant resistance to mefloquine has been documented in Thailand, Myanmar, Vietnam, Laos, and Cambodia (**Fig. 203-10**), mefloquine is usually effective against multidrug-resistant strains of *P. falciparum* outside these areas and, in combination with artesunate, achieves cure rates exceeding 90% nearly everywhere. Atovaquone-proguanil is also highly effective. In areas with more drug-sensitive isolates, atovaquone-proguanil, mefloquine, artesunate-amodiaquine, or artesunate-sulfadoxine/pyrimethamine can be used, depending on the prevailing drug susceptibility pattern. These 3-day regimens are all well tolerated, although mefloquine is associated with increased rates of vomiting and dizziness. As second-line treatment for recrudescence following first-line therapy, a 7-day course of either artesunate or quinine plus tetracycline, doxycycline, or clindamycin is effective. Tetracycline and doxycycline cannot be given to pregnant women or to children <8 years of age. Oral quinine is extremely bitter and regularly produces cinchonism comprising tinnitus, high-tone deafness, nausea, vomiting, and dysphoria. Adherence is poor with the required 7-day regimens of quinine.

Patients should be monitored for vomiting for 1 h after the administration of any oral antimalarial drug. If there is vomiting, the dose should be repeated. Symptom-based treatment, with tepid sponging and acetaminophen administration, lowers fever and thereby reduces the patient's propensity to vomit these drugs. Minor central nervous system reactions (nausea, dizziness, sleep disturbances) are common. The incidence of serious adverse neuropsychiatric reactions to mefloquine treatment is ~1 in 1000 in Asia but may be as high as 1 in 200 among Africans and Caucasians. All the antimalarial quinolines (chloroquine, mefloquine, and quinine) exacerbate the orthostatic hypotension associated with malaria, and all are tolerated better by children than by adults. Pregnant women, young children, patients unable to tolerate oral therapy, and nonimmune subjects (e.g., travelers) with suspected malaria should be evaluated carefully and hospitalization considered. If there is any doubt as to the identity of the infecting malarial species, treatment for falciparum malaria should be given. A negative blood smear does not rule out malaria; thick blood films should be checked 1 and 2 days later to exclude the diagnosis. Nonimmune patients receiving treatment for malaria should have daily parasite counts performed until negative thick films indicate clearance of the parasite. If the level of parasitemia does not fall below 25% of the admission value in 48 h or if parasitemia has not cleared by 7 days (and adherence is assured), drug resistance is likely and the regimen should be changed. If treatment failures occur with commonly used antimalarial agents, alternative drugs should be used.

To eradicate persistent liver stages and prevent relapse (radical treatment), primaquine (0.25–0.5 mg of base/kg, adult dose) should be given daily for 14 days to patients with *P. vivax* or *P. ovale* infections after laboratory tests for G6PD deficiency have proved negative. A total dose of 22.5–30 mg for an adult is recommended for infections acquired in Southeast Asia and Oceania. If the patient has a mild variant of G6PD deficiency, primaquine can be given in a dose of 0.75 mg of base/kg (45 mg maximum) once weekly for 6 weeks.

COMPLICATIONS **Acute Renal Failure** If the level of BUN or creatinine rises despite adequate rehydration, fluid administration should be restricted to prevent volume overload. As in other forms of hypercatabolic acute renal failure, renal replacement is best performed early (Chap. 273). Hemofiltration and hemodialysis are more effective than peritoneal dialysis and are associated with lower mortality. Some patients with renal impairment pass small volumes of urine sufficient to allow control of fluid balance; these cases can be managed conservatively if other indications for dialysis do not arise. Renal function usually improves within days, but full recovery may take weeks.

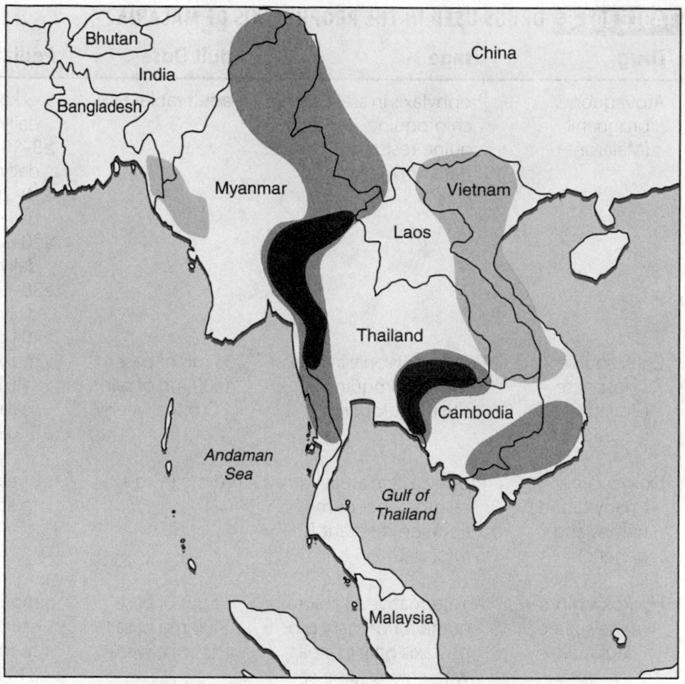

FIGURE 203-10 Mefloquine resistance in *Plasmodium falciparum* in Southeast Asia: high-level mefloquine resistance (*brown*), low-level mefloquine resistance (*red*), and mefloquine sensitivity (failure rate, <20%; *green*). There is insufficient information for the other areas.

Acute Pulmonary Edema Patients should be positioned with the head of the bed at a 45° elevation and given oxygen and IV diuretics. Pulmonary artery occlusion pressures may be normal, indicating increased pulmonary capillary permeability. Positive-pressure ventilation should be started early if the immediate measures fail (Chap. 228).

Hypoglycemia An initial slow injection of 50% dextrose (0.5 g/kg) should be followed by an infusion of 10% dextrose (0.10 g/kg per hour). The blood glucose level should be checked regularly thereafter as recurrent hypoglycemia is common, particularly among patients receiving quinine or quinidine. In severely ill patients, hypoglycemia commonly occurs together with metabolic (lactic) acidosis and carries a poor prognosis.

Other Complications Patients who develop spontaneous bleeding should be given fresh blood and IV vitamin K. Convulsions should be treated with IV or rectal benzodiazepines and, if necessary, respiratory support. Aspiration pneumonia should be suspected in any unconscious patient with convulsions, particularly with persistent hyperventilation; IV antimicrobial agents and oxygen should be administered, and pulmonary toilet should be undertaken. Hypoglycemia or gram-negative septicemia should be suspected when the condition of any patient suddenly deteriorates for no obvious reason during antimalarial treatment. Systemic *Salmonella* infections are common complications among African children with falciparum malaria. Antibiotics should be considered for severely ill patients not responding to antimalarial treatment.

PREVENTION

These are halcyon days for malaria prevention and control. New drugs have been discovered and developed; highly effective drugs, insecticide-treated nets, and insecticides for spraying dwellings are being purchased for endemic countries by the Global Fund to Fight HIV/AIDS, Tuberculosis, and Malaria and the President's Malaria Initiative; and even stronger support is being advocated by the Roll Back Malaria Partnership, the Global Health Council, and other supporters of malaria control and research. Still, the eradication of malaria is not yet feasible because of the widespread distribution of *Anopheles* breeding

TABLE 203-8 DRUGS USED IN THE PROPHYLAXIS OF MALARIA

Drug	Usage	Adult Dose	Pediatric Dose	Comments
Atovaquone/ proguanil (Malarone)	Prophylaxis in areas with chloroquine- or mefloquine-resistant *Plasmodium falciparum*	1 adult tablet PO[a]	5–8 kg: ½ pediatric tablet[b] daily ≥8–10 kg: ¾ pediatric tablet daily ≥10–20 kg: 1 pediatric tablet daily ≥20–30 kg: 2 pediatric tablets daily ≥30–40 kg: 3 pediatric tablets daily ≥40 kg: 1 adult tablet daily	Begin 1–2 days before travel to malarious areas. Take daily at the same time each day while in the malarious area and for 7 days after leaving such areas. Atovaquone-proguanil is contraindicated in persons with severe renal impairment (creatinine clearance rate <30 mL/min). It is not recommended for children weighing <5 kg, pregnant women, or women breast-feeding infants weighing <5 kg. Atovaquone/proguanil should be taken with food or a milky drink.
Chloroquine phosphate (Aralen and generic)	Prophylaxis only in areas with chloroquine-sensitive *P. falciparum*[c]	300 mg of base (500 mg of salt) PO once weekly	5 mg/kg of base (8.3 mg of salt/kg) PO once weekly, up to a maximum adult dose of 300 mg of base	Begin 1–2 weeks before travel to malarious areas. Take weekly on the same day of the week while in the malarious areas and for 4 weeks after leaving such areas. Chloroquine phosphate may exacerbate psoriasis.
Doxycycline (many brand names and generic)	Prophylaxis in areas with chloroquine- or mefloquine-resistant *P. falciparum*[c]	100 mg PO qd	≥8 years of age: 2 mg/kg, up to adult dose	Begin 1–2 days before travel to malarious areas. Take daily at the same time each day while in the malarious areas and for 4 weeks after leaving such areas. Doxycycline is contraindicated in children <8 years of age and in pregnant women.
Hydroxychloroquine sulfate (Plaquenil)	An alternative to chloroquine for primary prophylaxis only in areas with chloroquine-sensitive *P. falciparum*[c]	310 mg of base (400 mg of salt) PO once weekly	5 mg of base/kg (6.5 mg of salt/kg) PO once weekly, up to maximum adult dose of 310 mg of base	Begin 1–2 weeks before travel to malarious areas. Take weekly on the same day of the week while in the malarious areas and for 4 weeks after leaving such areas. Hydroxychloroquine may exacerbate psoriasis.
Mefloquine (Lariam and generic)	Prophylaxis in areas with chloroquine-resistant *P. falciparum*	228 mg of base (250 mg of salt) PO once weekly	≤9 kg: 4.6 mg of base/kg (5 mg of salt/kg) PO once weekly 10–19 kg: ¼ tablet once weekly 20–30 kg: ½ tablet once weekly 31–45 kg: ¾ tablet once weekly ≥46 kg: 1 tablet once weekly	Begin 1–2 weeks before travel to malarious areas. Take weekly on the same day of the week while in the malarious areas and for 4 weeks after leaving such areas. Mefloquine is contraindicated in persons allergic to this drug or related compounds (e.g., quinine and quinidine) and in persons with active or recent depression, generalized anxiety disorder, psychosis, schizophrenia, other major psychiatric disorders, or seizures. Use with caution in persons with psychiatric disturbances or a history of depression. Mefloquine is not recommended for persons with cardiac conduction abnormalities.
Primaquine	An option for prophylaxis in special circumstances	30 mg of base (52.6 mg of salt) PO qd	0.5 mg of base/kg (0.8 mg of salt/kg) PO qd, up to adult dose; should be taken with food	Begin 1–2 days before travel to malarious areas. Take daily at the same time each day while in the malarious areas and for 7 days after leaving such areas. Primaquine is contraindicated in persons with G6PD1 deficiency. It is also contraindicated during pregnancy and in lactation unless the infant being breast-fed has a documented normal G6PD level. Use in consultation with malaria experts.
Primaquine	Used for presumptive antirelapse therapy (terminal prophylaxis) to decrease risk of relapses of *P. vivax* and *P. ovale.*	30 mg of base (52.6 mg of salt) PO qd for 14 days after departure from the malarious area	0.5 mg of base/kg (0.8 mg of salt/kg), up to adult dose, PO qd for 14 days after departure from the malarious area	This therapy is indicated for persons who have had prolonged exposure to *P. vivax* and/or *P. ovale.* It is contraindicated in persons with G6PD1 deficiency as well as during pregnancy and in lactation unless the infant being breast-fed has a documented normal G6PD level.

[a]An adult tablet contains 250 mg of atovaquone and 100 mg of proguanil hydrochloride.
[b]A pediatric tablet contains 62.5 mg of atovaquone and 25 mg of proguanil hydrochloide.
[c]Very few areas now have chloroquine-sensitive malaria (Fig. 203-2).

Source: CDC: *http:/wwwn.cdc.gov/travel/contentMalariaDrugsHC.aspx*, accessed September 13, 2007.

sites; the great number of infected persons; the continued use of ineffective antimalarial drugs; and inadequacies in human and material resources, infrastructure, and control programs. Malaria may be contained by judicious use of insecticides to kill the mosquito vector, rapid diagnosis, appropriate patient management, and—where effective and feasible—administration of intermittent presumptive treatment or chemoprophylaxis to high-risk groups. Malaria researchers are intensifying their efforts to gain a better understanding of parasite-human-mosquito interactions and to develop more effective control and prevention interventions. Despite the enormous investment in efforts to develop a malaria vaccine, no safe, effective, long-lasting vaccine is likely to be available for general use in the near future (Chap. 116). While there is promise for one or more malaria vaccines on the more distant horizon, prevention and control measures continue to rely on antivector and drug-use strategies.

PERSONAL PROTECTION AGAINST MALARIA

Simple measures to reduce the frequency of mosquito bites in malarious areas are very important. These measures include the avoidance of exposure to mosquitoes at their peak feeding times (usually dusk and dawn) and throughout the night as well as the use of insect repellents containing DEET (10–35%) or picaridin (7%; if DEET is unacceptable), suitable clothing, and insecticide-impregnated bed nets or other materials. Widespread use of bed nets treated with residual pyrethroids reduces the incidence of malaria in areas where vectors bite indoors at night and has been shown to reduce mortality rates in western and eastern Africa.

CHEMOPROPHYLAXIS

(Table 203-8; *http://wwwn.cdc.gov/travel/contentMalariaDrugsHC.aspx*; accessed September 13, 2007) Recommendations for prophylaxis depend on knowledge of local patterns of plasmodial drug sensitivity and the likelihood of acquiring malarial infection. When there is uncertainty, drugs effective against resistant *P. falciparum* should be used [atovaquone-proguanil (Malarone), doxycycline, mefloquine, or primaquine]. Chemoprophylaxis is never entirely reliable, and malaria should always be considered in the differential diagnosis of fever in patients who have traveled to endemic areas, even if they are taking prophylactic antimalarial drugs.

Pregnant women traveling to malarious areas should be warned about the potential risks. All pregnant women at risk in endemic areas should be encouraged to attend regular antenatal clinics. Mefloquine is the only drug advised for pregnant women traveling to areas with drug-resistant malaria; this drug is generally considered safe in the second and third trimesters of pregnancy, and the limited data on first-trimester exposure are reassuring. The safety of other prophylactic antimalarial agents in pregnancy has not been established. Antimalarial prophylaxis has been shown to reduce mortality rates among children between the ages of 3 months and 4 years in malaria-endemic areas; however, it is not a logistically or economically feasible option in many countries. The alternative—to give intermittent treatment doses [intermittent preventive treatment (IPT)]—shows promise for more widespread use in infants, young children, and pregnant women. Children born to nonimmune mothers in endemic areas (usually expatriates moving to malaria-endemic areas) should receive prophylaxis from birth.

Travelers should start taking antimalarial drugs 2 days to 1–2 weeks before departure so that any untoward reactions can be detected and so that therapeutic antimalarial blood concentrations will be present when needed (Table 203-8). Antimalarial prophylaxis should continue for 4 weeks after the traveler has left the endemic area, except if atovaquone-proguanil or primaquine has been taken; these drugs have significant activities against the liver stage of the infection (causal prophylaxis) and can be discontinued 1 week after departure from the endemic area. Presumptive self-treatment for malaria with atovaquone-proguanil (for 3 consecutive days) or another drug can be considered under special circumstances; medical advice on self-treatment should be sought before departure for malarious areas and as soon as possible after illness begins.

Atovaquone-proguanil (Malarone; 3.75/1.5 mg/kg or 250/100 mg, daily adult dose) is a fixed-combination, once-daily prophylactic agent that is very well tolerated by adults and children, with fewer adverse gastrointestinal effects than chloroquine-proguanil and fewer adverse central nervous system effects than mefloquine. It is proguanil itself, rather than the antifolate metabolite cycloguanil, that acts synergistically with atovaquone. This combination is effective against all types of malaria, including multidrug-resistant falciparum malaria. Atovaquone-proguanil is best taken with food or a milky drink to optimize absorption. There are insufficient data on the safety of this regimen in pregnancy.

Mefloquine (250 mg of salt weekly, adult dose) has been widely used for malarial prophylaxis because it is usually effective against multidrug-resistant falciparum malaria and is reasonably well tolerated. Mild nausea, dizziness, fuzzy thinking, disturbed sleep patterns, vivid dreams, and malaise are relatively common. Approximately 1 in every 10,000 recipients develops an acute reversible neuropsychiatric reaction manifested by confusion, psychosis, convulsions, or encephalopathy. The role of mefloquine prophylaxis during pregnancy remains uncertain; in studies in Africa, mefloquine prophylaxis was found to be effective and safe during pregnancy. However, in one study from Thailand, treatment of malaria with mefloquine was associated with an increased risk of stillbirth.

Daily administration of doxycycline (100 mg daily, adult dose) is an effective alternative to atovaquone-proguanil or mefloquine. Doxycycline is generally well tolerated but may cause vulvovaginal thrush, diarrhea, and photosensitivity and cannot be used by children <8 years old or by pregnant women.

Chloroquine remains the drug of choice for the prevention of infection with drug-sensitive *P. falciparum* (now found in very few areas of the world) and with the other human malarial species (although chloroquine-resistant *P. vivax* has been reported from parts of eastern Asia, Oceania, and Central and South America). Chloroquine is generally well tolerated, although some patients cannot take the drug because of malaise, headache, visual symptoms (from reversible keratopathy), gastrointestinal intolerance, or (in dark-skinned patients) pruritus. A concomitant filarial infection may provoke or aggravate chloroquine-induced pruritus. Chloroquine is considered safe in pregnancy. With chronic administration for >5 years, a characteristic dose-related retinopathy may develop, but this condition is rare at the doses used for antimalarial prophylaxis. Idiosyncratic or allergic reactions are also rare. Skeletal and cardiac myopathy are potential problems with protracted prophylactic use; they are more likely to occur with the high doses used in the treatment of rheumatoid arthritis. Neuropsychiatric reactions and skin rashes are unusual. When used continuously, amodiaquine, a related aminoquinoline, is associated with a high risk of agranulocytosis (~1 person in 2000) and hepatotoxicity (~1 person in 16,000) and should not be used for prophylaxis.

Primaquine (0.5 mg of base/kg or 30 mg, daily adult dose taken with food) has proved safe and effective in the prevention of drug-resistant falciparum and vivax malaria in adults. This drug can be considered for persons who are traveling to areas with or without drug-resistant *P. falciparum* and who are intolerant to other recommended drugs. Abdominal pain and oxidant hemolysis—the principal adverse effects—are not common as long as the drug is taken with food and is not given to G6PD-deficient persons. Primaquine should not be given to pregnant women or neonates. Travelers must be tested for G6PD deficiency and be shown to have a level in the normal range before receiving primaquine. In G6PD deficiency, primaquine can cause hemolysis that is sometimes fatal.

In the past, the dihydrofolate reductase inhibitors pyrimethamine and proguanil (chloroguanide) have been administered widely, but the rapid selection of resistance in both *P. falciparum* and *P. vivax* has limited their use. Whereas antimalarial quinolines such as chloroquine act on the erythrocyte stage of parasitic development, the dihydrofolate reductase inhibitors also inhibit preerythrocytic growth in the liver (causal prophylaxis) and development in the mosquito (sporontocidal activity). Proguanil is safe and well tolerated, although mouth ulceration occurs in ~8% of persons using this drug; it is considered safe for antimalarial prophylaxis in pregnancy. The prophylactic use of the combination of pyrimethamine and sulfadoxine is not recommended because of an unacceptable incidence of severe toxicity, principally exfoliative dermatitis and other skin rashes, agranulocytosis, hepatitis, and pulmonary eosinophilia (incidence, 1:7000; fatal reactions, 1:18,000). The combination of pyrimethamine with dapsone (0.2/1.5 mg/kg weekly; 12.5/100 mg, adult dose) is a third-line alternative available in some countries. Dapsone may cause methemoglobinemia and allergic reactions and (at higher doses) may pose a significant risk of agranulocytosis. Proguanil and the pyrimethamine-dapsone combination are not available in the United States.

Because of the increasing spread and intensity of antimalarial drug resistance (Figs. 203-2 and 203-10), the Centers for Disease Control and Prevention (CDC; *http://www.cdc.gov/malaria/index.htm*), which recommends a daily dose of atovaquone-proguanil for all travelers, maintains an updated 24-h travel and malaria information audiotape that can be accessed by touch-tone telephone (877-FYI-TRIP). Regional and disease-specific documents may be requested from the CDC Fax Information Service (888-232-3299). Consultation for the evaluation of prophylaxis failures or treatment of malaria can be obtained from state and local health departments and the CDC Malaria Hotline (770-488-7788) or the CDC Emergency Operations Center (770-488-7100).

FURTHER READINGS

BAIRD JK et al: Prevention and treatment of vivax malaria. Curr Infect Dis Rep 9:39, 2007

CENTERS FOR DISEASE CONTROL AND PREVENTION: Treatment of malaria (guidelines for clinicians). Atlanta, Department of Health and Human Services, 2000; available online at *http://www.cdc.gov/malaria/diagnosis_treatment/tx_clinicians.htm*

DONDORP A et al: Artesunate versus quinine for treatment of severe falciparum malaria: A randomised trial. Lancet 366:717, 2005

PHU NH et al: Hemofiltration and peritoneal dialysis in infection-associated acute renal failure in Vietnam. N Engl J Med 347:895, 2002

WHITE NJ: The assessment of antimalarial drug efficacy. Trends Parasitol 18:865, 2002

World Health Organization: Severe falciparum malaria. Trans R Soc Trop Med Hyg 94(Suppl 1):51, 2000

———: Guidelines for the treatment of malaria. Geneva, World Health Organization, 2006

———: Assessment and monitoring of antimalarial drug efficacy for the treatment of uncomplicated falciparum malaria. WHO/HTM/RBM/2003.50; available online at *http://www.who.int/malaria/docs/ProtocolWHO.pdf*

204 Babesiosis

Jeffrey A. Gelfand, Edouard Vannier

Babesiosis is an emerging infection transmitted by ticks and caused by intraerythrocytic protozoa of the genus *Babesia*. Wild and domestic animals are natural reservoirs of *Babesia* species. Only in the past 50 years has *Babesia* been appreciated to be a pathogen in humans. Usually a mild flulike illness in young and healthy people, babesiosis may develop into a life-threatening malaria-like syndrome in asplenic, immunocompromised, or elderly patients.

ETIOLOGY AND NATURAL CYCLE

In the northeastern United States, *Babesia microti* is transmitted to humans by the hard-bodied tick *Ixodes scapularis* (*I. dammini*). In the fall, adult ticks feed primarily on white-tailed deer. Deer are incompetent reservoirs for *B. microti* but are essential for the maintenance of *I. scapularis*. Adult ticks overwinter and lay eggs in the spring. The eggs hatch into larvae in late July. In August and September, larvae become infected as they feed on *B. microti*–infected white-footed mice. In the spring of the following year, larvae molt into nymphs that remain infected with *B. microti* (transstadial transmission). Early in the summer, these nymphs feed on white-footed mice that become reservoirs of *B. microti*. Transmission of *B. microti* to humans is incidental and occurs primarily at the nymphal stage.

In Europe, *I. ricinus* is regarded as the main vector for infection of humans with *B. divergens*, a pathogen of cattle. *B. divergens* is maintained in the life cycle of the tick by transstadial and transovarial transmission. Nymphs and adults are considered the primary vectors in bovine and human babesiosis.

As ticks feed, *Babesia*-infected red blood cells (RBCs) accumulate in their gut. Gametes fuse into zygotes that translocate across the epithelium, enter the hemolymph, and become kinetes. Some kinetes reach salivary acini and undergo hypertrophy to become dormant sporoblasts. Upon attachment of the tick to the host, sporogony is initiated. In the last hours of feeding, sporozoites are deposited in the host dermis. Once in the blood, sporozoites invade erythrocytes to become trophozoites. Trophozoites undergo asynchronous schizogony, resulting in the budding of two or four merozoites. Tetrads ("Maltese crosses") are pathognomonic of *B. microti* and other small *Babesia* species (e.g., *B. duncani*) but are seen only rarely in blood smears during infection.

EPIDEMIOLOGY

United States Babesiosis due to *B. microti* is an emerging infection in the United States. Most of the >300 documented cases have occurred in coastal southern New England (from eastern Connecticut to Cape Cod, MA) and the chain of islands off the coast, particularly Nantucket Island and Martha's Vineyard (MA); Block Island (RI); and eastern Long Island, Shelter Island, and Fire Island (NY). Several cases have been reported from upstate New York, New Jersey, and Pennsylvania and from the upper Midwest (Wisconsin, Minnesota). Because babesiosis is not a notifiable disease in every state and asymptomatic infection is common, the incidence of *B. microti* infection is greatly underestimated. In New York state alone, >800 cases have been reported in the past decade. In Washington state and northern California, nine cases have been attributed to *B. duncani* (isolates WA1 and CA5), *B. duncani*–type parasites (WA2 and CA6), and other closely related babesial parasites (CA1–4). These organisms are antigenically distinct from *B. microti* and belong to the clade of piroplasms found in dogs (*B. conradae*) and wild animals in the western United States. As asymptomatic infection may persist for months without detectable parasitemia, babesiosis may be transmitted by blood transfusion, especially in endemic areas. More than 50 transfusion-transmitted cases have been attributed to *B. microti* and two to *B. duncani* (WA1 and WA2). Neonatal babesiosis is rare and has been acquired by vertical transmission, blood transfusion, or tick bite. Lastly, *B. divergens*–like parasites have been implicated in three cases of acute babesiosis (one each in Missouri, Kentucky, and Washington state).

Other Countries Babesiosis is rare in Europe, with half of the >35 cases documented in France and the British Isles. In addition to the original case from Croatia, cases have been reported from the central Alpine region (Austria, Italy, Switzerland) and from southern Europe (Spain, Portugal). Most cases have involved asplenic patients and have been attributed to *B. divergens*. *B. microti* has been implicated in only a handful of cases, although serologic evidence of *B. microti* infection has emerged from Switzerland and midwestern Germany. A study of two patients from Austria and Italy has identified *Babesia* EU1 as a novel pathogen that belongs to the *B. divergens* clade and is closely related to *B. odocoilei*, a parasite of white-tailed deer.

Sporadic cases of human babesiosis have been described in Mexico, Colombia, the Canary Islands, Ivory Coast, Egypt, Mozambique, South Africa, and India. Cases due to *B. microti*–like piroplasms have been reported from Taiwan and Japan.

CLINICAL PRESENTATION

Infections with *B. microti* vary in severity. Asymptomatic infection or self-limiting flulike illness occurs in ~25% of adults and ~50% of children. The incubation period lasts 1–6 weeks. Onset is gradual. The most common manifestations are fever (intermittent or sustained, with temperatures sometimes reaching 40°C), fatigue, malaise, shaking chills, sweats, myalgias, and arthralgias. Less frequent symptoms include shortness of breath, headache, anorexia, and nausea. Malaise, myalgias, arthralgias, and shortness of breath may help differentiate babesiosis from other febrile illnesses. Fever is the salient feature on physical examination. Mild splenomegaly and hepatomegaly may be noted. Jaundice is rare.

Low hematocrit, low hemoglobin, and hemoglobinuria are consistent with hemolytic anemia. The parasitemia level is usually 1–10% in immunocompetent hosts but can reach 85% in asplenic patients. Reticulocyte counts are elevated, white blood cell (WBC) counts are normal or slightly low, and thrombocytopenia is common. Levels of liver enzymes (including alkaline phosphatase, lactate dehydrogenase, aspartate and alanine aminotransferases, and bilirubin) are elevated. With hemolysis, the serum haptoglobin concentration is low, and urinalysis may show hemoglobinuria and proteinuria.

Complications of babesiosis include acute respiratory failure, disseminated intravascular coagulation, congestive heart failure, and renal failure. *B. microti* infection may be fatal in 5–10% of cases in hospitalized patients. Severe anemia (hemoglobin concentration, <10 g/dL) and high-level parasitemia (>10%) are risk factors for complications. Alkaline phosphatase levels of >125 U/L, WBC counts of >5 × 10^9/L, and male gender are strong predictors of severe disease, as defined by death, hospitalization for >2 weeks, or admission to an intensive care unit for >2 days. Severe babesiosis is common among asplenic patients, patients co-infected with *Borrelia burgdorferi* (i.e., those with Lyme disease), persons >50 years of age, and individuals with comorbidities, including HIV infection, cancer, and other diseases associated with immunosuppression. Infection may recrudesce after splenectomy or immunosuppressive therapy.

Babesiosis due to *B. divergens* occurs most often in asplenic patients. After an incubation period of 1–3 weeks, disease suddenly appears. Hemoglobinuria—the presenting symptom—is followed by jaundice, persistent high fever (40°–41°C), myalgias, shaking chills, and drenching sweats. Babesiosis may evolve into a shocklike syndrome, with renal failure and pulmonary edema. The parasitemia level can reach 80%. Hemoglobin levels may plunge to 4–8 g/dL. The mortality rate remains high (42%).

Infections with *B. duncani* and related parasites range from asymptomatic to severe and are sometimes fatal.

DIAGNOSIS

A diagnosis of babesiosis should be considered for any symptomatic patient who resides or travels in endemic areas. The tick bite often goes unnoticed. Because symptoms are nonspecific, the diagnosis requires laboratory testing. Babesiosis is diagnosed by microscopic examination of Giemsa-stained thin blood smears. *Babesia* spp. appear annular, oval, or piriform. Ring forms are most common and do not contain the central brownish deposits (hemozoin) typical of *Plasmodium falciparum*. Tetrads are indicative of small babesial parasites, such as *B. microti* and *B. duncani*. An indirect immunofluorescent antibody test (IFAT) for *B. microti* is available from the Centers for Disease Control and Prevention. A serum IgG titer of ≥1:64 is diagnostic. The latter test has good predictive value for infection but must be interpreted in the clinical context; antibodies do not develop until at least 1 week into the illness, and serologic testing does not distinguish prior infection from active infection. Thus, IFAT is ideal for detection of past or persistent infection but not of fulminant acute infection. Antibodies to *B. microti* do not react with *B. divergens* or *B. duncani*. The persistence of low-grade infection is best diagnosed by polymerase chain reaction (PCR)–based amplification of the babesial 18S rRNA gene in blood samples. As primers are species-specific, this assay is a valuable adjunct in the diagnosis of babesiosis.

TABLE 204-1 ANTIBIOTIC REGIMENS FOR THE TREATMENT OF BABESIOSIS

Organism	Severity	Adults	Children
B. microti	Mild[a]	Atovaquone (750 mg q12h PO) *plus* Azithromycin (500–1000 mg/d PO on day 1, 250 mg/d PO thereafter)	Atovaquone (20 mg/kg q12h PO; maximum, 750 mg/dose) *plus* Azithromycin [10 mg/kg qd PO on day 1 (maximum, 500 mg/dose), 5 mg/kg qd PO thereafter (maximum, 250 mg/dose)]
	Severe[a]	Clindamycin (300–600 mg q6h IV or 600 mg q8h PO) *plus* Quinine (650 mg q6–8h PO) *plus* Consider RBC exchange transfusion	Clindamycin (7–10 mg/kg q6–8h IV or 7–10 mg/kg q6–8h PO; maximum, 600 mg/dose) *plus* Quinine (8 mg/kg q8h PO; maximum, 650 mg/dose) *plus* Consider RBC exchange transfusion
B. divergens	Mild or severe[b]	Immediate complete RBC exchange transfusion *plus* Clindamycin (600 mg q6–8h IV) *plus* Quinine (650 mg q8h PO)	Immediate complete RBC exchange transfusion *plus* Clindamycin (7–10 mg/kg q6–8h IV; maximum, 600 mg/dose) *plus* Quinine (8 mg/kg q8h PO; maximum, 650 mg/dose)

[a]Treatment duration: 7–10 days.
[b]Treatment duration: generally 7–10 days, but may vary.
Note: RBC, red blood cell.

℞ BABESIOSIS

(See **Table 204-1**) Whether *B. microti* infection should be treated depends on the clinical context. Asymptomatic infections need not be treated, but if *Babesia* organisms continue to be seen on blood smear or by PCR for >3 months, treatment should be considered. Symptomatic infections should not be treated if blood smear and PCR are both negative for *Babesia*. If *Babesia* is detected in blood samples from symptomatic patients, treatment should be initiated.

A combination of atovaquone and azithromycin, given for 7–10 days, constitutes initial therapy for non-life-threatening (mild) babesiosis due to *B. microti*. For immunocompromised patients, higher doses of azithromycin (600–1000 mg/d) than those listed in the table are used. A combination of clindamycin and quinine is given for 7–10 days to patients with severe *B. microti* babesiosis; whenever possible, clindamycin should be given IV rather than PO. Partial or complete RBC exchange transfusion is advised in severe babesiosis, which is defined as a parasitemia level of >10%; significant hemolysis; or renal, hepatic, or pulmonary compromise. Treatment failures have been described with the recommended medical regimens. Other combination therapies may be used. A combination of azithromycin and quinine was effective in two patients with infection refractory to clindamycin plus quinine. One patient with AIDS and chronic babesiosis was treated successfully with a combination of clindamycin, doxycycline, and azithromycin after becoming allergic to quinine.

In patients with mild *B. microti* babesiosis, symptoms should improve within the first 48 h of therapy and should resolve within 3 months. In patients with severe babesiosis, hematocrit and parasitemia should be monitored each day or every other day until symptoms recede and the parasitemia level is <5%. Re-treatment may be required if the babesial parasite or amplifiable babesial DNA is detected for >3 months after initial therapy, but routine testing is not needed for immunocompetent patients who are asymptomatic. Underlying immunodeficiency (such as malignancy or HIV infection) should be considered in patients with severe or prolonged episodes of babesiosis. There is increasing evidence that immunosuppressed patients may need treatment for considerably longer periods.

Patients with babesiosis should be evaluated for Lyme disease (Chap. 166) and human granulocytotropic anaplasmosis (Chap. 167), as all three infections may be acquired from the same tick vector. In endemic areas for these infections, relevant antimicrobial therapy should be considered when an intercurrent infection is strongly suspected.

B. divergens infection is often severe and progresses rapidly. The recommended treatment is immediate complete blood exchange transfusion and medical therapy with IV clindamycin plus oral quinine. Exchange transfusion ensures a complete and rapid removal of parasitized RBCs, RBC debris, and inflammatory mediators. Although uninfected RBCs are introduced by exchange transfusion, anemia may persist for >1 month. If so, additional transfusion is needed.

PREVENTION

Individuals who live or travel in endemic areas, especially those at increased risk for severe babesiosis, should be advised to avoid tick exposure by wearing protective clothing (long sleeves/long pants, with pants tucked into socks); applying tick repellents (such as DEET) to clothing; and limiting outdoor activities, especially between May and September, when infection risk is highest. Thorough skin examination after outdoor exposure allows removal of ticks within 24 h of attachment—i.e., before transmission can occur.

FURTHER READINGS

AGUILAR-DELFIN I et al: Resistance to acute babesiosis is associated with interleukin-12 and gamma interferon–mediated responses and requires macrophages and natural killer cells. Infect Immun 71:2002, 2003

HOLMAN PJ: Phylogenetic and biologic evidence that *Babesia divergens* is not endemic in the United States. Ann NY Acad Sci 1081:518, 2006

THOMPSON C et al: Coinfecting deer-associated zoonoses: Lyme disease, babesiosis, and ehrlichiosis. Clin Infect Dis 33:676, 2001

YOKOYAMA N et al: Erythrocyte invasion by *Babesia* parasites: Current advances in the elucidation of the molecular interactions between the protozoan ligands and host receptors in the invasion stage. Vet Parasitol 138:22, 2006

205 Leishmaniasis

Barbara L. Herwaldt

The term *leishmaniasis* encompasses multiple clinical syndromes. Most notable are visceral, cutaneous, and mucosal leishmaniasis, which result from infection of macrophages throughout the reticuloendothelial system, in the dermis, and in the naso-oropharyngeal mucosa, respectively.

Leishmaniasis, a vector-borne disease caused by obligate intracellular protozoa, is characterized by vast diversity and by specificity within that diversity. The disease is endemic in focal areas of ~90 countries in the tropics, subtropics, and southern Europe, in settings that range from deserts to rain forests and from rural to urban areas. Infection in humans is caused by ~20 *Leishmania* species (*Leishmania* and *Viannia* subgenera) (Table 205-1), which are transmitted by ~30 species of phlebotomine sandflies [*Phlebotomus* (Old World) and *Lutzomyia* (New World)]. Amid this diversity, particular parasite, vector, and host species maintain the transmission cycle in a given setting.

Both the diversity and the specificity of the disease confound attempts to generalize about any aspect of leishmaniasis, including control measures and clinical management. The multitudinous possible combinations of *Leishmania* species/strains, syndromes, and geographic areas—modified by host factors and immunoinflammatory responses—may be associated with clinically relevant differences, such as diverse manifestations of infection and diverse responses to particular therapies. It is essential that clinicians understand the dangers associated with extrapolating data from one setting to another and the importance of individualizing patient care, with expert consultation.

TABLE 205-1 *LEISHMANIA* SPECIES THAT CAUSE DISEASE IN HUMANS

Species[a]	Clinical Syndrome[b]	Geographic Distribution[c]
Subgenus *Leishmania*		
L. donovani complex		
L. donovani sensu stricto	VL (PKDL, OWCL)	China, Indian subcontinent (southern Asia), southwestern Asia, Ethiopia,[d] Kenya, Somalia, Sudan, Uganda; possibly sporadic elsewhere in sub-Saharan Africa
L. infantum sensu stricto[e]	VL (OWCL)	China, central and southwestern Asia, Middle East, southern Europe, northern Africa, Ethiopia,[d] Sudan; sporadic elsewhere in sub-Saharan Africa
L. chagasi[e]	VL (NWCL)	Central and South America
L. mexicana complex		
L. mexicana	NWCL (DCL)	Mexico, Central and South America; sporadic in Texas and Oklahoma
L. amazonensis	NWCL (ML, DCL, VL)	Panama and South America
L. tropica	*OWCL (VL)*[f]	*Central Asia, India, Pakistan, southwestern Asia, Middle East, Turkey, Greece, northern Africa, Ethiopia,*[d] *Kenya, Namibia*
L. major	OWCL	Central Asia, India, Pakistan, southwestern Asia, Middle East, Turkey, northern Africa, Sahel region of north-central Africa, Ethiopia,[d] Sudan, Kenya
L. aethiopica	OWCL (DCL)	Ethiopia,[d] Kenya, Uganda
Subgenus *Viannia*		
L. (V.) braziliensis	NWCL (ML)	Central and South America
L. (V.) guyanensis	NWCL (ML)	South America
L. (V.) panamensis	NWCL (ML)	Central America, Venezuela, Colombia, Ecuador, Peru
L. (V.) peruviana	NWCL[g]	Peru (western slopes of Andes)

[a]Species other than those listed here have been reported to infect humans.
[b]DCL, diffuse cutaneous leishmaniasis; ML, mucosal leishmaniasis; NWCL, New World (American) cutaneous leishmaniasis; OWCL, Old World cutaneous leishmaniasis; PKDL, post–kala-azar dermal leishmaniasis; VL, visceral leishmaniasis. Clinical syndromes less frequently associated with the various species are shown in parentheses.
[c]The geographic distribution is highly focal within countries/regions, and the order in which areas are listed does not reflect the level of endemicity. (See text for further information.) The geographic distribution of cases evaluated in countries such as the United States reflects travel and immigration patterns.
[d]Cutaneous and visceral leishmaniasis also are endemic in parts of Eritrea, but the causative species have not been well established.
[e]"*L. infantum*" and "*L. chagasi*" are considered synonymous.
[f]*L. tropica* also causes leishmaniasis recidivans and viscerotropic leishmaniasis.
[g]The cutaneous leishmaniasis syndrome caused by this species is called *uta*.

LIFE CYCLE AND IMMUNOREGULATION

Leishmania parasites, which target and persist in tissue macrophages, are transmitted by the bite of female phlebotomine sandflies. While probing for a blood meal, sandflies regurgitate the parasite's flagellated promastigote stage into the host's skin; sandfly salivary components with immunomodulating effects have been shown to promote experimental infection. Promastigotes bind to receptors on macrophages, are phagocytized, and transform within phagolysosomes into nonflagellated amastigotes (Fig. 205-1), which replicate and infect additional macrophages. Amastigotes ingested by sandflies transform back into infective promastigotes. Other modes of transmission include congenital and parenteral (e.g., by blood transfusion or needle sharing).

Leishmaniasis is viewed as a model system for exploring immunoregulatory responses to intracellular pathogens. Murine models of *L. major* infection exemplify the T_H1/T_H2 paradigm, in which polarized T_H1 and T_H2 responses govern resistance and susceptibility, respectively. Production of interferon γ (IFN-γ) by T_H1 and natural killer cells confers resistance; interleukin (IL) 12 induces naïve T cells to differentiate into T_H1 cells and induces T cells and natural killer cells to produce IFN-γ. In contrast, expansion of IL-4-producing T_H2 cells and IL-10 mediate susceptibility.

Although the immunoregulatory responses are more complex and less polarized in humans than in inbred mice, key principles are evident. The immunoinflammatory response is central to pathogenesis, healing is associated with activation of macrophages to kill intracellular amastigotes, and persistent infection is characteristic. Although the correlates of immunity are not fully defined and may differ between treated and untreated persons, nonsterile cure is a mixed blessing: quiescent parasites may help the host maintain a protective T cell–mediated immune response but may also serve as a source for activation of latent or clinically cured infection if the protective mechanisms fail.

EPIDEMIOLOGY, PREVENTION, AND CONTROL

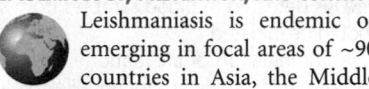

Leishmaniasis is endemic or emerging in focal areas of ~90 countries in Asia, the Middle East, southern Europe, and Africa (Old World disease) and the Americas (New World disease) (Table 205-1). Upwards of several hundred thousand cases of visceral leishmaniasis and 1–1.5 million cases of cutaneous leishmaniasis occur annually. Leishmaniasis is associated with the loss of ~2.4 million disability-adjusted life-years.

More than 90% of the world's cases of visceral leishmaniasis occur in three regions: (1) southern Asia or the Indian subcontinent, particularly in Bihar State in northeastern India and in foci in Bangladesh and Nepal; (2) eastern Africa (Sudan and neighboring countries); and (3) the Americas, particularly in periurban areas of northeastern Brazil.

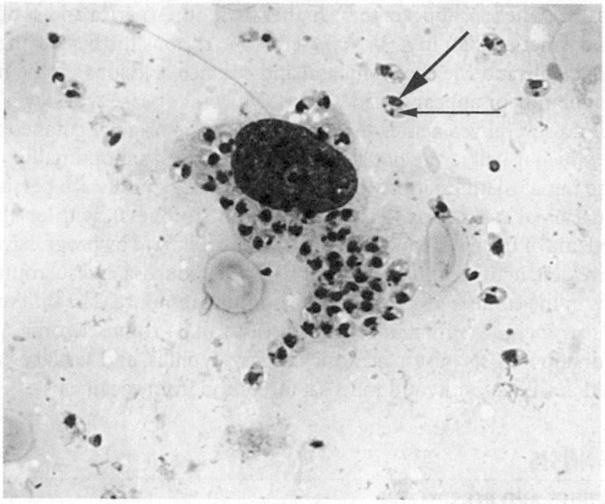

FIGURE 205-1 Amastigotes (the tissue stage of *Leishmania* parasites) in a Giemsa-stained impression smear of tissue from a patient with cutaneous leishmaniasis. Amastigotes are oval or egg shaped and ~2–4 μm in length. Their internal organelles include a nucleus (*larger arrow*) and rod-shaped kinetoplast (*smaller arrow*). In particular, the kinetoplast, a specialized mitochondrial structure that contains extranuclear DNA, should be visualized. The extracellular amastigotes probably were released from macrophages during manipulation of the specimen. Magnification: ×1000, obtained using a ×100 oil-immersion objective. *(Photograph courtesy of H. Bishop; with permission.)*

The predominant etiologic agents are *L. donovani* in southern Asia and eastern Africa and *L. infantum/L. chagasi* elsewhere in the Old and New Worlds. These organisms can also cause cutaneous leishmaniasis.

More than 90% of the world's cases of cutaneous leishmaniasis occur in Afghanistan (Fig. 205-2), Algeria, Iran, Iraq, Pakistan, Saudi Arabia, and Syria (Old World) and in Brazil and Peru (New World). The predominant etiologic agents are *L. tropica*, *L. major*, and *L. aethiopica* (Old World) and species of the *L. mexicana* complex and the *Viannia* subgenus (New World).

In general, prevention and control measures are difficult to sustain and must be tailored to the setting. Vaccine strategies are being explored. Vector characteristics contribute to the focality of transmission in time and place and have implications for preventive measures. Sandflies are nocturnal (i.e., most active from dusk to dawn), have a limited flight range (usually remaining within a few hundred meters of their breeding site), and are small (about one-third the size of mosquitoes). Personal protective measures include minimizing nocturnal outdoor activities, wearing protective clothing, and applying insect repellent to exposed skin. In settings with domiciliary transmission, spraying dwellings with residual-action insecticides and using bed nets treated with long-lasting insecticides may be protective.

Most transmission cycles traditionally have been classified as zoonotic, except for the anthroponotic cycles of *L. donovani* (in southern Asia and potentially in eastern Africa) and *L. tropica*. However, some zoonotic cycles may be partially anthroponotic (and vice versa), and transmission patterns can evolve (e.g., from predominantly sylvatic to include domiciliary transmission) in the context of environmental and epidemiologic changes.

If transmission is exclusively or partially anthroponotic, treatment of infected persons can serve as a control measure, and suboptimal treatment can lead to dissemination of drug resistance. In southern Asia, which arguably carries ~70% of the global burden of visceral leishmaniasis, transmission of *L. donovani* is anthroponotic and largely intra- or peridomiciliary. In 2005, India, Nepal, and Bangladesh resolved to collaborate to reduce the annual incidence of visceral leishmaniasis to <1 case per 10,000 persons by the year 2015. For areas where canids are reservoir hosts (*L. infantum/L. chagasi*–endemic regions), various control strategies are being explored (e.g., insecticide-impregnated dog collars and vaccine candidates).

CLINICAL MANIFESTATIONS AND DIFFERENTIAL DIAGNOSIS

VISCERAL LEISHMANIASIS

The general term *visceral leishmaniasis* encompasses a broad spectrum of severity and manifestations, with a chronic, subacute, or acute onset and an incubation period of weeks, months, or sometimes years. In contrast, the term *kala-azar* typically is reserved for advanced, life-threatening disease. Although *kala-azar* means black [*kala*] fever [*azar*] in Hindi, darkening of the skin is uncommon. The classic manifestations of advanced disease include prolonged fever; cachexia (malnutrition being both a risk factor for and a sequela of visceral leishmaniasis); hepatosplenomegaly (with splenomegaly usually predominant and the spleen sometimes massive); anemia; leukopenia (neutropenia, marked eosinopenia, and relative lymphocytosis and monocytosis); thrombocytopenia, sometimes associated with bleeding; hypergammaglobulinemia (chiefly IgG, from polyclonal B cell activation); and hypoalbuminemia. The differential diagnosis includes tropical and infectious diseases that cause fever or organomegaly (e.g., typhoid fever, subacute bacterial endocarditis, miliary tuberculosis, brucellosis, histoplasmosis, tropical splenomegaly syndrome, and schistosomiasis) and myeloproliferative diseases (e.g., leukemia and lymphoma).

Post–kala-azar dermal leishmaniasis (PKDL) is a syndrome characterized by skin lesions (including macules, papules, nodules, and patches) that are typically most prominent on the face and that develop during or after therapy for visceral leishmaniasis. In Sudan, PKDL is noted in ~50% of patients from 0 to 6 months after therapy and usually heals spontaneously. In contrast, in India, PKDL is noted in ~5–10% of patients, occurring several years after treatment and usually requiring further therapy. PKDL can be confused with miliaria rubra, syphilis, yaws, and leprosy.

The diagnosis of visceral leishmaniasis should be considered for HIV-infected patients who have ever been in leishmaniasis-endemic areas and have manifestations consistent with visceral infection. The leishmanial infection may have been acquired recently (e.g., from a contaminated syringe) or may represent activation of latent infection acquired in

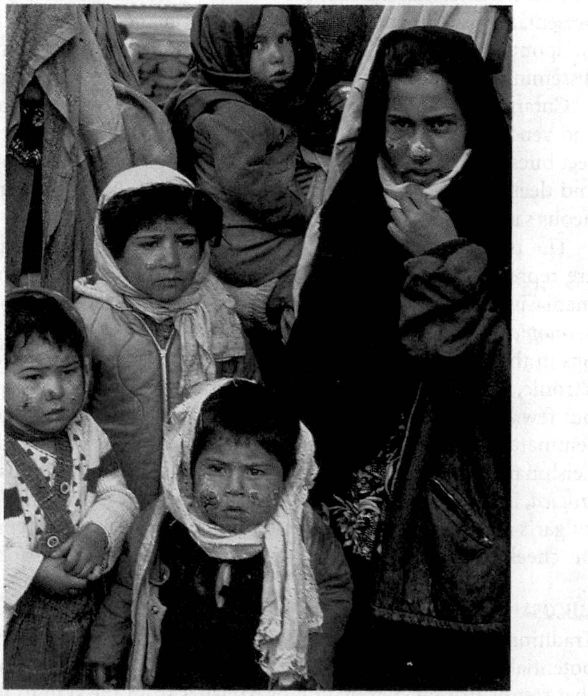

FIGURE 205-2 People in Kabul, Afghanistan, standing in line for hours on a bitterly cold day in February 1997 at a treatment center for cutaneous leishmaniasis. Kabul is experiencing a prolonged epidemic of anthroponotic cutaneous leishmaniasis caused by *Leishmania tropica*. *[Photograph courtesy of Dr. R. Ashford and reprinted with permission from Elsevier Science (Lancet 354:1193, 1999).]*

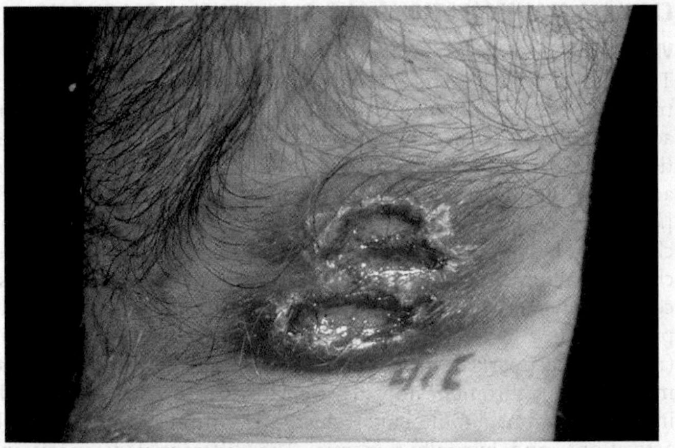

FIGURE 205-3 Ulcerative skin lesions with raised outer borders on the arm of a patient with New World (American) cutaneous leishmaniasis acquired in Costa Rica. *(Photograph courtesy of Dr. A. Wright, with permission.)*

the distant past; most co-infected patients with clinically evident visceral infection have CD4+ T lymphocyte counts of <200/μL.

Most cases of *Leishmania*-HIV co-infection have been reported from southern Europe (particularly Spain, France, Italy, and Portugal). Whereas antiretroviral therapy has decreased the incidence of clinically manifest leishmanial infection in Europe, increasing numbers of co-infected cases are being reported in resource-poor countries.

CUTANEOUS LEISHMANIASIS

Typically, the incubation period of cutaneous leishmaniasis ranges from weeks to months. Lesions progress from papules to plaques (which can be smooth or scaly and develop central ulceration; Fig. 205-3) to atrophic scars. The spectrum includes papulonodular, nodular, and noduloulcerative lesions. Multiple primary lesions, satellite lesions, regional adenopathy, nodular lymphangitis, secondary bacterial infection, and thick hemorrhagic crusts or verrucous (wart-like) scale are variably present. Both active and healed lesions can cause considerable morbidity. Spontaneous resolution does not preclude reactivation of infection, dissemination to mucous membranes (see below), or reinfection.

Cutaneous leishmaniasis can be confused with tropical, traumatic, and venous-stasis ulcers; foreign-body reactions; myiasis; infected insect bites; impetigo, ecthyma, and pyoderma gangrenosum; superficial and deep fungal, mycobacterial, and spirochetal infections; and cutaneous sarcoidosis and neoplasms.

The polyparasitic and oligoparasitic ends of the disease spectrum are represented by diffuse cutaneous leishmaniasis (DCL) and leishmaniasis recidivans, respectively. DCL, which typically is caused by *L. aethiopica* (Old World) and *L. mexicana* species (New World), develops in the context of *Leishmania*-specific anergy and is manifested by chronic, disseminated, nonulcerative lesions, with abundant parasites but few lymphocytes. DCL should be differentiated from benign disseminated cutaneous leishmaniasis, lepromatous leprosy, and PKDL. Leishmaniasis recidivans, which most characteristically is caused by *L. tropica*, is a hyperergic variant with scarce parasites. It resembles lupus vulgaris and is characterized by a chronic, solitary plaque (typically on the cheek) that heals centrally but slowly expands at the periphery.

MUCOSAL LEISHMANIASIS

Traditionally, the term *mucosal leishmaniasis* (or *espundia*) refers to a potentially disfiguring sequela of New World cutaneous leishmaniasis that results from dissemination of parasites from the skin to the naso-oropharyngeal mucosa. Mucosal leishmaniasis is caused by species in the *Viannia* subgenus [especially *L. (V.) braziliensis* and *L. (V.) panamensis* but also *L. (V.) guyanensis*] and by *L. amazonensis* (Table 205-1).

The magnitudes and the determinants (both parasite- and host-related) of the risks for mucosal dissemination and mucosal disease are poorly defined. Overall risk estimates for mucosal disease typically are ≤5% (~1–10%). The risk appears to be higher in South America and southern Central America than in *L. Viannia*–endemic regions further north (e.g., in Guatemala and Mexico). Mucosal and cutaneous lesions can be noted concomitantly or appear decades apart. Mucosal disease typically is noted within several years after the resolution of the original cutaneous lesions, which usually were not treated or were treated suboptimally.

The initial manifestations of mucosal disease typically are persistent, unusual nasal symptoms (e.g., epistaxis and stuffiness), with erythema and edema of the nasal mucosa, which can be followed by progressive, ulcerative destruction of the naso-oropharyngeal mucosa and surrounding tissues in the context of a hyperactive immune response. The differential diagnosis includes other infectious diseases (e.g., rhinoscleroma, paracoccidioidomycosis, histoplasmosis, leprosy, syphilis, and tertiary yaws), sarcoidosis, neoplasms, and mucosal ulceration from cocaine use.

DIAGNOSIS

PRINCIPLES AND PERSPECTIVE

Leishmaniasis often is diagnosed presumptively by clinical and epidemiologic criteria. Definitive diagnosis requires demonstration of the parasite in specimens from infected sites, which typically relies on classic microbiologic methods—i.e., detection of amastigotes by light microscopic examination of stained slides or detection of promastigotes by in vitro culture. In general, amastigotes, including their characteristic internal organelles (Fig. 205-1), are more easily recognizable on Giemsa-stained smears (e.g., thin smears of dermal scrapings or bone marrow aspirates and impression smears of biopsy specimens) than in tissue sections, particularly if organisms are rare.

Leishmania species can be distinguished by isoenzyme analysis of cultured promastigotes or determination of monoclonal antibody specificity. Molecular techniques of assorted types, with diverse genetic markers, are at various stages of development and validation for diagnosis of leishmaniasis and identification of species. Analyses of the genomes and the proteome profiles of *Leishmania* species may lead to novel diagnostic approaches.

Immunologic diagnostic methods include serologic assays and tests for *Leishmania*-specific cell-mediated immunity (e.g., skin testing for delayed-type hypersensitivity reactions). The utility of such methods depends in part on the syndrome. Most serologic assays do not reliably distinguish active from quiescent infection. No leishmanin skin-test preparation has been approved for use in the United States.

VISCERAL LEISHMANIASIS

Patients with advanced visceral leishmaniasis commonly have relatively heavy parasite burdens and high-level antibody responses that are not protective but are useful diagnostically; skin-test reactivity develops after recovery. Aspirates and biopsy specimens (e.g., of spleen, bone marrow, liver, or lymph node) are useful for parasitologic confirmation by traditional and molecular methods. Although the diagnostic yield is highest for splenic aspirates (>95%), bone marrow aspiration is safer.

In the appropriate setting, seropositivity is often the diagnostic standard. Although test performance can vary by region, approaches that offer the potential for improved field applicability include direct agglutination testing with freeze-dried antigen and immunochromatographic dipstick testing of fingerstick blood for antibody to recombinant antigens or synthetic peptides (e.g., rK39). In addition, assays for detection of leishmanial antigen in urine are being evaluated.

The sensitivity of serologic methods is lower in HIV-infected patients than in persons not infected with HIV (~50% vs. >90%). In contrast, the parasites may be abundant in typical sites (e.g., bone marrow), in atypical sites (e.g., gastrointestinal tissue), and in circulating monocytes—a circumstance that facilitates parasitologic diagnosis. The sensitivities of peripheral-blood smear and buffy-coat culture are ~50% and ~70%, respectively. PCR may be even more sensitive.

CUTANEOUS AND MUCOSAL LEISHMANIASIS

Aspirates and biopsy specimens of skin lesions and lymph nodes are useful for parasitologic confirmation of cutaneous and mucosal leishmaniasis by traditional and molecular methods. Parasitologic confirmation of mucosal leishmaniasis—a pauciparasitic syndrome—by traditional methods can be difficult. Serologic testing usually is not helpful for patients with cutaneous leishmaniasis; except in patients with DCL and some patients with mucosal leishmaniasis, antibody is either undetectable or present at low levels. In contrast, skin-test reactivity usually develops during active infection except in patients with DCL.

℞ LEISHMANIASIS

PRINCIPLES AND PERSPECTIVE **(Table 205-2)** Decisions about whether and how to treat leishmaniasis should be individualized. For cases in which systemic treatment is indicated, the parenterally administered pentavalent antimonial (Sb^V) compounds sodium stibogluconate and meglumine antimonate have been the mainstays of therapy for more than half a century. Manifestations of toxicity (e.g., body aches, malaise, elevated aminotransferase levels, chemical pancreatitis, and electrocardiographic abnormalities) are commonly noted but usually do not limit therapy and are reversible.

Conventional amphotericin B deoxycholate and pentamidine isethionate, the traditional parenteral alternatives to Sb^V, were previously relegated to second-line status, largely because of less experience with their use for the treatment of leishmaniasis and greater concern about their induction of potentially serious or irreversible toxicities (e.g., renal impairment). Amphotericin B, which has high-level, broad-spectrum antileishmanial activity, has been upgraded to first-line status in settings in which its benefits outweigh its risks (e.g., for Sb^V-resistant visceral leishmaniasis).

Lipid formulations of amphotericin B passively target the agent to macrophage-rich organs, resulting in less renal and other toxicity and permitting the use of higher daily doses and shorter courses of therapy. Targeting of drug to the reticuloendothelial system is ideal for visceral leishmaniasis but may not be advantageous for other syndromes. For amphotericin B and other antileishmanial agents, various delivery/targeting mechanisms and formulations are being explored.

Although some alternative therapies may have utility in particular settings, even data from well-conducted clinical trials cannot necessarily be generalized to other contexts. Of particular note, data from the many clinical trials of therapy for visceral leishmaniasis in foci in northeastern India are not necessarily directly applicable to visceral leishmaniasis caused by *L. donovani* in other foci in southern Asia or elsewhere (e.g., eastern Africa) or to visceral infection caused by *L. infantum/chagasi*—let alone to other leishmanial syndromes.

Except for the development of resistance to Sb^V and pentamidine, Indian kala-azar typically is easier to treat than visceral leishmaniasis elsewhere: i.e., it is more responsive to therapy, even with lower total doses. Counterintuitively, visceral leishmaniasis often is easier to treat than cutaneous or mucosal leishmaniasis. Achieving adequate drug levels in the phagolysosomes of dermal and mucosal macrophages can be challenging, and the difficulty can be compounded by the fact that some dermotropic species are intrinsically less sensitive than *L. donovani* to particular drugs.

Some of these issues are exemplified by miltefosine, the first highly active oral agent for visceral leishmaniasis. Both experimental (in vitro) and clinical data indicate that *L. donovani* (the agent of Indian visceral leishmaniasis) is highly sensitive to miltefosine, whereas other species are variably responsive. In addition, the long half-life of the drug and suboptimal treatment predispose to the development of resistance. The most common side effects of therapy include gastrointestinal symptoms and reversible elevations in creatinine and aminotransferase levels. Miltefosine's teratogenicity in animals has implications for its use in women of child-bearing age (Table 205-2).

TABLE 205-2 PARENTERAL AND ORAL DRUG REGIMENS FOR TREATMENT OF LEISHMANIASIS[a]

Clinical Syndrome, Drug	Route of Administration	Regimen
Visceral Leishmaniasis		
Parenteral therapy		
Pentavalent antimony[b]	IV, IM	20 mg Sb^V/kg qd for 28 days
Amphotericin B, lipid formulation[c]	IV	2–5 mg/kg qd (total: usually ~15–21 mg/kg)
Amphotericin B (deoxycholate)	IV	0.5–1 mg/kg qod or qd (total: usually ~15–20 mg/kg)
Paromomycin sulfate[d]	IV, IM	15–20 mg/kg qd for ~21 days
Pentamidine isethionate	IV, IM	4 mg/kg qod or thrice weekly for ~15–30 doses
Oral therapy		
Miltefosine[d,e]	PO	2.5 mg/kg qd for 28 days
Cutaneous Leishmaniasis		
Parenteral therapy		
Pentavalent antimony[b]	IV, IM	20 mg Sb^V/kg qd for 10–20 days (standard recommendation: 20 days)
Pentamidine isethionate	IV, IM	2 mg/kg qod for 7 doses
Amphotericin B (deoxycholate)	IV	0.5–1 mg/kg qod or qd (total: up to ~20 mg/kg)
Oral therapy		
Fluconazole	PO	200 mg qd for 6 weeks[f]
Ketoconazole	PO	600 mg qd for 28 days[f]
Itraconazole	PO	200 mg bid for 28 days[f]
Miltefosine[d,e]	PO	2.5 mg/kg qd for 28 days
Mucosal Leishmaniasis		
Pentavalent antimony[b]	IV, IM	20 mg Sb^V/kg qd for 28 days
Amphotericin B (deoxycholate)	IV	1 mg/kg qod or qd (total: usually ~20–40 mg/kg)
Pentamidine isethionate	IV, IM	2–4 mg/kg qod or thrice weekly for ≥15 doses

[a]See text for additional details and perspective about the drugs and regimens in this table and about treatment of leishmaniasis in general. Some of the listed drugs are effective only against certain *Leishmania* species/strains and only in certain areas of the world. Classification of drugs/regimens in such categories as first-line, alternative, (in)effective, investigational, (un)available, and cost-prohibitive is highly dependent on the setting. Ranges shown for doses and durations of therapy reflect variability both in dosage regimens among clinical trials and in responsiveness in different settings. To maximize effectiveness and minimize toxicity, the listed regimens should be individualized according to the particularities of the case and in consultation with an expert. Children may need different dosage regimens. Except for liposomal amphotericin B (see footnote c), as of this writing, none of the drugs listed is licensed by the U.S. Food and Drug Administration (FDA) for the treatment of leishmaniasis per se.

[b]The Centers for Disease Control and Prevention (CDC) provides the pentavalent antimonial (Sb^V) compound sodium stibogluconate (Pentostam; Glaxo Operations UK Limited, Barnard Castle, United Kingdom; 100 mg Sb^V/mL) to U.S.-licensed physicians through the CDC Drug Service (404-639-3670) under an IND mechanism with the FDA. The other widely used Sb^V compound, meglumine antimonate (Glucantime; typically, ~85 mg Sb^V/mL), is available primarily in Spanish- and French-speaking areas of the world. Locally made (generic) Sb^V preparations may have different Sb^V concentrations and may vary in quality and safety.

[c]The lipid formulations of amphotericin B include liposomal amphotericin B and amphotericin B lipid complex. In 1997, the FDA approved the following regimen of liposomal amphotericin B for immunocompetent patients with visceral leishmaniasis: 3 mg/kg qd on days 1–5, 14, and 21, for a total of 21 mg/kg. For immunosuppressed patients, the approved regimen is 4 mg/kg qd on days 1–5, 10, 17, 24, 31, and 38, for a total of 40 mg/kg. Many alternative regimens have been proposed for immunocompetent patients in various regions of the world; the regimens vary with respect to total and daily doses, number of doses, and intervals between doses. See text for perspective on the use of lipid formulations of amphotericin B for treatment of cutaneous and mucosal leishmaniasis.

[d]Not commercially available in the United States as of this writing.

[e]Miltefosine, which is teratogenic in animals, should not be used to treat pregnant women. Women of child-bearing age should use effective birth control during treatment and for 2 months thereafter. See text regarding the treatment of mucosal leishmaniasis.

[f]Adult dosage.

VISCERAL LEISHMANIASIS The primary goal of treatment for visceral leishmaniasis is to prevent death. Highly effective antileishmanial therapy is essential, as is supportive care (e.g., therapy for malnutrition, anemia, bleeding, and intercurrent infections). In most regions, Sb^V therapy remains highly effective. However, use of an alternative agent should be considered if high-level Sb^V resistance is prevalent or if non-Sb^V therapy is advantageous for other reasons (e.g., duration, cost, or tolerability). In general, most patients feel better and become afebrile during the first week of therapy; resolution of splenomegaly and hematologic abnormalities may require weeks or months.

In northeastern India, districts of Bihar State north of the Ganges River constitute the epicenter of the epidemic of Sb^V resistance, which is spreading—to varying degrees—to contiguous areas of India and southern Nepal. Conventional amphotericin B has become first-line therapy where Sb^V and pentamidine are no longer effective. Lipid formulations of amphotericin B, which are cost-prohibitive where they are most needed, are increasingly being used in southern Europe.

The anthroponotic transmission of *L. donovani* in southern Asia is both a blessing and a curse: a blessing because treatment can serve as a control measure, and a curse because suboptimal treatment can and does lead to the development and dissemination of drug resistance and thereby to the elimination of drugs from the limited armamentarium and to the demise of patients who cannot afford or access the few alternatives. In this context, the oral agent miltefosine, which is registered for commercial use in India and some other countries, has great potential but also is highly vulnerable. The advent of oral therapy translates into unsupervised outpatient treatment, in which patients buy the quantity of drug they can afford and prematurely stop therapy when their supply is depleted or their symptoms are alleviated. Unless protective measures are implemented (e.g., with directly observed or multidrug therapy), drug resistance almost assuredly will develop and spread. The oral agent sitamaquine, an 8-amino-quinoline, is being field-tested in various regions but appears to have a narrow therapeutic window and can cause nephrotoxicity.

The aminoglycoside paromomycin (the chemical equivalent of aminosidine) is a candidate parenteral agent for use alone or in drug combinations. To date, the rates of response in field tests have been variable; response rates may be higher in India than in eastern Africa.

Patients who are co-infected with HIV may initially respond well to standard therapy but typically experience more toxicity. Antiretroviral therapy delays but does not prevent relapses. Consensus approaches to treatment and secondary prophylaxis have not been established.

CUTANEOUS LEISHMANIASIS Decisions about clinical management of cutaneous leishmaniasis should be based on consideration of goals (e.g., accelerating the healing of skin lesions, decreasing morbidity, decreasing risks for local and mucosal dissemination and relapse), parasite factors (e.g., tissue tropisms and drug sensitivities), and the extent to which the lesions are of concern or are bothersome because of their location (e.g., on the face or near joints), number, size, persistence, or other features (e.g., nodular lymphangitis). When optimal effectiveness is important, parenteral Sb^V therapy is generally recommended. The first sign of a clinical response typically is decreasing induration, and relapses usually are noted first at the margins of healed lesions.

Although clinical trials of conventional amphotericin B for cutaneous leishmaniasis have not been conducted and standard dosage regimens have not been established, this agent almost assuredly is highly and broadly effective, albeit potentially toxic. Conflicting, limited data are available for lipid formulations. Pentamidine was effective in Colombia [predominantly against *L. (V.) panamensis*] but not in Peru [against *L. (V.) braziliensis*].

The effectiveness of the oral agent miltefosine is species and strain dependent. For example, this drug has been effective against *L. (V.) panamensis* in Colombia but ineffective against *L. (V.) braziliensis* in Guatemala. At best, azoles have shown modest activity against particular species in isolated studies—e.g., ketoconazole and itraconazole against *L. mexicana* in Guatemala, ketoconazole against *L. (V.) panamensis* in Panama, and fluconazole against *L. major* in Saudi Arabia. Itraconazole has been ineffective against *L. (V.) panamensis* in Colombia.

Local therapy can be considered for some cases without demonstrable local dissemination or risk of mucosal dissemination (e.g., for relatively benign lesions caused by *L. mexicana* or *L. major*). Examples of approaches being used or evaluated in some settings include intralesional Sb^V, various formulations of paromomycin ointments, topical immunomodulators, thermotherapy, and cryotherapy.

MUCOSAL LEISHMANIASIS The traditional treatment options for mucosal leishmaniasis include Sb^V and conventional amphotericin B; conflicting, limited data are available for lipid formulations of the latter drug. The response rates approach those for cutaneous leishmaniasis if mucosal disease is detected and treated at early stages, whereas advanced disease may be unresponsive or relapse repeatedly. Oral miltefosine therapy shows promise, on the basis of a clinical trial in Bolivia. Adjunctive immunotherapy is being evaluated. Concomitant glucocorticoid therapy is indicated if respiratory compromise develops after initiation of therapy.

FURTHER READINGS

ALVAR J et al: Chemotherapy in the treatment and control of leishmaniasis. Adv Parasitol 61:223, 2006

COLER RN, REED SG: Second-generation vaccines against leishmaniasis. Trends Parasitol 21:244, 2005

CROFT SL et al: Drug resistance in leishmaniasis. Clin Microbiol Rev 19:111, 2006

CRUZ I et al: *Leishmania*/HIV co-infections in the second decade. Indian J Med Res 123:357, 2006

HERWALDT BL: Leishmaniasis. Lancet 354:1191, 1999

MURRAY HW et al: Advances in leishmaniasis. Lancet 366:1561, 2005

SMITH DF et al: Comparative genomics: From genotype to disease phenotype in the leishmaniases. Int J Parasitol 37:1173, 2007

206 Trypanosomiasis

Louis V. Kirchhoff

The genus *Trypanosoma* contains many species of protozoans. *Trypanosoma cruzi*, the cause of Chagas' disease in the Americas, and the two trypanosome subspecies that cause human African trypanosomiasis, *Trypanosoma brucei gambiense* and *T. brucei rhodesiense*, are the only members of the genus that cause disease in humans.

CHAGAS' DISEASE

DEFINITION

Chagas' disease, or American trypanosomiasis, is a zoonosis caused by the protozoan parasite *T. cruzi*. Acute Chagas' disease is usually a mild febrile illness that results from initial infection with the organism. After spontaneous resolution of the acute illness, most infected persons remain for life in the indeterminate phase of chronic Chagas' disease, which is characterized by subpatent parasitemia, easily detectable antibodies to *T. cruzi*, and an absence of symptoms. In a minority of chronically infected patients, cardiac and gastrointestinal lesions develop that can result in serious morbidity and even death.

LIFE CYCLE AND TRANSMISSION

T. cruzi is transmitted among its mammalian hosts by hematophagous triatomine insects, often called *reduviid bugs*. The insects become infected by sucking blood from animals or humans who have circulating parasites. Ingested organisms multiply in the gut of the triatomines, and infective forms are discharged with the feces at the time of subsequent blood meals. Transmission to a second vertebrate host occurs when breaks in the skin, mucous membranes, or conjunctivae become contaminated with bug feces that contain infective parasites. *T. cruzi* can also be transmitted by the transfusion of blood donated by infected persons, by organ transplantation, from mother to fetus, and in laboratory accidents.

PATHOLOGY

An indurated inflammatory lesion called a *chagoma* often appears at the parasites' portal of entry. Local histologic changes include the presence of parasites within leukocytes and cells of subcutaneous tissues and the development of interstitial edema, lymphocytic infiltration, and reactive hyperplasia of adjacent lymph nodes. After dissemination of the organisms through the lymphatics and the bloodstream, muscles (including the myocardium) may become heavily parasitized (Fig. 206-1). The characteristic pseudocysts present in sections of infected tissues are intracellular aggregates of multiplying parasites.

In the minority of persons with chronic *T. cruzi* infections who develop related clinical manifestations, the heart is the organ most commonly affected. Changes include thinning of the ventricular walls, biventricular enlargement, apical aneurysms, and mural thrombi. Widespread lymphocytic infiltration, diffuse interstitial fibrosis, and atrophy of myocardial cells are often apparent, but parasites are difficult to find in myocardial tissue. Conduction-system involvement often affects the right branch and the left anterior branch of the bundle of His. In chronic Chagas' disease of the gastrointestinal tract (megadisease), the esophagus and colon may exhibit varying degrees of dilatation. On microscopic examination, focal inflammatory lesions with lymphocytic infiltration are seen, and the number of neurons in the myenteric plexus may be markedly reduced. Accumulating experimental evidence implicates the persistence of parasites and the accompanying chronic inflammation—rather than autoimmune mechanisms—as the basis for the pathology in patients with chronic *T. cruzi* infection.

EPIDEMIOLOGY

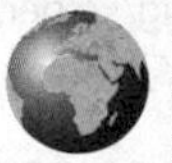

T. cruzi is found only in the Americas. Wild and domestic mammals harboring *T. cruzi* and infected triatomines are found in spotty distributions from the southern United States to southern Argentina. Humans become involved in the cycle of transmission when infected vectors take up residence in the primitive wood, adobe, and stone houses common in much of Latin America. Thus human *T. cruzi* infection is a health problem primarily among the poor in rural areas of Mexico and Central and South America. Most new *T. cruzi* infections in rural settings occur in children, but the incidence is unknown because most cases go undiagnosed. Historically, transfusion-associated transmission of *T. cruzi* has been a serious public health problem in many endemic countries. However, with some notable exceptions, transmission by this route has been markedly reduced as effective programs for the screening of donated blood have been implemented. Several dozen patients with HIV and chronic *T. cruzi* infections who underwent acute recrudescence of the latter have been described. These patients generally presented with *T. cruzi* brain abscesses, a manifestation of the illness that does not occur in immunocompetent persons. Currently, it is estimated that 12 million people are chronically infected with *T. cruzi* and that 25,000 deaths due to the illness occur each year. Of chronically infected persons, 10–30% eventually develop symptomatic cardiac lesions or gastrointestinal disease. The resulting morbidity and mortality make Chagas' disease the most important parasitic disease burden in Latin America.

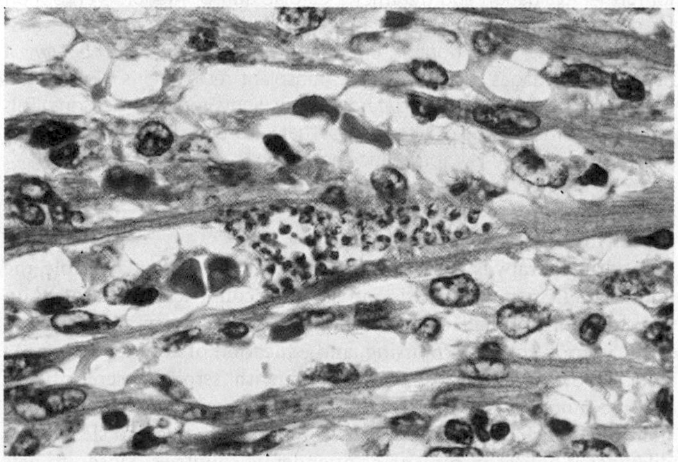

FIGURE 206-1 *Trypanosoma cruzi* in the heart muscle of a child who died of acute Chagas' myocarditis. An infected myocyte containing several dozen *T. cruzi* amastigotes is in the center of the field (hematoxylin and eosin, ×900).

In recent years, the rate of *T. cruzi* transmission has decreased markedly in several endemic countries as a result of successful programs involving vector control, blood-bank screening, and education of at-risk populations. A major program begun in 1991 in the "southern cone" nations of South America (Uruguay, Paraguay, Bolivia, Brazil, Chile, and Argentina) has provided the framework for much of this progress. Uruguay and Chile were certified transmission-free in the late 1990s, and Brazil was declared free of transmission in 2006. Transmission has been reduced markedly in Argentina as well. Similar control programs have been initiated in the countries of northern South America and in the Central American nations.

Acute Chagas' disease is rare in the United States. Five cases of autochthonous transmission and five instances of transmission by blood transfusion have been reported. Moreover, *T. cruzi* was transmitted to five recipients of organs from three *T. cruzi*–infected donors. Two of these recipients became infected through cardiac transplants. Acute Chagas' disease has not been reported in tourists returning to the United States from Latin America, although two such instances have been reported in Europe. In contrast, the prevalence of chronic *T. cruzi* infections in the United States has increased considerably in recent years. Data from the 2000 census indicate that >12 million immigrants from Chagas'-endemic countries currently live in the United States, ~8 million of whom are Mexicans. The prevalence of *T. cruzi* infection in Mexico is 0.5–1.0%, and most of the 4 million immigrants from Chagas'-endemic nations who are not Mexicans come from countries in which the prevalence of *T. cruzi* infection is greater than it is in Mexico. The total number of *T. cruzi*–infected persons living in the United States can be estimated reasonably to be 80,000–120,000. The number of instances of transfusion-associated transmission in this country is likely to be considerably greater than the number reported. Screening of the U.S. blood supply for evidence of *T. cruzi* infection has recently begun (see "Diagnosis," below).

CLINICAL COURSE

The first signs of acute Chagas' disease develop at least 1 week after invasion by the parasites. When the organisms enter through a break in the skin, an indurated area of erythema and swelling (the chagoma), accompanied by local lymphadenopathy, may appear. *Romaña's sign*—the classic finding in acute Chagas' disease, which consists of unilateral painless edema of the palpebrae and periocular tissues—can result when the conjunctiva is the portal of entry (Fig. 206-2). These initial local signs may be followed by malaise, fever, anorexia, and edema of the face and lower extremities. A morbilliform rash may also appear. Generalized lymphadenopathy and hepatosplenomegaly may develop. Severe myocarditis develops rarely; most deaths in acute Chagas' disease are due to heart failure. Neurologic signs are not common, but meningoencephalitis occurs occasionally. The acute symptoms resolve spontaneously in virtually all patients, who then enter the asymptomatic or indeterminate phase of chronic *T. cruzi* infection.

Symptomatic chronic Chagas' disease becomes apparent years or even decades after the initial infection. The heart is commonly involved, and symptoms are caused by rhythm disturbances, dilated cardiomyopathy, and thromboembolism. Right bundle-branch block is a common electrocardiographic abnormality, but other types of atrioventricular block, premature ventricular contractions, and tachy- and bradyarrhythmias occur frequently. Cardiomyopathy often results in right-sided or biventricular heart failure. Embolization of mural thrombi to the brain or other areas may take place. Patients with megaesophagus suffer from dysphagia, odynophagia, chest pain, and regurgitation. Aspiration can occur (especially during sleep) in patients with severe esophageal dysfunction, and repeated episodes of aspiration pneumonitis are common. Weight loss, cachexia, and pulmonary infection can result in death. Patients with megacolon are

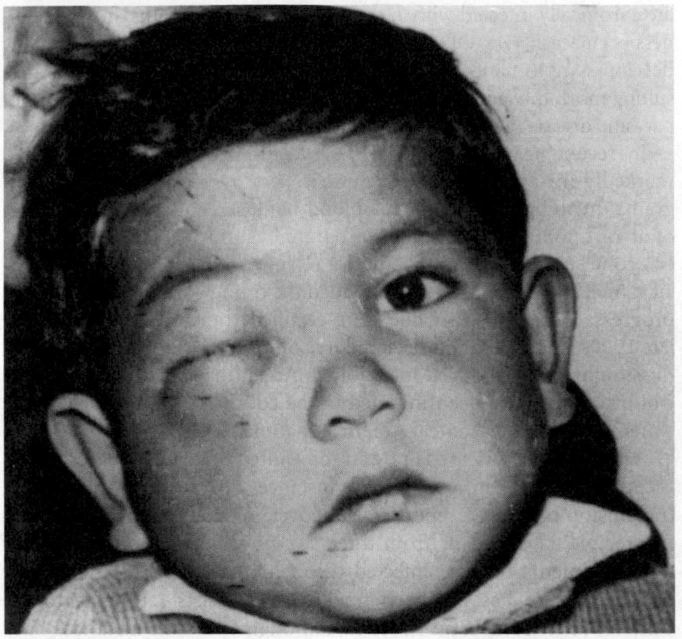

FIGURE 206-2 Romaña's sign in an Argentinean patient with acute *T. cruzi* infection. *(Courtesy of Dr. Humberto Lugones, Centro de Chagas, Santiago del Estero, Argentina; with permission.)*

plagued by abdominal pain and chronic constipation, and advanced megacolon can cause obstruction, volvulus, septicemia, and death.

DIAGNOSIS

The diagnosis of acute Chagas' disease requires the detection of parasites. Microscopic examination of fresh anticoagulated blood or of the buffy coat is the simplest way to see the motile organisms. Parasites also can be seen in Giemsa-stained thin and thick blood smears. Microhematocrit tubes containing acridine orange as a stain can be used for the same purpose. When repeated attempts to visualize the organisms are unsuccessful, polymerase chain reaction (PCR) or hemoculture in special media can be performed. When used by experienced personnel, all of these methods yield positive results in a high proportion of cases of acute Chagas' disease. Hemoculture has the disadvantage of taking several weeks to give positive results. Serologic testing plays no role in diagnosing acute Chagas' disease.

Chronic Chagas' disease is diagnosed by the detection of specific antibodies that bind to *T. cruzi* antigens. Demonstration of the parasite is not of primary importance. In Latin America, ~20 assays are commercially available, including several based on recombinant antigens. Unfortunately, these tests have varying levels of sensitivity and specificity, and false-positive reactions are a particular problem—typically with samples from patients who have other infectious and parasitic diseases or autoimmune disorders. In addition, confirmatory testing has presented a persistent challenge. For these reasons, it is generally recommended that specimens be tested in at least two assays and that well-characterized positive and negative comparison samples be included in each run. The radioimmune precipitation assay (Chagas' RIPA) is a highly sensitive and specific confirmatory method for detecting antibodies to *T. cruzi* [approved under the Clinical Laboratory Improvement Amendment (CLIA) and available in the author's laboratory]. In December 2006, the U.S. Food and Drug Administration (FDA) approved a test to screen blood and organ donors for *T. cruzi* infection (Ortho *T. cruzi* ELISA Test System, Ortho-Clinical Diagnostics, Raritan, NJ). In late January 2007, the American Red Cross and Blood Systems, Inc.—blood-collection agencies that together account for ~65% of the U.S. blood supply—initiated screening of all the donations they process for *T. cruzi*. The Chagas' RIPA is being used as the confirmatory assay. Data generated during the first 2 months of screening suggest that if 65% of the blood supply continues to be tested, ~1500 Ortho-reactive donors will be identified annually, ~350 of whom will be RIPA-positive; these figures reflect an overall prevalence of ~1 in 30,000 donors. The use of PCR assays to detect *T. cruzi* DNA in chronically infected persons has been studied extensively. The sensitivity of this approach has not been shown to be reliably greater than that of serology, and no PCR assays are commercially available.

Rx CHAGAS' DISEASE

Therapy for Chagas' disease is unsatisfactory. For many years, only two drugs—nifurtimox and benznidazole—have been available for this purpose. Unfortunately, both drugs lack efficacy and often cause severe side effects.

In acute Chagas' disease, nifurtimox markedly reduces the duration of symptoms and parasitemia and decreases the mortality rate. Nevertheless, limited studies have shown that only ~70% of acute infections are cured parasitologically by a full course of treatment. Despite its limitations, treatment with nifurtimox should be initiated as early as possible in acute Chagas' disease. Common adverse effects of nifurtimox include abdominal pain, anorexia, nausea, vomiting, and weight loss. Neurologic reactions to the drug may include restlessness, disorientation, insomnia, twitching, paresthesia, polyneuritis, and seizures. These symptoms usually disappear when the dosage is reduced or treatment is discontinued. The recommended daily dosage is 8–10 mg/kg for adults, 12.5–15 mg/kg for adolescents, and 15–20 mg/kg for children 1–10 years of age. The drug should be given orally in four divided doses each day, and therapy should be continued for 90–120 days. Nifurtimox is available from the Drug Service of the Centers for Disease Control and Prevention (CDC) in Atlanta (telephone number, 770-639-3670).

The efficacy of benznidazole is similar to that of nifurtimox; a cure rate of 90% among congenitally infected infants treated before their first birthday has been reported. Adverse effects include peripheral neuropathy, rash, and granulocytopenia. The recommended oral dosage is 5 mg/kg per day for 60 days. Benznidazole is generally considered the drug of choice in Latin America.

The question of whether patients in the indeterminate or chronic symptomatic phase of Chagas' disease should be treated with nifurtimox or benznidazole has been debated for years. The fact that parasitologic cure rates in chronically infected persons may be <10% is central to this controversy. There is no convincing evidence from properly controlled trials that treatment of adults with long-standing *T. cruzi* infections with either of the drugs is beneficial. The current consensus of Latin American authorities is that all *T. cruzi*–infected persons up to 18 years old should be given benznidazole or nifurtimox.

The usefulness of allopurinol, fluconazole, and itraconazole for the treatment of acute Chagas' disease has been studied in laboratory animals and to a lesser extent in humans. None of these drugs has exhibited a level of anti–*T. cruzi* activity that warrants its use in patients. Several newer antifungal azoles have shown promise in animal studies but have not yet been tested in humans.

Patients who develop cardiac and/or gastrointestinal disease in association with *T. cruzi* infection should be referred to appropriate subspecialists for further evaluation and treatment. Cardiac transplantation is an option for patients with end-stage chagasic cardiopathies, and >100 such transplantations have been done in Brazil and the United States. The survival rate among Chagas' disease cardiac transplant recipients is higher than that among persons receiving cardiac transplants for other reasons. This better outcome may be due to the fact that lesions are limited to the heart in most patients with symptomatic chronic Chagas' disease.

PREVENTION

Since drug therapy is unsatisfactory and vaccines are not available, the control of *T. cruzi* transmission in endemic countries must depend on reduction of domiciliary vector populations by spraying of insecticides, improvements in housing, and education of at-risk persons. As noted above, these measures, coupled with serologic screening of blood donors, have markedly reduced transmission of the parasite in many endemic countries. Tourists would be wise to avoid sleeping in dilapidated houses in rural areas of endemic countries. Mosquito nets and insect repellent provide additional protection.

In view of the possibly serious consequences of chronic *T. cruzi* infection, it would be prudent for all immigrants from endemic regions living in the United States to be tested for evidence of infection. Identification of persons harboring the parasite would permit periodic electrocardiographic monitoring, which can be important because pacemakers benefit some patients who develop ominous rhythm disturbances. The possibility of congenital transmission is yet another justification for screening. Guidance for the evaluation and long-term monitoring of *T. cruzi*–infected persons is being developed by staff at the CDC.

Laboratory personnel should wear gloves and eye protection when working with *T. cruzi* and infected vectors.

SLEEPING SICKNESS

DEFINITION

Sleeping sickness, or human African trypanosomiasis (HAT), is caused by flagellated protozoan parasites that belong to the *T. brucei* complex and are transmitted to humans by tsetse flies. In untreated patients, the trypanosomes first cause a febrile illness that is followed months or years later by progressive neurologic impairment and death.

THE PARASITES AND THEIR TRANSMISSION

The East African (*rhodesiense*) and the West African (*gambiense*) forms of sleeping sickness are caused, respectively, by two trypanosome subspecies: *T. brucei rhodesiense* and *T. brucei gambiense*. These subspecies are morphologically indistinguishable but cause illnesses that are epidemiologically and clinically distinct (Table 206-1). The parasites are transmitted by blood-sucking tsetse flies of the genus *Glossina*. The insects acquire the infection when they ingest blood from infected mammalian hosts. After many cycles of multiplication in the midgut of the vector, the parasites migrate to the salivary glands. Their transmission takes place when they are inoculated into a mammalian host during a subsequent blood meal. The injected trypanosomes multiply in the blood (Fig. 206-3) and other extracellular spaces and evade immune destruction for long periods by undergoing antigenic variation, a process driven by gene switching in which the antigenic structure of the organisms' surface coat of glycoproteins changes periodically.

PATHOGENESIS AND PATHOLOGY

A self-limited inflammatory lesion (trypanosomal chancre) may appear a week or so after the bite of an infected tsetse fly. A systemic febrile illness then evolves as the parasites are disseminated through the lymphatics and bloodstream. Systemic HAT without central nervous system (CNS) involvement is generally referred to as *stage I disease*. In this stage, widespread lymphadenopathy and splenomegaly reflect marked lymphocytic and histiocytic proliferation and invasion of morular cells, which are plasmacytes that may be involved in the production of IgM. Endarteritis, with perivascular infiltration of both parasites and lymphocytes, may develop in lymph nodes and the spleen. Myocarditis develops frequently in patients with stage I disease and is especially common in *T. b. rhodesiense* infections.

TABLE 206-1 COMPARISON OF WEST AFRICAN AND EAST AFRICAN TRYPANOSOMIASES

Point of Comparison	West African (*Gambiense*)	East African (*Rhodesiense*)
Organism	*T. b. gambiense*	*T. b. rhodesiense*
Vectors	Tsetse flies (palpalis group)	Tsetse flies (morsitans group)
Primary reservoir	Humans	Antelope and cattle
Human illness	Chronic (late CNS disease)	Acute (early CNS disease)
Duration of illness	Months to years	<9 months
Lymphadenopathy	Prominent	Minimal
Parasitemia	Low	High
Diagnosis by rodent inoculation	No	Yes
Epidemiology	Rural populations	Workers in wild areas, rural populations, tourists in game parks

Abbreviation: CNS, central nervous system.
Source: Reprinted with permission from LV Kirchhoff in GL Mandell et al (eds): *Principles and Practice of Infectious Diseases*, 6th ed. Philadelphia, Elsevier Churchill Livingstone, 2005.

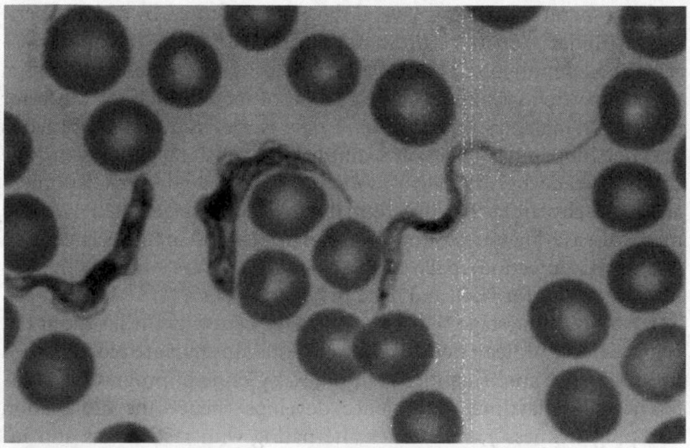

FIGURE 206-3 *Trypanosoma brucei rhodesiense* forms in rat blood. The slender parasite is thought to be the form that multiplies in mammalian hosts, while the stumpy forms are nondividing and are capable of infecting insect vectors (Giemsa, ×1200). *(Courtesy of Dr. G. A. Cook, Madison, WI; with permission.)*

Hematologic manifestations that accompany stage I HAT include moderate leukocytosis, thrombocytopenia, and anemia. High levels of immunoglobulins, consisting primarily of polyclonal IgM, are a constant feature, and heterophile antibodies, antibodies to DNA, and rheumatoid factor are often detected. High levels of antigen-antibody complexes may play a role in the tissue damage and increased vascular permeability that facilitate dissemination of the parasites.

Stage II disease involves invasion of the CNS. The presence of trypanosomes in perivascular areas is accompanied by intense infiltration of mononuclear cells. Abnormalities in cerebrospinal fluid (CSF) include increased pressure, elevated total protein concentration, and pleocytosis. In addition, trypanosomes are frequently found in CSF.

EPIDEMIOLOGY

The trypanosomes that cause sleeping sickness are found only in Africa. Approximately 50 million persons are at risk of acquiring HAT, and tens of thousands of new cases occur every year. Precise data are not available because health statistics are often incomplete in the developing countries where HAT is endemic. Sleeping sickness has undergone a resurgence in recent years, with major epidemics in the Sudan, Ivory Coast, Chad, the Central African Republic, and several other endemic countries.

Humans are the only reservoir of *T. b. gambiense*, which occurs in widely distributed foci in tropical rain forests of Central and West Africa. *Gambiense* trypanosomiasis is primarily a problem in rural populations; tourists rarely become infected. Trypanotolerant antelope species in savanna and woodland areas of Central and East Africa are the principal reservoir of *T. b. rhodesiense*. Cattle can also be infected with this and other trypanosome species but generally succumb to the infection. Since risk results for the most part from contact with tsetse flies that feed on wild animals, humans acquire *T. b. rhodesiense* infection only incidentally, usually while visiting or working in areas where infected game and vectors are present. Roughly one or two patients with HAT acquired in East African game parks (and typically caused by *T. b. rhodesiense*) are reported to the CDC each year.

CLINICAL COURSE

A painful trypanosomal chancre appears in some patients at the site of inoculation of the parasite. Hematogenous and lymphatic dissemination (stage I disease) is marked by the onset of fever. Typically, bouts of high temperatures lasting several days are separated by afebrile periods. Lymphadenopathy is prominent in *T. b. gambiense* trypanosomiasis. The nodes are discrete, movable, rubbery, and nontender. Cervical nodes are often visible, and enlargement of the nodes of the posterior cervical triangle, or *Winterbottom's sign*, is a classic finding. Pruritus and maculopapular rashes are common. Inconstant findings include malaise, headache, arthralgias, weight loss, edema, hepatosplenomegaly, and tachycardia. The differential diagnosis of stage I HAT includes many diseases that are common in the tropics and are associated with fevers. HIV infection, malaria, and typhoid fever are common in populations at risk for HAT and need to be considered.

CNS invasion (stage II disease) is characterized by the insidious development of protean neurologic manifestations that are accompanied by progressive abnormalities in the CSF. A picture of progressive indifference and daytime somnolence develops (hence the designation "sleeping sickness"), sometimes alternating with restlessness and insomnia at night. A listless gaze accompanies a loss of spontaneity, and speech may become halting and indistinct. Extrapyramidal signs may include choreiform movements, tremors, and fasciculations. Ataxia is frequent, and the patient may appear to have Parkinson's disease, with a shuffling gait, hypertonia, and tremors. In the final phase, progressive neurologic impairment ends in coma and death.

The most striking difference between the West African and East African trypanosomiases is that the latter illness tends to follow a more acute course. Typically, in tourists with *T. b. rhodesiense* disease, systemic signs of infection, such as fever, malaise, and headache, appear before the end of the trip or shortly after the return home. Persistent tachycardia unrelated to fever is common early in the course of *T. b. rhodesiense* trypanosomiasis, and death may result from arrhythmias and congestive heart failure before CNS disease develops. In general, untreated *T. b. rhodesiense* trypanosomiasis leads to death in a matter of weeks to months, often without a clear distinction between the hemolymphatic and CNS stages. In contrast, *T. b. gambiense* disease can smolder for many months or even for years.

DIAGNOSIS

A definitive diagnosis of HAT requires detection of the parasite. If a chancre is present, fluid should be expressed and examined directly by light microscopy for the highly motile trypanosomes. The fluid also should be fixed and stained with Giemsa. Material obtained by needle aspiration of lymph nodes early in the illness should be examined similarly. Examination of wet preparations and Giemsa-stained thin and thick films of serial blood samples is also useful. If parasites are not seen initially in blood, efforts should be made to concentrate the organisms; the simplest method involves the use of microhematocrit tubes containing acridine orange. In these tubes the parasites are separated from blood cells by centrifugation and are easily seen under light microscopy because of the stain. Alternatively, the buffy coat from 10–15 mL of anticoagulated blood can be examined directly under a microscope. The likelihood of finding parasites in blood is higher in stage I than in stage II disease and in patients infected with *T. b. rhodesiense* rather than *T. b. gambiense*. Trypanosomes may also be seen in material aspirated from the bone marrow; the aspirate can be inoculated into liquid culture medium, as can blood, buffy coat, lymph node aspirates, and CSF. Finally, *T. b. rhodesiense* infection can be detected by inoculation of these specimens into mice or rats, which—when positive—results in patent parasitemias in a week or two. Although this method is highly sensitive for the detection of *T. b. rhodesiense*, it does not detect *T. b. gambiense* because of host specificity.

It is essential to examine CSF from all patients in whom HAT is suspected. Abnormalities in the CSF that may be associated with stage II disease include an increase in the CSF mononuclear cell count as well as increases in opening pressure and in levels of total protein and IgM. Trypanosomes may be seen in the sediment of centrifuged CSF. Any CSF abnormality in a patient in whom trypanosomes have been found at other sites must be viewed as pathognomonic for CNS involvement and thus must prompt specific treatment for CNS disease. In patients with CSF pleocytosis in whom parasites are not found, tuberculous meningitis and HIV-associated CNS infections such as cryptococcosis should be considered in the differential diagnosis.

A number of serologic assays are available to aid in the diagnosis of HAT, but their variable sensitivity and specificity mandate that decisions about treatment be based on demonstration of the parasite. These tests are of value for epidemiologic surveys. PCR assays for detecting African trypanosomes in humans have been developed, but none is commercially available.

TABLE 206-2 TREATMENT OF HUMAN AFRICAN TRYPANOSOMIASES[a]

Causative Organism	Clinical Stage: I (Normal CSF)	Clinical Stage: II (Abnormal CSF)
T. brucei gambiense (West African)	Pentamidine Alternative: Suramin	Eflornithine Alternative: Melarsoprol
T. brucei rhodesiense (East African)	Suramin	Melarsoprol

[a]For doses and duration, see text.
Note: CSF, cerebrospinal fluid.

℞ SLEEPING SICKNESS

The drugs used for treatment of HAT are suramin, pentamidine, eflornithine, and the organic arsenical melarsoprol. In the United States these drugs can be obtained from the CDC. Therapy for HAT must be individualized on the basis of the infecting subspecies, the presence or absence of CNS disease, adverse reactions, and occasionally drug resistance. The choices of drugs for the treatment of HAT are summarized in **Table 206-2**.

Suramin is highly effective against stage I East African disease. However, it can cause serious adverse effects and must be administered under the close supervision of a physician. A 100- to 200-mg IV test dose should be given to detect hypersensitivity. The dosage for adults is 20 mg/kg on days 1, 5, 12, 18, and 26. The drug is given by slow IV infusion of a freshly prepared 10% aqueous solution. Approximately 1 patient in 20,000 has an immediate, severe, and potentially fatal reaction to the drug, developing nausea, vomiting, shock, and seizures. Less severe reactions include fever, photophobia, pruritus, arthralgias, and skin eruptions. Renal damage is the most common important adverse effect of suramin. Transient proteinuria often appears during treatment. A urinalysis should be done before each dose, and treatment should be discontinued if proteinuria increases or if casts and red cells appear in the sediment. Suramin should not be given to patients with renal insufficiency.

Eflornithine is highly effective for treatment of both stages of West African trypanosomiasis. In the trials on which the FDA based its approval, this agent cured >90% of 600 patients with stage II disease. The recommended treatment schedule is 400 mg/kg per day, given intravenously in four divided doses, for 2 weeks. Adverse reactions include diarrhea, anemia, thrombocytopenia, seizures, and hearing loss. The high dosage and duration of therapy required are disadvantages that make widespread use of eflornithine difficult.

Pentamidine is the first-line drug for patients with stage I West African HAT. The dose for both adults and children is 4 mg/kg per day, given intramuscularly or intravenously, for 10 days. Frequent, immediate adverse reactions include nausea, vomiting, tachycardia, and hypotension. These reactions are usually transient and do not warrant cessation of therapy. Other adverse reactions include nephrotoxicity, abnormal liver function tests, neutropenia, rashes, hypoglycemia, and sterile abscesses.

The arsenical melarsoprol is the drug of choice for the treatment of East African trypanosomiasis with CNS involvement and is an alternative agent for stage II West African disease. Melarsoprol cures both stages of the disease and therefore is also indicated for the treatment of stage I disease in patients who fail to respond to or cannot tolerate suramin or pentamidine. However, because of its relatively high toxicity, melarsoprol is never the first choice for the treatment of stage I disease. For East African disease, the drug should be given to adults in three courses of 3 days each. The dosage is 2–3.6 mg/kg per day, given intravenously in three divided doses for 3 days, followed 1 week later by 3.6 mg/kg per day, also in three divided doses and for 3 days. The latter course is repeated 7 days later. In debilitated patients, suramin is administered for 2–4 days before therapy with melarsoprol is initiated; an 18-mg initial dose of the latter drug, followed by progressive increases to the standard dose, has been recommended. For children, a total of 18–25 mg/kg should be given over 1 month. An IV starting dose of 0.36 mg/kg should be increased gradually to a maximum of 3.6 mg/kg at 1- to 5-day intervals, for a total of 9 or 10 doses. The regimen for West African disease is 2.2 mg/kg per day, given intravenously for 10 days.

Melarsoprol is highly toxic and should be administered with great care. To reduce the likelihood of drug-induced encephalopathy, all patients receiving melarsoprol should be given prednisolone at a dose of 1 mg/kg (up to 40 mg) per day, beginning 1–2 days before the first dose of melarsoprol and continuing through the last dose. Without prednisolone prophylaxis, the incidence of reactive encephalopathy has been reported to be as high as 18% in some series. Clinical manifestations of reactive encephalopathy include high fever, headache, tremor, impaired speech, seizures, and even coma and death. Treatment with melarsoprol should be discontinued at the first sign of encephalopathy but may be restarted cautiously at lower doses a few days after signs have resolved. Extravasation of the drug results in intense local reactions. Vomiting, abdominal pain, nephrotoxicity, and myocardial damage can occur.

PREVENTION

HAT poses complex public-health and epizootic problems in Africa. Considerable progress has been made in some areas through control programs that focus on eradication of vectors and drug treatment of infected humans; however, there is no consensus on the best approach to solving the overall problem, and major epidemics continue to occur. Individuals can reduce their risk of acquiring trypanosomiasis by avoiding areas known to harbor infected insects, by wearing protective clothing, and by using insect repellent. Chemoprophylaxis is not recommended, and no vaccine is available to prevent transmission of the parasites.

FURTHER READINGS

Chang CD et al: Evaluation of a prototype *Trypanosoma cruzi* antibody assay with recombinant antigens on a fully automated chemiluminescence analyzer for blood donor screening. Transfusion 46:1737, 2006

Fiorelli AI et al: Later evolution after cardiac transplantation in Chagas' disease. Transplant Proc 37:2793, 2005

Kirchhoff LV et al: Transfusion-associated Chagas' disease (American trypanosomiasis) in Mexico: Implications for transfusion medicine in the United States. Transfusion 46:298, 2006

Lambert N et al: Chagasic encephalitis as the initial manifestation of AIDS. Ann Intern Med 144:941, 2006

Mascola L et al: Chagas disease after organ transplantation—Los Angeles, California, 2006. MMWR 55:798, 2006

Rassi A Jr et al: Development and validation of a risk score for predicting death in Chagas' heart disease. N Engl J Med 355:799, 2006

Sartori AM et al: Exacerbation of HIV viral load simultaneous with asymptomatic reactivation of chronic Chagas' disease. Am J Trop Med Hyg 67:521, 2002

Schmunis GA, Cruz JR: Safety of the blood supply in Latin America. Clin Microbiol Rev 18:12, 2005

Welburn SC et al: Crisis, what crisis? Control of Rhodesian sleeping sickness. Trends Parasitol 22:123, 2006

207 *Toxoplasma* Infections

Lloyd H. Kasper

DEFINITION

Toxoplasmosis is caused by infection with the obligate intracellular parasite *Toxoplasma gondii*. Acute infection acquired after birth may be asymptomatic but frequently results in the chronic persistence of cysts in the host's tissues. In both acute and chronic toxoplasmosis, the parasite is responsible for clinically evident disease, including lymphadenopathy, encephalitis, myocarditis, and pneumonitis. Congenital toxoplasmosis is an infection of newborns that results from the transplacental passage of parasites from an infected mother to the fetus. These infants usually are asymptomatic at birth but later manifest a wide range of signs and symptoms, including chorioretinitis, strabismus, epilepsy, and psychomotor retardation.

ETIOLOGY

T. gondii is an intracellular coccidian that infects both birds and mammals. There are two distinct stages in the life cycle of *T. gondii* (Fig. 207-1). In the *nonfeline* stage, tissue cysts that contain bradyzoites or sporulated oocysts are ingested by an intermediate host (e.g., a human, mouse, sheep, pig, or bird). The cyst is rapidly digested by the acidic-pH gastric secretions. Bradyzoites or sporozoites are released, enter the small-intestinal epithelium, and transform into rapidly dividing tachyzoites. The tachyzoites can infect and replicate in all mammalian cells except red blood cells. Once attached to the host cell, the parasite penetrates the cell and forms a parasitophorous vacuole within which it divides. Parasite replication continues until the number of parasites within the cell approaches a critical mass and the cell ruptures, releasing parasites that infect adjoining cells.

As a result of this process, an infected organ soon shows evidence of cytopathology. Most tachyzoites are eliminated by the host's humoral and cell-mediated immune responses. Tissue cysts containing many bradyzoites develop 7–10 days after systemic tachyzoite infection. These tissue cysts occur in various host organs but persist principally within the central nervous system (CNS) and muscle. The development of this chronic stage completes the nonfeline portion of the life cycle. Active infection in the immunocompromised host is most likely to be due to the spontaneous release of encysted parasites that undergo rapid transformation into tachyzoites within the CNS.

The principal (*feline*) stage in the life cycle takes place in the cat (the definitive host) and its prey. The parasite's sexual phase is defined by the formation of oocysts within the feline host. This enteroepithelial cycle begins with the ingestion of the bradyzoite tissue cysts and culminates (after several intermediate stages) in the production of gametes. Gamete fusion produces a zygote, which envelops itself in a rigid wall and is secreted in the feces as an unsporulated oocyst. After 2–3 days of exposure to air at ambient temperature, the noninfectious oocyst sporulates to produce eight sporozoite progeny. The sporulated oocyst can be ingested by an intermediate host, such as a person emptying a cat's litter box or a pig rummaging in a barnyard. It is in the intermediate host that *T. gondii* completes its life cycle.

EPIDEMIOLOGY

T. gondii infects a wide range of mammals and birds. Its seroprevalence depends on the locale and the age of the population. Generally, hot arid climatic conditions are associated with a low prevalence of infection. In the United States and most European countries, the seroprevalence increases with age and exposure. For example, in the United States, 5–30% of individuals 10–19 years old and 10–67% of those >50 years old have serologic evidence of exposure; seroprevalence increases by ~1% per year. In Central America, France, Turkey, and Brazil, the seroprevalence is higher. There may be as many as 2100 cases of toxoplasmic encephalitis (TE) each year in the United States.

TRANSMISSION

Oral Transmission The principal source of human *Toxoplasma* infection remains uncertain. Transmission usually takes place by the oral route and can be attributable to ingestion of either sporulated oocysts from contaminated soil or bradyzoites from undercooked meat. During

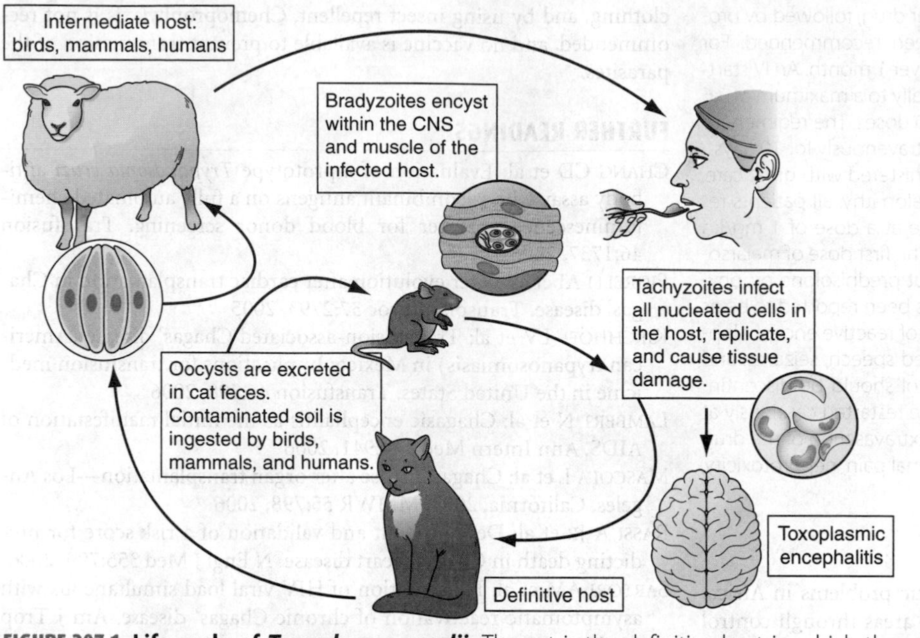

FIGURE 207-1 Life cycle of *Toxoplasma gondii*. The cat is the definitive host in which the sexual phase of the cycle is completed. Oocysts shed in cat feces can infect a wide range of animals, including birds, rodents, grazing domestic animals, and humans. The bradyzoites found in the muscle of food animals may infect humans who eat insufficiently cooked meat products, particularly lamb and pork. Although human disease can take many forms, congenital infection and encephalitis from reactivation of latent infection in the brains of immunosuppressed persons are the most important manifestations. CNS, central nervous system. *(Courtesy of Dominique Buzoni-Gatel, Institut Pasteur, Paris; with permission.)*

acute feline infection, a cat may excrete as many as 100 million parasites per day. These very stable sporozoite-containing oocysts are highly infectious and may remain viable for many years in the soil. Humans infected during a well-documented outbreak of oocyst-transmitted infection develop stage-specific antibodies to the oocyst/sporozoite.

Children and adults also can acquire infection from tissue cysts containing bradyzoites. The ingestion of a single cyst is all that is required for human infection. Undercooking or insufficient freezing of meat is an important source of infection in the developed world. In the United States, 10–20% of lamb products and 25–35% of pork products show evidence of cysts that contain bradyzoites. The incidence in beef is much lower—perhaps as low as 1%. Direct ingestion of bradyzoite cysts in these various meat products leads to acute infection.

Transmission via Blood or Organs In addition to oral transmission, direct transmission of the parasite by blood or organ products during transplantation takes place at a low rate. Viable parasites can be cultured from refrigerated anticoagulated blood, which may be a source of infection in individuals receiving blood transfusions. *T. gondii* infection also has been reported in kidney and heart transplant recipients who were uninfected before transplantation.

Transplacental Transmission About one-third of all women who acquire infection with *T. gondii* during pregnancy transmit the parasite to the fetus; the remainder give birth to normal, uninfected babies. Of the various factors that influence fetal outcome, gestational age at the time of infection is the most critical (see below). Few data support a role for recrudescent maternal infection as the source of congenital disease. Thus, women who are seropositive before pregnancy usually are protected against acute infection and do not give birth to congenitally infected neonates.

The following general guidelines can be used to evaluate congenital infection. There is essentially no risk if the mother becomes infected ≥6 months before conception. If infection is acquired <6 months before conception, the likelihood of transplacental infection increases as the interval between infection and conception decreases. In pregnancy, if the mother becomes infected during the first trimester, the incidence of transplacental infection is lowest (~15%), but the disease in the neonate is most severe. If maternal infection occurs during the third trimester, the incidence of transplacental infection is greatest (65%), but the infant is usually asymptomatic at birth. Infected infants who are normal at birth may have a higher incidence of learning disabilities and chronic neurologic sequelae than uninfected children. Only a small proportion (20%) of women infected with *T. gondii* develop clinical signs of infection. Often the diagnosis is first appreciated when routine postconception serologic tests show evidence of specific antibody.

PATHOGENESIS

Upon the host's ingestion of either tissue cysts containing bradyzoites or oocysts containing sporozoites, the parasites are released from the cysts by a digestive process. Bradyzoites are resistant to the effect of pepsin and invade the host's gastrointestinal tract. Within enterocytes (or other gut-associated cells), the parasites undergo morphologic transformation, giving rise to invasive tachyzoites. These tachyzoites induce a parasite-specific secretory IgA response. From the gastrointestinal tract, parasites are disseminated to a variety of organs, particularly lymphatic tissue, skeletal muscle, myocardium, retina, placenta, and the CNS. At these sites, the parasite infects host cells, replicates, and invades the adjoining cells. In this fashion, the hallmarks of the infection develop: cell death and focal necrosis surrounded by an acute inflammatory response.

In the immunocompetent host, both the humoral and the cellular immune responses control infection; parasite virulence and tissue tropism may be strain specific. Tachyzoites are sequestered by a variety of immune mechanisms, including induction of parasiticidal antibody, activation of macrophages with radical intermediates, production of interferon γ (IFN-γ), and stimulation of cytotoxic T lymphocytes of the CD8+ phenotype. These antigen-specific lymphocytes are capable of killing both extracellular parasites and target cells infected with parasites. As tachyzoites are cleared from the acutely infected host, tissue cysts containing bradyzoites begin to appear, usually within the CNS and the retina. In the immunocompromised or fetal host, the immune factors necessary to control the spread of tachyzoite infection are lacking. This altered immune state allows the persistence of tachyzoites and gives rise to progressive focal destruction that results in organ failure (i.e., necrotizing encephalitis, pneumonia, and myocarditis).

Persistence of infection with cysts containing bradyzoites is common in the immunocompetent host. This lifelong infection usually remains subclinical. Although bradyzoites are in a slow metabolic phase, cysts do degenerate and rupture within the CNS. This degenerative process, with the development of new bradyzoite-containing cysts, is the most probable source of recrudescent infection in immunocompromised individuals and the most likely stimulus for the persistence of antibody titers in the immunocompetent host.

PATHOLOGY

Cell death and focal necrosis due to replicating tachyzoites induce an intense mononuclear inflammatory response in any tissue or cell type infected. Tachyzoites rarely can be visualized by routine histopathologic staining of these inflammatory lesions. However, immunofluorescent staining with parasitic antigen–specific antibodies can reveal either the organism itself or evidence of antigen. In contrast to this inflammatory process caused by tachyzoites, bradyzoite-containing cysts cause inflammation only at the early stages of development, and even this inflammation may be a response to the presence of tachyzoite antigens. Once the cysts reach maturity, the inflammatory process can no longer be detected, and the cysts remain immunologically quiescent within the brain matrix until they rupture.

Lymph Nodes During acute infection, lymph node biopsy demonstrates characteristic findings, including follicular hyperplasia and irregular clusters of tissue macrophages with eosinophilic cytoplasm. Granulomas rarely are evident in these specimens. Although tachyzoites are not usually visible, they can be sought either by subinoculation of infected tissue into mice, with resultant disease, or by polymerase chain reaction (PCR). PCR amplification of DNA fragments representing either p30 (SAG-1) or p22 (SAG-2) surface antigen or B1 antigen is an effective and sensitive assay for establishing lymph node infection by tachyzoites.

Eyes In the eye, infiltrates of monocytes, lymphocytes, and plasma cells may produce uni- or multifocal lesions. Granulomatous lesions and chorioretinitis can be observed in the posterior chamber after acute necrotizing retinitis. Other ocular complications include iridocyclitis, cataracts, and glaucoma.

Central Nervous System During CNS involvement, both focal and diffuse meningoencephalitis can be documented, with evidence of necrosis and microglial nodules. Necrotizing encephalitis in patients without AIDS is characterized by small diffuse lesions with perivascular cuffing in contiguous areas. In the AIDS population, polymorphonuclear leukocytes may be present in addition to monocytes, lymphocytes, and plasma cells. Cysts containing bradyzoites frequently are found contiguous with the necrotic tissue border. As stated previously, it is estimated that there are as many as 2100 cases of TE in the United States each year.

Lungs and Heart Among patients with AIDS who die of toxoplasmosis, 40–70% have involvement of the lungs and heart. Interstitial pneumonitis can develop in neonates and immunocompromised patients. Thickened and edematous alveolar septa infiltrated with mononuclear and plasma cells are apparent. This inflammation may extend to the endothelial walls. Tachyzoites and bradyzoite-containing cysts have been observed within the alveolar membrane. Superimposed bronchopneumonia can be caused by other microbial agents. Cysts and aggregates of parasites in cardiac muscle tissue are evident in patients with AIDS who die of toxoplasmosis. Focal necrosis surrounded by inflammatory cells is associated with hyaline necrosis and disrupted myocardial cells. Pericarditis is associated with toxoplasmosis in some patients.

Gastrointestinal Tract Acute infection in certain strains of inbred mice (B6) results in lethal ileitis within 7–9 days. This inflammatory bowel disease has been recognized in several mammalian species, including pigs and nonhuman primates. The association between human inflammatory bowel disease and either acute or recurrent *Toxoplasma* infection has not been established.

Other Sites Pathologic changes during disseminated infection are similar to those described for the lymph nodes, eyes, and CNS. In patients with AIDS, the skeletal muscle, pancreas, stomach, and kidneys can be involved, with necrosis, invasion by inflammatory cells, and (rarely) tachyzoites detectable by routine staining. Large necrotic lesions may cause direct tissue destruction. In addition, secondary effects from acute infection of these various organs, including pancreatitis, myositis, and glomerulonephritis, have been reported.

HOST IMMUNE RESPONSE

Acute *Toxoplasma* infection evokes a cascade of protective immune responses in the immunocompetent host. *Toxoplasma* enters the host at the gut mucosal level and evokes a mucosal immune response that includes the production of antigen-specific secretory IgA. Titers of serum IgA antibody directed at p30 (SAG-1) are a useful marker for congenital and acute toxoplasmosis. Milk-whey IgA from acutely infected mothers contains a high titer of antibody to *T. gondii* and can block infection of enterocytes in vitro. In mice, IgA intestinal secretions directed at the parasite are abundant and are associated with the induction of mucosal T cells.

Within the host, *T. gondii* rapidly induces detectable levels of both IgM and IgG serum antibodies. Monoclonal gammopathy of the IgG class can occur in congenitally infected infants. IgM levels may be increased in newborns with congenital infection. The polyclonal IgG antibodies evoked by infection are parasiticidal in vitro in the presence of serum complement and are the basis for the Sabin-Feldman dye test. However, cell-mediated immunity is the major protective response evoked by the parasite during host infection. Macrophages are activated after phagocytosis of antibody-opsonized parasites. This activation can lead to death of the parasite by either an oxygen-dependent or an oxygen-independent process. If the parasite is not phagocytosed and enters the macrophage by active penetration, it continues to replicate, and this replication may represent the mechanism for transport and dissemination to distant organs. *Toxoplasma* stimulates a robust interleukin (IL) 12 response by human dendritic cells. The requirement for costimulation via CD40/154 has been established. The CD4+ and CD8+ T cell responses are antigen-specific and further stimulate the production of a variety of important lymphokines that expand the T cell and natural killer cell repertoire. *T. gondii* is a potent inducer of a T_H1 phenotype, with IL-12 and IFN-γ playing an essential role in the control of the parasites' growth in the host. Regulation of the inflammatory response is at least partially under the control of a T_H2 response that includes the production of IL-4 and IL-10 in seropositive individuals. Both asymptomatic patients and those with active infection may have a depressed CD4+ to CD8+ ratio. This shift may be correlated with a disease syndrome but is not necessarily correlated with disease outcome. Human T cell clones of both the CD4+ and the CD8+ phenotypes are cytolytic against parasite-infected macrophages. These T cell clones produce cytokines that are "microbistatic." IL-18, IL-7, and IL-15 upregulate the production of IFN-γ and may be important during acute and chronic infection. The effect of IFN-γ may be paradoxical, with stimulation of a host downregulatory response as well.

Although in patients with AIDS *T. gondii* infection is believed to be recrudescent, determination of antibody titers is not helpful in establishing reactivation. Because of the severe depletion in CD4+ T cells, quite frequently there is no observed increase in antibody titer during exacerbation of infection. T cells from AIDS patients with reactivation of toxoplasmosis fail to secrete both IFN-γ and IL-2. This alteration in the production of these critical immune cytokines contributes to the persistence of infection. *Toxoplasma* infection frequently develops late in the course of AIDS, when the loss of T cell–dependent protective mechanisms, particularly CD8+ T cells, becomes most pronounced.

CLINICAL MANIFESTATIONS

In persons whose immune systems are intact, acute toxoplasmosis is usually asymptomatic and self-limited. This condition can go unrecognized in 80–90% of adults and children with acquired infection. The asymptomatic nature of this infection makes diagnosis difficult in mothers infected during pregnancy. In contrast, the wide range of clinical manifestations in congenitally infected children includes severe neurologic complications such as hydrocephalus, microcephaly, mental retardation, and chorioretinitis. If prenatal infection is severe, multiorgan failure and subsequent intrauterine fetal death can occur. In children and adults, chronic infection can persist throughout life, with little consequence to the immunocompetent host.

Toxoplasmosis in Immunocompetent Patients The most common manifestation of acute toxoplasmosis is cervical lymphadenopathy. The nodes may be single or multiple, are usually nontender, are discrete, and vary in firmness. Lymphadenopathy also may be found in suboccipital, supraclavicular, inguinal, and mediastinal areas. Generalized lymphadenopathy occurs in 20–30% of symptomatic patients. Between 20 and 40% of patients with lymphadenopathy also have headache, malaise, fatigue, and fever [usually with a temperature of <40°C (<104°F)]. A smaller proportion of symptomatic individuals have myalgia, sore throat, abdominal pain, maculopapular rash, meningoencephalitis, and confusion. Rare complications associated with infection in the normal immune host include pneumonia, myocarditis, encephalopathy, pericarditis, and polymyositis. Symptoms associated with acute infection usually resolve within several weeks, although the lymphadenopathy may persist for some months. In one epidemic, toxoplasmosis was diagnosed correctly in only 3 of the 25 patients who consulted physicians. If toxoplasmosis is considered in the differential diagnosis, routine laboratory and serologic screening should precede node biopsy.

The results of routine laboratory studies are usually unremarkable except for minimal lymphocytosis, an elevated erythrocyte sedimentation rate, and a nominal increase in liver aminotransferases. Evaluation of cerebrospinal fluid (CSF) in cases with evidence of encephalopathy or meningoencephalitis shows an elevation of intracranial pressure, mononuclear pleocytosis (10–50 cells/mL), a slight increase in protein concentration, and (occasionally) an increase in the gamma globulin level. PCR amplification of the *Toxoplasma* DNA target sequence in CSF may be beneficial. The CSF of chronically infected individuals is normal.

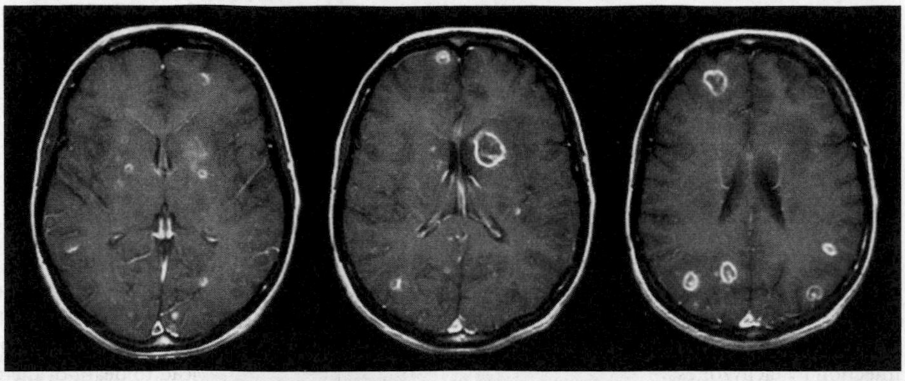

FIGURE 207-2 Toxoplasmic encephalitis in a 36-year-old patient with AIDS. The multiple lesions are demonstrated by magnetic resonance scanning (T1 weighted with gadolinium enhancement). *(Courtesy of Clifford Eskey, Dartmouth Hitchcock Medical Center, Hanover, NH; with permission.)*

Infection of Immunocompromised Patients Patients with AIDS and those receiving immunosuppressive therapy for lymphoproliferative disorders are at greatest risk for developing acute toxoplasmosis. This predilection may be due either to reactivation of latent infection or to acquisition of parasites from exogenous sources such as blood or transplanted organs. In individuals with AIDS, >95% of cases of TE are believed to be due to recrudescent infection. In most of these cases, encephalitis develops when the CD4+ T cell count falls below 100/μL. In immunocompromised hosts, the disease may be rapidly fatal if untreated. Thus accurate diagnosis and initiation of appropriate therapy are necessary to prevent fulminant infection.

Toxoplasmosis is a principal opportunistic infection of the CNS in persons with AIDS. Although geographic origin may be related to frequency of infection, it has no correlation with the severity of disease in immunocompromised hosts. Individuals with AIDS who are seropositive for *T. gondii* are at very high risk for encephalitis. In the United States, about one-third of the 15–40% of adult AIDS patients who are latently infected with *T. gondii* develop TE.

The signs and symptoms of acute toxoplasmosis in immunocompromised patients principally involve the CNS (Fig. 207-2). More than 50% of patients with clinical manifestations have intracerebral involvement. Clinical findings at presentation range from nonfocal to focal dysfunction. CNS findings include encephalopathy, meningoencephalitis, and mass lesions. Patients may present with altered mental status (75%), fever (10–72%), seizures (33%), headaches (56%), and focal neurologic findings (60%), including motor deficits, cranial nerve palsies, movement disorders, dysmetria, visual-field loss, and aphasia. Patients who present with evidence of diffuse cortical dysfunction develop evidence of focal neurologic disease as infection progresses. This altered condition is due not only to the necrotizing encephalitis caused by direct invasion by the parasite but also to secondary effects, including vasculitis, edema, and hemorrhage. The onset of infection can range from an insidious process over several weeks to an acute confusional state with fulminant focal deficits, including hemiparesis, hemiplegia, visual-field defects, localized headache, and focal seizures.

Although lesions can occur anywhere in the CNS, the areas most often involved appear to be the brainstem, basal ganglia, pituitary gland, and corticomedullary junction. Brainstem involvement gives rise to a variety of neurologic dysfunctions, including cranial nerve palsy, dysmetria, and ataxia. With basal ganglionic infection, patients may develop hydrocephalus, choreiform movements, and choreoathetosis. Because *Toxoplasma* usually causes encephalitis, meningeal involvement is uncommon, and thus CSF findings may be unremarkable or may include a modest increase in cell count and in protein—but not glucose—concentration.

Cerebral toxoplasmosis must be differentiated from other opportunistic infections or tumors in the CNS of AIDS patients. The differential diagnosis includes herpes simplex encephalitis, cryptococcal meningitis, progressive multifocal leukoencephalopathy, and primary CNS lymphoma. Involvement of the pituitary gland can give rise to panhypopituitarism and hyponatremia from inappropriate secretion of vasopressin (antidiuretic hormone). AIDS-dementia complex may present as cognitive impairment, attention loss, and altered memory. Brain biopsy in patients who have been treated for TE but who continue to exhibit neurologic dysfunction often fails to identify organisms.

Autopsies of *Toxoplasma*-infected patients have demonstrated the involvement of multiple organs, including the lungs, gastrointestinal tract, pancreas, skin, eyes, heart, and liver. *Toxoplasma* pneumonia can be confused with *Pneumocystis* pneumonia (PcP). Respiratory involvement usually presents as dyspnea, fever, and a nonproductive cough and may rapidly progress to acute respiratory failure with hemoptysis, metabolic acidosis, hypotension, and (occasionally) disseminated intravascular coagulation. Histopathologic studies demonstrate necrosis and a mixed cellular infiltrate. The presence of organisms is a helpful diagnostic indicator, but organisms can also be found in healthy tissue. Infection of the heart is usually asymptomatic but can be associated with cardiac tamponade or biventricular failure. Infections of the gastrointestinal tract and the liver have been documented.

Congenital Toxoplasmosis Between 400 and 4000 infants born each year in the United States are affected by congenital toxoplasmosis. Infection of the placenta leads to hematogenous infection of the fetus. As stated earlier, the proportion of fetuses that become infected increases but the clinical severity of the infection declines as gestation proceeds. Persistence of *T. gondii* can ultimately result in reactivation and further damage decades later. Factors associated with relatively severe disabilities include delays in diagnosis and in initiation of therapy, neonatal hypoxia and hypoglycemia, profound visual impairment (see "Ocular Infection," below), uncorrected hydrocephalus, and increased intracranial pressure. If treated appropriately, upwards of 70% of children have normal developmental, neurologic, and ophthalmologic findings at follow-up evaluations. Treatment for 1 year with pyrimethamine and a sulfonamide is tolerated with minimal toxicity (see "Treatment," below).

Ocular Infection Infection with *T. gondii* is estimated to cause 35% of all cases of chorioretinitis in the United States and Europe. Most ocular involvement is believed to be due to congenital infection, with a very low incidence following acquired infection. Between 1 and 3% of all patients with AIDS develop debilitating chorioretinitis due to *T. gondii*. A variety of ocular manifestations are documented, including blurred vision, scotoma, photophobia, and eye pain. Macular involvement occurs with loss of central vision, and nystagmus is secondary to poor fixation. Involvement of the extraocular muscles may lead to disorders of convergence and to strabismus. Ophthalmologic examination should be undertaken in newborns with suspected congenital infection. As the inflammation resolves, vision improves, but episodic flare-ups of chorioretinitis, which progressively destroy retinal tissue and lead to glaucoma, are common.

The ophthalmologic examination reveals yellow-white, cotton-like patches with indistinct margins of hyperemia. As the lesions age, white plaques with distinct borders and black spots within the retinal pigment become more apparent. Lesions usually are located near the posterior pole of the retina; they may be single but are more commonly multiple. Congenital lesions may be unilateral or bilateral and show evidence of massive chorioretinal degeneration with extensive fibrosis. Surrounding these areas of involvement are a normal retina and vasculature. In patients with AIDS, retinal lesions are often large, with diffuse retinal necrosis, and include both free tachyzoites and cysts containing bradyzoites. Toxoplasmic chorioretinitis may be a prodrome to the development of encephalitis.

DIAGNOSIS

Tissue and Body Fluids The differential diagnosis of acute toxoplasmosis can be made by appropriate culture, serologic testing, and PCR (Table 207-1). Although difficult, the isolation of *T. gondii* from blood or other body fluids can be accomplished after subinoculation of the sample into the peritoneal cavity of mice. Mice should be tested for organisms in the peritoneal fluid 6–10 days after inoculation. If no parasites are found in the mouse's peritoneal fluid, its anti-*Toxoplasma* serum titer can be evaluated 4–6 weeks after inoculation. Isolation of *T. gondii* from the patient's body fluids reflects acute infection, whereas isolation from biopsied tissue is an indication only of the presence of tissue cysts and should not be misinterpreted as evidence of acute toxoplasmosis. Persistent parasitemia in patients with latent, asymptomatic infection is rare. Histologic examination of lymph nodes may suggest the characteristic changes described above. Demonstration of tachyzoites in lymph nodes establishes the diagnosis of acute toxoplasmosis. Like subinoculation into mice, histologic demonstration of cysts containing bradyzoites confirms prior infection with *T. gondii* but is nondiagnostic for acute infection.

TABLE 207-1 DIFFERENTIAL LABORATORY DIAGNOSIS OF TOXOPLASMOSIS

Clinical Setting	Alternative Diagnosis	Distinguishing Characteristics
Mononucleosis syndrome	Epstein-Barr virus	Serologic test
	Cytomegalovirus	Serologic test
	HIV	Serologic test
Congenital infection	Cytomegalovirus	Viral culture
	Herpes simplex virus	Viral culture
	Rubella virus	Viral culture/serologic test
	Syphilis	Serologic test
	Listeriosis	Bacterial culture
Retinochoroiditis in immunocompetent individual	Tuberculosis	Bacterial culture
	Syphilis	Serologic test
	Histoplasmosis	Serologic test/culture
Retinochoroiditis in AIDS	Cytomegalovirus	Viral culture/PCR
	Syphilis	Serologic test
	Herpes simplex virus	Viral culture/PCR
	Varicella-zoster virus	Viral culture/PCR
	Fungal infection	Culture
CNS lesions in AIDS	Lymphoma or metastatic tumor	Tissue biopsy
	Brain abscess	Bacterial culture
	Progressive multifocal leukoencephalopathy	PCR
	Fungal/mycobacterial infection	Biopsy and culture

Source: Adapted from Schwartzman JD: Toxoplasmosis, in *Principles and Practice of Clinical Parasitology*. Hoboken, Wiley, 2001.

Serology The procedures just described have great diagnostic value but are limited by difficulties encountered either in the growth of parasites in vivo or in the identification of tachyzoites by histochemical methods. Serologic testing has become the routine method of diagnosis. A wide range of serologic tests that can be used to measure antibody to *T. gondii* are available commercially.

Diagnosis of acute infection with *T. gondii* can be established by detection of the simultaneous presence of IgG and IgM antibodies to *Toxoplasma* in serum. The presence of circulating IgA favors the diagnosis of an acute infection. The Sabin-Feldman dye test, the indirect fluorescent antibody test, and the enzyme-linked immunosorbent assay (ELISA) all satisfactorily measure circulating IgG antibody to *Toxoplasma*. Positive IgG titers (>1:10) can be detected as early as 2–3 weeks after infection. These titers usually peak at 6–8 weeks and decline slowly to a new baseline level that persists for life. It is necessary to measure the serum IgM titer in concert with the IgG titer to better establish the time of infection. The methods currently available for this determination are the double-sandwich IgM-ELISA and the IgM-immunosorbent assay (IgM-ISAGA). Both of these assays are specific and sensitive, and their use precludes the false-positive results associated with tests for rheumatoid factor and antinuclear antibody. The double-sandwich IgA-ELISA is more sensitive than the IgM-ELISA for detecting congenital infection in the fetus and newborn.

Recently, the results obtained with PCR have suggested high sensitivity, specificity, and clinical utility in the diagnosis of TE in resource-poor settings.

Molecular Diagnostics Molecular approaches can directly detect *T. gondii* in biologic samples independent of the serologic response. Specific molecular analysis for either the B1 gene or the 529-bp sequence is useful. Real-time PCR is a promising technique that can provide quantitative results. Isolates can be genotyped and polymorphic sequences can be obtained, with the consequent identification of the precise strain. Knowledge of the correct sequence is important in studies on the correlation of clinical signs and symptoms of disease with the *T. gondii* genotype.

The Immunocompetent Adult or Child For the patient who presents with lymphadenopathy only, a positive IgM titer is an indication of acute infection—and an indication for therapy, if that is clinically warranted (see "Treatment," below). The serum IgM titer should be determined again in 3 weeks. An elevation in the IgG titer without an increase in the IgM titer suggests that infection is present but is not acute. If there is a borderline increase in either IgG or IgM, the titers should be reassessed in 3–4 weeks.

The Immunocompromised Host A presumptive clinical diagnosis of TE in patients with AIDS is based on clinical presentation, history of exposure (as evidenced by positive serology), and radiologic evaluation. To detect latent infection with *T. gondii*, HIV-infected persons should be tested for IgG antibody to *Toxoplasma* soon after HIV infection is diagnosed. When these criteria are used, the predictive value is as high as 80%. More than 97% of patients with AIDS and toxoplasmosis have IgG antibody to *T. gondii* in serum. IgM serum antibody usually is not detectable. Attempts to evaluate rising IgG titers or to determine whether IgM is present are not productive. Serologic evidence of infection virtually always precedes the development of TE. It is therefore important to determine the *Toxoplasma* antibody status of all patients infected with HIV. Antibody titers may range from negative to 1:1024 in patients with AIDS and TE. Fewer than 3% of patients have no demonstrable antibody to *Toxoplasma* at diagnosis. Intrathecal antibody to *T. gondii* may be present; determination of the titer may help identify prior infection.

Patients with TE have focal or multifocal abnormalities demonstrable by CT or MRI. Neuroradiologic evaluation should include double-dose contrast CT of the head. By this test, single and frequently multiple contrast-enhancing lesions (<2 cm) may be identified. MRI usually demonstrates multiple lesions located in both hemispheres, with the basal ganglia and corticomedullary junction most commonly involved; MRI provides a more sensitive evaluation of the efficacy of therapy than does CT (Fig. 207-2). These findings are not pathognomonic of *Toxoplasma* infection, since 40% of CNS lymphomas are multifocal and 50% are ring-enhancing. For both MRI and CT scans, the rate of false-negative results is ~10%. The finding of a single lesion on an MRI scan increases the likelihood of primary CNS lymphoma (in which solitary lesions are four times more likely than in TE) and strengthens the argument for the performance of a brain biopsy. A therapeutic trial of anti-*Toxoplasma* medications is frequently used to assess the diagnosis. Treatment of presumptive TE with pyrimethamine plus clindamycin results in quantifiable clinical improvement in >50% of patients by day 3. By day 7, >90% of treated patients show evidence of improvement. In contrast, if patients fail to respond or have lymphoma, clinical signs and symptoms worsen by day 7. Patients in this category require brain biopsy with or without a change in therapy. This procedure can now be performed by a stereotactic CT-guided method that reduces the potential for complications. Brain biopsy for *T. gondii* identifies organisms in 50–75% of cases. PCR amplification of genetic material of the parasite found in the CSF may prove diagnostically beneficial in the future.

Now used in some centers, single-photon emission CT (SPECT) has been touted as a definitive means of detecting or ruling out *Toxoplasma* infection when a CNS lesion is suspected. In the future, SPECT may well be widely used for this purpose.

As in other conditions, the radiologic response may lag behind the clinical response. Resolution of lesions may take from 3 weeks to 6 months. Some patients show clinical improvement despite worsening radiographic findings.

Congenital Infection The issue of concern when a pregnant woman has evidence of recent *T. gondii* infection is obviously whether the fetus is infected. PCR analysis of the amniotic fluid for the B1 gene of *T. gondii* has replaced fetal blood sampling. Serologic diagnosis is based on the persistence of IgG antibody or a positive IgM titer after the first week of life (a time frame that excludes placental leak). The IgG determination should be repeated every 2 months. An increase in IgM beyond the first week of life is indicative of acute infection. However, up to 25% of infected newborns may be seronegative and have normal routine physical examinations. Thus assessment of the eye and the brain, with ophthalmologic testing, CSF evaluation, and radiologic studies, is important in establishing the diagnosis.

Ocular Toxoplasmosis Because of the congenital nature of ocular toxoplasmosis, the serum antibody titer may not correlate with the presence of active lesions in the fundus. In general, a positive IgG titer (measured in undiluted serum if necessary) in conjunction with typical lesions establishes the diagnosis. Antibody production is expressed in terms of the Goldmann-Witmer coefficient (C), in which $C = $ [anti-*Toxoplasma* IgG (aqueous humor/serum)]/[total IgG (serum/aqueous humor)]. The positive cutoff of 3 is the generally accepted discrimination level. The sensitivity of this index as a diagnostic tool lies between 60 and 85%, with a specificity close to 90% in persons of European or North American origin. Confirmation of local specific antibody production in the eye indicates that the site of inflammatory activity is localized to this organ. However, two-thirds of patients without evidence of specific antibody production at initial clinical presentation later develop a detectable titer. If lesions are atypical and the titer is in the low-positive range, the diagnosis is presumptive. The parasitic antigen–specific polyclonal IgG assay as well as parasitic antigen–specific PCR may facilitate the diagnosis. Accordingly, the clinical diagnosis of ocular toxoplasmosis can be supported in 60–90% of cases by laboratory tests, depending on the time of anterior chamber puncture and the panel of antibody analyses used. In the remaining cases, the possibility of a falsely negative laboratory diagnosis or of an incorrect clinical diagnosis cannot be clarified further.

℞ TOXOPLASMOSIS

CONGENITAL INFECTION Congenitally infected neonates are treated with daily oral pyrimethamine (0.5–1 mg/kg) and sulfadiazine (100 mg/kg) for 1 year. In addition, therapy with spiramycin (100 mg/kg per day) plus prednisone (1 mg/kg per day) is efficacious for congenital infection.

INFECTION IN IMMUNOCOMPETENT PATIENTS Immunologically competent adults and older children who have only lymphadenopathy do not require specific therapy unless they have persistent, severe symptoms. Patients with ocular toxoplasmosis should be treated for 1 month with pyrimethamine plus either sulfadiazine or clindamycin. Prenatal antibiotic therapy can reduce the number of infants severely affected by *Toxoplasma* infection.

INFECTION IN IMMUNOCOMPROMISED PATIENTS **Primary Prophylaxis** Patients with AIDS should be treated for acute toxoplasmosis; in immunocompromised patients, toxoplasmosis is rapidly fatal if untreated. Before the introduction of antiretroviral therapy (ART), the median survival time was >1 year for patients who could tolerate treatment for TE. Despite their toxicity, the drugs used to treat TE were required for survival prior to ART. The incidence of TE has declined as survival of patients with HIV infection has increased as a result of ART.

In Africa, many patients are diagnosed with HIV infection only after developing opportunistic infections such as TE. Hence, the optimal management of these opportunistic infections is important if the benefits of subsequent ART are to be realized. AIDS patients who are seropositive for *T. gondii* and who have a CD4+ T lymphocyte count of <100/μL should receive prophylaxis against TE. A recent Cochrane analysis of clinical trials of TE treatment failed to document the superiority of any one regimen. Of the currently available agents, trimethoprim-sulfamethoxazole (TMP-SMX) appears to be an effective alternative for TE in resource-poor settings where the preferred combination of pyrimethamine plus sulfadiazine is not available. The daily dose of TMP-SMX recommended as the preferred regimen for PcP prophylaxis (one double-strength tablet) is effective against TE. If patients cannot tolerate TMP-SMX, the recommended alternative is dapsone-pyrimethamine, which is also effective against PcP. Atovaquone with or without pyrimethamine also can be considered. Prophylactic monotherapy with dapsone, pyrimethamine, azithromycin, clarithromycin, or aerosolized pentamidine is probably insufficient. AIDS patients who are seronegative for *Toxoplasma* and are not receiving prophylaxis for PcP should be retested for IgG antibody to *Toxoplasma* if their CD4+ T cell count drops to <100/μL. If seroconversion has taken place, then the patient should be given prophylaxis as described above.

Discontinuing Primary Prophylaxis Some current studies indicate that prophylaxis against TE can be discontinued in patients who have responded to ART and whose CD4+ T lymphocyte count has been >200/μL for 3 months. Although patients with CD4+ T lymphocyte counts of <100/μL are at greatest risk for developing TE, the risk that this condition will develop when the count has increased to 100–200/μL has not been established. Thus, prophylaxis should indeed be discontinued only when the count has increased to >200/μL. Continued prophylaxis at a CD4+ count of >200/μL has only a limited preventive effect against TE. Discontinuation of therapy reduces the pill burden; the potential for drug toxicity, drug interaction, or selection of drug-resistant pathogens; and cost. Prophylaxis should be recommenced if the CD4+ T lymphocyte count again decreases to <100–200/μL.

Individuals who have completed initial therapy for TE should receive treatment indefinitely unless immune reconstitution, with a CD4+ T cell count of >200/μL, occurs as a consequence of ART. Combination therapy with pyrimethamine plus sulfadiazine plus leucovorin is effective for this purpose. An alternative to sulfadiazine in this regimen is clindamycin. Unfortunately, only the combination of pyrimethamine plus sulfadiazine provides protection against PcP as well.

Discontinuing Secondary Prophylaxis (Chronic Maintenance Therapy) Patients receiving secondary prophylaxis for TE are at low risk for recurrence when they have completed initial therapy for TE, remain asymptomatic, and have a CD4+ T lymphocyte count of >200/μL for at least 6 months after ART. This recommendation is based on recent observations in a large cohort (381 patients) and is consistent with more extensive data indicating the safety of discontinuing secondary prophylaxis for other opportunistic infections during advanced HIV disease. Discontinuation of chronic maintenance therapy among these patients appears reasonable. A repeat MRI brain scan is recommended. Secondary prophylaxis should be reintroduced if the CD4+ T lymphocyte count decreases to <200/μL.

PREVENTION

All HIV-infected persons, including those who lack IgG antibody to *Toxoplasma*, should be counseled regarding sources of *Toxoplasma* infection. The chances of primary infection with *Toxoplasma* can be reduced by not eating undercooked meat and by avoiding oocyst-contaminated material (i.e., a cat's litter box). Specifically, lamb, beef, and pork should be cooked to an internal temperature of 165°–170°F; from a more practical perspective, meat cooked until it is no longer pink inside usually satisfies this requirement. Hands should be washed thoroughly after work in the garden, and all fruits and vegetables should be washed. If the patient owns a cat, the litter box should be cleaned or changed daily, preferably by an HIV-negative, nonpregnant person; alternatively, patients should wash their hands thoroughly after changing the litter box. Patients should be encouraged to keep their cats inside and not to adopt or handle stray cats. Cats should be fed only canned or dried commercial food or well-cooked table food, not raw or undercooked meats. Patients need not be advised to part with their cats or to have their cats tested for toxoplasmosis. Blood intended for transfusion into *Toxoplasma*-seronegative immunocompromised individuals should be screened for antibody to *T. gondii*. Although such serologic screening is not routinely performed, seronegative women should be screened for evidence of infection several times during pregnancy if they are exposed to environmental conditions that put them at risk for infection with *T. gondii*. HIV-positive individuals should adhere closely to these preventive measures.

FURTHER READINGS

DEDICOAT M: Management of toxoplasmic encephalitis in HIV-infected adults (with an emphasis on resource-poor settings). Cochrane Database Syst Rev 3:CD005420, 2006

GARWEG JG: Determinants of immunodiagnostic success in human ocular toxoplasmosis. Parasite Immunol 27:61, 2005

LEHMANN T et al: Globalization and the population structure of *Toxoplasma gondii*. Proc Natl Acad Sci USA 103:11423, 2006

MASUR H et al: Guidelines for preventing opportunistic infections among HIV-infected persons—2002. Ann Intern Med 137:435, 2002

MCLEOD R et al: Outcome of treatment for congenital toxoplasmosis, 1981–2004: The National Collaborative Chicago-Based, Congenital Toxoplasmosis Study. Clin Infect Dis 42:1383, 2006

MIRO JM et al: Discontinuation of primary and secondary *Toxoplasma gondii* prophylaxis is safe in HIV-infected patients after immunological restoration with highly active antiretroviral therapy: Results of an open, randomized, multicenter clinical trial. Clin Infect Dis 43:79, 2006

MOCROFT A et al: Decline in the AIDS and death rates in the EuroSIDA study: An observational study. Lancet 362:22, 2003

SCHMIDT DR et al: The national neonatal screening programme for congenital toxoplasmosis in Denmark: Results from the initial four years, 1999–2002. Arch Dis Child 91:661, 2006

SWITAJ K et al: Recent trends in molecular diagnostics for *Toxoplasma gondii* infections. Clin Microbiol Infect 11:170, 2005

208 Protozoal Intestinal Infections and Trichomoniasis

Peter F. Weller

PROTOZOAL INFECTIONS

GIARDIASIS

Giardia lamblia (also known as *G. intestinalis*) is a cosmopolitan protozoal parasite that inhabits the small intestines of humans and other mammals.

Giardiasis is one of the most common parasitic diseases in both developed and developing countries worldwide, causing both endemic and epidemic intestinal disease and diarrhea.

Life Cycle and Epidemiology (Fig. 208-1) Infection follows the ingestion of environmentally hardy cysts, which excyst in the small intestine, releasing flagellated trophozoites (Fig. 208-2) that multiply by binary fission. *Giardia* remains a pathogen of the proximal small bowel and does not disseminate hematogenously. Trophozoites remain free in the lumen or attach to the mucosal epithelium by means of a ventral sucking disk. As a trophozoite encounters altered conditions, it forms a morphologically distinct cyst, which is the stage of the parasite usually found in the feces. Trophozoites may be present and even predominate in loose or watery stools, but it is the resistant cyst that survives outside the body and is responsible for transmission. Cysts do not tolerate heating, desiccation, or continued exposure to feces but do remain viable for months in cold fresh water. The number of cysts excreted varies widely but can approach 10^7 per gram of stool.

Ingestion of as few as 10 cysts is sufficient to cause infection in humans. Because cysts are infectious when excreted, person-to-person transmission occurs where fecal hygiene is poor. Giardiasis, as symptomatic or asymptomatic infections, is especially prevalent in day-care centers; person-to-person spread also takes place in other institutional settings with poor fecal hygiene and during anal-oral contact. If food is contaminated with *Giardia* cysts after cooking or preparation, foodborne transmission can occur. Waterborne transmission accounts for episodic infections (e.g., in campers and travelers) and for major epidemics in metropolitan areas. Surface water, ranging from mountain streams to large municipal reservoirs, can become contaminated with fecally derived *Giardia* cysts; outmoded water systems are subject to cross-contamination from leaking sewer lines. The efficacy of water as a means of transmission is enhanced by the small infectious inoculum of *Giardia*, the prolonged survival of cysts in cold water, and the resistance of cysts to killing by routine chlorination methods that are adequate for controlling bacteria. Viable cysts can be eradicated from water by either boiling or filtration. In the United States, *Giardia* (like *Cryptosporidium*; see below) is a common cause of waterborne epidemics of gastroenteritis. *Giardia* is common in developing countries, and infections may be acquired by travelers.

The importance of animal reservoirs as sources of infection for humans is unclear. *Giardia* parasites morphologically similar to those in humans are found in many mammals, including beavers from reservoirs implicated in epidemics, dogs, and cats.

Giardiasis, like cryptosporidiosis, creates a significant economic burden because of the costs incurred in the installation of water filtration systems required to prevent waterborne epidemics, in the management of epidemics that involve large communities, and in the evaluation and treatment of endemic infections.

Pathophysiology The reasons that some, but not all, infected patients develop clinical manifestations and the mechanisms by which *Giardia* causes alterations in small-bowel function are largely unknown. Although trophozoites adhere to the epithelium, they do not cause invasive or locally destructive alterations. The lactose intolerance and, in a minority of infected adults and children, significant malabsorption that develop are clinical signs of the loss of brush-border enzyme activities. In most infections, the morphology of the bowel is unaltered; however, in a few cases (usually in chronically infected, symptomatic patients), the histopathologic findings (including flattened villi) and the clinical manifestations resemble those of tropical sprue and gluten-sensitive enteropathy. The pathogenesis of diarrhea in giardiasis is not known.

The natural history of *Giardia* infection varies markedly. Infections may be aborted, transient, recurrent, or chronic. Parasite as well as host factors may be important in determining the course of infection and disease. Both cellular and humoral responses develop in human infections, but their precise roles in the control of infection and/or dis-

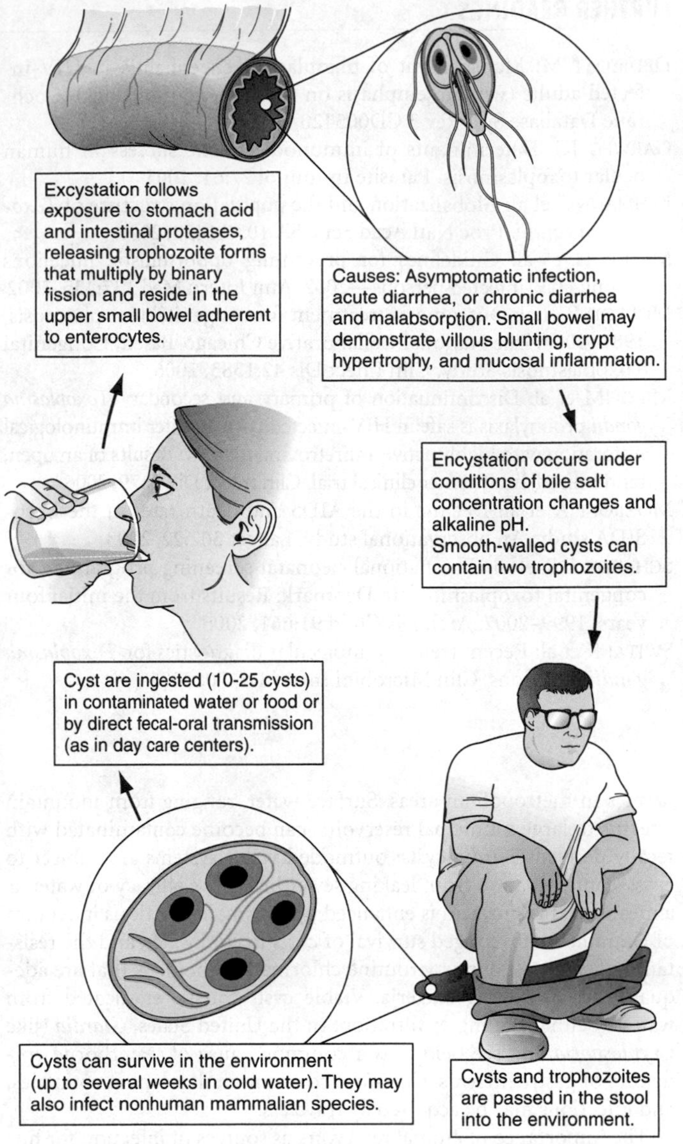

Excystation follows exposure to stomach acid and intestinal proteases, releasing trophozoite forms that multiply by binary fission and reside in the upper small bowel adherent to enterocytes.
Causes: Asymptomatic infection, acute diarrhea, or chronic diarrhea and malabsorption. Small bowel may demonstrate villous blunting, crypt hypertrophy, and mucosal inflammation.
Encystation occurs under conditions of bile salt concentration changes and alkaline pH. Smooth-walled cysts can contain two trophozoites.
Cyst are ingested (10-25 cysts) in contaminated water or food or by direct fecal-oral transmission (as in day care centers).
Cysts can survive in the environment (up to several weeks in cold water). They may also infect nonhuman mammalian species.
Cysts and trophozoites are passed in the stool into the environment.

FIGURE 208-1 Life cycle of *Giardia*. *(Reprinted from RL Guerrant et al: Tropical Infectious Disease: Principles, Pathogens and Practice, 2d ed, 2006, p 987, with permission from Elsevier Science.)*

ease are unknown. Because patients with hypogammaglobulinemia suffer from prolonged, severe infections that are poorly responsive to treatment, humoral immune responses appear to be important. The greater susceptibility of the young than of the old and of newly exposed persons than of chronically exposed populations suggests that at least partial protective immunity may develop. *Giardia* isolates vary genotypically, biochemically, and biologically, and variations among isolates may contribute to different courses of infection.

Clinical Manifestations Disease manifestations of giardiasis range from asymptomatic carriage to fulminant diarrhea and malabsorption. Most infected persons are asymptomatic, but in epidemics the proportion of symptomatic cases may be higher. Symptoms may develop suddenly or gradually. In persons with acute giardiasis, symptoms develop after an incubation period that lasts at least 5–6 days and usually 1–3 weeks. Prominent early symptoms include diarrhea, abdominal pain, bloating, belching, flatus, nausea, and vomiting. Although diarrhea is common, upper intestinal manifestations such as nausea, vomiting, bloating, and abdominal pain may predominate. The duration of acute giardiasis is usually >1 week, although diarrhea often subsides. Individuals with chronic giardiasis may present with or without having experienced an antecedent acute symptomatic episode. Diarrhea is not necessarily prominent, but increased flatus, loose stools, sulfurous belching, and (in some instances) weight loss occur. Symptoms may be continual or episodic and can persist for years. Some persons who have relatively mild symptoms for long periods recognize the extent of their discomfort only in retrospect. Fever, the presence of blood and/or mucus in the stools, and other signs and symptoms of colitis are uncommon and suggest a different diagnosis or a concomitant illness. Symptoms tend to be intermittent yet recurring and gradually debilitating, in contrast with the acute disabling symptoms associated with many enteric bacterial infections. Because of the less severe illness and the propensity for chronic infections, patients may seek medical advice late in the course of the illness; however, disease can be severe, resulting in malabsorption, weight loss, growth retardation, and dehydration. A number of extraintestinal manifestations have been described, such as urticaria, anterior uveitis, and arthritis; whether these are caused by giardiasis or concomitant processes is unclear.

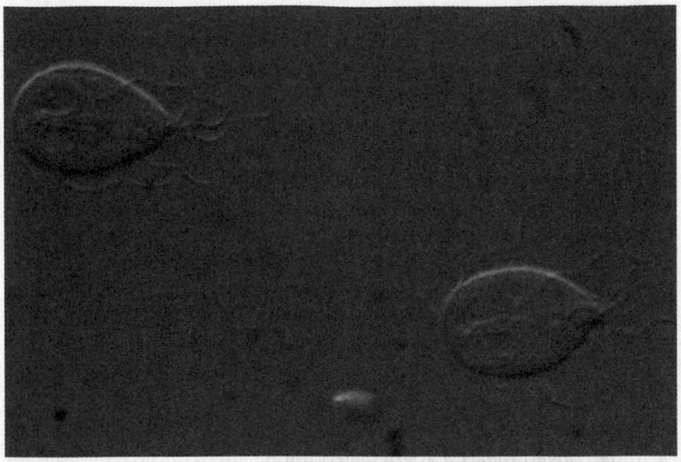

FIGURE 208-2 Flagellated, binucleate ***Giardia* trophozoite.**

Giardiasis can be severe in patients with hypogammaglobulinemia and can complicate other preexisting intestinal diseases, such as that occurring in cystic fibrosis. In patients with AIDS, *Giardia* can cause enteric illness that is refractory to treatment.

Diagnosis (Table 208-1) Giardiasis is diagnosed by detection of parasite antigens in the feces or by identification of cysts in the feces or of trophozoites in the feces or small intestines. Cysts are oval, measure 8–12 μm × 7–10 μm, and characteristically contain four nuclei. Trophozoites are pear-shaped, dorsally convex, flattened parasites with two nuclei and four pairs of flagella (Fig. 208-2). The diagnosis is sometimes difficult to establish. Direct examination of fresh or properly preserved stools as well as concentration methods should be used. Because cyst excretion is variable and may be undetectable at times, repeated examination of stool, sampling of duodenal fluid, and biopsy of the small intestine may be required to detect the parasite. Tests for parasitic antigens in stool are at least as sensitive and specific as good microscopic examinations and are easier to perform. All of these methods occasionally yield false-negative results.

TABLE 208-1 DIAGNOSIS OF INTESTINAL PROTOZOAL INFECTIONS

Parasite	Stool O+P[a]	Fecal Acid-Fast Stain	Stool Antigen Immunoassays	Other
Giardia	+		+	
Cryptosporidium	−	+	+	
Isospora	−	+		
Cyclospora	−	+		
Microsporidia	−			Special fecal stains, tissue biopsies

[a]O+P, ova and parasites.

℞ GIARDIASIS

Cure rates with metronidazole (250 mg thrice daily for 5 days) are usually >90%. Tinidazole (2 g once by mouth) is reportedly more effective than metronidazole. Nitazoxanide (500 mg twice daily for 3 days) is an alternative agent for treatment of giardiasis. Paromomycin, an oral aminoglycoside that is not well absorbed, can be given to symptomatic pregnant patients, although information is limited on how effectively this agent eradicates infection.

Almost all patients respond to therapy and are cured, although some with chronic giardiasis experience delayed resolution of symptoms after eradication of *Giardia*. For many of the latter patients, residual symptoms probably reflect delayed regeneration of intestinal brush-border enzymes. Continued infection should be documented by stool examinations before treatment is repeated. Patients who remain infected after repeated treatments should be evaluated for reinfection through family members, close personal contacts, and environmental sources as well as for hypogammaglobulinemia. In cases refractory to multiple treatment courses, prolonged therapy with metronidazole (750 mg thrice daily for 21 days) has been successful.

Prevention Although *Giardia* is extremely infectious, disease can be prevented by consumption of noncontaminated food and water and by personal hygiene when caring for infected children. Boiling or filtering potentially contaminated water prevents infection.

CRYPTOSPORIDIOSIS

The coccidian parasite *Cryptosporidium* causes diarrheal disease that is self-limited in immunocompetent human hosts but can be severe in persons with AIDS or other forms of immunodeficiency. Two species of *Cryptosporidium, C. hominis* and *C. parvum,* cause most human infections.

Life Cycle and Epidemiology *Cryptosporidium* species are widely distributed in the world. Cryptosporidiosis is acquired by the consumption of oocysts (50% infectious dose: ~132 oocysts in nonimmune individuals), which excyst to liberate sporozoites that in turn enter and infect intestinal epithelial cells. The parasite's further development involves both asexual and sexual cycles, which produce forms capable of infecting other epithelial cells and of generating oocysts that are passed in the feces. *Cryptosporidium* species infect a number of animals, and *C. parvum* can spread from infected animals to humans. Since oocysts are immediately infectious when passed in feces, person-to-person transmission takes place in day-care centers and among household contacts and medical providers. Waterborne transmission (especially that of *C. hominis*) accounts for infections in travelers and for common-source epidemics. Oocysts are quite hardy and resist killing by routine chlorination. Both drinking water and recreational water (e.g., pools, waterslides) have been increasingly recognized as sources of infection.

Pathophysiology Although intestinal epithelial cells harbor cryptosporidia in an intracellular vacuole, the means by which secretory diarrhea is elicited remain uncertain. No characteristic pathologic changes are found by biopsy. The distribution of infection can be spotty within the principal site of infection, the small bowel. Cryptosporidia are found in the pharynx, stomach, and large bowel of some patients and at times in the respiratory tract. Especially in patients with AIDS, involvement of the biliary tract can cause papillary stenosis, sclerosing cholangitis, or cholecystitis.

Clinical Manifestations Asymptomatic infections can occur in both immunocompetent and immunocompromised hosts. In immunocompetent persons, symptoms develop after an incubation period of ~1 week and consist principally of watery nonbloody diarrhea, sometimes in conjunction with abdominal pain, nausea, anorexia, fever, and/or weight loss. In these hosts, the illness usually subsides after 1–2 weeks. In contrast, in immunocompromised hosts (especially those with AIDS and CD4+ T cell counts <100/µL), diarrhea can be chronic, persistent, and remarkably profuse, causing clinically significant fluid and electrolyte depletion. Stool volumes may range from 1 to 25 L/d. Weight loss, wasting, and abdominal pain may be severe. Biliary tract involvement can manifest as midepigastric or right upper quadrant pain.

Diagnosis (Table 208-1) Evaluation starts with fecal examination for small oocysts, which are smaller (4–5 µm in diameter) than the fecal stages of most other parasites. Because conventional stool examination for ova and parasites does not detect *Cryptosporidium*, specific testing must be requested. Detection is enhanced by evaluation of stools (obtained on multiple days) by several techniques, including modified acid-fast and direct immunofluorescent stains and enzyme immunoassays. Cryptosporidia can also be identified by light and electron microscopy at the apical surfaces of intestinal epithelium from biopsy specimens of the small bowel and, less frequently, the large bowel.

℞ CRYPTOSPORIDIOSIS

Nitazoxanide is approved by the U.S. Food and Drug Administration for the treatment of cryptosporidiosis and is available in tablet form for adults (500 mg twice daily for 3 days) and as an elixir for children. To date, however, this agent has not been effective for the treatment of HIV-infected patients, in whom improved immune status due to antiretroviral therapy can lead to amelioration of cryptosporidiosis. Otherwise, treatment includes supportive care with replacement of fluids and electrolytes and administration of antidiarrheal agents. Biliary tract obstruction may require papillotomy or T-tube placement. Prevention requires minimizing exposure to infectious oocysts in human or animal feces. Use of submicron water filters may minimize acquisition of infection from drinking water.

ISOSPORIASIS

The coccidian parasite *Isospora belli* causes human intestinal disease. Infection is acquired by the consumption of oocysts, after which the parasite invades intestinal epithelial cells and undergoes both sexual and asexual cycles of development. Oocysts excreted in stool are not immediately infectious but must undergo further maturation.

Although *I. belli* infects many animals, little is known about the epidemiology or prevalence of this parasite in humans. It appears to be most common in tropical and subtropical countries. Acute infections can begin abruptly with fever, abdominal pain, and watery nonbloody diarrhea and can last for weeks or months. In patients who have AIDS or are immunocompromised for other reasons, infections often are not self-limited but rather resemble cryptosporidiosis, with chronic, profuse watery diarrhea. Eosinophilia, which is not found in other enteric protozoan infections, may be detectable. The diagnosis (Table 208-1) is usually made by detection of the large (~25-µm) oocysts in stool by modified acid-fast staining. Oocyst excretion may be low-level and intermittent; if repeated stool examinations are unrevealing, sampling of duodenal contents by aspiration or small-bowel biopsy (often with electron-microscopic examination) may be necessary.

℞ ISOSPORIASIS

Trimethoprim-sulfamethoxazole (TMP-SMX; 160/800 mg four times daily for 10 days, and for HIV-infected patients, then three times daily for 3 weeks) is effective. For patients intolerant of sulfonamides, pyrimethamine (50–75 mg/d) can be used. Relapses can occur in persons with AIDS and necessitate maintenance therapy with TMP-SMX (160/800 mg three times per week).

CYCLOSPORIASIS

Cyclospora cayetanensis, a cause of diarrheal illness, is globally distributed: illness due to *C. cayetanensis* has been reported in the United States, Asia, Africa, Latin America, and Europe. The epidemiology of this parasite has not yet been fully defined, but waterborne transmission and food-borne transmission by basil and imported raspberries have been recognized. The full spectrum of illness attributable to *Cyclospora* has not been delineated. Some patients may harbor the infection without symptoms, but many have diarrhea, flulike symptoms, and flatulence and belching. The illness can be self-limited, can wax and wane, or in many cases can involve prolonged diarrhea, anorexia, and upper gastrointestinal symptoms, with sustained fatigue and weight loss in some instances. Diarrheal illness may persist for >1 month. *Cyclospora* can cause enteric illness in patients infected with HIV.

The parasite is detectable in epithelial cells of small-bowel biopsy samples and elicits secretory diarrhea by unknown means. The absence of fecal blood and leukocytes indicates that disease due to *Cyclospora* is not caused by destruction of the small-bowel mucosa. The diagnosis (Table 208-1) can be made by detection of spherical 8- to 10-μm oocysts in the stool, although routine stool O and P examinations are not sufficient. Specific fecal examinations must be requested to detect the oocysts, which are variably acid-fast and are fluorescent when viewed with ultraviolet light microscopy. Cyclosporiasis should be considered in the differential diagnosis of prolonged diarrhea, with or without a history of travel by the patient to other countries.

Rx CYCLOSPORIASIS

Cyclosporiasis is treated with TMP-SMX (160/800 mg twice daily for 7 days). HIV-infected patients may experience relapses after such treatment and thus may require longer-term suppressive maintenance therapy.

MICROSPORIDIOSIS

Microsporidia are obligate intracellular spore-forming protozoa that infect many animals and cause disease in humans, especially as opportunistic pathogens in AIDS. Microsporidia are members of a distinct phylum, Microspora, which contains dozens of genera and hundreds of species. The various microsporidia are differentiated by their developmental life cycles, ultrastructural features, and molecular taxonomy based on ribosomal RNA. The complex life cycles of the organisms result in the production of infectious spores (**Fig. 208-3**). Currently, eight genera of microsporidia—*Encephalitozoon, Pleistophora, Nosema, Vittaforma, Trachipleistophora, Brachiola, Microsporidium,* and *Enterocytozoon*—are recognized as causes of human disease. Although some microsporidia are probably prevalent causes of self-limited or asymptomatic infections in immunocompetent patients, little is known about how microsporidiosis is acquired.

Microsporidiosis is most common among patients with AIDS, less common among patients with other types of immunocompromise, and rare among immunocompetent hosts. In patients with AIDS, intestinal infections with *Enterocytozoon bieneusi* and *Encephalitozoon* (formerly *Septata*) *intestinalis* are recognized to contribute to chronic diarrhea and wasting; these infections are found in 10–40% of patients with chronic diarrhea. Both organisms have been found in the biliary tracts of patients with cholecystitis. *E. intestinalis* may also disseminate to cause fever, diarrhea, sinusitis, cholangitis, and bronchiolitis. In patients with AIDS, *Encephalitozoon hellem* has caused superficial keratoconjunctivitis as well as sinusitis, respiratory tract disease, and disseminated infection. Myositis due to *Pleistophora* has been documented. *Nosema*, *Vittaforma*, and *Microsporidium* have caused stromal keratitis associated with trauma in immunocompetent patients.

Microsporidia are small gram-positive organisms with mature spores measuring 0.5–2 μm × 1–4 μm. Diagnosis of microsporidial infections in tissue often requires electron microscopy, although intracellular spores can be visualized by light microscopy with hematoxylin and eosin, Giemsa, or tissue Gram's stain. For the diagnosis of intestinal microsporidiosis, modified trichrome or chromotrope 2R-based staining and Uvitex 2B or calcofluor fluorescent staining reveal spores in smears of feces or duodenal aspirates. Definitive therapies for microsporidial infections remain to be established. For superficial keratoconjunctivitis due to *E. hellem*, topical therapy with fumagillin suspension has shown promise (Chap. 201). For enteric infections with *E. bieneusi* and *E. intestinalis* in HIV-infected patients, therapy with albendazole may be efficacious (Chap. 201).

OTHER INTESTINAL PROTOZOA

Balantidiasis *Balantidium coli* is a large ciliated protozoal parasite that can produce a spectrum of large-intestinal disease analogous to amebiasis.

The parasite is widely distributed in the world. Since it infects pigs, cases in humans are more common where pigs are raised. Infective cysts can be transmitted from person to person and

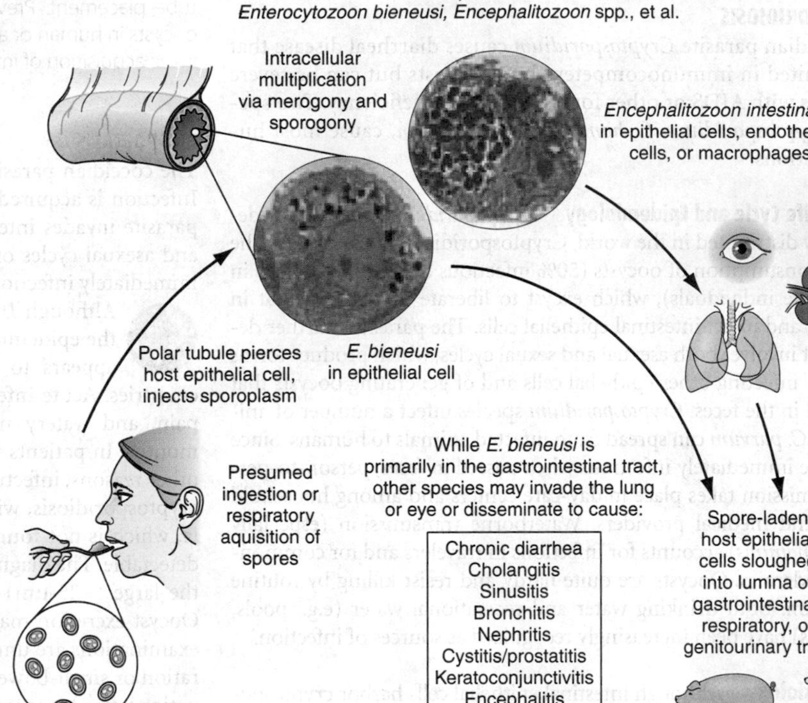

Polar tubule pierces host epithelial cell, injects sporoplasm

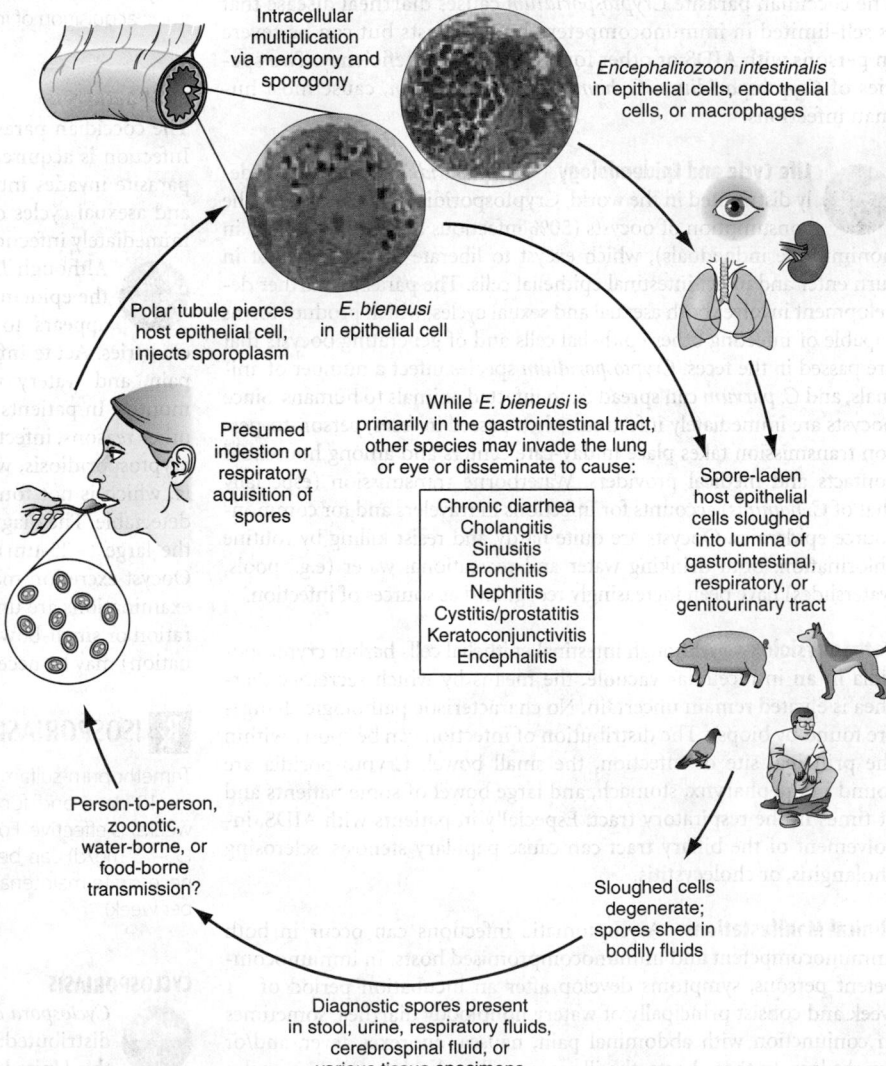

Sloughed cells degenerate; spores shed in bodily fluids
Diagnostic spores present in stool, urine, respiratory fluids, cerebrospinal fluid, or various tissue specimens

FIGURE 208-3 Life cycle of microsporidia. *(Reprinted from RL Guerrant et al: Tropical Infectious Disease: Principles, Pathogens and Practice, 2d ed, 2006, p 1128, with permission from Elsevier Science.)*

through water, but many cases are due to the ingestion of cysts derived from porcine feces in association with slaughtering, with use of pig feces for fertilizer, or with contamination of water supplies by pig feces.

Ingested cysts liberate trophozoites, which reside and replicate in the large bowel. Many patients remain asymptomatic, but some have persisting intermittent diarrhea, and a few develop more fulminant dysentery. In symptomatic individuals, the pathology in the bowel—both gross and microscopic—is similar to that seen in amebiasis, with varying degrees of mucosal invasion, focal necrosis, and ulceration. Balantidiasis, unlike amebiasis, does not spread hematogenously to other organs. The diagnosis is made by detection of the trophozoite stage in stool or sampled colonic tissue. Tetracycline (500 mg four times daily for 10 days) is an effective therapeutic agent.

***Blastocystis hominis* Infection** *B. hominis*, while believed by some to be a protozoan capable of causing intestinal disease, remains an organism of uncertain pathogenicity. Some patients who pass *B. hominis* in their stools are asymptomatic, whereas others have diarrhea and associated intestinal symptoms. Diligent evaluation reveals other potential bacterial, viral, or protozoal causes of diarrhea in some but not all patients with symptoms. Because the pathogenicity of *B. hominis* is uncertain and because therapy for *Blastocystis* infection is neither specific nor uniformly effective, patients with prominent intestinal symptoms should be fully evaluated for other infectious causes of diarrhea. If diarrheal symptoms associated with *Blastocystis* are prominent, either metronidazole (750 mg thrice daily for 10 days) or TMP-SMX (160 mg/800 mg twice daily for 7 days) can be used.

***Dientamoeba fragilis* Infection** *D. fragilis* is unique among intestinal protozoa in that it has a trophozoite stage but not a cyst stage. How trophozoites survive to transmit infection is not known. When symptoms develop in patients with *D. fragilis* infection, they are generally mild and include intermittent diarrhea, abdominal pain, and anorexia. The diagnosis is made by the detection of trophozoites in stool; the lability of these forms accounts for the greater yield when fecal samples are preserved immediately after collection. Since fecal excretion rates vary, examination of several samples obtained on alternate days increases the rate of detection. Iodoquinol (650 mg three times daily for 20 days), paromomycin (25–35 mg/kg per day in three doses for 7 days), metronidazole (500–750 mg three times daily for 10 days), or tetracycline (500 mg four times daily for 10 days) is appropriate for treatment.

TRICHOMONIASIS

Various species of trichomonads can be found in the mouth (in association with periodontitis) and occasionally in the gastrointestinal tract. *Trichomonas vaginalis*—one of the most prevalent protozoal parasites in the United States—is a pathogen of the genitourinary tract and a major cause of symptomatic vaginitis.

LIFE CYCLE AND EPIDEMIOLOGY

T. vaginalis is a pear-shaped, actively motile organism that measures about 10 × 7 μm, replicates by binary fission, and inhabits the lower genital tract of females and the urethra and prostate of males. In the United States, it accounts for ~3 million infections per year in women. While the organism can survive for a few hours in moist environments and could be acquired by direct contact, person-to-person venereal transmission accounts for virtually all cases of trichomoniasis. Its prevalence is greatest among persons with multiple sexual partners and among those with other sexually transmitted diseases (Chap. 124).

CLINICAL MANIFESTATIONS

Many men infected with *T. vaginalis* are asymptomatic, although some develop urethritis and a few have epididymitis or prostatitis. In contrast, infection in women, which has an incubation period of 5–28 days, is usually symptomatic and manifests with malodorous vaginal discharge (often yellow), vulvar erythema and itching, dysuria or urinary frequency (in 30–50% of patients), and dyspareunia. These manifestations, however, do not clearly distinguish trichomoniasis from other types of infectious vaginitis.

DIAGNOSIS

Detection of motile trichomonads by microscopic examination of wet mounts of vaginal or prostatic secretions has been the conventional means of diagnosis. Although this approach provides an immediate diagnosis, its sensitivity for the detection of *T. vaginalis* is only ~50–60% in routine evaluations of vaginal secretions. Direct immunofluorescent antibody staining is more sensitive (70–90%) than wet-mount examinations. *T. vaginalis* can be recovered from the urethra of both males and females and is detectable in males after prostatic massage. Culture of the parasite is the most sensitive means of detection; however, the facilities for culture are not generally available, and detection of the organism takes 3–7 days.

Rx TRICHOMONIASIS

Metronidazole, given either as a single 2-g dose or in 500-mg doses twice daily for 7 days, is usually effective. Tinidazole (a single 2-g dose) is also effective. All sexual partners must be treated concurrently to prevent reinfection, especially from asymptomatic males. In males with persistent symptomatic urethritis after therapy for nongonococcal urethritis, metronidazole therapy should be considered for possible trichomoniasis. Alternatives to metronidazole for treatment during pregnancy are not readily available, although use of 100-mg clotrimazole vaginal suppositories nightly for 2 weeks may cure some infections in pregnant women. Reinfection often accounts for apparent treatment failures, but strains of *T. vaginalis* exhibiting high-level resistance to metronidazole have been encountered. Treatment of these resistant infections with higher oral doses, parenteral doses, or concurrent oral and vaginal doses of metronidazole or with tinidazole has been successful.

FURTHER READINGS

CHEX XM et al: Cryptosporidiosis. N Engl J Med 346:1723, 2002

CDC DIVISION OF PARASITIC DISEASES. *http://www.cdc.gov/ncidod/dpd/default.htm*

DIDIER ES: Microsporidiosis: An emerging and opportunistic infection in humans and animals. Acta Trop 94:61, 2005

LEDER K et al: No correlation between clinical symptoms and *Blastocystis hominis* in immunocompetent individuals. J Gastroenterol Hepatol 20:1390, 2005

ROXSTROM-LINDQUIST K et al: Giardia immunity—an update. Trends Parasitol 22:26, 2006

VANDENBERG O et al: Clinical and microbiological features of dientamoebiasis in patients suspected of suffering from a parasitic gastrointestinal illness: A comparison of *Dientamoeba fragilis* and *Giardia lamblia* infections. Int J Infect Dis 10:255, 2006

VAN DER POL B et al: Prevalence, incidence, natural history, and response to treatment of *Trichomonas vaginalis* infection among adolescent women. J Infect Dis 192:2039, 2005

WEISS LM, SCHWARTZ DA: Microsporidiosis, in *Tropical Infectious Diseases: Principles, Pathogens and Practice*, 2d ed, RL Guerrant et al (eds). Elsevier, Philadelphia, 2006, pp 1126–1140

WEITZEL T et al: Epidemiological and clinical features of travel-associated cryptosporidiosis. Clin Microbiol Infect 12:921, 2006

YODER JS, BEACH MJ: Cryptosporidiosis surveillance—United States, 2003–2005. MMWR Surveill Summ 56:1, 2007

——— et al: Giardiasis surveillance—United States, 2003–2005. MMWR Surveill Summ 56:11, 2007

209 *Trichinella* and Other Tissue Nematodes

Peter F. Weller

Nematodes are elongated, symmetric roundworms. Parasitic nematodes of medical significance may be broadly classified as either predominantly intestinal or tissue nematodes. This chapter covers trichinellosis, visceral and ocular larva migrans, cutaneous larva migrans, cerebral angiostrongyliasis, and gnathostomiasis. All are zoonotic infections caused by incidental exposure to infectious nematodes. The clinical symptoms of these infections are due largely to invasive larval stages that (except in the case of *Trichinella*) do not reach maturity in humans.

TRICHINELLOSIS

Trichinellosis develops after the ingestion of meat containing cysts of *Trichinella*—for example, pork or other meat from a carnivore. Although most infections are mild and asymptomatic, heavy infections can cause severe enteritis, periorbital edema, myositis, and (infrequently) death.

Life Cycle and Epidemiology Eight species of *Trichinella* are recognized as causes of infection in humans. Two species are distributed worldwide: *T. spiralis*, which is found in a great variety of carnivorous and omnivorous animals, and *T. pseudospiralis*, which is found in mammals and birds.

T. nativa is present in Arctic regions and infects bears; *T. nelsoni* is found in equatorial eastern Africa, where it is common among felid predators and scavengers such as hyenas and bush pigs; and *T. britovi* is found in Europe, western Africa, and western Asia among carnivores but not among domestic swine. *T. murrelli* is present in North American game animals.

After human consumption of trichinous meat, encysted larvae are liberated by digestive acid and pepsin (Fig. 209-1). The larvae invade the small-bowel mucosa and mature into adult worms. After ~1 week, female worms release newborn larvae that migrate via the circulation to striated muscle. The larvae of all species except *T. pseudospiralis*, *T. papuae*, and *T. zimbabwensis* then encyst by inducing a radical transformation in the muscle cell architecture. Although host immune responses may help to expel intestinal adult worms, they have little effect on muscle-dwelling larvae.

Human trichinellosis is often caused by the ingestion of infected pork products and thus can occur in almost any location where the meat of domestic or wild swine is eaten. Human trichinellosis also may be acquired from the meat of other animals, including dogs (in parts of Asia and Africa), horses (in Italy and France), and bears and walruses (in northern regions). Although cattle (being herbivores) are not natural hosts of *Trichinella*, beef has been implicated in outbreaks when contaminated or adulterated with trichinous pork. Laws that prohibit the feeding of uncooked garbage to pigs have greatly reduced the transmission of trichinellosis in the United States. About 12 cases of trichinellosis are reported annually in this country, but most mild cases probably remain undiagnosed. Recent U.S. and Canadian outbreaks have been attributable to consumption of wild game (especially bear meat) and, less frequently, of pork.

Pathogenesis and Clinical Features Clinical symptoms of trichinellosis arise from the successive phases of parasite enteric invasion, larval migration, and muscle encystment (Fig. 209-1). Most light infections (those with <10 larvae per gram of muscle) are asymptomatic, whereas heavy infections (which can involve >50 larvae per gram of muscle) can be life-threatening. Invasion of the gut by large numbers of parasites occasionally provokes diarrhea during the first week after infection. Abdominal pain, constipation, nausea, or vomiting also may be prominent.

Symptoms due to larval migration and muscle invasion begin to appear in the second week after infection. The migrating *Trichinella* larvae provoke a marked local and systemic hypersensitivity reaction, with fever and hypereosinophilia. Periorbital and facial edema is common, as are hemorrhages in the subconjunctivae, retina, and nail beds ("splinter" hemorrhages). A maculopapular rash, headache, cough, dyspnea, or dysphagia sometimes develops. Myocarditis with tachyarrhythmias or heart failure—and, less commonly, encephalitis or pneumonitis—may develop and accounts for most deaths of patients with trichinellosis.

Upon onset of larval encystment in muscle 2–3 weeks after infection, symptoms of myositis with myalgias, muscle edema, and weakness develop, usually overlapping with the inflammatory reactions to

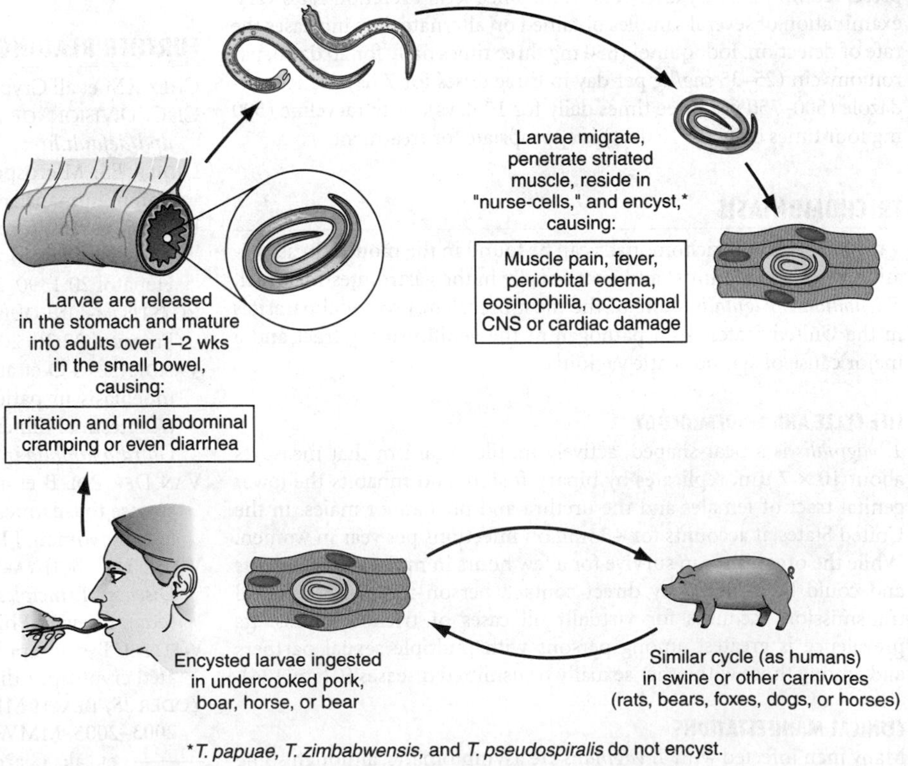
Larvae migrate, penetrate striated muscle, reside in "nurse-cells," and encyst,* causing:
Muscle pain, fever, periorbital edema, eosinophilia, occasional CNS or cardiac damage
Larvae are released in the stomach and mature into adults over 1–2 wks in the small bowel, causing:
Irritation and mild abdominal cramping or even diarrhea
Encysted larvae ingested in undercooked pork, boar, horse, or bear
Similar cycle (as humans) in swine or other carnivores (rats, bears, foxes, dogs, or horses)
*T. papuae, T. zimbabwensis, and T. pseudospiralis do not encyst.

FIGURE 209-1 Life cycle of *Trichinella spiralis* (cosmopolitan); *nelsoni* (equatorial Africa); *britovi* (Europe, western Africa, western Asia); *nativa* (Arctic); *murrelli* (North America); *papuae* (Papua New Guinea); *zimbabwensis* (Tanzania); and *pseudospiralis* (cosmopolitan). *[Reprinted from Guerrant RL et al (eds): Tropical Infectious Diseases: Principles, Pathogens and Practice, 2d ed, p 1218. © 2006, with permission from Elsevier Science.]*

migrating larvae. The most commonly involved muscle groups include the extraocular muscles; the biceps; and the muscles of the jaw, neck, lower back, and diaphragm. Peaking ~3 weeks after infection, symptoms subside only gradually during a prolonged convalescence. Uncommon infections with *T. pseudospiralis*, whose larvae do not encapsulate in muscles, elicit prolonged polymyositis-like illness.

Laboratory Findings and Diagnosis Blood eosinophilia develops in >90% of patients with symptomatic trichinellosis and may peak at a level of >50% between 2 and 4 weeks after infection. Serum levels of muscle enzymes, including creatine phosphokinase, are elevated in most symptomatic patients. Patients should be questioned thoroughly about their consumption of pork or wild-animal meat and about illness in other individuals who ate the same meat. A presumptive clinical diagnosis can be based on fevers, eosinophilia, periorbital edema, and myalgias after a suspect meal. A rise in the titer of parasite-specific antibody, which usually does not occur until after the third week of infection, confirms the diagnosis. Alternatively, a definitive diagnosis requires surgical biopsy of at least 1 g of involved muscle; the yields are highest near tendon insertions. The fresh muscle tissue should be compressed between glass slides and examined microscopically (Fig. 209-2), because larvae may be overlooked by examination of routine histopathologic sections alone.

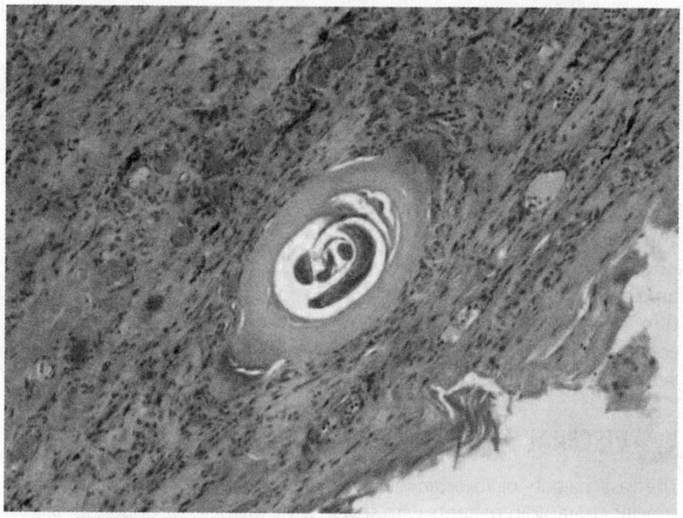

FIGURE 209-2 ***Trichinella* larva** encysted in a characteristic hyalinized capsule in striated muscle tissue. *(Photo/Wadsworth Center, New York State Department of Health. Reprinted from CDC MMWR 53:606, 2004; public domain.)*

Rx TRICHINELLOSIS

Most lightly infected patients recover uneventfully with bed rest, antipyretics, and analgesics. Glucocorticoids like prednisone **(Table 209-1)** are beneficial for severe myositis and myocarditis. Mebendazole and albendazole are active against enteric stages of the parasite, but their efficacy against encysted larvae has not been conclusively demonstrated.

Prevention Larvae may be killed by cooking pork until it is no longer pink or by freezing it at –15°C for 3 weeks. However, Arctic *T. nativa* larvae in walrus or bear meat are relatively resistant and may remain viable despite freezing.

VISCERAL AND OCULAR LARVA MIGRANS

Visceral larva migrans is a syndrome caused by nematodes that are normally parasitic for nonhuman host species. In humans, the nematode larvae do not develop into adult worms but instead migrate through host tissues and elicit eosinophilic inflammation. The more common form of visceral larva migrans is toxocariasis due to larvae of the canine ascarid *Toxocara canis*, less commonly to the feline ascarid *T. cati*, and even less commonly to the pig ascarid *Ascaris suum*. Rare cases with eosinophilic meningoencephalitis have been caused by the raccoon ascarid *Baylisascaris procyonis*.

Life Cycle and Epidemiology The canine roundworm *T. canis* is distributed among dogs worldwide. Ingestion of infective eggs by dogs is followed by liberation of *Toxocara* larvae, which penetrate the gut wall and migrate intravascularly into canine tissues, where most remain in a developmentally arrested state. During pregnancy, some larvae resume migration in bitches and infect puppies prenatally (through transplacental transmission) or after birth (through suckling). Thus, in lactating bitches and puppies, larvae return to the intestinal tract and develop into adult worms, which produce eggs that are released in the feces. Humans acquire toxocariasis mainly by eating soil contaminated by puppy feces that contains infective *T. canis* eggs. Visceral larva migrans is most common among children who habitually eat dirt.

Pathogenesis and Clinical Features Clinical disease most commonly afflicts preschool children. After humans ingest *Toxocara* eggs, the larvae hatch and penetrate the intestinal mucosa, from which they are carried by the circulation to a wide variety of organs and tissues. The larvae invade the liver, lungs, central nervous system (CNS), and other sites, provoking intense local eosinophilic granulomatous responses. The degree of clinical illness depends on larval number and tissue distribution, reinfection, and host immune responses. Most light infections are asymptomatic and may be manifest only by blood eosinophilia. Characteristic symptoms of visceral larva migrans include fever, malaise, anorexia and weight loss, cough, wheezing, and rashes. Hepatosplenomegaly is common. These features are often accompanied by extraordinary peripheral eosinophilia, which may approach 90%. Uncommonly, seizures or behavioral disorders develop. Rare deaths are due to severe neurologic, pneumonic, or myocardial involvement.

The ocular form of the larva migrans syndrome occurs when *Toxocara* larvae invade the eye. An eosinophilic granulomatous mass, most commonly in the posterior pole of the retina, develops around the entrapped larva. The retinal lesion can mimic retinoblastoma in appearance, and mistaken diagnosis of the latter condition can lead to unnecessary enucleation. The spectrum of eye involvement also in-

TABLE 209-1 THERAPY FOR TISSUE NEMATODE INFECTIONS

Infection	Severity	Treatment
Trichinellosis	Mild	Supportive
	Moderate	Albendazole (400 mg bid × 8–14 days) *or* Mebendazole (200–400 mg tid × 3 days, then 400 mg tid × 8–14 days)
	Severe	Add glucocorticoids (e.g., prednisone, 1 mg/kg qd × 5 days)
Visceral larva migrans	Mild to moderate	Supportive
	Severe	Glucocorticoids (as above)
	Ocular	Not fully defined; albendazole (800 mg bid for adults, 400 mg bid for children) with glucocorticoids × 5–20 days has been effective
Cutaneous larva migrans		Ivermectin (single dose, 200 μg/kg) *or* Albendazole (200 mg bid × 3 days)
Angiostrongyliasis	Mild to moderate	Supportive
	Severe	Glucocorticoids (as above)
Gnathostomiasis		Ivermectin (200 μg/kg per day × 2 days) *or* Albendazole (400 mg bid × 21 days)

cludes endophthalmitis, uveitis, and chorioretinitis. Unilateral visual disturbances, strabismus, and eye pain are the most common presenting symptoms. In contrast to visceral larva migrans, ocular toxocariasis usually develops in older children or young adults with no history of pica; these patients seldom have eosinophilia or visceral manifestations.

Diagnosis In addition to eosinophilia, leukocytosis and hypergammaglobulinemia may be evident. Transient pulmonary infiltrates are apparent on chest x-rays of about half of patients with symptoms of pneumonitis. The clinical diagnosis can be confirmed by an enzyme-linked immunosorbent assay for toxocaral antibodies. Stool examination for parasite eggs, while important in the evaluation of unexplained eosinophilia, is worthless for toxocariasis, since the larvae do not develop into egg-producing adults in humans.

℞ VISCERAL AND OCULAR LARVA MIGRANS

The vast majority of *Toxocara* infections are self-limited and resolve without specific therapy. In patients with severe myocardial, CNS, or pulmonary involvement, glucocorticoids may be employed to reduce inflammatory complications. Available anthelmintic drugs, including mebendazole and albendazole, have not been shown conclusively to alter the course of larva migrans. Control measures include prohibiting dog excreta in public parks and playgrounds, deworming dogs, and preventing pica in children. Treatment of ocular disease is not fully defined, but the administration of albendazole in conjunction with glucocorticoids has been effective (Table 209-1).

CUTANEOUS LARVA MIGRANS

Cutaneous larva migrans ("creeping eruption") is a serpiginous skin eruption caused by burrowing larvae of animal hookworms, usually the dog and cat hookworm *Ancylostoma braziliense*. The larvae hatch from eggs passed in dog and cat feces and mature in the soil. Humans become infected after skin contact with soil in areas frequented by dogs and cats, such as areas underneath house porches. Cutaneous larva migrans is prevalent among children and travelers in regions with warm humid climates, including the southeastern United States.

After larvae penetrate the skin, erythematous lesions form along the tortuous tracks of their migration through the dermal-epidermal junction; the larvae advance several centimeters in a day. The intensely pruritic lesions may occur anywhere on the body and can be numerous if the patient has lain on the ground. Vesicles and bullae may form later. The animal hookworm larvae do not mature in humans and, without treatment, will die after an interval ranging from weeks to a couple of months, with resolution of skin lesions. The diagnosis is made on clinical grounds. Skin biopsies only rarely detect diagnostic larvae. Symptoms can be alleviated by ivermectin or albendazole (Table 209-1).

ANGIOSTRONGYLIASIS

Angiostrongylus cantonensis, the rat lungworm, is the most common cause of human eosinophilic meningitis (Fig. 209-3).

Life Cycle and Epidemiology This infection occurs principally in Southeast Asia and the Pacific Basin but has spread to other areas of the world. *A. cantonensis* larvae produced by adult worms in the rat lung migrate to the gastrointestinal tract and are expelled with the feces. They develop into infective larvae in land snails and slugs. Humans acquire the infection by ingesting raw infected mollusks; vegetables contaminated by mollusk slime; or crabs, freshwater shrimp, and certain marine fish that have themselves eaten infected mollusks. The larvae then migrate to the brain.

Pathogenesis and Clinical Features The parasites eventually die in the CNS, but not before initiating pathologic consequences that, in heavy infections, can result in permanent neurologic sequelae or death. Migrating larvae cause marked local eosinophilic inflammation and hemorrhage, with subsequent necrosis and granuloma formation around dying worms. Clinical symptoms develop 2–35 days after the ingestion of larvae. Patients usually present with an insidious or abrupt excruciating frontal, occipital, or bitemporal headache. Neck stiffness, nausea and vomiting, and paresthesias are also common. Fever, cranial and extraocular nerve palsies, seizures, paralysis, and lethargy are uncommon.

Laboratory Findings Examination of cerebrospinal fluid (CSF) is mandatory in suspected cases and usually reveals an elevated opening pressure, a white blood cell count of 150–2000/μL, and an eosinophilic pleocytosis of >20%. The protein concentration is usually elevated and the glucose level normal. The larvae of *A. cantonensis* are only rarely seen in CSF. Peripheral-blood eosinophilia may be mild. The diagnosis is generally based on the clinical presentation of eosinophilic meningitis together with a compatible epidemiologic history.

℞ ANGIOSTRONGYLIASIS

Specific chemotherapy is not of benefit in angiostrongyliasis; larvicidal agents may exacerbate inflammatory brain lesions. Management consists of supportive measures, including the administration of analgesics, sedatives, and—in severe cases—glucocorticoids (Table 209-1). Repeated lumbar punctures with removal of CSF can relieve symptoms. In most patients, cerebral angiostrongyliasis has a self-limited course, and recovery is complete. The infection may be prevented by adequately cooking snails, crabs, and prawns and inspecting vegetables for mollusk infestation. Other parasitic or fungal causes of eosinophilic meningitis in endemic areas may include gnathostomiasis (see below), paragonimiasis (Chap. 212), schistosomiasis (Chap. 212), neurocysticercosis (Chap. 213), and coccidioidomycosis (Chap. 193).

GNATHOSTOMIASIS

Infection of human tissues with larvae of *Gnathostoma spinigerum* can cause eosinophilic meningoencephalitis, migratory cutaneous swellings, or invasive masses of the eye and visceral organs.

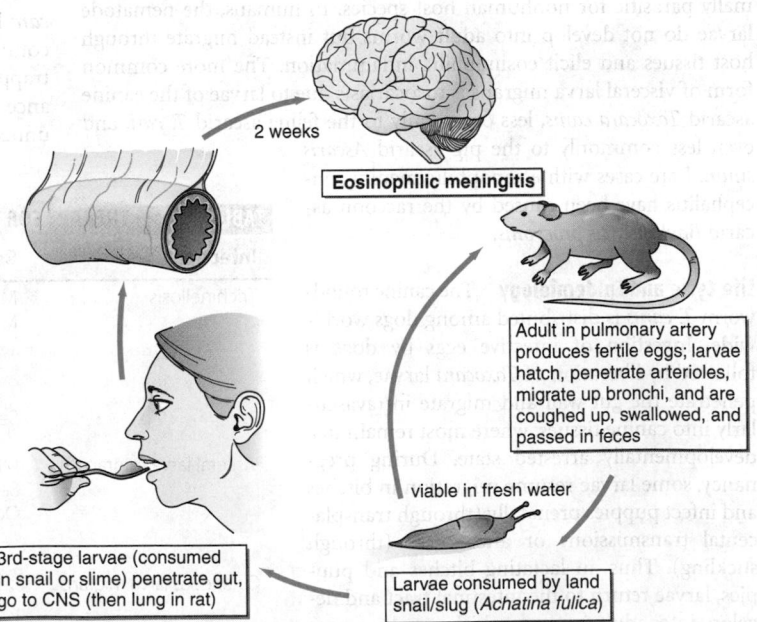

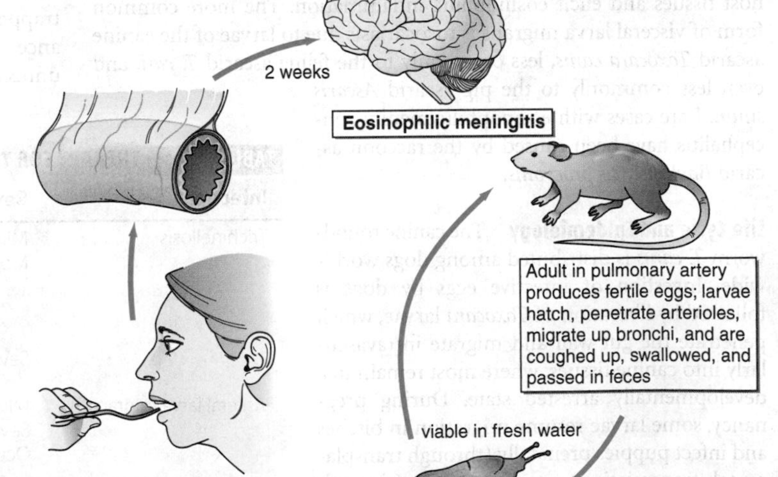
2 weeks
Eosinophilic meningitis
Adult in pulmonary artery produces fertile eggs; larvae hatch, penetrate arterioles, migrate up bronchi, and are coughed up, swallowed, and passed in feces
viable in fresh water
3rd-stage larvae (consumed in snail or slime) penetrate gut, go to CNS (then lung in rat)
Larvae consumed by land snail/slug (*Achatina fulica*)

FIGURE 209-3 Life cycle of *Angiostrongylus cantonensis* (rat lung worm). Also found in Southeast Asia, Pacific Islands, Cuba, Australia, Japan, China, Mauritius, and U.S. ports. *[Reprinted from Guerrant RL et al (eds): Tropical Infectious Diseases: Principles, Pathogens and Practice, 2d ed, p 1225. © 2006, with permission from Elsevier Science.]*

Life Cycle and Epidemiology Human gnathostomiasis occurs in many countries and is notably endemic in Southeast Asia and parts of China and Japan. In nature, the mature adult worms parasitize the gastrointestinal tract of dogs and cats. First-stage larvae hatch from eggs passed into water and are ingested by *Cyclops* species (water fleas). Infective third-stage larvae develop in the flesh of many animal species (including fish, frogs, eels, snakes, chickens, and ducks) that have eaten either infected *Cyclops* or another infected second intermediate host. Humans typically acquire the infection by eating raw or undercooked fish or poultry. Raw fish dishes, such as *som fak* in Thailand and *sashimi* in Japan, account for many cases of human gnathostomiasis. Some cases in Thailand result from the local practice of applying frog or snake flesh as a poultice.

Pathogenesis and Clinical Features Clinical symptoms are due to the aberrant migration of a single larva into cutaneous, visceral, neural, or ocular tissues. After invasion, larval migration may cause local inflammation, with pain, cough, or hematuria accompanied by fever and eosinophilia. Painful, itchy, migratory swellings may develop in the skin, particularly in the distal extremities or periorbital area. Cutaneous swellings usually last ~1 week but often recur intermittently over many years. Larval invasion of the eye can provoke a sight-threatening inflammatory response. Invasion of the CNS results in eosinophilic meningitis with myeloencephalitis, a serious complication due to ascending larval migration along a large nerve track. Patients characteristically present with agonizing radicular pain and paresthesias in the trunk or a limb, which are followed shortly by paraplegia. Cerebral involvement, with focal hemorrhages and tissue destruction, is often fatal.

Diagnosis and Treatment Cutaneous migratory swellings with marked peripheral eosinophilia, supported by an appropriate geographic and dietary history, generally constitute an adequate basis for a clinical diagnosis of gnathostomiasis. However, patients may present with ocular or cerebrospinal involvement without antecedent cutaneous swellings. In the latter case, eosinophilic pleocytosis is demonstrable (usually along with hemorrhagic or xanthochromic CSF), but worms are almost never recovered from CSF. Surgical removal of the parasite from subcutaneous or ocular tissue, though rarely feasible, is both diagnostic and therapeutic. Albendazole or ivermectin may be helpful (Table 209-1). At present, cerebrospinal involvement is managed with supportive measures and generally with a course of glucocorticoids. Gnathostomiasis can be prevented by adequate cooking of fish and poultry in endemic areas.

FURTHER READINGS

BARISANI-ASENBAUER T et al: Treatment of ocular toxocariasis with albendazole. J Ocul Pharmacol Ther 17:287, 2001

BOUCHARD O et al: Cutaneous larva migrans in travelers: A prospective study, with assessment of therapy with ivermectin. Clin Infect Dis 31:493, 2000

CDC DIVISION OF PARASITIC DISEASES. *www.cdc.gov/ncidod/dpd/default.htm*

CIANFERONI A et al: Visceral larva migrans associated with earthworm ingestion: Clinical evolution in an adolescent patient. Pediatrics 117:e336, 2006

LIGON BL: Gnathostomiasis: A review of a previously localized zoonosis now crossing numerous geographical boundaries. Semin Pediatr Infect Dis 16:137, 2005

MAGANA M et al: Gnathostomiasis: Clinicopathologic study. Am J Dermatopathol 26:91, 2004

MENARD A et al: Imported cutaneous gnathostomiasis: Report of five cases. Trans R Soc Trop Med Hyg 97:200, 2003

PULJIZ I et al: Electrocardiographic changes in trichinellosis: A retrospective study of 154 patients. Ann Trop Med Parasitol 99:403, 2005

SAKAI S et al: Pulmonary lesions associated with visceral larva migrans due to *Ascaris suum* or *Toxocara canis*: Imaging of six cases. AJR Am J Roentgenol 186:1697, 2006

SLOM TJ et al: An outbreak of eosinophilic meningitis caused by *Angiostrongylus cantonensis* in travelers returning from the Caribbean. N Engl J Med 346:668, 2002

TSAI HC et al: Outbreak of eosinophilic meningitis associated with drinking raw vegetable juice in southern Taiwan. Am J Trop Med Hyg 71:222, 2004

210 Intestinal Nematodes

Peter F. Weller, Thomas B. Nutman

More than a billion persons worldwide are infected with one or more species of intestinal nematodes. Table 210-1 summarizes biologic and clinical features of infections due to the major intestinal parasitic nematodes. These parasites are most common in regions with poor fecal sanitation, particularly in resource-poor countries in the tropics and subtropics, but they have also been seen with increasing frequency among immigrants and refugees to resource-rich countries. Although nematode infections are not usually fatal, they contribute to malnutrition and diminished work capacity. It is interesting that these helminth infections may protect some individuals from allergic disease. Humans may on occasion be infected with nematode parasites that ordinarily infect animals; these zoonotic infections produce diseases such as trichostrongyliasis, anisakiasis, capillariasis, and abdominal angiostrongyliasis.

Intestinal nematodes are roundworms; they range in length from 1 mm to many centimeters when mature (Table 210-1). Their life cycles are complex and highly varied; some species, including *Strongyloides stercoralis* and *Enterobius vermicularis*, can be transmitted directly from person to person, while others, such as *Ascaris lumbricoides*, *Necator americanus*, and *Ancylostoma duodenale*, require a soil phase for development. Because most helminth parasites do not self-replicate, the acquisition of a heavy burden of adult worms requires repeated exposure to the parasite in its infectious stage, whether larva or egg. Hence, clinical disease, as opposed to asymptomatic infection, generally develops only with prolonged residence in an endemic area. In persons with marginal nutrition, intestinal helminth infections may impair growth and development. Eosinophilia and elevated serum IgE levels are features of many helminthic infections and, when unexplained, should always prompt a search for occult helminthiasis. Significant protective immunity to intestinal nematodes appears not to develop in humans, although mechanisms of parasite immune evasion and host immune responses to these infections have not been elucidated in detail.

ASCARIASIS

A. lumbricoides is the largest intestinal nematode parasite of humans, reaching up to 40 cm in length. Most infected individuals have low worm burdens and are asymptomatic. Clinical disease arises from larval migration in the lungs or effects of the adult worms in the intestines.

Life Cycle Adult worms live in the lumen of the small intestine. Mature female *Ascaris* worms are extraordinarily fecund, each producing up to 240,000 eggs a day, which pass with the feces. Ascarid eggs, which are remarkably resistant to environmental stresses, become infective after several weeks of maturation in the soil and can remain infective for years. After infective eggs are swallowed, larvae hatched in the intestine invade the mucosa, migrate through the circulation to the lungs, break into the alveoli, ascend the bronchial tree, and return via

TABLE 210-1 MAJOR HUMAN INTESTINAL PARASITIC NEMATODES

	Parasitic Nematode				
Feature	***Ascaris lumbricoides* (Roundworm)**	***Necator americanus*, *Ancylostoma duodenale* (Hookworm)**	***Strongyloides stercoralis***	***Trichuris trichiura* (Whipworm)**	***Enterobius vermicularis* (Pinworm)**
Global prevalence in humans (millions)	1221	740	50	795	300
Endemic areas	Worldwide	Hot, humid regions	Hot, humid regions	Worldwide	Worldwide
Infective stage	Egg	Filariform larva	Filariform larva	Egg	Egg
Route of infection	Oral	Percutaneous	Percutaneous or autoinfection	Oral	Oral
Gastrointestinal location of worms	Jejunal lumen	Jejunal mucosa	Small-bowel mucosa	Cecum, colonic mucosa	Cecum, appendix
Adult worm size	15–40 cm	7–12 mm	2 mm	30–50 mm	8–13 mm (female)
Pulmonary passage of larvae	Yes	Yes	Yes	No	No
Incubation period[a] (days)	60–75	40–100	17–28	70–90	35–45
Longevity	1 y	*N. americanus*: 2–5 y *A. duodenale*: 6–8 y	Decades (owing to autoinfection)	5 y	2 months
Fecundity (eggs/day/worm)	240,000	*N. americanus*: 4000–10,000 *A. duodenale*: 10,000–25,000	5000–10,000	3000–7000	2000
Principal symptoms	Rarely gastrointestinal or biliary obstruction	Iron-deficiency anemia in heavy infection	Gastrointestinal symptoms; malabsorption or sepsis in hyperinfection	Gastrointestinal symptoms, anemia	Perianal pruritus
Diagnostic stage	Eggs in stool	Eggs in fresh stool, larvae in old stool	Larvae in stool or duodenal aspirate; sputum in hyperinfection	Eggs in stool	Eggs from perianal skin on cellulose acetate tape
Treatment	Mebendazole Albendazole Pyrantel pamoate Ivermectin	Mebendazole Pyrantel pamoate Albendazole	1. Ivermectin 2. Albendazole	Mebendazole Albendazole Ivermectin	Mebendazole Pyrantel pamoate Albendazole

[a]Time from infection to egg production by mature female worm.

swallowing to the small intestine, where they develop into adult worms. Between 2 and 3 months elapse between initial infection and egg production. Adult worms live for 1–2 years.

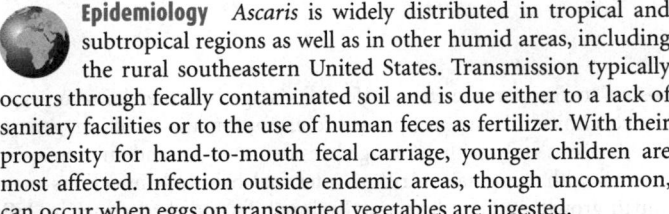

Epidemiology *Ascaris* is widely distributed in tropical and subtropical regions as well as in other humid areas, including the rural southeastern United States. Transmission typically occurs through fecally contaminated soil and is due either to a lack of sanitary facilities or to the use of human feces as fertilizer. With their propensity for hand-to-mouth fecal carriage, younger children are most affected. Infection outside endemic areas, though uncommon, can occur when eggs on transported vegetables are ingested.

Clinical Features During the lung phase of larval migration, ~9–12 days after egg ingestion, patients may develop an irritating nonproductive cough and burning substernal discomfort that is aggravated by coughing or deep inspiration. Dyspnea and blood-tinged sputum are less common. Fever is usually reported. Eosinophilia develops during this symptomatic phase and subsides slowly over weeks. Chest x-rays may reveal evidence of eosinophilic pneumonitis (Löffler's syndrome), with rounded infiltrates a few millimeters to several centimeters in size. These infiltrates may be transient and intermittent, clearing after several weeks. Where there is seasonal transmission of the parasite, seasonal pneumonitis with eosinophilia may develop in previously infected and sensitized hosts.

In established infections, adult worms in the small intestine usually cause no symptoms. In heavy infections, particularly in children, a large bolus of entangled worms can cause pain and small-bowel obstruction, sometimes complicated by perforation, intussusception, or volvulus. Single worms may cause disease when they migrate into aberrant sites. A large worm can enter and occlude the biliary tree, causing biliary colic, cholecystitis, cholangitis, pancreatitis, or (rarely) intrahepatic abscesses. Migration of an adult worm up the esophagus can provoke coughing and oral expulsion of the worm. In highly endemic areas, intestinal and biliary ascariasis can rival acute appendicitis and gallstones as causes of surgical acute abdomen.

Laboratory Findings Most cases of ascariasis can be diagnosed by microscopic detection of characteristic *Ascaris* eggs (65 by 45 μm) in fecal samples. Occasionally, patients present after passing an adult worm—identifiable by its large size and smooth cream-colored surface—in the stool or through the mouth or nose. During the early transpulmonary migratory phase, when eosinophilic pneumonitis occurs, larvae can be found in sputum or gastric aspirates before diagnostic eggs appear in the stool. The eosinophilia that is prominent during this early stage usually decreases to minimal levels in established infection. Adult worms may be visualized, occasionally serendipitously, on contrast studies of the gastrointestinal tract. A plain abdominal film may reveal masses of worms in gas-filled loops of bowel in patients with intestinal obstruction. Pancreaticobiliary worms can be detected by ultrasound and endoscopic retrograde cholangiopancreatography; the latter method also has been used to extract biliary *Ascaris* worms.

℞ ASCARIASIS

Ascariasis should always be treated to prevent potentially serious complications. Albendazole (400 mg once), mebendazole (500 mg once), or ivermectin (150–200 μg/kg once) is effective. These medications are contraindicated in pregnancy, however. Pyrantel pamoate (11 mg/kg once; maximum, 1 g) is safe in pregnancy. Mild diarrhea and abdominal pain are uncommon side effects of these agents. Partial intestinal obstruction should be managed with nasogastric suction, IV fluid administration, and instillation of piperazine through the nasogastric tube, but complete obstruction and its severe complications require immediate surgical intervention.

HOOKWORM

Two hookworm species (*A. duodenale* and *N. americanus*) are responsible for human infections. Most infected individuals are asymptomatic. Hookworm disease develops from a combination of factors—a heavy worm burden, a prolonged duration of infection, and an inadequate iron intake—and results in iron-deficiency anemia and, on occasion, hypoproteinemia.

Life Cycle Adult hookworms, which are ~1 cm long, use buccal teeth (*Ancylostoma*) or cutting plates (*Necator*) to attach to the small-bowel mucosa and suck blood (0.2 mL/d per *Ancylostoma* adult) and interstitial fluid. The adult hookworms produce thousands of eggs daily. The eggs are deposited with feces in soil, where rhabditiform larvae hatch and develop over a 1-week period into infectious filariform larvae. Infective larvae penetrate the skin and reach the lungs by way of the bloodstream. There they invade alveoli and ascend the airways before being swallowed and reaching the small intestine. The prepatent period from skin invasion to appearance of eggs in the feces is ~6–8 weeks, but it may be longer with *A. duodenale*. Larvae of *A. duodenale*, if swallowed, can survive and develop directly in the intestinal mucosa. Adult hookworms may survive over a decade but usually live ~6–8 years for *A. duodenale* and 2–5 years for *N. americanus*.

Epidemiology *A. duodenale* is prevalent in southern Europe, North Africa, and northern Asia, and *N. americanus* is the predominant species in the western hemisphere and equatorial Africa. The two species overlap in many tropical regions, particularly Southeast Asia. In most areas, older children have the highest incidence and greatest intensity of hookworm infection. In rural areas where fields are fertilized with human feces, older working adults also may be heavily affected.

Clinical Features Most hookworm infections are asymptomatic. Infective larvae may provoke pruritic maculopapular dermatitis ("ground itch") at the site of skin penetration as well as serpiginous tracks of subcutaneous migration (similar to those of cutaneous larva migrans; Chap. 209) in previously sensitized hosts. Larvae migrating through the lungs occasionally cause mild transient pneumonitis, but this condition develops less frequently in hookworm infection than in ascariasis. In the early intestinal phase, infected persons may develop epigastric pain (often with postprandial accentuation), inflammatory diarrhea, or other abdominal symptoms accompanied by eosinophilia. The major consequence of chronic hookworm infection is iron deficiency. Symptoms are minimal if iron intake is adequate, but marginally nourished individuals develop symptoms of progressive iron-deficiency anemia and hypoproteinemia, including weakness and shortness of breath.

Laboratory Findings The diagnosis is established by the finding of characteristic 40- by 60-μm oval hookworm eggs in the feces. Stool-concentration procedures may be required to detect light infections. Eggs of the two species are indistinguishable by light microscopy. In a stool sample that is not fresh, the eggs may have hatched to release rhabditiform larvae, which need to be differentiated from those of *S. stercoralis*. Hypochromic microcytic anemia, occasionally with eosinophilia or hypoalbuminemia, is characteristic of hookworm disease.

Rx HOOKWORM INFECTION

Hookworm infection can be eradicated with several safe and highly effective anthelmintic drugs, including albendazole (400 mg once), mebendazole (500 mg once), and pyrantel pamoate (11 mg/kg for 3 days). Mild iron-deficiency anemia can often be treated with oral iron alone. Severe hookworm disease with protein loss and malabsorption necessitates nutritional support and oral iron replacement along with deworming.

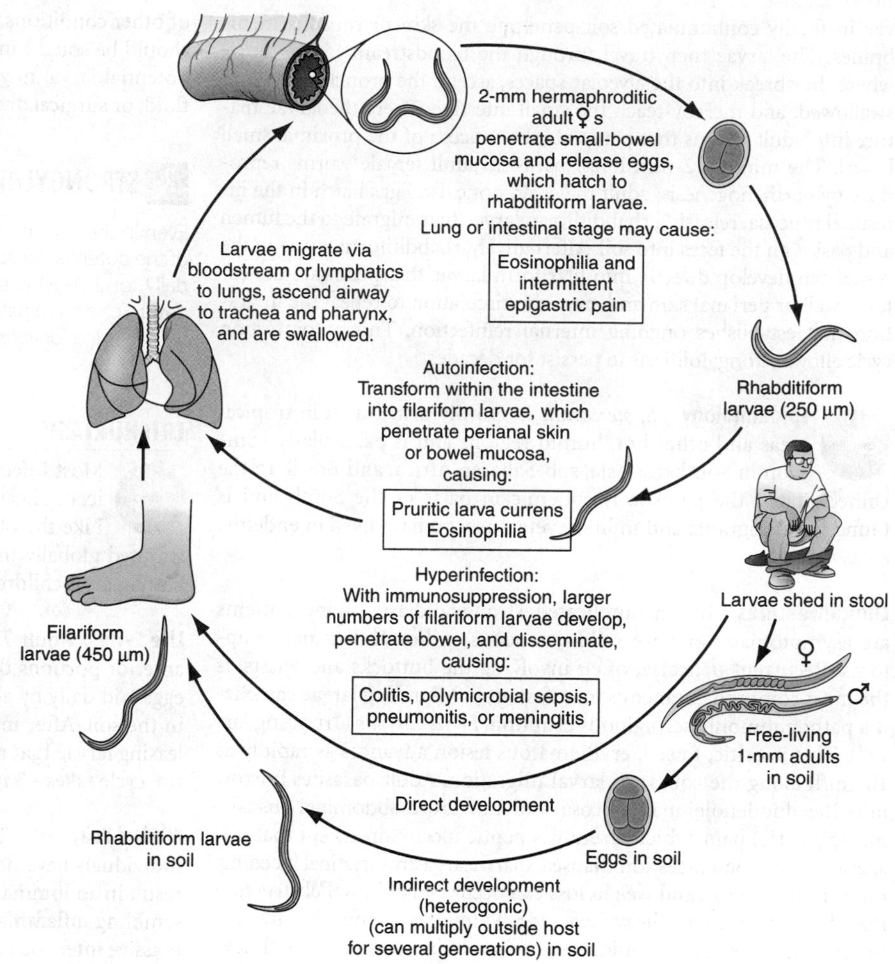

FIGURE 210-1 Life cycle of *Strongyloides stercoralis*. *[Adapted from Guerrant RL et al (eds): Tropical Infectious Diseases: Principles, Pathogens and Practice, 2d ed, p 1276. © 2006, with permission from Elsevier Science.]*

Ancylostoma caninum* and *Ancylostoma braziliense *A. caninum*, the canine hookworm, has been identified as a cause of human eosinophilic enteritis, especially in northeastern Australia. In this zoonotic infection, adult hookworms attach to the small intestine (where they may be visualized by endoscopy) and elicit abdominal pain and intense local eosinophilia. Treatment with mebendazole (100 mg twice daily for 3 days) or albendazole (400 mg once) or endoscopic removal is effective. Both of these animal hookworm species can cause cutaneous larva migrans ("creeping eruption"; Chap. 209).

STRONGYLOIDIASIS

S. stercoralis is distinguished by its ability—unusual among helminths—to replicate in the human host. This capacity permits ongoing cycles of autoinfection as infective larvae are internally produced. Strongyloidiasis can thus persist for decades without further exposure of the host to exogenous infective larvae. In immunocompromised hosts, large numbers of invasive *Strongyloides* larvae can disseminate widely and can be fatal.

Life Cycle In addition to a parasitic cycle of development, *Strongyloides* can undergo a free-living cycle of development in the soil (Fig. 210-1). This adaptability facilitates the parasite's survival in the absence of mammalian hosts. Rhabditiform larvae passed in feces can transform into infectious filariform larvae either directly or after a free-living phase of development. Humans acquire strongyloidiasis when filariform larvae in fecally contaminated soil penetrate the skin or mucous membranes. The larvae then travel through the bloodstream to the lungs, where they break into the alveolar spaces, ascend the bronchial tree, are swallowed, and thereby reach the small intestine. There the larvae mature into adult worms that penetrate the mucosa of the proximal small bowel. The minute (2-mm-long) parasitic adult female worms reproduce by parthenogenesis; adult males do not exist. Eggs hatch in the intestinal mucosa, releasing rhabditiform larvae that migrate to the lumen and pass with the feces into soil. Alternatively, rhabditiform larvae in the bowel can develop directly into filariform larvae that penetrate the colonic wall or perianal skin and enter the circulation to repeat the migration that establishes ongoing internal reinfection. This autoinfection cycle allows strongyloidiasis to persist for decades.

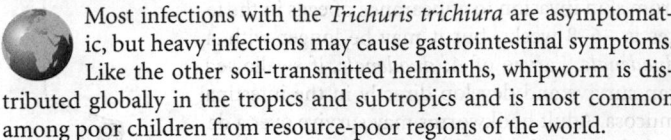

Epidemiology *S. stercoralis* is spottily distributed in tropical areas and other hot, humid regions and is particularly common in Southeast Asia, sub-Saharan Africa, and Brazil. In the United States, the parasite is endemic in parts of the South and is found in immigrants and military veterans who have lived in endemic areas abroad.

Clinical Features In uncomplicated strongyloidiasis, many patients are asymptomatic or have mild cutaneous and/or abdominal symptoms. Recurrent urticaria, often involving the buttocks and wrists, is the most common cutaneous manifestation. Migrating larvae can elicit a pathognomonic serpiginous eruption, *larva currens* ("running larva"). This pruritic, raised, erythematous lesion advances as rapidly as 10 cm/h along the course of larval migration. Adult parasites burrow into the duodenojejunal mucosa and can cause abdominal (usually midepigastric) pain, which resembles peptic ulcer pain except that it is aggravated by food ingestion. Nausea, diarrhea, gastrointestinal bleeding, mild chronic colitis, and weight loss can occur. Small-bowel obstruction may develop with early, heavy infection. Pulmonary symptoms are rare in uncomplicated strongyloidiasis. Eosinophilia is common, with levels fluctuating over time.

The ongoing autoinfection cycle of strongyloidiasis is normally contained by unknown factors of the host's immune system. Abrogation of host immunity, especially with glucocorticoid therapy and much less commonly with other immunosuppressive medications, leads to hyperinfection, with the generation of large numbers of filariform larvae. Colitis, enteritis, or malabsorption may develop. In disseminated strongyloidiasis, larvae may invade not only gastrointestinal tissues and the lungs but also the central nervous system, peritoneum, liver, and kidneys. Moreover, bacteremia may develop because of the passage of enteric flora through disrupted mucosal barriers. Gram-negative sepsis, pneumonia, or meningitis may complicate or dominate the clinical course. Eosinophilia is often absent in severely infected patients. Disseminated strongyloidiasis, particularly in patients with unsuspected infection who are given glucocorticoids, can be fatal. Strongyloidiasis is a frequent complication of infection with human T cell lymphotropic virus type I, but disseminated strongyloidiasis is not common among patients infected with HIV.

Diagnosis In uncomplicated strongyloidiasis, the finding of rhabditiform larvae in feces is diagnostic. Rhabditiform larvae are ~250 μm long, with a short buccal cavity that distinguishes them from hookworm larvae. In uncomplicated infections, few larvae are passed and single stool examinations detect only about one-third of cases. Serial examinations and the use of the agar plate detection method improve the sensitivity of stool diagnosis. In uncomplicated strongyloidiasis (but not in hyperinfection), stool examinations may be repeatedly negative. *Strongyloides* larvae may also be found by sampling of the duodenojejunal contents by aspiration or biopsy. An enzyme-linked immunosorbent assay for serum antibodies to antigens of *Strongyloides* is a sensitive method of diagnosing uncomplicated infections. Such serologic testing should be performed for patients whose geographic histories indicate potential exposure, especially those who exhibit eosinophilia and/or are candidates for glucocorticoid treatment of other conditions. In disseminated strongyloidiasis, filariform larvae should be sought in stool as well as in samples obtained from sites of potential larval migration, including sputum, bronchoalveolar lavage fluid, or surgical drainage fluid.

Rx STRONGYLOIDIASIS

Even in the asymptomatic state, strongyloidiasis must be treated because of the potential for subsequent fatal hyperinfection. Ivermectin (200 μg/kg daily for 2 days) is more effective than albendazole (400 mg daily for 3 days). For disseminated strongyloidiasis, treatment with ivermectin should be extended for at least 5–7 days or until the parasites are eradicated.

TRICHURIASIS

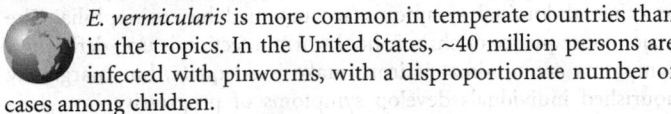

Most infections with the *Trichuris trichiura* are asymptomatic, but heavy infections may cause gastrointestinal symptoms. Like the other soil-transmitted helminths, whipworm is distributed globally in the tropics and subtropics and is most common among poor children from resource-poor regions of the world.

Life Cycle Adult *Trichuris* worms reside in the colon and cecum, the anterior portions threaded into the superficial mucosa. Thousands of eggs laid daily by adult female worms pass with the feces and mature in the soil. After ingestion, infective eggs hatch in the duodenum, releasing larvae that mature before migrating to the large bowel. The entire cycle takes ~3 months, and adult worms may live for several years.

Clinical Features Tissue reactions to *Trichuris* are mild. Most infected individuals have no symptoms or eosinophilia. Heavy infections may result in abdominal pain, anorexia, and bloody or mucoid diarrhea resembling inflammatory bowel disease. Rectal prolapse can result from massive infections in children, who often suffer from malnourishment and other diarrheal illnesses. Moderately heavy *Trichuris* burdens also contribute to growth retardation.

Diagnosis and Treatment The characteristic 50- by 20-μm lemon-shaped *Trichuris* eggs are readily detected on stool examination. Adult worms, which are 3–5 cm long, are occasionally seen on proctoscopy. Mebendazole (500 mg once) or albendazole (400 mg daily for 3 doses) is safe and effective for treatment. Ivermectin (200 μg/kg daily for 3 doses) is also safe but is not quite as efficacious as the benzimidazoles.

ENTEROBIASIS (PINWORM)

E. vermicularis is more common in temperate countries than in the tropics. In the United States, ~40 million persons are infected with pinworms, with a disproportionate number of cases among children.

Life Cycle and Epidemiology *Enterobius* adult worms are ~1 cm long and dwell in the cecum. Gravid female worms migrate nocturnally into the perianal region and release up to 10,000 immature eggs each. The eggs become infective within hours and are transmitted by hand-to-mouth passage. From ingested eggs, larvae hatch and mature into adults. This life cycle takes ~1 month, and adult worms survive for ~2 months. Self-infection results from perianal scratching and transport of infective eggs on the hands or under the nails to the mouth. Because of the ease of person-to-person spread, pinworm infections are common among family members.

Clinical Features Most pinworm infections are asymptomatic. Perianal pruritus is the cardinal symptom. The itching, which is often worse at night as a result of the nocturnal migration of the female worms, may lead to excoriation and bacterial superinfection. Heavy infections have been claimed to cause abdominal pain and weight loss. On rare occasions, pinworms invade the female genital tract, causing vulvovaginitis and pelvic or peritoneal granulomas. Eosinophilia is uncommon.

Diagnosis Since pinworm eggs are not released in feces, the diagnosis cannot be made by conventional fecal ova and parasites tests. Instead, eggs are detected by the application of clear cellulose acetate tape to the perianal region in the morning. After the tape is transferred to a slide, microscopic examination will detect pinworm eggs, which are oval, measure 55 by 25 μm, and are flattened along one side.

℞ ENTEROBIASIS

Infected children and adults should be treated with mebendazole (100 mg once), albendazole (400 mg once), or pyrantel pamoate (11 mg/kg once; maximum, 1 g), with the same treatment repeated after 2 weeks. Treatment of household members is advocated to eliminate asymptomatic reservoirs of potential reinfection.

TRICHOSTRONGYLIASIS

Trichostrongylus species, which are normally parasites of herbivorous animals, occasionally infect humans, particularly in Asia and Africa. Humans acquire the infection by accidentally ingesting *Trichostrongylus* larvae on contaminated leafy vegetables. The larvae do not migrate in humans but mature directly into adult worms in the small bowel. These worms ingest far less blood than hookworms; most infected persons are asymptomatic, but heavy infections may give rise to mild anemia and eosinophilia. *Trichostrongylus* eggs in stool examinations resemble those of hookworms but are larger (85 by 115 μm). Treatment consists of mebendazole or albendazole (Chap. 201).

ANISAKIASIS

Anisakiasis is a gastrointestinal infection caused by the accidental ingestion in uncooked saltwater fish of nematode larvae belonging to the family Anisakidae. The incidence of anisakiasis in the United States has increased as a result of the growing popularity of raw fish dishes. Most cases occur in Japan, the Netherlands, and Chile, where raw fish—sashimi, pickled green herring, and ceviche, respectively—are national culinary staples. Anisakid nematodes parasitize large sea mammals such as whales, dolphins, and seals. As part of a complex parasitic life cycle involving marine food chains, infectious larvae migrate to the musculature of a variety of fish. Both *Anisakis simplex* and *Pseudoterranova decipiens* have been implicated in human anisakiasis, but an identical gastric syndrome may be caused by the red larvae of eustrongylid parasites of fish-eating birds.

When humans consume infected raw fish, live larvae may be coughed up within 48 h. Alternatively, larvae may immediately penetrate the mucosa of the stomach. Within hours, violent upper abdominal pain accompanied by nausea and occasionally vomiting ensues, mimicking an acute abdomen. The diagnosis can be established by direct visualization on upper endoscopy, outlining of the worm by contrast radiographic studies, or histopathologic examination of extracted tissue. Extraction of the burrowing larvae during endoscopy is curative. In addition, larvae may pass to the small bowel, where they penetrate the mucosa and provoke a vigorous eosinophilic granulomatous response. Symptoms may appear 1–2 weeks after the infective meal, with intermittent abdominal pain, diarrhea, nausea, and fever resembling the manifestations of Crohn's disease. The diagnosis may be suggested by barium studies and confirmed by curative surgical resection of a granuloma in which the worm is embedded. Anisakid eggs are not found in the stool, since the larvae do not mature in humans. Anisakid larvae in saltwater fish are killed by cooking to 60°C, freezing at –20°C for 3 days, or commercial blast freezing, but not usually by salting, marinating, or cold smoking. No medical treatment is available; surgical or endoscopic removal should be undertaken.

CAPILLARIASIS

Intestinal capillariasis is caused by ingestion of raw fish infected with *Capillaria philippinensis*. Subsequent autoinfection can lead to a severe wasting syndrome. The disease occurs in the Philippines and Thailand and, on occasion, elsewhere in Asia. The natural cycle of *C. philippinensis* involves fish from fresh and brackish water. When humans eat infected raw fish, the larvae mature in the intestine into adult worms, which produce invasive larvae that cause intestinal inflammation and villus loss. Capillariasis has an insidious onset with nonspecific abdominal pain and watery diarrhea. If untreated, progressive autoinfection can lead to protein-losing enteropathy and severe malabsorption and ultimately to death from cachexia, cardiac failure, or superinfection. The diagnosis is established by identification of the characteristic peanut-shaped (20- by 40-μm) eggs on stool examination. Severely ill patients require hospitalization and supportive therapy in addition to prolonged anthelmintic treatment with mebendazole or albendazole (Chap. 201).

ABDOMINAL ANGIOSTRONGYLIASIS

Abdominal angiostrongyliasis is found in Latin America and Africa. The zoonotic parasite *Angiostrongylus costaricensis* causes eosinophilic ileocolitis after the ingestion of contaminated vegetation. *A. costaricensis* normally parasitizes the cotton rat and other rodents, with slugs and snails serving as intermediate hosts. Humans become infected by accidentally ingesting infective larvae in mollusk slime deposited on fruits and vegetables; children are at highest risk. The larvae penetrate the gut wall and migrate to the mesenteric artery, where they develop into adult worms. Eggs deposited in the gut wall provoke an intense eosinophilic granulomatous reaction, and adult worms may cause mesenteric arteritis, thrombosis, or frank bowel infarction. Symptoms may mimic those of appendicitis, including abdominal pain and tenderness, fever, vomiting, and a palpable mass in the right iliac fossa. Leukocytosis and eosinophilia are prominent. A barium enema may reveal ileocecal-filling defects, but a definitive diagnosis is usually made surgically with partial bowel resection. Pathologic study reveals a thickened bowel wall with eosinophilic granulomas surrounding the *Angiostrongylus* eggs. In nonsurgical cases, the diagnosis rests solely on clinical grounds because larvae and eggs cannot be detected in the stool. Medical therapy for abdominal angiostrongyliasis (mebendazole, thiabendazole; Chap. 201) is of uncertain efficacy. Careful observation and surgical resection for severe symptoms are the mainstays of treatment.

FURTHER READINGS

BETHONY J et al: Soil-transmitted helminth infections: Ascariasis, trichuriasis, and hookworm. Lancet 367:1521, 2006

HOTEZ PJ et al: Hookworm infection. N Engl J Med 351:799, 2004

KEISER PB et al: *Strongyloides stercoralis* in the immunocompromised population. Clin Microbiol Rev 17:208, 2004

LAM CS et al: Disseminated strongyloidiasis: A retrospective study of clinical course and outcome. Eur J Clin Microbiol Infect Dis 25:14, 2006

LIM S et al: Complicated and fatal *Strongyloides* infection in Canadians: Risk factors, diagnosis and management. CMAJ 171:479, 2004

LU LH et al: Human intestinal capillariasis (*Capillaria philippinensis*) in Taiwan. Am J Trop Med Hyg 74:810, 2006

SHAH OJ et al: Biliary ascariasis: A review. World J Surg 30:1500, 2006

211 Filarial and Related Infections

Thomas B. Nutman, Peter F. Weller

Filarial worms are nematodes that dwell in the subcutaneous tissues and the lymphatics. Eight filarial species infect humans (Table 211-1); of these, four—*Wuchereria bancrofti*, *Brugia malayi*, *Onchocerca volvulus*, and *Loa loa*—are responsible for most serious filarial infections. Filarial parasites, which infect an estimated 170 million persons worldwide, are transmitted by specific species of mosquitoes or other arthropods and have a complex life cycle including infective larval stages carried by insects and adult worms that reside in either lymphatic or subcutaneous tissues of humans. The offspring of adults are microfilariae, which, depending on their species, are 200–250 μm long and 5–7 μm wide, may or may not be enveloped in a loose sheath, and either circulate in the blood or migrate through the skin (Table 211-1). To complete the life cycle, microfilariae are ingested by the arthropod vector and develop over 1–2 weeks into new infective larvae. Adult worms live for many years, whereas microfilariae survive for 3–36 months. The *Rickettsia*-like endosymbiont *Wolbachia* has been found intracellularly in all stages of *Brugia*, *Wuchereria*, *Mansonella*, and *Onchocerca* and is viewed as a possible target for antifilarial chemotherapy.

Usually, infection is established only with repeated, prolonged exposures to infective larvae. Since the clinical manifestations of filarial diseases develop relatively slowly, these infections should be considered to induce chronic diseases with possible long-term debilitating effects. In terms of the nature, severity, and timing of clinical manifestations, patients with filarial infections who are native to endemic areas and undergo lifelong exposure may differ significantly from those who are travelers or who have recently moved to these areas. Characteristically, filarial disease is more acute and intense in newly exposed individuals than in natives of endemic areas.

LYMPHATIC FILARIASIS

Lymphatic filariasis is caused by *W. bancrofti*, *B. malayi*, or *B. timori*. The threadlike adult parasites reside in lymphatic channels or lymph nodes, where they may remain viable for more than two decades.

EPIDEMIOLOGY

W. bancrofti, the most widely distributed human filarial parasite, affects an estimated 115 million people and is found throughout the tropics and subtropics, including Asia and the Pacific Islands, Africa, areas of South America, and the Caribbean basin. Humans are the only definitive host for the parasite. Generally, the subperiodic form is found only in the Pacific Islands; elsewhere, *W. bancrofti* is nocturnally periodic. (Nocturnally periodic forms of microfilariae are scarce in peripheral blood by day and increase at night, whereas subperiodic forms are present in peripheral blood at all times and reach maximal levels in the afternoon.) Natural vectors for *W. bancrofti* are *Culex fatigans* mosquitoes in urban settings and anopheline or aedean mosquitoes in rural areas.

Brugian filariasis due to *B. malayi* occurs primarily in China, India, Indonesia, Korea, Japan, Malaysia, and the Philippines. *B. malayi* also has two forms distinguished by the periodicity of microfilaremia. The more common nocturnal form is transmitted in areas of coastal rice fields, while the subperiodic form is found in forests. *B. malayi* naturally infects cats as well as humans. *B. timori* exists only on islands of the Indonesian archipelago.

PATHOLOGY

The principal pathologic changes result from inflammatory damage to the lymphatics, which is typically caused by adult worms and not by microfilariae. Adult worms live in afferent lymphatics or sinuses of lymph nodes and cause lymphatic dilatation and thickening of the vessel walls. The infiltration of plasma cells, eosinophils, and macrophages in and around the infected vessels, along with endothelial and connective tissue proliferation, leads to tortuosity of the lymphatics and damaged or incompetent lymph valves. Lymphedema and chronic-stasis changes with hard or brawny edema develop in the overlying skin. These consequences of filariasis are due both to direct effects of the worms and to the inflammatory response of the host to the parasite. Inflammatory responses are believed to cause the granulomatous and proliferative processes that precede total lymphatic obstruction. It is thought that the lymphatic vessel remains patent as long as the worm remains viable and that the death of the worm leads to enhanced granulomatous reaction and fibrosis. Lymphatic obstruction results, and, despite collateralization of the lymphatics, lymphatic function is compromised.

CLINICAL FEATURES

The most common presentations of the lymphatic filariases are asymptomatic (or subclinical) microfilaremia, hydrocele (Fig. 211-1), acute adenolymphangitis (ADL), and chronic lymphatic disease. In areas where *W. bancrofti* or *B. malayi* is endemic, the overwhelming majority of infected individuals have few overt clinical manifestations of filarial infection despite large numbers of circulating microfilariae in the peripheral blood. Although they may be clinically asymptomatic, virtually all persons with *W. bancrofti* or *B. malayi* microfilaremia have some degree of subclinical disease that includes microscopic hematuria and/or proteinuria, dilated (and tortuous) lymphatics (visualized

TABLE 211-1 CHARACTERISTICS OF THE FILARIAE

Organism	Periodicity	Distribution	Vector	Location of Adult	Microfilarial Location	Sheath
Wuchereria bancrofti	Nocturnal	Cosmopolitan areas worldwide, including South America and Africa	*Culex* (mosquitoes)	Lymphatic tissue	Blood	+
		Mainly India	*Anopheles* (mosquitoes)			
		China, Indonesia	*Aedes* (mosquitoes)			
	Subperiodic	Eastern Pacific	*Aedes* (mosquitoes)	Lymphatic tissue	Blood	+
Brugia malayi	Nocturnal	Southeast Asia, Indonesia, India	*Mansonia, Anopheles* (mosquitoes)	Lymphatic tissue	Blood	+
	Subperiodic	Indonesia, Southeast Asia	*Coquillettidia, Mansonia* (mosquitoes)	Lymphatic tissue	Blood	+
B. timori	Nocturnal	Indonesia	*Anopheles* (mosquitoes)	Lymphatic tissue	Blood	+
Loa loa	Diurnal	West and Central Africa	*Chrysops* (deerflies)	Subcutaneous tissue	Blood	+
Onchocerca volvulus	None	South and Central America, Africa	*Simulium* (blackflies)	Subcutaneous tissue	Skin, eye	–
Mansonella ozzardi	None	South and Central America Caribbean	*Culicoides* (midges) *Simulium* (blackflies)	Undetermined site	Blood	–
M. perstans	None	South and Central America, Africa	*Culicoides* (midges)	Body cavities, mesentery, perirenal tissue	Blood	–
M. streptocerca	None	West and Central Africa	*Culicoides* (midges)	Subcutaneous tissue	Skin	–

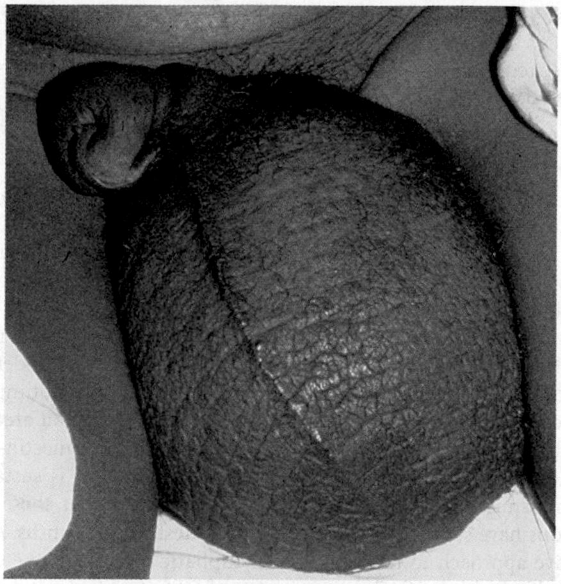

FIGURE 211-1 Hydrocele associated with *Wuchereria bancrofti* infection.

by imaging), and—in men—scrotal lymphangiectasia (detectable by ultrasound). In spite of these findings, the majority of individuals appear to remain clinically asymptomatic for years; relatively few progress to either acute or chronic disease.

ADL is characterized by high fever, lymphatic inflammation (lymphangitis and lymphadenitis), and transient local edema. The lymphangitis is retrograde, extending peripherally from the lymph node draining the area where the adult parasites reside. Regional lymph nodes are often enlarged, and the entire lymphatic channel can become indurated and inflamed. Concomitant local thrombophlebitis can occur as well. In brugian filariasis, a single local abscess may form along the involved lymphatic tract and subsequently rupture to the surface. The lymphadenitis and lymphangitis can involve both the upper and lower extremities in both bancroftian and brugian filariasis, but involvement of the genital lymphatics occurs almost exclusively with *W. bancrofti* infection. This genital involvement can be manifested by funiculitis, epididymitis, and scrotal pain and tenderness. In endemic areas, another type of acute disease—dermatolymphangioadenitis (DLA)—is recognized as a syndrome that includes high fever, chills, myalgias, and headache. Edematous inflammatory plaques clearly demarcated from normal skin are seen. Vesicles, ulcers, and hyperpigmentation may also be noted. There is often a history of trauma, burns, radiation, insect bites, punctiform lesions, or chemical injury. Entry lesions, especially in the interdigital area, are common. DLA is often diagnosed as cellulitis.

If lymphatic damage progresses, transient lymphedema can develop into lymphatic obstruction and the permanent changes associated with elephantiasis (Fig. 211-2). Brawny edema follows early pitting edema, and thickening of the subcutaneous tissues and hyperkeratosis occur. Fissuring of the skin develops, as do hyperplastic changes. Superinfection of these poorly vascularized tissues becomes a problem. In bancroftian filariasis, in which genital involvement is common, hydroceles may develop (Fig. 211-1); in advanced stages, this condition may evolve into scrotal lymphedema and scrotal elephantiasis. Furthermore, if there is obstruction of the retroperitoneal lymphatics, the increased renal lymphatic pressure leads to rupture of the renal lymphatics and the development of chyluria, which is usually intermittent and most prominent in the morning.

The clinical manifestations of filarial infections in travelers or transmigrants who have recently entered an endemic region are distinctive. Given a sufficient number of bites by infected vectors, usually over a 3- to 6-month period, recently exposed patients can develop acute lymphatic or scrotal inflammation with or without urticaria and localized angioedema. Lymphadenitis of epitrochlear, axillary, femoral, or inguinal lymph nodes is often followed by retrogradely evolving lymphangitis. Acute attacks are short-lived and are not usually accompanied by fever. With prolonged exposure to infected mosquitoes, these attacks, if untreated, become more severe and lead to permanent lymphatic inflammation and obstruction.

DIAGNOSIS

A definitive diagnosis can be made only by detection of the parasites and hence can be difficult. Adult worms localized in lymphatic vessels or nodes are largely inaccessible. Microfilariae can be found in blood, in hydrocele fluid, or (occasionally) in other body fluids. Such fluids can be examined microscopically, either directly or—for greater sensitivity—after concentration of the parasites by the passage of fluid through a polycarbonate cylindrical pore filter (pore size, 3 μm) or by the centrifugation of fluid fixed in 2% formalin (Knott's concentration technique). The timing of blood collection is critical and should be based on the periodicity of the microfilariae in the endemic region involved. Many infected individuals do not have microfilaremia, and definitive diagnosis in such cases can be difficult. Assays for circulating antigens of *W. bancrofti* permit the diagnosis of microfilaremic and cryptic (amicrofilaremic) infection. Two tests are commercially available: an enzyme-linked immunosorbent assay (ELISA) and a rapid-format immunochromatographic card test. Both assays have sensitivities of 96–100% and specificities approaching 100%. There are currently no tests for circulating antigens in brugian filariasis.

Polymerase chain reaction (PCR)–based assays for DNA of *W. bancrofti* and *B. malayi* in blood have been developed. A number of studies indicate that this diagnostic method is of equivalent or greater sensitivity compared with parasitologic methods, detecting patent infection in almost all infected individuals.

In cases of suspected lymphatic filariasis, examination of the scrotum or the female breast by means of high-frequency ultrasound in conjunction with Doppler techniques may result in the identification of motile adult worms within dilated lymphatics. Worms may be visualized in the lymphatics of the spermatic cord in up to 80% of infected men. Live adult worms have a distinctive pattern of movement within the lymphatic vessels (termed the *filaria dance sign*). Radionuclide lymphoscintigraphic imaging of the limbs reliably demonstrates widespread lymphatic abnormalities in both asymptomatic microfilaremic persons and those with clinical manifestations of lymphatic pathology. While of potential utility in the delineation of anatomic changes associated with

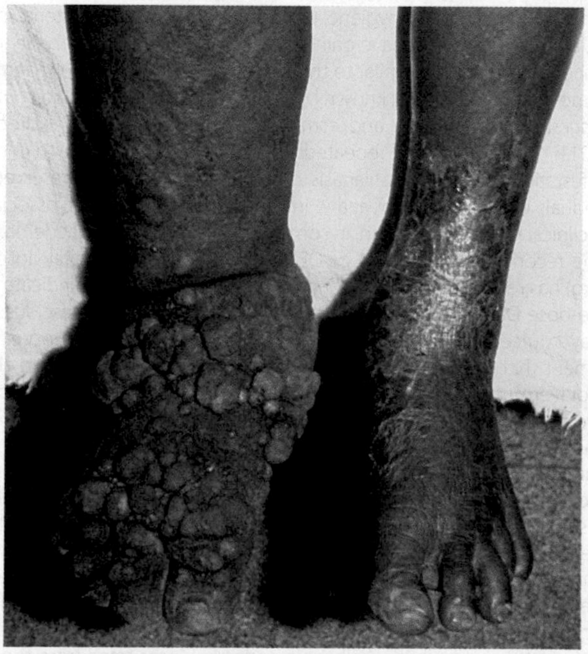

FIGURE 211-2 Elephantiasis of the lower extremity associated with *Wuchereria bancrofti* infection.

infection, lymphoscintigraphy is unlikely to assume primacy in the diagnostic evaluation of individuals with suspected infection; it is principally a research tool, although it has been used more widely for assessment of lymphedema of any cause. Eosinophilia and elevated serum concentrations of IgE and antifilarial antibody support the diagnosis of lymphatic filariasis. There is, however, extensive cross-reactivity between filarial antigens and antigens of other helminths, including the common intestinal roundworms; thus, interpretations of serologic findings can be difficult. In addition, residents of endemic areas can become sensitized to filarial antigens (and thus be serologically positive) through exposure to infected mosquitoes without having patent filarial infections.

The ADL associated with lymphatic filariasis must be distinguished from thrombophlebitis, infection, and trauma. Retrogradely evolving lymphangitis is a characteristic feature that helps distinguish filarial lymphangitis from ascending bacterial lymphangitis. Chronic filarial lymphedema must also be distinguished from the lymphedema of malignancy, postoperative scarring, trauma, chronic edematous states, and congenital lymphatic system abnormalities.

Rx LYMPHATIC FILARIASIS

With newer definitions of clinical syndromes in lymphatic filariasis and new tools to assess clinical status (e.g., ultrasound, lymphoscintigraphy, circulating filarial antigen assays, PCR), approaches to treatment based on infection status can be considered. Diethylcarbamazine (DEC, 6 mg/kg daily for 12 days), which has both macro- and microfilaricidal properties, remains the treatment of choice for the individual with active lymphatic filariasis (microfilaremia, antigen positivity, or adult worms on ultrasound). An alternative treatment is albendazole (400 mg bid for 21 days), although this drug's macrofilaricidal efficacy may be less than that of DEC. An 8-week course of daily doxycycline (targeting the intracellular *Wolbachia* endosymbiont) has significant macrofilaricidal activity, as does a 7-day course of daily DEC/albendazole.

As has already been mentioned, a growing body of evidence indicates that, although they may be asymptomatic, virtually all persons with *W. bancrofti* or *B. malayi* microfilaremia have some degree of subclinical disease (hematuria, proteinuria, abnormalities on lymphoscintigraphy). Thus, early treatment of asymptomatic persons is recommended to prevent further lymphatic damage. For ADL, supportive treatment (including the administration of antipyretics and analgesics) is recommended, as is antibiotic therapy if secondary bacterial infection is likely. Similarly, because lymphatic disease is associated with the presence of adult worms, treatment with DEC is recommended for microfilaria-negative adult-worm carriers.

In persons with chronic manifestations of lymphatic filariasis, treatment regimens that emphasize hygiene, prevention of secondary bacterial infections, and physiotherapy have gained wide acceptance for morbidity control. These regimens are similar to those recommended for lymphedema of most nonfilarial causes and known by a variety of names, including *complex decongestive physiotherapy* and *complex lymphedema therapy*. Hydroceles (Fig. 211-1) can be drained repeatedly or managed surgically. With chronic manifestations of lymphatic filariasis, drug treatment should be reserved for individuals with evidence of active infection; therapy has been associated with clinical improvement and, in some cases, reversal of lymphedema.

The recommended course of DEC treatment (12 days; total dose, 72 mg/kg) has remained standard for many years. However, data indicate that single-dose DEC treatment with 6 mg/kg may be equally efficacious. The 12-day course provides more rapid short-term microfilarial suppression. Regimens that use combinations of single doses of albendazole and either DEC or ivermectin all have a sustained microfilaricidal effect. As mentioned above, an 8-week course of daily doxycycline (200 mg/d) or a 7-day course of daily DEC/albendazole has both significant macrofilaricidal activity and sustained microfilaricidal activity.

Side effects of DEC treatment include fever, chills, arthralgias, headaches, nausea, and vomiting. Both the development and the severity of these reactions are directly related to the number of microfilariae circulating in the bloodstream. The adverse reactions may represent either an acute hypersensitivity reaction to the antigens being released by dead and dying parasites or an inflammatory reaction induced by lipopolysaccharides from the intracellular *Wolbachia* endosymbionts freed from their intracellular niche. Ivermectin has a side effect profile similar to that of DEC when used in lymphatic filariasis. In patients infected with *L. loa*, who have high levels of *Loa* microfilaremia, DEC—like ivermectin (see "Loiasis," below)—can elicit severe encephalopathic complications. When used in single-dose regimens for the treatment of lymphatic filariasis, albendazole is associated with relatively few side effects.

PREVENTION AND CONTROL

Avoidance of mosquito bites usually is not feasible for residents of endemic areas, but visitors should make use of insect repellent and mosquito nets. Impregnated bednets have a salutary effect. DEC can kill developing forms of filarial parasites and is useful as a prophylactic agent in humans.

Community-based intervention is the current approach to elimination of lymphatic filariasis as a public health problem. The underlying tenet of this approach is that mass annual distribution of antimicrofilarial chemotherapy—albendazole with either DEC (for all areas except those where onchocerciasis is coendemic) or ivermectin—will profoundly suppress microfilaremia. If the suppression is sustained, then transmission can be interrupted. As an added benefit, these combinations have secondary effects on gastrointestinal helminths. An alternative approach to the control of lymphatic filariasis is the use of salt fortified with DEC. Community use of DEC-fortified salt dramatically reduces microfilarial density with no apparent adverse reactions. Community education and clinical care for persons already suffering from the chronic sequelae of lymphatic filariasis are important components of filariasis control and elimination programs.

TROPICAL PULMONARY EOSINOPHILIA

Tropical pulmonary eosinophilia (TPE) is a distinct syndrome that develops in some individuals infected with lymphatic filarial species. This syndrome affects males and females in a ratio of 4:1, often during the third decade of life. The majority of cases have been reported from India, Pakistan, Sri Lanka, Brazil, Guyana, and Southeast Asia.

CLINICAL FEATURES

The main features include a history of residence in filarial-endemic regions, paroxysmal cough and wheezing (usually nocturnal and probably related to the nocturnal periodicity of microfilariae), weight loss, low-grade fever, adenopathy, and pronounced blood eosinophilia (>3000 eosinophils/μL). Chest x-rays or CT scans may be normal but generally show increased bronchovascular markings. Diffuse miliary lesions or mottled opacities may be present in the middle and lower lung fields. Tests of pulmonary function show restrictive abnormalities in most cases and obstructive defects in half. Characteristically, total serum IgE levels (10,000–100,000 ng/mL) and antifilarial antibody titers are markedly elevated.

PATHOLOGY

In TPE, microfilariae and parasite antigens are rapidly cleared from the bloodstream by the lungs. The clinical symptoms result from allergic and inflammatory reactions elicited by the cleared parasites. In some patients, trapping of microfilariae in other reticuloendothelial organs can cause hepatomegaly, splenomegaly, or lymphadenopathy. A prominent, eosinophil-enriched, intraalveolar infiltrate is often reported, and with it comes the release of cytotoxic proinflammatory granular proteins that may mediate some of the pathology seen in TPE. In the absence of successful treatment, interstitial fibrosis can lead to progressive pulmonary damage.

DIFFERENTIAL DIAGNOSIS

TPE must be distinguished from asthma, Löffler's syndrome, allergic bronchopulmonary aspergillosis, allergic granulomatosis with angiitis (Churg-Strauss syndrome), the systemic vasculitides (most notably periarteritis nodosa and Wegener's granulomatosis), chronic eosinophilic pneumonia, and the idiopathic hypereosinophilic syndrome. In addition to a geographic history of filarial exposure, useful features for distinguishing TPE include wheezing that is solely nocturnal, very high levels of antifilarial antibodies, and a rapid initial response to treatment with DEC.

℞ TROPICAL PULMONARY EOSINOPHILIA

DEC is used at a daily dosage of 4–6 mg/kg for 14 days. Symptoms usually resolve within 3–7 days after the initiation of therapy. Relapse, which occurs in ~12–25% of cases (sometimes after an interval of years), requires re-treatment.

ONCHOCERCIASIS

Onchocerciasis ("river blindness") is caused by the filarial nematode *O. volvulus*, which infects an estimated 13 million individuals. The majority of individuals infected with *O. volvulus* live in the equatorial region of Africa extending from the Atlantic coast to the Red Sea. About 70,000 persons are infected in Guatemala and Mexico, with smaller foci in Venezuela, Colombia, Brazil, Ecuador, Yemen, and Saudi Arabia. Onchocerciasis is the second leading cause of infectious blindness worldwide.

ETIOLOGY AND EPIDEMIOLOGY

Infection in humans begins with the deposition of infective larvae on the skin by the bite of an infected blackfly. The larvae develop into adults, which are typically found in subcutaneous nodules. About 7 months to 3 years after infection, the gravid female releases microfilariae that migrate out of the nodule and throughout the tissues, concentrating in the dermis. Infection is transmitted to other persons when a female fly ingests microfilariae from the host's skin and these microfilariae then develop into infective larvae. Adult *O. volvulus* females and males are ~40–60 cm and ~3–6 cm in length, respectively. The life span of adults can be as long as 18 years, with an average of ~9 years. Because the blackfly vector breeds along free-flowing rivers and streams (particularly in rapids) and generally restricts its flight to an area within several kilometers of these breeding sites, both biting and disease transmission are most intense in these locations.

PATHOLOGY

Onchocerciasis primarily affects the skin, eyes, and lymph nodes. In contrast to the pathology in lymphatic filariasis, the damage in onchocerciasis is elicited by microfilariae and not by adult parasites. In the skin, there are mild but chronic inflammatory changes that can result in loss of elastic fibers, atrophy, and fibrosis. The subcutaneous nodules, or onchocercomata, consist primarily of fibrous tissues surrounding the adult worm, often with a peripheral ring of inflammatory cells. In the eye, neovascularization and corneal scarring lead to corneal opacities and blindness. Inflammation in the anterior and posterior chambers frequently results in anterior uveitis, chorioretinitis, and optic atrophy. Although punctate opacities are due to an inflammatory reaction surrounding dead or dying microfilariae, the pathogenesis of most manifestations of onchocerciasis is still unclear.

CLINICAL FEATURES

Skin Pruritus and rash are the most frequent manifestations of onchocerciasis. The pruritus can be incapacitating; the rash is typically a papular eruption (Fig. 211-3) that is generalized rather than localized to a particular region of the body. Long-term infection results in exaggerated and premature wrinkling of the skin, loss of elastic fibers, and epidermal atrophy that can lead to loose, redundant skin and hypo- or hyperpigmentation. Localized eczematoid dermatitis can cause hyperkeratosis, scaling, and pigmentary changes. In an immunologically hyperreactive form of onchodermatitis (commonly termed *sowdah*, from the Yemeni word meaning "black"), the affected skin darkens as a consequence of the profound inflammation that occurs as microfilariae in the skin are cleared.

Onchocercomata These subcutaneous nodules, which can be palpable and/or visible, contain the adult worm. In African patients, they are common over the coccyx and sacrum, the trochanter of the femur, the lateral anterior crest, and other bony prominences; in patients from South and Central America, nodules tend to develop preferentially in the upper part of the body, particularly on the head, neck, and shoulders.

FIGURE 211-3 Papular eruption as a consequence of onchocerciasis.

Nodules vary in size and characteristically are firm and not tender. It has been estimated that, for every palpable nodule, there are four deeper nonpalpable ones.

Ocular Tissue Visual impairment is the most serious complication of onchocerciasis and usually affects only those persons with moderate or heavy infections. Lesions may develop in all parts of the eye. The most common early finding is conjunctivitis with photophobia. Punctate keratitis—acute inflammatory reactions surrounding dying microfilariae and manifested as "snowflake" opacities—is common among younger patients and resolves without apparent complications.

Sclerosing keratitis occurs in 1–5% of infected persons and is the leading cause of onchocercal blindness in Africa. Anterior uveitis and iridocyclitis develop in ~5% of infected persons in Africa. In Latin America, complications of the anterior uveal tract (pupillary deformity) may cause secondary glaucoma. Characteristic chorioretinal lesions develop as a result of atrophy and hyperpigmentation of the retinal pigment epithelium. Constriction of the visual fields and frank optic atrophy may occur.

Lymph Nodes Mild to moderate lymphadenopathy is common, particularly in the inguinal and femoral areas, where the enlarged nodes may hang down in response to gravity ("hanging groin"), sometimes predisposing to inguinal and femoral hernias.

Systemic Manifestations Some heavily infected individuals develop cachexia with loss of adipose tissue and muscle mass. Among adults who become blind, there is a three- to fourfold increase in the mortality rate.

DIAGNOSIS

Definitive diagnosis depends on the detection of an adult worm in an excised nodule or, more commonly, of microfilariae in a skin snip. Skin snips are obtained with a corneal-scleral punch, which collects a blood-free skin biopsy sample extending to just below the epidermis, or by lifting of the skin with the tip of a needle and excision of a small (1- to 3-mm) piece with a sterile scalpel blade. The biopsy tissue is incubated in tissue culture medium or in saline on a glass slide or flat-bottomed microtiter plate. After incubation for 2–4 h (or occasionally overnight in light infections), microfilariae emergent from the skin can be seen by low-power microscopy.

Eosinophilia and elevated serum IgE levels are common but, because they occur in many parasitic infections, are not diagnostic in themselves. Assays to detect specific antibodies to *Onchocerca* and PCR to detect onchocercal DNA in skin snips are used in specialized laboratories and are highly sensitive and specific.

The *Mazzotti test* is a provocative technique that can be used in cases where the diagnosis of onchocerciasis is still in doubt (i.e., when skin snips and ocular examination reveal no microfilariae). A small dose of DEC (0.5–1.0 mg/kg) is given orally; the ensuing death of any dermal microfilariae elicits the development or exacerbation of pruritus or dermatitis within hours—an event that strongly suggests onchocerciasis.

Rx ONCHOCERCIASIS

The main goals of therapy are to prevent the development of irreversible lesions and to alleviate symptoms. Surgical excision is recommended when nodules are located on the head (because of the proximity of microfilaria-producing adult worms to the eye), but chemotherapy is the mainstay of management. Ivermectin, a semisynthetic macrocyclic lactone active against microfilariae, is the first-line agent for the treatment of onchocerciasis. It is given orally in a single dose of 150 μg/kg, either yearly or semiannually. Recently, more frequent ivermectin administration (every 3 months) has been suggested to ameliorate pruritus and skin disease. Moreover, quadrennial administration of ivermectin has some macrofilaricidal activity.

After treatment, most individuals have few or no reactions. Pruritus, cutaneous edema, and/or maculopapular rash occurs in ~1–10% of treated individuals.

In areas of Africa co-endemic for *O. volvulus* and *L. loa*, however, ivermectin is contraindicated (as it is for pregnant or breast-feeding women) because of severe posttreatment encephalopathy seen in patients, especially children, who are heavily microfilaremic for *L. loa* (2000–5000 microfilariae/mL). Although ivermectin treatment results in a marked drop in microfilarial density, its effect can be short-lived (<3 months in some cases). Thus, it is occasionally necessary to give ivermectin more frequently for persistent symptoms. A 6-week course of doxycycline is macrofilaristatic, rendering female adult worms sterile for long periods. Because this agent targets the *Wolbachia* endosymbiont of the filarial parasite, new approaches for definitive treatment (i.e., cure) may become available.

PREVENTION

Vector control has been beneficial in highly endemic areas in which breeding sites are vulnerable to insecticide spraying, but most areas endemic for onchocerciasis are not suited to this type of control. Community-based administration of ivermectin every 6–12 months is being used to interrupt transmission in endemic areas. This measure, in conjunction with vector control, has already helped reduce the prevalence of disease in endemic foci in Africa and Latin America. No drug has proved useful for prophylaxis of *O. volvulus* infection.

LOIASIS

ETIOLOGY AND EPIDEMIOLOGY

Loiasis is caused by *L. loa* (the African eye worm), which is present in the rain forests of West and Central Africa. Adult parasites (females, 50–70 mm long and 0.5 mm wide; males, 25–35 mm long and 0.25 mm wide) live in subcutaneous tissues. Microfilariae circulate in the blood with a diurnal periodicity that peaks between 12:00 noon and 2:00 P.M.

CLINICAL FEATURES

Manifestations of loiasis in natives of endemic areas may differ from those in temporary residents or visitors. Among the indigenous population, loiasis is often an asymptomatic infection with microfilaremia. Infection may be recognized only after subconjunctival migration of an adult worm (Fig. 211-4) or may be manifested by episodic Calabar swellings—evanescent localized areas of angioedema and erythema developing on the extremities and less frequently at other sites. Nephropathy, encephalopathy, and cardiomyopathy are rare. In patients who are not residents of endemic areas, allergic symptoms predominate, episodes of Calabar swelling tend to be more frequent and debilitating, microfilaremia is rare, and eosinophilia and increased levels of antifilarial antibodies are characteristic.

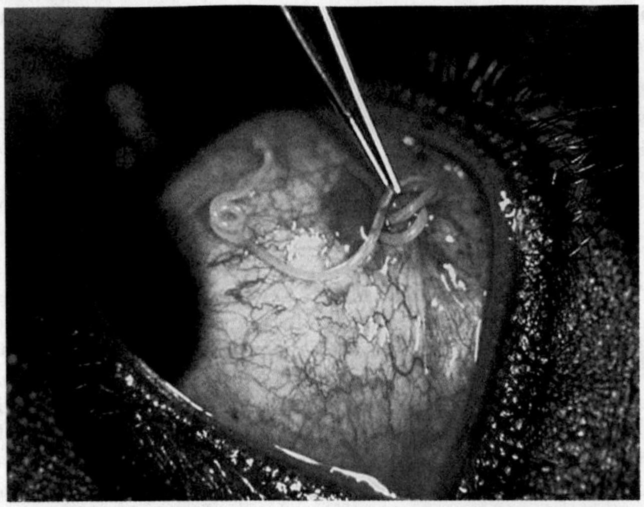

FIGURE 211-4 Adult *Loa loa* being surgically removed after its subconjunctival migration.

PATHOLOGY

The pathogenesis of the manifestations of loiasis is poorly understood. Calabar swellings are thought to result from a hypersensitivity reaction to adult worm antigens.

DIAGNOSIS

Definitive diagnosis of loiasis requires the detection of microfilariae in the peripheral blood or the isolation of the adult worm from the eye (Fig. 211-4) or from a subcutaneous biopsy specimen from a site of swelling developing after treatment. PCR-based assays for the detection of *L. loa* DNA in blood are available in specialized laboratories and are highly sensitive and specific. In practice, the diagnosis must often be based on a characteristic history and clinical presentation, blood eosinophilia, and elevated levels of antifilarial antibodies, particularly in travelers to an endemic region, who are usually amicrofilaremic. Other clinical findings in the latter individuals include hypergammaglobulinemia, elevated levels of serum IgE, and elevated leukocyte and eosinophil counts.

Rx LOIASIS

DEC (8–10 mg/kg per day for 21 days) is effective against both the adult and the microfilarial forms of *L. loa*, but multiple courses are frequently necessary before loiasis resolves completely. In cases of heavy microfilaremia, allergic or other inflammatory reactions can take place during treatment, including central nervous system involvement with coma and encephalitis. Heavy infections can be treated initially with apheresis to remove the microfilariae and with glucocorticoids (40–60 mg of prednisone per day) followed by doses of DEC (0.5 mg/kg per day). If antifilarial treatment has no adverse effects, the prednisone dose can be rapidly tapered and the dose of DEC gradually increased to 8–10 mg/kg per day.

Albendazole or ivermectin is effective in reducing microfilarial loads, although neither is approved for this purpose by the U.S. Food and Drug Administration. DEC (300 mg weekly) is an effective prophylactic regimen for loiasis.

STREPTOCERCIASIS

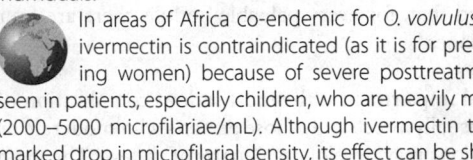

Mansonella streptocerca, found mainly in the tropical forest belt of Africa from Ghana to the Democratic Republic of the Congo, is transmitted by biting midges. The major clinical manifestations involve the skin and include pruritus, papular rashes, and pigmentation changes. Many infected individuals have inguinal adenopathy, although most are asymptomatic. The diagnosis is made by detection of the characteristic microfilariae in skin snips. DEC (6 mg/kg per day in divided doses for 14–21 days) effectively kills both microfilariae and adult worms. As in onchocerciasis, treatment is sometimes accompanied by urticaria, arthralgias, myalgias, headaches, and abdominal discomfort. Ivermectin at a single dose of 150 μg/kg leads to sustained suppression of microfilariae in the skin and is likely to assume primacy in the treatment of streptocerciasis.

MANSONELLA PERSTANS INFECTION

Mansonella perstans, distributed across the center of Africa and in northeastern South America, is transmitted by midges. Adult worms reside in serous cavities—pericardial, pleural, and peritoneal—as well as in the mesentery and the perirenal and retroperitoneal tissues. Microfilariae circulate in the blood without periodicity. The clinical and pathologic features of the infection are poorly defined. Most patients appear to be asymptomatic, but manifestations may include transient angioedema and pruritus of the arms, face, or other parts of the body (analogous to the Calabar swellings of loiasis); fever; headache; arthralgias; and right-upper-quadrant pain. Occasionally, pericarditis and hepatitis occur. The diagnosis is based on the demonstration of microfilariae in blood or serosal effusions. Perstans filariasis is often associated with peripheral-blood eosinophilia and antifilarial antibody elevations. Although DEC (8–10 mg/kg per day for 21 days) is the standard therapeutic agent, there is little evidence that it is effective. Cure is indicated by the disappearance of symptoms and eosinophilia; multiple courses of therapy are usually required. Ivermectin, used in frequent repeated doses, can reduce blood microfilarial levels. Both mebendazole (100 mg bid for 30 days) and albendazole (400 mg bid for 10 days) have occasionally been reported to be effective.

MANSONELLA OZZARDI INFECTION

The distribution of *Mansonella ozzardi* is restricted to Central and South America and certain Caribbean islands. Adult worms are rarely recovered from humans. Microfilariae circulate in the blood without periodicity. Although this organism has often been considered nonpathogenic, headache, articular pain, fever, pulmonary symptoms, adenopathy, hepatomegaly, pruritus, and eosinophilia have been ascribed to *M. ozzardi* infection. The diagnosis is made by detection of microfilariae in peripheral blood. Ivermectin (a single dose of 6 mg) is effective in treating this infection.

DRACUNCULIASIS (GUINEA WORM INFECTION)

ETIOLOGY AND EPIDEMIOLOGY

The incidence of dracunculiasis, caused by *Dracunculus medinensis*, has declined dramatically because of global eradication efforts. Current estimates suggest that there are slightly more than 10,000 cases worldwide, the majority in Sudan, Ghana, and Mali. Asia has now been deemed dracunculiasis-free.

Humans acquire *D. medinensis* when they ingest water containing infective larvae derived from *Cyclops*, a crustacean that is the intermediate host. Larvae penetrate the stomach or intestinal wall, mate, and mature. The adult male probably dies; the female worm develops over a year and migrates to subcutaneous tissues, usually in the lower extremity. As the thin female worm, ranging in length from 30 cm to 1 m, approaches the skin, a blister forms that, over days, breaks down and forms an ulcer. When the blister opens, large numbers of motile, rhabditiform larvae can be released into stagnant water; ingestion by *Cyclops* completes the life cycle.

CLINICAL FEATURES

Few or no clinical manifestations of dracunculiasis are evident until just before the blister forms, when there is an onset of fever and generalized allergic symptoms, including periorbital edema, wheezing, and urticaria. The emergence of the worm is associated with local pain and swelling. When the blister ruptures (usually as a result of immersion in water) and the adult worm releases larva-rich fluid, symptoms are relieved. The shallow ulcer surrounding the emerging adult worm heals over weeks to months. Such ulcers, however, can become secondarily infected, the result being cellulitis, local inflammation, abscess formation, or (uncommonly) tetanus. Occasionally, the adult worm does not emerge but becomes encapsulated and calcified.

DIAGNOSIS

The diagnosis is based on the findings developing with the emergence of the adult worm, as described above.

Rx DRACUNCULIASIS

Gradual extraction of the worm by winding of a few centimeters on a stick each day remains the common and effective practice. Worms may be excised surgically. The administration of metronidazole (250 mg tid for 10 days) may relieve symptoms but has no proven activity against the worm.

PREVENTION

Prevention, which remains the only real control measure, depends on the provision of safe drinking water.

ZOONOTIC FILARIAL INFECTIONS

Dirofilariae that affect primarily dogs, cats, and raccoons occasionally infect humans incidentally, as do *Brugia* and *Onchocerca* parasites that affect small mammals. Because humans are an abnormal host, the parasites never develop fully. Pulmonary dirofilarial infection caused by the canine heartworm *Dirofilaria immitis* generally presents in humans as a solitary pulmonary nodule. Chest pain, hemoptysis, and cough are uncommon. Infections with *D. repens* (from dogs) or *D. tenuis* (from raccoons) can cause local subcutaneous nodules in humans. Zoonotic *Brugia* infection can produce isolated lymph node enlargement, whereas zoonotic *Onchocerca* can cause subconjunctival masses. Eosinophilia levels and antifilarial antibody titers are not commonly elevated. Excisional biopsy is both diagnostic and curative. These infections usually do not respond to chemotherapy.

FURTHER READINGS

BOCKARIE MJ et al: Mass treatment to eliminate filariasis in Papua New Guinea. N Engl J Med 347:1841, 2002

BOUSSINESQ M et al: Clinical picture, epidemiology and outcome of *Loa*-associated serious adverse events related to mass ivermectin treatment of onchocerciasis in Cameroon. Filaria J 2(Suppl 1):S4, 2003

DREYER G et al: Acute attacks in the extremities of persons living in an area endemic for bancroftian filariasis: Differentiation of two syndromes. Trans R Soc Trop Med Hyg 93:413, 1999

GARDON J et al: Serious reactions after mass treatment of onchocerciasis with ivermectin in an area endemic for *Loa loa* infection. Lancet 350:18, 1997

HOERAUF A et al: Onchocerciasis. BMJ 326:207, 2003

——— et al: Depletion of *Wolbachia* endobacteria in *Onchocerca volvulus* by doxycycline and microfilaridermia after ivermectin treatment. Lancet 357:1415, 2001

MCPHERSON T et al: Interdigital lesions and frequency of acute dermatolymphangioadenitis in lymphoedema in a filariasis-endemic area. Br J Dermatol 154:933, 2006

OTTESEN EA: Lymphatic filariasis: Treatment, control and elimination. Adv Parasitol 61:395, 2006

WALTHER M, MULLER R: Diagnosis of human filariases (except onchocerciasis). Adv Parasitol 53:149, 2003

WHO EXPERT COMMITTEE ON ONCHOCERCIASIS: Onchocerciasis and its control: Fourth report. Tech Rep Ser No 852. Geneva, World Health Organization, 1995

212 Schistosomiasis and Other Trematode Infections

Adel A.F. Mahmoud

Trematodes, or flatworms, are a group of morphologically and biologically heterogeneous organisms that belong to the phylum Platyhelminthes. Human infection with trematodes occurs in many geographic areas and can cause considerable morbidity and mortality. For clinical purposes, significant trematode infections of humans may be divided according to tissues invaded by adult flukes: blood, biliary tree, intestines, and lungs (Table 212-1).

Trematodes share some common morphologic features, including macroscopic size (from 1 cm to several cm); dorsoventral, flattened, bilaterally symmetric bodies (adult worms); and the prominence of two suckers. Except for schistosomes, all human parasitic trematodes are hermaphroditic. Their life cycle involves a definitive host (mammalian/human), in which adult worms initiate sexual reproduction, and an intermediate host (snails), in which asexual multiplication of larvae occurs. More than one intermediate host may be necessary for some species of trematodes. Human infection is initiated either by direct penetration of intact skin or by ingestion. Upon maturation within humans, adult flukes initiate sexual reproduction and egg production. Helminth ova leave the definitive host in excreta or sputum and, upon reaching suitable environmental conditions, they hatch, releasing free-living miracidia that seek specific snail intermediate hosts. After asexual reproduction, cercariae are released from infected snails. In certain species, these organisms infect humans; in others, they find a second intermediate host to allow encystment into metacercariae—the infective stage.

The host-parasite relationship in trematode infections is a product of certain biologic features of these organisms: they are multicellular, undergo several developmental changes within the host, and usually result in chronic infections. In general, the distribution of worm infections in human populations is *overdispersed*; i.e., it follows a negative binomial mathematical relationship in which most infected individuals harbor low worm burdens while a small percentage are heavily infected. It is the heavily infected minority who are particularly prone to disease sequelae and who constitute an epidemiologically significant reservoir of infection in endemic areas. Equally important is an appreciation that worms do not multiply within the definitive host and that they have a relatively long life span, ranging from a few months to a few years. Morbidity and death due to trematode infections reflect a multifactorial process that results from the tipping of a delicate balance between intensity of infection and host reactions, which initiate and modulate immunologic and pathologic outcome. Furthermore, the genetics of the parasite and of the human host contribute to the outcome of infection and disease. Infections with trematodes that migrate through or reside in host tissues are associated with a moderate to high degree of peripheral blood eosinophilia; this association is of significance in protective and immunopathologic sequelae and is a useful clinical indicator of infection.

APPROACH TO THE PATIENT: Trematode Infection

The approach to individuals with suspected trematode infection begins with a question: Where have you been? Details of geographic history, exposure to freshwater bodies, and indulgence in local eating habits without ensuring safety of food and drink are all essential elements in the history. The workup plan must include a detailed physical examination and tests appropriate for the suspected infection. Diagnosis is based either on detection of the relevant stage of the parasite in excreta, sputum, or (rarely) tissue samples or on sensitive and specific serologic tests. Consultation with physicians familiar with these infections or with the U.S. Centers for Disease Control and Prevention (CDC) is helpful in guiding diagnosis and selecting therapy.

TABLE 212-1 MAJOR HUMAN TREMATODE INFECTIONS

Trematode	Transmission	Endemic Area(s)
Blood Flukes		
Schistosoma mansoni	Skin penetration by cercariae released from snails	Africa, South America, Middle East
S. japonicum	Skin penetration by cercariae released from snails	China, Philippines, Indonesia
S. intercalatum	Skin penetration by cercariae released from snails	West Africa
S. mekongi	Skin penetration by cercariae released from snails	Southeast Asia
S. haematobium	Skin penetration by cercariae released from snails	Africa, Middle East
Biliary (Hepatic) Flukes		
Clonorchis sinensis	Ingestion of metacercariae in freshwater fish	Far East
Opisthorchis viverrini	Ingestion of metacercariae in freshwater fish	Far East, Thailand
O. felineus	Ingestion of metacercariae in freshwater fish	Far East, Europe
Fasciola hepatica	Ingestion of metacercariae on aquatic plants or in water	Worldwide
F. gigantica	Ingestion of metacercariae on aquatic plants or in water	Sporadic, Africa
Intestinal Flukes		
Fasciolopsis buski	Ingestion of metacercariae on aquatic plants	Southeast Asia
Heterophyes heterophyes	Ingestion of metacercariae in freshwater or brackish-water fish	Far East, North Africa
Lung Flukes		
Paragonimus westermani	Ingestion of metacercariae in crayfish or crabs	Global except North America and Europe

BLOOD FLUKES: SCHISTOSOMIASIS

Human schistosomiasis is caused by five species of the parasitic trematode genus *Schistosoma*: the intestinal species *S. mansoni*, *S. japonicum*, *S. mekongi*, and *S. intercalatum* and the urinary species *S. haematobium*. Infection may cause considerable morbidity in the intestines, liver, and urinary tract, and a proportion of affected individuals die. Other schistosomes (e.g., avian species) may invade human skin but then die in subcutaneous tissue, producing only self-limiting cutaneous manifestations.

ETIOLOGY

Human infection is initiated by penetration of intact skin with infective cercariae. These organisms, which are released from infected snails in freshwater bodies, measure ~2 mm in length and possess an anterior and a ventral sucker that attach to the skin and facilitate penetration. Once in subcutaneous tissue, cercariae transform into schistosomula, with morphologic, membrane, and immunologic changes. The cercarial outer membrane changes from a trilaminar to a heptalaminar structure that is then maintained throughout the organism's life span in humans. This transformation is thought to be the schistosome's main adaptive mechanism for survival in humans. Schistosomula begin their migration within 2–4 days via venous or lymphatic vessels, reaching the lungs and finally the liver parenchyma. Sexually mature worms descend into the

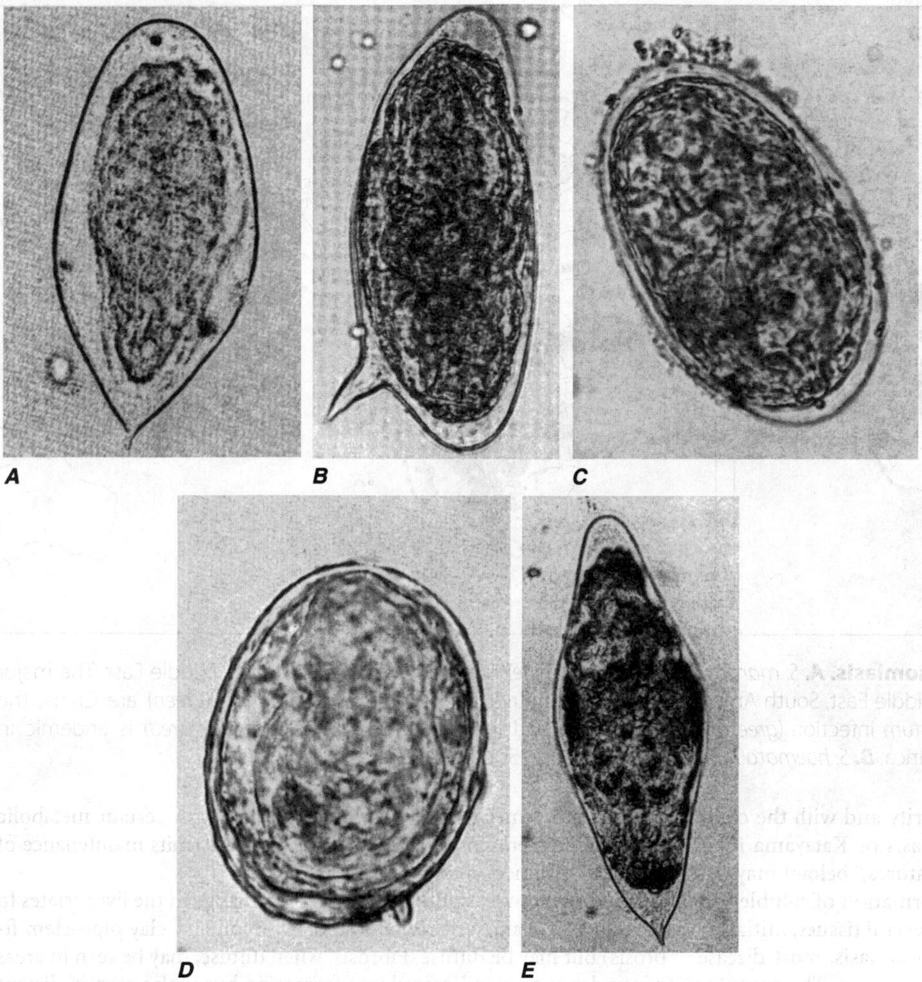

FIGURE 212-1 Morphology of schistosome eggs, the diagnostic stage of the parasite's life cycle. ***A.*** *S. haematobium* egg found in urine sample. Egg is large (~140 μm long), with a terminal spine. ***B.*** *S. mansoni* egg found in feces. Egg is large (~150 μm long), with a thin shell and lateral spine. ***C.*** *S. japonicum* egg found in feces. Egg is smaller than that of *S. mansoni* (~90 μm long), with a small spine or hooklike structure. ***D.*** *S. mekongi* egg found in feces. Egg is similar to that of *S. japonicum* but smaller (~65 μm long). ***E.*** *S. intercalatum* egg found in feces. Egg is larger than that of *S. haematobium* (~190 μm long), with a longer, sharply pointed spine. *(From LR Ash, TC Orihel: Atlas of Human Parasitology, 3d ed. Chicago, ASCP Press, 1990; with permission.)*

venous system at specific anatomic locations: intestinal veins (*S. mansoni, S. japonicum, S. mekongi*, and *S. intercalatum*) and vesical veins (*S. haematobium*). After mating, adult gravid females travel against venous blood flow to small tributaries, where they deposit their ova intravascularly. Schistosome ova (Fig. 212-1) have specific morphologic features that vary with the species. Aided by enzymatic secretions through minipores in eggshells, ova move through the venous wall, traversing host tissues to reach the lumen of the intestinal or urinary tract, and are voided with stools or urine. Approximately 50% of ova are retained in host tissues locally (intestines or urinary tract) or are carried by venous blood flow to the liver and other organs. Schistosome ova that reach freshwater bodies hatch, releasing free-living miracidia that seek the snail intermediate host and undergo several asexual multiplication cycles. Finally, infective cercariae are shed from snails.

Adult schistosomes are ~1–2 cm long. Males are slightly shorter than females, with flattened bodies and anteriorly curved edges forming the gynecophoral canal, in which mature adult females are usually held. Females are longer, slender, and rounded in cross-section. The precise nature of biochemical and reproductive exchanges between the two sexes is unknown, as are the regulatory mechanisms for pairing. Adult schistosomes parasitize specific sites in the host venous system. What guides adult intestinal schistosomes to branches of the superior or inferior mesenteric veins or adult *S. haematobium* worms to the vesical plexus is unknown. In addition, adult worms inhibit the coagulation cascade and evade the effector arms of the host immune responses by still-undetermined mechanisms. The genome of schistosomes is relatively large (~270 Mb) and is arrayed on seven pairs of autosomes and one pair of sex chromosomes. For *S. mansoni*, a total of ~14,000 genes have been estimated; some are species-conserved. The complete sequence of the schistosome genome should be available soon.

EPIDEMIOLOGY

The global distribution of schistosome infection in human populations (Fig. 212-2) is dependent on both parasite and host factors. Information on prevalence and global distribution is inexact. The five *Schistosoma* species are estimated to infect 200–300 million individuals in South America, the Caribbean, Africa, the Middle East, and Southeast Asia. The total population living under conditions favoring transmission approximates double or triple that number—a fact reflecting the public health significance of schistosomiasis.

In endemic areas, the rate of yearly onset of new infection, or incidence, is generally low. Prevalence, on the other hand, starts to be appreciable by the age of 3–4 years and builds to a maximum that varies by endemic region (up to 100%) in the 15- to 20-year age group. Prevalence then stabilizes or decreases slightly in older age groups (>40 years). Intensity of infection (as measured by fecal or urinary egg counts, which correlate with adult worm burdens in most circumstances) follows the increase in prevalence up to the age of 15–20 years and then declines markedly in older age groups. This decline may reflect acquisition of resistance or may be due to changes in water contact patterns, since older people have less exposure. Furthermore, the overdispersed distribution of schistosomes in human populations may be due to the heterogeneity of worm populations, with some more invasive than others; alternatively, it may be due to the demonstrated differences in genetic susceptibility of host populations.

Disease due to schistosome infection is the outcome of parasitologic, host, and additional infectious, nutritional, and environmental factors. Most disease syndromes relate to the presence of one or more of the parasite stages in humans. Disease manifestations in the populations of endemic areas correlate, in general, with the intensity and duration of infection as well as with the age and genetic susceptibility of the host. Overall, disease manifestations are clinically relevant in only a small proportion of persons infected with any of the intestinal schistosomes. In contrast, urinary schistosomiasis manifests clinically in most infected individuals. Recent estimates of total morbidity due to chronic schistosomiasis indicate a significantly greater burden than was previously appreciated.

Patients with both HIV infection and schistosomiasis excrete far fewer eggs in their stools than those infected with *S. mansoni* alone; the mechanism underlying this difference is unknown. Treatment with praziquantel may result in reduced HIV replication and increased CD4+ T lymphocyte counts.

PATHOGENESIS AND IMMUNITY

Cercarial invasion is associated with dermatitis arising from dermal and subdermal inflammatory responses, both humoral and cell-me-

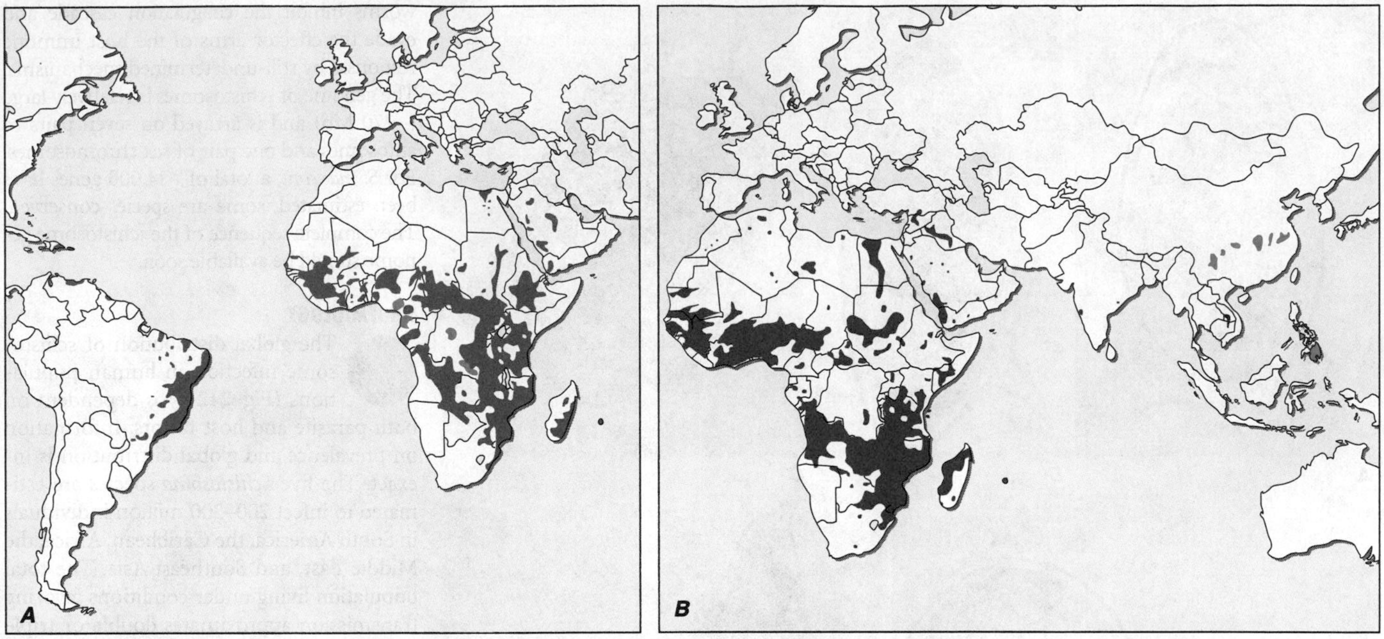

FIGURE 212-2 Global distribution of schistosomiasis. *A.* *S. mansoni* infection (*dark blue*) is endemic in Africa, the Middle East, South America, and a few Caribbean countries. *S. intercalatum* infection (*green*) is endemic in sporadic foci in West and Central Africa. ***B.*** *S. haematobium* infection (*purple*) is endemic in Africa and the Middle East. The major endemic countries for *S. japonicum* infection (*green*) are China, the Philippines, and Indonesia. *S. mekongi* infection (*red*) is endemic in sporadic foci in Southeast Asia.

diated. As the parasites approach sexual maturity and with the commencement of oviposition, acute schistosomiasis or Katayama fever (a serum sickness–like illness; see "Clinical Features," below) may occur. The associated antigen excess results in formation of soluble immune complexes, which may be deposited in several tissues, initiating multiple pathologic events. In chronic schistosomiasis, most disease manifestations are due to eggs retained in host tissues. The granulomatous response around these ova is cell-mediated and is regulated both positively and negatively by a cascade of cytokine, cellular, and humoral responses. Granuloma formation begins with recruitment of a host of inflammatory cells in response to antigens secreted by the living organism within the ova. Cells recruited initially include phagocytes, antigen-specific T cells, and eosinophils. Fibroblasts, giant cells, and B lymphocytes predominate later. These lesions reach a size many times that of parasite eggs, thus inducing organomegaly and obstruction. Immunomodulation or downregulation of host responses to schistosome eggs plays a significant role in limiting the extent of the granulomatous lesions—and consequently disease—in chronically infected experimental animals or humans. The underlying mechanisms involve another cascade of regulatory cytokines and idiotypic antibodies. Subsequent to the granulomatous response, fibrosis sets in, resulting in more permanent disease sequelae. Because schistosomiasis is also a chronic infection, the accumulation of antigen-antibody complexes results in deposits in renal glomeruli and may cause significant kidney disease.

The better-studied pathologic sequelae in schistosomiasis are those observed in liver disease. Ova that are carried by portal blood embolize to the liver. Because of their size (~150 × 60 μm in the case of *S. mansoni*), they lodge at presinusoidal sites, where granulomas are formed. These granulomas contribute to the hepatomegaly observed in infected individuals. Schistosomal liver enlargement is also associated with certain class I and class II human leukocyte antigen (HLA) haplotypes and markers; its genetic basis appears to be multigenic. Presinusoidal portal blockage causes several hemodynamic changes, including portal hypertension and associated development of portosystemic collaterals at the esophagogastric junction and other sites. Esophageal varices are most likely to break and cause repeated episodes of hematemesis. Because changes in hepatic portal blood flow occur slowly, compensatory arterialization of the blood flow through the liver is established. While this compensatory mechanism may be associated with certain metabolic side effects, retention of hepatocyte perfusion permits maintenance of normal liver function for several years.

The second most significant pathologic change in the liver relates to fibrosis. It is characteristically periportal (Symmers' clay pipe–stem fibrosis) but may be diffuse. Fibrosis, when diffuse, may be seen in areas of egg deposition and granuloma formation but is also seen in distant locations such as portal tracts. Schistosomiasis results in pure fibrotic lesions in the liver; cirrhosis occurs when other nutritional factors or infectious agents (e.g., hepatitis B or C virus) are involved. In recent years, it has been recognized that deposition of fibrotic tissue in the extracellular matrix results from the interaction of T lymphocytes with cells of the fibroblast series; several cytokines, such as interleukin (IL) 2, IL-4, IL-1, and transforming growth factor β (TGF-β), are known to stimulate fibrogenesis. The process may be dependent on the genetic constitution of the host. Furthermore, regulatory cytokines that can suppress fibrogenesis, such as interferon γ (IFN-γ) or IL-12, may play a role in modulating the response.

While the above description focuses on granuloma formation and fibrosis of the liver, similar processes occur in urinary schistosomiasis. Granuloma formation at the lower end of the ureters obstructs urinary flow, with subsequent development of hydroureter and hydronephrosis. Similar lesions in the urinary bladder cause the protrusion of papillomatous structures into its cavity; these may ulcerate and/or bleed. The chronic stage of infection is associated with scarring and deposition of calcium in bladder wall.

Studies on immunity to schistosomiasis, whether innate or adaptive, have expanded our knowledge of the components of these responses and target antigens. The critical question, however, is whether humans acquire immunity to schistosomes. Epidemiologic data suggest the onset of acquired immunity during the course of infection in young adults. Curative treatment of infection divides populations in endemic areas into those who acquire reinfection rapidly (susceptible) and those who follow a protracted course (resistant). This difference may be explained by differences in transmission, immunologic response, or genetic susceptibility. The mechanism of acquired immunity involves antibodies, complement, and several effector cells, particularly eosinophils. Furthermore, the intensity of schistosome infection has been correlated with a region in chromosome 5. In several studies, a few protective schistosome antigens have been identified as vaccine candidates, but none has been evaluated in human populations to date.

CLINICAL FEATURES

In general, disease manifestations of schistosomiasis occur in three stages, which vary not only by species but also by intensity of infection and other host factors, such as age and genetics. During the phase of cercarial invasion, a form of dermatitis may be observed. This so-called swimmers' itch occurs most often with *S. mansoni* and *S. japonicum* infections, manifesting 2 or 3 days after invasion as an itchy maculopapular rash on the affected areas of the skin. The condition is particularly severe when humans are exposed to avian schistosomes. This form of cercarial dermatitis is also seen around freshwater lakes in the northern United States, particularly in the spring. Cercarial dermatitis is a self-limiting clinical entity. During worm maturation and at the beginning of oviposition (i.e., 4–8 weeks after skin invasion), acute schistosomiasis or Katayama fever—a serum sickness–like syndrome with fever, generalized lymphadenopathy, and hepatosplenomegaly—may develop. Individuals with acute schistosomiasis show a high degree of peripheral blood eosinophilia. Parasite-specific antibodies may be detected before schistosome eggs are identified in excreta. Acute schistosomiasis has become an important clinical entity worldwide because of increased travel to endemic areas. Travelers are exposed to parasites while swimming or wading in freshwater bodies and upon their return present with the acute manifestations. The course of acute schistosomiasis is generally benign, but deaths are occasionally reported in association with heavy exposure to schistosomes.

The main clinical manifestations of chronic schistosomiasis are species-dependent. Intestinal species (*S. mansoni*, *S. japonicum*, *S. mekongi*, and *S. intercalatum*) cause intestinal and hepatosplenic disease as well as several manifestations associated with portal hypertension. During the intestinal phase, which may begin a few months after infection and may last for years, symptomatic patients characteristically have colicky abdominal pain, bloody diarrhea, and anemia. Patients may also report fatigue and an inability to perform daily routine functions and may show evidence of growth retardation. It has been demonstrated that schistosomiasis morbidity is generally underappreciated. The severity of intestinal schistosomiasis is often related to the intensity of the worm burden. The disease runs a chronic course and may result in colonic polyposis, which has been reported from some endemic areas, such as Egypt.

The hepatosplenic phase of disease manifests early (during the first year of infection, particularly in children) with liver enlargement due to parasite-induced granulomatous lesions. Hepatomegaly is seen in ~15–20% of infected individuals; it correlates roughly with intensity of infection, occurs more often in children, and may be related to specific HLA haplotypes. In subsequent phases of infection, presinusoidal blockage of blood flow leads to portal hypertension and splenomegaly. Moreover, portal hypertension may lead to varices at the lower end of the esophagus and at other sites. Patients with schistosomal liver disease may have right-upper-quadrant "dragging" pain during the hepatomegaly phase, and this pain may move to the left upper quadrant as splenomegaly progresses. Bleeding from esophageal varices may, however, be the first clinical manifestation of this phase. Patients may experience repeated bleeding but seem to tolerate its impact, since an adequate total hepatic blood flow permits normal liver function for a considerable duration. In late-stage disease, typical fibrotic changes occur along with liver function deterioration and the onset of ascites, hypoalbuminemia, and defects in coagulation. Intercurrent viral infections of the liver (especially hepatitis B and C) or nutritional deficiencies may well accelerate or exacerbate the deterioration of hepatic function.

The extent and severity of intestinal and hepatic disease in schistosomiasis mansoni and japonica have been well described. While it was originally thought that *S. japonicum* might induce more severe disease manifestations because the adult worms can produce 10 times more eggs than *S. mansoni*, subsequent field studies have not supported this claim. Clinical observations of individuals infected with *S. mekongi* or *S. intercalatum* have been less detailed, partly because of the limited geographic distribution of these organisms.

The clinical manifestations of *S. haematobium* infection occur relatively early and involve a high percentage of infected individuals. Up to 80% of children infected with *S. haematobium* have dysuria, frequency, and hematuria, which may be terminal. Urine examination reveals blood and albumin as well as an unusually high frequency of bacterial urinary tract infection and urinary sediment cellular metaplasia. These manifestations correlate with intensity of infection, the presence of urinary bladder granulomas, and subsequent ulceration. Along with local effects of granuloma formation in the urinary bladder, obstruction of the lower end of the ureters results in hydroureter and hydronephrosis, which may be seen in 25–50% of infected children. As infection progresses, bladder granulomas undergo fibrosis, which results in typical sandy patches visible on cystoscopy. In many endemic areas, an association between squamous cell carcinoma of the bladder and *S. haematobium* infection has been observed. Such malignancy is detected in a younger age group than is transitional cell carcinoma. In fact, *S. haematobium* has now been classified as a human carcinogen.

Significant disease may occur in other organs during chronic schistosomiasis. Most important are the lungs and central nervous system (CNS); other locations, such as the skin and the genital organs, are far less frequently affected. In pulmonary schistosomiasis, embolized eggs lodge in small arterioles, producing acute necrotizing arteriolitis and granuloma formation. During *S. mansoni* and *S. japonicum* infection, schistosome eggs reach the lungs after the development of portosystemic collateral circulation; in *S. haematobium* infection, ova may reach the lungs directly via connections between the vesical and systemic circulation. Subsequent fibrous tissue deposition leads to endarteritis obliterans, pulmonary hypertension, and cor pulmonale. The most common symptoms are cough, fever, and dyspnea. Cor pulmonale may be diagnosed radiologically on the basis of prominent right side of the heart and dilation of the pulmonary artery. Frank evidence of right-sided heart failure may be seen in late cases.

CNS schistosomiasis is important but less common than pulmonary schistosomiasis. It characteristically occurs as cerebral disease due to *S. japonicum* infection. Migratory worms deposit eggs in the brain and induce a granulomatous response. The frequency of this manifestation among infected individuals in some endemic areas (e.g., the Philippines) is calculated at 2–4%. Jacksonian epilepsy due to *S. japonicum* infection is the second most common cause of epilepsy in these areas. *S. mansoni* and *S. haematobium* infections have been associated with transverse myelitis. This syndrome is thought to be due to eggs traveling to the venous plexus around the spinal cord. In schistosomiasis mansoni, transverse myelitis is usually seen in the chronic stage after the development of portal hypertension and portosystemic shunts, which allow ova to travel to the spinal cord veins. This proposed sequence of events has been challenged because of a few reports of transverse myelitis occurring early in the course of *S. mansoni* infection. More information is needed to confirm these observations. During schistosomiasis haematobia, ova may travel through communication between vesical and systemic veins, resulting in spinal cord disease that may be detected at any stage of infection. Pathologic study of lesions in schistosomal transverse myelitis may reveal eggs along with necrotic or granulomatous lesions. Patients usually present with acute or rapidly progressing lower-leg weakness accompanied by sphincter dysfunction.

DIAGNOSIS

Physicians in areas not endemic for schistosomiasis face considerable diagnostic challenges. In the most common clinical presentation, a traveler returns with symptoms and signs of acute syndromes of schistosomiasis—namely, cercarial dermatitis or Katayama fever. Central to correct diagnosis is a thorough inquiry into travel history and exposure to freshwater bodies, whether slow or fast running. Differential diagnosis of fever in returned travelers includes a spectrum of infections whose etiologies are viral (e.g., Dengue fever), bacterial (e.g., enteric fever, leptospirosis), rickettsial, or protozoal (e.g., malaria). In cases of

Katayama fever, prompt diagnosis is essential and is based on clinical presentation, high-level peripheral blood eosinophilia, and a positive serologic assay for schistosomal antibodies. Two tests are available at the CDC: the Falcon assay screening test/enzyme-linked immunosorbent assay (FAST-ELISA) and the confirmatory enzyme-linked immunoelectrotransfer blot (EITB). Both tests are highly sensitive and ~96% specific. In some instances, examination of stool or urine for ova may yield positive results.

Individuals with established infection are diagnosed by a combination of geographic history, characteristic clinical presentation, and presence of schistosome ova in excreta. The diagnosis may also be established with the serologic assays mentioned above or with those that detect circulating schistosome antigens. These assays can be applied either to blood or to other body fluids (e.g., cerebrospinal fluid). For suspected schistosome infection, stool examination by the Kato thick smear or any other concentration method generally identifies all but the most lightly infected individuals. For *S. haematobium,* urine may be examined by microscopy of sediment or by filtration of a known volume through Nuclepore filters. Kato thick smear and Nuclepore filtration provide quantitative data on the intensity of infection, which is of value in assessing the degree of tissue damage and in monitoring the effect of chemotherapy. Schistosome infection may also be diagnosed by examination of tissue samples, typically rectal biopsies; other biopsy procedures (e.g., liver biopsy) are not needed, except in rare circumstances.

Differential diagnosis of schistosomal hepatomegaly must include viral hepatitis of all etiologies, miliary tuberculosis, malaria, visceral leishmaniasis, ethanol abuse, and causes of hepatic and portal vein obstruction. Differential diagnosis of hematuria in *S. haematobium* infection includes bacterial cystitis, tuberculosis, urinary stones, and malignancy.

Rx SCHISTOSOMIASIS

Treatment of schistosomiasis depends on stage of infection and clinical presentation. Other than topical dermatologic applications for relief of itching, no specific treatment is indicated for cercarial dermatitis caused by avian schistosomes. Therapy for acute schistosomiasis or Katayama fever needs to be adjusted appropriately for each case. While antischistosomal chemotherapy may be used, it does not have a significant impact on maturing worms. In severe acute schistosomiasis, management in an acute-care setting is necessary, with supportive measures and consideration of glucocorticoid treatment. Once the acute critical phase is over, specific chemotherapy is indicated for parasite elimination. For all individuals with established infection, treatment to eradicate the parasite should be administered. The drug of choice is praziquantel, which—depending on the infecting species **(Table 212-2)**—is administered PO as a total of 40 or 60 mg/kg in two or three doses over a single day. Praziquantel treatment results in parasitologic cure in ~85% of cases and reduces egg counts by >90%. Few side effects have been encountered, and those that do develop usually do not interfere with completion of treatment. Dependence on a single chemotherapeutic agent has raised the possibility of development of resistance in schistosomes; to date, such resistance does not seem to be clinically significant. The effect of antischistosomal treatment on disease manifestations varies by stage. Early hepatomegaly and bladder lesions are known to resolve after chemotherapy, but the late established manifestations, such as fibrosis, do not recede. Additional management modalities are needed for individuals with other manifestations, such as hepatocellular failure or recurrent hematemesis. The use of these interventions is guided by general medical and surgical principles.

PREVENTION AND CONTROL

Transmission of schistosomiasis is dependent on human behavior. Since the geographic distribution of infections in endemic regions of the world is not clearly demarcated, it is prudent for travelers to avoid contact with all freshwater bodies, irrespective of the speed of water flow or unsubstantiated claims of safety. Some topical agents, when applied to skin, may inhibit cercarial penetration, but none is currently available. If exposure occurs, a follow-up visit with a health care provider is strongly recommended. Prevention of infection in inhabitants of endemic areas is a significant challenge. Residents of these regions use freshwater bodies for sanitary, domestic, recreational, and agricultural purposes. Several control measures have been used, including application of molluscicides, provision of sanitary water and sewage disposal, chemotherapy, and health education. Current recommendations to countries endemic for schistosomiasis emphasize the use of multiple approaches. With the advent of an oral, safe, and effective antischistosomal agent, chemotherapy has been most successful in reducing intensity of infection and reversing disease. The duration of this positive impact depends on transmission dynamics of the parasite in any specific endemic region. The ultimate goal of research on prevention and control is development of a vaccine. Although there are a few promising leads, this goal is probably not within reach during the next decade or so.

TABLE 212-2 DRUG THERAPY FOR HUMAN TREMATODE INFECTIONS

Infection	Drug of Choice	Adult Dose and Duration
Blood Flukes		
S. mansoni, S. intercalatum, S. haematobium	Praziquantel	20 mg/kg, 2 doses in 1 day
S. japonicum, S. mekongi	Praziquantel	20 mg/kg, 3 doses in 1 day
Biliary (Hepatic) Flukes		
C. sinensis, O. viverrini, O. felineus	Praziquantel	25 mg/kg, 3 doses in 1 day
F. hepatica, F. gigantica	Triclabendazole	10 mg/kg once
Intestinal Flukes		
F. buski, H. heterophyes	Praziquantel	25 mg/kg, 3 doses in 1 day
Lung Flukes		
P. westermani	Praziquantel	25 mg/kg, 3 doses per day for 2 days

LIVER (BILIARY) FLUKES

Several species of biliary fluke infecting humans are particularly common in Southeast Asia and Russia. Other species are transmitted in Europe, Africa, and the Americas. On the basis of their migratory pathway in humans, these infections may be divided into the *Clonorchis* and *Fasciola* groups (Table 212-1).

CLONORCHIASIS AND OPISTHORCHIASIS

Infection with *Clonorchis sinensis,* the Chinese or oriental fluke, is endemic among fish-eating mammals in Southeast Asia. Humans are an incidental host; the prevalence of human infection is highest in China, Vietnam, and Korea. Infection with *Opisthorchis viverrini* and *O. felineus* is zoonotic in cats and dogs. Transmission to humans occurs occasionally, particularly in Thailand (*O. viverrini*) and in Southeast Asia and eastern Europe (*O. felineus*). Data on the exact geographic distribution of these infectious agents in human populations are rudimentary.

Infection with any of these three species is established by ingestion of raw or inadequately cooked freshwater fish harboring metacercariae. These organisms excyst in the duodenum, releasing larvae that travel through the ampulla of Vater and mature into adult worms in bile canaliculi. Mature flukes are flat and elongated, measuring 1–2 cm in length. The hermaphroditic worms reproduce by releasing small operculated eggs, which pass with bile into the intestines and are voided with stools. The life cycle is completed in the environment in specific freshwater snails (the first intermediate host) and encystment of metacercariae in freshwater fish.

Except for late sequelae, the exact clinical syndromes caused by clonorchiasis and opisthorchiasis are not well defined. Since most infected individuals harbor a low worm burden, many are asymptomatic. Moderate to heavy infection may be associated with vague right-upper-quadrant pain. In contrast, chronic or repeated infection is associated with manifestations such as cholangitis, cholangiohepatitis, and biliary obstruction. Cholangiocarcinoma is epidemiologically related to *C. sinensis* infection in China and to *O. viverrini* infection in northeastern Thailand. This association has resulted in classification of these infectious agents as human carcinogens.

FASCIOLIASIS

Infections with *Fasciola hepatica* and *F. gigantica* are worldwide zoonoses that are particularly endemic in sheep-raising countries. Human cases have been reported in South America, Europe, Africa, Australia, and the Far East. Recent estimates indicate a worldwide prevalence of 17 million cases. High endemicity has been reported in certain areas of Peru and Bolivia. In most endemic areas the predominant species is *F. hepatica*, but in Asia and Africa a varying degree of overlap with *F. gigantica* has been observed.

Humans acquire fascioliasis by ingestion of metacercariae attached to certain aquatic plants, such as watercress. Infection may also be acquired by consumption of contaminated water or ingestion of food items washed with such water. Acquisition of human infection through consumption of freshly prepared raw liver containing immature flukes has been reported. Infection is initiated when metacercariae excyst, penetrate the gut wall, and travel through the peritoneal cavity to invade the liver capsule. Adult worms finally reach bile ducts, where they produce large operculated eggs, which are voided in bile through the gastrointestinal tract to the outside environment. The flukes' life cycle is completed in specific snails (the first intermediate host) and encystment on aquatic plants.

Clinical features of fascioliasis relate to the stage and intensity of infection. Acute disease develops during parasite migration (1–2 weeks after infection) and includes fever, right-upper-quadrant pain, hepatomegaly, and eosinophilia. CT of the liver may show migratory tracks. Symptoms and signs usually subside as the parasites reach their final habitat. In individuals with chronic infection, bile duct obstruction and biliary cirrhosis are infrequently demonstrated. No relation to hepatic malignancy has been ascribed to fascioliasis.

DIAGNOSIS

Diagnosis of infection with any of the biliary flukes depends on a high degree of suspicion, elicitation of an appropriate geographic history, and stool examination for characteristically shaped parasite ova. Additional evidence may be obtained by documenting peripheral blood eosinophilia or imaging the liver. Serologic testing is helpful, particularly in lightly infected individuals.

Rx BILIARY FLUKES

Drug therapy (praziquantel or triclabendazole) is summarized in Table 212-2. Patients with anatomic lesions in the biliary tract or malignancy are managed according to general medical guidelines.

INTESTINAL FLUKES

Two species of intestinal flukes cause human infection in defined geographic areas worldwide (Table 212-1). The large *Fasciolopsis buski* (adults measure 2 × 7 cm) is endemic in Southeast Asia, while the smaller *Heterophyes heterophyes* is found in the Nile Delta of Egypt and in the Far East. Infection is initiated by ingestion of metacercariae attached to aquatic plants (*F. buski*) or encysted in freshwater or brackish-water fish (*H. heterophyes*). Flukes mature in human intestines, and eggs are passed with stools. Most individuals infected with intestinal flukes are asymptomatic. In heavy *F. buski* infection, diarrhea, abdominal pain, and malabsorption may be encountered. Heavy infection with *H. heterophyes* may be associated with abdominal pain and mucous diarrhea. Diagnosis is established by detection of characteristically shaped ova in stool samples. The drug of choice for treatment is praziquantel (Table 212-2).

LUNG FLUKES

Infection with the lung fluke *Paragonimus westermani* (Table 212-1) and related species (e.g., *P. africanus*) is endemic in many parts of the world, excluding North America and Europe. Endemicity is particularly noticeable in West Africa, Central and South America, and Asia. In nature, the reservoir hosts of *P. westermani* are wild and domestic felines. In Africa, *P. africanus* has been found in other species, such as dogs. Adult lung flukes, which are 7–12 mm in length, are found encapsulated in the lungs of infected persons. In rare circumstances, flukes are found encysted in the CNS (cerebral paragonimiasis) or abdominal cavity. Humans acquire lung fluke infection by ingesting infective metacercariae encysted in the muscles and viscera of crayfish and freshwater crabs. In endemic areas, these crustaceans are consumed either raw or pickled. Once the organisms reach the duodenum, they excyst, penetrate the gut wall, and travel through the peritoneal cavity, diaphragm, and pleural space to reach the lungs. Mature flukes are found in the bronchioles surrounded by cystic lesions. Parasite eggs are either expectorated with sputum or swallowed and passed to the outside environment with feces. The life cycle is completed in snails and freshwater crustacea.

When maturing flukes lodge in lung tissues, they cause hemorrhage and necrosis, resulting in cyst formation. The adjacent lung parenchyma shows evidence of inflammatory infiltration, predominantly by eosinophils. Cysts usually measure 1–2 cm in diameter and may contain one or two worms each. With the onset of oviposition, cysts usually rupture in adjacent bronchioles—an event allowing ova to exit the human host. Older cysts develop thickened walls, which may undergo calcification. During the active phase of paragonimiasis, lung tissues surrounding parasite cysts may contain evidence of pneumonia, bronchitis, bronchiectasis, and fibrosis.

Pulmonary paragonimiasis is particularly symptomatic in persons with moderate to heavy infection. Productive cough with brownish sputum or frank hemoptysis associated with peripheral blood eosinophilia is usually the presenting feature. Chest examination may reveal signs of pleurisy. In chronic cases, bronchitis or bronchiectasis may predominate, but these conditions rarely proceed to lung abscess. Imaging of the lungs demonstrates characteristic features, including patchy densities, cavities, pleural effusion, and ring shadows. Cerebral paragonimiasis presents as either space-occupying lesions or epilepsy.

DIAGNOSIS

Pulmonary paragonimiasis is diagnosed by detection of parasite ova in sputum and/or stools. Serology is of considerable help in egg-negative cases and in cerebral paragonimiasis.

Rx LUNG FLUKES

The drug of choice for treatment is praziquantel (Table 212-2). Other medical or surgical management may be needed for pulmonary or cerebral lesions.

CONTROL AND PREVENTION OF TISSUE FLUKES

For residents of nonendemic areas who are visiting an endemic region, the only effective preventive measure is to avoid ingestion of local plants, fish, or crustaceans; if their ingestion is necessary, these items should be washed or cooked thoroughly. Instruction on water and food preparation and consumption should be included in physicians' advice to travelers (Chap. 117). Interruption of transmission among residents of endemic areas depends on avoiding ingestion of infective stages and disposing of feces and sputum appropriately to prevent hatching of eggs in the environment. These two approaches rely greatly on socioeconomic development and health education. In countries where economic progress has resulted in financial and social improvements, transmission has decreased. The third approach to control in endemic communities entails selective use of chemotherapy for individuals posing the highest risk of transmission—i.e., those with heavy infections. The availability of praziquantel—a broad-spectrum, safe, and effective anthelmintic agent—provides a means for reducing the reservoirs of infection in human populations. However, the existence of most of these helminths as zoonoses in several animal species complicates control efforts.

FURTHER READINGS

Alves Oliveira LF et al: Cytokine production associated with peripheral fibrosis during chronic schistosomiasis mansoni in humans. Infect Immun 74:1215, 2006

Caffrey CR: Chemotherapy of schistosomiasis: Present and future. Curr Opin Chem Biol 11:433, 2007

Centers for Disease Control and Prevention: *http://www.cdc.gov/ncidod/dpd*

Drugs for Parasitic Infections. Med Lett Drugs Ther, August 1, 2004

Jia TW et al: Assessment of the age-specific disability weight of chronic schistosomiasis japonica. Bull World Health Organ 85:458, 2007

Kallestrup P et al: Schistosomiasis and HIV-1 infection in rural Zimbabwe: Effect of treatment of schistosomiasis on CD4 cell count and plasma HIV-1 RNA load. J Infect Dis 192:1956, 2005

King CH: Lifting the burden of schistosomiasis—defining elements of infection-associated disease and the benefits of antiparasite treatment. J Infect Dis 196:653, 2007

Lim JH et al: Parasitic diseases of the biliary tract. AJR Am J Roentgenol 188:1596, 2007

Lun ZR et al: Clonorchiasis: A key foodborne zoonosis in China. Lancet Infect Dis 5:31, 2005

Mahmoud AAFM (ed): Schistosomiasis, in *Tropical Medicine: Science and Practice*, G Pasvol, S Hoffman (eds). London, Imperial College Press, 2001, pp 1–510

Stauffer WM et al: Biliary liver flukes (opisthorchiasis and clonorchiasis) in immigrants in the United States: Often subtle and diagnosed years after arrival. J Travel Med 11:157, 2004

213 Cestodes

A. Clinton White, Jr., Peter F. Weller

Cestodes, or tapeworms, are segmented worms. The adults reside in the gastrointestinal tract, but the larvae can be found in almost any organ. Human tapeworm infections can be divided into two major clinical groups. In one group, humans are the definitive hosts, with the adult tapeworms living in the gastrointestinal tract (*Taenia saginata, Diphyllobothrium, Hymenolepis,* and *Dipylidium caninum*). In the other, humans are intermediate hosts, with larval-stage parasites present in the tissues; diseases in this category include echinococcosis, sparganosis, and coenurosis. For *Taenia solium*, the human may be either the definitive or the intermediate host.

The ribbon-shaped tapeworm attaches to the intestinal mucosa by means of sucking cups or hooks located on the scolex. Behind the scolex is a short, narrow neck from which proglottids (segments) form. As each proglottid matures, it is displaced further back from the neck by the formation of new, less mature segments. The progressively elongating chain of attached proglottids, called the *strobila*, constitutes the bulk of the tapeworm. The length varies among species. In some, the tapeworm may consist of more than 1000 proglottids and may be several meters long. The mature proglottids are hermaphroditic and produce eggs, which are subsequently released. Since eggs of the different *Taenia* species are morphologically identical, differences in the morphology of the scolex or proglottids provide the basis for diagnostic identification to the species level.

Most human tapeworms require at least one intermediate host for complete larval development. After ingestion of the eggs or proglottids by an intermediate host, the larval oncospheres are activated, escape the egg, and penetrate the intestinal mucosa. The oncosphere migrates to tissues and develops into an encysted form known as a *cysticercus* (single scolex), a *coenurus* (multiple scolices), or a *hydatid* (cyst with daughter cysts, each containing several protoscolices). Ingestion by the definitive host of tissues containing a cyst enables a scolex to develop into a tapeworm.

TAENIASIS SAGINATA

The beef tapeworm *T. saginata* occurs in all countries where raw or undercooked beef is eaten. It is most prevalent in sub-Saharan African and Middle Eastern countries. *T. saginata asiatica* is a variant of *T. saginata* that is found in Asia and for which pigs are the intermediate host.

Etiology and Pathogenesis Humans are the only definitive host for the adult stage of *T. saginata*. This tapeworm, which can reach 8 m in length, inhabits the upper jejunum and has a scolex with four prominent suckers and 1000–2000 proglottids. Each gravid segment has 15–30 uterine branches (in contrast to 8–12 for *T. solium*). The eggs are indistinguishable from those of *T. solium*; they measure 30–40 μm, contain the oncosphere, and have a thick brown striated shell. Eggs deposited on vegetation can live for months or years until they are ingested by cattle or other herbivores. The embryo released after ingestion invades the intestinal wall and is carried to striated muscle, where it transforms into a cysticercus. When ingested in raw or undercooked beef, this form can infect humans. After the cysticercus is ingested, it takes ~2 months for the mature adult worm to develop.

Clinical Manifestations Patients become aware of the infection most commonly by noting passage of proglottids in their feces. The proglottids are often motile, and patients may experience perianal discomfort when proglottids are discharged. Mild abdominal pain or discomfort, nausea, change in appetite, weakness, and weight loss can occur with *T. saginata* infection.

Diagnosis The diagnosis is made by the detection of eggs or proglottids in the stool. Eggs may also be present in the perianal area; thus, if proglottids or eggs are not found in the stool, the perianal region should be examined with use of a cellophane-tape swab (as in pinworm infection; Chap. 210). Distinguishing *T. saginata* from *T. solium* requires examination of mature proglottids or the scolex. Serologic tests are not helpful diagnostically. Eosinophilia and elevated levels of serum IgE may be detected.

Rx TAENIASIS SAGINATA

A single dose of praziquantel (10 mg/kg) is highly effective.

Prevention The major method of preventing infection is the adequate cooking of beef; exposure to temperatures as low as 56°C for 5 min will destroy cysticerci. Refrigeration or salting for long periods or freezing at –10°C for 9 days also kills cysticerci in beef. General preventive measures include inspection of beef and proper disposal of human feces.

TAENIASIS SOLIUM AND CYSTICERCOSIS

The pork tapeworm *T. solium* can cause two distinct forms of infection in humans: adult tapeworms in the intestine or larval forms in the tissues (cysticercosis). Humans are the only definitive hosts for *T. solium*; pigs are the usual intermediate hosts, although other animals may harbor the larval forms.

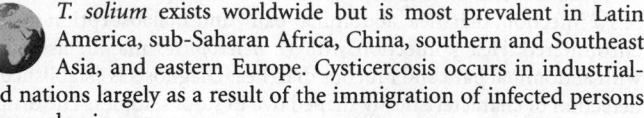

T. solium exists worldwide but is most prevalent in Latin America, sub-Saharan Africa, China, southern and Southeast Asia, and eastern Europe. Cysticercosis occurs in industrialized nations largely as a result of the immigration of infected persons from endemic areas.

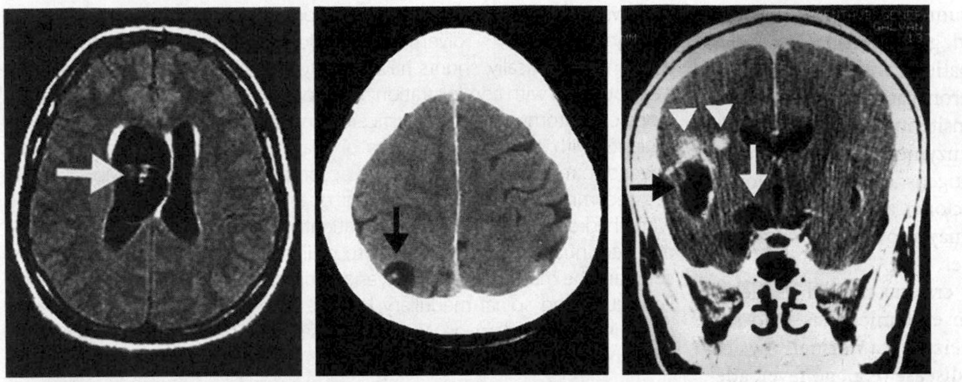

FIGURE 213-1 Neurocysticercosis is caused by *Taenia solium*. Neurologic infection can be classified on the basis of the location and viability of the parasites. When the parasites are in the ventricles, they often cause obstructive hydrocephalus. ***Left:*** MRI showing a cysticercus in the lateral ventricle, with resultant hydrocephalus. The arrow points to the scolex within the cystic parasite. ***Center:*** CT showing a parenchymal cysticercus, with enhancement of the cyst wall and an internal scolex (*arrow*). ***Right:*** Multiple cysticerci, including calcified lesions from prior infection (*arrowheads*), viable cysticerci in the basilar cisterns (*white arrow*), and a large degenerating cysticercus in the Sylvian fissure (*black arrow*). (*Modified with permission from JC Bandres et al: Clin Infect Dis 15:799, 1992. © The University of Chicago Press.*)

Etiology and Pathogenesis The adult tapeworm generally resides in the upper jejunum. The scolex attaches by both sucking disks and two rows of hooklets. Often only one adult worm is present, but that worm may live for years. The tapeworm, usually ~3 m in length, may have as many as 1000 proglottids, each of which produces up to 50,000 eggs. Groups of 3–5 proglottids are generally released and excreted into the feces, and the eggs in these proglottids are infective for both humans and animals. The eggs may survive in the environment for several months. After ingestion of eggs by the pig intermediate host, the larvae are activated, escape the egg, penetrate the intestinal wall, and are carried to many tissues, with a predilection for striated muscle of the neck, tongue, and trunk. Within 60–90 days, the encysted larval stage develops. These cysticerci can survive for months to years. By ingesting undercooked pork containing cysticerci, humans acquire infections that lead to intestinal tapeworms. Infections that cause human cysticercosis follow the ingestion of *T. solium* eggs, usually from close contact with a tapeworm carrier. Autoinfection may occur if an individual with an egg-producing tapeworm ingests eggs derived from his or her own feces.

Clinical Manifestations Intestinal infections with *T. solium* may be asymptomatic. Fecal passage of proglottids may be noted by patients. Other symptoms are infrequent.

In cysticercosis, the clinical manifestations are variable. Cysticerci can be found anywhere in the body but are most commonly detected in the brain, cerebrospinal fluid (CSF), skeletal muscle, subcutaneous tissue, or eye. The clinical presentation of cysticercosis depends on the number and location of cysticerci as well as the extent of associated inflammatory responses or scarring. Neurologic manifestations are the most common (Fig. 213-1). Seizures are associated with inflammation surrounding cysticerci in the brain parenchyma. These seizures may be generalized, focal, or Jacksonian. Hydrocephalus results from obstruction of CSF flow by cysticerci and accompanying inflammation or by CSF outflow obstruction from arachnoiditis. Signs of increased intracranial pressure, including headache, nausea, vomiting, changes in vision, dizziness, ataxia, or confusion, are often evident. Patients with hydrocephalus may develop papilledema or display altered mental status. When cysticerci develop at the base of the brain or in the subarachnoid space, they may cause chronic meningitis or arachnoiditis, communicating hydrocephalus, or strokes.

Diagnosis The diagnosis of intestinal *T. solium* infection is made by the detection of eggs or proglottids, as described for *T. saginata*. In cysticercosis, diagnosis can be difficult. A consensus conference has delineated absolute, major, minor, and epidemiologic criteria for diagnosis (Table 213-1). Diagnostic certainty is possible only with definite demonstration of the parasite (absolute criteria). This task can be accomplished by histologic observation of the parasite in excised tissue, by funduscopic visualization of the parasite in the eye (in the anterior chamber, vitreous, or subretinal spaces), or by neuroimaging studies demonstrating cystic lesions containing a characteristic scolex. In most cases, diagnostic certainty is not possible. Instead, a clinical diagnosis is made on the basis of a combination of clinical presentation, radiographic studies, serologic tests, and exposure history.

Neuroimaging findings suggestive of neurocysticercosis constitute the primary major diagnostic criterion. These findings include cystic lesions with or without enhancement (e.g., ring enhancement), one or more nodular calcifications (which may also have associated enhancement), or focal enhancing lesions. Cysticerci in the brain parenchyma are usually 5–20 mm in diameter and rounded. Cystic lesions in the subarachnoid space or fissures may enlarge up to 6 cm in diameter and may be lobulated. For cysticerci within the subarachnoid space or ventricles, the walls may be very thin and the cyst fluid is often isodense with CSF. Thus, obstructive hydrocephalus or enhancement of the basilar meninges may be the only finding on CT in extraparenchymal neurocysticercosis. Cysticerci in the ventricles or subarachnoid space are usually visible to an experienced neuroradiologist on MRI or on CT with intraventricular contrast injection. CT is more sensitive than MRI in identifying calcified lesions, whereas MRI is better for identifying cystic lesions and enhancement.

The second major diagnostic criterion is detection of specific antibodies to cysticerci. While most tests employing unfractionated antigen have high rates of false-positive and false-negative results, this problem

TABLE 213-1 DIAGNOSTIC CRITERIA FOR HUMAN CYSTICERCOSIS[a]

1. Absolute criteria
   a. Demonstration of cysticerci by histologic or microscopic examination of biopsy material
   b. Visualization of the parasite in the eye by funduscopy
   c. Neuroradiologic demonstration of cystic lesions containing a characteristic scolex
2. Major criteria
   a. Neuroradiologic lesions suggestive of neurocysticercosis
   b. Demonstration of antibodies to cysticerci in serum by enzyme-linked immunoelectrotransfer blot
   c. Resolution of intracranial cystic lesions spontaneously or after therapy with albendazole or praziquantel alone
3. Minor criteria
   a. Lesions compatible with neurocysticercosis detected by neuroimaging studies
   b. Clinical manifestations suggestive of neurocysticercosis
   c. Demonstration of antibodies to cysticerci or cysticercal antigen in cerebrospinal fluid by ELISA
   d. Evidence of cysticercosis outside the central nervous system (e.g., cigar-shaped soft tissue calcifications)
4. Epidemiologic criteria
   a. Residence in a cysticercosis-endemic area
   b. Frequent travel to a cysticercosis-endemic area
   c. Household contact with an individual infected with *Taenia solium*

[a]Diagnosis is confirmed by either one absolute criterion or a combination of two major criteria, one minor criterion, and one epidemiologic criterion. A probable diagnosis is supported by the fulfillment of (1) one major criterion plus two minor criteria; (2) one major criterion plus one minor criterion and one epidemiologic criterion; or (3) three minor criteria plus one epidemiologic criterion.

Note: ELISA, enzyme-linked immunosorbent assay.

Source: Modified from Del Brutto et al.

can be overcome by using the more specific immunoblot assay. An immunoblot assay using lentil-lectin purified glycoproteins has >99% specificity and is highly sensitive. However, patients with single intracranial lesions or with calcifications may be seronegative. With this assay, serum samples provide greater diagnostic sensitivity than CSF. All of the diagnostic antigens have been cloned, and enzyme-linked immunosorbent assays (ELISAs) using recombinant antigens are being developed. Antigen detection assays employing monoclonal antibodies to detect parasite antigen in the blood or spinal fluid may also facilitate diagnosis. However, these assays are not widely available.

Studies have demonstrated that clinical criteria can aid in the diagnosis in selected cases. In patients from endemic areas who had single enhancing lesions presenting with seizures, a normal physical examination, and no evidence of systemic disease (e.g., no fever, adenopathy, or abnormal chest radiograph), the constellation of rounded CT lesions 5–20 mm in diameter with no midline shift was almost always caused by neurocysticercosis. Finally, spontaneous resolution or resolution after therapy with albendazole alone is consistent with neurocysticercosis.

Minor diagnostic criteria include neuroimaging findings consistent with but less characteristic of cysticercosis, clinical manifestations suggestive of neurocysticercosis (e.g., seizures, hydrocephalus, or altered mental status), evidence of cysticercosis outside the central nervous system (CNS; e.g., cigar-shaped soft tissue calcifications), or detection of antibody in CSF by ELISA. Epidemiologic criteria include exposure to a tapeworm carrier or household member infected with *T. solium*, current or prior residence in an endemic area, and frequent travel to an endemic area.

Diagnosis is confirmed in patients with either one absolute criterion or a combination of two major criteria, one minor criterion, and one epidemiologic criterion (Table 213-1). A probable diagnosis is supported by the fulfillment of (1) one major criterion plus two minor criteria; (2) one major criterion plus one minor criterion and one epidemiologic criterion; or (3) three minor criteria plus one epidemiologic criterion. While the CSF is usually abnormal in neurocysticercosis, CSF abnormalities are not pathognomonic. Patients may have CSF pleocytosis with a predominance of lymphocytes, neutrophils, or eosinophils. The protein level in CSF may be elevated; the glucose concentration is usually normal but may be depressed.

℞ TAENIASIS SOLIUM AND CYSTICERCOSIS

Intestinal *T. solium* infection is treated with a single dose of praziquantel (10 mg/kg). However, praziquantel occasionally evokes an inflammatory response in the CNS if concomitant cryptic cysticercosis is present. Niclosamide (2 g) is also effective but is not widely available.

The initial management of neurocysticercosis should focus on symptom-based treatment of seizures or hydrocephalus. Seizures can usually be controlled with antiepileptic treatment. If parenchymal lesions resolve without development of calcifications and patients remain free of seizures, antiepileptic therapy can usually be discontinued after 1–2 years. Placebo-controlled trials are beginning to clarify the clinical advantage of antiparasitic drugs for parenchymal neurocysticercosis. Trends toward faster resolution of neuroradiologic abnormalities have been observed in most studies. The clinical benefits are less dramatic and consist mainly of shortening the period during which recurrent seizures occur and decreasing the number of patients who have many recurrent seizures. For the treatment of patients with brain parenchymal cysticerci, most authorities favor antiparasitic drugs, including praziquantel (50–60 mg/kg daily in three divided doses for 15–30 days) or albendazole (15 mg/kg per day for 8–28 days). Both agents may exacerbate the inflammatory response around the dying parasite, thereby exacerbating seizures or hydrocephalus as well. Thus, patients receiving these drugs should be carefully monitored, and high-dose glucocorticoids should be used during treatment. Since glucocorticoids induce first-pass metabolism of praziquantel and may decrease its antiparasitic effect, cimetidine should be coadministered to inhibit praziquantel metabolism.

For patients with hydrocephalus, the emergent reduction of intracranial pressure is the mainstay of therapy. In the case of obstructive hydrocephalus, the preferred approach is removal of the cysticercus via endoscopic surgery. However, this intervention is not always possible. An alternative approach is initially to perform a diverting procedure, such as ventriculoperitoneal shunting. Historically, shunts have usually failed, but low failure rates have been attained with administration of antiparasitic drugs and glucocorticoids. Open craniotomy to remove cysticerci is now required only infrequently. For patients with subarachnoid cysts or giant cysticerci, glucocorticoids are needed to reduce arachnoiditis and accompanying vasculitis. Most authorities recommend prolonged courses of antiparasitic drugs and shunting when hydrocephalus is present. In patients with diffuse cerebral edema and elevated intracranial pressure due to multiple inflamed lesions, glucocorticoids are the mainstay of therapy, and antiparasitic drugs should be avoided. For ocular and spinal medullary lesions, drug-induced inflammation may cause irreversible damage. Most patients should be managed surgically, although case reports have described cures with medical therapy.

Prevention Measures for the prevention of intestinal *T. solium* infection consist of the application to pork of precautions similar to those described above for beef with regard to *T. saginata* infection. The prevention of cysticercosis involves minimizing the opportunities for ingestion of fecally derived eggs by means of good personal hygiene, effective fecal disposal, and treatment and prevention of human intestinal infections. Mass chemotherapy has been administered to human and porcine populations in efforts at disease eradication.

ECHINOCOCCOSIS

Echinococcosis is an infection caused in humans by the larval stage of the *Echinococcus granulosus* complex, *E. multilocularis*, or *E. vogeli*. *E. granulosus* complex parasites, which produce unilocular cystic lesions, are prevalent in areas where livestock is raised in association with dogs. These parasites are found on all continents, with areas of high prevalence in China, central Asia, the Middle East, the Mediterranean region, eastern Africa, and parts of South America. Molecular evidence suggests that *E. granulosus* strains may actually belong to more than one species; specifically, strains from sheep, cattle, pigs, horses, and camels probably represent separate species. *E. multilocularis*, which causes multilocular alveolar lesions that are locally invasive, is found in Alpine, sub-Arctic, or Arctic regions, including Canada, the United States, and central and northern Europe; China; and central Asia. *E. vogeli* causes polycystic hydatid disease and is found only in Central and South America.

Like other cestodes, echinococcal species have both intermediate and definitive hosts. The definitive hosts are canines that pass eggs in their feces. After the ingestion of eggs, cysts develop in the intermediate hosts—sheep, cattle, humans, goats, camels, and horses for the *E. granulosus* complex and mice and other rodents for *E. multilocularis*. When a dog (*E. granulosus*) or fox (*E. multilocularis*) ingests infected meat containing cysts, the life cycle is completed.

Etiology The small (5-mm-long) adult *E. granulosus* worm, which lives for 5–20 months in the jejunum of dogs, has only three proglottids: one immature, one mature, and one gravid. The gravid segment splits to release eggs that are morphologically similar to *Taenia* eggs and are extremely hardy. After humans ingest the eggs, embryos escape from the eggs, penetrate the intestinal mucosa, enter the portal circulation, and are carried to various organs, most commonly the liver and lungs. Larvae develop into fluid-filled unilocular hydatid cysts that consist of an external membrane and an inner germinal layer. Daughter cysts develop from the inner aspect of the germinal layer, as do germinating cystic structures called *brood capsules*. New larvae, called *protoscolices*, develop in large numbers within the brood capsule. The cysts expand slowly over a period of years.

The life cycle of *E. multilocularis* is similar except that wild canines, such as foxes, serve as the definitive hosts and small rodents serve as the intermediate hosts. The larval form of *E. multilocularis*, however, is quite different in that it remains in the proliferative phase, the parasite is always multilocular, and vesicles without brood capsule or protoscolices progressively invade the host tissue by peripheral extension of processes from the germinal layer.

Clinical Manifestations Slowly enlarging echinococcal cysts generally remain asymptomatic until their expanding size or their space-occupying effect in an involved organ elicits symptoms. The liver and the lungs are the most common sites of these cysts. The liver is involved in about two-thirds of *E. granulosus* infections and in nearly all *E. multilocularis* infections. Since a period of years elapses before cysts enlarge sufficiently to cause symptoms, they may be discovered incidentally on a routine x-ray or ultrasound study.

Patients with hepatic echinococcosis who are symptomatic most often present with abdominal pain or a palpable mass in the right upper quadrant. Compression of a bile duct or leakage of cyst fluid into the biliary tree may mimic recurrent cholelithiasis, and biliary obstruction can result in jaundice. Rupture of or episodic leakage from a hydatid cyst may produce fever, pruritus, urticaria, eosinophilia, or anaphylaxis. Pulmonary hydatid cysts may rupture into the bronchial tree or peritoneal cavity and produce cough, dyspnea, chest pain, or hemoptysis. Rupture of hydatid cysts, which can occur spontaneously or at surgery, may lead to multifocal dissemination of protoscolices, which can form additional cysts. Other presentations are due to the involvement of bone (invasion of the medullary cavity with slow bone erosion producing pathologic fractures), the CNS (space-occupying lesions), the heart (conduction defects, pericarditis), and the pelvis (pelvic mass).

The larval forms of *E. multilocularis* characteristically present as a slowly growing hepatic tumor, with progressive destruction of the liver and extension into vital structures. Patients commonly report upper quadrant and epigastric pain. Liver enlargement and obstructive jaundice may be apparent. The lesions may infiltrate adjoining organs (e.g., diaphragm, kidneys, or lungs) or may metastasize to the spleen, lungs, or brain.

Diagnosis Radiographic and related imaging studies are important in detecting and evaluating echinococcal cysts. Plain films will define pulmonary cysts of *E. granulosus*—usually as rounded masses of uniform density—but may miss cysts in other organs unless there is cyst wall calcification (as occurs in the liver). MRI, CT, and ultrasound reveal well-defined cysts with thick or thin walls. When older cysts contain a layer of hydatid sand that is rich in accumulated protoscolices, these imaging methods may detect this fluid layer of different density. However, the most pathognomonic finding, if demonstrable, is that of daughter cysts within the larger cyst. This finding, like eggshell or mural calcification on CT, is indicative of *E. granulosus* infection and helps to distinguish the cyst from carcinomas, bacterial or amebic liver abscesses, or hemangiomas. In contrast, ultrasound or CT of alveolar hydatid cysts reveals indistinct solid masses with central necrosis and plaquelike calcifications.

A specific diagnosis of *E. granulosus* infection can be made by the examination of aspirated fluids for protoscolices or hooklets, but diagnostic aspiration is not usually recommended because of the risk of fluid leakage resulting in either dissemination of infection or anaphylactic reactions. Serodiagnostic assays can be useful, although a negative test does not exclude the diagnosis of echinococcosis. Cysts in the liver elicit positive antibody responses in ~90% of cases, whereas up to 50% of individuals with cysts in the lungs are seronegative. Detection of antibody to specific echinococcal antigens by immunoblotting has the highest degree of specificity.

Rx ECHINOCOCCOSIS

Therapy for cystic echinococcosis is based on considerations of the size, location, and manifestations of cysts and the overall health of the patient. Surgery has traditionally been the principal definitive method of treatment. Currently, ultrasound staging is recommended for *E. granulosus* infections (**Fig. 213-2**). For CE1 lesions, uncomplicated CE3 lesions, and some CE2 lesions, PAIR (*p*ercutaneous *a*spiration, *i*nfusion of scolicidal agents, and *r*easpiration) is now recommended instead of surgery. PAIR is contraindicated for superficially located cysts (because of the risk of rupture), for cysts with multiple thick internal septal divisions (honeycombing pattern), and for cysts communicating with the biliary tree. For prophylaxis of secondary peritoneal echinococcosis due to inadvertent spillage of fluid during PAIR, the administration of albendazole (15 mg/kg daily in two divided doses) should be initiated at least 4 days before the procedure and continued for at least 4 weeks afterward. Ultrasound- or CT-guided aspiration allows confirmation of the diagnosis by demonstration of protoscolices in the aspirate. After aspiration, contrast material should be injected to detect occult communications with the biliary tract. Alternatively, the fluid should be checked for bile staining by dipstick. If no bile is found and no communication visualized, the contrast material is reaspirated, with subsequent infusion of scolicidal agents (usually 95% ethanol; alternatively, hypertonic saline). Daughter cysts within the primary cyst may need to be

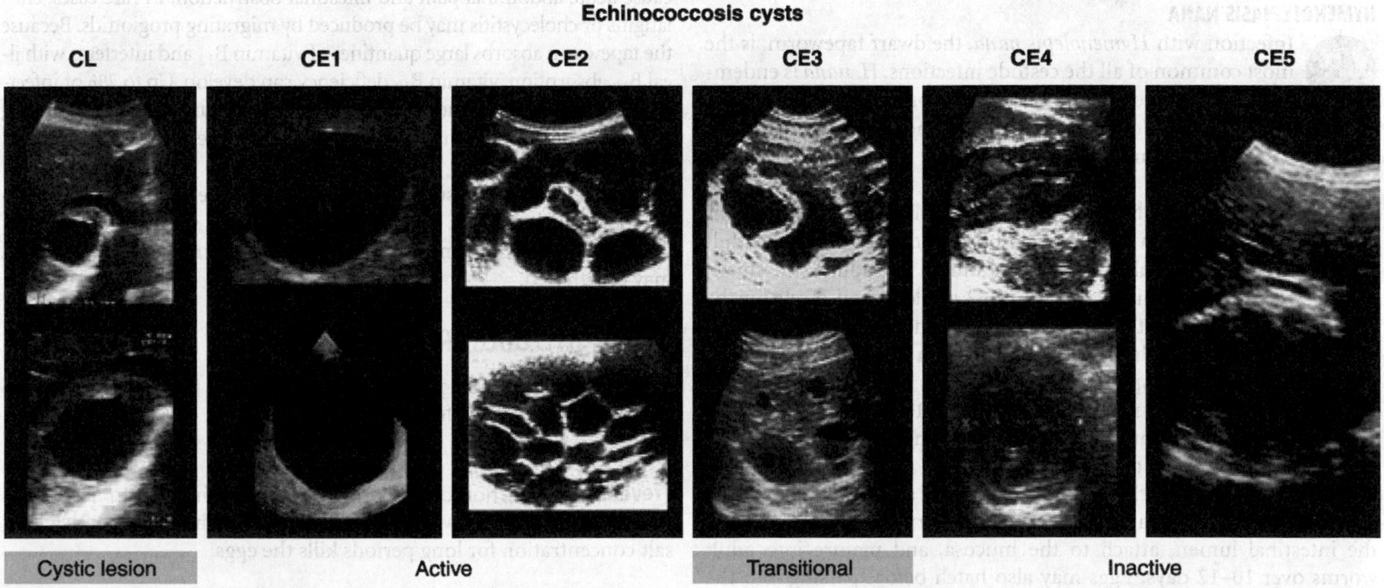

FIGURE 213-2 Management of cystic hydatid disease caused by *Echinococcus granulosus* should be based on viability of the parasite, which can be estimated from radiographic appearance. The ultrasound appearance includes lesions classified as active, transitional, and inactive. *Active* cysts include types CL (with a cystic lesion and no visible cyst wall), CE1 [with a visible cyst wall and internal echoes (snowflake sign)], and CE2 (with a visible cyst wall and internal septation). *Transitional cysts* (CE3) may have detached laminar membranes or may be partially collapsed. *Inactive cysts* include types CE4 (a nonhomogeneous mass) and CE5 (a cyst with a thick calcified wall). *[Adapted from RL Guerrant et al (eds): Tropical Infectious Diseases: Principles, Pathogens and Practice, 2d ed, p 1312. © 2005, with permission from Elsevier Science.]*

punctured separately. In experienced hands, this approach yields rates of cure and relapse equivalent to those following surgery, with less perioperative morbidity and shorter hospitalization.

Surgery remains the treatment of choice for complicated *E. granulosus* cysts (e.g., those communicating with the biliary tract) or for areas where PAIR is not possible. For *E. granulosus*, the preferred surgical approach is pericystectomy, in which the entire cyst and the surrounding fibrous tissue are removed. The risks posed by leakage of fluid during surgery or PAIR include anaphylaxis and dissemination of infectious protoscolices. The latter complication has been minimized by careful attention to the prevention of spillage of the cyst and by soaking of the drapes with hypertonic saline. Infusion of scolicidal agents is no longer recommended because of problems with hypernatremia, intoxication, or sclerosing cholangitis. Albendazole, which is active against *Echinococcus*, should be administered adjunctively, beginning several days before resection and continuing for several weeks for *E. granulosus*. Praziquantel (50 mg/kg daily for 2 weeks) may hasten the death of the protoscolices. Medical therapy with albendazole alone for 12 weeks to 6 months results in cure in ~30% of cases and in improvement in another 50%. In many instances of treatment failure, *E. granulosus* infections are subsequently treated successfully with PAIR or additional courses of medical therapy. Response to treatment is best assessed by serial imaging studies, with attention to cyst size and consistency. Some cysts may not demonstrate complete radiologic resolution even though no viable protoscolices are present. Some of these cysts with partial radiologic resolution (e.g., CE4) can be managed with observation only.

Surgical resection remains the treatment of choice for *E. multilocularis* infection. Complete removal of the parasite continues to offer the best chance for cure. Ongoing therapy with albendazole for at least 2 years after presumptively curative surgery is recommended. Most cases are diagnosed at a stage at which complete resection is not possible; in these cases, albendazole treatment should be continued indefinitely, with careful monitoring. In some cases, liver transplantation has been used because of the size of the necessary liver resection. However, continuous immunosuppression favors the proliferation of *E. multilocularis* larvae and reinfection of the transplant. Thus, indefinite treatment with albendazole is required.

Prevention In endemic areas, echinococcosis can be prevented by administering praziquantel to infected dogs, by denying dogs access to infected animals, or by vaccinating sheep. Limitation of the number of stray dogs is helpful in reducing the prevalence of infection among humans.

HYMENOLEPIASIS NANA

Infection with *Hymenolepis nana*, the dwarf tapeworm, is the most common of all the cestode infections. *H. nana* is endemic in both temperate and tropical regions of the world. Infection is spread by fecal/oral contamination and is common among institutionalized children.

Etiology and Pathogenesis *H. nana* is the only cestode of humans that does not require an intermediate host. Both the larval and adult phases of the life cycle take place in the human. The adult—the smallest tapeworm parasitizing humans—is ~2 cm long and dwells in the proximal ileum. Proglottids, which are quite small and are rarely seen in the stool, release spherical eggs 30–44 μm in diameter, each of which contains an oncosphere with six hooklets. The eggs are immediately infective and are unable to survive for >10 days in the external environment. *H. nana* can also be acquired by the ingestion of infected insects (especially larval meal-worms and larval fleas). When the egg is ingested by a new host, the oncosphere is freed and penetrates the intestinal villi, becoming a cysticercoid larva. Larvae migrate back into the intestinal lumen, attach to the mucosa, and mature into adult worms over 10–12 days. Eggs may also hatch before passing into the stool, causing internal autoinfection with increasing numbers of intestinal worms. Although the life span of adult *H. nana* worms is only ~4–10 weeks, the autoinfection cycle perpetuates the infection.

Clinical Manifestations *H. nana* infection, even with many intestinal worms, is usually asymptomatic. When infection is intense, anorexia, abdominal pain, and diarrhea develop.

Diagnosis Infection is diagnosed by the finding of eggs in the stool.

Rx HYMENOLEPIASIS NANA

Praziquantel (25 mg/kg once) is the treatment of choice, since it acts against both the adult worms and the cysticercoids in the intestinal villi. Nitazoxanide (500 mg bid for 3 days) may be used as an alternative.

Prevention Good personal hygiene and improved sanitation can eradicate the disease. Epidemics have been controlled by mass chemotherapy coupled with improved hygiene.

HYMENOLEPIASIS DIMINUTA

Hymenolepis diminuta, a cestode of rodents, occasionally infects small children, who ingest the larvae in uncooked cereal foods contaminated by fleas and other insects in which larvae develop. Infection is usually asymptomatic and is diagnosed by the detection of eggs in the stool. Treatment with praziquantel results in cure in most cases.

DIPHYLLOBOTHRIASIS

Diphyllobothrium latum and other *Diphyllobothrium* species are found in the lakes, rivers, and deltas of the northern hemisphere, Central Africa, and Chile.

Etiology and Pathogenesis The adult worm—the longest tapeworm (up to 25 m)—attaches to the ileal and occasionally to the jejunal mucosa by its suckers, which are located on its elongated scolex. The adult worm has 3000–4000 proglottids, which release ~1 million eggs daily into the feces. If an egg reaches water, it hatches and releases a free-swimming embryo that can be eaten by small freshwater crustaceans (*Cyclops* or *Diaptomus* species). After an infected crustacean containing a developed procercoid is swallowed by a fish, the larva migrates into the fish's flesh and grows into a plerocercoid, or sparganum larva. Humans acquire the infection by ingesting infected raw or smoked fish. Within 3–5 weeks, the tapeworm matures into an adult in the human intestine.

Clinical Manifestations Most *D. latum* infections are asymptomatic, although manifestations may include transient abdominal discomfort, diarrhea, vomiting, weakness, and weight loss. Occasionally, infection can cause acute abdominal pain and intestinal obstruction; in rare cases, cholangitis or cholecystitis may be produced by migrating proglottids. Because the tapeworm absorbs large quantities of vitamin B_{12} and interferes with ileal B_{12} absorption, vitamin B_{12} deficiency can develop. Up to 2% of infected patients, especially the elderly, have megaloblastic anemia resembling pernicious anemia and may exhibit neurologic sequelae of B_{12} deficiency.

Diagnosis The diagnosis is made readily by the detection of the characteristic eggs in the stool. The eggs possess a single shell with an operculum at one end and a knob at the other. Mild to moderate eosinophilia may be detected.

Rx DIPHYLLOBOTHRIASIS

Praziquantel (5–10 mg/kg once) is highly effective. Parenteral vitamin B_{12} should be given if B_{12} deficiency is manifest.

Prevention Infection can be prevented by heating fish to 54°C for 5 min or by freezing it at –18°C for 24 h. Placing fish in brine with a high salt concentration for long periods kills the eggs.

DIPYLIDIASIS

Dipylidium caninum, a common tapeworm of dogs and cats, may accidentally infect humans. Dogs, cats, and occasionally humans become infected by ingesting fleas harboring cysticercoids. Children are more likely to become infected than adults. Most infections are asymptomatic, but abdominal pain, diarrhea, anal pruritus, urticaria, eosinophilia, or passage of segments in the stool may occur. The diagnosis is made by the detection of proglottids or ova in the stool. As in *D. latum* infection, therapy consists of praziquantel. Prevention requires anthelmintic treatment and flea control for pet dogs or cats.

SPARGANOSIS

Humans can be infected by the sparganum, or plerocercoid larva, of a diphyllobothrid tapeworm of the genus *Spirometra.* Infection can be acquired by the consumption of water containing infected *Cyclops*; by the ingestion of infected snakes, birds, or mammals; or by the application of infected flesh as poultices. The worm migrates slowly in tissues, and infection commonly presents as a subcutaneous swelling. Periorbital tissues can be involved, and ocular sparganosis may destroy the eye. Surgical excision is used to treat localized sparganosis.

COENUROSIS

This rare infection of humans by the larval stage (coenurus) of the dog tapeworm *Taenia multiceps* or *T. serialis* results in a space-occupying cystic lesion. As in cysticercosis, involvement of the CNS and subcutaneous tissue is most common. Both definitive diagnosis and treatment require surgical excision of the lesion. Chemotherapeutic agents generally are not effective.

WEBSITE OF INTEREST: *CDC Division of Parasitic Diseases. www.cdc.gov/ncidod/dpd/default.htm*

FURTHER READINGS

DEL BRUTTO OH et al: Proposed diagnostic criteria for neurocysticercosis. Neurology 57:177, 2001

ECKERT J, DEPLAZES P: Biological, epidemiological, and clinical aspects of echinococcosis, a zoonosis of increasing concern. Clin Microbiol Rev 17:107, 2004

GARCIA HH et al: A trial of antiparasitic treatment to reduce the rate of seizures due to cerebral cysticercosis. N Engl J Med 350:249, 2004

——— et al: Current consensus guidelines for treatment of neurocysticercosis. Clin Microbiol Rev 15:747, 2002

NASH TE et al: Treatment of neurocysticercosis: Current status and future research needs. Neurology 67:1120, 2006

PAWLOWSKI ZS et al: Echinococcosis in humans: Clinical aspects, diagnosis, and treatment, in *WHO/OIE Manual on Echinococcosis in Humans and Animals: A Public Health Problem of Global Concern*, J Eckert et al (eds). Paris, World Organization for Animal Health, 2001

SCHANTZ PM et al: Echinococcosis, in *Tropical Infectious Diseases: Principles, Pathogens and Practice*, 2d ed, RL Guerrant et al (eds). Philadelphia, Churchill Livingstone, 2005, p 1304

SINGH G, PRABHAKAR S: *Taenia solium Cysticercosis: From Basic Science to Clinical Science.* Wallingford, UK, CABI Publishing, 2002

WORLD HEALTH ORGANIZATION INFORMAL WORKING GROUP ON ECHINOCOCCOSIS: International classification of ultrasound images in cystic echinococcosis for application in clinical and field epidemiological settings. Acta Tropica 85:253, 2003

———: PAIR puncture, aspiration, injection, re-aspiration: An option for the treatment of cystic echinococcosis. WHO/CDS/CSR/APH/2001.6. Geneva, WHO, 2001

214 Microbial Bioterrorism

H. Clifford Lane, Anthony S. Fauci

Descriptions of the use of microbial pathogens as potential weapons of war or terrorism date from ancient times. Among the most frequently cited of such episodes are the poisoning of water supplies in the sixth century B.C. with the fungus *Claviceps purpurea* (rye ergot) by the Assyrians, the hurling of the dead bodies of plague victims over the walls of the city of Kaffa by the Tartar army in 1346, and the efforts by the British to spread smallpox via contaminated blankets to the native American population loyal to the French in 1767. Although the use of chemical weapons in wartime took place in the not-too-distant past (Chap. 215), the tragic events of September 11, 2001, followed closely by the anthrax attacks through the U.S. Postal System, dramatically changed the mindset of the American public regarding both our vulnerability to microbial bioterrorist attacks and the seriousness and intent of the Federal government to protect its citizens against future attacks. Modern science has revealed methods of deliberately spreading or enhancing disease in ways not appreciated by our ancestors. The combination of basic research, good medical practice, and constant vigilance will be needed to defend against such attacks.

Although the potential impact of a bioterrorist attack could be enormous, leading to thousands of deaths and extensive morbidity, acts of bioterrorism would be expected to produce their greatest impact through the fear and terror they generate. In contrast to biowarfare, where the primary goal is destruction of the enemy through mass casualties, an important goal of bioterrorism is to destroy the morale of a society through fear and uncertainty. While the actual biologic impact of a single act may be small, the degree of disruption created by the realization that such an attack is possible may be enormous. This was readily apparent with the impact on the U.S. Postal System and the functional interruption of the activities of the legislative branch of government following the anthrax attacks noted above. Thus, the key to the defense against these attacks is a highly functioning system of public health surveillance and education so that attacks can be quickly recognized and effectively contained. This is complemented by the availability of appropriate countermeasures in the form of diagnostics, therapeutics, and vaccines, both in response to and in anticipation of bioterrorist attacks.

The Working Group for Civilian Biodefense has put together a list of key features that characterize the elements of biologic agents that make them particularly effective as weapons (Table 214-1). Included among these are the ease of spread and transmission of the agent as well as the presence of an adequate database to allow newcomers to the field to quickly apply the good science of others to bad intentions of their own. Agents of bioterrorism may be used in their naturally occurring forms or they can be deliberately modified to provide maximal impact. Among the approaches to maximizing the deleterious effects of biologic agents are the genetic modification of microbes for the purposes of antimicrobial resistance or evasion by the immune system, creation of fine-particle aerosols, chemical treatment to stabilize and prolong infectivity, and alteration of host range through changes in surface proteins. Certain of these approaches fall under the category of *weaponization*, which is a term generally used to describe the processing of microbes or toxins in a manner that would ensure a devastating effect of a release. For example, weaponization of anthrax by the Soviets comprised the production of vast amounts of spores in a form that maintained aerosolization for prolonged periods of time; the spores were of appropriate size to reach the lower respiratory tract easily and could be delivered in a massive release, such as via widely dispersed bomblets.

The U.S. Centers for Disease Control and Prevention (CDC) classifies potential biologic threats into three categories, A, B, and C (Table 214-2). Category A agents are the highest-priority pathogens. They pose the greatest risk to national security because they (1) can be easily disseminated or transmitted from person to person, (2) result in high mortality rates and have the potential for major public health impact, (3) might cause public panic and social disruption, and (4) require special action for public health preparedness. Category B agents are the second highest priority pathogens and include those that are moderately easy to disseminate, result in moderate morbidity rates and low mortality rates, and require specifically enhanced diagnostic capacity. Category C agents are the third highest priority. These include certain emerging pathogens, to which the general population lacks immunity, that could be engineered for mass dissemination in the future because of availability, ease of production, ease of dissemination, potential for high morbidity and mortality, and major public health impact. A potential pandemic strain of influenza, such as avian influenza, is one such example. It should be pointed out, however, that these designations are empirical, and, depending on evolving circumstances such as intelligence-based threat assessments, the priority rating of any given microbe or toxin could change. The CDC classification system also largely reflects the severity of illness produced by a given agent, rather than its accessibility to potential terrorists.

TABLE 214-1 KEY FEATURES OF BIOLOGIC AGENTS USED AS BIOWEAPONS

1. High morbidity and mortality
2. Potential for person-to-person spread
3. Low infective dose and highly infectious by aerosol
4. Lack of rapid diagnostic capability
5. Lack of universally available effective vaccine
6. Potential to cause anxiety
7. Availability of pathogen and feasibility of production
8. Environmental stability
9. Database of prior research and development
10. Potential to be "weaponized"

Source: From L Borio et al: JAMA 287:2391, 2002; with permission.

TABLE 214-2 CDC CATEGORY A, B, AND C AGENTS

Category A
- Anthrax (*Bacillus anthracis*)
- Botulism (*Clostridium botulinum* toxin)
- Plague (*Yersinia pestis*)
- Smallpox (*Variola major*)
- Tularemia (*Francisella tularensis*)
- Viral hemorrhagic fevers
  - Arenaviruses: Lassa, New World (Machupo, Junin, Guanarito, and Sabia)
  - Bunyaviridae: Crimean Congo, Rift Valley
  - Filoviridae: Ebola, Marburg

Category B
- Brucellosis (*Brucella* spp.)
- Epsilon toxin of *Clostridium perfringens*
- Food safety threats (e.g., *Salmonella* spp., *Escherichia coli* 0157:H7, *Shigella*)
- Glanders (*Burkholderia mallei*)
- Melioidosis (*B. pseudomallei*)
- Psittacosis (*Chlamydophila psittaci*)
- Q fever (*Coxiella burnetii*)
- Ricin toxin from *Ricinus communis* (castor beans)
- Staphylococcal enterotoxin B
- Typhus fever (*Rickettsia prowazekii*)
- Viral encephalitis [alphaviruses (e.g., Venezuelan, eastern, and western equine encephalitis)]
- Water safety threats (e.g., *Vibrio cholerae*, *Cryptosporidium parvum*)

Category C
- Emerging infectious diseases threats such as Nipah, hantavirus, SARS coronavirus, and pandemic influenza.

Centers for Disease Control and Prevention and the National Institute of Allergy and Infectious Diseases.

ANTHRAX

See also Chap. 131.

Bacillus anthracis as a Bioweapon Anthrax may be the prototypic disease of bioterrorism. Although rarely, if ever, spread from person to person, the illness embodies the other major features of a disease introduced through terrorism, as outlined in Table 214-1. U.S. and British government scientists studied anthrax as a potential biologic weapon beginning approximately at the time of World War II (WWII). Offensive bioweapons activity including bioweapons research on microbes and toxins in the United States ceased in 1969 as a result of two executive orders by President Richard M. Nixon. The 1972 Biological and Toxin Weapons Convention Treaty outlawed research of this type worldwide. Clearly, the Soviet Union was in direct violation of this treaty until at least the Union dissolved in the late 1980s. It is well documented that during this post-treaty period, the Soviets produced and stored tons of anthrax spores for potential use as a bioweapon. At present there is suspicion that research on anthrax as an agent of bioterrorism is ongoing by several nations and extremist groups. One example of this is the release of anthrax spores by the Aum Shrinrikyo cult in Tokyo in 1993. Fortunately, there were no casualties associated with this episode because of the inadvertent use of a nonpathogenic strain of anthrax by the terrorists.

The potential impact of anthrax spores as a bioweapon was clearly demonstrated in 1979 following the accidental release of spores into the atmosphere from a Soviet Union bioweapons facility in Sverdlosk, Russia. While actual figures are not known, at least 77 cases of anthrax were diagnosed with certainty, of which 66 were fatal. These victims were exposed in an area within 4 km downwind of the facility, and deaths due to anthrax were also noted in livestock up to 50 km further downwind. Based on recorded wind patterns, the interval between the time of exposure and development of clinical illness ranged from 2–43 days. The majority of cases were within the first 2 weeks. Death typically occurred within 1–4 days following the onset of symptoms. It is likely that the widespread use of postexposure penicillin prophylaxis limited the total number of cases. The extended period of time between exposure and disease in some individuals supports the data from nonhuman primate studies suggesting the anthrax spores can lie dormant in the respiratory tract for at least 4–6 weeks without evoking an immune response. This extended period of microbiologic latency following exposure poses a significant challenge for management of victims in the postexposure period.

In September 2001, the American public was exposed to anthrax spores as a bioweapon delivered through the U.S. Postal System. The CDC identified 22 confirmed or suspected cases of anthrax as a consequence of this attack. These included 11 patients with inhalational anthrax, of whom 5 died, and 11 patients with cutaneous anthrax (7 confirmed), all of whom survived (Fig. 214-1). Cases occurred in individuals who opened contaminated letters as well as in postal workers involved in the processing of mail. A minimum of five letters mailed from Trenton, NJ, served as the vehicles for these attacks. One of these letters was reported to contain 2 g of material, equivalent to 100 billion to 1 trillion weapon-grade spores. Since studies performed in the 1950s using monkeys exposed to aerosolized anthrax suggested that ~10,000 spores were required to produce lethal disease in 50% of animals exposed to this dose (the LD_{50}), the contents of one letter had the theoretical potential, under optimal conditions, of causing illness or death in up to 50 million individuals when one considers an LD_{50} of 10,000 spores. The strain used in this attack was the Ames strain. Although it was noted to have an inducible beta-lactamase and to constitutively express a cephalosporinase, it was susceptible to all antibiotics standard for *B. anthracis.*

Microbiology and Clinical Features Anthrax is caused by *B. anthracis*, a gram-positive, nonmotile, spore-forming rod that is found in soil and predominantly causes disease in herbivores such as cattle, goats, and sheep. Anthrax spores can remain viable for decades. The remarkable stability of these spores makes them an ideal bioweapon, and their destruction in decontamination activities can be a challenge. Naturally occurring human infection is generally the result of contact with anthrax-infected animals or animal products such as goat hair. While an LD_{50} of 10,000 spores is a generally accepted number it has also been suggested that as few as one to three spores may be adequate to cause disease in some settings. Advanced technology is likely to be necessary to generate spores of the optimal size (1–5 μm) to travel to the alveolar spaces as a bioweapon.

The three major clinical forms of anthrax are gastrointestinal, cutaneous, and inhalational. *Gastrointestinal anthrax* typically results from the ingestion of contaminated meat; the condition is rarely seen and is unlikely to be the result of a bioterrorism event. The lesion of *cutaneous an-*

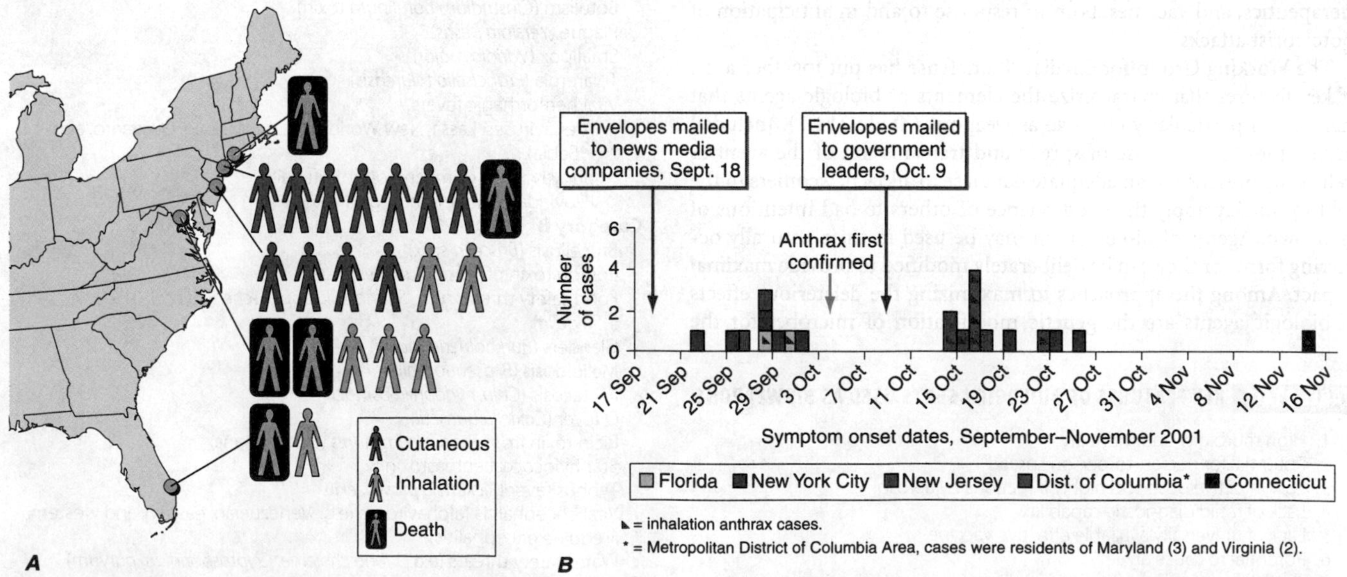

FIGURE 214-1 Confirmed anthrax cases associated with bioterrorism: United States, 2001. *A.* Geographic location, clinical manifestation, and outcome of the 11 cases of confirmed inhalational and 11 cases of confirmed cutaneous anthrax. ***B.*** Epidemic curve for 18 confirmed cases of inhalational and cutaneous anthrax and additional 4 cases of suspected cutaneous anthrax. (*From DB Jernigan et al: Investigation of bioterrorism-related anthrax, US 2001: Epidemiologic findings. Emerg Infect Dis 8:1019, 2002; with permission.*)

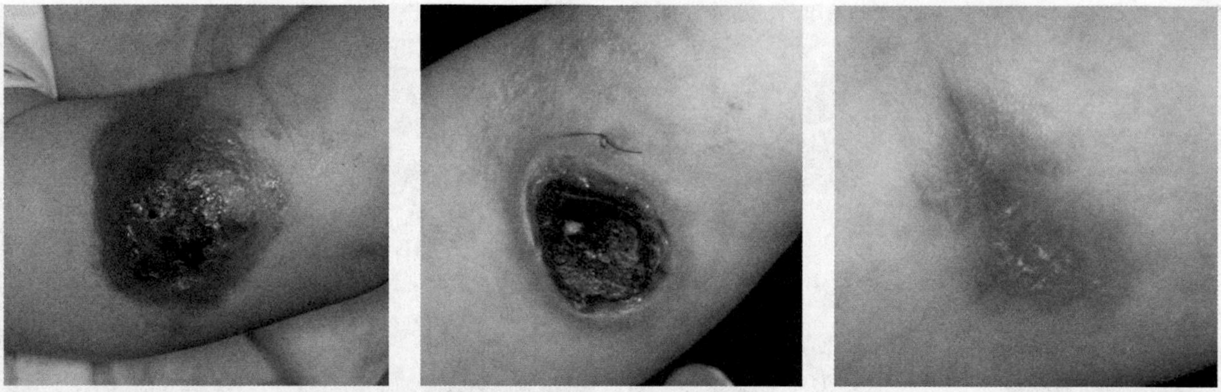

A B C

FIGURE 214-2 Clinical manifestations of a pediatric case of cutaneous anthrax associated with the bioterrorism attack of 2001. The lesion progresses from vesicular on day 5 ***(A)*** to necrotic with the classic black escar on day 12 ***(B)*** to a healed scar 2 months later ***(C)***. *(Photographs provided by Dr. Mary Wu Chang and (A) reprinted with permission of the New England Journal of Medicine.)*

thrax typically begins as a papule following the introduction of spores through an opening in the skin. This papule then evolves to a painless vesicle followed by the development of a coal-black, necrotic eschar (Fig. 214-2). It is the Greek word for coal (*anthrax*) that gives the organism and the disease its name. Cutaneous anthrax was ~20% fatal prior to the availability of antibiotics. *Inhalational anthrax* is the form most likely to be responsible for death in the setting of a bioterrorist attack. It occurs following the inhalation of spores that become deposited in the alveolar spaces. These spores are phagocytosed by macrophages and transported to the mediastinal and peribronchial lymph nodes where they germinate, leading to active bacterial growth and elaboration of the bacterial products edema toxin and lethal toxin. Subsequent hematogenous spread of bacteria is accompanied by cardiovascular collapse and death. The earliest symptoms are typically a viral-like prodrome with fever, malaise, and abdominal and/or chest symptoms that progress over the course of a few days to a moribund state. A characteristic finding is mediastinal widening and pleural effusions on chest x-ray (Fig. 214-3). While initially thought to be 100% fatal, the experiences at Sverdlosk in 1979 and in the United States in 2001 (see below) indicate that with prompt initiation of antibiotic therapy survival is possible. The characteristics of the 11 cases of inhalational anthrax diagnosed in the United States in 2001 following exposure to contaminated letters postmarked September 18 or October 9, 2001, followed the classic pattern established for this illness, with patients presenting with a rapidly progressive course characterized by fever, fatigue or malaise, nausea or vomiting, cough, and shortness of breath. At presentation, the total white blood cell counts were ~10,000 cells/μL; transaminases tended to be elevated, and all 11 had abnormal findings on chest x-ray and CT. Radiologic findings included infiltrates, mediastinal widening, and hemorrhagic pleural effusions. For cases in which the dates of exposure were known, symptoms appeared within 4–6 days. Death occurred within 7 days of diagnosis in the five fatal cases (overall mortality rate 55%). Rapid diagnosis and prompt initiation of antibiotic therapy were key to survival.

℞ ANTHRAX

Anthrax can be successfully treated if the disease is promptly recognized and appropriate therapy is initiated early. While penicillin, ciprofloxacin, and doxycycline are the currently licensed antibiotics for this indication, clindamycin and rifampin also have in vitro activity against the organism and have been used as part of treatment regimens. Until sensitivity results are known, suspected cases are best managed with a combination of broadly active agents **(Table 214-3)**. Patients with inhalational anthrax are not contagious and do not require special isolation procedures.

Vaccination and Prevention The first successful vaccine for anthrax was developed for animals by Louis Pasteur in 1881. At present, the single vaccine licensed for human use is a product produced from the cell-free culture supernatant of an attenuated, nonencapsulated strain of *B. anthracis* (Stern strain), referred to as *anthrax vaccine adsorbed* (AVA). Clinical trials for safety in humans and efficacy in animals are currently under way to evaluate the role of recombinant protective antigen (one of the major components, along with lethal factor and edema factor, of *B. anthracis* toxins) as an alternative to AVA. In a postexposure setting in non-human primates a 2-week course of AVA + ciprofloxacin was found to be superior to ciprofloxacin alone in preventing the development of clinical disease and death. While the current recommendation for postexposure prophylaxis is 60 days of antibiotics, it would seem prudent to include immunization with anthrax vaccine if available. Given the potential for *B. anthracis* to be engineered to express penicillin resistance, the empirical regimen of choice in this setting is either ciprofloxacin or doxycycline.

PLAGUE

See also Chap. 152.

***Yersinia pestis* as a Bioweapon** Although it lacks the environmental stability of anthrax, the highly contagious nature and high mortality of plague make it a close to ideal agent of bioterrorism, particularly if delivered in a weaponized form. Occupying a unique place in history, plague has been alleged to have been used as a biologic weapon for centuries. The catapulting of plague-infected corpses into besieged fortresses is a practice that was first noted in 1346 during the assault of the city of Kaffa by the Tartars. Although unlikely to have resulted in disease transmission, some believe that this event may have played a role in the start of the Black Death pandemic of the fourteenth and fifteenth centuries in Europe. Given that plague was already moving across Asia toward Europe at this time, it is unclear whether such an allegation is accurate. During WWII, the infamous Unit 731 of the Japanese army was reported to have repeatedly dropped plague-infested fleas over parts of China, including Manchuria. These drops were associated with subsequent outbreaks of plague in the targeted areas. Following WWII, the United States and the Soviet Union conducted programs of research on how to create aerosolized *Y. pestis* that could be used as a bioweapon to cause primary pneumonic plague. As mentioned above, plague was thought to be an excellent bioweapon due to the fact that in addition to causing infection in those inhaling the aerosol, significant numbers of secondary cases of primary pneumonic plague would likely occur due to the contagious nature of the disease and person-to-person transmission via respiratory aerosol. Secondary reports of research conducted during that time suggest that organisms remain viable for up to 1 h and can be dispersed for distances up to 10 km. While the offensive bioweapons program in the United States was terminated prior to production of sufficient quantities of plague organisms for use as a weapon, it is believed that Soviet scientists did manufacture quantities sufficient for such a purpose. It has also been

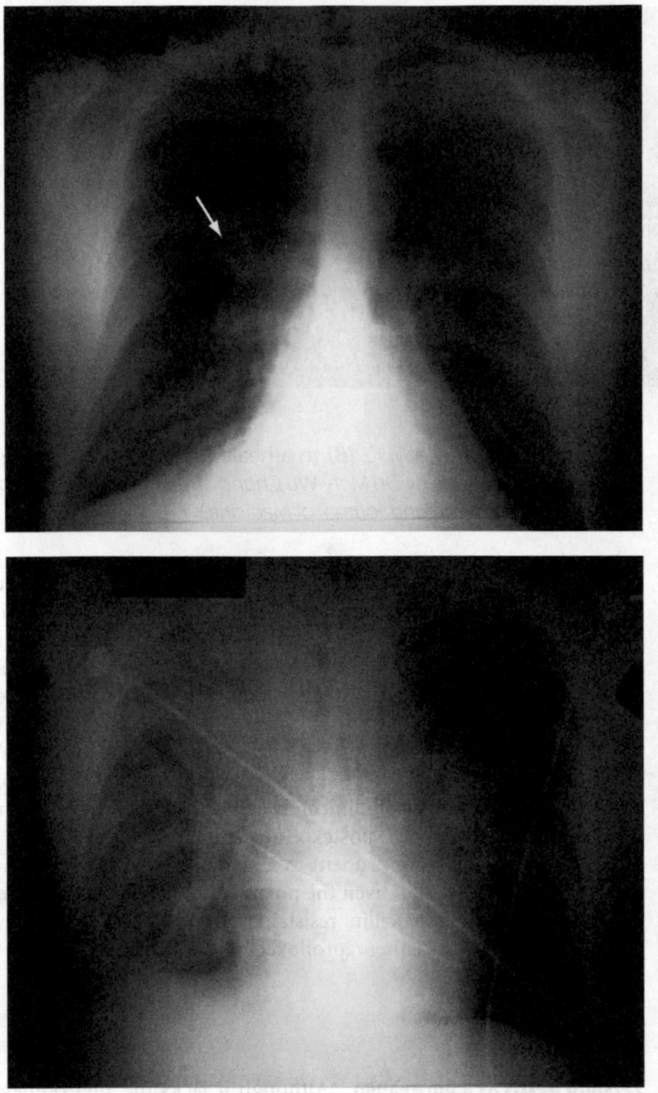

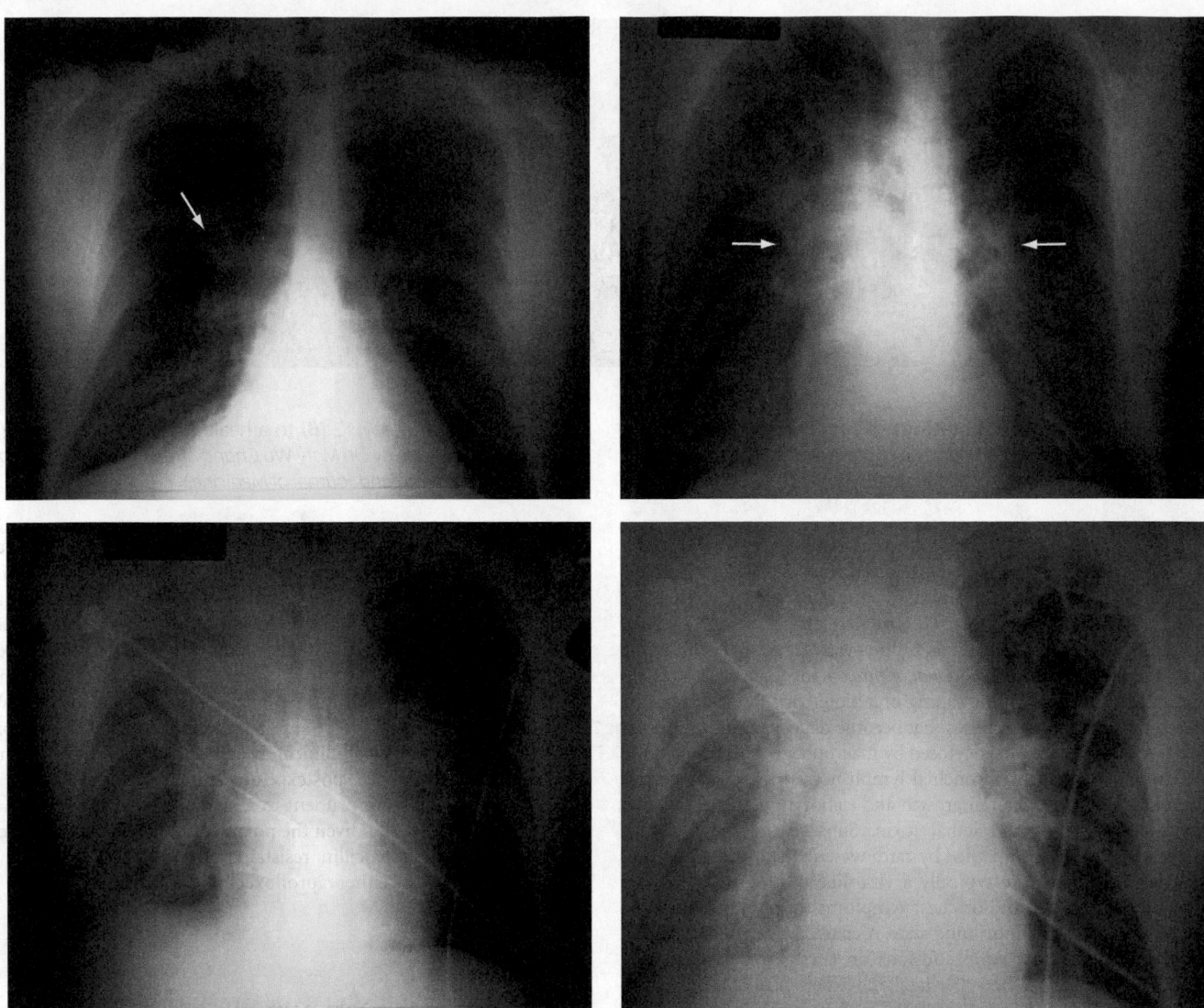

FIGURE 214-3 Progression of chest x-ray findings in a patient with inhalational anthrax. Findings evolved from subtle hilar prominence and right perihilar infiltrate to a progressively widened mediastinum, marked perihilar infiltrates, peribronchial cuffing, and air bronchograms. (*From L Borio et al: Death due to bioterrorism-related inhalational anthrax. JAMA 286:2554, 2001; with permission.*)

reported that more than 10 Soviet Institutes and >1000 scientists were working with plague as a biologic weapon. Of concern is the fact that in 1995 a microbiologist in Ohio was arrested for having obtained *Y. pestis* in the mail from the American Type Culture Collection, using a credit card and a false letterhead. In the wake of this incident, the U.S. Congress passed a law in 1997 requiring that anyone intending to send or receive any of 42 different agents that could potentially be used as bioweapons first register with the CDC.

Microbiology and Clinical Features Plague is caused by *Y. pestis*, a nonmotile, gram-negative bacillus that exhibits bipolar, or "safety pin," staining with Wright, Giemsa, or Wayson stains. It has had a major impact on the course of history, thus adding to the element of fear evoked by its mention. The earliest reported plague epidemic was in 224 B.C. in China. The most infamous pandemic began in Europe in the fourteenth century, during which time one-third to one-half of the entire population of Europe was killed. During a plague outbreak in India in 1994, even though the number of confirmed cases was relatively small, it is estimated that 500,000 individuals fled their homes in fear of this disease.

The clinical syndromes of plague generally reflect the mode of infection. *Bubonic plague* is the consequence of an insect bite; primary *pneumonic plague* arises through the inhalation of bacteria. Most of the plague seen in the world today is bubonic plague and is the result of a bite by a plague-infected flea. In part as a consequence of past pandemics, plague infection of rodents exists widely in nature, including in the southwestern United States, and each year thousands of cases of plague occur worldwide through contact with infected animals or fleas. Following inoculation of regurgitated bacteria into the skin by a flea bite, organisms travel through the lymphatics to regional lymph nodes, where they are phagocytized but not destroyed. Inside the cell, they multiply rapidly leading to inflammation, painful lymphadenopathy with necrosis, fever, bacteremia, septicemia, and death. The characteristic enlarged, inflamed lymph nodes, or *buboes*, give this form of plague its name. In some instances, patients may develop bacteremia without lymphadenopathy following infection, a condition referred to as *primary septicemic plague*. Extensive ecchymoses may develop due to disseminated intravascular coagulation, and gangrene of the digits and/or nose may develop in patients with advanced septicemic plague. It is thought that this appearance of some patients gave rise to the term *Black Death* in reference to the plague epidemic of the fourteenth and fifteenth centuries. Some patients may develop pneumonia (secondary pneumonic plague) as a complication of bubonic or septicemic plague. These patients may then transmit the agent to others via the respiratory route, causing cases of primary pneumonic plague. Primary pneumonic plague is the manifestation most likely to occur as the result of a bioterrorist attack, with an aerosol of bacteria spread over a wide area or a particular environment that is densely populated. In this setting patients would be expected to develop fever, cough with hemoptysis, dyspnea, and gastrointestinal

TABLE 214-3 CLINICAL SYNDROMES, PREVENTION, AND TREATMENT STRATEGIES FOR DISEASES CAUSES BY CATEGORY A AGENTS

Agent	Clinical Syndrome	Incubation Period	Diagnosis	Treatment	Prophylaxis
Bacillus anthracis (anthrax)	Cutaneous lesion: Papule to eschar Inhalational disease: Fever, malaise, chest and abdominal discomfort Pleural effusion, widened mediastinum on chest x-ray	1–12 days 1–60 days	Culture, Gram stain, PCR, Wright stain of peripheral smear	*Postexposure:* Ciprofloxacin, 500 mg, PO bid × 60 d *or* Doxycycline, 100 mg PO bid × 60 d also (Amoxicillin, 500 mg PO q8h, likely to be effective if strain penicillin sensitive) *Active disease:* Ciprofloxacin, 400 mg IV q12h *or* Doxycycline, 100 mg IV q12 *plus* Clindamycin, 900 mg IV q8h and/or rifampin, 300 mg IV q12h; switch to PO when stable ×60 d total *Antitoxin strategies:* Neutralizing monoclonal and polyclonal antibodies are under study	Anthrax vaccine adsorbed Recombinant protective antigen vaccines are under study
Yersinia pestis (pneumonic plague)	Fever, cough, dyspnea, hemoptysis Infiltrates and consolidation on chest x-ray	1–6 days	Culture, Gram stain, direct fluorescent antibody, PCR	Gentamicin, 2.0 mg/kg IV loading then 1.7 mg/kg q8h IV *or* Streptomycin, 1.0 g q12h IM or IV Alternatives include doxycycline, 100 mg bid PO or IV; chloramphenicol 500 mg qid PO or IV	Doxycycline, 100 mg PO bid (ciprofloxacin may also be active) Formalin-fixed vaccine (FDA licensed; not available)
Variola major (smallpox)	Fever, malaise, headache, backache, emesis Maculopapular to vesicular to pustular skin lesions	7–17 days	Culture, PCR, electron microscopy	Supportive measures; consideration for cidofovir, antivaccinia immunoglobulin	Vaccinia immunization
Francisella tularensis (tularemia)	Fever, chills, malaise, myalgia, chest discomfort, dyspnea, headache, skin rash, pharyngitis, conjunctivitis Hilar adenopathy on chest x-ray	1–14 days	Gram stain, culture, immunohistochemistry, PCR	Streptomycin, 1 g IM bid *or* Gentamicin, 5 mg/kg per day div q8h IV for 14 days *or* Doxycycline, 100 mg IV bid *or* Chloramphenicol, 15 mg/kg IV qid *or* Ciprofloxacin, 400 mg IV bid	Doxycycline, 100 mg PO bid × 14 days *or* Ciprofloxacin, 500 mg PO bid × 14 days
Viral hemorrhagic fevers	Fever, myalgia, rash, encephalitis, prostration	2–21 days	RT-PCR, serologic testing for antigen or antibody Viral isolation by CDC or U.S. Army Medical Institute of Infectious Diseases (USAMRIID)	Supportive measures Ribavirin 30 mg/kg up to 2 g × 1, followed by 16 mg/kg IV up to 1 g q6h for 4 days, followed by 8 mg/kg IV up to 0.5 g q8h × 6 days	No known chemoprophylaxis Consideration for ribavirin in high-risk situations Vaccine exists for yellow fever
Botulinum toxin (*Clostridium botulinum*)	Dry mouth, blurred vision, ptosis, weakness, dysarthria, dysphagia, dizziness, respiratory failure, progressive paralysis, dilated pupils	12–72 h	Mouse bioassay, toxin immunoassay	Supportive measures including ventilation 5000–9000 IU equine antitoxin	Administration of antitoxin

Note: CDC, U.S. Centers for Disease Control and Prevention; FDA, U.S. Food and Drug Administration; PCR, polymerase chain reaction; RT-PCR, reverse transcriptase PCR.

symptoms 1–6 days following exposure. Clinical features of pneumonia would be accompanied by pulmonary infiltrates and consolidation on chest x-ray. In the absence of antibiotics, the mortality of this disease is on the order of 85%, and death usually occurs within 2–6 days.

Rx PLAGUE

Streptomycin, tetracycline, and doxycycline are licensed by the U.S. Food and Drug Administration (FDA) for the treatment of plague. Multiple additional antibiotics licensed for other infections are commonly used and are likely effective. Among these are aminoglycosides such as gentamicin, cephalosporins, trimethoprim/sulfamethoxazole, chloramphenicol, and ciprofloxacin (Table 214-3). A multidrug-resistant strain of *Y. pestis* was identified in 1995 from a patient with bubonic plague in Madagascar. While this organism was resistant to streptomycin, ampicillin, chloramphenicol, sulfonamides, and tetracycline, it retained its susceptibility to other aminoglycosides and cephalosporins. Given the subsequent identification of a similar organism in 1997 coupled with the fact that this resistance is plasmid-mediated, it seems likely that genetically modifying *Y. pestis* to a multidrug resistant form is possible. Unlike patients with inhalational anthrax (see above), patients with pulmonary plague should be cared for under conditions of strict respiratory isolation comparable to that used for multidrug-resistant tuberculosis.

Vaccination and Prevention A formalin-fixed, whole-organism vaccine was licensed by the FDA for the prevention of plague. That vaccine is no longer being manufactured, but its potential value as a current countermeasure against bioterrorism would likely have been modest at best as it was ineffective against animal models of primary pneumonic plague. Efforts are under way to develop a second generation of vaccines that will protect against aerosol challenge. Among the candidates being tested are recombinant forms of the F1 and V antigens of *Y. pestis*. It is likely that doxycycline or ciprofloxacin would provide coverage in a chemoprophylaxis setting. Unlike the case with anthrax, in which one has to be concerned about the persistence of ungerminated spores in the respiratory tract, the duration of prophylaxis against plague need only extend to 7 days following exposure.

SMALLPOX

See also Chap. 176.

Variola Virus as a Bioweapon Given that most of the world's population was vaccinated against smallpox, variola virus would not have been considered a good candidate as a bioweapon 30 years ago. However, with the cessation of immunization programs in the United States in 1972 and throughout the world in 1980 due to the successful global eradication of smallpox, close to 50% of the U.S. population is fully susceptible to smallpox today. Given its infectious nature and the 10–30% mortality in unimmunized individuals, the deliberate spread of this virus could have a devastating effect on our society and unleash a previously conquered deadly disease. It is estimated that an initial infection of 50–100 persons in a first-generation of cases could expand by a factor of 10–20 with each succeeding generation in the absence of any effective containment measures. While the likely implementation of an effective public health response makes this scenario unlikely, it does illustrate the potential damage and disruption that can result from a smallpox outbreak.

In 1980, the World Health Organization (WHO) recommended that all immunization programs be terminated; that representative samples of variola virus be transferred to two locations: one at the CDC in Atlanta, GA, in the United States and the other at the Institute of Virus Preparations in the Soviet Union; and that all other stocks of smallpox be destroyed. Several years later, it was recommended that these two authorized collections be destroyed. However, these latter recommendations were placed on hold in the wake of increased concerns on the use of *variola virus* as a biologic weapon and thus the need to maintain an active program of defensive research. Many of these concerns were based upon allegations made by former Soviet officials that extensive programs had been in place in that country for the production and weaponization of large quantities of smallpox virus. The dismantling of these programs with the fall of the Soviet Union and the subsequent weakening of security measures led to fears that stocks of *V. major* may have made their way to other countries or terrorist organizations. In addition, accounts that efforts had been taken to produce recombinant strains of *Variola* that would be more virulent and more contagious than the wild-type virus have led to an increase in the need to be vigilant for the reemergence of this often fatal infectious disease.

Microbiology and Clinical Features Smallpox is caused by one of two variants of variola virus, *V. major* and *V. minor*. Variola is a double-strand DNA virus and member of the Orthopoxvirus genus of the Poxviridae family. Infections with *V. minor* are generally less severe than those of *V. major*, with milder constitutional symptoms and lower mortality rates; thus *V. major* is the only one considered to be a viable bioweapon. Infection with *V. major* typically occurs following contact with an infected person from the time that a maculopapular rash appears on the skin and oropharynx, through the resolution and scabbing of the pustular lesions. Infection occurs principally during close contact, through the inhalation of saliva droplets containing virus from the oropharyngeal exanthem. Aerosolized material from contaminated clothing or linen can also spread infection. Several days after exposure, a primary viremia is believed to occur that results in dissemination of virus to lymphoid tissues. A secondary viremia occurs ~4 days later that leads to localization of infection in the dermis. Approximately 12–14 days following the initial exposure the patient develops high fever, malaise, vomiting, headache, backache, and a maculopapular rash that begins on the face and extremities and spreads to the trunk (centripetal) with lesions in the same developmental stage in any given location. This is in contrast to the rash of varicella (chickenpox) that begins on the trunk and face and spreads to the extremities (centrifugal) with lesions at all stages of development. The lesions are initially maculopapular and evolve to vesicles that eventually become pustules and then scabs. The oral mucosa also develops maculopapular lesions that evolve to ulcers. The lesions appear over a period of 1–2 days and evolve at the same rate. Although virus can be isolated from the scabs on the skin, the conventional thinking is that once the scabs have formed the patient is no longer contagious. Smallpox is associated with a 10–30% mortality, with patients typically dying of severe systemic illness during the second week of symptoms. Historically, ~5–10% of naturally occurring smallpox cases take either of two highly virulent atypical forms, classified as *hemorrhagic* and *malignant*. These are difficult to recognize because of their atypical presentations. The hemorrhagic form is uniformly fatal and begins with the relatively abrupt onset of a severely prostrating illness characterized by high fevers and severe headache and back and abdominal pain. This form of the illness resembles a severe systemic inflammatory syndrome, in which patients have a high viremia, but die without developing the characteristic rash. Cutaneous erythema develops accompanied by petechiae and hemorrhages into the skin and mucous membranes. Death usually occurs within 5–6 days. The malignant, or "flat," form of smallpox is frequently fatal and has an onset similar to the hemorrhagic form, but with confluent skin lesions developing more slowly and never progressing to the pustular stage.

℞ SMALLPOX

Given the infectious nature of smallpox and the extreme vulnerability of contemporary society, patients who are suspected cases should be handled with strict isolation procedures. While laboratory confirmation of a suspected case by culture and electron microscopy is essential, it is equally important that appropriate precautions be employed when obtaining samples for culture and laboratory testing. All health care and laboratory workers caring for patients should have been recently immunized with vaccinia, and all samples should be transported in doubly sealed containers. Patients should be cared for in negative-pressure rooms with strict isolation precautions.

There is no licensed specific therapy for smallpox, and historic treatments have focused solely on supportive care. While several antiviral agents, including cidofovir, that are licensed for other diseases have in vitro activity against *V. major*, they have never been tested in the setting of human disease. For this reason it is difficult to predict whether or not they would be effective in cases of smallpox and, if effective, whether or not they would be of value in patients with advanced disease. Research programs studying the efficacy of new antiviral compounds against *V. major* are currently under way.

Vaccination and Prevention In 1796 Edward Jenner demonstrated that deliberate infection with cowpox virus could prevent illness on subsequent exposure to smallpox. Today, smallpox is a preventable disease following immunization with vaccinia. The current dilemma facing our society regarding assessment of the risk and/or benefit of smallpox vaccination is that the degree of risk that someone will deliberately and effectively release smallpox into our society is unknown. As a prudent first step in preparedness for a smallpox attack, virtually all members of the U.S. armed services have received primary or booster immunizations with vaccinia. In addition, tens of thousands of civilian health care workers who comprise smallpox-response teams at the state and local public health level have been vaccinated.

Initial fears regarding the immunization of a segment of the American population with vaccinia when there are more individuals receiving

TABLE 214-4 COMPLICATIONS FROM 438,134 ADMINISTRATIONS OF VACCINIA DURING THE UNITED STATES DEPARTMENT OF DEFENSE (DOD) SMALLPOX IMMUNIZATION CAMPAIGN INITIATED IN DECEMBER 2002

Complication	Number of Cases	DoD Rate per Million Vaccinees (95% Confidence Interval)	Historic Rate Per Million Vaccinees
Mild or temporary:			
Generalized vaccinia, mild	35	67 (52, 85)	45 to 212[a]
Inadvertent inoculation, self	62	119 (98, 142)	606[a]
Vaccinia transfer to contact	28	53 (40, 69)	8 to 27[a]
Moderate or serious:			
Encephalitis	1	2.2 (0.6, 7.2)	2.6 to 8.7[a]
Acute myopericarditis	69	131 (110, 155)	100[b]
Eczema vaccinatum	0	0 (0, 3.7)	2 to 35[a]
Progressive vaccinia	0	0 (0, 3.7)	1 to 7[a]
Death[c]	1	1.9 (0.2, 5.6)	1 to 2[a]

[a]Based on adolescent and adult smallpox vaccinations from 1968 studies, both primary and revaccinations.
[b]Based on case series in Finnish military recruits given the Finnish strain of smallpox vaccine.
[c]Potentially attributable to vaccination; after lupus-like illness.
Source: From JD Grabenstein and W Winkenwerder: *http://www.smallpox.mil/event/SPSafetySum.asp*

immunosuppressive drugs and other immunocompromised patients than ever before have largely been dispelled as data are generated from the current military and civilian immunization campaigns. Adverse event rates for the first 450,000 immunizations are similar to and, in certain categories of adverse events, even lower than those from historic data, in which most severe sequelae of vaccination occurred in young infants (Table 214-4). In addition, 11 patients with early stage HIV infection have been inadvertently immunized without problem. One significant concern during the recent immunization campaign, however, has been the description of a syndrome of myopericarditis, which was not appreciated during prior immunization campaigns with vaccinia.

TULAREMIA

See also Chap. 151.

Francisella tularensis as a Bioweapon Tularemia has been studied as an agent of bioterrorism since the mid-twentieth century. It has been speculated by some that the outbreak of tularemia among German and Soviet soldiers during fighting on the Eastern Front during WWII was the consequence of a deliberate release. Unit 731 of the Japanese Army studied the use of tularemia as a bioweapon during WWII. Large preparations were made for mass productive of *F. tularensis* by the United States, but no stockpiling of any agent took place. Stocks of *F. tularensis* were reportedly generated by the Soviet Union in the mid-1950s. It has also been suggested that the Soviet program extended into the era of molecular biology and that some strains were engineered to be resistant to common antibiotics. *F. tularensis* is an extremely infectious organism, and human infections have occurred from merely examining an uncovered petri dish streaked with colonies. Given these facts, it is reasonable to conclude that this organism might be utilized as a bioweapon through either an aerosol or contamination of food or drinking water.

Microbiology and Clinical Features While similar in many ways to anthrax and plague, tularemia, also referred to as rabbit fever or deer fly fever, is neither as lethal nor as fulminant as either of these other two category A bacterial infections. It is, however, extremely infectious, and as few as 10 organisms can lead to establishment of infection. Despite this fact, it is not spread from person to person. Tularemia is caused by *F. tularensis*, a small, nonmotile, gram-negative coccobacillus. Although it is not a spore-forming organism, it is a hardy bacterium that can survive for weeks in the environment. Infection typically comes from insect bites or contact with organisms in the environment. Large waterborne outbreaks have been recorded. It is most likely that the outbreak among German and Russian soldiers and Russian civilians noted above during WWII represented a large waterborne tularemia outbreak in a *Tularensis*-enzootic area devastated by warfare.

Humans can become infected through a variety of environmental sources. Infection is most common in rural areas where a variety of small mammals may serve as reservoirs. Human infections in the summer are often the result of insect bites from ticks, flies, or mosquitoes that have bitten infected animals. In colder months infections are most likely the result of direct contact with infected mammals and are most common in hunters. In these settings infection typically presents as a systemic illness with an area of inflammation and necrosis at the site of tissue entry. Drinking of contaminated water may lead to an oropharyngeal form of tularemia characterized by pharyngitis with cervical and/or retropharyngeal lymphadenopathy (Chap. 151). The most likely mode of dissemination of tularemia as a biologic weapon would be as an aerosol, as has occurred in a number of natural outbreaks in rural areas, including Martha's Vineyard in the United States. Approximately 1–14 days following exposure by this route one would expect to see inflammation of the airways with pharyngitis, pleuritis, and bronchopneumonia. Typical symptoms would include the abrupt onset of fever, fatigue, chills, headache, and malaise (Table 214-3). Some patients might experience conjunctivitis with ulceration, pharyngitis, and/or cutaneous exanthems. A pulse-temperature dissociation might be present. Approximately 50% of patients would show a pulmonary infiltrate on chest x-ray. Hilar adenopathy might also be present, and a small percent of patients could have adenopathy without infiltrates. The highly variable presentation makes acute recognition of aerosol-disseminated tularemia very difficult. The diagnosis would likely be made by immunohistochemistry or culture of infected tissues or blood. Untreated, mortality rates range from 5–15% for cutaneous routes of infection and 30–60% for infection by inhalation. Since the advent of antibiotic therapy, these rates have dropped to <2%.

℞ TULAREMIA

Both streptomycin and doxycycline are licensed for treatment of tularemia. Other agents likely to be effective include gentamicin, chloramphenicol, and ciprofloxacin (Table 214-3). Given the potential for genetic modification of this organism to yield antibiotic-resistant strains, broad-spectrum coverage should be the rule until sensitivities have been determined. As mentioned above, special isolation procedures are not required.

Vaccination and Prevention There are no vaccines currently licensed for the prevention of tularemia. While a live, attenuated strain of the organism has been used in the past with some reported success, there are inadequate data to support its widespread use at this time. Development of a vaccine for this agent is an important part of the current biodefense research agenda. In the absence of an effective vaccine, post-exposure chemoprophylaxis with either doxycycline or ciprofloxacin appears to be a reasonable approach (Table 214-3).

VIRAL HEMORRHAGIC FEVERS

See also Chaps. 189 and 190.

Hemorrhagic Fever Viruses as Bioweapons Several of the hemorrhagic fever viruses have been reported to have been weaponized by the Soviet Union and the United States. Nonhuman primate studies indicate that infection can be established with very few virions and that infectious aerosol preparations can be produced. Under the guise of wanting to aid victims of an Ebola outbreak, members of the Aum Shrinrikyo cult in Japan were reported to have traveled to central Africa in 1992 in an attempt to obtain Ebola virus for use in a bioterrorist attack. Thus, while there has been no evidence that these agents have ever been used in a biologic attack, there is clear interest in their potential for this purpose.

Microbiology and Clinical Features The viral hemorrhagic fevers are a group of illnesses caused by any one of a number of similar viruses (Table 214-2). These viruses are all enveloped, single-strand RNA viruses that are thought to depend upon a rodent or insect host reservoir for long-term survival. They tend to be geographically restricted according to the migration patterns of their hosts. Great apes are not a natural reservoir for Ebola virus, but large numbers of these animals in sub-Saharan Africa have died from Ebola infection over the past decade. Humans can become infected with hemorrhagic fever viruses if they come into contact with an infected host or other infected animals. Person-to-person transmission, largely through direct contact with virus-containing body fluids, has been documented for Ebola, Marburg and Lassa virus and rarely for the New World arenaviruses. While there is no clear evidence of respiratory spread among humans, these viruses have been shown in animal models to be highly infectious by the aerosol route. This, coupled with mortality rates as high as 90%, makes them excellent candidate agents of bioterrorism.

The clinical features of the viral hemorrhagic fevers vary depending upon the particular agent (Table 214-3). Initial signs and symptoms typically include fever, myalgia, prostration, and disseminated intravascular coagulation with thrombocytopenia and capillary hemorrhage. These findings are consistent with a cytokine-mediated systemic inflammatory syndrome. A variety of different maculopapular or erythematous rashes may be seen. Leukopenia, temperature-pulse dissociation, renal failure, and seizures may also be part of the clinical presentation. Outbreaks of most of these diseases are sporadic and unpredictable. As a consequence, most studies of pathogenesis have been performed using laboratory animals. The diagnosis should be suspected in anyone with temperature >38.3°C for <3 weeks who also exhibits at least two of the following: hemorrhagic or purpuric rash, epistaxis, hematemesis, hemoptysis, or hematochezia in the absence of any other identifiable cause. In this setting, samples of blood should be sent after consultation to the CDC or the U.S. Army Medical Research Institute of Infectious Diseases (USAMRIID) for serologic testing for antigen and antibody as well as reverse transcriptase polymerase chain reaction (RT-PCR) testing for hemorrhagic fever viruses. All samples should be handled with double-bagging. Given how little is known regarding the human-to-human transmission of these viruses, appropriate isolation measures would include full barrier precautions with negative-pressure rooms and use of N95 masks or powered air-purifying respirators (PAPRs). Unprotected skin contact with cadavers has been implicated in the transmission of certain hemorrhagic fever viruses such as Ebola, so it is recommended that autopsies be performed using the strictest measures for protection and that burial or cremation be performed promptly without embalming.

Rx VIRAL HEMORRHAGIC FEVERS

There are no approved and effective antiviral therapies for this class of viruses (Table 214-3). While there are anecdotal reports of the efficacy of ribavirin, interferon-α, or hyperimmune immunoglobulin, definitive data are lacking. The best data for ribavirin are in arenavirus (Lassa and New World) infections. In some in vitro systems specific immunoglobulin has been reported to enhance infectivity, and thus these potential treatments must be approached with caution.

Vaccination and Prevention A live attenuated virus vaccine is available in limited quantities for prevention of yellow fever. There are no other licensed and effective vaccines for these agents. Studies are currently underway examining the potential role of DNA, recombinant viruses, and attenuated viruses as vaccines for several of these infections. Among the most promising at present are vaccines for Argentine, Ebola, Rift Valley, and Kayasanur Forest viruses.

BOTULISM TOXIN (*CLOSTRIDIUM BOTULINUM*)

See also Chap. 135.

Botulinum Toxin as a Bioweapon In a bioterrorist attack, botulinum toxin would likely be dispersed as an aerosol or as contamination of a food supply. While contamination of a water supply is possible, it is likely that any toxin would be rapidly inactivated by the chlorine used to purify drinking water. Similarly, toxin can be inactivated by heating any food to >85°C for >5 min. Without external facilitation, the environmental decay rate is estimated at 1% per minute, and thus the time interval between weapon release and ingestion or inhalation needs to be rather short. The Japanese biologic warfare group, Unit 731, is reported to have conducted experiments on botulism poisoning in prisoners in the 1930s. The United States and the Soviet Union both acknowledged producing botulinum toxin, and there is some evidence that the Soviet Union attempted to create recombinant bacteria containing the gene for botulinum toxin. In records submitted to the United Nations, Iraq admitted to having produced 19,000 L of concentrated toxin—enough toxin to kill the entire population of the world three times over. By many accounts, botulinum toxin was the primary focus of the pre-1991 Iraqi bioweapons program. In addition to these examples of state-supported research into the use of botulinum toxin as a bioweapon, the Aum Shrinrikyo cult unsuccessfully attempted on a least three occasions to disperse botulism toxin into the civilian population of Tokyo.

Microbiology and Clinical Features Unique among the category A agents for not being a live microorganism, botulinum toxin is one of the most potent toxins ever described and is thought by some to be the most poisonous substance in existence. It is estimated that 1 g of botulinum toxin would be sufficient to kill 1 million individuals if adequately dispersed. Botulinum toxin is produced by the gram-positive, spore-forming anaerobe *C. botulinum* (Chap. 135). Its natural habitat is soil. There are seven antigenically distinct forms of botulinum toxin, designated A–G. The majority of naturally occurring human cases are of types A, B, and E. Antitoxin directed toward one of these will have little to no activity against the others. The toxin is a 150-kDa zinc-containing protease that prevents the intracellular fusion of acetylcholine vesicles with the motor neuron membrane, thus preventing the release of acetylcholine. In the absence of acetylcholine-dependent triggering of muscle fibers, a flaccid paralysis develops. Although botulism does not spread from person to person, the ease of production of the toxin coupled with its high morbidity and 60–100% mortality make it a close to ideal bioweapon.

Botulism can result from the presence of *C. botulinum* infection in a wound or the intestine, the ingestion of contaminated food, or the inhalation of aerosolized toxin. The latter two forms are the most likely modes of transmission for bioterrorism. Once toxin is absorbed into the bloodstream it binds to the neuronal cell membrane, enters the cell, and cleaves one of the proteins required for the intracellular binding of the synaptic vesicle to the cell membrane, thus preventing release of the neurotransmitter to the membrane of the adjacent muscle cell. Patients initially develop multiple cranial nerve palsies that are followed by a descending flaccid paralysis. The extent of the neuromuscular compromise is dependent upon the level of toxemia. The majority of patients experience diplopia, dysphagia, dysarthria, dry mouth, ptosis, dilated pupils, fatigue, and extremity weakness. There are minimal true central nervous system effects, and patients rarely show significant alterations in mental status. Severe cases can involve complete muscular collapse, loss of the gag reflex, and respiratory failure, requiring weeks or months of ventilator support. Recovery requires the regeneration of new motor neuron synapses with the muscle cell, a process that can take weeks to months. In the absence of secondary infections, which may be common during the protracted recovery phase of this illness, patients remain afebrile. The diagnosis is suspected on clinical grounds and confirmed by a mouse bioassay or toxin immunoassay.

Rx BOTULISM

Treatment for botulism is mainly supportive and may require intubation, mechanical ventilation, and parenteral nutrition (Table 214-3). If diagnosed early enough, administration of equine antitoxin may reduce the extent of nerve injury and decrease the severity of disease. At present antitoxins are available on a limited basis as a licensed bivalent product with activity against toxin types A and B and as an experimental product with activity against toxin type E. In the event of attack with another toxin type, an investigational antitoxin with activity against all seven toxin types is also available through the U.S. Army. A single dose of antitoxin is usually adequate to neutralize any circulating toxin. Given that these preparations are all derived from horse serum, one needs to be vigilant for hypersensitivity reactions, including serum sickness and anaphylaxis following their administration. Once the damage to the nerve axon has been done, however, there is little possible in the way of specific therapy. At this point vigilance for secondary complications such as infections during the protracted recovery phase is of the utmost importance. Due to their ability to worsen neuromuscular blockade, aminoglycosides and clindamycin should be avoided in the treatment of these infections.

Vaccination and Prevention A botulinum toxoid preparation has been used as a vaccine for laboratory workers at high risk of exposure and in certain military situations; however, it is not currently available in quantities that could be used for the general population. At present, early recognition of the clinical syndrome and use of appropriate equine antitoxin is the mainstay of prevention of full-blown disease in exposed individuals. The development of human monoclonal antibodies as a replacement for equine antitoxin antibodies is an area of active research interest.

CATEGORY B AND C AGENTS

The category B agents include those that are easy or moderately easy to disseminate and result in moderate morbidity and low mortality rates. A listing of the current category B agents is provided in Table 214-2. As can be seen, it includes a wide array of microorganisms and products of microorganisms. Several of these agents have been used in bioterrorist attacks, although never with the impact of the agents described above. Among the more notorious of these was the contamination of salad bars in Oregon in 1984 with *Salmonella typhimurium* by the religious cult Rajneeshee. In this outbreak, which many consider to be the first bioterrorist attack against U.S. citizens, >750 individuals were poisoned and 40 were hospitalized in an effort to influence a local election. The intentional nature of this outbreak went unrecognized for more than a decade.

Category C agents are the third highest priority agents in the biodefense agenda. These agents include emerging pathogens to which little or no immunity exists in the general population, such as the severe acute respiratory syndrome (SARS) coronavirus or pandemic-potential strains of influenza that could be obtained from nature and deliberately disseminated. These agents are characterized as being relatively easy to produce and disseminate and as having high morbidity and mortality rates as well as a significant public health impact. There is no running list of category C agents at the present time.

PREVENTION AND PREPAREDNESS

As noted above, a large and diverse array of agents has the potential to be used in a bioterrorist attack. In contrast to the military situation with biowarfare, where the primary objective is to inflict mass casualties on a healthy and prepared militia, the objectives of bioterrorism are to harm civilians as well as to create fear and disruption among the civilian population. While the military needs only to prepare their troops to deal with the limited number of agents that pose a legitimate threat of biowarfare, the public health system needs to prepare the entire civilian population to deal with the multitude of agents and settings that could be utilized in a bioterrorism attack. This includes anticipating issues specific to the very young and the very old, the pregnant patient, and the immunocompromised individual. The challenges in this regard are enormous and immediate. While military preparedness emphasizes vaccines toward a limited number of agents, civilian preparedness needs to rely upon rapid diagnosis and treatment of a wide array of conditions.

The medical profession must maintain a high index of suspicion that unusual clinical presentations or the clustering of cases of a rare disease may not be a chance occurrence but rather the first sign of a bioterrorist event. This is particularly true when such diseases occur in traditionally healthy populations, when surprisingly large numbers of rare conditions occur, and when diseases commonly seen in rural settings appear in urban populations. Given the importance of rapid diagnosis and early treatment for many of these conditions, it is essential that the medical care team report any suspected cases of bioterrorism immediately to local and state health authorities and/or to the CDC (888-246-2675). Recent enhancements have been made to the public health surveillance network to facilitate the rapid sharing of information among public health agencies.

At present a series of efforts are taking place to ensure the biomedical security of the civilian population of the United States. The Public Health Service is moving toward a larger, more highly trained, fully deployable force. A Strategic National Stockpile (SNS) has been created by the CDC to provide rapid access to quantities of pharmaceuticals, antidotes, vaccines, and other medical supplies that may be of value in the event of biologic or chemical terrorism. The SNS has two basic components. The first of these consists of "push packages" that can be deployed anywhere in the United States within 12 h. These push packages are a preassembled set of supplies, pharmaceuticals, and medical equipment ready for immediate delivery to the field. They provide treatment for a variety of conditions given the fact that an actual threat may not have been precisely identified at the time of stockpile deployment. The contents of the push packs are constantly updated to ensure that they reflect current needs as determined by national security threat assessments; they include antibiotics for treatment of anthrax, plague, and tularemia as well as a cache of vaccine to deal with a smallpox threat. The second component of the SNS comprises inventories managed by specific vendors and consists of the provision of additional pharmaceuticals, supplies, and/or products tailored to the specific attack.

The number of FDA-approved and -licensed drugs and vaccines for category A and B agents is currently limited and not reflective of the pharmacy of today. In an effort to speed the licensure of additional drugs and vaccines for these diseases, the FDA has proposed a new rule for the licensure of such countermeasures against agents of bioterrorism when adequate and well-controlled clinical efficacy studies cannot be ethically conducted in humans. Thus, for indications in which field trials of prophylaxis or therapy for naturally occurring disease are not feasible, the FDA is proposing to rely on evidence solely from laboratory animal studies. For this rule to apply it must be shown that (1) there are reasonably well-understood pathophysiologic mechanisms for the condition and its treatment; (2) the effect of the intervention is independently substantiated in at least two animal species, including species expected to react with a response predictive for humans; (3) the animal study endpoint is clearly related to the desired benefit in humans; and (4) the data in animals allow selection of an effective dose in humans.

Finally, an initiative referred to as Project BioShield has been established to facilitate biodefense research within the federal government, create a stable source of funding for the purchase of countermeasures against agents of bioterrorism, and create a category of "emergency use authorization" to allow the FDA to approve the use of unlicensed treatments during times of extraordinary unmet needs, as might be present in the context of a bioterrorist attack.

While the prospect of a deliberate attack on civilians with disease-producing agents may seem to be an act of incomprehensible evil, history shows us that it is something that has been done in the past and will likely be done again in the future. It is the responsibility of health care providers to be aware of this possibility, to be able to recognize early signs of a potential bioterrorist attack and alert the public health system, and to respond quickly to provide care to the individual patient. Among the web sites with current information on microbial bioterrorism are *www.bt.cdc.gov, www.niaid.nih.gov, www.jhsph.edu/preparedness*, and *www.cns.miis.edu/research/cbw/index.htm*.

ALIBEK K, HANDELMAN S: *Biohazard: The Chilling True Story of the Largest Covert Biological Weapons in the World, Told from the Inside by the Man Who Ran It.* New York, Random House, 1999

BEIGEL JH et al: Avian influenza A (H5N1) infection in humans. N Engl J Med 353:1375, 2005

CRODDY E (WITH C PEREY-ARMENDARIZ AND J HART): *Chemical and Biological Warfare: A Comprehensive Survey for the Concerned Citizen.* New York, Copernicus Books, 2001

HENDERSON DA et al (eds): *Bioterrorism: Guidelines for Medical and Public Health Management.* JAMA and Archives Journals, AMA Press, 2002

JERNIGAN JA et al: Bioterrorism-related inhalational anthrax: The first 10 cases reported in the United States. Emerg Infect Dis 7:933, 2001

WILKENING DA: Sverdlovsk revisited: Modeling human inhalation anthrax. Proc Natl Acad Sci USA 103:20, 2006

215 Chemical Bioterrorism

Charles G. Hurst, Jonathan Newmark, James A. Romano, Jr.

The use of chemical warfare agents (CWAs) in modern warfare dates back to World War I (WWI). Most recently, sulfur mustard and nerve agents were used by Iraq against the Iranian military and Kurdish civilians. Since the Japanese sarin attacks in 1994–1995 and the terrorist strikes of September 11, 2001, the all too real possibility of chemical or biological terrorism against civilian populations anywhere in the world has attracted increased attention.

Military planners consider the WWI blistering agent, sulfur mustard, and the organophosphorus nerve agents as the most likely agents to be used on the battlefield. In a civilian or terrorist scenario, the choice widens considerably. Cyanide, a common chemical, causes symptoms within seconds and death in 5–10 min if not treated rapidly. Chlorine and phosgene have no specific antidotes but can require intensive care for weeks to months. These agents or one of the industrial HAZMATs will be the likely choice of terrorists. Table 215-1 gives antidote recommendations following exposure to cyanide.

Many mistakenly believe that chemical attacks will always be so severe that little can be done except to bury the dead. History proves the opposite. Even in WWI, when IV fluids, endotracheal tubes, and antibiotics were unavailable, the mortality rate in U.S. forces on the battlefield from chemical warfare agents, chiefly sulfur mustard and the pulmonary intoxicants, was only 1.9%. This was far less than the 7% mortality rate from conventional wounds. In the 1995 Tokyo subway sarin incident, of the 5500 patients who sought medical attention at hospitals, 80% of whom were not actually symptomatic, only 12 died. Recent events should produce not a fatalistic attitude but a realistic wish to understand the pathophysiology of the syndromes these agents cause, with a view to treating expeditiously all patients who present for care and an expectation of saving the vast majority. As we prepare to defend our civilian population from the effects of chemical terrorism, we must also consider the fact that terrorism itself can produce sequelae such as physiologic or neurologic effects that may resemble the effects of nonlethal exposures to CWAs. These effects are due to a general fear of chemicals, fear of decontamination, fear of protective ensemble, or other phobic reactions.

Many writers have pointed out the increased difficulty in differentiating between stress reactions and nerve agent–induced organic brain syndromes. Knowledge of the behavioral effects of CWAs and their medical countermeasures is imperative to ensure that military and civilian medical and mental health organizations can deal with possible incidents involving weapons of mass destruction.

The chemical warfare agents, their NATO codes, and initial effects are listed in Table 215-2.

VESICANTS

Sulfur Mustard Sulfur mustard has been a military threat since it first appeared on the battlefield in Belgium during WWI. In modern times it remains a threat on the battlefield as well as a potential terrorist threat for bioterrorism because of simplicity of manufacture and extreme effectiveness. Sulfur mustard accounted for 70% of the 1.3 million chemical casualties in WWI.

MECHANISM Sulfur mustard constitutes both a vapor and a liquid threat to all exposed epithelial surfaces. Mustard's effects are delayed, appearing hours after exposure. Organs most commonly affected are the skin (with erythema and vesicles), eyes (ranging from mild conjunctivitis to severe eye damage), and airways (ranging from mild upper airway irritation, to severe bronchiolar damage). Following exposure to large quantities of mustard, precursor cells of the bone marrow are damaged, leading to pancytopenia and secondary infection. The gastrointestinal mucosa may be damaged, and there are sometimes central nervous system (CNS) signs of unknown mechanism. No specific antidotes exist; management is entirely supportive. Immediate decontamination of the liquid is the only way to reduce damage. Complete decontamination in 2 min stops clinical injury; decontamination at 5 min will reduce skin injury by ~50%. Table 215-3

TABLE 215-1 ANTIDOTE RECOMMENDATIONS FOLLOWING EXPOSURE TO CYANIDE

Patient	Mild (Conscious)	Severe (Unconscious)	Other Treatment
Child	If patient is conscious and has no other signs or symptoms, antidotes may not be necessary.	Sodium nitrite[a]: 0.12–0.33 mL/kg, not to exceed 10 mL of 3% solution[b] slow IV over no less than 5 min, or slower if hypotension develops *and* Sodium thiosulfate: 1.65 mL/kg of 25% solution IV over 10–20 min	For sodium nitrite–induced orthostatic hypotension, normal saline infusion and supine position are recommended. If still apneic after antidote administration, consider sodium bicarbonate for severe acidosis.
Adult	If patient is conscious and has no other signs or symptoms, antidotes may not be necessary.	Sodium nitrite[a]: 10–20 mL of 3% solution[b] slow IV over no less than 5 min, or slower if hypotension develops *and* Sodium thiosulfate: 50 mL of 25% solution IV over 10–20 min	

[a]If sodium nitrite is unavailable, administer amyl nitrite by inhalation from crushable ampules.
[b]Available in Pasadena Cyanide Antidote Kit, formerly Lilly Cyanide Kit.
Note: Victims whose clothing or skin is contaminated with hydrogen cyanide liquid or solution can secondarily contaminate response personnel by direct contact or through off-gassing vapors. Avoid dermal contact with cyanide-contaminated victims or with gastric contents of victims who may have ingested cyanide-containing materials. Victims exposed only to hydrogen cyanide gas do not pose contamination risks to rescuers. *If the patient is a victim of recent smoke inhalation (may have high carboxyhemoglobin levels), administer only sodium thiosulfate.*
Source: State of New York, Department of Health.

TABLE 215-2 RECOGNIZING AND DIAGNOSING HEALTH EFFECTS OF CHEMICAL TERRORISM

Agent	Agent Name	Unique Characteristics	Initial Effects
Nerve	Cyclohexyl sarin (GF) Sarin (GB) Soman (GD) Tabun (GA) VX	Miosis (pinpoint pupils) Copious secretions Muscle twitching/fasciculations	Miosis (pinpoint pupils) Blurred/dim vision Headache Nausea, vomiting, diarrhea Copious secretions/sweating Muscle twitching/fasciculations Breathing difficulty Seizures
Asphyxiant/blood	Arsine Cyanogen chloride Hydrogen cyanide	Possible cherry red skin Possible cyanosis Possible frostbite[a]	Confusion Nausea Patients may gasp for air, similar to asphyxiation but more abrupt onset Seizures prior to death
Choking/pulmonary-damaging	Chlorine Hydrogen chloride Nitrogen oxides Phosgene	Chlorine is a greenish-yellow gas with pungent odor Phosgene gas smells like newly mown hay or grass Possible frostbite[a]	Eye and skin irritation Airway irritation Dyspnea, cough Sore throat Chest tightness
Blistering/vesicant	Mustard/Sulfur mustard (HD, H) Mustard gas (H) Nitrogen mustard (HN-1, HN-2, HN-3) Lewisite (L) Phosgene oxime (CX)	Mustard (HD) has an odor like burning garlic or horseradish Lewisite (L) has an odor like penetrating geranium Phosgene oxime (CX) has a pepperish or pungent odor	Severe irritation Redness and blisters of the skin Tearing, conjunctivitis, corneal damage Mild respiratory distress to marked airway damage May cause death
Incapacitating/behavior-altering	Agent 15/BZ	May appear as mass drug intoxication with erratic behaviors, shared realistic and distinct hallucinations, disrobing and confusion Hyperthermia Mydriasis (dilated pupils)	Dry mouth and skin Initial tachycardia Altered consciousness, delusions, denial of illness, belligerence Hyperthermia Ataxia (lack of coordination) Hallucinations Mydriasis (dilated pupils)

[a]Frostbite may occur from skin contact with liquid arsine, cyanogen chloride, or phosgene. **Source:** State of New York, Department of Health.

TABLE 215-3 DECONTAMINATION AND TREATMENT OF CHEMICAL TERRORISM

Agent	Decontamination	First Aid	Other Patient Considerations
Nerve	Remove clothing immediately Gently wash skin with soap and water Do not abrade skin For eyes, flush with plenty of water or normal saline	Atropine before other measures Pralidoxime (2-PAM) chloride	Onset of symptoms from dermal contact with liquid forms may be delayed Repeated antidote administration may be necessary
Asphyxiant/blood	Remove clothing immediately if no frostbite[a] Gently wash skin with soap and water Do not abrade skin For eyes, flush with plenty of water or normal saline	Rapid treatment with oxygen For cyanide, use antidotes (sodium nitrite and then sodium thiosulfate)	Arsine and cyanogen chloride may cause delayed pulmonary edema
Choking/pulmonary-damaging	Remove clothing immediately if no frostbite[a] Gently wash skin with soap and water Do not abrade skin For eyes, flush with plenty of water or normal saline	Fresh air, forced rest Semi-upright position If signs of respiratory distress are present, oxygen with or without positive airway pressure may be needed Other supportive therapy, as needed	May cause delayed pulmonary edema, even following a symptom-free period that varies in duration with the amount inhaled
Blistering/vesicant	Immediate decontamination is essential to minimize damage Remove clothing immediately Gently wash skin with soap and water Do not abrade skin For eyes, flush with plenty of water or normal saline	Immediately decontaminate skin Flush eyes with water or normal saline for 10–15 min If breathing difficulty, give oxygen Supportive care	Mustard has an asymptomatic latent period There is no antidote or treatment for mustard Lewisite has immediate burning pain, blisters later Specific antidote British Anti-Lewisite (BAL) may decrease systemic effects of Lewisite Phosgene oxime causes immediate pain Possible pulmonary edema
Incapacitating/behavior-altering	Remove clothing immediately Gently wash skin with water or soap and water Do not abrade skin	Remove heavy clothing Evaluate mental status Use restraints as needed Monitor core temperature carefully Supportive care	Hyperthermia and self-injury are largest risks Hard to detect because it is an odorless and non-irritating substance Possible serious arrhythmias Specific antidote (physostigmine) may be available

[a]For frostbite areas, do NOT remove any adhering clothing. Wash area with plenty of warm water to release clothing. **Source:** State of New York, Department of Health.

 lists approaches to decontamination of mustard and other CWAs.

Mustard dissolves slowly in aqueous media, such as sweat, but once dissolved, it rapidly forms extremely reactive cyclic ethylene sulfonium ions, which react with cell proteins, cell membranes, and especially DNA in rapidly dividing cells. The ability of mustard to react with and alkylate DNA gives rise to the effects by which it has been characterized as "radiomimetic," similar to radiation injury. Mustard has many biologic actions, but its actual mechanism of action is largely unknown. Much of the biologic damage from mustard results from DNA alkylation and crosslinking in rapidly dividing cells: corneal epithelium, basal keratinocytes, bronchial mucosal epithelium, gastrointestinal mucosal epithelium, and bone marrow precursor cells. This may lead to cellular death and inflammatory reactions. In the skin, proteolytic digestion of anchoring filaments at the epidermal-dermal junction may be the major mechanism of action resulting in blister formation. Mustard also possesses mild cholinergic activity, which may be responsible for effects such as early gastrointestinal and CNS symptoms.

Mustard reacts with tissue within minutes of entering the body. Its circulating half-life in unaltered form is extremely brief.

CLINICAL FEATURES Topical effects of mustard occur in the skin, airways, and eyes, with the eyes being most sensitive, followed by the airways. Absorbed mustard may produce effects in the bone marrow, gastrointestinal tract, and CNS. Direct injury to the gastrointestinal tract may also occur following ingestion of the compound through contamination of water or food.

Erythema is the mildest and earliest form of mustard skin injury. It resembles sunburn and is associated with pruritus, burning, or stinging pain. Erythema begins to appear within 2 h to 2 d after vapor exposure. Time of onset depends on severity of exposure, ambient temperature and humidity, and type of skin. The most sensitive sites are the warm moist locations and thin delicate skin, such as the perineum, external genitalia, axillae, antecubital fossae, and neck.

Within the erythematous areas, small vesicles can develop, which may later coalesce to form bullae (Fig. 215-1). The typical bulla is large, dome-shaped, flaccid, thin-walled, translucent, and surrounded by erythema. The blister fluid, a transudate, is clear to straw-colored, which becomes yellow tending to coagulate. The fluid does not contain mustard and is not itself a vesicant. Lesions from high-dose liquid exposure may develop a central zone of coagulation necrosis with blister formation at the periphery. These lesions take longer to heal and are more prone to secondary infection than the uncomplicated lesions seen at lower exposure levels. Severe lesions might require skin grafting.

The primary airway lesion is necrosis of the mucosa with possible damage to underlying smooth muscle. The damage begins in the upper airways and descends to the lower airways in a dose-dependent manner. Usually the terminal airways and alveoli are affected only as a terminal event. Pulmonary edema is not usually present unless the damage is very severe, and then it becomes hemorrhagic.

The earliest effects from mustard and perhaps the only effects from a low concentration involve the nose, sinuses, and pharynx. There may be irritation or burning of the nares, epistaxis, sinus pain, and pharyngeal pain. As the concentration increases, laryngitis, voice changes, and nonproductive cough develop. Damage to the trachea and upper bronchi leads to a productive cough. Lower airway involvement causes dyspnea, severe cough, and increasing quantities of sputum. Terminally, there may be necrosis of the smaller airways with hemorrhagic edema into surrounding alveoli. Hemorrhagic pulmonary edema is rare.

Necrosis of airway mucosa causes "pseudomembrane" formation. These membranes may cause obstruction of the bronchi. During WWI, high dose mustard exposure caused acute death via this mechanism in a small minority of cases (Fig. 215-2).

The eyes are the organs most sensitive to mustard vapor injury. The latent period is shorter for eye injury than for skin injury and is also exposure concentration–dependent. After low-dose vapor exposure, irritation evidenced by reddening of the eyes may be the only effect. As the dose increases, the injury includes progressively more severe conjunctivitis, photophobia, blepharospasm, pain, and corneal damage (Fig. 215-3).

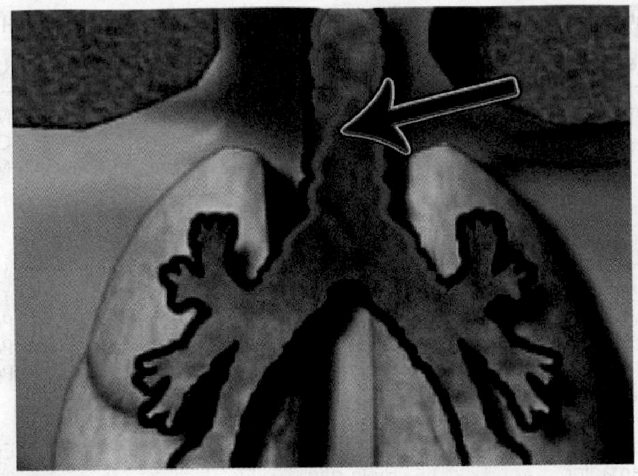

FIGURE 215-2 Schematic diagram of pseudomembrane formation as is seen in high-dose sulfur mustard vapor inhalation exposure. In World War I, severe inhalation exposure often caused death via large airways obstruction.

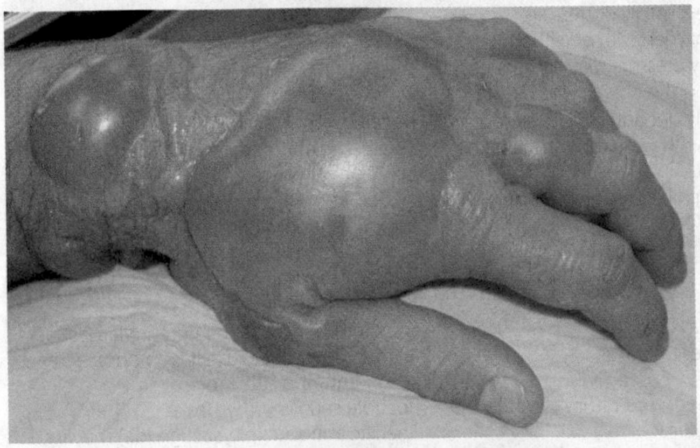

FIGURE 215-1 Large bulla formation from mustard burn in Iranian patient. Although the blisters on this patient's hand involve only 7% of the body surface area, this patient still required hospitalization in a burn intensive care unit.

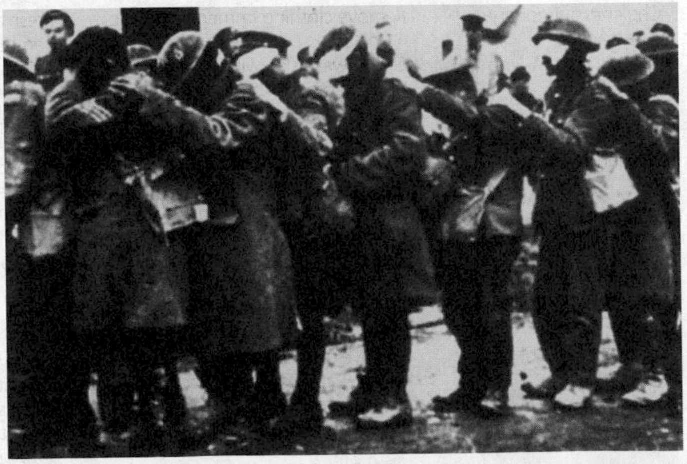

FIGURE 215-3 World War I photograph of troops exposed to sulfur mustard vapor. The vast majority of these troops survived with no long-term damage to the eyes; however, they were effectively rendered blind for days to weeks.

About 90% of eye injuries related to mustard heal in 2 weeks to 2 months without sequelae. Scarring between the iris and lens may follow severe effects; this scarring may restrict pupillary movements and may predispose victims to glaucoma. The most severe damage is caused by liquid mustard. After extensive eye exposure, severe corneal damage with possible perforation of the cornea and loss of the eye can occur. In some individuals, a latent chronic keratitis sometimes associated with corneal ulcerations has been described as early as 8 months and as late as 20 years after initial exposure.

The mucosa of the gastrointestinal tract is susceptible to mustard damage, either from systemic absorption or ingestion of the agent. Mustard exposure in small amounts will cause nausea and vomiting lasting up to 24 h. The mechanism of the nausea and vomiting is not understood, but mustard does have a cholinergic-like effect. The CNS effects of mustard, likewise, remain poorly defined. Large exposures can cause seizures in animals. Reports from WWI, and again from the Iran-Iraq war, described people exposed to small amounts of mustard acting sluggish, apathetic, and lethargic. These reports suggest that minor psychological problems could linger for a year or longer.

The cause of death in the majority of mustard poisoning cases is sepsis and respiratory failure. Mechanical obstruction via pseudomembrane formation and agent-induced laryngospasm is important in the first 24 h, but only in cases of severe exposure. From the third through the fifth day after exposure, expect a secondary pneumonia due to bacterial invasion of denuded necrotic mucosa. The third wave of death is caused by agent-induced bone marrow suppression, which peaks 7–21 days after exposure and causes death via sepsis.

℞ SULFUR MUSTARD

A patient severely ill from mustard poisoning requires the general supportive care provided for any severely ill patient, as well as the specific care given to a burn patient. Liberal use of systemic analgesics, maintenance of fluid and electrolyte balance, nutrition, appropriate antibiotics, and other supportive measures are necessary (Table 215-3).

The management of a patient exposed to mustard may range from simple, as in the provision of symptomatic care for a sunburn-like erythema, to complex, as in providing total management for a severely ill patient with burns, immunosuppression, and multi-system involvement. Before raw denuded areas of skin develop, especially with less severe exposures, topical cortisone creams or lotions may be of benefit. Some very basic research data point to the early use of anti-inflammatory preparations. Small blisters (<1–2 cm) should be left intact. Because larger bullae will eventually break, they should be carefully unroofed. Denuded areas should be irrigated three to four times daily with saline, other sterile solutions, or soapy water and then liberally covered with the topical antibiotic of choice, such as silver sulfadiazine or mafenide acetate to a thickness of 1–2 mm. Some physicians advocate sterile needle drainage of large blisters, collapsing the blister roof to form a sterile dressing. Mustard blister fluid does not contain sulfur mustard, only sterile tissue fluid. Health care staff should not fear possible contamination. If an antibiotic cream is not available, sterile petrolatum will be useful. Modified Dakins solution (sodium hypochlorite 0.5%) was used both in WWI and in Iranian casualties (1984–1987) for field-expedient irrigation and antisepsis. Large areas of vesication require hospitalization, IV therapy, and whirlpool bath irrigation.

Systemic analgesics should be used liberally, particularly before manipulation of the patient. Monitoring of fluids and electrolytes is important in any sick patient, but it must be recognized that fluid loss is not of the magnitude seen with thermal burns. Overly rigorous hydration seems to have precipitated pulmonary edema in a few Iranian casualties sent to European hospitals.

Conjunctival irritation from a low vapor exposure will respond to any of a number of available ophthalmic solutions after the eyes are thoroughly irrigated. A topical antibiotic applied several times a day will reduce the incidence and severity of infection. Animal laboratory data have shown remarkable results with commercially available topical antibiotic/glucocorticoid ophthalmologic ointments applied early. An ophthalmologist should be consulted. Topical glucocorticoids are not of proven value, but their use during the first few hours or days might significantly reduce inflammation and subsequent damage. Further use should be relegated to an ophthalmologist.

Vaseline or a similar substance should be applied regularly to the edges of the lids to prevent them from sticking together. Topical analgesics may be useful initially if blepharospasm is too severe to permit an adequate examination; however, topical analgesics have limited value.

A productive cough and dyspnea accompanied by fever and leukocytosis occurring within 12–24 h is indicative of a chemical pneumonitis. The clinician must resist the urge to use prophylactic antibiotics for this process. Infection often occurs on the third to fifth day and is signaled by an increased fever, pulmonary infiltrate, and an increase in sputum production with a change in color. Appropriate antibiotic therapy should await confirmation by Gram stain, and later, positive culture and sensitivity.

Intubation may be necessary if laryngeal spasm or edema makes it difficult or becomes life-threatening. Intubation permits better ventilation and facilitates suction of the necrotic and inflammatory debris. Early use of positive end-expiratory pressure (PEEP) or continuous positive airway pressure (CPAP) may be beneficial. Pseudomembrane formation may require fiberoptic bronchoscopy for suctioning of the necrotic debris.

Bronchodilators are of benefit for bronchospasm. If additional relief of bronchospasm is needed, glucocorticoids should be used. There is little evidence that the routine use of glucocorticoids is beneficial, except for additional relief of bronchospasm.

Leukopenia begins around day 3 with major systemic absorption. Marrow suppression peaks at 7–14 days. In the Iran/Iraq war, a white blood count of ≤200/μL usually resulted in death of the patient. Sterilization of the gut by nonabsorbable antibiotics should be considered to reduce the possibility of sepsis from enteric organisms. Cellular replacement (bone marrow transplants or transfusions) may be successful. Granulocyte colony-stimulating factor (G-CSF) produced a 50% reduction in the time for the bone marrow to recover in non-human primates exposed to sulfur mustard. Medication for nausea and vomiting may be necessary for gastrointestinal side effects.

Excellent assessments of the contributions of DNA alkylation, inflammation, activation of proteolytic enzymes, or lipid peroxidation to the mustard injury have been developed in the past 15–20 years. Some examples include (1) the demonstration of up to 75% reduction of inflammation and tissue damage in the mouse ear swelling test by vanilloid compounds, and (2) the demonstration of 50–60% protection by *N*-acetylcysteine in the generation of free radicals within guinea pig lung exposed to mustard. In many cases, the demonstration of protection is dependent on the availability of sufficient amounts of drug with adequate half-lives. Strategies to enhance bioavailability include attachment of polyethylene glycol to the antioxidant drug/enzyme or delivery of the drug/enzyme in a liposome (or both).

NERVE AGENTS

The organophosphorus nerve agents are the deadliest of the CWAs. They work by inhibition of tissue synaptic acetylcholinesterase, creating an acute cholinergic crisis. Death ensues because of respiratory depression, and can occur within seconds to minutes.

The nerve agents tabun and sarin were first used on the battlefield by Iraq against Iran during the first Persian Gulf War (1984–1987). Estimates of casualties from these agents range from 20,000–100,000. In 1994 and 1995, the Japanese cult Aum Shinrikyo used sarin in two terrorist attacks in Matsumoto and Tokyo.

The "classic" nerve agents include tabun (GA), sarin (GB), soman (GD), cyclosarin (GF), and VX. VR, similar to VX, was manufactured in the former Soviet Union (Table 215-2). The two-letter codes were established by a North Atlantic Treaty Organization (NATO) international convention and convey no clinical implications. All of the nerve agents are organophosphorus compounds, which are liquid at standard temperature and pressure. The "G" agents evaporate at about the rate of water, except for GF, which is oily, and thus will probably have evaporated within 24 h after deposition on the ground. Their high volatility thus makes a spill of any amount a serious vapor hazard. In the Tokyo subway attack where sarin was used, 100% of the symptomatic patients inhaled sarin vapor that spilled out on the floor of the subway cars. VX, an oily liquid, is the exception. Its low vapor pressure makes it much less of a vapor hazard but potentially a greater environmental hazard because it persists in the environment far longer.

MECHANISM Acetylcholinesterase inhibition accounts for the major life-threatening effects of nerve agent poisoning. Reversal of this inhibition by antidotal therapy is effective, proving that this is the primary toxic action of these poisons. At cholinergic synapses, acetylcholinesterase, bound to the postsynaptic membrane, functions as a turn-off switch to regulate cholinergic transmission. Inhibition of acetylcholinesterases causes the released neurotransmitter, acetylcholine, to accumulate abnormally. End-organ overstimulation, recognized by clinicians as cholinergic crisis, ensues (Fig. 215-4).

CLINICAL FEATURES Clinical effects of nerve agent exposure are identical for vapor and liquid exposure routes if the dose is sufficiently large. The speed and order of symptom onset will differ (Table 215-2).

Exposure of a patient to nerve agent vapor, overwhelmingly the more likely route of exposure in both battlefield and terrorist scenarios, will cause cholinergic symptoms in the order that the toxin encounters cholinergic synapses. The most exposed synapses on the integument of the human are in the pupillary muscles. Nerve agent vapor easily crosses the cornea, interacts with these synapses, and produces miosis, described by Tokyo subway victims as "the world going black." Rarely this can also cause eye pain and nausea. Exocrine glands located in the nose, mouth, and pharynx next become exposed to the vapor, and cholinergic overload here causes increased secretions, rhinorrhea, excess salivation, and drooling. Next, toxin interacts with exocrine glands in the upper airway, causing bronchorrhea, and with bronchial smooth muscle, causing bronchospasm. This combination of events can cause hypoxia.

Once the victim has inhaled, vapor can passively cross the alveolar-capillary membrane, enter the bloodstream, and, incidentally and asymptomatically, inhibit circulating cholinesterases, particularly free butyrylcholinesterase and erythrocyte acetylcholinesterase, both of which can be assayed. Unfortunately, the assay may not be easily interpreted without a baseline, since cholinesterase levels vary enormously between subjects and over time in an individual healthy patient.

Usually the first organ system to become symptomatic from bloodborne nerve agent exposure is the gastrointestinal tract, where cholinergic overload causes abdominal cramping and pain, nausea, vomiting, and diarrhea. After the gastrointestinal tract is involved, nerve agents will affect the heart, distant exocrine glands, muscles, and brain. Because there are cholinergic synapses on both the vagal (parasympathetic) and sympathetic sides of the autonomic input to the heart, one cannot predict how heart rate and blood pressure will change once intoxicated. Remote exocrine activity will include oversecretion in the salivary, nasal, respiratory, and sweat glands—the patient will be "wet all over." Bloodborne nerve agents will overstimulate neuromuscular junctions in skeletal muscles, causing fasciculations followed by frank twitching. If the process goes on long enough, eventually ATP in muscle will be depleted and flaccid paralysis will ensue.

In the brain, since the cholinergic system is so widely distributed, bloodborne nerve agents will, in sufficient doses, cause rapid loss of consciousness, seizures, and central apnea leading to death within minutes. If respiration is supported, status epilepticus, which does not respond to usual anticonvulsants, may ensue (Chap. 363). If status epilepticus persists, neuronal death and permanent brain dysfunction may occur. Even in mild nerve agent intoxication, patients may recover but may experience weeks of irritability, sleep disturbance, and nonspecific neurobehavioral symptoms.

The time from exposure to development of the full-blown cholinergic crisis from nerve agent vapor inhalation can be minutes or even seconds, yet there is no depot effect. Since nerve agents have a short circulating half-life, if the patient is supported and, ideally, treated with antidotes, improvement should be rapid without subsequent deterioration.

Liquid exposure to nerve agents differs in speed and order of symptom onset. A nerve agent on intact skin will partially evaporate and partially begin to travel through the skin, causing localized sweating

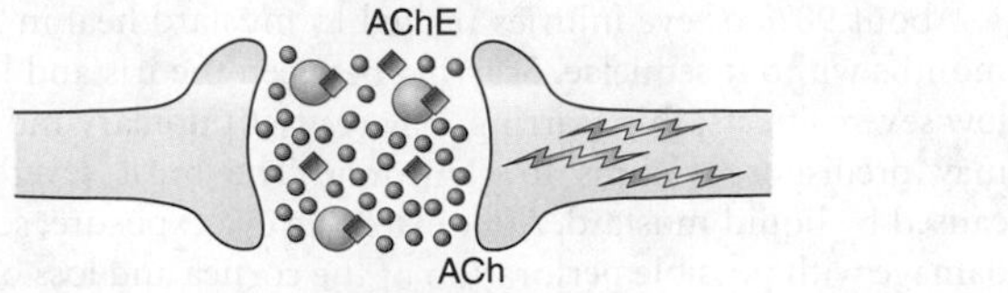

FIGURE 215-4 Schematic diagram of the pathophysiology of nerve agent exposure. Nerve agent (◆) binds to the active site of acetylcholinesterase (AChE), which is shown as floating free in space but is in reality a postsynaptic membrane-bound enzyme. As a result, acetylcholine (●), which is normally released from presynaptic membrane but normally degraded, accumulates, and this leads (↯) to organ overstimulation and cholinergic crisis.

and then localized fasciculations when it encounters neuromuscular junctions. Once in muscle, it will cross into the circulation and cause gastrointestinal discomfort, respiratory distress, heart rate changes, generalized fasciculations and twitching, loss of consciousness, seizures, and central apnea. The time course will be much longer than with vapor inhalation; even a large, lethal droplet can take up to 30 min to have an effect, and a small, sublethal dose could continue to take effect over 18 h. Clinical worsening that occurs hours after treatment has started is far more likely with liquid than with vapor exposure. Additionally, miosis, practically unavoidable with vapor exposure, is not always present with liquid exposure and may be the last symptom to present in this situation. This is due to the relative insulation of the pupillary muscle from the systemic circulation.

Unless removed by specific therapy (oximes), binding of a nerve agent to cholinesterase is essentially irreversible. Erythrocyte acetylcholinesterase activity recovers at about 1% per day. Plasma butyrylcholinesterase recovers more quickly and is a better guide to recovery of tissue enzyme activity.

℞ NERVE AGENTS

Acute nerve agent poisoning is treated by decontamination, respiratory support, and three antidotes—an anticholinergic, an oxime, and an anticonvulsant (Tables 215-3 and **215-4**). In acute cases, all of these forms of therapy may be given simultaneously.

DECONTAMINATION Decontamination of a vapor is formally not necessary, but in the Tokyo subway attack, sarin vapor trapped in the patients' clothing caused miosis in 10% of emergency personnel. Removal of clothing would have obviated most of this problem. Decontamination of liquid is accomplished in the military using the M291 skin decontamination kit, containing an Ambergard resin capable of absorbing liquid off the skin. Civilian agencies now stockpile this product approved by the U.S. Food and Drug Administration (FDA). At hospitals, soap and copious amounts of water should suffice. Physical removal of the agent is superior to all known decontamination solutions and lotions. In any event, decontamination must be accomplished before the patient enters the hospital facility to avoid contaminating the facility and its staff. In patients with contaminated wounds, extract potentially contaminated clothing and other foreign material that may serve as a depot for the liquid agent.

RESPIRATORY SUPPORT Death from nerve agent poisoning is almost always from respiratory causes. Ventilation will be complicated by increased resistance and secretions. Atropine should be given before ventilation or as ventilation begins, since it will make ventilation far easier.

ANTIDOTAL THERAPY **Atropine** In theory, any anticholinergic could be used to treat nerve agent poisoning, but worldwide the choice is invariably atropine due to its wide temperature stability, rapid effectiveness either IM or IV, and because inadvertent administration of this drug usually causes little CNS dysfunction (Table 215-4). Atropine rapidly reverses cholinergic overload at muscarinic synapses but has little effect at nicotinic synapses. Practically, this implies that atropine can quickly treat the life-threatening respiratory effects of nerve agents but will probably not help neuromuscular and possibly sympathetic effects. In the field, military personnel are given MARK I kits **(Fig. 215-5*A*)** containing 2 mg atro-

TABLE 215-4 ANTIDOTE RECOMMENDATIONS FOLLOWING EXPOSURE TO NERVE AGENTS

	Antidotes		
Patient Age	**Mild/Moderate Effects[a]**	**Severe Effects[b]**	**Other Treatment**
Infants (0–2 yrs)	Atropine: 0.05 mg/kg IM, *or* 0.02 mg/kg IV; *and* 2-PAM chloride: 15 mg/kg IM *or* IV slowly	Atropine: 0.1 mg/kg IM, *or* 0.02 mg/kg IV; *and* 2-PAM chloride: 25 mg/kg IM, *or* 15 mg/kg IV slowly	Assisted ventilation after antidotes for severe exposure.
Child (2–10 yrs)	Atropine: 1 mg IM, *or* 0.02 mg/kg IV; *and* 2-PAM chloride[c]: 15 mg/kg IM *or* IV slowly	Atropine: 2 mg IM, *or* 0.02 mg/kg IV; *and* 2-PAM chloride[c]: 25 mg/kg IM, *or* 15 mg/kg IV slowly	Repeat atropine (2 mg IM, or 1 mg IM for infants) at 5- to 10-min intervals until secretions have diminished and breathing is comfortable or airway resistance has returned to near normal.
Adolescent (>10 yrs)	Atropine: 2 mg IM, *or* 0.02 mg/kg IV; *and* 2-PAM chloride[c]: 15 mg/kg IM *or* IV slowly	Atropine: 4 mg IM, *or* 0.02 mg/kg IV; *and* 2-PAM chloride[c]: 25 mg/kg IM, *or* 15 mg/kg IV slowly	
Adult	Atropine: 2 to 4 mg IM *or* IV; *and* 2-PAM chloride: 600 mg IM, *or* 15 mg/kg IV slowly	Atropine: 6 mg IM; *and* 2-PAM chloride: 1800 mg IM, *or* 15 mg/kg IV slowly	Phentolamine for 2-PAM-induced hypertension: (5 mg IV for adults; 1 mg IV for children). Diazepam for convulsions: (0.2 to 0.5 mg IV for infants <5 years: 1 mg IV for children >5 years; 5 mg IV for adults).
Elderly, frail	Atropine: 1 mg IM; *and* 2-PAM chloride: 10 mg/kg IM, *or* 5 to 10 mg/kg IV slowly	Atropine: 2 to 4 mg IM; *and* 2-PAM chloride: 25 mg/kg IM, *or* 5 to 10 mg/kg IV slowly	

[a]Mild/moderate effects include localized sweating, muscle fasciculations, nausea, vomiting, weakness, dyspnea.
[b]Severe effects include unconsciousness, convulsions, apnea, flaccid paralysis.
[c]If calculated dose exceeds the adult IM dose, adjust accordingly.
Note: 2-PAM chloride is pralidoxime chloride or protopam chloride.
Source: State of New York, Department of Health.

pine in autoinjector form for IM use. Civilian agencies are now stockpiling this FDA-approved product as well. One can only give full autoinjector doses and not divide them. The field-loading dose is 2, 4, or 6 mg, with retreatment every 5–10 min until the patient's breathing and secretions improve. The Iranians used larger doses initially during the Iran-Iraq war where oximes were in short supply. When the patient reaches a level of medical care where drugs can be given IV, this is the preferred route; in small children this may be the initial form of atropine therapy. However, pediatric autoinjectors of 0.5 mg and 1.0 mg are now manufactured. There is no upper limit to atropine therapy in a patient either IM or IV; however, a total average adult dose for a severely afflicted patient would usually be 20–30 mg.

In a mildly afflicted patient with miosis and no other systemic symptoms, atropine or homatropine eye drops may suffice for therapy. This will produce ~24 h of mydriasis. Frank miosis or imperfect accommodation may persist for weeks or even months after all other signs and symptoms have resolved.

Oxime Therapy Oximes are nucleophiles that reactivate the cholinesterase whose active site has been occupied and bound to nerve agent (Table 215-4). Therapy with oximes therefore restores normal enzyme function. Oxime therapy is limited by a second side reaction, called "aging," in which a side chain on nerve agents falls off the complex at a characteristic rate. "Aged" complexes are negatively charged, and oximes cannot reactivate negatively charged complexes. The practical effect of this differs from one nerve agent to another since each ages at a characteristic rate. VX, for practical purposes, never ages, sarin ages in 3–5 h, and tabun ages over a longer period. All of these are so much longer than the patient's expected lifespan after acute nerve agent toxicity that they may be ignored. Soman, on the other hand, ages in 2 min. Thus, after only a few minutes following exposure, oximes are useless in treating soman poisoning. The oxime used varies by country; the United States has approved and fielded 2-pralidoxime chloride (2-PAM Cl). MARK I kits (Fig. 215-5*A*) contain autoinjectors of 600 mg 2-PAM Cl. Initial field loading doses are 600, 1200, or 1800 mg. Since blood pressure elevation may occur after administration of 45 mg/kg in adults, field use of 2-PAM Cl is restricted to 1800 mg, IM, per hour. During the time when more oxime cannot be given, atropine alone is recommended. In the hospital setting, 2.5–25 mg/kg IV 2-PAM Cl has been found to reactivate 50% of inhibited cholinesterase. The usual recommendation is 1000 mg through slow IV drip over 20–30 min, with ≤2500 mg over a period of 1–1.5 h.

Anticonvulsants Nerve agent–induced seizures do not respond to the usual anticonvulsants used for status epilepticus, including phenytoin, phenobarbital, carbamazepine, valproic acid, and lamotrigine (Chap. 363). The only class of anticonvulsants that has been shown to stop this form of status are the benzodiazepines. Diazepam is the only benzodiazepine approved for seizures in humans, although other FDA-approved benzodiazepines work well against nerve agent–induced seizures in animal models. Diazepam, therefore, is manufactured in 10-mg injectors for IM use and given to U.S. forces for this purpose **(Fig. 215-5*B*)**. Civilian agencies are stockpiling this field product (convulsive antidote for nerve agent, "CANA"), which is not generally used in hospital practice. Extrapolation from animal studies indicates that adults will probably require 30–40 mg diazepam, IM, to stop nerve agent–induced status epilepticus. In the hospital, or in a small child unable to receive the autoinjector, IV diazepam may be used at similar doses. The clinician may confuse seizures with the neuromuscular signs of nerve agent poisoning. In the hospital, early electroencephalography is advised to distinguish between nonconvulsive status epilepticus, actual seizures, and postictal paralysis. Recent animal studies have shown that the most effective benzodiazepine in this situation is midazolam, which is not FDA-approved for seizures.

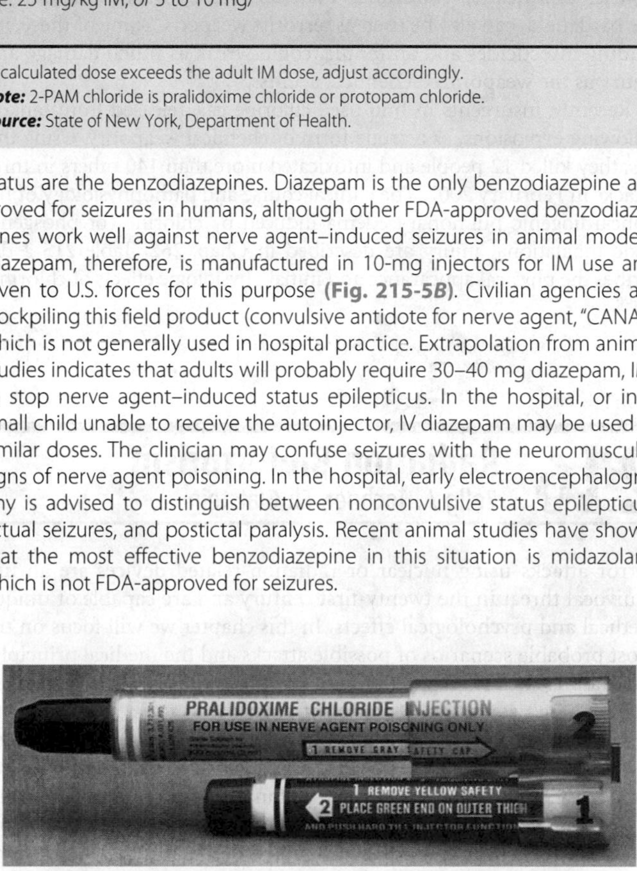

A

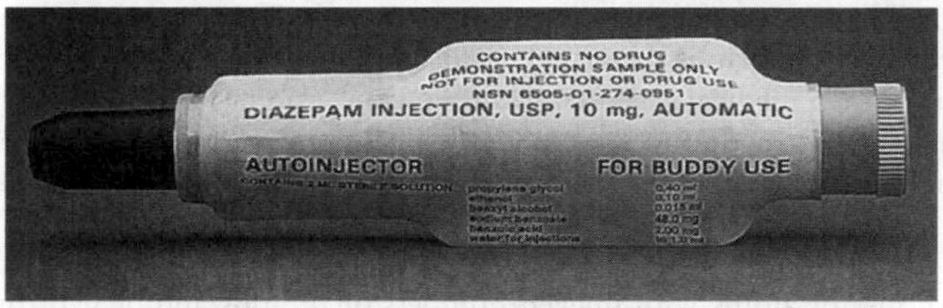

B

FIGURE 215-5 Antidotes to nerve agents. *A.* MARK I autoinjector set containing one 600-mg dose of 2-pralidoxime chloride and one 2-mg dose of atropine. Such sets are carried by all U.S. military forces in a potentially chemical battlefield and are now being stockpiled by civilian first responders. ***B.*** Diazepam 10-mg autoinjector. These are carried by all U.S. military forces in a potential chemical battlefield and are being stockpiled by civilian first responders.

Peripheral neuropathy and the so-called intermediate syndrome, prominent long-term effects of insecticide poisoning, are not described in nerve agent survivors.

Recent research has explored approaches leading to a transient "immunity," or drugs that would provide protection against lethal nerve agents yet be devoid of side effects. A novel approach is to use enzymes to scavenge these highly toxic nerve agents before they attack their intended targets. The accumulated work has shown that if a scavenger is present at the time of nerve agent exposure, rapid reduction of toxicant levels is observed. This reduction is so rapid and profound that the need to administer a host of pharmacologically active drugs as antidotes is, in theory, eliminated.

INDUSTRIAL CHEMICALS IN TERRORISM

Many of the chemical warfare agents of WWI, including chlorine, phosgene, and cyanide, are used today in large amounts in industry. They are produced in chemical plants, stockpiled in large tanks, and travel up and down highways and railways in large tanker cars. The rupture of any of these by accident or purposefully could cause many injuries and deaths. Hazardous materials (HAZMATs), not used on the battlefield, can also be used as terrorist weapons. Some of these, including insecticides and ammonia, could wreak as much damage and injury as the weaponized chemical agents.

Recently, insurgents in Iraq used chlorine gas, released from tankers following explosions, as a crude form of chemical weaponry. Using this gas, they killed 12 people and intoxicated more than 140 others in three attacks in February 2007. The clinical course and pathophysiology of the noncardiogenic pulmonary edema induced by chlorine (or phosgene) toxic inhalational injury are described in Chap. 262. Table 215-2 describes the physical appearance and initial physiologic effects of chlorine.

FURTHER READINGS

BROOMFIELD CA et al: Progress on the road to new nerve agent treatments. J Appl Toxicol 21:S43, 2001

GUNDERSON CH et al: Nerve agents: A review. Neurology 42:946, 1992

KARALLIEDDE L et al: Possible immediate and long-term health effects following exposure to chemical warfare agents. Public Health 114:238, 2000

MCDONOUGH JH et al: Anticonvulsant treatment of nerve agent seizures: Anticholinergics versus diazepam in soman-intoxicated guinea pigs. Epilepsy Res 38:1, 2000

OKUMURA T et al: Report on 640 victims of the Tokyo subway sarin attack. Ann Emerg Med 28:129, 1996

SIDELL FR: Clinical considerations in nerve agent intoxication, in *Chemical Warfare Agents*, SM Somani (ed). San Diego, California, Academic Press, 1992, pp 156–194

——— et al (eds.): *Medical Aspects of Chemical and Biological Warfare, Volume I of Textbook of Military Medicine*, Walter Reed Army Medical Center, Washington, DC, Borden Institute, 1997. [Available on the website: *http://ccc.apgea.army.mil*]

SMITH WJ: Vesicant agents and antivesicant medical countermeasures: Clinical toxicology and psychological implications. Mil Psychol 14:145, 2002

US ARMY MEDICAL RESEARCH INSTITUTE OF CHEMICAL DEFENSE, CHEMICAL CASUALTY CARE DIVISION: *Medical Management of Chemical Casualties Handbook*, 3d ed. Aberdeen Proving Ground, Maryland, 1999. [Available on the website: *http://ccc.apgea.army.mil*]

WILLEMS JL: Clinical management of mustard gas casualties. Ann Med Milit Belg 3S:1, 1989

216 Radiation Bioterrorism

Zelig A. Tochner, Eli Glatstein

Terror attacks using nuclear or radiation-related devices are an unequivocal threat in the twenty-first century and are capable of unique medical and psychological effects. In this chapter we will focus on the most probable scenarios of possible attacks and the medical principles of handling such threats.

There are two major categories of potential terrorist incidents with widespread radiologic consequences. The first is the use of radiologic dispersal devices. This could cause a purposeful dissemination of radioactive material without nuclear detonation by using conventional explosives with radionuclides, attacking fixed nuclear facilities, or attacking nuclear-powered surface vessels or submarines. Malfunctioning nuclear weapons that are detonated with no nuclear yield (nuclear "duds") and/or installation of radionuclides in food or water are also a possible means of generating a terror attack. The second, and less probable, scenario is the actual use of nuclear weapons. Each scenario has its own medical aspects, including "conventional" blast or thermal injury, introduction to a radiation field, and exposure to either external or internal contamination from a radioactive explosion.

TYPES OF RADIOISOTOPIC RADIATION

Isotopes of atoms with uneven numbers of protons and/or neutrons are typically unstable; such isotopes discharge particles or energy to matter, a process that we define as *radiation*. The main radiation types are alpha, beta, gamma, and neutrons.

Alpha (α) radiation consists of heavy, positively charged particles containing two protons and two neutrons. Alpha particles are usually emitted from isotopes with an atomic number of ≥82, such as uranium or plutonium. Due to their large size, alpha particles have limited penetrating power. Fine obstacles such as cloth or human skin can usually stop them from penetrating into the body, and they represent a small risk to external exposure due to their limited penetration. If they somehow are internalized, then alpha particles can cause significant cellular damage within their immediate proximity.

Beta (β) radiation consists of electrons, which are small, light, negatively charged particles (about 1/2000 the mass of a neutron or proton). They can travel only a short finite distance in tissue, depending on their energy. Exposure to beta particles is common in many radiation accidents. Radioactive iodine, released in nuclear plant accidents, is the best known member of this group. Plastic layers and clothing can stop most beta particles, and their penetration is measured to be a few millimeters. A large quantum of energy to the basal stratum of the skin can cause a burn that is similar to a thermal burn and is treated as such.

Gamma (γ) rays and *x-rays* (both photons) are similar. Gamma rays are uncharged electromagnetic radiation discharged from a nucleus as a wave or photons of energy. X-rays are the product of abrupt mechanical deceleration of electrons striking a heavy target such as tungsten. Gamma and x-rays have similar properties, i.e., no charge and no mass, just energy. Both travel easily through matter, sometimes called *penetrating radiation*, and are the principal type of radiation to cause total-body exposure. If the energy of gamma rays and x-rays is the same, then their biological effects will be the same.

Neutron (η) particles are heavy and uncharged, often emitted during nuclear detonation. They possess a wide energy range; their ability to penetrate tissues is variable, depending upon their energy. They are less likely to be present in most scenarios of radiation bioterrorism.

The ionization resulting from protons, electrons, and gamma rays is either a direct or indirect (i.e., mediated through water) effect of particles or photons on DNA. Ionization of DNA resulting from neutrons is secondary to the neutrons knocking electrons out of their atomic orbit and the formation of free radicals, which can also damage DNA directly.

The commonly used units of radiation are the rad and the gray (Gy). The rad (radiation absorbed dose) is energy deposited within living matter and is equal to 100 ergs/g of tissue.

The traditional rad has been replaced by the Système Internationale (SI) unit of the gray; 100 rad = 1 Gy.

TYPES OF EXPOSURE

Whole-body exposure represents deposition of radiation energy over the entire body. Alpha and beta particles have limited penetration and do not cause significant noncutaneous injury unless emission results from an internalized source. Whole-body exposure from gamma rays, x-rays, or neutrons, which can penetrate through the body (depending on their energy), can result in damage to multiple tissues and organs. The tissue damage is proportional to the radiation exposure of that organ or tissue.

External contamination is a result of fallout of radioactive particles that land on the body surface, clothing, skin, and hair. This is the dominant element to consider in the mass casualty situation resulting from a radioactive terrorist strike. The common contaminants will primarily emit alpha and beta radiation. Alpha particles do not penetrate beyond the skin and thus have minimal systemic effects. Beta emitters can cause significant cutaneous burns and scarring. Gamma emitters may not only cause local damage but can also cause whole-body radiation exposures and injury. The medical treatment is primarily decontamination of the body, including wounds and burns, to prevent the contamination from becoming internalized. Removing the contaminated clothing reduces the contamination significantly and is a first step in the decontamination process. Generally patients will not constitute a significant radiation hazard to health care providers, and life-saving treatment should not be delayed for fear of secondary contamination of the medical team. Any damage to health care personnel will depend directly on the duration of exposure and will be inversely proportional to the square of the distance from any radioactive source. Gowns that can be easily removed are essential to protect health care personnel.

Internal contamination will occur when radioactive material is inhaled, ingested, or able to enter the body through open wounds or burns or via skin absorption. In principle, any externally contaminated casualty should be evaluated for internal contamination. Some isotopes may have toxic effects on specific target organs due to their chemical properties, in addition to radiologic injury. The respiratory system is the main portal of entrance for internal contamination, and the lung is the organ at greatest risk. Aerosol particles <5 μm can reach the alveoli, whereas larger particles will remain in proximal airways. The tiny particles can be absorbed by the lymphatic system or the bloodstream, continuing to irradiate (depending on their biologically active half-life) until being exhaled. Bronchial lavage is often helpful treatment in this situation. Radioactive material entering the gastrointestinal (GI) tract will be absorbed according to its chemical structure and solubility. The insoluble radionuclides may affect the lower GI tract. Intact skin is normally a good barrier to most radionuclides. Penetration through the skin usually takes place when wounds or burns have altered the skin barriers. Therefore, any skin erosion should be cleaned and decontaminated promptly.

Absorbed radioactive materials will travel throughout the body. Liver, kidney, adipose tissue, and bone tend to bind and retain the radioactive material more than other tissues. The medical treatment includes preventing absorption, reducing incorporation, and enhancing elimination (see below).

Localized exposure means close contact between a highly radioactive source and a part of the body, causing discrete damage to the skin and deeper tissues, similar to a thermal burn. Later signs include epilation, erythema, moist desquamation, ulceration, blistering, or necrosis in proportion to exposure. Alopecia, transient or permanent, is dose-related and starts at cutaneous doses >3 Gy. Overt tissue damage can take weeks and even months to develop; the healing process can also be very slow and last for months. Long-term cutaneous changes, including keratosis, fibrosis, and telangiectasias, may appear years after the exposure. Treatment is based on analgesia and infection prophylaxis. Nevertheless, severe burns can often require grafting or even amputation. Long-term radiation effects are characterized by cell loss and cell death.

RADIOLOGIC DISPERSAL EVENTS

Radiologic dispersal incidents are generally of two types resulting from: (1) small, usually localized sources; or (2) wide dispersals over large areas. The radioactive materials can take the form of solid state, aerosol, gas, or liquid. They can be put into food or water, released from vehicles, or be spread by explosion. The principal route of exposure is usually by direct contact between the victim's skin and the radioactive particles, although internal contamination could occur if the material were inhaled or ingested. The radiation field is also a potential source of whole-body exposure. The psychosocial effects that accompany such an event are significant and are beyond the scope of this chapter. A list of radioactive materials, including information on their major properties and medical treatment, is shown in Table 216-1.

In a localized event, the amount and spread of the radioactive materials are usually limited and can be treated like a spill of hazardous material. Protective clothing prevents or minimizes the contamination of emergency responders.

The use of explosives coupled with a large amount of radioactive materials can result in wide dispersion of radiation, which is of far greater concern. Other potential sources of radiation are nuclear reactors, spent nuclear fuel, and transport vehicles. Less probable but still possible is the use of a large source of penetrating radiation without explosion. It is expected that most exposures would be low, and the principal health and psychosocial effects would be similar to the former scenario but on a larger scale.

Whenever an explosion is involved, conventional life-saving treatment should be given first priority. Only then should decontamination and specific treatment be given for the radiation exposure.

Silent exposure represents a scenario in which a powerful radiologic source could be hidden in a crowded place or radiologic materials spread without any awareness or announcement. It might take a long time to recognize the event and the source of exposure. One of the major clues to this situation is the appearance of unusual clinical manifestations in many individuals; such manifestations are often nonspecific and include symptoms of acute radiation sickness (see below) such as headache, fatigue, malaise, and opportunistic infections. GI phenomena such as diarrhea, nausea, vomiting, and anorexia may occur. Dermatologic symptoms (burns, ulceration, and epilation) and hematopoietic manifestations such as bleeding tendency, thrombocytopenia, purpura, lymphopenia, or neutropenia are also possible and dose-related. Careful epidemiologic studies may be necessary to identify the source of such exposure.

NUCLEAR WEAPONS

The most likely scenario of nuclear terror would be the detonation of a single low-yield device. The estimated yield of such device is anywhere between 0.01 and 10 kiloton of TNT, although the probability would more likely be toward the lower yield. Coping with such an event is certainly possible. The effects of such an explosion are a combination of several components: ground shock, air blast, thermal radiation, initial nuclear radiation, residual nuclear radiation, crater formation, and radioactive fallout.

The nuclear detonation, like a conventional explosion, will produce a shock wave that can further damage structures and cause many casualties. In addition, the detonation can produce an extremely hot fireball that can ignite materials and cause severe burns. The detonation also releases an intense pulse of ionizing radiation, mainly gamma rays and neutrons. The radiation produced in the first minute is termed *initial radiation*, while the ongoing radiation due to fallout is termed *residual radiation*. Both types of radiation can cause acute radiation sickness (ARS; see below). The $LD_{50/30}$ (i.e., a dose that causes 50% mortality at 30 days) is ~4 Gy for whole-body exposure without medical support; with medical support, the $LD_{50/30}$ ranges between 8 and 10 Gy. Winds can carry fallout and contaminate large areas.

On top of its effects, a massive blast forms a crater in the soil and usually produces a ground shock compounding the damage and number of casualties. Inhalation of large amounts of radioactive dust causes pneu-

TABLE 216-1 INTERNAL CONTAMINANT RADIONUCLIDES: PROPERTIES AND TREATMENT

Isotope Name	Symbol	Common Usage	Radiation Type $t_{1/2}$ Radiologic $t_{1/2}$ Biologic, days	Exposure Type	Mode of Contamination	Focal Accumulation in Body	Treatment
Manganese	Mn-56	Reactors, research laboratories	β, γ 2.6 h 5.7	External, internal	N/A	Liver	N/A
Cobalt	Co-60	Medical radiotherapy devices, commercial food irradiators	β, γ 5.26 y 9.5	External, internal	Lungs	Liver	Gastric lavage, purgatives; penicillamine in severe cases
Strontium	Sr-90	Fission product of uranium	β 28 y 18,000	Internal	Moderate GI tract	Bones—similar to calcium	Strontium, calcium, ammonium chloride
Molybdenum	Mo-99	Hospitals—scans	β, γ 66.7 h 3	External, internal	N/A	Kidneys	N/A
Technetium	Tc-99m	Hospitals—scans	β, γ 6.049 h 1	External, internal	IV administration	Kidneys, total body	Potassium perchlorate to reduce thyroid dose
Cesium	Cs-137	Medical radiotherapy devices	β, γ 30 y 70	External, internal	Lungs, GI tract, wounds, follows potassium	Renal excretion	Ion-exchange resins, Prussian blue
Gadolinium	Gd-153	Hospitals	β, γ 242 d 1000	External, internal	N/A	N/A	N/A
Iridium	Ir-192	Commercial radiography	β, γ 74 d 50	External, internal	N/A	Spleen	N/A
Radium	Ra-226	Instrument illumination, industrial applications, old medical equipment, former Soviet Union military equipment	α, β, γ 1602 y 16,400	External, internal	GI tract	Bones	$MgSO_4$ lavage, ammonium chloride, calcium alginates
Tritium	H-3	Luminescent gun sights, muzzle-velocity detectors, nuclear weapons	β 12.5 y 12	Internal	Inhalation, GI tract, wounds	Total body	Dilution with controlled water intake, diuretics
Iodine	I-131	Reactor accidents, thyroid ablators	β, γ 8.1 d 138	Internal	Inhalation, GI tract, wounds	Thyroid	Potassium/sodium iodide, propylthiouracil, methimazole
Uranium	U-235	Depleted uranium, natural uranium, fuel rods, weapons-grade material	α, (α, β, γ) 7.1×10^8 y 15	Internal	GI tract	Kidneys, bones	$NaHCO_3$, chelation with EDTA
Plutonium	Pu-239	Produced from uranium in reactors, nuclear weapons	α 2.2×10^4 y 73,000	Internal	Limited lung absorption, high retention	Lungs, bones, bone marrow, liver, gonads	Chelating with DTPA or EDTA
Americium	Am-241	Smoke detectors, nuclear weapon detonation fallout	α 458 y 73,000	Internal	Inhalation, skin wounds	Lungs, liver, bones, bone marrow	Chelating with DTPA or EDTA
Polonium	Po-210	Calibration source	α 138.4 d 60	Internal	Inhalation, wounds	Spleen, kidneys	Lavage, dimercaprol
Thallium	Th-232	Calibration source	α 1.41×10^{10} y 73,000	Internal	N/A	N/A	N/A
Phosphorus	P-32	Research laboratories, medical facilities	β 14.3 d 1155	Internal	Inhalation, GI tract, wounds	Bones, bone marrow, rapidly replicating cells	Lavage, aluminum hydroxide, phosphate

Note: N/A, not available; h, hours; y, years; GI, gastrointestinal.

monitis that can lead to pulmonary fibrosis. Use of a mask covering the mouth and nose can be very helpful. The intense flash of infrared and visible light can cause either temporary or permanent blindness. Cataracts can develop months to years later among those who survive.

ACUTE RADIATION SICKNESS

Radiation interactions with atoms can result in ionization and the formation of free radicals that damage tissue by disrupting chemical bonds and molecular structures in the cell, including DNA. Radiation damage can lead to cell death; those cells that recover may be mutated and at higher risk for subsequent cancer. Cell sensitivity increases as the replication rate increases and the cell differentiation decreases. Bone marrow and mucosal surfaces of the GI tract, which have vast mitotic activity, are significantly more sensitive to radiation than slowly dividing tissues such as bones and muscles. Following exposure of either all or most of the human body to ionizing radiation, ARS can develop. The clinical manifestations of ARS reflect the dose and type of radiation as well as the part of the body exposed.

Clinical Manifestations ARS manifests as three major groups of signs and symptoms: hematopoietic, gastrointestinal, and neurovascular. There are four major stages in ARS: prodrome, latent phase, illness, and either recovery or death. The higher the radiation doses, the shorter and more severe each stage. The prodrome appears within minutes to 4 days postexposure; lasts between a few hours to a few days; and can include nausea, vomiting, anorexia, and diarrhea. At the end of the prodrome, ARS progresses to the latent phase. Minimal or no symptoms are present during the latent phase, which commonly lasts up to 2.5 weeks, but can last up to 6 weeks. The duration depends on the radiation dose, the health of the patient, and the coexisting illness or injury. Following the latent phase, the exposed person manifests illness that may eventuate in recovery or lead to death.

With exposure to doses <1 Gy, ARS is generally mild. At this dose symptoms can be minimal or nonexistent, even if the entire body is exposed to penetrating radiation. The clinical picture will mainly be transient depression of bone marrow (lymphopenia) that lasts up to 2 to 3 weeks and then recovers.

ARS is significantly more acute and severe with exposure to very high doses—>30 Gy. At this dose the prodrome appears in minutes and is followed by 5 to 6 h of latency before a cardiovascular collapse occurs secondary to irreversible damage to the microcirculation.

The type and dose of radiation and the part of the body exposed will determine not only the timing of the different stages of ARS but also the dominant clinical picture. At low radiation doses of 0.7 to 4 Gy, hematopoietic depression due to bone marrow suppression takes place and constitutes the main illness. The patient may develop infections and bleeding secondary to low leukocyte and platelet counts, respectively. The bone marrow will eventually recover in almost all patients if they are supported with transfusions and fluids; antibiotics are often needed in addition. With exposure to 6 to 8 Gy, the clinical picture is significantly more complicated. At these doses the bone marrow will not always recover and death may ensue. A GI syndrome may also accompany the hematopoietic manifestations and further worsen the patient's condition. Compromise of the absorptive layer of the gut alters absorption of fluids, electrolytes, and nutrients. GI injury can lead to vomiting, diarrhea, GI bleeding, sepsis, and electrolyte and fluid imbalance in a patient whose blood counts are compromised for a period of weeks, often leading to death. Whole-body exposure to doses >9–10 Gy is almost always fatal. Crucial elements of the bone marrow simply will not recover. In addition to the GI syndrome associated with very large exposures, patients may develop a neurovascular syndrome; the latter dominates with whole-body doses >20 Gy. Vascular collapse, seizures, confusion, and death usually occur within days. In this variant the prodrome and latent phase both shorten to a few hours.

℞ ACUTE RADIATION SICKNESS

The treatment of ARS is focused on maintaining homeostasis, giving damaged organs the chance to recover. Aggressive support is given to every damaged system. Treatment for the hematopoietic system includes mainly therapy for neutropenia and infection, transfusion and blood products as needed, and hematopoietic growth factors. The value of bone marrow transplantation in this situation is questionable. None of the transplants that were performed among the victims of the nuclear reactor accident in Chernobyl proved successful. Another major component of the treatment of ARS is partial or total parenteral nutrition, to bypass the damaged GI system. For blast and thermal injuries, standard therapy for trauma is given. Psychological support is essential in many cases.

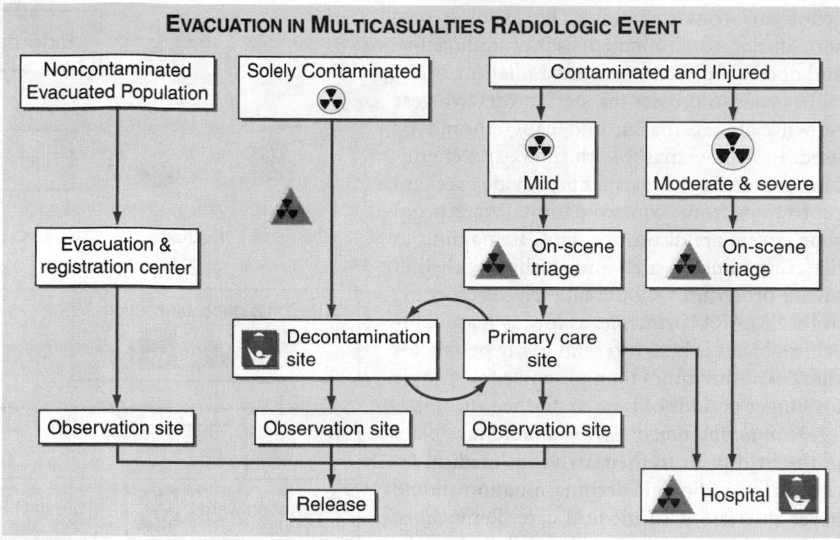

FIGURE 216-1 Algorithm for evacuation in a multicasualties radiologic event.

MEDICAL MANAGEMENT OF RADIATION BIOTERRORISM

Victims of radiation bioterrorism can suffer from conventional thermal or blast injuries, exposure to radiation, and contamination by radioactive materials. Many will have combinations of the above, which can be synergistic and cause higher morbidity and mortality than when they occur alone. The number of casualties will be a major factor in determining the response of the medical system to an act of radiation bioterrorism. If only a few persons are affected, then no significant changes and adaptation of the system are needed to treat the victims. However, if a terror attack results in a large number (dozens, or more) of casualties, then an organized disaster plan at the local and state levels must be invoked to deal with the crisis properly. Medical personnel should have a prior assignment and training and be prepared to function in a scenario with which they are familiar. Stockpiles of specific equipment and medications have to be preplanned (see the Centers for Disease Control and Prevention website—*http://www.bt.cdc.gov*). One of the terrorists' goals is to overwhelm medical facilities and to minimize the salvage of casualties.

Initial management consists of *primary triage and transportation* of the wounded to emergency rooms for treatment. The rationale behind the triage is to sort patients into classes according to the severity of injury, for the purpose of expediting clinical care and maximizing the use of the available clinical services and facilities. Triage requires determination of the level of emergency care needed. The higher the number and range of casualties, the more complex and difficult triage becomes. The mildly wounded and victims of contamination only can be sent to evacuation, registration with disaster response teams, and decontamination and treatment centers. Figure 216-1 illustrates evacuation in a multicasualties radiologic event. In this way, the hospitals themselves can avoid being directly overwhelmed, and those who are severely wounded can receive better treatment. Emergency treatment will be administered initially according to the presence of conventional injuries such as wounds, trauma, and thermal or chemical burns. Individuals with such injuries should be stabilized, if possible, and immediately transported to a medical facility. Removing the victim's clothes and wrapping him or her in clean blankets or nylon sheets reduces both the exposure of the patient and the contamination risk to the staff. However, the possibility of contamination needs to be determined. Less severely injured victims should receive a preliminary decontamination before or during evacuation to a hospital.

One must remember that radionuclide contamination of the skin is commonly not an acute life-threatening situation to the patient or the personnel who care for the patient. Only powerful gamma emitters are likely to cause real damage from contamination. It is important to emphasize that exposure to a radiation field alone does not necessarily create any contamination. The exposed person, if not contaminated, is not radioactive and does not directly emit any radiation.

In order to protect the staff, protective gear (gowns, gloves, masks, and caps) should be used. Protective masks with filters and chemically protective overgarments provide excellent protection from contamination. Waterproof shoe covers are also important. Remaining in the contaminated area and dealing with lifesaving procedures should take place according to the "ALARA" principle: as low as reasonably achievable. It is better to send many people for short exposure times than to send a few people for longer periods of time to do the same job.

Decontamination of victims should take place in the field prior to their arrival at medical facilities, but radiologic decontamination should never interfere with medical care. Removal of outer clothing and shoes will usually reduce the patient's contamination by 80–90%. Contaminated clothes should be carefully removed by rolling them over themselves, placing them in marked plastic bags, and removing them to a predefined area for contaminated clothes and equipment. A radiation detector should then be used to check for the presence of any residual radiologic contamination on the patient's body. In order to prevent internalization of the radioactive materials, one should cover open wounds prior to decontamination. Showering or washing of the entire skin and hair is very important. The skin is dried and reassessed for residual contamination until no radiation is found. Contamination-removing chemical agents are more than sufficient to remove radiologic contamination.

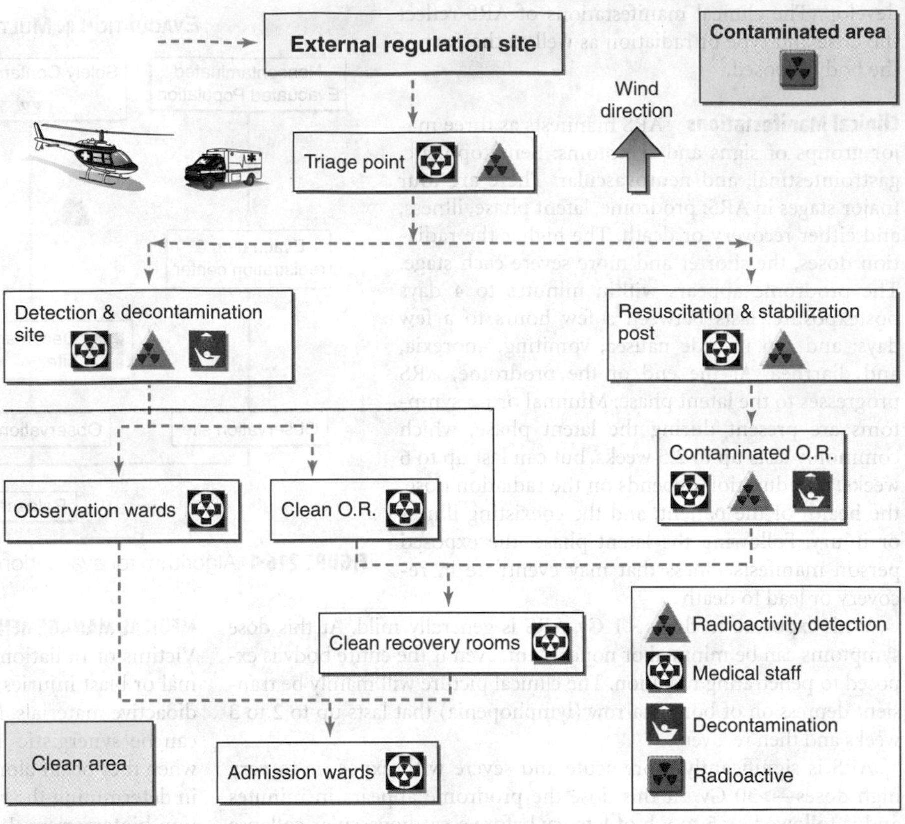

FIGURE 216-2 Flow chart of hospital triage. O.R., operating room.

Wound decontamination should be as conservative as possible. The main goal is to prevent both extensive local damage and internal contamination through lacerated skin. The bandages should be removed and the wounds flushed. The wound should then be dried and assessed for radiation. This procedure can be repeated again and again until contamination is undetectable. Excision of contaminated wounds should be attempted only when surgically necessary.

In the hospital, staff can wear normal hospital barrier clothing, including two pairs of gloves, a gown, shoe covers, a head cover, and a face mask. Eye protection is recommended. Decontamination of medical personnel is obligatory following emergency treatment and decontamination of the patient. All protective clothing should be placed after use in a designated container for contaminated clothing.

Radiation intensity decays rapidly with the square of the distance from the source, and increasing the distance from the source and decreasing the time spent near it are basic principles of radiation safety. Shielding with lead can be used as protection from small radioactive gamma sources. Geiger counters can detect gamma and beta radiation. Pocket chamber (pencil) dosimeters, film badges, and thermoluminescent dosimeters can measure accumulated exposure to gamma radiation. All of these detectors are in common use in medical facilities and should be used to help and define the level of contamination. Alpha radiation is harder to detect due to its poor penetration. An alpha scintillation counter, which is capable of detecting alpha radiation, is not commonly used in medical facilities.

GUIDELINES FOR HOSPITAL MANAGEMENT

Figure 216-2 illustrates a model for hospital arrangement for triage. Persons contaminated either externally or internally should be identified, externally decontaminated, and, if needed, treated immediately and specifically for internal contamination. In all other cases, the need for treatment of radiation injuries does not constitute a medical emergency. Early actions, such as blood sampling both for assessing the degree of severity of the exposure and for blood type and cross-matching for possible transfusion, need to be promptly taken if ARS is evident or if exposure is suspected.

In the hospital entrance, a distinct decontamination area should be set up promptly. Separation between clean and contaminated areas is essential. Medical personnel in this area should wear protective gear as noted above. They also should be rotated in their assignments every 1 to 2 h to ensure minimal exposure to radiation. If patients are critically wounded and require either surgery or resuscitation, they need to pass directly to "contaminated" operating rooms or resuscitation sites for life-saving procedures. Once such patients are stable, they should then be decontaminated. It is important to obtain details concerning the exposure, to look for prodromal signs of radiation sickness, and to do a physical examination. One of the best ways to estimate exposure clinically is to measure the time of prodromal appearance. The earlier the prodromal signs and symptoms appear, the higher the dose of radiation exposure. A few laboratory tests need to be routinely taken, such as complete blood count and urinalysis. If internal contamination is suspected, specific treatment should be given, as outlined below.

Rx RADIONUCLIDE CONTAMINATION

Treatment for internal radionuclide contamination should be started as soon as possible after suspected or known exposure. The goal is to leave the smallest amount of radionuclides as possible in the body. Treatment is given in order to reduce absorption and to enhance elimination and excretion.

Clearance of the GI tract may be achieved by stomach lavage; emetics (such as apomorphine, 5 to 10 mg, or ipecac, 1- to 2-g capsules or 15 mL in syrup); or by using purgatives, laxatives, ion exchangers, and aluminum antacids. Prussian blue, 1 g tid for a minimum of 3 weeks, is an ion exchanger used to treat cesium 137 internal contamination. Aluminum antacids (such as aluminum phosphate gel) may reduce strontium uptake in the gut if given immediately after exposure. Aluminum hydroxide is less effective.

Prevention or reversal of radionuclide interaction with tissues can be done by blocking, diluting, mobilizing, and chelating agents. *Blocking agents* prevent entrance of radioactive materials. A good example is potassium iodide (KI), which blocks the uptake of radioactive iodine (^{131}I) by the thyroid. KI is most effective if taken within the first hour after exposure and is still effective 6 h after exposure. The effectiveness subsequently declines until 24 h after exposure; however, it is recommended that KI be taken up to 48 h postexposure. The KI dose is based on age, predicted thyroid exposure, and pregnancy and lactation status. Adults between the ages of 18–40 should receive 130 mg/d for 7–14 days if exposed to ≥10 cGy of radioactive iodine. Other thyroid-blocking agents include prophylthiouracil, 100 mg tid for 8 days, or methimazole, 10 mg tid for 2 days followed by 5 mg tid for 6 days, but they are somewhat less effective.

Diluting agents decrease the absorption of the radionuclide; for example, water may be used as a diluting agent in the treatment for tritium (^{3}H) contamination. The recommended amount is 3–4 L/d for at least 3 weeks.

Mobilizing agents are most effective when given immediately; however, they may be effective for up to 2 weeks after exposure. These include antithyroid drugs, parathyroid extract, glucocorticoids, ammonium chloride, diuretics, expectorants, and inhalants. All of them should induce the release of radionuclides from tissues.

Chelating agents can bind many radioactive materials, after which the complexes are excreted from the human body. In this regard, diethylenetriaminepentaacetic acid (DTPA) either as Ca-DTPA or Zn-DTPA is superior to ethylenediamine tetraacetic acid (EDTA); it was approved by the U.S. Food and Drug Administration (FDA) to treat internal contamination with plutonium, americium and curium, but it also chelates berkelium, californium, or any material with an atomic number >92. Ca-DTPA is more effective than Zn-DTPA during the first 24 h after internal contamination, and both drugs are equally effective after the initial 24 h. If both drugs are available, then Ca-DTPA should be given as the first dose. If additional treatment is needed, treatment should be switched to Zn-DTPA. The dose is 1 g Ca-DTPA or Zn-DTPA, dissolved in 250 mL of normal saline or 5% glucose, given IV over 1 h daily. The duration of chelation treatment depends on the amount of internal contamination and individual response to treatment. DTPA can also be administrated by nebulized inhalation; 1 g is given in 1:1 dilution with water or saline over 15–20 min. Nebulized Zn-DTPA is recommended if the internal contamination is only by inhalation. The IV route is recommended and should be used if the route of internal contamination

TABLE 216-2 COMMON DRUGS[a] FOR TREATMENT OF INTERNAL CONTAMINATION

Medication	Administered for Radionuclides	Route of Administration	Dosage	Duration	Mechanism of Action
KI	Iodine-131	PO	130 mg/d for adults >40 with thyroid exposure >500 cGy 130 mg/d for adults 18–40 with thyroid exposure >10 cGy 130 mg/d for pregnant or lactating women with thyroid exposure >5 cGy 65 mg/d for children and adolescents 3–18 with thyroid exposure >5 cGy 32.5 mg/d for infants 1 month to 3 years with thyroid exposure >5 cGy 16 mg/d for neonates from birth to 1 month with thyroid exposure >5 cGy	7–14 days	Blocking agent
Zn-DTPA	Plutonium, transplutonium, yttrium, americium, curium	IV	1 g in 250 mL NS or 5% glucose, given in 1–2 h, *or* bolus over 3–4 min	Up to 5 days	Chelating agent
		Inhalation	1 g in 1:1 dilution with water or NS over 15–20 min		
		IM	1 g; not recommended because of pain		
Ca-DTPA	Plutonium, *trans*-plutonium, yttrium, americium, curium	IV	1 g in 250 mL NS or 5% glucose, given in 1–2 h, *or* bolus over 3–4 min	Up to 5 days	Chelating agent
		Inhalation	1 g in 1:1 dilution with water or NS over 15–20 min		
		IM	1 g; not recommended because of pain		
Bicarbonate	Uranium	IV	2 ampules sodium bicarbonate (44.3 meq each, 7.5%) in 1000 mL NS, 125 mL/L, *or* 1 ampule of sodium bicarbonate (44.3 meq, 7.5%) in 500 mL NS, 500 mL/h	Usually IV for the first 24 h, PO for additional 2 days; continuation of treatment for >3 days is rare and can be done according to titration of uranium amounts in the body	Increased excretion via the kidneys
		PO	2 tablets every 4 h until urine pH = 7–8, *or* 4 g (8 tablets) 3 tid		
Prussian blue	Cesium-137	PO	1 g tid with 100–200 mL water, up to 10 g/d	≥3 weeks titrated by urine and fecal bioassay and whole-body counting	Ion exchanger
Water	Tritium (H-3)	PO	>3–4 L per day	3 weeks	Excretion of water
Aluminum phosphate gel	Strontium	PO	100 mL immediately after exposure	Once	Decreased gut absorption
Aluminum hydroxide		PO	60–100 mL	Once	Decreased gut absorption

[a]Excluding KI, these drugs have not been approved for this purpose by the U.S. Food and Drug Administration at the time of publication.

Note: NS, normal saline.

is not known or if multiple routes of internal contamination are likely. Treating uranium contamination with DTPA is contraindicated, due to its synergistic damage to the kidneys.

Lung lavage can reduce radiation-induced pneumonitis and is indicated only when a large amount of radionuclide enters the lungs and has the potential for acute radiation injury. The procedure requires anesthesia. **Table 216-2** summarizes the common treatment regimens for internal radionuclide contamination.

MEDICAL ASSAY OF THE RADIATION-EXPOSED PATIENT

One of the major difficulties in treating victims exposed to radiation is the determination of the amount of exposure. Clinical assessment of the patient is the best approach. Appearance of an early prodrome indicates high exposure to radiation. Victims who arrive at the hospital complaining of severe weakness, nausea, vomiting, diarrhea, or seizures probably will not survive despite support measures. Decontamination and the use of radiation-detection equipment are both very important. Few tests can be performed in order to estimate the radiation exposure and the contamination. Baseline laboratory tests should include a complete blood count with differential and platelet count, renal evaluation, and determination of electrolytes. Urine and stool samples should be obtained if internal contamination is suspected. Nasal swabs should be taken from each nostril for determination of inhalation of radionuclides. After exhalation, each swab is labeled and sealed in a plastic bag and sent for analysis to appropriate laboratories. Patients exposed to 0.7–4 Gy will develop pancytopenia from as early as 10 days to as long 8 weeks postexposure. Lymphocytes show the most rapid decline, while other leukocytes and platelets decline less rapidly. Erythrocytes are the least vulnerable blood elements.

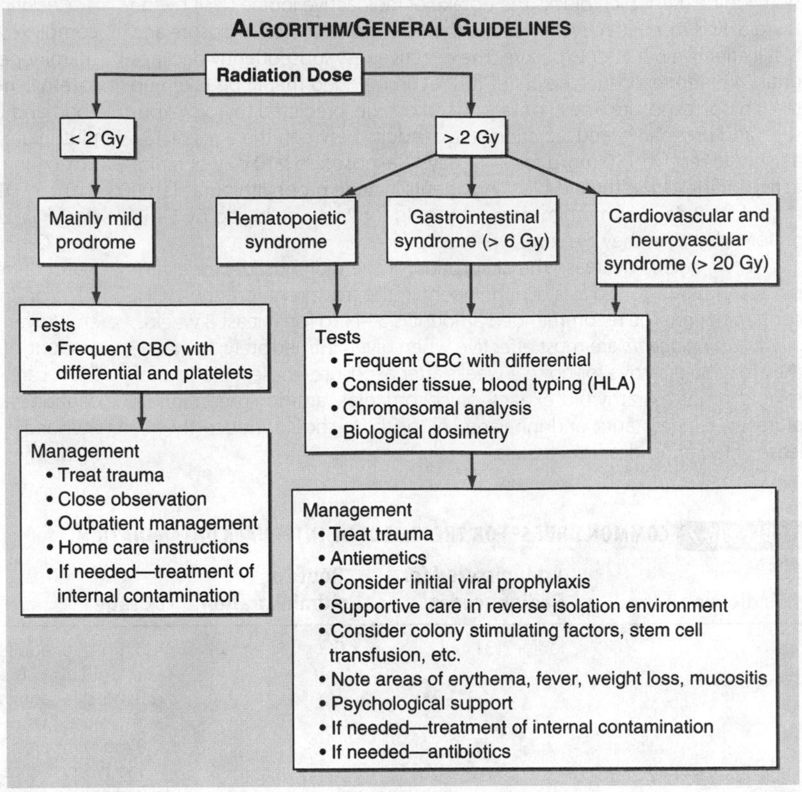

FIGURE 216-3 General guidelines for treatment of radiation casualties. CBC, complete blood count.

Absolute lymphocyte counts should be taken every 4–6 h for 5–6 days; they are the most valuable early indicator because they are recognized to be a sensitive marker for radiation damage and correlate with both the exposure and prognosis. A 50% drop in absolute lymphocyte count within the first 24 h indicates a signficant injury. HLA typing is necessary whenever there is suspicion of irreversible bone marrow damage. Lymphocyte chromosomal analysis can detect radiation exposure as low as 0.03–0.06 Gy, and 15 mL of blood should be drawn as early as possible in a heparinized collection tube and kept cool. Radiation-induced chromosomal aberrations in peripheral blood lymphocytes include dicentric chromosomes and ring forms that last for a few weeks. By calibrating a dose-response curve, the radiation dose can be assessed.

Another method for estimating exposure is the micronucleus (MN/Mni) scoring, which is simple and fast but still empirical. An algorithm for the treatment of radiation casualties is shown in Fig. 216-3.

FOLLOW-UP

It is desirable to continue follow-up in some circumstances. In general, only persons who are exposed to <8–10 Gy whole-body irradiation have a chance to survive long term, and they are at risk of developing cataracts; sterility; and lung, kidney, and bone marrow problems. Based on their age, gender, and amount and type of exposure, they should be followed for many years. A major public health issue is the risk of secondary malignancy in individuals and populations who were exposed to low doses of radiation. Leukemia, breast, brain, thyroid, and lung cancer are the most common, but the exposed population is at increased risk for many other cancers as well. Appropriate follow-up protocols should be developed based on the type of exposure and the exposed population. In cases of internal contamination, the long-term follow-up should be focused on the organ at risk. Such is the case with uranium contamination, with its nephrotoxic properties.

FURTHER READINGS

DAINIAK N: Hematologic consequences of exposure to ionizing radiation. Exp Hematol 30:513, 2002

GUIDANCE FOR RADIATION ACCIDENT MANAGEMENT, OAK RIDGE–ASSOCIATED UNIVERSITIES: *http://www.orau.gov/reacts/guidance.htm*, updated 03/22/2002

JARRETT D et al (eds): *Medical Management of Radiation Casualties: Handbook*. AFRRI special publication 99-2. Bethesda, MD, Armed Forces Radiobiology Research Institute, 1999 (also available at *http://www.afrri.usuhs.mil.*)

Management of Terrorist Events Involving Radioactive Material. NCRP report no. 138. Bethesda, MD, National Council on Radiation Protection, 2001

METTLER FA JR, VOELZ GL: Major radiation exposure—what to expect and how to respond. N Engl J Med 346:1554, 2002

MOULDER JE: Report on an interagency workshop on the radiobiology of nuclear terrorism. Molecular and Cellular Biology of Moderate Dose (1–10 Sv) Radiation and Potential Mechanisms of Radiation Protection (Bethesda, MD, December 17–18, 2001). Radiat Res 158: 118, 2002

Appendix: Laboratory Values of Clinical Importance

Alexander Kratz, Michael A. Pesce, Daniel J. Fink

INTRODUCTORY COMMENTS

The following are tables of reference values for laboratory tests, special analytes, and special function tests. A variety of factors can influence reference values. Such variables include the population studied, the duration and means of specimen transport, laboratory methods and instrumentation, and even the type of container used for the collection of the specimen. The reference or "normal" ranges given in this appendix may therefore not be appropriate for all laboratories, and these values should only be used as general guidelines. Whenever possible, reference values provided by the laboratory performing the testing should be utilized in the interpretation of laboratory data. Values supplied in this Appendix reflect typical reference ranges in adults. Pediatric reference ranges may vary significantly from adult values.

In preparing the Appendix, the authors have taken into account the fact that the system of international units (SI, système international d'unités) is used in most countries and in some medical journals. However, clinical laboratories may continue to report values in "conventional" units. Therefore, both systems are provided in the Appendix. The dual system is also used in the text except for (1) those instances in which the numbers remain the same but only the terminology is changed (mmol/L for meq/L or IU/L for mIU/mL), when only the SI units are given; and (2) most pressure measurements (e.g., blood and cerebrospinal fluid pressures), when the conventional units (mmHg, mmH_2O) are used. In all other instances in the text the SI unit is followed by the traditional unit in parentheses.

REFERENCE VALUES FOR LABORATORY TESTS

TABLE 1 HEMATOLOGY AND COAGULATION

Analyte	Specimen[a]	SI Units	Conventional Units
Activated clotting time	WB	70–180 s	70–180 seconds
Activated protein C resistance (Factor V Leiden)	P	Not applicable	Ratio > 2.1
$Alpha_2$ antiplasmin	P	0.87–1.55	87–155%
Antiphospholipid antibody panel			
PTT-LA (Lupus anticoagulant screen)	P	Negative	Negative
Platelet neutralization procedure	P	Negative	Negative
Dilute viper venom screen	P	Negative	Negative
Anticardiolipin antibody	S		
IgG		0–15 arbitrary units	0–15 GPL
IgM		0–15 arbitrary units	0–15 MPL
Antithrombin III	P		
Antigenic		220–390 mg/L	22–39 mg/dL
Functional		0.7–1.30 U/L	70–130%
Anti-Xa assay (heparin assay)	P		
Unfractionated heparin		0.3–0.7 kIU/L	0.3–0.7 IU/mL
Low-molecular-weight heparin		0.5–1.0 kIU/L	0.5–1.0 IU/mL
Danaparoid (Organ)		0.5–0.8 kIU/L	0.5–0.8 IU/mL
Autohemolysis test	WB	0.004–0.045	0.4%–4.50%
Autohemolysis test with glucose	WB	0.003–0.007	0.3%–0.7%
Bleeding time (adult)		<7.1 min	<7.1 min
Bone marrow: see Table 8			
Clot retraction	WB	0.50–1.00/2 h	50–100%/2 h
Cryofibrinogen	P	Negative	Negative
D-Dimer	P	0.22–0.74 μg/mL	0.22–0.74 μg/mL
Differential blood count	WB		
Neutrophils		0.40–0.70	40–70%
Bands		0.0–0.05	0–5%
Lymphocytes		0.20–0.50	20–50%
Monocytes		0.04–0.08	4–8%
Eosinophils		0.0–0.6	0–6%
Basophils		0.0–0.02	0–2%
Eosinophil count	WB	150–300/μL	$150–300/mm^3$
Erythrocyte count	WB		
Adult males		$4.30–5.60 \times 10^{12}/L$	$4.30–5.60 \times 10^6/mm^3$
Adult females		$4.00–5.20 \times 10^{12}/L$	$4.00–5.20 \times 10^6/mm^3$
Erythrocyte life span	WB		
Normal survival		120 days	120 days
Chromium labeled, half life ($t_{1/2}$)		25–35 days	25–35 days
Erythrocyte sedimentation rate	WB		
Females		0–20 mm/h	0–20 mm/h
Males		0–15 mm/h	0–15 mm/h
Euglobulin lysis time	P	7200–14400 s	120–240 min
Factor II, prothrombin	P	0.50–1.50	50–150%
Factor V	P	0.50–1.50	50–150%
Factor VII	P	0.50–1.50	50–150%
Factor VIII	P	0.50–1.50	50–150%
Factor IX	P	0.50–1.50	50–150%
Factor X	P	0.50–1.50	50–150%
Factor XI	P	0.50–1.50	50–150%
Factor XII	P	0.50–1.50	50–150%
Factor XIII screen	P	Not applicable	Present
Factor inhibitor assay	P	< 0.5 Bethesda Units	< 0.5 Bethesda Units

(continued)

TABLE 1 **HEMATOLOGY AND COAGULATION (CONTINUED)**

Analyte	Specimen[a]	SI Units	Conventional Units
Fibrin(ogen) degradation products	P	0–1 mg/L	0–1 μg/mL
Fibrinogen	P	2.33–4.96 g/L	233–496 mg/dL
Glucose-6-phosphate dehydrogenase (erythrocyte)	WB	< 2400 s	<40 min
Ham's test (acid serum)	WB	Negative	Negative
Hematocrit	WB		
Adult males		0.388–0.464	38.8–46.4
Adult females		0.354–0.444	35.4–44.4
Hemoglobin			
Plasma	P	6–50 mg/L	0.6–5.0 mg/dL
Whole blood	WB		
Adult males		133–162 g/L	13.3–16.2 g/dL
Adult females		120–158 g/L	12.0–15.8 g/dL
Hemoglobin electrophoresis	WB		
Hemoglobin A		0.95–0.98	95–98%
Hemoglobin A_2		0.015–0.031	1.5–3.1%
Hemoglobin F		0–0.02	0–2.0%
Hemoglobins other than A, A_2, or F		Absent	Absent
Heparin-induced thrombocytopenia antibody	P	Negative	Negative
Joint fluid crystal	JF	Not applicable	No crystals seen
Joint fluid mucin	JF	Not applicable	Only type I mucin present
Leukocytes			
Alkaline phosphatase (LAP)	WB	0.2–1.6 μkat/L	13–100 μ/L
Count (WBC)	WB	$3.54–9.06 \times 10^9$/L	$3.54–9.06 \times 10^3$/mm^3
Mean corpuscular hemoglobin (MCH)	WB	26.7–31.9 pg/cell	26.7–31.9 pg/cell
Mean corpuscular hemoglobin concentration (MCHC)	WB	323–359 g/L	32.3–35.9 g/dL
Mean corpuscular hemoglobin of reticulocytes (CH)	WB	24–36 pg	24–36 pg
Mean corpuscular volume (MCV)	WB	79–93.3 fL	79–93.3 μm^3
Mean platelet volume (MPV)	WB	9.00–12.95 fL	9.00–12.95 μm^3
Osmotic fragility of erythrocytes	WB		
Direct		0.0035–0.0045	0.35–0.45%
Index		0.0030–0.0065	0.30–0.65%
Partial thromboplastin time, activated	P	26.3–39.4 s	26.3–39.4 s
Plasminogen	P		
Antigen		84–140 mg/L	8.4–14.0 mg/dL
Functional		0.70–1.30	70–130%
Plasminogen activator inhibitor 1	P	4–43 μg/L	4–43 ng/mL
Platelet aggregation	PRP	Not applicable	> 65% aggregation in response to adenosine diphosphate, epinephrine, collagen, ristocetin, and arachidonic acid
Platelet count	WB	$165–415 \times 10^9$/L	$165–415 \times 10^3$/mm^3
Platelet, mean volume	WB	6.4–11 fL	6.4–11.0 μm^3
Prekallikrein assay	P	0.50–1.5	50–150%
Prekallikrein screen	P		No deficiency detected
Protein C	P		
Total antigen		0.70–1.40	70–140%
Functional		0.70–1.30	70–130%
Protein S	P		
Total antigen		0.70–1.40	70–140%
Functional		0.65–1.40	65–140%
Free antigen		0.70–1.40	70–140%
Prothrombin gene mutation G20210A	WB	Not applicable	Not present
Prothrombin time	P	12.7–15.4 s	12.7–15.4 s
Protoporphyrin, free erythrocyte	WB	0.28–0.64 μmol/L of red blood cells	16–36 μg/dL of red blood cells
Red cell distribution width	WB	< 0.145	< 14.5%
Reptilase time	P	16–23.6 s	16–23.6 s
Reticulocyte count	WB		
Adult males		0.008–0.023 red cells	0.8–2.3% red cells
Adult females		0.008–0.020 red cells	0.8–2.0% red cells
Reticulocyte hemoglobin content	WB	>26 pg/cell	>26 pg/cell
Ristocetin cofactor (functional von Willebrand factor)	P		
Blood group O		0.75 mean of normal	75% mean of normal
Blood group A		1.05 mean of normal	105% mean of normal
Blood group B		1.15 mean of normal	115% mean of normal
Blood group AB		1.25 mean of normal	125% mean of normal
Sickle cell test	WB	Negative	Negative
Sucrose hemolysis	WB	<0.1	<10% hemolysis
Thrombin time	P	15.3–18.5 s	15.3–18.5 s
Total eosinophils	WB	$150–300 \times 10^6$/L	150–300/mm^3
Transferrin receptor	S, P	9.6–29.6 nmol/L	9.6–29.6 nmol/L
Viscosity			
Plasma	P	1.7–2.1	1.7–2.1
Serum	S	1.4–1.8	1.4–1.8

(continued)

TABLE 1 HEMATOLOGY AND COAGULATION (CONTINUED)

Analyte	Specimen[a]	SI Units	Conventional Units
Von Willebrand factor (vWF) antigen (factor VIII:R antigen)	P		
Blood group O		0.75 mean of normal	75% mean of normal
Blood group A		1.05 mean of normal	105% mean of normal
Blood group B		1.15 mean of normal	115% mean of normal
Blood group AB		1.25 mean of normal	125% mean of normal
Von Willebrand factor multimers	P	Normal distribution	Normal distribution
White blood cells: see "leukocytes"			

[a]P, plasma; JF, joint fluid; PRP, platelet-rich plasma; S, serum; WB, whole blood.

TABLE 2 CLINICAL CHEMISTRY AND IMMUNOLOGY

Analyte	Specimen[a]	SI Units	Conventional Units
Acetoacetate	P	20–99 μmol/L	0.2–1.0 mg/dL
Adrenocorticotropin (ACTH)	P	1.3–16.7 pmol/L	6.0–76.0 pg/mL
Alanine aminotransferase (AST, SGPT)	S	0.12–0.70 μkat/L	7–41 U/L
Albumin	S		
Female		41–53 g/L	4.1–5.3 g/dL
Male		40–50 g/L	4.0–5.0 g/L
Aldolase	S	26–138 nkat/L	1.5–8.1 U/L
Aldosterone (adult)			
Supine, normal sodium diet	S, P	55–250 pmol/L	2–9 ng/dL
Upright, normal sodium diet	S, P		2–5-fold increase over supine value
Supine, low-sodium diet	S, P		2–5-fold increase over normal sodium diet level
	U	6.38–58.25 nmol/d	2.3–21.0 μg/24 h
Alpha fetoprotein (adult)	S	0–8.5 μg/L	0–8.5 ng/mL
Alpha$_1$ antitrypsin	S	1.0–2.0 g/L	100–200 mg/dL
Ammonia, as NH_3	P	11–35 μmol/L	19–60 μg/dL
Amylase (method dependent)	S	0.34–1.6 μkat/L	20–96 U/L
Androstenedione (adult)	S	1.75–8.73 nmol/L	50–250 ng/dL
Angiotensin-converting enzyme (ACE)	S	0.15–1.1 μkat/L	9–67 U/L
Anion gap	S	7–16 mmol/L	7–16 mmol/L
Apo B/Apo A-1 ratio		0.35–0.98	0.35–0.98
Apolipoprotein A-1	S	1.19–2.40 g/L	119–240 mg/dL
Apolipoprotein B	S	0.52–1.63 g/L	52–163 mg/dL
Arterial blood gases			
$[HCO_3^-]$		22–30 mmol/L	22–30 meq/L
P_{CO_2}		4.3–6.0 kPa	32–45 mmHg
pH		7.35–7.45	7.35–7.45
P_{O_2}		9.6–13.8 kPa	72–104 mmHg
Aspartate aminotransferase (AST, SGOT)	S	0.20–0.65 μkat/L	12–38 U/L
Autoantibodies			
Anti-adrenal antibody	S	Not applicable	Negative at 1:10 dilution
Anti-double-strand (native) DNA	S	Not applicable	Negative at 1:10 dilution
Anti–glomerular basement membrane antibodies	S		
Qualitative		Negative	Negative
Quantitative		<5 kU/L	<5 U/mL
Anti-granulocyte antibody	S	Not applicable	Negative
Anti-Jo-1 antibody	S	Not applicable	Negative
Anti-La antibody	S	Not applicable	Negative
Anti-mitochondrial antibody	S	Not applicable	Negative
Antineutrophil cytoplasmic autoantibodies, cytoplasmic (C-ANCA)	S		
Qualitative		Negative	Negative
Quantitative (antibodies to proteinase 3)		< 2.8 kU/L	< 2.8 U/mL
Antineutrophil cytoplasmic autoantibodies, perinuclear (P-ANCA)	S		
Qualitative		Negative	Negative
Quantitative (antibodies to myeloperoxidase)		< 1.4 kU/L	< 1.4 U/mL
Antinuclear antibody	S	Not applicable	Negative at 1:40
Anti–parietal cell antibody	S	Not applicable	Negative at 1:20
Anti-Ro antibody	S	Not applicable	Negative
Anti-platelet antibody	S	Not applicable	Negative
Anti-RNP antibody	S	Not applicable	Negative
Anti-Scl 70 antibody	S	Not applicable	Negative
Anti-Smith antibody	S	Not applicable	Negative
Anti-smooth-muscle antibody	S	Not applicable	Negative at 1:20
Anti-thyroglobulin	S	Not applicable	Negative
Anti-thyroid antibody	S	< 0.3 kIU/L	<0.3 IU/mL

(continued)

TABLE 2 **CLINICAL CHEMISTRY AND IMMUNOLOGY (CONTINUED)**

Analyte	Specimen[a]	SI Units	Conventional Units
B type natriuretic peptide (BNP)	P	Age and gender specific: < 167 ng/L	Age and gender specific: < 167 pg/mL
Bence Jones protein, serum	S	Not applicable	None detected
Bence Jones protein, urine, qualitative	U	Not applicable	None detected in 50× concentrated urine
Bence Jones Protein, urine, quantitative	U		
Kappa		<25 mg/L	<2.5 mg/dL
Lambda		<50 mg/L	<5.0 mg/dL
β_2-Microglobulin			
	S	<2.7 mg/L	<0.27 mg/dL
	U	<120 μg/d	<120 μg/day
Bilirubin	S		
Total		5.1–22 μmol/L	0.3–1.3 mg/dL
Direct		1.7–6.8 μmol/L	0.1–0.4 mg/dL
Indirect		3.4–15.2 μmol/L	0.2–0.9 mg/dL
C peptide (adult)	S, P	0.17–0.66 nmol/L	0.5–2.0 ng/mL
C1-esterase-inhibitor protein	S		
Antigenic		124–250 mg/L	12.4–24.5 mg/dL
Functional		Present	Present
CA 125	S	0–35 kU/L	0–35 U/mL
CA 19-9	S	0–37 kU/L	0–37 U/mL
CA-15-3	S	0–34 kU/L	0–34 U/mL
CA27-29	S	0–40 kU/L	0–40 U/mL
Calcitonin	S		
Male		3–26 ng/L	3–26 pg/mL
Female		2–17 ng/L	2–17 pg/mL
Calcium	S	2.2–2.6 mmol/L	8.7–10.2 mg/dL
Calcium, ionized	WB	1.12–1.32 mmol/L	4.5–5.3 mg/dL
Carbon dioxide content (TCO_2)	P (sea level)	22–30 mmol/L	22–30 meq/L
Carboxyhemoglobin (carbon monoxide content)	WB		
Nonsmokers		0–0.04	0–4%
Smokers		0.04–0.09	4–9%
Onset of symptoms		0.15–0.20	15–20%
Loss of consciousness and death		>0.50	>50%
Carcinoembryonic antigen (CEA)	S		
Nonsmokers		0.0–3.0 μg/L	0.0–3.0 ng/mL
Smokers	S	0.0–5.0 μg/L	0.0–5.0 ng/mL
Ceruloplasmin	S	250–630 mg/L	25–63 mg/dL
Chloride	S	102–109 mmol/L	102–109 meq/L
Cholesterol: see Table 5			
Cholinesterase	S	5–12 kU/L	5–12 U/mL
Complement			
C3	S	0.83–1.77 g/L	83–177 mg/dL
C4	S	0.16–0.47 g/L	16–47 mg/dL
Total hemolytic complement (CH50)	S	50–150%	50–150%
Factor B	S	0.17–0.42 g/L	17–42 mg/dL
Coproporphyrins (types I and III)	U	150–470 μmol/d	100–300 μg/d
Cortisol			
Fasting, 8 A.M.–12 noon	S	138–690 nmol/L	5–25 μg/dL
12 noon–8 P.M.		138–414 nmol/L	5–15 μg/dL
8 P.M.–8 A.M.		0–276 nmol/L	0–10 μg/dL
Cortisol, free	U	55–193 nmol/24 h	20–70 μg/24 h
C-reactive protein	S	0.2–3.0 mg/L	0.2–3.0 mg/L
Creatine kinase (total)	S		
Females		0.66–4.0 μkat/L	39–238 U/L
Males		0.87–5.0 μkat/L	51–294 U/L
Creatine kinase-MB	S		
Mass		0.0–5.5 μg/L	0.0–5.5 ng/mL
Fraction of total activity (by electrophoresis)		0–0.04	0–4.0%
Creatinine	S		
Female		44–80 μmol/L	0.5–0.9 ng/mL
Male		53–106 μmol/L	0.6–1.2 ng/mL
Cryoproteins	S	Not applicable	None detected
Dehydroepiandrosterone (DHEA) (adult)			
Male	S	6.2–43.4 nmol/L	180–1250 ng/dL
Female		4.5–34.0 nmol/L	130–980 ng/dL
Dehydroepiandrosterone (DHEA) sulfate	S		
Male (adult)		100–6190 μg/L	10–619 μg/dL
Female (adult, premenopausal)		120–5350 μg/L	12–535 μg/dL
Female (adult, postmenopausal)		300–2600 μg/L	30–260 μg/dL
Deoxycorticosterone (DOC) (adult)	S	61–576 nmol/L	2–19 ng/dL
11-Deoxycortisol (adult) (compound S) (8:00 A.M.)	S	0.34–4.56 nmol/L	12–158 ng/dL
Dihydrotestosterone			
Male	S, P	1.03–2.92 nmol/L	30–85 ng/dL
Female		0.14–0.76 nmol/L	4–22 ng/dL

(continued)

TABLE 2 **CLINICAL CHEMISTRY AND IMMUNOLOGY (CONTINUED)**

Analyte	Specimen[a]	SI Units	Conventional Units
Dopamine	P	< 475 pmol/L	< 87 pg/mL
Dopamine	U	425–2610 nmol/d	65–400 μg/d
Epinephrine	P		
Supine (30 min)		< 273 pmol/L	< 50 pg/mL
Sitting		< 328 pmol/L	< 60 pg/mL
Standing (30 min)		< 491pmol/L	< 90 pg/mL
Epinephrine	U	0–109 nmol/d	0–20 μg/d
Erythropoietin	S	4–27 U/L	4–27 U/L
Estradiol	S, P		
Female			
Menstruating:			
Follicular phase		74–532 pmol/L	<20–145 pg/mL
Mid-cycle peak		411–1626 pmol/L	112–443 pg/mL
Luteal phase		74–885 pmol/L	<20–241 pg/mL
Postmenopausal		217 pmol/L	<59 pg/mL
Male		74 pmol/L	< 20 pg/mL
Estrone	S, P		
Female			
Menstruating:			
Follicular phase		55–555 pmol/L	15–150 pg/mL
Luteal phase		55–740 pmol/L	15–200 pg/mL
Postmenopausal		55–204 pmol/L	15–55 pg/mL
Male		55–240 pmol/L	15–65 pg/mL
Fatty acids, free (nonesterified)	P	<0.28–0.89 mmol/L	<8–25 mg/dL
Ferritin	S		
Female		10–150 μg/L	10–150 ng/mL
Male		29–248 μg/L	29–248 ng/mL
Follicle stimulating hormone (FSH)	S, P		
Female			
Menstruating:			
Follicular phase		3.0–20.0 IU/L	3.0–20.0 mIU/mL
Ovulatory phase		9.0–26.0 IU/L	9.0–26.0 mIU/mL
Luteal phase		1.0–12.0 IU/L	1.0–12.0 mIU/mL
Postmenopausal		18.0–153.0 IU/L	18.0–153.0 mIU/mL
Male		1.0–12.0 IU/L	1.0–12.0 mIU/mL
Free testosterone, adult			
Female	S	2.1–23.6 pmol/L	0.6–6.8 pg/mL
Male		163–847 pmol/L	47–244 pg/mL
Fructosamine	S	<285 μmol/L	<285 μmol/L
Gamma glutamyltransferase	S	0.15–0.99 μkat/L	9–58 U/L
Gastrin	S	<100 ng/L	<100 pg/mL
Glucagon	P	20–100 ng/L	20–100 pg/mL
Glucose (fasting)	P		
Normal		4.2–6.1 mmol/L	75–110 mg/dL
Impaired glucose tolerance		6.2–6.9 mmol/L	111–125 mg/dL
Diabetes mellitus		>7.0 mmol/L	>125 mg/dL
Glucose, 2 h postprandial	P	3.9–6.7 mmol/L	70–120 mg/dL
Growth hormone (resting)	S	0.5–17.0 μg/L	0.5–17.0 ng/mL
Hemoglobin A_{Ic}	WB	0.04–0.06 Hb fraction	4.0–6.0%
High-density lipoprotein (HDL) (see Table 5)			
Homocysteine	P	4.4–10.8 μmol/L	4.4–10.8 μmol/L
Human chorionic gonadotropin (hCG)	S		
Non-pregnant female		< 5 IU/L	< 5 mIU/mL
1–2 weeks postconception		9–130 IU/L	9–130 mIU/mL
2–3 weeks postconception		75–2600 IU/L	75–2600 mIU/mL
3–4 weeks postconception		850–20,800 IU/L	850–20,800 mIU/mL
4–5 weeks postconception		4000–100,200 IU/L	4000–100,200 mIU/mL
5–10 weeks postconception		11,500–289,000 IU/L	11,500–289,000 mIU/mL
10–14 weeks postconception		18,300–137,000 IU/L	18,300–137,000 mIU/mL
Second trimester		1400–53,000 IU/L	1400–53,000 mIU/mL
Third trimester		940–60,000 IU/L	940–60,000 mIU/mL
β-Hydroxybutyrate	P	0–290 μmol/L	0–3 mg/dL
5-Hydroindoleacetic acid [5-HIAA]	U	10.5–36.6 μmol/d	2–7 mg/d
17-Hydroxyprogesterone (adult)	S		
Male		0.15–7.5 nmol/L	5–250 ng/dL
Female			
Follicular phase		0.6–3.0 nmol/L	20–100 ng/dL
Midcycle peak		3–7.5 nmol/L	100–250 ng/dL
Luteal phase		3–15 nmol/L	100–500 ng/dL
Postmenopausal		≤ 2.1 nmol/L	≤ 70 ng/dL
Hydroxyproline	U, 24 hour	38–500 μmol/d	38–500 μmol/d
Immunofixation	S	Not applicable	No bands detected

(continued)

TABLE 2 CLINICAL CHEMISTRY AND IMMUNOLOGY (CONTINUED)

Analyte	Specimen[a]	SI Units	Conventional Units
Immunoglobulin, quantitation (adult)			
IgA	S	0.70–3.50 g/L	70–350 mg/dL
IgD	S	0–140 mg/L	0–14 mg/dL
IgE	S	24–430 μg/L	10–179 IU/mL
IgG	S	7.0–17.0 g/L	700–1700 mg/dL
IgG_1	S	2.7–17.4 g/L	270–1740 mg/dL
IgG_2	S	0.3–6.3 g/L	30–630 mg/dL
IgG_3	S	0.13–3.2 g/L	13–320 mg/dL
IgG_4	S	0.11–6.2 g/L	11–620 mg/dL
IgM	S	0.50–3.0 g/L	50–300 mg/dL
Insulin	S, P	14.35–143.5 pmol/L	2–20 μU/mL
Iron	S	7–25 μmol/L	41–141 μg/dL
Iron-binding capacity	S	45–73 μmol/L	251–406 μg/dL
Iron-binding capacity saturation	S	0.16–0.35	16–35%
Joint fluid crystal	JF	Not applicable	No crystals seen
Joint fluid mucin	JF	Not applicable	Only type I mucin present
Ketone (acetone)	S, U	Negative	Negative
17 Ketosteroids	U	0.003–0.012 g/d	3–12 mg/d
Lactate	P, arterial	0.5–1.6 mmol/L	4.5–14.4 mg/dL
	P, venous	0.5–2.2 mmol/L	4.5–19.8 mg/dL
Lactate dehydrogenase	S	2.0–3.8 μkat/L	115–221 U/L
Lactate dehydrogenase isoenzymes	S		
Fraction 1 (of total)		0.14–0.26	14–26%
Fraction 2		0.29–0.39	29–39%
Fraction 3		0.20–0.25	20–26%
Fraction 4		0.08–0.16	8–16%
Fraction 5		0.06–0.16	6–16%
Lipase (method dependent)	S	0.51–0.73 μkat/L	3–43 U/L
Lipids: see Table 5			
Lipoprotein (a)	S	0–300 mg/L	0–30 mg/dL
Low-density lipoprotein (LDL) (see Table 5)			
Luteinizing hormone (LH)	S, P		
Female			
Menstruating			
Follicular phase		2.0–15.0 U/L	2.0–15.0 U/L
Ovulatory phase		22.0–105.0 U/L	22.0–105.0 U/L
Luteal phase		0.6–19.0 U/L	0.6–19.0 U/L
Postmenopausal		16.0–64.0 U/L	16.0–64.0 U/L
Male		2.0–12.0 U/L	2.0–12.0 U/L
Magnesium	S	0.62–0.95 mmol/L	1.5–2.3 mg/dL
Metanephrine	P	<0.5 nmol/L	<100 pg/mL
Metanephrine	U	30–211 mmol/mol creatinine	53–367 μg/g creatinine
Methemoglobin	WB	0.0–0.01	0–1%
Microalbumin urine	U		
24-h urine		0.0–0.03 g/d	0–30 mg/24 h
Spot urine		0.0–0.03 g/g creatinine	0–30 μg/mg creatinine
Myoglobin	S		
Male		19–92 μg/L	19–92 μg/L
Female		12–76 μg/L	12–76 μg/L
Norepinephrine	U	89–473 nmol/d	15–80 μg/d
Norepinephrine	P		
Supine (30 min)		650–2423 pmol/L	110–410 pg/mL
Sitting		709–4019 pmol/L	120–680 pg/mL
Standing (30 min)		739–4137 pmol/L	125–700 pg/mL
N-telopeptide (cross linked), NTx	S		
Female, premenopausal		6.2–19.0 nmol BCE	6.2–19.0 nmol BCE
Male		5.4–24.2 nmol BCE	5.4–24.2 nmol BCE
Bone collagen equivalent (BCE)			
N-telopeptide (cross linked), NTx	U		
Female, premenopausal		17–94 nmol BCE/mmol creatinine	17–94 nmol BCE/mmol creatinine
Female, postmenopausal		26–124 nmol BCE/mmol creatinine	26–124 nmol BCE/mmol creatinine
Male		21–83 nmol BCE/mmol creatinine	21–83 nmol BCE/mmol creatinine
Bone collagen equivalent (BCE)			
5′ Nucleotidase	S	0.02–0.19 μkat/L	0–11 U/L
Osmolality	P	275–295 mOsmol/kg serum water	275–295 mOsmol/kg serum water
	U	500–800 mOsmol/kg water	500–800 mOsmol/kg water
Osteocalcin	S	11–50 μg/L	11–50 ng/mL
Oxygen content	WB		
Arterial (sea level)		17–21	17–21 vol%
Venous (sea level)		10–16	10–16 vol%
Oxygen percent saturation (sea level)	WB		
Arterial		0.97	94–100%
Venous, arm		0.60–0.85	60–85%

(continued)

TABLE 2 CLINICAL CHEMISTRY AND IMMUNOLOGY (CONTINUED)

Analyte	Specimen[a]	SI Units	Conventional Units
Parathyroid hormone (intact)	S	8–51 ng/L	8–51 pg/mL
Phosphatase, alkaline	S	0.56–1.63 μkat/L	33–96 U/L
Phosphorus, inorganic	S	0.81–1.4 mmol/L	2.5–4.3 mg/dL
Porphobilinogen	U	None	None
Potassium	S	3.5–5.0 mmol/L	3.5–5.0 meq/L
Prealbumin	S	170–340 mg/L	17–34 mg/dL
Progesterone	S, P		
Female			
Follicular		<3.18 nmol/L	<1.0 ng/mL
Midluteal		9.54–63.6 nmol/L	3–20 ng/mL
Male		<3.18 nmol/L	< 1.0 ng/mL
Prolactin	S	0–20 μg/L	0–20 ng/mL
Prostate-specific antigen (PSA)	S		
Male			
<40 years		0.0–2.0 μg/L	0.0–2.0 ng/mL
>40 years		0.0–4.0 μg/L	0.0–4.0 ng/mL
PSA, free; in males 45–75 years, with PSA values between 4 and 20 μg/mL	S	>0.25 associated with benign prostatic hyperplasia	>25% associated with benign prostatic hyperplasia
Protein fractions	S		
Albumin		35–55 g/L	3.5–5.5 g/dL (50–60%)
Globulin		20–35 g/L	2.0–3.5 g/dL (40–50%)
$Alpha_1$		2–4 g/L	0.2–0.4 g/dL (4.2–7.2%)
$Alpha_2$		5–9 g/L	0.5–0.9 g/dL (6.8–12%)
Beta		6–11 g/L	0.6–1.1 g/dL (9.3–15%)
Gamma		7–17 g/L	0.7–1.7 g/dL (13–23%)
Protein, total	S	67–86 g/L	6.7–8.6 g/dL
Pyruvate	P, arterial	40–130 μmol/L	0.35–1.14 mg/dL
	P, venous	40–130 μmol/L	0.35–1.14 mg/dL
Rheumatoid factor	S, JF	<30 kIU/L	<30 IU/mL
Serotonin	WB	0.28–1.14 μmol/L	50–200 ng/mL
Serum protein electrophoresis	S	Not applicable	Normal pattern
Sex hormone binding globulin (adult)	S		
Male		13–71 nmol/L	13–71 nmol/L
Female		18–114 nmol/L	18–114 nmol/L
Sodium	S	136–146 mmol/L	136–146 meq/L
Somatomedin-C (IGF-1) (adult)	S		
16–24 years		182–780 μg/L	182–780 ng/mL
25–39 years		114–492 μg/L	114–492 ng/mL
40–54 years		90–360 μg/L	90–360 ng/mL
>54 years		71–290 μg/L	71–290 ng/mL
Somatostatin	P	<25 ng/L	<25 pg/mL
Testosterone, total, morning sample	S		
Female		0.21–2.98 nmol/L	6–86 ng/dL
Male		9.36–37.10 nmol/L	270–1070 ng/dL
Thyroglobulin	S	0.5–53 μg/L	0.5–53 ng/mL
Thyroid-binding globulin	S	13–30 mg/L	1.3–3.0 mg/dL
Thyroid-stimulating hormone	S	0.34–4.25 mIU/L	0.34–4.25 μIU/mL
Thyroxine, free (fT_4)	S	10.3–21.9 pmol/L	0.8–1.7 ng/dL
Thyroxine, total (T_4)	S	70–151 nmol/L	5.4–11.7 μg/dL
(Free) thyroxine index	S	6.7–10.9	6.7–10.9
Transferrin	S	2.0–4.0 g/L	200–400 mg/dL
Triglycerides (see Table 5)	S	0.34–2.26 mmol/L	30–200 mg/dL
Triiodothyronine, free (fT_3)	S	3.7–6.5 pmol/L	2.4–4.2 pg/mL
Triiodothyronine, total (T_3)	S	1.2–2.1 nmol/L	77–135 ng/dL
Troponin I	S		
Normal population, 99 %tile		0–0.08 μg/L	0–0.08 ng/mL
Cut-off for MI		>0.4 μg/L	>0.4 ng/mL
Troponin T	S		
Normal population, 99 %tile		0–0.1 μg/L	0–0.01 ng/mL
Cut-off for MI		0–0.1 μg/L	0–0.1 ng/mL
Urea nitrogen	S	2.5–7.1 mmol/L	7–20 mg/dL
Uric acid	S		
Females		0.15–0.33 μmol/L	2.5–5.6 mg/dL
Males		0.18–0.41 μmol/L	3.1–7.0 mg/dL
Urobilinogen	U	0.09–4.2 μmol/d	0.05–25 mg/24 h
Vanillylmandelic acid (VMA)	U, 24h	<30 μmol/d	<6 mg/d
Vasoactive intestinal polypeptide	P	0–60 ng/L	0–60 pg/mL

[a]P, plasma; S, serum; U, urine; WB, whole blood; JF, joint fluid.

TABLE 3 **TOXICOLOGY AND THERAPEUTIC DRUG MONITORING**

	Therapeutic Range		Toxic Level	
Drug	**SI Units**	**Conventional Units**	**SI Units**	**Conventional Units**
Acetaminophen	66–199 μmol/L	10–30 μg/mL	>1320 μmol/L	>200 μg/mL
Amikacin				
Peak	34–51 μmol/L	20–30 μg/mL	>60 μmol/L	>35 μg/mL
Trough	0–17 μmol/L	0–10 μg/mL	>17 μmol/L	>10 μg/mL
Amitriptyline/nortriptyline (total drug)	430–900 nmol/L	120–250 ng/mL	>1800 nmol/L	>500 ng/mL
Amphetamine	150–220 nmol/L	20–30 ng/mL	>1500 nmol/L	>200 ng/mL
Bromide				
Sedation	1.3–6.3 mmol/L	10–50 mg/dL		
Epilepsy	9.4–18.8 mmol/L	75–150 mg/dL		
Mild toxicity			6.4–18.8 mmol/L	51–150 mg/dL
Severe toxicity			>18.8 mmol/L	>150 mg/dL
Lethal			>37.5 mmol/L	>300 mg/dL
Carbamazepine	17–42 μmol/L	4–10 μg/mL	85 μmol/L	>20 μg/mL
Chloramphenicol				
Peak	31–62 μmol/L	10–20 μg/mL	>77 μmol/L	>25 μg/mL
Trough	15–31 μmol/L	5–10 μg/mL	>46 μmol/L	>15 μg/mL
Chlordiazepoxide	1.7–10 μmol/L	0.5–3.0 μg/mL	>17 μmol/L	>5.0 μg/mL
Clonazepam	32–240 nmol/L	10–75 ng/mL	>320 nmol/L	>100 ng/mL
Clozapine	0.6–2.1 μmol/L	200–700 ng/mL	>3.7 μmol/L	>1200 ng/mL
Cocaine			>3.3 μmol/L	>1.0 μg/mL
Codeine	43–110 nmol/mL	13–33 ng/mL	>3700 nmol/mL	>1100 ng/mL, lethal
Cyclosporine				
Renal transplant				
0–6 months	208–312 nmol/L	250–375 ng/mL	>312 nmol/L	>375 ng/mL
6–12 months after transplant	166–250 nmol/L	200–300 ng/mL	>250 nmol/L	>300 ng/mL
>12 months	83–125 nmol/L	100–150 ng/mL	>125 nmol/L	>150 ng/mL
Cardiac transplant				
0–6 months	208–291 nmol/L	250–350 ng/mL	>291 nmol/L	>350 ng/mL
6–12 months after transplant	125–208 nmol/L	150–250 ng/mL	>208 nmol/L	>250 ng/mL
>12 months	83–125 nmol/L	100–150 ng/mL	>125 nmol/L	>150 ng/mL
Lung transplant				
0–6 months	250–374 nmol/L	300–450 ng/mL	>374 nmol/L	>450 ng/mL
Liver transplant				
0–7 days	249–333 nmol/L	300–400 ng/mL	>333 nmol/L	>400 ng/mL
2–4 weeks	208–291 nmol/L	250–350 ng/mL	>291 nmol/L	>350 ng/mL
5–8 weeks	166–249 nmol/L	200–300 ng/mL	>249 nmol/L	>300 ng/mL
9–52 weeks	125–208 nmol/L	150–250 ng/mL	>208 nmol/L	>250 ng/mL
>1 year	83–166 nmol/L	100–200 ng/mL	>166 nmol/L	>200 ng/mL
Desipramine	375–1130 nmol/L	100–300 ng/mL	>1880 nmol/L	>500 ng/mL
Diazepam (and metabolite)				
Diazepam	0.7–3.5 μmol/L	0.2–1.0 μg/mL	>7.0 μmol/L	>2.0 μg/mL
Nordiazepam	0.4–6.6 μmol/L	0.1–1.8 μg/mL	>9.2 μmol/L	>2.5 μg/mL
Digoxin	0.64–2.6 nmol/L	0.5–2.0 ng/mL	>3.1 nmol/L	>2.4 ng/mL
Disopyramide	>7.4 μmol/L	2.5 μg/mL	20.6 μmol/L	>7 μg/mL
Doxepin and nordoxepin				
Doxepin	0.36–0.98 μmol/L	101–274 ng/mL	>1.8 μmol/L	>503 ng/mL
Nordoxepin	0.38–1.04 μmol/L	106–291 ng/mL	>1.9 μmol/L	>531 ng/mL
Ethanol				
Behavioral changes			>4.3 mmol/L	>20 mg/dL
Legal limit			≥17 mmol/L	≥80 mg/dL
Critical with acute exposure			>54 mmol/L	>250 mg/dL
Ethylene glycol				
Toxic			>2 mmol/L	>12 mg/dL
Lethal			>20 mmol/L	>120 mg/dL
Ethosuximide	280–700 μmol/L	40–100 μg/mL	>700 μmol/L	>100 μg/mL
Flecainide	0.5–2.4 μmol/L	0.2–1.0 μg/mL	>3.6 μmol/L	>1.5 μg/mL
Gentamicin				
Peak	10–21 μmol/mL	5–10 μg/mL	>25 μmol/mL	>12 μg/mL
Trough	0–4.2 μmol/mL	0–2 μg/mL	>4.2 μmol/mL	>2 μg/mL
Heroin (diacetyl morphine)			>700 μmol/L	>200 ng/mL (as morphine)
Ibuprofen	49–243 μmol/L	10–50 μg/mL	>97 μmol/L	>200 μg/mL
Imipramine (and metabolite)				
Desimipramine	375–1130 nmol/L	100–300 ng/mL	>1880 nmol/L	>500 ng/mL
Total imipramine + desimipramine	563–1130 nmol/L	150–300 ng/mL	>1880 nmol/L	>500 ng/mL
Lidocaine	5.1–21.3 μmol/L	1.2–5.0 μg/mL	>38.4 μmol/L	>9.0 μg/mL
Lithium	0.5–1.3 mmol/L	0.5–1.3 meq/L	>2 mmol/L	>2 meq/L
Methadone	1.3–3.2 μmol/L	0.4–1.0 μg/mL	>6.5 μmol/L	>2 μg/mL
Methamphetamine	1.3–4.0 μmol/L	2–6 μg/dL	4.0–33.5 μmol/L 67.0–268.0 μmol/L	60-500-1.0 μg/dL, toxic 1000–4000 μg/dL, lethal

(continued)

TABLE 3 TOXICOLOGY AND THERAPEUTIC DRUG MONITORING (CONTINUED)

Drug	Therapeutic Range		Toxic Level	
	SI Units	**Conventional Units**	**SI Units**	**Conventional Units**
Methanol			>6 mmol/L >16 mmol/L >28 mmol/L	>20 mg/dL, toxic >50 mg/dL, severe toxicity >89 mg/dL, lethal
Methotrexate				
Low-dose	0.01–0.1 μmol/L	0.01–0.1 μmol/L	>0.1 mmol/L	>0.1 mmol/L
High-dose (24 h)	<5.0 μmol/L	<5.0 μmol/L	>5.0 μmol/L	>5.0 μmol/L
High-dose (48 h)	<0.50 μmol/L	<0.50 μmol/L	>0.5 μmol/L	>0.5 μmol/L
High-dose (72 h)	<0.10 μmol/L	<0.10 μmol/L	>0.1 μmol/L	>0.1 μmol/L
Morphine	35–250 μmol/L	10–70 ng/mL	180–14000 μmol/L	50–4000 ng/mL
Nitroprusside (as thiocyanate)	103–499 μmol/L	6–29 μg/mL	860 μmol/L	>50 μg/mL
Nortriptyline	190–569 nmol/L	50–150 ng/mL	>1900 nmol/L	>500 ng/mL
Phenobarbital	65–172 μmol/L	15–40 μg/mL	>215 μmol/L	>50 μg/mL
Phenytoin	40–79 μmol/L	10–20 μg/mL	>118 μmol/L	>30 μg/mL
Phenytoin, free	4.0–7.9 μmol/L	1–2 μg/mL	>13.9 μmol/L	>3.5 μg/mL
% Free	0.08–0.14	8–14%		
Primidone and metabolite				
Primidone	23–55 μmol/L	5–12 μg/mL	>69 μmol/L	>15 μg/mL
Phenobarbital	65–172 μmol/L	15–40 μg/mL	>215 μmol/L	>50 μg/mL
Procainamide				
Procainamide	17–42 μmol/L	4–10 μg/mL	>51 μmol/L	>12 μg/mL
NAPA (*N*-acetylprocainamide)	22–72 μmol/L	6–20 μg/mL	>126 μmol/L	>35 μg/mL
Quinidine	6.2–15.4 μmol/L	2.0–5.0 μg/mL	>31 μmol/L	>10 μg/mL
Salicylates	145–2100 μmol/L	2–29 mg/dL	>2172 μmol/L	>30 mg/dL
Sirolimus (trough level)				
Kidney transplant	4.4–13.1 nmol/L	4–12 ng/mL	>16 nmol/L	>15 ng/mL
Tacrolimus (FK506) (trough)				
Kidney and liver				
0–2 months posttransplant	12–19 nmol/L	10–15 ng/mL	>25 nmol/L	>20 ng/mL
> 2 months posttransplant	6–12 nmol/L	5–10 ng/mL		
Heart				
0–2 months posttransplant	19–25 nmol/L	15–20 ng/mL	>25 nmol/L	>20 ng/mL
3–6 months posttransplant	12–19 nmol/L	10–15 ng/mL		
>6 months posttransplant	10–12 nmol/L	8–10 ng/mL		
Theophylline	56–111 μmol/L	10–20 μg/mL	>140 μmol/L	>25 μg/mL
Thiocyanate				
After nitroprusside infusion	103–499 μmol/L	6–29 μg/mL	860 μmol/L	>50 μg/mL
Nonsmoker	17–69 μmol/L	1–4 μg/mL		
Smoker	52–206 μmol/L	3–12 μg/mL		
Tobramycin				
Peak	11–22 μmol/L	5–10 μg/mL	>26 μmol/L	>12 μg/mL
Trough	0–4.3 μmol/L	0–2 μg/mL	>4.3 μmol/L	>2 μg/mL
Valproic acid	350–700 μmol/L	50–100 μg/mL	>1000 μmol/L	>150 μg/mL
Vancomycin				
Peak	14–28 μmol/L	20–40 μg/mL	>55 μmol/L	>80 μg/mL
Trough	3.5–10.4 μmol/L	5–15 μg/mL	>14 μmol/L	>20 μg/mL

TABLE 4 **VITAMINS AND SELECTED TRACE MINERALS**

Specimen	Analyte[a]	Reference Range SI Units	Reference Range Conventional Units
Aluminum	S	<0.2 μmol/L	<5.41 μg/L
	U, random	0.19–1.11 μmol/L	5–30 μg/L
Arsenic	WB	0.03–0.31 μmol/L	2–23 μg/L
	U, 24 h	0.07–0.67 μmol/d	5–50 μg/d
Cadmium	WB	<44.5 nmol/L	<5.0 μg/L
Coenzyme Q10 (ubiquinone)	P	433–1532 μg/L	433–1532 μg/L
B carotene	S	0.07–1.43 μmol/L	4–77 μg/dL
Copper			
	S	11–22 μmol/L	70–140 μg/dL
	U, 24 h	<0.95 μmol/d	<60 μg/d
Folic acid	RC	340–1020 nmol/L cells	150–450 ng/mL cells
Folic acid	S	12.2–40.8 nmol/L	5.4–18.0 ng/mL
Lead (adult)	S	<0.5 μmol/L	<10 μg/dL
Mercury			
	WB	3.0–294 nmol/L	0.6–59 μg/L
	U, 24 h	<99.8 nmol/L	<20 μg/L
Selenium	S	0.8–2.0 μmol/L	63–160 μg/L
Vitamin A	S	0.7–3.5 μmol/L	20–100 μg/dL
Vitamin B_1 (thiamine)	S	0–75 nmol/L	0–2 μg/dL
Vitamin B_2 (riboflavin)	S	106–638 nmol/L	4–24 μg/dL
Vitamin B_6	P	20–121 nmol/L	5–30 ng/mL
Vitamin B_{12}	S	206–735 pmol/L	279–996 pg/mL
Vitamin C (ascorbic acid)	S	23–57 μmol/L	0.4–1.0 mg/dL
Vitamin D_3, 1,25-dihydroxy	S	60–108 pmol/L	25–45 pg/mL
Vitamin D_3, 25-hydroxy	P		
Summer		37.4–200 nmol/L	15–80 ng/mL
Winter		34.9–105 nmol/L	14–42 ng/mL
Vitamin E	S	12–42 μmol/L	5–18 μg/mL
Vitamin K	S	0.29–2.64 nmol/L	0.13–1.19 ng/mL
Zinc	S	11.5–18.4 μmol/L	75–120 μg/dL

[a]P, plasma; RC, red cells; S, serum; WB, whole blood; U, urine.

TABLE 5 **CLASSIFICATION OF LDL, TOTAL, AND HDL CHOLESTEROL**

LDL cholesterol, mg/dL (mmol/L)	
<70 (<1.81)	Therapeutic option for very high risk patients
<100 (<2.59)	Optimal
100–129 (2.59–3.34)	Near optimal/above optimal
130–159 (3.36–4.11)	Borderline high
160–189 (4.14–4.89)	High
≥190 (≥4.91)	Very high
Total cholesterol, mg/dL (mmol/L)	
<200 (<5.17)	Desirable
200–239 (5.17–6.18)	Borderline high
≥240 (≥6.21)	High
HDL cholesterol, mg/dL (mmol/L)	
<40 (<1.03)	Low
≥60 (≥1.55)	High

Note: LDL, low-density lipoprotein; HDL, high-density lipoprotein

Source: Executive summary of the third report of the National Cholesterol Education Program (NCEP) expert panel on detection, evaluation, and treatment of high blood cholesterol in adults (adult treatment panel III). JAMA 285:2486, 2001; and Implications of recent clinical trials for the National Cholesterol Education Program Adult Treatment Panel III Guidelines: SM Grundy et al for the Coordinating Committee of the National Cholesterol Education Program. Circulation 110:227, 2004.

TABLE 6 CEREBROSPINAL FLUID (CSF)[a]

	Reference Range	
Constituent	SI Units	Conventional Units
Osmolarity	292–297 mmol/kg water	292–297 mosmol/L
Electrolytes		
Sodium	137–145 mmol/L	137–145 meq/L
Potassium	2.7–3.9 mmol/L	2.7–3.9 meq/L
Calcium	1.0–1.5 mmol/L	2.1–3.0 meq/L
Magnesium	1.0–1.2 mmol/L	2.0–2.5 meq/L
Chloride	116–122 mmol/L	116–122 meq/L
CO_2 content	20–24 mmol/L	20–24 meq/L
P_{CO_2}	6–7 kPa	45–49 mmHg
pH	7.31–7.34	
Glucose	2.22–3.89 mmol/L	40–70 mg/dL
Lactate	1–2 mmol/L	10–20 mg/dL
Total protein		
Lumbar	0.15–0.5 g/L	15–50 mg/dL
Cisternal	0.15–0.25 g/L	15–25 mg/dL
Ventricular	0.06–0.15 g/L	6–15 mg/dL
Albumin	0.066–0.442 g/L	6.6–44.2 mg/dL
IgG	0.009–0.057 g/L	0.9–5.7 mg/dL
IgG index[b]	0.29–0.59	
Oligoclonal bands	<2 bands not present in matched serum sample	
Ammonia	15–47 μmol/L	25–80 μg/dL
Creatinine	44–168 μmol/L	0.5–1.9 mg/dL
Myelin basic protein	<4 μg/L	
CSF pressure		50–180 mmH_2O
CSF volume (adult)	~150 mL	
Red blood cells	0	0
Leukocytes		
Total	0–5 mononuclear cells per μL	0–5 mononuclear cells per mm^3
Differential		
Lymphocytes	60–70%	
Monocytes	30–50%	
Neutrophils	None	

[a]Since cerebrospinal fluid concentrations are equilibrium values, measurements of the same parameters in blood plasma obtained at the same time are recommended. However, there is a time lag in attainment of equilibrium, and cerebrospinal levels of plasma constituents that can fluctuate rapidly (such as plasma glucose) may not achieve stable values until after a significant lag phase.

[b]IgG index = CSF IgG(mg/dL) × serum albumin(g/dL)/Serum IgG(g/dL) × CSF albumin(mg/dL).

TABLE 7 URINE ANALYSIS

	Reference Range	
	SI Units	Conventional Units
Acidity, titratable	20–40 mmol/d	20–40 meq/d
Ammonia	30–50 mmol/d	30–50 meq/d
Amylase		4–400 U/L
Amylase/creatinine clearance ratio [(Cl_{am}/Cl_{cr}) × 100]	1–5	1–5
Calcium (10 meq/d or 200 mg/d dietary calcium)	<7.5 mmol/d	<300 mg/d
Creatine, as creatinine		
Female	<760 μmol/d	<100 mg/d
Male	<380 μmol/d	<50 mg/d
Creatinine	8.8–14 mmol/d	1.0–1.6 g/d
Eosinophils	<100,000 eosinophils/L	<100 eosinophils/mL
Glucose (glucose oxidase method)	0.3–1.7 mmol/d	50–300 mg/d
5-Hydroxyindoleacetic acid (5-HIAA)	10–47 μmol/d	2–9 mg/d
Iodine, spot urine		
WHO classification of iodine deficiency		
Not iodine deficient	>100 μg/L	>100 μg/L
Mild iodine deficiency	50–100 μg/L	50–100 μg/L
Moderate iodine deficiency	20–49 μg/L	20–49 μg/L
Severe iodine deficiency	<20 μg/L	<20 μg/L
Microalbumin		
Normal	0.0–0.03 g/d	0–30 mg/d
Microalbuminuria	0.03–0.30 g/d	30–300 mg/d
Clinical albuminuria	>0.3 g/d	>300 mg/d
Microalbumin/creatinine ratio		
Normal	0–3.4 g/mol creatinine	0–30 μg/mg creatinine
Microalbuminuria	3.4–34 g/mol creatinine	30–300 μg/mg creatinine
Clinical albuminuria	>34 g/mol creatinine	>300 μg/mg creatinine
Oxalate		
Male	80–500 μmol/d	7–44 mg/d
Female	45–350 μmol/d	4–31 mg/d
pH	5.0–9.0	5.0–9.0
Phosphate (phosphorus) (varies with intake)	12.9–42.0 mmol/d	400–1300 mg/d
Potassium (varies with intake)	25–100 mmol/d	25–100 meq/d
Protein	<0.15 g/d	<150 mg/d
Sediment		
Red blood cells	0–2/high power field	
White blood cells	0–2/high power field	
Bacteria	None	
Crystals	None	
Bladder cells	None	
Squamous cells	None	
Tubular cells	None	
Broad casts	None	
Epithelial cell casts	None	
Granular casts	None	
Hyaline casts	0–5/low power field	
Red blood cell casts	None	
Waxy casts	None	
White cell casts	None	
Sodium (varies with intake)	100–260 mmol/d	100–260 meq/d
Specific gravity	1.001–1.035	1.001–1.035
Urea nitrogen	214–607 mmol/d	6–17 g/d
Uric acid (normal diet)	1.49–4.76 mmol/d	250–800 mg/d

Note: WHO, World Health Organization.

TABLE 8 DIFFERENTIAL NUCLEATED CELL COUNTS OF BONE MARROW ASPIRATES[a]

	Observed Range, %	95% Confidence Intervals, %	Mean, %
Blast cells	0–3.2	0–3.0	1.4
Promyelocytes	3.6–13.2	3.2–12.4	7.8
Neutrophil myelocytes	4–21.4	3.7–10.0	7.6
Eosinophil myelocytes	0–5.0	0–2.8	1.3
Metamyelocytes	1–7.0	2.3–5.9	4.1
Neutrophils			
Males	21.0–45.6	21.9–42.3	32.1
Females	29.6–46.6	28.8–45.9	37.4
Eosinophils	0.4–4.2	0.3–4.2	2.2
Eosinophils plus eosinophil myelocytes	0.9–7.4	0.7–6.3	3.5
Basophils	0–0.8	0–0.4	0.1
Erythroblasts			
Male	18.0–39.4	16.2–40.1	28.1
Females	14.0–31.8	13.0–32.0	22.5
Lymphocytes	4.6–22.6	6.0–20.0	13.1
Plasma cells	0–1.4	0–1.2	0.6
Monocytes	0–3.2	0–2.6	1.3
Macrophages	0–1.8	0–1.3	0.4
M:E ratio			
Males	1.1–4.0	1.1–4.1	2.1
Females	1.6–5.4	1.6–5.2	2.8

[a]Based on bone marrow aspirate from 50 healthy volunteers (30 men, 20 women).

Source: From BJ Bain: The bone marrow aspirate of healthy subjects. Br J Haematol 94(1):206, 1996.

TABLE 9 STOOL ANALYSIS

	Reference Range	
	SI Units	Conventional Units
Amount	0.1–0.2 kg/d	100–200 g/24 h
Coproporphyrin	611–1832 nmol/d	400–1200 μg/24 h
Fat		
Adult		<7 g/d
Adult on fat-free diet		<4 g/d
Fatty acids	0–21 mmol/d	0–6 g/24 h
Leukocytes	None	None
Nitrogen	<178 mmol/d	<2.5 g/24 h
pH	7.0–7.5	
Occult blood	Negative	Negative
Trypsin		20–95 U/g
Urobilinogen	85–510 μmol/d	50–300 mg/24 h
Uroporphyrins	12–48 nmol/d	10–40 μg/24 h
Water	<0.75	<75%

Source: Modified from FT Fishbach, MB Dunning III: *A Manual of Laboratory and Diagnostic Tests*, 7th ed., Lippincott Williams & Wilkins, Philadelphia, 2004.

TABLE 10 RENAL FUNCTION TESTS

	Reference Range	
	SI Units	Conventional Units
Clearances (corrected to 1.72 m^2 body surface area)		
Measures of glomerular filtration rate		
Inulin clearance (Cl)		
Males (mean ± 1 SD)	2.1 ± 0.4 mL/s	124 ± 25.8 mL/min
Females (mean ± 1 SD)	2.0 ± 0.2 mL/s	119 ± 12.8 mL/min
Endogenous creatinine clearance	1.5–2.2 mL/s	91–130 mL/min
Measures of effective renal plasma flow and tubular function		
p-Aminohippuric acid clearance (Cl_{PAH})		
Males (mean ± 1 SD)	10.9 ± 2.7 mL/s	654 ± 163 mL/min
Females (mean ± 1 SD)	9.9 ± 1.7 mL/s	594 ± 102 mL/min
Concentration and dilution test		
Specific gravity of urine		
After 12-h fluid restriction	>1.025	>1.025
After 12-h deliberate water intake	≤1.003	≤1.003
Protein excretion, urine	<0.15 g/d	<150 mg/d
Specific gravity, maximal range	1.002–1.028	1.002–1.028
Tubular reabsorption, phosphorus	0.79–0.94 of filtered load	79–94% of filtered load

TABLE 11 CIRCULATORY FUNCTION TESTS

	Results: Reference Range	
Test	SI Units (Range)	Conventional Units (Range)
Arteriovenous oxygen difference	30–50 mL/L	30–50 mL/L
Cardiac output (Fick)	2.5–3.6 L/m^2 of body surface area per min	2.5–3.6 L/m^2 of body surface area per min
Contractility indexes		
Max. left ventricular *dp/dt(dp/dt)*/DP when DP = 5.3 kPa (40 mmHg) (DP, diastolic pressure)	220 kPa/s (176–250 kPa/s) (37.6 ± 12.2)/s	1650 mmHg/s (1320–1880 mmHg/s) (37.6 ± 12.2)/s
Mean normalized systolic ejection rate (angiography)	3.32 ± 0.84 end-diastolic volumes per second	3.32 ± 0.84 end-diastolic volumes per second
Mean velocity of circumferential fiber shortening (angiography)	1.83 ± 0.56 circumferences per second	1.83 ± 0.56 circumferences per second
Ejection fraction: stroke volume/end-diastolic volume (SV/EDV)	0.67 ± 0.08 (0.55–0.78)	0.67 ± 0.08 (0.55–0.78)
End-diastolic volume	70 ± 20.0 mL/m^2 (60–88 mL/m^2)	70 ± 20.0 mL/m^2 (60–88 mL/m^2)
End-systolic volume	25 ± 5.0 mL/m^2 (20–33 mL/m^2)	25 ± 5.0 mL/m^2 (20–33 mL/m^2)
Left ventricular work		
Stroke work index	50 ± 20.0 (g•m)/m^2 (30–110)	50 ± 20.0 (g•m)/m^2 (30–110)
Left ventricular minute work index	1.8–6.6 [(kg•m)/m^2]/min	1.8–6.6 [(kg•m)/m^2]/min
Oxygen consumption index	110–150 mL	110–150 mL
Maximum oxygen uptake	35 mL/min (20–60 mL/min)	35 mL/min (20–60 mL/min)
Pulmonary vascular resistance	2–12 (kPa•s)/L	20–130 (dyn•s)/cm^5
Systemic vascular resistance	77–150 (kPa•s)/L	770–1600 (dyn•s)/cm^5

Source: E Braunwald et al: *Heart Disease*, 6th ed, Philadelphia, Saunders, 2001.

TABLE 12 GASTROINTESTINAL TESTS

Test	Results: SI Units	Results: Conventional Units
Absorption tests		
D-Xylose: after overnight fast, 25 g xylose given in oral aqueous solution		
Urine, collected for following 5 h	25% of ingested dose	25% of ingested dose
Serum, 2 h after dose	2.0–3.5 mmol/L	30–52 mg/dL
Vitamin A: a fasting blood specimen is obtained and 200,000 units of vitamin A in oil is given orally	Serum level should rise to twice fasting level in 3–5 h	Serum level should rise to twice fasting level in 3–5 h
Bentiromide test (pancreatic function): 500 mg bentiromide (chymex) orally; *p*-aminobenzoic acid (PABA) measured		
Plasma		>3.6 (±1.1) μg/mL at 90 min
Urine	>50% recovered in 6 h	>50% recovered in 6 h
Gastric juice		
Volume		
24 h	2–3 L	2–3 L
Nocturnal	600–700 mL	600–700 mL
Basal, fasting	30–70 mL/h	30–70 mL/h
Reaction		
pH	1.6–1.8	1.6–1.8
Titratable acidity of fasting juice	4–9 μmol/s	15–35 meq/h
Acid output		
Basal		
Females (mean ± 1 SD)	0.6 ± 0.5 μmol/s	2.0 ± 1.8 meq/h
Males (mean ± 1 SD)	0.8 ± 0.6 μmol/s	3.0 ± 2.0 meq/h
Maximal (after SC histamine acid phosphate, 0.004 mg/kg body weight, and preceded by 50 mg promethazine, or after betazole, 1.7 mg/kg body weight, or pentagastrin, 6 μg/kg body weight)		
Females (mean ± 1 SD)	4.4 ± 1.4 μmol/s	16 ± 5 meq/h
Males (mean ± 1 SD)	6.4 ± 1.4 μmol/s	23 ± 5 meq/h
Basal acid output/maximal acid output ratio	≤0.6	≤0.6
Gastrin, serum	0–200 μg/L	0–200 pg/mL
Secretin test (pancreatic exocrine function): 1 unit/kg body weight, IV		
Volume (pancreatic juice) in 80 min	>2.0 mL/kg	>2.0 mL/kg
Bicarbonate concentration	>80 mmol/L	>80 meq/L
Bicarbonate output in 30 min	>10 mmol	>10 meq

TABLE 13 NORMAL VALUES OF DOPPLER ECHOCARDIOGRAPHIC MEASUREMENTS IN ADULTS

	Range	Mean
RVD (cm), measured at the base in apical 4-chamber view	2.6–4.3	3.5 ± 0.4
LVID (cm), measured in the parasternal long axis view	3.6–5.4	4.7 ± 0.4
Posterior LV wall thickness (cm)	0.6–1.1	0.9 ± 0.4
IVS wall thickness (cm)	0.6–1.1	0.9 ± 0.4
Left atrial dimension (cm), antero-posterior dimension	2.3–3.8	3.0 ± 0.3
Aortic root dimension (cm)	2.0–3.5	2.4 ± 0.4
Aortic cusps separation (cm)	1.5–2.6	1.9 ± 0.4
Percentage of fractional shortening	34–44%	36%
Mitral flow (m/s)	0.6–1.3	0.9
Tricuspid flow (m/s)	0.3–0.7	0.5
Pulmonary artery (m/s)	0.6–0.9	0.75
Aorta (m/s)	1.0–1.7	1.35

Note: RVD, right ventricular dimension; LVID, left ventricular internal dimension; LV, left ventricle; IVS, interventricular septum.

Source: From A Weyman: *Principles and Practice of Echocardiography*, 2d ed., Philadelphia, Lea & Febiger, 1994.

TABLE 14 SUMMARY OF VALUES USEFUL IN PULMONARY PHYSIOLOGY

	Symbol	Typical Values: Man, Age 40, 75 kg, 175 cm Tall	Typical Values: Woman, Age 40, 60 kg, 160 cm Tall
Pulmonary Mechanics			
Spirometry—volume-time curves			
Forced vital capacity	FVC	5.1 L	3.6 L
Forced expiratory volume in 1 s	FEV_1	4.1 L	2.9 L
FEV_1/FVC	FEV_1%	80%	82%
Maximal midexpiratory flow	MMF (FEF 25–27)	4.8 L/s	3.6 L/s
Maximal expiratory flow rate	MEFR (FEF 200–1200)	9.4 L/s	6.1 L/s
Spirometry—flow-volume curves			
Maximal expiratory flow at 50% of expired vital capacity	V_{max} 50 (FEF 50%)	6.1 L/s	4.6 L/s
Maximal expiratory flow at 75% of expired vital capacity	V_{max} 75 (FEF 75%)	3.1 L/s	2.5 L/s
Resistance to airflow			
Pulmonary resistance	RL (R_L)	<3.0 (cmH_2O/s)/L	
Airway resistance	Raw	<2.5 (cmH_2O/s)/L	
Specific conductance	SGaw	>0.13 cmH_2O/s	
Pulmonary compliance			
Static recoil pressure at total lung capacity	Pst TLC	25 ± 5 cmH_2O	
Compliance of lungs (static)	CL	0.2 L cmH_2O	
Compliance of lungs and thorax	C(L + T)	0.1 L cmH_2O	
Dynamic compliance of 20 breaths per minute	C dyn 20	0.25 ± 0.05 L/cmH_2O	
Maximal static respiratory pressures			
Maximal inspiratory pressure	MIP	>90 cmH_2O	>50 cmH_2O
Maximal expiratory pressure	MEP	>150 cmH_2O	>120 cmH_2O
Lung Volumes			
Total lung capacity	TLC	6.7 L	4.9 L
Functional residual capacity	FRC	3.7 L	2.8 L
Residual volume	RV	2.0 L	1.6 L
Inspiratory capacity	IC	3.3 L	2.3 L
Expiratory reserve volume	ERV	1.7 L	1.1 L
Vital capacity	VC	5.0 L	3.4 L
Gas Exchange (Sea Level)			
Arterial O_2 tension	Pa_{O_2}	12.7 ± 0.7 kPa (95 ± 5 mmHg)	
Arterial CO_2 tension	Pa_{CO_2}	5.3 ± 0.3 kPa (40 ± 2 mmHg)	
Arterial O_2 saturation	Sa_{O_2}	0.97 ± 0.02 (97 ± 2%)	
Arterial blood pH	pH	7.40 ± 0.02	
Arterial bicarbonate	HCO_3^-	24 + 2 meq/L	
Base excess	BE	0 ± 2 meq/L	
Diffusing capacity for carbon monoxide (single breath)	DL_{CO}	0.42 mL CO/s per mmHg (25 mL CO/min per mmHg)	
Dead space volume	V_D	2 mL/kg body wt	
Physiologic dead space; dead space-tidal volume ratio	V_D/V_T		
Rest		≤35% V_T	
Exercise		≤20% V_T	
Alveolar-arterial difference for O_2	$P(A - a)_{O_2}$	≤2.7 kPa ≤20 kPa (≤20 mmHg)	

TABLE 15 BODY FLUIDS AND OTHER MASS DATA

	Reference Range	
	SI Units	**Conventional Units**
Ascitic fluid: See Table 44-1		
Body fluid,		
Total volume (lean) of body weight	50% (in obese) to 70%	
Intracellular	0.3–0.4 of body weight	
Extracellular	0.2–0.3 of body weight	
Blood		
Total volume		
Males	69 mL per kg body weight	
Females	65 mL per kg body weight	
Plasma volume		
Males	39 mL per kg body weight	
Females	40 mL per kg body weight	
Red blood cell volume		
Males	30 mL per kg body weight	1.15–1.21 L/m^2 of body surface area
Females	25 mL per kg body weight	0.95–1.00 L/m^2 of body surface area
Body mass index	18.5–24.9 kg/m^2	18.5–24.9 kg/m^2

TABLE 16 RADIATION-DERIVED UNITS

Quantity	Old Unit	SI Unit	Name for SI Unit (and Abbreviation)	Conversion
Activity	curie (Ci)	Disintegrations per second (dps)	becquerel (Bq)	1 Ci = 3.7×10^{10} Bq 1 mCi = 37 mBq 1 μCi = 0.037 MBq or 37 GBq 1 Bq = 2.703×10^{-11} Ci
Absorbed dose	rad	joule per kilogram (J/kg)	gray (Gy)	1 Gy = 100 rad 1 rad = 0.01 Gy 1 mrad = 10^{-3} cGy
Exposure	roentgen (R)	coulomb per kilogram (C/kg)	—	1 C/kg = 3876 R 1 R = 2.58×10^{-4} C/kg 1 mR = 258 pC/kg
Dose equivalent	rem	joule per kilogram (J/kg)	sievert (Sv)	1 Sv = 100 rem 1 rem = 0.01 Sv 1 mrem = 10 μSv

ACKNOWLEDGMENT

The authors acknowledge the contributions of Dr. Patrick M. Sluss, Dr. James L. Januzzi, and Dr. Kent B. Lewandrowski to this chapter in previous editions.

FURTHER READINGS

KRATZ A et al: Case records of the Massachusetts General Hospital. Weekly clinicopathological exercises. Laboratory reference values. N Engl J Med 351(15):1548, 2004

LEHMAN HP, HENRY JB: SI units, in *Henry's Clinical Diagnosis and Management by Laboratory Methods*, 21st ed, RC McPherson, MR Pincus (eds). Philadelphia, Elsevier Saunders, 2007, pp 1404–1418

PESCE MA: Reference ranges for laboratory tests and procedures, in *Nelson's Textbook of Pediatrics*, 18th ed, RM Klegman et al (eds). Philadelphia, Elsevier Saunders, 2007, pp 2943–2949

SOLBERG HE: Establishment and use of reference values, in *Tietz Textbook of Clinical Chemistry and Molecular Diagnostics*, 4th ed, CA Burtis et al (eds). Philadelphia, Elsevier Saunders, 2006, pp 425–448

Bold number indicates the start of the main discussion of the topic; numbers followed by "f" or "t" refer to pages of figures and tables; numbers preceded by "e" refer to the e-chapter pages on the DVD; "V" refers to the videos on the DVD; numbers preceded by "A" refer to the Appendix.

INDEX

INDEX

INDEX

INDEX

INDEX

INDEX

INDEX

INDEX

INDEX

INDEX

INDEX

INDEX

INDEX

INDEX

INDEX

INDEX

INDEX

INDEX

INDEX

INDEX

INDEX

INDEX

INDEX

INDEX

INDEX

INDEX

INDEX